M000290966

Cummings Otolaryngology
Head & Neck Surgery

VOLUME ONE

Part 1: Basic Principles
Paul W. Flint, Editor

Part 2: General Otolaryngology
Paul W. Flint, Editor

Part 3: Facial Plastic and Reconstructive Surgery
J. Regan Thomas, Editor
- Section 1: Facial Surgery
- Section 2: Rhinoplasty

Part 4: Sinus, Rhinology, and Allergy/Immunology
Valerie J. Lund, Editor

Part 5: Laryngology and Bronchoesophagology
Paul W. Flint, Editor
- Section 1: Evaluation and Management of Laryngeal and Pharyngeal Disorders
- Section 2: Management of Unilateral Vocal Fold Paralysis
- Section 3: Management of Acquired Disorders and Trauma
- Section 4: Bronchoesophagology

VOLUME TWO

Part 6: Head and Neck Surgery and Oncology
Bruce H. Haughey and K. Thomas Robbins, Editors
- Section 1: General Considerations
- Section 2: Salivary Glands
- Section 3: Oral Cavity
- Section 4: Pharynx and Esophagus
- Section 5: Larynx
- Section 6: Neck
- Section 7: Thyroid/Parathyroid

Part 7: Otology, Neuro-otology, and Skull Base Surgery
John K. Niparko, Editor
- Section 1: Basic Science
- Section 2: Diagnostic Assessment
- Section 3: External Ear
- Section 4: Middle Ear, Mastoid, and Temporal Bone

VOLUME THREE

Part 7: Otology, Neuro-otology, and Skull Base Surgery—*cont'd*
John K. Niparko, Editor
- Section 5: Inner Ear
- Section 6: Auditory Prosthetic Stimulation, Devices, and Rehabilitative Audiology
- Section 7: Vestibular Disorders
- Section 8: Facial Nerve Disorders
- Section 9: Cranial Base

Part 8: Pediatric Otolaryngology
Mark A. Richardson, Editor
- Section 1: General
- Section 2: Craniofacial
- Section 3: Hearing Loss and Pediatric Otology
- Section 4: Infections and Inflammation
- Section 5: Head and Neck
- Section 6: Pharynx, Larynx, Trachea, and Esophagus

Cummings Otolaryngology Head & Neck Surgery

FIFTH EDITION

Paul W. Flint, M.D.
Professor and Chair
Department of Otolaryngology–Head and Neck Surgery
Oregon Health and Science University
Portland, Oregon

Bruce H. Haughey, M.B.Ch.B., F.A.C.S., F.R.A.C.S.
Professor and Director
Head and Neck Surgical Oncology
Department of Otolaryngology–Head and Neck Surgery
Washington University School of Medicine
St. Louis, Missouri

Valerie J. Lund, C.B.E., M.S., F.R.C.S., F.R.C.S.Ed.
Professor of Rhinology
University College London
Honorary Consultant ENT Surgeon
Royal National Throat, Nose, and Ear Hospital
Royal Free Hospital
Moorfields Eye Hospital
London, United Kingdom

John K. Niparko, M.D.
George T. Nager Professor
Department of Otolaryngology–Head and Neck Surgery
Director
Divisions of Otology, Neurotology, Skull Base Surgery, and Audiology
Johns Hopkins University School of Medicine
Baltimore, Maryland

Mark A. Richardson, M.D.
Professor
Department of Otolaryngology–Head and Neck Surgery
Dean
School of Medicine
Oregon Health and Science University
Portland, Oregon

K. Thomas Robbins, M.D.
Director
SimmonsCooper Cancer Institute at Southern Illinois University
Professor
Division of Otolaryngology–Head and Neck Surgery
Southern Illinois University School of Medicine
Springfield, Illinois

J. Regan Thomas, M.D.
Francis L. Lederer Professor and Chairman
Department of Otolaryngology–Head and Neck Surgery
University of Illinois at Chicago
Chicago, Illinois

Illustrator:

Tim Phelps, M.S., F.A.M.I.
Associate Professor and Medical Illustrator
Art as Applied to Medicine
Johns Hopkins University School of Medicine
Baltimore, Maryland

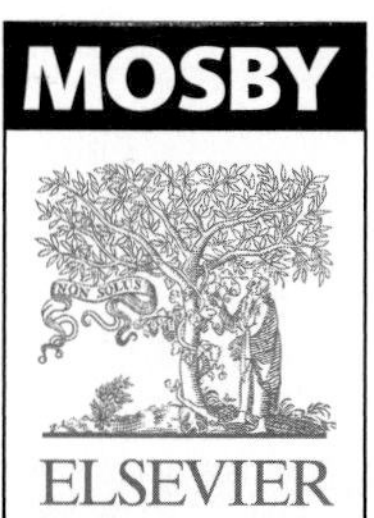

VOLUME THREE

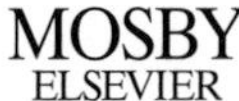

MOSBY
ELSEVIER

1600 John F. Kennedy Blvd
Suite 1800
Philadelphia, PA 19103-2899

CUMMINGS OTOLARYNGOLOGY–HEAD AND NECK SURGERY
FIFTH EDITION
ISBN: 978-0-323-05283-2
IE ISBN: 978-0-8089-2434-0

Library of Congress Cataloging-in-Publication Data
Cummings otolaryngology–head & neck surgery / [edited by] Paul W. Flint ... [et al.] ; illustrator, Tim Phelps.–5th ed.
p. ; cm.
Rev. ed. of: Otolaryngology–head & neck surgery / edited by Charles W. Cummings ... [et al.]. 4th ed. c2005.
Includes bibliographical references and index.
ISBN 978-0-323-05283-2
1. Otolaryngology, Operative. I. Flint, Paul W. II Cummings, Charles W. (Charles William).
III. Otolaryngology–head & neck surgery. IV. Title: Otolaryngology–head & neck surgery.
[DNLM: 1. Otorhinolaryngologic Surgical Procedures. WV 168 C971 2010]
RF51.086 2010
617.5′1059—dc22 2009010493

Acquisitions Editor: Rebecca S. Gaertner
Developmental Editor: Roxanne Halpine
Publishing Services Manager: Frank Polizzano
Project Management: Rachel Miller, Robin E. Hayward
Design Direction: Lou Forgione
Marketing Manager: Radha Mawrie

Printed in China.

Last digit is the print number: 9 8 7 6 5 4 3 2

Contributors

Waleed M. Abuzeid, M.B.B.S.
Resident
Department of Surgery
University of Michigan Health System
Ann Arbor, Michigan

Meredith E. Adams, M.D.
Fellow
Division of Otology and Neurotology
Department of Otolaryngology
University of Michigan Medical Center
Ann Arbor, Michigan

Peter A. Adamson, M.D., F.R.C.S.C., F.A.C.S.
Professor and Head
Division of Facial Plastic and Reconstructive Surgery
Department of Otolaryngology–Head and Neck Surgery
University of Toronto Faculty of Medicine
Staff Surgeon
University Health Network
Toronto General Hospital
Toronto, Ontario, Canada

Antoine Adenis, M.D., Ph.D.
Professor of Medical Oncology
Catholic University
Chief
Department of Gastrointestinal Oncology
Centre Oscar Lambret
Lille, France

Seth Akst, M.D.
Assistant Professor
Department of Anesthesiology and Critical Care Medicine
George Washington University School of Medicine and Health Sciences
Washington, D.C.

Sheri L. Albers, D.O.
Fellow
Pain Management and Spinal Interventional Neuroradiology
University of California, San Diego, School of Medicine
UC San Diego Medical Center
La Jolla, California
VA San Diego Medical Center
San Diego, California

David Albert, M.B.B.S., F.R.C.S.
Honorary Senior Lecturer
University College London Institute of Child Health
Lead Clinician
ENT Department
Great Ormond Street Hospital for Children
London, United Kingdom

Ronda E. Alexander, M.D.
Assistant Professor
Department of Otolaryngology–Head and Neck Surgery
University of Texas Health Science Center at Houston
Houston, Texas

Sue Archbold, M.Phil.
CEO
The Ear Foundation
Nottingham, United Kingdom

William B. Armstrong, M.D.
Associate Professor
Department of Otolaryngology–Head and Neck Surgery
University of California, Irvine, School of Medicine
Irvine, California

Moisés A. Arriaga, M.D., F.A.C.S.
Clinical Professor and Director
Division of Otology and Neuro-otology
Department of Otolaryngology and Neurosurgery
Louisiana State University Health Sciences Center School of Medicine at New Orleans
New Orleans, Louisiana
Director
Hearing and Balance Center
Our Lady of the Lake Regional Medical Center
Baton Rouge, Louisiana
Director
Department of Cochlear Implants and Neurotology
Children's Hospital New Orleans
New Orleans, Louisiana

H. Alexander Arts, M.D.
Professor
Department of Otolaryngology and Neurosurgery
University of Michigan Medical School
Ann Arbor, Michigan

Yasmine A. Ashram, M.D., D.A.B.N.M.
Assistant Professor
Department of Physiology
University of Alexandria School of Medicine
Surgical Neurophysiologist
Alexandria University Hospital
Alexandria, Egypt

Jonathan E. Aviv, M.D., F.A.C.S.
Clinical Professor
Department of Otolaryngology
Mount Sinai School of Medicine
Clinical Director
Voice and Swallowing Center
ENT and Allergy Associates
New York, New York

Nafi Aygun, M.D.
Assistant Professor
Department of Radiology
Neuroradiology Division
Johns Hopkins University School of Medicine
Baltimore, Maryland

Douglas D. Backous, M.D., F.A.C.S.
Director
Listen For Life Center
Virginia Mason Medical Center
Seattle, Washington
Department of Otolaryngology–Head and Neck Surgery
Madigan Army Medical Center
Fort Lewis, Washington

Shan R. Baker, M.D.
Professor
Department of Otolaryngology–Head and Neck Surgery
University of Michigan Medical School
Ann Arbor, Michigan
Chief
Facial Plastic and Reconstructive Surgery
University of Michigan Center for Facial Cosmetic Surgery
Livonia, Michigan

Thomas J. Balkany, M.D., F.A.C.S., F.A.A.P.
Hotchkiss Professor and Chair
Department of Otolaryngology
Professor of Neurological Surgery and Pediatrics
University of Miami Miller School of Medicine
Chief of Service
Division of Otology
Jackson Memorial Hospital
Miami, Florida

Robert W. Baloh, M.D.
Professor
Department of Neurology and Otolaryngology
David Geffen School of Medicine at UCLA
Director
Neuro-otology Program
Department of Neurology
Ronald Reagan UCLA Medical Center
Los Angeles, California

Julie Barkmeier-Kraemer, Ph.D.
Associate Professor
Department of Speech, Language, and Hearing Sciences
University of Arizona College of Medicine
Tucson, Arizona

Fuad M. Baroody, M.D., F.A.C.S.
Professor
Department of Otolaryngology–Head and Neck Surgery
Department of Pediatrics
University of Chicago Pritzker School of Medicine
Chicago, Illinois

Nancy L. Bartlett, M.D.
Professor
Department of Medicine
Division of Oncology
Washington University in St. Louis School of Medicine
Medical Oncologist
Siteman Cancer Center
St. Louis, Missouri

Jonathan Z. Baskin, M.D.
Assistant Professor
Department of Otolaryngology
Case Western Reserve University School of Medicine
Section Chief
Department of Otolaryngology–Head and Neck Surgery
Cleveland VA Medical Center
Attending Physician
Rainbow Babies and Children's Hospital
Cleveland, Ohio

Robert W. Bastian, M.D.
Clinical Professor
Department of Otolaryngology
Loyola University School of Medicine
Chicago, Illinois
Founder and Director
Bastian Voice Institute
Downers Grove, Illinois

Carol A. Bauer, M.D.
Professor of Surgery
Division of Otolaryngology–Head and Neck Surgery
Southern Illinois University School of Medicine
Springfield, Illinois

Michael S. Benninger, M.D.
Professor
Cleveland Clinic Lerner School of Medicine
Case Western Reserve University
Chairman
Head and Neck Institute
The Cleveland Clinic
Cleveland, Ohio

Prabhat K. Bhama, M.D.
Resident and Research Fellow
University of Washington Medical Center
Seattle, Washington

Nasir Islam Bhatti, M.D., F.A.C.S., F.R.C.S.
Associate Professor
Department of Otolaryngology–Head and Neck Surgery
Johns Hopkins University School of Medicine
Baltimore, Maryland

Andrew Blitzer, M.D., D.D.S.
Professor
Department of Clinical Otolaryngology
Columbia University College of Physicians and Surgeons
Director
New York Center for Voice and Swallowing Disorders
Attending
Department of Otolaryngology
St. Luke's Roosevelt Hospital Center
New York, New York

Simone Boardman, M.B.B.S., F.R.A.C.S.(OHNS)
Great Ormond Street Hospital
London, United Kingdom

Emily F. Boss, M.D.
Assistant Professor
Department of Otolaryngology
Division of Pediatric Otolaryngology
Johns Hopkins University School of Medicine
Baltimore, Maryland

Derald E. Brackmann, M.D.
Clinical Professor
Department of Otolaryngology–Head and Neck Surgery
David Geffen School of Medicine at UCLA
Clinical Professor
Department of Neurological Surgery
University of Southern California Keck School of Medicine
President
House Ear Clinic
Los Angeles, California

Carol R. Bradford, M.D., F.A.C.S.
Professor and Chair
Department of Otolaryngology–Head and Neck Surgery
University of Michigan Medical School
Ann Arbor, Michigan

Barton F. Branstetter, IV, M.D.
Associate Professor
Departments of Radiology, Otolaryngology, and Biomedical Informatics
University of Pittsburgh School of Medicine
Director
Head and Neck Imaging
University of Pittsburgh Medical Center
Pittsburgh, Pennsylvania

Edward B. Braun, M.D.
Assistant Professor
Department of Anesthesiology
University of Kansas School of Medicine
University of Kansas Hospital
Kansas City, Kansas

Robert J. S. Briggs, M.B.B.S., F.R.A.C.S.
Clinical Associate Professor
Department of Otolaryngology
The University of Melbourne Faculty of Medicine
Melbourne, Australia

Hilary A. Brodie, M.D., Ph.D.
Professor and Chair
Department of Otolaryngology
University of California, Davis, School of Medicine
UC Davis Medical Center
Sacramento, California

Carolyn J. Brown, Ph.D.
Professor
Department of Communication Sciences and Disorders
Department of Otolaryngology–Head and Neck Surgery
University of Iowa Carver College of Medicine
Iowa City, Iowa

David J. Brown, M.D.
Assistant Professor of Otolaryngology
Medical College of Wisconsin
Children's Hospital of Wisconsin
Milwaukee, Wisconsin

Kevin D. Brown, M.D., Ph.D.
Assistant Professor
Department of Otolaryngology
Weill Cornell Medical College
Assistant Attending Otorhinolaryngologist
NewYork–Presbyterian Hospital
New York, New York

J. Dale Browne, M.D, F.A.C.S.
Professor and Chair
Department of Otolaryngology–Head and Neck Surgery
Wake Forest University School of Medicine
Winston-Salem, North Carolina

John M. Buatti, M.D.
Professor and Head
Department of Radiation Oncology
University of Iowa Carver College of Medicine
University of Iowa Hospitals and Clinics
Iowa City, Iowa

Luke Buchmann, M.D.
Assistant Professor
Department of Otolaryngology–Head and Neck Surgery
University of Utah School of Medicine
Salt Lake City, Utah

Patrick J. Byrne, M.D.
Associate Professor
Departments of Otolaryngology–Head and Neck Surgery and Dermatology
Johns Hopkins University School of Medicine
Director
Division of Facial Plastic and Reconstructive Surgery
Johns Hopkins Hospital
Baltimore, Maryland

Gabriel G. Galzada, M.D.
Department of Head and Neck Surgical Oncology
Kaiser Permanente
Downey, California

John P. Carey, M.D.
Associate Professor
Department of Otolaryngology–Head and Neck Surgery
Division of Otology, Neurotology, and Skull Base Surgery
Johns Hopkins University School of Medicine
Baltimore, Maryland

Margaretha L. Casselbrant, M.D., Ph.D.
Eberly Professor of Pediatric Otolaryngology
Department of Otolaryngology
University of Pittsburgh School of Medicine
Director
Department of Pediatric Otolaryngology
Children's Hospital of Pittsburgh of UPMC
Pittsburgh, Pennsylvania

Paolo Castelnuovo, M.D.
Professor
University of Insubria
Chairman
Ospedale di Circolo e Fondazione Macchi
Varese, Italy

Steven Chang, M.D.
Resident
Department of Otolaryngology–Head and Neck Surgery
Johns Hopkins Medical Institutions
Baltimore, Maryland

Burke E. Chegar, M.D.
Clinical Assistant Professor
Department of Dermatology
Indiana University School of Medicine
Indianapolis, Indiana
Director
Center for Facial Plastic Surgery–Head and Neck Surgery
Fayette Regional Health System
Connersville, Indiana

Amy Chen, M.D., M.P.H.
Associate Professor
Department of Otolaryngology–Head and Neck Surgery
Emory School of Medicine
Atlanta, Georgia

Eunice Y. Chen, M.D., Ph.D.
Assistant Professor
Dartmouth Medical School
Hanover, New Hampshire
Pediatric Otolaryngologist
Dartmouth Hitchcock Medical Center
Lebanon, New Hampshire

Theodore Chen, M.D.
Department of Head and Neck Surgery
Kaiser Permanente Los Angeles Medical Center
Los Angeles, California

Douglas B. Chepeha, M.D., M.P.H.
Associate Professor
Department of Otolaryngology–Head and Neck Surgery
University of Michigan Medical School
Director
Microvascular Program
A. Alfred Taubman Health Care Center
Ann Arbor, Michigan

Alice Cheuk, M.D.
Resident Physician
Los Angeles County Hospital and USC Medical Center
Los Angeles, California

Neil N. Chheda, M.D.
Assistant Professor
Department of Otolaryngology
Division of Laryngology
University of Florida College of Medicine
Shands at the University of Florida
Gainesville, Florida

Wade Chien, M.D.
Clinical Fellow
Department of Otolaryngology
Johns Hopkins University School of Medicine
Johns Hopkins Hospital
Baltimore, Maryland

Sukgi S. Choi, M.D.
Professor
Departments of Otolaryngology and Pediatrics
George Washington University School of Medicine and Health Sciences
Vice Chief
Department of Pediatric Otolaryngology
Children's National Medical Center
Washington, D.C.

Richard A. Chole, M.D., Ph.D.
Lindburg Professor and Head
Department of Otolaryngology–Head and Neck Surgery
Washington University in St. Louis School of Medicine
Chief of Staff
Department of Otolaryngology
Barnes-Jewish Hospital
St. Louis, Missouri

James M. Christian, D.D.S., M.B.A.
Visiting Associate Professor
Department of Otolaryngology–Head and Neck Surgery
Johns Hopkins University School of Medicine
Director
Division of Dentistry and Oral Surgery
Johns Hopkins Hospital
Baltimore, Maryland

Eugene A. Chu, M.D.
Clinical Instructor in Rhinology and Sinus Surgery
Department of Otolaryngology–Head and Neck Surgery
Johns Hopkins University School of Medicine
Baltimore, Maryland

Martin J. Citardi, M.D.
Professor and Chair
Department of Otolaryngology–Head and Neck Surgery
University of Texas Medical School at Houston
Chief
Otorhinolaryngology
Memorial Hermann–Texas Medical Center
Houston, Texas

Marc A. Cohen, M.D.
Resident
Department of Otorhinolaryngology–Head and Neck Surgery
University of Pennsylvania Health System
Philadelphia, Pennsylvania

Savita Collins, M.D.
Physician
Departments of Otolaryngology–Head and Neck Surgery and Audiology
South Bend Clinic
South Bend, Indiana

Nancy A. Collop, M.D.
Professor
Department of Medicine
Division of Pulmonary/Critical Care Medicine
Johns Hopkins University School of Medicine
Medical Director
Sleep Disorders Center
Johns Hopkins Hospital
Baltimore, Maryland

Philippe Contencin, M.D., Ph.D.
Senior Consultant
Department of Otorhinolaryngology
Hôpital Necker
Paris, France

Raymond Cook, M.D.
Assistant Professor
Department of Otolaryngology–Head and Neck Surgery
University of North Carolina at Chapel Hill School of Medicine
Chapel Hill, North Carolina
WakeMed Health and Hospitals
Raleigh, North Carolina

Jacquelynne Corey, M.D.
Professor of Surgery
Department of Otolaryngology–Head and Neck Surgery
University of Chicago Pritzker School of Medicine
Director
ENT Allergy Program
University of Chicago Medical Center
Chicago, Illinois

Robin T. Cotton, M.D., F.A.C.S., F.R.C.S.C
Professor
Department of Otolaryngology–Head and Neck Surgery
University of Cincinnati College of Medicine
Director
Pediatric Otolaryngology–Head and Neck Surgery
Cincinnati Children's Hospital
Cincinnati, Ohio

Marion Everett Couch, M.D., Ph.D.
Associate Professor
Department of Otolaryngology–Head and Neck Surgery
University of North Carolina at Chapel Hill School of Medicine
Chapel Hill, North Carolina

Mark S. Courey, M.D.
Professor
Department of Otolaryngology–Head and Neck Surgery
Director
Division of Laryngology
University of California, San Francisco, School of Medicine
Director
UCSF Voice and Swallowing Center
San Francisco, California

Benjamin T. Crane, M.D., Ph.D.
Assistant Professor
Departments of Otolaryngology and Neurobiology
University of Rochester School of Medicine and Dentistry
Department of Otolaryngology
Strong Memorial Hospital
Rochester, New York

Roger L. Crumley, M.D.
Professor and Chair
Department of Otolaryngology–Head and Neck Surgery
University of California, Irvine, School of Medicine
Orange, California

Oswaldo Laércio M. Cruz, M.D.
Associate Professor and Chief
Division of Otology-Neurotology
Department of Otolaryngology
Federal University of São Paulo
São Paulo, Brazil

Frank Culicchia, M.D.
Professor and Chair
Department of Neurosurgery
Louisiana State University Health Sciences Center
New Orleans, Louisiana

Charles W. Cummings, M.D.
Distinguished Professor
Johns Hopkins University School of Medicine
Executive Medical Director
Johns Hopkins International
Baltimore, Maryland

Calhoun D. Cunningham, III, M.D.
Assistant Consulting Professor of Surgery
Division of Otorhinolaryngology–Head and Neck Surgery
Duke University School of Medicine
Durham, North Carolina
Associate Physician
Carolina Ear and Hearing Clinic
Raleigh, North Carolina

Greg E. Davis, M.D., M.P.H.
Assistant Professor
Department of Otolaryngology–Head and Neck Surgery
University of Washington School of Medicine
Seattle, Washington

Larry E. Davis, M.D.
Distinguished Professor of Neurology
Research Professor
Departments of Neuroscience and Molecular Genetics and Microbiology
University of New Mexico School of Medicine
Chief
Neurology Service
New Mexico VA Health Care System
Albuquerque, New Mexico

Terry A. Day, M.D.
Professor and Clinical Vice Chair
Department of Otolaryngology–Head and Neck Surgery
Medical University of South Carolina
Charleston, South Carolina

Antonio De la Cruz, M.D.
Clinical Professor
Department of Otolaryngology–Head and Neck Surgery
University of Southern California Keck School of Medicine
Director of Education
House Ear Clinic
Los Angeles, California

Charles C. Della Santina, M.D., Ph.D.
Associate Professor
Departments of Otolaryngology–Head Neck Surgery and Biomedical Engineering
Director
Vestibular NeuroEngineering Laboratory
Division of Otology, Neurotology, and Skull Base Surgery
Johns Hopkins School of Medicine
Baltimore, Maryland

Chadrick Denlinger, M.D.
Assistant Professor
Department of Surgery
Medical University of South Carolina
Charleston, South Carolina

Craig S. Derkay, M.D., F.A.A.P., F.A.C.S.
Professor of Otolaryngology and Pediatrics
Vice Chair
Department of Otolaryngology
Eastern Virginia Medical School
Director of Pediatric Otolaryngology
Children's Hospital of the King's Daughters
Norfolk, Virginia

Rodney C. Diaz, M.D.
Assistant Professor of Otology, Neurotology, and Skull Base Surgery
Department of Otolaryngology–Head and Neck Surgery
University of California, Davis, School of Medicine
Sacramento, California

Robert A. Dobie, M.D.
Professor
Department of Otolaryngology–Head and Neck Surgery
University of California, Davis, School of Medicine
Sacramento, California

Suzanne K. Doud Galli, M.D., Ph.D.
Department of Otolaryngology
Inova Fairfax Hospital
Washington, D.C.

Newton O. Duncan, M.D.
Clinical Assistant Professor
Departments of Otorhinolaryngology and Pediatrics
Baylor College of Medicine
Attending Surgeon
Texas Children's Hospital
Houston, Texas

Scott D. Z. Eggers, M.D.
Assistant Professor
Department of Neurology
Mayo Medical School
Ann Arbor, Michigan
Associate
Department of Neurology
Mayo Clinic
Rochester, Minnesota

Avraham Eisbruch, M.D.
Professor
Department of Radiation Oncology
University of Michigan Medical School
Associate Chair of Clinical Research
University of Michigan Health System
Ann Arbor, Michigan

David W. Eisele, M.D., F.A.C.S.
Professor and Chair
Department of Otolaryngology–Head and Neck Surgery
University of California, San Francisco, School of Medicine
San Francisco, California

Hussam K. El-Kashlan, M.D.
Associate Professor
Department of Otolaryngology
University of Michigan Medical School
Medical Director
Vestibular Testing Center
University of Michigan Health System
Ann Arbor, Michigan

Ravindhra G. Elluru, M.D., Ph.D.
Associate Professor
Department of Otolaryngology–Head and Neck Surgery
University of Cincinnati College of Medicine
Division of Pediatric Otolaryngology
Cincinnati Children's Hospital
Cincinnati, Ohio

Kevin H. Ende, M.D.
Clinical Instructor
Plastic Surgery and Facial Surgery
University of California, San Francisco, School of Medicine
San Francisco, California

Audrey B. Erman, M.D.
Resident
Department of Otolaryngology
University of Michigan Health System
Ann Arbor, Michigan

Samer Fakhri, M.D.
Associate Professor
Department of Otolaryngology–Head and Neck Surgery
University of Texas Medical School at Houston
Houston, Texas

Carole Fakhry, M.D., M.P.H.
Resident
Department of Otolaryngology–Head and Neck Surgery
Johns Hopkins Hospital
Baltimore, Maryland

Edward H. Farrior, M.D.
Visiting Clinical Associate Professor
Department of Otolaryngology
University of Virginia School of Medicine
Charlottesville, Virginia
Founder and Physician
Farrior Facial Plastic and Cosmetic Surgery Center
Tampa, Florida

Richard T. Farrior, M.D.
Boca Grande, Florida

Russell A. Faust, M.D., Ph.D.
Assistant Professor
Department of Otolaryngology, College of Medicine
Department of Oral Triology, College of Dentistry
The Ohio State University
Staff Attending Physician
Department of Otolaryngology
Nationwide Children's Hospital
Columbus, Ohio

Berrylin J. Ferguson, M.D.
Associate Professor
Department of Otolaryngology
University of Pittsburgh School of Medicine
Director
Division of Sino-Nasal Disorders and Allergy
University of Pittsburgh Medical Center
Pittsburgh, Pennsylvania

Paul W. Flint, M.D.
Professor and Chair
Department of Otolaryngology–Head and Neck Surgery
Oregon Health and Science University
Portland, Oregon

Howard W. Francis, M.D.
Associate Professor
Residency Program Director
Department of Otolaryngology–Head and Neck Surgery
Johns Hopkins University School of Medicine
Baltimore, Maryland

Marvin P. Fried, M.D.
Professor and University Chairman
Albert Einstein College of Medicine
Department of Otorhinolaryngology–Head and Neck Surgery
Montefiore Medical Center
Bronx, New York

David R. Friedland, M.D., Ph.D.
Associate Professor
Department of Otolaryngology and Communication Sciences
Chief
Division of Otology and Neuro-otologic Skull Base Surgery
Medical College of Wisconsin
Milwaukee, Wisconsin

Oren Friedman, M.D.
Assistant Professor
Department of Otolaryngology
Mayo Medical School
Director
Facial Plastic and Reconstructive Surgery
Mayo Clinic
Rochester, Minnesota

John L. Frodel, Jr., M.D., F.A.C.S.
Clinical Professor
Department of Otolaryngology–Head and Neck Surgery
Temple University School of Medicine
Philadelphia, Pennsylvania
Associate
Geisinger Medical Center
Danville, Pennsylvania

Gerry F. Funk, M.D., F.A.C.S.
Professor
Department of Otolaryngology–Head and Neck Surgery
University of Iowa Carver College of Medicine
Director
Division of Head and Neck Oncology
University of Iowa Hospitals and Clinics
Iowa City, Iowa

Bruce J. Gantz, M.D.
Professor
Department of Otolaryngology–Head and Neck Surgery
University of Iowa Carver College of Medicine
Head
Department of Otolaryngology–Head and Neck Surgery
University of Iowa Hospitals and Clinics
Iowa City, Iowa

C. Gaelyn Garrett, M.D.
Professor
Vanderbilt University School of Medicine
Medical Director
Vanderbilt Voice Center
Nashville, Tennessee

Jackie Gartner-Schmidt, Ph.D.
Assistant Professor
Department of Otolaryngology
University of Pittsburgh School of Medicine
Associate Director
University of Pittsburgh Voice Center
UPMC Mercy Hospital
Pittsburgh, Pennsylvania

William Donald Gay, D.D.S.
Hawes Professor of Maxillofacial Prosthetics (retired)
Department of Otolaryngology
Washington University in St. Louis School of Medicine
Attending Dentist
Barnes Hospital
St. Louis, Missouri

Norman N. Ge, M.D., M.S.E.E., F.A.C.S.
Associate Professor
Department of Otolaryngology
University of California, Irvine, School of Medicine
Orange, California
Chief
Department of Head and Neck Surgery
VA Long Beach Healthcare System
Long Beach, California

M. Boyd Gillespie, M.D., M.S.
Associate Professor
Department of Otolaryngology–Head and Neck Surgery
Medical University of South Carolina
Charleston, South Carolina

Douglas A. Girod, M.D., F.A.C.S.
Professor and Russell E. Bridwell Chair
Department of Otolaryngology–Head and Neck Surgery
Senior Associate Dean for Clinical Affairs
University of Kansas School of Medicine
University of Kansas of Medical Center
Kansas City, Kansas

George S. Goding, Jr., M.D.
Associate Professor
Department of Otolaryngology
University of Minnesota Medical School
Faculty
Department of Otolaryngology
Hennepin County Medical Center
Minneapolis, Minnesota

Andrew N. Goldberg, M.D., F.A.C.S.
Professor
Departments of Otolaryngology–Head and Neck Surgery and Neurological Surgery
University of California, San Francisco, School of Medicine
Director
Rhinology and Sinus Surgery
UCSF Medical Center
San Francisco, California

David Goldenberg, M.D.
Associate Professor
Department of Surgery
Division of Otolaryngology–Head and Neck Surgery
Penn State University College of Medicine
Director
Head and Neck Surgery
Penn State Milton S. Hershey Medical Center
Director
Head and Neck Cancer Program
Penn State Cancer Institute
Hershey, Pennsylvania

Daniel O. Graney, Ph.D.
Professor
Department of Biological Structure
University of Washington School of Medicine
Seattle, Washington

Nazaneen N. Grant, M.D.
Assistant Professor
Department of Otolaryngology–Head and Neck Surgery
Georgetown University School of Medicine and Health Sciences
Georgetown University Hospital
Washington, D.C.

Vincent Grégoire, M.D., Ph.D., Hon.F.R.C.R.
Professor of Radiation Oncology
Catholic University of Louvain
Louvain-la-Neuve, Belgium
Head of Clinics
St. Luc University Hospital
Brussels, Belgium

Heike Gries, M.D., Ph.D.
Assistant Professor of Anesthesiology and Pediatrics
Division of Pediatric Anesthesiology
Department of Anesthesiology and Peri-Operative Medicine
Oregon Health and Science University School of Medicine
Portland, Oregon

Samuel P. Gubbels, M.D.
Assistant Professor
Department of Surgery
University of Wisconsin–Madison School of Medicine and Public Health
Madison, Wisconsin

Joel Guss, M.D.
Attending Physician
Department of Head and Neck Surgery
Kaiser Permanente Medical Center
Walnut Creek, California

Patrick Ha, M.D., F.A.C.S.
Assistant Professor
Department of Otolaryngology–Head and Neck Surgery
Johns Hopkins University School of Medicine
Physician
Johns Hopkins Head and Neck Surgery at the Greater Baltimore Medical Center
Milton J. Dance, Jr., Head and Neck Center
Baltimore, Maryland

Grant S. Hamilton, III, M.D.
Assistant Professor
University of Iowa Carver College of Medicine
University of Iowa Hospitals and Clinics
Iowa City, Iowa

Ehab Y. Hanna, M.D., F.A.C.S.
Lecturer
University of Arkansas for Medical Sciences
Little Rock, Arkansas
Professor and Vice Chairman
Department of Head and Neck Surgery
Director of Skull Base Surgery
Medical Director of Head and Neck Center
University of Texas M.D. Anderson Cancer Center
Houston, Texas

Lee A. Harker, M.D.
Formerly Deputy Director
Boys Town National Research Hospital
Vice Chair
Department of Otolaryngology and Human Communication
Omaha, Nebraska

Uli Harréus, Dr.Med.
Assistant Professor
Department of Otolaryngology–Head and Neck Surgery
Ludwig-Maximilians University
Grosshadern Clinic
Munich, Germany

Robert V. Harrison, Ph.D.
Professor and Director of Research
Department of Otolaryngology–Head and Neck Surgery
University of Toronto Faculty of Medicine
Senior Scientist
Neuroscience and Mental Health
Hospital for Sick Children
Toronto, Ontario, Canada

Bruce H. Haughey, M.B.Ch.B., F.A.C.S., F.R.A.C.S.
Professor and Director
Head and Neck Surgical Oncology
Department of Otolaryngology–Head and Neck Surgery
Washington University in St. Louis School of Medicine
St. Louis, Missouri

John W. Hellstein, D.D.S.
Clinical Professor of Oral and Maxillofacial Pathology
University of Iowa Carver College of Medicine
Iowa City, Iowa

Kurt Herzer
Marshall Scholar
Department of Social Policy and Social Work
University of Oxford
Oxford, United Kingdom
Woodrow Wilson Fellow
Departments of Public Health Studies and Anesthesiology and Critical Care Medicine
Johns Hopkins University School of Medicine
Baltimore, Maryland

Michael S. Hildebrand, Ph.D.
Postdoctoral Fellow
Department of Otolaryngology
University of Iowa Carver College of Medicine
University of Iowa Hospitals and Clinics
Iowa City, Iowa

Frans J. M. Hilgers, M.D., Ph.D.
Professor
Amsterdam Center for Language and Communication (Institute of Phonetic Sciences)
Academic Medical Center
University of Amsterdam
Emeritus Chairman
Department of Head and Neck Oncology and Surgery
The Netherlands Cancer Institute–Antoni van Leeuwenhoek Hospital
Amsterdam, The Netherlands

Justin D. Hill, M.D.
Physician
Central Oregon Ear, Nose & Throat
Bend, Oregon

Michael L. Hinni, M.D.
Associate Professor and Residency Program Director
Mayo Clinic College of Medicine
Consultant
Department of Otolaryngology–Head and Neck Surgery
Mayo Clinic
Phoenix, Arizona

Henry T. Hoffman, M.D., F.A.C.S.
Professor
Department of Otolaryngology–Head and Neck Surgery
University of Iowa Carver College of Medicine
Director
Voice Clinic
University of Iowa Hospitals and Clinics
Iowa City, Iowa

Eric H. Holbrook, M.D., M.S.(Anat.)
Assistant Professor
Department of Otology and Laryngology
Harvard Medical School
Associate Surgeon
Department of Otolaryngology
Massachusetts Eye and Ear Infirmary
Boston, Massachusetts

Lauren D. Holinger, M.D.
Professor
Department of Otolaryngology–Head and Neck Surgery
Northwestern University Feinberg School of Medicine
Head
Division of Pediatric Otolaryngology
Children's Memorial Hospital
Chicago, Illinois

Allison MacGregor Holzapfel, M.D.
Volunteer Clinical Professor
Department of Otolaryngology–Head and Neck Surgery
University of Cincinnati College of Medicine
Cincinnati, Ohio

David B. Hom, M.D., F.A.C.S.
Professor
Department of Otolaryngology–Head and Neck Surgery
University of Cincinnati College of Medicine
Director
Facial Plastic and Reconstructive Surgery
University of Cincinnati Medical Center
Cincinnati Children's Hospital Medical Center
Cincinnati, Ohio

John W. House, M.D.
Clinic Professor
Department of Otorhinolaryngology–Head and Neck Surgery
University of Southern California Keck School of Medicine
Associate Physician
House Clinic
President
House Ear Institute
Los Angeles, California

Joyce Colton House, M.D.
Chief Resident
Boston Medical Center
Boston, Massachusetts

Timothy E. Hullar, M.D.
Assistant Professor
Department of Otolaryngology–Head and Neck Surgery
Washington University in St. Louis School of Medicine
St. Louis, Missouri

Murad Husein, M.D.
Assistant Professor
London Health Sciences Centre
Victoria Hospital
Children's Hospital of Western Ontario
London, Ontario, Canada

Steven Ing, M.D.
Assistant Professor of Medicine
The Ohio State University College of Medicine
Columbus, Ohio

Tim A. Iseli, M.B.B.S., F.R.A.C.S.
Staff Surgeon
Royal Melbourne Hospital
Melbourne, Victoria, Australia

Stacey Ishman, M.D.
Assistant Professor
Department of Pediatrics
Department of Otolaryngology–Head and Neck Surgery
Johns Hopkins University School of Medicine
Director
Center for Snoring and Sleep Surgery
Johns Hopkins Hospital
Baltimore, Maryland

Robert K. Jackler, M.D.
Edward C. and Amy H. Sewall Professor and Chair
Department of Otolaryngology–Head and Neck Surgery
Associate Dean
Stanford University School of Medicine
Attending Physician
Lucile Packard Children's Hospital at Stanford
Stanford, California

Brian Jameson, D.O.
Clinical Assistant Professor
Temple University School of Medicine
Philadelphia, Pennsylvania
Attending Endocrinologist
Geisinger Wyoming Valley Medical Center
Wilkes-Barre, Pennsylvania

Herman A. Jenkins, M.D.
Professor and Chair
Department of Otolaryngology
University of Colorado, Denver, School of Medicine
University of Colorado Hospital
Aurora, Colorado

Hong-Ryol Jin, M.D., Ph.D.
Professor
Department of Otolaryngology–Head and Neck Surgery
Seoul National University College of Medicine
Seoul, Korea

John K. Joe, M.D.*
Assistant Professor
Department of Surgery
Division of Otolaryngology–Head and Neck Surgery
Yale University School of Medicine
New Haven, Connecticut

Stephanie A. Joe, M.D.
Assistant Professor
Department of Otolaryngology–Head and Neck Surgery
University of Illinois at Chicago College of Medicine
Director
Sinus and Nasal Allergy Center
Codirector
Skull Base Surgery
University of Illinois Hospital
Chicago, Illinois

*Deceased

Gary Johnson, M.D.
Professor
Department of Obstetrics and Gynecology
Director of Gynecologic Oncology
Clerkship Director
Southern Illinois University School of Medicine
Springfield, Illinois

Rhonda Johnson, M.Ed., Ph.D.
Assistant Professor
Department of Psychiatry
Southern Illinois University School of Medicine
Psychologist
SimmonsCooper Cancer Institute
St. John's Hospital
Memorial Medical Center
Springfield, Illinois

Tiffany A. Johnson, Ph.D.
Assistant Professor
Department of Speech-Language-Hearing: Sciences and Disorders
University of Kansas
Lawrence, Kansas

Timothy M. Johnson, M.D.
Professor
Department of Dermatology and Otorhinolaryngology–Head and Neck Surgery
University of Michigan Medical School
Ann Arbor, Michigan

Nick S. Jones, M.D., F.R.C.S., F.R.C.S.(ORC)
Professor
Department of Otorhinolaryngology–Head and Neck Surgery
University of Nottingham
Queens Medical Centre
University Hospital
Nottingham, United Kingdom

Sheldon S. Kabaker, M.D.
Professor
Department of Otolaryngology
University of California, San Francisco, School of Medicine
San Francisco, California

Lucy H. Karnell, Ph.D.
Research Scientist
University of Iowa Hospitals and Clinics
Iowa City, Iowa

Matthew L. Kashima, M.D., M.P.H.
Assistant Professor
Johns Hopkins University School of Medicine
Chair
Department of Otolaryngology–Head and Neck Surgery
Johns Hopkins Bayview Medical Center
Baltimore, Maryland

Robert M. Kellman, M.D.
Professor and Chair
Department of Otolaryngology and Communication Sciences
SUNY Upstate Medical University
Syracuse, New York

Paul E. Kelly, M.D.
Staff Surgeon
Eastern Long Island Hospital
Greenport, New York
Peconic Bay Medical Center
Riverhead, New York

David W. Kennedy, M.D.
Professor of Rhinology
Department of Otolaryngology–Head and Neck Surgery
Vice Dean for Professional Services
University of Pennsylvania School of Medicine
Philadelphia, Pennsylvania

Ayesha N. Khalid, M.D.
Clinical Instructor
Oregon Health and Science University School of Medicine
Portland, Oregon

Merrill S. Kies, M.D.
Professor of Medicine
University of Texas M.D. Anderson Cancer Center
Houston, Texas

Paul R. Kileny, Ph.D.
Professor
Departments of Otolaryngology and Pediatrics
University of Michigan Medical School
Academic Program Director
Audiology and Hearing Rehabilitation
University of Michigan Health System
Ann Arbor, Michigan

David W. Kim, M.D.
Clinical Associate Professor
Department of Otolaryngology–Head and Neck Surgery
Division of Facial Plastic Surgery
University of California, San Francisco, School of Medicine
San Francisco, California

Jason H. Kim, M.D., F.A.C.S.
Assistant Professor
Department of Otolaryngology–Head and Neck Surgery
University of California, Irvine, School of Medicine
Orange, California

Theresa B. Kim, M.D.
Resident
Department of Otolaryngology–Head and Neck Surgery
UCSF Medical Center
San Francisco, California

William J. Kimberling, Ph.D.
Professor of Ophthalmology
Departments Ophthalmology and Visual Sciences and Otolaryngology
University of Iowa Carver College of Medicine
Iowa City, Iowa
Senior Scientist
Boys Town National Research Hospital
Omaha, Nebraska

Jeffrey Koh, M.D., M.B.A.
Professor of Anesthesiology and Pediatrics
Oregon Health and Science University School of Medicine
Chief
Division of Pediatric Anesthesiology and Pain Management
Doernbecher Children's Hospital
Portland, Oregon

Niels Kokot, M.D.
Assistant Professor
Department of Otolaryngology–Head and Neck Surgery
University of Southern California Keck School of Medicine
Los Angeles, California

Peter J. Koltai, M.D., F.A.C.S., F.A.A.P.
Professor of Otolaryngology
Department of Otolaryngology–Head and Neck Surgery
Stanford University School of Medicine
Chief
Division of Pediatric Otolaryngology
Lucile Packard Children's Hospital at Stanford
Stanford, California

Frederick K. Kozak, M.D.
Clinical Professor
University of British Columbia Faculty of Medicine
Head
Division of Pediatric Otolaryngology
Medical/Surgical Director
Cochlea Implant Program
B.C. Children's Hospital
Vancouver, British Columbia, Canada

Paul R. Krakovitz, M.D.
Assistant Professor
Department of Surgery
Cleveland Clinic Lerner College of Medicine of Case Western Reserve University
Section Head, Pediatric Otolaryngology
Head and Neck Institute
Cleveland Clinic
Cleveland, Ohio

Russell W. H. Kridel, M.D., F.A.C.S.
Clinical Professor
Department of Otolaryngology–Head and Neck Surgery
Division of Facial Plastic and Reconstructive Surgery
University of Texas Medical School at Houston
Houston, Texas

Parvesh Kumar, M.D.
Professor and Chair
Department of Radiation Oncology
University of Southern California Keck School of Medicine
Chair
Department of Radiation Oncology
Los Angeles County Hospital–USC Medical Center
Director
Division of Radiation Oncology
USC Norris Cancer Center Hospital
Los Angeles, California

Melda Kunduk, Ph.D.
Assistant Professor
Department of Communication Sciences and Disorders
Louisiana State University School of Medicine at New Orleans Health Sciences Center
Speech Pathologist
Department of Otolaryngology–Head Neck Surgery
Louisiana State University Health Sciences Center New Orleans, Lourisiana
Our Lady of the Lake Voice Center
Baton Rouge, Louisiana

Ollivier Laccourreye, M.D.
Professor
Department of Otorhinolaryngology–Head and Neck Surgery
Paris Descartes University
Hôpital Européen Georges Pompidou
Paris, France

JoAnne Lacey, M.D.
Assistant Professor
Department of Radiology
Division of Neuroradiology
Washington University in St. Louis School of Medicine
Neuroradiologist
Barnes-Jewish Hospital
St. Louis, Missouri

Stephen Y. Lai, M.D., Ph.D.
Assistant Professor
Department of Head and Neck Surgery
University of Texas M.D. Anderson Cancer Center
Houston, Texas

Devyani Lal, M.D.
Chief Resident
Department of Otolaryngology–Head and Neck Surgery
Loyola University Medical Center
Maywood, Illinois

Anil K. Lalwani, M.D.
Mendik Foundation Professor and Chair
Department of Otolaryngology
New York University School of Medicine
New York, New York

Paul R. Lambert, M.D.
Professor and Chair
Department of Otolaryngology–Head and Neck Surgery
Medical University of South Carolina
Charleston, South Carolina

Amy Anne Lassig, M.D.
Assistant Professor
Department of Otolaryngology–Head and Neck Surgery
University of Minnesota Medical School
Minneapolis, Minnesota

Richard E. Latchaw, M.D.
Professor
Department of Radiology
University of California, Davis, School of Medicine
Director
Neuroradiology Division
Department of Radiology
UC Davis Medical Center
Sacramento, California

Kevin P. Leahy, M.D., Ph.D.
Assistant Professor
Department of Otorhinolaryngology–Head and Neck Surgery
University of Pennsylvania School of Medicine
Philadelphia, Pennsylvania

Daniel J. Lee, M.D.
Assistant Professor
Department of Otology and Laryngology
Harvard Medical School
Department of Otolaryngology
Massachusetts Eye and Ear Infirmary
Boston, Massachusetts

Ken K. Lee, M.D.

Associate Professor
Departments of Dermatology, Surgery, and Otolaryngology
Director
Department of Dermatologic and Laser Surgery
Oregon Health and Science University School of Medicine
Portland, Oregon

Nancy Lee, M.D.

Associate Attending
Department of Radiation Oncology
Memorial Sloan-Kettering Cancer Center
New York, New York

Jean-Louis Lefebvre, M.D.

Professor and Chief
Head and Neck Cancer
Center Oscar Lambret
Lille, France

Maureen A. Lefton-Greif, Ph.D.

Associate Professor
Department of Otolaryngology–Head and Neck Surgery
Department of Pediatrics
Johns Hopkins University School of Medicine
Speech-Language Pathologist
Johns Hopkins Hospital
Baltimore, Maryland

Donald A. Leopold, M.D., M.S.(Bus.)

Professor and Chair
Department of Otolaryngology–Head and Neck Surgery
University of Nebraska School of Medicine
Omaha, Nebraska

James S. Lewis, Jr., M.D.

Assistant Professor of Pathology and Immunology
Department of Anatomic and Molecular Pathology
Director, Research Histology and Tissue Microarray Laboratory
Washington University in St. Louis School of Medicine
St. Louis, Missouri

Daqing Li, M.D.

Associate Professor
Department of Otorhinolaryngology–Head and Neck Surgery
University of Pennsylvania School of Medicine
Director
Gene and Molecular Therapy Laboratory
Director
Temporal Bone Laboratory
Hospital of the University of Pennsylvania
Philadelphia, Pennsylvania

Timothy S. Lian, M.D.

Associate Professor
Department of Otolaryngology–Head and Neck Surgery
Residency Program Director
Louisiana State University Health Sciences Center School of Medicine Shreveport
Shreveport, Louisiana

Greg R. Licameli, M.D., M.H.C.M., F.A.C.S.

Assistant Professor
Department of Otology and Laryngology
Harvard Medical School
Interim Chief
Department of Otolaryngology
Children's Hospital
Boston, Massachusetts

Charles J. Limb, M.D.

Associate Professor
Department of Otolaryngology–Head and Neck Surgery
Johns Hopkins University School of Medicine
Johns Hopkins Hospital
Baltimore, Maryland

Jeri A. Logemann, Ph.D.

Ralph and Jean Sundin Professor
Department of Communication Sciences and Disorders
Northwestern University
Evanston, Illinois
Professor
Departments of Neurology and Otolaryngology–Head and Neck Surgery
Northwestern University Feinberg School of Medicine
Director
Voice, Speech, and Language Service and Swallowing Center
Northwestern Memorial Hospital
Chicago, Illinois

Thomas Loh, M.B.B.S., F.R.C.S.

Associate Professor
Department of Otolaryngology
National University of Singapore
Senior Consultant
Department of Otolaryngology–Head and Neck Surgery
National University Hospital
Singapore

Brenda L. Lonsbury-Martin, Ph.D.

Professor
Department of Otolaryngology–Head and Neck Surgery
Loma Linda University School of Medicine
Senior Research Scientist
VA Loma Linda Healthcare System
Loma Linda, California

Manuel A. Lopez, M.D.

Chief
Facial Plastic Surgery
Wilford Hall Medical Center
San Antonio, Texas

Rodney P. Lusk, M.D.

Director
Ear, Nose, and Throat Institute
Boys Town National Research Hospital
Omaha, Nebraska

Lawrence R. Lustig, M.D.

Francis A. Sooy, M.D., Chair in Otolaryngology
Chief
Division of Otology and Neurotology
Department of Otolaryngology–Head and Neck Surgery
University of California, San Francisco, School of Medicine
San Francisco, California

Anna Lysakowski, Ph.D.

Professor
Department of Anatomy and Cell Biology
University of Illinois at Chicago College of Medicine
Chicago, Illinois

Carol J. MacArthur, M.D.

Associate Professor
Department of Otolaryngology–Head and Neck Surgery
Oregon Health and Science University School of Medicine
Portland, Oregon

Robert H. Maisel, M.D.
Professor
Department of Otolaryngology
University of Minnesota Medical School
Chief of Otolaryngology
Hennepin County Medical Center
Minneapolis, Minnesota

James P. Malone, M.D.
Associate Professor
Division of Otolaryngology
Southern Illinois University School of Medicine
Springfield, Illinois

Ellen M. Mandel, M.D.
Associate Professor
Department of Otolaryngology
University of Pittsburgh School of Medicine
Children's Hospital of Pittsburgh
Pittsburgh, Pennsylvania

Susan J. Mandel, M.D., M.P.H.
Professor and Associate Chief
Division of Endocrinology, Diabetes and Metabolism
Department of Medicine
University of Pennsylvania Health System
Philadelphia, Pennsylvania

Scott C. Manning, M.D.
Professor
Department of Otolaryngology
University of Washington in St. Louis School of Medicine
Chief
Division of Pediatric Otolaryngology
Seattle Children's Hospital
Seattle, Washington

Lynette Mark, M.D.
Associate Professor
Departments of Anesthesiology and Critical Care Medicine and Otolaryngology–Head and Neck Surgery
Johns Hopkins University School of Medicine
Johns Hopkins Hospital
Baltimore, Maryland

Jeffery C. Markt, D.D.S.
Associate Professor and Director
Department of Otolaryngology–Head and Neck Surgery
Division of Oral Facial Prosthetics/Dental Oncology
University of Nebraska School of Medicine
Omaha, Nebraska

Michael Marsh, M.D.
Physician
Arkansas Center for Ear, Nose, Throat and Allergy
Fort Smith, Arkansas

Glen K. Martin, Ph.D.
Professor
Department of Otolaryngology–Head and Neck Surgery
Loma Linda School of Medicine
Loma Linda, California

Douglas E. Mattox, M.D.
Professor and William Chester Warren, Jr., M.D., Chair
Department of Otolaryngology–Head and Neck Surgery
Emory School of Medicine
Atlanta, Georgia

Thomas V. McCaffrey, M.D., Ph.D.
Professor and Chair
Department of Otolaryngology–Head and Neck Surgery
University of South Florida College of Medicine
Program Leader and Senior Member
Head and Neck Oncology
H. Lee Moffitt Cancer Center
Tampa, Florida

Timothy M. McCulloch, M.D., F.A.C.S.
Professor
Department of Surgery
University of Wisconsin School of Medicine and Public Health
Chair
Division of Otolaryngology–Head and Neck Surgery
University of Wisconsin Hospitals and Clinics
Madison, Wisconsin

JoAnn McGee, Ph.D.
Scientist
Developmental Auditory Physiology Laboratory
Boys Town National Research Hospital
Omaha, Nebraska

John F. McGuire, M.D.
Attending Physician
Department of Otolaryngology
Fallbrook Hospital
Fallbrook, California

Jonathan McJunkin, M.D.
Resident
Department of Otolaryngology–Head and Neck Surgery
Washington University Medical Center
St. Louis, Missouri

J. Scott McMurray, M.D.
Associate Professor
Departments of Surgery and Pediatrics
University of Wisconsin School of Medicine and Public Health
American Family Children's Hospital
Madison, Wisconsin

Albert L. Merati, M.D.
Associate Professor and Chief
Division of Laryngology
Department of Otolaryngology–Head and Neck Surgery
Department of Speech and Hearing Sciences
University of Washington School of Medicine
Adjunct Associate Professor
Seattle, Washington

Saumil N. Merchant, M.D.
Gudrun Larsen Eliasen and Nels Kristian Eliasen Professor of Otology and Laryngology
Harvard Medical School
Surgeon in Otolaryngology
Massachusetts Eye and Ear Infirmary
Boston, Massachusetts

Anna H. Messner, M.D.
Professor
Departments of Otolaryngology–Head and Neck Surgery and Pediatrics
Stanford University School of Medicine
Stanford, California
Vice Chair
Department of Otolaryngology–Head and Neck Surgery
Lucile Packard Children's Hospital at Stanford
Palo Alto, California

James Michelson, M.D.
Professor
Department of Orthopedics and Rehabilitation
University of Vermont College of Medicine
Medical Informaticist
Fletcher Allen Health Care
Burlington, Vermont

Henry A. Milczuk, M.D.
Associate Professor of Pediatric Otolaryngology
Oregon Health and Science University School of Medicine
Portland, Oregon

Lloyd B. Minor, M.D.
Andelot Professor and Director
Department of Otolaryngology–Head and Neck Surgery
Johns Hopkins University School of Medicine
Johns Hopkins Hospital
Baltimore, Maryland

Steven Ross Mobley, M.D.
Associate Professor
Facial Plastic and Reconstructive Surgery
Department of Otolaryngology
University of Utah School of Medicine
Salt Lake City, Utah

Harlan Muntz, M.D., F.A.C.S., F.A.A.P.
Professor
Department of Otolaryngology–Head and Neck Surgery
University of Utah School of Medicine
Director
Department of Pediatric Otolaryngology
Primary Children's Medical Center
Salt Lake City, Utah

Craig S. Murakami, M.D.
Clinical Associate Professor
Department of Otolaryngology–Head and Neck Surgery
University of Washington School of Medicine
Director
Department of Facial Plastic Surgery
Virginia Mason Medical Center
Seattle, Washington

Charles M. Myer, III, M.D.
Professor and Vice Chair
Department of Otolaryngology
University of Cincinnati College of Medicine
Director
Hearing Impaired Clinic
Cincinnati Children's Hospital Medical Center
Cincinnati, Ohio

Robert M. Naclerio, M.D.
Professor and Chief
Department of Otolaryngology–Head and Neck Surgery
University of Chicago Pritzker School of Medicine
Chicago, Illinois

Joseph B. Nadol, Jr., M.D.
Walter Augustus Lecompte Professor and Chair
Department of Otology and Laryngology
Harvard Medical School
Chief
Department of Otolaryngology
Massachusetts Eye and Ear Infirmary
Boston, Massachusetts

Paul S. Nassif, M.D., F.A.C.S.
Assistant Clinical Professor
Department of Otolaryngology
University of Southern California Keck School of Medicine
Los Angeles, California
Partner
Spalding Drive Cosmetic Surgery and Dermatology
Beverly Hills, California

Julian Nedzelski, M.D.
Professor
Department of Otolaryngology
University of Toronto Faculty of Medicine
Otolaryngologist-in-Chief
Sunnybrook Health Sciences Centre
Toronto, Ontario, Canada

Piero Nicolai, M.D.
Professor
University of Brescia School of Medicine
Chairman
Spedali Civili
Brescia, Italy

David R. Nielsen, M.D.
Executive Vice President and CEO
American Academy of Otolaryngology–Head and Neck Surgery
Alexandria, Virginia

John K. Niparko, M.D.
George T. Nager Professor
Department of Otolaryngology–Head and Neck Surgery
Director
Divisions of Otology, Neurotology, Skull Base Surgery, and Audiology
Johns Hopkins University School of Medicine
Baltimore, Maryland

Susan J. Norton, Ph.D.
Professor
Department of Otolaryngology–Head and Neck Surgery
Adjunct Professor
Department of Speech and Hearing Sciences
University of Washington School of Medicine
Chief
Department of Pediatric Audiology
Seattle Children's Hospital
Seattle, Washington

S. A. Reza Nouraei, M.A.(Cantab.), M.B.B.Chir., M.R.C.S.
Researcher
The Laryngology Research Group
University College London
Academic Specialist Registrar
Charing Cross Hospital
London, United Kingdom

Daniel W. Nuss, M.D., F.A.C.S.
G. D. Lyons Professor and Chair
Department of Otolaryngology–Head and Neck Surgery
Louisiana State University Health Sciences Center School of Medicine at New Orleans
New Orleans, Louisiana

Brian Nussenbaum, M.D.
Associate Professor of Otolaryngology
Vice Chair for Clinical Affairs
Patient Safety Officer
Washington University in St. Louis School of Medicine
Attending Surgeon
Barnes-Jewish Hospital
St. Louis, Missouri

Rick M. Odland, M.D., Ph.D.
Associate Professor
Department of Otolaryngology
University of Minnesota Medical School
Staff Surgeon
Departmental of Otolaryngology
Hennepin County Medical Center
Minneapolis, Minnesota

Gerard O'Donoghue, M.Ch., F.R.C.S.
Professor of Otology and Neurotology
University of Nottingham
Codirector
National Biomedical Unit in Hearing
Department of Otolaryngology
Queen's Medical Centre
Nottingham, United Kingdom

Eric R. Oliver, M.D.
Chief Resident
Department of Otolaryngology–Head and Neck Surgery
MUSC University Hospital
Charleston, South Carolina

Bert W. O'Malley, Jr., M.D.
Gabriel Tucker Professor and Chairman
Department of Otorhinolaryngology–Head and Neck Surgery
Professor of Neurosurgery
Abramson Cancer Center
University of Pennsylvania School of Medicine
Codirector
Center for Cranial Base Surgery
Codirector
Head and Neck Cancer Center
University of Pennsylvania Health System
Philadelphia, Pennsylvania

Robert C. O'Reilly, M.D.
Clinical Associate Professor
Department of Otolaryngology and Pediatrics
Jefferson Medical College
Thomas Jefferson University
Philadelphia, Pennsylvania
Pediatric Otology/Neurotology
A. I. duPont Hospital for Children
Wilmington, Delaware

Juan Camilo Ospina, M.D.
Assistant Professor
Javeriana University School of Medicine
Head
Division of Otorhinolaryngology and Maxillofacial Surgery
San Ignacio University Hospital
Director
Division of Otorhinolaryngology
Roosevelt Institute
Bogota, Colombia

Robert H. Ossoff, D.M.D., M.D.
Guy M. Maness Professor of Laryngology and Voice
Department of Otolaryngology–Head and Neck Surgery
Vanderbilt University School of Medicine
Assistant Vice Chancellor for Compliance and Corporate Integrity
Vanderbilt Medical Center
Nashville, Tennessee

Kristen J. Otto, M.D.
Assistant Professor
Department of Otolaryngology and Communicative Sciences
University of Mississippi School of Medicine
Jackson, Mississippi

Mark D. Packer, M.D.
Assistant Clinical Professor
University of Texas Health Science Center at San Antonio School of Medicine
San Antonio Uniformed Services Health Education Consortium
San Antonio, Texas
Staff Neurotologist
Wilford Hall Medical Center
Lackland Air Force Base, Texas

John Pallanch, M.D.
Assistant Professor
Department of Otolaryngology
Mayo School of Graduate Medical Education
Chair
Division of Rhinology
Department of Otorhinolaryngology
Mayo Clinic
Rochester, Minnesota

James N. Palmer, M.D.
Associate Professor
Department of Otorhinolaryngology–Head and Neck Surgery
University of Pennsylvania School of Medicine
Director
Division of Rhinology
Hospital of the University of Pennsylvania
Philadelphia, Pennsylvania

Stephen S. Park, M.D.
Professor and Vice Chair
Department of Otolaryngology
Director
Division of Facial Plastic Surgery
University of Virginia School of Medicine
Charlottesville, Virginia

Sundip Patel, M.D.
Resident
Department of Otolaryngology–Head Neck Surgery
University of Illinois Hospital
Chicago, Illinois

G. Alexander Patterson, M.D.
Professor
Department of Surgery
Washington University in St. Louis School of Medicine
Barnes-Jewish Hospital
St. Louis, Missouri

Bruce W. Pearson, M.D.

Emeritus Professor
Department of Otolaryngology–Head and Neck Surgery
Mayo Clinic College of Medicine
Jacksonville, Florida

Phillip K. Pellitteri, D.O., F.A.C.S.

Clinical Professor
Department of Otolaryngology–Head and Neck Surgery
Temple University School of Medicine
Philadelphia, Pennsylvania
Chief, Section of Head, Neck, and Endocrine Surgery
Department of Otolaryngology–Head and Neck Surgery
Geisinger Health System
Danville, Pennsylvania

Jonathan A. Perkins, D.O.

Associate Professor
Department of Otolaryngology–Head and Neck Surgery
University of Washington School of Medicine
Attending Pediatric Otolaryngologist
Seattle Children's Hospital
Seattle, Washington

Stephen W. Perkins, M.D.

Clinical Associate Professor
Department of Otolaryngology
Indiana University School of Medicine
President
Meridian Plastic Surgeons
Meridian Plastic Surgery Center
Indianapolis, Indiana

Colin D. Pero, M.D.

Volunteer Clinical Faculty
University of Texas Southwestern Medical School
Dallas, Texas
Private Practice
Plano, Texas

Shirley S. N. Pignatari, M.D., Ph.D.

Associate Professor
Department of Otolaryngology–Head and Neck Surgery
Federal University of São Paulo
Head
Pediatric ENT Division
ENT Center of São Paulo
Professor
Edmundo Uasconcelos Hospital
São Paulo, Brazil

Steven D. Pletcher, M.D.

Assistant Professor
Department of Otolaryngology–Head and Neck Surgery
University of California, San Francisco, School of Medicine
San Francisco, California

Aron Popovtzer, M.D.

Physician
Davidoff Comprehensive Cancer Center
Consultant
Department of Otolaryngology
Rabin Medical Center
Petah-Tikva, Israel

Gregory N. Postma, M.D.

Professor
Department of Otolaryngology
Medical College of Georgia
Director
Center for Voice and Swallowing Disorders
Augusta, Georgia

William P. Potsic, M.D., M.M.M.

Professor
Department Otolaryngology–Head and Neck Surgery
University of Pennsylvania School of Medicine
Senior Surgeon
Division of Otolaryngology
The Children's Hospital of Philadelphia
Philadelphia, Pennsylvania

Sheri A. Poznanovic, M.D.

Clinical Instructor
University of Colorado School of Medicine
Clinical Staff
The Children's Hospital
Denver, Colorado
Pediatric Otolaryngologist
Colorado Otolaryngology Associates
Colorado Springs, Colorado

Vito C. Quatela, M.D.

Clinical Associate Professor
Department of Otolaryngology
University of Rochester School of Medicine and Dentistry
Quatela Center for Plastic Surgery
Rochester, New York

C. Rose Rabinov, M.D.

Bakersfield, California

Virginia Ramachandran, Au.D

Senior Staff Audiologist
Department of Otolaryngology–Head and Neck Surgery
Division of Audiology
Henry Ford Hospital
Detroit, Michigan

Gregory W. Randolph, M.D., F.A.C.S

Associate Professor
Department of Otolaryngology–Head and Neck Surgery
Harvard Medical School
Director
Endocrine Surgery, General Otolaryngology, and General and Thyroid Services
Massachusetts Eye and Ear Infirmary
Boston, Massachusetts

Christopher H. Rassekh, M.D., F.A.C.S

Associate Professor
Department of Otolaryngology–Head and Neck Surgery
Chief
Division of Head and Neck Oncology
West Virginia University School of Medicine
Co-Director, Center for Cranial Base Surgery
Morgantown, West Virginia

Steven D. Rauch, M.D.
Associate Professor
Department of Otology and Laryngology
Harvard Medical School
Coordinator
Medical Student Education
Department of Otolaryngology–Head and Neck Surgery
Massachusetts Eye and Ear Infirmary
Boston, Massachusetts

Lou Reinisch, Ph.D.
Professor of Physics and Head
Department of Physical and Earth Sciences
Jacksonville State University
Jacksonville, Alabama

Mark, A. Richardson, M.D.
Professor
Department of Otolaryngology–Head and Neck Surgery
Dean
School of Medicine
Oregon Health and Science University
Portland, Oregon

Gresham T. Richter, M.D.
Assistant Professor
Department of Otolaryngology–Head and Neck Surgery
The University of Arkansas for Medical Sciences College of Medicine
Division of Pediatric Otolaryngology
Vascular Anomalies Center
Arkansas Children's Hospital
Little Rock, Arkansas

James M. Ridgway, M.D.
Fellow
Facial Plastic and Reconstructive Surgery
Department of Otolaryngology–Head and Neck Surgery
University of Washington School of Medicine
Seattle, Washington

K. Thomas Robbins, M.D.
Director
SimmonsCooper Cancer Institute at Southern Illinois University
Professor
Division of Otolaryngology–Head and Neck Surgery
Southern Illinois University School of Medicine
Springfield, Illinois

Frederick C. Roediger, M.D.
Resident
Department of Otolaryngology–Head and Neck Surgery
UCSF Medical Center
San Francisco, California

Jeremy Rogers, M.D.
Chief Resident
Department of Otolaryngology–Head and Neck Surgery
USF Medical Center
Head and Neck Program
H. Lee Moffitt Cancer Center
Tampa, Florida

Ohad Ronen, M.D., F.A.C.S.
Attending Surgeon
Department of Otolaryngology–Head and Neck Surgery
Lady Davis Carmel Medical Center
Haifa, Israel

Richard M. Rosenfeld, M.D., M.P.H.
Professor and Chairman
Department of Otolaryngology
SUNY Downstate School of Medicine
Chairman
Department of Otolaryngology
Long Island College Hospital
Brooklyn, New York

Bruce E. Rotter, D.M.D.
Professor
Oral and Maxillofacial Surgery
Associate Dean for Academic Affairs
Southern Illinois University School of Dental Medicine
Alton, Illinois
Consultant
Oral and Maxillofacial Surgeon
John Cochrane VA Medical Center
St. Louis, Missouri

Jay T. Rubinstein, M.D., Ph.D.
Professor
Departments of Otolaryngology and Bioengineering
University of Washington School of Medicine
Seattle, Washington

Michael J. Ruckenstein, M.D., F.A.C.S., F.R.C.S.C.
Professor
Residency Program Director
Department of Otorhinolaryngology–Head and Neck Surgery
Vice Chair for Education and Academic Affairs
University of Pennsylvania School of Medicine
Philadelphia, Pennsylvania

Zoran Rumboldt, M.D.
Associate Professor
Department of Radiology
Medical University of South Carolina
Charleston, South Carolina

Christina L. Runge-Samuelson, Ph.D.
Associate Professor
Department of Otolaryngology and Communication Sciences
Medical College of Wisconsin
Director
Koss Cochlear Implant Program
Children's Hospital of Wisconsin
Froedtert Hospital
Milwaukee, Wisconsin

Leonard P. Rybak, M.D., Ph.D.
Professor
Department of Surgery
Division of Otolaryngology
Southern Illinois University School of Medicine
Springfield, Illinois

Babak Sadoughi, M.D.
Resident and House Officer
Department of Otorhinolaryngology–Head and Neck Surgery Montefiore Medical Center
Bronx, New York

John R. Salassa, M.D.
Associate Professor
Department of Otolaryngology–Head and Neck Surgery
Mayo Clinic College of Medicine
Jacksonville, Florida

Thomas J. Salinas, D.D.S.
Associate Professor of Dentistry
Department of Dental Specialties
Mayo Clinic
Rochester, Minnesota

Sandeep Samant, M.D., F.R.C.S.
Associate Professor and Chief
Division of Head and Neck Surgery
Department of Otolaryngology–Head and Neck Surgery
University of Tennessee College of Medicine
Director
Multidisciplinary Head and Neck Clinic
University of Tennessee Cancer Institute
Memphis, Tennessee

Robin A. Samlan, M.S., M.B.A.
Doctoral Student
University of Arizona College of Medicine
Tucson, Arizona

Ravi N. Samy, M.D.
Assistant Professor
Department of Otolaryngology
University of Cincinnati College of Medicine
Cincinnati, Ohio

Henry D. Sandel, IV, M.D.
Medical Director
The Sandel Center for Facial Plastic Surgery
Annapolis, Maryland

Guri S. Sandhu, M.B.B.S., F.R.C.S.(ORL-HNS)
Honorary Senior Lecturer
University College London
Consultant Otolaryngologist/Head and Neck Surgeon
Charing Cross Hospital
London, United Kingdom

Isamu Sando, M.D.
Professor Emeritus
Department of Otolaryngology
University of Pittsburgh School of Medicine
Pittsburgh, Pennsylvania

Cara Sauder, M.A., CCC-SLP
Adjunct Instructor
Division of Otolaryngology–Head and Neck Surgery
University of Utah School of Medicine
Clinical Director
Voice Disorders Clinic
University Hospital
Salt Lake City, Utah

Jeremy A. Scarlett, M.D.
Assistant Professor
Department of Anesthesiology
Medical College of Wisconsin
Milwaukee, Wisconsin

Richard L. Scher, M.D., F.A.C.S.
Associate Professor and Associate Chief
Division of Otolaryngology–Head and Neck Surgery
Duke University School of Medicine
Durham, North Carolina

David A. Schessel, M.D.
Assistant Professor
Department of Otolaryngology
Stony Brook University Medical Center School of Medicine
Stony Brook, New York

Cecelia E. Schmalbach, M.D.
Head and Neck–Microvascular Surgery
Wilford Hall Medical Center
Lackland Air Force Base
San Antonio, Texas

Todd J. Schwedt, M.D.
Assistant Professor of Neurology and Anesthesiology
Washington University in St. Louis School of Medicine
Director
Washington University Headache Center
St. Louis, Missouri

James J. Sciubba, D.M.D., Ph.D.
Professor (Retired)
Otolaryngology, Head and Neck Surgery, Dermatology, Pathology
Johns Hopkins University School of Medicine
Oral Medicine and Oral Pathology
Milton J. Dance, Jr., Head and Neck Center
Baltimore, Maryland

Sunitha Sequeira, M.D.
Resident
Department of Otolaryngology–Head and Neck Surgery
Washington University Medical Center
St. Louis, Missouri

Meena Seshamani, M.D., Ph.D.
Resident
Department of Otolaryngology–Head and Neck Surgery
Johns Hopkins Hospital
Baltimore, Maryland

Clough Shelton, M.D.
Professor and Chair
Department of Otolaryngology
Hetzel Presidential Endowed Chair in Otolaryngology
University of Utah School of Medicine
Salt Lake City, Utah

Neil T. Shepard, Ph.D.
Professor of Audiology
Department of Otolaryngology
Mayo Medical School College of Medicine
Rochester, Minnesota

Jonathan A. Ship, D.M.D.*
New York University College of Dentistry
New York, New York

W. Peyton Shirley, M.D.
Assistant Clinical Professor
Department of Otolaryngology
University of Alabama at Birmingham School of Medicine
The Children's Hospital of Alabama
Birmingham, Alabama

*Deceased.

Yelizaveta Shnayder, M.D., F.A.C.S.
Assistant Professor
Department of Otolaryngology–Head and Neck Surgery
University of Kansas School of Medicine
Kansas City, Kansas

Joseph Shvidler, M.D.
Attending Physician
Department of Otolaryngology
Madigan Army Medical Center
Tacoma, Washington

Kathleen C. Y. Sie, M.D.
Professor
Department of Otolaryngology–Head and Neck Surgery
University of Washington School of Medicine
Director
Childhood Communication Center
Seattle Children's Hospital
Seattle, Washington

Daniel B. Simmen, M.D.
Center for Rhinology and Facial Plastic Surgery, Skull Base Surgery, and Otology
Zurich, Switzerland

Marshall E. Smith, M.D., F.A.C.S., F.A.A.P.
Professor
Division of Otolaryngology–Head and Neck Surgery
University of Utah School of Medicine
Attending Physician and Medical Director
Voice Disorders Clinic
Primary Children's Medical Center
University Hospital
Salt Lake City, Utah

Richard J. H. Smith, M.D.
Professor
Department of Otolaryngology
University of Iowa Carver College of Medicine
Iowa City, Iowa

Robert A. Sofferman, M.D.
Professor and Chief
Department of Otolaryngology–Head and Neck Surgery
University of Vermont School of Medicine
Burlington, Vermont

Marlene Soma, M.B.B.S., F.R.A.C.S.
ENT Clinical Fellow
Great Ormond Street Hospital for Children
London, United Kingdom

Brad A. Stach, Ph.D.
Head
Division of Audiology
Department of Otolaryngology–Head and Neck Surgery
Henry Ford Hospital
Detroit, Michigan

Hinrich Staecker, M.D., Ph.D.
Associate Professor
Otolaryngology–Head and Neck Surgery
University of Kansas School of Medicine
Kansas City, Kansas

Aldo Cassol Stamm, M.D., Ph.D.
Affiliate Professor
Department of Otolaryngology–Head and Neck Surgery
Federal University of São Paulo
Director
ENT Center of São Paulo
Edmundo Vasconcelos Hospital
São Paulo, Brazil

James A. Stankiewicz, M.D.
Professor and Chair
Department of Otolaryngology–Head and Neck Surgery
Loyola University School of Medicine
Senior Attending Staff Surgeon
Loyola University Medical Center
Maywood, Illinois

Rose Stavinoha, M.D.
Chief Resident
Department of Otolaryngology–Head and Neck Surgery
USF Medical Center
Tampa, Florida

Laura M. Sterni, M.D.
Assistant Professor
Department of Pediatrics
Johns Hopkins University School of Medicine
Director
Johns Hopkins Pediatric Sleep Center
Johns Hopkins Children's Center
Baltimore, Maryland

David L. Steward, M.D.
Associate Professor
Department of Otolaryngology–Head and Neck Surgery
Director of Thyroid/Parathyroid Surgery
University of Cincinnati College of Medicine
Cincinnati, Ohio

Rose Mary S. Stocks, M.D., Pharm.D.
Professor and Residency Program Director
Department of Otolaryngology–Head and Neck Surgery
University of Tennessee College of Medicine
Memphis, Tennessee

Holger H. Sudhoff, M.D., Ph.D.
Professor
Ruhr University Bochum School of Medicine
Bochum, Germany
Chairman and Medical Director
Department of Otorhinolaryngology–Head and Neck Surgery
Klinikum Bielefeld
Bielefeld, Germany

John B. Sunwoo, M.D.
Assistant Professor
Department of Otolaryngology–Head and Neck Surgery
Stanford University School of Medicine
Stanford Cancer Center
Stanford University Hospitals and Clinics
Stanford, California

Neil A. Swanson, M.D.
Professor of Dermatology, Surgery, and Otolaryngology
Chair
Department of Dermatology
Oregon Health and Science University School of Medicine
Portland, Oregon

Veronica C. Swanson, M.D.
Associate Professor
Departments of of Anesthesiology and Pediatrics
Oregon Health and Science University School of Medicine
Director
Pediatric Cardiac Anesthesia
Doernbecher Children's Hospital
Portland, Oregon

Robert A. Swarm, M.D.
Professor
Department of Anesthesiology
Washington University in St. Louis School of Medicine
Director
Barnes-Jewish Hospital–Washington University Pain Management Center
St. Louis, Missouri

Jonathan M. Sykes, M.D., F.A.C.S.
Professor
University of California, Davis, School of Medicine
Director
Facial Plastic Surgery
UC Davis Medical Center
Sacramento, California

Luke Tan, M.B.B.S., F.R.C.S., M.Med.Sci.
Associate Professor (Adjunct)
National University of Singapore
Senior Consultant
Head and Neck Surgeon
Gleneagles Medical Centre
Singapore

M. Eugene Tardy, Jr., M.D., F.A.C.S.
Professor of Clinical Otolaryngology
Division of Facial Plastic and Reconstructive Surgery
Department of Otolaryngology–Head and Neck Surgery
University of Illinois at Chicago College of Medicine
Chicago, Illinois

Sherard A. Tatum, III, M.D.
Associate Professor
Department of Otolaryngology–Head and Neck Surgery
SUNY Upstate Medical University
Director
Division of Facial Plastic and Reconstructive Surgery
Director
Cleft and Craniofacial Center
University Hospital
Syracuse, New York

S. Mark Taylor, M.D., F.R.C.S.C., F.A.C.S.
Associate Professor
Division of Otolaryngology–Head and Neck Surgery
Head
Section of Head and Neck Surgery
Dalhousie University Faculty of Medicine
Halifax, Nova Scotia, Canada

Natacha Teissier, M.D., Ph.D.
Senior Consultant
Department of Otorhinolaryngology
R. Debre Hospital
Paris, France

Steven A. Telian, M.D.
John L. Kemink Professor of Neurotology
Department of Otolaryngology–Head and Neck Surgery
University of Michigan Medical School
Ann Arbor, Michigan

David J. Terris, M.D.
Porubsky Distinguished Professor and Chairman
Department of Otolaryngology
Medical College of Georgia
Surgical Director
Medical College of Georgia Thyroid Center
Augusta, Georgia

Karen B. Teufert, M.D.
House Ear Institute
Los Angeles, California

J. Regan Thomas, M.D.
Francis L. Lederer Professor and Chairman
Department of Otolaryngology–Head and Neck Surgery
University of Illinois at Chicago
Chicago, Illinois

James N. Thompson, M.D., F.A.C.S.
Clinical Professor
Department of Otolaryngology
University of Texas Southwestern Medical School
Dallas, Texas
President and CEO
Federation of State Medical Boards of the United States

Dean M. Toriumi, M.D.
Professor
Department of Otolaryngology–Head and Neck Surgery
Division of Facial Plastic Surgery
University of Illinois at Chicago College of Medicine
Chicago, Illinois

Alejandro I. Torres, B.S.
Department of Biology
Seattle Pacific University
Virginia Mason Medical Center
Seattle, Washington

Joseph B. Travers, Ph.D.
Professor
Section of Oral Biology
Department of Dentistry
Associate Professor
Department of Psychology
The Ohio State University
Columbus, Ohio

Susan P. Travers, Ph.D.
Professor
Section of Oral Biology
Department of Dentistry
Associate Professor
Department of Psychology
The Ohio State University
Columbus, Ohio

Terance T. Tsue, M.D., F.A.C.S.

Associate Dean of Graduate Medical Education
Douglas A. Girod, M.D. Professor of Head and Neck Surgical Oncology
Vice Chair
Department of Otolaryngology–Head and Neck Surgery
University of Kansas School of Medicine
University of Kansas Hospital
Kansas City, Kansas

Ralph P. Tufano, M.D.

Associate Professor
Department of Otolaryngology–Head and Neck Surgery
Johns Hopkins University School of Medicine
Director
Thyroid and Parathyroid Surgery
Johns Hopkins Hospital
Baltimore, Maryland

David E. Tunkel, M.D.

Associate Professor of Otolaryngology–Head and Neck Surgery, Pediatrics, and Anesthesia–Critical Care Medicine
Johns Hopkins University School of Medicine
Director
Pediatric Otolaryngology
Johns Hopkins Hospital
Baltimore, Maryland

Michael D. Turner, D.D.S., M.D.

New York University College of Dentistry
New York University School of Medicine
NYU Medical Center
New York, New York

Ravindra Uppaluri, M.D., Ph.D.

Assistant Professor
Department of Otolaryngology–Head and Neck Surgery
Washington University in St. Louis School of Medicine
St. Louis, Missouri

Michael F. Vaezi, M.D., Ph.D.

Professor of Medicine and Clinical Director
Division of Gastroenterology and Hepatology
Department of Medicine
Vanderbilt University School of Medicine
Director
Clinical Research
Director
Center for Esophageal and Mobility Disorders
Vanderbilt University Medical Center
Nashville, Tennessee

Thierry Van den Abbeele, M.D., Ph.D.

Professor
Department of Otorhinolaryngology
Paris Diderot University
Head
Department of Otorhinolaryngology
R. Debre Hospital
Paris, France

Michiel W. M. van den Brekel, M.D., Ph.D.

Professor
Academic Medical Center
University of Amsterdam
Chair
Department of Head Neck Oncology and Surgery
The Netherlands Cancer Institute–Antoni van Leeuwenhoek Hospital
Amsterdam, The Netherlands

Mikhail Vaysberg, D.O.

Assistant Professor
Department of Otolaryngology
University of Florida College of Medicine
Gainesville, Florida

David E. Vokes, M.B.Ch.B., F.R.A.C.S.

Consultant Otolaryngologist
Head and Neck Surgeon
Auckland City Hospital
Auckland, New Zealand

P. Ashley Wackym, M.D.

Vice President for Research
Legacy Health System
President
Ear and Skull Base Institute
Portland, Oregon

Tamekia L. Wakefield, M.D.

Clinical Assistant Professor
Department of Otolaryngology
University of Kansas School of Medicine
Pediatric Otolaryngologist
University of Kansas Hospital
Kansas City, Kansas
Children's Mercy Hospital
Kansas City, Missouri

David L. Walner, M.D.

Assistant Professor of Pediatric Otolaryngology
Rush Medical College
Chicago, Illinois
Staff
Lutheran General Children's Hospital
Park Ridge, Illinois

Edward J. Walsh, Ph.D.

Director
Developmental Auditory Physiology Laboratory
Boys Town National Research Hospital
Omaha, Nebraska

Rohan R. Walvekar, M.D.

Assistant Professor
Department of Otolaryngology–Head and Neck Surgery
Louisiana State University Health Sciences Center School of Medicine at New Orleans
New Orleans, Louisiana

Tom D. Wang, M.D.

Professor of Facial Plastic Surgery
Department of Otolaryngology–Head and Neck Surgery
Oregon Health and Science University School of Medicine
Portland, Oregon

Frank M. Warren, III, M.D.

Assistant Professor
Department of Surgery
Division of Otolaryngology–Head and Neck Surgery
University of Utah School of Medicine
Salt Lake City, Utah

Randal S. Weber, M.D.

Professor and Chair
Department of Head and Neck Surgery
University of Texas M.D. Anderson Cancer Center
Houston, Texas

Richard O. Wein, M.D., F.A.C.S.
Assistant Professor
Tufts University School of Medicine
Tufts Medical Center
Boston, Massachusetts

Gregory S. Weinstein, M.D.
Professor and Vice Chair
Department of Otorhinolaryngology–Head and Neck Surgery
University of Pennsylvania School of Medicine
Director
Division of Head and Neck Surgery
Department of Otorhinolaryngology–Head and Neck Surgery
Hospital of the University of Pennsylvania
Philadelphia, Pennsylvania

Erik Kent Weitzel, M.D.
Adjunct Assistant Professor
F. Edward Hébert School of Medicine
Uniformed Services University of the Health Sciences
Chief
Department of Rhinology
Wilford Hall USAF Medical Center
Lackland Air Force Base, Texas

D. Bradley Welling, M.D., Ph.D., F.A.C.S.
Professor and Chair
Department of Otolaryngology
The Ohio State University College of Medicine
Columbus, Ohio

Richard D. Wemer, M.D.
Clinical Faculty
University of Minnesota
Minneapolis, Minnesota Medical School
Associate Physician
Park Nicolette Hospitals and Clinics
Saint Louis Park, Minnesota

Ralph F. Wetmore, M.D.
Professor
Department of Otorhinolaryngology–Head and Neck Surgery
University of Pennsylvania School of Medicine
Chief
Division of Otolaryngology
The Children's Hospital of Philadelphia
Philadelphia, Pennsylvania

Ernest A. Weymuller, Jr., M.D.
Professor
Department of Otolaryngology–Head and Neck Surgery
University of Washington School of Medicine
Seattle, Washington

Brian J. Wiatrak, M.D.
Clinical Associate Professor of Surgery
University of Alabama at Birmingham School of Medicine
Chief
Pediatric Otolaryngology
Children's Hospital of Alabama
Birmingham, Alabama

Gregory J. Wiet, M.B.S., M.D.
Associate Professor
Departments of Otolaryngology and Biomedical Informatics
The Ohio State University College of Medicine
Department of Otolaryngology
Nationwide Children's Hospital
Columbus, Ohio

Richard H. Wiggins, III, M.D.
Associate Professor
Departments of Radiology, Otolaryngology–Head and Neck Surgery, and Biomedical Informatics
Director
Imaging Informatics
University of Utah School of Medicine
Department of Oncological Sciences–Head and Neck Imaging
Huntsman Cancer Institute
Salt Lake City, Utah

Andrea Willey, M.D.
Assistant Clinical Professor
Department of Dermatology
University of California, Davis, School of Medicine
Physician
Mohs and Reconstructive Surgery and Laser Surgery
Laser and Skin Surgery Center of Northern California
Sacramento, California
Solano Dermatology Associates
Vacaville, California

William N. William, Jr., M.D.
Assistant Professor
Department of Thoracic/Head and Neck Medical Oncology
University of Texas M.D. Anderson Cancer Center
Houston, Texas

Glenn B. Williams, M.D.
Resident
Department of Otolaryngology–Head and Neck Surgery
University of Tennessee College of Medicine
Memphis, Tennessee

Franz J. Wippold, II, M.D., F.A.C.R.
Professor of Radiology
Washington University in St. Louis School of Medicine
Chief of Neuroradiology
Mallinckrodt Institute of Radiology
St. Louis, Missouri
Adjunct Professor
Department of Radiology/Radiologic Sciences
F. Edward Hébert School of Medicine
Uniformed Services University of the Health Sciences
Bethesda, Maryland
Attending Neuroradiologist
Barnes-Jewish Hospital
St. Louis Children's Hospital
St. Louis, Missouri

Gayle Ellen Woodson, M.D.
Professor and Chair
Division of Otolaryngology
Southern Illinois University School of Medicine
Springfield, Illinois

Audie L. Woolley, M.D.
Associate Clinical Professor of Surgery
Department of Otolaryngology
University of Alabama at Birmingham School of Medicine
Birmingham, Alabama

Christopher T. Wootten, M.D.
Assistant Professor
Department of Otolaryngology–Head Neck Surgery
Vanderbilt University School of Medicine
Division of Pediatric Otolaryngology
Vanderbilt Children's Hospital
Nashville, Tennessee

Peter-John Wormald, M.D., F.R.A.C.S., F.C.S.(SA), F.R.C.S.
Chair
Department of Otolaryngology–Head and Neck Surgery
University of Adelaide and Flinders University
Professor and Head
Department of Otolaryngology–Head and Neck Surgery
Queen Elizabeth Hospital
Adelaide, Australia

Charles D. Yingling, Ph.D., D.A.B.N.M.
Clinical Professor
Department of Otolaryngology–Head and Neck Surgery
Stanford University School of Medicine
Stanford, California
Chief
Surgical Neuromonitoring Services
Sausalito, California

Bevan Yueh, M.D., M.P.H.
Professor and Chair
Department of Otolaryngology–Head and Neck Surgery
University of Minnesota Medical School
Minneapolis, Minnesota

Rex C. Yung, M.D.
Assistant Professor of Medicine and Oncology
Johns Hopkins University School of Medicine
Director
Pulmonary Oncology and Bronchology
Johns Hopkins Hospital
Baltimore, Maryland

Renzo A. Zaldívar, M.D.
Fellow
Ophthalmic Plastic and Reconstructive Surgery
Mayo Clinic
Rochester, Minnesota

George H. Zalzal, M.D.
Professor
Departments of Otolaryngology and Pediatrics
George Washington University School of Medicine and Health Sciences
Chief
Department of Pediatric Otolaryngology
Children's National Medical Center
Washington, D.C.

David S. Zee, M.D.
Professor
Department of Neurology
Johns Hopkins University School of Medicine
Johns Hopkins Hospital
Baltimore, Maryland

Marc S. Zimbler, M.D., F.A.C.S.
Assistant Professor
Department of Otolaryngology–Head and Neck Surgery
Albert Einstein College of Medicine
Director
Facial Plastic and Reconstructive Surgery
Department of Otolaryngology–Head and Neck Surgery
Beth Israel Medical Center
New York, New York

S. James Zinreich, M.D.
Professor
Department of Radiology
Division of Neuroradiology
Johns Hopkins University School of Medicine
Baltimore, Maryland

Teresa A. Zwolan, Ph.D.
Associate Professor
Department of Otolaryngology
University of Michigan Medical School
Director
Cochlear Implant Program
University of Michigan Health System
Ann Arbor, Michigan

Preface

The fifth edition of *Cummings Otolaryngology–Head and Neck Surgery* is written in response to the vast expansion of medical knowledge and technological advancements impacting our specialty and presents the most up-to-date information, covering new topics from surgical robotics and image guidance to evidence-based performance measurements. Nonetheless, we have worked hard to keep the fifth edition concise, removing overlapping content to make for easier reading, yet still covering in detail all major developments in the field.

Building on the success of the past four editions, the fifth edition also reflects a technology-driven change in curriculum, featuring access to the Expert Consult website, with text and images from the book as well as online video demonstrating the ACGME Key Indicator Procedures. The video component provides residents with a new opportunity to better understand the critical elements of these core procedures.

As with past editions, the field of otolaryngology–head and neck surgery is represented in all of its diversity. The table of contents has been restructured to reflect the extensive interrelationship of its various components. Every chapter contains Key Points at the start and a "most relevant" Suggested Readings list. A full reference list for each chapter is available online to supplement the overall content. Combined with the online version, the fifth edition remains the definitive resource for our specialty.

In acknowledgement of all those who have contributed to the specialty, the list of authors includes worldwide representation. Adding to excellence at the editorship level, Drs. Valerie Lund and John Niparko have assumed leadership roles, and Dr. Howard Francis has assumed an associate editorship position for the online video content. Through the combined effort of all contributors, our goal is to further the education of those now associated with otolaryngology–head and neck surgery and provide a foundation for continued progress by the generations to follow.

Acknowledgments

For those individuals privileged to serve and train under Dr. Charles Cummings, we recognize him as mentor, colleague and friend, physician and healer; we are grateful for his leadership and everlasting imprint on our mission in academic medicine.

Charlie, thank you. From your student, colleague, and friend,

Paul W. Flint

It has been a distinct honor and pleasure to be part of the editorial and publishing team assembled for this edition of *Cummings Otolaryngology–Head and Neck Surgery*. The authors have been tireless in their efforts and have worked strongly to produce chapters that are truly comprehensive in scope and depth. My sincere thanks goes to each one of them and their families, who inevitably have put up with liberal amounts of "burning the midnight oil." My loyal assistant of 20 years, Debbie Turner, has kept us to our deadlines and liaised with both authors and publishers in a highly organized way, while my office nurses have provided generous amounts of patient care to cover for my time away from the front lines during this textbook's creation. Similarly, the residents and fellows at Washington University in St. Louis have "held the fort" when necessary.

The ability to purvey knowledge starts, and continues, with one's education, for which thanks goes to my parents, the late Thomas and Marjorie Haughey, my teachers, medical professors, Otolaryngology residency mentors in Auckland, New Zealand, and at the University of Iowa, and colleagues in the specialty, from whom I have and will continue to learn.

My family has unswervingly endorsed the time required for this project, so heartfelt love and thanks go to my wife, Helen, as well as to Rachel and Jack, Chris, Will and Rachel, and Gretchen.

Finally, as we enjoy the teaching of this book and its ensuing online components, I try to keep in mind the source of all knowledge and truth: in the words of Proverbs 2 v.6 "…the Lord gives wisdom and from his mouth come knowledge and understanding." My sincere hope is that the readers everywhere will benefit from this textbook, better accomplishing our specialty's common goal of top quality patient care.

Bruce H. Haughey

I would like to thank Paul Flint and his colleagues for inviting me to participate in this prestigious project, the publishers for their exemplary efficiency in its management, and my partner, David Howard, for his constant support and encouragement.

Valerie J. Lund

Otolaryngology is a specialty of immense power. Scholarly work such as this text shows that in the tools of our specialty is the potential to address unmet challenges. I am grateful to Drs. Charles Cummings and Paul Flint, who showed confidence in me in inviting me to join a marvelously collaborative editorial team, and to the many chapter authors who have given their very best efforts in composing this essential resource.

My work is dedicated to those who have provided my guidance. To my parents, my family, my colleagues, and my ever thoughtful patients, you have taught me the importance of dedication to others and that true compassion is shown in action. Through you I've learned that this is not a world of scarcity but one of abundance that is to be shared.

John K. Niparko

The process of learning is truly lifelong. Participating in the creation of this text allows another way for me to continue to become invigorated and inspired by my specialty field. To my invaluable support mechanism, my wife, children, and family: Thank you.

Mark A. Richardson

I am deeply appreciative and honored to again serve as an editor of this important book. I would like to take this opportunity to recognize some individuals who have influenced my career: John Fredricksen; Douglas Bryce; the late Sir Donald Harrison; Robert Byers; Oscar Guillamondegui; Helmuth Goepfert; Robert Jahrsdoerfer; Charles Cummings; and the late Edwin Cocke. Also, I would like to remember and honor my parents, the late Elizabeth and Wycliffe Robbins, for the values they instilled in me. Finally, and most of all, I cherish the love and support of my wife, Gayle Woodson, and the children, Phil, Nick, Greg, and Sarah, who together provide the caring background for making it all meaningful.

K. Thomas Robbins

It is a great privilege and honor to serve as an editor for this outstanding textbook. Although the knowledge base for our specialty and indeed all of medicine is continually evolving and growing, this contribution serves otolaryngologists and their patients throughout the world with the current expertise required for best ultimate treatment. As an academic department head, I treasure the wealth of information available to my resident physicians in training. As an individual who has centered his career in a subspecialty of Otolaryngology, I am especially proud to help enhance the information available to the reader in the area of Facial Plastic and Reconstructive Surgery.

On a personal note, I want thank and acknowledge the great help and assistance I received from my administrative assistant, Denise McManaman, in editing this textbook. Her tireless work ethic is always admirable and appreciated. Finally, thank you to my wife, Rhonda, and my children, Ryan, Aaron, and Evan, for their enthusiastic and never-wavering support in my professional activities.

J. Regan Thomas

Video Contents

Available online at www.expertconsult.com

Key Indicator Videos

Howard W. Francis, M.D., Associate Editor
Nasir Bhatti, M.D., Assistant Editor
Kulsoom Laeeq, M.D., Assistant Editor
Jay Corey, Videographer
Johns Hopkins University, Baltimore, Maryland

1 Parotidectomy, *Joseph Califano, M.D.*
2 Selective Neck Dissection–Levels II-IV, *Sandeep Samant, M.D.**
3 Laryngectomy, *Jeremy Richmon, M.D., and Patrick Ha, M.D.*
4 Thyroid/Parathyroidectomy, *Ralph Tufano, M.D., and Kavita Pattani, M.D.*
5 Tympanoplasty, *Charles Limb, M.D.*
6 Mastoidectomy, *Howard W. Francis, M.D.*[†]
7 Stapedectomy, *Howard W. Francis, M.D.*[†]
8 Rhinoplasty, *Ira D. Papel, M.D., and Taha Shipchandler, M.D.*
9 Ethmoidectomy, *James A. Stankiewicz, M.D., Devyani Lal, M.D., and Kevin Welch, M.D.**

Note: Additional videos will be added to the website as they become available.

Videos Submitted by Chapter Authors

Chapter 4B Validation/Dissemination of Temporal Bone Dissection Simulation

Chapter 49 Fronto-Ethmoidal Osteoma

Chapter 51 Primary Endoscopic Sinus Surgery (see Key Indicator Video 9)
Preoperative CT Review
Injections
Maxillary Antrostomy
Complete Ethmoidectomy
Sphenoidotomy
Skull Base Dissection

Chapter 55 Endoscopic DCR without Tubes

Chapter 57 HSDI vs. STROBE: Normal Voice with HSDI
HSDI vs. STROBE: Normal Phonation Onset with HSDI Playback Rate 30 fps
HSDI vs. STROBE: Normal Phonation Onset with HSDI Playback Rate 150 fps
HSDI vs. STROBE: Normal Voice with Strobe
HSDI vs. STROBE: Patient 1 with Hx of Cancer—HSDI Playback Rate 20 fps
HSDI vs. STROBE: Patient with Hx of Cancer—STROBE: T1ca1
NBI 1

Chapter 113 Primary TEP
Secondary TEP Standard
Secondary TEP Alternative
Short Myotomy of Upper Esophageal Sphincter
Sectioning of SCM Muscles
Replacement of Provox2
Patient Speaking with an Automatic Valve (counting, telling days of the week in Dutch)
Videofluoroscopy of Tracheoesophageal Voicing

Chapter 121 Selective Neck Dissection–Levels II-IV (see Key Indicator Video 2)

Chapter 129 Left Superior Canal Dehiscence Repair

*This Key Indicator Video was submitted by the chapter author(s) and was not produced by Johns Hopkins University.
[†]Copyright Howard W. Francis, M.D.

Contents

Volume One

Part 1: Basic Principles

Editor: Paul W. Flint

CHAPTER 1 **Genetics and Otolaryngology** 3
William J. Kimberling

CHAPTER 2 **Fundamentals of Molecular Biology and Gene Therapy** 11
Bert W. O'Malley, Jr., Daqing Li, Waleed M. Abuzeid, and Hinrich Staecker

CHAPTER 3 **Laser Surgery: Basic Principles and Safety Considerations** 25
C. Gaelyn Garrett, Robert H. Ossoff, and Lou Reinisch

CHAPTER 4A **Surgical Robotics in Otolaryngology** 38
David J. Terris

CHAPTER 4B **Simulation and Haptics in Otolaryngology Training** 45
Marvin P. Fried, Gregory J. Wiet, and Babak Sadoughi

CHAPTER 5 **Outcomes Research** 52
Amy Anne Lassig and Bevan Yueh

CHAPTER 6 **Interpreting Medical Data** 59
Richard M. Rosenfeld

CHAPTER 7 **Evidence-Based Performance Measurement** 76
David R. Nielsen

Part 2: General Otolaryngology

Editor: Paul W. Flint

CHAPTER 8 **History, Physical Examination, and the Preoperative Evaluation** 93
Marion Everett Couch

CHAPTER 9 **General Considerations of Anesthesia and Management of the Difficult Airway** 108
Lynette Mark, Kurt Herzer, Seth Akst, and James Michelson

CHAPTER 10 **Surgical Management of the Difficult Adult Airway** 121
Nasir Islam Bhatti

CHAPTER 11 **Overview of Diagnostic Imaging of the Head and Neck** 130
Nafi Aygun and S. James Zinreich

CHAPTER 12 **Odontogenic Infections** 177
James M. Christian

CHAPTER 13 **Pharyngitis in Adults** 191
Brian Nussenbaum and Carol R. Bradford

CHAPTER 14 **Deep Neck Space Infections** 201
Eric R. Oliver and M. Boyd Gillespie

CHAPTER 15 **Head and Neck Manifestations in the Immunocompromised Host** 209
Theresa B. Kim, Steven D. Pletcher, and Andrew N. Goldberg

CHAPTER 16 **Special Considerations in Managing Geriatric Patients** 230
Meena Seshamani and Matthew L. Kashima

CHAPTER 17 **Pain Management in the Head and Neck Patient** 239
Edward B. Braun, Jeremy A. Scarlett, Todd J. Schwedt, and Robert A. Swarm

CHAPTER 18 **Sleep Apnea and Sleep Disorders** 250
Stacey L. Ishman, Tamekia L. Wakefield, and Nancy A. Collop

Part 3: Facial Plastic and Reconstructive Surgery

Editor: J. Regan Thomas

Section 1: Facial Surgery

CHAPTER 19 **Aesthetic Facial Analysis** 269
Marc S. Zimbler

CHAPTER 20 **Recognition and Treatment of Skin Lesions** 281
Andrea Willey, Neil A. Swanson, and Ken K. Lee

CHAPTER 21 **Scar Revision and Camouflage** 295
J. Regan Thomas and Steven Ross Mobley

CHAPTER 22 **Facial Trauma: Soft Tissue Lacerations and Burns** 302
Justin D. Hill and Grant S. Hamilton, III

CHAPTER 23 **Maxillofacial Trauma** 318
Robert M. Kellman

CHAPTER 24 **Reconstruction of Facial Defects** 342
Shan R. Baker

CHAPTER 25 **Nasal Reconstruction** 364
Norman N. Ge, C. Rose Rabinov, and Roger L. Crumley

CHAPTER 26 **Hair Restoration: Medical and Surgical Techniques** 373
Kevin H. Ende and Sheldon S. Kabaker

CHAPTER 27 **Management of Aging Skin** 390
Stephen W. Perkins and Henry D. Sandel

CHAPTER 28 **Rhytidectomy** 405
Shan R. Baker

CHAPTER 29 **Rejuvenation of the Aging Brow and Forehead** 428
Paul S. Nassif

CHAPTER 30 **Blepharoplasty** 439
Oren Friedman, Renzo A. Zaldívar, and Tom D. Wang

CHAPTER 31 **Liposuction** 452
Edward H. Farrior and Stephen S. Park

CHAPTER 32 **Mentoplasty and Facial Implants** 461
Jonathan M. Sykes and John L. Frodel, Jr.

CHAPTER 33 **Otoplasty** 475
Peter A. Adamson, Suzanne K. Doud Galli, and Theodore Chen

Section 2: Rhinoplasty

CHAPTER 34 **The Nasal Septum** 481
Russell W. H. Kridel, Paul E. Kelly, and Allison MacGregor Holzapfel

CHAPTER 35 **Nasal Fractures** 496
Burke E. Chegar and Sherard A. Tatum, III

CHAPTER 36 **Rhinoplasty** 508
M. Eugene Tardy, Jr., and J. Regan Thomas

CHAPTER 37 **Special Rhinoplasty Techniques** 545
Richard T. Farrior, Edward H. Farrior, and Raymond Cook

CHAPTER 38 **Noncaucasian Rhinoplasty** 568
Stephen S. Park and Hong Ryul Jin

CHAPTER 39 **Revision Rhinoplasty** 580
David W. Kim, Manuel A. Lopez, and Dean M. Toriumi

Part 4: Sinus, Rhinology, and Allergy/Immunology

Editor: Valerie J. Lund

CHAPTER 40 **Immunology of the Upper Airway and Pathophysiology and Treatment of Allergic Rhinitis** 597
Fuad M. Baroody and Robert M. Naclerio

CHAPTER 41 **Physiology of Olfaction** 624
Donald A. Leopold and Eric H. Holbrook

CHAPTER 42 **Evaluation of Nasal Breathing Function with Objective Airway Testing** 640
Jacquelynne Corey and John Pallanch

CHAPTER 43 **Nasal Manifestations of Systemic Diseases** 657
Rose Stavinoha and Thomas V. McCaffrey

CHAPTER 44 **Radiology of the Nasal Cavity and Paranasal Sinuses** 662
Nafi Aygun and S. James Zinreich

CHAPTER 45 **Epistaxis** 682
Daniel B. Simmen and Nick S. Jones

CHAPTER 46 **Nonallergic Rhinitis** 694
Stephanie A. Joe and Sundip Patel

CHAPTER 47 **The Pathogenesis of Rhinosinusitis** 703
Michael S. Benninger

CHAPTER 48 **Fungal Rhinosinusitis** 709
Berrylin J. Ferguson

CHAPTER 49 **Benign Tumors of the Sinonasal Tract** 717
Piero Nicolai and Paolo Castelnuovo

CHAPTER 50 **Medical Management of Nasosinus Infectious and Inflammatory Disease** 728
Scott C. Manning

CHAPTER 51 **Primary Sinus Surgery** 739
Devyani Lal and James A. Stankiewicz

CHAPTER 52 **Concepts of Endoscopic Sinus Surgery: Causes of Failure** 759
James N. Palmer and David W. Kennedy

CHAPTER 53 **Management of the Frontal Sinuses** 775
Nick S. Jones

CHAPTER 54 **Cerebrospinal Fluid Rhinorrhea** 785
Martin J. Citardi and Samer Fakhri

CHAPTER 55 **Endoscopic Dacryocystorhinostomy** 797
Erik Kent Weitzel and Peter-John Wormald

Part 5: Laryngology and Bronchoesophagology

Editor: Paul W. Flint

Section 1: Evaluation and Management of Laryngeal and Pharyngeal Disorders

CHAPTER 56 **Laryngeal and Pharyngeal Function** 805
Gayle Ellen Woodson

CHAPTER 57 **Visualization of the Larynx** 813
Robin A. Samlan, Jackie Gartner-Schmidt, and Melda Kunduk

CHAPTER 58 **Voice Evaluation** 825
Robin A. Samlan and Julie Barkmeier-Kraemer

CHAPTER 59 **Neurologic Evaluation of the Larynx and Pharynx** 832
Gayle Ellen Woodson, Andrew Blitzer, Ronda E. Alexander, and Nazaneen N. Grant

CHAPTER 60 **Neurologic Disorders of the Larynx** 837
Andrew Blitzer, Ronda E. Alexander, and Nazaneen N. Grant

CHAPTER 61 **The Professional Voice** 844
Mark S. Courey, Gregory N. Postma, and Robert H. Ossoff

CHAPTER 62 **Benign Vocal Fold Mucosal Disorders** 859
Robert W. Bastian

CHAPTER 63 **Acute and Chronic Laryngitis** 883
Albert L. Merati

CHAPTER 64 **Laryngeal and Tracheal Manifestations of Systemic Disease** 889
Kevin P. Leahy

CHAPTER 65 **Upper Aerodigestive Manifestations of Gastroesophageal Reflux Disease** 894
Jonathan E. Aviv and Savita Collins

Section 2: Management of Unilateral Vocal Fold Paralysis

CHAPTER 66 **Medialization Thyroplasty** 904
Carole Fakhry, Paul W. Flint, and Charles W. Cummings

CHAPTER 67 **Arytenoid Adduction** 912
Gayle Ellen Woodson

CHAPTER 68 **Laryngeal Reinnervation** 917
George S. Goding, Jr.

Section 3: Management of Acquired Disorders and Trauma

CHAPTER 69 **Chronic Aspiration** 925
Steven D. Pletcher and David W. Eisele

CHAPTER 70 **Laryngeal and Esophageal Trauma** 933
Guri S. Sandhu and Reza S. A. Nouraei

CHAPTER 71 **Surgical Management of Upper Airway Stenosis** 943
Ayesha N. Khalid and David Goldenberg

Section 4: Bronchoesophagology

CHAPTER 72 **The Esophagus: Anatomy, Physiology, and Diseases** 953
Michael F. Vaezi

CHAPTER 73 **Transnasal Esophagoscopy** 981
Neil N. Chheda and Gregory N. Postma

CHAPTER 74 **Zenker's Diverticulum** 986
Richard L. Scher

CHAPTER 75 **Tracheobronchial Endoscopy** 998
Rex C. Yung and Emily F. Boss

Index i

Volume Two

Part 6: Head and Neck Surgery and Oncology

Editors: Bruce H. Haughey and K. Thomas Robbins

Section 1: General Considerations

CHAPTER 76 **Biology of Head and Neck Cancer** 1015
Steven Chang and Patrick Ha

CHAPTER 77 **Radiotherapy for Head and Neck Cancer: Radiation Physics, Radiobiology, and Clinical Principles** 1030
Aron Popovtzer and Avraham Eisbruch

CHAPTER 78 **Chemotherapy and Targeted Biologic Agents for Head and Neck Cancer** 1051
William N. William, Jr., and Merrill S. Kies

CHAPTER 79 **Skin Flap Physiology and Wound Healing** 1064
Eugene A. Chu, Patrick J. Byrne, Rick M. Odland, and George S. Goding, Jr.

CHAPTER 80 **Free Tissue Transfer** 1080
Douglas A. Girod, Terance T. Tsue, and Yelizaveta Shnayder

CHAPTER 81 **Integrating Palliative and Curative Care Strategies in the Practice of Otolaryngology** 1100
Rhonda Johnson and Gary Johnson

CHAPTER 82 **Management of Head and Neck Melanoma and Advanced Cutaneous Malignancies** 1106

Cecelia E. Schmalbach, Timothy M. Johnson, and Carol R. Bradford

CHAPTER 83 **Malignancies of the Paranasal Sinus** 1121

Ernest A. Weymuller, Jr., and Greg E. Davis

Section 2: Salivary Glands

CHAPTER 84 **Physiology of the Salivary Glands** 1133

Ravindhra G. Elluru

CHAPTER 85 **Diagnostic Imaging and Fine-Needle Aspiration of the Salivary Glands** 1143

JoAnne Lacey

CHAPTER 86 **Inflammatory Disorders of the Salivary Glands** 1151

Jeremy Rogers and Thomas V. McCaffrey

CHAPTER 87 **Benign Neoplasms of the Salivary Glands** 1162

Gabriel G. Calzada and Ehab Y. Hanna

CHAPTER 88 **Malignant Neoplasms of the Salivary Glands** 1178

John B. Sunwoo, James S. Lewis, Jr., Jonathan McJunkin, and Sunitha Sequeira

Section 3: Oral Cavity

CHAPTER 89 **Physiology of the Oral Cavity** 1200

Joseph B. Travers, Susan P. Travers, and James M. Christian

CHAPTER 90 **Mechanisms of Normal and Abnormal Swallowing** 1215

Jeri A. Logemann

CHAPTER 91 **Oral Mucosal Lesions** 1222

James J. Sciubba

CHAPTER 92 **Oral Manifestations of Systemic Diseases** 1245

Jonathan A. Ship and Michael D. Turner

CHAPTER 93 **Odontogenesis, Odontogenic Cysts, and Odontogenic Tumors** 1259

John W. Hellstein

CHAPTER 94 **Temporomandibular Joint Disorders** 1279

Bruce E. Rotter

CHAPTER 95 **Benign Tumors and Tumor-Like Lesions of the Oral Cavity** 1287

Timothy S. Lian

CHAPTER 96 **Malignant Neoplasms of the Oral Cavity** 1293

Richard O. Wein, James P. Malone, and Randal S. Weber

CHAPTER 97 **Reconstruction of the Mandible** 1319

Brian Nussenbaum

CHAPTER 98 **Prosthetic Management of Head and Neck Defects** 1329

Jeffery C. Markt, Thomas J. Salinas, and William Donald Gay

Section 4: Pharynx and Esophagus

CHAPTER 99 **Benign and Malignant Tumors of the Nasopharynx** 1348

Luke Tan and Thomas Loh

CHAPTER 100 **Malignant Neoplasms of the Oropharynx** 1358

Uli Harréus

CHAPTER 101 **Reconstruction of the Oropharynx** 1375

S. Mark Taylor and Bruce H. Haughey

CHAPTER 102 **Diagnostic Imaging of the Pharynx and Esophagus** 1393

Barton F. Branstetter, IV

CHAPTER 103 **Neoplasms of the Hypopharynx and Cervical Esophagus** 1421

Ravindra Uppaluri and John B. Sunwoo

CHAPTER 104 **Radiotherapy and Chemotherapy of Squamous Cell Carcinomas of the Hypopharynx and Esophagus** 1441

Jean-Louis Lefebvre and Antoine Adenis

CHAPTER 105 **Reconstruction of the Hypopharynx and Esophagus** 1448

Douglas B. Chepeha

Section 5: Larynx

CHAPTER 106 **Diagnostic Imaging of the Larynx** 1462

Franz J. Wippold, II

CHAPTER 107 **Malignant Tumors of the Larynx** 1482

William B. Armstrong, David E. Vokes, and Robert H. Maisel

CHAPTER 108 **Management of Early Glottic Cancer** 1512

Henry T. Hoffman, Tim A. Iseli, Lucy H. Karnell, Timothy M. McCulloch, John M. Buatti, and Gerry F. Funk

CHAPTER 109 **Transoral Laser Microresection of Advanced Laryngeal Tumors** 1525

Michael L. Hinni, John R. Salassa, and Bruce W. Pearson

CHAPTER 110 **Conservation Laryngeal Surgery** 1539

Gregory S. Weinstein, Ollivier Laccourreye, Christopher H. Rassekh, Ralph P. Tufano, and Niels Kokot

CHAPTER 111 **Total Laryngectomy and Laryngopharyngectomy** 1563

Christopher H. Rassekh and Bruce H. Haughey

CHAPTER 112 **Radiation Therapy for the Larynx and Hypopharynx** 1577

Alice Cheuk and Parvesh Kumar

CHAPTER 113 **Vocal and Speech Rehabilitation Following Laryngectomy** 1594
Frans J. M. Hilgers and Michiel W. M. van den Brekel

CHAPTER 114 **Diagnosis and Management of Tracheal Neoplasms** 1611
Chadrick Denlinger and G. Alexander Patterson

Section 6: Neck

CHAPTER 115 **Penetrating and Blunt Trauma to the Neck** 1625
David B. Hom and Robert H. Maisel

CHAPTER 116 **Differential Diagnosis of Neck Masses** 1636
Amy Chen and Kristen J. Otto

CHAPTER 117 **Ultrasound Imaging of the Neck** 1643
Mikhail Vaysberg and David L. Steward

CHAPTER 118 **Neoplasms of the Neck** 1656
Terry A. Day, Luke Buchmann, Zoran Rumboldt, and John K. Joe

CHAPTER 119 **Lymphomas Presenting in the Head and Neck** 1673
Nancy L. Bartlett

CHAPTER 120 **Radiation Therapy and Management of the Cervical Lymph Nodes and Malignant Skull Base Tumors** 1682
Vincent Grégoire and Nancy Lee

CHAPTER 121 **Neck Dissection** 1702
K. Thomas Robbins, Sandeep Samant, and Ohad Ronen

CHAPTER 122 **Complications of Neck Surgery** 1726
Frederick C. Roediger and David W. Eisele

Section 7: Thyroid/Parathyroid

CHAPTER 123 **Disorders of the Thyroid Gland** 1735
Phillip K. Pellitteri, Steven Ing, and Brian Jameson

CHAPTER 124 **Management of Thyroid Neoplasms** 1750
Stephen Y. Lai, Susan J. Mandel, and Randal S. Weber

CHAPTER 125 **Management of Parathyroid Disorders** 1773
Phillip K. Pellitteri, Robert A. Sofferman, and Gregory W. Randolph

CHAPTER 126 **Management of Thyroid Eye Disease (Graves' Ophthalmopathy)** 1806
Douglas A. Girod and Richard D. Wemer

Part 7: Otology, Neuro-otology, and Skull Base Surgery

Editor: John K. Niparko

Section 1: Basic Science

CHAPTER 127 **Anatomy of the Temporal Bone, External Ear, and Middle Ear** 1821
Howard W. Francis

CHAPTER 128 **Anatomy of the Auditory System** 1831
Christina L. Runge-Samuelson and David R. Friedland

CHAPTER 129 **Physiology of the Auditory System** 1838
Wade Chien and Daniel J. Lee

CHAPTER 130 **Anatomy of the Vestibular System** 1850
Anna Lysakowski

CHAPTER 131 **Anatomy and Physiology of the Eustachian Tube** 1866
Robert C. O'Reilly and Isamu Sando

CHAPTER 132 **Neural Plasticity in Otology** 1876
Robert V. Harrison

Section 2: Diagnostic Assessment

CHAPTER 133 **Diagnostic Audiology** 1887
Paul R. Kileny and Teresa A. Zwolan

CHAPTER 134 **Electrophysiologic Assessment of Hearing** 1904
Carolyn J. Brown and Tiffany A. Johnson

CHAPTER 135 **Neuroradiology of the Temporal Bone and Skull Base** 1916
Frank M. Warren, Clough Shelton, and Richard H. Wiggins, III

CHAPTER 136 **Interventional Neuroradiology of the Skull Base, Head, and Neck** 1932
Richard E. Latchaw and Sheri L. Albers

Section 3: External Ear

CHAPTER 137 **Infections of the External Ear** 1944
Joel Guss and Michael J. Ruckenstein

CHAPTER 138 **Topical Therapies of External Ear Disorders** 1950
Joyce Colton House and Daniel J. Lee

Section 4: Middle Ear, Mastoid, and Temporal Bone

CHAPTER 139 **Chronic Otitis Media, Mastoiditis, and Petrositis** 1963
Richard A. Chole and Holger H. Sudhoff

CHAPTER 140 **Complications of Temporal Bone Infections** 1979
Hussam K. El-Kashlan, Lee A. Harker, Clough Shelton, Nafi Aygun, and John K. Niparko

CHAPTER 141 **Tympanoplasty and Ossiculoplasty** **1999**
Meredith E. Adams and Hussam K. El-Kashlan

CHAPTER 142 **Mastoidectomy** **2009**
Paul R. Lambert

CHAPTER 143 **Clinical Assessment and Surgical Treatment of Conductive Hearing Loss** **2017**
Alejandro I. Torres and Douglas D. Backous

CHAPTER 144 **Otosclerosis** **2028**
John W. House and Calhoun D. Cunningham, III

CHAPTER 145 **Management of Temporal Bone Trauma** **2036**
Hilary A. Brodie

Index **i**

Volume Three

Part 7: Otology, Neuro-otology, and Skull Base Surgery—*cont'd*

Editor: John K. Niparko

Section 5: Inner Ear

CHAPTER 146 **Cochlear Transduction and the Molecular Basis of Auditory Pathology** **2049**
JoAnn McGee and Edward J. Walsh

CHAPTER 147 **Genetic Sensorineural Hearing Loss** **2086**
Michael S. Hildebrand, Murad Husein, and Richard J. H. Smith

CHAPTER 148 **Otologic Manifestations of Systemic Disease** **2100**
Saumil N. Merchant and Joseph B. Nadol, Jr.

CHAPTER 149 **Sensorineural Hearing Loss in Adults** **2116**
H. Alexander Arts

CHAPTER 150 **Tinnitus and Hyperacusis** **2131**
Carol A. Bauer

CHAPTER 151 **Noise-Induced Hearing Loss** **2140**
Brenda L. Lonsbury-Martin and Glen K. Martin

CHAPTER 152 **Infections of the Labyrinth** **2153**
Larry E. Davis

CHAPTER 153 **Autoimmune Inner Ear Disease** **2164**
Steven D. Rauch, Marc A. Cohen, and Michael J. Ruckenstein

CHAPTER 154 **Vestibular and Auditory Ototoxicity** **2169**
Leonard P. Rybak

CHAPTER 155 **Pharmacologic and Molecular Therapies of the Cochlear and Vestibular Labyrinth** **2179**
Anil K. Lalwani and John F. McGuire

CHAPTER 156 **Otologic Symptoms and Syndromes** **2194**
Carol A. Bauer and Herman A. Jenkins

Section 6: Auditory Prosthetic Stimulation, Devices, and Rehabilitative Audiology

CHAPTER 157 **Implantable Hearing Aids** **2203**
Lawrence R. Lustig and Charles C. Della Santina

CHAPER 158 **Cochlear Implantation: Patient Evaluation and Device Selection** **2219**
P. Ashley Wackym and Christina L. Runge-Samuelson

CHAPTER 159 **Cochlear Implantation: Medical and Surgical Considerations** **2234**
Thomas J. Balkany, Kevin D. Brown, and Bruce J. Gantz

CHAPTER 160 **Cochlear Implants: Results, Outcomes, Rehabilitation, and Education** **2243**
Charles J. Limb, Howard W. Francis, Sue Archbold, Gerard O'Donoghue, and John K. Niparko

CHAPTER 161 **Central Neural Auditory Prosthesis** **2258**
Robert J. S. Briggs

CHAPTER 162 **Hearing Aids: Strategies of Amplification** **2265**
Brad A. Stach and Virginia Ramachandran

Section 7: Vestibular Disorders

CHAPTER 163 **Principles of Applied Vestibular Physiology** **2276**
John P. Carey and Charles C. Della Santina

CHAPTER 164 **Evaluation of the Patient with Dizziness** **2305**
Timothy E. Hullar, David S. Zee, and Lloyd B. Minor

CHAPTER 165 **Peripheral Vestibular Disorders** **2328**
Benjamin T. Crane, David A. Schessel, Julian Nedzelski, and Lloyd B. Minor

CHAPTER 166 **Central Vestibular Disorders** **2346**
Benjamin T. Crane, Scott D. Z. Eggers, David S. Zee, and Robert W. Baloh

CHAPTER 167 **Surgery for Vestibular Disorders** **2359**
Steven A. Telian

CHAPTER 168 **Vestibular and Balance Rehabilitation: Program Essentials** **2372**
Neil T. Shepard, Steven A. Telian, and Audrey B. Erman

Section 8: Facial Nerve Disorders

CHAPTER 169 **Tests of Facial Nerve Function** 2381
Rodney C. Diaz and Robert A. Dobie

CHAPTER 170 **Clinical Disorders of the Facial Nerve** 2391
Douglas E. Mattox

CHAPTER 171 **Intratemporal Facial Nerve Surgery** 2403
Bruce J. Gantz, Jay T. Rubinstein, Ravi N. Samy, and Samuel P. Gubbels

CHAPTER 172 **Rehabilitation of Facial Paralysis** 2416
James M. Ridgway, Roger L. Crumley, and Jason H. Kim

Section 9: Cranial Base

CHAPTER 173 **Surgical Anatomy of the Lateral Skull Base** 2434
Oswaldo Laércio M. Cruz

CHAPTER 174 **Surgery of the Anterior and Middle Cranial Base** 2442
Colin D. Pero, Frank Culicchia, Rohan R. Walvekar, Bert W. O'Malley, Jr., and Daniel W. Nuss

CHAPTER 175 **Transnasal Endoscopic-Assisted Surgery of the Anterior Skull Base** 2471
Aldo Cassol Stamm and Shirley S. N. Pignatari

CHAPTER 176 **Temporal Bone Neoplasms and Lateral Cranial Base Surgery** 2487
Michael Marsh and Herman A. Jenkins

CHAPTER 177 **Neoplasms of the Posterior Fossa** 2514
Derald E. Brackmann and Moisés A. Arriaga

CHAPTER 178 **Intraoperative Monitoring of Cranial Nerves in Neurotologic Surgery** 2542
Yasmine A. Ashram and Charles D. Yingling

CHAPTER 179 **Stereotactic Radiation Therapy of Benign Tumors of the Cranial Base** 2557
D. Bradley Welling and Mark D. Packer

Part 8: Pediatric Otolaryngology

Editor: Mark A. Richardson

Section 1: General

CHAPTER 180 **General Considerations in Pediatric Otolaryngologic Surgery** 2569
J. Scott McMurray

CHAPTER 181 **Anatomy and Developmental Embryology of the Neck** 2577
Daniel O. Graney and Kathleen C. Y. Sie

CHAPTER 182 **Anesthesia in Pediatric Otolaryngology** 2587
Veronica C. Swanson, Heike Gries, and Jeffrey Koh

CHAPTER 183 **Obstructive Sleep Apnea Syndrome** 2602
Laura M. Sterni and David E. Tunkel

Section 2: Craniofacial

CHAPTER 184 **Characteristics of Normal and Abnormal Postnatal Craniofacial Growth and Development** 2613
Frederick K. Kozak and Juan Camilo Ospina

CHAPTER 185 **Craniofacial Surgery for Congenital and Acquired Deformities** 2638
Jonathan Z. Baskin and Sherard A. Tatum, III

CHAPTER 186 **Cleft Lip and Palate** 2659
Oren Friedman, Tom D. Wang, and Henry A. Milczuk

CHAPTER 187 **Velopharyngeal Dysfunction** 2676
Harlan Muntz, Marshall E. Smith, and Cara Sauder

CHAPTER 188 **Congenital Malformations of the Nose** 2686
Ravindhra G. Elluru and Christopher T. Wootten

CHAPTER 189 **Pediatric Facial Fractures** 2697
Peter J. Koltai and Paul R. Krakovitz

Section 3: Hearing Loss and Pediatric Otology

CHAPTER 190 **Early Detection and Diagnosis of Infant Hearing Impairment** 2718
Susan J. Norton, Prabhat K. Bhama, and Jonathan A. Perkins

CHAPTER 191 **Congenital Malformations of the Inner Ear** 2726
Robert K. Jackler

CHAPTER 192 **Microtia Reconstruction** 2741
Craig S. Murakami, Vito C. Quatela, Kathleen C. Y. Sie, and Joseph Shvidler

CHAPTER 193 **Reconstruction of the Auditory Canal and Tympanum** 2752
Antonio De la Cruz and Karen B. Teufert

CHAPTER 194 **Acute Otitis Media and Otitis Media with Effusion** 2761
Margaretha L. Casselbrant and Ellen M. Mandel

Section 4: Infections and Inflammation

CHAPTER 195 **Pediatric Chronic Sinusitis** 2778
Rodney P. Lusk

CHAPTER 196 **Pharyngitis and Adenotonsillar Disease** 2782
W. Peyton Shirley, Audie L. Woolley, and Brian J. Wiatrak

CHAPTER 197 **Infections of the Airway in Children** 2803
Newton O. Duncan

Section 5: Head and Neck

CHAPTER 198 **Differential Diagnosis of Neck Masses** 2812
Ralph F. Wetmore and William P. Potsic

CHAPTER 199 **Vascular Anomalies of the Head and Neck** 2822
Jonathan A. Perkins and Eunice Y. Chen

CHAPTER 200 **Pediatric Head and Neck Malignancies** 2835
Carol J. MacArthur and Richard J. H. Smith

CHAPTER 201 **Salivary Gland Disease in Children** 2850
Gresham T. Richter, David L. Walner, and Charles M. Myer, III

Section 6: Pharynx, Larynx, Trachea, and Esophagus

CHAPTER 202 **Congenital Disorders of the Larynx** 2866
Anna H. Messner

CHAPTER 203 **Voice Disorders** 2876
Sukgi S. Choi and George H. Zalzal

CHAPTER 204 **Recurrent Respiratory Papillomatosis** 2884
Craig S. Derkay and Russell A. Faust

CHAPTER 205 **Evaluation and Management of the Stridulous Child** 2896
David Albert, Simone Boardman, and Marlene Soma

CHAPTER 206 **Glottic and Subglottic Stenosis** 2912
George H. Zalzal and Robin T. Cotton

CHAPTER 207 **Diagnosis and Management of Tracheal Anomalies and Tracheal Stenosis** 2925
Greg R. Licameli and Mark A. Richardson

CHAPTER 208 **Foreign Bodies of the Airway and Esophagus** 2935
Lauren D. Holinger and Sheri A. Poznanovic

CHAPTER 209 **Gastroesophageal Reflux and Laryngeal Disease** 2944
Philippe Contencin, Thierry Van den Abbeele, and Natacha Teissier

CHAPTER 210 **Aspiration and Swallowing Disorders** 2948
David J. Brown, Maureen A. Lefton-Greif, and Stacey Ishman

CHAPTER 211 **Caustic Ingestion** 2956
Glenn B. Williams, Rose Mary S. Stocks, J. Dale Browne, and James N. Thompson

Index i

SECTION FIVE

Inner Ear

CHAPTER ONE HUNDRED AND FORTY-SIX

Cochlear Transduction and the Molecular Basis of Auditory Pathology

JoAnn McGee

Edward J. Walsh

Key Points

- Animal models have played a key role in the effort to elucidate the role of gene products in peripheral auditory physiology and the molecular basis of deafness.
- Congenital hearing loss generally is inherited, and the phenotypic spectrum produced by mutations in a particular gene can be attributed to the severity of the mutation, allelic heterogeneity, alternative splicing, and the contribution of modifier genes. In addition, some genes interact with the environment (e.g., noise, aminoglycoside antibiotics) to increase susceptibility to hearing loss.
- The physical characteristics of the cochlear partition (i.e., its mass and stiffness) vary from one end of the cochlea to the other, creating a basoapical gradient that results in a mechanical system with resonant properties that are continuously distributed and span the audiometric range of hearing from high to low frequency.
- The tectorial membrane, a gelatinous extracellular matrix overlying the organ of Corti, provides the necessary structure to convert basilar membrane displacement to radial shearing forces, which in turn influence hair bundle deflection and subsequent mechanoelectrical transduction. Defects in genes encoding extracellular matrix proteins that are components of the tectorial membrane (e.g., TECTA, COL11A2, COL9A1) result in hearing deficits.
- Cochlear amplification refers to a physiologically vulnerable mechanism that increases sensitivity to sound, enhances frequency selectivity, and broadens the dynamic operating range. Cochlear amplification is the result of unique voltage-dependent contractile properties of outer hair cells, which rely on the *SLC26A5* gene that encodes the essential motor protein prestin.
- Numerous proteins that are localized to sensory hair cells are critical for the normal development and/or maintenance of the intricate structure and/or function of the hair bundle and when defective are responsible for various forms of deafness. These include motor proteins (e.g., myosin IIIa, VI, VIIa, XVa), cytoskeletal proteins (e.g., espin, γ-actin, TRIOBP, radixin, diaphanous 1), adhesion proteins (e.g., cadherin 23, protocadherin 15, usherin, Vlgr1), scaffolding proteins (e.g., harmonin, SANS, whirlin), and other necessary proteins of unknown function (e.g., TMC1, TMHS, TMIE).
- Hearing impairments categorized as "auditory neuropathy" include those associated with defective inner hair cell ribbon synapse function (e.g., those caused by mutations in the genes *OTOF* and *VGLUT3*), as well as neuropathies involving faulty conduction along auditory nerve fibers, which often occur when components of the Schwann cell myelin sheath are defective (e.g., MPZ, GJB1, PMP22).
- Development of the epithelial barrier forming the endolymphatic compartment within the cochlear duct requires the vital tight junction components claudin-14 and tricellulin. In addition, the gap junction proteins connexin 26, connexin 30, and connexin 31 (encoded by *GJB2*, *GJB6*, and *GJB3*, respectively) are essential for ion homeostasis, as are numerous ion channel subunits (e.g., KCNQ4, BSND, KCNE1, KCNQ1) and ion pumps and transporters (e.g., ATP6B1, SLC26A4 [PDS, pendrin]).
- Many other proteins, including transcription factors and regulators, enzymes, ligands and receptors, and proteins produced by mitochondrial genes, have been associated with human deafness. Moreover, many genes underlying deafness in mouse models have been identified for which human deafness has not yet been established, and vice versa.
- A thorough, comprehensive understanding of the role that distinctive proteins play in normal cochlear development and peripheral auditory function will require a continuing aggressive effort on the part of the scientific community, and the knowledge gained from the use of animal models will help guide clinical diagnoses and provide direction for appropriate treatment strategies.

The work on which this chapter is based was supported in part by NIH Grant NIDCD R01 #DC04566 and NEI R01 #EY016247.

Deafness, in all of its forms, affects an estimated 186 of every 100,000 newborns in the United States[372] and increases in prevalence with advancing age. For example, by the age of 60 years, one of every three people in the United States experiences communication difficulties as a consequence of lost hearing, and by the age of 85 years, one half of the population has some degree of hearing disability. In most cases, peripheral auditory disease involves some form of cochlear abnormality that disrupts sensory transduction, and various etiologic factors have been recognized, including genetic abnormalities, trauma (acoustic and mechanical), ototoxic agents, bacterial and viral infections, and disturbances in other organ systems that influence cochlear physiology indirectly. This chapter describes the physiologic mechanisms underlying cochlear transduction at both the systemic and molecular levels. In addition, basic mechanisms of cochlear transduction are correlated with a subset of inner ear disorders that are representative of various classes of disease.

Significant breakthroughs in the identification of genes and gene products that serve as integral elements of cochlear transduction have been made beginning in the mid to late 1990s. Clearly, pathogenic mutations of many of these genes are implicated in various forms of deafness (Table 146-1). Although numerous cases of inherited deafness had been identified historically on the basis of phenotype, the etiopathogenic mechanisms responsible for deafness remained unknown before technologic advances allowed for the identification and cloning of genes associated with normal hearing. By comparing human genes with orthologous genes that are known to cause deafness in animals, the cell biology and disease associated with particular gene mutations can be studied, leading to an understanding of the role of gene products in sensory transduction. Although a variety of nonhuman species have played indispensable roles in the study of cochlear transduction and sensory pathology, in recent years the mouse model has emerged as particularly useful (Table 146-2; see also Table 146-1). This movement is fueled, in large part, by the highly successful, comprehensive investigation of the murine genome and the ever-expanding availability of tools that allow the targeting and manipulation of specific genes, technologic changes that greatly extend the capability of researchers to examine the role of gene products in the transduction process. However, although much has been learned about the molecular and genetic basis of cochlear function, or malfunction as the case may be, much work remains to be done in the ongoing effort to unravel the intricacies associated with cochlear transduction and deafness.

Approximately 68% of all cases of congenital hearing loss are inherited, and of these, at least 70% are nonsyndromic—that is, auditory disability is the only manifestation of the disorder.[372] Nonsyndromic hearing losses are grouped according to their inheritance mode: DFNA refers to autosomal dominant cases, DFNB to autosomal recessive, and DFN to X-linked or mitochondrial cases; a unique numeral following each acronym has been used to identify each chromosomal locus discovered in chronologic order. As a consequence of a major effort to identify and classify inherited hearing disabilities, it is clear that the nonsyndromic basis of inherited deafness is highly heterogeneous. Many loci known to produce autosomal dominant forms of deafness when mutated have been genetically mapped, although only a subset of the genes responsible for autosomal dominant forms have been identified and cloned. Autosomal recessive forms of inherited hearing loss account for most nonsyndromic abnormalities (approximately 80%). It has become increasingly clear, however, that different mutations in a given gene may be responsible for differences in the severity of hearing loss, different patterns of inheritance, and susceptibility to environmental factors such as noise or aminoglycoside antibiotics, as well as the involvement of other organ systems. For example, mutations in a number of genes (e.g., *COL11A2, ESPN, GJB2, GJB3, GJB6, MYO6, MYO7A, PJVK, TECTA, TMC1*) are responsible for both autosomal dominant and autosomal recessive forms of nonsyndromic deafness. Moreover, mutations in several genes (e.g., *CDH23, COL11A2, GJB2, GJB3*, GJB6, *MYH9, MYO7A, MYO15A, PCDH15, SLC26A4, USH1C, WFS1, WHRN*) are responsible for both nonsyndromic and syndromic forms of deafness (see Table 146-1). The phenotypic spectrum produced by mutations in a gene has been attributed to the severity of the mutation, allelic heterogeneity, alternative splicing, and the contribution of modifier genes.[60,136,171,254,336,362,486]

This chapter reviews basic mechanisms underlying sensory transduction associated with hearing and integrates contemporary models of transduction with the latest acquired information regarding the molecular structure and organization of key inner ear systems. Because of the sheer number of factors now known to be necessary for normal inner ear development, maintenance, and function, a comprehensive accounting is not possible here—not all such factors are addressed. Of note, the stated biologic role of most of the proteins discussed here remains speculative, and substantial work is needed to determine their precise role in the inner ear, as well as the nature of their interactions with other proteins. Excellent reviews that are relevant to the subject of this chapter are listed in the Bibliographic References.[29,61,170,187,215,236,310,320,443,453,585,588,631]

Passive Cochlear Mechanics

The cochlea, and the organ of Corti in particular, constitute an evolutionary marvel of biologic engineering as intricate, microscaled mechanical systems. Although the hallmark of peripheral auditory function in mammals may be the evolutionary adaptation of a relatively simple, passive resonant system into an active one that consumes energy and efficiently detects and amplifies vibratory energy, it is useful to note that the fundamental nature of cochlear mechanics is evident even in cadavers, as so elegantly demonstrated by Nobel prize winner Georg von Békésy.[586] Because cochlear mechanics at this level of function are independent of other factors—neither requiring nor consuming adenosine triphosphate (ATP), for example—the sound-driven motion of the organ of Corti observed by von Békésy and others is commonly referred to as passive.

The primary elements of passive cochlear transduction are hydromechanical in character, and the integrated contributions of many structural elements are known to determine the resonant character of cadaveric and therefore mechanically passive cochleae (Fig. 146-1). The cochlear partition is composed of an epithelial sheet known as the tympanic cover layer that supports the fibroelastic basilar membrane, itself the central structure of the end organ both functionally and anatomically. This partition supports, in turn, both the sensory and nonsensory supporting epithelium. The fluid-filled major chambers of the cochlea—specifically, the scala vestibuli and scala tympani, which are filled with perilymph, and the scala media, which is filled with endolymph—also play an important role in transduction. These structural elements, together with the tectorial membrane (an extracellular gelatinous structure secreted by nonsensory inner ear epithelial cells) that extends from the spiral limbus radially over the apical surface of the organ of Corti, comprise the principal elements that give rise to passive mechanical transduction. Although Reissner's membrane separates scala media from scala vestibuli and therefore plays an important homeostatic role in the maintenance of cochlear electrochemistry, it does not seem to play a significant role as an element of passive cochlear mechanics.

Because the focus of this chapter is on cochlear transduction, we will only remind the reader that sound waves collected in the external ear canal produce vibrations of the tympanic membrane, which in turn vibrate middle ear ossicles (Fig. 146-2A). It is, of course, the vibratory motion of the stapedial footplate that transmits the mechanical energy of the ossicular chain directly through the oval window of the cochlea, effectively delivering sound pressure waves to the scala vestibuli and translating mechanical motion into pressure waves that propagate through the virtually incompressible cochlear fluids at a velocity approximating 1.5 km/sec. At this rate of propagation, the spread of the pressure wave throughout the volume of the cochlea is nearly instantaneous. Because the bony walls of the cochlea are rigid and its fluid contents incompressible, the higher pressure (or lower, depending on the direction of motion of the stapedial footplate) in scala vestibuli relative to scala tympani produces a pressure differential across the cochlear partition that creates intracochlear forces that set the partition into motion (see Fig. 146-2D). As described in more detail in a later section, the physical makeup of the organ of Corti, and of the basilar

Text continues on p. 2060

Table 146-1

Selected Genes Underlying Various Forms of Deafness in Humans

Gene	Name/Protein	Human Disorder	Murine Disorder	Type of Molecule	Localization
ACTG1	Actin γ1	DFNA20, DFNA26[572,639]	Targeted null[406]	Intracellular protein, cytoskeletal nonmuscle actin isoform	Hair cell stereocilia, cuticular plate, and adherens junctions
ATP2B2 (*PMCA2*)	Ca^{2+}-ATPase 2, Ca^{2+}-transporting, plasma membrane 2	Increased severity of autosomal recessive hearing loss associated with a missense mutation in *CDH23*[486]	Deafwaddler (*dfw*), targeted null—increased susceptibility to noise-induced hearing loss[297,298,532]	Calcium pump	Hair cells
ATP6B1	β-Subunit of renal apical H^+-ATPase pump	Renal tubular acidosis with deafness[265]	Targeted null—normal hearing[131]	Ion pump, ATPase	Interdental cells, endolymphatic sac, kidney
BSND	Barttin (NKCC2)	Bartter syndrome type IV (with sensorineural deafness)[53,145]	Bsnd conditional knockout[447]	Cl^- channel β-subunit	Strial marginal cells
CCDC50	Coiled-coil domain–containing protein 50/Ymer	DFNA44[369]		Cytoplasmic protein (associated with microtubule-based cytoskeleton and mitotic apparatus); effector of EGF-mediated cell signaling	Pillar cells, stria vascularis; during development also expressed in cells lining cochlear duct, spiral ganglion, spiral limbus, OHCs, spiral ligament, Deiters cells
CDH23	Cadherin 23, otocadherin	DFNB12, Usher syndrome type 1D[58,60]	Waltzer (v), age-related hearing loss (*ahl*), modifier of deafwaddler (*mdfw*)[120,384]	Cell adhesion protein	Hair cells, retina
CLDN14	Claudin-14	DFNB29[606]	Targeted null[45]	Tight junction component	Hair cells, Deiters cells, inner and outer phalangeal cells, epithelial cells lining inner spiral sulcus
COCH	Coagulation factor C homology/cochlin	DFNA9[452]	Targeted null—not deaf; targeted missense—late-onset hearing loss[348,451]	Extracellular matrix component	Spiral ligament, spiral limbus, and osseous spiral lamina
COL1A1	Type I collagen α1 chain	Osteogenesis imperfecta[37]	Mov13, transgene[19,59]	Extracellular matrix component	Mineralized and nonmineralized connective tissue
COL2A1	Type II collagen α1 chain	Stickler syndrome type I[7]	Disproportionate micromelia (*Dmm*); spondyloepiphyseal dysplasia congenita (*sedc*); mutant transgenes[48,126,347]	Extracellular matrix component	Spiral ligament and limbus, tectorial membrane, basilar membrane, cartilage

Continued

Table 146-1

Selected Genes Underlying Various Forms of Deafness in Humans—cont'd

Gene	Name/Protein	Human Disorder	Murine Disorder	Type of Molecule	Localization
COL4A3	Type IV collagen α3 chain	Alport syndrome[368]	Targeted null[89]	Extracellular matrix component	Basal lamina of cochlear duct and strial blood vessels, kidney
COL4A4	Type IV collagen α4 chain	Alport syndrome[368]		Extracellular matrix component	Basal lamina of cochlear duct and strial blood vessels, kidney
COL4A5	Type IV collagen α5 chain	Alport syndrome, X-linked[36]		Extracellular matrix component	Basal lamina of cochlear duct and strial blood vessels, kidney
COL9A1	Type IX collagen α1 chain	Stickler syndrome[566]	Targeted null[537]	Extracellular matrix component	Tectorial membrane, fibrocytes of spiral ligament
COL11A1	Type XI collagen α1 chain	Stickler, syndrome type II, Marshall, syndrome[198,442]	Chondrodysplasia (*cho*)[74,326]	Extracellular matrix component	Greater epithelial ridge and lateral wall of the cochlea early in development; inner sulcus, Claudius cells, and Boettcher cells during development
COL11A2	Type XI collagen α2 chain	DFNB53, DFNA13, Stickler syndrome type III (nonocular), otospondylomega-epiphyseal dysplasia (OSMED) syndrome[71,361,581]	Targeted null[361]	Extracellular matrix component	Tectorial membrane
CRYM	μ-Crystallin (NADP-regulated thyroid hormone–binding protein)	DFNAi[2]	Targeted null—normal hearing[538]	Involved in K^+ recycling?	Lateral region of spiral ligament and fibrocytes of spiral limbus
DFNA5	Deafness, autosomal dominant 5, ICERE-1	DFNA5[569]	Targeted null—normal hearing[570]		Organ of Corti, limbus, stria (RT-PCR only)
DIAPH1 (*HDIA1*)	Diaphanous homolog 1	DFNA1[346]	Targeted null—hearing not assessed[404]	Cytoplasmic protein regulating actin polymerization	Inner ear (RT-PCR only)
DSPP	Dentin sialophosphoprotein	DFNA39 associated with dentinogenesis imperfecta type 1[620]			
EDN3	Endothelin 3	Waardenburg syndrome type IV, Waardenburg-Hirschsprung disease[138]	Lethal spotting (*ls*)[39]	Ligand	Strial intermediate cells, pigmentation, gut
EDNRB	Endothelin receptor type B	Waardenburg syndrome type IV, Waardenburg-Hirschsprung disease[34]	Piebald (s)[232]	Receptor	Widespread in pigmentation, gut

Table 146-1

Selected Genes Underlying Various Forms of Deafness in Humans—cont'd

Gene	Name/Protein	Human Disorder	Murine Disorder	Type of Molecule	Localization
ESPN	Espin	DFNB36, DFNAi[129,381]	Jerker (*je*)[634]	Actin-bundling protein	Hair cell stereocilia
ESRRB (*NR3B2*)	Estrogen-related receptor β	DFNB35[80]	Targeted conditional null[69]	Orphan nuclear receptor; alters cell fate of strial epithelial cells	Strial marginal cells
EYA1	Eyes-absent 1 homolog (*Drosophila*)	Branchio-oto-renal syndrome type 1[1]	Targeted null, spontaneous mutant[250,621]	Transcriptional coactivator	Neuroepithelia, ganglia, otic capsule and middle ear mesenchyme, kidney, jaw
EYA4	Eyes-absent 4 homolog (*Drosophila*)	DFNA10[599]	Targeted null[116]	Transcriptional coactivator	Eustachian tube and middle ear?
FGFR3	Fibroblast growth factor receptor 3	Craniosynostosis with deafness, Muenke syndrome[125,224]	Targeted null[81]	Growth factor receptor; affects support cell fate	Pillar cells, Deiters cells, hair cells during development, skull
FOXI1 (*FKH10*)	Forkhead box I1	Pendred syndrome[625]	Targeted null[242,243]	Transcriptional activator of SLC26A4	Endolymphatic duct/sac
GATA3	GATA-binding protein 3	Hypoparathyroidism, sensorineural deafness, and renal dysplasia (HDR) syndrome[567]	Targeted null[266,571]	Enhancer-binding protein (for T-cell antigen receptor gene activation); zinc finger transcription factor	Otocyst and periotic mesenchyme; developing sensory epithelia, OHCs, spiral ganglion neurons, olivocochlear efferent neurons
GJB1 (*CMT*) (*CX32*)	Gap junction membrane channel protein β1, connexin 32	Charcot-Marie-Tooth type 1X syndrome (X-linked)[49]		Gap junction component	Schwann cells of auditory nerve and other peripheral nerves
GJB2 (*CX26*)	Gap junction membrane channel protein β2, connexin 26	DFNB1, DFNA3, keratitis-ichthyosis-deafness syndrome, palmoplantar hyperkeratosis, palmoplantar keratoderma[269,439,441]	Targeted, conditional null; dominantnegative transgene[79,305]	Gap junction component	Fibrocytes of the spiral ligament and spiral limbus; nonsensory epithelial cells in the region of the organ of Corti
GJB3 (*CX31*)	Gap junction membrane channel protein β3, connexin 31	DFNA2, DFNBi; erythrokeratodermia variabilis, peripheral neuropathy[340,342,440,618]	Targeted null—no hearing loss[421]	Gap junction component	Fibrocytes of the spiral ligament and spiral limbus; Schwann cells of auditory nerve and other peripheral nerves
GJB6 (*CX30*)	Gap junction membrane channel protein β6, connexin 30	DFNB1, DFNA3, Clouston syndrome[108,197]	Targeted null[544]	Gap junction component	Cells of the spiral limbus, the spiral ligament, the stria vascularis, and in supporting cells of the organ of Corti
KCNE1 (*IsK*, *MinK*)	Potassium voltage-gated channel, IsK-related subfamily, member 1	Jervell and Lange-Nielsen syndrome locus 2[487,561]	Targeted null; spontaneous mutant (*pkr*)[323,580]	K^+ channel β-subunit	Strial marginal cells, heart

Continued

Table 146-1

Selected Genes Underlying Various Forms of Deafness in Humans—cont'd

Gene	Name/Protein	Human Disorder	Murine Disorder	Type of Molecule	Localization
KCNQ1 (*KvLQT1*, *KCNA9*)	Potassium voltage-gated channel, subfamily Q, member 1	Jervell and Lange-Nielsen syndrome locus 1[382]	Targeted null[66,315]	K^+ channel subunit	Strial marginal cells, heart
KCNQ4	Potassium voltage-gated channel, subfamily Q, member 4	DFNA2[304]	Targeted null, targeted knock-in[275]	K^+ channel subunit	Hair cells, spiral ganglion neurons
Kit	Kit proto-oncogene	Piebald syndrome[183]	Dominant spotting (*W*)[180,528]	Transmembrane protein, receptor for tyrosine kinase	Developing melanocytes (including strial intermediate cells)
LRTOMT	Leucine-rich transmembrane *O*-methyltransferase	DFNB63[9]		Fusion gene that gives rise to *LRTOMT1* and *LRTOMT2*	Hair cells and supporting cells
MITF	Microphthalmia transcription factor	Waardenburg syndrome type IIA, Tietz syndrome[20,541]	Microphthalmia (*mi*)[222]	Transcription factor	Strial intermediate cells during development, pigmentation
MPZ (P_0)	Myelin protein zero (P_0)	Charcot-Marie-Tooth syndrome type 1B with sensorineural deafness (auditory neuropathy), Déjérine-Sottas syndrome, congenital hypomyelinating neuropathy[212,213]	Transgenic mouse line[638]	Cell adhesion molecule and main component of compact myelin in peripheral nervous system	Schwann cells of auditory nerve and other peripheral nerves
MYH9	Myosin heavy chain IX, nonmuscle heavy chain IIA (NMHC IIA)	DFNA17, May-Hegglin anomaly, Sebastian, Fechtner, and Epstein syndromes[309,497]	Gene-trapping, homozygotes—embryonic lethal, heterozygotes—normal hearing[400]	Motor protein	Hair cells, spiral ligament, spiral limbus, spiral ganglion
MYH14	Myosin heavy chain XIV, nonmuscle heavy chain IIC (NMHC IIC)	DFNA4[128]		Motor protein	Organ of Corti, stria vascularis, Hensen cells, Claudius cells, external sulcus cells, epithelium of the spiral prominence
MYO1A	Myosin IA	DFNA48[127]	Targeted null—normal startle response[560]	Motor protein	
MYO3A	Myosin IIIA	DFNB30[591]		Motor protein	Hair cells
MYO6	Myosin VI	DFNB37, DFNA22[10,363]	Snell's waltzer (*sv*), tailchaser (*tlc*) (ENU)[35,219]	Motor protein	Hair cells
MYO7A	Myosin VIIA	DFNB2, DFNA11, Usher syndrome type 1B[338,339,600]	Shaker 1 (*sh1*)[182]	Motor protein	Hair cells, retina
MYO15A	Myosin XVa	DFNB3; Smith-Magenis syndrome[330,592]	Shaker 2 (*sh2*)[422]	Motor protein	Hair cells

Table 146-1

Selected Genes Underlying Various Forms of Deafness in Humans—cont'd

Gene	Name/Protein	Human Disorder	Murine Disorder	Type of Molecule	Localization
ND	Norrie disease protein, norrin	Norrie disease[46,72]	Targeted null[47,429]	Extracellular matrix component	Stria, spiral ganglion, eye, brain
OTOA	Otoancorin	DFNB22[640]		Glycosylphosphatidylinositol-linked membrane protein	Apical surface of interdental cells; apical surface of border epithelial cells lying adjacent and medial to IHCs during development
OTOF	Otoferlin	DFNB9[626]	Targeted null[455]	Synaptic vesicle–trafficking protein	IHCs
PAX2	Paired box gene 2	Renal-coloboma syndrome[137]	Targeted null[552]	Transcription factor	
PAX3	Paired box gene 3	Waardenburg syndrome types I, III[234,542]	Splotch (*Sp*)[141,530]	Transcription factor	Developing dorsal neural tube, pigmentation
PCDH15	Protocadherin-15	DFNB23, Usher syndrome types 1F[11,12,15]	Ames waltzer (*av*)[14]	Cell adhesion protein	Hair cells
PJVK	Pejvakin	DFNB59, DFNAi[109,488]	DFNB59 knock-in, sirtaki (ENU)[109,488]		Hair cells, spiral ganglion, brainstem auditory neurons
PMP22	Peripheral myelin protein 22	Charcot-Marie-Tooth syndrome type 1A with sensorineural deafness (auditory neuropathy)[296]	Trembler (*Tr*)[536,638]	Hydrophobic intrinsic membrane protein of myelin sheaths in peripheral nervous system	Schwann cells of auditory nerve and other peripheral nerves
POU3F4 (*BRN4*.0)	POU domain, class 3, transcription factor 4	DFN3 (X-linked)[107]	Targeted null, sex-linked fidget (*slf*)[366,412,414]	Transcription factor	Mesoderm around otic vesicle and lateral wall; spiral ligament, Reissner's membrane
POU4F3 (*BRN3c*)	POU domain, class 4, transcription factor 3	DFNA15[564]	Targeted null, dreidel (*ddl*)[143,619]	Transcription factor	Hair cells
RDX	Radixin	DFNB24[273]	Targeted null[289]	Cross-link actin filaments to plasma membrane	Hair cells
SALL1 (*HSAL1*)	Sal-like 1	Townes-Brocks syndrome[292]	Targeted mutation producing truncated protein[280]	Transcription factor (repressor)	
SANS	Scaffolding protein containing ankyrin repeats and SAM (sterile alpha motif) domain	Usher syndrome type 1G[377,601]	Jackson shaker (*js*)[283]	Scaffold protein	Hair cells
SIX1	Homolog of *Drosophila* sine oculis homeobox 1 gene	Branchio-oto-renal or branchio-otic syndrome type 3[458]	Targeted null[637]	Transcriptional regulator	Embryonic development of ear, kidney, muscle; branchial arch

Continued

Table 146-1

Selected Genes Underlying Various Forms of Deafness in Humans—cont'd

Gene	Name/Protein	Human Disorder	Murine Disorder	Type of Molecule	Localization
SIX5	Homolog of *Drosophila* sine oculis homeobox 5 gene	Branchio-oto-renal syndrome type 2[231]	Targeted null[291,479]	Transcriptional regulator	Embryonic development of ear, kidney; branchial arch
SLC17A8 (*VGLUT3*)	Solute carrier family 17 (sodium phosphate cotransporter), member 8; vesicular glutamate transporter-3	DFNA25[457]	Targeted null[457,490]	Vesicular glutamate transporter	IHCs (synaptic vesicles)
SLC19A2	Solute carrier family 19 (thiamine transporter), member 2; high-affinity thiamine transporter 1 (Thtr1)	Thiamine-responsive megaloblastic anemia syndrome (diabetes mellitus, megaloblastic anemia, sensorineural deafness)[121,158,308]	Targeted null[390]	Thiamine transporter	Hair cells, greater expression in IHCs than in OHCs
SLC26A4 (*PDS*)	Solute carrier family 26, member 4 (pendrin)	DFNB4, Pendred syndrome, enlarged vestibular aqueduct, Mondini dysplasia[151,325]	Targeted null[150]	Anion transporter (pumps bicarbonate into endolymph and maintains pH homeostasis)	Spiral prominence epithelial cells, root cells, endolymphatic duct and sac, thyroid gland
SLC26A5 (*PRES*)	Solute carrier family 26, member 5 (prestin)	DFNB61[337]	Targeted null, targeted knock-in[103,328]	Cl^- translocator/motor protein	OHCs
SLUG, *SNAI2*	Snail homolog 2	Waardenburg syndrome type II[474]	Targeted null[474]	Transcription factor	Embryonic neural crest
SOX2	Sex-determining region of the Y chromosome–related (SRY-related) high-mobility group (HMG) box gene 2	Syndromic: anophthalmia or microphthalmia, sensorineural hearing loss, anterior pituitary hypoplasia, hypogonadism[268]	Light coat and circling (*lcc*); yellow submarine (*ysb*)[130,281]	Transcription factor	Developing CNS and placodes—involved in hypothalamopituitary and reproductive axes; prosensory domain of cochlear epithelium
SOX10	SRY-box containing gene 10	Waardenburg syndrome type IV[419]	Dominant megacolon (*dom*)[217,521]	Transcription factor	Otocyst, pigmentation, gut
STRC	Stereocilin	DFNB16[576]	Targeted null[577]	Transmembrane or extracellular protein?	Hair cells (component of horizontal top connectors between adjacent stereocilia and the tops of the tallest OHC stereocilia that attach to the tectorial membrane)
TBX1	T-box 1	DiGeorge syndrome[73]	Transgene overexpression, targeted null[172,582]	Transcription factor	Otocyst
TCOF1	Treacle	Treacher Collins syndrome[123]	Targeted null heterozygotes[122]	Nucleolar trafficking protein	Neural crest cells

Table 146-1

Selected Genes Underlying Various Forms of Deafness in Humans—cont'd

Gene	Name/Protein	Human Disorder	Murine Disorder	Type of Molecule	Localization
TECTA	α-Tectorin	DFNB21, DFNA8/ DFNA12[378,574]	Targeted null, targeted missense[317,318]	Extracellular matrix component	Tectorial membrane; also in inner sulcus and Hensen cells during development
TFCP2L3 (*GRHL2*)	Transcription factor cellular promotor 2-like 3 (grainyhead-like 2)	DFNA28, age-related hearing loss[408,568]		Transcription factor	Organ of Corti, stria vascularis, Reissner's membrane, interdental cells, cells lining the scala media
THRB	Thyroid hormone receptor β	Thyroid hormone resistance[473]	Targeted null[167]	Transcription factor	Cochlear sensory epithelium, Kolliker's organ, spiral ganglion, Hensen cells, stria vascularis
TIMM8A (*DDP1*)	Translocase of mitochondrial inner membrane 8A; DDP1 (deafness dystonia peptide 1)	Mohr-Tranebjaerg syndrome/Jensen syndrome (X-linked)[248,553,554]		Mitochondrial protein	Widespread including muscle
TMC1	Transmembrane channel-like gene 1	DFNB7/DFNB11, DFNA36[306]	Deafness (*dn*); Beethoven (*Bth*)[306,587]	Transmembrane protein	Hair cells
TMHS (*LHFPL5*)	Tetraspan membrane protein of hair cell stereocilia; lipoma HMGIC fusion partner-like 5	DFNB66/ DFNB67[263,498]	Hurry-scurry (hscy)[341]	Transmembrane protein	Transient expression in hair cells (especially stereocilia) during development
TMIE	Transmembrane inner ear expressed gene	DFNB6[380]	Spinner (*sr*), circling (*cir*)[75,367]	Transmembrane protein	Hair cells
TMPRSS3 (*ECHOS1*)	Type II transmembrane protease, serine 3	DFNB8/DFNB10[489]		Transmembrane serine protease	Stria vascularis, inner and outer pillar cells, Deiters cells, Hensen cells, epithelial cells lining the inner spiral sulcus, spiral ganglion
TRIC (*MARVELD2*)	Tricellulin (Marvel domain–containing protein 2)	DFNB49[435]		Tight junction membrane protein at tricellular contacts	Tricellular tight junctions in sensory epithelium, including among hair cells and supporting cells, and among strial marginal cells
TRIOBP (*TARA*)	TRIO (triple functioning domain) and filamentous actin [F-actin]–binding protein (TRIO-associated repeat on actin)	DFNB28[436,499]		F-actin–binding protein	Hair cells

Continued

Table 146-1

Selected Genes Underlying Various Forms of Deafness in Humans—cont'd

Gene	Name/Protein	Human Disorder	Murine Disorder	Type of Molecule	Localization
USH1C	Usher 1C, harmonin	DFNB18, Usher syndrome type 1C[13,575]	Deaf circler, (*dfcr*), targeted null, targeted knock-in[252,316,321]	Scaffold protein	Hair cells, photoreceptors
USH2A	Usherin	Usher syndrome type 2A[147]	Targeted null[335]	Transmembrane protein (component of ankle links of hair cell stereocilia)	Hair cells, photoreceptors
USH3A (*CLRN1*)	Clarin-1	Usher syndrome type 3[6,249]	Targeted null (unpublished)	Transmembrane protein	Hair cells, photoreceptors
VLGR1 (*MASS1*; *GPR98*)	Very large G-protein–coupled receptor 1	Usher syndrome type 2C[603]	Targeted mutation producing truncated protein, targeted null, frings, rueda (ENU)[255,359,623]	Transmembrane protein (component of ankle links of hair cell stereocilia)	Hair cells, photoreceptors
WFS1	Wolfram syndrome gene 1, wolframin	DFNA6/DFNA14/DFNA38, Wolfram syndrome[51,534,629]		Transcellular ion movement (component of endoplasmic reticulum, especially canalicular reticulum)	Hair cells, Deiters cells, Hensen cells, Claudius cells; epithelial cells lining the external spiral sulcus, spiral prominence, spiral ligament; interdental cells; Reissner's membrane
WHRN	Whirlin	DFNB31; Usher syndrome type 2D[136,358]	Whirler (*wi*)[358]	Scaffold protein involved in elongation and maintenance of hair cell stereocilia	Hair cells, photoreceptors

ATPase, adenosine triphosphatase; CNS, central nervous system; EGF, epithelial growth factor; HMGIC, high mobility group I-C proteins; IHC, inner hair cell; NADP, nicotinamide-adenine dinucleotide phosphate; OHC, outer hair cell; RT-PCR, reverse transcriptase–polymerase chain reaction.

Table 146-2

Selected Genes Underlying Murine Deafness for Which Human Deafness Has Not Been Determined

Gene	Name/Protein	Murine Disorder	Type of Molecule	Localization
Bsn	Bassoon	Targeted disruption—Bassoon (*Bsn*) mice exhibit characteristics of auditory neuropathy; anchoring of ribbons in inner hair cells is impaired[277]	Presynaptic scaffolding protein	Hair cells
Cacna1D ($Ca_V1.3$)	Calcium channel, voltage-dependent, L type, α1D subunit	Targeted null mice are deaf[420]	Voltage-sensitive calcium channel	Hair cells
Cdkn2d (*Ink4D*)	Cyclin-dependent kinase inhibitor 2D	Targeted null mice—the postmitotic state of sensory hair cells is disrupted: they reenter the cell cycle and subsequently undergo apoptosis, resulting in progressive hearing loss[70]	Cell cycle regulation	Hair cells
Cldn11	Claudin-11	Targeted null mice are hearing-impaired; endocochlear potential is reduced[195,290]	Tight junction protein	Strial basal cells

Table 146-2

Selected Genes Underlying Murine Deafness for Which Human Deafness Has Not Been Determined—cont'd

Gene	Name/Protein	Murine Disorder	Type of Molecule	Localization
Clic5	Chloride intracellular channel 5	Jitterbug (*jbg*) mice are hearing-impaired; hearing loss is progressive[175]	May associate with radixin and stabilize connection between actin core of stereocilia and plasma membrane	Hair cells
Gfi1	Growth factor–independent 1	Targeted null mice lack an acoustic startle reflex; outer hair cells degenerate[218,590] Humans with a missense mutation show no evidence of hearing loss[407]	Transcriptional repressor oncoprotein; regulated by POU4F3	Hair cells, spiral ganglion cells
Itga8	Integrin α8β1	Targeted null mice die soon after birth; utricular hair cells lack stereocilia or have malformed stereocilia[334]	Cell surface glycoprotein that mediates cell-cell and cell–extracellular matrix interactions (signaling molecule)	Apical hair cell surface where stereocilia form
Kcnj10 (*Kir4.1*)	Potassium channel, inwardly rectifying, subfamily J, member 10	Targeted null mice are deaf (absent endocochlear potential; reduced endolymph volume and K^+ concentration)[353]	K^+ channel	Strial intermediate cells
Math1 (*Atoh1*)	Mouse homolog of atonal 1	Targeted null mice are deaf (hair cells do not develop)[50]	Basic helix-loop-helix transcription factor	Hair cells
Otog	Otogelin	Twister (*twt*), targeted null mice are hearing-impaired[508,509]	Extracellular matrix component	Tectorial membrane
Otos	Otospiralin	Targeted null mice are moderately hearing-impaired; type II and IV fibrocytes degenerate[112]		Fibrocytes of the spiral limbus and spiral ligament
Ptprq	Protein tyrosine phosphatase receptor Q	Transgenic mice are hearing-impaired and have progressive hair cell loss in the base of the cochlea[190]	Receptor-like protein tyrosine phosphatase	Hair cells
Slc4a7 (*Nbc3*)	Solute carrier family 4 (sodium bicarbonate cotransporter), member 7; Nbc3	Targeted null mice develop hearing impairment[57]	Sodium bicarbonate cotransporter (Nbc); pH regulation	Type I and II fibrocytes
Slc12a2 (*Nkcc1*)	Solute carrier family 12 (sodium-potassium-chloride transporter), member 2	Shaker-without-syndactylism (*sy-ns*)[124]; Targeted null mice are deaf[110,157]	Na^+-K^+-$2Cl^-$ cotransporter	Strial marginal cells, distal nephron
Slc12a6 (*Kcc3*)	Solute carrier family 12 (potassium-chloride cotransporter), member 6; Kcc3	Targeted null mice develop a slowly progressive hearing loss[56]	K^+-Cl^- cotransporter	Supporting cells of hair cells, epithelial cells of organ of Corti, type I and III fibrocytes, neurons, renal proximal tubule
Slc12a7 (*Kcc4*)	Solute carrier family 12 (potassium-chloride cotransporter), member 7; Kcc4	Targeted null mice are deaf, develop renal tubular acidosis[55]	K^+-Cl^- cotransporter	Deiters cells, supporting cells of inner hair cells

Continued

Table 146-2

Selected Genes Underlying Murine Deafness for Which Human Deafness Has Not Been Determined—cont'd

Gene	Name/Protein	Murine Disorder	Type of Molecule	Localization
Spnb4	β-Spectrin 4	Quivering (*qv*) mice have moderate to severe abnormalities in ABR wave I; later peaks generally are absent[401]	Ion channel localization in myelinated nerves	Spiral ganglion neurons (axons)
Tbx18	T-box transcription factor 18	Transgenic mice are deaf; endocochlear potential is absent; stria vascularis is disrupted[555]	Transcription factor	Otic mesenchyme that differentiates into fibrocytes
Tectb	β-Tectorin	Targeted null mice have significantly elevated thresholds below 20 kHz and sharper tuning at high frequencies[462]	Extracellular matrix component	Tectorial membrane
Tmprss1 (*Hpn*)	Transmembrane protease serine 1 (hepsin)	Targeted null mice exhibit profound hearing loss[201]	Transmembrane serine protease	Inner ear
Trpml3 (*Mcoln3*)	Transient receptor potential cation channel, mucolipin subfamily member 3	Varitint-waddler (*Va*) mice are deaf, have reduced endocochlear potential and pigmentation defects[65,119]	Transmembrane protein; ion channel protein of intracellular endosomes and lysosomes	Hair cells (cytoplasmic vesicles, stereocilia, plasma membrane), strial intermediate cells

ABR, auditory brainstem response.

membrane in particular, establishes a space-frequency map that determines the limits of hearing and the capacity of the subject to resolve frequency differences among vibrations that contain energy in the audible range.

Physical Dimensions

At the basal end of the cochlea near the round window, the width of the basilar membrane, as measured between the tympanic lip of the spiral limbus and the basilar crest of the spiral ligament, is narrow relative to dimensions representing more apical locations (Fig. 146-3). In fact, the width of the basilar membrane progressively increases along a base-to-apex gradient in mammals, such that in humans, for example (see Fig. 146-3 E), the width at the base is approximately 100 μm and approaches 500 μm near the apex.[604] In association with graded basilar membrane width, the number of mesothelial cells, or tympanic border cells, lining the basilar membrane increases along the basoapical length of the end organ, as does the length of outer hair cells (OHCs) and associated stereocilia. Conversely, the thickness of the basilar membrane and the density of radial filaments embedded in the homogenous ground matrix of the partition decrease progressively from base to apex (see Fig. 146-3C). It is notable that radial filaments are composed primarily of collagen type II,[132,545,558] whereas the ground matrix of the partition itself is composed primarily of fibronectin, tenascin, proteoglycans containing keratin sulfate and chondroitin sulfate, and emilin-2 (*e*lastin *m*icrofibril *i*nterface-*l*ocated prote*in*-2).[21,375,475,539,611] Consequently, the basilar membrane and organ of Corti complex is stiffer and less massive at the base than at the apex (see Fig. 146-3F). The result is an end organ with resonant properties that are continuously distributed from base to apex that supports a mechanical system that separates, or filters, complex fluid waves into sinusoidal constituents. As a result, high-frequency acoustic events are preferentially transduced in the base (see Fig. 146-3G), because it is stiff and less massive. The inverse is true in the case of low-frequency acoustic events.

Another physical characteristic of the cochlea that exerts influence over the mechanics of transduction is the relative volume of perilymphatic fluid compartments that are larger at the base than at the apex (see Fig. 146-1). Consequently, there is a clear difference in fluid-mass loading of basilar membrane motion along the length of the end organ. The magnitude of the intracochlear fluid load is thought to dominate longitudinal coupling along the length of the cochlea. Of note, very little coupling occurs otherwise between adjacent regions of the basilar membrane—beyond, that is, simple stretching and compression forces.[204,394,395,583] At rest, therefore, the basilar membrane seems to be under very little tension, and without direct mechanical coupling, the traveling wave cannot propagate further apically after reaching its resonant peak, or place. Moreover, the viscous friction between the basilar membrane and cochlear fluids produces a damping effect that limits its displacement.

The Traveling Wave

The hydromechanical consequences of introducing a pressure pulse, or wave, into perilymphatic fluids is a traveling wave that propagates along the organ of Corti from the base to the apex (see Fig. 146-2). The traveling wave propagates basoapically, because the stiffness of the cochlear partition decreases longitudinally from the base to the apex (see Fig. 146-3F) as its mass increases. The motion and direction of the wave that travels along the basilar membrane are independent of the location of the vibratory source. von Békésy[586] observed this feature of cochlear mechanics by introducing a pressure pulse through an artificial window carved into the bony labyrinth near the cochlear apex. Traveling waves created under these conditions are essentially indistinguishable from traveling waves triggered by ossicular vibration. The basoapical propagation of the traveling wave is an outcome of the end organ's physical makeup, with the stiffer and less massive elements forming the base of the organ of Corti being set into motion by an instantaneous pressure difference between the major scalae before the more compliant and massive sections of the apical cochlea. The resultant traveling wave reflects the more or less independent, yet orderly, sequential movement of loosely coupled basilar membrane segments that form a frequency decomposition system generally thought of as the *space-frequency* or *tonotopic map* (see Fig. 146-3G).

As the traveling wave propagates toward the apex, traveling initially at a high rate of speed, the velocity of the wave decreases, with production of progressively shorter wavelengths for any given input frequency as a consequence (see Fig. 146-2E). As the amplitude of the propagating wave steadily increases as it passes toward the apex,

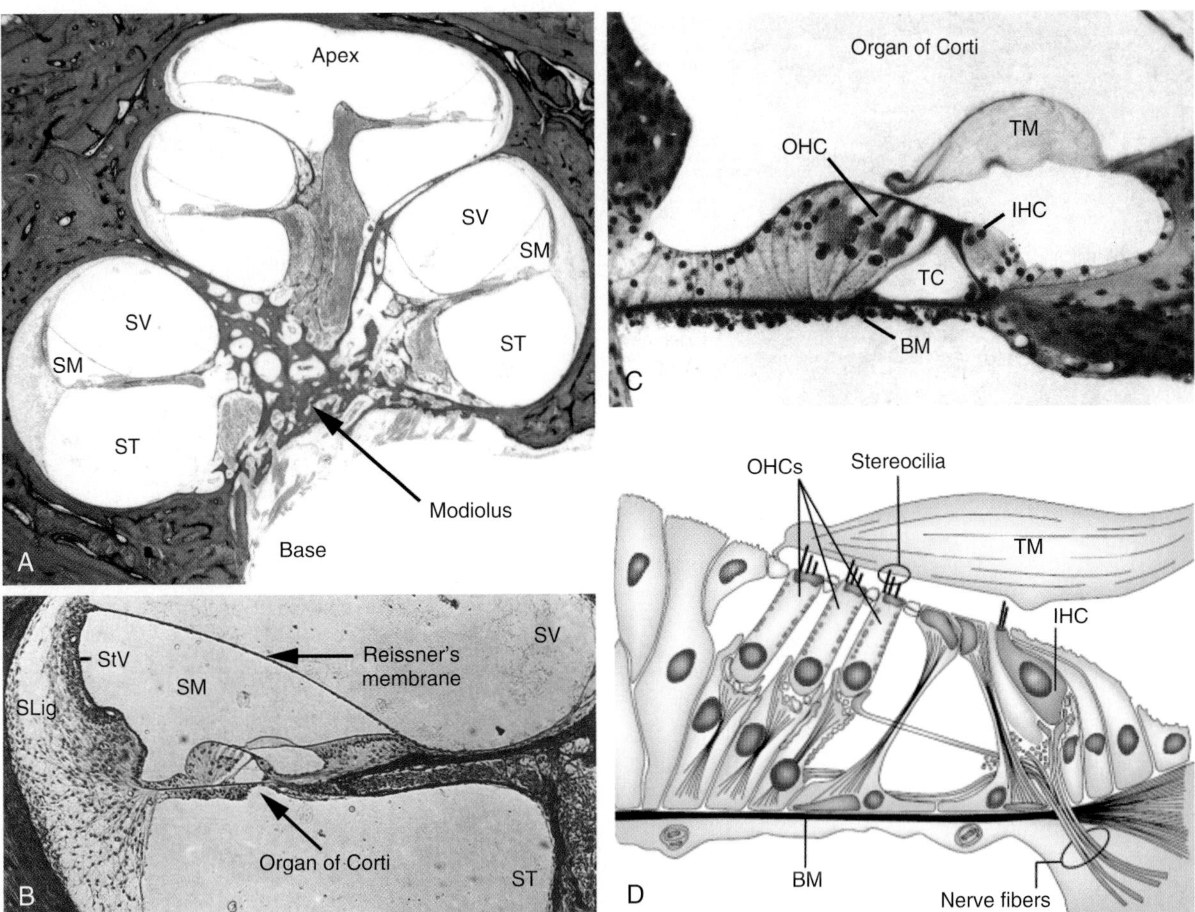

Figure 146-1. **A,** Midmodiolar section through a human cochlea showing the basal *(lower)*, middle, and apical *(upper)* turns. The modiolus is the central core of the cochlea and houses spiral ganglion neurons. The cochlear duct, otherwise known as the scala media (SM), contains endolymph and is separated from the perilymphatic fluid chambers, scala tympani (ST), and scala vestibuli (SV) by the cochlear partition and Reissner's membrane, respectively. At the cochlear apex, the fluids of the ST and SV mix through an opening called the helicotrema. **B,** Higher-magnification image of a modiolar section through the basal turn of the cochlea of a Rhesus monkey. The organ of Corti rests on the cochlear partition, a structure that includes the basilar membrane (BM) and a layer of mesothelial cells lining the BM and facing the ST. The stria vascularis (StV) and spiral ligament (SLig) form the lateral boundary of SM. **C,** Cross section of the organ of Corti from the middle turn of a cat cochlea. The triangular-shaped tunnel of Corti (TC), formed by the inner and outer pillar cells, separates the inner hair cell (IHC) from the outer hair cells (OHCs). The tectorial membrane (TM) can be seen pulled away from the sensory cells. **D,** Representation of the organ of Corti, showing the one row of IHCs and three rows of OHCs. Note the fluid spaces surrounding the OHCs, and that the tallest stereocilia of OHCs are embedded in the tectorial membrane, whereas the stereocilia of IHCs do not reach the tectorial membrane. *(**A,** Courtesy of Dr. William B. Warr; **B,** from Engstrom H, Angelborg C. Morphology of the walls of the cochlear duct. In: Zwicker E, Terhardt E, eds.* Facts and Models in Hearing. *New York: Springer-Verlag; 1974:3; **C,** from Engstrom H, Ades HW, Andersson A.* Structural Pattern of the Organ of Corti. *Baltimore: Williams & Wilkins; 1966; **D,** from Dallos P, Fakler B. Prestin, a new type of motor protein.* Nat Rev Mol Cell Biol. *2002;3:104.)*

partition displacement reaches a maximum value at its characteristic place—where intrinsic resonance meets, and nearly matches, the vibratory frequency of the triggering acoustic event (see Fig. 146-2F). As pointed out previously, the stiffness of the basilar membrane decreases exponentially with distance from the stapes,[205,394,395,586] so it is not surprising that the resonant frequency also decreases exponentially as a function of distance from the stapes, because the characteristic place is determined by the stiffness of the cochlear partition. Thus, the aforementioned space-frequency, or tonotopic, map is created, whereby the peak in vibration amplitude is located at the base of the cochlea for high frequencies and at progressively apical regions for lower frequencies.

Just as stiffness dominates the physics of the traveling wave as it travels toward its characteristic place, basilar membrane motion at and just above the characteristic place is dominated by the mass of the system. It is important to point out that the actual peak of the traveling wave occurs at a location just basal to the true resonant place, characterized by a match between intrinsic resonance and the triggering vibratory energy. At the place of peak displacement, the traveling wave slows to an essential standstill (i.e., it stalls) before remaining energy is completely dissipated, and the partition is completely and rapidly restored to its resting position slightly apical to the resonant place. Near the characteristic place for a given stimulus frequency, the pressure wave returns to the basal end of the cochlea through the fluids of the scala tympani, where the flexible round window membrane is displaced in an equal but opposite direction to that of the volume displacement of the stapes footplate.

At the apical end of the cochlea, the endolymphatic space terminates just short of the bony labyrinthine wall and maintains a firm physical boundary between endolymph and perilymph, allowing the fluids in the scala vestibuli and scala tympani to communicate directly by way of a small duct called the helicotrema (see Fig. 146-3B). The helicotrema acts as an acoustic shunt across the cochlear partition that reduces the pressure difference between the scalae produced by very-low-frequency stimulation.[96] The size of the helicotrema is thought to determine the low frequency cutoff of the system; that is, large

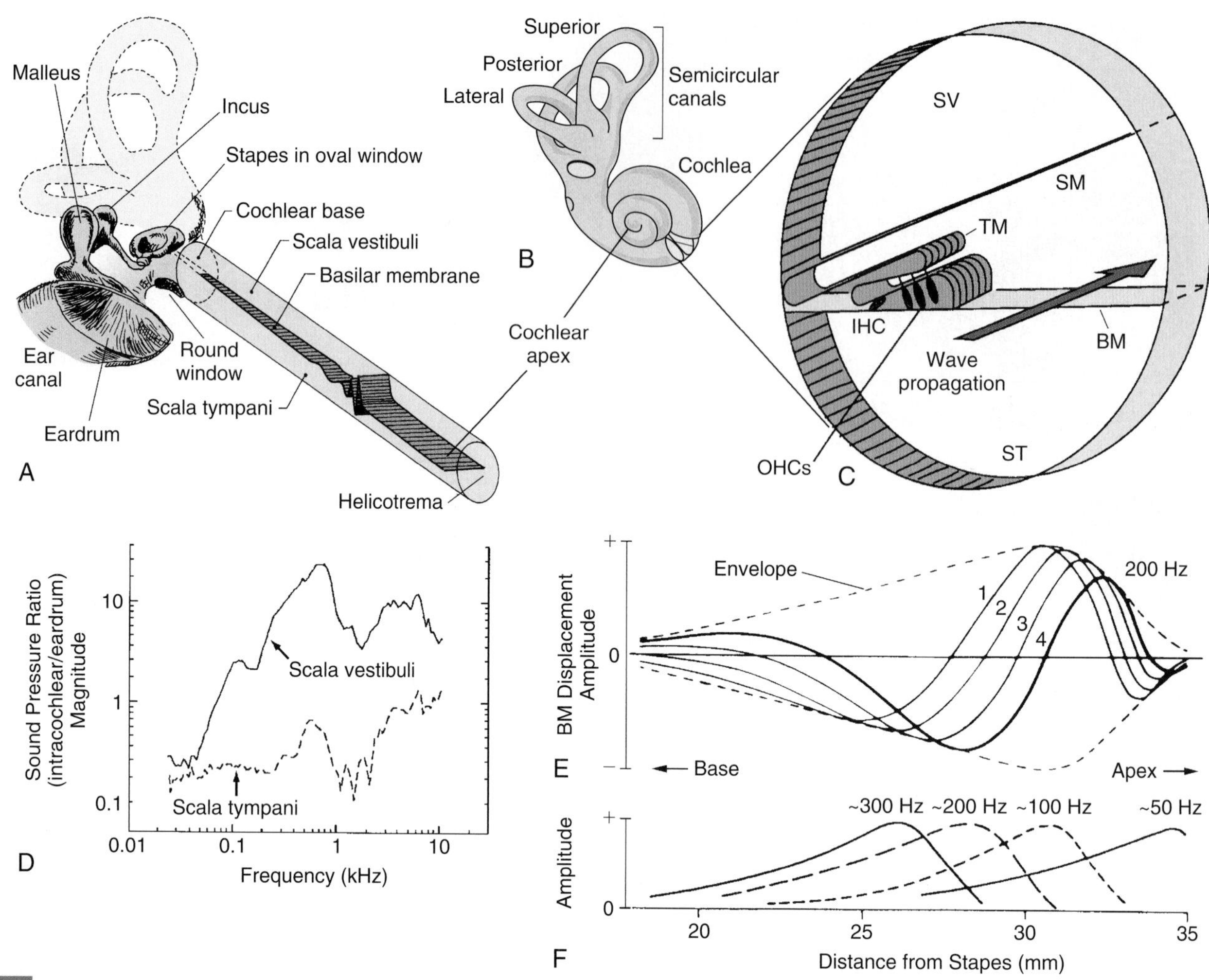

Figure 146-2. **A,** Schematic illustration of the inner ear with the cochlea uncoiled revealing the basilar membrane (BM) and a traveling wave at one instant in time in response to a pure tone. The eardrum (tympanic membrane) and middle ear ossicles also are shown in relation to the semicircular canals. The oval window opens into scala vestibuli (SV) and the round window to scala tympani (ST). **B,** Drawing of the inner ear with a segment of a cochlear turn extracted to expose the scalae. **C,** Diagram of a section through the cochlea showing the location of inner and outer hair cells (IHC and OHCs, respectively) in relation to the BM and TM and the direction of wave propagation. SM, scala media. **D,** The ratio of pressures measured within the SV and ST to the pressure at the eardrum produced in response to tone bursts are plotted as a function of stimulus frequency; responses were recorded from a cat. The difference between SV and ST pressures is responsible for displacement of the basilar membrane. **E,** BM displacements produced in a cadaveric human cochlea in response to 200 Hz at four separate points in time. The envelope of the traveling wave also is indicated. **F,** Envelopes of traveling waves measured along the BM in a cadaveric human cochlea in response to four stimulus frequencies, showing the relationship between the location of peak displacement and frequency (higher frequencies produce peaks at locations progressively closer to the base). *(**A,** From Dallos P, Fakler B.* Nat Rev Md Cell Biol. *2002;3:104; **B,** from Holme RH, Steel KP. Genes involved in deafness.* Curr Opin Genet Dev. *1999;9:309; **C,** adapted from Ashmore JF, Kolston PJ. Hair cell based amplification in the cochlea.* Curr Opin Neurobiol. *1994;4:503; **D,** from Nedzelnitsky V. Sound pressures in the basal turn of the cat cochlea.* J Acoust Soc Am. *1980;68:1676; **E** and **F,** from von Bekesy G.* Experiments in Hearing. *New York: McGraw-Hill; 1960.)*

openings shunt pressure waves extending to higher frequencies than those associated with small helicotrema. The shunting effect of helicotrema reduces the pressure differential across the cochlear partition, and it is this aspect of cochlear design that is thought to decrease damage to the cochlea produced by intense low-frequency pressure fluctuations.[403]

Active Cochlear Mechanics

Von Békésy recognized more than half a century ago that the envelope of the traveling wave measured in cochleae from human cadavers is broadly tuned—so broadly tuned as to be inconsistent with a living person's ability to discriminate closely spaced frequencies. Numerous groups of investigators have since confirmed the findings of von Békésy and have shown with clarity that sharp tuning and high sensitivity are lost in physiologically compromised cochleae or cochleae from cadavers.[432,494] Only after mechanical measurements were made in vivo with nonhuman species did it become clear that the peak of the traveling wave in living animals is, in fact, very sharply tuned at low levels of stimulation and exhibits nonlinear growth as sound levels increase.[274,314,433,454,494] The seminal study of Rhode,[433] which showed the amplitude of basilar membrane vibration relative to stapes displacement to be as much as two to three orders of magnitude greater under low-stimulus-level conditions than at higher levels in normal animals, led most directly to the contemporary understanding of cochlear mechanics as a nonlinear phenomenon (i.e., high sensitivity to changes in stimulus pressure at low levels, marked compression in the midlevel range, and linear growth at high levels) (Fig. 146-4).

Active mechanics associated with basilar membrane amplification is a metabolically labile, energy-consuming process that is, consequently, physiologically vulnerable. It is of particular importance to

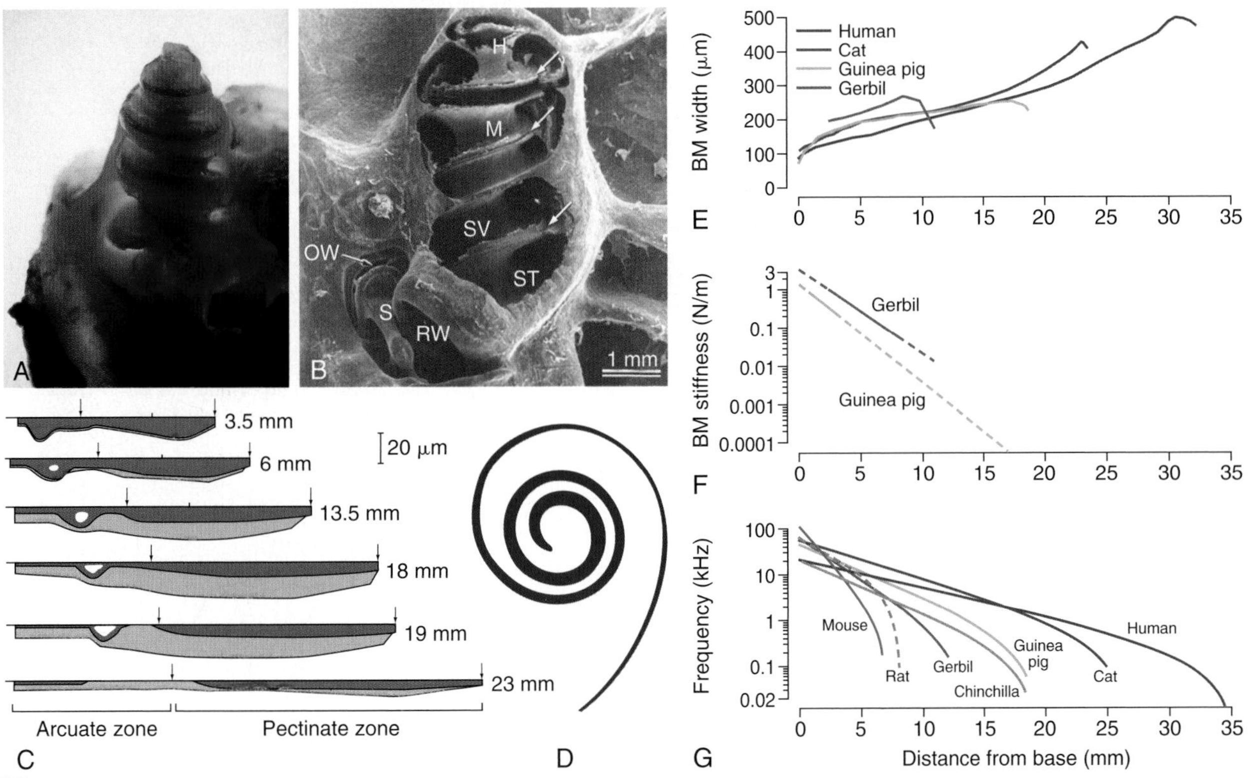

Figure 146-3. **A,** Photograph of the cochlea of a guinea pig after the outer bony shell has been thinned. **B,** Scanning electron micrograph (SEM) of a chinchilla cochlea after the bone on one side has been removed. The bony modiolus (M) is shown in the center, and the fluid-filled scala tympani (ST) and scala vestibuli (SV) are indicated in the basal turn. The helicotrema (H) is shown at the apex, and the *arrows* indicate the osseous spiral lamina to which the cochlear partition is attached at its medial extent. The round window (RW) and the stapes (S) are indicated, and the footplate of the stapes has been pulled away slightly, exposing the oval window (OW). **C,** Schematic illustration of the variation in thickness of the basilar membrane *(dark blue area)* and the associated mesothelial layer *(light blue area)* and the width of the basilar membrane *(horizontal axis)* at six locations along the cochlear spiral of the cat; specified locations are relative to the base. The demarcation between the arcuate and pectinate zones is indicated by the *left arrow* at each location; the arcuate zone (pars tecta) extends from the lip of the osseous spiral lamina to the foot of the outer pillar cell (OPC) and the pectinate zone from the OPC to the basilar crest of the spiral ligament *(right arrows)*. **D,** Scaled representation of the ribbon-like nature of the human basilar membrane indicating its width relative to its length. **E,** Quantitative relationship between the width of the basilar membrane (BM) and the distance from the base for the human,[604] cat,[64] guinea pig,[154] and gerbil.[445] **F,** Estimates of the stiffness of the basilar membrane in the guinea pig[205] and gerbil[139] as a function of location. **G,** Maps of the characteristic frequency (CF) of a cochlear location (i.e., peak of the envelope of the traveling wave) as a function of position along the basilar membrane for several species. Note that the lengths of the basilar membrane for each species can be estimated by the distance that each curve occupies along the x-axis. Frequency-position maps were based on a formulation developed by Greenwood[196] using empirical fits to data for the species shown here, except for rat, which was developed by Muller.[374] *(**A,** From Wasterstrom SA. Accumulation of drugs on inner ear melanin. Therapeutic and ototoxic mechanisms.* Scand Audiol Suppl. *1984;23:1;* ***B,*** *from Harrison RV, Hunter-Duvar IM. An anatomical tour of the cochlea. In: Jahn AF, Santos-Sacchi J, eds.* Physiology of the Ear. *New York: Raven Press; 1988:160;* ***C,*** *from Cabezudo LM. The ultrastructure of the basilar membrane in the cat.* Acta Otolaryngol. *1978;86:160;* ***D,*** *from Wever EG.* Theory of Hearing. *New York: Dover Publications; 1949.)*

recognize that the active mechanical event underlying amplification is highly localized. That is, the principle of active mechanics applies to a circumscribed portion of the cochlear partition that is limited to the immediate vicinity of the characteristic place for a given stimulus frequency (see Fig. 146-4A and B). At frequencies removed from the characteristic place, the properties of cochlear partition vibration in a living animal follow linear rules of growth, as in cadaverous tissue (Fig. 146-5).[179] Another important point is that the traveling wave peaks at increasingly apical regions of the cochlear partition with increasing stimulus level, shifting the cochlear place-frequency map toward lower frequencies at any given place.

Role of Outer Hair Cells in Active Mechanics

Many early studies indicated that OHCs play a fundamental role in active cochlear mechanics, as indicated by estimates of diminished cochlear sensitivity and frequency selectivity and loss of nonlinear operating properties when OHCs are missing from the end organ (see Fig. 146-4). The identification of specializations that distinguish inner hair cells (IHCs) from OHCs of the mammalian cochlea offered early clues that the contribution of OHCs to the transduction process is unique (Fig. 146-6). For example, only approximately 5% of all auditory nerve fibers innervate OHCs,[371,525,524] yet there are at least three times as many OHCs as IHCs (Fig. 146-7). These findings suggested that the transmission of sensory information to the central nervous system (CNS) probably is not the primary function of OHCs. In studies of acute preparations, investigators noted that the cochlea, and OHCs in particular, are highly vulnerable to hypoxia or other forms of insult.[76,148,293,432,433,448,449,494] In animal models of chronic damage, OHCs were found to be more susceptible to noise-induced or aminoglycoside-induced damage than IHCs, and when OHCs were lost, with IHCs appearing unaffected, cochlear sensitivity was significantly reduced, as was frequency selectivity, and input-output curves acquired a more linear character in the region of OHC damage.[77,97,101,149,208,278,279,329,450,465] In addition, other cochlear nonlinearities, such as two-tone suppression (i.e., the reduction in the response to one tone elicited by the presence of another) and distortion tones (i.e., the appearance of additional tones not present in the stimulus produced by the interaction of two or more primary tones, such as $2f_1$-f_2 or f_2-f_1, where f_1 and f_2 represent the

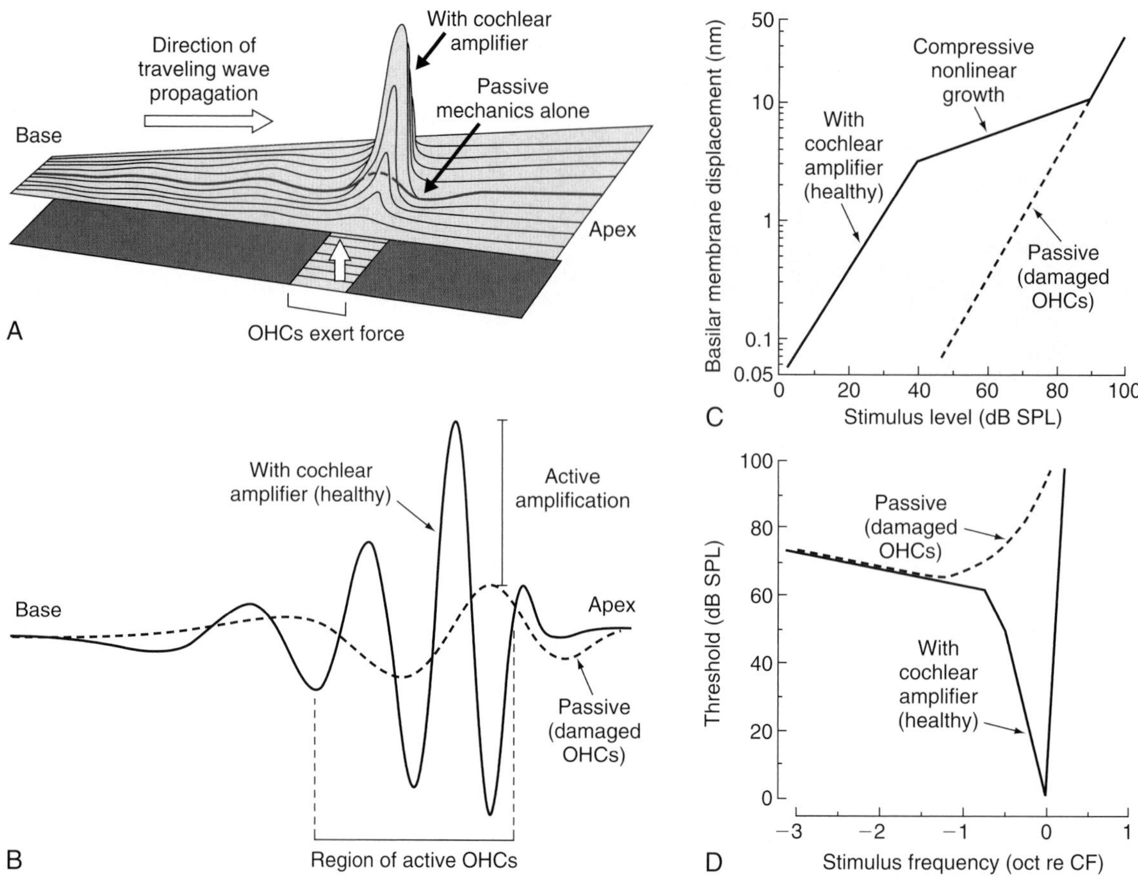

Figure 146-4. A, Schematic representation of traveling waves propagating along the basilar membrane (BM) in response to a pure tone. When the cochlear amplifier is functioning, outer hair cells (OHCs) within a restricted region of the traveling wave peak exert a force that enhances BM motion relative to that observed during passive mechanics alone for low-level stimuli. **B,** Similar to **A,** except note that the peak of the traveling wave produced with cochlear amplification is much narrower than the peak produced during passive mechanics alone, which is important for frequency discrimination. Also note that during active amplification, the peak of the traveling wave occurs slightly more basal than that produced during passive mechanics. **C,** Schematic relationship between stimulus level and BM displacement. When OHCs are normal, stimulus level increments of less than 40 dB sound pressure level (SPL) produce a linear increase in BM displacement. Between approximately 40 and 80 dB SPL, OHC responses saturate, producing a compressed response and nonlinear growth. Above 80 dB SPL, growth becomes linear again. When OHCs are damaged, displacements occur only to higher level stimuli and exhibit linear growth. **D,** The relationship between stimulus frequency (measured in octaves relative to the characteristic frequency [oct re CF] at that location) and the level required to elicit a criterion or "threshold" response at a given point along the BM (e.g., tuning curves). When the cochlear amplifier is operational, thresholds may be 40 to 60 dB lower and frequency selectivity greatly enhanced compared with a passive cochlea. *(**A,** From Ashmore JF, Kolston PJ. Hair cell based amplification in the cochlea.* Curr Opin Neurobiol. *1994;4:503. **B,** from Gummer AW, Preyer S. Cochlear amplification and its pathology: emphasis on the role of the tectorial membrane.* Ear Nose Throat J. *1997;76:151.)*

primary tones, with f_1 less than f_2), are either lost or diminished when OHCs are traumatized.[102,480] The discovery of sound-evoked otoacoustic emissions, sounds that are generated by the end organ during transduction and are measured in the external ear canal,[270] along with spontaneous otoacoustic emissions,[608] and their dependence on OHCs provided additional evidence that an active, OHC-driven mechanism operates within the cochlea, which is capable of producing energy and propagating it in the reverse direction. The influence of OHCs on cochlear mechanics was further suggested on the basis of observations made after stimulating the crossed olivocochlear bundle (OCB), a brainstem pathway populated by large, myelinated fibers that arise among neurons located in the medial region of the superior olivary complex that cross the brainstem at the floor of the fourth ventricle and terminate in calyx-like presynaptic terminals on OHCs.[200,287,427,428,518,597,598] Specifically, OCB activation altered cochlear output,[118,155,156,176,605] as well as otoacoustic emissions[373,505] and basilar membrane displacement,[376] supporting the notion that OHCs directly influence cochlear mechanics. Further support for the view that OHCs play an essential role in active mechanics comes from the work of Mammano and Ashmore,[349] who demonstrated that outer hair cell motility induced by electrical stimulation of the excised cochlea displaced both the reticular lamina and the basilar membrane.

Prestin (SLC26A5) Is Essential for Outer Hair Cell Motility and Active Transduction

The finding that OHCs contract or elongate at very high rates (up to at least 70 kHz) along the length of their longitudinal axes when depolarized or hyperpolarized, respectively,[30,62,63,98,99,168,177,261,478,630] led to the suggestion that OHCs may amplify the displacement of the basilar membrane if forces generated by their motility are produced on a cycle-by-cycle basis and precisely timed relative to passive mechanical events (see Fig. 146-6E). Somatic length changes of up to 5% of the total length of OHCs are determined directly by the magnitude of the transmembrane voltage and not by ionic currents. In addition, the voltage-motility relationship observed among OHCs is highly nonlinear (Fig. 146-8B). Unlike in IHCs, the lateral wall of OHCs is densely packed with particles that are integral components of the plasma membrane,[165,202,264,470] and these particles are thought to be oligomers of the protein recently identified as the molecular motor underlying fast somatic motility (see Fig. 146-6C and E).

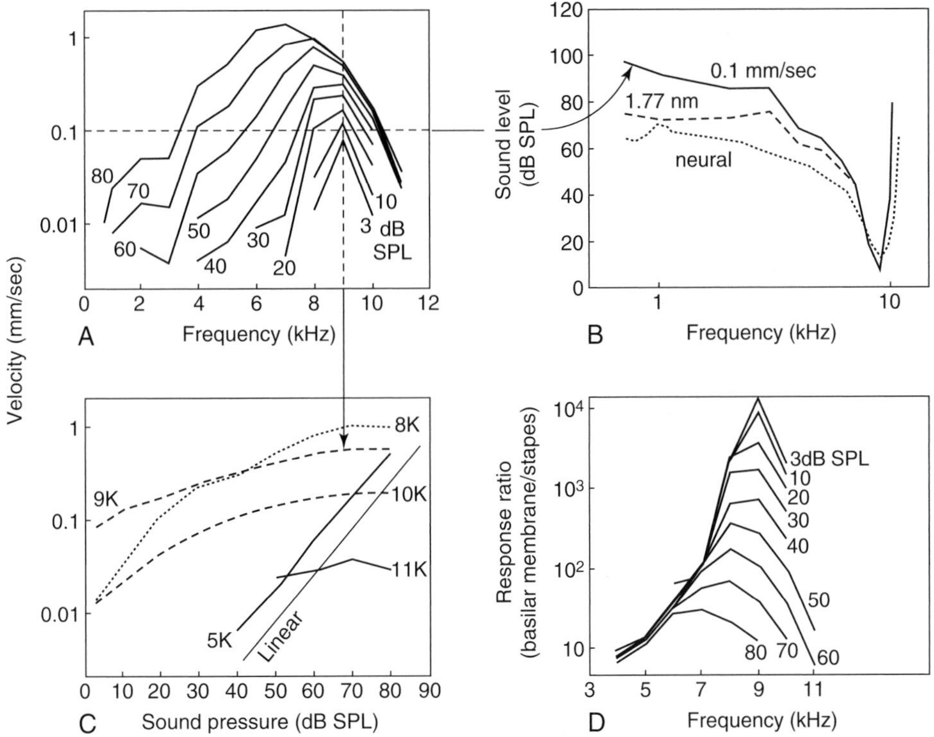

Figure 146-5. Measurements of basilar membrane (BM) motion in a healthy chinchilla cochlea at one location near the base in response to tone bursts. **A,** Measurement of BM velocity in response to tone bursts of different frequencies *(abscissa)* at various levels (parameter). The characteristic frequency (CF) at this location is 9 kHz. SPL, sound pressure level. **B,** Tuning curves (i.e., stimulus levels required to generate a criterion response as a function of stimulus frequency) are shown for a criterion BM velocity of 0.1 mm/sec and for a criterion displacement amplitude of 1.77 nm. Data were taken from **A.** A tuning curve from an auditory nerve fiber that innervates this BM location is also shown. **C,** BM velocities as a function of stimulus level for various frequencies. A line showing a linear relationship between velocity and level also is shown. **D,** The ratio between BM velocity and stapes velocity (i.e., gain) as a function of stimulus frequency. Note the high gain (i.e., amplification) at low stimulus levels near the CF location that is reduced as a stimulus level increases. *(**A** and **B,** From Ruggero MA, Rich MC. Application of a commercially-manufactured Doppler-shift laser velocimeter to the measurement of basilar-membrane vibration.* Hear Res. *1991;51:215; **C,** from Ruggero MA. Responses to sound of the basilar membrane of the mammalian cochlea.* Curr Opin Neurobiol. *1992;2:449; **D,** from Ruggero MA, Robles L, Rich NC, Recio A. Basilar membrane responses to two-tone and broadband stimuli.* Philos Trans R Soc Lond B Biol Sci. *1992;336. The figure was prepared by Geisler CD.* From Sound to Synapse: Physiology of the Mammalian Ear. *New York: Oxford University Press; 1998.)*

The discovery that OHC motility is accompanied by gating currents that reflect a nonlinear capacitance led to the suggestion that it was the movement of charged particles within the domain of the plasma membrane that operates as the motive force of contractility.[31,476] The voltage-sensitive motor protein underlying the process was identified in 2000 and given the name prestin (SLC26A5). Prestin (Fig. 146-8A) is a modified anion-transporter protein belonging to the solute carrier 26 (SLC) family of proteins.[633] Antibodies to prestin have been localized in OHC membranes, and developmental changes in the expression of prestin immunoreactivity follow a temporal profile that overlaps the development of electromotility, providing further support for the view that prestin is the motor protein.[42] Although the precise location of the voltage sensor remains unknown, and although it may be an integral component of the prestin molecule itself, findings from recent studies suggest that intracellular Cl^- ions act as extrinsic charged voltage sensors (see Fig. 146-8B, inset). In this model, Cl^- ions occupy a position in the intracellular domain of the membrane-bound prestin protein and move along an inward electrical gradient away from the extracellular domain during depolarization. This charge movement produces, in turn, a conformational change in the protein that reduces its surface area and shortens the cell; the opposite action occurs during hyperpolarization, when Cl^- ions move toward the extracellular space within the domain of the protein (although the anion is never translocated to the extracellular space), causing an increase in surface area and lengthening of the cell.[100,391] Salicylates, which are known to cause temporary hearing loss when administered at high doses,[535] are permeable to the plasma membrane and act as competitive antagonists of Cl^-, thereby reducing electromotility and, presumably, diminishing sensitivity.[391] The role of prestin in transduction was studied directly in a mouse strain in which prestin was deleted. The knockout mouse exhibited a loss of OHC electromotility in homozygous mutant animals (see Fig. 146-8D), a 40- to 60-dB loss in sensitivity, and loss of OHCs in the base of the cochlea (see Fig. 146-8C).[328] In addition, the frequency selectivity of individual auditory nerve fibers is diminished in knockout mice.[68] Although the length and stiffness of OHCs are reduced in the knockout mouse, these findings collectively suggest that active transduction is a direct product of OHC somatic motility. Confirmation of prestin's role in cochlear amplification was recently established in a study of a "knock-in" mouse model, in which the protein's function was diminished but OHCs exhibited normal length and stiffness.[103] Natural mutations of the prestin gene have been identified in humans, and the resulting condition is transmitted as a recessive, nonsyndromic form of congenital deafness. In this case, however, hearing loss is in the severe to profound category (i.e., on the order of 90 dB or greater) and exists as a bilateral form of deafness among persons who are homozygous for the trait. The degree of hearing loss is more variable among heterozygotes, ranging from normal in one case to mild (40 dB) and even moderate to profound (60 dB) in others, suggesting the semidominance of the abnormal allele through haploinsufficiency.[337]

Conversion of Basilar Membrane Displacement to Radial Shearing Forces

All existing models of transduction center on the idea that displacement of the basilar membrane results in a radial shearing motion between

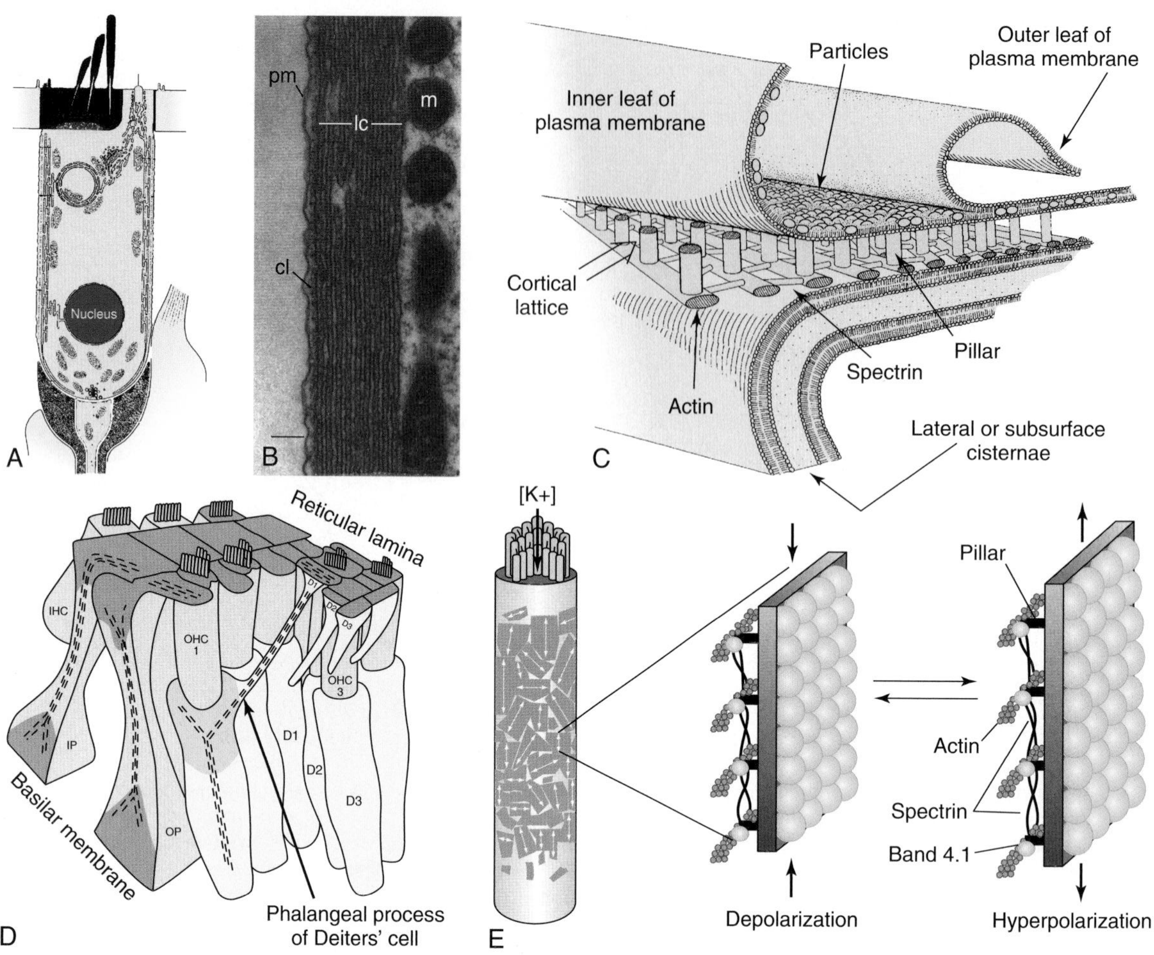

Figure 146-6. **A,** Drawing of an outer hair cell (OHC) showing the cylindrical soma; the nucleus located near the basal end of the cell; the cuticular plate at the apex of the cell where the rootlets of the stereocilia insert; the subsurface cisternae, which are stacks of smooth endoplasmic reticulum that line the lateral sides of the cell; and Hensen's body, which is a continuation of the endoplasmic reticulum, located beneath the cuticular plate. This structure probably functions as a Golgi apparatus. **B,** Transmission electron microscopy of the lateral membrane of a guinea pig OHC, showing the plasma membrane (pm), the cortical lattice (cl) just beneath the membrane, the lateral cisterns (lc), and mitochondria (m) just inside the cisterns. Scale bar is 200 nm. **C,** Diagram of the OHC lateral membrane, where the inner and outer leaflets of the plasma membrane have been separated revealing a high density of membrane particles not present in IHCs, which presumably are oligomers of the motor protein prestin. The cortical lattice is composed of many subdomains of parallel actin filaments oriented circumferentially around the cell that are cross-linked by spectrin. The actin filaments are bound to the plasma membrane by pillar molecules (composition unknown), and the subsurface cisternae lie just inside the cortical lattice. **D,** Illustration of the expanded apical surfaces of the inner and outer pillar cells (IP and OP, respectively) in relation to the apical surfaces of OHCs and the phalangeal processes of Deiters cells (D1, D2, D3) forming the reticular lamina. **E,** Diagram of the orientation of several subdomains of membrane particles *(left)* and an array of particles that undergo conformational changes that alter particle packing density associated with a change in transmembrane voltage. During depolarization, tighter packing results in shortening of the subdomain, as well as the hair cell itself, and during hyperpolarization, elongation occurs. *(**A,** from Lim DJ. Functional structure of the organ of Corti: a review.* Hear Res. *1986;22:117; **B,** from Holley MC. Outer hair cell motility. In: Dallos P, Popper AN, Fay RR, eds.* The Cochlea. *New York: Springer-Verlag; 1996:386; **C,** adapted from Oghalai, et al.* J Neurosci. *1998;18:48; **D,** from Slepecky NB. Structure of the mammalian cochlea. In: Dallos P, Popper AN, Fay RR, eds.* The Cochlea. *New York: Springer-Verlag; 1996:44; **E,** from Frolenkov GI, Atzori M, Kalinec F, Mammano F, Kachar B. The membrane-based mechanism of cell motility in cochlear outer hair cells.* Mol Biol Cell. *1998;9:1961.)*

the reticular lamina and the tectorial membrane, a motion that serves as the mechanical trigger of transduction currents. The reticular lamina consists of the interdigitating heads of the inner and outer pillar cells, the apical surfaces of the phalangeal processes of Deiters cells, and the apical surfaces of the hair cells through which the stereocilia project (see Fig. 146-6D). The apical surfaces of the supporting cells are flattened and are composed of microtubules and actin microfilaments, lending support to the idea that the reticular lamina is a relatively rigid structure that moves in concert with basilar membrane motion. The tectorial membrane is firmly attached to the spiral limbus and overlies the reticular lamina, with its tip or marginal zone connected to Hensen cells. The tallest row of stereocilia protrude from the apical surface of each outer hair cell and embed within the inferior surface of the tectorial membrane along the entire length of the cochlear spiral.[288,333] Bundles of radially oriented filaments, consisting of type II, V, IX, and XI collagens, are embedded within the gelatinous matrix of the mammalian tectorial membrane (see Fig. 146-10A and B).[209,361,444,514,515,545,546] The presence of collagen enhances the rigidity of the structure, making it less compressible and less elastic, particularly in the radial dimension.[3,199,446] These features support a system in which the shearing motion between the reticular lamina and the tectorial membrane causes stereocilia to bend in the direction of the modiolus or the spiral limbus, depending on whether the basilar membrane is displaced toward the scala tympani or scala vestibuli, respectively.

In contrast with OHCs, the stereocilia of IHCs do not appear to firmly contact the tectorial membrane (see Fig. 146-1D). Therefore,

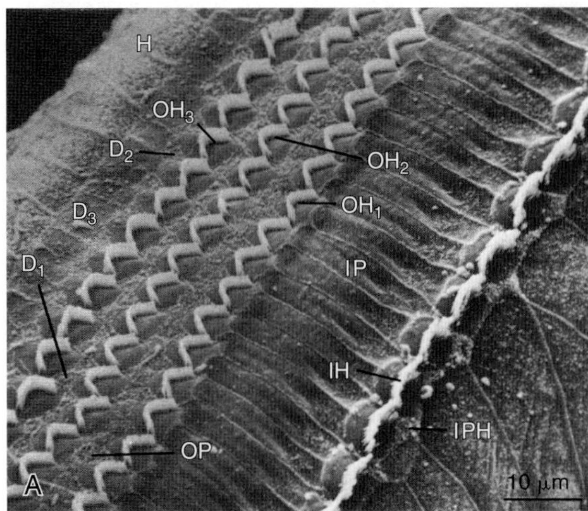

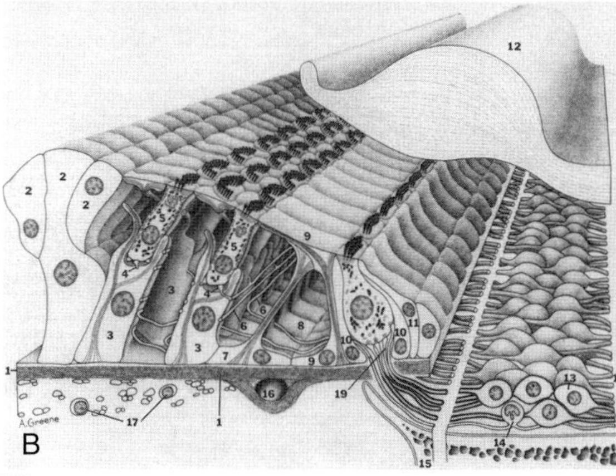

Figure 146-7. A, Scanning electron micrograph of the surface of the organ of Corti of a chinchilla showing the three rows of outer hair cells (OH_1, OH_2, OH_3), one row of inner hair cells (IH), inner and outer pillar cells (IP and OP, respectively), inner phalangeal cell (IPH), Deiters cells (D_1, D_2, D_3), and Hensen cells (H). **B,** Schematic illustration of the structure of the organ of Corti: 1, basilar membrane; 2, Hensen cells; 3, outer phalangeal cells; 4, nerve endings; 5, outer hair cells; 6, outer spiral fibers; 7, outer pillar cells; 8, tunnel of Corti; 9, inner pillar cells; 10, inner phalangeal cells; 11, border cells; 12, tectorial membrane; 13, type I spiral ganglion cell (SGC); 14, type II SGC; 15, bony spiral lamina; 16, spiral blood vessel; 17, spindle cells; 18, auditory nerve fibers; 19, radial fiber. *(**A,** From Lim DJ. Functional structure of the organ of Corti: a review.* Hear Res. *1986;22:117; **B,** from Kiang NY: Peripheral neural processing of auditory information. In: Darian-Smith I, ed.* Handbook of Physiology. *New York: Oxford; 1984:639.)*

during basilar membrane vibration, the relevant mechanical stimulus to IHC stereocilia is thought to be the flow of endolymph within the subtectorial space, the narrow channel between the reticular lamina and tectorial membrane into which the stereocilia protrude.[387] Fluid coupling is then thought to lead directly to the displacement of IHC stereocilia in proportion to basilar membrane velocity at low frequencies (less than 500 Hz) and to basilar membrane displacement at higher frequencies; sustained displacements of the basilar membrane, or very-low-frequency displacements, do not effectively bend IHC stereocilia.[403]

Radial Displacement Patterns of the Basilar Membrane

The dynamics of basilar membrane displacement at the characteristic frequency place are more complex when examined radially. Inner and outer pillar cells that form the fluid-filled tunnel of Corti are packed with bundles of microtubules and actin microfilaments arranged in parallel that are cross-linked and are thought to produce structural rigidity within the cochlear partition.[25,140,244] The foot of the inner pillar cell lies near the bony spiral lamina, whereas the foot of the outer pillar cell lies over the basilar membrane and is not supported by bone (Fig. 146-9). Therefore, when the basilar membrane is displaced in a passive cochlea, movement occurs maximally near the foot of the outer pillar cell, with the basilar membrane pivoting at the foot of the inner pillar cell.[104] When OHCs contract, the reticular lamina pivots at the apex of the tunnel of Corti, and the basilar membrane and reticular lamina are pulled together, enhancing overall basilar membrane displacement.[168,349,350,383] Furthermore, unlike in passive mechanical events, in which the full width of the basilar membrane moves uniformly (synchronously), during active mechanics, the magnitude and phase of displacement vary in the radial dimension.[83,383,388,395,396,431,495,563,609,622] Although differences among studies from different laboratories are significant regarding the precise pattern of basilar membrane movement in the radial direction after displacement, many workers suggest that the position of greatest motion is in the domain of the OHC, and that motion in the OHC region is out of phase relative to the foot of the outer pillar cell. This finding has significant implications in the ongoing effort to understand the relationship between inner and outer hair cell responses during the transduction process.

Tectorial Membrane Pathophysiology

The tectorial membrane is composed of two primary matrix elements: a group of radially oriented collagen fibrils and a striated sheet matrix that is made up of tightly packed, small-diameter filaments that are interlinked by cross-bridges to give it a striated appearance.[209,288,300,333,559] In addition to the variety of collagens making up the core structure, a collection of glycoproteins—α-tectorin, β-tectorin, and otogelin—also are constituent elements of the tectorial membrane.[78,193,285,319,444] Otogelin, a glycoprotein that is found in essentially all of the acellular membranes of the inner ear, is associated with the large collagen fibrils, whereas α-tectorin and β-tectorin are components of the striated sheet matrix.

The mass and stiffness of the tectorial membrane are important variables that together determine the resonant properties of the structure that, in turn, affects its displacement pattern during acoustic stimulation. Much like dimensional changes that have been measured along the length of the basilar membrane, the cross-sectional area of the tectorial membrane has been shown to increase from the base to the apex as indicated by morphometric measurements of fully hydrated tissue specimens (Fig. 146-10C).[445] Moreover, base-to-apex stiffness gradients in both the transverse and radial axes of the tectorial membrane have been observed,[199,446] and they are similar to those reported for basilar membrane stiffness gradients (see Fig. 146-10C).[139,205] Taken together, basoapical gradients in the physical properties of the tectorial membrane suggest the possibility that the structure may support longitudinally propagating traveling waves,[181] giving rise to a second cochlear frequency-place map. Some investigators have suggested that the resonant frequency of the tectorial membrane lies approximately one-half octave below that of the basilar membrane's characteristic or resonant frequency at any given position along the cochlear spiral.[17,18,203,641] However, until the opportunity to study mutant mice in which the tectorial membrane is completely detached from the spiral limbus and the surface of the organ of Corti[317] presented itself, direct evidence regarding the precise role of the tectorial membrane as an element of transduction was largely unavailable.

Targeted disruption of the gene that encodes α-tectorin (*Tecta*) in mice (*Tecta*$^{\Delta ENT/\Delta ENT}$) leads to loss of not only α-tectorin but also β-tectorin and otogelin.[317] In addition, the striated sheet matrix is absent, and collagen fibrils are disorganized in the tectorial membranes of mice that are homozygous for the deletion, not to mention that the structure is detached from the spiral limbus and floats freely in scala media. Like the IHC stereocilia of normal animals, the stereocilia of OHCs in α-tectorin–mutant mice are fluid-coupled to end organ motion, and mice exhibit elevated thresholds that reflect that condition (i.e., generally elevated neural thresholds decrease at a rate of approximately 6 dB/octave with increasing frequency). Mechanical input-output curves constructed from responses to tone bursts presented at characteristic frequency also are more linear (although approximately 35 dB less sensitive), and frequency selectivity is normal, or at least

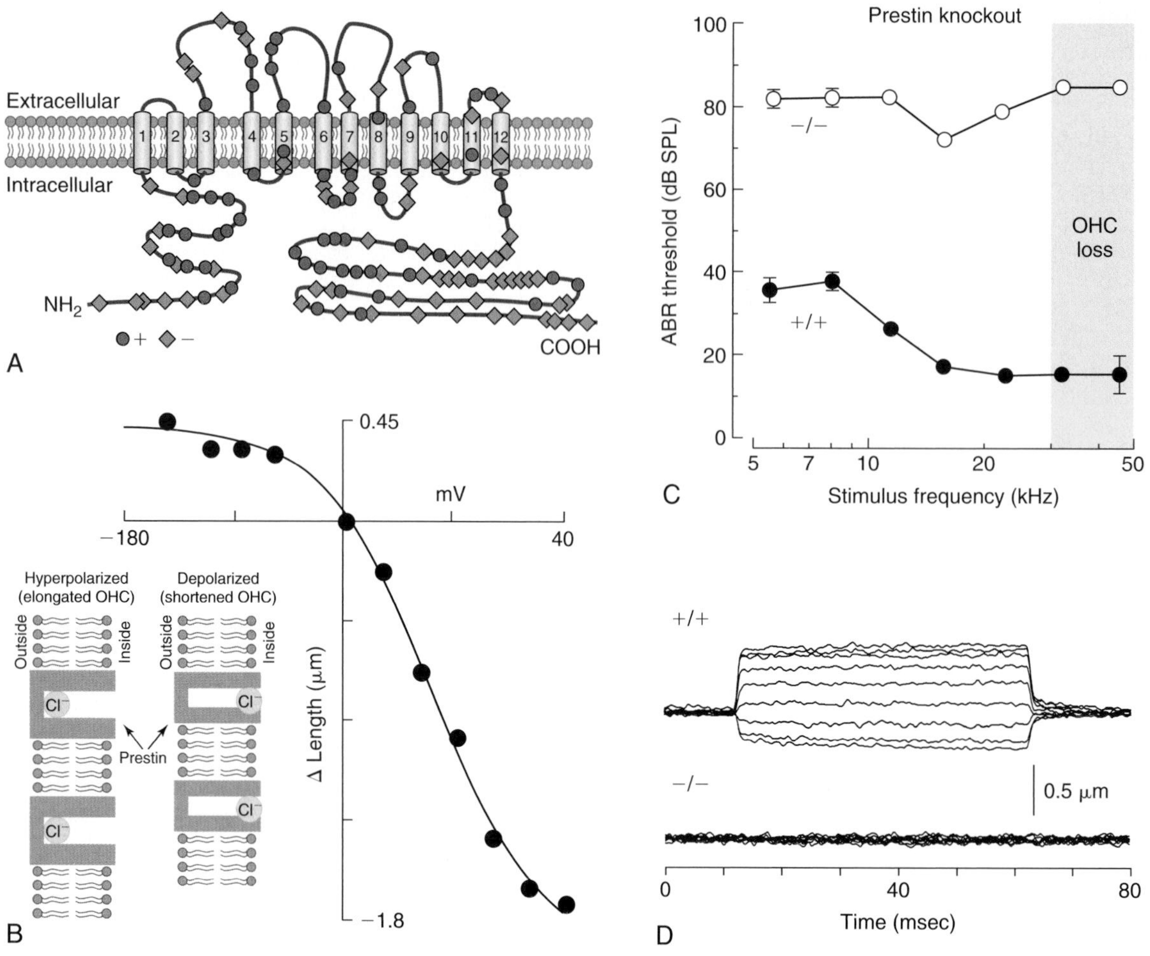

Figure 146-8. **A,** Schematic representation of the membrane topology of prestin (SLC26A5). Prestin consists of 744 amino acids and is predicted to have 12 transmembrane domains and intracellular amino-terminal (NH_2) and carboxyl-terminal (COOH) ends. *Circles* and *diamonds* represent positively and negatively charged amino acids, respectively. **B,** Change in the length of an isolated outer hair cell (OHC) as a function of voltage stepped from a holding potential of −68.4 mV. The *inset* is an illustration of single prestin molecules located in the plasma membrane that can toggle between two conformational states, depending on transmembrane voltage. The larger the depolarization, the greater likelihood that the shorter state will be adopted, and vice versa. The nonlinear capacitance associated with length changes may be due to the translocation of anions, such as Cl^- *(yellow circles)*, that move closer to the extracellular side during hyperpolarization and toward the intracellular side during depolarization. **C,** Targeted disruption of prestin results in severely elevated auditory brainstem response (ABR) thresholds in homozygous mice, and somatic motility is absent in isolated OHCs (**D**). *(**A,** From Dallos P, Fakler B. Prestin, a new type of motor protein.* Nat Rev Mol Cell Biol. *2002;3:104; Reprinted by permission from Macmillan Publishers Ltd. **B,** from Santos-Sacchi J. On the frequency limit and phase of outer hair cell motility: effects of the membrane filter.* J Neurosci. *1992;12:1906;* inset, *prepared by M. Walsh; **C,** and **D,** adapted from Liberman MC, Gao J, He DZ, et al. Prestin is required for electromotility of the outer hair cell and for the cochlear amplifier.* Nature. *2002;419:300.)*

nearly so. Of interest, a second region of sensitivity in basilar membrane tuning curves that is approximately 0.5 octave below the best frequency in normal mice is not observed in α-tectorin mutant mice, suggesting that the tectorial membrane may be responsible for that second resonance.

These findings suggest that the tectorial membrane is required for OHCs to amplify displacement of the basilar membrane at low stimulus levels. In humans, mutations in the *TECTA* gene are responsible for both recessive and dominant forms of deafness—DFNB21, DFNA8, and DFNA12.[378,574] In patients with DFNA8 or DFNA12, hearing loss is congenital and nonprogressive[574] and can be more severe in the midfrequency than other frequency ranges, whereas patients with DFNB21 experience severe-to-profound deafness, and the onset can be either prelingual or postlingual.[378]

Further insight into the tectorial membrane's role in transduction can be found by studying a strain of mice in which the *Tecta* gene is disrupted at the same location (Y1870C)[318] as a mutation found in patients with autosomal dominant hearing loss associated with a missense mutation in the *TECTA* gene.[574] The tectorial membrane is detached and individuals exhibit a phenotype similar to that observed in *Tecta*$^{\Delta ENT/\Delta ENT}$ mice in the case of homozygotes, whereas the tectorial membrane remains attached in heterozygous mice, although the striated sheet matrix is disrupted, Hensen's stripe is lost, and the subtectorial space in the region of IHCs is enlarged. Although basilar membrane thresholds are minimally elevated (approximately 10 dB) in heterozygotes, neural thresholds are elevated by approximately 55 dB, suggesting that the precise spatial relationship between the tectorial membrane and reticular lamina in the region of the IHCs is a critical factor associated with fluid coupling between IHCs and OHCs.

As with mice expressing an abnormal *Tecta* gene, loss of β-tectorin in the tectorial membrane is associated with the loss of the striated sheet matrix and Hensen's stripe, although the tectorial membrane itself remains attached to the spiral limbus.[462] Both α-tectorin and otogelin have been detected in the tectorial membrane of mutant animals, and imprints of the tallest row of outer hair cell stereocilia have been observed on the underside of the membrane. Although basilar membrane sensitivity is just slightly diminished at the base of the cochlea in affected animals (i.e., tuning curve tips are elevated approximately 10 dB), tuning curve sharpness is enhanced, and the second resonance normally observed below the best frequency is lost. In contrast with

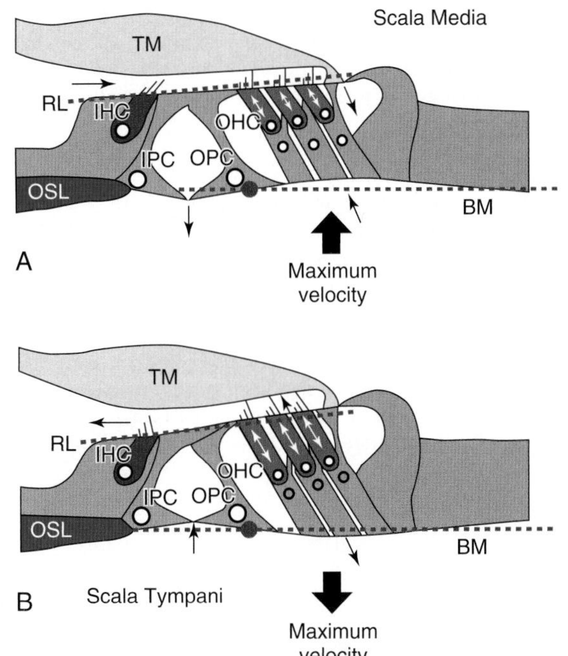

Figure 146-9. Model of basilar membrane (BM) vibration across the radial extent of the membrane. **A,** As the BM moves toward scala vestibuli, at the point of maximum BM velocity, the shearing motion between the BM and tectorial membrane (TM) causes the stereocilia to bend in the excitatory direction, producing depolarization and contraction or shortening of the outer hair cells (OHCs), pulling the reticular lamina (RL) toward the BM. IHC, inner hair cell; IPL, inner pillar cell; OPC, outer pillar cell; OSL, osseus spiral lamina. **B,** As the BM moves toward the scala tympani, and at the point of maximum BM velocity, hair bundles are deflected in the inhibitory direction, causing hyperpolarization and elongation of the OHCs. *Dotted lines* indicate the positions of the BM and RL at rest. Note that the *large red dot* along the BM located at the foot of the OPC represents a pivot point, which allows the displacement of the BM beneath the tunnel of Corti to be out of phase with the displacement that occurs under the OHCs. *(Redrawn from Nilsen KE, Russell IJ. The spatial and temporal representation of a tone on the guinea pig basilar membrane.* Proc Natl Acad Sci U S A. *2000;97:11751.)*

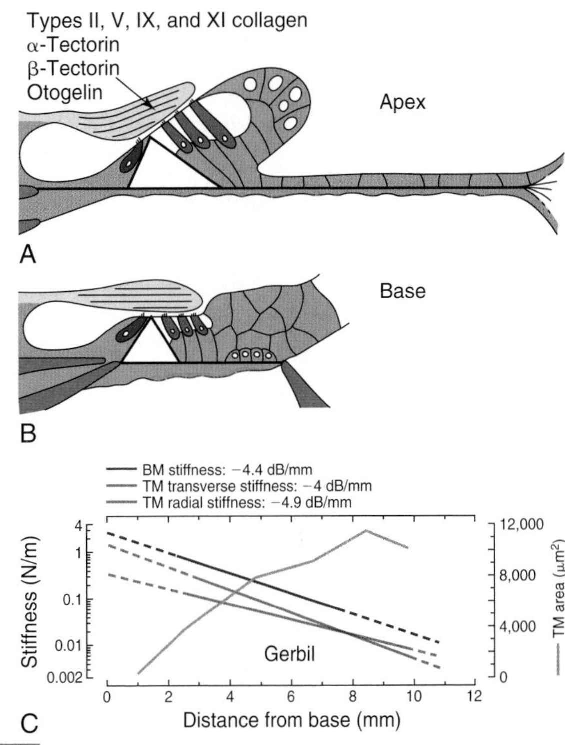

Figure 146-10. A and **B,** Schematic representation of the organ of Corti from the apical (**A**) and basal turns (**B**) of the cochlea showing the location of the tectorial membrane (TM) in relation to the surface of the organ of Corti. Major proteins of the TM include types II, V, IX, and XI collagen, α- and β-tectorin, and otogelin. Note the differences in basilar membrane (BM) width and thickness and outer hair cell lengths at the two locations. **C,** The cross-sectional area of the TM[445] and its stiffness,[446] measured in both the transverse and radial directions, are shown as a function of distance from the base of the cochlea for the gerbil. Stiffness of the gerbil's basilar membrane[139] is plotted for comparison. *(**A** and **B,** Adapted from Spoendlin H. Innervation densities of the cochlea.* Acta Otolaryngol. *1972;73:235.)*

findings observed in the base, neural sensitivities were elevated by 40 to 50 dB at frequencies below 20 kHz. The enhanced frequency selectivity observed in the base of the cochlea in β-tectorin–deficient mice may be a consequence of the loss of the striated sheet matrix in that region and the concomitant reduction of longitudinal elastic coupling that reduces, in turn, the spread of excitation, although this explanation remains speculative.

Mice with a targeted disruption of the gene that encodes otogelin (Otog) exhibit abnormalities in the tectorial membrane, primarily in the region near the spiral limbus. The tectorial membrane of these animals lacked normal fibrils, and anomalous rodlike structures within the limbal zone of the tectorial membrane were observed in the apex of the cochlea in some cases and along its entire length in others.[508] The degree of hearing loss in otogelin-null mutants is highly variable, even within individual mice. Some animals seemed to experience mild, frequency-independent deficits, whereas others seemed to be profoundly deaf and have a progressive loss of hearing. Heterozygous mice, on the other hand, had normal phenotypes. Although mutations in the human otogelin gene have not been reported, results from mouse studies suggest that abnormalities in otogelin mutants may increase susceptibility of the tectorial membrane to mechanical stress.

Absence of the α2 chain of collagen type XI (Col11a2) also produces defects in the tectorial membrane, as well as moderate to severe hearing loss.[361] In mutant mice, the tectorial membrane is slightly thicker than normal, and collagen fibrils seem to be less densely and evenly packed and more disorganized than in control animals. Col11a2 is thought to play an important role in the maintenance of the tectorial membrane by influencing the spacing of interfibrillar distances among type II fibrils, which are present in large numbers. It is interesting that phenotypic differences are observed between heterozygous mice and wild-type mice. In patients expressing *COL11A2* mutations, a continuum of defects is observed, the mildest form being an autosomal dominant, nonsyndromic form of deafness (DFNA13),[361] whereas autosomal recessive, nonsyndromic deafness (DFNB53),[71] Stickler's syndrome locus 3 (without eye involvement), and autosomal dominant or autosomal recessive otospondylomegaepiphyseal dysplasia (OSMED) syndrome[418,510,581] represent the most severe forms. Hearing loss in patients with DFNA13 occurs prelingually, is nonprogressive, and primarily affects the midfrequency range of hearing[361]; hearing loss in patients with DFNB53 is prelingual, nonprogressive, and profound.[71]

It is noteworthy that type IX collagen forms heterotypic fibrils with type II collagen in the tectorial membrane.[514] In this regard, a mutation in the *COL9A1* gene has been identified that causes Stickler's syndrome.[566] The condition is inherited as an autosomal recessive trait and is characterized by moderate to severe hearing loss, with greater insensitivity in the high-frequency domain. Although type IX collagen has been detected in fibrocytes of the spiral ligament, abnormalities, including disorganized collagen fibril patterns, are limited to the tectorial membrane of *Col9a1*-targeted null mice. However, auditory brainstem response (ABR) thresholds are elevated on P30, and sensitivity is progressively diminished with age in this mouse strain.[537]

Hair Cell Transduction

Although hydromechanical events produce organ of Corti vibration patterns that serve as the effective sensory stimulus for hearing and form the basis of the relationship between cochlear place and characteristic frequency (i.e., tonotopy), the hair cell is the central element of sensory transduction because it is the receptor cell, a mechanoreceptor that converts mechanical to electrical energy. In the human cochlea there are approximately 3500 IHCs and 12,000 OHCs, with densities corresponding to approximately 86 IHCs/mm and 343 OHCs/mm, although considerable variability exists within the population generally.[562,614] The lengths of OHCs increase continuously from the base of the cochlea to the apex, whereas the lengths of IHCs remain fairly consistent (Fig. 146-11C). Unlike some sensory systems (e.g., olfactory and somatosensory systems), in which primary afferent fibers display specialized peripheral endings designed to sense external stimuli and transmit that information directly to the CNS, the statoacoustic system, as well as the visual and gustatory systems, senses its environment by means of specialized epithelial cells, the receptor cells, that are housed in specialized peripheral organs (e.g., the cochlea, the semicircular canals, the otolith organs). Furthermore, receptor cells serving the statoacoustic system are innervated by primary afferents and do not enter the CNS directly.

Hair Cell Stereocilia

To understand the dynamics of transduction, it is necessary to look carefully at the apical surface of statoacoustic receptor cells (see Fig. 146-11A and B). In doing so, it is immediately apparent that they are highly differentiated. Numerous shaft-like protrusions, referred to individually as "hairs" and collectively as "hair bundles" by early anatomists, project from each receptor cell. These apical extensions came to be known as stereocilia, even though they clearly are not true cilia (i.e., they do not conform to the well-defined organizational plan of true cilia, in which two central tubules are surrounded by nine doublet microtubules) and are more appropriately thought of as specialized

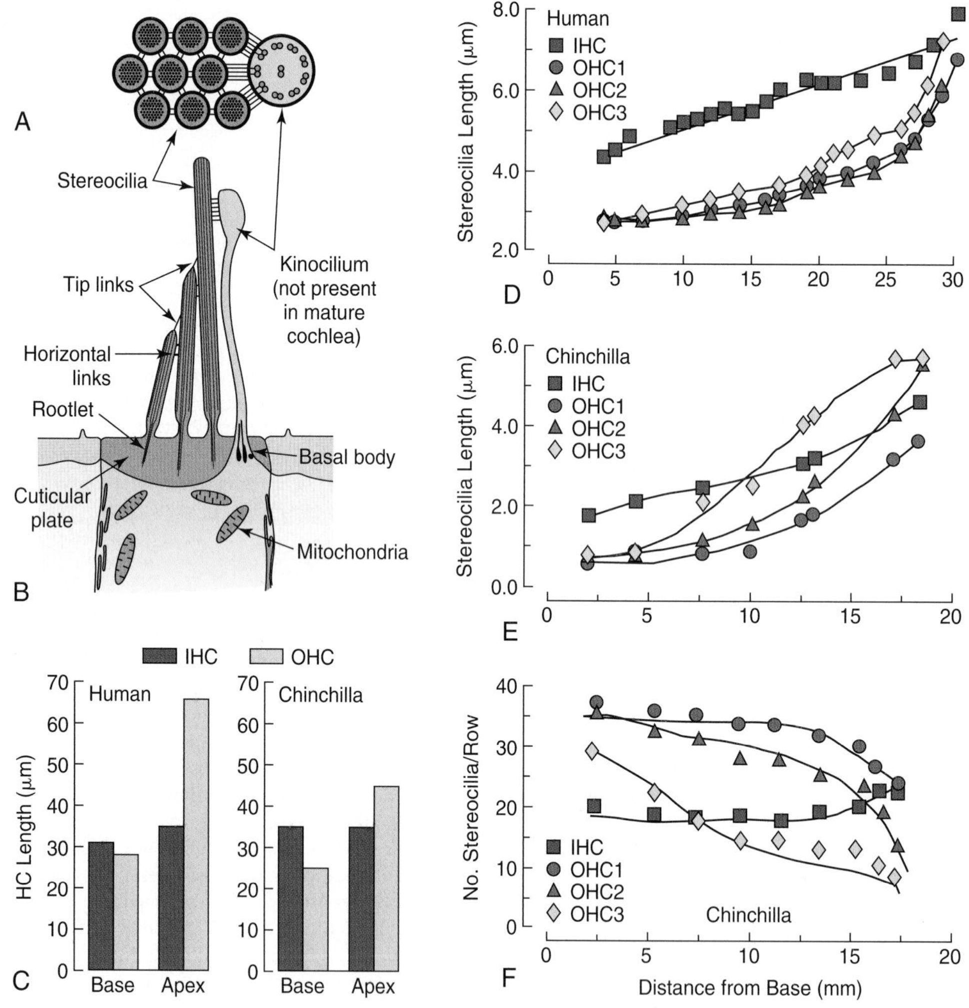

Figure 146-11. **A,** Drawing of a cross section through hair cell stereocilia and the kinocilium, which is present on auditory hair cells only during early development, showing the dense, regular packing of actin filaments that constitute the central core of each stereocilium and the single doublet surrounded by nine pairs of microtubules that make up kinocilia. **B,** Representation of the apical region of hair cells, illustrating tip links that connect the tips of shorter stereocilia with the adjacent taller stereocilia and horizontal links that cross-link all adjacent stereocilia, as well as the kinocilium (also shown in **A**). **C,** The lengths of inner hair cells (IHCs) populating the base and apex are similar, as are IHCs from humans and chinchilla, whereas outer hair cell (OHC) lengths increase from base to apex—quite dramatically in the case of human OHCs. Data for human hair cells are from Nadol[379] and those for chinchillas are from Lim.[331] **D** and **E,** The length of the stereocilia in the tallest row of a hair bundle increases progressively from base to apex in humans (**D**) and chinchillas (**E**). Data for humans were obtained by Wright,[612] and those for chinchillas by Lim.[332] **F,** The number of stereocilia per row as a function of distance along the cochlear partition. Data from Lim.[332] *(**A,** From Thurm U, et al. Studies of mechanoelectric transduction in concentric hair bundles of invertebrates. In: Lewis ER, et al, eds.* Diversity in Auditory Mechanics. *Singapore: World Scientific; 1997:119;* ***B,*** *from Pickles JO.* An Introduction to the Physiology of Hearing. *2nd ed. London: Academic Press; 1988.)*

microvilli. All vestibular hair cells and all auditory hair cells of lower vertebrates are equipped with a single kinocilium, a true cilium that protrudes from the apical surface of each receptor cell. The functional role of kinocilia is uncertain, in no small measure owing to the observation that hair cell transduction remains unchanged after its microsurgical ablation.[241] It also is interesting that kinocilia project from the surface of immature auditory hair cells of mammals but are lost during the final stages of differentiation.

Approximately 50 to 70 stereocilia protrude from each IHC and approximately 150 from each OHC, although toward the apex of the cochlea, the number of stereocilia on OHCs decreases to less than half of the number found on OHCs populating the basal turn of the cochlea in humans,[613] as in other mammals (see Fig. 146-11F). Stereociliary lengths for both IHCs and OHCs progressively increase from the base to the apex of the cochlea (see Fig. 146-11D and E). The orientation and pattern of stereocilia within a bundle are highly stereotypical, and the overall configuration for auditory hair cells is conserved among mammals. Individual hair bundles are organized into approximately three rows of stereocilia that are arranged according to a nearly linear motif in the case of IHCs and in the form of a W in the case of OHCs, with the base of the W facing the lateral wall of the cochlea (Fig. 146-12). Stereocilia within each row are approximately the same height, and the longest row is located on the side of the cell that is proximal to the spiral ligament and adjacent to the kinocilium, or the basal body in the case of mature auditory hair cells. The length of stereocilia decreases in an orderly manner in rows that are located progressively proximal to the modiolus, producing what is commonly described as a stairstep configuration. As a result of this arrangement, the hair bundle has a plane of bilateral symmetry, providing the foundation for directional sensitivity (see the following).

The stereocilium tapers near its point of insertion into the surface of the receptor cell (see Figs. 146-11B and 146-12C), and only a small fraction of the total number of actin filaments penetrate the cuticular plate, itself a dense network of randomly oriented, interconnected actin filaments packed into the apical fraction of the receptor cell body.[117,160,220,549] The rootlets of actin filaments projecting from the base of stereocilia are anchored firmly within the cuticular plate and are linked to the actin filaments within the plate, enhancing the rigidity of the structure. The protein spectrin is a major actin linkage element within the overall assembly,[133] and along with fimbrin, α-actinin (which attaches to the ends of the actin filaments), tropomyosin, profilin (a protein that regulates actin polymerization and sequesters actin monomers), myosin, calmodulin, and calbindin, these compounds are the major proteinaceous components of the cuticular plate.[513,516,517,627] The stereociliary neck produced by the constriction of the stereocilium at its insertion point allows the structure to pivot, as opposed to flexing, near the surface of the receptor cell, acting like a stiff lever when mechanically distorted.

Much of what is known about the receptor cell trigger mechanism, an event characterized by the deformation or bending of stereocilia, comes from studies in which stereocilia are physically displaced throughout their dynamic range. In that context, it is remarkable to note that the deflection of a hair bundle by 30 to 60 nm generates a receptor potential equal to approximately 90% of a receptor cell's dynamic range,[463] reflecting a very steep and very sensitive deflection-response relationship. This deflection is less than the typical diameter of a single stereocilium (i.e., approximately 200 nm). It is in this dimension that we can begin to appreciate the intrinsic value of the elaborate design of the cochlea. The ability to detect acoustic events as faint as 0 dB sound pressure level (SPL) clearly requires the sensory cell to perform optimally, and optimization is achieved by placing the cell in a highly stable environment (a fluid-filled bony labyrinth) and supporting it within a rigid but flexible infrastructure (the organ of Corti). The need for such architectural sophistication becomes apparent with the recognition that the sensitivity of hearing is ultimately limited by the Brownian motion of hair bundles, estimated to be on the order of 1 nm[52] but reduced to approximately 0.1 nm as a consequence of inherent mechanical filtering.[95] It is relatively easy to gain perspective on this matter by considering the observation that the absolute threshold of hearing requires a displacement of the basilar membrane of a mere 0.1 nm,[494] a motion that would be reduced to approximately 0.001 nm were it not for the basilar membrane amplification provided by actively motile OHCs. The amplified motion of the basilar membrane at threshold translates into displacement of hair cell stereocilia of approximately 1 nm and sensitivities on the order of 30 mV per degree of rotation, corresponding to approximately 0.4 mV per nm of displacement at the tip of a 3- to 4-μm-long bundle.[463]

Hair Bundle Deflections and Receptor Potentials

Statoacoustic receptor cell potentials, like receptor cells in sensory systems in general, are graded in response to stimulation, and the displacement-voltage curve associated with the movement of a stereociliary bundle throughout its dynamic range generally is sigmoidal.[91,240,460,463] The nature of this relationship is consistent with the observation that the magnitude of the receptor potential is proportional to the degree of stereociliary deflection in the most sensitive region of its operating range but saturates with larger deflections in either direction (see Fig. 146-12G). When the bundle is deflected toward the tallest stereocilia, the hair cell depolarizes, and deflections of the bundle in the direction opposite the tallest stereocilia hyperpolarize the cell (see Fig. 146-12G, inset). These findings support the view that hair bundle polarity is an essential element of normal hair cell function.[343] In addition, the displacement-voltage curve is highly asymmetrical relative to its resting state, such that responses saturate with smaller deflections directed away from the taller stereocilia than in the excitatory or depolarizing direction, and that deflection of the hair bundle in a direction perpendicular to this axis produces no response. Furthermore, displacement along an intermediate or oblique axis elicits a response that is proportional to its vectorial projection along the axis of symmetry.[159,503]

Hair Cell Transduction Channels

Conductance changes in hair cells associated with mechanically evoked responses indicate that when stereocilia are deflected in the excitatory direction, transduction channels in the membrane open, producing current flow leading to membrane depolarization, whereas movement of the stereocilia in the inhibitory direction causes the closure of transduction channels.[240] The latency of hair cell responses to bundle displacement is remarkably fast, on the order of 40 μsec at 22° C,[86] and kinetic analyses of the receptor current have shown that it takes approximately 100 μsec to reach steady-state currents at 4° C in response to large bundle displacements.[85] Activation time is inversely related to the magnitude of bundle displacement and is temperature-dependent, and fast offset times associated with receptor current follow positive voltage steps.[85] Because enzymatic systems or second messengers would be too slow to underlie the transducer response, these data suggest that transducer channel activation is directly coupled to displacement of the stereocilia.[85] Additional studies support a two-state model, whereby transduction channels operate in either an open or a closed state, with the probability of being in one or the other state depending on the degree of hair bundle deflection.[90,230,389] Moreover, the concept of an elastic mechanical linkage, or gating spring, associated with the transduction channel was established on the basis of the observation that the offset dynamic of transducer currents after a positive prepulse is independent of bundle position for negative stereociliary bundle displacements beyond a certain critical limit. According to this model, these linkages relax at negative displacements and therefore do not influence the state of the channel.[85]

On the basis of this model, the asymmetrical displacement-voltage curve described previously is explained by the fact that a small population of transduction channels, roughly 10% to 15%, is in the open state at rest. When stereocilia are bent toward the tallest stereocilia, the probability that channels will open increases, driving membrane resistance to lower values. Conversely, during maximal deflection of stereocilia in the inhibitory direction, transduction channels that were open at rest close and hyperpolarize the cell. The proportion of time spent in the open or the closed state is a function of the degree of mechanical displacement of stereocilia. Moreover, it is known that the stiffness of the hair bundle is at its minimum at the point of maximum sensitivity of the displacement-receptor potential curve

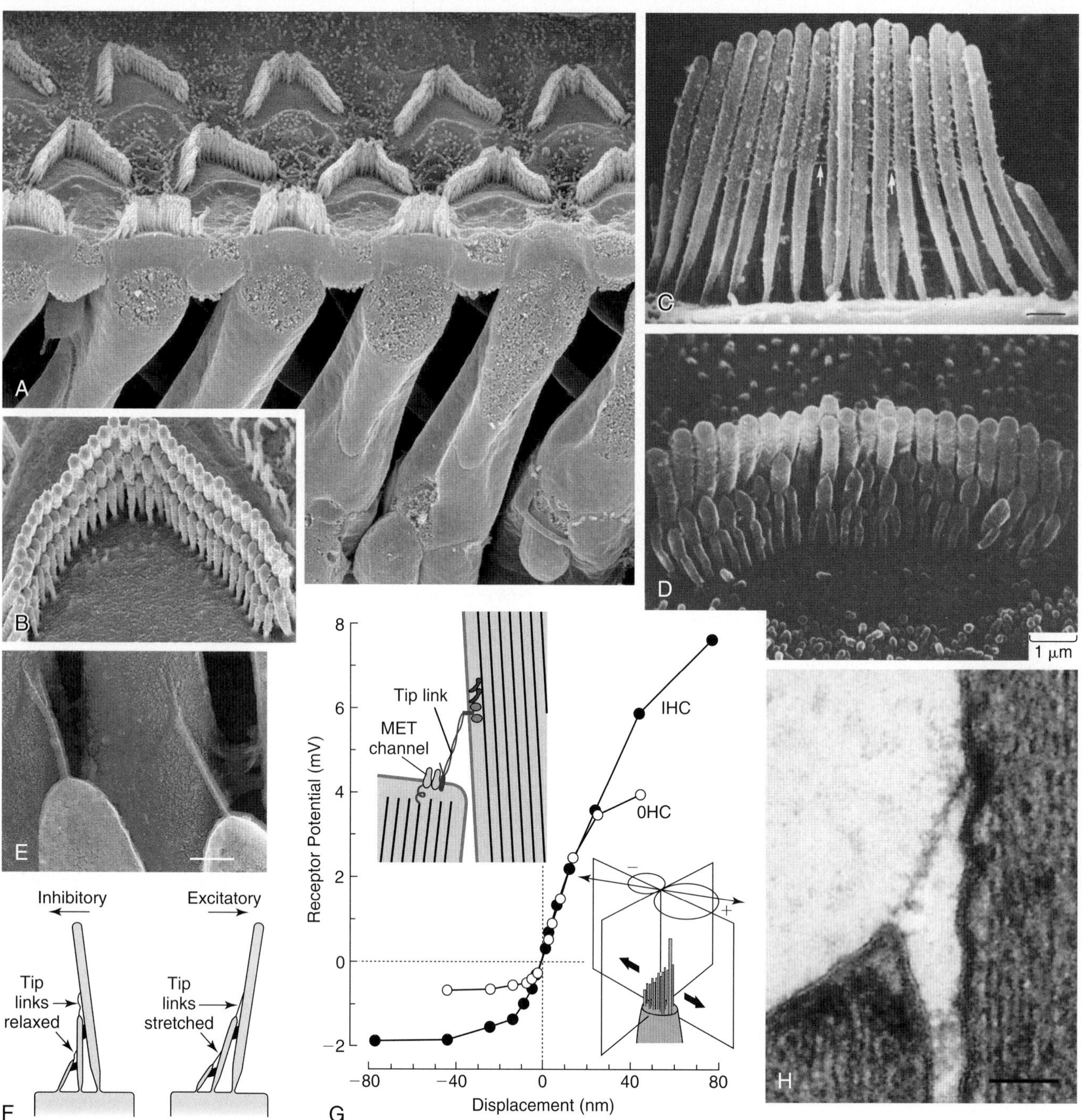

Figure 146-12. **A,** Scanning electron micrograph (SEM) of the outer hair cell (OHC) region of a mouse cochlea after the tectorial membrane and pillar cells have been removed, showing the large intercellular chamber that OHCs occupy in situ. **B,** Higher magnification of an SEM showing the highly ordered hair bundle of a single OHC. **C,** SEM of the tallest row of stereocilia of an inner hair cell (IHC) from a guinea pig cochlea. The view is looking toward the modiolus. Note the horizontal links adjoining adjacent stereocilia *(arrows)* and the narrowing of each stereocilium as each approaches the apical surface of the hair cell. Scale bar is 500 nm. **D,** SEM of an IHC from a guinea pig cochlea showing the nearly straight alignment of stereocilia compared with the V-shape or W-shape arrangement characteristic of OHCs. **E,** High-resolution images of tip links in a hair cell from a guinea pig cochlea showing splaying of the link at the upper insertion point on the taller stereocilium. Scale bar is 100 nm. **F,** Schematic illustration showing deflection of the hair bundle toward the taller stereocilia causes stretching of tip links *(right)* and opening of transduction channels, and hair bundle deflection toward the shorter stereocilia, produces tip link compression *(left)*, closing any transduction channels that were open. **G,** Receptor potential for an IHC and an OHC from the apical turn of a mouse cochlea maintained in vitro in response to hair bundle displacement. *Upper inset*, Illustration of a tip link and associated mechanoelectrical transduction (MET) channel at each end of the link. *Lower inset*, Directional sensitivity of a hair bundle showing that movements of the hair bundle perpendicular to the axis of symmetry produce no responses, and displacements at angled directions produce reduced responses. **H,** Transmission electron micrograph showing a tip link under tension. Note the electron densities at each end of the tip link and the pulling of the stereocilium's membrane to a point at which tension is high (see **B, C,** and **E**). *(**A** and **B**, From Friedman TB, Hinnant JT, Fridell RA, et al. DFNB3 families and Shaker-2 mice: mutations in an unconventional myosin, myo 15.* Adv Otorhinolaryngol. *2000;56:131; **C, D,** and **F**, from Pickles JO.* An Introduction to the Physiology of Hearing. *2nd ed. London: Academic Press; 1988; **E** and **H**, from Kachar B, Parakkal M, Kurc M, et al. High-resolution structure of hair-cell tip links.* Proc Natl Acad Sci U S A. *2000;97:13336; **G**, data from Russell IJ, Richardson GP, Cody AR. Mechanosensitivity of mammalian auditory hair cells in vitro.* Nature. *1986;321:517;* upper inset, *adapted from Holt JR, Corey DP. Two mechanisms for transducer adaptation in vertebrate hair cells.* Proc Natl Acad Sci U S A. *2000;97:11730;* lower inset, *from Flock A. Transducing mechanisms in the lateral line canal organ receptors.* Cold Spring Harb Symp Quant Biol. *1965;30:133.)*

when approximately 50% of the channels are open, a finding that supports the gating spring model.[238,461]

Focal measurements of extracellular potentials at various locations in the vicinity of hair bundles during the activation phase of transduction,[239] along with studies designed to block transduction by the local application of an aminoglycoside antibiotic[299] at different sites around the hair bundle,[246] revealed that the transduction channels are situated near the tips of the stereocilia. Additional support for this view has been advanced through imaging studies in which calcium was identified in the tips of stereocilia initially after bundle deflection and later in the base of the structure,[113] a finding that supports the view that Ca^{2+} enters the stereocilia through a transduction channel located at the tip.

Estimates indicate that the number of transduction channels per cell corresponds roughly to the number of stereocilia in a hair bundle (see Fig. 146-11F),[230,238,460] and transduction channels seem to be present in stereocilia of all heights within a bundle.[113]

Because of the small number of transduction channels present on hair cells, the effort to identify their molecular composition has been difficult at best.[84,94] However, results from invertebrate studies in *Drosophila melanogaster* and from studies of nonmammalian vertebrates (zebrafish) suggest that the best candidates for the transduction channel gene in mammalian hair cells belong to the transient receptor potential (TRP) gene family.[286,504] Nonetheless, it remains clear that additional studies are necessary to answer the question.

Transduction Channel Ion Selectivity

Hair cell transduction channels are permeable to a large number of monovalent and divalent cations, including small organic cations, such as choline and tetramethylammonium, suggesting that the internal diameter of the channel is relatively large, on the order of 0.7 nm, and the channel is relatively nonselective.[87,389] It is known that K^+ carries the major portion of the receptor current in vivo, as indicated by three observations: (1) the high concentration of K^+ in endolymph[27,259,519]; (2) the reversal potential of the transducer current is the same as the endocochlear potential[459]; and (3) that the concentration of K^+ found in perilymph increases after stimulation.[257] As a result of the combined positive endocochlear potential (+80 mV) and the negative intracellular potential of hair cells (−40 to −60 mV), a large potential gradient (greater than 120 mV) is established across the apical hair cell membrane (Figure 146-13). When hair bundles are deflected and transduction channels open, K^+ ions in the endolymph are flushed down a large electrochemical gradient through stereociliary transduction channels. This inward transducer current flows across the basolateral membrane, producing the receptor potential, and voltage-gated Ca^{2+} channels are activated, resulting in an influx of Ca^{2+} and release of neurotransmitter from the base of the hair cell.

Gating of Transduction Channels

Anatomic support for the presence of mechanical linkages that gate the opening and closing of transduction channels was acquired with the

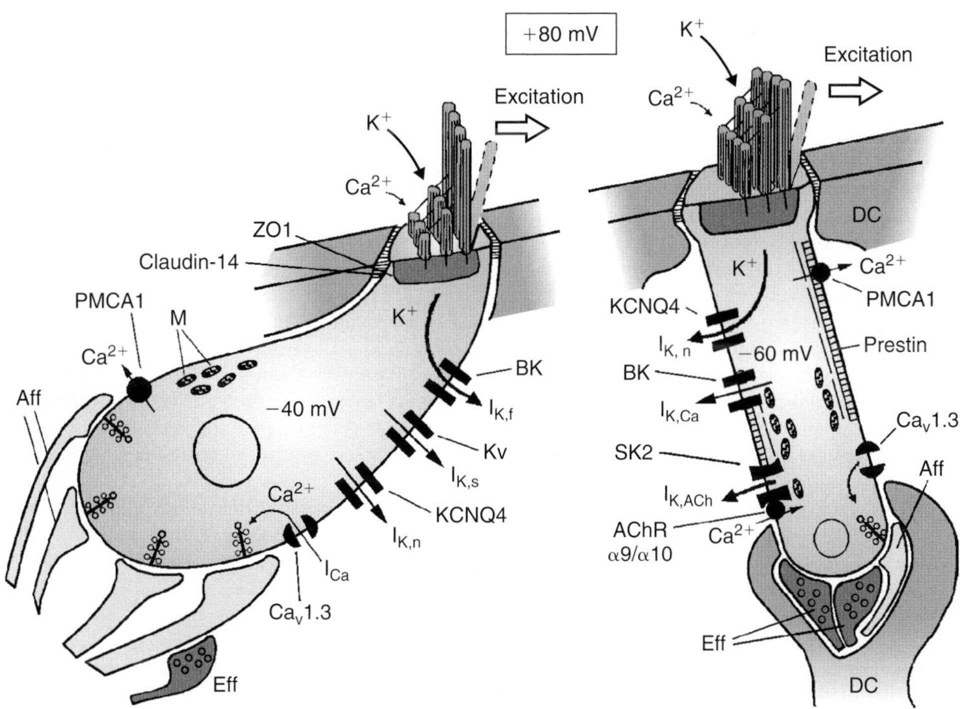

Figure 146-13. Drawing of an inner hair cell (IHC) *(left)* and an outer hair cell (OHC) *(right),* illustrating some of the basolateral membrane ion channels, pumps, and contacts by nerve endings. Three potassium currents in the IHC are shown: The K^+ current with fast kinetics, $I_{K,f}$, is carried by the large-conductance Ca^{2+}-dependent and voltage-dependent K^+ channel, BK; the $I_{K,s}$ current with slow kinetics is carried by a voltage-gated potassium channel (Kv). Both of these are outwardly rectifying. A slow delayed rectifier activated at negative potentials, $I_{K,n}$, carried by KCNQ4 channels also is shown. In OHCs, the major basolateral membrane K^+ current is $I_{K,n}$, which is active at negative potentials and carried by voltage-dependent KCNQ4 channels. A smaller voltage-dependent and Ca^{2+}-dependent current, $I_{K,Ca}$, carried by BK channels also is present. In addition, acetylcholine (ACh) released by efferent nerve terminals binds to acetylcholine receptors (AChR α9/α10) on OHCs that activate Ca^{2+}-permeable excitatory channels, which evoke a hyperpolarizing potassium current ($I_{K,ACh}$) mediated by a small-conductance Ca^{2+}-activated potassium channel (SK2). Both IHCs and OHCs have voltage-gated Ca^{2+} currents (I_{Ca}) mediated by L-type Ca^{2+} channels ($Ca_V1.3$) that open during depolarization, causing Ca^{2+} to enter the cell and trigger neurotransmitter release. Ca^{2+} is extruded from both hair cell types through plasma membrane Ca^{2+}-ATPase isoform 1 (PMCA1) pumps, and PMCA3 is localized to the cuticular plate region of IHCs (PMCA2a is concentrated in the stereocilia). Note that most channels are actually located in the basal portion of the membrane. In addition, claudin-14 is localized to the tight junctions near the apical membrane, and zona occludens-1 (ZO-1) is located near the tight junctions and cuticular plate of both hair cell types, as well as supporting cells. Prestin is present along the lateral cytoplasmic membrane of OHCs. Aff, afferent nerve ending; Eff, efferent nerve ending; DC, Deiters cell; M, mitochondria. *(Modified from Geisler CD.* From Sound to Synapse: Physiology of the Mammalian Ear. *New York: Oxford University Press; 1998.)*

discovery of tip links that stretch between shorter stereocilia and adjacent taller stereocilia (see Fig. 146-11B), connecting the distal tip of each stereocilium with the side of the longer adjacent stereocilium (Fig.e 146-12).[415] Tip links are aligned parallel to the axis of polarization of the hair bundle[82] and therefore play a role in the mechanism that determines the sensitivity of hair bundles to direction of displacement. When the bundle is deflected toward the taller stereocilia, tip links are stretched, which physically opens transduction channels, causing excitation (see Fig. 146-12G). When the bundle is deflected away from the taller stereocilia, tip links relax, causing the channel to close. Movement of the bundle perpendicular to the axis of symmetry produces little or no response, because the tension on tip links does not change. Orthogonal displacement of stereociliary bundles, on the other hand, produces reduced responses that are proportional to the exerted force.

The presence of tip links also may account for the rapid response of the transduction channel, and elastic linkages, like those considered previously, also may explain why transduction channels can be pulled open but not pushed shut. Moreover, the arrangement of tip links may explain why the number of transduction channels per hair cell is so small. Finally, although still an outstanding question, some studies suggest that transduction channels may be located at each end of the tip link,[113] as depicted schematically in Figure 146-12G.

The chemical composition of tip links is glycoproteinaceous, and glycoproteins seem to organize as two intertwined helical filaments that bifurcate and attach at two points on the side of the taller stereocilium (see Fig. 146-12E) by way of an electron-dense insertional plaque (see Fig. 146-12H) and at the level of an electron-dense region at the tip of the shorter stereocilium by way of three anchor filaments.[262] The molecular integrity of the tip link depends on the presence of calcium, as demonstrated by treating preparations with the Ca^{2+} chelator BAPTA (1,2-bis(*o*-aminophenoxy)ethane-*N,N,N′,N′*-tetraacetic acid), which breaks tip links and eliminates mechanoelectrical transduction.[33] Acoustic overstimulation can also cause tip link breakage.[416,540] Zhao and colleagues[632] made the important observation that tip links broken as a result of exposure to BAPTA regenerate within 24 hours, restoring mechanoelectrical transduction in the process. Perhaps a similar dynamic is operative in the case of recovery from temporary threshold shifts associated with acoustic overstimulation.

Recent studies have shown that tip links are composed of the extracellular domains of two proteins belonging to the cadherin superfamily of proteins, which generally mediate adhesion between cells—cadherin 23 (CDH23) and protocadherin 15 (PCDH15).[8,507,520] Tip links appear to form as an asymmetrical complex, consisting of homodimers of CDH23 localized to the upper segment of the tip link and homodimers of PCDH15 localized to the lower segment, with the two proteins interacting in the trans configuration at their NH_2 termini (see Fig. 146-15C).[267]

The gene that encodes cadherin 23 is defective in both patients with DFNB12[60] and persons with Usher syndrome type 1D,[58,60] as well as the waltzer (*v*) mouse[120,589,610] and the mutant zebrafish sputnik.[520] Usher syndrome type 1D is characterized by a constellation of signs and symptoms, including congenital sensorineural hearing loss, retinitis pigmentosa, and vestibular dysfunction.[58] Persons in the DFNB12 category exhibit profound, prelingual sensorineural hearing impairment.[67] Stereociliary abnormalities observed in waltzer mice during the late embryonic and early postnatal period include misplacement of the kinocilium and the presence of multiple stereociliary bundle islets on individual hair cells.[120,589,610] Although stereocilia are properly oriented early in development among waltzer mice, the characteristic polarization found in normal stereociliary bundles is lost, and orientation becomes chaotic as they degenerate. ABRs to intense acoustic stimuli cannot be detected in homozygous $Cdh23^{v\text{-}2J}$- or $Cdh23^{v\text{-}6J}$-mutant animals at the age of 3 to 4 weeks[120] and have not been detected at any age in yet another allelic variant of a waltzer mutant, $Cdh23^{v\text{-}Bus}$.[628]

Genetic complementation tests have shown that the locus for age-related hearing loss (AHL), a common characteristic of inbred mouse strains,[144,251,253,607,636] is allelic with Cdh23.[384] In addition, a predisposition to noise-induced hearing loss has been linked to this locus.[105,226,635] Thus, although certain mutations of Cdh23 are directly associated with deafness, others may enhance susceptibility to hearing loss associated with aging, environmental factors such as acoustic trauma, or other genetic factors, possibly as a consequence of altered binding capacity or decreased stability of Cdh23.

Defects in the gene that encodes protocadherin 15 cause deafness in patients with Usher syndrome type 1F,[12,15] in DFNB23,[11] and in the Ames waltzer (*av*) mouse.[14] In addition to congenital deafness, persons affected by Usher syndrome type 1F exhibit signs of vestibular dysfunction and suffer the consequences of retinitis pigmentosa.[12,15] The stereociliary bundles of hair cells in various mutant strains of Ames waltzer mice consistently display abnormal morphology followed by hair cell death and degeneration of the organ of Corti.[12,15,16,207,398,426] Stereocilia of both IHCs and OHCs become disorganized early in postnatal life, with loss of the stereotypical staircase profile of normal hair bundles as the clearest expression of stereociliary abnormality. Similar pathology has been observed in vestibular hair cells.[426] Acoustic stimuli fail to elicit responses in mice that are homozygous for several of the alleles that have been studied,[16,398,426] although mice that are homozygous for the $Pcdh15^{av\text{-}Jfb}$ allele appear to respond to high-level acoustic stimulation.[207] Of note, some of the hair cell abnormalities observed in Cdh23- and Pcdh15-mutant mice may be the result of other roles played by these proteins (see later on).

Composition of Stereocilia

As mentioned previously, stereocilia are not true cilia—they are microvillous extensions of the apical plasma membrane of hair cells. These extensions are tightly packed with microfilaments that run the length of each specialized villus.[163] Like microvilli of other epithelial cells (e.g., the brush border of intestinal epithelial cells), the longitudinally arrayed microfilaments of stereocilia are composed of hexagonally organized, tightly compacted actin filament bundles. Filamentous actin monomers are polar molecules, and individual filaments within a bundle are arranged in parallel and exhibit common polarity (Fig. 146-14A).[161,548] This organizational scheme provides a framework for the renewal of stereocilia, because actin monomers are incorporated into actin filaments at the tips of stereocilia as older components of actin filaments cycle toward the cell body at a rate of approximately 2.5 μm/day.[467,482] These data suggest that the actin core of the tallest stereocilia turns over completely every 2 days, approximately, in the base and every 3 days in the apex of the human cochlea. These rates are considerably slower than the overall turnover rates for shorter, conventional microvilli, like those found on Hensen cells and outer phalangeal cells.[194] The continuous renewal of actin filaments within stereocilia appears to play an important role in repair and recovery from acoustic overstimulation, and the failure of this system to operate properly may have significant otopathologic consequences.

The hexagonal pattern of actin bundles comprising the stereociliary core is maintained by actin-bundling proteins, including plastin/fimbrin and espin that form cross-linkages and fasten together individual actin filaments (see Fig. 146-14B). These bridging proteins occur at frequent and uniform intervals along the shafts of actin filaments[133,160,501,548,551] and, in keeping with the stereotypical association with crossover points of the α-helical subunits, are highly organized and coaligned.[548] The extensive cross-linking among adjacent actin filaments imparts a high degree of stiffness to each stereocilium (see Fig. 146-14C)[533] and consequently minimizes independent movement of actin elements during deflection such that an individual stereocilium moves as a rigid rod, one that will fracture much like glass if excessively deflected.[162] Moreover, actin filaments are neither stretched nor compressed during bundle deflection but appear to slide past one another as a result of the flexibility of the bond between the actin cross-linking proteins and the actin filaments.[549,584] It is noteworthy that cross-bridges between stereociliary actin filaments are reduced in number after acoustic overstimulation resulting in temporary threshold elevation, a condition that reduces stereocilia stiffness as a consequence.[550]

Defects in Cytoskeletal Proteins Lead to Deafness

Cytoskeletal actin exists in one of two highly conserved forms, either the β- or the γ-form, and the proteins differ from one another by a mere four amino acids located at the NH_2-terminal ends of the

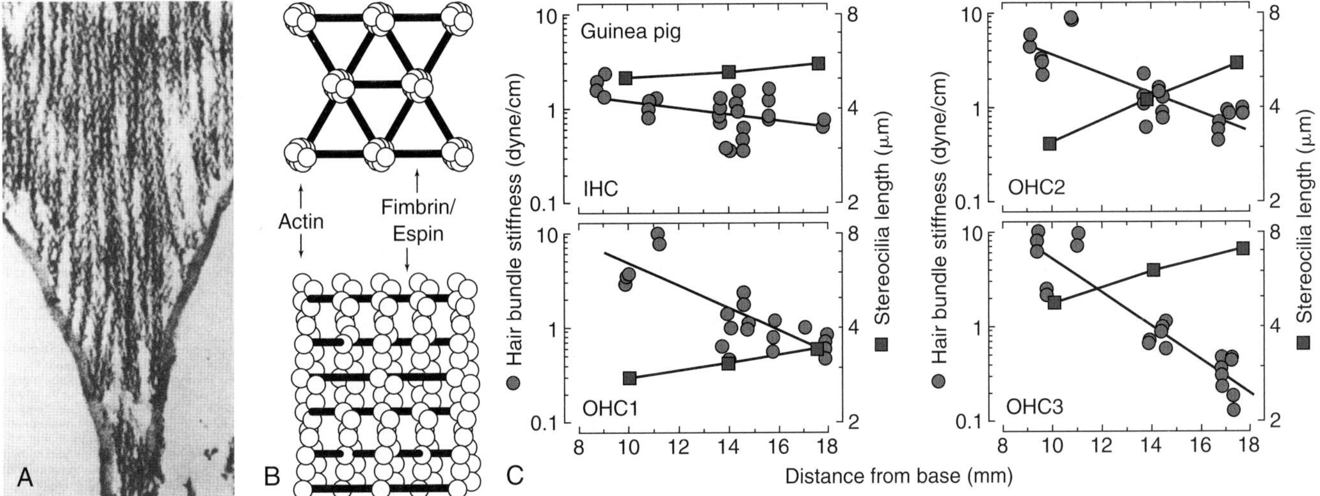

Figure 146-14. **A,** The uniform polarity of actin filaments within the stereocilium is demonstrated in a lizard cochlea by incubating preparations with the S1 fragment of myosin, thereby marking the polarity of the filament. The arrowhead-like appearance of actin filaments indicates that their pointed ends are located proximal to the hair cell body and that the barbed ends of actin filaments are located at the stereocilia tips. **B,** Paracrystalline array of actin filaments depicted in the longitudinal orientation *(bottom)* and in cross section *(top)*, showing the cross-linkages composed of fimbrin and espin. **C,** Stiffness of hair bundles of guinea pig hair cells as a function of distance along the cochlear partition *(circles)*. Also shown are lengths of the tallest row of stereocilia for each hair cell row at three basilar membrane locations *(squares)*. IHC, inner hair cell; OHC, outer hair cell. *(**A,** From Tilney LG, DeRosier DJ, Mulroy MJ. The organization of actin filaments in the stereocilia of cochlear hair cells.* J Cell Biol. *1980;86:244; **B,** from Tilney LG, Egelman EH, DeRosier DJ, Saunder JC. Actin filaments, stereocilia, and hair cells of the bird cochlea. II. Packing of actin filaments in the stereocilia and in the cuticular plate and what happens to the organization when the stereocilia are bent.* J Cell Biol. *1983;96:822; **C,** data from Strelioff D, Flock A. Stiffness of sensory-cell hair bundles in the isolated guinea pig cochlea.* Hear Res. *1984;15:19.)*

molecule.[142] Both forms generally are coexpressed in mammalian nonmuscle cells[272]; however, unlike in most nonmuscle cells, in which β-actin is expressed as the principal form, in auditory hair cells γ-actin is the principal variant of the protein, and it is distributed ubiquitously within the cell.[223] β-Actin expression, on the other hand, is restricted to stereocilia.[482] Mutations in the γ-actin gene (*ACTG1*) lead to autosomal dominant progressive hearing loss (DFNA20/26)[572,639] that presumably is the consequence of a diminished ability to repair the actin cytoskeleton (Fig. 146-15) among affected persons. A mouse model expressing a functional null mutation in the gene encoding γ-actin is available, and animals from this strain acquire normal hearing during the early postnatal period.[41] However, this relatively brief period of normalcy gives way to progressive hearing loss, as indicated by ABR and distortion product otoacoustic emission (DPOAE) recordings.[406] The first morphologic sign of pathology appears in the form of hair bundle disruption and is followed shortly thereafter by the loss of hair and supporting cells. These data suggest that whereas β-actin is sufficient for the normal development of stereociliary bundles, γ-actin is required for their normal maintenance. Insight into the role that γ-actin may play in maintenance can be gleaned from noise exposure studies. It turns out that occasional gaps appear in phalloidin-stained F-actin filaments forming the core of stereocilia after noise exposure, and that these gaps are labeled by an antibody to γ-actin. These findings suggest, naturally enough, that γ-actin may be required to repair traumatized hair bundles. Similar gaps have been observed in mature actin filaments associated with $Actg1^{-/-}$ mice, again suggesting that γ-actin is a necessary player in the maintenance of stereociliary structural integrity.[41]

An essential role for the actin-bundling protein espin in the maintenance of stereociliary infrastructure also has been identified in deaf mice that are homozygous for the jerker (*je*) mutation,[634] a finding that led to the identification of mutations in the *ESPN* gene in autosomal recessive, prelingual and profound hearing loss (DFNB36) in humans.[381] The jerker trait arose spontaneously, and homozygous mutant animals exhibit stereociliary abnormalities, hair cell degeneration, deafness, and vestibular system dysfunction.[26,115,511,512,529] Although stereocilia seem to develop normally, they are shorter than normal as a rule, and degenerative changes occur during the early postnatal period. Homozygous mutant animals are unresponsive to acoustic stimuli throughout life. Of interest, overexpression of espin in hair cells results in abnormally long stereocilia, suggesting that the level of espin expression is critical for normal stereocilia development.[466] Espin is expressed primarily in hair bundles and is distributed along the entire stereociliary length (see Fig. 146-15),[634] although light espin staining has been observed in the cuticular plate and soma in chicks.[324] Although fimbrin also plays a role cross-linking actin filaments, in contrast with espin, its activity is inhibited by Ca^{2+}.[38] Thus, in the absence of espin, Ca^{2+} entry into stereocilia may destabilize the actin core and serve to trigger pathologic changes as a consequence.[634] Also of note is that espin binds to actin with higher affinity than does fimbrin and may play a role as an important stabilizing factor after formation,[38] although data from studies in the chick suggest that espin is expressed early on when stereocilia first begin to elongate.[324] Autosomal dominant forms of hearing loss resulting from mutations in ESPN in humans also have been identified.[129]

In the context of linkage proteins that have a clear role in peripheral auditory function, a gene family of integral membrane proteins that appear to link the actin cytoskeleton to the plasma membrane and are essential elements of audition have been identified, and include proteins in the ezrin-radixin-moesin family. The highest concentration of the protein radixin is found at the base of hair cell stereocilia in a variety of species, including frog, chicken, zebrafish, and mouse (see Fig. 146-15A). Radixin appears to anchor the pointed ends of actin filaments to the plasma membrane in the region of the stereocilium taper.[402] In the absence of radixin, mice are profoundly deaf, and both IHC and OHC stereocilia become progressively disarrayed and hair cells subsequently degenerate, even though the system appears to develop normally.[289] Of interest, whereas radixin alone is detectable in cochlear hair cells from normal adult mice, both radixin and, to a lesser extent, ezrin are found in adult vestibular hair cells. In radixin-null mice, ezrin appears to compensate for radixin, promoting development of both cochlear and vestibular hair cell stereociliary bundles. However, unlike vestibular hair cells, cochlear hair cells require radixin for continued maintenance beyond early postnatal life. As in the mouse, radixin is required for normal hearing in humans as well, with pathogenic mutations producing prelingual, bilateral, and profound hearing loss that is inherited as an autosomal recessive trait (DFNB24).[273] Moreover, immunoreactiv-

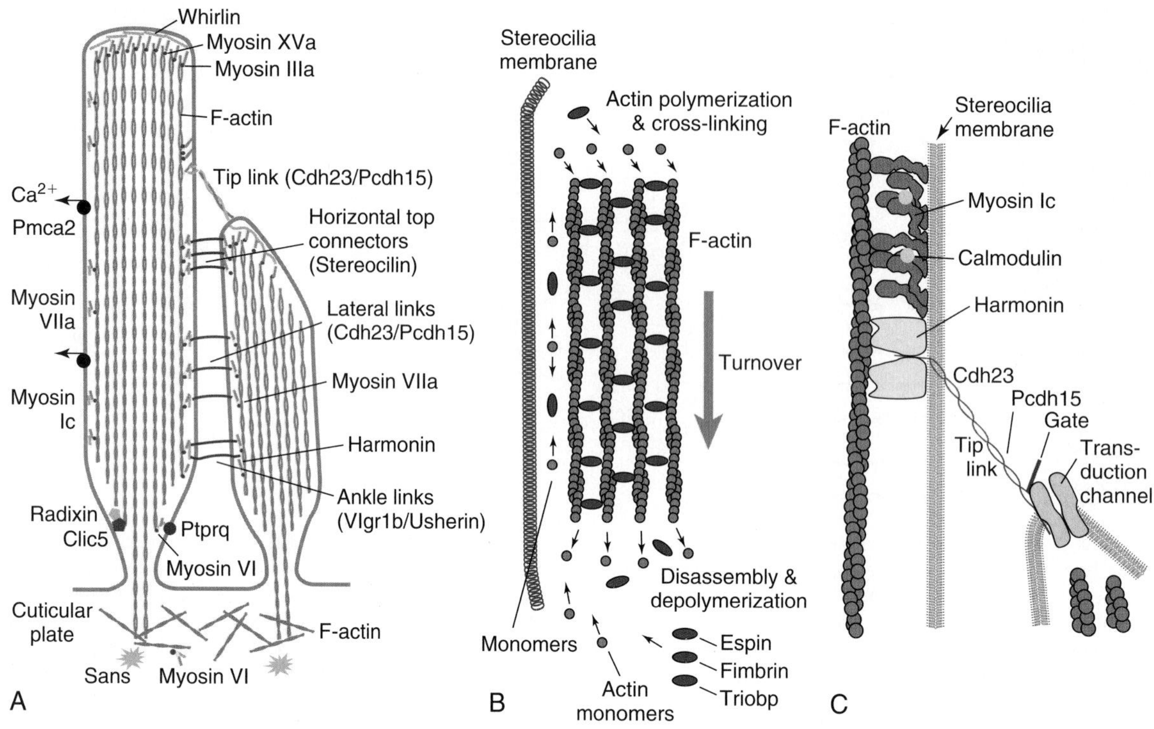

Figure 146-15. **A,** Schematic illustration of a longitudinal section through two stereocilia located in adjacent rows, connected by a tip link, and other linkages. Note that lateral links and ankle links are found only in developing cochlear hair cells. Unconventional myosins found in the mature hair cell include myosin XVa and myosin IIIa, which concentrate at stereocilia tips; myosin VIIa and myosin 1c, which are are found along the shafts of stereocilia; and myosin VI, the only known member of the myosin superfamily that moves toward the pointed end of actin filaments, found at the base of stereocilia and in the cuticular plate. Whirlin also concentrates at tips of stereocilia, whereas radixin, Clic5, and Ptprq concentrate near the base of stereocilia. Transmembrane proteins with long extracellular domains include cadherin 23, protocadherin 15, Vlgr1b, and usherin, which appear to be components of specific interstereociliary linkages, along with stereocilin, which may be an extracellular protein. The intracellular scaffolding protein, harmonin, may serve to anchor the transmembrane proteins with long extracellular domains to the F-actin core. **B,** The treadmill model of actin turnover within a stereocilium depicting actin polymerization and cross-linking occurring at the barbed ends of actin filaments located at the tips of stereocilia, and disassembly and depolymerization of actin filaments occurring at the base of stereocilia. **C,** Schematic illustration of the transduction channel, including the tip link complex, myosin motors for adaptation, and harmonin. *(**A** and **B**, Adapted from Rzadzinska AK, Schneider ME, Davies C, et al. An actin molecular treadmill and myosins maintain stereocilia functional architecture and self-renewal.* J Cell Biol. *2004;164:887;* ***C**, adapted from Gillespie PG, Cyr JL. Myosin-1c, the hair cell's adaptation motor.* Annu Rev Physiol. *2004;66:521.)*

ity to radixin is reduced in mice carrying the spontaneous mutation Jitterbug, responsible for a mutation in Clic5, an intracellular chloride channel that is expressed in normal hair cell stereocilia, particularly at the stereociliary base.[175] Stereocilia of mice deficient in Clic5 develop normally but show progressive degeneration after the onset of hearing. Studies suggest that Clic5 may associate with a radixin-actin cytoskeletal complex that appears to be necessary for stereocilia maintenance.

Other proteins associated with actin and that are critical for hearing include TRIOBP and diaphanous 1. Mutations in a long isoform of TRIOBP have been shown to cause autosomal recessive deafness (DFNB28),[436,499] whereas mutations in DIAPH1 are associated with autosomal dominant hearing loss.[346] TRIOBP is associated with filamentous actin, is relatively resistant to the F-actin destabilizer latrunculin B, and is thought to regulate the organization of the actin cytoskeleton.[492] Numerous isoforms of TRIOBP are present in the cochlea, in both IHCs and OHCs, and the protein colocalizes with F-actin along the length of stereocilia (see Fig. 146-15B).[436,499] Diaphanous belongs to the formin family of proteins, which are known to interact with the growing, or barbed, end of actin and recently have been shown to act as effectors for Rho GTPases, key regulators of actin dynamics. Although its role remains unproved, diaphanous is thought to participate in the regulation of cytoskeletal actin turnover, but the protein also may be involved in endosome motility.[397] Diaphanous has been identified within the cochlea by use of a reverse transcription–polymerase chain reaction (RT-PCR) approach,[346] but its precise localization remains unknown. As with many other proteins, the role of both TRIOBP and diaphanous 1 in transduction requires additional investigation.

Dynamic Regulation of Stereocilia Length

In addition to *Espn*, other genes that are required for the development of normal stereocilia height include *Myo15a* and *Whrn* (see Fig. 146-15A). *Myo15a* encodes myosin XVa, an unconventional myosin that is localized near the site of actin polymerization at the tip of each stereocilium in both auditory and vestibular hair cells.[43] *MYO15A* is indispensable for hearing, and pathogenic mutations result in a form of nonsyndromic deafness, DFNB3, in humans,[592] and persons who are homozygous for the mutation are congenitally deaf. The shaker 2 (*sh2*) mutant mouse strain also carries a defect in *Myo15*.[422] The condition is inherited as an autosomal recessive trait, and 1-month-old homozygous mutant mice are unresponsive to acoustic stimulation.[327] Although hair cells are present at this age and stereociliary bundles are present, stereocilia of both IHCs and OHCs are notably shorter than normal, and the normal gradation in stereociliary height is less prominent among adjacent hair cell rows.[422] The stereocilia of vestibular hair cells in both otolith organs and semicircular canals also are abnormally short in mutant mice.[22] It is noteworthy that myosin XVa immunoreactivity is first detected in mice at about the time that stereocilia begin to grow differentially and establish the row-dependent stereociliary bundle height gradation that is characteristic of normal mammals.[43] Labeling also is more intense in the tallest stereocilia, suggesting that formation of the graded stereociliary row pattern requires the presence of myosin XVa.[43,467] Thus, although normal development of the hair bundle is arrested in the absence of functional myosin XVa, the precise mechanism of its action will be the subject of continued investigation.

Whrn encodes a putative scaffolding protein known as whirlin, and genetic abnormalities of the gene, *WHRN*, are the source of deafness in persons with DFNB31; likewise, *Whrn* abnormalities are responsible for deafness in mice designated whirler mutants.[358] DFNB31 is characterized by profound, prelingual sensorineural hearing loss, and mutant whirler (*wi*) mice also exhibit profound deafness, as well as vestibular abnormalities. Hair bundles associated with both IHCs and OHCs in homozygous mutant whirler mice are abnormal.[225] Specifically, IHC stereocilia are significantly shorter than normal as early as embryonic day 18.5. However, stereociliary shaft lengths do continue to increase until approximately 1 day after birth, when the process actually reverses and individual stereociliary lengths begin to decrease. During this period, the organization of stereocilia within hair bundles remains normal, and although relative height gradations are normal, height differences between rows are clearly less prominent than in normal mice. Likewise, overall stereociliary height along the length of the cochlear spiral, a morphologic feature that normally is characterized as a gradient in which height increases continuously from base to apex, is notably reduced in mutant mice.

As with IHCs, OHC stereociliary lengths generally are smaller than normal in whirler mutants, although OHC defects appear slightly later than in IHCs in affected animals. However, an interesting variation in the pattern of stereociliary anomaly has been described in whirler-mutant mice: Specifically, abnormally short stereocilia are located on the edges of each row, although the number of rows appears normal, and stereociliary rows are graded in height. Also of note is that hair bundles do not conform to the classic V- or W-shape observed in normal hair cells. Instead, bundle patterns exhibit a more curvilinear profile. Hair cell degeneration, starting with OHCs, is first observed at approximately the 60th postnatal day and is followed by IHC degeneration,[225] and extensive degeneration generally occurs by the 90th postnatal day, particularly in the basal and middle turns of the cochlea.[358]

In addition to the independent roles played by whirlin and myosin XVa, normal hair bundle development appears to depend on their interaction. Indirect evidence supporting this view suggests that myosin XVa may guide whirlin to stereociliary tips, thereby promoting length enhancement. The rationale for this scenario, speculative as it is, is driven by the observation that the amount of whirlin measured at stereociliary tips is directly proportional to the amount of myosin XVa measured at the same location.[44,111,282] Of interest in this regard is that whirlin expression is down-regulated after stereociliary maturation, whereas myosin XVa expression continues throughout life.[282] In addition to whirlin and myosin XVa, differences in hair bundle morphology between *sh2* and *wi* mice, reviewed earlier,[370] suggest that other interacting proteins are likely to be involved in the development and maintenance of stereocilia.[357] One such protein may be myosin VIIa (see later). Specifically, Prosser and colleagues made the observation that stereocilia grow abnormally long in the absence of myosin VIIa and that whirlin expression persists at the tips of mature stereocilia, rather than undergoing naturally programmed down-regulation. In addition, when either whirlin or myosin XVa is absent from hair cells, myosin VIIa is expressed at the tips of the abnormally short stereocilia, suggesting that myosin VIIa is critically important in regulating the dynamics of stereocilia elongation during maturation.[423]

Another unconventional myosin that is expressed in stereociliary tips is myosin IIIa. This myosin variant appears to concentrate around the tips of stereocilia in a "thimble-like" pattern, in contrast with the "caplike" pattern of myosin XVa expression.[483] Although myosin IIIa does not appear to play a role in development, it has been shown to cause bilateral, autosomal recessive nonsyndromic hearing impairment that begins in the second decade of life. The pattern of hearing loss associated with this condition is such that high-frequency sensitivity is affected initially, with losses occurring progressively in the case of middle- and low-frequency sensitivity.[591]

Interstereociliary Linkages

Like actin-binding proteins, which cross-link actin filaments and help form the core of individual stereocilia, stereocilia are themselves interconnected by way of a complex array of extracellular fibrous cross-linkages (see Fig. 146-15A). At the most fundamental level of organization, filamentous links bind stereocilia within a bundle into a mechanical unit by connecting a stereocilium with neighboring stereocilia on all sides.[173,399,415,434] In adult animals, these proteinaceous links run parallel to the apical surface of the cell connecting different rows of stereocilia, as well as stereocilia of the same row (see Fig. 146-11A), and are thought to contribute to the overall cohesiveness and stiffness of the hair bundle.

Numerous morphologically and biochemically distinct* interstereociliary linkages are recognized; however, some are permanent features of the system, whereas others appear transiently during development.[173,189,191,192,193,415,417,434,547,556,557] For example, although horizontal top connectors are present in both IHCs and OHCs of adults, shaft connectors, located beneath the top connectors in roughly the middle section of the shaft, are found in inner hair cells throughout life but are expressed in outer hair cells only during development. Lateral links, which are located along stereocilia sides, and ankle links, which are located at the stereociliary base, are expressed transiently in both IHCs and OHCs during hair bundle development. Linkages between the kinocilium and two to three adjacent stereocilia from the tallest row are present during the developmental period when kinocilia are a feature of IHCs and OHCs.

Like tip links, kinocilial links are sensitive to BAPTA and resistant to the protease subtilisin. These linkage proteins appear to be composed of both Cdh23 and Pcdh15.[8,192,365] Of interest, transient lateral links also appear to be composed of Cdh23; however, in sharp contrast with tip links, these lateral linkages are insensitive to BAPTA and sensitive to subtilisin.[365] Links resistant to both BAPTA and subtilisin treatment include horizontal top connectors. Stereocilin (STRC) appears to be a primary constituent of top connectors, as well as being present in the attachments between the tallest row of OHC stereocilia and the tectorial membrane.[576,577] Mutations in STRC are associated with nonsyndromic autosomal recessive deafness (DFNB16),[576] and stereocilin-null mice show progressive hearing loss, suggesting that horizontal top connectors are an essential hair bundle feature.[577] The formation of shaft connectors, which are resistant to BAPTA but sensitive to subtilisin, requires protein tyrosine phosphatase receptor Q (Ptprq), and when the *Ptprq* gene is disrupted in mice, stereocilia of hair cells located in the base of the cochlea become disorganized during the early postnatal period and are sporadically lost—an event that leads to hair cell death.[190] Finally, ankle links, which are sensitive to both BAPTA and subtilisin, appear to be composed of both Vlgr1 (*v*ery *l*arge *G*-protein–coupled *r*eceptor 1) and usherin.[4,359] Gene mutations affecting these proteins in humans result in Usher syndrome type 2C and type 2A, respectively.[147,603] Mice carrying functional null alleles for Vlgr1 are profoundly hearing impaired by the age of 3 weeks and lack ankle links at the base of hair cell stereocilia, with progressive disorganization of hair bundles, eventually leading to hair cell loss.[359] By contrast, auditory deficits in usherin-null mice are mild and limited to high frequencies and are not progressive.[335]

Usher syndrome is a genetically heterogeneous disease and the leading cause of combined deafness and blindness around the world. No fewer than 10 forms of the syndrome are recognized, many of which are associated with well-characterized gene defects that produce a group of abnormal gene products collectively referred to as the Usher proteins. Included in that collection is the unconventional myosin VIIa (Usher syndrome type IB [USHIB]),[600] the scaffold protein harmonin (USH1C),[13] the novel cytoplasmic protein sans (USH1G),[377,601] and the transmembrane protein clarin-1 (USH3).[6,249] Spontaneous mutations in orthologous murine genes also have been identified and include shaker-1 (*sh1*),[182] deaf circler (*dfcr*),[252] and Jackson shaker (*js*),[283] representing mutations in *Myo7a, Ush1c,* and *Sans,* respectively. Persons affected by Usher syndrome type I exhibit severe to profound congenital hearing loss, vestibular system dysfunction, and early-onset, progressive retinitis pigmentosa, whereas those affected by Usher syndrome type II have moderate to severe high-frequency hearing impairment, normal vestibular function, and progressive retinitis pigmentosa.

*Differing sensitivities to the Ca^{2+}-chelating agent BAPTA and the protease subtilisin are commonly used to distinguish biochemical differences among interstereociliary linkages being considered in this chapter.

The clinical phenotypes of patients suffering with Usher syndrome type III are highly variable, often leading to misdiagnosis of the disorder as either type I or type II.[405]

Like mice exhibiting abnormalities Cdh23, Pcdh15, or Vlgr1, mice with defective genes encoding myosin VIIa, harmonin, or Sans also are deaf, and hair bundle abnormalities that appear during development constitute a common feature in all three animal models.[182,252,283] The common morphologic phenotype shared by affected animals suggests that these proteins interact with one another, each satisfying a unique role with respect to hair bundle development. Furthermore, the proteins in question do not appear to compensate for one another; pathology ensues when any one of the group is lost or is defective.

Predictably, in keeping with the close functional association of the Usher proteins, numerous interprotein interactions have been identified in recent years. For example, harmonin has been shown to bind with both Cdh23 and Pcdh15, as well as actin filaments, and on the basis of the molecular characteristics of Cdh23 and Pcdh15, some investigators have suggested that harmonin anchors Cdh23 and Pcdh15 to the actin core of stereocilia.[5,54,506] Harmonin also binds to myosin VIIa, and it is especially informative that harmonin cannot be found in the hair bundles of *sh1*-mutant mice, animals exhibiting an abnormal version of Myo7a. This finding suggests that myosin VIIa transports harmonin from the cytoplasmic compartment of the cell body to the stereocilia.[54] Likewise, protocadherin 15 binds to myosin VIIa, and neither protein is "correctly" localized when one of the partners is lost or disrupted, a finding that supports a model in which the two proteins interact critically to ensure the proper spatial maintenance of the protein complex as the hair bundle matures.[496]

Harmonin also binds with both Vlgr1 and usherin,[4,430] as does whirlin,[4,573] and myosin VIIa binds with Vlgr1, usherin, and whirlin.[111,364] Vezatin, a transmembrane protein that also is localized to the basal region of stereocilia,[307] binds to usherin and may be a constituent of the ankle link complex,[364] an idea that is supported by the finding that vezatin, in addition to usherin and whirlin, cannot be detected in the stereocilium of *Vlgr1*-null animals.[364] In an especially revealing study, Vlgr1, usherin, and whirlin, as well as vezatin, cannot be detected in hair cell stereocilia in animals without functional myosin VIIa. This observation suggests that proteins associated with the ankle links are transported to the stereocilia by myosin VIIa,[364] an actin-based motor that is capable of transporting cargo toward the plus, or barbed, ends of actin filaments (i.e., toward stereocilia tips).[565] These findings—that is, the absence of usherin, vezatin, and Vlgr1 in stereocilia of whirler-mutant animals—implicate whirlin as a scaffold protein supporting the ankle link complex.[364] The protein Sans is unusual among the Usher proteins in that it is localized not in stereocilia but in the region beneath the cuticular plate.[5] Sans interacts with harmonin,[5,601] as well as myosin VIIa, and it may regulate the trafficking of at least some of the Usher proteins to the stereocilium, as supported by its location at the interface of the cell body and the hair bundle.[5] Finally, it has been shown that harmonin, Vlgr1b, and usherin are found together in the synapse between hair cells and afferent or efferent fibers in adult cochleae. This observation suggests that Usher proteins may play yet another functional role in mammals, one that influences neural processing within the auditory pathway.[430]

Myosin VI

Numerous unconventional myosins are essential for normal hair cell function, including myosin VI. Mutations in the *MYO6* gene are responsible for autosomal dominant hearing loss, DFNA22[363]; autosomal recessive deafness, DFNB37[10]; and the phenotype observed in Snell's waltzer (*sv*) and tailchaser (*tlc*) mice,[35,219] as well as mutant satellite zebrafish.[491] People affected with DFNB37 have profound congenital sensorineural hearing loss with complementary vestibular dysfunction, whereas hearing deficits in persons affected with DFNA22 are sensorineural in nature, but the onset of the condition is postlingual, and the anomaly develops progressively, unlike in the case of DFNB37-mediated deafness. The degree of hearing loss in these patients ranges from moderate to profound, and affected persons show no signs of vestibular dysfunction.

Like other myosin proteins, myosin VI is a molecular motor that binds to actin filaments or microtubules; however, it is unique as the only myosin thus far identified that moves backward toward the pointed end of actin filaments.[210,602] Of interest, the phenotype of the myosin VI mutant is limited to hair cell dysfunction.

Myosin VI is localized at the base of the stereocilia,[35,211] where the pointed ends of core stereociliary actin filaments project into the cuticular plate and rootlets of stereociliary actin filaments terminate (see Fig. 146-15A). More specifically, myosin VI is located in the circumferential region surrounding the lateral margins of the cuticular plate, an area that is rich in cytoplasmic vesicles, a finding that is particularly evident in amphibian hair cells. More recent localization studies suggest that myosin VI may be found along the length of stereocilia.[219] Unlike with the mutations in mice causing an Usher-like phenotype, the basal aspect of adjacent stereociliary membranes in *Myo6*-mutant animal models appears to fuse, reducing the numbers of individual stereocilia and leading to the formation of "giant" stereocilia that are both longer and wider than normal and often display swollen or bulbous tips, and branching of stereocilia also is observed occasionally. Sequentially, giant stereocilia collapse onto the apical surface of the organ of Corti and appear to fuse with the apical membranes of hair cells and supporting cells, and the organ of Corti undergoes degeneration. During the period of stereocilia fusion, stereocilia branching also is observed, and the apical surfaces of hair cells appear to bulge outward. Ultrastructural examination indicates the presence of extraneous material within the fused stereocilia, possibly components normally found in the apical cytoplasm of hair cells.[219,472,491,493]

Although numerous hypotheses have been advanced to explain hair cell abnormalities observed in *Myo6*-mutant animals, recent studies suggest that the protein may serve to tether Ptprq to the actin cytoskeleton at the base of the stereocilia, maintaining the stereocilia taper and preventing fusion between adjacent stereocilia.[472] In that regard, unlike with the focal localization of Ptprq in the stereociliary base of normal animals, the protein is distributed throughout the stereocilium in Snell's waltzer mice, suggesting that the proteins normally interact with one another directly.[472] Moreover, as an inositol lipid phosphatase, Ptprq would be in a key position to regulate the phosphoinositide phospholipid content of the hair cell membrane.[190] The reciprocal distribution of phosphatidylinositol 4,5-bisphosphate (PIP_2) and Ptprq in stereocilia[221] suggests that Ptprq may play a role in the regulation of actin and membrane turnover, a process that is disrupted in the absence of functional myosin VI.[472]

Adaptation of Mechanoelectrical Transduction Currents

It is well known that receptor currents adapt after sustained deflection of hair bundles (Fig. 146-16A). Adaptation is associated with a horizontal shift in input-output curves after bundle displacement (see Fig. 146-16B), without a change in the slope of the steepest portion of the curve. Shifts in the horizontal position of input-output curves, like those described here, reflect the actions of a dynamic system in which the central operating point is restored after sustained depolarization, re-establishing the sensitivity of the system. The prevailing model used most often to explain adaptation entails a reduction in tip link tension when the bundle is deflected in the excitatory direction and an increase in tension for deflections in the inhibitory direction.[85,88,135,227,502]

Two mechanisms of adaptation have been described: one that underlies rapid adaptation, a phenomenon characterized by a time constant of less than a few milliseconds, and another with a time constant greater than 10 msec, which can achieve values as high as several hundred milliseconds under some circumstances. In the case of *rapid* adaptation, Ca^{2+} ions entering the cell through transduction channels bind directly to an intracellular site that is part of the transduction channel itself (see Fig. 146-16D), which in turn modifies the relationship between tension and the probability that the channel is in the open state.[90,438] In the case of *slow* adaptation, an active motor is thought to slide the transduction channel associated with the taller stereocilium down the actin filament core of the stereocilium (see Fig. 146-16C), thereby reducing tension on the tip link and decreasing the probability that the channel will be in the open state.[32,184,237] Conversely, moving

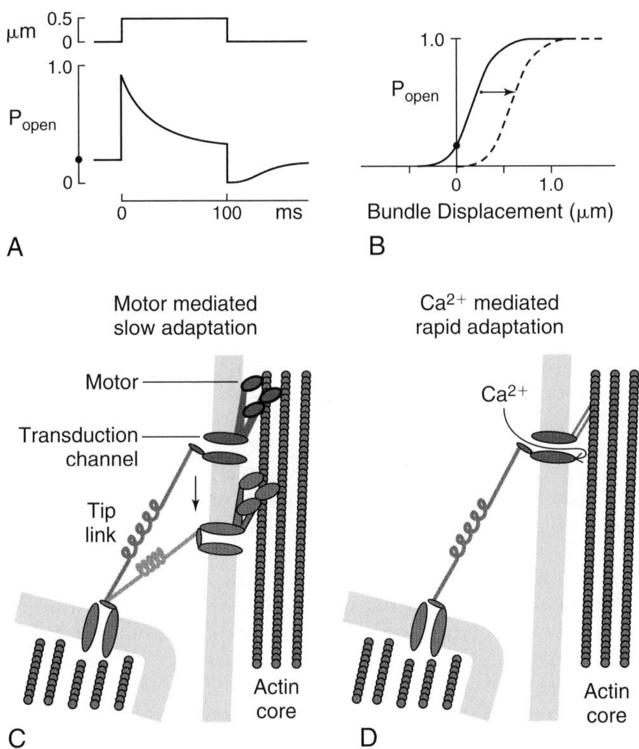

Figure 146-16. A, Diagram depicting positive (depolarizing) deflection of a hair bundle and the resulting adaptation observed as a decrease in the probability (*P*) of transduction channel opening over time during sustained bundle deflection. **B,** During the adapted state, the bundle displacement–versus–open probability curve is shifted horizontally along the x-axis, such that still larger bundle displacements are required to evoke a response comparable to that observed at the onset of stimulation. Two models have been proposed to account for adaptation: a motor-mediated slower process that requires resetting tip link tension by slippage of the entire transduction channel along the actin filaments (**C**) and a direct Ca^{2+}-mediated adaptation (**D**) that results from Ca^{2+} entry through the transduction channel and binding to an intracellular site of the channel, altering it to prefer the closed state. *(**A** and **B**, From Pickles JO, Corey DP. Mechanoelectrical transduction by hair cells.* Trends Neurosci. *1992;15:254; **C** and **D**, adapted from Holt JR, Corey DP. Two mechanisms for transducer adaptation in vertebrate hair cells.* Proc Natl Acad Sci U S A. *2000;97:11730.)*

the hair bundle in the inhibitory direction is thought to cause tip links to relax and close channels that were open at rest. During the adaptation phase, transduction channels are thought to climb along the actin core, resetting the operating point and increasing the probability of channel opening. In addition to Ca^{2+}, the latter mechanism requires an active motor, presumably an unconventional myosin that interacts directly with the actin core. Although both forms of adaptation exist in individual hair cells, rapid adaptation is much faster in mammalian IHCs and OHCs than in nonmammalian hair cells.[214,247,271,303,526]

Myosin 1c (myosin 1β) may be the best candidate for the adaptation motor associated with slow adaptation (see Fig. 146-15C).[184,185,228] This view is supported by the observation that slow adaptation profiles are altered when myosin 1c mutations occur.[228] Recent studies suggest that myosin 1c also may influence fast adaptation profiles.[527] In addition, binding between the tip link–associated protein cadherin 23 and myosin 1c has been reported,[507] and the binding character is modulated by calmodulin and is sensitive to calcium chelators, which are known to break tip links.[411] Furthermore, although myosin 1c is detected in stereocilia from mice with abnormal copies of cadherin 23 or myosin VIIa, only in *Cdh23*-mutant mice is its stereociliary binding profile disrupted, suggesting that myosin 1c regulates the gating characteristics of the transduction channel by interacting with cadherin 23.[411] Finally, myosin 1c associates with PIP_2, which normally concentrated in the upper two thirds of the stereocilia, and agents that deplete or sequester PIP_2 significantly reduce the rates of fast and slow adaptation, suggesting that the complex has a role in the regulation of the adaptation process.[221]

Although in early studies it was determined that myosin 1c was localized in the tips of stereocilia, or near each end of the tip link in vestibular hair cells,[178,185,211,531] more recent studies of mammalian auditory hair cells suggest that myosin 1c is distributed throughout the entire stereocilium, and not at the very tip.[483] Accordingly, the protein may play different or additional roles in hair cells of the mammalian auditory system. In that regard, abnormal adaptation profiles have been observed in auditory hair cells of *Myo7a*-mutant mice, indicating that myosin VIIa may anchor or play a role in anchoring transduction channels to the actin core.[302] Moreover, as indicated by the observation that myosin IIIa is localized in the lower insertion site of the tip link, this protein may influence adaptation indirectly by exerting tension at the tip of the stereociliary membrane.[483] Further experimentation is clearly needed to identify the motor of adaptation and to determine the precise role(s) of myosin 1c in auditory hair cells.

Effects of Deficiencies of Other Hair Cell Channels on Hearing

Numerous K^+ channels have been identified in the basolateral membrane of vertebrate hair cells (Fig. 146-13), including BK (large-conductance, Ca^{2+}-activated K^+ channels), SK2 (small conductance Ca^{2+}-activated K^+ channels), and KCNQ4. It is notable that mutations in the gene that encodes KCNQ4 result in the autosomal dominant (DFNA2) form of deafness,[304] a finding that implicates the channel as a particularly important factor in inner ear potassium homeostasis. Persons carrying the mutant allele gradually acquire hearing loss, first in the high-frequency portion of the audible spectrum and slowly progressing to include lower frequencies, suggesting that the mutation leads to slow degeneration of hair cells. KCNQ4 is strongly expressed in OHCs but also has been detected in IHCs.[40,276,392] It appears that the protein is an essential component of the channel that carries the major K^+ current in OHCs, the outwardly rectifying $I_{K,n}$ current,[229,235,275,351] because targeted mutations of *Kcnq4* result in loss of $I_{K,n}$ in OHCs, both in vivo[275] and in organotypic cultures of transfected hair cells.[229] Although response thresholds of mutant mice improve during the first 3 postnatal weeks of life, normal sensitivity is never achieved, and thresholds progressively deteriorate thereafter, reaching a plateau loss of approximately 60 dB, the rate of loss being dependent on which specific mutation is expressed.[275] Hair cell degeneration is the expected histologic correlate of the hearing loss in mutant animals, and the process starts in the base of the cochlear spiral and progresses apically. IHCs are preserved throughout the cochlea and OHCs are preserved in the apical turn. Whereas IHCs from mutant animals are slightly more depolarized at rest when compared with control subjects, OHCs from mutant animals are more significantly depolarized at rest, suggesting that the hearing loss of DFNA2 is the consequence of chronic OHC depolarization resulting from loss of the ability to extrude K^+, which leads in turn to OHC degeneration.[275]

The principal K^+ current in IHCs, on the other hand, is the fast, voltage- and Ca^{2+}-activated current, $I_{K,f}$, which is carried by BK channels[301] composed of α-, β1-, and β4-subunit.[311] Of interest, cochlear thresholds in mice lacking the BKβ1- or the BKβ4-subunit, or both, are normal, strongly suggesting that neither subunit is critical for hearing.[424,464] Nevertheless, an early report suggested that OHCs do indeed degenerate in *BKα*-deficient mice, a condition leading to high-frequency hearing loss[464]; other studies suggest that cochlear thresholds and frequency selectivity are normal in mutant animals.[393,424] However, although IHCs from *BKα*-deficient mice are slightly depolarized at rest, maximum driven discharge rates are reduced, and timing, measured as both increased jitter in first-spike latency and reduced phase-locking, is impaired in many auditory nerve fiber responses. These findings clearly indicate that BK channels play a key role in the temporal processing of acoustic signals.[393]

Although the impact of SK2 channel abnormalities per se on hearing has not been studied, affected animals exhibit Preyer's reflex, and voltage-gated ionic currents (other than those produced by SK2) in hair cells generally are unaffected.[256,294] However, SK2 channels are known to play an essential role in the maintenance of repetitive spiking activity of immature IHCs,[256] which may have a long-term influence on the normal maturation of the end organ. Of interest, efferent-mediated synaptic currents are absent in OHCs of SK2 mutants, as well as in immature IHCs, which are known to receive a transient cholinergic innervation during maturation.[294] In addition, the absence of SK2 leads to a significant reduction in the efferent innervation of OHCs, and OHC responses to cholinergic agents are absent, suggesting that the SK2 channel regulates or maintains the functional status of acetylcholine receptors.[294] Olivocochlear innervation also is disrupted in mice with deficiencies in the α9- or α10-subunit of nicotinic acetylcholine receptors, although these subunits are not necessary for the development of normal cochlear thresholds.[578,579]

Because the transduction channel is highly permeable to Ca^{2+},[87,113,345,389,437] a mechanism must exist for its extrusion after depolarization. This generally is accomplished by means of the action of plasma membrane Ca^{2+}-ATPases.[344] Pmca2 (also known as Atp2b2) is the primary Ca^{2+}-ATPase isoform expressed in hair bundles,[93,134] where it is found in high concentrations, with estimates reaching approximately 2000 molecules/μm^2 of stereocilia membrane.[28,93,532,624] Mutations in the *Pmca2* gene produce the phenotype observed in deafwaddler (*dfw*) mice, and the consequences of targeted deletion of the gene are deafness and vestibular abnormality.[298,532] In addition, heterozygous $Pmca2^{+/-}$ mice are more susceptible to noise-induced hearing loss,[297] and the severity of age-related hearing loss in mice carrying the mutant *ahl* allele of *Cdh23* (i.e., modifier of deafwaddler [*mdfw*]) is increased by heterozygosity for dysfunctional Pmca2.[384,385] A similar exacerbation in the severity of autosomal recessive hearing loss associated with a missense mutation in *CDH23* by a hypofunctional variant of PMCA2 is observed in humans and underlines the importance of Ca^{2+} homeostasis in the inner ear.[486]

Finally, mice that are deficient in voltage-gated L-type Ca^{2+} channels ($Ca_V1.3$, Cacna1D, or D-LTCC), which are responsible for most of the voltage-gated Ca^{2+} entry into IHCs by way of the basolateral membrane, are congenitally deaf.[420] It generally is thought that the current carried by these L-type Ca^{2+} channels control neurotransmitter release. Degenerative changes in both IHCs and OHCs, as well as spiral ganglion cells, have been observed early in postnatal life,[188] suggesting that this channel is indispensable for normal hearing.

Defects in Hair Cell–Afferent Dendrite Synapses Lead to Deafness

In addition to the requirement for calcium entry into IHCs for normal synaptic transmission, an event that is dependent on the Ca^{2+} channels composed of $Ca_V1.3$ subunits reviewed earlier, the hair cell–afferent dendrite synapse is distinct from other synapses in several ways. First, and perhaps foremost, the synapse in question is characterized by a large presynaptic dense body commonly referred to as a "ribbon." Each afferent dendrite receives input from a single "ribbon synapse" (Fig. 146-17A). The physical arrangement of vesicles attached to the ribbon is thought to provide a readily and continuously available pool of synaptic vesicles that can support a highly efficient and coordinated process of vesicular exocytosis that leads in turn to the synchronous release of neurotransmitter when hair cell depolarization occurs. Such a system is optimally designed to support fine temporal coding of acoustic stimuli.[386] IHC–afferent ribbon synapses also exhibit molecular specializations that differ in some ways from conventional synapses, as well as ribbon synapses found in association with other pathways. For example, IHC ribbon synapses lack synaptophysin, synapsin, and synaptotagmins I and II,[322] and they contain the proteins Ribeye and Piccolo, as well as the presynaptic scaffolding protein Bassoon (see Fig. 146-17B). It is thought that Bassoon is required to anchor the ribbon to the presynaptic membrane.[277] Mice deficient in Bassoon exhibit abnormal ABRs, elevated thresholds, a reduced rate of "fast" exocytosis, and normal DPOAEs—a constellation of characteristics that satisfy the definition of auditory neuropathy.[277]

When depolarized, $Ca_V1.3$ channels open and allow calcium to rapidly enter the cell, and intracellular Ca^{2+} activates the protein otoferlin, which in turn triggers the fusion of synaptic vesicles with the presynaptic membrane and subsequent vesicular exocytosis at the hair

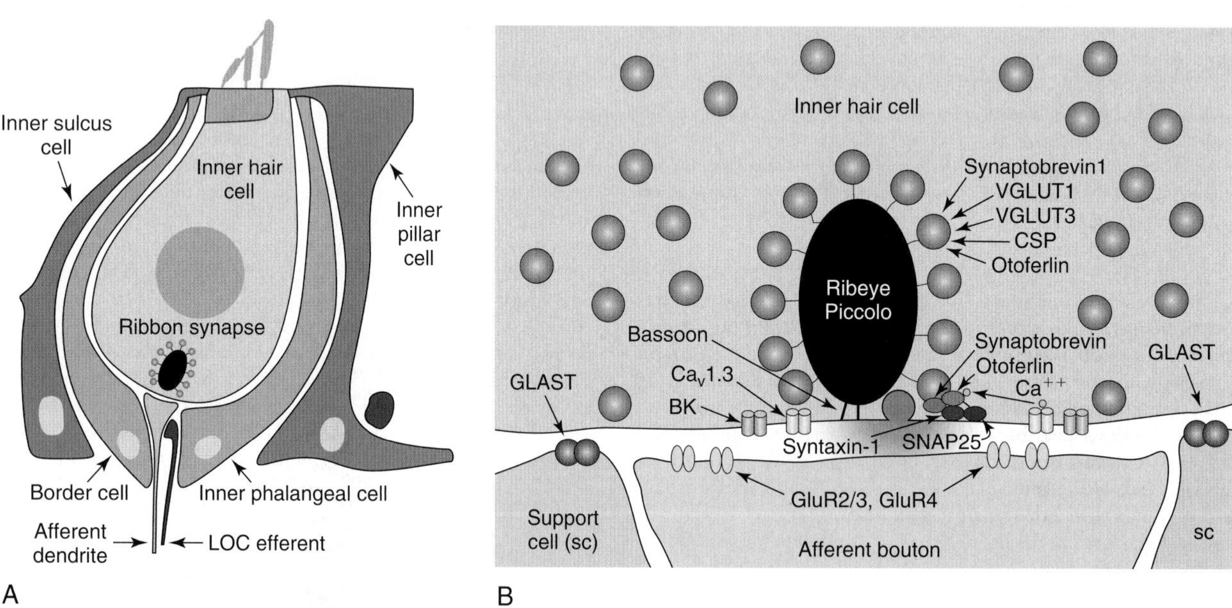

Figure 146-17. A, Schematic illustration of an inner hair cell (IHC) and a ribbon synapse with a type I radial afferent dendrite. Supporting cells shown include a border cell located adjacent to the modiolar side of the IHC and an inner phalangeal cell located on the opposite side; an inner sulcus cell and inner pillar cell also are illustrated. A lateral olivocochlear efferent fiber (LOC) is depicted making an axodendritic contact with the radial afferent fiber. **B,** Drawing of a single IHC ribbon synapse and proteins associated with the synapse. The synaptic ribbon is an electron dense body, holding numerous synaptic vesicles *(blue spheres)*, anchored to the presynaptic membrane. BK, large-conductance Ca^{2+}-activated K^+ channel; CSP, cystein-string protein; GluR, glutamate receptor; GLAST, glutamate-aspartate transporter; SNAP-25, synaptosomal-associated protein 25kDa; VGLUT, vesicular glutamate transporter. *(**A,** Adapted from Ruel J, Wang J, Rebillard G, et al. Physiology, pharmacology and plasticity at the inner hair cell synaptic complex.* Hear Res. *2007;227:19; **B,** adapted from Fuchs PA, Glowatzki E, Moser T. The afferent synapse of cochlear hair cells.* Curr Opin Neurobiol. *2003;13:452 and Nouvian R, Beutner D, Parsons TD, Moser T. Structure and function of the hair cell ribbon synapse.* J Membr Biol. *2006;209:153.)*

cell–afferent bouton synapse. Like synaptotagmin in conventional synapses, otoferlin acts as a Ca^{2+} sensor and interacts, in a calcium-dependent manner, with the t-SNARE proteins syntaxin-1 and SNAP-25, which are integrated into the presynaptic plasma membrane. The v-SNARE protein synaptobrevin (the vesicle-associated membrane protein [VAMP]) is located within the synaptic vesicle[468] and when activated initiates fusion of the exocytic vesicle with the presynaptic plasma membrane and subsequent release of neurotransmitter into the synaptic cleft. Mutations in otoferlin result in autosomal recessive, prelingual deafness (DFNB9) in humans,[626] and otoferlin-deficient mice also are congenitally deaf.[455] Although ABRs cannot be elicited from targeted null mice, presumably a consequence of failed vesicular exocytosis, ribbon synapses appear intact from a histologic perspective, and DPOAEs are normal; a clear case of auditory neuropathy. Interestingly, however, ABRs can be elicited electrically in null mice, suggesting that DFNB9 patients may be prime candidates for cochlear implants.

Other vesicular proteins of interest include the cysteine-string protein (CSP) is also found in hair cell vesicles[153] and is thought to act as a co-chaperone and protect tonically active synapses from neurodegeneration.[481] The vesicular glutamate transporters VGLUT1[174] and VLGUT3, the latter an unconventional but essential transporter, are located in the synaptic vesicle membrane and are responsible for loading L-glutamate into synaptic vesicles. Mutations in VGLUT3 (SLC17A8) lead to progressive deafness (DFNA25) in humans,[457] as well as in targeted null mice.[457,490] The glutamate-aspartate transporter (GLAST), or excitatory amino acid transporter 1 (EAAT1), is located on adjacent support cells (border and inner phalangeal cells) and is responsible for uptake and recycling of glutamate.[174,186] GLAST-deficient mice accumulate excess glutamate in the perilymph and are more susceptible than normal to acoustic overstimulation. This finding is consistent with the view that GLAST has a significant role to play in the clearance of glutamate from the extracellular milieu and, in doing so, protecting dendrites from glutamate neurotoxity.[206] Neurotransmitter-induced activation of the ionotropic AMPA-type receptors GluR2/3 and GluR4, located in postsynaptic afferent boutons,[355] leads to depolarization of the primary afferent dendrite and transmission of encoded acoustic information to the central nervous system.

Auditory Neuropathy

Auditory neuropathy–type pathologic conditions have been associated with a number of mutated genes that encode proteins located in the presynaptic compartment of the IHC–afferent dendrite synapse, as shown in the previous section. Perhaps those pathologic conditions should be thought of as auditory "synaptopathy"–type pathologic processes because of their locus of origin. These proteins prominently include the $Ca_V1.3$ subunit, Bassoon, otoferlin, and VGLUT3 (SLC71A8). In the following discussion, pathologic conditions associated with synaptic protein abnormalities are differentiated from those that fit more neatly into the "true" auditory neuropathy category—those that are associated with the nerve fiber itself. A good representative of a true auditory neuropathy model is the spontaneous mutant mouse *quivering*, in which defects in the protein β-spectrin 4 (Spnb4) lead to the abnormal distribution of ion channels in spiral ganglion axons, as well as axons of other peripheral and central neurons.[401] In mutant mice, the voltage-gated potassium channel Kcna1 is abnormally distributed along the length of auditory nerve axons, rather than being localized in a juxtaparanodal cluster as in normal animals. β-Spectrin 4 normally is detected in axonal initial segments and the nodes of Ranvier of nerve fibers, and it is generally suspected that the protein may serve to anchor ion channels to the juxtaparanodal region in myelinated nerve fibers and thereby influence saltatory nerve fiber conduction. Response amplitudes and latencies of ABR wave I are distinctly abnormal in β-spectrin 4–mutant mice, and later occurring peaks generally are absent from the response waveform. Likewise, disruption of the myelin sheath of the auditory nerve due to defects in peripheral myelin protein 22 (PMP22) or myelin protein zero (MPZ), also denoted P_0, as observed in Charcot-Marie-Tooth syndrome types 1A[296] and 1B,[212] respectively, leads to true auditory neuropathy in both humans and mice.[638] As in the case of β-spectrin 4–mutant mice, ion channel distributions in auditory nerve fiber axons are disrupted in these animal models as well.[233,593]

Perilymphatic-Endolymphatic Barrier

Normal mechanoelectrical transduction requires the separation of the endolymphatic and perilymphatic inner ear compartments, and the barrier that divides the major perilymph filled scalae from scala media is fashioned by tight junctions that form at the boundaries between cells that limit the endolymphatic space (Fig. 146-18A). These barriers, naturally, prevent the passage of water, ions, and molecules through intercellular spaces (see Fig. 146-18B), thereby maintaining a unique endocochlear milieu and separating the environment of the hair cells' apical surface from the basolateral plasma membrane of the cell by virtue of tight junctions formed between cells that make up the reticular lamina. To maintain this separate endolymphatic compartment, tight junctions are found in all epithelial cells lining the boundaries of the scala media, including the sensory epithelium, supporting cells within the sensory epithelium, cells lining the inner and outer sulci and the spiral limbus, marginal cells of the stria vascularis, and cells of Reissner's membrane. In addition, tight junctions are found in basal cells of the stria vascularis, forming an intrastrial compartment that is separate from both endolymph and perilymph.

Proteins of the claudin family (see Fig. 146-18C) are essential tight junction elements that form connections with the actin cytoskeleton by way of the protein zona occludens 1 (ZO-1), which has been identified as a component of the reticular lamina,[425] the scaffold protein shroom2, and myosin VIIa (see Fig. 146-18D).[146] Mutations in the gene (*CLDN14*) that encodes claudin 14, which is localized in the sensory epithelium, are responsible for an autosomal recessive form of deafness known as DFNB29.[606] Targeted deletion of *Cldn14* in the mouse leads to deafness associated with OHC degeneration that is followed by IHC degeneration. It generally is presumed that cellular death observed under these conditions is due to the increased permeability of cations through cells composing the paracellular pathway of the reticular lamina.[45] Although the endocochlear potential is normal in affected animals, claudin 14 is nonetheless required for the maintenance of the endolymphatic-perilymphatic ionic barrier, which breaks down in its absence. By contrast, tight junctions between strial basal cells are composed of claudin 11, and animals with null mutations in the encoding gene have reduced endocochlear potentials and elevated thresholds, although potassium recycling appears to be normal.[195,290] Moreover, specialized tight junctions connecting tricellular contact points composed of the protein tricellulin (see Fig. 146-18E) are essential for hearing and are responsible for autosomal recessive deafness (DFNB49) when dysfunctional.[435] Mutations associated with other components of tight junction–adherens junction complexes will almost certainly prove to be responsible for as yet unknown statoacoustic abnormalities in both human and nonhuman animals.

Endolymph Homeostasis

Homeostatic mechanisms involving the maintenance of separate endolymphatic and perilymphatic compartments, as well as preservation of the normal ionic environments within each scala, are essential for normal auditory function. Numerous genes, including several genes encoding gap junction proteins (Fig. 146-19), that alter homeostasis and are responsible for hereditary hearing impairments when mutated have been identified. The functions of a subset of these proteins are described in the following paragraphs.

It generally is understood that extrusion and recycling of K^+ after the depolarization of sensory cells are necessary components of mechanoelectrical transduction (Fig. 146-20). As described earlier, after entering hair cells through transduction channels, K^+ ions are extruded through channels located in the basolateral membrane, and enter the extracellular perilymphatic space. Once extruded, the K^+-Cl^- cotransporters Kcc3 and Kcc4, proteins that are encoded by *Slc12a6* and *Slc12a7*, respectively, take K^+ up by way of Deiters cells, which are situated underneath OHCs, and phalangeal cells that surround IHCs.[55,56] Kcc3 also is found in other epithelial cells of the organ of Corti, as well as type I and type III fibrocytes of the spiral ligament.[56] Absence of either protein produces a progressive form of deafness

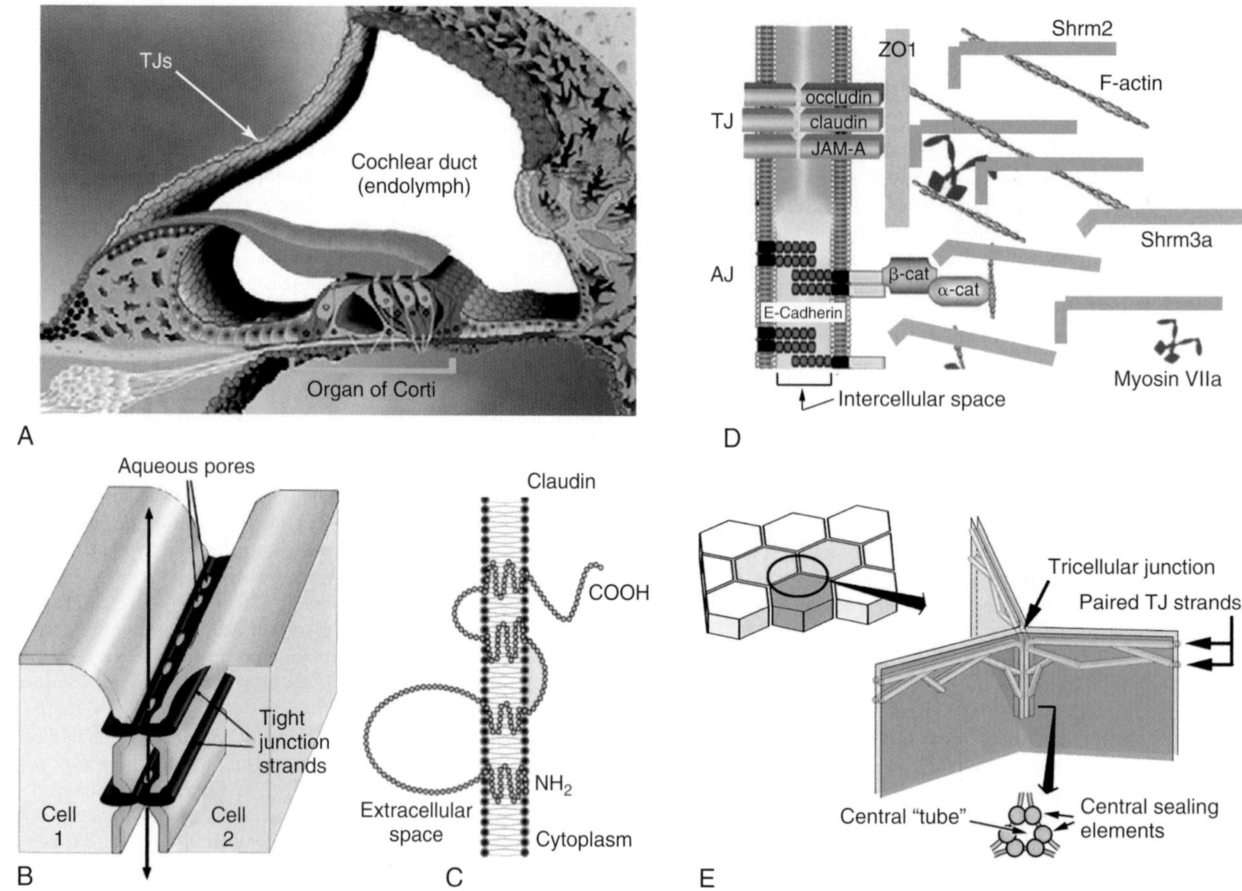

Figure 146-18. A, Schematic representation of the location of tight junctions (TJs), composed of claudin-14 within the epithelial barrier forming the cochlear duct, and those composed of claudin-11 between strial intermediate cells forming the barrier between intrastrial fluid and perilymph. **B,** Representation of bicellular TJ strands connecting the most apical region of the lateral membrane of two adjacent cells. TJs function as barriers to establish distinct fluid compartments separating the apical surface of the epithelial cells from the basolateral compartment by preventing admixture of molecules located above the apical surface of the cells from those surrounding the lateral membranes. TJ strands associate laterally with those in apposing membranes, forming paired strands. The aqueous pores regulate the passive paracellular passage *(arrow)* of ions, water, and various molecules, and these vary among epithelial cells in terms of size and charge selectivity. **C,** Proteins in the claudin family are integrally responsible for the formation of TJ strands and have four transmembrane domains and two extracellular loops, and both the amino and carboxyl termini are located on the intracellular side of the membrane. **D,** Claudins located on adjacent cells can form homotypic as well as heterotypic associations, resulting in intercellular adhesion, and they connect to the actin cytoskeleton by means of the scaffolding protein zona occludens 1 (ZO-1), as well as other members of the ZO family. Occludin and the junctional adhesion molecule (JAM-A) also are transmembrane components of TJs, sealing the paracellular space. Shroom 2 and 3a (Shrm2, Shrm3a) are proteins associated with TJs and adherens junctions (AJs), respectively, that may form a network between the actin cytoskeleton and unconventional myosins, such as myosin VIIa, which also is located at the site of TJs. **E,** Schematic illustration of the organization of tricellular TJs, composed of the essential protein tricellulin, as well as occludin. TJs between two adjacent cells become discontinuous at tricellular contact zones and extend basolaterally, forming a central tube; the tricellular TJs become vertically oriented and are composed of three pairs of TJ strands called "central sealing elements," forming a paracellular barrier at tricellular contacts. *(**A** and **D,** Adapted with permission from Etournay R, Zwaenepoel I, Perfettini I, et al. Shroom2, a myosin-VIIa- and actin-binding protein, directly interacts with ZO-1 at tight junctions.* J Cell Sci. *2007;120:2838; **B** and **C,** adapted from Tsukita S, Furuse ML. The structure and function of claudins, cell adhesion molecules at tight junctions.* Ann NY Acad Sci. *2000;915:129; **E,** from Ikenouchi J, Furuse M, Furuse K, et al. Tricellulin constitutes a novel barrier at tricellular contacts of epithelial cells.* J Cell Biol. *2005;171:939.)*

in mice beginning near the onset of hearing. Pathology progresses faster in the case of Kcc4 null mice. Hair cell loss is observed in affected animals, and loss of Kcc4 also is associated with renal tubular acidosis.

K^+ taken up by support cells then diffuses through gap junctions to other epithelial cells of the outer sulcus that include Hensen and Claudius cells and into root cells of the spiral ligament,[245,284,477] where the ion is extruded into the extracellular space within the connective tissue of the spiral ligament. Type II fibrocytes, which express Na^+,K^+-ATPase (ATPA1 and ATPB1) and the Na^+-K^+-$2Cl^-$ (Slc12a2, Nkcc1) transporter,[92,484,485,522] take up K^+, which then passes through gap junctions to type I fibrocytes and into basal cells and intermediate cells of the stria vascularis. Intermediate cells that contain KCNJ10 channels extrude K^+ into the intrastrial space,[23,353] where it is taken up by the basolateral membranes of marginal cells, through Na^+-K^+-$2Cl^-$ (Slc12a2, Nkcc1) transporters[295,354,594] and Na^+-K^+-ATPase, including the ATP1A1, ATP1B1, and ATP1B2 subunits.[360,409,484,485,543] In addition, the marginal cell basolateral membrane contains Cl^- channels that associate with a protein called Barttin, encoded by *BSND* (*B*artter syndrome with *s*ensori*n*eural *d*eafness, or Bartter syndrome type IV), which forms the β-subunit required to transport ClC-Ka and ClC-Kb channels to the plasma membrane.[24,53,145,216,469] These channels are responsible for passive diffusion of Cl^- into the intrastrial space. Marginal cells secrete K^+ from their apical membrane by way of heteromeric K^+ channels composed of KCNQ1 (KvLQT1) and KCNE1 (IsK) subunits into scala media.[352,471,500,594,596]

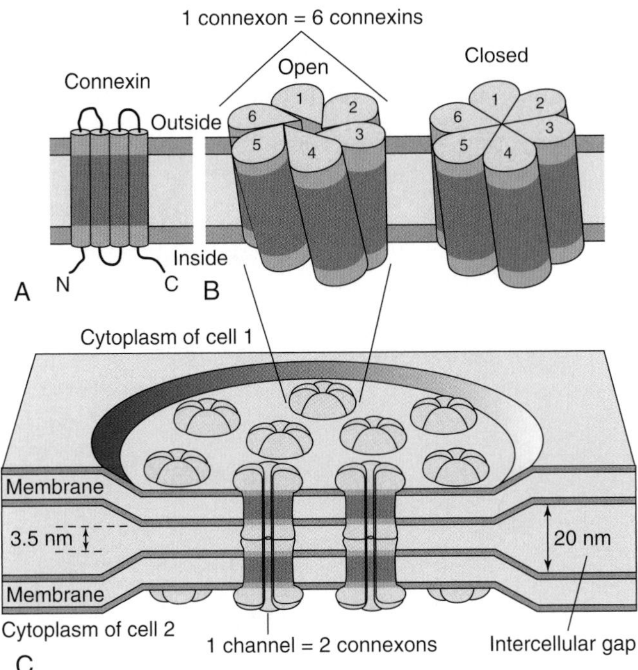

Figure 146-19. A, Gap junctions, which allow the direct passage of low-molecular-weight ions, second messengers, and metabolites (less than 1 kDa in size) between the cytoplasm of adjacent cells, are formed by the connexin family of proteins. Each connexin molecule has four transmembrane α-helical domains, and the amino and carboxyl termini are located intracellularly. Six connexins assemble to form a connexon or hemichannel (**B**). Connexons of adjacent cells form apposing partners to form a gap junction (**C**). Different types of channels can be formed, depending upon the combination of connexin proteins assembling to form the connexon, and depending upon the combination of connexons forming the channel. The channel pore can be regulated by protein kinase C, Ca^{2+}, calmodulin, cyclic adenosine monophosphate (cAMP), and pH, as well as other factors. Aggregates of gap junctions form large semicrystalline arrays where the apposing plasma membranes are in close proximity (3.5 nm) compared with the typical extracellular distance between cells (20 nm). *(**A** to **C**, Modified from Kandel ER, Siegelbaum SA, Schwartz JH. Synaptic transmission. In: Kandel ER, Schwartz JH, Jessel TM, eds.* Principles in Neural Science. *New York: Elsevier; 1991:123.)*

Numerous proteins that are components of gap junctions have been identified in the cochlea, including the connexins CX26 (GJB2), CX30 (GJB6), and CX31 (GJB3). These proteins are particularly evident in supporting cells, interdental cells of the spiral limbus, root cells, and fibrocytes, as well as in basal and intermediate cells of the stria vascularis.[164,166,169,258,284,312,313,615-617] Mutations of the *GJB2* gene cause autosomal recessive and autosomal dominant forms of deafness (DFNB1, DFNA3), in addition to syndromic conditions that include deafness.[114,269,439,441] Mutations of *GJB6* also are responsible for autosomal recessive (DFNB1)[108] and autosomal dominant (DFNA3)[197] forms of deafness, and mutations in *GJB3* are associated with autosomal dominant (DFNA2)[618] and autosomal recessive forms of hearing loss.[340]

Similarly, genetically targeted ablation or mutation of CX26[79,305] or CX30[544] in mice results in hearing impairment, with associated degeneration of supporting cells in the organ of Corti, initially in the region of IHCs, followed by hair cell loss. These findings suggest that both CX26 and CX30 play a particularly important role in organ of Corti homeostasis. Similar degeneration of the sensorineural epithelium was observed in a human temporal bone associated with CX26-related hearing loss.[260]

Mutations in KCNQ1 (KVLQT1) or KCNE1 cause deafness associated with Jervell and Lange-Nielsen syndrome, as well as cardiac manifestations including a prolonged QT interval.[382,487,561] In addition, the endolymphatic compartment of transgenic mice lacking Kcnq1[66,315] or KCNE1,[580] or mice carrying spontaneous mutations of *Kcne1*,[323] is collapsed, and affected animals are deaf. Mutations in *BSND* cause Bartter syndrome, which is associated with sensorineural deafness and kidney failure,[53] suggesting that Cl^- extrusion from marginal cells into the intrastrial fluid space is essential for hearing. Similarly, mice with targeted disruption of *Bsnd* in the inner ear exhibit congenitally elevated thresholds as a result of a reduction in endocochlear potential, although the K^+ concentration in endolymph remains normal.[447] Of interest, mice lacking the ClC-Ka subunit are not deaf,[356] suggesting that the channel formed by the ClC-Kb subunit is sufficient for hearing. Targeted deletion of the *Nkcc1* (Slc12a2) gene that encodes the Na^+-K^+-$2Cl^-$ transporter protein in mice leads to deafness,[110,157] and a spontaneously occurring mutation in the gene is responsible for deafness in the mouse mutant called no syndactylism (*sy-ns*), which is transmitted as an autosomal recessive trait.[124] These findings suggest that abnormalities of this protein may cause human deafness as a consequence of defective endolymph secretion. In transgenic mice lacking the KCNJ10 (Kir4.1) channel, the endocochlear potential is eliminated, endolymphatic K^+ concentration is reduced, and Reissner's membrane is partially collapsed, producing deafness as assessed by absent Preyer's reflexes,[353] and sensory cells degenerate early in the postnatal period,[456] suggesting that KCNJ10 is necessary for providing the force for endocochlear potential generation.

Ablation of the *Pou3f4* gene, located on the X chromosome and known to encode a POU transcription factor expressed in fibrocytes of the spiral ligament, results in a reduced endocochlear potential and profound deafness in mice,[366,414] as does a spontaneous mutation named sex-linked fidget (*slf*).[412] Not surprisingly, developmental defects in the formation of the cochlea also are known to occur in affected animals, including an enlarged internal auditory meatus, stapes malformation, a reduction in the number of cochlear turns, thinning of the bony capsule and spiral limbus, and reduced scala tympani volume. Pou3f4 is expressed extensively in cochlear tissues of mesenchymal origin during development.[413] In humans, mutations of *POU3F4* are associated with X-linked (DFN3) deafness, resulting from both a conductive hearing loss caused by stapes fixation and progressive sensorineural pathology.[106] Reports also indicate that persons carrying this mutation seem to produce large volumes of perilymphatic flow (perilymphatic "gusher") during stapes surgery and exhibit abnormally large internal auditory meatuses.

Other ion transporters involved with homeostasis include pendrin (SLC26A4, PDS), an anion exchanger associated with Pendred's syndrome and prelingual profound deafness, and DFNB4,[325] which involves enlargement of the vestibular aqueduct.[410] Pendrin is expressed in cells of the spiral prominence and in the endolymphatic duct and sac,[152] where it may function to secrete bicarbonate into endolymph[595] and maintain pH homeostasis. Targeted disruption of the *Pds* gene in mice results in deafness and hair cell degeneration.[150,595] Although essential components of the proposed pathway described here remain to be identified, it is clear that homeostasis within the endolymphatic compartment is essential for hearing.

Summary

In the 21st century, the prospect of rescuing the victims of deafness from a life of relative isolation is bright, but the challenge to make sense of the complex interplay between genes and environment that shape the peripheral auditory system is more than significant. As has been emphasized throughout this chapter, the molecular and genetic basis of transduction is complex, and the molecular and cellular mechanisms for both transduction and deafness require further elucidation. Despite the steep learning curve for scientists around the world, reflecting an enormous and an emerging database centered on the role of integral proteins in the development and maintenance of inner ear anatomy and physiology, the precise mechanism of action is understood for only a small number of the known gene products that work harmoniously to support effective mechanoelectrical transduction, we are

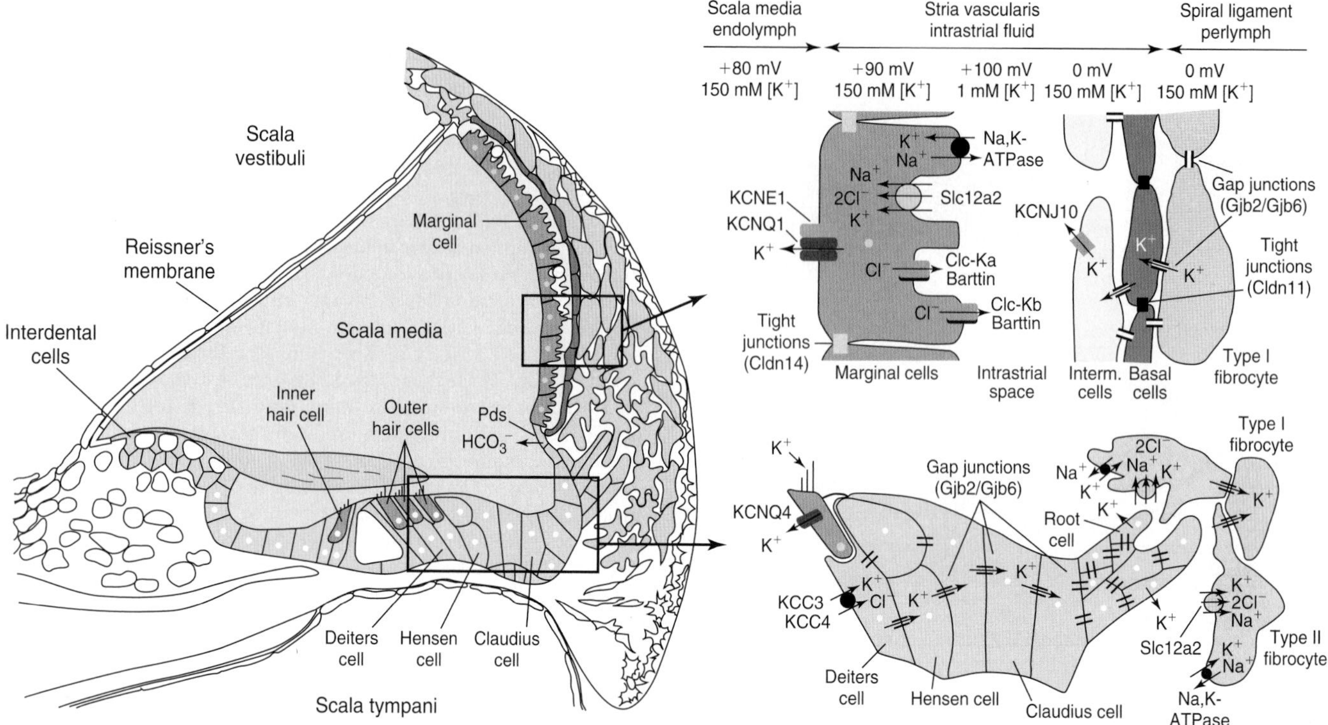

Figure 146-20. A proposed scheme for ion transport within the cochlea focused on K^+ circulation from cells within the stria vascularis *(upper right)* to the endolymphatic compartment *(left)*, through the sensory cells, and transportation back to the stria vascularis through the epithelial cell gap junction network into the outer spiral sulcus, and then through the connective tissue gap junction network of the spiral ligament *(lower right)*. Although the illustrated scheme is focused on a laterally oriented pathway from the organ of Corti toward the spiral ligament, a medial pathway has been proposed as well.[523] Several key proteins within this pathway have been identified as essential for normal hearing. See text for details. *(Modified from Heller S. Application of physiological genomics to the study of hearing disorders.* J Physiol. *2002;543:3.)*

nonetheless on the brink of what promises to be a breathtaking period of achievement.

Acknowledgments

We thank Michael Walsh and Skip Kennedy for their assistance with figure development.

SUGGESTED READINGS

Brown SD, Hardisty-Hughes RE, Mburu P. Quiet as a mouse: dissecting the molecular and genetic basis of hearing. *Nat Rev Genet.* 2008;9:277.

Dallos P. Cochlear amplification, outer hair cells and prestin. *Curr Opin Neurobiol.* 2008;18:370.

Friedman LM, Dror AA, Avraham KB. Mouse models to study inner ear development and hereditary hearing loss. *Int J Dev Biol.* 2007;51:609.

Glowatzki E, Grant L, Fuchs P. Hair cell afferent synapses. *Curr Opin Neurobiol.* 2008;18:389.

Hudspeth AJ. Making an effort to listen: mechanical amplification in the ear. *Neuron.* 2008;59:530.

Jentsch TJ. CLC chloride channels and transporters: from genes to protein structure, pathology and physiology. *Crit Rev Biochem Mol Biol.* 2008;43:3.

Kelley MW. Cellular commitment and differentiation in the organ of Corti. *Int J Dev Biol.* 2007;51:571.

Kochhar A, Hildebrand MS, Smith RJ. Clinical aspects of hereditary hearing loss. *Genet Med.* 2007;9:393.

Kremer H, van Wijk E, Märker T, et al. Usher syndrome: molecular links of pathogenesis, proteins and pathways. *Hum Mol Genet.* 2006;15(Spec No 2):R262.

Kros CJ. How to build an inner hair cell: challenges for regeneration. *Hear Res.* 2007;227:3.

Lang F, Vallon V, Knipper M, et al. Functional significance of channels and transporters expressed in the inner ear and kidney. *Am J Physiol Cell Physiol.* 2007;293:C1187. Erratum in: *Am J Physiol Cell Physiol.* 2007;293: C2001.

Leibovici M, Safieddine S, Petit C. Mouse models for human hereditary deafness. *Curr Top Dev Biol.* 2008;84:385.

Manor U, Kachar B. Dynamic length regulation of sensory stereocilia. *Semin Cell Dev Biol.* 2008;19:502.

McHugh RK, Friedman RA. Genetics of hearing loss: allelism and modifier genes produce a phenotypic continuum. *Anat Rec A Discov Mol Cell Evol Biol.* 2006;288:370.

Morton CC, Nance WE. Newborn hearing screening—a silent revolution. *N Engl J Med.* 2006;354:2151.

Nayak GD, Ratnayaka HS, Goodyear RJ, et al. Development of the hair bundle and mechanotransduction. *Int J Dev Biol.* 2007;51:597.

Patuzzi R. Cochlear micromechanics and macromechanics. In: Dallos P, Popper AN, Fay RR, eds. *The Cochlea.* New York: Springer; 1996:186.

Richardson GP, Lukashkin AN, Russell IJ. The tectorial membrane: one slice of a complex cochlear sandwich. *Curr Opin Otolaryngol Head Neck Surg.* 2008;16:458.

Robles L, Ruggero MA. Mechanics of the mammalian cochlea. *Physiol Rev.* 2001;81:1305.

Sabag AD, Dagan O, Avraham KB. Connexins in hearing loss: a comprehensive overview. *J Basic Clin Physiol Pharmacol.* 2005;16:101.

Scherer SS, Wrabetz L. Molecular mechanisms of inherited demyelinating neuropathies. *Glia.* 2008;56:1578.

Tachibana M, Kobayashi Y, Matsushima Y. Mouse models for four types of Waardenburg syndrome. *Pigment Cell Res.* 2003;16:448.

Vollrath MA, Kwan KY, Corey DP. The micromachinery of mechanotransduction in hair cells. *Annu Rev Neurosci.* 2007;30:339.

Xing G, Chen Z, Cao X. Mitochondrial rRNA and tRNA and hearing function. *Cell Res.* 2007;17:227.

Zhao HB, Kikuchi T, Ngezahayo A, et al. Gap junctions and cochlear homeostasis. *J Membr Biol.* 2006;209:177.

For complete list of references log onto www.expertconsult.com.

CHAPTER ONE HUNDRED AND FORTY-SEVEN

Genetic Sensorineural Hearing Loss

Michael S. Hildebrand

Murad Husein

Richard J. H. Smith

Key Points

- It is estimated that at least 50% of congenital hearing impairment has a genetic origin.
- A hearing loss can be defined by numerous clinical criteria, including causality, time of onset, age of onset, clinical presentation, anatomic defect, severity, and frequency loss.
- The worldwide rate of profound hearing loss is 4 in every 10,000 infants born.
- The term *homozygosity* means that a person carries two identical alleles of a gene; *heterozygosity* represents the state in which a person carries two different variants of a given gene.
- The basic forms of inheritance can be mendelian (single-gene inheritance—autosomal or X-linked), mitochondrial, or complex (chromosomal, new mutations, germline mosaicism, genomic imprinting, polygenic, and multifactorial inheritance).
- Nonsyndromic hearing impairment in the absence of other phenotypic manifestations accounts for 70% of hereditary hearing loss.
- Mutations in *GJB2* have been shown to cause 50% of autosomal recessive nonsyndromic deafness in many world populations.
- Syndromic hearing impairment refers to deafness that cosegregates with other features, forming a recognizable constellation of findings known as a syndrome. Sensorineural deafness has been associated with more than 400 syndromes.
- The most common syndromic form of hereditary sensorineural hearing loss, Pendred syndrome, is inherited in an autosomal recessive fashion; affected individuals also have goiter.
- A well-performed patient history, physical examination, and audiologic evaluation are keys to assessing the cause of hearing loss, and may aid in ascertaining etiology.
- Prenatal diagnosis for some forms of hereditary hearing loss is technically possible by analysis of DNA extracted from fetal cells.
- Cochlear implantation is becoming an increasingly important option for individuals with severe to profound deafness.

It was famously put by Terry Savage that "… a child will hear his mother's voice for the rest of his life…." Many children never hear their mother's voice, however, and others do not hear it very well throughout their lives. Hearing loss is a common human sensory defect. The incidence of congenital hearing impairment is at least 1 child in every 1000 born.[1] A hearing impairment commonly involves damage to or loss of cochlear hair cells; this is referred to as a sensorineural hearing loss (SNHL). Individuals with SNHL are often referred to as deaf (lower case "d") by the community. The term *Deafness* (capital "D") is used to describe an individual with SNHL who is part of a cultural group based on their use of sign language for communication. Members of this group tend to be the offspring of Deaf parents and generally have congenital SNHL. In contrast, individuals who acquire SNHL later in childhood or adulthood generally do not use sign language and persist with oral communication. These individuals are usually not part of the Deaf community.

It is estimated that at least 50% of congenital hearing impairment has a genetic origin.[1] Late-onset hearing loss can also be caused by genetic defects. As understanding of the genetics of deafness increases, the role of the otolaryngologist in diagnosing, interpreting, and managing this form of hearing loss has mandated a basic understanding of genetics. This chapter provides an introduction to the genetics of hearing loss. An overview of hearing loss is followed by discussion of the fundamentals of genetics and a synopsis of syndromic and nonsyndromic deafness. The final section focuses on the clinical approach to a child with suspected genetic deafness and potential therapies for genetic hearing loss.

Background

Classification of Hearing Impairment

A hearing loss can be defined by numerous clinical criteria, including causality, time of onset, age of onset, clinical presentation, anatomic

Table 147-1

Hearing Loss Classification

Criteria	Classification	Comment
Causality	Genetic Environmental Multifactorial	Hereditary Nonhereditary
Time of onset	Congenital Acquired	At birth Late-onset
Age of onset	Prelingual Postlingual	Before speech development After speech development
Clinical presentation	Nonsyndromic Syndromic	Hearing loss only symptom Hearing loss and other symptoms
Anatomic defect	Conductive Sensorineural Mixed	Dysfunction of outer or middle ear Dysfunction of inner ear
Severity	Mild Moderate Moderately severe Severe Profound	Range 20-40 dB Range 41-55 dB Range 56-70 dB Range 71-90 dB Range >90 dB
Frequency loss	Low-frequency Midfrequency High-frequency	Range <500 Hz Range 501-2000 Hz Range >2000 Hz
Ears affected	Unilateral Bilateral	One ear affected Both ears affected
Prognosis	Stable Progressive	Severity remains unchanged Severity increases over time

defect, severity, and frequency loss (Table 147-1). Etiologically based classifications can be broadly divided into genetic versus nongenetic factors. This distinction is important because hereditary deafness does not imply congenital deafness; the latter describes a condition present from birth regardless of causality. Hereditary deafness may be present at birth or develop any time thereafter.

It is well known that heritable and environmental factors can make strong contributions to hearing loss. There are three types of anatomic defects—conductive, sensorineural, or a combination of both (mixed)—and these defects may arise from syndromic or nonsyndromic conditions. Generally, when discussing hereditary deafness, a clinically based classification reflecting the presence or absence of coinherited anomalies—that is, syndromic or nonsyndromic deafness—is most useful. Syndromic and nonsyndromic conditions can be subclassified by inheritance pattern as autosomal dominant, autosomal recessive, X-linked, mitochondrial, or complex. Hearing loss can also be distinguished by differences in severity and frequency loss. Additional features of a hearing loss that are assessed include whether one or both ears are affected, and the prognosis for the condition (see Table 147-1).

Although these classifications assist clinicians in their assessment of patients and lead to better clinical outcomes, they do not adequately represent the complex interactions that underlie most forms of hearing loss. This limitation is exemplified in hearing loss that is attributable to exposure to the ototoxic antibiotics, aminoglycosides. Although at high concentration these antibiotics interfere with the normal function of the cochlea, individuals with an A1555G mutation in their mitochondrial 12S rRNA gene are more susceptible to the ototoxic effect of these drugs.[2] In some cases, hearing loss is attributable to genetic and environmental factors, and this dual causality can make classifying hearing loss less informative.

Table 147-2

Quantification of Hearing Impairment

Impairment (%)	Pure Tone Average (dB)*	Residual Hearing (%)
100	91	0
80	78	20
60	65	40
30	45	70

*Pure tone average of 500 Hz, 1000 Hz, 2000 Hz, and 3000 Hz.

Diagnosis of Hearing Impairment

The primary diagnosis of hearing loss is by auditory testing to detect loss in hearing acuity. Hearing function is measured in decibels and is considered normal if the lowest level (threshold) a sound can be perceived is between 0 and 20 dB. The value of 0 dB is defined as the point at which a tone burst of a given frequency is perceived 50% of the time by a young adult. The severity and frequency loss sustained during a hearing impairment are given in Tables 147-1 and 147-2. Hearing acuity can be readily measured quantitatively and objectively by numerous physiologic tests, including auditory brainstem response (ABR) measurements, auditory steady-state responses, impedance testing (tympanometry), and otoacoustic emissions. For all these auditory tests except tympanometry, normal middle ear function is required for a normal response to be generated.

ABR testing records the electrophysiologic response of the auditory nerve (eighth cranial nerve) and brainstem to tone bursts (sound wave trains consisting of several cycles of the same frequency) or clicks (unidirectional rectangular voltage pushes) applied to the outer ear.[3,4] The waveform patterns are detected by electrodes connected to the skin, with maximal obtainable values at 94 to 100 dB sound pressure level. Sound pressure level refers to the ratio of the pressure of a sound wave to the standard air pressure level. Otoacoustic emissions are distinct from ABRs in that they are sounds generated only from the cochlea, and represent the activity of outer hair cells in response to transient or continuous stimulation. The emissions are measured in the external auditory canal, and are usually absent in individuals with hearing loss greater than 40 to 50 dB.[4]

The audiometry steady-state response has some similarity to the ABR, but the stimulus is continuous. A continuous tonal stimulus generates a higher sound pressure level than is possible with click stimuli, and allows a better estimation of hearing acuity in profoundly deaf individuals.[4] Impedance audiometry is used in conjunction with ABR, otoacoustic emissions, or auditory steady-state response testing because it does not measure hearing. This technique is used routinely to determine middle ear pressure, movement of the tympanic membrane and middle ear ossicles, and eustachian tube activity.[4]

Epidemiology of Hearing Impairment

Hearing loss is a prevalent human sensory defect. The worldwide rate of profound hearing loss is 4 in every 10,000 infants born.[5,6] The rate of SNHL determined in universal newborn screening programs in developed countries of 2 to 4 children per 1000 born compares favorably with this figure.[7,8] The incidence of congenital SNHL in developing countries is likely to be much higher,[9,10] although more data are required. The implications for the personal and social development of these children are significant.

Historical Background of Genetics

Mendel is considered the father of modern genetics. His work formulating the fundamentals of heredity by experimenting on the garden pea is well known to all school students. From this work, he postulated the principles of segregation and independent assortment, publishing these concepts in 1865. In the early 1900s, the impact of these ideas was recognized. Johannsen described the basic unit of heredity as the gene in 1909, and Avery showed that genes are composed of deoxyribonucleic acid (DNA) in 1944. In 1953, Watson and Crick described the physical structure of DNA, and 3 years later, the correct number of human chromosomes was confirmed to be 46. Sequencing these chromosomes was the goal of the Human Genome Project, initiated in 1991 and completed with first-pass data in 2001. The impact of this project on medicine has been tremendous, with the field of genetic deafness being just one of many areas of medical science to have flourished. A list of the current known deafness genes can be found on the Hereditary Hearing Loss Homepage.[11]

Fundamentals of Genetics

Each person has 46 chromosomes—22 pairs of autosomes and one pair of sex chromosomes (XY in males or XX in females). According to Mendel's principle of segregation, in sexually reproducing organisms, each partner contributes only one member of each chromosome pair to an offspring. This fact means that each individual has inherited one copy of each chromosome from each parent. Carried on these chromosomes are genes, estimated to number approximately 30,000. Variations in these genes impart uniqueness to each individual. These variations, termed *alleles,* can sometimes be deleterious.

If a mutation occurs in the normal or wild-type sequence of a gene expressed in the inner ear, and if the protein translated from this new allele variant does not function as well as the normal protein, deafness may result. If the remaining normal protein (recall that each gene is represented in duplicate) is able to cover for the abnormal protein, however, deafness manifests only in the individuals who carry two copies of the abnormal gene. This scenario is an example of autosomal recessive inheritance. If the abnormal protein interferes with the normal protein function, deafness manifests in an individual carrying a single abnormal gene. This scenario is an example of autosomal dominant inheritance.

In describing these inheritance patterns, we are describing a person's genotype or genetic makeup. The term *homozygosity* means that a person carries two identical alleles of a gene; *heterozygosity* represents the state in which a person carries two different variants of a given gene. The observable consequence that derives from an individual's genotype is his or her *phenotype.* Often individuals carrying identical genetic mutations exhibit a spectrum of different phenotypic features. Not every person with Waardenburg's syndrome type 1 has synophrys, premature graying of the hair, or heterochromia irides, a phenomenon called *variable expressivity.* In some cases, the phenotype can be so subtle as to be entirely absent, and the causative genetic mutation is said to be incomplete or nonpenetrant. This occurrence can give the impression that a disease "skips" generations.

Patterns of Inheritance

The basic forms of inheritance can be mendelian (single-gene inheritance—autosomal or X-linked), mitochondrial, or complex (chromosomal, new mutations, germline mosaicism, genomic imprinting, polygenic, and multifactorial inheritance). Pedigrees for these inheritance patterns are shown in Figure 147-1. Mendelian and mitochondrial forms of inheritance are discussed in this chapter; for the reader who is interested in complex forms of inheritance, we recommend more appropriate texts.[12,13] Punnett squares are used to show inheritance patterns by displaying the outcomes of crosses with both parents and allowing probability estimates for the offspring (Fig. 147-2).

Autosomal Dominant

In autosomal dominant diseases, heterozygotes express the disease phenotype. The affected parent can pass either a disease allele or a normal allele to offspring, with the likelihood of each event being 0.5, or 50%. This fact means that 50% of offspring inherit the normal allele, and

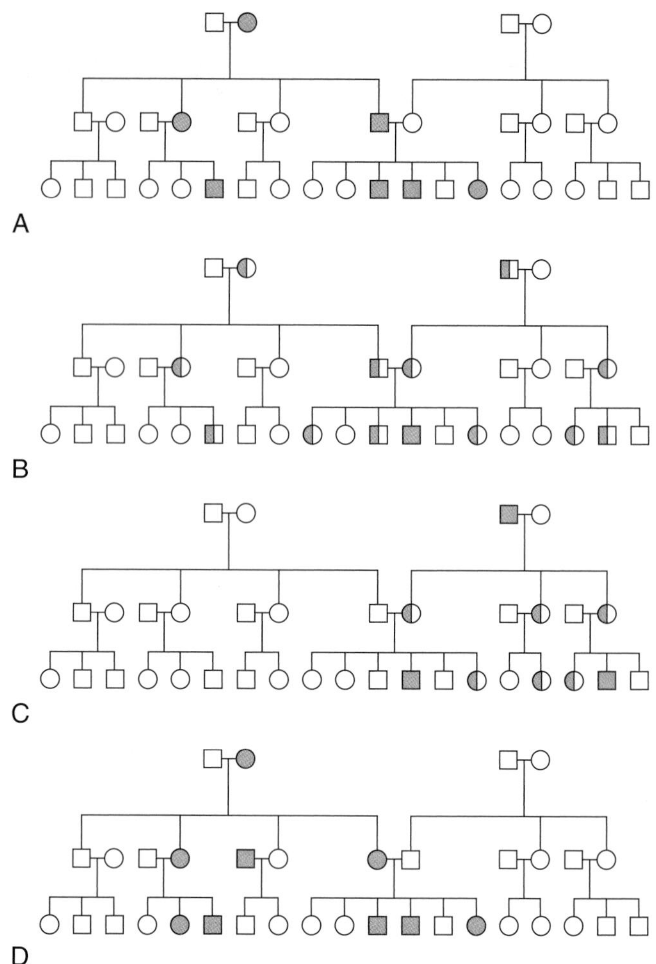

Figure 147-1. Inheritance patterns. **A,** Pedigree illustrating autosomal dominant inheritance. The inheritance pattern shows vertical transmission of the affected phenotype including father-to-son transmission. There are no skipped generations. **B,** Pedigree of autosomal recessive inheritance. Note the disease phenotype is not usually seen in the parents or other ancestors. Likelihood of affected males to females is equal. Refer to Punnett square in Figure 147-2 for estimating risks for recessive inheritance in heterozygous parents. **C,** Pedigree of X-linked recessive inheritance. The disease phenotype is present with one disease allele in the male, but requires a homozygous genotype to be expressed in the female. **D,** Pedigree illustrating mitochondrial inheritance. Note the maternal transmission of the affected phenotype. There is no paternal transmission.

50% inherit the disease allele. In the case of dominant diseases, 50% of offspring express the disease.

There are several implications of autosomal dominant transmission. First, there is no sexual predilection for the disease phenotype; males and females are equally likely to be affected, and to transmit the disease allele to their offspring. Second, unless the disease gene is nonpenetrant, the disease does not skip generations. This type of transmission is called *vertical transmission.* Third, male-to-male (father-son) transmission is seen. This observation in a pedigree rules out mitochondrial or X-linked inheritance.

Autosomal Recessive

In contrast to autosomal dominant inheritance, in autosomal recessive inheritance, a homozygous genotype is necessary for expression of the disease phenotype. A homozygous parent transmits the disease allele to all offspring, but offspring do not show the disease phenotype unless the other parent carries at least one mutant copy of the same gene. More frequently, however, neither parent is affected, but both carry a single

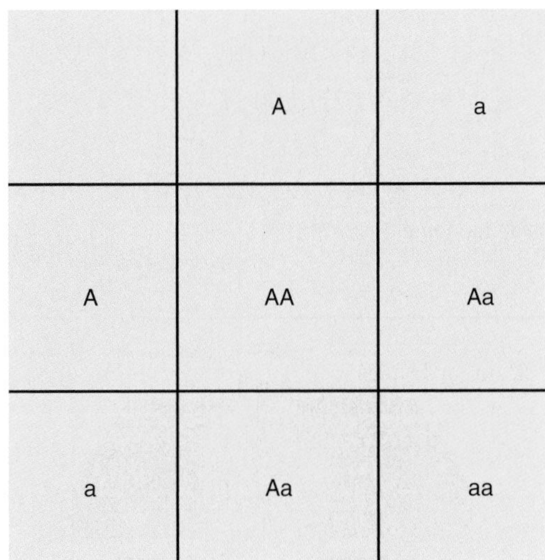

Figure 147-2. Punnett squares may be used to estimate inheritance probabilities for mendelian inheritance patterns. This Punnett square illustrates the mating of two individuals who are heterozygous carriers of an autosomal recessive gene, showing that there is a 25% chance of having a child with the recessive phenotype (aa), a 50% chance of having a child who carries the recessive allele but is not affected (Aa), and a 25% chance of having a child who does not carry the recessive allele (AA).

mutant gene, and by chance each passes this mutant copy on to the offspring. In this scenario, 25% of offspring carry two mutant copies of the gene and express the disease phenotype, 50% of offspring are carriers of a mutant copy (similar to the parents), and 25% of offspring have two wild-type copies of the gene. As with autosomal dominant diseases, there is no sexual predilection—males and females are equally likely to be affected—but vertical transmission is rarely seen. Recessive diseases tend to be generation specific. If the disease is exceptionally rare, the likelihood of parental consanguinity, albeit distant, is high.

X-Linked Inheritance

X-linked inheritance may be either recessive or dominant. In recessive X-linked inheritance, females are unlikely to be affected because a homozygous disease genotype is needed for the disease phenotype to manifest. Heterozygous females do occasionally exhibit subtle aspects of the disease phenotype, however, because of the phenomenon of X chromosome inactivation (the Lyon hypothesis). In each cell, only one of the two X chromosomes in females is active, and if X chromosome inactivation is entirely random, 50% of cells in a heterozygous female express the disease-carrying X chromosome. Through mechanisms that are not clearly understood, this process is not random, and inactivation of the mutated X chromosome is much higher than is inactivation of the normal X chromosome. Males have only a single X chromosome, and always express the disease phenotype.

In a pedigree showing X-linked recessive inheritance, the trait is seen more frequently in males; there is no father-son transmission; affected fathers transmit the disease allele to all female offspring, who may have affected males ("skipped generation"); and heterozygous females transmit the disease allele to half of all sons, who manifest the disease, and half of all daughters, who are heterozygous and phenotypically normal. In X-linked dominant inheritance, affected fathers transmit the disease allele to all daughters who exhibit the disease phenotype (with complete penetrance); there is no father-son transmission. Heterozygous females are affected and transmit the trait to half of all sons and to half of all daughters.

Mitochondrial Inheritance

Mitochondria are the "powerhouses" of the human cell and the site of oxidative phosphorylation, the process that leads to the production of adenosine triphosphate (ATP). Mitochondria possess their own

Table 147-3

Prevalence of Different Forms of Congenital Hearing Loss

Form	Prevalence (%)
Environmental	50
Genetic	50
Syndromic	15
Nonsyndromic	35
Autosomal recessive	28
Autosomal dominant	7
X-linked and mitochondrial	<1

intrinsic DNA, with several copies of the mitochondrial genome in each mitochondrion. The mitochondrial genome is a 16,569 base pair circular molecule that encodes two ribosomal RNAs, 22 transfer RNAs, and 13 polypeptides.[14] The remaining mitochondrial proteins required for oxidative phosphorylation are encoded by the nuclear genome.

Mitochondrial DNA (mtDNA) is inherited solely through the maternal lineage, reflecting the presence of large amounts of mtDNA in the cytoplasm of the egg. If all of the mtDNA molecules are abnormal, a condition known as *homoplasmy,* all progeny cells contain abnormal mitochondria. If normal and abnormal mtDNA molecules coexist, a condition known as *heteroplasmy,* there is a wide range of expression of the mutant phenotype, reflecting the random distribution of mitochondria to progeny cells. Because mitochondria lack a DNA repair mechanism, mtDNA accumulates mutations at a higher rate than nuclear DNA.

Genetic Hearing Impairment

Nonsyndromic Hearing Impairment

Genetic hearing loss is common in humans. Nonsyndromic hearing impairment in the absence of other phenotypic manifestations accounts for 70% of hereditary hearing loss.[15] More than half of SNHL that occurs in neonates is attributable to simple mendelian inherited traits (Table 147-3). In most cases, the inheritance pattern is recessive (75% to 80% of cases), and consequently the parents of affected children generally do not exhibit the phenotype. Congenital nonsyndromic hearing loss is inherited in an autosomal dominant (approximately 20%), X-linked (2% to 5%), or mitochondrial (approximately 1%) mode. Nomenclature is based on the prefix "DFN" to designate *nonsyndromic deafness.* DFN followed by an "A" implies dominant inheritance, a "B" implies recessive inheritance, and no letter means X-linked inheritance. The integer suffix denotes the order of locus discovery. DFNA1 and DFNB1 were the first autosomal dominant and recessive nonsyndromic deafness loci to be identified. Table 147-4 lists the genes included in clinical screens for nonsyndromic SNHL.

Autosomal Recessive Nonsyndromic Hearing Impairment

Autosomal recessive nonsyndromic hearing impairment is usually prelingual and severe to profound across all frequencies.[16] To date, 67 loci have been mapped, and 23 causative genes have been cloned (Table 147-5).[11] Although autosomal recessive SNHL is heterogeneous, mutations in the connexin 26 (*GJB2*) gene at the DFNB1 locus contribute about half of all hereditary cases in Australia, the United States, Israel, and many European countries.

DFNB1

In 1994, Guilford and coworkers[17] mapped the first autosomal recessive nonsyndromic deafness locus to 13q12-13 and called it DFNB1. Three

Table 147-4

Hearing Loss Genes Currently Screened for Clinical Diagnostics

Syndromic Hearing Loss	Gene
Branchio-oto-renal (BOR) syndrome	*EYA1*
Mohr-Tranebjaerg syndrome (deafness–dystonia–optic atrophy syndrome)	*TIMM8A*
Pendred syndrome	*SLC26A4*
Usher syndrome type 1B	*USH1B*
Usher syndrome type 2A	*USH2A*
Usher syndrome type 3	*USH3A* (one mutation)
Wolfram syndrome	*WFS1*
Nonsyndromic Hearing Loss	
DFNA3 and DFNB1	*GJB2* and *GJB6*
DFN3	*POU3F4*
DFNB4	*SLC26A4*
DFNA 6/14	*WFS1*
DFNA8/12	*TECTA*
DFNA9	*COCH*
DFNB9	*OTOF*
DFNB21	*TECTA*
Mitochondrial Hearing Loss	
	MTRNR1, MTTS1, MTTL1

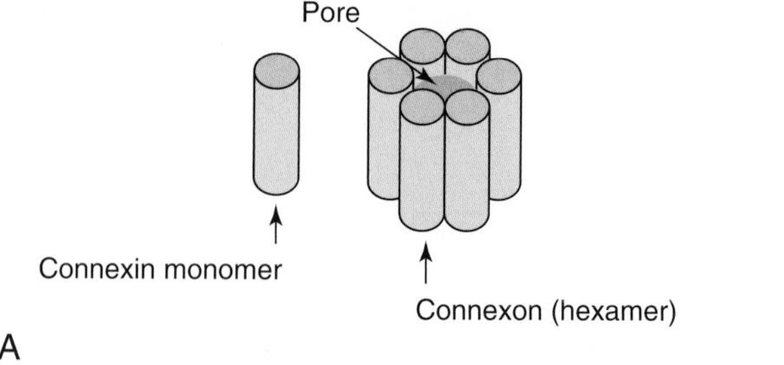

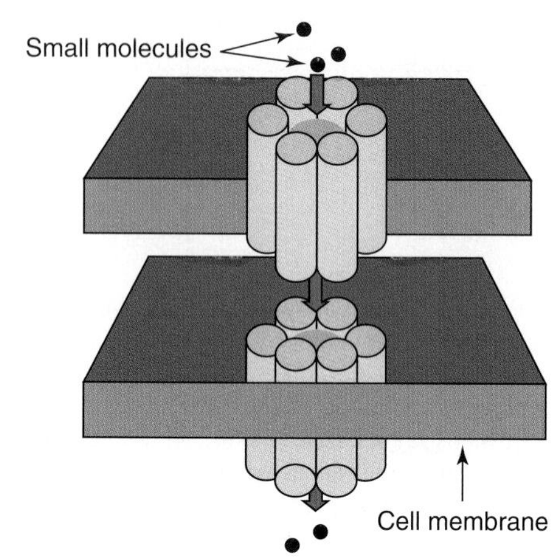

Figure 147-3. Diagram of a gap junction and its constituents. **A,** Three-dimensional view of a connexon hexamer composed of six connexin monomers. **B,** Three-dimensional view of a gap junction composed of two connexons in adjacent cells. Small molecules can pass through the gap junction from one cytoplasm to another without having to cross two cell membranes.

years later, Kelsell and colleagues[18] identified the DFNB1 gene as a gap junction gene called *GJB2*. The encoded protein, connexin 26 (Cx26), oligomerizes with five other connexin proteins to form a connexon; the docking of two connexons in neighboring cells results in a gap junction (Fig. 147-3). These gap junctions are thought to be conduits through which potassium ions are recycled from the outer hair cells back through the supporting cells and spiral ligament to the stria vascularis.[19] The ions are pumped into the endolymph to perpetuate the mechanosensory transduction of hair cells. Mutations in *GJB2* may disrupt this recycling process and prevent normal mechanosensory transduction.[18] This role is consistent with the expression of *GJB2* in the stria vascularis, nonsensory epithelial cells, spiral ligament, and spiral limbus of the inner ear.[18]

Mutations in *GJB2* have been shown to cause 50% of autosomal recessive nonsyndromic deafness in many world populations.[20] More than 90 deafness-causing mutations are described, with several being very common in specific ethnic groups.[21] The 35delG mutation predominates in populations of European descent[22]; this mutation has a carrier frequency in the Midwestern United States of 2.5%.[23] In the Ashkenazi Jewish population, the most common mutation is the 167delT; its carrier frequency is approximately 4%.[24] In Japanese populations, the 235delC mutation is the most common deafness-causing allele variant of *GJB2*.[25]

The DFNB1 auditory phenotype is varied, although homozygosity for protein-truncating mutations is generally associated with impaired gap junction activity and moderate to profound deafness.[21,26] With missense mutations, the degree of residual hearing can be substantially greater.[21] Most frequently, the loss is symmetric between ears, and does not progress over the long-term. Temporal bone anomalies are not part of the DFNB1 phenotype, obviating the need for routine temporal bone imaging.

Genetic testing is available to diagnose *GJB2*-related deafness and is warranted because the relative contribution of this gene to the total genetic deafness mutation load is high. Mutation screening facilitates genetic counseling and prediction of the chance of recurrence. It also provides prognostic information because several studies have shown that cochlear implant recipients with *GJB2*-related deafness do very well.[27]

Autosomal Dominant Nonsyndromic Hearing Impairment

To date, 54 loci for autosomal dominant nonsyndromic deafness have been mapped, and 21 causative genes have been cloned (Table 147-6).[11] Generally, the onset of deafness is postlingual, progressive, and milder than recessive forms, with several loci having characteristic audioprofiles.[28,29] Several common forms of dominant hearing impairment have unique or characteristic audioprofiles. One of the most common types of autosomal dominant nonsyndromic deafness is high-frequency hearing loss resulting from *KCNQ4* mutations at the DFNA2 locus.[30]

DFNA2 (High-Frequency Hearing Loss)

Autosomal dominant high-frequency hearing loss can be the consequence of mutations in numerous different genes (i.e., *KCNQ4* [DFNA2], *DFNA5* [DFNA5], *COCH* [DFNA9], *POU4F3* [DFNA15]). Mutations in some of these genes cause autosomal dominant deafness through a dominant-negative mechanism of action.[30-32] One example is deafness at the DFNA2 locus, which is caused by dominant-negative mutations in *KCNQ4*.[30,32] *KCNQ4* is organized into 14 exons that encode a protein with six transmembrane domains and a P-loop to confer K^+ ion selectivity to the channel pore.[32] A voltage sensor in the fourth transmembrane domain drives a conformational

Table 147-5
Autosomal Recessive Nonsyndromic Hearing Loss

Locus Name	Chromosomal Locus	Gene Symbol	Phenotype*
DFNB1	13q11q12 13q12	*GJB2* *GJB6*	Prelingual† hearing loss that remains stable[17,18]
DFNB2	11q13.5	*MYO7A*	Prelingual or postlingual hearing loss of unspecified type[164,165]
DFNB3	17p11.2	*MYO15*	Prelingual hearing loss that remains stable[166,167]
DFNB4	7q31	*SLC26A4*	Prelingual or postlingual hearing loss that may be stable or progressive. May also be associated with dilation of vestibular aqueduct[102,103]
DFNB5	14q12		Prelingual hearing loss that remains stable[168]
DFNB6	3p21	*TMIE*	Prelingual hearing loss that remains stable[169,170]
DFNB7/11	9q13-q21	*TMC1*	Prelingual hearing loss that remains stable[171,172]
DFNB8/10	21q22.3	*TMPRSS3*	Postlingual (DFNB8)† or prelingual (DFNB10) hearing loss that may be progressive or stable[173,174]
DFNB9	2p22-p23	*OTOF*	Prelingual hearing loss that remains stable[175,176]
DFNB12	10q21-q22	*CDH23*	Prelingual hearing loss that remains stable[177,178]
DFNB16	15q15	*STRC*	Prelingual hearing loss that remains stable and is more pronounced in higher frequencies[179]
DFNB18	11p15.1	*USH1C*	Prelingual hearing loss that remains stable[180,181]
DFNB21	11q22-q24	*TECTA*	Prelingual severe to profound isolated SNHL[41]
DFNB22	16p12.2	*OTOA*	Prelingual moderate to severe SNHL[182]
DFNB23	10q21.1	*PCDH15*	Prelingual severe to profound SNHL[183]
DFNB28	22q13.1	*TRIOBP*	Prelingual severe to profound SNHL[184,185]
DFNB29	21q22.3	*CLDN14*	Prelingual profound SNHL[186]
DFNB30	10p11.1	*MYO3A*	Progressive hearing loss that first affects high frequencies and begins in the 2nd decade; is severe in high and middle frequencies and moderate at low frequencies by age 50[187]
DFNB31	9q32-q34	*DFN31*	Prelingual profound SNHL[188,189]
DFNB36	1p36.31	*ESPN*	Prelingual hearing loss of unspecified or unknown type[190]
DFNB37	6q13	*MYO6*	Prelingual hearing loss of unspecified or unknown type[191]
DFNB67	6p21.1-p22.3	*TMHS*	Prelingual profound SNHL[192-194]

*Most important references are cited.
†Prelingual deafness also includes congenital deafness.
†The onset of DFNB8 hearing loss is postlingual (10-12 years old), whereas the onset of DFNB10 hearing loss is prelingual (congenital). This phenotypic difference reflects a genotypic difference—the DFNB8-causing mutation is a splice site mutation, suggesting that inefficient splicing is associated with a reduced amount of normal protein, which is sufficient to prevent prelingual deafness, but insufficient to prevent eventual hearing loss.
SNHL, sensorineural hearing loss.
Adapted from Van Camp G, Smith RJ. Hereditary Hearing Loss Homepage. Available at http://webh01.ua.ac.be/hhh/. 2009.

change that leads to channel opening. *KCNQ4* subunits are typically organized into homotetramers to form functional channels.[32]

The G285S allele was the first DFNA2 mutation identified, and a knockout mouse model of this variant has been generated.[33] The substitution of a serine for a glycine affects the first highly conserved glycine in a GYG signature sequence of the P-loop of the channel pore, and abolishes channel function by preventing correct subunit assembly. Impaired *KCNQ4* function in the inner ear affects K^+ ion recycling. Normally, mechanosensory transduction leads to an increase in cytosolic K^+ in the outer hair cells of the cochlea, the major site of *KCNQ4* expression. *KCNQ4* channels expressed in the base of these cells transport K^+ extracellularly, where the ion is taken up by supporting cells and cycled back into the scala media.[30] The consequence of abnormal *KCNQ4* function is apoptosis of the outer hair cells. The clinical

Table 147-6
Autosomal Dominant Nonsyndromic Hearing Loss

Locus Name	Chromosomal Locus	Gene Symbol	Phenotype*
DFNA1	5q31	*DIAPH1*	Postlingual low-frequency hearing loss (1st decade)[195,196]
DFNA2	1p35.1 1p34	*GJB3* *KCNQ4*	Postlingual high-frequency hearing loss (2nd decade)[30,32,197]
DFNA3†	13q11-q12 13q12	*GJB2* *GJB6*	Prelingual high-frequency hearing loss[31,198,199]
DFNA4	19q13	*MYH14*	Postlingual hearing loss with flat/gently downsloping audioprofile[200]
DFNA5	7p15	*DFNA5*	Postlingual high-frequency hearing loss (1st decade)[201,202]
DFNA6/14/38‡	4p16.1	*WFS1*	Prelingual low-frequency hearing loss[45,203,204]
DFNA8/12†	11q22-q24	*TECTA*	Prelingual midfrequency hearing loss[36]
DFNA9	14q12-q13	*COCH*	Postlingual high-frequency hearing loss (2nd decade)[205,206]
DFNA10	6q23	*EYA4*	Postlingual hearing loss with flat/gently downsloping audioprofile (3rd/4th decade)[207,208]
DFNA11	11q13.5	*MYO7A*	Postlingual hearing loss (1st decade)[165,209]
DFNA13	6p21.3	*COL11A2*	Postlingual midfrequency hearing loss (2nd decade)[42,43]
DFNA15 DFNA17 DFNA20/26 DFNA22	5q31 22q11.2 17q25 6q13	*POU4F3* *MYH9* *ACTG1* *MYO6*	Postlingual high-frequency hearing loss[210-214]
DFNA28 DFNA36	8q22 9q13-q21	*TFCP2L3* *TMC1*	Postlingual hearing loss with flat/gently downsloping audioprofile[171,215]
DFNA39	4q21.3	*DSPP*	Postlingual high-frequency hearing loss[216]
DFNA48	12q13-q14	*MYO1A*	Postlingual hearing loss[217,218]

*Most important references are cited.
†Most autosomal dominant loci cause postlingual hearing impairment. Some exceptions are DFNA3, DFNA8, and DFNA12.
‡DFNA6/14 is noteworthy because the hearing loss primarily affects the low frequencies.
Adapted from Van Camp G, Smith RJ. Hereditary Hearing Loss Homepage. Available at http://webh01.ua.ac.be/hhh/. 2008.

manifestation of this damage is hearing loss that is progressive and biased to the high frequencies.[30]

DFNA8/12 and DFNA13 (Midfrequency Hearing Loss)

Identification of phenotype-genotype correlations is crucial in determining the etiology of autosomal dominant sensorineural hearing loss (ADSNHL),[34] and has implications for prognostic and therapeutic outcomes. Some correlations are very robust, such as the low-frequency audioprofile associated with *WFS1*-related hearing loss (DFNA6/14/38)[35] and the "cookie-bite" (midfrequency) audioprofile associated with *TECTA*-related hearing loss (DFNA8/12),[36] whereas other correlations, such as high-frequency hearing loss, are more difficult to define. Hearing loss at the DFNA8/12 locus is unusual among dominant forms because midfrequencies are predominantly affected, it is congenital, and it is nonprogressive.[37] The causative gene at this locus, α-tectorin (*TECTA*), was identified in Austrian DFNA8[37] and Belgian DFNA12[36,38] families. In both families, missense mutations were identified that are thought to have a dominant-negative effect leading to disruption of the structure of the tectorial membrane.[36]

α-Tectorin is the major noncollagenous component of the tectorial membrane of the inner ear. A mouse mutant generated with a *TECTA* missense mutation showed elevated neural thresholds, broadened neural tuning, and decreased sensitivity of the tip of the neural tuning curve, indicating that the tectorial membrane enables the motion of the basilar membrane optimally to drive the inner hair cells at their best frequency.[39] *TECTA* has also been implicated in recessive deafness at the DFNB21 locus.[40,41] Hearing loss in these families was also congenital, but severe to profound across all frequencies rather than restricted to the midfrequencies.

DFNA13 is a related form of dominant hearing impairment that is also characterized by initial midfrequency loss and disruption of the tectorial membrane. In this case, missense mutations were identified in the *COL11A2* gene of American and Dutch DFNA13 families, and were predicted to affect the triple helical domain of the collagen protein.[42,43] A $Col11a2^{-/-}$ mouse model displayed moderate to severe hearing loss and an enlarged tectorial membrane attributable to disorganized and widely spaced collagen fibrils.[43] Defects in genes encoding components of the collagenous and noncollagenous regions of the tectorial membrane can induce autosomal dominant midfrequency hearing impairment.

DFNA6/14/38 (Low-Frequency Hearing Loss)

Mutations in the Wolfram syndrome 1 gene (*WFS1*) at the DFNA6/14/38 locus are a common cause of low-frequency sensorineural hearing loss. *WFS1* was originally identified in human disease as a cause of Wolfram syndrome, an autosomal recessive neu-

Table 147-7

X-Linked Nonsyndromic Hearing Loss

Locus Name	Chromosomal Locus	Gene Symbol	Phenotype*
DFN2	Xq22	—	Prelingual profound SNHL in all frequencies[219]
DFN3	Xq21.1	*POU3F4*	Mixed variable prelingual hearing loss that progresses to profound in all frequencies[50]
DFN4	Xp21	—	Stable prelingual profound SNHL in all frequencies[54]
DFN5	Withdrawn	—	—
DFN6	Xp22	—	Progressive severe to profound postlingual (1st decade) SNHL that begins with high-frequency hearing loss that evolves to include all frequencies by adulthood[53]
DFN7	Withdrawn	—	—
DFN8	Reserved	—	—

*Most important references are cited.
SNHL, sensorineural hearing loss.
Adapted from Van Camp G, Smith RJ. Hereditary Hearing Loss Homepage. Available at http://webh01.ua.ac.be/hhh/. 2009.

rodegenerative disorder comprising diabetes mellitus, optic atrophy, and often deafness.[44] Later, *WFS1* was implicated in autosomal dominant, nonsyndromic hearing loss at the DFNA6/14 locus in six families segregating delayed-onset, slowly progressive, low-frequency SNHL.[45] These families all carried missense mutations located in a region of exon 8 that encodes the C-terminal domain.[45] Although the protein is known to contain nine putative transmembrane domains, its function and role in causing low-frequency SNHL remain unclear. One of the original *WFS1* mutations, V779M, was identified in 1 of 336 control individuals.[45] This frequency is comparable to that of heterozygous carriers of Wolfram syndrome, which has been estimated to be 0.3% to 1%.[46] Because an increased risk of SNHL had been reported for these carriers,[46] it was predicted that *WFS1* was a common cause of low-frequency SNHL. This assumption has been supported by the subsequent discovery of *WFS1* mutations at high frequency in families with low-frequency SNHL from different populations.[47,48]

X-Linked Nonsyndromic Hearing Impairment

X-linked nonsyndromic hearing impairment accounts for less than 2% of nonsyndromic hearing loss.[1] Five loci and one causative gene have been identified (Table 147-7). Re-examination of the original family used to map DFN1 has revealed other cosegregating features, including mental retardation. This type of deafness is now recognized as a form of X-linked syndromic hearing loss.[49] Of the remaining DFN loci, DFN3 is most common. It is due to mutations in a transcription factor called POU3F4,[50] and manifests as congenital stapes fixation with radiologic findings that include widening of the lateral internal auditory canal and dilation of the vestibule.[51] Hearing loss is usually mixed, and stapedectomy is typically attended by a perilymph gusher.[52] The hearing impairment associated with the other loci is variable.[53,54]

Mitochondrial Nonsyndromic Hearing Impairment

Mitochondrial nonsyndromic deafness can be caused by various mtDNA mutations, although the 1555 A-to-G mtDNA has been characterized best (Table 147-8). As mentioned earlier, this mutation is also associated with aminoglycoside ototoxicity. As a cause of nonsyndromic deafness, the phenotype is similar to aminoglycoside ototoxicity with a mild, high-frequency loss that shows progression.[55] The loss is generally of later onset in individuals who have not been exposed to aminoglycosides.[2]

Presbycusis, or age-related hearing loss, also may have a mitochondrial basis.[56-59] Because mtDNA mutations accumulate at several times the rate of nuclear DNA mutations, mitochondrial function ultimately may be impaired, resulting in age-related cochlear dysfunction.[57] In support of this hypothesis, an increase in the mtDNA mutation load has been shown in aged cochlea.[59]

Table 147-8

Mitochondrial Nonsyndromic Hearing Loss

Gene Symbol	Mutation	Phenotype*
MTRNR1	961 different mutations	Commonly secondary to aminoglycoside use with variable severity and highly variable penetrance[138,220]
	c.1494 C>T	
	c.1555 A>G	
MTTS1	c.7445 A>G	Variably severe hearing loss with highly variable penetrance[221-224]
	c.7472 ins C	
	c.7510 T>C	
	c.7511 T	

*Most important references are cited.

Syndromic Hearing Impairment

Syndromic forms of hereditary SNHL are less common than nonsyndromic forms (Table 147-9). Syndromic hearing impairment refers to deafness that cosegregates with other features, forming a recognizable constellation of findings known as a syndrome. Sensorineural deafness has been associated with more than 400 syndromes. A discussion of a few of the more common syndromes follows.

Autosomal Dominant Syndromic Hearing Impairment

Branchio-oto-renal Syndrome

Melnick coined the term *branchio-oto-renal (BOR) syndrome* in 1975 to describe the cosegregation of branchial, otic, and renal anomalies in

Table 147-9

Syndromic Forms of Hearing Loss

Syndrome	Chromosomal Locus	Gene*
Autosomal Dominant		
Branchio-oto-renal		
BOR1	8q13.3	*EYA1*[65]
BOR2	1q31	Unknown[225]
BOR3	14q	*SIX1*[66]
	19q13.3	*SIX5*[67]
Waardenburg's		
WS1	2q35	*PAX3*[85]
WS2†	3p14.1-p12.3	*MITF*[86]
		SNAI2[87]
WS3 (Klein-Waardenburg)	2q35	*PAX3*[88]
WS4†	13q22	*EDNRB*[89]
Shah-Waardenburg or Waardenburg-Hirschsprung	20q13.2-q13.3	*EDN3*[90]
	22q13	*SOX10*[91]
Stickler		
STL1	12q13.11-13.2	*COL2A1*[76]
STL2	6p1.3	*COL11A1*[77]
STL3	1p21	*COL11A2*[79]
STL4	6q13	*COL9A1*[78]
Neurofibromatosis		
NF2	22q12	*NF2*[226]
Treacher Collins		
TCOF1	5q32-q33.1	*TCOF1*[227]
Autosomal Recessive		
Pendred		
PDS	7q21-34	*SLC26A4/PDS*[96]
Foxi1	5q34	*Foxi1*[104]
Usher		
USH1A	14q32	Unknown[228,229]
USHIB	11q13.5	Unknown[115]
USH1C	11p15.1	*MYO7A*[230]
		USH1C[231-233]
USH1D	10q22.1	*CDH23*[177]
USH1E	21q21	Unknown[234,235]
USH1F	10Q21-22	*PCDH15*[183]
USH1G	17Q24-25	*SANS*[236-239]
USH2A	1q41	*USH2A*[116]
USH2B	3p23-24.2	Unknown[240,241]
USH2C	5q14.3-q21.3	*VLGR1*[242]
USH3	3q21-q25	*USH3A*[243,244]
Jervell and Lange-Nielsen		
JLNS1	11p15.5	*KCNQ1*[106,107]
JLNS2	21q22.1-q22.2	*KCNE1*[108]
Biotinidase deficiency	3p25	*BTD*[245]
Refsum disease	10pter-p11.2	*PAHX*[246]
	6q22-q24	*PEX7*[119]
Alport syndrome	2q36-2q37	*COL4A3*[247]
	2q36-2q37	*COL4A4*[247]
X-Linked		
Alport syndrome	Xq22	*COL4A5*[123]
Mohr-Tranebjaerg syndrome	Xq22	*TIMM8A*[248]
Norrie's disease	Xp11.3	*NDP*[249]
Mitochondrial		
MELAS	mtDNA	tRNA(Leu)(UUR)[133]
NIDDM	mtDNA	tRNA(Leu)(UUR)/deletions[250]
MERRF	mtDNA	Large deletions[251]

*Most important references are cited.

†Although Waardenburg's syndrome (WS) is usually inherited in an autosomal dominant manner, sometimes WS2 can be inherited in an autosomal recessive manner. WS4 is always inherited in an autosomal recessive manner.

deaf individuals.[60] Inheritance is autosomal dominant, penetrance is nearly 100%, and prevalence is estimated at 1 in 40,000 newborns.[61] BOR affects 2% of profoundly deaf children.[61] Otologic findings can involve the external, middle, or inner ear. External ear anomalies include preauricular pits (82%), preauricular tags, auricular malformations (32%), microtia, and external auditory canal narrowing[62,63]; middle ear anomalies include ossicular malformation (fusion, displacement, underdevelopment), facial nerve dehiscence, absence of the oval window, and reduction in size of the middle ear cleft[62]; and inner ear anomalies include cochlear hypoplasia and dysplasia.[64] Enlargement of the cochlear or vestibular aqueducts may be seen,[63] or merely hypoplasia of the lateral semicircular canal.[64]

Hearing impairment is the most common feature of BOR syndrome and is reported in almost 90% of affected individuals.[61] The loss can be conductive (30%) or sensorineural (20%), but is most often mixed (50%). It is severe in one third of individuals and is progressive in one quarter.[61] Branchial anomalies occur in the form of laterocervical fistulas, sinuses, and cysts, and renal anomalies ranging from agenesis to dysplasia are found in 25% of individuals.[61] Less common phenotypic findings include lacrimal duct aplasia, short palate, and retrognathia.[61]

One causative gene is *EYA1,* the human homologue of the *Drosophila* eyes absent gene.[65] The gene contains 16 exons encoding for 559 amino acids.[65] *EYA1* mutations are found in approximately 25% of patients with a BOR phenotype, and this phenotype is hypothesized to reflect a reduction in the amount of the EYA1 protein. Mutations in two additional genes, *SIX1* and *SIX5,* also have been shown more recently to cause BOR syndrome.[66,67] Both genes act within the genetic network of the *EYA* and *PAX* genes to regulate organogenesis.

Neurofibromatosis Type 2

Neurofibromatosis type 2 (NF2) is characterized by the development of bilateral vestibular schwannomas and other intracranial and spinal tumors (schwannomas, meningiomas, gliomas, and ependymomas). In addition, patients may have posterior subcapsular lenticular opacities. Diagnostic criteria include (1) bilateral vestibular schwannomas that usually develop by the second decade of life, or (2) a family history of NF2 in a first-degree relative, plus one of the following: unilateral vestibular schwannomas at less than 30 years of age, or any two of meningioma, glioma, schwannoma, or juvenile posterior subcapsular lenticular opacities/juvenile cortical cataract. The causative gene is a 17 exon gene that codes for a 595-amino acid protein named merlin on chromosome 22q12.[68] Merlin is a tumor suppressor that regulates the actin cytoskeleton.[69,70] Although its mechanism of action is not completely understood, microarray analysis has identified numerous other genes that become deregulated during tumorigenesis.[71]

The incidence of NF2 is 1:40,000 to 1:90,000.[70] Hearing loss is usually high frequency and sensorineural; vertigo, tinnitus, and facial nerve paralysis may be associated findings. The diagnosis rests on the clinical and family history, physical examination, and imaging studies (magnetic resonance imaging [MRI]). Treatment of the vestibular schwannomas usually consists of surgery, although Gamma knife surgery is considered in selected cases.[72] Auditory brainstem implants have been used with success in patients with vestibular schwannomas, although their use is limited if there is a history of Gamma knife treatment.[72,73]

Stickler Syndrome

In 1965, Stickler described a family followed at the Mayo Clinic for five generations that segregated syndromic features, including myopia, clefting, and hearing loss.[74] The disease, now known eponymously as Stickler syndrome (SS), has a prevalence of 1:10,000,[75] and is caused by mutations in *COL2A1, COL11A2,* or *CO11A1* genes that encode for the constituent proteins of type II and type XI collagen.[76-79] On the basis of criteria set forth by Snead and Yates,[80] the diagnosis of SS requires (1) congenital vitreous anomaly, and (2) any three of myopia with onset before age 6 years, rhegmatogenous retinal detachment or paravascular pigmented lattice degeneration, joint hypermobility with abnormal Beighton score, SNHL (audiometric confirmation), or midline clefting. Other manifestations include craniofacial anomalies such as midfacial flattening, mandibular hypoplasia, short upturned nose, or a long philtrum. Micrognathia is common, and if severe leads to the Robin sequence with cleft palate (28% to 65%).[81] Clefting may be complete, with a U-shaped cleft palate secondary to Robin sequence, but is more commonly limited to a submucous cleft.[82]

SS type 1 is caused by mutations in *COL2A1.*[76] The phenotype includes the classic ocular findings with a "membranous" vitreous. SS type 2 is due to missense or in-frame deletion mutations in *COL11A2,*[79] and is unique in that there are no ocular abnormalities because *COL11A2* is not expressed in the vitreous. SS type 3 is caused by mutations in *COL11A1.*[77] The vitreous in these patients shows irregularly thickened fiber bundles that may be visualized on slit-lamp examination.[77,80]

The hearing loss associated with SS can be conductive, sensorineural, or mixed. If it is conductive, the loss typically reflects the eustachian tube dysfunction that commonly occurs with palatal clefts. SNHL is more common in the older age groups. Its pathogenesis is incompletely understood, but possible mechanisms include primary neurosensory deficits because of alterations in the pigmented epithelium of the inner ear or abnormalities of inner ear collagen.[81] Computed tomography (CT) has not shown gross structural abnormalities. Patients with SS type 3 tend to have moderate to severe hearing loss, patients with SS type 1 have either normal hearing or only a mild impairment, and patients with SS type 2 fall in between.[75]

The ocular findings in SS are the most prevalent feature and warrant special discussion.[82] Most affected individuals are myopic,[80] but also may have vitreoretinal degeneration, retinal detachment, cataract, and blindness.[74] Retinal detachment leading to blindness is the most severe ocular complication and affects approximately 50% of individuals with SS.[81] Detachment typically occurs in adolescence or early adulthood.

Waardenburg Syndrome

Waardenburg published an article defining a auditory-pigmentary disease in 1951.[83] The association, now known as Waardenburg syndrome (WS), is classified under four types and has an aggregate prevalence of 1:10,000 to 1:20,000.[84] WS type 1 is recognized by SNHL, white forelock, pigmentary disturbances of the iris, and dystopia canthorum, a specific displacement of the inner canthi and lacrimal puncti.[83] Other features include synophrys, broad nasal root, hypoplasia of the alae nasi, patent metopic suture, and a square jaw. WS type 1 is caused by mutations in *PAX3,* a DNA-binding transcription factor homologous to mouse Pax-3, the gene implicated in the Splotch mouse mutant.[85] *PAX3* is expressed in neural crest cells in early development, and strial melanocytes are absent in affected individuals.[85]

WS type 2 is distinguished from WS type 1 by the absence of dystopia canthorum. Approximately 15% of WS type 2 cases are caused by mutations in *MITF,* a transcription factor also involved in melanocyte development.[86] Mutations in *SNAI2,* a zinc-finger transcription factor expressed in migratory neural crest cells, have also been shown to cause WS type 2.[87] WS type 3 is called Klein-Waardenburg syndrome, and is characterized by WS type 1 features with the addition of hypoplasia or contracture of the upper limbs. *PAX3* is the causative gene.[88] WS type 4 is also known as Waardenburg-Shah syndrome, and involves the association of WS with Hirschsprung disease. Three genes have been implicated: endothelin 3 (*EDN3*), endothelin receptor B gene (*EDNRB*), and *SOX10.*[89-91] Although WS types 1 to 3 are inherited as dominant diseases, WS type 4 is autosomal recessive (see Table 147-9).

The hearing loss in WS shows considerable variability between and within families. Congenital hearing impairment is present in 36% to 66.7% of cases of WS type 1 versus 57% to 85% of cases of WS type 2.[84] Most commonly, the loss affects individuals with more than one pigmentation abnormality and is profound, bilateral, and stable over time. Audiogram configuration varies, with low-frequency loss being more common. Nadol and Merchant[92] examined the inner ear of a 76-year-old woman with WS type 1 and found intact neurosensory structures only in the basal turn of the cochlea. Temporal bone imaging is typically normal, although malformation of the semicircular canals and cochlear hypoplasia can be found.[93] Risk chance prediction of the findings associated with WS is difficult because of variability in disease expression.

Treacher-Collins Syndrome

Treacher-Collins syndrome is an autosomal dominant syndrome characterized by abnormalities of craniofacial development. The phenotype includes maldevelopment of the maxilla and mandible, with abnormal canthi placement, ocular colobomas, choanal atresia, and conductive hearing loss secondary to ossicular fixation.[94] The causative gene is *TCOF,* which encodes for the protein treacle.[94]

Autosomal Recessive Syndromic Hearing Impairment

Pendred Syndrome

The most common syndromic form of hereditary SNHL, Pendred syndrome (PS) was described by Pendred in 1896.[95] The condition is autosomal recessive, and affected individuals also have goiter.[96] The prevalence of PS is estimated at 7.5 to 10 per 100,000 individuals, suggesting that the syndrome may account for 10% of hereditary deafness.[96] The hearing loss is usually congenital and severe to profound, although progressive mild to moderate SNHL is sometimes seen.[96] Bilateral dilation of the vestibular aqueduct is common, and may be accompanied by cochlear hypoplasia. Most cases of PS result from mutations in the *SLC26A4* gene that encodes an anion transporter known as pendrin that is expressed in the inner ear, thyroid, and kidney.[97] Expression of *SLC26A4* has been shown throughout the endolymphatic duct and sac, in distinct areas of the utricle and saccule, and in the external sulcus region within the developing cochlea.[98] Pendrin is thought to be involved in chloride and iodide transport and not sulfate transport.[99]

Affected individuals have thyroid goiter develop in their second decade, although they usually remain euthyroid.[97] Thyroid dysfunction can be shown with a perchlorate discharge test, in which radioactive iodide and perchlorate are administered. Mutations in *SLC26A4* prevent rapid movement of iodide from the thyrocyte to the colloid, and perchlorate blocks the Na/I symporter that moves iodide from the bloodstream into the thyrocyte. The net effect is that iodide in the thyrocyte washes back into the bloodstream in affected individuals, with a release of greater than 10% radioactivity considered diagnostic for PS.[95,100] The sensitivity of this test is low, making genetic testing the preferred diagnostic method.[95] The hearing impairment is usually prelingual, bilateral, and profound, although it can be progressive.[95] Radiologic studies always show a temporal bone anomaly, either dilated vestibular aqueducts or Mondini dysplasia.[95,101]

Mutations in *SLC26A4* also cause a type of nonsyndromic autosomal recessive deafness called DFNB4.[102,103] Whether the phenotype is syndromic or nonsyndromic may reflect the degree of residual function in the abnormal protein. PS and DFNB4 can be diagnosed by screening this gene for mutations. More recently, mutations in the transcription factor *FOXI1* have also been shown to cause PS in patients heterozygous for a mutation in *SLC26A4.*[104]

Jervell and Lange-Nielsen Syndrome

In 1957, Jervell and Lange-Nielsen described a syndrome characterized by congenital deafness, prolonged Q-T interval, and syncopal attacks.[105] Long Q-T syndrome itself can be dominantly or recessively inherited. The dominant disease is called Romano-Ward syndrome. It is more common and does not include the deafness phenotype.[105] The recessive disease is known as Jervell and Lange-Nielsen syndrome (JLNS).

JLNS is genetically heterogeneous with mutations in *KVLQT1* and *KCNE1* causing this phenotype.[106-108] These genes encode for subunits of a potassium channel expressed in the heart and inner ear. Hearing impairment is due to changes in endolymph homeostasis caused by malfunction of this channel and is congenital, bilateral, and severe to profound.[106-108] Although the prevalence of JLNS among children with congenital deafness is only 0.21%,[109] it is an important diagnosis to consider because of its cardiac manifestations. The prolonged Q-T interval can lead to ventricular arrhythmias, syncopal episodes, and death in childhood.[109] Effective treatment with β-adrenergic blockers reduces mortality from 71% to 6%.[109]

Usher Syndromes

The Usher syndromes (US) are a genetically and clinically heterogeneous group of diseases characterized by SNHL, retinitis pigmentosa, and often vestibular dysfunction.[110] Prevalence is estimated at 4.4 : 100,000 in the United States with 3% to 6% of congenitally deaf individuals carrying this diagnosis.[111] It is the cause of 50% of deaf-blindness in the United States.[111]

Three clinical variants of US are recognized. Type 1 is phenotypically distinguished by the presence of severe to profound congenital hearing loss, vestibular dysfunction, and retinitis pigmentosa that develops in childhood[112]; type 2 is distinguished by moderate to severe congenital hearing loss, with uncertainty related to progression, no vestibular dysfunction, and retinal degeneration that begins in the third to fourth decade[112,113]; and type 3 is characterized by progressive hearing loss, variable vestibular dysfunction, and variable onset of retinitis pigmentosa.[112] Within each subtype, there is genetic heterogeneity, and numerous subtypes are recognized, although the two most common forms are US type 1B (USH1B) and US type 2A (USH2A), which account for 75% to 80% of the Usher syndromes.[114] USH1B accounts for 75% of US type 1 and is caused by mutations in an unconventional myosin called *MYO7A.*[115] USH2A is the most common form, and the causative gene encodes a 1551-amino acid protein named usherin that is a putative extracellular matrix molecule.[116] Numerous other genes have been implicated in US subtypes, and these are listed in Table 147-9.

Biotinidase Deficiency

Biotinidase deficiency is secondary to an absence in the water-soluble B-complex vitamin biotin. Biotin covalently binds to four carboxylases that are essential for gluconeogenesis, fatty acid synthesis, and catabolism of several branched-chain amino acids. If biotinidase deficiency is not recognized and corrected by daily addition of biotin to the diet, affected individuals develop neurologic features such as seizures, hypertonia, developmental delay, ataxia, and visual problems. In at least 75% of children who become symptomatic, SNHL develops, and can be profound and persistent even after treatment is initiated.[117] Cutaneous features are also present and include a skin rash, alopecia, and conjunctivitis. With treatment that consists of biotin replacement, the neurologic and cutaneous manifestations resolve; however, the hearing loss and optic atrophy are usually irreversible. If a child presents with episodic or progressive ataxia and progressive sensorineural deafness, with or without neurologic or cutaneous symptoms, biotinidase deficiency should be considered. To prevent metabolic coma, diet and treatment should be initiated as soon as possible.[117,118] If untreated, 75% of affected infants develop hearing loss, which can be profound, and persists despite the subsequent initiation of treatment.[117]

Refsum Disease

Refsum disease is a postlingual severe progressive SNHL associated with retinitis pigmentosa, peripheral neuropathy, cerebellar ataxia, and elevated protein levels in the cerebrospinal fluid without an increase in the number of cells.[119] It is caused by defective phytanic acid metabolism, and the diagnosis is established by determining serum concentration of phytanic acid. Two genes, *PHYH* and *PEX7,* have been implicated in most cases of Refsum disease, although a few patients exist in whom mutations have not been found.[119] Although extremely rare, it is important that Refsum disease be considered in the evaluation of a deaf person because it can be easily treated with dietary modification and plasmapheresis.

X-Linked Syndromes

Alport Syndrome

Alport syndrome (AS) is a disease of type IV collagen that is manifested by hematuric nephritis, hearing impairment, and ocular changes. The inheritance pattern, although predominantly X-linked (approximately 80%), can be autosomal recessive or dominant.[120] Prevalence is estimated at 1 : 5000 in the United States; a significant proportion of renal transplant patients have AS.[121] Diagnostic criteria include at least three of the following four characteristics[122]: (1) positive family history of hematuria with or without chronic renal failure, (2) progressive high-tone sensorineural deafness, (3) typical eye lesion (anterior lenticonus or macular flecks or both), and (4) histologic changes of the glomerular basement membrane of the kidney.

Mutations in *COL4A5* are the cause of X-linked AS.[123] Type IV collagen is the major component of basement membranes and is formed by the trimerization of various combinations of six type IV collagen genes. Deficiency of this protein results in complete or partial deficiency of the trimerized 3-4-5 complex in the basement membranes of the kidney, cochlea, and eye.[123] More than 300 disease-causing mutations of 5 have been identified with 9.5% to 18% arising de novo.[121,124]

The disease phenotype is more pronounced in males, as expected for X-linked diseases. Gross or microscopic hematuria is the hallmark of disease, and all males ultimately have end-stage renal disease, although the rate of progression depends on the underlying mutation.[125] Ocular manifestations are present in one third of patients and are characterized by anterior lenticonus, an anomaly in which the central portion of the lens protrudes into the anterior chamber of the eye, causing myopia.[125] End-stage renal disease develops before age 30 in patients with anterior lenticonus.[121] Maculopathy and corneal lesions may also be found in patients with AS. Diffuse esophageal leiomyomatosis has been associated with deletion mutations of *COL4A5* and *COL4A6*.[122,125]

Hearing impairment is common in AS and is usually a symmetric, high-frequency sensorineural loss that can be detected by late childhood and progresses to involve all frequencies.[125] Pathogenesis is thought to be related to the loss of the 3-4-5 network, which is important for radial tension on the basilar membrane. Diagnosis currently relies on clinical and histopathologic confirmation, although genetic confirmation can allow the stratification and prediction of severity of the disease phenotype.

Mohr-Tranebjaerg Syndrome

Mohr-Tranebjaerg syndrome was first described in a large Norwegian family with apparent progressive postlingual nonsyndromic hearing impairment and classified as DFN1.[126] Re-evaluation of this family revealed additional findings, however, including visual disability, dystonia, fractures, and mental retardation, indicating that this form of hearing impairment is syndromic, rather than nonsyndromic.[49] The gene for this syndrome, *TIMM8A,* is involved in the translocation of proteins from the cytosol across the inner mitochondrial membrane (TIM) system and into the mitochondrial matrix.[127,128]

Mitochondrial Syndromes

Mitochondrial diseases typically cause a phenotype in tissues with high energy demands, such as muscle, retina, brainstem, pancreas, and cochlea.[55,57] The process by which mitochondrial diseases lead to SNHL is debated and is confounded by the demonstration that nuclear modifier genes have an impact on the outcome.[129] Syndromic mitochondrial diseases are usually multisystemic, with hearing loss present in 70% of affected individuals.[57] Examples include MELAS (mitochondrial encephalopathy, lactic acidosis, and strokelike episodes) syndrome, MERRF (myoclonic epilepsy and red ragged fibers) syndrome, and Kearns-Sayre syndrome (KS) (see Table 147-9).

In MELAS syndrome, hearing loss is sensorineural, progressive, and bilateral, and more severely affects the higher frequencies[130-132]; temporal bone histopathologic findings show severe atrophy of the stria vascularis.[92] MERRF syndrome is characterized by hearing loss, ataxia, dementia, optic nerve atrophy, and short stature. In contrast to MELAS and MERRF, which are caused by point mutations in mtDNA, KS is caused by large duplications and deletions.[133] First described in 1958, KS involves progressive external ophthalmoplegia, atypical retinal pigmentation, and heart block typically starting before age 20.[134,135] SNHL is present in 50% of patients with KS,[57,131] and temporal bone histopathologic findings show cochleosaccular degeneration.[132]

Maternally inherited diabetes and deafness is another syndromic mitochondrial disease. It affects an estimated 0.5% to 2.8% of diabetic patients.[136] The hearing loss occurs late, and is progressive, bilateral, and high frequency; its presence is correlated with the level of heteroplasmy for the 3243 A-to-G mtDNA mutation.[57,130]

Susceptibility to aminoglycoside ototoxicity is also maternally inherited. It is caused by the 1555 A-to-G mtDNA mutation, a nucleotide change found in 17% to 33% of individuals with aminoglycoside-induced hearing loss.[137,138] This mutation changes the 12S rRNA gene, altering its structure to make it more similar to bacterial rRNA, the natural target of aminoglycosides.[137,138] Hearing loss develops even when aminoglycosides are administered at normal doses, with residual thresholds varying widely among individuals. Hearing losses can be seen months after aminoglycoside exposure. Outer hair cells in the basal turn of the cochlea are affected first, but damage eventually extends to include apical outer hair cells and inner hair cells.[139] The same mutation causes nonsyndromic mitochondrial hearing loss.[2]

PATIENT MANAGEMENT

Diagnosis

The evaluation of a deaf patient should involve a team of health care professionals that includes an audiologist, clinical geneticist, ophthalmologist, and otolaryngologist, with the otolaryngologist most frequently coordinating overall care. A well-performed history, physical examination, and audiologic evaluation are keys to assessing the cause of hearing loss.[140]

The American College of Medical Genetics more recently released genetic evaluation guidelines for the diagnosis of congenital hearing loss.[141] Specific details of the family history that should be covered include a pedigree with attention to consanguinity and hearing status of first-degree relatives. Ethnicity, inheritance patterns, audiometric characteristics, and an inquiry of syndromic versus nonsyndromic features are necessary.[141] To assess for the presence of a syndrome related to hearing loss, questions and physical examination regarding endocrine abnormalities (diabetes, thyroid nodules), pigmentary anomalies (white forelock, heterochromic irides), visual anomalies (retinitis pigmentosa, retinal detachment), craniofacial anomalies (dystopia canthorum, aural atresia, cleft palate, branchial anomalies), cardiac manifestations (syncope, arrhythmias, sudden death), and renal anomalies should be performed.[141,142] The patient history and physical examination also should include a search for acquired causes of hearing loss, such as intrauterine infections, meningitis, hypoxia, and ototoxic drugs.

The audiologic evaluation is a crucial part of the initial diagnostic workup. In infants, behavioral testing is often impossible. Electrophysiologic tests such as ABR and otoacoustic emissions provide a means of objectively documenting hearing impairment, and can be used to provide information regarding auditory thresholds. Behavioral tests can be used when infants reach 6 months of age. A trained pediatric audiologist can measure hearing losses of 20 dB in the better hearing ear. The frequency of testing is usually decided on a case-by-case basis, although Tomaski and Grundfast[143] recommend a more rigid schedule in cases of confirmed SNHL in children. They recommend testing every 3 months in the first year of life, followed by every 6 months during the preschool years, and once a year while in school.

No cause of hearing loss may be apparent in 30% of cases even after a thorough history and physical examination.[141] To increase the yield further, additional investigations are necessary. In the past, a battery of tests including thyroid function studies, urinalysis, electrocardiogram, and temporal bone imaging was routinely ordered. Today, genetic screening should supplant these tests. Screening for *GJB2* mutations should be completed; if the diagnosis of DFNB1 is made, further testing is not required.[144] If CT shows dilated vestibular aqueducts or Mondini dysplasia, mutation screening of *SLC26A4* is warranted. Additional known deafness genes may be screened depending on the clinical presentation and the gene testing available at some institutions (see Table 147-4).

Acquired congenital deafness must also be considered. The most frequent cause is in utero cytomegalovirus infection, a diagnosis that can be made definitively only in the neonatal period before the possibility of postnatally acquired cytomegalovirus, which can confound the diagnosis of a congenital infection.[145] MRI has a place in the evaluation of hereditary hearing impairment if a patient is suspected to have NF2, if the hearing loss is progressive, and if the audiologic battery suggests retrocochlear pathology.[143] Other potential investigations include thyroid function studies, electrocardiogram, urinalysis, renal ultrasonography, and electroretinography.

Genetic Testing

In the United States, congenital SNHL occurs about three times more frequently than Down syndrome, six times more frequently than spina bifida, and more than 50 times more frequently than phenylketonuria, making it the most frequently occurring birth defect.[146] An estimated 4000 infants are born each year with severe to profound bilateral hearing loss,[147,148] and another 8000 are born with unilateral or mild to moderate bilateral SNHL.[5] At least 50% of congenital hearing loss has an underlying genetic cause; this is a compelling reason to provide genetic testing services to all children diagnosed with congenital hearing loss. The implementation of the Early Hearing Detection and Intervention (EHDI) program in the United States and similar universal hearing screening programs around the world has facilitated increased detection, genetic diagnosis, and intervention for these children.[149] In addition, advances in genetic technologies have led to an increase in the availability of genetic diagnostic services for infants with hearing loss.[149]

Despite the fact that genetic SNHL is heterogeneous, mutations in the *GJB2* gene (DFNB1) have been shown to account for at least half of all severe to profound congenital nonsyndromic SNHL in the United States, many European countries, Israel, and Australia.[150-153] *GJB2*-related SNHL also has been repeatedly described in several Asian, Latin American, and African countries, but it is less common in these regions. Based on this frequency, first-pass screening of all individuals with congenital hearing loss for *GJB2* mutations is warranted.

For individuals not diagnosed with DFNB1, US should be the next consideration because it accounts for approximately 3% to 6% of all children who have severe to profound hearing loss and is second to *GJB2* mutations as a cause of deafness in the congenitally deaf cochlear implant population.[154] The three different types of US are caused by mutations in at least nine different genes.[155] Determining which genes to screen can be based on the onset and severity of the hearing loss and the presence or absence of vestibular dysfunction.

The third most common genetic cause of early childhood hearing loss is the PS-DFNB4 deafness spectrum. PS accounts for approximately 10% of all syndromic forms of hearing loss and is present in approximately 3% of individuals with hereditary hearing loss.[156] A diagnostic feature of PS is enlarged vestibular aqueducts with or without cochlear dysplasia (Mondini's dysplasia) that is detectable by CT scanning or MRI; the presence of thyroid goiter differentiates PS from DFNB4. Most cases of PS-DFNB4 are due to mutations in the *SLC26A4* gene, and individuals with diagnosed enlarged vestibular aqueducts should be screened for mutations in this gene. More recently, mutations in another gene, *Foxi1,* have also been found to cause PS-DFNB4, and this gene should also be considered in genetic analyses of these families.[104]

ADNSHL is a genetically heterogeneous disorder that is typically postlingual in onset and progressive. It accounts for approximately 15% of inherited hearing loss. To date, 21 genes for nonsyndromic ADNSHL have been identified, and a further 30 dominant loci have been mapped to chromosomal regions.[157] Individuals with apparent ADNSHL should be considered for genetic screening, with criteria for gene selection based on their audioprofile. Identification of phenotype-genotype correlations is crucial in determining the etiology of ADNSHL,[34] and has implications for prognostic and therapeutic outcomes. Some phenotype-genotype correlations are very robust, such as the low-frequency audioprofile associated with *WFS1*-related hearing loss (DFNA6/14/38)[35] and the "cookie-bite" audioprofile associated with *TECTA*-related hearing loss (DFNA8/12)[36]; other correlations are more difficult to define. Autosomal dominant high-frequency hearing loss can be the consequence of mutations in numerous different genes (e.g., *KCNQ4* [DFNA2], *DFNA5* [DFNA5], *COCH* [DFNA9], *POU4F3* [DFNA15]).

Current recommendations for genetic testing are to screen individuals with low-frequency ADNSHL for mutations in *WFS1* and individuals with midfrequency ADNSHL for mutations in *TECTA*. *WFS1* mutations account for approximately 75% of all cases of low-frequency ADNSHL.[45] For individuals with high-frequency hearing loss, because of the number of potential candidate genes, mutation screening is offered only on a research basis. Computer algorithms are being developed, however, to analyze audiograms and to construct audioprofiles as a method of selecting genes for mutation screening for all types of ADNSHL.

Prenatal Testing

Prenatal diagnosis for some forms of hereditary hearing loss is technically possible by analysis of DNA extracted from fetal cells. Fetal material can be obtained by amniocentesis at 15 to 18 weeks' gestation or chorionic villus sampling at 10 to 12 weeks' gestation. Gestational age is expressed as menstrual weeks calculated from the first day of the last normal menstrual period or by ultrasound measurements. The deafness-causing allele of a deaf family member must be identified before prenatal testing can be performed.

Requests for prenatal testing for conditions such as hearing loss are uncommon. Differences in perspective may exist among medical professionals and within families regarding the use of prenatal testing, particularly if the testing is being considered for the purpose of pregnancy termination, rather than early diagnosis. Although most centers would consider decisions about prenatal testing to be the choice of the parents, careful discussion of these issues is appropriate. Preimplantation genetic diagnosis may be available for families in which the deafness-causing mutation has been identified in a deaf family member.

Treatment

When a diagnosis is made, directed treatment is possible. Appropriate consultation and management of the associated conditions should be considered. A diagnosis of JLNS may necessitate therapy with β-blockers to reduce the chance of life-threatening arrhythmias. If US is considered, close ophthalmologic follow-up is mandatory. In contrast, a genetic diagnosis of *GJB2*-related deafness requires no other consultation because there is no associated comorbidity.

Genetic counseling should be offered to patients and their families by a professional trained in clinical genetics. Most otolaryngologists do not have an adequate understanding of recurrence chances to provide accurate data.[158] Green and coworkers[23] have estimated the recurrence chance for a normal-hearing couple with a deaf child to have a second deaf child at 17.5%, much higher than earlier estimates of 9.8%. Factors that explain this increase include an improved ability to identify syndromic forms of deafness and a decrease in congenital acquired deafness.[23] A well-trained genetic counselor can also help to interpret medical data and potential treatment options. Counseling sessions should occur before and after genetic testing has been done.

Management of hearing loss should be directed at providing appropriate amplification as soon as possible. Hearing aids provide significant benefits to individuals with mild to moderate hearing loss. Cochlear implantation is becoming an increasingly important option for individuals with severe to profound deafness.[27] The Joint Committee on Infant Hearing recommends that diagnosis and rehabilitation be instituted by 6 months of age to minimize delays in communicative language development. Coupled with this recommendation, universal screening is becoming a reality throughout the United States. For the detection of congenital hearing loss, the U.S. government has facilitated the creation of EHDI programs for early newborn hearing screening (http://www.infanthearing.org). EHDI programs aim to screen neonates for hearing loss immediately after birth or before hospital discharge. The programs include a follow-up arm to confirm hearing loss in neonates who do not pass the initial screening test so that intervention can be initiated to prevent delayed language acquisition.[159]

EHDI program guidelines include three phases: screening, audiologic evaluation, and intervention. In the first phase, newborns are screened with otoacoustic emissions and ABR to detect permanent bilateral or unilateral sensory or conductive hearing loss averaging 30 to 40 dB SPL (sound pressure level) or more in the frequency region important for speech recognition. In the second phase, all infants who do not pass the initial screen are evaluated with a series of diagnostic audiologic tests, preferably before age 3 months. In the third phase, early intervention services are implemented before age 6 months for all infants with confirmed hearing loss.[159]

Prevention of Hearing Impairment

Although experimental methodologies to restore auditory function are currently being developed and tested,[160,161] no effective therapy is clinically available. Existing measures must focus on the prevention of hearing loss to decrease the frequency of acquired and genetic hearing loss.[4] Improved implementation of vaccination programs in developing nations, avoidance of exacerbating factors such as noise, and focused genetic counseling and health education in populations with a high prevalence of consanguinity are several methods that if implemented would reduce the incidence of acquired and hereditary hearing loss.

Cultural Considerations

Having discussed the management of a patient with hearing loss, a mention of the Deaf (written with a capital "D") culture is necessary. Individuals who identify with the Deaf culture consider themselves as culturally Deaf and understandably wish to preserve their culture. Generally, members of the Deaf community look on genetics negatively.[162,163] A study by Middleton and colleagues[163] found that 55% of deaf respondents at a conference on the "Deaf Nation" thought genetics would do more harm than good. Of respondents, 46% thought that the use of genetics may devalue deaf people. This response may represent sample bias, however, because a study by Stern and associates[162] found that most deaf individuals have a positive view of the field of genetics. These studies highlight an important point—that attitudes about hearing loss, or more specifically deafness, are culturally dependent. The medical community must understand and appreciate this perspective, and try to offer advances in diagnosis, counseling, and treatment in a nonjudgmental manner.

Acknowledgment

The authors thank Katy Nash Krahn, MS, CGC, in the Department of Pediatrics, University of Iowa Hospitals and Clinics, for her help in preparing the pedigrees of the various forms of hearing impairment. This work was supported in part by NIH grants DC02842 and DC03544 (R.J.H.S.).

SUGGESTED READINGS

Abdelhak S, Kalatzis V, Heilig R, et al. A human homologue of the Drosophila eyes absent gene underlies branchio-oto-renal (BOR) syndrome and identifies a novel gene family. *Nat Genet.* 1997;15:157-164.

Chang EH, Van Camp G, Smith RJ. The role of connexins in human disease. *Ear Hear.* 2003;24:314-323.

Der Kaloustian VM. Congenital anomalies of ear, nose and throat. In: Tewfik TL, Der Kaloustian VM, eds. *Introduction to Medical Genetics and Dysmorphology.* New York: Oxford University Press; 1997.

Duncan RD, Prucka S, Wiatrak BJ, et al. Pediatric otolaryngologists' use of genetic testing. *Arch Otolaryngol Head Neck Surg.* 2007;133:231-236.

For complete list of references log onto www.expertconsult.com.

Ensink RJ, Huygen PL, Cremers CW. The clinical spectrum of maternally transmitted hearing loss. *Adv Otorhinolaryngol.* 2002;61:172-183.

Everett LA, Glaser B, Beck JC, et al. Pendred syndrome is caused by mutations in a putative sulphate transporter gene (PDS). *Nat Genet.* 1997;17:411-422.

Fischel-Ghodsian N. Genetic factors in aminoglycoside toxicity. *Ann N Y Acad Sci.* 1999;884:99-109.

Green GE, Scott DA, McDonald JM, et al. Performance of cochlear implant recipients with GJB2-related deafness. *Am J Med Genet.* 2002;109:167-170.

Gross O, Netzer KO, Lambrecht R, et al. Meta-analysis of genotype-phenotype correlation in X-linked Alport syndrome: impact on clinical counselling. *Nephrol Dial Transplant.* 2002;17:1218-1227.

Joint Committee on Infant Hearing, American Academy of Audiology, American Academy of Pediatrics, American Speech-Language-Hearing Association, and Directors of Speech and Hearing Programs in State Health and Welfare Agencies. Year 2000 position statement: principles and guidelines for early hearing detection and intervention programs. Joint Committee on Infant Hearing, American Academy of Audiology, American Academy of Pediatrics, American Speech-Language-Hearing Association, and Directors of Speech and Hearing Programs in State Health and Welfare Agencies. *Pediatrics.* 2000;106:798-817.

Jorde L. *Medical Genetics.* St Louis: Mosby-Year Book; 1995.

Kelsell DP, Dunlop J, Stevens HP, et al. Connexin 26 mutations in hereditary non-syndromic sensorineural deafness. *Nature.* 1997;387:80-83.

Kubisch C, Schroeder BC, Friedrich T. KCNQ4, a novel potassium channel expressed in sensory outer hair cells, is mutated in dominant deafness. *Cell.* 1999;96:437-446.

Morton NE. Genetic epidemiology of hearing impairment. *Ann N Y Acad Sci.* 1991;630:16-31.

Nowak CB. Genetics and hearing loss: A review of Stickler syndrome. *J Commun Disord.* 1998;31:437-453.

Pennings RJ, Wagenaar M, van Aarem A, et al. Hearing impairment in Usher's syndrome. *Adv Otorhinolaryngol.* 2002;61:184-191.

Read AP, Newton VE. Waardenburg syndrome. *J Med Genet.* 1997;34:656-665.

Smith RJ, Bale JF Jr, White KR. Sensorineural hearing loss in children. *Lancet.* 2005;365:879-890.

Strachan T, Read AP. Genes in pedigrees. In: Kingston F, ed. *Human Molecular Genetics.* 2nd ed. New York: John-Wiley & Sons; 1999.

Tekin M, Arnos KS, Pandya A. Advances in hereditary deafness. *Lancet.* 2001;358:1082-1090.

Van Camp G, Smith RJ. Hereditary Hearing Loss Homepage. http://webh01.ua.ac.be/hhh/; 2007.

Yang T, Vidarsson H, Rodrigo-Blomqvist S, et al. Transcriptional control of SLC26A4 is involved in Pendred syndrome and nonsyndromic enlargement of vestibular aqueduct (DFNB4). *Am J Hum Genet.* 2007;80:1055-1063.

CHAPTER ONE HUNDRED AND FORTY-EIGHT

Otologic Manifestations of Systemic Disease

Saumil N. Merchant

Joseph B. Nadol, Jr.

Key Points

- A wide variety of systemic diseases can affect the temporal bone, including granulomatous and infectious diseases, neoplasms, disorders of bone, storage and metabolic diseases, and autoimmune and immunodeficiency disorders.
- Otologic manifestations of a particular systemic disease are determined by location and extent of involvement within the temporal bone, and the nature of the disease. Any part of the temporal bone may be affected, and the clinical features may include conductive or sensorineural hearing loss, vestibular manifestations, otalgia, and facial nerve paralysis.
- Systemic disease may mimic more common otologic disorders, such as acute or chronic otitis media, sudden idiopathic deafness, and Bell's palsy.
- Otologic manifestations may constitute a small part of a wider constellation of symptoms and signs, or may be the sole and initial presenting feature of a systemic disease.
- Diagnosis may be challenging, requiring a high level of suspicion, with use of ancillary tests such as laboratory studies, radiographic evaluation, and biopsy.
- Management of otologic symptoms must be individualized and often requires coordinated care across multiple disciplines.

Systemic diseases that may involve the ear include granulomatous and infectious processes, tumors, bone disorders, storage diseases, collagen vascular and autoimmune diseases, and immunodeficiency disorders (Table 148-1). In some of these diseases, the initial clinical symptoms may occur in the temporal bone and be confused with other diseases that are limited to the ear.

Granulomatous and Infectious Diseases

Chronic otitis media with otorrhea, inflammation, and granulation of the middle ear and mastoid is one of the most common entities treated by otolaryngologists. Several more generalized disease entities, such as the Langerhans cell histiocytosis (LCH), tuberculosis, Wegener's granulomatosis (WG), and mycotic diseases, may closely mimic the symptoms of chronic suppurative otitis media, whereas others, such as Lyme disease and sarcoidosis, may mimic idiopathic cranial neuropathy.

Langerhans Cell Histiocytosis

LCH (formerly called histiocytosis X) refers to a group of disorders that are characterized by a proliferation of cytologically benign histiocytes. The term *histiocytosis X* was proposed by Lichtenstein,[1] who considered eosinophilic granuloma, Hand-Schüller-Christian disease, and Letterer-Siwe disease to be related disorders because of the similarity of their pathologic lesions. The severity of these diseases and prognosis and treatment differ greatly, however. Histopathologically, the primary lesion of LCH is formed by collections of pathologic Langerhans cells with variable numbers of eosinophils, macrophages, and lymphocytes. Diagnostic characteristics of the pathologic Langerhans cells include nuclei that are deeply indented and elongated on light microscopy, cytoplasm that is pale and abundant, Birbeck granules on electron microscopy, expression of CD1 on the cell surface, and positive immunostaining for S100 protein and for the so-called Langerin protein.[2,3] The etiology and pathogenesis of LCH remain unknown, although more recent research has begun to shed some light on these.[2,4,5] Current thinking favors the notion that LCH results from immunologic dysfunction, resulting in unchecked proliferation of pathologic Langerhans cells.[5]

Unifocal eosinophilic granuloma, which occurs in children and young adults, shows a male predominance. It appears as a solitary osteolytic lesion in the femora, pelvis, scapulae, vertebrae, ribs, mandible, maxilla, or skull (including the temporal bone). The lesion may be asymptomatic, or it may cause pain, local swelling, or pathologic fracture. There are no systemic manifestations. The clinical course is typically benign, the prognosis is excellent, and spontaneous regression may occur. Local curettage with or without low-dose irradiation (approximately 60 Gy)[6] is usually curative. Temporary splinting or casting may be necessary for weight-bearing bones. Follow-up examination with a radiographic skeletal survey should be performed to detect lesions at other sites; such lesions are almost always found within 1 year.

Hand-Schüller-Christian disease may be best understood as a multifocal form of LCH. It usually occurs in children younger than 5 years old, and it is characterized by multifocal osteolytic lesions with limited extraskeletal involvement of skin, lymph nodes, and viscera. Multiple lesions are evident at diagnosis or develop within 6 months after a unifocal lesion appears. Systemic manifestations include fever, anorexia, recurrent upper respiratory infections, anterior cervical lymphadenopathy, otitis media, and hepatosplenomegaly. The classic triad

Table 148-1

Systemic Diseases That Affect the Ear

Granulomatous and infectious diseases
Langerhans cell histiocytosis
Tuberculosis
Wegener's granulomatosis
Sarcoidosis
Syphilis
Lyme disease
Mycotic diseases
Neoplastic diseases
Multiple myeloma
Leukemia
Metastatic neoplasms
Diseases of bone
Paget's disease (osteitis deformans)
Osteogenesis imperfecta
Fibrous dysplasia
Osteopetroses
Osteitis fibrosa cystica
Storage and metabolic diseases
Mucopolysaccharidoses
Gout
Ochronosis
Collagen vascular and autoimmune diseases
Immunodeficiency disorders
Primary or congenital
Humoral immunodeficiency disorders
Cellular immunodeficiency disorders
Disorders of phagocyte function
Complement system defects
Acquired
Acquired immunodeficiency syndrome
Genetically determined defects

of osteolytic skull lesions, exophthalmos as a result of orbital bone involvement, and diabetes insipidus secondary to pituitary disease may be seen in 25% of patients.[7] Chest radiograph may show diffuse pulmonary infiltration, particularly in central and perihilar areas. Hilar lymphadenopathy is rare. Diagnosis requires biopsy of an accessible lesion. Spontaneous regression may occur, but the disease is typically chronic, and low-dose chemotherapy may be required to control systemic manifestations.

Letterer-Siwe disease is a disseminated form of LCH that occurs in children younger than 3 years old and manifests with the diffuse involvement of multiple organs. Manifestations include fever, seborrheic or eczema-like rash, oral lesions, lymphadenopathy, hepatosplenomegaly, multiple bony lesions, diffuse replacement of marrow with resulting blood dyscrasias, and pulmonary infiltration with respiratory failure. The disease is virulent, with a poor prognosis and a high mortality rate. Treatment consists of varying combinations of corticosteroids and cytotoxic drugs such as methotrexate, mercaptopurine, vincristine, vinblastine, chlorambucil, cyclophosphamide, and etoposide. High-dose chemotherapy and radiation followed by bone marrow transplantation or hematopoietic stem cell transplantation has been reported to be successful in a few advanced refractory cases of LCH.[8]

Otologic Manifestations

The mastoid is a common site of involvement in LCH. When small, the lesion is asymptomatic. As it expands, the lesion may manifest in several ways: by erosion of the posterior bony canal wall; by erosion through the cortex of the mastoid, zygomatic, or squamosal portions; or by secondary infection.[9] The otic capsule and facial nerve are relatively resistant. Although sensorineural hearing loss (SNHL), vertigo, and facial nerve paralysis can occur, they are infrequent. Similarly, extension beyond the temporal bone involving the jugular fossa and skull base is rare.

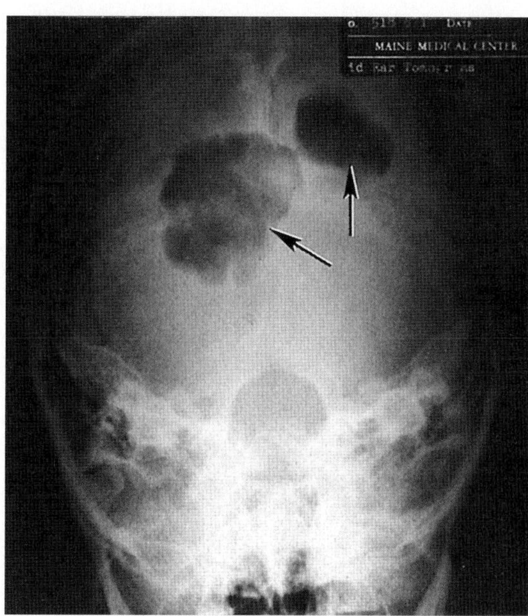

Figure 148-1. Multiple eosinophilic granulomas in a 32-year-old woman. There are two lytic lesions of the skull showing beveled edges *(arrows)* and nonsclerotic margins, which are typical of this disease.

The reported incidence of otologic manifestations in patients with LCH is 15% to 61%,[7] and they may be the initial presentation of the disease. The most common symptom is otorrhea, followed by postauricular swelling, hearing loss, and vertigo.[10,11] The most common sign is granulation tissue or aural polyps in the external auditory canal. The disease may manifest with perforation of the tympanic membrane, otitis media, otitis externa, fistula between the mastoid and the external canal, or nontender postauricular swelling. Occasionally, inner ear symptoms and a positive fistula test are found in the presence of an intact tympanic membrane. The disease often mimics chronic otitis media, and mastoid surgery is frequently performed before the diagnosis is made.[9]

Diagnosis of LCH is suggested by an inflammatory disorder of the middle ear and mastoid that does not respond to routine antibiotic therapy, bilateral destructive ear disease, an elevated erythrocyte sedimentation rate in the absence of acute infection, exuberant granulation tissue after mastoid surgery with a persistently draining cavity, and associated skin and systemic lesions. Radiographs show destructive lesions in the mastoid and temporal bones (Figs. 148-1 and 148-2).[9,10,12] The diagnosis is established by biopsy; because the surface of the granulation tissue often shows infection, necrosis, and fibrosis, tissue should be acquired from deeper parts of the lesion.[13] Microscopic findings include sheets of histiocytes with a variable number of eosinophils, plasma cells, polymorphonuclear leukocytes, and multinucleated cells (Figs. 148-3, 148-4, and 148-5). Areas of hemorrhage and necrosis are common. A definitive diagnosis of LCH is usually made on the basis of immunostaining and electron microscopic studies.[2,4]

Tuberculosis

The incidence of tuberculous otitis media has decreased dramatically. During the early part of the 20th century, 1.3% to 18.6% of all cases of chronic otitis media were reportedly caused by tuberculosis, whereas more recent studies report tuberculous otitis media rates of 0.05% to 0.9%.[14] The last 20 years have witnessed an increase in incidence of tuberculosis, however, which is caused in part by the aggressive nature of tuberculosis in individuals infected with human immunodeficiency virus (HIV), and by an emerging resistance to antituberculosis drugs.[15]

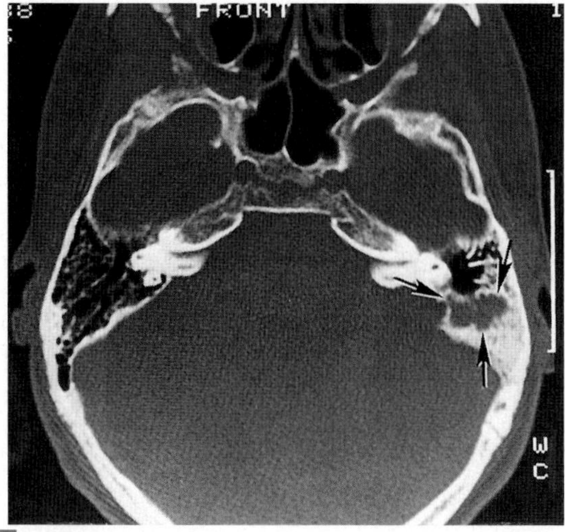

Figure 148-2. Irregular lytic lesion in the mastoid bone *(arrows)* of a 13-year-old boy with unifocal eosinophilic granuloma.

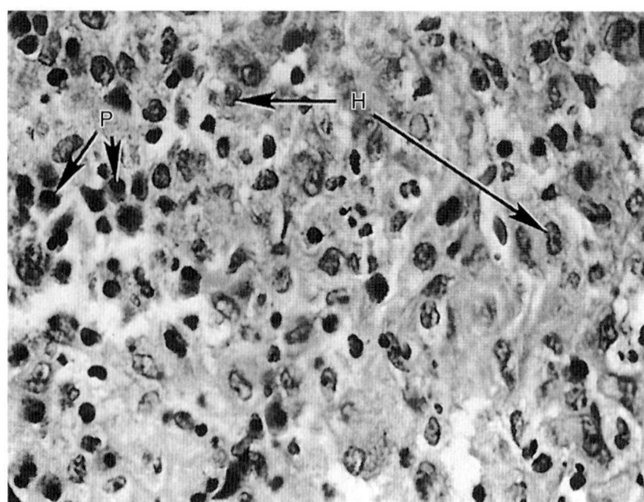

Figure 148-5. Eosinophilic granuloma of the external ear canal with plasma cells (P), eosinophils, and histiocytes (H), which show "folded" nuclei, a morphology that is peculiar to the histiocytoses (×640).

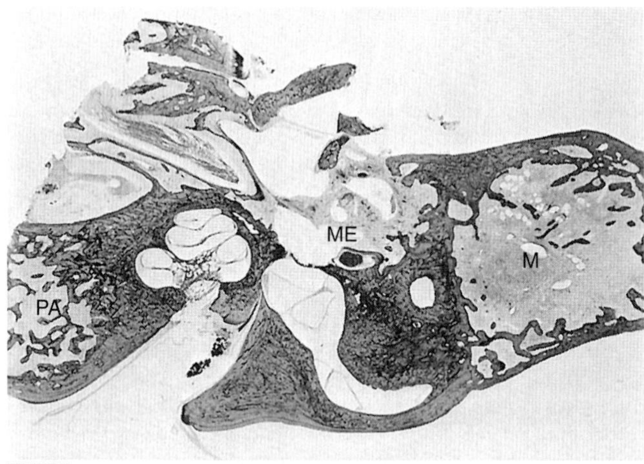

Figure 148-3. Letterer-Siwe disease affecting the temporal bone of a 4-year-old boy. Granulation tissue typical of histiocytosis can be seen in lytic lesions within the mastoid (M), middle ear (ME), and petrous apex (PA) (×4).

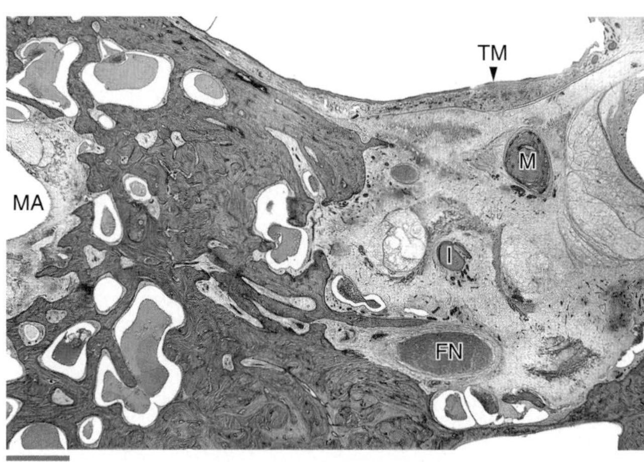

Figure 148-6. Tuberculous granulation tissue filling the middle ear of a 57-year-old man who died of miliary tuberculosis (×12.35). FN, facial nerve; I, incus; M, malleus; MA, mastoid; TM, tympanic membrane.

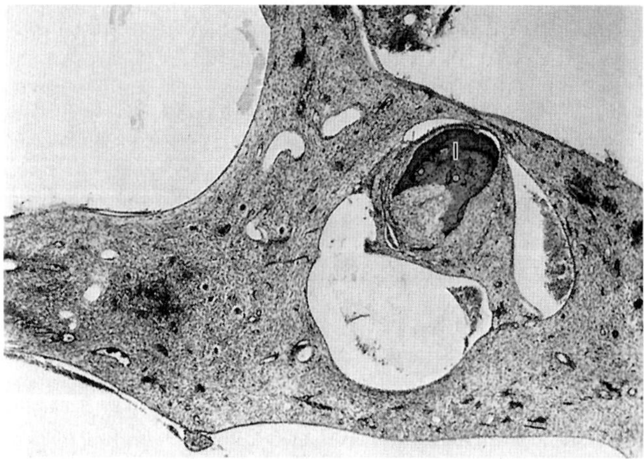

Figure 148-4. A higher power view of part of the middle ear area seen in Figure 148-3. The infiltrate consists of histiocytes, eosinophils, and multinucleated cells. The incus (I) has been partially resorbed (×45).

Mycobacterium tuberculosis is the infective organism in most cases; occasionally, atypical mycobacteria (e.g., *Mycobacterium avium* and *Mycobacterium fortuitum*) are responsible.[16]

Tuberculosis of the middle ear and mastoid may occur as a result of hematogenous or lymphatic spread, or by extension to the middle ear cleft through the eustachian tube. Direct inoculation through a perforation of the tympanic membrane is also possible. Middle ear involvement in the absence of active pulmonary disease is rare, but may occur.

During the early stages of tuberculous otitis media, the tympanic membrane becomes thickened, and the otoscopic landmarks become obliterated. There is a conductive hearing loss as a result of middle ear effusion, a thickening of the tympanic membrane and middle ear mucosa, and a destruction of the ossicles (Figs. 148-6 and 148-7). There is no characteristic pain or tenderness, but lymphadenopathy in the high jugular chain occurs early. Multiple small perforations of the tympanic membrane may occur, with seropurulent drainage. The perforations quickly coalesce to cause loss of the tympanic membrane. Likewise, a myringotomy site in an intact tympanic membrane may enlarge quickly. The middle ear mucosa appears to be hyperemic with polypoid granulation. Osseous involvement results in the sequestration of bone and the destruction of the inner ear, the facial nerve, or both.

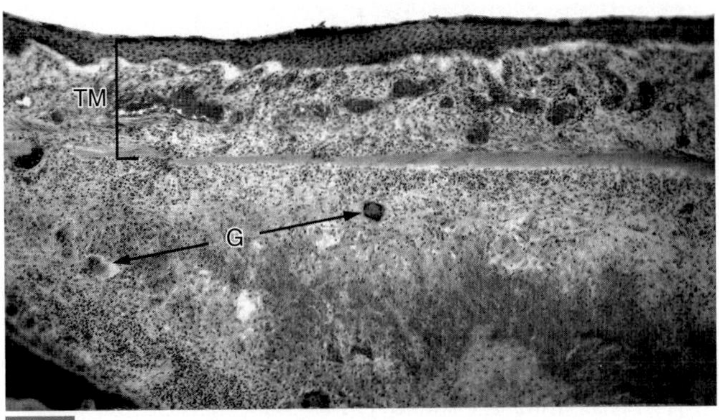

Figure 148-7. A higher power view of the tympanic membrane (TM) seen in Figure 148-6. The TM is intact, but greatly thickened by tuberculous granulation tissue containing the typical epithelioid cells, round cells, and multinucleated giant cells (G) (×100).

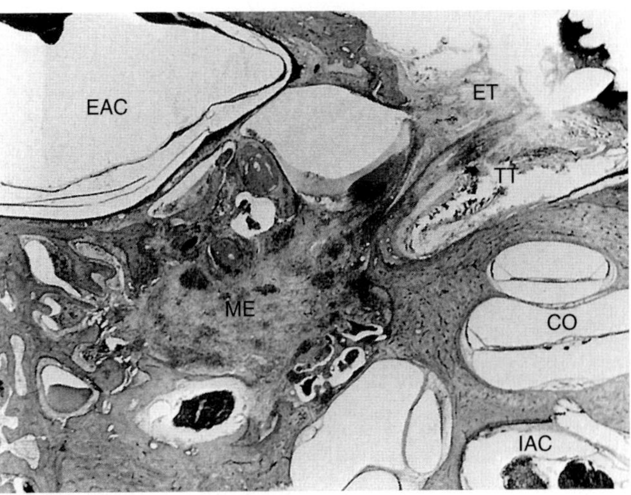

Figure 148-8. Wegener's granulomatosis causing blockage of the eustachian tube (ET) and infiltration of the middle ear (ME) in a 41-year-old man (×10). CO, cochlea; EAC, external auditory canal; IAC, internal auditory canal; TT, tensor tympani. *(Courtesy of Leslie Michaels, MD, Institute of Laryngology and Otology, London.)*

Destruction of the mastoid tip may result in an asymptomatic, nontender Bezold's abscess (i.e., a "cold" abscess). Rarely, tuberculosis can also manifest as primary tuberculous petrositis,[17] or as SNHL caused by chronic labyrinthitis and tuberculous meningitis.[18]

The diagnosis of tuberculous involvement of the middle ear is usually delayed. The characteristic signs and symptoms include multiple perforations of the tympanic membrane that quickly coalesce to form total tympanic membrane loss, nontender cervical lymphadenopathy, intractable otitis media with polypoid granulation, and bony sequestration; these should alert the physician to this possible diagnosis. Otic capsule involvement with resultant loss of auditory and vestibular function may be the first symptom, which indicates a process that differs from the more typical chronic otitis media. Definitive diagnosis is made by histopathologic examination of tissue from the middle ear or mastoid showing a granulomatous process with multinucleated giant cells (Langhans cells) (see Figs. 148-6 and 148-7) and histologic demonstration of acid-fast organisms of tuberculosis. The accurate identification of the mycobacterial species and drug-resistant isolates by culture is still the gold standard. Culture takes several weeks, however, and is time-consuming. The process is facilitated by the use of several different types of nucleic acid amplification tests that have been approved by the U.S. Food and Drug Administration for rapid identification of *M. tuberculosis*.[15,19]

Multiple perforations of the tympanic membrane, exuberant polypoid granulation within the middle ear, and early loss of inner ear function also are seen in WG. These two diseases are distinguished on the basis of skin tests for tuberculosis and the histologic demonstration of acid-fast organisms of tuberculosis in granulation tissue, cultures of the middle ear, the presence of antineutrophil cytoplasmic antibodies (ANCAs) in WG, and the systemic manifestations of each process.

The mainstay of management of tuberculosis of the middle ear and mastoid is the systemic use of standard antituberculous chemotherapy.[14] Mastoid surgery may be required to remove sequestrated bone. Reconstructive surgery of the ossicles and tympanic membrane is feasible after the infection has been controlled.

Wegener's Granulomatosis

WG is a granulomatous inflammatory process with necrotizing vasculitis. It primarily affects the upper and lower respiratory tracts and kidneys, but WG can involve essentially any organ in the body. The disease occurs equally in men and women, and the mean age of onset is 40 years. Common presenting symptoms include headache, sinusitis, rhinorrhea, otitis media, fever, and arthralgia.[20,21] Upper airway and sinus involvement occurs in 75% to 90% of cases. Pulmonary manifestations include cough, pleuritic chest pain, hemoptysis, and nodular or cavitary infiltrates on chest radiography. Pulmonary manifestations occur in 65% to 85% of cases. Other manifestations include glomerulonephritis (60% to 75% of cases); eye involvement in the form of conjunctivitis, iritis, scleritis, or proptosis (15% to 50% of cases); and dermatologic findings of necrotic ulcerations, vesicles, or petechiae.

Laboratory findings in WG may include normochromic, normocytic anemia; thrombocytosis; positive rheumatoid factor; and hyperglobulinemia, particularly of IgA. The erythrocyte sedimentation rate is almost always elevated. The discovery in 1985 of autoantibodies directed against the cytoplasmic constituents of neutrophils (ANCA, c-ANCA) in patients with WG was a major advance in the diagnosis and understanding of WG.[22] A positive ANCA test, especially proteinase 3–specific c-ANCA, is very helpful in establishing or supporting a diagnosis of WG. The specificity of positive c-ANCA testing in WG is greater than 95%; the sensitivity is variable and depends on the phase and type of WG. c-ANCA is positive in more than 90% of patients with systemic and active WG, whereas in limited WG (e.g., ear or head and neck only or inactive disease), the sensitivity of c-ANCA is only 65% to 70%. In addition, the antibody titer parallels the activity of the disease, although there have been conflicting data about the value in using the titer as a guide for immunosuppressive therapy.

The diagnosis of WG is made histologically by the presence of necrosis, granulomatous inflammation with multinucleated giant cells, vasculitis, and microabscess formation (Figs. 148-8 and 148-9). Small biopsy specimens (e.g., from the ear or upper airways) may lack all of the various diagnostic features, however. In such cases, a diagnosis of WG can be made on the basis of the clinical presentation, ANCA testing, and repeat biopsy specimens taken from the same or related sites.

The etiology and pathogenesis of WG are unknown. Infectious, genetic, and environmental risk factors and combinations thereof have been proposed. The evidence to date suggests that WG is a complex, immune-mediated disorder in which tissue injury results from the interplay of an initiating inflammatory event and a highly specific immune response.[23] Part of this response consists of the production of ANCA, directed against antigens present within the primary granules of neutrophils and monocytes; these antibodies produce tissue damage by interacting with primed neutrophils and endothelial cells.

The prognosis of WG has dramatically improved from a mortality rate of 82% before the era of immunosuppressive therapy to the current remission rate of more than 75% with appropriate medical therapy.[24] Induction of remission is usually achieved with high doses of corticosteroids, cyclophosphamide, or methotrexate given for 3 to 6 months. Maintenance of remission is achieved with lower doses of corticosteroids and less toxic alternatives to cyclophosphamide, such as azathioprine, methotrexate, trimethoprim-sulfamethoxazole, or other drug

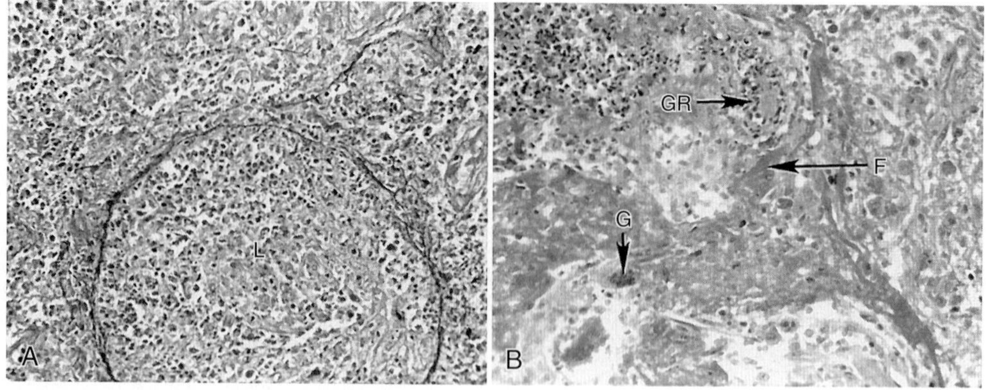

Figure 148-9. Wegener's granulomatosis in lung biopsy specimen. **A,** Arteriole showing necrotizing vasculitis with obliteration of the lumen (L) and infiltration of the vessel wall with polymorphonuclear leukocytes (elastic stain; ×256). **B,** Vessel wall showing fibrin deposit (F), giant cells (G), and granuloma (GR) (hematoxylin-eosin stain; ×256).

combinations. Other therapies that have been used include leflunomide, mycophenolate mofetil, and the tumor necrosis factor inhibitors etanercept and infliximab.

Otologic Manifestations

The middle ear and mastoid are the most common sites within the temporal bone that are involved in patients with WG.[20,25] WG may cause obstruction of the eustachian tube with resultant serous otitis media and conductive hearing loss (see Fig. 148-8). Some patients also have purulent otitis media, and others may have frank granulomatous involvement of the middle ear and mastoid. The process can extend to involve the facial nerve and the inner ear, which is usually manifested as rapidly progressive SNHL and loss of vestibular function. Otologic disease may be the sole and initial presenting feature in some patients with WG.

Sarcoidosis

Sarcoidosis is a chronic multisystem disorder of unknown etiology that is characterized by the presence of noncaseating granulomas. It most frequently affects the lungs, although almost all body parts can be affected. The disease shows a female predominance, and is 10 times more common in blacks than in whites. The onset of disease is usually during the third to fourth decade of life. Common presenting manifestations include bilateral hilar adenopathy on chest radiography, cough, and granulomatous skin rash. Other manifestations include iridocyclitis, keratoconjunctivitis, peripheral lymphadenopathy, hepatosplenomegaly, cardiac failure, myalgia, and arthralgia. Neurologic involvement includes central and peripheral manifestations. The facial and optic nerves are the most commonly affected cranial nerves. Either peripheral mononeuritis or polyneuritis may be seen. Laboratory findings may include hilar adenopathy on chest radiography (Fig. 148-10), hypercalcemia, and elevated serum angiotensin-converting enzyme. The histopathologic feature of the sarcoid lesion is noncaseating epithelioid granulomas (Fig. 148-11).

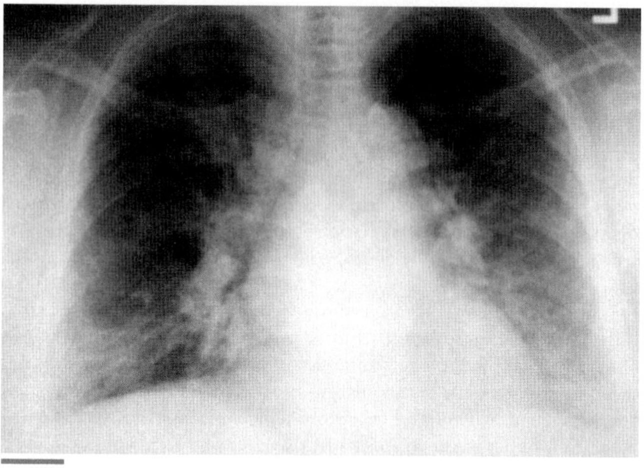

Figure 148-10. Bilateral hilar adenopathy and linear parenchymal densities in a 56-year-old woman with pulmonary sarcoidosis.

The etiology and pathogenesis of sarcoidosis are unknown. The initial pulmonary lesion is an alveolitis characterized by the accumulation of $CD4^+$ T cells, followed by development of noncaseating granulomas. The antigenic stimulus that initiates the disease process remains elusive. Several possible associations have been investigated, including mycobacteria, certain HLA complexes, abnormalities of T cells and the T-cell antigen receptor, and involvement of several different cytokines.[26]

Spontaneous resolution occurs in many patients. Corticosteroids are beneficial for patients with progressive symptoms or with ocular, cardiac, or central nervous system involvement. For patients who cannot tolerate or do not respond to corticosteroids, alternative drugs include methotrexate, cyclophosphamide, azathioprine, chlorambucil, cyclosporine, chloroquine, pentoxifylline, and antagonists of human tumor necrosis factor-α such as etanercept (Enbrel) and infliximab (Remicade).[27]

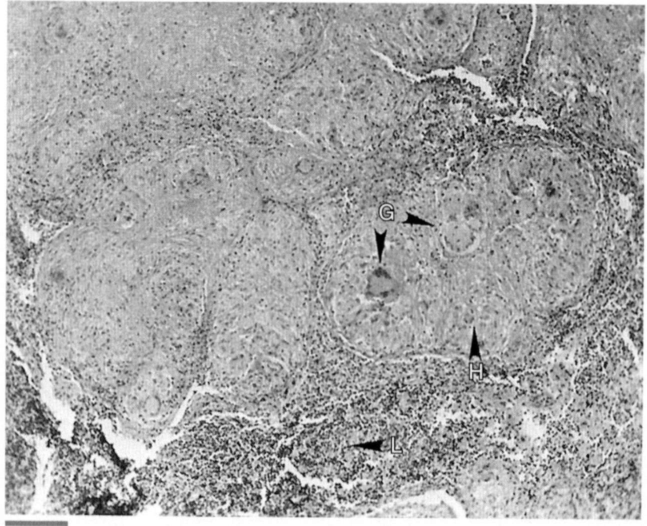

Figure 148-11. Sarcoidosis in a lymph node specimen. There are noncaseating granulomas with giant cells (G), histiocytes (H), and lymphocytes (L) (×79).

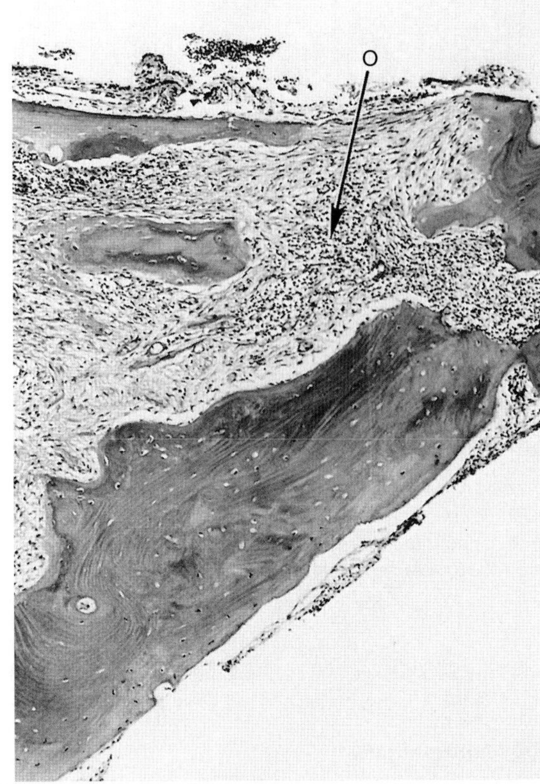

Figure 148-12. Section of the incus in a patient with acquired syphilis. There is an active round cell osteitis (O), with involvement of the periosteum (×120).

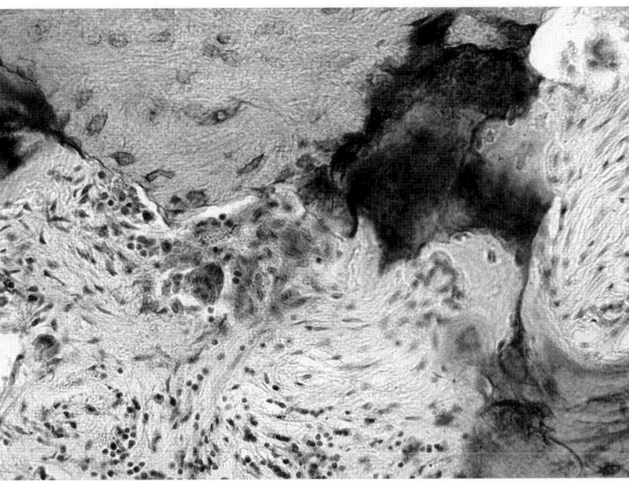

Figure 148-13. Area of active bone resorption in a 43-year-old patient with congenital syphilis. The inflammatory infiltrate includes lymphocytes, plasma cells, and multinucleated giant cells (×396).

Otologic Manifestations

Otologic manifestations of sarcoidosis include SNHL, vestibular dysfunction, and facial nerve paralysis, and occasionally granulomatous disease of the external or middle ear and mastoid.[28-31] The facial nerve is the most commonly affected cranial nerve and is usually involved as part of the triad of uveoparotid fever (Heerfordt's syndrome) that is characterized by parotitis, uveitis, facial nerve paralysis, and mild pyrexia. The facial paralysis may be sudden in onset, it is often bilateral, and it may resolve spontaneously. Histopathology of the temporal bone in sarcoidosis has been reported in only one case; the main findings were perivascular lymphocytic infiltration and granulomatous inflammation involving the cochlear, vestibular, and facial nerves within the internal auditory canal.[32]

Syphilis

Congenital and acquired syphilis may affect the middle ear in the late latent and tertiary forms. In the late latent form, the middle ear and mastoid may be affected by a rarefying osteitis with leukocytic infiltration of the ossicles and mastoid bone (Figs. 148-12 and 148-13). A similar but larger lesion of tertiary syphilis, the gumma, shows obliterative arteritis and central necrosis. A gumma of the ear canal or middle ear may result in perforation of the tympanic membrane and a granulomatous appearance of the middle ear mucosa. Definitive diagnosis of syphilis of the middle ear requires a positive serologic test and a histologic demonstration of *Treponema pallidum*. Syphilitic involvement of the tympanic membrane and middle ear may mimic tuberculosis, and superinfection may result in chronic otitis media.

Inner ear involvement may occur in the absence of macroscopic changes in the tympanic membrane or middle ear. Hennebert's sign, which is the induction of ocular deviation with positive or negative pressure in the external auditory canal, was believed to indicate a true fistula between the middle and inner ear because of rarefying osteitis of the otic capsule. The more probable cause is fibrous adhesions, however, between the stapes footplate and the membranous labyrinth as a result of endolymphatic hydrops.[33] Combined antibiotic and corticosteroid therapy is beneficial for the management of SNHL.[34]

Lyme Disease

Lyme disease is a multisystem inflammatory disorder that primarily affects the skin, nervous system, heart, and joints. It is caused by a spirochete, *Borrelia burgdorferi,* that is transmitted to humans by certain *Ixodes* ticks that are part of the *Ixodes ricinus* complex. The known primary reservoirs of the disease are white-footed mice and white-tailed deer. The disease was initially recognized in 1975 because of a clustering of patients with arthritis in Lyme, Connecticut, but it is now known that Lyme disease has been present for several decades in Europe, where it is called Bannwarth's syndrome.

Infection is usually acquired in the summer, and individuals of all ages and both sexes can be affected. Three clinical stages that are similar to the stages seen with cases of syphilis are recognized.[35] The first stage (early, localized infection) begins 3 to 33 days after a tick bite with a characteristic skin lesion (erythema migrans). This lesion occurs in 60% to 80% of patients and may be accompanied by minor constitutional symptoms. The second stage (early, disseminated infection) occurs within days or weeks after inoculation and begins with hematogenous dissemination of the organism from the site of inoculation. The symptoms, which mimic a systemic viral illness, include fever, migratory arthralgia, myalgia, headache, meningismus, generalized lymphadenopathy, malaise, fatigue, and secondary annular skin lesions.

After hematogenous spread, *B. burgdorferi* seems to be able to sequester itself in certain niches and cause localized inflammation in the nervous system, heart, or joints. Neurologic involvement is manifested by meningitis, encephalitis, cerebrospinal fluid lymphocytosis, peripheral neuropathy, myelitis, or cranial neuropathy (including facial nerve paralysis). Cardiac manifestations include atrioventricular block or other arrhythmias, myocarditis, and pericarditis. Joint disease manifests as brief attacks of asymmetrical oligoarticular arthritis, primarily in large joints (especially the knee). The third stage (late or persistent infection) occurs more than 1 year after onset, and can result in chronic, prolonged arthritis; chronic encephalomyelitis; chronic axonal peripheral polyradiculopathy; keratitis (similar to syphilis); acrodermatitis chronica atrophicans; and localized scleroderma-like lesions. A patient may experience one or all of the stages and the infection may not become symptomatic until the second or third stage. Affected tissues show infiltration by lymphocytes and plasma cells. Mild vasculitis and hypercellular vascular occlusion can occur. There is generally no tissue necrosis. In contrast to the findings in patients with syphilis, granulomas, gummas, multinucleated giant cells, and fibrinoid necrosis have not been observed as yet.[36]

In recent years, the complete genome of the spirochete has been sequenced, and animal models have been developed for studying the pathogenesis of Lyme disease using mice and primates. The animal models have shown that inflammatory innate immune responses are critical in the pathogenesis of the disease, and that genetic factors may be important in determining the severity of some of the manifestations.

The diagnosis of Lyme disease is usually based on the recognition of the characteristic clinical features, a history of exposure in an area where the disease is endemic, and detection of a specific antibody to *B. burgdorferi* by enzyme-linked immunosorbent assay and Western blotting.[35] The antibody test must be interpreted properly using the criteria of the Centers for Disease Control and Prevention because false-negative and false-positive results can occur. In addition, *B. burgdorferi* may cause asymptomatic infection, in which case the symptoms caused by another disease may be wrongly attributed to Lyme borreliosis.

The spirochete is highly sensitive to doxycycline, but only moderately so to penicillin. Other effective antibiotics include amoxicillin, erythromycin, cefuroxime, ceftriaxone, and imipenem. Steroids have been used for severe carditis and arthritis. Among patients managed early in the course of the disease, the specific antibody response usually disappears within months, and patients may become reinfected in the future. Among patients with late manifestations such as arthritis, titers decline after successful management, but patients remain seropositive. Although two vaccines were developed and found to be effective in clinical trials, they are not currently being marketed.[37]

Otologic Manifestations

Facial nerve paralysis is the most common otologic manifestation, with a reported incidence of 3% to 11%[38,39]; it may be bilateral in 25% of cases. This type of paralysis is seen in the second stage of the disease, and it affects patients of all ages and both sexes. The onset is acute, the duration is weeks to a few months, and the return of function is spontaneous and is usually complete. There may be a history of preceding otalgia, ipsilateral facial pain, or paresthesias.[40] Although other neurologic features of the second stage may be seen, facial nerve paralysis can occur as the sole neurologic abnormality (including normal cerebrospinal fluid).

Antibiotics or steroids do not seem to influence the duration or outcome of facial paralysis,[38] but they are recommended to treat concurrent symptoms and to prevent the more serious late complications. There is no role for surgery. The precise cause and histopathology of facial nerve palsy have not been elucidated. Histology from other involved peripheral nerves shows perineural and perivascular infiltration by lymphocytes and plasma cells. In chronic and severe neuropathies, demyelination and loss of nerve fibers similar to wallerian degeneration occur.[36] It is unclear whether neural lesions result from an inflammatory response to the spirochete or an immune-mediated epiphenomenon.

A well-documented otologic manifestation is an unusual skin lesion called a lymphocytoma, in which intensely red and violet nodules occur on the earlobe during the second stage of disease.[35] The lesion consists of benign but hyperplastic lymphocytic follicles in the dermis.[36]

Auditory and vestibular manifestations, such as SNHL, sudden hearing loss, positional vertigo, and Meniere's-like symptoms have been described.[41-44] More clinical data and temporal bone studies are needed to substantiate these preliminary observations.

Mycotic Diseases

Fungi are ubiquitous in the environment and are of low intrinsic virulence. Systemic invasive clinical disease reflects some defect in host defenses, such as diabetic ketoacidosis, chemotherapy for malignancy, corticosteroid therapy, or acquired immunodeficiency syndrome (AIDS). Aspergillosis, mucormycosis, candidiasis, cryptococcosis, coccidioidomycosis, and histoplasmosis are systemic mycoses that can cause disseminated disease, including involvement of the temporal bone. Diagnosis is made by biopsy and culture. Treatment consists of control of the underlying predisposing condition, surgical débridement of necrotic tissues, and systemic chemotherapy, usually with amphotericin B.

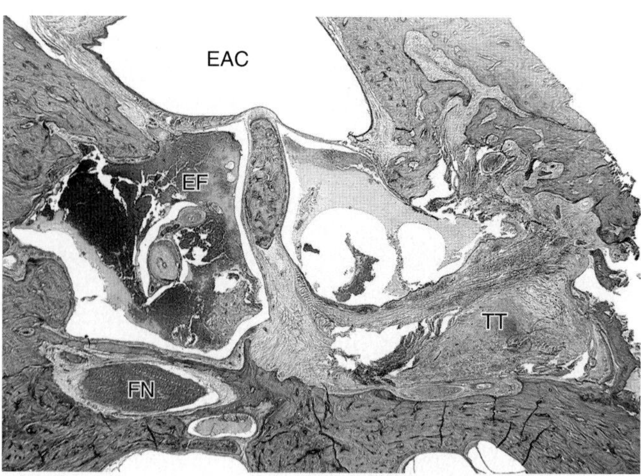

Figure 148-14. Mucormycosis in a 37-year-old man with diabetes. Inflammatory cells have invaded and destroyed the tensor tympani muscle (TT), and there is a hemorrhagic effusion (EF) in the mesotympanum (×12.35). EAC, external auditory canal; FN, facial nerve.

Otologic Manifestations

The middle ear and mastoid can be involved as a result of ascending infection along the eustachian tube and tensor tympani (often seen in mucormycosis) (Fig. 148-14) or through superinfection of existing chronic otitis media.[45] Destruction of the middle ear cleft ensues, often with extension to the surrounding structures, including thrombosis or rupture of the internal carotid artery.[46] Other routes of infection include hematogenous embolic dissemination, which can result in multiple granulomas throughout the temporal bone, and through cryptococcal involvement of the central nervous system, which can cause invasion and degeneration of the nerve trunks in the internal auditory canal.[47]

Neoplastic Diseases

Although neoplasms of the temporal bone are discussed elsewhere (see Chapters 176 and 177), three neoplasms—multiple myeloma, leukemia, and metastatic tumors—warrant mention here because temporal bone manifestations can occur with these diseases.

Multiple Myeloma

Multiple myeloma is a malignancy of plasma cells derived from B lymphocytes, and its major feature is the demonstration of an abnormal monoclonal protein (M component) in blood, urine, or both. There is a slight male predominance, and the median age of onset is 60 years. Clinical manifestations are the result of multiple plasma cell tumors, and consist of severe bone pain, pathologic fractures, failure of the bone marrow, renal failure, hypercalcemia, and recurrent infections.

Laboratory findings include the demonstration of the M component on serum or urine electrophoresis; normochromic, normocytic anemia; hypercalcemia; and elevated blood urea nitrogen levels. Typical radiographic findings include punched-out osteolytic lesions, which are particularly well seen on lateral skull radiography. Bone marrow aspirates show infiltration by plasma cells. For decades, the mainstay of therapy has been the use of alkylating agents, such as melphalan and corticosteroids; with this regimen, the median survival is approximately 3 years. Important advances have been made more recently that have substantially altered therapy for patients with myeloma. These advances include the use of hematopoietic cell transplantation; improved supportive care measures such as the use of bisphosphonates and erythropoietin; and novel agents such as thalidomide, lenalidomide, and bortezomib.[48,49]

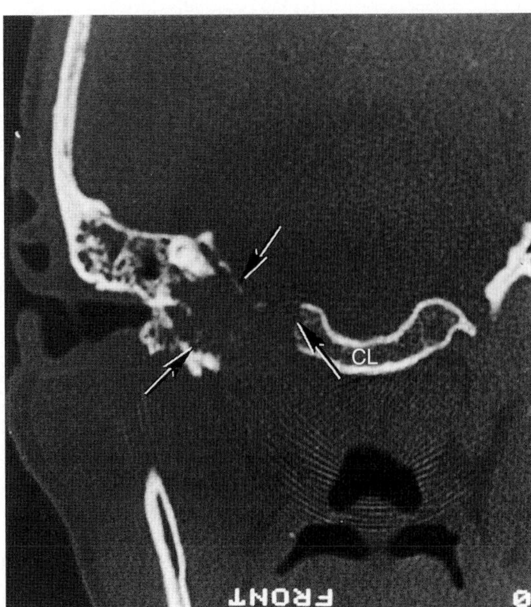

Figure 148-15. Coronal CT scan showing a large lytic destructive lesion *(arrows)* of the clivus (CL), petrous temporal bone, middle ear, and jugular foramen area caused by multiple myeloma in a 72-year-old man. The presenting symptoms were facial nerve paralysis and otorrhea.

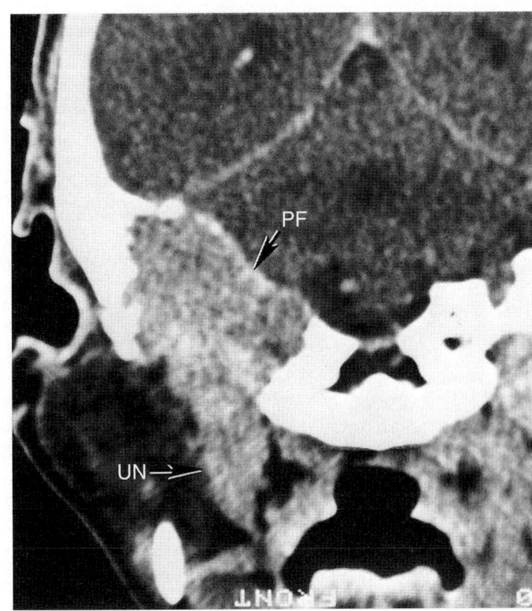

Figure 148-16. Coronal CT scan with contrast enhancement and a soft tissue technique in the same patient from Figure 148-15 shows a slightly enhancing mass that has destroyed the mastoid bone and extends to the posterior fossa (PF) and upper neck (UN).

Occasionally, only one plasma cell tumor (without marrow plasmacytosis) can be found. These lesions can occur in bone (solitary bone plasmacytoma) or soft tissue (extramedullary plasmacytoma), including the temporal bone. Both lesions can affect younger individuals, are associated with an M component in less than 30% of the cases, and have an indolent course with survival rates of 10 years or more. Local radiotherapy (40 Gy) is usually sufficient management. Periodic evaluation of serum and urine globulins and a skeletal radiographic survey should be performed to detect conversion to multiple myeloma.

Otologic Manifestations

The temporal bone is frequently involved in cases of multiple myeloma. Radiography may show rounded lytic lesions of the calvaria and temporal bone (Figs. 148-15 and 148-16). At a microscopic level, the marrow spaces of the petrous bone are commonly replaced by myeloma cells, and discrete lytic bone lesions may be seen in the otic capsule (Fig. 148-17).[50] Symptoms referable to temporal bone involvement are usually overshadowed by manifestations of diffuse disease. Occasionally, these may be the presenting feature of myeloma,[51] or they may be the only evidence of disease (plasmacytoma of the temporal bone).[52] Symptoms are nonspecific and include hearing loss, tinnitus, vertigo, otalgia, and facial paralysis.[53]

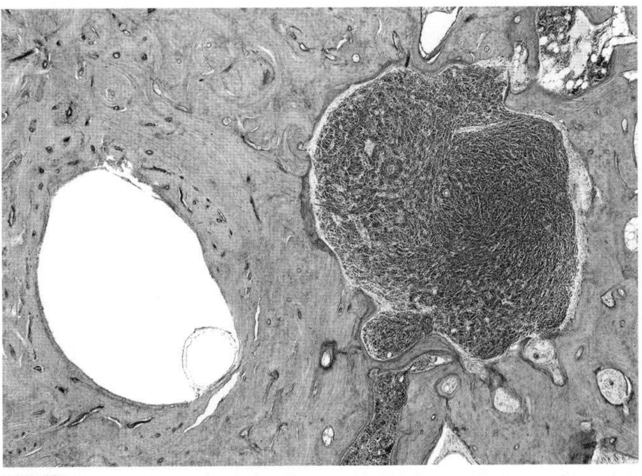

Figure 148-17. One of several osteolytic lesions of the temporal bone of a 69-year-old woman with multiple myeloma. The lesion shows sharp bony margins and consists of immature plasma cells (×39.6).

Leukemia

Leukemic infiltrates may occur in the temporal bone. They are common in the submucosa of the pneumatized areas of the middle ear and mastoid, including the tympanic membrane (Fig. 148-18), and in the bone marrow of the petrous apex (Fig. 148-19).[54,55] Secondary bacterial infection of the middle ear and mastoid often results from an immunocompromised state that is a result of either the disease itself or chemotherapy. Hemorrhage commonly occurs in association with infiltrates and can occur in the middle ear, mastoid, or inner ear. Clinical manifestations include middle ear effusion, acute and chronic suppuration in the middle ear and mastoid, thickening of the tympanic membrane, conductive hearing loss, SNHL (including sudden SNHL), vertigo, facial paralysis, and skin lesions in the auricle or external auditory canal.[56,57]

Granulocytic sarcoma or chloroma is a localized extramedullary tumor that is composed of immature myeloid cells. It is related to acute or chronic myelogenous leukemia, and its appearance may precede, coincide with, or follow the diagnosis of leukemia. Such a lesion can occur in the temporal bone,[58-60] and otologic manifestations can constitute the initial presentation. Management is by local irradiation and systemic chemotherapy.

Metastatic Neoplasms

Secondary malignant tumors usually involve the temporal bone through hematogenous dissemination. The most common sites of origin, in order of decreasing frequency, are the breast, the lung, the prostate, and the skin.[61] The lesions are usually destructive and osteolytic (Fig. 148-20); however, some lesions, such as from the prostate or breast, may be osteoblastic. The petrous apex and internal auditory canal seem to be sites of predilection for metastases, although any part of the temporal bone may be involved (Fig. 148-21). The otic capsule seems to be resistant to neoplastic invasion.[62]

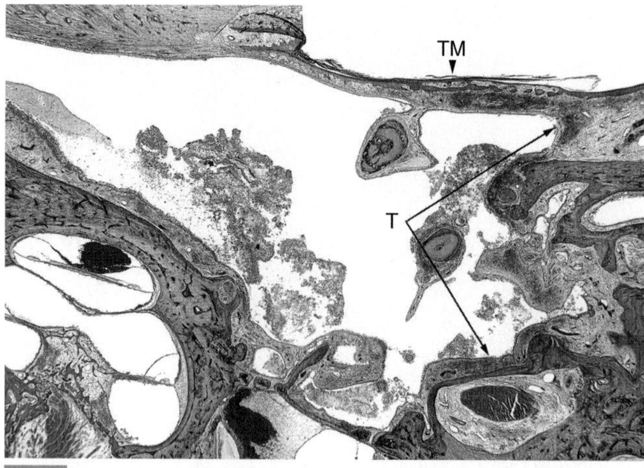

Figure 148-18. Acute lymphocytic leukemia in a 9-year-old boy. Ten days before his death, the patient complained of ear pain. Otoscopic examination revealed a hyperemic tympanic membrane (TM). The TM and mucosa of the middle ear are infiltrated by tumor cells (T), and the middle ear space contains a purulent exudate (×12.35).

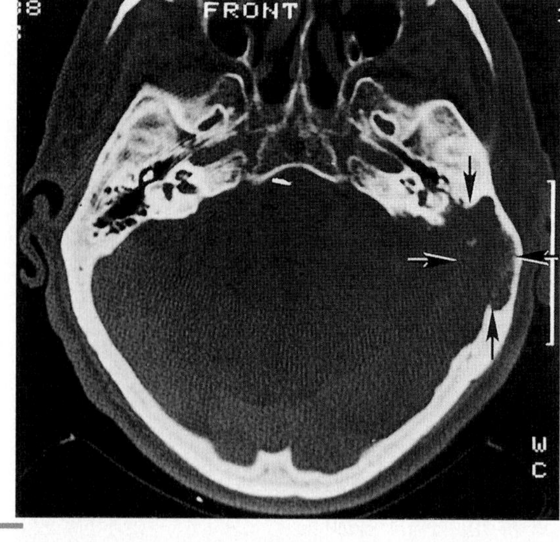

Figure 148-20. Axial CT scan of an 82-year-old woman with metastatic breast adenocarcinoma showing a large lytic lesion *(arrows)* destroying the mastoid, squamosa, otic capsule, and labyrinth.

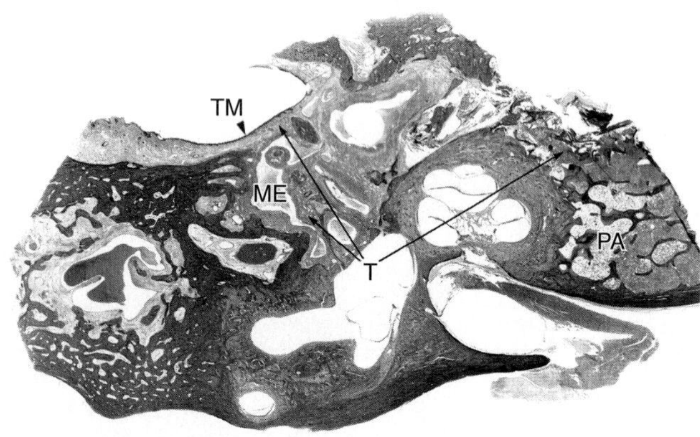

Figure 148-19. Acute myelogenous leukemia in a 38-year-old man. Leukemic infiltrates (T) are seen in the tympanic membrane (TM), middle ear (ME), and marrow spaces of the petrous apex (PA) (×6.7).

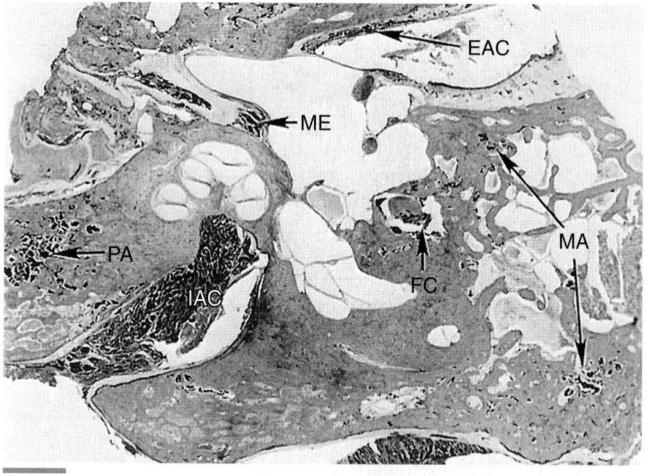

Figure 148-21. Metastatic breast adenocarcinoma in a 75-year-old woman involving the nerve trunks in the internal auditory canal (IAC), petrous apex (PA), subcutaneous tissues of the external auditory canal (EAC), facial canal (FC), middle ear (ME), and mastoid (MA) (×4.5).

Although otologic manifestations infrequently are the first evidence of malignant disease, more often they are preceded by other systemic symptoms. Involvement of the external canal, the middle ear cleft, or the eustachian tube may cause conductive hearing loss and pain; involvement of the otic capsule may produce SNHL, vertigo, and facial nerve paralysis. In meningeal carcinomatosis, rapidly progressive unilateral or bilateral SNHL is a common presenting symptom.[63] Unilateral SNHL may mimic a cerebellopontine angle tumor, and bilateral SNHL may mimic immune-mediated inner ear disease. Diagnosis is made by cytology of the cerebrospinal fluid.

Diseases of the Bone

Several generalized bone diseases affect the middle ear and temporal bone, and occasionally the initial symptoms of the disease occur in the temporal bone. Paget's disease, osteogenesis imperfecta (OI), and osteopetrosis can sometimes mimic the clinical features of otosclerosis.

Paget's Disease

Paget's disease of bone (osteitis deformans) is a chronic and sometimes progressive disease of unknown etiology. It is characterized by osteolytic and osteoblastic changes that mainly affect the axial skeleton. Genetic factors play a role in the pathogenesis of Paget's disease, which may be inherited in an autosomal dominant manner with high penetrance. Four susceptibility loci have been identified, one on chromosome 18, one on chromosome 6, and two on chromosome 5.[64] Mutations in the *SQSTM1* gene encoding the sequestosome 1 protein have been found in some individuals. Viral infection also seems to play a role in the etiology of Paget's disease, based on electron microscopy and immunohistochemical studies.[65,66] It is possible that the disease develops from a slow virus infection in susceptible individuals who have an underlying genetic predisposition.

Paget's disease affects 3% of the population that is 40 years old and older and 11% of the population that is 80 years old and older.[67] Men are affected more commonly than women. The onset of clinical manifestations is usually in the sixth decade of life, and includes enlarging skull; progressive kyphosis; and deformities of the pelvis, femur, and tibia. Radiographic findings (Figs. 148-22 and 148-23) include a thickened skull table; patchy, ill-defined densities of the skull; and poor definition of the cortical margins of the inner ear and internal auditory canal, particularly in the lytic phase of the disease. The bisphosphonates, which inhibit the resorption of bone, constitute the mainstay of medical therapy for symptomatic Paget's disease.[68] Other antipagetic drugs include calcitonin, mithramycin, ipriflavone, and gallium nitrate.

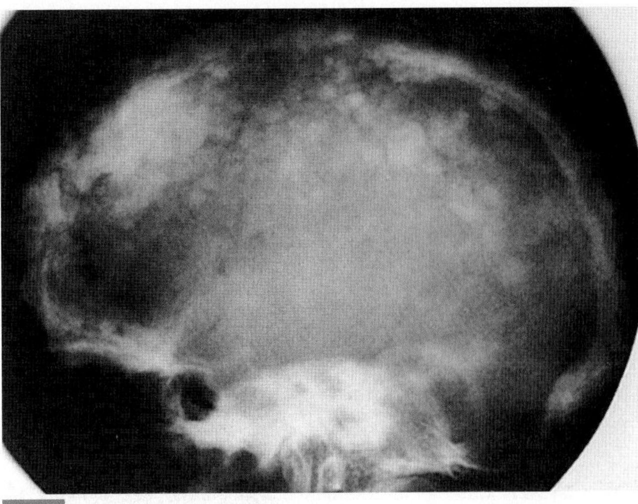

Figure 148-22. Lateral skull radiograph in a patient with Paget's disease. Findings include thickening of the skull table, multiple patchy densities, and platybasia.

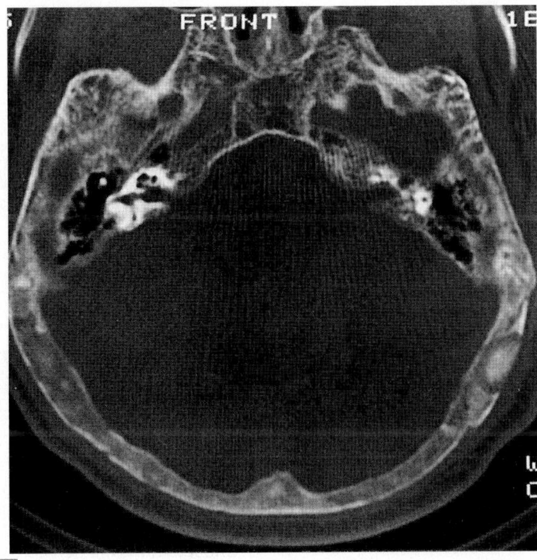

Figure 148-23. Axial CT scan of a 75-year-old man with Paget's disease. There is diffuse expansion of the skull table and involvement of both temporal bones, with patchy demineralization.

Otologic Manifestations

Clinical manifestations include hearing loss, tinnitus, and mild vestibular dysfunction. The facial nerve is spared. Hearing loss occurs in 5% to 44% of patients,[67] and may be sensorineural, mixed, or, rarely, conductive only. Most often, there is a mixed loss, with a descending pattern for bone conduction and relatively flat air conduction thresholds. Hearing losses are progressive and greater than hearing losses of age-matched healthy subjects. Distinguishing features of Paget's disease (compared with otosclerosis, which is the most common differential diagnosis) include a later age of onset (sixth decade), greater SNHL (with a descending pattern), enlarged calvaria, enlargement and tortuosity of the superficial temporal artery and its anterior branches,[67] elevated serum alkaline phosphatase level, and radiographic evidence of pagetic changes in the temporal bones.

None of the many published clinical and histologic reports has clearly identified a consistent pathologic basis for these hearing losses[69]; specifically, the apparent conductive hearing loss is not caused by ossicular fixation, and SNHL is not caused by the compression of cochlear nerve fibers. Attempts at the surgical correction of conductive

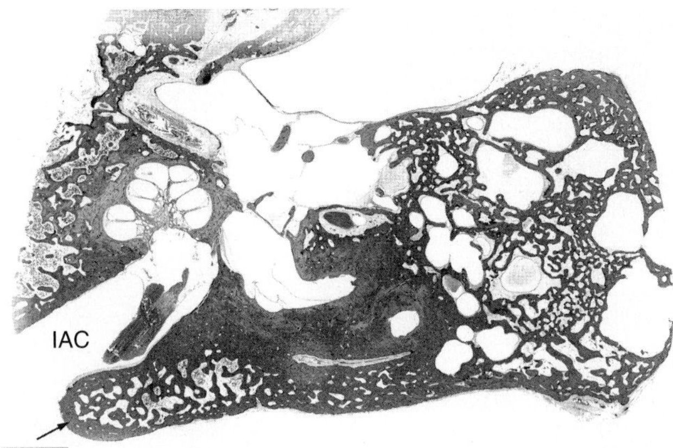

Figure 148-24. Pagetic involvement of the temporal bone in a 70-year-old man. The pagetic bone encroaches on the posterior margin *(arrow)* of the internal auditory canal (IAC). The mastoid is largely replaced by pagetic bone (×6.7).

loss are generally not considered worthwhile. Monsell and colleagues[70,71] reported a statistically significant correlation between the bone mineral density of the cochlear capsule (measured in vivo by quantitative computed tomography [CT]) and the high-frequency pure-tone air-conduction thresholds and the air-bone gap in patients with Paget's disease of the skull. It is unclear whether this finding is only a marker of disease effect, or a phenomenon that is closely related to the mechanism of hearing loss.

The histopathologic appearance of pagetic bone is variable, and depends on the relative osteoclastic and osteoblastic activity. Typical findings include osteoclastic resorption of marrow-containing bone, with an increase in vascularity and formation of fibrous tissue. New bone formation occurs in an irregular manner and produces its typical mosaic pattern as a result of irregular and curved cement lines (Fig. 148-24). Pagetic bone changes occur in three phases: an initial osteolytic phase, a mixed or combined phase, and an osteoblastic or "burnt-out" phase. In the temporal bone, a fourth phase can be identified, which is the remodeling of inactive pagetic bone into normal-appearing lamellar bone.[69] The disease usually begins in periosteal bone and extends to involve enchondral and endosteal bone.

Osteogenesis Imperfecta

OI (also known as van der Hoeve–de Kleyn syndrome) is a genetically determined disorder of the connective tissue that is characterized clinically by fragile bones that break with minor trauma. Approximately 80% to 90% of patients with OI have mutations of one of the two type I collagen genes (*COL1A1* and *COL1A2*). Many hundreds of unique mutations of *COL1A1* and *COL1A2* have been identified in individuals with OI. The older terms OI congenita and tarda have been replaced by a classification system (OI types I through IV) that is based on clinical features, radiologic criteria, and mode of inheritance.

OI type I has an autosomal dominant mode of inheritance. It is the mildest form and is associated with blue sclerae, nondeforming fractures, and normal stature. Hearing loss is common, occurring in 30% to 50% of cases. OI type II is the most severe form, with multiple fractures occurring in utero and often resulting in stillbirth. This type either is acquired as a sporadic new mutation or is inherited in an autosomal recessive manner. OI type III is characterized by multiple fractures, progressive bone deformity during childhood and adolescence, and sclerae that are bluish at birth but white later in life. Hearing loss occurs in about 50% of individuals. The long bones may be slender and bowed, with abrupt widening near the epiphyses. Kyphoscoliosis, pectus excavatum, weak joints, dental abnormalities, and wormian bone in the skull table are common (Figs. 148-25 and 148-26). The mode of inheritance varies; it may be autosomal dominant, autosomal recessive, or due to a new mutation. OI type IV is a dominantly inher-

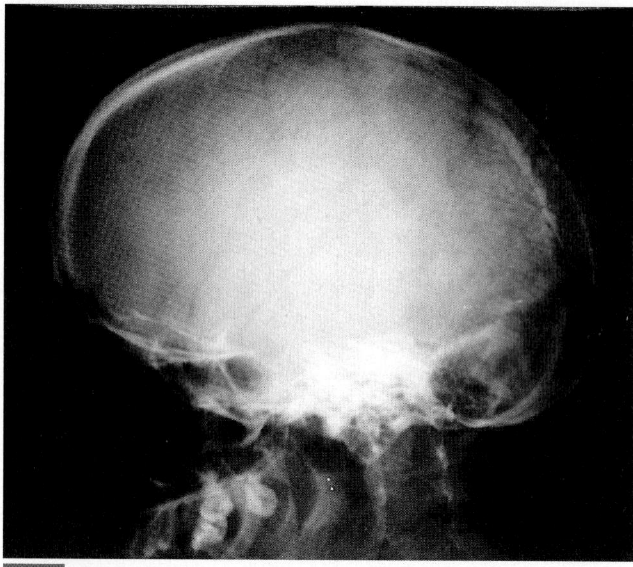

Figure 148-25. Lateral radiograph of the skull in a patient with osteogenesis imperfecta. Wormian bone is seen, particularly in the posterior table.

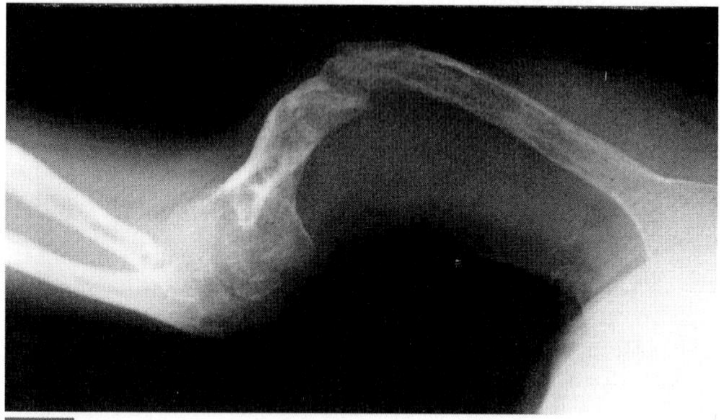

Figure 148-26. Radiograph of the arm of a patient with osteogenesis imperfecta. There is a pathologic fracture, demineralization of the humerus, and gross abnormalities of the elbow joint.

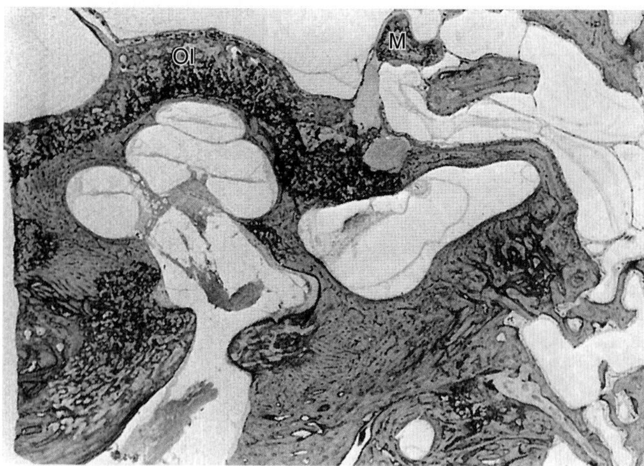

Figure 148-27. Osteogenesis imperfecta (OI) in a 15-year-old girl. The osteogenesis has replaced the enchondral and periosteal layers of the otic capsule. The neck of the malleus (M) is also involved (×8.5).

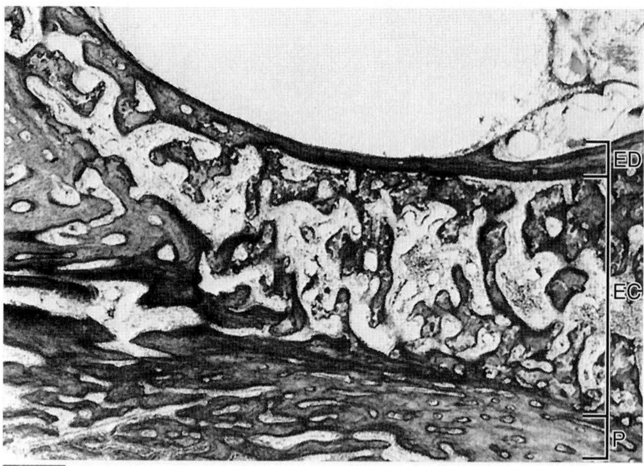

Figure 148-28. Osteogenesis imperfecta involving the otic capsule of a newborn boy. The enchondral (EC) and periosteal (P) layers have been replaced by finely trabeculated bone with an increase in fibrous tissue and vascular spaces. The endosteal layer (ED) is normal (×60).

ited form; it is similar to OI type I except that the sclerae are white (normal). Hearing loss is less common than it is with type I, occurring in 10% to 30% of cases.[72,73]

Management consists of treatment of fractures, orthopedic surgery to correct deformities, use of orthotic devices, and physical and occupational therapy. Bisphosphonate therapy is being increasingly used because these drugs are potent inhibitors of bone resorption and bone turnover.[74] Other therapies under investigation include use of growth hormone and allogeneic bone marrow transplantation.

Otologic Manifestations

Conductive hearing loss and SNHL occur in patients with OI. Severe SNHL has been estimated to occur in approximately 40% of patients, and has a high correlation with gray or white sclerae. Conductive hearing loss usually accompanies blue sclerae, which first becomes apparent by 20 to 25 years of age, and then becomes severe enough to cause the patient to seek medical attention 15 to 20 years later.[75] There is no relationship between hearing loss and frequency or severity of fractures.[73] Some patients with mild OI present with conductive hearing loss similar to that seen with otosclerosis. Early age of onset of hearing loss, high compliance values on tympanometry, a history of fractures after minor trauma in childhood that ceased after puberty, a family history of OI, and blue sclerae are helpful diagnostic clues.

The conductive loss reflects structural changes in the ossicles. Microfractures of the manubrium,[76] fragility of the long process of the incus, and fracture or resorption of the crura of the stapes have been reported.[75,77,78] The stapedial footplate is typically described as thick, soft, and chalklike or granular, and is usually fixed.[79] Rehabilitation can be accomplished by amplification or surgery.[80-82] A stapedectomy can give results similar to those seen with otosclerosis, but the procedure is extremely delicate. Crimping the prosthesis around the incus may cause a pathologic fracture, and a platinum ribbon is preferred to stainless steel wire.[75]

Histopathology of the temporal bone (Figs. 148-27 and 148-28) in cases of OI type II has shown deficient ossification of the endochondral layer of the otic capsule, which shows increased amounts of fibrous tissue with numerous blood vessels. The periosteal layer is often thin and deficient (see Fig. 148-28). The stapes crura are often thin and incomplete. The otopathology in cases of OI type I is very similar if not identical to that seen in cases of otosclerosis.[83,84] The abnormal bone involves the periosteal and endochondral layers of the otic capsule (see Fig. 148-27), and may result in the fixation of the stapes footplate.

Fibrous Dysplasia

Fibrous dysplasia is a benign, chronic, slowly progressive bone disorder of unknown etiology that is characterized by the replacement of normal

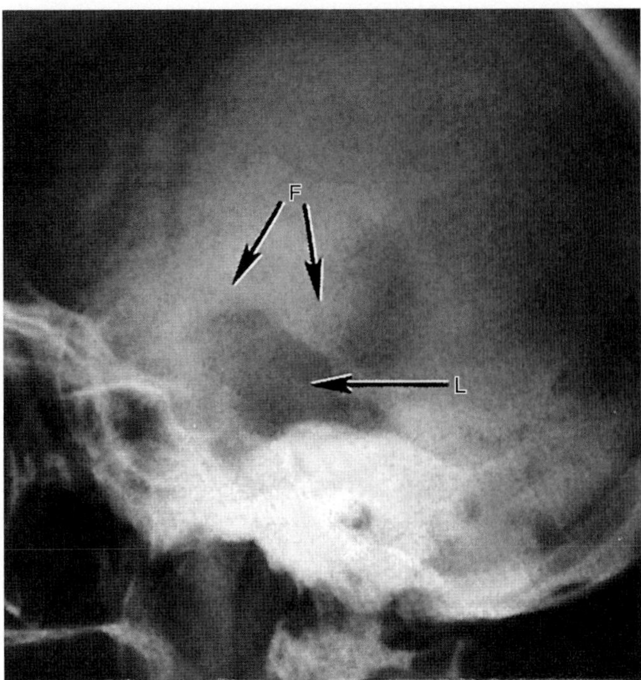

Figure 148-29. Lateral radiograph of the skull of a patient with fibrous dysplasia showing lytic (L) and fibrous (F) phases of disease. Spicules of new bone are responsible for the ground-glass appearance of the fibrous phase.

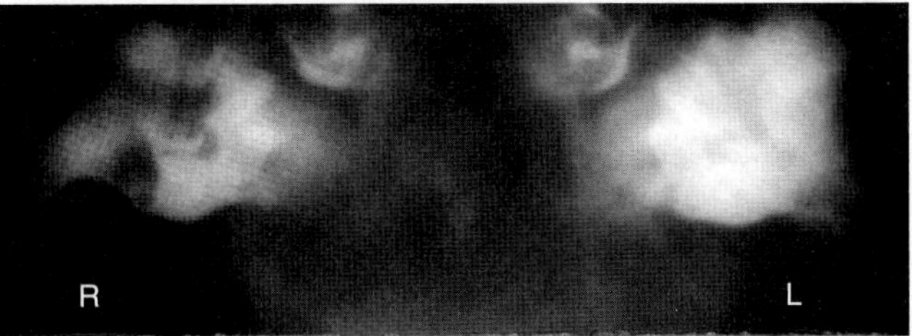

Figure 148-30. Coronal tomographic radiograph of a patient with fibrous dysplasia. New bone formation causes a dense appearance of the involved left temporal bone.

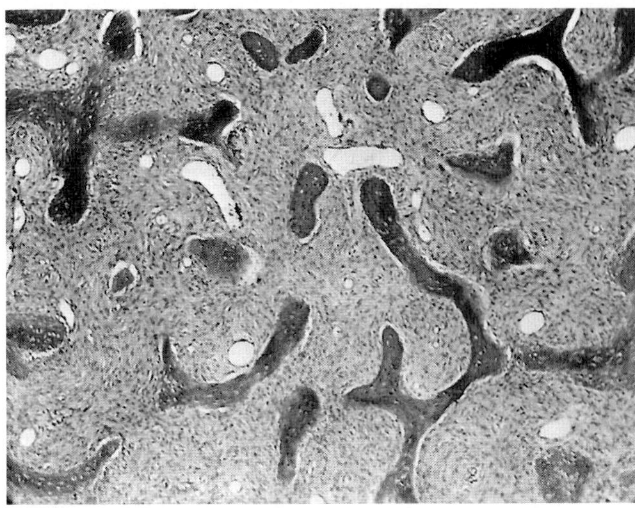

Figure 148-31. Fibrous dysplasia. The irregularly arranged spicules of woven bone in a fibrovascular stroma show a whorled pattern (×64).

bone with a variable amount of fibrous tissue and woven bone. It may occur as part of Albright's syndrome (characterized by multiple bony lesions, abnormal pigmentation, endocrine dysfunction, and precocious puberty in girls), or it may exist alone as the monostotic or polyostotic form. The monostotic form is more common and usually occurs in the skull, ribs, proximal femur, or tibia. In the polyostotic form, skull lesions are seen in more than 50% of patients.

Clinical manifestations of fibrous dysplasia include bony deformity, pathologic fracture, and cranial nerve palsies. The disease starts early in life, usually in childhood; the monostotic form may become quiescent at puberty, whereas the polyostotic form can continue to progress. Sarcomatous transformation can occur, with an estimated incidence of 0.4%.[85] Laboratory findings include elevated serum alkaline phosphatase level in 30% of patients with polyostotic fibrous dysplasia, with usually normal serum calcium and phosphorus levels. The typical radiographic findings include a radiolucent area with a well-defined smooth or scalloped edge and a ground-glass appearance. Areas of increased radiodensity may also be seen (Figs. 148-29 and 148-30). The histopathology of fibrous dysplasia consists of the replacement of normal cancellous bone by a fibrous stroma arranged in a whorled pattern. A variable amount of irregularly arranged spicules of woven bone cause the ground-glass radiographic changes (Fig. 148-31).

Advances have been made toward understanding the cellular and molecular basis of fibrous dysplasia. The lesion is composed of immature mesenchymal osteoblastic precursor cells. There is an activating mutation in the gene that encodes the α subunit of stimulatory G protein.[86] Elevated levels of cyclic adenosine monophosphate result that affect the transcription and expression of multiple downstream genes, which ultimately result in the pathologic lesion.[87] Treatment consists of bisphosphonate therapy and orthopedic surgery for correction of deformities and treatment of pathologic fractures.[88]

Otologic Manifestations

The temporal bone occasionally may be involved in cases of fibrous dysplasia, with about 100 cases reported to date.[89-91] Of these, the monostotic form occurred in 70%, the polyostotic form occurred in 23%, and Albright's syndrome occurred in 7%. All parts of the temporal bone can be involved, but the process generally begins as a painless, slowly progressive swelling that involves the mastoid or squama. Progressive narrowing of the external auditory canal with conductive hearing loss is the most common manifestation and occurs in about 80% of cases. This narrowing may be mistaken for exostoses, but fibrous dysplasia is encountered during the second or third decade of life; at surgery, it is vascular with a characteristic soft, spongy, and gritty consistency. Entrapment of keratin debris medial to a stenotic canal can cause an external canal cholesteatoma. Involvement of the middle ear and ossicles or obstruction of the eustachian tube also can cause conductive hearing loss. Erosion of the fallopian canal with facial nerve paralysis or erosion of the otic capsule with SNHL and vertigo is seen occasionally. An isolated lesion of the mesotympanic bone can simulate a glomus tympanicum tumor and manifest as a reddish mass behind an intact tympanic membrane with pulsatile tinnitus and hearing loss.

Management of fibrous dysplasia is symptomatic. Operative procedures should be limited to biopsy and relief of functional deficits. Stenosis of the external canal often requires surgical removal with canalplasty and meatoplasty. Restenosis as a result of regrowth of fibrous dysplasia occurs, and multiple procedures are sometimes needed. Compared with simple canalplasty, a postauricular canal wall down mastoidectomy with wide canalplasty and skin grafting gives better results, with long-term canal patency. Radiotherapy is contraindicated because of an increased rate of malignant degeneration.[85] Long-term follow-up is indicated because of the potential for facial nerve involvement and for the progression of conductive hearing loss to profound SNHL.[90]

Osteopetroses

Osteopetroses are rare genetic disorders that are characterized by greatly increased bone density.[92-94] Osteopetroses result from the defective function of osteoclasts, which results in a failure of normal bone resorption while normal bone formation by osteoblasts continues, with deposition of excessive mineralized osteoid and cartilage. Four types of osteopetrosis have been defined, although patients with atypical symptoms are frequent, which suggests that there are additional types.

Malignant osteopetrosis is an autosomal recessive form that manifests in infancy and is rapidly progressive, with a high mortality rate. Many cases have been shown to be due to mutations in the gene encoding for the TCIRG1 subunit of the vacuolar proton pump within osteoclasts. The disease is characterized by the encroachment of bone marrow that leads to anemia, thrombocytopenia, hepatosplenomegaly, increased susceptibility to infection, and encroachment of the neural foramina, which causes neural degeneration. Optic atrophy, facial paralysis, SNHL, hydrocephalus, and mental retardation are common, and death usually occurs during the first or second decade of life. The only effective treatment is bone marrow transplantation. Another type of autosomal recessive osteopetrosis is due to a mutation in the gene for cytoplasmic carbonic anhydrase II. This type is very rare (approximately 50 cases have been reported), and it is associated with distal renal tubular acidosis.

Autosomal dominant type II osteopetrosis (also known as Albers-Schönberg disease and marble bone disease) is the most frequent type. It is associated with normal life expectancy and may be asymptomatic. Many cases have been shown to result from mutations in the *CLCN7* chloride-channel gene.[92] Clinical manifestations include an increased incidence of fractures (osteopetrotic bone is fragile despite its solid appearance); osteomyelitis of the mandible from dental infection; progressive enlargement of the head and mandible; clubbing of the long bones; and cranial neuropathies such as progressive optic atrophy, trigeminal hypesthesia, recurrent facial paralysis, and SNHL. Patients may have syndactyly of the fingers or toes and abnormal fingernails; these abnormalities can aid the physician in making the clinical diagnosis. Radiographic evaluation reveals a great increase in the density of all bones.

Autosomal dominant osteopetrosis type I is an extremely rare type (it has been reported in only three families), and it seems to be linked to a locus on chromosome 11q12-13.[94] Patients with this type of osteopetrosis are often asymptomatic, but some have pain and hearing loss. This is the only type of osteopetrosis that is not associated with an increased rate of fractures.

Otologic Manifestations

The endochondral layer of the otic capsule and ossicles in the temporal bones of infants and children with the malignant recessive form of osteopetrosis consist mainly of dense calcified cartilage.[95] The mastoid is not pneumatized, and the stapes persists in fetal form (Figs. 148-32 and 148-33). The inner ears appear normal. Dehiscence of the tympanic segment of the facial nerve (often with herniation of the nerve into the oval window niche) has been a consistent finding.[95-97] There seems to be no observable nerve compression, however. These children often have recurrent episodes of acute otitis media, serous otitis media, stenosis of the external auditory canal, conductive hearing loss or SNHL, and unilateral or bilateral facial nerve paralysis.[98,99]

In the more benign adult (autosomal dominant type II) form, the temporal bone is markedly sclerotic, with obliteration of the mastoid air cells and a narrowing of the eustachian tube and the external and internal auditory canals. Exostotic overgrowth of the periosteal bone surrounding the tympanic cavity can occur (Fig. 148-34), with ankylosis of the ossicles and obliteration of the oval and round window niches (Fig. 148-35). These changes explain the common finding of conductive hearing loss. SNHL also occurs, but the inner ears appear normal. Narrowing of the eustachian tube predisposes a patient to serous otitis media.[100] Recurrent acute facial nerve paralysis that is similar to Bell's palsy (involving one or both sides) is a frequent manifestation. There is a tendency toward progressive residual weakness with each episode. Radiographic studies should be performed in any child or young adult with recurrent facial nerve paralysis to determine the possibility of osteopetrosis. Total decompression of the facial nerve has been advocated to ameliorate recurrent palsies.[101,102]

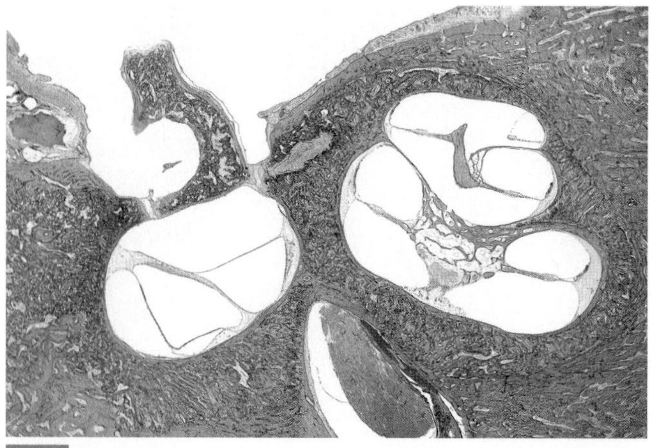

Figure 148-32. Recessive osteopetrosis of the temporal bone of a 15-month-old boy. The endochondral layer of the otic capsule and stapes is composed of calcified cartilage (×12.3).

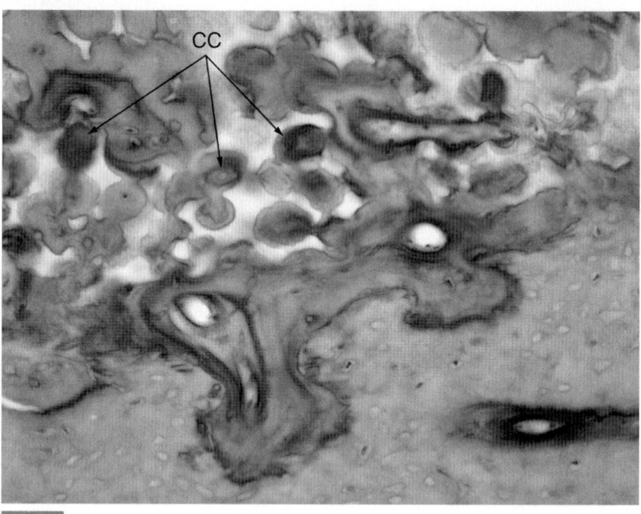

Figure 148-33. Higher magnification of the temporal bone seen in Figure 148-32. The calcified cartilage (CC) of endochondral bone appears as densely staining, round-to-ovoid profiles (×396).

Osteitis Fibrosa Cystica

Osteitis fibrosa cystica (von Recklinghausen's disease) is a bone lesion caused by excess parathyroid hormone, and it is characterized in classic cases by osteoclastic bone resorption, marrow fibrosis, bone cysts, bone pain, and fractures. In most cases, it is caused by primary hyperparathyroidism, which is usually due to an adenoma. Other manifestations relate to hypercalcemia and hypercalciuria. Although the temporal bone can be affected in this disorder,[103,104] it is very rare in clinical practice. The otic capsule is replaced by abnormal bone composed of loosely arranged trabeculae of varying size and shape that are interspersed with marrow spaces that contain fibrous tissue. SNHL has been attributed to osteitis fibrosa involving the temporal bone.

Storage and Metabolic Diseases

Mucopolysaccharidoses

The mucopolysaccharidoses (MPS) are a group of diseases that are caused by an inherited deficiency of one of several lysosomal enzymes that degrade mucopolysaccharides. As a result, undergraded mucopolysaccharides accumulate intracellularly, which gives rise to large cells

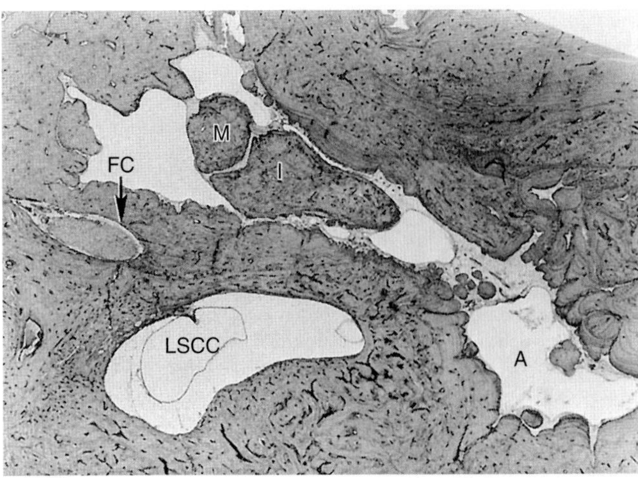

Figure 148-34. Osteopetrosis in a 30-year-old man showing overgrowth of dense lamellar bone around the epitympanum, with jamming of the malleus (M) and incus (I). The facial nerve canal (FC) is narrowed (×9). A, antrum; LSCC, lateral semicircular canal.

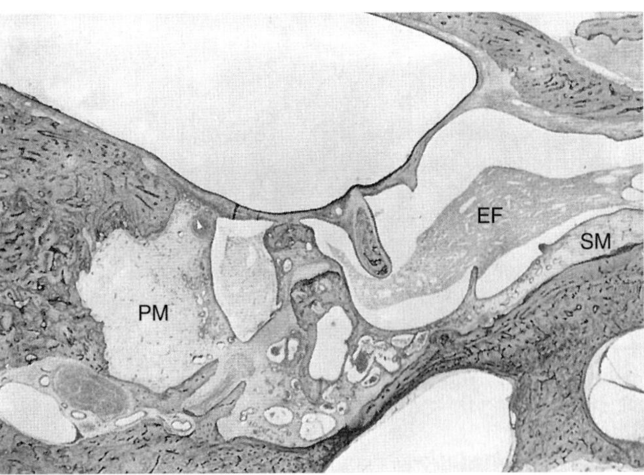

Figure 148-36. Hunter's syndrome in a 24-year-old man. The middle ear contains an effusion (EF) as a result of eustachian tube dysfunction. The submucosa (SM) is thickened, and the posterior mesotympanum (PM) contains unresorbed mesenchymal tissue (×11).

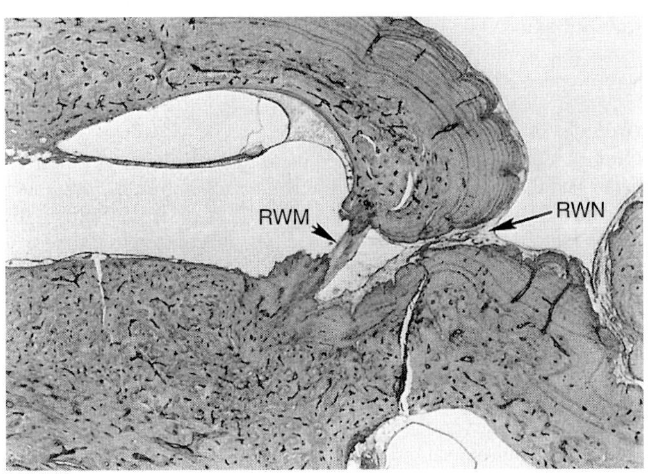

Figure 148-35. Osseous obliteration of the round window niche (RWN) of the same patient as seen in Figure 148-34. There is fluid in the niche adjacent to the round window membrane (RWM) (×18).

with vacuolated cytoplasm. Ten enzyme deficiencies have been identified to date and are classified into seven types or syndromes. All are transmitted as autosomal recessive traits except for Hunter's syndrome (MPS II), which is X-linked recessive. Diagnosis is made either by an assay of the specific enzyme in plasma or serum or by tissue culture using fibroblasts or leukocytes. Management is mainly supportive and symptomatic. MPS are potentially amenable, however, to enzyme replacement therapy and to procedures such as bone marrow transplantation or gene transfer.[105]

Hurler's syndrome (MPS I) is caused by a deficiency of L-iduronidase that leads to the accumulation of heparan sulfate and dermatan sulfate. Clinical manifestations include corneal clouding, abnormal facies, hepatosplenomegaly, mental retardation, dysostosis multiplex, joint stiffness, and hernias. Radiographic features include a broadening and shortening of long bones; hypoplasia and fractures of the lumbar vertebrae, causing kyphosis; and enlargement of the sella turcica. Death usually occurs during the first decade of life.

Hunter's syndrome (MPS II) results from a deficiency of iduronate-2-sulfatase, which leads to an accumulation of heparan sulfate and dermatan sulfate. The syndrome is similar to Hurler's syndrome, but corneal clouding is not seen. Survival to adulthood may occur.

Morquio's syndrome (MPS IV) is attributable to a deficiency of *N*-acetylgalactosamine-6-sulfatase or of β-galactosidase, resulting in excessive urinary excretion of keratan sulfate. Clinical manifestations include spondyloepiphyseal dysplasia. Spinal cord compression caused by hypoplasia of the odontoid process and cervical dislocation are common and may be the cause of death.

Otologic Manifestations

Hearing loss in MPS is usually conductive and sensorineural. The conductive component is attributable to serous otitis media as a result of dysfunction of the eustachian tube and chronic thickening of the mucosa of the middle ear (Fig. 148-36). Unresorbed mesenchyme has been described in the middle ear and mastoid in Hurler's syndrome.[106] Large cells with vacuolated cytoplasm have been described in the middle ear mucosa in both Hunter's syndrome[107] and Hurler's syndrome.[108] The cause of SNHL is unknown, but it has been attributed to abnormal metabolism within neural elements.[107-110]

Gout

Gout is a metabolic disease that results from the deposition of crystals of monosodium urate within joint spaces and cutaneous structures.[111,112] The crystals stimulate production of interleukin-1 and other cytokines by monocytes and macrophages, leading to inflammation and tissue damage. Patients with gout invariably have hyperuricemia (serum urate level >7 mg/dL). Genetic factors influence the renal clearance of uric acid and may be involved in the familial incidence of hyperuricemia and gout. More recent studies have implicated loci on the X chromosome and on chromosome 16 in the pathogenesis of hyperuricemia.[113] Other risk factors for gout include alcohol use, exposure to lead, diuretics, hypertension, and renal insufficiency.

The clinical manifestations of gout include acute gouty arthritis, aggregates of crystal in connective tissue (tophi), urate urolithiasis, and, rarely, gouty nephropathy. Laboratory abnormalities include hyperuricemia, leukocytosis, and an elevated erythrocyte sedimentation rate. The diagnosis of gout depends on the identification of urate crystals within joint fluid or within tophi under polarized light. The treatment of acute gouty arthritis includes bed rest, nonsteroidal anti-inflammatory agents, and colchicine. Uricosuric drugs such as probenecid are useful for patients with hyperuricemia as a result of the decreased renal clearance of uric acid. Xanthine oxidase inhibitors such as allopurinol are useful if excess production of uric acid is the basis of the hyperuricemia.

Otologic Manifestations

Tophaceous deposits can occur in multiple areas in the head and neck.[111] The helical rim of the pinna is the classic site of involvement. Such tophi are usually asymptomatic and do not require any treatment.

Ochronosis

Ochronosis is a rare disease that is caused by an inherited lack of the enzyme homogentisic acid oxidase. The presence of homogentisic acid in urine is called *alkaptonuria.* The result of this inborn error of metabolism is the deposition of a dark pigment in tissues that are rich in collagen. Patients often present with symptoms and signs during the third decade of life. Manifestations include ochronotic arthropathy, ocular and cutaneous pigmentation, obstruction of the genitourinary tract by ochronotic calculi, and cardiovascular manifestations as a result of ochronosis affecting the aortic valve. There is no effective management or cure for the condition. Treatment is based on symptomatic therapy.[114]

Otologic Manifestations

Ochronosis has manifestations in the external ear; cartilage is a site of predilection for the deposition of the pigment of ochronosis. Blue or mottled-brown macules can appear on the pinna and in other areas of the head and neck, including the nose, buccal mucosa, tonsils, pharynx, larynx, and esophagus.

Collagen Vascular and Autoimmune Diseases

The ear may be a target organ in several systemic (non–organ-specific) diseases that are thought to be autoimmune in nature (e.g., polyarteritis nodosa, relapsing polychondritis, Cogan's syndrome), or it may be the sole target of an immune-mediated (organ-specific) inner ear process that causes progressive SNHL with or without vestibular dysfunction. The latter was described by McCabe,[115] although the theoretical concept was proposed by Lehnhardt in 1958.[116] Histopathologic findings in the temporal bone in both groups of disorders are similar and include destruction and degeneration of the inner ear tissues; scattered infiltrates of lymphocytes, plasma cells, and macrophages; focal or diffuse proliferation of fibrous tissue and bone; and a variable degree of endolymphatic hydrops.[117] The otologic manifestations of these diseases are discussed in Chapter 153 and in published reviews.[118-120]

Immunodeficiency Disorders

Infections of the middle ear and mastoid can occur as part of the clinical spectrum of congenital and acquired immunodeficiency disorders. Occasionally, otologic manifestations may constitute the presenting feature of the disease.

Primary or Congenital Immunodeficiency Disorders

Primary or congenital immunodeficiency disorders constitute a diverse group of conditions that can be subdivided into four broad categories. Humoral immunodeficiency disorders are characterized by the inability to produce antigen-specific antibodies. Patients commonly have recurrent and chronic respiratory tract infections owing to high-grade extracellular bacteria, such as *Haemophilus influenzae, Streptococcus pneumoniae,* and *Streptococcus pyogenes*. Diagnosis is based on the analysis of immunoglobulin subtypes and the assessment of specific antibody production. Management is symptomatic with appropriate antibiotics and replacement therapy with immune human serum globulin. Individual syndromes within the group are classified according to the type of immunoglobulin deficiency, the mode of genetic transmission, and the specific clinical features, including X-linked infantile agammaglobulinemia (Bruton's), autosomal recessive agammaglobulinemia, acquired agammaglobulinemia (common variable immunodeficiency), X-linked immunodeficiency with hyper-IgM, and selective IgA deficiency.

Cellular immunodeficiency disorders exhibit partial or severe deficiencies in the function of T lymphocytes. Patients with these disorders typically have recurrent infections owing to intracellular, low-grade, opportunistic pathogens including viruses, fungi, protozoa, and some bacteria. Diagnosis is based on quantitative and qualitative tests of T-cell function, and there is often an associated deficiency of antibody production. Syndromes include thymic hypoplasia (DiGeorge's syndrome), Wiskott-Aldrich syndrome, ataxia-telangiectasia, chronic mucocutaneous candidiasis, hyperimmunoglobulinemia E (Job's syndrome), and severe combined immunodeficiency.

Disorders of phagocyte function are primarily disorders of neutrophils that leave patients vulnerable to pyogenic bacterial or fungal infections of varying severity and chronicity. This group includes neutropenia, which may be inherited or acquired; if severe, it can cause fulminant sepsis, chemotactic defects that result in pyogenic respiratory infections, and microbicidal disorders such as chronic granulomatous disease and Chédiak-Higashi syndrome. Therapy includes antibiotics, neutrophil transfusions, and bone marrow transplantation.

Complement system defects include deficiencies of the individual components or of the regulatory proteins. Clinical features vary with the type of defect and include recurrent *Neisseria* infections (C5, C6, C7, and C9 deficiency), recurrent staphylococcal infections (C3b inactivator deficiency), lupus-like syndromes (C1, C4, and C2 deficiency), and angioedema (C1 esterase-inhibitor deficiency). All complement defects are inherited (generally autosomal recessive); management is symptomatic and supportive.

Major advances in the understanding of the genetic basis and molecular mechanisms of immunodeficiency disorders have occurred.[121,122] As a result, most of the more than 100 primary immunodeficiency diseases can be diagnosed by molecular techniques. These molecular approaches have also resulted in significant insight into the pathophysiology of the various conditions, which has permitted early diagnosis of many of these conditions by neonatal screening of umbilical cord blood. The immunodeficiency syndromes have also played a major role in the development of human gene therapy, which is being actively pursued in many centers.

Otologic Manifestations

Otologic disease has been described in all four categories of immunodeficiency disorders. Humoral immune defects result in recurrent and persistent acute and serous otitis media. Chronic suppurative otitis media (with all its attendant complications) may develop and is often refractory to medical and surgical therapy.[123,124] A subgroup consists of children with selective IgG subclass 2 deficiency who have been shown to be susceptible to recurrent episodes of otitis media.[125] DiGeorge's syndrome (T-cell deficiency as a result of thymic hypoplasia) can manifest varying degrees of anomalies of the external, middle, and inner ears with conductive, sensorineural, or mixed hearing losses[126]; there is also a high incidence of Mondini's dysplasia in these ears. Recurrent episodes of acute and chronic otitis media have also been described with neutrophil chemotactic defects,[127] microbicidal disorders (chronic granulomatous disease),[128] and complement system defects.[129]

Acquired Immunodeficiency Syndrome

AIDS, which was first recognized in 1981, is caused by HIV. HIV is lymphotropic and attacks primarily T-helper lymphocytes, rendering the patient susceptible to numerous opportunistic infections (see Chapter 15).

Otologic Manifestations

Otologic manifestations are infrequent in patients with AIDS except in children, in whom serous otitis media is common.[130] When otologic disease does occur, the microbiology is similar to that of non-AIDS patients, with the addition of unusual opportunistic organisms (protozoa, fungi, viruses, and mycobacteria).

Middle ear and mastoid manifestations include acute otitis media, acute mastoiditis, serous otitis media, and bullous myringitis; the severity of these infections varies and depends on the immune status of the patient. External ear disease such as otitis externa and Kaposi's sarcoma can also occur. Tissue diagnosis by biopsy or tympanocentesis is indicated to identify the causative agent before initiating therapy.

Pneumocystis jiroveci is an unusual opportunistic protozoan that is a common cause of middle ear and external ear disease in patients with AIDS. Subcutaneous masses in the external canal or aural polyps arising from the canal, the tympanic membrane, or the mesotympanum can result in conductive hearing loss, otorrhea, or otalgia. Presumed routes of infection include hematogenous spread from another source (e.g., pulmonary), ascending infection through the eustachian tube from pharyngeal colonization, or airborne transmission of the aerosolized organism directly to the external canal.[131,132] A biopsy specimen shows the characteristic organism, and the infection responds to treatment with oral trimethoprim-sulfamethoxazole. Otologic disease resulting from *P. jiroveci* may be the only and the initial presenting symptom of AIDS.[131-133] Inner ear symptoms such as SNHL (including fluctuating and sudden hearing loss), vertigo, and tinnitus can occur.[134,135] SNHL is ascribed to various causes, including otosyphilis, cryptococcal meningitis, tuberculous meningitis, central nervous system toxoplasmosis, and ototoxic medication.[133,136] HIV is neurotropic and may itself be the primary cause of SNHL. The facial nerve can be involved by herpes zoster (Ramsay Hunt syndrome).

In a study of 49 temporal bones from 25 patients with AIDS, Michaels and colleagues[137] found low-grade otitis media in 60% of cases, severe otitis media in 20%, cytomegalovirus inclusion-bearing cells in the inner and middle ears in 24%, labyrinthine cryptococcosis in 8%, and Kaposi's sarcoma deposit in the eighth cranial nerve in 4%. They concluded that the ear is no less susceptible to AIDS-associated diseases than any other organ, and that it is particularly prone to cytomegalovirus infection. The spectrum of otologic manifestations and their pathophysiologic mechanisms in AIDS is most likely to expand as more clinical and histopathologic data accrue.

Genetically Determined Defects

Numerous syndromic disorders secondary to genetic defects may have otologic manifestations consisting of hearing loss or vestibular dysfunction or both. Examples include syndromes caused by mutations in single genes (autosomal or sex-linked), mutations in mitochondrial genes, or chromosomal abnormalities. Such disorders are beyond the scope of this chapter, and the reader is referred to Chapter 147 or other sources.[138]

SUGGESTED READINGS

Agrup C, Luxon LM. Immune-mediated inner-ear disorders in neuro-otology. *Curr Opin Neurol.* 2006;19:26-32.

Cunningham MJ, Curtin HD, Jaffe R, et al. Otologic manifestations of Langerhans' cell histiocytosis. *Arch Otolaryngol Head Neck Surg.* 1989; 115:807.

Harris JP, South MA. Immunodeficiency diseases: head and neck manifestations. *Head Neck Surg.* 1982;5:114.

Khetarpal U, Schuknecht HF. In search of pathologic correlates of hearing loss and vertigo in Paget's disease: a clinical and histopathologic study of 26 temporal bones. *Ann Otol Rhinol Laryngol Suppl.* 1990;145:1.

McCabe BF. Autoimmune sensorineural hearing loss. *Ann Otol Rhinol Laryngol.* 1979;88:585.

McCaffrey TV, McDonald TJ, Facer GW, DeRemee RA. Otologic manifestations of Wegener's granulomatosis. *Otolaryngol Head Neck Surg.* 1980;88: 586.

McGill TJI. Mycotic infection of the temporal bone. *Arch Otolaryngol Head Neck Surg.* 1978;104:140.

McKenna MJ, Kristiansen AG, Bartley ML, et al. Association of COL1A1 and otosclerosis: evidence for a shared genetic etiology with mild osteogenesis imperfecta. *Am J Otol.* 1998;19:604.

Megerian CA, Sofferman RA, McKenna MJ, et al. Fibrous dysplasia of the temporal bone: ten new cases demonstrating the spectrum of otologic sequelae. *Am J Otol.* 1995;16:408.

Michaels L, Suocek S, Liang J. The ear in the acquired immunodeficiency syndrome, 1: temporal bone histopathologic study. *Am J Otol.* 1994;15:515.

Monsell EM. The mechanism of hearing loss in Paget's disease of bone. *Laryngoscope.* 2004;114:598-606.

Nadol JB Jr. Positive "fistula sign" with an intact tympanic membrane. *Arch Otolaryngol Head Neck Surg.* 1974;100:273.

Rinaldo A, Brandwein MS, Devaney KO, et al. AIDS-related otological lesions. *Acta Otolaryngol.* 2003;123:672-674.

Ryan AF, Harris JP, Keithley EM. Immune-mediated hearing loss: basic mechanisms and options for therapy. *Acta Otolaryngol Suppl.* 2002;548:38-43.

Schuknecht HF. *Pathology of the Ear.* 2nd ed. Philadelphia: Lea & Febiger; 1993.

Skolnik PR, Nadol JB Jr, Baker AS. Tuberculosis of the middle ear: review of the literature with an instructive case report. *Rev Infect Dis.* 1986;8:403.

Zoller M, Wilson WR, Nadol JB Jr. Treatment of syphilitic hearing loss, combined penicillin and steroid therapy in 29 patients. *Ann Otol Rhinol Laryngol.* 1979;88:160.

For complete list of references log onto www.expertconsult.com.

CHAPTER ONE HUNDRED AND FORTY-NINE

Sensorineural Hearing Loss in Adults

H. Alexander Arts

Key Points

- Sensorineural hearing loss (SNHL) is one of the most common clinical disorders, and is associated with a multitude of etiologies.
- Because of the wide range of genetic, infectious, vascular, neoplastic, traumatic, toxic, iatrogenic, degenerative, and immunologic and inflammatory pathologies that can affect the cochlea, a systematic approach to assessment is crucial to identifying the responsible etiology. Audiologic, serologic, blood chemistry, and radiologic testing can be used strategically for a cost-effective approach to diagnosis of SNHL.
- SNHL results from cochlear hair cell or auditory nerve dysfunction. Psychophysical abnormalities that result from impaired auditory physiology combine to challenge effective listening.
- Sudden SNHL is a clinical syndrome with a lengthy differential diagnosis. Prompt assessment and management of sudden SNHL may offer the opportunity to reverse or ameliorate the hearing loss using more recently developed therapeutic protocols.

Sensorineural hearing loss (SNHL) is an extremely common disorder, with a spectrum of effect ranging from an almost undetectable degree of disability to a profound alteration in the ability to function in society. Because its onset is frequently insidious, and because it is frequently accompanied by subtle compensatory strategies, hearing loss is frequently overlooked by physicians and patients. The auditory system is complex, depending on the performance of many different systems for its continued function. Normal hearing function depends on the mechanical integrity of the middle ear mechanism and cochlear duct, micromechanical and cellular integrity of the organ of Corti, homeostasis of the inner ear biochemical and bioelectric environment, and adequate function of the central nervous system (CNS) pathways and nuclei. These depend on normal vascular, hematologic, metabolic, and endocrine function. As a result, disease of almost any human physiologic system has the potential to affect auditory function.

This chapter addresses the clinical evaluation, differential diagnosis, natural history, and pathogenesis of SNHL in adults, and provides a systematic review of the broad array of etiologies of SNHL. There is inevitably some overlap with other chapters in this text, and in these cases the reader is referred elsewhere for a more detailed discussion.

Clinical Evaluation of the Patient with Hearing Loss

History

Evaluation of patients with sudden SNHL begins with a careful history. The degree of loss from the patient's perspective and its laterality (unilateral or bilateral) and chronicity (sudden onset, rapidly progressive, slowly progressive, fluctuating, or stable) should be assessed. Patients should be questioned for associated symptoms, such as tinnitus, vertigo, dysequilibrium, otalgia, otorrhea, or headache, and ophthalmologic or neurologic complaints should be sought. A sensation of aural fullness or pressure may be present, and may be the patient's only complaint.

A thorough medical history should be obtained with particular attention to cardiovascular, rheumatologic, endocrine, neurologic, and renal disorders, and to any exposure to potentially ototoxic drugs. Surgical history should be evaluated, and a history of skull trauma, penetrating trauma to the ear canal, and compressive force applied to the ear canal (e.g., slap injury) should be queried. The patient's history of exposure to noise, occupational and otherwise, should be specifically addressed. The type of noise, its estimated level, duration of exposure, and use of hearing protection should be documented. Patients and physicians frequently underestimate the importance of a patient's occupational noise exposure, and avocational exposures, such as hunting and power tool use. Finally, family history with regard to hearing loss is particularly important and frequently overlooked.

Physical Examination

Physical examination of the ears in patients with SNHL is frequently unrevealing. The whisper test and tuning fork testing can be used to estimate the degree of hearing loss and to determine whether the loss is predominantly conductive or sensorineural. With the exception of these findings, no abnormality generally is seen in patients with SNHL. Otoscopic examination of the ears should exclude the possibility of acute or chronic otitis media. Neoplasm within the middle ear may rarely be noted. Pulsatile tinnitus may be heard by the examiner with a standard or Toynbee stethoscope. Other cranial nerve abnormalities and stigmata of associated systemic disease or hereditary abnormalities should be specifically sought. The nonotologic portion of the physical examination is more likely to reveal positive findings.

Audiometric Testing

Only a brief discussion of audiometric testing is presented here. Conventional audiometric testing is discussed more thoroughly in Chapter 133, and electrophysiologic testing is addressed in Chapter 134.

Audiometric testing serves to verify and to quantify the degree of hearing loss. Air-conduction, bone-conduction, and speech audiometry and tympanometry constitute the minimum test battery in patients with suspected SNHL. Bone-conduction and air-conduction pure-tone audiometry helps to determine the type of hearing loss (conductive, sensorineural, or mixed). Speech audiometry verifies the pure-tone audiometric results. Speech discrimination testing with assessment of the performance-intensity function helps to define further the nature of the SNHL (cochlear vs. retrocochlear) and provides essential prognostic information regarding the potential benefits of amplification. Tympanometry with acoustic reflex testing verifies the conductive or sensorineural nature of the hearing loss and provides additional clues regarding etiology. Tympanometry can be especially helpful in excluding the possibility of a conductive component in patients with profound losses or bilateral losses in the presence of a masking dilemma.

Basic audiologic tests also can provide essential diagnostic clues as to whether SNHL is cochlear or "retrocochlear" in origin. By "retrocochlear," we mean a lesion proximal to the cochlea, the most common retrocochlear lesion being vestibular schwannoma. The examiner should have a high degree of suspicion for retrocochlear etiologies when there is asymmetry of loss, abnormally reduced or asymmetric speech discrimination, abnormal performance-intensity relationships ("rollover") on speech discrimination testing, or acoustic reflex abnormalities. Other cranial nerve findings, asymmetric tinnitus, or vestibular complaints (even if mild) should increase the level of suspicion.

Auditory brainstem response (ABR) testing is useful in evaluating the possibility of a retrocochlear etiology, and for establishing thresholds in difficult-to-test patients (young children or malingerers). In the past, the ABR was believed to be a highly sensitive test for the presence of a retrocochlear lesion. It is less commonly used in this role today because of reduced sensitivity in patients with small vestibular schwannomas—tumors that are readily detected with the high accuracy offered by magnetic resonance imaging (MRI).[1-3] New modifications of the ABR may increase this study's sensitivity.[4]

Electrocochleography differs from ABR testing in that the reference electrode is placed closer to the cochlea (on or close to the tympanic membrane or promontory). This allows measurement of the cochlear microphonic potential, the summating potential, and the auditory nerve action potential. Wave I of the ABR corresponds to the action potential of electrocochleography. Approximately two thirds of patients with classic Meniere's disease have an elevated summating potential-to-action potential ratio. It is believed that such a finding suggests the presence of endolymphatic hydrops.[5,6] Electrocochleography can also be useful in patients in whom wave I of the ABR is weak or not present because the location of the reference electrode inherently enlarges wave I.

Otoacoustic emissions consist of acoustic energy generated by the cochlea and recorded with a microphone in the external auditory canal. These emissions can be spontaneous in onset or, more commonly, evoked by an acoustic stimulus delivered to the ear canal. If the acoustic stimulus consists of a transient sound (a click or tone pip), the resulting emission is termed a transient-evoked otoacoustic emission. If the stimulus consists of continuous pure tones of two separate frequencies (F1, F2), the resulting emission is a continuous tone of frequency 2F1-F2, and is termed a distortion product otoacoustic emission. Otoacoustic emissions are clearly generated within the cochlea and are believed to be a by-product of the "cochlear amplifier," which is dependent on outer hair cell function. They depend highly on the physiologic state of the cochlea and, if present, suggest normal cochlear function. Otoacoustic emissions are rarely present with hearing thresholds greater than 30 dB HL, regardless of etiology. In addition, for an otoacoustic emission to be present, the middle ear mechanism must be functioning normally because the stimulus and the response must traverse the middle ear. The presence of an otoacoustic emission in an ear with SNHL suggests a retrocochlear etiology or possible pseudohypacusis. Because these etiologies are extremely rare in neonates, otoacoustic emissions also have been useful in neonatal hearing screening programs.

Vestibular Testing

Vestibular testing can be a useful adjunct in the evaluation of SNHL in selected patients. Evidence of ipsilateral peripheral vestibular hypofunction in a patient with unilateral progressive SNHL suggests the presence of a retrocochlear lesion.

Laboratory Testing

Laboratory testing rarely proves to be helpful in determining the etiology of SNHL. In most patients, either the fluorescent treponemal antibody absorption test or the microhemagglutination test for *Treponema pallidum* should be obtained because the prevalence of syphilis is relatively high, it is frequently asymptomatic, it is important to manage, and it is a potentially treatable cause of SNHL. The Venereal Disease Research Laboratory (VDRL) test is not helpful in this regard because it frequently becomes negative with inadequate management, in the latent phase of the disease, or in neurosyphilis. Routinely obtaining hematologic, metabolic, and endocrine studies does not seem to be necessary or cost-effective. Similarly, routine screening for autoimmune disorders does not seem warranted. If these disorders are clinically significant, they typically are apparent from the history and physical examination. In addition, there seems to be no clear relationship between the results of any of these tests and the presence of autoimmune hearing loss.

Radiographic Testing

Radiographic imaging is warranted in selected patients with SNHL. MRI with gadolinium enhancement is currently the gold standard in evaluating potential retrocochlear hearing losses. The role of MRI versus ABR testing in this regard is controversial. It is clear, however, that MRI with gadolinium is much more sensitive than ABR for diagnosis of small lesions.[1-3] Selective T2-weighted fast spin-echo MRI may be almost as sensitive as gadolinium-enhanced standard MRI and is less expensive.[7] Computed tomography (CT) is useful in patients with suspected labyrinthine anomalies, such as large vestibular aqueduct syndrome or Mondini dysplasia. CT may also be useful in patients with suspected labyrinthine fistula or temporal bone fractures. High-resolution CT with reformatted images in the plane of, and perpendicular to, the semicircular canals is the study of choice for showing semicircular canal dehiscence syndrome.[8]

Etiology of Sensorineural Hearing Loss

Developmental and Hereditary Disorders

Hereditary Disorders of Adult Onset

The discussion of hereditary causes of hearing loss in this chapter is limited to the more common etiologies primarily presenting in adulthood. Hereditary factors frequently play a role in SNHL, and research in this area is expanding rapidly. For a complete categorization and review of these disorders, the reader is referred to an excellent and encyclopedic work by Toriello and colleagues.[9]

Nonsyndromic Hereditary Hearing Loss

Most hereditary SNHL is not associated with other hereditary abnormalities. Hereditary hearing loss without associated abnormalities is much more common than generally appreciated and frequently is overlooked. It is likely that genetic factors play a role in presbycusis and in susceptibility to noise-induced hearing loss (NIHL).[10-13] Distinct patterns of hereditary hearing loss transmitted in autosomal-dominant, autosomal-recessive, and X-linked fashion have been well described. Recessive or dominant isolated SNHL can be progressive or static, and may be congenital, present first at birth, manifest in childhood, or manifest in adulthood. Approximately 90% of inherited SNHL is recessive.

Waardenburg's Syndrome

Waardenburg's syndrome is transmitted in an autosomal-dominant fashion and consists of a constellation of findings, including (1) dysto-

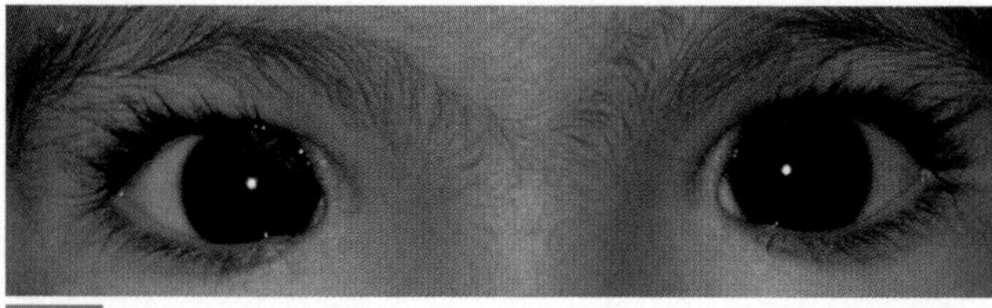

Figure 149-1. Ocular findings in Waardenberg's syndrome. Note the dystopia canthorum, the broad nasal root, the confluence of the eyebrows, and the heterochromia iridis.

pia canthorum (lateral displacement of the medial canthi), (2) broad nasal root, (3) confluence of the medial portions of the eyebrows, (4) partial or total heterochromia iridis, (5) a white forelock, and (6) SNHL (Fig. 149-1). There is extreme variability in the expression of this disorder, and the hearing loss can vary from profound to none at all. The hearing loss can be unilateral or bilateral, and can be associated with vestibular abnormalities.

Alport's Syndrome

Alport's syndrome is characterized by interstitial nephritis, SNHL, and, much less commonly, ocular manifestations.[14] This disease is unique because it is more common in women, but typically is much more severe in men. In the past, it has been thought to be transmitted in an autosomal-dominant fashion. It is now clear that there is significant genetic heterogeneity. Hearing loss is progressive and variable, usually beginning in the second decade of life. By age 20 to 40 years, 50% to 75% of men develop end-stage renal failure.

Usher's Syndrome

Usher's syndrome consists of the combination of retinitis pigmentosa and SNHL, with or without vestibular deficits. Three distinct groups have been defined. Usher's syndrome type I accounts for 85% of all cases, and is characterized by profound congenital hearing loss, absent vestibular response, and the development of retinitis pigmentosa by age 10 years. Type II accounts for 10% of cases, and is characterized by congenital moderate to severe stable hearing loss, normal vestibular responses, and onset of retinitis pigmentosa in patients 17 to 23 years old. Type III is typified by progressive hearing loss with onset in childhood or late adolescence and variable onset of retinitis pigmentosa. Approximately 5% of patients have type III. The disease is transmitted in an autosomal-recessive fashion, and it is estimated that 1 of 100 people is a carrier of the trait.

Inner Ear Anomalies

Many patterns of dysplasia of the inner ear have been described, and most have been associated with SNHL. These dysplastic patterns of development may be inherited, sporadic, or the result of chromosomal abnormalities. Commonly used descriptive terms for these dysplasias include Scheibe dysplasia (cochleosaccular dysplasia, involving membranous labyrinth only), Mondini dysplasia (dysplasia of bony and membranous labyrinth), and common cavity deformity (otocyst-like labyrinth with no cochlea or clear vestibular organs). Patterns of labyrinthine dysplasias form a spectrum with all manner of anomalies and patterns of hearing loss.[15]

Large Vestibular Aqueduct Syndrome

One form of inner ear dysplasia is unique because it has been associated with delayed onset of SNHL. An enlarged vestibular aqueduct is commonly seen in combination with other inner ear dysplasias, but more recently, it has been noted as an isolated finding in many ears. These patients may have any level of hearing from normal to a profound loss. Frequently, both ears are affected, and the losses are asymmetric. Fluctuation of hearing is common and usually affects one ear at a time; this may manifest as anacusis in one ear with fluctuation in the other. There is often evidence of a conductive component to the low-frequency portion of hearing loss. In patients who have been followed over time, a progressive stepwise loss has been noted in many.[15] This syndrome

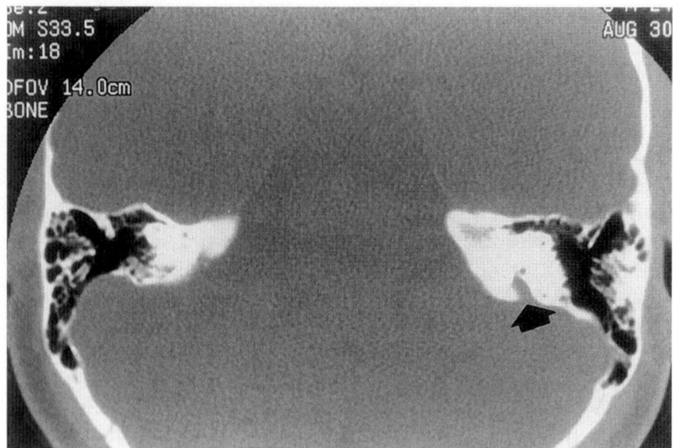

Figure 149-2. CT scan of the temporal bone showing the large vestibular aqueduct syndrome. *Arrow* indicates the enlarged vestibular aqueduct.

has been found to be familial in some cases, and probably occurs much more commonly than generally appreciated.[16] It is seen in isolation, as part of the Mondini malformation, and in patients with branchio-oto-renal syndrome[17] and Pendred syndrome.[18] It is well shown on high-resolution CT imaging of the temporal bone (Fig. 149-2).

Infectious Disorders

Infectious disease is a leading cause of SNHL in children and less so in adults. Infectious etiologies causing SNHL primarily in adults are discussed.

Labyrinthitis

An infectious or inflammatory process within the labyrinth can take two forms pathologically: serous (sometimes referred to as "toxic") or suppurative. Serous labyrinthitis is defined as an abnormal process within the labyrinth, caused by the degradation of the tissue-fluid environment within the inner ear.[19] It may be caused by bacterial toxins or contamination of perilymph with blood, products of tissue injury, or air at surgery. Bacterial toxins may enter the inner ear during the course of acute or chronic otitis media, presumably through either the oval or the round window membranes. Because both acute and chronic suppurative otitis media are common, and because SNHL associated with either condition is rare, these membranes seem to provide an excellent barrier preventing transmission of bacteria or their toxins to the inner ear. The principal abnormal finding in patients with serous labyrinthitis is endolymphatic hydrops, and the hearing loss and vestibular dysfunction associated with this state can be permanent or transient.

Commonly, a clinical diagnosis of labyrinthitis is made when patients present with sudden onset of SNHL and acute vertigo. The exact etiology in cases such as this is uncertain, but it is probably identical or similar to the etiology of sudden SNHL. The evidence tends to support the theory that this is most commonly caused by a viral labyrinthitis.[20,21]

Suppurative labyrinthitis is caused by bacterial invasion of the inner ear, and it is manifested by profound hearing loss and acute vertigo. The route of invasion can be otogenic, from acute or chronic otitis media, most commonly caused by a fistula between the middle ear and the labyrinth. Alternatively, the route of invasion can be meningogenic, through the cochlear aqueduct or internal auditory canal. This is the most common etiology of deafness associated with meningitis.

Otitis Media

SNHL is rarely associated with acute otitis media. No study has shown a relationship between SNHL and frequency of acute otitis media.[22] Patients with long-standing chronic otitis media commonly have a mixed hearing loss. Whether the sensorineural component of this loss is a result of the infectious process itself, or a result of other factors such as surgery or chronic use of ototoxic topical antibiotics, has been a long-standing controversy. When controlled for sensorineural losses associated with surgery, there seems to be no increase in SNHL in patients with chronic otitis media.[23]

Viral Infections

Herpes zoster oticus is a varicella-zoster infection most commonly associated with facial paralysis and a herpetic skin eruption over the auricle or within the external auditory canal. Although facial paralysis is the most frequent finding, hearing loss and vertigo can occur singly or in combination.

Measles is now rare in the developed world because of widespread vaccination. In the past, measles was a common cause of deafness in children. The hearing loss usually is bilateral and moderate to profound in degree. Vestibular function can be similarly affected.

Similar to measles, mumps is uncommon in the developed world because of widespread vaccination. Mumps is a paramyxovirus infection causing parotitis. Complications of mumps include orchitis, pancreatitis, SNHL, prostatitis, nephritis, myocarditis, and meningoencephalitis. SNHL resulting from mumps is unique because it is almost always unilateral. Bilateral involvement is rare. Unilateral deafness in otherwise healthy children or sudden deafness in adults may be caused by subclinical mumps infection in individuals without previous immunity.

Cytomegalovirus infection is thought by some authors to be a common cause of congenital and progressive hearing loss in children.[24-27] It has been proposed to be a cause of sudden SNHL in adults.[28] Hearing loss associated with acquired immunodeficiency syndrome (AIDS) may represent reactivation of latent cytomegalovirus infections.[29]

Syphilis

Congenital or acquired syphilis has been well established as a cause of SNHL. Although hearing loss is not associated with primary acquired syphilis, its incidence has been estimated to be 80% in patients with symptomatic neurosyphilis, 29% in patients with asymptomatic neurosyphilis, 25% in patients with late latent syphilis, and 17% in patients with congenital syphilis.[19] The mechanism of hearing loss in syphilis is either a meningolabyrinthitis as seen in neurosyphilis, or an osteitis of the temporal bone with secondary involvement of the labyrinth as seen in late congenital, late latent, or tertiary syphilis.[30] Pathologically, a resorptive osteitis is seen in the temporal bone, with progressive endolymphatic hydrops noted within the labyrinth. Clinically, the presentation of syphilitic hearing loss often is indistinguishable from Meniere's disease, with fluctuating hearing loss, tinnitus, aural fullness, and episodic vertigo. Hennebert's sign (a positive fistula test without middle ear disease) and Tullio's phenomenon (vertigo or nystagmus on exposure to high-intensity sound) have been strongly associated with otosyphilis.[19] The generally recommended treatment consists of an antibiotic protocol adequate for neurosyphilis with the addition of systemic corticosteroids.[31]

Rocky Mountain Spotted Fever

Rocky Mountain spotted fever is a tickborne infection caused by *Rickettsia rickettsii*. Headache, fever, myalgias, and an expanding petechial rash follow the tick bite by approximately 1 week. The disease results in systemic vasculitis, resulting in encephalitis, nephritis, and hepatitis. Rapidly progressive SNHL has been associated with Rocky Mountain spotted fever and may be transient.[32,33] Vasculitis involving the auditory system has been postulated to be the etiology of the hearing loss. Diagnosis is made primarily by clinical presentation and is confirmed by serologic titers. Treatment is with broad-spectrum antibiotics.

Lyme Disease

Lyme disease is a tickborne spirochetal illness caused by *Borrelia burgdorferi*. Although the most well-known otolaryngologic manifestation of the disease is facial paralysis, there is some evidence that the disease can be a cause of SNHL.[34-37] Although its true significance remains unclear, Lyme disease should be considered a possible etiology of SNHL in endemic areas.

Pharmacologic Toxicity

Aminoglycosides

At least 96 different pharmacologic agents have potential ototoxic side effects.[38,39] Among these, aminoglycoside antibiotics are perhaps the most common offending agents. This group of antibiotics includes streptomycin, dihydrostreptomycin, kanamycin, neomycin, amikacin, gentamicin, tobramycin, and netilmicin. Drugs that are ototoxic frequently are also nephrotoxic and vice versa (aminoglycosides, loop diuretics, potassium bromates, and nonsteroidal anti-inflammatory drugs [NSAIDs]). Alport's syndrome, described earlier, is a hereditary disorder affecting the kidneys and the inner ear, and there are developmental disorders resulting in renal and inner ear abnormalities. The strong association between pathology of the renal and auditory systems has not been well explained.

Aminoglycosides target the hair cells and enter the hair cell in an energy-dependent process. The end result is death of the hair cell. The reader is referred to excellent reviews of the current understanding of the mechanism of aminoglycoside ototoxicity (see Chapter 154).[40-42] The final common pathway of hair cell damage consists of the generation of reactive oxygen species. Different aminoglycosides have affinities for differing groups of hair cells, which result in different patterns of ototoxicity with different aminoglycosides. Kanamycin, tobramycin, amikacin, neomycin, and dihydrostreptomycin are more cochleotoxic than vestibulotoxic. Others, such as streptomycin and gentamicin, are more vestibulotoxic than cochleotoxic. The time course of the toxicity can vary.[39] Neomycin toxicity is typically rapid and profound, whereas a significant delayed effect has been noted for systemically administered streptomycin, dihydrostreptomycin, tobramycin, amikacin, and netilmicin, and for gentamicin administered through the middle ear.[43]

The hearing loss may be unilateral or asymmetric and can progress during or after cessation of therapy. Some degree of reversibility of the hearing loss sometimes is noted weeks to months after treatment.[39] Protective agents, including antioxidants, show promise for preventing or reducing aminoglycoside toxicity. More recently, the use of salicylates has been proposed.[44] A placebo-controlled clinical trial in China has shown a beneficial effect from the use of aspirin during aminoglycoside administration.[45]

Well-defined risk factors for aminoglycoside-induced ototoxicity have been established and include (1) presence of renal disease; (2) longer duration of therapy; (3) increased serum levels (either peak or trough levels); (4) advanced age; and (5) concomitant administration of other ototoxic drugs, particularly the loop diuretics. Peak and trough serum levels should be routinely monitored when these drugs are being used, and particular attention should be paid to avoidance of dosing intervals that are too short. With the more recent increased use of prolonged home-based intravenous antibiotic therapy, an increase in ototoxic complications has been noted, possibly a result of reduced attentiveness to serum levels and dosing intervals.

Ototopical Preparations

Topical preparations containing neomycin, gentamicin, and tobramycin have long been used directly in the ear for treatment of otitis externa and chronic otitis media. Placement of aminoglycosides within a healthy middle ear space frequently results in cochlear or vestibular ototoxicity as shown in experimental animals and in patients. This effect is now used to perform a titrated chemical labyrinthectomy for patients with Meniere's disease.[46,47] These same drugs have been used extensively over the years in countless ears with chronic otitis media with little to no apparent clinically significant effect on hearing or vestibular function.[48,49] Reduced permeability of the inflamed round and oval window membranes and dilution of the toxic drugs by purulent fluids and increased absorption into the vascular system by the hyperemic mucosa probably account for this decreased toxicity in the presence of otitis media.

It is clear, however, that use of aminoglycosides in the middle ear of animals does cause significant and predictable cochlear and vestibular toxicity in animals.[50] Based on this toxicity, and on the now widespread effective use of aminoglycosides to create a chemical labyrinthectomy, it is now generally regarded as unwise to use topical aminoglycoside antibiotics for treatment of otitis media. The American Academy of Otolaryngology–Head and Neck Surgery convened a consensus panel in 2004 that, after careful review of the literature, recommended against the use of aminoglycosides in topical form in the middle ear unless no alternative was available.[51] Other ingredients of older ototopical preparations also have ototoxic potential (e.g., polymyxin B, propylene glycol, acetic acid, and antifungal agents).[52,53] It seems prudent to use only agents specifically designed and approved for use in the middle ear for treatment of chronic otitis.

Loop Diuretics

The loop diuretics ethacrynic acid, bumetanide, and furosemide exert their diuretic effect by blocking sodium and water reabsorption in the proximal portion of the loop of Henle. The use of these drugs has been associated with a reversible SNHL and with the potentiation of aminoglycoside-induced hearing loss. The loss typically is bilateral and symmetric, and may be sudden in onset.[54,55] These drugs seem to alter metabolism in the stria vascularis, resulting in alteration of endolymphatic ion concentration and endocochlear potential.[56] Risk factors for loop diuretic–induced ototoxicity include (1) renal failure, (2) rapid infusion, and (3) concomitant aminoglycoside administration.[125]

Antimalarials

Quinine has long been known to be associated with the development of tinnitus, SNHL, and visual disturbances.[57] The drug, derived from the bark of the cinchona tree, has a colorful history as an antipyretic. It was dispensed by quacks and in secret remedies in the 17th and 18th centuries. The syndrome of tinnitus, headache, nausea, and disturbed vision is termed *cinchonism*. Larger doses may cause a more severe form of the syndrome, which also includes gastrointestinal, CNS, cardiovascular, and dermatologic manifestations. Quinine is used as an adjunct in the treatment of malaria and nocturnal leg cramps.[58] The ototoxic effect of quinine seems to be primarily on hearing and usually is transient. Permanent hearing loss may occur with large doses or in sensitive patients. Chloroquine and hydroxychloroquine (Plaquenil) are currently used antimalarial drugs structurally related to quinine. They have also been associated with ototoxicity and retinopathy. Ototoxicity with these drugs seems to be rare and possibly reversible.[59,60]

Salicylates

Aspirin and other salicylates are strongly associated with tinnitus and reversible SNHL. The hearing loss is dose-dependent and can be in the moderate-to-severe range. On discontinuation of the drug, hearing returns to normal within 72 hours.[57] Tinnitus consistently occurs at a dose of 6 to 8 g/day of aspirin and at lower doses in some patients.[61,62] Caloric responses also can be reduced by salicylates.[63] The site of the ototoxic effect seems to be at the level of basic cochlear mechanics, as evidenced by SNHL, loss of otoacoustic emissions, reduced cochlear action potentials, and alteration of the "tips" of auditory nerve fiber tuning curves.[64] These effects may be a result of alteration in turgidity and motility of outer hair cells.[65]

Nonsteroidal Anti-inflammatory Drugs

NSAIDs share many of the therapeutic actions and side effects of salicylates. Although there are isolated reports of hearing loss caused by naproxen,[66] ketorolac,[67] and piroxicam,[68] ototoxicity resulting from use of NSAIDs generally is rare compared with salicylates.[57,69] Similar to salicylates, animal models of NSAID ototoxicity show only reversible physiologic changes, without major morphologic changes.

Vancomycin

Vancomycin generally is believed to be ototoxic, but the available data are difficult to evaluate.[70] In clinical reports of vancomycin ototoxicity, patients almost always also received loop diuretics or aminoglycosides. Vancomycin has been associated with ototoxicity when administered intravenously, but not when given orally. Auditory impairment has been reported to be permanent or transient and is extremely unusual if serum concentrations are less than 30 mg/mL. In animals, vancomycin ototoxicity does not occur, unless toxic levels are administered.[71] Vancomycin is nephrotoxic and excreted by the kidneys. Renal failure can prolong vancomycin half-life and increase the likelihood of ototoxicity. Ototoxicity and nephrotoxicity are reputed to be less common with newer, more purified formulations of vancomycin.[72] When given orally, or in appropriate intravenous doses, vancomycin ototoxicity seems to be very rare, but vancomycin may potentiate other ototoxic drugs.[73,74] There is one reported case of severe, irreversible hearing loss associated with intrathecal administration of vancomycin.[75]

Erythromycin

Numerous case reports document SNHL associated with erythromycin administration.[76] In almost all reports, the drug was given intravenously rather than orally. The hearing loss seems to be uncommon and, in most cases, recovers within 1 to 3 weeks after the drug is stopped. The risk of erythromycin ototoxicity seems to be greater in patients with renal or hepatic insufficiency. There have also been reports of ototoxicity associated with the newer macrolide antibiotic azithromycin.[77] Limited histologic data suggest that the site of lesion in erythromycin toxicity is the stria vascularis.[78]

Cisplatin and Carboplatin

cis-Diamminedichloroplatinum (cisplatin) is a cell cycle–nonspecific cancer chemotherapeutic agent that produces dose-limiting SNHL and peripheral neuropathy, and a dose-related cumulative renal toxicity, hematologic toxicity, and gastrointestinal toxicity.[79] The incidence of hearing loss varies in adults (25% to 86%) and children (84% to 100%). Children seem to be significantly more susceptible to ototoxicity.[80] The hearing loss initially is worse at high frequencies, bilateral, and irreversible. It occasionally is accompanied by tinnitus or vertigo. The degree of hearing loss is dose-related, but there is considerable variability. Occasionally, severe hearing loss can occur after a single dose.[81] If ultra-high-frequency hearing is tested, 100% of patients show a loss. Many factors influence this variability, including mode of drug administration, tumor site, age, renal function, diet, cranial irradiation, interaction with aminoglycosides and loop diuretics, preexisting hearing loss, cumulative dose, and total dose per treatment.[79,82,83]

Carboplatin is a cisplatin analogue with a similar spectrum of antineoplastic activity. Carboplatin is less nephrotoxic than cisplatin. Myelosuppression is the dose-limiting toxicity with carboplatin. It was initially thought that carboplatin was less ototoxic than cisplatin. More recent studies have shown higher rates of ototoxicity than initially appreciated, however. In a series of children, high-dose carboplatin therapy was associated with a very high rate of ototoxicity.[84]

Cisplatin and carboplatin ototoxicity seems to be due to the creation of reactive oxygen species within the inner ear that target the hair cells. Cisplatin results in greater outer than inner hair cell damage, whereas carboplatin seems to affect the inner hair cells preferentially.[85]

Nitrogen Mustards

Nitrogen mustards are antineoplastic agents that include mechlorethamine (Mustargen), chlorambucil (Leukeran), cyclophosphamide (Cytoxan), melphalan (Alkeran), and ifosfamide (Ifex). Of these drugs, only mechlorethamine has ototoxicity as a serious adverse effect, and it has limited usefulness today because of its severe toxic profile. Animal and human studies with mechlorethamine ototoxicity have revealed severe loss of outer hair cells.[69] Other studies have shown shrinkage of the organ of Corti and loss of inner and outer hair cells.[86]

Vincristine and Vinblastine

The vinca alkaloids vincristine and, to a lesser extent, vinblastine are notable for their potent neurotoxicity. Peripheral neuropathy is common. Cranial neuropathies, ataxia, and hearing loss have been reported. Vincristine has been shown in animals to cause loss of hair cells and primary auditory neurons, whereas vinblastine has been shown to result in only hair cell loss.[79]

Eflornithine

Eflornithine (difluoromethylornithine) is a potent inhibitor of ornithine decarboxylase and is very effective in the treatment of trypanosomiasis. It also has proven useful in some patients with *Pneumocystis carinii* pneumonia, cryptosporidiosis, leishmaniasis, and malaria. It has shown potential as an antineoplastic agent. This drug has been reported to cause major and dose-related SNHL.[87]

Deferoxamine

Deferoxamine is an iron-chelating agent used in some patients with chronic iron overload or acute, severe iron intoxication. Auditory and visual neurotoxicity have been reported, particularly with larger doses in younger patients. SNHL is reversible in some patients when the dosage is reduced.[88]

Lipid-Lowering Drugs

Although optic and vestibulocochlear nerve degeneration (wallerian-like degeneration) have been seen in dogs given high doses of 3-hydroxy-3-methylglutaryl-coenzyme A (HMG-CoA) reductase inhibitors, no clinically significant effect on vision or hearing has been found.

Renal Disorders

Numerous genetic causes of SNHL are associated with renal abnormalities; Alport's syndrome is the most well recognized.[9] Acquired renal disorders have an unclear association with SNHL. Chronic renal failure, especially when managed with hemodialysis or renal transplantation, has been associated with progressive, fluctuating, or sudden SNHL. Oda and coworkers[89] found that 15% of 290 hemodialysis and renal transplantation patients developed SNHL. The etiology of the SNHL is difficult to determine precisely and probably is multifactorial. In addition to the electrolyte and metabolic abnormalities caused by the renal failure and subsequent hemodialysis, these patients typically receive frequent doses of loop diuretics, aminoglycoside antibiotics, and vancomycin. Because of the altered pharmacodynamics of these drugs caused by renal failure, their ototoxic potential is increased.

Trauma

Head Injury

Blows to the head can cause labyrinthine injury and resultant SNHL, either directly through fracture of the labyrinth resulting from temporal bone fracture or indirectly through labyrinthine concussion. The most common type of temporal bone fracture, longitudinal fracture, uncommonly extends through the labyrinth. The hearing loss associated with longitudinal fractures typically is similar to that of acoustic trauma (i.e., limited to the high frequencies and worse at 4 kHz). Similarly, blunt head injury alone, without temporal bone fracture, can result in concussive injury of the labyrinth, resulting in SNHL. Transverse fractures almost always traverse the labyrinth, resulting in complete loss of auditory and vestibular function. Penetrating injuries to the inner ear are rare, but they most commonly involve subluxation of the stapes into the vestibule, with resultant profound SNHL.

Noise-Induced Hearing Loss and Acoustic Trauma

The fact that excessive noise exposure could cause hearing loss was first recognized in the 18th century. In the early 20th century, NIHL was termed "boilermaker's deafness." Careful descriptions of the hearing loss sustained in industry would await development of the audiometer and were first published in the 1930s.[90] NIHL is now recognized as one of the most common occupationally induced disabilities, and noise exposure is now regulated by the Occupational Health and Safety Administration.[91]

Noise can be defined loosely as "unwanted sound," and subdivided by intensity, time course (continuous, fluctuating, intermittent, impact, impulse), and spectral content (pure-tone, narrow-band, broad-band). Impact noise is noise caused by collision of two objects and is common in industry. Impulse noise is noise resulting from sudden release of energy, such as an explosion or weapon fire.

Hearing loss caused by noise is sensorineural in nature. Rarely, extremely intense impulse exposures can result in tympanic membrane perforations, causing a conductive component. Most hazardous noise exposure produces a temporary SNHL that recovers over the next 24 to 48 hours. This reversible loss is termed a *temporary threshold shift* (TTS). If the noise is of high enough intensity or is repeated often enough, a permanent loss of hearing results, and is referred to as a *permanent*

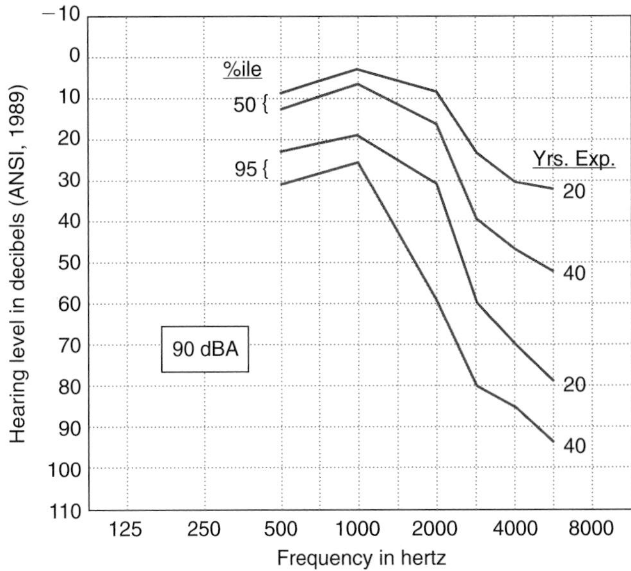

Figure 149-3. Predicted hearing thresholds (median and extreme values) after 20 years and 40 years of occupational noise exposure at 90 dBA. *(ISO-1999, from Dobie RA.* Medical-Legal Evaluation of Hearing Loss. *New York: Van Nostrand Reinhold; 1993.)*

threshold shift (PTS). Two distinct types of hearing loss are caused by excessive noise exposure: NIHL versus acoustic trauma. NIHL is caused by repeated exposures to sound that is too intense or too long in duration. Each exposure is followed by a TTS, which recovers, but eventually a PTS develops. Acoustic trauma consists of a single exposure to a hazardous level of noise, resulting in a PTS without an intercurrent TTS.

NIHL almost always results in a symmetric, bilateral hearing loss. It almost never results in a profound loss. Early in the course of NIHL, the loss usually is limited to 3 kHz, 4 kHz, and 6 kHz. The greatest loss usually occurs at 4 kHz. As the loss progresses, lower frequencies become involved, but the loss at 3 to 6 kHz is always far worse. The loss progresses most rapidly during the first 10 to 15 years of exposure and thereafter grows at a much-reduced rate. Figure 149-3 shows the 50% and 95% confidence limits for 20-year and 40-year exposures to 90 dBA (decibel, with "A"-weighting that fully weights 700-9000 Hz) sound. Figure 149-4 shows an example of the rate of growth of NIHL over time. The International Organization for Standardization has established standards for determining and quantifying occupational hearing loss and noise-induced hearing impairment.[92]

The hearing loss from acoustic trauma is similar to that from NIHL (i.e., worse at high frequencies with a 4-kHz "notch"), although other patterns also are seen. The other, most common patterns include flat losses and downsloping losses. Acoustic trauma frequently is unilateral or asymmetric. There is considerable variability in hearing loss among subjects with identical exposure. Age, gender, race, and coexisting vascular disease have been carefully studied, and when adequately controlled for other factors, they have not been shown to correlate with susceptibility to NIHL. An attractive theory suggests that patients who are more susceptible to TTS would be more susceptible to PTS and NIHL; this has not been shown to be the case. At present, there is no known way to predict susceptibility to NIHL.

There are three exceptions. Conductive hearing losses are clearly protective for NIHL in the same way that earplugs or earmuffs would be. The lack of an acoustic reflex has been shown to predispose patients to NIHL (the protective effect of the acoustic reflex is primarily ≤2 kHz).[19] Finally, patients with an unusually large PTS already should be considered to be more susceptible. TTS and PTS are commonly accompanied by tinnitus, and tinnitus after a noise exposure should be considered a warning sign.

There is little a clinician can do in the management of NIHL or acoustic trauma. The primary role of otolaryngologists and audiologists is in prevention and early identification. Many hazardous noise expo-

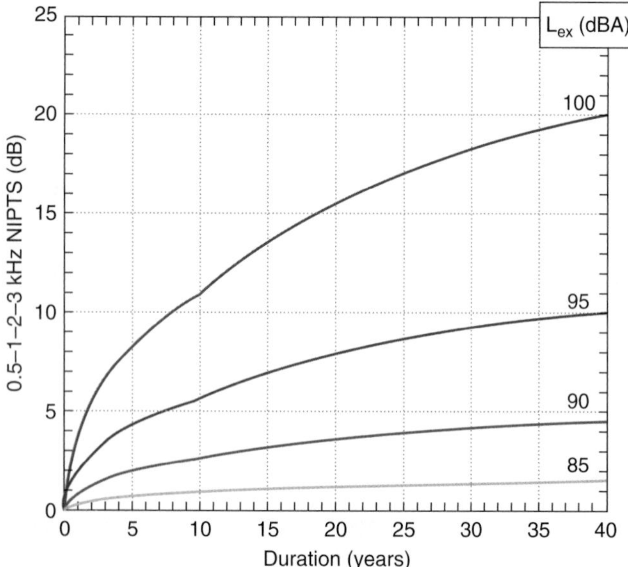

Figure 149-4. Speech frequency average noise-induced permanent threshold shift (NIPTS) as a function of level of exposure (in dBA-TWA) and duration. *(ISO-1999, from Dobie RA.* Medical-Legal Evaluation of Hearing Loss. *New York: Van Nostrand Reinhold; 1993.)*

sures are not occupational in origin. Many companies either are unable or unwilling to provide hearing conservation programs.

Barotrauma and Perilymphatic Fistula

Otitic barotrauma consists of traumatic injury of the tympanic membrane and middle ear caused by unequalized pressure differentials between the middle and external ears. The injury typically occurs during flying or underwater diving, and consists of pain, hyperemia, and possible perforation of the tympanic membrane, and edema and ecchymosis of the middle ear mucosa. These symptoms can be followed by the development of a hemotympanum or a transudative middle ear effusion. Conductive hearing loss may result. Any abnormality resulting in compromised eustachian tube function may predispose to barotrauma.

A perilymphatic fistula consists of a pathologic communication between the perilymphatic space of the inner ear and the middle ear. Perilymphatic fistulas can be congenital or acquired in origin. The fistulas can occur at either the round or the oval windows.[93]

Congenital defects can occur in the stapes footplate in patients with labyrinthine anomalies such as Mondini dysplasia.[94,95] These fistulas can communicate with the subarachnoid space and result in cerebrospinal fluid leak and possible meningitis. Typically, these ears have a profound hearing loss. This phenomenon should be a consideration in the differential diagnosis of patients with recurrent meningitis.[96-98]

Acquired perilymphatic fistulas can result from barotrauma, direct or indirect trauma to the temporal bone, or a complication of stapedectomy surgery. A typical history attributed to perilymphatic fistula consists of the sudden development of SNHL and vertigo after a head injury, barotrauma, or heavy lifting or straining. The event is sometimes associated with an audible "pop." Patients may have a positive Hennebert sign and positional nystagmus when the involved ear is placed in a dependent position.[99] Some authors believe that perilymphatic fistulas develop spontaneously.[100,101]

Diagnosis is made by middle ear exploration. Visualization of fluid in the region of the oval or round windows is not definitive evidence of a fistula because serous fluid can ooze from the middle ear mucosa, or lidocaine from the local anesthetic can collect in the vicinity.[102,103] Treatment consists of packing the area in question with tissue. Because of the lack of a definitive diagnostic test for the presence of a fistula, and because even surgical exploration does not reliably diagnose or exclude the possibility of a fistula, there is considerable controversy with regard to the management of this entity.[93,100,104,105] In the 1980s and early 1990s, it was commonly believed that spontaneous perilymphatic fistulas were a common cause of otherwise unexplained hearing loss and vertigo. Many surgical fistula repairs were performed as a result of this belief. It has since become clear that spontaneous perilymphatic fistula is rare.[106] No clear consensus exists regarding diagnosis or management.

Finally, labyrinthine fistula can result from erosion by cholesteatoma, or may develop spontaneously as in the superior semicircular canal dehiscence syndrome. The reader is referred to Chapters 140, 163, and 165 of this book for detailed descriptions of these entities.

Irradiation

The cochlea seems to be resistant to radiation injury at doses less than 45 Gy. At doses greater than 45 Gy, there is a clear, dose-dependent toxicity that manifests as hearing loss.[107-109] Radiation also seems to cause a dose-dependent toxicity to the auditory nerve and brainstem.[110] The latency period from radiation exposure to clinical hearing loss can be 12 months or more. One report notes that early-onset SNHL after radiation can recover to some degree.[111] Fractionated irradiation has been used to a limited extent in the past to treat vestibular schwannoma. Whether it has had an effect on hearing in these patients is difficult to determine because of the limited data available.[112] More recently, there has been much more extensive experience with stereotactic irradiation (radiosurgery) for vestibular schwannoma. This modality seems to be associated with substantial risk of SNHL, at least as high as with microsurgical removal.[113]

There is a relative paucity of published literature on the experimental effects of radiation on hearing. In a histologic study in chinchillas, sacrificed 2 years after fractionated irradiation of the cochlea, Bohne and coworkers[114] showed a dose-dependent loss of inner and outer hair cells. Early studies of the effects of radiotherapy involving the cochlea on human hearing were flawed because lack of controls, inadequate follow-up, and the retrospective nature of the studies. Many well-designed studies now have shown that radiotherapy involving the cochlea causes SNHL in 50% of patients.[107-109,115-117] The hearing loss occurs in a dose-dependent fashion, and seems to increase significantly at doses greater than 45 Gy. Advanced age, preexisting hearing loss, and adjuvant ototoxic chemotherapeutic agents are likely to amplify the effects of radiation. The hearing loss occurs with a latency of 0.5 to 2 years post-treatment and is probably progressive.[111] This delayed onset, and the fact that many patients do not survive for sufficient follow-up, results in underestimation of the frequency and severity of this complication. Dose-dependent injury to the auditory nerve and brainstem also occurs; however, the frequency in the absence of other neurologic complications is difficult to determine.[110]

An understanding of the effects of radiation on hearing has become much more clinically relevant more recently because of the popularity of stereotactic radiotherapy for the treatment of vestibular schwannoma and other similar lesions. Although many reports suggest that the risk of hearing loss is minimal, these studies are limited by (1) their retrospective design, (2) lack of long-term follow-up, and (3) incomplete audiologic characterization. In addition, it is difficult to compare the studies that are available because of differences in tumor size, radiation dose, radiation field, technique of radiation administration, and follow-up. There is a wealth of literature on the treatment outcomes after stereotactic radiotherapy; however, almost all of them are limited by one of the above-mentioned shortcomings. More recent studies report hearing preservation rates (defined in different ways and with different follow-up periods) between 36% and 61%.[118-121] The time course of hearing loss after stereotactic radiotherapy is poorly characterized; available data would suggest that the loss is progressive, and that early results may not predict later outcomes.

Neurologic Disorders

Multiple Sclerosis

Multiple sclerosis is a chronic disease characterized pathologically by multiple areas of CNS demyelination, inflammation, and glial scarring. The clinical course is variable, ranging from a benign, almost symptom-free disease to a rapidly progressive, disabling disorder. Early in the patient's course, the disease is characterized by remissions and relapses.

The disease is said to result in dissemination of neurologic lesions in time (remissions and relapses) and in space (variability of multiple deficits). The age at onset is typically between 20 and 30 years, rarely occurring before age 10 years or after age 60 years. Multiple sclerosis is more common in women than in men. There are striking racial and geographic differences in prevalence, with the disease being most common in whites and in individuals living at higher latitudes. The cause is unknown, but seems to be related to genetic factors, autoimmune mechanisms, and viral infection.

SNHL develops in 4% to 10% of patients with multiple sclerosis.[122,123] The hearing loss can be progressive or sudden in onset, and can be bilateral, unilateral, symmetric, or asymmetric.[124-128] Frequently, the loss is sudden and unilateral, and can recover after days or weeks.[125,129] Audiometrically, speech discrimination can be normal or reduced out of proportion to the increase of pure-tone thresholds. Abnormal patterns of acoustic reflexes can be seen in some patients.[126,130,131] Abnormalities of the ABR frequently are seen and are a diagnostic criterion for multiple sclerosis. Patterns of abnormality vary and include latency prolongation of wave I or the later waves, absence or poor morphology of waveforms, and waveform abnormalities with increased stimulus presentation rate.[124,128,130,132-134] MRI frequently is abnormal in multiple sclerosis and typically reveals periventricular white matter plaques on T2-weighted images. Plaques can be seen in the cochlear nucleus or inferior colliculus in patients with SNHL.[135-138]

Benign Intracranial Hypertension

Benign intracranial hypertension, also known as pseudotumor cerebri, probably is better termed *idiopathic intracranial hypertension* because it is not always benign in nature. The disorder consists of increased intracranial pressure without evidence of mass lesion, obstructive hydrocephalus, intracranial infection, or hypertensive encephalopathy. It is associated with a long list of medical disorders, but frequently manifests as an isolated phenomenon. The underlying pathophysiology is poorly understood. The most common presenting symptoms are headache and visual blurring. Pulsatile tinnitus, SNHL, and vertigo also may be present. It is more commonly seen in obese women.[139,140]

The pulsatile tinnitus is usually objective and is eliminated by jugular venous compression.[141,142] SNHL typically is a fluctuating, low-frequency loss that is unilateral or bilateral. Vertigo and aural fullness also may be present. The most serious manifestation of the disorder is progressive visual loss caused by optic atrophy. The disease is characterized by remissions and relapses. The diagnosis is confirmed by documentation of papilledema on funduscopy or cerebrospinal fluid pressure greater than 200 mm H_2O. ABR and electrocochleography abnormalities can be seen. Management consists of weight loss, acetazolamide, furosemide, and occasionally, lumbar-peritoneal shunting.[142,143]

Vascular and Hematologic Disorders

Migraine

Migraine is a common disorder, usually restricted to headache and sometimes the neurologic symptoms of an aura. Numerous subtypes of migraine are associated with different neurologic deficits. Basilar migraine has been associated with numerous auditory and vestibular symptoms and signs, including episodic vertigo, SNHL, tinnitus, aural fullness, distortion, and recruitment. Fairly complex and specific diagnostic criteria have been established for basilar migraine.[144] In a series of 50 patients meeting the criteria for basilar migraine, 46% had bilateral, low-frequency SNHL, and an additional 34% had unilateral low-frequency SNHL.[145] The hearing loss frequently fluctuated and occasionally was severe. Basilar migraine has been implicated as an occasional cause of SNHL. Because of their similarity, there has been considerable speculation in the literature of an etiologic association between basilar migraine and Meniere's disease.

Migraine headache can be managed with β-blockers, calcium channel blockers, acetazolamide, NSAIDs, and antiserotonin agents. No systematic study evaluating the use of these drugs in patients with basilar migraine is currently available. The reader is referred to the excellent reviews of Olsson[145] and Harker,[146] and to Chapter 165 for a more detailed discussion.

Vertebrobasilar Arterial Occlusion

Several eponyms have been applied to brainstem syndromes, but all apply to neoplasms with the exception of Wallenberg's syndrome (lateral medullary syndrome). Classic brainstem infarction patterns are seen less often than incomplete or mixed clinical pictures. To result in SNHL, the occlusion generally has to involve the anterior inferior cerebellar artery (AICA). Occlusion of the AICA results in ischemic infarction of the regions of the brainstem supplied by this artery. The occlusion typically results from thrombosis or embolism, and rarely from other vascular disorders or surgical occlusion of the vessel. The area infarcted includes the inferior pons, and many of the findings are similar to Wallenberg's syndrome. In addition, the AICA usually gives rise to the internal auditory artery, which is the principal blood supply to the labyrinth. The findings in patients with acute AICA infarction include acute vertigo with associated nausea and vomiting, facial paralysis, SNHL, tinnitus, ipsilateral gaze paralysis, ipsilateral loss of pain and temperature sensation on the face, contralateral partial loss of pain and temperature sensation on the trunk and extremities, and ipsilateral Horner's syndrome. The vertigo and hearing loss are caused by ischemic injury of the cochlear and vestibular nuclei in the brainstem and in the labyrinth itself.[19] Isolated cerebellar infarction can result in hearing loss, vertigo, facial pain or numbness, headache, or ataxia.[147]

Rheologic Disorders and Blood Dyscrasias

Waldenström's macroglobulinemia is a plasma cell disorder in which abnormally large amounts of IgM are synthesized and circulate in the plasma. The result is increased blood viscosity and subsequent ischemic lesions. Progressive and sudden hearing losses caused by this disorder have been reported, and some patients with SNHL have responded to treatment with alkylating agents or plasmapheresis.[148]

Cryoglobulinemia results from immune-complex disease, in which the resulting immune complexes are soluble at body temperature and precipitate at lower temperatures. The deposition of these complexes results in glomerulonephritis, vasculitis, and arthritis. The disorder can be associated with progressive or sudden SNHL.[149]

Sickle cell disease is associated with an increased incidence of SNHL.[150-152] It has been estimated that SNHL is present in 22% of patients with sickle cell disease.[153] The hearing loss may be progressive or sudden, and associated with sickle cell crises.[154-156] Leukemias and lymphomas also have been associated with SNHL caused by either leukemic infiltrates or hemorrhage within the inner ear or by vascular occlusion and resulting labyrinthine ischemia.[19]

Cardiopulmonary bypass has been associated with a slightly increased risk of SNHL.[157-159] The loss most often is sudden, but one study suggests an increased incidence of bilateral high-frequency loss postoperatively.[160] The etiology would seem to be either embolic phenomenon or reduced perfusion of the inner ear.

Vascular loops within the cerebellopontine angle or internal auditory canal have been proposed to be a cause not only of SNHL, but also of tinnitus, vertigo, and Meniere's disease.[161-164] Although the concept of vascular compression of cranial nerves causing intermittent neurologic dysfunction has been reasonably well accepted in trigeminal neuralgia and hemifacial spasm, it has achieved far less support in auditory and vestibular dysfunction. Vessel loops are found in contact with these nerves routinely during cerebellopontine angle surgery for other reasons, and these patients seem to be suffering no ill effects as a result. The entire CNS is subjected to such pulsation continuously. To date, nothing other than anecdotal evidence has been published supporting this theory.

Immune Disorders

Systemic Autoimmune Disorders

Various systemic (non–organ-specific) autoimmune disorders have been associated with SNHL.

Cogan's Syndrome

Cogan's syndrome is perhaps the prototypical autoimmune disorder affecting the inner ear. It consists of attacks of acute nonsyphilitic interstitial keratitis together with auditory and vestibular dysfunction. SNHL may be unilateral or bilateral, and associated with severe vertigo, nausea, vomiting, and tinnitus. If untreated, the hearing loss frequently progresses to a profound loss over months. Other ophthalmologic findings may be present. If treated early enough, SNHL typically is responsive to aggressive treatment with steroids. Immunosuppressive agents sometimes are required.[165]

Polyarteritis Nodosa

Polyarteritis nodosa consists of a necrotizing vasculitis of small-sized and medium-sized arteries. It can manifest with myriad findings, including weight loss, fatigue, fever, anorexia, arthritis, neuropathy, hypertension, renal failure, abdominal pain, and SNHL. Diagnosis is made by demonstration of the necrotizing vasculitis on biopsy specimen of involved tissue. SNHL may precede the development of systemic symptoms or occur late in the disease. It may be unilateral or bilateral, and either rapidly or slowly progressive. Facial paralysis also may be seen. Aggressive doses of steroids and immunosuppressive drugs are given for management.[166,167]

Relapsing Polychondritis

Relapsing polychondritis consists of an inflammatory reaction in multiple cartilages. The auricles usually are the first cartilages to be affected. Arthritis and eye findings are commonly present. The disorder frequently is present in conjunction with other autoimmune diseases. The associated hearing loss may be conductive, sensorineural, or mixed. SNHL can be sudden or progressive in onset, and may be associated with vestibular disturbances. Therapy includes steroids, immunosuppressive drugs, or dapsone.[168,169]

Wegener's Granulomatosis

Wegener's granulomatosis is a syndrome of necrotizing granulomatous vasculitis involving principally the lungs, airway, and kidneys. Hearing loss usually is conductive because of involvement of the eustachian tube or middle ear. SNHL may be present if the granulomatous disease or secondary infection extends into the inner ear.[170-172]

Other Autoimmune Disorders

Other systemic autoimmune disorders less commonly associated with SNHL include scleroderma,[173] temporal arteritis,[174] systemic lupus erythematosus,[175,176] sarcoidosis,[177,178] and Vogt-Koyanagi-Harada syndrome.

Primary Autoimmune Inner Ear Disease

McCabe[179] first described patients with bilateral SNHL responsive to immunosuppressive drugs. The loss can be sudden or progressive in onset. The loss usually involves both ears, either simultaneously or alternately. The hearing loss frequently is associated with vestibular symptoms and can strongly mimic Meniere's disease. Myriad nonspecific tests of humoral autoimmunity may be abnormal. The hallmark of the disease is the responsiveness of the hearing loss to steroids or cytotoxic drugs. In some patients, a course of drug treatment can produce a long-lasting improvement in hearing, and in others, the hearing improvement depends on continued use of the medications.[180] In these patients, methotrexate is sometimes used to reduce the need for continued high-dose steroids and their resultant side effects.[181] In still others, SNHL progresses despite aggressive treatment.

Sera of many of these patients have been shown to contain an antibody to a 68-kD protein of bovine or guinea pig inner ear extracts. The responsiveness of SNHL to steroid treatment correlates with the presence of this antibody.[182-185] This 68-kD protein has been shown to be a member of the heat shock protein 70 family (HSP70).[186,187] A significant percentage of patients with Meniere's disease show similar reactivity, suggesting that autoimmunity may play a role in at least a subset of patients with Meniere's disease.[188,189] Chapter 153 contains a full discussion of autoimmune inner ear disease.

Acquired Immunodeficiency Syndrome

SNHL is among the numerous neurologic manifestations of AIDS. The hearing loss may be a result of an infectious complication of AIDS, particularly cryptococcal meningitis or syphilis, or as a primary neurologic manifestation of the disease. Human immunodeficiency virus (HIV) should be a consideration in patients with otherwise unexplained SNHL when risk factors are present.[190-197]

Paraneoplastic Syndromes

Neurologic paraneoplastic syndromes consist of neurologic abnormalities associated with malignant neoplasms not metastatic to the nervous system. Rarely, the abnormality may involve the auditory or vestibular system.[198]

Bone Disorders

Otosclerosis

Otosclerosis primarily causes a conductive hearing loss, but it is commonly associated with a progressive SNHL, especially later in the course of the disease. The precise mechanism remains unclear. CT images of the cochlea in these patients frequently reveal a radiolucent area immediately surrounding the cochlea. Histologically, otosclerotic bone frequently involves the endosteum, but the degree of endosteal involvement does not clearly correlate with the degree of SNHL.[199] It is doubtful that isolated cochlear otosclerosis without stapedial involvement (and conductive hearing loss) occurs with any clinically significant frequency.[200] Treatment with sodium fluoride has been reported to retard the progression of hearing loss in these patients.[200-203] The efficacy of this treatment remains controversial.[204-207] Patients with very advanced otosclerosis can have a bilateral profound mixed hearing loss, which can be audiometrically indistinguishable from a profound SNHL. In these patients, stapedectomy can result in useful hearing improvement.[30,208,209]

Paget's Disease

Paget's disease (osteitis deformans) is a common but poorly understood disorder of bone. It is most common in older individuals, with an estimated incidence ranging from 1% in individuals 40 to 49 years old to 19% in individuals 80 to 89 years old. Approximately 50% of patients with Paget's disease manifest hearing loss. The loss can be conductive, sensorineural, or mixed. The stapes footplate is rarely fixed, and surgical ossicular chain reconstruction is rarely beneficial.[210] The treatment of Paget's disease consists of calcitonin or etidronate disodium. Some evidence indicates that medical treatment may stabilize or reverse SNHL.[211,212]

Neoplasms

When patients are initially seen with unilateral or asymmetric SNHL, particularly when the presentation is not typical for Meniere's disease, neoplasm should be a principal diagnostic consideration. All patients with asymmetric or progressive SNHL should be evaluated for a neoplastic etiology. Lesions resulting in SNHL usually are located within the internal auditory canal or cerebellopontine angle, but tumors located anywhere in the skull base or temporal bone can result in SNHL if the labyrinth is invaded.

Vestibular schwannoma is the most common neoplasm resulting in SNHL (Fig. 149-5). Best known as acoustic neuroma, vestibular schwannomas originate from the vestibular nerves, within the cerebellopontine angle or the internal auditory canal. Acoustic neuroma is common, constituting 6% of all intracranial neoplasms.[213] It has been estimated that 2500 new acoustic neuromas are diagnosed in the United States annually.[214] Acoustic neuromas account for approximately 80% of all cerebellopontine angle neoplasms.[213] The most common presenting feature of acoustic neuroma is progressive unilateral SNHL. Any pattern of hearing loss can occur, but most frequently the loss initially involves principally the high frequencies. Commonly, speech discrimination is reduced out of proportion to the pure-tone thresholds. Acoustic neuroma can manifest as a sudden loss in 10% of patients, although most sudden losses are not a result of acoustic neuroma.[215] Unilateral or asymmetric tinnitus, with or without hearing loss, also is a common manifestation of acoustic neuroma. Patients may have mild or severe vestibular symptoms or may have none. Bilateral acoustic neuromas are pathognomonic for neurofibromatosis type 2 (Fig. 149-6). The reader is referred to Chapter 177 in this text for a

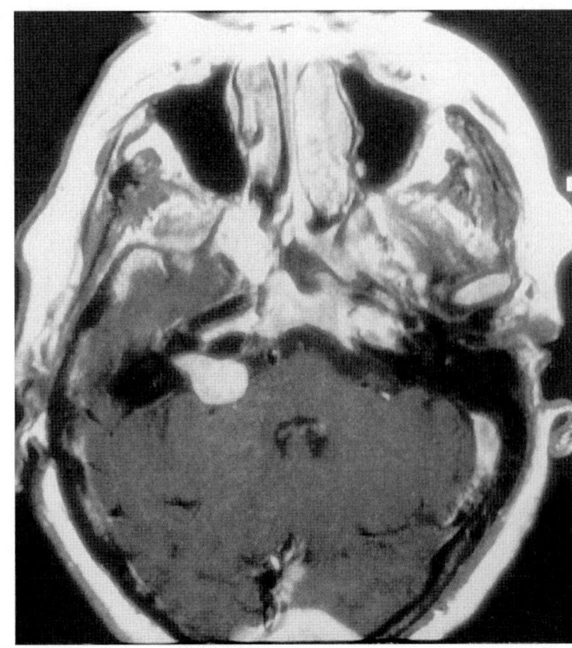

Figure 149-5. Gadolinium-enhanced MR image showing a medium-sized vestibular schwannoma.

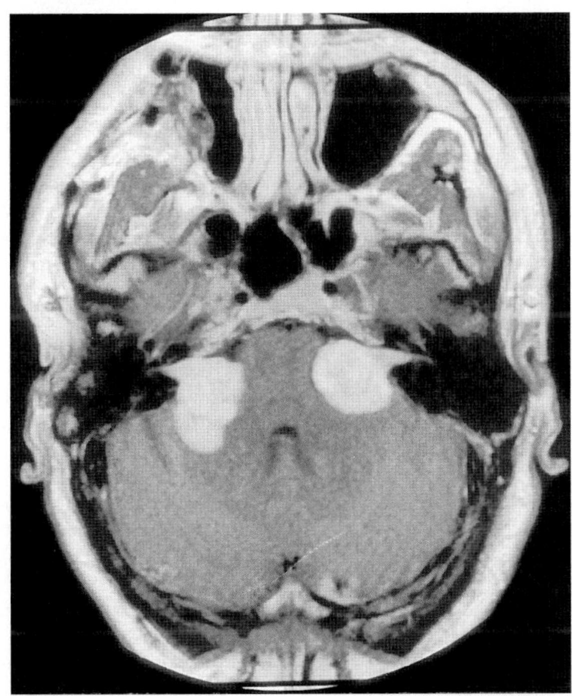

Figure 149-6. Gadolinium-enhanced MR image showing bilateral vestibular schwannomas pathognomonic for neurofibromatosis type 2.

more complete discussion of the pathogenesis, evaluation, and management of these common lesions.

Meningiomas account for approximately 15% of cerebellopontine angle neoplasms. The manifestation of cerebellopontine angle meningiomas is very similar to that of acoustic neuromas. For reasons that are unclear, meningiomas generally have less effect on hearing for a given size than do acoustic neuromas (Fig. 149-7). The remaining 5% of cerebellopontine angle lesions include dermoid cysts (congenital cholesteatoma), lipomas, arachnoid cysts, cholesterol granulomas, and hemangiomas. Metastatic lesions, particularly adenocarcinoma, also

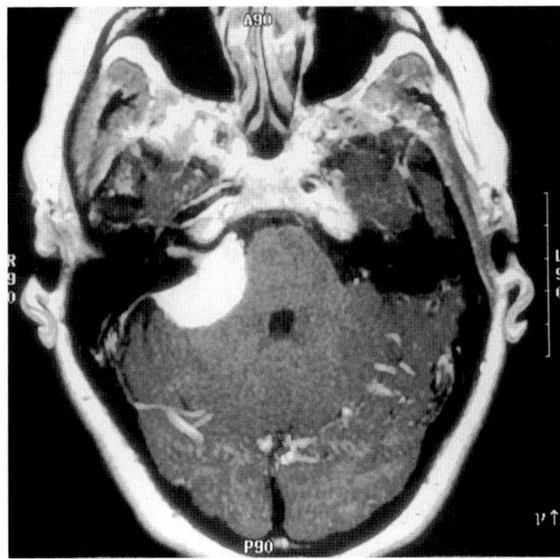

Figure 149-7. Gadolinium-enhanced MR image showing a large cerebellopontine angle meningioma. This patient had tinnitus and normal hearing, and had normal hearing after surgical removal of the lesion.

can occur in the internal auditory canal. Tumors occurring elsewhere in the skull base that can cause SNHL by involvement of the labyrinth include paragangliomas, chondrosarcoma, hemangioma, middle ear adenoma, rhabdomyosarcoma, lymphoma, and leukemia.[19]

Endocrine and Metabolic Disorders

It would seem logical that the diffuse large and small vessel atherosclerotic disease resulting from diabetes would be associated with an increased incidence of SNHL; however, this has not proven to be the case. There seems to be no significant association between the presence of diabetes and SNHL, when adjusted for expected hearing loss as a result of age.[216]

Although there is a definite association between SNHL and congenital hypothyroidism, there is little to no evidence that adult-onset acquired hypothyroidism can result in SNHL.[217-220] Similarly, reports have suggested that there is an association between hypoparathyroidism and hyperlipidemia. No convincing studies have shown either association.[221-223]

Pseudohypacusis

Pseudohypacusis is simply a factitious or exaggerated hearing loss and is common, especially in situations in which there is secondary gain to patients. Pseudohypacusis should be considered whenever the pattern of loss does not fit the clinical picture. Discordance between the speech reception threshold and the pure-tone average is a strong indicator of a factitious loss. Other audiometric studies, such as the Stenger test, ABR, and otoacoustic emissions, are helpful in clarifying such situations.

Disorders of Unknown Etiology

Presbycusis

SNHL associated with the aging process is termed *presbycusis*. In the strictest sense, only SNHL specifically caused by the aging process, and not by genetic factors, accumulated noise injury, vascular and metabolic factors, and so on, should be attributed to presbycusis. Because of the limitations of controlled studies in such a situation, it is difficult, if not impossible, to establish absolutely the existence of presbycusis. A better term for such a loss is age-related hearing loss, and this applies to any loss associated with age without other apparent etiology. Age-related hearing loss is a major public health issue. Actual prevalence of age-related hearing loss depends on its definition and is difficult to determine. It has been difficult in large epidemiologic studies to exclude

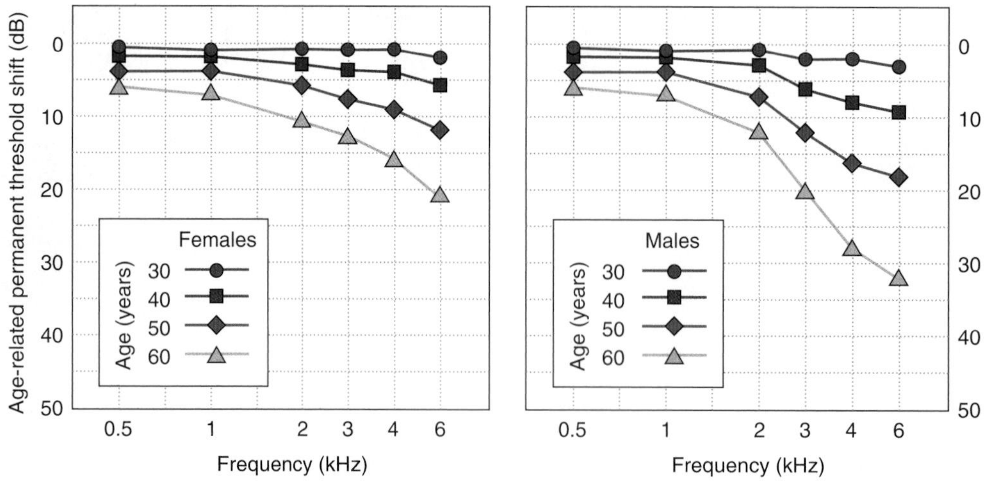

Figure 149-8. Median audiograms for patients with little to no noise exposure as a function of gender, frequency, and age. *(From Dobie RA.* Medical-Legal Evaluation of Hearing Loss. *New York: Van Nostrand Reinhold; 1993.)*

NIHL from study groups. Approximately 30% of individuals older than 65 years admit to a hearing loss.[91] Because at least 12% of the population is older than 65 years, there probably are more than 9 million people in the United States with age-related hearing loss.

Age-related hearing loss typically is worse for high frequencies and is more severe in men.[224] The rate of loss accelerates with time, so that the older patient is, the greater the threshold shift that can be expected in the future. Many large studies document the degree and prevalence of age-related hearing loss. Figure 149-8 shows the median pure-tone thresholds of a group "highly screened" to exclude noise exposure.

Schuknecht[19] has defined four separate types of presbycusis on the basis of pathologic findings in human temporal bones. In sensory presbycusis, hair cells are progressively lost beginning at the base of the cochlea. Patients with this abnormal pattern tend to have steeply sloping high-frequency hearing losses. Neural presbycusis implies a loss of auditory nerve fibers. These patients tend to have reduced speech discrimination out of proportion to their pure-tone thresholds. Atrophy of the stria vascularis was seen in strial presbycusis, and these patients have relatively flat audiograms. Finally, Schuknecht[19] described a fourth type of presbycusis termed *cochlear conductive* or *mechanical presbycusis*. No light microscopic abnormalities are seen in these specimens, and Schuknecht theorized that an age-related change in the stiffness of the basilar membrane resulted in the hearing loss. These patients have gradually descending (approximately 25 dB/octave) pure-tone thresholds.[19] These patterns are not useful clinically because there is variability of audiometric shape and severity in individuals with age-related hearing loss, and clinically the losses do not fall naturally into these patterns.[225]

Meniere's Disease and Endolymphatic Hydrops

Meniere's disease is a common disorder consisting of fluctuant SNHL, tinnitus, episodic vertigo, and aural fullness. The hearing loss typically begins as a fluctuating low-frequency loss, but progresses, gradually or quickly, to a permanent loss involving any or all frequencies. The tinnitus is most commonly described as "buzzing" or "roaring," and can fluctuate in loudness and character. The aural fullness perhaps is the most consistent and stable complaint, but it also typically fluctuates. The vertigo of Meniere's disease is the most disabling aspect of the disorder.

The typical presentation consists of episodic, spontaneous attacks of severe, spinning vertigo that lasts for several hours. The attacks frequently are associated with nausea, vomiting, and diaphoresis. After the attacks, patients usually are fatigued for 24 hours or more. The attacks of vertigo may be associated with a concomitant or preceding change in their hearing loss, tinnitus, or aural fullness. Many patients also have various combinations of dysequilibrium or motion-provoked vertigo between the classic attacks. Subtypes of Meniere's disease are described that have only vestibular symptoms (vestibular Meniere's) or auditory symptoms (cochlear Meniere's).

The hallmark of Meniere's disease is variability and unpredictability, and this holds true for the hearing loss associated with the disease. The hearing loss may fluctuate wildly or be quite stable over many years. It also may manifest as a sudden, permanent loss. Although most patients progress over the years to a moderate to severe loss, many do not, and progression to a profound loss is rare. The low frequencies are more commonly involved than middle or high frequencies, especially in the early stages of the disease, but there is considerable variability. The disease is bilateral in perhaps 30% of cases.[226-229] Patients who have bilateral disease usually develop bilaterality early in the course of the disease. Patients who maintain hearing loss in only one ear for the first few years rarely develop it in the contralateral ear. This finding supports the idea that the syndrome we have labeled as Meniere's disease is actually the manifestation of several different pathologies.

Although vestibular destructive therapy (chemical or surgical labyrinthectomy, vestibular nerve section) is effective in controlling the episodic vertigo associated with Meniere's disease, no therapy to date has been proven to be effective in the treatment of the hearing loss. The most widely accepted medical therapy for Meniere's disease, a sodium-restricted diet and diuretic administration, is based on the hypothesis that the hydropic distention of the membranous labyrinth can be reduced by altering body water distribution, as in the management of hypertension. This regimen of sodium restriction and diuretics was first proposed by Furstenberg and has gained wide acceptance.[230,231] Despite this wide acceptance, few studies have been able to show definitively that there is a beneficial therapeutic effect with regard to improvement or preservation of hearing.[232-234]

The creation of an intralabyrinthine shunt (cochleosacculotomy) has been proposed as a mechanism to control the hydrops and prevent the recurrent membrane ruptures thought to traumatize the organ of Corti. This procedure has been shown to be beneficial in controlling vertigo, but has been associated with an unacceptably high incidence of severe hearing loss.[235,236] Surgical decompression of the endolymphatic sac, with or without shunting of the sac into the mastoid or the subarachnoid space, has been proposed as a way to correct the presumed defective sac physiology. Although excellent results have been reported, double-blind, randomized studies comparing endolymphatic sac with mastoid shunt procedures with mastoidectomy alone have failed to show any significant difference in maintenance of hearing or control of vertigo.[237-241] The unpredictable, fluctuating nature of Meniere's disease, the lack of an objective diagnostic test, and the high incidence of spontaneous resolution of symptoms make it extremely difficult to come to valid statistical conclusions with regard to therapeutic efficacy in Meniere's disease.

Meniere's disease may be considered to be idiopathic endolymphatic hydrops. Although it is the most common cause of endolymphatic hydrops, many other entities result in similar clinical presentations and pathologic findings. The syndrome of delayed endolymphatic hydrops consists of the initial development of a profound SNHL in one ear, followed by development of symptoms of endolymphatic hydrops years later in either the ipsilateral ear (ipsilateral delayed endolymphatic hydrops) or the contralateral ear (contralateral delayed endolymphatic hydrops).[242] Other pathologic processes have been associated with development of endolymphatic hydrops, including syphilis, temporal bone trauma, serous labyrinthitis, stapedectomy, and autoimmune disease.[19] The reader is referred to Chapter 165 for a more extensive discussion of Meniere's disease.

Sudden Sensorineural Hearing Loss

A subset of patients with SNHL develop hearing loss rapidly, frequently awakening with it in the morning or developing a progressive loss over 12 hours or less. This commonly is a frightening experience for the patient, who might assume that this is a life-threatening disorder or will lead to profound, bilateral deafness. Neither scenario typically is the case. The etiology and appropriate evaluation and management of this common syndrome have been the subject of much debate over the years, illustrated by the fact that there have been more than 100 proposed etiologies for this disorder.[243]

Prevalence, Natural History, and Prognosis

Sudden SNHL is a syndrome and not a diagnosis. Most commonly, the syndrome has been referred to as sudden deafness or sudden SNHL and has many possible etiologies. In most patients, the cause is idiopathic. Among patients with no identifiable etiology, there seem to be several different pathogenetic mechanisms. In reviewing the natural history of the disorder, one should keep in mind that the described natural history is most likely the sum of the histories of patients with differing abnormalities. Because of this, and because of the difficulty of studying such an entity, either in clinical trials or in animal models, much remains to be learned about sudden SNHL.

A universal definition of sudden SNHL does not exist, and the rate of progression of SNHL can vary from seconds to days. For purposes of this discussion, sudden SNHL develops over 12 hours or less. This rate of progression can sometimes be unclear in the history because some patients notice their loss only on using a telephone. In other patients, sensation of fullness or tinnitus is the patient's primary initial complaint. The incidence of sudden SNHL has been estimated to range from 5 to 20 per 100,000 persons per year.[244] In a typical otologic practice, this may account for 2% to 3% of unselected outpatient visits. Any age group can be affected, but the peak incidence seems to be in the sixth decade. The male/female distribution is essentially equal.[245] Bilateral involvement is rare, and simultaneous bilateral involvement is very rare.[246]

The most common presentation is a patient noticing a unilateral hearing loss on awakening. Others notice a sudden, stable hearing loss or a rapidly progressive loss. Occasionally, patients note a fluctuating hearing loss, but most patients have a stable loss. A sensation of aural fullness in the affected ear is common and frequently is the only complaint. Tinnitus is present in the ear to a variable degree, and the hearing loss sometimes is preceded by the onset of tinnitus. Vertigo or dysequilibrium is present to a variable degree in approximately 40% of patients.[247]

Four variables seem to affect the prognosis of untreated idiopathic sudden SNHL: severity of loss, audiogram shape, presence of vertigo, and age. The more severe the loss, the lower the prognosis for recovery, and profound losses have an exceptionally poor prognosis. Upsloping and midfrequency losses recover more frequently than downsloping and flat losses. The presence of vertigo, particularly with a downsloping loss, is a poor prognostic indicator, although not all studies concur on this point. Reduced speech discrimination carries a poor prognosis. Finally, most studies show that children and adults older than 40 years have a poorer prognosis than others.[244,245,247,248] Most recovery occurs within the first 2 weeks after onset; as a corollary, the prognosis for recovery decreases the longer the loss persists. Without treatment of any kind, a significant proportion (30% to 65%) of patients experience complete or partial recovery.[247,248]

Etiology of Sudden Sensorineural Hearing Loss

The management of sudden SNHL should be focused on excluding known causes of the syndrome, especially conditions that require treatment. Similar to causes of SNHL in general, these disorders can be conveniently broken down into infectious, neoplastic, traumatic, ototoxic, immunologic, vascular, developmental, psychogenic, and idiopathic etiologies. Despite a thorough search for an etiology, most cases remain idiopathic. There has been, and continues to be, considerable debate regarding the pathogenesis of the disease in these patients. Principal theories include viral infection, vascular occlusion, intracochlear membrane breaks, and autoimmunity.

Infectious Disorders

Viral Infection

Viral neuritis or cochleitis has long been thought to be the most common cause of sudden SNHL, although much of the evidence for this is circumstantial. SNHL can complicate clinically evident infections with mumps, measles, herpes zoster, and infectious mononucleosis and with congenital rubella and cytomegalovirus. Of patients presenting with sudden SNHL, 28% report a viral-like upper respiratory infection within 1 month before the onset of their hearing loss.[245,249] With the possible exception of mumps parotitis and herpes zoster infections, however, the clinical diagnosis of viral infections is unreliable. Azimi and colleagues[250] reported that 53% of mumps meningoencephalitis occurs without parotitis. Other evidence for a viral etiology for sudden SNHL includes studies documenting increased viral titers in such patients,[249] pathology consistent with viral infection,[251-254] and viral seroconversion studies.[255-258] These seroconversion studies showed a mixture of viruses, including herpes simplex, herpes zoster, cytomegalovirus, influenza, parainfluenza, mumps, measles, and adenovirus. The studies failed to show a relationship between titer results and severity of hearing loss or frequency of recovery.

For some viruses, the evidence of a causative relationship is more convincing. The mumps virus has been isolated from the perilymph of patients with sudden SNHL,[259] and experimental mumps labyrinthitis has been reproduced in hamsters by inoculation of the subarachnoid space with mumps virus.[259,260] Lassa fever, an arenavirus infection endemic in West Africa, has been shown to be associated with sudden SNHL in approximately two thirds of the patients.[261] The time course, the results of audiometric testing, and the patterns of recovery in Lassa fever are very similar to that in idiopathic sudden SNHL.[262] Measles and rubella also are well-documented causes of labyrinthitis,[253] but these cases rarely manifest in a manner typical of sudden SNHL. Herpes zoster oticus also can cause sudden SNHL, although it is a clinical entity distinct from idiopathic sudden SNHL. The evidence that herpes zoster may be associated with idiopathic sudden SNHL is limited to viral seroconversion studies. Sudden hearing loss associated with infectious mononucleosis is rare but has been reported.[263] For a few viruses, there seems to be strong evidence that they may be an occasional cause of idiopathic sudden SNHL. For most other viruses, there is an association with idiopathic sudden SNHL, although convincing evidence of a causal relationship is lacking.

Meningitis

Meningitis is a well-recognized and common etiology of acquired severe to profound SNHL. It is possible that rare cases of idiopathic sudden SNHL may be caused by subclinical meningoencephalitis.

Syphilis

It has been estimated that the incidence of syphilis in patients with sudden SNHL is 2% or less. Syphilitic hearing loss may manifest at any stage of the disease, and may be associated with other manifestations of syphilis, with vestibular symptoms, or alone. It may manifest with unilateral or bilateral sudden SNHL. More typical presentations of syphilitic hearing loss are discussed in other sections of this chapter.

It is important to consider the possibility of reactivation of syphilis in patients with HIV infection.[194,196]

Lyme Disease

Lyme disease is a well-established etiology of acute facial paralysis, and it would not be unreasonable to assume that it could also cause SNHL. Hearing loss has not been strongly associated with Lyme disease, however. The literature contains several descriptions of associations between positive Lyme titers and acute or chronic SNHL, but a causal relationship seems doubtful. In one large study, Lyme titers were found in 21% of patients with sudden SNHL, and there was no difference in outcome between patients with or without positive titers, despite antibiotic treatment of all seropositive patients.[264] Reports of hearing loss in patients with Lyme disease with improved hearing after antibiotic treatment are limited to a few case reports.[35,265]

Acquired Immunodeficiency Syndrome

At autopsy, 88% of HIV-positive patients have evidence of CNS involvement,[266] and approximately 10% of patients with AIDS present because of neurologic symptoms.[190] It is not surprising that sudden SNHL may be associated with HIV infection. Sudden SNHL is not a common manifestation of AIDS, but it has been well documented in the literature.[191-194,197,267] In the presence of HIV infection, sudden SNHL may occur with or without the presence of opportunistic infection, and may occur without clinical evidence of AIDS. Sudden SNHL caused by reactivation of latent syphilis may complicate any stage of HIV infection.[193,194,196] As previously mentioned, some cases of sudden SNHL associated with AIDS may be the result of reactivation of latent cytomegalovirus infection.

Neoplasms

Acoustic Neuroma

It is common for a sudden SNHL to be the initial manifestation of a vestibular schwannoma (acoustic neuroma). According to Moffat and associates,[215] 10.2% of acoustic neuromas initially manifest with sudden SNHL. The prevalence of acoustic neuroma among patients with sudden SNHL is less clear. Estimates range from 0.8%[246] to 3%.[268,269] There are no clear criteria that suggest that sudden SNHL may be a result of an acoustic neuroma. The presence of tinnitus in the ipsilateral ear before sudden SNHL is suggestive, but not present in most cases.[269] In addition, midfrequency and high-frequency hearing loss are more commonly associated with acoustic neuroma than are low-frequency losses, and electronystagmography abnormalities are more common with acoustic neuroma.[269]

Responsiveness of the hearing loss to treatment with steroids is an unreliable indicator that a retrocochlear lesion is not present. There have been many reported cases of steroid-responsive SNHL and SNHL with spontaneous recovery, which have been found to be caused by acoustic neuroma.[269,270] One should have a high level of suspicion for acoustic neuroma in any patient with SNHL. Most investigators recommend that ABR or gadolinium-enhanced MRI be obtained in patients with sudden SNHL.[271] There is no relationship between tumor size and SNHL.[269] Because of this and the numerous more recent reports of false-negative ABR tests in patients with small acoustic neuromas,[3,272-274] it seems warranted to evaluate all patients with sudden SNHL with gadolinium-enhanced MRI.

Other Neoplasms

Neoplasms of the cerebellopontine angle or internal auditory canal other than acoustic neuromas have been associated with SNHL. These include meningioma,[275] cholesteatoma, hemangioma,[276] arachnoid cyst, and metastatic neoplasms. In addition, skull base neoplasms eroding into the inner ear can rarely manifest with SNHL.

Trauma and Membrane Ruptures

Head Injury

Sensorineural hearing loss of any degree can occur after closed or open head injury. The mechanism of injury in such patients has been shown pathologically to vary from mild loss of outer or inner hair cells or cochlear membrane breaks to fracture across the labyrinth or intralabyrinthine hemorrhage.[19] Many of these injuries are pathologically indistinguishable from injuries of acoustic trauma.[277] Some patients experience a variable degree of recovery from head injury–induced hearing loss, a process probably equivalent to the temporary threshold shift seen with acoustic trauma.

Perilymphatic Fistula

Round or oval window fistulas can occur congenitally, after stapedectomy, or after barotrauma. SNHL is well described after events causing barotrauma.[278,279] Some investigators theorize that these fistulas can occur after heavy lifting or straining or even spontaneously. Patients with such fistulas can have sudden or fluctuating SNHL and varying degrees of vestibular symptoms. There is no reliable test for the presence of such a fistula, and even surgical exploration is subject to error.[280] Except in poststapedectomy patients, it is doubtful that perilymph fistula is a significant cause of SNHL.

Intracochlear Membrane Breaks

Intracochlear membrane ruptures and fistulas have been documented pathologically in patients with endolymphatic hydrops.[19] Such breaks have been proposed to be an etiology of SNHL.[281] Schuknecht and Donovan[253] found no evidence of such breaks in a series of temporal bones from patients with sudden SNHL. Gussen[282-284] found evidence to support the membrane break theory in a few temporal bones, however.

Pharmacologic Toxicity

Toxicity from any of the drugs discussed in the previous section on ototoxic causes of SNHL may result in the relatively sudden onset of hearing loss. In addition to these drugs, others have been associated with sudden SNHL. Interferon has been associated with SNHL, which has been reversible in most patients.[285,286] The insecticides malathion and methoxychlor have been associated with bilateral SNHL.[287]

Immunologic Disorders

The finding that many patients with SNHL seem to benefit from glucocorticoid therapy, and the finding of cross-reacting circulating antibodies in many patients with sudden and rapidly progressive SNHL suggest that at least a subset of SNHL cases are caused by inner ear autoimmunity.[185] In addition, many well-known autoimmune diseases have been associated with SNHL, including Cogan's syndrome,[288,289] systemic lupus erythematosus,[175] temporal arteritis, and polyarteritis nodosa.

Vascular Disorders

Sudden hearing loss can occur with occlusion of the cochlear blood supply. Because of the abruptness of onset of SNHL, and the fact that the cochlea depends on a single terminal branch of the posterior cerebral circulation, vascular occlusion has been thought by some authors to be an attractive hypothetical etiology for idiopathic sudden hearing losses. Other aspects arguing against a circulatory etiology include high incidence of spontaneous recovery, significant incidence in young patients, lack of an apparent increased incidence in diabetics, the fact that the loss frequently is limited to just a few frequencies, and the fact that most patients do not have vertigo. Similar to viral etiologies, a few cases of SNHL are clearly a result of vascular occlusion, but most cases remain idiopathic. Temporal bone studies have not found evidence of vascular occlusion in cases of idiopathic SNHL.[19] Series of patients with idiopathic SNHL have been evaluated for hemostatic abnormalities, and no significant association has been found.[290] The role of vascular occlusion versus viral infection in these idiopathic cases has been the subject of extensive debate over the years. At this point, it seems doubtful that a significant proportion of cases of idiopathic sudden SNHL have a vascular etiology.

Migraine,[145,291,292] hemoglobin SC disease,[151,153-156] and macroglobulinemia[148,149] have been documented to be associated with sudden SNHL. Rare cases of thromboangiitis obliterans (Buerger's disease) have been associated with sudden SNHL.[293] Small cerebellar infarctions may mimic labyrinthine lesions, including sudden onset of hearing loss.[294] Cardiopulmonary bypass[158,159] and noncardiac surgery[157] have been associated with an increased risk of sudden SNHL. Sudden SNHL has been reported after spinal manipulation with probable injury to the vertebrobasilar arterial system.[295]

It has long been believed that patients with diabetes have a higher incidence of idiopathic sudden SNHL than nondiabetics. This belief has been based on the higher incidence of other acute cranial neuropathies and on the diffuse vascular abnormality found in patients with diabetes. Histologic studies of human temporal bones from patients with diabetes mellitus have not consistently found any abnormal alterations.[19,296] In a careful study of the relationship of idiopathic sudden SNHL to diabetes, Wilson[28] found that diabetic patients with idiopathic sudden SNHL were less likely to recover hearing at higher frequencies. There was no significant difference in audiologic pattern between diabetic and nondiabetic patients with idiopathic sudden SNHL. An attempt to compare the incidence of diabetes in patients with idiopathic sudden SNHL with a control population was inconclusive.

Developmental Abnormalities

Large vestibular aqueduct syndrome is associated with SNHL, which frequently occurs in a stepwise fashion associated with minor head trauma. It seems plausible that other, as yet undefined, developmental abnormalities may predispose individuals to sudden SNHL, either spontaneously or after minor head trauma.

Idiopathic Disorders

Meniere's Disease

Some patients seen with typical sudden SNHL ultimately may develop a history more suggestive of endolymphatic hydrops or even frank Meniere's syndrome; this probably constitutes only 5% of all patients with sudden SNHL. In a review of 1270 patients with Meniere's disease, Hallberg[297] found that only 4.4% had initially been seen with sudden SNHL. A subset of these patients very likely have an autoimmune etiology of their hearing loss.

Multiple Sclerosis

Multiple sclerosis is a demyelinating disorder of the CNS manifested by differing neurologic lesions separated by space and time. Sudden SNHL is a rare initial manifestation of multiple sclerosis.[124,137,298] Among patients with multiple sclerosis, auditory abnormalities are common.[127,130]

Sarcoidosis

CNS manifestations are rare (incidence of 1% to 5%), although among patients with neurosarcoidosis, 20% have eighth cranial nerve findings. This eighth cranial nerve involvement may manifest as sudden SNHL, although it only rarely is an isolated finding.[178]

Psychogenic Disorders

Pseudohypacusis frequently manifests as a sudden loss. In most patients, malingering is readily apparent after initial audiologic studies.

Treatment

Treatment of sudden SNHL should be based on its etiology. If an etiology is apparent, the appropriate treatment should follow: appropriate antibiotics for infectious causes, withdrawal of the offending drug for ototoxicity, and so on. Most cases are idiopathic, and treatment decisions should be made on the basis of empirical guidelines. Because of the poor understanding of idiopathic sudden SNHL, controversy surrounds its treatment. Because of the dictum, "first, do no harm," new or unconventional treatment protocols should be well reasoned and carefully applied. It seems prudent to avoid the use of potentially harmful treatment protocols outside of controlled clinical trials because serious complications and deaths have been reported after treatment of idiopathic sudden SNHL.[299]

Steroids in moderate doses have become the most widely accepted treatment option for idiopathic sudden SNHL. Wilson and associates[248] performed a double-blind randomized trial of steroids versus placebo for idiopathic sudden SNHL. Their active drug group was treated with either a 10-day or 12-day course of orally administered dexamethasone or methylprednisolone at tapering doses. They found that all patients ($n = 14$) with midfrequency losses (loss at 4 kHz better than 8 kHz) had a complete recovery regardless of treatment. They noted that among patients with losses greater than 90 dB HL at all frequencies, there was no difference in recovery between the steroid-treated versus placebo-treated groups. Among the remaining patients (nonprofound losses with hearing at 4 kHz better than 8 kHz), there was a significant increase in recovery in the steroid-treated group. Of patients, 78% in the steroid-treated group experienced complete or partial recovery compared with 38% in the placebo-treated group.

In a similar study, Moskowitz and colleagues[300] confirmed a significantly improved recovery rate in a steroid-treated group compared with a nontreated control group. Direct steroid treatment to the inner ear, via middle ear instillation or round window microcatheter, has seen increasing use on an empiric basis. This treatment has the potential advantage of very high steroid concentrations within the inner ear without the associated systemic side effects. Anecdotal reports indicate that this treatment may be more effective than orally administered steroids, and that local complications are infrequent.[301] Refer to Chapter 153 for a more complete discussion.

An alternative management regimen proposed by some investigators involves attempts to improve blood flow or oxygenation to the inner ear. Vasodilators have been used extensively in the treatment of sudden SNHL. Any proposed vasodilator would have to cross the blood-brain barrier and have an effect on intracranial circulation. Intravenous histamine infusion, oral papaverine, and oral nicotinic acid have been used most frequently. Fisch and others[302,303] have shown that breathing a gas mixture with increased partial pressures of oxygen and carbon dioxide (carbogen) results in increased perilymph oxygen tension in cats and humans.

Other agents proposed to improve cochlear blood flow include low-molecular-weight dextran, mannitol, pentoxifylline, and heparin. In addition, the iodinated radiographic contrast agent diatrizoate (Hypaque) was serendipitously noted during a vertebral angiogram to improve the hearing in patients with sudden SNHL. Morimitsu and coworkers[304] showed in the same report that, in a small series, 54% of patients treated with diatrizoate had a complete recovery compared with 19% of a control group treated with vasodilators. It was later shown that triiodinated benzoic acid derivatives such as diatrizoate had a specific effect on the stria vascularis, protecting the endocochlear potential from furosemide-induced depression.[305]

Clinical studies that used the previously mentioned agents have shown poor to mixed results. The varying definition of recovery used by different authors complicates the interpretation of these results. No controlled study has shown a beneficial effect from papaverine, nicotinic acid, or pentoxifylline. Donaldson[306] found no improvement with aggressive heparin therapy in a series of patients. In a prospective, randomized double-blind study, Probst and colleagues[307] found no difference in outcome between placebo and treatment with low-molecular-weight dextran, pentoxifylline, or both. In a randomized prospective trial comparing papaverine/dextran infusion treatment with inhaled carbogen, the average hearing improvement in the carbogen group was better, although no significant difference in hearing recovery was seen between the two groups after 5 days of treatment.[302] After 1 year of treatment, there was a statistically significant improvement in hearing in the carbogen-treated group.[308]

Redleaf and coworkers[309] reviewed their 10-year experience with diatrizoate and dextran, and noted that 74% of their 36 patients showed audiometric improvement with treatment. Only 36% improved to 50% of their premorbid hearing levels, however, very close to the 32% recovery noted in the placebo group of the Wilson study.[248] Another, even more empirical, treatment protocol is the so-called shotgun regimen, which uses most of the proposed agents in hopes that one or more will be beneficial. Wilkins and associates[310] reviewed their results with a protocol of dextran, histamine, diatrizoate, diuretics, steroids, oral vasodilators, and carbogen inhalation. Although it was a retrospective study and limited by methodologic problems, these authors were unable to show any difference in recovery between patients who had the "full" protocol versus patients who had only portions of the total regimen. Their overall results were no better than the results expected for spontaneous recovery.

Still other treatment ideas are directed at other presumed etiologies. Because endolymphatic hydrops is a common final pathology for many inner ear injuries and may be associated with some cases of sudden SNHL, some authors have advocated treatment with a sodium-restricted diet and a diuretic.[311] Because of the evidence for a viral etiology and specifically evidence of herpesvirus, treatment with oral antiviral medications has been proposed. Because these drugs rarely have adverse side effects, many practitioners routinely treat patients with sudden hearing loss with antivirals in addition to steroids. In a double-blind, randomized, placebo-controlled multicenter trial, Tucci and colleagues[312] found no difference in hearing recovery outcome between patients treated with steroids and valaciclovir versus steroids and placebo. Some authors have advocated aggressive management with very large (mega) doses of steroids or even cytotoxic medications. Clinical studies supporting the efficacy of any of these treatments have yet to be published.

The author believes that a reasonable treatment approach to sudden SNHL is as follows: Sudden SNHL is regarded as an otologic emergency, and patients are evaluated audiometrically and by an otolaryngologist on an urgent basis. Known etiologies are excluded by a thorough history; physical examination; and appropriate laboratory, special audiologic, and radiologic studies. Gadolinium-enhanced MRI of the internal auditory canal and cerebellopontine angle is obtained in all patients. A 10-day course of prednisone, approximately 1 mg/kg/day, is prescribed, followed by a slow taper. If a partial recovery is noted at the end of the 10 days, the full dose is extended another 10 days, and the cycle is repeated until no further improvement is noted. Valaciclovir, 1000 mg three times daily for 10 days, also is considered because it may be beneficial, and because the risks and side effects are minimal. A 2-g sodium diet is recommended with a hydrochlorothiazide-triamterene diuretic combination. Despite the possible efficacy of carbogen treatment, it is not routinely offered to patients with sudden SNHL. The treatment requires inpatient hospitalization, which renders it expensive and inconvenient. Insurers typically regard carbogen as investigational, which results in significant expense to patients. Because of these issues and its controversial nature, most patients do not accept carbogen if it is offered. It would be more strongly considered in exceptional situations, such as a patient with sudden SNHL in an only-hearing ear or in a particularly motivated patient.

SUGGESTED READINGS

Arts HA, Kileny PR, Telian SA. Diagnostic testing for endolymphatic hydrops. *Otolaryngol Clin North Am.* 1997;30:987.

Bakthavachalam S, Driver MS, Cox C, et al. Hearing loss in Wegener's granulomatosis. *Otol Neurotol.* 2004;25:833.

Bretlau P, Thomsen J, Tos M, et al. Placebo effect in surgery for Meniere's disease: nine-year follow-up. *Am J Otol.* 1989;10:259.

For complete list of references log onto www.expertconsult.com.

Byl FM Jr. Sudden hearing loss: eight years' experience and suggested prognostic table. *Laryngoscope.* 1984;94:647.

Dobie RA. *Medical-Legal Evaluation of Hearing Loss.* 2nd ed. San Diego: Singular; 2001.

Friedland DR, Wackym PA. A critical appraisal of spontaneous perilymphatic fistulas of the inner ear. *Am J Otol.* 1999;20:261.

Grau C, Overgaard J. Postirradiation sensorineural hearing loss: a common but ignored late radiation complication. *Int J Radiat Oncol Biol Phys.* 1996;36:515.

Jackler RK, Luxford WM, House WF. Congenital malformations of the inner ear: a classification based on embryogenesis. *Laryngoscope.* 1987;97:2.

Matz G, Rybak L, Roland PS, et al. Ototoxicity of ototopical antibiotic drops in humans. *Otolaryngol Head Neck Surg.* 2004;130:S79.

Moscicki RA, San Martin JE, Quintero CH, et al. Serum antibody to inner ear proteins in patients with progressive hearing loss: correlation with disease activity and response to corticosteroid treatment. *JAMA.* 1994;272:611.

Musiek FE, Gollegly KM, Kibbe KS, et al. Electrophysiologic and behavioral auditory findings in multiple sclerosis. *Am J Otol.* 1989;10:343.

Paek SH, Chung H-T, Jeong SS, et al. Hearing preservation after gamma knife stereotactic radiosurgery of vestibular schwannoma. *Cancer.* 2005;104:580.

Pan CC, Eisbruch A, Lee JS, et al. Prospective study of inner ear radiation dose and hearing loss in head-and-neck cancer patients. *Int J Radiat Oncol Biol Phys.* 2005;61:1393.

Rybak LP, Ramkumar V. Ototoxicity. *Kidney Int.* 2007;72:931.

Saunders JE, Luxford WM, Devgan KK, et al. Sudden hearing loss in acoustic neuroma patients. *Otolaryngol Head Neck Surg.* 1995;113:23.

Schacht J. Biochemical basis of aminoglycoside ototoxicity. *Otolaryngol Clin North Am.* 1993;26:845.

Schuknecht HF. *Pathology of the Ear.* 2nd ed. Philadelphia: Lea & Febiger; 1993.

Schweitzer VG. Ototoxicity of chemotherapeutic agents. *Otolaryngol Clin North Am.* 1993;26:759.

Sismanis A. Otologic manifestations of benign intracranial hypertension syndrome: diagnosis and management. *Laryngoscope.* 1987;97:1.

Sismanis A, Smoker WR. Pulsatile tinnitus: recent advances in diagnosis. *Laryngoscope.* 1994;104:681.

Toriello HV, Reardon W, Gorlin RJ. *Hereditary Hearing Loss and Its Syndromes.* 2nd ed. Oxford: Oxford University Press; 2004.

Torok N. Old and new in Meniere disease. *Laryngoscope.* 1977;87:1870.

Tucci DL, Farmer JC Jr, Kitch RD, et al. Treatment of sudden sensorineural hearing loss with systemic steroids and valacyclovir. *Otol Neurotol.* 2002;23:301.

Wilkins SA Jr, Mattox DE, Lyles A. Evaluation of a "shotgun" regimen for sudden hearing loss. *Otolaryngol Head Neck Surg.* 1987;97:474.

Wilson WR, Byl FM, Laird N. The efficacy of steroids in the treatment of idiopathic sudden hearing loss: a double-blind clinical study. *Arch Otolaryngol.* 1980;106:772.

CHAPTER ONE HUNDRED AND FIFTY

Tinnitus and Hyperacusis

Carol A. Bauer

Key Points

- Tinnitus is common, affecting 30% of people older than age 55, with an annual incidence of 5%.
- Disturbing tinnitus that impairs daily life activity affects 3% to 5% of individuals with tinnitus.
- Auditory deprivation from hearing loss induces central neural changes that result in tinnitus. Mechanisms responsible for tinnitus involve peripheral triggers and central plasticity.
- Sound therapy is an effective form of tinnitus treatment, and benefits most patients when combined with education and adjunct treatments directed toward factors that exacerbate tinnitus.
- Tinnitus that can be modulated with somatic manipulation may respond to therapy targeting temporomandibular joint and cervical spine disorders.
- Medications are helpful for specific forms of tinnitus.
- Functional imaging studies suggest that temporoparietal cortex and cortical association areas may be important targets for electric and magnetic modulation of tinnitus.
- Clinicians knowledgeable in auditory function and head and neck physiology are well equipped to provide most tinnitus patients with effective treatment, including education, rehabilitation of hearing loss, and identification and treatment of exacerbating factors.

Tinnitus

Tinnitus is the perception of sound without an external source. Although 30 million Americans are estimated to have chronic tinnitus, for most it is not a problem sufficient for them to seek treatment. Tinnitus is a chronic sensation virtually all would prefer not to experience, but for most it is not disabling. Disturbing tinnitus occurs in 3% to 5% of individuals with tinnitus.[1] Until more recently, treatments available for disturbing tinnitus were limited. Significant advances in auditory neuroscience have advanced the treatment of tinnitus beyond the traditional recommendation instructing the patient to "learn to live with it." This chapter reviews current theories and mechanisms of idiopathic subjective tinnitus. It also outlines a clinical strategy for evaluating tinnitus and determining tinnitus subtypes, and reviews current management strategies for tinnitus.

Tinnitus can be classified as objective or subjective. Objective tinnitus can be detected by an observer using a stethoscope or ear canal microphone. Objective tinnitus arises from vascular or muscular sources. Objective tinnitus usually has a pulsatile quality. Table 150-1 lists the causes of pulsatile tinnitus. Many of these causes are uncommon and are not responsible for most instances of tinnitus. Because there are excellent reviews of treatments for objective tinnitus, this uncommon form is not addressed further.[2]

In contrast to objective tinnitus, subjective tinnitus is not audible to an observer. This form is more common, with a 5-year incidence of 5.7%.[3] Estimates of subjective tinnitus prevalence range from 8% to 30%, depending on the definition of tinnitus, tinnitus severity, the population sampled, and assessment methodology.[3-5] In a large population-based study of participants 55 to 99 years old, combining detailed tinnitus questionnaires with audiologic assessment, 30% reported experiencing tinnitus, with prevalence related to audiometric threshold, but not age or gender.[5] Mildly annoying tinnitus was reported in 50% of respondents, and extremely annoying tinnitus was reported in 16%. Tinnitus prevalence in individuals with normal hearing was 26.6% compared with 35.1% in individuals with hearing loss. An estimated 20% of individuals with profound hearing loss do not experience tinnitus.[6] These data illustrate that chronic tinnitus is associated with, and may be triggered by, hearing loss, but they also indicate that hearing loss is not an invariable cause of tinnitus. The pathology necessary to initiate tinnitus may be quite subtle. The survey data also confirm that as a clinical problem tinnitus is more than the presentation of its sensory features.

Idiopathic Subjective Tinnitus

Idiopathic subjective tinnitus is the most common form affecting adults, and is the focus of this chapter. By definition, this form of tinnitus excludes known objective causes, such as conductive hearing loss, endolymphatic hydrops, and cerebellopontine angle neoplasms. Historically, the pathology underlying idiopathic tinnitus was unknown, and the symptom was generally viewed as refractory to intervention. Advances in tinnitus research have revealed mechanisms likely responsible for some forms of idiopathic tinnitus. Two examples are tinnitus-associated pathology of the cochlea or head and neck, and tinnitus susceptible to somatic modulation. Both mechanisms are discussed subsequently.

Subjective tinnitus can be subtyped based on etiology, the pattern of associated hearing loss, psychoacoustic features (simple versus complex), exacerbating factors, psychological comorbidities, and the presence of somatic modulators. Tinnitus subtype classification schemes can be useful in identifying forms of tinnitus that are responsive to specific targeted treatment programs. Table 150-2 lists some useful features for subtyping tinnitus.

Hearing Loss Subtypes

The two most common types of hearing loss associated with tinnitus are noise-induced hearing loss (NIHL) and presbycusis. NIHL is a

Table 150-1

Objective Tinnitus

Objective Tinnitus
Pulsatile
Synchronous with pulse
Arterial etiologies
Arteriovenous fistula or malformation
Paraganglioma (glomus tympanicum or jugulare)
Carotid artery stenosis
Other atherosclerotic disease (subclavian, external carotid)
Arterial dissection (carotid, vertebral)
Persistent stapedial artery
Intratympanic carotid artery
Vascular compression of cranial nerve VIII
Increased cardiac output (pregnancy, thyrotoxicosis)
Intraosseous (Paget's disease, otosclerosis)
Venous etiologies
Pseudotumor cerebri
Venous hum
Jugular bulb anomalies
Asynchronous with pulse
Palatal myoclonus
Tensor tympani or stapedius muscle myoclonus
Nonpulsatile
Spontaneous otoacoustic emission
Patulous eustachian tube

Table 150-2

Subjective Tinnitus Subtypes

Subjective Tinnitus Subtypes
Pattern of hearing loss
Noise-induced hearing loss
Presbycusis
Unilateral
High-frequency hearing loss
Outer hair cell dysfunction
Somatic tinnitus
Temporomandibular joint dysfunction
Cervical dysfunction
Gaze-evoked
Cutaneous-evoked
General somatosensory modulated
Typewriter tinnitus
Exacerbated by sleep or rest
Musical/complex
Associated affective disorder
Intrusive (versus habituated)

significant and growing health problem. Although reduction of exposure to occupational noise has been effective in the last several decades, there has been a notable increase in the incidence of NIHL from recreational and leisure activity in children and adolescents, and military combat–related noise exposure in young adults.[7-9] A Web-based survey of 9693 adolescents determined that 61% of respondents experienced hearing loss and temporary tinnitus after attending concerts.[10] Acute transient tinnitus is nearly universal immediately after unprotected exposure to loud acoustic stimuli such as gunfire and amplified music. Tinnitus prevalence among Army personnel evaluated for hearing complaints after deployment was 30% compared with 1.5% in personnel not deployed.[8]

The prevalence of chronic tinnitus associated with NIHL is 50% to 70%.[11] Subjectively, the sensory aspects of acute and chronic tinnitus can be very similar. Chronic tinnitus occurs in a delayed time course for a significant portion of individuals with a history of exposure to damaging sounds. It is unknown if the pathology of transient acoustic trauma–induced tinnitus is the same as the pathology responsible for chronic tinnitus associated with permanent noise-induced threshold shifts. Chronic tinnitus induced by acoustic trauma occurs at a younger age than tinnitus associated with other types of hearing loss. Consequently, acoustic trauma–induced tinnitus is experienced for a longer portion of the life span than other forms of tinnitus.

NIHL and associated tinnitus are preventable. In addition to obvious proactive methods, such as wearing ear protective hardware, intervention in the periexposure period may prove useful in preventing the onset or progression of NIHL, and possibly the incidence of tinnitus. Intense sound exposure triggers a reduction of blood flow and a cascade of metabolic events in the cochlea, with formation of reactive oxygen and nitrogen species that damage cellular lipids, proteins, and DNA, culminating in increased cell death.[12] Interventions targeting these molecular mechanisms of NIHL include antioxidant therapy such as vitamin E, salicylate, and *N*-acetylcysteine.[13] *Ginkgo biloba* extract contains multiple compounds with vasotropic, potential neuroprotective, and antioxidant effects. Although uncontrolled trials and anecdotal reports have suggested the efficacy of ginkgo, a more recent review failed to show efficacy in treating tinnitus.[14]

Serum magnesium levels have been correlated with NIHL in animals.[15] Controlled studies in humans have shown the prophylactic efficacy of oral magnesium in preventing temporary and permanent NIHL.[16,17] It is unknown, however, if these interventions are also effective in decreasing the risk of immediate or delayed onset of tinnitus after traumatic injury.

Presbycusis is sensorineural hearing loss related to aging. Most cases of presbycusis cannot be strictly and solely attributed to aging, but rather involve some combination of cochlear injury from additional sources, such as cumulative noise injury, metabolic or vascular dysfunction, and genetic predisposition. Elderly patients with diabetes have significantly higher pure-tone thresholds, lower otoacoustic emission amplitude, and lower speech recognition in noise[18] than age-matched individuals without diabetes.[19] Interactions between age and other factors affecting the cochlea and auditory pathway make identification of a single mechanism for presbycusis-associated tinnitus and an effectively targeted intervention a challenge.

Somatic Tinnitus Subtype

Somatic tinnitus is a unique form of tinnitus in which the loudness, laterality, or tonality of the tinnitus can by modulated by somatic stimuli. This form of tinnitus was originally observed in a small group of patients after surgical removal of large vestibular schwannomas.[20,21] Postoperatively, these patients had the ability to modulate their chronic tinnitus by exaggerated eye movements, leg motion, or gentle cutaneous stimulation of the hands or face.[22,23] The presumed mechanism of action for this unusual form of tinnitus is neural sprouting or aberrant reinnervation after auditory deafferentation. Subsequent to these observations, however, a more general form of somatosensory modulation has been found in patients with idiopathic tinnitus. In these cases, tinnitus is modulated by maneuvers or stimulation of the head and neck region. It has been reported that forceful isometric contraction of the head and neck muscles can modify the loudness and pitch of tinnitus in 65% to 80% of patients with mild, idiopathic tinnitus.[24-26] Tinnitus can be induced by strong contractions of muscles in the jaw, head, or neck in 58% of subjects without a history of tinnitus.[25]

The association between tinnitus and somatic pathology of the head and neck is underscored by the reported higher incidence of tinnitus in individuals with temporomandibular joint dysfunction and normal audiometric thresholds compared with controls.[27] One third of patients with symptoms of temporomandibular joint dysfunction reported modulation of tinnitus with jaw movement or pressure applied to the temporomandibular joint.[28] When tinnitus occurs in association with disorders of the head and neck, such as temporomandibular joint dysfunction, unilateral facial pain, otalgia, and occipital or temporal headache, successful tinnitus alleviation may be possible using interventions targeting the somatic dysfunction.

Animal research has established that multimodal and in particular somatic inputs to the auditory pathway are evident from auditory brainstem to cortex.[29-33] These inputs allow integration of information from vision, head position, and internal sound (e.g., vocalization) to be used in important functions, such as sound localization and auditory selective attention. It has been hypothesized that aberrations in these multimodal connections can either trigger tinnitus or modulate existing tinnitus. Reduction of normal afferent input to the auditory brainstem (e.g., cochlear nuclei) may trigger inappropriate compensatory up-regulation of somatosensory inputs to these regions. Stimulus-driven or spontaneous activity within the nonauditory somatic pathways may be perceived as an audible "sound."[33]

Recognition of somatic tinnitus is important because it may be amenable to targeted intervention. Levine and colleagues[34] systematically reviewed the efficacy of treatments targeting somatosensory systems. They defined somatic tinnitus syndrome as tinnitus that is (1) perceived in the ear and (2) ipsilateral to the somatic trigger and (3) not associated with any new hearing complaints. Tinnitus that is strongly lateralized to one ear in the presence of symmetric hearing (including symmetric hearing loss) would theoretically have a somatic etiologic component by the definition of Levine and colleagues.[34] The review by these authors presents evidence that somatic tinnitus is often responsive to acupuncture, electric stimulation of the scalp and auricle, trigger point treatment, and treatment of temporomandibular joint dysfunction.[34]

Typewriter Tinnitus Subtype

Typewriter tinnitus is defined, as its name implies, by a characteristic sensation. The tinnitus has a staccato quality, similar to a typewriter tapping, popcorn popping, or Morse code signal. Its presence is intermittent and chronic. It may be confused with tinnitus arising from a muscular source, such as spasm of the tensor tympani or stapedius muscle, or palatal myoclonus. That typewriter tinnitus is a condition distinct from these somatic sources is supported by a case history of a patient with typewriter tinnitus that failed to respond to multiple treatments, including tensor tympani and stapedius resection. The patient was successfully treated, however, with carbamazepine (Tegretol). This case illustrates the importance of accurate recognition and diagnosis of typewriter tinnitus.[35] A small case series reporting successful treatment with carbamazepine suggested that typewriter tinnitus may be caused by vascular compression of the auditory nerve ipsilateral to the tinnitus.[36]

Tinnitus Treatment Strategies

Auditory Deprivation and Neural Plasticity

Acoustic-based tinnitus treatments encompass a range of delivery systems and types of sound. The rationale for using external sound to treat tinnitus derives from the hypothesis that hearing loss leads to deafferentation-induced reorganization of the auditory pathway. Hearing loss decreases the afferent stream of neural activity from the cochlea to the auditory cortex. Chronic deafferentation alters activity in the auditory brainstem and midbrain, and may change the tonotopic organization of the auditory cortex. Brainstem spontaneous activity may increase, and midbrain patterns may change (e.g., with aberrant synchronization or bursting) because of compensatory down-regulation of inhibition. Altered activity in the auditory pathway may be responsible for the tinnitus percept. Stimulus interventions that restore afferent input to more normal levels may act through improved inhibition. They may also restore cortical tonotopic organization to normative levels and reduce tinnitus.

A related phenomenon that illustrates the concept and treatment of deafferentation-induced cortical plasticity is phantom limb pain.[37] The phantom limb syndrome is the continued sensation of the presence of an absent limb, in a distorted or painful manner, after amputation. Amputation of a limb is an extreme form of deafferentation. The parallels between tinnitus and phantom limb pain, in terms of onset rate, persistence, and affected ages, are striking. Greater than 90% of amputees experience a vivid limb phantom immediately after amputation.[37] Phantoms are more likely to occur in adults than in children.[38] In many cases, the phantom sensation fades after days or weeks, but it persists chronically for decades in 30% of patients.[37]

It is well known that the adult and the immature brain can undergo plastic change. Neural plasticity is the ability of a neuron or neural network to change its function, organization, and connectivity through long-term alterations in synaptic efficiency.[39] Neurons can significantly alter their response to inputs, and receptive field sizes change, as a consequence of either decreased or increased input and training procedures.[40] The changes can be extensive. Magnetoencephalographic studies have shown that stimulation of intact body areas distant from the amputation site is perceived, with corresponding central neural activity, at the cortical site of the amputated limb.[41] Similar changes of auditory cortical representation may underlie tinnitus.[42] Primary auditory cortex steady-state evoked magnetic fields were enhanced in tinnitus patients compared with controls, and the degree of enhancement correlated with the perceived intensity and intrusiveness of the tinnitus.[43] Functional imaging studies in humans have suggested that expanded representation of frequency regions in the auditory cortex may underpin tinnitus.[44-47]

Animal models have been important in studying the deafferentation-loss-of-inhibition hypothesis of tinnitus, and have been used to evaluate sound therapy for reversal of pathologic neural plasticity. A key study by Norena and Eggermont[48] illustrates the effect of noise trauma and therapeutic sound stimulation on receptive fields of primary and secondary auditory cortex. Cats exposed to a traumatizing noise were evaluated for changes in the location and responsiveness of auditory cortex neurons to acoustic stimuli. The frequency tuning of cortical neurons was altered after the trauma, distorting the overall representation of sound and over-representing frequencies surrounding the exposure sound. A second cohort of cats, exposed to the same traumatizing sound, was subsequently reared in an enriched acoustic environment for several weeks before mapping the auditory cortex. The enriched environment was spectrally composed to compensate for the anticipated frequency distortions induced by hearing loss.

Two important outcomes were obtained in the cats raised in the enriched environment: (1) Their hearing loss was significantly reduced compared with the cats with similar sound exposure raised in a quiet environment, and (2) there was no evidence of plastic reorganization of the auditory cortex. The tonotopic organization of the exposed and treated cats was similar to that of unexposed control cats. These results suggest that tinnitus may be partly the result of abnormal reorganization of the auditory cortex. These results show that therapeutic acoustic intervention may be effective in reducing or eliminating the abnormal cortical organization associated with, and potentially responsible for, tinnitus. The implications for tinnitus treatment using sound therapy are obvious.

Using Sound to Decrease Loudness and Annoyance of Tinnitus

Acoustic stimulation is an important component of successful management of tinnitus in many patients. A wide range of acoustic delivery strategies are currently available. Most patients with tinnitus, including patients with minimal threshold shift on standard audiometric testing, can benefit from acoustic stimulation. Patients with severe to profound hearing loss that is not amenable to conventional amplification can achieve tinnitus relief from other modes of auditory pathway stimulation, such as cochlear implantation or cortical stimulation (discussed later).

Ambient Stimulation

The simplest method of increasing afferent input to reverse putative central reorganization and tinnitus is environmental sound enrichment. Use of supplemental environmental sound to treat tinnitus has been recommended for more than 50 years.[49] Enrichment can be achieved using background music, relaxation tapes or CDs, tabletop nature sound machines, or waterfalls or fountains. Patients are typically instructed to use a source of constant background sound to decrease attention to their tinnitus. Sound enrichment is not intended to mask the tinnitus in the conventional sense of completely eliminating the tinnitus percept (discussed subsequently). Rather, by elevating the level of ambient sound using a constant, spectrally rich stimulus, the tinnitus sensation becomes less noticeable.

Hearing loss is present in more than 90% of patients with tinnitus. Conversely, epidemiologic studies have reported tinnitus prevalence of 50% in hearing-impaired patients.[50] Effective use of sound stimulation for managing tinnitus in hearing-impaired patients can be achieved only with appropriate amplification. Typically, amplification is achieved with hearing aids. Even without supplemental sound, the therapeutic effect of hearing aids for tinnitus patients is well documented.[51,52] Hearing aids reduce the awareness of tinnitus through amplification of ambient sound and reduce the perception that tinnitus masks hearing and impedes communication.

Surr and coworkers[53] reviewed the initial effect of hearing aid use on tinnitus in 124 patients. Approximately one half of patients reported that the hearing aid reduced (26%) or eliminated (29%) the tinnitus. Folmer and Carroll[54] reviewed their clinical experience with 50 patients with mild to moderate sensorineural hearing loss fitted with hearing aids for tinnitus management. Patients were re-evaluated 6 to 48 months after initial fitting (mean 18 months), and 70% reported significant improvement in their tinnitus. Similar results were obtained in a larger study of 1440 patients fitted with hearing aids for unilateral or bilateral hearing loss.[55] In this study, digital hearing aids provided significantly greater tinnitus relief than analog hearing aids. Of patients fitted with digital hearing aids for unilateral hearing loss, 65% reported greater than 50% improvement in tinnitus compared with 39% reporting a similar degree of improvement after fitting with an analog aid. An even greater therapeutic effect was obtained with bilateral digital hearing aids: 85% of patients reported greater than 50% improvement in tinnitus compared with 30% fitted with bilateral analog aids.

Programmable digital hearing aids can selectively amplify within the high-frequency range, a region where most tinnitus patients typically have some measurable threshold loss. Current-generation digital aids have significant output gain up to 10 kHz, which significantly benefits tinnitus patients with hearing loss in the high-frequency range. An open-fit, nonoccluding ear mold is crucial to minimize the occlusion effect, which can amplify the tinnitus percept.[56]

Personal Listening Devices

Tinnitus management can be implemented through the use of personal listening devices, such as flash-memory music players. Miniaturization, data storage, and digital software have greatly expanded the available tools that clinicians and patients can use to produce a customized sound library. Inexpensive online sources are also available for downloading digital sound specifically developed for tinnitus therapy (e.g., http://www.vectormediasoftware.com). Patients can build and use a small library of sounds, which may include music to their liking, nature sounds, and noise bands of different spectral composition. Important key features of any regimen of amplified sound therapy are (1) use of open-fit, nonoccluding ear level drivers, (2) long-term exposure to the sounds, (3) sound spectral composition that is reasonably broad, and (4) sound levels below that of the perceived tinnitus.

Appropriate patient education is crucial to successful treatment. Many treatment failures occur because patients erroneously expect complete elimination of tinnitus after a few days to weeks of treatment. Patients must be counseled about the typical slow time course of improvement, and must be encouraged to have realistic expectations about the benefits of sound therapy. Sound therapy can decrease the subjective loudness and significantly decrease the annoyance of tinnitus, but this may require weeks to months of daily application.[57,58]

Total Masking Therapy

Total masking therapy is the use of sound with spectral characteristics and sufficient volume to render the tinnitus inaudible. This form of sound therapy has likely been used for centuries, and derives from empirical experience that certain environmental sounds are efficient tinnitus maskers. The clinical use of total masking therapy has a long history.[59] A formal masking therapy program was first proposed by Vernon and Schleuning.[60] Patients are fitted with ear-level devices that generate sound. The devices can be adjusted to have outputs with different frequency spectra and levels. There is no codified scheme for selecting effective masker characteristics. The general fitting principle is to determine the minimum level of broadband noise that masks the tinnitus without interfering with communication. The fitting is empirical because there is a wide range of patient preference in the type and level of sound that masks the tinnitus and is not perceived as annoying.[61,62] Two significant benefits likely attend the successful application of total masking therapy: (1) Patients have control over their tinnitus, and (2) patients experience immediate relief with complete elimination of tinnitus.[63]

Benefits from masking therapy have been shown in a large prospective controlled study of chronic significant tinnitus in U.S. veterans.[64] Validated standardized tinnitus severity questionnaires were used to screen and enroll 123 subjects with clinically significant tinnitus. Subjects were quasirandomly assigned to either the total masking group or a tinnitus retraining therapy (TRT) group. Subjects in the total masking group received hearing aids, maskers, or combination instruments, and all received information counseling over an 18-month follow-up period. Subjects in the TRT group received standardized TRT treatment (see later). All subjects were evaluated for response to treatment at 6, 12, and 18 months. Subjects in both treatment groups showed improvement on multiple measures of tinnitus over the course of the study. Subjects in the total masking group who rated their tinnitus as a "moderate" problem had effect sizes between 0.27 and 0.48 compared with effect sizes for the TRT group of 0.77 and 1.26 at 18 months. Mean effect sizes in subjects with tinnitus rated as a "very big problem" were 0.64 in the total masking group and 1.08 in the TRT group. Although both therapies resulted in clinically significant improvement in tinnitus with medium (>0.5) to large (>0.8) effect sizes, optimal outcomes were obtained with long-term TRT treatment.

Acoustic Stimulation Combined with Education and Counseling

TRT combines sound therapy with a formalized program of directive counseling to achieve habituation to tinnitus.[65] TRT is based on the assumption that tinnitus distress derives from activation of an emotional and an autonomic response to tinnitus.[66] Within this theoretical framework, tinnitus emerges as a result of damage or dysfunction within the auditory pathway, and is detected at subcortical levels of the brain. The critical event that leads to clinically significant tinnitus is not its sensory features, but rather the perception and evaluation of the tinnitus-related neural activity that occurs in the auditory cortex, and subsequent cortical interaction with the limbic system, prefrontal cortex, and cortical association areas.[65] According to Jastreboff and Hazell,[65] tinnitus becomes clinically significant when a negative affective response to the tinnitus has been established.

The goals of TRT are to remove, decrease, or change the perception of tinnitus by promoting habituation of the reactions to the tinnitus sensation. Habituation of the reaction to tinnitus would reduce the derived annoyance, anxiety, and stress. A key feature of TRT involves behavioral retraining of the associations induced by the tinnitus sensation. TRT uses five distinct levels of therapy, aimed at stratified patient groups. Stratification is based on tinnitus distress, associated hearing impairment, presence of sound-induced exacerbation of tinnitus, and comorbid hyperacusis (see later). The five strata are (1) patients with tinnitus that causes minimal distress (category 0); (2) patients with tinnitus causing distress (category 1); (3) patients with distressing tinnitus and hearing loss (category 2); (4) patients with distressing tinnitus, normal hearing, and hyperacusis (category 3); and (5) patients with distressing tinnitus, normal hearing, hyperacusis, and prolonged sound-induced exacerbation of tinnitus (category 4). Treatment is specific for each patient category, and uses directive counseling, auditory enrichment, hearing aids, and sound generators.

Jastreboff and Hazell[65] described directive counseling as a teaching session in which patients are instructed on the mechanisms of tinnitus generation. Directive counseling demystifies tinnitus for the patient, and attempts to eliminate anxiety and fear of tinnitus through education. Auditory enrichment is typically achieved through the use of broadband noise generators. Ear-level devices physically similar in design to maskers are used, but sound output is distinctly lower than that used in masking therapy where sound levels render the tinnitus inaudible. In TRT, the volume of noise is set at a partial masking level, which allows continued perception of the tinnitus. The concept is that habituation would normally occur to the noise, much as one habituates to the background sound of a running air conditioner. Because the external noise and the internal tinnitus are equivalent in loudness, or "mixed," habituation generalizes to the tinnitus and its attendant emotional reactions.

Retrospective clinical trials evaluating the efficacy of TRT have generally been positive with a consensus that TRT reduces the annoyance and impact of tinnitus within a time frame of 12 to 18 months. Sheldrake and associates[67] reported a retrospective review of clinical outcomes on 224 patients completing a course of TRT. Outcome measures were percentage of time of tinnitus awareness, tinnitus distress, and the number of life factors affected by tinnitus. A successful outcome was defined as either a 40% improvement in tinnitus annoyance and awareness or 40% improvement in annoyance or awareness plus an improvement or facilitation of one life factor. At 6 months, 70% of patients had a successful outcome, and this percentage increased to 84% by 18 months. The mean awareness of and distress related to tinnitus before therapy were 63% and 45%, whereas after 18 months of therapy these percentages were 15% and 5%.

Bartnik and colleagues[68] retrospectively reviewed the 12-month outcomes of 108 clinic patients treated with TRT for chronic tinnitus. Significant improvement was defined as a minimum decrease of 20% in at least three of these parameters (impact on daily life, time aware of tinnitus, degree of annoyance, and tinnitus intensity). Significant improvement was reported for patients treated with counseling alone (79%), counseling combined with noise generators (73%), and counseling combined with hearing aids (88%).

Berry and coworkers[69] reported the 6-month results of a nonrandomized, prospective analysis of 32 patients treated with TRT. Treatment outcomes included psychophysical measures of loudness discomfort levels; minimal masking levels; and a standardized, validated measure of tinnitus severity and disability (Tinnitus Handicap Inventory [THI]; see later). Average THI score (pretreatment total score 52) significantly improved after 6 months of therapy (post-treatment total score 24; $P < .001$). Nine patients with sound sensitivity (hyperacusis) before treatment had a significant ($P < .05$) increase in sound tolerance after therapy, indicated by a 14 dB HL improvement in loudness discomfort level.

TRT is derived from a reasonable set of assumptions about the mechanism of disruptive chronic tinnitus, and may provide an effective therapeutic option for some patients. Evaluation of TRT effectiveness using the gold standard of a randomized controlled trial with multiple outcome measures is yet to be reported, however.

Acoustic Desensitization Protocol

The acoustic desensitization protocol is a proprietary tinnitus treatment program (Neuromonics, Bethlehem, PA) that combines features of sound therapy; systematic desensitization; directive counseling; and supportive intervention for stress management, sleep disruption, and coping strategies. Systematic desensitization is a psychological technique originally developed for the treatment of phobias. Progressive gradual controlled exposure to the phobic stimulus within the context of a deeply relaxed state of mind results in a gradual desensitization of the phobic response to the stimulus.[70] This technique has been adapted to the treatment of tinnitus, by targeting the individual's tinnitus as the stimulus that provokes the phobic, or at least negative emotional, response.

Patients listen to their tinnitus in gradual, progressive increments within a background context of pleasant, relaxing therapeutic sound. The therapeutic sound has three key features that are fundamental to the protocol. The sound used is music spectrally modified in accord with the patient's hearing loss, with enhancement of loudness levels of frequencies where hearing loss is pronounced, re-establishing stimulation of the auditory pathway over a wide frequency range. Music that is nonintrusive and has a slow rhythm is used to maximize relaxation during treatment. The music has a dynamic component that permits intermittent tinnitus perception alternating with tinnitus masking. The gradual exposure to one's tinnitus in the context of therapeutic music is achieved using a staged treatment program. In the initial stage, the spectrally modified music is embedded within a background sound of high-frequency noise that masks the tinnitus. In the second stage, the masking noise is removed, and the tinnitus percept becomes gradually and progressively more audible.

A Neuromonics-sponsored outcome study of the acoustic desensitization protocol has shown positive effects.[71] In the study, 35 patients with moderate to severe tinnitus received Neuromonics tinnitus treatment and were tested for subjective (distress, awareness) and objective (minimum masking levels, loudness discomfort levels) changes at four time points, including 1 year, after therapy. Within the first 6 months of treatment, 91% of participants reported an improvement in tinnitus distress, reflecting a mean improvement of 65% in the Tinnitus Reaction Questionnaire. The reported "percent of time aware of tinnitus" before therapy was 90%, which was significantly reduced to 30% after 12 months of therapy.

Cognitive-Behavioral Therapy for Tinnitus

Cognitive-behavioral therapy (CBT) is a well-established psychotherapy based on identification of maladaptive behaviors and their modification using therapist-mediated cognitive restructuring. The technique has been successfully applied to tinnitus for many years, and forms the basis of another type of habituation therapy for tinnitus.[66] CBT for tinnitus is based on the concept that the normal response to meaningless stimuli is habituation, and tinnitus distress results from a failure to habituate. Jakes and associates[72] summarized the causes of habituation failure to include emotional responses, orientation to stimuli, arousal, and unfavorable signal-to-noise ratio. When a normal subject is presented repeatedly with a meaningless stimulus, responses to the stimulus, such as orientation, attention, and cognitive processing, soon habituate (i.e., the responses drop out). When the same subject is presented repeatedly with a noxious stimulus (e.g., the cry of a baby), sensitization occurs (i.e., the response to the stimulus becomes more pronounced and may have an emotional component). CBT uses techniques of reassurance, relaxation training, and selective attention distraction to induce habituation to tinnitus. It may be, as suggested by some, that defusing the emotional component of tinnitus, with or without concomitant changes in tinnitus loudness, is sufficient for improving patient outlook and perception.[72]

A review of CBT as a tinnitus treatment by the Cochrane Collaboration evaluated six trials comprising 285 participants.[73] The primary outcome measure was subjective tinnitus loudness, and the secondary outcome measures were improvement in symptoms of mood disturbance and quality-of-life evaluation. The pooled results for the five trials reporting subjective loudness before and after treatment showed no significant difference between treatment with CBT and either a waiting list control or an alternative treatment. There was also no significant treatment effect for the secondary outcome measures of depression and mood disturbance. There was a significant improvement, however, in the quality of life of CBT participants, as measured by a global decrease in tinnitus severity, with a standardized mean difference of 0.70 (95% CI 0.33 to 1.08). The reviewers conclude that CBT has a significant impact on the qualitative aspects of tinnitus and contributes positively to the management of tinnitus.

Nevertheless, controversy continues regarding the relative benefits of CBT and sound stimulation in promoting psychological and physiologic habituation in patients who have chronic tinnitus. Hiller and Haerkotter[74] followed 124 outpatients with chronic tinnitus, randomly assigned to either CBT alone or CBT combined with sound stimulation using noise generators. Tinnitus-related distress and psychosocial functioning were significantly improved in both groups, with no additive benefit observed in the sound-stimulation group.

Transcranial Magnetic Stimulation

The more recently developed diagnostic and treatment technique of transcranial magnetic stimulation (TMS) has opened a novel avenue for investigating the causal and associational aspects of tinnitus-related cortical activity, and may provide an effective tinnitus therapy for some patients. TMS uses a brief intense current in a surface coil applied to the scalp to induce a magnetic field in the underlying brain. The magnetic pulse induces a temporary focal disruption of neural activity in a discrete area of cortex. This "virtual lesion" briefly, and reversibly, disrupts cortical activity and allows the investigator to determine if the cortical region of interest contributes to a specific behavior or perception.[75] The effect of a single pulse-induced magnetic field is short-lived, on the order of milliseconds. Repetitive TMS over seconds to minutes causes neuronal depolarization within the superficial cortex. Low-frequency (<1 Hz) repetitive TMS decreases cortical excitability,[76] whereas high-frequency (5 to 20 Hz) repetitive TMS increases cortical excitability.[77] All repetitive TMS frequency parameters can induce long-term plastic changes in cortical function that reportedly outlast the stimulation period by hours to days.[78]

TMS can be combined with functional imaging techniques to locate regions of interest for TMS application, and to examine the effect of cortical stimulation on distant structures. The combined techniques of TMS and functional brain imaging may be useful for investigating cortical mechanisms of tinnitus, and may be of clinical value as a treatment for some forms of tinnitus. Enhanced cerebral blood flow in temporoparietal cortex was shown using positron emission tomography (PET) imaging in patients who could modulate their tinnitus with orofacial movement[46] or eye position.[45] The association between tinnitus loudness and temporoparietal cortical blood flow was also observed in studies using lidocaine as a tinnitus modulator.[47,79,80] To date, there have been no studies correlating changes in regional cerebral blood flow and altered tinnitus sensation modulated by repetitive TMS, although combining these methods might be revealing.

The functional relevance of temporoparietal cortex activity to tinnitus was first suggested by studies examining the effect of repetitive TMS on auditory hallucinations. Three patients with schizophrenia and persistent auditory hallucinations were studied in a double-blind crossover design using low-frequency (1 Hz) repetitive TMS to the left temporoparietal cortex versus sham stimulation. All three subjects reported significant improvement in severity of hallucinations after active treatment compared with sham stimulation. Two subjects had near-complete cessation of hallucinations for 2 weeks after treatment.[81] Meta-analysis of the effect of repetitive TMS on auditory hallucinations in schizophrenic patients has supported these early results, and shows a significant positive effect.[82]

Plewnia and coworkers[83] showed short-term suppression of idiopathic subjective tinnitus after high-frequency (10 Hz) TMS stimulation of temporoparietal cortex. Fourteen adults with chronic tinnitus were stimulated at 12 cortical locations with 10 Hz repetitive TMS for 3 seconds, repeated five times, and at two control locations for sham stimulation. Eight of the 14 subjects reproducibly reported on more than one trial an immediate decrease in tinnitus loudness after repetitive TMS, ranging from slight decrease to complete suppression. Five subjects did not perceive a reproducible attenuation of tinnitus, and one subject reported transient increase in tinnitus loudness that persisted for 2 weeks. Post-hoc analysis showed that the strongest tinnitus attenuation was obtained with stimulation of left temporal and left temporoparietal cortex.

Long-term inhibition of cortical hyperactivity can be induced using low-frequency repetitive TMS.[76,84] In a double-blind, crossover, placebo-controlled (sham stimulation) trial of low-frequency repetitive TMS, PET-guided neuronavigation was used to target hyperactive areas within the superior temporal gyrus of 14 patients with chronic tinnitus (tinnitus durations of 1 to 30 years). The left temporal lobe was targeted in 12 patients, and the right lobe was targeted in 2 patients. After 5 days of treatment (2000 stimuli/day) there was a 7-day nontreatment interval, followed by 5 days of sham treatment. A significant reduction in standardized tinnitus questionnaire score was observed after active treatment ($P < .005$), but not after sham stimulation ($P = .336$).[85] At 6-month follow-up, five patients reported worse tinnitus, with a mean increase in tinnitus questionnaire score of 5, and eight patients had an average 12. 4 decrease in tinnitus questionnaire score. Three of the eight patients had a clinically significant reduction in score of 16 to 34 points. There was no correlation between initial tinnitus severity or tinnitus duration and the response to active treatment.

Plewnia and coworkers[86] subsequently examined the immediate effect of neuronavigated low-frequency repetitive TMS and sham stimulation on tinnitus loudness in another eight subjects in a single-blind crossover trial. Tinnitus loudness was assessed using an 11-point visual analog scale, with −5 indicating suppression of tinnitus, 0 no change, and +5 indicating increased loudness. Areas shown to be correlated with the tinnitus percept on PET imaging were primarily in sensory association cortex, but not primary auditory cortex. These included the left middle and inferior temporal cortex, the right gyrus angularis, and the posterior cingulum. Two of the eight subjects showed a decrease in tinnitus loudness (−3 and −5) after active low-frequency repetitiveTMS, and no change after sham stimulation. Three subjects were nonresponders during active and sham stimulation, and the three remaining subjects reported moderate (−2) to significant (−5) reduction in tinnitus loudness after active stimulation and sham stimulation. The outcomes of these evaluations of TMS were very mixed.

If TMS is effective in reversing neurogenic pathology, its mechanism of action remains unclear. High-frequency repetitive TMS can result in long-lasting clinical improvement in cases of chronic neurogenic pain, suggesting that the therapeutic effect may not be related to a reduction in cortical excitability, but rather be through reversal of chronic maladaptive plastic changes.[87] The long-term effect of different repetitive TMS stimulation rates delivered to the left temporoparietal cortex was assessed in 39 subjects with chronic tinnitus (duration 6 months to 25 years).[88] Subjects were randomly assigned to one of four stimulation groups (1 Hz, 10 Hz, 25 Hz, or sham stimulation) and treated with five sessions over a 2-week period. All subjects in the active repetitive TMS groups reported significant improvement ($P < .05$) in tinnitus severity on the standardized THI questionnaire at 4 months after completing treatment compared with the sham treatment group. Tinnitus improvement occurred regardless of stimulation rate for active repetitive TMS. A greater proportion of subjects experienced an 80% or greater improvement in THI score after treatment with 10 Hz (29%) and 25 Hz (35%), however, than after 1 Hz (6%). As reported in other studies, there was a negative correlation between tinnitus duration and percent improvement 4 months after treatment.

Further work is needed in this area to understand the mechanisms of TMS and its efficacy in treating tinnitus. It is unknown if the tinnitus-associated hyperactivity in secondary auditory cortex normalizes after subjectively successful treatment with repetitive TMS. There currently is no consensus on the relationship of hemispheric dominance and metabolic hyperactivity to tinnitus. Some studies have shown left temporoparietal activity is associated with tinnitus,[45,46] and others have shown right-sided dominance.[47,80] Finally, there are conflicting results on the effect of tinnitus duration on responsiveness to TMS.

Electric Stimulation

Electric stimulation has been used to treat tinnitus since the advent of Volta's battery in the early 19th century.[89] Although anodal direct current has been used by multiple investigators to suppress tinnitus, practical use is limited by tissue damage induced by chronic stimulation with direct current.[90] Nondestructive methods of delivering electric current required the development of improved noninvasive techniques, such as transcutaneous electric stimulation, and surgically implanted devices using alternating current, such as cochlear implants and cortical stimulators.

Transcutaneous Electric Stimulation

Initial systematic attempts to decrease tinnitus using transcutaneous electric stimulation used the Audimax Theraband, a device that delivers inaudible, transdermal electric current to the mastoid eminence. Lyttkens and colleagues[91] showed complete tinnitus suppression in one of five patients treated with transcutaneous stimulation. In a larger double-blind crossover study, 20 patients were treated first using the active device followed by a placebo device in which the internal circuitry was deactivated. Four patients (20%) reported reduction with the placebo, whereas two patients (10%) reported tinnitus reduction with the active device. One of the responders was examined further with random trials of either active or placebo stimulation, and reported a median 70% tinnitus decrease during active stimulation and 16% decrease during placebo stimulation.[92] A subsequent single-blind crossover study of 30 patients showed a similar proportion of patients responded to stimulation.[93] Levine and coworkers[34] reviewed the characteristics of tinnitus patients who respond to transcutaneous electric stimulation and concluded that the common finding present in all cases is tinnitus with features of somatic modulation.

Herraiz and associates[94] prospectively studied the effect of transcutaneous electric nerve stimulation in 26 patients with tinnitus categorized as somatically modulated. Although the trial lacked a placebo control, a striking effect was obtained in this sample from a selected population, with tinnitus elimination in 23% and tinnitus improvement in 23%. Further analysis by tinnitus type showed that the group most responsive to transcutaneous electric nerve stimulation treatment had typewriter tinnitus, with 88% experiencing improved or eliminated tinnitus.

Cochlear Implants

Suppression of tinnitus as a secondary benefit of cochlear implantation was noted in the early days of cochlear implant development.[95] Although there is a large variability in the methods of assessing and reporting tinnitus, most studies report a consistent and clinically significant beneficial effect of cochlear implantation on tinnitus suppression.[96] A significant proportion of patients (38% to 85%) report either a decrease or complete suppression of tinnitus after intracochlear electrode insertion before initial stimulation.[97] Although there have not been extensive studies, there does not seem to be a significant difference in effective tinnitus suppression with different device manufacturers. Cochlear stimulation has been reported to reduce tinnitus intensity perceived in the ear contralateral and ipsilateral to the implant.[97] This is not paradoxical because the brainstem cochlear nuclei have contralateral connections, and bilateral elevation of spontaneous activity in the dorsal cochlear nucleus has been shown in animals with tinnitus induced by unilateral acoustic trauma.[98]

The effectiveness of cochlear stimulation on decreasing tinnitus loudness increases over time. Tinnitus was suppressed in 65% of patients on initial stimulation, but after a 2-month period, stimulation suppressed tinnitus in 93% of patients. These observations suggest that the mechanism responsible for tinnitus suppression by cochlear implants may relate to reversal of maladaptive central plastic changes associated with auditory deprivation.

Multiple factors may contribute to the efficacy of tinnitus suppression after cochlear implantation, including etiology, duration, and extent of hearing loss, and stimulation strategy. Potentially, there is much to be learned about tinnitus mechanisms from patients with cochlear implants. Studies that systematically investigate the impact of these factors are few, however.

Pharmacologic Tinnitus Treatments

Written accounts indicate medical treatment of tinnitus dates back to the Egyptians (2660-2160 B.C.E.).[99] An ear that was bewitched or humming would be infused with oil, frankincense, tree sap, herbs, and soil. Mesopotamian writings considered the psychological aspects of tinnitus, possibly the earliest recognition that stress and emotional factors are significant components of tinnitus dysfunction. These early attempts at treatment contained elements that presage modern views of tinnitus pathology.

Until more recently, most pharmacologic interventions for tinnitus were empirically determined. Anecdotal experience and fortuitous observations of tinnitus relief were the primary sources of innovation. Over the past 50 years, pharmacologic treatment of tinnitus has become more rational. Anesthetics (lidocaine, tocainide, mexiletine), anticonvulsants (carbamazepine, gabapentin), and tranquilizers (diazepam, clonazepam, oxazepam) have been investigated as tinnitus treatments. They have in common the general property of facilitating neural inhibition. Antidepressants such as trimipramine, nortriptyline, amitriptyline, and selective serotonin reuptake inhibitors have been tested for their ability to ameliorate the comorbid mood disturbance associated with tinnitus. Considering only well-controlled trials, mixed results have been obtained for all drugs tested to date.

The hypothesis that tinnitus emerges from increased central neural activity after loss of inhibition can be used to guide pharmacologic intervention. Animal models of tinnitus support the loss of inhibition and enhanced neural activity hypothesis.[98,100,101] The loss-of-inhibition hypothesis provides a rational basis for numerous pharmacologic interventions, including lidocaine, carbamazepine, alprazolam, and gabapentin.

Despite the increase in targeted tinnitus drug trials, using a single agent to treat a heterogeneous large sample of subjects has been for the most part unsuccessful. Several reasons, not mutually exclusive, may account for this lack of success. Most tinnitus clinical trials randomly select and assign participants to treatment groups. There is emerging evidence, however, that tinnitus is a heterogeneous disorder with variable pathologic features.[34,102,103] Testing drugs with a single mechanism of action is unlikely to succeed when using randomly determined heterogeneous sample groups. For the same reason, trials using small dose ranges may fail.

Studies that enroll subjects with a single tinnitus etiology may be more likely to identify successful treatments. A study that examined the effect of gabapentin on tinnitus in two specific patient subpopulations obtained positive results.[104] The study was designed to test the hypothesis that acoustic trauma leads to a loss of inhibition in the auditory pathway mediated by the inhibitory neurotransmitter γ-aminobutyric acid (GABA). The hypothesis was advanced after an animal experiment that showed gabapentin, a GABA analogue, to be effective in reducing the loudness of tinnitus in rats.[100] This study used a very wide dose range, and tested one group of patients with objective and historical evidence of traumatic sound exposure, and a second group without such evidence. Gabapentin was found to reduce tinnitus annoyance significantly in the trauma group at a daily dose level of 1800 to 2400 mg. In contrast, a subsequent clinical trial studying the effect of only a single dose in a randomly selected group of patients did not obtain a significant effect.[105] The therapeutic effect was likely missed because only a single dose level was used, and the treatment group included various tinnitus etiologies. Drugs with a specific mechanism of action are unlikely to be effective in all subjects characterized by such heterogeneity. Stratified study designs with segregation of tinnitus types, etiology, and hearing characteristics should be more successful in identifying effective drug therapies.

The most extensively used drugs for tinnitus treatment are antidepressants. Attempting to treat tinnitus with antidepressants is sensible for two reasons. There is a well-recognized association between severe tinnitus and mood disorders. The pharmacologic mechanism of action of many antidepressants involves receptors and neurotransmitters that are located in the auditory pathway.[106] Although GABA deficiency seems to contribute to tinnitus pathology,[104,107-109] the role of other neurotransmitter systems in triggering or maintaining tinnitus is currently unknown. Serotonin is known to function as a modulator of sensory systems, learning, and memory. Along with acetylcholine, serotonin can affect behavioral conditioning and associated plastic changes in auditory cortex. Both neurotransmitters may be important in the distress associated with tinnitus.

Treatment with sertraline, a selective serotonin reuptake inhibitor, improved tinnitus loudness (P = .014) and severity (P = .024) in a group of tinnitus patients with an associated depressive or anxiety disorder.[110] Despite this positive evidence, it is unclear whether selective serotonin reuptake inhibitor treatment improved tinnitus directly or indirectly through alleviation of mood disorder. A placebo-controlled trial of the selective serotonin reuptake inhibitor paroxetine in a group of subjects without coexisting mood or anxiety disorder did not produce improvement in any tinnitus measure over placebo.[111]

Clinical Evaluation of Tinnitus

Clinical treatment of a patient with tinnitus should begin with a general medical evaluation followed by a complete head and neck examination. Objectives of the evaluation include a descriptive characterization of the tinnitus (psychoacoustic properties, impact on daily life, reactive components); determination of etiology; and identifying factors that exacerbate, ameliorate, or trigger the tinnitus. At a minimum, the results of the examination educate the patient about the tinnitus. Patient education is a powerful therapeutic component of the clinical process, which should not be undervalued or underestimated. A thorough examination also facilitates development of a directed individual treatment plan.

Tinnitus can be described in terms of its psychoacoustic properties and in terms of the affective or reactive responses to the tinnitus. The psychoacoustic properties of tinnitus can be determined from psychophysical assessment of its features. Important features include tonality; noise aspects such as hissing, buzzing, humming, sizzling, and roaring; unilateral-bilateral localization in the head; temporal features (e.g., pulsatile vs. steady); and interaction with external sounds, including masking, inhibition, and exacerbation. The affective or reactive components include the comorbid problems of depression, sleep disruption, difficulty with concentration, sadness, anxiety, and fear. The reactive components of tinnitus are highly individual and are significant factors in tinnitus disability. Careful evaluation of both components is important for the clinician to appreciate fully the impact of the tinnitus on the individual, and to formulate a directed treatment plan.

The auditory qualities of tinnitus can be assessed using standardized questionnaires and psychophysical measurements. Basic information about the auditory characteristics of tinnitus includes localization (left, right, in the head, outside of the head), constancy (episodic, fluctuating, constant, pulsatile), pitch, loudness, and sound quality (tonal, hissing, buzzing, clicking, ringing). This information can be useful in determining etiology. Pulsatile tinnitus can imply a vascular source. Fluctuating tinnitus may be linked to specific triggers, such as foods, illnesses, stress, or acoustic trauma. Episodic tinnitus may relate to unstable hearing thresholds deriving from cochlear dysfunctions, such as hydrops or perilymph fistulas. Clicking or tapping tinnitus may occur with mechanical disorders affecting either the middle ear muscles (stapedial or tensor tympani spasm) or the auditory nerve (vascular loop or demyelination). Identification of tinnitus with specific characteristics such as these is very useful, and can lead to a directed course of therapy.

Standardized Outcome Measures

Numerous standardized questionnaires are available for measuring tinnitus severity and perceived disability. Standardized assessment is useful for documenting clinical outcomes and reporting the results of clinical trials. Standardized measures are also crucial for determining the subjective impact of tinnitus. Finally, standardized questionnaires are useful for stratifying patients according to the severity and impact of their tinnitus, which facilitates identification of specific problems, and serves to triage patient care from minimal counseling to intensive rehabilitation.

The THI is a widely used self-assessment tool.[112] It is a 25-item questionnaire that has good construct validity, strong internal consistency, and good test-retest reliability. The THI yields a total score and three subscale scores. The subscales encompass functional limitations in mental (e.g., difficulty concentrating), social, occupational and physical domains (e.g., difficulty sleeping); emotional responses to tinnitus (e.g., anger, depression, anxiety); and catastrophic reactions to tinnitus (e.g., desperation, loss of control, failure to cope). In addition to its good internal consistency and test-retest reliability, the THI has high convergent validity with the 27-item Tinnitus Handicap Questionnaire and the 52-item Tinnitus Questionnaire.[113] The 95% confidence interval for the THI is 20 points, suggesting that a difference in scores of 20 points or greater represents a statistically and clinically significant change.[112]

Tinnitus Comorbidities

As previously mentioned, severe debilitating tinnitus is frequently associated with depression, anxiety, and other mood disorders.[114-116] Comorbid emotional disturbance is not unique to tinnitus, and has been shown to accompany many chronic illnesses.[117,118] It is well recognized that coexisting mood disorders hamper improvement and interfere with treatment of conditions such as chronic pain and tinnitus. Identifying and treating comorbid conditions in tinnitus patients is an important aspect of the clinical evaluation. Tools are available to screen for mood disorders in an outpatient setting (e.g., Beck Depression Inventory, Hamilton Anxiety Scale). An important therapeutic adjunct is teaching coping skills through behavior modification and cognitive therapy.[119]

Tinnitus and Insomnia

Patients commonly report that tinnitus interferes with their ability to fall asleep, and sleep disruption is a significant comorbid condition in adults and children.[120,121] A robust correlation has been shown between the reported loudness and severity of tinnitus and degree of sleep disruption.[122,123] A positive feedback loop may exist in which tinnitus leads to sleep deprivation, and the sleep deprivation exacerbates somatic complaints, tinnitus among them. Depression and anxiety exacerbated by sleep loss may significantly interact with and compound the cycle of tinnitus and poor quality sleep. Coping ability may also deteriorate as a result of sleep deprivation or lack of restorative sleep. Interventions that break this cycle by improving sleep have been shown to improve tinnitus.

Pharmacologic sleep aids such as melatonin can reduce tinnitus severity, particularly in patients with pronounced sleep difficulties.[14,125] Bedside sound generators have also been shown to improve sleep quality significantly and lessen tinnitus distress. The bedside sounds most frequently chosen are often selected for their perceived positive emotional effect.[126]

Sleep difficulties include insufficient sleep, poor quality sleep, and nonrestorative sleep. Psychological and behavioral management of sleep disturbance is an effective treatment modality.[127] McKenna and Daniel[128] have outlined a treatment strategy that addresses tinnitus and insomnia as components adversely affected by anxiety.

Hyperacusis

There is no single, universally accepted definition of hyperacusis, and there is no consensus on the physiologic mechanisms that cause the condition. Hyperacusis has been defined as noise intolerance, annoyance caused by ordinary sounds, and abnormal discomfort for suprathreshold sound.[129] These definitions distinguish hyperacusis, considered by many to be a central phenomenon, from recruitment. Recruitment is the rapid growth of perceived loudness with increasing stimulus level, and is observed in association with cochlear hearing loss and outer cell dysfunction. Hyperacusis frequently occurs in association with tinnitus, but can be present without tinnitus or any associated hearing loss. Hyperacusis can occur after the loss of the stapedial reflex in association with acute facial paralysis,[130] in association with general conditions such as migraine attacks,[131] in association with Lyme disease,[132] as a result of benzodiazepine withdrawal,[133] or as part of a syndrome.[134] Patients with tinnitus and hyperacusis frequently have loudness discomfort levels that are lower than loudness discomfort levels of individuals with similar levels of sensorineural hearing loss, indicating that these phenomena are distinctly different from recruitment.[135]

Andersson and associates[136] assessed the prevalence of hyperacusis in the general population in two surveys of the adult Swedish population. The point prevalence of hyperacusis was 5.9% (postal survey) and 7.7% (Internet survey). Participants reporting hearing impairment were excluded from the prevalence calculations, minimizing the inclusion of patients with cochlear damage and reduced dynamic range in the sample. Other reports of hyperacusis prevalence in the general population are 22%.[137] The prevalence of hyperacusis within the tinnitus population is unknown. Estimates range from 40% to 80%, but no systematic survey has been conducted for accurate estimation.[138,139] In the general population and the tinnitus population, the adopted operational definition of hyperacusis would determine its estimated prevalence.

Objective tests of loudness discomfort or sound intolerance in patients with hyperacusis have been adapted from procedures developed for assessing recruitment.[140,141] There are several variations on the technique for measuring loudness discomfort levels, but no consensus or standardization has been established. In addition, issues of intersubject and intrasubject variability,[142] test-retest reliability,[143] operator dependency, and poor face validity for test stimuli all limit the utility of adapting measures of loudness intolerance to patients with hyperacusis.

There are very few validated, well-established self-report questionnaires that specifically target hyperacusis. Two questionnaires developed in France are available, but have not yet been validated in English translation. Dauman and Bouscau-Faure[139] have developed a scale for assessing hyperacusis in patients with tinnitus: The Multiple-Activity Scale for Hyperacusis (MASH). MASH employs a structured interview for rating the annoyance induced by sound exposure from different physical and social activities. Dauman and Bouscau-Faure[139] reported hyperacusis was present in 197 of 249 (79%) clinical patients screened with the instrument, with substantial to severe annoyance from hyperacusis present in 42%. There was no correlation between the severity of hyperacusis, as indicated by MASH, and audiometric threshold shift, indicating that hyperacusis is a phenomenon distinct from loudness recruitment. The Hyperacusis Questionnaire is a 14-item instrument, also developed in French, in which hyperacusis is assessed using a four-alternative Likert scale.[144]

The impact of hypersensitivity to sound can range from general avoidance of social situations such as concerts and restaurants to specific sound aversions (e.g., vacuum cleaners, traffic, clinking dishes, children playing). In extreme cases, patients with severe hypersensitivity become housebound in an effort to control acoustic exposure, wearing ear plugs and ear muffs for extended periods. In all cases of sound hypersensitivity, it is important to address the physiologic component of loudness discomfort and reduced dynamic range, and the psychological component of fear, anxiety, social withdrawal, and maladaptation that accompanies the condition. The cognitive influence on sound sensitivity has been shown by the high correlation of loudness tolerance with anxiety.[99]

The efficacy of sound therapy for treating hyperacusis has had mixed results. Dauman and Bouscau-Faure[139] reported that TRT was more effective in improving hyperacusis (63%) than tinnitus (47%) in 32 patients evaluated at three time points after therapy. They reported that hyperacusis remains a problem for a significant proportion of patients treated with TRT. Gold and associates[145] reported a retrospective study on the effect of TRT on selected patients with reduced sound tolerance. Hyperacusis was defined as average loudness discomfort levels for 1 kHz, 2 kHz, 4 kHz, and 8 kHz below 100 dB HL and patient reports of physical discomfort with exposure to sounds. Hearing thresholds were unchanged between initial measures and follow-up after 9 months of therapy; however, mean loudness discomfort levels were improved 12.48 dB, and the dynamic range was significantly increased by a mean 11.32 dB. A corresponding improvement in the number of activities avoided because of sound tolerance problems was noted as well.

SUGGESTED READINGS

Aydemir G, Tezer MS, Borman P, et al. Treatment of tinnitus with transcutaneous electrical nerve stimulation improves patients' quality of life. *J Laryngol Otol.* 2006;120:442-445.

Bauer CA, Brozoski TJ. Effect of gabapentin on the sensation and impact of tinnitus. *Laryngoscope.* 2006;116:675-681.

Bauer CA, Brozoski TJ, Myers K. Primary afferent dendrite degeneration as a cause of tinnitus. *J Neurosci Res.* 2007;85:1489-1498.

Bauer CA, Brozoski TJ, Myers KS. Acoustic injury and TRPV1 expression in the cochlear spiral ganglion. *Int Tinnitus J.* 2007;13:21-28.

For complete list of references log onto www.expertconsult.com.

Davis PB, Paki B, Hanley PJ. Neuromonics tinnitus treatment: third clinical trial. *Ear Hear.* 2007;28:242-259.

Folmer RL, Griest SE. Tinnitus and insomnia. *Am J Otolaryngol.* 2000;21:287-293.

Hebert S, Carrier J. Sleep complaints in elderly tinnitus patients: a controlled study. *Ear Hear.* 2007;28:649-655.

Herraiz C, Toledano A, Diges I. Trans-electrical nerve stimulation (TENS) for somatic tinnitus. *Prog Brain Res.* 2007;166:389-553.

Jakes SC, Hallam RS, Rachman S, et al. The effects of reassurance, relaxation training and distraction on chronic tinnitus sufferers. *Behav Res Ther.* 1986;24:497-507.

Kirsch CA, Blanchard EB, Parnes SM. Psychological characteristics of individuals high and low in their ability to cope with tinnitus. *Psychosom Med.* 1989;51:209-217.

Levine RA. Typewriter tinnitus: a carbamazepine-responsive syndrome related to auditory nerve vascular compression. *ORL J Otorhinolaryngol Relat Spec.* 2006;68:43-46.

Lockwood AH, Salvi RJ, Coad ML, et al. The functional neuroanatomy of tinnitus: evidence for limbic system links and neural plasticity. *Neurology.* 1998;50:114-120.

Mardini MK. Ear-clicking "tinnitus" responding to carbamazepine. *N Engl J Med.* 1987;317:1542.

Martinez Devesa P, Waddell A, Perera R, et al. Cognitive behavioural therapy for tinnitus. *Cochrane Database Syst Rev.* 2007;(1)CD005233.

Norena AJ, Eggermont JJ. Enriched acoustic environment after noise trauma reduces hearing loss and prevents cortical map reorganization. *J Neurosci.* 2005;25:699-705.

Robinson SK, Viirre ES, Bailey KA, et al. Randomized placebo-controlled trial of a selective serotonin reuptake inhibitor in the treatment of nondepressed tinnitus subjects. *Psychosom Med.* 2005;67:981-988.

Rosenberg SI, Silverstein H, Rowan PT, et al. Effect of melatonin on tinnitus. *Laryngoscope.* 1998;108:305-310.

Rubinstein B, Axelsson A, Carlsson GE. Prevalence of signs and symptoms of craniomandibular disorders in tinnitus patients. *J Craniomandib Disord.* 1990;4:186-192.

Shulman A, Goldstein B. Pharmacotherapy for severe, disabling, subjective, idiopathic tinnitus: 2005-2006. *Int Tinnitus J.* 2006;12:161-171.

Trotter MI, Donaldson I. Hearing aids and tinnitus therapy: a 25 year experience. *J Laryngol Otol.* 122:1052-1056, 2008.

Tyler RS, ed. *Tinnitus Treatment: Clinical Protocols.* New York: Thieme Medical Publishers; 2006.

Zoger S, Svedlund J, Holgers KM. The effects of sertraline on severe tinnitus suffering—a randomized, double-blind, placebo-controlled study. *J Clin Psychopharmacol.* 2006;26:32-39.

CHAPTER ONE HUNDRED AND FIFTY-ONE

Noise-Induced Hearing Loss

Brenda L. Lonsbury-Martin

Glen K. Martin

Key Points

- Noise-induced hearing loss (NIHL) is second only to age-related hearing loss as the most prevalent form of hearing loss.
- NIHL resulting from relatively brief noise exposures can be reversible, as happens with exposure occurring at an evening spent in a loud entertainment venue.
- Permanent NIHL is caused by either an acoustic trauma (i.e., a brief exposure to a very intense blastlike sound) or a chronic long-term exposure to the loud sounds associated with a noisy occupation.
- An accelerating incidence of high-frequency hearing loss in younger individuals points to early, chronic noise exposure, possibly from personal entertainment devices.
- NIHL is a complex condition that is influenced by environmental and genetic factors.
- Genetic association studies have identified genetic factors primarily related to oxidative stress that influence an individual's susceptibility to NIHL.
- Current research on the administration of certain antioxidants before or after noise exposure shows promise for developing a pharmacologic treatment for NIHL in the near future.
- NIHL is a preventable condition and the otolaryngologist plays a critical role in educating patients about protecting their ears from the adverse effects of noise overexposure.

One of the most common causes of permanent hearing impairment is exposure to excessive sounds. Millions of individuals worldwide have noise-induced hearing loss (NIHL), resulting in a reduced quality of life because of social isolation, and possible inexorable tinnitus and impaired communication with family members, coworkers, and friends.[1] The costs in terms of compensation and early retirement payments for work-related NIHL are immense. The U.S. Department of Veterans Affairs spends approximately $700 million a year on disability compensation and treatments for NIHL. NIHL is the single largest disability expenditure of the Veterans Benefits Administration.[2]

This chapter presents and discusses more recent perspectives on the effects of excessive noise on hearing that address the scientific and practical aspects of NIHL. Although NIHL has been studied experimentally for more than a century, only in the last few decades have some major breakthroughs occurred in our basic understanding of the ear's reaction to damaging sounds, along with a better understanding of the environmental and genetic factors that contribute to NIHL. This steady progression in the knowledge base about NIHL promises to improve significantly the detection and treatment of this disorder over the coming years.

Measurement of Noise

The term *noise* is commonly used to designate an undesirable sound. In the scientific and clinical fields that deal with hearing, this term has come to mean any excessively loud sound that has the potential to harm hearing. The temporal patterns of environmental noise are typically described as continuous, fluctuating, intermittent, or impulsive.[3] Continuous or steady-state noise remains relatively constant, whereas fluctuating noise increases and decreases in level over time, and intermittent sounds are interrupted for varying time periods. Impulsive or impact noises caused by explosive or metal-on-metal mechanical events have rapidly changing pressure characteristics consisting of intense, short-lasting (i.e., milliseconds) wave fronts, followed by much smaller reverberations and echoes that occur over many seconds. The amount of noise, usually referred to as the sound pressure level (SPL), is conventionally measured by a sound-level meter in decibel (dB) units using a frequency-weighting formula called the A-scale. The dBA-scale metric of sound level essentially mimics the threshold-sensitivity curve for the human ear, so the low-frequency and high-frequency components are given less emphasis as auditory hazards. Standard sound-level meters have electronic networks designed to measure noise magnitude automatically in dBA, whereas to measure impulse or impact noise, a more intricate peak-reading sound-level meter is needed that is capable of accurately measuring sounds with essentially instantaneous onset times.

The personal noise dosimeter is typically used to measure noise exposure in the workplace. This instrument provides readout of the noise dose or the percent exposure experienced by a single worker, typically over a specific shift. The logging dosimeter integrates a function of sound pressure over time and calculates the daily (8-hour) dose with respect to the current permissible noise level for a continuous noise of less than or equal to 85 dBA lasting 8 hours. More recently, personal noise dosimeters have been offered to the consumer as a portable, compact, and affordable device that can be used as hearing protectors. The instrument measures and displays noise dose continuously for 16 hours. The dosimeter provides an early warning that the user is approaching overexposure and should use hearing protection. A particular noise (e.g., from power tools, music concerts, sporting events) can also be measured for 2 minutes, and then the estimated dose per hour is calculated and displayed to determine if permissible exposure levels would be exceeded. By putting valuable health information into the hands of consumers, such easy-to-use, inexpensive (<$100) dosimeters empower them to take appropriate steps to prevent NIHL.

Nature of the Hearing Loss

Depending on the level of the sound exposure, either reversible or permanent damage can occur to the peripheral auditory end organ. The reversible loss, typically referred to as a *temporary threshold shift* (TTS), results from exposures to moderately intense sounds, such as might be encountered at a philharmonic orchestra concert. Hearing problems associated with TTS include elevated thresholds, particularly for the higher midfrequency region that includes the 3- to 6-kHz frequencies. The TTS condition is often accompanied by many other common symptoms of hearing impairment, including tinnitus, loudness recruitment, muffled sounds, and diplacusis. Depending on the duration of the exposure, recovery from TTS can occur over periods ranging from minutes to hours and days. After exposure, if TTS does not recover before the ear is re-exposed to excessive sound, a permanent change in hearing can occur, which is referred to as a *permanent threshold shift* (PTS).

In PTS, the elevation in hearing thresholds is irreversible because lasting structural damage occurs to the critical elements of the cochlea. The precise relationship between the TTS and PTS stages of hearing loss caused by noise exposure is unknown. Although it seems logical to assume that repeated episodes of TTS would eventually lead to PTS, experimental findings imply that the fundamental processes underlying the development of reversible versus permanent NIHL are unrelated. Nordmann and colleagues[4] using a survival fixation approach showed that the histopathologic manifestations of TTS and PTS noise damage to the chinchilla cochlea are distinct. Specifically, TTS was correlated with a buckling of the supporting pillar cell bodies in the frequency region of the maximal exposure effect. The morphologic abnormality that was consistently correlated with PTS was a focal loss of hair cells, and a complete degeneration of the corresponding population of nerve fiber endings. Because PTS eventually develops from repeated exposures to stimuli that initially produce only TTS, it is likely that the latter condition is also associated with subtle changes to the sensitive outer hair cell (OHC) system that go undetected by conventional light microscopy.

Traditionally, PTS caused by acoustic overstimulation has been separated in two distinct classes. One type, called *acoustic trauma,* is caused by a single, short-lasting exposure to a very intense sound (e.g., an explosive blast), and results in a sudden, usually painful, loss of hearing. The other type of hearing loss is commonly referred to as NIHL, and results from chronic exposure to less intense levels of sound. A great deal more is known about the anatomic processes underlying the symptoms of and recovery from acoustic trauma than is known about NIHL. Consequently, it is well established that a single exposure to a severe sound causing violent changes in air pressure can produce direct mechanical damage to the delicate tissues of the peripheral auditory apparatus, including components of the middle ear (tympanic membrane, ossicles) and inner ear (organ of Corti). In contrast, regular exposure to less intense but still noisy sounds involves the insidious destruction of cochlear components that eventually and unavoidably leads to an elevation in hearing levels, along with other common symptoms of hearing impairment.

Acoustic trauma was previously a relatively rare event that was typically associated with accidental explosions in industrial settings. Military servicemen and servicewomen caught in roadside bomb explosions in the current armed conflicts in Iraq and Afghanistan are returning home in epidemic numbers, however, with profound permanent hearing losses and tinnitus.[5] Consequently, acoustic trauma is a hearing problem that is increasing, at least in combat troops. Because many of these postdeployment cases are being treated in the private sector, all otolaryngologists may see acoustic trauma in increasing numbers.

Irreversible NIHL is a specific pathologic state exhibiting a recognized set of symptoms and objective findings.[6] NIHL includes (1) a permanent sensorineural hearing loss with damage principally to cochlear hair cells, and primarily to OHCs; (2) a history of a long-term exposure to dangerous noise levels (i.e., >90 dBA for 8 hours/day) sufficient to cause the degree and pattern of hearing loss described by audiologic findings; (3) a gradual loss of hearing over the first 5 to 10 years of exposure; (4) a hearing loss involving initially the higher frequencies from 3 to 8 kHz before including frequencies less than or equal to 2 kHz; (5) speech-recognition scores that are consistent with the audiometric loss; and (6) a hearing loss that stabilizes after the noise exposure is terminated.

A patient with NIHL commonly consults a physician because of difficulties in hearing and understanding ordinary speech, especially in the presence of background noise. Many variations can be found in the detailed configuration of the audiogram of a noise-damaged ear, depending on the temporal and spectral distribution of the noise stimulus, and on the stage of hearing loss. The pattern of hearing loss most commonly associated with the earlier stages of NIHL is illustrated in Figure 151-1A. The beginning region of impairment involves the sensitive midfrequency range, primarily 3 to 6 kHz, and the corresponding hearing loss is classically described as the "4-kHz notch." This pattern of maximal hearing loss, with little or no loss at less than 2 kHz, typically occurs regardless of the noise-exposure environment. The audiogram results in Figure 151-1A also show the sensorineural aspect of NIHL in that thresholds for bone-conducted stimuli are essentially identical to the thresholds for air conduction. The profile of noise-induced threshold hearing is usually symmetric for both ears, particularly for individuals who have been working in noisy industrial settings in which there are "surround" sounds.

Commonly, other forms of noxious sound, such as the gunfire associated with sport shooting, cause an asymmetric pattern of hearing loss similar to the one illustrated in Figure 151-1B. In this case, the ear pointed toward the source of noise (gun barrel), which is the right ear of the left-handed shooter depicted in Figure 151-1B, would have worse hearing than the ear directed away from the source (in this example, the left or protected ear) by 15 to 30 dB or more, and particularly at higher frequencies because of the absence of the protective head-shadow effect.

The development of a hearing loss caused by habitual exposure to moderately intense levels of noise typically consists of two stages. Initially, the middle to high frequencies exhibit the resulting hearing loss. As the length of time of exposure to loud noise increases, hearing loss becomes greater and begins to affect adjacent higher and lower frequencies. In a classic cross-sectional study of occupational NIHL, Taylor and colleagues[7] showed the gradual loss of hearing sensitivity in workers caused by habitual exposure to the intense sounds of dropforging tools that are commonly used in foundries. Figure 151-2 illustrates the progressive effects of exposure to the wideband noise (Fig. 151-2A) of two types of forging tools, presses and hammers, on the magnitude of hearing loss as the length of exposure increased. For the operators of the press and hammer equipment (Fig. 151-2B and C), the approximate 10- to 20-dB threshold shifts, typically observed at the higher frequencies during the first 1 to 2 years of exposure, grew to be a 20-dB or greater loss, from 3 to 6 kHz, after a 3-year exposure. There was a 40-dB or greater threshold shift after an 8-year exposure.

Detailed comparisons of the NIHL growth curves of Figure 151-2B and C reveal that with continuing exposure, hearing loss worsened at the higher frequencies and spread to the lower frequencies. In addition, for average exposure times of less than 10 years, hearing levels for the press and hammer operators who were exposed to mean levels of 108 and 99 dB SPL deteriorated similarly. For long-term exposures of 10 years or more, the results of Taylor and colleagues[7] indicated that hearing losses resulting from the hammer-induced impact noise were greater than the losses resulting from the more continuous noise of the press equipment. Finally, a characteristic feature of NIHL, which is clearly documented in Figure 151-2B and C, is that hearing levels are increased rarely beyond about 70 to 90 dB of hearing loss, on average, even after more than 31 years of continuous noise exposure.

Cochlear Damage

The primary site of anatomic damage is at the level of the mechanosensory receptors of the auditory system's end organ. Loud sound damages the inner hair cells and OHCs of the organ of Corti, with the

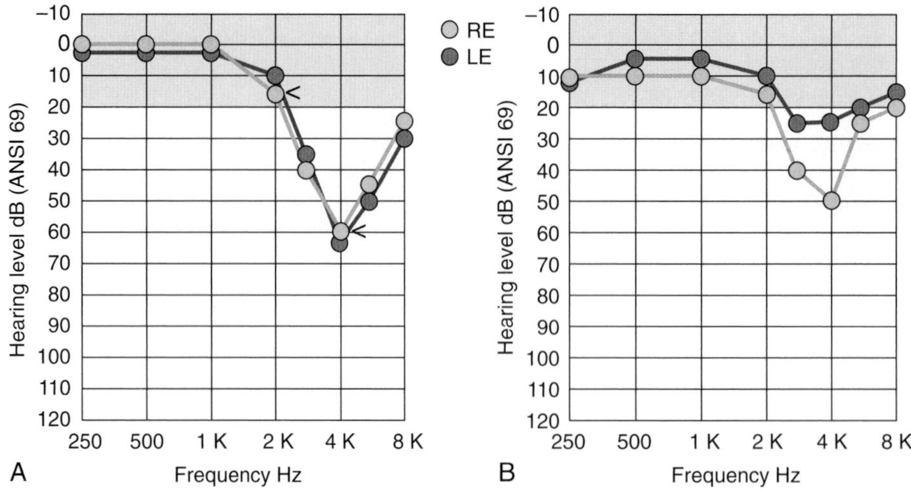

Figure 151-1. Audiometric patterns of hearing levels from patients in beginning stages of noise-induced hearing loss. **A,** A "4-kHz notch" symmetric pattern for a 44-year-old male factory worker. Thresholds for bone-conducted stimuli *(arrows)* were similar to thresholds determined with routine air-conduction methods. **B,** Asymmetric pattern for a 45-year-old man who was a recreational rifle shooter. For this left-handed patient, note greater impairment in the right (*yellow circles*) rather than the left (*red circles*) ear because of protective head-shadow effect. <, unmasked right ear.

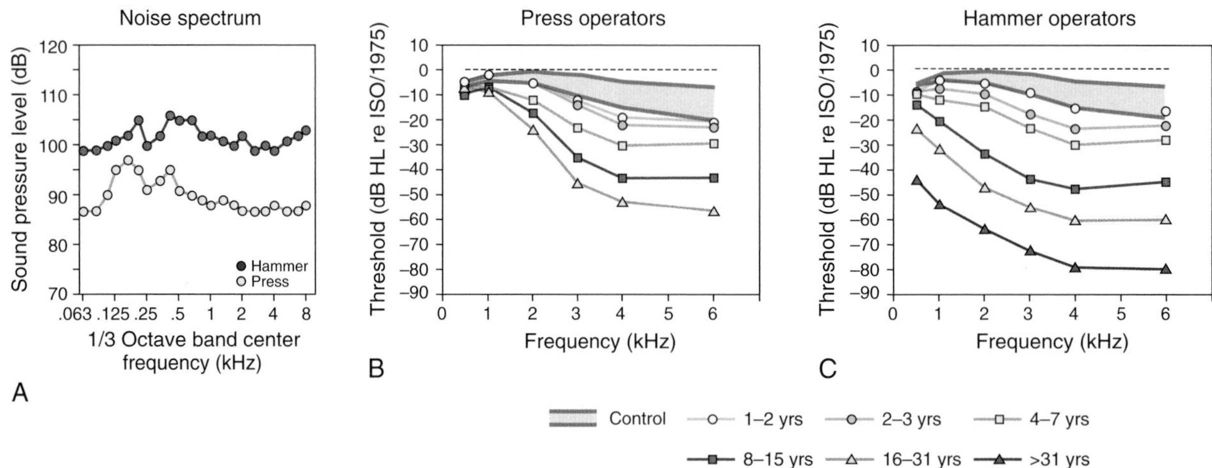

Figure 151-2. Development of the audiometric pattern of noise-induced hearing loss as a function of years of exposure to constant occupational noises. **A,** Spectra of noise produced by hammer *(red circles)* and press *(yellow circles)* equipment, with maximal energy centered in 0.2- to 1-kHz and 0.125- to 0.5-kHz regions. **B** and **C,** Resulting hearing losses for press **(B)** and hammer **(C)** operators. Noise-induced hearing losses occurred at frequencies above peak energy in the exposure. *Geometric symbols* represent experimental subjects according to years of noise exposure. *Shaded areas* indicate effects of aging on hearing levels in control subjects of similar age (i.e., 23 to 54 years old), who worked in non-noisy parts of the same drop-forging plants. *(Adapted from Taylor W, Lempert B, Pelmear P, Hemstock I, Kershaw J. Noise levels and hearing thresholds in the drop forging industry.* J Acoust Soc Am. *1984;76:807-819.)*

OHCs in particular being most affected in the initial stages. In instances involving very intense acoustic stimulation, supporting-cell elements also can be directly affected. Depending on the physical attributes of the exposure stimulus (e.g., time-varying characteristics or the intensity, frequency, or spectral content, duration, or schedule), noise can cause damage to hair cells ranging from total destruction to effects evident only in the ultrastructure of specialized subcellular regions (e.g., the fusing or bending of the individual cilia that make up the stereociliary bundle). Whenever degenerative processes or structural modifications to the cochlea reach a significant level, an associated reduction in hearing capability can be detected.

Johnsson and Hawkins[8] were among the first investigators to describe the typical patterns of cochlear injury for humans with chronic exposure to different types of loud sound. The photomicrograph of the cochlear tissue in Figure 151-3A depicts some common histopathologic consequences of NIHL for a patient with a lengthy history of noise exposure. The authors reported that the 50-year-old patient had worked intermittently over a 5- to 6-year period in an automotive body–stamping plant, and that he had a long history of using recreational firearms. The sharp transition in the basal end (following the uncoiling to the right) from the normal-looking organ of Corti (a darkish stripe corresponding to the region of inner hair cells and OHCs), with its dense network of nerve fibers, to the complete absence of hair cells and their corresponding nerve fibers (the much lighter adjacent area) can be noted. Figure 151-3B graphically reconstructs the histopathologic features of this cochlea as a cytocochleogram by depicting the number of remaining hair cells, in the form of percentages, averaged over 1-mm sections. A typical finding in individuals exposed to the occupational noise exemplified in this case is the almost symmetric pattern of degeneration observed for the two ears. The *inset* at the top right of the cytocochleogram shows the patient's audiogram obtained about 1 year before his death, which shows the severity of the anatomic damage in functional terms by revealing an abrupt hearing loss for test frequencies greater than 2 kHz.

Examination of human temporal bone specimens by numerous laboratories[8-10] has yielded documentation of the progressive stages of

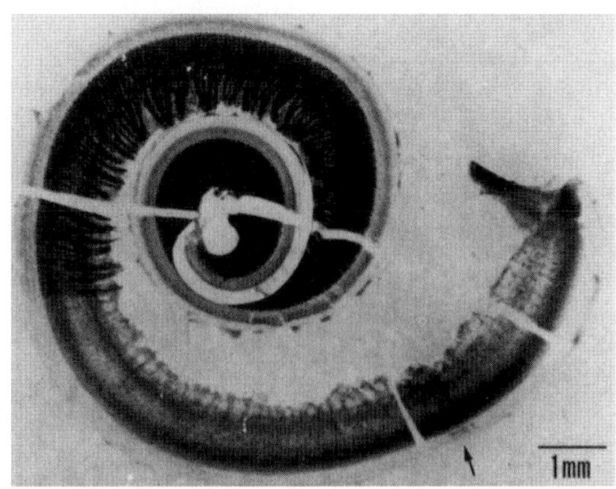

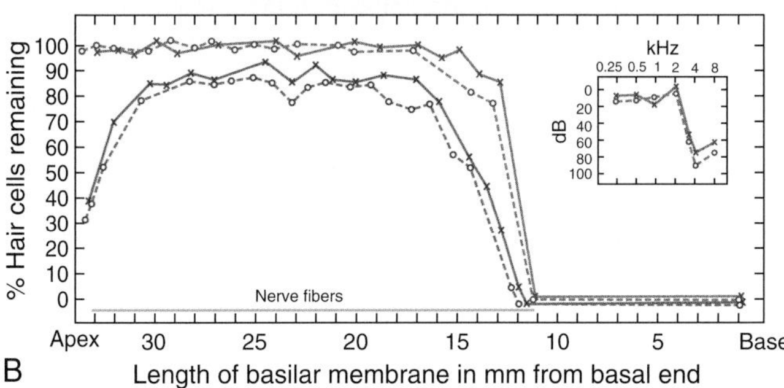

Figure 151-3. **A,** Low-power photomicrograph of a soft surface preparation of organ of Corti from the left cochlea of a 50-year-old man exposed extensively to occupational noise, showing a pattern of abrupt degeneration of basal region. *Arrow* indicates a small patch of remaining organ of Corti near basal end. **B,** Modified cytocochleograms for two ears along with an audiogram that was measured 1 year earlier, showing sharp pattern of hair cell degeneration (expressed as percentage remaining per millimeter of length of basilar membrane measured from basal end) and nerve fiber degeneration. Note relative symmetry of corresponding abrupt high-frequency loss of cochlear elements. Separate curves represent inner *(solid lines)* and outer *(dashed lines)* hair cells (averaged over three rows of outer hair cells) for left *(X)* and right *(O)* ears. *Yellow horizontal line* along abscissa indicates presence of nerve fibers in osseous spiral lamina. *(Adapted from Johnsson LG, Hawkins JE. Degeneration patterns in human ears exposed to noise.* Ann Otol Rhinol Laryngol. *1976;85:725-739.)*

noise damage as depicted by epidemiologic data such as those of Figure 151-2. First, in the predictable sequence of events, a small region of hair cell and nerve fiber degeneration appears bilaterally at a cochlear region corresponding to the 4-kHz notch. Typically, these discrete lesions gradually grow in the basal-ward direction (i.e., toward the high-frequency extent of the cochlea) to involve a greater portion of the organ of Corti. Finally, as exposure to noise continues over years, the remaining sensory and neural elements in the basal end of the cochlea are destroyed, resulting in an abrupt loss of midfrequency to high-frequency hearing, such as that depicted by the clinical audiogram of Figure 151-3.

Research on Noise-Induced Hearing Loss

Scientific interest in the damaging effects of excessive sound on hearing has a long history for many reasons. First, the experimental strategy of exposing animals to noise and examining their ears for the sites of the resulting acoustic injury was used in the past as the independent variable in establishing some of our basic knowledge about hearing. Particularly, with the use of intense tones as the damaging agents, frequency information relating physical distance along the basilar membrane to the "best" frequency of the injured region provided an initial basis for understanding the tonotopicity of the cochlea and the central projection of such frequency-related information.[11] Additionally, noise-damage strategies have been used to contribute to our understanding of the function of inner hair cells and OHCs by permitting differences in their central terminations in the ventral and dorsal cochlear nuclei to be distinguished.[12]

Although useful as an analytic strategy, the major impetus behind the more contemporary interest in the effects of noise on hearing originates from a desire to understand the fundamental processes by which exposure to loud sound leads to acoustic injury. The reward of achieving an appreciation of the basic processes underlying NIHL lies in the ability to prevent, or at least predict, an individual's susceptibility to PTS, or perhaps even to initiate regeneration of damaged or lost critical cellular components, which would eventually lead to the recovery of hearing.

The research literature on the effects of noise on hearing and the anatomic elements of the ear is voluminous. Early experiments performed more than 65 years ago were straightforward anatomic studies based on the strategy of exposing various animal models to intense noises, followed by a general description of the resulting histopathology at the cellular level. More modern noise studies in animal models have attempted to establish a structure/function relationship between noise-induced morphologic damage and the inability to detect auditory signals.

In this extensive literature, a great disparity in the experimental findings relating the effects of missing hair cells to the corresponding hearing sensitivity is frequently apparent. Such contrasting findings and the confusion they have caused are related to numerous confounding variables, including poor analysis of the problem, experimental error, and a failure to understand the limitations of the functional and anatomic techniques used. Also, such disparate studies typically exposed animal subjects to a single noise at levels much greater than 100 dB SPL in an attempt to mimic, within a relatively brief study interval, damage patterns that develop in humans from intermittent exposure to much less intense noises over many years. Consequently, although early noise studies showed that the longer an animal was exposed to extreme levels of sound, the greater was the resulting cochlear injury, they contributed little to our knowledge concerning how NIHL develops in humans working for long periods in noisy work settings.

In contrast, research conducted over the past few decades has made use of more realistic experimental protocols that incorporate intermittent exposure stimuli of intensities and durations designed to approximate the effects of a working lifetime of exposure to occupational noise. Additionally, most more recent studies have been developed sequentially within a program of research, so that a thorough understanding of a particular effect is achieved.

Anatomic Mechanisms Underlying Noise Damage

Experimental studies have led to an increased understanding of some major features of NIHL. It is well-accepted that the origin of the 4-kHz notch in the NIHL audiogram is related to the resonator function of the external auditory ear canal,[13] rather than to indeterminable innate properties of the cochlea, such as a reduced vascular supply to this region of the organ of Corti.[14] The primary research interest has always been, however, in the fundamental mechanism by which the sensory cell degenerates or is damaged after exposure. Numerous mechanisms[15] have been proposed, including mechanical injury caused by severe motion of the basilar membrane, metabolic exhaustion of activated cells, activity-induced vascular narrowing that causes ischemia, and ionic poisoning from interruption of the normal chemical gradients of the cochlea owing to minuscule disruptions in the organization of sensory and supporting cells.

Although the many years of experimental research have not yet produced a major breakthrough in understanding of damage mechanisms, the current most convincing morphologic evidence supports a combination of the mechanochemical theories. First, at the ultrastructural level, it is likely that alterations in the stereocilia in the form of shortened or broken rootlets are involved in the initial pathologic processes that lead to TTS and, if such injuries are not repaired, then PTS.[16-18] More recent findings showed that hair bundles are capable of rebuilding their ultrastructure from top to bottom over a 48-hour period.[19,20] If damage is so severe that it overwhelms this self-repair mechanism as exposure continues, a discrete but direct mechanical disruption likely results in a toxic mixing of endolymph and perilymph through microbreaks in the structural framework of the cochlear duct,[21] which leads to secondary effects, including loss of hair cells and their corresponding nerve fibers.

New Knowledge about Cellular and Molecular Mechanisms of Noise-Induced Hearing Loss

The research frontiers that promise to provide fresh insights into the fundamental basis of NIHL and eventually into the development of a cure for this disorder consist of hair cell regeneration or repair or both, "training" protocols that target the cochlear-efferent system to make hair cells more resistant, the use of protective agents before and after noise exposure, and understanding the genetic basis of susceptibility and resistance to the adverse effects of sound overexposure.

Hair Cell Regeneration and Repair

In the late 1980s, several seminal reports on hair cell regeneration in avian species established that hair cells in neonatal and adult birds regenerate after exposure to either damaging levels of sound[22-24] or ototoxic antibiotics.[25] Additionally, follow-up studies showed that recovery of cochlear function accompanied the cellular-recovery process.[26-28] In the best-studied model for hair cell regeneration, the neonatal chick, it was shown that new hair cells arose as progeny from an otherwise nondividing supporting-cell population that was induced to proliferate by the damaging insult.[29]

Generally, noise-induced hair cell loss in the mammalian cochlea is irreversible. Experimental findings using in vitro cultures of neonatal mouse cochleas showed, however, that overexpression of mammalian atonal homolog 1 (Atoh1), also known as Math 1, a basic helix-loop-helix transcription factor known to be necessary for hair cell differentiation during development, leads to an increase in the production of extranumerary hair cells.[30] Consequently, it seems that certain cells in the mammalian organ of Corti, at least in young animals, can be redirected toward a hair cell fate by the overexpression of Math 1.[31] In addition, a most exciting finding was the discovery that new hair cells can be grown in a mature mammalian ear using the Math 1 gene. Kawamoto and colleagues[32] injected an adenovirus carrying the Math 1 gene into the endolymph of mature guinea pigs. Using scanning electron microscopy, 1 to 2 months after the inoculation of the Math 1 gene insert, immature hair cells within the nonsensory supporting cells of the organ of Corti were detected. Most importantly, follow-up studies in the deafened guinea pig showed that not only did Math 1 induce regeneration of hair cells in the adult, deafened guinea pig, but also substantially improved hearing thresholds were measured.[33] These findings that Math 1 (Atoh1) can direct hair cell differentiation and induce hearing function in mature nonsensory cells support the notion that adenoviral gene therapy based on expressing crucial developmental genes for cellular and functional restoration in damaged auditory epithelium may lead some day to a new treatment for NIHL.

Protection from Conditioning the Cochlear Efferent System

The outcomes of other experiments indicate that the mammalian cochlea may be capable of actively adapting to certain high-level sounds by receiving "exposure experience." The notion that the cochlea can become resistant over time to the consequences of excessive sound was reported initially by noting "conditioning" effects in several animal models.[34-37] The typical conditioning paradigm consists of providing a pre-exposure training experience using a moderate-level stimulus that, at a more intense level, becomes the subsequent overexposure stimulus. Together, these findings in animal models suggested that the mammalian cochlea might be capable under certain conditions of dynamically adapting to excessive sound.

For humans, the practical implications of the capacity to develop a "resistance" to loud sounds are obvious. A follow-up study in teenagers used a TTS-type paradigm to show the relevance of resistance training to humans. In this experiment,[38] the investigators provided a pre-exposure training period in which the young subjects were exposed to 6 hours of pop/rock music at around 70 dBA. Threshold shifts in response to a 10-minute exposure to a 105-dB SPL, one-third octave-band noise centered at 1 kHz were compared for pretraining versus post-training intervals. The major result was that the "trained" ears exhibited significant decreases in TTS compared with their baseline values, showing that the "conditioning" effect, or the development of "resistance," can be shown in human subjects, at least under brief TTS-exposure conditions.

Such human studies of the relationship between noise exposure and permanent hearing loss are more difficult to perform for many reasons including the ethical issues involved in the deliberate exposure of study subjects to noises, even though they are thought to be reversibly damaging. More recent research into the protective role of cochlear efferents in NIHL has depended more on the benefits of diagnostic testing with evoked otoacoustic emissions (OAEs) to predict potential susceptibility to the aftereffects of noise exposure.[39] This simple, noninvasive, and objective procedure is based on the systematic measurement of a class of cochlear responses (i.e., the OAEs) that are primarily generated by the OHCs.[40] Not only are OHCs exquisitely sensitive to the initial effects of acoustic overstimulation, which makes them excellent indicators of sound-induced ultrastructural damage, but also the final common pathway of the descending auditory-efferent system preferentially innervates the OHCs.

To take advantage of the ability of OAEs to measure efferent activity, several experimental paradigms were developed including a common one[41] that uses contralateral acoustic stimulation to elicit medial olivocochlear-induced reductions of OAEs from the ipsilateral test ear. The other procedure[42] is based on measurements of a subtype of evoked emissions represented by distortion product OAEs (DPOAEs) at $2f_1$-f_2. In this strategy, long-lasting f_1 and f_2 primary tones of approximately 1 second are applied binaurally to elicit an efferent-based fast adaptation response that tests the ability of the combined medial and lateral cochlear-efferent systems to suppress DPOAEs in the test ear.

Experiments in guinea pigs documented the ability of the fast-adaptive DPOAE response to predict vulnerability to acoustic injury based on the vigor of efferent activity.[43] The robustness of the olivocochlear efferents was inversely correlated with the degree of cochlear dysfunction after subsequent noise exposure, in that animals exhibiting large adaptive effects showed smaller postexposure losses than animals displaying small amounts of efferent-induced adaptation. It is clear from these findings that a modification of this assay could easily be applied to human populations to screen for individuals most at risk in noisy environments.

Some studies[44] simply relating the presence or absence of the contralateral acoustic stimulation–induced reduction of emissions in human ears have reported such suppression is absent in most industrial workers who otherwise have normal OAEs. One implication of such observations is that a lack of efferent-related activity may be an early indication of cochlear damage from exposure to noise. Experimental studies such as these will eventually determine whether inherent efferent processes can account for and predict the remarkable individual variation in susceptibility to NIHL. The use of efferent-induced suppression of evoked OAEs in predicting susceptibility to NIHL, or in monitoring of noise effects in hearing-conservation programs, represents a promising line of future investigation.

Pharmacologic Protection from Noise-Induced Hearing Loss

It has long been recognized that hypoxia is a major pathogenic factor in NIHL. Based on the assumption that oxidative stress plays a substantial role in the genesis of noise-induced cochlear injuries that lead to permanent hearing loss, numerous pharmacologic strategies have been developed primarily in animal models to enhance the intrinsic defense mechanisms of the cochlea against this condition.[45] Kopke and colleagues[46] postulated several causes of noise-induced oxidative stress, all of which are amenable to pharmacologic treatments. Specifically, these investigators proposed that noise-induced oxidative stress leading to cochlear injury was related to (1) impaired mitochondrial function with respect to bioenergetics and biogenesis; (2) glutamate-induced excitotoxicity, which is the main excitatory neurotransmitter in the peripheral and central auditory systems; and (3) depletion of glutathione (GSH), an antioxidant that protects cells from toxins such as free radicals.

Related experimental work showed a reduction in NIHL and hair cell loss in the chinchilla model after application of pharmacologic agents specific to these oxidative stress–related states. Acetyl-L-carnitine, an endogenous mitochondrial membrane compound that helps maintain mitochondrial bioenergetics and biogenesis in the face of oxidative stress; carbamathione, which acts as a glutamate antagonist for cochlear *N*-methyl-D-aspartate (NMDA) receptors; and the GSH-repletion drug, D-methionine (MET), all improved hearing in noise-exposed animals as indexed by auditory brainstem responses, along with reductions in inner hair cell and OHC loss compared with counterpart measures in saline-treated control subjects.[46]

Based on the assumption that a potential mechanism of NIHL is the generation of damaging free radicals through the activation of reactive oxygen species such as hydrogen peroxide, hydroxyl radicals, and superoxide, many other studies have tested the influence of antioxidants and related compounds on noise-induced cochlear dysfunction and organ of Corti morphology. Such candidate substances include GSH,[47] the xanthine oxidase blocker allopurinol,[48] *N*-L-acetylcysteine (L-NAC),[49] and GSH peroxidase and superoxide dismutase.[50] Together, all these findings support the notion that combating cellular oxidative stress, principally with prophylactic administration of antioxidant compounds, eliminates noise-induced cochlear injury in animal models. More recently, Kopke and colleagues[51] reported on some promising results using L-NAC in military recruits to reduce the NIHL sometimes associated with the basic training related to military operations. The success of such a pharmacologic approach essentially ensures the development in the near future of a therapeutic intervention that reduces NIHL clinically.

Susceptibility

A long-standing observation in NIHL has been that some ears are more easily damaged by noise than others. Individually varying susceptibilities to noise-induced hearing impairment have been found in humans and research animals. Because of the widespread interest in NIHL and its prevention, it is important to develop valid and reliable indices to predict human susceptibility to various noise levels. It is commonly assumed that such variability in susceptibility is a manifestation of biologic factors unique to each subject. A genetically based imperfection in the physical characteristics of the cochlea (e.g., stiffness of the cochlear partition) and variability in cochlear ultrastructure (e.g., density of hair cells) have been proposed as contributing to susceptibility.[52]

Identifying individual differences among various factors has long been a focus of interest. Numerous potentially important variables that have been investigated in the past and continue to be examined include age[53]; gender[54]; race[55]; previous damage to the cochlea[56]; efficiency of the acoustic reflex[57]; smoking habits[58]; and the influence of certain disease states such as hypercholesterolemia[59] or hypertriglyceridemia,[60] diabetes,[61] and cardiovascular disease represented by hypertension.[62] Although many pertinent factors have been uncovered, most data are inconclusive. In addition, although a few factors, such as pigmentation,[63] seem to have some relationship to potentiating noise damage, others, such as age, simply produce additive effects,[64] although this latter relationship remains controversial.[65] Possibly, as McFadden and Wightman[66] suggested in their review of the contribution of the psychoacoustic method toward understanding the symptoms of clinical hearing disorders, the orthogonally based research approach, which assumes a causal relationship between factors, will not reveal meaningful relationships. Perhaps the uncovering of interrelationships among myriad individual differences by application of a multivariate test battery would be more successful in identifying the basic factors that predict susceptibility to NIHL.

One of the most exciting areas in current experimental research is aimed at examining the genetic origin of differences in susceptibility to noise damage using the mouse model. A clear benefit of the mouse as an experimental animal is the great amount of knowledge that exists about the mouse genome. Additionally, mice from the same inbred strain are considered to be genetically identical. Consequently, assessing individual variability to noise damage in subjects that are homozygous at all chromosomal loci offers a unique opportunity to isolate genetic factors responsible for susceptibility to NIHL. To date, several studies[67,68] have shown that the inbred, mutant C57BL/6J (C57) strain, often used as a model of early age-related hearing loss, is more susceptible to noise damage than the CBA/CaJ (CBA) strain, which is frequently used as a model of normal hearing. Other observations supporting the potentiation of noise damage by the age-related hearing loss gene, *Ahl*, relate to the finding that when C57 (B6) mice are backcrossed with a mouse strain (e.g., CAST/Ei) exhibiting normal aging, the B6/CAST progeny display neither age-related hearing loss nor susceptibility to noise exposure aftereffects.[69]

Just as susceptible mutant mouse strains are readily available, there are also strains with normal cochlear function that are exceptionally resistant to acoustic overstimulation, such as wild-type inbred MOLF/Ei (MOLF) mice. Figure 151-4 compares the effects of an intense noise exposure (105-dB SPL, octave-band noise centered at 10 kHz, for 8 hours) on control CBA and MOLF mice at 2 months of age.[70] Although CBA mice showed only an expected minor recovery of DPOAEs to baseline levels at 2 days and 1 and 2 weeks postexposure, MOLF DPOAEs had essentially returned to their pre-exposure levels by 1 to 2 weeks postexposure. In combination, findings in inbred mouse models of NIHL provide the basis for applying suitable molecular techniques that permit the mapping of an NIHL gene to specific chromosomal loci (e.g., identifying differentially expressed genes using DNA microarrays and suppressive subtractive hybridization). Successful identification of this gene and perhaps its related modifier genes would have great implications for developing a diagnostic indicator of the susceptibility of a particular human ear to the adverse effects of sound overexposure.

Genetic association studies on oxidative stress genes have identified the first heritable factors that likely influence an individual's susceptibility to NIHL. Konings and coworkers[71] investigated whether variations in the form of single nucleotide polymorphisms of the catalase gene, which is one of the genes involved in oxidative stress, influenced noise susceptibility. By comparing audiometric data and DNA samples from the 10% most susceptible and 10% most resistant Swedish and Polish noise-exposed workers, significant interactions were observed between noise-exposure levels and several single nucleotide polymorphisms in both populations. These findings indicate that catalase is potentially a noise susceptibility gene.

Although the findings of more recent studies in particular have resulted in advancing our scientific knowledge of the sound-damage process, many major empirical issues remain to be satisfied. These issues include development of low-cost technical methods for controlling noise at the source, physical protection of individuals from excessive exposure, identification of individuals who are in the early stages of NIHL, prediction of the degree of risk from potentially hazardous noises, and determination of whether particular individuals or ears already damaged by noise are more susceptible to injury.

Ethical issues prevent the deliberate exposure of human subjects to extreme noises as a means of studying NIHL experimentally. The complexity of measurements demanded by the alternate cross-sectional study design that describes the hearing of humans exposed occupationally is considerable, however. These difficulties include differences inherent in the population (e.g., race, gender, presence of ear disease); problems involved in controlling concomitant exposure to no occupational noise or past exposure history; and technical problems with the descriptive techniques themselves, ranging from variability in audiometric measures to difficulties in performing valid measurements of the noise environment itself. Because of the complicated experimental designs demanded by all of these controls, there have been few faultless clinical, epidemiologic, or experimental studies of the effects of excessive noise on hearing in humans.

The importance of performing longitudinal field studies of communities or particular population segments, such as elderly individuals, children, and chronically ill individuals, who are habitually exposed to loud environmental noises produced by road traffic or aircraft, is obvious to determine effective health criteria for controlling such

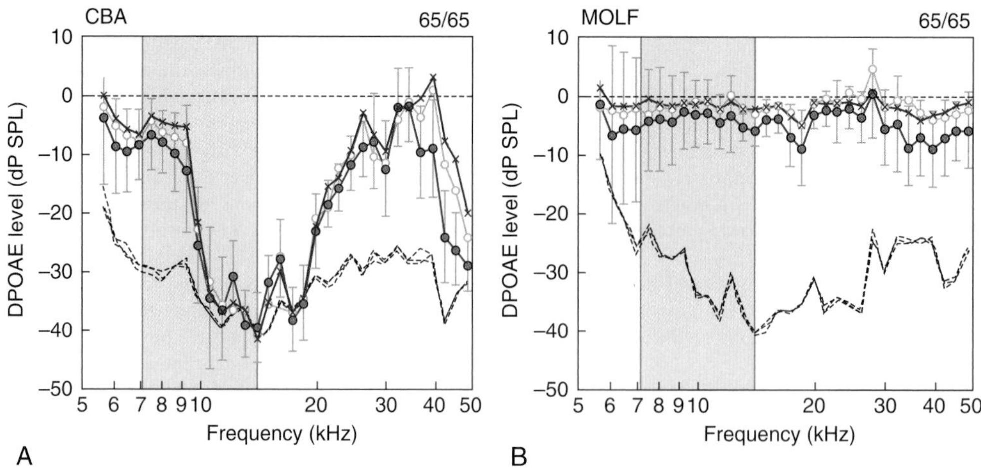

Figure 151-4. **A** and **B,** Mean difference DP-grams (i.e., pre-exposure distortion product otoacoustic emission [DPOAE] levels – postexposure DPOAE levels) for 65-dB SPL primary tones comparing effects of an extreme 8-hour exposure to a 10-kHz octave band of noise (*shaded region* from approximately 7 to 14 kHz) at 105 dB SPL for 2-month-old CBA **(A)** compared with 7-month-old MOLF **(B)** mice. *Bold horizontal dotted line* at 0 indicates no change between pre-exposure baseline DPOAE levels and postexposure counterparts measured at 2 days *(filled circles)*, 1 week *(open circles)*, and 2 weeks *(x)* after overexposure session. Note only minor recovery of DPOAEs for CBA mice between 2 days and 2 weeks postexposure, especially for frequencies greater than 30 kHz. In contrast, DPOAEs for MOLF mice essentially returned to baseline values. Although not shown here, immediately after exposure, both strains exhibited essentially no DPOAEs greater than approximately 10 kHz. Noise-floor differences *(dashed lines without symbols in lower portion of plots)* represent pre-exposure DPOAEs subtracted from postexposure noise floors to indicate maximum possible DPOAE loss. *Vertical bars* represent ±1 SD for 2 days postexposure. CBA, n = 10, 19 ears; MOLF, n = 8, 15 ears.

noises. Most notably, a great disadvantage in gaining a more complete understanding of NIHL in humans is that there have been no more recent studies of the hearing status of contemporary workers, at least in the countries of North America and Europe. Reliance on data collected 30 or more years ago, such as those illustrated in Figure 151-2,[7] has likely resulted in underestimates of the amount of hearing loss that is due to occupational noise, especially for individuals with intermittent or impulsive noise exposures.

Early Detection of Noise-Induced Hearing Loss

One aspect of NIHL that has not received a great deal of research attention is the development of more sensitive measures that are capable of detecting small acoustically induced injuries to the organ of Corti (i.e., the beginning stages of NIHL) so that individuals vulnerable to the long-term damage caused by continuous exposure can be identified. In recent years, evidence has been accumulating that the routine audiometric testing of behavioral thresholds to pure tones at octave intervals does not meet this need because by the time such a loss is identified using methods that test behavioral hearing sensitivity, permanent cochlear damage has occurred. Many threshold and suprathreshold psychoacoustic tests to detect subtle deteriorations in hearing acuity, including psychophysical tuning curves and frequency discrimination tasks, either have not proved to be of general usefulness or have proved to be too cumbersome methodologically to implement in a clinical or workplace setting because of the limitations associated with the necessarily brief evaluation periods.

The diagnostic technique incorporating OAEs is ideal for assessing the normality of cochlear processing in ears suspected of being overstimulated by loud sound because of its well-recognized sensitivity to the OHC class of receptor cell, which is primarily involved in the initial stages of NIHL. The functional status of OHCs in established instances of NIHL has been well described in many more recent studies on the practical applicability of evoked OAE testing in the audiology clinic.[72] Numerous reports in the literature have shown that in groups of noise-exposed humans who have been followed serially, reductions in OAE levels are more sensitive than pure-tone audiometric thresholds in detecting the early states of permanent noise-induced cochlear damage.[73-77] In these studies, decreases in emission magnitudes were measured in the absence of any change in the corresponding audiometric threshold frequencies.

In Figure 151-5, the ability of the two major types of evoked OAEs, the DPOAE, in its DP-gram form depicting emission level as a function of the f_2 test frequency (*lower left* in Fig. 151-5), and the transient-evoked OAE (TEOAE), elicited by clicks, in its spectral form (*right plots* in Fig. 151-5), to describe the configuration of a developing NIHL is illustrated. The 43-year-old woman in this example had participated in recreational rifle shooting for 3 years before OAE testing, and she claimed to have worn protective headphone devices continuously during this period. This right-shouldered shooter presented in the otology clinic with complaints of hearing loss, tinnitus, muffled hearing, and difficulty in understanding speech in background noise. It is clear from the test results that the magnitude and frequency extents of the TEOAEs reflected the pattern of normal hearing illustrated by the clinical audiogram at top left of Figure 151-5. The DP-gram clearly shows abnormal activity, however, with the right ear showing below-average response levels and the left ear exhibiting a significant reduction in emitted responses for frequencies greater than 3 kHz. True to classic principles, the left ear, which was exposed more to the muzzle end of the gun, went unprotected by the head-shadow effect. This example of the ability of evoked OAEs to detect cochlear pathology caused by noise exposure attests to the potential usefulness of emission procedures in identifying the primary site of pathology associated with hearing complaints secondary to a sensorineural loss, and in monitoring the development of potential hearing impairments in hearing-conservation programs.

Other evidence supporting the usefulness of evoked OAEs in examining patients with noise damage is illustrated in Figures 151-6 and 151-7. In Figure 151-6, the results of OAE testing in a 21-year-old man, who had just completed 3 years of military service in the infantry, show the precision of DPOAEs in particular in tracking the asymmetric pattern of hearing loss for this left-handed shooter. Additionally, the OAE findings presented in Figure 151-7 show the ability of evoked emissions to reflect accurately the magnitude and frequency extent of the more severe, but essentially symmetric hearing loss experienced by a 49-year-old man who had been working for more than 20 years in a fish cannery.

Both examples attest to several other benefits of OAE testing in NIHL patients. A significant advantage of the digital hearing aid over

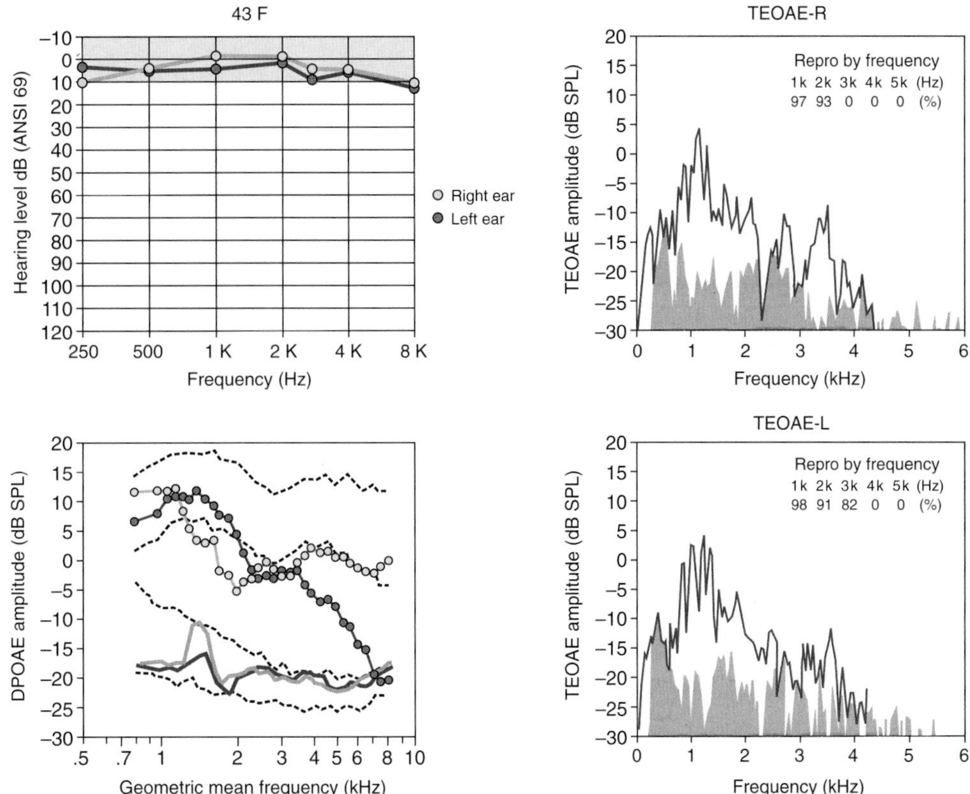

Figure 151-5. Early detection of noise-induced hearing loss in a 43-year-old female rifle shooter who complained of muffled hearing, tinnitus, and difficulty hearing speech in background noise. Note normal pure-tone audiogram bilaterally *(top left)*. In corresponding DP-grams at *lower left,* greater functional loss in the left *(red circles)* compared with the right *(yellow circles)* ear, particularly for frequencies greater than 3 kHz, was due to protective head-shadow effect for this right-handed individual. Emission levels for $2f_1$-f_2 distortion product otoacoustic emission (DPOAE) are plotted in response to 75-dB SPL primary tones as a function of geometric mean of two eliciting stimuli (f_1, f_2). Spectral plots of click-evoked otoacoustic emissions are shown on the *right* (transient-evoked otoacoustic emission [TEOAE]). Emitted response *(open area)* for the better-functioning right (R) ear was more prominently distributed above related noise floor *(shaded area)* than were emissions for the left (L) ear for frequencies greater than 3 kHz. In addition, higher "Repro" values for the right ear *(top right of each plot)* reflected its more robust activity levels. In DP-gram plot, variability of emission level (±1 SD) in normal-hearing ears is represented by *bold dashed lines in top portion of plot*. Similar variability of related noise floor is indicated by pair of *shorter dashed lines along bottom of plot.*

the older analog models is its ability to provide frequency-specific amplification based on the configuration of a particular patient's hearing loss. Knowledge of the pattern of surviving OHCs in an impaired ear based on tests of OAEs and particularly the DP-gram can assist the clinician in achieving an optimal match between the patterns of hearing-aid amplification and hearing loss.

Also, especially important to hearing conservation is the correct identification of individuals exhibiting pseudohypacusis, who seek monetary compensation for a purported work-related hearing impairment. An example of this application is illustrated in Figure 151-8 for a 42-year-old man who was referred to the audiology clinic for assessment by a local worker's compensation committee. In this case, the patient claimed to have poor hearing caused by on-the-job exposure to intense noise to the extent that he could not hear frequencies greater than about 4 kHz. According to the OAE findings, it is likely that the patient, a wood-lathe operator, had an asymmetric noise-related hearing loss that was worse in the ear (right) that was more exposed to the tool. Based on the type of hearing-loss data presented in Figure 151-1A for an industrial worker, however, it is unlikely that lathe-related noises could cause such a profound deafness for frequencies greater than 4 kHz. Additionally, the normal levels of DPOAEs and TEOAEs for frequencies less than 2 kHz do not support the patient's claim that the elevated audiometric hearing levels over the low-frequency to midfrequency regions were due to noise overexposure. Findings such as these support the use of objective tests of evoked OAEs in determining the authenticity of compensation claims for work-related hearing problems.

Interactive Effects

It is well established that noise in combination with certain chemical agents produces stronger reactions than each stimulus applied singly. The four major categories of ototoxic drugs are aminoglycoside antibiotics, platinum derivative antitumor agents, "loop" diuretics, and salicylates. The latter two classes of drug cause reversible effects, whereas aminoglycosides and platinum derivatives cause permanent damage to the inner ear and to hearing. Many laboratories have established in animal models that kanamycin, neomycin, or amikacin applied in combination with different types of noise produces a marked potentiating interaction.[78,79] Other studies of the temporal aspects of interactive effects indicate that the degree of potentiating interaction is the same whether the drug is given concurrently with the noise exposure or several months later.[80] Other evidence from humans[81] and controlled laboratory research in a rat model[82] indicates that additional loss may occur when subjects are treated with aspirin and exposed to noise concomitantly, although other findings infer that the combination of salicylate plus noise does not produce greater effects than noise alone.[83] Finally, experimental evidence in several animal models showed that the heavy-metal, antineoplastic agent *cis*-diamminedichloroplatinum, commonly known as cisplatin, significantly increased the amount of hearing and sensory cell losses from exposure to noise.[84,85]

In recent years, the interactive effects of noise with chemical agents common to industry and the environment have been reported. In a series of experimental studies in the rat model, Fechter and colleagues[86] discovered that the simultaneous exposure to noise and the environ-

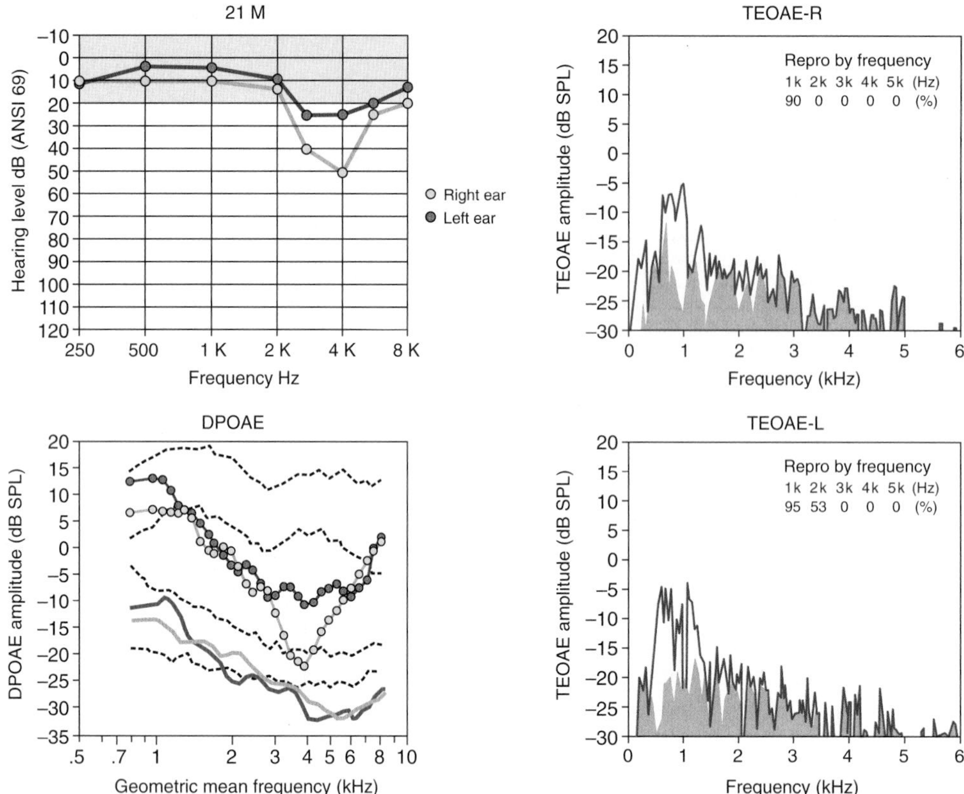

Figure 151-6. Early stages of noise-induced hearing loss in a 21-year-old military veteran, who had just completed a 3-year tour of duty. For this left-handed infantryman, note greater hearing loss from approximately 3 to 4 kHz for the right ear *(yellow circles)* depicted in the audiogram *(top left)*. In corresponding DP-gram, note abnormally low levels of distortion product otoacoustic emission (DPOAE) activity for frequencies greater than 1.5 kHz, which were poorer for the right ear. Click-evoked otoacoustic emission spectra on the *right* (transient-evoked otoacoustic emission [TEOAE]) also show poorer emitted responses from 1 to 2 kHz and lower "Repro" values for the right (R) ear. There is no emitted response for either ear greater than 2 kHz. See legend for Figure 151-5 for an explanation of click-evoked spectra and two sets of *dashed lines* in DP-gram.

mental pollutants carbon monoxide or hydrogen cyanide produced more permanent hearing loss at the high frequencies than the sum of the losses produced by each agent administered alone. Various other chemicals present in the environment as commercial products or chemical intermediaries and contaminants, such as the organic solvents toluene and hexane, the pollutants methyl mercury and lead acetate, and the organic compounds trimethyltin chloride and styrene used in the manufacture of plastics and polyurethane foam and rubber, have been identified as potent ototoxic agents that potentially interact synergistically with excessive noises. The ototoxicity of environmental agents such as metals, solvents, and asphyxiants and their interaction with noise are issues that have received a great deal of attention in the literature.[87] Although many of these environmental toxicants have been associated with direct injury to inner ear structures, possible additional anatomic damage to more central auditory pathways is also very likely.

Other Adverse Effects Caused by Noise

Damage to the vestibular system is a potential problem with noise because balance receptors are coupled physically with the auditory receptors; that is, they share the membranous labyrinth. In addition to the anatomic proximity of the vestibular labyrinth to the acoustic-energy delivery system, the great similarity in cochlear and vestibular hair cell ultrastructure, and the common arterial blood supply of the cochlea and vestibular end organs via the same end artery support the possibility of vestibular damage associated with NIHL. Theoretically, the limiting membrane, the membranous partition that separates the utricle and semicircular canals from the rest of the vestibule, protects most vestibular sensory cells from the adverse effects of intensive stapes vibration.

Nevertheless, some studies of industrial workers and military personnel have reported a high occurrence of vestibular symptoms and signs, and complaints of dysequilibrium.[88] Such simple correlations between noise exposure and vestibular disturbances are highly controversial because of the typical low incidence of clinical vestibular symptoms associated with gradually developing NIHL.[89] A study of military personnel with mild to severe NIHL using sophisticated vestibular testing in the form of a computerized rotatory-chair system along with routine electronystagmographic measures of caloric responses showed more direct correlations between hearing loss and vestibular upset.[90] In combination, the results showed a symmetrically centrally compensated decrease in the response of the vestibular end organ that was associated with a symmetric hearing loss. A more recent study[91] combining caloric testing with vestibular-evoked myogenic potentials in patients with chronic NIHL showed absent or delayed electrophysiologic potentials, indicating that the vestibular system, especially the sacculocollic reflex pathway, was damaged in addition to the cochlear portion of the inner ear.

Together, these findings imply that a subclinical, well-compensated malfunction of the vestibular system is associated with NIHL. Beyond the medicolegal implications is the daunting possibility that a currently asymptomatic vestibulopathy produced by noise exposure might progress to a disturbing vertigo under certain environmental conditions.[92]

There has been considerable interest more recently in the interaction of vibration and noise, which are common cofactors in the workplace. Although most research shows that vibration alone does not affect hearing, the results of epidemiologic studies in humans and controlled laboratory studies in animal models indicate a synergistic

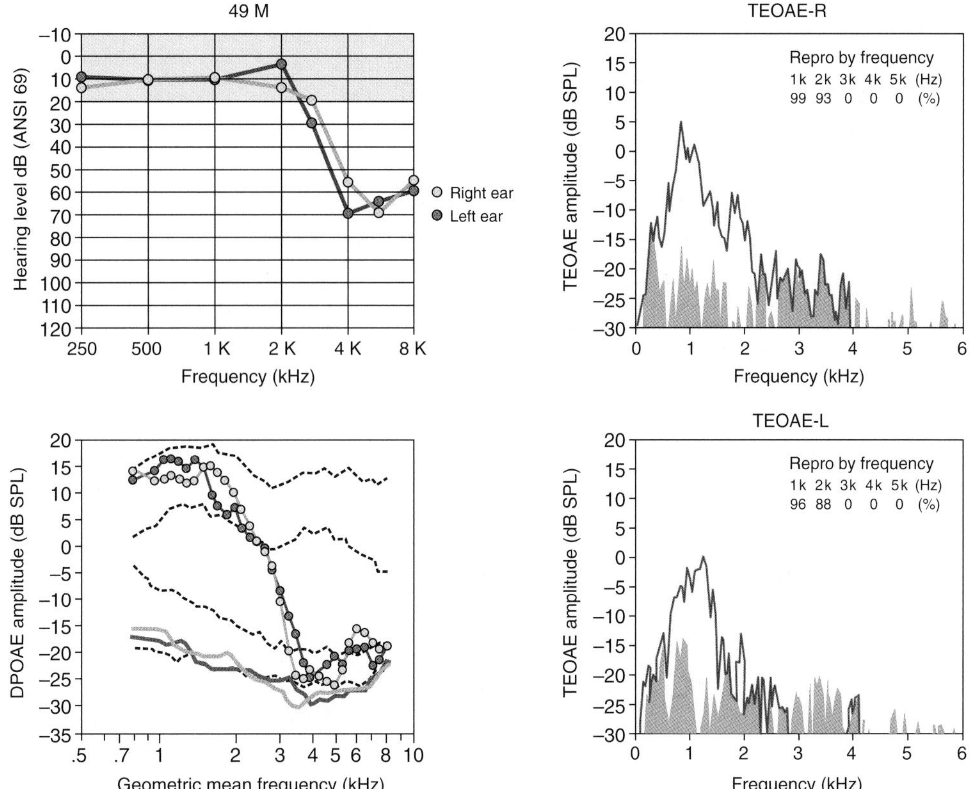

Figure 151-7. More advanced stage of noise-induced hearing loss for a 49-year-old man, who had worked for more than 20 years in a fish cannery. Audiograms at *top left* exhibit symmetric hearing loss for frequencies greater than 2 kHz. DP-grams indicate symmetric pattern of dysfunction in a similar manner. Click-evoked otoacoustic emission spectra on the *right* (transient-evoked otoacoustic emission [TEOAE]) also show a lack of emitted responses for frequencies greater than 2 kHz. See legend for Figure 151-5 for an explanation of click-evoked spectra and two sets of *dashed lines* in DP-grams. DPOAE, distortion product otoacoustic emission.

interaction of concomitant vibration (either whole-body or hand-arm) and noise that results in an increase in the degree of NIHL.[93]

Exposure to infra-frequency and ultra-frequency sounds outside of the human hearing range has also been studied. Infrasonic or vibratory stimuli are defined as sounds in the range of 0.1 to 20 Hz. There are no known instances in which infrasound alone clearly caused permanent damage to the human cochlea. Studies in the chinchilla model showed, however, that the presence of intense sounds in the audible frequency range along with simultaneous infrasound increases cochlear damage.[94]

In contrast, some reports have shown detrimental effects of microwaves on hearing.[95] The thermal properties of ultra-high-frequency sound waves in the gigahertz range, rather than mechanical energy, seem to have produced these adverse experimental effects. Overall, it is probably safe to conclude that the auditory system's built-in, middle ear filter limits the extreme frequencies of sound that are hazardous to the inner ear.[96]

Magnetic resonance imaging (MRI) systems have acoustic noise associated with their clinical scanning actions. For specific protocols that are incorporating faster and noisier sequences, peaks of 120 to 130 dBA have been measured, particularly during high-speed echoplanar imaging.[97] Early on, Brummett and associates[98] showed that sounds generated by MRI are sufficiently intense to cause some TTS in a significant number of patients. Their results also showed, however, that earplugs help attenuate the noise sufficiently to prevent TTS in most patients undergoing MRI evaluation. The use of the higher gradient fields that are applied at faster slew rates, which are used in current functional MRI, demands increased hearing protection systems to minimize the risk of noise trauma.[99]

Other nonauditory problems concern the general bothersome or fatiguing effects of noise, which may lead to nonspecific health disorders because of interference with the restorative processes associated with rest and sleep. In conditions of chronic exposure, noise is considered to act as a biologic stressor that can lead to prolonged activation of the autonomic nervous system and the pituitary-adrenal complex, resulting in general health impairment.[100] Noise has also been related to disorders involving gastrointestinal motility, such as peptic ulcers,[101] and, as noted earlier, to circulatory problems such as hypertension.[102] Certain types of noise can be annoying and lead to emotional unrest.[103] Finally, noise can have a deleterious effect on task performance, especially if speech understanding is involved.[104] Generally, data relevant to the nonauditory effects of noise tend to be inconclusive because the variables are difficult to identify and isolate for objective study.

Legal Issues

One practical issue that the lawmakers of industrialized societies have had to consider concerns the balancing of two conflicting goals: How can laborers be protected against the hazards of the workplace without placing an enormous financial burden on society, either by satisfying compensatory obligations or by preventing such work-related effects through costly engineering modifications of the industrial process? Over the years, concerns about protecting the public and work force from environmental insults such as noise have been written into a combination of law and governmental regulations. Federal, state, and community legislative and regulatory actions are continually being reviewed and altered. Although the purpose of this review is not to detail such legal controls, regarding either their historical development or their current status, a brief discussion is appropriate. For a lucid analysis of governmental statutes and regulations pertaining to noise control, see the review by Dobie.[6]

The major difficulty encountered in composing regulatory control has been in defining in practical terms what constitutes a hazardous noise. The equal-energy principle[105] embodies one popular approach toward expressing the danger of a particular noise by a simple number.

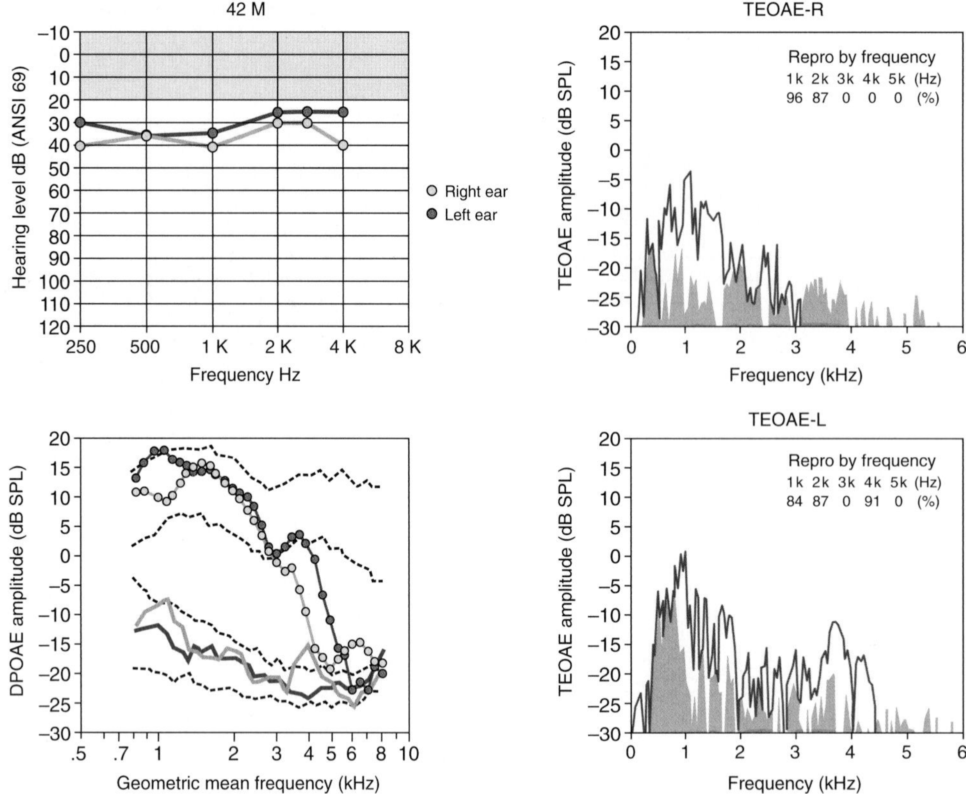

Figure 151-8. A possible case of pseudohypacusis in a 42-year-old male factory worker, who operated a wood lathe. Audiograms at *top left* show a relatively flat hearing loss up to approximately 4 kHz. For frequencies greater than 4 kHz, the patient claimed that test tones were inaudible. DP-grams show normal-like function up to approximately 3 to 4 kHz, when reductions in distortion product otoacoustic emission (DPOAE) levels are evident, occurring initially for the right ear *(yellow circles)*, which was more exposed to the lathe. Spectral plots on the *right* (transient-evoked otoacoustic emission [TEOAE]) also show poorer click-evoked otoacoustic emissions for the right ear. Together, normal levels of evoked emissions for frequencies less than 3 kHz and asymmetric pattern of reduction in otoacoustic emissions suggest that exposure to noise and aging contributed to decreased levels of activity for frequencies greater than 3 kHz. See legend for Figure 151-5 for an explanation of click-evoked spectra and two sets of *dashed lines* in DP-grams.

The equal-energy principle assumes that permanent damage to hearing is related to total sound energy, which is a product of the noise level in dBA and the duration of exposure. One tenet of this postulate is that an equal amount of noise energy causes an equal amount of hearing loss.

Burns and Robinson,[106] who investigated the hearing loss of thousands of industrial workers, concluded that the equal-energy principle could be applied to determine daily exposure doses because hearing loss caused by work-related noise exposure seemed to be a simple function of noise energy. Atherley and Martin[107] extended the concept to impulse noise by application of the equivalent continuous sound level (L_{eq}) principle. The L_{eq} is defined as the A-weighted level of a continuous, steady sound that produces, in a specified interval, an exposure that has the same total acoustic energy as that of an actual time-varying sound over the identical interval.[108] In other words, if one sound contains twice as much energy as a second sound but lasts half as long, both sounds would be characterized by the same equivalent sound level. The L_{eq} concept holds that these two exposures produce the same damage to the ear.

Although notions such as the equal-energy principle have proved useful in the practical definition of noise-control variables, their validity has been more difficult to establish. Over the years, experimental evidence has been conflicting in that it has tended to be either for or against the equal-energy rule. Generally, it seems that the principle cannot be generalized indiscriminantly to stimuli throughout the range of noise parameters because exposure to impulse or intermittent noises may lead to more or less degeneration in the organ of Corti than would be expected according to the equal-energy principle. Some aspect of the equal-energy concept has been adopted by most industrialized nations, however, including the United States, as a means of measuring the potential hazard of a particular noise exposure. Present regulations use a 5-dB exchange rate, along with a 90-dBA time-weighted average to define the permissible exposure limit over an 8-hour work day.[109] Consequently, exposure to 90 dBA for 8 hours is equivalent in sound-energy terms to an exposure of 85 dBA for half that time (i.e., 4 hours).

Currently, industries that employ laborers who work where noise is greater than 85 dB SPL implement a hearing-conservation program consisting of several components as dictated by the U.S. Occupational Safety and Health Administration (OSHA).[109] First, pre-employment audiometric assessment and annual audiometric monitoring are required so that noise-induced cochlear impairment can be detected before becoming too severe. When a hearing loss is identified, the worker must be notified of the disorder and counseled about the use of personal hearing protectors. The second portion of the conservation program requires workers in areas of high-noise levels (≥85 dBA) to wear ear protectors and to participate in a noise education program that informs the employee of the hazardous effects and the correct fitting of personal protectors. An important part of hearing conservation is the otologic referral (see next), which is essential when in-plant audiometry has detected a substantial hearing loss.

Role of the Otolaryngologist

Patients with NIHL constitute a notable portion of an otolaryngologist's patient population, particularly for otolaryngologists who are in private practice. With the increase in the population older than 65 years, the psychological, economic, and social impact of NIHL is still growing. Modern stereo systems in the form of personal music players such as the MP3 and iPod systems have sufficient noise levels and listening durations to put consumers at risk for developing NIHL.[110,111] The widespread use of these devices, particularly among children and adolescents, is a growing worry,[112] particularly as reported by the mainstream media. Such concern is supported by the finding uncovered in the audiometric database of a large-scale national cross-sectional survey of an accelerating prevalence of sensorineural hearing loss in young adults 20 to 29 years old.[113] This growing prevalence of a high-frequency hearing loss in young adults may relate to an increase in personal stereo player use. The outcome of at least one relevant experimental study using similarly aged subjects, who were systematically exposed to music from an MP3 player at their preferred listening levels, does not agree with this explanation, however.[114] In any case, otolaryngologists are expected to continue to be conspicuously involved with the problem of NIHL.

Although a known prevention exists, it is unlikely for fiscal and technical reasons that the general loud sound levels of our environment will be reduced. Although the inhalation of hyperoxygenated air as a prophylaxis[115] has been proposed, and, as noted previously, clinical trials on the safety and efficacy of certain antioxidant compounds to prevent or reverse NIHL are currently in progress, to date, no proven treatment or cure for noise damage exists. Consequently, detecting the early stages of NIHL is important to prevent further injury to the crucial sensory-cell receptors of the organ of Corti.

The role of the otolaryngologist is first to identify the cause and extent of a reported hearing loss through systematic medical and audiometric evaluation. As part of the course of otologic management, the patient should be educated about the hazards of noise, and about preventive measures to preserve remaining hearing. The physician should make basic decisions about the appropriate aural rehabilitative course of action. Finally, the otolaryngologist should be sensitive to any emotional problems the patient may have in accepting a hearing impairment, which may be dealt with by counseling or special provisions.

Although NIHL is not medically or surgically treatable, it is almost entirely preventable. Its prevention requires education, engineering, and administrative controls, and the proper use of hearing protection. One of the otolaryngologist's most important contributions is in teaching the patient to guard against further losses.[116] When recommending the use of personal hearing protectors or reinforcing compliance with ongoing hearing-protection measures, the physician should be aware that the commonly used personal protectors in the form of inserted earplugs or earmuffs vary considerably in effectiveness, and produce an attenuation that is highly frequency dependent.[117,118] When sealed correctly into the ear canal, earplugs reduce the noise reaching the middle ear by 15 to 30 dB, and work best for the midfrequency to higher frequency range (i.e., 2 to 5 kHz). Earmuffs are more effective protectors, especially for frequencies between 500 Hz and 1 kHz, where noise is attenuated by 30 to 40 dB.[119] In areas with extremely high noise levels, earplugs do not afford sufficient protection, and individuals should be advised to wear both earplugs and earmuffs. Also, sound energy associated with high noise levels may reach the inner ear by passing through vibrating bone and tissues adjacent to the ear. Bone-conduction and tissue-conduction thresholds set a practical limit to the possible attenuation provided by hearing-protection devices.

A final point concerning the use of hearing protectors should be impressed on the patient. When data relating the maximal protection in dBA to the percentage of time that the devices are worn are considered, it is clear that hearing protectors should be worn all the time because if they are removed for even a few minutes, their effective cumulative attenuation capability is severely reduced. Removing hearing protection for only 15 minutes of an 8-hour work shift can cut protection efficacy in half. Similarly, a poorly fitting hearing protector does not prevent hearing loss.[1]

In many states, compensation is available for occupational NIHL. Physicians are required sometimes to serve as expert witnesses as to the probable cause of a claimant's hearing loss. Such medicolegal testimony requires that the patient undergo careful otologic and audiometric evaluation so that hearing losses caused by unrelated ear disorders, such as cerumen impaction, middle ear effusion, aging, genetic deficits, otosclerosis, and an array of other ear diseases (e.g., Meniere's disease, acoustic neuroma), can be excluded. To permit the reversible (i.e., TTS) effects to recover, most states require a recovery time (ranging from 14 "quiet" hours to 24 weeks) away from the occupational noise source before audiometric assessment. By ruling out organic disease, giving careful attention to the history of job-related and recreation-related noise exposure, and documenting the extent and degree of involvement of both ears, an informed decision concerning any causal relationship between the noted disability and the work environment can be made.

Hearing impairment is the medical term used to refer to the hearing level at which individuals begin to experience difficulties in everyday life. Hearing impairment manifests in practical terms, such as a difficulty in understanding speech. By the time an individual becomes aware of decreased speech intelligibility, considerable damage to the organ of Corti likely has occurred because speech reception is not altered greatly until a hearing loss is more than 40 dB. The amount of loss at frequencies most important to speech (i.e., at 2 kHz, 3 kHz, and 4 kHz) is used by OSHA[108] as a basis for calculating amounts of compensation because NIHL occurs initially at greater than or equal to 2 kHz. The measure of hearing impairment is called the hearing handicap, which is always based on the functional state of both ears. An official guide devised by the American Academy of Otolaryngology–Head and Neck Surgery[120] provides a detailed explanation of how to evaluate and compute an NIHL handicap. Generally, the disability benefits of the U.S. Social Security Administration[121,122] are less generous than are the benefits for either military veterans or typical worker's compensation programs.

Because of an increasingly noisy environment and the probability that many individuals will unwittingly sustain hearing losses because of exposure to loud sounds at home, on the job, and during recreational activity, otolaryngologists, along with other health care professionals dealing with hearing problems, should educate the public about hearing conservation. Such education is needed especially for children and adolescents, who, as noted previously, are regularly exposed to the amplified music associated with personal music players, stereos, dance clubs, and live concerts. A common image that can be used to motivate the public and workers in industry to be aware of the insidious damage of noise exposure is the grass metaphor representing the sensory cells of the inner ear. Typically, blades of grass straighten up after they have been bent by being walked on. If one continues to tread on the same patch day after day, however, the grass eventually dies, leaving a bare spot; this is similar to what happens to the ear's hair cells when assaulted continually by high-intensity sounds.

The physician can be particularly effective in teaching individuals how to recognize the danger signals of potential NIHL including the need to shout to be heard and the development of the sensation of pain, muffled sound, and tinnitus.[123,124] The influence of otolaryngologists as hearing experts in the areas of education and motivation can be a major force in preventing NIHL.

Summary

We know more now than ever about the workings of the human ear, including how it responds initially to excessive sound, and how it eventually fails to reverse the progressive damage. We also know how much more we need to learn about basic ear processes before such damage can be corrected. As understanding of the fundamental mechanisms involved in the process of NIHL progresses, developing a medical intervention to minimize permanent injury seems achievable. In the meantime, we know what needs to be done to prevent or check the damage process. In light of the economic impracticability of noise control at the engineering or administrative level, especially in industry, it seems that education of the public about the potential hazards of excessive sound and the beneficial use of protective devices will be the major weapons against NIHL. Consequently, the educational role of otolaryngologists is paramount for the conservation of hearing that is threatened by habitual noise exposure.

Acknowledgments

The authors acknowledge the long-time support of the National Institutes of Health (NIDCD) to their programs of research (DC00613,

DC03114), and Barden B. Stagner, for conducting data analysis and assisting with assembling the illustrations used here.

SUGGESTED READINGS

Bogoch II, House RA, Kudla I. Perceptions about hearing protection and noise-induced hearing loss of attendees of rock concerts. *Can J Public Health.* 2005;96:69-72.

Carlsson PI, Van Laer L, Borg E, et al. The influence of genetic variation in oxidative stress genes on human noise susceptibility. *Hear Res.* 2005;202:87-96.

Darrat I, Ahmad N, Seidman K, et al. Auditory research involving antioxidants. *Curr Opin Otolaryngol Head Neck Surg.* 2007;15:358-363.

Davis RR, Kozel P, Erway LC. Genetic influences in individual susceptibility to noise: a review. *Noise Health.* 2003;5:19-28.

Dobie RA. The burdens of age-related and occupational noise-induced hearing loss in the United States. *Ear Hear.* 2008;29:565-577.

Fechter LD. Promotion of noise-induced hearing loss by chemical contaminants. *J Toxicol Environ Health A.* 2004;67:727-740.

Folmer RL, Griest SE, Martin WH. Hearing conservation education programs for children: a review. *J Sch Health.* 2002;72:51-57.

Kanzaki S, Kawamoto K, Oh SH, et al. From gene identification to gene therapy. *Audiol Neurootol.* 2002;7:161-164.

For complete list of references log onto www.expertconsult.com.

Kujawa SG, Liberman MC. Acceleration of age-related hearing loss by early noise exposure: evidence of a misspent youth. *J Neurosci.* 2006;26:2115-2123.

Lefebvre PP, Malgrange B, Lallemend F, et al. Mechanisms of cell death in the injured auditory system: otoprotective strategies. *Audiol Neurootol.* 2002;7:165-170.

Le Prell CG, Dolan DF, Schacht J, et al. Pathways for protection from noise induced hearing loss. *Noise Health.* 2003;5:1-17.

Lynch ED, Kil J. Compounds for the prevention and treatment of noise-induced hearing loss. *Drug Discov Today.* 2005;10:1291-1298.

Niu X, Canlon B. Protective mechanisms of sound conditioning. *Adv Otorhinolaryngol.* 2002;59:96-105.

Ohlemiller KK. Contributions of mouse models to understanding of age- and noise-related hearing loss. *Brain Res.* 2006;1091:89-102.

Rosenhall U. The influence of ageing on noise-induced hearing loss. *Noise Health.* 2003;5:47-53.

Sisto R, Chelotti S, Moriconi L, et al. Otoacoustic emission sensitivity to low levels of noise-induced hearing loss. *J Acoust Soc Am.* 2007;122:387-401.

Toppila E, Pyykko I, Starck J. Age and noise-induced hearing loss. *Scand Audiol.* 2001;30:236-244.

Wagner W, Heppelmann G, Kuehn M, et al. Olivocochlear activity and temporary threshold shift-susceptibility in humans. *Laryngoscope.* 2005;115:2021-2028.

Williams W. Noise exposure levels from personal stereo use. *Int J Audiol.* 2005;44:231-236.

Infections of the Labyrinth

Larry E. Davis

Key Points

- RNA and DNA viruses, bacteria, and fungi cause infections of the human labyrinth in fetuses, children, and adults.
- Selective vulnerability of inner ear structures varies by the virus, and results in different inner ear pathologies.
- Some viruses and bacteria primarily destroy sensorineural epithelium causing permanent hearing loss, whereas other viruses, such as cytomegalovirus, cause little direct damage to cochlear sensorineural structures, and apparently cause deafness by another mechanism.
- The precise role viral infections play in sudden sensorineural hearing loss, vestibular neuritis, and Meniere's disease is unclear.
- There is increasing evidence that hearing loss from otosclerosis is associated with a persistent rubeola virus infection of the stapes footplate.
- There currently are no good antiviral agents for most viruses that infect the inner ear.
- Administration of mumps, rubella, rubeola, and varicella-zoster vaccines is the best method to prevent viral inner ear infections.
- Placement of cochlear implants is successful treatment for children born with congenital deafness from cytomegalovirus or rubella.

Infectious agents, particularly viruses and bacteria, are thought to play a direct or indirect role in causing several inner ear disorders.[1] Each year, several thousand infants are born deaf or with impaired hearing. At least 18% of these cases are proven to be caused by congenital viral infection, and a greater percentage are suspected to have an infectious cause.[2] Each year, about 10 out of every 100,000 individuals are stricken by so-called sudden deafness, which occurs as unilateral or bilateral sensorineural hearing loss (SNHL) of varying degrees.[3] Infectious agents are often suspected as the cause. Bacterial labyrinthitis with profound hearing loss occurs in 10% of patients with bacterial meningitis.[4] Thousands of individuals each year have vestibular neuritis, which many authors think has an infectious origin.[5]

Although many infectious agents are thought to play important etiologic roles in labyrinthine disorders, there are many difficulties in proving that a given infectious agent infects the human labyrinth.[1]

1. Otologic examination shows the degree of functional deficit of the inner ear, but seldom establishes the cause.

2. Cranial computed tomography (CT) shows the shape of the bony labyrinth, but does not show the membranous labyrinth or facial nerve.

3. Resolution of cranial magnetic resonance imaging (MRI) is presently insufficient to show clearly details of the membranous labyrinth.

4. The inner ear is encased within a dense temporal bone, making viral culture of inner ear fluids or tissue from the spiral or vestibular ganglia difficult and seldom done.

5. Acute hearing loss or vertigo is rarely fatal; acute inner ear tissue is rarely available from autopsies.

6. The temporal bone is seldom removed at routine autopsies, so inner ear tissue seldom becomes available for histologic examination even when the illness was remote.

7. Decalcification of temporal bones is slow (months), and often involves agents such as nitric acid that damage the inner ear tissue morphology, often making the tissue inadequate for immunohistochemical studies.

8. Serologic studies can determine that an individual was infected by a given virus, but do not prove the virus caused the labyrinthine damage.

9. Serologic studies of herpes simplex virus (HSV) are difficult to interpret because studies of healthy individuals show that fourfold increases and decreases in HSV antibody titers commonly occur without disease.[6]

10. Isolation of virus from the mouth or nasopharynx does not imply that the virus caused the inner ear damage. HSV and adenoviruses are commonly latent in humans and are intermittently shed in the oropharynx.[7] Other viruses, such as enteroviruses, can be isolated from the throats or stool of asymptomatic individuals, especially when the virus is prevalent in the community.[7]

11. HSV and varicella-zoster virus (VZV) (and likely other herpesviruses) can establish viral latency in neuronal populations and never reactivate during the life of the individual. Detection of viral nucleic acid by polymerase chain reaction (PCR) within neurons does not in itself prove that the latent virus was the cause of the tissue damage.

Establishing whether a given virus is the cause of the patient's deafness or vertigo is difficult. The criteria in Box 152-1 are proposed for determining causality.

Box 152-1

Optimal Proof for Infectious Cause of Inner Ear Infection

1. Clinical association of infectious agent with a specific cochlear or vestibular syndrome
   Epidemiologic studies of infectious agent and syndrome
   Clinical studies of syndrome and isolation of infectious agent at other sites or serologic antibody titer rise
2. Clear evidence of infectious agent presence within inner ear tissue
   Isolation of infectious agent RNA (vRNA) or messenger RNA (mRNA) (excluding mRNA latency-associated transcripts) in inner ear tissue
   Histologic demonstration in inner ear tissue by electron microscopy of infectious agent or by light microscopy finding of inclusion bodies or characteristic cell morphology plus isolation of infectious agent at other body sites
3. In experimental animals, demonstration that suspect infectious agent can cause similar auditory or vestibular signs and inner ear pathology

Modified from Davis LE. Neurovirology of deafness, labyrinthitis and Bell's palsy. In: Johnson RT, ed. *Neurovirology*. Minneapolis: American Academy of Neurology; 2002.

PCR has become a powerful tool in the detection of nucleic acid from infectious agents in human tissues. PCR is difficult to use, however, when tissues, such as temporal bones, have been fixed in formalin and decalcified for weeks with nitric acid. Formalin fixation cross-links DNA and RNA, and nitric acid harms nucleic acids. PCR has been helpful in analyzing small amounts of fresh perilymph removed during surgery and detecting cytomegalovirus (CMV).[8-10]

At present, an unresolved controversy exists regarding the significance of detection of latent herpesvirus DNA in human tissue. Several PCR studies have detected HSV DNA in neurons at autopsy from previously healthy patients from several sites, including the brainstem and cerebral cortex[11] and spiral and vestibular ganglia.[12-14] To date, culture of neuronal explants from these sites has not yielded isolation of HSV similar to culture of trigeminal or sacral ganglia.[15] Clear evidence for the breaking of viral latency and subsequent viral replication currently is lacking. It is unclear whether vestibular and cochlear neurons are dead-end cells, capable of developing latency, but incapable or poorly capable of breaking latency. The latter possibility might allow for occasional patients developing a solitary episode of vestibular neuritis or sudden hearing loss, whereas many patients develop repeated episodes of lip or genital HSV blisters from repeated breakage of latency in the trigeminal and sacral ganglia.

To date, only a few infectious agents have been recovered from or identified within human labyrinthine tissues. CMV[8,9,16] and mumps virus[17] have been isolated from perilymph. CMV antigen has been detected by immunohistochemistry within inner ear tissues.[16,18] Morphologic identification of infectious agents within the labyrinth has been accomplished for several bacteria,[19,20] fungi,[20,21] and *Treponema pallidum*.[22] A multinucleated giant cell, typical of rubeola (measles) virus infection, has been seen within the scala vestibuli.[22] HSV DNA[10,12,23] has been identified within vestibular and cochlear ganglia neurons by PCR assay. One study reported detection of HSV DNA by PCR in vestibular labyrinth tissue.[24] To date, intranuclear inclusion bodies or viral antigens have not been identified within inner ear tissues.

Although rubella has been closely associated epidemiologically with congenital deafness, and has been isolated from many sites in congenitally deaf infants, the virus has never been isolated from or viral antigens have never been identified within inner ear tissues. Histopathologic changes of the temporal bone are not specific for rubella. Nevertheless, available evidence strongly argues that rubella can cause congenital deafness.

Box 152-2

Infectious Agents Associated with Acquired Sudden Sensorineural Hearing Loss or Vertigo*

Viruses
Mumps
Herpes simplex
Epstein-Barr
Varicella zoster
Hepatitis viruses
Adenovirus
Enterovirus
Lassa fever
Rubella
Yellow fever
Variola (smallpox)
Measles (rubeola)
Influenza B virus
Influenza A virus
Parainfluenza
Western equine encephalitis
St. Louis encephalitis
Encephalomyocarditis
Russian-spring-summer encephalitis
Tick-borne encephalitis
Lymphocytic choriomeningitis
Hantavirus

Bacteria
Borrelia burgdorferi
Treponema pallidum
Mycoplasma pneumoniae
Brucella sp
Mycobacterium tuberculosis

Fungi
Cryptococcus neoformans

Rickettsia
Rickettsia prowazekii

***Bold** indicates the most common causes.

It is assumed that infectious agents are not normally present in the membranous labyrinth or adjacent ganglia; isolation of an infectious agent from the inner ear carries considerable etiologic significance. This assumption is not based on comprehensive bacteriologic or virologic studies, however. Healthy guinea pigs may harbor herpeslike viruses in the spiral ganglia neurons.[25,26]

Many infectious agents have been reported to be associated with deafness or vertigo. For some infectious agents, the association has been based on case reports that describe acute deafness or vertigo that developed during a systemic infection. For other infectious agents (e.g., rubella), the epidemiologic association has been strong between systemic infection of the individual or mother, and subsequent deafness or vertigo. Box 152-2 lists infectious agents that have been associated with deafness or vertigo, but have yet to fulfill the criteria for optimal proof of causality.

Congenital Hearing Loss

Cytomegalovirus

Clinical Features

CMV is the most common infectious cause of congenital hearing loss in the United States, accounting for 2600 to 4000 cases of SNHL each year.[27,28] The incidence of congenital CMV infection is about 0.3 to 1 case/100 live births.[29-31] Less than 5% of all congenital CMV infections result in the severe infection termed *cytomegalic inclusion disease*. In this multiorgan infection, the incidence of SNHL is 50% in infants who survive the neonatal period.[32] Hearing loss when measured years later is bilateral, symmetric, and often severe.[33] High-frequency hearing loss is usually greater than lower frequency hearing loss.

Most (>95%) congenital CMV infections are silent, and the newborn appears normal at birth. When 12,371 newborns were screened for the presence of CMV in urine that would indicate a congenital infection, the incidence of SNHL was found to be 1.1/1000 live births.[30] Another study of 307 infants with asymptomatic congenital CMV infection reported 7.2% had SNHL that ranged from mild to profound.[28] Fifty percent had bilateral hearing loss, and 20% had late-onset hearing loss. Other studies have reported that 5% to 15% of children born with silent congenital CMV infection and normal hearing in the neonatal period subsequently developed mild to moderate bilateral SNHL that may be progressive.[31,34-36] Occasionally, these children progress to profound hearing loss in one or both ears. Studies estimate the prevalence of moderate or worse SNHL caused by congenital CMV to be 0.2 to 0.6 case/1000 live births.[29]

Diagnosis

Congenital CMV is diagnosed in symptomatic and asymptomatic infants by isolation of CMV from fresh urine during the first 1 to 2 weeks of life. CMV DNA can also be detected by PCR from urine, blood, cerebrospinal fluid (CSF), and infected tissues.[37] Of congenitally infected infants, 60% to 75% have detectable IgM antibodies to CMV in the umbilical cord or infant serum. Antibodies of the IgM class imply fetal synthesis because maternal IgM antibody normally does not cross the placenta. This serologic test is difficult to perform and should be done only in qualified laboratories. CMV has been isolated from the amniotic fluid of mothers with a congenitally infected fetus.[38,39] After 1 year of age, diagnosis of congenital CMV infection is very difficult. Healthy infants may acquire the virus infection asymptomatically, shedding the virus in their urine and developing antibody titers. Because most maternal infections are asymptomatic, no reliable history can be obtained retrospectively from the mother.

Temporal Bone Pathology

Limited histologic studies of infants dying with cytomegalic inclusion disease show labyrinthitis of the endolymphatic system.[18,40-43] Inclusion-bearing cells have been identified in the auditory and vestibular portions of the inner ear (Fig. 152-1). Within the cochlea, damage is most severe along the basal turn. Evaluating the condition of the organ of Corti has been difficult because of postmortem autolysis, but it seems that the major hair cell degeneration seldom occurs, and that the tectorial membrane remains normal. There is little histologic damage to the auditory and vestibular nerves along with the spiral and vestibular ganglia. Hydrops of the cochlea and saccule and collapse of Reissner's membrane have been observed. In one patient with cytomegalic inclusion disease, a thick layer of these inclusion-bearing cells was found inside the membranous walls of the utricle in the regions where dark cells are located.[41]

The temporal bones of an infant with severe cytomegalic inclusion disease and bilateral deafness who survived 14 years were studied.[44] Chronic pathologic changes were seen in the cochlear and vestibular and nonsensory tissues. Reissner's membrane was collapsed in the more apical turns. Strial atrophy and a loss of cochlear hair cells were observed along the entire length of the basilar membrane. Vestibular neuroepithelial regions were degenerated, and fibrosis was seen within the vestibular perilymphatic tissue spaces. In cochlear and vestibular spaces, isolated regions of calcifications were present. The fibrosis and calcifications suggest that late pathologic changes developed months to years after the acute viral damage had subsided.

In infants dying of cytomegalic inclusion disease, CMV antigen has been identified within cells lining the membranous labyrinth by immunofluorescent antibody staining.[41] Virus particles belonging to the herpesvirus family have been seen within cells of the membranous labyrinth by electron microscopy.[40,41]

CMV has been isolated from perilymph obtained at autopsy from an infant with cytomegalic inclusion disease.[41] CMV also has been isolated from the perilymph of a 5-month-old infant who died with asymptomatic congenital CMV infection whose inner ear morphology was normal by light microscopy.[42] CMV has been detected by PCR in perilymph removed during placement of cochlear implants in children 4½ years old with congenital CMV,[8] but CMV was not isolated from perilymph, or cytomegalic inclusion body–containing cells were not

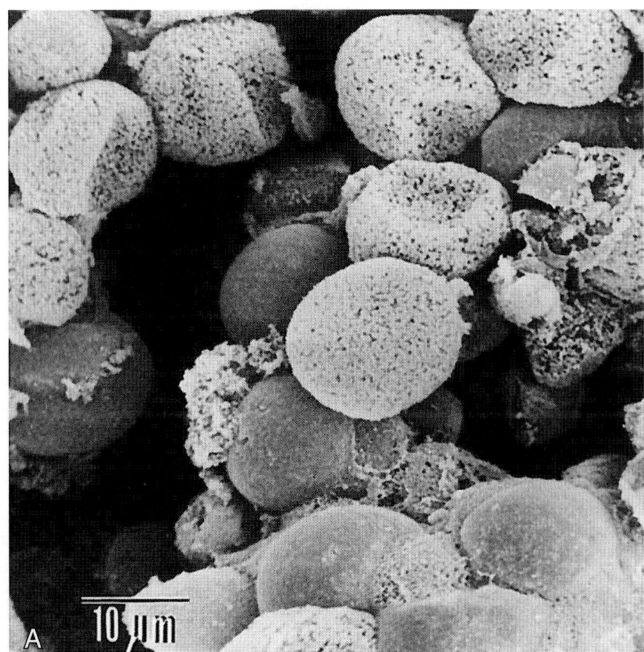

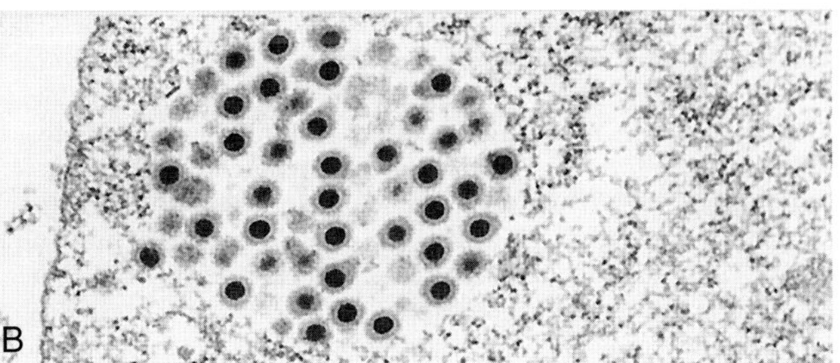

Figure 152-1. Congenital cytomegalovirus infection in a 1-month-old infant. **A,** Scanning electron micrograph shows large osmiophilic cytomegalovirus inclusion-bearing cells lining the membranous wall of utricle. **B,** Transmission electron micrograph shows cytomegalovirus particles with dense cores forming aggregates in the cytoplasm of utricular epithelium (×34,500). *(From Davis LE, Johnsson L-G, Kornfeld M. Cytomegalovirus labyrinthitis in an infant: morphological, virological, and immunofluorescent studies.* J Neuropathol Exp Neurol. *1981;40:9.)*

seen in a child with cytomegalic inclusion disease and bilateral deafness who survived 14 years.[44] It seems that CMV can persist for years in children with congenital viral infections. What role CMV persistence plays in the delayed hearing loss of asymptomatically infected children is unclear.

Management and Prevention

Four approaches have had limited success in preventing or treating SNHL in congenital CMV. Toward prevention of primary CMV infection in a CMV-seronegative woman of childbearing age, several experimental CMV vaccines have been developed and are in clinical testing. These include protein subunit vaccines, DNA vaccines, vectored vaccines using viral vectors, peptide vaccines, and live attenuated vaccines.[45,46]

Treatment of pregnant women with primary CMV infection has been tried by passive immunization using hyperimmune CMV gamma globulin. A nonrandomized study of pregnant women with primary CMV infections showed a significant reduction in symptomatic infected newborn infants at 2 years of age.[47] Valacyclovir at 8 g/day given to pregnant women with primary CMV infection has been shown to achieve therapeutic levels in maternal and fetal blood with a reduction in fetal viral load.[39] Mixed clinical outcomes occurred in the 21 fetuses treated at 28 weeks of gestation, however.

The antiviral drugs, ganciclovir and valganciclovir, have had some success in treating infants with cytomegalic inclusion disease.[48-52] Ganciclovir requires phosphorylation to ganciclovir triphosphate in part by enzymes from CMV. The triphosphate molecule inhibits viral DNA polymerase with inhibition of CMV replication.[48] In a randomized controlled trial, intravenous ganciclovir begun in the neonatal period of symptomatically infected infants was effective in preventing hearing deterioration at 6 months, and may prevent hearing deterioration past 1 year.[49]

Ganciclovir can be delivered only by the intravenous route, and so creates a major problem for extended delivery of the agent. Valganciclovir, a monovalyl ester of ganciclovir, is an oral prodrug of ganciclovir, and in small studies seems to have similar efficacy in treating congenital CMV infections.[50,51] Both drugs reduce CMV viral load in blood and urine, but rarely eliminate the virus from the host. Both drugs also frequently cause neutropenia, so dosages must be carefully monitored.

There is increasing evidence that deafness from congenital CMV is not a contraindication for cochlear implantation. Studies of these children have shown hearing improvement results similar to other congenitally deaf children, and no unusual complications have developed.[53,54]

Experimental Cytomegalovirus Inner Ear Infections

The human strain of CMV has not been shown to infect the labyrinth of small animals. The mouse and guinea pig strains of CMV have been shown to infect primarily perilymphatic structures of the cochlea and vestibule with variable secondary degeneration of the organ of Corti.[55] In guinea pigs, guinea pig CMV has been inoculated directly into the basal turn of the cochlea, resulting in inflammation and cytomegalic cells within the perilymphatic duct along with variable secondary degeneration of the organ of Corti.[56,57] These strains are also capable of infecting neurons in the spiral and vestibular ganglia. Guinea pig CMV has been shown to reach the cochlea by the intravenous route, and to cross the placenta to infect the fetal cochlea.[58] Electrophysiologic recordings of cochlea microphonic and eighth cranial nerve have shown objective hearing loss in N1 compound action potential thresholds of infected guinea pigs.[59-61] To date, all experimental models differ from human inner ear infection in that the animal viruses have primarily infected cells of the perilymphatic system, whereas human CMV primarily infects cells of the endolymphatic system.

Congenital Rubella Deafness

Clinical Features

Rubella infection of the pregnant mother as a cause of neonatal deafness was first recognized during the 1939 Australian rubella epidemic.[62] From 1964 to 1965 during the U.S. rubella epidemic, more than 12,000 infants were found with hearing loss and congenital rubella.[63] Since the introduction of rubella vaccine, the number of cases in developed countries has dramatically decreased, but not disappeared. The World Health Organization estimates that more than 100,000 infants are born each year with congenital rubella syndrome with 50% having hearing impairment.[64] In many developed countries, it is estimated that 15% to 20% of women in childbearing years are susceptible to rubella infection, a number that is similar to that in industrialized countries in the prevaccination era.[65] Since 2001 in the United States, there have been less than 25 cases of rubella each year, and no reported cases of congenital rubella syndrome.[66]

Maternal rubella infection during the first trimester of pregnancy places the fetus at the highest risk of congenital infection and subsequent hearing loss. In addition to the hearing loss, infants are often born with cardiac malformations, vision loss, and mental retardation.[67] Approximately 50% of infants born with symptomatic congenital rubella have hearing loss. Infants infected with rubella during the second and third trimesters often are born with silent rubella infection and appear healthy at birth. Ten percent to 20% of these children are subsequently identified as hearing impaired.[68]

Hearing Loss

Congenital rubella infection involving the inner ear usually results in bilateral, often asymmetric, hearing loss. In a series of 8168 children with hearing loss from congenital rubella, 55% had profound hearing loss (≥91 dB ISO [International Standards Organization]), 30% had severe hearing loss (71 to 90 dB), and 15% had mild to moderate hearing loss (<70 dB).[63] The audiograms of most children were usually flat, with hearing deficits occurring in all frequencies, but some had the greatest hearing loss in the midfrequency range of 500 to 2000 Hz, which is the range of voice.[69] Children with rubella deafness may have poor speech discrimination, and a few may experience progressive hearing loss. Some children have had delayed or impaired speech development, but still have healthy pure tone hearing, which suggests a central auditory imperception.[70] Adults who experience rubella infection rarely develop hearing loss.[71]

The vestibular system seems to be involved to a lesser extent than the auditory system.[72] Caloric stimulation with 1 mL of ice water has suggested that some children have reduced caloric responses in one or both ears.[73]

Diagnosis

Congenital rubella may be diagnosed by (1) isolation of rubella or detection of rubella-specific RNA from urine or throat cultures during the first weeks of life, (2) identification of IgM antibodies against rubella in serum from the neonate, or (3) increased antibody titer to rubella in an infant during the first few months of life who did not receive the rubella vaccine. Identification of IgM antibodies against rubella is difficult and should be performed only in qualified laboratories. In children older than 1 year, congenital rubella is difficult to diagnose because many children have received the rubella vaccine. A maternal history of rash during pregnancy is unreliable for establishing or ruling out the diagnosis. Congenital rubella has been diagnosed in utero by isolation of rubella from amniotic fluid. No specific management for children exists because no antirubella virus drugs are available. Management should be directed toward minimizing the consequences of the hearing loss and possible use of a cochlear implant.

Temporal Bone Pathology

Histopathologic changes seen in the temporal bones of congenital rubella deafness show characteristic changes, but the histopathologic findings are not specific for a rubella infection. The predominant abnormality is cochleosaccular degeneration and strial atrophy of varying degrees.[74,75] Reissner's membrane and the wall of the saccule may sag and even collapse (Fig. 152-2). The tectorial membrane is frequently abnormal, often displaced from the organ of Corti toward the limbus. The stria vascularis shows varying degrees of atrophy. Inflammatory cells in the cochlea are seldom seen. Cells with inclusion bodies do not occur. The vestibular neuroepithelia and their nerves

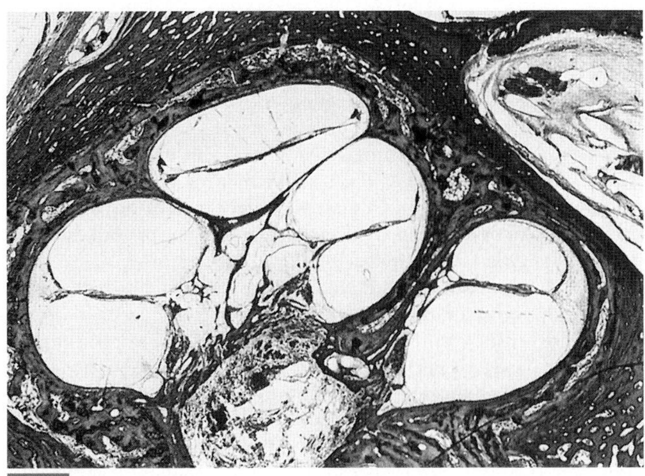

Figure 152-2. Congenital rubella infection in a premature infant. Cochlea shows partial collapse of Reissner's membrane onto the organ of Corti in all turns (hematoxylin-eosin stain, ×40.) *(Courtesy of G. Nagar, Baltimore, MD.)*

usually appear healthy. There are no animal models for congenital rubella or rubella deafness.

Acquired Sensorineural Hearing Loss

Sudden Sensorineural Hearing Loss

Clinical Features

Many causes of SNHL have been described in children[76,77] and adults.[78] Although several definitions exist, most require a loss of greater than 30 dB in three contiguous frequencies that occurs in less than 3 days in the absence of a skull fracture.[79] The incidence of severe SNHL is about 10/100,000 persons per year.[3,80] The incidence of mild cases is unknown because many individuals do not seek medical attention. Most patients awaken with the hearing loss, or the loss develops within minutes to several hours. The hearing loss is unilateral in more than 90% of cases. Approximately half of the patients note accompanying vertigo or imbalance. Recovery of hearing ranges from 45% to 60%.[3,81] The usual recovery period is days to weeks. After 1 month, little recovery occurs.[3] The extent of recovery is related to age and severity of initial hearing loss. Untreated patients younger than 40 years of age have a better recovery rate. For individuals older than 40 years, the recovery rate may be only 30%.[79]

Temporal Bone Pathology

The mechanisms involved in the sudden hearing loss have not been fully clarified because there are few available temporal bone studies from patients during the acute period. A viral infection of the cochlear endolymphatic structures or spiral ganglia is one of several theories that has been postulated as the cause. Schuknecht[82,83] examined the temporal bones of 12 patients with idiopathic sudden SNHL in his series and reviewed 9 additional published cases. Vertigo was noted in 47% of cases. Histologic abnormalities were identified in the organ of Corti (76%), tectorial membrane (53%), stria vascularis (62%), cochlear neurons (48%), saccule (43%), fibrosis with ectopic bone formation (10%), and tears in Reissner's membrane or oval or round windows (10%). Schuknecht[82,83] concluded that a viral infection of the endolymphatic labyrinth was the most tenable pathogenesis. Another study of 15 temporal bones from patients with SNHL reported the most prominent histologic findings to be loss of hair cells and supporting cells of the organ of Corti (with or without atrophy of the tectorial membrane), stria vascularis, spiral limbus, and cochlear neurons.[84] This study reported examination of one temporal bone from a patient who died 9 days after unilateral sudden hearing loss and failed to find evidence of cochlear inflammation.

Several studies have attempted to define the infectious causes of idiopathic SNHL. Two viruses, mumps and measles (rubeola), have been recognized for centuries as a cause of acquired hearing loss in children. For other viruses, associations generally have been made on the basis of fourfold elevations in viral antibody titers in convalescence or case reports with isolation of the candidate virus from the nasopharynx or mouth. In addition to viruses, syphilis is recognized to cause acute hearing loss[85]; Lyme disease may also be a cause.[86] Box 152-2 lists these candidate infectious agents. To date, associations of infectious agents have represented only a small fraction of the total SNHL cases.

Management

Administration of high-dose corticosteroids shortly after the onset of SNHL has been shown to have a significant benefit in recovery of hearing.[87-89] More recently, nonrandomized studies of repeat treatment with intratympanic dexamethasone in patients who failed systemic corticosteroids reported that occasionally additional hearing recovery ensued.[90-92] Because of the possibility that SNHL might be due to reactivation of HSV, a prospective, randomized, double-blind clinical trial of systemic prednisolone versus corticosteroids and acyclovir was performed on 91 patients.[93] The investigators reported no additional benefit of the acyclovir over prednisolone only. If the sudden severe hearing loss permanently involved both ears, these patients may be candidates for cochlear implants.

Major Causes of Acquired Deafness from Viruses

Mumps Deafness

Clinical Features

Mumps was first recognized to cause deafness in 1860. Since then, it is estimated that 5 of every 10,000 patients with mumps have hearing loss develop.[94] The widespread use of the mumps vaccine in developed countries has dramatically reduced the incidence. Mumps deafness continues to occur, however, in developing countries that do not have major vaccination programs. A study of 115 children with profound bilateral deafness reported that mumps was responsible for 7% of the cases.[95] There has been a more recent increase in mumps in college-aged individuals in the United States (>2600 cases) and United Kingdom.[96] Many of these individuals had previously received two doses of the mumps vaccine. It is unclear how often the mumps caused hearing loss in these patients.

Deafness associated with mumps usually develops in children toward the end of the parotitis, but can occur from a subclinical infection in the absence of parotitis.[97-100] The onset of the deafness is usually rapid and unilateral in 80%. Hearing loss is maximal at high frequencies. Tinnitus and fullness in the involved ear are common. In two patients with acute mumps deafness, MRI showed enhancement of the labyrinth and CN VIII[101] and the cochlea and vestibule.[102]

The hearing loss is often profound and usually permanent. A prospective study by Vuori and colleagues[103] found the hearing loss to be transient in some patients, however. Some patients have vertigo develop that usually resolves over several weeks, but the patient may be left with permanent diminished or absent caloric responses in that ear. Absent caloric responses have also been found in patients with deafness associated with mumps, but without a history of vertigo.

Diagnosis

Mumps is diagnosed by (1) isolation of mumps virus from the saliva or CSF, or detection of mumps virus RNA, or (2) a fourfold or greater serologic increase in mumps antibodies between acute and convalescent serum samples. Sensitive real-time reverse transcriptase PCR assays are available for rapid detection of mumps virus from saliva.[104] Mumps virus has been isolated from the perilymphatic fluid in one patient with acute unilateral deafness associated with parotitis.[17] Currently, no specific antiviral drugs for mumps deafness exists, and it is unclear whether administration of corticosteroids improves hearing recovery. Administration of mumps vaccine in infancy effectively prevents subsequent mumps infections in childhood and adulthood.

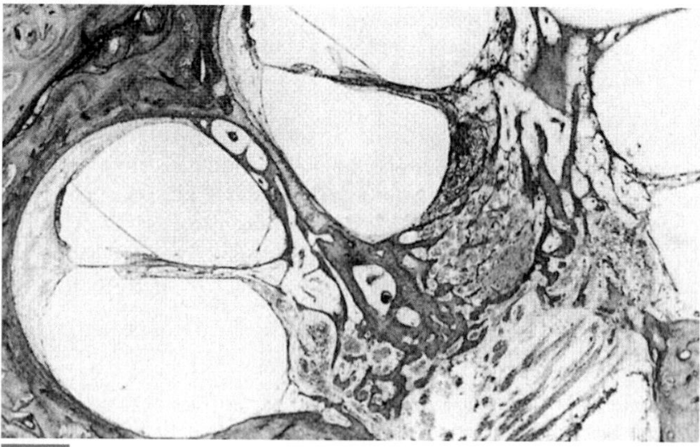

Figure 152-3. Acquired mumps virus deafness 13 years previously. Cochlea shows absent organ of Corti in the basal turn with secondary degeneration of some ganglion cells and severe degeneration of their distal processes in osseous lamina (hematoxylin-eosin stain, ×22.) *(From Smith GA, Gussen R. Inner ear pathologic features following mumps infection: report of a case in an adult.* Arch Otolaryngol. *1976;102:108. Copyright © 1976, American Medical Association.)*

Temporal Bone Pathology

Temporal bones from two patients with mumps-associated deafness have been examined.[105,106] The cochlea showed severe atrophy of the organ of Corti and the stria vascularis, with partial collapse of Reissner's membrane in the basal turn (Fig. 152-3). The tectorial membrane in one case was folded, thickened, and displaced from the organ of Corti. The upper turns of the cochlea showed less damage with occasional loss of hair cells. Cochlear ganglion neurons may be decreased in the area of the basal turn. Minimal vestibular abnormalities were seen.

Experimental Mumps Viral Labyrinthitis

Mumps virus inoculated into the inner ear of hamsters, guinea pigs, and monkeys principally infected non-neuroepithelial cells of the membranous labyrinth, which included cells of Reissner's membrane, stria vascularis, and supporting cells of the organ of Corti.[73,107,108] In the cochlear basal turn, degeneration of the organ of Corti and damage to the stria vascularis developed. Cells of the inner ear could be infected if the virus was inoculated directly into the inner ear, or if the virus entered the perilymphatic fluid of the scala tympani by way of the cochlear aqueduct after intracerebral inoculation.

Because the virus could reach the perilymph from the CSF in the model, the question arises as to whether this route of infection could occur in humans. Support for this hypothesis is severalfold. Mumps viral meningitis occurs in one third of infected children.[109] The cochlear aqueduct is more often patent in children than adults, and dilated cochlear aqueducts have been recognized by CT in 6% of children with SNHL.[76,110] Finally, deafness often develops toward the end of the first week of parotitis, a time consistent with spread of mumps virus from the infected CSF because of the meningitis from the cochlear aqueduct to the scala tympani. Spread of virus from CSF to the inner ear could also occur by way of the CN VIII pathway through the internal auditory canal to the spiral ganglion. Against both hypotheses is one study that did not find a correlation between mumps meningitis and deafness.[103]

Measles Deafness

Clinical Features

Rubeola virus is the cause of measles and continues to be an important cause of acquired hearing loss in developing countries. The incidence of deafness after measles is slightly less than 1 out of every 1000 cases of measles. Before the introduction of rubeola virus vaccine in developed countries, rubeola virus caused 3% to 10% of all acquired deafness in children. Now rubeola deafness occurs primarily in developing countries without measles vaccination programs.

Measles virus involvement of the labyrinth usually is seen with the abrupt onset of bilateral hearing loss at the time of the rash, but occasional children have only unilateral hearing loss develop. In one large study, 45% of the children were left with severe bilateral hearing loss, and 55% had mild to moderate hearing loss.[111] The typical audiogram shows bilateral loss that is often asymmetric and maximal at higher frequencies. The hearing loss is usually permanent and acutely may be accompanied by vertigo and tinnitus. Seventy percent of patients are left with absent or diminished caloric responses in one or both ears even though the vertigo has subsided.[111]

Conductive hearing loss from otosclerosis is becoming highly associated with persistent rubeola virus infection of the stapes footplate. Rubeola virus RNA has been detected by PCR in the stapes footplate removed at stapedectomy from patients with otosclerosis, but not stapes footplates of other diseases.[104,112,113] Tissue culture explants of the stapes footplates also showed rubeola virus RNA.[114] In addition, filamentous structures in osteoblast-like cells resembling nucleocapsids of rubeola virus were seen by electron microscopy.[115] One laboratory was unable, however, to detect by PCR or immunofluorescence rubeola RNA or antigen in stapes footplates or their explants.[116] Epidemiology studies in Denmark and Germany have shown a significant reduction in stapedectomies, particularly in younger patients, since the rubeola vaccination campaign began.[117] The pathogenesis of how measles virus can persistently infect the stapes footplate in healthy individuals and cause otosclerosis is still unclear.

Diagnosis

Measles can be diagnosed by (1) isolation of rubeola virus from throat cultures; (2) detection of rubeola viral RNA from clinical specimens; (3) identification of rubeola viral antigen by immunofluorescent staining of exfoliated epithelial cells obtained by swabbing of the pharynx, conjunctiva, or buccal cavity; or (4) demonstration of a fourfold or greater serologic increase in measles antibody titer between acute and convalescent serum samples. At present, no antiviral medication has shown benefit in the treatment of deafness from measles. It is unclear whether administration of steroids is beneficial.

Temporal Bone Pathology

Only a few temporal bones have been examined from patients with deafness associated with measles.[22,82,118] The major histopathology was a sensorineural degeneration seen in the cochlear and vestibular system. The cochlear degeneration was most severe in the basal turn. The tectorial membrane was often thickened and distorted. Atrophy of the stria vascularis was seen and was maximal at the basal turn. The saccule had collapsed, and the membranous wall adhered to the degenerated macular epithelium. The macula utriculi and the crista ampullaris frequently showed minimal changes. In one case, a subacute inflammatory process with granulomas and a giant cell was seen in the endolymphatic fluid attached to the stria vascularis.[22] Multinucleated giant cells are characteristic of rubeola virus infections.

Experimental Rubeola Virus Labyrinthitis

Experimental rubeola virus infections of hamsters have been shown to cause an inner ear infection with viral antigen principally seen within sensory structures of the cochlea, utricle, saccule, and semicircular canals.[119,120] Cochlear and vestibular ganglion cells were infected, and viral antigen could be identified in their distal nerve processes. Giant cells typical for rubeola virus were seen within the organ of Corti and spiral ganglion neurons. No experimental studies of rubeola infection of stapes have been reported.

Lassa Fever Hearing Loss

Lassa fever is an arenavirus that is endemic throughout West Africa, where 100,000 cases occur each year.[121] The virus is spread to humans from infected urine of rodents. The disease is characterized by an insidious onset of fever, weakness, and malaise followed by cough, back pain, and pharyngitis.[121-123] The mortality rate is estimated at 15% of hospitalized patients. Survivors have hearing loss develop with an incidence of approximately 30%, the highest incidence of hearing loss of any acquired viral illness.[7,124] The hearing loss usually develops during the convalescent phase of the illness; hearing loss is unrelated to severity of the acute disease. The mean auditory threshold of affected patients is 55 dB. Approximately half the patients show improvement in hearing over 3 to 4 months, but the other half are left with a moderate to severe SNHL. Of 24 patients with imported Lassa fever, only one has developed sudden SNHL, and that was during convalescence.[125] Because temporal bones from these patients have not been examined, the pathology is unclear. The pathogenesis of cochlear damage could be from direct arenavirus infection, from vascular thrombosis or hemorrhage, or most likely secondary from an immune response to the arenavirus in the inner ear.[121,126]

Varicella-Zoster Virus Deafness and Vertigo

Clinical Features

Hearing loss occasionally occurs after chickenpox, but this is usually caused by secondary viral or bacterial otitis media producing a conductive hearing loss. Herpes zoster oticus, or Ramsay Hunt syndrome, is caused by a VZV infection that became latent in the geniculate ganglia during the period of acute chickenpox. Decades later, the VZV breaks latency and replicates first in the geniculate ganglion and then travels down the peripheral facial nerve, causing a peripheral facial palsy that resembles Bell's palsy. Approximately 25% of patients experience vestibular or cochlear symptoms (or both) apparently caused by spread of inflammatory cells from the geniculate ganglion to the inner ear, spiral, and vestibular ganglia.[127-130] Occasionally, patients develop prominent vertigo or hearing loss before or along with the facial palsy that may be mild.[131,132]

Vesicles, which may be painful, usually develop on the skin of the pinna of the ear, behind the pinna, and along the external auditory canal (Fig. 152-4). This development is followed 1 to 2 days later by unilateral facial paralysis and deep ear pain.[133] The facial weakness usually improves over weeks, but is occasionally permanent. In one fourth of patients, symptoms also include vertigo, nystagmus, tinnitus, and hearing loss. Although patients may complain of auditory symptoms, SNHL occurs in only approximately 6% of patients. Audiograms vary, and may suggest primary cochlear involvement or cochlear nerve damage.[35] Caloric tests often show decreased to absent responses in the involved ear.

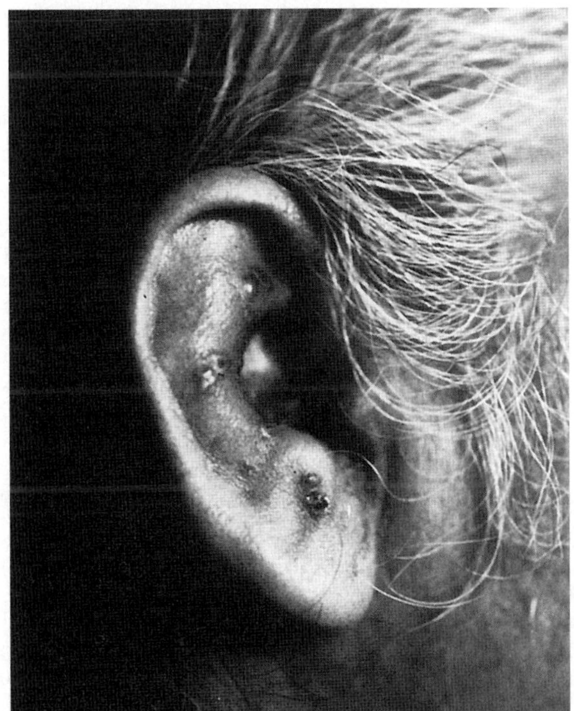

Figure 152-4. Right ear pinna of a 50-year-old woman with herpes zoster oticus. Intense vertigo followed 1 day later with right facial weakness. Multiple vesicles are seen over the pinna, from which varicella-zoster virus was isolated.

Diagnosis

The diagnosis of herpes zoster oticus can be suspected in a patient with acute facial weakness and vesicles on the auricle or in the external canal.[134] Gadolinium-enhanced MRI of the temporal bone of patients with only herpes zoster oticus show enhancement of the involved geniculate ganglion and facial nerve.[135] One MRI report from a patient with herpes zoster oticus and inner ear symptoms found enhancement in the distal internal auditory canal and labyrinthine segments of patients.[136] The diagnosis can be confirmed by isolation of VZV from vesicle fluid; detection of VZV DNA by PCR assay in vesicle fluid, facial nerve sheath, or CSF[134,137-139]; or histologic presence of multinucleated giant cells in vesicle scrapings.

Management

Acute treatment with high-dose acyclovir (800 mg PO five times daily for 7 days), famciclovir (500 mg PO three times daily for 7 days), or valaciclovir (1 g PO three times daily for 7 days) plus a tapering 6-day course of prednisone (beginning usually at 1 mg/kg PO) is widely administered for herpes zoster oticus.[140] One retrospective study compared patients given treatment within the first 3 days of onset with others starting 4 to 7 days after onset or later than 7 days.[141] Patients beginning steroids and acyclovir early did significantly better than patients starting later. Other studies support their use.[142-144] No prospective randomized study has been done, however.

The hearing loss, vertigo, and facial weakness slowly improve over weeks to several months.[145] Serial audiograms showed complete hearing recovery in 66% of children and 38% of adults. Some patients have permanently reduced caloric responses.

A new adult varicella vaccine (Zostavax) has been approved by the U.S. Food and Drug Administration for the prevention of shingles. A randomized, double-blind, placebo-controlled study of more than 38,000 adults older than 60 years showed a 51% reduction in the incidence of shingles.[146] Widespread administration of this vaccine in elderly individuals should reduce the incidence of herpes zoster oticus.

Temporal Bone Pathology

In patients with auditory and vestibular symptoms, the inflammation seems to spread to involve CN VIII and the labyrinth.[78,147] Temporal bones of patients with herpes zoster oticus show facial nerves with active neuritis, including inflammatory cells, edema, hemorrhages, and axon degeneration throughout the facial nerve sheath, but maximally near the geniculate ganglion. The geniculate ganglion usually shows inflammation, edema, and neuronal degeneration. The facial nerve nucleus in the brainstem is not involved.

Pathologic changes in the auditory nerve and labyrinth also have been reported. In all cases, patients had vertigo and hearing loss associated with facial nerve paralysis. Several months after acute paralysis, inflammatory cells have been seen along CN VIII, particularly the vestibular branches. Inflammatory cells have also been seen in the macula of the utricle and saccule. In one case, the branch of the vestibular nerve going to the lateral and superior semicircular canals was atrophic.[78,148,149] Corresponding atrophy and loss of hair cells of the cristae of the corresponding semicircular canal were also seen.

Herpes Simplex Virus Deafness

Infants surviving HSV encephalitis may have permanent hearing loss.[150] Even infants surviving the milder HSV infection of skin occasionally have subsequent hearing loss. An adult with HSV encephalitis has also been reported to have severe bilateral SNHL develop.[151] To date, there have been no histopathologic studies of temporal bone from patients dying after HSV encephalitis. One elderly woman was reported who first developed vertigo and jerk nystagmus with normal MRI followed 3 days later with proven ipsilateral HSV encephalitis.[152] The authors speculate that HSV vestibular neuritis first developed followed by the encephalitis.

For more than 30 years, there has been clinical suspicion that HSV can cause SNHL. To date, the evidence remains inconclusive. In favor of HSV as a cause of SNHL, HSV DNA has been detected by PCR assay in spiral ganglia in 50% of specimens obtained at routine autopsies.[13,23] HSV seems capable of becoming latent in the spiral ganglia. HSV has been isolated from the oropharynx of patients with sudden hearing loss. Acute and convalescent antibody studies of patients with sudden hearing loss have shown some patients have an increase in antibody titer to HSV. Other studies have shown a higher prevalence of HSV antibodies in children and adults with SNHL than control children.[153,154] In experimental animals, HSV can infect cells of the inner ear of hamsters, guinea pigs, mice, and monkeys.[119,155-157] The resulting infections usually involve cells of the endolymphatic labyrinth and corresponding vestibular and spiral ganglia.

There is also evidence against HSV as a cause of sudden hearing loss. HSV has not been isolated from perilymphatic fluid or inner ear tissues, and Cowdry type A inclusion bodies (typical for HSV infection) have not been identified in inner ear tissue. Several studies have not found the percentage of patients with HSV antibodies or HSV titer elevations different from controls.[158-160] No study has found differences in the clinical features of patients with presumed HSV SNHL compared with other patients with SNHL. HSV can be isolated from the mouth in 10% of normal children[7] and 7.4% of healthy adults without herpes vesicles.[161] The occasional HSV isolation from the mouth of patients with SNHL easily could be coincidental. Likewise, interpretation of increases in HSV antibody titers cited by some authors is problematic because increases and decreases in HSV antibody titer are common in healthy individuals.[6]

The known biology of HSV makes the virus a poor candidate for SNHL. Labial and genital herpes frequently recur, but SNHL rarely does, and the age distribution of SNHL does not match that of HSV recurrences from the trigeminal ganglia or the sacral ganglia. Finally, one randomized, double-blind study assessed the value of acyclovir treatment in patients with SNHL and found no beneficial effect on hearing recovery from combining acyclovir and prednisone compared with administering prednisone alone.[162]

Bacterial and Fungal Labyrinthitis

Bacteria and fungi can damage the peripheral auditory and vestibular systems through (1) suppurative labyrinthitis, (2) toxic labyrinthine damage from bacterial or fungal toxins or inflammatory cell cytokines that reach the perilymph through the round window or modiolus, (3) purulent exudate enveloping CN VIII with nerve infarction or entrapment, (4) purulent exudate or infectious agent reaching the cochlear perilymphatic space by way of the cochlear aqueduct from an infected CSF subarachnoid space, and (5) ototoxic antibiotics to manage infection with elevated concentrations in blood. In most cases, suppurative labyrinthitis seems to be the most important mechanism, with bacteria or fungi reaching the cochlea from blood, the subarachnoid space (meningitis), temporal bone (osteomyelitis), or middle ear (otitis media). In meningitis, bacteria or fungi reach the scala tympani from the subarachnoid space by way of a patent cochlear aqueduct or up the internal auditory canal passing through perineural and perivascular spaces.[19]

Temporal Bone Pathology

When bacteria infect the labyrinth, suppurative labyrinthitis ensues.[163] The acute bacterial infection elicits an acute inflammatory response of neutrophils that results in severe destruction of the membranous labyrinth.[164] Usually, severe hearing loss and acute vertigo occur. The hearing loss is usually permanent, whereas the vertigo slowly resolves over weeks to months. There is often permanent loss of caloric responses.

After appropriate antibiotic management, the acute inflammation slowly resolves. Macrophages may invade from the bloodstream, giving rise to granulomas. Over months to years, fibroblasts may invade the membranous labyrinth to cause permanent scarring of endolymphatic structures.[20] Primitive multipotential mesenchymal cells invade and proliferate from the adjacent modiolus, the bony endosteum lining, and other sites to become osteoblasts. The osteoblasts may form ectopic ossification sites with bony spicules in the perilymphatic space. Eventually, the spicules and trabeculae become vascularized to become new ectopic bone that may partially obliterate the old membranous labyrinthine space.[20] When fungal infections such as mucormycosis[21] and coccidioidomycosis[19] infect the labyrinth, the pathologic changes are similar except that ectopic bone formation seems to be less common.

Bacterial Meningitis Hearing Loss

Approximately one third of all hearing deficits acquired after birth are caused by complications of bacterial meningitis.[165] In a careful prospective study of acute bacterial meningitis in children, Dodge and colleagues[4] found persistent SNHL in 10% of patients. The incidence of deafness in a meta-analysis found the average to be 10%, with a range from 2.4% to 20%.[166] In the study by Dodge and colleagues,[4] SNHL was bilateral in 5% and unilateral in 5%. A transient conductive hearing loss was found in 16%. In adults, pneumococcal meningitis is also associated with a 20% incidence of hearing loss.[167] The incidence of hearing loss varies by strain of bacteria isolated from the CSF: *Streptococcus pneumoniae,* 20%; *Haemophilus influenzae,* 12%; and *Neisseria meningitidis,* greater than 5%.[166] The incidence of hearing loss does not seem to increase when the pneumococcus is penicillin-nonsusceptible.[168]

The hearing loss usually results from purulent exudate damage to the cochlea and spiral ganglia. A histologic study of 41 temporal bones from patients dying of bacterial meningitis reported suppurative labyrinthitis in the cochlea in 49% and in vestibular organs in 25%.[169] The scala tympani of the basal turn had the most inflammation. The sensory and neural structures often appeared intact, but in 12% the spiral ganglia showed extensive degeneration. A study of seven adults with bacterial meningitis that used high-resolution MRI with gadolinium also found abnormal contrast enhancement, mainly in the first cochlear turn, distal CN VIII, and vestibular structures.[170] Over time, damage to the organ of Corti and the membranous labyrinth may progress, with labyrinthitis ossificans developing.

On the basis of the preceding observations, the pathogenesis of hearing loss from bacterial meningitis seems to develop from inflammatory cells and bacteria traversing a patent cochlear aqueduct from the subarachnoid space to enter perilymph in the basal turn of the scala tympani,[171] or by extension of inflammation into the internal auditory canal reaching the cochlear modiolus.[169] The cochlear aqueduct is often patent in small children and progressively closes as the head grows.[172]

Clinical Features

Deafness generally occurs early in the course of the meningitis, but may develop at any time in the clinical course. Early diagnosis and management of the meningitis may not prevent deafness.[154] Children of all ages seem equally susceptible to deafness developing, which may be unilateral or bilateral. The hearing loss usually involves all frequencies and is often profound. Although most patients with SNHL after meningitis have a permanent loss of hearing, clinical hearing improvement occurs in occasional patients, especially if the initial hearing loss was partial.[19] One study of 124 children with bacterial meningitis that conducted repeated audiologic assessments found 10.5% of the children had a transient hearing loss that began within 6 hours and resolved within 24 hours.[173] More recent studies have reported that the incidence of postmeningitis hearing loss is similar for all the commonly involved bacteria.[174]

Evoked-response audiometry is sensitive in detecting SNHL and helpful in diagnosing hearing loss in young uncooperative children.[4] Vestibular symptoms (vertigo, nausea, vomiting, and ataxia) often develop in children regardless of whether hearing loss is present.

Management

Treatment of bacterial meningitis with appropriate antibiotics is essential. Broad-spectrum antibiotics should be given early and modified when bacteria are isolated and antibiotic sensitivities are determined. Evidence that administration of corticosteroids reduces the incidence of hearing loss in children and adults is accumulating.[72,166,175-177] A more recent MEDLINE survey concluded, however, that the benefit of corticosteroids remains unclear.[178] Maximal benefit occurs when the corticosteroids are given early in the course of meningitis in individuals from developed countries.[179]

When hearing loss has developed, no management modifies its severity or permanency. Because hearing deficits are common in patients with bacterial meningitis, a hearing evaluation of all patients during recovery is recommended. If the child is young or uncooperative, evoked-response audiometry should be used.[154]

Vaccines to Prevent Hearing Loss

Bacterial and viral vaccines are playing an increasing role in prevention of hearing loss in adults and children through prevention of meningitis and acute otitis media. The pneumococcal vaccines have significantly reduced the incidence of invasive pneumococcal disease, including pneumococcal meningitis in elderly individuals[180] and children.[180,181] *H. influenzae* type B used to be the most common cause of bacterial meningitis in children.[182] Since the introduction of *H. influenzae* type B vaccine for children, the incidence of *H. influenzae* meningitis has dramatically decreased.[182] Several studies have recommended the administration of these vaccines to children receiving cochlear implants to reduce to risk of bacterial meningitis.[183,184]

Acute otitis media is responsible for conductive hearing loss and SNHL in children. Bacteria are responsible for about 70% of cases of acute otitis media, with *S. pneumoniae,* nontypable *H. influenzae,* and *Moraxella catarrhalis* as the most common causes.[185] Viruses including influenza, respiratory syncytial, rhinovirus, and parainfluenza account for the remaining 30%. Immunization of young children with vaccines that contain *S. pneumoniae*[181,186] or killed influenza virus[187,188] have been shown in some studies to reduce the incidence of acute otitis media. Other studies report less benefit, however.[189,190] The creation of specific childhood vaccines to prevent otitis media are being considered.[185]

Cochlear Implant Infections

Placement of cochlear implants is associated with several types of infections involving the inner ear or meninges. Since 2003, an average of 4% of cochlear implants develop a delayed major infectious complication requiring hospitalization, intravenous antibiotics, and often removal of the device.[191] The risk of infectious complications does not vary whether the cause was congenital or postmeningitis, and cochlear implants seem to improve patient communication equally.[192] Studies have varied regarding whether children or adults are more prone to device infections. The most common bacteria encountered are *Staphylococcus aureus* and *Pseudomonas aeruginosa.* Repeated episodes of otitis media and poor chronic health conditions increase the risk of infection. Some cochlear implant infections are associated with *S. aureus* biofilms on the implanted device that are difficult to cure with antibiotics.[193]

Bacterial meningitis from *S. pneumoniae* and *H. influenzae* occurs about 30 times more often in children with cochlear implants than in normal children.[194,195] About half the infections have been associated with a device positioner that has been discontinued. The risk of meningitis continues for many years, however, and argues that these children should receive the pneumococcal and *H. influenzae* B vaccines repeatedly.[196]

Congenital and Acquired Syphilitic Deafness

Clinical Features

SNHL can be a complication of congenital and acquired syphilis.[197] Hearing loss from congenital syphilis can occur early (birth to 3 years old) or late (8 to 20 years old). In 2002, 450 cases of congenital syphilis were reported to the Centers for Disease Control and Prevention, an incidence of 11 cases per 100,000 live births.[198] Extensive multisystem damage from syphilitic infections of other organs usually accompanies early congenital syphilitic hearing loss, which is a bilateral profound symmetric SNHL. Relatively few vestibular symptoms and signs are noted.

Patients with late congenital syphilitic hearing loss are usually 8 to 20 years old when symptoms first appear, but occasionally the hearing loss takes longer to occur. These patients usually have a progressive but fluctuating hearing loss that is asymmetric. Audiograms show a flat sensorineural type of hearing loss. Frequently, there are low speech discrimination scores that are disproportionate to the loss in pure tone thresholds. Tinnitus may occur intermittently. These patients also may experience episodes of acute vertigo similar to episodes of Meniere's disease. Hennebert's sign (a positive fistula test with intact tympanic membranes) may be present. Frequently, decreased caloric responses are found.

Acquired syphilitic deafness usually occurs during secondary syphilis.[85] The hearing loss usually has an abrupt onset, tends to be bilateral, and is progressive. Usually minimal vestibular symptoms exist. Patients may have headaches, stiff necks, cranial nerve palsies, optic neuritis, secondary syphilitic rashes, and lymphadenopathy. The CSF shows lymphocytic pleocytosis, elevated protein, and normal glucose.

Acquired syphilitic hearing loss can also develop during the tertiary stage of syphilis.[199] Similar to the late congenital form, the hearing loss is progressive, fluctuating, asymmetric, and sensorineural. Tinnitus may occur. Episodes of vertigo similar to those in Meniere's disease may be experienced. Loss of speech discrimination may be disproportionate to the pure tone hearing loss. Decreased caloric responses and a positive fistula test with an intact tympanic membrane may exist. The CSF may show minimal pleocytosis and elevated or normal protein. Electrocochleographic features of endolymphatic syphilitic lesions generally resemble the features found in Meniere's disease.[200]

Diagnosis

The diagnosis of all types of syphilitic hearing loss requires recent SNHL in the presence of a positive serum rapid plasma reagin test and a positive fluorescent treponemal antibody absorption test or a positive CSF Venereal Disease Research Laboratory test. Spirochetes have been shown by dark-field examination of perilymph obtained from a diagnostic stapes footplate labyrinthotomy.

Management

The Centers for Disease Control and Prevention recommends aqueous crystalline penicillin G, 3 to 4 million U by intravenous injection every 4 hours for 10 days, to treat neurosyphilis.[201] In addition, administration of prednisone, 30 to 60 mg by mouth every day or every other day, is usually given for the first week unless contraindicated.[202] If hearing loss recurs after tapering, long-term maintenance of prednisone (10 to 20 mg every other day) may be necessary. This complication occurs most commonly in the late congenital and late acquired forms of the disease.

The prognosis is poor in the early congenital form; bilateral profound permanent hearing loss usually results. In the late congenital or acquired forms of syphilitic hearing loss, the prognosis is better. Overall, 50% of patients show minor to considerable improvement after management.

Temporal Bone Pathology

The pathology in cases of early congenital syphilitic hearing loss is primarily that of a labyrinthitis with lymphocytic infiltration and destruction of the labyrinth and CN VIII. Spirochetes have been shown in temporal bones obtained at autopsy and stained with a silver stain.[203] In late congenital syphilis, an osteitis of the otic capsule exists with secondary involvement of the membranous labyrinth[204]; this may give rise to endolymphatic hydrops. In early acquired syphilis, the predominant finding is a basilar meningitis affecting CN VIII, particularly its auditory branch. In late acquired syphilitic deafness, temporal bone osteitis is seen, resulting in secondary degeneration of the cochlear end organ.[199] Damage to the membranous labyrinth may occur, giving rise to endolymphatic hydrops.

Hearing Loss in Immunocompromised Patients

Immunocompromised patients are particularly susceptible to middle ear or inner ear infections. Most commonly, chronic fungal or bacterial middle ear infections spread to the inner ear by way of the oval or round window or from osteomyelitis of the petrous bone. Approximately 30% of patients with acquired immunodeficiency syndrome (AIDS) have otologic complaints that include dizziness, hearing loss, tinnitus, and

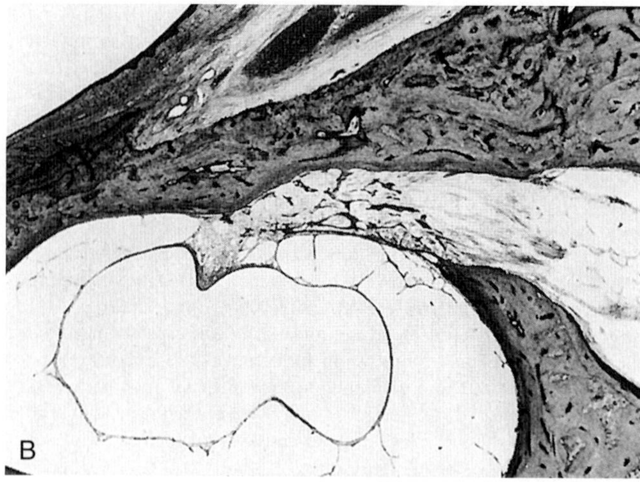

Figure 152-5. Vestibular neuritis developed in this man at ages 55 and 60 years, reducing caloric responses in the left ear. **A,** Right semicircular canal; nerve and crista are normal. **B,** Left semicircular canal; atrophy of nerve and partial atrophy of crista. *(From Schuknecht HF, Kitamura K. Vestibular neuritis.* Ann Otol Rhinol Laryngol. *1981;90[Suppl]:1.)*

otalgia.[205,206] CMV, adenovirus, and HSV have been recovered from perilymphatic fluid of patients with AIDS at death.[207] Histologic damage to the cochlea in viral infections was minimal, suggesting viral entry occurred immediately before death, or the inability of the patient to mount an immune inflammatory response resulted in little inner ear damage.[140,208] Other organisms implicated in SNHL include *Pneumocystis carinii, Candida albicans, S. aureus, Mycobacterium tuberculosis, Toxoplasma gondii, T. pallidum,* and *Cryptococcus neoformans.*[209] Some antiretrovirus medications, including azidothymidine, dideoxyinosine, and dideoxycytidine, have also been associated with SNHL.[209]

Vestibular Neuritis

Clinical Features

Vestibular neuritis has also been called epidemic vertigo, acute labyrinthitis, vestibular paralysis, vestibular neuropathy, and vestibular ganglionitis. The name *vestibular neuritis* is currently used because available pathology suggests that the vestibular nerve is the most common site of damage.[5,210]

The incidence of vestibular neuritis is unknown, but a Japanese questionnaire survey reported 35 cases per 100,000 population.[211] The peak onset of vestibular neuritis is between 30 and 60 years of age. Most patients experience an abrupt onset with a single, severe attack of prolonged vertigo.[212-215] Patients occasionally experience a flurry of attacks over several weeks.[213] Vestibular neuritis should not be accompanied by acute hearing loss or severe tinnitus, although some patients complain of "stuffiness" in the ear. Other neurologic signs or symptoms should not be present. Patients usually have a vigorous spontaneous nystagmus toward the uninvolved side, usually of a horizontal or horizontal-rotary type. Usually only one ear is involved. Caloric responses are diminished or absent in the involved ear in about 50% of patients, and the canal paresis may be permanent.[211,216] CSF examination and electroencephalograms are normal. The diagnosis is made on the basis of characteristic clinical signs. Unilateral diminished or absent caloric tests support the diagnosis.

Management

Early treatment of the patient with methylprednisolone has been shown in a randomized double-blind, placebo-controlled study to improve outcome.[217] Patients were given a 21-day tapering course of methylprednisolone beginning at 100 mg/day. The addition of acyclovir or valaciclovir in two studies did not improve outcome, however.[162,217] During the acute phase, nausea and vomiting may be severe enough to cause clinical dehydration and require hospitalization of the patient and the administration of intravenous fluids. The acute vertigo usually lasts many hours to 1 to 2 weeks.[218]

Spontaneous recovery occurs over weeks to months. There has been concern on the basis of animal studies that prolonged administration of antivertiginous medications may prolong the time to recovery.[219] Many physicians ask patients to stop medication as soon as they can tolerate it. By 6 months, most patients have fully recovered, but may still experience transient positional vertigo triggered by sudden head movements. With recovery, the caloric responses may return to normal or remain diminished or absent.

Temporal Bone Pathology

Studies of temporal bones have been reported from only a few patients with vestibular neuritis.[5,199,214] No patient who died during the acute illness has had his or her temporal bones studied. Most studies from patients dying in the subacute stage have shown primary damage to a branch of the vestibular nerve.[5] Partial to total loss of the superior division of the vestibular nerve supplying the horizontal and superior ampullae has been reported (Fig. 152-5). Associated degeneration of the hair cells occurs in the corresponding sensory organ.

Infectious Causes

Infectious illness, especially colds, sinusitis, and other respiratory tract infections, precede or occur with vestibular neuritis approximately 50% of the time.[211,212] Several viruses have been suggested to be a cause.[220] Patients with mumps may experience vertigo. In a study of proven mumps meningoencephalitis, 37% had impairment of balance, 13% experienced vertigo, and only 2% had an associated hearing loss.[147] In herpes zoster oticus caused by VZV, approximately 25% of patients have vertigo, and may have diminished or absent caloric responses on the ipsilateral side. Some patients have vertigo without an accompanying hearing loss. Patients with influenza often have transient dizziness and vertigo.[221,222] Enterovirus infections have been associated with vestibular neuritis, and the virus has been detected by PCR in CSF in one patient.[223,224] Patients with infectious mononucleosis from an infection with Epstein-Barr virus may have transient vertigo with vertical or horizontal nystagmus.[225] Human herpesvirus type 7 has been associated with one case of vestibular neuritis.[149]

HSV is also associated with vestibular neuritis. Evidence in favor of this association is severalfold. HSV-1 DNA has been identified in vestibular ganglia from tissue obtained at routine autopsies. In some vestibular ganglia, latency-associated transcripts to HSV-1 have been found by reverse transcriptase PCR.[14] Latency-associated transcripts are thought to be responsible for maintaining latency in neurons. Another study could not identify HSV latency-associated transcripts in vestibular ganglia, however.[12]

Studies using a nested PCR assay of 21 randomly selected temporal bones at autopsy reported finding HSV DNA in 62% of vestibular ganglia and 48% of tissue taken from semicircular canals and macular organs.[226,227] The finding of HSV DNA within vestibular tissue suggests that a focal labyrinthine HSV recurrence could occur. Bacteria (*Borrelia burgdorferi* [Lyme disease] and *T. pallidum* [syphilis]) have also been associated with vertigo attacks similar to vestibular neuritis.[228,229]

Experimental Viral Infections of the Vestibular System

Several other viruses, including rubeola, HSV, mumps, and reoviruses, have been shown to infect the endolymphatic cells in the vestibular system and the vestibular ganglia after intracerebral, intravenous, or direct inoculation through the round window.[119] Generally, these viruses also infected the cochlea. When HSV-1 virus was inoculated into the auricle of 99 mice, 5% developed ataxia 6 to 8 days later.[230] Degeneration of Scarpa's ganglia was found in four of the five mice, and HSV viral antigen was identified in two ganglia. To date, there has been no experimental model that selectively damages branches of the vestibular nerve.

Meniere's Disease

Clinical, diagnostic, and management aspects of Meniere's disease are discussed in Chapters 149 and 164. The cause of Meniere's disease or endolymphatic hydrops remains elusive. Available temporal bone pathologic studies suggest an abnormality of endolymphatic overproduction or underabsorption.[231] Various pathophysiologic mechanisms have been proposed, with several suggesting an abnormal immune mechanism or persistence of a viral infection.[232,233]

In previous years, otitic syphilis was identified as a cause,[234] but more recently syphilis has rarely been found. Viruses have received considerable attention as a possible cause of Meniere's disease.[83,233,235] To date, viral associations have been mainly based on serologic studies.[236] No virus has been isolated from endolymphatic fluid or inner ear structures, and histologic studies have not identified characteristic viral inclusion bodies or viral antigens.

The herpesviruses have gained considerable interest because these viruses establish latency and could recur, causing repeated attacks of vertigo. CMV has been considered because approximately 1 in 100 to 200 infants are born with asymptomatic congenital CMV infection.[30] Some congenitally infected children subsequently have hearing loss that can occur more than 10 years after birth.[18] Evidence for persistence of CMV in the inner ear into adulthood is negligible, however. To date, CMV or its latent state has rarely been found in histologic material of inner ear tissue obtained at autopsy or endolymphatic shunt surgery from patients with Meniere's disease. Experimental inoculation of guinea pig CMV into adult seronegative or seropositive guinea pig endolymphatic sacs has produced the histologic picture of endolymphatic hydrops.[237]

HSV infections have also been considered to cause Meniere's disease.[236,238] Patients with Meniere's disease have been reported to have higher HSV serum antibody titers than controls.[233,236,239] HSV IgG antibody has been reported in perilymph of patients with Meniere's disease and in patients with otosclerosis.[238] One study reported HSV DNA in 100% of 25 vestibular ganglia from patients with Meniere's disease versus 81% of 37 vestibular ganglia from control patients.[240] Another study performed PCR assays for HSV, CMV, and VZV on 22 endolymphatic sacs obtained from patients with Meniere's disease.[241] On finding only two endolymphatic sacs positive for HSV DNA, the authors concluded that ongoing herpesvirus infection in the endolymphatic sac was an infrequent factor in the development of Meniere's disease. Another study using in situ hybridization on 10 endolymphatic sac specimens obtained at surgery for Meniere's disease reported VZV in 7, Epstein-Barr virus in 3, CMV in 1, and HSV in 0.[242]

The two aforementioned studies are difficult to interpret because, except for Epstein-Barr virus, DNA of the other herpesviruses is known to be latent only in neuronal cell bodies, which would not be expected to be present in endolymphatic sacs. Additional evidence against HSV as the etiology comes from several studies. HSV DNA has not been found in the vestibular ganglia of 11 individuals with Meniere's disease.[243] Palva and coworkers[244] were unable to culture HSV from Scarpa's ganglia of patients with Meniere's disease. Cowdry type A intranuclear inclusion bodies or HSV-like viral particles have not been identified in inner ear tissue of patients with Meniere's disease. Finally, Meniere's disease occurs usually in older adults, whereas recurrent herpetic infections occur typically in children and young adults. The current weight of evidence does not support a role for HSV, CMV, or VZV as an important cause of Meniere's disease.

SUGGESTED READINGS

Adler SP, Nigro G, Pereira L. Recent advances in the prevention and treatment of congenital cytomegalovirus infections. *Semin Perinatol.* 2007;31:10.

Bang HO, Bang J. Involvement of the central nervous system in mumps. *Acta Med Scand.* 1943;113:487.

Brookhouser PE, Bordley JE. Congenital rubella deafness: pathology and pathogenesis. *Arch Otolaryngol Head Neck Surg.* 1973;98:252.

Davis LE. Viruses and vestibular neuritis: review of human and animal studies. *Acta Otolaryngol Suppl.* 1993;503:70.

Davis LE, Johnsson L-G, Kornfeld M. Cytomegalovirus labyrinthitis in an infant: morphological, virological, and immunofluorescent studies. *J Neuropathol Exp Neurol.* 1981;40:9.

Everberg G. Deafness following mumps. *Acta Otolaryngol (Stockh).* 1957;48:397.

Frame JD. Clinical features of Lassa fever in Liberia. *Rev Infect Dis.* 1989;11(Suppl 4):S783.

Gacek RR, Gacek MR. Vestibular neuronitis: a viral neuropathy. *Adv Otorhinolaryngol.* 2002;60:54.

Gurney TA, Murr AH. Otolaryngologic manifestations of human immunodeficiency virus infection. *Otolaryngol Clin North Am.* 2003;36:607.

Hopfenspirger MT, Levine SC, Rimell FL. Infectious complications in pediatric cochlear implants. *Laryngoscope.* 2007;117:1825.

Kimberlin DW, Lin CY, Sánchez PJ, et al. Effect of ganciclovir therapy on hearing in symptomatic congenital cytomegalovirus disease involving the central nervous system: a randomized, controlled trial. *J Pediatr.* 2003; 143:16.

Linstrom CJ, Gleich LL. Otosyphilis: diagnostic and therapeutic update. *J Otolaryngol.* 1993;22:401.

Pass RF. Congenital cytomegalovirus infection and hearing loss. *Herpes.* 2005;12:50.

Reefhuis J, Honein MA, Whitney CG, et al. Risk of bacterial meningitis in children with cochlear implants. *N Engl J Med.* 2003;349:435.

Richardson MP, Reid A, Tarlow MJ, et al. Hearing loss during bacterial meningitis. *Arch Dis Child.* 1997;76:134.

Sekitani T, Imate Y, Noguchi T, et al. Vestibular neuronitis: epidemiological survey by questionnaire in Japan. *Acta Otolaryngol Suppl.* 1993;503:9.

Shambaugh GE, Hagens EW, Holderman JW, et al. Statistical studies of the children in the public schools for the deaf. *Arch Otolaryngol Head Neck Surg.* 1928;7:424.

Wellman MB, Sommer DD, McKenna J. Sensorineural hearing loss in postmeningitic children. *Otol Neurotol.* 2003;24:907.

Westerlaken BO, Stokroos RJ, Dhooge IJ, et al. Treatment of idiopathic sudden sensorineural hearing loss with antiviral therapy: a prospective randomized, double-blind clinical study. *Ann Otol Rhinol Laryngol.* 2003;112:993.

For complete list of references log onto www.expertconsult.com.

CHAPTER ONE HUNDRED AND FIFTY-THREE

Autoimmune Inner Ear Disease

Steven D. Rauch

Marc A. Cohen

Michael J. Ruckenstein

Key Points

- Autoimmune inner ear disease (AIED) is a rare entity characterized by bilateral sensorineural hearing loss that progresses over weeks to months, and is responsive to steroids.
- Primary AIED refers to pathology restricted to the ear, and secondary AIED refers to inner ear involvement of multisystemic autoimmune diseases.
- Autoimmune diseases associated with the inner ear include Cogan's syndrome, Wegener's granulomatosis, systemic lupus erythematosus, rheumatoid arthritis, scleroderma, Sjögren's syndrome, and celiac disease.
- Approximately 50% of patients with AIED have vestibulopathy.
- Studies have shown that the inner ear does not represent an immune-privileged site, but can generate a local immune response after either local or systemic immunization of antigen.
- Studies suggest that there is likely B-cell and T-cell involvement in AIED, but the pathogenesis has not been elucidated.
- Diagnosis of AIED relies on clinical evaluation and a comprehensive assessment of immunologic markers; Western blot for an antibody to a 68-kD protein that binds heat shock protein 70 is not the standard of care in the evaluation of AIED.
- Treatment of AIED is not urgent because there is a 6- to 12-month period in which a significant recovery of hearing is possible with administration of high-dose corticosteroids.
- Initial therapy for AIED is 60 mg of prednisone per day for 4 weeks.
- Response to steroids varies, and treatment is tailored to the initial response.
- Neither etanercept nor methotrexate has been shown to be efficacious in improving hearing loss in patients with AIED.
- Research regarding AIED is important because this is a reversible cause of sensorineural hearing loss; protocols must be informed by expanding knowledge of the pathophysiology of the disorder, and multicenter studies are necessary to evaluate the best use of immunosuppressive drugs.

Otologists and otologic researchers have long believed that the immune system might be capable of damaging the inner ear or eighth cranial nerve, leading to symptoms of hearing loss or dizziness. Some well-documented examples in which systemic autoimmune disease can do this include systemic lupus erythematosus, ulcerative colitis, Cogan's syndrome, and multiple sclerosis. There are some inner ear diseases, such as Meniere's disease and idiopathic sudden sensorineural hearing loss (SNHL), in which an immune-mediated mechanism has been hypothesized but not shown.

One condition—characterized by the clinical presentation of idiopathic, rapidly progressive, bilateral SNHL—has come to be known as autoimmune inner ear disease (AIED), immune-mediated inner ear disease, or immune-mediated cochleovestibular disease. Whether all patients with this presentation have the same underlying pathophysiology, and whether the pathophysiology is autoimmune are unknown. Research regarding AIED is important because the disease represents one of the few medically reversible causes of SNHL.

Definition

Defense against microorganisms is the prevalent concept explaining the evolution and need for the immune system. The immune system must possess the capacity to respond to potential environmental pathogens, and must maintain mechanisms that allow it to distinguish between foreign constituents and the host's own tissue. An autoimmune reaction ensues when the immune system's ability to distinguish between self and nonself is disturbed.

The classic definition of AIED, as provided by McCabe,[1] is that of rapidly progressive (over weeks to months) bilateral SNHL that responds to the administration of immunosuppressive agents. Although McCabe is often credited as the first to describe AIED, the concept of autoimmune hearing loss was first described in the German literature by Lehnhardt in 1958,[2] who described an "antigen-antibody reaction" in the "hearing organs," which improved with steroids. Although this entity is likely an immune-mediated disorder, there is no direct evidence that it is autoimmune in etiology. Nonetheless, the nomenclature coined by McCabe has become established and accepted in the literature.

The disorder defined earlier as AIED refers to a pathology restricted to the ear (primary AIED). Multisystemic, organ-nonspecific autoimmune diseases may involve the inner ear (secondary AIED), however. Such disorders include Cogan's syndrome, Wegener's granulomatosis, systemic lupus erythematosus, and the various systemic vasculitides.

Epidemiology

Primary AIED is a rare disorder. Because of the lack of a definitive diagnostic test for AIED, the precise incidence cannot be determined. It is less common, however, than sudden SNHL, which occurs with an incidence of 1 case per 5000 to 10,000 population per year.[3]

With several exceptions, inner ear involvement is rare in multisystemic autoimmune disorders. Cogan's syndrome, the archetypal AIED, is defined by the presence of labyrinthine and ocular pathology (described in more detail later). Wegener's granulomatosis manifests a significant incidence of ear disease (30% to 50%), with most patients having middle ear pathology, such as chronic otitis media and conductive hearing loss.[4] The presence of concomitant SNHL in patients with middle ear involvement is approximately 30%.[4,5] AIED has been associated with other systemic diseases of the immune system, including rheumatoid arthritis, scleroderma, Sjögren's syndrome, and celiac disease.

Pathology and Pathogenesis

Animal Studies

Various experimental approaches have been used to gain insight into the pathogenesis of AIED. None of these studies has yielded an animal model that is definitively analogous to the human condition, however.

Harris and colleagues[6-8] have contributed significant information to the literature pertaining to the processes mediating inflammation in the inner ear. Using a sterile labyrinthitis, Harris and colleagues[6-8] showed in these studies that the inner ear does not represent an immune-privileged site, but can generate a local immune response after either local or systemic immunization of antigen. These immune responses depend on the presence of an intact endolymphatic sac.[9] Cells that mediate the labyrinthitis enter the scala tympani via the spiral modiolar vein.[10] The ensuing labyrinthitis results in physiologic dysfunction, loss of sensory cells, and, ultimately, fibrosis and osteoneogenesis within the cochlea.[11]

Although these studies shed light on the mechanisms by which an immune-mediated response can be elicited within the cochlea, they do not specifically address the issues of an autoimmune response. To that end, a model of AIED was proposed in which heterologous (bovine) temporal bone antigen and immune adjuvant were used to immunize guinea pigs systemically.[12] This model showed modest changes in physiologic measures of hearing and cochlear morphology. The model has proven to be difficult to replicate, however. The main contribution of this work pertains to the detection of a specific antibody that binds to a 68-kD bovine inner ear antigen on Western blot analysis. This antibody has been found in the guinea pig model, and in humans with AIED.[13] The same antibody also binds to the inducible form of bovine (but not human) heat shock protein 70 (HSP-70), although it does not seem that this antibody is primarily directed against HSP-70 in the in vivo setting. The primary antigenic epitope against which this antibody is directed is unknown, and its role in mediating AIED is unclear.

Another approach to understanding the etiology of this disorder was taken by Nair and coworkers.[14-18] They immunized mice with chick and guinea pig inner ear extracts and created monoclonal antibodies against inner ear cells. One particular antibody, KHRI-3, binds to supporting cells of the organ of Corti, creating a characteristic wine-glass staining pattern when observed through immunofluorescence.[15-18] Infusion of KHRI-3 into live guinea pigs produces hearing loss.[15,16] The KHRI-3 antibody also binds to a 68- to 72-kD antigen on a Western blot of inner ear extract.[18] Sera from some humans with AIED strongly stained a 68- to 72-kD inner ear antigen immunoprecipitated from guinea pig inner ear extract with KHRI-3, and these same patient sera stained organ of Corti–supporting cells in a wine-glass pattern.[19] This is strong evidence that KHRI-3 and human antibodies recognize the same inner ear–supporting cell antigen.

More recent data suggest that KHRI-3 targets multiple peptides similar to those present in the highly conserved protein CTL2, which is abundantly expressed in the guinea pig and human inner ear.[14] CTL2 coprecipitates with the protein cochlin, which is one of the most expressed proteins in the inner ear. Cochlin is critical to the structure and function of the inner ear, and mutations are known to cause cochleovestibular pathology. More recent work reveals that cochlin-specific serum antibody titers are significantly elevated in individuals with AIED compared with age-matched controls.[20] The same study also implicates T-cell response to this specific protein, supporting cochlin as a possible target antigen susceptible to B-cell and T-cell influence.

A third approach has incorporated the study of animal models of multisystemic, organ-nonspecific autoimmune disease. These mouse models of systemic lupus erythematosus spontaneously develop autoimmune disease; they do not require any experimental manipulation. Various strains have been examined, with the most detailed studies focusing on the MRL-Fas^{lpr} and C3H-Fas^{lpr} mice. These strains develop elevations in auditory thresholds, degeneration of the stria vascularis, and antibody deposition within the strial capillaries.[5,21-25] These changes occur in the absence of inflammatory response. The etiology of the observed strial degeneration is unknown. The administration of corticosteroids improves cochlear function in these animals without impeding the development of the morphologic changes.[24,25] Studies have shown that there is similar efficacy in resolution of hearing loss with glucocorticoid and mineralocorticoid administration. These results suggest that the mechanism of reversal of hearing loss occurs as a result of alterations in local ion transport in the cochlea.[25-27]

These studies illustrate that immune-mediated and autoimmune pathology can affect the inner ear. The various pathologies observed in these models do not correlate well, however, with the clinical entity known as AIED.

Human Temporal Bone Studies

A few studies have been performed on human temporal bones derived from patients with autoimmune disease, specifically Wegener's granulomatosis, polyarteritis nodosa, Cogan's syndrome, and systemic lupus erythematosus.[5,21-23] Morphologic changes show findings consistent with two different pathogenic mechanisms. Some bones show fibrosis and osteoneogenesis within the scalae, findings consistent with the end stages of inflammation, as described earlier. Other bones show changes more consistent with ischemia, including cellular atrophy in the absence of inflammation. In cases of ischemia, the vascular compromise is likely secondary to a nonspecific vasculopathy in which the labyrinthine artery becomes occluded in the absence of vascular inflammation and necrosis associated with vasculitis.

Clinical Presentation

The hallmark of AIED, as originally described by McCabe,[1] is the presence of bilateral SNHL that progresses over weeks to months. The hearing loss may initially be unilateral, and it may take months for the bilaterality to emerge. Fluctuations in hearing may occur, but the overall course is one of a relentless deterioration in auditory function. Approximately 50% of patients have symptoms of vestibular dysfunction, with 20% of patients experiencing episodes of vertigo consistent with those seen in Meniere's disease.[5]

Cogan's syndrome represents the classic autoimmune disorder leading to inner ear dysfunction.[21,22] The original definition included the presence of nonsyphilitic interstitial keratitis, SNHL, vertigo, and tinnitus. Labyrinthine pathology may be coincident with the ocular manifestations, or may occur 6 months before or after the onset of eye disease. Other forms of ocular inflammation, including uveitis, iritis, episcleritis, or conjunctivitis, may occur instead of the keratitis, in which case the disorder may be defined as atypical Cogan's syndrome.[21,22] Many patients with Cogan's syndrome note a prodrome with symptoms of an upper respiratory tract infection, symptoms often seen with autoimmune disorders.[28]

Vogt-Koyanagi-Harada syndrome manifests with symptoms similar to those seen in Cogan's syndrome. It also includes depigmentation of the hair and skin around the eyelashes, loss of eyelashes, and onset of aseptic meningitis. This syndrome may represent an autoimmune reaction to melanin-containing cells.[4]

Wegener's granulomatosis is another multisystemic autoimmune disease associated with inner ear dysfunction. The disease is characterized by the granuloma formation and vasculitis typically initially affecting the upper and lower respiratory tracts. Ultimately, it may progress to a more diffuse granulomatous vasculitis with renal involvement. As noted earlier, the disorder is more commonly associated with middle ear disease resulting in a conductive hearing loss. Approximately 10% of patients may manifest an SNHL.[5]

Antiphospholipid antibody syndrome is a disorder of the immune system that causes coagulopathy and is defined by recurrent thrombosis, spontaneous abortions in women, and the presence of antiphospholipid antibodies (anticardiolipin or antilupus anticoagulant antibody). Investigators have noted the association of this autoimmune disorder with SNHL, likely related to microthrombus formation; 25% of all patients who fit the diagnostic criteria for Meniere's disease and idiopathic SNHL have at least one positive antiphospholipid antibody marker.[29]

Systemic vasculitides, such as polyarteritis nodosa, may rarely result in a rapidly progressive hearing loss.[30] In one prospective controlled study, the incidence of SNHL in patients with systemic lupus erythematosus was noted to be 58%.[31] Confounding variables in this study included the administration of potentially ototoxic medications and the presence of renal failure. One temporal bone derived from a patient with lupus did manifest evidence of intracochlear inflammation, including fibrosis and osteoneogenesis.[32]

Differential Diagnosis

AIED may initially manifest in a fashion similar to that seen in sudden SNHL. AIED and idiopathic sudden SNHL are two distinct disorders, however. AIED is considerably rarer than sudden SNHL. AIED is by definition bilateral, although at initial presentation AIED may not have affected both ears, whereas sudden hearing loss is virtually always unilateral. Sudden hearing loss develops in 72 hours or less. In contrast, AIED progresses over days to months; serial audiograms on a monthly basis show continued decline. Sudden hearing loss is an otologic emergency with a treatment window of perhaps 2 to 4 weeks, during which a short burst and taper of corticosteroids must be administered to achieve optimal recovery.

AIED is not urgent. Patients with hearing loss progression over 6 to 12 months can still achieve significant recovery with administration of a long course of high-dose corticosteroids or other immunosuppressive drugs. Throughout the otolaryngology community, there is general awareness that some cases of SNHL are potentially reversible with corticosteroids. There is little awareness, however, that these two entities are quite different in etiology, presentation, workup, and management. Hasty administration of a short tapering course of steroids can delay diagnosis of AIED, and can confuse interpretation of serologic testing.

The clinical presentation of AIED may closely mimic the presentation of Meniere's disease. During the first months of evaluation, the two entities may be difficult to differentiate. Both can manifest fluctuations in hearing and episodic vertigo. If corticosteroids are administered, a spontaneous recovery in hearing, as seen in Meniere's disease, may be mistaken for a positive response to immunosuppressive therapy. Ultimately, the more aggressive course of AIED allows for the differentiation of these two disorders. It has been suggested that a subgroup of patients with symptoms of Meniere's disease may share a common pathophysiology with patients who have AIED. This association is based on studies that have noted that approximately one third of patients with Meniere's disease may have a positive Western blot assay for anti-HSP-70 antibodies.[33,34] This finding was not supported by a later study, however, in which the commercially available assay was used.[35]

Otosyphilis is a disorder that can closely mimic AIED, and must be ruled out as part of the workup. An acoustic neuroma may manifest with sudden or progressive unilateral SNHL. Rarely, meningitis, multiple sclerosis, or malignancy (e.g., metastatic disease, lymphoma) involving the dura may manifest as rapidly progressive bilateral hearing loss.

Diagnosis

In patients suspected to have AIED, an appropriate review of systems would include questions pertaining to recurrent or chronic ocular disease, nephritis, arthritis, pneumonitis, sinusitis, and inflammatory bowel disease. Routine serologic tests in patients who may have AIED include a complete blood count with differential white blood cell count, erythrocyte sedimentation rate, rheumatoid factor, antinuclear antibody test, anti–double-stranded DNA antibodies, anti-SSA/B antibodies, antiphospholipid antibodies, C3 and C4 complement levels, antigliadin antibodies, and Raji cell assay for circulating immune complexes. A fluorescent treponemal antibody absorption test (or a *Treponema pallidum* hemagglutination test) must be obtained to rule out otosyphilis. A human immunodeficiency virus test may be considered to rule out hearing loss associated with acquired immunodeficiency syndrome. This workup is aimed at detecting evidence of systemic immunologic dysfunction. None of these tests has been shown to correlate with the diagnosis of primary AIED. Magnetic resonance imaging with paramagnetic enhancement must be obtained to rule out the retrocochlear lesions discussed earlier in this chapter.

Diagnosis of primary AIED can be difficult. No serologic or immunologic test has yet shown sufficient diagnostic accuracy to allow for the establishment of a definitive diagnosis. Tests of cellular immunity have been advocated by McCabe[23] (lymphocyte migration-inhibition assay), and Hughes and coworkers[36] (lymphocyte transformation test). These tests have never been adequately validated, and their diagnostic accuracy has not been determined. During the 1990s, most attention was focused on the role of Western blotting for detection of an antibody that binds to a 68-kD antigen derived from bovine temporal bone extract and to the inducible form of HSP-70.[5,13,37,38] As noted earlier, these antibodies were first determined to be significant when they were detected in guinea pigs immunized with bovine inner ear extract and in humans manifesting AIED.[13]

In a prospective controlled study, with well-defined entry criteria, Moscicki and colleagues[39] showed that 89% of patients with active, rapidly progressive hearing loss did have detectable levels of this antibody, whereas none of the control patients had positive Western blots. Subsequently, 66 additional cases of possible immune-mediated inner ear disease were studied using the same diagnostic criteria of Moscicki and colleagues.[39] Five patients were excluded from analysis because they had Cogan's syndrome, an autoimmune vasculitis characterized by SNHL, vertigo, and interstitial keratitis of the eyes, leaving 61 patients with AIED. Results are shown in Table 153-1. Demographic features and trends in the correlation of Western blot assay with steroid response in this group of patients are essentially the same as Moscicki's original cohort. The proportion of patients with positive Western blot assay and the proportion of Western blot–positive patients who responded to steroids are lower than in the retrospective study by Moscicki and colleagues.[39]

More recent studies have evaluated the use of positron emission tomography (PET) scan as a tool for the diagnosis of AIED. Although initial observations suggested an association between AIED and positive PET scans, the more recent work fails to show any diagnostic benefit to PET scan.[40,41] At this time, there is no role for PET in diagnosis of AIED.

The diagnosis of primary AIED is based on clinical evaluation, the demonstration of progressive SNHL on audiometric assessment done at monthly intervals, and, most importantly, a positive response to the administration of corticosteroids. The presence of a positive Western blot may support the diagnosis of AIED, but can neither confirm nor rule out the diagnosis.

Treatment

Corticosteroid therapy for AIED evolved during the mid-1980s through the 1990s as a result of clinical experience. Niparko and associates[42] reported a prospective, randomized trial that showed most patients with suspected AIED responded to corticosteroids, although the response was highly variable. These data seem to substantiate the current practice of most otologists. Initial therapy for adults consists of a therapeutic trial of prednisone (60 mg daily for 4 weeks). Pediatric patients receive 1 mg/kg/day of prednisone for 4 weeks. Although patients may occasionally respond early in the 4-week period, many do not begin to improve until late in the month; shorter courses of treatment usually result in relapse.

Table 153-1

Relationship of Western Blot Assay for Anti–Heat Shock Protein 70 Antibodies and Response to Corticosteroid Therapy in 61 Patients with Autoimmune Inner Ear Disease

	Steroid Response		
Western Blot	Positive	Negative	No Prescription
Positive	14	11	7
Negative	5	12	8
Undetermined	2	2	—

From Moscicki RA, San Martin JE, Quintero CH, et al. Serum antibody to increase ear proteins in patients with progressive hearing loss, correlation with disease activity and response to corticosteroid treatment. *JAMA*. 1994;272:611.

Patients' hearing is tested at the initiation of therapy and again at 4 weeks. If the threshold has improved by 15 dB or more at one frequency or 10 dB at two or more consecutive frequencies, or if the discrimination is significantly improved, patients are considered steroid responders. Nonresponders are tapered off their medication in 12 days. Responders continue full-dose therapy until monthly audiograms confirm that they have reached a plateau of recovery. Their medication is slowly tapered over 8 weeks to a maintenance dose of 10 to 20 mg every other day. This maintenance dose is continued for a variable time. Clinical observation suggests that patients with a treatment duration of less than 6 months are at increased risk of relapse compared with patients treated for 6 months or longer.

Patterns of response to corticosteroid therapy vary. Some patients have improvement in threshold, some have improvement in discrimination only, and some experience improvement in both areas. Some patients with hearing loss fluctuation and progression before therapy show stabilization in hearing without actual improvement. Historically, these cases have been considered nonresponders, but this issue is currently being reassessed. Most responders slowly taper off the steroid dose, wean from steroids, and do well. A subset of AIED patients relapses while tapering or after discontinuing the medication. In some instances, additional corticosteroid therapy is effective. Occasionally, the hearing loss becomes refractory to corticosteroids. In such cases, alternative immunosuppressive drugs are considered. Some patients, especially children, may occasionally show steroid-dependent hearing loss. In other words, they cannot be weaned below a certain level of steroid dosage without decline in hearing. Such patients often develop unacceptable side effects of long-term steroid administration. Methotrexate has been used as part of a prednisone-sparing regimen; however, a more recent randomized, prospective controlled, multicenter trial has shown methotrexate to be no better than placebo at maintaining a remission in these patients.[43]

Corticosteroid therapy has limitations. The risks of long-term administration include gastritis and ulcers, fluid retention and weight gain, blood pressure lability, altered blood glucose metabolism and diabetes, avascular necrosis of the hip, mood changes or psychiatric problems, sleep disturbance, accelerated cataract formation, osteoporosis, and cushingoid habitus. Overall steroid response rate is approximately 60% in AIED patients. Some initial responders become refractory at the time of relapse. Despite these limitations, corticosteroid therapy remains the mainstay of AIED treatment on the basis of the extensive clinical experience with its use.

Alternatives to systemic corticosteroids include methotrexate, etanercept, and cyclophosphamide. Low-dose methotrexate seemed to be useful as an adjunct in management of steroid-dependent hearing loss.[44] As noted earlier, a more recent large trial indicates that methotrexate may not serve an effective role as a prednisone-sparing drug.

Etanercept, an inhibitor of tumor necrosis factor-α, has been used to treat AIED. Anecdotally, it seems to work well in combination with methotrexate because of its steroid-sparing effect. As seen in rheumatoid arthritis, etanercept alone does not seem to be nearly as effective. In an open-label and blinded, prospective study, etanercept was shown not to be efficacious in improving hearing loss in patients with AIED.[40,45] A more recent study of nine patients showed, however, that the administration of transtympanic tumor necrosis factor-α inhibitor may aid in the tapering of high-dose steroids in AIED.[46] Although this is a pilot study, the results are promising and warrant further investigation.

Cyclophosphamide is a potent cytotoxic agent generally used for cancer chemotherapy and treatment of Wegener's granulomatosis. Although some authors advocate its use as a first-line drug,[23] the high risk of toxicity makes it a better choice as a salvage drug or treatment of last resort. An initial dose of 1 mg/kg/day orally for 4 to 6 weeks may be instituted. When no response is apparent, the dose is doubled to 2 mg/kg/day. Responders are treated for 6 to 12 months. Toxicity includes severe myelosuppression, opportunistic infection, hair loss, cystitis, infertility, and increased risk of malignancies. Weekly monitoring of hematologic status is mandatory. Many patients, when confronted with the risk of this medication, would rather consider cochlear implantation.

Intratympanic steroid therapy, intratympanic tumor necrosis factor-α inhibitor, systemic IgG injections, and plasmapheresis are possible treatments with sound theoretic justification. Intratympanic steroid therapy is particularly appealing because it is minimally invasive and enables direct application of the drug to the affected site with low risk of systemic effects. There are, however, no published series in which these treatments have been systematically applied. The best role for any of these treatment modalities remains to be determined.

The only drugs of proven utility in the management of AIED are the corticosteroids. All other immunosuppressants currently employed have not been systematically evaluated and carry with them serious toxicity risks. In a patient who cannot be maintained on corticosteroids because of complications, the possibility of withdrawing treatment, with the intention of inserting a cochlear implant when hearing becomes significantly impaired, must be considered.

Summary and Future Directions

The story of AIED from the initial description by McCabe to current therapy practices has been presented here as a simple and direct path. That has not been the actual case. It has been a broad and meandering path with significant contributions by many investigators and numerous important digressions. It is a story that still has far to go. The clinical description of this disorder is confined to its auditory manifestations. As noted earlier, 50% of AIED patients have vestibular symptoms. This aspect of the illness has not been well characterized clinically. Just as there are many AIED patients with auditory symptoms exclusively, there may be an equal number with vestibular symptoms exclusively. Such a presentation has not yet been reported.

Little is understood about the underlying pathophysiology of AIED. That SNHL can be reversible flies in the face of accepted dogma that, after SNHL, hearing cannot be restored. It is interesting to consider what pathophysiologic mechanism could disable neural signal transduction or transmission in the auditory system, yet be reversed months later by anti-inflammatory or immunosuppressive drugs. A solution to this puzzle is expected to come from systematic research into the nature of the humoral and cell-mediated immune response of affected patients. Although the Carey model using KHRI-3 is promising, as yet there is no widely accepted animal model of the AIED phenomenon in which to carry out such research, and human studies progress slowly because of the lack of the clinical material. This scarcity does not diminish the significance of the topic, however.

Understanding the mechanism of AIED would provide a new level of insight into the role of systemic and organ-specific immune reactions in disease of the inner ear. The fact that 20% of AIED patients have a clinical presentation overlapping with Meniere's disease, and 33% of Meniere's disease patients have evidence of antibodies to the 68- to 72-kD antigen by Western blot assay is strong evidence of a shared pathophysiologic mechanism. Although AIED is rare, Meniere's disease is not. In the United States alone, there are an estimated 125,000 cases yearly. New ways of understanding Meniere's disease could have great public health benefit.

Diagnosis of AIED currently relies on clinical factors alone. As stated earlier, the observation that many AIED patients carry serum antibodies reactive with HSP-70 does not seem to implicate HSP-70 in the pathophysiology of AIED. HSP-70 may carry an epitope shared with the true target antigen, or may otherwise colocalize with it biochemically. Despite poor understanding of AIED pathophysiology, detection of this, CTL2, cochlin, or other marker antibodies may become clinically useful. The utility of an assay would be greatly enhanced by development of a quantitative measure that enables clinicians to follow antibody titers by serial testing. In addition, estimation of sensitivity and specificity of the assay must be made by its broad application to a wide variety of ear diseases and immunologic disorders.

Current AIED therapy is based on empiric experience gathered during the late 1980s and through the 1990s, and validated by more recent clinical studies; this is despite a clear understanding of the underlying pathophysiology. Future therapeutic protocols must be informed by expanding knowledge of the pathophysiology of the disorder. Large multicenter studies are necessary to evaluate carefully the best use of corticosteroids and other immunosuppressive drugs. Consensus must be achieved on the clinical diagnostic criteria and treatment regimens to enable comparison between studies. Even with strict adherence to rigorous methodology, it may take many years to address these questions. For the foreseeable future, AIED will remain one of the most interesting, important, and challenging problems confronting otologists and otologic researchers.

SUGGESTED READINGS

Baek MJ, Park HM, Johnson JM, et al. Increased frequencies of cochlin-specific T cells in patients with autoimmune sensorineural hearing loss. *J Immunol.* 2006;177:4203.

Harris JP, Weisman MH, Derebery JM, et al. Treatment of corticosteroid-responsive autoimmune inner ear disease with methotrexate: a randomized controlled trial. *JAMA.* 2003;290:1875.

Matteson EL, Choi HK, Poe DS, et al. Etanercept therapy for immune-mediated cochleovestibular disorders: a multicenter, open-label, pilot study. *Arthritis Rheum.* 2005;53:337.

McCabe BF. Autoimmune sensorineural hearing loss. *Ann Otol Rhinol Laryngol.* 1979;88:585.

Moscicki RA, San Martin JE, Quintero CH, et al. Serum antibody to inner ear proteins in patients with progressive hearing loss: correlation with disease activity and response to corticosteroid treatment. *JAMA.* 1994;272:611.

Nair TS, Kozma KE, Hoefling NL, et al. Identification and characterization of choline transporter like protein 2, an inner ear glycoprotein of 68 and 72 kDa that is the target of antibody-induced hearing loss. *J Neurosci.* 2004;24:1772.

Niparko JK, Wang NY, Rauch SD, et al. Serial audiometry in a clinical trial of AIED treatment. *Otol Neurotol.* 2005;26:908.

For complete list of references log onto www.expertconsult.com.

CHAPTER ONE HUNDRED AND FIFTY-FOUR

Vestibular and Auditory Ototoxicity

Leonard P. Rybak

Key Points

- Measurement of peak and trough serum levels of aminoglycosides provides rough guidelines for therapeutic efficacy, but is not an absolute guarantee for prevention of ototoxicity, particularly vestibular ototoxicity.
- Bacteremia, fever, hepatic dysfunction, the presence of another ototoxic, and renal dysfunction have been associated with increased incidence or severity of ototoxicity of aminoglycosides.
- Aminoglycosides seem to form an ototoxic complex with iron.
- Ototoxicity from aminoglycosides may be reduced by pretreatment with salicylates.
- Although some clinical improvement can be seen beginning 2 months after onset of symptoms, recovery from oscillopsia resulting from aminoglycoside ototoxicity is rarely complete.
- Cisplatin and aminoglycoside antibiotics damage outer hair cells in the base of the cochlea, resulting in high-frequency sensorineural hearing loss that may later involve lower frequencies.
- There is a genetic predisposition to aminoglycoside-induced hearing loss that involves a mutation of mitochondrial DNA.
- Ototoxicity caused by aminoglycosides and cisplatin seems to be related to the production of reactive oxygen species that damage the hair cells, resulting in cell death and hearing loss.
- Hearing loss caused by cisplatin seems to be highly variable, and seems to be related to dose; age of the patient; and other factors such as noise exposure, exposure to other ototoxic drugs, depleted nutritional state including low serum albumin and anemia, and cranial irradiation.
- Ototoxicity with difluoromethylornithine, salicylates, and erythromycin is nearly always reversible.
- Hearing loss caused by abuse of hydrocodone does not respond to corticosteroids.

Ototoxicity refers to the tendency of a drug or chemical agent to cause inner ear dysfunction, producing symptoms of hearing loss, dizziness, or both. Inner ear tissues may be damaged either temporarily or permanently. Many agents can cause ototoxicity. This chapter discusses some common drugs that can cause hearing loss or injury to the cochleovestibular apparatus.

Aminoglycoside Antibiotics

The aminoglycoside antibiotics are an important class of anti-infectious agents. They were developed to combat tuberculosis and other life-threatening infections. The first members of this class of drugs were streptomycin and dihydrostreptomycin. Initial clinical trials showed that these compounds could damage the kidneys and the inner ear. Since then, many new aminoglycosides have been developed. Dihydrostreptomycin proved to be too toxic and was taken off the market. Neomycin was found to be too toxic for systemic use and has been relegated to local application. Other members of this group of drugs include kanamycin, gentamicin, tobramycin, amikacin, netilmicin, and sisomicin. Some of these agents are more toxic to either the cochlea or the vestibular apparatus, although their ototoxicity is not completely selective. Toxicity generally occurs only after days or weeks of exposure. The overall incidence of aminoglycoside auditory toxicity is estimated to be approximately 20%, whereas vestibulotoxicity may occur in about 15%.[1]

Pharmacokinetics

Aminoglycosides are highly charged molecules and are poorly absorbed orally. Only approximately 3% of an orally administered dose is absorbed from the gastrointestinal tract. Aminoglycosides are normally used parenterally for severe systemic infections. The concentrations of aminoglycosides in tissues are usually approximately one third of the corresponding serum concentration. Penetration of the blood-brain barrier is generally poor, so aminoglycosides are injected intrathecally to treat meningitis. Previous studies have suggested that aminoglycosides are not metabolized. A toxic metabolite may be formed in the inner ear, however.[1] Aminoglycosides are excreted primarily by the kidney by glomerular filtration, and high concentrations of drug in the urine may be achieved. Impaired renal function reduces the rate of excretion. Renal failure is a risk factor for ototoxicity, and dosing of aminoglycosides must be modified to compensate for delayed renal excretion.

Measurement of peak and trough serum levels of aminoglycosides provides rough guidelines for therapeutic efficacy, but is not an absolute guarantee for prevention of ototoxicity, particularly vestibular ototoxicity. An association between trough levels of aminoglycosides and ototoxicity has been pointed out.[2] Ototoxicity is likely related to the area under the curve of blood levels over time, rather than individual peak and trough measurements.[3] An animal study showed no relationship between ototoxicity and plasma level of aminoglycoside. The total dose or area under the curve was a much better predictor of amikacin ototoxicity in this animal model.[4]

Suggested guidelines for monitoring serum levels of aminoglycosides are as follows:

1. In patients with normal kidney function, the peak level is measured within the first 1 or 2 days of treatment, the trough level is measured within 1 week, and peak and trough levels are measured about every week after that.

2. In patients with impaired but stable renal function, the peak level is determined within the first 2 days of treatment, the trough and another peak level are determined within 1 week, and peak and trough levels are measured about twice weekly thereafter.

3. In the presence of impaired and unstable kidney function, peak and trough levels are obtained within the first 2 days of therapy. Serum levels may need to be measured every day as long as renal function is unstable.

4. After any changes in dosage, peak and trough levels are determined within the next 2 days.[5]

Aminoglycoside ototoxicity may be detected, but because of a life-threatening infection and a lack of suitable alternative antibiotic therapy, it may be necessary to continue treatment. Antibiotic ototoxicity may continue even after cessation of aminoglycoside therapy.[5]

More recent studies in animals and in humans have shown the presence of a metabolite of streptomycin in the serum of patients with tuberculosis treated with streptomycin. Five male patients treated with streptomycin for 35 to 90 days with 1 g/day presenting with mild to severe inner ear malfunction were found to have streptidine present. Streptidine may represent an ototoxic metabolite of streptomycin.[6]

Histopathology

Animal and human temporal bone histopathologic studies show that the cochlear and vestibular hair cells serve as primary targets for injury. In the organ of Corti, the outer hair cells of the basal turn are damaged first. As drug treatment is continued, the damage may spread to more apical regions. Inner hair cells seem to be more resistant to injury than outer hair cells. This difference could be a result of the higher concentration of the natural antioxidant, glutathione, in the inner hair cells and in the apical turn outer hair cells compared with in the outer hair cells of the basal turn.[7] Progressive destruction of spiral ganglion cells has been shown in animal studies and in human temporal bone reports.[8,9] In some patients, spiral ganglion cells may be damaged directly by aminoglycosides without injury to outer hair cells.[10] The stria vascularis may become thinner as a result of marginal cell death.[11] In the vestibular system, the hair cell damage may begin in the apex of the cristae and in the striola regions of the maculi.[12] Hair cell destruction may extend to the periphery of the vestibular sensory epithelium, where type I hair cells are primarily affected.[13]

A quantitative study of 17 temporal bones was carried out in patients with well-documented clinical evidence of aminoglycoside ototoxicity, and the results were compared with age-matched controls. Streptomycin caused a significant loss of type I and type II hair cells in all vestibular organs, with a greater loss of type I hair cells in the cristae, but not in the maculae. The vestibular toxic effects of kanamycin seemed to be similar to streptomycin, but neomycin did not cause the loss of any vestibular hair cells. There was no significant loss of Scarpa's ganglion cells for any of the aminoglycosides.[14]

Clinical Manifestations

High-frequency hearing loss tends to occur first and may be detectable before it becomes clinically noticeable.[15] Continued exposure to aminoglycosides may result in hearing loss that progresses to lower frequencies, including the important speech range, interfering with communication skills. A hearing loss of 20 dB or more at two or more adjacent frequencies should be documented to confirm the diagnosis of drug-related hearing loss after exclusion of other causes of hearing loss.

Delayed ototoxicity may occur after cessation of treatment with aminoglycoside antibiotics. Delayed onset of hearing loss usually manifests within 1 to 3 weeks after the end of therapy.[16]

Onset of vestibular ototoxicity is unpredictable, and may not correlate with cumulative dose of ototoxic medication.[17] Ambulatory patients are asymptomatic until they notice the presence of imbalance and ataxia, dramatically worsened by motion, with relative freedom from symptoms during periods of complete immobility. Patients change from being normal to being symptomatic during an easily identifiable 1- or 2-day period, after which symptoms are always present during motion or ambulation. The severity of symptoms varies, ranging from imbalance and staggering to complete inability to walk without assistance. Severely affected individuals also usually experience oscillopsia. Although some clinical improvement can be seen beginning 2 months after onset of symptoms, it is rarely complete.[18]

Rotational vestibular testing in a few patients indicated that results were normal in patients receiving aminoglycoside therapy who were asymptomatic. When abnormalities were observed, as they always were in symptomatic patients, the low-frequency rotational responses were affected first and most severely. When responses to all frequencies were absent, oscillopsia and severe imbalance were usually present. Improvement in function sometimes could be shown by rotational testing. This improvement was always greatest in the high frequencies, and clinical recovery was often not as great as the improvements in test results would have suggested.[18]

Various risk factors have been studied to determine whether they play a role in increasing the likelihood of ototoxicity in various patient populations. Bacteremia, fever, hepatic dysfunction, and renal dysfunction have been associated with ototoxicity in prospective, double-blind clinical trials of gentamicin, tobramycin, and amikacin.[19] Combinations of another ototoxic drug and an aminoglycoside may increase the risk and severity of ototoxicity. Ethacrynic acid was reported to exacerbate the ototoxicity of aminoglycosides in patients with uremia.[3] Furosemide was reported to result in severe sensorineural hearing loss (SNHL) in a patient who had received only five doses of gentamicin for pneumonia.[20] An extremely important risk factor is a mitochondrial RNA mutation, which dramatically increases the risk of ototoxicity. This mutation may sensitize a patient to even a single dose of aminoglycoside. This mutation follows a maternal inheritance pattern, and has been described in Chinese, Arab-Israeli, Japanese, and North American families.[21] Seventeen percent of patients with aminoglycoside-induced hearing loss may have this mutation.[1]

Mutations in mitochondrial 12S ribosomal RNA render patients highly susceptible to aminoglycoside ototoxicity. The first described mutation was an A1555G mutation in the 12S rRNA gene. Mutations in the mitochondrial 12S rRNA make this mammalian RNA more similar to the bacterial rRNA, the primary target of the bactericidal activity of aminoglycosides.[22] This mutation has been associated with spontaneous and aminoglycoside-induced hearing loss. In China, where this mutation seems to occur in 5% to 6% of sporadic patients, approximately one third of patients with aminoglycoside ototoxicity seem to have the A1555G mutation.[22] For an unknown reason, only the auditory system, but not the vestibular part of the inner ear, is sensitized to the toxic effects of aminoglycosides in patients with this mutation.[1]

The risks of intratympanic therapy for Meniere's disease and the use of potential otoprotective agents to prevent or reduce aminoglycoside ototoxicity are discussed in greater detail in Chapters 149, 155, and 165.

Mechanisms of Ototoxicity

Aminoglycosides, such as dihydrostreptomycin, enter the mouse outer hair cell through the mechanoelectrical transduction channel and act as a permeant blocker.[23,24] This channel can act as a one-way valve for aminoglycoside entry, promoting the accumulation of aminoglycoside within the cell. There seems to be a competition between the aminoglycoside and calcium for entry into the outer hair cell. The normal low endolymph concentration of calcium promotes intracellular accumulation of aminoglycosides.[24]

The aminoglycoside reacts with inner ear tissues to form an active, ototoxic metabolite. The drug in its inactive form combines with iron to form an ototoxic complex. This complex reacts with oxygen to produce reactive oxygen species (ROS). These ROS can react with various cell components, primarily in the outer hair cell.

ROS formation by aminoglycosides in vitro requires iron and the presence of polyunsaturated lipids as electron donors. Electron spray ionization mass spectrometry showed that gentamicin strongly binds to L-R-phosphatidylinositol 4,5-bisphosphate (PIP_2), a membrane lipid rich in arachidonic acid. Studies using lipid-coated membranes confirmed that iron ions and gentamicin can form ternary complexes among gentamicin, iron, and phospholipids. Peroxidation of PIP_2 by ferrous ions significantly increased in the presence of gentamicin, and oxidative damage to PIP_2 was accompanied by the release of arachidonic acid. Arachidonic acid also forms a ternary complex with Fe^{2+}/Fe^{3+}-gentamicin. This complex reacts with lipid peroxides and molecular oxygen, leading to arachidonic acid peroxidation.[25] These ROS can react with various cell components, including the phospholipids in the cell membrane, proteins, and DNA to disrupt the function, primarily in the outer hair cell. This process can trigger programmed cell death, resulting in apoptosis.[1]

Data from experimental studies strongly suggest that aminoglycosides trigger apoptosis at clinically relevant doses,[26] whereas higher doses may trigger necrotic cell death.[27] The ototoxic effects of neomycin[28,29] seem to be mediated by c-Jun N-terminal kinase (JNK). JNK[30] and extracellular regulated kinase (ERK) 1/2 mitogen-activated protein kinases seem to be associated with gentamicin-induced apoptosis in the inner ear.[31] Gentamicin seems to trigger apoptosis by ROS and to be mediated by Ras/Rho GTPases.[30]

Inhibitors of apoptosis proteins play an important role in regulating apoptosis by preventing activation of effector caspases. The effects of specific inhibitors of the X-linked inhibitor of apoptosis (XIAP) on hair cell death caused by gentamicin were examined in basal turn organ of Corti explants from postnatal day 3 or 4 rats in tissue culture exposed to gentamicin. XIAP inhibitors increased gentamicin-induced hair cell loss, but an inactive analog had no effect. A caspase-3 inhibitor decreased caspase-3 activation and hair cell loss from gentamicin plus an XIAP, but caspase-8 and caspase-9 inhibitors did not. These findings indicate that XIAP acts normally to decrease caspase-3 activation and hair cell loss during gentamicin ototoxicity.[32]

Apoptosis may be related to the enzyme protein kinase C zeta. Amikacin treatment in animals induced the cleavage of this enzyme and nuclear translocation, leading to chromatin condensation and decreased nuclear factor kappa B (NFκB) levels in the nucleus. These deleterious effects were prevented by pretreatment with aspirin, resulting in protection of hair cells and spiral ganglion neurons.[33]

Concentration-dependent protection against the ototoxicity of kanamycin combined with ethacrynic acid was found in guinea pigs receiving dexamethasone by intracochlear administration with an osmotic minipump before and after the ototoxic treatment. A statistically significant preservation of outer hair cell counts and lower auditory brainstem evoked potential threshold shifts were found in the dexamethasone-infused ears. No significant rescue was observed.[34]

Antineoplastic Agents

Cisplatin

Cisplatin is a potent antineoplastic agent that is used to treat various malignant tumors, including ovarian, testicular, bladder, lung, and head and neck carcinomas. Side effects include nausea and vomiting, neurotoxicity, ototoxicity, and nephrotoxicity.

Pharmacokinetics

The pharmacokinetics of cisplatin follow a biphasic clearance pattern. After a 1-hour intravenous infusion of 70 mg/m^2, the plasma half-lives in patients were 23 minutes and 67 hours; 17% ± 2.7% of the dose administered was excreted in the urine within the first 24 hours, primarily by glomerular filtration. Cisplatin is extensively bound to serum proteins. This bound form is inactive against tumor cells. The half-lives of free cisplatin in serum are much shorter than the total platinum, with half-lives of 8 minutes (free cisplatin) and 40 to 45 hours (total platinum).[35] The liver rapidly converts cisplatin into nontoxic metabolites within 1 hour after administration. The cytosol of the liver cells seems to form adducts of cisplatin with glutathione and cysteine. Cisplatin is taken up into the cells of the cortex and outer medulla of the kidney during the time when nephrotoxicity begins.[36]

Clinical Ototoxicity

Hearing loss caused by cisplatin seems to be highly variable, and seems to be related to dose; age of the patient; and other factors such as noise exposure,[37] exposure to other ototoxic drugs, depleted nutritional state including low serum albumin and anemia,[38] and cranial irradiation.[39] Children seem to be more susceptible than adults.[40] Hearing loss tends to be permanent and bilaterally symmetric. Symptoms of ototoxicity include subjective hearing loss, ear pain, and tinnitus.[41] Tinnitus has been reported in 2% to 36% of patients treated with cisplatin, and may be transient or permanent.[41] Although higher frequencies are affected first, hearing impairment may extend into the middle frequency range when doses greater than 100 mg/m^2 are used. When ultra-high-frequency audiometric testing is used, 100% of patients receiving high-dose cisplatin (150 to 225 mg/m^2) may show some degree of hearing loss.[38] Dose-related ototoxicity is illustrated by a report that 20% of patients treated with cisplatin for testicular cancer experienced permanent ototoxicity, but more than 50% of patients who received cisplatin in doses of greater than 400 mg/m^2 cumulative dose had permanent hearing loss.[37]

Pediatric patients were studied for cisplatin ototoxicity by use of otoacoustic emissions. A good correlation between transient otoacoustic emissions and pure-tone audiometric threshold was shown in children with normal middle ear function. In this series, 90.5% of patients had a significant SNHL at 8 kHz. The magnitude of the hearing loss was associated with young age at first dose of cisplatin administration, large number of cycles of chemotherapy, and high cumulative dose of cisplatin.[42]

The incidence and severity of hearing loss are reportedly enhanced by cranial irradiation.[39] Patients with nasopharyngeal carcinoma seem to be particularly susceptible to the interaction of cochlear irradiation and cisplatin chemotherapy. The required dose of radiation that acts on the cochlea is greater than 48 Gy in such patients.[43] A more recent study reported that radiation therapy for brain tumors, such as medulloblastoma, can be modified to reduce the doses of radiation to the cochlea, while still delivering full doses to the desired target volume of tissue. Using the technique of intensity-modulated radiation therapy for these tumors, far fewer patients had hearing loss. Only 13% of patients receiving the intensity-modulated radiation therapy protocol with cisplatin had grade 3 or 4 hearing loss compared with 64% of the conventional radiation therapy group.[39]

Whether hearing loss progresses after cessation of cisplatin chemotherapy has been a matter of controversy. It has been reported that 8 years after cisplatin therapy for testicular cancer, elevated urinary and serum platinum levels can be measured; nevertheless, no long-term toxicity was detected in these patients.[44] Long-term audiometric studies of 26 women treated with moderate-dose cisplatin (50 mg/m^2 body surface area every 4 weeks) for gynecologic cancer showed progressive hearing loss equal to or greater than 15 dB at long-term (59 to 115 months after treatment) follow-up in 14 patients (54%). These changes were considered to be small and restricted to three frequencies or fewer in one ear. Only two patients (8%) showed more severe threshold changes. The authors concluded that adult patients who receive treatment with moderate-dose cisplatin have a negligible long-term risk of drug-induced social disability from hearing.[45]

Delayed ototoxicity from cisplatin seems to be much more significant in children. Pediatric patients treated with cisplatin at cumulative doses approaching 400 mg/m^2 showed worsening of hearing with time after treatment. Audiograms showed hearing loss in 5% of patients before the end of therapy. After more than 2 years of follow-up, 44%

had significant hearing loss.[46] A more recent study found that the median time for first significant decrease in hearing was 135 days in children. Additional follow-up for 6 to 44 months showed mild further progression of hearing loss of 10 to 15 dB after completion of therapy.[47]

Studies of vestibular function in patients receiving cisplatin chemotherapy have suggested vestibulotoxic effects, especially in patients with preexisting vestibular problems.[48] With the vestibular autorotation test to study the vestibulo-ocular reflex, patients receiving cisplatin were screened for vestibulotoxicity. Vestibulo-ocular reflex gains at 3.1 Hz, 3.9 Hz, and 5.1 Hz were decreased, and phase lags at 3.1 Hz and 3.9 Hz were increased.[49]

Because chemoradiation protocols with intra-arterial cisplatin include thiosulfate protection, one may think that there would be less ototoxicity with this regimen than with intravenous cisplatin. This does not seem to be the case, however. A prospective study[50] evaluated 146 patients receiving high-dose intra-arterial cisplatin chemotherapy (150 mg/m^2 for four courses) with sodium thiosulfate rescue and concurrent radiation therapy (70 Gy) for locally advanced head and neck cancer. After treatment, 23% of the ears were recommended to need hearing aids. With multivariate analysis, cumulative dose of cisplatin and radiation, and young age were found to have a causal relationship with increased SNHL during and after therapy. In the multivariate prediction analysis, the pretreatment hearing level of the involved ear was found to be an independent predictive factor for hearing capability after therapy.

Maximum threshold shifts occurred after the second cisplatin infusion, and occurred at 8 kHz. Hearing loss seemed to reach a plateau at higher levels (75 to 80 dB hearing loss) for frequencies greater than compared with frequencies less than 8 kHz (45 to 60 dB hearing loss). Recovery was detected after therapy in 27 ears that had extensive losses at 1 kHz, 2 kHz, and 4 kHz.[51]

Risk Factors

There seems to be considerable individual variation in susceptibility to cisplatin ototoxicity. The severity of hearing loss seems to be related to the cumulative dose.[43] Age seems to be an important risk factor for ototoxicity. Children younger than 5 years and elderly adults are more susceptible to cisplatin-induced hearing loss than younger adults.[52,53] Additional factors, such as renal insufficiency and preexisting hearing loss and noise exposure, may increase the probability of cisplatin ototoxicity.[37]

Genetic Predisposition

Genetic predisposition to cisplatin-induced hearing loss may be related to mitochondrial mutations. Five of 20 cancer survivors with cisplatin ototoxicity were clustered in a rare European J mitochondrial haplogroup that is also associated with Leber's hereditary optic atrophy.[54] Other genetic factors may render patients susceptible to cisplatin ototoxicity. Testicular cancer survivors who received cisplatin chemotherapy showed differences in functional polymorphisms for glutathione-S-transferase. Having both alleles of 105Val-GSTP1 seemed to offer protection against hearing loss from cisplatin. The risk of having a poor hearing result was more than fourfold greater in patients with 105Ile/105Ile-GSTP1 or 105Val/105Ile-GSTP1. Genotypes associated with poorer hearing after cisplatin could indicate patients with a limited amount of glutathione for detoxification of cisplatin.[55]

Another potential genetic variant that could influence cisplatin susceptibility is megalin. Megalin is a member of the low-density lipoprotein family that is highly expressed in kidney proximal tubular cells and in marginal cells of the inner ear. Marginal cells have been shown in experimental animal studies to accumulate high levels of platinum-DNA adducts.[56] Twenty-five patients who developed hearing loss after cisplatin therapy were compared with 25 patients who received cisplatin chemotherapy without hearing loss, and were tested for nonsynonymous single nucleotide polymorphisms of megalin. A higher frequency of the A-allele of rs2075252 was observed in patients with hearing impairment compared with patients with normal hearing after cisplatin treatment. These findings suggest that single nucleotide polymorphisms at the megalin gene may affect individual susceptibility to cisplatin ototoxicity.[57]

Histopathology

Human temporal bone histopathology studies have shown the effects of cisplatin on the inner ear. The cochlea of a 9-year-old child with a brain tumor who sustained hearing loss after cisplatin showed degeneration of outer hair cells in the lower turns of the cochlea, spiral ganglia, and cochlear nerve. The vestibular ganglion cells and vestibular nerve were reportedly normal.[58] Scanning electron microscopic studies of the inner ear tissues of five patients with cisplatin ototoxicity revealed fusion of stereocilia of the outer hair cells, with damage to the cuticular plate.[59] Another study of patients receiving cisplatin with or without irradiation revealed a decreased number of inner and outer hair cells and spiral ganglion cells. The stria vascularis was also found to be atrophic.[60]

Experimental Studies

Histopathologic studies of the inner ear in animals mirror the findings reported in humans. The outer hair cells of the basal turn of the cochlea are damaged first, which extends to the more apical cells when dosing is continued.[41,61] The first row of outer hair cells seems to be most vulnerable.[41] Damage progresses to the outer hair cells, with dilation of the parietal membrane, softening of the cuticular plate, vacuole formation, and increased number of lysosome-like bodies in the apical portion of the hair cells. Stereocilia abnormalities, including fusion, on inner and outer hair cells are visible.[62] Damage to the stria vascularis can also occur, especially after exposure to high-dose cisplatin.[63] Electrophysiologic studies have shown that cisplatin ototoxicity can be manifested by a decrease in the endocochlear potential,[64] by elevation in auditory brainstem response thresholds,[64-67] and by elevations of the distortion product otoacoustic emissions (DPOAE).[65,68,69] The DPOAE input/output protocol is most sensitive for early detection of hair cell damage.[65] Elevations of DPOAE thresholds 4 days after cisplatin infusion in dogs could not be attributed to differences in peak plasma platinum levels. The variability in susceptibility in individual animals could not be explained by variations in plasma concentration of filterable platinum between animals.[69]

Mechanisms of Ototoxicity

The ototoxicity of cisplatin seems to be mediated by the production of ROS. Reactive oxygen molecules such as superoxide anion, hydrogen peroxide, and reactive nitrogen species such as nitric oxide can cause cell damage by reacting with cellular lipids, proteins, and DNA. The inner ear has an antioxidant defense system, consisting of the tripeptide glutathione and its related antioxidant enzymes, such as glutathione peroxidase, glutathione reductase, and the other antioxidant enzymes catalase and superoxide dismutase. Glutathione and the antioxidant enzymes have been shown to be decreased in association with cisplatin-induced ototoxicity in the rat.[66,67] Cisplatin has been shown to increase the formation of ROS in the cochlea by use of electron paramagnetic resonance spectrometry[70] and fluorescent dyes.[71] The production of superoxide anions inside the cochlear hair cells has been shown in vitro by use of the nitroblue tetrazolium reduction assay.[72] Superoxide dismutates to hydrogen peroxide either spontaneously or by means of superoxide dismutase. Increased hydrogen peroxide formation has been detected in the inner ear after cisplatin exposure.[70]

One of the enzymes that can produce superoxide radicals is an isoform of nicotinamide adenine dinucleotide phosphate (NADPH) oxidase, NOX-3, which is unique to the cochlea. Cisplatin has been shown to activate this enzyme, leading to a dramatic increase in superoxide production[73] not only in cochlear cell lines, but also in the cochlea of rats exposed to cisplatin.[74] Superoxide can lead to the formation of hydrogen peroxide, as just shown. The latter can be catalyzed by iron to form the very reactive hydroxyl free radical, which can react with polyunsaturated fatty acids in membranes to form the extremely toxic aldehyde, 4-hydroxynonenal. Superoxide can also react with nitric oxide to form peroxynitrite, which reacts with proteins to form nitrotyrosine. Cochlear hair cells of cisplatin-treated guinea pigs show immunoreactivity for 4-hydroxynonenal, but auditory neurons were found to be immunopositive for 4-hydroxynonenal and nitrotyrosine.[75]

Because iron chelators have been shown to provide partial protection to hair cells exposed to cisplatin in vitro, it has been proposed that part of the ototoxic mechanism of cisplatin includes an iron-dependent pathway.[72] The reaction of ROS with the plasma membrane leads to the formation of membrane lipid peroxidation products such as 4-hydroxynonenal, which are highly reactive and can lead to cellular damage and cell death.[76] The primary target of cisplatin ototoxicity seems to be the outer hair cells, with the hair cells in the basal turn being most susceptible. This increased susceptibility may result from the relatively low stores of glutathione in the outer hair cells of the basal turn compared with the inner hair cells and the outer hair cells in the more apical turns.[7] The ROS and reactive nitrogen species can attack cellular components as discussed previously, and superoxide anion can react with nitric oxide to form the highly toxic peroxynitrite, which can also attack cellular components.

A partial scheme for the mechanism for cisplatin ototoxicity has been shown in vitro. The reactive molecules, such as superoxide anion, nitric oxide, and others, can activate a cellular protein, p53. This activation can activate enzymes in the cell death pathway, the caspases. Caspase-8 has been shown to be activated, which converts a cellular protein BID from an inactive to an active form, truncated BID. Activated BID acts on a cytosolic protein, BAX, which translocates to the mitochondria. Activated BAX makes the mitochondrial membrane leaky, and the mitochondrial enzyme cytochrome-*c* leaks out into the cytoplasm. Cytosolic cytochrome-*c* interacts with another cell death enzyme, caspase-9, which activates caspase-3 and caspase-7, resulting in apoptosis or death of hair cells.[77] The application of caspase inhibitors to organ of Corti explants before and during exposure to cisplatin in vitro prevented apoptosis of hair cells.[78] This finding provides further evidence that cisplatin ototoxicity may be mediated by the cell death pathways, resulting in hair cell death and permanent hearing loss. These results need to be confirmed by the use of in vivo models of cisplatin ototoxicity. Additional research may provide clinically useful drugs that can block parts of these pathways and protect against ototoxicity of cisplatin.

A more recent study in rats treated with cisplatin confirmed that cisplatin induces an intrinsic apoptotic pathway in the cochlea. Cisplatin significantly increased the levels of caspase-3 and caspase-7 activity, active caspase-3 protein expression, and caspase-9 activity, and increased BAX protein expression accompanied by a decrease in the anti-apoptotic protein Bcl-2 expression in the cochlea. These changes were accompanied by elevation of auditory brainstem response threshold measurements.[79]

Cisplatin-induced cell death may be independent of p53 and caspases. A more recent study using the OC-k3 cell line exposed to cisplatin suggested that the mitogen-activated protein kinase cascade may be involved in induction of cell death by cisplatin. Cells exposed to cisplatin were found to express an increased phosphorylation of ERK 1/2 that was inhibited by PD98059 and suramin. Both of these inhibitors protected these cells from cisplatin-induced cytotoxicity. Activated ERK 1/2 may be a main effector of cell death, causing nuclear fragmentation, actin cytoskeleton rearrangement, and cell death. Cell death from cisplatin apparently occurred in a p53-independent and caspase-independent manner because these cell lines are functionally depleted of p53.[80]

Inflammatory cytokines may also play a role in cisplatin ototoxicity. These cytokines (tumor necrosis factor [TNF], interleukin-1β, and interleukin-6) may be up-regulated by activation of ERK and NFκB; this was shown in HEIOC1 cells in vitro. Neutralization of these cytokines by antibodies and pharmacologic inhibition of ERK significantly reduced the death of these cells exposed to cisplatin. These in vitro studies were confirmed in vivo using rats treated with cisplatin. TNF was immunolocalized to the spiral ligament, spiral limbus, and organ of Corti. NFκB protein expression was very strong in cells where TUNEL-positive staining was observed—the organ of Corti, spiral ligament, and stria vascularis. These findings suggest that proinflammatory cytokines, especially TNF-α, play a significant role in cochlear damage caused by cisplatin.[81]

A more recent review of potential protective agents tested against cisplatin ototoxicity pointed out that no successful clinical trials of protective agents against cisplatin had yet been published. Although numerous successful experiments showed protection in animal models, it is important to try to translate these results to the patients. One concern about the use of systemic protective agents, such as antioxidants, is the possible interference with the therapeutic effect of cisplatin. This problem could be circumvented with intratympanic administration of the protective agent, provided that it diffuses through the round window membrane and penetrates into the inner ear. Positive results with otoprotective regimens in clinical practice may increase the efficacy of cisplatin, and improve the quality of life in survivors of chemotherapy with cisplatin.[82]

Intratympanic dexamethasone has been reported to protect against cisplatin ototoxicity in guinea pigs and mice. In the study of guinea pigs, intratympanic saline also seemed to be protective.[83] In the mouse study, dexamethasone provided significant protection against auditory brainstem response threshold shifts with clicks, 8 kHz and 16 kHz compared with the contralateral, saline-injected ear.[84] A clinical study reported that, contrary to previous studies in the literature, amifostine (600 mg/m^2), given as an intravenous bolus immediately before and 3 hours after cisplatin and craniospinal irradiation in children with medulloblastoma, provided significant protection against hearing loss. One year after treatment initiation, 13 (37.1%) controls compared with 9 (14.5%) amifostine-treated patients had hearing loss sufficient to require a hearing aid in at least one ear ($P = .005$ chi-square one-sided test). There was no evidence that the amifostine interfered with the efficacy of the cisplatin, and the side effects of amifostine therapy were mild and well tolerated.[85]

Carboplatin

Carboplatin is a newer platinum compound that has been found to be less nephrotoxic than cisplatin. Preliminary data suggested that carboplatin was less ototoxic than cisplatin. The primary dose-limiting toxic side effect of carboplatin is bone marrow suppression. The latter effect can be overcome by autologous stem cell rescue and the use of hematopoietic growth factors; this has allowed the administration of higher doses of carboplatin to improve its antitumor efficacy and its therapeutic index. Carboplatin may be more ototoxic than initial studies indicated. High-dose carboplatin (2 g/m^2 total dose) was associated with hearing loss in 9 of 11 children (82%), with hearing losses in the speech frequencies that were sufficiently severe that hearing aids were recommended.[86] These children had each received prior treatment with cisplatin, and several of them had been treated with aminoglycoside antibiotics.

Carboplatin is highly effective in treating malignant brain tumors when given in conjunction with mannitol to open the blood-brain barrier. Fifteen of 19 patients (79%) had high-frequency hearing loss develop when this treatment regimen was used.[87] Patients with ovarian cancer were treated with combination therapy of carboplatin and cisplatin for six courses. A retrospective study of the first course area under the curve (AUC) concentration-time data for carboplatin was carried out. No patients with a low AUC had ototoxicity, but 12% of patients in the high AUC group were found to have hearing loss, and 45% had thrombocytopenia.[88]

Nearly half of a group of children undergoing hematopoietic stem cell transplantation were found to have deterioration in hearing. Children with neuroblastoma receiving carboplatin "conditioning" and children with renal dysfunction were found to be at higher risk for ototoxicity associated with hematopoietic stem cell transplantation[89]; all nine patients receiving high-dose carboplatin for cisplatin-resistant germ cell tumors were reported to develop a clinically manifested hearing loss.[90] A study of 30 children with unresectable neuroblastoma reported only one mild case of hearing loss at 6 years of follow-up.[91] The ototoxicity of carboplatin seems to vary according to the dose administered.

Carboplatin seems to be unique in that it has been shown to damage inner hair cells preferentially in the chinchilla.[92] The mechanisms of ototoxicity of carboplatin may be related to the production of ROS and reactive nitrogen species.[93] This idea is supported by the finding that pretreatment with butathione sulfoximine (BSO) enhances the ototoxicity of carboplatin in the chinchilla. BSO inhibits the synthesis of glutathione. Animals treated with BSO by continuous intracochlear infusion had significantly greater losses of inner and outer hair cells than animals treated with carboplatin alone. DPOAE and evoked potentials recorded from the inferior colliculus were found to be significantly reduced in amplitude in animals receiving BSO in combination with carboplatin compared with animals receiving carboplatin alone.[94]

Difluoromethylornithine

Clinical Studies

D,L-α-difluoromethylornithine (DFMO) was developed as an irreversible inhibitor of the enzyme ornithine decarboxylase. It was hoped to be effective in chemotherapy for hyperproliferative diseases, including cancer and certain infectious processes. DFMO was found to cause treatment-limiting, but reversible ototoxicity at high doses.[95] DFMO is an antitumor agent and a chemoprotective compound that reduces the incidence and frequency of tumors, and is useful clinically in treating infections with *Trypanosoma brucei gambiense* (West African sleeping sickness).

In phase I studies, doses of 12 g/m^2/day for 28 days resulted in thrombocytopenia and gastrointestinal disturbances. Larger doses (64 g/m^2/day intravenously for 25 to 43 days by continuous infusion) caused diarrhea and metabolic acidosis. In phase II studies, hearing loss was observed. A clinical trial of DFMO administered orally daily for 6 months was carried out in 27 patients after surgery for cancer or who were at high risk for development of cancer. The dose-limiting toxicity was defined as high-tone hearing loss on audiogram. Hearing loss was determined in seven patients. It was not stated whether the hearing loss was reversible or irreversible. The total drug dose that resulted in ototoxicity was highly variable among patients studied.[96]

A clinical trial was carried out in 66 volunteer subjects with previously treated bladder, prostate, or colon cancer without evidence of recurrent or residual disease or healthy individuals at increased risk for developing colon cancer who were tested for potential ototoxicity of DFMO. Predictable shifts in auditory thresholds occurred that were related to the dose of DFMO. As the dose of drug increased, the magnitude and incidence of hearing threshold shift increased, and the time of its onset decreased. Threshold changes were greater in the lower frequencies than in the higher frequencies. No association could be made between the gender, age, or renal function of the subjects and hearing loss. Threshold shifts were reversible with discontinuation of DFMO.[97]

A prospective, placebo-controlled phase II clinical trial of DFMO in patients with a prior history of adenomatous colon polyp was carried out with long-term, low-dose administration of DFMO to assess the effects on hearing. Volunteers ($N = 123$) with normal hearing for frequencies between 250 Hz and 2000 Hz were tested for audiometric thresholds at baseline and 1, 3, 6, 9, and 12 months after starting treatment with either DFMO or placebo, and follow-up testing was done 3 months after cessation of treatment if there was a suggestion of audiometric changes at the 12-month measurement. Subjects receiving doses of 0.075 to 0.4 g/m^2/day for 12 months had little evidence for shifts in auditory pure-tone thresholds, and there were no statistically significant shifts in DPOAEs. There was only a subtle, approximately 2- to 3-dB hearing threshold elevation at the two lowest frequencies of 250 Hz and 500 Hz. The authors concluded that the administration of low-dose DFMO for 12 months did not produce hearing loss, in contrast to other studies that examined the ototoxicity of higher doses.[98]

Irreversible hearing loss has been reported in a patient treated with DFMO as a chemopreventive for Barrett's esophagus. After taking 0.5 g/m^2/day of DFMO for approximately 13 weeks, hearing loss of 15 dB was noted at 250 Hz, 2000 Hz, and 3000 Hz in the right ear, and hearing loss of greater than 20 dB was noted at 4000 to 6000 Hz in the left ear. These threshold shifts persisted for 7 months after DFMO was discontinued. This was the first reported case of irreversible ototoxicity related to DFMO administration.[99]

Animal Studies

Studies of DFMO ototoxicity in guinea pigs revealed that DFMO administered for 12 weeks resulted in loss of hair cells in the hook and first turn. Inner hair cell loss was greater than loss of outer hair cells. Hearing loss was confirmed by brainstem audiometry.[100]

Daily intragastric administration of D,L-DFMO did not produce any auditory dysfunction in rats given doses of 200 mg/kg/day to 1.2 g/kg/day for 8 weeks. In contrast, substantial ototoxicity was found in guinea pigs given intraperitoneal doses of D,L-DFMO of 500 mg/kg/day to 1 g/kg/day. Damage to inner and outer hair cells in the cochlea, with greater loss of inner hair cells, especially in the basal turn, occurred. These histologic findings corresponded to loss of compound action potential sensitivity. The ototoxicity of the enantiomers was also studied in the guinea pig. It was found that 1 g/day of the D-enantiomer of DFMO did not produce any evidence of hearing impairment; 1 g/kg/day of the L-enantiomer of DFMO produced a threshold shift greater than the same dose of the racemic mixture.[101]

Studies in neonatal gerbils at 21 days of age were designed to test DFMO ototoxicity. Click-evoked auditory brainstem response testing was carried out before and 3 weeks after completion of an 18-day regimen of daily subcutaneous injections of DFMO at 1 g/kg/day. DFMO administration resulted in click threshold elevations of 20 to 60 dB, which recovered by 3 weeks after cessation of the drug.[102] This study was repeated using tone pips at 2 kHz, 4 kHz, 8 kHz, 16 kHz, and 32 kHz in neonatal gerbils to see whether specific frequencies were affected, and to examine cochlear tissues after DFMO administration. Dosing regimens of 750 mg/kg/day or 1 g/kg/day subcutaneously administered were employed in two groups of gerbils. Hearing threshold shifts of 21 to 29 dB were found in the higher dose group, whereas threshold elevations of 11 to 17 dB were observed in gerbils receiving the lower dose. Higher thresholds were shown at the higher frequencies, although a broad frequency range was affected. No significant cochlear abnormalities were observed at the light microscopic level, consistent with the fact that the hearing threshold changes were reversible after 3 weeks of recovery.[102] The ototoxicity of DFMO may be mediated by alteration of the inward rectification of Kir4.1 channels, leading to a marked reduction in endocochlear potential and elevation of auditory brainstem response thresholds in mice.[103]

Conclusions

From the animal studies reported to date, it seems that DFMO has species-specific ototoxicity that apparently is dose related, but variable, depending on the rodent model used. The rat is resistant to DFMO ototoxicity, perhaps because DFMO may not inhibit polyamine synthesis in the rat cochlea to a critical level. The rat may not be used as a reliable animal model for the study of DFMO ototoxicity.[101] The guinea pig seems to be quite sensitive to DFMO ototoxicity. DFMO, particularly the L-enantiomer, caused hearing threshold changes and hair cell loss in the high-frequency region. Inner hair cells seem to be more sensitive to damage from DFMO than do outer hair cells. The neonatal gerbil apparently has an intermediate sensitivity to DFMO. Long-term administration of DFMO resulted in temporary threshold elevations, which recovered within 3 weeks after cessation of treatment, and no evidence of cochlear tissue damage was ascertained with light microscopy.[102] In mice, DFMO seemed to affect primarily the stria vascularis by altering the inward-rectification of potassium channels (Kir4.1). This alteration resulted in a concomitant elevation of auditory brainstem response thresholds. It was not specified whether this effect was temporary or permanent, and no histology was reported.[103]

Clinical studies have shown that DFMO administration is associated with reversible hearing loss. One article reported permanent hearing loss in one patient that persisted for 7 months.[99] It seems appropriate to warn patients about potential ototoxicity of this chemopreventive agent before its use. Future human temporal bone studies may shed additional light on the effects of DFMO on human cochlear tissues.

Loop Diuretics

The loop diuretics are potent synthetic drugs that exert therapeutic effects through their action on the loop of Henle of the kidney. They inhibit the reabsorption of sodium, potassium, and chloride ions by blocking an Na/K/2Cl carrier.[104] Through this action on the kidney, loop diuretics produce a rapid and dramatic increase in the volume of urine output. The most commonly used loop diuretics are furosemide and bumetanide. Ethacrynic acid is used less frequently. These drugs are used to treat congestive heart failure in infants and adults, to reduce high blood pressure, to remove excess fluid from the lungs in newborns with immature lungs, and to assist in the control of edema from liver or kidney failure.

Ethacrynic acid can be administered either orally or by intravenous injection. It was soon discovered to cause hearing loss after it was introduced into clinical medicine in the 1960s. Numerous cases of transient and permanent deafness have been reported.[105] Permanent, profound midfrequency and high-frequency SNHL has been reported in a kidney transplant patient who was treated with ethacrynic acid. This patient was successfully rehabilitated with binaural hearing aids.[106]

Furosemide can be administered orally or by intravenous injection. Approximately 65% of an oral dose is absorbed after oral ingestion.[107] This diuretic follows a three-compartment pharmacokinetic model with an average half-life of 29.5 minutes for renal elimination. The half-life of furosemide increases dramatically in patients with severe renal failure, in whom the half-life may be 10 to 20 hours.[105] Furosemide has also been found to cause temporary and some permanent cases of hearing loss. Permanent hearing loss has been reported in certain adults[105] and in high-risk premature infants treated with furosemide.[108] Plasma levels of furosemide greater than 50 mg/L have been associated with hearing loss.[109,110] SNHL may be accompanied by tinnitus and vertigo. The incidence of ototoxicity with furosemide was reported to be approximately 6% in a small series of patients.[111]

Bumetanide, a more potent sulfonamide loop diuretic, has been reported to cause a much smaller incidence of hearing loss than furosemide.[111,112] A related loop diuretic, piretanide, was found to be equally effective as furosemide in treating patients with congestive heart failure in a study of a small group of patients, and no patients were found to have hearing loss.[113]

Studies of experimental animal and human temporal bones[114] show that the primary target of loop diuretics is the stria vascularis, where extensive edema develops in conjunction with loss of auditory function.[105] The primary target in the stria vascularis seems to be the Na/2Cl/K transporter (SLC12A2),[115] which may be similar to or identical to the transporter that furosemide and bumetanide inhibit in the kidney.[116] Mice lacking this transporter are deaf,[117] but it is unknown whether mutations of SLC12A2 contribute to human deafness.[118] The action of loop diuretics on the stria vascularis results in a reduction of the endocochlear potential, with an elevation of the threshold for the compound action potential.[119] Immature rats[120] and rats with low albumin[121] are more susceptible to the ototoxic effects of furosemide. This finding suggests that the ototoxic action of loop diuretics depends on the unbound fraction of drug in the serum.[121]

Clinical studies suggested that the ototoxicity of furosemide may be reduced by infusing the drug at rates of less than 15 mg/min.[110] Studies in the chinchilla have suggested that the ototoxicity of ethacrynic acid may be caused by impaired blood flow in the lateral wall of the cochlea. In these experiments, the blood vessels to the modiolus, spiral lamina, and vestibular end organs seemed normal. The vessels supplying the spiral ligament and stria vascularis had poor flow at 2 minutes after ethacrynic acid injection, however, and the vessels seemed to lack red blood cells 30 minutes after injection. The compound action potential, cochlear microphonics, and summating potential all declined without recovery after the microcirculatory changes in the lateral wall vessels, and reperfusion was delayed in the stria vascularis arterioles to other blood vessels in the lateral wall. Ischemia followed by reperfusion generates large quantities of oxygen free radicals that could cause structural and functional damage to the stria vascularis and organ of Corti.[122] Outer hair cell loss in the basal turn of the cochlea has been observed in temporal bone studies of patients experiencing ethacrynic acid ototoxicity.[114]

Torsemide, a new loop diuretic, was found to cause reversible hearing loss in cats at a dose that was similar to that of furosemide.[123] No evidence of ototoxicity has been shown in humans to date.[124]

Analgesics

Hydrocodone

Hydrocodone is a narcotic analgesic. It is often combined with acetaminophen, and is frequently prescribed for the relief of acute and chronic pain.[125] Common adverse reactions to this combination analgesic drug include dizziness, nausea, vomiting, drowsiness, and euphoria. More severe side effects include respiratory depression and mood disturbances. Because hydrocodone is a narcotic, abuse can lead to psychological and physical dependence. It is the most widely prescribed opioid narcotic analgesic in the United States, and is one of the most widely abused prescription drugs.[125]

Hearing loss from hydrocodone abuse has been reported in a few cases, but the incidence may be much greater than previously suspected. Two cases of rapidly progressive sensorineural deafness with relative sparing of the vestibular system and normal magnetic resonance imaging scans were reported in two patients taking huge doses of this combination. One patient took 15 tablets four times a day, and the second patient took up to 35 tablets per day. Neither patient responded to high-dose oral prednisone therapy. The first patient received a cochlear implant, with restoration of functional hearing, but no information was provided about auditory rehabilitation in the second patient, who progressed to profound bilateral SNHL.[126]

Hydrocodone abuse was associated with rapidly progressive SNHL in 12 patients reported from the House Ear Clinic. In four patients, the initial presentation was unilateral, and two patients also experienced vestibular symptoms. High-dose prednisone therapy was unsuccessful in improving hearing in any of the patients. Seven of eight patients who underwent cochlear implantation had early success with these devices. An additional series of five patients with a history of chronic ingestion of hydrocodone in doses ranging from 10 to 300 mg/day was reported. The duration of use varied from months to years. The initial audiogram showed typically a moderate SNHL. Subsequent audiograms showed rapid progression of hearing loss. Communication was severely affected. There was no spontaneous recovery of hearing in any patient reporting cessation of drug use. Hearing loss was asymmetric in three patients. Tinnitus was reported by three patients. The only significant comorbidity in this series was hepatitis C. All five patients underwent cochlear implantation and became successful users.[125]

The mechanisms of ototoxicity of hydrocodone/acetaminophen are unknown. Opioid receptors of the mu type have been shown in spiral and Scarpa's ganglia,[127,128] whereas delta and kappa receptors have been shown in hair cells.[127] Genetic abnormalities of drug-metabolizing enzymes and comorbidities such as hepatitis C infection may be factors in development of ototoxicity from this drug combination. More research is required to confirm or refute this theory, however.[125]

The following guidelines have been recommended:

1. The clinician should document rapidly progressive SNHL that is bilateral.
2. There should be no vestibular symptoms (although this is contradicted in a previous series).[129]
3. There should be no response to steroid therapy.
4. There should be no symptoms or laboratory evidence of intracranial infection or concurrent autoimmune disease with the exception of possible hepatitis C–induced autoimmune hepatitis.
5. The clinician should document prolonged daily use of hydrocodone or oxycodone, or high doses over a short interval preceding the onset of hearing loss.[125]

Salicylates

Salicylates are derivatives of benzoic acid that have been used to treat mild to moderate pain, such as headache, dental pain, and arthritis. These drugs have an anti-inflammatory and an analgesic effect. Salicylates are tightly bound to serum proteins after oral absorption, and only a small percentage of the concentration of salicylate in blood is unbound or free.

In animal experiments, it has been reported that after systemic administration, salicylates rapidly enter the perilymph. The percentage of the corresponding blood level achieved in the perilymph can be 25% to 33%[130,131] in chinchillas,[130] and in rats,[132] the relationship between serum and perilymph concentrations is nearly linear. Serum levels of 25 to 50 mg/dL were reported in chinchillas receiving 450 mg/kg of salicylate intraperitoneally. The chinchillas were found to have threshold elevations for auditory brainstem response of 30 dB, on the average, primarily at the higher frequencies.[130] Guinea pigs receiving the same dose were found to have increased spontaneous activity of inferior colliculus neurons, which may be a neural correlate of tinnitus.[132] The effects of salicylates on the cochlea may be caused by changes in blood flow, and by changes in the stiffness of the lateral membrane of the outer hair cells.[133]

Hearing loss in humans may be related to the concentration of salicylates in blood. Patients with blood levels of 20 to 50 mg/dL can have hearing losses of 30 dB.[134] Lower concentrations of salicylate may correlate with hearing loss. At concentrations of 11 mg/dL, hearing loss was 12 dB. There seems to be a linear relationship between hearing loss and free salicylate concentrations.[135] Site of lesion testing in patients with salicylate-induced hearing loss shows a cochlear site of lesion.[136] Tinnitus seems to increase continuously with increasing plasma concentrations of salicylate over 40 to 320 mg/dL. Histopathologic studies of animal and human temporal bones from patients with documented hearing loss after receiving salicylates do not show significant hair cell damage or injury to the stria vascularis.[137] No damage to the spiral ganglion cells or myelin sheath of the eighth cranial nerve has been shown.[138]

Experiments in rats suggest that salicylate induces tinnitus throughout activation of *N*-methyl-D-aspartate (NMDA) receptors in the cochlea. The application of NMDA antagonists into the perilymph blocked the increase in pole-jumping behavior induced by salicylate, a behavioral procedure to measure tinnitus.[139] Salicylates probably cause a reversible SNHL by altering the function of the motor protein, prestin, in outer hair cells.[140]

Quinine and Related Drugs

Quinine is an alkaloid drug that is used to treat malaria and leg cramps. It is also present in tonic drinks. Quinine toxicity can manifest as a syndrome termed *cinchonism*. The symptoms include deafness, vertigo, tinnitus, headache, visual loss, and nausea. Twenty percent of patients may complain of high-frequency hearing loss with prolonged courses of treatment. There may be a 4-kHz notch, and speech discrimination score may be less than 30%, but the hearing loss may be reversible.[141] If hearing loss occurs within the speech frequencies, the loss may be permanent.[142] Guinea pigs were found to have increasing hearing loss with increasing blood concentrations of quinine.[143] Chinchillas receiving a single intramuscular injection of quinine, 150 mg/kg, were found to have a reversible 20-dB threshold elevation of auditory brainstem response, and similar shifts were observed after application of quinine to the round window.[144] Perceptual tinnitus may occur after quinine administration. A conditioned-suppression study of rats revealed a dose-dependent induction of behavioral tinnitus after quinine treatment. These effects were blocked by nimodipine, a calcium channel blocker.[145] Nimodipine did alter the threshold elevation of compound action potential observed after quinine, however.[146]

Chloroquine is an aminoquinoline drug initially used to treat malaria. In the 1950s, it began to be used to treat rheumatoid arthritis, then later other connective tissue diseases. It is chemically related to quinine. It seems to be ototoxic, but only a few cases have been reported. The ototoxicity may be reversible if detected early by auditory brainstem evoked response audiometry followed by cessation of therapy with chloroquine and administration of steroids and plasma expanders.[147,148]

Hydroxychloroquine is also a quinoline compound used to treat rheumatoid arthritis and lupus. It rarely causes ototoxicity. It has been reported to cause reversible SNHL in an adult with rheumatoid arthritis after 5 months of treatment.[149] Permanent SNHL was reported in two adults with lupus erythematosus[150] and in a 7-year-old girl after 2 years of treatment for idiopathic pulmonary hemosiderosis.[151]

Erythromycin and Related Macrolide Antibiotics

Erythromycin was introduced into clinical medicine in the 1950s. This antibiotic has been found to be useful in the treatment of various infections, including pneumonia caused by *Legionella pneumophila,* which has resulted in increased use of erythromycin by the intravenous route. It was screened for possible ototoxicity early on, but only vestibular testing was carried out. Nevertheless, it was concluded that erythromycin was not ototoxic. In 1973, the first case of ototoxicity in patients was reported.[152] Many cases of bilateral SNHL have been reported after intravenous or oral administration. Most of these patients were elderly and had liver or kidney disease, or had been treated with high-dose erythromycin for legionnaires' disease.

Ototoxic symptoms include "blowing" tinnitus, loss of hearing, and vertigo in some cases. Some patients complained of confusion, fear, psychiatric disturbances,[153] visual changes, slurred speech, a sensation of having been drugged, or lack of control.[154] Most cases of hearing loss and tinnitus have been transient. Recovery of normal hearing usually occurs within 1 to 2 weeks after stopping erythromycin.[155] Two cases of permanent ototoxicity have been reported, however: one with permanent tinnitus[156] and one with permanent hearing loss.[157] Hearing loss from erythromycin has been reported in liver or kidney transplant patients. The incidence of hearing loss in these patients seems to be dose related. Hearing loss was observed in 16% of patients receiving 2 g daily, but increased to 53% in patients treated with 4 g daily. Complete reversal of hearing loss occurred after modification of therapy.[158] In a separate series of three liver transplant recipients, it was believed that an interaction occurred between erythromycin and cyclosporine that may have caused the hearing loss.[159]

The audiometric pattern in patients with erythromycin ototoxicity can be a flat type of SNHL, although some patients manifest a high-frequency loss. Auditory brainstem response testing in two patients with erythromycin ototoxicity showed absence of waves I to III during erythromycin therapy, when pure-tone audiograms documented SNHL. The auditory brainstem response pattern and the audiograms normalized after cessation of erythromycin.[160]

Several guidelines have been recommended for the prevention of erythromycin ototoxicity: (1) Pretreatment audiograms should be obtained in elderly patients and in patients who have impaired liver or kidney function. (2) Caution should be used in combining erythromycin with other potentially ototoxic drugs. (3) If the serum creatinine is greater than 180 mol/L, the daily dose of erythromycin should not be greater than 1.5 g.[161]

Azithromycin is a newer antibiotic related to erythromycin. Similar to erythromycin, it is also ototoxic. This side effect was first reported in patients with acquired immunodeficiency syndrome undergoing long-term treatment for disseminated *Mycobacterium avium* infections. Three patients complained of hearing loss, and audiograms confirmed mild to moderate SNHL, which resolved within 2 to 4 weeks after cessation of treatment.[162] Another series of patients had reversible ototoxicity associated with high-dose oral azithromycin therapy (2400 mg/day). It took an average of 5 weeks for hearing to recover after cessation of treatment.[163] Two additional cases of reversible SNHL with azithromycin have been reported.[164] Two cases of apparently permanent hearing loss have been reported. A 47-year-old woman became completely deaf after 8 days of treatment with azithromycin.[165] A 39-year-old woman had tinnitus develop bilaterally within 24 hours of taking the drug and subjective hearing loss after the second day when she stopped taking the medication. An audiogram revealed moderate to severe high-frequency SNHL in the right ear and mild to moderate high-frequency loss on the left side. The tinnitus and hearing loss were still present 12 months later, although the tinnitus was less severe.[166] Guinea pigs treated with azithromycin or a related drug, clarithromycin, were found to have a reversible alteration of transiently evoked otoacoustic emissions.[167] The mechanisms of ototoxicity of these macrolide antibiotics are unknown.

Deferoxamine

Among a group of 153 children with β-thalassemia and treated with regular blood transfusions and iron overload chelation with deferoxamine, 38% were found to have a significant SNHL at high frequencies with recruitment. Younger patients had a greater hearing loss. The hearing loss was apparently correlated with mean and peak doses of deferoxamine, and was more severe in patients with lower iron load.[168]

In a population of 75 adult transfusion-dependent patients with thalassemia major and other hematologic diseases treated with regular transfusions, 93% (70 of 75) had a history of long-term subcutaneous or intravenous deferoxamine therapy. Audiometric testing revealed hearing loss that was attributed to deferoxamine therapy in 22 of 75 patients (29%). Of patients with thalassemia, 35% (21 of 59) had hearing loss attributable to deferoxamine ototoxicity. These patients with deferoxamine ototoxicity had high-frequency SNHL. Seven of the 21 patients had a notch at 6 kHz, and 1 had a notch at 3 kHz. Few of the hearing losses were considered as disabling, however. Audiologic monitoring was recommended for patients undergoing deferoxamine therapy.[169]

Hearing loss was attributed to deferoxamine therapy in 6 of 30 patients 7 to 25 years old. Most of the patients with hearing loss had Cooley's anemia requiring regular blood transfusions and deferoxamine therapy in a dose of 40 to 50 mg/kg subcutaneously overnight for 8 to 10 hours by pump, 4 to 7 days per week. The hearing loss was sensorineural, mild to moderate, and involved the high frequencies (3 to 12.5 kHz). Only one patient had hearing loss at less than 6 kHz. Only one patient reported tinnitus. Transient evoked otoacoustic emissions and DPOAEs were abnormal in 27% and 33% of patients.[170]

Wide variations in the incidence of ototoxicity in transfusion-dependent patients receiving deferoxamine have been reported, ranging from 3.8% to 57%.[170] Although it has been reported that patients with deferoxamine ototoxicity were younger and had received higher doses of deferoxamine than patients who were not affected,[171] the doses of deferoxamine used in the 1980s were higher than the doses used in more recent years.[170] The latter study found no association between age and ototoxicity. Twenty-two patients had abnormal audiograms in the 4- to 8-kHz region, with thresholds of 30 to 100 dB. Of the 22 patients, 18 received deferoxamine doses greater than the recommended dose of 50 mg/kg subcutaneously. When deferoxamine was discontinued, audiograms in seven cases reverted to normal or near-normal in 2 to 3 weeks, and 9 of 13 patients who had symptomatic hearing losses became asymptomatic. When therapy was restarted with lower doses, no further ototoxicity was shown except in two cases. It was recommended that in patients with symptomatic hearing loss, the drug should be stopped for 4 weeks, and when the repeat audiograms were stable or improved, therapy could be restarted at 10 to 25 mg/kg per dose. The authors recommended serial audiograms every 6 months in asymptomatic patients receiving deferoxamine, and more frequent audiograms in young patients with normal serum ferritin values and in patients with hearing loss shown on audiograms.[172]

A therapeutic index has been recommended to avoid deferoxamine ototoxicity. This index is obtained by dividing the daily deferoxamine dose (mg/kg) by the serum ferritin level (ng/mL). A therapeutic index of 0.025 was considered safe.[173] For a patient with a ferritin level greater than 2000 ng/mL, deferoxamine doses of less than 50 mg/kg are considered as safe.[170] Audiometric screening for ototoxicity should include measurements of pure-tone thresholds at 6 kHz, which is the frequency most affected in patients with deferoxamine ototoxicity.[170] A more recent study showed that DPOAE testing was extremely sensitive and superior to pure-tone audiometry.[174]

Vancomycin

Vancomycin is a glycopeptide antibiotic that is used to treat methicillin-resistant infections caused by *Staphylococcus aureus* and *Staphylococcus epidermidis,* and other difficult-to-treat infections, such as enterococcal endocarditis in patients with penicillin allergies. It has been reported to be ototoxic. Vancomycin is used orally to treat pseudomembranous colitis caused by *Clostridium difficile.* Because of poor oral absorption, vancomycin is usually given intravenously. Multicompartment pharmacokinetic models have been described.[175,176] It is usually given every 12 hours in patients with normal renal function, but a once-daily regimen has been described more recently that has equivalent efficacy and a similar safety profile.[182]

As mentioned previously, vancomycin is given orally to treat pseudomembranous colitis. Usually, no significant absorption occurs after oral dosing.[9] It is sometimes administered intrathecally to treat bacterial meningitis, and severe SNHL has been reported in a patient receiving vancomycin by this route.[177] Elderly patients, even if they have normal renal function, have reduced renal clearance of vancomycin.[176] The half-life is significantly longer in premature infants; careful monitoring of blood levels in premature infants has been recommended.[178] Vancomycin administered to pregnant women did not cause hearing loss in their infants who were tested after birth.[179] In a large-scale newborn hearing screening, vancomycin was not associated with failure on automated auditory brainstem response.[180]

Vancomycin given in near-lethal doses in guinea pigs was found to be not ototoxic, but potentiation of gentamicin ototoxicity in guinea pigs was found.[181] A critical review of previously reported cases of permanent ototoxicity attributed to vancomycin suggested that most cases could be explained by concomitant aminoglycoside exposure.[181] Vancomycin seems to have a low probability of causing permanent ototoxicity if it is not given in combination with another ototoxic agent. Although the incidence of audiometrically proven hearing loss was 1 in 31 (3.2%) and 5 in 32 (15.6%) in patients receiving once-daily or twice-daily vancomycin therapy, these findings were based on a single post-treatment audiogram compared with the pretreatment baseline. It is unknown whether these hearing losses were temporary or permanent.[182]

Ototoxicity Monitoring for Hearing Loss

Audiometric monitoring for ototoxicity depends on the risk of the treatment regimen. For a low-dosage or short-duration treatment protocol for aminoglycosides with no clinical risk factors, the use of a pretreatment and post-treatment audiogram with a weekly self-assessment checklist monitoring may be adequate, but would not provide an early warning of potential hearing loss. For a high-risk, long-duration course of therapy with a high-risk agent such as amikacin, pretreatment and post-treatment testing with intervening weekly or biweekly monitoring of conventional audiometry and high-frequency audiometry may be advisable. For aminoglycosides, the final audiogram after treatment should not be performed until a few weeks after conclusion of therapy because additional delayed effects on hearing may occur.[183] For cisplatin treatment protocols, monitoring at baseline, just before beginning each cycle, when the patient is less ill and is able to cooperate better, and after the conclusion of therapy may be sufficient to document hearing loss and provide guidelines for rehabilitation because lifesaving therapy may impossible to modify.

As protective agents progress into clinical use, high-frequency audiometry may help to monitor the efficacy of the protective protocols.[183] DPOAEs seem to be more sensitive and superior to pure-tone audiometry in detecting early hearing loss caused by cisplatin[65,184] and deferoxamine.[174]

SUGGESTED READINGS

Cheng AG, Cunningham LL, Rubel EW. Mechanisms of hair cell death and protection. *Curr Opin Otolaryngol Head Neck Surg.* 2005;13:343-348.

Clerici WJ, Hensley K, DiMartino DL, et al. Direct detection of ototoxicant-induced reactive oxygen species generation in cochlear explants. *Hear Res.* 1996;98:116-124.

Fischel-Ghodsian N. Genetic factors in aminoglycoside toxicity. *Pharmacogenomics.* 2005;6:27-36.

Ho T, Vrabec JT, Burton AW. Hydrocodone use and sensorineural hearing loss. *Pain Physician.* 2007;10:467-472.

Kushner BH, Budnick A, Kramer K, et al. Ototoxicity from high-dose use of platinum compounds in patients with neuroblastoma. *Cancer.* 2006;107:417-422.

Lallemend F, Lefebvre PP, Hans G, et al. Molecular pathways involved in apoptotic cell death in the injured cochlea: cues to novel therapeutic strategies. *Curr Pharmaceut Design*. 2005;11:2257-2275.

Oldenburg J, Kraggerud SM, Cvancarova M, et al. Cisplatin-induced long-term hearing impairment is associated with specific glutathione-S-transferase genotypes in testicular cancer survivors. *J Clin Oncol*. 2007;25: 708-714.

Rizzi MD, Hirose K. Aminoglycoside ototoxicity. *Curr Opin Otolaryngol Head Neck Surg*. 2007;15:352-357.

Rybak LP. Mechanisms of cisplatin ototoxicity and progress in otoprotection. *Curr Opin Otolaryngol Head Neck Surg*. 2007;15:364-369.

Rybak LP, Whitworth CA. Ototoxicity: therapeutic opportunities. *Drug Discov Today*. 2005;10:1313-1321.

Rybak LP, Whitworth CA, Mukherjea D, et al. Mechanisms of cisplatin-induced ototoxicity and prevention. *Hear Res*. 2007;226:157-167.

Yorgason JG, Fayad JN, Kalinec F. Understanding drug ototoxicity: molecular insights for prevention and clinical management. *Expert Opin Drug Saf*. 2006;5:383-399.

For complete list of references log onto www.expertconsult.com.

CHAPTER ONE HUNDRED AND FIFTY-FIVE

Pharmacologic and Molecular Therapies of the Cochlear and Vestibular Labyrinth

Anil K. Lalwani

John F. McGuire

Key Points

- The round window membrane (RWM) is a three-layered dynamic biologic structure capable of active and passive transport. Key features of RWM permeability have been described.
- The kinetics of RWM drug delivery are primarily affected by the method of delivery, the permeability of the substance applied, and the rate of clearance from the perilymph.
- Adhesions over the RWM may significantly alter delivery of therapeutics. Some clinicians advocate microscopic removal of adhesions before the administration of therapeutics.
- The concentration of steroids in perilymph is much higher after intratympanic application than after oral administration.
- The two principal indications of intratympanic steroids are Meniere's disease and sudden sensorineural hearing loss. Data are mixed on the use of intratympanic steroids for Meniere's disease. There are strong data for the use of intratympanic steroids as a salvage therapy after failure to respond to oral steroids. Results of salvage intratympanic steroid administration for sudden sensorineural hearing loss are best when steroids are applied as early as possible after the onset of symptoms.
- The use of intratympanic gentamicin has been studied extensively for its ability to relieve vertigo symptoms in Meniere's disease, but the incidence of hearing loss with this therapy is also high. There is currently no consensus on the intratympanic gentamicin protocol that best relieves vertigo, while preserving hearing.
- The pharmacodynamics of intratympanic gentamicin injections are much more variable than the pharmacodynamics of sustained-release intratympanic administration. Variability in pharmacodynamics may be responsible for the unpredictable incidence of hearing loss.
- Otoprotective therapies of the cochlea and labyrinth are in the experimental phase. Many of the new otoprotective strategies employ the use of neurotrophins.
- Gene therapy for the cochlea and labyrinth is also in the experimental phase. The primary mechanical issues with gene therapy for the cochlea and labyrinth are the choice of vector for gene transfer and the method of delivery of this vector to the cochlea. Optimizing safety of gene transfer continues to be a research priority.
- Most attempts at gene therapy to date involve up-regulating the production of neurotrophins. There have also been attempts to up-regulate apoptosis inhibitors, and to stimulate hair cell regeneration through gene therapy.

Protected by one of the hardest bones in body, the cochlea is nearly an impenetrable structure, frustrating bacteria and humans trying to gain access to it. Were it not for its windows, delivery of therapeutic agents to the inner ear would always necessitate traumatic disruption of the bony walls and fearful consequences to hearing. In the past 20 years, there has been a resurgence of interest in directed therapy to address inner ear disorders because indirect, systemic therapy has shown limited success and significant morbidity. Experimentally, as reviewed later, investigators have shown that intratympanic and intracochlear therapy is feasible and efficacious. The direct intracochlear application of therapeutic agents, previously feared, may become the standard therapy of the future. Inner ear "surgery" is expected to be developed to the fullest to prevent hearing loss and to restore hearing. This chapter reviews the knowledge regarding delivery of material into the inner ear and its therapeutic consequences. The dawning of a new era in ototherapy is here.

Round Window Membrane

Anatomy

The round and oval windows sit on the medial wall of the middle ear. The conduction apparatus of the middle ear converges on the oval window, an arrangement designed to transfer the mechanical energy of sound waves into fluid waves that pass through the cochlea. Although situated at the tail end of this apparatus, the round window membrane (RWM) plays an essential role in acoustic dynamics because the compliance of the membrane allows for this mechanical energy to be released from the cochlea; without this outlet, no waves could travel through the perilymph. The actual RWM sits in the round window niche (fossula fenestrae cochleae) just posteroinferior to the promontory. When viewed from the intact tympanic membrane, the round window niche can be found an average of 3.44 mm (±0.68 mm) from the umbo, at an average angle of 113.2 degrees (±9.8 degrees) from the long process of the malleus.[1]

The RWM is a three-layered structure designed to protect the inner ear from middle ear pathology and to facilitate active transport. There is an outer epithelial layer that faces the middle ear, a central connective tissue layer, and an inner epithelial layer interfacing with the scala tympani. The outer epithelial layer is continuous with the promontory. Mucoperiosteal folds from the neighboring epithelium sometimes can obstruct the round window niche, forming a "false" RWM. The most prominent feature of the outer epithelial layer is the extensive interdigitations and tight junctions of its cells; in addition, there is a continuous basement membrane layer. This architecture, with tight junctions and a continuous basement membrane, functions as a defensive shield designed to protect the inner ear from middle ear infections. The cells also feature a well-developed rough endoplasmic reticulum and Golgi complex with occasional microvilli, suggesting that active transport of elements across the middle and inner ear compartments may occur.

The connective tissue core contains fibroblasts, collagen, and elastic fibers, and houses blood and lymph vessels. The connective tissue layer is divided roughly into thirds, differing by fiber type and cellular material. Closest to the middle ear epithelium are coarse, loosely arranged collagen fibers, devoid of elastic fibers. In the middle of this layer, these fibers are joined by fibroblasts and ground substance, with occasional blood vessels and elastic fibers. Bordering the inner ear epithelium, there is a gradual increase in fibroblasts, collagen, and elastic fibers. As a whole, the connective tissue layer is responsible for providing compliance to the RWM. A discontinuous inner epithelial layer bathes in the perilymph of the scala tympani. Cells in this layer house pinocytotic vesicles and amorphous intracellular components, and feature long lateral extensions that bathe in the perilymph, suggesting that the RWM participates in some form of active transport.[2] Figure 155-1 depicts the histologic complexity of the RWM.

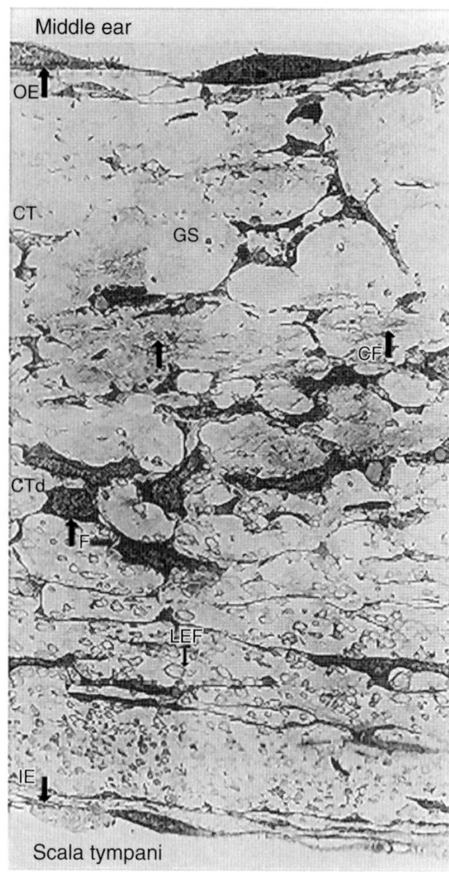

Figure 155-1. Normal human round window membrane in a 70-year-old individual. CF, collagen fibers; CT, area of loose connective tissue; CTd, area of dense connective tissue; F, fibroblasts; LEF, large elastic fibers; GS, ground substance (uranyl acetate–lead citrate); IE, inner epithelium; OE, outer epithelium. ×3000. *(From Goycoolea MV. Clinical aspects of round window membrane permeability under normal and pathological conditions.* Acta Otolaryngol. *2001;121:437.)*

Physiology

The RWM is a dynamic biologic membrane. All three layers of the RWM participate in a defensive response to pathogen insult. In the context of otitis media, the outer epithelial cells become hyperplastic, whereas blood vessels within the connective tissue layer become edematous and dilated, permitting extravasation of neutrophils and macrophages. Fibroblasts also become hyperplastic, displaying an increased volume of basophilic cytoplasm.[2] Yoon and Hellstrom[3] found that although all layers of the RWM are involved in the defense response, the most dramatic changes are seen in the subepithelial space close to the basement membrane (Fig. 155-2). Certain toxins can also initiate these metaplastic changes, resulting in a thicker RWM. The thickness of the RWM doubles after exposure to *Pseudomonas* exotoxin.[4] Streptolysin O has been shown to cause breakdown of the RWM, increasing its permeability to substances in the middle ear space.[5]

Another dynamic aspect of the RWM is its ability to transport macromolecules. This process seems to be receptor mediated.[6] Transport starts at the outer layer, where molecules are taken up by pinocytosis and are brought into the connective tissue layer. From there, substances either are absorbed by blood or lymphatic vessels or are mobilized further to the inner epithelial layer, where they are released by pinocytosis into the perilymph. The RWM may also participate in the absorption of perilymph because experimental evidence has shown the passage of tracer substances from the perilymph compartment into the RWM.[2]

The RWM displays dynamic changes as it ages. Although there is no change in the thickness of the RWM with aging, changes in cellular density and elastic fiber patterns can be seen. These changes may decrease the compliance of the membrane and compromise the overall function of the auditory system.[7]

Permeability

A large range of materials are able to cross the RWM, including various antimicrobials, steroids, anesthetics, tracers, albumin, horseradish peroxidase, latex spheres, germicidal solutions, water, ions, and macromolecules (including bacterial toxins).[8] Several factors contribute to the permeability of the RWM, including size, charge, the morphology of the compound, and the thickness of the RWM. Size has proved to be a factor in permeability because 1-μm microspheres cross the RWM, but 3-μm microspheres do not.[9] Substances with a molecular weight of less than 1000 kD diffuse across the RWM rapidly, whereas substances greater than 1000 kD are transported by pinocytosis.[10] Charge of the molecule can also affect its ability to traverse the RWM: cationic ferritin crosses the RWM, but anionic ferritin does not.[9] The implication is that liposolubility is a factor in RWM permeability, a feature that is important in the design of liposome vectors for gene therapy.[8] The morphologic features of the compound can stimulate pinocytosis, presumably by a receptor-mediated mechanism.[8,10] Increased thickness of the RWM decreases permeability of substances.[8] Although the average thickness of the human RWM is 10 to 30 μm, this thickness can double in inflammatory conditions.[11,12]

RWM permeability can be altered with the use of exogenous adjuvants. Chandrasekhar and colleagues[6] compared the ability of three exogenous adjuvants to increase the perfusion of dexamethasone applied to the round window niche. These compounds included hista-

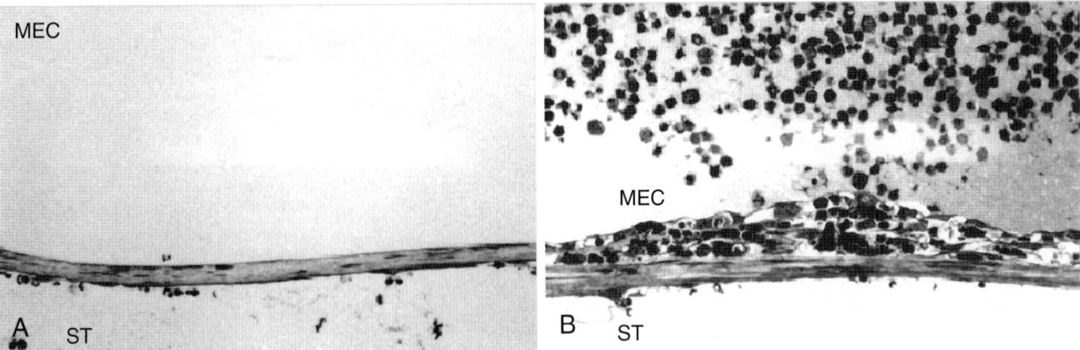

Figure 155-2. **A** and **B,** Light microscopic changes in the thickness of the round window membrane stained for toluidine blue on normal control **(A)** and day 1 in pneumococcus-induced otitis media **(B)**. The change was most prominent on day 1, which was most evident in the outer epithelium and subepithelial space of the round window membrane. MEC, middle ear cavity; ST, scala tympani. ×200. *(From Yoon YJ, Hellstrom S. Ultrastructural characteristics of the round window membrane during pneumococcal otitis media in rat.* J Korean Med Sci. *2002;17:230.)*

mine (for its vasodilatory effects), hyaluronic acid (for its proposed osmotic effect), and dimethyl sulfoxide (for its ability to increase medication solubility in perilymph). Histamine adjuvant with dexamethasone resulted in significantly higher perilymph steroid levels than all other combinations, whereas hyaluronic acid and dimethyl sulfoxide had no significant effect. Although this study failed to show an increase in steroid perfusion with the use of hyaluronic acid, several practitioners advocate use of hyaluronic acid in their intratympanic steroid protocols.[1,13]

Kinetics

Delivery of therapeutic agents across the RWM displays a nonuniform distribution in the perilymph. Concentrations of the delivered agent are usually high in the basal turns in close proximity to the RWM, and are low at the apical turns. The permeability characteristics of the substance across the RWM and the rate of its clearance from the perilymph are the two major factors that determine the dispersal characteristics of substances in perilymph; this can include a combination of clearance to blood, clearance to any other scala, uptake or binding by cells, or metabolism by any of the cochlear tissues.[14] Knowing the RWM permeability and clearance rates of a given agent permits the simulation of its perilymphatic distribution with reasonable accuracy.

With these observations, Salt and Ma[14] described the development of a computer-simulated model of drug distribution in the perilymphatic space (Fig. 155-3). Their model, the Washington University Cochlear Fluids Simulator, is a public-domain program that is available on the Internet at http://otowustl.edu/cochlea/. An example of the power of this program is provided in the study by Plontke and coworkers,[15] in which a model of gentamicin kinetics in the perilymph was closely approximated to published in vivo kinetics data by adjusting input parameters defining RWM permeability, clearance, and interscala drug exchange. These investigators were able to establish that intratympanically administered gentamicin spreads from the RWM to the vestibule by communication through the scala, rather than by diffusion through the helicotrema. The study also suggested that drug concentrations and distribution in the perilymph were substantially influenced by the delivery method and the duration of exposure of the drug to the RWM. These computer-generated simulations are useful because they permit the optimization of different treatment protocols in humans, without resorting to simple trial and error or costly animal trials.

Another important finding from this simulated research is that the distribution of substances in perilymph is dramatically altered after perforation of the otic capsule. This finding is important because many previous pharmacokinetic studies have perforated the otic capsule to access perilymph for drug concentration sampling; their findings may be distorted by this phenomenon.[14]

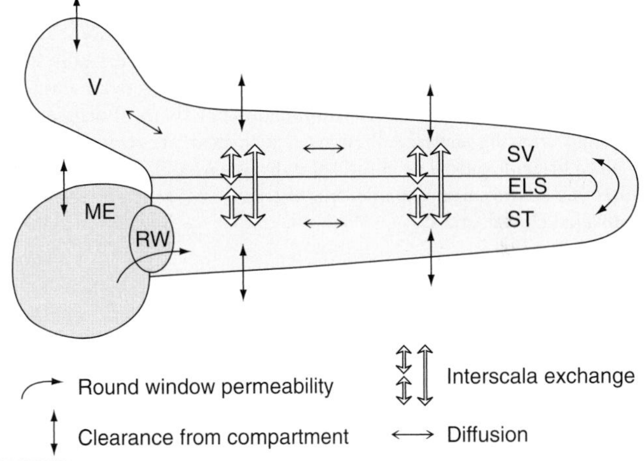

Figure 155-3. Schematic of the physical processes incorporated into the simulation program (the Washington University Cochlear Fluids Simulator, version 1.6, a public-domain computer program available at http://oto.wustl.edu/cochlea/). The compartments shown include the middle ear (ME), scala tympani (ST), cochlear endolymphatic space (ELS), scala vestibuli (SV), and vestibule (V). Drug enters through the round window (RW) in an amount depending on the permeability, and spreads longitudinally by diffusion. Local interscala exchange allows drug to spread to the endolymphatic space and the scala vestibuli, and from there to the vestibule. Drug clearance (losses to other compartments such as to blood) occurs from each compartment. Diffusion, clearance, and interscala exchange are calculated for each 0.1-mm segment of the fluid space. *(From Plontke SKR, Wood AW, Salt AN. Analysis of gentamicin kinetics in fluids of the inner ear with round window administration.* Otol Neurotol. *2002;23:967.)*

Adhesions

As noted previously, the epithelium that neighbors the round window niche sometimes can create a veil that separates the RWM from the middle ear. Other reactive changes, such as scarring from repeated middle ear infections or from prior middle ear surgery, may also lead to adhesions that obstruct the RWM.[16] In a cadaveric study of 202 ears to determine the rate and nature of RWM obstruction, Alzamil and Linthicum[17] identified RWM obstruction in one third of ears. In their series, 21% had false RWMs, 10% had fibrous plugs, and 1.5% had fatty plugs. In cases in which temporal bones came from the same cadaver, 57% had no obstruction, 22% had bilateral obstruction, and 21% had unilateral obstruction. These investigators noted that the plugs filling the round window niche are 1 mm (in contrast to the RWM, which is approximately 20 μm thick).

Silverstein and coworkers[16] provided further evidence of RWM obstruction. In a series of 41 patients, they found that 17% of ears had partial obstruction and 12% had total obstruction of the round window niche. Because these adhesions may cause significant variability in the

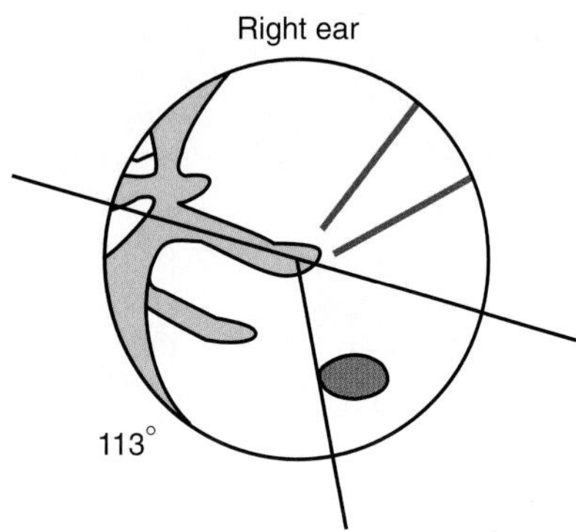

Figure 155-4. Illustration shows how the angle between the handle of the malleus and the round window (shown in the supine operative position) was calculated. *(From Silverstein H, Durand B, Jackson LE, et al. Use of the malleus handle as a landmark for localizing the round window membrane.* Ear Nose Throat J. *2001;80:444.)*

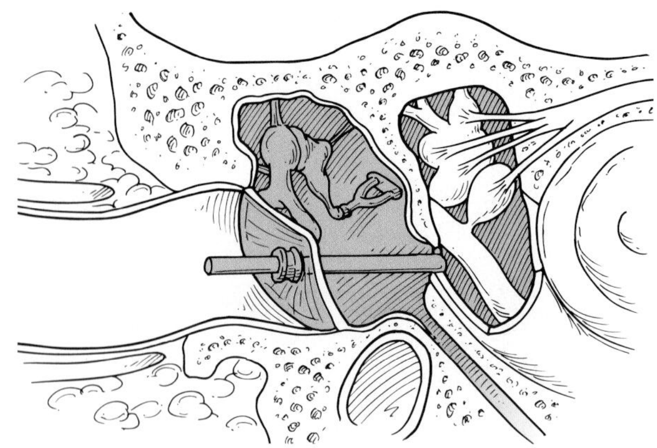

Figure 155-5. Silverstein MicroWick. *(Reprinted with permission of Micromedics, Inc.)*

pharmacokinetics of intratympanically applied medications, these authors recommended that endoscopic removal of these adhesions should be performed before any intratympanic drug treatments. In their practice, they use a 1.7-mm endoscope with 0-degree and 30-degree viewing angles. Adhesions, if identified, are removed with a small right-angle pick. The clinical and therapeutic advantages of lysing adhesions before intratympanic drug therapy have yet to be shown in controlled clinical trials.

Delivery Method

Following is a description of how typical intratympanic injections are performed. The patient lies flat with the affected ear facing the ceiling. The external ear canal is cleaned of debris, and the tympanic membrane is visualized with an operating microscope. The round window niche can be found an average of 3.44 mm (±0.68 mm) from the umbo, at an average angle of 113.2 degrees (±9.8 degrees) from the long process of the malleus (Fig. 155-4).[18] Local anesthetic is applied to the tympanic membrane. Anesthetic preparations include topical tetracaine with alcohol, topical 15% phenol preparation, or ear canal injection of 1% lidocaine with 1 : 100,000 epinephrine.[19] If endoscopy is to be performed, a generous myringotomy incision is made from the umbo posteriorly to the anulus, large enough to pass the endoscope (with scope diameters of approximately 1.7 to 2.4 mm). If simple injection is performed, myringotomy may still be necessary because there needs to be a vent for air to escape the middle ear space as it is filled with fluid.

If endoscopic examination is performed, the round window niche is identified, and any mucosal adhesions are removed by use of an angled pick. The injection follows with a 1-mL tuberculin syringe and a spinal needle. Cutting 2 inches off of the tip shortens the needle and dulls the tip, decreasing the risk of a traumatic puncture of surrounding tissue. The injection should be administered slowly and directed so that the solution pools around the round window niche. Because the solution often drains into deeper air cells after the first injection, a second injection can be applied. The patient should remain with the injected ear toward the ceiling for approximately 15 to 30 minutes. It is important to instruct the patient to refrain from swallowing, talking, or yawning during this time.

Some protocols call for multiple injections over a short time. In these cases, it is useful to place a tympanostomy tube after the initial myringotomy. Montandon and colleagues[20] found that placement of tympanostomy tubes resulted in resolution of vertigo in 71% of patients with Meniere's disease in their study; if tubes are going to be used in a study, they should be acknowledged as a confounding variable.

Advances in microendoscopes may significantly increase the ease and accuracy of intratympanic drug delivery. Plontke and associates[21] described the development of a 1.2-mm endoscope that incorporates a thin fiberoptic, a working/laser channel (0.3 mm), and a suction/irrigation channel (0.27 mm). This new device would allow for several manipulations to occur at once, including direct observation of the RWM, lysis of adhesions (if present), and application of medications directly to the RWM.

Intratympanic injection is inherently inaccurate because the injected medication can leak down the eustachian tube, escape out of the external canal, or be sequestered in the middle ear. The amount of medication delivered potentially changes with each patient and each dose.[22] In an attempt to address this problem, several static sustained-release vehicles have been developed. A dry 2 mm × 3 mm Gelfoam (Upjohn, Kalamazoo, MI) pledget can be placed directly in the round window niche against the RWM. The treatment compound can be injected directly onto the Gelfoam pad. Because of the slow dissipation of Gelfoam, this injection can be repeated several times (as in titration protocols for gentamicin treatment of Meniere's disease).[19] Gelfoam slurry can also be used to suspend the medicine. This slurry can be directly injected into the middle ear space. This method has the advantage of the Gelfoam being easily removed from the middle ear in the case of an adverse reaction to the applied medicine.[23]

A two-component fibrin glue system also can be used (developed by Red Cross–Holland Lab, College Park, MD). The first component of the glue is deposited in the round window niche. The other component is mixed with the medicine and is added to the first (which is already in the round window niche). The two are mixed in situ and subsequently solidified, allowing the medicine to be slowly released from the glue onto the RWM.[23]

The ultimate degree of pharmacokinetic control is achieved with the use of mechanical sustained-release devices. These devices allow researchers to manipulate inner ear kinetic curves reliably by changing the rate and amount of dose delivered to the RWM.[22] Two devices are currently approved for use in humans and have been studied in clinical trials: the Silverstein MicroWick (Micromedics, Eaton, MN) and the IntraEar Microcatheter (Durect, Cupertino, CA). The Silverstein MicroWick (Fig. 155-5) is made from polyvinyl acetate and measures 1 mm × 9 mm long, small enough to fit through a tympanostomy tube. The wick absorbs medication (which can be administered by the patient at home) that has been applied to the external ear canal and delivers it to the RWM. The advantage of this system is that fitting the device is a simple, minimally invasive procedure (only nominally more invasive than tympanostomy tube placement), and the device can be removed without anesthesia. Long-term use is not advised because the wick material may become adherent to the mucosa of the round window niche. This device has been used to deliver steroids and gentamicin treatments in human clinical trials.[19]

The IntraEar Microcatheter (Fig. 155-6) consists of an electronic pump (Disetronics, Minneapolis, MN) connected to a catheter tip that is placed directly on the RWM. Implantation of the microcatheter is more invasive and requires the elevation of a tympanomeatal flap. Several sizes are available to secure a good fit of the catheter tip into the round window niche. The rate and dose of drug delivery are set by the practitioner at the time of implantation, but can be adjusted in the

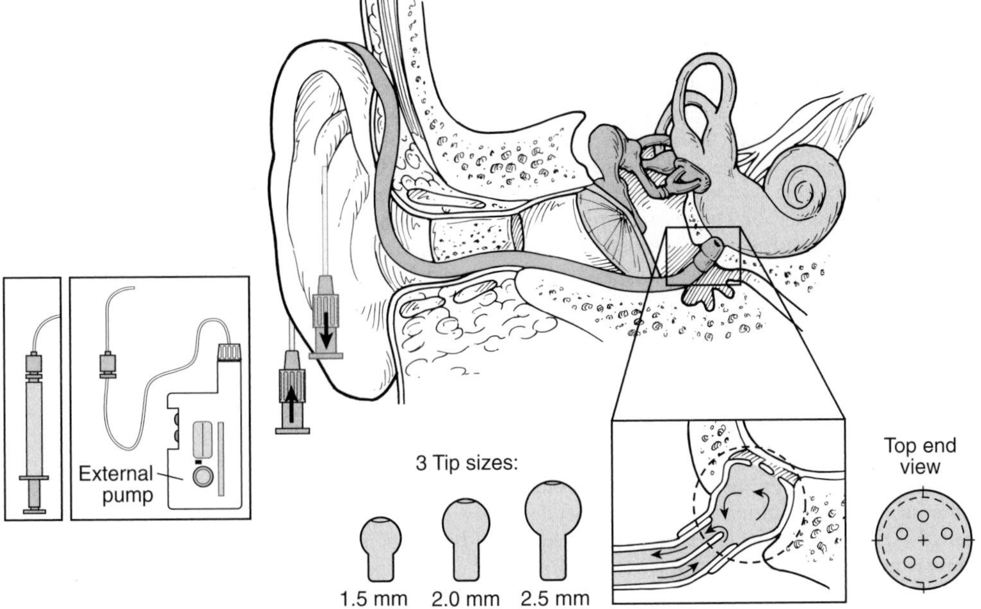

Figure 155-6. IntraEar Microcatheter. *(Reprinted with permission of the DURECT corporation.)*

middle of the treatment period. This device has also been extensively tested in human subjects for steroid and gentamicin therapy to the inner ear.[24]

Several new therapeutic agents (e.g., neurotrophins) require long-term or continuous application, which presents a serious challenge from a delivery point of view. In an attempt to address the need for a long-term delivery device, Praetorius and colleagues[25] developed a fully implantable micropump system. The device is made from pure titanium, polyethylene, and silicone, and is designed for lifelong implantation in humans. To place the device, a cavity is drilled out of the mastoid bone to house the pump and reservoir system, a procedure that is similar to the one used to place cochlear implants or implantable hearing devices. The catheter tip is placed into the round window niche. The design allows for variation in kinetics, enabling bolus and continuous infusions. The device is designed so that it can be refilled by a simple procedure without the need for reimplantation.

Steroids

The two principal indications for intratympanic steroids are sudden sensorineural hearing loss (SNHL) and Meniere's disease. The pathogenesis, pathophysiology, and diagnostic criteria for these indications are subject to controversy, making a comprehensive evaluation of the use of intratympanic steroids as a treatment for these conditions exceedingly difficult. The mechanism of action of steroids in the inner ear is incompletely understood. We review what is known about how steroids affect the inner ear, their systemic use for treatment of inner ear diseases, and the reported clinical outcomes of intratympanic steroid therapy.

Mechanism of Action

Steroids mitigate the destructive processes caused by the immune response by decreasing the number of circulating blood leukocytes and inhibiting the formation and liberation of inflammatory mediators.[26] They also inhibit the release of chemoattractive and vasoactive factors, decrease the secretion of lipolytic and proteolytic enzymes, and inhibit the release of proinflammatory cytokines, such as interferon-γ, granulocyte/monocyte colony-stimulating factor, interleukins, and tumor necrosis factor-α.[27] These actions decrease the damage from an inflammatory response, whether the insult is secondary to mechanic, hypoxic, ischemic, infectious, or autoimmunologic causes.[28]

Several studies have established how steroids attenuate pathogen-induced immune responses in the ear. On exposure to lipopolysaccharide, cultured endothelial modiolar cells and tissue exhibit a generic response and release proinflammatory cytokines.[29] These proinflammatory cytokines cause vasculitis, vascular leakage syndrome, entry of immunocompetent cells, and perivasculitis, ultimately leading to cochlear ischemia, intracochlear tissue damage, and hearing loss. Administration of dexamethasone can inhibit this cytokine immune response, and can potentially interrupt the beginnings of the inflammatory cascade at the level of cytokine expression.

Several other studies support the role of steroids in ion homeostasis in the inner ear. Serum glucocorticoid levels are directly correlated with activity and concentration of Na^+,K^+-ATPase in the inner ear.[30] Lee and Marcus[31] found that potassium secretion by marginal cells is immediately increased after the administration of steroids. Because the kinetics are too rapid for transcriptional activation to cause this change (it takes at least 30 minutes for RNA polymerase to be activated), a nongenomic mechanism is implicated. Modern theories of steroid pharmacology include not only nongenomic and genomic pathways of steroid hormone action, but also a nongenomic modulation of the genomic effects.[32] These relationships in the inner ear are just beginning to be understood.

Pharmacokinetics

Intratympanic administration yields much higher concentrations of steroids in the inner ear than either intravenous or oral administration.[6,33] Parnes and colleagues[33] compared intravenous and intratympanic administration of hydrocortisone, methylprednisolone, and dexamethasone (short-acting, intermediate-acting, and long-acting steroids). Although all three steroids successfully penetrated the blood-labyrinthine barrier, there was a much higher concentration of steroids in inner ear tissues with intratympanic administration. Other investigators have shown that the metabolism of steroids, including uptake and elimination, is different in cochlear tissues compared with other organs.[34] Methylprednisolone had the highest concentration and longest duration in perilymph and endolymph of the three compounds.[33] Similar concentrations of steroids were found in the scala tympani and scala vestibuli. The authors argue that the concentration of steroids in the endolymph implies some form of active transport through the membranous labyrinth.

The findings regarding the superior concentrations of methylprednisolone are controversial. First, other forms of steroids have been tolerated much better by middle ear tissues. Dexamethasone seems to be better tolerated and less irritative to middle ear tissues. Second, higher concentrations have not led to superior clinical results. It may be that higher perilymph and endolymph concentrations do not translate into greater efficacy. In addition, although high methylprednisolone concentrations and high anti-inflammatory activity associated with attainable levels are observed with methylprednisolone, therapeutic efficacy may rely on other mechanisms of action. One possibility relates to Na^+-K^+ channel activity. The mineralocorticoid and glucocorticoid classes of steroids induce markedly different responses in Na^+-K^+ channel activity.[31] At this point, it is reasonable to use the less morbid middle ear therapeutic agents (i.e., dexamethasone) until more definitive studies can determine whether the higher concentrations in the study by Parnes and colleagues[33] translate into better clinical results, despite decreased tolerability.

Systemic Steroids

Currently, systemic steroids are the treatment of choice for sudden SNHL[35,36] and acute vestibular vertigo.[37] The most frequently used protocol of oral steroids for inner ear disease is 60 mg of prednisone (or 1 mg/kg/day for adults) taken for 10 to 14 days in idiopathic sudden SNHL or for 1 month in suspected autoimmune inner ear disease.[38] Both indications call for a gradual taper after the initial treatment period is finished. If hearing loss returns during the taper, a higher dose of prednisone is restarted. Relapse of hearing loss is often preceded by tinnitus.[39] Shea[40] recommended that in addition to oral steroids, 16 mg of intravenous dexamethasone should be perfused over 3 hours. The value of adjunctive intravenous delivery of steroids in addition to oral therapy remains to be established.

Meniere's Disease

Meniere's disease may be due in some cases to immune dysfunction. Steroids are often used in Meniere's disease treatment protocols.[1] Itoh and Sakata[41] reported the first intratympanic steroid protocol in 1987, in which four to five weekly injections of 2 mg of dexamethasone were administered to 61 patients with unilateral Meniere's disease. This protocol resulted in relief of vertigo in 80% of patients and reduction in tinnitus in 74% of patients. Subsequently, additional studies have used intratympanic steroids to treat Meniere's disease, some with more promising results than others.

Sennaroglu and colleagues[42] placed tympanostomy tubes in 24 patients with Meniere's disease with intractable vertigo and applied 5 drops of 1 mg/mL dexamethasone solution into the middle ear space every other day for 3 months (administered at home by the patient). This protocol resulted in a vertigo control rate of 72%, improved hearing in 17%, decreased tinnitus in 75%, and reduced aural fullness in 75%. This protocol is attractive because the drug is self-administered, the entire procedure can be accomplished under local anesthesia, and the delivery method provides flexibility to titrate the dose. The authors acknowledge that their results may be confounded by a placebo effect secondary to the tympanostomy tubes. They cite a study by Montandon and associates[20] that reported that tympanostomy tube placement prevented vertigo attacks in 71% of patients.

Barrs and coworkers[43] also used tympanostomy tubes to administer intratympanic dexamethasone. They used a dose of 0.3 to 0.5 mL of 4 mg/mL dexamethasone. Injections were given daily for the first 2 days and weekly thereafter for a total of 1 month and five treatments. The vertigo control responses were reported in time intervals, with an 86% response at less than 3 months, a 52% response at 3 months, and a 43% response at 6 months. There was an average of 2.7-dB hearing loss, but one patient had a 35-dB hearing loss. The authors propose that intratympanic steroid treatment is effective for short-term management of vertigo, but is less successful for long-term vertigo control.

Shea[40] reported on a protocol that uses a combination of intravenous, intratympanic, and oral dexamethasone to treat patients with Meniere's disease. A mixture of 0.5 mL hyaluronan containing 16 mg/mL of dexamethasone is injected into the middle ear after argon laser myringotomy and removal of RWM adhesions. The patient sits with the injected ear up for 3 hours while receiving 16 mg of intravenous dexamethasone. This treatment is performed for 3 consecutive days. Then 0.25 mg of oral dexamethasone is taken for 30 to 90 days, depending on the response to treatment. This protocol resulted in a vertigo control rate of 77%, hearing improvement in 35.4%, and hearing loss in 6.3%. With the 6-point functional level score recommended by the American Academy of Otolaryngology–Head and Neck Surgeons (AAO-HNS) guidelines,[44] 61.3% of patients were improved, 32.3% were unchanged, and 6.4% were worse after treatment.

In a rare controlled trial, Silverstein and colleagues[1] conducted a prospective, randomized, double-blind, crossover trial of intratympanic dexamethasone and placebo in 17 patients with Meniere's disease. All patients had stage IV Meniere's disease by the Shea classification (they no longer had vertigo, had poor hearing, and had significant fullness and tinnitus). Patients received intratympanic injection of either placebo (0.2 to 0.3 mL of 1 : 1 normal saline and sodium hyaluronate) or 0.2 to 0.3 mL of a 1 : 1 mixture of 16 mg/mL dexamethasone and sodium hyaluronate. This treatment was performed for 3 consecutive days. Three weeks after the initial treatment, the groups received the crossover treatment (the placebo group received intratympanic steroids and vice versa). The parameters recorded were audiometric data, electronystagmography recordings, and tinnitus evaluations; several questionnaires and telephone interviews were included. Intratympanic steroids provided no significant benefit over placebo in any of the parameters recorded, and patients could not guess which arm of the study they were in. This study would seem to confirm the lack of benefit of intratympanic steroid use for Meniere's disease. The severely diseased patient population (all stage IV) may be a selection bias not present in other studies, however, leaving open the possibility that intratympanic steroids may be useful in less severe cases. Also, most successful intratympanic steroid protocols involve steroid treatments that last longer than 3 days.

In another well-designed study, Garduño-Anaya and associates[45] conducted a prospective, placebo-controlled, double-blind, randomized study with 2-year follow-up, and found dramatically different results than Silverstein and colleagues.[1] A regimen of 5 consecutive days of intratympanic dexamethasone (4 mg/mL) versus saline for placebo control was administered to 11 study patients and 11 controls, all having unilateral disease as outlined by the 1995 AAO-HNS Committee on Hearing and Equilibrium. In the dexamethasone group at 2-year follow-up, complete control of vertigo (class A) was achieved in 9 of 11 patients (82%), and substantial control of vertigo (class B) was achieved in the remaining 2 patients. In the control group, only 7 of 11 patients finished the trial, and of these, 4 patients (57%) achieved class A vertigo control, 2 patients (29%) achieved class C, and 1 patient (14%) achieved class F. These results were statistically significant. There were several other outcome measures with variable results, with significant improvement in AAO-HNS 6-point functional level; Dizziness Handicap Inventory; and subjective vertigo, tinnitus, and aural fullness scores in the treatment group, but no significant changes in the Tinnitus Handicap Score, pure-tone average, speech discrimination score, electronystagmography, or electrocochleography tests between the two groups. The final verdict on intratympanic steroid use for Meniere's disease is still pending, and more data on optimal dosing and protocols are needed.

Sudden Sensorineural Hearing Loss

Systemic and intratympanic steroid therapy has also been used for treatment of sudden SNHL. The major prognostic factors predicting response to treatment for sudden SNHL are initial severity of hearing loss and time between onset and treatment.[6,46] There is a high spontaneous recovery rate of 30% to 60%; treatment efficacy of any intervention has to be greater than the spontaneous recovery rate. Oral steroid therapy within the first 2 weeks has shown recovery rates approaching 80% and decreasing thereafter.[46,47] Because of the high initial response to oral steroids, few practitioners have attempted to use intratympanic steroids, and most intratympanic steroid trials enroll patients who had oral treatment fail. That being said, numerous studies, mostly retrospective, have shown that intratympanic steroids do provide an excellent method for salvage of hearing in the case of systemic steroid treatment failure.

Gianoli and Li[35] reported results of a trial of intratympanic steroids for patients with sudden SNHL who had failed to improve after high-dose systemic steroids (1 mg/kg/day of prednisone for a minimum of 1 week). The protocol consisted of tympanostomy tube placement followed by instillation of 0.5 mL of steroid solution consisting of either

25 mg/mL of dexamethasone or 62.5 mg/mL of methylprednisolone. Four treatments were administered over 10 to 14 days, and audiometric data were recorded 1 to 2 weeks after treatment. The results showed a pure-tone average improvement of 10 dB or greater in 44% of patients. The authors argued that although this improvement seems modest, this is in a cohort of patients who would otherwise be considered refractory to steroid treatment. Although there was a trend toward better outcomes for methylprednisolone, there was no significant difference between the two steroid solutions.

Kopke and colleagues[46] reported results of the use of methylprednisolone perfusion by means of an RWM microcatheter in patients with sudden SNHL who failed oral prednisone therapy. The catheter delivered 62.5 mg/mL of methylprednisolone at a continuous rate of 10 µL/hour for 14 days with an electronic pump. Audiometric changes were the main outcome measures recorded. Of the six patients who had catheter placement 6 weeks or less after the onset of hearing loss, five had improvements of 10 dB or more in pure-tone averages, and four of these had a return to baseline pure-tone averages. Results were less promising for patients receiving treatment more than 6 weeks after onset of symptoms; in one patient, there was additional hearing loss associated with vertigo.

Several other, smaller reports have been published. Chandrasekhar[47] reported results from a series of 10 patients treated with intratympanic dexamethasone. The dexamethasone concentration and number of intratympanic injections varied among patients, and several patients were taking oral medications in addition to intratympanically administered steroids, making outcomes difficult to assess. Of the 10 patients treated, 6 experienced hearing improvements greater than 10 dB, however. Parnes and colleagues[33] reported results from a similar series of 13 patients with sudden SNHL treated with intratympanic steroids. Because there was considerable variation in the number of treatments applied and the drug administered (dexamethasone vs. methylprednisolone), the results are difficult to assess. Of the 13 patients treated, 6 showed hearing improvements of 10 dB or more.

One point of consensus about these studies is that they show that the longer between the insult and the administration of intratympanic steroid treatment after oral steroid failure, the lower are the chances of salvaging hearing. If intratympanic steroids are to be used, they should be used as soon as possible after it becomes clear that oral steroids are not improving hearing, preferably within the first 2 weeks of the original insult.[48]

Dosing

The most widely used steroid for intratympanic protocols is dexamethasone, followed by methylprednisolone. Intratympanic dexamethasone preparations vary from 1 to 25 mg/mL.[49,50] Some studies use a hyaluronic acid preparation consisting of a 1 : 1 mixture of 16 mg/mL of dexamethasone and 0.5 mg/mL of hyaluronate sodium.[1,40] Most intratympanic methylprednisolone studies use a solution of 62.5 mg/mL.[22,46] The amount of solution injected in each protocol is designed to fill the middle ear space (which is 0.3 to 0.5 mL). The interval of dosing depends mostly on the instillation method. Protocols that include self-administration through tympanostomy tubes have every-other-day dosing.[49] Intratympanic injection protocols are much less frequent, and often include "shotgun" dosing with multiple injections over the first 2 weeks of treatment.[1,51]

Side Effects

The side effects of long-term systemic steroid use are well known and include compromise of the immune system leading to infections, osteoporosis, peptic ulcers, hypertension, myopathy, ocular effects, impaired healing, psychologic effects, and avascular necrosis.[52] In contrast, intratympanic steroids are characterized by minor local morbidities. Several preclinical studies have documented that intratympanic steroids cause no morphologic or functional compromise in animal models.[27,53] Human clinical trials have reported benign side-effect profiles, even after multiple and long-term treatments.[33] There are several reports of decreased hearing in human clinical trials of patients with Meniere's disease,[40,43] but it is unclear whether this is a side effect of treatment or part of the natural course of the disease.[51,54] There are some reports of tympanic membrane perforations and otitis media secondary to the perfusion process.[35] Some patients experience a mild burning sensation in the ear after injection of methylprednisolone. This side effect has been avoided by combining 0.1 mL of 1% lidocaine with 0.9 mL of standard intravenous methylprednisolone solution (40 mg/mL).[33]

Summary

There is currently no consensus on the mechanism of action of steroids in the inner ear. Experience with intratympanic steroids is insufficient to recommend their routine use in autoimmune hearing loss, sudden SNHL, or Meniere's disease. Intratympanic steroid use is proving to have a role as a salvage therapy, however, for sudden SNHL unresponsive to oral steroids.

Gentamicin

Fowler[55] first described the use of aminoglycosides for chemical ablation of the labyrinth in 1948, using systemic streptomycin to treat patients with Meniere's disease with intractable vertigo. Bilateral cochlear damage led to the abandonment of this effort, but in 1957, Schuknecht[56] revived interest in chemical ablation with the introduction of intratympanic administration of aminoglycosides. Although loss of hearing was almost as common as the resolution of vertigo, his work set the stage for the development of modern intratympanic chemical ablation protocols. In the mid-1970s, Beck and Schmidt[57] described a low-dose strategy that departed from the goal of total vestibular ablation. They compared a high-dose ablative protocol with a low-dose, low-injection-frequency protocol, and found that although vertigo control was essentially the same, the hearing loss rate decreased from 58% to 15%. This improvement rekindled interest in intratympanic gentamicin therapy, and led to the development of strategies that maximize vertigo control, while minimizing hearing loss.

Mechanism of Action

Despite the widespread belief that gentamicin is selectively toxic to vestibular hair cells, this assertion is not fully supported by the literature. Several researchers have shown that gentamicin and streptomycin cause parallel and dose-dependent damage to vestibular and cochlear hair cells.[58,59] Wanamaker and colleagues[59] stated, "When the vestibular system was severely damaged, the cochlea was severely damaged; when loss in the vestibular system was mild, loss in the cochlea was mild. We did not observe any dose-related selectivity for the vestibular system over the cochlea." The clinical finding of significant correlation between loss of caloric response and hearing loss after gentamicin exposure further betrays the notion of selective vestibular toxicity.[60,61]

If there is no selective vestibular toxicity, how is it that clinicians have achieved good vertigo control with minimal hearing loss? In part, the answer may lie in pharmacokinetics.[22,62,63] Hoffer and colleagues[22] compared the kinetic profiles of intratympanic injection versus microcatheter delivery of gentamicin, and correlated these data with the functional and morphologic changes observed in the inner ear. Despite the fact that the total dose in both methods was roughly equal, the resulting morphologic changes were quite different. Intratympanic injection led to erratic changes, sometimes causing obliteration of auditory functioning within 4 hours, and in other cases showing significantly delayed ototoxic effects. In contrast, controlled perfusion by microcatheter caused predictable and uniform damage.

Hoffer and colleagues[22] explained that these different morphologic changes may be due to two different patterns of hair cell loss, patterns that correlate with the timing and concentration of aminoglycoside delivery. These patterns include a necrotic pattern that is associated with rapid and high-dose perfusion, and an apoptotic pattern that is associated with slower or chronic perfusion.[53,64] This complicated relationship may be secondary to saturation of anionic binding sites on the cell membrane or to modifiable active uptake patterns that depend on gentamicin kinetics.[65] In addition to the amount of gentamicin that accumulates in the perilymph over time, the nature of the distribution curve, timing of the peak, and total dose determine morphologic and functional consequences of aminoglycoside exposure.

There is overwhelming clinical evidence that vestibular ablation is not required for vertigo control. These observations have caused a shift in strategy from vestibular ablation to *chemical alteration* or *subablation*. These terms describe the clinical goal of balancing vertigo control and hearing loss. This quest has spawned numerous clinical trials with various dosing protocols and delivery methods, all designed to achieve this goal.

What is the histologic and physiologic correlate of partial ablation? It is known that gentamicin damages type I hair cells more rapidly and severely than type II hair cells.[66] In the chinchilla, investigators showed that type II hair cells regenerated to approximately 55% of the baseline population, whereas type I hair cells showed no regeneration at all. It may be that these patterns of hair cell destruction and regeneration describe the partial vestibular ablation seen in intratympanic gentamicin clinical trials. Carey and associates[67] examined the changes in the angular vestibulo-ocular reflex after a single dose of intratympanic gentamicin, and found that in all cases there was a decreased, but not abolished, angular vestibulo-ocular reflex gain. These authors concluded that this finding provides evidence of incomplete hair cell destruction, which may account for the phenomenon of "partial ablation." Minor[68] speculated that there may be a critical level of vestibular activity required to initiate an episode of vertigo, and that the regions of vestibular epithelium or groups of afferent nerve fibers responsible for vertigo may be more susceptible to gentamicin toxicity than others. Minor[68] also speculated that hair cell regeneration may explain the phenomenon of recurrent vertigo after initial control with intratympanic gentamicin.

Although selective hair cell destruction and regeneration have yet to be established in humans, this may explain some of the more puzzling findings documented in clinical trials. Numerous trials have reported that there is an increase in hearing after gentamicin treatment.[61,69,70] In addition, in the microdose infusion trials by Hoffer and colleagues,[71] vestibular function improved in 78% of patients. These findings are hard to reconcile with traditional models of aminoglycoside toxicity.

The alternative explanation for how gentamicin achieves a selective vestibular effect is the proposal that gentamicin primarily affects secretory, rather than sensory, cells; this is known as the dark cell theory. Although cited in almost every article related to intratympanic gentamicin treatment, there is no firm documented scientific evidence showing how the effect actually occurs. Vestibular dark cells are important (but not essential) in creating and maintaining ion homeostasis in the inner ear.[72-74] Several studies have documented that aminoglycosides induce structural and functional alteration of these dark cells.[19,75] This damage is thought to alter the ionic homeostasis of the inner ear in such a way that it brings the ionic dysregulation in endolymphatic hydrops back into balance.[76,77] This theory helps explain how the hearing restoration and vestibular improvement referenced earlier might occur; re-establishment of ionic homeostasis would restore baseline function in the cochlea and labyrinth. There is uncertainty, however, whether this dark cell damage occurs before damage to sensory cells. Chen and colleagues[58] looked at secretory and sensory cells in response to aminoglycoside challenge, and found no significant changes in dark cells, despite extensive damage in cochlear and vestibular hair cells in the same animal. If dark cells are responsible for the selective effect of gentamicin, this has yet to be established in any preclinical models. Explanation of this mechanism, if it exists, would be a great advance in otology.

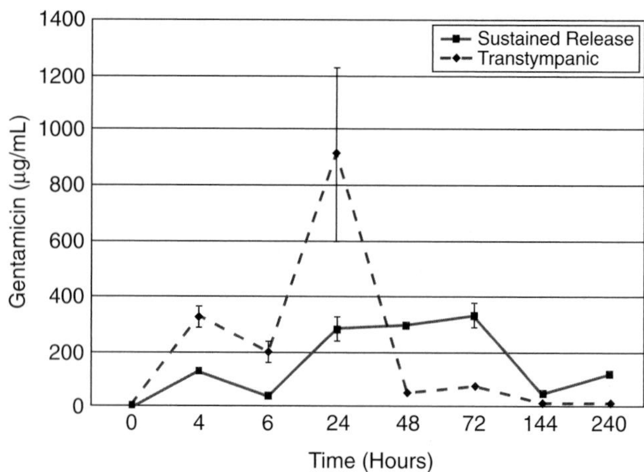

Figure 155-7. Perilymph gentamicin kinetics after sustained-release and transtympanic local delivery. Kinetic curves of perilymphatic gentamicin concentrations after sustained-release and transtympanic delivery are depicted. *Solid line* shows the sustained-release curve. The transient 4-hour peak followed by sustained delivery from 24 to 72 hours with the presence of gentamicin at 6 and 10 days is also depicted. *Dashed line* is the transtympanic curve with rapid uptake and almost total elimination within 48 hours. The SEM bars are much larger for transtympanic delivery than for sustained-release delivery. *Note*: The *x*-axis (time) is not to scale. *(From Hoffer ME, Allen K, Kopke RD, et al. Transtympanic versus sustained-release administration of gentamicin: kinetics, morphology, and function.* Laryngoscope. *2001;111:1343.)*

Pharmacokinetics

Intratympanic gentamicin kinetics in the perilymph follow a one-compartment model.[22,78] Gentamicin rapidly diffuses across the RWM; the kinetics of gentamicin in perilymph are largely determined by the method of delivery.[22,78,79] Intratympanic injection has a faster absorption phase, shows higher peak concentrations, and exhibits significantly more variability in all measurements than sustained-release delivery methods.[22,80] In pharmacokinetic studies, large value ranges and standard deviations are characteristic of intratympanic injection delivery (Fig. 155-7).[22]

Elimination of gentamicin from the perilymph compartment is rapid and dose-dependent.[78] Because of this rapid elimination, a sustained-release vehicle for drug delivery, such as a fibrin-based glue[80] or delivery by microcatheter, is the only way to maintain high concentrations of gentamicin in perilymph.[22] Although elimination in perilymph is rapid, there seems to be significant uptake of gentamicin in inner ear tissues, essentially constituting a second, "deeper" compartment. Access of aminoglycosides to the organ of Corti is probably directly from the perilymph, rather than from the endolymph.[81] That gentamicin appears in the endolymph at all seems to be a function of it being slowly released from inner ear tissues. This delayed release may explain why aminoglycosides are not immediately toxic when applied into the perilymph, whereas toxicity in vitro (without compartments) is seen immediately.[82] Hiel and coworkers[83] showed that gentamicin is rapidly and specifically captured by hair cells, such that there is significant uptake of gentamicin before morphologic ototoxic changes occur. Hair cells store aminoglycosides in lysosomes, essentially constituting the "deep" intracellular compartment referred to previously. This compartment provides prolonged exposure of these cells to aminoglycosides, and may be the basis for the delayed morphologic and functional effects seen clinically.

The pharmacokinetic data generated in animal models seem to fit what occurs in humans. Becvarovski and colleagues[79] devised an in vivo human pharmacokinetic study by recruiting patients who were undergoing either translabyrinthine surgery or labyrinthectomy and exposing them to gentamicin intraoperatively through the facial recess. In these patients, there was rapid diffusion of gentamicin into the perilymph that peaked after 30 minutes. After this peak, concentrations were in a stable range until the limit of the experiment at 110 minutes. Although there was no evidence of gentamicin in the cerebrospinal fluid, gentamicin was detected in serum shortly after administration (1 to 2 hours). This study confirms that rapid diffusion of gentamicin across the RWM occurs in humans. This study indicates that the elimination of gentamicin involves crossing the blood-labyrinthine barrier because gentamicin was detected in the serum shortly after administration.

As mentioned previously, progress in understanding gentamicin pharmacokinetics has been made with computer simulations. Plontke and colleagues[15] approximated published in vivo kinetics data by adjusting input parameters defining RWM permeability, clearance, and interscala drug exchange. The results are shown in Figure 155-8. They were able to establish that intratympanically administered gentamicin spreads from the RWM to the vestibule by communication through the scala,

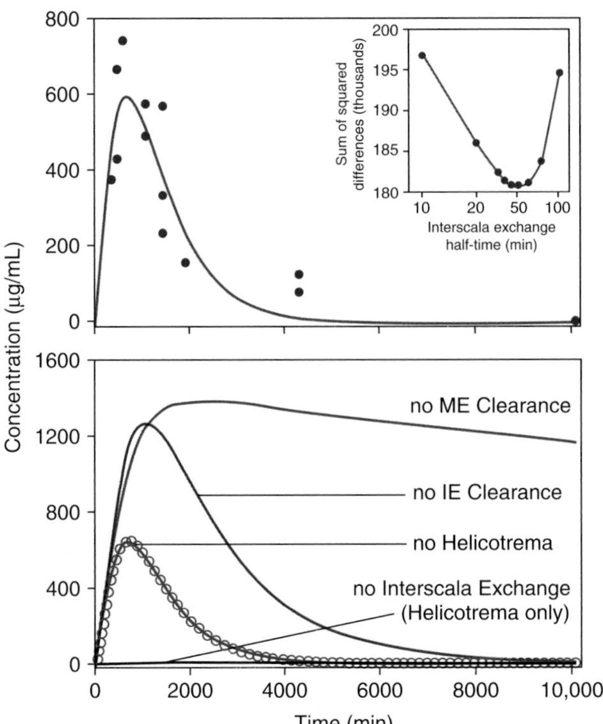

Figure 155-8. *Top,* Experimental measurements of gentamicin levels in perilymph samples taken from the vestibule after application to the round window *(solid circles).* Data are replotted from Hoffer and colleagues and Balough.[23,80,169] *Solid line* shows best fit of the concentration time course established by the simulator (the Washington University Cochlear Fluids Simulator, version 1.6) based on physical processes of solute movement. The curve represents the calculated concentration of a simulated 15-μL sample taken from the vestibule (as described in the text). *Inset graph,* A unique best fit (using methods described in the text) was found to occur with an interscala exchange half-time of 45 minutes. *Bottom,* Calculated gentamicin time course in the vestibule with best-fit parameters *(open circles)* and with specific processes in the simulator disabled *(solid lines). (From Plontke SKR, Wood AW, Salt AN. Analysis of gentamicin kinetics in fluids of the inner ear with round window administration.* Otol Neurotol. *2002;23:967.)*

rather than by diffusion through the helicotrema. The study also suggested that drug concentrations and distribution in the perilymph were substantially influenced by the delivery method and the duration of exposure of the drug to the RWM.

Clinical Protocols

Although many studies that used intratympanic gentamicin have been published, because of extreme differences in the quality of data, comparison of the different intratympanic gentamicin protocols is exceedingly difficult. Instead, several studies representing various strategies are discussed, and their results are summarized. There are three basic strategies used in intratympanic gentamicin therapy: fixed protocols, titrated protocols, and sustained-release protocols. Fixed protocols use a specific dose and number of injections in all patients. Titration protocols adjust the total dose delivered to a predetermined end point, such as paralytic nystagmus, decreased tandem gait, subjective dysequilibrium, or, more simply (and more commonly), relief from vertigo.[76] Sustained-release protocols work on various principles, depending on the delivery mechanism.

There is little difference between fixed and titration protocols because most fixed protocols can be repeated if no clinical response is seen, and most titration protocols deliver a fixed number of injections in the beginning of the protocol, and then repeat them as necessary. The supposed advantage of fixed protocols is that each patient receives the same treatment, making outcomes easier to interpret across individuals. Fixed protocols can be more cost-effective because excessive testing and clinical visits are avoided.[61] The flexible structure of titrated protocols supposedly allows for more control of the ototoxic effects of gentamicin, decreasing the risk of hearing loss.[84] Close monitoring for ototoxic symptoms does not confer the ability to reverse these symptoms, however.[85]

Much of the controversy in intratympanic gentamicin therapy in the 1990s concerned a form of fixed protocol known as a "shotgun" protocol. The classic "shotgun" protocol was popularized by Nedzelski and colleagues in 1992.[86] There have been periodic reports on this original "shotgun" protocol, and it is now one of the largest series in the literature, spanning a decade and including more than 90 patients. The protocol calls for three daily injections for 4 consecutive days of 26.7 mg/mL of gentamicin, and results in a vertigo control rate of 94% and hearing loss rate of 26%.[60,61,86] The main argument against "shotgun" protocols is that they lead to higher rates of hearing loss,[87] and that the hearing loss realized is profound.[69] Toth and Parnes[87] followed the classic "shotgun" protocol outlined previously, but encountered an unacceptable rate of hearing loss (57%) following 18 patients. After they changed to a titration protocol that involved weekly injections, the hearing loss rate decreased to 19%. Altlas and Parnes[69] pointed out that in "shotgun" protocols, the proportion of patients who experience hearing loss greater than 30 dB (10% to 24%) is much higher than the proportion seen in titration protocols (0% to 4%).

More recently, "hybrid" protocols have been introduced. Quaranta and associates[88] used a fixed schedule of two 0.5-mL intratympanic injections of 20 mg/mL of gentamicin solution spaced 1 week apart. Patients who did not achieve vertigo control after the first two doses were offered additional doses to a total of four doses. This was a prospective study that included a control group of patients with Meniere's disease who refused treatment. At the 2-year follow-up point, the vertigo control rate was 93% versus 47% for the untreated group. Hearing loss was 7% for the treated group versus 47% for the untreated group. Tinnitus rate and aural pressure relief were 20% and 40% for the treated group versus 27% and 27% for the untreated group. In the protocol, 47% of patients had residual vertigo after two doses and went on to receive a third dose, and 27% went on to receive a fourth dose. This study illustrates the paradoxic effect that intratympanic gentamicin actually improves hearing outcomes of patients with Meniere's disease. Improvement in hearing from the baseline decline encountered in untreated Meniere's disease is not a logical outcome if the mechanism of action of intratympanic gentamicin is merely the selective ablation of vestibular hair cells.

The microcatheter delivery method has been recommended to provide sustained gentamicin levels in the perilymph. Schoendorf and associates[89] used a high-precision insulin pump and a microcatheter to deliver 40 mg/day of gentamicin to the RWM. The treatment was continued at this fixed rate until vestibular symptoms appeared (in essence, a titration protocol). Although vertigo control was achieved in most patients, 8 of 11 patients treated became deaf. The authors claim that the occurrence of deafness was not correlated with dose because one deafened patient received 720 mg and another received only 60 mg, and hearing was unchanged in a patient who received 240 mg. The authors noted that continuous perfusion protocols should not use titration strategies because the adequate dose for vertigo control may be quickly exceeded. This study highlights the notion that kinetics can have a larger impact on morphologic and functional outcomes than dose-related effects.

In contrast to the preceding study, most continuous-delivery protocols use microdose, slow-infusion strategies. Seidman and colleagues[90] reported retrospective data from a multi-institutional trial that compared results of different microcatheter infusion rates. The vertigo control rate was 90% in the group receiving infusions of 1 μL/hr versus 79% in the group receiving infusions of greater than 10 μL/hr, a nonsignificant difference. The hearing loss rate was 23% in the group receiving 1 μL/hr versus 50% in the group receiving greater than 10 μL/hr, however, and this difference was statistically significant. The authors recommended the slow infusion rate and suggested that infusion rates less than 1 μL/hr might have even lower hearing loss rates, while maintaining equal clinical efficacy.

In a study that epitomizes the microdose, slow perfusion rate strategy, Hoffer and colleagues[91] reported the 2-year results of 27 patients who underwent microcatheter gentamicin therapy. The study used a pediatric solution of 10 mg/mL, with the pump set at 1 μL/hr for 10 days, resulting in total dose of 2.4 mg. This strategy achieved vertigo control in 93% of patients, hearing loss in only 4%, tinnitus relief in 63%, and elimination of aural pressure in 74%. The protocol included a wide variety of vestibular tests, including vestibulo-ocular gain, phase, and symmetry; posturography score; and step velocity testing. Ninety-six percent of patients had no decrease in vestibular function; however, caloric testing was not performed. The investigators found that vestibular function was improved in 79% of patients.[71] These results represent some of the most impressive results of intratympanic gentamicin therapy.

Chia and coworkers[92] conducted a meta-analysis of intratympanic gentamicin trials. The study included seven studies ($N = 218$) that used multiple daily dosing technique (delivery three times per day for ≥4 days), two studies ($N = 84$) that used weekly dosing technique (weekly injections for four total doses), eight studies ($N = 253$) that used the low-dose technique (one to two injections with re-treatment for recurrent vertigo), four studies ($N = 156$) that used continuous microcatheter delivery, and six studies ($N = 269$) that used the titration technique (daily or weekly doses until onset of vestibular symptoms, change in vertigo, or hearing loss). The titration method of gentamicin delivery showed significantly better complete (81.7%; $P = .001$) and effective (96.3%; $P < .05$) vertigo control compared with other methods. The low-dose method of delivery showed significantly worse complete vertigo control (66.7%; $P < .001$) and trended toward worse effective vertigo control (86.8%; $P = .05$) compared with other methods. The weekly method of delivery trended toward less overall hearing loss (13.1%; $P = .08$), and the multiple daily method showed significantly more overall hearing loss (34.7%; $P < .01$) compared with other groups. No significant difference in profound hearing loss was found between groups, and the degree of vestibular ablation after gentamicin therapy was not significantly correlated with the resulting vertigo control or hearing loss status.

As with all meta-analyses, caution needs to be used when interpreting these results. Differences in patient profiles, dose and concentration of gentamicin delivered, quality of follow-up analysis, and multiple other factors are necessarily bracketed for the sake of getting a reasonable idea of what treatments are best for patients. Perhaps the best outcome of this effort is that it can guide a rational design for a well-run, controlled trial that would provide a new level of evidence regarding superior treatment for patients with vertigo.

Practical Considerations

The argument for the use of intratympanic injection is that it is the simplest, most cost-effective, and least invasive method of delivery, and from published studies, it provides comparative vertigo control and hearing preservation rates to sustained-release protocols. Blakely[93,94] argued that even though there are no head-to-head comparisons of these methods, the published results suggest that there is no reason to use anything but the simplest administration protocols. The argument for using sustained-release mechanisms, particularly continuous infusion devices, is that they seem to produce lower rates of hearing loss, allow for standardization across individuals, lead to more predictable and uniform results, and improve vestibular and auditory functioning.[71]

Dose

Eklund and coworkers[95] found that frequency of deafness was dose-dependent in their intratympanic injection study. There is no minimum safe dose, however, because the lowest documented intratympanic gentamicin dose to produce hearing loss is 0.24 mg.[96] The method of delivery is as important as dose in terms of ototoxicity; this was illustrated earlier in the trial by Schoendorf and colleagues,[89] in which a microcatheter delivered a severely ototoxic dose of gentamicin, a dose that would be considered to be a "low dose" in intratympanic injection protocols. Per the pharmacokinetic studies of Hoffer and colleagues[22] mentioned previously, functional and morphologic end organ damage depends less on the total dose delivered to the inner ear than on the kinetics of how the drug reaches inner ear tissues.

Concentration

The concentration of gentamicin used varies among different studies. Low-dose protocols use the pediatric formulation of gentamicin, which comes in a preparation of 10 mg/mL.[96] The adult preparation of 40 mg/mL is often diluted to 30 mg/mL. Abou-Halawa and Poe[76] compared outcomes between intratympanic gentamicin preparations of 30 mg/mL and 40 mg/mL, and found that although both cohorts had similar vertigo control and hearing loss rates, the cohort receiving 40 mg/mL required fewer injections to achieve these results. Several other studies have confirmed that with low-dose protocols, more periodic treatments are needed, and there is an increase in the recurrence rate.[71]

Interval

The injection interval depends on the end point chosen for the study. There is increasing support for spacing the injections over at least a week, primarily because of the delayed onset of gentamicin toxicity. The typical deafferentation syndrome occurs only 3 to 5 days after injection.[88,97] Other advocates say that if a patient has Meniere's disease with episodes that are only every other week, it is unreasonable to check for results on a weekly basis.[98] In Blakely's review of intratympanic gentamicin protocols,[93,94] he argued that differences in injection intervals have little impact, if any, on outcomes.

Number of Injections

The general belief in the literature is that the fewer intratympanic gentamicin injections, the better. Youssef and Poe[70] found that the chances of gentamicin being effective after three injections are significantly reduced. Other reasons to limit the number of injections include an increased risk of permanent perforation of the tympanic membrane with each injection (unless tympanostomy tubes are placed), the increased cost and inconvenience to the patient and the physician, and an increase in the risk of hearing loss (although this is not supported by all studies).[87]

Complications

The most notorious complication of intratympanic gentamicin treatment is hearing loss. Risk factors for hearing loss have been inconsistently identified across studies; this is partially due to the substantial differences in protocols between studies. Kaplan and associates[60] found that the only factor related to hearing loss was poor hearing before treatment. Although some series have reported that the rate of hearing loss increases after multiple daily injections,[87] others have found no correlation between the number of injections and hearing loss.[70,72,95] There may be a genetic disposition to hearing loss after aminoglycoside treatment because of a maternally inherited 1555 A-to-G nucleotide substitution in the 12s mitochondrial ribosomal RNA.[99] Several patients who experienced hearing loss secondary to intratympanic gentamicin have been tested for this substitution, and, to date, not one has been positive for this substitution.[60,93,94,100]

One issue that has been raised in assessing hearing loss across studies is the extent of the hearing loss. Most studies document hearing loss as being greater than 10-dB pure-tone average loss or greater than 15% decrease in speech discrimination scores (1995 AAO-HNS guidelines[44]). This may be a poor reporting format, however, because it does not indicate whether hearing loss is serviceable or profound. As noted previously, Altlas and Parnes[69] argued that "shotgun" protocols result in substantial rates of hearing loss greater than 30 dB (range 10% to 24%[84,86,97,101]), whereas titration methods report low rates of substantial hearing loss (range 0% to 3.5%[69,96,98,102]). Although scientifically valid comparisons of these studies are impossible because of substantial difference in protocols, this trend is a troubling feature of "shotgun" protocols.

Reporting of hearing loss n gentamicin trials does not distinguish whether the deficit is due to drug-induced toxicity or the natural consequence of Meniere's disease. The long-term hearing outcome for untreated Meniere's disease has been reported to be approximately 30% with medical therapy.[68] This figure is close to the hearing loss rates reported by most intratympanic gentamicin trials. The implication is that any intratympanic gentamicin trial that reports rates significantly better than 30% hearing loss rate of untreated patients may represent an actual prevention of hearing loss.

Determination of when hearing loss occurs in the course of therapy may be just as important as if hearing loss occurs. Several studies reported that if severe hearing loss occurs, it is noticed within 24 hours of gentamicin administration.[96] Kaplan and associates[60] reported updated data from patients who underwent the classic "shotgun" protocol, including statistics on the hearing loss rates at 1 month and 2 years. Of the 22 patients with worse hearing at 2 years, 80% realized this loss in the first month after treatment. Similarly, 91% of patients whose hearing was unchanged at the 1-month checkup had unchanged hearing at the 2-year checkup. Of the patients who experienced early hearing loss, 14 of 17 had profound hearing loss (defined as >50 dB or <50% word discrimination score), whereas of the patients who experienced late hearing loss, 4 of 5 had nonprofound hearing loss. These findings imply that the 1995 AAO-HNS guidelines[44] might be improved if they asked clinicians to report hearing results immediately after treatment and at the 2-year interval. This information also supports efforts to use otoprotective agents to salvage hearing after toxic gentamicin treatment. Finally, although no formal data have been published to date, Jackson and Silverstein[19] described initial efforts to use steroids as a salvage treatment for hearing loss secondary to ototoxic side effects of gentamicin treatment in patients with Meniere's disease.

Acute vestibular deafferentation syndrome should be an anticipated outcome of treatment, and in this sense it is not strictly a complication. Acute vestibular deafferentation syndrome, also known as acute chemical labyrinthine upset, is the consequence of unilaterally insulting the vestibular apparatus.[103] This phenomenon usually occurs 3 to 5 days after the injection. Symptoms include vertigo, nausea, oscillopsia, and dysequilibrium. Patients can readily distinguish these symptoms from symptoms typically related to Meniere's disease. These symptoms become progressively worse until they peak 1 week after onset. During this peak, patients usually require 2 to 3 days of bed rest. Gradual resolution is achieved in 2 to 4 weeks in most patients.[88,97] Because acute vestibular deafferentation syndrome is an expected outcome of therapy, some authors recommend that a vestibular rehabilitation team be available to work with severely affected patients.[104]

Other vestibular-related side effects include constant unsteadiness and dizziness, insecure gait in dark rooms, instability of the field of vision when turning the head, and very short episodes of losing control over balance or gait (or so-called Tumarkin attacks, which characterize the symptoms of some patients with Meniere's disease). Tumarkin attacks may not depend on the vestibular function because these attacks have been reported in patients with no caloric response after treatment.[89] Visual vestibular mismatch is currently being investigated as a possible side effect of gentamicin therapy. Visual vestibular mismatch is a syndrome in which visual and vestibular information is poorly coordinated in the brain, resulting in complaints of malaise and "dizziness." Classic complaints include feeling uneasy, nauseous, or unsteady in supermarket aisles or in shopping malls, new-onset motion sickness, a dislike of fluorescent lights, or an aversion to elevator and escalator rides. This syndrome is believed to result from an overreliance on visual signals. Longridge and colleagues[105] found that 17 of 28 patients with Meniere's disease who had previous gentamicin therapy had visual vestibular mismatch. Currently, visual vestibular mismatch is a clinical diagnosis, does not correlate with posturography or caloric tests, and is a relatively new diagnostic category; conclusions about visual vestibular mismatch and gentamicin therapy should be interpreted with caution.

Indications and Contraindications

Intratympanic gentamicin treatment is indicated in patients with Meniere's disease who have had conservative therapy fail and have recurrent vertigo. Conservative therapy consists of a diuretic and diet restrictions (salt, caffeine), and is effective in 70% of cases. Some patients try additional medical treatments, including vasodilators, vestibular suppressants, tranquilizers, calcium antagonists, betahistine, antidepressants, histamine, and steroids.[72] Most practitioners consider intratympanic gentamicin therapy only after conservative therapy has failed after being tried for at least 1 year. At this junction, intratympanic steroids, endolymphatic sac surgery, and intratympanic gentamicin therapy are considered.

Sennaroglu and coworkers[42] argued that it is reasonable to try to use intratympanic steroids before using intratympanic gentamicin. In a prospective study that compared intratympanic dexamethasone (n = 24) and gentamicin (n = 16), they found that vertigo control rates were 72% and 75%. Intratympanic gentamicin was considerably more cochleotoxic than intratympanic steroids, however. Vestibular nerve section and labyrinthectomy are reserved for only the most severe and refractory cases with and without residual hearing.

Some practitioners recommend that elderly patients should be treated with caution because central compensation for peripheral vestibular loss is less effective in elderly patients.[104] Bilateral Meniere's disease (incidence of 15% to 30%) is considered by some practitioners to be a contraindication for unilateral intratympanic gentamicin treatment because if hearing loss results from treatment the remaining ear may be vulnerable to hearing loss as a natural course of the disease.[106] If bilateral disease is treated, some authors advocate that an intramuscular streptomycin protocol, rather than an intratympanic protocol, be used.[107] Patients with no serviceable hearing in the problematic ear are generally considered candidates for labyrinthectomy, but some authors recommend that the low-morbidity, low-cost intratympanic gentamicin protocol should be attempted in these patients before surgery is considered.[108]

There is some debate as to whether otologic surgery is a contraindication to intratympanic gentamicin treatment. Minor[68] reported that of patients with prior otologic surgery, only one of six achieved vertigo control. Eklund and colleagues[95] also noted that patients with prior endolymphatic sac surgery had poorer hearing outcomes. Other authors have found that prior otologic surgery does not affect either vertigo or hearing outcomes.[24] The importance of this debate is that several practitioners advocate endolymphatic shunt procedures before resorting to intratympanic gentamicin when treating intractable vertigo in patients with Meniere's disease.[68]

Summary

Gentamicin has complex pharmacokinetics, depending on the dose and route of delivery. Its toxicity is related to peak dosage, dosage interval, and route of delivery. For some practitioners, intratympanic gentamicin therapy, using low doses with long intertherapy intervals, has become the treatment of choice for medically recalcitrant Meniere's disease. The primary complication of intratympanic gentamicin is permanent hearing loss.

Otoprotective Agents

Several otologic conditions may benefit from protective or preventive treatment, including noise-induced hearing loss, exposure to ototoxic medications, and salvage of spiral ganglion neurons (SGNs) for the purposes of maximizing the effectiveness of cochlear prostheses. Otoprotective agents can be categorized as either primary or secondary interventions to the overall pathophysiologic process. Primary interventions act directly at the site of insult, whereas secondary interventions act on the intracellular sequelae of primary insults (i.e., apoptosis). Examples of primary interventions include MK801, an *N*-methyl-D-aspartate receptor antagonist, which has shown protection against acoustic trauma and aminoglycoside toxicity,[109,110] and methionine for gentamicin and cisplatin toxicity.[111,112] Secondary interventions include steroids,[28] apoptosis inhibitors,[95] and neurotrophins.[113]

There is a sort of "intermediate intervention" that is possible with noise-induced hearing loss and the use of antioxidants. The contribution of free radical damage in noise-induced hearing loss results from metabolic and oxidative stress, ionic flux and dysregulation of calcium homeostasis, and mitochondrial injury. A more recent example of antioxidant treatment for noise-induced hearing loss is the use of *N*-acetyl cysteine.[114] We focus here mainly on neurotrophins as otoprotective agents because these are most cogent to the emerging pharmacology of the cochlea and labyrinth.

Apoptosis has been shown to be the major pathway of cell death in various conditions, including aminoglycoside toxicity,[53] cisplatin toxicity,[115] hypoxia,[116] acoustic trauma,[77] neurotrophin withdrawal,[113,115] and presbycusis.[117] Neurotrophic support may be crucial in preventing apoptosis. Malgrange and associates[113] prevented apoptosis in explanted outer hair cells by administering various neurotrophins. In the same experiment, these investigators prevented apoptosis by administering protein synthesis inhibitors. These observations imply that neurotrophic support (among other things) provides tonic suppression of proteins in the apoptotic cascade. Rong and colleagues[118] provided proof of this notion by showing that nerve growth factor (NGF) promotes cell survival by regulating proteins that are essential to the apoptotic cascade.

Free radicals also play an important role in hearing loss. They are primary inducers of apoptosis (as in free radical–generating aminoglycoside-iron compounds) and secondary consequences of cochlear insult (as in the oxidative stress of excitotoxicity). The generation of free radicals may be a required step in apoptosis. There is a strong connection between free radicals and neurotrophins. Dugan and coworkers[119] showed that removal of NGF from cultured auditory neurons caused a rapid increase in intracellular free radical generation and subsequent apoptosis. Reapplying NGF rapidly diminished the concentration of these free radicals and decreased apoptotic cell death. Shulz and coworkers[4] showed that inhibition of caspases (proteases associated with apoptosis) not only blocked apoptosis, but also blocked the formation of free radicals, implying that the formation of free radicals is downstream from caspases in the apoptotic cascade. Likewise, exogenous brain-derived neurotrophic factor (BDNF) not only protects cisplatin-exposed neuronal cultures from apoptosis, but also reduces the free radical species in the culture.[120] These results have led researchers to believe that free radicals are effector molecules in the apoptotic cascade, and that they can be regulated not only by antioxidants, but also by neurotrophins.

Neurotrophins modulate calcium homeostasis,[94] regulate apoptotic proteins,[118] and alter expression of endogenous free radical scavengers,[4,119,120] and any of these functions may account for their otoprotective effects. Several specific neurotrophins have been used for in vivo models of noise-induced hearing loss with variable success. Glial cell line–derived neurotrophic factor (GDNF) greatly enhances the survival of guinea pig cochlear neurons (but not hair cells) if administered 4 days after noise-induced trauma.[121] Keithley and associates[122] showed that hair cells are preserved if GDNF is administered before or immediately after toxic noise exposure. Damage was attenuated if GDNF was applied after 2 hours, but not after 4 hours. The method of delivery in this experiment was topically to the RWM.

Shoji and coworkers[123] found that GDNF provides bilateral protection even when administered in only one ear. Because their experiment used long-term application of GDNF, it may have diffused through the cerebrospinal fluid. Another possibility is that GDNF influences higher cortical centers in the auditory pathway, which has a rich efferent projection and is highly bilateral. Yamasoba and colleagues[124] combined GDNF with antioxidants to determine whether synergistic protection could be achieved. They found that additional functional, but not morphologic, protection was achieved, implying that the interventions in antioxidant and neurotrophin therapy are additive, not synergistic. Neurotrophin-3 (NT-3) showed equal or greater physiologic and histologic protection from acoustic trauma relative to GDNF (with the same animal model).[125] BDNF and fibroblastic growth factor show no protective effect against toxic noise.[125]

Many experimental otoprotective treatments have been shown to be effective only if administered prophylactically or immediately after injury. Many of these injuries clinically manifest long after the initial insult, precluding any hope of salvaging hair cells. There is a much larger window of opportunity to salvage the auditory neurons after injury, however. Although there is rapid degeneration of the peripheral processes of the auditory nerve after inner hair cell loss (within hours or days), the degeneration of SGN soma and central auditory projections takes much longer (weeks to years).[126] There is intense interest in the use of neurotrophic agents to enhance SGN survival, mostly in anticipation of future cochlear implantation. This is because the hearing benefits of cochlear implants are directly related to the number of surviving auditory neurons[127] and their proximity to stimulating electrodes.[126,128]

Neurotrophins are essential not only for the normal development of the central and peripheral nervous systems, but also for their maintenance and normal function.[126] The destruction of cochlear hair cells and supporting cells because of exogenous insults (e.g., ototoxicity, acoustic trauma) results in the de facto withdrawal of trophic support. The ensuing degeneration of SGNs after cochlear insult is most likely a result of the loss of cochlear trophic support, rather than from direct toxic insult.[126] Withdrawal of neurotrophins in vitro causes apoptosis in SGNs.[116] The application of antisense oligonucleotides to inhibit expression of BDNF and NT-3 induces programmed cell death in explanted auditory neurons.[115] Apoptosis inhibitors have been shown to block neurotrophin withdrawal–induced cell death.[116]

Numerous neurotrophins have been shown to be effective in preventing SGN demise after experimental destruction by various insults. Exogenously applied NT-3,[129,130] BDNF,[130-132] BDNF in combination with a ciliary neurotrophic factor analogue,[133] NGF,[134] and 4-methylcatechol (an inducer of NGF synthesis)[135] enhance SGN survival after aminoglycoside insult. BDNF and GDNF enhance SGN survival after acoustic trauma[121]; BDNF[136] and GDNF[137] enhance SGN survival after cisplatin exposure. The enhancement of SGN survival with electric stimulation may also involve neurotrophins because depolarization induces an autocrine neurotrophin loop.[138] A strategy to use neurotrophins to enhance SGN survival before implantation and electric stimulation to promote autocrine neurotrophin release after implantation may be effective in enhancing hearing outcomes in patients receiving cochlear implants.

Aside from neuronal salvage, numerous studies have documented the ability of neurotrophins to stimulate innate regenerative and repair capabilities in auditory cells. Enfors and colleagues[129] showed that NT-3 induced neurofilament growth after aminoglycoside ototoxicity, as evidenced by the appearance of Gap 43, a growth cone marker. Lefebvre and colleagues[139] showed that NGF is a potent stimulator of repair and reinnervation in auditory neurons. Ylikoski and coworkers[121] showed that GDNF has potent trophic effects on the cochlear-neuron perikarya. Fibroblastic growth factor alone[140] or in combination with BDNF[141] produces a dose-dependent increase in the number and length of SGNs. These and other similar findings are significant because closer contact between stimulating electrodes on cochlear implants and auditory neurons leads to reduced stimulation thresholds, increased dynamic range of responsiveness, and potentially enhanced specificity of excitation.[126,128] It is possible that these growth-stimulating properties of neurotrophins could be exploited to engineer intimate contact with implanted electrodes, such that increasingly focused tonotopic stimulation could be matched to advanced signal-processing strategies.[126]

Preliminary studies on the interactions between auditory neurons and alloplastic cochlear implant materials have been performed, paving the way for the development of implant-tissue interfaces for the next generation of cochlear prostheses.[142] Neurotrophins are expected to play a role in this effort to unite biologic and synthetic materials, an effort that may lead to the development of a fully functional artificial cochlea. Neurotrophins have also been tested as a secondary intervention after aminoglycoside toxicity. Ruan and colleagues[143] used long-term infusion of NT-3 and BDNF in the setting of aminoglycoside challenge, and found that NT-3, and to a much lesser extent BDNF, protected hair cells from aminoglycoside toxicity. Although the mechanism of action is unclear, the authors speculate that just as SGNs rely on trophic support from hair cells, these hair cells may have trophic dependence on SGNs. This notion is supported by an increasing body of evidence showing that there is anterograde transport, transcytosis, and recycling of neurotrophic factors in neural networks.[144] Hair cell survival is partly determined by neurotrophin support. Malgrange and colleagues[113] tested a panel of 13 different growth factors and found that acidic fibroblastic growth factor, insulin-like growth factor-1, epidermal growth factor, transforming growth factor-β1, and GDNF were able to sustain adult explanted outer hair cells (which otherwise experience rapid demise in in vitro culture media).

Table 155-1
Features of Various Gene Therapy Vectors

Vector	Genome	Insert Size	Site	Efficiency	Cell Division	Expression	Advantages	Disadvantages
AAV	ssDNA	4.5 kB	Genome	Variable	Not required	Permanent	No human disease	Difficult to produce
Retrovirus	RNA	6-7 kB	Genome	Low	Required	Permanent	Suited for neoplastic cells	Insertional mutagenesis
Adenovirus	dsDNA	7.5 kB	Episome	Moderate	Not required	Transient	Ease of production	Inflammatory response
Herpesvirus	dsDNA	10-100 kB	Episome	Moderate	Not required	Transient	Neural tropism	Human disease
Plasmid	RNA/DNA	Unlimited	Episome	Very low	Not required	Transient	Safe, easy production	Low transfection
Liposome	RNA/DNA	Unlimited	Episome	Very low	Not required	Transient	Safe, easy production	Low transfection

Summary

One of the goals of rational drug discovery is to dissect the specific molecular mechanisms in a given pathophysiologic process, and determine where they are redundant and where they are independent. If nonredundant mechanisms can be identified, synergistic strategies to treat the pathologic process can be devised. In the context of hearing loss, multiple interventions can be constructed that are nonredundant and synergistic, as in the combination of an antioxidant, a neurotrophin, and an apoptosis inhibitor. The new understanding of the molecular mechanisms of hearing loss is creating quantum advances in otopharmacology by supplying researchers with a multitude of potential targets for therapeutic intervention and prosthetic augmentation.

Gene Therapy

Although gene therapy of the inner ear is a technology still in its infancy, advances in pharmacologic and gene therapy offer prospects to manage degenerative disorders of the labyrinth. Much of the experimental data so far concern the development of suitable vectors for gene transfer and methods of delivering these vectors to their target. Some teams have reported successful gene transfer of therapeutic genes, however. These advances may be able to stimulate hair cell regeneration and, ultimately, restoration of the transduction potential within the organ of Corti.

Otologic science was revolutionized by the observation that avian hair cells regenerate after insult.[145,146] Since then, barriers to inducing regeneration within the mammalian cochlea have been elucidated, including strategies that can address mature and damaged inner ear.[147] Beyond hair cell regeneration, there is the related problem of inducing synaptogenesis and nerve regrowth to these newly created hair cells.[148] These and a host of other concerns are currently being investigated. The ultimate vision is to orchestrate through pharmacology and gene therapy a recapitulation of the embryonic events that lead to a functioning auditory system. Although this section deals mainly with gene therapy, there are exciting new stem cell therapies that address similar topics on the horizon as well.[149]

Vectors

There is no single ideal vector for gene transfer because each vector has characteristics that make it more or less suitable to each application (Table 155-1). The length of the gene to be transferred, the specific inner ear tissue that is targeted, the desired method of delivery, and the duration of transgene expression are all factors that determine the most suitable vectors. Various viral and nonviral vectors are available to the gene therapist. The variability in the transgene expression pattern with different gene transfer vectors is likely a consequence of numerous factors, including the size of the viral particle, presence or absence of viral receptors, and mode of delivery. Inspection of Table 155-1 allows for some generalization about the ability of various viral vectors in transfecting cochlear tissues. The spiral ganglion cells, spiral ligament, and Reissner's membrane were transfected by every virus tested. Only adenovirus showed transgene expression within the stria vascularis. Immune response was present in the cochlea after transfection with adenovirus, herpes simplex virus, and vaccinia virus.

Delivery

Local gene therapy to the inner ear is feasible because of its relatively closed anatomy. Developing a delivery method for genetic vectors to the inner ear without causing local destruction is a significant obstacle. Several delivery methods have been used, including mini–osmotic pump infusion (either through cochleostomy or through the RWM), microinjection into the RWM, injection into the endolymphatic sac, and diffusion across the RWM after local Gelfoam placement. Cochleostomy has been shown to cause histopathologic alterations (including localized surgical trauma and inflammation), and may lead to hearing loss.[150]

Introduction of viral vector by means of infusion with a mini–osmotic pump was characterized by evidence of trauma at the basal turn adjacent to the cochleostomy associated with an inflammatory response and connective tissue deposition. Carvalho and Lalwani[150] showed preservation of preoperative auditory brainstem response thresholds in the lower frequencies (1 to 2 kHz), mild postoperative elevation of thresholds (<10 dB) in the midfrequencies (4 to 8 kHz), and marked increase (>30 dB) in auditory brainstem response thresholds at higher frequencies (>16 kHz) after mini–osmotic pump infusion by way of a cochleostomy.

Several studies have documented that direct microinjection through the RWM can be accomplished without causing permanent hearing loss or tissue destruction seen with cochleostomy.[56,124] Histologically, cochleae microinjected through the RWM showed intact cochlear cytoarchitecture and an absence of inflammatory response 2 weeks after microinjection through the RWM. Microinjection through the RWM did not cause permanent hearing dysfunction.[151]

The potential for surgical trauma, inflammation, and hearing loss associated with these infusion or microinjection techniques led to the investigation of a less invasive delivery method. Diffusion across the RWM has been shown to be an effective, atraumatic, but vector-dependent method of delivery for gene transfer vectors. Jero and coworkers[152] investigated the potential to deliver various vectors across an intact RWM by loading vectors onto a Gelfoam patch that was placed in the round window niche. Adenovirus and liposome vectors, but not the AAV vector, effectively infected inner ear tissues, as evidenced by detection of reporter genes. Lipocomplexed plasmid vectors have also been shown to cross the RWM effectively.[153]

Preclinical Applications

Most of the preclinical applications for gene therapy in the inner ear have concerned neurotrophin therapy. This is because for some applications of exogenous neurotrophins (e.g., to maintain SGN survival or to induce neurite outgrowth), the neurotrophins must be applied long-term. In this sense, gene therapy is being used as a long-term drug delivery strategy, rather than to replace defective or missing genes.

Staecker and colleagues[130] used a herpes simplex virus-1 vector to deliver BDNF to the inner ear. After neomycin injection, the gene therapy group showed a 94.7% salvage rate for SGNs, in contrast to a 64.3% loss of SGNs in control animals. Although BDNF staining was ubiquitous in inner ear tissues, this was not the case for the reporter gene, β-galactosidase. Although only 50% of cells were transfected (as determined by the number of β-galactosidase cells), this was enough to cause cochlea-wide BDNF distribution and to ensure 95% SGN survival. The authors speculate that SGNs must require only a few BDNF-producing cells to ensure the survival of the entire ganglion.

Lalwani and colleagues[154] used in vitro and in vivo models to test effectiveness of an AAV vector for BDNF transfer. They found a significant survival effect from controls after aminoglycoside challenge in cochlear explants. Although direct measurements of BDNF could not be recorded, the vector's ability to salvage SGNs was tested against a gradient of known BDNF concentrations. They found that the vector system was able to achieve the same protective effects as 0.1 ng/mL of BDNF. This dose is subtherapeutic because the most efficient dose was determined to be 50 ng/mL, a concentration of BDNF that results in almost total SGN protection. In the in vivo experiment, animals infused with AAV-BDNF with a mini-osmotic pump displayed enhanced SGN survival. The protection from AAV-BDNF therapy was region specific; there was protection at the basal turn of the cochlea, but not the middle or apical turn. The authors propose that this regional selectivity is a pharmacokinetic phenomenon.

NT-3 gene transfer for protection against cisplatin-induced ototoxicity has been achieved by the use of a herpes simplex virus-1 amplicon–mediated delivery system.[155,156] Chen and associates[156] established efficacy of the vector in an in vitro study, in which amplicon-mediated transfer of NT-3 (shown by production of NT-3 mRNA proteins and by reporter gene expression) conferred increased survival to cochlear explants after cisplatin exposure. Bowers and colleagues[155] confirmed these effects in an in vivo model, in which amplicon-mediated transfer of NT-3 to SGNs suppressed cisplatin-induced apoptosis and necrosis. The authors suggest that these findings not only may be useful to prevent cisplatin-related injury, but also may provide preventive treatment for hearing degeneration because of normal aging.

Several studies have established the efficacy of an Ad vector carrying the GDNF gene (Ad.GDNF) to protect against various ototoxic insults. When administered before aminoglycoside challenge, Ad.-GDNF significantly protects cochlear[157] and vestibular[158] hair cells from cell death. Pretreatment with Ad.GDNF also provides significant protection against noise-induced trauma.[50] Finally, Ad.GDNF enhances SGN survival when administered 4 to 7 days after ototoxic deafening with aminoglycosides.[159]

Some studies have used gene therapy to induce the expression of target proteins other than neurotrophins. Several studies have transduced genes that express proteins that inhibit the apoptosis cascade, and protect against ototoxic insult. Liu and associates[160] used an AAV vector to induce Bcl-x(L), an apoptosis inhibitor to mitigate aminoglycoside toxicity. Chan and colleagues[161] successfully induced the expression of the X-linked apoptosis inhibitor using an AAV virus, and this proved to be protective against cisplatin toxicity. In another line of research, attempts are being made to overexpress *Math1* through gene transfer. The significance of *Math1* gene is that it is intimately associated with cochlear and vestibular stem cells, and the overexpression of the *Math1* protein stimulates hair cell regeneration. Izumikawa and colleagues[162] used an adenovirus vector to induce overexpression of *Math1* after aminoglycoside deafening, and showed cellular and functional repair in the organ of Corti. Similarly, Staecker and coworkers[163] used an adenovirus vector to induce expression of *Math1* after vestibulotoxic aminoglycoside exposure, and successfully induced the regeneration of vestibular hair cells. These and other studies are adding to the list of potential targets for gene therapy for the inner ear.

Safety Concerns

Early investigations in the development of gene transfer in the cochlea identified potential safety concerns. Through use of AAV as the gene therapy vector, Lalwani and associates[164] observed transgene expression within the contralateral cochlea of the AAV-perfused animal, albeit much weaker than within the directly perfused cochlea. Subsequently, Stover and colleagues[165] showed transgene expression in the contralateral cochlea using adenovirus. This finding of transgene expression in the contralateral cochlea raises concern about dissemination of the virus from the target tissue. The appearance of the virus, distant from the site of infection, may be due to its hematogenous dissemination to near and distant tissues; however, this is unlikely.[165,166] Other possible explanations include migration of AAV by way of the bone marrow space of the temporal bone[166] or the cerebrospinal fluid space to the contralateral ear.[165,166] The perilymphatic space into which the virus is perfused is directly connected to the cerebrospinal fluid by way of the cochlear aqueduct; transgene expression within the contralateral cochlear aqueduct has been shown after introduction of the viral vector in the ipsilateral cochlea. Collectively, these results suggest potential routes for AAV dissemination from the infused cochlea through the cochlear aqueduct, or by extension through the temporal bone marrow spaces. Subsequent investigations have shown that dissemination outside the target cochlea can largely be eliminated by the use of microinjection or RWM application of vector, and avoidance of the infusion technique.[152,167,168]

Summary

A crucial step forward toward the eventual application of gene therapy for hearing disorders has been accomplished: viral and nonviral vectors have been shown to introduce and express exogenous genes capably into the peripheral auditory system. Future refinements will include the development of newer hybrid vectors that assimilate the infectivity and stability of the viral vectors and the safety of liposomes. The hybrid vectors will largely replace the current generation of vectors. The preferred mode of introduction of gene therapy vectors will be one that minimizes tissue damage and hearing loss, such as microinjection or application of the vector at the RWM. Safety concerns, especially regional and distant dissemination of the therapeutic agent, will need to be monitored and minimized.

SUGGESTED READINGS

Chandrasekhar SS. Intratympanic dexamethasone for sudden sensorineural hearing loss: clinical and laboratory evaluation. *Otol Neurotol.* 2001;22:18.

Chandrasekhar SS, Rubinstein RY, Kwartler JA, et al. Dexamethasone pharmacokinetics in the inner ear: comparison of route of administration and use of facilitating agents. *Otolaryngol Head Neck Surg.* 2000;122:521.

Chen JM, Kakigi A, Harakawa H, et al. Middle ear instillation of gentamicin and streptomycin in chinchillas: morphological appraisal of selective ototoxicity. *J Otolaryngol.* 1999;28:121.

Chia SH, Gamst AC, Anderson JP, et al. Intratympanic gentamicin therapy for Ménière's disease: a meta-analysis. *Otol Neurotol.* 2004;25:544-552.

Fitzgerald DC, McGuire JF. Intratympanic steroids for idiopathic sudden sensorineural hearing loss. *Ann Otol Rhinol Laryngol.* 2007;116:253-256.

Garduño-Anaya MA, Couthino De Toledo H, Hinojosa-González R, et al. Dexamethasone inner ear perfusion by intratympanic injection in unilateral Ménière's disease: a two-year prospective, placebo-controlled, double-blind, randomized trial. *Otolaryngol Head Neck Surg.* 2005;133:285-294.

Goycoolea MV, Lundman L. Round window membrane: structure function and permeability: a review. *Microsc Res Tech.* 1997;36:201.

Hoffer ME, Allen K, Kopke RD, et al. Transtympanic versus sustained-release administration of gentamicin: kinetics, morphology, and function. *Laryngoscope.* 2001;111:1343.

Hoffer ME, Kopke RD, Weisskopf P, et al. Microdose gentamicin administration via the round window microcatheter. *Ann N Y Acad Sci.* 2001;942:46-51.

Izumikawa M, Minoda R, Kawamoto K, et al. Auditory hair cell replacement and hearing improvement by Atoh1 gene therapy in deaf mammals. *Nat Med.* 2005;11:271-276.

Kopke RD, Hoffer ME, Wester D, et al. Targeted topical steroid therapy in sudden sensorineural hearing loss. *Otol Neurotol.* 2001;22:475.

Lalwani AK, Jero J, Mhatre AN. Current issues in cochlear gene transfer. *Audiol Neurotol.* 2002;7:146.

Malgrange B, Rigo JM, Coucke P, et al. Identification of factors that maintain mammalian outer hair cells in adult organ of Corti explants. *Hear Res.* 2002;170:48.

Montandon P, Guillemin P, Hausler R. Prevention of vertigo in Ménière's syndrome by means of transtympanic ventilation tubes. *Otorhinolaryngology.* 1988;50:377.

Parnes LS, Sun AH, Freeman DJ. Corticosteroid pharmacokinetics in the inner ear fluids: an animal study followed by clinical application. *Laryngoscope.* 1999;109(Suppl 9):1.

Plontke SKR, Wood AW, Salt AN. Analysis of gentamicin kinetics in fluids of the inner ear with round window administration. *Otol Neurotol.* 2002;23:967.

Salt AN, Ma Y. Quantification of solute entry into cochlear perilymph through the round window membrane. *Hear Res.* 2001;154:88.

Schuknect H. Ablation therapy in Ménière's disease. *Acta Otolaryngol (Stockh).* 1957;132(Suppl):1.

Sennaroglu L, Sennaroglu G, Gursel B, et al. Intratympanic dexamethasone, intratympanic gentamicin, and endolymphatic sac surgery for intractable vertigo in Ménière's disease. *Otolaryngol Head Neck Surg.* 2001;125:537.

Shinohara T, Bredberg G, Ulfendahl M, et al. Neurotrophic factor intervention restores auditory function in deafened animals. *Proc Natl Acad Sci U S A.* 2002;99:1657.

Shirwany NA, Seidman MD, Tang W. Effects of transtympanic injection of steroids on cochlear blood flow, auditory sensitivity, and histology in the guinea pig. *Am J Otol.* 1998;19:230.

Silverstein H, Isaacson JE, Olds MJ, et al. Dexamethasone inner ear injection for the treatment of Ménière's disease: a prospective, randomized, double blind crossover trial. *Am J Otol.* 1998;19:196.

Silverstein H, Rowan PT, Olds MJ, et al. Inner ear perfusion and the role of round window patency. *Am J Otol.* 1997;18:586.

Staecker H, Praetorius M, Baker K, et al. Vestibular hair cell regeneration and restoration of balance function induced by math1 gene transfer. *Otol Neurotol.* 2007;28:223-231.

Wilson WR, Byl FM, Laird N. The efficacy of steroids in the treatment of idiopathic sudden hearing loss: a double blind clinical study. *Arch Otolaryngol Head Neck Surg.* 1980;106:772.

For complete list of references log onto www.expertconsult.com.

CHAPTER ONE HUNDRED AND FIFTY-SIX

Otologic Symptoms and Syndromes

Carol A. Bauer

Herman A. Jenkins

Key Points

- Otalgia in the absence of detectable ear pathology can arise from a wide range of sources and requires a complete head and neck examination for accurate diagnosis.
- Chronic painful bloody otorrhea should prompt an evaluation for malignant otitis externa or neoplasia of the external auditory canal.
- The most informative features in evaluating hearing loss are the time course of the loss, associated symptoms, and age of the patient.
- The most common bacterial pathogens causing otitis externa are *Pseudomonas aeruginosa* and *Staphylococcus aureus*.
- Radiographic imaging of the temporal bone with high-resolution CT is essential in the evaluation of clear watery otorrhea.
- A complete history with a careful description of the symptoms is needed to discriminate between central and peripheral causes of vertigo.

Various symptoms can be either suggestive or diagnostic of ear disease. Accurate clinical assessment is facilitated by understanding the significance of symptom combinations and the relative frequency of specific otologic diseases in different patient populations. This chapter reviews the common symptoms associated with otologic diseases and the diagnoses to be considered when evaluating these symptoms. Common symptoms that indicate an otologic problem are otorrhea, otalgia, aural fullness, hearing loss, vertigo, and tinnitus. The symptoms of hearing loss, vertigo, and tinnitus are discussed in other chapters, and are addressed only briefly here.

Otorrhea

In adults and children, otorrhea can arise from numerous sources (external ear canal, middle ear, mastoid) and may have a variety of etiologies (Box 156-1). Diagnostic considerations and subsequent treatment plans are directed by the source of the otorrhea; the age of the patient; the type of otorrhea (clear, mucoid, purulent, or bloody); the nature of the drainage (acute, chronic, or pulsatile); and the presence of other symptoms, such as otalgia, neurologic deficits, or associated systemic disease or symptoms. Evaluation requires meticulous suctioning of secretions under a microscope to identify the source of the drainage, and to differentiate between a primary infection or purulent drainage occurring secondary to an underlying inflammatory process.

Common causes of otorrhea differ between adults and children. In children, otorrhea is caused most commonly by either acute otitis media with tympanic membrane rupture or chronic otitis media in the presence of a tympanic membrane perforation. In adults, otorrhea results most commonly from either external otitis or chronic otitis media with a perforation. The initial history and physical examination should be directed toward establishing the time course of the symptom and the source of the otorrhea (ear canal, middle ear, mastoid).

The diagnosis of external otitis as the source of purulent otorrhea is suggested by a history of ear trauma or swimming-related water contamination of the canal. Trauma resulting in external otitis may occur from the use of cotton-tip swabs, irrigators for cerumen removal, in-the-canal hearing aids, or digital ear thermometers. A history of otalgia and drainage after swimming easily leads to a diagnosis of external otitis. Although typically painful, there are usually no additional systemic symptoms associated with this localized infection. The typical findings on physical examination include an exquisitely tender ear canal that is partially to completely obstructed by edematous skin, and associated with preauricular tenderness.

Purulent otorrhea may develop secondarily in patients with chronic dermatitis or eczema of the ear canal, without any prior history of trauma or water contamination. Bacterial or fungal infections may complicate this chronic skin condition. Symptoms of chronic dermatitis of the ear canal include complaints of dry, itchy ears. Secondary infection of chronic dermatitis of the ear canal is usually painless. Important points include a history of recent use of topical antibiotic ointments or solutions that may cause an localized allergic skin reaction with canal pruritus, edema, and purulent drainage. Physical examination should document the presence of fungal hyphae in the canal, keratin debris from chronic dermatitis, or, uncommonly, a canal cholesteatoma or keratoma. After suctioning all purulent material from the canal, the tympanic membrane must be examined for evidence of a retained foreign body, such as a pressure equalizing tube with localized granulation tissue, as the source of the otorrhea.

The most common bacterial pathogens causing external otitis are *Pseudomonas aeruginosa* and *Staphylococcus aureus*. Less commonly, other aerobic, facultative, and anaerobic organisms have been cultured from infected ears. Rarely, external otitis results from a local or regional infection that involves the ear secondarily. *Actinomyces israelii* is an

Box 156-1

Sources of Otorrhea

External Canal

Otitis externa (fungal, bacterial, viral)
Necrotizing otitis externa
Acute dermatitis
Keratosis obturans
Canal cholesteatoma
Neoplasm
Regional infection (parotid)

Tympanic Membrane

Granulation tissue
Granular myringitis
Bullous myringitis
Retraction pocket with cholesteatoma

Middle Ear

Acute otitis media with perforation
Chronic otitis media with perforation
Neoplasm

Mastoid

Mastoiditis, acute or chronic, with perforation
Granulomatous disease
Cholesteatoma
Neoplasm

Cerebrospinal Fluid

Temporal bone fracture
Tegmen defect
Cochlea deformity
Hyrtl's fissure

anaerobic gram-positive bacterium that can cause external otitis from a primary dental or parotid infection. This infection may manifest as refractory otitis externa with granulation tissue in the ear canal and thick yellow otorrhea. Recognition of this entity is important because treatment involves surgical débridement and prolonged antibiotic therapy.[1]

Malignant or necrotizing external otitis is a locally aggressive, potentially progressive form of otitis externa. Inflammation and necrosis can extend beyond the ear canal skin to involve underlying cartilage and bone. Extensive disease involves local and regional osteomyelitis of the temporal bone, resulting in severe, deep ear pain. Malignant otitis externa occurs most commonly in adults. The diagnosis should be considered, however, in children with poor general health or concurrent systemic disease with acute onset of painful otorrhea. Fifteen cases of malignant external otitis occurring in infants and children 2 months to 15 years old have been reported in the literature.[2,3] Risk factors in these patients included poor general health, immunosuppression, and diabetes mellitus. Common presenting findings on physical examination include granulation tissue within the external auditory canal, preauricular and auricular edema and erythema, tympanic membrane necrosis, and facial nerve paralysis. *P. aeruginosa* is the most common causative organism in children and adults with malignant external otitis.

Fungal infections of the ear (otomycoses) are typically limited to the external ear canal as a superficial infection. Rarely, these infections are invasive and involve the temporal bone. Common fungal species infecting the external ear canal are *Aspergillus niger* and *Candida albicans*. The former is easily recognized as pigmented fungal tufts atop a tangle of hyphal threads resembling a ball of cotton. *Candida* spp. also may colonize the ear canal, especially in patients previously treated with prolonged courses of antibiotic eardrops. A canal infected with *Candida* appears wet and macerated, filled with soft, curdlike debris. If the fungal infection has an associated bacterial component, the fungal elements may not be immediately evident. Rarely, the external ear canal and mastoid are primarily involved with coccidioidomycosis, which may resemble eczema or an allergic dermatitis.[4]

Secondary mycosis of the temporal bone is quite rare and may arise from a primary focus of infection involving the meninges or the paranasal sinuses. Causative agents include *Cryptococcus, Candida, Blastomyces,* and *Mucor*. Primary otogenic invasive fungal infections can occur in immunocompromised hosts who are human immunodeficiency virus positive, elderly individuals, and patients with diabetes mellitus. These cases may develop invasive fungal disease within the mastoid and temporal bones, resulting in rapidly progressive hearing loss and facial paralysis. *Aspergillus fumigatus* and *Aspergillus flavus* are sources of invasive fungal mastoiditis with serious morbidity and mortality.

An uncommon cause of purulent otorrhea arising from the external canal in children is infection of a first branchial cleft cyst. In some forms of this congenital anomaly, there is a sinus tract adjacent to the external canal causing localized edema, whereas in others a fistula may be present with an external opening into the external ear canal. The anomaly may not be recognized until drainage and swelling of the ear canal occur. An even rarer source of secondary external canal otorrhea in children and adults is a primary infection of the parotid gland that extends into the external ear canal through the fissures of Santorini. These fibrous channels within the cartilaginous ear canal can serve as a direct route of disease extension.

Severe otalgia associated with bloody or serous otorrhea should prompt examination of the canal and tympanic membrane for evidence of vesicles. Bullous external otitis and myringitis result in hemorrhagic vesicles on the bony external canal and tympanic membrane. This uncommon infection causes exquisite ear pain out of proportion to the physical examination. The infection may be viral, but *Mycoplasma pneumoniae* and *Haemophilus influenzae* have also been cultured from the vesicles. Conductive hearing loss secondary to an associated middle ear effusion often accompanies the localized infection. A mixed loss with a significant sensorineural component has been shown in 30% to 65% of cases of bullous myringitis in which audiometric assessment was performed. The hearing loss completely resolved in 60% of cases.[5,6]

Herpes zoster oticus (Ramsay Hunt syndrome) should be considered if vesicles with an erythematous base are evident on the external canal, pinna, or soft palate. Significant otalgia described as a burning sensation is present with this infection, along with hearing loss, vertigo, and facial paralysis.

Tympanic Membrane, Middle Ear, and Mastoid Sources of Otorrhea

If the physical examination shows a normal-appearing external ear canal, the source of the otorrhea is the tympanic membrane, the middle ear, or the mastoid. Acute otitis media, chronic otitis media, and cholesteatoma are the most common sources of purulent or mucoid drainage from the middle ear and mastoid. Less common causes of chronic otorrhea from the middle ear and mastoid are neoplasms that become secondarily infected and systemic diseases with otologic manifestations.

If a patient with chronic otorrhea has undergone prior mastoid surgery, the physical examination should be directed toward establishing whether the drainage is from a superficial infection of the mastoid cavity or is caused by recurrent or residual mastoid disease. When the mastoid cavity is inspected, any anatomic factors should be noted that predispose toward poor aeration and bowl hygiene, such as a small meatus, high facial ridge, or large dependent mastoid tip. In these cases, the tympanic membrane may appear normal, and the middle ear may be aerated, but because of poor hygiene the mastoid bowl collects debris, and a superficial infection develops. The infection may be fungal or bacterial in nature; examination with meticulous cleaning under a microscope establishes the diagnosis.

In most cases, débridement and treatment with topical antifungal or antimicrobial eardrops or acidifying and drying agents, such as boric acid and alcohol solution, or dilute vinegar solution, suffice as management. In chronic infection, granulation tissue and mucosalized epithelium in the bowl can develop, however, requiring more aggressive treatment with chemical cauterization. Meticulous inspection of the mastoid bowl also reveals evidence of retained mastoid air cells or recurrent cholesteatoma debris as the cause of recurrent otorrhea. Revision mastoid surgery is usually required to eliminate these sources of infection.

In the case of otorrhea from acute otitis media, the drainage may be bloody, mixed with mucus, or mucopurulent, and is typically short-lived. Bloody or purulent otorrhea associated with pain also may occur either immediately or in a delayed fashion after placement of pressure equalization tubes. This otorrhea may occur because of granulation tissue obstructing the tube lumen, middle ear contamination after bathing or swimming, acute otitis media, or reflux of nasopharyngeal secretions through the eustachian tube into the middle ear.

Neglected or inadequately treated acute or chronic otitis media may progress to acute coalescent mastoiditis or chronic bacterial otomastoiditis. Typically, acute otomastoiditis manifests with otalgia, mastoid tenderness, and purulent drainage from the middle ear. Uncommonly, mastoiditis may result from obstruction of the aditus ad antrum; the tympanic membrane and middle ear appear normal in this situation. In acute mastoiditis, the ear canal typically is edematous and tender, resembling external otitis with retroauricular extension. In addition to external canal edema, patients with acute mastoiditis may have auricle protrusion, mastoid tenderness, and swelling, and possibly systemic symptoms of fever. Additional symptoms may be present if there are aural or intracranial complications of the acute or chronic infection. Aural complications include subperiosteal abscess, petrositis, facial paralysis, and labyrinthitis. Intracranial complications include extradural abscess; thrombosis or thrombophlebitis of the sigmoid sinus, transverse sinus, or sagittal sinus; subdural abscess; brain abscess; meningitis; and otitic hydrocephalus. A high index of suspicion and a thorough neurologic examination are required to detect possible aural and intracranial complications of a mastoid infection.

Acquired cholesteatoma is a common cause of painless, recurrent purulent otorrhea in adults and children. The otorrhea may be scant or profuse depending on the extent of the disease, and whether the keratin debris is infected. There is usually an associated long-standing hearing loss. Vestibular symptoms are typically not present, unless there is extensive bone destruction by the cholesteatoma. Erosion of the lateral semicircular canal with formation of a labyrinthine fistula may occur, and the patient may note dysequilibrium that is either spontaneous or induced by loud sounds (Tullio's phenomenon) or positive pressure applied to the external ear canal. Diagnosis of cholesteatoma as the source of otorrhea is evident after meticulous cleaning of the ear canal and examination with binocular microscopy. Typically, a retraction pocket is seen in the posterosuperior quadrant of the tympanic membrane or in the pars flaccida region. The otorrhea and keratin debris emanating from the abnormal retraction are indicative of the acquired cholesteatoma.

Granular myringitis is an uncommon, idiopathic, inflammatory process involving the tympanic membrane. Granulation tissue and mucosalized epithelium extend over patchy areas of the tympanic membrane. In extensive cases, the entire tympanic membrane is thickened, and the granulation tissue exudes a thin transudate that may become secondarily infected.[7]

Systemic Disease Associated with Otorrhea

Noninfectious Causes

Granulomatous diseases of the temporal bone are uncommon. Presenting symptoms can mimic acute or chronic mastoiditis. Children with histiocytosis of the temporal bone can present with symptoms of painful purulent or bloody otorrhea. The three forms of histiocytosis (eosinophilic granuloma, Letterer-Siwe disease, and Hand-Schüller-Christian disease) all may involve the temporal bone.[8] In addition to complaints of localized ear pain, there is evidence of suppurative drainage from the middle ear and mastoid, granulation tissue within the external auditory canal, local swelling of the postauricular or preauricular region, and bone destruction on radiographic imaging. Auditory and vestibular deficits, facial palsy, and lower cranial nerve deficits also may be present.[9]

Wegener's granulomatosis is a granulomatous disorder consisting of inflammatory vasculitis of the upper and lower respiratory tracts and kidney. Almost one fourth of patients have otologic disease at some point during their illness. Otologic involvement may manifest as a serous otitis media or a suppurative otitis media with either thickening or perforation of the tympanic membrane. Granulation tissue may be present within the middle ear and mastoid, causing a painless chronic otorrhea that is associated with conductive, sensorineural, or mixed hearing loss.[10] A high index of suspicion and confirmation with an elevated cytoplasmic antineutrophil cytoplasmic autoantibody titer facilitate the diagnosis.

Churg-Strauss syndrome is an autoimmune disease that may have otologic manifestations in the late stages of the disease. Asthma, recurrent sinusitis, peripheral neuropathy, eosinophilic infiltrates, systemic vasculitis, and peripheral eosinophilia are hallmarks of the disease. In advanced disease, otologic involvement may include a dense aural discharge, granulomatous eosinophilic infiltrates of the middle ear and mastoid, and severe to profound mixed hearing loss. Recognition of this entity is important because the disease is highly responsive to systemic steroids.[11]

Infectious Causes

Aural tuberculosis and nontuberculous mycobacterial mastoiditis are granulomatous infections with presentations that may mimic either otitis externa or chronic otomastoiditis in adults or children. The typical history is that of an indolent infection of the external canal or middle ear with chronic painless otorrhea that is thin, watery, or serous in nature. In documented cases of aural tuberculosis, patients have had acute otalgia with purulent drainage when a bacterial superinfection is present. Typically, patients with aural tuberculosis do not have a history of pulmonary infection or exposure to a known source of tuberculosis. The diagnosis of tuberculous or atypical mycobacterial otomastoiditis is suspected when the infection fails to clear after multiple treatments with antibiotics. The ear canal and middle ear have granulation tissue, polyps, and inflammatory tissue, all of which may be diffusely destructive. In addition, there may be associated cervical, postauricular, or occasionally preauricular adenopathy and systemic symptoms of fever and malaise. The physical examination findings of a postauricular fistula associated with preauricular adenopathy, a denuded malleus, and multiple tympanic membrane perforations are reported to be pathognomonic of aural tuberculosis. Facial palsy associated with aural tuberculosis has been reported in 45% of patients.[12-14]

Neoplastic Disease Causing Otorrhea

The presenting signs and symptoms of neoplastic involvement of the temporal bone include conductive and sensorineural hearing loss, otalgia, mastoiditis, facial nerve paralysis, and purulent or bloody otorrhea. The chronic purulent or bloody otorrhea can arise from neoplasms in the ear canal, middle ear, or mastoid. In adults, the most common neoplasms of the external canal causing otorrhea are squamous cell carcinoma, basal cell carcinoma, and ceruminous gland tumors. In the early stages of disease, these neoplasms may remain asymptomatic and unnoticed until a secondary bacterial infection develops. Advanced disease with temporal bone destruction is associated with chronic deep otalgia. Examination of the ear canal with binocular microscopy after removal of purulent debris may reveal the tumor as an erosive or fungating lesion. These lesions also may manifest as persistent granulation tissue that is refractory to routine management. Biopsy of the granulation tissue is indicated to rule out an underlying neoplastic process. Glomus tumors may be isolated to the middle ear or jugular foramen region and usually do not result in otorrhea. Large tumors may fill the mesotympanum and extend into the ear canal, however, resulting in bloody or purulent otorrhea. Performing a biopsy of glomus tumors extending into the ear canal can result in profuse bleeding and should be avoided.

Metastatic lesions to the temporal bone rarely manifest with otorrhea as an initial symptom. Primary tumors from the breast, lung, kidney, prostate, and stomach are the common sources of temporal bone metastatic lesions.[15] These tumors metastasize predominantly to the petrous apex marrow through hematogenous dissemination. Metastatic involvement of the mastoid air cells and the tympanic cavity may occur. Lymphoma and leukemia also may infiltrate the petrous apex and subsequently involve mastoid air cells. Infiltration into the middle ear cleft along mucosal folds and into the fallopian canal and internal auditory canal is common.[16]

Acute myelogenous leukemia may involve the temporal bone by chloroma formations, which are masses of leukemic cells seen as discrete green collections within the mastoid or internal auditory canal. In children, uncommon neoplasms that result in otorrhea include histiocytosis, rhabdomyosarcoma, leukemia, and lymphoma. Because the presenting symptoms can resemble chronic otitis media with purulent or bloody otorrhea, granulation tissue, and aural polyps, diagnosis of the underlying neoplasm is often delayed.

Intracranial Sources of Otorrhea

The unique presentation of continuous or intermittent clear otorrhea may represent cerebrospinal fluid (CSF). Clear otorrhea may manifest spontaneously through a perforated tympanic membrane or through a pressure equalizing tube. It may be caused by an underlying congenital anomaly or an idiopathic dural dehiscence within the temporal bone. CSF otorrhea may occur as a direct result of trauma or as a complication of neoplasia, infection, or previous surgery. Regardless of the etiology, all cases of clear otorrhea must be investigated because of the risk of meningitis associated with a persistent CSF leak. If possible, the clear fluid should be collected and the sample analyzed for the presence of β_2-transferrin. This is a protein found in CSF and perilymph, but not in blood, nasal secretions, or inflammatory effusions.[17] If the fluid is identified as CSF, immunization for *Streptococcus pneumoniae* should be considered to prevent meningitis, in addition to pursuing appropriate measures directed to stop the CSF leakage. Occasionally, serous discharge from chronic mastoiditis (or through a ventilating tube) can be profuse and mimic CSF leakage.

Radiographic imaging using high-resolution computed tomography (CT) is essential in the diagnostic evaluation of patients with clear otorrhea. Axial and coronal views should be obtained and evaluated for evidence of congenital labyrinthine abnormalities, erosive changes within the mastoid air cells, dehiscence of the middle or posterior cranial fossa dural plates, or temporal bone fractures.

Congenital labyrinthine abnormalities are an uncommon cause of CSF otorrhea. The most common labyrinthine anomaly associated with spontaneous CSF leak is a Mondini malformation. The leak may manifest as recurrent meningitis in childhood or as intermittent leakage of clear fluid from a tympanic membrane perforation or myringotomy tube. CSF leakage occurs through a defect in the lamina cribrosa of the internal auditory canal in association with a defect in the stapes footplate. A high index of suspicion should be maintained when evaluating a child with a history of recurrent clear otorrhea and sensorineural hearing loss. A much rarer source of CSF in the middle ear is through a persistently patent perilabyrinthine pathway, such as a persistent Hyrtl's fissure. This bony cleft extends medially from below the round window niche to the posterior fossa and normally ossifies during development.[18] In the absence of normal ossification, this tympanomeningeal fissure may persist as an abnormal connection between the middle ear and the subarachnoid space, resulting in a CSF fistula.

Spontaneous CSF leaks also may occur from the middle or posterior cranial fossae secondary to progressive erosion and weakening of the dura by aberrant arachnoid granulations. These leaks typically occur after the fifth decade, and manifest as a persistent unilateral effusion or profuse clear otorrhea after myringotomy.[19,20] The leakage site often is evident on CT scan as a dehiscent area of either the superior or the posterior surface of the temporal bone.

Temporal bone CSF leaks can also occur after mastoidectomy, skull base surgery, or any surgical approach to the internal auditory canal or cerebellopontine angle (e.g., translabyrinthine, middle cranial fossa, posterior cranial fossa). Inadequate dural closure at the time of surgery results in CSF leakage. Occasionally, the CSF leak occurs weeks, months, or years after temporal bone surgery in which dura was exposed but not damaged. In open mastoid cavities with exposed dura, subsequent infections may incite the formation of granulation tissue with subsequent weakening of the underlying dura. The weakened dura allows prolapse of either the temporal lobe or the cerebellum into the mastoid cavity. Over time, intracranial pressure results in erosion and exposure of the subarachnoid space with leakage of CSF. When this occurs, surgical exploration and direct dural repair with tissue grafts and supporting packing is necessary.

In an ear previously known to be normal, watery otorrhea after severe head trauma almost certainly represents meningeal laceration and CSF leakage. Egress of fluid from the ear canal occurs most commonly in cases of longitudinal temporal bone fractures because the tympanic membrane often is disrupted in these situations. Leakage of CSF from the external auditory canal occurs in 21% to 44% of temporal bone fractures.[21,22] Because the drainage typically is mixed with blood, the presence of CSF should always be suspected. If profuse clear otorrhea follows trauma that is confined to the external auditory canal and tympanic membrane, stapes dislocation and a congenital abnormality of the labyrinth are suggested. Prompt surgical exploration and, if appropriate, oval window sealing are necessary.

A rare source of clear, painless otorrhea that is not CSF in origin is gustatory otorrhea or Frey's syndrome of the external ear canal.[23] Excisional biopsy of the canal skin showing thickened skin with sudomotor gland hyperplasia is diagnostic. A parotid fistula to the external canal is another diagnostic consideration for symptoms of gustatory otorrhea.

Otalgia

Otalgia most commonly reflects either localized otologic pathology or a problem within a contiguous, periauricular structure. The physical examination usually reveals the source of the pain. It is common, however, for a patient to complain of ear pain and have no identifiable pathology within the ear. Evaluation of patients with otalgia is facilitated by a thorough understanding of the innervation of the ear. Appreciation of the anatomy underlying shared neural pathways and the potential causes of referred otalgia arising from a distant site enables an astute physician to reach a diagnosis when evaluating a patient with the complaint of ear pain.

The auricle, periauricular region, external canal, and middle ear are supplied with sensory afferents from the trigeminal, facial, glossopharyngeal, and vagal nerves, and the cervical plexus. The auriculotemporal branch of the mandibular division of the trigeminal nerve provides sensation to the tragus, anterior pinna, anterior lateral surface of the tympanic membrane, and anterosuperior external auditory canal wall. The vagus nerve provides sensation to the larynx, hypopharynx, trachea, esophagus, and thyroid gland. The auricular branch of the vagus nerve (Arnold's nerve) provides sensation to the concha, inferoposterior external auditory canal, tympanic membrane, and postauricular skin. The glossopharyngeal nerve provides sensory innervation to the oropharynx, tonsils, and tongue base. Jacobson's nerve is the tympanic branch of the glossopharyngeal nerve that provides sensation to the medial surface of the tympanic membrane, mucosa of the middle ear, eustachian tube, and mastoid air cells. The cervical roots C2 and C3 provide sensation to the postauricular region. The facial nerve innervates the skin of the lateral concha and antihelix, lobule, mastoid, posterior external auditory canal, and posterior portion of the tympanic membrane.

Primary Otalgia

Primary otalgia arises from local or regional pathology. Sources of primary otalgia include acute otitis media, otitis externa, mastoiditis, eustachian tube dysfunction, cerumen impaction, inflammation or infection of the auricle, or ear trauma. Regional causes include temporomandibular joint dysfunction and periauricular lymphadenopathy from scalp or neck infections.

Referred Otalgia

Pain may be referred to the ear from distant sources, such as periodontal or dental disease, parotitis, sinusitis, thyroiditis, tonsillitis, laryngitis, or hiatal hernia with gastroesophageal reflux. Referred pain to the ear can arise from any structure within the head and neck that shares a common neural pathway with the temporal bone and periauricular region. In the initial assessment, examination of the ear indicates whether the otalgia is local or regional in origin. If the ear examination is normal, it is helpful to ask the patient to point with one finger to the area of maximal pain.

The trigeminal nerve has a wide sensory distribution throughout the head and neck. Infection and neoplasms within the nasal cavity or paranasal sinuses, particularly the sphenoid or maxillary sinuses, can cause irritation of the vidian nerve, resulting in referred otalgia. Contact points between the turbinates and septal spurs can cause a similar type of pain. Nasopharyngeal surgery and neoplasms and infections in this region are common sources of referred otalgia. In children, erupting dentition is the most common cause of referred ear pain, which is recognized as ear pulling in preverbal children. Similarly, an impacted molar in an adult may cause symptoms of ear pain. Dental malocclusion resulting from temporomandibular joint dysfunction (Costen's syndrome) can cause referred ear pain from masticator muscle spasms. A history of excessive gum chewing, malocclusion, and bruxism may suggest this diagnosis. Sluder's neuralgia consists of lancinating pain in the lower face that radiates to the orbit, temple, forehead, and upper neck. The sphenopalatine branch of the trigeminal nerve is the source of this pain.

The facial nerve can be involved in referred ear pain in cases of geniculate neuralgia, Bell's palsy, and herpes zoster oticus. The ear pain of herpes zoster oticus can occur even in the absence of a significant vesicular eruption. The otalgia associated with Bell's palsy frequently occurs before the onset of facial paralysis.

The glossopharyngeal and vagus nerves can transmit referred ear pain as a result of pathology originating from anywhere within the upper aerodigestive tract. The ninth cranial nerve can be stimulated from pathology in the pharynx, such as tonsillitis, postoperative tonsillectomy, peritonsillar abscess, and neoplasms. Lingual tonsillitis and impacted foreign bodies within the tongue can also cause otalgia. Eagle's syndrome consists of ear pain secondary to stretching and irritation of the glossopharyngeal nerve from elongation of the styloid process. Glossopharyngeal neuralgia is similar to tic douloureux or trigeminal neuralgia. The pain is sharp and lancinating in quality, and originates in the tongue base, soft palate, or tonsillar fossa and radiates to the ear. Rosenmüller's fossa may be the trigger zone with this form of neuralgia.

Neoplasms within the larynx and esophagus have long been recognized as causes of referred otalgia. Ulcerations, foreign bodies, and reflux also can be seen in this manner. Chronic or subacute inflammation of the thyroid gland may cause referred ear pain through stimulation of the vagus nerve.

Aural Fullness

Patients often describe aural fullness as a stuffy feeling in the ear, ear pressure, or a clogged sensation. This subjective symptom may be associated with various ear disorders.

Aural fullness may occur because of obstruction of the external ear canal by cerumen, debris, or a foreign body. A sensation of fullness also may result from a soft tissue mass either in the middle ear or arising from the tympanic membrane. Cholesteatoma and neoplastic disease can manifest in this manner. If the patient's history reveals associated ear pain, drainage, or hearing loss, the physical examination easily establishes the diagnosis.

An abnormally patent or an obstructed eustachian tube also may elicit the sensation of aural fullness. Patients complain of autophony and of hearing breath sounds in the ear. A history of weight loss, steroid use, or hormonal therapy may precede the onset of symptoms. Evidence for an abnormally patent eustachian tube includes relief of symptoms (1) when the patient is supine or bending over, (2) during periods of nasal congestion, and (3) with sniffing. Evidence for a chronically obstructed eustachian tube orifice includes the inability to insufflate the ear with Valsalva's maneuver, chronic retraction of the tympanic membrane, and a history of nasal congestion and allergic disorder.

Aural fullness is part of the symptom complex of Meniere's disease. When the fullness is associated with fluctuating hearing and discrete spells of vertigo, its significance is apparent. Aural fullness also may occur as the result of a perilymphatic fistula. Seltzer and McCabe[24] noted that 25% of patients with fistulas confirmed at exploratory tympanotomy had aural fullness.

Box 156-2

Hearing Loss in Adults

Acute

- Sudden idiopathic sensorineural hearing loss
- Infection (acute otitis media, external otitis, syphilis, Lyme disease, viral)
- Perilymphatic fistula
- Ischemia of retrocochlear structures
- Multiple sclerosis
- Autoimmune disease
- Traumatic
- Metabolic (chronic renal failure)
- Hematologic (sickle cell anemia)

Gradual

- Presbycusis
- Noise-induced
- Familial
- Retrocochlear neoplasm
- Chronic otitis media, cholesteatoma
- Otosclerosis
- Endocrine (hypothyroidism, diabetes mellitus)
- Paget's disease
- Metabolic (chronic renal failure, hyperlipoproteinemia)
- Mucopolysaccharidosis

Fluctuating

- Perilymphatic fistula
- Meniere's disease
- Multiple sclerosis
- Migraine-associated hearing loss
- Infection (syphilis)
- Autoimmune (Cogan's syndrome, systemic lupus, polyarteritis nodosa, Wegener's syndrome, temporal arteritis, scleroderma)
- Sarcoidosis

Rapidly Progressive

- Autoimmune inner ear disease
- Meningeal carcinomatosis
- Vasculitis secondary to infection (Rocky Mountain spotted fever)
- Lyme disease
- Ototoxic exposure (aminoglycosides, diuretics, chemotherapy)

Hearing Loss

A complaint of hearing loss can reflect a wide variety of abnormalities (Box 156-2), and diagnostic considerations are different in pediatric and adult patients. Evaluation should determine whether the loss is unilateral or bilateral or fluctuating in nature. The time course of the hearing loss should be established, and associated symptoms should be documented. The medical history should investigate current and past treatments with oral and intravenous medications, and nonprescription drug use. The patient should be screened for systemic diseases, including cardiovascular, metabolic, endocrine, neurologic, hematologic, infectious, and autoimmune diseases. Prior ear surgery, cardiac bypass surgery, and lumbar puncture also may be relevant to the current complaint of hearing loss.[25] A family history of hearing loss, neoplasms, renal disease, and balance disorders should be obtained. Finally, previous sharp or blunt head trauma, noise trauma, or barotrauma should be noted.

The most informative features that facilitate determining the etiology of hearing loss are the time course of the loss, associated symptoms, and age of the patient. It should be determined whether the loss is acute or gradual in onset, long-standing, fluctuating, rapidly progressive, or of unknown duration. Associated symptoms of aural fullness, pain, otorrhea, vertigo, tinnitus, or cranial neuropathies can assist diagnosis. The clinical feature of unilateral or bilateral hearing loss is less revealing in determining the etiology of hearing loss.

Acute Hearing Loss

Acute unilateral hearing loss may result from a range of disease states. Sudden or acute sensorineural hearing loss may be idiopathic; iatrogenic; a complication of a viral or bacterial infection, labyrinthine fluid abnormality, vascular event, trauma, neoplasm, autoimmune abnormality, or neurologic disease; or a side effect of medication.

Viral infections such as mumps, rubella, rubeola, and Epstein-Barr virus may involve the ear directly by causing varying degrees of transient or permanent hearing loss with or without associated vertigo. These infections may also cause a serous labyrinthitis, causing sensorineural hearing loss from toxins affecting the inner ear. Ramsay Hunt syndrome is an example of a viral polyneuropathy that typically involves facial and cochleovestibular dysfunction. Bacterial and fungal meningitis may also extend to the labyrinth, causing sudden hearing loss. Other infectious causes of sudden hearing loss are acute otitis media, suppurative labyrinthitis from acute or chronic otitis media, and syphilis. In most of these cases, the history, physical examination, and appropriate serology establish the etiology of the hearing loss.

Abnormalities of labyrinthine fluid include hydrops and perilymphatic fistula. Both of these conditions typically cause fluctuating hearing loss, but sudden, permanent loss also is possible. A history of recent heavy lifting or straining, head trauma, or barotrauma suggests a possible perilymphatic fistula. Hydrops typically causes low-frequency hearing loss. The presence of diplacusis and recruitment on examination and associated spells of recurrent vertigo support the diagnosis.

Sudden hearing loss may occur as the result of a vascular event involving the cochlea. Thrombosis or embolic occlusion of the labyrinthine and cochlear arteries is an uncommon but well-recognized cause of hearing loss. Hyperviscosity states such as polycythemia vera may result in cochlear ischemia. Obstruction of small vessels as a result of diabetes mellitus, atherosclerosis, and sickle cell anemia should also be considered when no other causes of hearing loss can be identified.

Head trauma, barotrauma, and noise trauma all can result in acute hearing loss that may be transient or permanent. Direct head trauma resulting in temporal bone fracture may cause either a conductive or a sensorineural hearing loss. Hearing loss also may occur because of a concussive injury to labyrinthine membranes without an associated temporal bone fracture. The history is usually sufficient in these cases to establish the cause of the hearing loss.

Sudden transient or permanent hearing loss is an atypical presentation of a retrocochlear neoplasm in the cerebellopontine angle. This diagnosis can be difficult to make because associated symptoms from a tumor manifesting in this manner are uncommon, particularly in the case of small tumors. Radiographic imaging should always be performed in cases of sudden hearing loss without any identifiable etiology.

When evaluating a patient with sudden or rapidly progressive hearing loss, the presence or absence of other neurologic symptoms should be investigated. Hearing loss that is unilateral, bilateral, sudden, subacute, or insidious may be the presenting symptom for multiple sclerosis.[26,27] Presentation of hearing loss associated with ophthalmologic disease should prompt investigation of Susac's syndrome. First described in 1979, Susac's syndrome is characterized by the triad of retinal arterial occlusions, encephalopathy, and cochlear microangiopathy. The neurotologic features are frequently misdiagnosed as multiple sclerosis, delaying the effective treatment and control of symptoms with systemic immunosuppression.[28]

In adults, a gradual or long-standing hearing loss may reflect various disorders (see Box 156-2). Bilateral gradual hearing loss may reflect presbycusis, noise-induced hearing loss, or familial sensorineural

Table 156-1

Lower Cranial Nerve Deficits Associated with Jugular Foramen Syndromes

	Cranial Nerve			
Syndrome	**IX**	**X**	**XI**	**XII**
Avellis		X		
Tapia		X		X
Vernet	X	X	X	
Jackson		X	X	X
Collet-Sicard	X	X	X	X

hearing loss. A history of exposure to ototoxic medication should also be investigated. If the sensorineural hearing loss is unilateral, a retrocochlear lesion should be investigated as the cause of the loss. If the loss has a conductive component, diagnoses such as otosclerosis, chronic otitis media with effusion, malleus head fixation, tympanosclerosis, myringosclerosis, tympanic membrane perforation, cholesteatoma, or ossicular chain disruption should be considered.

Patients with tumors of the jugular foramen commonly present with unilateral hearing loss. This loss may be conductive because of a mass effect of the tumor impinging on the tympanic membrane and ossicles, or sensorineural secondary to erosion of the cochlea or compression of the eighth cranial nerve within the internal auditory canal and cerebellopontine angle. Although symptoms related to these tumors may be subtle, diagnostic suspicion should be high when evaluating a patient with a middle ear or external auditory canal mass associated with pulsatile tinnitus. Dysfunction of the lower cranial nerves may occur in many combinations (Table 156-1), depending on the size and location of the tumor.

Fluctuating Hearing Loss

Fluctuating hearing loss can reflect various diseases. The most common causes are Meniere's disease, perilymphatic fistula, and luetic labyrinthitis. Less commonly, systemic diseases such as multiple sclerosis, tuberculosis, and sarcoidosis cause fluctuating hearing loss. Meniere's disease is usually easily recognized because of the associated vestibular symptoms. Diagnosis of a perilymphatic fistula can be challenging because the symptoms can be quite variable. A history of prior ear surgery, head trauma, barotrauma, or straining may increase suspicion for perilymphatic fistula. Syphilitic inner ear disease also can be an elusive diagnosis because of the various possible presenting symptoms. When hearing loss is associated with either autoimmune disorders or sarcoid, the patient typically has other systemic symptoms relating to the primary disorder that facilitate recognition of the nature of the hearing loss.[29] Autoimmune diseases with cochlear involvement can mimic Meniere's disease early in the course of the disease, before permanent nonfluctuating sensorineural hearing loss occurs.

An uncommon cause of fluctuating hearing loss is an endolymphatic sac tumor. These tumors originate from the epithelium of the vestibular aqueduct and endolymphatic sac. A high index of suspicion is needed to diagnose these tumors, which manifest with symptoms similar to Meniere's disease.[30]

Rapidly Progressive Hearing Loss

Rapidly progressive hearing loss may occur as a result of isolated autoimmune inner ear disease or systemic autoimmune disease with otologic involvement. The hearing loss may be unilateral initially, but progresses to bilateral involvement. Less commonly, the loss may fluctuate or manifest as a sudden sensorineural hearing loss. Autoimmune diseases associated with hearing loss are Cogan's syndrome (nonsyphilitic interstitial keratitis with audiovestibular involvement),[31,32] polyarteritis nodosa, relapsing polychondritis, sarcoid, ulcerative colitis, systemic lupus erythematosus, Wegener's disease, Churg-Strauss syndrome, and Behçet's disease.

An unusual cause of rapidly progressive or sudden hearing loss is neoplastic disease metastatic to the brain or temporal bone from a distant primary site. Hearing loss is usually associated with additional symptoms, such as tinnitus, vertigo, dysequilibrium, and facial nerve paralysis. Metastatic disease may involve the brain and skull base by several mechanisms. Metastatic disease may involve the temporal bone directly through hematogenous spread to petrous bone marrow. Metastases may be single or multiple intraparenchymal or epidural lesions. Diffuse multifocal seeding of the leptomeninges (meningeal carcinomatosis) also may occur. The most common sources of metastatic disease directly affecting the temporal bone are breast, lung, kidney, stomach, bronchus, and prostate neoplasms. The most common tumor type that causes intraparenchymal lesions is carcinoma of the lung. Generally, 20% of intraparenchymal brain metastases occur in the cerebellum and brainstem. Prostate carcinoma and breast cancer have a propensity to metastasize to the dura. Non-Hodgkin's lymphoma, breast carcinoma, and melanoma are the most common tumor types associated with leptomeningeal metastasis. A high index of suspicion for metastatic disease should always be maintained when evaluating a patient with a known history of cancer who presents with new cranial nerve deficits.[15,33,34]

Pediatric Sensorineural Hearing Loss

Pediatric hearing loss can be categorized as congenital (present at birth) or acquired (auditory function was present initially with subsequent loss of hearing). Congenital and acquired hearing loss may result from an abnormality in the genetic code (syndromic or nonsyndromic, single gene or chromosomal abnormality), or may result from perinatal insults that are infectious, toxic, or systemic in nature. The Joint Committee on Infant Hearing[35] has outlined the identifiable risk factors associated with neonatal hearing loss. These risk factors include a family history of hereditary childhood sensorineural hearing loss; perinatal infection with cytomegalovirus, rubella, syphilis, herpes, or toxoplasmosis; evidence of craniofacial abnormalities; birth weight less than 1500 g; significant hyperbilirubinemia requiring exchange transfusion; treatment with ototoxic medications; history of bacterial meningitis; history of Apgar scores between 0 and 4 at 1 minute, or 0 and 6 at 5 minutes; history of prolonged mechanical ventilation in the postnatal period; or any other findings on physical examination suggestive of a syndrome associated with hearing loss.

Diagnostic considerations for nongenetic causes of hearing loss include kernicterus, prematurity with low birth weight, birth trauma, postnatal anoxia requiring mechanical ventilation, use of extracorporeal membrane oxygenation therapy, and treatment with ototoxic medications in the postnatal period. Perinatal infections can result in congenital and delayed hearing loss. Young children are particularly vulnerable to bacterial meningitis, and the incidence of hearing loss after such an infection is 3.5% to 37%.[36] Prenatal exposure to toxoplasmosis, rubella, cytomegalovirus, herpes simplex virus, and syphilis can result in mild to profound sensorineural hearing loss. Box 156-3 lists the 10 most common syndromes associated with hearing loss and some rare disorders in which hearing loss is a major feature.[37]

Approximately 20% of patients with congenital sensorineural hearing loss have radiographic evidence of an inner ear malformation.[38] Malformations of the inner ear may occur in isolation or associated with other physical abnormalities as part of a syndrome. The malformation may result from exposure to teratogens (chemical or viral) during embryogenesis, or may be idiopathic in nature. Congenital inner ear abnormalities constitute a spectrum of recognized malformations that are associated with various hearing loss patterns. Complete aplasia of the labyrinthine capsule (Michel's aplasia) is associated with profound deafness. The most common malformation is cochleosaccular dysgenesis (Scheibe's aplasia), which is a malformation limited to the membranous portion of the pars inferior. The Mondini deformity derives from arrested development of the labyrinthine capsule during the 7th week of gestation, resulting in a small cochlea with an incomplete partition and an abnormally dilated vestibular aqueduct and vestibule.

Box 156-3

Hearing Loss in Congenital and Genetic Conditions

Syndromes Most Commonly Associated with Hearing Loss

1. Oculoauriculovertebral spectrum (hemifacial microsomia, Goldenhar's syndrome)
2. Stickler's syndrome (hereditary arthro-ophthalmopathy)
3. Congenital cytomegalovirus
4. Usher's syndrome
5. Branchio-oto-renal syndrome
6. Pendred's syndrome
7. CHARGE association (*c*oloboma [of eyes], *h*earing deficit, choanal *a*tresia, *r*etardation of growth, *g*enital defects [males only], *e*ndocardial cushion defect)
8. Neurofibromatosis type 2
9. Mitochondrial disorders
10. Waardenburg's syndrome

Rare Disorders with Hearing Loss as a Major Feature

1. Otopalatal-digital syndromes
2. Skeletal dysplasias (osteogenesis imperfecta)
3. Metabolic storage diseases (mucopolysaccharidoses, Refsum's disease)
4. Townes-Brock syndrome
5. Wildervanck's syndrome
6. Biotinidase deficiency

Variable degrees of hearing loss and vestibular dysfunction are associated within the spectrum of labyrinthine developmental abnormalities. Generally, the more severe the malformation, the greater the associated hearing loss.

More than half of all cases of prelingual sensorineural hearing loss are the result of a genetic abnormality. Autosomal recessive patterns of inheritance are responsible for almost three quarters of these cases, and most are nonsyndromic. Most of these inherited forms of hearing loss are permanent and irreversible. An exception is the sensorineural hearing loss associated with biotinidase deficiency. This is an autosomal recessive disorder of failure to recycle the vitamin biotin, resulting in mental retardation, hypotonia, seizure disorder, alopecia, and skin rash. Sensorineural hearing loss is now recognized to occur in 75% of children with a symptomatic biotinidase deficiency. Early recognition in the neonatal period is crucial for initiating appropriate therapy.[39]

One third of the inherited forms of congenital hearing loss occur as part of a syndrome.[40] Recognition of these forms of hereditary hearing loss is assisted by the identification of associated physical and metabolic abnormalities. The presence of renal abnormalities suggests the possibility of Alport's syndrome, which can be inherited in an autosomal dominant, autosomal recessive, and X-linked pattern. Branchio-oto-renal syndrome should be considered if there are structural abnormalities, such as auricular pits, malformed pinnae, or branchial cleft fistulas or cysts, in association with conductive, mixed, or sensorineural hearing loss. A complete eye examination, including electroretinography, is crucial to early identification of retinitis pigmentosa associated with Usher's syndrome.[41] Associated metabolic dysfunction may be obvious, as in inherited mucopolysaccharidoses, or more subtle, as in Pendred's syndrome. A family history of fatal cardiac arrhythmias should suggest the possibility of Jervell-Lange-Nielsen syndrome. Pigmentary abnormalities such as a bicolored iris, white eyelashes, or piebald skin are associated with Waardenburg's syndrome.

Pediatric Conductive Hearing Loss

Most pediatric conductive hearing loss is the result of acute or chronic otitis media and the sequelae of these diseases. Noninfectious causes of congenital conductive hearing loss include congenital cholesteatoma, external auditory canal atresia,[42] and labyrinthine structural abnormalities such as ossicular chain fixation and congenital absence of the oval window.[43-45] A rare developmental abnormality that results in a prominent conductive hearing loss in children is a salivary gland choristoma of the middle ear. Twenty-six cases of heterotopic salivary gland tissue in the middle ear have been documented in the literature. Patients are seen at a young age with a persistent conductive hearing loss and a middle ear mass. Often the mass is adherent to the tympanic or descending portions of the facial nerve. Associated malformations of the ossicular chain and external ear also have been found.[46-48]

Vertigo

The sensations of vertigo and dysequilibrium in children and adults may reflect disease within the labyrinth, a retrocochlear abnormality involving either the eighth cranial nerve or more central structures, or the effects of a systemic abnormality. A thorough and well-directed history discriminates otologic from nonotologic causes of vertigo in most cases. Identification of associated symptoms, the time course of the vertigo or dysequilibrium, precipitating and alleviating factors, and the general medical history should be assessed in patients with vertigo.

The patient's description of symptoms helps in discriminating between central and peripheral causes of vertigo. A sensation of spinning or motion commonly results from acute vestibular dysfunction, such as viral neuronitis, labyrinthitis, and Meniere's disease. Nonvestibular causes of imbalance, such as cardiogenic, metabolic, neurogenic, or psychogenic dysfunction, are often described as a more nonspecific sensation of light-headedness. Encouraging the patient to describe the symptoms or spells in detail without using the word *dizzy* can be helpful.

The time course of the patient's symptoms is crucial to distinguish between otologic and nonotologic causes of vertigo (Box 156-4). Vertigo that is continuously present for weeks without fluctuation is generally not the result of a peripheral vestibular abnormality. Acute injury to the inner ear or eighth cranial nerve initially results in severe and prolonged vertigo. As central compensation progresses, the vertigo subsides over days to weeks. Persistent vertigo indicates an uncompensated labyrinthine or eighth cranial nerve lesion, or a central abnormality.

Vertigo in discrete isolated spells should be characterized by the frequency and duration of symptoms. Vertigo that lasts for less than 1 minute can represent benign paroxysmal positional vertigo. Spells lasting several minutes may represent migraine-associated vertigo or transient ischemia of the vertebrobasilar circulation. Vertigo that is prolonged for hours is typical of Meniere's disease or endolymphatic hydrops. Vertigo that persists for days but gradually subsides is seen with vestibular neuritis.

Box 156-4

Time Course of Vertigo

Seconds to Minutes to Hours

- Perilymphatic fistula
- Benign paroxysmal positional vertigo
- Otosclerosis
- Vascular
- Migraine
  - Vertebrobasilar insufficiency (anterior inferior cerebellar artery)
  - Wallenberg's syndrome
  - Hyperviscosity syndromes

Hours

- Meniere's disease
- Migraine
- Metabolic
- Iatrogenic
- Syphilis

Days

- Labyrinthitis
- Temporal bone trauma
- Iatrogenic
- Viral neuronitis
- Vertebrobasilar infarction
- Cerebellar/brainstem hemorrhage
- Autoimmune neurolabyrinthitis
- Multiple sclerosis

Labyrinthine Vertigo

Diseases affecting the labyrinth that result in vertigo may be categorized as infectious, post-traumatic, metabolic, autoimmune, ischemic, drug-induced, hydropic, or multifactorial in character. The most common infectious cause of acute vertigo is viral labyrinthitis. Most patients with viral labyrinthitis have isolated vestibular dysfunction of sudden onset, without associated hearing loss. In some cases, identification of the inciting agent is evident because of systemic manifestation of the disease, such as with measles, mumps, infectious mononucleosis, herpes zoster, and cytomegalovirus. Bacterial infection from acute or chronic otitis media also may result in a toxic or serous labyrinthitis with vestibular symptoms. A more severe infection can result in suppurative labyrinthitis either from direct bacterial invasion into the inner ear from chronic otomastoiditis (through a labyrinthine fistula from a cholesteatoma) or from bacterial meningitis contaminating the perilymphatic space of the labyrinth through the cochlear aqueduct or internal auditory canal. Chronic infections such as syphilis and Lyme disease may cause persistent or recurring symptoms of vertigo and dysequilibrium through direct invasion of the otic capsule or by leptomeningeal involvement.

Traumatic causes of vertigo include temporal bone fractures, labyrinthine concussion, and perilymphatic fistula. Transverse fractures of the temporal bone extend from the posterior fossa across the petrous portion of the temporal bone into the vestibule. Rupture of the membranous labyrinth and laceration of the cochleovestibular nerve in these cases result in profound deafness and severe vertigo. Longitudinal temporal bone fracture without violation of the labyrinth and blunt head trauma without associated temporal bone fracture also may cause hearing loss and vertigo because of a concussive injury to the membranous labyrinth.

Metabolic causes of vertigo should always be considered when a labyrinthine or central etiology is absent. Systemic metabolic abnormalities that can affect vestibular function include hyperviscosity syndromes (hyperlipidemia, polycythemia, macroglobulinemia, and sickle cell anemia), diabetes mellitus, hyperlipoproteinemia, and hypothyroidism. Hormonal fluctuations occurring in the premenstrual and perimenopausal periods and oral contraceptives and estrogen replacement therapy also may cause neurotologic symptoms, including vertigo. Metabolic dysfunction isolated to the labyrinth may occur because of cochlear otosclerosis. In addition to sensorineural hearing loss, cochlear otosclerosis may cause vestibular symptoms of dysequilibrium or vertigo. Altered cochlear microvascularization, direct otosclerotic degeneration of vestibular nerve fibers, and humoral toxicity secondary to proteolytic enzymes within the perilymph all have been proposed as mechanisms for vertigo associated with otosclerosis.

Numerous collagen vascular disorders have been associated with vestibular dysfunction as a form of autoimmune inner ear disease. Common disorders of this type include rheumatoid arthritis, polyarteritis nodosa, temporal arteritis, nonsyphilitic interstitial keratitis, lupus, sarcoid, relapsing polychondritis, dermatomyositis, and scleroderma.

Ischemia of small labyrinthine vessels causes isolated infarction of the vestibular labyrinth and vertigo. Occlusion of larger vessels, such as the anterior inferior cerebellar artery or its branches, causes sudden and profound loss of auditory and vestibular function and regional infarction of the brainstem.[49]

Aminoglycoside ototoxicity is a well-recognized cause of drug-induced vertigo. The degree of cochlear and vestibular toxicity of these drugs varies with each drug, the duration of treatment, concomitant exposure to noise, and genetic susceptibility of the individual.[50]

Endolymphatic hydrops or Meniere's disease is defined by the well-recognized symptoms of vertigo, hearing loss, tinnitus, and aural fullness. The underlying mechanism that causes abnormal homeostasis of endolymph resulting in distention and rupture of the membranous labyrinth is unknown. Histopathologic findings suggest that fibrosis of the endolymphatic sac, altered glycoprotein metabolism, and viral infections may be pathogenic mechanisms, but further study in this area is needed.[51]

Retrocochlear Vertigo

Retrocochlear causes of vertigo can be categorized as neoplastic, paraneoplastic, vascular (infarction or ischemia), and demyelinating in origin. Diagnosis relies on a thorough history and physical examination documenting other associated cranial nerve or neurologic deficits, evidence of malignancy, and identification of risk factors for vascular disturbances.

Cerebellopontine angle tumors such as acoustic neuroma and meningioma more commonly cause a sense of dysequilibrium or unsteadiness rather than true vertigo. Because these tumors are slow-growing, central compensation occurs over time for the unilateral loss of vestibular function. In addition, these space-occupying lesions of the posterior fossa may cause dysequilibrium and positional vertigo because of cerebellar compression. Brainstem tumors such as gliomas and medulloblastomas commonly manifest with vestibular and cochlear symptoms in addition to long tract signs, cranial nerve deficits, ataxia, and headache.

Although paraneoplastic syndromes associated with carcinoma are uncommon causes of vertigo, they are worthy of mention because the vestibular symptoms may precede the diagnosis of underlying malignancy.[52] Paraneoplastic encephalomyelitis is an autoimmune process most commonly associated with small cell carcinoma of the lung. Inflammatory changes may occur throughout the neuraxis, with subsequent neuronal destruction and glial activation. When the brainstem is involved, degeneration of the vestibular nuclei and the lower cranial nerves is common. Paraneoplastic cerebellar degeneration has been associated with lymphoma and with carcinoma of the ovary, breast, and lung. Paraneoplastic cerebellar degeneration may manifest as sudden-onset vertigo or progressive truncal and extremity ataxia with nystagmus, dysarthria, and diplopia.

Cerebellar atrophy and diffuse small vessel ischemia associated with aging may cause mild unsteadiness, but rarely true vertigo. The coexistence of multisensory deficits with decreased peripheral sensitivity and proprioception and poor visual acuity exacerbates any central or vestibular hypofunction resulting in dysequilibrium.

Acute vascular events affecting the cerebellum and brainstem usually produce more pronounced and severe symptoms. Transient ischemia of the vertebrobasilar system may cause acute onset of vertigo that lasts only minutes and resolves without sequelae. Occlusion of the vertebral artery or the posterior inferior cerebellar artery results in infarction of the dorsolateral medulla (Wallenberg's syndrome). Cerebellar ataxia, vertigo with nausea and vomiting, Horner's syndrome, conjugate gaze paresis, and contralateral loss of pain and temperature sensation are the associated signs and symptoms.

Episodic vertigo may be a component of a migraine aura. The vertigo may occur in conjunction with or precede the migraine headache. Vertigo also may occur without headache; this is known as migraine equivalent.

Demyelinating disorders of the central nervous system are uncommon causes of vertigo and dysequilibrium. Unusual causes of demyelination include exposure to toxins (carbon monoxide, lead, and methotrexate), nutritional disorders (vitamin B_{12} deficiency), postviral syndromes (measles and papovavirus), and hereditary degeneration. Multiple sclerosis is the most common demyelinating disorder encountered by otolaryngologists assessing cochleovestibular dysfunction. Although vertigo is the presenting symptom in only 5% of patients with multiple sclerosis, dysequilibrium and unsteadiness are common in most of these patients at some point in their disease.

SUGGESTED READINGS

Aran JM. Current perspectives on inner ear toxicity. *Otolaryngol Head Neck Surg.* 1995;112:133.

Bachor E, Just T, Wright CG, et al. Fixation of the stapes footplate in children: a clinical and temporal bone histopathologic study. *Otol Neurotol.* 2005; 26:866.

Berlinger NT, Koutroupas S, Adams G, et al. Patterns of involvement of the temporal bone in metastatic and systemic malignancy. *Laryngoscope.* 1980;90:619.

Brihaye P, Halama AR. Fluctuating hearing loss in sarcoidosis. *Acta Otorhinolaryngol Belg.* 1993;47:23.

Brodie HA, Thompson TC. Management of complications from 820 temporal bone fractures. *Am J Otol.* 1997;18:188.

Butman JA, Kim HJ, Baggenstos M, et al. Mechanisms of morbid hearing loss associated with tumors of the endolymphatic sac in von Hippel-Lindau disease. *JAMA.* 2007;298:41.

Commins DJ, Chen JM. Multiple sclerosis: a consideration in acute cranial nerve palsies. *Am J Otol.* 1997;18:590.

Ferguson BJ, Wilkins RH, Hudson W, et al. Spontaneous CSF otorrhea from tegmen and posterior fossa defects. *Laryngoscope.* 1986;96:635.

Fortnum HM. Hearing impairment after bacterial meningitis: a review. *Arch Dis Child.* 1992;67:1128.

Gacek RR, Gacek MR, Tart R. Adult spontaneous cerebrospinal fluid otorrhea: diagnosis and management. *Am J Otol.* 1999;20:770.

Gorlin RJ, Toriello HV, Cohen MM, eds. *Hereditary Hearing Loss and Its Syndromes.* New York: Oxford University Press; 1995.

Gulya AJ. Neurologic paraneoplastic syndromes with neurotologic manifestations. *Laryngoscope.* 1993;103:754.

Hariri MA. Sensorineural hearing loss in bullous myringitis: a prospective study of eighteen patients. *Clin Otolaryngol.* 1990;15:351.

Jackler RK, Luxford WM, House WF. Congenital malformations of the inner ear: a classification based on embryogenesis. *Laryngoscope.* 1987;97(Suppl 40):2.

Lambert PR, Dodson EE. Congenital malformations of the external auditory canal. *Otolaryngol Clin North Am.* 1996;29:741.

McDonald TJ, Vollertsen RS, Younge BR. Cogan's syndrome: audiovestibular involvement and prognosis in 18 patients. *Laryngoscope.* 1985;95:650.

Ndiaye IC, Rassi SJ, Wiener-Vacher SR. Cochleovestibular impairment in pediatric Cogan's syndrome. *Pediatrics.* 2002;109:E38.

Oas JG, Baloh RW. Vertigo and the anterior inferior cerebellar artery syndrome. *Neurology.* 1992;42:2274.

Saw VP, Canty PA, Green CM, et al. Susac syndrome: microangiopathy of the retina, cochlea and brain. *Clin Exp Ophthalmol.* 2000;28:373.

Schaefer GB. Ten syndromes most commonly associated with hearing impairment. *Natl Inst Deafness Commun Disord.* 1995;2:1.

Seltzer S, McCabe BF. Perilymph fistula: the Iowa experience. *Laryngoscope.* 1986;94:37.

Skedros DG, Cass SP, Hirsch BE, et al. Beta-s transferrin assay in clinical management of cerebral spinal fluid and perilymphatic fluid leaks. *J Otolaryngol.* 1993;22:341.

Stoney P, Kwok P, Hawke M. Granular myringitis: a review. *J Otolaryngol.* 1992;21:129.

Wolf B, Spencer R, Gleason T. Hearing loss is a common feature of symptomatic children with profound biotinidase deficiency. *J Pediatr.* 2002;140:242.

Zeifer B, Sabini P, Sonne J. Congenital absence of the oval window: radiologic diagnosis and associated anomalies. *AJNR Am J Neuroradiol.* 2000;21:322.

For complete list of references log onto www.expertconsult.com.

Auditory Prosthetic Stimulation, Devices, and Rehabilitative Audiology

CHAPTER ONE HUNDRED AND FIFTY-SEVEN

Implantable Hearing Aids

Lawrence R. Lustig

Charles C. Della Santina

Key Points

- Limitations of conventional hearing aids compared with newer implantable hearing aids include insufficient amplification, acoustic feedback, distortion of spectral shape and phase shifts, nonlinear sound distortion, occlusion effects, poor auditory transduction, and cosmetic appearance. Abnormalities in the ear canal also prevent the use of a conventional hearing aid.
- All middle ear implantable hearing aids include a transducer (either piezoelectric or electromagnetic) and couple to one of the three middle ear bones in one of many ways to drive the ossicular chain directly. Some newer designs also couple directly to the round window.
- Economic factors have limited the availability of middle ear implantable hearing aids in the United States; there is more widespread application in Europe.
- Bone-anchored hearing aids are useful for patients with conductive hearing loss who cannot use a conventional hearing aid for a variety of reasons, including patients with chronically draining ears despite multiple corrective attempts, patients with discomfort from the sound levels required from a traditional hearing aid, and patients with a large mastoid bowl or meatoplasty.
- Bone-anchored hearing aids are beneficial in patients with otosclerosis, tympanosclerosis, or canal atresia, and in patients who have undergone external auditory canal closure after extensive skull base surgery.
- Patients with unilateral deafness benefit from a bone-anchored hearing aid through improved hearing in noise, although objective evidence of improved sound localization is unavailable.

Hearing aids are the principal means of auditory rehabilitation for patients with sensorineural hearing loss (SNHL). Hearing aids may also play a role in the management of patients with conductive hearing losses (CHL), particularly losses that result from pathologies that are not amenable to medical and surgical treatment. Improvements in signal processing capabilities and increasing miniaturization of hearing aids have increased their acceptance among patients. Hearing aids remain a "tough sell" to many patients who could potentially benefit from them, however, owing to lack of sufficient perceived benefit, expense, complications of external auditory canal occlusion, and cosmetic concerns. In a restaurant, multiple competing sound sources, such as conversations, the ventilation system, and music, can undermine the ability to detect and resolve speech cues. Many other patients simply cannot wear a hearing aid because of problems with the external auditory canal, chronic infections, or extreme discomfort. Although newer hearing aid technologies have tried to address many of these difficulties, many patients still find that hearing aids fall short in meeting expectations in a variety of situations (Box 157-1). Partly for these reasons, less than one in eight eligible adults actually use a hearing aid.[1]

These inherent limitations in hearing aids, combined with the social stigma of their use, have led to the development of implantable hearing aids (Figs. 157-1 and 157-2). Implantable hearing aids offer patients with hearing loss several potential advantages over conventional hearing aids, including increased gain and dynamic range, reduced feedback, reduced maintenance, improved appearance, and freedom from ear canal occlusion. These potential benefits must be weighed against the possible downsides of their use, including the risk of surgical implantation, difficulty of maintenance, and increased initial device cost (Table 157-1). Complicating this risk-benefit calculation is the uncertain future of corporations marketing and supporting various implantable hearing aids. Before discussing each of the implantable hearing aids currently available or in development, it is important to review in more detail *why* there is a desire for their implementation in the first place.

Limitations of Auditory Rehabilitation Using Traditional Hearing Aids

Physical Factors

Traditional hearing aids are limited in their ability to amplify sound without imparting distortion or generating feedback, in part because these three aspects of performance are physically interrelated.

Insufficient Gain

For patients with severe to profound hearing loss, sound amplification (or *gain*) is a primary concern. For a patient with air-conduction thresholds of 80 dB hearing level (HL) to perceive quiet sounds at a normal threshold of 0 dB HL, a hearing aid must amplify sound intensity by 80 dB, generating a 10,000-fold increase in sound pressure wave amplitude and a 100,000,000-fold increase in sound power intensity.[2] This represents the limit of existing traditional hearing aids. The maximum amplification at 1 kHz for a behind-the-ear (BTE) Phonak SuperFront PPCL4 power digital hearing aid is about 75 to 82 dB.[3] Gain generally scales with hearing aid size, so that cosmetically less

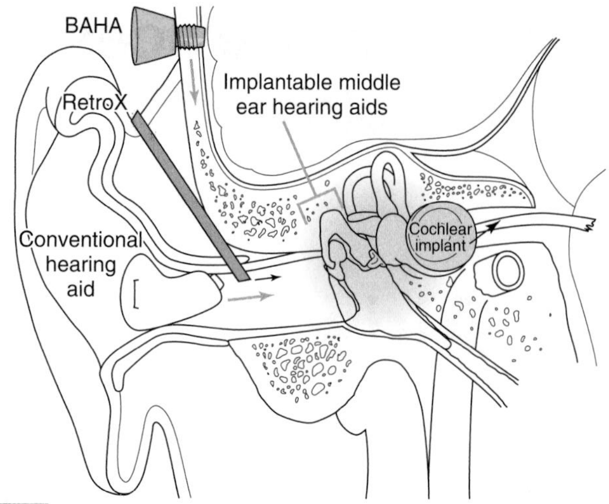

Figure 157-1. Overview of how various implantable hearing aids interface with the auditory system. Conventional hearing aids amplify from within the canal, whereas bone-anchored conductive devices are applied to the retroauricular skull to provide hearing via bone conduction. The RetroX sits behind the ear, but delivers sound through a channel that emerges in the external auditory canal. Implantable middle ear hearing aids interface at the level of the ossicles, bypassing the eardrum. In contrast, cochlear implants directly stimulate the remaining neural elements within the cochlea. BAHA, bone-anchored hearing device. *(Adapted from Nikolas Blevins, MD.)*

Box 157-1

Nonideal Features of Conventional Aids

- Insufficient amplification
- Acoustic feedback
- Spectral distortion
- Nonlinear/harmonic distortion
- Occlusion of external auditory canal
- Appearance/visibility
- Lack of directionality

obtrusive hearing aids offer less gain. The maximum gains for digital in-the-ear (ITE), in-the-canal (ITC), and completely-in-canal (CIC) hearing aids currently are about 55 to 65 dB, 45 to 55 dB, and 35 to 50 dB.[3]

Acoustic Feedback

In practice, feedback often limits the useful gain of traditional hearing aids to less than the above-listed maximum gains. Acoustic waves from the hearing aid speaker leak through the air space between the hearing aid body and the external auditory canal wall back to the microphone, where (for a subset of frequencies) they add to existing microphone input and are amplified further. The resulting positive feedback loop causes the familiar squealing and hum that signify a poorly fitting or overamplified aid. Potential for feedback is worst for CIC aids, in which the microphone is closest to the speaker, and for ears with mastoid bowls, in which an air seal is difficult to obtain. At very high amplification, it is a problem even for BTE aids. Fitting aids tightly into the external auditory canal can decrease feedback, but at the cost of increased discomfort, and the risk of otitis externa, autophony, and blockage of natural sound input.

Distortion of Spectral Shape and Phase Shifts

Traditional hearing aids are limited in the frequency range over which they amplify sound. Most are optimized for performance in the speech band (500 to 2000 Hz) and cannot provide much amplification at less than 100 to 200 Hz or greater than 5000 to 6000 Hz. Although the most important spectral components for speech recognition are amplified, the loss of "bass" and "treble" can give the resultant sound percept an artificial character. Isolated severe hearing loss at low frequencies (e.g., in Meniere's disease) or high frequencies (e.g., in presbycusis or ototoxic exposure) can be difficult to remediate with traditional hearing aids without overamplifying the midrange frequencies at which a patient may have normal hearing. Even in the 500- to 2000-Hz band, steep changes in audiometric threshold at neighboring frequencies (e.g., noise-induced hearing loss) cannot be perfectly fit because of inherent limitations in the rate of change of gain across frequencies. Too steep a change in amplifier gain across frequencies typically imparts phase shifts that distort sound percepts such as pitch and timbre. Digital signal processing technology has greatly improved spectral shaping options compared with analog aids, but these fundamental limitations persist.

Nonlinear Distortion

Similar to most other amplifiers, hearing aids are designed under assumption of linearity—that is, if a given sound input at the microphone leads to some output at the speaker (amplified and spectrally shaped by the aid), doubling the sound input's magnitude should exactly double the output, without changes in spectral content or phase shifts. For high-intensity speaker output, this assumption breaks down as the speaker is driven into the range of movements for which it begins to saturate or clip. An input sinusoid can appear at the output as a waveform with blunted peaks. This nonlinear distortion imparts aberrant spectral components into the sound percept, giving it an artificial or robotic character. Although digital signal processing can mitigate distortion effects within an aid's amplification circuitry, distortion produced by a speaker generating loud sounds in air remains a fundamental limitation of traditional hearing aids.

Occlusion Effects

To minimize feedback, most traditional hearing aids are fit to create an airtight seal with the external auditory canal wall, with the hearing aid's speaker being isolated in the occluded ear canal. Canal occlusion has several undesirable effects. First, it can be uncomfortable because of pressure on canal skin. Second, it increases the likelihood of otitis externa because of disturbance of wax egress and air circulation. Some patients with chronic suppurative otitis media cannot tolerate hearing aids because of exacerbation of otorrhea. Third, it causes autophony and a sense of aural fullness that can worsen with changes in ambient barometric pressure. Fourth, it blocks the normal pathway for sound entry to the ear. Finally, canal occlusion disrupts the spectral shaping that normally occurs as a result of external auditory canal resonances.

Poor Appearance

Many patients reject hearing aids because of the social stigma of being seen as old or infirm. Eight percent of hearing aid candidates wearing the less noticeable ITC hearing aids listed poor cosmetic appearance as a major contributing factor in their decision not to use a hearing aid.[4] Hearing aids are difficult to conceal in patients who are balding or who wear their hair short. Miniaturization of electronics continues to improve hearing aids in this regard, and CIC hearing aids are essentially invisible to the casual observer. Miniaturization comes at the cost of lower gain, more feedback, and higher cost, however. Ultimately, battery size becomes the limiting factor, with smaller batteries costing more and requiring more frequent replacement.

Poor Transduction Efficiency

Loss of energy because of impedance mismatching and transduction losses is another inherent drawback of conventional hearing aids. The mechanical impedance (change in pressure for a given displacement flow) of the air-filled external auditory canal differs from that of the fluid-filled cochlea. Without a middle ear mechanism, most of the acoustic energy striking the stapes footplate reflects back into the air. When the tympanic membrane and ossicular chain are functioning normally, they act as an impedance-matching transformer by virtue of

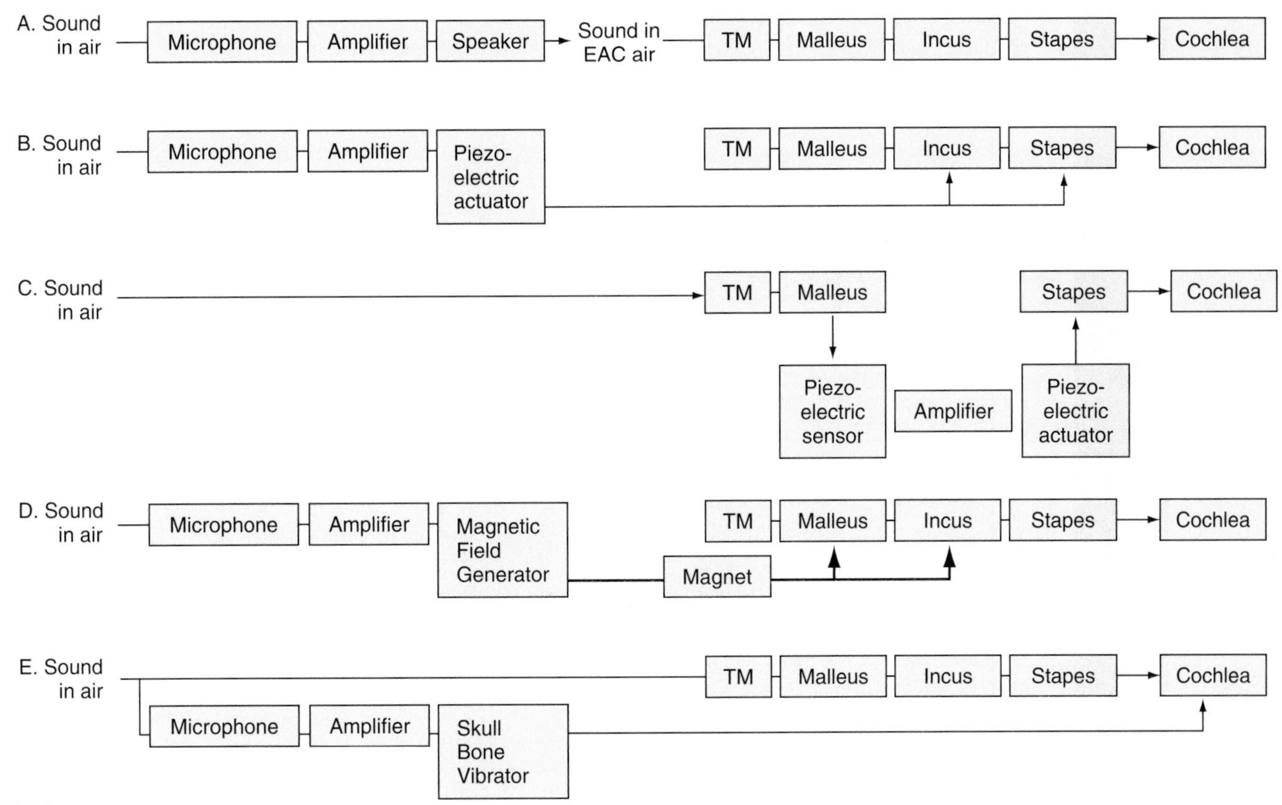

Figure 157-2. Sound transduction and coupling to the auditory system for different classes of hearing aids. **A,** Conventional air-conducting hearing aid. **B,** Implantable aids with piezoelectric actuator (e.g., Rion-E, Otologics MET, and Implex TICA). **C,** Implantable aids with piezoelectric sensor and actuator (e.g., St. Croix Envoy). **D,** Implantable aids with magnetic actuator (e.g., Vibrant Med-El Soundbridge, Soundtec DDHS). **E,** Bone-anchored hearing aid (e.g., Cochlear/Entific BAHA). EAC, external auditory canal; TM, tympanic membrane.

the relative areas of the tympanic membrane and stapes footplate, and by the lever action of the ossicular chain.[5] The relatively large-displacement, low-pressure movements of air against the tympanic membrane are transduced to the relatively small-displacement, high-pressure movements of the footplate. Except for bone-conducting hearing aids, all traditional hearing aids use a speaker to output an (amplified) acoustic wave into the air of the external auditory canal. When this middle ear apparatus is malfunctioning, as occurs in otosclerosis, tympanic membrane perforation, or a canal wall down mastoidectomy, traditional hearing aids must overcome the impedance mismatch. The result is reduced effective gain, increased distortion, or both.

Even when the ossicular chain is functioning normally, the transduction of acoustic energy from air at the input of a traditional hearing aid to stapes footplate motion is imperfect. Whenever a signal flows from one physical realm (e.g., electric current in a speaker) to another (e.g., acoustic waves in air), some energy is lost (e.g., to heat) and noise or distortion can add to the desired signal. There are several transduction steps for a traditional hearing aid—from acoustic waves in ambient air, to electric current in a microphone, to a larger electrical current in a speaker wire or piezoelectric driver, to acoustic waves in air within the external auditory canal, to movement of the tympanic membrane and ossicular chain, to acoustic waves in perilymph, to hair cell stereociliary deflection and depolarization. Most steps are unavoidable (although cochlear implants bypass these steps through direct cochlear nerve stimulation). Directly coupling a hearing aid actuator movement of the ossicular chain can delete some of these transduction steps, however, boosting gain and reducing distortion. Nearly all implantable hearing aids make use of this approach.

Human Factors

Although not specific to traditional hearing aids, SNHL imposes additional constraints on the degree to which sound amplification can overcome hearing deficits. These factors must be considered when evaluating whether technical improvements such as increased amplification gain are worth pursuing for a given patient.

Recruitment and Compression of Dynamic Range

A primary source of frustration of patients with SNHL is reduced speech intelligibility. The common complaint, "I can hear, but I cannot understand," underscores this point. This problem relates to abnormal frequency resolution and aberrant patterns of growth in loudness, each of which reduces speech intelligibility in challenging listening conditions such as noisy surroundings.[6,7]

SNHL also imposes severe constraints on the dynamic range of perceived sound. For normal listeners, the dynamic range from sensing soft sounds to the loudest tolerable noise is more than 100 dB. Within this wide dynamic range of hearing lies an approximately 35-dB dynamic range of conversational speech. In contrast, the dynamic range of patients with SNHL is often narrowed by an increase in the threshold of audibility and a lowering of the ceiling of tolerance to high-intensity sounds. This compaction of dynamic range leads to "recruitment," an abnormal growth in loudness as sound intensity increases.[8,9] What sounds normal for someone with normal hearing may be too soft for someone with recruitment, whereas what is too loud for someone with normal hearing is *also* too loud for a patient with recruitment. In effect, there is a much narrower range of sound intensity that a patient with recruitment can tolerate. Further adding to the difficulty, recruitment is observed in frequencies that are most impaired, in the high frequencies, which also carry crucial information for speech understanding.

Recruitment remains one of the principal challenges of hearing aid rehabilitation, and is responsible for a common phenomenon most clinicians dealing with hearing loss have witnessed or experienced: At average speaking levels, an individual with recruitment may ask a speaker to talk more loudly, yet with even a slight increase in intensity the speech becomes intolerably loud, and the speaker is told not to

Table 157-1

Comparison of Implantable and Nonimplantable Hearing Aids

Device (Manufacturer)	Sensor	Actuator	Regulatory Approval	Totally/Partially Implanted	Surgical Placement	Audiologic Indications	MRI	Special Advantages/ Disadvantages	EAC Occlusion
Envoy (St. Croix Medical, Intl., St. Paul, MN)	Piezoelectric, coupled to malleus/ TM	Piezoelectric, to stapes	In clinical trials	Total	Transmastoid, mandatory incus removal	Figure 157-9		Very high power; requires incus removal	No
MET Middle Ear Transducer (Otologics, LLC, Boulder, CO)	Piezoelectric, coupled to malleus	Piezoelectric, to incus	FDA clinical trials Phase 2	Partial	Transmastoid	Moderate to severe		High-powered output; fully implantable; ossicles remain intact; adjustable for ossicular abnormalities	No
Vibrant Soundbridge (Vibrant-Med-El, Innsbruck, Austria*)	External BTE microphone	Magnetic, clipped to incus	Approved, U.S. FDA and CE Mark	Partial	Transmastoid and endaural	Figure 157-4		First FDA approved, largest install base	No
Bone-anchored device (BAHA) (Cochlear Corp., Lane Cove, Australia)	External microphone	Electromagnetic vibrator, coupled to titanium screw in skull	Approved, U.S. FDA and CE Mark	Partial	Cortical skull bone screw	CHL unable to tolerate conventional HA	+	Simple placement, nothing in ear or mastoid	No
RetroX (Auric Hearing Systems, Rheine, Germany)	External BTE microphone	Acoustic, to TM	Approved U.S. FDA and CE Mark	Partial	Transconcha	Mild to severe CHL or SNHL	+	Noninvasive placement; acoustic coupling	Yes
Conventional Digital BTE (many manufacturers)	External BTE microphone	Acoustic, to TM	Yes	NA	NA	Mild to severe CHL or SNHL	NA	No surgery required; visible, EAC occlusion	Yes
Conventional Digital CIC (many manufacturers)	External microphone at lateral end of CIC device	Acoustic, to TM	Yes	NA	NA	Mild to moderate CHL or SNHL	NA		

*Symphonix Devices, Inc., San Jose, CA, until 2003.

BTE, behind-the-ear; CHL, conductive hearing loss; CIC, completely-in-canal; EAC, external auditory canal; HA, hearing aid; MRI, magnetic resonance imaging; NA, not applicable; SNHL, sensorineural hearing loss; TM, tympanic membrane.

shout. Although many hearing aids can be programmed to prevent sound from amplifying into a range that is uncomfortable, even the most advanced aids cannot fully replicate the complex, nonlinear response patterns of a healthy cochlea.[9]

Disordered Perception of Pitch and Sound Localization

Another challenge faced by conventional hearing aids relates to impaired pitch resolution and sound localization. Although simple amplification strategies can compensate for this loss of sensitivity, they do little to restore the exquisite selectivity of the cochlea in organizing pitch information. Much of the benefit provided by the normal auditory system is based on the presence of two ears that independently sample the acoustic environment and send this information to the brain for comparison and analysis. Sound detection is an important first step in hearing, and can be performed reasonably well by one sensitive ear. There is significant additional auditory benefit, however, when sound input occurs through both ears. When only one ear functions, or when there is a drastic difference in hearing levels between ears, the ability to locate the source of sound decreases, as does suppression of background echoes and the ability to "block out" background noise.

All of the aforementioned factors play a role to various degrees in patients, and combine to increase the noncompliance rate in hearing aid users. For most patients, these are the principal reasons why hearing aids are unacceptable.[10] With all these challenges concerning conventional hearing aids, it is not surprising that many hearing aid users feel frustrated when hearing aids fail to perform to expectations.

Promise of Implantable Hearing Aids

The limitations of traditional air-conduction hearing aids have constituted the driving force behind the new generation of implantable hearing aids. Can implantable hearing aids solve these difficult challenges? Implantable hearing aids face most of these same challenges, but also have the added obstacle of requiring surgery for their placement, and being potentially much more costly. Their appeal includes the possibility of improved signal-to-noise ratios, greater amplification/gain potential, invisibility, loss of distortion and feedback, getting the aid out of the canal with the associated occlusion effect, greater dynamic range, and improved cosmetics. For some patients who simply cannot wear a hearing aid because of underlying medical problems or extreme discomfort, implantable hearing aids may be the only option.

It is widely accepted that implantable hearing aids should provide distinct advantages over conventional hearing aids, including better cosmetics, improved fidelity, broader frequency response, less distortion, reduction or elimination of feedback, and better speech understanding, without reducing residual hearing, limiting patient activities, or predisposing patients to infection.[11,12] In other words, implantable hearing aids should be at least as good as, and preferably better than, the best available noninvasive method of hearing rehabilitation: binaural amplification with the best available aid.[13]

Although significant strides have been made in many of these areas, implantable hearing aids have yet to deliver on all these features. There also remain questions regarding candidacy for implantation and willingness of patients to accept the costs and surgical risks. As noted by Junker and colleagues,[14] the number of patients in a fairly typical population of hearing-impaired individuals who would be considered realistic candidates is limited, on the order of 0.09%. The market for implantable hearing aids may not be sufficiently large to support the current array of device manufacturers. The 2002 financial failing of Symphonix Corp., the first company to gain U.S. Food and Drug Administration (FDA) approval and market their implantable middle ear hearing aid in the United States, strongly underscores this point, as do the subsequent withdrawal of the Soundtec and TICA devices described subsequently in the review of technologies.

The focus of the remainder of this chapter is on critical reviews of the advantages and disadvantages of each of the implantable hearing aids that are either in development or already in clinical use. A different type of implantable hearing aid, the bone-anchored hearing aid (BAHA), is widely used in hearing rehabilitation for some very specific indications, and this also is discussed.

Middle Ear Implants

Basic Design Features

Transducer Design

Conventional hearing aids function by receiving acoustic energy through a microphone, processing and amplifying the signal (in either an analog or a digital fashion), and transmitting the signal through a speaker adjacent to the eardrum. This amplified sound travels through the normal auditory pathway of the tympanic membrane and ossicles to the inner ear. Implantable middle ear hearing aids also employ a microphone that senses sounds and a signal processor that amplifies and alters the sound signal, just as in a conventional hearing aid. From here, they differ from conventional hearing aids. In one of several mechanisms unique to each device, the implantable middle ear hearing aids convert the electric signal into a mechanical energy that is coupled directly to the ossicular chain (see Fig. 157-1).The critical components of these systems are the transducer, which enables the device to output a signal that can be received by the ossicles, and the mechanism by which the transducer is coupled to the ossicles, which can either be a direct or indirect contact.[15] Variations in these critical components distinguish the various implant designs (see Fig. 157-2). Goode and colleagues[11] previously outlined the history of the development of implantable middle ear hearing aids.

Two basic types of transducers have been incorporated into middle ear implantable hearing aids: *piezoelectric* and *electromagnetic*. Piezoelectric implantable hearing aids function by connecting the ossicles to an amplifier using a piezoelectric crystal vibrator. Piezoelectric materials are dielectric materials with coupled electrical and mechanical properties. Applying a voltage across an appropriately designed piezoelectric rod causes it to bend or lengthen, with a predictable change in deflection based on the voltage applied. Within the implant, sounds picked up by a microphone are converted by the signal processor to an electrical signal, and sent to the piezoelectric rod. As this rod vibrates in response to the converted auditory signal, it lies in direct contact with the ossicles. In this manner, sound waves are transferred directly to the ossicles, which travel along the normal auditory pathway. A critical feature of implants that use a piezoelectric transducer is direct contact between the piezoelectric unit and the ossicles.

Implantable middle ear hearing aids may also incorporate an electromagnetic transducer. These transducers generate a magnetic field using a coil carrying a current that encodes the microphone output. This magnetic field from the coil can cause motion in a ferromagnetic substance that is nearby, causing it to vibrate.[15] As applied to middle ear implants, sound received from a microphone is converted by the signal processor, amplified, and sent to the electromagnetic transducer. The electromagnetic field that is set up vibrates a ferromagnetic unit coupled directly to the ossicles. In contrast to the piezoelectric unit that must be in direct contact with the ossicles, electromagnetic transducers need only to be near the ossicles, which have attached to them the ferromagnetic device that transmits the auditory signal to the ossicles.

These two types of amplification have different advantages for use in an implantable hearing aid. Electromagnetic transducers do not directly contact the ossicular chain, but rely on electromagnetic transmission to a ferromagnetic unit that is attached to the ossicles. Electromagnetic transducers can be packaged in a smaller housing, an important factor in the ear. In contrast, piezoelectric devices are larger and couple directly to the ossicular chain. The advantage of this type of transducer is its ability to deliver more distortion-free amplification directly to the ossicular chain.[15] In either event, to accommodate patients with moderate to severe SNHL in the 55- to 90-dB hearing level range, any implant, whether electromechanical or piezoelectric, should be able to deliver a maximum mechanical stimulation output equivalent to 120 to 130 dB sound pressure level (SPL).[16,17] How each implant achieves this output level is described subsequently.

Ossicular Coupling

As noted by Huttenbrink,[18] to obtain optimal efficiency in implantable hearing aids, they must adapt to the mechanics of the middle ear and ossicular chain. As the third ossicle in the chain, and the one in conti-

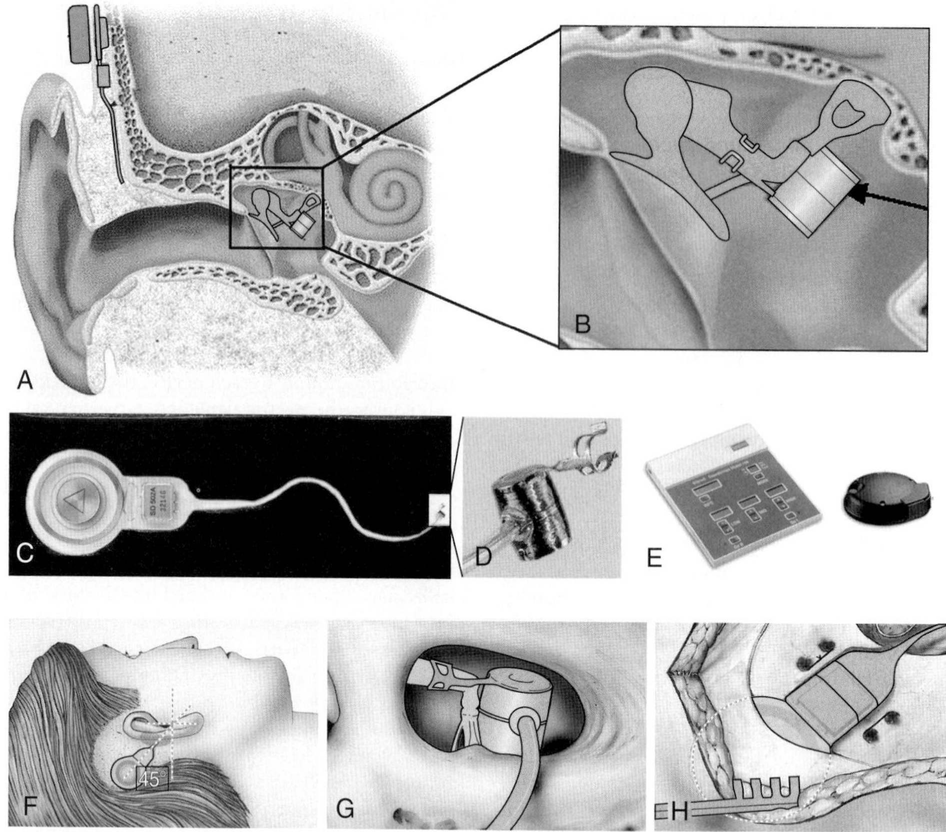

Figure 157-3. **A-H,** Med-El Vibrant Soundbridge semi-implantable hearing aid. **A** and **B,** External microphone couples via an inductive transcutaneous link to the actuator, a vibrating ossicular prosthesis (VORP) that couples to the incus long process **(B)**. **C,** Implanted component of device. **D,** VORP actuator. **E,** Programming unit and external circuitry. **F-G,** Inductive link is implanted against retromastoid cortical bone, similar to a cochlear implant **(F** and **H)**. VORP is clipped to the incus via a facial recess approach **(G)**.

nuity with the inner ear, the motion of the stapes is crucial in sound transmission. The stapes moves in a piston-like fashion.[19] The ideal motion of the stapes by a prosthesis would be in this piston-like fashion. Any implant that directly attached to the stapes would function best by mimicking this motion.[20,21]

Various implants employ numerous ways to couple vibration stimuli to the inner ear. Some employ a piezoelectric transducer to contact either the stapes head directly (e.g., St. Croix Envoy/Esteem-Hearing Implant) or the incus body (e.g., Implex TICA). Others use an electromagnetic transducer typically attached to the incus (e.g., Med-El Vibrant Soundbridge, Otologics Carina/MET), but sometimes adapted to contact the stapes capitulum, stapes footplate, or round window membrane. Others clip to the incudostapedial joint (e.g., Soundtec Direct Drive System). Each of these systems is described in greater detail individually.

Total versus Partially Implantable Hearing Aids

Implantable middle ear hearing devices may be either totally or partially implantable. Partially implantable devices consist of an external microphone and speech processor that are connected to a transmitter with an external coil that transmits electrical energy transcutaneously to the internal device, in much the same way cochlear implants are now powered. The battery-powered system is contained within the external device, decreasing the size of the implanted component. The internal device consists of an internal receiving coil, which provides electric energy to the mechanical driver connected to the ossicular chain.

In contrast, the fully implantable systems house all of the above-mentioned components within the implanted portion of the device, including the battery pack. Although the size and complexity of the implanted components are increased, the visibility of the device is reduced, a feature that is desirable among hearing aid users. Because of the finite life of the rechargeable batteries, the totally implantable designs employed in clinical settings so far require reoperation at approximately 5-year intervals to exchange the spent device with one containing a new battery.

Electromagnetic Middle Ear Implantable Hearing Aids

Vibrant Soundbridge

To date, the implantable middle ear hearing aid with the most clinical data is the Vibrant Soundbridge, manufactured by Symphonix Corporation until 2002, when Symphonix was dissolved and the Vibrant technology was bought and later re-released by a subsidiary of the Med-El Corporation (Innsbruck, Austria), which resumed Vibrant Soundbridge sales in 2004. Because it was the first commercially available, FDA-approved middle ear hearing aid, a thorough review of this device is instructive.

The Vibrant Soundbridge is a semi-implantable hearing aid that was first introduced in 1997 (Fig. 157-3). Since its introduction in 1997, more than 2300 patients have been implanted worldwide.[14] The device was approved for commercial availability in Europe in 1998, and in the United States in 2000. The electromagnetic transducer uses a proprietary vibrating ossicular prosthesis (VORP), which typically is attached to the long process of the incus. The VORP contains a rare earth magnet surrounded by a receiving coil, a demodulator package, a conductor link, and a proprietary floating mass transducer (FMT).[22,23] The transducer was developed by Ball, and incorporated prior conceptual work performed by Goode and colleagues.[11,22,24] The VORP is electrically connected to the internal receiver.[25] These internal components are coupled to the audio processor via a telemetry link, similar to a cochlear implant. The processor, which is worn behind the ear, contains the microphone, audio processing electronics, magnet, telemetry transmission equipment, and room for a standard 675 zinc battery to power the implant.

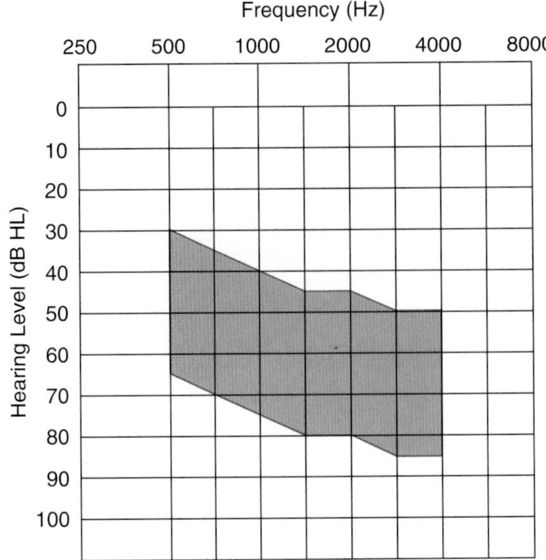

Soundbridge Clinical Indications:
Pure-tone air-conduction thresholds within selection criteria
Normal middle ear anatomy
Word recognition score of ≥50% using recorded material
Absence of retrocochlear or central involvement
≥18 years old

Figure 157-4. Audiologic selection criteria for the Soundbridge. The Soundbridge is indicated in patients with moderate to severe sensorineural hearing loss of 70 dB pure-tone average hearing thresholds. The shaded area of the figure corresponds to the pure-tone audiometric implant criteria.

The function of the externally worn processor is similar to a conventional hearing aid. Sound is picked up by the microphone and processed by the external receiver by the electronics. The signal is sent via telemetry to the internal receiver. From here it is sent to the demodulator, which provides a safety feature to limit maximum power output and prevent overstimulation. The demodulator generates a current encoding the sound, and this current travels to the FMT, causing the FMT to vibrate through inductive interaction with the magnet. Because the FMT is firmly attached to the incus using a titanium clip, amplified sound is transmitted directly to the ossicular chain. Because the FMT includes a magnetic component, implantation of this device prevents a patient from undergoing magnetic resonance imaging (MRI) without device removal.

The Vibrant Soundbridge is indicated in patients with moderate to severe SNHL and desire for an alternative to an acoustic hearing aid (Fig. 157-4).[23] Studies have indicated that it may be suitable for patients with hearing loss of 70 dB pure-tone average (PTA) hearing thresholds.[26] When first introduced, the externally worn audio processor was an analog device that incorporated a wide dynamic range compression. Because of inadequate gain of the device, particularly at lower frequencies and with low sound levels,[27] a newer, more powerful digital audio processor was introduced in 1999. Studies done shortly after its introduction failed to show superior hearing results compared with conventional aids, although patients preferred the device, in part because of ability to wear it for a much longer time without discomfort.[26]

The device typically is implanted using a standard transmastoid, facial recess approach to the middle ear. The VORP is crimped into the long process of the incus. The internal receiver is placed in a bony trough in the retrosigmoid bone several centimeters behind the ear, in a location similar to the receiver placed during cochlear implantation. One potential drawback of this design concerns the size of the VORP. Because of the confined space between the eardrum and the incus, the dimensions and mass of the FMT are limited, restricting its output.[28] A second potential drawback is erosion of the incus long process, owing to ischemia at the clip attachment site. Modifications of the typical surgical approach allow treatment of mixed hearing losses resulting from otosclerosis or ossicular erosion or agenesis through direct placement of the VORP on the stapes superstructure, round window, or oval window.[29-32]

Owing to its primacy in regulatory approval processes and patient availability, to date more clinical data are available for the Vibrant Soundbridge than for all other middle ear implants. Results from the phase III clinical trial of 53 patients were sufficiently favorable to merit FDA approval of the device (phase I trials typically test feasibility and safety in a small group of subjects, phase II trials typically test effectiveness in a slightly larger group, and phase III trials assess safety and effectiveness in a large group).[23] Patients in the study were analyzed with conventional analog hearing aids, digital hearing aids, and the Vibrant Soundbridge. Standard audiologic tests included pure-tone air-conduction and bone-conduction thresholds (250 to 8000 Hz), functional gain, speech recognition tests, the Profile of Hearing Aid Performance, and the Hearing Device Satisfaction Scale.

Although one patient had a shift of 18 dB after device placement, the effect of implantation on residual, native hearing was believed not to be significant (<10 dB PTA at 500 to 2000 Hz). This finding corroborated earlier studies that showed little to no effect of the presence of the FMT on hearing sensitivity.[33] When compared with presurgical conventional hearing aid test scores, the implant showed a statistically significant improvement in functional gain at all frequencies and greater than 10 dB improvement at 2 kHz, 4 kHz, and 6 kHz. No significant difference was noted in speech recognition (NU-6 word list) between the preoperative hearing aid and the implant. On the revised speech reception in noise score, 7 patients (13%) showed significantly better scores, 70% showed no change, and 17% had worsening of their scores. As an entire group, there were no significant differences between the conventional hearing aid and implant group test scores on speech reception scores. Significant improvements were noted in the implanted group on the two self-assessment questionnaires (Profile of Hearing Aid Performance and Hearing Device Satisfaction Scale).

It seemed from the results of this phase III study that there were some objective gains in auditory scores with the implants compared with conventional hearing aids, and patient perceptions of the implant were better than conventional aids. Most of the subjective benefits of the implant centered around the ability to wear the device all day without the discomfort afforded by conventional aids.

The European experience with the Vibrant Soundbridge seems similar to the experience in the United States.[24,25,34] A multicenter study from Europe, which included 63 patients, focused on the gain provided by the implant and attempted to assess the quality of the amplified speech.[25] In contrast to the U.S. FDA phase III study, the European study did not compare results with a conventional hearing aid, but used the unaided condition as a comparison. The study noted a large variability in gain for each patient. For most patients, the greatest gain was in the 1- to 2-kHz region, where the transducer has its resonance.[22] The authors reasoned that an inefficient coupling in some patients (e.g., the FMT may be loose) may be responsible for the wide variability seen, and highlighted the importance of effective placement of the VORP on the incus.

When the authors compared gain at threshold and gain at normal speech, there was only a small difference noted (6 dB), indicating that the gain is effective at normal speech levels. The authors also concluded that the amplified sound from the Vibrant Soundbridge had adequate quality for speech intelligibility. Overall, the authors believed that there was clear benefit from the Vibrant Soundbridge, but there was a subgroup of patients with low gain, secondary to the limited bandwidth of the amplified signal. Other work from this same multicenter European group has shown a significant improvement in communication in various listening conditions with the Vibrant Soundbridge compared with conventional aids.[24,34]

A more recent report relates the Belgian experience with the Vibrant Soundbridge.[35] In a study of 13 patients, the average functional gain between 500 Hz and 4000 Hz was 30 dB, similar to prior European and American studies published. The authors noted, however, that not all of their patients studied were able to afford the best possible digital hearing aid preoperatively, and they could not adequately compare satisfaction levels. The cost of the implant is severalfold higher than for the top-of-the-line digital aids, and it is likely that these patients could not afford the implant on their own. The authors reported high satisfaction of all the users of the device, and the "impressive" functional gains, particularly at higher frequencies.

One study that has specifically addressed the functional gain of the Vibrant Soundbridge with conventional hearing aids is from Todt and associates.[36] Examining five patients first fit with an analog and then digital conventional processor, the authors compared results with a digital processor of the Vibrant Soundbridge. As with previous studies, no significant differences were noted in underlying, residual hearing as a result of implant placement. Their data showed a significant improvement of hearing compared with conventional aids in quiet (approximately 10 dB PTA), and a better functional gain in noise for the Soundbridge compared with conventional aids. Subjective outcomes of a hearing aid questionnaire (Abbreviated Profile of Hearing Aid Benefit) also showed significant improvement of the Symphonix implant compared with conventional aids. As with other studies, the greatest gains were noted in the higher frequencies.

Placement of the Vibrant Soundbridge on the round window for treatment of conductive and mixed hearing loss has become commonplace in Europe. FDA approval in the United States for this approach and indication is still under investigation in a clinical trial that started in 2008.

The Vibrant Soundbridge story provides a cautionary insight into potentially the future of all implantable hearing aids. In late 2002, before the ultimate purchase of Symphonix by Med-El Corp., the Symphonix corporate website abruptly announced dissolution of the company. The Symphonix announcement raised poignant medical and ethical questions not just for the more than 600 patients already implanted with Symphonix devices, but also for the middle ear implantable hearing aid field as a whole. When novel implantable technologies are championed by small companies dependent on venture capital for continued support of operations, the longevity of corporate support of a device must be in question. Should there arise a serious liability issue with the device in the future, would implanted patients have any recourse? In this instance, an established company (Med-El Corporation, a manufacturer of cochlear implants) bought the technology and offered to provide patient support. Would a similar bailout occur if another of the middle ear implantable hearing aid companies fails? Surgeons and patients must consider these issues before implanting a middle ear hearing aid from a company without a proven track record of product reliability and financial stability.

MET (Middle Ear Transducer) and Carina

The Otologics MET (Middle Ear Transducer) is an electromechanical middle ear hearing aid using a mechanism initially developed by a group headed by Fredrickson in collaboration with Storz Instrument Co. It is now manufactured by Otologics LLC.[16] Although the original MET (on which most data reviewed here are based) was semi-implantable, that design has been replaced by a fully implantable version marketed as the Carina (Fig. 157-5).

The MET implantable unit consists of the transducer coupled to an electronic receiver.[16,37] The transducer vibrates a probe that is in direct contact with the incus. For the semi-implantable version, two external devices were developed. The device initially used in clinical trials was a modified version of Oticon's JUMP-1 hearing aid (Oticon Inc., Copenhagen, Denmark), and comprised a BTE signal processor, microphone, amplifier, and battery. This device was attached to a transmitter coil via a short cable. A newer unit housed the transmitter coil together with the BTE components. These semi-implantable designs enabled the MET to deliver the equivalent of greater than 135 dB SPL over a frequency range of 250 to 6250 Hz.[16] This output should theoretically provide adequate gain for patients with moderate to severe SNHL.

Placement of the MET Ossicular Stimulator requires a general anesthetic and approximately a 2-hour operation (Fig. 157-6). Using a standard, postauricular approach to the mastoid cortex, the root of the zygoma, posterior canal, and linea temporalis are clearly delineated (see Fig. 157-6).[16] A limited mastoidectomy (antrostomy) is performed directly superior to the external canal and inferior to the tegmen tympani using a 6-mm bur, and extended until the incus body (approximately a 10-mm width) and head of malleus are exposed. When complete, a mounting system is attached over the opening using bone screws. The MET Ossicular Stimulator is maneuvered into the mounting system with the transducer probe tip fully retracted. A laser is used to make a small hole in the incus body to accept the probe tip. The tip is advanced into position using a micrometer screw, and ultimately becomes firmly attached to the incus from fibrous tissue. The receiver capsule and transducer electronics are placed in a recess drilled in the mastoid, similar to cochlear implant electronics.

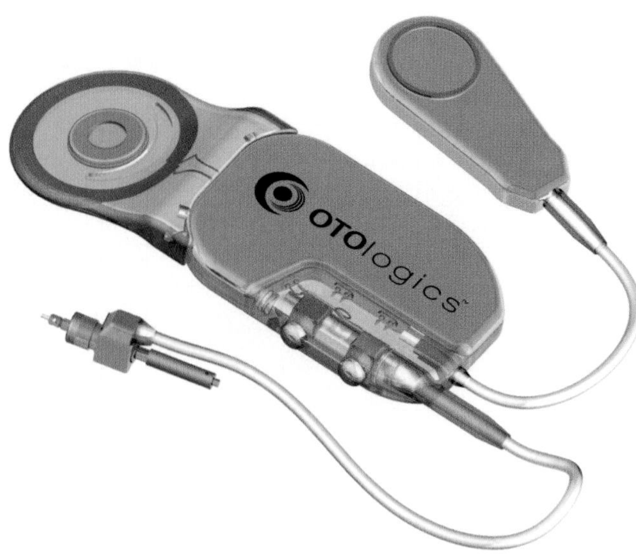

Figure 157-5. Otologics Carina fully implantable system. *(Courtesy of Otologics, LLC, Boulder, CO.)*

Ultimately, 282 patients were implanted with the semi-implantable MET in Europe and the United States during phase I and II trials.[16] Pure-tone audiometry, speech recognition, and subjective assessment of benefit were tested before the surgery and 12 months after. Group mean postoperative bone-conduction and air-conduction thresholds were not significantly changed from preoperative levels compared with a well-fit digital hearing aid used preoperatively. A slight (approximately 5 dB) increase in CHL was attributed to mass loading by the transducer on the ossicles. Sufficient gain was available to make the device useful for subjects with moderate to severe SNHL. Speech and subjective assessment of patient preference indicated that patients did as well or better with the MET compared to their "walk-in" aid or the standardized digital hearing aid (Fig. 157-7).[37]

The Otologics Carina fully implantable hearing system is similar to the original MET except that it requires no external components apart from a charger and remote.[38] It uses a subcutaneous microphone rather than an external microphone, and it is designed to work for waking hours of 1 day between charging sessions that require 1 hour. Phase I trial results in the United States showed 10 to 20 dB of functional gain across audiometric frequencies at 3 months postoperatively.[39,40] Pure-tone bone averages were minimally changed from preoperative values. Pure-tone air averages and monaural word recognition scores were initially slightly worse with the device than measured preoperatively with the walk-in aid, but patients reported greater subjective benefit with the implanted device.

Within 12 months postoperatively, a high rate of device failure was observed, leading to explantation in 5 of the 20 adult study subjects as of early 2008. Failure modes included partial device extrusion, inability to communicate to external components, and failure of the recharging mechanism. Even among devices that did not require explantation, degradation in hearing performance commonly occurred at approximately 6 months after implantation and was attributed to movement of the subcutaneous microphone. These observations led to a redesign

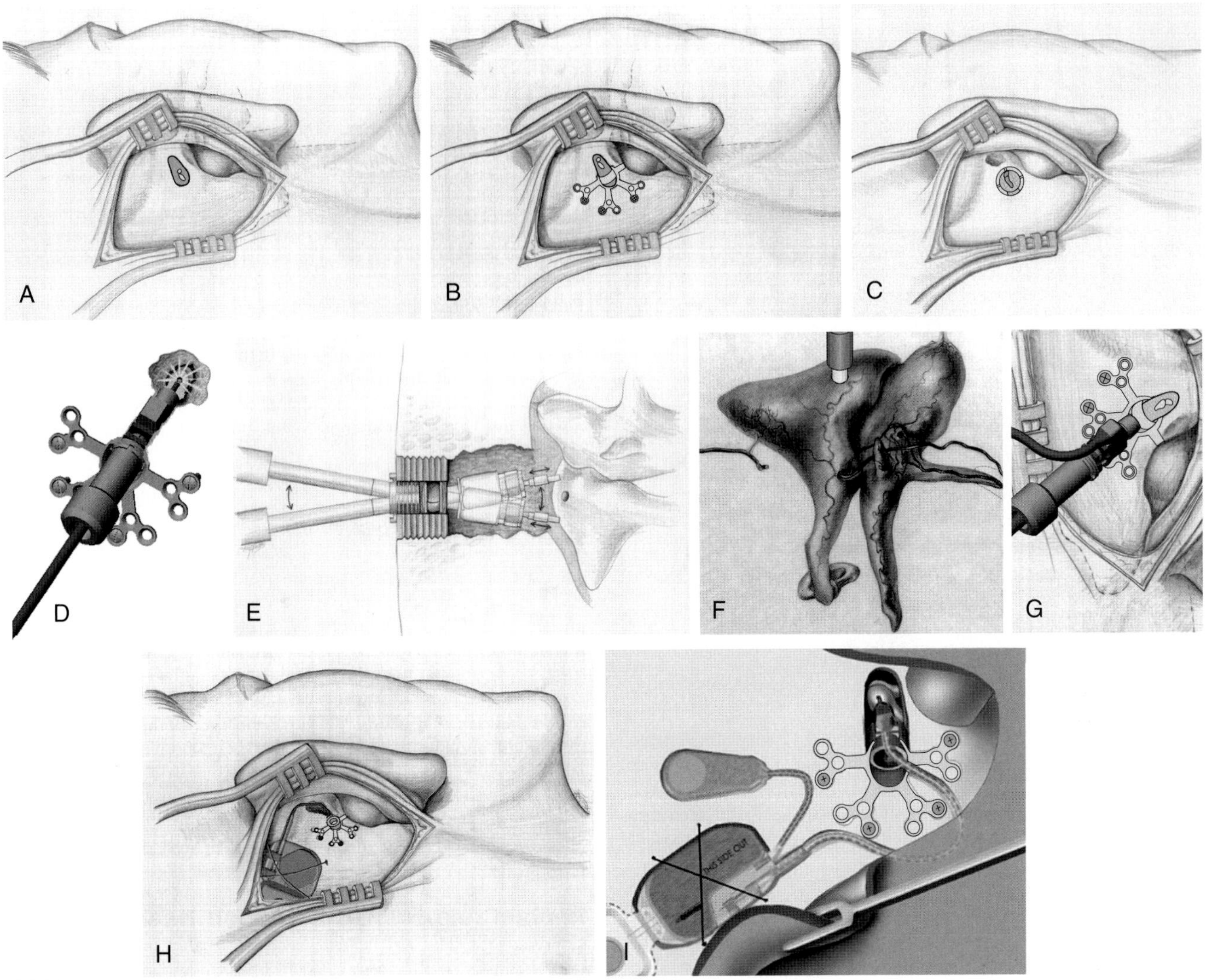

Figure 157-6. **A-I,** Surgical implantation of the Otologics MET or Carina begins with a limited antrostomy **(A)** sparing cortical bone ledges for attachment of a metallic stage **(B, C)**, which is used to steady a laser **(D)** for creation of a small hole in the posterosuperior incus **(E)**. The laser is removed and replaced with the MET actuator, the tip of which inserts into the incudotomy **(F)**. The actuator is secured to the stage **(G)**, and the remainder of the implanted device is secured to retromastoid cortical bone **(H)**. In the Carina totally implantable version of this device **(I)**, a subcutaneous microphone beneath the skin covering the mastoid replaces the external microphone and inductive link used in the MET, but the implantation procedure is otherwise similar.

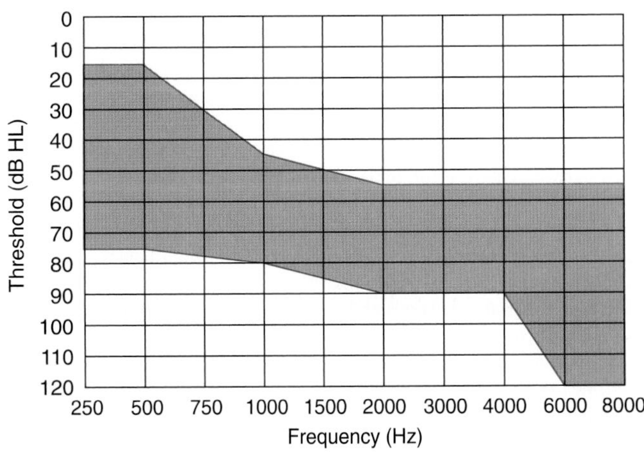

Figure 157-7. Audiologic selection criteria for Otologics MET. The shaded area of the figure corresponds to the pure-tone audiometric implant criteria.

and revision in surgical technique emphasizing creation of a well adequately deep to prevent device extrusion and a tie-down mechanism to prevent microphone migration. Intraoperative measurement and optimization of ossicular coupling compression resulted in more consistent and better coupling efficiency of the transducer to the ossicles.[41,42]

The Carina has received the CE Mark for clinical use in Europe, and phase II trials are under way in the United States. As of early 2008, more than 50 patients had been implanted with the redesigned device, and the failure modes identified during the phase I trial had not recurred.[39] Variations on the size and length of the ossicular coupling have expanded the application of the Carina to patients with aural atresia and ossicular discontinuity, via direct attachment of the device on the stapes capitulum, stapes footplate, and round window.[41,43]

Piezoelectric Middle Ear Implantable Hearing Aids

Esteem-Hearing Implant

A piezoelectric bimorph placed on the malleus head can effectively use the tympanic membrane as a microphone, offering a viable alternative to a subcutaneously implanted microphone. Studies in cadaveric temporal bones have shown that such a device had a dynamic range of

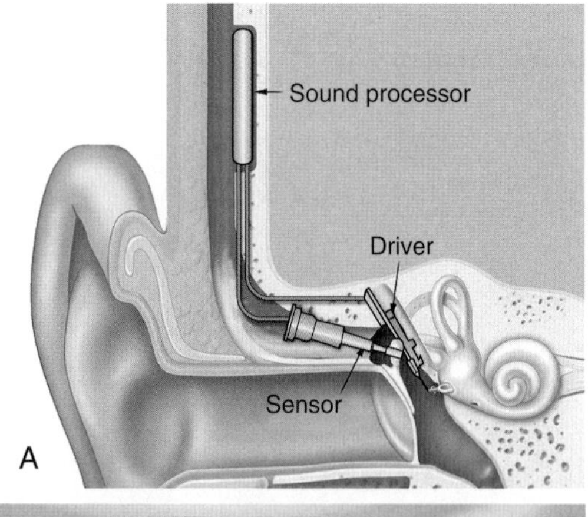

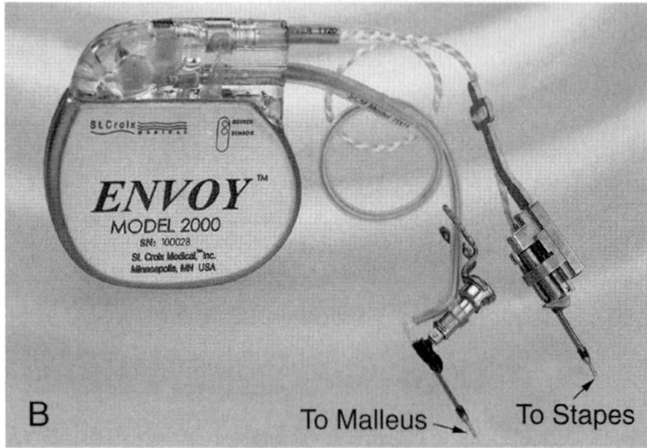

Figure 157-8. The Envoy/Esteem piezoelectric totally implantable hearing aid. **A,** Implantation schematic. Instead of a microphone, sound enters the device via a piezoelectric transducer coupled to the malleus and tympanic membrane. A piezoelectric actuator produces amplified stapes motion. The incus has been removed to prevent feedback. **B,** Complete device.

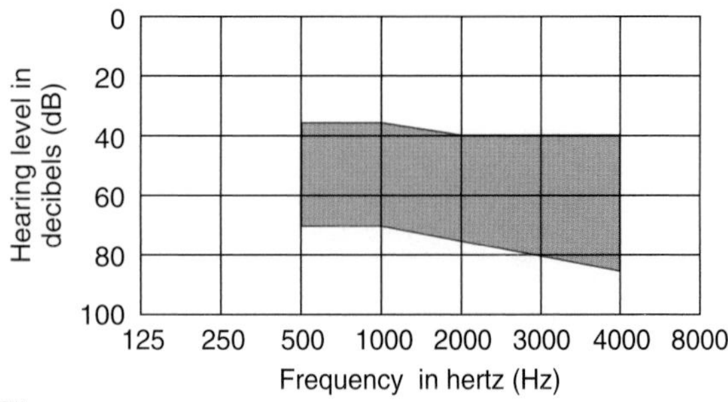

Figure 157-9. Audiologic selection criteria for the Envoy. The Envoy is designed for patients with moderate to severe hearing loss (35 to 85 dB) between 500 Hz and 4000 Hz in the implanted ear that is equal to or worse than the hearing loss in the nonimplanted ear, normal tympanometry, and speech discrimination 60% or greater. The shaded area of the figure corresponds to the pure-tone audiometric implant criteria.

80 dB at 1000 Hz, with precise ossicular tracking out to 4000 Hz.[44] The Esteem-Hearing Implant developed by Envoy Medical (formerly called the Envoy device and developed by St. Croix Medical, Inc., Minneapolis, MN) is a fully implantable piezoelectric device that uses this approach (Fig. 157-8). It received the CE Mark in Europe in 2006 and as of 2008 was in a phase II clinical trial in the United States.

Similar to all passive transducers, piezoelectric devices are bidirectional. The Esteem/Envoy uses a piezoelectric crystal to convert malleus vibrations (owing to sound waves impinging on the tympanic membrane) into a voltage encoding sound. After amplification, this electric signal is applied to a piezoelectric output transducer, which converts from the applied voltage to mechanical vibration coupled to the stapes. Power is provided by a nonrechargeable lithium-iodine battery designed to last 5 years between replacements, according to the manufacturer.[45] Programming and control of the device are accomplished through a radiofrequency transcutaneous link to a hand-held device or laptop computer.

By using acoustic input measured at the malleus, the Esteem/Envoy should maintain the spectral shaping and sound-localizing characteristics of the pinna, external auditory canal, and tympanic membrane. Implantation of the Esteem/Envoy requires partial removal of the incus, however, to prevent feedback from actuator to sensor; this ensures a maximal CHL in the event of device failure or removal, unless an ossiculoplasty is performed. This drawback has presented a significant hurdle to acceptance of the Envoy, which has not yet obtained FDA approval for routine clinical use in the United States despite earning a CE Mark in 2006. The internal battery must be replaced approximately every 5 years, and this requires repeated surgeries.

The Esteem/Envoy is designed for patients with moderate to severe hearing loss. Indications include age 18 years or old, mild to severe (35 to 85 dB) SNHL between 500 Hz and 4000 Hz in the implanted ear that is equal to or worse than the hearing loss in the nonimplanted ear, a healthy ear with normal pneumatization and adequate space for device implantation on computed tomography (CT), normal tympanometry, and speech discrimination 60% or greater (Fig. 157-9). A phase I trial in the United States and Germany was completed in 2003. By 1 year after implantation, three of seven subjects continued to use the implant, three had been revised and then explanted, and one was awaiting revision surgery. For the three subjects with functioning implants, there was no significant change in bone thresholds, and the 4-frequency (500 Hz, 1000 Hz, 2000 Hz, and 3000 Hz) average functional gain was 17 dB ± 6 dB, which was comparable to conventional hearing aids except at 3000 Hz, where the Envoy performed less well than conventional hearing aids. The decline in performance was attributed to a gradual ingress of moisture in the transducers.[46]

Implantable Bone-Conduction Hearing Aids

Conductive and mixed hearing losses are highly prevalent disorders that often may be effectively treated using standard surgical techniques or rehabilitated with traditional hearing aids. For a variety of reasons, a large subset of these patients are not suitable surgical candidates for correction of their deficit, however, or are unable to tolerate a conventional hearing aid. This group includes patients with chronically draining ears despite multiple corrective attempts, patients with discomfort from the sound levels required from a traditional hearing aid, and patients unable to tolerate a hearing aid because of a large mastoid bowl or meatoplasty after chronic ear surgery. Additionally, patients with otosclerosis, tympanosclerosis, or canal atresia, and who have a contraindication to surgical repair may also fall into this category of patients who defy traditional attempts at hearing restoration. Patients who have undergone external auditory canal closure after extensive skull base surgery also are not amenable to traditional hearing aid rehabilitation. The osseointegrated BAHA device was originally intended for this group of patients.[47-49] The BAHA device now has also been used extensively for patients with unilateral deafness with good results.[49]

Conventional bone-conducting hearing aids have been advocated as an alternative for patients with conductive or mixed hearing loss who cannot benefit from a traditional hearing aid. The utility of these devices is constrained, however, by several physical factors. Because the bone conductor must be applied with steady pressure to the mastoid cortex (usually via a headband or eyeglasses), patients often experience pain, headache, and skin irritation at the contact site. Sound fidelity is limited by soft tissue attenuation, variable placement of the vibrator, and flaccidity of the securing device (usually eyeglass frames).[50,51] Coupling the bone vibrator to an osseointegrated implant, as originally performed by Tjellstrom and colleagues[51] at the Institute of Applied Biotechnology in Sweden in 1977, circumvents many of these drawbacks. This new generation of osseointegrated conductive hearing aids now offers an effective alternative to hearing rehabilitation for this difficult subset of hearing-impaired patients.

Osseointegration

Background

In the 1960s, Branemark and associates[52] from Gothenburg, Sweden, discovered that titanium had a unique ability to become firmly anchored in bone without interposed soft tissue, while at the same time achieving a reaction-free epithelial penetration of the implant. In these permanent fixtures, Branemark presciently foresaw the ability of implanted titanium to support functional prostheses, and termed this state *osseointegration*. Osseointegration is considered to be successful if the implant became rigidly anchored into adjacent bone with no reaction at the implant-bone interface.[53] This concept was initially applied to dental implants, but in 1975, Branemark's group began studying the possibility of creating a *skin*-penetrating implant. By the 1980s, Branemark and colleagues, including Albrektsson, Jacobsson, and Tjellstrom,[54] had developed a clinical program with percutaneous titanium implants to provide an anchor for facial prosthetics (pinna, eye, or nose), and an attachment for a BAHA device.

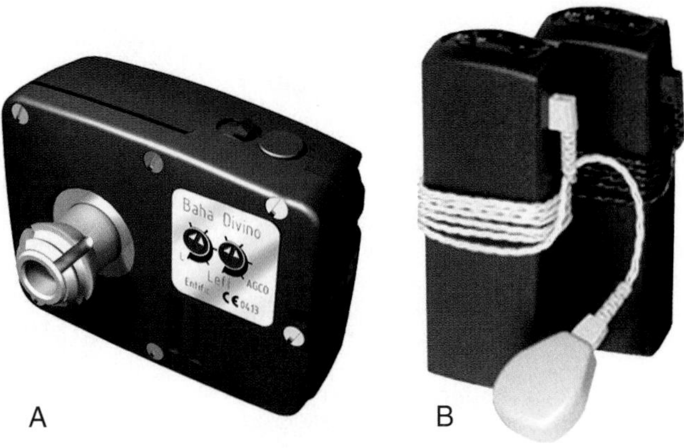

Figure 157-10. Osseointegrated bone-anchored hearing aid (BAHA). **A,** BAHA Divino is shown with its schematic attachment to the abutment and titanium implant. **B,** For patients with a more severe sensorineural component, the Cordelle offers increased amplification. *(Courtesy of Cochlear Corp, Lane Cove, Australia.)*

Biophysical Principles

Implant Material

One initial determinant of successful osseointegration is the chemical composition of the implant. Titanium has survived osseointegration's "test of time," and now represents the standard by which all other biomaterials are measured. Titanium is available commercially as "pure" titanium, which is 99.75% pure titanium, and titanium alloy, containing 90% titanium, 6% aluminum, and 4% vanadium. Titanium, similar to all other metals, forms several types of oxides on exposure to oxygen. In contrast to many of its metallic counterparts, however, titanium has the ability to create a tightly bonded and corrosion-resistant oxide layer on the surface of the implant. This oxide coating of the implant is in contact with the host tissue, which seems most important in determining the biocompatibility of titanium.[55,56] Because the implant may be worn for several decades or longer, the toxicity and carcinogenicity of the oxide coating take on particular importance.[53] Reports have shown that titanium is superior to stainless steel, lacking steel's high potential for corrosion or the toxicity of its components.[56] To date, pure titanium has shown none of these adverse sequelae, and continues to represent an ideal implant material.[55]

Implant Design

Implant microstructure and macrostructure also impact the likelihood of osseointegration. Although a rough-surfaced implant would theoretically better distribute a weight-bearing load, a rough, porous surface less than 100 μm would greatly increase the surface area and increase the risk of implant corrosion, even with a relatively corrosion-free material such as titanium. According to Eriksson and Branemark,[53] it is important that the microarchitecture of the implant surface features a topography with micropits that fit the dimensions of the cell membrane and large biomolecules; this facilitates direct bonding of the implant's oxide surface with the bone matrix. Parametric studies also show that *threaded*, screw-shaped implants have a greater likelihood of osseointegrating, and seem to distribute stress more efficiently than T-shaped or cylindric types of implants.[53,57] The threaded design success is probably most critical in conferring stability in the initial healing phase. If an implant is not absolutely stable after placement, connective tissue may form between the implant and the bone, preventing sufficient osseointegration.

Biology and Histology

Various studies have addressed the biologic correlates of osseointegration. First, there must be *direct* contact between the bone matrix and the implant, without interposed fibrous or soft tissue.[52] Pure (99.75%) titanium has shown this capability histologically, whereas titanium alloys, despite some clinical success, have not. Additionally, for successful osseointegration to occur, there should be no evidence of inflammation at the implantation site, including an infiltrate surrounding the implant or evidence of osteolysis with bone loss.[58] Pure titanium, as opposed to alloyed titanium, has also been shown to be superior in this regard.[51,55] Lastly, there should ideally be no evidence of a connective tissue capsule on the implant surface, although studies have shown that an implant with a capsule less than 30 μm in thickness may achieve osseointegration.[59] By all the above-mentioned criteria, pure titanium seems superior in every category for successful osseointegration compared with alloyed titanium. This superiority is borne out by several clinical studies as well.[50,60,61] Most authors continue to recommend pure titanium for implant material.

Radiologic Implications

A chief disadvantage of any metallic implant is interference with subsequent radiologic studies. Many osseointegration implant candidates are considered for implantation because of surgical defects caused by tumor extirpation, or other medical problems that require long-term surveillance with repeated postoperative CT or MRI scans. The presence of an implant that diminishes the quality of these scans, by introducing echo artifact, takes on increased importance. Pure titanium produces little degradation of images on either CT or MRI. Because of backscatter emissions, a radiation dose delivers 11% of the radiation dose in front of the implant, and 89% behind it.[62] This scatter effect produces little effect on the quality of CT images produced. Similarly, MRI is not contraindicated with the presence of a titanium implant. Any attached components must be removed before the MRI scan, however.

Operative Technique

Complete insertion of osseointegrated implants for the BAHA generally is done in a single stage (Figs. 157-10 and 157-11).[63] Although most surgeons perform the BAHA application in the operating room, there are reports of performing the procedure in an outpatient clinic setting.[64] Because of the importance of the implant's surface-bone interface, the surgeon must use a meticulous and precise method of implant insertion. This method sets the stage for osseointegration with minimal surrounding tissue damage. Only a single implant is needed for a BAHA. According to Branemark's original studies, insertion of the implant *must* be performed meticulously and as gently as possible to minimize thermal damage to surrounding bone.[65] This insertion is optimally performed with a high-torque drill at slow speeds (1500 to 3000 rpm) with sharp drill bits. The use of disposable drill bits avoids the possibility of worn cutting surfaces that damage the implant bed. Maximal irrigation is employed to prevent temperature elevations greater than 33° C. Previous studies have shown that heating tissue to 47° C for 1 minute obviates osseointegration because osteocytes are lost.

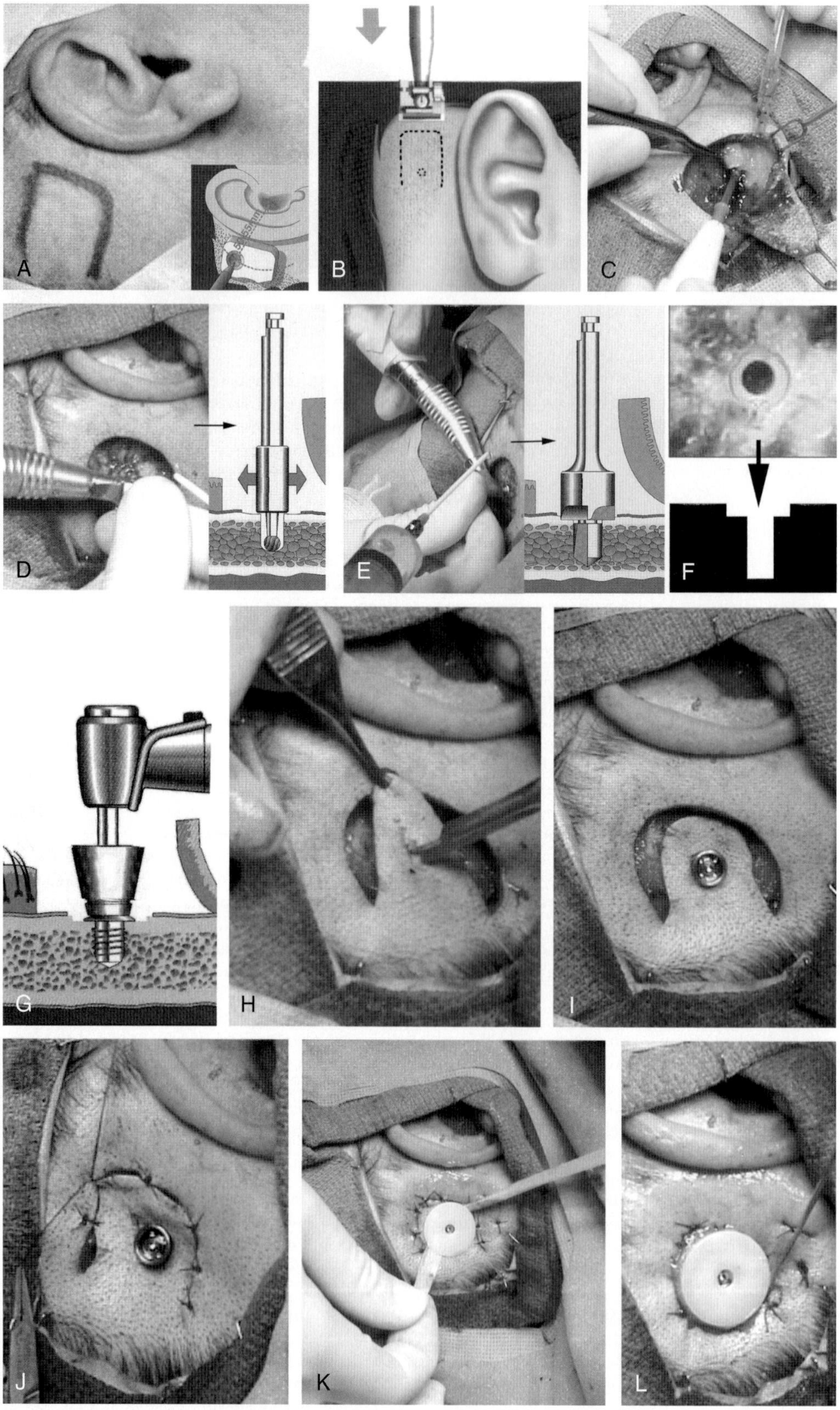

Figure 157-11. **A-L,** Operative technique for placement of Entific BAHA. **A,** Posterior-based skin flap is outlined. **B,** BAHA dermatome is used to elevate a thin flap (in this schematic the flap is inferiorly based). **C,** Soft tissues beneath and adjacent to flap are excised to create a smooth transition from surrounding tissue to thin central skin flap. **D,** A 3- to 4-mm hole is drilled in mastoid or retromastoid cortex. **E** and **F,** Countersink creates a recessed surface for implant placement. **G,** In the single-stage procedure used most commonly, the titanium implant with attached abutment is drilled into the skull at low torque. For a staged procedure, the abutment is removed, and the implant is closed laterally with a sealing screw (not shown). **H** and **I,** Skin flap is replaced, and a hole punch is used to create an opening to transmit the abutment. **J,** Flap is sutured closed. **K** and **L,** Healing cap is placed with gauze wrapped medially to apply pressure to the skin flap. *(Courtesy of Cochlear Corp, Lane Cove, Australia.)*

High-speed drilling typically used in surgery causes temperature elevations to 89° C.[66]

During the surgery, the postauricular skin surrounding the implant must be prepared for percutaneous attachment. The cutaneous-implant interface, as originally conceived by Branemark, is based on biologic principles found elsewhere in the body and throughout nature. Teeth and nails in humans, and talons, tusks, or claws as found in other species, all interface with a thin, firmly attached cutaneous or mucosal border, with little to no hair. This arrangement limits tissue mobility and increases stability of the area, while inhibiting the penetration of microbes with subsequent inflammation or infection.[67,68]

To recreate surgically a reaction-free implant-cutaneous junction, two preconditions *must* be met: The skin penetrated by the implant must be hairless, to facilitate keeping the implant site clean, and subcutaneous tissue should be aggressively thinned to minimize skin mobility in relation to the implant. The dermal layer is allowed to heal directly on the mastoid periosteum, creating a solid, immobile foundation for the implant.[63] To achieve these prerequisites in the temporal bone, hair-bearing skin overlying the implant is aggressively thinned, and hair follicles are removed from the level of the dermis. Some authors originally advocated removal of skin and replacement with a full-thickness skin graft, but this was associated with an increased incidence of skin breakdown surrounding the implant.[69] More recently, a dermatome has been developed specifically for use with the BAHA that has decreased the incidence of skin necrosis.[70] The final skin flap or graft should be less than 1 mm thick at the implant site and adjacent area. The edges of the surrounding skin flaps are sutured down to the periosteum to minimize tension on the flap.

After cutaneous work, disposable 3- and 4-mm drill bits are used to drill a hole in the skull corresponding to the central region of the flap, located at a distance approximately 5.5 cm posterior to the external auditory canal. This hole may be moved for specific anatomic irregularities or the presence of a plate from a prior skull base operation, ensuring that the placement of the abutment would not allow the hearing aid to contact the auricle. After the pilot drill hole, the countersink of the appropriate depth is used, again using maximal irrigation. Subsequently, the titanium implant with attached abutment is drilled into the skull under low torque until secured.

A hole is punched in the skin directly over each implant, and the abutment is screwed into the implant. A healing cap is placed over the abutment with antibiotic ointment–soaked gauze wrapped underneath, which helps prevent hematoma formation during the healing phase by anchoring the flap or graft to the mastoid cortex. After allowing for 12 weeks (adults) or 16 weeks (children) for osseointegration, the BAHA is simply snapped onto the abutment.

Bone-Anchored Hearing Aid in Young Children

The manufacturer of the BAHA recommends the osseointegration procedure in children older than 5 years. For children younger than 5 years in need of bone-conduction hearing rehabilitation, the BAHA-Softband is available.[71] Similar to a conventional bone-conduction hearing aid, the Softband allows bone-conduction hearing by coupling a standard BAHA device to a soft headband, providing hearing that is nearly equivalent to the osseointegrated hearing aid.

Some groups have advocated a traditional osseointegrated implant in this younger age group.[72,73] One complication that must be overcome, however, is the higher incidence of nonintegration in this younger age group, reported to be 15%.[74] Several recommendations have been proposed to avoid this complication. One is to use a two-stage procedure, whereby the implant is placed into the bone without the abutment, and the skin closed directly over this.[72,73] At a later second stage (6 months later if the skull is particularly thin), the skin flap is re-elevated, the abutment is placed, and the remainder of the procedure is finished as with the single stage. One can also leave the abutment in place during the first stage.[72] During the second stage when elevating the skin flap, a scalpel is used rather than the dermatome when the skin is tented by the healing screw, or the flap is infiltrated with local anesthetic to balloon it before using the dermatome. A final recommendation is to create an extremely thin flap to prevent cellulitis during the healing period.[72] Studies have shown that equal hearing results can be obtained when applying this staged approach in children younger than 5 years.[73]

Complications Associated with Osseointegration

The most frequently encountered complication associated with osseointegration is a soft tissue reaction at the percutaneous implant site. Soft tissue and skin reactions associated with percutaneous attachments were studied during the initial development phases of osseointegration technology. In one of the first large studies to address this issue specifically, Holgers and coworkers[75] monitored the soft tissue reactions of 67 patients who underwent osseointegrated implantation. With an average follow-up of 3 to 96 months, 14 of the 67 patients eventually developed adverse tissue reactions. One patient required removal of the abutment because of an infection, 5 patients developed redness and moisture at the abutment site requiring surgical revision (usually subcutaneous tissue thinning), 2 patients had redness with moisture requiring only local treatment, and 13 patients had developed minor erythema requiring temporary local treatment.

Jacobsson and colleagues[76] also published a case report of a patient who developed a soft tissue infection at an abutment site, eventually necessitating implant removal. Despite the presence of an ongoing infection, the implant showed histologic evidence of osseointegration. Niparko and associates[61] reported the first U.S. results with extraoral osseointegrated implants in 14 patients, noting a 3.5% incidence of symptomatic soft tissue reactions, with no implant extrusion. In the largest series to date, Tjellstrom and Hakansson[63] reported implant results on 456 patients, noting a 3.4% incidence of adverse tissue reactions; 3 patients required implant removal for infection, 3 required revision surgery for continued erythema and moisture, and 23 had tissue reactions requiring local treatment only. In the first large U.S. survey of BAHA devices, soft tissue complications were minimal and consisted of local inflammation at the percutaneous-implant junction (three patients).[47] A study of 149 consecutive cases showed that skin overgrowing the abutment was the most common complication (7%), which occurred on average 1 year after the initial surgery.[77]

Observations from these studies indicate that soft tissue reactions with percutaneous implants are largely prevented by soft tissue reduction and attachment of dermis to subjacent bone, to achieve immobility, and patient compliance with routine cleaning of the abutment site and close monitoring of skin attachment of the implant to the abutment. Complications other than adverse skin reactions are rare. Osseointegration failure is the second most common complication of the technique. In the study by Tjellstrom and Hakansson,[63] of 149 patients, 5 were considered failures; 4 failed to osseointegrate, whereas the fifth implant was lost through direct trauma. The first large U.S. series had only one patient with osseointegration failure,[47] whereas a more recent study by House and Kutz[77] had a 3.4% rate of implant extrusion. A rarely described complication is an intracerebral abscess.[78] Overall, studies consistently show that when Branemark's original surgical guidelines are followed, osseointegrated implantation is associated with high surgical success, and a low rate of morbidity and subsequent complications.

Results

In the largest series to date, Hakansson and colleagues[79] reported on their 10-year experience in 147 patients who received the BAHA. Patients were divided into three groups based on their PTA bone thresholds: 0 to 45 dB, 46 to 60 dB, and greater than 60 dB. The authors noted a strong relationship between PTA thresholds and successful rehabilitation. In the group with the best cochlear reserve (PTA <45 dB), 89% of patients' hearing was subjectively improved by the implant, whereas 8% believed their hearing was worse. Conversely, in the groups with progressively less cochlear function, 46 to 60 dB and greater than 60 dB, 61% and 22% of patients reported subjective hearing improvement. On average, speech discrimination scores improved from 14% unaided and 67% with a traditional hearing aid to 81% with the BAHA. This number increased to 85% if subjects with SNHL less than 60 dB HL were excluded, and to 89% if subjects with PTA less than 45 dB were excluded. Based on these results, the authors recommended that to be in consideration for a "high success

Table 157-2

Indications and Contraindications for Bone-Anchored Hearing Aid

Indications	Contraindications
Any patient using a conventional BC hearing aid	PTA BC thresholds (0.5-3.0 kHz) worse than 45 dB HL, SDS >60%
Any AC hearing aid user with chronic otorrhea	Emotional instability, development delay, or drug abuse
Any AC hearing aid user experiencing too much discomfort because of chronic otitis media or otitis externa	Age <5 yr
Any AC hearing aid user experiencing uncontrollable feedback because of a radical mastoidectomy or large meatoplasty	
Otosclerosis, tympanosclerosis, canal atresia with a contraindication to repair, such as in an only-hearing ear. Also, otosclerosis in combination with second, third, and fourth indications	

AC, air conduction; BC, bone conduction; HL, hearing loss; PTA, pure-tone average; SDS, speech discrimination score.

rate" with the BAHA, patients should have a PTA less than 45 dB, although improvements in hearing should still be expected for a PTA of 60 dB (Table 157-2).

In describing the Birmingham experience, Stevenson and colleagues[80] reported on the BAHA in seven children. Four children obtained improvements in PTA by 5 dB or more compared with their previous hearing aid, whereas four had changes in their thresholds of less than 5 dB. Only one of the six children tested for speech discrimination postoperatively had a significant improvement over his prior hearing aid, although the average speech discrimination score in this group was about 90% compared with 0% unaided. Liepert and DiToppa,[81] citing the Edmonton experience in 15 patients, reported an average gain of 30 dB SRT with the NAS compared with unaided speech. In the 10 patients queried, all reported that the BAHA was "better" to "much better" than their previous hearing, with or without their prior hearing aid, in all situations. Overall, the BAHA seems to offer patients with a PTA less than 45 dB a high degree of hearing rehabilitation, and excellent patient satisfaction with the device.

In the initial review of the U.S. experience with the BAHA,[47] the most common indications for implantation included chronic otitis media or draining ears and external auditory canal stenosis or aural atresia. Patients who had undergone skull base surgery and had complete closure of the external auditory canal were also included. Overall, each patient had an average improvement of 32 dB ± 19 dB with the use of the BAHA. Closure of the air-bone gap to within 10 dB of the preoperative bone-conduction thresholds occurred in 80% of patients, and closure to within 5 dB occurred in 60%. Nearly one third of patients showed "overclosure" of the preoperative bone-conduction threshold of the better hearing ear.

The BAHA Compact and the older BAHA Classic 300, on which these earlier studies are based, use an analog technology. A newer device, termed the Divino, featuring more contemporary signal processing has been developed. A more recent review comparing the Compact and Divino showed roughly equivalent results, with an average improvement over all frequencies of 27 to 28 dB for each device.[82] For speech understanding in noise, an advantage of 2.3 dB for the BAHA Divino versus the BAHA Compact was found, if noise was emitted from a loudspeaker to the rear of the listener, and the directional microphone noise reduction system was activated. Subjectively, the Divino was rated better in terms of overall sound quality by the patients.[82]

The BAHA Cordelle is the device with the most powerful gain. Although the recommended levels of hearing loss for the traditional BAHA (Classic, Compact, and Divino) encompass a PTA bone-conduction loss at 500 Hz, 1000 Hz, 2000 Hz, and 3000 Hz at less than 40 dB HL, the body-worn BAHA Cordelle is recommended for patients with a more compromised cochlear reserve. Studies have shown that bone-conduction PTAs of less than 65 dB are acceptable for fitting.[83] There is also the BAHA Intenso, and similar to the Divino, but with additional power for an intermediate sensorineural component.

Bone-Anchored Hearing Aid for Unilateral Sensorineural Hearing Loss

BAHA is gaining increasing popularity for the rehabilitation of unilateral SNHL.[49,84,85] It is hypothesized that using the BAHA device on the deafened ear can expand the sound field for the patient and improve the patient's speech understanding in noise, similar to a contralateral routing of signal (CROS) hearing aid or transcranial CROS system. A prospective trial of subjects with unilateral deafness using benefit surveys, source identification testing, and hearing in noise testing was undertaken by Niparko and colleagues.[84] This study consisted of 10 adults with unilateral deafness (PTA >90 dB, SD <20%) for a variety of etiologies, including acoustic neuroma, meningitis, sudden SNHL, and sudden SNHL with chronic suppurative otitis media. Patients were fitted with contralateral routing of offside signal amplification devices (CROS) for 1 month and tested with contralateral routing of offside signal before mastoid implantation of the deaf ear, fitting, and testing for BAHA.

The results of this study showed that there was consistent satisfaction with BAHA implantation and amplification, and poor acceptance of CROS amplification. Sound localization was poor at baseline and with BAHA and contralateral routing of offside signal. Relative to baseline, CROS and the BAHA produced significantly better speech recognition in noise under most conditions. The BAHA enabled significantly better speech recognition than CROS in quiet and in a composite of noise conditions, a result that may have been related to averting the interference of speech signals delivered to the better ear, as occurs with conventional CROS amplification. The study showed that the BAHA, when placed on the side of a deaf ear, yielded greater benefit in subjects with normal monaural hearing than did CROS amplification.

Another study by Wazen and colleagues[85] has also evaluated the BAHA for unilateral SNHL. This prospective study of nine patients included hearing loss from congenital aural atresia or mastoidectomies secondary to chronic ear infections with or without cholesteatoma, or temporal bone tumor excision. Comparing BAHA-aided with the unaided condition, the authors showed that all patients had tonal and spondee threshold improvement with BAHA compared with thresholds before treatment. Speech recognition performance in BAHA-aided conditions was comparable to the patient's best score in unaided condition, and patients reported a significant improvement in their hearing handicap scores with the BAHA.

A more recent study by Lin and coworkers[86] for patients with unilateral SNHL showed consistent satisfaction with BAHA amplification and poor acceptance of CROS amplification. Sound localization was worse when using the CROS aid, but showed no benefit with the BAHA. In keeping with prior studies, the BAHA produced significantly better speech recognition in noise. Similar findings have been borne out by other studies.[87] These studies show that the BAHA is an excellent tool for rehabilitation of unilateral SNHL, and seems to outperform the only other rehabilitative option available for this difficult problem, the CROS hearing aid. The primary benefit seems to be improved hearing in noise, whereas the BAHA provides no objective benefit of sound localization.

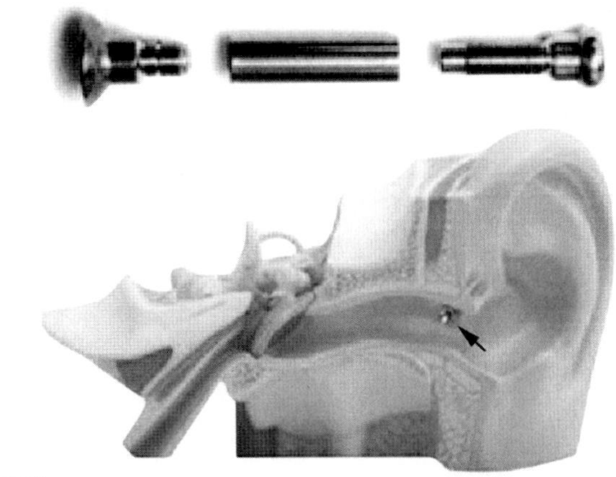

Figure 157-12. Auric metallic tube and transcutaneous placement from retroauricular sulcus to external auditory canal.

Implantable Adjuncts to Conventional Hearing Aids

RetroX

The RetroX (Auric Hearing Systems, Rheine, Germany) consists of an inert titanium metal tube that passes from the postauricular sulcus to the posterior aspect of the external auditory canal, passing just lateral to the mastoid cortical bone and external auditory canal bone (Fig. 157-12). Its major purported advantages are that it does not block the external auditory canal, and it does decrease feedback by separating the device microphone (which lies in a BTE unit) and the output of the speaker in the external auditory canal. Secondarily, there is a cosmetic advantage over traditional BTE aids in that the device is largely hidden behind the pinna, with no speaker tube visibly entering the external auditory canal. According to the manufacturer, the device is appropriate for patients with SNHL or CHL to 30 dB HL at 1 kHz and less and 30 to 80 dB HL loss at 3 to 8 kHz, and is especially suitable for cases of high-frequency SNHL with a steep slope (ski-slope audiogram).

To date, few peer-reviewed reports of device results have appeared in the literature. In one study of 10 patients, all were satisfied with the hearing improvement provided by the RetroX.[88] There was an improvement of pure-tone thresholds at 1 kHz, 2 kHz, and 4 kHz, whereas in quiet, the speech reception threshold improved by 9 dB. Speech audiometry in noise showed that intelligibility improved by 26% for a signal-to-noise ratio of −5 dB, by 18% for a signal-to-noise ratio of 0 dB, and by 13% for a signal-to-noise ratio of +5 dB. Complications included one patient with acoustic feedback and one patient with a granulomatous reaction to the foreign body that necessitated removing the implant. Refinements to the surgical process of placing the titanium tube seem to have diminished the rate of this complication.[89]

A subsequent study of 25 patients by this same group was reported after 2.5 to 15 months of use.[90] Of 25 patients, 23 were satisfied with the device, whereas 4 patients developed a persistent granulomatous reaction that disappeared after explantation, and 2 patients complained of acoustic feedback and needed supplementary fitting. The authors of this study observed a statistically significant improvement of the pure-tone thresholds, with similar speech in quiet and noise scores as their initial study. A study in 2005 by Barbara and colleagues[91] showed that the RetroX provided better hearing in noise with higher rates of satisfaction compared with a CIC hearing aid.[91]

Conclusion

Technology has brought about new and revolutionary means of rehabilitating patients with SNHL and CHL. Totally implanted and semi-implanted hearing aids have the potential to deliver improved sound quality, greater amplification, less distortion, better directional hearing, and better cosmetic appearance than conventional hearing aids. Whether this potential will be fully realized depends on further refinements of their design, acceptance by patients and third-party payers, and the financial viability of the corporations promoting them. Although current economic and financial obstacles may make the short-term outlook for these devices unclear, they will undoubtedly continue to be improved, and ultimately may prove to be a critical part of the armamentarium of devices used for rehabilitation of hearing loss.

SUGGESTED READINGS

Barbara M, Bandiera G, Serra B, et al. Digital hearing aids for high-frequency sensorineural hearing loss: preliminary experience with the RetroX device. *Acta Otolaryngol.* 2005;125:693-696.

Chen DA, Backous DD, Arriaga MA, et al. Phase 1 clinical trial results of the Envoy System: a totally implantable middle ear device for sensorineural hearing loss. *Otolaryngol Head Neck Surg.* 2004;131:904-916.

Colletti V, Soli SD, Carner M, et al. Treatment of mixed hearing losses via implantation of a vibratory transducer on the round window. *Int J Audiol.* 2006;45:600-608.

Davids T, Gordon KA, Clutton D, et al. Bone-anchored hearing aids in infants and children younger than 5 years. *Arch Otolaryngol Head Neck Surg.* 2007;133:51-55.

Goode RL, Rosenbaum ML, Maniglia AJ. The history and development of the implantable hearing aid. *Otolaryngol Clin North Am.* 1995;28:1-16.

Hol MK, Cremers CW, Coppens-Schellekens W, et al. The BAHA Softband: a new treatment for young children with bilateral congenital aural atresia. *Int J Pediatr Otorhinolaryngol.* 2005;69:973-980.

House JW, Kutz JW Jr. Bone-anchored hearing aids: incidence and management of postoperative complications. *Otol Neurotol.* 2007;28:213-217.

Jenkins HA, Atkins JS, Horlbeck D, et al. Otologics fully implantable hearing system: Phase I trial 1-year results. *Otol Neurotol.* 2008;29:534-541.

Jenkins HA, Atkins JS, Horlbeck D, et al. U.S. Phase I preliminary results of use of the Otologics MET Fully-Implantable Ossicular Stimulator. *Otolaryngol Head Neck Surg.* 2007;137:206-212.

Jenkins HA, Niparko JK, Slattery WH, et al. Otologics Middle Ear Transducer Ossicular Stimulator: performance results with varying degrees of sensorineural hearing loss. *Acta Otolaryngol.* 2004;124:391-394.

Kiefer J, Arnold W, Staudenmaier R. Round window stimulation with an implantable hearing aid (Soundbridge) combined with autogenous reconstruction of the auricle—a new approach. *ORL J Otorhinolaryngol Relat Spec.* 2006;68:378-385.

Kompis M, Krebs M, Hausler R. Speech understanding in quiet and in noise with the bone-anchored hearing aids Baha Compact and Baha Divino. *Acta Otolaryngol.* 2007;127:829-835.

Lin LM, Bowditch S, Anderson MJ, et al. Amplification in the rehabilitation of unilateral deafness: speech in noise and directional hearing effects with bone-anchored hearing and contralateral routing of signal amplification. *Otol Neurotol.* 2006;27:172-182.

Luetje CM, Brackmann D, Balkany TJ, et al. Phase III clinical trial results with the Vibrant Soundbridge implantable middle ear hearing device: a prospective controlled multicenter study. *Otolaryngol Head Neck Surg.* 2002;126:97-107.

Lustig LR, Arts HA, Brackmann DE, et al. Hearing rehabilitation using the BAHA bone-anchored hearing aid: results in 40 patients. *Otol Neurotol.* 2001;22:328-334.

Niparko JK, Cox KM, Lustig LR. Comparison of the bone anchored hearing aid implantable hearing device with contralateral routing of offside signal amplification in the rehabilitation of unilateral deafness. *Otol Neurotol.* 2003;24:73-78.

Siegert R, Mattheis S, Kasic J. Fully implantable hearing aids in patients with congenital auricular atresia. *Laryngoscope.* 2007;117:336-340.

Snik AF, Mylanus EA, Proops DW, et al. Consensus statements on the BAHA system: where do we stand at present? *Ann Otol Rhinol Laryngol Suppl.* 2005;195:2-12.

Todt I, Seidl RO, Gross M, et al. Comparison of different Vibrant Soundbridge audioprocessors with conventional hearing aids. *Otol Neurotol.* 2002;23: 669-673.

For complete list of references log onto www.expertconsult.com.

Venail F, Lavieille JP, Meller R, et al. New perspectives for middle ear implants: first results in otosclerosis with mixed hearing loss. *Laryngoscope.* 2007;117:552-555.

Yellon RF. Bone anchored hearing aid in children—prevention of complications. *Int J Pediatr Otorhinolaryngol.* 2007;71:823-826.

CHAPTER ONE HUNDRED AND FIFTY-EIGHT

Cochlear Implantation: Patient Evaluation and Device Selection

P. Ashley Wackym

Christina L. Runge-Samuelson

Key Points

- Cochlear implants are auditory prostheses designed to link an internal device interfaced with the auditory nerve to an external device that uses a specific speech coding strategy to translate acoustic information into electric stimulation.
- Prelingually deafened children acquire speech and language through central plasticity resulting from stimulation by auditory prostheses.
- Postlingually deafened children and adults, as well as those with severe to profound hearing loss, who derive marginal benefit from hearing aids, are appropriate cochlear implant candidates.
- The medical evaluation begins with a detailed collection of the patient's history including age of onset, progression, and bilaterality of the hearing loss; risk factors for hearing loss (e.g., noise exposure, ototoxicity, trauma); and ear infection and surgery.
- Congenital deafness occurs in approximately 1 in every 1000 children, and at least 60% of these children have hereditary causes of the deafness.
- The diagnosis of auditory neuropathy/auditory dys-synchrony has been specified as a hearing disorder where preserved outer hair cell function exists with abnormal auditory neural responses; some of these patients may be cochlear implant candidates.
- Preoperative imaging using CT and/or MRI is essential.
- Current adult selection criteria in the most recent clinical trials include (1) severe or profound hearing loss with a pure-tone average of 70 dB HL, (2) use of appropriately fit hearing aids or a trial with amplification, (3) aided scores on open-set sentence tests of less than 50%, (4) no evidence of central auditory lesions or lack of an auditory nerve, and (5) no evidence of contraindications for surgery in general or cochlear implant surgery in particular.
- With the benefits of binaural cochlear implantation being realized, current candidacy decisions now include whether to receive two implants rather than one.
- We suggest the following referral criteria for cochlear implant evaluation for adults: (1) unaided thresholds of 70 dB HL or poorer at 1000 Hz and above in the better ear, even if hearing levels at 250 and 500 Hz are better; (2) unaided word discrimination less than 70%; and (3) frustration on the part of the patient because of communication difficulties, even with appropriate hearing aid use.
- Cochlear implant evaluation for children can be considered with (1) unaided thresholds of greater than 90 dB HL at 2000 Hz and above in the better ear, even if hearing levels at 250 and 500 Hz are better; (2) aided thresholds in the better ear are greater than 35 dB HL, especially at 4000 Hz; (3) no response for ABR testing in both ears or no response for one ear and responses at elevated levels in the other ear; (4) parents are frustrated with their child's development of auditory and/or communication skills; (5) progressive hearing loss with detection levels at or near the profound range at 2000 Hz and above; or (6) evidence of severely impairing auditory neuropathy/dys-synchrony. There is no lower age limit for evaluation.
- Signal-processing strategies may affect device selection for a given patient (e.g., patients who are music enthusiasts may be interested in comparing aspects of fine structure strategies, whereas other patients with neurologic processing issues may benefit from having strategies that offer slower stimulation rates).

The development and improvement of cochlear auditory prostheses have radically improved the management of children and adults with profound hearing loss. Rapid evolution in the candidacy criteria and the technology itself has resulted in large numbers of individuals who have benefited from implantation. Likewise, the introduction of three device manufacturers into the U.S. marketplace has accelerated the research and development of these auditory prostheses. In this chapter, the evaluation and expectations for both children and adults are presented, as are the similarities and differences among all three available devices in the United States.

General Background

Cochlear implants are auditory prostheses designed to link an internal device interfaced with the auditory nerve to an external device that uses a specific speech coding strategy to translate acoustic information into electrical stimulation. For the majority of causes of deafness, the auditory hair cells are lost or dysfunctional. The bipolar spiral ganglion neurons and their primary afferent dendrites remain intact, to varying degrees on the basis of etiology, and are available for direct electrical stimulation by the cochlear implant. The tonotopic organization of the cochlea is emulated by orienting the electrode contacts toward the modiolus within the scala tympani and assigning frequencies to specific electrodes along the length of the electrode array such that electrical stimulation corresponding to the highest pitches are delivered within the basal region of the cochlea while electrical stimulation corresponding to the lowest pitches are delivered within the apical region of the cochlea. The electrical impulses directly depolarize the primary afferent neurons, effectively bypassing the dysfunctional hair cells. All three device manufacturers use an external processor that encodes speech on the basis of features that are critical for word understanding in normal listeners, and these features are discussed later in this chapter. More than 70,000 individuals have received cochlear implants, and these devices are now reliably enabling speech comprehension in the vast majority of appropriate cochlear implant recipients.

Prelingually deafened children acquire speech and language through central plasticity resulting from stimulation by auditory prostheses. Some prelingually deafened adults are appropriate cochlear implant recipients but have limited central plasticity that is required for auditory pathway development and processing. Postlingually deafened children and adults, as well as those with severe to profound hearing loss, who derive marginal benefit from hearing aids, are appropriate cochlear implant candidates.

Patient Evaluation

Otologic/Medical Evaluation and Imaging

The medical evaluation begins with a detailed collection of the patient's history, followed by physical examination. The otologic history includes age of onset, progression, bilaterality of the hearing loss; risk factors for hearing loss (e.g., noise exposure, ototoxicity, trauma), and ear infection and surgery. History of possible vestibular dysfunction includes delayed walking, difficulty in riding a bicycle, or difficulty maintaining balance while walking with eyes closed or in the dark. A thorough family history is important including the age of onset, severity, and rate of progression of any hearing loss.

GENETIC HEARING LOSS. The etiology of the hearing loss is an important consideration. Profound hearing loss and deafness, although clear symptoms, have a heterogeneous group of causes. Of the genetic causes, more than 400 forms of syndromic hearing loss have been described, and the list of nonsyndromic loci now exceeds 80,[1] many of which are discussed elsewhere in this book.

Congenital deafness occurs in approximately 1 in every 1000 children, and at least 60% of these children have hereditary causes of the deafness.[2] It is estimated that 70% of all hereditary hearing losses are nonsyndromic, nearly 80% of which are inherited in an autosomal recessive fashion.[3] To date, 54 autosomal recessive, 24 autosomal dominant, and 8 X-linked loci have been characterized for nonsyndromic sensorineural hearing loss (NSHL).[1] Several mitochondrial DNA variants have also been implicated.[1] Studies indicate that up to 50% of all NSHL cases are due to a mutation in a single gene encoding connexin 26 (Cx26).[4] The gene coding for Cx26 (gap junction protein beta 2 or *GJB2*) is located at locus DFNB1 on human chromosome 13q12. The coding sequence of the protein is contained in a single exon that can be easily analyzed using sequencing methods.[5] Children with nonsyndromic genetic hearing loss, if implanted early, are typically excellent performers with their devices.

Genetic syndromal deafness represents a small proportion of all profound hearing impairment; however, there are typically other considerations to be made when these individuals are being considered for cochlear implantation. Although there are more than 400 genetic syndromes that include hearing loss, most syndromic deafness is confined to a limited number of syndromes.[6] Only two common autosomal recessive forms of syndromic deafness exist: Pendred's syndrome (deafness, wide vestibular aqueduct, and thyroid dysfunction) and Usher's syndrome (deafness, blindness due to retinitis pigmentosa, with or without vestibular dysfunction). Jervell and Lange-Nielsen syndrome (deafness and sudden death syndrome due to prolonged QT interval) occurs in families with strong histories or in population isolates. It is, however, important to consider when preparing to bring a child to the operating room when there is a family history of deafness and cardiac death. Unfortunately, the electrocardiogram (ECG) is not entirely sensitive or specific for this syndrome[7]; however, referral to a cardiologist for evaluation and treatment is essential for any deaf child with prolongation of the QT interval on an ECG, history of syncopal episodes, or a family history of prolonged QT interval. Neurofibromatosis type 2 (NF2) is usually diagnosed between the ages of 10 and 30 years, and these individuals can express the phenotype of bilateral acoustic neuromas, which is an important issue to consider when developing a management algorithm. If one of the tumors is removed while small and if the cochlear nerve is preserved, despite losing functional hearing, cochlear implantation is appropriate if a several-year interval has been observed indicating that a recidivistic tumor will not compromise the cochlear nerve. Otherwise, auditory brainstem implantation is an appropriate alternative.

The previous four syndromic disorders are not readily diagnosed at birth by history and physical examination. The most common dominant syndromes resulting in deafness are Stickler syndrome, branchio-oto-renal syndrome, and Waardenburg syndrome. When physical examination or history suggests a syndromic hearing loss, online resources have been developed to help the physician during the evaluation process.[8]

AUDITORY NEUROPATHY/AUDITORY DYS-SYNCHRONY. Over several years evidence has emerged regarding the existence of a hearing disorder that does not fit into the standard conductive, mixed, or sensorineural hearing loss categories. Relatively recently, the diagnosis of auditory neuropathy/auditory dys-synchrony (AN/D) has been specified as a hearing disorder in which present cochlear outer hair cell function is found in conjunction with absent or abnormal auditory neural responses, which is indicative of poor neural synchrony.[9] Reports on the incidence of AN/D symptoms range from 0.5[10] to 1.3%[11] of the population suspect for hearing loss, and 15% of those with absent auditory brainstem response,[11] which is otherwise consistent with severe to profound sensorineural hearing loss. Behavioral audiometric thresholds may or may not be within normal limits and can fluctuate over time, and speech perception in AN/D patients is often much poorer than the behavioral thresholds would predict. There are many possible reasons for poor auditory neural synchrony including, but not limited to, dysfunction of cochlear inner hair cells, of the inner hair cell/spiral ganglion nerve synapse, or of the auditory nerve itself.

The variety of etiologies in AN/D results in a heterogeneous population. Starr[12] reported the diagnoses from 70 patients with AN/D as fitting into the following categories: 40% hereditary, often associated with Charcot-Marie-Tooth disease; 20% with a mix of etiologies including toxic-metabolic (i.e., anoxia, hyperbilirubinemia), immunologic, and infectious; and 40% idiopathic. Transient AN/D has also been documented with temperature fluctuation in cases of severe illness.[13,14] In addition, AN/D may coexist with peripheral neuropathy, which has been observed as a loss of myelin and neural fibers in the cross section of sural nerves from some AN/D patients.[12]

Fitting AN/D patients with hearing aids may not provide sufficient benefit for communication because amplification provides increased sound intensity but does not have the capability to contribute to improved neural synchrony. After careful evaluation and when recommended, electrical stimulation with cochlear implants holds promise as a treatment option for individuals who are severely hearing impaired from AN/D,[15,16] and has been successful in our clinical experience. However, cochlear implantation may be contraindicated in cases in which neural function is significantly compromised or the auditory nerve is deficient or absent.[17]

ACQUIRED DEAFNESS. In young children, many acquired forms of deafness cannot be easily differentiated from genetic deafness. Prenatal infection with TORCH microorganisms (toxoplasmosis, syphilis, rubella, cytomegalovirus [CMV], and herpes) is commonly associated with deafness. This spectrum of infections can result in reduced ganglion cell counts, cognitive dysfunction, and abnormal position of the facial nerve, all issues limiting the effectiveness of cochlear implants or increasing the risk of cochlear implant surgery. Prematurity and low birth weight, low Apgar scores, and hyperbilirubinemia can all be associated with deafness and, because of the central auditory processing abnormalities associated with these conditions, expectations for performance outcome following cochlear implantation should be tempered. Similarly, there can be rehabilitation needs and problems with these multiply disabled children.

Autoimmune inner ear disease (see Chapter 153) is typically rapidly progressive and often associated with highly favorable outcomes in postlingual patients receiving cochlear implants, likely due to the well-preserved primary afferent neuron population and the short duration of deafness. Although it is unusual for patients with bilateral Meniere disease to lose enough hearing to require cochlear implantation, such patients typically perform at excellent levels with an implant, likely due to significant residual hearing and auditory memory.

Many inherited or acquired diseases affect the temporal bone, which can produce severe to profound hearing loss requiring cochlear implantation. Otosclerosis, Paget disease, Camurati-Engelmann disease,[18] and meningitis with secondary labyrinthitis ossificans are a few examples of diseases that can present management challenges with cochlear implantation. Aside from the potential difficulty in electrode insertion, the reduction in bone density often leads to unwanted sequelae such as facial nerve stimulation due to current spread outside of the cochlea, affecting the postoperative programming of the device.

Although rare, bilateral temporal bone fractures resulting in deafness can be rehabilitated with cochlear implants. Early implantation should be performed to avoid cochlear fibrosis. If imaging studies suggest trauma to the auditory nerve, it is important to determine if the auditory nerve is functional using promontory electrical stimulation while recording electrically evoked auditory brainstem potentials (ABR). The use of auditory brainstem implantation in this clinical setting has been reported in Europe[19]; however, the first such application of this technology in the United States occurred only recently.

PHYSICAL EXAMINATION. All adults or children with profound hearing loss should have a complete physical examination. Clinical correlates of specific etiologies of sensorineural hearing loss are addressed in Chapters 147, 148, and 149 of this text.

CHRONIC SUPPURATIVE OTITIS MEDIA. Cochlear implantation was initially viewed as contraindicated in young children with chronic suppurative otitis media (CSOM) because of the potential risk of infection.[20] However, selective retrospective studies have shown that the prevalence and severity of OM does not increase following implantation,[21,22] leading surgeons to advocate cochlear implantation if the ear is dry at the time of implantation.

Some surgeons advocate a two-stage operative approach; the first operation involves a radical mastoidectomy (if not already performed), eustachian tube obliteration, and mastoid cavity obliteration with oversewing of the ear canal. Cochlear implantation is performed at a later time, usually 2 to 6 months postobliteration.[23] The major risk of mastoid obliteration is the formation of cholesteatoma, which must be carefully monitored on a long-term basis. Other authors advocate an individualized management strategy: (1) patients with a dry tympanic membrane perforation receive a first-stage myringoplasty followed by implantation in 3 months; (2) patients with cholesteatoma or an unstable mastoid cavity receive a radical mastoidectomy and obliteration followed months later by a second stage cochlear implantation; (3) patients with a stable cavity receive one-stage cavity obliteration and electrode implantation.[24] Finally, some practitioners advocate treating radical mastoid cavities with a one-stage operative approach that includes oversewing the external auditory canal and cochlear implantation without obliteration or reduction of the cavity.[25,26] Luntz and colleagues[27] have described a treatment algorithm with multiple steps aimed at resolving the draining ear. Using this strategy, cochlear implantation is performed at the completion of any step if the ear is dry. The existence of multiple protocols for managing cochlear implant candidates with CSOM reflects the problematic nature of this disease process. Regardless of the management protocol, all patients currently receive selected antimicrobial prophylaxis immediately before implantation.

Microbial biofilms are a common if not normal phenomena in nature; however, in the clinical arena biofilm formation is associated with increased morbidity and mortality.[28,29] Biofilms are characterized by a complex three-dimensional architecture with a network of adherent cells connected by water channels and encapsulated within an extracellular matrix.[30] Biofilms are recalcitrant to antibiotics, antiseptics, and industrial biocides. Possible mechanisms include (1) restricted penetration of drugs through the matrix; (2) phenotypic changes resulting from a decreased growth rate or nutrient limitation; and (3) surface-induced expression of resistance genes. Although there is an extensive literature on bacterial biofilms, little attention has been paid to medically relevant fungal biofilms, despite the fact that yeasts are the third leading cause of catheter-related infections, with the second highest colonization to infection rate and the highest crude mortality. Transplantation procedures, immunosuppression, use of chronic indwelling catheters, and prolonged intensive care unit stays are salient risk factors for fungal disease.[31] Biomedical devices including stents, shunts, and prostheses (voice, heart valve, knee, etc.); implants (breast, lens, dentures, etc.); endotracheal tubes; pacemakers; and various types of catheters have been shown to support colonization and biofilm formation by *Candida*.[32] Antifungal therapy alone has been shown to be insufficient for cure, requiring removal of the biomedical device.[33]

Since the advent of antibiotics in the 1940s, many authors have reported fungal overgrowth following antibacterial therapy.[34] Although bacteria usually cause CSOM, fungal infection or overgrowth is surprisingly common. One prospective study in CSOM patients reported growth of *Candida* species in 10% of ears with purulent otorrhea and in 35% of ears treated for purulence with topical ciprofloxacin for 3 weeks.[35] Furthermore, another study in which cultures were obtained from ears with ventilation tubes and otorrhea before and after a 10-day course of topical ofloxacin ear drops (Floxin) or oral amoxicillin/clavulanate demonstrated a 5% incidence of *Candida* superinfections in the amoxicillin/clavulanate group but negligible incidence in the ofloxacin group.[36] These results confirm the findings of an earlier study in which the incidence of *Candida* was significantly greater for patients treated with amoxicillin/clavulanate compared with a group treated with topical ofloxacin. We have had one case of fungal colonization of a cochlear implant with *Candida albicans*.[37] No guidelines have been proposed for dealing with episodes of otitis media in the early postoperative period. During this time interval, the physical barrier created by the fibrous sealing of the cochleostomy is in the process of being laid down, and thus the electrode array provides direct access to the inner ear. An infection of the middle ear during this period may easily extend along the electrode array, induce damage to the auditory nerve, and possibly lead to biofilm formation, requiring immediate removal of the implant. In addition, this puts the patient at higher risk for further spread of infection into the intracranial space and subsequent meningitis.[38] The high prevalence of bacterial biofilms in chronic otitis media have been recently demonstrated,[39] and bacterial biofilms have also been demonstrated in cases of infected cochlear implants that required explantation.[40]

IMAGING. Preoperative high-resolution temporal bone computed tomography (CT) scans, without contrast, should be performed on all cochlear implant candidates. Determination of intact internal auditory canals, normalcy of the cochlea, primary or secondary bone diseases affecting the cochlea, and presence of a wide vestibular aqueduct represent an important data set to complete. Many children with congenital deafness will be found to have an associated cochlear malformation, typically dilated vestibule, wide vestibular aqueduct, cochlear hypoplasia, or a common cavity.[41] When congenital or acquired narrow internal auditory canals are identified on preoperative CT scanning, primary afferent innervation may be lacking and cochlear implantation is therefore contraindicated.[18,42] Another important finding to identify is a wide vestibular aqueduct, which, when present, is an indication to perform preoperative magnetic resonance imaging

(MRI). This is an important preoperative consideration because this abnormality is associated with an abnormal communication between the cerebrospinal fluid (CSF) space and the cochlea. Clinically, this is often associated with a "perilymph gusher," and sealing of the cochleostomy with pericranium or fascia is particularly important to avoid meningitis following acute suppurative otitis media. Hypoplastic cochleas are associated with shorter length and range in character from a common cavity to an incomplete partition at the apical region of the cochlea. In children with auditory neuropathy/auditory dys-synchrony, MRI should be performed because up to 18% of these children can have small or absent cochlear nerves despite normal internal auditory canal size as demonstrated with CT.[17] Other anomalies such as the abnormal course or position of the facial nerve and round window niche occur. With the exception of an absent auditory nerve or internal auditory canal, most malformed cochleas can be implanted with a sufficient number of electrodes to provide open-set (unlimited word or sentence possibilities) speech perception.

Labyrinthitis ossificans can occur after meningitis, particularly when *Streptococcus pneumoniae* is the infecting mocroorganism.[38] Whereas temporal bone CT can show complete ossification well, MRI can provide complementary information when partial ossification has occurred. T2-weighted MRI sequences are particularly useful in determining whether a scala tympani with partial ossification or fibrosis contains perilymph.

High-resolution temporal bone CT scanning can also be helpful in sorting out issues related to device dysfunction or when unexpectedly poor outcome occurs. Figure 158-1 shows the temporal bone containing a Med-El C40+ device in a patient who has otosclerosis and the new onset of facial nerve stimulation. The reduced bone density and lucency seen around the otic capsule resulting from her advanced cochlear otosclerosis allowed current to spread from the cochlea to the facial nerve. Figure 158-2 shows the temporal bone of a young child whose performance was unexpectedly low and who was also noted to have facial nerve stimulation with cochlear implant use. After his referral to our center for evaluation, a high-resolution temporal bone CT was obtained. The CT scan showed a malformed cochlea with an incomplete partition at the apex and the electrode tip leaving the cochlea and extending into the internal auditory canal. This type of cochlear malformation is typically associated with a thin partition between the modiolus and the internal auditory canal.

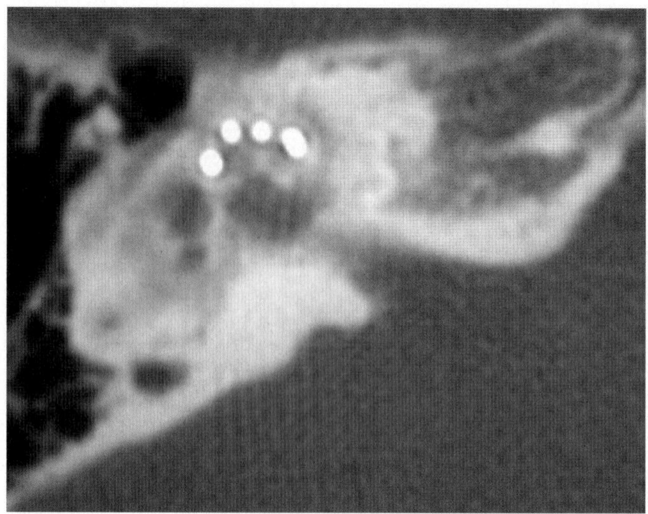

Figure 158-1. High-resolution temporal bone axial computed tomography scan using a bone window algorithm shows a right ear with a well-positioned electrode array (Med-El C40+) within a cochlea affected by otosclerosis. Note the reduced density of the otic capsule bone and the lucency surrounding the otic capsule *(center, top right).* This patient was experiencing facial nerve stimulation with cochlear implant use due to current spread through the otic capsule to the facial nerve *(Published with permission, copyright © 2009 P.A. Wackym, MD.)*

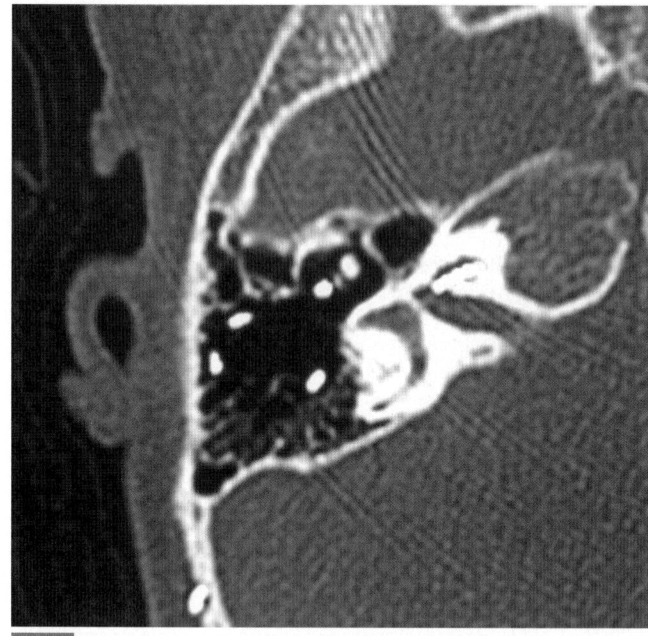

Figure 158-2. High-resolution temporal bone axial computed tomography (CT) using a bone window algorithm shows a right ear with a cochlear implant electrode array that has broken through the cochlea/modiolar wall to enter the internal auditory canal (CII Bionic Ear with HiFocus 1j electrode). The implanting surgeon, at another institution, did not recognize that the child had an incomplete partition at the apex of the cochlea. This malformation can be associated with a thin bony wall between the cochlea and the modiolus. This child was performing at a level lower than expected with his cochlear implant and had facial nerve activation with implant use, which led to the CT scan to evaluate the electrode position. The child's second side was implanted with a HiRes 90K device, and the initial device was removed and replaced with a HiRes 90K device, resolving his facial nerve stimulation problem. *(Published with permission, copyright © 2009 P.A. Wackym, MD.)*

Evaluation of Adult Cochlear Implant Candidates

The benefits of cochlear implantation have increased substantially over the past quarter century due to changes in technology and expanded candidate criteria. Consideration for cochlear implantation in adults still requires careful assessment to (1) determine preimplant hearing aid fitting and performance, (2) compare a candidate's preimplant performance with that of current implant recipients, (3) provide a recommendation for or against cochlear implantation, (4) select an ear for implantation, and (5) determine appropriate expectations that will guide the counseling of prospective patients, which is critical for user satisfaction.

Current Adult Selection Criteria

Food and Drug Administration (FDA) approved guidelines for cochlear implantation vary slightly with different clinical trials depending on the manufacturer's submission and labeling aims. Guidelines also change over time, in part, because cochlear implant recipients' average scores have been found to be higher than individuals with better hearing or word recognition. Current adult selection criteria in the most recent clinical trials include (1) severe or profound hearing loss with a pure-tone average (PTA) of 70 dB HL, (2) use of appropriately fit hearing aids or a trial with amplification, (3) aided scores on open-set sentence tests of less than 50%, (4) no evidence of central auditory lesions or lack of an auditory nerve, and (5) no evidence of contraindications for surgery in general or cochlear implant surgery in particular. Additionally, cochlear implant centers generally recommend at least 1 to 3 months of hearing aid use, realistic expectations by the patient and family members, and willingness to comply with follow-up procedures as defined by the center.

The goal of the evaluation process is to determine whether an individual would perform as well with appropriately fit hearing aids as with a cochlear implant. In addition to comparing the candidate's performance with average cochlear implant users, it is important to compare the candidate with cochlear implant users who are matched for such factors as length of profound hearing loss or useable residual hearing, which are known factors that contribute to the variance in patient performance. In other words, if a candidate has had recent onset of profound hearing loss, it is more appropriate to compare him or her to the top 25% of cochlear implant users. Likewise, if a candidate has had no hearing aid use for 20 years and long-term deafness, it is more appropriate to compare that individual with the lower 25% of implant recipients' performance. However, even with the most educated guess of cochlear implant outcome for a given individual and the knowledge that detection levels can be improved, specific postimplant results cannot be guaranteed, and this principle must be effectively communicated to candidates.

ADULT AUDIOLOGIC PROTOCOL. For adults, sound detection and speech perception abilities are assessed to determine candidacy. Preoperatively, patients are evaluated with a battery of measures while using hearing aids, and the results are compared with the most recent average and range of cochlear implant performance. Preoperative measures are also repeated postimplant for longitudinal monitoring of patient performance. Single-subject research designs are often implemented in clinical trials in which each patient serves as his or her control, primarily due to the large variability within the population of cochlear implant candidates and users. The selection of preoperative test measures, therefore, should also take into consideration comparative postimplant measures.

Preimplant audiologic tests include unaided and aided detection thresholds for pure-tone and warble-tone stimuli, respectively. Unaided thresholds are obtained in each ear individually, and aided detection thresholds may be obtained monaurally and binaurally. Although there are no aided detection level criteria, it is helpful to determine aided levels as one aspect of appropriate hearing aid fitting and for comparison with expected postimplant sound field detection thresholds. For some patients, aided testing can also reveal recruitment (i.e., unusual sensitivity to loud sounds), which may limit benefit from amplification due to the inability to incorporate needed hearing aid gain.

Aided speech perception abilities are often assessed in both monaural and binaural conditions, depending on the use of amplification in each ear. Speech perception measures are conducted in the sound field, typically at a presentation level of 60 dB SPL and include open-set recorded presentations of words and sentences in quiet, and if appropriate, in noise. In the best-aided condition, the assessment of individual ears provides critical information for determining which ear to implant for unilateral implantation. In addition, the best-aided condition, whether it be either ear alone or both ears together, provides information about the candidate's maximum performance for comparison with cochlear implant performance.

Word and sentence recognition tests included in the Minimum Speech Test Battery for Adult Cochlear Implant Users (MSTB) are used at many cochlear implant centers to assess performance. The MSTB is a set of compact disc recordings designed to provide word and sentence tests for the preimplant and postimplant evaluation of speech recognition, regardless of implant device. The Consonant-Nucleus-Consonant (CNC) Monosyllable Word Test[43] assesses single-syllable word recognition. One CNC list contains 50 monosyllabic words presented in an open-set format. The CNC Words were among the original set of words from which the Northwestern University Auditory Test 6 (NU6) Monosyllabic Word Test[44] were taken.

The presentation of auditory-only sentence lists from the Hearing in Noise Test (HINT)[45] evaluates each patient's ability to understand sentence material in quiet or in the presence of background noise. Each HINT list is phonemically balanced and contains 10 sentences recorded by a male speaker that are equivalent in the features of length, intelligibility, and naturalness. When the sentences are presented in noise, the signal-to-noise ratio typically used is +10 dB, although this ratio can be adjusted to make the test condition more or less difficult. For patients with some open-set speech recognition for words and/or sentences preoperatively, the BKB (Bamford-Koval-Bench) Sentences[46] may be administered in an adaptive procedure (i.e., BKB SIN; sentences-in-noise). In this condition the sentences are presented at a fixed presentation level (e.g., 65 dB SPL), and the noise is varied for signal-to-noise (S/N) ratios between +20 and −5. Clinical observations suggest that, when testing adults, scores on open-set word and sentence measures, particularly in the presence of noise, are more reflective of patient satisfaction with hearing aids and more useful for determining cochlear implant candidacy than unaided and/or aided detection thresholds.

As performance with cochlear implants continues to improve because of advances in technology and broadening candidacy criteria, it is recommended that speech perception performance be assessed with measures that approximate everyday listening. Study findings by Skinner and colleagues[47] and our cochlear implant team[48] suggest that speech recognition tests be presented at 60 rather than 70 dB SPL to determine implant candidacy. These findings have resulted in the use of 60 dB SPL in U.S. clinical trials and general clinical practice across centers. Additional steps toward the use of measures that approximate everyday listening include the presence of background noise, variation in speaker gender and rate, and variation in the location of the speaker.

Following the evaluation of sound detection and speech perception, other areas of assessment may include vestibular testing, tinnitus assessment, and patient satisfaction or quality-of-life questionnaires.

OUTCOME EXPECTATIONS FOR ADULTS. Almost all patients demonstrate improved sound detection with their cochlear implants compared with their preoperative performance with hearing aids, and this is especially evident in the high-frequency range. Average postoperative sound-field detection thresholds for warble-tone stimuli are approximately 25 to 30 dB HL for frequencies 250 through 4000 Hz.[48]

When determining patient's expectations for cochlear implant performance and when counseling patients preimplant, it is important to stay abreast of both the average speech perception performance of cochlear implant recipients and the range of performance. In a recent study of 78 of adult cochlear implant users, 26 each with the Clarion, Nucleus, and Med-El device, the average CNC word scores at 70, 60, and 50 dB SPL were 42%, 39%, and 24%, respectively.[48] In this same group of subjects the mean HINT scores at 70, 60, and 50 dB SPL were 72%, 73%, and 57%, respectively. When the HINT was presented at 60 dB SPL in the presence of speech spectrum noise at an S/N ratio of +10, the average score for this subject sample was 48%. These results represent average performance; however, there was a great deal of variation in scores for individuals, ranging from 0% to 100% for most measures. In general, patients perform less well on single syllable word tests compared with sentence tests, and less well in the presence of noise than in quiet. Many cochlear implant users can understand sentences without lipreading cues and can therefore converse on the telephone. Although the primary objective of speech coding strategies is the perception of speech, some patients also enjoy music.

The majority of postlingually deafened adults demonstrate significant preoperative to postoperative improvements on open-set speech perception measures, often as early as 1 month postimplant. Compared with postlingual affected adults, some prelingually affected adults, defined as having onset of profound or severe-to-profound hearing loss at younger than 3 to 6 years of age (depending on the respective study), demonstrate open-set speech recognition, although the percentage is smaller and often the length of device use needed to achieve this is longer. Although the average postoperative scores for individuals with prelingual hearing loss are generally lower compared with those with postlingual hearing loss, there have been significant preoperative to postoperative improvements in speech perception reported for this group.[49] Therefore adults with prelingual onset of severe-to-profound hearing loss may be appropriate candidates for cochlear implantation.

Providing that older patients are enjoying relatively good health, there is presently no upper age limit for cochlear implantation. Audiologic results for cochlear implant users ages 65 to 80 years indicate significant improvements for both preoperative to postoperative comparisons[50,51] and for varied speech stimulus presentation levels.[48]

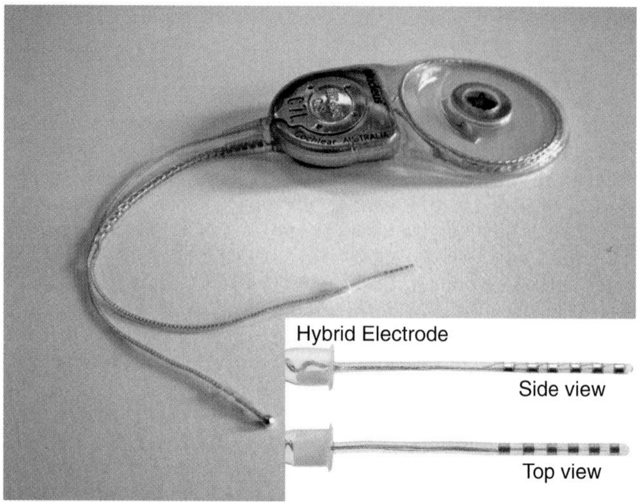

Figure 158-3. General appearance of the Nucleus Hybrid device for electroacoustic stimulation. Note the receiver/stimulator, removable magnet, loop antenna, separate ground electrode, and 10-mm electrode array. Inset shows the side and top view of the array that is designed to minimize electrode insertion trauma and preserve residual hearing. *(Published with permission, copyright © 2007 Cochlear Americas.)*

Current Trends That Affect Adult Cochlear Implant Candidacy

COMBINED ELECTRIC AND ACOUSTIC STIMULATION. For patients with more residual hearing preimplant than the average cochlear implant candidate, performance is expected to be better. In addition, some patients have considerable residual hearing in the lower frequencies (i.e., 250 and 500 Hz) but little measurable hearing for frequencies at 1000 Hz and above. In these patients it is difficult to obtain good aided benefit in the high frequencies with a hearing aid while maintaining appropriate gain in the lower frequencies where little, if any, amplification is necessary. The ability to understand speech is consequently compromised by the inability to detect and/or discriminate important high frequency sounds. Also, low-frequency sounds may be masked or distorted by the power needed in the high frequencies. These findings have led to the investigation of combined electrical and acoustic stimulation (EAS), such that the basal end of the cochlea receives electrical signals that are complemented by acoustic signals received at the apical portion of the cochlea. To use EAS, the low-frequency residual hearing must be preserved when the electrode array is inserted in the cochlea (Fig. 158-3). This is obtained by using shortened electrode arrays (20 mm for the Med-El device, and 10 mm for the Nucleus Hybrid device) inserted into the scala tympani and specific surgical techniques designed to make the electrode insertion as atraumatic as possible. These modifications include controlled opening and no direct suctioning of perilymph from the scala tympani; avoidance of perilymph contamination by blood and debris; use of nonototoxic topical antibiotics, corticosteroids, and lubricant (hyaluronic acid) during insertion; and immediate sealing of the cochleostomy after insertion using fascia. Speech perception findings reported thus far suggest improved performance in the combined EAS condition compared with either stimulation condition alone and compared with preimplant performance.[52] Additionally, recent data suggest that speech perception performance while listening in the presence of noise including multitalker babble is superior in the combined EAS condition compared with that of traditional cochlear implant users under the same adverse listening conditions.[53] It is likely that future candidacy may include patients with more low-frequency hearing, which is therefore a consideration during patient evaluation.

REHABILITATION OF ASYMMETRIC HEARING LOSS. A large number of patients who have lost hearing in one ear are not traditional cochlear implant candidates. These patients vary in the amount of hearing in their functional ear, ranging from normal hearing to severe hearing loss associated with marginal hearing aid benefit. As more experience has been gained with implantation of patients with more residual hearing and patients who benefit from hearing aid use in the nonimplanted ear,[52] the concept of cochlear implantation to rehabilitate asymmetric hearing loss is being considered.

BINAURAL COCHLEAR IMPLANTS. Historically, individuals received cochlear implants in one ear only. With the completion of clinical trials with bilateral implantation and the benefits of binaural implantation being realized, current candidacy decisions now include whether to receive two implants rather than one. Outcomes data regarding the benefits of binaural implantation continue to be published, and clear benefits in sound localization and listening in noise have been demonstrated.[54] Specifically, studies have shown that binaural implants provide a "head shadow" effect for listening to speech in the presence of other noise or competing speakers. This occurs because one ear is "shadowed" from the noise source when speech and noise come from different directions, allowing the ear with the better signal-to-noise ratio to do the listening. Other binaural advantages occur when information from both ears is combined to improve listening. Binaural summation effects have been reported whereby performance is improved in the binaural condition compared with monaural condition when speech and noise are in the front.[55] Binaural squelch effects have been reported less frequently to date, but in some cases, improvement in performance has been shown by adding the ear nearer the noise source.[56] Both binaural summation and binaural squelch effects rely on successful bilateral interaction of the brainstem and central auditory system nuclei, whereas the head shadow effect is simply a physical phenomenon created by the listener's head. We have found that presentation of more difficult auditory stimuli helps to demonstrate the improved benefit obtained by patients tested in the binaural condition compared with the benefit from their better-performing cochlear implant.[57]

Binaural implantation in adults recently completed clinical trials at a number of centers and with each of the cochlear implant manufacturers in the United States. Because results have been generally positive and the majority of bilateral recipients indicate a strong preference for bilateral over unilateral implant use, it is now the case that binaural implantation has become a part of the candidacy decision.

Recommendations for Referral for Adult Cochlear Implant Evaluation

At our center, we suggest the following referral criteria for cochlear implant evaluation for adults. Referral to a cochlear implant center does not mean that the individual is necessarily going to receive a cochlear implant, but that an evaluation is recommended to determine whether a cochlear implant would be beneficial. If the individual meets the following criteria, an evaluation is suggested. The criteria are (1) unaided thresholds of 70 dB HL or poorer at 1000 Hz and above in the better ear, even if hearing levels at 250 and 500 Hz are better; (2) unaided word discrimination less than 70%; and (3) frustration on the part of the patient due to communication difficulties, even with appropriate hearing aid use.

Evaluation of Pediatric Cochlear Implant Candidates

Cochlear implants have been available for children ages 2 to 17 years since 1990. Originally, children who were candidates for cochlear implantation typically had profound bilateral sensorineural hearing loss with pure-tone average thresholds of 100 dB HL or greater, often with corner audiograms. These children also displayed aided sound-field thresholds well below the range of average conversational speech and typical speech detection thresholds at and above 60 dB HL. During early clinical trials, pediatric candidates were not able to understand words when using their hearing alone, even with high-gain hearing aids and well-fitted earmolds. Since then, candidacy criteria have changed and technology has improved, both of which have influenced benefit. As with adults, consideration for cochlear implantation still requires careful assessment to (1) determine preimplant fitting of hearing aids and baseline performance, (2) compare a candidate's preimplant performance with that of current implant users, (3) provide a recommendation for or against cochlear implantation, (4) select an ear for implantation, and (5) determine appropriate expectations that will guide the counseling of prospective families.

Current Pediatric Selection Criteria

The selection criteria for children vary slightly depending on the respective FDA-approved clinical trial and/or criteria recommended by the cochlear implant center. Generally speaking, the subject selection criteria include the following: (1) 12 months through 17 years of age; (2) profound sensorineural hearing loss (unaided PTA thresholds of ≥ 90 dB HL); (3) minimal benefit from hearing aids, defined as less than 20% to 30% on single-syllable word tests, or for younger children, lack of developmentally appropriate auditory milestones measured using parent report scales; (4) no evidence of central auditory lesions or lack of an auditory nerve; and (5) no evidence of contraindications for surgery in general or cochlear implant surgery in particular. Additionally, cochlear implant centers generally recommend at least 3 to 6 months of hearing aid use, unless cochlear ossification is noted or anticipated; realistic expectations by family members; enrollment in a postoperative rehabilitation program that supports the use of cochlear implants and the development of auditory skills; and willingness on the part of the family to comply with follow-up procedures as defined by the center.

PEDIATRIC AUDIOLOGIC PROTOCOL. As with adults, children are assessed preoperatively with a battery of sound detection and speech perception measures while using hearing aids, and this baseline is compared with the most recent average and range of cochlear implant performance. For children, speech perception measures assess a wide range of auditory skills from sound detection to recognition of words and sentences. Measures are selected that are developmentally appropriate for the child's age, language level, and auditory ability. Although the audiologic assessment will play a key role in candidacy, with children other factors may influence the candidacy decision and/or postimplant outcome, and therefore a multidisciplinary team approach is advised.

Before cochlear implant evaluation, most children will have an ABR test as an objective measure of the status of the peripheral and brainstem auditory system. With an ABR, acoustic click stimuli are presented to assess auditory sensitivity to each ear. Children who are implant candidates typically have no response to acoustic stimuli at the limits of the testing equipment, suggesting with reasonable accuracy hearing loss in the profound range. Another group of children that can display absent or abnormal ABR findings are those with auditory neuropathy.[9] In these cases of absent or abnormal ABR, comparison of positive (condensation) and negative (rarefaction) polarity stimuli will show an inversion of the peaks of the cochlear microphonic. The cochlear microphonic appears as an early latency response on the ABR waveform and is indicative of outer hair cell function. Otoacoustic emission testing can also be used as a measure of outer hair cell function. Due to the prevalence of children diagnosed with AN/AD[15] and the number of these children who have received cochlear implants,[58] our current protocols for electrophysiologic assessment include otoacoustic emission and ABR testing because these measures are sensitive to cochlear and auditory nerve function, respectively. The diagnosis of auditory neuropathy does not necessarily preclude a child from cochlear implant candidacy.

Unaided detection thresholds for pure-tone stimuli are obtained in individual ears using standard clinical procedures. Aided thresholds are obtained in the binaural condition, and if possible, the monaural conditions. For young children who are unable to participate in speech perception tasks, both unaided threshold testing and electrophysiologic measures become important criteria for cochlear implantation. Because we know the limitations of hearing aids, if we are confident in the reliability of the unaided threshold levels, we can predict with some certainty the eventual aided benefit. Using hearing aids, the measurement of sound detection levels, and when possible, speech perception abilities, can provide confirmation of the unaided thresholds. Although one criterion for pediatric candidacy is profound hearing loss, published reports and clinical experience both indicate that adults with severe hearing losses perform well with cochlear implants. Therefore we might expect the same outcome for children with similar severe hearing losses. With respect to children with AN/AD, unaided detection levels vary considerably and may not be predictive of aided levels or speech perception abilities.

Tests of speech perception assess a range of skills depending on the child's auditory abilities and language level. Closed-set measures include a small number of choices that are provided to the child either as objects or pictures (e.g., Early Speech Perception Test or ESP).[59] Monosyllable, spondee, and/or trochee words are spoken with audition alone (no visual cues), and the child is asked to select the object or picture that represents the stimulus. With open-set measures of word and sentence recognition, no choices are provided. The child repeats the words or sentences presented in quiet or in the presence of background noise. For example, using the Lexical Neighborhood Test (LNT),[60] 50 monosyllabic words are presented that are either "easy," occurring with high frequency in the English language and having few lexical neighbors, or "hard," occurring less frequently and with many lexical neighbors. For children with vocabulary levels that approximate those of a 5-year old, the Phonetically Balanced Kindergarten (PBK) Test[61] can be administered. It includes 50 words and has been in clinical use for many years. Recordings of the BKB Sentences[46] and the HINT-C Sentences[45] are typically used in the evaluation process for children who have some language and auditory experience. For children who are too young to participate in speech perception measures, parent interview scales are administered. The Meaningful Auditory Integration Scale (MAIS)[62] asks questions of parents or family members related to the child's spontaneous awareness of sound and use of audition in a meaningful way at home, school, or other natural environments.

OTHER EVALUATIONS FOR PEDIATRIC COCHLEAR IMPLANT CANDIDATES. For children, the results of speech production assessments are good indicators of hearing history and whether the child has learned to use his or her residual hearing. Language evaluations are also important because the ultimate goal of cochlear implantation is effective communication. Neither of these areas of assessment dictates candidacy, but they contribute to the confirmation of hearing levels and expected preimplant communication coincident with auditory experience. Results are also used to monitor either preimplant or postimplant performance over time and to develop rehabilitation goals for educators, clinicians, and parents.

A psychologic evaluation is obtained to assess the child's verbal and nonverbal intelligence, attention and memory skills, and visual-motor integration. When considering a child for a cochlear implant, counseling the family preimplant, and planning for possible rehabilitative needs postimplant, it is important to know the cognitive abilities of the child. If the child is gifted, for example, then expecting average cochlear implant performance may be an underestimation. Likewise, if the child has a developmental delay, this will affect rate and eventual level of performance with the implant and counseling may be directed toward more conservative expectations. Differentiating the influence of deafness and cochlear implantation from other disabilities or diagnoses such as developmental delay, autism, attention deficit disorder, or learning disabilities can be difficult. These issues are addressed in the psychologic evaluation preimplant and influence the recommendation for or against cochlear implantation, provide guidance for counseling families, and assist in rehabilitative planning.

Success with a cochlear implant can be influenced by the collaboration of individuals working with the child (parents, educators, and therapists). A team effort is best initiated during the preimplant process and sets the stage for later communication between the individuals on the implant team and the child's educators and family. Early cultivation of communication is important for a variety of reasons including confirmation of the child's test results and use of residual hearing, discussion of areas of concern, sharing effective test-taking and rehabilitative strategies, setting expectations, and identification of postimplant rehabilitation resources and goals.

OUTCOME EXPECTATIONS FOR CHILDREN. Auditory detection levels with a cochlear implant are expected to be similar to those for adults, which are approximately 25 dB HL for frequencies 250 through 4000 Hz. These detection levels allow access to information that is important for the development of auditory skills and communication.

As with adults, when determining expectations, it is important to stay informed of the average and range of pediatric cochlear implant performance.

In a publication by Geers and colleagues,[63] the results of 181 prelingual deaf children, implanted before 5 years of age who had used their cochlear implants for an average of 5 years, were reported for the outcome areas of speech perception, speech production, spoken language, total language, and reading. The average scores reported for several measures are as follows: ESP-spondee 85%, ESP-monosyllable 79%, LNT-easy 48%, LNT-hard 44%, and BKB sentences 57%. Children who were good speech perceivers were also the children who exhibited superior performance for measures of speech intelligibility, language, and reading. Half of the children were enrolled in oral communication programs, and the other half were enrolled in programs using total communication. Those children enrolled in educational environments that emphasized auditory and spoken language development had the highest scores on speech perception, speech production, and language measures. In this study, subjects were implanted between 1992 and 1994, mostly using the Nucleus 22 and SPEAK coding strategy; therefore the most recent cochlear implant technology and candidacy criteria were not represented.

Studies conducted with children indicate that earlier implantation is associated with higher performance for a given time period postimplant,[64] that preimplant unaided residual hearing influences performance and the development of speech perception skills postimplant,[65] and that there is a steady increase in performance over time that does not plateau during the first 3 to 5 years of implant use.[66]

On the basis of research studies and clinical experience, we describe in this section general expectations for children with onset of deafness of less than 1 year on the basis of their age at implantation. Expectations for children implanted at age 2 years and before include the potential for communication skill development at rates similar to normal-hearing peers, potential for speech to be easily understood by strangers, reduced or possible elimination of language delay, attendance at a neighborhood school with minimal support services by kindergarten or first grade, and increased likelihood of becoming an auditory/oral communicator. Expectations for children implanted before the age of 4 years include substantial improvement in speech perception, increased vocalizations/verbalizations at early stages postimplant, auditory behaviors evident before they can be formally measured, speech production skills reflective of auditory abilities, and language delays that are reduced. For children implanted between 4 and 5 years, expectations include improvement in speech perception with excellent closed-set performance and varied open-set abilities, improvements in speech production, use of hearing to support improvements in language, and reduced dependence on visual cues for communication. For children implanted at or after age 6 years, we expect improved auditory detection abilities, improvements in speech perception that entail good closed-set abilities but limited open-set skills, possible improvements in speech production, and continued dependence on visual cues for communication. Generally, children implanted at an older age require more time to reach their potential with the device than those implanted at younger ages.

In addition, for children with progressive or sudden onset of hearing loss, we expect excellent progress with cochlear implantation and achievement of these skills with a shorter duration of cochlear implant use. Likewise, for children with some residual hearing preimplant, we also expect higher levels of performance in relatively shorter periods of time. As discussed regarding adults, it is important to match expectations with reasonable appropriate outcomes for children on the basis of their hearing history, age at implantation, and nonaudiologic factors.

Current Trends That Affect Pediatric Cochlear Implant Candidacy

BINAURAL COCHLEAR IMPLANTS. Far beyond what has been experienced with adult patients, the majority of major cochlear implant centers are now performing bilateral cochlear implantation in the majority of children. Reports in children have followed similar trends as those for adults, with improvements in the ability to recognize speech in noise and to localize a sound source. The ability to follow large spatial changes in speaker location is a critical skill for academic learning in the classroom setting, as is the ability to follow rapid changes between speakers in a smaller space such as in a small group setting at school or during a conversation with multiple speakers at home. Bilateral implantation is desirable for young children during the critical period for the development of spoken communication. To study the observed clinical benefits reported by parents and teachers and observed by clinicians caring for these children, there are several multicenter investigations of bilateral cochlear implantation in children currently under way in North America and Europe. Due to the longer periods required for speech language development in young children, these trials are designed to extend a minimum of 5 years. On the basis of the findings in these trials, the circumstances for which we would recommend bilateral implants for children will be evident.

Factors That Affect Pediatric Cochlear Implant Performance

The most common preimplant factors that affect performance for children include age at implantation, hearing experience (age at onset of profound hearing loss, amount of residual hearing, progressive nature of the hearing loss, aided levels, consistency of hearing aid use), training with amplification (in the case of some residual hearing), presence of other disabilities, and parent and family support. Postimplant factors that contribute to performance levels include length of cochlear implant use, rehabilitative training, and family support. Communication mode is also a documented variable that affects postimplant outcome because children in programs and homes that focus on the development of spoken language perform higher than children in programs without this emphasis.[63] Children using total communication at school and home can achieve substantial levels of performance; however, this achievement will be less likely if an emphasis on auditory skill development and spoken communication is not included with the use of sign language.

Ear Selection in Pediatric Cochlear Implant Candidates

For children whose parents elect for their child to receive a single cochlear implant, the selection of the ear for unilateral implantation follows the same logic as discussed earlier for adults. At our center, the pediatric population differs from the adults in that fewer children have an etiology of progressive hearing loss (22%), compared with those with congenital bilateral hearing loss (65%) or sudden onset of bilateral hearing loss (13%). In general, this results in fewer children having ear asymmetries or patterns of change in hearing over time. Therefore fewer children have ear differences. Because we encourage the use of a contralateral hearing aid postimplant if at all possible, we select the ear for implantation that is least likely to benefit from amplification. All things being equal, we select the right ear to capture the possible advantage of contralateral, left hemisphere specialization for speech recognition.[67]

Recommendations for Referral for Pediatric Cochlear Implant Evaluation

At our center, we suggest the following referral criteria for cochlear implant evaluation for children. As mentioned previously with adults, referral to a cochlear implant center does not mean that a child is necessarily going to receive a cochlear implant, but that an evaluation is recommended to determine whether a cochlear implant would be beneficial. If the child meets one or more of the following criteria, an evaluation is suggested. The criteria are (1) unaided thresholds of 90 dB HL or poorer at 2000 Hz and above in the better ear, even if hearing levels at 250 and 500 Hz are better; (2) aided levels in the better ear poorer than 35 dB HL, especially at 4000 Hz; (3) no response for ABR testing in both ears or no response for one ear and responses at elevated levels in the other ear; (4) parents are frustrated with their child's development of auditory and/or communication skills; (5) progressive hearing loss with detection levels at or near the profound range at 2000 Hz and above; or (6) evidence of severely impairing auditory neuropathy/dys-synchrony. Evaluation has no lower age limit; age at implantation is a critical factor that influences postimplant performance, and children who may be too young for the operation are not too young for evaluation.

Device Selection

All cochlear implant systems include external and internal hardware. The external equipment includes a microphone, speech processor, and transmission system. The internal device includes a receiver/stimulator and an electrode array.

In general, an external microphone picks up sound and speech in the environment and sends the information to a speech processor, either the body-worn (BW) or ear-level type. The speech processor converts the sounds into electric signals, which are sent across the skin via radio frequency transmission to the internal receiver/stimulator. The transmission of the signal occurs when there is successful alignment of the external magnet housed in the transmitter with the internal magnet housed in the receiver/stimulator. The receiver/stimulator decodes the signals and delivers them to the electrodes positioned within the cochlea. The electrodes stimulate the auditory nerve, and the signal is sent along the auditory pathway to the auditory cortex. A description of the most recent available equipment for each cochlear implant manufacturer used by patients in the United States is provided as follows.

Internal Receiver Stimulators and Electrode Designs

NUCLEUS FREEDOM WITH CONTOUR ADVANCE ELECTRODE. The Nucleus Freedom device with Contour Advance electrode (CI24RE[CA]) consists of an internal receiver/stimulator that uses a flexible silicone housing surrounding a titanium case. The Nucleus Freedom device with the Contour Advance electrode is shown in Figures 158-4 and 158-5. The magnet is removable/replaceable and allows for MRI studies with magnets up to 1.5 tesla (T), after removal of the magnet. The electrode design is a perimodiolar electrode and is preformed to conform to the modiolus. A stylet is positioned within this electrode array and maintains the electrode in a straight configuration until its removal during the operation. The electrode array is curved, consisting of 22 half-banded platinum electrodes, variably spaced over 15 mm. The diameter of the intracochlear portion ranges from 0.5 mm to 0.8 mm. Overall, the length of the electrode array distal to the first of three silicon marker rings is 24 mm; however, the electrode is designed to be inserted 22 mm, and a platinum band is present at this position to use as a guide for depth of insertion. The half-banded electrodes face the modiolus with a width of 0.3 mm and a geometric area ranging from 0.28 mm^2 to 0.31 mm^2. Of all available electrodes on the market, this is the stiffest electrode and consequently is relatively easy to insert. The greatest disadvantage of this current electrode design is that once the stylet has been removed, it cannot be replaced. This is problematic should the electrode insertion be difficult because of anatomic variations, in which case the back-up device would be required. Manual positioning of the electrode tip within the opening of the cochleostomy is performed, and guiding the tip into this position is assisted by the use of a claw-shaped instrument held in the dominant hand. Once the electrode tip is retained within the opening of the cochleostomy, bimanual advancement of the electrode array using two claw-shaped instruments held opposing each other, as close to the cochleostomy as possible, assists advancement of the electrode array within the scala tympani. There is a white marker incorporated along the electrode that is used to determine when the electrode array should be advanced off of the stylet until complete insertion has been achieved. The Nucleus Contour electrode array has three Silastic bands outside of the electrode array that represent the proximal limit, and these should remain outside of the cochleostomy. Once this level is reached, the remainder of the stylet is withdrawn and discarded. The electrode is then maintained in a perimodiolar position.[68]

The Nucleus device also has a second electrode design, a double electrode array to be used for implantation of severely ossified cochleas (Fig. 158-6). The configuration for this includes two electrode arrays, each with 11 contacts within a length of 8.5 mm.

HiRes 90K. The Advanced Bionics Corporation system includes the HiRes 90K receiver/stimulator (Fig. 158-7) and a choice of two electrodes; the HiFocus 1j array or the Helix array. The HiRes 90K system has a removable magnet that has been approved by the FDA to allow for an MRI with a field strength of up to 1.5T, providing that the magnet has been removed. The HiFocus 1j electrode system is shown in Figure 32-14. This electrode is "banana shaped" and curved toward the modiolus, consisting of 16 contacts, spaced every 1.1 mm over 17 mm. The length of the electrode array inserted into the cochlea is 23 mm. The electrodes face the modiolus with a width of 0.4 mm and length of 0.5 mm. The HiFocus 1j electrode system uses an insertion tube through which the insertion tool allows advancement of the electrode array. Both a metal (outer diameter of 1.5 mm) insertion tube and a Teflon (outer diameter of 2 mm) insertion tube are included, and selection is based on surgeon preference; however, the metal tube provides greater stability. Gentle pressure along a thumb-driven advancement mechanism is required to insert the electrode. Should errors occur during electrode insertion, the electrode is easily reloaded into the insertion tube, and additional electrode insertion attempts can be completed until the electrode insertion has been achieved.

The HiFocus Helix electrode system is shown in Figure 158-8. This electrode is designed to be perimodiolar in location after insertion. The array consists of 16 contacts, spaced every 0.85 mm over 13 mm.

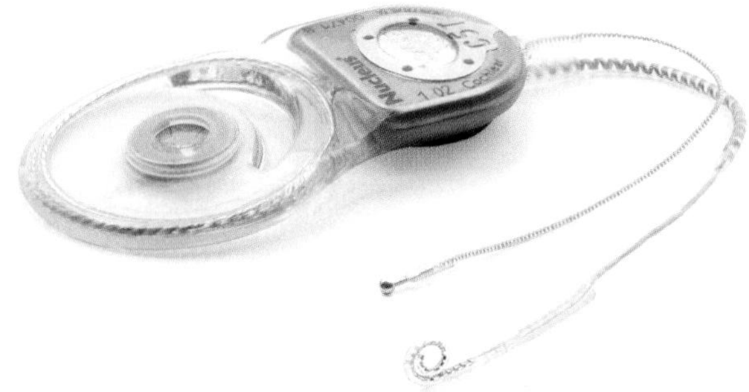

Figure 158-4. General appearance of the Nucleus Freedom device with the Contour Advance electrode. Note the receiver/stimulator, removable magnet, loop antenna, separate ground electrode, and electrode array. *(Published with permission, copyright © 2008 Cochlear Americas.)*

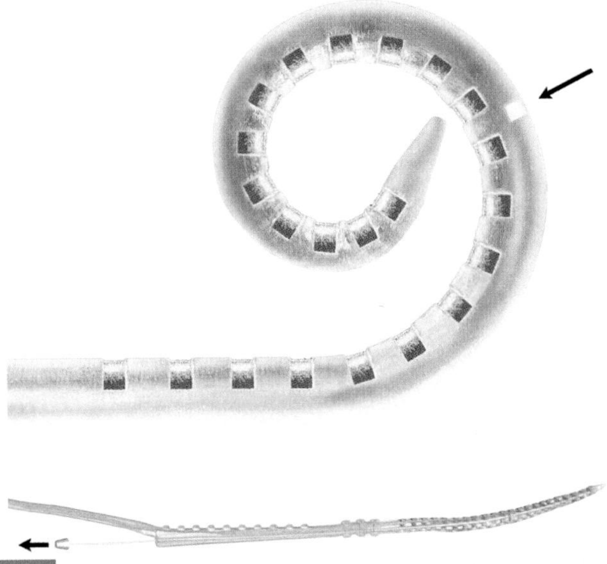

Figure 158-5. Nucleus Contour Advance electrode after *(top)* and before *(bottom)* stylet removal. The electrode array has a more linear configuration before stylet removal. The electrode is advanced until the white marker *(long arrow)* is located at the level of the cochleostomy. The electrode is then advanced off of the stylet by holding the stylet with a forceps and inserting the electrode. Removal of the stylet *(short arrow)* allows the electrode to return to the precurved configuration of the array, which places the electrode contacts in a perimodiolar position. *(Published with permission, copyright © 2008 Cochlear Americas.)*

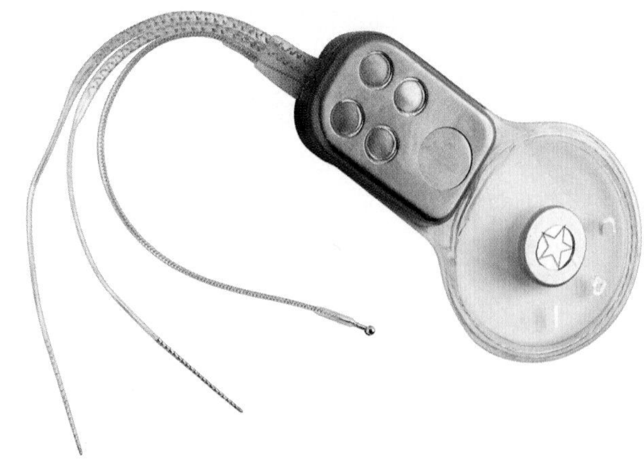

Figure 158-6. General appearance of the Nucleus device with double electrodes for use in patients with cochlear ossification. Note the receiver/stimulator, removable magnet, loop antenna, separate ground electrode, and the dual electrode arrays, each with 11 contacts over a length of 8.5 mm. *(Published with permission, copyright © 2008 Cochlear Americas.)*

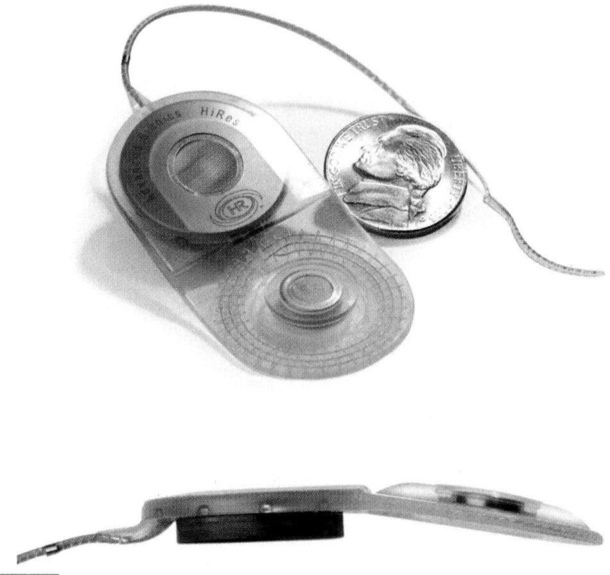

Figure 158-7. General appearance of the HiRes 90K Bionic Ear device with the 1j electrode. Note the receiver/stimulator with tapered edge at the front of the implant, removable magnet, loop antenna, and electrode array *(top)*. The side view shows the low profile of the portion of the device that is located on the surface of the skull *(bottom)*. *(Published with permission, copyright © 2008 Advanced Bionics Corporation.)*

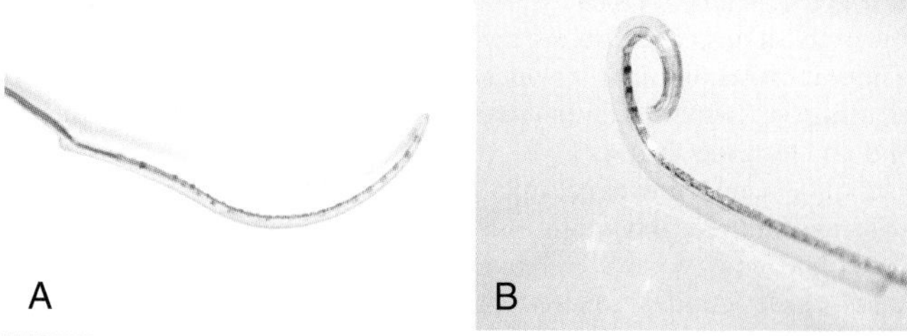

Figure 158-8. Photographs of the HiFocus 1j and Helix electrodes. **A,** The 1j electrode is banana shaped and has flat contacts oriented toward the modiolus. The raised partitions shown in the inset, between electrode contacts, are designed to reduce electrode interactions. **B,** The Helix electrode uses the same flat contact configuration with the raised partitions but is precurved to place the electrode array in a perimodiolar position after insertion. *(Published with permission, copyright © 2008 Advanced Bionics Corporation.)*

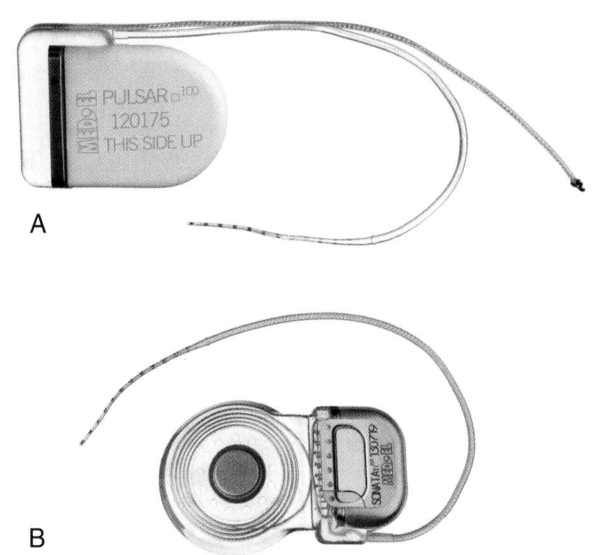

Figure 158-9. **A,** General appearance of the Med-El PulsarCI100 device. The internal device is housed in a ceramic case containing the receiver/stimulator, internal magnet, and loop antenna. **B,** General appearance of the Med-El SonataTI100 device. The internal device is housed in Silastic and has a similar configuration for the receiver/stimulator, internal magnet, and loop antenna as does the Nucleus Freedom and HiRes 90K devices. *(Published with permission, copyright © 2008 Med-El Corporation.)*

The diameter of the intracochlear portion ranges from 0.6 mm to 1.1 mm. The length of the electrode array inserted into the cochlea is 24.5 mm. The electrodes face the modiolus with a width of 0.4 mm and length of 0.5 mm. The HiFocus Helix electrode system uses a preloaded stylet assembly by which the electrode array is advanced. Should errors occur during electrode insertion, the electrode is easily reloaded into the insertion stylet assembly, and additional electrode insertion attempts can be completed until the electrode insertion has been achieved. This is in contrast to the Nucleus Contour Advance perimodiolar electrode, which cannot be reloaded after removal of the stylet.

MED-EL PULSARCI100 AND SONATATI100. The Med-El PulsarCI100 system uses a receiver/stimulator that is housed in a ceramic case (Fig. 158-9). The PulsarCI100 system has FDA approval for use with MRI at 0.2 T causing no additional risk to the patient or significant impact on the device or image quality, except for the magnet-induced artifact surrounding the internal magnet. In Europe many patients with Med-El implants have safely undergone MRI studies with 1.0 and 1.5 T scanners.[69] The Med-El system has six separate electrode designs (see Figs. 158-12 and 158-13). The standard electrode is the longest electrode available in the marketplace and is tapered in design. Twelve pairs of electrode bands are distributed over the 31.5 mm electrode array length. A FLEXeas array (20.9 mm) is also available for applications such as EAS; for cochleas that are partially ossified, a compressed electrode is available; and for severely ossified cochleas, a split electrode array is available. In July 2007 FDA approval was granted for the Med-El SonataCI100 internal device (see Fig. 158-9). The SonataCI100 Cochlear Implant contains the same electronics as the PulsarCI100 device, but the electronics are encased in a titanium housing that is smaller and thinner than the PulsarCI100 ceramic casing. All Med-El electrode arrays are compatible with the SonataTI100. The receiver coil and internal magnet are positioned outside of the electronics package in flexible silicone, although the magnet is not removable for MRI. The SonataTI100 is also MRI compatible in the United States at 0.2T without magnet removal.

If ossification of the cochlea is encountered during the opening of the cochleostomy, the use of the Med-El Insertion Test Device (ITD) can be helpful to determine which of their various electrode options should be used. If the ITD can be inserted to the small flanges present 17.8 mm from the tip, the standard array should be used; if less than that, the medium or compressed array should be used. The medium electrode array (PulsarCI100M) has all 12 pairs of electrodes distributed over 21 mm spaced 1.9 mm apart. The PulsarCI100 compressed electrode (PulsarCI100S) is designed with the same number of electrode contacts ($n = 12$ pairs), but arranged closer together on the apical end of the array and spaced over 12.1 mm. With ossification present, the ITD is advanced through the cochleostomy and the depth of insertion is determined. If it is apparent that insertion of the standard electrode array would result in electrodes being extracochlear in location, the compressed or medium electrode array should be used and fully inserted.

For more severely ossified cochleas, the Med-El split electrode design (PulsarCI100GB) has two compressed electrode arrays with five and seven pairs of electrode contacts, respectively (Fig. 158-10). These electrode arrays are inserted via two cochleostomies. When the two arrays are in place, the electrode contacts provide more sites of potential stimulation than a single standard array incompletely inserted into the cochlea. The sixth electrode design is for applications in patients who have a common cochlear cavity (see Figs. 158-10 and 158-11). This electrode uses the basic PulsarCI100S array with 3 to 5 mm of Silastic and a distal nonfunctional platinum ball.

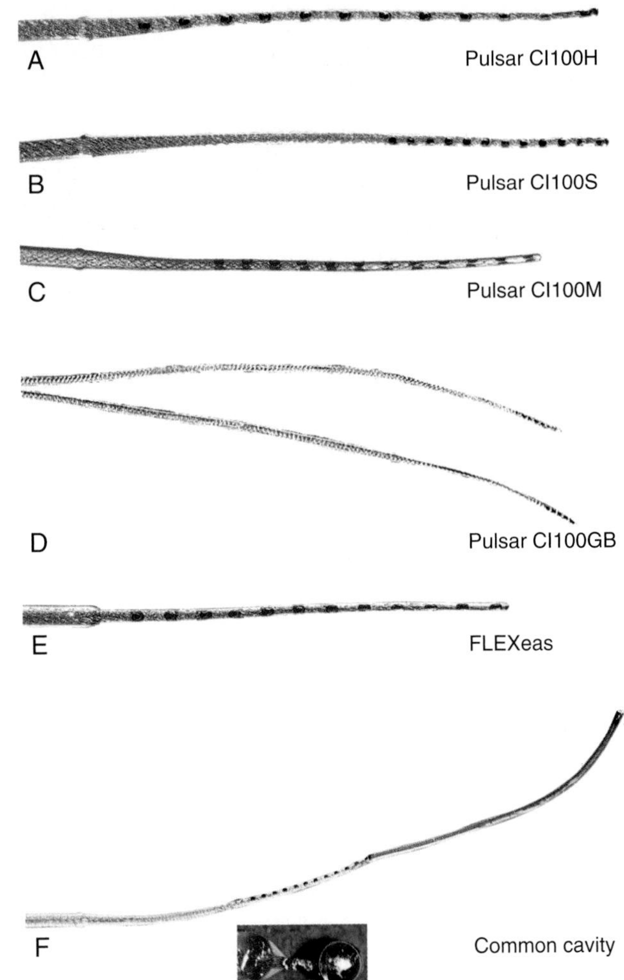

Figure 158-10. Six electrode designs available for the Med-El PulsarCI100 and SonataTI100 cochlear implants. **A,** Standard 31.5 mm electrode with the electrode contacts distributed over 26.4 mm. When ossification is encountered during creation of the cochleostomy, use of the insertion test device allows determination of whether to open the standard electrode array or one of the two shorter arrays or the split electrode array. **B,** The compressed array distributes the electrode contacts over 13 mm. **C,** The medium array distributes the electrode contacts over 21 mm. **D,** The split array has one with five pairs of electrode contacts, while the other has seven pairs of electrode contacts. **E,** For hearing preservation and application of electroacoustic stimulation, the FLEXeas electrode is designed to be thin and 20.9 mm in length. **F,** For severe cochlear malformations such as a common cavity, the custom-manufactured common cavity electrode can be used. This electrode array uses the basic compressed electrode with a nonfunctional Silastic extension terminating in a platinum ball *(inset),* which is used to place the electrode array via a double labyrinthotomy technique as shown in Figure 158-11. *(Published with permission, copyright © 2009 P.A. Wackym, MD.)*

External Speech Processors

Each manufacturer offers a body-worn (BW) and behind-the-ear (BTE) processor. The BW processors were the first wearable devices for each implant type, followed by the introduction of BTE processors, which are generally preferred by adults and some children/parents. Both BW and BTE processors have program switches, volume and/or sensitivity controls, batteries (rechargeable or alkaline), and accessories. External processor wear options vary from one device to another but may include, for example, a remote battery pack worn off the ear or a rechargeable battery pack worn on the processor at the ear. A variety of mechanisms (e.g., earhooks, indicator lights) perform functions such as alerting parents to a low battery or a disconnected headpiece. External auditory input sources can be connected to the processors such as auxiliary microphones, telephone adaptors, tape recorders, television audio amplifiers, or FM systems. Other cosmetic considerations include a variety of processor and transmission coil colors, decorative caps, processor belt clips, and harnesses or hip packs for daily wear. Because the external equipment changes regularly, the specifics for each manufacturer are reviewed at the time of device discussion and selection, which occurs once cochlear implantation has been recommended.

Current Signal Processing Strategies

Each device manufacturer provides a selection of signal processing strategies that may affect device selection for a given patient. For example, patients who are music enthusiasts may be interested in comparing aspects of fine structure strategies, whereas other patients with neurologic processing issues may benefit from having strategies that offer slower stimulation rates. Below are summaries of currently available signal processing strategies.

Temporal Strategies

CONTINUOUS INTERLEAVED SAMPLING. Continuous interleaved sampling (CIS) is a speech processing strategy that has been implemented in cochlear implant devices in recent years. One problem encountered with early speech processing strategies was interaction between electrical fields when electrodes were stimulated simultaneously, particularly with broad, monopolar stimulation. This is referred to as channel interaction, and it is thought to result in a degradation of the intended signal. CIS was introduced by Wilson and colleagues[70] as a way to minimize overlap between monopolar electric fields across stimulated electrodes, thereby preserving the integrity of the electrical signal. In CIS, biphasic pulses are delivered to electrodes with timing offsets so that none of the electrodes are stimulated simultaneously. This sequential stimulation pattern results in increased electrical channel independence, which, in addition to decreasing channel interaction, allows for the possible advantage of using more channels.

Although several versions of CIS are implemented across devices, the pulse amplitudes in CIS are generally determined by several steps. First, at a given point in time, the acoustic input signal is bandpass filtered, with the lower frequency information allocated to apical channels and higher-frequency information allocated to basal channels.

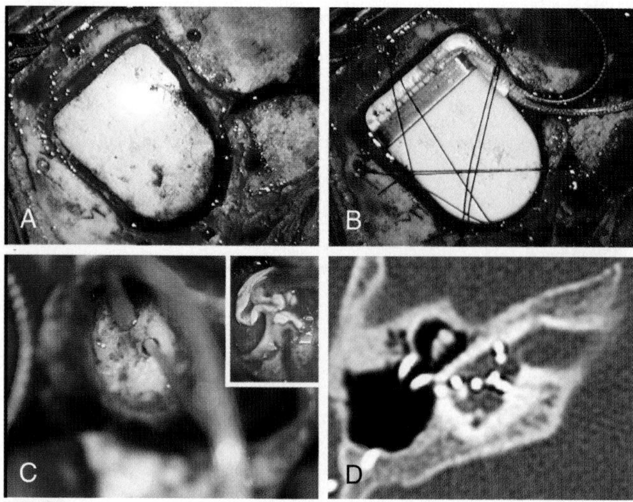

Figure 158-11. Cochlear implantation in a common cavity malformation. **A,** Craniotomy with the bone island technique. **B,** The Med-El internal receiver/stimulator secured with three 3-0 nylon sutures. **C,** the common cavity electrode was inserted via a double labyrinthotomy technique. Inset shows fascia sealing both labyrinthotomies. **D,** Postoperative computed tomography scan shows the position of the electrode array within the common cavity. *(Published with permission, copyright © 2009 P.A. Wackym, MD.)*

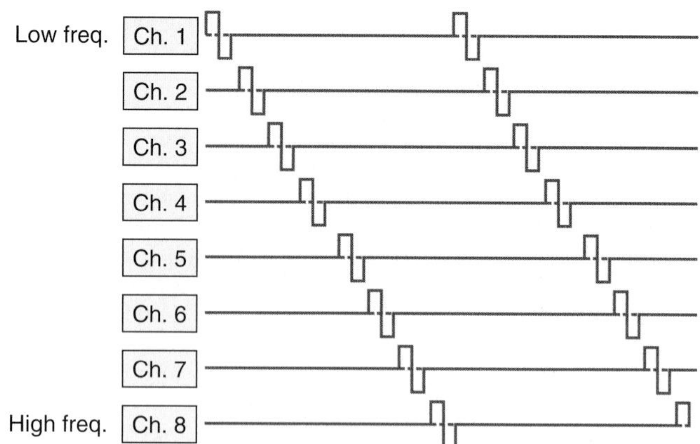

Figure 158-12. Analog stimulation. Each electrode is stimulated continuously and simultaneously. In this example, electrode 1 carries the lowest frequency information and electrode 7 carries the highest frequency information. The Simultaneous Analog Stimulation (SAS) implemented by Advanced Bionics Corporation uses a bipolar electrode configuration to reduce electrode interaction. *(Published with permission, copyright © 2008 Advanced Bionics Corporation.)*

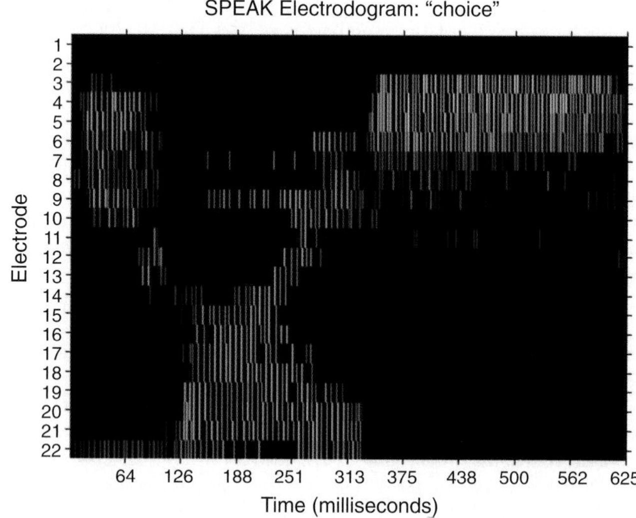

Figure 158-13. Spectral Peak Extraction (SPEAK). An electrodogram is shown for the word "choice" encoded by the SPEAK strategy. Time is plotted on the abscissa and electrode number on the ordinate, and the more intense stimuli are indicated by brighter bars. The relatively low stimulation rate of 250 Hz is apparent. *(Published with permission, copyright © 2008 Cochlear Americas.)*

Next, within each frequency band, the amplitude of the input signal is determined, and this envelope amplitude is compressed to fit into the appropriate dynamic range of electrical hearing for each channel. The compressed amplitude calculated from the input signal is used to determine the amplitude of the stimulus pulses that are sent to the designated electrodes. In this way, CIS primarily conveys temporal information from the input signal. All three devices available in the United States have a CIS strategy option.

ANALOG STIMULATION. Electric analog stimulation is a digitized representation of the original acoustic signal that is presented continuously over time and simultaneously to the different electrodes in a tonotopic manner. Preservation of the original acoustic signal would presumably be beneficial for electrical hearing, but limitations to this stimulation paradigm warrant consideration. An early analog speech processing strategy, compressed analog (CA),[71] was presented using a monopolar electrode configuration. The combination of broad current spread and continuous, simultaneous stimulation resulted in extensive channel interaction. Current spread can be reduced by changing the electrode configuration from monopolar to bipolar mode, which localizes the electric field by stimulating between a pair of electrodes on the array.[72] Using a bipolar coupling mode, the analog strategy available in the Clarion 1.2, CI Bionic Ear, CII Bionic Ear, and HiRes 90K devices is referred to as Simultaneous Analog Stimulation (SAS). An example of SAS is shown in Figure 158-12, with the low-frequency analog stimulation sent to the apical channel (channel 1 in the Advanced Bionics Corporation devices) and the highest frequency stimulation to the basal channel (channel 7).

Spectral Emphasis Strategies

SPECTRAL PEAK EXTRACTION. Spectral peak extraction, or SPEAK, is implemented in the Nucleus device.[73] SPEAK includes a bandpass filter analysis of the input signal, and the outputs selected for stimulation are those with the highest amplitude components, or the largest spectral peaks. The corresponding electrodes are activated sequentially in a basal-to-apical direction at a relatively low rate (≈250 Hz). Typically, the number of electrodes stimulated, or maxima, is 6 to 8, although it may range from 1 to 10, with the more electrodes stimulated, the slower the rate. Figure 158-13 shows an example of the stimulus output pattern for the SPEAK strategy in the Nucleus device. The plot, referred to as an *electrodogram,* shows the electrodes stimulated over time for the word "choice," with intensity indicated by the relative brightness of the lines.

ADVANCED COMBINATION ENCODER. The Advanced Combination Encoder (ACE) strategy was designed for the Nucleus device to incorporate the spectral representation benefits of SPEAK with a high rate CIS.[74] ACE provides a range of stimulation rates per channel, from 500 to 3500 pulses per second, and allows for a maxima range from 1 to 20. An electrodogram for the word "choice" processed with ACE is shown in Figure 158-14. The rapid stimulation rate and increased number of stimulated electrodes is apparent when compared with the SPEAK strategy.

Fine Structure Signal Processing

Fine structure signal processing combines both temporal and spectral cues, is typically presented using high pulse rates, and may incorporate a recently implemented "virtual channel" paradigm. The higher rate

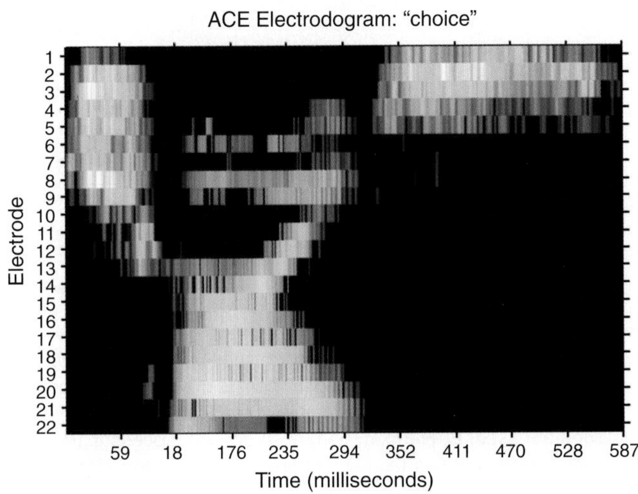

Figure 158-14. Advanced Combination Encoder (ACE). An electrodogram for the word "choice" (as plotted in Fig. 158-17) is shown for coding with the ACE strategy. Compared with SPEAK, the stimulation rate is faster and the number of electrodes stimulated is greater. *(Published with permission, copyright © 2008 Cochlear Americas.)*

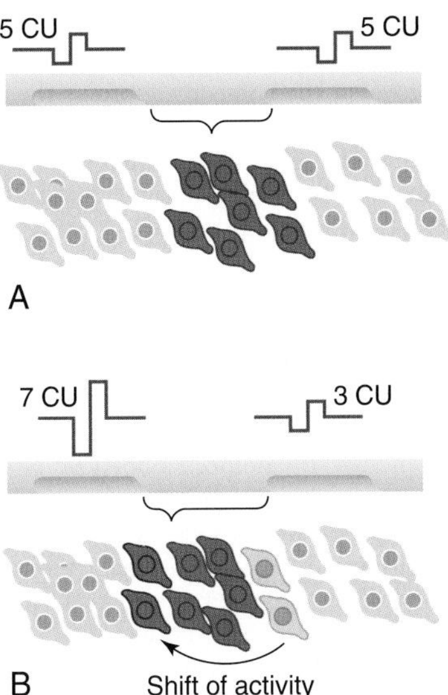

Figure 158-15. Schematic illustration of current steering between adjacent electrodes and stimulation of neural elements. **A** shows equal proportions of current presented to the electrodes, which effectively focuses stimulation halfway between the contacts. **B** shows a shift in the current proportions between electrodes and the resulting shift of activity toward the more heavily weighted contact. *(Published with permission, copyright © 2008 Advanced Bionics Corporation.)*

strategies generally use short duration pulses and increased filter update rates. It is theorized that this results in electrical stimulation that more accurately represents the input signal.

Improving delivery of spectral cue information with coding strategies has become of particular interest with advances in device design and evolving patient expectations such as music appreciation and listening in noise. Stimulation of different electrodes along the array typically elicits different pitch percepts in cochlear implant users. The number of different pitch percepts a person has reflects that individual's spectral resolution abilities. Until recently, spectral resolution with cochlear implants was limited by the number of stimulating electrodes. A method of stimulus current delivery has been developed to increase the number of pitch percepts given a finite number of electrodes. This stimulation paradigm is referred to as "current steering," and the resulting additional pitch percepts are called "virtual channels."

Current steering is accomplished when two adjacent electrodes are stimulated simultaneously, subsequently eliciting a pitch percept that falls between the pitches from each electrode when stimulated alone.[75,76] This effect has also been shown with sequential stimulation of adjacent electrodes.[77] Figure 158-15 shows a schematic example of equal proportions of current presented simultaneously to two electrodes *(top),* thus stimulating the neural population halfway between the contacts. By changing the proportion of current delivered to each electrode, the responding neural population likewise shifts (Fig. 158-15, *bottom*) and thus creates an additional pitch percept without changing the loudness.[78] Algorithms for current steering between electrodes and across the array have been developed by all three manufacturers, for use with their recent-generation devices.

Factors That Affect Device Choice

NEED FOR SPECIAL ELECTRODE ARRAYS. When individuals have hearing loss that is appropriate for cochlear implantation, it is possible that the cochlea may be malformed, depending on the etiology of the hearing loss. This includes varying degrees of Mondini malformation, in which there may be fewer cochlear turns or dehiscent cochleae. The cochlea may be ossified, to varying degrees, which may occur with meningitis, Paget disease, or otosclerosis. In addition, there are types of hearing loss that may necessitate preservation of hearing with implantation. In any of these cases, it may be necessary to have special electrode arrays available such as short, compressed, split, or custom arrays, all of which have been described earlier.

TECHNOLOGY DIFFERENCES IN SPEECH CODING STRATEGY AND ELECTRODE CONFIGURATION. Device selection is also influenced by changes in technology that may make one device more appealing than another for a given individual. For example, a speech coding strategy that emphasizes both temporal and spectral cues may be desirable for a patient who has a great love of music. Depending on an individual's work or other daily life environment, certain noise reduction features may become relevant. As discussed previously, in some cases a patient may be limited to selecting a given device on the basis of his or her cochlear anatomy or hearing status that requires the use of a particular electrode array design.

MAGNETIC RESONANCE IMAGING COMPATIBILITY. MRI is a powerful noninvasive diagnostic tool that uses magnetic fields and pulses of radio waves to generate images. The components of an MRI unit include a static magnetic field (0.5 to 4T); magnetic fields caused by switched gradients (0 to 20T/s at ≈ 15 Hz); and radiofrequency energy (0 to 6 kW peak at 64 MHz [for 1.5T]).[79,80] It is an imaging modality with an already wide range of clinical applications that continues to expand. Ideally, this diagnostic tool should be available for the benefit of cochlear implant (CI) recipients. The Cochlear Corporation's CI24M, CI24R(CA), and CI24ABI devices, as well as the Advanced Bionics Corporation's HiRes 90K device, were all designed so that the internal magnet could be removed and replaced to complete an MRI study.

Studies with the Med-El Combi 40/40+ and Clarion 1.2 (Advanced Bionics) cochlear implants have delineated many of the factors in CI/MRI interactions.[81,82] The factors that have been studied include demagnetization, artifacts, induced voltages, temperature increases, torque, and force. These investigations have used both the 0.3T and 1.5T MRI units. The force and torque exerted by the MRI unit on the internal magnet of the cochlear implant receiver are of particular concern. The potential for a catastrophic force on the implant to fracture the inner table of skull and exert pressure on the brain demands full investigation of cochlear implant/MRI compatibility. Previous studies concluded that a 0.2T MRI evaluation force and torque remained within "acceptable limits."[81,82] There have been several in vivo studies performed in Europe using 1.0T MRI.[69] In this largest series of 30 patients with Med-El cochlear implants who underwent 1.0T MRI evaluations with a variety of MRI sequences, none suffered pain, burning, auditory sensation, deterioration of their auditory abilities, or other adverse sequelae. Presently, patients with the

Med-El C40+, PulsarCI100, or SonataTI100 devices in place greater than 6 months are approved by the FDA to undergo MRI studies with a 0.2T scanner, provided the company approves the protocol for the radiologist.

We have completed studies to determine the magnitude of force required to fracture the floor of a cochlear implant receiver bed.[83] The testing protocol was designed to create a physical worst-case scenario yet approximate the in vivo condition. Several considerations went into attaining this dual goal. Each recessed cochlear implant bed was drilled to a maximum uniform thinness rather than drilling just deep enough to accommodate the cochlear implant. A stainless steel template was chosen for impacting the specimens because the arc of its edge would closely approximate that of the cochlear implant affecting the skull in vivo. In addition, a line load system more realistically approximated the in vivo condition than a point load system. The center of the specimen was chosen for contact with the template. This placement minimized the risk of the template touching any surface other than the floor of the recessed cochlear implant bed. It also assisted identical placement of the template for each specimen. Finally, this placement allowed the template to affect the specimen at its least reinforced site, thereby providing a worst-case scenario. Since the in vivo system had the thinned bone in continuity with the native skull and it is this region that receives the force vector during the cochlear implant magnet/MRI magnet interaction, it is anticipated that the biomechanical forces required to produce failure at this interface would be much greater than those measured in the study referenced earlier.[83] In an earlier investigation of cochlear implant/MRI compatibility, 0.3 to 1.0 newtons (N) was used as an acceptable level of force exerted on a cochlear implant during MRI evaluation.[81] The researchers recommended this range because it represents the magnitude of force that a cochlear implant may experience during a regular day in the life of a cochlear implant recipient. More specifically, this is the magnitude of the force exerted on the internal magnet of a cochlear implant when the external transmitter and magnet are removed. In these prior studies, the measured force vectors ranged from 0.17 to 0.42 N. Calculations using these measured force vectors and appropriate geometry resulted in maximum forces of approximately 8 N exerted on the cochlear implant during 1.5 T MRI evaluation in a worst-case scenario. The results of our biophysics studies showed that the load-carrying capacity of a recessed cochlear implant bed drilled into fresh frozen human calvaria specimens, with bone thickness of 0.3 to 0.6 mm (S.D. 0.11 mm), is more than an order of magnitude greater than this force (mean = 134.13 *N*).[83] When a bone island with exposed dura is necessary to inset the internal device, titanium or resorbable mesh has been shown in vitro to provide even greater mechanical support beneath a cochlear implant and this approach also has the advantage of providing immediate support.[84] Moreover, we have demonstrated that no demagnetization of the internal device magnet occurs after 15 successive MRI scans in a 1.5 T unit.[85] Further studies in patients will be necessary to demonstrate the safety of this practice using cochlear implants with the internal magnet remaining in place. However, for all candidates, and particularly those who are in need of frequent MRI scans, the options and limitations of each device should be discussed so that the patient can make an informed decision.

EXTERNAL SPEECH PROCESSOR SIZE, WEIGHT AND AESTHETICS. Often, the design and aesthetics of the external components, specifically the speech processor, have a great deal of influence on device selection (Figs. 158-16 to 158-18). Individuals tend to prefer a BTE processor because it is lighter, smaller, and does not have a cord that runs down the back of the neck. For young children, it may be desirable to use a BW processor that can be worn on the child's back and out of reach. In addition, some BTE processors may be too large or heavy to stay on a child's ear. However, some manufacturers have introduced smaller, lighter BTE wear options designed specifically for children. Patients with dexterity or vision problems often select a processor with larger, more accessible controls. Color choice of the external components is also relevant. Some prefer to match hair and/or skin tone, and others like interesting designs or colors that they can change to match their clothing.

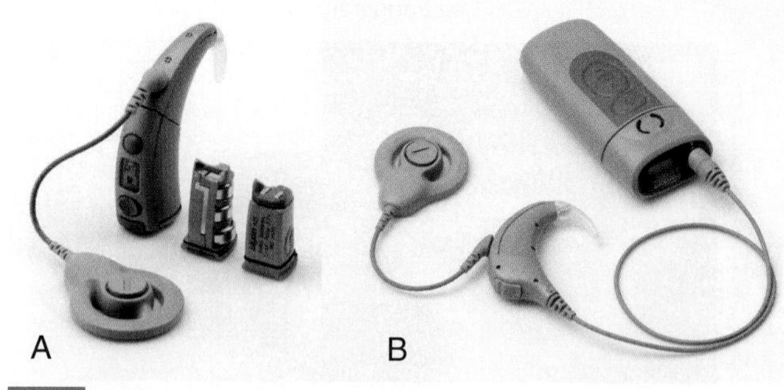

Figure 158-16. Ear-level and body-worn speech processors for the Nucleus Freedom System. **A,** Freedom behind-the-ear speech processor. Multiple colors are also available. Disposable or rechargeable batteries are used. **B,** Freedom body-worn speech processor. Note the ear hook, which contains the microphone and the magnet/transmitter coil. *(Published with permission, copyright © 2008 Cochlear Americas.)*

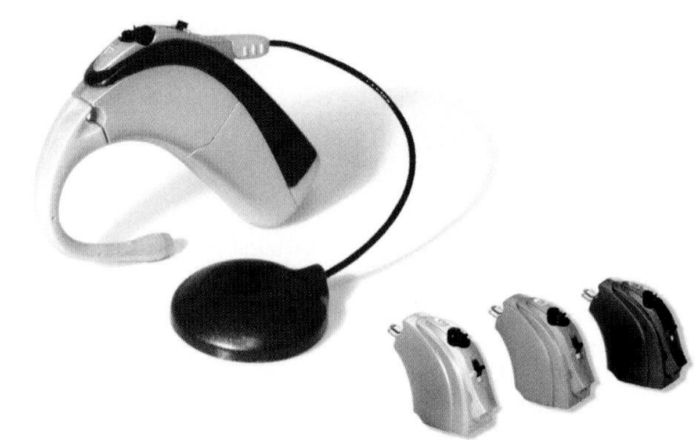

Figure 158-17. Harmony ear-level speech processor. Multiple colors are available, *lower right,* as well as multiple-colored accent strips. A separate body-worn battery pack is also available for infants with cochlear implants. *(Published with permission, copyright © 2008 Advanced Bionics Corporation.)*

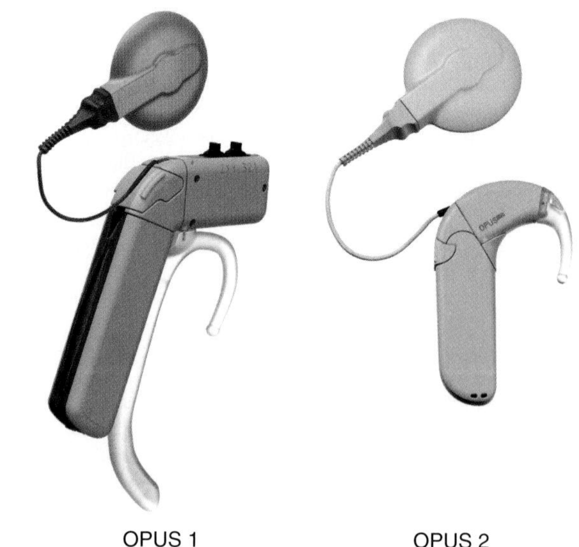

Figure 158-18. Ear-level speech processors for the Med-El cochlear implant systems. The OPUS 1 has a modular design with two small switches, whereas the OPUS 2 has a more ergonomic switch-free design. Multiple colors are available. A separate body-worn battery pack is also available for infants with cochlear implants. *(Published with permission, © 2007 Med-El Corporation.)*

BATTERIES. The type, cost, and lifespan of batteries are important to some patients when choosing a device. Body-worn speech processors can use either disposable alkaline or rechargeable batteries. BTE processors use either disposable high power 675 hearing aid batteries or proprietary rechargeable batteries, depending on the manufacturer of the device. The specific processor, battery type, speech coding strategy, and patient programming needs each affect battery life. However, the generally expected battery life and ease of changing the batteries may cause a patient or family to choose one implant design over another.

SUGGESTED READINGS

Balkany T, Hodges A, Telischi F, et al. William House Cochlear Implant Study Group: position statement on bilateral cochlear implantation. *Otol Neurotol.* 2008;29:107-108.

Brown KD, Balkany TJ. Benefits of bilateral cochlear implantation: a review. *Curr Opin Otolaryngol Head Neck Surg.* 2007;15:315-318.

Chorost M. *Rebuilt: How Becoming Part Computer Made Me More Human.* Boston: Houghton Mifflin; 2005:1-232.

For complete list of references log onto www.expertconsult.com.

Geers AE. Factors influencing spoken language outcomes in children following early cochlear implantation. *Adv Otorhinolaryngol.* 2006;64:50-65.

Jöhr M, Ho A, Wagner CS, et al. Ear surgery in infants under one year of age: its risks and implications for cochlear implant surgery. *Otol Neurotol.* 2008;29:310-313.

Karen Pedley K, Giles E. *Adult Cochlear Implant Rehabilitation.* Malden, Mass: Wiley-Blackwell; 2005:1-330.

Nelson HD, Bougatsos C, Nygren P; 2001 US Preventive Services Task Force. Universal newborn hearing screening: systematic review to update the 2001 US Preventive Services Task Force Recommendation. *Pediatrics.* 2008;122: e266-e276.

Niparko JK. *Cochlear Implants: Principles & Practices.* Philadelphia: Lippincott Williams & Wilkins; 2000:1-396.

Papsin BC, Gordon KA. Bilateral cochlear implants should be the standard for children with bilateral sensorineural deafness. *Curr Opin Otolaryngol Head Neck Surg.* 2008;16:69-74.

Wackym PA (guest ed). Cochlear and brainstem implantation. *Oper Tech Otolaryngol Head Neck Surg.* 2005;16:73-163.

Wilson BS, Dorman MF. Cochlear implants: a remarkable past and a brilliant future. *Hear Res.* 2008;242(1-2):3-21.

CHAPTER ONE HUNDRED AND FIFTY-NINE

Cochlear Implantation: Medical and Surgical Considerations

Thomas J. Balkany

Kevin D. Brown

Bruce J. Gantz

Key Points

- Diagnostic therapy, including auditory verbal therapy with appropriate hearing aids, is critical before implanting devices in children with severe to profound hearing loss.
- MRI offers numerous advantages over CT, including direct visualization of the cochlear nerve, assessment of the patency of the cochlea, and visualization of the cerebellar pontine angle and brainstem for other abnormalities.
- Children and adults should be immunized against *Streptococcus pneumoniae* according to the high-risk schedule before cochlear implantation.
- Auditory neuropathy is not a contraindication to cochlear implantation.
- Cochlear implantation in children is ideally performed before 12 months of age.
- Michel's aplasia or absence of the cochlear nerve are absolute contraindications to cochlear implantation.
- Patients who require revision implant surgery (reimplantation) generally perform as well with their second implant as with their first.
- A second cochlear implant (implanted sequentially or simultaneously) improves sound localization and speech recognition in noise over a single implant.

Cochlear implantation has become a standard medical procedure for the rehabilitation of hearing-impaired adults and children. The medical and surgical decision to undertake cochlear implantation is based on the doctor-patient relationship. Candidacy issues, device selection, and planning for postoperative habitation are more complex than for other otologic surgeries, and they require a dedicated cochlear implant team. Decisions about whether to operate and which ear and device to select are made on the basis of input from the cochlear implant team, a detailed medical history and physical examination, and laboratory and imaging studies.

The physical characteristics of receiver stimulators and electrode arrays vary among manufacturers, thus necessitating surgical techniques that are specific to the device to minimize complications.[1-4] The facial nerve monitor is recommended in all cases as an adjunct for preventing overheating or other damage to the facial nerve while working within the facial recess and the middle ear.

Cochlear implant surgery—like technology and candidate evaluation—has evolved since the mid 1980s. During that time, techniques have been developed to reduce complications, to safely place implants in children who are younger than 12 months old, to insert electrodes in ossified and dysplastic cochlea, and to replace failed devices. The implantation procedure includes elements of mastoid and middle ear surgery, as well as cochleostomy, electrode insertion, and securing of the receiver stimulator.

Medical and Surgical Evaluation

This evaluation includes all aspects of cochlear implant candidacy, including critical analysis of hearing tests, motivation of the patient and family, and status of language development (Box 159-1). It should also focus on the patient's general health, especially with regard to his or her ability to undergo general anesthesia. A complete history and physical examination is followed by appropriate laboratory tests. Imaging studies play a particularly important role in this evaluation. When necessary, consultation with appropriate specialists is indicated.

During the physical examination, special attention is paid to the ear and central nervous system. Extensive laboratory evaluations such as thyroid function studies, lipid profiles, and viral screens are expensive and have not been found to be helpful unless specifically indicated by the history and physical examination.

Hearing tests with ear-specific auditory information in both aided and unaided conditions must be obtained. It is critically important to be certain that the patient's hearing aids are appropriate for the hearing loss. In young, prelinguistically deafened children, it may not be possible to accurately assess hearing during a single session or even a series of sessions within a sound booth. In very young children, a combination of diagnostic audiometric strategies may be necessary, including auditory brainstem response (ABR), auditory steady-state response (ASSR), and behavioral observation. The ABR is limited in its ability to obtain tone-specific information (limited frequency specificity).

Box 159-1

Candidacy Criteria for Children

- Severe to profound bilateral sensorineural hearing loss
- Benefits from hearing aids less than that expected from cochlear implants
- Medical clearance to undergo general anesthesia
- Family support, motivation, and appropriate expectations
- Rehabilitation/educational support for the development of aural language, speech, and hearing in children

ASSR uses a continuous tone with a carrier frequency that is amplitude and frequency modulated. Similar to an ABR, the ASSR is recorded from scalp electrodes, but the recordings show primary energy at the carrier frequency and two sidebands separated from the carrier by the modulation frequency. Recent studies have demonstrated correlation between the degree of hearing loss measured by standard PTA and ASSR at 500, 1000, 2000, and 4000 Hz.[5]

In diagnostic therapy, the patient is fit with the appropriate hearing aids, placed in a program of auditory-verbal or auditory-oral therapy, and followed up for a period of months. During that time, it is typical to see hearing-impaired children make some gains with regard to receptive language function, and these may be compared with the expected gains that typically occur with cochlear implants.

Genetic testing continues to evolve as an important adjunct in the diagnosis of hearing loss. Approximately half of the estimated 1 in 1000 infants born with bilateral severe to profound deafness are thought to have genetic factors. There are more than 46 genes currently identified that contribute to hearing loss, but one gene, *GJB2*, which encodes the protein connexin 26 and maps to the autosomal recessive deafness gene (*DFNB1*) locus, is responsible for a significant proportion of these cases. When mutations in *GJB2* and *GJB6* (connexin 30) are screened together, the cause of 50% of bilateral severe to profound hearing loss is identified in certain populations. Four main benefits of genetic testing have been identified.[6] First, the identification of a specific genetic cause precludes further costly testing. It also defines the chance of transmission by understanding the specific genetic cause of the hearing loss and its method of inheritance. Testing also provides parental reassurance that it was nothing done during the pregnancy that contributed to the hearing loss, thus helping to prevent unnecessary guilt. It also provides prognostic information with respect to the possible development of other medical problems and can help in predicting outcomes with hearing rehabilitation such as cochlear implantation.[7]

Both high-resolution computed tomography (HRCT) and magnetic resonance imaging (MRI) may be used in the preoperative evaluation of patients with profound deafness who are candidates for cochlear implantation. HRCT may assist in the evaluation of inner ear morphology (Fig. 159-1), patency of the cochlea (Fig. 159-2), position of the facial nerve, location of large mastoid emissary veins, size of the facial recess, thickness of the parietal bone, and height of the jugular bulb (Box 159-2). MRI has been used more frequently for preimplantation evaluation in recent years. Although MRI is not as effective in visualizing the fallopian canal or the bony structure of the otic capsule, it is more effective in identifying fibrosis of the cochlea by assessing its patency, in identifying the presence and caliber of the cochlear nerve (especially on sagittal T2 imaging of the internal auditory canal), and in providing information about brainstem and cortical lesions. A study compared the ability of HRCT and MRI for identifying abnormalities of the cochlea and modiolus, and MRI was found to be superior.[8] For these reasons, it has subsequently become the preferred means for preoperative evaluation of children undergoing cochlear implantation at many institutions. It is recommended, however, that HRCT still be performed in cases in which there are malformations of the external canal, semicircular canals, or vestibule due to the higher incidence of an anomalous facial nerve.[8] Both tests may be indicated in the presence of labyrinthine anomaly.

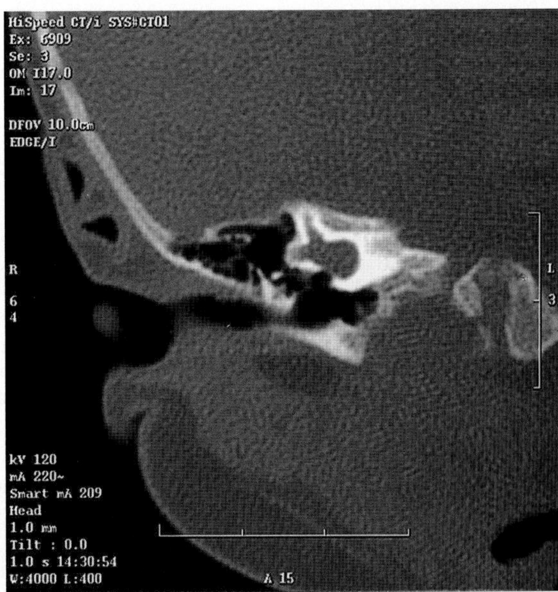

Figure 159-1. Cochlear dysplasia, absence of modiolus and bony partition. This coronal high-resolution computed tomography scan of a child with congenital deafness demonstrates a cystic cochlea without bony partition, the absence of a partition from the vestibule, and a wide, stubby, horizontal, semicircular canal. A large oval window niche can also be seen in this view.

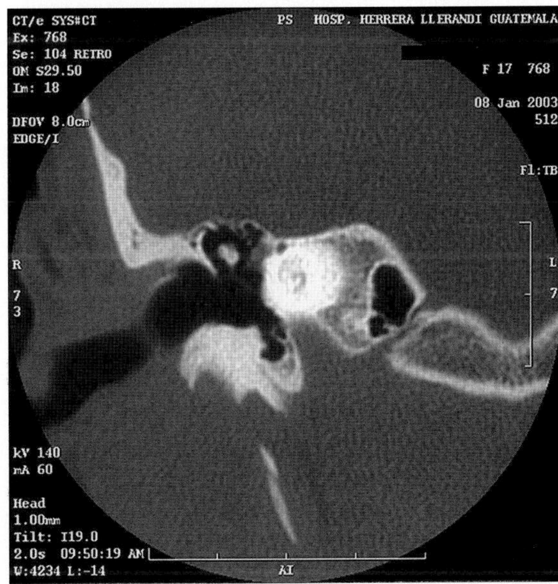

Figure 159-2. Coronal high-resolution computed tomography scan demonstrating nearly complete cochlear ossification. This scan demonstrates nearly complete ossification of the labyrinth. A small portion of the upper turns may remain patent. Note that ossification generally begins in the basal turn and proceeds apically.

Ear Selection

Selection of the ear to be operated on is somewhat complex and prescriptive for the individual patient. The factors to be considered include the following.

Physical Characteristics

Physical characteristics of the temporal bone that are used for ear selection include the presence of the cochlea and the auditory nerve, the degree of dysplasia, the degree of ossification, prior surgical procedures (e.g., canal-wall-down mastoidectomy), facial nerve anomalies, and chronic otitis media.

Residual Hearing Level

At this time, the risk of losing residual hearing during electrode insertion is estimated at 50% to 70%, although recent techniques may reduce the risk to 20%.[9] Thus, if there is significant aided benefit from the better ear, the worse ear is often favored. Conversely, it is widely held that patients with more residual hearing have better outcomes from cochlear implantation. For this reason, if a patient is anacusic, the ear that has more residual hearing may be favored. Fig. 159-3 presents an algorithm that may be helpful when considering these issues.

If one ear has had profound deafness for more than 10 to 15 years, the ear with better hearing is usually selected, because duration of deafness is one of the few measures that correlate with performance outcome. If the individual can use a hearing aid for sound awareness, preserving the ear with better hearing may assist with binaural localization and may assist with competing noise.

Box 159-2

Computed Tomography and Magnetic Resonance Imaging Information

- Inner ear morphology
- Cochlear patency
- Position of fallopian canal
- Presence of cochlear nerve
- Size of facial recess
- Location of large mastoid emissary veins
- Height of jugular bulb
- Thickness of parietal bone

Vaccination for Meningitis

In 2003, a *New England Journal of Medicine* article highlighted an increased incidence of pneumococcal meningitis in cochlear implant recipients in comparison to an age-matched general population.[10] A total of 4264 children were evaluated and 26 children were identified with streptococcal meningitis, representing an incidence of 0.6% in cochlear implant recipients. This was a 30-fold increase over their age-matched convenience sample cohort. Two major limitations of the study were that, first, 11.5% of children receiving an implant have a previous history of meningitis, and these children have an increased risk of recurrence. Second, 8.5% of children receiving implants have labyrinthine dysplasia, which also places them at an increased risk for meningitis. The degree to which an increase in meningitis is due to a cochlear implant, versus high risk factors such as prior meningitis or dysplasia, requires an adequate control group of deaf children rather than normal children as used in this study.

In order to test whether this risk was theoretical or actual in nature, animal experiments were performed in rats to determine whether placement of a cochlear implant increases the risk of meningitis.[11] In this study, rats receiving a cochlear implant were at a significantly increased risk of developing bacterial meningitis when inoculated with *S. pneumoniae* by any route (intraperitoneal, middle ear, inner ear) in comparison to surgical controls. In a later companion study, vaccination with 23-valent pneumococcal capsular polysaccharide vaccine (PPV23, Pneumovax) prevented the development of meningitis in rats inoculated by an intraperitoneal route and significantly reduced the frequency of meningitis in rats inoculated by a middle ear route. There was a nonsignificant reduction in frequency of meningitis

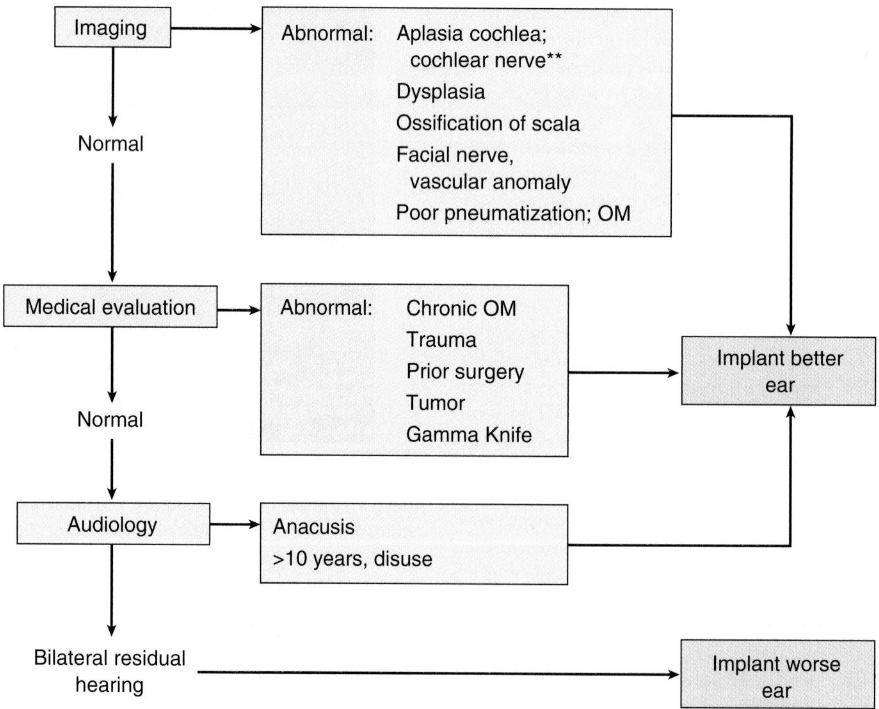

Figure 159-3. Ear selection algorithm. Selection of the ear to receive a cochlear implant is not a simple matter and must be prescribed specifically for each patient. The three general considerations are imaging, otologic history, and residual hearing level. Individual considerations such as lifestyle (driver vs. passenger), handedness (regarding ability to place the external device), and the patient's preferences must also be taken into consideration. OM, otitis media.

in rats inoculated via the inner ear. This suggested PPV23 can protect healthy rats from meningitis caused by a vaccine-covered *S. pneumoniae* serotype.[12]

There are currently two vaccines available that both generate antibodies to the polysaccharide capsule of *S. pneumoniae.* These include the PPV23 vaccine, which is a 23-valent vaccine composed of pure capsular antigen, and the heptavalent pneumococcal conjugated vaccine (PCV7, Prevnar), which contains seven pneumococcal serotypes conjugated to a nontoxic variant of diphtheria toxin. Both of these generate an antibody response, although PPV23 is not recommended for children younger than 2 years of age because of immaturity of their immune systems that may lead to a potentially poor response to pure capsular antigen.[13] It is the current recommendation of the Centers for Disease Control and Prevention (CDC) to ensure that children receiving a cochlear implant are immunized according to age-appropriate pneumococcal vaccination with PCV7, PPV23, or both according to the Advisory Committee on Immunization Practices (ACIP) schedules for persons at high risk (Box 159-3).[14]

Surgical Technique

Preparation and Draping

Under general anesthesia, the patient is placed supine with the head turned 45 to 60 degrees away from the surgeon. With very young children, care should be taken to avoid excessive rotation of the head so as to avoid subluxation of the cervical spine when the child is relaxed under general anesthesia. Long-lasting neuromuscular blockade is avoided to allow the use of the facial nerve monitor. Minimal shaving is used to reduce the psychologic impact of the procedure. The ear is prepped in a sterile manner, and a povidone-iodine–impregnated occlusive drape is used to retract the pinna anteriorly and to seal off the external auditory meatus. Using the appropriate implant guides provided by the manufacturer, the location of the implantable receiver stimulator may be marked on underlying parietal bone transcutaneously using methylene blue. A single intravenous injection of prophylactic antibiotics within 30 minutes of surgery is recommended, although this has not been subject to a prospective trial.

Incisions and Flap Design

Cochlear implant incisions have evolved over time (Fig. 159-4), but the principles of incision design remain constant. The resulting flap should cover the implant with margins of at least 1 cm in all directions, and a good blood supply should be maintained. Access to the linea temporalis, mastoid tip, and spine of Henle, without undue retraction, is necessary.

The original postauricular C-shaped incision used with single-channel implants was effective and had a low rate of complications. However, as multichannel devices came into use, the larger receiver stimulators required a larger flap. These larger postauricular C-shaped incisions were associated with a higher rate of complications—mainly device extrusion—and were subsequently replaced by an inferiorly based "inverted U" flap. This has undergone further modification (see Fig. 159-4), to an extended postauricular incision that has gradually become shortened and remains the most commonly used incision at this time. An extended endaural incision has also been used, but early experience with this incision demonstrated an unacceptably high incidence of skin breakdown at the external auditory meatus.

Box 159-3

ACIP Recommendations for Persons Receiving a Cochlear Implant

- Children younger than 24 months with cochlear implants should receive PCV7, as is universally recommended; children with a lapse in vaccination should be vaccinated according to the catch-up scheduled after the PCV7 shortage resolved.
- Children 24 to 59 months old with cochlear implants who have not received PCV7 should be vaccinated according to the high-risk schedule; children with a lapse in vaccination should be vaccinated according to the catch-up scheduled after the PCV7 shortage resolved; children who have completed the PCV7 series should receive PPV23 2 months or more after vaccination with PCV7.
- Persons 5 to 64 years with cochlear implants should receive PPV23 according to the schedule used for persons with chronic illnesses; a single dose is indicated.
- Persons planning to receive a cochlear implant should be up-to-date on age-appropriate pneumococcal vaccination at least 2 weeks before surgery, if possible.

ACIP, Advisory Committee on Immunization Practices.

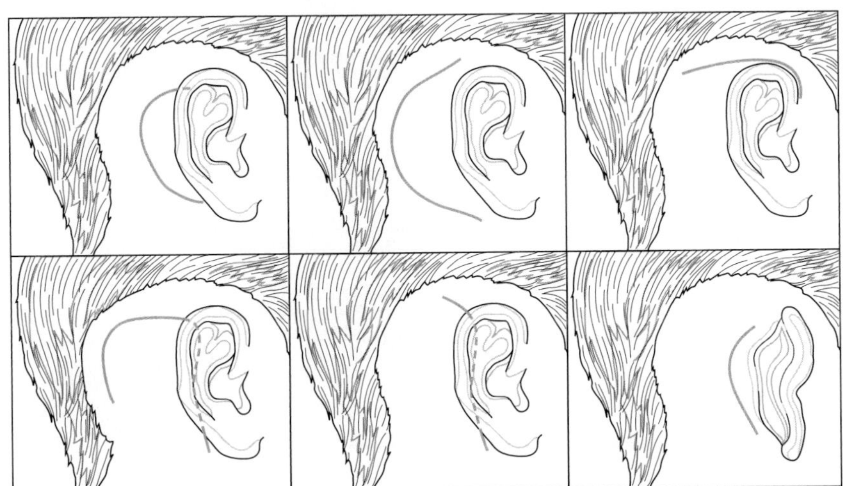

Figure 159-4. Cochlear implant incisions. Since the 1970s, a number of incisions have been used for cochlear implantation. The original small C-shaped incision was used for the relatively small, single-channel cochlear implant. When multichannel cochlear implants came into wide use in the 1980s, the C-shaped incision was simply enlarged. At that time, most complications had to do with flap breakdown. The large C-shaped incision had to be extended superiorly and inferiorly to allow for adequate arterial and venous blood supply. In response to the wound problems, an extended endaural incision was widely used in Europe, and an inferiorly based or U-shaped incision was developed in Australia. This gradually evolved into a simple extension of the standard postauricular incision. At the present time, a minimal incision is used in many centers for children and, in some centers, for adults as well.

A "minimal incision" has also been used for cochlear implantation. This incision is approximately 3 to 4 cm long and situated 1 cm posterior to the retroauricular crease. The advantages of this incision are that it requires minimal hair shaving, it heals faster and with less swelling than larger incisions, and it allows for initial stimulation at 2 weeks in most cases. Disadvantages include the need for additional skin retraction, reduced visibility, and somewhat limited access when drilling a bone seat and tie-down holes for securing the device.

Before incision, the intracutaneous infiltration of 1 to 3 mL of 1 : 100,000 epinephrine may be used to obtain better hemostasis. Similarly, a monopolar cautery knife may be used for both incision and flap elevation. It should be noted, however, that in cases of simultaneous or sequential cochlear implantation, monopolar cautery is contraindicated due to potential current interaction with the circuitry of the receiver-stimulator. In these cases, it is advisable to perform the approach for both sides before placing the implant (simultaneous implants)[15] to use a nonconducting means of dissection to provide hemostasis, including the bipolar, Shaw scalpel, and most recently the Plasma Knife in cases of sequential implantation.[16]

Skin Flap

The skin flap is elevated, along with subcutaneous tissue, in the plane of the temporalis fascia. By splitting the fascia, the flap may be raised in an avascular plane; this plane is most easily identified in the superior area of the flap and carried inferiorly.

Because the receiver stimulator will be situated at an angle of 30 to 45 degrees from vertical (it is more vertical in younger children), the skin and subcutaneous tissue flap are usually not elevated inferiorly to the lamdoidal suture. If dissection is carried below this point, large branches of the occipital artery and vein may be encountered, thereby causing unnecessary blood loss and delaying the procedure.

Because the external processor must transmit across the skin, the efficiency of both power and information transmission is governed by the thickness of the skin flap. The stability of the external transmitting coil, which is held in place magnetically, is similarly affected by skin thickness. Current devices require that the flap be less than 10 to 12 mm thick. Significant risk is inherent whenever a skin flap must be thinned. It is recommended to avoid thinning the skin flap to less than 0.8 cm and to prevent thinning to the level of hair follicles in all cases. When hair follicles are exposed, the risks of infection around the receiver/stimulator and of eventual extrusion are heightened.

After the skin/subcutaneous tissue flap has been elevated, a separate anteriorly based pericranial flap is then elevated. This flap extends along the linea temporalis posteriorly from a point just above the exterior auditory canal to a point that will cover at least the anterior portion of the receiver stimulator. The subcutaneous pericranial flap should be 2 to 3 cm in the cephalocaudal dimension and at least 2 cm in length. The pericranial incision is then carried inferiorly to a point just above the occipital crest and then anteroinferiorly, staying above the attachment of strap muscles, to the mastoid tip. In young children, the usual precautions to avoid the facial nerve in the absence of a mastoid tip are exercised. This flap is elevated anteriorly and retained in fishhooks or with a self-retaining retractor to expose the mastoid cortex and the area of the receiver/stimulator seat and tie-down sutures.

It is important to carry the soft tissue dissection anteriorly to expose and thin the bony wall of the posterior external auditory canal. In young children, care must be taken when placing the retractor, because it can tear the skin of the external auditory canal, thereby contaminating the surgical area.

A subperiosteal pocket for the receiver-stimulator is elevated beneath the pericranium posterosuperior to the mastoid using a periosteal elevator. The dimensions of the pocket depend on the design of the receiver-stimulator.

Bony Seat

A custom-fit bony seat and tie-down holes may be drilled into the parietal bone to recess and immobilize the receiver/stimulator; this reduces its profile and protects it from trauma as well as making it less noticeable to the patient and family. Drilling the seat and bone holes in young children often exposes dura, and care must be taken to avoid complications. Cerebrospinal fluid (CSF) leak, subdural hematoma, epidural hematoma, lateral sinus thrombosis, and cerebral infarct have all been reported.[17-19] At this time, techniques are being developed that do not require bone seats or bone tie-down holes.

The anterior edge of the receiver/stimulator should be at least 1 cm behind the skin incision. In addition, the location of the internal magnet should be far enough posterior so that the patient will not have a problem wearing an ear-level processor. Each manufacturer provides a mock implant and guide to help determine the site of the receiver-stimulator seat. Bony tie-down holes are drilled superior and inferior to the seat (Fig. 159-6). In young children, the bony fixation holes are often epidural and require that the dura be slightly elevated to avoid damage. Later, the receiver-stimulator will be secured with a single nonreabsorbable suture. The knot should be rotated into an inferior tie-down hole using two mosquito clamps.

Mastoidectomy

A complete mastoidectomy is performed, but, unlike in chronic ear surgery, the mastoid cortex is not marsupialized but rather is left slightly overhanging superiorly, posteriorly, and inferiorly to help retain and control the electrode cable. Likewise, it is not necessary to exenterate all retrosigmoid or tip cells.

The facial recess is widely opened. Care is taken to preserve a layer of bone overlying the facial nerve. It may be necessary to remove bone on the anterior medial surface of the fallopian canal just below the pyramidal process to provide adequate access to the round window. The bony external auditory canal wall should be thinned maximally, but it should never be penetrated. The chorda tympani can usually be preserved. Thinning the posterior canal wall allows the microscopic view to vector from anterolateral to posteromedial, because the round window niche is a posterior structure of the mesotympanum.

The incus bridge that separates the fossa incudis from the facial recess may be divided between the short process of the incus and the horizontal semicircular canal (Fig. 159-5). Although this requires only a few seconds with a 0.5-mm diamond burr, it allows the electrode cable to be passed under the short process into the epitympanum and firmly lodges it in position. Another benefit of this procedure is to direct

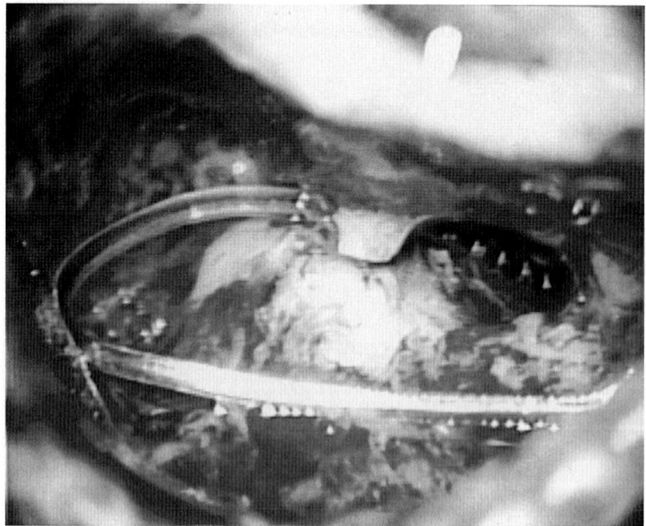

Figure 159-5. Split bridge. The incus bridge is divided using a 0.5-mm diamond burr between the short process of the incus anteriorly and the horizontal, semicircular canal. In doing this, the posterior incudal ligament is sacrificed. A cochlear implant electrode is seen after it has been placed inside the split bridge; this fixes the electrode in place, prevents extrusion, and directs the electrode away from the drill-exposed segment of the fallopian canal and the tympanic membrane (in the event that it should retract).

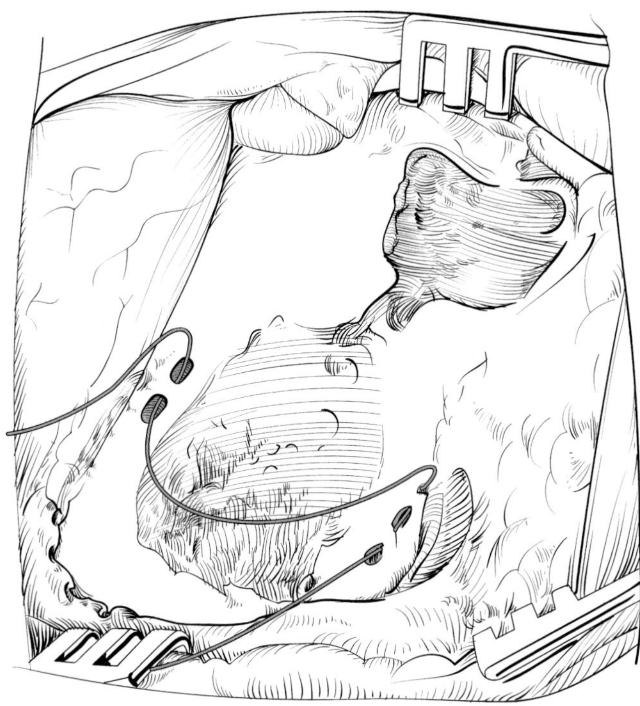

Figure 159-6. Bony seat and tie-down sutures with mastoid cavity. A custom-designed bony seat is made to recess the implantable receiver stimulator, thereby reducing its profile, providing a degree of protection from trauma, and minimizing mobility, which could result in work hardening of the electrode lead. A 2-mm diamond drill bit is used to create connecting suture holes superiorly and inferiorly, and a 2-0 nonabsorbable monofilament suture is used to secure the device into its seat. A trough is drilled to connect the seat to the mastoid cavity.

the cable away from the tympanic membrane in cases in which retraction or the need for myringotomy may arise.[20]

Cochleostomy

In the past, there have been instances in which the electrode was inadvertently placed into a hypotympanic air cell. It is important to identify the round window membrane to be certain that the cochleostomy and electrode insertion will proceed properly. The round window membrane is rarely more than 1- to 1.5-mm inferior to the stapedius tendon.

As with other aspects of the surgery, the placement and size of the cochleostomy varies somewhat depending on the implant to be used. In general terms, the cochleostomy is drilled through the promontory just anterior and inferior to the round window membrane. Care is taken to prevent bleeding into the cochleostomy by elevating the mucoperiosteum away from the selected site and using topical epinephrine on Gelfoam pledgets (Pharmacia & Upjohn Co., Kalamazoo, MI), if necessary. Good hemostasis should be obtained before opening the cochlea. If necessary, large Gelfoam pledgets may be placed in the epitympanum or mastoid cavity to prevent the drip down of blood. Bone dust should also be kept out of the cochlea.

A 1.5-mm diamond burr is used to thin the bone anteroinferior to the round window membrane. The overhanging niche is removed, if necessary, to positively identify the round window membrane. A 1-mm burr is used to remove remaining bone down to the endosteum itself. As the endosteum is approached, meticulous drilling is necessary to avoid inadvertent penetration. As a correlate, exposure of the endosteum of the scala tympani should be treated like a stapedotomy because penetration into the scala exposes the inner ear to significant acoustic trauma of up to 130 dB.[21] Endosteum is continuous with and found at the level of the round window membrane, which is used as a guide to the depth of the drilling. After this, the middle ear is carefully irrigated to remove all bone dust. It is imperative to prevent the rotating drill shaft from contacting the facial recess bone that overlies the facial nerve while drilling the cochleostomy. Overheating may result in delayed or immediate postoperative facial weakness.

The size of the cochleostomy is determined by the manufacturer and varies from 1.0 to 1.4 mm. The endosteum may be opened with a 25-gauge spinal needle, straight pick, or Beaver 59-10 cataract knife (Becton Dickinson Co., Franklin Lakes, NJ) just before insertion of the electrode.

Recent research has focused on the benefit of preserving low-frequency hearing in patients with predominantly high-frequency (speech frequencies) hearing loss by atraumatic insertion of the cochlear implant electrode. Low-frequency hearing may be preserved because the typical electrode does not extend into the distal apex of the cochlea, the frequency place of low tones. Use of a short/hybrid electrode has resulted in improved patient word understanding, particularly in noise, as well as improved music perception.[22,23] This has also been investigated using standard electrode insertion through the round window as opposed to performing the previous standard cochleostomy. In a noncontrolled case series, five of nine children were shown to have preserved low-frequency hearing after surgery, and eight of nine demonstrated a benefit of combined electric and acoustic stimulation.[24] Patients undergoing implantation by a round window approach may also have reduced postoperative vertigo.[25]

The round window approach to cochlear implant insertion has support in anatomic studies as well. Reduced damage to intracochlear structures has been directly demonstrated and/or suggested by multiple cadaveric temporal bone studies.[26-28] In addition, temporal bone studies have revealed the potential for significant acoustic trauma while drilling the cochleostomy, with up to 130 dB levels experienced by the inner ear.[21] The round window approach also is technically less difficult than cochleostomy and uses easily visible landmarks in many cases.[28]

Receiver Stimulator

The pocket for the receiver stimulator is copiously irrigated with dilute bacitracin solution, and any final hemostasis necessary is undertaken. Monopolar electrocoagulation systems are turned off and unplugged. The receiver stimulator is then placed into its bony seat/pocket and tied down with suture.

Electrode Insertion

The electrode tip is placed in the cochleostomy using specially adapted instruments or jeweler's forceps. It is important to direct the natural curvature of the electrode away from the basilar membrane and to insert it into the principal axis of the scala. Hyaluronic acid or 50% glycerine may be used to keep blood out of the scala during electrode insertion and to lubricate the electrode. Specialized instruments provided by the manufacturer may then be used to slowly and gently insert the electrode.

The electrode cable may be stabilized by placing it into the split bridge, if desired. Then, 1- to 2-mm pieces of temporalis fascia, pericranium, or muscle are used to pack 360 degrees around the electrode at the cochleostomy. Alternatively, a 3-mm piece of tissue may be buttonholed and slipped up the electrode array past all of the contacts. After near total insertion, it is then slipped back into the cochleostomy, and the electrode is advanced 1 mm farther.

The entire area is then copiously irrigated, and the incision is closed in layers. A light mastoid pressure dressing is applied overnight and removed after a wound check in the morning. Typically, drains are not used.

Special Considerations for Children

Hearing loss during the first few years of life is known to delay the development of language and to lead to serious developmental consequences. During the language-sensitive first years of life, loss of peripheral hearing has been shown to cause central auditory system abnormalities in experimental animals and to cause auditory perceptual disorders in children.[29-32] Cochlear implants, on the other hand, have shown a protective effect when electrical stimulation is delivered to the developing auditory system of deafened animals.[33-35] These issues have led to the initial perception that the restriction of cochlear implantation to children older than the age of 2 years may limit potential development and linguistic outcomes. Children who have received implants by the age of 2 years acquire language at approximately the same rate as children without implants.[36] When implanted at this age, however, the child may not be able to overcome the original language gap caused by a lack of auditory input during the preimplant years. This has led to an increased interest in earlier implantation. A number of studies have demonstrated the safety and benefit of cochlear implantation in children younger than 12 months of age as well as the benefit to the children with respect to preverbal communication.[37-40] One study that evaluated children who had received their implants before 12 months of age revealed language comprehension and expressive development comparable to hearing peers. Their levels of language comprehension and expressive development was significantly better than those of children receiving implants between 12 and 24 months of age, thus supporting the practice of earlier implantation.[41] This has led to recommendations for implantation in appropriate candidates as young as 6 months of age. It is difficult to perform surgery much earlier, because approximately 6 months is needed for diagnostic testing, medical evaluations, and trials with hearing aids.

As the age of implantation has decreased, the acceptable levels of residual hearing of cochlear implant candidates has increased. Thus, although cochlear implants were originally restricted to children who were nearly anacusic, experience has shown that children with more residual hearing often perform better with implants. Hearing results in children with some measurable open-set speech recognition ability before implantation are better than those in children with none at all.[42-46]

Because the cochlea is full size at birth, there is no anatomic difficulty with electrode insertion in infants. However, deliberate surgical techniques for stimulator fixation and mastoidectomy and accommodation for head growth have been necessary for successful implantation. In very young children, it is often necessary to expose small areas of dura for the placement of tie-down sutures or seating of the implant. The skin incision must avoid the exposed facial nerve at the stylomastoid foramen. Redundancy of the electrode cable has been sufficient to prevent the extrusion of implants placed in very young children.

No specific complications associated with putting implants into very young children have been reported.

Otitis Media

The increased incidence of otitis media in very young children was once considered a relative contraindication to implantation. However, a number of studies have demonstrated that, after the ear infections are controlled medically or with ventilation tubes, implantation may proceed. Cochlear implantation is associated with neither increased incidence of otitis media nor complications such as labyrinthitis.[47-53] Some evidence has in fact suggested that mastoidectomy when combined with the improved ventilation of the middle ear afforded by performing a facial recess may decrease the incidence of otitis media.[54]

Otitis media should be managed aggressively to avoid delay in cochlear implantation. Treatment may require acute and prophylactic antibiotics, insertion of ventilation tubes, and in some cases, mastoidectomy with obliteration. The latter is usually performed as a staged preliminary step toward implantation in patients with chronic otitis media. It has been suggested that ventilation tubes be placed before implantation in children with unremitting otitis media with effusion and left in place for spontaneous extrusion.[55]

The recent association of meningitis and cochlear implantation has altered the thinking of some physicians regarding the management of recurrent otitis media, active otitis media with effusion, and an ear with a perforation. If severe chronic eustachian tube dysfunction is evident, a subtotal petrosectomy and closure of the eustachian tube and ear canal is advocated by some. This procedure should be performed 2 to 3 months before implantation of the internal stimulator receiver.

Auditory Neuropathy

Auditory neuropathy (AN) or dyssynchrony is associated with hearing loss in which outer hair cells function but inner hair cells or the cochlear nerve are dysfunctional. The diagnosis is made when otoacoustic emissions or cochlear microphonics are recordable (thus indicating outer hair cell function to be present) and the auditory brainstem response is absent. AN is suspected when the audiogram shows disproportionately low word recognition scores and the MRI is normal. It is critical in this population to provide an adequate trial of hearing aids and auditory verbal therapy because, despite an absent ABR, some children will have adequate benefit from hearing aids alone. Our experiences (as well as that of others) with AN implantees have been excellent in both adults and children.[56-58] The diagnosis of AN should not preclude consideration of a child for implantation. However, receipt of cochlear implants in many children has been delayed after a diagnosis of AN is made.

Meningitis and the Ossified Cochlea

Deafness caused by meningitis is associated with a reduction in spiral ganglion cells and often with ossification of the fluid spaces of the cochlea.[32] Because children who are deafened by meningitis may regain some of the hearing that was initially lost, immediate implantation is not recommended. However, fibrosis and ossification of the cochlea may occur within a few months after meningitis, and follow-up with serial MRIs performed at 2- to 3-month intervals may be done. If the perilymph/endolymph signature is lost, it indicates that fibrosis and eventual ossification may be occurring. In such cases, hearing does not return, and early implantation may be indicated. In some cases, the horizontal semicircular canal may show ossification earlier than the cochlea.

Meningitic patients generally require higher stimulation levels and more adaptive changes in their programming modes over time as compared with other patients.[59] This population has also been found to be at an increased risk of stimulation of the facial nerve (as have otosclerotic patients); however, this may be due to the higher stimulation amplitudes that are necessary, and it is usually controlled by inactivation of the offending electrodes or decreasing maximum stimulation levels. This may result in reduced performance of the implant. Nonetheless, patients with postmeningitic deafness and cochlear ossification can receive their implants via a variety of techniques,[60,61] and they can be electrically stimulated with generally good outcomes.[62] In the decade of the 1990s, approximately 3% to 9% of pediatric cochlear implant candidates had some degree of cochlear ossification, but in nearly 90% of these patients, the ossification is limited to the area that is adjacent to the round window membrane.[61] This may be drilled through to reach the open lumen of the basilar turn. When there is more extensive ossification of the scala tympani, the scala vestibuli may be patent and used for insertion. In both of these instances, a standard, full-length electrode is used, and results are similar to those of patients with no ossification.[61,63]

When both scala are ossified beyond the ascending turn of the cochlea, a complete drill out procedure or the use of a special electrode may be implemented.[64,65] Med-El Corporation (Innsbruck, Austria) manufactures a compressed electrode that has all of its contacts within a 10-mm distance for insertion into the inferior segment tunnel of the basal turn. Both Med-El and Cochlear Corporation (Melbourne, Australia) produce a split electrode array in which some contacts are placed in the inferior segment tunnel and others in the superior segment of the basal turn or in the second turn of the cochlea (see Fig. 159-7).

Labyrinthine Dysplasia

Deformities of the cochlea were once considered an absolute contraindication to cochlear implantation. However, at this time, deafness as a result of cochlear dysplasia is routinely managed with cochlear implants. Results vary directly with the degree of abnormal development. The majority of cases—including Mondini's dysplasia (incomplete partition), large vestibular aqueduct, and other, less severe forms of dysplasia—are associated with excellent results.[66,67]

The common cavity deformity, however, has highly variable results that are generally not as good as those seen in children with normal cochlea. Aplasia of the cochlea (Michel's deformity) or absence of the auditory nerve are absolute contraindications to implantation of the affected ear.

Absence of the cochlear nerve is suspected in anacusic patients with internal auditory canal (IAC) diameters of 1.5 mm or less. When a stenotic bony IAC is found, sagittal high-resolution MRI with heavily T2-weighted images is indicated to identify the presence of nerve bundles. The normal cochlear nerve may be seen coursing anteriorly toward the base of the modiolus. When facial nerve function is normal, one of the visible nerve bundles is considered to be the seventh cranial nerve. If the child has vestibular responses to calorics, another bundle may be considered the vestibular nerve; however, this nerve may be combined with the cochlear nerve. Electrical auditory brainstem responses may be performed to document the presence of the auditory nerve when there is doubt. In adults and children who are 6 years old and older, simple promontory testing may be performed in the office with topical anesthesia to obtain the same information.

CSF gushers should be expected in all cases of labyrinthine dysplasia. When a gusher occurs, implantation may proceed through the clear fluid, or the surgeon may elect to elevate the head of the table by 15 degrees and wait until no further fluid emerges. After the electrode is inserted, muscle and fascia are tightly packed into the cochleostomy to prevent further CSF leakage. A lumbar drain should not be used before sealing the cochleostomy, because it reduces the CSF pressure head, thereby making it impossible to determine whether the tissue seal is adequate.

Patients with Compromised Healing

Patients with reduced wound-healing capabilities because of underlying medical conditions or who are immunosuppressed by medications are considered to be at increased risk for postoperative infection and device extrusion. Nonetheless, in a review of patients with systemic autoimmune disorders as well as after liver and kidney transplantation, after high-dose radiation to the surgical field, or who were taking relatively high-dose immunosuppressive medications, implantation has been accomplished without significant complications.[68]

Older Patients

Some unique changes associated with aging must be considered in patients older than age 70 years. These include degeneration of all elements of the auditory system, the likelihood of prolonged duration of deafness, diminished central auditory function and communication ability, and coexisting medical and psychosocial problems.

Nonetheless, cochlear implantation in older adults has been successful, with results comparable to those in younger adults overall.[69] In our experience, patients up to the age of 87 years have obtained excellent results as evaluated by audiometric and quality-of-life measures. Nonetheless, in patients who are older than 80 years, these outcomes are not as good overall as they are in younger patients. Perioperative attention to medical and surgical details has allowed for safe insertion and a minimum of postoperative problems. Patients at this age are generally observed overnight in the hospital after surgery and are discharged the following morning.

Older patients may have difficulty understanding and recalling the information necessary for proper operation of their external device. Difficulties associated with arthritis and fine motor abilities may lead to problems changing batteries or adjusting the controls of the device. Older adults may also progress less rapidly with the use of their device if they live alone and are not exposed to verbal communication on a consistent basis.[69] Extensive counseling is required to address all of these issues and limitations. The ability to retain and use the relatively large amount of technical information by older patients must be kept in mind during counseling.

Bilateral Cochlear Implantation

The psychoacoustic literature has demonstrated improved auditory function when normal-hearing people listen with both ears and when hearing-impaired subjects use bilateral hearing aids.[70] This finding extends to bilateral implant recipients who have been clearly demonstrated to have improved speech recognition in noise compared with unilateral conditions.[15,71-74] This binaural advantage is predominantly from the head shadow effect in which speech and noise are spatially separated such that one ear is protected from the noise due to an acoustic shadow, and therefore has a better signal-to-noise ratio. Binaural summation and squelch have variable effects.[75] Because much social discourse occurs within a background of noise (classroom, party, busy restaurant), this advantage is of paramount importance to patients.

Sound localization is better in patients with bilateral implants than in patients with unilateral listening conditions. Unilateral localization accuracy has been identified between 50 and 67 degrees, whereas bilateral accuracy was determined to be between 24 and 29 degrees.[76-78] Sound localization is of critical importance in avoiding a potentially dangerous situation (e.g., locating an ambulance speeding down the street); it also permits the listener to focus on source and position of sound to improve the signal-to-noise ratio in daily situations.

In 2008, a position statement from the William House Cochlear Implant Study Group formally advocated bilateral cochlear implantation in children and adults because their review of literature supported the conclusion that both children and adults performed better with two implants than with one.[79]

Complications

Drilling the internal cochlear stimulator (ICS) seat and tie-down holes engenders the possibility of damage to the dura or the underlying dural blood vessels. Performing the mastoidectomy and opening the facial recess have the same risks as are present in other transmastoid procedures. However, because of the absence of chronic disease in most cases, the risks are somewhat reduced. Nonetheless, when operating on children with congenital deformities, there is a greater risk that the facial nerve may follow an aberrant course within the temporal bone.

Cochlear implantation also includes the insertion of a very delicate electrode, and the incidence of damaged or misplaced electrodes has declined from 1.74% to 1.18% since the late 1990s. The risk of postoperative facial paresis has also decreased from 1.74% in 1995 to 0.41%.[80,81]

Revision cochlear implantation surgery is not an uncommon occurrence after initial surgery. Reported rates of revision surgery vary, but recently revision surgery in adults has been reported at 5.4% to 7%.[81,82] The rate of revision implantation in children has typically been higher, with reports placing the rate between 8% and 12.5%.[81-83] The most common indications for revision surgery in a 2008 report was "hard failure" or device malfunction that occurred in 46% of the cases of revision surgery.[83] Medical-surgical reasons (e.g., wound healing, electrode malposition, cholesteatoma) were the second most common cause, occurring in 37% of cases. A "soft failure" (decrease in auditory performance or aversive symptoms in a device that performs within manufacturer specifications) occurred in 15% of cases. In general, patients performed as well after reimplantation as their best performance before surgery.[83,84]

Reimplantation may also be necessary when technology advances to the point that the device in use is outmoded (e.g., the transition from single-channel to multichannel implants). Studies of repeat electrode insertion depth show results that are generally equal to the original, although cases of both improved and diminished function have been reported.[84,85]

SUGGESTED READINGS

Brown KD, Balkany TJ. Benefits of bilateral cochlear implantation: a review. *Curr Opin Otolaryngol Head Neck Surg.* 2007;15(5):315-318.

Cullen RD, Fayad JN, Luxford WM, Buchman CA. Revision cochlear implant surgery in children. *Otol Neurotol.* 2008;29(2):214-220.

Dettman SJ, Pinder D, Briggs RJ, et al. Communication development in children who receive the cochlear implant younger than 12 months: risks versus benefits. *Ear Hear.* 2007;28(Suppl 2):11S-18S.

Gantz BJ, Tyler RS, Rubenstein JT, et al. Binaural cochlear implants placed during the same operation. *Otol Neurotol.* 2002;23(2):169-180.

Parry DA, Booth T, Roland PS. Advantages of magnetic resonance imaging over computed tomography in preoperative evaluation of pediatric cochlear implant candidates. *Otol Neurotol.* 2005;26(5):976-982.

Skarzynski H, Lorens A, Piotrowski A, Anderson I. Partial deafness cochlear implantation in children. *Int J Pediatr Otorhinolaryngol.* 2007;71(9):1407-1413.

For complete list of references log onto www.expertconsult.com.

Wei BP, Robins-Browne RM, Shepherd RK, et al. Assessment of the protective effect of pneumococcal vaccination in preventing meningitis after cochlear implantation. *Arch Otolaryngol Head Neck Surg.* 2007;133(10):987-994.

CHAPTER ONE HUNDRED AND SIXTY

Cochlear Implants: Results, Outcomes, Rehabilitation, and Education

Charles J. Limb

Howard W. Francis

Sue Archbold

Gerard O'Donoghue

John K. Niparko

Key Points

- Performance of cochlear implants is affected by baseline factors that should be assessed as implant candidacy is considered. A multidisciplinary team enables simultaneous input from multiple perspectives, and is the most effective approach to assessing a candidate's needs and desires and the potential for an implant to meet them.
- In the 1980s, candidacy requirements for a cochlear implant required total or near-total sensorineural hearing loss as characterized by a pure-tone average of 100 dB or greater; amplified thresholds that failed to reach 60 dB; and an absence of open-set speech recognition despite the use of powerful, best-fit hearing aids. Because clinical experience has indicated that the mean speech reception scores of implant recipients generally exceed the aided results of individuals with lesser impairments, the audiologic criteria have been progressively relaxed since the early stages of multichannel implants to include a range of pure-tone averages, focusing instead on functional benefits provided by amplification.
- Although a cochlear implant facilitates sensitive hearing reliably, actual "listening" capabilities are less easily characterized.
- Speech recognition remains the standard metric of cochlear implant candidacy and performance. Speech recognition results show high variability, however, and awareness is increasing that epiphenomena surrounding implantation and the postimplant experience affect performance.
- For children, the extent to which the implant experience assists oral language development is a key reflection of the effectiveness with which developmental learning is normalized. Children with early-onset deafness lack the base of auditory memory needed to pair implant-mediated precepts with meaning. They may harbor other disabilities that may prevent instinctive language learning. Such conditions can produce a wide range of individual variability, particularly when intervention with a cochlear implant is delayed.
- In children, initial reports suggested that implantation before age 3 years provides distinct advantages over later implantation in cases of early-onset deafness. More recent data suggest that speech recognition and language skills are facilitated with implantation in earlier toddler and even infancy stages. Whether earlier implantation may yield greater benefits requires longitudinal follow-up of the development of ever younger infants undergoing implantation.
- Adults with cochlear implants exhibit a similarly wide range of results, often owing to factors outside of the device per se.
- To improve the accuracy of predicting an implant's outcome and to counsel patients effectively, comprehensive preimplant assessment is necessary.
- Screening for other handicapping conditions, particularly conditions that would impair the acquisition of receptive and productive communication skills, helps determine candidacy and direct rehabilitative strategies.
- Postimplantation rehabilitation can be important for some adult implant recipients, but is crucial for children to optimize the usefulness of an implant. It is often assumed that effective interactive skills and language comprehension directly result from the sensitivity with which sound is perceived through a cochlear implant. Hearing is not a sufficient condition for these higher skills, however, and a high priority should be placed on auditory rehabilitation to enhance fundamental skills in verbal communication.

Three decades of clinical experience with cochlear implantation suggest that notions of "success" or "failure" are highly nonspecific. There is a wide spectrum of the effects of cochlear implantation, which span a range of communication, psychosocial, and cognitive outcomes. Assessment of "success" with a cochlear implant is complex. The sense of hearing is pivotal to the phonologic awareness and processing that supports speech and language, including the development of visual language reception (reading) and production (writing), and a range of communicative behaviors and cognitive functions. This chapter examines the broad effects of cochlear implants in children and adults. We have drawn information from reports of clinic-based results and patient-based surveys. Basic assessment of physiologic response to auditory nerve stimulation, measures of receptive and productive benefit, and surveys of life effects as reflected in measures of quality of life and economic outcomes are described.

Although we characterize the effects of the implant per se, clinicians caring for hearing-impaired patients are increasingly aware that *clinical practices* related to cochlear implantation—especially practices related to candidate selection and rehabilitation—modify expectations and observed results. The most obvious effect of severe to profound sensorineural hearing loss is that there is insufficient phonologic access to encode complex information contained in speech streams. Cochlear implants seem to enable a level of phonologic access that can reliably overcome barriers to speech recognition. It has been tempting to assume that restored audition through a cochlear implant would provide sufficient input for a child to achieve a normal trajectory of developmental learning or an adult to reacquire the skills of verbal communication fully. The tasks of developmental learning and spoken communication require more than basic perceptive capacity, however.

A child or adult with an implant must attempt to process information conveyed by a prosthetic device using afferent tracts that may be altered consequent to early deafferentation. The ability to assimilate auditory information in facilitating communication tasks cannot be assumed because of well-recognized deprivation effects inherent in advanced sensorineural hearing loss. Environment and developmental experience are likely important, if not determinative, of implant benefit in some domains. Through a fuller understanding of the elements of success and failure with cochlear implants, clinicians can gain insight into criteria for candidate selection, and for the services and environments that would optimize use of an implant as a communication tool.

Results of Implantation

Factors Related to the Measurement of Auditory Performance

Auditory performance is measured at preimplant and postimplant intervals. Preimplant assessments form the basis of evaluating patient candidacy. Postimplant measures document the progress of the patient, while allowing the clinician to monitor for device-related and environmental factors that can influence long-term outcomes. Measurement variables associated with auditory testing should be standardized as much as possible. Clinicians can choose between closed-set tests (e.g., forced choice of one answer from a list of four) and open-set tests (auditory alone without context) of words or sentences. Closed-set tests are easier for patients than open-set tests, and are susceptible to "ceiling effects," reflecting high contextual information available when word and sentence material are presented.[188] The method of presentation can also affect speech perception scores.[1a] Live presentation typically produces higher rates of correct responses than taped presentations.

Trends toward higher rates of open-set speech recognition with newer implant technology and longer implant experience have prompted more stringent assessments. Increasing the difficulty of a speech perception test has the effect of limiting the "ceiling effect" that results from testing with simple, everyday phrases. To generate meaningful comparative data, increasing test difficulty normalizes distributions of scores, enabling more powerful statistical tests of differences between groups.

Tests of Implant Performance

The Minimum Speech Test Battery (MSTB) was developed for adult cochlear implant users. The MSTB is a set of high-fidelity disc recordings that provide a standardized set of comprehensive tests of preoperative and postoperative speech recognition.[2] To minimize the effects of learning and memorization, MSTB word and sentence tests have different lists for at least six testing trials. The average and range of performance of cochlear implant users are crucial to defining audiologic performance boundaries for implant candidacy.

The major components of the MSTB are the Hearing in Noise Test (HINT) and the Consonant/Nucleus/Consonant Test (CNC). The HINT[2] provides a measure of speech recognition ability for sentences in quiet and in noise. The background noise is filtered to match the long-term average spectrum of the sentences. In the MSTB, the HINT sentence lists are presented at 70 +dB in quiet and at 10 +dB signal-to-noise ratio (i.e., noise at 60 +dB). Smaller signal-to-noise ratios (e.g., 5 +dB or 0 +dB) may also be used to avoid ceiling effects. Although normal-hearing listeners can comprehend sentences effectively with signal-to-noise ratios of 3 +dB, implant recipients typically show degraded speech recognition when signal-to-noise ratios are reduced beyond 10 +dB.

The CNC consists of lists of monosyllabic words with equal phonemic distribution, with each list having approximately the same phonemic distribution as the English language.[3] Such lists provide material for performance testing that is more likely to represent daily experience with speech stimuli. These tests measure percentage of words correctly recognized. Open-set conditions for monosyllabic word recognition are considered the most difficult challenge to a listener with a cochlear implant, and such tests are useful to compare outcomes in adults.[4] Revised CNC lists[5] were developed to eliminate uncommon words and proper nouns. Ten lists of 50 words contain monosyllabic words that are employed with a frequency of greater than 4 per 1 million, as calculated in word-frequency tables. As part of the MSTB protocol, during each preoperative and postoperative evaluation, one CNC and one HINT list should be presented in quiet at 70 dB(A). In addition, if the patient performs greater than 30% under quiet conditions, HINT sentences can be presented in noise at 10 +dB signal-to-noise ratio.

Implant Performance in Adults

Improved speech perception is the primary goal of cochlear implantation. Although initial clinical series judged implant efficacy mostly on environmental sound perception and performance on closed-set tests, greater emphasis is now placed on measures of open-set speech comprehension. Speech-perception results from early clinical trials have served to guide the evolution of cochlear implantation. Gantz and colleagues[6] provided early comparative data in their assessment of environmental sound and speech perception in a large cohort of nonrandomized single-channel and multichannel implant users. Multichannel implants provided significantly higher levels of performance on all measures. Cohen and associates[7] performed the first prospective, randomized trial of cochlear implants through the U.S. Veterans' Administration hospital system. The trial provided high-quality clinical data and convincing evidence of open-set speech recognition, and established the clear superiority of multichannel over single-channel designs. The study was the first to report a low complication rate and high device reliability in individuals deafened after language acquisition from multiple centers with varying levels of prior programmatic implant experience.

Cohen and Waltzman,[8] Skinner and colleagues,[9,10] and Wilson and associates[11] assessed effects of changing external processing capabilities. They compared the performance of subjects fitted with processors designed to increase the rate of information transfer through higher rates of pulsed stimulation. Each study assessed a different processor, and study design and processing strategy also differed among studies. In each study, the use of a more sophisticated speech processor led to significantly better performance in open-set speech recognition.

Clinical observations in patients with current processors indicate that for patients with implant experience longer than 6 months, the mean score on open-set word testing approximates 25% to 40% (range 0% to 100%).[7,12-14] Results achieved with the most recently developed speech processing strategies reveal mean scores greater than 75% on words-in-sentence testing (range 0% to 100%). Although subjects perform substantially poorer on single-word testing, these mean scores continue to improve as speech-processing strategy evolves.[10] After implantation, speech recognition by telephone[15] and music appreciation are often observed.

Benefits are enhanced through the use of more recently developed processing strategies. Spahr and colleagues[16] observed that differences in implant design affect performance, especially in difficult listening situations. Input dynamic range and the method by which compression is implemented seem to be the major factors that account for results in difficult listening situations, with greater performance associated with the expanded dynamic range offered by current processing strategies employed by the Advanced Bionics and MedEl devices.

Predictors of Benefit in Adults

Assessments of speech recognition in adults with cochlear implants offer the opportunity to develop models of benefit prediction. As investigators identify the salient predictive factors, candidacy, device and processing strategy, and the degree of postoperative auditory rehabilitation necessary, they can be better informed. The contributions of modifiers to differences in performance (multivariate analysis) have been addressed in several large studies.[6,7,12-14,17-19] The following factors have been evaluated:

- *Subject variables*: age of onset, age of implantation, deafness duration, etiology, preoperative hearing, survival and location of spiral ganglion cells, patency of the scala tympani, cognitive skills, personality, visual attention, motivation, engagement, communication mode, and auditory memory
- *Device variables*: processor, implant, electrode geometry, electrode number, duration and pattern of implant use, and strategy employed by the speech processing unit

Although the significance of the above-listed factors varies across different populations, multiple regression analysis has identified variables with high predictive value for speech comprehension. Length of implant use accounts for a high degree of variance in speech perception measured postoperatively. When length of use is controlled, preoperative hearing (particularly with respect to speech recognition) also accounts for a high degree of variance. Duration of deafness, age of implantation, cochlear patency, subject engagement with the therapeutic regimen, and processor type also carry high predictive values for speech understanding.

In addition to the factors in the list, the choice of ear to implant is a highly compelling issue. Other studies have emphasized the utility of implanting the better hearing ear.[13] At Johns Hopkins Hospital, we have long advocated the implantation of the poorer hearing ear. Although more data are needed, our studies so far reveal no significant difference in implant performance based on whether the better or worse hearing ear is implanted. Figure 160-1 shows a regression plot of the predicted postoperative word scores for each patient as modeled by the Johns Hopkins (implant poorer ear) and Iowa formulas (better ear).[17] Virtually identical scores are predicted on the basis of each patient's duration of deafness and preoperative sentence recognition scores. These data suggest that results obtained through cochlear implantation of the poorer hearing ear are statistically equivalent to results obtained through implantation of the better hearing ear. The similarity of results obtained through both methods suggests that implantation may have a beneficial effect on central auditory pathway development regardless of sidedness.

Another variable that influences speech perception is technologic sophistication of the implanted device. Improvements in speech perception have been associated with generational improvements in signal processing strategies, speech processors, and electrode arrays,[20] but may reflect clinical trends and technologic advances.[13] Criteria for cochlear implant candidacy are constantly expanding. Research has shown that patients with greater residual hearing show even more promising results. Identification of monosyllabic words for individuals using early generations of the Nucleus (Cochlear Corp., Sydney, Australia) multichannel cochlear implant averaged 16%,[6] whereas performance exceeds 50% on similar measures with current technology.[10,16] Earlier

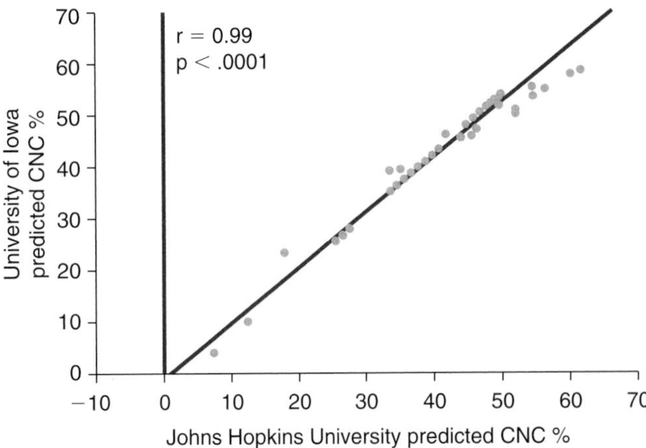

Figure 160-1. Regression plot of the predicted postoperative word scores for each patient as modeled by the Johns Hopkins (implant poorer ear) and Iowa formulas (better ear). There are virtually identical scores predicted on the basis of each patient's duration of deafness and preoperative sentence recognition scores. These data suggest that results obtained through cochlear implantation of the poorer hearing ear are statistically equivalent to results obtained through implantation of the better hearing ear. The similarity of results obtained through both methods suggests that implantation may have a beneficial effect on central auditory pathway development regardless of sidedness. CNC, Consonant/Nucleus/Consonant Test.

studies have contrasted performance across different manufacturers of devices. Differences in performance seem more closely related, however, to general demographic differences across patient populations, tests used, and length of experience with the devices than to differences in characteristics of like-generation devices per se.[21,22]

Cochlear Implantation with Hearing Preservation in Adults

There has been considerable interest in clinical strategies that combine residual acoustic hearing with electric hearing provided by a cochlear implant. Two strategies have been developed, depending on baseline hearing status. A *combined* mode uses a cochlear implant in one ear and a hearing aid in the other ear.[23] A *hybrid* strategy uses a hearing aid and a cochlear implant in the same ear.[24,25]

The goal of combining amplification with a cochlear implant in the opposite ear is to preserve perceptual advantages inherent in (predominantly low frequency) acoustic hearing in an attempt to capture at least some binaural cues. In fact, binaural advantages are observed in some patients.[23] Tests of speech perception in noise reveal trends toward a binaural advantage for word recognition depending on the direction of origin of noise (with advantages obviated when noise is on the hearing aid side). Localization ability improved with both devices. These data support the use of a hearing aid opposite a cochlear implant for appropriate patients.

Success with hearing preservation[26,27] in ears implanted with scala tympani electrodes has encouraged the development of hybrid modes of stimulation—electroacoustic hearing. Various surgical strategies have been adopted in attempts to limit cochlear trauma with scala tympani electrode insertion, enhancing opportunities for preserving residual (typically, <1 kHz) hearing. Hearing preservation procedures are designed to avert basilar membrane rupture and attendant spiral ganglion cell loss. Optimal preservation seems to be achieved with placement of the cochleostomy in a strategic location (away from the basilar membrane) along with cautious insertion of adapted, smaller arrays in a manner that limits impact on the endosteal and basilar membrane surfaces.[28]

Electroacoustic hearing seems to confer distinct advantages in speech perception and in music listening.[25,29] Improvements in speech-in-noise understanding and melody recognition are linked to the ability to distinguish fine pitch differences through preserved, low-frequency acoustic hearing. There may be expanded spectral representation that more faithfully supports higher frequency hearing over time.[30] These observations suggest that the preservation of residual low-frequency hearing should be considered in selected patients. Observations of advantages in electroacoustic hearing may expand candidate selection criteria for cochlear implantation.

Although electroacoustic stimulation is a promising treatment for patients with residual low-frequency hearing, a small subset lose residual hearing despite best attempts with preservation. Such patients may obtain expected levels of benefit using the electric mode of the hybrid implant alone. For patients unable to achieve this benefit from an electroacoustic strategy after losing residual hearing, reimplantation with a standard array seems to provide higher levels of speech recognition.[31]

Implant Performance in Children

Pediatric cochlear implantation began with House-3M, single-channel implants in 1980. Investigational trials with multichannel cochlear implants began with adolescents (10 to 17 years old) in 1985 and with children (2 to 9 years old) in November 1986. Implantation of infants and toddlers younger than 2 years began in 1995.[32] Although clinical experience with cochlear implantation is shorter in children than in adults, a large body of clinical reports is now available.[33,34] Investigators have evaluated the hearing and speech receptive benefit of cochlear implants in children since 1985.

Auditory Performance Assessments for Children

Auditory performance in children is assessed with a battery of audiologic tests that can address the wide range of perceptual skills exhibited by children with severe-to-profound sensorineural hearing loss. Although substantial auditory gains are apparent in implanted children, the range of quantifiable improvement varies widely among children, and depends heavily on the duration of use of the device, preoperative conditions, and longitudinal experience and training effects. For this reason, testing should survey a range of levels of speech recognition, including simple awareness of sound, pattern perception (discrimination of time and stress differences of utterance), closed-set (multiple choice) speech recognition, and open-set (auditory only) recognition.

Methodologic variables must be considered when attempting to rate objectively the effect of cochlear implants on the development of speech perception in deaf children. Difficulties are inherent in objectively rating communication competence in very young children. Older children may exhibit advantages by virtue of greater familiarity with a test's context, independent of perceptual skills. Objective assessment mandates a structured setting that is not always conducive to eliciting a child's best cooperative effort. Investigators must also account for discontinuity in the age-appropriate measures necessary for longitudinal assessment.[34] Methodologic challenges and developmental considerations inherent in pediatric implant assessment have been examined in detail by Kirk and Diefendorf,[35] who categorized variables as relating to the following:

- *Internal variables*: the child's age and level of language and cognitive development
- *External variables*: the child's ability and willingness to respond as influenced by reinforcement and required memory task
- *Methodologic variables*: the procedure of voice presentation, the test administered, and the available options from which to choose a response

Tests of speech perceptions typically used for childhood assessment have been described in detail,[1a,35-37] and usually consist of closed-set tests that assess word identification among a limited set of options with auditory cues only, open-set tests (scored by percentage of individual words correctly repeated), and structured interviews of parents using criteria-based surveys[38] to assess response to sound in everyday situations and behaviors related to spoken communication.

Early Studies of Speech Reception in Children with Cochlear Implants

House and colleagues[39] found that children with cochlear implants obtain substantial improvement in auditory thresholds, closed-set speech recognition, and limited open-set speech recognition with the House-3M single-channel implant. Miyamoto and coworkers[40] provided systematic, well-controlled assessments of childhood cohorts and consistently showed performance advantages of multichannel over single-channel implants. Other early studies by Fryauf-Bertschy,[41] Gantz,[42] Miyamoto,[18] and Waltzman[43] and their colleagues observed that implanted children gain substantial speech perceptive capabilities for 5 years after implantation. Because many of the implanted children tracked in these studies were congenitally or prelingually deaf, there are compelling data to indicate that implantation can provide auditory access during critical developmental stages to form the early correlates of spoken language.

The studies we have cited have shown implant benefit in children with total or near-total hearing loss. An important issue for candidacy of children with lesser degrees of hearing impairment is the study of implant benefit relative to controls who have not received implants. Classification of children according to preoperative hearing levels can provide a common ground for comparison. Miyamoto and associates[44] described the following candidacy scale for stratifying children according to aided pure-tone detection thresholds: "Gold" class hearing aid users have unaided thresholds of 90 to 100 dB at two of three frequencies (0.5 kHz, 1 kHz, 2 kHz), with a mean of 94 dB. "Silver" class hearing aid users have unaided thresholds of 101 to 110 dB at two of three frequencies, with a mean of 104 dB. "Bronze" class users have unaided thresholds of greater than 110 dB at two of three frequencies, with a mean greater than 110 dB.

Hearing aid users in the "gold" category generally fall into Boothroyd's[45] category of "considerable residual hearing." In many such cases, hearing aid users that function at this level show substantial capabilities for near-normal trajectories of speech and oral language acquisition. This particular group of profoundly hearing-impaired children sets a comparative standard for speech perception performance. "Silver" category hearing aid users receive few spectral cues and rely heavily on temporal cues for speech perception. "Bronze" category users are considered "totally deaf," and receive only low-frequency percepts and restricted or no temporal cues.

Most hearing-impaired children who have received cochlear implants fell into or were eventually moved into the "bronze" category. Compared with children using amplification, children with implants have shown the following:

- After 2 years of implant experience, mean speech intelligibility scores of implanted children surpass those of "silver" category hearing aid users and approach within 10% scores of "gold" category users, particularly on more stringent tests of speech comprehension.[44,46] Longitudinal tracking of implanted children shows no evidence of a plateau effect in mean scores of speech comprehension. In conjunction with evidence based on multivariate analysis, this observation suggests that length of implant use is the primary determinant of receptive benefit.
- Trends toward continued improvement in speech reception are also associated with improved intelligibility of speech.[47] Although the measured proficiency of speech produced remains low through the first 2 years after implantation, intelligibility scores thereafter show dramatic gains and surpass those of hearing aid users in the "silver" category.[48] These observations are consistent with observations of gains in speech intelligibility in other childhood cohorts.[49,50]

More Recent Studies of Speech Reception in Children with Cochlear Implants

Between 1994 and 2004, numerous reports documented various levels of gains in speech recognition in young deaf children using multichannel cochlear implants. Miyamoto and coworkers[18] noted that in 29 children with 1 to 4 years of experience with a cochlear implant, approximately one half achieved open-set speech recognition. Waltzman and Cohen[51] found that 14 children implanted before age 3 years attained high levels of speech perception performance with only 2 years of experience. Fryauf-Bertschy and coworkers[52] examined speech perception in cochlear-implanted children over 4 years, and noted significant increases in pattern perception and results of closed-set speech perception tests.

Variability in speech-perception performance across subjects is widely recognized, and is related to several variables, including age of implantation,[33,42,52-54] mode of communication,[43,55] family support,[52] and length of deafness.[56,57] Miyamoto and colleagues[40] found that duration of deafness, communication mode, age at onset of deafness, and type of processor accounted for approximately 35% of variance in closed-set testing. The length of implant use alone accounted for a larger percentage of variance on all speech perception measures. In a 5-year follow-up study, O'Donoghue and associates[53] found that age at implantation was the most significant covariant, and that mode of communication was the most significant between-individuals factor. The latter study showed that young age at implantation and oral communication mode are the most important known determinants of later speech perception in young children after cochlear implantation.

Waltzman and colleagues[43] and Brackett and Zara[58] reported improved speech reception in children implanted at age 2 to 3 years compared with children implanted at an older age. Multicenter data reported by Osberger and associates[59] indicated that implant performance of children implanted before age 2 years is significantly better than implant performance of children implanted between age 2 and 3 years. The authors also identified an important confounding variable, however, that exists in the children who receive a cochlear implant at a younger age: they are more likely to use an oral mode of communication. This, by itself, may be a predictor of higher implant performance—an observation borne out in early studies of a national childhood cohort assembled by Geers and colleagues.[55]

Osberger and coworkers[59] also found that children with more residual hearing relative to earlier cohorts were undergoing implantation. Gantz and colleagues[60] compiled data from across centers that indicate children with some degree of preoperative open-set speech recognition obtain substantially higher levels of speech comprehension. Taken together, these studies suggest the strongest potential for benefit exists with implantation at a young age, when intervention is provided early and, in the case of a progressive loss, before auditory input is lost completely.

Cheng and associates[33] performed a meta-analysis of relevant literature on speech recognition in children with cochlear implants. Of 1916 reports on cochlear implants published since 1966, 44 contained sufficient patient data to compare speech recognition results between published (n = 1904 children) and unpublished (n = 261) trials.[33] Meta-analysis was complicated by the diversity of tests required to address the full spectrum of speech reception in children with cochlear implants. An expanded format of the Speech Perception Categories[61] was designed to integrate results across studies. The main conclusions of this meta-analysis were that earlier implantation is associated with a greater trajectory of gain in speech recognition (Fig. 160-2), performance comparing deafness of congenital and acquired etiologies levels out over time, and there is an absence of reaching a plateau of speech recognition benefits over time. More than 75% of the children with cochlear implants reported in peer-reviewed publications have achieved substantial open-set speech recognition after 3 years of implant use.

Implantation of Infants

New diagnostic approaches and improved treatment options have enhanced real-life outcomes and transformed clinical approaches to the treatment of early-onset hearing loss. Universal newborn hearing screening now routinely identifies hearing loss that might have gone unnoticed in years past until a child had failed to develop language skills. Such early identification affords the opportunity to provide clinical intervention during a brief and critical growth period when neural connections develop physiologic support needed for children to achieve verbal communication.

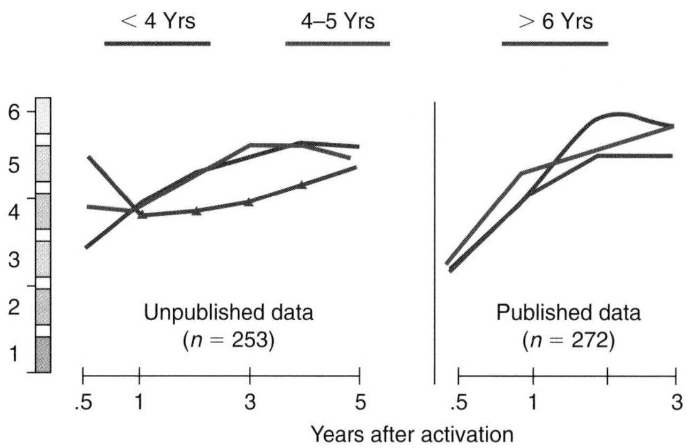

Figure 160-2. Meta-analysis of speech perception results with cochlear implantation in children, showing effects of age at implantation on speech perception. Published and unpublished data are shown. Three different ages at implantation groups are compared (<4 years, 4 to 5 years, and >6 years). The ordinal scale represents levels of speech perception: 1, detection; 2, pattern; 3, limited closed-set; 4, substantial closed-set; 5, limited open-set; and 6, substantial open-set.

A growing body of evidence supports the early application of cochlear implantation in congenitally deaf children. Meta-analyses of the effects of age at implantation have shown that children undergoing implantation at younger ages achieve greater progress in speech perception skills than children implanted at older ages.[33,62,63] Because the development of language follows the same trajectory as that reflecting speech perception, language growth is more favorable in children who receive cochlear implants early in life.[64] To the extent that higher language ability results in greater independence in school settings,[65] earlier intervention would enhance the cost-effectiveness of the cochlear implant.

Cochlear implantation has been shown to be a safe procedure in children younger than 12 months old.[66,67] The motivation to pursue implantation when a child has been deemed an appropriate candidate is supported by compelling data showing the benefits of earlier intervention. Tait and colleagues[68] showed that preverbal skills develop much more rapidly in children who receive cochlear implants before 2 years of age compared with children implanted between 2 and 3 years old, or between 3 and 4 years old. Connor and colleagues[69] examined latent growth curves and showed the value of very early implantation as it translated into more favorable outcomes. Dettman and colleagues[70] in Australia and Lesinski-Schiedat and associates[71] in Germany have convincingly shown with longitudinal assessment that the language trajectories of children implanted before age 12 months are greater than those achieved with implantation after 12 months of age.

Nicholas and Geers[72] showed that language outcomes for deaf children for whom appropriate intervention occurs within the first months of life are far superior to outcomes associated with later intervention. They noted that the first 3 years in a child's life are crucial for acquiring information about the world, communicating with family, and developing a cognitive and linguistic foundation from which all further development unfolds.

Because of the demonstrated safety of early implantation and the effectiveness of early linguistic intervention, cochlear implantation in younger children (12 months old) has been approved by the Food and Drug Administration in the United States. The current approval for implantation at age 12 months should be interpreted with caution. The intent of that approval is based on open market applications from manufacturers; delaying intervention results and the risk of prolonged auditory deprivation and adverse consequences for development should be weighed in each individual case.

Bilateral Cochlear Implantation

In an effort to expand the benefits obtained with unilateral cochlear implantation, bilateral implantation has been pursued in increasing numbers of patients, either simultaneous or sequential. As of this writing, approximately 20% of all implant users have bilateral devices based on generally positive subjective experiences with low rates of complication. An important development within the field of cochlear implantation is to assess fully the impact of bilateral intervention.

Normal listeners possess a range of auditory capabilities owing to binaural processing, as follows:

Localization: Normal listeners are able to tell where sound is coming from in the horizontal plane (at ear level) with an accuracy of ±14 degrees.[73] The brain uses differences in intensity and time between the two ears to determine the location of a sound source. To localize sound in the vertical plane (up and down), or when time and intensity cues between the two ears are ambiguous, spectral (pitch) information is important.[74] The shapes of the outer ear and ear canal change the intensities of all of the pitches arriving at the ear (by reflecting them differently) to determine the location of sounds in the vertical plane.[75]

Head shadow: When listening to speech in noise, the head acts as a sound barrier that makes noise quieter on the side away from the speech. When one ear is close to the noise source, adding the other ear (away from the noise) provides a second ear where the speech is louder than the competing noise.

Squelch: When signals and noise come from different directions, the brain is able to separate them by comparing time, intensity, and pitch differences between the two ears. The practical effect is that the brain is able to suppress signals that the listener does not wish to hear.

Summation: When identical signals are presented to the two ears, there is an advantage when hearing with both ears instead of just one alone. The brain has a special ability to use the signals from both ears to produce this binaural advantage.

Studies of subjects with unilateral hearing loss illustrate some of the problems that a listener with only one "good" ear may encounter. Background noise often interferes with word recognition in quiet and noisy conditions even when the speech is directed to the good ear. People have reported difficulty hearing and understanding speech even in relatively quiet situations that include low-level noise (e.g., car radios, air conditioners).[76] Children with unilateral hearing loss not only have difficulty in noise,[77] but also show delays in language development and academic performance relative to their peers with normal hearing.[78]

In addition to the general advantages of binaural hearing, there may be other compelling reasons for considering bilateral implantation in very young children. Congenitally deaf children depend on their cochlear implants for learning spoken language. Children with normal hearing acquire language through incidental learning—that is, through participation in everyday communication and social experiences, which are often unintended and incidental. Although studies have shown improved language acquisition in children with unilateral implants relative to their preimplant performance with hearing aids,[64,79] children still lag behind their peers with normal hearing in mastery of more complex language structures that are requisites for academic success.[80] If a young deaf child has two implants, the rate of incidental language learning is likely to be accelerated because they would be better able to understand speech in everyday situations (most of which are noisy), and to localize to the most relevant (speech) events in their environment. The improved benefits with bilateral implants in young deaf children have important implications for language acquisition, academic success, and educational and occupational opportunities.

Providing sound input to both ears in a young deaf child ensures that sound is processed on both sides of the brain. The right and left auditory cortices can develop in a more normal sequence. If a child is implanted on only one side, the parts of the brain that would have been stimulated by the nonimplanted ear do not develop, and eventually plasticity is greatly diminished. Ryugo and colleagues[81] reported that electric stimulation of the auditory system largely prevents or reverses the synaptic abnormalities seen in congenitally deaf white cats.

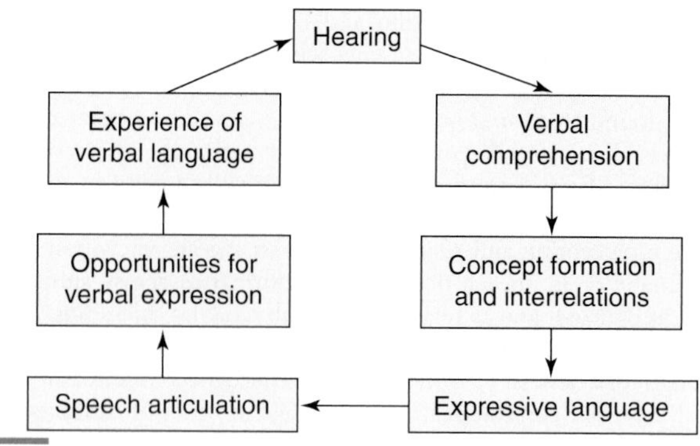

Figure 160-3. The cycle of verbal communication. Hearing is crucial to the process of verbal communication and allows for verbal comprehension. Concept formation gives rise to expressive language and speech articulation capabilities, which are applied as verbal language in appropriate situations. Successful verbal communication ultimately depends on hearing. *(Modified from the Reynell Developmental Scales Manual. Los Angeles: Western Psychological Services.)*

Reports of the bilateral benefits experienced by adult and pediatric patients with two implants continue to increase.[82-91] There are few prospective studies of children who receive two implants during early childhood, however.

Although the "era of bilateral implantation" has been introduced, there are few controlled trials to date.[92] Preliminary results reveal evidence of an expanded sound field and loudness summation, and some level of sound localization ability to most bilateral recipients. In a few patients, benefits attributable to effective squelch are noted. Such findings show central integration of electric stimulation from the two ears despite an absence of precise tonotopic matching of binaural inputs. Systems that enable integrated speech processing of inputs from the bilateral sound fields have yet to be introduced clinically. It is uncertain whether potential benefits of bilateral implantation could be expanded through such processing.

Language Development in Children

A primary goal of implantation in children is to assist comprehension and expression through the use of spoken language. Language is defined as a vehicle for shaping and relating abstractions for communication.[93] The meaning of language-mediated abstraction is independent of the immediate situation. Practical use of language is based on the assignment of a single name to various appearances and situations under varying conditions. Information exchange via spoken language involves a conversion of thought into speech. This conversion relies on mental representations of phonologic (sound) structure and syntactic (phrase) structure.

All fundamental models of language development propose that the acquisition of language is the result of progressive organization from an initially undifferentiated state. As incremental differentiation occurs, language skills become more sophisticated and hierarchically integrated. The child first must learn to form internal representations of acoustic speech patterns (Fig. 160-3). These experiences enable a child to identify consistent patterns in phonologic inputs and to develop associations between context and semantic and syntactic patterns. Through increased familiarity, these associations between spoken language and their actual counterparts build a child's semantic awareness.[94] Social cognition and emotional needs are likely to encourage such development, as supported by observations that infants become "tuned" to their language environment in the form of "perceptual maps" (Fig. 160-4),[95] and show protolinguistic behaviors with caretakers that are bidirectional.[96-98]

Early communication between infants and caregivers forms a critical foundation for development. This foundation provides a base on which cognition, affect, and social interaction may evolve.[99] If communication is hindered, development fails to proceed normally, with

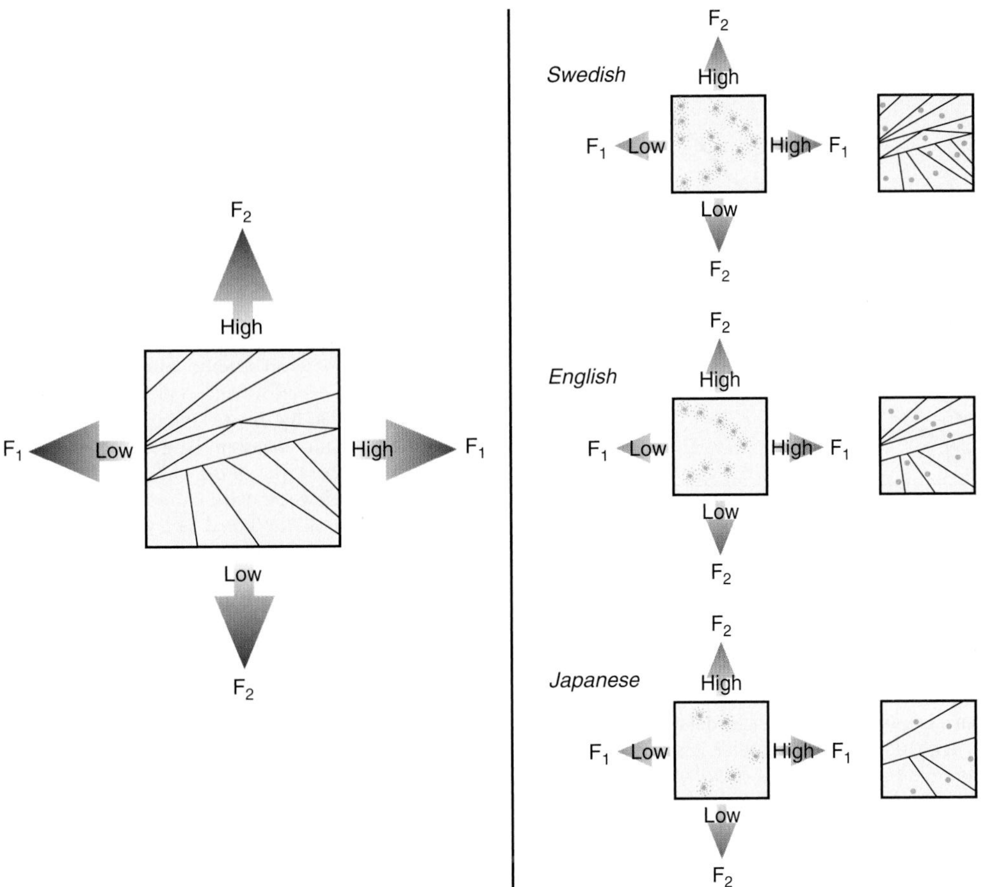

Figure 160-4. *Left,* Schematic figure shows natural auditory boundaries according to F_1 and F_2 formant frequencies. These boundaries are thought to provide a framework by which infants process incoming sound streams into gross categories. Intrinsic phonetic differences separate boundary regions from one another. *Right,* The ability to partition auditory input according to these boundaries is independent of linguistic experience, and is present throughout various languages. Examples of vowel processing in three different languages (Swedish, English, and Japanese) are shown. *(Adapted from Kuhl PK, Meitzoff A. Speech as an intermodal object of perception. In: Yonas A, ed. Perceptual Development in Infancy. Hillsdale, NJ: Lawrence Erlbaum Associates; 1988:235-266; and Kirk KI. Challenges in the clinical investigation of cochlear implant outcomes. In: Niparko JK, ed.* Cochlear Implants: Principles and Practices. *Philadelphia: Lippincott Williams & Wilkins; 2000:225-259.)*

detrimental sequelae in terms of cognitive, behavioral, and social development. Hearing loss and subsequent obstacles to communication threaten optimal development.[100-102] Because most children who have sensorineural hearing loss are born to hearing parents, a "mismatch" may exist between child and parent[103] that prevents effective communication.[104,105] Because sign language skills in hearing parents tend to be absent or basic, such children are at further risk for developmental delay.[106,107] Additional evidence confirms that children with sensorineural hearing loss who engage in linguistic interactions with their parents show age-appropriate cognitive, social, and behavioral development.[100] More recent theories suggest the processes linking language to cognition, affect, and behavior are dynamic and bidirectional, rather than discrete or independent.[108,109]

For successful bidirectional communication to occur within the family unit, language must be linked to cognition, affect, and behavior. Visual attention, which may be reliably assessed at 4 months of age, is crucial for guiding development.[99,110] Data suggest that visual attention is highly relevant to the development of emotional bonds to caregivers, language learning, and the processing of perceptual information.[111-114] In normal development, much of this early visual attention is actually directed by sound. Infants look longer in the direction of sound and longer at visual events whose temporal rhythms match what they hear.[115,116] When sound perception is impaired, visual and auditory integration is similarly disrupted, forcing a child with sensorineural hearing loss to rely on vision for communication and cues about when and where to direct attention.[117,118] This notion has been confirmed in studies of hearing-impaired children using computerized task performance measures.[117,119,120] These impairments have been found to contribute to behavioral problems.[120] By comparison, two studies found that children with cochlear implants perform better on this computerized task than children without cochlear implants.[117,119]

In addition to visual attention, other types of preverbal communication underlie the acquisition of verbal language. Substantial gains in prelinguistic behaviors, including eye contact and turn-taking,[121] and in verbal spontaneity[122] are observed as early correlates of implant benefit, developing within 6 months of implantation in young children.[123] Tait and associates[124] found that preverbal measures obtained 12 months after implantation are predictive of late performance on speech perception tasks. They observed a significant association between the preverbal measure of "autonomy" obtained before implantation and later speech perception performance. This latter finding has important theoretic implications for understanding of language development, and suggests that intervention that promotes autonomy in adult-child interaction may lead to improved outcomes. Such intervention can be introduced as soon as deafness is discovered.

Language Acquisition in Children with Cochlear Implants

By improving auditory access, cochlear implants augment sound and phrase structure. Although difficult to characterize, benefits in receptive language skills and language production after implantation are the crucial measure by which effectiveness of implants in young children should be assessed. One approach is to compare language performance on standardized tests. The Reynell Developmental Language Scale evaluates receptive and expressive skills independently.[125] These scales

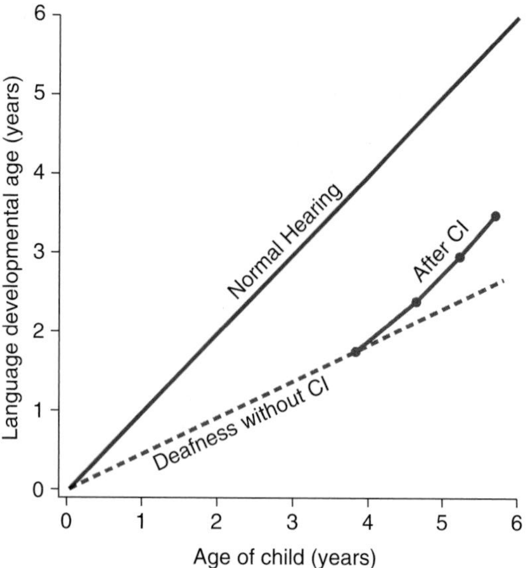

Figure 160-5. The effect of cochlear implantation (CI) in children on language development. *Solid line* depicts normal language development as it correlates to chronologic age. *Dashed line* shows the developmental delay that occurs in deafness before CI. After CI, language development progresses at the same rate as children with normal hearing. This suggests that language delay is a product of cumulative deficits acquired before CI, rather than from impaired progress after CI. *(Modified from Svirsky MA, Teoh SW, Neuburger H. Development of language and speech perception in congenitally, profoundly deaf children as a function of age at cochlear implantation.* Audiol Neurootol. *2004;9:224-233.)*

have been normalized on the basis of performance levels of hearing children in an age range of 1 to 8 years, and have been used extensively in populations of deaf children. Although deaf children without cochlear implants achieved language competence at half the rate of normal-hearing peers, implanted subjects exhibited language-learning rates that matched, on average, those of their normal-hearing peers.[125,126] In a study of 23 children who became deaf before 3 years of age, Svirsky and colleagues[126] studied language development after cochlear implantation. The average age of implantation in this cohort was approximately 4 years. These investigators found that speech development progressed at a decreased rate before implantation, but that after implantation, language development in implanted children was parallel to that of normal-hearing children (Fig. 160-5). The implication of this study is that differences in language delay between implanted and normal-hearing children could be explained by the initial period of deafness before implantation, rather than performance or progress after implantation. These findings also emphasize the importance of early implantation. Data are rapidly being gathered to confirm that earlier implantation might limit early language delays to enable more age-appropriate language acquisition.

Robbins and associates[125] noted that implantation improved language-learning rates for children in oral communication and total communication settings based on the Reynall Developmental Language Scale. Geers and coworkers,[55] also assessing language skills in implanted children enrolled in oral communication and total communication settings, found that the groups did not differ in language level, although the oral group showed significantly better intelligibility in their speech production.

Delays in receptive and expressive language among hearing-impaired children have consistently been documented in the literature, although such delays are not strongly related to degree of hearing loss.[127,128] Performance on language measures can be influenced by the child's mode of communication such that results may not directly reflect the influences of auditory perception or prosthetic intervention. Clinical findings support the hypothesis, however, that some deaf children are able to use the acoustic-phonetic cues provided by the implant in ways that may reduce the language gap between normal-hearing and deaf children.

Central nervous system processing is a primary determinant of the level of verbal language ultimately attained after cochlear implantation.[129] Pisoni[129] assessed performance in two groups of pediatric cochlear implant users: "Stars" were children whose phonetically balanced kindergarten scores placed them in the top 20%. The second group, children with scores in the bottom 20%, comprised the control group. Speech perception, spoken word recognition, speech intelligibility, and language level were compared between the two groups at preimplantation and at yearly postimplant intervals. Children in the "Stars" group did not score consistently better on all behavioral measures than children in the control group. Differences between the groups were manifest only on specific tests and task demands. Children with superior implant performance were consistently better on measures of speech perception (i.e., vowel and consonant recognition), spoken word recognition, comprehension, language development, and speech intelligibility than were the control children. The two groups did not differ, however, in their vocabulary knowledge, nonverbal intelligence, visuomotor integration, or visual attention. It was concluded that "Star performance" on measures of spoken language processing and speech intelligibility was not attributed to global differences in overall performance, but to differences specifically in the task of processing auditory information provided by the cochlear implant.

The authors also examined the differential performance on various behavioral tests of communicative ability administered after 1 year of cochlear implant use. Strength of correlation revealed a significant association between spoken word recognition, language development, and speech intelligibility for the "Stars" group, but not for the control group. "Star performance" seemed to result from an enhanced language processing ability and the development of phonologic and lexical representations.

The strong relationship between spoken word recognition and speech intelligibility for superior implant performers suggests that (1) a transfer of knowledge exists between speech perception and production, and (2) that speech perception and production share a common system of internal representation. According to Pisoni and Geers,[130] the exceptional performance of the "Stars" seems to be a result of their superior abilities to perceive, encode, and retrieve information about spoken words from lexical memory. They described the capacity for processing tasks that require the manipulation and transformation of the phonologic representations of spoken words as "working memory." Pisoni and Geers[130] then investigated the impact of working memory on measures of speech perception, speech intelligibility, language processing, and reading in implanted children with prelingual deafness. The investigators evaluated correlations between children's ability to recall lists of orally presented digits and their performance on these measures. The authors observed correlations between auditory memory and performance in each outcome area, suggesting that working memory plays an important role in mediating performance across these higher communication tasks.[130]

Promising clinical studies have generally supported wider application of cochlear implants in children. Childhood implant research has often relied, however, on case-series design, based in a single center that evaluated children who used different generations of implant technology. Few studies have examined the impact of cochlear implants on the "whole" child, particularly when one considers the importance of understanding longitudinal measures of cognitive, social, and behavioral development. There is also little information available on the perceived benefit of childhood implantation from a perspective of cost-effectiveness.

The need and significance of this information is underscored by the fact that clinical decisions to pursue early cochlear implantation are often prompted by parental choice. Parents of deaf children choose among options which have vastly different implications for the use of medical, (re)habilitative, educational, and other societal resources. A pressing issue concerns the validity of generalizing from early observations of benefit from cochlear implantation to the decision to implant younger children. Should very young infants identified with severe to profound sensorineural hearing loss undergo cochlear implantation within weeks of diagnosis?

An ongoing multicenter study is examining the clinical modifiers of postimplant developmental outcomes, including oral language acquisition, speech recognition skills, selective attention and problem-solving skills, behavioral and social development, parent-child interactions, and quality-of-life measures in children undergoing implantation in six U.S. implant centers.[131] It is hoped that a detailed assessment of communicative and psychosocial results will contribute to an understanding of the factors predicting implant-associated language use, communication competence in early childhood, and the perceived value of early cochlear implantation in light of associated costs. It is hoped that conclusions will enable an informed approach to implant candidacy when considering (re)habilitative strategies designed to enhance developmental learning in children with severe to profound sensorineural hearing loss.

Outcomes after Cochlear Implantation

Educational Placement and Support of Implanted Children

A hearing-impaired child is at substantial risk for educational underachievement.[132,133] Educational achievement by a hearing-impaired child can be enhanced by verbal communication. Traditional methods of speech instruction are more successful with children who have enough residual hearing to benefit from early devices of hearing rehabilitation.[134] Improved speech perception and production provided by cochlear implants offer the possibility of increased access to oral-based education and enhanced educational independence.

Francis[135] and Koch[136] and their colleagues tracked the educational progress of implanted children by using an educational resource matrix to map educational and rehabilitative resource use. The matrix was developed on the basis of observations that changes in classroom settings (e.g., into a mainstream classroom) are often compensated by an initial increase in interpreter and speech-language therapy. Follow-up of 35 school-aged children with implants indicated that, relative to age-matched hearing aid users with equivalent baseline hearing, implanted students are mainstreamed at a substantially higher rate, although this effect is not immediate, and requires rehabilitative support to be achieved. Within 5 years after implantation, the rate of full-time assignment to a mainstream classroom increases from 12% to 75% (Fig. 160-6).

Quality of Life and Cost-Effectiveness

Prior studies of the cost-utility of cochlear implants have assessed quality of life and health status to determine the utility gained from cochlear implants.[19,137,138] *Utility* is a concept that reflects the true value of a good or service. Cost-utility methods determine the ratio of monetary expenditure to change in utility as defined by a change in quality of life over a given period. The assessment of cost-utility is based on the following:

$$\text{Cost-utility} = \text{costs (in \$)/(quality-adjusted life-years)} = \text{costs (in \$)/(life-years} \times \text{health utility)}$$

Life-years is the mean anticipated number of years of implant experience based on a life-expectancy analysis of the participating cohort. The change in health utility reflects the difference between preimplant and postimplant scores on survey instruments that have been designed and validated to reflect quality of life. In the United States, England, and Canada, health interventions with a cost-utility ratio less than $20,000 (U.S.) are generally considered to represent acceptable value for money expended (i.e., they are "cost-effective").[139-141]

Quality-of-Life Studies in Adults and the Elderly

Costs per quality-adjusted life-year (QALY) for cochlear implants in adult users were determined using cost data that account for the preoperative, postoperative, and operative phases of cochlear implantation.[19,138] Benefits were determined on the basis of functional status and quality of life. The precise cost-utility results varied among studies, mostly because of methodologic differences in the determination of benefit, level of benefit obtained, and differences in costs associated with the intervention. Nonetheless, these appraisals consistently indicated that the multichannel cochlear implant in adult populations is associated with cost-utility ratios in the range of $14,000 to $18,000/QALY, indicating a highly favorable position in terms of cost-effectiveness (Table 160-1).

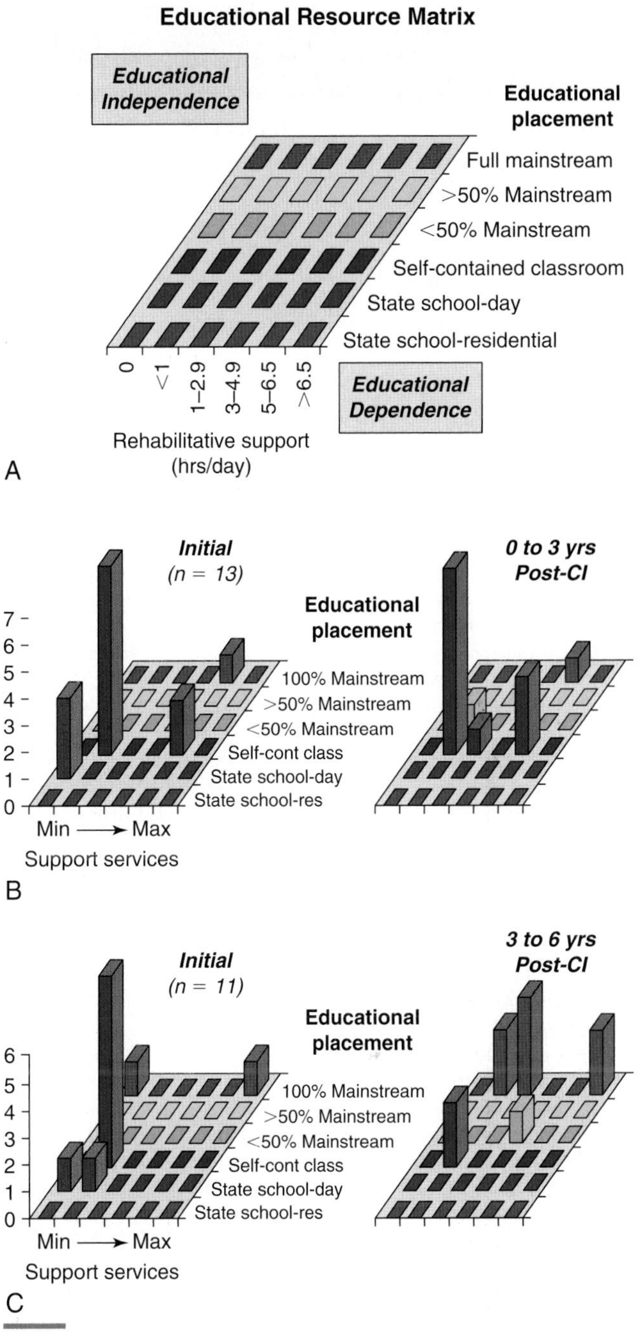

Figure 160-6. Matrix of educational resource usage by children with cochlear implantation (CI). **A,** The Educational Resource Matrix (ERM) plot classroom placement *(ordinate)* versus rehabilitative (speech-language and interpretive) support *(abscissa)*. **B,** Patterns of change in use of educational resources in a cohort of children within 3 years of CI. **C,** Patterns of change in use of educational resources in a cohort of children 3 to 6 years after CI. Note the higher levels of mainstreaming, and reduced use of support services with prolonged use of the cochlear implant. *(**A,** From Koch ME, Wyatt JR, Francis HW, Niparko JK. A model of educational resource use by children with cochlear implants.* Otolaryngol Head Neck Surg. *1997;117:174-179; **B,** from Francis HW, Koch ME, Wyatt JR, Niparko JK. Trends in educational placement and cost-benefit considerations in children with cochlear implants.* Arch Otolaryngol Head Neck Surg. *1999;125:499-505.)*

Table 160-1
Cost-Utility Ratio of Cochlear Implantation in Adults

Source; Year	Instrument	Country	No. Patients	Health Utility Gain	Cost-Utility Ratio, S/QALY
Palmer et al; 1999	HUI	U.S.	37	+0.20	14,670
Wyatt et al; 1996	HUI	U.S.	229	+0.204	15,928
Wyatt and Niparko; 1995	VAS—without*	U.S.	229	+0.304	9,000
Summerfield and Marshall; 1995	VAS—without*	United Kingdom	105	+0.41	7,405
Summerfield and Marshall; 1995	VAS—before†	United Kingdom	103	+0.23	13,200
Harris et al; 1995	QWB	U.S.	7	+0.072	31,711
Fugain et al; 1998	VAS	France	30	+0.22	6,848
Overall			**511**	**+0.26**	**12,787**

Meta-analysis of studies of cost-effectiveness of cochlear implantation in adults. The overall cost-utility ratio was calculated to be $12,787 per quality-adjusted life-years (QALYs). In the United States, England, and Canada, a threshold of $25,000/QALY or less is considered an acceptable cost-utility ratio for a given health intervention.

*Patient rating of health utility if cochlear implant were taken away.

†Patient rating of health utility before implantation.

HUI, Health Utilities Index; QWB, Quality of Well-Being Scale; VAS, Visual Analog Scale.

Hearing impairment is one of the most common clinical conditions affecting elderly individuals in the United States.[142] Hearing loss is so profound in 10% of elderly hearing-impaired individuals that little or no benefit is gained with conventional amplification.[143] Assessing the effectiveness of cochlear implants in elderly patients requires consideration of audiologic and psychosocial factors. The social isolation associated with acquired hearing loss in elderly individuals[144] is accompanied by a significant decline in quality of life and an increase in emotional handicap.[145] The rehabilitation of hearing loss is an important goal in this vulnerable population, providing functional and psychologic contributions to quality of life.

Age-related degeneration of the spiral ganglion[146,147] and progressive central auditory dysfunction[148,149] raise potential concerns about the efficacy of cochlear prostheses in the elderly. Comparable gains in speech understanding have been reported for elderly and younger groups of implant recipients,[150] but the implications of these functional gains on the quality of life of older adults have not been well characterized. The determination of auditory efficacy and quality of life is crucial to any cost-benefit analysis in elderly patients, and may help guide clinical resource allocation, particularly in light of the high costs associated with cochlear implantation as a nonlifesaving intervention.

Reports of quality of life gains in elderly patients with cochlear implants have been favorable,[151-153] but are based on questionnaires that are difficult to correlate with function and cost-utility. Francis and colleagues[151] evaluated 47 patients with multichannel cochlear implants, 50 to 80 years old, who completed the Ontario Health Utilities Index Mark 3 (HUI3) survey and a quality-of-life survey. This study assessed preimplantation and postimplantation (6 months and 1 year after implantation) responses to questions related to device use and quality of life. A significant mean gain occurred in health utility of 0.24 (SD 0.33) associated with cochlear implantation ($P < .0001$) (Fig. 160-7). Improvements in hearing and emotional health attributes were primarily responsible for this increase in health-related quality-of-life measure. A significant increase occurred in speech perception scores at 6 months after surgery ($P < .0001$ for Central Institute for the Deaf sentence and monosyllabic word tests), and there was a strong correlation between the magnitude of health utility gains and postoperative enhancement of speech perception ($r = 0.45$, $P < .05$). Speech perception gain was also correlated with improvements in emotional status and the hours of daily implant use. The authors concluded that cochlear implantation has a statistically significant and cost-effective impact on the quality of life of older deaf patients.

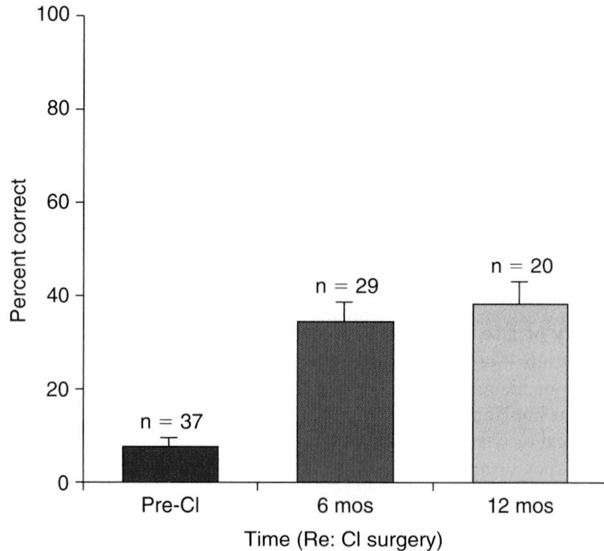

Figure 160-7. Mean monosyllabic word scores obtained in older adult subjects with postlingual hearing impairment just before cochlear implantation (CI) and at 6 and 12 months afterward (error bar = 1 SE). Monosyllabic word scores, which are generally considered one of the most difficult tests of speech perception, clearly increase during the first year after CI.

Quality-of-Life Studies in Children

Published cost-utility analyses of the cochlear implant in children have been limited by using either health utilities obtained from adult patients[19,139,154] or hypothetically estimated utilities of a deaf child.[155-158] These studies yielded cost-utility ratios that spread over a wide range ($3141 to $25,450/QALY). Utility assessments derived from adult patient surveys may not capture the impact of issues unique to childhood deafness.[33] To address this issue more rigorously, Cheng and coworkers[137] surveyed parents of a cohort of 78 children (average age 7.4 years, with 1.9 years of cochlear implant use) who received multichannel implants at the Johns Hopkins Hospital to determine direct and total cost to society per QALY. Parents of profoundly deaf children

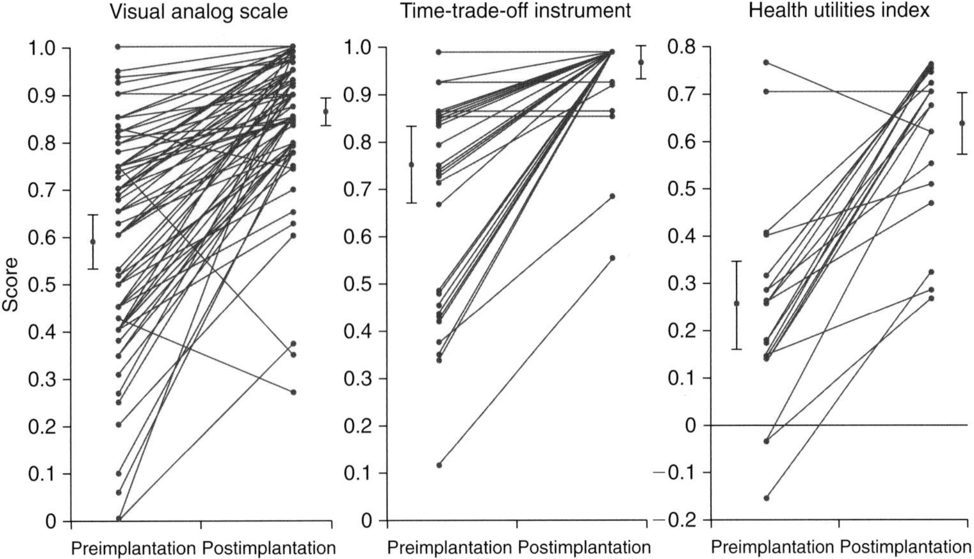

Figure 160-8. Retrospective health utility scores from parents of children with cochlear implants. Three different methods of assessing health utility scores are shown. The mean change in utility (postintervention—preintervention scores) was 0.27 for the visual analog scale, 0.22 for the time-trade-off instrument, and 0.39 for the health utilities index. The error bars on the side of each graph show mean scores with 95% confidence intervals.

($n = 48$) awaiting cochlear implantation served as a comparison group to assess the validity of recall. Using the Time-Trade-Off (TTO), Visual Analog Scale (VAS), and HUI3, parents rated their child's health state "now," "immediately before," and "1 year before" the cochlear implant. Mean VAS scores increased 0.27 on a scale of 0 to 1 (from 0.59 to 0.86), TTO scores increased 0.22 (from 0.75 to 0.97), and HUI scores increased 0.39 (from 0.25 to 0.64) (Fig. 160-8). Discounted direct medical costs were $60,228, yielding cost-utility ratios of $9029/QALY using the TTO, $7500/QALY using the VAS, and $5197/QALY using the HUI3. Including indirect costs, such as reduced educational expenses, the cochlear implant yielded a calculated net savings of $53,198 per child. Based on assessments of this cohort from a single center, childhood cochlear implantation produces a positive impact on quality of life at reasonable direct costs and results in societal savings.

The educational resource matrix used by Francis[135] and Koch[136] and their colleagues offers a basis for assessing overall cost-benefit ratios of the cochlear implant in children. Although educational costs for all implanted students remain static or initially increased, ultimate achievement of educational independence for most implanted children produces net savings that range from $30,000 to $100,000 per child, including the costs associated with initial cochlear implantation and postoperative rehabilitation. Language-related and education-related outcomes in children with cochlear implants have been supplemented with parental perspectives of quality-of-life effects to yield cost-utility ratings.[137,154] Despite conservative assumptions, results show that cochlear implantation is, relative to other medical and surgical interventions, highly cost-effective in profoundly hearing-impaired young children.

Auditory Rehabilitation after Cochlear Implantation

The uniqueness of the listening experience enabled by a cochlear implant is underscored by qualitative differences in how sound perception is elicited compared with other strategies of auditory rehabilitation. A hearing aid filters, amplifies, and compresses the acoustic signal, delivering a processed signal to the cochlea for transduction. In contrast, a cochlear implant receives, processes, and transmits acoustic information by generating electric fields. Electric hearing bypasses nonfunctional cochlear transducers by directly depolarizing auditory nerve fibers. Implant systems convey an electric code based in selected features of speech that are crucial to phoneme and word understanding in normal listeners, without the advantages of signal preparation provided by cochlear mechanisms of sound processing that render complex sounds listenable and discriminable. The listening experience with the cochlear implant also differs from normal audition in the timing of when that experience begins.

Either through a process of learning in the early, formative years in children, or by virtue of "auditory memory" in adults, capabilities for meaningful listening develop for most implant recipients. A central clinical question relates to the potential benefit to be derived from dedicated sensory training, commonly referred to as "auditory training." Can such training enable a cochlear implant user to apply latent skills and adaptive strategies to listening tasks that offset deprivation effects and the limitations of cochlear implant listening to capitalize on the device capabilities?

Exposure to conversational speech likely provides insight otherwise unavailable. Language learning may be too complex to be acquired using didactic methods alone. Consistent, frequent exposure may offer the greatest prospects of refining oral language skills. Through tracking the temporal, spectral, and intensity parameters of sound, the cochlear implant provides cues of voicing and articulation patterns that are not visually detectable. For deaf children who experience difficulty in developing their language skills, the possibilities afforded by early implantation, before the onset of changes consequent to deafferentation, seem to be substantial. The best method of achieving such outcomes are yet to be determined, however.

Efficacy of Auditory Training in Cochlear Implant Rehabilitation

Auditory training that provides real-world utility to restored audition in implant recipients is necessarily highly individualized. That is, the goals for a patient's auditory, speech, language, and cognitive development rely on a host of influences unique to the individual. Because of the need for such an individualized approach, studies of treatment efficacy of auditory training with high internal validity are difficult to construct. Carney and Moeller[159] noted that earlier efficacy studies target specific treatment areas of perceptual skill development, language development, speech production, academic performance, and social-emotional growth. Treatment goals within various treatment areas often vary, limiting the ability to assess the impact within any single category.

Prior studies have systematically assessed the development of speech perception with training in implant listeners. Watson[160] noted that studies of the perception of complex nonspeech sounds have shown that individual parts of spectral-temporal waveforms can become more salient through selective training. One consequence of training is that the same sound can be perceived quite differently, depending on earlier experience as it affects a listener's expectancy and the psychologic mindset brought to the task. The time course of learning to identify initially unfamiliar speech sounds by normal-hearing listeners extends through months, possibly even years, before reaching a stable level of performance. If implant users are required to learn to interpret sounds as unfamiliar to them as the nonspeech sounds used in research are to normal-hearing listeners, a similar lengthy experience may be required to reach a plateau of maximum performance. Why this has not been the case in some clinical studies is a puzzle.

Watson[160] offered an explanation in that speech perception may depend heavily on abilities other than sensory acuity or tonal resolution. Studies of individual differences in auditory temporal and spectral acuity have not shown strong correlations between individual differences in those abilities and individual differences in speech perception. It is argued that one way to interpret this observation is that differences in the ability to hear speech (as by two hearing-impaired listeners with the same audiogram) may be the result of differences in the way in which central pathways generate the ability to infer an original stimulus from its fragments.

Dawson and Clark[161] tested whether the ability to use place-coded vowel formant information would be subject to training effects in a group of congenitally deafened patients with limited speech perception ability. They investigated the relationship between electrode position difference limens and vowel recognition. Young subjects were assessed with synthesized versions of the words "hid," "head," "had," "hud," "hod," and "hood." Performance during a nontraining period was compared with the change in performance after 10 training sessions. Two of four subjects showed significant gains, and improvements were consistent with their electrode discrimination ability. Difference limens ranged from one to three electrodes for these patients, and for two other patients who showed minimal to no improvements. Minimal gains shown by one subject could be partly explained by poorer apical electrode position difference limen. The authors concluded that significant gains in vowel perception occurred after training, and suggested the need for children to continue prolonged aural rehabilitation for a period after implantation. Despite intensive efforts, minimal improvements can sometimes occur, however, and such limited success is not always accounted for by limitations at the level of the auditory periphery.

Svirsky and coworkers[162] examined two possible reasons underlying longitudinal improvements in vowel identification by cochlear implant users: improved labeling of vowel sounds and improved electrode discrimination. Improvements in vowel identification were attributed to improved labeling, suggesting cortical learning effects were responsible for the observed changes, as opposed to enhanced electrode discrimination.

Rehabilitation in Adults with Cochlear Implants

After implant activation, adult users must adjust to the novel signals transmitted by the speech processor. Recipients must learn to associate electrically elicited sound patterns with perceptions that were previously meaningful sound sensations. Rehabilitative needs differ in implant recipients depending on their auditory experience before the onset of deafness. For a prelinguistically deafened implant recipient, auditory and speech (articulation) training are crucial in facilitating communication change. For a postlinguistically deafened patient, auditory training often focuses on more complex listening skills—understanding speech in noise, telephone use, and music appreciation.[163]

Auditory Training in Children with Cochlear Implants

Programs of auditory training in children with implants are often organized with a hierarchic approach by which the child learns to associate meaning with unfamiliar and possibly unnatural sounds.[122,164] After showing awareness of sounds (detection), the child is taught to determine whether sounds are the same or different (discrimination), to recognize sounds and to associate meaning with them (identification), and to respond appropriately in verbal discourse (comprehension). Expressively, the child learns to imitate phonemes and syllables and to coarticulate these sounds to produce progressively more difficult words and phrases. Imitation or approximation of speech sounds and words is a strategy used for developing an "auditory feedback loop"—the interrelated function of perception of sound and production of speech. Functional use of spoken language depends on the child's ability to produce meaningful linguistic utterances spontaneously. This process begins with a single word and progresses through sequential stages to complex phrases and entire stories.[165] Boothroyd[166] stressed the need for flexibility in guidelines for therapy sessions, noting that "the structure needs to exist in the mind of the teacher, and not be so obvious in the activities done with the child."

Boothroyd and colleagues[167] provided a model of auditory development that highlights the time course of development and identifies component skills that are crucial to effective auditory perception in children. They defined auditory perception as the interpretation of sensory evidence that is derived from sound and is reflective of objects and events that caused the sound. Similar to other perceptual events, auditory perception involves not only sensory evidence, but also contextual evidence, prior knowledge, memory, attention, and processing skills. Auditory speech perception is special because the events to be perceived are those of language. Similarly, the listener's knowledge base and processing skills must include those related to language in general and to spoken language in particular.

The normal auditory system is complete and functional at birth, but myelination continues for several years in the higher auditory pathways. Correspondingly, infants display increasingly sophisticated discrimination and recognition ability. Psychoacoustic performance does not reach adult levels for several years, however. Infants at 6 months of age show the beginnings of phonemic classification. Their capacity of performance improves during childhood, including phonetic contrast perception, phoneme recognition, perception of speech in noise, selective attention, and the use of linguistic context. Because experience plays a key role in the development of the knowledge and skills required for auditory perception in general, and for auditory speech perception in particular, intensifying that experience in hearing loss and with prosthetic devices is theoretically attractive.

Boothroyd and colleagues[167] noted that it is tempting to assume that the sensory evidence available to a developing child is determined only by the functional integrity of the peripheral auditory system, independent of auditory experience. Basic science investigations document the influence of auditory experience on the organization of auditory pathways,[168] however, and observe that better organization through experience could increase the sensory evidence made available from patterns of neural excitation produced in the cochlea.

Cochlear implants provide profoundly deaf children with a level of hearing sensitivity that enables them to perceive most of the sounds of spoken language, even when presented at low levels of intensity. Rehabilitative practices are designed to build on this level of sound awareness. In the case of a child who developed an audition-based language system before the onset of deafness, the cochlear implant restores access to spoken language—in many cases with expanded phonemic access. In the case of children who have never heard or who lost their hearing before the establishment of spoken language, access to sound provided by the cochlear implant initially lacks meaningful associations.

Current cochlear implant technology also provides the potential for deaf children to make use of generalization and incidental learning. Benefits of "hearing" extend well beyond contexts of one-on-one repartees with predictable discourse. Age of onset, degree of hearing loss, and amplification history[47] determine the quantity and quality of auditory stimulation received before implantation and readiness to interpret acoustic information. A child experienced in using residual hearing from an early age through amplification is likely to adapt to the sounds provided by the implant more quickly than a child with limited experience in listening.[167] The close scrutiny afforded by regular interaction with an auditory training therapist allows for the early detection of either the need for device reprogramming or failure of components of the implant system.

Components of auditory training in children with cochlear implants are designed to foster the development of auditory and speech skills in a manner that simulates a hearing child's acquisition of spoken language, while addressing remedial needs that arise as a consequence of auditory deprivation during early development.[169] Rehabilitative strategies related to auditory, speech, and language skills should seek to achieve overall communicative competence.[50] Ideally, rehabilitative strategies do not teach specific, isolated auditory, speech, or language subskills. Because subskills are only a means to an end that is multimodal communicative competence, training in any one individual subskill should not be given too much weight. Programs are most effective when they take an integrated approach to rehabilitation and avoid rote, drill-oriented approaches.

Maintenance of the Device

An important role in developing auditory skills and using a cochlear implant successfully is maintenance of the device itself.[155,156] This maintenance includes keeping all external parts in good functioning order, and working with an audiologist who specializes in cochlear implants on a regularly scheduled basis for device programming. In most cochlear implant centers, the audiologist serves as the case manager for the patient during the cochlear implant candidacy process and postimplantation.

Programming the device requires software and hardware from the cochlear implant manufacturer. For an adult patient, programming the cochlear implant involves numerous perception judgments, such as threshold of hearing, loudness level, loudness balancing, and in some cases pitch ranking. The patient's hearing history can determine the ease or difficulty of these tasks. Other factors, such as tinnitus, can come into consideration when establishing threshold levels of hearing with an electric stimulus. These measurements are necessary to program a patient's dynamic range of hearing with the cochlear implant. These settings are individual and can vary from patient to patient. The program that is saved to the external components is referred to as the cochlear implant map. Changes in the stimulus levels are most frequently seen in the initial stages of activation of the device. Many appointments are involved in the activation process to keep up with the physiologic changes involved with an individual learning to hear with the electric input. Through time, the stimulus levels become more stable, and primarily fine-tuning adjustments are made. Little research is available to explain the physiologic changes that induce needed map changes. Anecdotal reports are available that also suggest various program changes are needed when the patient is undergoing hormonal changes, such as pregnancy, puberty, or menopause.

If the patient is unable to participate in the judgments needed to create a cochlear implant map, some objective measures may be used. Cochlear implant manufacturers have created software that can measure an electrically evoked compound action potential through the cochlear implant: Neural Response Telemetry (NRT), by the Cochlear Corporation of Englewood, Colorado (manufacturer of the N24 device), and Neural Response Imaging (NRI), by the Advanced Bionics Corporation of Sylmar, California (manufacturer of the Clarion/Hi-Res devices). NRT measures are found at levels between threshold and maximal comfort in an individual's map. Limitations exist when using these measurements.[170,171] Although direct nerve responses seem to have value in some populations, behavioral testing is the tried and true method of programming.

Another objective measurement that has been previously used in device programming is electric acoustic reflex thresholds. Studies have found that the electric acoustic reflex threshold highly correlates with comfort levels on a cochlear implant map.[172,173] These measurements are not present in all patients, however, so this option may not always be available. If the reflex is measurable, this can provide valuable information for the audiologist when programming a child. Some children have high tolerance levels for the electric stimulus and do not react negatively if the map is created using inappropriately high levels. If the cochlear implant program is too loud, it can prevent the child from developing auditory skills or responding appropriately.

Audiograms may also be used to check the validity of a cochlear implant map. Using the audiogram has limitations, however, when determining the integrity of a cochlear implant program. The audiogram is going to show the patient's responses to the perception of soft stimuli. It does not tell you, however, whether the program is at an appropriate comfort level, or whether the sound quality of the map is good. Most cochlear implant audiograms are in the 20- to 30-dB range. It is possible to have a good audiogram with inappropriate map settings in the external device. A strength of the audiogram is that it can flag equipment malfunction or gross changes needed in the cochlear implant settings.

Intensive follow-up is required for successful outcomes after cochlear implantation. The adult cochlear implant patient should have his or her external devices reprogrammed at least annually. Pediatric patients should, at a minimum, come on a biannual basis. Many children are seen more frequently than a twice a year if any questions arise on how their listening skills are developing, and to ensure that their devices are programmed appropriately. Regularly scheduled program checks also offer an opportunity for the audiologist to track the development of the patient's speech understanding scores using the MSTB protocol explained previously. Conducting speech perception measures at regular intervals can provide the cochlear implant audiologist or therapist with valuable information on what the patient is hearing and understanding. This information can be used to change the patient's map or as an indication of where to focus therapy goals. Also, if the patient reports a sudden change in performance, this change can be documented by showing a decrease in speech perception abilities. This documentation validates the patient's concerns and assists the audiologist and therapist to help return the patient to baseline functioning.

The cochlear implant should not be considered a "fix" for severe to profound hearing loss. This device requires intensive rehabilitation to use it effectively and requires regular follow-up and maintenance. Although the learning process with the cochlear implant seems complex and unpredictable, the cochlear implant can provide an opportunity for deaf individuals to hear sounds that would never be possible with conventional amplification. This is especially true for deaf children, who can use the cochlear implant as a tool for receptive and expressive oral speech abilities and, most importantly, language learning.

Educating Children with Cochlear Implants

Deaf education has long been concerned with the necessity of overcoming the devastating effect profound deafness has on language acquisition and on educational attainments. Normally hearing children come to education and the development of literacy and numeracy skills with language already acquired through the channel of hearing in interaction with their care providers. For children deaf from birth, this normal process is disrupted with consequent effects on language acquisition. Deaf education is concerned not only with the processes of educational attainments of literacy and numeracy, but also with the processes of linguistic development and how to overcome the problem of lack of hearing in the normal communicative development.

The two major questions that have challenged educators for years have been which communication method to use (oral or sign language), and where to educate children (in special or mainstream schools). Visual means of communication were promoted, with sign language being seen as the solution by some, and oral language using visual support of lip-reading and other clues as the way forward. In 1880, the Milan conference on deaf education promulgated the opinion that oral language was "superior" to that of sign language. This statement, at a time when there was little amplification available, began the predominance of oralism throughout the world, and a polarization of views between individuals who believed that all deaf children should communicate by spoken language alone, and individuals who believed that all deaf children should communicate by sign language.

Although the oral view was held strongly in the 19th century and first half of the 20th century, reports of poor linguistic and educational attainments and speech intelligibility of deaf children began to challenge it. The increasing voice of the deaf community, wanting recognition of its own language and culture, also began to be heard. Signed methods of communication were increasingly introduced to educational systems in many countries, often taking the form of total, or simultaneous, communication, where spoken language is used with signed support. This method does not use the grammar of sign language, however, and in the 1980s interest grew in the use of sign bilingualism, where the languages of the deaf community and the hearing community are used to varying degrees and emphases. In the United States, the term "bi-bi" is often used to describe bilingual and bicultural approaches. Although terminology may vary, communication approaches may be grouped into three broad categories:

- Oral/aural—spoken language alone
- Use of speech and sign simultaneously (total communication)
- Bilingualism

There are subcategories within each category; oral communication methods include natural oralism, the use of cued speech, and auditory verbal approaches. These subcategories make comparison of the effectiveness of differing communication choices complex, and make the appropriate communication choices challenging for parents.

Another major choice for parents pertains to the setting in which their deaf child should be educated. Historically, deaf children were educated in special schools for the deaf. These schools were often residential and in remote areas, requiring children to leave home and obtain their education away from their families. Large schools for the deaf were established in many countries in the 19th century, and deaf culture and language thrived in these institutions. During the second half of the 20th century, there was an increasing trend for children with any disability to be educated in mainstream schools with appropriate support. For deaf children, the development of more effective hearing aids and the provision of FM systems facilitated the greater possibility of participation in mainstream education.

The closure of many schools for the deaf has been a worldwide phenomenon, which may be seen by the deaf community as a threat to their culture and language. With more children in mainstream schools, a reduction in special schools may also mean greater difficulty in providing specialist educational support to deaf children, and greater difficulty in accessing individuals working with deaf children in mainstream schools for continuing professional development and attaining the knowledge and expertise they need.

The options for educational placement today are the following:

- A school for the deaf (residential or day)
- A unit or resource base in a mainstream school (with varying degrees of integration into the mainstream school)
- A mainstream school (with varying degrees of support in quality and quantity)

These situations are not mutually exclusive, but overlap to a large degree, with wide variations in practice, particularly in degree of support. This overlap makes comparisons about educational independence in varying educational settings complex, and comparing the effectiveness of differing educational settings complex. Francis and colleagues[135] produced a useful matrix of educational resource use, illustrating the continuum of support; a child in a mainstream school with full-time support in class may have less educational independence than a child in a class of 10 in a special school.

Historically, the education of deaf children has been the subject of great controversy, often fed by rhetoric rather than fact, and with few data about the comparative efficacy of various alternatives, or information about making such important choices for parents. Into this already controversial area, the advent of cochlear implantation has added another dimension.

Advent of Cochlear Implantation

The advent of cochlear implantation was hoped to ameliorate the educational challenges produced by profound deafness.[80] In providing useful hearing across the speech frequencies, cochlear implantation facilitates the development of early communication skills and spoken language through interaction with care providers. Early reports of encouraging levels of spoken language perception and production led many authors to predict that mainstream education would be the likelihood for most profoundly deaf children. The success of cochlear implantation has often been measured in terms of access to mainstream education, not least because it has been seen as a means of measuring cost-benefit from cochlear implantation.[135,154] Children with implants are attending mainstream schools in greater numbers after implantation,[174] and this has been thought to be associated with potential savings in educational costs.[154]

What are the needs of children with implants, and are they different from the needs of users of traditional hearing aids? Children with implants need the implant system working well and worn consistently, good listening conditions, and good communication opportunities. These needs are not so different from the needs of hearing aid wearers. What cochlear implants have done is enable profoundly deaf children to function as moderately deaf—and many with a unilateral loss, despite the trend to bilateral implantation. Cochlear implants provide useful hearing to enable profoundly deaf children to acquire language through hearing,[169] to hear all the grammatical features of speech, and to develop wholly intelligible speech. Cochlear implants require complex technology, which requires a surgical procedure and long-term maintenance. How to ensure that children with implants obtain the maximum benefit from this technology remains a challenge.

It has long been recognized that the long-term management of deaf children with implants is in the hands of educators, and there is a major need for educators responsible for the children on a daily basis to have training and regular updates on this complex technology and the expectations they can have. In a survey of parents, community-based implant professionals, and implant professionals in Europe,[175] the most common thread in the responses was the need for long-term support in education for the implant system and for educational services to become more flexible in meeting the needs of this growing group of children. Parents expressed great frustration that their children did not receive the support they needed particularly as they went to secondary or high school, and frustration that there were not greater links between the implant centers and the local educational services. A survey of European teachers of the deaf showed that they were highly interested in receiving information and training about cochlear implants.[176]

To be successful in mainstream education, it must be ensured that the classroom situation is appropriate, with good acoustics, and that the technology is successfully managed, with high expectations of its use. We know the educational implications of a unilateral or moderate hearing loss in the busy mainstream classroom environment[177,178]; children would mishear or misunderstand in noise and not follow the fast-moving discourse around the classroom. For some children, implants may work too well: their speech intelligibility may be such that they appear as normally hearing children, and their needs may be overlooked, and for the children themselves it is difficult to articulate their needs. In such situations, misunderstandings would continue, and children would be unlikely to realize their academic potential. For other children, the implant may not have provided the outcomes expected; the range of outcomes from implantation is large. For these children, an auditory processing disorder or a language learning difficulty may be present, which affects the development of spoken language. The educational needs of these children may not be met in mainstream provision, as had been predicted.

Educational Outcomes

With regard to these educational decisions that parents make for their children, there is evidence that cochlear implantation has had an influence. More children with cochlear implants are going to mainstream schools than to schools for the deaf compared with a group of profoundly deaf children with hearing aids of the same age.[174] These were children 5 to 7 years old; Thoutenhoofd[179] did not find such a trend long-term toward mainstream placement, and there is anecdotal evidence that children with implants are findin g challenges in managing in the secondary or high school environment. Geers and colleagues[180] also found a trend toward mainstream education, but again this was in children at the primary stage.

With regard to communication mode and choices of communication after implantation, there is varying evidence of the influence of oral and signing environments. On the whole, the trend is to support the use of oral input,[180] but the context in which this is best provided in the long-term is still debated, and the situation is complex. Archbold and colleagues[181] showed that the outcomes in terms of speech perception and production 3 years after implantation were not different in children who had begun with some form of signed input and changed to oral, and children who had used oral communication only. Further study showed that children implanted before age 3 change from using signed communication to oral communication,[182] and children implanted at a younger age change communication mode faster.[68] There is evidence that although young people with implants develop intelligible spoken language, they also value the use of sign language, or signed support.[183] If children are to develop spoken language, however, they need to be in an educational environment that values it and promotes its use.

With regard to educational attainments, Stacey and coworkers[184] and Thoutenhoofd[179] showed that children with cochlear implants had improved educational attainments compared with children with hearing aids. Increasing evidence is showing that children with implants have better reading skills than comparative groups with hearing aids,[185] and that children implanted younger are continuing to read at improved rates.[186] In providing access to the grammatical features of spoken language through hearing, cochlear implants have enabled profoundly deaf children to have a greater awareness than previously of the phonology of language before coming to the written word. Spencer and Marschark[187] stated, "Spoken language development of deaf children may be more possible today than ever before. We are poised on a threshold of what often seem like unlimited possibilities." This statement reflects the ways in which new hearing technologies, and cochlear implantation in particular, have transformed educational opportunities for deaf children.

SUGGESTED READINGS

Cheng AK, Rubin HR, Powe NR, et al. Cost-utility analysis of the cochlear implant in children. *JAMA*. 2000;284:850-856.

Francis HW, Buchman CA, Visaya JM, et al. Surgical factors in pediatric cochlear implantation and their early effects on electrode activation and functional outcomes. *Otol Neurotol*. 2008;29:502-508.

Limb CJ. Cochlear implant-mediated perception of music. *Curr Opin Otolaryngol Head Neck Surg*. 2006;14:337-340.

Lin FR, Wang NY, Fink NE, et al. Assessing the use of speech and language measures in relation to parental perceptions of development after early cochlear implantation. *Otol Neurotol*. 2008;29:208-213.

Rubinstein JT. Paediatric cochlear implantation: prosthetic hearing and language development. *Lancet*. 2002;360:483-485.

Wilson B, Dorman M. Cochlear implants: a remarkable past and a brilliant future. *Hearing Res*. 2008;242:3-21.

For complete list of references log onto www.expertconsult.com.

CHAPTER ONE HUNDRED AND SIXTY-ONE

Central Neural Auditory Prosthesis

Robert J. S. Briggs

Key Points

- The concept of auditory brainstem implantation was introduced in 1979 by House and Hitselberger at the House Ear Institute.
- The biocompatibility of direct electric stimulation of the auditory brainstem has been shown in experimental preparations and clinical experience. The electric threshold for tissue damage, relating most specifically to charge density, is typically orders of magnitude greater than the threshold for activating the auditory pathway.
- The auditory brainstem implant (ABI) is now established as an effective method of partial hearing restoration in patients with neurofibromatosis type 2 (NF2). The ABI can provide environmental sound awareness and an aid to lip reading; however, open set speech perception is achieved only rarely.
- The most common indication for ABI is in patients with NF2. The current criteria for use in the United States are NF2 patients 12 years old or older, undergoing first or second side vestibular schwannoma removal. There are no specific audiologic criteria.
- The ABI consists of a multielectrode surface array that is placed over the cochlear nucleus within the lateral recess of the fourth ventricle. Intraoperative electrically evoked auditory brainstem responses are measured to confirm and refine correct position.
- Although some pitch differentiation is achieved between electrodes on the surface array, the tonotopic orientation of cochlear nucleus neurons is unfavorable for surface stimulation. Electric stimulation from individual electrodes may activate a broad area of neurons; in addition, adjacent electrodes may activate overlapping regions of neurons, so provision of independent spectral information by electric stimulation is very limited. The cochlear nucleus comprises a variety of specialized neurons with extrinsic and intrinsic projections that are either excitatory or inhibitory in function. In addition to losing the degree of peripheral tonotopic stimulation achieved with a cochlear implant, direct stimulation of the cochlear nucleus with an ABI may mean loss of specialized neural function within the cochlear nucleus.
- Because the tonotopicity of the cochlear nucleus is not adequately accessed with a surface electrode, it is proposed that a penetrating array might allow more selective tonotopic stimulation of the cochlear nucleus. A clinical trial has been undertaken at House Ear Institute, with 10 NF2 patients implanted with a prototype penetrating ABI in combination with a surface array. The outcomes are not proving any better than the surface electrode ABI, in terms of the reliability of achieving auditory sensations or of the speech perception levels achieved. In the cases where the penetrating ABI provided little benefit, the surface electrode array was successful in providing auditory benefit.
- The inferior colliculus is an obligatory synaptic terminus in the ascending auditory system. The central nucleus of the inferior colliculus also has a clearly defined tonotopic map, and so has been proposed as an alternative site for stimulation with a penetrating electrode. Clinical trials with a prototype auditory midbrain implant electrode are currently under way.
- Improved speech perception outcomes have been shown in ABI recipients without NF2—patients with cochlear nerve avulsion or injury or cochlear ossification who cannot benefit from a cochlear implant. These improved outcomes have led to the hope that children with cochlear nerve aplasia, who are unsuitable for cochlear implants, might benefit from ABI.

Multichannel cochlear implantation is now well established as an extremely effective method of hearing restoration for congenital and acquired sensorineural hearing loss. When conditions involving the cochlear nerve make peripheral intracochlear stimulation ineffective, some patients cannot benefit from cochlear implantation. Most commonly, this situation occurs in patients with neurofibromatosis type 2 (NF2), where bilateral vestibular schwannoma growth or surgical removal results in loss of cochlear nerve function. In this situation, direct electric stimulation of the cochlear nucleus at the brainstem using an auditory brainstem implant (ABI) is possible. Although the hearing outcomes with ABIs are limited compared with cochlear implants, the ABI is currently the most sophisticated and successful central neural prosthesis.

There is now a large experience with the use of ABIs in NF2 patients. Although some auditory benefit is usually achieved, it is generally limited to perception of environmental sound and an aid to lip reading. Rarely, open set speech understanding is achieved.

More recently, there has been increased interest in the use of ABIs for conditions where cochlear implants are ineffective, in particular, postmeningitic cochlear ossification or bilateral eighth cranial nerve injury from temporal bone fractures or avulsion. Better hearing outcomes have been observed in these patients without NF2, suggesting that NF2 is associated with intrinsic dysfunction of the cochlear nucleus. This suggestion has led investigators to attempt stimulation higher up the auditory pathway at the inferior colliculus with auditory midbrain implants (AMIs). The improved performance with ABIs in patients without NF2 has also provided hope that children with cochlear aplasia, who are unsuitable for cochlear implants, might benefit from ABIs.

Biocompatibility

Direct stimulation of the central nervous system entails unique safety concerns. The mechanisms of tissue damage resulting from the direct injection of current into brain parenchyma have been extensively studied.[1-3] Charge transfer from an electrode to biologic tissue depends on two independent electrochemical mechanisms, as follows:

1. The first mechanism is a simple capacitive mechanism of current that flows when a relatively high dielectric boundary exists between electrode and tissue. When an alternate voltage is created across the interface, charges accumulate differentially on each side of the dielectric boundary, alternating in polarity as dictated by the stimulus. Charging and discharging on either side of the dielectric boundary induces current flow in the biologic medium *without* the direct transfer of the carriers of the charge between electrode and tissue.

2. A second mechanism is one without a dielectric boundary. Charge carriers transfer between electrode and tissue as a result of reduction-oxidation reactions. Reversible reactions are confined to the electrode-tissue interface. Irreversible reactions generate new chemical species, however, which migrate into the tissue and may cause damage.

Safety thresholds of neuroprosthetic stimulation depend on several factors. Yuen and colleagues[4] have shown that the extent of neural injury with contemporary electroprosthetic materials producing direct stimulation closely correlates with the *charge density per phase*. Charge density directly relates to stimulation intensity, stimulation duration, and the effective area of the electrode terminus. The effective area of an electroprosthesis can differ from its geometric area. Brummer and Turner[5] measured the real surface area and suggested that surface roughness factors would range from 1.4 to 30.

The threshold for damage to the cerebral cortex found by Agnew and associates[6] was 320 μA, with a corresponding charge density of 3200 μcoul/cm^2/phase. Niparko and colleagues[7] found that the threshold for tissue damage within the cochlear nucleus (with a penetrating electrode) was 150 μA, a current that corresponded with a charge density of 600 μcoul/cm^2/phase. Stimulation at intensities of 150 μA and 200 μA (approximately 600 μcoul/cm^2/phase and 800 μcoul/cm^2/phase) produced significant tissue response at the site of the electrode terminus with neuronal loss, fiber necrosis, and reactive cells present. The injury threshold was found to exceed the threshold for functional activation, however, by a factor of at least five across all animals studied.

Differences between the damage thresholds determined across studies of central nervous system stimulators may relate to differences in implantation sites and variance in calculations that relate to effective versus geometric surface area. Differences also may be attributable to differences in microelectrode design (e.g., percentage of iridium) and fabrication that affect real charge densities at the electrode terminus for the same stimulation intensities.

History of Clinical Approaches

The concept of auditory brainstem implantation was introduced by House and Hitselberger at the House Ear Institute (HEI, Los Angeles, CA). In 1979, they implanted a two-ball electrode in a woman with NF2 undergoing acoustic neuroma removal. This first ABI was stimulated with a modified hearing aid, and the patient received useful auditory sensations.[8] Nonauditory stimulus occurred, which limited use of the electrode. Subsequently, this original electrode was replaced with a specially designed two-electrode surface array, which used a Dacron mesh carrier. This electrode was attached to a percutaneous pedestal connector and was stimulated by a modified 3M-House cochlear implant speech processor. This patient has continued to achieve acoustic percepts with electric stimulation, and has continued to use the device successfully 10 to 12 hours a day.[9] Between 1984 and 1992, 24 NF2 patients were implanted at HEI, with the single-channel, initially two-electrode, and subsequently three-electrode, ABI under an investigational device exemption from the U.S. Food and Drug Administration (FDA).

The first fully implantable ABI was manufactured by Cochlear Pty Ltd, based on the CI 22 mini–cochlear implant. The electrode array was modified to an eight-electrode pad, developed by HEI in collaboration with Cochlear Ltd and Huntington Medical Research Institute (Pasadena, CA). After initial trials at HEI, a multicenter clinical trial, based in North America, was undertaken. In Europe, a 21-electrode array was also developed by Cochlear Ltd and used with the same receiver stimulator.[10-13] Clinical experience from these trials led to the best features of both electrode arrays being combined to create the current Nucleus ABI electrode, a 21-electrode array connected to the CI 24M receiver stimulator (Fig. 161-1). The system functions similar to a cochlear implant with a fully implantable receiver stimulator package and an externally worn speech processor and transmitting coil. The receiver stimulator package has a removable magnet because

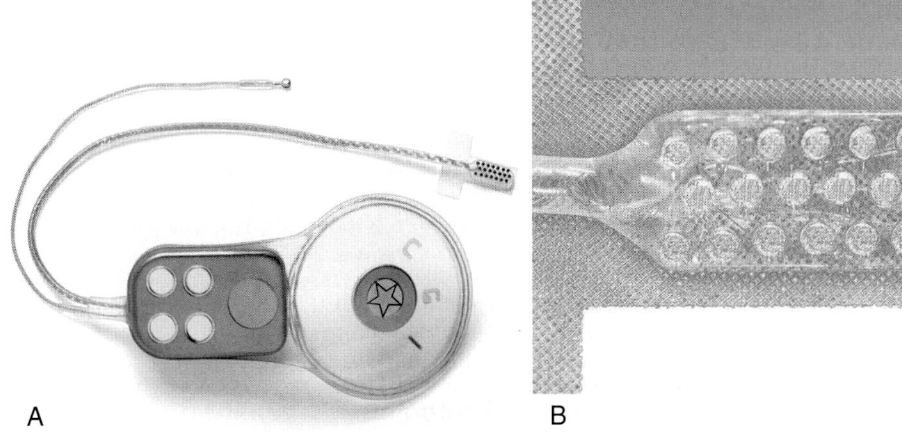

Figure 161-1. The current auditory brainstem implant (ABI) is a 21-electrode array that is stimulated similar to a cochlear implant through a transcutaneous radiofrequency transmitter and receiver. **A,** Internal component of ABI. **B,** Enlarged view of electrode array. *(Courtesy of Cochlear Ltd.)*

many recipients require repeated postoperative cranial magnetic resonance imaging examinations.

ABIs have also been produced by Med El in Europe and Advanced Bionics in the United States. The function of all these devices is the same as a cochlear implant with variation only in the size of the electrode pad and number of electrode contacts.

The Nucleus 24 ABI is the multichannel 21-electrode surface array, which remains commercially available with FDA and CME approval. Studies have been undertaken at HEI with a penetrating electrode array with limited success. The most recent development is the use of an AMI, in an attempt at inferior colliculus stimulation, either with a surface array or with a penetrating electrode.

With respect to biocompatibility, there is no clinical evidence for neuronal injury occurring as a result of chronic electric stimulation, as evidenced by the demonstrated gradual improved performance over time.

Indications

The most common indication for an ABI is in patients with NF2. In the United States, the ABI is approved only for use in NF2 patients. The current criteria for use in the United States are postlingual NF2 patients 12 years old or older, undergoing first or second side vestibular schwannoma removal. There are no specific audiologic criteria.

Auditory brainstem implantation should be considered in all NF2 patients undergoing vestibular schwannoma removal, in whom there is no expectation of ipsilateral residual hearing. ABIs are indicated particularly if contralateral hearing is absent or poor, or if there is a contralateral tumor that is likely to result in hearing loss in the foreseeable future.

Usually, the ABI is placed at the time of second side vestibular schwannoma removal, when the patient either has a preoperative profound-to-total hearing loss or will have one postoperatively. Some patients choose to have an ABI placed at the time of first side tumor removal (if hearing preservation is not attempted), as a so-called sleeper, in the expectation that the patients will not use the device while they have useful residual hearing in the contralateral ear.

An ABI can be successfully placed as a second-stage procedure after previous vestibular schwannoma surgery. There may be an advantage in delayed implantation if, at the first surgery, there is a large tumor deforming the brainstem and distorting the lateral recess anatomy and position. There is potential, however, for fibrosis and loss of brainstem landmarks occurring after initial tumor surgery that would make placement of the ABI difficult at a second procedure. Prior stereotactic radiotherapy, particularly by gamma knife, is a relative contraindication to ABI placement because of the potential for radiation necrosis of the cochlear nucleus region or fibrous tissue preventing proper device placement. There have been reports where this has been a problem, and where successful ABI use after radiotherapy was achieved.[14,15] The use of ABIs in patients without NF2 is discussed later in this chapter.

Anatomy and Surgical Approaches

Much of the early ABI research focused on gaining a better understanding of the three-dimensional anatomy of the cochlear nerve root, foramen of Luschka, and cochlear nucleus, and potential surgical approaches.[16-23] The cochlear nucleus comprises ventral and dorsal components, situated in the pons where the eighth cranial nerve enters the brainstem at the pontomedullary junction, medial to the cerebellar peduncle. The surfaces of the ventral and dorsal cochlear nuclei are exposed in the anterosuperior aspect of the lateral recess of the fourth ventricle. The ABI electrode is placed into this recess. The foramen of Luschka is the lateral opening of the recess and contains choroid plexus.

The surface landmarks for the lateral recess are the adjacent lower cranial nerves. The foramen of Luschka is situated immediately posterior to the origin of the ninth glossopharyngeal and tenth vagal nerve rootlets, inferior to the eighth nerve root entry zone and posteroinferior to the seventh nerve origin. The flocculus of the cerebellum overlies the foramen. The recess runs in a posteromedial direction from the foramen of Luschka to enter the fourth ventricle.

The translabyrinthine approach has been favored by most surgeons for ABI placement in NF2 patients undergoing tumor removal.[10] Some centers have used a retrosigmoid approach for recipients with NF2 and without NF2.[24] The translabyrinthine approach provides a more lateral view of the brainstem and better view into the foramen of Luschka. Possibly this better view assists in atraumatic electrode array placement; however, translabyrinthine and retrosigmoid approaches can be used effectively. Cerebellar retraction is reduced or avoided by the translabyrinthine approach. If a retrosigmoid or lateral suboccipital approach is used, it is important that the exposure is made as far forward and inferiorly as possible, skeletonizing and retracting the sigmoid sinus anteriorly, to allow a low anterior approach to give the most direct access to the region of the foramen, with the least cerebellar retraction.

The cochlear nucleus is identified within the lateral recess of the fourth ventricle. The cochlear nucleus is identified by following the eighth and ninth cranial nerves medially. The flocculus is retracted posteriorly, and the foramen of Luschka is identified, immediately posterior to the origin of the ninth cranial nerve. The cochlear nerve is followed medially, as it enters the lateral recess of the fourth ventricle. Dissection is carried between the eighth cranial nerve and the choroid plexus, which may need to be removed or shrunk with bipolar cautery. Within the lateral recess, as the cochlear nerve is followed medially, two prominent structures can be visualized anterosuperiorly curving around the brainstem caudally to the pontobulbar sulcus. The cranial structure is the bulging of the cochlear nucleus, and the caudal structure is the pontobulbar body. Between them, a small straight vein is a constant finding and important landmark. The taenia of the choroid plexus is a fibrous band at the entrance of the fourth ventricle. This band usually needs to be divided to allow visualization within the lateral recess and create room for the electrode array insertion. The location of the lateral recess usually can be confirmed by observing flow of cerebrospinal fluid as the anesthesiologist induces a Valsalva maneuver in the patient.

Positioning the electrode array within the lateral recess is crucial to successful auditory stimulation. If the array is too lateral, stimulation of the glossopharyngeal and facial nerves or other lower cranial nerves and cerebellar flocculus can occur. If the array is too deep, the medial electrode contacts would lie within the fourth ventricle and be ineffective. Similarly, caudal or cranial rotation of the electrode array can significantly affect position over the cochlear nucleus. Figure 161-2 shows a schematic representation of the electrode array position.

Intraoperative Monitoring

Successful positioning of the electrode array and final adjustment of position is confirmed by the use of intraoperative electric evoked auditory brainstem response (ABR) testing. The technique of intraoperative recording of short latency auditory potentials induced by electric stimulation of the cochlear nucleus was developed by Waring[25] at HEI. When the electrode array is initially positioned within the lateral recess using anatomic landmarks, electrodes within the array are stimulated, and the evoked ABR response is recorded. Initially, stimulation is performed across the entire length of the electrode array. If a response is achieved, a selection of distal, proximal, and lateral electrode combinations is used in forward and reserve polarity to differentiate stimulus artifact from real response. Presence or absence of response at different electrode combinations allows careful manipulation of the electrode array, such as deeper insertion or caudal or cranial rotation, to identify optimal position and improve the ABR responses.

Typically, either two or three wave responses are seen, as shown in Figure 161-3. The electric evoked ABR response waves are of short latency (0.7 to 3.6 ms). If large late potentials greater than 4 ms are observed, this is usually an indication of motor cranial nerve stimulation. While electric evoked ABR testing is undertaken, monitoring of cranial nerves V, VII, and IX should be continued. This monitoring helps identify inadvertent nonauditory stimulation, and may assist electrode positioning further.

Outcomes

Complications

Because the ABI is usually placed at the time of vestibular schwannoma removal, the occurrence of postoperative problems, including bleeding

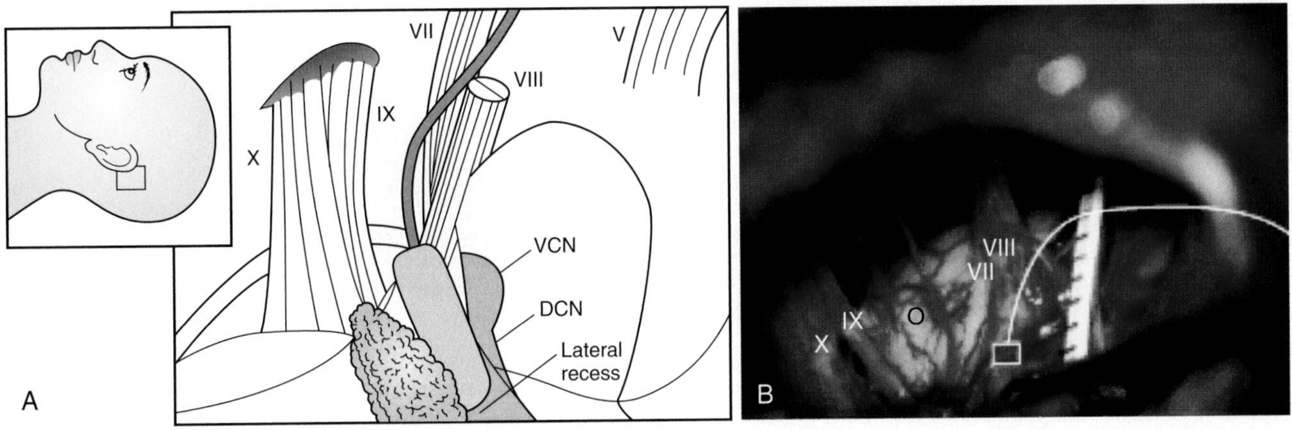

Figure 161-2. The region for placement of the auditory brainstem implant (ABI). **A,** Schematic of the left brainstem. The ABI electrode pad is being placed in the lateral recess. DCN, dorsal cochlear nucleus; VCN, ventral cochlear nucleus; V, trigeminal nerve; VII, facial nerve; VIII, cochleovestibular nerve (cut); IX, glossopharyngeal nerve; X, vagus nerve. **B,** Photograph of the left brainstem and cochlear nucleus region as seen from the lateral suboccipital approach. *Rectangle* indicates position of electrode array. O, inferior olive; VII, facial nerve; VIII, cochleovestibular nerve; IX, glossopharyngeal nerve; X, vagus nerve.

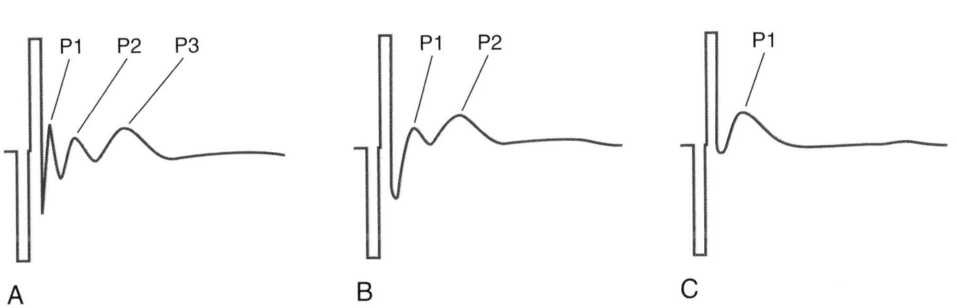

Figure 161-3. Idealized evoked auditory brainstem responses produced by electric stimulation of the cochlear nucleus. **A,** Three-wave response. **B,** Two-wave response. **C,** One-wave response.

and cranial nerve deficit, particularly facial nerve and cerebellar dysfunction, is generally attributed to the tumor removal and not specifically to the ABI placement. Similarly, postoperative cerebrospinal fluid fistula is well recognized after vestibular schwannoma surgery, and it is not thought that the presence of the electrode cable or subcutaneous receiver stimulator increases this risk. Cerebrospinal fluid fistula through the wound and the attendant risk of infection in the presence of the ABI is a potentially disastrous problem, however. As with cochlear implants, meticulous care must be taken with planning of incisions and placement of the receiver stimulator package to avoid problems with wound breakdown and infection. There have been anecdotal reports of hydrocephalus after surgery and ABI placement, possibly resulting from obstruction of cerebrospinal fluid flow through the lateral recess of the fourth ventricle by the electrode array position.

For patients without NF2, in whom there is no indication for surgery to remove a tumor, the potential risks of a craniotomy, cerebellar retraction, brainstem and lower cranial nerve manipulation, and electrode placement all need to be weighed against the potential hearing benefit with the ABI.

Long-term follow-up of ABI recipients, particularly the initial multicenter clinical trial subjects, has involved extensive neurologic examination, and no changes in neurologic status have been identified that seem to be related to the ABI electrode and electric stimulation. Probably the most specific ABI complication is the failure to achieve auditory stimulation and sensation. The normal anatomy of the fourth ventricle lateral recess allows the electrode array with its Dacron mesh backing to be held securely. Displacement of the electrode array can occur, however. This displacement is more likely when there has been distortion of the brainstem by a large tumor. The foramen of Luschka and lateral recess is often widely effaced, and so secure positioning of the array is difficult. Despite packing with fat or oxidized cellulose (Surgicel), migration of the array may occur in the early postoperative period. If there is absence of auditory perception on electrode stimulation, nonauditory stimulation, particularly of the facial, trigeminal, or lower cranial nerves, is more likely.

Even with accurate stable electrode positioning within the lateral recess, there is a high incidence of nonauditory or somatic sensations occurring with stimulation of at least some electrodes across the array. Otto and coworkers[26] reported results from a multicenter study in which 42% of all electrodes resulted in noticeable nonauditory sensations. The most commonly reported nonauditory sensations are ipsilateral facial tingling or throat discomfort or sensation of jittering of the visual field. Less commonly, discomfort or tingling occurs in the limbs or trunk, either ipsilateral or contralateral. Only rarely are motor responses (muscle twitch) in the arm or leg reported; and cardiorespiratory changes have been reported very rarely with electrode stimulation.

It is presumed that nonauditory sensation occurs from stimulation of adjacent anatomic structures, in particular (1) cerebellar flocculus (visual jitter), (2) facial nerve, (3) glossopharyngeal nerve (throat discomfort), and (4) retrograde activation of cerebellar peduncle (ipsilateral tingling and motor activation). Usually, the nonauditory sensation occurs together with an auditory percept, on a particular electrode or pair of electrodes. The nonauditory effect can usually be reduced or eliminated by increasing the pulse width of stimulus, referencing the electrode to a different stimulation ground, or turning off that electrode.[12] It has been observed that there is a decrease in nonauditory sensations over time. Possibly this decrease is due to fibrous encapsulation of the electrode array or, perhaps, alteration of brainstem shape after removal of a compressive tumor.

Auditory Performance

The auditory performance achieved with the ABI in NF2 patients has been very encouraging with similar outcomes reported from different centers and patient groups. Although useful auditory perception is usually achieved, the hearing level does not compare with that of current cochlear implant recipients. When auditory sensations are achieved with the ABI, the hearing has generally been limited to perception of environmental sound and an aid to lip reading. Ebinger and colleagues[27] reported the results of the U.S. multicenter ABI clinical trial. Of 92 subjects, 85% showed auditory sensation, of whom 93% showed improvement in speech understanding using audition with ABI and lip reading compared with the ABI alone or lip reading alone. Significant open set speech understanding in the audition alone condition (e.g., telephone use) is rare.[28] Remarkably similar outcomes have been reported from various centers in Europe and Australia.[11,29-31]

The ABI provides subjects with auditory percepts sufficient to give environmental sound awareness (as shown by the Sound Effects Recognition Test).[32] Information is also provided on the stress and rhythm in speech, which assists subjects with lip reading. Why ABI performance is limited compared with cochlear implant speech perception outcomes is unclear. On psychophysical testing, there is limited pitch variation between separate electrodes or channels on the ABI array.[33] This means limited tonotopic stimulation and limited independent channels of spectral information can be provided. The first step in mapping the ABI is the pitch ranking of the electrodes with auditory percepts. Most ABI patients exhibit a rising pitch percept from lateral to medial across the array, a few have a falling pitch pattern, and some have a variable or flattened pitch pattern.

The tonotopic orientation of neurons within the cochlear nucleus is suboptimal for surface electrode stimulation. The frequency change is from superficial to deep, rather than across the cochlear nucleus surface. Electric stimulation from individual electrodes or channels may activate a broad area of neurons; in addition, adjacent electrodes may activate overlapping regions of neurons, so provision of independent spectral information by electric stimulation is very limited.

The cochlear nucleus is composed of various specialized neurons with extrinsic and intrinsic projections that are either excitatory or inhibitory in function. In addition to losing the degree of peripheral tonotopic stimulation achieved with a cochlear implant, direct stimulation of the cochlear nucleus with an ABI may mean loss of specialized neural function within the cochlear nucleus.

Penetrating Auditory Brainstem Implant

Because the tonotopicity of the cochlear nucleus is not adequately accessed with a surface electrode, it is proposed that a penetrating array might allow more selective tonotopic stimulation of the cochlear nucleus.[34] Animal studies have shown that selective neural stimulation is possible with proximal recording in the inferior colliculus.[35]

A prototype human penetrating ABI (PABI) has been developed at HEI. There have been two generations of PABI with each being a combination of penetrating and surface arrays (Fig. 161-4). In the first, there were 8 penetrating electrodes and 14 surface electrodes. The second contained 10 penetrating electrodes and 12 surface electrodes. Placement of the PABI presents a greater surgical challenge than a surface array. The electrode needs to be accurately inserted into the cochlear nucleus for auditory stimulation to be successful. A stimulating probe has been used to generate an evoked ABR in an attempt to confirm the site of the cochlear nucleus before PABI insertion. This probe has not proven specific enough in site of stimulation to identify the cochlear nucleus definitely. The penetrating array must also be inserted rapidly to avoid any shearing effect on neural tissue because of brainstem movement during the insertion. To facilitate accurate rapid placement, a pneumatic insertion tool has also been developed.

A clinical trial has been undertaken at HEI, with 10 NF2 patients implanted with the two generations of PABI. The outcomes are not proving any better than the surface electrode ABI in terms of the reliability of achieving auditory sensations or of the speech perception levels achieved. In the cases where the PABI provided little benefit, the surface electrode array was successful in providing auditory benefit (Brackmann D, Otto S, personal communication).

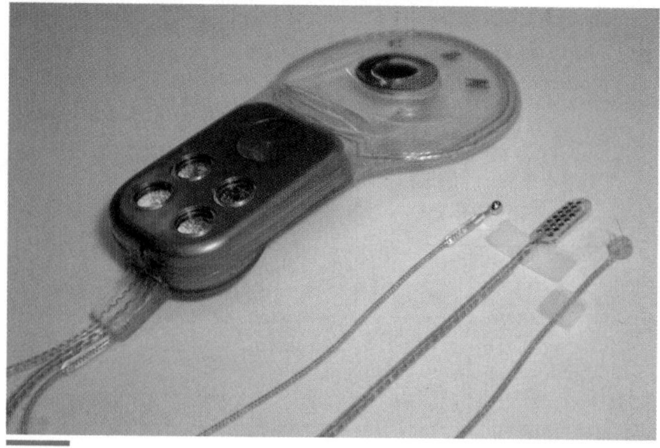

Figure 161-4. Combined penetrating auditory brainstem implant and surface electrode array. *(Courtesy of Cochlear Ltd. and House Ear Institute.)*

Outcome of Auditory Brainstem Implants in Patients without Neurofibromatosis Type 2

Although the ABI has been predominantly implanted in NF2 patients, there is increasing international experience with ABI use in patients without NF2 who are unsuitable for, or have failed, cochlear implantation. Typically, these subjects have loss of eighth cranial nerve integrity because of skull base fracture or traumatic avulsion, or have severe postmeningitis cochlear ossification.

The hearing outcomes achieved in these patients are significantly better than the outcomes in NF2 patients. Some non-NF2 ABI recipients achieve speech perception at levels comparable to successful cochlear implant recipients. Colletti and colleagues[36] reported 63% open set sentence recognition in the audition alone mode in nontumor patients compared with 12% in NF2 patients. Similar outcomes have been reported Grayeli and associates.[37]

This difference in performance between the tumor and nontumor groups implies that the NF2 condition and presence of bilateral vestibular schwannomas has an intrinsic effect on cochlear nucleus function that adversely effects the speech perception achieved with electric stimulation. Colletti and Shannon[38] examined two groups of ABI recipients, 10 NF2 and 10 non-NF2 patients. Parameters studied included electric stimulation thresholds, electrode selectivity, and amplitude modulation and speech perception. These investigators showed that the NF2 patients have significantly worse modulation detection and speech discrimination than non-NF2 recipients. Both groups had similar range of pitch perception and loudness percepts, and so the investigators postulated that the poorer amplitude detection may be due to damage to a specific cell type or region within the cochlear nucleus. Possibly the chopper cells are more susceptible to damage because of their large size and large metabolic requirements. Alternatively, the small cell cap of the cochlear nucleus may be specifically damaged. These cells receive projections from the vestibular nerve root, and so may be affected by vestibular schwannoma growth or surgical removal.

It is unclear why the presence of the vestibular schwannoma has an adverse effect. It may be neural damage associated with progressive sensorineural hearing loss, brainstem distortion owing to the mass effect of a large tumor, or direct brainstem trauma or alteration in vascularity associated with surgical tumor removal. It does not seem to be simply a tumor mass effect or brainstem manipulation that limits ABI outcomes. Some NF2 patients lose hearing with only small tumors that do not contact the brainstem. In the author's experience, these patients do not perform better with an ABI than patients who had large tumors and significant brainstem compression.

Penetrating Auditory Midbrain Implant

The fact that the ABI can produce high levels of speech perception in non-NF2 patients, presumably owing to intrinsic cochlear nucleus dysfunction, raises the possibility that stimulating the auditory midbrain proximal to the damaged cochlear nucleus may be a better alternative in NF2 patients. Lenarz and coworkers[39] suggested the central nucleus of the inferior colliculus as the potential site.

Colletti and colleagues[40] reported placement of an electrode array (Med El ABI) on the dorsal surface of the inferior colliculus in an NF2 patient. The patient was considered unsuitable for an ABI because of prior surgery and radiation therapy for vestibular schwannomas. The electrode array was placed via a median infratentorial, supracerebellar approach. All 12 electrodes on the array produced auditory sensations without nonauditory responses. Postoperatively, some electrodes apparently developed higher thresholds, presumably because of movement of the array. Seven electrodes were activated with discernible pitch differentiation, measured on only three of the seven electrodes. Apparently, the patient could discriminate multisyllabic words in a five-choice test, and achieved an aid to lip reading with audition via the AMI.

To achieve useful speech perception with multielectrode AMI stimulation, pitch differentiation between electrodes is necessary. The inferior colliculus is an obligatory synaptic terminus in the ascending auditory system.[41] It consists of the central nucleus, the external nucleus, and the dorsal nucleus. The central nucleus contains a clearly defined tonotopic map with preserved tonotopic projections to the ipsilateral auditory thalamus and cortex and to the contralateral inferior colliculus.[42] Most of the tonotopic structures of the inferior colliculus are internally oriented along a dorsolateral to ventromedial axis. A penetrating electrode array has been developed by MHH and Cochlear Limited to access the tonotopic orientation of the inferior colliculus. The penetrating AMI array is 6.2 mm long and 0.4 mm in diameter with 20 platinum ring electrodes. The array is constructed of soft silicon with a central removable stainless steel stylet to facilitate insertion into the inferior colliculus (Fig. 161-5).

Samii and associates[43] reported use of the lateral suboccipital approach for combined vestibular schwannoma removal and supracerebellar access to the inferior colliculus for insertion of the penetrating AMI. Three NF2 patients were implanted in Hannover, Germany, using this approach with intraoperative stereotactic navigation to identify the appropriate trajectory for electrode insertion. All three subjects got auditory percepts; however, postoperative imaging and the presence of nonauditory sensations showed that proper electrode placement was achieved in only one case with the other two electrodes being in the dorsal cortex of the inferior colliculus and the surface of the lateral lemniscus. Each subject showed various pitch, temporal, loudness, and directional percepts. They achieved environmental sound perception and obtained an aid to lip reading, but at 6 months did not get open set speech perception.[44] The hearing obtained apparently improves over time, as is observed in cochlear implant and ABI patients over several years.

The hearing result in the patient with accurate central nucleus inferior colliculus placement was superior to the other two. The electrophysiologic properties of the inferior colliculus neurons are different from the peripheral auditory nerve or cochlear nucleus. Modified stimulation and speech processing strategies may be necessary to activate neurons more effectively across the frequency and isofrequency dimensions of the central nucleus of the inferior colliculus and to optimize speech perception outcomes.

Alternative Strategies in Patients with Neurofibromatosis Type 2

Because the speech perception outcomes achieved with ABIs and AMIs remain limited, tumor management strategies that preserve an intact cochlear nerve should be considered. Successful cochlear implantation has been reported in patients after vestibular schwannoma removal.[45-47] Cochlear implantation after long-term vestibular schwannoma growth control by stereotactic radiation therapy can also provide open set speech perception (Briggs RJS, personal experience). Planned partial tumor removal preserving the cochlear nerve, possibly with radiation therapy if necessary, in association with cochlear implantation rather than ABI may give better hearing outcomes in selected NF2 patients.

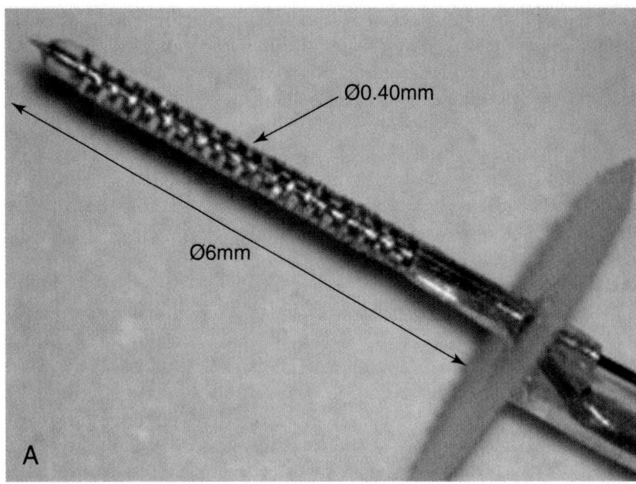

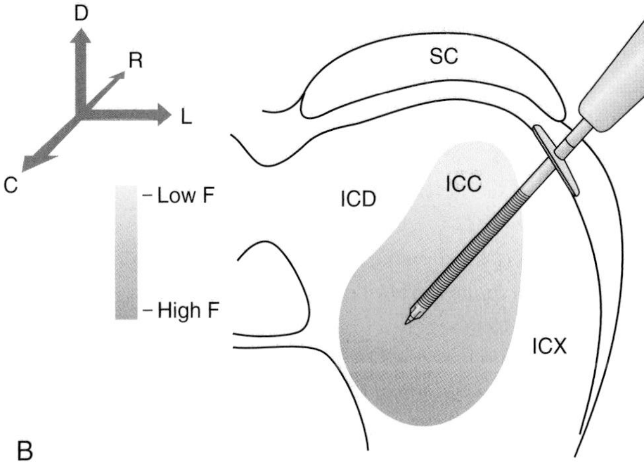

Figure 161-5. A, Image of the human prototype auditory midbrain implant (AMI) electrode array. **B,** Schematic of inferior colliculus showing AMI electrode in situ. ICC, central inferior colliculus; ICD, dorsal inferior colliculus; ICX, lateral inferior colliculus; SC, superior colliculus. *(**A**, Courtesy of Cochlear Ltd. and Medical University of Hannover.)*

Auditory Brainstem Implants in Children with Cochlear Nerve Aplasia

Because of the improved outcomes in non-NF2 ABI recipients, there is hope that the same improved level of hearing may be possible in children with cochlear dysplasia or cochlear nerve aplasia who are unsuitable for cochlear implantation. There is limited experience in numerous centers with ABI placement in children with various cochlear dysplasias and cochlear nerve aplasia or hypoplasia. Colletti and colleagues[48] showed that ABI placement is technically feasible, and that some auditory rehabilitation is possible with children showing environmental sound awareness and limited speech detection.

Although the ABI electrode array can be placed in children younger than 2 years, the subsequent programming of the ABI to achieve potentially useful sound detection is an enormous challenge. As discussed earlier, the successful use of an ABI depends on programming the device to use electrodes that produce auditory sensation without significant nonauditory stimulation, and to use pitch ranking of electrodes across the array. Although electric evoked ABR recording can give some indication of which electrodes produce an auditory response, it is extremely difficult to differentiate auditory from nonauditory responses, and virtually impossible to pitch rank electrodes in prelingual children who cannot give meaningful feedback. Device programming is undertaken on an empiric basis, using cautious and lengthy stepwise programming sessions.

Although initial reports of sound detection and device use in these children have been encouraging, it will be some time before it is shown whether the hearing achieved is sufficient for useful speech and language development. Of three young children implanted in Manchester, one had a potentially life-threatening postoperative posterior fossa bleed, but made a good recovery and shows benefit with the ABI (Ramsden R, personal communication). Presumably, as with cochlear implantation, the younger the age of intervention, the better the hearing outcome will be; however, the potential hearing benefits need to be well shown and carefully weighed against the potential risks of such major surgery in young children.

Summary

The ABI is now established as an effective method of partial hearing restoration in patients with NF2. The ABI can provide environmental sound awareness and an aid to lip reading; however, open set speech perception is achieved only rarely. Trials of a penetrating ABI and penetrating inferior colliculus AMI have not provided improved hearing outcomes yet. Better speech perception outcomes have been shown in ABI recipients without NF2. These improved outcomes have led to hope that children with cochlear nerve aplasia, who are unsuitable for cochlear implants, might benefit from ABI.

SUGGESTED READINGS

Brackmann DE, Hitselberger WE, Nelson RA, et al. Auditory brainstem implant, 1: issues in surgical implantation. *Otolaryngol Head Neck Surg.* 1993;108:624-633.

Colletti V, Carner M, Fiorino F, et al. Hearing restoration with auditory brainstem implant in three children with cochlear nerve aplasia. *Otol Neurotol.* 2002;23:682-693.

Colletti V, Sacchetto L, Giarbini N, et al. Retrosigmoid approach for auditory brainstem implant. *J Laryngol Otol.* 2000;114(Suppl 27):37-40.

Colletti V, Shannon RV. Open set speech perception with auditory brainstem implant? *Laryngoscope.* 2005;115:1974-1978.

Ebinger K, Otto S, Arcaroli J, et al. Multichannel auditory brainstem implant: US clinical trial results. *J Laryngol Otol.* 2000;114(Suppl 27):50-53.

Grayeli AB, Bouccara D, Kalamarides M, et al. Auditory brainstem implant in bilateral and completely ossified cochlea. *Otol Neurol.* 2003;24:79-82.

House WF, Hitselberger WE. Twenty-year report of the first auditory brainstem nucleus implant. *Ann Otol Rhinol Laryngol.* 2001;110:103.

Kalamarides M, Grayeli AB, Bouccara D, et al. Hearing restoration with auditory brainstem implants after radiosurgery for neurofibromatosis type 2. *J Neurosurg.* 2001;95:1028-1033.

Klose AK, Sollmann WP. Anatomical variations of landmarks for implantation at the cochlear nucleus. *J Laryngol Otol Suppl.* 2000;27:8.

Lenarz T, Lim H, Reuter G, et al. The auditory midbrain implant: a new auditory prosthesis for neural deafness—concept and device description. *Otol Neurotol.* 2006;27:838-843.

Lim HH, Lenarz T, Joseph G, et al. Electrical stimulation of the midbrain for hearing restoration: insight into the functional organization of the human central auditory system. *J Neurosci.* 2007;27:13541-13551.

Malmierca MS, Rees A, Le Beau FE, et al. Laminar organization of frequency defined local axons within and between the inferior colliculi of the guinea pig. *J Comp Neurol.* 1995;357:124-144.

McCreery DB, Shannon RV, Moore JK, et al. Accessing the tonotopic organization of the ventral cochlear nucleus by intranuclear microstimulation. *IEEE Trans Rehabil Eng.* 1998;6:391-399.

McElveen JT, Hitselberger WE, House WF. Surgical accessibility of the cochlear nuclear complex in man: surgical landmarks. *Otolaryngol Head Neck Surg.* 1987;96:135.

Monsell EM, McElveen JT Jr, Hitselberger WE, et al. Surgical approaches to the human cochlear nuclear complex. *Am J Otol.* 1987;8:450-455.

Nevison B, Laszig R, Sollmann WP, et al. Results from a European clinical investigation of the Nucleus multichannel auditory brainstem implant. *Ear Hear.* 2002;23:170-183.

Otto SR, Brackmann DE, Hitselberger WE, et al. Multichannel auditory brainstem implant: update on performance in 61 patients. *J Neurosurg.* 2002;96:1063-1071.

Samii A, Lenarz M, Majdani O, et al. Auditory midbrain implant: a combined approach for vestibular schwannoma surgery and device implantation. *Otol Neurotol.* 2007;28:31-38.

Shannon RV, Otto SR. Psychophysical measures from electrical stimulation of the human cochlear nucleus. *Hear Res.* 1990;47:159.

Shannon RV, Fayad J, Moore JK, et al. Auditory brainstem implant, II: postsurgical issues and performance. *Otolaryngol Head Neck Surg.* 1993;108:634.

Sinha UK, Terr LI, Galey FR, Linthicum RH Jr. Computer-aided three-dimensional reconstruction of the cochlear nerve root. *Arch Otolaryngol Head Neck Surg.* 1987;113:651-655.

Terr LI, Edgerton BJ. Three-dimensional reconstruction of the cochlear nuclear complex in humans. *Arch Otolaryngol.* 1985;111:495.

Terr LI, Sinha UK, House WF. Anatomical relationships of the cochlear nuclei and the pontobulbar body: possible significance for neuroprosthesis placement. *Laryngoscope.* 1987;97:1009.

Tono T, Ushisako Y, Morimitsu T. Cochlear implantation in an intralabyrinthine acoustic neuroma patient after resection of an intracanalicular tumour. *J Laryngol Otol.* 1996;110:570.

Waring MD. Electrically evoked auditory brainstem response monitoring of auditory brainstem implant integrity during facial nerve tumour surgery. *Laryngoscope.* 1992;102:1293-1295.

For complete list of references log onto www.expertconsult.com.

CHAPTER ONE HUNDRED AND SIXTY-TWO

Hearing Aids: Strategies of Amplification

Brad A. Stach

Virginia Ramachandran

Key Points

- Hearing aid technology is advancing at a rapid pace, resulting in an expansion of candidacy and enhancement in benefit from hearing aid use.
- Resulting in large part from the adaptability of modern technology, indications for successful hearing aid use relate more to a patient's communication needs and challenges than to the specifics of degree or configuration of hearing loss.
- Most modern hearing aids use digital signal processing, with high-fidelity signal reproduction and considerable flexibility for matching hearing loss and communication needs.
- Input to the hearing aid is ordinarily received by microphones with variable directionality that may change as a function of the listening environment. Signals may also be received by various wireless transmitter/receiver technologies.
- Directional microphones enhance signal-to-noise ratios, allowing for improved speech perception in noise.
- The digital amplifier allows for variable control in the frequency, amplitude, and time domains to permit programming to fit an individual's hearing loss and ability.
- Hearing aid selection involves matching hearing loss and communication needs with style, technology, and features.
- Type, degree, and configuration of hearing loss are the most important determinants of the style and type of signal processing and features that are indicated.
- Hearing aid validation is carried out by in situ measurement of speech and other signals being delivered to the tympanic membrane.
- Outcome measures provide valuable information regarding satisfaction with and benefit from hearing aid use.

The most common treatment for sensorineural hearing loss is the use of conventional hearing aid amplification. Despite substantial strides in the implementation of implantable technology, hearing aids remain the most widely used and appropriate treatment solution for most patients with hearing loss. Although hearing devices implanted worldwide during a year now number in the thousands, more than 2.4 million hearing aids were dispensed last year in the United States alone.[1]

Previously, hearing aid amplifiers used analog circuits with limited flexibility to fit a patient's hearing loss. Modern hearing aids incorporate digital signal processing (DSP), sophisticated noise and feedback reduction, adaptable directionality, and wireless connectivity. These advances permit accurate fitting over a broader range of hearing loss degree and configurations, and lead to noticeable enhancement in quality of amplified sound and listening performance. This chapter provides a general overview of hearing aids, including indications for their use; amplification technologies; and the selection, fitting, and verification process.

Indications for Hearing Aid Use

Whether a patient is a candidate for a hearing aid is determined by three primary factors and several secondary considerations. Assuming that surgical or other medical management of the hearing loss has been exhausted, candidacy is based on the interaction of degree and configuration of hearing loss, the extent of the communication disorder resulting from the loss, motivation of the patient to address the communication disorder, and attitude toward hearing aid use.[2] Generally, most patients who seek hearing aids can benefit from their use. Even in cases in which the prognosis for successful hearing aid use is guarded, an amplification solution is usually available if the patient is sufficiently motivated.

Hearing Loss Considerations

A primary consideration in successful hearing aid use is the nature, degree, and configuration of hearing sensitivity loss. Although no firm criteria exist about how much hearing loss is too little or too much to preclude successful hearing aid use, some general rules guide prognosis.

In an effort to provide a realistic view of the characteristics of hearing aid users, we evaluated data from 1860 ears of 1049 consecutive patients who were fitted with hearing aids at the Henry Ford Hospital during 2007. Patients ranged in age from 1 to 101 years old. The distribution of ages is shown in Figure 162-1. Of all patients, 81% were at least 60 years old, and 61% were 70 years or older. These percentages are typical of the hearing aid population in general. The prevalence of hearing loss is progressively greater with age, as is the use of hearing aids. Hearing aids are predominantly fitted on ears with sensorineural (88%) or mixed (11%) hearing loss. In this sample, less than 1% of

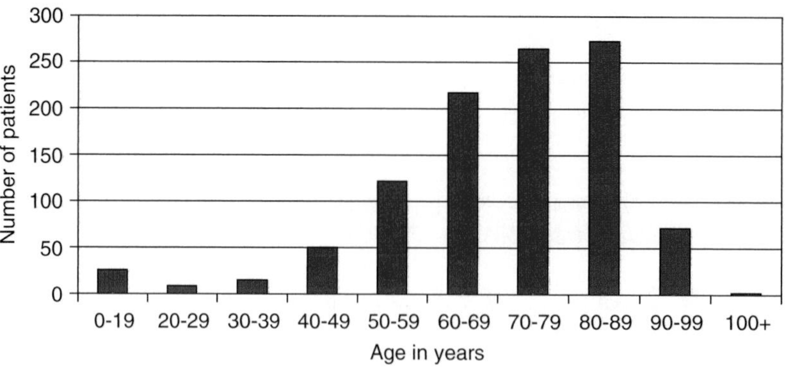

Figure 162-1. Distribution of hearing aid patients by age.

hearing aid devices were fitted on ears with pure conductive hearing loss.

Among people with hearing loss, there are significantly more individuals with mild hearing loss than severe or profound loss. Among this group of hearing aid users, most patients who choose to use hearing aids have hearing loss that is at least moderate in degree. The proportion of patients who have hearing loss and use hearing aids increases substantially with increasing severity of hearing loss. Stated the other way, the penetration of hearing aids into the potential market is low for mild hearing loss and considerably greater as hearing loss increases.

Slope of the audiometric configuration is another factor that influences hearing aid usage. Most patients have flat or sloping hearing loss—that is, hearing sensitivity that is similar across frequencies, or that is better in the low frequencies than the high frequencies. For some audiometric configurations, it is very challenging to provide appropriate amplification. One difficult configuration is a high-frequency precipitous loss, where hearing sensitivity is normal through 500 Hz and decreases dramatically at higher frequencies. There may even be dead regions in the cochlea, where hair cell loss is so complete that no transduction occurs. Depending on the frequency at which the loss begins and the slope of the loss, this type of hearing loss can be very difficult to fit effectively. The other extreme is the rising audiogram, a relatively unusual audiometric configuration in which a hearing loss occurs at the low frequencies, but not the high frequencies. Although this type of loss seldom causes enough of a communication problem to warrant hearing aid use, when it does, certain aspects of the fitting can be troublesome, and the prognosis for successful fitting is limited. In the present sample, less than 2% of ears had rising audiograms.

Although degree of loss is associated with hearing aid use, the audiogram offers only one piece of information needed to determine candidacy. Most patients with minimal to mild hearing loss do not pursue hearing aids, although some do. This fact indicates that the presence of hearing loss alone may be insufficient to compel a patient to hearing aid use, but that a mild degree of hearing loss does not contraindicate hearing aid use. Even patients with minimal hearing losses can wear mild gain hearing aids with benefit. Generally, if the hearing impairment is enough to cause a problem in communication, the patient is a candidate for hearing aids.

Some patients have too much hearing loss for hearing aid use. Severe or profound loss can limit the usefulness of even the most powerful hearing aids. In many cases of profound hearing loss, a hearing aid can provide only environmental awareness or some rudimentary perception of speech. Many patients do not consider this benefit to be valuable enough to warrant the use of hearing aids. In these cases, cochlear implantation is often the most beneficial treatment strategy.

Another audiometric consideration in hearing aid use is suprathreshold speech recognition ability. In most patients, speech recognition is commensurate with degree of hearing loss and is simply a reflection of audibility of spoken speech. In these patients, amplification of the sound that is missing can provide significant enhancement of speech recognition. In other patients, speech recognition is poorer than expected for a given hearing loss. For example, cochlear hearing loss secondary to endolymphatic hydrops can cause substantial distortion of sound, resulting in very poor speech recognition ability. If it is sufficiently poor, hearing aid amplification may contribute to audibility but will be unsatisfactory overall.

Auditory processing disorders in young children and in aging adults can also reduce the benefit from conventional hearing aid amplification. It is not unusual for geriatric patients who were previously successful hearing aid users to experience increasingly less success as their central auditory nervous systems change with age.[3] The problem is seldom extreme enough to preclude hearing aid use, but these patients may benefit more from assistive technology to complement hearing aid use.[4] Prognosis for hearing aid benefit in these patients is guarded.

Communication Disorder and Motivation

The impact of a hearing loss can vary considerably among patients and is an important factor in hearing aid candidacy. Some patients with slow onset presbycusis, of even moderate degree, perceive no difficulty with communication. Such patients effectively use communication strategies such as speech reading and manipulation of the environment to minimize the impact of hearing loss. The prognosis for successful hearing aid use is limited by the patient's lack of recognition of the hearing loss. Other patients, who have considerably less hearing loss but greater communication demands or less success with coping strategies, might perceive communication difficulties and be anxious to quantify the hearing loss for the purpose of obtaining hearing instruments.

Patient motivation is another key factor in predicting success with hearing aids. A patient who is internally motivated to hear better is an excellent candidate for successful hearing aid use. The breadth of amplification options for such a patient is substantial. In contrast, an unwilling patient who gives in to the requests of a spouse or other family members to seek hearing aid amplification often finds numerous reasons why hearing aid amplification is unsatisfactory.

Candidacy for hearing aid amplification is fairly straightforward. If a patient has a sensorineural or other nontreatable hearing loss that is causing a communication disorder, the patient is a candidate for amplification. Even when a hearing impairment is mild, if it is causing difficulty with communication, and the patient is motivated to do something about it, the patient is a candidate for hearing aid amplification and is likely to benefit from its use.

Otologic and Other Factors

Other factors can influence hearing aid candidacy, although they are more likely to influence the selection of type and style of device than to preclude its use. Although a progressive or fluctuating hearing loss does not rule out conventional hearing aid use, the selected hearing instrument must be sufficiently flexible to allow for alterations in programming to accommodate the patient's changing hearing. Patients with microtia or other anomalies may have ear canals or pinnae that prevent fitting with a conventional custom hearing instrument or the ear mold used with a behind-the-ear (BTE) hearing aid. More commonly, the size of the ear canal of a patient sometimes limits the use of certain in-the-ear (ITE) hearing aids. Other physical and medical limitations can make conventional hearing aid use difficult. Occasionally, a patient with hearing loss has external otitis or ear drainage that cannot be controlled medically. Placing a hearing aid in such an ear can be a constant source of problems. Certain rare pain disorders may also limit access to the ear canal.

Physical and cognitive limitations may influence hearing aid candidacy. Physical limitations are primarily limitations pertaining to dexterity issues from arthritis and other conditions that affect a patient's ability to manipulate certain styles of hearing aids.[5,6] Limited cognitive ability can be a barrier to successful hearing aid use when a patient has difficulty remembering how to operate a hearing aid and its components.

Hearing Aid Technology

Evolution of Hearing Aid Technology

Hearing aid technology has advanced rapidly. Modern hearing aids use DSP for high-fidelity sound reproduction. They have adaptive directionality, feedback control, noise reduction, and low battery drain. They are readily programmable, providing substantial flexibility for precise fitting. Modern hearing aids also have advanced amplification strategies that reduce distortion and enhance listening comfort.[7]

One early step in the progress of technology was component miniaturization. Microphones, amplifier circuits, loudspeakers, and batteries all have been reduced in size. This miniaturization has allowed sophisticated signal processing circuits to be fitted into a completely-in-the-canal (CIC) style of hearing aid. It has also allowed for more technology components, such as wireless receivers, to be incorporated into smaller sized devices worn over or in the ear.

Programmability of hearing aids was a major step in the advancement of hearing aid technology. This programmability provided flexible control of hearing aid characteristics. In the recent past, a hearing aid circuit had to be matched carefully to a patient's audiogram at the time of hearing aid selection. Now hearing aids are available that can be programmed over a wide fitting range so that the matching is done at the time of hearing aid fitting, rather than at the time of selection. Programmability also provides multiple memories for a single hearing aid, allowing the potential for use of different response parameters for different listening situations.

Hearing aids have progressed since the late 1990s from analog to DSP. In analog hearing aids, acoustic signals followed an analog path that was under analog control, wherein an acoustic signal was converted by a microphone into electric energy in a continuously variable manner. In DSP hearing aids, acoustic signals are converted from analog to digital and back again, with digital control over various amplification parameters. DSP eliminated many of the barriers faced in trying to design analog circuits to fit in a small hearing aid and run on low-powered batteries. Along with flexibility inherent in enhanced programmability, modern devices provide more precise and flexible frequency shaping, more sophisticated compression algorithms, better acoustic feedback reduction, and enhanced noise reduction algorithms.[8,9] The degree of sophistication of signal processing that is used in modern hearing aids seems limited only by the conceptual framework of how hearing aid amplification should work.

The most recent technologic advance in hearing aids is the growing opportunity of wireless connectivity, permitting communication from one hearing aid to another and from hearing aids to other electronic devices and signal sources.[10]

Hearing Instrument Components

A hearing aid is an amplification device that consists of three basic components: a microphone, an amplifier, and a receiver. The power source for the amplifier is a battery. Most hearing aids also have some external controls, such as a program button or volume control on the hearing aid, or a remote control. A schematic of the basic components is shown in Figure 162-2.

The most common input transducer in a hearing aid is a microphone, which converts acoustic energy into electric energy. As a sound source vibrates, it creates pressure waves of expanding and compressing air molecules. The membrane of the microphone vibrates in response to these pressure changes, creating an electric energy flow that corresponds to the amplitude, frequency, and phase of the acoustic signal.

Sound can also be delivered to the amplifier of a hearing aid via direct audio input, wherein a sound source reaches the hearing aid directly via a wire connector or "boot" that connects to a BTE hearing aid. One of the most common alternative input transducers is the telecoil, or t-coil. A telecoil allows the hearing aid to receive electromagnetic signals directly, bypassing the hearing aid microphone. The telecoil is often used with the telephone to reduce background noise, and to minimize the potential for feedback that occurs when placing a device near the microphone. A telecoil can be activated by a manual control on the hearing aid, by remote control, or automatically when the hearing aid senses an electromagnetic field.[11]

The telecoil can also be used to provide input for remote-microphone sources. The signal from the remote microphone is transmitted in some form to a loop of wire, which transmits the signal electromagnetically to the telecoil of the hearing aid.[11] This type of technology is often used in a classroom situation, to allow the signal delivered from the remote-microphone worn by a teacher to be directly input to the hearing aid worn by the student.[12] This technology minimizes the degradation of the auditory signal caused by background noise and distance.

A hearing aid may have some other form of wireless transducer, such as a frequency-modulated (FM) receiver or Bluetooth or other modern wireless connectivity. An FM receiver can be built into a hearing aid or attached as a boot on a BTE hearing aid. The FM receiver acts like an FM radio, receiving signals from a transmitter and directing them to the amplifier of the hearing aid.[13] Increasingly, modern hearing aids are equipped with other wireless connectivity solutions, so that the hearing aid amplifier can receive signals directly from mobile phones, computers, or personal music players.[10]

The function of a hearing aid is to amplify sound. This amplification is accomplished through the power amplifier of the hearing aid. The amplifier adds gain to the level of the electric signal that is delivered to the hearing aid's transducer. The amplifier can differentially enhance higher or lower frequency and higher or lower intensity sounds. It also has a limiting function so that it does not deliver excessive energy to the ear.

The output transducer of a hearing aid is its receiver, or loudspeaker. The loudspeaker receives an amplified electric signal from the hearing aid amplifier and converts it back into acoustic energy. Hearing aid receivers have a broad, flat frequency response to reproduce accurately the signals being processed by the hearing aid amplifier.

Electroacoustic Characteristics

The acoustic response characteristics of hearing aids are described in terms of frequency gain, input-output, and output limiting. Gain is the amount of energy that is added to the input signal. The amount of gain

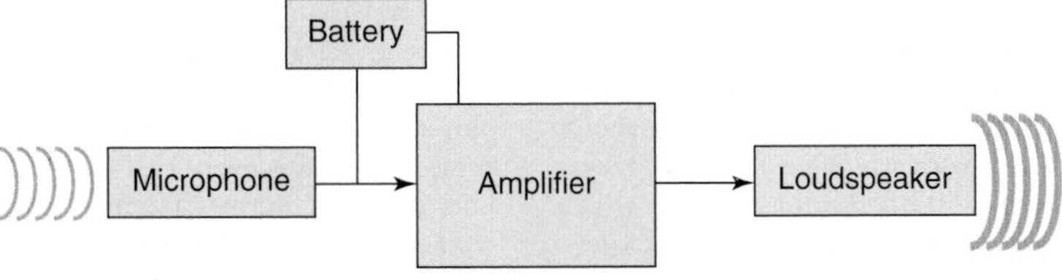

Figure 162-2. The components of a hearing aid.

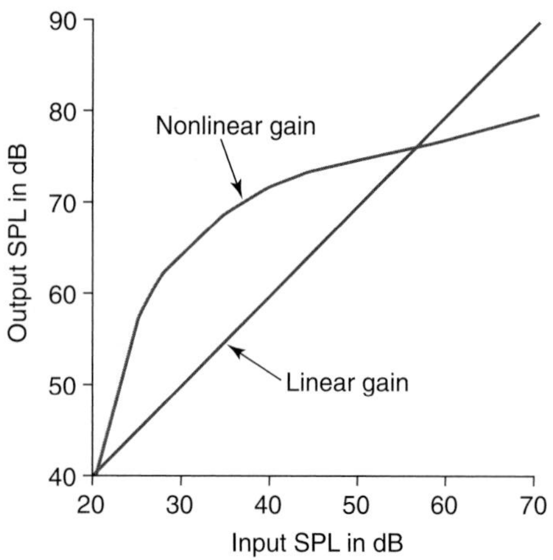

Figure 162-3. Relationship of sound input to output in linear and nonlinear hearing aid circuits. For the linear circuit, gain remains at a constant 20 dB, regardless of input level. For the nonlinear circuit, amount of gain changes as a function of input level. SPL, sound pressure level.

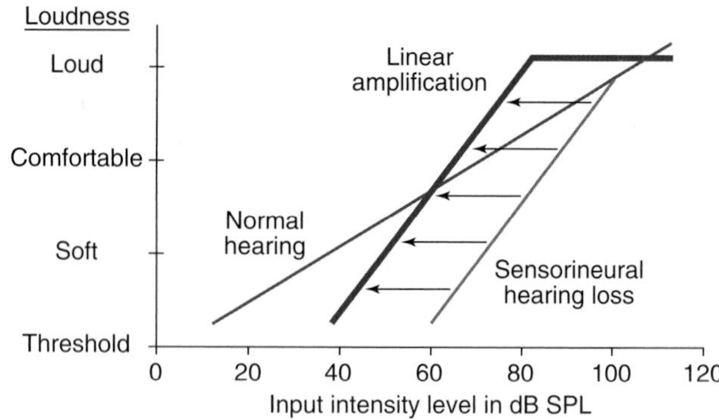

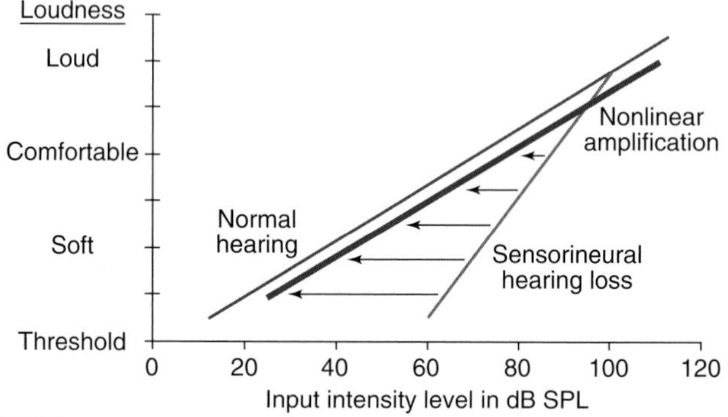

Figure 162-4. The difference between linear and nonlinear amplification in an ear with sensorineural hearing loss and nonlinear loudness growth. SPL, sound pressure level. *(From Stach B.* Clinical Audiology: An Introduction. *2nd ed. Clifton Park, NY: Delmar Cengage Learning: 2010, 583.)*

varies as a function of frequency to accommodate varying hearing loss configurations. The relationship of gain as a function of frequency is the frequency gain response of a hearing aid. The frequency gain response represents the gain produced by a hearing aid to a specified intensity level of a signal presented across the frequency range. It reflects the difference between the intensity level of the output of the hearing aid and the intensity level of the input. Most methods used for prescribing a hearing aid are based on providing a specified amount of gain at a given frequency, based on a patient's pure-tone audiogram.

The amount of gain also varies as a function of intensity level. The input-output characteristic of a hearing aid describes this relationship. The input-output function can be linear or nonlinear.

With linear amplification, the same amount of amplification, or gain, is applied to an input signal regardless of the intensity level of the signal so that low-intensity sounds are amplified to the same extent as high-intensity sounds. Figure 162-3 shows an example of a linear input-output function. In this example, for every dB increase in the input, there is a corresponding dB increase in the output. Fitting of linear hearing aids was a standard approach in the early years of hearing aids and remains applicable for conductive hearing loss and some mild sensorineural hearing losses. A problem with this type of amplification is that it does not address the nonlinearity of loudness growth that occurs with sensorineural hearing impairment. Many patients with sensorineural hearing loss do not hear low-intensity sounds, but can hear high-intensity sounds normally or even excessively loud owing to recruitment phenomena. Because a linear device amplifies soft and loud sounds identically, if a low-intensity sound is made loud enough to be audible, a high-intensity sound is likely to be too loud for the listener.[14]

In nonlinear amplification, the relationship between input and output is not constant, so that low-intensity sounds are amplified to a greater extent than high-intensity sounds; this is shown schematically in Figure 162-3. The overall effect is to make low-intensity sounds audible; moderate sounds comfortable; and high-intensity sounds loud, but not too loud.

Nonlinear amplification is designed to address two problems with sensorineural hearing loss: reduced dynamic range, and loudness growth that is different from that of a normal ear. *Dynamic range* in this case is a term used to describe the decibel difference between the level of a person's threshold of hearing sensitivity and the level that causes discomfort. In an individual with normal hearing, this range is 0 to about 100 dB hearing level (HL). In a patient with sensorineural hearing loss, the range is reduced. A patient with a 50-dB hearing loss and a discomfort level of 100 dB has a dynamic range of only 50 dB. Compression circuitry is used to boost the gain of low-intensity sounds so that they are audible, but to limit the gain of high-intensity sounds so that they are not uncomfortable. Figure 162-4 illustrates the difference between linear output and dynamic-range compression as it relates to an ear with sensorineural hearing loss and nonlinear loudness growth.

Nonlinear amplification is achieved with compression circuitry. *Compression* is a term that is used to describe how the amplification of a signal is changed as a function of its intensity. Compression techniques are used to limit the maximum output of a hearing aid and to provide nonlinear amplification across a wide range of inputs.[14,15]

Numerous nonlinear compression strategies have been developed to address the dynamic-range issue, and they vary in approach and complexity. Some strategies are designed to provide compression over a portion of the dynamic range. Partial dynamic-range compression typically provides linear amplification for low input signals and some level of compression when the input reaches a certain level. Other strategies are designed to provide compression over a wider portion of the dynamic range. Wide dynamic-range compression has as its basis the enhanced amplification of quiet sounds and reduced amplification of loud sounds, and is designed to package speech into a listener's residual dynamic range. For most systems, dynamic-range compression can be altered in multiple frequency bands. In this way, if a patient's dynamic range is reduced in one frequency range and nearly normal in another, the compression can be tailored to the frequency band where it is needed, and the other band can act as more of a linear amplifier.[14-16]

An amplifier also contains circuitry that limits its output. It is important that the output level of a hearing aid be limited to some maximum because high-intensity sounds can be damaging to the ear and uncomfortable to the listener. The classic method of limiting output, known as *peak clipping,* does not allow the peaks of signals to exceed a certain level. This method commonly causes distortion for high-intensity inputs. Compression limiting, the current standard method of output limiting, allows the amplifier to become nonlinear as input signals reach a predetermined level, so that the amount of gain is diminished significantly near the maximum output level.[14,15]

Other Hearing Aid Features

Today's hearing aids include many features that make an important contribution to successful hearing aid fitting: directionality, noise reduction, feedback reduction, program management, automatic adaptivity, and data logging. During normal hearing, sound pressure waves reach the tympanic membrane after the acoustic signal has been modified by the resonance characteristics of the pinna, concha, and ear canal. These changes to the acoustic signal greatly aid the localization of a sound source in space, and contribute to the ability to hear in the presence of background noise.[17] With hearing aid use, sound is received by the microphone, which is removed from the location of the tympanic membrane. The signal from the microphone does not include the spatial cues provided by the ear, reducing the ability to hear in background noise.

One important strategy for restoring some of these spatial cues is the use of directional microphones. A directional microphone is one that is designed to be more sensitive to sounds emanating from one direction than another. In most listening situations, the signal of interest is in front of the listener, and background noise is separated spatially, often from behind the listener. A directional microphone is designed to enhance the signal from the front and reduce the signal from behind or from wherever else it might be detected.

In its simplest form, a microphone is equally sensitive to sounds coming from all directions, or is omnidirectional in nature. A microphone can be made to be more directional by using two ports, one on the front and one on the back of the hearing aid. Each port leads to the opposite side of the diaphragm of the microphone. The rear port of the microphone is filtered in a way that causes a phase shift, or time delay, between sounds reaching each side of the microphone. In this way, sounds emanating from behind the listener are delayed so that they arrive at the back of the diaphragm simultaneously with their arrival at the front of the diaphragm. Equal sound pressure levels at both sides of the diaphragm essentially cancel those from behind because the diaphragm cannot move. The directional response pattern can be manipulated by changing the spacing of the ports or the time delay or both.

The modern version of the directionality feature uses two or more directional microphones in an array within the hearing aid. The directionality is created by subtracting the sound at the rear microphone from that at the front. The time delay is manipulated acoustically and electronically based on the number of microphones, the physical nature of the array, and the filters used to optimize the directionality pattern.

Most hearing aids can be changed from an omnidirectional to a directional setting. Typically, omnidirectional microphones are used in quiet environments.[18] Directional microphones are beneficial in background noise so that the microphone sensitivity is focused in a desired direction. In some instruments, the directionality feature is activated manually by the patient. In other instruments, it can be activated automatically and adaptively when the hearing aid senses background noise, changing the amount of directionality based on the extent of the noise.[19]

Noise reduction circuitry is available in most modern hearing aids to reduce unwanted background noise in an effort to improve patient comfort and speech recognition. The sophistication of noise reduction strategies has advanced dramatically,[20] and a thorough description is beyond the scope of this chapter. A simple example might serve to illustrate how the problem can be approached. The frequency and intensity of ongoing speech is highly variable and of short duration, whereas some background noise is relatively constant in nature. A DSP hearing aid can easily detect the difference in time constant and reduce the gain of the hearing aid in the frequency band of constant noise. Modern strategies use increasingly sophisticated algorithms to improve comfort and audibility in noise.

Acoustic feedback occurs when the amplified sound emanating from a receiver is directed back into the microphone of the same amplifying system. Physical separation of the microphone and receiver is the most effective way to reduce feedback. Another feedback reduction mechanism is feedback suppression circuitry. With feedback suppression, the hearing aid recognizes the occurrence of feedback based on frequency, intensity, and temporal characteristics. It reduces amplification in the offending frequency range to reduce feedback or uses phase cancellation of the feedback signal to eliminate audible feedback.[21,22]

All listening situations are not equal. As a result of modern programming capabilities of hearing aids, different responses can be programmed for different situations. One hearing aid response may be appropriate for a certain acoustic environment, such as telephone use, whereas a different type of response may be more appropriate for listening in a noisy environment. Most modern hearing aids have multiple memories that contain different acoustic responses or programs. Multiple memories have the potential to make many programmed responses available in the same hearing device. These programs can be manually accessed through push-button or other types of switches to change settings, or can be changed automatically by the hearing aid as it responds adaptively to the acoustic environment.

The more recent trend in hearing aids is to reduce user control of the response in favor of adaptive control by the hearing aid itself. In such cases, the device continuously samples the acoustic environment and makes changes based on what it measures. This type of automatic control of the hearing aid is beneficial because changes can be made without users needing to monitor the environment themselves. The willingness and ability to use the various programs and features of the hearing aid effectively varies among hearing aid users. These differences can be addressed with adaptivity, as the hearing aid algorithms dictate when the acoustic environment calls for changes to the hearing aid function. In some cases, patients may choose to retain control over the hearing aid, even when adaptive features are available, owing to very specific listening requirements.

Data logging is a feature available in most modern digital hearing aids. The programming software of the hearing aid is designed to track and record user settings and changes to provide statistics that characterize hearing aid use. Commonly accrued information includes time of hearing aid use by the patient, use of automatic or manually controlled hearing aid programs and features, and classification of the listening environments of the user. Data logging is typically used for counseling of patients regarding hearing aid use. If data logging indicates that a patient has used a hearing aid only for a limited time each day, the patient can be effectively counseled regarding the benefit of consistent hearing aid use. Data logging can also be used for troubleshooting of patient complaints. In addition, based on the changes that are typically made by the user and the examination of the typical listening environments of the user, changes can be made to hearing aid programming by the provider.[23] Many data logging systems suggest changes based on listener preferences and experiences. Some data logging systems allow for changes to be automatically made to programming based on these factors and with input by the user when hearing aid characteristics are optimal for a particular listening environment.[24]

Hearing Aid Styles

Hearing aids are available in several styles and with a range of functionality. Each style type has characteristic advantages and disadvantages that must be weighed against user needs and preferences. The most common styles of hearing aids are BTE and ITE hearing aids.

Behind-the-Ear Hearing Aids

A BTE hearing aid consists of the microphone and amplifier in a case that is worn behind the ear. The receiver may be located behind the ear or in the ear canal. Amplified sound is delivered to the ear canal through a tube that leads to a custom-fitted ear mold, a standard open-canal coupler, or a receiver in the canal. External controls for patient manipulation, usually volume control or program button or both, are located on the back side. Figure 162-5 shows BTE hearing aids.

One method for delivery of sound to the ear canal is to channel sound from the ear hook through tubing that terminates in a custom ear mold that fits in the auricle. Ear molds are custom-made in a variety of styles. The resonance characteristics of the ear mold and tubing significantly alter the acoustic properties of amplified sound. The frequency gain characteristics of the hearing aid output can be modified by ear mold and tubing selection and modifications.[25]

Another method of coupling the BTE to the external canal is known as *open-fit technology* or *open-canal fittings*. With these fittings, the ear canal coupler is typically nonoccluding so that it does not completely fill the ear canal. It typically uses thinner tubing than that found with traditional custom-made ear molds, and it is usually a standard, rather than custom-made, coupler. Open-canal fittings are especially useful for high-frequency hearing loss. Low-frequency sound is free to pass through the ear canal in an unobstructed manner, permitting natural hearing in the lower frequencies.[25]

Another BTE variation is the receiver-in-the-canal (RIC) fitting. The RIC fitting can be an open-canal fit, or a conventional, occluded BTE fit. The use of the RIC fitting reduces potential for acoustic feedback by increasing the separation of the receiver from the microphone, creating opportunity for more hearing aid gain when using an occluded fit. When using an open-canal fit, the opportunity for acoustic feedback is similar to that of an open-canal fit with the receiver in the BTE.[26] With an RIC device, the tubing that is used with other BTE devices is replaced by a thin wire that directs the amplifier output to the receiver.

In-the-Ear Hearing Aids

An ITE hearing aid has all of the components contained in a custom-fitted case that fits into the outer ear or ear canal. A device that fills the outer ear concha is referred to as an ITE hearing aid. A device that is smaller and fits into the ear canal is known as an in-the-canal (ITC) hearing aid. Another device, a CIC hearing aid, is even smaller and fits deeply in the canal. Figure 162-6 shows ITE hearing aids.

Style Considerations

The choice of hearing aid style is based on several important factors. The first consideration is acoustic feedback. The higher the intensity of output, the more likely it is that sound will escape from the ear canal, and feedback will occur. Potential for acoustic feedback is lowest in BTE hearing aids, where the distance between the microphone and loudspeaker is greatest. Feedback potential is also reduced by sealing off the ear canal with a tightly fitting aid or ear mold.[27] Although electronic feedback control has reduced these problems,[22] smaller ITE hearing aids are generally restricted to milder hearing losses.

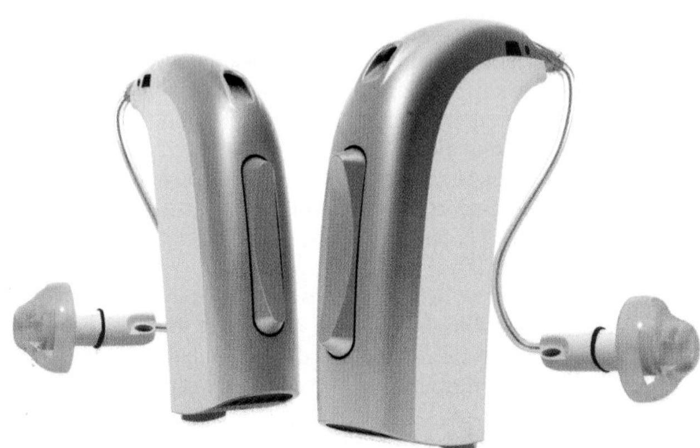

Figure 162-5. Behind-the-ear hearing aids. *(Courtesy of Oticon, Inc., Somerset, NJ.)*

Occlusion of the ear canal creates problems in some patients, and may influence style consideration. Occlusion of the ear canal results in reduced aeration of the external auditory meatus, which may lead to problems associated with external otitis. In addition, a certain amount of hearing loss, known as *insertion loss,* occurs with occlusion of the ear canal while the hearing aid is in place. This occlusion creates hearing loss for patients who have normal low-frequency hearing. Occlusion of the ear canal also causes a phenomenon referred to as the *occlusion effect,* wherein a patient's own voice is perceived as loud and "echoing."[28]

One solution to occlusion problems is the placement of a vent. A vent is simply a passageway for exchange of air and sound around or through a hearing aid or ear mold. The acoustic characteristics of the hearing aid response can be manipulated by the size and type of vent used.[29] Low-frequency amplification can be eliminated, and natural sound can be allowed to pass through the hearing aid for patients with normal low-frequency hearing. Generally, the larger the vent, the more pronounced is the effect. A vent also creates opportunity for acoustic feedback to occur, however, because sound is more likely to escape from the ear canal and be directed into the microphone.[25] The use of an open-canal fit also reduces problems associated with occlusion,[30] with the same feedback-related challenges encountered with venting.

The choice of hearing aid style has an impact on microphone placement. Our ability to localize sound benefits from the natural influences of the auricle and concha. In addition, the auricle and concha increase high-frequency hearing by collecting and resonating sound greater than 2000 Hz. The closer the microphone is to the tympanic membrane, the more the hearing aid can benefit from these natural influences. Conversely, the farther removed the microphone, the more the hearing aid would have to make up for the elimination of these influences. CIC hearing aids can have an advantage over other styles in terms of microphone location.[17] Placing the microphone deeply in the ear canal has other practical advantages, including reduction of wind noise, ease of telephone use, and enhanced listening with headsets and stethoscopes.

Hearing aid style also affects effectiveness of directional microphones. Directional effectiveness is greatest when there is sufficient distance between the microphones located on the hearing aid. Because larger devices such as BTEs and ITEs have microphones that are farther removed from the tympanic membrane, directionality is more of a necessity. Larger devices also have more space available to accommodate optimal microphone placement, so greater directionality is more easily achieved.

An important style consideration relates to durability of the instruments. In ITE instruments, all of the electronic components are placed within the ear canal and are subjected to the detrimental effects of perspiration and cerumen. As a result, repair rates and downtime can be considerably greater for these devices. In contrast, BTE hearing aids have these components housed away from the ear canal, minimizing these effects.

Hearing Assistive Technologies

Assistive technologies other than hearing aids are available for situation-specific hearing, including assistive listening devices (ALDs), alerting

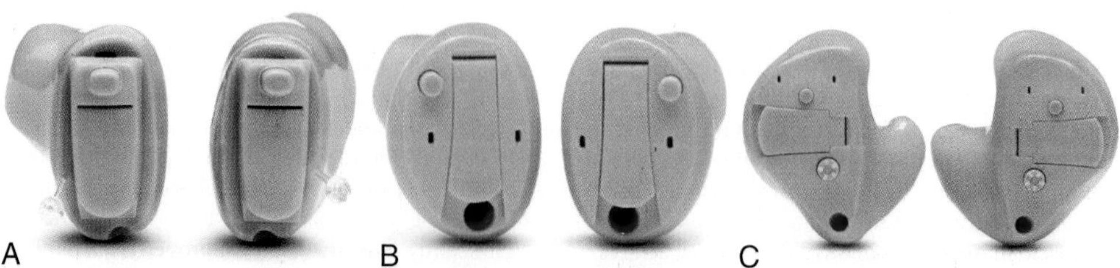

Figure 162-6. In-the-ear hearing aids. **A,** Completely-in-the-canal aids. **B,** In-the-canal aids. **C,** In-the-ear aids. *(Courtesy of Oticon, Inc., Somerset, NJ.)*

and signaling devices, and telephone amplifiers. ALDs include personal amplifiers, FM systems, and television listeners. These devices are designed to enhance an acoustic signal over background noise by the use of a remote microphone. The use of a remote microphone allows the signal to be received by the listener without the degrading effects of distance and reverberation.[13]

Several groups of patients benefit from use of ALDs. Some patients with severe hearing loss do not receive sufficient benefit from hearing aids and find that supplementing hearing aid use with ALDs is necessary. Other individuals with high communication demands in their workplace or social life also benefit from ALDs. Some patients may have communication limitations only in very specific situations, so that general use of a hearing aid is not indicated. An example is a patient who notes difficulty only with watching television or attending a meeting. ALDs tailored to particular needs are often a more appropriate solution in such cases. Some patients have auditory processing disorder that is not accompanied by a loss in hearing sensitivity. Communication difficulties for such patients are characterized by difficulty understanding speech in background noise. For these patients, use of a remote microphone for enhancement of signal-to-noise ratio is more appropriate than amplification from a hearing aid.

A personal FM system is an ALD designed to minimize the effects of noise and distance with a remote microphone. The system consists of two parts, a microphone-transmitter and an amplifier-receiver. The microphone and transmitter are worn by or are close to the speaker. Some transmitters have array microphones that are designed for directionality. The signal is transmitted to the receiver via FM radio waves. The amplifier and receiver are worn by the listener, usually integrated into the hearing aid or coupled to the listener's ear via earphones.[13] Newer forms of wireless coupling of transmitter and receiver are also emerging as a solution for enhancing spatial hearing.[10]

Other assistive technologies are available to provide solutions for specific listening situations. Telephone amplifiers, which are available in several forms, increase the ability to hear on the telephone for many patients. Another commonly used assistive technology is closed captioning of television shows, which allow the viewer to see the spoken dialogue in printed form. Alerting devices, such as alarm clocks, fire alarms, and doorbells, are designed to flash a light or vibrate a bed when activated.

Selection and Fitting Process

The process of hearing aid selection and fitting usually follows this course: selection, quality control, programming, verification, and adjustment. Hearing aids are selected based on the degree and configuration an individual's hearing loss, the individual's communication needs, and other factors relating to style choice. After hearing aid selection, impressions are made of the ear canal for custom ear molds or hearing aids. When the hearing aids are received from the manufacturer, the aids are subjected to quality control of form and electroacoustic function. The hearing aids are programmed based on the patient's audiometric outcomes and needs. Verification of the frequency response is usually made by probe-microphone measurement. A small microphone is placed near the tympanic membrane, and the responses of the hearing aids to speech or speechlike sounds are determined for different levels of input. The hearing aids are adjusted so that the responses approximate the desired targets. The electroacoustic performance is verified further with formal or informal assessment of quality, loudness, or speech perception. The hearing aids may be adjusted again if perceptual expectations are not met.

Target Gain

The fundamental way to specify a starting point for determining the response of a hearing aid is to prescribe frequency-gain characteristics based on audiometric measures.[31] Numerous prescriptive rules have been developed. Some are based on hearing thresholds alone and attempt to specify gain that would amplify average conversational speech to a comfortable or preferred listening level. The half-gain rule prescribes gain equal to one half the amount of hearing loss; the third-gain rule prescribes gain equal to one third of the loss. Most prescriptive rules have this simple approach as a basis, then adjust individual frequencies based on empirically determined correction factors. One popular early threshold-based procedure, which still serves as the basis for some current approaches, is that of the National Acoustic Laboratory.[32]

Another approach is to prescribe frequency-gain characteristics based on threshold and discomfort levels.[31] One notable effort is the desired sensation level (DSL) method.[33] The DSL was originally designed for fitting hearing aids in children, and it prescribed gain based on thresholds and predicted discomfort levels. A newer alternative, the DSL[i/o], is designed to ensure audibility of soft sounds[34] and is used in many modern fitting systems.

Prescriptive procedures were also developed in response to wide-dynamic range compression amplifiers. In these approaches, targets were determined for soft, moderate, and loud sound.[35] More recent procedures combine the linear approach of the early threshold-based prescription methods with different prescription requirements for soft and loud sounds.[31,36]

Other considerations for determining targets include the type of hearing loss and whether one or both ears are being fitted. When there is a conductive component to the hearing loss, target gain is usually increased by approximately 25% of the air-bone gap at a given frequency. When the hearing aid fitting is binaural, the target gain for each ear should be reduced by 3 to 6 dB for binaural summation.[31,37]

Hearing Aid Selection

The process of hearing aid selection first involves assessment of the patient's communication needs and other patient factors that may have an impact on hearing aid use. Appropriateness of the patient for hearing aid candidacy is assessed, and the determination is made whether to pursue hearing aid amplification. This decision is followed by determination of the style and features that would be most appropriate for the patient's hearing loss and communication needs.[38]

The fitting range of a hearing aid is used to determine appropriateness of a hearing aid circuit for a patient's degree and configuration of hearing loss. The fitting range shows the general response curve of the amplifier and is used to determine the ability of a particular hearing aid amplifier to provide necessary gain. This response curve can be manipulated with software controls to reduce or enhance specific frequency ranges to provide the necessary gain for a specific hearing sensitivity. An example is shown in Figure 162-7. Newer hearing aid circuits have a more generic frequency response that can be extensively manipulated, creating a "one-size-fits-many" concept of hearing aid circuitry.

Because of the inherent flexibility of the DSP platform of modern hearing aids, a given hearing aid can be programmed to fit a wide range of degree and configuration of hearing loss. Generally, the factors that separate one hearing aid from another are related to features and processor algorithms, rather than to the frequency gain response of the hearing aid.

Ear Considerations

For most patients, it is best to fit both ears with hearing aids because of the binaural advantage. The brain relies on differences in time and intensity of signals between the ears to localize the source of a sound in the environment.[39] Binaural processing of sound enhances the audibility of speech coming from different directions,[40] and the ability to focus on a desired sound source[41] while suppressing background noise. The use of two ears also improves the perception of sound quality[42] and enhances hearing sensitivity.[37] If a patient has relatively symmetric hearing loss, he or she would benefit more from two hearing aids than from one hearing aid.[41] Evidence suggests that unilateral hearing aid fitting places the unaided ear at a relative disadvantage, which may have a long-term negative effect on the speech perception ability of the unaided ear.[43,44]

Sometimes it is impossible to fit binaural hearing aids effectively. In cases where both ears have hearing loss, but there is significant asymmetry between ears, it is generally more appropriate to fit a hearing aid on the better hearing ear than on the poorer hearing ear.[45,46] This is because fitting the better ear would provide the best aided ability of either monaural fitting. Rarely, in cases of poor speech recognition in

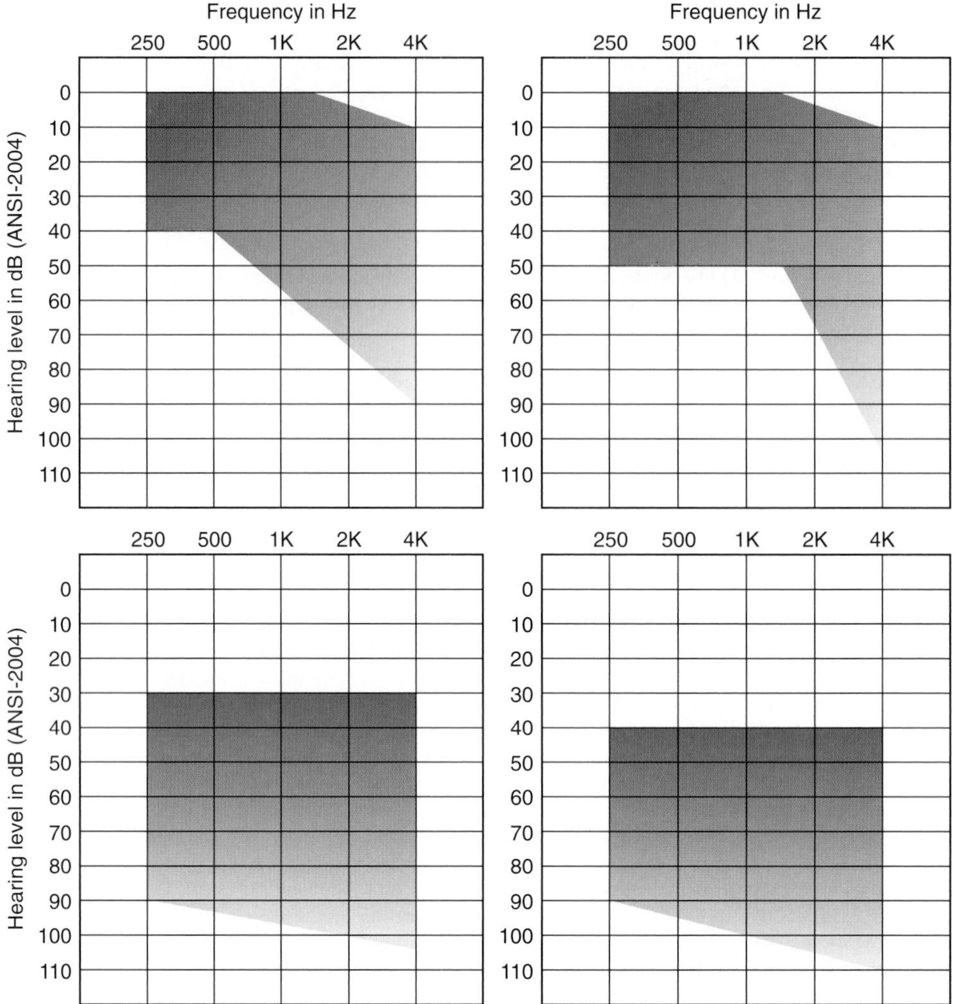

Figure 162-7. Fitting ranges for four different hearing aids, ranging from a mild gain to a power hearing device. ANSI, American National Standards Institute.

one ear, stimulation of the poorer ear can lead to a binaural interference effect, wherein speech understanding is decreased overall.[45,47]

If only one ear has hearing loss, and it can be effectively fitted with a hearing aid, a monaural fitting is indicated. If the poorer ear cannot be effectively fitted, the approach of contralateral routing of signals may be used. A microphone and hearing aid are placed on the poorer or nonhearing ear to deliver signals to the other ear either through bone conduction or via a receiving device worn on the normal-hearing ear.[48]

Other Considerations

Other factors that must be considered in the hearing aid selection process include hearing aid style, directional microphones, occlusion issues, feedback suppression, noise reduction, number and size of user controls, telecoil and other wireless options, and device costs.[38,49] Many of these factors interact with each other because hearing aid manufacturers tend to group availability of features into particular technology levels.

The selection process usually begins with a discussion of hearing aid style. In many cases, the hearing loss may dictate or at least influence this decision. The decision is also influenced by patient preference, which is often based on appearance, convenience issues, or past experience.

The feature/technology level of the hearing aid must also be determined. Grouping of hearing aid features varies among and within manufacturers. Higher levels of technology increase the financial cost of the device.

Some hearing aid selection decisions are made by the provider, and others are made by the patient. The selection of the appropriate feature/technology level involves negotiation with the patient about communication needs and the cost-effectiveness of the various solutions. The communication needs assessment plays a vital role in determination of the hearing aid characteristics that are most important for a given patient. When all of the decisions have been made, the selection is narrowed down to a set of device options. A decision is made regarding specific hearing aids for the patient by comparing these options against the knowledge of devices available from the hearing aid manufacturers.

Fitting and Verification

The general process of fitting and verification includes crafting ear impressions, quality control measures, device programming, verification of fit, and verification of function.

Fitting

The fitting process begins with making impressions of the outer ear and external auditory meatus. The impressions are used by the manufacturer to create custom-fitted ear molds or ITE hearing aids. The quality of the impression dictates the quality of the physical fit of the hearing instruments.

Impression making begins with otoscopic inspection of the ears and ear canals to ensure that they are healthy and suitable for the introduction of impression material. The ear canal is assessed for signs of external otitis and of the tympanic membranes for perforations or inflammation. The inspection process also includes an evaluation of the amount of cerumen in the canals to ensure that they are not impacted or would not become impacted as a result of the impression-making process.

Care must be taken to protect the tympanic membrane and middle ear from impression material. Significant complications have been reported from impression material entering the middle ear space or mastoid cavity.[50,51] For protection, a foam or cotton block is placed deep into the ear canal as a barrier between the tympanic membrane and the impression material. When ear impressions are being made for CIC hearing aids or ear molds for profound hearing loss, very deep impressions of the ear canal are taken, and extra precautions may be necessary. When the blocks are in place, impression material is mixed, and the ear canals are filled. Several types of materials are available for making impressions. Impressions that are silicone-based tend to be more viscous than the powder and liquid forms. It seems likely that additional viscosity should reduce the risk of complications. After the material has set, and the impressions are removed, the ear canals are inspected again to determine that all impression material has been removed, and no trauma has occurred during the impression-making process.

If the ear molds are to be used with BTE hearing aids, decisions are made about the style of ear mold, the material to be used, and the style and size of tubing and venting. Ear mold materials vary in softness and flexibility. Some materials are nonallergenic. The decisions regarding which material and style to use are based on issues relating to comfort and feedback.[27] Decisions regarding bore size, tubing, and venting affect the frequency gain of the hearing aid.

Electroacoustic analyses of the hearing aids are made before programming to ensure that their output meets specified design parameters. This is done with the hearing aid placed in a test chamber of a hearing aid analyzer, in a 2-cc coupler, attached to a microphone. The chamber has a loudspeaker to deliver test signals to the hearing aid. The amplified signal is sent to the analyzer, which is a sophisticated sound-level meter.[52]

Hearing aid analyzers measure the acoustic output of a hearing aid according to specifications of the American National Standards Institute's Standard for Characterizing Hearing Aid Performance (ANSI S3.2-2003).[53] Standard electroacoustic analysis of a hearing aid provides information about the hearing aid's gain, maximum output, and frequency response. It also provides a measure of circuit noise, distortion, and battery drain. Results of this analysis are compared with the hearing aid specifications provided by the manufacturer to ensure that the hearing aid is operating as expected.[52]

Programming of hearing aids is accomplished via computer software that is proprietary for each manufacturer. The basic response of the hearing aid is derived from the patient's audiogram based on a prescriptive target. Manufacturers usually use proprietary targets that match the assumptions underlying their signal processing strategy. Most parameters of the response can be adjusted as indicated. Some decisions are based on patient characteristics, such as age or experience using a hearing aid. New users typically initially prefer less gain than what might be prescribed for their hearing losses after they adjust to the amplification. For experienced users, response settings may vary depending on the type of processing used in the past.

During this initial stage, preliminary decisions are made about management of programming controls. A decision is made as to whether multiple memories are to be used for a given patient, and how the programs are organized among the memories. Decisions are also made regarding the activation of manual controls, telecoil preferences, noise and feedback reduction responses, and level of sensitivity or responsiveness for adaptive technology in hearing aids. The gain response, maximum output, and prescriptive formula are evaluated to determine appropriateness for the patient. These decisions are made based on the particular characteristics of the device and patient factors, including age and cognitive abilities, degree and configuration of hearing loss, patient experience with hearing aids, and communication needs.

After programming, the physical fit of the device is assessed. Appropriateness, comfort, and security of the fit are determined, as are the absence of feedback and appropriateness of the microphone location. If the fit is inadequate, the hearing aids or ear molds can be modified. Assessment of occlusion effect is typically made by patient perception of his or her own voice, and alterations are made if necessary. The patient's ability to insert and remove the devices and manipulate controls independently is also determined.

Verification

The overall process of verifying suitability of hearing aids includes objective measurements of gain and frequency response from the hearing aids in the ear canal, adjustment of parameters to meet targets for gain and frequency response, and subjective judgments from patients regarding sound quality.

As sound leaves the hearing aid, it is modified by the resonance characteristics of the physical features of the ear canal. The methods for prescriptive gain for the hearing aid take into account the physical characteristics of average ears and must be adjusted for individual variations. The characteristics of transducers can also vary slightly across hearing aids. The output of the hearing aid in the ear canal itself must be verified with real-ear testing. This testing assesses whether the targeted gains are achieved across the frequency range for a given input to the hearing aid. The most commonly used real-ear tests are probe-microphone measurements.

Probe-microphone measurements are made using a spectrum analyzer that delivers various types of signals to a loudspeaker located near the ears of a patient. A small thin tube is inserted into the ear canal down close to the tympanic membrane. The other end of the tube is attached to a sensitive microphone that records sound from deep in the ear canal. This tube allows for measurement of the acoustic changes that occur owing to the resonance of the patient's pinna and ear canal.[54-56]

With the probe tube in place, speech or speechlike sounds are presented through the loudspeaker at a given intensity level, and measurements are made of sound in the ear canal without a hearing aid in place. This measurement is called the real-ear unaided response or gain (REUR/G). Next, the same sounds are presented with the patient's hearing aid in place and functioning. This measurement is called the real-ear aided response or gain (REAR/G). The difference between the aided response and the unaided response (REAG – REUG) is the real-ear insertion gain (REIG). The REIG provides information about the amount of sound that the hearing aid adds when it is in place in the ear. This process is typically performed for low-intensity, average-intensity, and high-intensity signals. If the response does not match the expected target, programming changes are made to the hearing aid until the target is approximated.[54-57]

Another approach to probe-microphone measurements is known as *speech mapping*. In this case, the signal presented through the loudspeaker is low-intensity, average-intensity, and high-intensity speech. The response of the hearing aid is measured near the patient's tympanic membrane, and adjustments are made to approximate targets for speech input. Live speech, such as from a spouse, can also be used to examine the audibility of a particular voice with the hearing aid programming. This process results in verification that the amplified signal being delivered to a patient's tympanic membrane meets prescriptive targets for different input levels. If the targets are correct, when the patient is wearing the hearing aids, low-intensity sounds should be audible, average sounds should be comfortable, and high-intensity sounds should be loud but tolerable.[58]

After objective verification measures, the quality of the amplified sound is assessed with some form of subjective quality judgments or functional intelligibility procedures. Perceptual verification is done in many ways, informally and formally. Strategies include speech perception judgments, loudness judgment ratings, functional gain measurement, and speech recognition measures.

Orientation, Counseling, and Follow-up

After the completion of hearing aid fitting and verification, the patient is oriented to the hearing aid and its use. Areas addressed typically include components and functioning of the hearing aids, battery use, and care and maintenance of the hearing aids. One of the most crucial aspects of the hearing aid orientation is discussion of reasonable expectations of hearing aid use and strategies for adapting to different listening environments.[59] The goal of the hearing aid orientation is for the patient to learn how to use their hearing aid effectively.[60,61]

At the end of the orientation and counseling session, patients are typically scheduled for a follow-up visit. At the follow-up appointment, benefit and satisfaction with the hearing aid are assessed, and any necessary adjustments are made. It is often at this follow-up that outcome measures are made to ensure that the patient's communication needs are being met and to help in planning of any additional rehabilitative services.

Outcome Measurement

The goal of the hearing treatment process is to reduce the communication disorder imposed by a hearing loss. We generally define success at reaching this goal in terms of whether the patient understands speech better with the hearing aid, and whether the hearing aid helps to reduce the handicapping influence of hearing impairment. Outcome measures are designed to assess the impact of hearing aid use on communication. Self-assessment scales can be administered before and after amplification use to determine whether the hearing aids have had a positive impact in reducing communication disorder resulting from hearing loss.[62] Assessments may also be completed by spouses or other individuals who are affected by the hearing loss.

Patient perceptions of hearing ability and challenges are measured with self-assessment tools such as the Hearing Handicap Inventory for the Elderly (HHIE),[63] the Abbreviated Profile of Hearing Aid Benefit (APHAB),[64] and the Client Oriented Scale of Improvement (COSI).[65] Quality-of-life measures are used to determine how hearing aid amplification affects overall well-being. Measures such as the Glasgow Hearing Aid Benefit Profile (GHABP)[66] and the International Outcome Inventory—Hearing Aids (IOI-HA)[67] can help to measure the impact of audiologic treatment on quality of life.

Special Considerations Based on Patient Age

Infants and Children

Hearing aid selection and fitting for infants and children are more challenging than for adults for many reasons.[68-70] There is a smaller volume of space between the end of the ear mold and the tympanic membrane in children, owing to the smaller size of the ear canal, resulting in higher sound pressure levels delivered to the ear than in adults. Children also have different resonance characteristics than adults, which means that certain frequencies are emphasized more than others. In addition, because children are growing over time, these physical factors change, and must be regularly accounted for in hearing aid adjustments.[71]

Another major difference between hearing aid selection and fitting with children is that there is often considerably less information known about the hearing loss in a child compared with an adult.[70] This situation complicates the ability to prescribe gain in a hearing aid when fitting a child. Children are also less able to participate in the selection and fitting process and to provide useful information regarding perception of hearing aid sound quality and function.

There are important factors to consider regarding hearing aid use in children.[70] First, because children are still in the process of learning speech and language, it is crucial to provide consistent and undistorted auditory input.[72] Although adult knowledge of speech and language can fill in for missing or distorted input, children learning language through the auditory system have no linguistic basis for doing so. Second, children have less ability to control their listening environment than adults to maximize audibility. They also have less control over their hearing aids because most controls are disabled to protect against the child accidentally reducing the gain of the aid inappropriately.[71] Third, because of fluctuating hearing loss, such as that from otitis media with effusion, hearing may be more variable in young children.

Some general guidelines exist for fitting hearing aids on children. Children are always fitted with binaural hearing aids to maximize audibility, unless contraindicated by medical factors or extreme hearing asymmetry. BTE hearing aids are used in most cases because the auricle and ear canal grow in size, requiring that the custom portion of the hearing aid be changed frequently while the child is young; this is most appropriately accomplished by remaking the ear mold of a BTE, rather than an entire custom hearing aid. Soft material is used for ear molds, and the ear molds are connected to pediatric ear hooks for proper fitting.[71] BTE hearing aids are also indicated because flexibility in the fitting range of the hearing aid is necessary. Detailed information regarding the hearing loss may be incomplete at the time of the hearing aid fitting because of patient age. If the hearing loss fluctuates because of progressive hearing loss or otitis media with effusion, the BTE hearing aid allows for greater programming flexibility. Another advantage of BTE hearing aids for children is the nearly universal capacity for access to devices from remote microphones. The use of direct audio input, telecoils, and other wireless techniques are important for classroom and other listening environments to maximize the ability of the child to understand the teacher in a noisy classroom situation.[12]

The making of ear impressions can be challenging in a young child. If a child is sedated for the purpose of auditory brainstem response testing or surgical procedures, such as placement of pressure equalization tubes, this procedure can be readily accomplished at that time.

Prescriptive targets for hearing aid gain have been developed for children. An example is the DSL[i/o] approach.[34] These targets can be verified by probe-microphone measurements, which is even more important in pediatric ears because of the variability in ear canal size and its impact on the acoustic response of the hearing aid. Because of the difficulty of making real-ear measurements in children, a different measure, known as the real-ear coupler difference, is often useful. In this case, resonance characteristics of the child's ear are determined by making a single probe-tube measurement with a hearing aid in place. This measurement is compared with the resonance characteristics of a 2-cc coupler. Use of the coupler for measurement minimizes the impact of the patient's cooperation on verification procedures.[71,73,74]

Functional measures are more frequently made for pediatric patients than for adult patients to verify the appropriateness of hearing aid output.[75] Functional gain is the difference between the threshold with the hearing aid and without the hearing aid. Another useful functional measure is speech recognition with the hearing aids. Speech targets can be presented in the presence of background competition. The task of the child is to identify the correct speech stimulus, usually through a picture-pointing task. Aided results can be compared with unaided results and to expectations for normal hearing ability under similar circumstances.

Aging Patients

In some older patients, hearing loss sensitivity is compounded by changes in central auditory nervous system function. The consequence of such changes is typically reduction in speech recognition even in quiet, reduced temporal processing of auditory information, and reduced ability to hear speech in background noise because of diminished ability to use two ears to localize sound. Patients with significant changes in auditory nervous system function do not seem to benefit as much from hearing aid devices as their younger counterparts.[76] In fitting hearing aids for older patients, strategies designed to improve listening in background noise, such as the use of directional microphones,[19,77] noise-reduction processing, and use of remote microphones, are likely to improve patient benefit.

Another important consideration for fitting hearing aids in older patients is that there may be greater difficulty with physical manipulation of the hearing aid, owing to arthritis and other conditions.[6,78] Diminished vision may also be a problem.[79] Additionally, patients with cognitive decline may have difficulty remembering how to use or maintain their hearing aids effectively,[80] and in general may have greater difficulty understanding speech, even when speech is made audible with hearing aids.

Hearing Aids: Some Rules of Thumb

Most otolaryngologists encounter patients with medically intractable hearing loss on a daily basis in their clinics. Many clinicians do not have the opportunity to stay abreast of changes in hearing aid technology or fitting approaches. Patients seek their counsel about the appropriateness of devices. Although the details may change quickly, there are some rules of thumb that have withstood the test of time, as follows:

"Two ears are better than one." Most patients hear better with binaural amplification, are more satisfied with sound quality and with hearing in noise, and find better overall benefit.

"Bigger is better." BTE hearing aids are considerably more durable than ITEs, are often less conspicuous, are easier to get a comfortable fit, have fewer feedback issues, can have more features, have a longer battery life, and are easier to manipulate.

"It's about communication not the audiogram." If a patient is having difficulty communicating because of sensorineural hearing loss and is motivated for an amplification solution, one can be found.

"If you haven't tried a hearing aid in 2 years, you haven't tried a hearing aid." There is a technology arms race out there, and the result is higher quality devices, more flexible fitting opportunities, and better quality-of-life outcomes.

SUGGESTED READINGS

Aazh H, Moore BCJ. The value of routine real ear measurement of the gain of digital hearing aids. *J Am Acad Audiol.* 2007;18:653.

Byrne D, Dillon H, Ching T, et al. NAL-NL1 procedure for fitting nonlinear hearing aids: characteristics and comparisons with other procedures. *J Am Acad Audiol.* 2001;12:37.

Cornelisse LE, Seewald RC, Jamieson DG. The input/output [i/o] formula: a theoretical approach to the fitting of personal amplification devices. *J Acoust Soc Am.* 1995;97:1854.

Cox R, Alexander G. The International Outcome Inventory for Hearing Aids (IOI-HA): psychometric properties of the English version. *Int J Audiol.* 2002;41:30.

Dillon H. *Hearing Aids.* New York: Thieme; 2002.

Dillon H, James A, Ginis J. The Client Oriented Scale of Improvement (COSI) and its relationship to several other measures of benefit and satisfaction provided by hearing aids. *J Am Acad Audiol.* 1997;8:27.

Flamme GA. Localization, hearing impairment, and hearing aids. *Hear J.* 2002;55:10.

Jerger J, Silman S, Lew HL, et al. Case studies in binaural interference: converging evidence from behavioral and electrophysiologic measures. *J Am Acad Audiol.* 1993;4:122.

For complete list of references log onto www.expertconsult.com.

Kates JM. *Digital Hearing Aids.* San Diego: Plural Publishing; 2008.

Kricos PB. Audiologic management of older adults with hearing loss and compromised cognitive/psychoacoustic auditory processing capabilities. *Trends Amplification.* 2006;10:1.

Levitt H. A historical perspective on digital hearing aids: how digital technology has changed modern hearing aids. *Trends Amplification.* 2007;11:7.

Lewis DE. Hearing instrument selection and fitting in children. In: Valente M, Hosford-Dunn H, Roeser RJ, eds. *Audiology: Treatment.* New York: Thieme Medical Publishing; 2000:149.

Lybarger S. A historical overview. In: Sandlin RE, ed. *Handbook of Hearing Aid Amplification.* Vol I. Boston: College-Hill Press; 1988:1.

Moore BCJ. Dead regions in the cochlea: conceptual foundations, diagnosis, and clinical applications. *Ear Hear.* 2004;25:98.

Moore BCJ. Speech mapping is a valuable tool for fitting and counseling patients. *Hear J.* 2006;59:26.

Mormer E, Palmer C. A systematic program for hearing aid orientation and adjustment. In: Sweetow R, ed. *Counseling for Hearing Aid Fittings.* San Diego: Singular Publishing Group; 1999:165.

Revit LJ. Real-ear measures. In: Valente M, Hosford-Dunn H, Roeser RJ, eds. *Audiology Treatment.* New York: Thieme; 2000:105.

Ricketts TA, Hornsby BWY, Johnson EE. Adaptive directional benefit in the near field: competing sound angle and level effects. *Semin Hear.* 2005; 26:59.

Sammeth CA, Levitt H. Hearing aid selection and fitting in adults: history and evolution. In: Valente M, Hosford-Dunn H, Roeser RJ, eds. *Audiology Treatment.* New York: Thieme; 2000:213.

Silverman CA, Silman S. Apparent auditory deprivation from monaural amplification and recovery with binaural amplification. *J Am Acad Audiol.* 1990;1:175.

Stach BA. *Clinical Audiology: An Introduction.* San Diego: Singular Publishing Group; 1998.

Valente M, Valente M, Potts LG, et al. Earhooks, tubing, earmolds, and shells. In: Valente M, Hosford-Dunn H, Roeser RJ, eds. *Audiology Treatment.* New York: Thieme; 2000:59.

Venema TH. *Compression for Clinicians.* San Diego: Singular Publishing Group; 1998.

Wilson C, Stephens D. Reasons for referral and attitudes toward hearing aids: do they affect outcome? *Clin Otolaryngol Allied Sci.* 2003;28:81.

Wynne MK, Kahn JM, Abel DJ, et al. External and middle ear trauma resulting from ear impressions. *J Am Acad Audiol.* 2000;11:351.

SECTION SEVEN

Vestibular Disorders

CHAPTER ONE HUNDRED AND SIXTY-THREE

Principles of Applied Vestibular Physiology

John P. Carey

Charles C. Della Santina

Key Points

- The vestibular system primarily drives reflexes to maintain stable vision and posture.
- By modulating the non-zero baseline firing of vestibular afferent nerve fibers, semicircular canals encode rotation of the head, and otolith organs encode linear acceleration and tilt.
- Stimulation of a semicircular canal produces eye movements in the plane of that canal.
- A semicircular canal normally is excited by rotation in the plane of the canal bringing the head toward the ipsilateral side.
- Any stimulus that excites a semicircular canal's afferents will be interpreted as excitatory rotation in the plane of that canal.
- High-acceleration head rotation in the excitatory direction of a canal elicits a greater response than does the same rotation in the inhibitory direction.
- The response to simultaneous canal stimuli is approximately the sum of the responses to each stimulus alone.
- Nystagmus due to dysfunction of semicircular canals has a fixed axis and direction with respect to the head.
- Brainstem circuitry boosts low-frequency vestibulo-ocular reflex (VOR) performance through velocity storage and neural integration. Failure of these mechanisms suggests a central pathologic process.
- The utricle senses both head tilt and translation, but loss of unilateral utricular function is interpreted by the brain as a head tilt toward the opposite side.
- Sudden changes in saccular activity evoke changes in postural tone.
- The normal vestibular system can rapidly adjust the vestibular reflexes according to the context, but adaptation to unilateral loss of vestibular function may be slow and susceptible to decompensation.

This chapter presents an approach to the vestibular system that provides a basis for understanding the evaluation and management of vestibular disorders described in subsequent chapters. The chapter is organized around 12 basic principles of vestibular system function, reviewing the physiologic underpinnings of each and illustrating their importance in clinical findings when appropriate. This core set of organizing principles can help clinicians quickly recognize the significance of findings on the vestibular exam and precisely localize peripheral vestibular problems to the affected end organs.

Several reviews can be consulted for further explanations of vestibular physiology.[1-4]

Principles

Principle 1: The Vestibular System Primarily Drives Reflexes to Maintain Stable Vision and Posture

Anatomic and Physiologic Basis

The vestibular system's main function is to sense head movements, especially involuntary ones, and counter them with reflexive eye movements and postural adjustments that keep the visual world stable and keep us from falling. The labyrinth of the inner ear senses head rotation and linear acceleration and sends that information to secondary vestibular neurons in the brainstem vestibular nuclei. Secondary vestibular neuron signals diverge to other areas of the central nervous system to drive vestibular reflexes. Specifically, neurons encoding head movement form synapses within the ocular motor nuclei to elicit the patterns of extraocular muscle contraction and relaxation needed for the vestibulo-ocular reflex (VOR), which stabilizes gaze (eye position in space). Other secondary vestibular neurons synapse on cervical spinal motor neurons to generate the vestibulocolic reflex (VCR), or to lower spinal motor neurons to generate the vestibulospinal reflexes (VSRs). These reflexes stabilize posture and facilitate gait. Vestibular sensory input to autonomic centers, particularly information about posture with respect to gravity, is used to adjust hemodynamic reflexes to maintain cerebral perfusion. Finally, vestibular input to the cerebellum is essential for coordination and adaptation of vestibular reflexes when changes occur such as injury to a vestibular end organ or alteration in vision (e.g., a new pair of glasses).

Vestibular signals also reach cortical areas to mediate the perception of movement and orientation. Nevertheless, the common head movements of everyday life usually go unnoticed, which is why vestibular sensation is not included among the vernacular "five senses"—sight, smell, taste, touch, and hearing. Yet the loss of vestibular sensation causes distinct and often severe symptoms. This distress has perhaps been best captured in the first-hand account of J.C., a physician who lost his vestibular sense to an ototoxic aminoglycoside antibiotic: "By bracing my head between two of the metal bars at the head of the bed I found I could minimize the effect of the pulse beat that made the letters on the page jump and blur… In these corridors I had the peculiar sensation that I was inside a flexible tube, fixed at the end nearest me but swaying free at the far end."[5]

Like many other patients who have lost vestibular function, J.C. soon recovered and resumed most of his usual activities without the distressing sense of *oscillopsia*, the perception that the world is moving whenever the head is moved. This recovery is due to a combination of central adaptation to abnormal vestibular signals and the use of information from other sensory systems that provide information about movement and posture. For example, somatosensory information from proprioceptive sensors in the limbs contributes to the sense of vertical body orientation.[6] Proprioceptors in the neck mediate a cervico-ocular reflex that can augment the deficient VOR.[7,8] Likewise, postural information may be supplied by gravity receptors in the major blood vessels and abdominal viscera.[9] Because head movements may be also sensed by their impact on the retinal image, vision-based oculomotor systems can partly supplant a deficient VOR. For example, smooth pursuit is a type of reflexive eye movement that helps to stabilize images on the retina. During smooth pursuit, movement of a target image on the retina causes a conjugate following movement of the eyes to keep the target fixed on the fovea. The stimulus for this reflex is the difference between the velocity of the visual target and the velocity of the eye, which is called *retinal slip velocity*. This visual error is computed by the primary visual cortex; transmitted to the middle temporal, parietal, and frontal cortices; and forwarded to the brainstem and cerebellum to generate the oculomotor command signals. The multiple synapses involved in this reflex impose a long latency (approximately 100 msec), and the reflex breaks down at relatively modest velocities (more than approximately 50 degrees/second)[10] and frequencies (more than approximately 1 Hz).[11] Optokinetic nystagmus, which elicits eye rotation in response to optic flow of the visual scene, operates over a range of velocities and frequencies similar to smooth pursuit.[12] These limitations make these visually driven reflexes inadequate to stabilize vision during many common head movements. For example, the head pitches up and down at a frequency of approximately 2 Hz and velocity of approximately 90 degrees/second during walking, while during running head pitch harmonics may extend to 15 to 20 Hz. Voluntary head-on-body horizontal rotations can reach 800 degrees/second and can also have significant harmonics to 15 to 20 Hz.[13]

The limitations of smooth pursuit and optokinetic nystagmus illustrate the important concept that reflexive sensorimotor systems have optimal operating ranges. Smooth visual pursuit functions best for low-frequency and slow head movements. Autonomic gravity receptors function best for static and very-low-frequency conditions. These and other reflexes overlap with the vestibular system for part of its operating range, but nonvestibular systems largely break down during quick head movements. Therefore, the vestibular system is essential for gaze stabilization during *high-frequency*, *high-velocity*, and *high-acceleration* head movements.

Clinical Importance

The reflexive nature of the vestibular system is central to understanding vestibular pathophysiology. The brainstem interprets imbalances in vestibular input due to pathologic processes in the same way that it interprets imbalances due to physiologic stimuli. Therefore, the cardinal signs of vestibular disorders are reflexive eye movements and postural changes. These reflexive signs can largely be understood as the brainstem's responses to *perceived* rotation around a specific axis or *perceived* tilting or translation of the head, even though the head is still and upright. Knowing the effective stimulus for each vestibular end-organ allows determination of which end organ or combination of end organs must be stimulated to produce the observed motor output. Working backwards in this fashion, the end organs affected by pathology can usually be inferred.

In interpreting reflexive eye movements and postural changes in the search for vestibular dysfunction, an important consideration is that vestibular reflexes may be observed only in isolation under certain conditions. For many conditions, in fact, other reflexive systems can compensate for the loss of vestibular reflexes, thereby masking any deficit. For example, a patient with well-compensated, longstanding bilateral loss of vestibular function may surprisingly appear to have no problem keeping vision fixed on the examiner as the examiner rotates the patient's head slowly from side to side. In such persons, smooth pursuit, optokinetic nystagmus, and (to a lesser extent) the cervico-ocular reflex make up for the vestibular deficit. This is an example of a head movement that *can* be sensed by the vestibular system, but which is not in the range of frequencies and accelerations sensed *exclusively* by the vestibular system. However, when the examiner suddenly and rapidly rotates the head to either side, the eyes do not stay on target. The vestibular deficit can thus be unmasked by very dynamic head movements.

Principle 2: By Modulating the Non-Zero Baseline Firing of Vestibular Afferent Nerve Fibers, Semicircular Canals Encode Rotation of the Head, and Otolith Organs Encode Linear Acceleration and Tilt

Anatomic and Physiologic Basis

Sensory Transduction

The labyrinth of the inner ear houses a set of inertial sensors that detect rotary and linear acceleration. Each bony labyrinth encloses a membranous labyrinth consisting of three semicircular canals arrayed roughly at right angles to each other and two roughly orthogonal otolith organs, the utricle and saccule (Fig. 163-1). Semicircular canals primarily sense rotational acceleration of the head. The utricle and saccule primarily sense linear acceleration in horizontal and vertical (superoinferior) directions, respectively.

Sensation by semicircular canals works as follows. When the head accelerates in the plane of a semicircular canal, inertia causes the endolymph in the canal to lag behind the motion of the membranous canal, much as coffee in a mug initially remains in place as the mug is rotated about it. Relative to the canal walls, the endolymph effectively moves in the opposite direction as the head. Inside the ampulla, a swelling at the end of the canal where it meets the utricle, pressure exerted by endolymph deflects the cupula, an elastic membrane that spans a cross-section of the ampulla[14] (Fig. 163-2). Vestibular hair cells are arrayed beneath the cupula on the surface of the crista ampullaris, a saddle-shaped neuroepithelium. Hair cells are so named for tufts of stereocilia that project from their apical surfaces. These stereociliary bundles are coupled to the cupula so that its deflection creates a shearing stress between the stereocilia and the cuticular plates at the tops of the hair cells.

Stereocilia deflection is the common mechanism by which all hair cells transduce mechanical forces (Fig. 163-3). Stereocilia within a bundle are linked to one another by protein strands called "tip links" that span from the side of a taller stereocilium to the tip of its shorter neighbor in the array. The tip links are believed to act as gating springs for mechanically sensitive ion channels, meaning that the tip links literally tug at molecular gates in the stereocilia.[15,16] These gates, which are cation channels, open or close (or, more precisely, spend more or less time in the open state), depending on the direction in which the stereocilia are deflected. When deflected in the open or "on" direction, which is toward the tallest stereocilium, cations, including potassium ions from the potassium-rich endolymph, rush in through the gates, and the membrane potential of the hair cell becomes more positive (see Fig. 163-3B, C). This in turn activates voltage-sensitive calcium channels at the basolateral aspect of the hair cell, and an influx of calcium leads to an increase in the release of excitatory neurotransmitters, principally glutamate, from hair cell synapses onto the vestibular primary afferents (see Fig. 163-3D). All of the hair cells on a semicircular canal crista are oriented or "polarized" in the same direc-

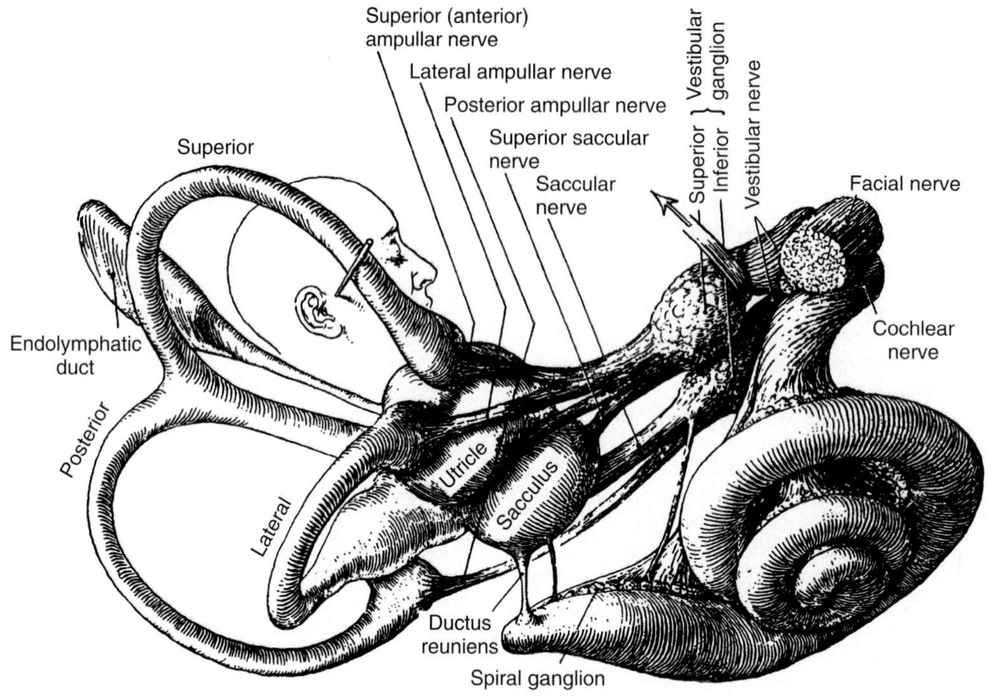

Figure 163-1. The vestibular end organs. *(From Brodel M.* Three Unpublished Drawings of the Anatomy of the Human Ear. *Philadelphia: WB Saunders; 1946.)*

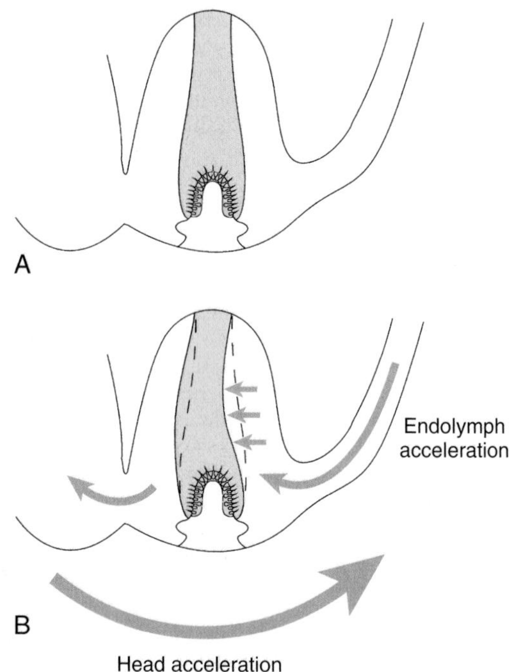

Figure 163-2. A, The cupula spans the lumen of the ampulla from the crista to the membranous labyrinth. **B,** Head acceleration exceeds endolymph acceleration. The relative flow of endolymph in the canal is therefore opposite to the direction of head acceleration. This flow produces a pressure across the elastic cupula, which deflects in response.

tion. That is to say that their stereociliary bundles all have the tall ends pointing the same way, so that the endolymph motion that is excitatory for one hair cell will be excitatory for all of the hair cells on that crista (Fig. 163-4).

The otolith organs sense linear accelerations. These organs contain sheets of hair cells on a sensory epithelium called a *macula* (Fig. 163-5). A gelatinous membrane sits atop the macula, and microscopic stones made of calcium carbonate, the *otoliths* (or *otoconia*), are embedded on the surface of this otolithic membrane. The *sacculus* (or *saccule*), located on the medial wall of the vestibule of the labyrinth in the spherical recess, has its macula oriented vertically. Gravity therefore tonically pulls the saccular otolithic mass inferiorly when the head is upright. The *utriculus* (or *utricle*) is located above the saccule in the elliptical recess of the vestibule. Its macula is oriented in roughly the same plane as the horizontal semicircular canal, although its anterior end curves upward. When the head tilts out of the upright position, the component of the gravitational vector that is tangential to the macula creates a shearing force on stereocilia of utricular hair cells. The cellular transduction process is identical to that described above for the crista. However, the hair cells of the maculae, unlike those of the cristae, are not all polarized in the same direction (Fig. 163-6). Instead, they are oriented relative to a curving central zone known as the *striola*. The utricular striola forms a C shape, with the open side pointing medially. The striola divides the utricular macula into a medial two thirds (polarized to be excited by downward tilt of the ipsilateral ear) and a lateral one third polarized in the opposite direction. Hair cells of the sacculus point away from its striola, which curves and hooks superiorly in its anterior portion. Each macula is essentially a linear accelerometer, with the saccular macula encoding acceleration roughly within a parasagittal plane (along the naso-occipital and superoinferior axes), and the utricular macula encoding linear acceleration roughly in an axial plane (along the naso-occipital and interaural axes). A given linear acceleration may produce a complex pattern of excitation and inhibition across the two maculas (Fig. 163-7), a pattern that encodes the direction and magnitude of the linear acceleration.[17] By contrast, each of the three semicircular canals senses just a one-dimensional component of rotational acceleration.

Modulation of neurotransmitter release from hair cells within each vestibular endorgan modulates the action potential frequency, or *firing rate*, of vestibular nerve afferent fibers (Fig. 163-8). The afferents have a baseline rate of firing, probably due to a baseline rate of release of neurotransmitter from the vestibular hair cells. Changes in vestibular nerve afferent firing are conveyed to secondary neurons in the brainstem. Baseline firing gives the system the important property of *bidirectional sensitivity*: Firing can increase for excitatory head movements and decrease for inhibitory head movements.[18] Thus, loss of one

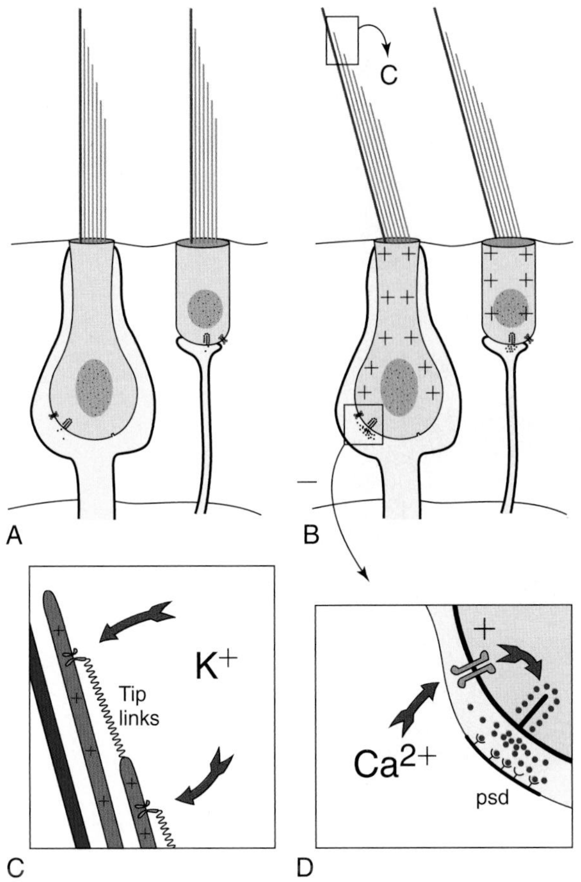

Figure 163-3. Sensory transduction by vestibular hair cells. **A,** At rest there is some baseline release of excitatory glutamate from the hair cell synapses onto the vestibular afferents. **B,** Hair cells are depolarized when the stereocilia are deflected in the "on" direction (toward the kinocilium, in dark blue). **C,** This occurs because the stretched tip links mechanically open cationic channels in the stereocilia membranes. The influx of potassium ions raises the hair cell's membrane potential. **D,** The increased membrane potential activates voltage-sensitive calcium channels in the basolateral membrane of the cell. Synaptic release of glutamate increases, and receptors in the postsynaptic (*psd*) density on the afferent increase its membrane potential, which in turn increases afferent firing rate.

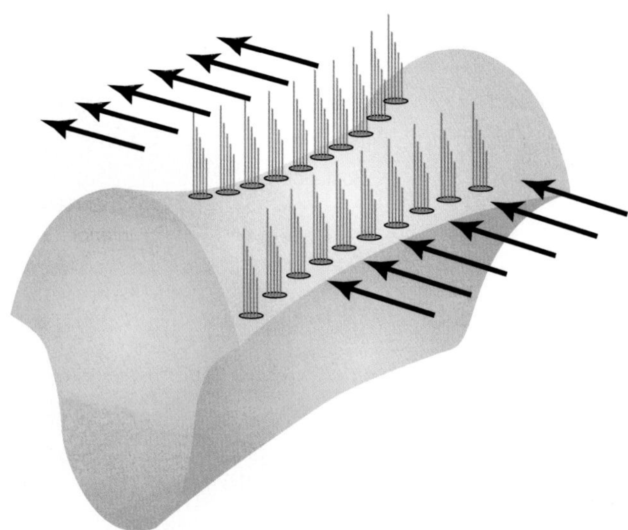

Figure 163-4. Morphologic polarization of the stereociliary bundles in the crista ampullaris. The "on" direction of deflection is always toward the kinocilium, which is next to the tallest stereocilium. Hair cells on the crista ampullaris of a given semicircular canal have all their stereocilia polarized in the same direction.

labyrinth does not mean loss of the ability to sense one half of the head's movements.

Response of the Cupula

How a semicircular canal encodes head rotation can be understood using a mathematical model of a fluid-filled *torsional pendulum*.[4] Figure 163-9 depicts the mechanical forces acting on the left horizontal semicircular canal seen from above during counterclockwise head rotation through angle $H(t)$ in the plane of the canal. Head rotation carries the membranous semicircular canal along with it, whereas the inertia of the endolymph and cupula tend to keep these elements stationary in space (like the coffee in a mug as the mug is quickly turned). Nevertheless, two things act to accelerate the endolymph in the same direction that the head is turning but through the smaller angle $X(t)$. The first is the elastic or spring-like push from the distended cupula as it pushes against the endolymph (deep blue in Fig. 163-9). The second is the viscous drag exerted on the endolymph at its interface with the walls of the membranous canal.

Recall that for linear motion, Newton's Second Law states that $\sum F = ma$, where $\sum F$ is the sum of all applied forces, m is mass, and a is the resultant acceleration. For rotational motion, the analogous equation is $\sum T = I\alpha$, where T is torque, I is the moment of inertia, and α is rotational acceleration. For the rotating semicircular canal, the equation can be written

$$\sum T = T_{elastic} + T_{viscous} = I\ddot{X}(t). \qquad \text{Eq. 163-1}$$

Equation 163-1 says that the sum of the elastic and viscous torques acts on the moment of inertia I of the endolymph and cupula to accelerate the endolymph through space by $\ddot{X}(t)$. (Overdots are used to denote time derivatives, so $X(t)$, $\dot{X}(t)$, and $\ddot{X}(t)$ are endolymph rotational position, velocity, and acceleration, respectively.)

The elastic torque exerted by the cupula is proportional to the deflection of the cupula from its resting position (light blue in Fig. 163-9). That deflection is given by the difference between how far the head moves in space and how far the endolymph moves in space:

$$\Theta(t) = H(t) - X(t). \qquad \text{Eq. 163-2}$$

Thus, the elastic torque is

$$T_{elastic} = K\Theta(t). \qquad \text{Eq. 163-3}$$

The viscous torque is proportional to the velocity of the endolymph relative to the walls of the canal. Differentiation of Equation 163-2 gives this relative endolymph velocity:

$$\dot{\Theta}(t) = \dot{H}(t) - \dot{X}(t). \qquad \text{Eq. 163-4}$$

Therefore,

$$T_{viscous} = B\dot{\Theta}(t). \qquad \text{Eq. 163-5}$$

Finally, to get endolymph acceleration, $\ddot{X}(t)$, we differentiate Equation 163-2 and rewrite it as

$$\ddot{X}(t) = \ddot{H}(t) - \ddot{\Theta}(t) \qquad \text{Eq. 163-6}$$

Now Equation 163-1 can be written as

$$K\Theta(t) + B\dot{\Theta}(t) = I\ddot{H}(t) - I\ddot{\Theta}(t). \qquad \text{Eq. 163-7}$$

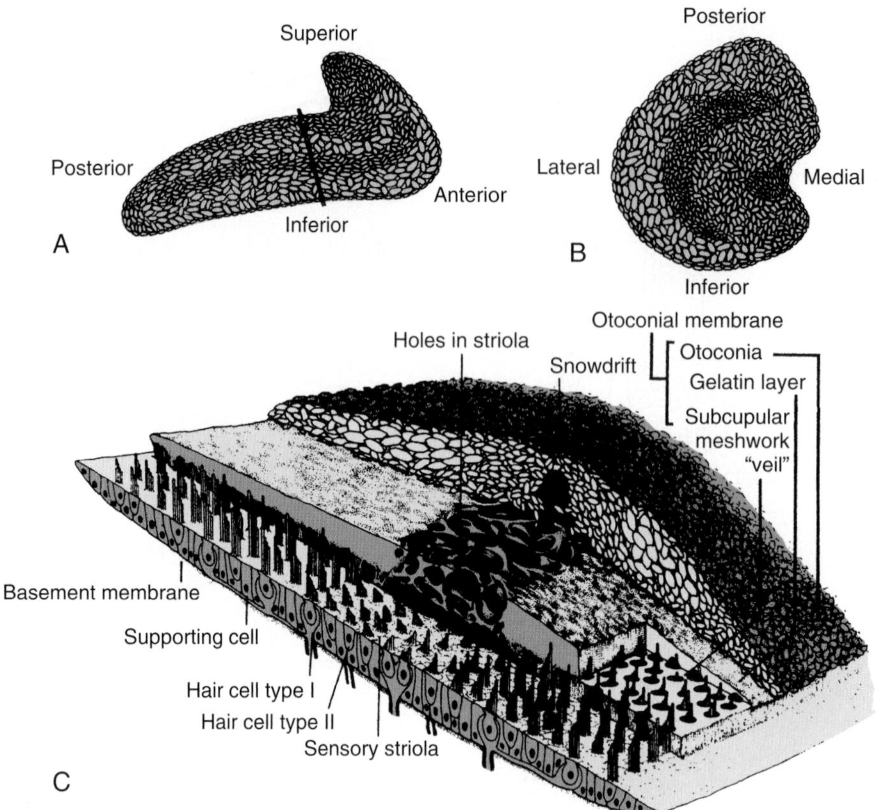

Figure 163-5. Arrangement of otoliths in the two maculae. **A,** Saccule. **B,** Utricle. **C,** Composition of the saccular otoconial membrane in a section taken at the level shown in **A.** *(From Paparella MM, Shumrick DA, eds.* Textbook of Otolaryngology. *Vol 1. Philadelphia: WB Saunders; 1980.)*

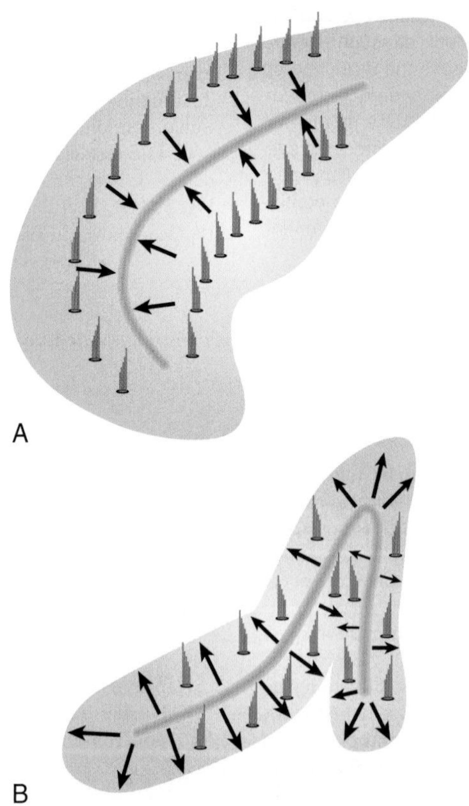

Figure 163-6. Morphologic polarizations of the stereociliary bundles in the maculae of the utricle (**A**) and saccule (**B**). The "on" direction of stereociliary deflection is indicated by the *arrows*. In the utricle (**A**), hair cells are excited by stereociliary deflection toward the striola *(curving central zone)*. In the saccule (**B**), hair cells are excited by stereociliary deflection away from the striola.

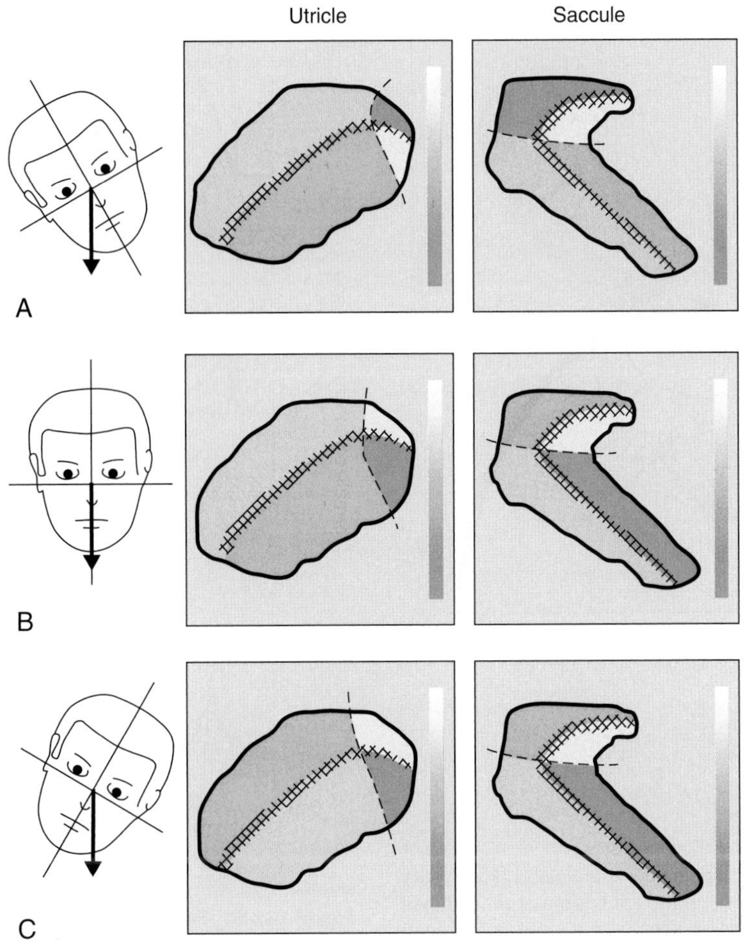

Utricle Saccule

A

B

C

Figure 163-7. Estimated patterns of excitation and inhibition for the left utricle and saccule when the head is (**A**) tilted with the right ear 30 degrees down, (**B**) upright, and (**C**) tilted with the left ear 30 degrees down. The utricle is seen from above, and the saccule from the left side. The nidpoint of the color scale represents baseline activity, whereas dark orange and white represent depolarization and hyperpolarization, respectively. *(Modified from Jaeger R, Takagi A, Haslwanter T. Modeling the relation between head orientations and otolith responses in humans.* Hear Res. *2002;173:29.)*

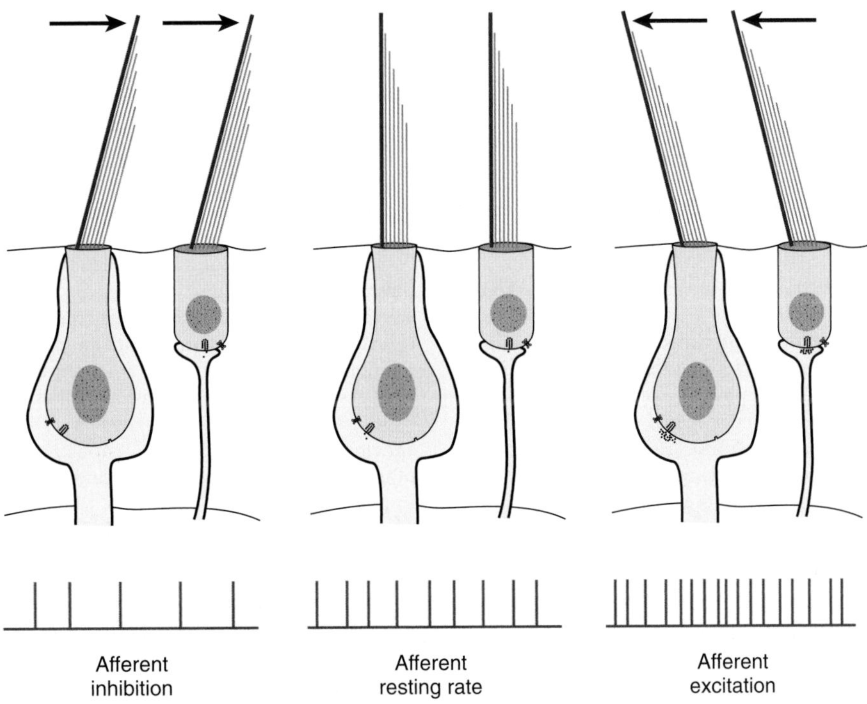

Figure 163-8. A vestibular afferent nerve fires actively at rest (*center*). Its firing rate is modulated by sensory transduction. The afferent is inhibited when its hair cells' stereocilia are deflected in the "off" direction (away from the kinocilium, in dark blue *left panel*) and excited when the stereocilia are deflected in the "on" direction (toward the kinocilium, *right panel*).

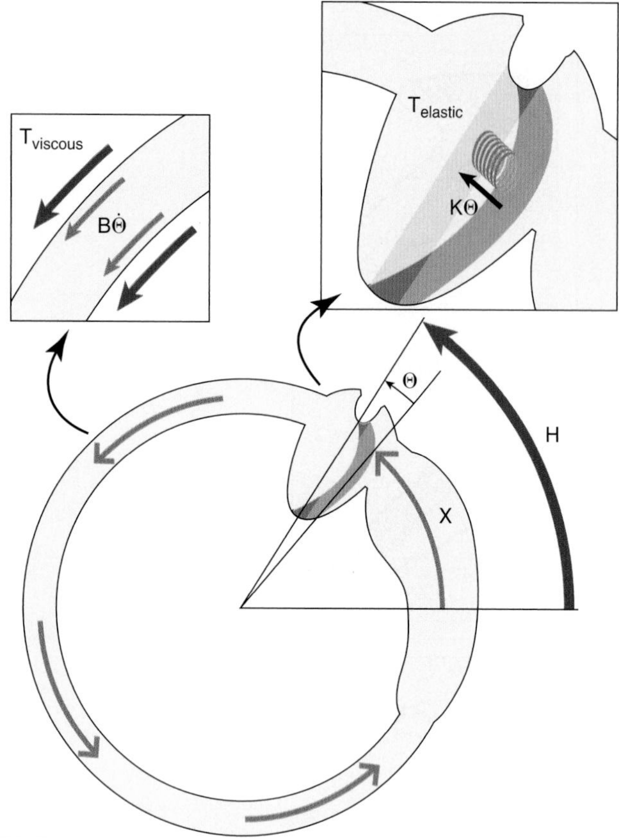

Figure 163-9. The torsional pendulum model of the mechanical forces acting on the cupula and endolymph of the left horizontal canal during leftward angular head acceleration as seen from above. As the head rotates through space over an angle H, endolymph inside the canal also rotates through space, but over a slightly smaller angle X. The difference between the angles through which the head and endolymph rotate in space is Θ, which approximates the angular deflection of the cupula. This creates an elastic torque proportional to the deflection: $T_{elastic} = K\Theta$. A viscous or drag torque is produced by the relative flow of endolymph along the walls of the canal and is proportional to the endolymph velocity relative to the canal: $T_{viscous} = B\dot{\Theta}$. The sum of these torques will equal the moment of inertia of the cupula and endolymph times their acceleration: $K\Theta + B\dot{\Theta} = I\ddot{X} = I\ddot{H} - I\ddot{\Theta}$.

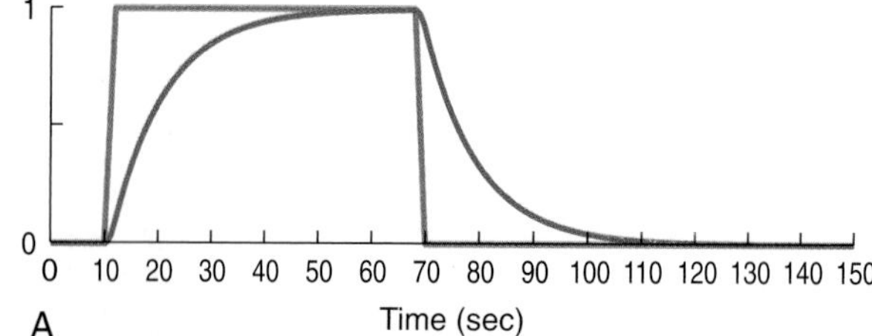

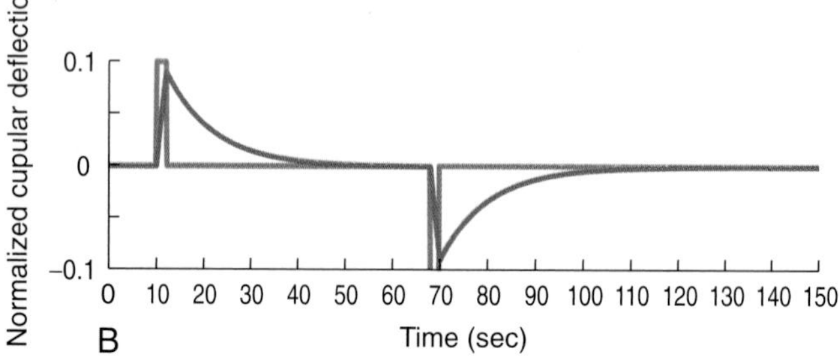

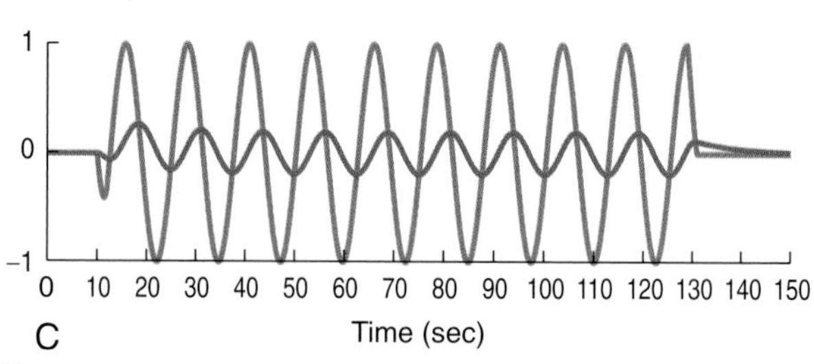

Figure 163-10. Patterns of cupular displacement in response to rotational head movements as predicted by the torsional pendulum model. **A,** A step of constant head acceleration *(red tracing)* results in a constant cupular deflection *(blue)* after an exponential increase in deflection with a time constant of about 10 sec. **B,** A step of constant velocity is produced by an impulse of acceleration in one direction followed by an impulse of deceleration in the opposite direction (acceleration impulses are shown in *red*). The cupula is transiently displaced, returning to its resting position with a decay time constant of about 10 sec. **C,** Sinusoidal *acceleration* of the head (*red*) yields a response in phase with head *velocity*.

The movement of the cupula can now be described as a function of head acceleration:

$$K\Theta(t) + B\dot{\Theta}(t) + I\ddot{\Theta}(t) = I\ddot{H}(t) \qquad \text{Eq. 163-8}$$

The full solution to Equation 163-8 is derived in the Appendix, but considerable insights can be gained without the full solution simply by inserting measured values for the physical constants in Equation 163-8 and considering the behavior under special circumstances.

For example, during a constant, low-acceleration head rotation (Fig.163-10A), cupular deflection eventually reaches a steady-state constant value. Because cupular velocity and acceleration eventually decay to zero under these circumstances, Equation 163-8 reduces to

$$K\Theta(t) \approx I\ddot{H}(t) \qquad \text{Eq. 163-9}$$

and cupular deflection (and afferent firing rate) is approximately proportional to head acceleration. The time course of cupular displacement in response to a constant acceleration approximates a single exponential growth, and the time constant with which cupular displacement reaches its maximum deflection is approximately 10 seconds, the time constant of the cupula (see Appendix). When the constant acceleration stops, the cupula returns to its zero position exponentially with the same time constant.

The same time constant governs the cupular response to very brief pulses of head acceleration. Figure 163-10B shows the predicted cupular deflection to an impulse of acceleration, which brings the head to a constant velocity plateau until an impulse of deceleration stops the rotation. Such "velocity steps" are often done as part of clinical rotary chair tests. However, the measured value of the time constant of the VOR in such testing is generally much longer than what would be anticipated by this calculated cupular response because of further processing by the brain (This is addressed later in the discussion of Principle 9.)

During sinusoidal head rotations in the range encompassing most natural head movements (approximately 0.1 to 15 Hz), viscous friction dominates the cupular response, and Equation 163-8 reduces to

$$B\dot{\Theta}(t) \approx I\ddot{H}(t) \qquad \text{Eq. 163-10}$$

This implies that

$$\Theta(t) \approx \frac{I}{B}\dot{H}(t), \qquad \text{Eq. 163-11}$$

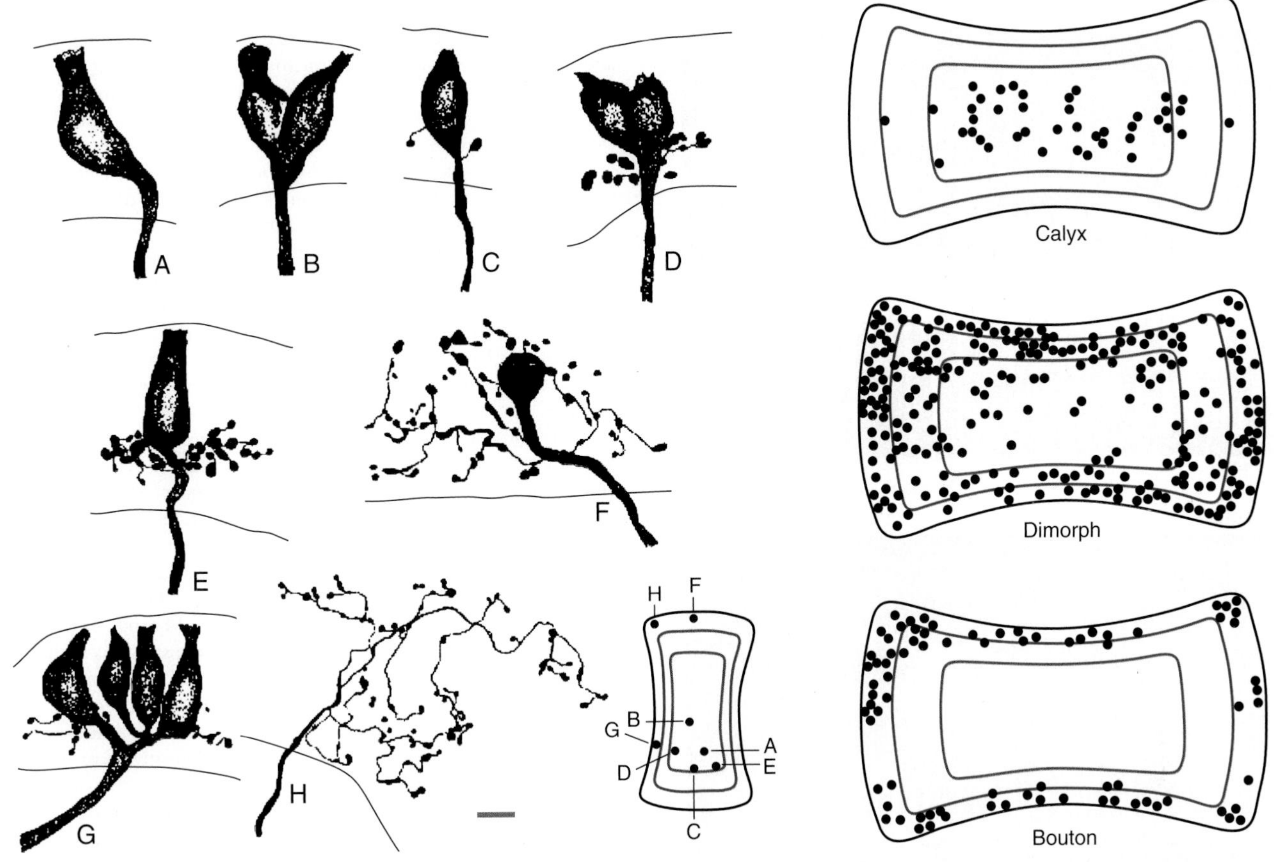

Figure 163-11. Morphology of mammalian vestibular afferents as revealed by horseradish peroxidase labeling of individual units in the chinchilla. **A,** Calyx fiber innervating a single type I hair cell. **B,** Calyx fiber innervating two type 1 hair cells. **C** to **G,** Dimorphic fibers innervate both type 1 and 2 hair cells. **H,** Bouton fiber. *Inset*: Locations of these afferents are placed on a standard map of the crista. *Right*: Three standard maps of the cristae divided into concentrically arranged central (*inside red border*), intermediate, and peripheral (*outside green*) zones of equal areas. Shown are the locations of calyx, dimorphic, and bouton fibers, with each colored dot representing a single dye-filled fiber. Dimorphic units make up 70% of the population, bouton units 20%, and calyx units 10%. *(From Fernandez C, Baird RA, Goldberg JM. The vestibular nerve of the chinchilla. I. Peripheral innervation patterns in the horizontal and superior semicircular canals.* J Neurophysiol. *1988;60:167.)*

so that cupular deflection is proportional to head *velocity*. This is demonstrated in Figure 163-10C: Note that the cupula's predicted response is not in phase with the sine wave that describes head acceleration (red). Rather, the cupula's motion appears to peak one-fourth cycle in advance of the head's motion. This 90-degree phase advance in the cupula's motion can be represented by a cosine wave, which is the integral of the sine wave. The endolymph and cupula thus act as a mechanical integrator of the input head acceleration. The integral of acceleration is velocity, so the important point here is that the cupula encodes head velocity over its physiologically relevant frequency range, even though the stimulus acting on the endolymph is head acceleration. Because of this, and because retinal image slip velocity is an important determinant of visual acuity, clinical and experimental tests conventionally report findings with respect to head velocity.

Response of the Otoconial Membrane

An approach similar to the analysis of cupular motion yields an equation relating the predicted movement of the otoconial membrane to head acceleration.[4] Unfortunately, the otoconial membrane is an inhomogeneous structure whose complexities make it difficult to estimate the physical parameters in the model that would predict its responses under different conditions. The membrane consists of the dense otoconial layer on top, a stiff mesh layer in the middle, and an elastic gel layer on the bottom.[19] At the macular surface it is presumably fixed. It is unclear how tightly otoconial displacement is coupled to the motion of the stereocilia. These uncertainties lead to models that variously predict that the otoconial membrane responds to linear acceleration or velocity, but the actual behavior remains unresolved.[17,20]

Encoding by the Afferents

Morphologically, mammalian vestibular afferents can be grouped into calyceal, bouton, and dimorphic fibers[21-23] (Fig. 163-11). Calyceal fibers (see Fig. 163-11A and B) form chalice-shaped calyx synapses on one or several neighboring type 1 hair cells. Each calyx engulfs the basolateral membrane of the enclosed type 1 hair cell(s). At the other end of the morphological spectrum, a bouton fiber (see Fig. 163-11H) forms 15 to 100 button-like synapses on multiple type 2 hair cells distributed over 25 to 75 μm. Dimorphic fibers (see Fig. 163-11C to G) include 1 to 4 calyceal synapses with type 1 hair cells and 1 to 50 bouton-type synapses with type 2 hair cells. The spatial distribution of afferent endings within the sensory neuroepithelium differs for these three different morphologic groups (shown to the right in Fig. 163-11). Calyceal afferents in the crista are found exclusively in the central zone (on the top of the crest) and in the macula exclusively in the striola. Bouton fibers mostly arborize in the peripheral zone of the crista and in the extrastriolar zones of the maculae. Dimorphic afferents innervate all regions of the vestibular sensory epithelia, and are the dominant fiber type.[22-24]

In mammals, physiologic response characteristics segregate vestibular nerve afferent fibers into two classes based on the regularity in the spacing of spontaneous action potentials[25] (as reviewed by Goldberg and Fernández[26]). *Regular afferents* (Fig. 163-12A) fire at 50 to 100 spikes/second at rest, with very little variation in resting rate for a given

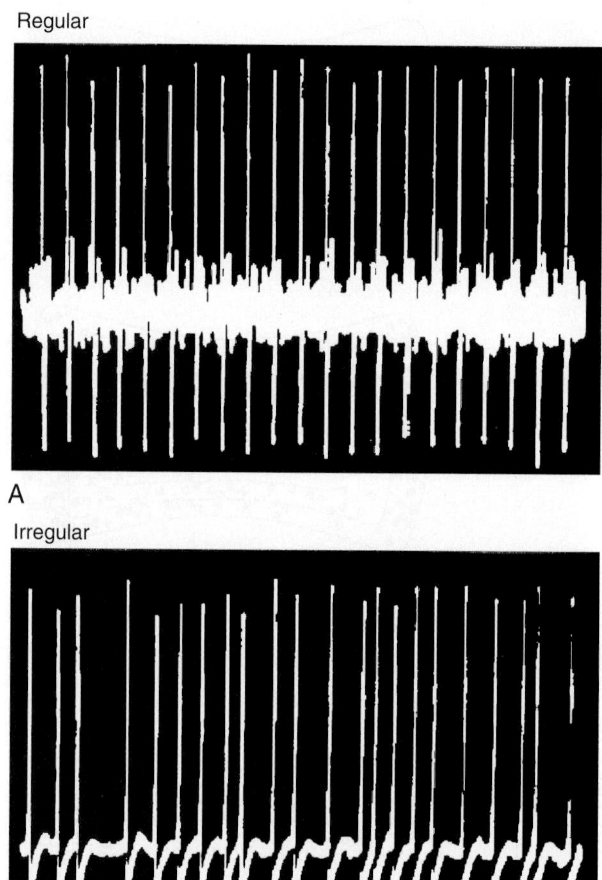

Figure 163-12. Regular (**A**) and irregular (**B**) discharge patterns in the spike trains recorded from two afferents from the superior canal crista in the squirrel monkey. *(From Goldberg JM, Fernandez C. Physiology of peripheral neurons innervating semicircular canals of the squirrel monkey. I. Resting discharge and response to constant angular accelerations.* J Neurophysiol. *1971;34:635.)*

fiber.[27,28] In general, they respond to vestibular stimulation with *tonic* responses. That is, their firing modulates about the baseline, going up and down in close approximation to the stimulus acting on the hair cells. For the otolith organs, the presumed stimulus acting on the hair cells is linear acceleration. The regular afferents in the macula fire in close approximation to linear acceleration.[29,30] For the semicircular canals, the effective stimulus acting on the hair cells turns out to be rotational *velocity*, not acceleration, as explained earlier and in the Appendix. Regular afferents innervating the crista respond with firing rate variations that closely approximate that head velocity signal. Regular units typically have a relatively low sensitivity (change in spike rate for a change in stimulus) to head rotation, to activation of efferent pathways, and to galvanic stimulation.[27,29,31,32] Regular afferents typically have medium or thin axons with bouton-only or dimorphic arborizations in the peripheral zones of cristae or otolithic maculae.[27,33-35]

In contrast with regular vestibular afferents, *irregular afferents* typically are thick to medium-sized axons that end in calyceal or dimorphic terminals in the central (or *striolar*) zones of vestibular endorgans.[27,32-35] Their interspike intervals are much more variable (see Fig. 163-12B). As a population, irregular afferents have a wider range of spontaneous rates than do regular fibers. Irregular units show *phasic* responses to the stimulus acting on the endorgan. That is, the response is more transient, and it approximates the rate of change of the stimulus acting on the endorgan rather than simply the stimulus itself. Thus, irregular units in the crista approximate the head's rotational *acceleration*, which is the rate of change of velocity.[27,29,31] Irregulars in the macula approximate the linear *jerk*, the derivative of linear acceleration.[29,30] Irregular units may have very high sensitivity to vestibular stimuli, except for a unique group of low-sensitivity calyx units in the crista, whose function is still unclear.[25] Sensitivities to activation by efferent pathways and to galvanic stimulation also are generally greater for irregular afferents.[26,36]

Smith and Goldberg[37] have described a model of vestibular nerve afferent spike-initiation dynamics that accounts for many of these observed differences between classes of afferent discharge (Fig. 163-13). After the peak of an action potential (caused by inward sodium currents), outward potassium currents briefly hyperpolarize the vestibular afferent membrane. The potassium conductance decays in a time-dependent manner, and the membrane potential rises again toward the threshold voltage for spike generation. Excitatory postsynaptic potentials (EPSPs) due to synaptic neurotransmitter release superimpose on this repolarization. The model assumes that variations in this potassium conductance between different afferents accounts for their regularity of discharge. In regularly discharging afferents, the model proposes that a

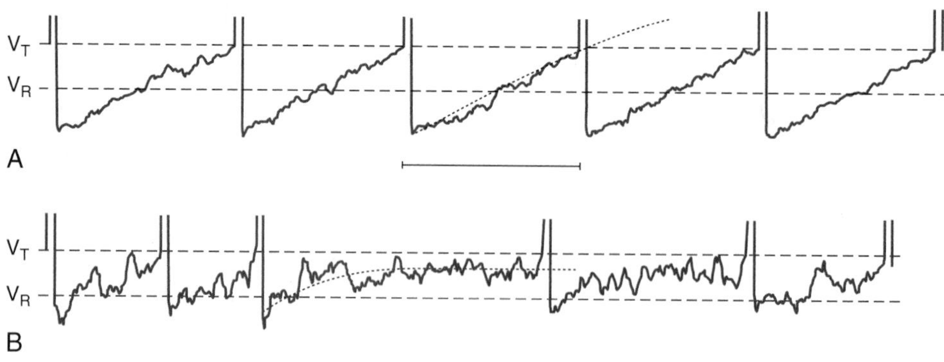

Figure 163-13. The stochastic afterhyperpolarization (AHP) model of repetitive discharge in vestibular afferents. V_R, resting potential; V_T, threshold for spike generation. Two model units are shown with their mean interspike trajectories *(dotted lines)*. **A,** The unit at the top has a regular discharge because of its deep and slow AHP and relatively small miniature excitatory postsynaptic potentials (EPSPs). **B,** The bottom unit is irregular because its AHP is shallow and fast, and its miniature EPSPs are somewhat larger than those in **A.** Note that regular discharge is associated with the mean trajectory eventually crossing V_T at regular intervals. For the irregular discharge, the mean trajectory does not cross V_T, and the actual unit potential crosses V_T only when sufficient EPSPs are added to the mean trajectory. As a result, the timing of spikes in the regular unit is largely determined by the mean trajectory, whereas timing for the irregular unit's spikes is largely determined by synaptic noise. *(Data from Smith CE, Goldberg JM. A stochastic afterhyperpolarization model of repetitive activity in vestibular afferents.* Biol Cybern. *1986;54:41.)*

large potassium conductance decays slowly but inexorably, so that the repolarization continues in a deterministic fashion until the membrane potential again reaches firing threshold (see Fig. 163-13A). The model assumes that quanta of neurotransmitter released from hair cells cause relatively little variation in the trajectory of the repolarization. This deterministic nature of the repolarization means that the membrane reaches the threshold for another spike at almost the same time for each spike. Thus, the interspike intervals are all similar, and the unit's discharge is regular. By contrast, in irregularly discharging afferents, the model assumes a potassium conductance that is high initially but decays rapidly so that it does not carry the membrane potential back up to the threshold for firing by itself (see Fig. 163-13B). These fibers sit just below threshold voltage until driven above it by the added potential due to EPSPs. Neurotransmitter release and EPSPs are quantal and random, so that the time at which the membrane reaches firing potential is highly variable from spike to spike. Thus, the unit's discharge is irregular.

These firing characteristics of the different classes of afferents may be dictated by morphologic and biochemical specializations of their membranes. The variation in discharge regularity is best correlated with the position of the afferent's endings in the neuroepithelium. Irregular units arise from the central zone of the crista or striola of the macula, and regular units arise from the peripheral zone of the crista or extrastriola of the macula. These variations may be due to regional variations in the ion channels that govern interspike intervals.[25] Alternatively, the correspondence between afferent discharge regularity and the number of hair cells with which an afferent forms synapses suggests that discharge regularity may be due in part to combining inputs from many stochastically independent synapses.[38]

Because regular and irregular vestibular nerve afferent fibers have distinct characteristics in so many respects, it seems likely that they mediate different functions.[25] One hypothesis holds that regular and irregular afferents may help compensate for different dynamic loads of the different vestibular reflexes. Regular afferents carry signals roughly in phase with head velocity, the expected output of the mechanics of the semicircular canals (as described; see also the Appendix). Irregular units with high gains have responses more in phase with head acceleration than velocity. The VOR for low-frequency head rotations requires a signal that approximates head velocity, and the regular afferents seem to provide an ideal input for this reflex.[39] By contrast, the VSRs involve very different mechanical loads and may require inputs from the labyrinth that better reflect the head's acceleration, a task to which the irregulars seem better suited.[40] Anatomically, regular and irregular afferents overlap extensively in their distributions to the central vestibular nuclei.[41-43] However, physiologic evidence suggests that there is some segregation of regular and irregular inputs between central projections to the ocular motor centers and the spinal motor centers.[44,45] Another role for the irregular afferents may be to initiate the vestibular reflexes with a very short latency for rapid head movements.[46] Finally, some evidence suggests that the dynamics of irregular afferents are better suited to provide the modifiable component of the VOR when gain must be changed rapidly. Examples are the higher gain needed when the eyes are verged on a near target,[47,48] the change needed to adapt to magnifying or "minifying" spectacles,[49,50] and the adaptation that must occur on one side when function is lost on the other side.[51,52]

In addition to more than 10,000 afferents, each labyrinth also receives efferent innervation from approximately 400 to 600 neurons that lie on either side of the brainstem adjacent to the vestibular nuclei.[53,54] Highly vesiculated efferent endings synapse onto type 2 hair cells and onto the axons of vestibular afferents.[55-57] In mammals, excitation of efferents causes an increase in the background discharge of vestibular afferents, particularly irregular ones.[26] Mammalian efferents can be activated by high head velocities.[58] In fish, vestibular efferents can be activated during behavioral arousal in which head movement would be anticipated.[36] These observations have led to the hypothesis that the efferents may serve to raise baseline afferent firing rates, particularly of irregular afferents, in anticipation of rapid head movements so as to prevent inhibitory silencing.[26,36] Yet Cullen and Minor[59] found that in alert monkeys, afferents responded identically to actively and passively generated rapid head-on-body rotations, making an efferent role in such brief movements unlikely. These investigators hypothesized that vestibular efferents may act to balance firing between the two labyrinths, a role that may be particularly important after some degree of loss of unilateral function.

Principle 3: Stimulation of a Semicircular Canal Produces Eye Movements in the Plane of that Canal

This important principle often is referred to as *Ewald's First Law*. Ewald cannulated the individual membranous canals in pigeons and observed the effects of endolymph motion on body, head, and eye movements. Although Ewald may have codified this principle on the basis of his work,[60] it is clear that earlier workers like Flourens and Mach recognized that manipulations of an isolated semicircular canal in experimental animals produced eye or head movements in the plane of that canal.[61]

Anatomic and Physiologic Basis

The anatomic basis of this principle begins with the anatomy of the semicircular canals. The arrangement of the canals places fluid motion sensors at the ends of relatively long, slender, fluid-filled, donut-shaped tubes. Each tube lies more or less in one plane. The most effective stimulus to move the fluid in such a planar semicircular tube is angular acceleration in that plane, about an axis perpendicular to the plane and through the center of the "donut hole."

The three semicircular canals of the labyrinth are roughly orthogonal to each other, so that one labyrinth can sense any rotation in three-dimensional space. Canals in the two labyrinths are arranged in complementary, coplanar pairs.[62] The two horizontal canals are roughly in one plane, which is nearly horizontal when the head is in an upright position. The left anterior canal is roughly coplanar with the right posterior canal in the *LARP* (left anterior–right posterior) plane, which lies approximately 45 degrees off the midsagittal plane with the anterior end toward the left and the posterior end toward the right. And the right anterior canal is roughly coplanar with the left posterior canal in the *RALP* (right anterior–left posterior) plane, again roughly 45 degrees off the sagittal plane and orthogonal to the LARP and horizontal planes (Fig. 163-14). These canal planes define the cardinal coordinate system for vestibular sensation.

The power of this principle goes beyond the notion that the canal planes simply provide a coordinate system for vestibular *sensation*. Canal planes also provide the coordinate system for the final *motor output* of the VOR (and for the vestibulo-colic neck reflex). The beauty of this canal-fixed (and thus head-fixed) coordinate system for eye movements is that it reduces the neural computation required for ocular motor output to exactly compensate for the head movement.

How is this coordinate system preserved in the central connections of the VOR? Figure 163-15 shows the connections from the left horizontal canal that mediate the VOR when that canal is excited. We have already seen how this movement excites the afferents from this canal; the inset demonstrates this increase in firing from the baseline rate. Secondary vestibular neurons in the ipsilateral vestibular (medial and superior) nuclei receive these afferent signals and connect to the ocular motor nuclei controlling the medial and lateral rectus muscles, which also lie roughly in a horizontal plane. Secondary vestibular neurons carry excitatory signals to the ipsilateral third nucleus and contralateral sixth nucleus to excite the ipsilateral medial rectus and contralateral lateral rectus, respectively. These muscles pull the eyes toward the right as the head turns toward the left, accomplishing the goal of keeping the eyes stable in space. Other secondary vestibular neurons carry inhibitory signals to the contralateral third and ipsilateral sixth nuclei to simultaneously relax the antagonist muscles, the contralateral medial rectus and the ipsilateral lateral rectus, respectively. This reciprocal activity is typical of the extraocular muscles, which work in contraction-relaxation pairs.[63]

Just as the extraocular muscles work in reciprocal pairs, so too do the coplanar semicircular canals. Like the left horizontal canal, the right horizontal canal is also stimulated by the horizontal head turn (Fig. 163-16). However, because the polarity of stereociliary bundles in the

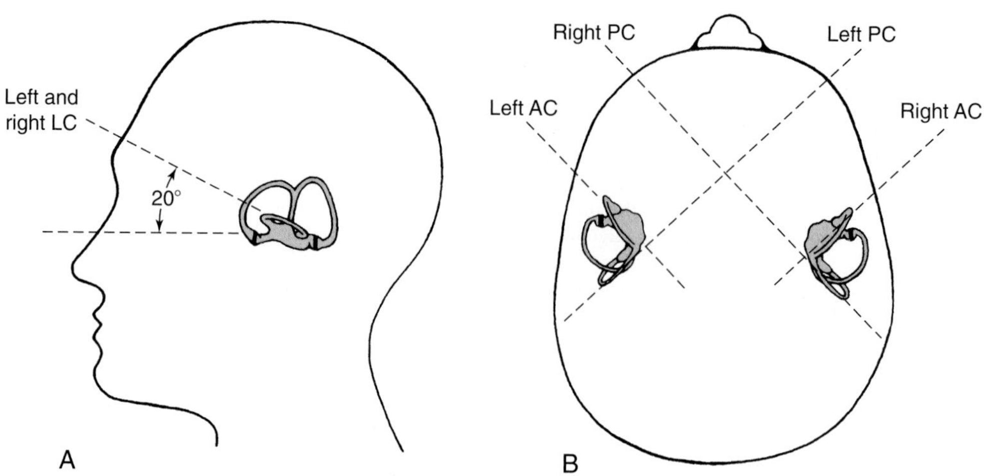

Figure 163-14. Orientation of the semicircular canals. **A,** When the head is upright, the horizontal canal (or lateral canal [LC]) is tilted approximately 20 degrees upward from the horizontal plane at its anterior end. **B,** The vertical canals are oriented in planes roughly 45 degrees from the midsagittal plane. The right anterior canal (AC) and left posterior canal (PC) lie in the same plane, the right anterior–left posterior (RALP) plane. The left anterior and right posterior canals lie in the left anterior–right posterior (LARP) plane. *(Adapted From Barber HO, Stockwell CW.* Manual of Electronystagmography. *St Louis: Mosby; 1976.)*

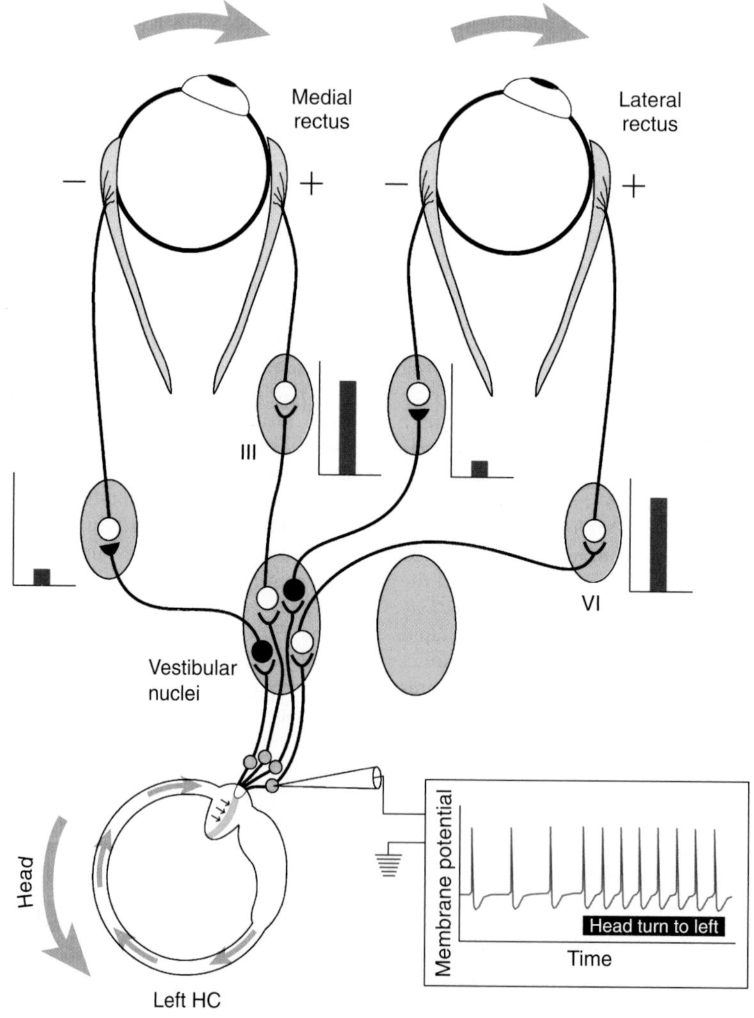

Figure 163-15. Neural connections in the direct pathway for the vestibulo-ocular reflex (VOR) from excitation of the left horizontal canal (HC). As seen from above, a leftward head rotation produces relative endolymph flow in the left HC that is clockwise and toward the utricle. The cupular deflection excites the hair cells in the left HC ampulla, and the firing rate in the afferents increases *(inset)*. Excitatory interneurons in the vestibular nuclei connect to motor neurons for the medial rectus muscle in the ipsilateral third nucleus (III) and lateral rectus muscle in the contralateral sixth nucleus (VI). Firing rates for these motor neurons increase *(mini bar graphs)*. The respective muscles contract and pull the eyes clockwise, opposite the head, during the slow phases of nystagmus. Inhibitory interneurons in the vestibular nuclei connect to motoneurons for the left lateral rectus and right medial rectus. Their firing rates decrease, and these antagonist muscles relax to facilitate the eye movement.

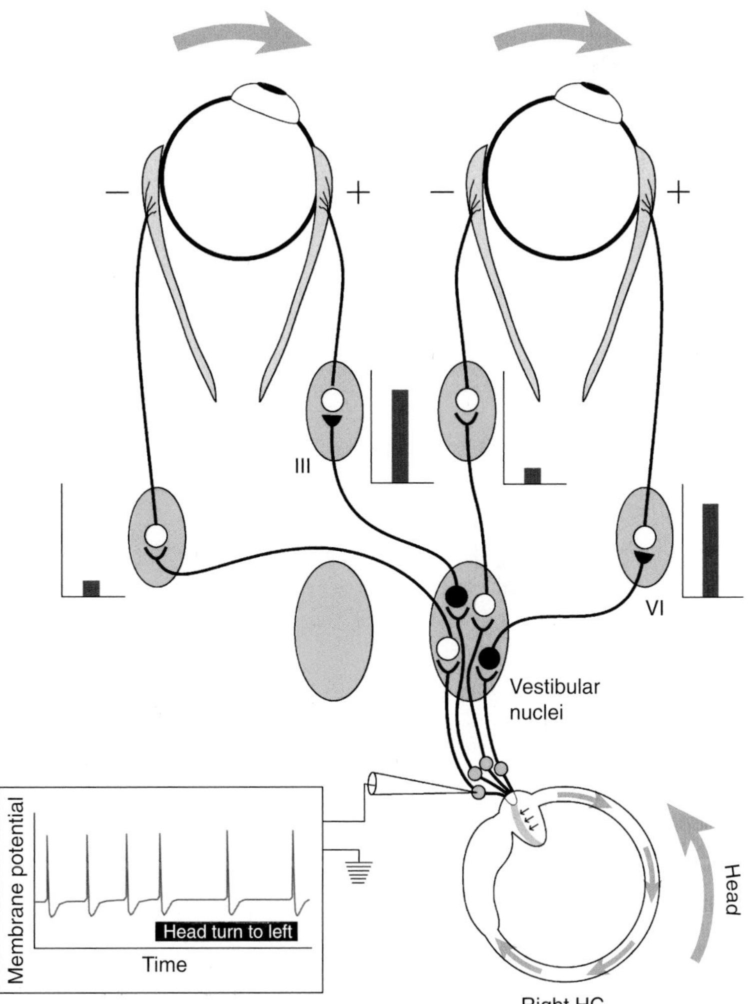

Figure 163-16. Complementary neural connections in the direct pathway for the vestibulo-ocular reflex (VOR) from inhibition of the right horizontal canal (HC). As seen from above, a leftward head rotation again produces relative endolymph flow that is clockwise in the canal. However, for the right HC, this flow is away from the utricle. The cupular deflection inhibits the hair cells in the right HC ampulla, and the firing rate in the afferents decreases *(inset)*. Inhibitory interneurons in the vestibular nuclei reverse this inhibition, sending further excitatory signals *(mini bar graphs)* to the motorneurons for the medial rectus muscle in the ipsilateral third nucleus (III) and lateral rectus muscle in the contralateral sixth nucleus (VI). The contraction of these muscles is augmented. Simultaneously, excitatory interneurons *(open circles)* in the vestibular nuclei preserve and convey inhibition *(mini bar graphs)* to motoneurons for the lateral rectus muscle in the left sixth nucleus (VI) and medial rectus muscle in the right third nucleus (III). The inhibitory signals further relax these antagonist muscles.

right horizontal canal is a mirror image of the arrangement on the left, the flow of endolymph with respect to the head, still clockwise as seen from above, has an *inhibitory* effect on the right horizontal canal afferents. Connections from the right vestibular nuclei to the ocular motor nuclei also mirror those on the left. With the inverse signals coming through this mirror-image circuit from the right side, the ocular motor nuclei receive greater excitatory stimuli for the right lateral and left medial rectus muscles, and more inhibition for their antagonists. Thus, head rotation produces an excitatory contribution to the VOR from one canal and an inhibitory contribution from its coplanar mate. This often is referred to as the "push-pull" arrangement of the canals. Thanks to the nonzero baseline firing rate of vestibular afferent neurons, both of the canals in a coplanar pair can encode rotational acceleration in that plane.

Like the horizontal canals and the lateral and medial recti, the vertical semicircular canals are linked to the vertical pairs of eye muscles, a fact that helps explain the pulling directions and insertions of the superior and inferior oblique muscles. Figure 163-17 demonstrates that the LARP plane aligns with the pulling directions of the left superior and inferior rectus muscles as well as the right superior and inferior oblique muscles. The connections from the secondary vestibular nuclei can be traced, just as shown in Figures 163-15 and 163-16. The important result is indicated by the contrast coding in Figure 163-17. Excitation of the left anterior canal (shading) and inhibition of the right posterior canal (shading) result in contraction of the muscles that pull the eyes upward in the LARP plane and relaxation of the muscles that pull them downward in that plane. Similarly, the RALP plane aligns with the pulling directions of those vertical eye muscles that move the eyes in the RALP plane.

The alignment of canal planes and extraocular muscle planes is not exact, and the excitation of a single canal pair does not solely produce activity in a dedicated pair of extraocular muscles. Other muscles must be activated to compensate for a head rotation even when it is purely in the plane of one semicircular canal. However, this arrangement between semicircular canals and extraocular muscles is remarkably constant across vertebrate species, even allowing for the shift between lateral-eyed species (e.g., rabbits) and frontal-eyed ones (e.g., humans). Because the vestibular labyrinth evolved before movable eyes,[64] extraocular muscles may have evolved to pull in the preexisting canal planes. Robinson[65] has argued that there is an evolutionary advantage to keeping the extraocular muscles aligned with the semicircular canals. Such an arrangement minimizes the brainstem processing

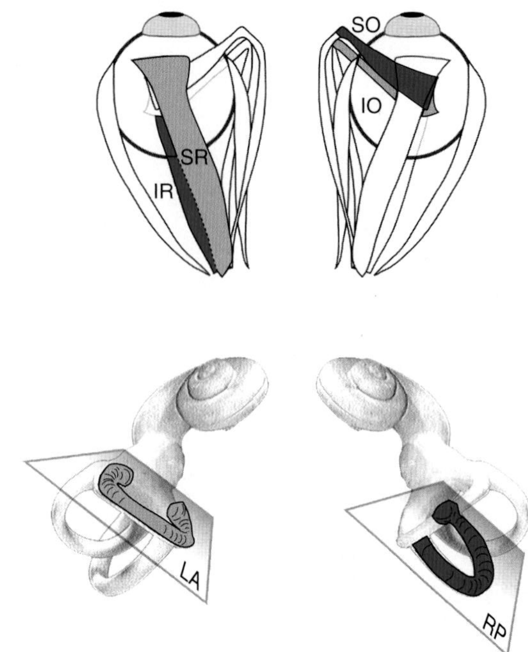

Figure 163-17. The left anterior–right posterior canal (LARP) plane aligns with the pulling directions of the left superior rectus (SR) and inferior rectus (IR) muscles, as well as the right superior oblique (SO) and inferior oblique (IO) muscles. As indicated by the shading, excitation of the left anterior canal (and inhibition of the right posterior canal) causes contraction of the left superior rectus and right inferior oblique muscles and relaxation of the darker-shaded antagonists. The result will be an upward movement of the eyes in the LARP plane. Excitation of the right posterior canal will produce the opposite effect.

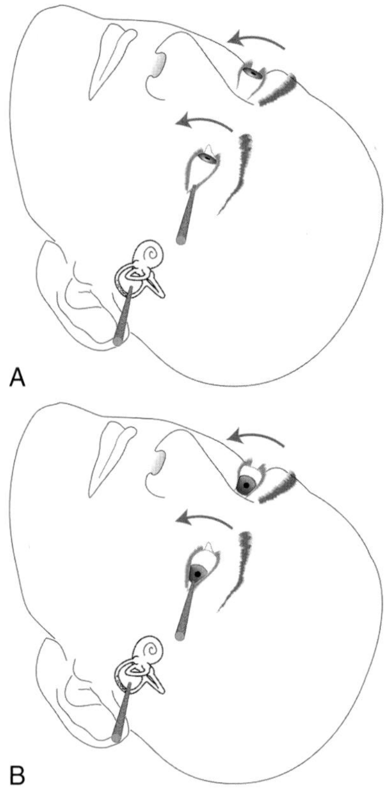

Figure 163-18. Excitation of the left posterior canal (PC) by moving canaliths in benign paroxysmal positional vertigo (PC-BPPV) causes slow phase eye movements downward in the plane of the affected PC. The eyes rotate around an axis parallel to the one going through the center of the affected PC. **A,** When gaze is directed perpendicular to the axis of eye rotation, the pupil appears to move up and down in an eye-fixed reference frame. **B,** When gaze is directed parallel to the axis of eye rotation, the pupil appears to move torsionally in an eye-fixed reference frame. In either case, the eyes rotate around the same axis when considered in a canal-fixed frame of reference.

needed to activate the appropriate ensemble of eye muscles to compensate for head movement. Minimizing the number of synapses involved in the reflex preserves its remarkably short latency of approximately 7 msec,[66] which in turn minimizes retinal image slip during very rapid head movements.

Clinical Importance

Because of the primacy of the canals in determining how the eyes move under vestibular stimulation, it is helpful to think about vestibular eye movements in a *canal-fixed frame of reference.* A good example of the power of this approach is in investigation of benign paroxysmal positional vertigo (BPPV). In the most widely accepted current model of BPPV, otolith crystals displaced from the utricular otoconial mass come to rest in one of the semicircular canals (typically the posterior semicircular canal).[67] When the patient lies down and turns the head toward the affected side, aligning the posterior canal (PC) with the pull of gravity (the left Dix-Hallpike maneuver), the otolith crystals fall toward what is now the "bottom" of the canal. As the otoliths fall, they push endolymph ahead of them, causing cupular deflection and exciting hair cells on the posterior canal crista. Nystagmus develops during the time that endolymph moves. Ewald's First Law predicts the direction of that nystagmus: It will be in the plane of the affected posterior canal, independent of pupil position or head position.

Trying to apply this principle to PC-BPPV confuses many novice examiners. They observe instead that the nystagmus seems to change direction depending on where the patient directs the gaze. When the patient looks out to the side (toward the affected ear), the examiner sees a primarily torsional movement of the eyes. When the patient looks up toward the ceiling (away from the affected ear), the eyes appear to move vertically (Fig. 163-18). With the eyes in a neutral position (straight-ahead gaze), the nystagmus is a mixture of vertical and torsional movements. How can the principle be valid if the nystagmus changes directions?

In reality, no change occurs in the direction of the nystagmus with respect to the canal planes; it is a figment of the wrong frame of reference. In examining eye movements, we are accustomed to thinking in an eye-fixed reference frame in which the line of sight (the line extending forward from the pupil) determines what is up, down, left, right, clockwise, and counterclockwise relative to that axis. But Ewald's First Law demands that we abandon this oculocentric view of eye movements and instead see them in a canal-centric view. In this view, the location of the pupil does not matter. The globe continues to rotate around the axis parallel to the one passing perpendicularly through the posterior canal that is being stimulated (shown in blue in Fig. 163-18). The pupil is simply a surface feature going along for the ride, wherever it happens to be directed. Ewald's First Law states that *the eyes will move in the plane of the stimulated canal no matter where gaze is directed.* In fact, the apparent variation in pupil movement with gaze direction during nystagmus can be used to an examiner's advantage in trying to discern which canal is affected in BPPV (or any other cause of single-canal dysfunction). By asking a patient to look parallel and perpendicular to the plane of the canal in question during periods of nystagmus, one should observe that when the pupil is in the plane of the affected canal, the nystagmus moves the pupil most obviously. This is because the pupil is at the equator of the rotating globe, where rotation will carry it the farthest. When the patient's gaze is directed perpendicular to the plane of the affected canal, the pupil is at the pole of the rotating globe, and eye movement is limited to cyclotorsion about the axis of rotation, which can be subtle to detect. Finding these two gaze directions can identify and confirm the canal (or at least the coplanar canal pair) causing the nystagmus.

Principle 4: A Semicircular Canal Normally Is Excited by Rotation in the Plane of the Canal Bringing the Head toward the Ipsilateral Side

Anatomic and Physiologic Basis

A semicircular canal crista is excited by rotation in its plane in one direction and is inhibited by rotation in its plane in the opposite direction. Another look at Figure 163-9 shows that turning the head toward the left in the horizontal canal plane produces endolymph rotation to the left *relative to space.* But that endolymph rotation is less than the head rotation by the angle Θ. Thus, *relative to the canal,* there is endolymph rotation of Θ to the right, and the cupula is deflected toward the utricle. The pattern of afferent activation results from the polarization of the stereocilia of the hair cells on the cristae. In the horizontal canal, the taller ends of the bundles point toward the utricle. Flow of endolymph (relative to the head) toward the ampulla-ampullopetal flow (from Latin *petere,* to seek), therefore excites the horizontal canal afferents, and flow of endolymph away from the ampulla—ampullofugal flow (from Latin *fugere,* "to flee")—inhibits these afferents. Thus, relative to the head, endolymph flow toward the ampulla occurs when the head is turning in the plane of the horizontal canal toward the same side.

The vertical canals, however, have the opposite pattern of hair cell polarization. The taller ends of the bundles point away from the utricle, so that flow away from the ampulla (ampullofugal) excites their afferents. For the left anterior canal, whose ampulla is at its anterior end, turning the head down and rolling it to the left in the plane of the left anterior canal results in relative endolymph flow that is ampullofugal. For the left posterior canal, whose ampulla is at its posterior end, turning the head up and rolling it to the left in the plane of the left posterior canal moves its endolymph away from the ampulla and excites its afferents. The mirror-image rotations would pertain to the right vertical canals.

Fortunately, keeping track of ampullopetal and ampullofugal flows is unnecessary. Instead, one need only recall that a semicircular canal is excited by rotation in the plane of the canal bringing the head toward the *ipsilateral* side. For example, the right horizontal canal is excited by turning the head rightward in the horizontal plane. The right anterior canal is excited by pitching the head nose down while rolling the head toward the right in a plane 45 degrees off of the midsagittal plane. The right posterior canal is excited by pitching the head nose up while rolling it toward the right in a plane 45 degrees off the midsagittal plane. In the case of each semicircular canal on the right, the rotation exciting that canal brings the head toward the right in the plane of the canal. In the case of the horizontal canals, the nose is turned toward the right. In the case of the vertical canals, the top of the head is rotated toward the right.

It should be obvious by now that a semicircular canal is inhibited by rotation in the plane of the canal toward the opposite side. As described previously, the arrangement of canals is such that when head rotation excites one, it inhibits its coplanar mate. Thus, the rotations explained in the last paragraph would produce inhibition of the left horizontal, posterior, and anterior canals, respectively.

Clinical Importance

This principle eliminates the need to memorize the orientations of stereocilia in particular ampullae and whether ampullopetal or ampullofugal flow excites a given canal. In fact, it is easier to deduce the basic anatomy and physiology from this principle than vice versa. For example, rolling the head toward the left and bringing the nose up excites the left posterior canal according to Principle 4. As noted earlier, endolymph flows relative to the membranous canal in a direction opposite to the head rotation. Thus, the left posterior canal is excited when endolymph flows upwards and toward the right in the canal—that is, ampullofugal. The stereocilia of this canal must be polarized with the tall ends away from the utricle. A considerable amount of anatomy and physiology is condensed into this simple principle.

Principle 5: Any Stimulus That Excites a Semicircular Canal's Afferents Will Be Interpreted as Excitatory Rotation in the Plane of That Canal

Anatomic and Physiologic Basis

Perhaps because the VOR is critical to the survival of any vertebrate that needs to see and move about its environment, evolution appears to have placed a high premium on maintaining parsimonious and rapid neural connections of head rotational sensors to eye muscles. This allows for optimal performance when the system is working normally. However, by devoting dedicated lines of communication from the canals to the extraocular muscles, nature has effectively made the eyes slaves to the vestibular system. Designed, as it is, to expeditiously and reliably produce the eye movements needed to counter a sensed head movement, the system cannot help but produce those eye movements when the vestibular afferent firing rate changes from some other cause. Likewise, the systems mediating postural reflexes and perception of spatial orientation will respond to pathologic alterations in peripheral vestibular input in the same way that they do to tilting or translational movement. An important point is that the brainstem (and patient) will interpret any change in firing rate from vestibular afferents as indicating head rotation, tilt, or translation that would normally produce that same change in firing rate. Secondary vestibular neurons relay the same misinformation to other reflex control centers and higher areas of conscious sensation. This leads to autonomic and postural disturbances as well as the noxious sensation of *vertigo,* an illusion of self-motion.

A pathologic asymmetry in input from coplanar canals causes the eyes to turn in an attempt to compensate for the "perceived" head rotation. However, given the mechanical constraints imposed by the extraocular muscles, the eyes cannot continue to rotate in the same direction that the canals command for very long. Instead, rapid, resetting movements occur, taking the eyes back toward their neutral positions in the orbits. The result is *nystagmus,* a rhythmic, slowly forward–quickly backward movement of the eyes. The quick resetting movements (similar to saccades) are *quick phases* of nystagmus, and the vestibular-driven slower movements are *slow phases.* Unfortunately, convention dictates that nystagmus direction is described according to the direction of the quick phases, because these are more dramatic and noticeable. However, an important pont is that the slow phases are the *components driven by the vestibular system.* By focusing on the direction of slow phases, one reduces the number of mental inversions required to identify the pathologic canal causing an observed nystagmus.

This principle holds almost universally true for brief, unpredictable changes in afferent firing, but not necessarily for persistent stable changes. Fortunately, the nystagmus caused by sustained imbalances in afferent vestibular tone eventually abates as brainstem and cerebellar neural circuitry adapt to the imbalance, as discussed later on (Principle 12). Still, this principle's explanation of responses to brief changes in labyrinthine activity provides a powerful clinical diagnostic tool in localizing disease processes to individual canals.

Clinical Importance

Posterior Canal Benign Paroxysmal Positional Vertigo

In the example of PC-BPPV introduced above, we saw how loose otoconia and endolymph flowed in an ampullofugal direction when the affected PC was oriented vertically in the Dix-Hallpike position. From Principle 4, this direction of endolymph flow excites the PC afferents. From Principle 3, the eye movements resulting from excitation of the PC will be in the plane of that PC. Principle 5 predicts the direction of the slow phases of the nystagmus in this plane. Excitation of the PC afferents will be interpreted as an excitatory rotation of the head in the plane of the PC, and the nystagmus generated would be compensatory for the perceived rotation. For the left PC, excitatory rotation consists rolling the head toward the left while bringing the nose up. To keep the eyes stable in space, the VOR generates slow phases that move the eyes down and roll them clockwise (with respect to the patient's head).

The quick phases are opposite; they beat up and counterclockwise with respect to the patient's head.

Superior Canal Dehiscence Syndrome

In another example of a disorder causing isolated stimulation of a single semicircular canal, a young woman complains that exposure of the left ear to loud sound "makes the world flutter up and down." Applying a loud sound to the left ear through a headphone causes her to develop vertigo and nystagmus. When she is directed to look 45 degrees to her left, one observes that the slow phases of her nystagmus move her pupils up and down. When she looks 45 degrees to her right, the slow phases appear to be cyclotorsional movements of her pupils clockwise (from her perspective). As she attempts straight-ahead gaze, the nystagmus becomes a mixture of these vertical and torsional movements. The examiner must think in a canal-fixed coordinate system and recognize that in each case, the eyes rotate around the same axis, or in the same plane. In this case, the eyes are moving in the LARP plane and in the direction anticipated for excitation of the left anterior canal or inhibition of the right posterior canal. Because only the left ear is receiving the sound stimulus, the problem must lie in the left anterior canal.

This is an example of *superior semicircular canal dehiscence syndrome* causing a *Tullio phenomenon*. Tullio[68] experimented with sound as a stimulus for the labyrinth in pigeons after he fenestrated their semicircular canals. He observed that this caused eye and head nystagmus in the plane of the fenestrated semicircular canal, another example of Ewald's First Law. Huizinga[69] proposed that the fenestra created a third "mobile window" in the labyrinth, in addition to the oval and round windows. This window opens another route for sound pressure dissipation in the labyrinth. This new route is along the affected canal, so endolymph moves through the semicircular canal under the influence of sound or other pressure changes applied to the oval or round windows (Fig. 163-19A). By Principle 5, the fenestrated superior canal exposed to loud sound encodes the resulting endolymph flow as it would a head rotation in the plane of the affected canal and toward the affected side. Superior canal dehiscence syndrome was only recently discovered.[70] It was the observation of nystagmus just as described here and the line of reasoning presented by Principles 1 to 5 that led investigators to suspect that the superior canal was the source of the nystagmus, which CT scanning confirmed (see Fig. 163-19B).

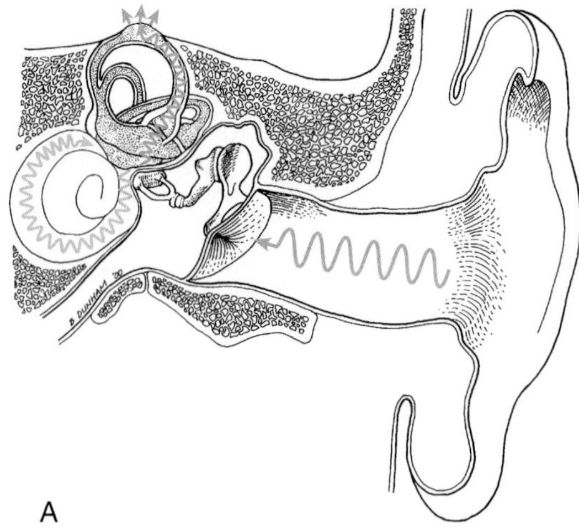

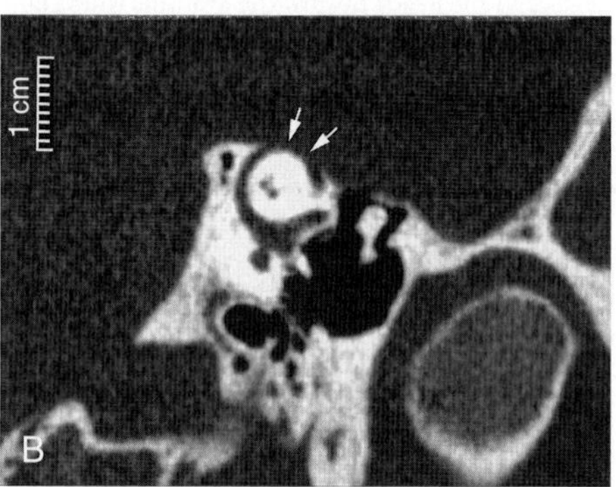

Figure 163-19. A, In superior canal dehiscence syndrome, sound waves can excite the superior canal because the "third mobile window" created by the dehiscence allows some sound pressure to be dissipated along a route through the superior canal in addition to the conventional route through the cochlea. **B,** CT scan demonstrating dehiscence *(arrows)* of the superior canal. *(Illustration courtesy of Dr. B. Dunham.)*

Nystagmus during Caloric Testing

In the caloric test, warm or cool water is irrigated in the external auditory canal. Thermal transfer across the mastoid and eardrum changes the temperature, and therefore density, of the endolymph in the lateral part of the horizontal semicircular canal. That endolymph becomes lighter (by heating) or heavier (by cooling) than the endolymph in the rest of the labyrinth. When the subject is placed supine (with the head up approximately 20 degrees) so as to bring the horizontal canal into a vertical plane, endolymph in the lateral part of the canal made lighter by warming rises toward the ampulla. This is equivalent to the movement caused by turning the head ipsilaterally in the head-horizontal plane. By Principle 4, this manuever excites that canal. By Principle 5, the compensatory eye movements, the slow phases of nystagmus, are in the horizontal canal plane and toward the contralateral side. The quick phases are directed toward the ipsilateral side. By reverse reasoning, for cool irrigation, the horizontal canal is inhibited, and the quick phases are directed toward the contralateral side. (The mnemonic COWS—*c*old *o*pposite, *w*arm *s*ame—can be used to recall the direction of the beating of the nystagmus.) A major advantage of the caloric test is that unlike rotational tests, it applies a truly unilateral stimulus. Diminished caloric responses on one side often help to localize a hypofunctional labyrinth. More details on the caloric test can be found in Chapter 164, Evaluation of the Patient with Dizziness.

Unfortunately, the caloric test has several disadvantages. Testing predominantly stimulates the horizontal semicircular canal, and little information is provided about other canals and the otolith end organs. Judging from the nystagmus it produces, a caloric stimulus is approximately equivalent to a 5- to 10 degrees/second squared (sec^2) acceleration to a sustained horizontal rotation of approximately 50 to 100 degrees/second. The nystagmus typically persists in one direction for 120 seconds or longer. A comparable head rotation would be a half-cycle of a sine wave with a period of 240 seconds, or a frequency of 1/240 second = 0.004 Hz. This stimulus is well below the ideal operating range of the semicircular canal (see Appendix). Nevertheless, the caloric test remains one of the cornerstones of vestibular evaluation because it gives information about one labyrinth in isolation, which low-frequency rotational tests cannot do.

Principle 6: High Acceleration Head Rotation in the Excitatory Direction of a Canal Elicits a Greater Response than the Same Rotation in the Inhibitory Direction

Anatomic and Physiologic Basis

Ewald made a second important observation in his experiments in which he moved endolymph in individual semicircular canals.[60] Movement of endolymph in the "on" direction for a canal produced greater nystagmus than an equal movement of endolymph in the "off" direction. This observation, *Ewald's Second Law*, indicates an *excitation-inhibition asymmetry*. Excitation-inhibition asymmetries occur at multiple levels in the vestibular system. First, in the hair cells there is an asymmetry in the transduction process. Figure 163-20 shows that in vestibular hair cells there is a larger receptor potential response for stereociliary deflection in the "on" direction than in the "off" direction. A second asymmetry is introduced by the vestibular nerve afferents. Recall that the afferents fire even when the head is at rest, and that this firing is modulated by the hair cell responses to head acceleration after the endolymph and cupula integrate the signal to yield one representing head velocity (Principle 2). Vestibular afferents in mammals

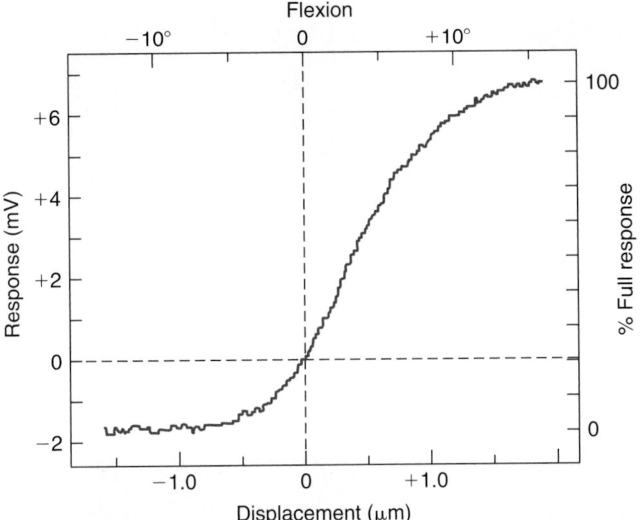

Figure 163-20. Excitation-inhibition asymmetry in the receptor potential of saccular hair cells from the bullfrog. Deflection of stereocilia in the "on" direction produces a larger change in receptor potential than does a comparable deflection in the "off" direction. *(From Hudspeth AJ, Corey DP. Sensitivity, polarity, and conductance change in the response of vertebrate hair cells to controlled mechanical stimuli.* Proc Natl Acad Sci U S A. *1977;74:2407.)*

have baseline firing rates ranging from 50 to 100 spikes/second.[25] Although these firing rates can be driven upwards to 300 to 400 spikes/second, they can be driven no lower than zero. This *inhibitory cutoff* is the most obvious and severe form of excitation-inhibition asymmetry in the vestibular system. Even in the range in which there is no inhibitory cutoff, responses for some vestibular afferents show excitation-inhibition asymmetry, with excitatory rotation causing a greater change in vestibular nerve afferent firing rate than does an equal and opposite inhibitory rotation. Using galvanic currents to stimulate vestibular afferents independent of their hair cells, Goldberg and coworkers[28] showed that this asymmetry is more marked for irregular afferents.

These peripheral asymmetries may be mostly eliminated in the central vestibular connections because of the reciprocal characteristics of signals from one side compared to another. In fact, such a combination of nonlinear sensors acting reciprocally on a symmetrical premotor system can increase the linear range of the vestibular reflexes when both sides are functioning appropriately.[72] However, nonlinearities in the VOR become pronounced when labyrinthine function is lost unilaterally.

Clinical Importance

Aw and colleagues[73] demonstrated that rapid passive rotary head movements elicit markedly asymmetrical VOR responses in humans after unilateral labyrinthectomy. These "head thrusts" are unpredictable, high-acceleration (3000 to 4000 degrees/sec^2) head rotations through amplitudes of 10 to 20 degrees. When the head is thrust in one of the semicircular canal planes so as to excite the canal on the intact side, the VOR that results is nearly compensatory for the head movement (Fig. 163-21, right panels). By contrast, when the head is thrust in one of

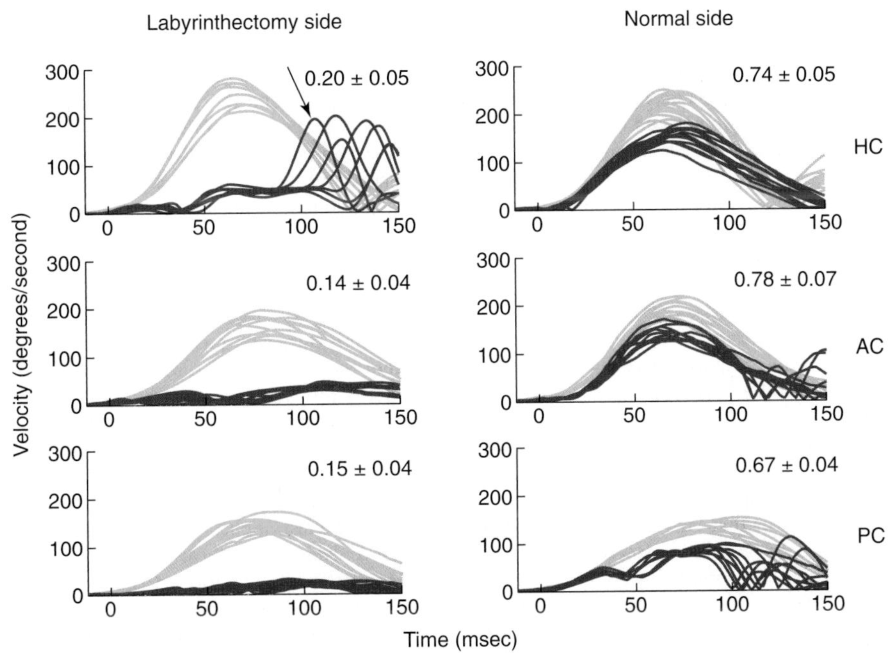

Figure 163-21. Results of head thrust testing of the angular vestibulo-ocular reflexes (aVORs) in a subject after unilateral labyrinthectomy. The examiner manually rotated the subject's head in one of the canal planes during each trial. The subject was instructed to keep his gaze fixed on a small stationary visual target 1.2 m directly in front of him. Eye and head velocities were measured with magnetic search coils. Each panel shows data for 8 to 15 trials exciting one canal. For example, the *top left panel* contains data for rotations in the plane of the horizontal canals (HCs) toward the side of the labyrinthectomy. Head velocity traces are shown in orange, and eye velocity traces are shown in red. For ease of comparison, all velocities are shown as positive values. Gain of the aVOR was defined as the peak eye velocity/peak head velocity ratio during a 30-msec window leading up to the peak head velocity. The gain (mean ± SD) for the respective canal is given in the *upper right corner* of each panel. Note that head thrusts that excited the canals on the normal side were accompanied by nearly compensatory eye movements. By contrast, head thrusts toward the labyrinthectomy side generated very minimal VORs in the period up to peak head velocity. After approximately 90 msec, the visual system registered the retinal slip and triggered a visually guided eye movement to reset gaze on the target *(arrow)*. AC, anterior canal; PC, posterior canal. *(Data from Carey JP, Minor LB, Peng GC, Della Santina CC, Cremer PD, Haslwanter T. Changes in the three-dimensional angular vestibulo-ocular reflex following intratympanic gentamicin for Meniere's disease. JARO. 2002;3:430.)*

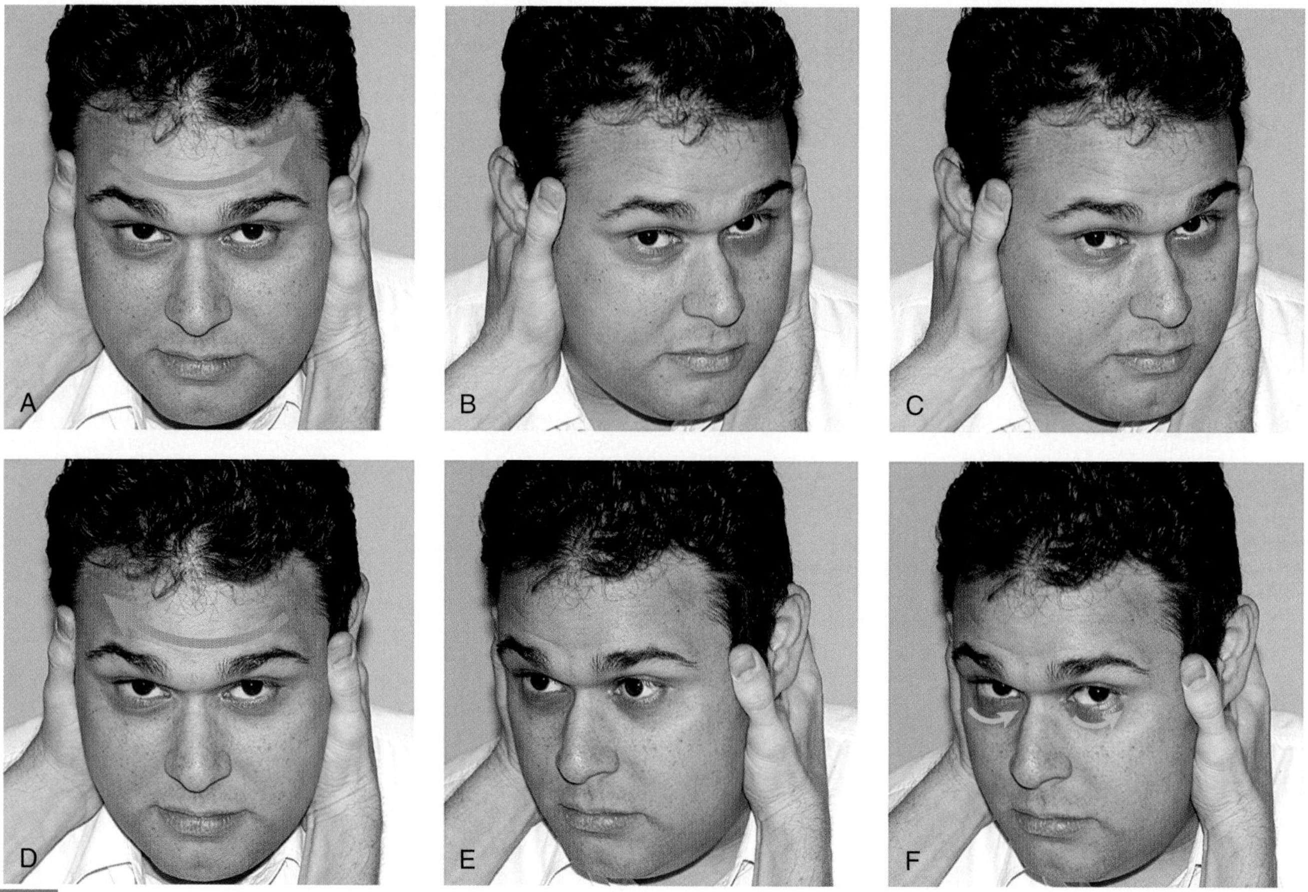

Figure 163-22. In the clinical version of the head thrust test, the examiner asks the subject to fix the gaze on the examiner's nose. The examiner rapidly turns the subject's head, but only by approximately 10 to 15 degrees; larger angles of rotation are unnecessary and may risk injury to the neck. The acceleration must be 3000 degrees/second squared (sec^2) or greater, and the peak velocity must be 150 to 300 degrees/second, meaning that the rotation must be finished in 150 msec. Photographs **A** to **C** show a head thrust to the left, exciting the left horizontal canal (HC). The eyes stay on the examiner's nose throughout the maneuver, indicating normal left HC function. Photographs **D** to **F** show a head thrust to the right, exciting the right HC. The eyes do not stay on target, but move with the head during the head thrust (**D** and **E**). A refixation saccade brings the eyes back on target after completion of the head movement (**F**). This is a "positive" head thrust sign for the right HC, indicating hypofunction of that canal.

the semicircular canal planes so as to excite the canal on the lesioned side, the VOR that results is markedly diminished (see Fig. 163-21, left panels). Although head rotation produces an excitatory contribution from the ipsilateral horizontal canal and an inhibitory contribution from the contralateral one, these contributions are markedly asymmetrical under these conditions. The inhibitory contribution from the intact canal is insufficient to drive a compensatory VOR when the head is thrust toward the lesioned side. Note that Figure 163-21 shows that there is a small VOR response for the head thrust toward the lesioned side. This is the inhibitory contribution from the intact canal. On the other hand, the excitatory contribution from the intact canal that is obtained when the head is thrust toward the intact side is almost adequate to drive a fully compensatory VOR by itself. Such a marked asymmetry may not be evident for low-frequency, low-velocity rotations, which are not dynamic enough to cut off responses in the inhibited nerve.[74]

The head thrust test (HTT) has become one of the most important tools in the clinical evaluation of vestibular function. In its qualitative, "bedside" form, the examiner simply asks the subject to stare at the examiner's nose while the examiner turns the subject's head quickly along the excitatory direction for one canal (Fig. 163-22). If the function of that canal is diminished, the VOR will fail to keep the eye on target, and the examiner will see the patient make a *refixation saccade* after the head movement is completed. If the patient has compensated well for the loss of function, the refixation saccade may even occur while the head is completing its movement, and it may take some experience to spot the saccade while the head is still in motion. By contrast, when the head thrust is in the excitatory direction of an intact canal (and nerve), the patient's gaze remains stable on the examiner's nose throughout the movement.

The HTT can localize isolated hypofunction of individual semicircular canals. Figure 163-23 shows an example of the quantitative head thrust test applied to all of the canals in a patient with a large (5-mm) dehiscence of the right superior canal. The VOR gain is reduced only for the affected superior canal, probably because large dehiscences allow the brain and dura to completely compress the membranous canal, thereby blocking endolymph motion in the canal.[75] The appearance of such a large dehiscence on computer tomographic (CT) scanning is shown in Figure 163-19B.

Principle 7: The Response to Simultaneous Canal Stimuli Is Approximately the Sum of the Responses to Each Stimulus Alone

This principle allows an intuitive approximation of the direction and magnitude of nystagmus caused by excitation (or inhibition) of any combination of semicircular canals.

Anatomic and Physiologic Basis

From Principle 3 and Principle 4, it should be clear that rotation of the head purely in one of the canal planes produces eye movements in

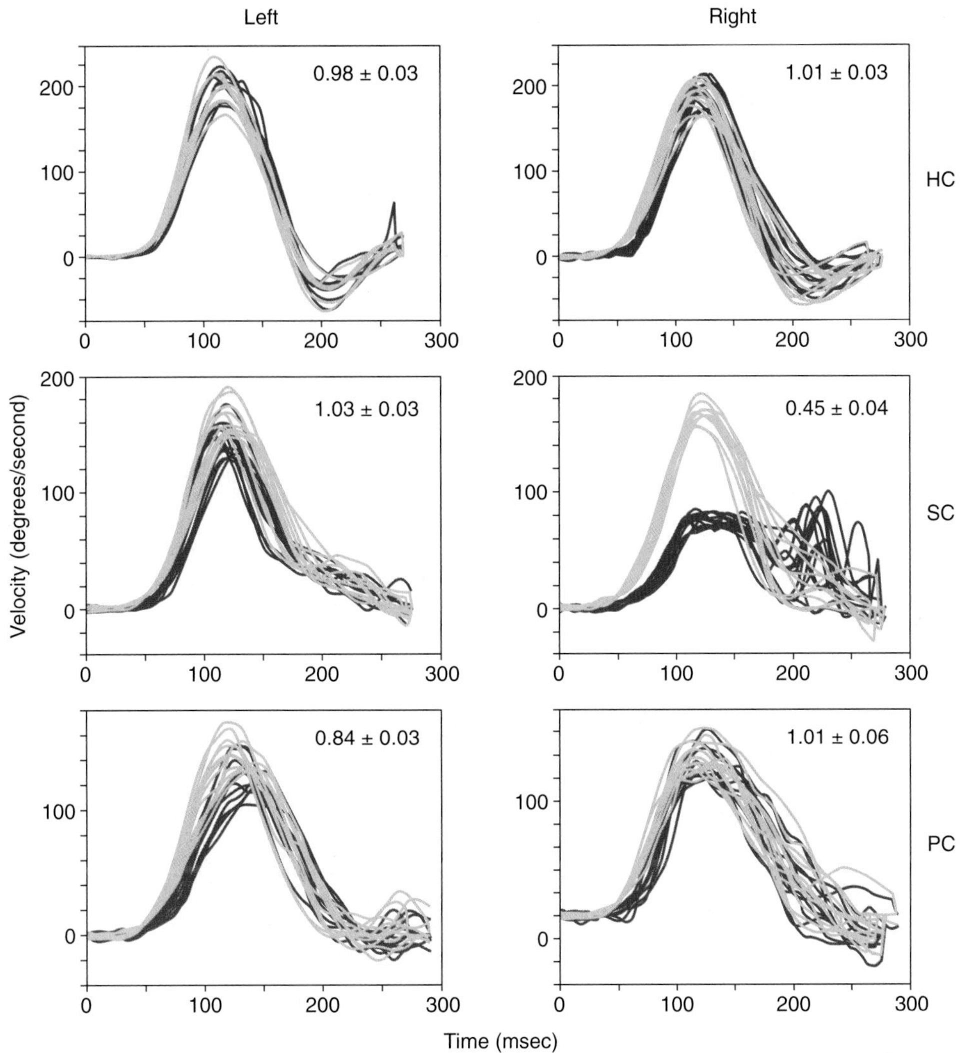

Figure 163-23. Results of head thrust testing of the aVOR in a subject with right superior semicircular canal (SC) dehiscence. Data are presented in the format described in Figure 163-21. Note the isolated loss of function in the right SC. This loss of rotary sensory function is presumably due to complete occlusion of the membranous canal by the brain and dura herniating into the lumen of the canal as shown on the CT scan *(inset)*. AC, anterior canal; HC, horizontal canal.

that canal plane. In reality, few natural head movements align solely with one canal plane, and most rotations stimulate two or even all three of the pairs of canals. How much is each canal stimulated in such a rotation? The motion of the endolymph in each canal (relative to the canal) will determine the degree to which the hair cells in that canal are stimulated. The endolymph motion in each canal is proportional to the component of the head's rotational velocity acting in the plane of that canal. A convenient way to view this is by the use of vector notation to describe the rotations.

The rotation of an object can be represented graphically with a vector that has direction and magnitude that uniquely describe the rotation. The vector lies along the axis about which the object is rotating. The direction of the vector along this axis is given by the right-hand rule (Fig. 163-24A). If the right hand were wrapped around that axis with the ends of the fingers pointing in the direction of the object's rotation, the thumb would point in the direction of the arrow of the vector. The length of the vector describes the magnitude of the rotation (e.g., degrees of angular displacement or degrees/second of angular velocity).

Using vector notation, the rotations that maximally excite each of the semicircular canals can be depicted as shown in Figure 163-24B to D. The axis of each of these rotations is perpendicular to the plane of the canal and is called its *sensitivity axis*. In the case of a head rotation that is not confined along one of these axes, the component of head velocity acting on each of the canals can be determined by graphically projecting the head velocity vector onto each of the sensitivity axes. For example, in Figure 163-24E, a head rotation to the left with the head upright mostly stimulates the left horizontal canal. The component of head rotation operating on the horizontal canal is the projection onto the horizontal canal's sensitivity axis. However, note that the projections onto the sensitivity axes of the superior and posterior canals indicate an excitatory stimulus acting on the ipsilateral superior canal and an inhibitory stimulus acting on the ipsilateral posterior canal. Mathematically, the magnitude of the stimulus projected onto the canal's sensitivity axis is the magnitude of the head velocity vector times the cosine of the angle between the axis around which the head rotates and the sensitivity axis of the canal.

Because the canal planes are approximately orthogonal to each other, the sensitivity axes are also approximately orthogonal. The pattern of activity induced in the ampullary nerves therefore effectively decomposes a head rotation into mutually independent simultaneous components along the sensitivity axes. The actions of pairs of extraocular muscles are similarly combined. The extraocular muscles are arranged in pairs that approximately rotate the eyes around axes in the orbit that parallel the sensitivity axes of the canals. Simultaneous activation of extraocular muscle pairs in proportions similar to the propor-

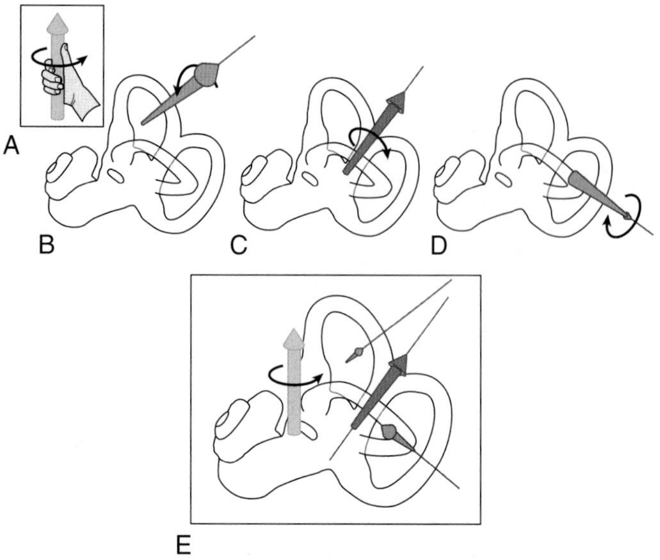

A B C D E

Figure 163-24. Vector representation of head velocity acting to stimulate the individual semicircular canals. **A,** The right-hand rule. The vector describing a rotation is oriented along the axis of rotation, pointing in the direction toward which the thumb of the right hand would point if the fingers wrapped around the axis and pointed in the direction of rotation. The magnitude of the vector represents a measure the rotation, either angular displacement or velocity. **B,** The sensitivity axis of the left superior canal lies perpendicular to the plane of that canal. Excitatory head rotation in that plane down and toward the left is depicted by a vector along the sensitivity axis. **C** and **D,** The sensitivity axes of the horizontal and posterior canals, each with a vector denoting the rotation that maximally excites it. **E,** The contribution of each canal in response to an upright horizontal head rotation to the left (orange vector). The bulk of the head velocity acts on the horizontal canal (HC), as shown by the projection (in red) along its sensitivity axis. The HC is not truly horizontal in this condition. Consequently, the rotation also acts on the superior canal (green vector) and posterior canal (blue vector). The SC receives a small excitatory stimulus. Note that the projection onto the PC's sensitivity axis is in its negative direction, meaning that the PC is inhibited under these circumstances.

tions of canal activation will result in eye rotation around an axis parallel to that about which the head rotates, but in the opposite direction. This, of course, is the goal of the angular VOR.

Given its ability to immediately sort incoming stimuli (head rotations) into spatially independent, minimally redundant channels of information, the labyrinth can be thought of as a "smart sensor" that not only measures stimuli but encodes them immediately in a maximally efficient way for downstream use in driving the angular VOR. In this respect, it is analogous to the cochlea, which segregates sounds into separate bins of the frequency spectrum, and the retina, which spatially maps the world into a retinotopic space.

Just as head rotations rarely stimulate only one pair of semicircular canals, labyrinthine pathology rarely affects only one canal. The brain perceives the simultaneous activation of several canals as the head rotation that would produce the same component of activation along each canal's sensitivity axis. These components are linearly combined to produce an eye movement that would compensate for the perceived head movement. By *observing the axis of the nystagmus*, the examiner can deduce which combination of canals are being excited (or inhibited). This *linear superposition* of the canal signals for simultaneous stimulation of multiple canals was confirmed in an elegant series of experiments by Cohen and associates.[63,76-78] These workers used both cineoculography of eye movements and electromyographic recordings from extraocular muscles in cats while electrically stimulating ampullary nerves alone and in combinations. They observed that even highly nonphysiologic combinations of ampullary nerve stimuli caused eye movements and extraocular muscle activity that could be predicted as the vector summation of responses to each stimulus alone (Fig. 163-25). Individual stimulation of the left semicircular canals caused eye movements that were rightward (for the left horizontal canal), upward and clockwise (for the left anterior canal), or downward and clockwise (for the left posterior canal) with respect to the animal's head. In a canal frame of reference, each of these eye movements is in the plane of the stimulated canal, as predicted by Ewald's First Law (Principle 3). Simultaneous stimulation of the left horizontal and anterior canals caused eye movements that were rightward, upward, and clockwise. In a canal frame of reference, the axis of these eye movements is a weighted vector sum of the responses of stimulated horizontal and anterior canals. Simultaneous stimulation of the left horizontal and posterior canals caused eye movements that were rightward, downward, and clockwise—that is, around an axis given by the sum of two equal vectors along the sensitivity axes of the horizontal and posterior canals. Simultaneous stimulation of the left anterior and left posterior canals caused eye movements that were clockwise, as would be expected from cancellation of the pitch (up and down) response components when vectors along the sensitivity axes of these two canals are summed. Finally, simultaneous stimulation of the all three left canals caused eye movements that were rightward and clockwise, again the prediction from a sum of equal vectors along the sensitivity axes of these canals.

Clinical Implications

This last experiment, by Suzuki and coworkers,[76] models what occurs when all of the canals on one side become excited from their baseline firing rates. The slow phase of the observed nystagmus has a horizontal component toward the contralateral side and a torsional component that moves the superior pole of the eye toward the contralateral side. The nystagmus beats to the ipsilateral side both horizontally and torsionally. There is no vertical component to this nystagmus. This *irritative nystagmus* can be seen when the labyrinth is irritated, for example, early in an attack of Meniere's disease, after stapedectomy procedures, and early in the course of viral labyrinthitis.

The same static imbalance in firing rates between sides occurs with unilateral labyrinthine hypofunction. Consider the case of left unilateral labyrinthectomy, in which case all three canals on that side are ablated. Unopposed activity of the right lateral canal contributes a leftward slow phase component. Unopposed activity of the right anterior canal contributes an upward and counterclockwise slow phase component. Finally, unopposed activity of the right posterior canal contributes a downward and counterclockwise slow phase component. These components combine, with the up and down components canceling each other, and with the net result being a leftward and counterclockwise slow phase (rightward- and clockwise-beating) nystagmus.

Quantitative application of this principle has yielded important information about the pathophysiology of vestibular neuritis. Fetter and Dichgans[79] measured three-dimensional eye movements in 16 patients with spontaneous nystagmus 3 to 10 days after the onset of vestibular neuritis. Their spontaneous nystagmus axes clustered between the direction expected from hypofunction of the horizontal canal and the direction expected from hypofunction of the anterior canal on the affected side. Hypofunction of the posterior canal did not seem to contribute to the nystagmus, and head thrusts in the plane of the ipsilateral posterior canal showed preserved function. These investigators proposed that vestibular neuritis is therefore usually a disorder of the organs innervated by the superior vestibular nerve—that is, the horizontal and anterior canals and the utricle. In support of this hypothesis is the observation that vestibular-evoked myogenic potentials (VEMPs) (a test of saccular function—see Principle 11) usually are preserved in these patients.[80] Furthermore, the frequent (approximately 21%) occurrence of ipsilateral posterior canal BPPV in these patients makes sense under this hypothesis: Function remains intact in the posterior canal, which can mediate BPPV if damage to the utricle releases otoconia into that canal.[80]

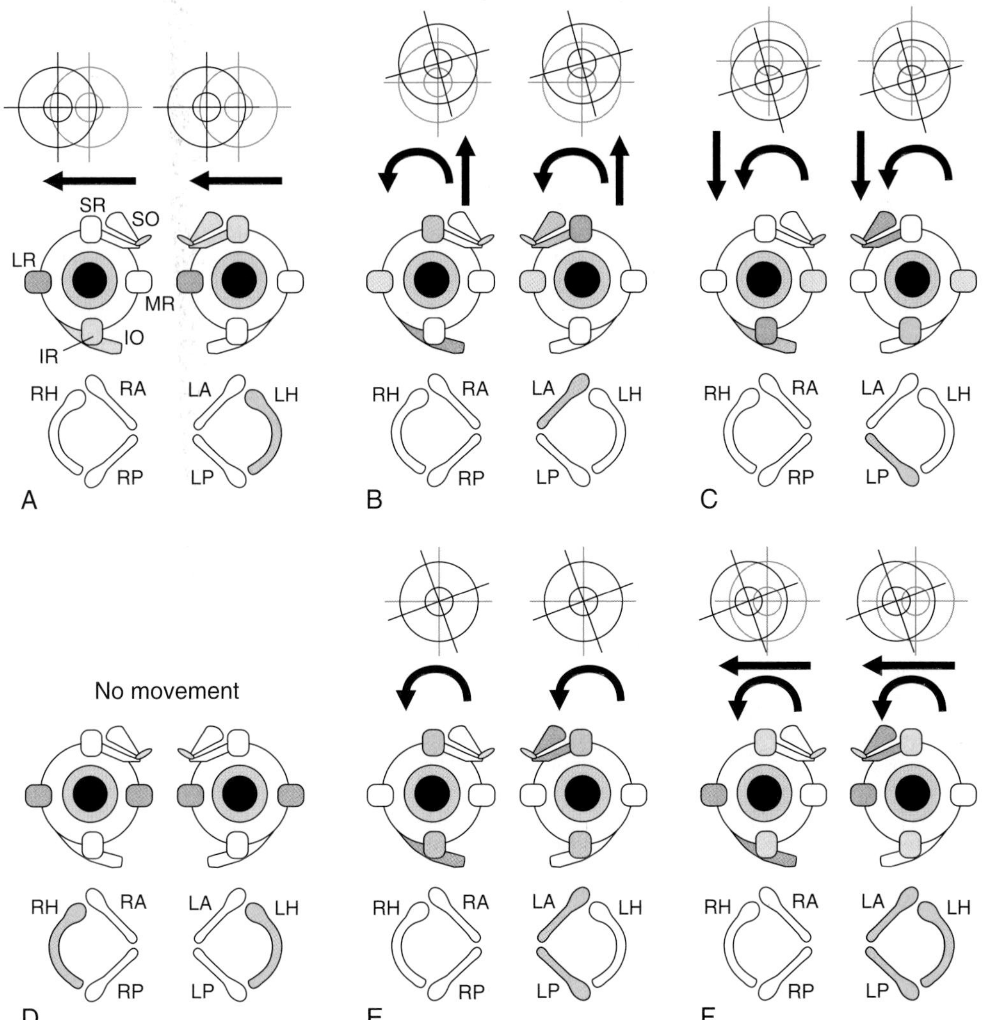

Figure 163-25. Nystagmus slow phases observed for excitation of individual semicircular canals. In the *bottom row* of each panel, *shading* indicates the excited canal(s). LA/LH/LP, left anterior, horizontal, and posterior canals; RA/RH/RP, right anterior, horizontal, and posterior canals. In the *middle row*, a cartoon of the extraocular muscles depicts which muscles are activated (darker shading indicates stronger activation). LR/MR/SR/IR, lateral, medial, superior, inferior rectus; SO/IO, superior/inferior oblique. In the *top row*, the resultant yaw, pitch, and/or roll eye movements are indicated. **A,** Excitation of the left horizontal canal causes rightward slow phases due mainly to strong activation of right LR and left MR. **B,** Excitation of the left anterior canal causes upward/clockwise (from patient's perspective) slow phases, due to combined action of the right IO and SR and the left SO and SR. **C,** Excitation of the left posterior canal causes downward/clockwise (from patient's perspective) slow phases, due to combined action of the right IO and IR and the left SO and IR. **D,** Equal stimulation of LH and RH canals elicits antagonistic contraction of MR and LR bilaterally, yielding no nystagmus. **E,** Combined equal excitation of LA and LP canals excites muscle activity that is the sum of each canal's individual effect; upward and downward pulls cancel, resulting in a purely clockwise nystagmus. **F,** Combined equal excitation of all three left canals causes a right-clockwise slow phase, the expected result of summing activity for each individual canal. *(Adapted from Cohen B, Suzuki J-I, Bender MB. Eye movements from semicircular canal nerve stimulation in the cat.* Ann Otol Rhinol Laryngol. *1964;73:153; data adjusted to human head frame of reference.)*

Principle 8: Nystagmus Due to Dysfunction of Semicircular Canals Has a Fixed Axis and Direction with Respect to the Head

Anatomic and Physiologic Basis

The concept of a fixed axis of nystagmus for stimulation of an isolated semicircular canal has already been demonstrated for posterior canal BPPV, under Principle 3. In that case, the eyes always rotated about the sensitivity axis of the affected posterior canal. Having the patient direct gaze orthogonal to and along the sensitivity axis of the posterior canal showed that there was really no change in the direction of nystagmus when considered in the canal-fixed reference frame (despite the dramatic change in the eye-fixed reference frame).

This principle extends that concept to any axis of rotation resulting from stimulation or inhibition of any combination of semicircular canals. Consider again the patient with acute unilateral hypofunction of all of the right semicircular canals. There is relative excitation of all the left canals. As demonstrated previously, the nystagmus will beat toward the left both horizontally and torsionally. Changing gaze direction does not change the leftward direction of the fast phases of this nystagmus. Thus, it is a *direction-fixed* nystagmus. In general, peripheral nystagmus has a fixed axis and direction.

Clinical Implications

This principle helps to distinguish nystagmus from a peripheral vestibular disorder from nystagmus due to a central disorder. In the case of the latter, the axis or direction of nystagmus may change depending on the direction of gaze.[81] It is important to note that the *magnitude* of the nystagmus is *not* fixed depending on gaze. The reason for this is discussed in the next principle.

Principle 9: Brainstem Circuitry Boosts Low-Frequency VOR Performance through Velocity Storage and Neural Integration; Failure of These Mechanisms Suggests Central Pathology

The description of the VOR up to this point has depicted little role for brainstem and cerebellar signal processing, other than passing on the vestibular signals to the appropriate ocular motor nuclei. This "direct pathway" is the classical three-neuron reflex arc. However, the brainstem does more than serve as a conduit for the vestibular afferent signals. An "indirect pathway" through the brainstem circuits also must account for the poor performance of the vestibular endorgans at low frequencies and the need for further integration of the incoming head velocity signal to generate fully compensatory eye movements. The brainstem accomplishes these tasks through processes called *velocity storage* and *velocity-to-position integration*. These two processes also lead to several important clinical phenomena, such as post-rotatory nystagmus, post–head-shaking nystagmus, and Alexander's Law. The last of these is another one of the cardinal signs that differentiates peripheral from central causes of nystagmus.

Anatomic and Physiologic Basis

Velocity Storage

For head rotations at frequencies below approximately 0.1 Hz, the vestibular nerve afferent firing rate gives a poor representation of head velocity (see Appendix). In response to a constant velocity rotation, the cupula initially deflects but then returns back to its resting position, with a time constant of approximately 13 seconds.[82] Thus, nystagmus in response to a constant-velocity rotation would be expected to disappear after approximately 30 seconds (see Fig. 163-10B).

In fact, the situation would be made somewhat worse because canal afferent neural responses also tend to decay for static or low frequency responses. This adaptation of afferent firing is a property of the neuron itself, and it is especially pronounced for irregular afferents. The effect of adaptation is to make afferents respond more transiently to static and low frequency cupular displacements. Thus, some canal afferents end up carrying a transient signal in response to low frequency and constant velocity rotations. This signal more closely reflects the rate of change of head velocity—that is, acceleration—than velocity itself.

Despite these tendencies for the peripheral vestibular signals to decay prematurely, experimental observations in humans have shown that the time constant of the decay of the angular VOR for constant velocity rotation is about 20 seconds, longer than would be expected based on the performance characteristics of the canals alone.[83] Neural circuits in the brainstem seem to perseverate canal signals, stretching them out in time. The important physiologic consequence of this effect (historically called *velocity storage*, because it appears to "store" the head velocity information for some period of time) is that it allows the vestibular system to function better at low frequencies. Because of velocity storage, the lower corner frequency of the system is extended to approximately 0.08 Hz. This allows sufficient overlap between the VOR and lower-frequency gaze-stabilizing systems (smooth pursuit and optokinetic nystagmus) to avoid having a region of frequency in which neither system works well.[12]

Robinson[84] proposed that velocity storage could be accomplished by a feedback loop operating in a circuit including the vestibular nuclei. Lesion studies in monkeys suggest that velocity storage arises from neurons in medial vestibular nucleus (MVN) and descending vestibular nucleus (DVN) whose axons cross the midline.[85]

Velocity-to-Position Integration

A second problem arises in matching the signals coming out of the semicircular canals to those needed to act on the eye muscles. For all eye movements, in order to move the eye, the contraction of an extraocular muscle must not only overcome the force of viscous drag (friction), which is proportional to eye velocity. It also must overcome the elastic restoring force that arises principally from stretch of the antagonistic extraocular muscle with which it is paired. This elastic restoring force is significant, even though the antagonist muscle receives an inhibitory command. This force, analogous to that produced by a spring, is proportional to the eye's displacement or position. Experimental evidence shows that the oculomotor neurons receive a signal that includes signal components for both the desired eye velocity $\dot{E}(t)$ and the instantaneous eye position $E(t)$:

$$\textit{firing rate} = kE(t) + r\dot{E}(t) \qquad \text{Eq. 163-12}^{86}$$

In making a horizontal saccade, for example, a velocity command is generated by an excitatory burst neuron in the paramedian pontine reticular formation (PPRF) (Fig. 163-26). This command is a pulse of neural activity, which is sent along a direct path to the abducens and oculomotor nuclei. Alone, it would provide only the term proportional to desired eye velocity, and the eye would slide back to its neutral position in the orbit without the ongoing pull from the muscle to overcome the elastic restoring force. The ongoing pull from the term proportional to eye position is obtained by way of an indirect path through neurons that mathematically time-integrate the pulse (a transient or phasic command) to yield a step (a tonic command). The final signal carried by the oculomotor neuron is thus a pulse-step (phasic-tonic) signal of the form of Equation 163-12.

For the VOR as well, the oculomotor neurons need to receive both an eye velocity and eye position command (Fig. 163-27). The desired eye velocity $\dot{E}(t)$ is easily obtained; it is simply equal and opposite to the head velocity $\dot{H}(t)$, a quantity approximately provided by the signals from the semicircular canals. The estimate of eye position $E(t)$ is provided by the brainstem *velocity-to-position integrator*, which integrates the velocity signal provided by the canals to give an estimate of position. All types of conjugate eye movements—the VOR, optokinetic nystagmus, saccades, and pursuit—are initiated as velocity commands that are passed both directly to the oculomotor neurons and indirectly through this shared neural integrator.[87] This brainstem integrator likely is a circuit of recurrently connected neurons in which signals reverberate and produce synaptic changes, a form of short-term memory.[88,89] For horizontal eye movements, the integrating neurons lie in the nucleus prepostitus hypoglossi region of the pons.[90,91] For torsional and vertical eye movements, they lie in the interstitial nucleus of Cajal.[92]

Clinical Implications

Pre- and Post-rotatory Nystagmus

Velocity storage is responsible for the prolonged nystagmus that occurs after sustained constant-velocity rotation in one direction (Fig. 163-28). Rotation to one side generates a positive change in afferent firing on the ipsilateral side and a negative change on the contralateral side. Because of the excitation-inhibition asymmetry inherent in the semicircular canal signals (Principle 6), the net result is not zero change in the afferent firing rate sensed by the brainstem, but rather a net excitation on the ipsilateral side. The velocity storage mechanism perseverates this net excitation beyond the time that the cupula deflection has returned to zero (see Fig. 163-10B). The brainstem thus perceives that the head continues to rotate toward the same side, and it generates an angular VOR for that perceived rotation. The slow phases of nystagmus are directed toward the contralateral side, and the fast phases are directed toward the ipsilateral side. This nystagmus decays exponentially as the velocity storage mechanism discharges with the time constant of approximately 20 seconds.

Head-Shake Nystagmus

If the head is rotated side to side in the horizontal plane in normal subjects, the velocity storage mechanism is charged equally on both sides. There is no post-rotatory nystagmus as the stored velocities decay at the same rate on either side. However, nystagmus does occur after head shaking in subjects with unilateral vestibular hypofunction.[93] In the clinical head-shaking test, the examiner passively rotates the subject's head horizontally at 1 to 2 Hz for 10 to 20 cycles of rotation. Once the rotation stops, the eyes are observed under Frenzel lenses in order to prevent visual suppression of the nystagmus. As the head is shaken from the lesioned side toward the intact side, net excitation is stored by the velocity storage mechanism. In fact, the *net* excitation

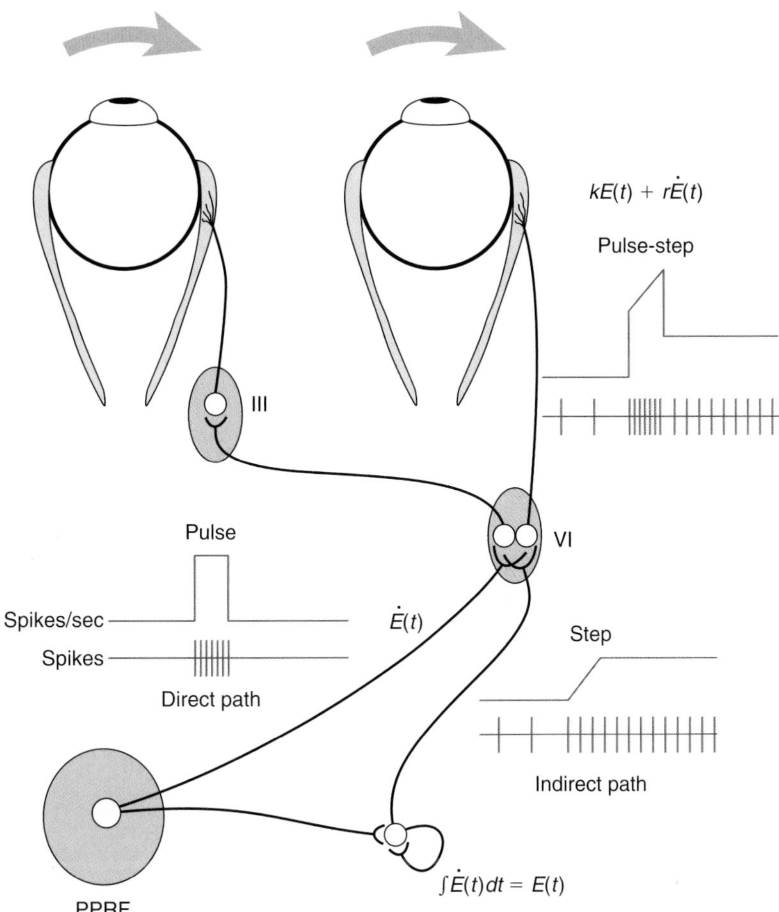

Figure 163-26. The motor command for the saccade originates in the paramedian pontine reticular formation (PPRF) as a pulse of neural firing. This activity is transmitted along a direct path to the ocular motor nuclei as a pulse. The pulse also is integrated into a step of neural discharge and transmitted to the ocular motor nuclei along an indirect path. The final motor signal is thus a pulse-step combination, as required by the dynamics of the eye muscles.

is greater than in normal subjects because there is no inhibitory signal coming from the lesioned labyrinth. When the head is turned and rotated toward the lesioned side, there is no excitatory stimulus sent to the brainstem from that side, and only a small inhibitory stimulus from the intact labyrinth. After multiple cycles of back-and-forth rotation, a marked asymmetry develops in the velocity storage mechanism, one that signals illusory continued rotation toward the intact side. As a result, when the head stops rotating, the nystagmus is as would be expected for continued rotation toward the intact side: The slow phases go toward the lesioned side, and the fast phases toward the intact side. This pattern may even reverse after several seconds, presumably because neurons affected by velocity storage adapt to the prolonged change in firing from their baseline rates.

The head shaking test provides another very useful means of localizing labyrinthine loss, one that complements the information derived from caloric testing and head thrust testing. As noted previously, caloric testing measures the function of an isolated semicircular canal at relatively low frequency. The head thrust test uses rapid, brief rotations with frequency content in the range of 3 to 5 Hz. By providing information about the function of the labyrinth at 1 to 2 Hz, the head-shaking test may provide information not available from the other two tests.

Alexander's Law

The brainstem integrator also manifests characteristic findings in vestibular pathology. In the acute period after loss of unilateral labyrinthine function, the integrator becomes dysfunctional or "leaky." In part, this may be an adaptive strategy by the brain to minimize nystagmus. As we have already seen, integration of the vestibular signal increases the drive to the extraocular muscles that pull the eye in the direction of the slow phases. By shutting down the integrator, the brain may decrease the slow-phase velocity of nystagmus. However, because the integrator is shared by other oculomotor systems, including the saccadic system, the ability to hold the eye in an eccentric position in the orbit is impaired when the integrator is leaky. As a result, the eyes tend to drift back to the center position in the orbits (Fig. 163-29). This centripetal drift has an important effect on the observed nystagmus. When the eyes look toward the direction of the fast phase of nystagmus, the drift due to the "leakiness" of the integrator adds to the slow-phase velocity due to the vestibular imbalance, and as a result the nystagmus slow-phase velocity increases. However, when the eyes look toward the direction of the slow phase, the centripetal drift due to the leaky integrator subtracts from the slow-phase velocity due to the vestibular imbalance, and the nystagmus slow-phase decreases or may disappear. This observation has come to be known as *Alexander's Law*.[94] Although occasionally seen in central lesions, peripheral types of nystagmus generally will obey Alexander's Law, making it an important neuro-otologic examination finding in distinguishing nystagmus of central origin from that of peripheral origin.

Interpreting Rotary Chair Tests

Dysfunction of the neural integrator and velocity storage can also be seen in the results of rotary chair testing. Rotary chair testing may consist of either steps of constant-velocity rotation or sinusoidal harmonic oscillations, typically from 0.01 to 0.6 Hz. Velocity steps may be delivered by suddenly starting the rotation of the chair from zero velocity to a sustained constant velocity in one direction (as in Fig. 163-8B). Alternatively, the equivalent stimulus may be obtained by braking the chair after a prolonged constant velocity rotation in the

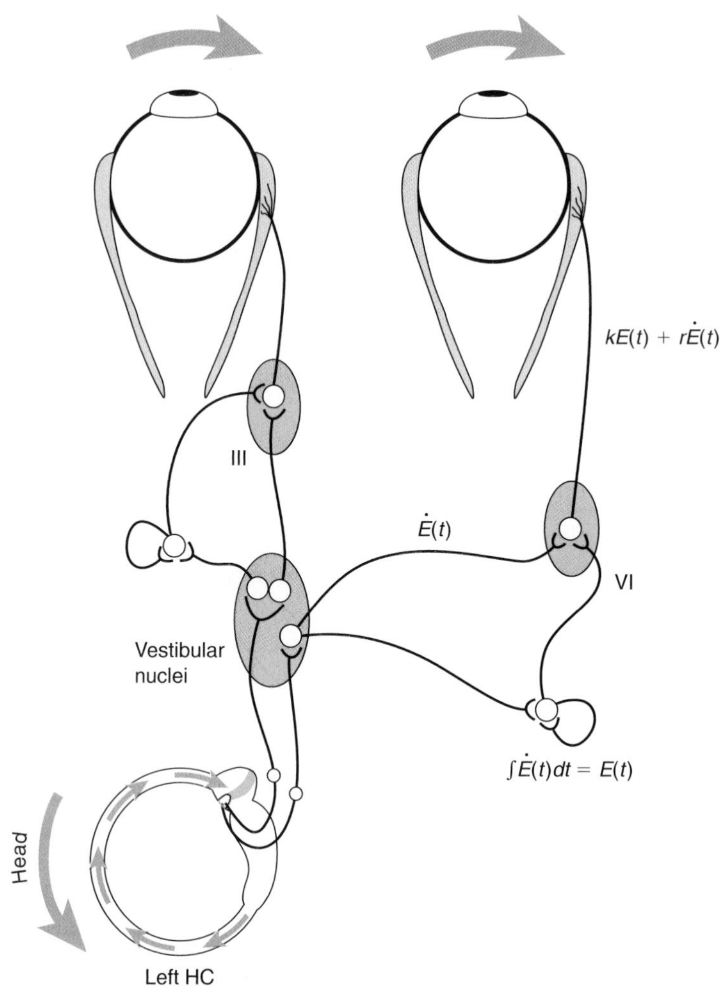

Figure 163-27. Signals from the canals also pass through direct and indirect pathways to the ocular motor nuclei. The direct excitatory pathway for the horizontal vestibulo-ocular reflex (VOR) is depicted in detail in Figure 163-15. The indirect pathway through the velocity-to-position integrator provides the final ocular motor signal with a component proportional to eye position. HC, horizontal canal.

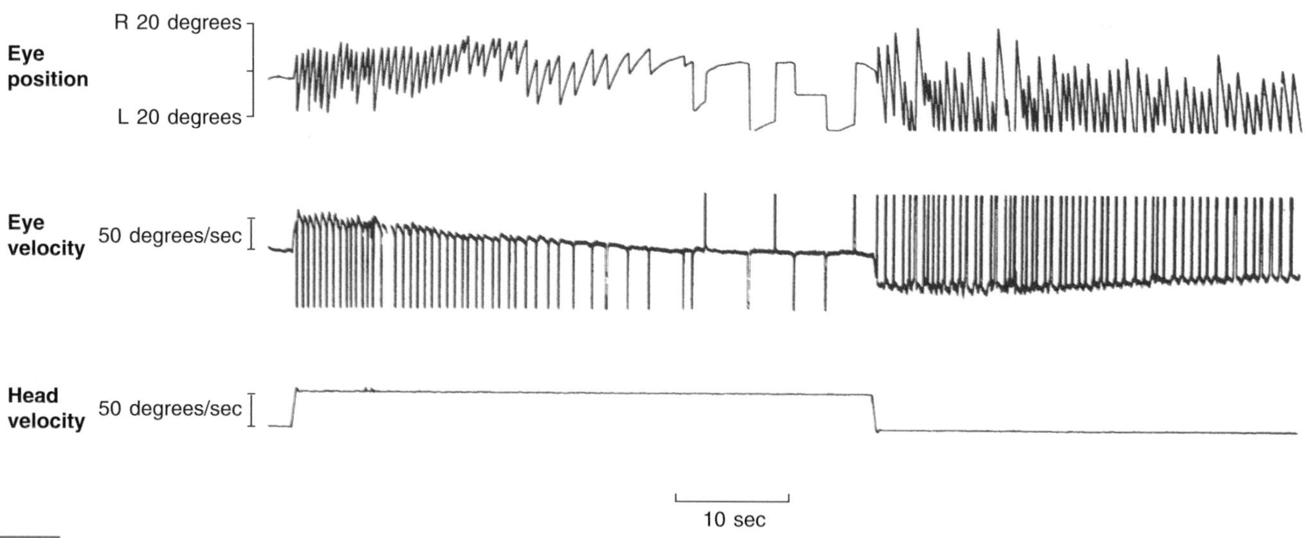

Figure 163-28. Per- and post-rotatory nystagmus in a monkey in response to a step of head velocity to 50 degrees/second. While the chair continues to rotate at 50 degrees/second constant velocity, the initial nystagmus decays more slowly than would be predicted based on the cupula's time constant. After the chair rotation stops, the nystagmus appears again but in the opposite direction. This after-nystagmus also decays more slowly than would be anticipated. The prolongation of the nystagmus after rotation is a manifestation of velocity storage. *(Modified from Cannon SC, Robinson DA. Loss of the neural integrator of the oculomotor system from brain stem lesions in monkey. J Neurophysiol. 1987;57:1383.)*

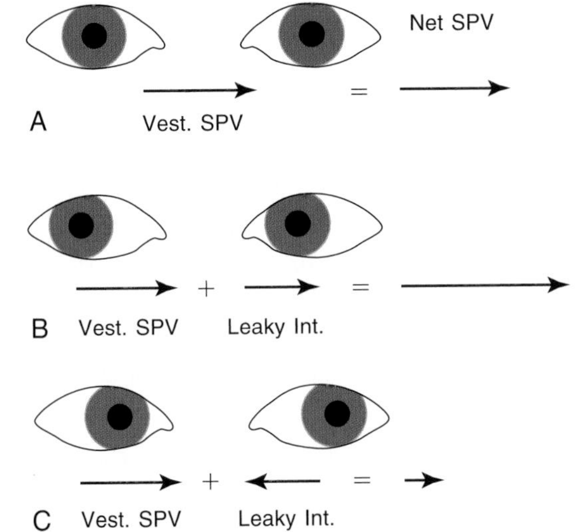

Figure 163-29. Alexander's law. The interactions of the vestibular slow phase velocity (Vest. SPV) and a leaky integrator (Int.) are demonstrated for a case of left acute vestibular hypofunction. In neutral gaze (**A**), the vestibular slow phase alone is manifest. When the gaze is in the direction of the fast phase (*right*, **B**), the leaky integrator causes the eyes to drift to the left. This drift adds to the vestibular slow-phase signal, and the net slow-phase velocity increases. When the gaze is in the direction of the slow phase (*left*, **C**), the leaky integrator causes the eyes to drift to the right. This drift subtracts from the vestibular slow-phase signal, and the net slow-phase velocity decreases.

other direction. The horizontal canals' endolymph and cupulae tend to keep moving in the direction that the chair had been moving, so that the stimulus is equivalent to a velocity step in the direction opposite to that in which the chair had been turning. In the case of unilateral loss of labyrinthine function, the magnitude of post-rotatory nystagmus in response to a velocity step expected to excite the lesioned horizontal canal may be low in comparison to that for velocity steps expected to excite the intact side. However, a decrement in nystagmus may not be detectable in subjects with compensated unilateral loss of labyrinthine function because, as explained in Principle 6, the relatively low frequencies and accelerations involved in rotary chair testing may not elicit much excitation-inhibition asymmetry. Instead, the only abnormality may be that the time constant of post-rotatory nystagmus is shortened. The impairment of the brainstem's velocity storage mechanism secondary to the loss of peripheral function decreases this time constant. For bilateral loss of labyrinthine function, nystagmus in response to steps is likely to show decreased gains and decreased time constants.

When sinusoidal rotary chair testing is performed in subjects with unilateral loss of labyrinthine function, the *gain* of the VOR (the ratio of eye velocity/head velocity; see Appendix) may be lower as the head is rotated toward the lesioned side. More commonly, however, the gain will be low bilaterally or even normal, especially once the individual has compensated for the loss of unilateral function. Often, however, the *phase* of the VOR will remain advanced relative to head velocity at low frequencies.[95] Again, this reflects the limitations of the semicircular canal in producing a response that encodes head velocity at low frequencies (see Appendix). These limitations, which are mitigated by velocity storage and neural integration, become manifest when velocity storage and integration are disrupted by a loss of peripheral vestibular function.

Principle 10: The Utricle Senses Both Head Tilt and Translation, but Loss of Unilateral Utricular Function Is Interpreted by the Brain as a Head Tilt toward the Opposite Side

Anatomic and Physiologic Basis

The utricle senses linear accelerations that are tangential to some portion of its curved surface. Most of the utricle is approximately in the plane of the horizontal canal, although its anterior end curves upward from this plane. The baseline firing of utricular afferent fibers is therefore best modulated by linear accelerations in the horizontal plane—that is, fore-and-aft or side-to-side. Hair cells in the utricle are polarized such that stereociliary deflections toward the striola excite the hair cells, and deflections away from the striola inhibit them. Because the orientations of the stereociliary bundles vary over the surface of the utricle, the organ's overall pattern of responses to a given linear acceleration can be quite complex (see Fig. 163-7). Linear accelerations in different directions probably activate unique ensembles of activity in the afferents of the utricle, with some areas being excited and others inhibited. These ensemble responses may encode the direction of head acceleration.[17]

Excitation or inhibition of *all* regions of the utricle does not occur under normal conditions of vestibular stimulation. Thus, predicting what the brain will perceive during pathologic conditions resulting in stimulation of the whole utricle is less straightforward than was the case for the semicircular canals, whose hair cells are all polarized in the same direction. However, studies in cats[96] and monkeys[97] have demonstrated a 3:1 predominance of afferents arising from the medial aspect of the utricle, which is sensitive to accelerations produced by ipsilateral tilts. Thus, the brain interprets a tonic increase in firing from the utricle on one side as a net acceleration of the otoconial mass toward the ipsilateral side. Conversely, the brain interprets a decrease or loss in firing from the utricle on one side as a net acceleration of the otoconial mass toward the contralateral or intact side.

However, the brain must still decide how to interpret this signal representing a net acceleration of the otoconial mass to one side. Such acceleration could be produced by an ipsilateral tilt or by a contralateral translational movement of the head. There is little physical difference between the shear forces acting on the hair cells of the otolith organs in these two circumstances, but the expected reflexive response of the vestibular system would be quite different depending on the interpretation. If tilt is perceived, then the appropriate compensatory reflexes would be counter rolling deviations of the eyes and head. If translation is perceived, the appropriate reflexes would be horizontal eye movements.

Just how the brain distinguishes utricular signals due to tilt from those due to translation remains one of the ongoing controversies in vestibular physiology. The equivalence of tilt and translation provides the brain a seemingly irresolvable ambiguity in the utricular afferent signals. Nevertheless, the brain is somehow able to correctly resolve the source of the ambiguous stimulus under normal conditions, so that an interaural translation produces horizontal eye movements with little or no roll movements. By contrast, when the same net acceleration acts on the utricles during tilting movements of the head, the eyes counter-roll appropriate to the tilt, but do not turn horizontally as they would for an interaural translation. One way to resolve these different stimuli might be based on the frequency content. Low-frequency or static linear accelerations acting on the otolith organs might be interpreted as gravitational accelerations resulting from tilt, whereas transient linear accelerations might be interpreted as linear translations.[98,99] An alternative hypothesis is that the central nervous system integrates information from the semicircular canals with information from the otolith organs to distinguish tilts (which also transiently activate canals) from translations (which activate only the otolith organs). In support of this hypothesis, experiments in rhesus monkeys in which the semicircular canals were inactivated by plugging demonstrated that in the absence of canal signals, modulation of otolith activity by roll tilts led to eye movements that would instead be compensatory for perceived interaural translations.[100] Thus, the brain appears to need the additional signals from the canals to distinguish tilts from translations.

Whether the brain uses the frequency content of the incoming utricular signal or the concomitant signals from the canals, the perception of a static decrease in the firing rates of utricular afferents on one side should be interpreted as tilt toward the opposite side, not translation toward the same side. From the point of view of frequency content, the static nature of the firing rate change would mimic the static (low-frequency) change due to a head tilt. From the point of view of the

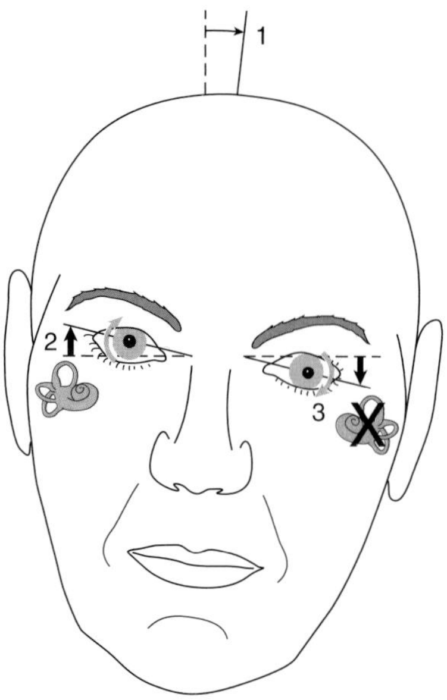

Figure 163-30. The otolith tilt reaction for loss of left utricular function consists of (1) head tilt to the left, (2) elevation of the right eye and depression of the left eye, and (3) roll of the superior pole of each eye to the patient's left.

canal signals, recall that loss of unilateral labyrinthine function leaves a relative excess of signals from the contralateral vertical canals that would be perceived as rolling of the head toward the intact side. This would be the expected concomitant canal signal for a head tilt toward the intact side. Thus, the loss of unilateral utricular function is interpreted by the brain as a head tilt toward the *opposite* side.

Clinical Importance

An isolated loss of utricular nerve activity elicits a stereotypical set of static responses called the *ocular tilt reaction*, which comprises (1) a head tilt toward the lesioned side, (2) a disconjugate deviation of the eyes such that the pupil on the intact side is elevated and the pupil on the lesioned side is depressed (a so-called skew deviation), and (3) a static conjugate counter-roll of the eyes rolling the superior pole of each eye away from the intact utricle[101] (Fig. 163-30). Each of these signs can be understood as the brain's compensatory response to a perceived head tilt toward the intact utricle. This perception arises from the excess of ipsilateral tilt information coming from the intact utricle. The ocular tilt reaction can also occur from interruption of central otolithic pathways as, for example, in multiple sclerosis.[102,103] The full ocular tilt reaction is not often observed with peripheral vestibular lesions because the brainstem compensates for some aspects very rapidly. However, the otolaryngologist will occasionally encounter the postoperative complaint of vertical diplopia after resection of an acoustic neuroma or sectioning of the vestibular nerve. By alternately covering the eyes and observing the opposite vertical shifts that occur for each eye, the skew deviation quickly becomes apparent.

Although the full ocular tilt reaction may not persist for very long after an acute lesion, the static roll of each eye toward the lesioned side may be detected for weeks to months afterward.[104,105] This can be shown with careful fundus photography, but a more practical method is with the perceptual test of subjective visual vertical (SVV) or subjective visual horizontal (SVH). Subjects with recent unilateral loss of otolith function will consistently displace a lighted line in a dark room so that it is tilted off the desired vertical or horizontal orientation toward the lesioned side. In fact, a close correlation has been noted between the absolute torsional deviation of the eyes and the angular displacement of the line from vertical or horizontal.[106] The tilt in SVV or SVH usually decreases over months after a loss of unilateral vestibular function, but for severe lesions such as vestibular nerve section some deviation persists permanently.[104]

Principle 11: Sudden Changes in Saccular Activity Evoke Changes in Postural Tone

Anatomic and Physiologic Basis

The saccule is almost planar and lies in a parasagittal orientation. Hair cells of the saccule, polarized so that they are excited by otoconial mass displacements away from the striola, can sense accelerations fore or aft (along the naso-occipital axis) or up and down. Most afferents from the saccule have a preferred up or down direction.[97] Moreover, only the sacculus can sense linear accelerations up or down, whereas naso-occipital accelerations will activate some utricular as well as saccular afferents. Thus, the sacculus has a unique role of sensing upward or downward accelerations.

When the head is upright in the gravitational field, the acceleration due to gravity (9.8 m/sec^2) constantly pulls the saccular otoconial mass toward the earth. Afferents in the inferior half of the saccule, whose hair cells are excited by this downward acceleration, have lower firing rates and lower sensitivities to linear accelerations than do those afferents in the upper half of the utricle.[97] The afferents in the upper half are excited by relative upward acceleration of the otoconial mass, such as might occur when the head drops suddenly, e.g., when one is falling. Thus, sudden excitation of hair cells across the saccular macula probably would be interpreted by the brain as a sudden loss of postural tone, as in falling. The appropriate compensatory reflex would be one that activates the trunk and limb extensor muscles and relaxes the flexors to restore postural tone. Accordingly, the saccular afferents project to the lateral portions of the vestibular nuclei, which give rise to the vestibulospinal tract, in contrast to the utricular afferents, which project more rostrally to areas involved in the VORs.[106]

Clinical Importance

Saccular excitation probably underlies the test of VEMPs. VEMPs are transient decreases in flexor muscle electromyographic (EMG) activity evoked by loud acoustic clicks or tones applied to the ear. Sufficiently loud sounds applied to the ear excite saccular afferents.[107,108] The predicted reflexive response as noted earlier would include relaxation of flexor muscles. The EMG activity averaged over multiple acoustic stimuli from a tonically contracting flexor muscle will demonstrate a biphasic short latency relaxation potential. The EMG activity can be recorded in many different flexor muscles, but the sternocleidomastoid (SCM) responses have been best described.[109] Because the saccule mediates sound-evoked VEMP responses in the normal labyrinth, absence of VEMP responses may indicate saccular dysfunction. However, transmission of the VEMP acoustic stimulus is very sensitive to any cause of conductive hearing loss in the middle ear, and VEMPs are usually absent in the presence of conductive hearing loss. Interestingly, the preservation of VEMP responses in the face of conductive hearing loss implies an abnormally low acoustic impedance of the labyrinth, such as occurs in superior canal dehiscence syndrome[110] or with enlarged vestibular aqueduct syndrome.[111]

Another example of the postural tone changes that may be related to saccular activity is the drop attack. Also known as the "otolithic crisis of Tumarkin," the drop attack is a dramatic loss of postural tone that can occur in Meniere's disease independent of other vestibular symptoms at the time of the fall.[112] It is not clear what causes the sudden loss of postural tone, but sudden deformations of the saccular macula associated with the hydropic changes of the labyrinth have been invoked.

Principle 12: The Normal Vestibular System Can Rapidly Adjust Vestibular Reflexes in Accordance with the Context, but Adaptation to Unilateral Loss of Vestibular Function May Be Slow and Susceptible to Decompensation

Anatomic and Physiologic Basis

As emphasized throughout this chapter, the vestibular system is efficiently designed to give stereotypical motor reflex outputs that compensate for the movements of the head. Yet a stereotypical output appropriate for one context may be inappropriate for another. For example, redirection of gaze is accomplished by turning first the eyes,

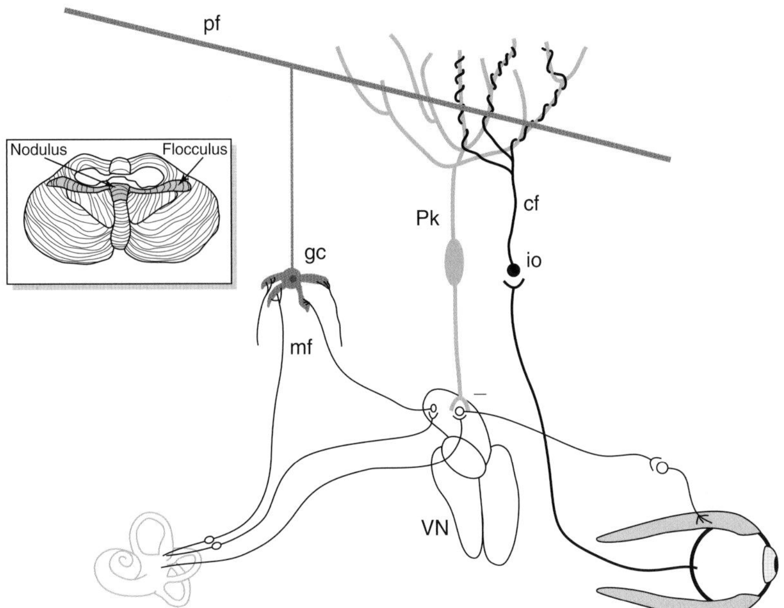

Figure 163-31. Circuitry of the cerebellum involved in modifying the vestibulo-ocular reflex (VOR). Inputs from primary vestibular afferents and secondary vestibular neurons (VN) form mossy fiber (mf) inputs to cerebellar granule cells (gc). Parallel fibers (pf) originating from these synapse weakly with Purkinje cells (Pk), causing a highly tonic inhibitory output of simple spikes from the Purkinje cells onto secondary vestibular neurons controlling the VOR. Climbing fiber (cf) input from the inferior olive (io) carries sensorimotor error information such as retinal slip. Climbing fibers make extensive and strong synapses onto Purkinje cells. Climbing fiber activity leads to complex spikes in the Purkinje cells, which can alter the efficacy of the parallel fibers' synapses onto the Purkinje cells—a form of learning.

then the head, toward a new visual target. During the gaze shift, there is a period during which both the eyes and head must move in the same direction. The VOR must actually be turned off during this period; otherwise, the eyes would stay fixed on the original target. This *cancellation* of the VOR is measurable in secondary vestibular neurons as a decrease in VOR gain when gaze is being redirected.[113,114] The mechanism by which the VOR can be canceled is not clear, but secondary vestibular neurons may receive "efference copies" of the commands going to the eye muscles. These oculomotor signals may, through inhibitory connections, decrease the responses of secondary vestibular neurons participating in the VOR reflex arc.

Under other circumstances, the VOR gain may need to be increased. For example, when the eyes are verged to view a target near the nose, they must rotate through a larger angle than that fore head rotation, in order to stay on target. In fact, as head rotation brings one eye closer to the target and takes the other eye farther away from it, each eye will require a *different* VOR gain value. Viirre and coworkers[115] showed that the VOR performs as needed under these demanding conditions to stabilize images on the retina, and it appears to do so within 10 to 20 msec of the onset of head movement—faster than could be explained by the use of any visual feedback information to correct the VOR. These investigators suggested that otolith interactions with canal signals could provide a means to constantly update an internal map of the visual target in space, allowing adjustments to the gain of the VOR for each eye.

Other contextual changes in the vestibular reflexes take place more slowly. For example, the VOR gain needs to be adjusted for changes in visual magnification when someone begins wearing spectacles. Long-term changes in vestibular reflexes, a form of motor learning, depend heavily on the cerebellum, specifically the flocculonodular lobe of the cerebellum. The basic wiring of the cerebellum as it relates to the VOR reflex arc is shown in Figure 163-31. The output of the cerebellar cortex comes from Purkinje cells, which have an inhibitory effect on their target neurons in the vestibular nuclei. Purkinje cells have two distinct patterns of activation. Simple spikes occur at high rates and are triggered by inputs from many parallel fibers. These parallel fibers arise from granule cells, which in turn receive inputs from mossy fibers. The latter convey a variety of motor and sensory signals. Input from many parallel fibers, each of which synapses weakly onto Purkinje cells, leads to a high tonic output of simple spikes from the Purkinje cells. By contrast, the climbing fibers from the inferior olive carry sensorimotor error signals—for example, retinal slip. Each climbing fiber makes numerous synapses with the dendrites of a Purkinje cell, so that one climbing fiber has a strong effect on the Purkinje cell. This effect generates complex spikes at low rates. In the classical model of cerebellar learning, repetitive and synchronous activation of climbing fiber and parallel fiber inputs causes a gradual reduction in the strength of parallel fiber synapses onto Purkinje cells—so-called long-term depression.[116] In the context of the VOR, weakening the parallel fiber input would diminish the tonic inhibition of the Purkinje cells on the secondary vestibular neurons. The VOR gain would increase as needed to correct the error signal carried by the climbing fibers. It is likely that learning in the cerebellum is much more complex than this, with changes occurring at multiple synapses. An important point is that error signals such as retinal slip may be necessary to drive the motor learning that underlies some compensatory changes in the vestibular system. This phenomenon is the basis for many physical therapy interventions for loss of unilateral vestibular function.

After unilateral loss of vestibular function (e.g., labyrinthectomy), a profound imbalance develops in the firing rates of the vestibular nuclei, with most second-order neurons on the ipsilateral side going silent.[116-125] The static imbalance results in the nystagmus and ocular tilt reaction described earlier. This static imbalance is corrected within 1 week of labyrinthectomy in alert guinea pigs[122] and within 3 weeks in the monkey.[126] Some component of the recovery of resting activity in secondary vestibular neurons is intrinsic.[127] On the other hand, subsequent lesions in other parts of the central nervous system (CNS), such as the spinal cord[128] or inferior olive,[129] can cause transient decompensation and recurrence of symptoms of static imbalance. Two important points emerge from these observations: First, an astonishing compensation for static vestibular imbalance can occur but may require a period of weeks. Second, this compensation may be disrupted by other changes in the CNS at later times, causing a recurrence of symptoms due to static vestibular imbalance. It bears repeating that despite the recovery of static central vestibular imbalance, asymmetries in dynamic responses to head movements persist, to some degree, permanently, after unilateral loss of vestibular function. This is exemplified by the head thrust test discussed in Principle 6.

Clinical Implications

Vestibular compensation requires there to be a stable (although reduced) level of peripheral vestibular function over time. The compensatory mechanisms must also be presented with sensory error signals, and their ability to sense and process these signals must not be compromised. These requirements have three important clinical consequences.

Static Loss of Vestibular Function Can Be Compensated, but Fluctuating Loss Cannot

There are important clinical correlates to the observations that the vestibular system adapts slowly to loss of unilateral function and that changes elsewhere in the CNS or further changes in vestibular function can cause decompensation. Disease states that cause static, stable loss of peripheral vestibular function are typically much less debilitating than are losses than fluctuate over minutes to hours. When there is an acute, fixed loss of unilateral vestibular function, such as after labyrinthectomy, vestibular neurectomy, or some cases of viral labyrinthitis, patients typically have several days of vertigo and nystagmus. Most patients with normal contralateral function compensate for unilateral loss remarkably well over 1 to 2 weeks.[130] Spontaneous nystagmus resolves within a few days, although nystagmus induced by head-shaking and lateral gaze toward the contralesional side may persist longer (see Principle 9). Again, it should be emphasized that sudden, rapid head rotations to the ipsilateral (nonfunctioning) side will always cause transient failure of the VOR if there is not recovery of ipsilateral peripheral function (see Principle 6). Within 2 weeks after acute unilateral loss of function, most patients no longer have vertigo at rest, and can walk, although they may require assistance. By 1 month later, most are walking unassisted and returning to normal daily activities.

In contrast to the relatively benign and predictable course after a permanent total unilateral loss of vestibular function, the fluctuating function typical in Meniere's disease and BPPV can cause intense and debilitating vertigo and nystagmus with each attack. These disorders cause a fluctuating perturbation of peripheral vestibular function on an hour-to-hour or even minute-to-minute basis. The brain simply cannot complete its compensatory work in this time frame, before peripheral function returns to normal. The compensatory mechanisms are effectively faced with a "moving target."

Perhaps the least symptomatic loss of vestibular function occurs with the slow growth of vestibular schwannomas. As the vestibular nerves are slowly infiltrated or compressed, the brain compensates for the gradual loss of function imperceptibly, and patients may have no symptoms save for the occasional off-balance feeling when turning the head rapidly toward the tumor side—a natural equivalent to the head thrust test. Patients with such loss of peripheral function may have little postoperative vertigo, whereas those with preserved function up until the time that one or both vestibular nerves are cut in removing the tumor often have severe vertigo, nystagmus, and the ocular tilt reaction.[130]

The disparity between typical responses to stable and fluctuating losses underlies the rationale behind use of ablative therapies such as intratympanic gentamicin, vestibular neurectomy, and labyrinthectomy for intractable Meniere's disease. After the initial period of compensation, patients who had previously suffered frequent bouts of vertigo usually have relatively few and tolerable vestibular symptoms, so long as contralateral function is intact and stable (reviewed by Blakley[131]).

The difference between stable and fluctuating losses also has diagnostic importance. Because stable vestibular deficits generally do not cause ongoing vertigo, recurrent vertigo in the setting of a well-compensated vestibular loss should be seen as a sign of further fluctuation in vestibular function. This fluctuation may be due to a reactivation of a quiescent disease process such as Meniere's disease, or the appearance of a new labyrinthine problem. A relatively common example of the latter is occurrence of posterior canal BPPV in 15% to 30% of patients who previously had vestibular neuritis.[132,133] As noted in the clinical implications of Principle 7, vestibular neuritis usually involves the superior vestibular nerve and its endorgans, sparing the saccule and posterior canal, which are supplied by the inferior vestibular nerve. It is thought that the damage to the labyrinth can cause release of otoconia from the utricle, and that these otoconia then settle in the posterior canal, precipitating BPPV. Typical posterior canal BPPV can develop in an ear that had vestibular neuritis even months after the onset of the neuritis.

The Effect of Suppressive Drugs on Vestibular Compensation

Patients with the acute syndrome of unilateral vestibular hypofunction are commonly given medications to alleviate their distressing symptoms: benzodiazepines (e.g., diazepam), anticholinergic agents (e.g., meclizine), and antiemetic agents (e.g., promethazine). Although these drugs are invaluable for the acute relief of these distressing symptoms, they can be counterproductive to vestibular compensation if continued for too long. Recall that central adaptation is partially driven by error signals, the sensory mismatch that occurs, for example, between the vestibular signals and visual signals when the VOR fails. These sensory mismatches cause a sense of vertigo in patients with recent-onset unilateral hypofunction as they begin moving once the static symptoms have abated. Suppressing this vertigo with the continued use of some medications can prolong or even prevent vestibular compensation. Studying the effects of medications on vestibular compensation after unilateral labyrinthectomy in cats, Peppard[134] found that the commonly used vestibular symptom suppressants diazepam, scopolamine and dimenhydrinate could hinder the rate and extent of compensation. Meclizine probably has similar effects. Conversely, a combination of a stimulant (amphetamine) and a general antiemetic (trimethobenzamide) had a beneficial effect in enhancing compensation, perhaps because increased physical activity corresponded to more head movements that challenged the system and drove compensation.

The Basis of Vestibular Rehabilitation

A variety of rehabilitation regimens have been constructed around the principle that vestibular compensation is driven by sensory mismatches, particularly between the visual and vestibular systems. Not only do these mismatches drive changes in the gain of remaining vestibular reflexes, but they also engender compensatory changes in other motor systems to replace lost vestibular functions. Examples are the central preprogramming of eye movements and of postural responses, the potentiation of the cervico-ocular reflex, and modification of saccadic eye movements. Sensory substitution of visual and somatosensory cues for the lost vestibular cues may also contribute to overall compensation.[135]

Although controlled studies of vestibular rehabilitation are difficult to perform, these programs generally do improve the subjective sense of balance in persons with fixed loss of vestibular function and often improve their objective performance on balance tests, as well as returning them to many of their activities of daily living.[136-138]

Appendix

Experimental and clinical vestibular tests often employ sinusoidal head rotations at different frequencies as stimuli, and report results in terms of VOR *gain*, *phase*, and *time constant*. These terms describe the *frequency response* of the system. The concept of the frequency response of a system is familiar to anyone who has used a graphic equalizer on a stereo system (Fig. 163-32A). Setting the sliders determines how much attenuation of the incoming signal is applied to each frequency band. The resulting output can be graphically described by the *Bode plot* (see Fig. 163-32B). In the example shown in Figure 163-32, the equalizer is set up as a low-pass filter, letting through low frequencies but attenuating high frequencies. The goal of the following analysis is to derive the frequency response—the Bode plot—for the semicircular canal.

Equation 163-8, which describes the movement of the cupula, can be written as

$$\ddot{\Theta}(t) = \ddot{H}(t) - \frac{B}{I}\dot{\Theta}(t) - \frac{K}{I}\Theta(t) \qquad \text{Eq. 163-13}$$

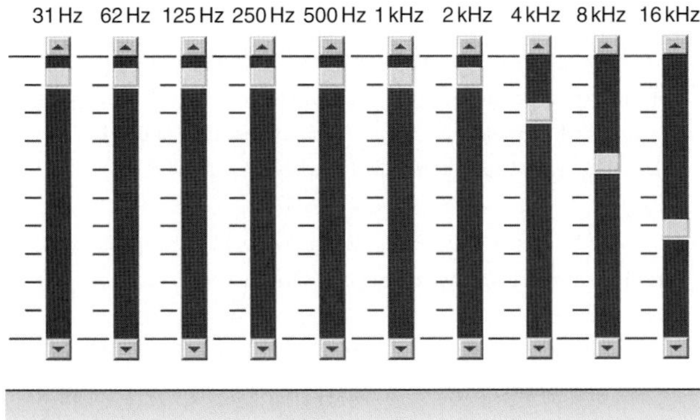

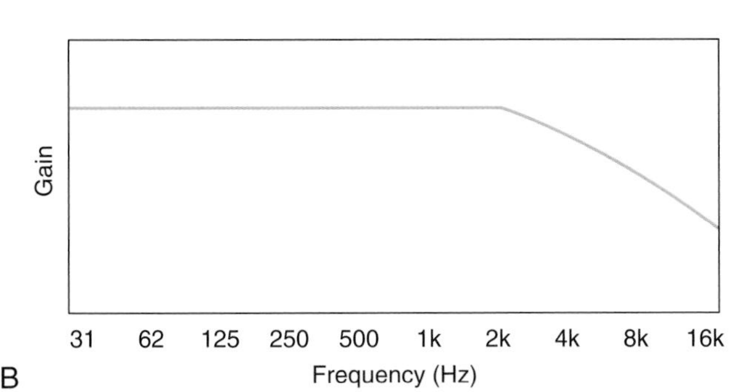

Figure 163-32. **A,** The graphic equalizer provides a means of setting signal strength (gain) across frequencies. **B,** The analytical expression of this is the Bode gain plot.

This differential equation is expressed as a function of time, or *in the time domain.* Although it can be solved as a function of time, our principal interest is to determine this system's frequency dependence. Thus, it is useful to transform this equation into the *frequency domain.* The French mathematician Laplace (1749-1827) devised a method to transform differential equations in the time domain to algebraic equations in the frequency domain. The latter are much easier to solve, and once the solution is obtained, tables can be used to look up the time-domain equivalent if it is needed. The power of Laplace's technique, however, is that it immediately gives the frequency response of the system in the form of a *transfer function* in the frequency domain. Transfer functions, which describe the input-output characteristics of systems across frequencies, are fundamental to the study of the auditory and vestibular systems.

The Laplace transform is

$$f(s)=L\{F(t)\}=\int_0^{\infty} e^{-st}F(t)dt, \text{ where } s=\sigma+j\omega. \qquad \text{Eq. 163-14}$$

The Laplace transform essentially converts signals that vary in time into those that vary in frequency by using complex exponentials. This works because most natural signals can be represented as some combination of functions that have exponential growth or decay and sinusoidal oscillations. Equations of the form $F(t) = Ae^{\sigma t}$ describe exponential growth or decay. Those of the form $F(t) = Ae^{j\omega t}$ describe sinusoidal oscillations, because

$$Ae^{j\omega t}=A(\cos\omega t+j\sin\omega t) \qquad \text{Eq. 163-15}$$

Thus, the complex exponential term $e^{-(\sigma+j\omega)t}$, encompasses most signals.

The following two features of the Laplace transform make it of such practical use in converting differential equations to algebraic ones. If $L\{Y(t)\} = y(s)$,

1. $$L\{\dot{Y}(t)\}=sy(s)-Y(0) \qquad \text{Eq. 163-16}$$

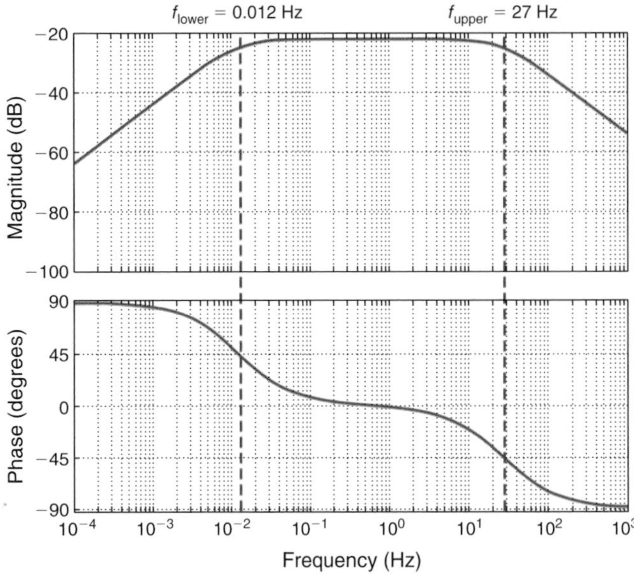

Figure 163-33. Gain (**A**) and phase (**B**) plots for the semicircular canal transfer function relative to head velocity as given in Equation 163-20. Upper and lower corner frequencies (*f*) are indicated.

That is, the Laplace transform of a derivative is just *s* times the Laplace transform of the function, minus the value of the function at time zero. The value at time zero often is 0. Thus, *differentiation* in the *time* domain becomes *multiplication* by *s* in the *frequency* domain.

2. $$L\left\{\int Y(t)dt\right\}=\frac{y(s)}{s} \qquad \text{Eq. 163-17}$$

That is, the Laplace transform of an integral is just the Laplace transform of the function divided by *s*. Thus, *integration in the time domain becomes division by s in the frequency domain.*

Using these features, Equation 163-13 can now be written in the frequency domain:

$$s^2\Theta(s)=s\dot{H}(s)-s\frac{B}{I}\Theta(s)-\frac{K}{I}\Theta(s) \qquad \text{Eq. 163-18}$$

or

$$\frac{\Theta(s)}{\dot{H}(s)}=\frac{s}{s^2+s\frac{B}{I}+\frac{K}{I}}=\frac{I}{K}\times\frac{s}{\frac{I}{K}s^2+\frac{B}{K}s+1} \qquad \text{Eq. 163-19}$$

Combining the different constants gives

$$\frac{\Theta(s)}{\dot{H}(s)}=\frac{\tau_1\tau_2 s}{(\tau_1 s+1)(\tau_2 s+1)} \qquad \text{Eq. 163-20}$$

where $\tau_1\tau_2 = I/K$ and $\tau_1 + \tau_2 = B/K$. Values for these time constants have been estimated at $\tau_1 \approx 0.006$ second and $\tau_2 \approx 13$ seconds.[82]

Note that Equation 163-20 gives the desired relationship between the motion of the endolymph (output) and the head velocity (input). This input-output relationship is the transfer function of the semicircular canal. The shown or frequency response of this transfer function can be obtained by standard engineering mathematics and is shown in Figure 163-33. This plot shows that the expected endolymph motion is indeed in phase with head velocity and has a constant gain over a wide frequency range, from approximately 0.012 to 27 Hz. Thus, over this frequency range, the *semicircular canal approximately encodes head velocity.*

Although this range encompasses most natural head movements, it should be noted that the canal is not a particularly good encoder of head velocity for very low frequency rotations. For example, whereas a slow turn at 0.02 Hz is sensed with little attenuation (1.4 dB below the flat midfrequency gain), the phase shift is approximately 32 degrees. This deficiency in the performance of the canals at low frequencies is improved by the central mechanism of *velocity storage* (see Principle 9).

Acknowledgments

We would like to thank Dr. Philip Cremer (Sydney, Australia) for the inspiration to explain vestibular physiology with a few fundamental principles. Principle 4 is directly attributed to him. We also thank Dr. Thomas Haslwanter (Linz, Austria) for comments on the manuscript.

SUGGESTED READINGS

Books

Baloh RW, Halmagyi GM. *Disorders of the Vestibular System.* New York: Oxford University Press; 1996.

Baloh RW, Honrubia V. *Clinical Neurophysiology of the Vestibular System.* New York: Oxford University Press; 2001.

Highstein SM, Fay RR, Popper AN, eds. *The Vestibular System.* New York: Springer; 2004.

Leigh RJ, Zee DS. *The Neurology of Eye Movements.* New York: Oxford University Press; 1999.

Wilson VJ, Melvill Jones G. *Mammalian Vestibular Physiology.* New York: Plenum Press; 1979.

Journal Articles

Carey JP, Minor LB, Peng GC, et al. Changes in the three-dimensional angular vestibulo-ocular reflex following intratympanic gentamicin for Meniere's disease. *J Assoc Res Otolaryngol.* 2002;3:430.

Goldberg JM, Fernández C. Physiology of peripheral neurons innervating semicircular canals of the squirrel monkey I. Resting discharge and response to constant angular accelerations. *J Neurophysiol.* 1971;34:635.

The Importance of Vestibular Reflexes

Crawford J. Living without a balancing mechanism. *N Engl J Med.* 1952;246:458.

(A classic paper describing first-hand the experience of oscillopsia from acute bilateral vestibular loss.)

Vestibular Afferent Physiology

Goldberg JM. Afferent diversity and the organization of central vestibular pathways. *Exp Brain Res.* 2000;130:277.

(This review summarizes decades of research into mammalian vestibular afferent physiology.)

Highstein SM, Rabbitt RD, Holstein GR, et al. Determinants of spatial and temporal coding by semicircular canal afferents. *J Neurophysiol.* 2005;93:2359.

(This work presents a novel explanation for why some semicircular canal afferents carry head acceleration information, even though endolymph motion in the canal approximates head velocity.)

Semicircular Canals

Aw ST, Halmagyi GM, Haslwanter T, et al. Three-dimensional vector analysis of the human vestibulo-ocular reflex in response to high acceleration head rotations. II. Responses in subjects with unilateral vestibular loss and selective semicircular canal occlusion. *J Neurophysiol.* 1996;76:4021.

(This paper lays the quantitative basis for the head thrust test.)

Aw ST, Todd MJ, Aw GE, et al. Benign positional nystagmus: a study of its three-dimensional spatio-temporal characteristics. *Neurology.* 2005;64:1897.

(This paper provides excellent examples of eye movements in the planes of individual semicircular canals.)

Cremer PD, Minor LB, Carey JP, et al. Eye movements in patients with superior canal dehiscence syndrome align with the abnormal canal. *Neurology.* 2000;55:1833.

(An example of Principle 5.)

Fetter M, Dichgans J. Vestibular neuritis spares the inferior division of the vestibular nerve. *Brain.* 1996;119:755.

(Illustrating Principle 7, this paper demonstrates that the spontaneous nystagmus of vestibular neuritis suggests a predominantly superior vestibular nerve lesion.)

Robinson DA. The use of matrices in analyzing the three-dimensional behavior of the vestibulo-ocular reflex. *Biol Cybern.* 1982;46:53.

(Robinson demonstrates how the anatomic alignment of semicircular canals and extraocular muscles simplifies the computational requirements of the angular VOR, making it the fastest reflex in the body.)

Otolith Organs

Murofushi T, Curthoys IS. Physiological and anatomical study of click-sensitive primary vestibular afferents in the guinea pig. *Acta Otolaryngol.* 1997;117:66.

(This work provides the cellular basis for vestibular sound-evoked myogenic potentials.)

Welgampola MS. Evoked potential testing in neuro-otology. *Curr Opin Neurol.* 2008;21:29.

(A review of vestibular-evoked potentials.)

Vestibular Compensation and Adaptation

De Zeeuw CI, Yeo CH. Time and tide in cerebellar memory formation. *Curr Opin Neurobiol.* 2005;15:667.

(This review summarizes recent insights into the molecular mechanisms of cerebellar adaptation of the vestibulo-ocular reflexes.)

Vibert N, Babalian A, Serafin M, et al. Plastic changes underlying vestibular compensation in the guinea-pig in isolated, in vitro whole brain preparations. *Neuroscience.* 1999;93:413.

(The investigators use innovative methods in vivo and in vitro to gain important insights into the mechanisms of compensation for loss of peripheral vestibular function.)

For complete list of references log onto www.expertconsult.com.

CHAPTER ONE HUNDRED AND SIXTY-FOUR

Evaluation of the Patient with Dizziness

Timothy E. Hullar

David S. Zee

Lloyd B. Minor

Key Points

- Imbalance can be due to dysfunction of either the peripheral or the central vestibular system.
- A careful clinical history is critical for determining the cause of imbalance; identification of symptom duration and triggers is key.
- The bedside examination often offers clues to the diagnosis, especially in patients who are asymptomatic at the time of the visit.
- Evaluation of eye movements and hearing assessment are the central parts of the physical examination.
- Laboratory tests must be used judiciously to investigate specific diagnostic entities suggested by the clinical history and bedside examination.
- Determination of treatment options depends on an accurate diagnosis.
- Specific exercises can help patients adapt to long-term balance deficits.

Background

Dizziness is the ninth most common complaint leading patients to visit their primary care physicians, rising to third among those 65 to 75 years of age and first among older patients.[1,2] Despite its frequency, symptoms of dizziness can be difficult for the patient to describe and for the physician to categorize. *Dysequilibrium*, *unsteadiness*, *vertigo*, and *lightheadedness* all are terms that patients may use to describe their sensations. Evaluation of balance signals from peripheral vestibular nerve afferents, the visual system, and somatosensory and proprioceptive receptors normally occurs below a patient's level of awareness, making symptoms particularly difficult to describe.

This chapter outlines an approach to the evaluation of patients with dizziness that builds on an understanding of the pathophysiology of dizziness to develop an organized method for history taking and physical examination leading to the identification of specific abnormalities. A description of some of the physiological and functional principles underlying the symptoms and signs of vestibular disorders is presented first. (A comprehensive description of these topics is provided in Chapter 163.) Using an approach based on these considerations, the clinical evaluation, including the history, physical examination, and quantitative tests of vestibular function, is described next. Finally, the adaptive capabilities of the vestibular system and principles of vestibular rehabilitation are reviewed.

Fundamentals of Vestibular Function

Peripheral Anatomy and Physiology

The vestibular receptors are located in the labyrinth and consist bilaterally of three orthogonally oriented semicircular canals and two otolith organs. The semicircular canals sense angular acceleration and are arranged in roughly parallel pairs: the two horizontal (also called "lateral") canals, the left anterior and right posterior canals, and the right anterior and left posterior canals. The orthogonal geometry of the semicircular canals in each labyrinth permits three-dimensional rotational head movements to be represented as the vector sum of components in each plane. Most vestibular nerve afferents have a spontaneous firing rate between 10 and 100 spikes/second. When the head is still, primary afferents in the right and left vestibular periphery discharge tonically at the same rate. During horizontal head rotation, the horizontal semicircular canal is stimulated in the ipsilateral labyrinth and inhibited in the opposite. During vigorous horizontal head rotations, many afferents and central vestibular neurons on the inhibited side are silenced.[3,4]

Over the physiologic range of head movements (0.1 to 15 Hz), the intrinsic mechanical properties of the semicircular canals integrate this acceleration signal into a velocity signal. This signal is further modified by individual afferents, providing central vestibular neurons with an array of signals carrying velocity and acceleration information. Activity in the vestibular nerve is the major source of sensory input to the vestibular nuclei, with almost 30,000 afferents projecting from each labyrinth to the brainstem in humans.[5] Neurons in the vestibular nuclei typically receive bilateral inputs from the coplanar semicircular canals (direct projections from afferent nerve fibers on the ipsilateral side and commissural projections from central vestibular neurons that cross from the contralateral side), with excitation of peripheral afferents causing increased firing rates of the neurons in the ipsilateral vestibular nucleus.

Eye Movements

Vestibular information is vital to controlling both eye movements and body posture, but eye movements are the more easily studied and the

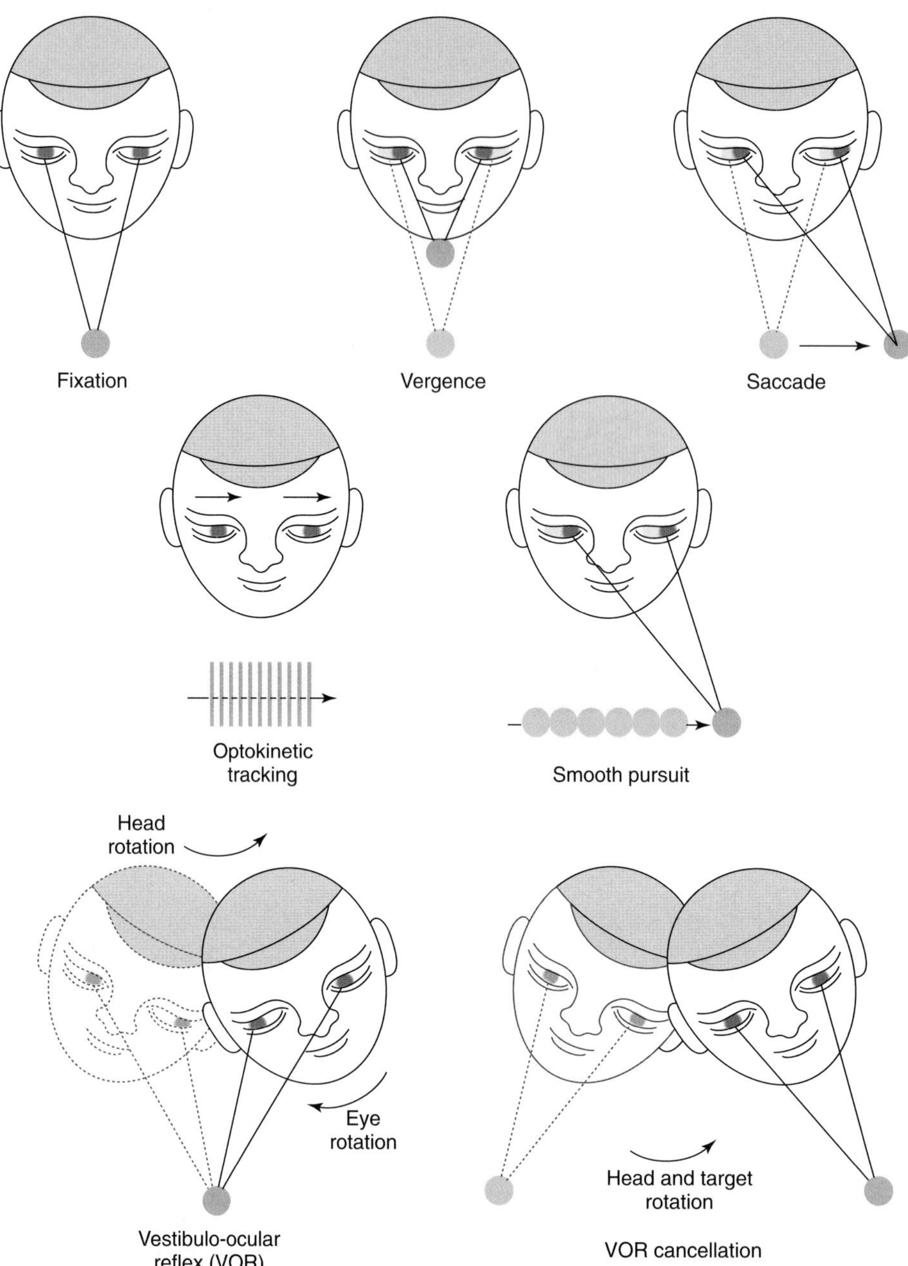

Figure 164-1. Schematic depiction of the functional classes of eye movements. Basic research in the neurophysiology of oculomotor control and clinical studies of eye movement disorders have been enhanced by the recognition of functionally distinct subsystems. Seven types of eye movements are shown.

better understood of the two. All eye movements are aimed at ensuring optimal visual acuity (Fig. 164-1). Vestibular and optokinetic eye movements work to hold eye position in space (i.e., *gaze*) constant by producing compensatory eye movements that keep images stable on the retina during head movements. Saccadic, pursuit, and vergence eye movements change gaze so that images of objects of interest are brought to or kept on the fovea, where visual resolution is highest. Saccades rotate the eye to bring an image onto the fovea, whereas pursuit maintains that image on the fovea as it moves across the visual field. Vergence movements are disjunctive, causing the eyes to move in opposite directions to place the image of an object simultaneously on both foveae during movements of the head or the object (Table 164-1).

Visual acuity is degraded if images slip across the retina even as slowly as 2 to 3 degrees/second.[6] Vestibulo-ocular reflexes (VORs) are responsible for maintaining binocular fixation and stabilizing binocular foveal images during head movements.[7] The VORs are divided into two types: angular and translational. *Angular* reflexes are initiated by activation of the semicircular canals. The canals are aligned with the pulling directions of the three pairs of extraocular muscles,[8] so that activation of a single semicircular canal (as in benign positional vertigo or canal dehiscence) leads to motion of the eyes about an axis that aligns with the axis of the semicircular canal (Fig. 164-2). The latency of the angular reflex is approximately 7 msec in humans.[9]

Translational VORs are driven by otolith afferents and can be grouped into two categories according to the eye movement responses: *tilt* responses, which compensate for lateral head tilt with respect to gravity, and *translational* responses, which produce eye movements compensatory for linear movements of the head (Fig. 164-3). Lateral head tilt produces ocular counter-rolling, a torsional movement of the eye about the line of sight. The torsional deviation of the eyes in response to 60- to 75-degree static head tilts is 6 to 8 degrees.[10] The small amplitude of eye movement produced by relatively large tilts of

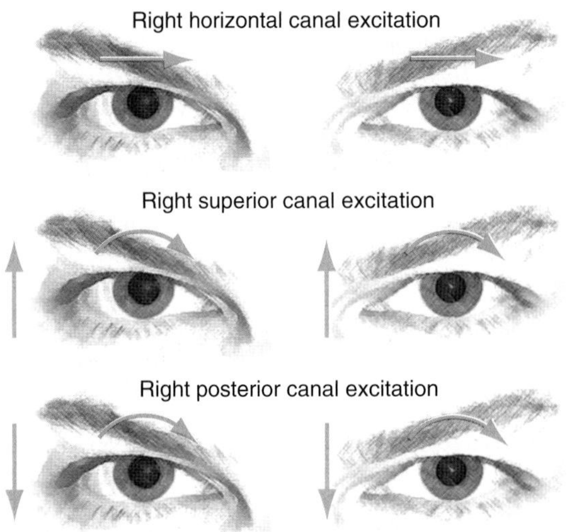

Figure 164-2. Relationship of individual canals and eye movements. Activation of individual canals leads to stereotypical eye movements. The horizontal canal is activated by head rotation in the horizontal plane, whereas pure activation of the posterior canal may be seen in benign positional vertigo, and pure activation of the superior canal is seen in superior canal dehiscence syndrome. All *arrows* represent direction of slow phase eye movements. *(From Hullar TE, Minor LB. The neurotologic examination. In: Jackler RK, Brackmann DE, eds.* Neurotology. *2nd ed. St Louis: Mosby; 2004:215-277.)*

Table 164-1

Functional Classes of Human Eye Movements

Class of Eye Movement	Main Function
Visual fixation	Holds the image of a stationary object on the fovea
Vestibular	Holds images of the seen world steady on the retina during brief head rotations
Optokinetic	Holds images of the seen world steady on the retina during sustained head rotations
Smooth pursuit	Holds the image of a moving target on the fovea
Nystagmus	The repetition of a compensatory slow phase and quick phase resetting movement of the eyes; in quick phases, gaze directed toward the oncoming visual scene
Saccades	Bring images of objects of interest onto the fovea
Vergence	Moves the eyes in opposite directions so that images of a single object are placed simultaneously on both foveas

the head appears to indicate that ocular counterrolling is a vestigial response with little compensatory function, but during lower-amplitude sinusoidal head rolls, the torsional gain is significantly greater. Compensatory eye movements in these situations seem to result largely from canal-related reflexes, although the otolith organs also are

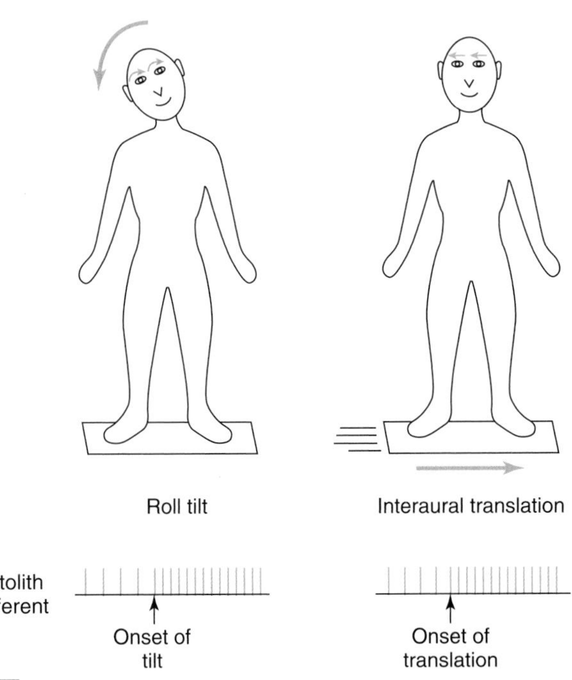

Figure 164-3. Otolith afferents respond to linear acceleration. Identical changes in otolith afferent activity can result from head movements that change the orientation of the head relative to gravity (roll tilt) and from linear translational movement (interaural translation). There is no way for otolith afferents to distinguish whether a translation or a tilt produced the modulation in otolith afferent activity. The compensatory eye movements evoked by these two types of head movements are quite different, as shown on the diagram. Central processing of signals in the brainstem must be responsible for resolution of the so-called translation-tilt ambiguity. *(From Minor LB. Physiological principles of vestibular function on earth and in space.* Otolaryngol Head Neck Surg. *1998;118:54.)*

activated.[11] Translational VORs produce eye movements that maintain the point of binocular fixation for each retina during linear head movements.

Otolith afferents cannot distinguish between tilt and translation. Information from the semicircular canals, comparison of the phasic and tonic components of modulation in otolith afferent activation, frequency-selective organization of otolith-mediated responses, or other sensory signals such as vision or proprioception must be involved in determining appropriate reflex responses. For example, tilting of the head involves both canal and otolith activation, and the combined activation of these receptors provides cues to the brain that the modulation in otolith activity is due to a tilt and not to a linear head movement. Frequency-selective filtering of otolith afferent signals provides another complementary mechanism. Head movements that change slowly with respect to gravity (frequency content less than 0.25 Hz) may be interpreted as tilt stimuli, whereas those with higher frequency content lead to responses that are directed to maintaining stable gaze during linear head movements.[12,13]

Head Movements

Compared with the relatively simple task of the six muscles moving each eye, the 20 muscles moving the neck must contend with more complicated planar relationships, the substantial inertia of the head, and the effect of stretch reflexes and muscular co-contraction. The situation is even more complicated because the trunk and lower extremities are involved in maintaining posture and upright stance. Two reflexes are important for stabilizing the head. The vestibulocollic reflex

(VCR) governs the activation of neck muscles in response to vestibular input,[14] and the cervicocollic reflex (CCR) governs the activation of neck muscles in response to stretch receptors.[15] Studies of head stability during locomotion in humans have shown that the peak velocity of these rotational head perturbations generally does not exceed 150 degrees/second, but their predominant frequency can be as high as 5 Hz, with a frequency for some components of head movements up to 15 Hz.[16-19] Studies of head movements in patients who have lost vestibular function indicate that head stability can be achieved by way of the mechanical properties of head and neck muscles, rather than neural reflexive factors.[20,21] The CCR, consisting of compensatory eye movements during head-on-body rotation caused by neck proprioception, contributes little to gaze stability in healthy people, although it may become more important if labyrinthine function is lost.[22,23]

Combinations of eye and head movements are used to acquire and track a target of interest, as well as to stabilize gaze in response to perturbations of the body. Voluntary eye-head movements can be thought of as either saccadic or pursuit in nature. During small eye-head saccades (less than 30 degrees), the shift of gaze may be achieved by superposition of an internal saccadic command and the VOR.[21] For larger eye-head saccades (more than approximately 40 degrees), the VOR appears to be "turned off" or "disconnected." Nevertheless, the vestibular signal caused by the head movement is still available so that an accurate gaze change can be achieved.[24] During smooth eye-head tracking, more than one mechanism may operate to override the VOR so that gaze follows the moving target smoothly. Evidence suggests that an internal smooth pursuit signal partly cancels the VOR, and that an additional mechanism may be reduction in the activity or partial suppression of the VOR during such eye-head tracking.[25-28] Disorders causing impairment of smooth pursuit usually, but not always, also cause deficits of smooth, combined, eye-head tracking.[29] Patients who have lost vestibular function, on the other hand, often show combined eye-head tracking that is superior to ocular pursuit.[26]

Posture

Active processes for control of the body's center of gravity are involved in maintaining postural stability in healthy subjects. The center of gravity is located in the lower abdominal area and slightly forward of the ankle joints in a healthy person standing erect. In humans, the goal of postural control is to maintain sway within the limits of stability for different body positions and activities. The limits of stability are defined by a horizontal ellipse measuring approximately 12.5 degrees from front to back. The lateral dimension of limits of stability depends on the subject's height relative to spacing between the feet. For a person 70 inches tall with feet placed 4 inches apart, the lateral dimension of the "limits of stability" ellipse is approximately 16 degrees from left to right.

Postural responses to perturbations (movement of the support surface or body) are organized into discrete patterns about the ankles and hips. The pattern(s) to be used depends on structure of the support surface and position of the center of gravity relative to limits of stability. Movements of the body about the ankle joints are the effectors of the *ankle strategy.* The ankle strategy is effective when the center of gravity moves slowly and within the limits of stability, and the support surface is longer than the feet and strong enough to resist torque about the ankles. When it is not possible to exert an adequate amount of torque around the ankle joint, healthy subjects invoke a *hip strategy.* This strategy consists of exerting a horizontal shear force on the support surface by counterphase leg and trunk movements about the hip. The hip strategy also is effective when the center of gravity moves rapidly or approaches the limits of stability.

Contributions of the Brainstem and Cerebellum

The cupula of the semicircular canal returns to neutral position with a time constant of approximately 6 seconds, but the associated decay in eye movements is closer to 15 seconds in normal humans because of the effect of a process termed *velocity storage.* The neural center responsible for this process is located in the brainstem. This mechanism improves the capability of the system to respond to low-frequency head motion[30] and to orient vestibulo-ocular responses to gravity.[31,32] Velocity storage is (transiently) lost in cases of acute unilateral vestibular loss and remains diminished in the long term.

The *neural integrator* is another brainstem mechanism vital for proper eye movements.[33] It produces a steady command to the extraocular muscles to hold the eyes eccentrically, instead of allowing them to drift back to neutral gaze position because of the elastic restoring forces of the orbital tissues. Proper function of the neural integrator also is necessary for the VOR to have the appropriate phase (timing) relationship to head rotation. The neural integrator is not able to hold gaze appropriately in cases of acute unilateral deafferentation.

The cerebellum plays an important role in immediate and long-term adaptive ocular motor control.[34] Lesions of the flocculus impair smooth pursuit and VOR cancellation, which normally allows the eyes to move with head rotations to follow a target.[35] Floccular lesions may cause horizontal gaze-evoked nystagmus, downbeat nystagmus, rebound nystagmus, increased or decreased amplitude (gain) of the VOR, and postsaccadic drift, or *glissades.*

The vestibulocerebellum also is important for ensuring that the eyes rotate in a plane parallel to head rotation so that images can be stabilized appropriately on the retina.[36] The dorsal vermis and underlying fastigial nuclei are important in the control of saccadic amplitude and smooth pursuit; lesions here produce saccadic inaccuracy (dysmetria) and impair the ability to make long-term adaptive adjustments in saccade accuracy.[37] Other "cerebellar" eye signs, which cannot be localized precisely, include square-wave jerks, defective convergence, divergence nystagmus, and alternating hyperdeviation (skew) on lateral gaze.[38]

Approach to the Patient with Dizziness

History

In many cases a specific cause for a patient's dizziness can be determined from an accurate history alone. Taking the history of a patient with a complaint related to dizziness must begin in an open-ended fashion, allowing the patient to describe the symptoms with minimal direction from the clinician. The process can be facilitated by asking the patient to complete and return a questionnaire about symptoms before the first appointment.

From the history, the clinician should have a general idea of whether the symptoms are attributable to a vestibular disorder and, if so, whether this disorder is central or peripheral in origin. An outline of diagnostic possibilities based on symptoms and signs is shown in Figure 164-4.

- Does the patient have vertigo? Vertigo is an illusory sense of motion. The patient can feel as if the motion is internal or that objects in the surroundings are moving or tilting. The sense of motion can be rotatory, linear, or a change in orientation relative to the vertical. Vertigo indicates a problem within the vestibular system, although the abnormality can be located anywhere within the system. Lightheadedness, as opposed to vertigo, may indicate presyncope. Although often related to neural factors, such as vasovagal syncope, it also can reflect cardiac disease, especially in older patients. Generalized imbalance may reflect more central processes, including mal de débarquement or migraine. Some conditions, such as migraine, can manifest with nonspecific imbalance symptoms in addition to acute vertigo.

- What happened the first time the imbalance occurred? The onset of symptoms with straining can be indicative of a disorder such as semicircular canal dehiscence or perilymphatic fistula. Straining also can lead to presyncope in a vasovagal reaction. In women, the association of symptoms with menstrual periods can indicate migraine. A correlation of symptoms with a large salt load should raise suspicion for Meniere's disease. The onset of symptoms after head trauma may indicate benign paroxysmal positional vertigo.

- Are the symptoms episodic or continuous, and if episodic, how long do they last? Most vestibulopathies cause fluctuating or episodic symptoms, although a constant sense of dysequilibrium may be

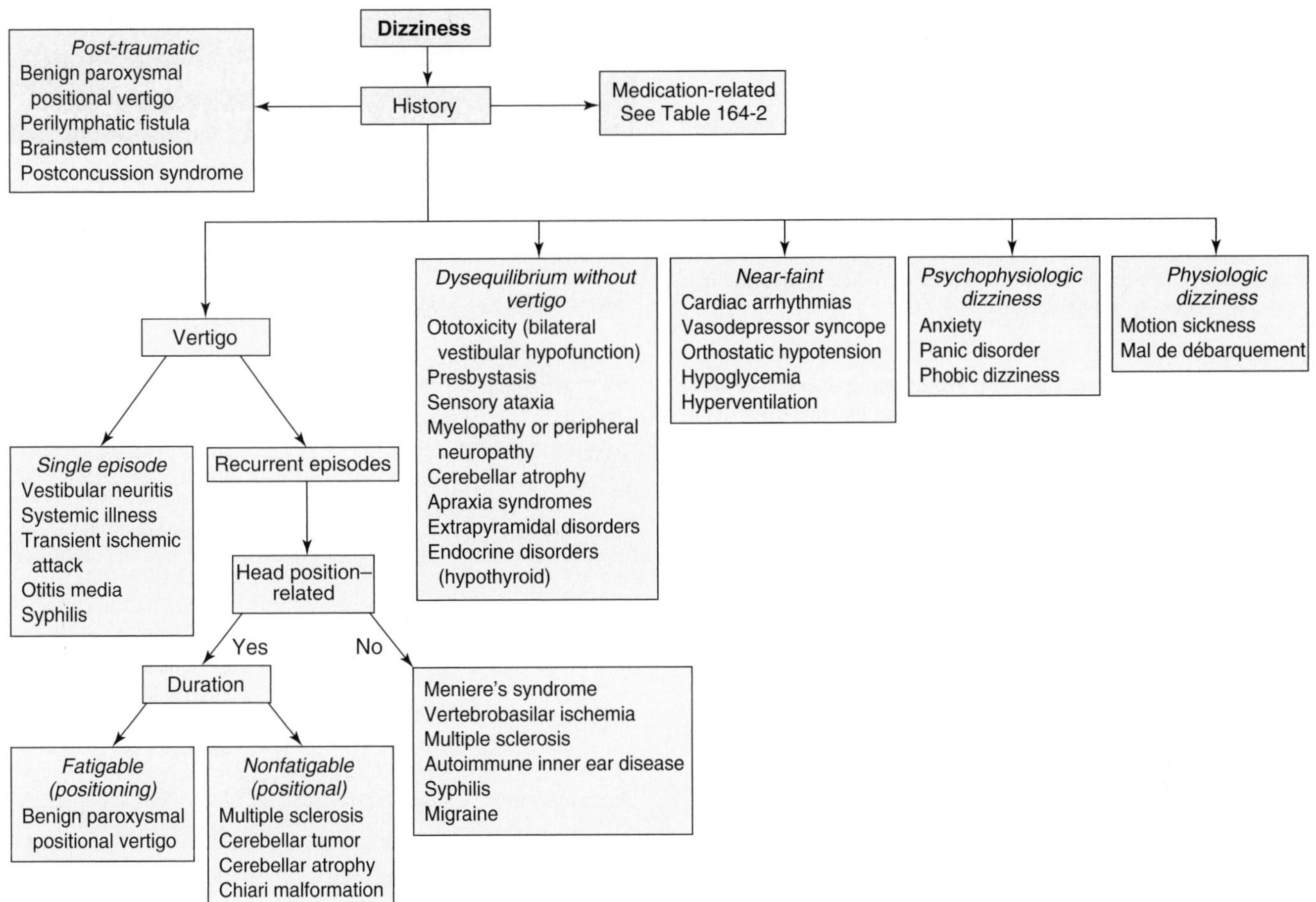

Figure 164-4. Algorithm for the differential diagnosis for dizziness, based on information from the patient's history. *(Modified from Baloh RW, Fife TD, Furman JM, Zee DS. The approach to the patient with dizziness. In: Mancall EL, ed.* Continuum: Lifelong Learning in Neurology. *Vol 2. Cleveland: Advanstar Communication; 1996:25-36.)*

present in addition to the more variable elements of the symptom complex. Migraine tends to be episodic, with each episode lasting hours to days. Benign paroxysmal positional vertigo (BPPV) is episodic but lasts a short time, although patients may note that they are "susceptible" to head motion for weeks and then not susceptible at other times. Continuous symptoms may reflect a condition such as mal de débarquement, migraine, or psychogenic dizziness.

- What brings on the problem? The diagnosis of certain vestibulopathies is strongly suggested from events or movements that trigger symptoms.
  - *Movement of the head.* BPPV of the posterior canal classically begins on rolling over in bed or tilting the head backward and toward the affected ear. BPPV of the horizontal canal can be brought on by lying with the head flat on the bed then turning it to the side. Rapid head movements may uncover vestibular hypofunction by producing a sensation of *oscillopsia* (an illusion of motion for objects that are known to be stationary). When induced by head movements, oscillopsia often is a sign of vestibular hypofunction. Brief (5 to 10 seconds) periods of vertigo, either spontaneous or sometimes induced by certain head movements, may be a sign of vascular compression of the eighth cranial nerve complex.
  - *Lifestyle.* Patients with vestibular migraine may report that certain foods such as caffeine, cheeses, wine, and other foodstuffs can bring on symptoms. The symptoms also may be induced by stress or lack of sleep.
  - *Environment.* Changes in the weather, menses, or motion stimulation such as ceiling fans or video games may bring on problems for patients who have vestibular migraine. Fluorescent lights also may cause a problem. In patients with canal dehiscence, symptoms may be brought on by loud sounds or by maneuvers that change middle ear or intracranial pressure. Changes in seasons also may provoke symptoms in patients with Meniere's disease or migraine, possibly as a result of allergy.
  - *Pressure.* Patients with semicircular canal dehiscence, perilymphatic fistula, or enlarged vestibular aqueduct may have problems with acute pressure changes such as in performing a Valsalva maneuver, coughing, or straining.

- What other signs and symptoms are associated with the dizziness or vertigo? A sensation of aural fullness and tinnitus can precede an attack of vertigo in patients with Meniere's disease. Sweating, dyspnea, and palpitations often accompany panic attacks but also may indicate a cardiogenic cause for presyncope manifesting as imbalance. Migraine-related vertigo may or may not be accompanied by an aura or headache. Other neurologic signs may indicate central mass effect or vascular pathology.

- Is there a family history of imbalance or headache? Migraine-related vertigo can run in families, and the same may be true for Meniere's disease. Otosclerosis, which can be accompanied by imbalance, also has a genetic component. Some genetic conditions, such as CHARGE syndrome (i.e., *c*oloboma, *h*eart anomalies, choanal *a*tresia, *r*etardation of growth and development, and *g*enital and *e*ar anomalies), have a prominent vestibular phenotype.

- Are there other, psychogenic disorders that may be responsible for the patient's symptoms? Anxiety disorders, panic syndromes, and agoraphobia can lead to episodic vertigo that mimics a vestibulopathy. These conditions are frequent in patients with dizziness. Patients with psychogenic dizziness often describe generalized imbalance that lasts for long periods.

- Are there underlying medical problems that may cause or exacerbate the patient's symptoms? Thyroid disease, diabetes mellitus, anemia, autoimmune diseases, infections such as syphilis or Lyme disease, hypoperfusion of the brain from postural hypotension, and cardiac arrhythmias all can lead to dizziness or vertigo. Patients with migraine are more likely to experience BPPV than are those who do not have migraine. Medications also can produce symptoms that mimic vestibular disorders (Table 164-2).

Physical Exam

The physical examination is goal-directed at testing hypotheses made from the history. Each physician will develop an individual approach, with elements of the examination tailored to specific symptoms reported by the patient. A careful bedside examination, including a general otolaryngologic exam, often can be sufficient for appropriate vestibular diagnosis. In some cases, laboratory tests or quantitative methods for evaluation of vestibular function, or both, are important to help make the diagnosis or to document pathophysiologic changes or recovery during the clinical course.

Bedside Exam

No clinical test can directly measure the function of the vestibular periphery. Instead, inferences must be made about vestibular function on the basis of the performance of "downstream" processes. The most important and well-studied of these are eye movements. Use of *Frenzel lenses* (magnifying lenses that prevent the patient from using visual fixation to suppress any spontaneous nystagmus) can increase the examiner's sensitivity for nystagmus and is vital to a thorough ocular examination.

Nystagmus

Eye movements indicative of a vestibular disorder commonly take the form of nystagmus. Several different types of nystagmus are recognized (Table 164-3). The most common is *jerk nystagmus*, which consists of

Table 164-2

Type and Mechanism of Dizziness Associated with Commonly Used Drugs

Drug(s)	Type(s) of Dizziness	Mechanism(s)
Aminoglycosides, cisplatin	Vertigo, dysequilibrium	Damage to vestibular hair cells
Tranquilizers	Intoxication	Central nervous system depression
Antiepileptics	Dysequilibrium	Cerebellar toxicity
Antihypertensives, diuretics	Near-syncope	Postural hypotension, reduced cerebral blood flow
Amiodarone	Dysequilibrium and oscillopsia	Unknown
Alcohol	Intoxication, dysequilibrium, positional vertigo	Central nervous system depression, cerebellar toxicity, change in cupular and endolymphatic specific gravity
Methotrexate	Dysequilibrium	Brainstem and cerebellar toxicity
Anticoagulants	Vertigo	Hemorrhage into inner ear or brain

From Baloh RW, Fife TD, Furman JM, Zee DS. The approach to the patient with dizziness. In: Mancall EI, ed. *Continuum: Lifelong Learning in Neurology*. Vol 2. Cleveland: Advanstar Communications; 1996:25-36.

Table 164-3

Clinical Observations and Causes of Nystagmus

Observation	Cause(s)
Sinusoidal oscillation without fast phases: "pendular nystagmus"	Multiple sclerosis, toluene intoxication, or brainstem infarction with inferior olivary hypertrophy (the syndrome of palatomyoclonus)[a,b] Acquired pendular nystagmus frequently disconjugate; may even be horizontal in one eye and vertical in the other May be responsive to memantine[c]
Purely torsional nystagmus	Intrinsic brainstem involvement within the vestibular nuclei; suggestive of syringomyelia[d]
Downbeat nystagmus	Arnold-Chiari deformity or degenerative lesions of the cerebellum[e] Treated with 4-aminopyridine
Upbeat nystagmus	Lesions at the pontomedullary or pontomesencephalic junction or within the fourth ventricle[f]
Horizontal jerk nystagmus that changes direction approximately every 2 minutes: "periodic alternating nystagmus"	Lesions in the nodulus of the cerebellum[g,h] Treated with baclofen
Nystagmus on attempted eccentric gaze and with slow phases that show a declining exponential time course	Side effect of certain medications, especially anticonvulsants, hypnotics, and tranquilizers, and in patients with disease of the vestibulocerebellum or its brainstem connections in the medial vestibular nucleus and nucleus prepositus hypoglossi[i]

Table 164-3

Clinical Observations and Causes of Nystagmus—cont'd

Observation	Cause(s)
Accelerating slow phases accentuated by attempted fixation, decreased by convergence or active eyelid closure, associated with a head turn, and sometimes accompanied by "reversed" smooth pursuit: "infantile" or "congenital" nystagmus	May be related to central or peripheral deficits[j] May be associated with albinism, retinal diseases, and early visual deprivation May be responsive to neurontin or memantine[j,k]
Gaze-evoked nystagmus that may dampen and actually change direction ("centripetal nystagmus") and often is followed by rebound nystagmus (slow phases are directed toward the previous position of eccentric gaze) when the eyes return to the primary position	Peripheral vestibular lesions, drug intoxication, and cerebellar lesions[l] Rebound nystagmus associated with many cerebellar lesions, including olivocerebellar atrophy[m]
Slow phases with exponentially increasing waveforms	Congenital nystagmus and acquired lesions of the cerebellum
Nystagmus of greater intensity or present only in the abducting eye: "dissociated nystagmus"	Commonly occurs in patients with internuclear ophthalmoplegia (INO) Mechanism unknown for abducting nystagmus in INO[n]
One eye goes up and the other goes down: "seesaw nystagmus"	Midbrain lesions May be related to an imbalance of activity in structures that receive projections from the labyrinthine otolith organs[o]
Slow phases directed centrally and with retraction of the eye into the orbit: "convergence-retraction nystagmus"	Midbrain lesions May be a failure of saccades or of vergence[p] Usually coexists with upgaze paralysis (Parinaud's syndrome)
Skew deviation and the ocular tilt reaction (one half-cycle of seesaw nystagmus)	Occurs with acute peripheral vestibular (otolith organ) lesions and with lesions in the medulla, the pons, and the midbrain Often associated with head tilt[q]
Nystagmus occurring in a plane other than that of vestibular stimulation: "perverted nystagmus"	Central vestibular disorders; multiple sclerosis[r]

[a]Data from Hain TC, Zee DS, Maria BL. Tilt suppression of vestibulo-ocular reflex in patients with cerebellar lesions. *Acta Otolaryngol.* 1988;105:13-20.

[b]Data from Nakada T, Kwee IL. Oculopalatal myoclonus. *Brain.* 1986;109(Pt 3):431-441.

[c]Data from Stahl JS, Rottach KG, Averbuch-Heller L, et al. A pilot study of gabapentin as treatment for acquired nystagmus. *Neuroophthalmology.* 1996;16:107-113.

[d]Data from Noseworthy JH, Ebers GC, Leigh RJ, et al. Torsional nystagmus: quantitative features and possible pathogenesis. *Neurology.* 1988;38:992-994.

[e]Data from Baloh RW, Yee RD. Spontaneous vertical nystagmus. *Rev Neurol (Paris).* 1989;145:527-532.

[f]Data from Ranalli PJ, Sharpe JA. Upbeat nystagmus and the ventral tegmental pathway of the upward vestibuloocular reflex. *Neurology.* 1988;38:1329-1330.

[g]Data from Leigh RJ, Robinson DA, Zee DS. A hypothetical explanation for periodic alternating nystagmus: instability in the optokinetic-vestibular system. *Ann N Y Acad Sci.* 1988;374:619-635.

[h]Data from Waespe W, Cohen B, Raphan T. Dynamic modification of the vestibulo-ocular reflex by the nodulus and uvula. *Science.* 1985;228:199-202.

[i]Data from Lewis RF, Zee DS. Ocular motor disorders associated with cerebellar lesions: pathophysiology and topical localization. *Rev Neurol (Paris).* 1993;149:665-677.

[j]Data from Jacobs JB, Dell'Osso LF. Congenital nystagmus: hypotheses for its genesis and complex waveforms within a behavioral ocular motor system model. *J Vis.* 2004;4:604-625.

[k]Data from McLean R, Proudlock F, Thomas S, Degg C, Gottlob I. Congenital nystagmus: randomized, controlled, double-masked trial of memantine/gabapentin. *Ann Neurol.* 2007;61:130-138.

[l]Data from Leech J, Gresty M, Hess K, Rudge P. Gaze failure, drifting eye movements, and centripetal nystagmus in cerebellar disease. *Br J Ophthalmol.* 1977;61:774-781.

[m]Data from Bondar RL, Sharpe JA, Lewis AJ. Rebound nystagmus in olivocerebellar atrophy: a clinicopathological correlation. *Ann Neurol.* 1984;15:474-477.

[n]Data from Zee DS, Hain TC, Carl JR. Abduction nystagmus in internuclear ophthalmoplegia. *Ann Neurol.* 1987;21:383-388.

[o]Data from Nakada T, Kwee IL. Seesaw nystagmus. Role of visuovestibular interaction in its pathogenesis. *J Clin Neuroophthalmol.* 1988;8:171-177.

[p]Data from Rambold H, Kompf D, Helmchen C. Convergence retraction nystagmus: a disorder of vergence? *Ann Neurol.* 2001;50:677-681.

[q]Data from Parulekar MV, Dai S, Buncic JR, Wong AM. Head position-dependent changes in ocular torsion and vertical misalignment in skew deviation. *Arch Ophthalmol.* 2008;126:899-905.

[r]Data from Minagar A, Sheremata WA, Tusa RJ. Perverted head-shaking nystagmus: a possible mechanism. *Neurology.* 2001;57:887-889.

so-called slow phases, which represent vestibular signals for eye movements, and fast phases, which represent resetting actions bringing the eyes back toward the center of the orbit but are not as relevant for diagnostic purposes. The direction of nystagmus often is named for the direction of the fast phases, because the fast phases are more obvious on clinical examination. The trajectory of the slow phases should be scrutinized for the following characteristics of individual slow phases: (1) an increase in velocity, as is commonly found with congenital nystagmus; (2) a decrease in velocity, as is seen in patients with cerebellar lesions; and (3) a constant velocity, as is typical for vestibular disturbances.

Spontaneous nystagmus of vestibular origin arises from an imbalance in tonic levels of activity mediating the VOR. The spontaneous nystagmus resulting from unilateral vestibular hypofunction is a jerk nystagmus and is present when the head is still, is reduced by visual fixation, and is increased or becomes apparent only when fixation is eliminated during use of Frenzel lenses. A horizontal-torsional nystagmus typically is observed acutely after unilateral loss of vestibular function. The horizontal component beats toward the "stronger" (intact) ear, and the torsional component involves beating of the superior poles of the eyes toward the intact ear.

The characteristics of nystagmus when the eyes are directed away from center often adds additional diagnostic information. The patient is asked to maintain eccentric horizontal and then vertical positions of gaze (approximately 30 degrees from center orientation). Minimal drift normally should be encountered for periods up to 15 seconds. Nystagmus arising from peripheral lesions and some central lesions is more intense (slow-phase velocity is higher) when the eyes are turned in the direction of the quick phase.[39] This effect, known as *Alexander's law* (Fig. 164-5), is due to the combination of gaze-evoked nystagmus (caused by the initial loss of the neural integrator after a peripheral lesion) and with the vestibular nystagmus caused by the static asymmetry of the lesion itself. The two factors add on looking away from the lesion and cancel each other on looking toward it. *Bruns' nystagmus,* found in patients with cerebellopontine angle tumors, is a combination of gaze-evoked nystagmus with low-frequency, large-amplitude, fast phases on looking toward the side of the lesion and jerk nystagmus with high-frequency, small-amplitude, fast phases on looking the other way.[40] The gaze-holding component of the nystagmus may represent an adaptation to the jerk nystagmus caused by vestibular imbalance.[41] Horizontal gaze–evoked nystagmus is a hallmark of lesions in the medial vestibular nucleus and nucleus prepositus hypoglossi complex. Low-amplitude gaze-evoked nystagmus often is a side effect of many types of medications, including hypnotics, sedatives, and anxiolytics. Many healthy persons may exhibit some physiologic, horizontal, end-gaze nystagmus. It usually disappears once the target is brought back into view of both eyes (i.e., at approximately 30 degrees of eccentricity).

The effect of vergence should be noted, because it may intensify or cause a change in direction of some central forms of vestibular nystagmus or may dampen congenital nystagmus.

Skew Deviation and Ocular Tilt Reaction

Skew deviation is a vertical misalignment of the eyes that cannot be explained on the basis of an ocular muscle palsy (Fig. 164-6). It is the hallmark of an imbalance in tonic levels of activity along peripheral or central pathways mediating otolith-ocular reflexes.[42] Patients with skew deviation often complain of vertical diplopia and sometimes torsional diplopia (one image tilted with respect to the other). The *alternate cover test* is used to detect skew deviation: The examiner covers one eye of the patient with a card and then moves the cover to the patient's other eye while looking for a vertical corrective movement as an index of a vertical misalignment. A skew deviation also can be detected by covering one eye with a red glass (Maddox rod) to dissociate images seen in the two eyes and inquiring whether the patient sees one image above the other, indicating vertical misalignment. The effect of position of the eye in the orbit and of left and right head tilt on the skew also should be examined. Skew deviations tend to be relatively comitant (i.e., the degree of misalignment changes little with different direction

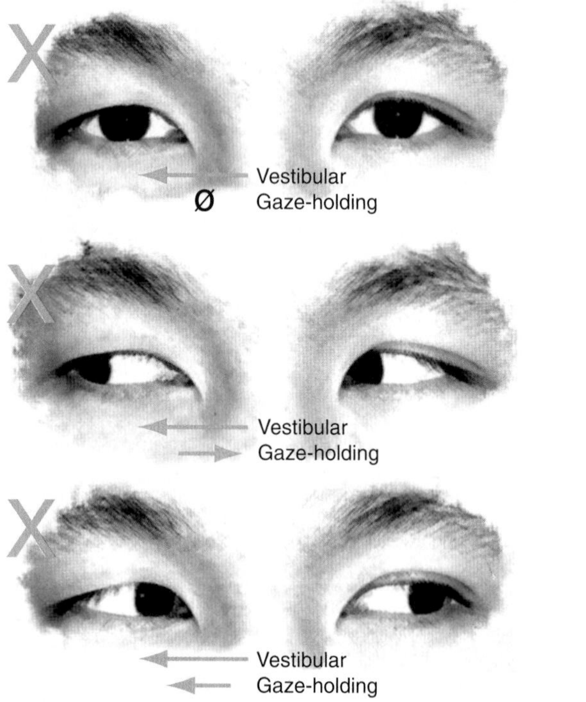

Figure 164-5. Alexander's law. With an acute deficit of the right labyrinth, vestibular input drives the eyes to the right (slow-phase component of nystagmus). A defective neural integrator (caused by the unilateral loss) tends to bring the eyes back to neutral position. With the eyes directed toward the lesion, the two effects cancel. With the eyes directed away from the lesion, they add. *(From Hullar TE, Minor LB. The neurotologic examination. In: Jackler RK, Brackmann DE, eds.* Neurotology. *2nd ed. St. Louis: Mosby: 2004:215-227.)*

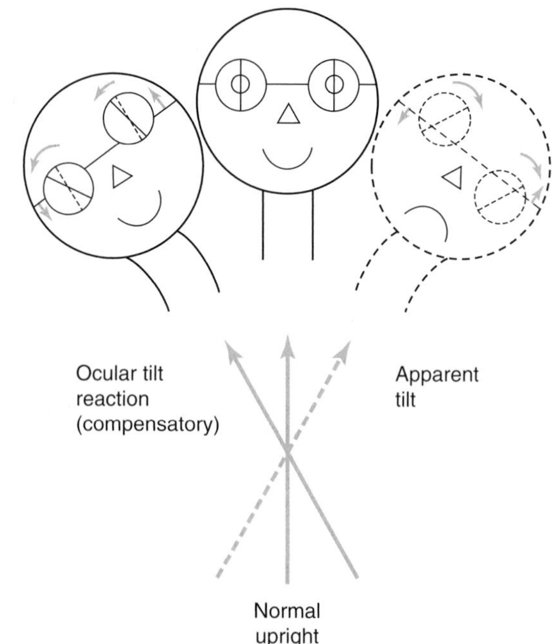

Figure 164-6. The ocular tilt reaction depicted as motor compensation to a lesion-induced apparent eye-head tile *(dashed line)*. The compensatory head tilt is in a direction opposite to the apparent head tilt *(solid line)*. Eyes and head are continuously adjusted to the orientation that the brain computes as being vertical. *(From Brandt T, Dieterich M. Pathological eye-head coordination in roll: tonic ocular tilt reaction in mesencephalic and medullary lesions.* Brain. *1987;110:649.)*

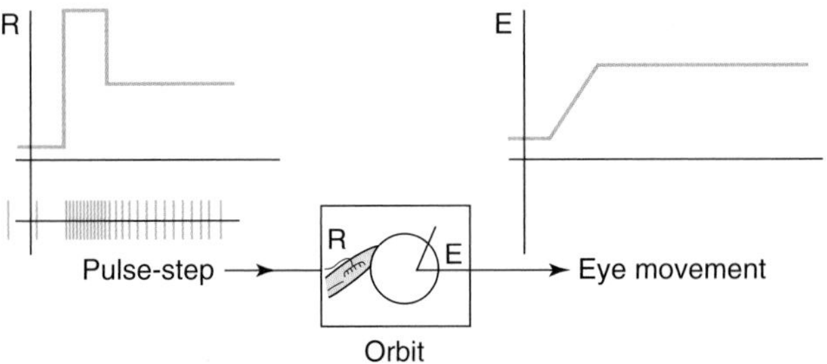

Figure 164-7. The neural signal for a saccade. At *right* is shown the eye movement: E is eye position in the orbit; the abscissa scale represents time. At *left* is shown the neural signal sent to the extraocular muscles to produce the saccade. The *vertical lines* indicate the occurrence of action potentials of an ocular motoneuron. The *graph* above plots the neuron's discharge rate (R) against time (firing frequency histogram). It shows the neurally encoded pulse (velocity command) and step (position command).

of gaze), whereas a fourth cranial nerve palsy causes a vertical misalignment that is greatest with the affected eye down and medial. The adducting eye is higher and the misalignment is greater with the head tilted toward the side of the higher eye. Skew deviations in otolith-ocular imbalance do not show such a clear relation to changes in eye and head position, although they may be decreased or disappear when the affected person is supine.[43] The lower eye is on the side of the lesion with peripheral or vestibular nucleus lesions. Otolith-ocular pathways cross at the level of the vestibular nucleus, so lesions above the decussation result in the higher eye being on the side of the lesion (such as with lesions of the medial longitudinal fasciculus causing internuclear ophthalmoplegia). The head usually is tilted toward the side of the lower eye. Skew deviations also can occur with cerebellar lesions.

Saccades

Rapid changes in gaze from one target to another are achieved by *saccades*. The neural signal for a saccade includes a *pulse* of activity, which brings the eye to its new position, and a *step*, which is a constant neural signal holding the eye at its new position in the orbit (Fig. 164-7). Saccades are examined by asking the patient to alternately fixate (with the head still) on the examiner's nose and then on the finger, held at different locations at approximately 15 degrees away from primary position. Measures of saccades such as accuracy, velocity, and stability represent the effects of the neural pulse, the step, and the match between pulse and step.[44] An error in the pulse amplitude creates overshoot or undershoot dysmetria. This is characteristic of disorders of the dorsal vermis or the fastigial nuclei of the cerebellum, although it appears with lesions in other parts of the nervous system. *Wallenberg's syndrome* produces a specific pattern of saccadic dysmetria: Saccades overshoot to the side of the lesion, undershoot away from the side of the lesion, and, with attempted purely vertical saccades, show an inappropriate horizontal component toward the side of the lesion. Lesions of the superior cerebellar peduncle produce just the opposite: Saccades overshoot when directed away from the side of the lesion.[45]

Normally, saccades follow a relatively invariant relationship between peak velocity and amplitude termed the *main sequence*.[46] A decrease in the height of the saccadic pulse causes slow saccades. Slow horizontal saccades usually imply disease of the pons such as olivopontocerebellar atrophy (spinal cerebellar atrophy type 2 [SCA2]). Slow vertical saccades usually imply disease affecting the midbrain such as progressive supranuclear palsy, Huntington's disease, or Niemann-Pick disease. A mismatch between the size of the pulse and step produces brief (several hundred milliseconds) postsaccadic drift, or glissades. Postsaccadic drift occurs with disease of the cerebellar flocculus. The combination of slow, hypometric saccades and postsaccadic drift also occurs in patients with internuclear ophthalmoplegia, oculomotor nerve palsies, myasthenia gravis, and ocular myopathies. Hypermetric saccades with macrosaccadic oscillations (large saccades about the position of the target) typically are found in patients with lesions in the midline deep cerebellar nuclei.[47] Saccadic oscillations without an intersaccadic interval (back-to-back, to-and-fro saccades) are called *ocular flutter* when they are limited to the horizontal plane and *opsoclonus* when they are multidirectional (horizontal, vertical, torsional). Either type of oscillation may occur in patients with various types of encephalitis or postinfectious immune-mediated processes, as a paraneoplastic remote effect of neuroblastoma or other tumors, or in association with toxins. Ocular flutter also may be voluntarily elicited by some normal people.[48]

The normal saccadic latency is approximately 200 msec, but this latency is increased by disorders of saccadic initiation. Impaired saccadic initiation has been reported in patients with a variety of conditions, including frontal lobe lesions, congenital or acquired oculomotor apraxia, Huntington's disease, progressive supranuclear palsy, and Alzheimer's disease. Patients with bilateral frontal lobe lesions or Parkinson's disease also have difficulty in rapidly alternating gaze between two stationary targets. Patients with Huntington's disease show a characteristic defect in initiating more voluntary, as opposed to more reflexive, saccades. They have particular difficulty in predictive tracking and are unable to suppress inappropriate saccades to the visual target.[49]

Inappropriate saccades disrupt steady fixation.[50] They include *square-wave jerks,* which are small-amplitude (up to 5 degrees) saccades that take the eyes off target and are followed within 200 msec by a corrective saccade. Square-wave jerks may occur in healthy elderly persons or in patients with cerebral hemisphere lesions but are especially prominent in patients with progressive supranuclear palsy and cerebellar disease. Square-wave jerks may be an exaggeration of the microsaccades that occur in healthy people during fixation and can be detected most easily by ophthalmoscopy when the patient is instructed to fixate on a target seen with the other eye. Macro square-wave jerks (10 to 40 degrees in amplitude, with a short intersaccadic interval) have been observed in patients with multiple sclerosis and olivopontocerebellar atrophy.

Smooth Pursuit

The tracking movements of the eyes used to follow an object moving across the field of view, caused by either motion of the object or motion of the viewer, are mediated by the smooth pursuit system. This requires that other gaze-stabilizing inputs, such as vestibular or optokinetic, be suppressed. Smooth pursuit is tested by having the patient follow targets moving no faster than 20 degrees/second. Asymmetries in horizontal tracking, as reflected by the presence of more corrective saccades in one direction, are more helpful in identification of an abnormality than is an overall symmetrical decrease in smooth tracking unless it is profound. Smooth pursuit mechanisms assist visual fixation, suppressing nystagmus from peripheral but not central lesions.

Patients with lesions affecting the temporo-occipital region have been reported to have selective defects in motion detection[24] and are unable to make accurate smooth pursuit or accurate saccadic eye movements because of this deficit.[51] Patients with posterior cortical lesions exhibit a unidirectional (ipsilateral) deficit for smooth pursuit and also a defect of motion detection in the contralateral hemifield.[51] Experimental lesions of dorsolateral pontine nuclei also cause an ipsilateral deficit of smooth pursuit tracking.[52] Lesions of frontal eye fields impair pursuit eye movements,[53] and lesions within the flocculus impair smooth pursuit, especially for ipsilateral tracking. The flocculus projects to the ipsilateral vestibular nuclei, and lesions of this area, including those associated with Wallenberg's syndrome, mainly impair contralateral smooth pursuit.[54]

In addition to the asymmetric deficits of pursuit that may occur with focal lesions, a variety of conditions may bilaterally impair smooth pursuit. A common cause of impaired smooth pursuit is the effect of medications such as anticonvulsants and sedatives. Smooth pursuit is performed less well by elderly persons and is impaired in patients with a variety of neurologic conditions such as Parkinson's disease, progressive supranuclear palsy, and Alzheimer's disease and in those with schizophrenia. In patients with congenital nystagmus, smooth pursuit may appear "reversed," with slow phases directed opposite to the motion of the target.[55] The pathomechanism for this apparent reversal of smooth pursuit is controversial.[56] Disease of the cerebral hemisphere may produce a low-amplitude horizontal nystagmus in primary position with constant-velocity slow phases directed toward the intact hemisphere. Slow-phase velocity is not decreased by fixation. This nystagmus may result from an imbalance of pursuit tone.

Optokinetic

During sustained rotations, the vestibular signal decays and becomes a poor indicator of head motion. This effect is well known to pilots, who are trained not to trust the vestibular system during prolonged turns. The optokinetic system drives the eyes to follow the visual surround during low-frequency (sustained) head movements. Optokinetic nystagmus (OKN) is a response to motion of the entire visual field, rather than to a particular target (for which the smooth pursuit system is used), and is responsible for effects such as automatic visual tracking of a picket fence seen from a moving car. Use of a bedside optokinetic tape is a convenient way to elicit OKN. Because smooth-pursuit tracking contributes to the generation of optokinetic responses, many of the abnormalities resulting in smooth pursuit deficits also lead to impaired OKN.

Vestibulo-Ocular Reflex Cancellation

The ability of a patient to maintain steady gaze on a target moving in tandem with the head is attributable to cancellation of the VOR. The patient is instructed to fixate on an object (such as the examiner's finger) that moves with the patient's head. A deficit of VOR cancellation is interpreted in conjunction with results obtained from evaluating VOR amplitude.

Vergence

Vergence eye movements, found in frontal-eyed animals such as humans, are disjunctive (opposite direction) responses to changes in gaze. They are necessary, for example, when a target is brought nearer to the viewer and the gaze of each eye converges to keep its image aligned on both retinas. Vergence can be generated volitionally or reflexively and, with accommodation of the lens and papillary constriction, is one element of the "near triad" for close viewing. Eye movements involved in vergence are under the control of several groups of neurons near the oculomotor nuclei.[57] Insufficient vergence causing diplopia at near viewing may be due to aging, stress, or head trauma.[58] Convergence spasm (which may be functional) or divergence paralysis has been mistakenly diagnosed as bilateral sixth nerve palsy. Divergence paralysis has been described with intracranial hypertension[59] or hypotension,[60] with lesions of the midbrain,[61] cerebellum, or in association with medication.[62]

Eye-Head Coordination

Unilateral labyrinthine loss may lead to a head tilt and counterrolling of the eyes.[42] Other disorders causing instability of the head include tremors such as those caused by Parkinson's disease and abnormal postures caused by dystonia and torticollis.[63] Patients with congenital nystagmus sometimes have a head tremor. Such head tremors usually do not compensate for the ocular oscillations, and both are likely to be caused by the same underlying disorder.[64] Intermittent head tremor also is a feature of spasmus nutans, which affects infants and young children.

Other features of this condition include head tilts and turns and nystagmus. The nystagmus is characteristically intermittent, of small amplitude and high frequency, and is typically asymmetric in the two eyes.[65] Any child seen with a monocular form of nystagmus requires a complete ophthalmologic examination and consideration of imaging studies to exclude a tumor of the anterior visual pathways. Disorders of eye-head saccades include involuntary head turning associated with focal epileptic seizures[66] and paresis of voluntary head turning associated with conjugate gaze palsy secondary to an acute lesion of one cerebral hemisphere. *Ocular motor apraxia*, which is characterized by the impaired ability to make voluntary eye movements, often is characterized by thrusting head movements by which the patient is able to shift gaze. These head movements are more conspicuous in the congenital form of ocular motor apraxia, which exclusively affects horizontal eye movements.[66,67] Acquired ocular motor apraxia is associated with bilateral frontoparietal hemispheral deficits, and horizontal and vertical head movements are affected.[68] Disorders causing impairment of smooth pursuit usually, but not always, cause commensurate deficits of smooth, combined, eye-head tracking.[29] Patients who also have lost vestibular function, on the other hand, often show combined eye-head tracking that is superior to smooth ocular pursuit, because no VOR occurs to cancel.[26]

Low-Frequency Vestibulo-Ocular Reflex

An abnormal VOR is indicated by the presence of corrective (catch-up) saccades during head rotations in the light. These can be identified by oscillating the patient's head smoothly left and right (yaw), followed by up and down (pitch) and then right-ear-down to left-ear-down positions (roll) at approximately 0.5 Hz. Because visual stimuli have little ability to generate torsional slow phases, responses to rotations of the head in roll reflect primarily labyrinthine (and possibly neck afferent) stimulation. Absence of torsional fast phases in one direction of head rotation in the roll plane points to a lesion in the rostral interstitial nucleus of the medial longitudinal fasciculus.[69]

Head-Shaking Nystagmus

Head-shaking nystagmus is a test of imbalance in dynamic vestibular function. With Frenzel lenses in place, the patient is instructed to shake the head vigorously approximately 30 times horizontally. Head shaking is stopped abruptly, and the examiner looks for any nystagmus. Healthy persons usually exhibit no or occasionally just a beat or two of head-shaking nystagmus. With a unilateral loss of labyrinthine function, however, a vigorous nystagmus is typical, with slow phases initially directed toward the lesioned side and then a reversal phase with slow phases directed oppositely.[70] The initial phase of head-shaking nystagmus arises because of asymmetry of peripheral inputs during high-velocity head rotations: More activity is generated during rotation toward the intact side than toward the affected side. This asymmetry leads to an accumulation of activity within central velocity storage mechanisms during head shaking. Nystagmus after head shaking reflects discharge of that activity.

The amplitude and duration of the initial phase of head-shaking nystagmus depend on the state of the velocity-storage mechanism. Because velocity storage typically is disabled during the immediate period after an acute unilateral vestibular loss, the primary phase of head-shaking nystagmus may be absent or attenuated in these circumstances. The reversal phase of head-shaking nystagmus reflects short-term adaptation, probably originating in the vestibular nerve and central pathways,[71] and may still be present in acute loss. With unilateral peripheral lesions, vertical head shaking may lead to a low-amplitude horizontal nystagmus, with slow phases directed toward the intact ear. Central lesions (such as those caused by cerebellar dysfunction) also may lead to head-shaking nystagmus, often with a vertical nystagmus after horizontal head shaking. It also is likely that head-shaking nystagmus may result from mechanical disturbances in the labyrinth (e.g., debris adherent to the semicircular canals) or an abnormality of the cupula itself.

Vibration

Vibration-induced nystagmus has been used as a diagnostic tool for patients with superior canal dehiscence. Application of a vibrator to the suboccipital area on the side of the dehiscence can induce a prominent vertical-torsional nystagmus consistent with activation of the dehiscent canal.[72] Vibration also has been shown to induce nystagmus with fast phases toward the intact side in patients with unilateral loss due to vestibular neuropathy or Meniere's disease.[73]

Head Impulse Test

The head impulse maneuver is uniquely able to examine individual canals and to test their responses to high-acceleration, high-frequency motions, whose pathology may be significantly different in genesis and effect from that in lower-frequency losses such as those identified on caloric testing.[74] Brief, high-acceleration horizontal head impulses in the excitatory direction of each canal are applied while the patient is instructed to look carefully at the examiner's nose (Fig. 164-8). A slow phase of abnormally low amplitude will be evoked in response to head

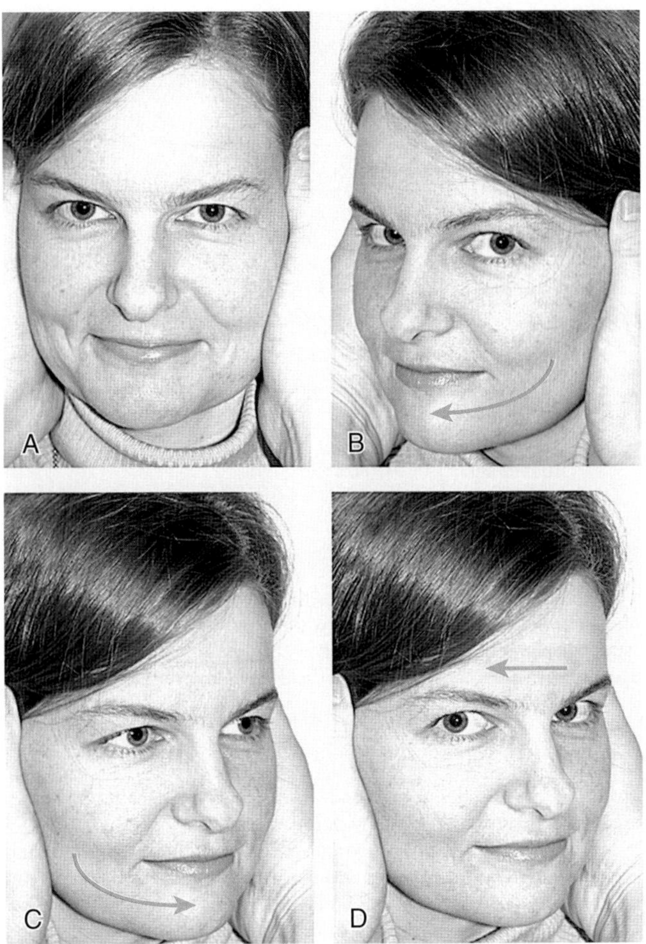

Figure 164-8. The head impulse sign. Starting from neutral position (**A**), a rapid head impulse to the right in the horizontal plane elicits compensatory eye movements to the left, and the patient's eyes remain stable on the examiner (**B**). With a similar movement to the left, a hypoactive labyrinth (**C**) results in a delayed catchup saccade (**D**) to maintain gaze. The *arrow* in **D** shows the direction of the catchup saccade. *(From Hullar TE, Minor LB. The neurotologic examination. In: Jackler RK, Brackmann DE, eds.* Neurotology. *2nd ed. St. Louis: Mosby: 2004:215-227.)*

impulse toward a lesioned or hypoactive labyrinth. A corrective rapid eye movement, required to bring the eyes back to the intended point of fixation, is seen in such cases. A full examination of the labyrinth involves head impulses in each of the three planes of the canals (horizontal, left anterior/right posterior, and right anterior/left posterior) in both directions for each plane. Detection of diminished function in the vertical canals through clinical observations on the head impulse test can be considerably more difficult than for the horizontal head impulse test.

Positional Testing

Positional (sustained) and positioning (transient) nystagmus are best observed with the patient wearing Frenzel lenses. Dix-Hallpike positioning for identification of posterior canal benign paroxysmal positional vertigo (BPPV) is performed first. The patient sits upright on an examination table. For testing to detect the presence of right posterior canal BPPV, the head is turned 45 degrees such that the chin is toward the right shoulder. The patient is then rapidly brought straight back into a right head-hanging position (Fig. 164-9). This position is maintained for at least 30 seconds. The nystagmus characteristic of BPPV begins after a latency of 2 to 10 seconds (although sometimes longer), increases in amplitude over approximately 10 seconds, and decreases in velocity over the next 30 seconds. Posterior canal BPPV results in a vertical-torsional nystagmus, with slow phases directed downward, with intorsion of the lower eye and extorsion of the higher eye. Because of the orientation of pulling directions for the oblique and vertical rectus muscles, the planar characteristics of the nystagmus relative to the orbit change with direction of gaze: on looking to the dependent ear, it appears more torsional and on looking to the higher ear, more vertical.

A horizontal canal variant of BPPV has been described. In these patients, a strong horizontal nystagmus builds up and declines over the same time course as for posterior canal BPPV. In some patients, the nystagmus beats toward the dependent ear (geotropic); in others, it beats away from the dependent ear (apogeotropic). The standard Dix-Hallpike maneuver may not elicit nystagmus in cases of horizontal canal BPPV. Such a nystagmus can be identified by bringing the patient backward into the supine, head-hanging position and then turning the head left-ear-down or right-ear-down. The nystagmus seen with horizontal canal BPPV may last longer than that seen in posterior canal BPPV. Such patients also may exhibit a small amount of spontaneous nystagmus when sitting upright, which varies as the head is pitched forward or backward. Anterior canal BPPV also has been described but is relatively rare. A sustained, usually horizontal positional nystagmus of low velocity is a common finding in patients with central or peripheral vestibular lesions and also may be present in asymptomatic human

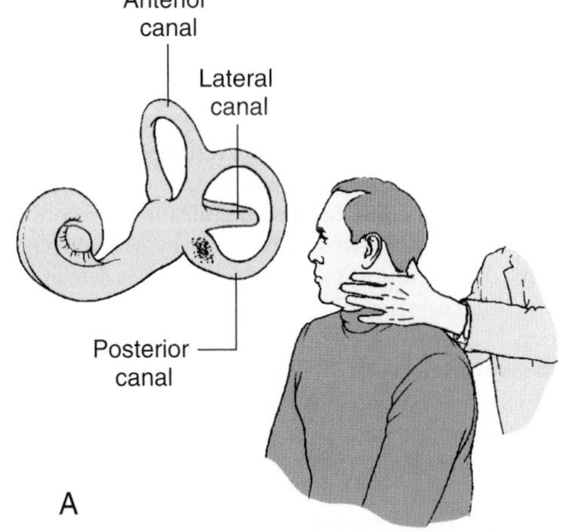

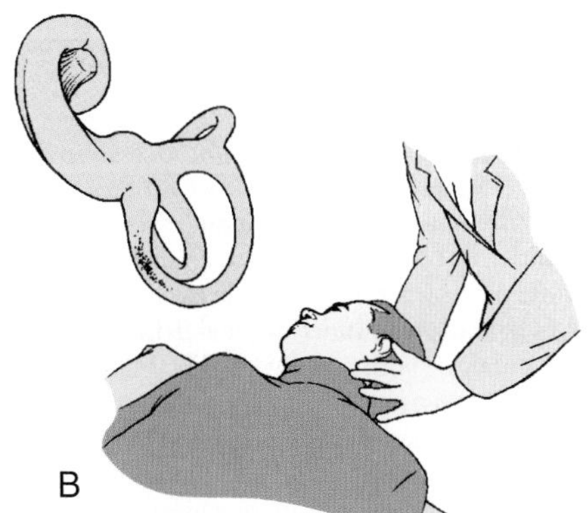

Figure 164-9. The Dix-Hallpike maneuver. Lowering the patient's head backwards and to the side allows debris in the posterior canal (**A**) to fall to its lowest position, activating the canal and causing eye movements and vertigo (**B**). *(From Hullar TE, Minor LB. Vestibular physiology and disorders of the labyrinth. In: Glasscock ME, Gulya AJ, eds.* Surgery of the Ear. *5th ed. Toronto: BC Decker; 2003.)*

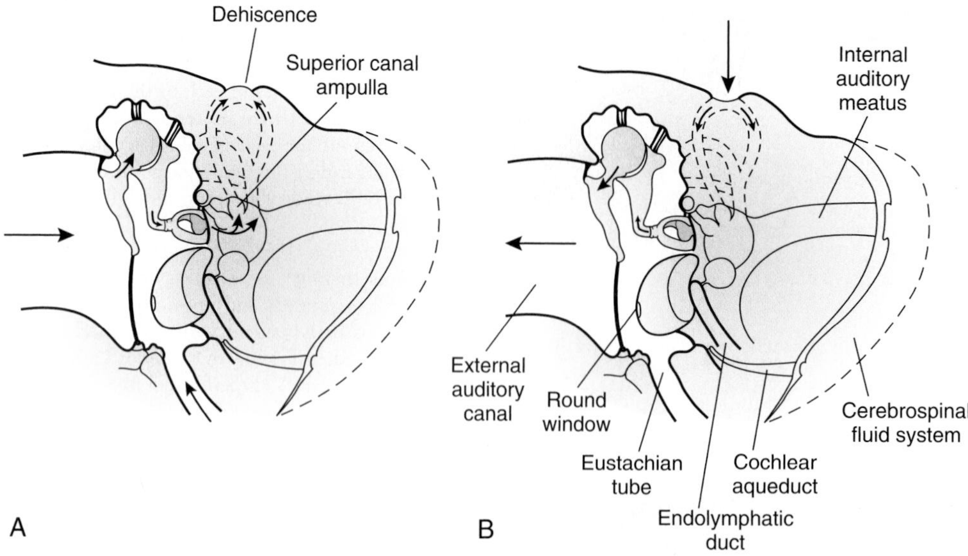

Figure 164-10. **A,** Pressure changes inducing eye movements in superior semicircular canal dehiscence syndrome. Positive pressure in the external auditory canal causes bulging of the membranous canal into the cranial cavity and ampullofugal flow (*arrows*). **B,** Negative pressure in the external auditory canal causes bulging of the cranial contents into the superior canal and ampullopetal flow (*arrows*). *(From Minor LB, Solomon D, Zinreich J, Zee DS. Sound- and/or pressure-induced vertigo due to bone dehiscence of the superior semicircular canal.* Arch Otolaryngol Head Neck Surg. *1998;124: 249-258.)*

subjects.[75] A central lesion is most likely when positional nystagmus is purely vertical or purely torsional or if the patient exhibits a sustained unidirectional horizontal positional nystagmus of high enough intensity to be observed without Frenzel lenses. Positional testing also may exacerbate a spontaneous nystagmus.

Dynamic Visual Acuity

Persons with normal vestibular function typically show no more than a one-line decline in visual acuity on the Snellen chart with head movement, whereas those with vestibular hypofunction (particularly bilateral hypofunction) may show up to a five-line decline in acuity with head movement.[23] To test for this effect, the patient's ability to read a Snellen chart with the head stationary is compared with acuity during horizontal head oscillations at a frequency of approximately 2 Hz. Patients with corrective lenses are instructed to wear their glasses or contact lenses during this testing. Quantitative analysis of dynamic visual acuity has revealed that retinal slip velocities of as little as 2 to 3 degrees/second result in oscillopsia and consequent loss of acuity.[6]

Vertical dynamic visual acuity also may be tested. The test can be improved by use of a computerized display, which prevents patients from seeing the Snellen chart when their head movements drop below a critical velocity at the ends of each oscillation.[76] Dynamic visual acuity also has been measured during rapid head movements and may, in some situations, serve as a useful proxy for quantitative measurement of angular VOR gain during these rapid head movements.

Eye Movements Evoked by Sound or Changes in Middle Ear Pressure

Changes in pressure in the inner ear can be induced by the Valsalva maneuver with the glottis closed (increasing intracranial pressure) and glottis open using a nose pinch (increasing middle ear pressure through the eustachian tube). In patients with superior canal dehiscence, nystagmus may be evoked by either or both maneuvers. The Valsalva maneuver with the glottis closed increases intracranial pressure and exerts force directly at the site of the dehiscence, causing deflection of the cupula of the superior canal toward the ampulla, in its "off" direction. On release of the pressure, the cupula is deflected in its preferred "on" direction, causing stimulatory nystagmus[77] (Fig. 164-10). The plane in which the eyes move during this nystagmus typically aligns with the plane of the affected superior canal. Craniocervical junction anomalies (e.g., Arnold-Chiari malformation), perilymph fistulas, and other abnormalities involving the ossicles, oval window, semicircular canals, or otolith organs also may cause vertigo with the Valsalva maneuver.

Tullio's phenomenon is the occurrence of vestibular symptoms and eye movements with exposure to sound. Motion of the tympanic membrane and ossicular chain can induce vertigo and nystagmus (*Hennebert's sign*) in patients with otic syphilis, perilymph fistula, and dehiscences of the semicircular canals. Superior semicircular canal dehiscence syndrome, caused by lack of bone covering the superior semicircular canal and arcuate eminence, may feature sound-evoked or pressure-evoked vertigo and conductive hearing loss.[78,79] If suspected, these causes should be investigated by moving the tympanic membrane with tragal compression or insufflation through a Siegle's speculum. Pure tones can be given over a range from 250 to 4000 Hz at intensities of 100 to 110 dB. The characteristic nystagmus evoked by activation of the superior canal is a vertical-torsional nystagmus with slow phases that are directed upward in the vertical plane and that involve motion of the superior pole of the eye away from the affected ear in the torsional plane. The eye movements evoked by sound or pressure stimuli in superior canal dehiscence typically are conjugate. Depending on the stimulus parameters and the effect of the dehiscence in individual patients, the evoked eye movements may be brief in duration and may not involve a sustained nystagmus.

Hyperventilation

Patients with anxiety or phobic disorders may sometimes hyperventilate and experience symptoms but usually do not show signs of nystagmus. Patients with demyelinating lesions on the vestibular nerve (such as an acoustic neuroma or compression by a small blood vessel) or with a central distribution (such as in multiple sclerosis) may show an excitatory (due to restoration of function) hyperventilation-induced nystagmus.[80] In the case of a peripheral lesion, the slow phase is away from the involved ear. Hyperventilation-induced nystagmus (usually a paretic nystagmus, with the slow phase toward the involved ear) rarely is noted in patients with pathologic conditions of the vestibular end organs alone.[81]

Vestibulospinal Function

Static imbalance in vestibulospinal reflexes is identified from Romberg testing, tandem walking, evaluation of past pointing, and the stepping test. The *Romberg test* is used to assess sway with feet together and tandem in eyes opened and closed condition. Falls during *tandem walking* are suggestive of horizontal canal dysfunction. *Past pointing* of the arms to previously seen targets with eyes closed also may be a sign of vestibulospinal imbalance. It is best elicited by having the patient repetitively raise both arms over the head, with index fingers extended, and then bring them down, with eyes closed, toward the examiner's index fingers (but without actually touching them) located at waist level. For the *stepping test,* the patient, with eyes closed and arms outstretched, steps in place for at least 30 seconds.[82,83] A patient with acute labyrinthine asymmetry may turn to the weak side, in the direction of the slow phase of the nystagmus. This test sometimes is augmented with caloric stimulation.[84] Dynamic vestibulospinal function is assessed by observing postural stability during rapid turns or in response to external perturbations imposed by the examiner (i.e., a gentle shove forward, backward, or to the side). A complete examination of (1) gait, (2) strength, reflexes, and sensation in the legs, and (3) cerebellar function is essential for the interpretation of postural instability and dysequilibrium.

Sensory Integration

Balance relies on collection of vestibular, visual, and proprioception information and also on their appropriate central integration. The Clinical Test of Sensory Integration and Balance (CTSIB) is a simple series of bedside tests designed to evaluate these processes.[85,86] This test simulates the test conditions of dynamic computed posturography, detailed later on, with the patient standing on foam to disrupt proprioception and wearing a large paper lantern over the head, to simulate posturography's sway-reference condition. Results of the CTSIB correspond with dynamic posturography findings.[87]

Quantitative Testing

Quantitative tests of physiologic processes under vestibular control can be useful in identifying the cause of a patient's symptoms, confirming clinical findings, planning therapy, and monitoring the response to treatment.

Methods of Eye Movement Recordings

Three techniques can be used for quantitative measurement of eye movements. *Electronystagmography* (ENG) remains the most practical laboratory test to evaluate patients with dizziness or imbalance.[88] ENG can be helpful when the clinical picture suggests unilateral or bilateral vestibular hypofunction; disorders of oculomotor control such as deficits of smooth pursuit, saccades, or optokinetic eye movements; Meniere's disease or endolymphatic hydrops; BPPV; recurrent vestibulopathy; or migraine-associated dizziness. The quantitative information from ENG enables the clinician to monitor progression of or recovery from disorders affecting vestibulo-ocular control.

Electro-oculography (EOG) is based on the corneoretinal potential (difference in electrical charge potential between the cornea and the retina). The eye acts as an electrical dipole oriented along its long axis. Movement of this dipole relative to the surface electrodes produces an electrical signal corresponding to eye position. Surface electrodes are placed about each eye as shown in Figure 164-11. Horizontal eye movements typically can be resolved to an accuracy of 0.5 degree. Even under optimal recording conditions, however, the sensitivity of EOG is less than that of direct visual inspection (approximately 0.1 degree). Visual inspection of small-amplitude eye movements either directly or with the aid of Frenzel lenses or an ophthalmoscope is important for documentation of low-amplitude nystagmus. Vertically aligned electrodes sense voltage associated with eye and lid movement, so EOG cannot be used in the quantitative assessment of *vertical* eye movements. It is adequate, in most instances, for qualitative clinical assessment of vertical eye movement disorders and provides a useful monitor of eye blinks.[89] Torsional eye movements cannot be measured with EOG. For this reason, it is important for the examiner to look at the patient's eyes, either directly or with Frenzel lenses in place, during positioning testing so that the vertical-torsional nystagmus caused by posterior canal BPPV is not missed.

The *magnetic search coil technique* is based on the principle that voltage changes are induced in a coil of wire moving in an oscillating magnetic field.[89a] A minute wire is embedded in a plastic annulus that is inserted surrounding, but not actually touching, the cornea. Eye movements in three dimensions—horizontal, vertical, and torsional—can be resolved to an accuracy of approximately 0.02 degree (1-minute arc) and at speeds of up to 1000 samples per second. The technique also can be used to measure combined eye and head movements. The main disadvantage of search coil recordings is the level of expertise, in comparison with other techniques, required to set up the apparatus and conduct the recording sessions. Topical anesthetic drops are required to insert the search coil on the patient's eye. The risk of corneal abrasion is low when proper coil insertion and removal techniques are used.

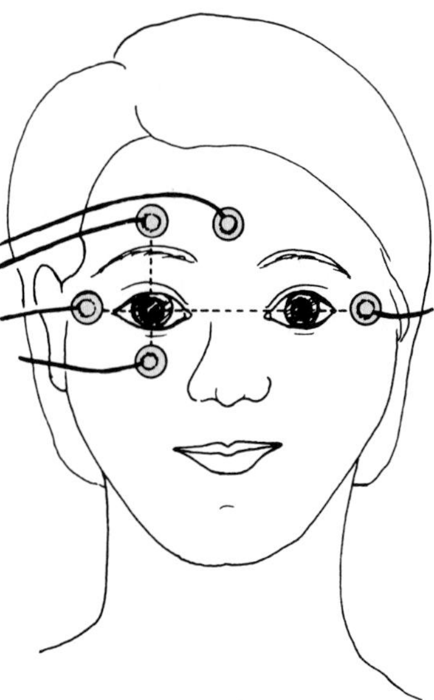

Figure 164-11. Surface electrodes are placed at outer canthi for recording horizontal eye movements and above and below one eye for recording vertical eye movements throughout the electronystagmographic procedure. A ground or reference electrode is placed on the forehead. If recordings are to be made of each eye independently, additional electrodes are placed at the inner canthus of the eye to be recorded.

Infrared video can monitor movement of the cornea or pupil. This technique can be used to record eye movements in three dimensions. Advantages are that the technique is noninvasive, requires little setup time, and is not associated with the position drifts (requiring repeated calibrations) seen with EOG. Disadvantages are that, although procedures and algorithms are improving at a rapid pace, image fitting and analysis techniques still do not work properly for some patients. The time resolution of these methods is poorer (lower sampling rates) than that available with search coil techniques.

Nystagmus

Eye movements are recorded with eyes closed and with eyes open and viewing a stationary visual target. A spontaneous nystagmus and effects of fixation suppression on this nystagmus are thereby determined. Effects of eye position on this nystagmus and the presence of gaze-evoked nystagmus are then assessed by asking the patient to look left, right, up, and down, much as in bedside testing as previously described. The recording of eye movements in darkness is a standard part of ENG testing.

Saccade Testing

The patient is instructed to fixate (with eye movements while keeping the head stationary) on a series of randomly displayed dots or lights at eccentricities of 5 to 30 degrees. Saccades typically begin with a latency of 180 to 200 msec after presentation of a target. Saccade velocity increases linearly with amplitude up to approximately 20 degrees but remains relatively constant for higher amplitudes (Fig. 164-12). Healthy persons consistently undershoot the target for saccades by more than 20 degrees. Asymmetries in saccade amplitude or peak

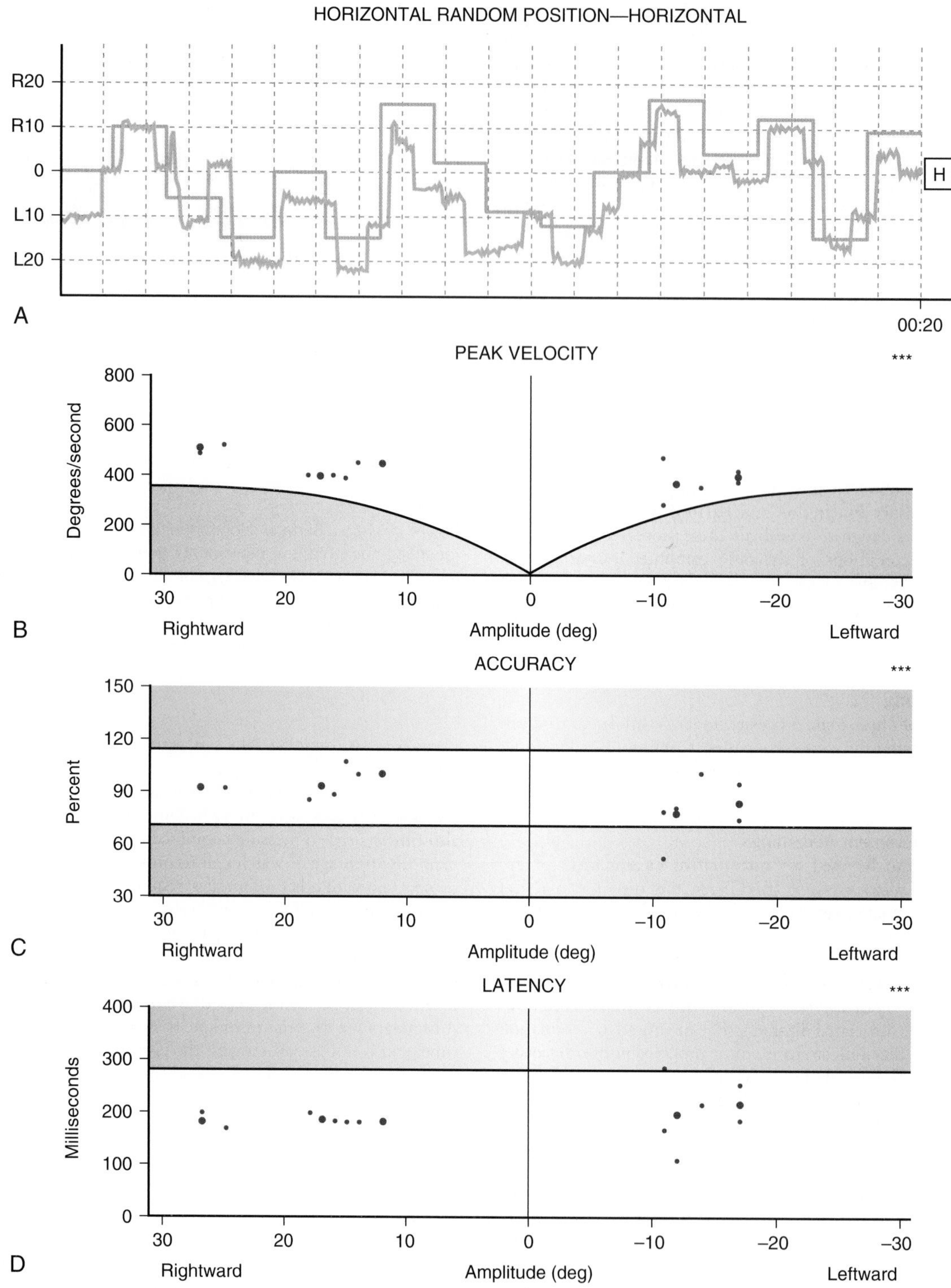

Figure 164-12. Electronystagmographic recordings of saccades. **A,** Eye tracings. **B,** Plot of speed versus amplitude. **C,** Accuracy. **D,** Latency. *Yellow* denotes areas of abnormal responses. See text for causes of inaccurate saccades.

velocity can provide localizing information. With EOG, the speed of abducting saccades seems to be lower than that of adducting saccades, although recordings with search coil and infrared techniques suggest the opposite.

Smooth Pursuit

The patient is asked to watch a target that moves horizontally in a sinusoidal fashion at a low frequency (0.2 to 0.7 Hz) with a position amplitude of 20 degrees in each direction. Inspection of the waveform of the tracking eye movement often is of greater diagnostic use than are absolute measures of gain and phase (Fig. 164-13). "Catch-up" saccades typically are seen when pursuit responses are decreased. Saccadic pursuit is characterized by the occurrence of these saccades in a "stair-step" pattern. Such patterns are seen in cerebellar disease and also may occur with the decreases in pursuit gain that occur with aging.

Optokinetic Testing

Testing is often performed with the subject surrounded by a visual scene that moves in one direction at velocities of 30 to 60 degrees/

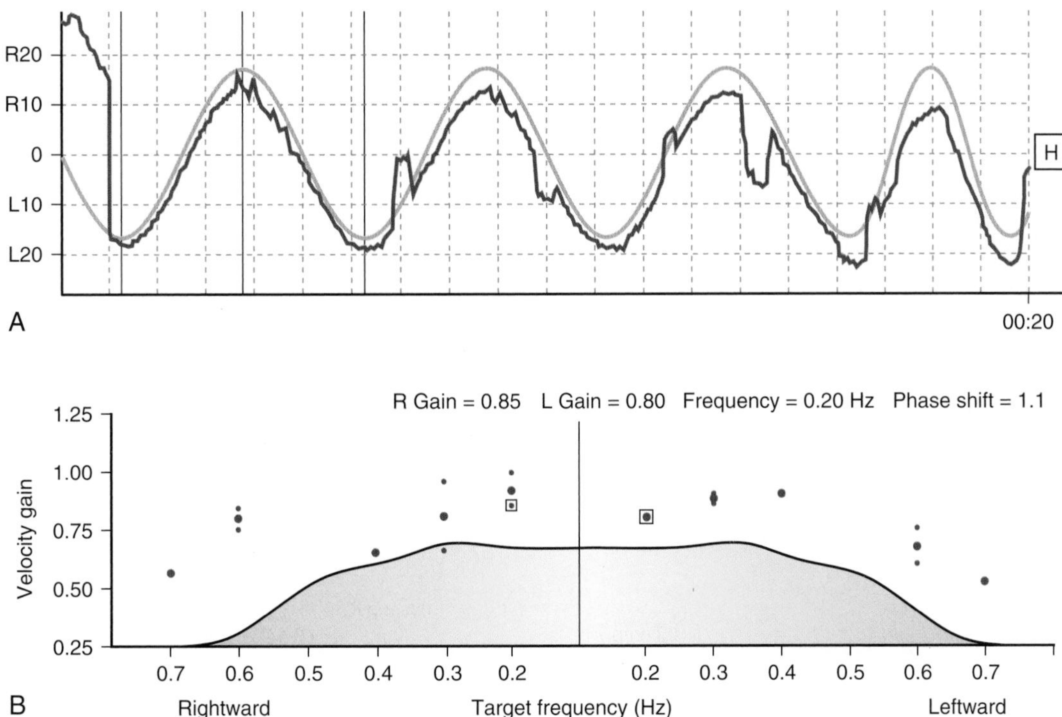

Figure 164-13. Electronystagmographic recordings of smooth pursuit. **A,** Smooth sinusoid, target motion; irregular tracing, eye movements. **B,** Gain in response to moving target at various frequencies. *Yellow shaded area* represents abnormally low responses.

second. The optokinetic tracking response is a nystagmus in the plane of motion of the visual scene. Response gain (the ratio of slow-phase eye velocity to velocity of the visual scene) is measured, and the profile of slow-fast component interaction is assessed. In general, slow-phase abnormalities on optokinetic tests parallel those detected with smooth pursuit testing, whereas fast-phase abnormalities are correlated with those detected on saccade testing. During sustained rotations, the vestibular signal decays and becomes a poor indicator of head motion. To maintain ocular fixation during low-frequency or sustained head movements, the optokinetic system drives the eyes to follow the visual surround. Optokinetic reflexes are a response to motion of the entire visual field rather than of a particular target (for which the smooth pursuit system is used) and are responsible for effects such as automatic tracking of a picket fence seen from a moving car.

Optokinetic afternystagmus (OKAN) is the perseveration of nystagmus after an optokinetic stimulus has been eliminated. OKAN is characterized by its initial eye velocity, time constant of declining eye velocity, cumulative eye position, and symmetry.[38] Velocity storage is believed to be the neural mechanism responsible for maintaining the nystagmus after an optokinetic stimulus. Because smooth pursuit tracking movements contribute to the generation of the slow phases of OKN and confound the assessment of the nystagmus response to optokinetic stimuli, OKAN is the best measure of the action of the portion of the optokinetic responses generated through the vestibular nuclei. If optokinetic reflexes are impaired, OKAN will not be generated even if smooth pursuit is preserved. Optokinetic reflexes are absent in persons with bilateral peripheral vestibular loss but also may be deficient in some normal subjects. OKAN declines with age,[90] and as with the effects of velocity storage caused by vestibular stimulation, its time constant can be reduced with repetition.[91] OKAN is modified in microgravity environments, and its duration is reduced by tilting the head, implying that the otolith organs are important to its genesis. Asymmetries in OKAN have been reported in patients with unilateral vestibular hypofunction induced by removal of an acoustic neuroma. Responses are greater in amplitude and longer in duration for stimulus and eye movement toward the side of the lesion.[92]

Caloric Testing

Caloric testing remains the most useful laboratory investigation for determining the responsiveness of the labyrinth. It is one of the few modalities that allow one labyrinth to be studied independently of the other. Caloric testing relies on stimulating (with a warm stimulus) or inhibiting (with a cool stimulus) the vestibular system by alternately changing the temperature of the external auditory canal with water or air. The horizontal canal is affected most by such temperature changes because it is located closest to the external auditory canal and is oriented in the plane of the temperature gradient that results in the temporal bone from irrigation with water.

Caloric testing causes a response in two ways. The first is a convective component, with the temperature gradient across the horizontal canal resulting in a density difference within the endolymph of the canal (Fig. 164-14). When the horizontal canal is oriented earth-vertically (by elevating the head 30 degrees from the supine position or 60 degrees backward from the upright position), the more dense fluid sinks to the lower position in the canal and the less dense fluid rises to the upper part of the canal. In the presence of gravity, a flow of endolymph occurs from the cooler (more dense) region to the warmer (less dense) region. This movement of fluid within the canal (convective flow) deflects the cupula, thereby leading to a change in the discharge rate of vestibular nerve afferents. Endolymph flows toward the ampulla (resulting in an increase in vestibular nerve afferent discharge) for warm irrigations and away from the ampulla (resulting in a decrease in afferent discharge) for cold irrigations. This effect depends on head position (Fig. 164-15).

The second component does not vary with head position and results in an excitation of the horizontal canal when the ear is warmed and in an inhibition when it is cooled. The nonconvective component may be a result of a direct temperature effect on hair cells or vestibular nerve afferents[93] or cupular displacement resulting from pressure changes in the membranous duct.[94] Direct evidence for the existence of a nonconvective component came from demonstration that a caloric nystagmus can be elicited in the microgravity environment of orbital space flight under conditions in which convection is absent.[95] The

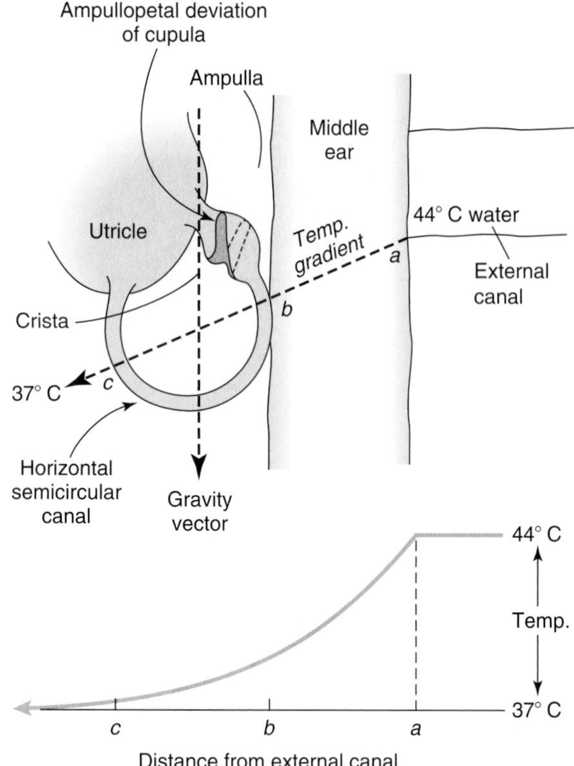

Figure 164-14. Top, Convective flow mechanism of the caloric response. Irrigation with warm or cold water (or air) results in a temperature gradient across the horizontal semicircular canal. With the horizontal canal oriented in the earth-vertical plane, gravity induces the convective flow of endolymph from the cooler area of the canal, in which endolymph is more dense, into the warmer area of the canal, in which endolymph is less dense. For the warm caloric irrigation used for this diagram, ampullopetal deflection of the cupula results from this flow of endolymph. Vestibular nerve afferents innervating the horizontal semicircular canal are excited, and a horizontal nystagmus with slow phase components directed toward the opposite ear is produced. A cold caloric stimulus results in an oppositely directed response with ampullofugal deflection to the cupula, inhibition of horizontal canal afferents, and a nystagmus with slow-phase components directed toward the ear to which the cold caloric is applied. **Bottom,** Graph showing temperature at locations *a*, *b*, and *c*, indicated above. *(From Baloh RW, Honorubia V. Clinical Neurophysiology of the Vestibular System. 2nd ed. Philadelphia: F.A. Davis; 1990.)*

convective component accounts for 75% of the caloric response in the conventional testing position. Convective and nonconvective components are, in the squirrel monkey, affected by a position-dependent, otolith-mediated modification of velocity storage mechanisms.[96]

An otoscopic examination should be performed before caloric testing. Cerumen should be removed to obtain clear visualization of the tympanic membrane. Testing of caloric nystagmus is performed with eyes opened in darkness, behind Frenzel lenses, or in a dimly illuminated room with the patient looking at a Ganzfeld or nonpatterned background. Concentration tasks such as mental arithmetic are used to maintain alertness. EOG calibrations typically are checked after each or every other stimulus. Water calorics should be avoided in cases of tympanic membrane perforation. Improved stimulus reproducibility can be obtained by direct visualization of the position of the irrigation source within the external canal at the time of the stimulus.

Alternate binaural, bithermal caloric testing is the most commonly used testing protocol.[97] Cool water (30° C) and warm water (44° C) are administered for 60 to 90 seconds to each ear in a set order such as right warm, left warm, right cold, left cold. Such a stimulus results in a heating effect in the temporal bone that lasts for 10 to 20 minutes, although nystagmus frequently decays over a much shorter time course (2 to 3 minutes) because of the effects of adaptation.[98] The prolonged heating effect of a single temperature irrigation requires that at least 10 minutes be allowed between successive irrigations. Biphasic caloric irrigations can reduce patient nausea and shorten the wait between stimuli to approximately 2 minutes by using irrigation with water at 43.5° C for 45 seconds, 30.5° C for 65 seconds, and 43.5° C for 23 seconds.[99,100]

Eye movements are recorded for a period of several seconds before onset of an irrigation, during the irrigation, and until the nystagmus has ended. Standard computer algorithms exist for distinguishing fast from slow components of nystagmus and for determining the velocity of each slow component. A plot of slow component velocity is then formed (Fig. 164-16), and the maximum slow component is determined on the basis of three to five slow components with highest velocity. Data are interpreted in terms of unilateral weakness (UW) and directional preponderance (DP), according to formulas described by Jongkees and colleagues[101]:

$$\mathrm{UW} = 100\% \times [(\mathrm{R}30° + \mathrm{R}44°) - (\mathrm{L}30° + \mathrm{L}44°)]/(\mathrm{R}30° + \mathrm{R}44° + \mathrm{L}30° + \mathrm{L}44°)$$

$$\mathrm{DP} = 100\% \times [(\mathrm{R}30° + \mathrm{L}44°) - (\mathrm{R}44° + \mathrm{L}30°)]/(\mathrm{R}30° + \mathrm{L}44° + \mathrm{R}44° + \mathrm{L}30°)$$

Normative values are established for each laboratory. A UW value greater than 20% and DP value greater than 25% usually are considered significant. UW is a sign of decreased responsiveness of the horizontal semicircular canal or the ampullary nerve that provides its innervation. DP commonly is seen in patients with spontaneous nystagmus. For example, a right-beating spontaneous nystagmus will commonly lead to a DP for right-beating responses on caloric testing. The spontaneous nystagmus simply adds to or subtracts from each response to caloric irrigation depending on its direction. In the absence of spontaneous nystagmus, DP may be a central sign indicating asymmetrical sensitivities of central vestibular neurons to inhibitory-excitatory stimuli or asymmetries in the inputs from these central vestibular neurons to extraocular motoneurons. An increased warm and a diminished cold response, as can occur in an ear affected with Meniere's disease, can result in a DP. Caloric nystagmus can be suppressed with visual fixation in healthy persons. Failure of fixation suppression of caloric nystagmus can be seen in central disorders such as cerebellar disease.

Rotatory Chair Testing

Unlike caloric tests, rotational tests analyze the responses of both semicircular canals together. They require a high-torque motor-driven chair and specific software to analyze the results. Rotatory chair testing is useful in assessing vestibular function in patients with suspected bilateral vestibular hypofunction, in patients receiving vestibulotoxic medications, and in children who may not tolerate caloric testing. Clinical situations in which findings on rotatory chair testing in pediatric patients may provide useful information include determining whether a failure to achieve normal developmental milestones is based in part on absent vestibular function, evaluating vestibular function after meningitis, and determining the presence or absence of vestibular function in patients undergoing a genetic evaluation for hearing loss.

Rotational testing does not depend on delivery of a stimulus directly to the inner ear, as with the caloric test, so results are therefore not susceptible to variables such as size or shape of the external auditory canal. Rotational testing is less bothersome to some patients than is caloric testing (although nausea and vertigo associated with calorics can be decreased considerably with the use of temperature switch techniques as described). Most commercially available rotational testing systems administer low-frequency sinusoidal rotations and analyze eye movement responses to the input stimulus. The patient's head typically is aligned with the chin pitched 30 degrees nose down such that horizontal semicircular canals are in the plane of rotation. Approximately 10 cycles of the sinusoidal head velocity stimulus are recorded for five to eight test frequencies over the range of 0.01 to 0.7 Hz, with the

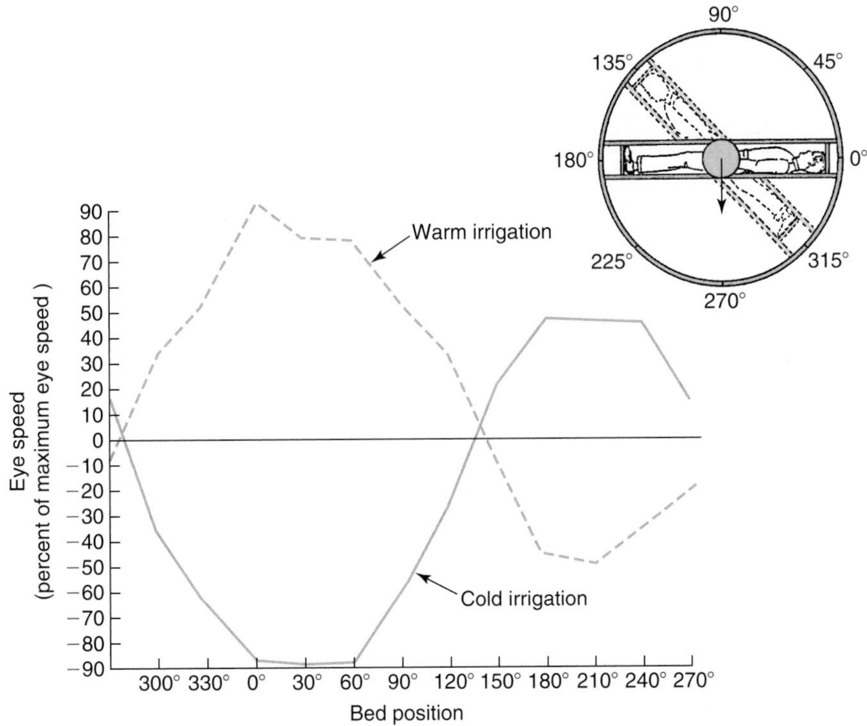

Figure 164-15. Average slow-phase eye velocity in response to warm (44° C) and cold (30° C) irrigations with subjects oriented in different bed positions. Subjects were lying on a Stryker bed that could be moved through 360 degrees in the pitch plane (see *inset*). For each subject, the percent of the maximum value in the curve (which usually occurred at the 30-degree position, at which the horizontal canal is in the earth-vertical plane) was determined at each of the positions tested. These percentages were then averaged for all subjects to obtain the composite plots shown. Four observations are apparent: (1) Caloric responses in the face-up positions are consistently greater in intensity than those in the face-down positions. (2) "Face-up" responses cover a larger segment of the 360-degree arc than the "face-down" responses. (3) The curves appear to approximate a sine function. (4) The findings are similar for warm and for cold irrigations. *(Modified from Coats AD, Smith SY. Body position and the intensity of caloric nystagmus.* Acta Otolaryngol (Stockh). *1967;63:515.)*

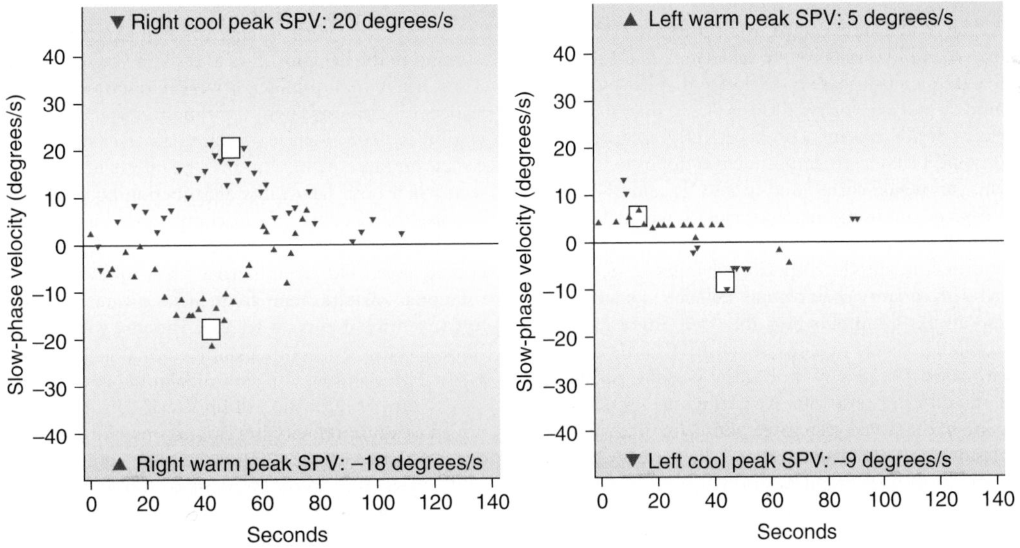

Figure 164-16. Caloric responses in a patient with unilateral labyrinthine hypofunction. The patient had no response in the left ear, although right ear responses to warm and cold irrigations were normal. SPV, slow component velocity.

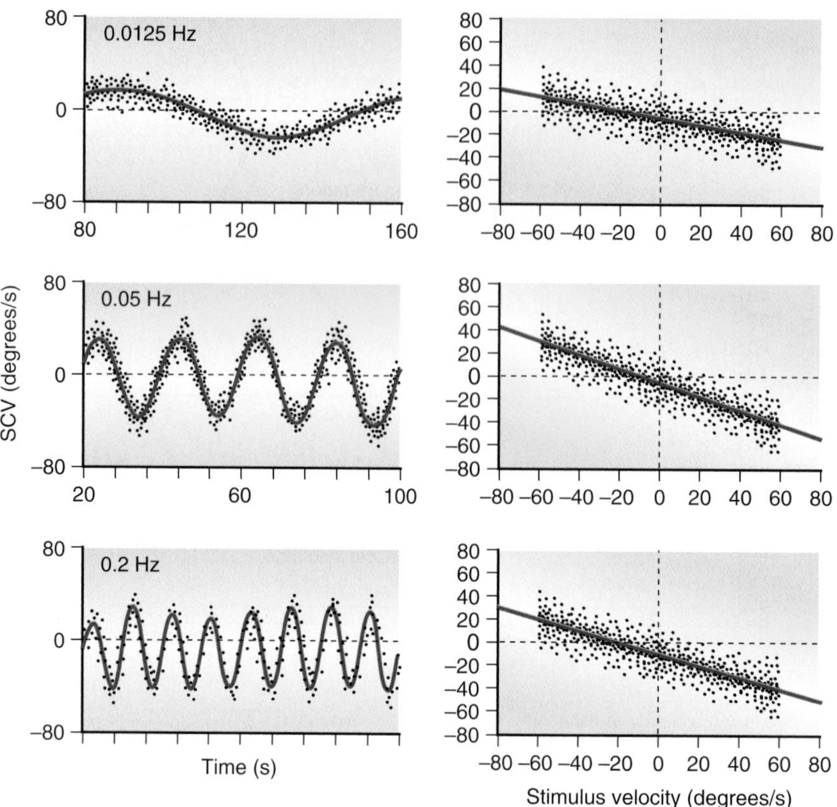

Figure 164-17. Rotational chair responses 3 months after unilateral vestibular deafferentation. Vertical axis = ocular response in degrees/second. Note that at the low frequencies tested here, the patient's responses *(dots)* closely follow the chair's movement *(solid line)*, indicating compensation from the lesion. Head impulse signs at this stage are likely to remain pathologic. The bottom stimulus-velocity curve *(lower right)* shows a slight bias (i.e., the line does not pass exactly through the origin). SPV, slow component velocity. *(From Jenkins HA. Long-term adaptive changes of the vestibulo-ocular reflex in patients following acoustic neuroma surgery.* Laryngoscope. *1985;95:1224.)*

patient in darkness. The results are averaged over successive cycles, and gain, phase, asymmetry, and bias velocity are calculated. *Gain* refers to amplitude of the maximum slow-phase eye velocity divided by amplitude of the maximum stimulus velocity. *Phase* is the temporal shift in eye velocity relative to head velocity. For a perfectly compensatory VOR, eye velocity should be equal in amplitude but opposite in direction to head velocity. This would correspond to a VOR gain of 1.0 and phase shift of 180 degrees (meaning that eye velocity would lag head velocity by 180 degrees).

Cerebellar abnormalities produce specific changes in responses that can be evaluated with rotatory chair testing. Velocity storage mechanisms that are responsible for prolonging the VOR time constant relative to that of vestibular nerve afferents are sensitive to the orientation of the head with respect to gravity. In healthy persons, tilting the head downward at the onset of post-rotatory nystagmus results in an immediate suppression of the stored velocity response, but patients with midline cerebellar lesions near the uvula and nodulus have VOR time constants that are normal in the upright position and are not affected by post-rotatory tilt.[102] Patients with cerebellar lesions such as caused by the Arnold-Chiari malformation exhibit tilt suppression intermediate between that of healthy persons and that of patients with midline cerebellar lesions. Abnormally high gain on rotational testing also has been noted in cases of cerebellar atrophy.[103] However, the presence of post-rotatory nystagmus evoked by this test is influenced by the level of vestibular function and by the status of velocity storage mechanisms, and the nystagmus can be suppressed by visual fixation. Because of the many processes involved, the test results have proved to be variable and difficult to correlate with specific pathologic processes.

Directionally dependent asymmetries can indicate relative weakness of function in one labyrinth compared with the other.[104] In the case of a patient with absence of vestibular function on the right, head rotation to the left continues to evoke a normal VOR, whereas rotations to the right may produce a weaker response, with gain decreasing as velocity increases. These asymmetries are thought to occur because vestibular neurons have an approximately three-fold higher range for excitation than for inhibition. The effects of these asymmetries are not seen when both labyrinths are functioning symmetrically, presumably because the brain is able to compensate for the loss of signals on the side being driven into inhibitory cutoff by use of signals from the excited side. The asymmetries are, however, more pronounced for rotational velocities and frequencies greater than those typically used in conventional clinical testing. Patients with compensated unilateral vestibular loss frequently exhibit normal gain and phase with minimal asymmetries on standard sinusoidal rotatory chair tests[105] (Fig. 164-17).

A further indication of unilateral deficiency of vestibular function is seen as a bias velocity in responses to sinusoidal rotations. Spontaneous nystagmus causes a bias velocity by adding the slow-phase velocity of the nystagmus to the response to sinusoidal stimulation, but such a bias also can be seen after spontaneous nystagmus has resolved. The direction of bias alone does not identify the affected ear, because both irritative lesions (such as Meniere's disease, serous labyrinthitis, labyrinthine fistulas, and acoustic neuromas) and ablative lesions can cause bias (but in opposite directions).

Step changes in head velocity can be used instead of sinusoidal rotations to identify vestibular hypofunction. The patient is seated in the rotatory chair apparatus, and eye movements are recorded with EOG. Testing is performed in darkness. The chair accelerates rapidly to the right or to the left, reaching its peak velocity (typically 60 or 240 degrees/second) in 1 second. A horizontal nystagmus is recorded. Response gain and VOR time constant are determined by the time after

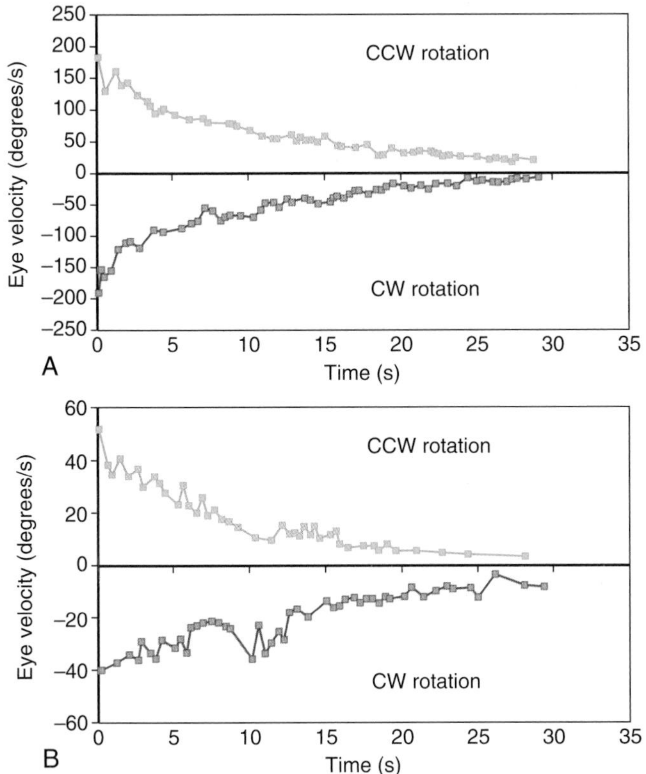

Figure 164-18. Velocity of horizontal slow-phase components of nystagmus evoked by velocity steps of 240 degrees/second (**A**) and 60 degrees/second (**B**). The subject is seated in a rotatory chair with the head positioned in approximately the horizontal canal plane (chin tilted downward 30 degrees from ambient position of the head) in **A** and in the ambient position (30 degrees upward from the horizontal canal plane) in **B.** Testing is conducted in darkness. Chair rotations in the counterclockwise (CCW) direction evoke slow phases to the right, whereas rotation in the clockwise (CW) direction evokes slow phases to the left. Gain is determined from the responses in **A** by dividing the velocity of the first slow phase in response to the stimulus by the head velocity. Gain measures approximately 0.80 in these data and is symmetrical for clockwise and counterclockwise rotations. Time constant is measured from responses to 60-degrees/second rotations as the time required for slow-phase velocity to decline by 63% of its initial value. In the data shown for CW rotation in **B,** the initial eye velocity is 40 degrees/second and falls to 15 degrees/second (a decline of 63% from the initial value) 20 seconds after the stimulus onset. The time constant of the response is therefore 20 seconds.

onset of the stimulus at which slow-phase eye velocity has decreased by 67% of its initial value (Fig. 164-18). A further procedure has been used to improve test sensitivity in identifying unilateral vestibular hypofunction: A rotation of 240 degrees/second is given with the patient's head aligned in the 30-degree chin-down position (to bring the horizontal canals into the plane of rotation) and with the head pitched 30 degrees upward.[106] The effect of the rotational stimulus on the horizontal semicircular canals varies with the cosine of the angle of the canal to the plane of rotation. Thus, the stimulus causes only approximately 60% of maximal activation with the head in the 30-degree pitched-upward position. Vertical semicircular canals are brought more into the plane of rotation in these pitched positions. In cases of unilateral vestibular hypofunction, gain asymmetries caused by the inhibitory cutoff effects are more likely to be seen with the horizontal canals aligned in the plane of rotation.

Electrocochleography

Electrocochleography (ECOG) may be useful in the diagnosis of Meniere's disease, although interpretation of the findings remains a

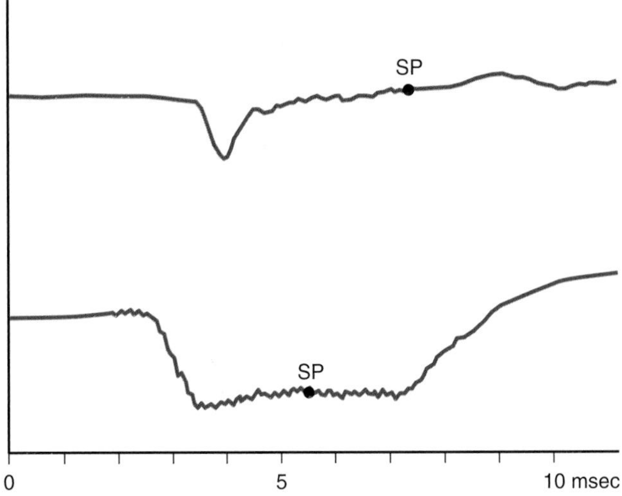

Figure 164-19. Transtympanic electrocochleography. *Top line*, Normal response to tone burst stimulus. *Bottom line*, Pathologic response, with shifted summating potential line (SP) relative to the baseline.

topic of controversy. The cochlea responds to repeated presentation of sound with auditory evoked potentials, which can be represented as an action potential (AP) and a summating potential (SP) (Fig. 164-19). A ratio between the two (SP/AP ratio) greater than 0.4 and an AP duration longer than 3 msec are indicative of endolymphatic hydrops.[107] This effect is believed to be due to the altered physical properties of the basilar membrane because of endolymphatic hydrops. ECOG can be performed with tone bursts or clicks. Recent studies regarding the safety and efficacy of transtympanic ECOG indicate that this technique may be superior to simply placing the electrode in the external canal.[108] The utility of ECOG in the identification of Meniere's disease has been questioned.

Subjective Visual Vertical

The subjective visual vertical is a useful measure of otolith function. Patients sit in a darkened area and focus on a line that they manipulate by use of a dial until they perceive it as vertical. Patients with acute utricular lesions usually leave the line tilted 10 to 15 degrees toward the side of the lesion. Deficits in subjective visual vertical also are seen in patients with brainstem infarctions.[109]

Quantitative Head Impulse Testing

Quantitative head impulse testing allows recording of responses for later analysis and detection of short-latency or small eye movements that may be missed under bedside conditions. Eye movements generally are recorded using scleral search coil technology. Quantitative head impulse testing allows accurate titration of intratympanic gentamicin treatment for intractable Meniere's disease[110,111] and to show that vestibular neuritis preferentially spares the inferior vestibular nerve serving the posterior semicircular canal.[112] These methods also have shown that plugging of the superior canal as used in the treatment of superior canal dehiscence typically causes reduction in function of the plugged canal with preservation of function in the other canals.[113]

Active Head Movement Analysis Techniques

Active head movement analysis techniques have been developed to evaluate the VOR in response to higher-frequency head rotations than those customarily used in rotatory chair testing. This broader range of stimulus frequencies is possible because the test subjects make the head movements actively, using their own neck musculature to rotate the head. In these cases, head velocity is measured by a transducer mounted directly to the head. In one of the more commonly used commercial systems (Vestibular Autorotation Test, Western Systems Research, Inc., Pasadena, California), a computer-generated metronome cues head movements for an 18-second trial period over a swept-frequency band from 2 to 6 Hz. Broad-band cross-spectral analysis is used to determine

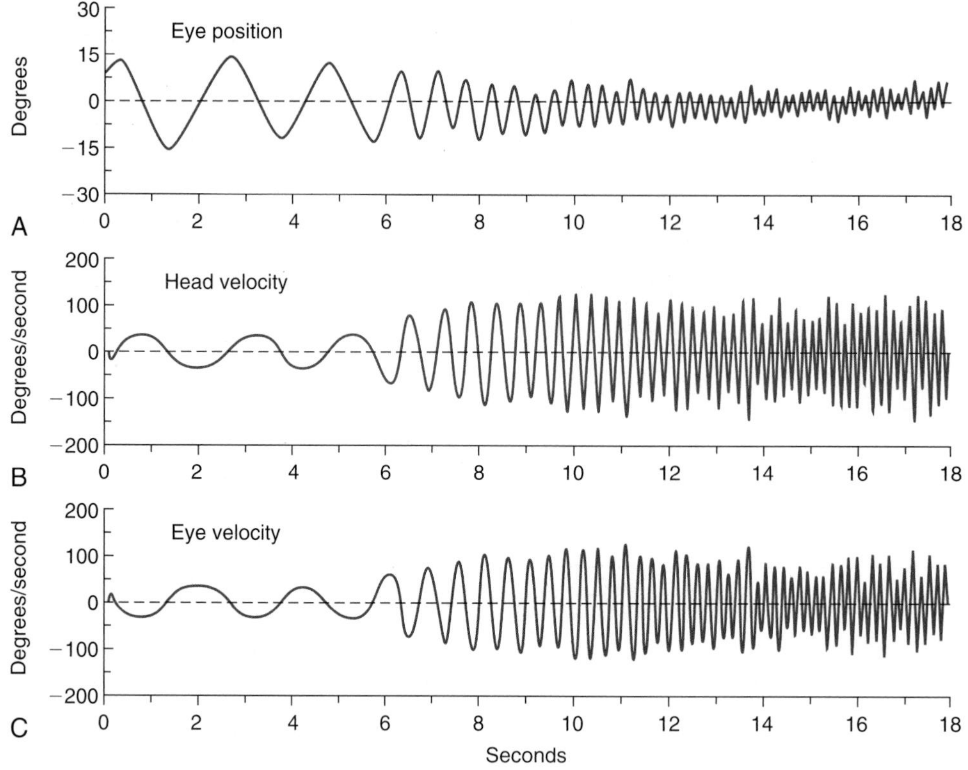

Figure 164-20. Horizontal eye position (**A**), head velocity (**B**), and eye velocity (**C**) during active head movement testing with the Vestibular Autorotation Test. *(From Fineberg R, O'Leary DP, Davis LL. Use of active head movements for computerized vestibular testing.* Arch Otolaryngol Head Neck Surg. *1987;113:1063.)*

all harmonic contributions that occur at each frequency. Results are computed and reported as gain and phase values at 12 selected frequencies over the range of 2 to 6 Hz (Fig. 164-20). Testing is performed with the room illuminated, while the patient fixates on a stationary target that does not move with the head. The range of frequencies tested exceeds that over which smooth pursuit typically is active, so responses are a result of the VOR. Normative data have been obtained for patients of various ages (see Fig. 164-20).[114,115] The vertical VOR can be evaluated in a similar fashion.

Active head movement testing of the VOR has been applied in monitoring patients receiving vestibulotoxic medications such as cisplatin.[116] Asymmetries in responses have been shown to be correlated directionally with the side of lesion in patients with unilateral labyrinthectomy and with the side of lesion in patients with acoustic neuroma.[115] Many patients with Meniere's syndrome also were noted to have abnormalities when these testing procedures were applied.[117] The sensitivity of active tests such as the vestibular autorotation test may be somewhat less than that of passive tests such as head impulse testing, because of the patient's ability to preprogram his or her eye movements during active head movements.[118]

Vestibular Evoked Myogenic Potentials

Recent studies have demonstrated that healthy subjects exhibit a relaxation of the ipsilateral sternocleidomastoid (SCM) muscle in response to auditory stimulation (100- to 200-msec rarefaction clicks, 95-dB sound pressure level [SPL] or tone bursts).[119] These cervical vestibular evoked myogenic potential (VEMP) responses are recorded with electromyelography (EMG) and occur at a short latency (12 msec) relative to onset of the click stimulus (Fig. 164-21). The responses are abolished on the side of surgery after unilateral vestibular neurectomy.[120] VEMP responses are a result of selective activation of vestibular nerve afferents innervating the sacculus. In addition to aiding in diagnosis of otolith function, patients with superior canal dehiscence syndrome also seem to have lower thresholds and increased amplitude[121] and patients with Meniere's disease may have higher thresholds for responses to VEMPs.[122]

Variants of the test include the use of a reflex hammer to produce a sharp tap on the patient's forehead. With this modification, VEMPs were evoked in a small series of patients with conductive hearing loss, while the selectivity of the test was maintained in patients with unilateral vestibular loss.[123] Bone-conducted stimulation with pure tones may be more sensitive than air-conducted sounds.[124] VEMPs also may be recorded from the extraocular musculature.[125] Ocular VEMPs may be superior to cervical VEMPs for detection of superior canal dehiscence.[126]

Posturography

Techniques for postural assessment in patients have been developed in an attempt to provide a quantitative assessment of processes involved in maintaining upright stance under static and dynamic conditions. These tests have conceptual appeal, because they provide a potential mechanism for evaluation of all sensory systems (vestibular, visual, and somatosensory) that provide information important for maintaining balance.

The most commonly used system for clinical postural assessment is computerized dynamic posturography (CDP) (e.g., Equitest, NeuroCom International, Clackamas, Oregon). The test subject stands on a computer-controlled movable platform with a movable visual surround. The platform and visual surround can be fixed or move independently or concomitantly with postural sway. Anterior-to-posterior sway of center of gravity is monitored with pressure-sensitive gauges located in each quadrant of the platform (Fig. 164-22). The standard CDP test battery includes assessment of automatic postural responses to platform movements—the motor control test—and determination of effects of manipulations of visual and somatosensory information on standing balance—the sensory organization test (SOT).

Motor Control Test

The platform administers sudden sagittal movements to the feet, and "toes-up" and "toes-down" platform rotations of 4.0 degrees in 500 msec also are presented. Strain gauges for each foot are then used to calculate the following: weight symmetry (distribution of weight over

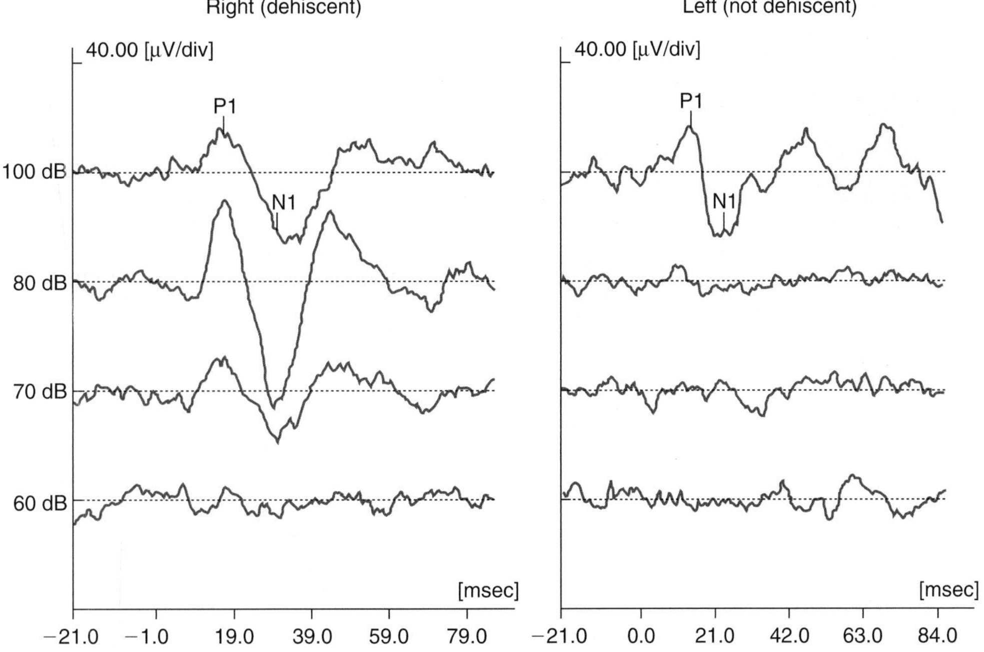

Figure 164-21. Vestibular evoked myogenic potentials (VEMPs) in a patient with unilateral semicircular canal dehiscence responding to clicks. Stimulus was presented at time = 0 msec. The evoked potential peaks at approximately 16 msec and is evident bilaterally at 100 dB *(top tracing)*. On the dehiscent side *(right)*, the potential is still present at 70 dB, but on the normal side *(left)*, no VEMP is present below 100 dB. div, division.

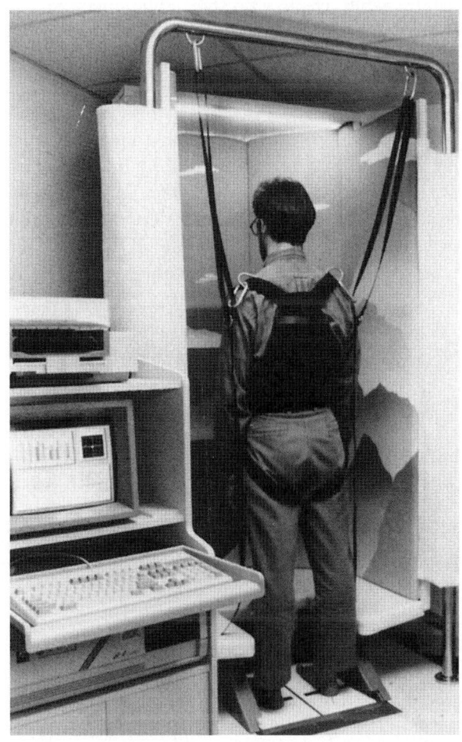

Figure 164-22. Photograph of the NeuroCom International Equitest system shows a subject standing on a platform surrounded by a visual scene. Pressure-sensing strain gauges beneath the platform surface detect patient sway by measuring vertical and horizontal forces applied to the surface. A safety harness is attached to the patient in case loss of balance occurs. The platform surface and the visual surround are capable of moving independently or simultaneously.

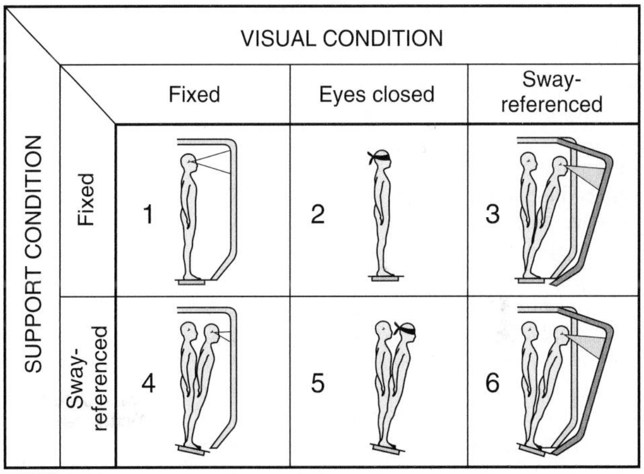

SUPPORT CONDITION	VISUAL CONDITION: Fixed	Eyes closed	Sway-referenced
Fixed	1	2	3
Sway-referenced	4	5	6

Figure 164-23. The sensory organization test protocol showing the six test conditions. *(From Nashner LM. Computerized dynamic posturography. In: Jacobson GP, Newman CW, Kartush JM, eds.* Handbook of Balance Function Testing. *St. Louis: Mosby; 1996:280-307.)*

both feet during movement), amplitude scaling (distribution of force through legs during platform movement), latency (time from onset of platform movement to discernible response and relationship to amplitude of movement), and adaptation (relationship between response amplitude and stimulus repetition).

Sensory Organization Test

Six test conditions comprise the SOT test battery (Fig. 164-23). The platform remains fixed under the first three test conditions, providing the patient with stable reference for somatosensory information. The visual surround also remains fixed in test condition 1, making this the condition for optimal stability. The patient's eyes are closed in test condition 2, and anteroposterior (AP) sway is controlled by vestibular and somatosensory information. Balance is controlled mainly by somatosensory information during this test condition, so patients with

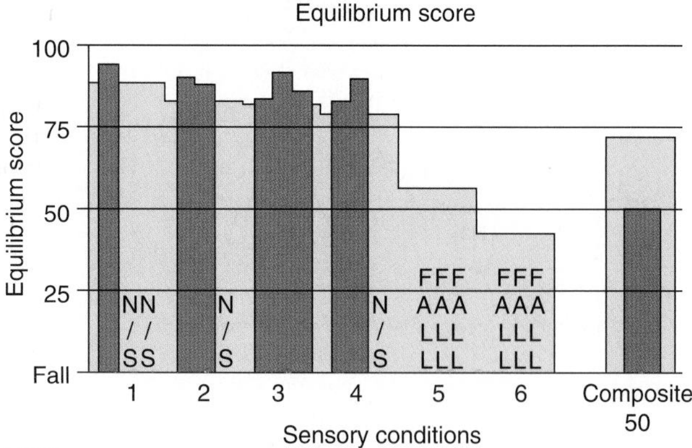

Figure 164-24. Vestibular dysfunction (5-6) pattern. Distortion of somatosensory cues (conditions 5 and 6) and distortion (condition 6) or elimination of visual cues (condition 5) force the patient to rely on vestibular information for balance and posture. This pattern can be seen with acute unilateral or bilateral vestibular lesions, in cases of poor compensation in response to peripheral vestibular lesions, and occasionally with central vestibular system disease. Patients with compensated unilateral peripheral vestibular lesions typically exhibit normal performance on the sensory organization test. During actual test conditions, a stimulus repetition may be deferred if the preceding presentation of that stimulus gives a normal response. The label FALL indicates trials in which the sway in response to the stimulus was outside the limits of stability and would have resulted in a fall had the patient not been secured with a harness. N/S, no stimulus.

deficient vestibular function typically show minimal unsteadiness on this test condition, provided that somatosensory function is normal.

The visual surround moves in reference to AP body sway in test condition 3. "Sway referencing" of the visual surround results in distorted visual inputs to systems controlling balance. Maintaining balance requires the brain to disregard these inaccurate visual inputs and select vestibular and somatosensory cues for balance. As in condition 2, somatosensory inputs are most important for postural control in these situations, so patients with vestibular deficits (but normal somatosensation) tend to do well.

The platform moves to follow the AP sway of the patient in test conditions 4, 5, and 6, thereby providing distorted somatosensory inputs to the brain. Inaccurate proprioceptive cues must be suppressed in these cases, with vestibular and visual inputs used to maintain postural stability. The visual surround remains fixed in condition 4, which permits visual and vestibular inputs to be used in maintaining balance. Patients with vestibular deficits tend to do well in this condition, provided that their vision is intact. The patient's eyes are closed in condition 5, and the platform is sway referenced. Only vestibular cues can be used to maintain balance in this condition, and patients with bilateral vestibular hypofunction or uncompensated unilateral vestibular hypofunction sway excessively. The platform and visual surround are sway referenced in condition 6. Vestibular inputs must now be selected over inaccurate somatosensory and visual cues to maintain balance in this situation. Responses are quantitatively assessed in each condition and compared with age-related norms. Balance strategies (hip or ankle) also are measured. Specific profiles for SOT findings are shown in Figure 164-24.

Use of Posturography

The role of CDP in the diagnosis and management of dizziness continues to be a topic of debate.[127] Rather than serving as a screening test for making a diagnosis in all patients with unidentified problems affecting posture or balance, CDP may be beneficial in three specifically defined clinical situations[128]:

1. *Planning and monitoring a course of postural rehabilitation.* Diagnoses for which posturography can be useful include unilateral or bilateral vestibular hypofunction, brainstem stroke, cerebellar ataxia, extrapyramidal disorders, and vestibular schwannomas and cerebellopontine angle neoplasms. Vestibular rehabilitation programs that are specifically designed for a patient's profile of deficits have been shown to be more effective at alleviating symptoms than generic physical therapy measures.[129] CDP can be useful in the selection of exercises included in a patient's rehabilitation program and in monitoring responses to the therapeutic regimen. For example, patients with dysequilibrium after a unilateral loss of vestibular function can demonstrate dependence on somatosensory or visual information to maintain balance. Patients with somatosensory reliance are given exercises that include walking on uneven surfaces to promote use of visual or vestibular cues to balance, whereas those with visual dependence do exercises that involve intermittently closing the eyes to promote use of somatosensory and vestibular cues.

   The organization of an exercise program on the basis of data obtained from posturography has been demonstrated to have a beneficial effect on functional outcome. Patients showed a significant reduction in postural sway on SOT conditions 5 and 6 in patients with peripheral vestibulopathy who received vestibular rehabilitation compared with those of a control group who only received vestibular-suppressant medication.[130] Patients with a variety of peripheral and central vestibular disorders show improvements in subjective and objective measures of functional outcome after receiving an exercise regimen organized around abnormalities on SOT.[131] Evaluation of CDP prelesion and postlesion can also be useful in defining the expected outcome and end point of vestibular rehabilitation for each patient. Patients undergoing vestibular neurectomy for intractable vertigo who showed preoperative abnormalities on CDP showed persisting abnormalities even after a postoperative recovery period, whereas patients with normal findings preoperatively returned to normal.[132]

2. *Determination of the need for high-volume cerebrospinal fluid (CSF) drainage with lumbar punctures or shunting in patients with dysequilibrium or gait disturbances caused by processes resulting in abnormal CSF pressure dynamics.* These patients develop dysequilibrium and ataxia with increased CSF accumulation. CDP is useful in quantifying their improvement after CSF draining and in predicting their response to ventriculoperitoneal shunting.[133]

3. *Documentation of postural responses when malingering, exaggeration of disability for compensation, or conversion disorder is suspected.* CDP can identify inconsistencies between symptoms and performance parameters that have been shown to indicate a functional deficit as in malingering or conversion disorder.[134,135] Patients with these disorders often show patterns on CDP that are described as aphysiologic (e.g., poorer performance on SOT conditions 1 and 2 than on 5 and 6). Identification of such patients can be useful in making recommendations about disability status and the need for psychiatric intervention.

Audiogram

Audiometric findings may indicate the cause of imbalance and guide its therapy. Sensorineural hearing loss may accompany peripheral vestibular loss caused by Meniere's disease or aminoglycoside vestibulotoxicity. A Stenger test may help identify malingering. Conductive hearing loss may accompany superior canal dehiscence and enlarged vestibular aqueduct syndrome. Auditory reflex testing helps distinguish these conditions from others, such as otosclerosis, that may have similar balance-related symptoms.

High-Resolution Temporal Bone Computed Tomography

Advances in radiologic techniques have allowed improved diagnosis of many otologic disorders. Superior canal dehiscence syndrome is characterized by sound-induced or pressure-induced vertigo or apparent conductive hearing loss, or both, due to incomplete covering of the superior semicircular canal in the arcuate eminence. In affected patients, eye movements in the plane of the superior semicircular canal often can be induced by loud noises and by maneuvers that change middle ear or intracranial pressure. Confirmation of this diagnosis requires thin-slice computed tomography (CT) images of the temporal bone in the plane of the superior semicircular canal. Scanners with 0.5-mm slice thickness had a 93% positive predictive value, compared with only 50% with a 1.0 mm slice thickness, because of partial volume averaging in the coarser scan.[136]

Magnetic Resonance Imaging

Dysarthria, diplopia, and paresthesias may accompany the vertigo seen in cases of vertebrobasilar insufficiency. Other neurologic signs including cranial neuropathies and seizure activity may indicate a primary intracranial process.

Serologic Tests

Serologic abnormalities are rare in patients with symptoms of imbalance but in some cases may indicate severe disease. Syphilis, Lyme disease, or Susac syndrome may manifest with hearing loss or imbalance. Antiphospholipid syndrome recently has been associated with inner ear disease, and treatment may prevent significant embolic events.[137] *Cogan's syndrome* is an inflammatory condition characterized by severe visual and vestibular symptoms. In some cases, life-threatening systemic vasculitis may develop.[138] Rare paraneoplastic syndromes associated with breast cancer or Hodgkin's lymphoma may be associated with imbalance.[139]

Adaptive Capabilities of the Vestibular System

The clinician must consider adaptive changes when evaluating the results of vestibular testing. Unilateral loss of vestibular function creates two general types of deficits for which a correction is required: *static imbalance*, related to differences in the levels of tonic activity of neurons in the vestibular nuclei, and *dynamic disturbances*, related to responsiveness to motion. For the VOR, spontaneous nystagmus with the head stationary is an example of the former type of disturbance, whereas decreased amplitude and asymmetry of eye rotation during head rotation are examples of the latter. For a fixed (nonfluctuating) unilateral loss of vestibular function, resolution of static signs such as spontaneous nystagmus and the ocular tilt reaction usually occurs within days, but dynamic processes return toward baseline levels over the course of several weeks. Some processes such as the function of velocity storage and responses to high-frequency, high-acceleration head movements toward the hypoactive labyrinth may not recover.

Adaptive mechanisms are most likely to involve increasing sensitivities of central vestibular neurons to signals they receive from the intact vestibular nerve or adjustments in the level of modulation in neurons that connect the vestibular nuclei from one side to the other. Experimental evidence indicates that once acquired, these adaptive and compensatory changes require continued sensory exposure for maintenance of appropriate responses. In addition to the central mechanisms that promote normalization of vestibular processes after labyrinthine or central injuries, the brain can substitute other strategies for generating responses involved in sensing and controlling motion. These substitutions can involve other sensory inputs for driving the same motor response (e.g., substitution of the cervico-ocular reflex or the optokinetic reflex for labyrinthine-evoked VOR). Other strategies can be based on prediction or anticipation of intended motor behavior (e.g., gaze overshoots during combined eye and head movements in labyrinthine-defective persons can be prevented by preprogramming compensatory slow phases and decreasing saccade size in anticipation of a head movement). A consequence of such an adaptive capability is that a vestibular disorder reflects the "pure" effects of a lesion only when history-taking and patient examination are done immediately after change in vestibular function.

Specific vestibular rehabilitation exercises constitute the appropriate treatment for patients with unilateral or bilateral vestibular loss. These exercises are designed to assist the brain's intrinsic adaptive processes to compensate for loss of peripheral function. A successful rehabilitation program usually is carried out in partnership with a physical therapist. Some exercises are designed to increase the gain of the hypoactive vestibular system by maintaining fixation on a target while moving the head. Others attempt to habituate the patient to disturbing symptoms by mildly and repetitively provoking them. Rehabilitation is effective in patients with acute vestibular loss, as well as in patients with more chronic symptoms. Patients with bilateral vestibular loss generally enjoy less benefit from rehabilitation than that observed in patients with unilateral loss. Despite the benefits of rehabilitation, many patients will never achieve the same level of activity that they had before their vestibular loss. Some patients who do not improve after vestibular exercises may have problems such as benign positional vertigo or superior canal dehiscence that are better treated with more specific therapies.

SUGGESTED READINGS

Baloh R, Honrubia V. *Clinical Neurophysiology of the Vestibular System*. 2nd ed. Philadelphia: F.A. Davis; 1990.

Furman JM, Cass SP. *Vestibular Disorders: A Case Study Approach*. 2nd ed. New York: Oxford University Press; 2003.

Goebel JA. *The Practical Management of the Dizzy Patient*. 2nd ed. Philadelphia: Lippincott Williams & Wilkins; 2008.

Highstein S. *The Vestibular System*. New York: Springer; 2004.

Leigh R, Zee D. *The Neurology of Eye Movements*. 4th ed. New York: Oxford University Press; 2006.

For complete list of references log onto www.expertconsult.com.

CHAPTER ONE HUNDRED AND SIXTY-FIVE

Peripheral Vestibular Disorders

Benjamin T. Crane

David A. Schessel

Julian Nedzelski

Lloyd B. Minor

Key Points

- The peripheral vestibular system transduces head movement, playing key roles in stabilizing vision and ambulation.
- The history of vertigo symptoms provides definitive insights into underlying diagnosis and pathophysiology; the first step is to differentiate peripheral from central vestibular disorders.
- Peripheral vestibular disorders are highly prevalent, affecting 1 in 13 people during their lifetime.
- Benign paroxysmal positional vertigo (BPPV) produces characteristic symptoms of position sensitivity and fatigability and often is effectively diagnosed with the Dix-Hallpike maneuver and treated with the Epley maneuver.
- The diagnosis of vestibular neuritis is suggested by dramatic, sudden-onset vertigo with vegetative symptoms.
- The diagnosis of Meniere's disease is based on a history of episodes of vertigo lasting up to 24 hours, fluctuating sensorineural hearing loss, tinnitus, and aural fullness. If followed for 2 years, more than half of Meniere's patients will have a spontaneous cessation of vertigo symptoms.
- Treatments for Meniere's disease include low-sodium diet, diuretics, and intratympanic injection of dexamethasone or gentamicin. More advanced cases not responsive to initial therapy may be treated with nerve section or labyrinthectomy.
- Superior canal dehiscence syndrome is caused by absence of bone over the superior canal. Symptoms include vertigo induced by loud sound or high pressure, conductive hearing loss, pulsatile tinnitus, and autophony.
- Cogan's syndrome is characterized by interstitial keratitis, hearing loss, and vestibular symptoms. Systemic steroids are the accepted treatment.
- Perilymph fistula is a controversial diagnosis with presenting symptoms of dizziness and hearing loss.
- Bilateral vestibular hypofunction can manifest with oscillopsia and gait disturbance. Aminoglycosides are the most common cause.
- Enlarged vestibular aqueduct syndrome usually manifests with hearing loss in childhood, but vertigo often develops later in life.

Basic Principles of Peripheral Vestibular Physiology

The peripheral vestibular system depends on the sensory receptor structures, which are responsible both for sensing motion and position of the head in space and for converting this sensory stimulus into an electrical signal. These sensory signals are carried to the central nervous system (CNS) in the form of neural activity.

Vestibular receptors are organized to detect head motion in a specific direction or plane. Horizontal head rotation (yaw) produces a stimulus to the horizontal semicircular canals. Pitching of the head from front to back, as well as roll from side to side, is detected by the superior and posterior semicircular canals. Linear acceleration such as gravity as well as motion along a straight trajectory are sensed by the otolith organs located in the utricle and saccule.

All receptors are tonically active. A resting, spontaneous, continual outflow of action potentials from the vestibular portion of the eighth cranial nerve has been recognized. With head motion, this spontaneous activity is modulated up or down. For example, turning the head to the right in the upright position produces an increase in activity in the nerve coming from the right horizontal semicircular canal, whereas left turns decrease activity below the resting rate from the same canal. These paired labyrinths (one in each ear) behave in a "push-pull" fashion. The CNS compares the inputs coming from both ears. When the inputs are equal, the system is balanced, with no sense of movement. When inputs are asymmetrical, the CNS interprets this finding as a head rotation and as a result generates compensatory eye movements and postural adjustments, all of which lead to a conscious sensation relative to the perceived movement of the head.

Of great importance, the CNS is capable of rebalancing itself—that is, compensating after an injury to the peripheral receptor. This compensation is thought to occur as a result of the organism's ability to compare other sensory, visual, and kinesthetic inputs to vestibular input and, when the inaccuracy of the latter has been recognized, to readjust the central response. As a consequence, the point of balance is reset. CNS compensation in an otherwise healthy person results in near-normal clinical recovery even if complete unilateral vestibular loss has occurred. However, compensation takes time, on the order of days.

Abrupt vestibular imbalance created by a labyrinthectomy leads to severe vertigo, nausea, and ataxia that gradually resolve over ensuing days. On the other hand, a slowly progressive lesion of the vestibular system, such as occurs with acoustic neuromas, rarely causes vertigo. Although vestibular function is destroyed, because the damage has been incurred gradually, ongoing central adaptation masks the developing asymmetry between the ears.

As opposed to acute unilateral peripheral vestibular loss, bilateral vestibular loss, exemplified in the patient who has suffered ototoxicity, results in permanent clinical disability. Because peripheral vestibular input is lacking, the CNS is unable to make the required adjustments to head movements. If the loss is simultaneous and symmetrical, no significant vertigo results. The patient complains of worsened balance, especially in the dark. Fixed objects appear to jump with any head movement (oscillopsia). The symptoms are due to a now inefficient vestibulo-ocular and vestibulospinal system. An important point is that so long as vestibular input is symmetrical, vertigo symptoms will not arise even in the case of complete absence of any vestibular activity.

Clinical Relevance

The lifetime prevalence of vestibular vertigo is 7.4%.[1] In 80% of affected persons, vertigo resulted in a medical consultation, interruption of daily activities, or sick leave. Of patients who present to emergency departments with falls of unknown cause, 80% have vestibular impairment, and 40% complain of vertigo.[2] Thus, peripheral vestibular disorders constitute a significant medical problem. The most important clinical feature in the diagnosis of peripheral vestibular dysfunction is its pattern of presentation or history.

Vertigo is the illusion of motion, either of self (subjective) or of the environment (objective). Although the thorough neuro-otologic examination is beyond the scope of this chapter, a minimum vertigo history should address the following: (1) the duration of the individual attack (e.g., hours vs. days); (2) frequency (e.g., daily versus monthly); (3) the effect of head movements (e.g., worse, better, or no effect); (4) specific position–induced (e.g., rolling onto the right side in bed); (5) associated aural symptoms (e.g., hearing loss and tinnitus); (6) concomitant ear disease (e.g., otorrhea, previous surgery, trauma).

One of the most important features of the pattern of presentation of peripheral vestibular disorders is the duration of vertigo. Based on this parameter, the following classification of peripheral vestibular disease can be used:

1. Vertigo lasting seconds (benign paroxysmal positional vertigo)

2. Vertigo lasting minutes to hours
   a. Meniere's disease
   b. Migraine-associated vertigo (covered in Chapter 166)
   c. Otic syphilis
   d. Cogan's disease

3. Vertigo lasting days to weeks (vestibular neuritis)

4. Vertigo of variable duration
   a. Inner ear fistula
   b. Labyrinthine concussion
   c. Blast trauma
   d. Barotrauma
   e. Familial vestibulopathy
   f. Superior semicircular canal dehiscence syndrome
   g. Bilateral vestibular hypofunction

Historical Background

Before the 1860s, dizziness and balance problems were thought to be exclusively central disorders, often referred to collectively as "cerebral congestion" or lumped in with epilepsy. As early as the 1820s, post-rotation nystagmus was observed in mental patients after rotation in cages as a means to subdue them. Jan E. Purkinje hypothesized that this effect was central in origin. Vertigo symptoms during this period often were treated with leaching, purging, and cupping. Around this time emerged the first hints that equilibrium may have a peripheral component. Pierre Flourens noticed that pigeons would fly in circles in the same orientation as an ablated semicircular canal.[3]

The existence of peripheral vestibular disorders was proposed by Prosper Meniere in 1861.[4] Meniere was the director of a large deaf-mute institution in Paris who probably saw patients in whom both vertigo and hearing loss developed immediately after trauma to the ear, allowing him to conclude that both symptoms have a common inner ear origin.[5] To support his conclusion he presented the results of an autopsy of a young girl in whom sudden hearing loss and acute vertigo developed after such injury. On autopsy, her brain was found to be normal but the inner ear was filled with blood. It is ironic that this patient probably had leukemia, and not endolymphatic hydrops. Because of this finding, it was commonly believed well into the 20th century that Meniere's disease was caused by hemorrhage. Before 1940, "Meniere's disease" was used as a generic term for any peripheral vertigo, especially if it involved hearing loss. The first insight into the true pathophysiology of Meniere's disease came a decade after his initial report, with Knapp's hypothesis that inner ear hydrops was similar to ocular glaucoma.[6]

Early treatments of peripheral vertigo focused on destruction of the end organ. In 1904 the techniques of both eighth cranial nerve section[7] and labyrinthectomy[8,9] were described. The concept of drainage of the endolymph was first reported by Portmann in 1926.[10] Dandy also proposed selective vestibular nerve sectioning using a suboccipital approach during the 1930s, by which he treated more than 600 patients.[11] In this early period these procedures carried a high risk of deafness and facial nerve paralysis, as well as significant mortality rates. It was not until 1938, after examination of nerve section specimens taken from two patients who died in the perioperative period, that Hallpike and Cairns were able to report dilatation of the endolymphatic system in patients with Meniere's disease. This finding was hypothesized to reflect a disruption of the resorptive mechanism.[12] This pathologic feature also was independently observed by Yamakawa.[13]

Treatment of Meniere's disease that focuses on reversing endolymphatic hydrops has continued to evolve through the present day, with several variations on the Portmann shunt being proposed, such as transmastoid decompression,[14] subarachnoid drainage,[15] and cochleosacculotomy.[16] All of these procedures have had incomplete success in treating vertigo symptoms and carry a risk of hearing loss. A randomized controlled trial has suggested that these procedures have an efficacy similar to that for the placebo effect of surgery,[17] although a more recent analysis of these data has suggested that endolymphatic shunts may have a real effect.[18] Accordingly, these procedures continue to evolve and be performed.

BPPV is the most common cause of peripheral vertigo. BPPV was first described by Bárány in 1921, and he attributed the disorder to otolith disease.[19] After Bárány's initial description, scattered contradictory and confusing reports of BPPV appeared in the literature.[20] The clinical diagnosis of this disorder was not well defined until Dix and Hallpike described the classic positioning which causes a characteristic nystagmus in 1952.[21] Like Bárány, however, they believed it was due primarily to otolith disease. It was noted that the disease could be cured by a chemical labyrinthectomy[22] and eighth nerve section.[23] Schuknecht observed granular deposits on the cupula of the posterior semicircular canal in temporal bone specimens and proposed the "cupulolithiasis" theory to explain the pathophysiology.[24] This theory provides a basis for understanding the disorder, although more recent work has shown that the disorder is more commonly due to free-floating particles in the semicircular canal ("canalithiasis"), rather than cupulolithiasis. Gacek proposed transection of only the posterior ampullary nerve for relief of BPPV, confirming the posterior canal origin.[25] In most patients, however, the Epley canalith repositioning maneuver is adequate treatment,[26] and no surgery is required.

The most recently described etiologic disorder with peripheral vertigo is superior canal dehiscence.[27] Affected patients often exhibit a

Tullio phenomenon (nystagmus with loud noise) or *Hennebert's sign* (eye movements caused by pressure on the external auditory canal). This dehiscence acts as a third window into the middle cranial fossa, which can be plugged using a middle cranial fossa approach[28] or a transmastoid approach.[29]

Tremendous progress has been made in understanding the causes of peripheral vertigo and developing treatments. However, even today, vertigo is a symptom whose cause often cannot definitely be attributed to a known single disease process. Further developments in our understanding will no doubt occur and will modify the medical and surgical treatments of peripheral vestibular disorders.

Benign Paroxysmal Positional Vertigo

The most common peripheral vestibular disorder generally is agreed to be BPPV. The hallmark of the disease is brief spells (lasting seconds) of often severe vertigo that are experienced after specific movements of the head. The head movements that most commonly cause symptoms are rolling over in bed and extreme posterior extension of the head as if looking under a sink. Current understanding of this disease has evolved such that specific therapies based on accepted theories have been developed and proved successful in controlling symptoms.

The disorder initially was described in 1921 by Bárány.[19] He recognized several of the cardinal manifestations of BPPV, including vertical and torsional components of the nystagmus, the brief duration of the nystagmus, and the fatigability of the nystagmus and vertigo. Bárány did not, however, correlate the onset of the nystagmus with the positioning maneuver. He erroneously concluded that an abnormality in the encoding of head position by the otoliths was responsible for the symptoms and signs that he had noted. In 1952, Dix and Hallpike[21] reported this entity in a large group of patients. They described their now well-known maneuver for eliciting the classic pattern of nystagmus and its associated symptoms. They recognized the important features of the nystagmus occurring in BPPV, including its latency, directional characteristics, brief duration despite maintaining the offending head position, reversibility upon returning the patient to a seated position, and fatigability from repeated testing. They correctly identified the offending labyrinth but incorrectly concluded that BPPV results from an otolithic disturbance.

Schuknecht[30] reviewed the previous studies of BPPV, including the temporal bone histology of several patients who had experienced the disorder. He noted extensive utricular destruction in these patients and damage to other structures supplied by the anterior vestibular artery. This observation and the failure of electrical stimulation of the utriculus or sacculus to produce discrete patterns of nystagmus in laboratory animals led Schuknecht to conclude that abnormal stimulation of the otoliths was not responsible for the disorder. He suggested that the posterior canal crista was the probable source of the dysfunction. According to Schuknecht, BPPV was caused by loose otoconia from the utricle that, in certain positions, displaced the cupula of the posterior canal. Deposition of otoconia on the cupula of the posterior canal, known as "cupulolithiasis," was later proposed by Schuknecht as the mechanism of BPPV.[24] However, this mechanism poorly explained the brief duration of the nystagmus and the reversal of the nystagmus on return to a sitting position.

The suggestion that the mechanism of BPPV could result from deflection of the posterior canal cupula by the movement of debris in the posterior canal was revisited by Hall and colleagues.[31] These investigators suggested that the nonfatigable form was due to fixed deposits on the cupula, whereas the fatigable form was attributed to the motion of free-floating material within the lumen of the posterior semicircular canal. In most cases, BPPV-associated nystagmus is most commonly due to motion of material in the lumen of the posterior canal.

This latter theory is consistent with the five typical features of posterior canal BPPV: (1) The canalithiasis mechanism explains the latency of nystagmus as a result of the time needed for motion of the material within the posterior canal to be initiated by gravity. (2) The nystagmus duration is correlated with the length of time required for the dense material to reach the lowest part of the canal. (3) The vertical (up-beating) and torsional (top of the eyes beating toward the lowermost ear) components of the nystagmus are consistent with eye movements evoked by stimulation of the posterior canal nerve in experimental animals. (4) The reversal of nystagmus when the patient returns to the sitting upright position is due to retrograde movement of material in the lumen of the posterior canal back toward the ampulla, with resulting ampullopetal deflection of the cupula. (5) The fatigability of the nystagmus evoked by repeated Dix-Hallpike positional testing is explained by dispersion of material within the canal.

Incidence

BPPV is the most common cause of vertigo in patients seen by the otolaryngologist, accounting for 20% to 40% of cases of peripheral vestibular disease[32]—making it almost twice as frequent as Meniere's disease. The incidence is difficult to estimate because of the benign, typically self-limited course of the disease. It is thought to range from 10.7 per 100,000 to 17.3 per 100,000 population in Japan[33] and has been reported as 64 per 100,000 in a population study from Minnesota.[34]

The mean age at onset is in the fourth and fifth decades, but BPPV also may occur in childhood.[35] In a study of pediatric patients with BPPV, an association with migraine was suggested, leading to the hypothesis that migraine-induced ischemia may be responsible for the release of otoconia in some cases.[36] Overall, the incidence increases with age,[37] and BPPV is twice as common in women.[35]

Diagnosis

History

The patient with BPPV experiences severe vertigo associated with change in head position. The most frequently cited occurrence of this symptom follows rolling over or getting into bed and assuming a supine position. Frequently a specific side is identified as being associated with symptom onset (e.g., "the dizziness comes when I roll over to my right side but not to the left"). Patients also will experience similar symptoms on arising from a bending position, looking up to take an object off a shelf, tilting the head back to shave, positioning the head in the hairdresser's chair, or turning rapidly.

Symptoms occur suddenly and last on the order of seconds but never in excess of a minute.[35] The subjective impression of attack reported by the patient frequently is longer.

Episodes of vertigo frequently are clustered in time and separated by remissions lasting months or more. The patient also may report that periods of active disease may be associated with constant feelings of lightheadedness, worsened by head movement.[38] These chronic balance problems may be worse on awakening.

In most cases of BPPV, no specific etiologic disorder can be identified. In a large survey by Baloh and colleagues, no cause was identified in 48% of cases.[35] The most common known cause was closed head injury, followed by vestibular neuritis. In our experience, BPPV will eventually develop in nearly 15% of patients suffering from vestibular neuritis. Other cited predisposing events include infections and certain surgical procedures, including stapedectomy[35] and insertion of a cochlear implant.[39] Prolonged bed rest and Meniere's disease also are predisposing factors.

Findings on Examination

The diagnosis of BPPV is made by observing the classic eye movements in association with the Dix-Hallpike maneuver, combined with a suggestive history. The *Dix-Hallpike maneuver* is carried out as follows (Fig. 165-1). The patient is positioned supine on an examination table with the head extending over the edge. The patient is lowered with the head supported and turned 45 degrees to one side. The eyes are carefully observed. If no abnormal eye movements are seen, the patient is returned to the upright position. The maneuver is repeated with the head turned in the opposite direction and finally with the head extended supine.[40]

The pattern of response consists of the following: (1) The nystagmus is a combined vertical up-beating and rotary (torsional) component beating toward the downward eye (the superior poles of the eyes beat toward the downward ear). Pure vertical nystagmus is not BPPV.[35] (2) A latency of onset of nystagmus (seconds) is common. (3) Duration

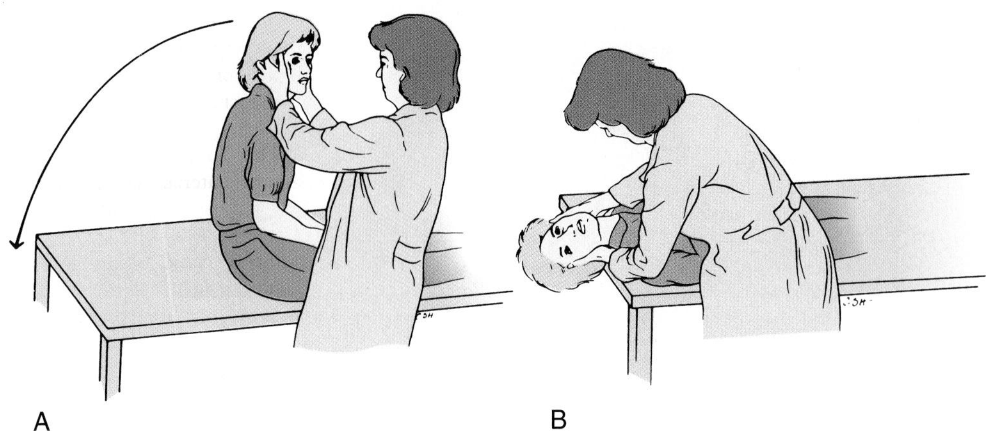

Figure 165-1. Right Dix-Hallpike maneuver for eliciting nystagmus and vertigo due to posterior canal benign paroxysmal positional vertigo (BPPV). The patient's head is first turned 45 degrees to the right (**A**). The patient's neck and shoulders are then brought into the supine position with the neck extended below the level of the examination table (**B**). The patient is observed for nystagmus and assessed for symptoms of vertigo. The patient is next returned to the upright position. *(From Herdman SJ, ed.* Vestibular Rehabilitation. *Philadelphia: F.A. Davis; 1994. Used with permission.)*

of nystagmus is short (less than 1 minute). (4) Vertiginous symptoms are invariably associated. (5) The nystagmus disappears with repeated testing (i.e., it is fatigable). (6) Symptoms often recur with the nystagmus in the opposite direction on return of the head to the upright position.[38]

Canalithiasis of the posterior semicircular canal is the most frequent cause of BPPV. Posterior canal BPPV rarely may be bilateral.[41] If the head is not positioned correctly during testing (i.e., not positioned with the head in the plane of the posterior canal during testing of the unaffected side), debris on the affected side may come to rest against the cupula, simulating an excitatory nystagmus from the unaffected ear.[42] The lateral semicircular canal has been identified as the affected structure in approximately 12% of cases, with a significant fraction of these being induced by the repositioning maneuver for posterior canal BPPV.[43] Lateral canal BPPV can be detected by a variation of the Dix-Hallpike maneuver: The patient is first brought to the supine position with the head resting on (not hyperextended below) the examining table. The head is then turned rapidly to the right so that the patient's right ear rests on the table. Eye movements are monitored with Frenzel lenses for 30 seconds. The patient is then returned to the supine position (looking upward) and the head is turned rapidly to the left so that the left ear rests on the table. Eye movements are again monitored.

The nystagmus with lateral canal BPPV is horizontal and may beat toward (geotropic) or away from (ageotropic) the downward ear. It often begins with a shorter latency, increases in magnitude while maintaining the test position, and is less susceptible to fatigue with repetitive testing than the vertical torsional nystagmus of posterior canal BPPV. The increased amplitude and duration of the horizontal nystagmus may reflect action of the central velocity storage mechanisms (which perseverate signals from the vestibular periphery, especially those arising from the lateral canal). Cupulolithiasis, arising either independently or in combination with canalithiasis, is more likely to be involved in the etiology of lateral canal BPPV than is the case for posterior canal BPPV. Cupulolithiasis can be differentiated from canalithiasis by minimal or absent latency to the onset of nystagmus. Cupulolithiaisis also can persist for minutes or even as long as the patient remains in the provocative position.[44] If the nystagmus is geotropic, the particles are likely to be in the long arm of the lateral canal relatively far from the ampulla. If the nystagmus is ageotropic, the particles may be in the long arm relatively close to the ampulla or on the opposite side of the cupula, either floating within the endolymph or embedded in the cupula.

The superior semicircular canal is affected in only 2% of cases of BPPV.[45] The nystagmus expected in cases of superior canal BPPV would be downbeat and torsional. Such a nystagmus can be elicited by standard Dix-Hallpike positioning testing. The right posterior canal lies in roughly the same plane as that of the left superior canal, and vice versa. Placement of the head into the right Dix-Hallpike position will therefore bring the left superior and right posterior canals into the plane of gravity. A nystagmus resulting from the left superior canal BPPV would, in this position, be expected to be downbeat, with a torsional component directed such that the superior part of each eye beats toward the upward ear. Note that this nystagmus is opposite in vertical and torsional direction from that resulting from right posterior canal BPPV.

Test Results

The bedside Dix-Hallpike test[21] combined with an appropriate history is key to making the diagnosis. Standard electro-oculography (EOG) and the many videonystagmography devices do not record the torsional eye movements associated with BPPV. The eye movement tracings obtained with these standard devices used for clinical testing reflect solely the associated vertical and horizontal components of the eye movements. The observation of these patterns may be facilitated by the use of Frenzel lenses.

Treatment with Repositioning

First-line therapy for BPPV is organized around repositioning maneuvers that, in cases of canalithiasis, use gravity to move canalith debris out of the affected semicircular canal and into the vestibule. For posterior canal BPPV, the maneuver developed by Epley[26] is particularly effective (Fig. 165-2). The maneuver begins with placement of the head into the Dix-Hallpike position, to evoke vertigo. The posterior canal on the affected side is in the earth-vertical plane with the head in this position. After the initial nystagmus subsides, a 180-degree roll of the head (in two 90-degree increments, stopping in each position until any nystagmus resolves) to the position in which the offending ear is up (i.e., the nose is pointed at a 45-degree angle toward the ground in this position) is performed. The patient is then brought to the sitting upright position. The maneuver is likely to be successful when nystagmus of the same direction continues to be elicited in each of the new positions (as the debris continues to move away from the cupula). The maneuver is repeated until no nystagmus is elicited. In our experience, when administered in this way, the Epley maneuver is effective in more than 90% of cases in eliminating BPPV. Medications are not usually given, but a low dose of meclizine or a benzodiazepine 1 hour before may be appropriate if the patient is unusually anxious or susceptible to nausea and vomiting with vestibular stimulation.

The Semont maneuver also is effective for posterior canal BPPV[46] but is more difficult to perform and is less effective than the simpler, more comfortable Epley maneuver.[47] The patient is moved quickly into the position that provokes the vertigo and remains in that position for 4 minutes. The patient is then turned rapidly to the opposite side, ear down, and remains in this second position before slowly sitting up.

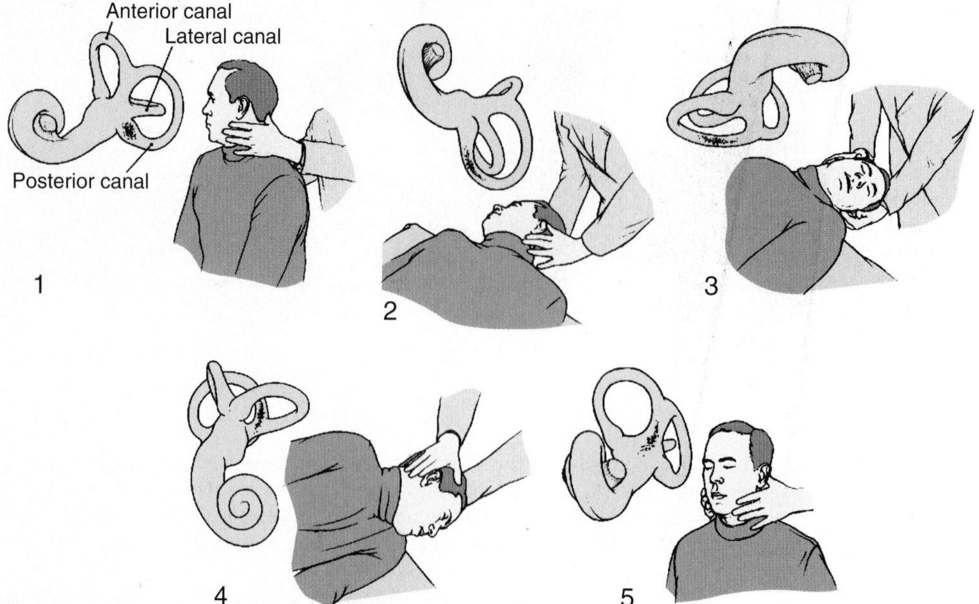

Figure 165-2. Canalith repositioning maneuver for treatment of benign paroxysmal positional vertigo (BPPV) affecting the posterior canal of the right ear. **1,** The patient's head is turned to the right at the beginning of the canalith repositioning maneuver. The *inset* shows the location of the debris near the ampulla of the posterior canal. The diagram of the head in each inset shows the orientation from which the labyrinth is viewed. **2,** The patient is brought into the supine position with the head extended below the level of the gurney. The debris falls toward the common crus as the head is moved backward. **3,** The head is moved approximately 180 degrees to the left while keeping the neck extended with the head below the level of the gurney. Debris enters the common crus as the head is turned toward the contralateral side. **4,** The patient's head is further rotated to the left by rolling onto the left side until the patient is face down. Debris begins to enter the vestibule. **5,** The patient is brought back to the upright position. Debris collects in the vestibule. *(Illustration by David Rini. From Hullar TE, Minor LB: Vestibular physiology and disorders of the labyrinth. In: Glasscock ME, Gulya AJ, eds.* Surgery of the Ear. *5th ed. Hamilton, Ontario: B.C. Decker; 2003.)*

For both Epley and Semont maneuvers, gravity is the stimulus that moves the particles within the canal, so turning the head on the body is unnecessary. En bloc movement of the head and body to the extent possible is the preferred treatment pattern. Some physicians also use a small handheld vibrator over the mastoid and claim slightly better results, although the results do not seem significantly different.[48] Mastoid vibration should be avoided in patients who have had retinal detachment or who may be susceptible to such a detachment because of high myopia. Some investigators recommend having the patient sleep with the head elevated for 1 to 2 days after the maneuver, but this has not been shown to have a significant effect.[49]

The following observations support the effectiveness of these maneuvers for treatment of posterior canal BPPV: (1) Patients who have been symptomatic for years can be cured; (2) BPPV involving one canal can convert to BPPV involving another canal as a result of treatment; (3) patients in whom the wrong side was treated and post-treatment instructions were given show no improvement; and (4) randomized trials have shown the effectiveness of the treatment maneuvers. Because BPPV commonly resolves in a few weeks to a month, a repositioning maneuver may seem to be no better than placebo in an unselected group of patients with BPPV in whom spontaneous recovery is common. In more intractable cases, however, the treatment will almost certainly be determined to be effective.

Treatment maneuvers also have been suggested for the lateral canal variant of BPPV. In cases that involve geotropic nystagmus, lying on one side with the affected ear up for 12 hours has been reported to be effective in the vast majority of cases.[50]

Treatment maneuvers for superior canal BPPV should follow the same principles. The head initially should be moved into a dependent position wherein the ampulla is superior, then rotated by 180 degrees, and then brought back to its initial position. Data on treatment of superior canal BPPV have not been reported, no doubt owing to its relative rarity.[51]

Some events that can occur during repositioning maneuvers are worthy of discussion. Posterior canal BPPV can be converted to lateral canal BPPV during the Epley maneuver. The lateral canal BPPV usually resolves in several days. Posterior canal BPPV can occasionally be converted into a presumed anterior canal BPPV (i.e., symptoms worsen when the offending ear is up). An obstruction of canalith material may occur at the common crus during the Epley maneuver, resulting in a sustained pure torsional nystagmus (both the superior and posterior canals are excited simultaneously, so the opposing vertical components cancel and the torsional components add).

Surgical Treatment

The vast majority of patients with BPPV will be cured by respositioning maneuvers, but surgical therapy remains an option for the rare patient with disabling persistent disease.

Singular neurectomy to treat refractory BPPV was proposed by Gacek.[25] During the three decades since it was described, the procedure has been performed at least 342 times, of which 252 were by Gacek himself.[52] Although the procedure generally is effective, it is technically difficult and the risk of hearing loss from the procedure may be as high as 41%.[53]

Posterior semicircular canal occlusion was introduced as a treatment for BPPV in 1990.[54] This technique blocks the canal lumen so that it becomes unresponsive to angular acceleration. At total of 97 cases have been reported in the literature. Although the procedure was associated with brief postoperative vertigo, 94 of the 97 patients were cured of their BPPV.[55] The procedure is associated with a postoperative hearing loss that usually recovers over several weeks.

Vestibular Neuritis

Vestibular neuritis typically manifests with dramatic, sudden onset of vertigo and attendant vegetative symptoms.[56] Typically, the dizziness lasts for days, with gradual, definite improvement throughout the course. Balance-related complaints, particularly caused by or related to rapid head movements, may be present for months after resolution of the acute disease. Paroxysmal positional vertigo occurs subsequently in a small percentage of patients.[57,58] Vestibular neuritis has been known to recur, with some patients reporting similar, usually less intense attacks for years.[58] Bilateral disease has been described and must be considered in the differential diagnosis for bilateral vestibular loss. Vestibular neuritis is not associated with subjective change in hearing or with any focal neurologic complaints.[21] Although historically the terms *vestibular neuritis* and *labyrinthitis* were used interchangeably, *vestibular neuritis* is now considered the more accurate term for cases that do not involve hearing loss. The term *epidemic vertigo* has also been used historically and is synonymous with vestibular neuritis; the term reflects the observation that the vertigo often is preceded by upper respiratory infection.[58]

Subjectively, hearing remains normal. When sudden sensorineural hearing loss accompanies vertigo with a vestibular neuritis–like pattern, classification as a sudden sensorineural hearing loss should be considered. In such cases, treatment appropriate for sudden sensorineural hearing loss should be instituted and the evaluation should include evaluation for a retrocochlear lesion, such as acoustic neuroma.

A documented caloric response reduction or positive head thrust test in the direction of the involved side can be used to identify the side of involvement.[56] Head thrust testing in the canal plane may have the advantage of localizing the pathology to the inferior or superior vestibular nerve.[59] However, inferior vestibular nerve involvement is unusual, so VEMP testing is rarely useful.[60] Lateralization also has been reported with use of magnetic resonance imaging (MRI) with gadolinium enhancement.[61]

Histopathologic studies of temporal bones from patients believed to have experienced this clinical entity reveals vestibular nerve degeneration with sparing of the peripheral receptor structure.[58] Human pathologic studies also have demonstrated signs of more chronic inflammation in the rare case manifesting a more chronic or recurrent course of disease. A postinfectious syndrome has been suggested in these cases. Opinion holds that the superior vestibular nerve is more commonly involved in this disease than the inferior. It is postulated that this predilection may be secondary to the longer and narrower bony canal traversed by the superior nerve, making it more susceptible to compressive swelling.[62] It also is possible that isolated inferior vestibular nerve neuritis is not diagnosed owing to normal horizontal head thrust and caloric testing.[63]

The cause of the degeneration is not established. Infection with one of the neurotropic viruses, such as herpesvirus, is thought to be responsible. *Borellia* infection also has been noted in some instances. In most cases, the responsible virus is never identified.

Treatment has historically been supportive and symptomatic for vertigo and related vegetative symptoms. Recently, methylprednisolone and valacyclovir have been investigated as possible therapeutic agents in a placebo-controlled, double-blind study.[64] Patients given methylprednisolone experienced significantly more improvement after 1 year. Valacyclovir was not shown to have any affect. As in all acute peripheral vestibular losses, early ambulation is encouraged.

Meniere's Disease

Meniere's disease (idiopathic endolymphatic hydrops) is a disorder of the inner ear associated with a symptoms consisting of spontaneous, episodic attacks of vertigo; sensorineural hearing loss which usually fluctuates; tinnitus; and often a sensation of aural fullness. Despite this well-known symptom complex, Meniere's disease remains a controversial and often difficult condition to diagnose and treat. This is in part due to the dramatic variability that is the hallmark of this disease. This discussion concentrates on current thought concerning Meniere's disease as well as indicates some of these underlying controversies.

History

Prosper Meniere first described the symptom complex in 1861 and proposed the pathologic site to be in the labyrinth. It was Meniere along with Flourens who recognized that vertiginous symptoms could originate in the inner ear. However, hemorrhage into the inner ear, which Meniere himself believed to be the pathophysiology, has proved to be erroneous. Knapp advanced the hypothesis that hydrops was similar to ocular glaucoma,[6] although this was not histologically demonstrated until 1938.[12,13] Before that time, "Meniere's disease" was used as a generic term for any peripheral vertigo. Understanding of Meniere's disease has advanced considerably since these initial descriptions, yet the cause of the underlying hydrops remains elusive and controversial despite seventy years of active research.

Incidence

Wide variation exists in the published rates for incidence of Meniere's disease. These range from 17 per 100,000 in the Japanese population[65] to a high of 513 per 100,000 in the population of southern Finland,[66] with several studies reporting intermediate values. Some of the variation may be explained by the diagnostic criteria used and by access to health care in a population. The disease seems to be more prevalent among whites,[67] with a male-to-female ratio of approximately 1. The peak age at onset is in the fourth and fifth decades of life, although presentation can be at almost any age.

The frequency of bilateral disease is unclear, and the incidence in published reports is from 2% to 78%.[68] The rate depends on the duration of follow-up and the diagnostic criteria. The studies at the extreme ends of this range were from before 1980, when standardized diagnostic criteria were not in use. The true incidence probably is in the range of 19% to 24%.[67,68] Symptoms of bilateral disease may appear many years or decades after onset of the unilateral symptoms.[69]

Familial occurrence of Meniere's disease has been reported in 10% to 20% of cases.[70] An autosomal dominant mode of inheritance has been suggested,[71] although the mode of inheritance can be variable. Migraine is strongly associated with Meniere's disease in familial cases.[72] The incidence is elevated in persons with specific major histocompatability complexes (MHCs). Human leukocyte antigens (HLA) B8/DR3 and Cw7 have been associated with Meniere's disease.[73,74] The etiology of the disease in persons with these HLAs may be autoimmune.[75]

Pathogenesis

Meniere's disease is characterized by recurring attacks of vertigo, sensorineural hearing loss, tinnitus, and, in some affected persons, a fluctuating sense of fullness in the ear. Acute attacks are superimposed on a gradual deterioration in sensorineural hearing in the involved ear, typically in the low frequencies initially. Over time, a reduction in responsiveness of the involved peripheral vestibular system occurs.

The pathologic basis thought to underscore these findings is a distortion of the membranous labyrinth. The hallmark of this distortion is endolymphatic hydrops.[12] This condition reflects the changes in the anatomy of the membranous labyrinth as a consequence of the overaccumulation of endolymph. Such changes occur at the expense of the perilymphatic space (Fig. 165-3).

Traditional thought has held that endolymph, which is produced by the stria vascularis in the cochlea and by the dark cells in the vestibular labyrinth, circulates in both a radial and a longitudinal fashion.[76] In the case of hydrops, the underlying pathophysiology is controversial, but inadequate absorption of endolymph by the endolymphatic sac is the prevalent theory.[77] The endolymphatic duct may act as a valve to regulate endolymph homeostasis.[78] Temporal bone histologic equivalents of hydrops have been produced in animals as a consequence of disruption of the endolymphatic sac, thereby supporting the above theory of pathogenesis.[79]

Histopathologic studies of the human sac in the hydrops patient remain controversial. Some investigators have reported perisaccular fibrosis[80] and decreased endolymphatic duct size.[81] However, the underlying cause of these histologic findings is not certain.

Imaging studies in patients with Meniere's disease also identify abnormalities of the endolymphatic drainage system. Such studies suggest hypoplasia of the endolymphatic sac and duct, reflected in the decreased visualization of the vestibular aqueduct and reduction in periaqueductal pneumatization on computed tomography (CT) imaging.[82] Persons with Meniere's disease have significantly smaller and shorter endolymph drainage systems, as measured by the distance between the posterior semicircular canal and the posterior fossa on magnetic resonance images.[83] These anatomic variations are apparent by the age of 3 years and may predispose affected persons to later development of Meniere's disease. Enhancement of the endolymphatic sac[84] (Fig. 165-4) and perilymphatic space[85] has been demonstrated on MRI after gadolinium enhancement. However, significant individual variation has been observed, so imaging studies are neither diagnostic or predictive for Meniere's disease. The main role of imaging in the diagnosis of Meniere's disease is to exclude other possible causes of dizziness and unilateral hearing loss, such as a vestibular schwannoma.

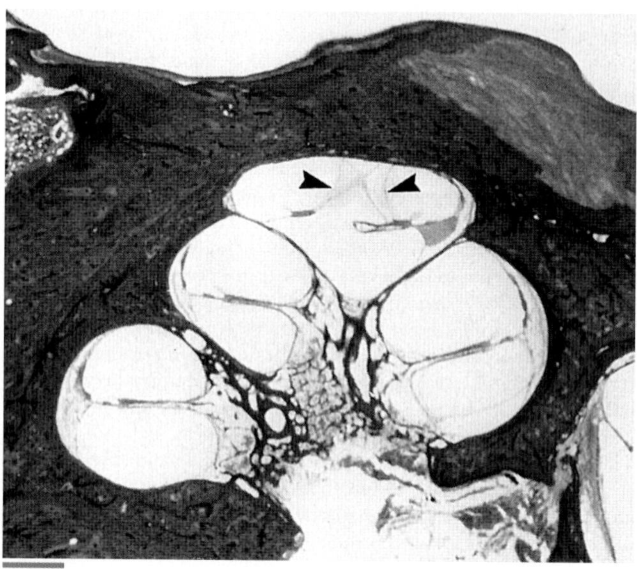

Figure 165-3. Photomicrograph of a cross section of human cochlea demonstrating endolymphatic hydrops in a patient with Meniere's disease. Note the distention of Reissner's membrane into the scala tympani in the apical turn of the cochlea *(arrowheads)*. *(Courtesy of Drs. J. Rutka and M. Hawke, University of Toronto.)*

Endolymphatic hydrops has been uniformly observed in the temporal bones from persons with Meniere's disease. However not all patients found to have hydrops, had a history of Meniere's disease.[86,87] Hydrops also is a postmortem finding after labyrinthitis, otitis media, head trauma, mumps, and meningitis. Asymptomatic hydrops also has been described.[88]

Ruptures in the membranous labyrinth of the patient with Meniere's disease are thought to be significant to the pathophysiology of the disorder. Membranous ruptures have been found in nearly all parts of the inner ear. Healed scars, presumably after rupture, also have been identified.[89,90] Their presence has supported one of the more prominent theories of the pathogenesis of Meniere's disease. Schuknecht postulated that ruptures in the membranous labyrinth allow leakage of the potassium-rich endolymph into the perilymph, bathing the eighth cranial nerve and lateral sides of the hair cells.[91] High concentrations of extracellular potassium depolarize the nerve cells, causing their acute inactivation. The result is a decrease in auditory and vestibular neuronal outflow consistent with the hearing loss and features of acute vestibular paralysis seen in a typical Meniere's attack. Healing of the membranes is presumed to allow restitution of the normal chemical milieu, with termination of the attack and improvement in vestibular and auditory function. The chronic deterioration in inner ear function presumably is the effect of repeated exposure to the effects of the potassium. This theory remains somewhat controversial, because some investigators have suggested that these ruptures rarely occur and do not adequately explain the observed symptoms.[92]

Etiology

The triad of hearing loss, tinnitus, and vertigo constitutes Meniere's syndrome. If the cause is unknown, it is defined as Meniere's disease.[93] However, if a disease entity that is known to cause endolymphatic hydrops is associated with the syndrome, the diagnosis is one of secondary endolymphatic hydrops (i.e., otosclerotic foci causing mechanical endolymphatic blockage[94]). Obstruction of the endolymphatic duct is the basis for development of hydrops in experimental animals. This is accomplished by any lesion that can produce failure of duct function, including mechanical blockage, chemical fibrosis, viral inoculation, immunologically induced inflammation, and ischemia.[95] However, these animal models cannot be interpreted to explain the actual cause of the human disease. These models also do not completely reproduce the clinical and pathologic entity experienced by humans.

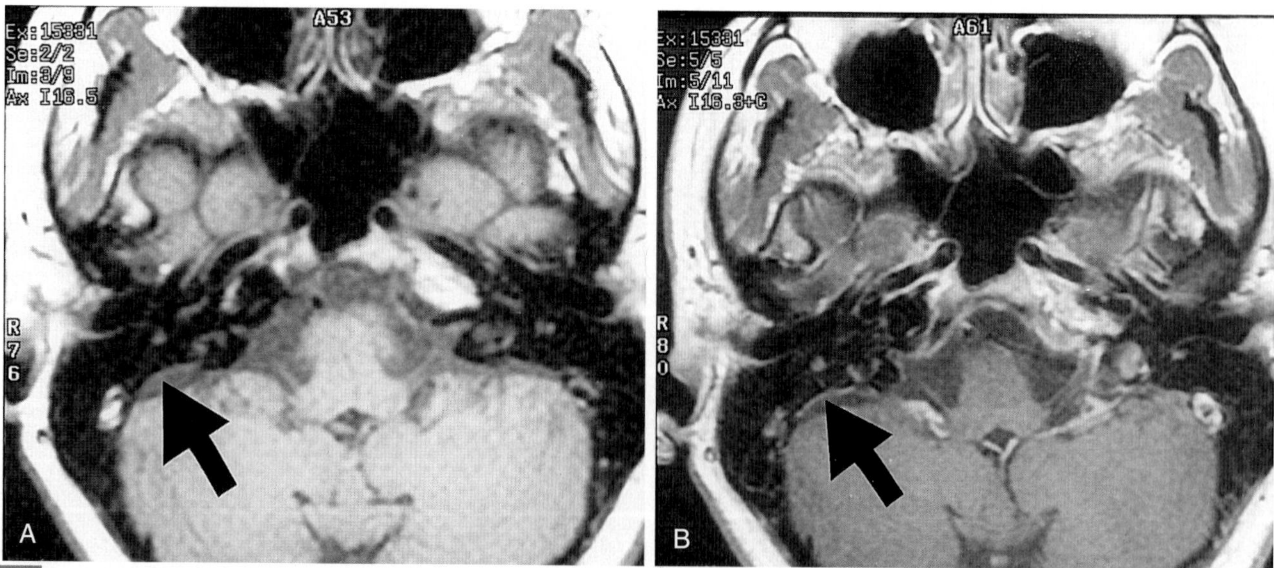

Figure 165-4. Magnetic resonance imaging for evaluating Meniere's disease. **A,** Nonenhanced axial T1-weighted image of right petrous bone demonstrating the nonenhancing endolymphatic sac *(arrow)* in a patient with Meniere's disease. **B,** Post-gadolinium T1-weighted image from the same patient. Note enhancement of the endolymphatic sac. *(Courtesy of Dr. D. Fitzgerald, Washington, DC.)*

Antibodies directed against normal inner ear elements have been suggested. Patients with Meniere's disease have an increased incidence of specific types of human leukocyte antigens.[70,96] However, most autoimmune processes, including those that affect the ear, such as Cogan's syndrome, have histopathologic findings including infiltration of white blood cells and cellular destruction. If an autoimmune mechanism is responsible, it would have to have a more indolent course or be intermittent and absent at the time of tissue sampling.

Viral infection also has been a suggested pathomechanism for Meniere's disease.[89] The observed occurrence of symptomatic hydrops many years after unexplained deafness, so-called delayed endolymphatic hydrops, suggests that subclinical viral infection could cause hydrops many decades later.[97] However, no virus has been conclusively identified, and comparison of patients with Meniere's disease with control subjects has demonstrated no difference in response to herpes simplex virus.[98]

Ischemia of the endolymphatic sac or inner ear has also been proposed as a underlying mechanism of Meniere's disease.[99] Such a common vascular mechanism may link migraine and Meniere's disease.[72,100,101]

Numerous factors have been implicated as causative for Meniere's disease. Although this lack of specificity in part reflects the current lack of understanding, it also suggests that Meniere's disease may be multifactorial or may represent the common end point of a variety of injuries or anatomic variables. A number of processes seem to be associated with the development of hydrops (e.g., trauma, acute otitis media, labyrinthitis, congenital inner ear deformity, idiopathic processes), but these are not always associated with the development of symptoms.[86] It is possible that Meniere's disease is precipitated by a variety of events such as autoimmune, viral, traumatic, or vascular or ischemic and may even be the result of congenital anatomic and molecular variations that may act as triggers for the later development of symptomatic hydrops (see Chapters 149 and 153).

Diagnosis

No single test is available to make the diagnosis of Meniere's disease. Rather, the most important aspect of the diagnostic process is a complete history, including a detailed description of the pattern of disease presentation, supported by quantitative testing. The most recent definition of the disease has been established by the Committee on Hearing and Equilibrium of the American Academy of Otolaryngology–Head and Neck Surgery (AAO-HNS) and is summarized in Table 165-1.[102]

Clinical Presentation

The typical history consists of recurring attacks of vertigo (96.2%) with tinnitus (91.1%) and ipsilateral hearing loss (87.7%).[103] Attacks often are preceded by an aura consisting of a sense of fullness in the ear, increasing tinnitus, and a decrease in hearing. The attacks may, however, be sudden in onset, with little or no warning. Acute attacks typically last from minutes to hours, most commonly 2 to 3 hours.[104] Attacks lasting longer than a day are unusual and if present should cast doubt on the diagnosis.

The classic presentation as just described is not always detailed by the patient. This is particularly true in the early phases of the disease. Often in retrospect, the disease seems to manifest with a predominance of either vestibular or auditory complaints.[105] In the series reported by Kitahara and associates, 50% of patients presented with vertigo and hearing loss together, 19% with vertigo only, and 26% with only deafness.[106] These variable initial presentations have led to the usage of the terms *cochlear* and *vestibular* Meniere's disease. These subtypes are not widely used, however, and are considered by the AAO-HNS Committee on Hearing and Equilibrium[102] to be an inappropriate application of the diagnosis.[106] Furthermore, no pathologic correlation for these subtypes has been found.[86] The terms *recurrent vestibulopathy* and *atypical Meniere's disease* have been used to describe the condition on persons with less than the classic triad of hearing loss, vertigo, and sensation of aural fullness or tinnitus.

The clinical course of Meniere's disease is highly variable. Patients often have a cluster of attacks separated by long remissions. Silverstein and coworkers[107] found that vertigo ceased spontaneously in 57% of patients in 2 years and in 71% after 8.3 years. Attacks often are clustered in time. Severity of symptoms ranges from minimal inconvenience to complete incapacitation; the AAO-HNS has provided staging guidelines[102] (Table 165-2). In addition to the incapacitating effects of the physical manifestations of Meniere's disease (vertigo, dysequilibrium, hearing loss, tinnitus, and pressure), the disease is emotionally disabling.[108]

Table 165-1

AAO-HNS Criteria for Meniere's Disease Diagnosis

Major Symptoms

Vertigo
- Recurrent, well-defined episodes of spinning or rotation
- Duration from 20 minutes to 24 hours.
- Nystagmus associated with attacks
- Nausea and vomiting during vertigo spells common
- No neurologic symptoms with vertigo

Deafness
- Hearing deficits fluctuate
- Sensorineural hearing loss
- Hearing loss progressive, usually unilateral

Tinnitus
- Variable, often low-pitched and louder during attacks
- Usually unilateral
- Subjective

Diagnosis

Possible Meniere's disease
- Episodic vertigo without hearing loss *or*
- Sensorineural hearing loss, fluctuating or fixed, with dysequilibrium, but without definite episodes
- Other causes excluded

Probable Meniere's disease
- One definitive episode of vertigo
- Hearing loss documented by audiogram at least once
- Tinnitus or sense of aural fullness in the presumed affected ear
- Other causes excluded

Definite Meniere's disease
- Two or more definitive spontaneous episodes of vertigo lasting at least 20 minutes
- Audiometrically documented hearing loss on at least one occasion
- Tinnitus or sense of aural fullness in the presumed affected ear
- Other causes excluded

Certain Meniere's disease
- Definite Meniere's disease, *plus* histopathologic confirmation

AAO-HNS, American Academy of Otolaryngology–Head and Neck Surgery.
From Committee on Hearing and Equilibrium guidelines for the diagnosis and evaluation of therapy in Meniere's disease. American Academy of Otolaryngology–Head and Neck Foundation, Inc. *Otolaryngol Head Neck Surg.* 1995;113:181.

History

Incapacitating, spinning vertigo, usually in the horizontal axis, is the most distressing complaint of the affected patient.[93] As is typical of peripheral vestibular dysfunction, the symptoms are exacerbated with any head movement. Accompanying symptoms and signs may include nausea, vomiting, diarrhea, and sweating. Between attacks, patients

Table 165-2

AAO-HNS Criteria for Meniere's Disease Severity

Vertigo

a. Any treatment should be evaluated after at least 24 months.
b. Formula to obtain numeric value for vertigo: ratio of average number of definitive spells per month after therapy divided by definitive spells per month before therapy (averaged over a 24-month period) × 100 = numeric value
c. Numeric value scale:

Numeric Value	Control Level	Class
0-40	Complete control of definitive spells	A
41-80	Limited control of definitive spells	B
81-120	Insignificant control of definitive spells	C
>120		D
Secondary treatment initiated		E

Disability

a. No disability
b. Mild disability: intermittent or continuous dizziness/unsteadiness that precludes working in a hazardous environment
c. Moderate disability: intermittent or continuous dizziness that results in a sedentary occupation
d. Severe disability: symptoms so severe as to exclude gainful employment

Hearing

a. Hearing is measured using a four-frequency pure-tone average (PTA) of 500 Hz, 1 kHz, 2 kHz, and 3 kHz.
b. Pretreatment hearing level: worst hearing level during 6 months before surgery
c. Post-treatment hearing level: poorest hearing level measured 18-24 months after institution of therapy
d. Hearing classification:
   i. Unchanged: ≤10-dB PTA improvement or worsening or ≤15% speech discrimination improvement or worsening
   ii. Improved: >10-dB PTA improvement or >15% discrimination improvement
   iii. Worse: >10-dB PTA worsening or >15% discrimination worsening

In 1996, the Committee on Hearing and Equilibrium reaffirmed and clarified the guidelines, adding initial staging and reporting guidelines:

Initial Hearing Level

Stage	Four-Tone Average (dB)
1	≤25
2	26-40
3	41-70
4	>70

Functional Level Scale

Regarding my current state of overall function, not just during attacks:

1. My dizziness has no effect on my activities at all.
2. When I am dizzy, I have to stop for a while, but it soon passes and I can resume my activities. I continue to work, drive, and engage in any activity I choose without restriction. I have not changed any plans or activities to accommodate my dizziness.
3. When I am dizzy I have to stop what I am doing for a while, but it does pass and I can resume activities. I continue to work, drive, and engage in most activities I choose, but I have had to change some plans and make some allowance for my dizziness.
4. I am able to work, drive, travel, and take care of a family or engage in most activities, but I must exert a great deal of effort to do so. I must constantly make adjustments in my activities and budget my energies. I am barely making it.
5. I am unable to work, drive, or take care of a family. I am unable to do most of the active things that I used to do. Even essential activities must be limited. I am disabled.
6. I have been disabled for 1 year or longer and/or I receive compensation because of my dizziness or balance problem.

AAO-HNS, American Academy of Otolaryngology–Head and Neck Surgery.
From Committee on Hearing and Equilibrium guidelines for the diagnosis and evaluation of therapy in Meniere's disease. American Academy of Otolaryngology–Head and Neck Foundation, Inc. *Otolaryngol Head Neck Surg.* 1995;113:181.

may be entirely asymptomatic or may describe periods of dysequilibrium, lightheadedness, and tilt.

Sudden unexplained falls without loss of consciousness or associated vertigo occasionally are described. Tumarkin[109] attributed these events to acute utriculosaccular dysfunction—so-called otolithic crises of Tumarkin, or drop attacks. It is thought that an abrupt change in otolithic input generates an erroneous vertical gravity reference. This in turn generates an inappropriate postural adjustment by way of the vestibulospinal pathway, resulting in a sudden fall.[110,111] Attacks are so sudden that injury can occur. The patient often describes a feeling of being pushed or "the world moving." The spells are brief with little associated vertigo. Drop attacks have been reported in 2% to 6% of persons with Meniere's disease. They tend to occur in clusters and then spontaneously remit.

Lermoyez described an unusual clinical presentation in which tinnitus and hearing loss precede and worsen with the onset of vertigo. When the vertiginous episode occurs, the tinnitus and hearing loss dramatically resolve. The temporal bone studies in a patient with such attacks noted hydrops and membrane ruptures isolated to the basal turns of the cochlea and the saccule.[112]

Acute Meniere's attacks are rarely observed by physicians. Horizontal nystagmus is the cardinal finding, but the direction varies over the course of the attack, so it is not useful in determining the involved ear.

Hearing Loss and Tinnitus

The sensorineural hearing loss in Meniere's disease typically is fluctuating and progressive. It often occurs coincident with the sensation of fullness or pressure in the ear. A pattern of low-frequency fluctuating loss and a coincident nonchanging, high-frequency loss is described, resulting in a "peaked" or "tent-like" tracing on the audiogram. This peak classically occurs at 2 kHz. Over time, the hearing loss normalizes across frequencies and becomes less variable.[105] In only 1% to 2% of patients does the hearing loss progress to profound deafness.

Additional features include diplacusis, a difference in the perception of pitch between the ears (43.6%) and recruitment (56%).[93]

Tinnitus tends to be nonpulsatile and variously described as whistling or roaring. It may be continuous or intermittent. Tinnitus often begins, gets louder, or changes pitch as an attack approaches. Frequently a period of improvement follows the attack.

Investigations

Electronystagmography

Electrooculographic recordings of eye movements after caloric and rotational stimulation are a commonly available and reliable method of assessing vestibular function. The caloric test often can localize the involved ear. A significant caloric response reduction is found in 48% to 73.5% of patients with Meniere's disease.[113] Complete absence of caloric response is reported in 6% to 11% of patients.

Head Thrust Testing

The head thrust test popularized by Halmagyi is very sensitive for detection of unilateral vestibular dysfunction.[114] However, in Meniere's disease, the asymmetry is subtle and present in only 29% of the patients.[115]

Electrocochleography

The summating potential (SP), as recorded by electrocochleography in patients with Meniere's disease, is larger and more negative. This is thought to reflect the distention of the basilar membrane into the scala tympani, causing an increase in the normal asymmetry of its vibration. The most commonly used value is the ratio of amplitudes of the SP and the eighth cranial nerve action potential (AP), the SP/AP ratio. This is based on the observed variability in the amplitude of the SP, considering variables such as recording technique and electrode placement. The SP/AP ratio has been used to reduce the intertest variability, resulting in a more linear response. The SP becomes relatively larger in hydrops; accordingly, the SP/AP ratio increases.[116] It is not a definitive test, because ratios are elevated in 62% of patients with Meniere's disease and in 21% of control subjects. Because of the difficulty in obtaining reproducible recordings and the variability of the wave amplitudes noted with patient age, hearing loss, and stage of disease, as well as the availability of reliable, less invasive diagnostic methods, electrocochleography is now infrequently used for this purpose.[117,118]

Dehydrating Agents

The assumption that an increase in endolymph volume, with its effect on labyrinthine membrane behavior, produces, in part, the hearing loss and vestibular deficit in Meniere's disease has led to the administration of dehydrating agents (e.g., urea, glycerol, furosemide). The goal is to reduce the volume abnormalities in the inner ear and produce a measurable change in response. Improvement has been measured with audiometrics, reduction in SP negativity (as recorded with electrocochleography), or a change in the gain of the vestibulo-ocular response to rotational stimulation. The reported sensitivity and specificity rates for the test vary widely. Klockhoff reports a 60% sensitivity in cases of known Meniere's disease.[119] Psychological factors constitute a significant source of variability, leading some authorities to question the usefulness of the test.[117,120]

Vestibular Evoked Myopotentials

VEMPs are generated by playing loud clicks in the ear, which move the stapes footplate and stimulate the saccule. This is the start of a disynaptic pathway that passes through the vestibular nuclei and then to synapses that relax the sternocleomastoid muscle. The saccule is the second most common site affected by hydrops, which has caused VEMPs to be investigated as a potential diagnostic tool. In the normal ear, the best response is near 500 Hz. Ears affected by Meniere's disease have elevated VEMP thresholds with flattened tuning.[121] The interaural amplitude difference in the response has been implicated as a staging tool for Meniere's disease.[122] Although these tests show differences between populations, they currently have limited diagnostic value owing to the large individual variation in responses.

Treatment

Therapy of Meniere's disease is aimed at the reduction of its associated symptoms. The optimal curative treatment should stop vertigo, abolish tinnitus, and reverse hearing loss. Unfortunately, long-term hearing impairment does not seem amenable to treatment.[108] Currently, almost all proven therapies are directed at relieving vertigo, which usually is the most distressing symptom.

Evaluating treatments for vertigo in patients with Meniere's disease has been made difficult by the natural history of the disease, which includes spontaneous improvement in 60% to 80% of cases, and because many treatments have a significant placebo effect.[96,123,124] This is further supported by the 71% reduction in symptoms by patients who refused surgery,[107] and placebo-controlled studies of endolymphatic sac surgery[17,125] and medical therapy.[126] The large variety of Meniere's disease treatments reflect the extreme variability in clinical response and the inherent difficulty in assessing effectiveness.

Dietary Modification and Diuretics

Salt restriction and diuresis may be the best initial therapy for Meniere's disease.[127,128] The goal of salt restriction and diuretics is to reduce endolymph volume by fluid removal or reduced production. Despite the popularity of these treatments, neither salt restriction[129] nor use of diuretics[130,131] has had its efficacy confirmed by double-blind, placebo-controlled studies. Carbonic anhydrase inhibitors such as acetazolamide were recommended on the basis of the localization of carbonic anhydrase to the dark cells and the stria vascularis. However, these agents have not proved to be clinically more effective than other diuretics.[132] Despite the lack of hard evidence of their efficacy, we feel that a low-salt diet and diuresis constitute an appropriate and effective treatment for Meniere's disease with a low risk of side effects.

Vasodilators

In the belief that Meniere's disease was the result of strial ischemia, vasodilating agents have been used. Betahistine, an oral preparation of histamine, is one such medication.[133] It has proved to be effective in treatment of Meniere's disease in a placebo-controlled study.[133,134] Such studies have flaws, however, which continues to raise doubts about the efficacy of betahistine over placebo.[135] The medication has become a popular treatment for Meniere's disease in Europe.[136] The drug is available through compounding pharmacies in the United States but often is not covered by insurance and is infrequently prescribed.

Symptomatic Treatment

Antivertiginous medications, antiemetics, sedatives, antidepressants, and psychiatric treatment have been reported to be beneficial in reducing the severity of the vertigo and vegetative symptoms and in improving tolerance of Meniere's symptoms.[137]

Local Overpressure Therapy

A relatively recent approach to decrease hydrops is by pulsing pressure in the middle ear. As long ago as 40 years, overpressure in the middle ear was reported to decrease Meniere's symptoms during acute vertigo attacks.[138] The mechanism of vertigo reduction is unclear, although it may facilitate endolymph absorption.[139]

Since 2000, the Meniett device has been approved for use by the U.S. Food and Drug Administration (FDA). This device is a handheld air pressure generator that the patient self-administers. The pressure is delivered in complex pulses of up to 20 cm of water, over a 5 minute period. The device requires a ventilation tube to be placed in the tympanic membrane before initiation of therapy. A randomized controlled trial demonstrated that patients using the Meniett device experienced a significant decrease in vertigo symptoms for the first 3 months of therapy but that findings afterward were similar to those with placebo.[140] The placebo device in these cases was an inactive device that did not administer pressure. Long-term treatment with the Meniett device has shown results similar to the natural course of Meniere's disease.[141]

Of note, simple placement of a ventilation tube with no additional therapy also has been reported to control vertigo symptoms in many patients with Meniere's disease.[142,143]

Intratympanic Injection

Intratympanic injection commonly is performed with either dexamethasone or gentamicin for control of vertigo symptoms. The term *chemical labyrinthectomy* often is applied to intratympanic gentamicin treatment, but it may not be an appropriate assessment of the effect of gentamicin on the labyrinth in titrated therapy. Instillation of aminoglycosides into the middle ear was described by Schuknecht in 1957 with streptomycin injection through a microcatheter placed through the tympanic membrane.[144] Control of vertigo was achieved in these patients, but severe hearing loss in the treated ear also occurred in most patients.

Gentamicin has a vestibulotoxicity that is high relative to its cochleotoxicity; accordingly, it can be used to control vestibular symptoms while sparing hearing. The gentamicin can be administered through either a tympanostomy tube or directly injected through the tympanic membrane. Peripheral vestibular deficits are evident on head thrust testing after even a single dose of gentamicin[145] (Fig. 165-5). The concentration of the medication used and frequency of injection vary by series. The risk of hearing loss also varies greatly by series, depending on the dose and frequency of treatment. Lange[146] reported elmination of vertigo in 90% of 92 patients, but the incidence of hearing loss and level of vestibular function were not specified. Beck and Schmit[147] sought to determine if complete ablation of vestibular function, as measured with ice water caloric response, was needed for vertigo control. They found that it was not, and that this end point led to severe to profound hearing loss in 58% of treated patients. Wu and Minor[148] found complete control of vertigo in 90%, with profound sensory neural hearing loss in only 3% of patients. Nedzelski and associates[149] found that control of vertigo was achieved in 83% of patients, with substantial control in the remaining subjects. A 10%

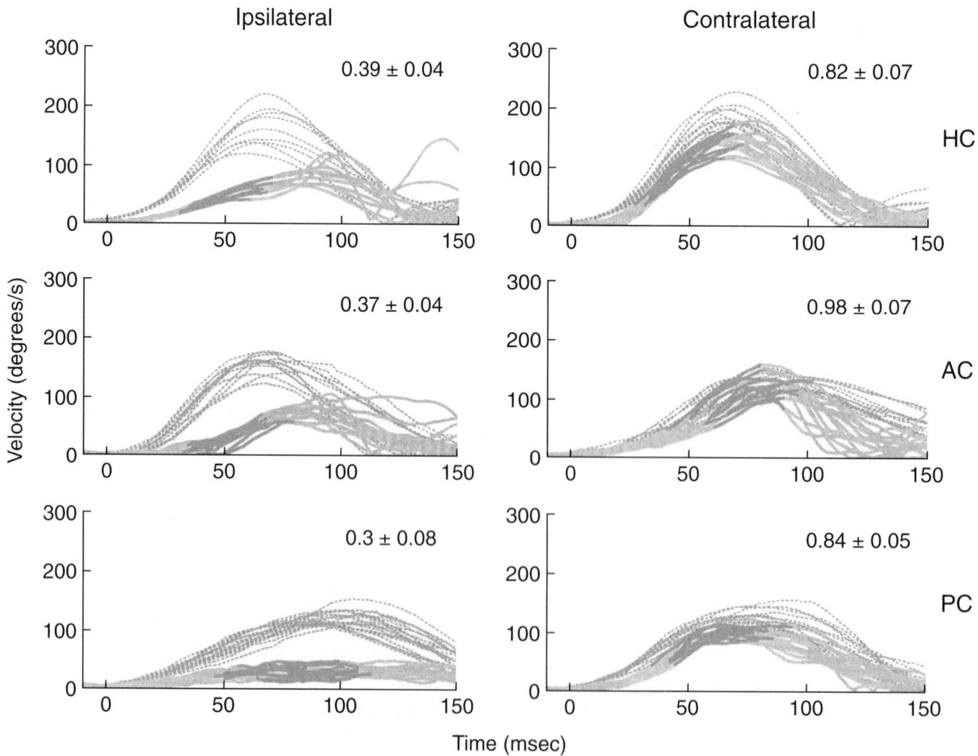

Figure 165-5. Response to head thrusts that excited each of the six semicircular canals in a typical subject measured 49 days after a single intratympanic injection of gentamicin in the right ear. AC, anterior canal; HC, horizontal canal; PC, posterior canal. *(Reproduced from Carey JP, Minor LB, Peng GC, et al. Changes in the three-dimensional angular vestibulo-ocular reflex following intratympanic gentamicin for Meniere's disease. J Assoc Res Otolaryngol. 2002;3:430.)*

incidence of profound hearing loss in the treated ear was noted. The current trend is away from multiple doses of gentamicin and toward a single-injection regimen, with additional doses only if needed to control symptoms (so-called titration therapy). The risk of hearing loss with gentamicin using many current protocols is similar to that with the natural history of Meniere's disease.[127,148]

Intratympanic injection of dexamethasone is considered by many experts to be a reasonable procedure to offer when vertigo is intractable but the patient still has some functional hearing. The mechanism for steroid effect on vertigo symptoms is not currently clear. Some evidence suggests that Meniere's disease has an autoimmune component, which the steroids may address. Several studies have reported a beneficial effect of intratympanic injection of dexamethasone in the control of vertigo from Meniere's disease,[150,151] although the effect on hearing loss and tinnitus is minimal. The risk of hearing loss or other complications from the steroid injection appears to be low. A small randomized trial has shown complete resolution of vertigo symptoms in 82% of patients receiving dexamethasone, compared with 57% receiving saline injection.[152] Dexamethasone injections may need to be repeated every 3 months to maintain the patient free of vertigo symptoms, although the optimal dosing frequency is variable and unknown. Concentrations used have varied from 2 to 24 mg/mL.

Endolymphatic Sac Surgery

Surgical decompression of the endolymph for Meniere's disease was first described by Portmann in 1926.[10] During the more than three fourths of a century during which this technique has been practiced, numerous variations on the concept have been devised. Despite significant investigation into techniques to decompress the endolymph, the etiology of endolymphatic hydrops as part of the pathophysiology of Meniere's disease is still an active area of controversy and debate. Several theories have been proposed: release of external compression on the sac, neovascularization of the perisaccular region, allowing passive diffusion of endolymph, and creation of an osmotic gradient out of the sac.[153]

Several variations of endolymphatic sac surgery have been described. Simple decompression, wide decompression that includes the sigmoid sinus,[154] cannulating the endolymphatic duct, endolymphatic drainage to the subarchnoid space, drainage to the mastoid, and removal of the extraosseous portion of the sac[155] all have been advocated. A variety of prostheses also have been proposed, ranging from simple Silastic sheets to tubes and one-way valves designed to allow flow selectively in either the mastoid or the subarachnoid direction.

In a double-blind, placebo-controlled study by Thomsen and coworkers, a mastoidectomy alone had the same efficacy as that of an endolymphatic shunt in a group of 30 patients, with 15 randomly selected for each operation.[17] The efficacy of the procedure remains controversial, with other workers re-examining the data of Thomsen and colleagues and claiming that a significant result would have been found if a different criterion for success had been used[156] or if different statistical methods were applied.[18]

Nerve Section

Several approaches to sectioning of the vestibular nerve have been described. The earliest approach was the retrosigmoid, with the first large series accumulated by Walter Dandy in the 1930s.[11] The terms *retrosigmoid* and *suboccipital* are now used interchangeably. The middle fossa approach to the internal auditory canal and superior vestibular nerve was developed by William House[157] and later modified to include sectioning of the inferior vestibular nerve.[158] A retrolabyrinthine approach has also been described.[159]

Vestibular nerve section achieves a complete vertigo control rate of approximately 85% to 95%, with 80% to 90% of patients maintaining their preoperative hearing after the procedure.[160-162] The procedure offers much greater vertigo control rates than those reported for endolymphatic shunt procedures but also is more invasive and technically challenging. Vestibular nerve section has been argued to carry a lower risk of hearing loss when compared with gentamicin injection,[161] although the risk of hearing loss with gentamicin seems to be most significant with high-dose protocols.

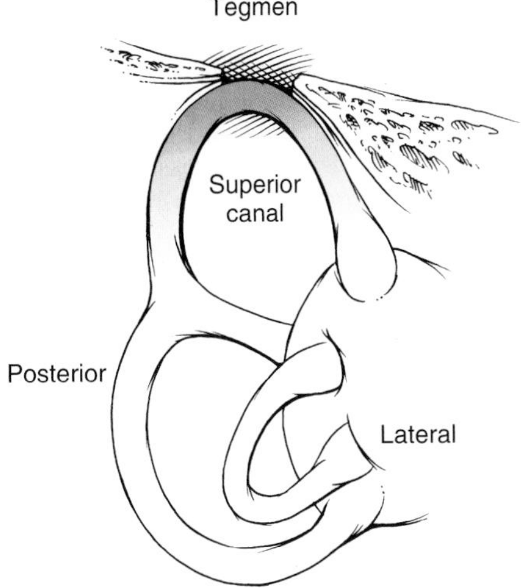

Figure 165-6. Superior canal dehiscence. *(© 2008 by Johns Hopkins University, Art as Applied to Medicine.)*

Labyrinthectomy

The most destructive procedure for treatment of Meniere's disease is labyrinthectomy, owing to the uniform destruction of hearing and vestibular function. Ideal candidates for the procedure are pateints who have no functional hearing and in whom more conservative treatments such as gentamicin injection have failed. Despite the associated morbidity, the procedure has a higher rate of vertigo control than that typical for vestibular neurectomy[163] and has been reported to improve quality of life in 98% of operated patients.[164] The procedure is most commonly performed through a transmastoid exposure but can be done using a transcanal approach.

Superior Canal Dehiscence Syndrome

Superior canal dehiscence syndrome (SCDS)[27] is the result of the absence of bone over the superior canal (Fig. 165-6). This bony dehiscence creates a third mobile window that allows the abnormal movement of endolymph during presentation of loud sounds (Tullio phenomenon[165]), tragal compression, nose-blowing, or other mechanisms for creation of a pressure gradient between the ear and middle fossa. Loud sound or increased pressure often causes nystagmus in the same plane as that of the superior canal on the affected side.[166] The nystagmus is a combination of vertical and torsional rotation aligning with the superior canal, as predicted by Ewald's first law.[167] When gaze shifts 45 degrees toward the side of the dehiscence, the pupil will move in a vertical direction. During gaze 45 degrees in the contralateral direction, the eye will rotate about an axis through the pupil. The Tullio phenomenon is not observed in all cases of SCDS. In addition to dizziness and nystagmus, SCDS may be characterized by autophony (sensation of increased loudness of the patient's own voice), conductive hearing loss that is not due to middle ear pathology, or pulsatile tinnitus.[168] High-resolution CT scans with reconstructions in the plane of the superior canal and orthogonal to that plane should be done to confirm the diagnosis.

The pathophysiology of superior canal dehiscence can be understood in terms of the effects of the dehiscence in creation of a third "mobile window" into the inner ear. Under normal circumstances, sound pressure enters the inner ear through the stapes footplate in the oval window and, after passing around the cochlea, exits through the round window. The presence of a dehiscence in the superior canal allows this canal to respond to sound and pressure stimuli. The direction of the evoked eye movements supports this mechanism. Loud sounds, positive pressure in the external auditory canal, and Valsalva maneuver against pinched nostrils cause ampullofugal deflection of the superior canal, which results in excitation of afferents innervating this canal. The evoked eye movements can include a nystagmus that has slow components directed upward with torsional motion of the superior pole of the eye away from the affected ear. Conversely, negative pressure in the external canal, Valsalva maneuver against a closed glottis, and jugular venous compression cause ampullopetal deflection of the superior canal, which results in inhibition of afferents innervating this canal. The evoked eye movements typically are in the plane of the superior canal but in the opposite direction (downward with torsional motion of the superior pole of the eye toward the affected ear) (Fig. 165-7).

The severity of a patient's symptoms and the impact of these symptoms on lifestyle are major determinants in the discussion of surgery for superior canal dehiscence.[168] Some patients are discovered to have SCDS as an incidental finding on CT scan and do not have symptoms. In other patients, only autophony or conductive hearing loss may be noted. A decision about surgical plugging of the superior canal to alleviate symptoms should be based on the impact of symptoms on a patient's lifestyle and a consideration of the risks of surgery.

Confirmation of dehiscence of bone overlying the superior canal in patients with the syndrome has been obtained with high-resolution CT scans of the temporal bones.[28,169-171] Conventional temporal bone CT scans are performed with 1.0-mm collimation, and images are displayed in the axial and coronal planes. These scans have a relatively low specificity (high number of false-positive results) in the identification of superior canal dehiscence because of the effects of partial volume averaging. The specificity and positive predictive value of these scans are improved when 0.5-mm-collimated helical CT scans are performed with re-formation of the images in the plane of the superior canal.[171] The scans also are reformatted radially around the canal in the plane perpendicular to the superior canal, so that the cross section of the canal can be evaluated (Fig. 165-8). Of note, even the best CT scan may be misleading, because very thin bone may be below the resolution of the scanner; accordingly, diagnosis should never be based on the CT scan alone.

CT studies have shown that the thickness of bone overlying the intact superior canal in a patient with unilateral dehiscence is significantly thinner than in patients without superior canal dehiscence.[172] This finding and observations from a review of 1000 histologically

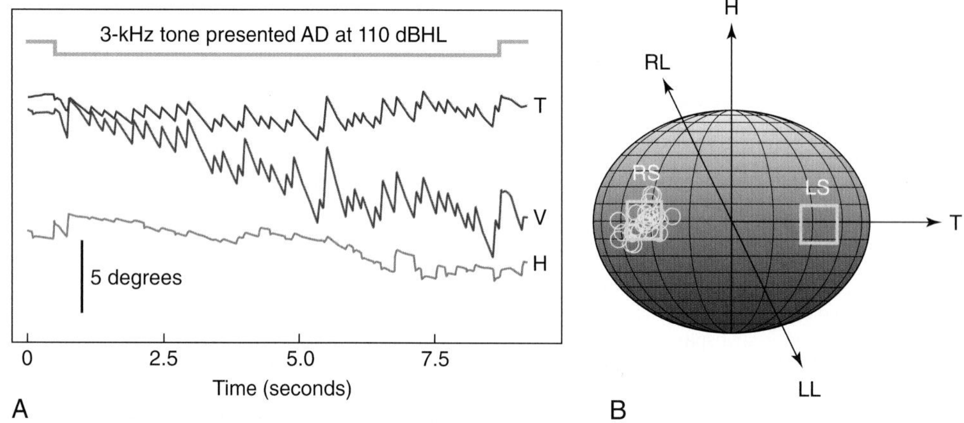

Figure 165-7. Ocular responses to sound in the superior canal dehiscence (SCD) syndrome. Nystagmus induced by a 3-kHz tone at an intensity of 100 dB in the right ear (AD [*auris dextra*]) of a 33-year-old woman with right SCD syndrome. **A,** Torsional (T), vertical (V), and horizontal (H) eye position recorded with the scleral search coil technique from the right eye. The time during which the tone was presented is indicated by the *yellow bar* at the top. Positive direction for horizontal is left, vertical is down, and torsional is clockwise (from the patient's perspective, so rotation of the superior pole of the patient's eye is to the patient's right). In response to the tone in her right ear, the patient developed a nystagmus with upward, counterclockwise slow phases consistent with excitation of the right superior canal. **B,** The axis of slow-phase eye velocity corresponded to the data plotted in **A.** The sphere represents the patient's head, as viewed from the right. The positive direction of the horizontal axis (H) travels upward from the top of the head, the torsional axis (T) straight ahead from the patient's nose, and the vertical axis (obscured by the sphere) from the patient's left ear. The anatomic axis of each of the right superior (RS), left superior (LS), right lateral (RL), and left lateral (LL) semicircular canals is shown. The box around the axis of each superior canal indicates the region (±2 SD) from the mean orientation of that axis. Each *light circle* represents the mean eye velocity axis for one slow phase of nystagmus. *(Reproduced with permission from Minor LB, Cremer PD, Carey JP, et al. Symptoms and signs in superior canal dehiscence syndrome.* Ann N Y Acad Sci. *2001;942:259-273.)*

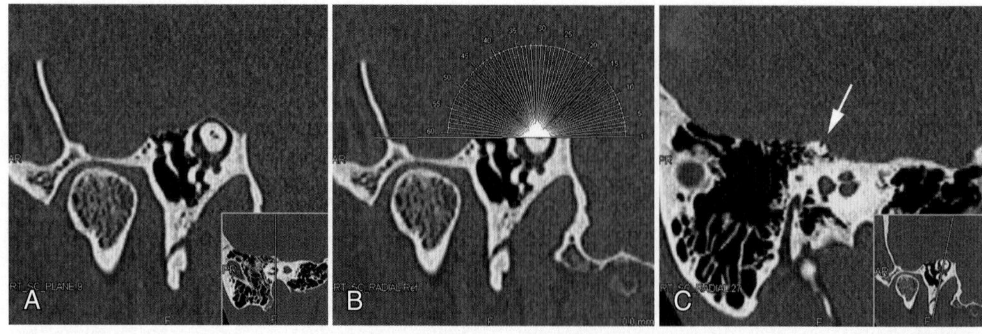

Figure 165-8. Computed tomography (CT) of the right superior semicircular canal demonstrating dehiscence. **A,** CT image is reconstructed in the plane of the torus of the right superior canal. **B,** The center of the superior canal is identified, and radial orthogonal reconstructions are performed at 3-degree intervals. **C,** The radial reconstructions are sequentially examined along the course of the superior canal, and dehiscence in the canal is identified if bone does not appear to completely cover the canal *(arrow)*. The *inset* at lower right in **A** and **C** shows the plane of section of this radial reconstruction relative to the superior canal plane.

processed temporal bones sectioned in a plane parallel to the petrous ridge[173] suggest an underlying developmental or congenital abnormality that leads to the development of the syndrome. The onset of symptoms and signs associated with this syndrome typically has been during adulthood. Patients in whom a normal thickness of bone fails to develop may then acquire the syndrome when the abnormally thin layer of bone is disrupted by trauma or is eroded over time as a consequence of the pressure from the overlying temporal lobe.

Vestibular evoked myogenic potentials (VEMP) responses have been useful in assessing for the presence of superior canal dehiscence syndrome.[174-176] In this test, short-latency relaxation potentials evoked by clicks or by tone bursts are recorded from surface EMG electrodes placed on the skin over the ipsilateral sternocleidomastoid muscle while that muscle is tonically contracted. These responses arise from the vestibular end organs, most likely the sacculus.[177,178] The threshold for eliciting the VEMP response is lower in an ear affected with superior canal dehiscence than in a normal ear.[174,176]

Some patients with the vestibular symptoms and signs indicative of superior canal dehiscence syndrome also have been noted to have auditory manifestations of the disorder. The Weber tuning fork test typically lateralizes to the affected ear, and patients also may hear a tuning fork placed on the lateral malleolus of the foot.[168,179] Patients may present with seemingly bizarre complaints, such as "hearing" their eye movements or their pulse. Bone conduction thresholds on audiometry can be below 0 dB normal hearing level (NHL). Therefore, an air-bone gap may be present even when air conduction thresholds are normal.[180] This conductive hearing loss may be caused by formation of a third window by the dehiscence, which causes a dissipation of acoustic energy transmitted through air conduction mechanisms. For some patients, autophony or a disturbing sound of their own voice can be the primary symptom.[181] The clinical manifestations of superior canal dehiscence include vestibular signs and symptoms in some patients, vestibular and auditory abnormalities in others, and exclusively auditory findings in others.

Patients who experience only mild effects of the symptoms and signs associated with superior canal dehiscence may not require any specific treatment other than avoidance of the stimuli that evoke these effects. Placement of a tympanostomy tube may be beneficial in some patients with principally pressure-induced symptoms. For patients who are debilitated by symptoms associated with the syndrome, surgical repair of the superior canal dehiscence by plugging the superior canal through a middle cranial fossa approach can be effective in alleviating or attenuating the vestibular signs and symptoms.[28,182]

Cogan's Syndrome

Cogan's syndrome was first described in 1945 and is characterized by interstitial keratitis, "low-frequency unilateral" hearing loss, and vestibular symptoms as well as nonreactive tests for syphilis.[183] The syndrome was later divided into typical and atypical forms on the basis of specific ocular findings.[184] The typical form includes interstitial keratitis, whereas the atypical form has ocular features of scleritis, episcleritis, papilledema, and retinal detachment.[185] Ten percent of patients with Cogan's syndrome have the atypical form. Multisystem involvement, including CNS manifestations and inflammatory vascular disease, is a feature of Cogan's disease. Of the two forms, systemic features are noted more commonly in atypical Cogan's disease. In the typical form, the heart and lungs are the usual site of systemic involvement, including aortitis, pleuritis, pericardial effusion, coronary arteritis, and myocardial infarction. In atypical Cogan's disease, systemic features arise from a systemic vasculitis (e.g., polyarteritis nodosa, arthritis, glomerulonephritis, gastrointestinal problems).

Ocular and inner ear changes appear concurrently or within 6 months of each other. Ocular complaints include photophobia, blurred vision, lacrimation, and pain. These symptoms and signs may be unilateral or bilateral. Onset usually is sudden, and resolution is gradual. Recurrences over years are not uncommon. Ocular pathologic changes include infiltration of the cornea with lymphocytes and plasma cells as well as corneal neovascularization.

Balance-related symptoms are similar to those of Meniere's disease and consist of sudden attacks of true vertigo with ataxia and vegetative symptoms. Progression to the complete absence of vestibular function, manifested by ataxia and oscillopsia, is common.

Hearing loss is sensorineural in type and is bilateral in 44% of patients.[186] The loss is progressive without spontaneous improvement, frequently becoming profound. In bilateral cases, hearing loss frequently begins on one side.

Cogan's syndrome is thought to be of autoimmune basis. This suspected etiology is based on lymphocyte transformation tests, migration inhibition to inner ear tissues, the association with rheumatologic diseases, and presence of lymphocytes and plasma cells in the ear and eye, as well as the clinical response to systemic steroids.

Clinically, patients often report having had an upper respiratory infection within 7 to 10 days of initial onset of Cogan's syndrome.[184] Raised IgG and IgM titers to *Chlamydia* are reported in association with active Cogan's syndrome. Furthermore, antibody titers are noted to decrease with remission of disease. For this reason, it has been suggested that an acute infection, perhaps with *Chlamydia*, promotes sensitization of the immune system to "self" and leads to immune-mediated disease.[184]

Systemic corticosteroids are the accepted treatment. An initial dose of 1 mg/kg per day of prednisone usually is recommended, followed by a slow taper. The probability of hearing improvement is thought to be better the sooner the steroids are started.[185] In addition, cyclophosphamide and methotrexate have been recommended by some authorities if systemic vasculitis is present.

Otosyphilis

Syphilis is a sexually transmitted disease that can become disseminated and affect almost any organ system. Although it is thought to be a rare condition in the modern era, the diagnosis is difficult to confirm, and many cases may be misdiagnosed as other conditions.[187] Thirty percent of patients suffering from congenital syphilis and 80% of symptomatic neurosyphilis patients experience significant hearing loss.[188]

Otologic involvement can be grouped into two categories: early syphilis, symptoms occurring within 2 years of exposure, and late otosyphilis, when the disease becomes symptomatic after 2 years. Vestibular symptoms are less frequent in early otosyphilis; they most commonly manifest as a sudden hearing loss. Late otosyphilis presents similar to Meniere's disease with episodes of vertigo combined with progressive hearing loss and tinnitus, which often is unilateral.[185,189] Late-stage otologic syphilis, whether acquired or congenital syphilis, can manifest up to 50 years or more after exposure. Systemic symptoms frequently overshadow the otologic ones and include signs of meningitis. In the case of early congenital syphilis, systemic involvement may prove to be fatal.

Interstitial keratitis is a feature of 90% of patients with late-onset otologic syphilis, whether congenital or acquired. The triad of sensorineural hearing loss, interstitial keratitis, and notched incisors—*Hutchinson's triad*—is an exclusive feature of late congenital syphilis.[188]

Hennebert's sign (nystagmus and vertigo produced by pressure change on the ear, thought to be due to deformation of a softened, gummatous otic capsule) and Tullio phenomenon (nystagmus and vertigo caused by loud noise), although often encountered in syphilis, are not pathognomonic for the disease and also are common findings in superior canal dehiscence.

The Venereal Disease Research Laboratory (VDRL) and the rapid plasma reagin (RPR) nontreponemal tests are easily performed and relatively inexpensive. Sensitivity varies with the stage of disease. In view of the fact that otologic symptoms occur in late-stage disease, nontreponemal tests detect only 70% of cases of otosyphilis.[190] These tests are useful in following therapeutic response, by change in titer and loss of reactivity. On the other hand, treponemal tests—such as free treponemal antigen absorption, FTA-ABS, and microhemagglutination *Treponema pallidum* [MHATP] assays, which detect the presence of the organism—are far more sensitive; these tests detect 95% or more of cases of late-stage disease. The FTA or MHATP and their variations are the tests of choice for the detection of otologic syphilis.[190] Lumbar puncture is not necessarily warranted because results are positive in only 5% of cases of otosyphilis.[185]

Treatment of otologic syphilis varies. Some investigators feel that in the early stages of the disease, treatment with antibiotics alone (i.e.,

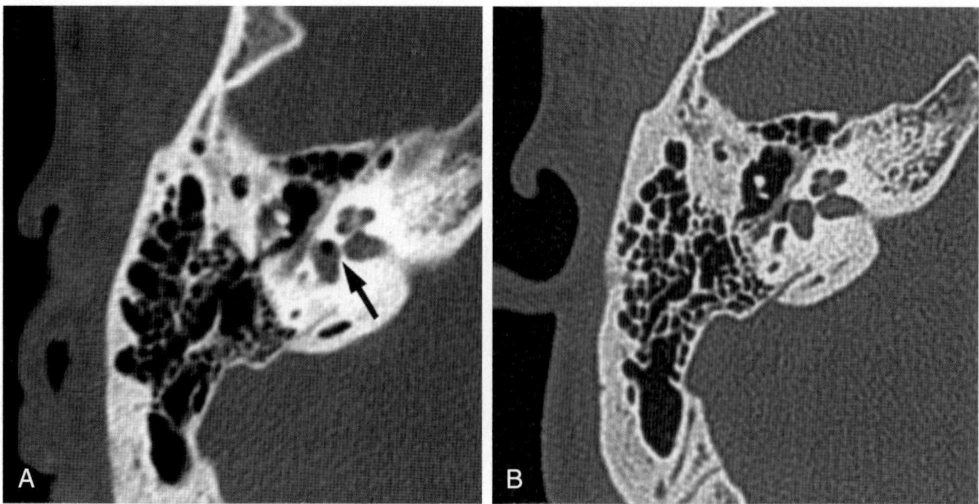

Figure 165-9. **A,** Axial CT scan of the temporal bone of a 15-year-old patient in whom pneumolabyrinth developed immediately after penetrating trauma to the left ear. This patient also presented with vertigo, a mixed hearing loss, nausea, and vomiting. The vestibular and auditory symptoms resolved with conservative management in the days after the injury, and no air was seen on a CT scan obtained 4 days later **(B)**. Within 5 months of the event, sensorineural hearing improved by 40 dB. *(Reproduced from Lao WW, Niparko JK. Assessment of changes in cochlear function with pneumolabyrinth after middle ear trauma.* Otol Neurotol. *2007;28:1013.)*

penicillin 2.4 million units IM) provides a cure, frequently resulting in hearing improvement.[188] Additional use of a 10-day course of steroids is advocated. Although consensus is lacking regarding exact drug treatment for late-stage disease, it generally is agreed that protracted therapy with both antibiotics and steroids is indicated. Difficulty in eradication of the infection, despite adequate antibiotic therapy, is ascribed to prolonged dividing time for the treponeme in late-stage disease. Antibiotic regimens of variable duration have been suggested. A recommended neurosyphilis treatment protocol consists of 1.8 million units of penicillin IM daily with 500 mg of oral probenicid four times daily for 3 weeks. It is suggested that otic syphilis and neurosyphilis are comparable with respect to response to treatment.[188] Prenisone (40 to 60 mg per day) is given for at least 2 weeks before tapering. Steroids are used in part to minimize the potential damage to the ear by the inflammatory response in the early treatment of syphilis. Improvement in hearing, particularly of speech discrimination, is noted in 35% to 50% of cases, along with resolution of vestibular symptoms.[188]

Perilymph Fistulas

Inner ear fistulas are abnormal communications between the labyrinth and surrounding structures. The labyrinth normally is covered by dense bone. Labyrinthine fistulas can be organized into three main categories: (1) leakage of perilymph from the inner ear to the middle ear, (2) disruption of the bony labyrinth by disease such as cholesteatoma, and (3) idiopathic bony dehiscence of the semicircular canals (i.e., superior semicircular canal dehiscence syndrome and posterior canal dehiscence). These disorders manifest with similar symptoms of hearing loss and episodic vertigo despite their differing etiology.[191] Idiopathic bony dehiscence of the semicircular canals creates problems of pressure transfer, as noted previously, but not fluid mixing.

The clinical presentation of inner ear fistula may range in severity from mild and inconsequential to severe and incapacitating. Sensorineural hearing losses vary from an isolated high-frequency loss to a low-frequency or flat one. Speech discrimination test results are not characteristic. Both the pure-tone threshold and speech discrimination scores have been noted to fluctuate. Isolated mild conductive losses have been noted.[192] Glasscock and colleagues, in a series of patients who had undergone surgical exploration for fistulas, were unable to identify differences in audiometric profile for patients with proven fistulas and those without.[193] Vestibular symptoms also are variable and may include episodic incapacitating vertigo (equivalent to a Meniere's disease attack), positional vertigo, motion intolerance, or occasional dysequilibrium. (Disequilibrium with increases in CSF pressure such as with nose blowing or lifting has been noted, as has Tullio's phenomenon (occurrence of vertigo during) exposure to loud noises).

Definitive leakage of perilymph from the inner ear to the middle ear can be caused by trauma[194] or may be noted after stapedectomy.[195] Spontaneous fistulas are rare except in cases of Mondini malformation and other congenital abnormalities.[196] CT may reveal pneumolabyrinth[194] (Fig. 165-9). In definitive cases of leakage, patching with a tissue graft can achieve the goal of hearing preservation and relief of vertigo, although even definitive cases can resolve with conservative management and without surgery.[194] However, many cases of vertigo or hearing loss alleged to be caused by perilymph fistula are much more ambiguous, with equivocal surgical findings.[197-199]

A fistula can be through fissula ante fenestram, or a fissure from the round window niche with the ampulla of the posterior canal may be seen. Fissures in these areas tend to be common, and their clinical significance is not clear.[200] It is difficult to ascertain whether small amounts of fluid seen during surgical exploration are truly perilymph. An assay for beta-2 transferrin (a protein unique to cerebrospinal fluid) has been suggested, but it has a low sensitivity for detection of small amounts of fluid.[201]

The absence of observed leakage during surgery has been interpreted to mean either that no fistula exists, that the fistula may be intermittent, or that the fistula may be present but too small to be detected. In cases of negative findings on exploration, it is unclear if patching of the oval and round windows is of any value. Criteria for determining when a middle ear exploration for perilymph fistula may be beneficial have been difficult to establish, because no definitive test is available to make the diagnosis and interobserver concordance is low.[202] Applying pressure in the external auditory canal to see if eye movements are evoked (Hennebert sign) has been used. Measuring postural sway during pressure to the external auditory canal also has been proposed as a diagnostic test for fistula.[202] Even if a fistula exists, spontaneous resolution may occur. Recently, many patients who initially were diagnosed with fistulas have been found to have superior canal dehiscence.[191]

Chronic ear disease can cause a bona fide fistula. Long-standing otitis media can lead to cholesteatoma formation, with consequent erosion of the dense bone around the labyrinth. Patients in whom fistulas develop usually have a multiyear history of chronic ear disease, sometimes requiring several operations. In a recent review of 375 surgical procedures done for chronic otitis media, labyrinthine fistulas were identified in 29 cases, 25 of which involved canal-wall-down mastoidectomies.[203] The overall incidence of fistulas after canal-wall-down mastoidectomies was 13%. All of these patients experienced vertigo symptoms. However, of the 19 tested, only 14 exhibited a Hennebert sign with positive pressure. The horizontal semicircular canal was the most common site of fistula formation (76%), followed by oval window and promontory. In these cases, surgical closure of the fistula is recommended.

Trauma

Vertigo and ataxia are common sequelae of head trauma. Vestibular-related complaints can arise from cervical trauma and CNS trauma, as well as peripheral vestibular damage. Only symptoms resulting from peripheral vestibular damage are considered here. Mechanisms by which damage can be inflicted include blunt concussive trauma, penetrating trauma, explosive blast, and barotrauma. Similar lesions can result with different mechanisms of injury. Hence, labyrinthine concussion can follow blunt trauma as well as barotraumas.

Nonpenetrating Trauma

Labyrinthine Concussion

Injuries of the labyrinth that do not result in violation of the otic capsule or the intralabyrinthine limiting membranes are classified as *labyrinthine concussion.*

Vestibular-related symptoms, although variable and not well characterized, generally are thought to include mild vertigo, imbalance, visual confusion, and vegetative symptoms (e.g., nausea and vomiting). These symptoms typically are short-lived and gradually subside over a period of days to weeks. Examination of the patient with active symptoms may demonstrate nystagmus directed toward the side of the lesion acutely (i.e., over hours), followed by more typical contralateral beating nystagmus. Past pointing and falling in the direction of the slow phase of nystagmus have been reported. Vestibular testing may demonstrate a reduction in the caloric response and abnormality of vestibulo-ocular reflex gain and phase after rotational testing.[204]

Benign positional vertigo also is a common sequel of blunt head trauma.[204] Diagnosis and management of this entity are discussed earlier in this chapter.

Hearing loss and tinnitus often are reported. When present, the most common pattern of hearing loss is similar to that of a noise-induced hearing loss, with a loss most apparent at 4 kHz.[205]

Both the vestibular and the auditory complaints usually are transient, with spontaneous resolution occurring over a matter of days to weeks.[204] However, symptoms also have been reported to persist and worsen over time.

Blast Trauma

Explosive blasts can produce pressure waves greater than 200 dB sound pressure level (SPL).[206] The ear, which exists to capture and amplify this energy, frequently is injured when exposed to such a noise. Blast trauma would include that incurred by such mechanisms as an open-handed slap to the ear, as well as actual explosions. Perforation of the tympanic membrane, ossicular disruption, or both may occur; however, inner ear damage is more likely when the conductive mechanism remains intact. Auditory loss is common and often recovers spontaneously but can be permanent.[207] Dizziness is present in 15% of patients.[208]

Penetrating Trauma

Acute vertigo and sensorineural hearing loss heralds inner ear damage. Nystagmus beats in the direction of the healthy ear owing to the acute loss on the affected side. Vegetative symptoms typically are present. Vertigo will gradually subside over the ensuing days to weeks. Hearing loss, when present, can range in severity from mild and transient to profound and permanent.

Barotrauma

Damage to the inner ear resulting from pressure changes is known as barotrauma. Historically thought to be a fairly rare problem, barotrauma is now believed to be a fairly frequent injury among divers. Inner ear dysfunction can be produced by rapidly changing air pressure, as in atmospheric barotrauma, by elevated or asymmetric middle ear pressure, as in alternobaric trauma, or by bubble formation within the labyrinth or its blood supply in the case of inner ear decompression sickness and isobaric gas counter diffusion sickness.

Alternobaric vertigo is most prominent in divers during ascent to the surface and in fliers during ascent of the aircraft. Both scenarios involve decreasing ambient pressure. Vertigo is relieved by equilibration of middle ear–ambient pressure differences, as well as by repressurization (i.e., by descending several meters in the case of divers). As many as 26% of divers and 10% to 17% of pilots have admitted to experiencing alternobaric-like vertigo.[209]

Susceptibility to alternobaric vertigo is thought to be a consequence of individual variations in the pressure required within the middle ear to force open the eustachian tube. Conditions that alter eustachian tube patency (e.g., mucosal turgescence) such as upper respiratory infection are known to contribute. The effects of alternobaric trauma on the inner ear are temporary. In most cases, vertigo, hearing loss, and tinnitus are described as resolving in 10 to 15 minutes. The occurrence of alternobaric trauma can be minimized by frequent equilibration of middle ear pressure during diving, the use of topical nasal decongestants before the dive, and the avoidance of diving during periods of increased upper respiratory obstruction (e.g., upper respiratory infection, sinusitis).[210]

Atmospheric barotrauma is caused by extremes of pressure or abrupt changes in middle ear pressure, which are capable of damaging middle ear and inner ear structures. Damage to the latter is reflected by auditory and vestibular dysfunction. As opposed to alternobaric trauma, barotraumatic injury frequently is long-lasting or permanent. Hearing loss and tinnitus are universal complaints, whereas vertigo tends to be less common (35%) and rarely is the primary complaint.[211] When present, vertigo resolves within a few weeks even without treatment. The hearing loss ranges in severity from a mild, high-frequency sensorineural type to complete deafness. Suggested treatment of inner ear barotrauma is similar to that recommended for perilymph fistula. Bed rest, head elevation, and close monitoring of hearing and balance-related symptoms are suggested. Symptoms usually resolve spontaneously in a matter of hours to days with conservative management.[212]

Inner ear decompression sickness (IEDS) has become more common as a consequence of the increased use of mixed gas, oxyhelium, for deep water diving. Although damage produced by these disorders is not restricted to the inner ear, it now represents the most common decompression injury experienced by persons diving to depths greater than 100 m.[213] In a recent series it was found to account for 33% of diving-related ear injuries.[214] In IEDS, vertigo is almost always the primary symptom, and hearing loss when present usually is unilateral and often manifests later, after the vertigo begins to resolve.[211] Otologic symptoms often are the sole feature of decompression sickness, particularly in cases in which oxyhelium is used. When the inner ear is affected, vestibular and auditory dysfunction often is permanent, particularly if treatment is delayed. One study claims that significant improvement is achieved only when hyperbaric oxygen therapy is started within 68 minutes.[215] In some reports, however, improvement has been obtained when hyperbaric oxygen was started 24 hours after the injury.[211]

Familial Vestibulopathy

The rare syndrome of familial vestibulopathy with autosomal dominant inheritance is characterized by sudden attacks of vertigo followed by chronic dysequilibrium. The vertigo typically lasts on the order of minutes, with several hours of subsequent dysequilibrium. These spells recur at variable intervals for many years. Some patients have reported that spells seemed to be triggered by stress. Patients also have described the gradual onset of chronic dysequilibrium and oscillopsia due to vestibular insufficiency.[216] Auditory symptoms including tinnitus are absent. It is notable that all affected persons also experience migraine headaches, although headache was not associated with the spells of vertigo. An autosomal dominant mode of inheritance was defined.

Findings on quantitative testing in these patients include imaging results that are normal except for bilateral vestibular responses on caloric testing and low gains with shortened time constants on rotary testing—all of which are consistent with damage to the peripheral vestibular system.

In all cases, spells of vertigo were successfully terminated with the administration of acetazolamide. The mechanism of action in this case is unknown; however, in a seemingly related condition, familial periodic vertigo and ataxia, the acetazolamide effect is presumed to be that of a reduction in acidity of the brain.

More recently, another familial syndrome associated with migraine headaches, essential tremor, and vertigo was identified.[217] In this syndrome, vertigo lasts minutes to hours. As in the familial vestibulopathy already described, headaches were unassociated with the spells of vertigo. Spells were triggered by stress, exercise, and lack of sleep. The long-term progressive vestibular deficit noted in the familial vestibulopathy syndrome was not noted in this latter disease. As in the former disease, acetazolamide was proved to be effective at curtailing spells of vertigo as well as the migraines. Although clustering of migraine and episodic vertigo occurs in many families, the search for a single gene remains elusive. It is likely that multiple genes and possible environmental factors are responsible.[218]

Migraine itself may contribute to permanent damage of the vestibular end organs. (Migraine-associated vertigo is discussed in Chapter 166). However, the disorder also may have a peripheral component in some patients. Caloric paresis in patients with migraine occurs at a rate of 15% to 35%.[218,219] Vasospasm and small artery infarction have been suggested as potential mechanisms.[220]

Bilateral Vestibular Hypofunction

Bilateral loss of vestibular function leads to oscillopsia with head movements, as well as to disturbances of gait of variable severity. Hypofunction most commonly is induced by the vestibulotoxic effects of aminoglycoside medications. In 1952, a physician published a classic description of the symptoms of vestibular hypofunction that developed 2.5 months into a course of intramuscular streptomycin injections to treat sepsis of his right knee.[221] He also described oscillopsia and dysequilibrium of sudden onset and worsening over 2 to 3 days. By then he had to stabilize his head on bars in order to read, because even his pulse induced enough head motion to produce oscillopsia. His balance improved as he learned how to use visual and somatosensory information to make up for his loss of vestibular function.

It is estimated that vestibular injury develops in up to 3% of patients who receive gentamicin.[222] The vestibulotoxicity usually is not detected until the patient leaves the hospital and does not correlate with peak or trough levels or with dosage levels.[223,224] A genetic predisposition to increased sensitivity for aminoglycoside toxicity has been identified as linked to mutation of a mitochondrial ribosomal protein.[225] Thus, aminoglycosides are not recommended when an alternative is practical. If gentamicin is used, bedside tests of vestibular function including assessment of dynamic visual acuity and the head thrust test should be performed daily, when feasible, so that the medication may be stopped at the first signs of vestibulotoxicity.[226]

Other causes of bilateral vestibular loss include degenerative diseases of the cerebellum, meningitis, systemic autoimmune diseases, trauma, and bilateral Meniere's disease. No underlying cause is identified in approximately 20% of cases.[227]

Enlarged Vestibular Aqueduct

The vestibular aqueduct is an aperture in the posterior ridge of the petrous bone that contains the endolymphatic duct and sac. Enlargement of this structure probably occurs as a result of dilation of the endolymphatic duct during embryogenesis.[228] Patients usually present with hearing loss that begins in early childhood and often progresses with minor head trauma. The onset of vestibular symptoms in these patients often is delayed until adulthood, with episodes of vertigo that last between 15 minutes and 3 hours.[229] Childhood vestibular symptoms also have been described.[230] On testing, patients have been found to have impaired vestibulo-ocular reflex function and decreased VEMP thresholds.[231] Diagnosis is based on the CT finding of a vestibular aqueduct width greater than 1.5 mm at the midpoint; in most patients, this is similar to the width of the horizontal semicircular canal (Fig. 165-10). Experience in treatment of vertigo associated with enlarged vestibular aqueduct has been limited, but symptomatic and supportive treatment is suggested.

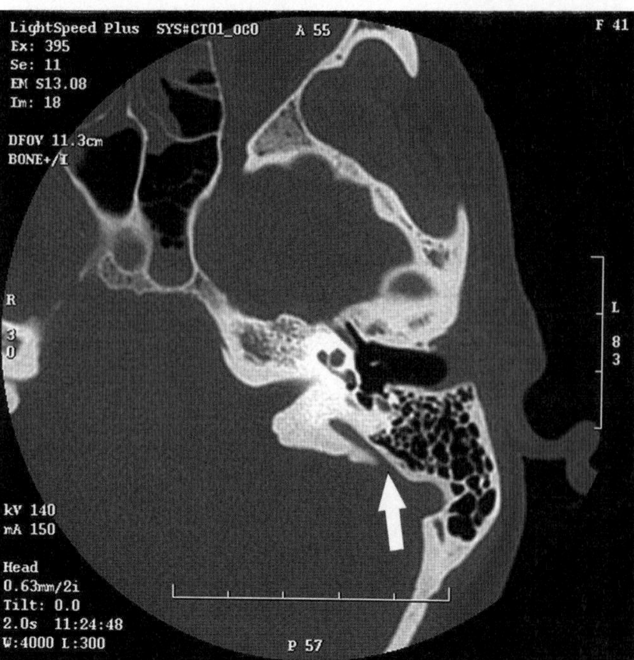

Figure 165-10. CT scan of the left temporal bone of a patient with enlarged vestibular aqueduct syndrome. *White arrow* points to the vestibular aqueduct. *(Courtesy of Dr. Howard Francis.)*

SUGGESTED READINGS

Albers FW, Van Weissenbruch R, Casselman JW. 3DFT–magnetic resonance imaging of the inner ear in Meniere's disease. *Acta Otolaryngol.* 1994;114:595.

Baloh RW, Jacobson K, Fife T. Familial vestibulopathy: a new dominantly inherited syndrome. *Neurology.* 1994;44:20.

Baloh RW. Charles Skinner Hallpike and the beginnings of neurotology. *Neurology.* 2000;54:2138.

Baloh RW. Clinical practice. Vestibular neuritis. *N Engl J Med.* 2003;348:1027.

Baloh RW. Prosper Meniere and his disease. *Arch Neurol.* 2001;58:1151.

Barrs DM, Keyser JS, Stallworth C, et al. Intratympanic steroid injections for intractable Meniere's disease. *Laryngoscope.* 2001;111:2100.

Carey JP, Minor LB, Nager GT. Dehiscence or thinning of bone overlying the superior semicircular canal in a temporal bone survey. *Arch Otolaryngol Head Neck Surg.* 2000;126:137.

Cha YH, Brodsky J, Ishiyama G, et al. The relevance of migraine in patients with Meniere's disease. *Acta Otolaryngol.* 2007;127:1241.

Cha YH, Kane MJ, Baloh RW. Familial clustering of migraine, episodic vertigo, and Meniere's disease. *Otol Neurotol.* 2008;29:93.

Garduno-Anaya MA, Couthino De Toledo H, Hinojosa-Gonzalez R, et al. Dexamethasone inner ear perfusion by intratympanic injection in unilateral Meniere's disease: a two-year prospective, placebo-controlled, double-blind, randomized trial. *Otolaryngol Head Neck Surg.* 2005;133:285.

Glasscock ME. Vestibular nerve section. *Arch Otolaryngol.* 1973;97:112.

Grasland A, Pouchot J, Hachulla E, et al. Typical and atypical Cogan's syndrome: 32 cases and review of the literature. *Rheumatology (Oxford).* 2004;43:1007.

Halmagyi GM, Curthoys IS. A clinical sign of canal paresis. *Arch Neurol.* 1988;45:737.

Halmagyi GM. Diagnosis and management of vertigo. *Clin Med.* 2005;5:159-165.

Hamill TA. Evaluating treatments for Meniere's disease: controversies surrounding placebo control. *J Am Acad Audiol.* 2006;17:27.

House JW, Doherty JK, Fisher LM, et al. Meniere's disease: prevalence of contralateral ear involvement. *Otol Neurotol.* 2006;27:355.

Lee H, Lopez I, Ishiyama A, et al. Can migraine damage the inner ear? *Arch Neurol.* 2000;57:1631.

Minor LB. Clinical manifestations of superior semicircular canal dehiscence. *Laryngoscope.* 2005;115:1717.

Minor LB. Gentamicin-induced bilateral vestibular hypofunction. *JAMA.* 1998;279:541.

For complete list of references log onto www.expertconsult.com.

Minor LB. Labyrinthine fistulae: pathobiology and management. *Curr Opin Otolaryngol Head Neck Surg.* 2003;11:340.

Minor LB, Carey JP, Cremer PD, et al. Dehiscence of bone overlying the superior canal as a cause of apparent conductive hearing loss. *Otol Neurotol.* 2003;24:270.

Minor LB, Solomon D, Zinreich JS, et al. Sound- and/or pressure-induced vertigo due to bone dehiscence of the superior semicircular canal. *Arch Otolaryngol Head Neck Surg.* 1998;124:249.

Rauch SD, Merchant SN, Thedinger BA. Meniere's syndrome and endolymphatic hydrops. Double-blind temporal bone study. *Ann Otol Rhinol Laryngol.* 1989;98:873.

Silverstein H, Norrel H. Retrolabyrinthine surgery: a direct approach to the cerebellopontine angle. *Otolaryngol Head Neck Surg.* 1980;88:462.

Thomsen J, Bretlau P, Tos M, et al. Placebo effect in surgery for Meniere's disease. A double-blind, placebo-controlled study on endolymphatic sac shunt surgery. *Arch Otolaryngol.* 1981;107:271.

CHAPTER ONE HUNDRED AND SIXTY-SIX

Central Vestibular Disorders

Benjamin T. Crane

Scott D. Z. Eggers

David S. Zee

Robert W. Baloh

Key Points

- Determining a central versus a peripheral origin for vertigo requires a careful assessment of symptoms and presenting circumstances, as well as physical findings.
- Appreciation of migraine as a common etiologic disorder in patients presenting with dizziness and other vestibular symptoms is essential to optimal clinical management of this highly prevalent disorder.
- The diagnosis of migraine-associated vertigo relies critically on the history and can be substantiated by monitoring the response over time to diet manipulation and medical management.
- Effective, definitive treatment of migraine-associated vertigo requires the patient's understanding of the importance of lifestyle modification to promote compliance.
- Migraine-associated vertigo is best treated with beta-blockers, tricyclic antidepressants, serotonin reuptake inhibitors, or anticonvulsants.
- Meniere's disease and benign paroxysmal positional vertigo (BPPV) are commonly associated with migraine.
- Vascular disorders are a common cause of vertigo in the elderly population.
- Several types of strokes can manifest with vertigo but almost always are associated with multiple neurologic deficits.
- Neoplasms can manifest with vertigo; vestibular schwannoma is the most likely tumor to present with this symptom, although tumors in the brain stem and cerebellum also can cause vertigo. Screening for neoplasm should be considered in patients with progression of symptoms, particularly when another cranial nerve or central nervous system disorder is present.
- Disorders of the craniovertebral junction can cause vertigo symptoms and should be considered when cervical motion is impaired or radiculopathy is suspected.
- The otolaryngologist should be aware that multiple sclerosis, normal pressure hydrocephalus, focal seizure disorders, and cerebellar ataxia syndromes can produce vertigo.

Dizziness can be classified into *vertigo* (a sense of motion, either of the person or of the visual surround), *dysequilibrium without vertigo*, *presyncope* (near-faint, lightheadedness), and *psychophysiologic dizziness* (often associated with extreme motion sensitivity, anxiety and panic, and phobic behavior). Dizziness, often with motion sickness, can occur in normal persons when they are exposed to unnatural patterns of motion—for example, during sea and car travel. Overlaid on all types of dizziness can be the psychological consequences of extremely distressing symptoms, and vice versa: Dizziness can be a symptom of a psychiatric disorder such as panic and anxiety syndromes and depression. Many conditions of central nervous system origin can cause each of these types of dizziness.

The first task of an otolaryngologist in examining a patient with dizziness is to determine if the symptom is of central or peripheral origin[1] (Table 166-1). Some central causes of acute vertigo can be life-threatening and may necessitate immediate intervention.[2] The differentiation can almost always be made by physical examination based on the type of nystagmus, result of head thrust test, severity of imbalance, and presence or absence of other neurologic signs.

Spontaneous nystagmus of peripheral origin typically is horizontal, or horizontal with a torsional component, and does not change direction with direction of gaze. Spontaneous nystagmus of central origin also can be purely horizontal but often is purely vertical or torsional and usually changes direction with changes in gaze.[1]

The *head thrust test* is performed as follows: The examiner grasps the patient's head and applies a brief, high-acceleration head rotation, first in one direction and then the other.[3] During these maneuvers, the patient fixates on the examiner's nose and the examiner watches for corrective rapid eye movements (saccades), which are a sign of decreased vestibular response (i.e., the eyes move with the head, rather than remaining fixed in space). If a "catch-up" saccade occurs after head thrusts in one direction but not in the other, a peripheral (including the labyrinth and the eighth cranial nerve on its course from the brainstem) lesion on that side is likely.

Patients with an acute peripheral vestibular lesion typically can stand but may demonstrate sway toward the side of a lesion. By contrast, patients with vertigo of central origin often are able to stand

Table 166-1

Differentiation of Central and Peripheral Vertigo

Feature	Central Origin	Peripheral Origin
Imbalance	Severe	Mild to moderate
Neurologic symptoms	Frequent	Rare
Nystagmus	Changes direction No change with fixation	Unidirectional Decreases with fixation
Hearing loss	Rare	Frequent
Nausea	Variable	Severe
Recovery	Slow	Rapid

Box 166-1

Diagnostic Criteria for Migraine

Migraine without Aura

A. At least five attacks fulfilling criteria B to D
B. Headache lasting 4 to 72 hours when untreated
C. Headache with at least two of the following characteristics: unilateral location, pulsating quality, moderate or severe intensity, aggravation by physical activity
D. During the headach, either nausea and vomiting or photophobia
E. Not attributable to another disorder

Typical Aura with Migraine Headache

A. At least two attacks fulfilling criteria B to D
B. Fully reversible visual, sensory, or aphasic aura symptoms with no motor weakness
C. At least two of the following: homonymous positive features or unilateral sensory symptoms; for at least one symptom, gradual development over more than 5 minutes; duration of 5 to 60 minutes for each symptom
D. Headache following aura after a symptom-free interval of less than 60 minutes
E. Not attributable to another disorder

without support. Associated neurologic signs such as dysarthria, incoordination, numbness, or weakness suggest a central origin.

Dizziness and vertigo can be caused by diverse pathologic conditions of the central nervous system (CNS). Differentiation of these disorders from those of peripheral labyrinthine origin requires familiarity with the associated signs and symptoms of CNS processes, their natural history, and their appearance. Definitive diagnostic evaluation and management usually involve cooperation with neurologists or neurosurgeons. A classification of CNS disorders associated with vestibular symptoms includes intracranial complications of suppurative otitis, vascular disorders, neoplasms, disorders of the craniovertebral junction, multiple sclerosis, familial ataxia syndromes, and focal seizure disorders.

Intracranial Complications of Otitic Infections

Epidural or subdural abscesses, as well as those of the temporal bone, petrous apex, or cerebellum, can cause vestibular signs and symptoms. Such processes usually are associated with other signs of infection, such as fever or sepsis, and are rare in the modern era of antibiotics.

Migraine

Migraine is characterized by recurrent headaches associated with nausea, vomiting, hypersensitivity to light, sound, and smell.[4] This clinical entity is an important consideration in the diagnosis because patients with migraine often present with dizziness. Neurologic aura symptoms are present in one third of migraine patients. Migraine affects nearly 25% of women, 15% of men,[5,6] and 5% of children.[7] In the prepubertal period, boys with migraine slightly outnumber girls, but at puberty, migraine decreases in boys and increases in girls, so that a 2:1 female preponderance is established by adulthood.[8] Migraine typically begins in young adulthood, with onset of symptoms after the age of 40 in only 10% of sufferers.

The diagnosis and classification of migraine and other headache disorders have been a controversial issue. The most recent effort of the Headache Classification Committee of the International Headache Society (IHS)[4] sets up criteria that allow meaningful comparisons of groups of patients between centers. The IHS classifies the most common type of migraine as migraine with and migraine without aura (Box 166-1); other classified types of migraine headache have been designated but are not considered in this chapter because they will only rarely be encountered by the otolaryngologist.

The definition of migrainous vertigo also has been controversial. Neuhauser and colleagues[9] proposed criteria for *definite migrainous vertigo* as follows: (1) episodic vestibular symptoms (rotational vertigo, other illusory self or object motion, positional vertigo, head motion intolerance) of at least moderate severity; (2) migraine according to IHS criteria; (3) at least one of the following migrainous symptoms during at least two vertiginous attacks: migrainous headache, photophobia, phonophobia, visual or other auras; and (4) other causes ruled out by appropriate investigations. *Probable migrainous vertigo* was the designation chosen for patients who did not meet definite criteria but were still believed to have migrainous vertigo as the most likely diagnosis. This definition requires criteria 1 and 4 from the foregoing list, plus at least one of the following: migraine according to IHS criteria; migrainous symptoms during vertigo; migraine-specific precipitants of vertigo (e.g., specific foods, sleep irregularities, hormonal changes); and response to antimigraine drugs. A diagnostic algorithm[10] for definite and probable migrainous vertigo (Fig. 166-1) has been proposed.

To elicit a history adequate to make the diagnosis, an understanding of the various components of the aura is essential. In descending order of frequency, these features are (1) scotoma or blind spots; (2) teichopsia, or fortification spectra (a zig-zag pattern in the visual field resembling a fort); (3) flashing or colored lights; and (4) paresthesias.

Vestibular Symptoms

Nonspecific Dizziness

Nonspecific dizziness occurs frequently in patients with either tension or migraine headaches and does not in itself differentiate between the two groups, although dizziness is more common and more severe in migraine sufferers.

Vertigo

Vertigo is extremely common in patients with migraine and occurred in 26.5% of Kayan and Hood's group of patients with migraine, compared with 7.8% of those with tension headache ($P < .001$).[11] Some studies have found the incidence of vertigo in classic migraine sufferers to be as high as 42%.[12] The severity of vertigo in patients with migraine tends to be greater than in those suffering from tension headaches. Vertigo severe enough for the patient to seek medical attention for relief occurred in 5% of those with migraine but in less than 1% of those with tension headache.[11]

The temporal relationship of vertiginous spells to migraine headaches is important to ascertain. Vertigo does not usually manifest as an aura immediately preceding the headache as a prodrome. Of the 53 patients with vertigo and migraine interviewed by Kayan and Hood,[11]

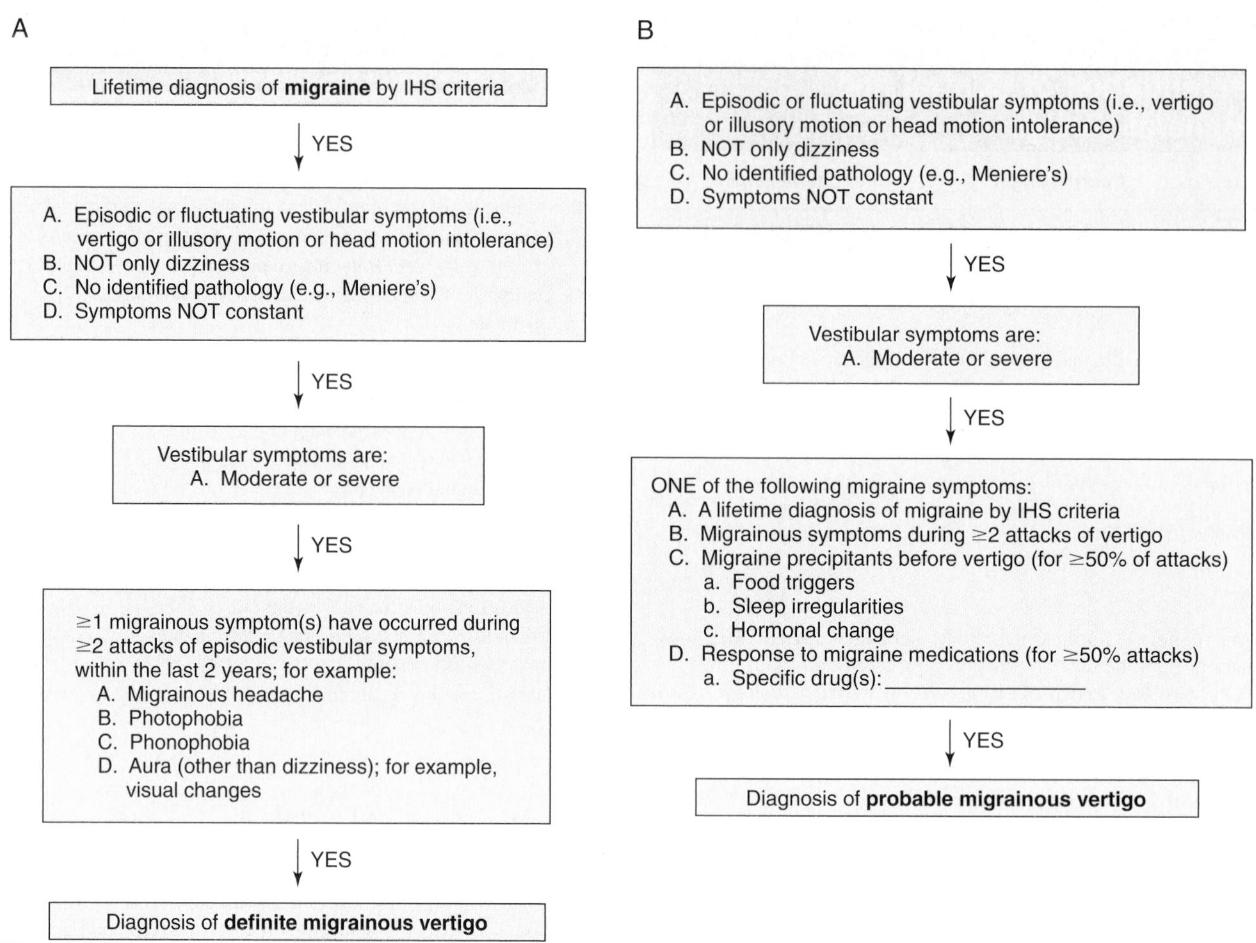

Figure 166-1. Diagnosis of definite (**A**) and probable (**B**) migrainous vertigo. "Moderate" vestibular symptoms interfere with daily activities, and "severe" vestibular symptoms prohibit daily activities. "Head motion intolerance" is the sensation of imbalance or illusory self or object motion provoked by head motion. IHS, International Headache Society. *(From Furman JM, Marcus DA, Balaban CD. Migrainous vertigo: development of a pathogenetic model and structured diagnostic interview.* Curr Opin Neurol. *2003;16:5-13. Adapted from Neuhauser H, Leopold M, von Brevern M, et al. The interrelations of migraine vertigo and migrainous vertigo.* Neurology. *2001;56:436-441.)*

the vertigo immediately preceded the headache in only 15%, whereas it occurred during the headache in 47% and during the headache-free interval in 36% of patients. In a series of 50 patients with basilar migraine, Olsson[13] and Cuttler and Baloh[14] also found vertigo to occur more often during the headache-free interval than as a prodrome before the headache.

Motion Sickness

The relationship between migraine and motion sickness is well established. In his seminal study of 9000 Swedish schoolchildren, Bille[15] matched children with more pronounced migraine to children in a similar group without migraine. Severe motion sickness was present in 49% of the children with migraine and in only 10% of the control group. Barabas and colleagues found that 45% of 60 children with migraine experienced at least three episodes of motion sickness culminating in vomiting, compared with 5% to 7% of three similar-sized control groups of subjects with non-migraine headaches, seizure disorders, and learning disabilities or neurologic perceptual impairments.[16] In adults, a similarly significantly greater incidence of motion sickness has been observed in patients with classic migraine than in patients with tension and cluster headaches.[12] In the Kayan and Hood[11] series of 200 unselected patients with migraine, 51% reported motion sickness, compared with 20% of the patients with tension headache.

A subset of migraine sufferers experience disabling motion sickness. These patients limit their head motion to a minimum, limit their daily activities accordingly, frequently rest during the day, and when symptomatic may need to remain motionless for up to an hour until symptoms abate. If they cannot avoid vestibular stimulation, a full-blown migraine attack can be triggered. Caloric responses in these patients tend to be symmetrical and very brisk, often culminating in emesis. If treatment provides a dramatic response, the patients often are surprised to recognize how much they had restricted their lifestyle. Often, neither the patient nor the physician suspects that the migraine had any relationship to the other symptoms. Patients often discuss only the vestibular symptoms and ignore or discount any effects of the underlying problem. Prophylactic migraine therapy often yields dramatic clinical improvement with a decrease in symptoms.

Auditory Symptoms

Of the patients studied by Kayan and Hood,[11] 20% complained of hearing loss, tinnitus, or pitch distortion, and one fourth of the 20% had multiple auditory symptoms. In descending order of frequency, the temporal patterns for occurrence of these symptoms were during the headache, during the headache-free interval, and immediately before the headache. The temporal relationship of these symptoms mirror the relationship of vertigo to headache in this same series.

Hearing Loss

The association of hearing loss to migraine is reported to be approximately 7%.[11] Hearing loss is a more prominent symptom in patients with basilar migraine. In Olsson's study,[13] 52% of the patients noticed a change in hearing as part of the aura immediately preceding the migraine headache and 50% had a fluctuating low-frequency sensorineural hearing loss. A group of migraine patients in whom hearing loss thought to be due to vasospasm has been reported.[17]

Tinnitus

Tinnitus was experienced by 15% of migraine patients, but none with tension headache,[11] and in more than 60% of basilar migraine patients.[13]

Distortion

Although distortion was noted by only 4% of patients in the Kayan and Hood series,[11] its actual prevalence may be higher. More attention may be given to more bothersome symptoms, and auditory distortion may be ignored by physicians and patients alike as unimportant.

Phonophobia

Loud noise aversion distinguishes patients with migraine from those suffering other types of headaches. Only 12% of tension headache sufferers experienced phonophobia, but 81% of those with migraine had the symptom.[11] Olsson[13] detected phonophobia in patients with basilar migraine at a rate of 70% during headache and 76% during headache-free intervals. Furthermore, he documented an abnormal loudness discomfort level in 78% of these patients, whereas only 14% had abnormal speech reception thresholds.

Migraine Associated with Neuro-otologic Symptoms

Basilar Migraine

Bickerstaff[18] described a form of migraine ascribed to ischemia in the distribution of the basilar artery. This syndrome currently is known as *basilar migraine*, replacing "basilar artery migraine" and "posterior fossa migraine," which occasionally appear in the older literature. This subtype of migraine was similar to classic migraine in that it consisted of an aura followed by a severe headache. However, a majority of affected patients were adolescent girls, in whom the migraine attacks often occurred premenstrually. Later observers emphasized other aspects of the clinical picture such as stupor,[19] loss of consciousness,[20] neurologic symptoms,[21] hearing loss, and vertigo.[22] These symptoms are thought to be due to involvement of the brainstem, cerebellum, cranial nerve nuclei, and occipital lobe cortex.

Migraine without Headache

Migraine should not be eliminated as a cause for vertigo just because headaches are not present. Whitty[23] reported on a series of patients with symptoms typically experienced during a migraine aura but no headaches. In these patients, typical headaches sometimes developed later in life, or auras that were only intermittently related to headaches were noted. Other observers have described similar patients using the term *migraine equivalent*[24-26] or *migraine accompaniments.*[27] A history of motion sickness, premenstrual clustering of attacks, or headaches associated with some of the attacks is frequent. Personal or family history of migraine also is helpful in diagnosing these patients.

Etiology

Historically migraine headache was thought to result from dilation of intracranial and dural arteries causing stretching of pain fibers in the walls of the arteries. The complex phenomena associated with migraine cannot be fully explained by a vascular theory. More recently, neurally based spreading of depression activity has been implicated,[28,29] although the neurophysiology is far from completely understood.

A family history of migraine is present in approximately 40% to 90% of affected persons, compared with 5% to 20% of unaffected subjects. When migraine sufferers with and without aura are examined separately, patients who have migraine with aura are more likely to have affected family members. When twins are studied, conconcordance rates for migraine are only 10% to 34%, depending on the country, suggesting that both genetic and environmental factors play a role.[30]

Familial hemiplegic migraine (FHM) is a rare type of migraine that affects only 0.01% of the general population.[31] However, the underlying cellular cause is relatively well understood. Unlike most types of migraine, FHM has a clear autosomal dominant pattern of inheritance. Thus far, mutations have been found in three different genes that determine neuronal excitability.

Management

Treatment of migraine has historically been focused on headache symptoms. Management of migraine headache can be divided into two categories: symptomatic and prophylactic. Some interventions are useful in ameliorating the symptoms of the acute attack, whereas others are designed to reduce the frequency or severity of attacks. Symptomatic management includes analgesics, antiemetics, antivertiginous drugs, sedatives, and vasoconstrictors. In many patients, over-the-counter analgesics such as ibuprofen, aspirin, or acetaminophen and rest are all that is needed to relieve headache symptoms. Decreased gastric motility occurs during and between migraine attacks, which may decrease absorption of oral drugs, contributing to nausea and vomiting.[32] Metocopramide promotes normal gastric motility and may improve absorption of oral medication.

Nutrition may play a significant role in the frequency and severity of migraine headaches and migraine-associated dizziness. Riboflavin (vitamin B_2) has been shown to be more effective than placebo in reducing the frequency of migraine headache when given in a dose of 400 mg daily.[33] High-dose magnesium also has been found to have a therapeutic effect on migraine; suggested mechanisms have included inhibiting platelet aggregation, counteracting vasospasm, stabilizing cell membranes, and anti-inflammatory effects.[34] Patients suffering from migraine symptoms have been found to have lower levels of magnesium, and infusion of magnesium can relieve symptoms.[35] Magnesium given orally in a dose of 600 mg daily also has been shown to decrease headache symptoms[36]; however, diarrhea is a potential side effect at these doses.

Food sensitivity may be a migraine trigger in a significant number of patients with migraine symptoms.[34] Although some patients have observed that consuming a certain food will reliably provoke a headache, the effect of diet is more subtle. Foods that should be avoided include red wine, aged cheeses, beer, chocolate, caffeine, and yogurt.[37] Alcohol itself does not seem to be a trigger, because vodka consumption does not provoke attacks.[38] Dietary modification may be considered as first-line therapy for migraine prophylaxis (Fig. 166-2).

Vestibular migraine symptoms often are not directly related to the headache symptoms, and in some cases, dizziness as a manifestation of migraine can be present nearly continuously. Treatment of vestibular migraine has tended to mirror that of traditional migraine symptoms, and medications that alleviate headache symptoms also tend to be effective for vertigo symptoms.[39] However, because the migraine-associated dizziness often is much more frequent than the headaches, prophylaxis usually is necessary.

Sumatriptan (Imitrex), a 5HT1D receptor agonist, has become the principal drug to abort severe migraine headache. Initial trials indicate that in 90% of cases the drug effectively aborts migraine headache symptoms within an hour of their onset when it is given subcutaneously; in 70% to 85%, symptoms may be aborted within 2 hours.[40] Common side effects include sensations of heaviness and pressure in the chest, with coronary artery vasospasm more rarely reported. Although sumatriptan is remarkably effective in relief of early migraine headaches, breakthrough is common, and the drug has limited efficacy for concurrent vestibular symptoms.

Propranolol (Inderal) is the drug most commonly used for preventing migraine episodes. Approximately 50% to 70% of patients with headache symptoms derive benefit from prophylactic propranolol therapy, which also may be beneficial for vertigo symptoms.[21] The medication is contraindicated in patients with asthma, congestive heart failure, peripheral vascular disease, diabetes, or hypothyroidism. Principal side effects include fatigue, lethargy, and dizziness, which usually occurs on rising from a seated or supine position. Side effects are minimized by slowly increasing the dose from a low starting level. Doses of 80 to 180 mg per day usually are effective. The medication should be continued for at least 2 to 3 months at the highest level of tolerance before it is considered a failure. On discontinuation, the drug should be gradually tapered over several days.

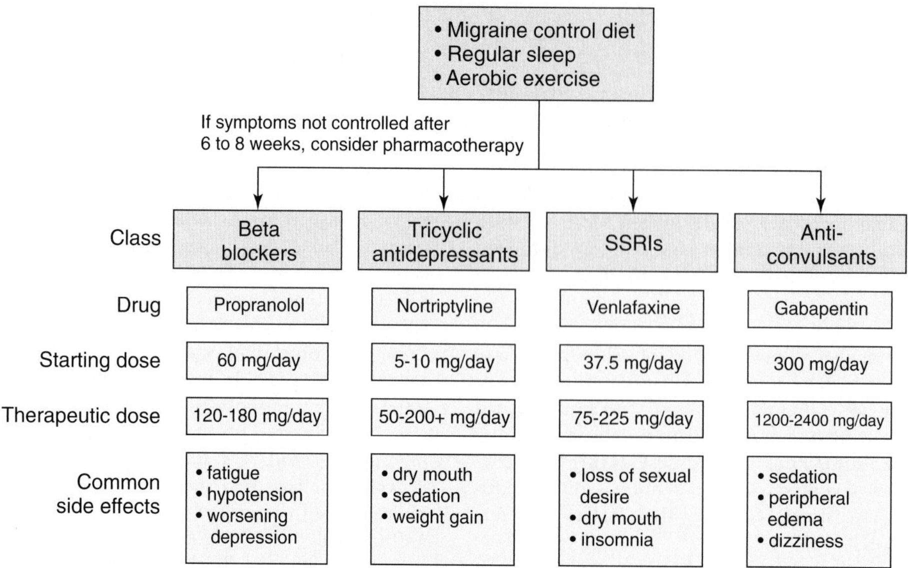

Figure 166-2. Flowchart of suggested migraine treatment. Lifestyle modification usually is a good first option because it is not associated with side effects and will provide symptomatic improvement in most patients. Pharmacotherapy should be considered if more conservative measures fail.

A variety of beta-adrenergic agents also have been used for migraine prophylaxis. Atenolol (Tenormin), metoprolol (Lopressor), nadolol (Corgard), and timolol (Blocadren) probably are as effective as propranolol. However, a number of other beta-adrenergic antagonists (e.g., acebutolol, oxprenolol, alprenolol) do not appear to be effective in migraine prophylaxis. It has been suggested that pure beta-adrenergic antagonism without intrinsic sympathomimetic activity is required for efficacy.

Calcium channel blockers (nifedipine, verapamil) also have been reported to reduce the frequency of migraine attacks, but the effect is likely to be only modest.[41] Diltiazem (Cardizem) does not seem to have any effect on migraine prevention.

Tricyclic antidepressants also have been shown to decrease the frequency and severity of migraine attacks. Amitriptyline is perhaps the most-studied drug in this category, with several studies showing its efficacy.[42] Starting doses usually are 10 to 25 mg, which usually is given at bedtime, to avoid the side effects of sedation and anticholinergic activity. Weight gain is a side effect that limits patient compliance with therapy in some populations. Therapeutic doses usually are 50 to 100 mg, with some patients who also suffer from depressive symptoms requiring doses of up to 400 mg. Nortriptyline is less sedating than amitriptyline and has a dosage profile similar to that of amitriptyline.

The role for selective serotonin reuptake inhibitors (SSRIs) for treatment of migraine remains controversial. Some evidence shows that they seem to be less effective than tricyclic antidepressants[43] for headache symptoms. However, in patients with chronic subjective dizziness as their primary symptom, SSRIs seem to be effective.[44]

Clinical trials have shown gabapentin (Neurontin) to be effective at dosages of 1200 to 2400 mg per day,[45] which usually is divided into three doses daily. Dizziness, peripheral edema, and somnolence are common side effects.

Valproic acid derivatives such as divalproex (Depakote) are effective in migraine prevention. However, the need to monitor levels and the side effect profile of these medications, which includes nausea, fatigue, weight gain, teratogenicity, hepatic toxicity, and tremor, have made them infrequently used.

Acetazolamide (Diamox) has been shown to be effective in preventing migraine headaches and episodic vertigo in families who also exhibit essential tremor.[46] However, it has not been shown to be of benefit in larger migraine headache populations.[47] It may be effective in ameliorating motion-induced vestibular symptoms in patients with migraine.

Vestibular Disorders Associated with Migraine

Benign Paroxysmal Positional Vertigo

BPPV is the most common cause of peripheral vertigo. The disorder probably is due to free-floating particles in the semicircular canal (canalithiasis), which usually collect in the posterior semicircular canal owing its low point with respect to gravity. Classic symptoms include brief episodes (lasting less than 1 minute) of vertigo when the head is tilted backwards or during rolling over in bed. An extensive discussion of diagnosis and treatment of this common disorder is outside the scope of this chapter. Of note, however, migraine and motion sickness are three times more common in patients with BPPV than in the general population, with 59% of patients having a family history of migraine.[48]

Meniere's Disease

Meniere's disease classically manifests with unilateral low-frequency fluctuating hearing loss, a sense of aural fullness, and dizziness lasting several minutes to hours.[49] However, the presence and severity of these symptoms are variable, which can overlap with those of migraine.[50] Unselected patients with migraine have a 7% incidence of hearing loss and 26% incidence of vertigo.[11] In patients with Meniere's disease, the lifetime incidence of migraine is 56%, versus only 25% in controls.[51] The frequent co-occurrence of Meniere's disease and migraine suggests a pathophysiologic link between the two syndromes.[52] Alternatively, the diseases may be separate processes that cause similar symptoms. It is likely that both Meniere's disease and migraine are not homogeneous disorders but may be caused by a spectrum of genetic and environmental influences—so both explanations may be correct: Migraine may be one of many risk factors for Meniere's disease, and vice versa.

Vestibular Disorders Related to Migraine

Benign Paroxysmal Vertigo of Childhood

Basser[53] described a clinical entity in children younger than 4 years of age that he called *benign paroxysmal vertigo*. This should not be confused with the much more common benign paroxysmal positional

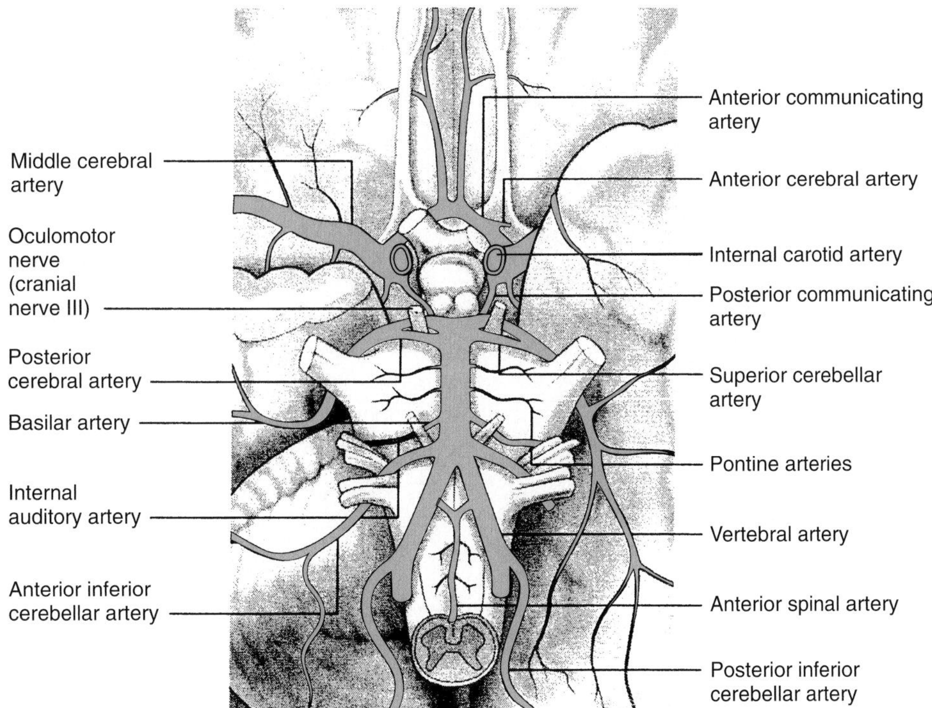

Figure 166-3. The blood vessels supplying the brain. The brainstem is supplied by branches of the vertebral arteries and basilar artery. Note that although this figure shows the internal auditory artery arising directly from the basilar artery, it more commonly branches off the anterior inferior cerebellar artery instead. *(Adapted from Kandel ER, Schwartz JH, Jessell TM.* Principles of Neural Science. *New York: McGraw-Hill; 2000:1303.)*

vertigo (BPPV), which also is referred to as benign positional vertigo. Children with this disorder usually become suddenly frightened, cry out, cling to the parent, stagger as though drunk, and exhibit pallor, diaphoresis, and frequent vomiting. Symptoms are worsened by head motion. The episodes last less than 5 minutes, after which the child is normal again. The symptoms usually manifest at the age of 2 to 3 years and gradually decrease until they resolve before age 8. When the clinical picture is clear, treatment is not needed. On long-term follow-up, classic migraine eventually developed in six of seven patients with this disorder.[54]

Paroxysmal Torticollis

Snyder[55] described a series of 12 infants who experienced recurrent attacks of head tilt before the age of 8 months. The spells lasted from a few hours to 3 days and occasionally were accompanied by pallor, vomiting, and agitation. Subsequent observers have suggested a familial occurrence[56] and that symptoms also may involve the trunk and extremities.[57] The spells usually stop spontaneously by age 5, and no treatment is needed.

Vascular Disorders

Abnormalities of blood flow to the vestibular system are relatively common causes of vestibular symptoms and often are difficult to distinguish from well-known end organ disorders. Clinical presentations vary for many reasons. Functional deficits may be restricted to one or both end organs or their structures or may involve the vestibular nuclei or other peripheral or central regions. Diverse abnormal processes can result in permanent or temporary loss of function. Permanent losses typically result from arterial occlusion or from hemorrhagic infarction. Transient effects may accompany arterial stenosis, vascular spasm, inadequate perfusion pressure, or reversed arterial flow with shunting such as in subclavian steal syndrome. Many symptom complexes are possible, but defined clinical entities are more common.

The blood supply to the inner ear, brainstem, and cerebellum arises from the vertebrobasilar system. Vertigo can occur from occlusion of any of the three major circumferential branches of the vertebral or basilar arteries: the posterior inferior cerebellar artery, the anterior inferior cerebellar artery, and the superior cerebellar artery (Fig. 166-3).

Specific Disorders

Vertebrobasilar Insufficiency

Vertebrobasilar insufficiency is a significant cause of vertigo in the elderly population.[58,59] Vertigo due to vertebrobasilar insufficiency is of abrupt onset, usually lasts several minutes, and frequently is associated with nausea and vomiting. Presentation with vertigo symptoms alone is extremely uncommon and occurs in less than 1% of patients.[60] Usually multiple symptoms are present, which often include headache, diplopia, ataxia, numbness, weakness, or oropharyngeal dysfunction. Repeated episodes of vertigo without other symptoms suggest another diagnosis.

Atherosclerosis of the subclavian, vertebral, or basilar arteries usually is the underlying cause of vertebrobasilar insufficiency. The distribution of large-artery atherosclerosis differs according to race and gender.[61] European men tend to have atherosclerosis at the origin of the vertebral arteries near the subclavian. Intercranial large-artery atherosclerosis is more common among African Americans, Asians, and women. Hypertension increases the risk of lipohyalinotic thickening of these vessels, which increases the risk of infarction.

Rarely, occlusion or stenosis of the subclavian or innominate artery just proximal to the origin of the vertebral artery results in *subclavian steal syndrome.* In patients with this syndrome, vertebral insufficiency results from siphoning of blood down the vertebral artery from the basilar system to supply the upper extremities. Vertigo and other symptoms are precipitated by exercise of the upper extremities.

If the patient is suspected to have had a stroke, a CT scan should be ordered to rule out the possibility of a hemorrhagic event. If a patient has presented within 3 hours after the onset of symptoms, the National Institute for Neurological Disorders and Stroke (NINDS) guidelines recommend administration of t-PA intravenously. However, recommendations in this area are rapidly evolving, and in the acute phase, patients should be treated by a neurologist familiar with stroke.

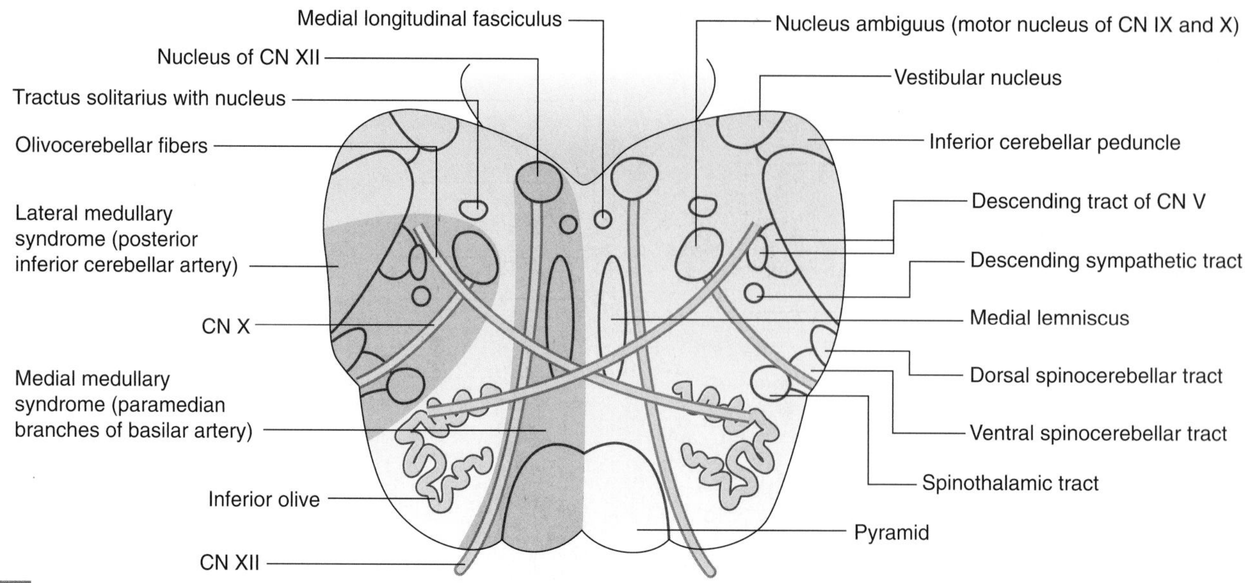

Figure 166-4. Medulla cross section with anatomic structures labeled on the *right* and vascular lesions on the *left*. CN, cranial nerve. *(Adapted from Kandel ER, Schwartz JH, Jessell TM.* Principles of Neural Science. *New York: McGraw-Hill; 2000:1303.)*

In most patients with nonacute presentations, treatment consists of controlling risk factors such as diabetes, hypertension, and hyperlipidemia. In patients with symptomatic intracranial stenosis with 50% to 99% occlusion, aspirin and warfarin are equally effective, but warfarin carries a higher risk of hemorrhagic events,[62] so aspirin is the agent of choice. Anticoagulation with warfarin should be considered if the patient has previously had an embolic stroke of cardiac origin.[58] Stenting of vertebral artery stenosis has been tried, with mixed results. Endarterectomy for extracranial vertebral artery disease also has been successfully performed, but indications for such procedures are still evolving.

Lateral Medullary Syndrome

The zone of infarction producing the lateral medullary syndrome (Wallenberg's syndrome) consists of a wedge of the dorsolateral medulla just posterior to the olive (Fig. 166-4). The syndrome usually results from occlusion of the ipsilateral vertebral artery and rarely from occlusion of the posterior inferior cerebellar artery.[63] The classic presentation includes sensory deficits affecting the trunk and extremities on the opposite side of the infarct and sensory and motor deficits affecting the face and cranial nerves ipsilateral to the infarct. Characteristic symptoms include vertigo, ipsilateral facial pain, diplopia, dysphagia, and dysphonia. Neurologic examination may reveal a ipsilateral Horner's syndrome, ipsilateral dysmetria, dysrhythmia, spontaneous nystagmus, and contralateral loss of pain and temperature sensation.

Hearing loss does not occur because the lesion is caudal to the cochlear nerve entry zone and cochlear nuclei.

Some patients exhibit a prominent motor disturbance that causes the body and extremities to deviate toward the lesion site as if being pulled by an invisible force.[64] This so-called lateral pulsion also affects the oculomotor system, producing excessively large saccades directed toward the side of the lesion and abnormally small saccades away from the lesion. Most patients with Wallenberg's syndrome have major residual neurologic deficits months or even years after the acute infarction.

Lateral Pontomedullary Syndrome

Ischemia in the distribution of the anterior inferior cerebellar artery results in infarction of the dorsolateral pontomedullary region and the inferolateral cerebellum.[65] The middle cerebellar peduncle typically is the core of the affected territory (Fig. 166-5). Because the labyrinthine artery originates from the anterior inferior cerebellar artery in 80% of patients, infarction of the membranous labyrinth is a common accompaniment. Severe vertigo, nausea, and vomiting are common initial symptoms. Other signs and symptoms include ipsilateral hearing loss, tinnitus, facial paralysis, and cerebellar asynergy. Spontaneous nystagmus is common. Contralateral loss of pain and temperature sensation may be caused by crossed spinothalamic fibers. Onset of symptoms is acute, followed by gradual improvement. Vertigo may persist for several weeks owing to damage of the central compensation mechanisms.

Cerebellar Infarction

Occlusion of the vertebral artery, the posterior inferior cerebellar artery, the anterior inferior cerebellar artery, or the superior cerebellar artery may result in infarction confined to the cerebellum without brainstem involvement[66] (Fig. 166-6). Initial signs and symptoms are severe vertigo, vomiting, and ataxia. Lack of typical brainstem signs may cause an incorrect diagnosis of an acute peripheral labyrinthine disorder. The key to the diagnosis is the presence of prominent cerebellar signs such as gait ataxia and paretic gaze nystagmus. The diagnostic modality of choice is magnetic resonance imaging (MRI). After a latent interval of 24 to 96 hours, some patients exhibit signs of progressive brainstem dysfunction caused by compression by a swelling cerebellum. Progression to quadriplegia, coma, and death may follow unless surgical decompression is performed.

Cerebellar Hemorrhage

Spontaneous intraparenchymal hemorrhage into the cerebellum causes neurologic symptoms that often rapidly progress to coma and death.[67-69] The initial manifestations are severe vertigo, vomiting, and ataxia. As with cerebellar infarction, brainstem signs may not initially be present, which may cause the condition to be confused with a peripheral vestibular problem. Modern imaging studies such as computed tomography (CT) and MRI have revolutionized the diagnosis of this condition (Fig. 166-7). Mortality rates range from as low as 20%[70] up to 74%, depending on the series. The value of and indications for surgical intervention remain controversial and probably depend on the size and location of the hematoma as well as the patient's symptoms.[67]

Evaluation and Management

Cerebrovascular disease is a primary consideration in the differential diagnosis for acute spontaneous vertigo, particularly if the patient has vascular risk factors. If the history and examination findings suggest a vascular disorder, immediate neuroimaging is necessary. CT of the brain without contrast often is the first imaging test because it is widely available and shows intraparenchymal or subarachnoid blood. Hemorrhage can mimic any of the ischemic stroke syndromes and must be

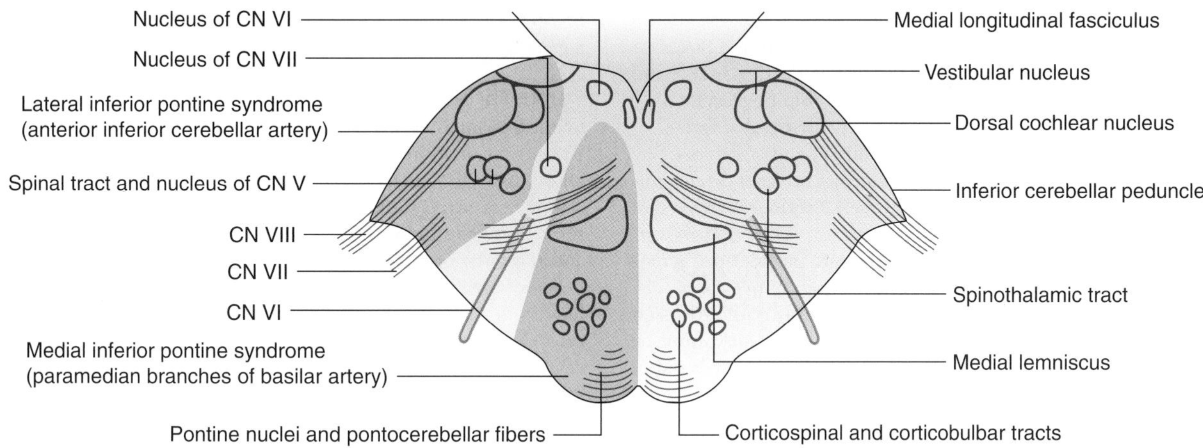

Figure 166-5. Lower pons cross section with anatomic structures labeled on the *right* and vascular lesions on the *left*. CN, cranial nerve. *(Adapted from Kandel ER, Schwartz JH, Jessell TM.* Principles of Neural Science. *New York: McGraw-Hill; 2000:1303.)*

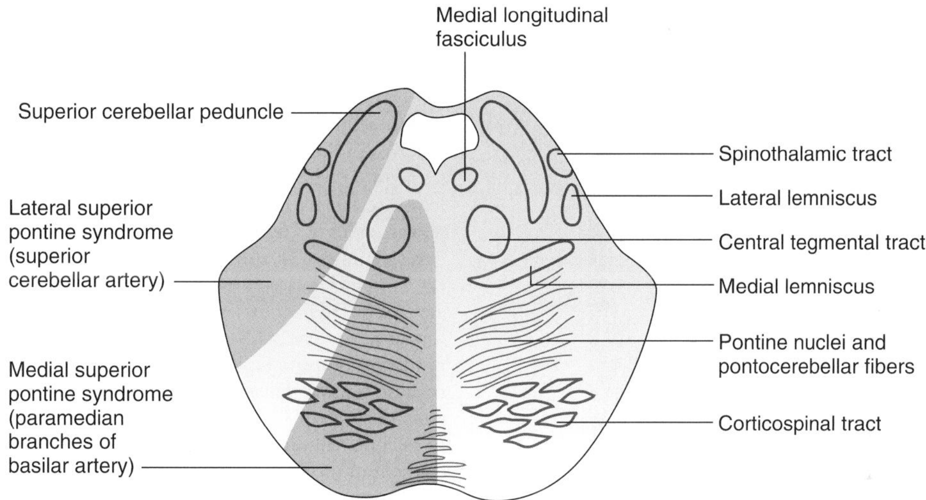

Figure 166-6. Upper pons cross section with anatomic structures labeled on the *right* and vascular lesions on the *left*. *(Adapted from Kandel ER, Schwartz JH, Jessell TM.* Principles of Neural Science. *New York: McGraw-Hill; 2000:1303.)*

excluded with thin-section CT through the cerebellum, brainstem, and fourth ventricle. MRI and magnetic resonance angiography (MRA) are superior to CT for viewing the vertebrobasilar vessels and their supplied structures, because CT scans often are normal in appearance with cerebellar or brainstem infarction. MRI, on the other hand, detects ischemic strokes in the brainstem and cerebellum early on, as well as edema. Diffusion-weighted imaging with MRI can now detect infarcts within the first hour of ischemia (Fig. 166-8). MRA has begun to replace conventional angiography in certain circumstances. Vertebral artery dissection and vertebral or basilar artery stenosis or occlusion generally can be identified with MRA of the cervical vessels performed with contrast (Fig. 166-9).

Neoplasms

Space-occupying lesions can induce vestibular symptoms by compressing or by destroying neural tissue within the temporal bone, in the cerebellopontine angle, or intra-axially within the brainstem and cerebellum. Symptoms also can be produced or increased by vascular compression.

Vestibular Schwannomas

Vestibular schwannomas can manifest with vertigo symptoms, which can be disabling in some patients,[71] although such symptoms are present in less than 20% of patients with these tumors.[72] Hyperventilation-induced vertigo also may occur in the absence of hearing loss.[73] Discussion of the diagnosis and treatment of vestibular neuromas can be found in Chapters 149 and 153.

Brainstem Neoplasms

Gliomas of the brainstem usually grow slowly and infiltrate the brainstem nuclei and fiber tracts, producing progressive symptoms and signs. The typical history is one of relentlessly progressive involvement of one brainstem center after another, often causing death with the destruction of the vital cardiorespiratory centers of the medulla. These tumors are 5 to 10 times more common in children than in adults. Vestibular and cochlear signs and symptoms occur in approximately one half of patients, but the spectrum of findings usually makes a brainstem origin clear. In the modern era, imaging studies such as CT or MRI usually are performed to investigate the initial manifestations, making the diagnosis obvious.

Tumors originating in the pons or midbrain initially are likely to cause long tract signs, cranial nerve deficits, and ataxia. Although uncommon, tumors that originate in the medulla are likely to cause recurrent vertigo and vomiting. Irradiation is the treatment of choice, because surgical resection of this area is associated with significant morbidity.

Tumors originating in the fourth ventricle and compressing the vestibular nuclei in its floor also can produce vestibular symptoms.

Medulloblastomas, occurring primarily in children and adolescents, are rapidly growing, highly cellular tumors that originate in the posterior midline or vermis of the cerebellum and invade the fourth ventricle and adjacent cerebellar hemispheres. Headaches and vomiting occur early from obstructive hydrocephalus and associated increased intracranial pressure. An attack of headache, vertigo, vomiting, and visual loss may result from a change in head position, producing transient cerebrospinal fluid (CSF) obstruction (Bruns' syndrome). Positional vertigo and nystagmus may be the presenting manifestations.[74,75] Other fourth ventricle tumors that produce a similar clinical picture include ependymomas, papillomas, teratomas, epidermoid cysts, and cysticercosis. The diagnosis of a fourth ventricular mass is made readily with MRI and CT scanning, but frequently the exact nature of the tumor cannot be determined before surgical exploration and biopsy. Complete removal of tumor should be achieved when possible. Medulloblastomas are particularly sensitive to radiotherapy.[76]

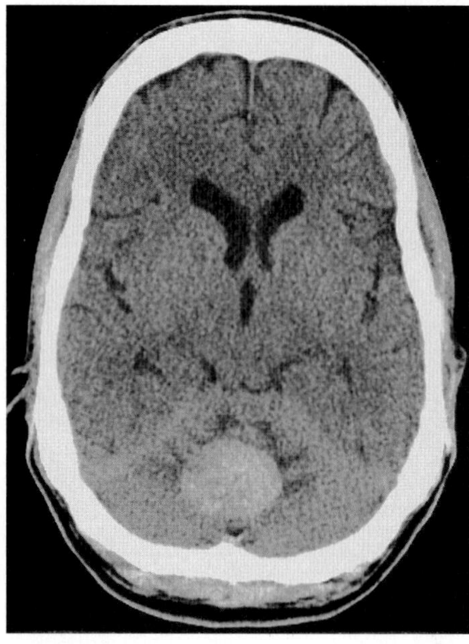

Figure 166-7. Noncontrast computed tomography scan of a cerebellar hematoma within the vermis. Surrounding edema and effacement of the superior aspect of the fourth ventricle are evident. Resulting obstruction of cerebrospinal fluid outflow may lead to hydrocephalus. *(Courtesy of K. D. Flemming.)*

Cerebellar Neoplasm

Clinical manifestations of posterior fossa tumors include dizziness in 81% and vertigo in 44% of patients.[77] One half of patients with posterior fossa tumors exhibit spontaneous nystagmus, and a third lack caloric responses. Other common symptoms and signs of cerebellar tumors include tinnitus, hearing loss, headache, nausea or vomiting, and ataxia. Gliomas of the cerebellum may be relatively silent until they become large enough to obstruct CSF circulation or compress the brainstem.[78] Positional vertigo occasionally is the initial symptom of a cerebellar tumor.[79,80] Paroxysmal positional nystagmus, when present, is atypical, because it can be induced in several different positions and is nonfatigable. Tumors that can produce these signs and symptoms include gliomas, teratomas, hemangiomas, and hemangioblastomas. Each of these tumors has a characteristic appearance on MRI and CT scans, although occasionally the exact tumor type cannot be determined before surgical biopsy.

Cervical Vertigo

Dizziness caused by disorders of the neck and cervical spine is poorly understood and relatively uncommon. Neck afferents are recognized to have a role in the coordination of eye, head, and body spatial orientation. Perception of head rotation can be driven by vestibular, proprioceptive, or visual inputs. Cervical vertigo must be by definition proprioceptive in nature, because the other inputs that cause vertigo do not exist in the neck. Laboratory experiments in humans that eliminate visual input with darkness and vestibular input by holding the head still have shown that trunk motion can produce the sensation of head turning[81]; however, this has not been shown to occur in more ordinary situations. Several studies have provided limited evidence for the existence of cervical vertigo. Unilateral local anesthesia of the cervical roots can cause ataxia and nystagmus in animals and ataxia without nystagmus in humans.[82] Patients with chronic cervicobrachial neck pain also have worse results on posturography tests.[83] These results are difficult to interpret because trauma that causes neck pain also can cause brain injury and damage to peripheral otolith organs. In clinical practice, it is necessary to exclude neurologic, vestibular, and psychosomatic disorders before a disorder of the craniovertebral junction can be given serious consideration. The diagnosis of cervical vertigo remains largely theoretical.[84,85]

Disorders of the Craniovertebral Junction

Disorders of the craniovertebral junction are poorly understood and relatively uncommon. The patients frequently are referred for

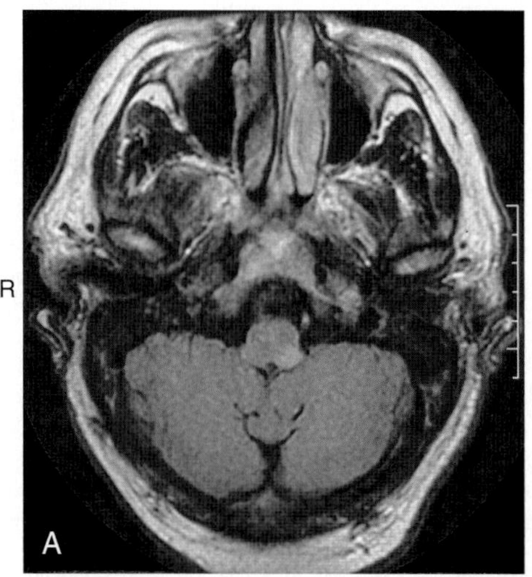

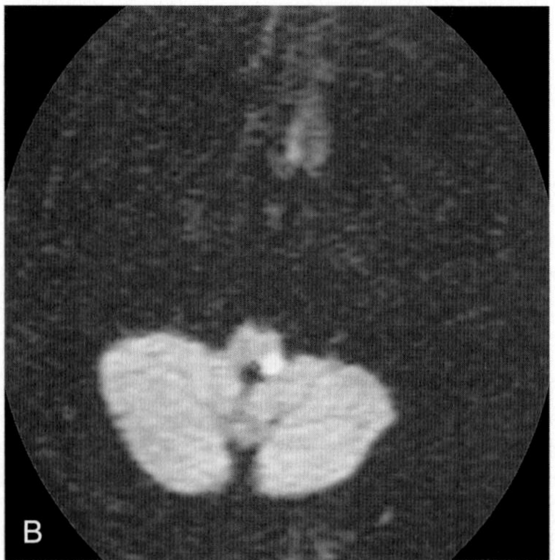

Figure 166-8. Magnetic resonance imaging of a lateral medullary infarction. **A,** Image obtained using the fluid-attenuated inversion recovery (FLAIR) sequence. **B,** Image obtained using a diffusion-weighted sequence. Both show changes of an acute infarction involving the left dorsolateral medulla. *(Courtesy of K. D. Flemming.)*

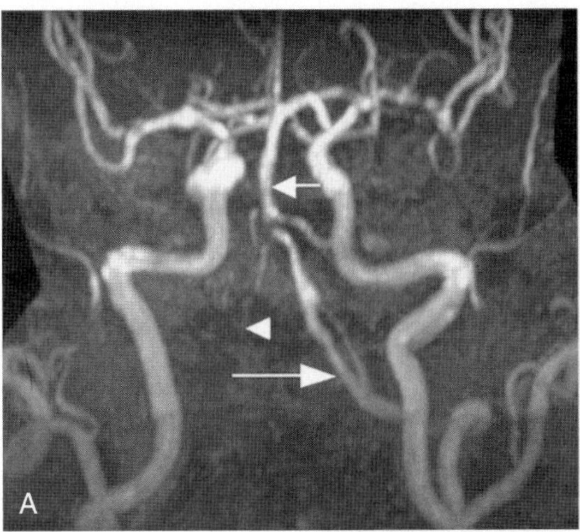

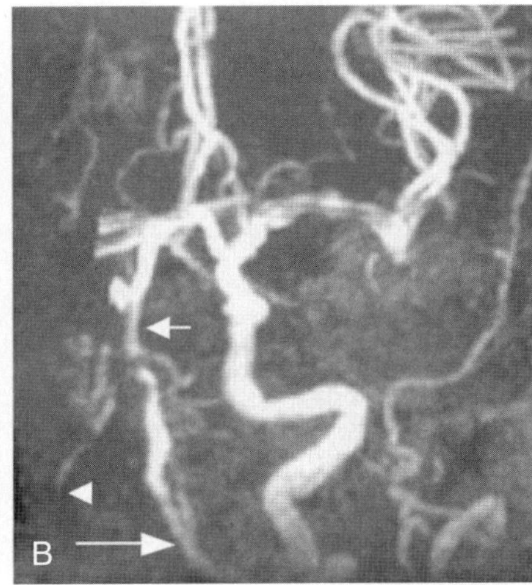

Figure 166-9. Contrast-enhanced magnetic resonance angiogram showing stenosis of the cervical vessels. **A,** Frontal view. **B,** Lateral view. Severe stenosis can be seen at the junction of the left vertebral artery *(long arrow)* and the basilar artery *(short arrow)*. The right distal vertebral artery also is occluded *(arrowhead)*. *(From Lee H. Sudden bilateral simultaneous deafness with vertigo as a sole manifestation of vertebrobasilar insufficiency.* J Neurol Neurosurg Psychiatry. *2003;74:540.)*

surgical evaluation because of brainstem or lower cranial nerve signs and symptoms such as tinnitus, vertigo, hearing loss, pharyngeal dysfunction, hoarseness, or airway obstruction. Physical examination can be difficult and misleading, and radiographic findings often are not sufficient to establish a diagnosis. An understanding of these disorders may facilitate appropriate evaluation and prevention of inappropriate management such as middle ear exploration and endolymphatic sac surgery.

Pathophysiology

The physiologic problem common to these disorders is physical compression of the CNS at the level of the upper spinal cord and medulla (cervicomedullary compression).[86-88] The rostrocaudal area of compression is variable, and the impingement can be ventral or dorsal, or (rarely) both. A second but uncommon potential mechanism is vascular insufficiency of the anterior spinal or vertebral arteries from angulation, stretching, or extrinsic obstruction.[89,90]

Classification

Basilar Impression

Basilar impression is an upward indentation or invagination of the clivus or posterior fossa floor.[86,91] This defect causes the upper cervical spine to migrate cephalad toward the brainstem, as the floor of the skull collapses under the weight of the head. The normal anatomy of the foramen magnum, first cervical vertebra (atlas), second cervical vertebra (axis), and its odontoid process (dens) can become altered by disease, trauma, or congenital deformities. When a softening of the skull base results, the skull literally descends onto the spinal column and odontoid. As the odontoid projects intracranially, it compresses the ventral aspect of the medulla.

Associated erosive changes of the occipital condyles and atlas accentuate the protrusion of the odontoid, narrow the diameter and circumference of the foramen magnum and spinal canal, and provide mechanisms for dorsal cervicomedullary compression. The odontoid not only projects above the foramen magnum but also occupies a large portion of its circumference.

Disorders known to cause basilar impression include Paget's disease, rheumatoid arthritis, osteomalacia, osteogenesis imperfecta, cretinism, and rickets.[86] The diagnosis is confirmed when lateral radiographic views of the skull demonstrate that the tip of the odontoid either extends above Chamberlain's line (a line extending from the posterior edge of the hard palate to the posterior lip of the foramen magnum)[92] or projects posterior to Wackenheim's clivus-canal line. The term *platybasia* has been used synonymously with *basilar artery impression* by some authors. Although the two conditions coexist, platybasia itself causes no symptoms.

Assimilation of the Atlas

Assimilation of the atlas (also called *occipitalization of the atlas*) is a bony union between the first cervical vertebra and the skull.[93] The amount of union varies, but motion between the two structures does not occur. As a result, the odontoid often impinges on the effective anteroposterior diameter of the foramen. A frequent associated finding is fusion of the axis to the third cervical vertebra. The condition is frequently developmental in origin and is found in association with abnormalities of the jaw, cleft palate, auricular deformities, cervical ribs, and urinary tract anomalies.[94] Klippel-Feil syndrome is one of the most common causes of cervical vertebral fusion.

Signs and symptoms of this syndrome are variable and typically appear fairly late and progress slowly. Symptoms may involve the brainstem, cerebellum, spinal cord, or lower cervical nerve roots or the vascular supply to these structures. These symptoms frequently precipitate a visit to a neurologist, but vertigo, facial paresis, dysphagia, hearing loss, and tongue atrophy may bring some patients to an otolaryngologist for initial evaluation. Although the disorder can be diagnosed with CT reconstructions, the key to diagnosis often is MRI, which allows direct coronal and sagittal imaging.[95]

Atlantoaxial Dislocation

During flexion and extension of the neck, congenital fusion of the occiput to the atlas increases the strain on the structures that normally restrict the motion of the atlas on the axis, especially if fusion of other cervical vertebrae also is present. The transverse ligaments that normally secure the odontoid against the anterior aspect of the arch of the atlas may weaken because of this repeated strain, and the resultant laxity allows the odontoid to move posteriorly into the lumen of the foramen magnum with neck flexion. Flexion or extension of the neck may then produce symptoms, depending on whether the predominant neural compression is anterior from the odontoid or posterior from the posterior arch of C1. When the atlas or congenital cervical fusion has been assimilated, the transverse odontoid ligament is sometimes hypoplastic, which makes laxity and atlantoaxial dislocation even more likely.

Atlantoaxial instability is associated with a number of congenital and acquired disease processes. It occurs in 10% to 30% of patients with Down syndrome when diagnosed radiographically, with an atlantodens interval of 4 to 5 mm.[96,97] The condition also is associated with spondyloepiphyseal dysplasia, Hurler's syndrome, and Morquio syndrome, and in those with achondroplastic dwarfism. A high incidence of atlantoaxial instability, resulting from destruction of the normal

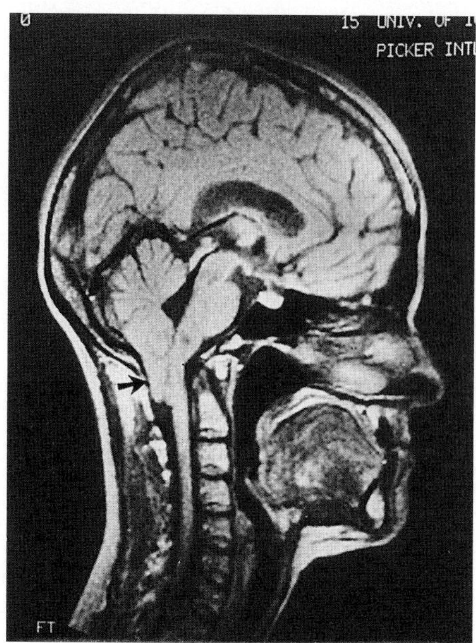

Figure 166-10. Magnetic resonance image of the head of a patient with Chiari type I malformation. Cerebellar tonsils *(arrow)* can be seen below the foramen magnum.

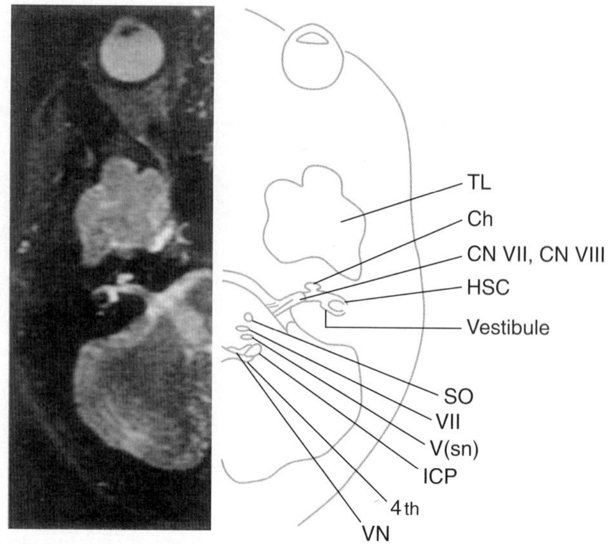

Figure 166-11. Axial T2-weighted brainstem magnetic resonance image showing high signal intensity in the region of the eighth nerve root-entry zone. Note that the vestibular nuclei appeared to be spared. Shown for comparison is a line drawing with major anatomic structures labeled. 4th, fourth ventricle; Ch, cochlea; CN VII, seventh cranial nerve; CN VIII, eighth cranial nerve; HSC, horizontal semicircular canal; ICP, inferior cerebellar peduncle; SO, superior olive; TL, temporal lobe; VII, facial nucleus; V(sn), spinal nucleus of the trigeminal tract; VN, vestibular nuclei. *(From Furman JM, Durrant JD, Hirsch WL. Eighth nerve signs in a case of multiple sclerosis.* Am J Otolaryngol. *1989;10:376-381.)*

stabilizing mechanisms by inflammatory tissue, has been reported in patients with rheumatoid arthritis.[98] Similarly, ligamentous laxity can result from inflammatory conditions affecting the retropharyngeal soft tissues or cervical bony structures, such as osteitis, retropharyngeal abscess, or lymphadenitis. Atlantoaxial instability in association with pharyngeal infection has come to be known as Grisel's syndrome.[99] It is rare in adults and associated with pain and dysphagia.

Most patients with atlantoaxial instability of developmental origin are asymptomatic, and the instability does not usually worsen with time.[97] Symptoms and signs develop in only 1% to 2% of patients with Down syndrome and usually appear between the ages of 5 and 15 years. Neck pain, sensory deficits, and difficulty with bladder control have been described; more subtle manifestations include decreased activity tolerance, changes in gait, and hyperreflexia.

Chiari Malformation

Chiari malformations are a group of developmental hindbrain and spinal cord abnormalities characterized by hernation of the contents of the posterior cranial fossa caudally through the foramen magnum into the upper cervical spine. These patients may present with symptoms related to the vestibular system such as ataxia, nystagmus, or vertigo.[100] Chiari malformation can be divided into two forms, type I and type II. The Chiari type I malformation is more common and more mild. Symptoms of Chiari type I usually are delayed until the age of 25 to 35 years. Affected persons often have subtle neurologic symptoms that are not associated with other developmental defects. Diagnosis is made by CT or MR images reconstructed in the sagittal plane, which may demonstrate deformation of the cerebellar tonsils more than 5 mm caudally through the foramen magnum (Fig. 166-10). The Chiari type II malformation manifests in the first few months of life with associated hydrocephalus and other CNS malformations such as meningomyelocele.

Classic presentation symptoms of Chiari type I malformation include upper extremity weakness, sensory loss, and pain. Occipital headaches that are exacerbated by coughing sneezing, bending over, or lifting also are a common presenting feature. Ataxia and nystagmus are reported in 24% of patients, with vertigo being a complaint in only 8%.[101] Patients also may have a vestibular test profile consistent with peripheral dysfunction but remain asymptomatic.[100] These patients also may present to the otolaryngologist with difficulty swallowing, aspiration, or hoarseness due to involvement of the lower cranial nerves (cranial nerves IX through XII).

Multiple Sclerosis

Multiple sclerosis (MS) is an inflammatory demyelinating CNS disorder of idiopathic origin with the onset in early adulthood. The disease affects women twice as often as men. The key to diagnosis is the presence of disseminated signs of CNS dysfunction manifested in an alternating and remitting and exacerbating course. Many symptoms can occur, depending on the location of the lesions. Vertigo is the initial symptom of MS in only approximately 5% of patients, although the symptom may be present in as many as one half of these patients at some point in the course of the disease.[102] Lesions within the vestibular nuclei and in the entry zone of cranial nerve VIII represent the most common locations for demyelinating activity to cause vertigo in patients with MS[103] (Fig. 166-11). However, benign paroxysmal positional vertigo remains the most common cause of vertigo in these patients,[104] as in the general population.

The diagnosis of MS remains a clinical one, with no definitive imaging study or laboratory tests.[105] Abnormalities in CSF can be identified in as many as 90% of patients with MS at some point in the course of the disease. Findings included increased gamma globulin level, oligoclonal banding of gamma globulin, and increased myelin basic protein. MRI demonstrates white matter lesions in more than 90% of patients, although similar lesions occasionally are seen in patients without MS.[106]

MS is treated with disease-modifying and symptomatic therapies. Intravenous methylprednisolone 500 to 1000 mg/day for 3 to 5 days is commonly used to hasten recovery from acute exacerbations. Drugs such as interferon-beta 1a and 1b and copolymer 1 are immunomodulating drugs that alter the natural history of MS. They reduce the relapse rate and the appearance of new MRI lesions and slow the progression. Other medications are used to treat symptoms of spasticity, neurogenic bladder, and fatigue.

Cerebellar Ataxia Syndromes

Recurrent or progressive ataxia is the primary neurologic deficit in several well-defined hereditary and sporadic degenerative disorders. Abnormal nystagmus is common and may be one of several categories, including gaze paretic nystagmus and rebound nystagmus. The central nature of this symptom is almost always clear owing to the gait disturbances, dysarthria, tremor, and bradykinesias; accordingly, these patients rarely present to otolaryngologists. Impaired vestibular function usually is not symptomatic, although it may be found on clinical tests.

Friedreich's ataxia, the most common hereditary ataxia, is of autosomal recessive inheritance and usually is caused by a GAA repeat expansion in the frataxin gene. The onset of symptoms usually is before 20 years but may be as late as the sixth decade. Classically, its distinguishing features include an axonal sensory neuropathy with areflexia, Babinski sign, dysarthria, diabetes, and cardiomyopathy, although genetic testing has expanded the phenotypic range. Reduced vestibulo-ocular reflex gain is common, and saccadic intrusions (square-wave jerks) are characteristic. Rarer causes of recessively inherited ataxias include ataxia-telangiectasia, abetalipoproteinemia, and Refsum's disease. Ataxia is a feature of many other inborn metabolic and mitochondrial disorders.

Spinocerebellar atrophy encompasses a group of disorders in which cerebellar ataxia is a prominent feature. Many different genetically inherited subtypes have been identified by genetic linkage analysis.[107]

Cerebellar atrophy is characterized by gradual onset of ataxia, without other associated signs, beginning later in life. The disorder can be genetic or sporadic. Vestibular testing often reveals rebound nystagmus and spontaneous vertical nystagmus.[108]

Familiar episodic ataxia is an uncommon ataxia with a dominant inheritance pattern characterized by recurrent vertigo and ataxia. Episodes of ataxia often are triggered by stress, last minutes to hours, and begin between early childhood and early adulthood. Symptoms are markedly reduced or eliminated by acetazolamide.[109]

Paraneoplastic cerebellar degeneration (PCD) typically manifests as a subacute, rapidly progressive cerebellar syndrome. The development of anti-Purkinje cell antibodies (PCAs) in patients with undiagnosed and otherwise asymptomatic malignancies may result in the syndrome of PCD. PCD typically begins fairly abruptly and progresses rapidly through several months, with cerebellar-type ocular motor and vestibular abnormalities, dysarthria, and severe appendicular and gait ataxia. The cerebellum is not directly invaded by tumor, but the tumor produces remote effects on the cerebellum that probably are immune-mediated. It most commonly occurs in patients with carcinoma of the lung (small cell), breast, ovary, and Hodgkin's lymphoma. However, the neurologic symptoms usually appear before the cancer is identified.[110]

Focal Seizure Disorders

Vertigo can be part of an aura of a focal seizure. Smith[111] studied a group of patients with vestibular symptoms as part of their aura. The most common vestibular symptom was a sense of spinning, which occurred in 55% of these patients, followed by a sense of linear translation in 30%. However, episodes of vertigo as isolated manifestations of a seizure disorder occur rarely, if ever.

Normal Pressure Hydrocephalus

Idiopathic normal pressure hydrocephalus classically manifests with the triad of dementia, urinary incontinence, and gait or balance disturbance. However, these symptoms represent the more severe end of the clinical spectrum, and more subtle cases can manifest with only mild gait or balance symptoms.[112] Cognitive symptoms also are common but may be mild. Patients usually become symptomatic after the age of 60 years. Diagnosis requires an imaging study that demonstrates nonobstructive ventricular enlargement disproportionate to the degree of cerebral atrophy.

Physiologic Dizziness

Physiologic dizziness refers to phenomena that occur in normal persons as a result of physiologic stimulation of the vestibular, visual, or somatosensory system. Typically a mismatch among sensory signals causes disorientation, imbalance, and vegetative symptoms.

Motion Sickness

Motion sickness is a common form of physiologic dizziness. The main symptoms are dizziness, fatigue, pallor, cold sweats, salivation, and finally nausea and vomiting. It usually is caused by prolonged vestibular stimulation but also may occur with visual stimulation. The key symptom is nausea, a term derived from the Greek *naus*, "ship." Motion sickness may develop aboard a ship, in a car, on an airplane, or in space. Symptoms generally are worse when subjects are not able to visualize the movement, thereby creating a visual-vestibular conflict. Relief may be gained on a ship by standing on the deck and focusing on the horizon or land, rather than sitting in an enclosed cabin. When riding in a car, riding in the back seat or reading may make symptoms worse than sitting in front and looking off into the distance. Susceptibility among affected persons varies considerably. Patients with migraine generally are more prone to motion sickness, and bouts of motion sickness during childhood may be the first symptom of migraine.

Physical measures may help prevent motion sickness. In the long term, repeated gradual exposure to motion causes protective habituation, which may be the most effective therapeutic measure. Minimizing conflicting sensory inputs by restricting unnecessary head movement (such as pressing the head firmly against the headrest of a car) is helpful, as is minimizing any visual-vestibular mismatch, as described earlier.

Anti–motion sickness drugs are aimed at modulating the histaminic, cholinergic, and noradrenergic neurotransmitters that are thought to be important in the neural processes of motion sickness. These drugs work by blocking the emetic response, reducing the size of the sensory mismatch by promoting habituation, or blocking conflicting sensory inputs.

Mal de Débarquement Syndrome

Mal de débarquement (MDD), "sickness of disembarkment," refers to inappropriate sensations of movement after exposure to motion. Although this unusual syndrome typically follows a sea voyage, MDD may occur after extended train, air, or car travel.[113] The characteristic symptom is a sensation of persistent rocking or swaying of the body without rotational vertigo. Vague dysequilibrium or unsteadiness also may be a feature. MDD is distinguished from motion sickness in that patients with MDD are mostly symptom-free during the period of motion. Although many normal persons experience similar symptoms of "land sickness" for up to 48 hours after exposure to prolonged motion, most experts define MDD as a syndrome persisting for at least a month. During symptomatic periods, patients typically report improvement while in a moving vehicle or while walking that is lost when they stop moving, when symptoms worsen. MDD affects predominantly women, with a mean age at onset in the 40s. Symptoms may last for months to years. Some investigators have hypothesized that MDD is caused by a multisensorimotor adaptation and habituation to a new or abnormal motion environment. Benzodiazepines such as clonazepam or diazepam or amitriptyline may have a beneficial effect, but meclizine and scopolamine were ineffective.[113]

SUGGESTED READINGS

Baloh RW. Clinical practice. Vestibular neuritis. *N Engl J Med.* 2003;348:1027-1032.

Baloh RW, Foster CA, Yue Q, et al. Familial migraine with vertigo and essential tremor. *Neurology.* 1996;46:458-460.

Bikhazi P, Jackson C, Ruckenstein MJ. Efficacy of antimigrainous therapy in the treatment of migraine-associated dizziness. *Am J Otol.* 1997;18:350-354.

Buchholz D, Reich SG. *Heal your headache.* New York: Workman Publishing; 2002.

Chen CC, et al. Posterior cranial fossa tumors in young adults. *Laryngoscope.* 2006;116:1678-1681.

Darnell RB, Posner JB. Paraneoplastic syndromes involving the nervous system. *N Engl J Med.* 2003;349:1543-1554.

Halmagyi GM, Curthoys IS. A clinical sign of canal paresis. *Arch Neurol.* 1988;45:737-739.

Harker LA, Rassekh CH. Episodic vertigo in basilar artery migraine. *Otolaryngol Had Neck Surg*. 1987;96:239.

Harker LA, Rassekh CH. Migraine equivalent as a cause of vertigo. *Laryngoscope*. 1988;98:160.

Hotson JR, Baloh RW. Acute vestibular syndrome. *N Engl J Med*. 1998;339:680-685.

Kentala E, Pyykko I. Vestibular schwannoma mimicking Meniere's disease. *Acta Otolaryngol Suppl*. 2000;543:17-19.

Neuhauser H, Leopold M, von Brevern M, et al. The interrelations of migraine, vertigo, and migrainous vertigo. *Neurology*. 2001;56:436-441.

Radtke A, Lempert T, Gresty MA, et al. Migraine and Meniere's disease: is there a link? *Neurology*. 2002;59:1700-1704.

Thomsen LL, Olesen J. Sporadic hemiplegic migraine. *Cephalalgia*. 2004; 24:1016-1023.

Viirre ES, Baloh RW. Migraine as a cause of sudden hearing loss. *Headache*. 1996;36:24.

For complete list of references log onto www.expertconsult.com.

CHAPTER ONE HUNDRED AND SIXTY-SEVEN

Surgery for Vestibular Disorders

Steven A. Telian

Key Points

- The otologist should recognize the vulnerability of patients with refractory vertigo, shelter them from nonvalidated treatments, and seek to guide them toward the most effective surgical options.
- Some operations seek to correct a pathologic process that is unique to a particular diagnosis, while preserving or restoring inner ear function. Success in this setting hinges on making an exact diagnosis and selecting procedures with proven efficacy.
- If a labyrinthine lesion is unstable or rapidly progressive in nature, central vestibular compensation is not possible unless the ear is first stabilized by medical or surgical management.
- The patient with recurrent vertigo refractory to conservative treatment is a candidate for a procedure that will ablate the residual vestibular function in the involved ear.
- Labyrinthectomy and vestibular nerve section will reliably ablate peripheral vestibular function and may be applied in the management of any unstable peripheral vestibular disorder.
- The endolymphatic sac is simply a specialized portion of the posterior fossa dura containing resorptive epithelium. Operations for decompression of the sac, with or without shunting, have a low efficacy rate but produce favorable results in some cases.
- It is not certain whether the observed benefits from sac decompression operations are due to a nonspecific effect of surgery or the decompression itself. Thus, if it is difficult to identify the sac, the prudent surgeon should never hesitate to terminate the procedure rather than risk a complication.
- Transmastoid labyrinthectomy is the gold standard procedure for surgical relief of vertigo from inner ear pathology but generally is reserved for patients who already have poor hearing in the involved ear.
- If hearing preservation is desired, selective vestibular nerve section procedures provide proven relief of vertigo for properly selected patients.
- If a patient describes a severe vestibular crisis at initial onset, without equally intense symptoms on any occasion since the original event, an uncompensated stable peripheral lesion is likely. Such patients are best treated with vestibular rehabilitation.
- Unilateral fluctuating or progressive sensorineural hearing loss is a strong indication of unstable inner ear function and is useful for lateralizing the offending ear.
- If uncertainty exists regarding which ear is causing vertigo, ablative surgery is not recommended. If the patient reports that vertigo spells are associated with auditory symptoms in the better ear, the second ear may have become involved, and surgery is ill-advised.

The otolaryngologist frequently is asked to evaluate a patient with intense vertigo or severe balance disturbance who has tried multiple medical treatments without success. Those who consider themselves disabled by their symptoms are eager, and often desperate, for relief. Although it is proper to consider surgical treatment in this setting, the physician should recognize that an unsuccessful surgical intervention may greatly aggravate the patient's discouragement regarding the disease, with the potential for alienation from the surgeon and from the medical profession in general. Recognizing the vulnerability of this patient population, the astute clinician seeks to guide the patient toward rational and effective surgical options when available, and to shelter them from nonvalidated medical or surgical treatments.

This chapter reviews the surgical procedures that are available for the management of vestibular disorders, with an emphasis on principles that promote understanding of the proper role and limitations of each procedure. Clinical application of these principles in patient selection can be expected to result in satisfactory outcomes in a high percentage of surgical procedures performed for dizziness.

Rationale for Surgery

When vertigo results from acute disturbances of the peripheral vestibular system, the patient will experience intense symptoms that gradually subside. If the lesion is self-limited and stable (e.g., acute viral labyrinthitis), it will not produce fluctuating or progressive dysfunction in the system. In this setting, the process of central vestibular compensation will reliably relieve dizziness in most patients by adjusting to the altered sensory inputs from the periphery. Similarly, ongoing vestibular compensation can minimize symptoms of vestibular loss from lesions that produce an insidious progressive deterioration, such as vestibular schwannoma. However, if the lesion is unstable or rapidly progressive in nature, central compensation is not possible unless the ear can be stabilized by medical or surgical management. Meniere's disease is the prototypical disorder in this category, wherein the ear fluctuates between normal labyrinthine function and dramatic cochleovestibular pathology. Accordingly, vestibular system surgery is most likely to succeed when it is undertaken to stabilize an unstable ear, either by correcting a defect that underlies the disorder or by ablating function in the pathologic ear.

Certain surgical procedures are applicable only for one particular diagnosis. Some of these operations are widely accepted as both rational and effective, such as repair of a superior semicircular canal dehiscence or operations for intractable benign paroxysmal positional vertigo. Other disease-specific operations, such as endolymphatic sac surgery for Meniere's disease, repair of perilymph fistula, and microvascular decompression of the eighth nerve, continue to generate controversy. All of these operations have as their unifying feature the goal of correcting a pathologic process that is unique to the particular diagnosis, while preserving or restoring inner ear function. Success in this setting hinges on making an exact diagnosis and selecting operations with proven efficacy. On the other hand, procedures such as labyrinthectomy and vestibular nerve section are designed to ablate unilateral vestibular function and may be applied in the management of any peripheral vestibular disorder. In this setting, an etiologic diagnosis is less critical. Instead, the physician must be certain that the problem is attributable to ongoing fluctuating or rapidly progressive labyrinthine dysfunction and that the pathologic ear has been correctly identified.

Procedures for Benign Paroxysmal Positional Vertigo

Benign paroxysmal positional vertigo (BPPV) most often affects the posterior semicircular canal. Variations of this condition affecting any of the three semicircular canals have now been recognized, as discussed in Chapters 164 and 165. BPPV seems to be caused by displaced otoconial debris within the membranous labyrinth. The original pathogenic hypothesis proposed that otoconial debris became lodged within the ampulla of the posterior semicircular canal (cupulolithiasis), rendering it sensitive to gravity. In the early 1990s, evidence accumulated to support the concept of otoconia floating freely in the membranous canal (canalithiasis).[1-3] These particles within the semicircular canal are purported to cause a transient flow of endolymph after a change in head position, producing a deviation of the cupula and triggering a change in the neural firing rate in the vestibular nerve. The brain perceives this change as rotation in the plane of the semicircular canal, with resulting vertigo and nystagmus. This theory is largely confirmed by the favorable results of particle repositioning maneuvers and the posterior canal occlusion procedure. It also better satisfies the conceptual framework for the biomechanics of BPPV originally suggested in the 1970s by McCabe and Ryu.[4] Although cupulolithiasis may certainly result in vestibular symptoms, this entity occurs much less frequently.

Before surgical procedures for BPPV are considered, it should be recognized that this condition has a high rate of spontaneous resolution and also is highly responsive to management by physical therapy interventions. Surgery is rarely required and should be reserved for refractory or multiply-recurrent cases. Nonsurgical management options[5] include traditional habituation exercises, Brandt-Daroff exercises, the liberatory maneuver of Semont, and particle repositioning techniques popularized by Epley and Parnes. A detailed discussion of these management options is provided in Chapters 163 and 165.

Singular Neurectomy

Gacek and Gacek[6] have advocated the singular neurectomy procedure for BPPV. This procedure involves selective transection of the branch of the inferior vestibular nerve innervating the posterior canal ampulla. The nerve is interrupted within the singular canal, which travels from the posterior portion of the internal auditory canal to the posterior canal ampulla (Fig. 167-1). This procedure is a highly rational choice for management of intractable posterior canal BPPV, because it is safer and more specific than a complete section of the vestibular nerve. However, this procedure is demanding technically and should not be undertaken unless the surgeon has mastered the approach in the temporal bone dissection laboratory. Gacek has performed 74% of the

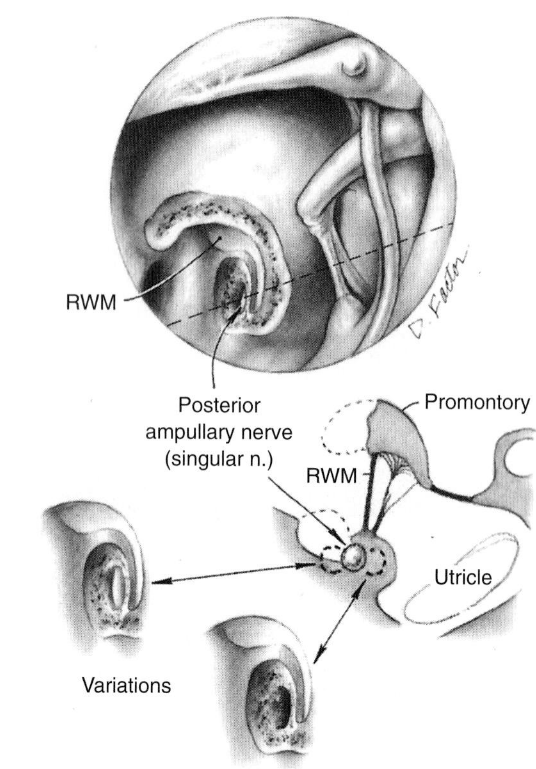

Figure 167-1. Singular neurectomy. After exposure of the round window membrane (RWM), the singular nerve is exposed inferior to the posterosuperior portion of RWM. Three variations in location of the nerve are illustrated in the vertical section taken along the broken line.

reported cases in the world literature, with preservation of hearing in 97% of the operated patients; other investigators report poor hearing results with this procedure.[7]

For this procedure, a tympanomeatal flap is elevated using a transcanal approach, and the bony lip of the round window niche is removed to visualize the round window membrane itself. The surgeon approaches the singular canal by drilling at a site inferior to the round window. Ideally, the nerve is transected just before its point of entry into the ampulla. The ampulla itself and the vestibule are at risk for injury during the procedure, and injury of either structure may result in severe vertigo and sensorineural hearing loss. One study suggested that the nerve measures approximately 5 mm in length and is best accessed by drilling approximately 0.7 mm posteroinferiorly to the posteromedial margin of the round window membrane after saucerization of the niche.[8] This study also found that whereas the average depth of the nerve was 1.5 mm, the posterior canal ampulla, the cochlear aqueduct, and the inferior cochlear vein were all within 2 mm of the preferred drilling point, which highlights the dangers of this approach. Another study showed that the nerve was always at least 0.7 mm from the edge of the exposed round window membrane, with an average depth of 1.3 mm.[9] Transtympanic access was believed to be straightforward in only 20% of specimens and impossible in 28%. This procedure has largely been supplanted by the technically simpler semicircular canal occlusion procedure.

Posterior Semicircular Canal Occlusion

Parnes and McClure[2] introduced the concept of surgical occlusion of the posterior semicircular canal for the relief of BPPV. Conceptually, the canal occlusion procedure is based on the assumption that otoconial debris, originally from the macula of the utricle, settles into the endolymphatic space of the posterior semicircular canal and produces the signs and symptoms of BPPV.

The surgery is conducted to obstruct the bony lumen of the dome of the posterior semicircular canal without disruption of the membra-

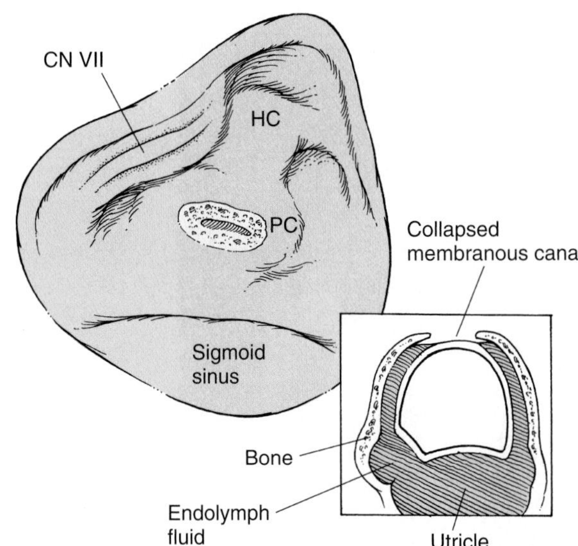

Figure 167-2. Posterior semicircular canal occlusion. After transmastoid exposure of the posterior semicircular canal, the bony lumen is opened and obstructed, with care to avoid disrupting the collapsed membranous canal (inset). CN VII, seventh cranial nerve; HC, horizontal semicircular canal; PC, posterior semicircular canal with fenestration.

nous labyrinth (see Fig. 167-2). After a complete mastoidectomy is performed, the horizontal semicircular canal is identified. The dome of the posterior semicircular canal is then identified between the horizontal canal and the posterior fossa dural plate. The lumen of the posterior canal is approached with a diamond drill until it is visible as a dark line through a thin layer of residual bone. The lumen is opened by removing the remaining thin bone over the canal lumen using delicate instrumentation, with care taken to avoid damaging the membranous canal or suctioning fluid from the perilymphatic space. The perilymph is gently removed by placing a wick of absorbent material near the labyrinthotomy site, causing the membranous semicircular canal to collapse against the deep wall of the bony canal lumen. The canal may then be occluded by placing small plugs of periosteum into the canal, one toward the ampulla and one toward the common crus. The labyrinthotomy is repaired by filling the lumen with wet bone dust harvested during the mastoidectomy. This material can be secured in position by placing bone wax or a piece of connective tissue over the dome of the canal.

The patient may have mild to moderate unsteadiness after the procedure but usually is fit for discharge from the hospital within 24 to 48 hours. A small risk of reactive labyrinthitis and sensorineural hearing loss is associated with the need to open the bony labyrinth. Approximately 15% of patients have protracted postoperative dysequilibrium, but vertigo control rates approach 100%, and hearing loss is uncommon.[10] Dizziness Handicap Inventory scores are reduced significantly, and patient satisfaction is 85%.[11]

Surgery for Superior Semicircular Canal Dehiscence

Minor[12] first described the syndrome of superior semicircular canal dehiscence (SSCD) in 2000. Further detailed characterization and recommendations for treatment have evolved since that ground-breaking report. Morphometric evidence indicates that SSCD may be associated with generalized reduction in the thickness of the squamous portion of the temporal bone,[13] which would predispose affected patients to middle fossa superior semicircular canal defects and explain the frequent association with natural dehiscences of the tegmen tympani and mastoideum. Aural pressure and unusual sensitivity to bone-conducted sounds are common complaints. Patients frequently report autophony, so this condition must be distinguished from the patulous eustachian tube. Vestibular symptoms typically are transient and are induced by loud sounds or any activity that leads to a transient increase in intracranial pressure. Some patients also report chronic dysequilibrium. Eye movements that are characteristic of superior semicircular canal stimulation may be seen in response to applied pressure stimuli—specifically, a torsional downward deviation of the eye. Vestibular evoked myogenic potential (VEMP) thresholds are reduced and amplitudes elevated in the setting of open dehiscence. Auditory findings include an apparent conductive or mixed hearing loss with a significant low-frequency conductive component. The apparent conductive hearing loss is believed to be caused by shunting of air-conducted acoustic energy away from the basilar membrance within the cochlea toward the dehiscence, which is functioning as a third mobile window.[14] It is essential to distinguish this condition audiometrically from otosclerosis by requesting testing for supranormal thresholds (often better than 0 dB) on bone conduction audiometry, and for the presence of acoustic reflexes.[15]

In cases in which clinical symptoms and test results suggest this diagnosis, high-resolution computed tomography (CT) of the temporal bone is indicated in an effort to visualize a dehiscence of the canal at the dural interface in the floor of the middle cranial fossa. These studies should be performed in a parasagittal plane orthogonal to the superior canal (Fig. 167-3). Generally, the dehiscence is repaired through a middle cranial fossa craniotomy, and evidence is mounting that disrupting the canal by obstructive plugging is superior to a simple repair ("resurfacing") of the defect.[16] Plugging of the SSCD reliably relieves vertigo symptoms and reduces the gain of the angular vestibulo-ocular reflex (VOR) by an average of 44% for the superior canal, along with a modest 10% reduction for the ipislateral posterior canal.[17] The procedure will resolve most of the auditory symptoms, but results are less predictable than those for vestibular symptoms. Care should be taken to avoid suctioning perilymph from the dehiscence during surgery; plugging may be accomplished with tissue plugs supported by bone chips or bone paté. In carefully selected patients, it may be possible to repair the dehiscence using a transmastoid approach, obviating the need for a craniotomy.[18]

Repair of Perilymphatic Fistula

Perilymphatic fistula is a controversial diagnosis that centers on the phenomenon of perilymph leaking from the inner ear into the middle ear cleft through the oval window, round window, or other abnormally patent fissures in the bony labyrinth.[19] A perilymph fistula may develop after stapedectomy surgery, penetrating middle ear trauma, head trauma, or barotrauma.[20] Uncertainty regarding the clinical criteria for the diagnosis and the inability to document the presence of a microfistula at surgery contribute to the problematic nature of this diagnosis.[21] Most authors agree that acute perilymph fistulas generally heal spontaneously, so a 2- to 3-day period of bedrest initially is appropriate. With suspected fistula after penetrating trauma, early exploration is indicated to preserve residual hearing, unless complete hearing loss is already present at diagnosis. In suspected chronic cases, a trial of vestibular rehabilitation before middle ear exploration may be appropriate if the diagnosis is uncertain, particularly if the hearing is stable.

Some investigators have attempted to use β-2 transferrin in fluids collected from the middle ear to support a clinical diagnosis of perilymph fistula, but results have been conflicting using this protein as a marker for perilymph.[22,23] Unpublished data from my laboratory suggest that assays for β-2 transferrin used for identification of cerebrospinal fluid leak are not sensitive enough to detect this protein in only 1 to 2 μL of perilymph. On the other hand, exquisitely sensitive assays will detect trace amounts that are present in serum, which could lead to false-positive results. Accordingly, use of this technique in an effort to confirm this diagnosis is not recommended.

An exploratory tympanotomy for perilymph fistula should be undertaken with use of local anesthesia and mild sedation whenever possible, so that the patient may be enlisted to perform the Valsalva maneuver to help identify perilymph leaks. After a tympanomeatal flap is elevated, bone is removed from the posterior superior wall of the bony external auditory canal until the oval window is completely visible. Likewise, it may be wise to remove any mucosal folds and the

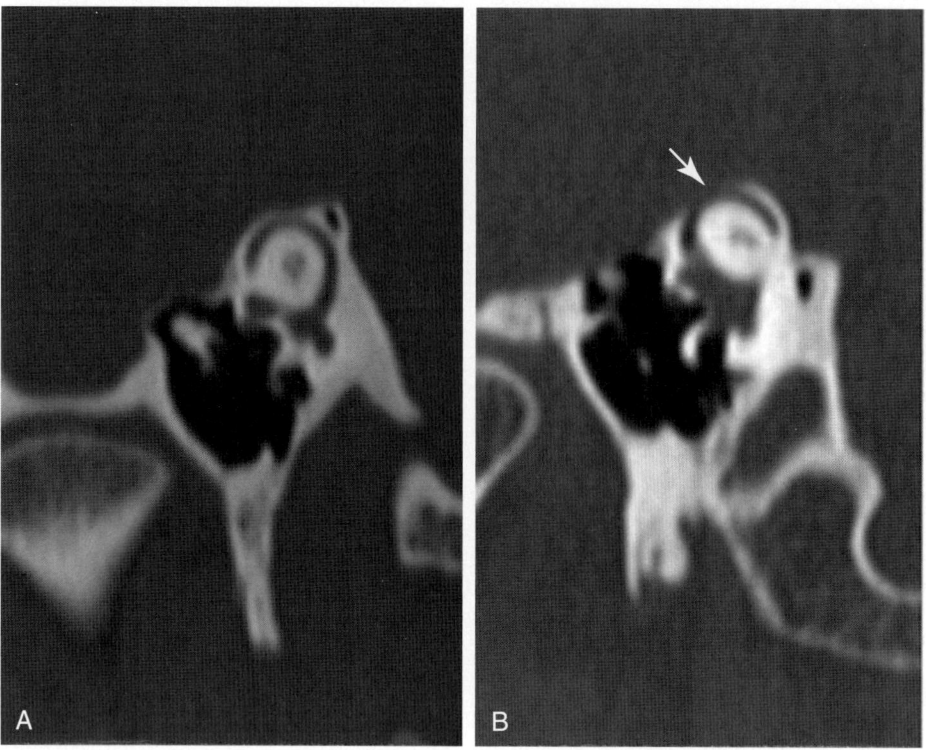

Figure 167-3. Superior canal dehiscence is best confirmed on a parasagittal computed tomography (CT) image obtained in the plane orthogonal to the superior canal. **A** shows a normal canal, with the *arrow* in **B** indicating a dehiscence.

bony overhang of the round window niche to better visualize the round window membrane. It is rare to see a dramatic defect in the oval or round window in routine perilymph fistula explorations. Fluid may be suctioned from the niche to see if it reaccumulates, although this phenomenon is common and does not verify that a perilymph fistula is present. Poe and Bottrill[24] have added credence to the suggestion that pooling of clear fluid in the oval or round window is due to transudation or to dependent accumulation of local anesthetic solutions. They performed transtympanic endoscopy of the middle ear before raising a tympanomeatal flap, and documented that fluid was not evident in the windows until after injection of the local anesthetic solution. In fact, endoscopic visualization of the middle ear could supplant formal tympanotomy for diagnosis of this disorder. The ear also should be inspected for abnormally patent fissures in the bony labyrinth, especially anterior to the oval window and inferior to the round window. Any suspicious defect should be repaired by removing surrounding mucosa and patching with connective tissue, secured by packing. My own practice is to routinely patch the round window niche in explorations with negative findings, but a more conservative approach is indicated in the oval window region to avoid the risk of an iatrogenic conductive hearing loss.

Specific Operations for Meniere's Disease

Meniere's disease is characterized clinically by the complex of recurrent episodic vertigo, fluctuating sensorineural hearing loss, tinnitus, and a subjective sense of aural fullness. If the diagnosis is uncertain, the indications for surgical procedures designed to address this specific disorder are less straightforward. The general teaching is that surgery is reserved for patients with "intractable vertigo in whom medical therapy has failed." Experience suggests that otologists differ significantly in their standards for determining medical failure. Some clinicians require that the patient experience 6 to 12 months of frequent and severe spells of vertigo before surgery is undertaken; others are willing to proceed more quickly. These differences are important to consider in evaluating uncontrolled clinical studies of surgical efficacy, especially in light of the spontaneous remissions that characterize this disorder.

A less invasive alternate treatment for Meniere's disease, intratympanic gentamicin injection, has become an accepted alternative to ablative surgery.[25-27] Uncontrolled reports of success with intratympanic corticosteroids are accumulating, but higher-quality studies of efficacy in this disorder are needed.[28] Therapy with a novel mechanical device, the Meniett device (Medtronic Xomed, Jacksonville, Florida), has demonstrated a significant reduction of episodic vertigo among surgical candidates in a placebo-controlled randomized clinical trial.[29] This therapy involves insertion of a tympanostomy tube in the affected ear, with subsequent application of intermittent pulsatile overpressure to the inner ear in 5-minute treatment cycles three times daily. Sustained remissions were typical, and only 24% elected to proceed to surgical treatment within 2 years.[30]

When a decision is made to proceed with surgery, questions arise regarding the choice of operation. Although vestibular nerve section or labyrinthectomy should reliably relieve vertigo related to Meniere's disease, these procedures ablate residual function in the affected ear. The ideal procedure for Meniere's disease would restore normal function, or at least preserve residual function, while stabilizing the ear. As discussed next, two operative procedures have been proposed to achieve this goal: cochleosacculotomy and endolymphatic sac surgery.

Cochleosacculotomy

The cochlear endolymphatic shunt procedure, usually referred to as *cochleosacculotomy*, is designed to create a permanent communication to equilibrate endolymphatic and perilymphatic pressures in the hydropic ear.[31] The goal is to create a small permanent fistula in the osseous spiral lamina within the basal turn of the cochlea. This is performed by elevating a tympanomeatal flap and exposing the round window niche. A 3-mm right-angle pick is inserted through the round window membrane and directed toward the oval window niche, hugging the lateral wall of the inner ear (Fig. 167-4), and fracturing the osseous spiral lamina. As might be expected, the operation has been associated with a 25% incidence of high-frequency sensorineural hearing loss and a 10% incidence of profound deafness.[32] Despite reports of 70% success with long-term relief of vertigo, the operation

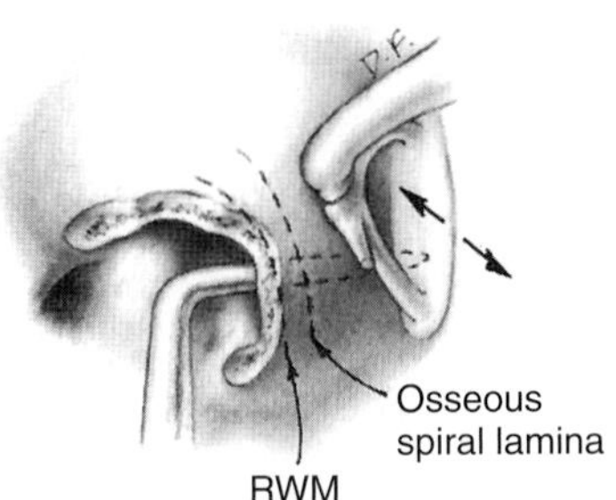

Figure 167-4. Cochleosacculotomy. Bony overhang of round window niche is removed to allow insertion of 3-mm, right-angle hook through the osseous spiral lamina of the basal end of the cochlea. Penetration of the tip of the hook can be monitored by movement of the stapes footplate. RWM, level of round window membrane.

has enjoyed only limited application. In one series of elderly patients with Meniere's disease, vertigo control was documented in almost every patient, but hearing was almost universally worse.[33] The study authors recommended that this operation be used as an alternative to labyrinthectomy in elderly patients with preexisting severe hearing loss.

Endolymphatic Sac Surgery

Although the specific physiologic defect causing Meniere's disease is unclear, many investigators report a beneficial effect in uncontrolled studies of surgical intervention directed toward the endolymphatic sac in patients with Meniere's disease. The first operative procedure on the endolymphatic sac was performed by Portmann.[34] Many modifications have been proposed, including bony decompression of the sac by Shambaugh,[35] placement of an endolymphatic-subarachnoid shunt by House,[36] and an endolymphatic-mastoid shunt by Shea.[37] Complications of endolymphatic sac procedures include hearing loss, cerebrospinal fluid leak, and facial nerve paralysis, although they are infrequent.

The efficacy of endolymphatic sac procedures has been widely questioned and debated. Some investigators suggest that the operation is ill-conceived and that the reported results may be biased or reflect a nonspecific effect of the operative undertaking or the natural history of this spontaneously remitting condition.[38,39] Evidence of a nonspecific effect of anesthesia on Meniere's disease has been provided by Gates,[40] who documented in a prospective observational trial that administration of a potent neuroleptic analgesic (Innovar) provided lasting relief of vertigo for most patients in whom medical management had failed to produce improvement. Advocates of sac surgery argue that a 50% to 70% success rate improves on the anticipated natural history in this patient population, making an endolymphatic sac procedure preferable to immediate use of an ablative procedure.[41] One uncontrolled observational study suggested that vertigo and vestibular disability could be largely corrected in 90% of patients evaluated 2 years after wide bony decompression of the sac and sigmoid sinus.[42] An important randomized clinical trial performed in Denmark during the 1970s compared endolymphatic sac decompression with a "sham" cortical mastoidectomy operation. The patients and those evaluating the outcomes were blinded to group assignment. Multiple subsequent reports were published, culminating with a 9-year follow-up report.[43] Both surgical groups demonstrated improvements that were not statistically different, and the investigators concluded that clinical improvement with decreased vertigo was attributable to a "placebo effect." The conclusions of this study have been widely debated, with proponents of sac surgery arguing that the sample size was too small to detect clinically important differences and pointing out that both groups did improve, thus arguing in favor of the operation even if the effect was nonspecific. Welling and Nagaraja[44] reanalyzed the data from this study by more sophisticated modern statistical methods. They demonstrated from the original data set that, even with the small sample size, the sac surgery group showed statistically significant reductions in postoperative vertigo, nausea and vomiting, and tinnitus compared with the mastoidectomy control group. Unfortunately, because the study did not include a nonsurgical control group, the potentially important influence of disease natural history on the reported efficacy could not be assessed. The Danish group performed another small controlled study comparing endolymphatic sac decompression and insertion of a tympanostomy tube, demonstrating that both groups had similar levels of improvement.[45] Again, a nonsurgical control group was not used.

One difficulty in performing vertigo outcome studies has been a lack of validated metrics for measuring treatment outcome. A previously validated medical quality-of-life instrument, the SF-36, has been demonstrated to correlate well with the 1995 disease reporting classification[44] proposed by the American Academy of Otolaryngology–Head and Neck Surgery (AAO-HNS).[46] The study showed that preoperative patients scored well below population norms, and that those achieving AAO-HNS class A or B outcomes (vertigo relief) normalized their scores. Alternative metrics have been proposed for future prospective studies that are more specific to Meniere's disease.[47,48]

In the absence of properly controlled clinical trials, the otologist should perform a critical review of the literature before recommending endolymphatic sac procedures. Several specific issues warrant consideration: Is endolymphatic sac surgery sufficiently efficacious for control of vertigo in patients who are eager for reliable results? If so, do the results deteriorate over time? Is the efficacy of sac surgery reported in uncontrolled observational studies inflated, in view of the retrospective nature of the studies? Is most of the observed benefit attributable to the placebo effect or to another nonspecific effect of surgery? The available evidence seems to indicate that endolymphatic sac surgery has not been demonstrated to be a sufficiently reliable surgical treatment for Meniere's disease. Continued uncertainty about these issues after decades of clinical experience underscores the need for properly controlled multi-institutional clinical trials to address the role of endolymphatic sac surgery in Meniere's disease.

The surgical approach to the endolymphatic sac begins with a cortical mastoidectomy. Once the antrum is exposed, it is wise to copiously irrigate the cavity and temporarily obstruct the aditus ad antrum to prevent bone dust from accumulating in the middle ear, which can result in a delayed conductive hearing loss from fixation of the ossicular chain. The bony labyrinth, particularly the posterior semicircular canal, should be positively identified before any bone is removed from the posterior fossa dura.

The endolymphatic sac is simply a specialized portion of the posterior fossa dura that contains the resorptive epithelium of the membranous labyrinth. It is connected to the vestibule by the endolymphatic duct, which travels in the vestibular aqueduct through the bony labyrinth medial to the posterior semicircular canal and then parallel to the common crus of the posterior and superior semicircular canals. The entrance of the endolymphatic sac into the vestibular aqueduct is a helpful surgical landmark in seeking to identify the sac. It is located roughly at the point where a hypothetical line parallel to the horizontal semicircular canal bisects the dome of the posterior semicircular canal (Donaldson's line). In seeking to identify the sac, this critical landmark should be remembered, because the endolymphatic sac is always inferior to this line. As indicated by my own experience performing surgical procedures after previous "endolymphatic sac decompression" failures, a not uncommon finding in such cases is that this area of the temporal bone was not previously dissected, so that the sac was never actually identified or decompressed.

The endolymphatic sac is bounded superiorly by Donaldson's line, posteriorly by the sigmoid sinus, anteroinferiorly by the jugular bulb, and laterally by the descending (mastoid) portion of the facial nerve. This region of the temporal bone may be poorly pneumatized, because there seems to be an association between Meniere's disease and underdevelopment of this portion of the mastoid process. Such an operative finding not only makes proper identification of the sac difficult but also increases the danger of injury to the facial nerve and the sigmoid sinus. To avoid injury to these structures, the surgeon should widely remove bone posterior and lateral to the sigmoid sinus. The digastric ridge should be identified inferiorly and followed toward the stylomastoid foramen. This will allow the surgeon to open any retrofacial air cell tract that is present and thus to identify the level of the facial nerve. After these structures are positively identified, the posterior

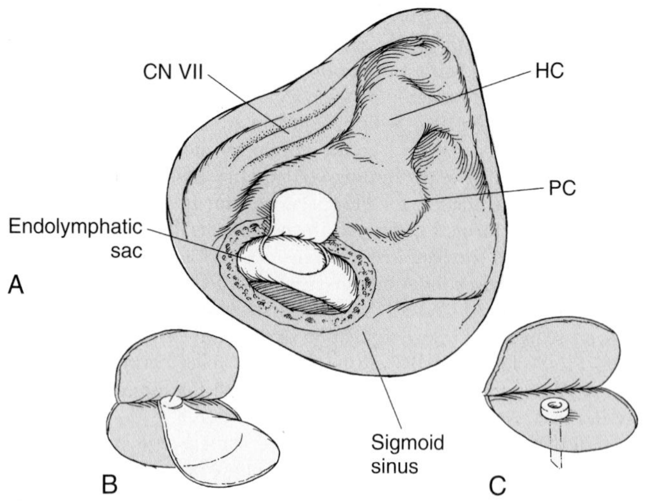

Figure 167-5. Endolymphatic sac surgery. **A,** Endolymphatic sac exposed by transmastoid approach and incised. **B,** Endolymphatic sac–mastoid shunt involves placing Silastic sheeting or a shunt into the lumen of the sac. **C,** Endolymphatic sac–subarachnoid shunt placement requires penetration of the deep layer of the sac lumen (posterior fossa dura) into the subarachnoid space. CN VII, seventh cranial nerve; HC, horizontal semicircular canal; PC, posterior semicircular canal.

fossa dura behind the sinus and the sinus itself should be decompressed with a large diamond drill. The surgeon then may retract the sinus and dissect bluntly between the bony dural plate and the presigmoid posterior fossa dura (containing the endolymphatic sac). After the sinus and the dura are safety retracted, the bony dural plate inferior to Donaldson's line can be removed down to the level of the jugular bulb. Dissection may proceed anteromedially into the retrofacial air cell tract until the site of the endolymphatic duct's entry into bone medial to the posterior semicircular canal is seen. Care should be taken not to injure the medial surface of the facial nerve or the dome of the posterior canal while drilling in this region. This portion of the dissection is greatly facilitated by the dural decompression that has already been accomplished.

Once the sac has been identified, the surgeon should decide whether to terminate the procedure, having accomplished a wide bony decompression, or to open the lumen and place a shunt. Reported series of wide bony decompression without shunting[49] compare favorably with those series that included shunt procedures. Some experts have recommended placing a pressure-sensitive valve into the endolymphatic duct after the sac lumen has been opened and followed into the duct.[50] Other surgeons have failed to achieve the positive results originally reported with this procedure.[51] It often is difficult or impossible to identify one predominant lumen of the sac, and foreign material placed into the sac has been shown to become rapidly encapsulated with fibrous tissue. Despite these considerations, most surgeons who perform endolymphatic sac surgery choose to place a shunt from the sac into the mastoid cavity (Fig. 167-5A and B). On the other hand, use of an endolymphatic sac–subarachnoid shunt[36] (Fig. 167-5C) carries a higher risk of cerebrospinal fluid leak. Beyond this consideration, the procedure seems to be conceptually flawed, because the pressure in the subarachnoid space will always exceed that in the endolymphatic space, even in an ear with significant endolymphatic hydrops. In general, the more the sac is surgically manipulated, the greater the risk of cerebrospinal fluid leak postoperatively. When it is difficult to identify the sac or its lumen, the prudent surgeon will never hesitate to terminate the procedure rather than risk a serious complication.

Patient Selection in Ablative Vestibular Surgery

The patient with recurrent vertigo that has been refractory to medical or conservative surgical treatment is a candidate to undergo a procedure that will ablate the residual vestibular function in the involved ear. In this setting, the patient willingly sacrifices the residual function in the diseased ear in order to eliminate the spontaneous episodes of vertigo that result from fluctuating inputs from the labyrinth to the central nervous system. A successful outcome hinges on the patient's ability to compensate centrally for the unilateral loss of function.

The transmastoid labyrinthectomy is the gold standard procedure for surgical relief of vertigo from inner ear pathology. Because complete loss of residual hearing is inevitable after this operation, it is reserved for those patients who have poor hearing in the affected ear. When hearing must be preserved, a selective vestibular nerve section procedure may be undertaken. Although more risky and slightly less reliable, vestibular neurectomy enjoys a proven track record in the surgical relief of vertigo in properly selected patients. Both of these procedures ideally will produce a total loss of afferent input from the offending vestibular periphery. Although these procedures are applied most often in persons with Meniere's disease, they may be effective in patients with any unstable peripheral vestibular disorder.[52,53]

The Priority of Distinguishing Poor Compensation from Unstable Labyrinthine Disease

Although the specific etiology of dizziness is at times elusive, it usually is possible to distinguish on clinical grounds those patients whose symptoms are caused by an uncompensated stable lesion from those with unstable or progressive disease in the vestibular system. It generally is believed that an operation designed to ablate unilateral vestibular function can effectively relieve vertigo caused by labyrinthine dysfunction of any cause. However, failure to recognize that the patient's symptoms result from poor vestibular compensation for a stable lesion may lead to inappropriate and fruitless surgical intervention.[54] This categorical distinction has important management implications, especially as current understanding of vestibular compensation has evolved. Before the availability of vestibular rehabilitation programs, surgery to ablate vestibular function was offered to any patient whose vestibular injuries were clearly peripheral in nature and could be lateralized to one ear. Subsequently, however, it was demonstrated that the results obtained with vestibular rehabilitation are markedly superior to those with vestibular nerve section for the control of symptoms caused by uncompensated vestibular neuritis (Table 167-1). Thus, surgery is rarely recommended for this indication today. With uncompensated lesions, both surgeon and patient should be aware that the prognosis for success is dramatically lower than that reported for disorders characterized by fluctuating or deteriorating unilateral labyrinthine function.

The methods available to help the clinician distinguish uncompensated patients with a stable vestibular lesion from those with unstable labyrinthine pathology include recognition of key features in the clinical history, the use of vestibular testing, and, when appropriate, the use of a therapeutic trial of vestibular rehabilitation.

Clues in the Clinical History

It often is argued that a complete neurotologic history is the most important component in the diagnostic evaluation of the patient with a balance disorder. This also is true in the assessment of the patient's compensation status. Certain clues in the history will suggest that the patient has incomplete compensation, despite the fact that the vestibular lesion is stable. If the patient describes a severe vestibular crisis at onset without equally intense symptoms on any occasion since that time, an uncompensated lesion is more likely, and the patient is best treated with vestibular rehabilitation. Poor compensation is particularly likely to be the cause of continuous unsteadiness or mild recurring motion-provoked vertigo after recovery from the severe crisis. However, if the current spells are just as severe or more severe than the initial insult, an unstable or progressive vestibular lesion is strongly suggested. In such cases, the patient is best treated with medical or surgical measures designed to stabilize labyrinthine function, once the possibility of a central pathologic process has been eliminated.

The documentation of fluctuating or progressive sensorineural hearing loss also provides a strong indication of unstable inner ear function. Sometimes the patient is uncertain about the nature of an

Table 167-1

University of Michigan Treatment Results in Uncompensated Vestibular Neuritis

Outcome	Vestibular Nerve Section (*n* = 16)	Vestibular Rehabilitation (*n* = 59)
Complete improvement	None	25%
Dramatic improvement	25%	47%
Mild improvement	45%	13%
No improvement	25%	15%
Worse	5%	None

associated hearing loss. A review of serial audiograms may be helpful in this setting. Occasionally, it is desirable to obtain an audiogram during an episode of vertigo to determine whether subtle changes in auditory function are occurring that may be imperceptible to the patient.

The Role of Vestibular Testing

A complete battery of vestibular tests may be helpful in assessing compensation status or in explaining poor compensation by identifying pathologic processes in the central nervous system. The specific vestibular test results that may be helpful in these distinctions are summarized in Box 167-1.

Clinically significant spontaneous nystagmus, positional nystagmus, or a directional preponderance on electronystagmography (ENG) or videonystagmography (VNG) studies provides evidence for failure of physiologic compensation in the VOR. Rotational chair phase or gain abnormalities may identify a pathologic change in the VOR but do not assess compensation within the central nervous system. However, persistent asymmetry in VOR responses strongly suggests that the peripheral lesion is physiologically uncompensated. For head rotation toward the paretic side, the maximum eye velocity induced by the VOR is reduced from normal. This fact results in the observed asymmetry of VOR gain for rightward versus leftward rotations. This asymmetry usually resolves as the compensation process proceeds, at least in the subphysiologic range tested by rotational chair technology. A persisting VOR asymmetry even in well-compensated patients may be identified using the head thrust test above frequencies of 1 Hz.

Dynamic posturography provides adjunctive functional information about the balance system. Sometimes a patient whose major complaints are related to the vestibular system will have normal findings on ENG and rotational chair testing. Posturography may help to demonstrate continued functional impairment despite relatively normal physiologic responses in both inner ears. Patient age and preoperative posturography score have been shown to correlate strongly with postoperative Dizziness Handicap Inventory score.[55] Any evidence of a malingering pattern on postural control testing also may inform the clinician of previously unsuspected psychosocial issues complicating the patient's care.

Box 167-1

Clinical Usefulness of Vestibular Test Results

Evidence for Peripheral Labyrinthine Dysfunction

Unilateral caloric weakness
Spontaneous or positional nystagmus with normal oculomotor findings
Rapid positioning nystagmus after Dix-Hallpike maneuver
Rotational chair phase or asymmetry abnormality
Reduced VOR gain on rotational chair (bilateral weakness)

Evidence for Central Nervous System Pathology

Vertical or perverted nystagmus
Oculomotor test abnormalities
Failure of visual fixation suppression of nystagmus
Motor coordination test abnormalities on dynamic posturography, without musculoskeletal disorder

Evidence for Uncompensated Status

Persistent spontaneous or positional nystagmus
Post–head-shaking nystagmus
Rotational chair asymmetry
Sensory organization test abnormalities on dynamic posturography

Evidence for Improved Compensation Status after Treatment

Resolution of nystagmus
Resolution of rotational chair asymmetry
Improved performance on posturography

VOR, vestibulo-ocular reflex.

Therapeutic Trial of Vestibular Rehabilitation

Ultimately, even with the best clinical history and vestibular test capabilities, the clinician often is faced with diagnostic uncertainty when treating patients with dizziness. As an extreme example, a head injury patient who has a mix of spontaneous and motion-provoked symptoms exhibits evidence of central and peripheral vestibular dysfunction; chronic headache, impairment of cognitive function, and reactive depression also are present. In such patients, it may be difficult or impossible to identify the primary cause of ongoing disability. In settings of diagnostic uncertainty, a program of supervised vestibular rehabilitation may be helpful from a diagnostic standpoint.[5] The patient may make outstanding progress, suggesting that the primary problem was poor compensation for a stable lesion in the vestibular system. If the patient fails to improve, or seems to be worse after 4 to 6 weeks of therapy, an unstable lesion of the labyrinth is considerably more likely. Such an outcome would add credibility to a clinical diagnosis such as post-traumatic endolymphatic hydrops or perilymphatic fistula.

Identification of the Offending Labyrinth

If if there is any uncertainty regarding the ear that is causing vertigo, ablative surgery should not be considered. Reliable lateralizing features include fluctuating or progressive unilateral sensorineural hearing loss and a consistently reproducible unilateral reduction of responsiveness to caloric irrigations. An asymmetrical hearing loss in one ear is the best indicator of the abnormal side.[56] Preexisting hearing loss of extended duration need not dissuade the physician from incriminating the involved ear as the cause of vertigo.[57,58] To illustrate the importance of this point, one study demonstrated 100% relief of vertigo in 13 patients with delayed-onset endolymphatic hydrops beginning up to 60 years after the onset of hearing loss.[59] Less reliable features include tinnitus, subjective sense of aural fullness, direction of observed spontaneous or positional nystagmus, and rotary chair asymmetries. Although audiologic and vestibular test results usually are reliable in determining the involved ear, they should always be interpreted in light of the entire clinical presentation, to avoid a serious error in diagnosis. For example, with significant unilateral sensorineural hearing loss and a unilateral vestibular weakness on the same side, the clinician usually can be confident that the suspect labyrinth is pathologic. However, if the patient reports that the vertigo spells are associated with roaring tinnitus or hearing fluctuations in the better ear, it is most likely that the second ear has become involved. In this case, surgery would be ill advised.

Identification of Intracranial Pathology

Acoustic neuroma and other lesions of the posterior fossa may manifest with clinical features indistinguishable from those of classic vertigo syndromes.[60] Therefore, it is appropriate to perform a definitive radiographic imaging study before vestibular surgery of any type is undertaken. Magnetic resonance imaging (MRI) of the posterior fossa with gadolinium enhancement provides a reliable means of detecting tumors of any size, early stages of demyelinating disease, and subtle ischemic lesions of the brainstem.

Consideration of Other Potential Treatments

Although labyrinthectomy and vestibular nerve section may be applied in any peripheral vestibular disorder, certain patients may be effectively treated by simpler procedures. The use of transtympanically injected aminoglycosides for chemical suppression or ablation of labyrinthine function is particularly appropriate for the management of Meniere's disease in those patients who would be poor surgical candidates.

Brackmann and associates[61] performed 25 eighth nerve microvascular decompression procedures for vertigo in 20 patients over one decade. This procedure was limited to patients who did not have episodic vertigo but had disabling motion-induced dizziness unrelieved by vestibular rehabilitation exercises or conventional medications. The diagnosis was confirmed when these symptoms were associated with radiographic evidence of a vessel loop impinging the nerve. The investigators reported significant improvement in 80% of patients. This procedure offers the potential to reduce vestibular symptoms without destruction of vestibular function in properly selected patients.

Residual Hearing and Selection of Procedure

Generally, labyrinthectomy is reserved for patients with extremely poor residual hearing in the involved ear. Rather than setting a specific hearing threshold or speech discrimination score as the criterion for suggesting a vestibular nerve section instead of a labyrinthectomy, most surgeons prefer to consider each case on an individual basis. Ultimately, the patient's perception of the usefulness of the residual hearing is the most important factor. Some patients insist that they receive benefit from hearing aid use in ears that the medical community would deem useless compared with the better ear. Others fail to recognize any functional utility from an ear that should provide benefit with proper amplification. Clearly, such perceptions must influence the choice of surgical procedure. It is appropriate to perform a labyrinthectomy instead of a selective vestibular nerve section if the contralateral ear is stable, if the patient is convinced that the involved ear is functionally useless, or if the incremental risks of intracranial surgery are unacceptable. A vestibular neurectomy is appropriate when hearing in the involved ear is deemed useful by the patient, especially when the hearing in the involved ear is unlikely to deteriorate in the near future. However, because the cochlear efferent fibers travel with the vestibular nerve, it must be recognized that a vestibular neurectomy may contribute to undesirable hearing symptoms in Meniere's disease: Sound intolerance and reduced speech discrimination in noise may be evident, even if the pure-tone detection and discrimination scores in quiet are unchanged.[62]

Some investigators argue that labyrinthectomy should never be performed if any hearing remains, fearing the unlikely scenario that the better ear may develop a hearing loss greater than the current loss in the diseased ear. If this rare outcome should occur, a cochlear implant in the most recently deafened ear would almost certainly rehabilitate the patient successfully. Insisting on the preservation of minimal residual hearing in a functionally useless poorer ear is too dogmatic to be practical, especially when the additional risks of vestibular nerve section, such as intracranial hemorrhage, meningitis, and cerebrospinal fluid leak, are considered. Beyond this, the available evidence suggests that preserved hearing often will continue to deteriorate and eventually provide no benefit for the patient.[63,64]

Ablative Procedures for the Control of Vertigo

Surgery for control of vertigo symptoms is virtually always elective. Patients should decide when their vertigo has produced sufficient disability in their lifestyle to outweigh the consequences and risks of surgery. A patient who has come to this decision without coercion by family or the physician is most prepared to face the surgery and the recovery period with a positive outlook.

Labyrinthectomy

Labyrinthectomy may be performed when persistent or recurrent labyrinthine symptoms of any etiology are attributed to dysfunction in an ear with severe to profound sensorineural hearing loss. All residual hearing sensitivity is sacrificed by this procedure. The operation may be undertaken using a transcanal or transmastoid approach. The transcanal labyrinthectomy, also known as oval window labyrinthectomy, retains some popularity. It can be performed quickly by approaching the inner ear through the external auditory canal, although complete ablation of vestibular neuroepithelium cannot reliably be accomplished.[65] The procedure begins by elevating a tympanomeatal flap to enter the middle ear and then accessing the vestibule of the bony labyrinth by removing the stapes from the oval window. Some surgeons advocate removing bone from the promontory below the oval window toward the round window to improve visualization of the vestibule (Fig. 167-6A). The saccule and utricle are identified and removed. An attempt may be made to reach and remove the ampullae of the horizontal and superior semicircular canals, although this step requires blind manipulation with a long right-angled instrument medial to the facial nerve. Augmenting this procedure by a selective section of the nerve to the posterior semicircular canal ampulla should help to prevent residual posterior canal function. To accomplish this, the bony exposure of the vestibule can be extended by drilling near the round window until the nerve to the posterior ampulla is identified and divided. Because the primary shortcoming of the transcanal labyrinthectomy is the inability to visualize all neuroepithelial elements of the inner ear, many surgeons supplement their mechanical efforts by filling the vestibule with absorbable packing soaked with an ototoxic aminoglycoside antibiotic, which enhances the likelihood of success. Although this procedure reliably eliminates vertigo, postoperative imbalance is seen in more than 60% of patients, a rate almost three times higher than after transmastoid labyrinthectomy in the elderly population.[66]

Transmastoid labyrinthectomy (Fig. 167-7) is the gold standard procedure for surgical ablation of vestibular function. The transmastoid approach allows complete visualization and removal of the entire semicircular canal system, utricle, and saccule, resulting in highly reliable relief of vertigo.[67,68] Success is nearly universal and the improvement in quality of life is remarkable for properly selected patients.[69] This transtemporal procedure requires precise knowledge of the anatomy of the bony vestibular labyrinth and other structures in the temporal bone that are medial to the tympanic and mastoid portions of the facial nerve. The neurotologic surgeon who is familiar with transtemporal surgical approaches generally is very proficient operating in this region and can be expected to safely accomplish a complete labyrinthectomy by way of a transmastoid approach. Those surgeons who are less familiar with the anatomy of the temporal bone medial to the facial nerve

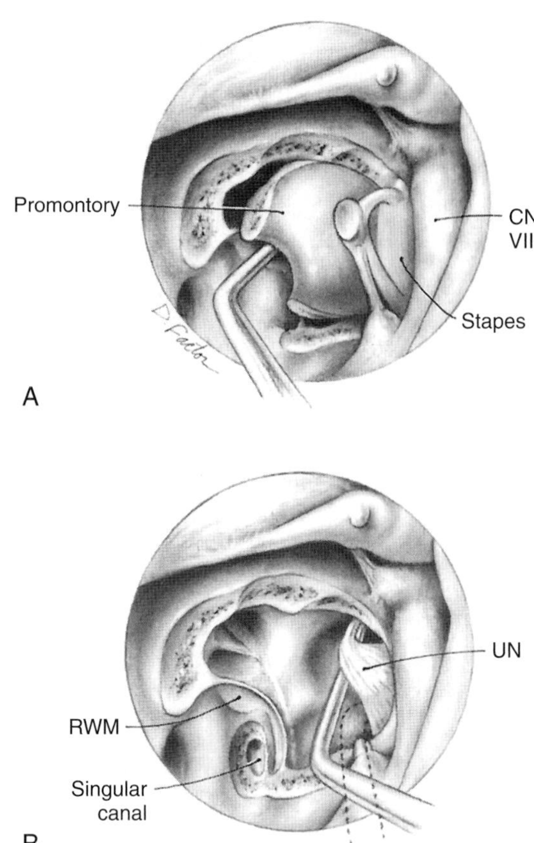

Figure 167-6. Transcanal labyrinthectomy. **A,** Removal of promontory bone and stapes provides wide exposure of vestibule. **B,** Right-angle hook is used to extract utricular neuroepithelium (UN) from the elliptical recess on the roof of the vestibule. Singular canal has been opened and the nerve to the posterior canal ampulla divided. CN VII, seventh cranial nerve; RWM, round window membrane.

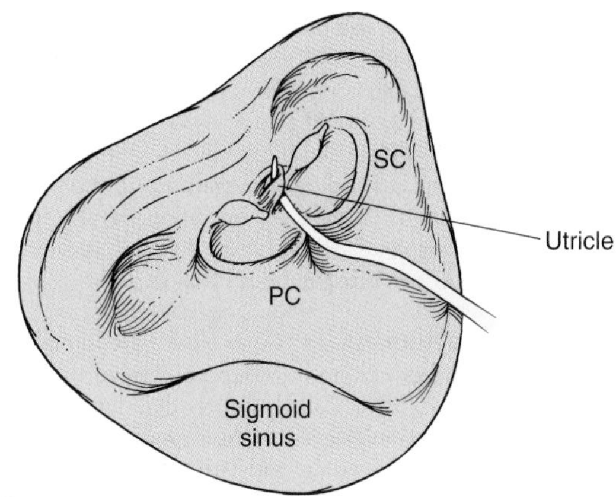

Figure 167-7. Transmastoid labyrinthectomy (left ear). Exposure of the ampullated ends of all three semicircular canals and the vestibule is accomplished, and all neuroepithelium is removed under direct vision. Care is taken to skeletonize but not expose the facial nerve. PC, posterior semicircular canal; SC, superior semicircular canal.

should familiarize themselves with this approach in the temporal bone laboratory before undertaking this procedure in the clinical setting.

The procedure begins with a cortical mastoidectomy performed through a postauricular approach. After the central mastoid air cell tract and the antrum are identified, the cavity should be widely beveled to improve exposure. Special attention should be paid to beveling the bone over the middle fossa dura and the sinodural angle; otherwise, the angle of visualization medial to the facial nerve may not be adequate to allow safe opening of the vestibule and the posterior canal ampulla. Rarely, a limited decompression of the middle fossa dura or the sigmoid sinus is required in a poorly pneumatized mastoid. After the mastoidectomy is completed, the dome of the horizontal semicircular canal is visible at the depth of the antrum. The largest burr or coarse diamond drill bit that will fit safely between the middle fossa dura and the dome of the horizontal canal (usually 4 mm) should be selected. Proper use of continuous suction-irrigation allows the surgeon to prevent injury to soft tissue structures that limit the margins of dissection, such as dura, the superior petrosal sinus, and the facial nerve. Drilling of the labyrinth should commence by deepening the "solid angle" between the three bony semicircular canals before the lumen of any canal is opened. The surgeon will then sequentially open the lumen of the bony semicircular canals, bivalving the internal surface of each canal toward the center of an ever deeper and wider bony cup that is developed as labyrinthine bone is removed.

Generally, the horizontal canal lumen is opened first and used as a landmark to protect the tympanic segment of the facial nerve. The equator of the rotating drill bit should never be allowed to come lateral to the inferior lip of the bony cup, because this would cause the drill to slip into the facial nerve. It is especially dangerous when a right-handed surgeon is operating in the right ear with the drill rotating clockwise. Some surgeons elect to reverse the direction of drill rotation for this part of the procedure in the right ear, to allow better control of the drill. After the horizontal canal lumen is identified, it is followed posteriorly toward the nonampullated end until the dome of the posterior canal is opened. This canal is then followed to the common crus, where the superior canal lumen can also be identified. By progressively deepening and widening the bony cup, it is possible to follow the superior canal toward its ampullated end. During this portion of the dissection, minor bleeding from the subarcuate artery is to be expected. Although this may be a nuisance, it is best to press ahead and completely open the arch of the superior canal and then control the vessel once in an definitive fashion, rather than stopping to address the bleeding several times.

The superior canal ampulla is adjacent to the horizontal canal ampulla, which is opened next. To approach the ampullated end of the posterior semicircular canal, the nonampullated end of the horizontal canal will have to be progressively transgressed until the posterior portion of the vestibule is open. The surgeon should stay within the cup and follow the internal surface of the posterior canal lumen as it passes medial to the second genu of the facial nerve. Care should be taken to avoid injury to the medial surface of the nerve by undercutting it with the drill. To prevent this injury, the surgeon should bevel the cup laterally over the second genu of the nerve and not allow an overhang of bone to develop that may potentially obscure visualization. It is safe and perhaps even desirable to carefully identify the nerve sheath through a thin layer of intact bone, a technique known as "skeletonizing" the nerve. This allows the surgeon to visualize and securely verify the position of the nerve. Whenever the nerve is being skeletonized, it is important to use a gentle polishing drill motion that parallels the direction of the nerve, along with copious irrigation so that the nerve can be seen through the bone before the sheath is exposed or injured. A smaller drill (usually 3 mm) is required to work safely between the skeletonized facial nerve and the posterior fossa dura. After the posterior canal ampulla has been opened, bone can be removed over the vestibule by connecting the three ampullated ends. Then sufficient access has been achieved so that all elements of the membranous labyrinth may be removed, including the cupula of each semicircular canal, the utricle, and the saccule. Care should be taken not to perforate the thin bone at the lateral end of the internal auditory canal during removal of neuroepithelium.

Disadvantages of labyrinthectomy include complete ipsilateral loss of hearing and a period of postoperative vertigo. Nystagmus usually is brisk and may persist for several days. Generally, the patient walks unassisted by the second or third postoperative day. Although vestibular compensation is mostly complete by 2 months postoperatively, further gradual improvement over 12 to 18 months may be anticipated. In some patients, significant dysequilibrium persists. Rare complications of labyrinthectomy that should be discussed with patients include facial nerve injury, cerebrospinal fluid leak, and disabling chronic dysequilibrium. In experienced hands, the overall occurrence of surgical complications is infrequent. Because the operation should not violate the dura of the posterior cranial fossa or the internal auditory canal, the risk of meningitis or cerebrospinal fluid leak is slight.

Vestibular Nerve Section

Success rates for control of vertigo by all approaches to the vestibular nerve ranges from 80% to 95%, notably poorer than with labyrinthectomy. In most cases, a vestibular nerve section procedure is selected in an effort to relieve episodic vertigo without sacrificing the patient's residual hearing. However, a complete discussion of the subject must at least mention two rarely used approaches for vestibular nerve section that, like labyrinthectomy, do sacrifice residual auditory function. These are the translabyrinthine vestibular neurectomy[70] (Fig. 167-8) and the transcochlear cochleovestibular neurectomy[71] (Fig. 167-9). Each of these operations supplements one of the two common labyrinthectomy procedures by adding an intradural dissection of the eighth cranial nerve within the internal auditory canal. The rationale used to justify adding a vestibular neurectomy after the labyrinthectomy has been completed is to accomplish division of the vestibular nerve medial to Scarpa's ganglion in the internal auditory canal. In the translabyrinthine vestibular neurectomy, a transmastoid labyrinthectomy is completed, and the internal auditory canal dura is then identified and opened, exposing the neural contents of the canal. Both the superior and inferior divisions of the vestibular nerve may then be avulsed from the lateral end of the canal and sectioned medial to the ganglion. Similarly, the transcochlear cochleovestibular neurectomy extends the transcanal labyrinthectomy to open the cochlea and the distal end of the internal auditory canal to section the cochlear nerve along with the vestibular nerve. The cochlear neurectomy is added in an effort to decrease tinnitus after the procedure. This approach currently has few adherents, because most reports of cochlear nerve section for tinnitus have shown a dismal success rate, thus failing to justify the additional risk associated with opening the internal auditory canal.

The rationale for these two extensions of labyrinthectomy procedures is dubious because of the excellent results obtained with transmastoid labyrinthectomy alone,[72] especially in view of the increased risk of cerebrospinal fluid leak and meningitis associated with intradural dissection.

Most often, vestibular nerve section is performed in an effort to eliminate disordered vestibular function while preserving useful hearing in the symptomatic ear. In this setting, selective section of the vestibular nerve is the primary goal, with intent to preserve the labyrinth, auditory nerve fibers, and cochlear blood supply. The best surgical approach for selective vestibular nerve section remains a controversial issue. The three conventional approaches that are used are the middle fossa approach, the retrolabyrinthine approach, and the retrosigmoid approach.

The middle fossa approach, popularized in the 1970s by Fisch[73] and Glasscock,[74] is the most technically demanding. It permits the most definitive section of the vestibular fibers by specifically identifying the superior and inferior vestibular nerves within the lateral portion of the internal auditory canal. In this location, they have separated anatomically from the auditory fibers of the eighth nerve (Fig. 167-10). Although this approach provides a better opportunity to avoid injury to the cochlear nerve fibers, it carries a risk for injury to the cochlear blood supply, because the labyrinthine artery ramifies in the distal portion of the internal auditory canal, in close proximity to the inferior vestibular nerve. If the surgeon elects to avoid this risk by choosing not to transect the inferior vestibular nerve, episodic vertigo may persist. In addition, this operation involves the highest rate of injury to the facial nerve among conventional approaches for vestibular neurectomy (with temporary paresis rates as high as 33%) and a significantly higher rate than in labyrinthectomy.[75,76]

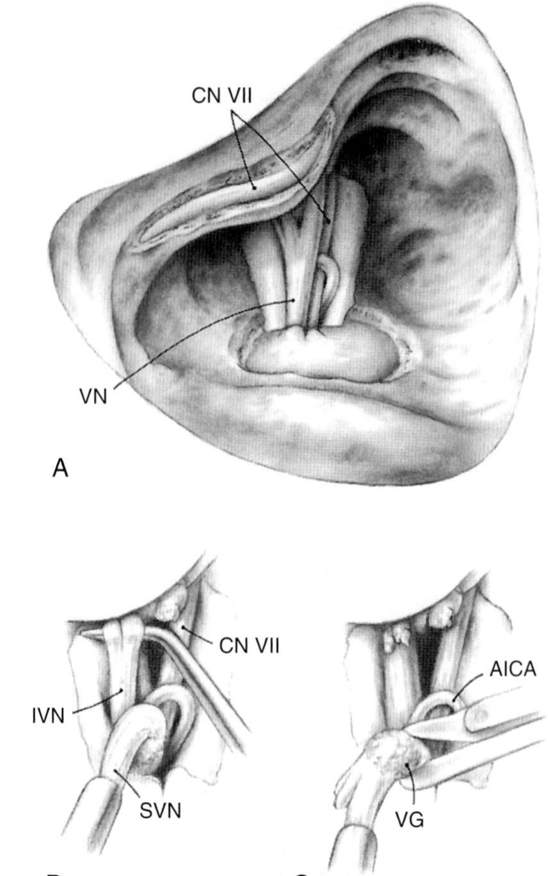

Figure 167-8. Translabyrinthine vestibular nerve transection. **A,** Nerves of internal auditory canal are exposed. **B,** Traction on the transected end of the superior division of the vestibular nerve (SVN) permits exposure of the inferior division of the vestibular nerve (IVN). **C,** Transection of the nerve trunk proximal to the vestibular ganglion (VG) completes excision of vestibular neurons. Anterior inferior cerebellar artery (AICA) is occasionally visualized. CN VII, seventh cranial nerve; VN, vestibular nerve.

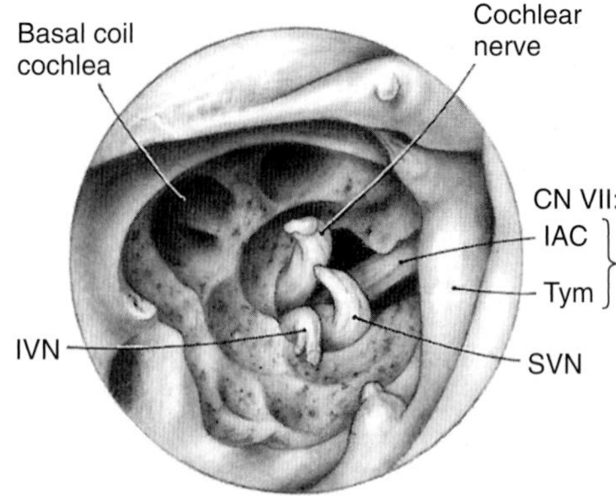

Figure 167-9. Transcochlear vestibular nerve transection. Medial wall of vestibule and lateral cochlear wall are removed to expose distal end of internal auditory canal (IAC). Cochlear and vestibular nerve branches are transected at their distal ends. SVN and IVN, superior and inferior divisions, respectively, of the vestibular nerve; Tym, tympanic segment of cranial nerve VII (CN VII).

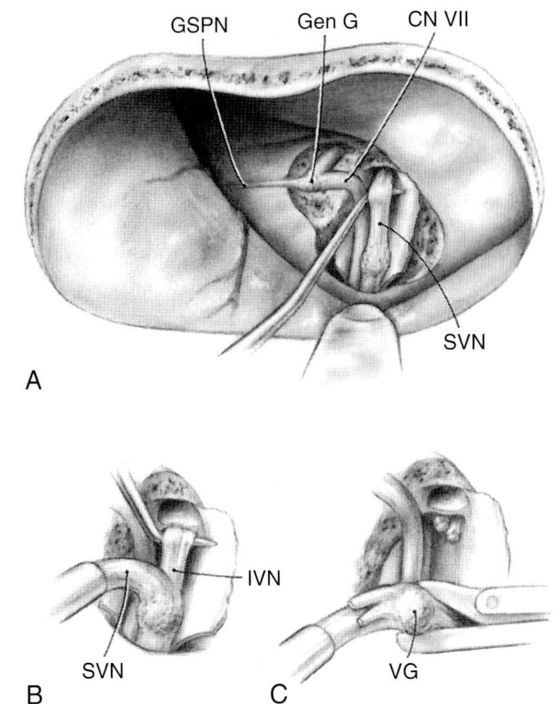

Figure 167-10. Selective transection of vestibular nerve (middle fossa approach). **A,** Vestibular and facial nerves are exposed in the superior compartment of the internal auditory canal. The superior division of the vestibular nerve (SVN) is avulsed distally with a right-angle hook. Gen G, geniculate ganglion; GSPN, greater superficial petrosal nerve. **B,** Traction on the distal end of the SVN with a suction tip permits exposure of the inferior division of the vestibular nerve (IVN). **C,** After lateral transection of the IVN, the vestibular nerve trunk is transected proximal to the vestibular ganglion (VG).

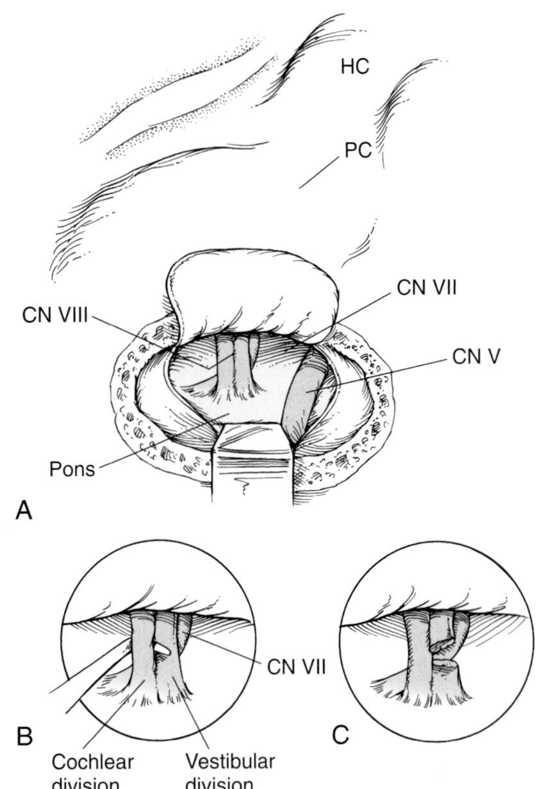

Figure 167-11. Retrolabyrinthine vestibular nerve transection. **A,** After a flap of posterior fossa dura including endolymphatic sac has been elevated, the retractor exposes the seventh and eighth cranial nerves (CN VII, CN VIII). **B,** Vestibular nerve fibers are separated from the cochlear nerve with sharp and blunt instruments. **C,** The vestibular nerve is transected. CN V, trigeminal nerve; HC, horizontal semicircular canal; PC, posterior semicircular canal.

With the middle fossa approach, the operation begins with a temporal craniotomy centered above the external auditory canal. The middle fossa dura is elevated from the surface of the temporal bone, and the temporal lobe is retracted extradurally with a specially designed retractor. Then the contents of the internal auditory canal are skeletonized, with care taken not to injure the cochlea, the superior semicircular canal, or the labyrinthine portion of the facial nerve. An effort should be made to dissect almost 180 degrees around the internal canal, so that its contents will be easily visible after the dura is opened (see Fig. 167-10A). It is not necessary to completely expose the labyrinthine segment of the facial nerve, although confirming its location will help with orientation. With continuous intraoperative monitoring of the facial nerve and auditory evoked potentials, the dura is incised, and the facial nerve is positively identified within the internal canal by electrical stimulation. The superior vestibular nerve then may be avulsed from its lateral attachments and sectioned (see Fig. 167-10B). The same procedure is repeated with the inferior division of the vestibular nerve, with care taken to avoid the cochlear blood supply and adjacent fibers of the auditory nerve that are traveling to the basal turn of the cochlea (see Fig. 167-10).

In the 1980s, several otologists reported series of retrolabyrinthine vestibular nerve section procedures, establishing this as a reliable approach with a lower incidence of hearing loss and facial nerve injury.[77-79] The retrolabyrinthine approach is also technically simpler than the middle fossa operation. The primary drawback is that the eighth cranial nerve (cranial nerve VIII) is exposed only in the cerebellopontine angle, between the porus acousticus and the brainstem, where it may be difficult to reliably separate auditory fibers from the vestibular fibers. The surgical view of cranial nerve VIII that is afforded by the retrolabyrinthine approach (Fig. 167-11) is somewhat constricted, particularly if the surgeon is not careful to follow several technical points designed to maximize exposure through the temporal bone.

The retrolabyrinthine exposure requires wide decompression of the posterior fossa dura both anterior and posterior to the sigmoid sinus. The dura should be exposed for approximately 1.5 cm posterior to the sinus to allow easy retraction. The bone anterior to the sinus then is removed until the bony labyrinth is outlined and until the entire endolymphatic sac area is exposed. The jugular bulb is the inferior limit of dissection. Because inferior bone removal is critical to satisfactory intracranial exposure, the surgeon should make every effort to open the retrofacial air cell tract and expose the sac until the jugular bulb is skeletonized. Care should be taken to prevent entry of bone dust into the middle ear while drilling, because this may lead to delayed fixation of the ossicular chain. The dura and the endolymphatic sac then are incised, and a flap of dura is retracted forward, exposing the posterior fossa. The cerebellum is gently retracted, and the cerebrospinal fluid of the cerebellopontine angle cistern is released by incising the arachnoid membrane. The trigeminal nerve and the tentorium cerebelli are identified superiorly for orientation. The eighth nerve complex then is identified inferiorly. Because the angle of vision is parallel to the posterior face of the petrous bone, the porus acousticus is not visible. If the inferior bony exposure is exceptionally good, the small multiple fibers of the intracranial portions of cranial nerves IX and X may be visible. Often, the flocculus of the cerebellum must be retracted to improve visualization of the eighth nerve. The facial nerve should be positively identified by electrical stimulation, which usually requires minor retraction of the eighth nerve. The superior (caudal) half of the eighth nerve complex contains the vestibular fibers, which should be divided from the inferior portion and then sharply sectioned. Ideally, the vestibular component is completely divided without injury to the nervus intermedius or facial nerve. The dura then is approximated, and the closure is augmented with a piece of temporalis fascia. The aditus ad antrum is blocked with an additional piece of fascia, and the mastoid defect is filled with an abdominal fat graft. It is best to place a small bone chip harvested during the mastoidectomy between the mastoid contents and the ossicle heads to prevent prolapse of the graft material into the middle ear.

A disadvantage of the retrolabyrinthine approach is uncertainty about the plane between the cochlear and vestibular nerve bundles. Thus, this approach is associated with a risk for incomplete vestibular neurectomy and some chance that auditory neurons may be inadvertently divided. Nevertheless, use of this approach is satisfactory if the hearing results are equivalent to those reported with other methods. A slightly higher risk of cerebrospinal fluid leak has been attributed to the difficulty of reliably closing the posterior fossa dura anterior to the sigmoid sinus.

In the 1930s, two neurosurgeons, Dandy[80] and McKenzie,[81] each reported a series of cranial nerve VIII section procedures for vertigo using a lateral suboccipital craniotomy approach. Long-term follow-up evaluation of Dandy's suboccipital vestibular nerve section procedures demonstrated a 90% rate of complete relief of vertigo.[82] This approach, now commonly called the retrosigmoid approach, allows for selective sectioning of the vestibular nerve in roughly the same location encountered in the retrolabyrinthine approach. Many neurotologists prefer this approach today, because no temporal bone dissection is required to expose the eighth nerve complex, improving the speed and perhaps the safety of the procedure. In addition, because a watertight closure of the retrosigmoid dura usually can be accomplished, the incidence of cerebrospinal fluid leak presumably will be lower. Disadvantages include poorer proximity to the nerve from the depth of the wound, the need for increased intradural retraction of the cerebellum, and a significant incidence of troublesome postoperative headaches. The headache problem may be ameliorated to some degree by avoiding intradural drilling, constraining the spread of bone dust in the subarachnoid space, and making efforts to prevent postoperative attachment of the deep skull base musculature to the exposed retrosigmoid dura.

One group of neurotologic surgeons reported a modification of the retrosigmoid approach in which 60 to 90 mL of cerebrospinal fluid is removed by means of a lumbar drain to decompress the posterior fossa before the operation.[83] They were then able to perform the procedure by use of a 2-cm craniotomy and reported a short operative time, no cerebrospinal fluid leaks, and a very low incidence of postoperative headache. Some surgeons prefer the retrosigmoid approach or even a combined retrolabyrinthine-retrosigmoid approach, because these provide the opportunity to remove bone behind the internal auditory canal to better distinguish between the auditory and vestibular fibers, providing a more reliable ablation of vestibular function.[84,85]

The infralabyrinthine approach[86] for vestibular nerve section is rarely used. As the name implies, the surgeon approaches the internal auditory canal by outlining the posterior semicircular canal and working through the retrofacial air cell tract inferior to the intact bony labyrinth. This approach offers the theoretical advantages of a highly selective vestibular nerve section, facial nerve safety, and a rather limited intradural dissection confined to the distal portion of the internal auditory canal. Of note, however, this technically demanding exposure can be accomplished only in extensively pneumatized temporal bones. It also requires substantial dural decompression and sigmoid sinus retraction inferiorly, where the sinus wall may be less durable.

Although intracranial approaches for the control of vertigo all are associated with the potential for catastrophic complications, the overall complication rate is low. Stroke, subdural hematoma, facial nerve paralysis, meningitis, and wound infection have been reported. Postoperative facial nerve paralysis is infrequent, especially with posterior fossa approaches. In most series, the incidence of sensorineural hearing loss is less than 10%. Vestibular nerve section should not be expected to eliminate the auditory symptoms of ongoing endolymphatic hydrops. The addition of a concurrent endolymphatic sac decompression procedure does not appear to increase the chance of a good hearing outcome after vestibular neurectomy.[87] After vestibular nerve section, most patients return to their usual activities within 2 to 4 months. Rates of control of vertigo by all approaches to the vestibular nerve range from 80% to 95%—notably poorer than with labyrinthectomy. In cases in which a neurectomy in the posterior fossa has failed to relieve the vertigo, a middle fossa approach may theoretically be used to accomplish a more selective vestibular neurectomy in the lateral portion of the internal auditory canal. One study reported only a 55% success rate in this setting, which again emphasizes the priority of differentiating disordered residual cranial nerve VIII function from inadequate compensation.[88]

Postoperative Vestibular Compensation

After any ablative vestibular procedure, there is always a requisite period of vestibular compensation. In counseling preoperative patients, an important point is that vestibular compensation is variable and somewhat unpredictable. Not all patients will compensate fully for the loss of unilateral vestibular function, and up to 30% may be left with considerable chronic dysequilibrium or motion-provoked vertigo. The phenomenon of incomplete or delayed postoperative compensation explains many of the unsatisfactory outcomes after vestibular surgery. One study documented that although most post-labyrinthectomy patients are relieved of vertigo, only 50% return to work.[89] This suggests that functional recovery is more complex than simply achieving relief of vertigo spells. It has long been the impression of some surgeons that recovery from vestibular nerve section is more protracted and more frequently incomplete than after labyrinthectomy.[75] One study showed that post-neurectomy patients had a higher incidence of prolonged postoperative ataxia (11%) than that experienced by post-labyrinthectomy patients (2%), as well as a longer delay of return to work.[75] Eisenman and colleagues[63] compared long-term compensation 3 to 10 years after these two operations in patients who had satisfactory relief of their episodic vertigo symptoms. No differences were found between the groups in self-assessment of balance abilities or functional balance performance. Both groups showed evidence of incomplete physiologic compensation in a majority of subjects, suggesting that recovery of vestibular function after seemingly successful ablative surgery is not as comprehensive as was previously believed.

The routine use of vestibular exercises may help to optimize balance function after any operation that results in unilateral loss of labyrinthine function. It is appropriate for the rehabilitation therapist to offer counseling and instruction in a generic exercise program to all postoperative patients, and any patients who demonstrate poor progress toward recovery should be promptly referred for a customized program of therapy. Persons at particular risk for poor recovery include patients with additional sensory deficits or other complicating neurologic conditions, those using centrally sedating medications, and any who may have a poor psychological motivation for recovery. Such patients should be encouraged to pursue a customized program of vestibular rehabilitation early in the postoperative course.

If a relapse of vestibular symptoms occurs beyond the acute phase of recovery, it may be difficult to distinguish among disease progression, involvement of the contralateral ear, and central decompensation. The phenomenon of decompensation may occur after an initially satisfactory recovery from any peripheral lesion, including vestibular surgery. Early failures after labyrinthectomy are best attributed to incorrect diagnosis, incomplete surgical removal of the neuroepithelium, or inadequate initial vestibular compensation. Late failures may be a result of central decompensation, which should respond briskly to vestibular rehabilitation.[54] Failures after vestibular nerve section may be caused by an incomplete division of the vestibular fibers. A labyrinthectomy or a revision procedure to complete the neurectomy may be required in this setting. However, a therapeutic trial of vestibular rehabilitation is always appropriate before additional surgery is considered if decompensation or incomplete compensation is a possibility.

SUGGESTED READINGS

Brackmann DE, Kesser BW, Day JD. Microvascular decompression of the vestibulocochlear nerve for disabling positional vertigo: the House Ear Clinic experience. *Otol Neurotol.* 2001;22:882.

Bretlau P, Thomsen J, Tos M, et al. Placebo effect in surgery for Meniere's disease: nine-year follow-up. *Am J Otol.* 1989;10:259.

Eisenman DJ, Speers R, Telian SA. Labyrinthectomy versus vestibular neurectomy: long-term physiologic and clinical outcomes. *Otol Neurotol.* 2001;22:539.

Friedland DR, Michel MA. Cranial thickness in superior canal dehiscence syndrome: implications for canal resurfacing surgery. *Otol Neurotol.* 2006;27:346.

Gacek RR, Gacek MR. Singular neurectomy in the management of paroxysmal positional vertigo. *Otolaryngol Clin North Am.* 1994;27:363.

Garcia-Ibanez E, Garcia-Ibanez JL. Middle fossa vestibular neurectomy: a report of 373 cases. *Otolaryngol Head Neck Surg.* 1980;88:486.

Gates GA, Green JD Jr, Tucci DL, et al. The effects of transtympanic micropressure treatment in people with unilateral Meniere's disease. *Arch Otolaryngol Head Neck Surg.* 2004;130:718.

Kemink JL, Hoff JT. Retrolabyrinthine vestibular nerve section: analysis of results. *Laryngoscope.* 1986;96:33.

Kemink JL, Telian SA, El-Kashlan H, et al. Retrolabyrinthine vestibular nerve section: efficacy in disorders other than Meniere's disease. *Laryngoscope.* 1991;101:523.

Kemink JL, Telian SA, Graham MD, et al. Transmastoid labyrinthectomy: reliable surgical management of vertigo. *Otolaryngol Head Neck Surg.* 1989;101:5.

Langman AW, Lindeman RC. Surgery for vertigo in the nonserviceable hearing ear: transmastoid labyrinthectomy or translabyrinthine vestibular nerve section. *Laryngoscope.* 1993;103:1321.

Leveque M, Labrousse M, Seidermann L, et al. Surgical therapy in intractable benign paroxysmal positional vertigo. *Otolaryngol Head Neck Surg.* 2007;136:693.

For complete list of references log onto www.expertconsult.com.

McKenna MJ, Nadol JB Jr, Ojemann RG, et al. Vestibular neurectomy: retrosigmoid-intracanalicular versus retrolabyrinthine approach. *Am J Otol.* 1996;17:253.

Minor LB. Clinical manifestations of superior semicircular canal dehiscence. *Laryngoscope.* 2005;115:1717.

Nadol JB Jr, Weiss AD, Parker SW. Vertigo of delayed onset after sudden deafness. *Ann Otol Rhinol Laryngol.* 1975;84:841.

Parnes LS, McClure JA. Posterior semicircular canal occlusion in the normal hearing ear. *Otolaryngol Head Neck Surg.* 1991;104:52.

Poe DS, Bottrill ID. Comparison of endoscopic and surgical explorations for perilymphatic fistulas. *Am J Otol.* 1994;15:735.

Schuknecht HF. Cochleosacculotomy for Meniere's disease: internal endolymphatic shunt. *Oper Techn Otolaryngol Head Neck Surg.* 1991;2:35.

Schuknecht HF. Transcanal labyrinthectomy. *Oper Techn Otolaryngol Head Neck Surg.* 1991;2:17.

Shea JJ. The myth of spontaneous perilymph fistula. *Otolaryngol Head Neck Surg.* 1992;107:613.

Shone G, Kemink JL, Telian SA. Prognostic significance of hearing loss as a lateralizing indicator in the surgical treatment of vertigo. *J Laryngol Otol.* 1991;105:618.

Silverstein H, Norrell H, Smouha EE. Retrosigmoid-internal auditory canal approach vs. retrolabyrinthine approach for vestibular neurectomy. *Otolaryngol Head Neck Surg.* 1987;97:300.

Silverstein H, Smouha E, Jones R. Natural history vs. surgery for Meniere's disease. *Otolaryngol Head Neck Surg.* 1989;100:6.

Telischi FF, Luxford WM. Long-term efficacy of endolymphatic sac surgery for vertigo in Meniere's disease. *Otolaryngol Head Neck Surg.* 1993;109:83.

Welling DB, Nagaraja HN. Endolymphatic mastoid shunt: a reevaluation of efficacy. *Otolaryngol Head Neck Surg.* 2000;122:340.

CHAPTER ONE HUNDRED AND SIXTY-EIGHT

Vestibular and Balance Rehabilitation: Program Essentials

Neil T. Shepard

Steven A. Telian

Audrey B. Erman

Key Points

- Vestibular compensation is the normal physiologic response of a healthy central nervous system to vestibular pathology.
- In many patients with chronic imbalance and dizziness, the symptom complex is a result of incomplete compensation after a vestibular insult.
- The compensation process hinges on the neurologic phenomenon of adaptive plasticity, with reorganization of perceptual and motor output responses to altered sensory inputs.
- Patients who avoid the inciting movements that provoke sensorimotor conflicts or continually use vestibular suppressant medications are at particular risk for delayed or incomplete compensation.
- Confounding central neurologic disease or an unstable peripheral lesion also can lead to ongoing symptoms.
- Individualized vestibular rehabilitation programs constitute a safe and effective treatment option for a large percentage of patients with complaints of imbalance and dizziness.
- Referrals are based on symptomatic complaints, rather than specific etiologic diagnoses or test results.
- Benign paroxysmal positional vertigo (BPPV) is an inner ear disorder that is particularly responsive to physical therapy interventions.

Vestibular exercises were first described in the early 1940s by Drs. Cooksey and Cawthorne for the treatment of surgically induced vestibulopathies. Their simple eye, head, and body movements assist in habituation and are still in use today. Modern vestibular and balance rehabilitation therapy (VBRT) programs have evolved into multidisciplinary efforts in which physicians and therapists collaborate in a team approach, frequently in association with sophisticated vestibular testing facilities. A sufficient number of prospective, controlled studies have now been conducted to demonstrate both the efficacy and cost-effectiveness of vestibular rehabilitation.[1] Accordingly, this treatment has become widely available and is the primary management technique for a large proportion of patients with complaints of imbalance and dizziness.

The two overall goals in a VBRT program are (1) to advance the central vestibular compensation process (Fig. 168-1), resulting in reduction in symptoms under static and dynamic conditions, and improvement in the function of the vestibulo-ocular reflex (VOR); and (2) improvement in the functionality of static and dynamic balance and gait. This second goal can be a process that is achievable independent of complete central compensation.

To accomplish these goals, a variety of different exercise techniques may be used. Each has specific subgoals within the overall structure of a VBRT program. Not all available techniques are used with every patient. The various techniques and their goals are as follows:

- *Adaptation exercises*: to improve the functional performance of the VOR[2-4] (Fig. 168-2).
- *Habituation exercises*: to reduce or eliminate dysphoric responses to a specific stimulus by repeated exposure to a sensory conflict situation.[5,6]
- *Sensory substitution exercises*: to allow for the use of alternative sensory inputs or central nervous system preprogramming and motor output paths in the acquisition of control for gaze stabilization during head movements, and for postural and gait control.[7-11]
- *Balance exercises*: improved performance in both static and dynamic postural control. Practice of tai chi or similar activities may be an effective adjunct in this setting, especially for patients with complaints of continuous imbalance when standing.

- *Gait exercises*: improvement in ambulation by use of both short and long courses. As the patient progresses in the program, these gait activities are combined with habituation and adaptation exercises through the use of head rotations during walking.

- *General conditioning*: to achieve lifestyle changes to increase activity and fitness.

- *Maintenance program*: to allow for continued exercise activity without the rigor of a formal program, yet to maintain the accomplishments achieved during the active treatment phase. This is especially important in certain central nervous system disorders.[12]

These elements form the basis for the programs discussed in this chapter. A full, in-depth discussion of all of the aspects of a VBRT program is available in Herdman's definitive work on vestibular rehabilitation.[13]

Physiologic Rationale for Vestibular and Balance Rehabilitation

A unique feature of the central nervous system is its ability to adjust to asymmetries in peripheral vestibular inputs and, to a lesser degree, to fix insults within the central vestibular pathways.[14] This adjustment process is referred to as vestibular compensation and occurs naturally after most vestibular insults, provided that the affected person resumes an active lifestyle. Such adaptive plasticity requires active neuronal changes in the cerebellum and the brainstem nuclei in response to the sensory conflicts produced by central or peripheral vestibular pathology. In most instances, this process will reliably relieve vestibular symptoms, provided that the lesion is either stable or producing only gradual progressive deterioration. The underlying physiologic components of this process are the foundations of vestibular and balance rehabilitation. At least four distinct components of vestibular compensation are recognized: *static compensation*, which occurs regardless of movement,

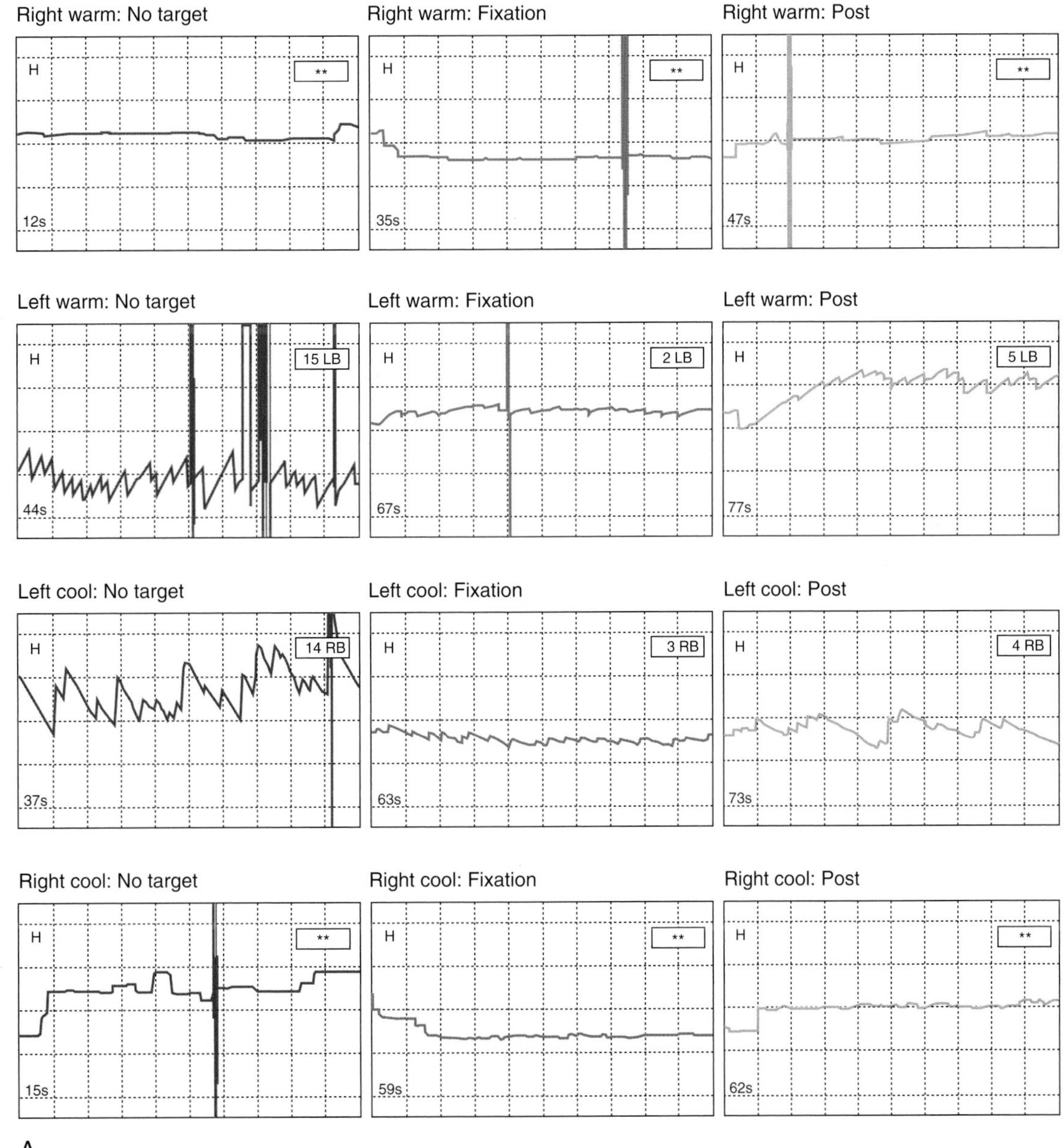

Figure 168-1. Videonystagmography test results from a patient with uncompensated right unilateral vestibular system hypofunction. **A,** Results of bithermal alternating open loop water irrigations. The *left column* shows the maximum nystagmus response to right warm, left warm, left cool, and right cool irrigations. The *center column* shows the suppression of nystagmus with a fixation target, and the *right column* shows return of nystagmus after ("post") suppression.

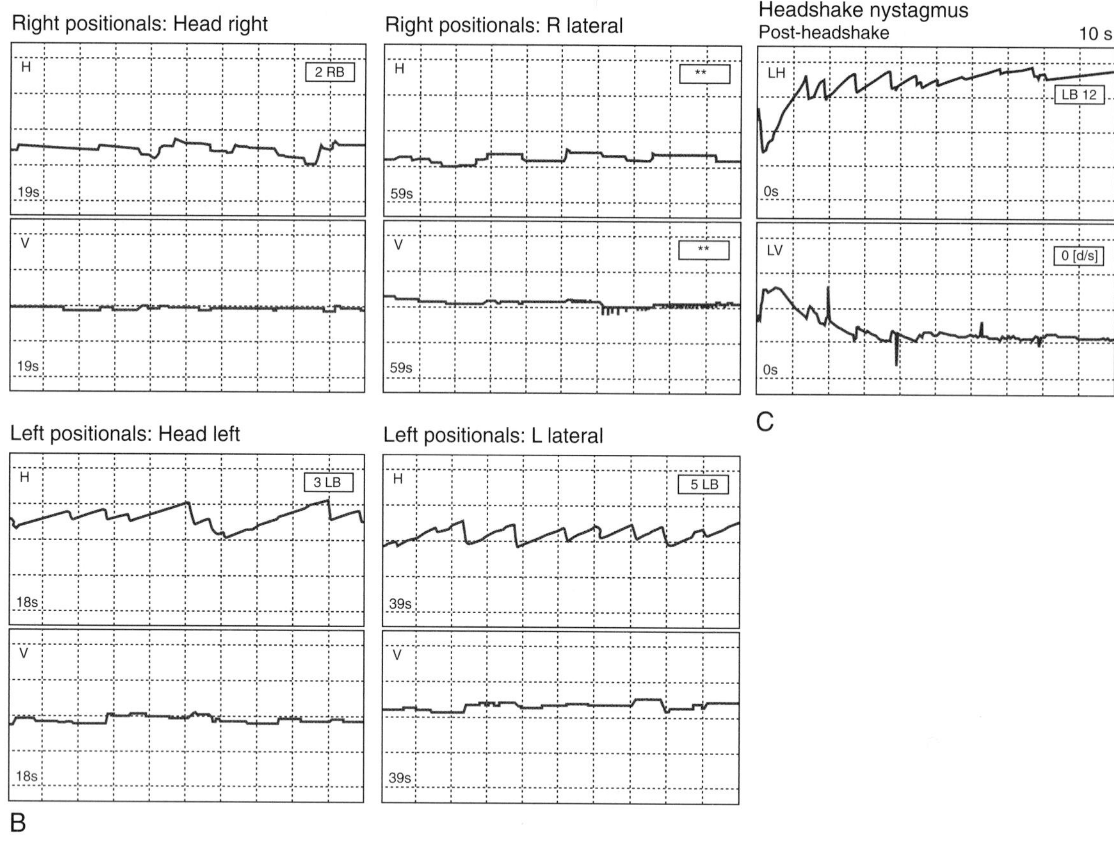

Figure 168-1. **B,** Results from positional testing. In the *top row*, the eye movement recordings for horizontal are shown in the *top box*, with vertical eye movements shown in the *lower box*, from positions of head turn right from supine and right lateral positions. In the *lower row*, the eye movement recordings are shown for the positions of head turn left and left lateral. Left-beating nystagmus ranging from 3 to 5 degrees/second slow-component eye velocity is noted, with no significant nystagmus in the head right and right lateral positions (not shown are three additional positions, also with left-beating nystagmus). **C,** Result of the post-headshake nystagmus test. The *top box* shows the significant left-beating nystagmus that resulted from horizontal headshaking. Minor up-beating nystagmus is seen in the *lower box*.

and three dynamic compensatory processes, *adaptation*, *habituation*, and *sensory substitution*, each of which is promoted by various exercise techniques targeted in VBFT.

Static Compensation for Peripheral Vestibular Lesions

Vertigo of acute onset is accompanied by nystagmus and a variety of neurovegetative symptoms, such as nausea and vomiting. This symptom complex is a result of a persistent asymmetry of vestibular input, often seen after ablative surgical procedures or with acute insults to the peripheral system. The acute or static phase of recovery is mediated by tonic rebalancing of the resting activity in the vestibular nuclei. These changes minimize side-to-side discrepancies between the tonic firing rates in the second-order neurons originating in the nuclei and occur without the need of head movement or vision.[14-18] This activity generally provides relief from the most intense symptoms of vertigo and vomiting within 24 to 72 hours. Nevertheless, the patient continues to experience considerable dysequilibrium, because the system is unable to respond appropriately to the dynamic aspects of vestibular input produced by normal head movements. Thus, even after the intense vertigo has been controlled, continued motion-provoked vertigo is common until dynamic compensation is achieved.

Dynamic Compensation

To eliminate persisting dysequilibrium and residual motion-provoked vertigo after a vestibular lesion, the system must adjust to produce accurate responses to head movements. The dynamic compensation phase seems to be accomplished by reorganization of brainstem and cerebellar pathways, without modulating the neural input to the vestibular nuclei from the peripheral system.[14] This process is much slower than static compensation and typically requires reprogramming of eye movements and postural control responses to head movements. The necessary reprogramming is accomplished by exposure to stimuli that challenge both the gaze stabilization and postural control systems. Because of the brainstem commissural pathways connecting the vestibular nuclei, appropriate central vestibular responses can be produced from inputs arriving from one functioning labyrinth. This feature of the compensation process is critical to recovery after extensive pathologic insults or ablative vestibular surgery, such as labyrinthectomy or vestibular nerve section. As discussed next, three major areas are active in the process of dynamic compensation: adaptation, habituation, and sensory substitution.

Adaptation is the neurologic mechanism that allows for long-term changes in the neuronal response to head movement-provoked gaze stabilization. The neural signals that induce the adaptation are generated primarily by "retinal slip" of the visual image on the retina. This phenomenon is generated by a disordered VOR response, when a head movement produces a perceived motion of a stable object in the visual environment. The resulting error signal can lead to fairly prompt and long-term changes in the functional performance of the VOR.[4] This process of adaptation produced by retinal slip seems to be context-dependent, so that specific adjustments must be made for movements of different frequency, directions of head movement, eye position in the orbit, and distances from the visual target.[3,19] The complexity of the adaptation process helps explain why residual symptoms are almost unavoidable even in a fairly well-compensated patient. Postural stability also is improved by reducing abnormal visual influences on postural control mechanisms secondary to retinal slip.

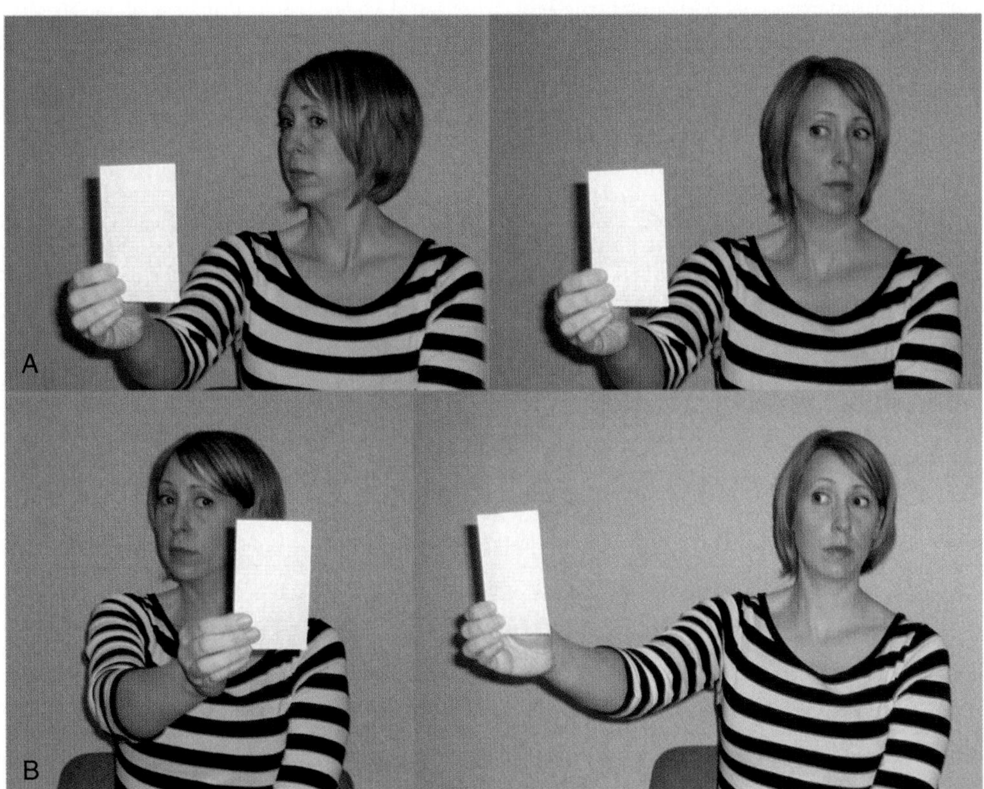

Figure 168-2. Adaptation exercises given to the patient whose videonystagmography results are shown in Figure 168-1. **A,** The "times 1" adaptation exercise. In the times 1 viewing, the target is held still and the patient focuses on a letter on the card and oscillates her head in a small arc in the horizontal plane as fast as she can while maintaining clear visual imaging of the target. **B,** Progression to a "times 2" viewing exercise. In the times 2 viewing, the task is the same, of maintaining clear visual imaging on the letter on the card; however, this time, as the head is moved to the right, the target is moved to the left, doubling the amount the eyes have to move for the same head movement shown in **A**.

Habituation is the long-term reduction of a response to a noxious stimulus resulting from repeated exposure to the stimulus.[20] This phenomenon seems to be context-dependent and does not generalize well from one head movement to another. This mechanism is essential for a variety of conditions that can produce sensitivity to head movement or motion in the visual surroundings. Although peripheral asymmetry is one common cause of these symptoms, other common causes are central lesions, anxiety disorders, and migraine disorders.[5] Although the adjustments produced by habituation are made fairly quickly and are reasonably accurate, the central system requires consistency in the inputs to use them properly for habituation. For this reason, it is essentially impossible to "compensate" for an unstable vestibular lesion such as Meniere's disease.

The primary goals of both adaptation and habituation are to produce gaze stability and postural stability in both static and dynamic situations. The response frequency ranges for gaze and postural stability are very different. To achieve gaze stability, the responsible mechanisms must function properly in a range from static position (no motion) up to movements that correlate with head motions as quick as 10 Hz. Postural stability is predominantly a task that requires responsiveness only below 4 Hz.[21,22]

In addition to adaptation and habituation, another critical component of dynamic compensation involves *sensory substitution*. This process requires the adoption of alternate strategies for gaze and postural control, in order to replace the compromised sensory function. For example, the patient with bilateral loss of peripheral vestibular function becomes dependent primarily on visual or proprioceptive inputs to maintain postural stability. Although these mechanisms may need to be fostered in a therapeutic setting, many patients will have developed some of these out of necessity before coming for evaluation. Although sensory substitution may be helpful, it may be maladaptive in some environmental settings. For example, a patient may be overly dependent on vision and therefore cannot use proprioceptive and residual vestibular inputs to successfully navigate in darkness. In addition to the common substitution of visual and proprioceptive inputs, some of the other mechanisms that may be invoked in the setting of vestibular loss include (1) activation of the cervico-ocular reflex, which is not particularly active in healthy persons[10]; (2) use of the smooth pursuit tracking system[11]; and (3) use of anticipatory or corrective saccades. Patients with both unilateral and bilateral vestibular deficits use corrective saccades to adjust for the reduction of VOR-induced eye movements after head movement. With central preprogramming through exposure to specific eye-head coordinated movements, these eye movements can be applied automatically to help maintain gaze stability when the VOR is deficient.[7,8]

Research findings suggest that initial central vestibular compensation for a peripheral lesion can be enhanced by head movement but is delayed by inactivity.[23-26] It also is hampered by central vestibular dysfunction of any cause.[27] Medications that typically are used for acute symptoms of vertigo, such as meclizine, scopolamine, and benzodiazepines, all cause sedation and central nervous system depression. Although they may provide helpful symptomatic relief during the initial stages of an acute labyrinthine crisis, their effects are potentially counterproductive with respect to vestibular compensation, especially with use over extended periods.[24,28] In addition, chronic anxiety or other psychiatric disorders may delay or disrupt the compensation process.[29,30]

Although remarkably reliable, vestibular compensation seems to be a somewhat fragile, energy-dependent process. Even after it is apparently complete, periods of symptomatic relapse may occur because of decompensation. A period of inactivity, extreme fatigue, change in medications, general anesthesia or an intercurrent illness may trigger these relapses. A relapse of vestibular symptoms in this setting does not imply ongoing, progressive, or new labyrinthine dysfunction.

These features of vestibular compensation suggest that avoidance of movements and body positions that provoke vertigo, as well as the traditional practice of prescribing vestibular suppressants, may be inappropriate. Because the stimulus for recovery seems to be repeated exposure to the sensory conflicts produced by movement, the patient's medications should be discontinued once the acute symptoms are resolved, and an active program geared toward recovery should be encouraged. For most affected persons, recovery will be rapid and nearly complete. For some, the symptoms of vestibular dysfunction may persist. Although the latter patients are candidates for vestibular rehabilitation programs, starting a formal vestibular rehabilitation program as early as possible for patients whose symptom presentation suggests a high likelihood of benefit from such programs can help to avoid the persistence of symptoms.

Assessment of Vestibular Compensation

Role of the Clinical History

A complete neuro-otologic history probably is the single most important component of the diagnostic evaluation of the patient with a balance disorder. Balance function study results must be interpreted in light of the presenting symptoms and medical history.[31] In general, the information sought should include the onset of symptoms and their characteristics at that time, the progression of symptoms over time, the nature and duration of typical spells, any predisposing factors in the medical history, and use of medications or other management strategies. Complicating features of anxiety, depression, or excessive dependence on medications should be addressed. Some effort should be extended to identify the degree of disability produced by the patient's vestibular complaints with respect to his or her professional and social activities. The stability and commitment of the patient's psychological support system also should be assessed.

Ongoing complaints after a peripheral vestibular insult indicate that compensation is incomplete. The history and presenting symptoms are used to determine whether these continuing sensations may be a result of a fluctuating or progressive labyrinthine disorder. In the case of the unstable lesion, poor compensation results because the central nervous system cannot react to unpredictable peripheral inputs. In the history, an unstable periphery is suspected if symptoms are spontaneous in onset. In the stable cases, the symptoms are much more likely to be consistently provoked by head or eye movements. It is the patients with stable lesions who are most likely to benefit from vestibular and balance rehabilitation. The patients in the group with unstable lesions may have VBRT as part of their management, but it is not likely to be the primary modality of treatment.

Role of Vestibular Testing

The most traditional purpose of balance function studies is site-of-lesion localization addressing the sensory inputs, motor output elements, and neural pathways that may be involved in producing the reported symptoms. Balance function studies also may assess the patient's functional ability to use sensory input systems in an integrated fashion, as in maintenance of stance before and after induced sway and coordination of head and eye movements during gaze activities. The third assessment goal is to evaluate, in a limited manner, the current degree of physiologic and functional compensation.[32]

Although a wide variety of studies may be used to assess the balance system in the broadest sense, tests that are used to determine the extent and site of vestibular lesions are unable to predict the type of vestibular symptoms, the magnitude of those symptoms, or the level of disability in an individual patient. When the predictive utility of the vestibular test battery is reviewed, no significant correlation is found between test results and performance of high-level activities of daily living in the chronically dizzy patient. Thus, a therapist can and must proceed with an evaluation of these factors, irrespective of the vestibular test results.

Although specific subtests within videonystagmography (VNG), rotary chair, and postural control testing can give indications of compensation status, the value of such tests is somewhat limited. Typically, the information obtained from these studies relates more to the static phase of compensation than that of the dynamic phase. Clinically significant spontaneous nystagmus, positional nystagmus, and a directional preponderance on the VNG provide evidence for failure of physiologic compensation in the control of eye movements. Rotational chair testing stimulates the horizontal semicircular canals and their afferent inputs over a broad range of frequencies and accelerations. Although this is a physiologic rather than a functional evaluation, it provides information about the vestibulo-ocular system that is not obtained from the VNG. In general, although abnormalities in the timing (phase lead) or amplitude (gain) of the eye movements produced by the VOR provide evidence for peripheral vestibular dysfunction, these physiologic measures do not assess the level of compensation within the central system.[14] On the other hand, persistent asymmetry (bias) in the slow-phase eye velocity responses produced by rightward versus leftward rotation strongly suggests that the peripheral lesion is physiologically uncompensated.

Dynamic posturography provides information about balance system function that is not available through the other vestibular testing modalities. The sensory organization portion of dynamic posturography is primarily a test of functional capabilities, rather than a site-of-lesion evaluation. By measuring the degree of postural sway under several test conditions, this test determines whether the patient is able to make proper use of sensory inputs from the visual, vestibular, and somatosensory systems for maintaining stable stance. By identifying difficulty in the use of one or more of the input informations, a quantitative estimate of functional compensation is obtained. It is not unusual to document normal sensory organization findings in patients who report motion-provoked symptoms exclusively and show no signs of pathologic nystagmus or significant asymmetry on rotational chair testing. By contrast, some patients will demonstrate significant abnormalities of postural control, reflecting inadequate functional compensation, even when the more physiologic measures (VNG and rotational chair) suggest a reasonably complete physiologic compensation process.

The movement coordination battery of dynamic posturography may be used to assess the automatic motor output responses from the central nervous system in response to perturbations of stance. Abnormalities detected may help to explain findings in the sensory organization test, especially the somatosensory and vestibular dysfunction pattern. It also may provide indications of previously undiagnosed peripheral neuropathy or biomechanical deficits resulting from known musculoskeletal conditions.[33,34] This protocol does not provide any information about the status of compensation.

Vestibular Rehabilitation: Patient Selection Criteria

Vestibular Rehabilitation as a Primary Treatment Modality

The use of VBRT in the treatment of BPPV is well accepted. The use of noncustomized programs such as Cawthorne exercises has a long and fairly successful history for the management of this problem.[19,23,35] However, for many patients, the commonly prescribed Cawthorne program is too intensive and often provokes intense vestibular symptoms, sometimes accompanied by nausea or vomiting. This discourages the patient from continuing. A preferred noncustomized program for BPPV that addresses the needs of most patients is the Brandt-Daroff program.[23] An alternate approach for the treatment of classic BPPV caused by otoconia floating free in one of the semicircular canals (canalithiasis) is to perform an appropriate particle repositioning maneuver.[36] When these techniques are insufficient to bring relief, the patient should be referred to a vestibular therapist for a customized program.[6] For a complete discussion of BPPV and particle repositioning maneuvers, please refer to Chapters 163-165.

The use of VBRT as the primary treatment recommendation is appropriate in any condition characterized by a stable unilateral peripheral or central vestibular deficit when the patient's natural compensation process is incomplete. This is a symptom-driven indication that is determined from the patient's presenting symptoms. The report of spontaneously occurring symptoms or documented fluctuations in hearing or vestibular function suggests an unstable lesion. If the patient's evaluation reveals no evidence of a progressive or fluctuant (unstable) process, it is likely that VBRT will produce a satisfactory resolution of symptoms. This intervention is certainly preferable to the protracted use of vestibular suppressants. In most patients with stable peripheral lesions, there is no role for the use of long-term vestibular suppressants. However, they may be useful at the outset of VBRT to reduce symptoms to a level that allows the patient to perform the prescribed exercise program.[37]

The final indication for the use of VBRT as a primary treatment modality is for disorders characterized by multifactorial balance difficulties, such as those seen in the elderly.[38] This option becomes especially important when other treatment options are unavailable or have been exhausted. These patients may benefit greatly from postural control exercises and individualized conditioning programs. Frequently, the relationship with the therapist assumes a strong counseling function, and the use of assistive devices for safety in ambulation can be introduced as needed.

Vestibular Rehabilitation as an Adjunctive Modality

Several situations may require the use of VBRT interventions as an adjunctive treatment modality. The use of routine or selective VBRT is helpful in optimizing the outcome after vestibular surgery, such as vestibular schwannoma removal, labyrinthectomy, or vestibular nerve section, and after intratympanic aminoglycoside administration for Meniere's disease. When a patient with an unstable vestibular condition undergoes an ablative procedure, a more profound, yet stable, unilateral vestibular lesion is created. The process of acute and chronic compensation must begin anew. It is possible that many of the unsatisfactory outcomes after vestibular surgery can be attributed to incomplete or delayed postoperative compensation. All patients should be instructed regarding the importance of central compensation for the success of any ablative vestibular procedure. Those individuals who are at particular risk for poor recovery because of complicating central nervous system conditions, sedating medications, or poor motivation for recovery should be encouraged to pursue a customized program of VBRT early in their postoperative course.

Vestibular rehabilitation may play a role in other conditions that include a component of balance complaints.[5,39] Frequently, patients who have had head injuries have significant disability from vestibular symptoms. Because their condition often includes cognitive and central vestibular involvement, along with the peripheral labyrinthine component, VBRT techniques are best used as a supplement to a comprehensive, multidisciplinary head injury program rather than as the primary rehabilitative measure. Similarly, patients with anxiety disorders often seek management of ill-defined vestibular symptoms. After a suitable evaluation is performed, VBRT may be recommended as an adjunctive measure for the anxiety disorder. If the anxiety is mild, VBRT functions as a behavioral intervention, similar to exposure therapy for treatment of phobias. If the anxiety component is significant, and particularly if panic attacks are frequent, psychiatric intervention will be required as well. The use of VBRT can be of assistance in situations of migraine-associated dizziness, provided that appropriate treatment for migraine is given concurrently.[5,13]

Patients with Meniere's disease may complain of positional vertigo or other chronic vestibular symptoms between their definitive attacks. Although such patients are candidates for VBRT, they need to recognize that the prognosis for lasting relief of chronic symptoms is reduced if the typical severe attacks of Meniere's disease occur more than monthly. If the attacks are rare, or the Meniere's disease is inactive, the prognosis is considerably improved.

Vestibular Rehabilitation as a Therapeutic Trial

At times, the physician may be uncertain whether a patient's complaints are due to stable vestibular disease with inadequate compensation or to an unstable labyrinthine disorder, such as perilymphatic fistula. In this setting, a trial of VBRT is appropriate if the hearing is stable and may assist in the diagnosis by clarifying this important distinction. Failure to improve in VBRT lends further credibility to the diagnostic impression that the lesion is unstable or progressive. It is then advisable to proceed with appropriate surgical management, provided that the symptoms are severe enough to warrant the procedure and they are believed to emanate from the end organ. This conservative treatment course is particularly appropriate before surgical interventions are considered for controversial diagnoses such as spontaneous perilymph fistula.[40]

It is sometimes difficult to determine whether a postoperative relapse of vestibular symptoms represents disease progression or merely central decompensation.[41] Decompensation may be observed as a late sequela after initially complete compensation for any peripheral lesion, including vestibular surgery. For example, many surgeons consider transmastoid labyrinthectomy to be a definitive procedure for the control of vertigo of peripheral origin. Thus, an explanation of why failures are reported to occur is warranted. Early failures are best attributed to incorrect diagnosis, incomplete removal of the neuroepithelium at the time of surgery, or inadequate initial central nervous system compensation. Late failures have been hypothesized to result from "post-labyrinthectomy neuromas."[42,43] Although there is little reason to expect that such lesions could produce symptoms, some surgeons would advocate performing a vestibular neurectomy in this setting. An alternate explanation for these recurrent symptoms after a complete labyrinthectomy would be late central decompensation, which should respond briskly to VBRT. Instead of proceeding to additional surgery, a therapeutic trial of VBRT is suitable whenever the possibility of incomplete compensation or decompensation remains.

Inappropriate Candidates

Patients whose symptoms occur strictly in spontaneous, discrete episodes, such as are seen with Meniere's disease, are unlikely to benefit from VBRT. If no provocative movements or body positions are found to reliably produce spells and no postural control abnormalities are noted during the evaluation, the patient is best managed with alternative medical or surgical strategies. Nonetheless, such patients should be encouraged to remain active and optimize their general health through physical activities performed at a level that is appropriate for their age and general health.

Role of Balance Function Studies in Patient Selection

It needs to be recognized that VBRT is a symptom-driven treatment program. The principal features that suggest use of VBRT for primary or adjunctive management are complaints related to motion-provoked symptoms or dysfunction with balance and gait. Is there a role for the use of balance function studies for determination of which patients would be appropriate candidates for VBRT? Do these tests play any role in the monitoring of the program's outcome?

Of the main balance function studies, *dynamic posturography* has the highest likelihood of suggesting that VBRT may be appropriate and guiding the treatment prescribed by the therapist. Some patients have a symptom presentation that does not suggest the use of therapy as a management option, yet performance on dynamic posturography shows clear deficits in maintenance of upright stance during challenging conditions. Such a patient would then be a highly appropriate candidate for VBRT to improve performance and reduce the potential for falls. Dynamic postural control evaluations in patients for whom VBRT is to be used can assist in the design and monitoring of the customized VBRT program.[19,33,37]

The VNG and rotary chair studies do not provide information that assists in deciding who is an appropriate candidate for VBRT. However, if a patient is otherwise an appropriate candidate for VBRT, these studies can be used to reinforce the use of a specific form of exercise in the therapy program. Indications of deficits in the VOR provide support for the use of adaptation exercises as a means for improving the VOR gain and, thereby, the functional performance of the VOR. Neither of these studies holds any significant utility with respect to the monitoring of the progress of a VBRT program. However, if the patient is not improving as expected, repeating portions of the VNG or rotary chair protocol may be useful in determining whether the vestibular system pathology has progressed in a way that would adversely affect the patient's progress.[44]

Table 168-1

Common Techniques for Vestibular Rehabilitation

Vestibulopathy	Rehabilitative Strategy
Acute uncompensated unilateral peripheral lesion *Example*: immediate postoperative status or recent crisis	Generic vestibular rehabilitation program to start Customized program if patient does not make satisfactory progress
Stable uncompensated unilateral peripheral lesion *Example*: previous crisis with continuous symptoms	Habituation and adaptation exercises Postural control activities if abnormalities detected during testing
Bilateral peripheral lesions	Sensory substitution with visual-vestibular interaction Postural control activities if abnormalities detected Screening for other comorbid conditions that may aggravate balance problems
BPPV	Particle repositioning maneuver Habituation exercises if repositioning fails
Vertiginous migraines Anxiety-provoked symptoms Head injury	Sensory substitution activities potentially of benefit with chronic dizziness related to vertiginous migraine Vestibular rehabilitative adjuvant treatment as part of a multidisciplinary approach

BPPV, benign paroxysmal positional vertigo.

Vestibular Rehabilitation: Common Techniques

The vestibular rehabilitation therapist uses a variety of techniques when providing a program customized to the needs of the individual patient (Table 168-1). For a complete discussion of the diagnostic and therapeutic interventions that may appropriately be performed by the therapist, the interested reader is referred to other resources for further reading.[13,45] This section of the chapter reviews several general categories of exercise techniques that are used in a customized program of VBRT.

Adaptation Exercises

The principal goal of adaptation exercises is improvement in the functional performance of the VOR and accompanying gaze stability for those who demonstrate a VOR deficit physiologically and who have predictable symptoms provoked by head movements. Evidence of a VOR deficit may include a caloric response asymmetry on VNG and/or an abnormal time constant on rotary chair testing. The functional impact of a physiologic VOR deficit is realized through the use of Dynamic Visual Acuity (DVA) testing, which assesses the ability to accurately resolve a visual target while the head is in motion.[13] The activities involve primarily eye-head coordinated movements called VOR *times 1* and *times 2* viewing exercises (see Fig. 168-2), described elsewhere.[5,13] Using eye movement recordings during the head thrust, test pilot data have been able to show an actual increase in the gain of the VOR correlating with functional improvement as reflected in the DVA in patients with unilateral hypofunction. However, the gain was more consistently increased for active (patient-initiated) head thrusts than for passive (unexpected examiner-initiated) head thrusts.[46] The implication of this work is that to appreciate an actual change in physiologic gain of the system, the task must have direct relevance to the patient. This is the first study to show a mechanistic change as a result of the vestibular rehabilitation adaptation exercises. Of interest is that even though the underlying mechanism for VOR adaptation may not as yet be well understood, the prescribed exercises do result in measurable changes in the VOR functional performance.[1,13,14]

Habituation Exercises

For most patients with positionally provoked symptoms, the primary goal is to extinguish residual pathologic responses after incomplete or disordered compensation.[47] The therapist identifies the typical movements that produce the most pronounced symptoms and provides the patient with a limited but progressive program of exercises that reproduce these movements. Typically, these are performed two to three times daily, with the duration and number of repetitions varying according to the severity of nausea or dizziness they produce. Patients are counseled that symptoms are aggravated by the exercises at first but that gradual improvement will follow. Patients often are encouraged by experiencing short-term habituation at the end of an exercise session. If they can persevere with their program, most patients will begin to note dramatic relief of positional vertigo within 4 to 6 weeks.

There is obviously significant overlap between these and the adaptation activities. Differences exist in the details of the techniques relative to speed, visual target, number of movements, and repetition. The underlying principle of habituation exercises is that of brief repeated exposures. This technique also can be used to reduce sensitivity to visual motion–provoked symptoms, although that is a more difficult task.

Substitution Exercises

As the name implies, substitution exercises teach the patient to use alternative strategies and sensory inputs to make up for those that are deficient or absent. There is clearly a limit to how much vision or proprioception can substitute for the vestibular system, or how much vestibular information can substitute for proprioception. These limits are secondary to the differences in the frequency range over which each of these inputs and the various motor and perceptual outputs function.[21,22] Notwithstanding the limitations, this technique can be successful in promoting changes in performance for both gaze stability and postural control by means of the mechanism of central preprogramming.[9,48]

Postural Control and Gait Exercises

When abnormalities of postural control are detected in the assessment, these may be specifically addressed in the prescribed exercise program. Programs can be designed to correct weight-bearing asymmetries, limited mobility about the center of gravity, and sensory input selection problems. For example, if the patient is found to depend on somatosensory input despite the availability of accurate visual cues, the program may involve exercises that require balancing on thick foam. This would be performed initially with eyes open and eventually with eyes closed.

Although working on static balance is one dimension of therapy, more complex gait activities over a short course (such as a 10- to 20-foot walk) often are prescribed and combined with other, more complex movements. These may involve specific activities such as stepping over objects or incorporating reciprocal head movements. The patient also may be asked to practice walking on different types of surfaces such as a compressible soft carpet or an irregular gravel parking lot. These activities are designed to enhance stability in daily activities. Patients with bilateral loss of vestibular function may be instructed to perform exercises that help with sensory substitution. These may include walking in progressively more challenging, dimly lit environments to facilitate somatosensory substitution and balancing on more challenging support services to facilitate visual substitution.[13]

Conditioning and Maintenance Activities

Most patients with vertigo and balance disorders have adopted a sedentary lifestyle to avoid precipitating their symptoms. Although such a response is understandable, the inactivity contributes to their ongoing disability and delays their recovery. Thus, all patients who receive customized VBRT programs also are provided with suggestions for a general exercise program that is suited to their age, health, and interests. For most patients, this would involve at least a graduated walking program. For many, a more strenuous program is suggested that may include jogging, treadmill, aerobics, or bicycling. Activities that involve coordinated eye, head, and body movements such as golf, bowling, handball, or racquet sports may be appropriate. Swimming is approached cautiously because of the disorientation experienced by many patients with vestibular dysfunction in the relative weightlessness of the aquatic environment.

Maintenance of Initial Results

Once the patient has completed the initial period of treatment, progress is assessed and adjustments are made in the program. Exercises that no longer produce symptoms are eliminated and replaced by others that were not originally included because of lower priority. This process is continued until the improvements begin to plateau. When this point is reached, it is important to provide the patient with counseling and a program of maintenance exercises to secure the benefits gained from the active treatment program. The maintenance program typically includes continuing the prescribed conditioning exercises, as well as any unique postural control activities that were required. The patient is instructed to resume exercises if a relapse of symptoms should occur. For central nervous system lesions involving the cerebellum, indications are that the active program needs to be continued indefinitely to maintain benefits.[12]

Role of Therapist in Patient Education

A key role of the therapist in the management of the patient with a balance disorder is to educate the patient about the illness.[12] The patient often has acquired considerable misinformation that must be addressed. This supportive function of the therapist is particularly essential for the management of patients with a less favorable prognosis. A patient who is well educated regarding the nature of vestibular or balance dysfunction will understand the rationale for vestibular rehabilitation. The patient will recognize that these measures are simply a management technique instead of a cure for the underlying deficits. This orientation takes the patient from a passive role toward an active role in his or her own recovery.

Vestibular Rehabilitation: Expected Results

A 2-year prospective clinical trial including all patients undergoing VBRT at the University of Michigan suggested that a reduction of symptoms can be expected in approximately 85% of cases. In this trial, 80% of patients also showed improved scores on a disability rating scale after therapy.[37] A subsequent randomized controlled clinical trial provided evidence that VBRT programs customized to the unique needs of the individual patient provided results that are superior to those obtained with generic programs of therapy.[49] A recent review from the Cochrane collaboration evaluated 21 randomized trials of vestibular rehabilitation for unilateral peripheral vestibular dysfunction. Overall, the results strongly support vestibular rehabilitation as an effective tool in the management for unilateral vestibular dysfunction over medications, placebo or sham interventions, or no intervention.[50] Whitney and Rossi[1] also have provided a useful review of multiple published studies of VBRT efficacy. In their review, they classify the works by the presence or absence of control groups and the prospective or retrospective nature of the studies. Overall, the studies reviewed demonstrate significant evidence supporting the efficacy of VBRT as a major management tool for patients with balance and vestibular disorders. This summary also demonstrates that VBRT is highly beneficial after unilateral surgical ablation of vestibular function. Similar results may be expected in treating fixed unilateral lesions such as vestibular neuritis and labyrinthitis. Treatment of canalithiasis causing classic BPPV with the particle-repositioning maneuver is effective in more than 90% of cases, but the condition may recur in up to 30% of patients. Habituation exercises have been reported to yield similar results but do not offer relief as promptly. Patients with bilateral vestibulopathy treated with VBRT show significant improvement in speed of ambulation and stair negotiation, postural stability, and reaching distance compared with control subjects.

In general, the patients who have a poorer prognosis for improvement with VBRT include those with severe bilateral peripheral lesions, combined central and peripheral vestibular deficits and headache syndromes after head injury, and those with established long-term disability. For those in whom migraine or anxiety disorders are the primary source for symptoms, VBRT can be effective if used with treatment for the primary disease process.[5] Although some elderly patients may progress poorly because of irreversible multisensory dysfunction, the overall experience with this age group has been favorable.

The concurrent use of vestibular suppressant medication or other centrally acting agents has been shown to delay the time course of recovery during VBRT. Whenever possible, these medications should be tapered to lower doses or discontinued completely. On the other hand, they may be continued if they are essential for treatment of complicating medical conditions or for relief of symptoms during the VBRT program, because their use does not seem to dramatically reduce the chances of a satisfactory ultimate outcome.

SUGGESTED READINGS

Baloh RW, Honrubia V. *Clinical Neurophysiology of the Vestibular System.* 2nd ed. Philadelphia: F.A. Davis; 1989.

Brandt T, Daroff RB. Physical therapy for benign paroxysmal positional vertigo. *Arch Otol Rhinol Laryngol.* 1980;106:484.

Cawthorne T. The physiological basis for head exercises. *J Chart Soc Physiother* 1944;30:106.

Cooksey FS. Rehabilitation in vestibular injuries. *Proc R Soc Med.* 1946;39:273.

Crane BT, Demer JL. Human gaze stabilization during natural activities: translation, rotation, magnification, and target distance effects. *J Neurophysiol.* 1997;78:2129.

Grossman GE, Leigh RJ. Instability of gaze during locomotion in patients with deficient vestibular function. *Ann Neurol.* 1990;27:528.

Grossman GE, Leigh RJ, Bruce EN, et al. Performance of the human vestibuloocular reflex during locomotion. *J Neurophysiol.* 1989;62:264.

Herdman S, ed. *Vestibular Rehabilitation.* 3rd ed. Philadelphia: F.A. Davis; 2007.

Herdman S, Tusa R. Assessment and treatment of patients with benign paroxysmal positional vertigo. In: Herdman S, ed. *Vestibular Rehabilitation.* 2nd ed. Philadelphia: F.A. Davis; 2000:451.

Hillier SL, Hollohan V. Vestibular rehabilitation for unilateral peripheral vestibular dysfunction. *Cochrane Database Syst Rev.* 2007;4:CD005397.

Horak FB, Nashner LM. Central programming of postural movements: adaptation to altered support surface configurations. *J Neurophysiol.* 1986;55:1369.

Igarashi M, Ishikawa M, Yamane H. Physical exercise and balance compensation after total ablation of vestibular organs. *Prog Brain Res.* 1988;76:395.

McCabe BF, Sekitani T. Further experiments on vestibular compensation. *Laryngoscope.* 1972;82:381.

Peppard SB. Effect of drug therapy on compensation from vestibular injury. *Laryngoscope.* 1986;96:878.

Schwarz DWF. Physiology of the vestibular system. In: Cummings C, Fredrickson J, Harker L, et al, eds. *Otolaryngology—Head and Neck Surgery.* Vol 3. St. Louis: Mosby; 1986.

Shepard NT, Asher A. Treatment of patients with nonvestibular dizziness and disequilibrium. In: Herdman S, ed. *Vestibular Rehabilitation.* 2nd ed. Philadelphia: F.A. Davis; 2000:534.

Shepard NT, Telian SA. Programmatic vestibular rehabilitation. *Otolaryngol Head Neck Surg.* 1995;112:173.

Shepard NT, Telian SA, Smith-Wheelock M, et al. Vestibular and balance rehabilitation therapy. *Ann Otol Rhinol Laryngol.* 1993;102:198.

Shumway-Cook A, Horak FB. Rehabilitation strategies for patients with vestibular deficits. *Neurol Clin.* 1990;8:441.

Smith-Wheelock M, Shepard NT, Telian SA, Boismer T. Balance retraining therapy in the elderly. In: Kashima H, Goldstein J, Lucente F, eds. *Clinical Geriatric Otolaryngology.* Philadelphia: B.C. Decker; 1992:71.

Smith-Wheelock M, Shepard NT, Telian SA. Physical therapy program for vestibular rehabilitation. *Am J Otol.* 1991;12:218.

Suarez H, Arocena M, Suarez A, et al. Changes in postural control parameters after vestibular rehabilitation in patients with central vestibular disorders. *Acta Otolaryngol.* 2003;123:143.

Telian SA, Shepard NT, Smith-Wheelock M, et al. bilateral vestibular paresis: diagnosis and treatment. *Otolaryngol Head Neck Surg.* 1991;104:67.

Whitney SL, Rossi MM. Efficacy of vestibular rehabilitation. *Otolaryngol Clin North Am.* 2000;33:659.

Yardley L. Overview of the psychologic effects of chronic dizziness and balance disorders. *Otolaryngol Clin North Am.* 2000;33:603.

Ylikoski J, Belal A. Human vestibular nerve morphology after labyrinthectomy. *Otolaryngol Head Neck Surg.* 1988;99:472.

Zee DS. Vestibular adaptation. In: Herdman S, ed. *Vestibular Rehabilitation.* 2nd ed. Philadelphia: F.A. Davis; 2000:77.

For complete list of references log onto www.expertconsult.com.

SECTION EIGHT

Facial Nerve Disorders

CHAPTER ONE HUNDRED AND SIXTY-NINE

Tests of Facial Nerve Function

Rodney C. Diaz

Robert A. Dobie

Key Points

- History and physical examination are the most important tools in evaluation of facial nerve function and in diagnosis of dysfunction.
- The House-Brackmann grading system is the most commonly used method of categorizing and documenting long-term facial nerve function after insult, injury, or surgery.
- Topognostic testing correlates specific functional deficits with corresponding anatomic branch points to determine the site of the lesion along the course of the facial nerve; it has been largely superseded by electrodiagnostic testing.
- The four types of electrodiagnostic testing are the nerve excitability test (NET), the maximum stimulation test (MST), electroneuronography (ENoG) (also called electroneurography), and electromyography (EMG). Each has its advantages and disadvantages.
- Electrodiagnostic testing of the facial nerve can differentiate neurapraxia from neural degeneration, but it cannot distinguish between different degrees of neural degeneration.
- Electrodiagnostic testing can provide prognostic information regarding the likelihood of complete or good recovery versus severely incomplete or poor recovery; threshold criteria for predicting poor recovery are used by some surgeons in patient selection for surgical exploration and decompression of the facial nerve.
- Intraoperative facial nerve monitoring has been shown to be a valuable adjunct in surgery for acoustic neuroma and other tumors of the cerebellopontine angle, as well as in revision parotidectomy for recurrent pleomorphic adenoma. Multiple factors can affect accuracy and performance; therefore, responses from a monitoring device should not supplant surgical knowledge and experience in intraoperative decision making.
- Unconventional forms of facial nerve monitoring, under development, may provide additional information for evaluating facial nerve integrity intraoperatively beyond standard methods of intraoperative monitoring.

In facial paralysis, as in most medical problems, history and physical examination usually provide more useful information than laboratory tests. Sometimes, however, a more objective evaluation of facial nerve function is indicated to detect a facial nerve lesion; to measure its severity; to localize it to a particular intracranial, intratemporal, or extratemporal site; to assess the prognosis for recovery; to assist in treatment decisions; or to detect and avoid surgical injury. Quantitative tests of facial nerve function are then used.

Useful diagnostic tests add information to what is already known, influence the choice of therapy, and ultimately improve clinical outcomes.[1] This chapter discusses several tests for evaluation of the facial nerve that can be helpful—as well as several that have not been shown to be helpful—in various clinical scenarios. Intraoperative monitoring of electrical activity of muscles innervated by the facial nerve is by far the most well-established, clinically useful means of assessing facial nerve function, other than physical examination. Outpatient electrical testing of facial nerve function makes sense in clinical settings in which surgical repair or decompression is under consideration, such as after temporal bone fracture or Bell's palsy. Of note, however, most of the tests described in this chapter have very limited proven clinical usefulness.

Facial nerve imaging also is briefly discussed. Although magnetic resonance imaging (MRI) is the modality of choice when a tumor is suspected to be the cause of facial paralysis, it seems not to be useful in Bell's palsy.

Physical Examination

Facial weakness can be extremely subtle, apparent only to a trained examiner (and perhaps to the patient). Paradoxically, mild unilateral facial weakness sometimes can be more easily detected by comparison with a normal contralateral side by having the patient perform nominal rather than maximal volitional movements. Rapid repetitive blinking also can unmask a mild facial weakness, which will manifest as slowed or reduced blink frequency compared with that on the normal side. By contrast, when facial paralysis is total or near-total, the diagnosis is obvious; such impairment can be devastating to the patient on functional, social, and psychologic levels.

Attempts have been made to standardize measurement of facial function, using techniques as simple as measurements with hand-held calipers and as complex as digital photographic and videographic documentation.[2,3] Whereas caliper methods have been shown to demonstrate a high intertest variability, digital photographic methods appear to be much more reliable.[4]

Several systems of clinical measurement of facial nerve function have been devised, but since the mid-1980s, the House-Brackmann system has been most widely used and has been endorsed by the

American Academy of Otolaryngology–Head and Neck Surgery.[5] In the House-Brackmann system, grade I is normal function, grade VI is complete absence of facial motor function, and grades II to V are intermediate (Table 169-1).

The House-Brackmann system is least ambiguous at its extremes and most prone to intertest variability at its intermediate grades II to V: Multiple regional descriptors of facial movement within each scale can overlap, leading to confusion in assigning the appropriate grade. Alternatively, major functional criteria can be used to create unambiguous categories of progression of deficit correlated with each grade (Fig. 169-1).

Similarly, examiners do not always agree among themselves, even when using the same formal grading system. In two studies, each with more than 100 patients with various degrees of facial weakness, examiners unanimously agreed on the House-Brackmann grade as often as 80% (three examiners in one study) and as seldom as 33% (five examiners in the other study).[6,7] Of course, the probability of disagreement should increase as more examiners are used; the probability of any two examiners disagreeing is as low as 13%[8] (on the assumption that in all cases of three-examiner disagreement, two choose one grade and the third choose another grade) and as high as 40% (on the assumption of maximum dispersion of examiner judgments across House-Brackmann categories).[9] It would be interesting to know how much of this variability is caused by individual examiners' test-retest variability (i.e., the tendency of an examiner to assign different scores to the same patient on repeated examination) and how much is attributable to consistent differences among examiners (e.g., between "strict" and "lax" graders).

The wide acceptance of the House-Brackmann system has not prevented many others from proposing new systems. For example, Burres and Fisch[10] described a method requiring multiple measurements of movement in different parts of the face; Croxson and colleagues[6] showed the expected correlation between Burres-Fisch and House-Brackmann in 42 patients, but considerable variability of Burres-Fisch scores was observed for House-Brackmann grades III and IV. Murtry and coworkers[9] proposed and tested the Nottingham system of subjective estimation of movement at each of several points on the face. This method correlated better with House-Brackmann than did Burres-Fisch, and it was simpler to perform. Newer systems include those devised by Ross and associates at Sunnybrook (Ontario, Canada)[11] and Coulson and colleagues in Sydney, Australia.[12] both of which place particular emphasis on the degree of synkinesis in facial movement. These systems demonstrate good overall test-intertest reliability and correlation with the House-Brackmann system, but subjective evaluation of degree of synkinesis is much more variable.[12,13]

Neely and associates[14] showed the feasibility of computer-assisted image analysis for measuring facial movement. Other objective measurement systems have been proposed by Johnson[15] and Jansen[16] and their coworkers. These methods are promising, particularly for research and for the assessment of weakness affecting only a single region of the face (e.g., forehead, lower lip).

An occasionally overlooked limitation of the House-Brackmann grading system is in the evaluation of acute facial paralysis. The differentiation among House-Brackmann grades II, III, IV, and V rests partly on the presence and severity of synkinesis, contracture, hemifacial spasm, and asymmetry at rest—all sequelae of long-term facial nerve dysfunction and hence all absent in the setting of acute facial paralysis. This inherent restriction extends to most other alternative grading systems as well.

The House-Brackmann system applied in its strictest sense is well suited for evaluation of long-standing facial nerve dysfunction but not acute facial paralysis.[17] Nonetheless, this system can be informally rethought for use in the acute setting, in terms of graduated degrees of facial weakness: grade I, normal or 100% function, grade II, mild weakness or 75% to 99% function; grade III, moderate weakness or 50% to 75% function; grade IV, moderately severe weakness or 25% to 50% function; grade V, severe weakness or 1% to 25% function; and grade VI, complete paralysis or zero function. The obvious disadvantage of this technique is in the reversion to a coarse, imprecise, unweighted method of scaling facial function. However, although not canonical, this method allows for continued use of a six-scale grading system to track facial nerve function through the entire clinical course, from acute onset of the paralysis to long-term outcome.

Table 169-1

House-Brackmann Facial Nerve Grading System

Grade	Description	Characteristics
I	Normal	Normal facial function in all areas
II	Mild dysfunction	Gross: slight weakness noticeable on close inspection; may have very slight synkinesis At rest: normal symmetry and tone Motion—Forehead: moderate to good function Motion—Eye: complete closure with minimum effort Motion—Mouth: slight asymmetry
III	Moderate dysfunction	Gross: Obvious but not disfiguring difference between two sides; noticeable but not severe synkinesis, contracture, or hemifacial spasm At rest: normal symmetry and tone Motion—Forehead: slight to moderate movement Motion—Eye: complete closure with effort Motion—Mouth: slightly weak with maximum effort
IV	Moderately severe dysfunction	Gross: obvious weakness and/or disfiguring asymmetry At rest: normal symmetry and tone Motion—Forehead: none Motion—Eye: incomplete closure Motion—Mouth: asymmetric with maximum effort
V	Severe dysfunction	Gross: only barely perceptible motion At rest: asymmetry Motion—Forehead: none Motion—Eye: incomplete closure Motion—Mouth: slight movement
VI	Total paralysis	No movement

The best system would be reliable, easy to use, and correlate well with patient self-assessment. Kahn and coworkers[18] developed a 15-item questionnaire for patient self-assessment of facial paralysis; questionnaire results in 76 patients correlated fairly well with both House-Brackmann and the Sunnybrook Facial Grading System.[11] The American Academy of Otolaryngology–Head and Neck Surgery committee on facial nerve disorders has been in the process of developing a standardized grading system for facial nerve function, but this has not yet been formalized.[19] For now, House-Brackmann still seems the most reasonable and widely used choice.

Topognostic Tests

Topognostic tests were intended to reveal the site of lesion by use of a simple principle: Lesions below the point at which a particular branch

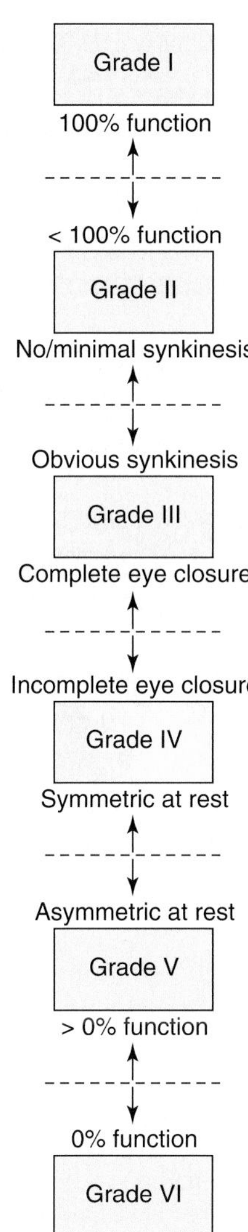

Figure 169-1. Schematic diagram of functional progression in assigning House-Brackmann grade to degree of facial paralysis.

leaves the facial nerve trunk will spare the function subserved by that branch. Accordingly, injury to the nerve in the face cannot affect lacrimation, salivation, taste, or the stapedius reflex. Conversely, the combination of facial paralysis and decreased lacrimation can theoretically be caused only by a lesion in the segment of the nerve in which voluntary motor fibers and parasympathetic fibers to the lacrimal gland run together (i.e., from the cerebellopontine angle to the geniculate ganglion).

In complete focal lesions, which often are the result of trauma, topognostic tests are reliable but usually are unnecessary, because clinical examination and imaging suffice to describe the site of lesion. Bell's palsy, on the other hand, usually is a mixed and partial lesion with varying degrees of conduction block and degeneration changes within different fibers and fascicles of the nerve trunk; therefore, topognostic tests are not expected to provide precise information about the level of the lesion. Many investigators have noted paradoxic and misleading results in applying topognostic testing principles in the evaluation of patients with Bell's palsy. In recent years, otologists use these tests only rarely.

Lacrimal Function

Schirmer's test has the advantages of simplicity, speed, and economy: The physician places a folded strip of sterile filter paper into the conjunctival fornix of each eye and compares the rate of tear production of the two sides. Normally, the portion of the filter paper in contact with the conjunctiva acts as an irritant, stimulating an increased flow of tears, which are then wicked along the filter paper strip by capillary action. The length of the wetted portion of the strip after a fixed interval (usually 5 minutes) is measured and is proportional to the volume of tears produced. A defect in the afferent (the trigeminal nerve along the opthalmic division, or V_1) or efferent (the facial nerve by way of the greater superficial petrosal nerve) limb of this reflex may cause a reduced flow. The reflex is consensual (i.e., a unilateral irritating stimulus in either eye causes tearing in both eyes, and a unilateral sensory deficit in either eye will reduce tearing bilaterally). However, unilateral corneal anesthesia reduces tearing asymmetrically, with a greater reduction on the anesthetized side; therefore, when a sensory deficit is present, presence of bilateral corneal anesthesia should be considered, and stimulation of lacrimation by other noxious stimuli (e.g., inhalation of ammonia) should be performed instead of the conventional Schirmer's test.[8]

Schirmer's test usually is considered positive if the affected side shows less than one-half the amount of lacrimation seen on the healthy side. This corresponds well to the normative data of Fisch,[20] who found that 95% of healthy persons had relatively symmetric responses (the lesser response was less than 54% of the greater response). Fisch[20] also pointed out that tearing often is reduced bilaterally in Bell's palsy (perhaps because of subclinical involvement of other cranial nerves). Thus, both the symmetry of the response and its absolute magnitude are important; a total response (sum of the lengths of wetted filter paper for both eyes) of less than 25 mm is considered abnormal.

Fisch[20] correlated the results of Schirmer's test and ENoG (see later under "Electrodiagnostic Testing") in patients with Bell's palsy and herpes zoster oticus and found that all cases with 90% or greater degeneration by ENoG had an abnormal result on Schirmer's test. However, the Schirmer's test result did not indicate degeneration earlier than ENoG and was abnormal in several cases in which ENoG correctly predicted a good spontaneous recovery.

May[21] added Schirmer's test to the salivary flow test and MST (see later under "Electrodiagnostic Testing") in a battery of prognostic tests. A decrease to 25% of normal in any of these was associated with a 90% chance of a poor recovery.

Stapedius Reflex

The nerve to the stapedius muscle branches off the facial trunk just past the second genu in the vertical (mastoid) part of the nerve. In patients with hearing loss, acoustic reflex testing is used to assess the afferent (auditory) limb of the reflex, but in cases of facial paralysis, the same test is used to assess the efferent (facial motor) limb. An absent reflex or a reflex that is less than one-half the amplitude of the contralateral side is considered abnormal.

The reflex can be elicited by ipsilateral or contralateral acoustic stimulation or, in cases of bilateral severe hearing loss, by tactile or electrical stimulation. It is absent in 69% of cases of Bell's palsy (in 84% when the paralysis is complete) at the time of presentation; the reflex recovers at about the same time as for clinically observed movements.[22] The prognostic value of this test therefore seems limited.

Taste

Because the chorda tympani carries fibers subserving taste from the anterior two thirds of the tongue, many investigators have studied abnormalities of taste in Bell's palsy. Psychophysical assessment can be performed with natural stimuli, such as filter paper disks impregnated with aqueous solutions of salt, sugar, citrate, or quinine, or with electrical stimulation of the tongue.[23] The latter modality, termed *electrogustometry* (EGM), has the advantages of speed and ease of quantification. EGM involves bipolar or monopolar electrical stimulation of the tongue, with current delivery on the order of 4 μA (−6 dB) to 4 mA (34 dB). Threshold responses are denoted by the current level's imparting a subjective sensation of one of the four cardinal tastes or of buzzing or tingling. In healthy persons, the two sides of the tongue have similar thresholds for electrical stimulation, rarely differing by greater than 25%.[24] Older studies demonstrated little usefulness of taste testing, because results were abnormal in almost all patients who were in the acute phase of Bell's palsy; accordingly, EGM could not be used to identify patients with a poor prognosis.[25,26] A newer study suggests better predictive value for the test: Of a cohort of 50 patients with complete idiopathic facial paralysis, 18 demonstrated abnormal EGM responses (defined as no response or a threshold difference greater than 20 dB across sides), and 7 demonstrated no response on NET, all of whom were in the abnormal EGM responses group. Of these 7, 5 demonstrated incomplete recovery of facial nerve function on long-term follow-up.[23] Taste function appears to recover before visible facial movement in some cases, so if the results of electrogustometry are normal in the second week or later, clinical recovery may be imminent.

Salivary Flow Test

The salivary flow test requires cannulation of the submandibular ducts and comparison of stimulated flow rates on the two sides. It is time-consuming and unpleasant for the patient, especially if performed repeatedly; this latter drawback is one good reason it is not widely used. Reduced submandibular flow implies a lesion at or proximal to the point at which the chorda tympani nerve leaves the main facial trunk; this is variable and may be anywhere in the vertical (mastoid) portion of the nerve.

Ekstrand[27] stated that reduced salivary flow (less than 45% of flow on the healthy side after stimulation with 6% citric acid) correlates well with worse outcome in Bell's palsy. Complete or incomplete recovery could be predicted with 89% accuracy. It is unclear whether these data, all collected within 10 days of onset of paralysis, provide an earlier or more reliable indication of prognosis than electrical or other tests.

May and Hawkins[28] noted that salivary flow decreases sooner than do threshold changes in NET (see under "Electrodiagnostic Testing" later on) in idiopathic facial paralysis. These workers argued that a flow rate of 25% or less of that on the contralateral, unaffected side is an indication for surgery.

Salivary pH

At least one report[29] showed that a submandibular salivary pH of 6.1 or less predicts incomplete recovery in cases of Bell's palsy. Presumably only the duct on the affected side needs to be cannulated, because in this study, all of the control sides had pH levels of 6.4 or more. The overall accuracy of prediction was 91%. Unfortunately, the reported experience with salivary pH is very limited; it is unknown whether this test gives an earlier prognosis than other tests.

Imaging

Magnetic resonance imaging (MRI) with intravenous gadolinium contrast has revolutionized tumor detection in the cerebellopontine angle and temporal bone and is currently the study of choice when a facial nerve tumor is suspected (e.g., in a case of slowly progressive or long-standing weakness).[30] However, enhancement also occurs in most cases of Bell's palsy and herpes zoster opticus, usually in the perigeniculate portions of the nerve.[31,32] This enhancement may persist for more than 1 year after clinical recovery; can be distinguished from neoplasm by its linear, unenlarged appearance; and has no apparent prognostic significance. Computed tomography (CT) is valuable for surgical planning in cholesteatomas and temporal bone trauma involving facial nerve paralysis but probably is less useful than MRI in the investigation of atypical idiopathic paralysis. Unfortunately, even MRI fails to detect a substantial number of malignant parotid tumors.[33]

MRI shows the greatest utility in predicting location and depth of parotid gland tumors, but even in this capacity it is no better than simple manual palpation alone. The MRI appearance of tumor indistinct from surrounding parotid parenchyma has a positive predictive value for malignancy of only 0.48; accordingly, fine needle aspiration biopsy continues to be the "gold standard" modality for preoperative evaluation of parotid masses.[34]

Pathophysiology

Sunderland[35] provided a simple, five-category histopathologic classification of peripheral nerve injury based on a schematic framework proposed by Seddon[36] (Fig. 169-2). Some investigators have since expanded this classification to include a sixth category involving mixed forms of injury proposed by MacKinnon and associates.[37] This classification of nerve trunk injury is helpful in understanding and interpreting the results of electrical tests.

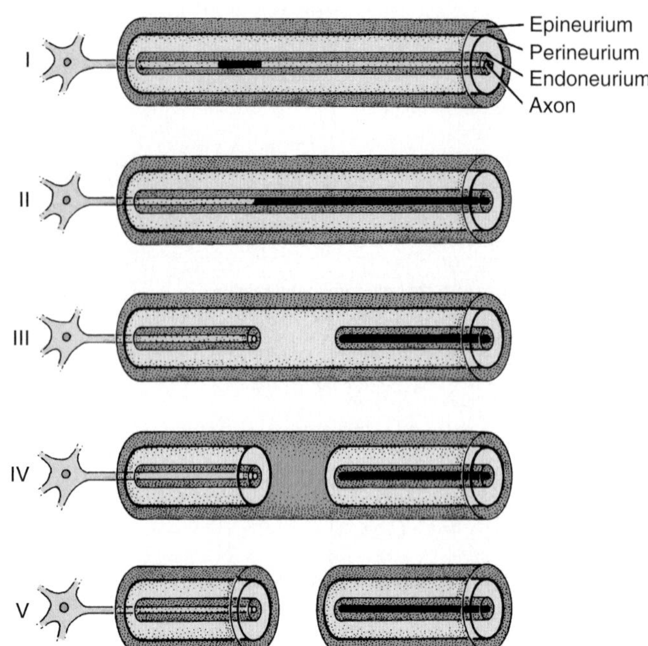

Figure 169-2. Sunderland histopathologic classification of peripheral nerve injury. Roman numerals I to V at *left* denote the Sunderland class corresponding to the degree of injury depicted in the diagram.

Class I: Pressure on a nerve trunk, provided that it is not too severe, causes conduction block, termed neurapraxia by Seddon. No physical disruption of axonal continuity occurs, and supportive connective tissue elements remain intact. When the pressure or other insult (e.g., local anesthetic infiltration) is removed, the nerve can recover quickly. During conduction block, no impulses can cross the area of the lesion, but electrical stimulation distal to the lesion still produces a propagated action potential and a visible muscle twitch at all times after injury. An example of a Sunderland class I injury is the neurapraxia of an arm or leg that has "gone to sleep."

Class II: A more severe lesion, whether caused by pressure or some other insult (e.g., viral inflammation), may cause axonal disruption without injury to supporting structures. Wallerian degeneration occurs and propagates distally from the site of injury to the motor end plate and proximally to the first adjacent node of Ranvier. In a class II injury, the connective tissue elements remain viable, so regenerating axons may return precisely to their original destinations. Removal of the original mechanism of insult permits complete recovery, but this is considerably delayed, because the axon must regrow from the site of the lesion to the motor end plate at a rate of approximately 1 mm/day before function returns. A class II injury is an *axonotmesis*.

Class III: If the lesion disrupts the endoneurium, wallerian degeneration occurs as in a class II injury, but the regenerating axons are free to enter the wrong endoneurial tubes or may fail to enter an endoneurial tube at all; this aberrant regeneration may be associated with incomplete recovery, manifested as an inability to make discrete movements of individual facial regions without involuntary movement of other parts of the face—an abnormality termed *synkinesis*. Sunderland class III to V nerve injuries, in which aberrant regeneration can occur, are *neurotmesis* injuries.

Class IV: Perineurial disruption implies an even more severe injury, in which the potential for incomplete and aberrant regeneration is greater. Intraneural scarring may prevent most axons from reaching the muscle, resulting in not only greater synkinesis but incomplete motor function recovery.

Class V: A complete transection of a nerve, including its epineurial sheath, carries almost no hope for useful regeneration, unless the ends are approximated or spanned and repaired.

Class VI: Insults to the facial nerve trunk, whether compressive, inflammatory, or traumatic in origin, can be heterogeneous in nature, with differing degrees of injury from fascicle to fascicle. Such mixed injury involving both neurapraxia and a variable degree of neurodegeneration has been advocated as an additional class of injury.

A patient with a conduction block (class I injury) cannot move the facial muscles voluntarily, but a facial twitch can be elicited by transcutaneous electrical stimulation of the nerve distal to the lesion. The twitch can be observed visually, or the electrical response of the facial muscles may be recorded. Because no wallerian degeneration occurs, this electrical stimulability distal to the site of lesion is preserved indefinitely in isolated class I injury.

In classes II to VI, once wallerian degeneration has occurred, electrical stimulation of the nerve distal to the lesion will fail to produce a propagated action potential and muscle contraction. However, before axonal degeneration, the distal segment is still electrically stimulable. Wallerian degeneration begins immediately after injury but progresses slowly. Histopathologic degeneration of the distal segment becomes apparent approximately 1 week after insult and continues for the ensuing 1 to 2 months.[38] In the case of the facial nerve, this delay in degeneration results in continued electrical stimulability of the distal segment for up to 3 to 5 days after injury.[39] Thus, during these first days after an insult, electrodiagnostic testing of any form cannot distinguish between neurapraxic and neurodegenerative injuries.

After wallerian degeneration, electrical testing can distinguish axonally intact but neurapraxic lesions (class I) from axonally disrupted and neurodegenerative lesions (classes II to V). It cannot, however, distinguish among the different classes of neurodegenerative lesions II, III, IV, and V. An important consideration in the use of such testing is its limited ability to distinguish between pure lesions associated with an excellent prognosis for perfect spontaneous recovery (class II) and those associated with a poor prognosis for useful recovery without surgical repair (class V).

It also is important to recognize that most facial nerve lesions are not pure but probably mixed, with some fibers in conduction block and others disrupted with varying degrees of connective tissue injury. Accordingly, a majority of insults to the facial nerve, whether compressive, inflammatory, or traumatic (except for complete transections), probably are class VI, with a variable threshold of electrical stimulability commensurate with the proportion of neural degeneration across the nerve trunk.

Electrodiagnostic Testing

Tests based on these two principles, electrical stimulation and recording of the electromyographic response, are useful in determining prognosis and sometimes in stratifying patients for nonsurgical versus surgical management. However, they are rarely useful in differential diagnosis. In Bell's palsy and traumatic facial nerve paralysis, electrical tests most often are used to identify patients whose nerves have begun to degenerate, because these patients may be candidates for decompression surgery. In this sense, outpatient evaluation of facial paralysis with electrical testing only needs to be performed if the physician is prepared to recommend decompression in the event that degeneration is discovered. However, intraoperative monitoring of facial nerve function (usually with electromyography) is in widespread use in many types of intracranial and intratemporal surgery.

Nerve Excitability Test

The simplest and best-known test for facial nerve degeneration is the NET introduced by Laumans and Jonkees.[40] The stimulating electrode is placed on the skin over the stylomastoid foramen or over one of the peripheral branches of the nerve, with a return electrode taped to the forearm. Beginning with the healthy side, electrical pulses, typically 0.3 msec in duration, are delivered at steadily increasing current levels until a facial twitch is noted. The lowest current eliciting a visible twitch is the threshold of excitation. Next, the process is repeated on the paralyzed side, and the difference in thresholds between the two sides is calculated.

In a simple conduction block (e.g., after infiltration of the perineural tissues with lidocaine proximal to the point of stimulation), no difference exists between the two sides; the paralyzed nerve is as easy to stimulate distal to the site of lesion as the healthy nerve. After a more severe injury (Sunderland classes II to V) in which distal axonal degeneration occurs, electrical excitability is gradually lost, over a period of 3 to 4 days—even after a total section of the nerve. Findings on the NET (and all other electrical tests involving distal stimulation), therefore, always lag several days behind the biologic events themselves.[41]

In most cases of Bell's palsy with complete paralysis, some degree of neural degeneration occurs, evolving over 1 to 2 weeks.[42] Accordingly, proponents of the NET urge frequent, even daily, examinations, so that severe degeneration can be detected as early as possible. A difference of 3.5 milliamperes (mA) or more in thresholds between the two sides has been proposed as a reliable sign of severe degeneration and has been used as an indicator for surgical decompression. With use of this criterion, complete versus incomplete recovery can be predicted with 80% accuracy.[40] Some investigators insist on conducting two consecutive tests showing differences greater than 3.5 mA to reduce the chance of test error. Lewis and colleagues[43] have reported thresholds in more than 10,000 NETs in cases of Bell's palsy, using the trunk and branches to the eye, forehead, and mouth.

The NET is useful only during the first 2 to 3 weeks of complete paralysis, before complete degeneration has occurred. This test is unnecessary in cases of incomplete paralysis, in which the prognosis is always excellent; in these cases, the test result will be normal when the segment of nerve distal to the lesion is stimulated. If the paralysis becomes total, the test can determine whether a pure conduction block exists or whether degeneration is occurring, as indicated by progressive loss of excitability. Total paralysis for longer than 1 month is almost invariably associated with total loss of excitability. Once excitability is lost and this result is confirmed by repeat testing, further excitability tests are pointless, because clinically evident recovery always begins before any apparent electrical excitability returns. This disparity results because the regenerating axons are smaller, more irregular in size, and fewer in number than before the lesion occurred. Electrical stimulation generally is ineffective in eliciting a synchronous and hence observable twitch in the early stages of regeneration. As these early fibers regenerate, they may regain electrical function individually, while group function, measured as a clinically apparent twitch on electrical stimulation, still is not evident. This phenomenon is termed *early deblocking*, or asynchronous firing of the facial nerve. Similarly, with complete paralysis, if clinical recovery begins before degeneration is noted, continuing testing is unnecessary, because recovery will be rapid and complete.

Partial degeneration and a bad outcome are not synonymous. In a Sunderland class II lesion, nearly complete recovery may occur without serious complications. Laumans and Jonkees[40] state that even patients who show degeneration (threshold difference greater than 3.5 mA) have a 38% chance for complete spontaneous recovery; in the remainder, development of complications such as permanent weakness (not total paralysis) and synkinesis is typical.

Because of relatively large intersubject variations in threshold compared with the small differences between the two sides of the face, stating NET results in proportional terms rather than in absolute threshold differences may be more appropriate. For example, Mechelse and associates[44] used as their criterion for decompression a 150% increase in threshold compared with the healthy side.

Maximum Stimulation Test

The MST is similar to the NET in that it involves visual (i.e., subjective) evaluation of electrically elicited facial movements. Instead of measuring threshold, however, maximal stimuli (current levels at which the greatest amplitude of facial movement is seen) or supramaximal stimuli (even higher current levels) are used. The electrode type and placement and the nerve-stimulating equipment are the same as in the NET. On the unaffected side, the stimulus current intensity is increased above the threshold level incrementally—with corresponding increases in subjective facial twitch magnitude—until the maximum stimulation level is reached. Stimulation above this level does not elicit any further increase in facial twitch magnitude. This maximum stimulation level is then used to stimulate the affected side, and the degree of facial contraction is subjectively assessed as either equal, mildly decreased, markedly decreased, or without response compared with that on the normal side. With MST as performed by May and coworkers,[45] peripheral branches are the preferred site of stimulation, and the movements on the paralyzed side are subjectively expressed as a percentage (0%, 25%, 50%, 75%, 100%) of the movements on the healthy side.

The theoretic basis of the MST is that by stimulating all intact axons, the proportion of fibers that have degenerated can be estimated; this information should more reliably guide prognosis and treatment than that obtained with the NET. Unfortunately, no good data comparing these or other electrical prognostic tests in the same patients are available, so this claim has not been proved.

According to May and coworkers,[46] when MST results remained normal in Bell's palsy, 88% of patients recovered completely. Reduced movement presaged only a 27% chance of complete recovery. An absence of electrically stimulated movement was always associated with incomplete recovery.

MST is painful for some patients; Molina[47] suggests that the use of a pulse duration less than 0.4 msec (as opposed to the 1 msec proposed by May and coworkers[46]) can eliminate this discomfort, although higher currents are required in some cases.

Electroneuronography

In ENoG, the facial nerve is stimulated transcutaneously at the stylomastoid foramen, as in the NET, although a bipolar stimulating electrode is used. Responses to maximal electrical stimulation of the two sides are compared, as in the MST, but they are recorded in a more objective fashion by measuring the evoked compound muscle action potential (CMAP) with a second bipolar electrode pair placed (usually) in the nasolabial groove. A supramaximal stimulus often is used, and peak-to-peak amplitude is measured in millivolts (mV). The average difference in response amplitude between the two sides in healthy patients has been said to be only 3%.[48] The term "electroneuronography" is actually a misnomer, because it is the facial muscle CMAP that is measured and recorded. Some workers use the term *evoked electromyography* synonymously with *electroneuronography*.

Clearly, this method offers the potential advantage of an objective registration of electrically evoked responses, and the amplitude of response on the paralyzed side can be expressed as a precise percentage of that on the healthy side. For example, if the amplitude of the response on the paralyzed side is only 10% of that on the normal side, an estimated 90% of fibers are said to have degenerated on the paralyzed side. However, this method has some practical difficulties that should be mastered before reliable results can be expected.[49,50] Test-retest errors in the 20% range have been reported by Raslan and associates,[51] despite standardization of electrode positions. Most investigators require a 30% or greater asymmetry (or change over time) for results to be considered abnormal.

The use of ENoG to prognosticate in Bell's palsy has become widespread, although Gates[52] points out the lack of comparative studies showing ENoG to be superior to NET or MST. For example, Coker and coworkers[53] showed good correlation between ENoG and NET (when NET threshold differences exceeded 2 mA, ENoG amplitude on the paralyzed side usually was less than 10% of the normal side), but their study provided no data on clinical outcomes to help choose one test over the other.

The most valid data supporting the use of ENoG would have to come from studies limited to cases of complete paralysis (because incomplete paralysis is known to have an excellent prognosis). In 37 such cases, May and colleagues[45] showed that severe ENoG amplitude reductions (to less than 10% of the unaffected side) were highly correlated with incomplete recovery. Although Canter and associates[54] could find no correlation of final outcome with ENoG in 23 patients with complete paralysis, they did not specifically test the predictive value of the 10% criterion widely used by other authors. More recently, Sillman and colleagues[25] found excellent correlations between ENoG and outcome in Bell's palsy ($n = 66$) but not in traumatic facial nerve palsy ($n = 29$).

Electrical recording of the muscle response also offers the possibility of measuring latency, which is the time elapsed between stimulus and response. Only slight interest in this variable has developed; although slow nerve conduction velocities might be expected to be an early indicator of degeneration, the available data are in conflict. Joachims and associates[55] stated that increased latency in the first 72 hours (before any observable change in threshold or response amplitude) was a reliable predictor of a poor outcome. However, Esslen[48] reported that in 145 patients, latency never increased before the 5th day, and latency changes never preceded changes in evoked potential amplitude; he concluded that latency measurements were of no clinical value. Danielides[42] and Ruboyianes[56] and their coworkers also suggested that latency adds nothing to information provided by ENoG amplitude or MST.

The limitation described for the NET, namely, its inapplicability in cases of partial paralysis after the beginning of clinical recovery and after excitability has been lost, also applies to the MST and to ENoG. In acute facial paralysis, all of these tests are useful only in tracking the early course of a completely paralyzed nerve until clinical recovery begins or the nerve shows complete loss of excitability.

Esslen[48] used ENoG to study the time course of Bell's palsy, finding that the acute phase rarely exceeds 10 days. Decreases in ENoG amplitude after the 10th day were associated with substantial latency increases and were attributed to desynchronization of surviving fibers, rather than to increased degeneration. Accordingly, the time elapsed since the onset of paralysis should be taken into account in the interpretation of ENoG results. Patients reaching 95% degeneration (amplitude of response equals 5% of that on the healthy side) within 2 weeks had a 50% chance of a poor recovery, whereas patients exhibiting a more gradual decrease in ENoG amplitude had a much better prognosis.[57]

Most proponents of ENoG use it mainly to obtain an early prognosis in acute facial paralysis (Bell's or post-traumatic) or to select patients for decompression surgery. Kartush[58] pointed out that ENoG also can document subclinical facial nerve involvement by tumors, especially acoustic neuromas. Patients with acoustic tumors who had ENoG evidence of nerve involvement (despite clinically normal facial movement) were more likely to have postoperative weakness. However, because ENoG amplitude reductions were highly correlated with increasing tumor size (which also predicts poorer facial nerve outcome), it is unclear whether ENoG really adds prognostic information when tumor size is known. ENoG also has demonstrated some success in preoperative detection of facial nerve infiltration by malignant parotid tumors, even when no paresis is seen on clinical examination.[59] Table 169-2 summarizes the three versions of electrodiagnostic testing and commonly accepted threshold criteria for consideration of facial nerve decompression for complete facial paralysis.

Electromyography

EMG is the recording of spontaneous and voluntary muscle potentials using needles introduced into the muscle. Its role in the early phase of Bell's palsy is limited, because it does not permit a quantitative estimate of the extent of nerve degeneration (the percentage of degenerated fibers). However, EMG may be helpful in certain situations. Several authorities who favor decompression for Bell's palsy base their decisions for surgery primarily on the NET or ENoG, but also require confirmatory EMG[40,49]; if it shows voluntarily active facial motor units despite loss of excitability of the nerve trunk, the prognosis for a good spontaneous recovery is excellent.[25,48] This application of EMG in Bell's palsy probably is underused.

After loss of excitability, tests requiring electrical stimulation such as NET and ENoG are no longer useful. However, EMG may give prognostically useful information during this phase of the illness. After 10 to 14 days, fibrillation potentials may be detected, confirming the presence of degenerating motor units; in 81% of patients with such findings, incomplete recovery is the rule.[60] More useful are the polyphasic reinnervation potentials that may be seen as early as 4 to 6 weeks

Table 169-2

Electrodiagnostic Testing Criteria

Test	Criteria to Consider Facial Nerve Decompression
Nerve excitability test (NET)	>3.5-mA threshold difference between sides
Maximal stimulation test (MST)	No response on injured side at maximal stimulation
Electroneurography (EnoG)	>90% degeneration within 14 days

after the onset of paralysis. Presence of these potentials precedes clinically detectable recovery and predicts a fair to good recovery.[48] Grosheva and coworkers noted that EMG performed after 14 days exhibited greater prognostic value for determining good versus poor recovery, with both higher specificity and positive predictive value, than ENoG performed before 14 days using a 75% degeneration cutoff criterion; however, their study included many patients with incomplete facial paralysis.[61]

Because few surgeons advocate decompression surgery for Bell's palsy late in the course of the disease, this use of EMG is uncommon. It may be helpful in the assessment of long-standing facial paralysis, along with muscle biopsy, to determine the possible success of substitution anastomosis or cross-facial anastomosis as a mechanism of restoring facial motion. EMG also can help assess whether a nerve repair (e.g., in the cerebellopontine angle) is unsuccessful. If no clinical recovery occurs and EMG shows no polyphasic reinnervation potentials at 15 months (or at 18 months at the latest), the anastomosis should be considered a failure, and another operation should be considered (e.g., hypoglossal-facial anastomosis).

Facial Nerve Monitoring

During the 1980s, audible EMG monitoring of facial nerve function during acoustic neuroma surgery became routine in many centers, and its application has spread to other operations involving risk to the facial nerve and other cranial nerves.[62] Although it is possible for the surgeon or an associate to watch for facial movements in response to mechanical or electrical stimulation of the nerve, simple observation fails to detect many small muscular contractions and in any case demands constant vigilance. By contrast, electrodes in or near the facial muscles record EMG potentials that can be amplified and made audible with a loudspeaker. Thus, the surgeon's ears can monitor the facial nerve while the hands and eyes operate. Harner and colleagues[63] pointed out that this technique is not really new but has only recently become popular.

Facial nerve monitoring can be performed in many different ways. One approach to categorizing the type of monitoring used is to consider if it is active versus passive.[64] Having a surgical assistant visually monitor the face for twitches during parotid surgery is technically a form of facial nerve monitoring, albeit a coarse and highly variable one. By applying needle electrodes to the facial muscles and recording CMAPs, the activity of the facial nerve can be monitored in a more standardized, precise, and sensitive fashion. Both of these examples are *passive* forms of facial nerve monitoing, whereby facial muscle movement is activated only with direct mechanical, stretch, caloric, or other nonelectrical stimulation of the facial nerve. Facial nerve monitoring electrodes typically are placed in a two-channel montage including the orbicularis oculi and orbicularis oris muscles, although four-channel arrangements can be used as well.

When electrical stimulation of the facial nerve is used along with measurement of facial CMAPs, the technique is termed *active* facial nerve monitoring. Electrical stimulation is delivered by a monopolar or bipolar electrode (e.g., similar to those used for bipolar electrocautery), which is insulated except at the tips. Commercially available monopolar electrodes are flexible with blunt tips, which makes them convenient for access to cramped areas. In addition, electrified instruments with insulated shafts are available that are shaped in the form of traditional otomicroscopic dissectors such as curved needles, sickle knives, round knives, gimmicks, and other elevators. On bipolar stimulation, the current is mostly confined to the tissue between the electrified tips; with wide tip separation, the stimulation is similar to that with use of a monopolar electrode, but with the tips close together, bipolar stimulation is quite specific. Both types are satisfactory if the user understands these differences.

Electrical stimulation activates a surrounding volume of tissue commensurate in size with the delivered current intensity, and modulation of current intensity can provide the surgeon with good sensitivity for locating and mapping the facial nerve. Early in the dissection before the facial nerve has been visually identified, initial stimulation with higher current levels allows the surgeon to stimulate the nerve from afar, without the need for direct contact on the nerve. As dissection is carried closer to the nerve, lowering the current level allows for more precise determination of nerve location. As dissection is continued and the facial nerve (or its candidates) are identified, low-level current stimulation directly on the nerve provides confirmation that the nerve has been positively identified.

When the surgeon stimulates the nerve electrically, a CMAP is recorded from the monitored facial muscles and can be plotted on an oscilloscope (if visual display is being used), and the loudspeaker emits a characteristic thump. Gentle mechanical stimulation (e.g., touching the nerve with an instrument) will produce a similar sound. Tension on the nerve from mechanical stretching or caloric or thermal stimulation of the nerve from irrigation often will produce a prolonged irregular series of discharges that sounds like popcorn popping. Prass and associates[65] termed these two characteristic sounds *bursts* and *trains*, respectively. Learning to identify these sounds is easy, providing instant feedback regarding the location of the facial nerve and concomitant surgical manipulation. Bursts imply near-instantaneous nerve stimulation; trains signify ongoing stimulation of the nerve, which can be potentially more damaging.

Kartush[58] stated that excessive intraoperative train activity predicts poor outcome; Prell and colleagues correlated total train time (the summation of online monitoring time during which trains were recorded) greater than 10 seconds with a higher likelihood of immediate and long-term deterioration in facial function.[66] Hone and associates[67] disagree. Conversely, if at the end of the surgical procedure the nerve can be stimulated successfully near the brainstem with low currents (0.05 to 0.1 mA), all investigators agree that the prognosis for postoperative function is excellent.[68-72] As seen in patients with Bell's palsy or traumatic facial paralysis, patients undergoing resection of acoustic neuromas in whom facial function is intact immediately postoperatively but a delayed paralysis develops subsequently have better long-term facial function than those with immediate weakness or paralysis.[73]

As with any technical aid, a number of pitfalls have been recognized. Failure to obtain audible facial nerve responses can be caused by any of a multitude of possible errors: detached or shorted electrodes, incorrect wiring of electrodes, malfunction of a nerve monitor or stimulator, inadvertent direct anesthesia of the facial nerve from local anesthetic infiltration to the stylomastoid foramen, pharmacologic muscular paralysis from induction agents used in anesthetic management, or even simply a muted speaker, as well as many other complications (including a nonfunctional nerve). Anesthesiologists have shown that the facial musculature is less susceptible to pharmacologic paralysis than somatic musculature and that a moderate degree of paralysis[74,75] (leading to 50% reduction of hypothenar muscle potentials or even "complete" neuromuscular blockage as measured in the thumb)[76] does not necessarily interfere with facial nerve monitoring.

Stimulation of the trigeminal nerve occasionally can cause electrical confusion, or crosstalk; the facial muscle electrodes may pick up EMG signals from the nearby masseter muscle. Similarly, stimulation of the adjacent vestibular or cochlear nerves can sometimes activate the facial nerve as well, leading to a false-positive identification.

Electrode position should always be checked by voluntary movement, transcutaneous electrical stimulation, or most commonly simply by tapping over the muscular area being monitored before the surgical site is draped. The most useful intraoperative check on the monitoring equipment is the stimulus artifact or warble tone, which is produced when the stimulating electrode touches tissue remote from the facial nerve. Standard neuromonitoring equipment can be set to produce an auditory flag such as a warble tone or a verbal phrase confirming current flow. This auditory notification confirms that the stimulator is delivering current, the electrodes are in place, and the loudspeaker is working and is to be distinguished from the audible bursts and trains indicating true facial nerve stimulation and facial muscle contraction.

The idea that audible EMG monitoring makes acoustic tumor surgery easier, faster, and probably more successful in terms of facial nerve preservation has become widely accepted anecdotally, and several investigators have shown that postoperative facial nerve function is better in patients who have been monitored (at least during operations for resection of large tumors).[77-79] These studies seem to have used historical control groups (i.e., monitoring was adopted for all patients at a particular point in time, with no monitoring for patients operated on before that time). This limitation makes it hard to be sure that some of the improvements were not caused by improvements over time in the surgeon's skill; indeed, one group acknowledged that the monitored group also had profited from evolving surgical techniques (more use of sharp dissection).[80] This finding highlights the role of the monitor as teacher; the surgeon rapidly learns to prefer medial-to-lateral over lateral-to-medial dissection and sharp over blunt dissection (when the tumor is adherent to the nerve). Although most surgeons use EMG monitoring, others have monitored facial contractions with a motion sensor connected to an electronic circuit that produces an audible signal or by the use of small bells that are sutured to facial skin.[72,81,82]

A panel discussion at a meeting of the American Otological Society produced consensus that electrical facial nerve monitoring is valuable in acoustic tumor surgery and may be useful in facial nerve rerouting in skull base surgery.[83,84] A consensus conference on acoustic tumors sponsored by the National Institutes of Health came to a similar conclusion that benefits of intraoperative facial nerve monitoring in acoustic neuroma surgery had been clearly established.[85]

Electrical facial nerve monitoring is now used by a majority of American otolaryngologists performing parotidectomies, although such monitoring has not been shown to improve postoperative facial paralysis rates after primary parotid gland surgery.[86-88] A retrospective study by Makeieff and colleagues did demonstrate an advantage in postoperative facial paralysis rates when intraoperative continuous facial nerve monitoring was used in 14 of 32 patients undergoing revision total parotidectomy for recurrent pleomorphic adenoma.[89]

In adjusting for the probabilities of facial nerve paralysis with or without monitoring, intraoperative facial nerve monitoring has been shown to be cost-effective for both primary and revision middle ear and mastoid surgical procedures, with a higher number of quality-adjusted life-years and lower average cost than for a no-monitoring strategy.[90]

Unconventional Tests of Facial Nerve Function

Acoustic Reflex Evoked Potentials

Hammerschlag and associates[91] reported a scalp-recorded potential at 12- to 15-msec latency in response to acoustic stimulation contralateral to the recording site and attributed this to facial motor pathway activation. The response persisted after paralysis during anesthesia, and these workers proposed its use for intraoperative monitoring of facial nerve function. However, the response was extremely small (much lower in amplitude than that of the auditory brainstem response), which would make it difficult and slow to record, requiring prolonged averaging. This response seems unlikely to be useful, because audible EMG monitoring gives essentially instantaneous feedback for intraoperative assessment of facial nerve function.

Antidromic Potentials

If a motor nerve is electrically or mechanically stimulated at some point between its cell body and its synapse on a muscle fiber, action potentials will be propagated in two directions: An orthodromic or antegrade impulse will travel distally toward the muscle, whereas an antidromic or retrograde impulse will travel proximally toward the cell body. The orthodromic impulse will cross the neuromuscular junction, resulting in an observable muscle contraction and a recordable compound muscle action potential. This *M-wave* is the same potential recorded in ENoG. Although the antidromic impulse will not cross a synapse, it can be recorded by electrodes on the proximal nerve (near field) or at a distance (far field). Tashima and coworkers[92] recorded electrical responses from the geniculate ganglion region in guinea pigs while stimulating the facial nerve at the stylomastoid foramen. These near-field antidromic responses were reliably altered by surgical lesions placed between the stimulating and the recording electrodes. Other modifications for improving the consistency and reliability in producing antidromic potentials involve stimulation of the buccal branch of the facial nerve through Stensen's duct, rather than percutaneous stimulation of the facial nerve branches.[93]

Far-field antidromic potentials have been recorded from the scalp after electrical stimulation near the stylomastoid foramen, in hopes that this would yield a noninvasive test of the integrity of the intratemporal or intracranial portions of the facial nerve. However, these responses are difficult to record and interpret. Metson[94] concluded, on the basis of studies in cats, that the intracranial nerve was the main generator, but Kartush and associates[95] found in dogs that the mastoid segment was primarily responsible.

As previously mentioned, the antidromic impulse will not travel farther "upstream" than the facial nucleus motor neuron, but it can be reflected back along that neuron's axon in an orthodromic direction, eventually reaching the muscle and stimulating a muscle action potential—the *F-wave*—that is delayed relative to the initial M-wave. These F-waves are unusually large in hemifacial spasm,[96] suggesting that facial nucleus hyperexcitability plays a role in that disorder. F-waves are easily disrupted by even the mildest degree of facial paresis.[97] They often are abnormal with delayed latency or decreased amplitude or are absent in patients with acoustic tumors, even when clinical examination of facial nerve function yields normal findings.[98] However, they do not predict postoperative function when tumor size is taken into consideration.[99]

Antidromic stimulation of peripheral branches of the facial nerve has been introduced into intraoperative monitoring, with continuous recording of either near-field potentials from the facial nerve near the brainstem[100] or F-waves from facial musculature.[89] Wedekind and Klug[98,101] believe that F-wave monitoring provides earlier and better prognostic information to the surgeon than that obtained with continuous EMG monitoring.

Blink Reflex

Electrical or mechanical stimulation of the supraorbital branch of the trigeminal nerve elicits a reflex contraction (blink) of the orbicularis oculi muscle, which is innervated by the facial nerve. Two studies found blink reflex abnormalities (recorded by EMG) in many patients with acoustic tumors (far more than were found by ENoG).[102,103] Although this finding suggests that subclinical facial nerve involvement is more common than has been clinically appreciated, neither study offered evidence that blink reflex testing added any prognostic information to that available from tumor size.

Magnetic Stimulation

A rapidly varying magnetic field produced by a surge of current in a coil placed over the skin will induce electrical currents in underlying tissue and can be used to stimulate nerves. This method offers two potential advantages over conventional electrical stimulation of the facial nerve: (1) the nerve can be maximally stimulated without pain or discomfort, and (2) if the coil is placed in the temporoparietal area (transcranial stimulation), the nerve seems to be stimulated in the region of the geniculate ganglion or the internal auditory canal. This functionality, when coupled with electrical stimulation of the facial nerve at the stylomastoid foramen, could obviously be useful for site-of-lesion determination, at least in the earliest phases of paralysis before electrical excitability distal to a lesion is lost.[104-108]

Patients with magnetically stimulable nerves, when tested up to 4 days after onset of Bell's palsy, had a better prognosis than those whose responses had been lost.[109] Unfortunately, it was unclear whether this test added prognostic information once the severity of the clinically assessed paresis was taken into account. Schriefer and colleagues[109] found no response to transcranial magnetic stimulation in serial follow-up evaluations of two patients with Bell's palsy, even after rapid and complete clinical recovery (2 and 3 weeks, respectively), suggesting that this technique may not be useful for prognostic purposes after the first few days. Rösler[110] and Duckert[111] and their coworkers found that magnetic stimulation offered no unique prognostic information in acoustic tumor cases once tumor size (the best predictor of facial nerve outcome) is considered.

Optical Stimulation

Another method of stimulating the facial nerve without direct tissue contact is by optical excitation. Contact-free optical excitation provides the important potential benefit of neural stimulation without mechanical trauma. Unfortunately, early efforts at optical nerve stimulation using ultraviolet-wavelength excimer laser were successful only at energy densities comparable to the photoablation threshold.[112] Wells and colleagues demonstrated successful optical stimulation of frog and rat sciatic nerve with pulsed short- and medium-wavelength infrared laser light, with neural tissue damage occurring at energy densities 2.5 times neural excitation threshold.[113] More recently, Teudt and coworkers used short-wavelength infrared pulsed laser light to successfully stimulate the extratemporal facial nerve without neural damage seen on histologic examination.[114] Neural tissue injury occurred at an energy density similar to that reported by Wells and colleagues,[113] approximately 1.3 to 3 times that of threshold.

Such optical excitation techniques would have an obvious advantage for use in locations in which mechanical dissection of the facial nerve must be kept to a minimum, such as at the cerebellopontine angle, where the nerve does not yet have a protective layer of epineurium for support. This specific application has not yet been reported.

Transcranial Electrical Stimulation–Induced Facial Motor Evoked Potentials

Current methods of intraoperative facial nerve monitoring allow for active stimulation of the nerve at the level of the hand-held stimulator. Although this technique is beneficial in identifying and confirming the integrity of the nerve at all points distal to the dissection, it cannot test the integrity of the nerve proximal to dissection, which may be vital to know during dissection of a large cranial base tumor, when the facial nerve root entry zone is not readily identified. Antidromic stimulation and F-wave monitoring of the facial nerve can theoretically overcome this drawback. Another more recently developed method involves transcranial electrical stimulation of the cortical facial motor pathway and measurement of the corresponding facial motor evoked potentials (MEPs).

In intraoperative transcranial electrical stimulation, spiral electrodes are placed at Cz and C3/C4 overlying the facial motor cortex contralateral to the side of the lesion being removed. Electrical stimulation of these facial corticobulbar neurons is propagated across the pyramidal decussation to stimulate facial nucleus neurons on the side ipsilateral to the lesion. Lower motor neuron stimulation propagates to the facial musculature, where a muscle action potential is recorded in the standard fashion; this corticobulbar-derived CMAP is the MEP. Thus, the integrity of the entire facial motor tract is tested by this technique. MEP recordings are performed before tumor microdissection (baseline), at regular intervals intraoperatively, and immediately after completion of dissection (final). The final-to-baseline MEP amplitude ratio is calculated to determine the likelihood of an intact or disrupted facial motor tract.[115]

Transcranial excitation of the facial motor cortex is dependent on multipulse stimulation, in contrast with facial nerve stimulation, which adds to the specificity of the technique. However, application of the transcranial electrical stimulation technique is characterized by multiple constraints, including the necessity for nonvolatile anesthesia (only propofol and narcotic infusions are used for maintenance of anesthesia, as volatile agents adversely affect corticobulbar stimulability), use of high stimulus voltages (on the order of 100 to 400 V) and subsequent need to pause surgical dissection during MEP acquisition, and the possibility of epileptic discharge during cortical stimulation.[116]

Nonetheless, the technique has been used with good success by several groups.[117-119] Final-to-baseline MEP amplitude ratios greater than 50% appear to correlate well with good immediate postoperative facial function (reported as House-Brackmann grade I or II); ratios less than 50% correlate with varying degrees of worse function (reported as House-Brackmann grades III to VI). This technique is in its infancy and is likely to undergo continued refinement, with its ultimate utility to be determined.

SUGGESTED READINGS

Akagami R, Dong CC, Westerberg BD. Localized transcranial electrical motor evoked potentials for monitoring cranial nerves in cranial base surgery. *Neurosurgery.* 2005;57(1 Suppl):78.

Beck DL, Atkins JS Jr, Benecke JE Jr, et al. Intraoperative facial nerve monitoring: prognostic aspects during acoustic tumor removal. *Otolaryngol Head Neck Surg.* 1991;104:780.

Brauer M, Knuettgen D, Quester R, et al. Electromyographic facial nerve monitoring during resection for acoustic neurinoma under moderate to profound levels of peripheral neuromuscular blockade. *Eur J Anaesthesiol.* 1996;13:612.

Brennan J, Moore EJ, Shuler KJ. Prospective analysis of the efficacy of continuous intraoperative nerve monitoring during thyroidectomy, parathyroidectomy, and parotidectomy. *Otolaryngol Head Neck Surg.* 2001;124:537.

Coker NJ, Fordice JO, Moore S. Correlation of the nerve excitability test and electroneurography in acute facial paralysis. *Am J Otol.* 1992;13:127.

Esslen E. *The Acute Facial Palsies: Investigations on the Localization and Pathogenesis of Meato-Labyrinthine Facial Palsies.* Berlin: Springer-Verlag; 1976.

Fisch U. Maximal nerve excitability testing vs electroneuronography. *Arch Otolaryngol Head Neck Surg.* 1980;106:352.

Fisch U. Prognostic value of electrical tests in acute facial paralysis. *Am J Otol.* 1984;5:494.

Harner SG, Daube JR, Beatty CW, et al. Intraoperative monitoring of the facial nerve. *Laryngoscope.* 1988;98:209.

Hone SW, Commins DJ, Rames P, et al. Prognostic factors in intraoperative facial nerve monitoring for acoustic neuroma. *J Otolaryngol.* 1997;26:374.

House JW. Facial nerve grading systems. *Laryngoscope.* 1983;93:1056.

Jessell TM. Reactions of neurons to injury. In: Kandel ER, Schwartz JH, Jessell TM, eds. *Principles of Neural Science.* 3rd ed. Norwalk, Conn: Appleton & Lange; 1991:1108-1112.

Kartush JM. Electroneurography and intraoperative facial nerve monitoring in contemporary neurotology. *Otolaryngol Head Neck Surg.* 1989;101:496.

Kartush JM. Intra-operative monitoring in acoustic neuroma surgery. *Neurol Res.* 1998;20:593.

Laumans EP, Jonkees LB. On the prognosis of peripheral facial paralysis of endotemporal origin. *Ann Otol Rhino Laryngol.* 1963;72:621.

May M, Blumenthal F, Klein S. Acute Bell's palsy: prognostic value of evoked electromyography, maximal stimulation, and other electrical tests. *Am J Otol.* 1983;5:1.

May M, Hardin WB, Sullivan J, et al. Natural history of Bell's palsy: the salivary flow test and other prognostic indicators. *Laryngoscope.* 1976;86:704.

National Institutes of Health. Acoustic neuroma. *Consensus Statement.* 1991;9:1.

Prass RL, Kinney SE, Hardy RW Jr, et al. Acoustic (loudspeaker) facial EMG monitoring. II. Use of evoked EMG activity during acoustic neuroma resection. *Otolaryngol Head Neck Surg.* 1987;97:541.

Seddon HJ. Three types of nerve injury. *Brain.* 1943;66:237.

Sittel C, Stennert E. Prognostic value of electromyography in acute peripheral facial nerve palsy. *Otol Neurotol.* 2001;22:100.

Sterkers JM, et al. Preservation of facial, cochlear, and other nerve functions in acoustic neuroma treatment. *Otolaryngol Head Neck Surg.* 1994;110:146.

Sunderland S. Some anatomical and pathophysiological data relevant to facial nerve injury and repair. In: Fisch U, ed. *Facial Nerve Surgery.* Birmingham, Ala: Aesculapius Publishing; 1977.

Wedekind C, Klug N. Facial F wave recording: a novel and effective technique for extra- and intraoperative diagnosis of facial nerve function in acoustic tumor disease. *Otolaryngol Head Neck Surg.* 2003;129:114.

Wilson L, Lin E, Lalwani A. Cost-effectiveness of intraoperative facial nerve monitoring in middle ear or mastoid surgery. *Laryngoscope.* 2003;113:1736.

For complete list of references log onto www.expertconsult.com.

CHAPTER ONE HUNDRED AND SEVENTY

Clinical Disorders of the Facial Nerve

Douglas E. Mattox

Key Points

- The term *Bell's palsy* should be reserved for abrupt-onset, idiopathic facial paralysis without other identified cause.
- Progressive facial paralysis is not Bell's palsy and should prompt an investigation for neoplasm.
- The etiology of Bell's palsy is reactivation of herpes simplex virus (HSV).
- The mainstay of treatment for Bell's palsy is corticosteroids.
- Ramsay Hunt syndrome (herpes zoster oticus) is caused by varicella-zoster virus (VZV).
- Bell's palsy is common during pregnancy and is managed as for any other facial palsy, in collaboration with the patient's obstetrician.
- Bilateral facial paralysis suggests the possibility of Lyme disease.
- When facial paralysis occurs in the setting of chronic otitis media (suppurative or cholesteatoma), the first line of treatment is to resolve the ear disease; subsequent recovery from the facial paralysis is the usual outcome in this setting.

This chapter describes clinical disorders of the facial nerve (Fig. 170-1). Most of the discussion is devoted to idiopathic paralysis (Bell's palsy); however, disorders of the facial nerve associated with other diseases also are presented. The usefulness of electrodiagnostic testing and the medical and surgical management of Bell's palsy are reviewed as well.

Bell's Palsy: Spontaneous Idiopathic Facial Paralysis

The term *Bell's palsy* should be reserved for cases of facial paralysis in which signs and symptoms are consistent with the disease and in which a diligent search fails to identify another cause for the clinical findings. Every experienced otolaryngologist has seen patients whose facial paralysis was caused by malignancy, facial neuroma, intracranial tumor, infection, or some other manageable cause but was misdiagnosed by another physician. The dictum that "all that palsies are not Bell's" cannot be overemphasized.

Although older literature relegated Bell's palsy to a diagnosis of exclusion, May and colleagues[1] emphasized the diagnosis on the basis of specific clinical features. Taverner[2] outlined the minimum diagnostic criteria for Bell's palsy: (1) paralysis or paresis of all muscle groups of one side of the face; (2) sudden onset; (3) absence of signs of central nervous system (CNS) disease; and (4) absence of signs of ear or cerebellopontine angle disease. The differential diagnosis of facial palsy is shown in Table 170-1.

Incidence

The annual estimated incidence of Bell's palsy is 20 to 30 patients per 100,000 population; it was 20.2 of 100,000 per year in the United Kingdom between 1992 and 1996.[3] The incidence is greater in patients older than 65 years (59 of 100,000) and lower in children younger than age 13 (13 of 100,000).[4-6] The male-to-female ratio for Bell's palsy is approximately equal, except for a predominance in women younger than 20 years of age and a slight predominance in men older than 40 years.[4] The left and right sides of the face are equally involved. Thirty percent of patients will have incomplete paralysis on presentation, and 70% will have a complete paralysis.[7] Bilateral paralysis occurs in 0.3% of patients, and 9% have a history of previous paralysis.[4] A family history of Bell's palsy can be elicited in 8% of patients.[4]

Etiology

Proposed causes of Bell's palsy include microcirculatory failure of the vasa nervorum,[8,9] viral infection, ischemic neuropathy, and autoimmune reactions.[10,11] Of these, the viral hypothesis has been the most widely accepted[4,12]; however, no virus has ever been consistently isolated from the serum of patients with Bell's palsy.[13] Thus, the evidence for the viral hypothesis is indirect, relying on clinical observations and changes in viral antibody titers. Furthermore, although the underlying cause may be viral, the immediate cause of the paralysis itself is debated to be viral neuropathy alone or ischemic neuropathy secondary to viral infection.[14]

Acute facial paralysis can occur as part of many viral illnesses, including mumps,[15] rubella,[16] herpes simplex,[17] and Epstein-Barr virus.[18,19] A viral cause for Bell's palsy also is supported by the finding that it seems to be part of a polyneuritis syndrome in which the facial palsy is the most obvious cranial nerve involved. Careful neurologic examination will reveal other cranial nerve weaknesses in more than 50% of patients with Bell's palsy.[20,21] Adour[22,23] found several affected cranial nerves in most patients (Table 170-2).

A direct link between Bell's palsy and viral infection has been difficult to establish. Serologic studies have examined both seroconversion and prevalence of antigens to suspected etiologic agents in patients with Bell's palsy, especially HSV and VZV. The results have been conflicting and have been dependent on techniques used and popula-

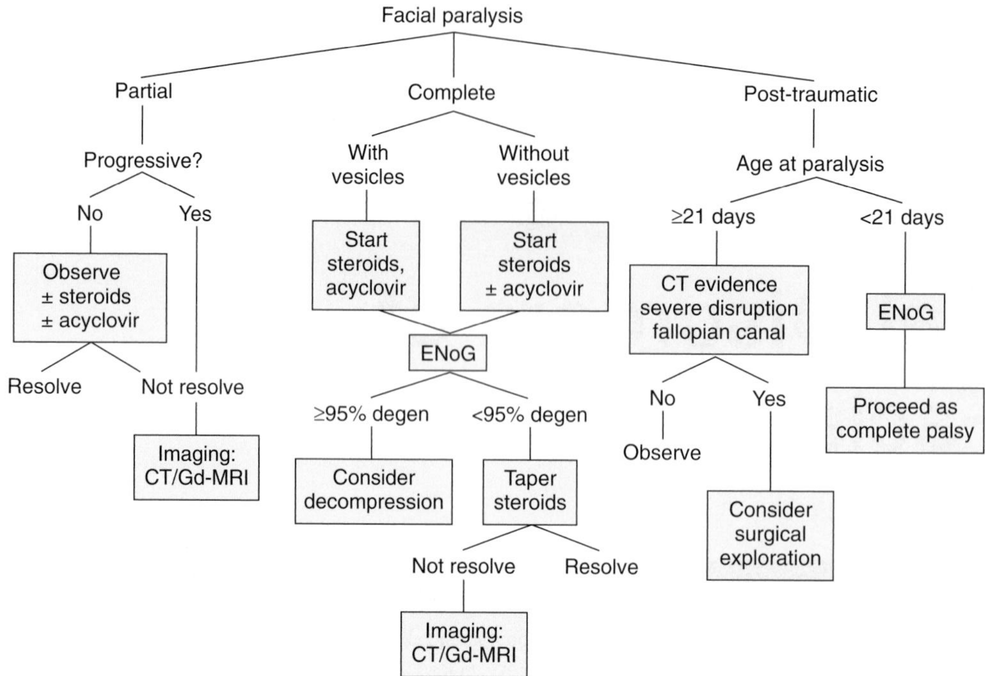

Figure 170-1. Facial paralysis: management algorithm.

Table 170-1

Differential Diagnosis of Facial Paralysis

Acute Paralysis	Chronic or Progressive Paralysis
Polyneuritis	Malignancies
· Bell's palsy	· Primary parotid tumor
· Herpes zoster	· Metastatic tumor
· Guillain-Barré syndrome	Benign tumors
· Autoimmune disease	· Schwannoma
· Lyme disease	· Glomus tumor
· Human immunodeficiency virus infection	Cholesteatoma
· Kawasaki's disease	
Trauma	
· Temporal bone fracture	
· Barotrauma	
· Birth trauma	
Otitis media	
· Acute bacterial	
· Chronic bacterial	
· Cholesteatoma	
Sarcoidosis	
Melkersson-Rosenthal syndrome	
Neurologic disorders	
· Human immunodeficiency virus infection	
· Cerebrovascular disorder—central or peripheral	

Modified from Adour KK, Hilsinger RL Jr, Callan EJ: Facial paralysis and Bell's palsy: a protocol for differential diagnosis. *Am J Otol.* 1985;Nov(Suppl):68.

Table 170-2

Polyneuropathy in Bell's Palsy

Symptom	Incidence (%)
Hypesthesia or dysesthesia of the glossopharyngeal or trigeminal nerve	80
Hypoesthesia of C2	20
Vagal motor weakness	20
Trigeminal motor weakness	3
Facial or retroauricular pain	60
Dysgeusia	57
Hyperacusis	30
Decreased tearing	17

From Adour KK: Current concepts in neurology: diagnosis and management of facial paralysis. *N Engl J Med.* 1982;307:348.

tions studied.[24,25] One reason for failure of these studies is that they sought for signs of an acute infection immediately preceding the onset of the Bell's palsy. No seasonal predilection or epidemic clustering has been documented, however, so it is much more likely that Bell's palsy is caused by reactivation of a latent virus rather than direct, communicable viral infection.

Morgan and colleagues[26,27] and Vahlne and coworkers[28] support the hypothesis that Bell's palsy is a reactivation of VZV that may be initiated by several stresses, including heterotopic viruses (viruses other than herpesviruses) or physical or metabolic stress. Activation by other agents may explain the diversity and inconsistency of the antibody titers reported in various studies, as well as the epidemicity or clustering of cases. This reactivation can occur without a measurable antibody response to HSV.

The best evidence for reactivation of HSV as the mechanism for Bell's palsy comes from several studies of the geniculate ganglion and facial nerve. Futura[29] and Takasu[30] and their coworkers have demonstrated HSV-1 DNA in both the trigeminal and geniculate ganglia of unselected autopsy specimens. Burgess and colleagues[31] reported a single of case of a patient who died shortly after Bell's palsy developed and in whom HSV-1 genomic DNA was identified in the geniculate ganglion of the facial nerve. Assay of archival control tissue for viral DNA yielded negative findings. In the most important study so far, Murakami and associates[32] looked at endoneurial fluid and postauricular muscle from patients with Bell's palsy or Ramsay Hunt syndrome and control subjects. Polymerase chain reaction (PCR) assay was used to test for HSV-1 DNA and VZV DNA, and the results were confirmed with Southern blot analysis. HSV DNA was detected in 11 of 14 patients with Bell's palsy, whereas VZV DNA was not recovered from any. Conversely, VZV DNA was recovered from all the patients with Ramsay Hunt syndrome, whereas none had HSV-1 DNA. Unaffected control subjects had neither virus DNA. This study suggests a clean distinction between Bell's palsy and Ramsay Hunt syndrome; however, other studies suggest more overlap.

Futura and coworkers[33] studied 142 patients with both clinical Ramsay Hunt syndrome and acute facial palsy. Thirteen were diagnosed as having Ramsay Hunt syndrome on the first visit, and in another eight, vesicular lesions developed subsequent to their initial evaluation. Of the 121 with nonvesicular acute facial paralysis, 35 had VZV DNA detected in their saliva or serologic evidence of VZV reactivation. Yamakawa and colleagues[34] demonstrated how technique-sensitive these studies are. Using two different PCR techniques, these investigators found high but differing rates of VZV DNA detection in patients with Ramsay Hunt symdrome.

A few animal studies also support a viral cause for Bell's palsy. Ishii and coworkers[35] induced facial paralysis in guinea pigs by inoculating the surface of the facial nerve with HSV-1. The severity of paralysis and subsequent degeneration were evaluated histologically and seemed to be worse if the epineurium was removed before inoculation. Of interest, these workers found greater extension of the virus centrally within the nerve than toward the periphery. Sugita and associates[36] induced an acute transient facial paralysis in mice by injecting HSV into the auricles and tongues of mice. The paralysis started 6 to 9 days after inoculation and resolved after 3 to 7 days. Viral antigens were detected in the facial nerve, geniculate ganglion, and facial nerve nucleus. A spontaneously recovering ischemic facial palsy also can be induced in cats by embolization of internal and external maxillary arteries. The onset of the paralysis is immediate after embolization and resolves after 2 months.[37]

Although it is likely that the underlying disease in Bell's palsy is viral polyneuropathy, an unresolved question is why such a profound effect on the facial nerve occurs, in contrast with the relatively minor and transient changes in the other cranial nerves. The major anatomic difference between the facial and other cranial nerves is in its long bony canal. Fisch[38] measured the diameter of the fallopian canal throughout the temporal bone and found that the narrowest point was at the junction of the internal auditory canal and the labyrinthine portion, which he called the *meatal foramen*. The meatal foramen averaged 0.68 mm in diameter, whereas the remainder of the fallopian canal measured 1.02 to 1.53 mm. Fisch reasoned that edema in this narrow segment of the fallopian canal could cause damming of the axoplasmic flow within the facial nerve. This site of lesion in Bell's palsy has been confirmed by clinical observation[39,40] and by intraoperative neuronography.[41,42] A similar site of lesion has been identified electrophysiologically in herpes zoster oticus.[43]

Histopathology

Fowler[16] reported autopsy findings in a patient who died shortly after Bell's palsy developed. The entire intratemporal nerve contained dilated and engorged veins and venules. Fresh hemorrhage was found within the internal auditory canal surrounding the facial nerve that extended as far as the geniculate ganglion. Fowler theorized that the ischemia resulted from microthrombi rather than vasospasm.

Reddy and associates[44] examined a facial nerve 17 days after the onset of spontaneous paralysis. The nerve showed scattered degeneration of the myelin sheaths and axons. From 10% to 30% of facial nerve fibers were surrounded by phagocytic cells. The perivascular areas also showed inflammatory reactive changes and hemorrhage.

Proctor and coworkers[45] examined a patient who died 13 days after the onset of facial paralysis. The facial nerve showed lymphocytic infiltration and phagocytosis of myelin by macrophages throughout the infratemporal course of the nerve. Initially, these findings were interpreted as evidence for a viral cause. However, when McKeever and colleagues[46] reexamined the case, they emphasized that the inflammatory cells were most prominent where the facial nerve was surrounded by bone, especially in the labyrinthine portion of the fallopian canal, but not within the internal auditory canal. These investigators theorized that the histopathologic features suggested a compression-type injury with no evidence of vascular occlusion.

O'Donoghue and Michaels[47] found degeneration of myelin sheaths and axon fibers throughout the intratemporal course of the facial nerve. The nerve was constricted at the meatal foramen, and an osteoclastic giant cell reaction caused resorption of bone around the geniculate ganglion. These workers interpreted the observed changes as consistent with a viral cause, but as pointed out by Jenkins and associates,[40] these findings do not preclude edema and constriction of the facial nerve as the final event leading to the paralysis.

Podvinec[48] found inflammatory infiltrates in the intratemporal portion of the facial nerve 6 months after the onset of the palsy, along with signs of wallerian degeneration and regeneration. He suggested that the persistence of infiltrates for this extended time may result from compromised circulation within the fallopian canal. Jackson and colleagues[49] reported the histopathologic findings from the labyrinthine segment of the facial nerve in a patient 1 year after the onset of a total facial paralysis secondary to herpes zoster. A portion of the nerve within the auditory canal was essentially healthy; however, at the meatal foramen, the nerve became a mixed fibrotic and necrotic acellular mass.

Michaels[50] described the histopathologic findings in an autopsy performed 11 days after the onset of Bell's palsy. As in other studies, histopathologic features included demyelination, compression, bone resorption, and lymphocytic infiltration in the proximal labyrinthine segment of the facial nerve. Michaels cautioned against the overinterpretation of bulging of the nerve in the distal internal auditory canal, because it was found on both the healthy and the pathologic sides.

Another approach to the histologic evaluation of Bell's palsy is with biopsy specimens obtained intraoperatively, including biopsy specimens of the chorda tympani and greater petrosal nerve. Chorda tympani specimens in acute Bell's palsy have shown degeneration of myelinated fibers but no inflammatory response.[51,52] Fisch and Felix[14] examined greater petrosal nerve specimens obtained during middle cranial fossa facial nerve decompression. Their findings included degeneration and demyelination of large axons and lymphocytic infiltration. They found these results to be consistent with wallerian degeneration starting proximal to the geniculate ganglion, probably from the meatal foramen.

In summary, most histologic studies show diffuse demyelination of the facial nerve throughout its intratemporal course, with the most severe changes in the labyrinthine segment and at the meatal foramen.

Central Nervous System Changes

Auditory symptoms, usually in the form of hyperacusis, may be present in up to 30% of patients with Bell's palsy.[53] The cause for these auditory symptoms is unknown. McCandless and Schumacher[54] did not find evidence of a lesion affecting the cochlear nerve in patients with facial paralysis. Many researchers have attributed the hyperacusis to decreased damping of sound secondary to dysfunction of the stapedius muscle. However, most investigators have not found reduced contralateral stapedius reflex thresholds, suggesting that an absence of stapedial damping is not the cause.[55]

On the basis of these observations, many investigators have concluded that the auditory dysfunction results from CNS involvement.[53] A few patients with Bell's palsy have auditory brainstem response (ABR) abnormalities compared with ABRs in age-matched control subjects. These abnormalities include an increase in the wave I to V interval and the interaural difference for wave V. These changes usually are present bilaterally and resolve with recovery from the facial paralysis.[55] These findings suggested a brainstem abnormality associated with Bell's palsy that the study authors hypothesized is related to the reactivation of HSV. These findings should be interpreted with caution. Other investigators did not confirm the presence of such ABR abnormalities,[56,57] and the findings have not been corroborated by somatosensory evoked potentials or visual evoked potentials.

Several investigators have looked for CNS changes in acute facial paralysis by studying the cerebrospinal fluid (CSF). Again the results are contradictory. Findings of elevated levels of myelin basic protein[58] and pleocytosis[59] in the CSF support CNS involvement in Bell's palsy. Weber and coworkers[60] found a normal total cell count, total protein concentration, blood-CSF permeability, and CSF–to–serum immunoglobulin ratios in most patients with Bell's palsy. Only approximately 10% of these patients demonstrated some pathologic feature of the CSF, including a mild increase in blood-CSF permeability or pleocytosis. These workers concluded that their findings did not support the hypothesis that Bell's palsy was a part of a cranial polyneuropathy.

CNS changes in Bell's palsy also have been suggested by magnetic resonance imaging (MRI). Jonsson and associates[61] found brain or brainstem changes in 5 of 19 patients with Bell's palsy. These areas of increased signal intensity did not correlate with the facial nerve brainstem nucleus or the supranuclear pathways and were interpreted as indicative of unrelated vascular disease.

Electrophysiology and Testing

The multiple branches from the facial nerve, including the greater petrosal nerve, stapedial nerve, chorda tympani, and muscular branches, led to the development of topodiagnostic testing to localize the site of a facial nerve lesion. Schirmer's test evaluates greater petrosal nerve function by measuring the lacrimal secretions accumulating on a piece of filter paper placed under the eyelid at the medial canthus.[62] Stapedial nerve function can be evaluated with stapedial reflex testing. The chorda tympani nerve can be evaluated with taste testing or with the submandibular salivary flow test described by Magielski and Blatt.[63] Unfortunately, the accuracy of localization with topodiagnostic testing has been disappointing.[42] This is not a surprising finding in Bell's palsy, in which the lesion is a diffuse demyelination throughout the nerve. However, topodiagnostic testing also has yielded disappointing results in investigation of tumors in which a sharply defined site of lesion was expected.[64]

Electrodiagnostic tests on the motor branches of the facial nerve also have been used to assess function and predict outcome. All of these tests have a similar shortcoming: Stimulation and recording are performed only distal to the lesion, rather than on opposite sides of the site of injury.[65] Accordingly, such testing should be delayed because it will not demonstrate abnormalities until nerve degeneration has reached the site of stimulation, usually 4 to 5 days after injury.

Nerve Excitability Threshold

The use of electricity as a neurodiagnostic test was described by Duchenne in 1892 and was adapted to the facial nerve by Laumans and Jongkees.[66] Application of the Hilger nerve stimulator is the method of facial nerve evaluation most commonly used by otolaryngologists. The extratemporal portion of the nerve is stimulated with a small-amplitude, pulsed direct current. The face is observed for the lowest current to produce a visible twitch. Although a threshold difference of more than 3.5 mA between the two sides has been considered to be suggestive of nerve degeneration, Gates[67] found that with careful technique, low thresholds were obtained with percutaneous stimulation. The thresholds increased slowly with age and body weight, but nerve excitability thresholds greater than 1.25 mA in the upper division and 2 mA in the lower division were statistically abnormal.

Maximal Stimulation Test

A modification of the minimal excitability test, the maximal stimulation test, attempted to determine the difference between the strength and amount of contraction of the facial musculature caused by a supramaximal electrical stimulus.[68,69] However, the maximal stimulation test is difficult to quantitate and is more subject to interobserver variation than is the minimal stimulation test.[65]

Electroneurography

Electroneurography (ENoG), also called electroneuronography, adds recording of the facial muscle action potential with surface or needle electrodes to the stimulation tests. Esslen[70] introduced the use of bipolar surface electrodes for stimulation and recording of responses. The two electrodes are moved independently to produce the maximum amplitude of response. The response is evaluated by comparing the peak-to-peak amplitude of the maximum response obtained for the two sides of the face.

Electromyography

Electromyography (EMG) measures muscle action potentials generated by spontaneous and voluntary activity. It is distinct from other electrodiagnostic tests in which the activity is generated by active stimulation of the nerve. Denervation potentials are seen 10 days or longer after onset of the palsy; therefore, they are of limited value in determining early prognosis of facial paralysis. However, the loss of voluntary motor unit potentials within the first 3 to 4 days of paralysis suggests a poor prognosis.[65] Conversely, retention of voluntary motor activity past the 7th day suggests that complete degeneration will not occur. Sittel and Stennert[71] found that the detection of spontaneous fibrillation by needle EMG had an 80% accuracy in predicting a poor outcome 10 to 14 days after onset of paralysis. Unfortunately, this is too late to be useful in surgical decision making.

Nerve Conduction Velocity

Nerve conduction velocity can be measured between the stylomastoid foramen and the mandibular branch of the facial nerve. A strong correlation has been found between decrease in nerve conduction velocity and decrease in the compound nerve action potential measured by ENoG during the first 2 weeks after the onset of paralysis.[72] Normal facial nerve conduction velocity ranges between 37 and 58 meters/second, and conduction velocities in this range were associated with uniformly good outcomes. Conduction velocities between 20 and 30 meters/second carry a 50% chance of significant residual paresis or synkinesis, and those less than 10 meters/second were associated with poor outcomes.

Interpretation of Electrical Tests

All electrical stimulation tests have the same fundamental weakness: inferences are made on the basis of tests on the nerve distal to the site of injury within the temporal bone. Therefore, there is an inherent delay between the onset of the injury and the development of sufficient degeneration of the distal segment of the nerve to be discovered by the tests. Only intraoperative monitoring, with stimulation proximal to the lesion, provides direct information about the state of the nerve at the site of the lesion. Newer experimental techniques, including antidromic stimulation and magnetic stimulation, hold some promise for circumventing this limitation.

Excellent recovery of facial function is invariable when the decline in the compound action potential (CAP) as measured by ENoG does not reach 90%, and one half of patients in whom this level of degeneration is documented also have excellent outcomes.[73,74] The problem is how to identify patients who will not achieve a good recovery, and at least a partial answer lies in the combination of ENoG with standard EMG. For patients who maintain recordable voluntary motor potentials despite a severe depression of the CAP, the prognosis is excellent.[74] This finding may be explained by severe desynchronization of the motor units, causing a reduced or absent CAP.

Electromagnetic Stimulation of the Facial Nerve

Facial nerve testing with electromagnetic stimulation also has been explored. Benecke and colleagues[75] were able to stimulate the nerve with cortical (supranuclear) electromagnetic discharges, demonstrating that the nerve could be stimulated trans-synaptically. Direct stimulation of the facial nerve with electromagnetic stimulation also has been described. On the basis of latencies of compound muscle action potentials from magnetic and electrical stimulation of the facial nerve, investigators concluded that the root entry zone of the facial nerve was the most likely site of excitation with magnetic stimulation.[76] These data are tantalizing because the ideal test of the facial nerve would stimulate the nerve medial to the presumed site of the conduction block in the labyrinthine segment. Meyer and coworkers[77] found an absence of electromagnetic responses to be the earliest sign of nerve conduction block in patients with Bell's palsy, and that electromagnetic stimulation could differentiate between central and peripheral nerve lesions.

It is not yet clear, however, whether magnetic stimulation will be a useful predictive test, because significant discrepancies have been noted between the response to magnetic stimulation and clinical findings. Patients with incomplete palsies may exhibit complete loss of response to magnetic stimulation.[78] Loss of response to electromagnetic stimulation occurs in more patients with Bell's palsy than does loss of electrical stimulation, and this finding may persist after facial function has clinically recovered.[75,79] Nowak and associates[80] tested 65 patients with facial paralysis with both transcranial magnetic stimulation and electrical stimulation of the facial nerve. A severe reduction in muscle action potiental response was observed in both Bell's palsy and herpes zoster and did not correlate with the clinical grade of the palsy. On the basis of current clinical information, electrical stimulation seems to add little to the diagnostic armamentarium in facial palsy.

Imaging of the Facial Nerve

Gadolinium-enhanced MRI has been used to study the peripheral facial nerve in Bell's palsy. Enhancement of the facial nerve is a common finding in healthy persons, making evaluation of facial nerve findings on MRI difficult. The most consistent area of enhancement in Bell's palsy and herpetic palsy is the distal meatal and labyrinthine segments.[81,82] Sartoretti-Schefer and associates[82] hypothesized that the gadolinium enhancement resulted from breakdown of the blood-brain barrier or from venous congestion in the epineurium. However, the location or degree of enhancement does not correlate with the recovery of facial movement.[81,83] In a recent report that used high-resolution gadolinium-enhanced MRI with surface coils, Kress and colleagues[84] were able to differentiate 3 patients with poor outcomes from 17 who recovered on the basis of the wide distribution and intensity of enhancement. The development of more detailed MRI techniques may prove useful in determining the prognosis of Bell's palsy.[85]

Prognosis and Statistics

The prognosis for most patients with Bell's palsy is excellent: 80% to 90% recover completely.[6,53] Peitersen[7] reported that none of 1505 patients followed without management had permanent complete paralysis, and that 17 had moderate to severe sequelae (contracture, synkinesis, palsy). Many large series of patients with Bell's palsy have been analyzed to identify prognostic factors that have a significant impact on outcome. The most important such factor is whether the paralysis is incomplete or complete. The prognosis for affected persons in whom complete facial paralysis never develops is excellent: 95% to 100% recover with no identifiable sequelae.[6,86]

The many reports available in the literature are difficult to compare, because they use different criteria for inclusion and evaluation of outcome. Stankiewicz[87] collated the outcomes from nine reports, including the large series of Park and Watkins[88] and Peitersen.[89] The overall results from these series were 53% complete recovery, 44% partial recovery, and only 3% no recovery. The results in the general population probably are better than those in these studies.

Other factors associated with poor outcome include hyperacusis; decreased tearing; age older than 60 years; diabetes mellitus; hypertension; and severe aural, anterior facial, or radicular pain.[4,90] Abraham-Inpijn and associates,[91] however, compared outcomes in 200 patients by use of several potential prognostic factors, including severity of the facial paralysis, mean arterial pressure, age, clinical or chemical diabetes mellitus, and history of hypertension. Only the severity of the paralysis at its maximum extent and the mean arterial pressure at presentation proved to be statistically significant. Peitersen[7] noted a correlation between sequelae (synkinesis, contracture) and the interval between paralysis and the onset of recovery.

Management

Management of Bell's palsy has had a long, complex evolution that is not yet complete. Methods currently advocated include observation, corticosteroids, surgical decompression, and antiviral agents.

The use of corticosteroids in Bell's palsy was first proposed by Rothendler.[92] Since then, corticosteroid therapy has become the most common approach to management of Bell's palsy.[93] Adour and Wingerd[94,95] stated that although prednisone does not reduce the number of patients with eventual partial denervation or contracture or synkinesis, it reduces the number of patients with eventual complete denervation, therefore making the disease less severe. Numerous prospective and retrospective studies on the effectiveness of corticosteroids in Bell's palsy have been reported. In a meta-analysis, Ramsey and colleagues[96] found two studies with sufficient numbers of patients and rigor for analysis and concluded that treated patients had a 17% better chance of complete recovery than placebo-managed or untreated patients. Their analysis of a larger number of studies concluded that the odds of recovery with steroid treatment ranged between 49% and 97%, versus 23% and 64% for untreated patients. Consensus is lacking regarding the dose or duration of steroid treatment.

The case for steroid treatment in children in less clear. Neither Prescott[97] nor Unüvar and coworkers[98] found a beneficial effect of corticosteroids for Bell's palsy in children. Salman and MacGregor[99] came to the same conclusion in their systematic review of the literature.

Patients with Bell's palsy commonly are treated with antiviral agents in addition to prednisone,[100] although once again, definitive proof of efficacy is lacking. Although initial enthusiasm was high for the use of a combination of steroids and antivirals[101,102] more recent studies have yielded negative results. Sullivan and colleagues[103] conducted a four-armed, multi-institutional trial of prednisolone, acyclovir, a combined regimen of both agents, and placebo. Significant improvement in outcome was observed in both arms containing prednisolone, but no additional benefit from antiviral treatment was found. A similar outcome was described in a study reported from Japan.[104] Current opinion does not support the use of antivirals in Bell's palsy.

Surgical therapy is more controversial, because unlike with corticosteroids, it is associated with the possibility of significant additional injury. Early enthusiasm for transmastoid decompression of the tympanic and mastoid segments of the facial nerve has waned,[105] and the procedure has been abandoned,[1] because randomized trials showed no benefit[1] and because of evidence that the site of the lesion is in the proximal labyrinthine portion of the facial nerve, which is inaccessible through the mastoid.[38]

The efficacy of surgical decompression of the meatal foramen and labyrinthine segment of the facial nerve in patients with poor prognosis as shown by ENoG testing is promising, but it has been difficult to assemble a large enough series to definitively establish its value in randomized trials. Fisch[38] compared outcomes in 14 surgical patients with 90% degeneration or greater as shown by ENoG within 3 weeks of the onset of paralysis with those in 13 similar patients who refused surgery. He found a subtle but statistically significant improvement in the long-term facial recovery in the operative group. Sillman[74] found a shift toward grade I and II recovery in patients with greater than 90% degeneration who underwent surgical decompression versus those managed with corticosteroids alone. In the most well-controlled study of middle fossa decompression of the facial nerve in Bell's palsy, Gantz and colleagues[106] evaluated the outcome when ENoG showed greater than 90% degeneration, and no voluntary motor unit potentials were found on electromyography performed within 2 weeks of onset of paralysis. Ninety-one percent of surgical patients achieved House-Brackmann grade I or II recovery, versus a 42% chance of these same results with steroids alone. Graham and Kartush[107] described six patients with recurrent facial paralysis, one of whom had Melkersson-Rosenthal syndrome. None of these patients experienced recurrent facial paralysis after total seventh nerve decompression from the stylomastoid foramen to the internal auditory canal. Thus, surgical decompression remains in the armamentarium for the management of facial paralysis, but timing and appropriate patient identification remain difficult.

Persistent synkinesis can be a problem for many patients recovering from severe degeneration of the facial nerve regardless of the cause. Chua and associates[108] performed a dose escalation study of botulinum toxin to determine the best treatment for reducing eyelid synkinesia and found the lowest dose, 40 units injected into the orbicularis oculi, to give the best reduction in synkinesia while avoiding ptosis. Borodic and coworkers[109] reported similar results with botulinum toxin in a multi-institutional study.

Special Cases of Facial Paralysis

Ramsay Hunt Syndrome

Ramsay Hunt syndrome (herpes zoster facial paralysis) differs from Bell's palsy, because it is associated with VZV infection (as shown by rising titers of antibodies to VZV) and the presence of skin vesicles on the pinna, retroauricular area, face, or mouth. Compared with Bell's palsy, Ramsay Hunt syndrome generally causes more severe symptoms, and patients are at higher risk for the development of complete nerve degeneration.[110]

Varicella, or chickenpox, is the manifestation of primary infection by VZV (HSV, varicellae) in a nonimmune host. Herpes zoster is the manifestation of this same virus infection in a partially immune host. Serologic and epidemiologic data strongly suggest that varicella-zoster represents the reactivation of a latent virus rather than reinfection. After the primary infection, the virus probably travels to the dorsal root to extramedullary cranial nerve ganglia, where it remains dormant until it is reactivated. Reactivation generally occurs during a period of decreased cell-mediated immunity. VZV infection is the second most common cause of facial paralysis. The incidence of herpes zoster in patients with peripheral facial palsy is 4.5% to 9%.[111] A Mayo Clinic study[112] estimated the annual incidence of herpes zoster as 130 cases per 100,000. The incidence increased dramatically in patients older than age 60; 10% of this population had identifiable risk factors for decreased cell-mediated immunity, including carcinoma, trauma, radiotherapy, and chemotherapy. The increased incidence in the elderly is explained by an age-related decrease in cellular immune response to VZV.[113]

The severity of the paralysis is worse and the prognosis poorer in herpes zoster oticus than in Bell's palsy. Peitersen[114] reported full recovery in only 22% of patients, and Devriese[115] found complete recovery in only 16%. As in Bell's palsy, the recovery is predicted in part by the severity of the paralysis. Complete recovery occurred in only 10% of patients after complete loss of facial function and in approximately 66% after incomplete loss.[111]

The timing of the appearance of the vestibular eruption may have prognostic significance. In most cases, eruption and paralysis occur simultaneously. In approximately 25% of cases, the eruption precedes the paralysis; these patients have a higher likelihood of recovery.[111] Patients with Ramsay Hunt syndrome also are more likely than patients with Bell's palsy to have associated cranial nerve symptoms, including hyperacusis, hearing loss, and pain.[116] Ramsay Hunt syndrome can be misdiagnosed on the basis of initial presentation. In approximately 10% of patients, the vesicular rash appears well after the initial facial paralysis, and many patients demonstrate a rise in antibody to VZV without ever exhibiting cutaneous or mucous membrane vesicles—so-called Ramsay Hunt sine herpete.

Severe ocular complications can occur with herpes zoster ophthalmicus. These complications include uveitis, keratoconjunctivitis, optic neuritis, and glaucoma and are almost always associated with involvement of the ophthalmic division of the trigeminal nerve. Herpes zoster ophthalmicus may be difficult to differentiate from the localized skin rash associated with HSV infection. Although both conditions may cause keratitis, differentiation between them is extremely important, because topical corticosteroids are used to manage herpes zoster but are contraindicated in HSV infection. Ophthalmologic consultation for biomicroscopy, staining, cytologic studies, and viral isolation studies may differentiate these two conditions.[117] Adour[94] stated that aside from concerns about ophthalmic involvement, the development of skin vesicles before or after initiation of prednisone does not contraindicate corticosteroid use.

Management of patients with herpes zoster, including cephalic zoster, consists of systemic corticosteroids.[118] A specific benefit of corticosteroid therapy is a reduction in postherpetic neuralgia. The usefulness of corticosteroids in fostering recovery from the facial paralysis is controversial; however, early institution of corticosteroids seems to relieve acute pain, reduce vertigo, and decrease the incidence of postherpetic neuralgia.[119,120]

The antiviral agent acyclovir also is recommended to treat herpes zoster facial paralysis.[121,122] Acyclovir is a nucleotide analog that interferes with herpes virus DNA polymerase and inhibits DNA replication. The drug is preferentially taken up by HSV-infected cells, making it nearly nontoxic to noninfected cells. Early return of facial function after acyclovir management has been reported by some investigators,[121,122] but no beneficial effects were reported by others.[123] At the least, treatment with acyclovir seems to lessen pain and promote resolution of the vesicles.

Box 170-1

Congenital versus Acquired Facial Paralysis

Congenital

Mononeural agenesis
Congenital facial paralysis
Congenital unilateral lower lip palsy
Facial paralysis with other deficits
Möbius syndrome (cranial nerves VI, VII; bilateral)
Hemifacial microsomia
Oculoauriculovertebral dysplasia
Poland's syndrome (agenesis of pectoralis major muscle)
Secondary to teratogens
Thalidomide
Rubella

Acquired

Birth trauma
Forceps injury
Pressure from maternal sacrum
Pressure from fetal shoulder
Intracranial hemorrhage
Idiopathic
Bell's palsy
Systemic or infectious disease
Melkersson-Rosenthal syndrome
Poliomyelitis
Infectious mononucleosis
Varicella
Acute otitis media
Meningitis

Modified from Harris JP, Davidson TM, May M, Fria T: Evaluation and treatment of congenital facial paralysis. *Arch Otolaryngol.* 1983;109:145.

Congenital Facial Paralysis

The incidence of facial paralysis in newborns has been estimated at 0.23% of live births.[124] The first dilemma in managing facial palsy in an infant or young child lies in differentiating true congenital paralysis from birth trauma. The differential diagnosis of congenital facial palsy is shown in Box 170-1. Birth trauma usually causes isolated facial paralysis and other signs of injury, including facial swelling, ecchymosis, and hemotympanum. Abnormalities of other cranial nerves or abnormalities on brainstem audiometry (prolongation of the I to III or I to V interval) suggest that the facial paralysis is congenital and not traumatic.[125]

Of facial paralysis cases in infants, 78% are related to birth trauma. These cases are equally divided between forceps deliveries and vaginal deliveries plus cesarean sections,[126,127] suggesting that intrauterine facial nerve injury can occur from pressure on the infant's face by the sacral prominence during birth. Supranuclear palsy secondary to intracranial hemorrhage also has been reported.[128]

The mildest form of congenital facial dysfunction is congenital unilateral lower lip palsy, in which the defect is limited to an absence of depressor labii inferioris muscle activity. It is associated with a lesion of the brainstem.[129]

Möbius' syndrome represents a broad spectrum of clinical and pathologic findings ranging from isolated unilateral facial paralysis (usually associated with sixth cranial nerve paralysis) to bilateral absence of facial and abducens nerve function. Multiple other cranial nerves, including the glossopharyngeal, vagus, hypoglossal, and other extraocular motor nerves, also may be affected.[129a] Forty-three percent of children with Möbius syndrome have a history of some significant event in utero.[130] A majority of patients with Möbius' syndrome demonstrate sparing of the lower face compared with the upper face. Verzijl and coworkers[131] performed electrophysiologic testing on 11 patients with Möbius syndrome and concluded that Möbius syndrome is not a primary developmental disorder of the facial musculature but is a disorder of the rhombencephalon including both motor nuclei and transversing long tracts. MRI evidence suggests evidence of absence of the seventh cranial nerve in the internal auditory canal, implying the lower face receives aberrant innervation from other nerves, including the trigeminal, glossopharyngeal, and hypoglossal nerves.

Multiple cranial nerve palsies including facial palsy are seen in the CHARGE association (*c*olobomata, *h*eart disease, *a*tresia of choanae, *r*etarded growth, *g*enital hypoplasia, *e*ar anomalies and deafness). Of CHARGE-associated cases, 75% have at least one cranial nerve involved, and 58% have two or more cranial nerves involved. The most frequently involved are the auditory nerve in 60%, the facial nerve in 43%, and the glossopharyngeal or vagus nerve in 30%.[132]

Habilitation of the face in congenital facial paralysis usually is accomplished with temporalis muscle transfer, tarsorrhaphy, upper eyelid gold weights, and free muscle transfers. Surgical exploration and decompression of the facial nerve are rarely useful.[133]

Spontaneous Facial Paralysis in Children

Bell's palsy is uncommon in children; 8% of patients in the series by Peitersen[89] and only 2% in the series by Adour and coworkers[4] were younger than 10 years of age. Manning and Adour[134] and Prescott[97] found a female preponderance in this group.

The prognosis for children with Bell's palsy is uncertain. Peitersen,[89] Taverner,[2] and Prescott[97] reported a high rate of spontaneous recovery in children with Bell's palsy, in part related to the high frequency of incomplete paralysis. Inamura and colleagues[135] found that 97% of 58 cases recovered completely and concluded that corticosteroids had no impact on recovery. However, Alberti and Biagioni[136] and Manning and Adour[134] reported that a significant percentage of children did not recover from their facial paralysis. Jenkins and colleagues[40] and Prescott[97] argued that the prognosis was determined by the amount of nerve degeneration revealed by electrophysiologic testing and noted that children and adults with similar electrical testing results had similar outcomes.

Familial Facial Paralysis

Adour and associates[4] reported that 8% of patients with Bell's palsy had a positive family history, and Willbrand and associates[137] reported a 6% incidence. In addition, sporadic reports describe families with several affected members, usually each experiencing several attacks. Cawthorne and Haynes[138] reported the cases of two brothers, one of whom had experienced five episodes of Bell's palsy and the other, three episodes. DeSanto and Schubert[139] reported 10 cases of Bell's palsy in a family over 83 years; Wilbrand and associates[137] reported a family with 29 cases of Bell's palsy over 40 years. Samuel[140] reported a child who experienced four episodes of Bell's palsy involving both sides of the face; the child's father had six episodes of unilateral Bell's palsy. Amit[141] described a family tree in which only women (the index patient and her mother, maternal aunt, and maternal grandmother) had Bell's palsy. In three of the four, onset was during puberty, suggesting that hormonal influence may have been important. The evidence from these sporadic cases is insufficient to determine conclusively a genetic influence. In such cases, however, the paralysis often has an early age at onset and is recurrent, and the prognosis is excellent.

Recurrent Paralysis

Adour and coworkers[4] found that 9.3% of patients with Bell's palsy had a history of previous paralysis. Similarly, Hallmo and colleagues[142] reported that 10.9% of patients had a history of a previous facial paralysis (approximately equally on the ipsilateral and contralateral sides). Prescott[97] reported that 20 of 228 children (9%) with Bell's palsy who were younger than 18 years had a history of previous paralysis on the same side, and 8 had contralateral paralysis. The interval between the two attacks usually was longer than 1 year.[143] Perhaps the record for recurrent facial paralysis was set by a woman who experienced more than 50 episodes of unilateral lower facial paralysis after exposure to the disinfectant chlorocresol.[144] The age distribution for patients with recurrent facial palsy was the same as that for the overall population with Bell's palsy,[4] except for those with ipsilateral recurrent palsies, which may be associated with a younger age at onset.[143] Several reports noted a slight female predominance in recurrent facial palsy.[143,145] Diabetes mellitus was present in 39% of patients with recurrent paralysis in one study[4] but only in 4% in another.[142]

Controversy continues regarding whether the prognosis for recovery from recurrent facial palsy is better or worse on subsequent attacks. Some investigators state that the second attack is associated with a poorer prognosis and therefore constitutes a stronger indication for surgical decompression.[146] Most other workers, however, found no prognostic difference between the primary and subsequent attacks of facial paralysis and no difference whether the second attack occurred on the ipsilateral or contralateral side.[142]

Recurrence of facial palsy should prompt a careful investigation for other etiologic disorders. May and associates[1] found a tumor in 8 of 40 of patients (20%) with a second palsy on the same side.

Bilateral Facial Paralysis

Bilateral idiopathic facial paralysis is much less common than unilateral paralysis and occurs in only 0.3% to 2% of patients.[147] Bilateral facial paralysis is associated with a much higher incidence of systemic causes than unilateral palsy and should spur a diligent search for an underlying disorder.[148] The diseases most commonly associated with bilateral facial paralysis are Guillain-Barré syndrome, Bell's palsy, multiple idiopathic cranial neuropathies, brainstem encephalitis, benign intracranial hypertension, syphilis, leukemia, sarcoidosis, Lyme disease, and bacterial meningitis.[149,150] The possibility of an intrapontine or prepontine tumor also should be excluded.[150] Most of these conditions are associated with other systemic or neurologic signs that suggest the appropriate diagnosis.

Guillain-Barré syndrome is a progressive ascending motor paralysis, occurring after a viral infection, that usually affects the lower limbs. However, rare bulbar, myelitic, and cerebral forms of Guillain-Barré do not affect the limbs. Of the cranial nerves, the facial nerve is the third most commonly affected, after the glossopharyngeal and vagus.[151] The diagnosis is based on the typical clinical picture and the presence of elevated CSF protein but a normal cell count. Other conditions associated with facial diplegia include influenza,[152] infectious mononucleosis,[153] other viral infections,[154] and diabetes.[155] Heerfordt's syndrome (parotid enlargement, iridocyclitis, and cranial nerve palsy) associated with sarcoidosis also can cause bilateral facial paralysis.

The workup for a patient with bilateral facial paralysis should include a careful neurologic examination to detect other cranial neuropathies, a lumbar puncture to obtain CSF for cytologic studies, chemistry, culture, a Venereal Disease Research Laboratory (VDRL) test for syphilis. An MRI scan should exclude space-occupying lesions.[156]

The disability caused by bilateral facial paralysis is dramatically more severe than that from unilateral paralysis. Aggressive eye care with ointment, taping, or patching usually is required, but this approach significantly interferes with visual function. Bilateral paralysis of the lower lip leads to a characteristic speech impairment, oral incompetence, and drooling. In severe cases, inadequate circulation of saliva may have dental sequelae.[157] The psychologic impact can be devastating, because these patients are incapable of voluntary or emotional expres-

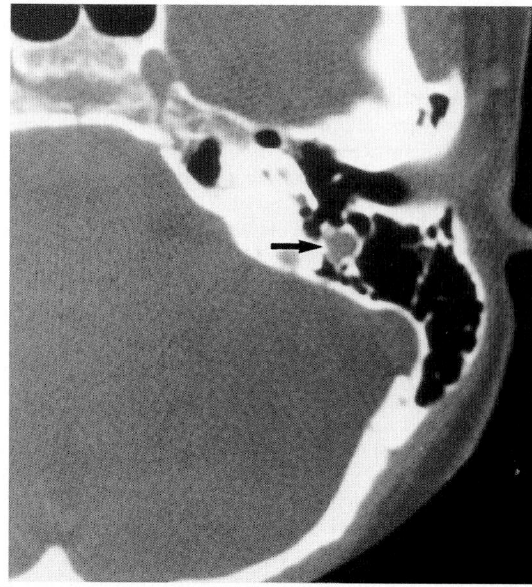

Figure 170-2. Axial CT scan of the right temporal bone shows enlargement of the mastoid segment of the fallopian canal *(arrow)* in the child with progressive facial paralysis. The lesion was a neuroma of the facial nerve.

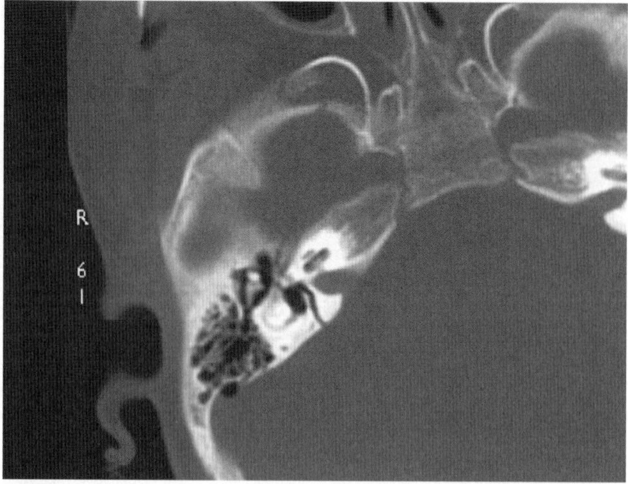

Figure 170-3. An axial CT scan of the temporal bone showing a transverse fracture of the temporal bone through the vestibule and geniculate ganglion.

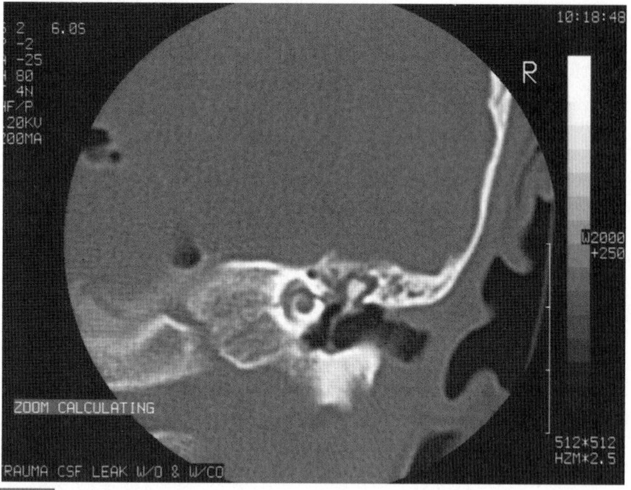

Figure 170-4. A coronal CT scan of the temporal bone showing a transverse fracture of the temporal bone through the cochlea and traversing the fallopian canal in the tympanic portion of the facial nerve.

sion.[158] Recovery in bilateral Bell's palsy is similar to that in unilateral palsy, although one side may recover before the other.[159]

Progressive Paralysis

Slowly progressive facial paralysis is not Bell's palsy. The differential diagnosis includes primary neuromas of the facial nerve (Fig. 170-2); metastases from squamous cell carcinomas and melanomas of the face and scalp; and occasionally distant metastases from kidney, breast, lung, and prostate.[160] Progressive facial paralysis also can occur from other primary temporal bone and cerebellopontine angle lesions and from carotid artery aneurysms.[161] A tumor should be excluded in all of these cases; the investigation should begin with physical examination for neuroma of the peripheral branches of the facial nerve and continue with computed tomography (CT) and gadolinium-enhanced MRI of the infratemporal and intracranial portions of the nerve. If results of these studies are negative, some authorities argue for exploration of the nerve from the peripheral branches through the temporal bone.[162] At the very least, patients with negative findings on initial evaluation require careful serial observation and imaging.

Traumatic Facial Paralysis

The most common causes of infratemporal facial nerve injury are temporal bone fracture, penetrating injuries (typically from a bullet), and iatrogenic injuries.

Injury of the facial nerve in temporal bone fractures can result from compression from bone fragments, intraneural hematomas, entrapment from compression, and loss of continuity. The distal labyrinthine segment and geniculate ganglion are the areas of the facial nerve most susceptible to injury in longitudinal and transverse temporal bone fractures[163] (Fig. 170-3). This portion of the facial nerve is particularly at risk because of its small size and lack of fibrous supporting tissue, and because of traction between the greater petrosal nerve and the geniculate ganglion caused by temporary distraction of the anterior and posterior portions of the temporal bone at the time of the injury.[163] Grobman and colleagues[164] presented a case that featured severe compression, demyelination, and edema of the facial nerve proximal to the site of the injury, with the most severe changes at the meatal foramen, in addition to direct injury to the nerve. These investigators pointed out that histologic changes in the facial nerve were similar to those in Bell's palsy, despite the fact that the initial insult to the nerve was different. High-resolution CT of the temporal bone is the most effective way to identify potential sites of injury of the facial nerve (Fig. 170-4).

Management of facial nerve injury in temporal bone fractures has been controversial. Some authorities recommend observation and symptomatic care only. Maiman and associates[165] followed 45 patients nonoperatively. Twenty-nine had injuries severe enough to be visible on polytomography. Of the 45, 44 achieved satisfactory recovery, and 65% had complete recovery. McKennan and Chole[166] reported excellent recovery in patients with delayed-onset paralysis managed nonsurgically.

In decisions about surgical decompression in specific cases, such cases traditionally have been divided into those with immediate onset and those with delayed onset after the injury; immediate-onset paralysis is associated with severe injuries and poorer outcomes.[166] Conversely, Adegbite and coworkers[167] found the outcome was predicted by the severity of the paralysis but not the time of onset. Fisch,[73] however, advocated surgical intervention on the basis of ENoG results rather than time of onset of the paralysis. He established a criterion of greater than 90% degeneration within 6 days of onset. The timing of surgery, however, does not have to be within 6 days; in fact, some advantage may lie in delaying surgery up to 3 weeks after an immediate paralysis, to allow resolution of edema and hematoma and to make the surgical field more discernible.[39] Chang and Cass[168] carefully reviewed the literature on surgical versus expectant management of facial paralysis after temporal bone fracture and concluded that the natural history, the appropriate timing, or reporting criteria exist to judge the true efficacy of facial nerve decompression in nonpenetrating injury of the temporal bone.

Long-standing paralysis also is a management problem, because electrical testing is not valid. In such cases, unless CT shows gross disruption of the fallopian canal, it is advisable to wait 12 months and then explore the nerve if clinical or EMG signs of recovery do not appear.

Penetrating injuries (gunshot wounds) often are accompanied by severe injuries, including dural tears, CSF otorrhea, damage of the otic capsule, and vascular injury. Evaluation includes high-resolution CT, carotid arteriography, and facial nerve electrical testing. Telischi and Patete[169] emphasize that extratemporal facial nerve blast injuries may not cause transection of the facial nerve; these workers recommend continued conservative management even if the nerve is severely hemorrhagic and contused.

Iatrogenic facial paralysis is a feared complication of ear surgery. For optimal management, the cases can be divided into those in which the integrity of the facial nerve was a concern intraoperatively and those in which the paralysis was unexpected. In the former group, the nerve should be positively identified by use of landmarks distant from the site of presumed injury. The nerve is traced to the site of injury, the local area decompressed, and disrupted nerve fibers reapposed. If loss of nerve tissue is serious, an onlay or interpositional facial graft can be used. If the landmarks are not discernible, the dissection should be terminated before further injury occurs and an appropriate colleague consulted. In the emotionally and medicolegally charged realm of iatrogenic injury, consultation is often beneficial to all involved. If the facial paralysis is unexpected, it is appropriate for the original surgeon to manage the case. Tight dressings and packing should be released immediately and time allowed for any local anesthetic effects to dissipate. If these measures do not result in recovery of function, urgent reexploration and decompression of the nerve should be performed.

Surgical exploration of the facial nerve after trauma requires the surgeon to be familiar with the entire temporal bone and to be prepared for mastoid, translabyrinthine, and middle fossa exploration and repair of the nerve. Caution is necessary for middle fossa exploration in patients with temporal bone trauma. Jones and associates[170] reported that 14 of 15 patients with CT evidence of temporal bone fracture also had MRI evidence of significant ipsilateral temporal lobe contusion.

Facial Paralysis Associated with Other Conditions

Pregnancy

The possible role of hormonal and fluid changes in the pathogenesis of Bell's palsy has been debated since Bell[171] first suggested an association between idiopathic paralysis and pregnancy in 1830. Bell's palsy is 3.3 times more frequent among pregnant women than among similarly aged nonpregnant women[172] and most commonly occurs in the third trimester or immediately post partum.[4,172] Recurrent palsy with repeated pregnancies and bilateral facial palsies during pregnancy also have been reported.[173]

In a series of 18 patients, Falco and Eriksson[174] reported that preeclampsia was six times more common among patients with facial palsy than in the general population of pregnant women. Facial palsy in pregnant women cannot be correlated with preterm labor, low birth weight, fetal congenital abnormality, or other perinatal abnormality. The prognosis and outcome compared with those in age-matched nonpregnant women are uncertain; some studies indicate no difference,[175] whereas others suggest decidedly worse results.[176] Gillman and coworkers[176] compared 77 women in whom Bell's palsy developed during pregnancy, or immediately post partum, with age-matched nonpregnant women and age-matched men. The pregnant patients had a statistically significant poorer result than either of the comparison groups.[176] Treatment with prednisone is the mainstay of management for the pregnant woman with Bell's palsy, although no significant difference in outcome with or without steroids was found in this study. Prednisone apparently poses minimal risk to the developing fetus, especially in the third trimester.[177]

Melkersson-Rosenthal Syndrome

Melkersson-Rosenthal syndrome consists of a triad of symptoms: recurrent orofacial edema, recurrent facial palsy, and lingua plicata (fissured tongue). The orofacial edema is the defining feature; lingua plicata and peripheral facial paralysis each occur in one half of the patients. The complete triad is present only in one fourth of the patients. Onset of the condition generally is in the second decade of life, and the manifestations usually occur sequentially and seldom appear simultaneously.

The major diagnostic criterion is persistent or recurring nonpitting facial edema that cannot be explained by infection, malignancy, or connective tissue disorder. The oral swelling usually involves the lips and buccal area, but the gingiva, palate, and tongue also can be affected. The swelling can extend to the supraorbital and infraorbital tissues of the cheek.[178] The edematous lips assume a chapped, fissured, red-brown appearance. The swelling usually is transient but may recur at regular intervals.

After numerous recurrences, the lips eventually become permanently deformed. They also may have chronic fissuring that is slow to heal and painful.[179] The extent of the facial swelling varies, ranging from unilateral involvement of the lower lip to bilateral total facial edema.[179] Chronic swelling constitutes a cosmetic problem and may interfere with speaking and eating. The chronic and recurrent nature of the edema distinguishes it from transient angioneurotic edema. Biopsy specimens of the lip reveal noncaseating epithelioid cell granulomas surrounded by histocytes, plasma cells, and lymphocytes.[179] The cause of Melkersson-Rosenthal syndrome is unknown. Some authorities consider it to be a variant of sarcoidosis, but others dispute this theory. Some experts suggest that it is a primary vasomotor disturbance,[180] whereas others suggest it has an allergic cause. Elevation of angiotensin-converting enzyme (ACE), seen in sarcoidosis and some other diseases, has been reported in some cases.[181]

Facial paralysis occurs in 50% to 90% of patients with Melkersson-Rosenthal syndrome, and it has an abrupt onset that is identical to that in Bell's palsy.[182] A history of bilateral sequential paralysis and relapse of paralysis after initial recovery is common. The site of the paralysis usually corresponds with the area of facial swelling.[179] Symptomatic management of the facial paralysis is indicated. No randomized trials of corticosteroids or surgery have been conducted, although cessation of the recurrent facial paralyses has been reported in several series after facial nerve decompression.[107,183]

Human Immunodeficiency Virus Infection

Acute facial palsy can occur at any stage of human immunodeficiency virus (HIV) infection. The palsy can be a direct result of or secondary to HIV disease (e.g., resulting from a secondary infection by herpes zoster virus). Most cases of facial palsy in patients with early-stage HIV infection resemble Bell's palsy in that (1) they have an abrupt onset and (2) no other cause is identifiable. These patients also are at risk for a craniocervical form of Guillain-Barré syndrome.

HIV is neurotropic and has been isolated from the CSF and neural tissues in all stages of HIV infection.[184] Acute facial palsy in acute and chronic HIV infection may result from invasion of the facial nerve or the facial ganglion by the virus.[185] Alternately, it has been suggested that acute facial palsy may be part of an acute inflammatory demyelinating polyneuropathy that occurs in other nerves in early stages of HIV.[186,187]

In later stages of HIV infection, facial nerve involvement may be related to the immunodeficiency, resulting in cephalic herpes zoster or systemic lymphoma. In addition, the facial nerve may be involved along with other nerves in a chronic peripheral polyneuropathy.[188]

The prognosis for idiopathic paralysis in patients with acquired immunodeficiency syndrome (AIDS) is similar to that in the general population.[189] The prognosis for facial paralysis from other causes in patients with AIDS depends on the underlying pathologic process.

Lyme Disease

Lyme disease (Bannwarth's syndrome in Europe) is caused by the tickborne spirochete *Borrelia burgdorferi*. The vectors for Lyme disease are several species of *Ixodes* ticks. The primary reservoirs of infection are the white-footed mouse and the white-tailed deer. The disease occurs in all parts of the United States.

Like syphilis, Lyme disease occurs in several stages. It begins with erythema migrans, an influenza-like illness, regional lymphadenopathy, and general malaise. The erythema migrans is an enlarging, annular, erythematous skin lesion, which may be multiple and is not limited to the site of the bite.[190] The second stage starts several weeks to months later when neurologic abnormalities develop, including meningitis, cranial nerve neuropathies, and other peripheral neuropathies. Early symptoms include headache, neck stiffness, and spinal pain. Stage three occurs months to years later with manifestations of chronic arthritis, neurologic deficits, recurrent meningitis, and subtle mental disorders.[191] Chronic neurologic complications occur in 18% of patients with untreated Lyme disease.[192]

Moscatello and coworkers[193] reviewed the head and neck symptoms in a large series of patients with Lyme disease. Headache, neck pain, and dizziness were the most common head and neck complaints. Facial paresis occurred in 4.5% of patients, may be unilateral or bilateral, and may be the sole neurologic abnormality. Halpern and Golightly[194] emphasized that the facial paralysis may precede serologic evidence of infection, and that facial paralysis may occur in the absence of either erythema migrans or identified tick bite.

Lyme disease is recognized as an increasingly important cause of facial paralysis, especially in children. In endemic areas, Lyme disease is responsible for one half of the cases of facial paralysis seen in children.[195] Facial weakness or paralysis usually resolves completely, although mild or, rarely, severe residual facial weakness has been described.[196] Reik and associates[197] reported the development of facial palsy in 6 of 18 patients with neurologic complications; 3 of these patints had residual weakness after 5 months. Puhakka and colleagues[198] found no difference in facial recovery between borreliosis and VZV infection.

The diagnosis of Lyme disease can be difficult.[199] Only 30% of patients have a recognized tick bite, and an erythema migrans rash fails to develop in 50%. Specific antibody tests may not yield a positive result for several weeks. MRI in children with neurologic symptoms may show hyperintense signal on T2-weighted images of the brain[200] and may be the best modality for following the effect of antibiotic therapy.[201]

Treatment of Lyme disease with neurologic symptoms is with ceftriaxone (2 g/day intravenously for 14 days).[201a] Improvement is not expected for several months after therapy, and recovery is seldom complete.[191]

Kawasaki's Disease

Kawasaki's disease, also known as infantile acute febrile mucocutaneous lymph node syndrome, is a multisystem disease occurring primarily in infants and young children. In addition to involvement of the mucous membranes, skin, lymph nodes, and cardiac system (coronary artery aneurysms), neurologic complications have been reported in up to 30% of patients.[202,203] Aseptic meningitis and irritability are the most common neurologic complications; however, facial palsy has been reported by several groups of investigators.[204-206]

In a review of 17 cases of well-documented facial palsy in the literature, Gallagher[204] reported the median age to be 13 months; no patient was older than 25 months. On average, onset of the paralysis occurred on day 16 of illness, and except for patients who died from cardiac complications, the palsy resolved in 1 to 12 weeks. Histologic examination of patients dying of Kawasaki's disease showed changes typical of arteritis,[207] leading Teresawa and associates[203] to conclude that the facial paralysis resulted from ischemia of the nerve. Treatment of Kawasaki's disease includes supportive care, appropriate management of cardiac failure, if present, and high-dose aspirin.

Sarcoid

Sarcoidosis is a chronic noncaseating granulomatous disease. Manifestations of systemic involvement usually include hilar or peripheral adenopathy (the lungs), polyarthralgias, anergy, hepatic dysfunction, and elevated serum calcium. Heerfordt's disease (uveoparotid fever), a variant of sarcoidosis, is characterized by nonsuppurative parotitis, uveitis, mild fever, and cranial nerve paralysis. Although only 5% of patients with sarcoidosis have cranial nerve involvement, the facial nerve is the most commonly affected.[208] By contrast, 50% of patients with uveoparotid fever have facial paralysis. The paralysis starts abruptly days to months after the onset of the parotitis. Paralysis is thought to be caused by direct invasion of the nerve by the granulomatous process[209] and not by pressure from the swollen parotid gland.[210] Sarcoidosis should be included in the differential diagnosis when the paralysis is bilateral.[147]

The diagnosis can be confirmed by an elevated serum ACE level, in contrast with tuberculosis, cancer, and pulmonary fungal diseases, in which ACE levels are low.[211] Sarcoidosis is treated with corticosteroids, after which the ACE levels are expected to return to normal.[212]

Otitis Media

Facial paralysis from otitis media is rare but can occur in acute or chronic cases. In a recent series, otitis media accounted for only 3.1% of acute facial palsies.[213] Of these 50 cases, only 5 were in children with acute otitis media. The remaining adult cases were divided equally between chronic purulent otitis media and cholesteatomas. Three additional cases were from tuberculous otitis.

Most paralyses were incomplete. Nearly all patients explored surgically were found to have a dehiscence of the bony canal of the facial nerve, usually in the tympanic segment, which presumably allowed spread of the inflammation from the middle ear to the nerve.

Facial paralysis associated with acute otitis media, especially in infants and children, should be treated with parenteral antibiotics and a wide myringotomy for drainage. Surgical manipulation of the facial nerve in acute otitis media is not recommended. Adour[94] also recommended the addition of a 10-day course of corticosteroids in conjunction with myringotomy and antibiotics.

Facial paralysis associated with chronic otitis media suggests a high probability of cholesteatoma, and surgical intervention is appropriate. The mechanism of facial paralysis associated with cholesteatoma may be compression or inflammation. Djeric[214] studied autopsy specimens from patients who had chronic otitis media but no antemortem evidence of facial paralysis. Two of 20 facial nerves had focal areas of demyelination, suggesting that adjacent inflammation may be more important than pressure. The most important hallmark of facial paralysis from cholesteatoma is a gradual onset, which distinguishes it from Bell's palsy. Removal of the cholesteatoma and decompression of the nerve without opening the perineurium will allow recovery from the paralysis in most cases.[215]

Barotrauma

Several investigators have described a curious phenomenon of recurrent facial paralysis with changes in barometric pressure. Woodhead[216] reported the case of a 50-year-old man who experienced repeated episodes of facial paralysis and ipsilateral loss of taste on ascending to 8000 to 10,000 feet while driving in mountainous regions or during air travel. His symptoms resolved on descent. Similar cases have been reported after commercial airline flights[217] and after scuba diving.[218,219] A brief facial palsy also has been reported after forceful nose blowing.[220] Barometric facial paralysis seems to be related to pressure changes in the middle ear transmitted directly to the facial nerve through natural dehiscences in the fallopian canal. Symptoms are relieved with placement of pressure equalization tubes or other means of improving eustachian tube function.[216]

Benign Intracranial Hypertension

The most common symptoms of benign intracranial hypertension are headache and visual disturbances, but occasionally it is associated with cranial nerve palsies, falsely suggesting a localized lesion. The abducens nerve is the most commonly involved, being affected in 10% to 60% of cases.[221] Unilateral and occasionally bilateral facial paralysis has been reported in a few cases of benign intracranial hypertension.[222] These cranial nerve palsies tend to resolve promptly after reestablishment of normal intracranial pressure through medical means or by shunting.

Metabolic Disorders

Adour and colleagues[223] reported that 17% of patients older than 40 years of age with Bell's palsy had abnormal results on glucose tolerance testing; on this basis, these workers calculated that the development of Bell's palsy is 4.5 times more likely in a person with diabetes than in a person without diabetes. The incidence of diabetes, or at least abnormal glucose tolerance curves, in patients with Bell's palsy is reportedly 10%[95] to 56%.[224] A case-control study by Paolino and associates[225] also found abnormal glucose tolerance curves in 24% of patients with Bell's palsy, compared with 13% of control subjects ($P < .005$). These findings warrant caution in prescribing corticosteroids to patients with Bell's palsy. Reversible facial paralysis has been reported with hypovitaminosis A.[226]

Central Facial Paralysis

Central facial paralysis is caused by a lesion in the parietal motor cortex or the connections between the cortex and the facial nucleus. Lesions in these areas usually are accompanied by other neurologic symptoms referable to the CNS. A supranuclear palsy of the face most severely affects the lower half of the face and spares the forehead. Another important sign is that emotional facial reaction remains intact even though voluntary motion may be severely affected.

Hyperkinetic Disorders

Hemifacial Spasm

Hemifacial spasm is an involuntary twitching and contraction of one side of the face. The spasm usually starts around the mouth and, as the disease develops, comes to involve the entire face.[48] These uncontrollable spasms cause severe functional, social, and psychologic impairment. Although the spasms usually are painless, a rare form of the disease also involves the trigeminal nerve.

The cause of hemifacial spasm is widely debated; in the past, hemifacial spasm was thought to originate somewhere in the peripheral facial nerve. Esslen hypothesized that pressure or ischemia within the fallopian canal could generate spontaneous action potentials.[227] Jannetta[228] thought that compression of the seventh nerve by aberrant blood vessels near its exit from the brainstem (root entry zone) was the cause, although other workers disagree with this conclusion.[229]

An unusual aspect of hemifacial spasm is the lateral spread response first described by Esslen, in which electrical stimulation of one branch of the facial nerve causes a response in muscle innervated by a different branch. This response disappears at the time of vascular decompression.[230] How could vascular compression of the facial nerve cause facial spasms? Two mechanisms have been hypothesized[231]: (1) ephaptic transmission of impulses (electrical side currents allowing the depolarization of adjacent nerve fibers) at the site of the compression or (2) hyperactivity of the facial nucleus secondary to continuous irritation at the site of the compression. Experiments by Kuroki and Møller[231] suggest that a combination of demyelination and arterial compression is required for generation of the symptoms of hemifacial spasm and that the facial nerve becomes hyperactive after long-term irritation of the demyelinated portion.[231]

The best management of hemifacial spasm also has been contested. Many surgeons advocate some form of partial destruction of the peripheral facial nerve—either partial resection of the three main branches[232,233] or resection of involved branches determined by EMG.[234] However, Jannetta and coworkers[235] and Møller and Jannetta[230] advocate separation of the aberrant vessels from the nerves through a posterior fossa craniotomy. The experience of other surgeons confirms the success of microvascular decompression; Samii[236] and Moffat[237] and their colleagues report that 92% of patients were spasm-free 6 months after decompression of the facial nerve. Selection of patients for surgery is difficult, but recent studies with MRI and magnetic resonance angiography suggest that neurovascular contact with the nerve at the root exit zone is producing the associated symptoms.[238]

Blepharospasm

Blepharospasm is an idiopathic progressive involuntary spasm of the orbicularis oculi and upper face (corrugator and procerus muscles). Extension of the spasms to include the lower face is not uncommon.[239] In advanced cases, the eyes may be closed for as much as one third of the patient's waking time, rendering the patient functionally blind.[48] Blepharospasm generally is considered to be central in origin, although the exact mechanism is not yet determined.[43]

Treatment is directed toward selective destruction of the peripheral nerve branches innervating the orbicularis oculi muscles. McCabe and Boles[240] recommend exposing the upper branches of the facial nerve, confirmation with nerve stimulation, and resection of all branches to the orbicularis oculi. Success has been obtained with injection of botulinum toxin. Botulinum A toxin, a neurotoxin produced by *Clostridium botulinum* that interferes with the presynaptic release of acetylcholine, has been used in the management of many facial dystonias, especially blepharospasm. More than 90% of patients have experienced some relief of symptoms, although the average duration of the maximum improvement is only 11 to 14 weeks.[241,242] Systemic complications after administration of botulinum toxin have not been reported. Local complications usually are transient and include lid ptosis, facial weakness, corneal exposure, and diplopia.[243] Long-term improvement is prevented by regeneration of axons after treatment.[244] Periorbital myectomy also may produce acceptable long-term results.[239]

SUGGESTED READINGS

Adour KK. Medical management of idiopathic (Bell's) palsy. *Otolaryngol Clin North Am.* 1991;24:663.

Adour KK, Wingerd J, Bell DN, et al. Prednisone treatment for idiopathic facial paralysis (Bell's palsy). *N Engl J Med.* 1972;287:1268.

Bellman AL, Coyle PK, Roque C, et al. MRI findings in children infected by *Borrelia burgdorferi. Pediatr Neurol.* 1992;8:428.

Borodic G, Bartley M, Slattery W, et al. Botulinum toxin for aberrant facial neve regeneration: double-blind, placebo-controlled trial using subjective endpoints. *Plast Reconstr Surg.* 2005;116:36.

Cook SP, Macartney KK, Rose CD, et al. Lyme disease and seventh nerve paralysis in children. *Am J Otolaryngol.* 1997;18:320.

Gantz BJ, Rubinstein JT, Gidley P, et al. Surgical management of Bell's palsy. *Laryngoscope.* 1999;109:1177.

Gillman GS, Schaitkin BM, May M, et al. Bell's palsy in pregnancy: a study of recovery outcomes. *Otolaryngol Head Neck Surg.* 2002;126:26.

Jackson C, Johnson GD, Hyams VJ, et al. Pathologic findings in the labyrinthine segment of the facial nerve in a case of facial paralysis. *Ann Otol Rhinol Laryngol.* 1990;99:327.

Moffat DA, Durvasula VS, Stevens King A, et al. Outcome following retrosigmoid microvascular decompression of the facial nerve for hemifacial spasm. *J Laryngol Otol.* 2005;119:779.

Nowak DA, Linder S, Topka H. Diagnostic relevance of transcranial magnetic and electric stimulation of the facial nerve in management of facial palsy. *Clin Neurophysiol.* 2005;116:2051.

Peitersen E. Natural history of Bell's palsy. *Acta Otolaryngol Suppl (Stockh).* 1992;492:122.

Ramsey MH, DerSimonian R, Holtel MR, et al. Corticosteroid treatment for idiopathic facial nerve paralysis: a meta-analysis. *Laryngoscope.* 2000;110:335.

Rowlands S, Hooper R, Hughes R, et al. The epidemiology and treatment of Bell's palsy in the UK. *Eur J Neurol.* 2002;9:63.

Salman MS, MacGregor DL. Should children with Bell's palsy be treated with corticosteroids? A systematic review. *J Child Neurol.* 2001;16:565.

Samii M, Günther T, Iaconetta G, et al. Microvascular decompression to treat hemifacial spasm: long term results for a consecutive series of 143 patients. *Neurosurgery.* 2002;50:712.

Sittel C, Stennert E. Prognostic value of electromyography in acute peripheral facial nerve palsy. *Otol Neurotol.* 2001;22:100.

Sullivan FM, Swan IR, Donnan PT, et al. Early treatment with prednisolone or acyclovir in Bell's palsy. *N Engl J Med.* 2007;357:1958.

Verzijl HT, Padberg GW, Zwarts MJ. The spectrum of Möbius' syndrome: an electrophysiological study. *Brain.* 2005;128:1728.

Yetiser S, Tosun F, Kazkayasi M. Facial nerve paralysis due to chronic otitis media. *Otol Neurotol.* 2002;23:580.

For complete list of references log onto www.expertconsult.com.

CHAPTER ONE HUNDRED AND SEVENTY-ONE

Intratemporal Facial Nerve Surgery

Bruce J. Gantz

Jay T. Rubinstein

Ravi N. Samy

Samuel P. Gubbels

Key Points

- Appropriate management of facial nerve disorders requires a thorough knowledge of the pathophysiology of the diseases affecting the facial nerve, experience in the interpretation of findings on radiologic and electrophysiologic tests of the nerve, and expertise in multiple neuro-otologic surgical approaches to the facial nerve.
- The middle fossa craniotomy surgical approach provides access to the canalicular, labyrinthine, geniculate and proximal tympanic segments of the nerve while preserving hearing but is technically challenging. The middle cranial fossa approach can be used for facial nerve decompression in palsy, facial nerve tumor decompression or removal, and facial nerve grafting in the internal auditory canal, and to address facial nerve impingement resulting from longitudinal temporal bone fractures.
- A transmastoid approach can be used to address pathologic processes involving the tympanic and mastoid segments of the facial nerve while preserving inner ear function. Total facial nerve decompression can be achieved using the transmastoid approach in combination with a middle fossa craniotomy.
- The translabyrinthine approach provides access to the entirety of the intratemporal facial nerve for decompression, mobilization, or grafting when no usable hearing remains.
- Retrolabyrinthine and retrosigmoid approaches provide access to the cisternal segment of the facial nerve while preserving hearing and can be used for vascular decompression and combined with other approaches for facial nerve grafting at the brainstem.
- Anterior rerouting of the facial nerve from the geniculate to the extratemporal segment, as in the Fisch type A approach, can be performed with normal facial function possible postoperatively.
- The most important element of successful facial nerve repair is a tension-free anastomosis. An interposition graft, using the great auricular or sural nerve, should be used for nerve repair in all cases in which a tension-free end-to-end anastomosis cannot be achieved.
- In general, facial nerve tumors should be observed in patients with House-Brackmann grade I or II function. Surgical decompression is a management option for patients with facial nerve tumors and House-Brackmann grade II or III function. Tumor resection with facial nerve grafting is recommended for patients with House-Brackmann grade IV function or worse due to a facial nerve tumor.

Advances in surgical instrumentation and refinements in surgical strategies have enabled the otologist to expose safely the entire course of the facial nerve from the brainstem to its exit from the temporal bone. Surgical management of facial nerve disorders, however, continues to be as controversial as it was in the days of Cawthorne and Kettel. Successful treatment of the disease processes that cause facial nerve dysfunction requires thorough knowledge of the pathophysiology of the disease process and accurate assessment of the degree of nerve injury. Newer diagnostic tools, such as electroneuronography (ENoG) (i.e., electroneurography), high-resolution computed tomography (CT), and magnetic resonance imaging (MRI), provide more precise assessment and localization of nerve injuries in many disorders. This advance has allowed more accurate preoperative planning and selection of the most expeditious surgical approach to the nerve injury site when surgery is appropriate.

This chapter describes surgical approaches in detail, including the advantages and disadvantages of each.

Surgical Anatomy

Thorough knowledge of the intricate, convoluted course of the facial nerve and its anatomic relationship to other vital structures is essential to the surgeon who plans to operate in this area. The facial nerve (cranial nerve VII) exits the brainstem at the pontomedullary junction approximately 1.5 mm anterior to the vestibulocochlear nerve (cranial

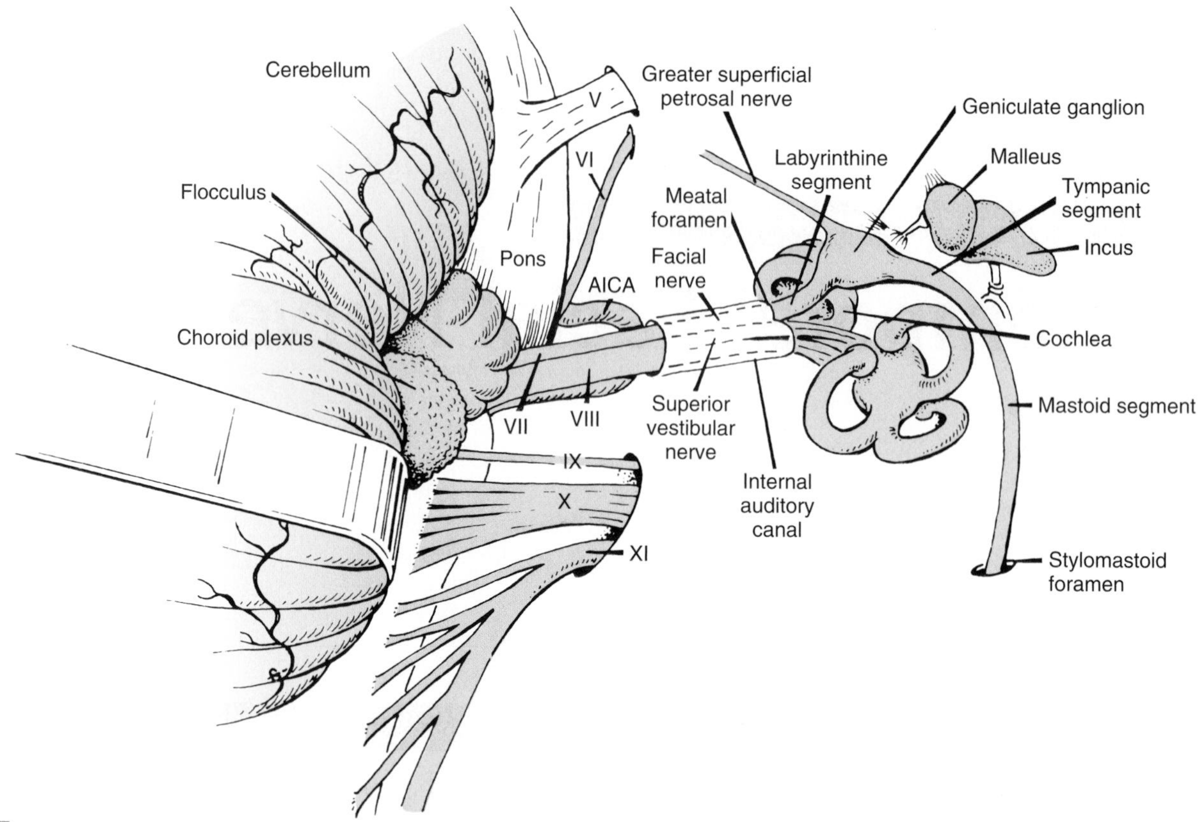

Figure 171-1. Course and relationships of the facial nerve from the pontomedullary junction to the stylomastoid foramen. AICA, anterior inferior cerebellar artery; Roman numerals designate cranial nerves.

nerve VIII). The facial nerve is smaller in diameter (approximately 1.8 mm) than the oval cranial nerve VIII (approximately 3 mm in the longer diameter). A third, smaller nerve, the nervus intermedius, emerges between cranial nerves VII and VIII and eventually becomes incorporated within the sheath of cranial nerve VII. After leaving the brainstem, cranial nerve VII follows a rostrolateral course through the cerebellopontine cistern for 15 to 17 mm, entering the porus of the internal auditory canal of the temporal bone (Fig. 171-1). Other important structures in the cerebellopontine cistern include the anterior inferior cerebellar artery (AICA) and the veins of the middle cerebellar peduncle. The AICA passes near or between cranial nerves VII and VIII; the veins are more variable in position and number. On entering the IAC, the facial nerve occupies the anterosuperior quadrant of this channel for 8 to 10 mm. Then it enters the fallopian canal at the fundus of the internal auditory canal. The internal auditory canal is anterior to the plane of the superior semicircular canal, with which it subtends an angle of approximately 60 degrees. At the entrance of the fallopian canal (meatal foramen), cranial nerve VII narrows to its smallest diameter, 0.61 to 0.68 mm.[1] Only the pia and arachnoid membranes form a sheath around the nerve at this point, because the dural investment terminates at the fundus of the internal auditory canal. Some investigators[2,3] identify the small diameter of the meatal foramen as an important contributory etiologic factor in facial paralysis associated with certain diseases, such as Bell's palsy and Ramsay Hunt syndrome.

Within its intratemporal course, the facial nerve has three distinct anatomic segments: labyrinthine, tympanic, and mastoid. The labyrinthine segment is shortest (approximately 4 mm), extending from the meatal foramen to the geniculate ganglion. This segment travels in an anterior, superior, and lateral direction, forming an anterior medial angle of 120 degrees with the internal auditory canal. Anteroinferior to the labyrinthine segment, the basal turn of the cochlea occupies a close relationship to the fallopian canal. At the lateral end of the labyrinthine segment, the geniculate ganglion is found, and the nerve makes an abrupt posterior change in direction, forming an acute angle of approximately 75 degrees. Anterior to the geniculate, the greater superficial petrosal nerve exits the temporal bone through the hiatus of the facial canal. The hiatus of the facial canal varies in distance from the geniculate ganglion. The greater superficial canal also contains the vascular supply to the geniculate ganglion region.

The tympanic segment of the nerve is approximately 11 mm long, running between the lateral semicircular canal superiorly and the stapes inferiorly, forming the superior margin of the fossa ovale. Between the tympanic and mastoid segments, the nerve gently curves inferiorly for approximately 2 to 3 mm.

The mastoid, or vertical, segment is the longest intratemporal portion of nerve: approximately 13 mm. As the nerve exits the stylomastoid foramen at the anterior margin of the digastric groove, an adherent fibrous sheath of dense vascularized connective tissue surrounds it. The stylomastoid artery and veins are within this dense sheath.

General Surgical Technique

Whenever the facial nerve is to be surgically exposed, several technical principles should be observed. First, a system for monitoring facial nerve function during the operation should be used.[4] One of the simplest monitoring methods is visual observation during critical stages of the operation. Needle electromyography also can be used if the equipment is available. No matter which monitoring technique is used, it is essential that the side of the face on which the nerve is to be exposed be draped in a manner that allows visual observation. The patient's forehead, eye, mouth, and chin should be visible. The endotracheal tube should be secured to the opposite side without taping on the side of the mouth to be observed. Towels drape the posterior, superior, and inferior margins; a fourth towel is placed along the anterior profile. An abdominal transparent plastic drape is placed over the face and operative area (Fig. 171-2). An observer can thus see the entire face during the procedure and determine whether any of the muscles move in response to surgical manipulation of the nerve. If the surgeon asks for

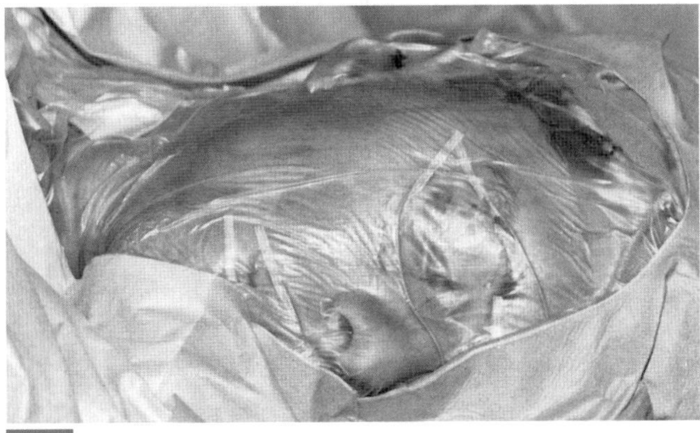

Figure 171-2. Plastic draping with exposure of hemiface allows visualization of facial movements in addition to electromyographic monitoring.

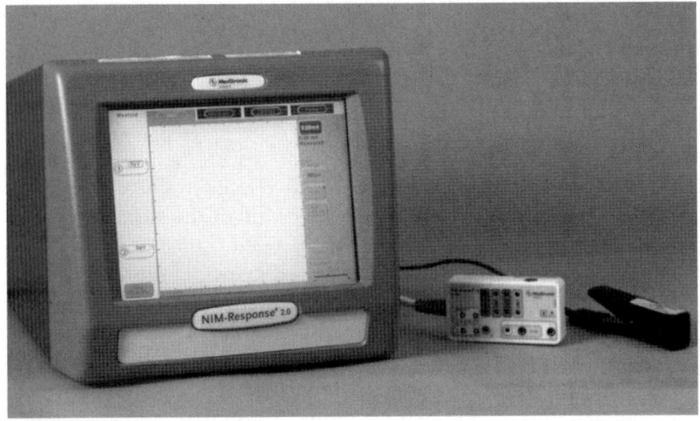

Figure 171-3. A popular commercially available nerve monitoring system. Stimulus intensity to the stimulator probe can be varied, as can the sensitivity of monitoring response.

observation during critical periods of the procedure, the circulating nurse is the best observer.

More precise intraoperative monitoring can be achieved using commercially available needle electromyographic systems (Fig. 171-3). Electromyographic needles are placed in the orbicularis oculi and orbicularis oris muscles, as shown in Figure 171-4. Stimulation of the facial nerve during the operation provides accurate localization of the nerve if the anatomy is distorted by a disease process or congenital abnormality. Constant current or constant voltage stimulators can be used. These systems allow auditory monitoring of facial nerve activity and alert the surgeon when the nerve has been stimulated. Auditory monitoring is especially useful during the removal of tumors adjacent to the facial nerve.

Instrumentation is crucial to successful exposure of the facial nerve. The largest diamond burr that the operative site can safely accommodate should be used when the operator is near the fallopian canal. Cutting burrs have a tendency to catch and jump unexpectedly, with the potential to cause severe injury to the nerve. Continuous suction-irrigation keeps the burr clean and also dissipates heat, which can induce neural damage.

The final layer of bone over the nerve should be removed by blunt elevators designed for this purpose. These instruments are thin but strong enough to remove a thin layer of bone. Stapes curettes usually are too large and can cause compression injury to the nerve. If neurolysis is to be performed, disposable microblades are available (Beaver No. 59-10). Sharp dissection is less traumatic than blunt elevation when the nerve must be lifted out of the fallopian canal. The medial surface of the nerve usually adheres to the bone and contains a rich vascular supply. Cauterization near the nerve should be performed only with bipolar electrocautery and insulated microforceps.

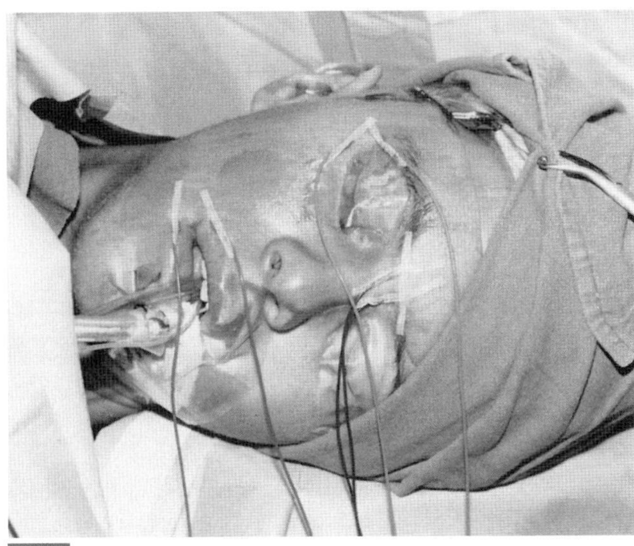

Figure 171-4. Placement of electromyographic electrodes in orbicularis oculi and orbicularis oris muscles. Ground electrodes are placed in the procerus muscle.

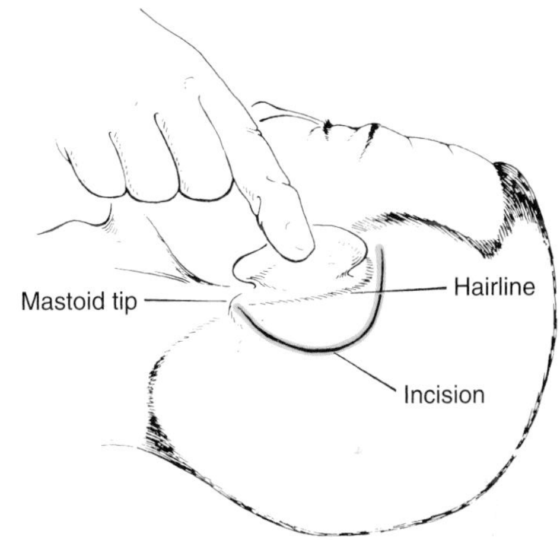

Figure 171-5. Skin incision for the retrolabyrinthine surgical approach.

Surgical Approaches

Retrolabyrinthine Approach: Brainstem to Internal Auditory Canal Porus

Technique

The patient is positioned on an operating table similar to that used for a mastoidectomy. Endotracheal anesthesia is administered, and the anesthetist is positioned at the foot of the table, allowing the surgical nurse to be opposite the surgeon. The hair is removed 4 cm superiorly and postauricularly, and the ear and the left lower abdominal quadrant (for the harvest of fat if necessary) are prepared and draped. An osmotic diuretic (250 mL of 20% mannitol) is administered intravenously at the start of the skin incision. The skin incision is made in the hairline 3 to 4 cm posterior to the postauricular crease and extended down over the mastoid tip (Fig. 171-5). Posterior placement of the skin incision provides access for occipital bone removal, which is necessary for posterior retraction of the sigmoid sinus.[5]

A complete mastoidectomy is performed. In addition, bone is removed over the sigmoid sinus from the sinodural angle to its most inferior extent. The dome of the jugular bulb also is identified. A large diamond burr and suction-irrigation are essential to prevent injury to the sinus and the posterior fossa dura. The cerebellar plate is removed

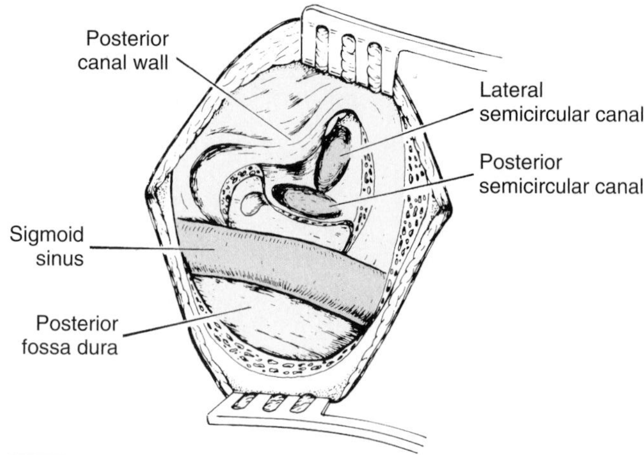

Figure 171-6. Exposure obtained through the left retrolabyrinthine approach before retraction and dural incision, as viewed by the surgeon.

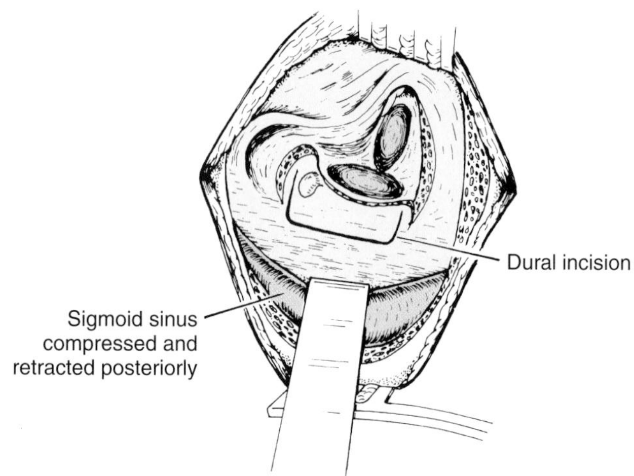

Figure 171-7. Dural incision for left retrolabyrinthine exposure.

from the tegmen mastoideum to the jugular bulb. Anteromedially, the posterior semicircular canal is identified, and inferior to the labyrinth (retrofacial area) the endolymphatic sac is exposed (Fig. 171-6). In a well-aerated mastoid, 2 to 3 mm of bone can be removed between the posterior semicircular canal and the cerebellar dura with the use of small diamond burrs. If the posterior canal is not evident, it should be blue-lined to locate its exact position.

An anteriorly based trapdoor cerebellar dural flap is fashioned with a sharp microscalpel and microscissors (Fig. 171-7). Care should be taken not to injure the small cerebellar arachnoid vessels when the dura is opened. A cuff of dura should be left adjacent to the bony margins, sigmoid sinus, and superior petrosal sinus for placement of sutures during closure. Sutures placed at the corners of the dural flap serve to retract it anteriorly. A malleable self-retaining retractor is used to retract the sigmoid sinus posteriorly. The cerebellum usually falls away from the temporal bone, and minimal, if any, retraction is required. Hyperventilation, in addition to an osmotic diuretic, is useful in obtaining brain shrinkage.

The cochleovestibular facial nerve complex is seen 2 to 3 mm inferior and parallel to Donaldson's line (a line extending posterior from the plane of the lateral semicircular canal). The arachnoid is incised sharply, releasing the cerebrospinal fluid (CSF) from the cistern. Other visible nerves are the trigeminal nerve (cranial nerve V) superiorly and the glossopharyngeal nerve (cranial nerve IX) and possibly the vagus nerve (cranial nerve X) inferiorly (Fig. 171-8). Visualization of cranial nerve VII may be completely blocked by cranial nerve VIII.

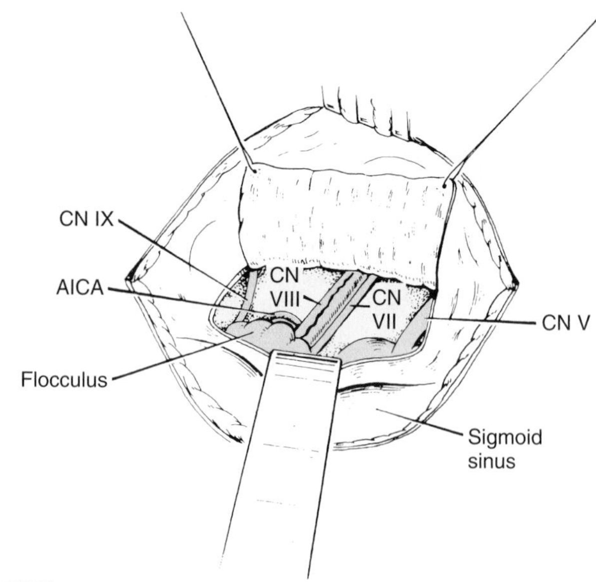

Figure 171-8. Left retrolabyrinthine exposure after retraction of the dural flap. AICA, anterior inferior cerebellar artery; CN, cranial nerve.

Cranial nerve VII usually arises 1.5 mm directly anterior to cranial nerve VIII. A Buckingham mirror aids identification of the facial nerve. The rostral division of the AICA may pass between cranial nerves VII and VIII, along with one or more veins. Approximately 15 mm of the nerve can be inspected in the cerebellopontine cistern.

At the end of the procedure, care should be taken to achieve watertight closure of the dura. Strips of abdominal fat (5 mm × 4 cm) are harvested from a lower abdominal incision, placed subdurally, and incorporated into the suture line. Braided nylon (4-0) sutures are used for closure of the dura. Fat can be placed in the mastoid but should not block the aditus or interfere with the ossicles. The subcutaneous tissues are closed in layers. A mastoid compression dressing is placed.

Retrosigmoid Approach

Technique

Another option for exposure of the facial nerve from the brainstem to the internal auditory canal is through a small retrosigmoid craniotomy. The preparation and incision are similar to those in the retrolabyrinthine approach (see Fig. 171-5). Instead of a complete mastoidectomy, the bone over the sigmoid sinus is removed to identify the posterior margin of the sinus. Bone is removed 4 cm posterior to the sigmoid sinus, exposing the posterior fossa dura (Fig. 171-9). The outline of the transverse sinus is exposed superiorly. A curvilinear incision in the posterior fossa dura is created to expose the cerebellum (Fig. 171-10). Care is taken to incise the dura without injuring the arteries and veins on the cerebellum. Cottonoid sponges lined with rubber glove strips are placed on the cerebellum. Slow, gentle retraction of the cerebellum over 5 to 10 minutes allows exposure of the posterior fossa face of temporal bone and internal auditory canal. Once the cerebellum has been slowly retracted, no external retraction is necessary. The cerebellum should fall away from the temporal bone, allowing viewing of the flocculus, choroid plexus, and the cranial nerve VII and VIII bundle (Fig. 171-11). The posterior lip of the internal auditory canal porus can be removed for additional lateral exposure, but the position of the posterior semicircular canal and its relationship to the posterior lip of the porus acusticus should be ascertained by CT.

Advantages and Uses

The retrolabyrinthine and retrosigmoid approaches provide access to the facial nerve in the cerebellopontine angle without sacrificing inner ear function. These approaches have an advantage over the routine suboccipital approach in that minimal or no cerebellar compression is needed. The procedure can be used in combination with middle fossa

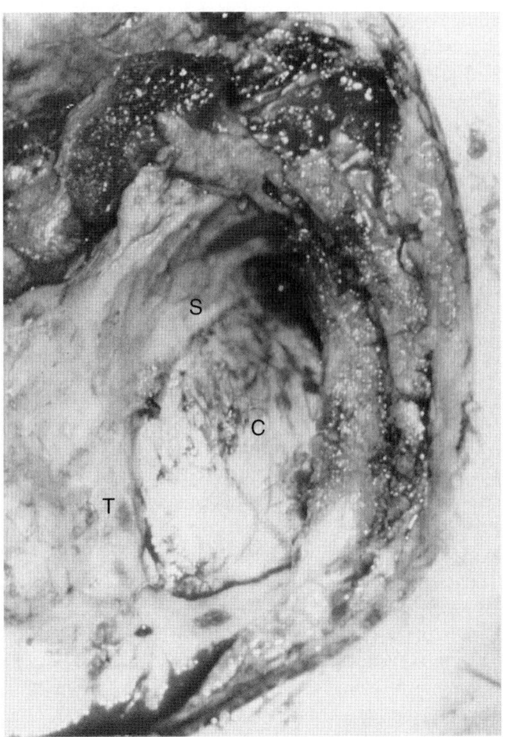

Figure 171-9. Retrosigmoid craniotomy. The skin flap is reflected anteriorly, exposing the mastoid and the cerebellar cortical bone. Craniotomy (approximately 4 × 4 cm), exposing the sigmoid sinus (S) anteriorly, transverse sinus (T) superiorly, and cerebellar dura (C).

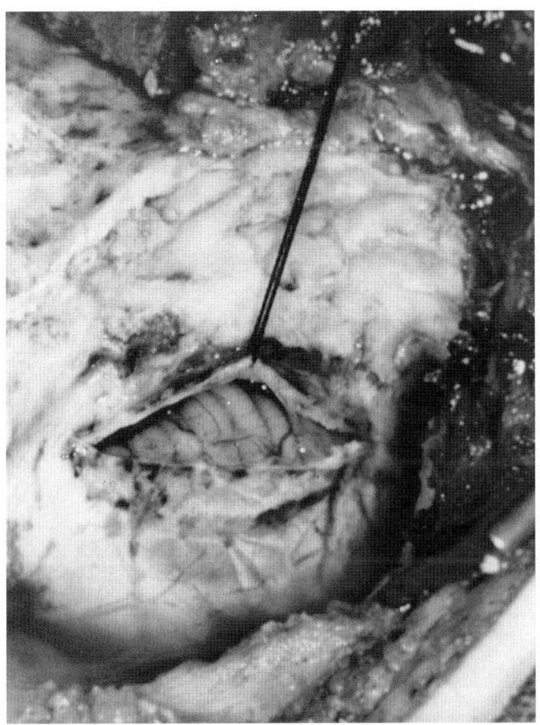

Figure 171-10. A dural incision (2 to 3 cm long) can be linear or curvilinear. Here, 4-0 Neurolon suture retracts the anterior leaf of the dural incision.

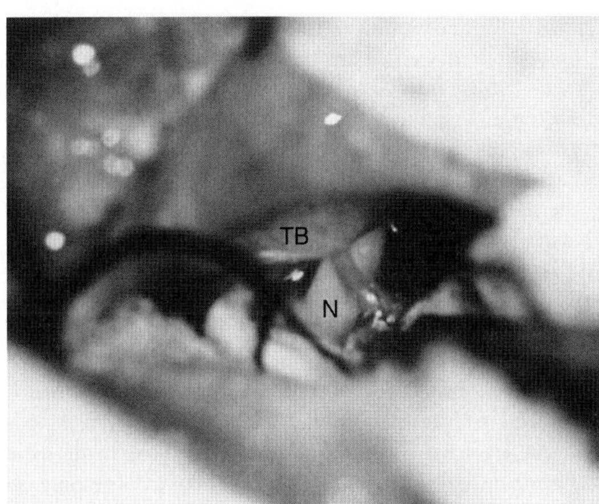

Figure 171-11. Retrosigmoid exposure. The cerebellum has been retracted from the cerebellar plate of the temporal bone (TB), exposing the neurovascular bundle (N). Cranial nerve VII is directly deep and slightly cephalic to cranial nerve VIII.

exposure for tumor removal and grafting of cranial nerve VII near the brainstem. For facial nerve surgery, the retrolabyrinthine technique is most commonly used in some practices for vascular decompression in hemifacial spasm. The AICA, posterior inferior cerebellar artery, and accompanying veins can be easily manipulated through this approach.

Limitations and Potential Complications

Visualization of the facial nerve often is hampered by the location of cranial nerve VIII. Gentle separation of the nerves with a blunt instrument can be accomplished but is associated with increased potential for hearing loss or vestibular complications. Because of the compromised exposure, management of any intracranial vascular complications is limited. If an intracranial complication occurs, rapid removal of suboccipital bone, in combination with a retrosigmoid dural opening, provides additional access.

CSF leakage is a potential problem with this approach, but careful dural reapproximation and use of subdural fat strips have decreased the incidence of this complication.

Middle Cranial Fossa (Transtemporal) Approach: Internal Auditory Canal Porus to Tympanic Segment

The middle cranial fossa approach[6] is used to expose the internal auditory canal and labyrinthine segments of the facial nerve when preservation of existing auditory function is desirable. The geniculate ganglion and tympanic portions of the nerve also can be decompressed using this approach.

Technique

The patient is placed supine on the operating table with the head turned so that the involved temporal bone is upward. The hair is shaved 6 to 8 cm above and anterior to the ear and 2 cm posterior to it. The surgeon is seated at the head of the table, with the instrument nurse at the anterior aspect of the patient's head.

A 6 cm × 8 cm posteriorly based trapdoor incision is marked in the hairline above the ear (Fig. 171-12). If exposure of the mastoid is necessary, the inferior limb of the incision can be extended postauricularly. The skin flap is elevated to expose the temporalis muscle. A 4 cm × 4 cm temporalis fascia graft is harvested for use during closure of the internal auditory canal dural defect. An anteriorly based trapdoor incision is used to elevate the temporalis muscle and periosteum. Staggering the levels of the muscle and skin incisions provides for a double-layer watertight closure at the end of the procedure.

The temporal root of the zygoma is exposed during elevation of the temporalis muscle. This landmark represents the level of the floor of the middle fossa. Stay sutures are placed in the skin and temporalis flaps to be used for retraction. A 3 cm × 5 cm bone flap centered above the temporal root of the zygoma is fashioned with a medium cutting burr. The anterior and posterior margins of the craniotomy should be parallel to facilitate placement of the self-retaining retractor.

Branches of the middle meningeal artery are occasionally embedded within the inner table of the skull; therefore, the bone flap should be elevated in a controlled manner. Bipolar coagulation and bone wax may be necessary to control bleeding. Elevation of the dura from the floor of the middle fossa can be one of the most difficult steps. Use of blunt dissection and magnification greatly facilitates dural elevation. The dura is elevated from posterior to anterior to prevent accidental injury to an exposed geniculate ganglion and greater superficial petrosal nerve. Bipolar coagulation is used to cauterize dural reflections within the petrosquamous suture before transection with scissors.

The elevation proceeds until the petrous ridge is identified medially and the arcuate eminence, meatal plane, and greater superficial petrosal nerve are revealed anteriorly. No attempt is made to identify the middle meningeal artery and accompanying troublesome bleeding veins. The tip of a self-retaining (House-Urban) retractor is placed at the petrous ridge anterior to the arcuate eminence. A medium diamond burr and a suction-irrigation apparatus are used to identify the blue line of the superior semicircular canal. Review of a Stenvers projection radiograph obtained preoperatively will help to determine the level of the superior semicircular canal in relation to the floor of the middle fossa.

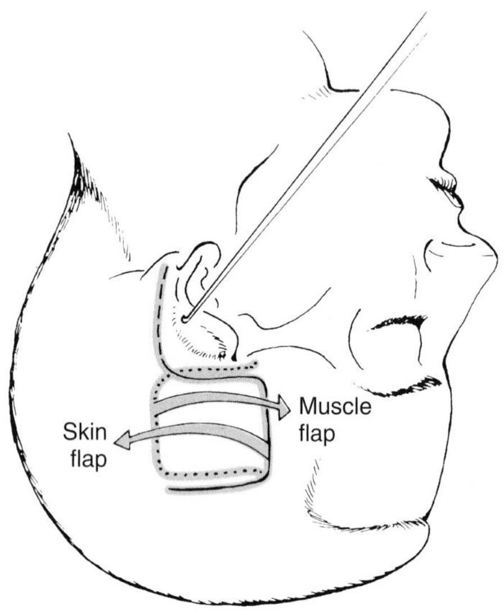

Figure 171-12. Surgical view of a skin incision *(solid line)* for the middle cranial fossa approach.Mastoid extension for total facial nerve exposure *(dashed line)* and extent of the muscle periosteal flap *(dotted line)* also are shown.

Drilling begins posterior to the arcuate eminence over the mastoid air cells and is continued until the dense yellow bone of the otic capsule is identified. Otic capsule bone is slowly removed until the blue outline of the superior semicircular canal is seen. The internal auditory canal is located by removing bone in a line 60 degrees anterior to the blue line of the superior semicircular canal and continuing until approximately 180 degrees of the canal is exposed (Fig. 171-13). Because of the close proximity of the superior semicircular canal and the basal turn of the cochlea, only approximately 120 degrees of the circumference of the internal auditory canal can be safely removed in its lateral 5 mm or more. The facial nerve occupies the anterosuperior portion of the internal auditory canal. Laterally, the vertical crest (Bill's bar) marks the division between the superior vestibular nerve and the meatal foramen.

The segment of the facial nerve at its entrance to the fallopian canal is the narrowest, most delicate portion of the nerve. At the meatal foramen, the facial nerve turns anterior and slightly superior. The basal turn of the cochlea can be within 1 mm inferiorly, and the ampulla of the superior semicircular canal can be directly posterior to the nerve. The labyrinthine segment is followed to the geniculate ganglion. The tegmen tympani is removed with care taken to avoid injury to the head of the malleus and incus. The tympanic segment is easily seen to turn abruptly posteriorly; it is followed to where it courses inferior to the lateral semicircular canal. It is advisable to leave a thin shell of bone covering the nerve until its entire course is identified. The final layer of bone is removed using small blunt elevators. The nerve is tightly confined within the labyrinthine segment of the fallopian canal; use of larger curettes should be avoided to prevent compression injury.

If the nerve is to be decompressed, neurolysis is the final step. A disposable microscalpel (Beaver No. 59-10) is used to slit the periosteum and epineural sheath.

Alternative methods to locate the facial nerve may be necessary, especially in traumatic cases. The greater superficial petrosal nerve can be traced posteriorly to the geniculate ganglion, or the tegmen tympani may be fractured to permit a view of the tympanic segment through the fracture. The tympanic segment is then used to locate the geniculate ganglion and labyrinthine segments.

At the end of the procedure, a corner piece of the bone flap is fashioned to cover the defects in the tegmen tympani and internal auditory canal (Fig. 171-14). This prevents herniation of the temporal lobe into the middle ear. The previously harvested temporalis fascia is placed over the bone plug to help seal the dural defect at the internal auditory canal. The squamous bone plug is replaced, and the temporalis muscle is closed with interrupted absorbable sutures. The skin is closed in layers. No drain is placed. A mastoid type of pressure dressing is applied.

Advantages and Uses

The middle cranial fossa approach is the only method that exposes the entire internal auditory canal and labyrinthine segment with preservation of hearing. In combination with the retrolabyrinthine and trans-

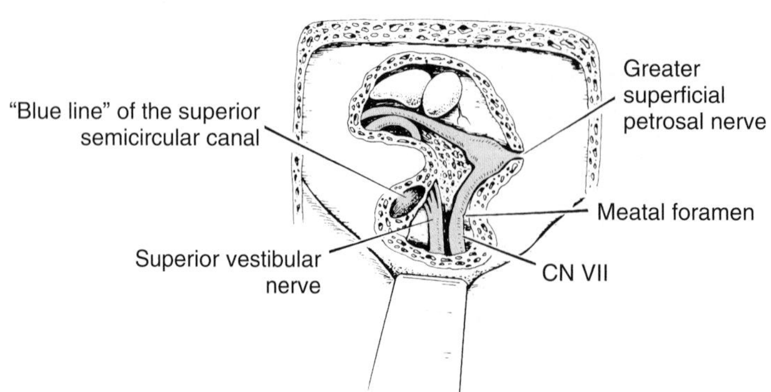

Figure 171-13. Surgical view of the left middle cranial fossa exposure after craniotomy, temporal lobe retraction, and bony exposure are complete. CN, cranial nerve.

mastoid approaches, this approach enables visualization of the entire course of the facial nerve and preserves function of the inner ear. The middle cranial fossa technique is most commonly used for decompression of the facial nerve in Bell's palsy[7,8] and with longitudinal temporal bone fractures.

Limitations and Potential Complications

The anatomy of the floor of the middle cranial fossa is variable and presents difficulty in identification of landmarks. The surgeon should have thorough knowledge of the three-dimensional anatomy of the temporal bone. Many hours in a temporal bone dissection laboratory are required to attain the delicate microsurgical skills necessary for this type of surgery.

Dural elevation can be difficult, especially in patients older than 60 years of age. The dura can adhere to the middle fossa floor and may be thin. A temporalis fascia patch should be used to repair any dural tears to prevent CSF leaks.

Conductive and sensorineural hearing losses can result from middle cranial fossa facial nerve decompression. Conductive hearing loss can be secondary to temporal lobe herniation or ossicular disruption during dissection in the attic. A free bone plug prevents temporal lobe herniation. Sensorineural hearing loss can result from direct injury to the inner ear from the drill during exposure of the cochlea or semicircular canals, or from translational injury incurred when the drill strikes an ossicle. Injury to the internal auditory vessels within the internal auditory canal also can result in loss of inner ear function. Loss of vestibular function can occur by the same mechanisms.

Persistent CSF leakage can lead to meningitis and should be controlled by a temporary lumbar drain. If CSF leakage continues despite an adequate period of lumbar drainage, surgical revision with dural repair may need to be performed.

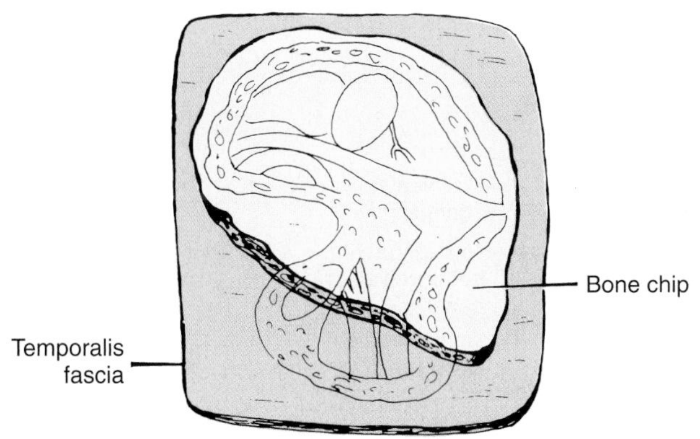

Figure 171-14. Bone chip and temporalis fascia placement for tegmen reconstruction and dural closure of the middle cranial fossa approach.

Uncontrolled bleeding or injury to the AICA poses the most serious complication during the operation. The middle cranial fossa approach does not provide adequate access to the cerebellopontine angle. The AICA and accompanying veins can loop into the internal auditory canal. Control of bleeding of these vessels may require a suboccipital exposure. Injury to the AICA results in brainstem and cerebellar infarction of variable degree, depending on the size and area of terminal arterial supply.

Results with Middle Cranial Fossa Decompression of Bell's Palsy

May and coworkers[9] showed the futility of transmastoid decompression for Bell's palsy. Only middle cranial fossa decompression of the meatal foramen, labyrinthine segment, and geniculate offers any benefit. Although the middle cranial fossa approach is used frequently for acoustic neuroma and vestibular nerve section with minimal morbidity, it is technically challenging even for experienced temporal bone surgeons and carries a significant potential for complications. A 30-dB conductive hearing loss constitutes minimal morbidity for a patient with an acoustic neuroma or intractable Meniere's disease, but it is significant for a patient who may have up to a 50% chance of spontaneous complete recovery. Thus, even with proof of efficacy, decompression is advocated only in centers experienced in the middle cranial fossa approach. As surgical series of middle cranial fossa decompression for Bell's palsy become available, honest appraisals of the statistical and clinical significance of improved facial function will be needed. Slight improvements in facial symmetry do not justify significant rates of conductive or neurosensory hearing loss or CSF leak, or the cost of the procedure and overnight postoperative stay in the intensive care unit.

In a study of middle cranial fossa decompression, Fisch[2] showed statistically significant improvements in outcome with surgery, but it is difficult to assess the degree of improvement in his subject population. Use of the House-Brackmann scale in subsequent reports will make this easier. Table 171-1 summarizes the published data available[3,10] and the experience at the University of Iowa Hospitals and Clinics through 1986 regarding outcome with middle cranial fossa decompression. All patients demonstrated more than 90% degeneration on ENoG within 14 days of onset of total paralysis and no voluntary electromyography potentials. The prognostic studies of Fisch[2] indicated, at best, a 50% rate of spontaneous satisfactory recovery when degeneration exceeded 90%.[11] Sillman and colleagues[12] and Marsh and Coker[13] studied ENoG prognostication using the House-Brackmann scale and verified Fisch's results, showing less than 50% recovery to grade I or II function when ENoG degeneration exceeded 90%.[12] Thus, patients managed with middle cranial fossa decompression are expected to return to grade I or II without surgery less than 50% of the time.

After at least a 7-month follow-up period, 23 of 26 patients returned to House-Brackmann grade I or II (see Table 171-1). Using a binomial distribution and assuming a 50% spontaneous recovery to grade I or II, this result is highly significant ($P < .00005$). No published study showed statistical significance, and none reported on morbidity

Table 171-1

Middle Cranial Fossa Decompression Outcomes in Patients with Bell's Palsy*

	No. of Patients			
House-Brackmann Grade	Iowa Cohort	Michigan Cohort[10]	Baylor Cohort[3]	Total
I	3	5	0	8
II	7	2	6	15
III	1	1	0	2
IV	0	1	0	1

*With >90% degeneration on electroneurography.

of the procedure, but all showed trends for the efficacy of middle cranial fossa decompression. Data for six of the Iowa patients appeared in a previous report.[14] With these additional cases, the Iowa patients had a highly significant recovery rate with middle cranial fossa decompression ($P < .006$). Table 171-2 shows outcome with corticosteroid management alone. Of the Iowa patients, five of eight who did not undergo prompt middle cranial fossa decompression but who met the electrophysiologic criteria for surgery did not recover to grade I or II (see Table 171-1). In the Michigan study, 14 of 25 patients who did not undergo decompression achieved grade III or IV recovery. Even if historical control subjects are not used, Iowa patients who underwent middle cranial fossa decompression improved to grade I or II significantly more often than those managed with corticosteroids alone ($P <.024$; Fisher's exact test).[15]

Table 171-2

Corticosteroid Treatment Outcomes in Patients with Bell's Palsy*

House-Brackmann Grade	No. of Patients		
	Iowa Cohort	Michigan Cohort[10]	Total
I	0	5	5
II	3	6	9
III	5	12	17
IV	0	2	2

*With >90% degeneration on electroneurography.

Transmastoid Approach: Geniculate Ganglion to Stylomastoid Foramen

Technique

A postauricular incision is used to expose the mastoid cortex. A complete mastoidectomy is performed, and the lateral semicircular canal, tegmen mastoideum, sigmoid sinus, and digastric ridge are identified. The lateral semicircular canal and digastric ridge are important landmarks for identification of the facial nerve. The tympanic segment of the nerve is immediately inferior to the lateral canal, and the anterior margin of the digastric ridge marks the location of the stylomastoid foramen. The short process of the incus is identified but should not be disturbed by an instrument or a rotating burr. The facial recess is opened with a small diamond burr (Fig. 171-15). This allows visualization of the tympanic segment of cranial nerve VII in the middle ear. With use of a medium-sized diamond burr and suction-irrigation, the fallopian canal is exposed from the lateral semicircular canal to the stylomastoid foramen. In the mastoid bone, the posterior 180 degrees of the circumference of the fallopian canal is removed. The retrofacial air cells can be removed if additional exposure is required. In the tympanum, a 1-mm diamond burr is used to remove bone to the geniculate ganglion. Again, the drill should not touch the incus. The final thin shell of bone covering the nerve is removed with blunt elevators (Fig. 171-16). Neurolysis is accomplished if desired. The wound is drained for 24 to 36 hours and closed in layers. A mastoid pressure dressing is placed.

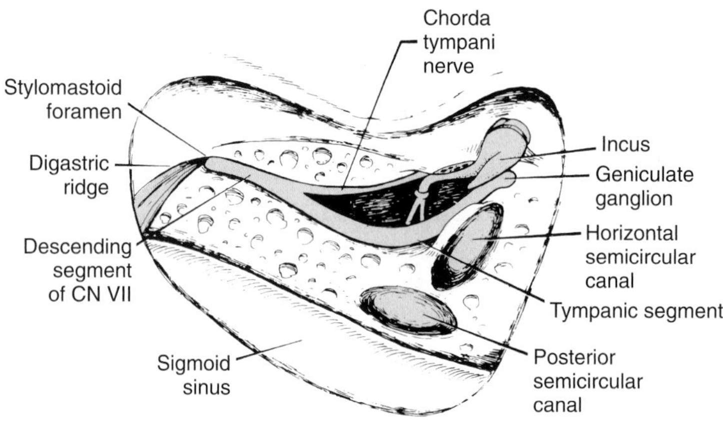

Figure 171-15. Transmastoid facial nerve exposure of the left ear after opening of the facial recess.

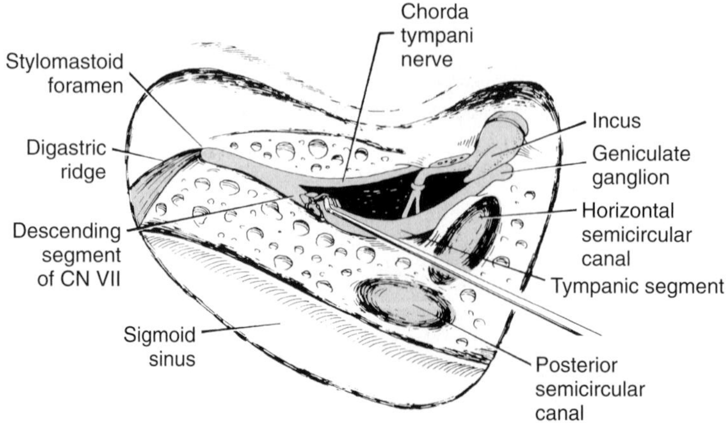

Figure 171-16. The final thin layer of bone covering the facial nerve is removed with a delicate but sturdy blunt elevator.

Advantages and Uses

Transmastoid decompression provides excellent exposure of the mastoid and tympanic segments of the facial nerve. Exposure of the geniculate ganglion requires removal of the incus, which can be replaced at the end of the operation. Conductive hearing loss may occur with this maneuver, and, in general, it is difficult to get adequate decompression of the geniculate segment without a middle fossa craniotomy. The labyrinthine segment cannot be reached through a transmastoid approach unless the ampulla of the lateral semicircular canal is sacrificed.

This route is used to explore the facial nerve when decompression is necessary for rerouting of the nerve and in cases of infection and fractures localized to the mastoid segment of the fallopian canal. Acute or chronic otitis media can induce facial paralysis. The most common sites of involvement are the tympanic segment (dehiscent in more than 25% of healthy persons) and the second genu as the nerve turns into the mastoid. With an isolated mastoid temporal bone fracture or a longitudinal temporal bone fracture that involves the distal geniculate ganglion and tympanic segments, adequate decompression can be accomplished through the mastoid. A longitudinal temporal bone fracture, however, is better managed with the improved exposure provided by a middle fossa approach. During removal of infratemporal fossa tumors, rerouting of the facial nerve frequently is required. Moving the facial nerve provides safer access to the jugular foramen and carotid canal. Transmastoid decompression is used in conjunction with middle fossa and retrolabyrinthine approaches if total facial nerve exposure is required and inner ear function is to be preserved.

Limitations and Complications

The major drawback with transmastoid exposure of the facial nerve is the limited access to the geniculate ganglion and the inability to reach the labyrinthine segment. The labyrinthine portion of the nerve commonly is the primary site of involvement in traumatic paralysis or Bell's palsy. Conductive or sensorineural hearing loss also can be a complication if the incus is removed or touched by a rotating burr during the procedure.

Translabyrinthine Approach: Total Facial Nerve Exposure

Technique

The patient is positioned on the operating table and the head and lower left abdominal quadrant are prepared and draped. An incision is made 3 cm behind the postauricular crease and carried inferiorly over the mastoid tip. Soft tissue is elevated forward off the mastoid cortex to the external auditory canal. A portion of the occipital bone posterior to the sigmoid sinus also should be exposed. An extended complete mastoidectomy is performed.

The bone over the sigmoid sinus is removed, along with 0.5 to 1.0 cm of bone posterior to this structure. The incus is removed, exposing the tympanic segment of the facial nerve inferior to the lateral semicircular canal. The facial recess is opened, further defining the position of the facial nerve in the middle ear and mastoid. A thin layer of bone should remain over the nerve while complete labyrinthectomy is performed. Inferior to the posterior semicircular canal, bone is removed, exposing the jugular bulb, posterior fossa dura, and endolymphatic sac (Fig. 171-17).

Medial to the posterior semicircular canal and lateral semicircular canal, the internal auditory canal appears blue compared with the surrounding yellow otic capsule bone. Bone is removed 180 degrees around the internal canal, exposing the porus acusticus. At the lateral margin of the internal auditory canal, the facial nerve is found medial and slightly superior to the superior vestibular nerve (Fig. 171-18). Bone is removed over the labyrinthine segment to the geniculate ganglion and then distally to the stylomastoid foramen at the anterior limit of the digastric groove. The final layer of bone is removed with blunt elevators.

The dura over the internal auditory canal and cerebellar plate can be opened to expose the cerebellopontine cistern and brainstem. Closure is accomplished with a 4 cm × 4 cm piece of temporalis fascia covering the dural defect and draped over the aditus to separate the mastoid from the middle ear (Fig. 171-19). Abdominal fat is harvested and used to obliterate the mastoid space.

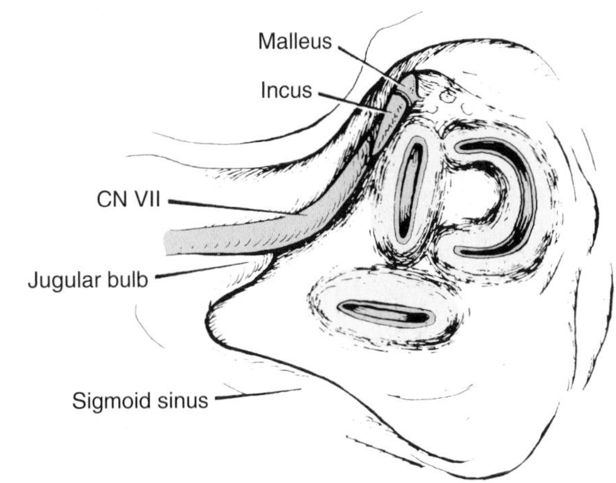

Figure 171-17. Left translabyrinthine exposure of the semicircular canals. CN, cranial nerve.

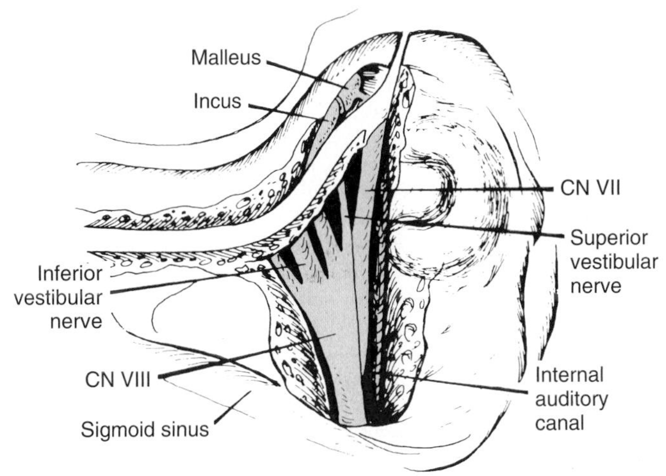

Figure 171-18. Completed left translabyrinthine exposure. CN, cranial nerve.

Advantages and Uses

The translabyrinthine exposure of the facial nerve is used primarily when the cochlear and vestibular functions have been lost preoperatively. The greatest advantage with this technique of facial nerve exposure is the ability to access the entire nerve using one approach. It most often is the approach of choice when facial paralysis has resulted from a transverse temporal bone fracture, an extensive facial neuroma, or a large congenital cholesteatoma that extends into the internal auditory canal. If an interpositional nerve graft is required, the translabyrinthine exposure provides enough working space for anastomosis at or near the brainstem.

Limitation and Complications

The greatest limitation of this procedure is that hearing and balance function must be sacrificed for total exposure of the nerve. When healthy cochlear and vestibular function exists, the surgeon should consider other approaches. Existing hearing and balance functions are destroyed, and the procedure may prevent future use of a cochlear implant device. CSF leakage and infection are the greatest risks with this operation, but the complication rate should be less than 2% if proper fascia graft and fat obliteration are performed.

Combination Approaches

It may be necessary to combine two or more of the approaches described to achieve the exposure dictated by the disease process. Occasionally, middle fossa exposure is combined with the transmastoid approach

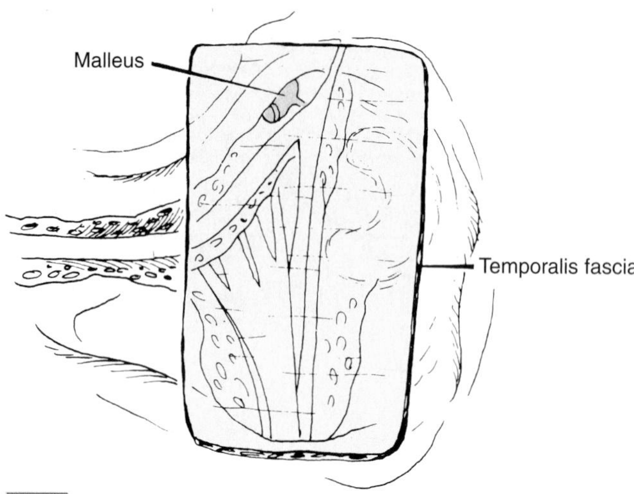

Figure 171-19. Placement of the temporalis fascia at the time of closure of the left translabyrinthine exposure.

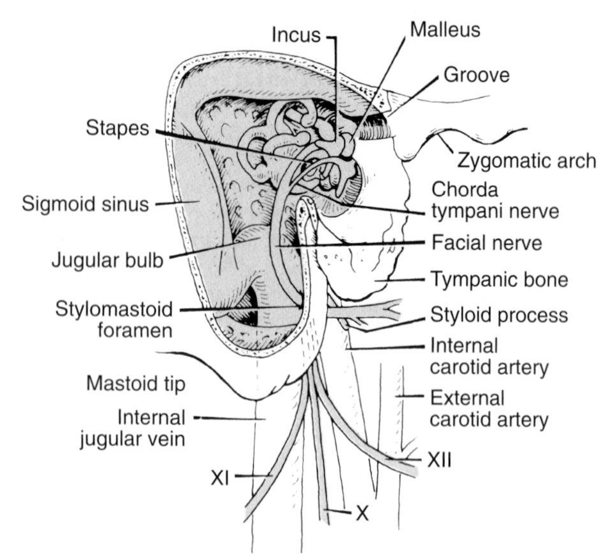

Figure 171-20. Facial nerve exposure for rerouting, as used in glomus jugulare tumor resection. Roman numerals denote cranial nerves.

when total decompression of the fallopian canal is needed. The middle fossa usually is exposed first. In most traumatic injuries, the area of facial nerve involvement is located at or just medial to the geniculate ganglion. If the injury extends distally, the lower limb of the skin incision is carried postauricularly, and a mastoid decompression is accomplished. The middle fossa retractor is left in place until the total nerve is exposed. A fascia graft is used to repair the dural defect in the internal auditory canal, and a portion of the craniotomy flap is placed over the tegmen tympani to prevent temporal lobe herniation. This combination also is useful in patients with facial nerve schwannoma and congenital cholesteatoma.

Retrolabyrinthine exposure also can be added if the disease extends medial to the porus of the internal auditory canal. During this portion of the procedure, the middle fossa retractor should be removed. Combination approaches are useful when a nerve graft is necessary and additional access is required.

Rerouting

Elevation of the facial nerve out of the fallopian canal may be necessary during nerve repair procedures and is essential for removal of sizable neoplasms in the proximity of the jugular foramen and carotid canal. Severe injury to the facial nerve at the geniculate ganglion occasionally occurs in longitudinal temporal bone fractures and can be managed by resecting the geniculate ganglion and reapproximating the labyrinthine and tympanic segments of the nerve through middle fossa exposure. Small tumors at the geniculate ganglion can be similarly managed.

To attain the necessary nerve length, the labyrinthine and transverse segments should be mobilized and elevated out of the fallopian canal. Extreme care should be taken during exposure of the labyrinthine segment of the nerve, because the basal turn of the cochlea can be less than 1 mm inferior and the ampulla of the posterior semicircular canal and lateral semicircular canal directly posterior. Small diamond burrs (0.4 to 0.8 mm) are used to remove the bone over the canal. It is safer to remove more bone anterior to the labyrinthine segment than posterior to it. The final thin layer of bone is removed with blunt microdissectors (Storz). When bone has been removed 180 degrees from the cephalic portion of the nerve, a microelevator is used to elevate the nerve gently out of the canal. Any adhesions to the bone are sharply separated with a microscalpel (Beaver No. 59-10). The tympanic segment of the nerve is mobilized in a similar manner. If the slightest tension would be necessary for reapproximation of the nerve ends, an interposition graft should be placed.

Surgical techniques have been developed to expose lesions near the jugular bulb, carotid canal, and parasellar regions.[8] The descending segment, stylomastoid foramen, and extratemporal course of the facial nerve are directly lateral to these structures. Rerouting the facial nerve greatly facilitates the surgical exposure and eliminates the need to transect the nerve in most instances. Commonly, the nerve is relocated anterior and superior to its original position, requiring the middle ear cleft to be obliterated and the posterior external bony canal to be removed.

A large, C-shaped postauricular skin incision is designed to allow exposure of the mastoid cortex and parotid gland. The skin flap is developed through the external ear canal at the bony cartilaginous junction and carried anteriorly, exposing the periparotid fascia. The extratemporal course of the facial nerve is exposed in the parotid gland in the usual fashion. The dissection of the nerve is carried distal to the pes anserinus, and the inferior division is freed from the surrounding gland for 1 to 2 cm. Additional dissection may be necessary, depending on the exposure required.

A complete mastoidectomy is performed, and the posterior external canal is lowered to the level of the lateral semicircular canal and the digastric ridge. The tympanic ring, malleus, and incus are removed. The tympanic and descending segments of the facial nerve are identified with a diamond burr (Fig. 171-20). Bone is removed 180 degrees around the nerve, leaving a thin shell that is removed with microelevators. Sharp dissection with a microscalpel frees the nerve sheath from the remaining fallopian canal.

An abundant vascular supply frequently is encountered during elevation of the nerve from the canal. Bleeding is controlled with a microtipped bipolar cautery at the lowest effective current.

At the stylomastoid foramen, a thick fibrous sheath strongly adheres to the bone. To prevent trauma to the nerve during elevation of this portion, it is suggested that the entire fibrous sheath be freed and moved with the nerve. Removal of the nerve from the sheath induces unnecessary trauma that may result in temporary paralysis. It also may be difficult to elevate the tympanic segment of the nerve because of the close proximity of the stapes superstructure. The crura and capitulum of the stapes can be removed with a crurotomy scissors. A groove that is larger than the nerve is then milled in the zygomatic root area of the epitympanum to accept the nerve as it is transposed anterosuperiorly at the level of the geniculate ganglion (Fig. 171-21).

Partial Rerouting

Partial rerouting of the facial nerve can be attempted for tumors that do not involve the protympanum, internal auditory canal, or eustachian tube. This procedure allows preservation of middle ear function. When hearing preservation is to be attempted, rerouting of only the mastoid segment of the facial nerve is more limited. The external auditory canal is transected 3 to 4 mm medial to the bony cartilaginous junction, allowing reconstruction of the external auditory canal at the end of the

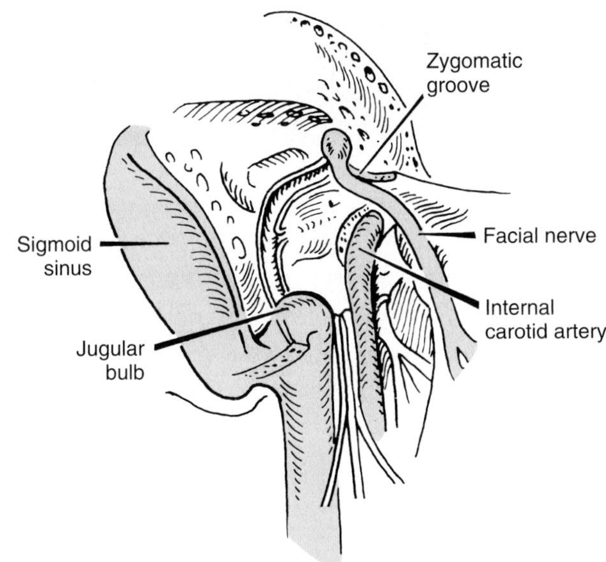

Figure 171-21. Appearance after rerouting of the facial nerve.

procedure. A canal wall-up mastoidectomy with an extended facial recess is created. In addition to thinning the posterior canal wall, the inferior wall or floor is thinned in a similar manner. The facial nerve is skeletonized to the tympanic segment and elevated out of the fallopian canal with sharp dissection. The nerve is sharply dissected with a cuff of tissue at the stylomastoid foramen, as in the total rerouting technique. The facial nerve is temporarily elevated laterally to allow exposure to the jugular foramen and the pars nervosa, containing cranial nerves IX, X, and XI. After tumor removal, the facial nerve is returned to its approximate position. A 1-mm burr is then used to create anchor holes at the lateral extent of the bony canal (one in the floor, two in the posterior wall, and one in the anterior wall). The external canal skin is secured to its position with 3-0 sutures. The sutures are placed into the thick subcutaneous tissue, rather than the skin. The canal is packed with antibiotic ointment–impregnated gauze strip for 1 week. Stenosis of the canal has not occurred in more than 30 partial rerouting procedures. Anchoring the canal skin to the bony canal prevents the formation of external canal mastoid fistula.

Nerve Repair

Whenever the continuity of the facial nerve has been disrupted by traumatic injury, iatrogenic injury, or tumor invasion, every effort should be made to restore its continuity. In some instances, an end-to-end reapproximation can be accomplished, but if any tension occurs at the anastomotic site, an interposition nerve graft confers a better chance of allowing facial movement. All nerve repair techniques produce synkinesis, but sphincteric function of the mouth and eye usually are restored. Newer microsuture techniques and instrumentation should be used to enhance return of function.

In general, the injured ends of the nerve should be freshened at a 45-degree angle. Experimental evidence has shown that cutting the nerve at this angle exposes more neural tubules, with consequently improved regrowth of the nerve.[16] In addition, a fresh razor blade induces less crush to the nerve than does a scalpel blade or scissors. Milesi[17] advocates removing a portion of the epineurium before suturing to prevent connective tissue growth at the anastomotic site. We have found that the perineurium of cranial nerve VII does not hold 10-0 sutures, and attempting to suture it increases trauma to the neural tubules. If the epineurium is cleaned from the end of the nerve for approximately only 0.5 mm, sutures can still be placed in the epineurium for reapproximating the nerve segments. Three or four sutures of 10-0 nylon are placed with jeweler's forceps or longer instruments (19-cm microforceps) for anastomosis in the cerebellopontine angle. At the brainstem, one or two sutures are placed. Within the fallopian canal, a nerve graft can be interposed without sutures if there is no chance of nerve end movement.

When an interposition graft is required, the great auricular nerve or the sural nerve is the preferred graft donor site. The great auricular nerve is readily available near the operative field if it is not involved in resection of a neoplasm and has approximately the same diameter as that of the facial nerve. It is easily located midway and perpendicular to a line drawn between the mastoid tip and the angle of the mandible. If a graft longer than 8 to 10 cm is required, the sural nerve should be used. The sural nerve has another advantage in that the peripheral portion of the nerve has many branches that can be used to reconstruct the branching pattern of the facial nerve. Little discomfort is associated with removal of the sural nerve, because it provides only a small area of sensation to the lateral lower leg. The sural nerve is found immediately posterior to the lateral malleolus, along the saphenous vein. The nerve graft should be 10% to 20% larger in diameter than the facial nerve and long enough to ensure tension-free anastomosis.

Facial Nerve Tumors

Tumors (both benign and malignant) can affect the facial nerve in the intracranial cavity, within the temporal bone, and in the parotid gland. Approximately 5% of cases of facial nerve dysfunction are due to the presence of a tumor. It is essential to differentiate intrinsic from extrinsic facial nerve tumors (e.g., a primary facial nerve tumor versus tumor contiguous with the facial nerve or metastatic disease). Extrinsic tumor involvement is much more common than intrinsic tumor involvement. Numerous benign and malignant neoplasms may occur in and around the temporal bone. Within the temporal bone itself, skull base tumors and metastases from the breast and lung are common neoplastic causes of facial paralysis in adults, whereas hematologic malignancies (leukemia, lymphoma) are common in children.[18] Management of these lesions is beyond the scope of this chapter. It is not possible to list all of the neoplasms, but common ones include facial schwannomas, congenital cholesteatomas, hemangiomas, glomus tumors, vestibular schwannomas (acoustic neuromas), squamous cell carcinomas, and parotid neoplasms. The following discussion is concerned primarily with those lesions of the facial nerve proximal to the stylomastoid foramen.

The classic symptom associated with tumors involving the facial nerve is a progressive paralysis of the face. In some benign lesions, this progression is extremely slow; months or even years may elapse before the paralysis becomes complete. The cause of a facial palsy progressive beyond 3 weeks after onset but with no return of function by 6 months is presumed to be a tumor until proven otherwise. Benign tumors produce facial paralysis by compressing the facial nerve, whereas malignant lesions invade the nerve itself. Therefore, in benign tumor removal, it is sometimes possible to dissect the mass away from the nerve without damage to the nerve itself. In dealing with malignant neoplasms, it is necessary to resect the nerve with the tumor and then perform a reconstruction of the nerve.

Early diagnosis of facial paralysis from a tumor is dependent on a high index of clinical suspicion. In addition to a slowly progressive paralysis, several other clinical features should heighten suspicion for a tumor involving the facial nerve. Twitching of the facial nerve in association with facial palsy is not seen with Bell's palsy. In addition, recurrent palsy also may be associated with a tumor. Pain, although frequently a feature of Bell's palsy or Ramsay Hunt syndrome, also is often a symptom with tumors involving the facial nerve. Involvement of other cranial nerves in addition to the facial nerve should raise concern that a neoplasm is present. A predilection for neoplasms to occur at the geniculate ganglion area, possibly owing to this area's embryologic diversity, has been suggested.[3] Evaluation for a neoplastic etiology for a facial palsy should include radiologic imaging (with both CT and MRI scans).

Acoustic neuromas are benign tumors and are the most common lesions of the internal auditory canal and cerebellopontine angle. Facial paralysis is an unusual manifestation of these tumors and generally signifies an advanced stage of tumor growth. Rarely does an acoustic neuroma actually invade the facial nerve. It also is possible for a patient with an acoustic neuroma and facial palsy to have a concomitant Bell's palsy as the true etiology of facial nerve dysfunction. In the absence of nerve sheath invasion, the facial nerve generally appears to tolerate gradual pressure stresses well. Facial dysfunction may also occur from local vascular compromise.[19]

Nerve sheath and vascular neoplasms make up the greatest percentage of intrinsic facial nerve tumors (although they are relatively rare as a group). These tumors typically are facial schwannomas (neuromas) but also may include meningiomas, hemangiomas, and glomus tumors.[18] These tumors may manifest relatively early with facial weakness.[19] Overall, facial nerve schwannomas are uncommon, slow-growing neoplasms arising from the nerve sheath, and they may occur anywhere from the cerebellopontine angle to the peripheral branches of the facial nerve.[20] A majority of facial nerve schwannomas are intratemporal, most often involving the labyrinthine segment and geniculate ganglion.[20,21] A retrospective review demonstrated that facial nerve schwannomas were more likely to involve multiple segments than a single segment.[21] One of the largest series of facial nerve tumors to date was published by McMenomey and colleagues in 1994.[22] They reviewed their experience with 32 primary facial nerve tumors between 1975 and 1992. Preoperatively, 38% were thought to be acoustic neuromas.

A facial nerve schwannoma may be misdiagnosed as an acoustic neuroma, especially when the tumor does not enter the meatal foramen or fallopian canal and is instead confined to the internal auditory canal.[22,23] Even with high-resolution MRI, it may be difficult to distinguish preoperatively between an acoustic neuroma and a facial schwannoma. Beyond the clinical examination and clinician suspicion, no useful preoperative evaluation tools are available that can definitively identify the precise nerve of origin of intracanalicular tumors. This limitation emphasizes the need to fully inform the patient preoperatively.[23]

Treatment decisions must be made based on the patient's desires, age, degree of facial function, tumor location, and hearing status.[8,24] The goal in the management of these tumors is to maximize long-term facial nerve function while minimizing morbidity. At most centers, the most common mode of treatment is tumor resection with grafting. Observation is another option for tumors that are not producing facial paresis or are generating minimal symptoms (House-Brackmann grade II). It also is possible that with observation or expectant management, complications such as total hearing loss may occur, particularly when the tumor involves the labyrinthine and internal auditory canal portions of the nerve.[25] Unfortunately, a majority of patients undergoing resection and grafting will have additional facial nerve deficits in the immediate postoperative period, and the long-term results with grafts generally are characterized by poor recovery of forehead motion and mass motion (grade C on the Repaired Facial Nerve Recovery Scale [RFNRS][26]).

A review of the records at House Ear Institute between 1977 and 1994 showed that 93 patients were diagnosed with facial neuromas and 3031 were diagnosed with acoustic neuromas.[27] In four patients in whom the diagnosis was made during surgery, the tumor was not completely resected.[27] Two of the patients underwent decompression using an middle cranial fossa or translabyrinthine approach. Two patients underwent a retrosigmoid craniotomy, one of whom also underwent decompression; for the other, postoperative management consisted of observation of her tumor. Follow-up for these patients ranged from 24 to 62 months. In three of the four tumors, no growth was noted on the MRI scan during the follow-up period (the other showed a 6-mm growth over 5 years). In one patient (who underwent translabyrinthine decompression), facial nerve function improved from grade V preoperatively to grade II postoperatively.

The medical records of 21 patients with facial nerve tumors treated between 1982 and 2002 at the University of Iowa Hospitals and Clinics were retrospectively reviewed. The ages of the patients ranged from 13 to 76 years. Follow-up ranged from 1 month to 22 years.

In 2 of the 21 patients, the tumor was identified on an MRI scan obtained for other medical reasons. Both have normal facial nerve function (House-Brackmann grade I) and undergo periodic MRI. One has been observed for longer than 20 years and continues to have grade I facial nerve function. Twenty-one procedures were performed on the other 19 patients. Of the 21 procedures performed, 11 consisted of resection followed by interposition grafting. Patients in this group presented with conditions classified as House-Brackmann grade IV or worse. All grafting was done using the greater auricular nerve. The other 10 procedures involved decompression, debulking, or both. *Decompression* included removal of the bony confines of the facial nerve either in the internal auditory canal or in the fallopian canal at the site of the tumor and some distance proximal and distal to the tumor. *Debulking* involved removal of portions of the tumor, with the use of intraoperative facial nerve monitoring to reduce the likelihood of inadvertent damage to normal facial nerve fibers.

Table 171-3

Repaired Facial Nerve Recovery Scale (RFNRS)

Score	Function
A	Normal facial function
B	Independent movement of eyelids and mouth, slight mass motion, slight movement of the forehead
C	Strong closure of eyelids and oral sphincter, some mass motion, no forehead movement
D	Incomplete closure of eyelids, significant mass motion, good tone
E	Minimal movement of any branch, poor tone
F	No movement

Facial nerve function was graded using the House-Brackmann scale for the observation and decompression-debulking group. However, owing to the limitations and inadequacies of this grading scale for nerve resections, a different scale, the RFNRS, was used to grade nerve function in the resection and grafting group (Table 171-3). A majority of the tumors in this series were facial nerve schwannomas. All 10 of the tumors in the decompression-debulking group were schwannomas, whereas 7 of the tumors in the resection group were schwannomas. Tumors in the resection group also included 3 hemangiomas and 1 meningioma. In the decompression-debulking group, five patients had grade I function. Three patients had grade II function, one patient had grade III function, and one had grade IV function. None of the patients in this group have had grade V or VI function.

In the resection and grafting group, the best facial function noted postoperatively was grade C, which is roughly equivalent to House-Brackmann grade III, in six patients. Three patients had grade D function. One patient had grade E function and one grade F function. Of significance, none of these patients achieved a preferred grade A or B function.

Observation of intrinsic facial nerve tumors is a possible management approach, especially for patients with House-Brackmann grade I or II facial function. Surgical decompression is an option for patients with House-Brackmann grade II or III facial function. Resection with grafting is recommended for those with grade IV function or worse. Conservative management with either observation or decompression often is an appropriate option, because the best facial nerve function result after resection and grafting is grade C on the RFNRS, owing to the presence of mass motion. Nonetheless, treatment is individualized.

SUGGESTED READINGS

Angeli SI, Brackmann DE. Is surgical excision of facial nerve schwannomas always indicated? *Otolaryngol Head Neck Surg.* 1997;117:S144.

Chiang CW, Chang YL, Lou PJ. Multicentricity of intraparotid facial nerve schwannomas. *Ann Otol Rhinol Laryngol.* 2001;110:871.

Fenton JE, Morrin MM, Smail M, et al. Bilateral facial nerve schwannomas. *Eur Arch Otorhinolaryngol.* 1999;256:133.

Fisch U. Current surgical treatment of intratemporal facial palsy. *Clin Plast Surg.* 1979;6:377.

Fisch U. Prognostic value of electrical tests in acute facial paralysis. *Am J Otol.* 1984;6:494.

Fisch U. Surgery for Bell's palsy. *Arch Otolaryngol Head Neck Surg.* 1981;107:1.

Fisch U, Pillsbury HC. Infratemporal fossa approach to lesions in the temporal bone and base of skull. *Arch Otolaryngol Head Neck Surg.* 1979;105:99.

Gantz BJ. Idiopathic facial paralysis. *Curr Ther Otolaryngol Head Neck Surg.* 1987;3:62.

Gantz BJ. Intraoperative facial nerve monitoring. *Am J Otol.* 1985; Nov(Suppl):58.

Gantz BJ, Gmur A, Fisch U. Intraoperative evoked electromyography in Bell's palsy. *Am J Otolaryngol.* 1982;3:273.

Gantz BJ, Rubinstein J, Gidley P, et al. Surgical management of Bell's palsy. *Laryngoscope.* 1999;109:1177.

Ge XX, Spector GJ. Labyrinthine segment and geniculate ganglion of the facial nerve in fetal and adult temporal bones. *Ann Otol Rhinol Laryngol.* 1981;90:1.

Gidley PW, Gantz BJ, Rubinstein J. Facial nerve grafts: from cerebellopontine angle and beyond. *Am J Otol.* 1999;20:781.

Glasscock ME, Shambaugh GE Jr. Facial nerve surgery. In: Glasscock ME, Shambaugh GE Jr. *Surgery of the Ear.* 4th ed. Philadelphia: WB Saunders; 1990:434-465.

For complete list of references log onto www.expertconsult.com.

House W. Surgical exposure of the internal auditory canal and its contents through the middle cranial fossa. *Laryngoscope.* 1961;71:1363.

Kertesz TR, Shelton C, Wiggins RH, et al. Intratemporal facial nerve neuroma: anatomical location and radiological features. *Laryngoscope.* 2001;111: 1250.

Marsh MA, Coker NJ. Surgical decompression of idiopathic facial palsy. *Otolaryngol Clin North Am.* 1991;24:675.

May M, Klein SR, Taylor FH. Idiopathic (Bell's) facial palsy: natural history defies steroid or surgical treatment. *Laryngoscope.* 1985;95:406.

McMenomey SO, Glasscock M, Minor L, et al. Facial nerve neuronal presenting as acoustic tumors. *Am J Otol.* 1994;15:307.

Milesi H. Facial nerve suture. In: Fisch U, ed. *Facial Nerve Surgery.* Birmingham, Ala: Aesculapius Publishing; 1977.

Perry BP, Gantz BJ. Diagnosis and management of acute facial palsies. In: Meyers EN, Bluestone CD, Bruckmann DE, et al, eds. *Advances in Otolaryngology–Head and Neck Surgery.* Vol 13. St Louis: Mosby; 1999:127-162.

Rubinstein JT, Gantz BJ. Facial nerve disorders. In: Hughes GB, Pensak ML, eds. *Clinical Otology.* New York: Thieme Medical Publishers; 1997: 367-380.

Sillman J, Niparko J, Lee S, et al. Prognostic value of evoked and standard electromyography in acute facial paralysis. *Otolaryngol Head Neck Surg.* 1992;107:377.

Silverstein H, Norrell H. Retrolabyrinthine surgery: a direct approach to the cerebellopontine angle. *Otolaryngol Head Neck Surg.* 1980;88:462.

Yamamoto E, Fisch U. Experiments on facial nerve suturing. *Otorhinolaryngol Relat Spec.* 1974;36:193.

CHAPTER ONE HUNDRED AND SEVENTY-TWO

Rehabilitation of Facial Paralysis

James M. Ridgway

Roger L. Crumley

Jason H. Kim

Key Points

- Paramount to the rehabilitation of facial nerve paralysis is a complete understanding of the nature of the injury, extent of the defect, viability of remaining facial nerve segments, integrity of potential donor nerves and tissues, and the overall patient's health status as well as personal desires and expectations for rehabilitation.
- A detailed history and physical examination should include a description of the mechanism of the injury, time of onset, duration of symptoms, previous surgery or radiation therapy, speech and swallowing function, and previous treatment and rehabilitation.
- Division of the face into upper, middle, and lower thirds allows for a more precise characterization of nerve defects and potential therapeutic options.
- Management of facial paralysis is dependent on the specific cause of the paralysis. Options for facial nerve rehabilitation include spontaneous nerve regeneration (observation), facial nerve neurorrhaphy, facial nerve cable graft, nerve transposition, muscle transposition, microneurovascular transfer, and static procedures.
- EMG is indispensable in determining the existence of denervation atrophy or subclinical innervation. EMG is the single most important test for determining the type of operative procedure to be performed.
- An operative electric nerve stimulator may be used only in acute injuries to identify severed distal nerve segments. Wallerian degeneration with impairment of nerve conduction has occurred by 72 hours after injury, and the surgeon is left to rely on visual identification after this point in time.
- The most desired source for rejuvenation of the paralyzed face is the ipsilateral facial nerve.
- Early protection of the eye in the setting of facial nerve paralysis is of the highest priority, because failure to recognize and treat eyelid dysfunction will result in devastating ocular complications that are entirely preventable.
- Tension-free repair of the facial nerve is critical to the success of nerve anastomosis. When operative circumstance does not permit such an end-to-end anastomosis, cable or interposition nerve grafting is the desired surgical approach to facial muscle reinnervation.
- When grafting to the proximal facial nerve segment is not an option in rehabilitation, attention is then shifted to the muscle (masseter or temporalis) or nerve (hypoglossal) transfer procedure.
- Static techniques are best used in debilitated patients with limited prognostic survival and in those for whom nerve or muscle is not available for dynamic procedures.
- Patients with incomplete recovery from facial nerve paralysis typically present with hyperkinetic, uncoordinated mass facial movements known as synkinesis. Botulinum toxin has dramatically improved the management of this condition and is the current first-line therapy.

Dealing with the consequences of unilateral facial paralysis usually is a devastating emotional ordeal for the patient. The ability to restore symmetry and motion to patients afflicted with facial paralysis is one of the most rewarding skills of the well-trained reconstructive surgeon. This chapter discusses rehabilitation of facial nerve injuries. Many of the diagnostic considerations and surgical techniques described are applicable to otogenic paralyses (intratemporal), as well as injuries and diseases that affect the parotid and facial portions of the facial nerve.

The facial nerve, once damaged, rarely attains full recovery of function. Given the challenges to the patient, counsultations regarding facial nerve paralysis require a clinician's fullest thought and compassion. A realistic approach yields the rewards of patient compliance, understanding, satisfaction, and acceptance of reality. A recent review of all state and federal civil trials alleging malpractice and facial nerve paralysis demonstrates the importance of careful explanation and documentation, as well as the importance of good patient rapport and bedside manner in preventing lawsuits.[1]

Patient Assessment

Complete patient assessment is critical to attain optimal rehabilitation of facial paralysis. It is critical to properly understand the nature of the injury and the resulting defect, to know the viability of the proximal and distal facial nerve segments, to properly assess the viability of potential donor nerves and facial musculature, and to thoroughly assess both the patient's health status and personal desires for rehabilitation.

An outline of assessment of facial nerve paralysis is presented in Box 172-1.

Box 172-1

Assessment of Facial Nerve Paralysis

History

Type of injury
Time since injury
Age, overall health, and life expectancy
Radiation therapy (past or planned)
Nutritional factors
Previous operative report

Physical Examination

Previous incisions and scars
Integrity of trigeminal, vagal, and hypoglossal nerves
Facial motion (e.g., complete versus partial paralysis)
Status of eye (e.g., lagophthalmos, ectropion)
Facial tone, structure (e.g., habitus)

Testing/Imaging

Electromyography: indicated in all patients who have had paralysis for more than 1 year
Computed tomography and magnetic resonance imaging of temporal bone and parotid: indicated if there is any question about the cause of paralysis

Assessment of the Deformity

Physical examination includes complete head and neck examination with attention to cranial nerve function and the presence of functional masseter and temporalis muscles. The degree of facial nerve function is recorded using the House-Brackmann Facial Grading System[2] (Table 172-1). A number of facial nerve grading scales have been developed, but the House-Brackmann scale was adopted by the Facial Nerve Disorders Committee of the American Academy of Otolaryngology–Head and Neck Surgery in 1985 because of its reproducibility and ease of use.[2] This scale is useful for evaluation of overall function, but it is insufficient for precise assessment of defects affecting one or more branches of the facial nerve, and it does not allow precise measurement of effectiveness of treatments isolated to one region of the face. Therefore, the examination should assess deformity of the upper, middle, and lower thirds of the face independently. This approach allows more precise characterization of defects, aids the decision-making process for rehabilitation, and allows more precise assessment of treatment results. Facial tone also is noted, as is the presence of any reinnervation. Thorough assessment of the eye also is performed. Visual acuity, corneal integrity, eyelid closure, tearing, Bell's phenomenon, lagophthalmos, lower lid laxity, position of the lacrimal puncta, and eyebrow position are noted. Nasal examination focuses on the position of the ala and nasal septum and the presence or absence of nasal obstruction. Oral competence and height and position of the lower lip are carefully reviewed. In long-term paralysis (of more than 1 year's duration), electromyography (EMG) of the facial muscles is performed before reinnervation procedures. Occasionally, muscle biopsy provides additional information about the presence of viable muscle for innervation. If nerve fibrosis is suspected, nerve biopsy occasionally is indicated.

Another important component of the assessment is evaluation of the patient's smile pattern. The smile is created by the muscles of the lips, and smile patterns can be classified into one of three types.[3] The "Mona Lisa" smile is the most common smile pattern (67%). It is

Table 172-1

House-Brackmann Grading System

Grade	Description	Characteristics
I	Normal	Normal facial function in all areas
II	Slight	Appearance: slight weakness noticeable on close inspection; may have very slight synkinesis At rest: normal symmetry and tone Forehead motion: moderate to good function Eyelid closure: complete with minimal effort Mouth motion: slight asymmetry
III	Moderate	Appearance: obvious but not disfiguring weakness between the two sides; noticeable but not severe synkinesis, contracture, and/or hemifacial spasm At rest: normal symmetry and tone Forehead motion: slight to moderate movement Eyelid closure: complete with effort Mouth motion: slightly weak with maximal effort
IV	Moderately severe dysfunction	Appearance: obvious weakness and/or disfiguring asymmetry At rest: normal symmetry and tone Forehead motion: none Eyelid closure: incomplete Mouth motion: asymmetric with maximal effort
V	Severe	Appearance: only barely perceptible motion At rest: asymmetric Forehead motion: none Eyelid closure: incomplete Mouth motion: slight movement
VI	Total	No facial function

From House JW, Brackmann DE. Facial nerve grading system. *Otolaryngol Head Neck Surg*. 1985;93:146.

dominated by action of the zygomaticus major muscle: The corners of the mouth move laterally and superiorly, with subtle elevation of the upper lip. The canine smile (31%) is dominated by levator labii superioris action, appearing as vertical elevation of the upper lip, followed by lateral elevation of the corner of the mouth. The least common smile is the full denture smile (2%), or "toothy smile," produced by simultaneous contraction of the elevators and depressors of the lips and angles of the mouth. Knowledge of facial muscle anatomy and the smile pattern exhibited by the patient is important in considering rehabilitation techniques other than nerve grafting to recreate a balanced facial appearance at rest and the simulation of a symmetric smile.

Considerations in Facial Nerve Rehabilitation

A number of factors come into play in designing a management plan for the patient with facial paralysis. In clinical situations requiring facial reanimation, the technique used often depends on the availability of a viable proximal facial nerve.

Tumor ablation with facial nerve sacrifice (as in radical parotidectomy for parotid malignancy) dictates immediate facial nerve restitution, usually by cable grafting. When the nerve's continuity and viability are in question, however, as may be seen during and after cerebellopontine angle surgery, it is wise to wait 9 to 12 months before an extratemporal facial nerve operative procedure is undertaken. Hence, no modality is universally appropriate for all afflictions of facial nerve function. Static procedures generally are used when no viable reinnervation options exist but also can be integrated with dynamic procedures to provide immediate restoration of facial symmetry.

Generally, however, the order of preference for rehabilitation procedures is as follows:

1. Spontaneous facial nerve regeneration (observation)
2. Facial nerve neurorrhaphy
3. Facial nerve cable graft
4. Nerve transposition
5. Muscle transposition
6. Microneurovascular transfer
7. Static procedures

Time since Transection

A chronic, long-standing paralysis with complete muscle degeneration poses several problems with regard to eventual reinnervation surgery. The facial muscles may undergo denervation atrophy. Severe atrophy renders the reasonably normal muscles incapable of reinnervation and contraction. Such severe atrophy may occur after 18 months of complete denervation, although in some clinical situations, muscles have been known to persist inexplicably for many years without incurring such atrophy.[4] EMG is the most helpful method for assessing facial muscle atrophy and is therefore a preoperative prerequisite for all reanimation candidates if the paralysis is of more than 12 months' duration. The presence of nascent, polyphasic, or normal voluntary action potentials in a patient with facial paralysis indicates the occurrence of reinnervation. If more than 12 months have passed since the facial nerve injury, the situation can be assumed to be stable, and an attempt at surgical reanimation may be warranted. Within the first 12 months, however, the presence of potentials may mean that reinnervation is occurring and that facial movements may return in the next few months. Reanimation surgery should therefore be postponed. Fibrillation or denervation potentials mean that the EMG electrode is positioned in denervated muscle. This is an optimal situation for cable nerve grafting or, when no viable proximal facial nerve is available, for hypoglossal-facial anastomosis.

One of the most significant EMG findings is electrical silence, reflecting denervation atrophy of the facial muscles. The surgical implication is that nerve grafting or transfer is futile and therefore contraindicated. If the facial muscles are absent or atrophied, muscle transfers are indicated.

Another effect of time includes endoneural scarring within distal nerve segments. It is not known whether endoneural scarring acts as an impediment to nerve regeneration, but when associated with muscular atrophy, it probably further precludes nerve grafting or transfer.

Presence of Partial Regeneration

Partial regeneration often is overlooked but is extremely important in determining which operation to perform. If the facial nerve has undergone enough regeneration to permit a few axons to reach the facial muscles, this partial innervation may be sufficient to preserve the muscles for many years, even though they may be totally paralyzed. In these clinical circumstances, results with hypoglossal-facial anastomosis, which generally is preferable to muscle transfer, will be optimized.

Status of the Proximal and Distal Facial Nerve

The optimal source for rejuvenation of the paralyzed face is the ipsilateral facial nerve. Anastomosis or grafting to the ipsilateral nerve has no donor consequence (other than the minor hypesthesia or anesthesia from the harvesting of a nerve graft) and facilitates natural voluntary and involuntary control. Exceptions to this general rule are those cases in which the patient needs prompt relief from corneal exposure or drooling, and a tissue transfer or sling technique may be preferred because its effects are immediate.

Accordingly, the integrity of the proximal facial nerve is critical. As with other motor nerves, no reliable electrical tests exist to confirm the viability of the proximal nerve when it is discontinuous with its distal portion. Factors that affect proximal nerve viability and are therefore important considerations in the clinical evaluation include (1) nature of the nerve injury (e.g., clean transection versus crush), (2) location of injury (proximal versus distal), (3) age (younger nerves tend to regenerate more quickly and fully), (4) nutritional status (which directly affects nerve regeneration), and (5) history of irradiation (which may impede neural regeneration).

The facial nerve distal to the injury site serves as a conduit for neural regeneration to the facial muscles after neurorrhaphy, grafting, or hypoglossal-facial anastomosis. With acute injuries (incurred less than 72 hours previous), the electrical stimulator may be used to identify the distal nerve and the muscular innervation of distal branches. After this "golden period," however, the surgeon must rely on visual identification of the divisions and branches of the distal nerve, because the capability of being stimulated electrically generally is lost after approximately 72 hours. For this reason, transected nerve branches in trauma or tumor cases should be tagged for identification by placing a small colored suture around or adjacent to each nerve branch. Any anatomic or surgical landmarks should be precisely dictated in the operative note. If no suture markers are available, and the golden period has elapsed, careful surgical searching (preferably with use of loupes or an operating microscope) may reveal each of the divisions or branches of the facial nerve. A topographic map is essential in guiding the dissection. A review by Bernstein and Nelson[5] describes the variability with which these branches are placed. The following landmarks are helpful (Fig. 172-1).

- The pes anserinus can be found 1.5 cm deep to a point 1 cm anterior and 2 cm inferior to the tragal cartilage.
- The superior division courses from the pes anserinus to the lateral corner of the eyebrow, convex posterosuperiorly (see Fig. 172-1). Bernstein and Nelson[5] stressed that these temporal branches may be multiple and reach as far posteriorly as the superficial temporal vessels.
- The buccal branch courses superiorly and then anteromedially, passing 1 cm inferior to the inferior border of the zygomatic arch (see Fig. 172-1).
- The marginal mandibular branch passes from the pes anserinus directly over the angle of the mandible and then under the inferior

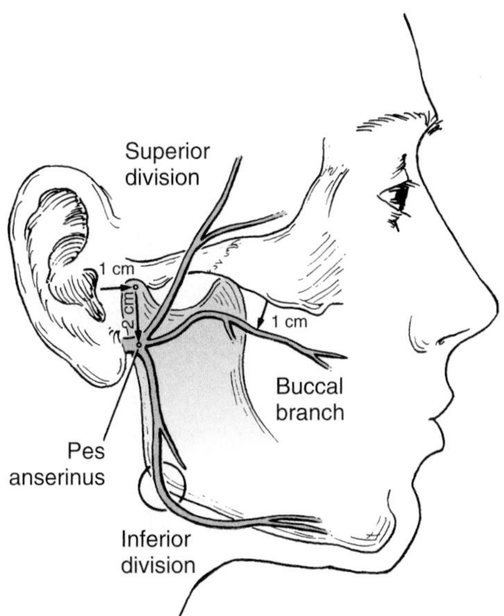

Figure 172-1. Topographic map of distal facial nerve anatomy, useful as a guide in finding nonstimulatable nerve branches for grafting. Pes anserinus is 2 cm inferior to a point 1 cm anterior to tragus. Marginal mandibular branch courses from the pes anserinus to the angle of the mandible: buccal branch parallels the zygomatic arch 1 cm below its inferior border. Superior division arcs from pes anserinus toward lateral end of the eyebrow, under a line that is convex superiorly. *(From House JW, Brackmann DE. Facial nerve grading system.* Otolaryngol Head Neck Surg. *1985;93:146.)*

border of the mandible for approximately 3 cm. It then crosses above the mandible at the level of the facial vessels. Any of several anatomic variations may exist, necessitating ingenuity in nerve grafting. When the facial nerve trunk and pes anserinus are intact, a cable graft (or hypoglossal nerve) should be sutured to that portion of the main nerve trunk. However, certain injuries and surgical procedures may sacrifice important individual portions of the nerve, requiring selective routing of reinnervation to specific divisions. The order of priority for reinnervation of facial nerve branches is as follows: (1) buccal and zygomatic branches (equal), (2) marginal mandibular, (3) frontal, and (4) cervical (the last may be disregarded or excluded).

As an example of selective routing, when a parotid tumor operation results in excision of the pes anserinus and the proximal facial branches, a branched nerve graft may be placed to reinnervate the zygomatic and the buccal branches, excluding unimportant branches. Fisch[6] advises clipping branches of cervical branches in order to route innervation to the more important portions of the face. Data confirming the efficacy of this technique, however, are very limited.

If no nerve branches are found, and EMG shows that denervated facial muscles are present, the nerve graft may be sutured directly to the muscles targeted for reinnervation (muscular neurotization). In these instances, the most important muscles are those of the midface (zygomaticus major and minor, levator labii superioris) and orbicularis oculi muscles. Reinnervation will not be as complete as in routine nerve grafting because the regenerating axons must form new connections to the old motor endplates, or they must create their own.[7]

Viability of Facial Muscles

Four types of EMG responses are observed[8]:

Normal voluntary action potentials indicate that functioning motor axons have connections with and are stimulating motor units of facial muscle.

Polyphasic potentials are seen during reinnervation and may precede visible evidence of reinnervation.

Denervation or *fibrillation potentials* indicate that otherwise normal denervated muscle exists.

Electrical silence, with no potentials seen, indicates atrophy or congenital absence of muscle, provided that the electromyographer has positioned the electrode correctly.

Donor Consequences

Many surgical procedures designed for facial reanimation borrow neural elements or signals from other systems (i.e., the hypoglossal and trigeminal systems). The consequences of sacrificing the donor nerve (known as donor deficit) are most important in planning for the overall needs of the patient. Certainly, the surgeon must assess the donor nerve preoperatively in all cases. The hypoglossal nerve must be tested for strength and vitality before it is transected and anastomosed to the distal facial nerve. Similarly, the trigeminal nerve must be intact and functional when its muscles, either masseter or temporalis, are considered for transposition into the facial muscle system.

The donor effects of facial reanimation surgery may be quite detrimental to the patient's welfare. For example, a patient with previous hypoglossal nerve injury on the opposite side could become an "oral cripple" if the remaining hypoglossal nerve were to be transected for use in a XII-VII anastomosis.

The ideal reanimation procedure is one that yields the following results: (1) no donor deficit; (2) immediate restitution of facial movement; (3) appropriate involuntary emotional response; (4) normal voluntary motion; and (5) facial symmetry. No currently available operative procedure satisfies all of these parameters. In fact, even with a bacteriologically sterile and precise surgical transection and immediate microsurgical repair of the facial nerve, completely normal neurologic function cannot be restored. Therefore, the surgeon must have a clear understanding of all operations available, including potential outcomes and sequelae.

Status of Donor Nerves

The hypoglossal nerve is the most frequently used nerve source for transfer. Reflex and physiologic similarities between the hypoglossal and facial nerves have been described.[9] The integrity of the hypoglossal nerve must be determined before it is transferred for reinnervation. Irradiation of the brainstem, lesions of the skull base and hypoglossal canal, and surgical procedures of the upper neck may affect the integrity and function of this nerve.

The trigeminal nerve has been used for facial reanimation in many ways. The methods currently used most often involve masseter or temporalis muscle transfer (necessitating that the motor portions of the trigeminal nerves be intact). Palpation of the muscle during jaw clenching confirms whether the muscle is functional.

The cross-face nerve graft procedure (faciofacial anastomosis) initially was thought to be the most appropriate and ingenious facial reanimation procedure.[10,11] The procedure is unique in that it borrows appropriate neural input from the contralateral normal side and routes it to the paralyzed side. Such a procedure requires a fully intact (contralateral) facial nerve.

Age

The proximal neuron's ability to regenerate declines with time because of denervation and aging-related changes. The etiologic mechanism probably involves diminishing regenerative vitality of the perikaryon (cell body), although peripheral scarring may play a role. The clinical implication is that facial reanimation surgery should always be performed as soon as possible, provided that the operative procedure does not interfere with or injure existing innervation or ongoing reinnervation.[12]

Health Status

Among patients with diabetes, regeneration of injured nerves is notoriously poor. Microangiopathy is an additional factor that may affect the grafted segment. These factors do not preclude a nerve graft procedure in a diabetic patient, but when combined with radiation, advancing age, and other factors, they may cause the surgeon to consider muscle transfer or a suspensory operation, rather than a neural anastomosis.

Prior Radiotherapy

Radiotherapy, a necessary component of treatment for certain salivary gland malignancies, appears to have a deleterious effect on reinnervation through facial nerve grafts. McCabe[13] demonstrated satisfactory muscle reinnervation from grafting despite irradiation in animals. These investigators subsequently have documented return of facial function in nine patients who received post-grafting radiotherapy. McGuirt and McCabe[13] and Conley and Miehlke[14] have published reports indicating that facial nerve grafts function well even though irradiated, and that nerves are among the most radioresistant tissues of the human body. Pillsbury and Fisch[15] found that radiotherapy reduced the average outcome from 75% to 25% of nerve function recovery in a review of 42 grafted patients. Irradiation probably affects the neovascularization of the nerve graft by decreasing vascularity of the tissue bed and probably injures the proximal and distal segments of the nerve as well. The most radiosensitive portion of the nerve—the pontine nucleus—should be assessed to determine whether it was present in the field of irradiation.

Congenital Paralysis

In a series of 95 infants with neonatal paralysis, Smith and associates[8] found 74 of the cases to be secondary to intrauterine injury or birth trauma, whereas 21 were thought to be congenital. These infants should be studied with nerve excitability and EMG testing early in life to ascertain the status of nerves and muscles. Most patients with injury-related neonatal paralysis recover rapidly, whereas the paralysis associated with other congenital anomalies (such as Möbius syndrome) is permanent. Nerve exploration or transfer generally is futile in the latter cases.

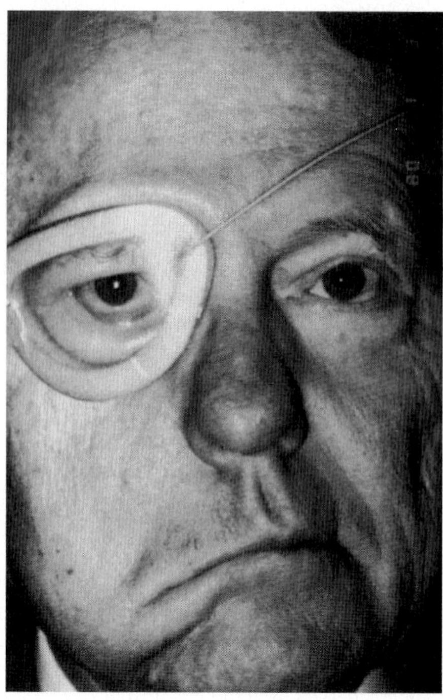

Figure 172-2. Occlusive bubble worn by a patient after acoustic neuroma surgery. The appliance has a foam rubber skin contact surface that is firmly attached to a thin Plexiglas lens. In our experience, patient compliance is relatively high with this type of device. *(Courtesy of Moisture Chamber, Pro-optics, Palatine, Illinois.)*

Early Care of Facial Nerve Injury

Failure to recognize and treat acute eyelid dysfunction will result in devastating ocular complications. The ability to prevent, diagnose, and treat paralytic eyelid sequelae before major complications occur is essential in the management of any patient with facial paralysis. An important point is that the outcome of the eyelid paralysis is directly related to patient education and compliance.

Eye Protection: Evaluation and Treatment of Eyelid Paralysis

Paralysis of the orbicularis oculi results in exposure and drying of the cornea. Patients at increased risk for exposure keratitis may be identified by applying the acronym BAD—*a*bsence of Bell's phenomenon, corneal *a*nesthesia, and history of *d*ry eye. An inability to protect the cornea is the result of incomplete eye closure, preventing effective distribution of the tear film across the surface of the eye, and ectropion occurs because the atonic lower lid and lacrimal punctum fail to appose the globe and bulbar conjunctiva. This causes faulty eyelid closure and improper distribution of tears across the cornea.

Epiphora may result from failure of tears to enter the lacrimal punctum, secondary to pooling of tears due to ectropion and the loss of the orbicularis oculi tear-pumping mechanism. The response to abnormal corneal sensation may be reflex tear hypersecretion, which will further increase the epiphora.

Any patient with facial paralysis who demonstrates a poor Bell's phenomenon is at risk for the development of exposure keratitis. Eye pain may herald the onset of keratitis. In patients with diminished corneal sensation, however, exposure keratitis may asymptomatically progress to corneal ulceration. Accordingly, all patients with diminished orbicularis oculi function require ophthalmologic consultation.

Initial eye care is directed toward moisturizing the dry eye and preventing exposure. It is important to communicate to the patient the potential consequences of failure to protect the eye, in hopes of improved compliance. If the eyelid paralysis is temporary or partial, these local measures may be all that are necessary to adequately protect the eye. Regular use of artificial tears commonly is the first-line method used to keep the eye moist. Ointments also may be used, but they are less practical in the daytime because they tend to blur vision.

Lacriserts, contact lenses, and occlusive bubbles commonly are used, although patient compliance may be problematic[16] (Fig. 172-2). The eyelids frequently are patched or taped, but if incorrectly used, these methods may result in corneal injuries. Tape should not be placed vertically across the eyelashes, but applied horizontally above the eyelashes on the upper eyelid, or supporting the lateral canthal portions of the lower eyelid.[17] When an eye patch is used, care must be taken to ensure that the eye cannot open, because this would allow contact between the patch and the cornea.

Procedures to Treat Paralysis of the Lower Lid (Ectropion)

Tarsorrhaphy

The temporary lateral tarsorrhaphy is an expeditious and effective method for protecting the eye in patients with mild lagophthalmos and mild corneal exposure. A horizontal mattress suture of 7-0 silk or nylon is placed laterally to approximate the gray line (mucocutaneous junction) of the upper and lower lids. Tarsorrhaphy sutures will remain effective longer if they are placed through bolsters made of rubber (Robinson) catheters.

For longer-lasting protection, the lid adhesion tarsorrhaphy is preferred. The lid margin (gray line) of each lid is denuded 4 to 6 mm from the lateral canthus, and a similar suture technique is used to approximate the denuded mucocutaneous junctions of upper and lower lids (Fig. 172-3). Like the temporary lateral tarsorrhaphy, this procedure can be reversed if function returns. The cosmetic deformity of tarsorrhaphy and the availability of improved, alternative techniques to rehabilitate the eyelids have reduced the use of tarsorrhaphies.

Wedge Resection and Canthoplasty for Paralytic Ectropion

Wedge resection of all layers of the lower lid is a simple and expeditious procedure, but it can result in notching of the eyelid margin. A more effective option for lower lid laxity is the lateral canthoplasty, which is more reliable, with a less noticeable defect. Several techniques have been described for lid shortening and resuspension. They share the goal of

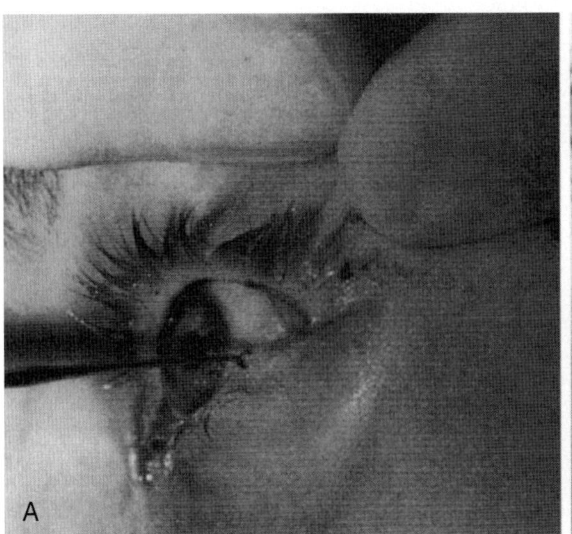

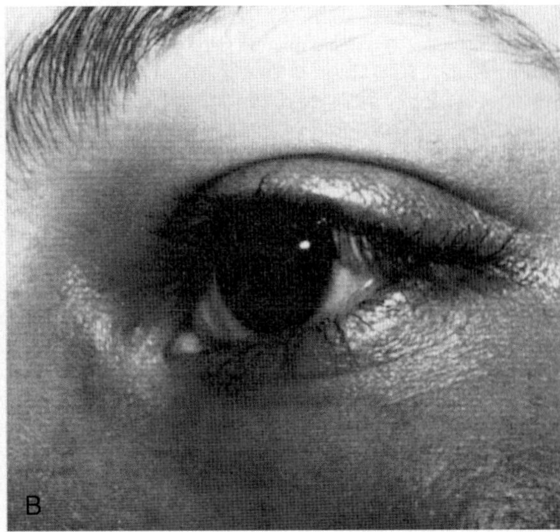

Figure 172-3. **A,** Tiny single skin hook being used to evert the lower lid for denuding of "gray line" (mucocutaneous junction). Note that a gray line of upper lid has been denuded. **B,** Healed tarsorrhaphy at 4 months. Increased eye closure may be achieved by extending the denudation and sutures medially.

eliminating laxity of the lateral canthal tendon by shortening or resuspending (or both) the tendon posteriorly behind and above Whitnall's tubercle.

The modified Bick procedure consists of lateral canthotomy and inferior cantholysis, followed by conservative resection of the lateral canthal tendon and fixation to the medial aspect of the lateral orbital wall above and posterior to Whitnall's tubercle.

The tarsal strip procedure described by Anderson and Gordy[18] modifies the previously described technique by denuding the conjunctiva over the lateral tendon and separating the posterior lamella and the tendon from the anterior lamella. The isolated tarsal strip is then suspended to the lateral orbital rim. In cases of severe ectropion, the lower lid punctum may be everted and displaced laterally after lateral canthoplasty. In these instances, a medial canthoplasty is used to restore the physiologic relationship of the punctum to the globe.[19,20] The lower lid also may be augmented with auricular cartilage to address inadequate support of the medial tarsal plate in cases not amenable to lateral tendon suspension alone.[21]

Procedures to Treat Paralysis of the Upper Lid (Lagophthalmos)

Weights, Springs, and Slings for Lagophthalmos

Gold weight insertion is extremely effective and very popular because of its reliability, minimal cosmetic deformity, and relative ease of insertion. The implant weight used is determined preoperatively by taping a weight to the upper eyelid and assessing eyelid closure. The smallest weight that allows comfortable eyelid closure and does not cause fatigue of the levator muscle is selected.

Under local anesthesia, an incision is made extending equally between the medial and middle thirds of the supratarsal crease, and the skin is elevated to the superior border of the tarsus. A pocket is formed immediately superficial to the tarsus to accommodate the dimensions of the weight. The weight is placed so that its inferior border is parallel to and just above the eyelash line. It is important to create a pocket directly on the tarsal plate, with care taken to preserve a thin cuff of tissue at the lid margin to prevent inferior extrusion of the implant. The implant is secured with clear nylon sutures superior and inferior to the tarsal plate, the orbicularis-levator complex is reapproximated, and the skin is closed.[16]

Gold weights have some disadvantages. A very low incidence of extrusion has been documented with their use even when they are inserted properly. In addition, weights depend on gravity and therefore do not effectively protect the cornea when the patient is supine, so a nighttime ointment is often required. If the weight is placed too far superior, it can result in paradoxical opening of the eye when the patient is in the supine position. Finally, the gold weight can occasionally be noticed by the casual observer as a bump in the eyelid.

Palpebral springs and silicone (Silastic) slings as described by Morel-Fatio and Lalardrie[22] and Arion,[23] respectively, also have been used for lagopththalmos. Silastic slings are used less frequently and are complicated by lateral ectropion.[24] Both types of implants share the disadvantage of extrusion, and they are more difficult to place than eyelid weights. Currently, titanium chain link implants are being used with greater frequency and with excellent results. These implants may be camouflaged to obtain a better cosmetic result, because they conform to the shape of the eyelid. Additionally, the titanium implants have been shown to result in less corneal astigmatism or cornea-altering effect on the globe itself than that typical with gold weights.[25]

Facial Nerve Grafting

Use of cable or interposition nerve grafts frequently is the desired approach to facial muscle reinnervation. The most common setting for this procedure is likely to be in combination with radical parotidectomy and facial nerve sacrifice. The clinical uses of interposition grafts are as follows: (1) radical parotidectomy with nerve sacrifice; (2) temporal bone resection; (3) traumatic avulsions; (4) cerebellopontine angle tumor resection; and (5) any other clinical situation in which viable proximal nerve can be sutured and distal elements of facial nerve can be identified. Tension-free repair is a critical element of successful nerve anastomosis. When tension-free apposition cannot be achieved using existing nerve ends, cable grafts are used.

Facial nerve grafting for acute causes such as parotid malignancy requires the surgeon to customarily identify the distal facial nerve trunk divisions or branches for the distal anastomosis. Nerve restitution should be performed at this time unless extenuating circumstances (e.g., anesthetic complications, intraoperative emergencies) rule out immediate grafting.[26] If grafting is not undertaken at the time of nerve sacrifice, it should be completed within 72 hours thereafter, so that the facial nerve stimulator may be used to identify the distal branches. Conversely, the nerve ends can be tagged for identification at a later time. When grafting is not done, the distal branch becomes nonstimulatable and thus much more difficult to locate and identify.

Surgical Planning

In planning the surgical procedure, the proximal site of nerve transection frequently is found to be in the intraparotid portion proximal to the pes anserinus. This location may present technical difficulties because the proximal stump may not be adequate for technical ease in suturing. In other instances, the nerve may be transected at the stylomastoid foramen. If it is seen to be transected at the stylomastoid foramen, a mastoidectomy should be performed. Distal to the mastoid portion, the nerve's sheath merges with periosteum of the stylomastoid foramen and temporal bone, making this portion difficult to dissect free for suture. This difficult region exists roughly from 1 cm above to 1 cm below the stylomastoid foramen. Use of the mastoid portion of the facial nerve may require use of the longer sural or medial antebrachial cutaneous nerve, rather than the greater auricular nerve, for a cable graft.

Distally, several situations may be encountered that require some ingenuity in effecting reanimation. When the distal anastomotic site is at or proximal to the pes anserinus, a simple nerve-to-nerve suture will suffice. More frequently, however, after resection for parotid malignancy, several branches or divisions may require anastomosis. In such cases, priority must be given to the zygomatic and buccal branches, sometimes to the exclusion of other, less important facial nerve branches. Frequently, a two-branch graft can be prepared from the greater auricular nerve or the sural nerve. This situation favors suturing of one branch of the nerve graft to the buccal branch and the other graft branch to the zygomatic branch or superior division. This technique will direct innervation to the important orbicularis oculi muscle and the muscles of the buccal-smile complex (Fig. 172-4).

Choosing a Donor Nerve

Four of the nerves most commonly used are the greater auricular nerve, the sural nerve, cervical plexus, and the medial antebrachial cutaneous nerve. Each has distinctive advantages and limitations; the reconstructive surgeon should be familiar with each.

When harvesting the greater auricular nerve, tumor considerations mandate that the ipsilateral nerve not be used. Consequently, the opposite neck should be prepped and draped for harvesting the contralateral nerve in parotid malignancy cases. The nerve is easily identified, arising from the posterior surface of the sternocleidomastoid muscle at Erb's point and traveling obliquely along the sternocleidomastoid muscle toward the ear. The surgical landmarks are well defined: a line drawn from the mastoid tip to the angle of the mandible is then bisected by a perpendicular line that crosses the sternocleidomastoid muscle from inferoposterior to anterosuperior, passing toward the parotid gland. A small horizontal incision in an upper neck skin crease is made along the path of the nerve. The nerve is identified in the subcutaneous tissues and followed superiorly to the parotid gland dissecting each of the three branches, and inferiorly to the posterior border of the sternocleidomastoid muscle. The greater auricular nerve has several advantages: its size and fascicular pattern are similar to the facial nerve, it is easily harvested in familiar anatomy, and it has a favorable distal branching pattern for facial nerve grafting. Unfortunately, the nerve is limited to a maximum of 10 cm for grafting.

In patients who have undergone neck dissection or parotidectomy and in whom the greater auricular nerve is not a viable grafting option, the cervical plexus is the next ideal donor nerve. The cervical plexus can be harvested in the similar fashion to the greater auricular nerve, but requires a longer neck incision. The nerve plexus can be located just posterior and deep to the sternocleidomastoid muscle.

The sural nerve is also commonly used for facial nerve grafting. In contrast to the greater auricular nerve, the sural nerve is the longest donor nerve available, with up to 70 cm of graft available when all branches are dissected into the popliteal fossa. The donor site is located distant from the surgical resection, allowing a second team to simultaneously harvest nerve tissue. Donor site morbidity is low. However, caution should be exercised when working with diabetics or patients with peripheral vascular disease as ischemic pressure necrosis could result in the area of sensory deficit along the lateral aspect of the foot. The sural nerve is of larger diameter than the greater auricular nerve or the facial nerve, and it has more prominent connective tissue than the greater auricular nerve or medial antebrachial cutaneous nerve.

The sural nerve is formed by the junction of the medial sural cutaneous nerve and the peroneal communicating branch of the lateral sural cutaneous nerve between the two heads of the gastrocnemius muscle. The nerve lies immediately deep to and behind the lesser saphenous vein with multiple nerve branches arising near the lateral malleolus. A pneumatic tourniquet should be applied to the thigh and a transverse incision made immediately behind the lateral malleolus. "Stair-step" horizontal incisions along the course of the nerve provide appropriate exposure during the harvesting procedure. The nerve should be harvested immediately before grafting and placed in physiologic solution after débriding away any small pieces of fat or other soft tissue that might interfere with graft revascularization. At all times care is taken to avoid stretching the nerve.

The medial antebrachial cutaneous nerve has been described in the orthopedic literature for peripheral nerve repairs and is used in situ with forearm microvascular flaps for sensory innervation in head and neck cancer reconstruction. This nerve has several properties that warrant consideration for use in facial nerve reconstruction[27]: It has a consistent anatomy, traveling in the bicipital groove immediately adjacent to the basilic vein. Nerve diameter and branching pattern are similar to those of the facial nerve, and donor site morbidity is minimal with nerve harvest. Cheney[27] has described the relevant anatomy in detail.

All of the aforementioned donor nerves are sensory nerves used to lead motor nerve regeneration. This is important as harvesting a motor nerve for grafting material would certainly incur some degree of morbidity to the donor area or muscle. Although there may be theoretic difference between using a sensory nerve versus a motor nerve, further investigation is required to determine if this is of any biologic implication.

Surgical Technique

For the surgical technique of neurorrhaphy, interrupted sutures using 9-0 or 10-0 monofilament nylon are preferred. A straight and a curved pair of jeweler's forceps as well as a Castroviejo needle holder are satisfactory instruments for performing the anastomosis. Both ends of the nerve graft and the proximal and distal stumps should be transected cleanly with a fresh sterile blade.[13] For nerve trunk anastomosis, four simple epineural sutures will usually coapt the nerve ends accurately. However, obvious discrepancies in size or other epineural gaps should be closed with additional sutures. The needle should pass through epineurium only to avoid injury to the fascicular neural contents. The nerve graft should lie in the healthiest possible bed of supporting tissue, with approximately 8 to 10 mm of extra length for each anastomosis. Thus, the graft should lie in a somewhat "lazy S" configuration (see Fig. 172-4), which appears to minimize tension during healing. Suction drainage systems should be placed away from any portions of the nerve graft.

When one division is excised or injured and other portions of the nerve remain intact, it may be desirable to graft from a fascicle within the pes anserinus to a distal branch. To accomplish this, fascicular dissection is performed in parallel and along the plane of the nerve fascicles with curved jewler's forceps into the pes anserinus (Fig. 172-5). The distal buccal branch often has several small filaments, so it may be necessary to select the larger of these for distal anastomosis.

Approximation of the nerve ends using an acrylic glue has been described (Histacryl or cyano-butyl-acrylate)[28] with subsequent investigators revealing that neural anastomosis with tissue adhesive yields results similar to nerve suture. This technique is most helpful in the confined surgical considerations of the temporal bone rather than in distal facial anastomosis.[29] Others have described using biodegradable nerve tubules.

Following temporal bone resection, the nerve may be routed from the tympanic or the labyrinthine portions directly to the face through a bony window near the posterior root of the zygomatic arch. This will shorten the necessary length of the nerve graft. However, when using this technique it is important to ensure the nerve graft's protection from trauma at the temporomandibular joint if the joint is preserved. Conley and Baker[30,31] have reported excellent results using similar techniques.

Millesi[32] introduced interfascicular nerve repair, reasoning that the exact microsurgical approximation of nerve fascicles or fascicle groups may minimize synkinesis or mass movement. It is well known

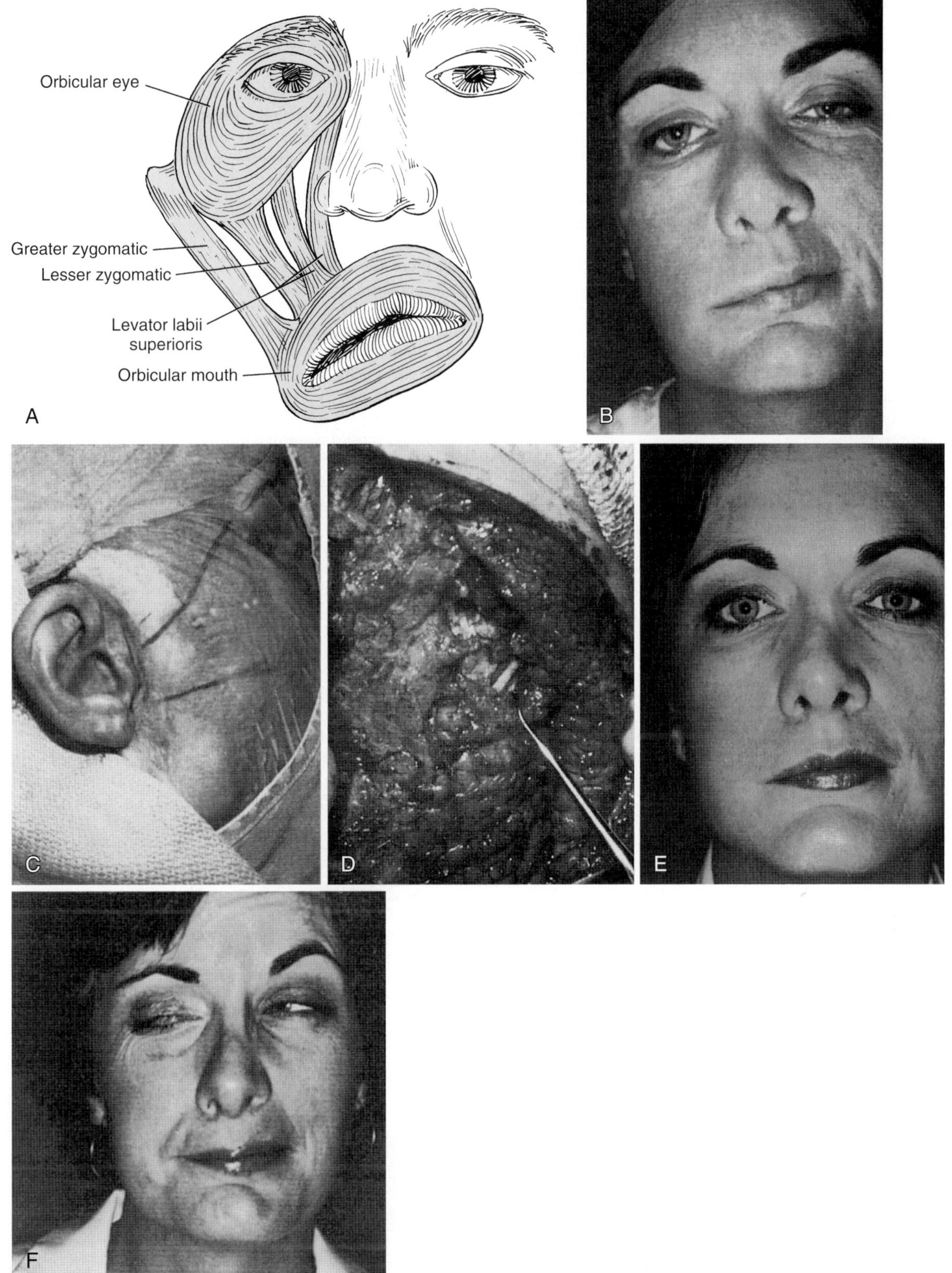

Figure 172-4. Facial muscles. **A,** The most important muscles for reanimation: The levator labii superioris, along with the lesser zygomatic muscle, probably is the most significant muscle for elevation of the upper lip. The greater zygomatic muscle also is critical as the strongest elevator of the oral commissura. **B** to **F,** Example of a delayed nerve graft in a patient in whom a parotid malignancy was removed without immediate reconstruction (because of intraoperative anesthesia considerations). **B,** The patient was referred for nerve grafting after 9 months elapsed. Note elongation of the buccal-smile complex of muscles (greater and lesser zygomatics, levator labii superioris) and paralysis of orbicular eye muscle. **C,** Preoperative surface markings for nerve branches. Nerve stimulator cannot be used to locate distal branches after 9-month time lapse. Markings are for the superior division and buccal branch, based on landmarks described in Figure 172-1 and the previous operative report. **D,** Superior division is found; it is ready for transection and anastomosis to sural graft (from midmastoid nerve segment). **E,** Result at 1 year after operation—typical for a delayed nerve graft. Orbicular eye and buccal branch muscle function is improved, but the muscles are not normally or completely reinnervated. **F,** Voluntary motion in both zygomatic and buccal branches, with synkinesia. This result also is typical for most nerve grafts in that the temporal branch (to occipitofrontal muscle) shows no reinnervation. Note the hairstyle designed to camouflage occipitofrontal muscle paralysis.

that this type of repair is preferred in nerve injuries in the extremities; however, such repairs have not been universally accepted for use in the facial nerve. Several reasons underlie this limited acceptance. The tympanic and, in many cases, the mastoid portions of the nerve have only one or two fascicles, and the intraneural topography is questionable. Few, if any, sensory fibers are present in the extratemporal portion of the facial nerve, so performing sensory-to-sensory fascicular repair is not of value.

Along with May and Miehlke, we have reported (independently) that discrete, spatially oriented fascicles are present in the nerve near the stylomastoid foramen.[33-35] Other authors, notably Sir Sidney Sunderland[36] and Tomander and colleagues,[37] have reported conflicting data demonstrating that various portions of the face are represented in a random fashion in the proximal nerve. At present, it probably is best to perform fascicular repair when the injury obviously lends itself to the technique (e.g., clean lacerations through the pes anserinus and branch nerve grafts that require fascicular dissection in the pes). Basic research has yet to reveal the exact neural topography of the more proximal portions of the nerve.

Cross-Face Nerve Grafting

Overview

The creative and physiologic method of cross-face nerve grafting provides the possibility for facial nerve control of previously paralyzed facial muscles. It is the only procedure with the theoretic capability for specific divisional control of facial muscle groups (e.g., the buccal branch controlling the buccal branch distribution, the zygomatic branch innervating the orbicularis oculi). Originally described by Scaramella[10] and Smith[11] in independent reports in 1971, the technique has not proved to be as advantageous as was first thought. Anderl[38] subsequently described his own results as good in 9 of 23 patients, whereas Samii[39] reported that only 1 of 10 patients had good movement as a result of this technique. A more recent update by Ferreira[40] indicates that those patients operated on within the first 6 months of the paralysis did better than those operated on at a later date. In some of these patients, however, partial spontaneous reinnervation may have occurred, because they appeared to have had lesions without total palsy, and the traditional waiting period of 1 year was not allowed to elapse.

Surgical Technique

The operative technique of cross-face grafting begins with transection of several fascicles, usually of the buccal branch, on the nonparalyzed side through a nasolabial fold incision. One to three sural nerve grafts are approximated to these normal contralateral branches. The nerve grafts are then passed through subcutaneous tunnels, usually in the upper lip. Cross-face grafts for the eye region often are passed above the eyebrow.

As described by most authors, this first surgical stage is performed during the first 6 months of paralysis. Surgery, of course, is not advised unless the paralysis is of known permanence. Tinel's sign often may be elicited after several months of neural ingrowth, because sensory fibers accompany the motor fibers through the cross-face graft. Anastomosis with the paralyzed facial nerve branches is performed by most surgeons during a second stage, 6 to 12 months after the first. At this time, the cross-face graft is explored and sutured to the appropriate branches of the paralyzed side. The approach is through a parotidectomy-rhytidectomy incision and usually is performed within the parotid portion of the paralyzed side.

The cross-face technique suffers from a lack of sufficient axon population and neural excitatory vitality. It is of marginal value when

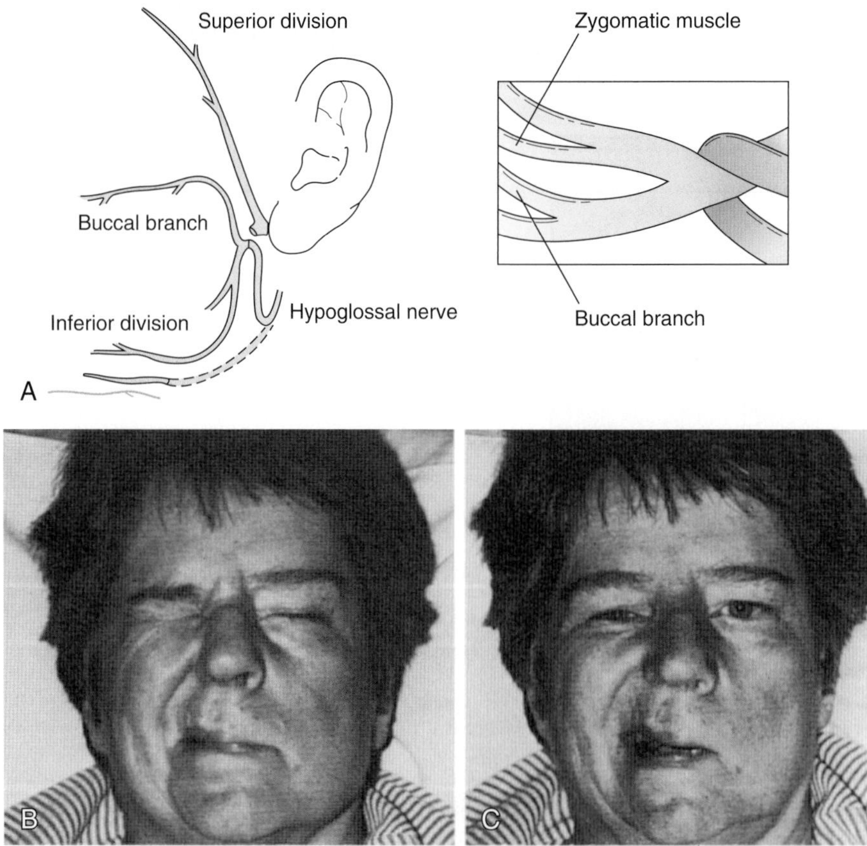

Figure 172-5. A, Hypoglossal-facial anastomosis showing selective reinnervation of the inferior division, leaving the superior division innervation intact. *Inset* shows fascicular dissection before anastomosis (see **D** and **E**). **B** and **C,** Preoperative photographs of patient with long-standing segmental paralysis of inferior division of facial nerve. Zygomatic branch to orbicular eye muscle shows preservation of innervation.

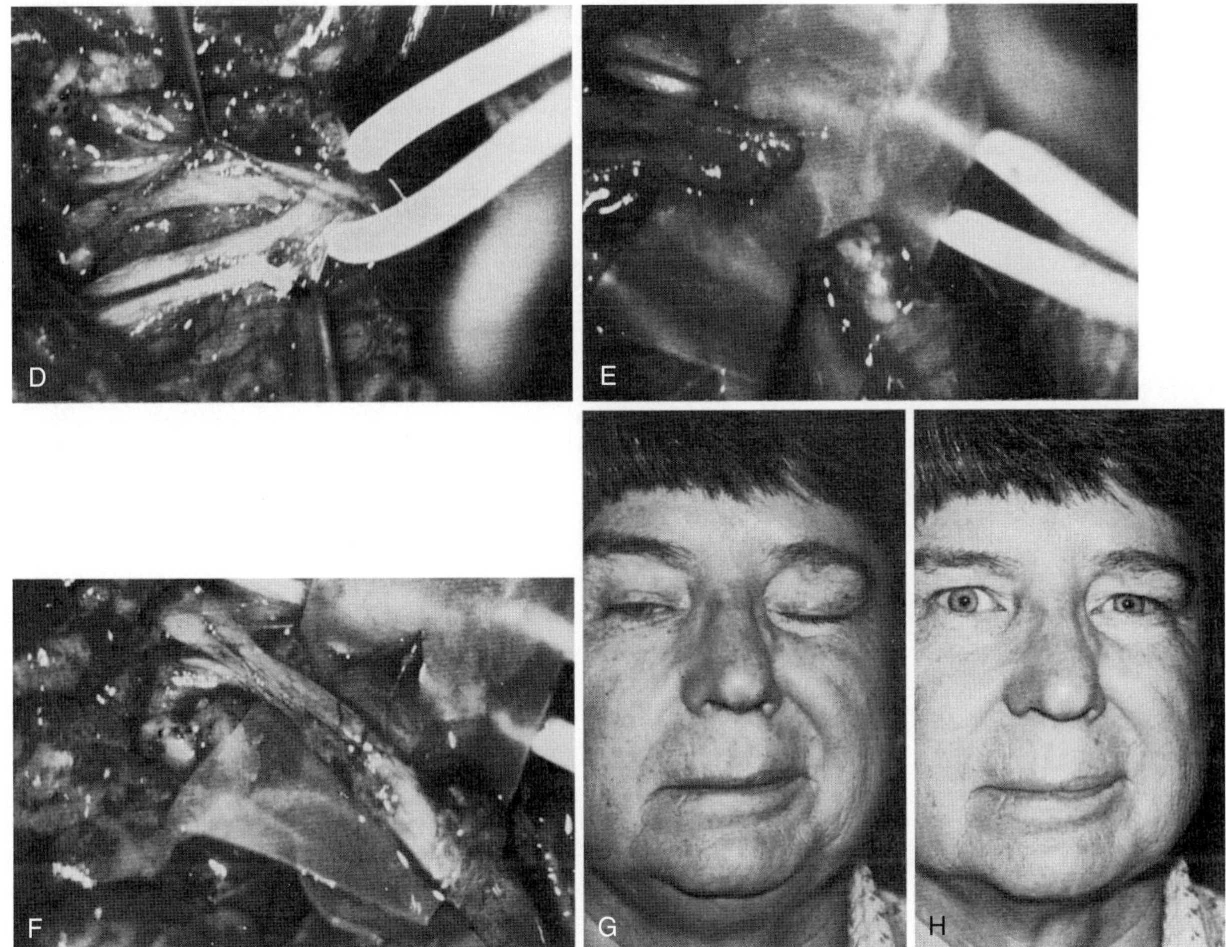

Figure 172-5, cont'd. D to F, Intraoperative photographs. **D,** Perineural dissection of pes anserinus reveals fascicles destined for zygomatic and buccal branches (see **A**). **E,** Buccal branch and inferior division transected. Neurosurgical loop protects intact superior division under background piece of polymeric silicone (Silastic). Hypoglossal nerve (at *lower right*) is ready for anastomosis. **F**, Completed anastomosis of hypoglossal nerve to the buccal branch and inferior division of the facial nerve. The superior division is intact and in continuity with proximal facial nerve. **G** and **H,** Strong reinnervation to entire face, 1 year after operation. **G,** Patient uses hypoglossal innervation to buccal branch muscles to enhance eye closure. **H,** Upward movement of oral commissura mediated by hypoglossal nerve, without associated or synkinetic eye closure.

used alone, but when combined with microvascular transfer of muscle (see below), it can provide suitable innervation. Conley[41] and Conley and Baker[42] have discussed the shortcomings and unproven status of cross-face grafting. Cross-face grafting currently is used only in conjunction with free muscle transfers. Reinnervation of paralyzed facial muscles has not been proved to be sufficient to justify use of this procedure without muscle transfer.

Nerve Transposition

Reinnervation by connecting an intact proximal facial nerve to the distal ipsilateral facial nerve generally is the preferred method for facial paralysis rehabilitation. Only when a proximal facial nerve stump is not viable or available should attention be turned to other strategies, such as muscle or nerve transfer.

Hypoglossal Nerve Transfer

Of the various nerves available for anastomosis with the facial nerve, the hypoglossal nerve is preferred, because an anatomic and functional relationship exists between the facial and the hypoglossal nerves. They both arise from a similar collection of neurons in the brainstem, and they also share similar reflex responses to trigeminal nerve stimulation.[9] In addition, the hypoglossal nerve is in close anatomic proximity and is readily available during other operations on the facial nerve. Hypoglossal nerve transection results in less donor disability than that typical with sacrifice of the spinal accessory, phrenic, or other regional nerves that have been used for facial reanimation. The most common criticism of hypoglossal nerve transfer is that it results in a lack of voluntary emotional control. Although this is true, ipsilateral facial nerve anastomosis often is associated with a similar drawback: Mass movements and spasms preclude any voluntary control of eye closure, smiling, or other emotional movements. In our practice, we have used hypoglossal nerve transfer for reanimation of the upper or lower division selectively by performing fascicular dissection in the pes anserinus to identify the specific fascicles that required reinnervation (see Fig. 172-5).

May and coworkers[43] attempted to decrease morbidity from tongue atrophy by performing partial transection of the hypoglossal nerve with use of a jump graft from the partially transected nerve to the distal facial nerve. Decreased effectiveness of partial transection with jump graft has been reported by some investigators.[44]

Recently, "pure" end-to-side anastomosis of the facial nerve or a jump graft into the donor hypoglossal nerve has been rediscovered[45] and reported in a small series of patients.[46] The study investigators performed anastomosis of facial nerve either mobilized from the mastoid or bridged by interposition graft into the intact hypoglossal nerve, without removal of epineurium or perineurium. This technique relies on the presumed axon sprouting across intact epineurium of the hypoglossal nerve. Some evidence indicates lateral axonal growth after

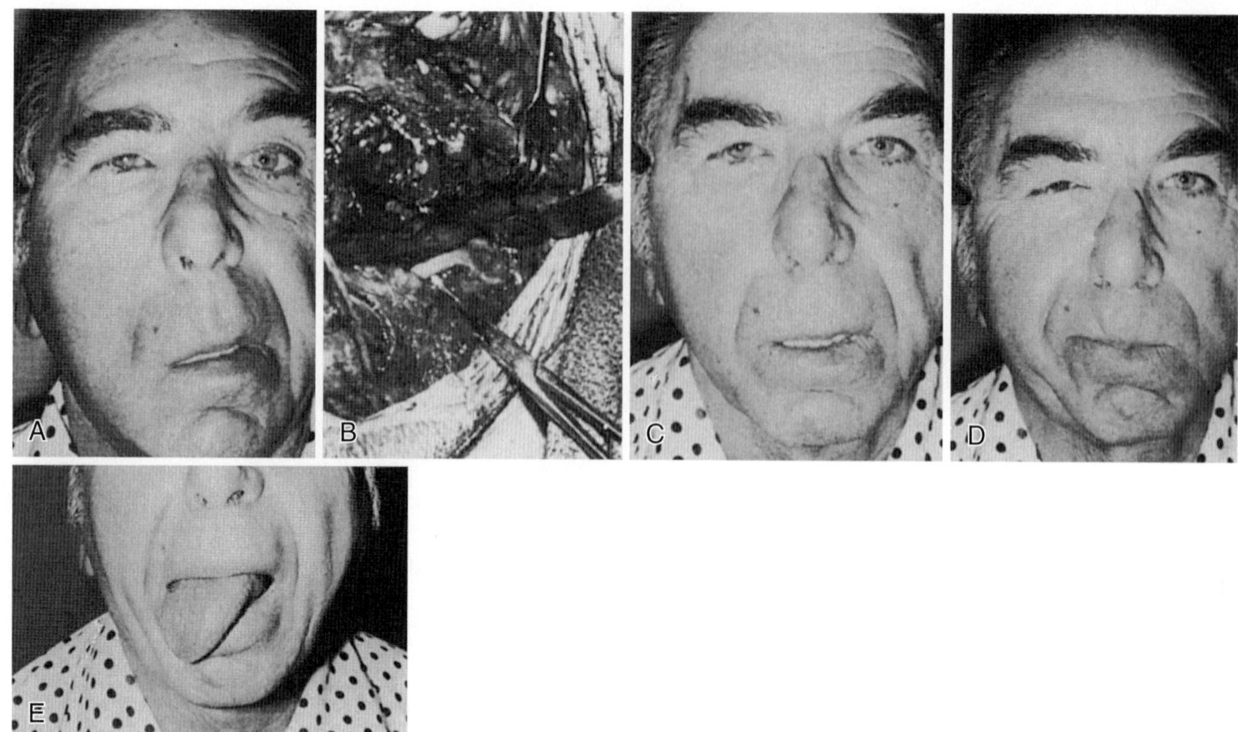

Figure 172-6. **A,** Patient with facial paralysis after acoustic neuroma excision. Lateral tarsorrhaphy is in place. **B,** Exposure of hypoglossal nerve. Note exit of ansa cervicalis branch at *lower right*. This may be transected and sutured to the distal hypoglossal, although preservation of tongue innervation usually is weak with this technique. **C,** Repose. Note elevated commissura and reconstitution of nasolabial fold. **D,** Movement instigated by pushing tongue tip against lingual aspect of mandible in canine region. This maneuver usually results in strongest facial movement after anastomosis of cranial nerves XII and VII. **E,** Typical lingual deviation after the procedure.

end-to-side nerve anastomosis occurs. Rat studies demonstrate axonal penetration of endoneurium, perineurium, and epineurium.[47-49] Whether this technique will be applicable in humans who have decreased nerve regenerative capacity and much thicker perineurium and epineurium than in the rat remains to be seen. It may be more effective to remove an epineurial window and perform the anastomosis without disruption of nerve fibers yet still induce enough axonal regrowth to provide tone and function. Further animal and human studies will be necessary to determine the usefulness and role of end-to-side neurorrhaphy for facial rehabilitation.

Surgical Technique

A modified facelift or parotidectomy incision with an extension made inferiorly toward the hyoid bone usually is used in hypoglossal nerve transfer. The parotid gland is dissected forward from the sternocleidomastoid muscle, and the facial nerve is identified in its trunk–pes anserinus region. The posterior belly of the digastric muscle is then identified, and the hypoglossal nerve is dissected free immediately medial to the tendon of the muscle. The ansa hypoglossi should be identified and dissected free so that, if desired, it may be sutured to the distal hypoglossal stump for reinnervation of the strap musculature. The hypoglossal nerve should be transected as far distally as possible to provide extra length for the anastomosis. After the nerve ends are prepared carefully under high power using a blade, four to eight epineural sutures of 10-0 monofilament nylon complete the anastomosis.

The procedure for the hypoglossal-facial nerve jump graft is similar to that for pure hypoglossal-facial nerve transfer. A greater auricular nerve graft is harvested for use as a jump graft. The facial nerve is transected on the main trunk. The hypoglossal nerve is incised in beveled fashion to expose approximately 30% of the nerve fibers. The jump graft is secured to the proximal edge of the hypoglossal nerve and to the distal end of the transected facial nerve. If the facial nerve is mobilized proximally from the mastoid, it can be directly anastomosed to the partially transected hypoglossal nerve, avoiding placement of a jump graft.

Results

In the largest series to date, involving 137 patients, approximately 95% regained satisfactory tone in repose and regained some mass facial movement.[50] Of these patients, 15% demonstrated hypertonia and excessive movement in the middle third of the face; however, none of these patients requested that the transferred nerve be reoperated. This excessive movement was found to decrease gradually over 10 to 20 years. However, Dressler and Schonle[51] and Borodic and coworkers[52] have had success treating facial hyperkinesia with selective injection of botulinum toxin. Seventy-eight percent of the patients had moderate to severe tongue atrophy, whereas 22% showed minimal atrophy; this wide variability in response of the tongue to hypoglossal nerve transection has been confirmed in other series[53] (Fig. 172-6). Use of the interpositional jump graft with partial hypoglossal nerve preservation preserved tongue function in a majority of patients and provided satisfactory function. In a series of 20 patients, good facial tone and symmetry were observed at follow-up evaluation in all patients, and 13 had "excellent" restoration of facial movement, with development of 12th nerve deficits noted in only 3 patients.[43]

Other Nerve Transfers

The spinal accessory nerve was used before the hypoglossal nerve in nerve transposition techniques. Drobnik performed the first anastomosis of cranial nerves XI and VII in 1879.[9] The phrenic nerve has been similarly used, but this technique causes paralysis of the diaphragm and induces undesirable involuntary inspiratory movements in the facial muscles.[54] The technique is now obsolete.

The neuromuscular pedicle technique described by Tucker transfers a branch of the ansa hypoglossi nerve and a small muscle bloc directly to paralyzed facial muscles. According to Tucker,[55] this procedure is valuable only for the perioral, depressor anguli oris, and zygomaticus muscles. The procedure is described as transferring innervated motor endplates to the denervated facial muscles without the usual delay period seen with free nerve grafts and nerve transfers. The technique allows limited reanimated strength because of the small number of axons present in the donor nerve. In addition, sound electrophysiologic confirmation that the technique produces reinnervation is somewhat lacking, despite a report by Anonsen and colleagues on this topic.[56] Until physiologic data are presented and confirmation by other surgeons is obtained, the procedure has potential but remains unproved.

Neurotropic Factors

With several growth factors known to promote neuronal survival, application and delivery of the these factors constitute an attractive therapy for nerve injury and surgical repair. The trophic effects of nerve growth factor (NGF), glial cell–derived neurotropic factor (GDNF), brain-derived neurotropic factor (BDNF), and insulin growth factors I and II all are under current investigation.[57] In ongoing rat experiments, embyronic stem cells are used to provide the trophic support factors to the host motor neurons in restitution of the neuromuscular junction.[58] These preliminary findings provide a model for motor unit restoration and a potential therapeutic intervention in the treatment of paralysis. However, these studies are limited to the rat model and require further basic and clinical investigation.

Muscle Transfers

Masseter Transfer

Although masseter and temporalis muscle transfer techniques are effective, generally they should be used only if ipsilateral cable nerve grafting is not possible. For most patients with viable facial muscle endplates, a nerve transfer such as hypoglossal facial anastomosis also is preferable to muscle transposition. However, when the proximal facial nerve and the hypoglossal nerve are unavailable, or when facial muscles are surgically absent or atrophied, new contractile muscle must be delivered into the face. A large group of patients who fit into this category are those whose complete paralysis has lasted 2 years or more. These patients usually are characterized by severe denervation atrophy as documented by EMG. In these situations, muscle transfer is the preferred technique of reanimation.

Since the masseter was first used for facial reanimation in 1908, many modifications have been described.[59] Many authors, notably Conley and Baker, prefer the masseter muscle for rehabilitation of the lower face and midface.[30]

The masseter transfer procedure generally is performed for rehabilitation of the sagging paralyzed oral commissure and the buccal-smile complex of muscles. The masseter's upper origin from the zygomatic arch allows a predominantly posterosuperior pull on the lower midface. Transfer of the muscle can be accomplished externally through a rhytidectomy-parotidectomy incision, or intraorally using a mucosal incision in the gingivobuccal sulcus lateral to the ascending ramus of the mandible (Fig. 172-7). The masseter's blood supply is medial and deep, and its nerve supply passes through the sigmoid notch between the condylar and the coronoid processes of the mandible to reach the upper deep surface of the muscle. The nerve supply then ramifies and courses distally and inferiorly, terminating near the periosteal attachments on the lateral aspect of the mandibular angle and body. In general, the external approach is preferred, insofar as the intraoral approach is associated with somewhat limited access, poorer muscle mobilization, and less vascular control.

A generous parotidectomy incision is made and extended inferiorly below the mastoid tip. The parotid gland and masseteric fascia are exposed. The posterior border of the muscle is freed from the mandible's ascending ramus and at the lower border of the mandible. The nerve supply courses along the deep surface approximately midway between the anterior and the posterior borders of the muscle (see Fig. 172-7). It is advisable to preserve the deep fascial layer in dissecting the muscle free from the mandible. Mobilization of the periosteal attachments along the inferior border will provide secure tissue for anchoring sutures and will provide greater length of the transposed muscle.

Dissection is then carried forward to the nasolabial fold in the subcutaneous plane using large Metzenbaum or rhytidectomy scissors. The external incisions are made at or just medial to the nasolabial fold, the lateral oral commissure, and the vermilion cutaneous junction of the lower lip. Each of these incisions is connected to the cheek tunnel, allowing transfer of the masseter muscle. The muscle may be divided into three slips for attachment at these sites, or the entire periosteal end of the muscle may be used to suture the remnants of the orbicularis oris muscle from the lateral upper lip to the commissure and below. These muscle slips are sutured to the dermis and the orbicularis oris muscle using 3-0 clear nylon sutures. The best results depend on gross overcorrection with hyperelevation of the oral commisure, preservation of masseteric nerve supply, secure suture stabilization of the transposed muscle, supportive tape dressing to maintain overcorrection of the oral commissure, and nasogastric feedings to minimize masseteric movement.

Results from the masseteric procedure are quite gratifying and usually yield a high degree of facial symmetry. However, the masseter's arc of rotation will not allow for rehabilitation around the orbit. For this reason, the temporalis transfer can be combined with masseter transfer, or the reanimation of the orbital region can be approached separately with such procedures as canthoplasty and gold weights.

Temporalis Transfer

Although Gillies[60] usually is given credit for introducing the temporalis procedure, Rubin[61,62] deserves much credit for refining the goals of the procedure and the operative technique in the United States. Like the masseter transfer, the temporalis transfer procedure requires an intact ipsilateral V_3 nerve. The nerve supply to the temporalis lies along the deep surface of the muscle. The blood supply comes from the deep temporal vessels from the external carotid artery. Thus, with total parotidectomy, extensive neck dissection, or infratemporal fossa dissection, the neurovascular supply may be tenuous at best. The upper origin of the temporalis muscle is fan-shaped and arises from the periosteum of the entire temporal fossa. The muscle belly converges on a short tendinous portion deep to the zygomatic arch and inserts on the coronoid process. The muscle is best exposed through an incision that passes above the ear, slightly posteriorly, and then in an anteromedial arc. This will expose the entire upper portion of the muscle (Fig. 172-8). A convenient aponeurotic dissection plane exists lateral to the temporalis fascia.

In Rubin's technique, the muscle is dissected free from the periosteum and attached to fascial strips, which are turned down inferiorly to reach the oral commissure and eyelid area. If these fascial strips are omitted, the transposed muscle's length will be insufficient to reach the lateral oral commissure. More recently, Rubin[62] refined his temporalis transfer technique by including a slip of masseter muscle that is sutured to the oral commissure and lower lip. The resulting masseteric pull improves results by providing more posterior and lateral vectors to the oral commissure.

We prefer to use the technique described by Baker and Conley,[50] who describe retaining the integrity of the upper muscle and its overlying fascia. The latter is dissected free and then turned inferiorly for suturing to the oral commissure.

A tunnel at least 1 to 1.5 inches wide must be made over the zygomatic arch to allow the muscle to turn inferiorly and eliminate an unsightly bulge. The attachment of the strip should be just medial to the nasolabial fold so that the natural crease is reproduced by the muscle pull. As with the masseteric procedure, a marked overcorrection is necessary on the operating table. A soft silicone block or a temporoparietal fascia flap may be used to fill the temporal hollow. A modification of this technique by Sherris[63] is performed by extending the transfer into the midregion of the upper and lower lips, to reduce stretching and thinning of the lips over time.

Several modifications of the temporalis transfer have been reported in attempts to avoid folding of the temporalis muscle over the zygomatic arch. Labbé and Huault[64] describe partial inferior mobilization of the temporalis muscle from the skull by elevation of the posterior and superior attachments of the muscle. The coronoid attachments of the muscle are detached, and the muscle is inferiorly mobilized toward the upper lip. The coronoid insertion of the inferiorly displaced muscle is secured to the perioral musculature.

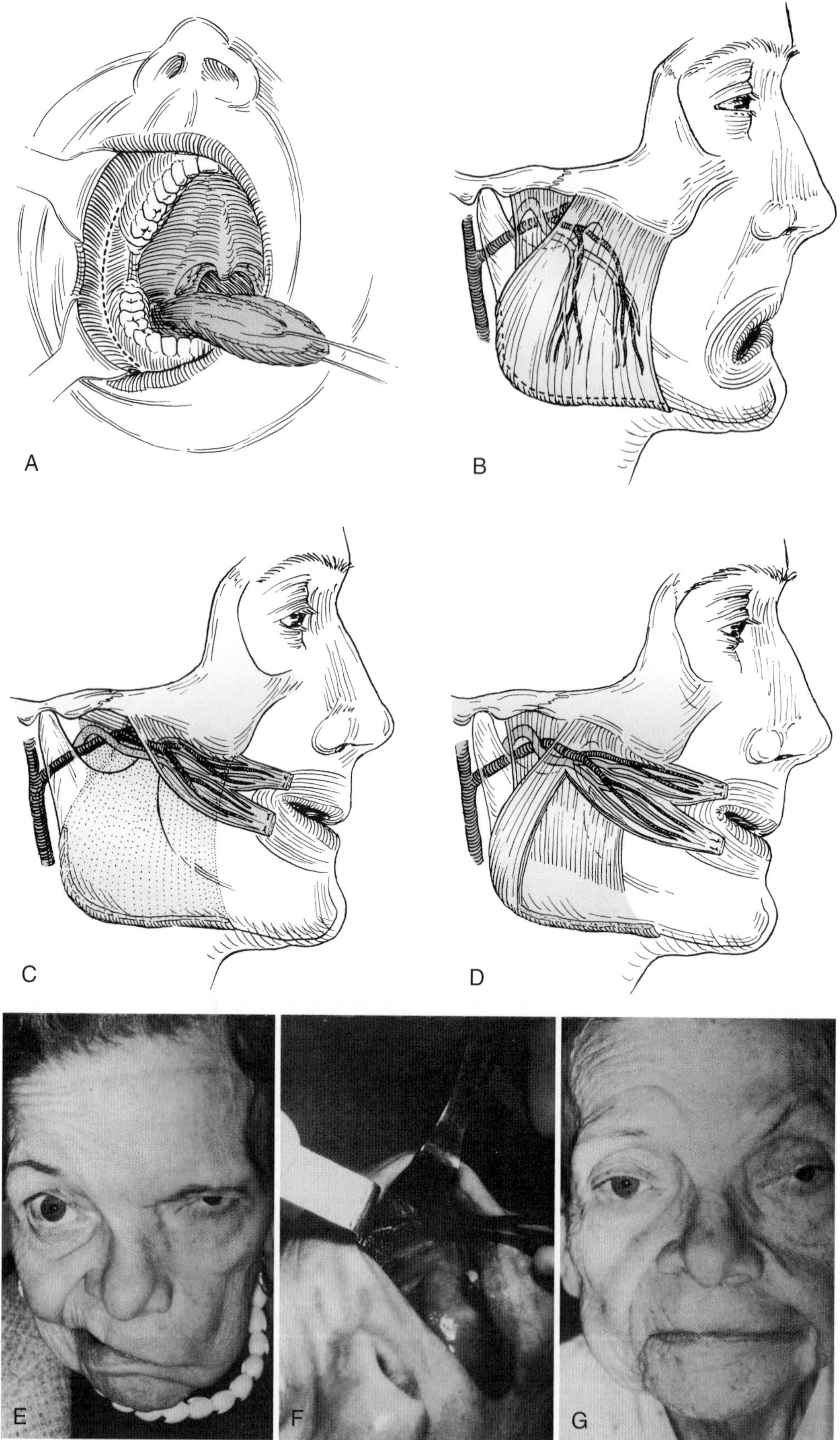

Figure 172-7. Masseter transfer procedure. **A** to **D,** Schematic depiction of key surgical principles. **A,** Intraoral approach to masseter. The procedure is more difficult when performed in this manner; an external approach is preferred. **B,** Correct incisions in muscle and periosteum. Periosteum must be incorporated in the lower portion of the muscle flap to leave the tissue secure for suturing to the lip region. **C** and **D,** Entire muscle, rather than only anterior elements, is transposed, so that the masseteric nerve supply is transferred intact with muscle belly. **E** to **G,** Use of intraoral masseter transfer for correction of complete left peripheral facial paralysis in an elderly woman. **E,** Note severe brow ptosis, medial tarsorrhaphy, and severe redundancy of cheek, paranasal, and lateral lip tissues on the left. **F,** Intraoperative photograph showing intraoral masseter transfer. Large Kelly clamp is used to grasp the inferior portion of the masseter, which will be passed through the cheek tissues to a nasolabial fold incision (see **A** through **D**). **G,** Photograph taken after browlift procedure (tarsorrhaphy has been left for eye safety). Masseter transfer has successfully raised the corner of the mouth and the nasolabial fold. The patient declined further excision of the nasolabial fold for improved cosmesis.

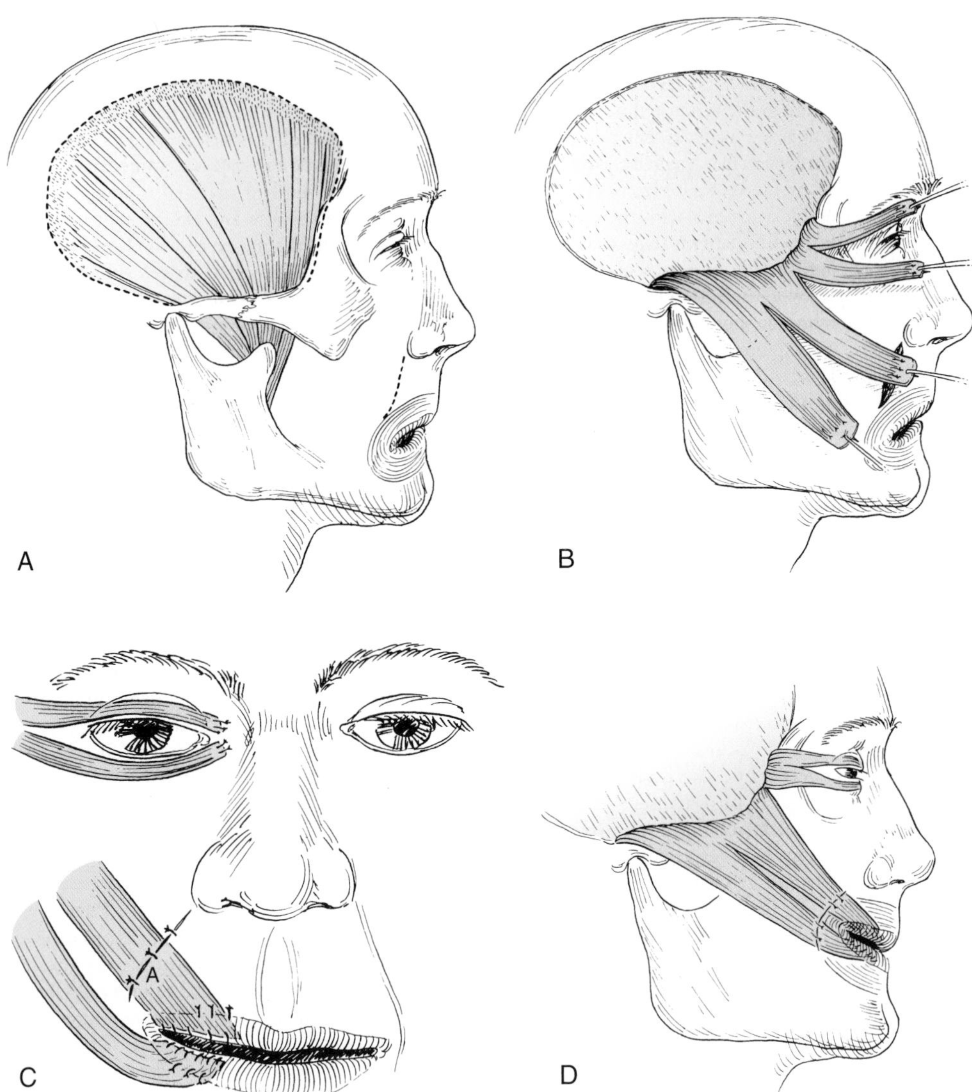

Figure 172-8. Temporalis muscle transposition. **A,** *Dotted line* illustrates the incision in the pericranium peripheral to the edge of the muscle. This results in strong periosteum to hold sutures in the transposed position. Nerve supply on deep side of muscle is not shown. **B,** Temporalis muscle divided into four slips. Note pericranium at the end of the slips sutured to the muscle to reinforce the suture site. Temporal fascia superficial to the muscle can be used in the same way. **C,** Transposed slips sutured to perioral muscles. Creativity and compulsivity are crucial during this portion of procedure. Overcorrection is mandatory. Sutures (A) must be placed in subdermis inferior to incision or in the submucosal portion of the wound deep to the orbicularis oris muscle. **D,** Completed procedure. Wide tunnel over the zygomatic arch precludes an unsightly bulge of muscle, which would otherwise be produced. Superior pull of temporalis muscle is somewhat preferred to posterolateral pull of masseter muscle (see Fig. 172-7).

Although the gold weight–canthoplasty technique often is preferred, the temporalis muscle can be used for orbital rehabilitation. The anterior third of the temporalis muscle is turned laterally into the eyelids (see Fig. 172-8). Subcutaneous tunnel dissection between the paralyzed orbicularis oculi and the eyelid skin allows passage of the fascial strips medially through both eyelids to the medial canthus, where they are sutured. As with any reconstructive procedure, adjustments and suture revisions should be checked carefully on the operating table to ensure proper eyelid contour.

With both masseter and temporalis transfer, facial muscle activation originates from the trigeminal nerve. Patients need to learn, through videotape, biofeedback, or similar methods, the proper way to contract the muscles by chewing or biting. Some younger patients may actually learn how to incorporate these movements into their own facial expressions (e.g., smiles, grimaces). However, patients should be told preoperatively that muscle transfer procedures will not allow any emotional or involuntary reanimation. When performed in the best hands, these techniques provide symmetry and tone in repose, with some learned and induced movements on attempted chewing.

Microneurovascular Muscle Transfer

Microneurovascular muscle transfer was popularized in the 1970s and has been combined with cross-face nerve grafting to restore some facial movement.[65] Because facial movements are highly complex and interrelated, enthusiasm for free muscle transfer was stimulated by the potential to use muscles that may provide isolated or independent segmental contractions, such as for superior elevation of the oral commissure. In patients with absence of facial musculature (such as those with congenital paralysis as in Möbius syndrome), microneurovascular muscle transfer seems to have strong potential.

A number of muscles and their respective nerve supply have been used for microneurovascular transfers. The most popular muscles include the gracilis, latissimus dorsi, and pectoralis minor muscle flaps.[66] Ideally, the proximal stump of the ipsilateral facial nerve is used, but this often is not possible. Traditionally, reinnervation has been accomplished in two stages, with a preliminary cross-face nerve graft performed approximately 1 year before muscle transfer. Neural ingrowth within the grafted nerve is monitored by recording progression of Tinel's sign along the path of the graft. When reinnervation of the graft has occurred, microvascular muscle transfer is then performed. One-stage procedures using long neurovascular pedicles connected directly to the contralateral facial nerve have been described.[67-70] A recent comparison study found favorable outcomes with the one-stage reconstruction compared to the more traditional two-stage reconstruction.[70] Muscle preservation using implantable intramuscular stimulators is under investigation and may allow preservation of facial muscles while reinnervation occurs.[71] This technique shows promise in management of peripheral nerve injuries, and exploratory studies on the facial nerve have been initiated. When facial nerve input is not available, alternative nerves can be used for input, including the masseteric branch of V_3, ansa hypoglossi, or the hypoglossal nerve.[66,72]

Composite tissue allograft procedures have gained considerable interest over the last 10 years. Devauchelle[73] and Dubernard[74] and their colleagues detailed the preliminary functional improvements of the first human partial face transplant, with the return of light touch, heat and cold perception, and mouth closure. These functional milestones were obtained by 10 months postoperatively; a normal smile was observed at 18 months. As with all tissue transplantation, however, immunosuppression is an essential adjunct and not without consequence. After transplantation, the patient suffered two episodes of acute rejection, two infectious complications (type 1 herpes simplex virus infection and molluscum contagiosum), renal failure, moderate thrombotic microangiopathy, and hemolytic anemia. These preliminary findings reveal a new dimension of reconstructive surgery while also underscoring the inherent benefits of native tissues in facial reconstruction.

Significant advances in microvascular techniques and one-stage microneurovascular facial rehabilitation have greatly improved the functional outcome for appropriately selected patients. These techniques are complex, requiring expertise in both microvascular techniques and facial reconstruction. In general, patients with absent distal facial nerve fibers or intact facial musculature who are motivated to attain dynamic function are potential candidates for these procedures.

Static Procedures

Although reinnervation techniques and dynamic slings (muscular transfers) generally provide the best functional outcomes, a number of static procedures still constitute an appropriate option for selected patients. Use of static techniques is indicated in debilitated persons with poor prognosis for survival and in those for whom nerve or muscle is not available for dynamic procedures. The primary benefit of static procedures is immediate restoration of symmetry in the midface. Success depends on mastering several techniques and selective application using sound clinical judgment. Static suspension relies on elevation and positioning the soft tissues of the oral commissure or nasal ala (or both), most commonly by attaching graft materials, which are elevated and secured to the temporal-zygomatic region. Several major benefits arise from the use of static slings. First, facial symmetry at rest can be achieved immediately. Second, better control of problems associated with ptosis of the oral commissure (e.g., drooling, disarticulation with air escape, difficulty with mastication) is achieved. Finally, nasal obstruction caused by alar soft tissue collapse can be dramatically relieved by resuspension and fixation of the nasal alar complex.

Several materials have been used for static suspension. The most common have been fascia lata[75] and acellular human dermis (Alloderm).[76] In the past, expanded polytetrafluoroethylene (PTFE) (i.e., Gore-Tex) has been used more frequently.[77] The acellular dermis preparation and PTFE have the advantage of avoiding donor site morbidity, but use of foreign materials carries a small risk of infection, which is of greater concern in persons undergoing radiation therapy.

Static Facial Sling

Technique

The implant can be placed through a preauricular or temporal incision. In patients with a well-developed contralateral nasolabial fold, a nasolabial incision may be used instead. Additional incisions are made at the vermilion border of the upper and lower lips, adjacent to the commissure. A subcutaneous dissection plane is created to connect the temporal region to the oral commissure. In selected patients with nasal alar collapse and nasal obstruction from soft tissue ptosis, the dissection is extended to include the midface immediately adjacent to the nasal ala. A single strip of implant material is adequate for the procedure. This is cut to appropriate size and can be split near the end to include slips for attachment to the upper and the lower lips. Permanent sutures are placed to secure the implant to the orbicularis oris muscle and deep dermis. Resorbable sutures are placed in the deep dermis to secure the material just medial to the proposed nasolabial fold. Similar fixation is performed for a strip to the ala if desired. The sling is then suspended and secured with permanent suture to the temporalis fascia, or to the periosteum of the zygoma or zygomatic arch. If fascia lata or acellular human dermis (AHD) is used, overcorrection of the smile is achieved before fixation. Current interest has been developed in the suspension of implant materials along the nasolabial fold with suture anchoring to the deep temporal fascia.[78] In similar fashion, mimicking of the contralateral crease is achieved through suture tension along various points.

Adjunctive Procedures

A number of adjunctive procedures are available to "fine-tune" the results in persons undergoing facial rehabilitative procedures. Optimizing the care of patients with facial paralysis requires a full range of techniques in the surgical armamentarium. Although reinnervation techniques and measures to protect the eye take precedence, a number of options allow "fine-tuning" of results for the patient with facial paralysis. These can be broadly subdivided into procedures to rehabilitate the upper, middle, and lower thirds of the face. Finally, synkinesis can be a major concern, and treatment options for synkinesis are available as well.

Procedures for Upper Third of the Face

Paralysis of the upper third of the face produces significant functional and cosmetic deformities. Brow ptosis may cause superior visual field deficits as well significant facial asymmetry. This asymmetry may be further accentuated after procedures to address the lower face. Browlift techniques to manage paralytic ptosis are the same as for a cosmetic browlift, the only significant technical difference being exercise of restraint to avoid further compromising eyelid closure. Direct, midforehead, endoscopic, and indirect browlifts are all effective. When not overdone, a browlift in conjunction with lid loading or lower eyelid tightening, or both, generally produces satisfactory cosmetic and functional results. Brow ptosis associated with normal aging may be accentuated unnaturally by a unilateral lift, and in older patients, improved results are seen when bilateral browlifts are performed.[79]

Many patients with facial paralysis, particularly older persons, will express interest in additional adjunctive procedures in the periocular region. In patients with excessive redundant eyelid skin, conservative blepharoplasty can decrease superior visual field defects while cosmetically addressing brow ptosis and excessive tissue folds. Extreme caution is necessary in performing blepharoplasty in conjunction with browlift procedures. The risk of further impairing eye closure mandates a conservative approach. A maneuver to help assess the amount of skin to be safely removed consists of manually holding the paralyzed brow in the normal position with observation for impairment of eyelid closure. Similarly, it also is helpful to pinch together the excessive eyelid skin to be resected while holding the brow superiorly and observing its effect on eye closure.

Procedures for Middle Third of the Face

The middle third of the face is most commonly rehabilitated using reinnervation techniques, dynamic slings, or static slings. A number of additional procedures are available to fine-tune the results obtained with these procedures, and selection of the appropriate procedure(s) is determined by both the defect and the desires of the patient.

Nasal obstruction after facial paralysis can occur because of collapse of the alar sidewall from adjacent soft tissue ptosis and loss of intrinsic dilator naris tone. As described, a properly designed static

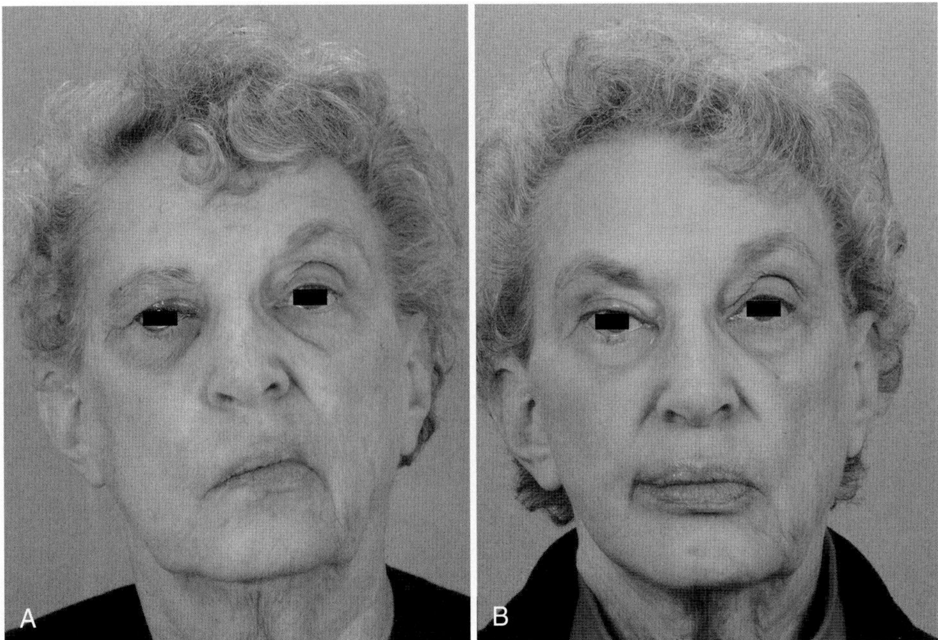

Figure 172-9. Result with static rehabilitation techniques in a patient with right facial paralysis:. Preoperative **(A)** and postoperative **(B)** photographs. Patient underwent direct browlift, lateral transorbital canthopexy, alloderm facial sling repair, and gold weight placement.

sling may alleviate this problem. Alar batten grafting also may provide relief.

Midface soft tissue laxity and sagging, characteristic of the aging midface, is abnormally pronounced in the paralyzed face. In older patients with significant skin laxity, performing a facelift enhances the results of other treatments for midface deformity. Facelifts can be performed concurrently with other procedures, whether dynamic or static, and some patients will benefit from and prefer a bilateral facelift (Fig. 172-9).

Like the aging patient, the patient with facial paralysis acquires ptotic palpebral-malar and nasojugal sulci, producing a hollowed-out appearance to these areas. The lower eyelid fat may bulge, and the suborbicularis oculi fat (SOOF) and midface complex descend, producing a "double convexity" sign on lateral view. In the youthful patient, the suborbicularis oculi fat typically lies at the inferior orbital rim between the orbicularis oculi muscle and the periosteum. The midface lift repositions the SOOF and associated midface soft tissue superior to its preexisting position. The lift has become a popular technique in facial rejuvenation surgery, and also has shown utility in the treatment of facial paralysis. The midface lift can be performed through a transconjunctival incision, with a lateral canthotomy and inferior cantholysis. The periosteum is incised near the orbital rim and is elevated down to the inferior maxilla, where it is released. It also is important to release the attachment to the masseter muscle. Care is taken to avoid injury to the infraorbital nerve. The periosteum and overlying soft tissue are then elevated and secured superiorly to the deep temporal fascia.

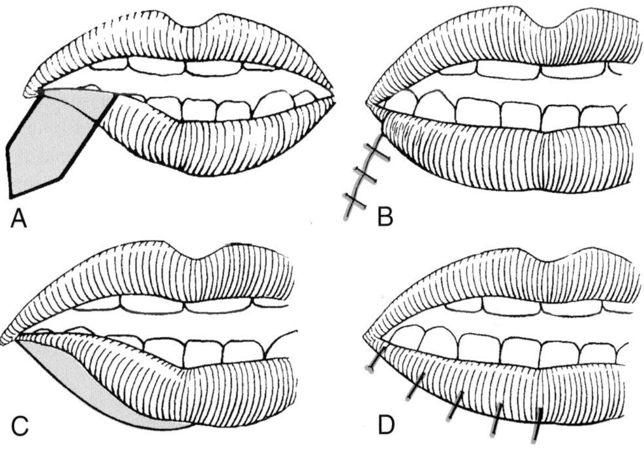

Figure 172-10. Lip wedge excision and cheiloplasty. **A,** Outline of incisions for lip wedge excision. Excision tightens the lower lip and removes part of the denervated muscle. **B,** Appearance after lip resection. Note the intentional asymmetry of vermilion border during closure to evert the lower lip. **C,** Outline of incisions for cheiloplasty. **D,** Appearance of cheiloplasty after resection. Note lowering and outward rotation of the lower lip *(Adapted from Glenn MG, Goode RL. Surgical treatment of the "marginal mandibular lip" deformity.* Otolaryngol Head Neck Surg. *1987;97:464-465.)*

Procedures for Lower Third of the Face

The functional deficits with paralysis of the lower face are dominated by manifestations of oral incompetence. Drooling, air escape with speech, and difficulty with mastication may be present. The asymmetry also produces a significant aesthetic deformity. This is due to the lack of a smile (loss of zygomaticus function) as well as the lack of depressor anguli oris (marginal mandibular nerve) function. These defects can be worsened by performance of static procedures on the middle third of the face, which can produce a troublesome gap in the region of the commissure from elevation of the upper lip.

Reinnervation, free tissue transfer, dynamic slings, and to some degree even static slings assist in repositioning the oral commissure to re-create a more symmetric smile. The asymmetry of depressor function, the so-called "marginal mandibular lip," is more troublesome and difficult to improve. The most commonly used procedures are wedge resection and transposition of the posterior belly of the digastric muscle. The wedge resection, with or without supplemental cheiloplasty technique to improve symmetry and oral competence, has been described by Glenn and Goode.[80] A 2- to 2.5-cm full-thickness excision is performed 7 to 10 mm lateral to the commissure (Fig. 172-10).

The most common dynamic technique for depressor dysfunction is the digastric transposition, first described by Conley and colleagues.[81] The digastric tendon is identified using a submandibular approach. It is released from the hyoid bone, transected near the mastoid tip, transposed superiorly, and attached to the orbicularis oris through a separate vermilion border incision. Care is taken to preserve the mylohyoid nerve innervating the anterior belly of the digastric muscle. The anterior belly of the digastric muscle may not be available after extirpative cancer surgery, however.[82]

Management of Synkinesis

Patients with incomplete recovery from facial paralysis typically are troubled by both weakness and hyperkinesis, or synkinesis. Synkinesis develops in many patients after facial paralysis of any cause. These uncoordinated mass movements may begin within weeks after paralysis as regeneration occurs. Although the classic description of synkinesis places the etiologic mechanism in aberrant axonal regeneration, it is now known that the sites of pathology are multiple. Synaptic stripping also occurs in the facial nucleus of the brainstem, and ephaptic (nonsynaptic) transmission among axons contributes to synkinesis. Future efforts to prevent or treat synkinesis will require addressing each of these areas. Synkinesis ranges in severity from a mild, barely noticeable tic to painful and debilitating mass facial movements.

Careful assessment of each region of the face is performed. It is esssential to identify the patient's most troublesome symptoms and then determine which symptoms result from decreased function and which from synkinesis. The treatment plan can then be individualized to address the patient's needs.

Traditionally, neurolysis has been a mainstay in the management of synkinesis, but it has been largely abandoned as safer and more conservative yet effective techniques have evolved. Such techniques include chemodenervation with botulinum A toxin injections and selective myectomies to target affected muscles.

Botulinum A Toxin

Botulinum A toxin is the most potent poison known to humankind, yet it has been used effectively for more than 2 decades to treat a variety of hyperfunctional disorders including torticollis,[52] blepharospasm,[83] spasmodic dysphonia,[84] strabismus,[85] hyperhidrosis,[86] hyperdynamic skin creases,[87] palatal myoclonus,[88] hemifacial spasm,[89] and facial synkinesis.[90,91] Botulinum toxin causes paralysis by blocking the presynaptic release of acetylcholine at the neuromuscular junction. This typically results in paralysis of the treated muscle for approximately 3 to 6 months. Systemic weakness can occur with doses greater than 200 units. The lethal dose is approximately 40 units/kg.[92]

Botulinum toxin has dramatically improved the management of patients with facial movement disorders. It is now a first-line agent for treatment of facial synkinesis. In most persons, surgical treatment is not necessary or desired. Synkinesis after facial nerve injury can occur in any region of the face, and botulinum toxin can be used to denervate specific muscle groups. The location of the injections is targeted to the muscles causing synkinesis. Typically, 1 to 5 units is injected per site. Initial treatments use conservative doses, which subsequently can be titrated upwards. No anesthesia generally is necessary, but many patients prefer pretreatment of the area with ice or a topical anesthetic. Drug effects are first seen several days after the injection, with a maximal effect observed at 5 to 7 days. Additional toxin can be injected after this time if the initial effect is insufficient.

Adverse effects can occur, related to the diffusion of toxin into surrounding muscles. An example is the development of ptosis after periocular injection. This problem is uncommon, occurring in perhaps 5% of cases. It can be treated with apraclonidine 0.5% drops administered to the affected eye three or four times a day until the ptosis resolves.[93] Apraclonidine causes contraction of Müller's muscle to elevate the upper eyelid. Other complications from botulinum toxin treatment of the face include diplopia, further impairment of eyelid closure, lower eyelid ectropion, brow ptosis, and drooling.

In some patients, the effectiveness of botulinum toxin decreases over time. This diminishing effect may be the result of resprouting of motor endplates or the development of neutralizing antibodies and cannot be overcome with increased doses of the toxin.[94] Patients who do not benefit from botulinum toxin treatments or demonstrate the development of resistance, or who desire a more permanent solution, may be candidates for selective myectomy.

Selective Myectomy

The development of botulinum toxin has significantly expanded the options available to the surgeon caring for a patient with synkinesis. Some patients, however, will prefer something more permanent or may exhibit unsatisfactory results with botulinum toxin injection. These patients may be candidates for selective myectomy.

Neurolysis was for many years the procedure of choice for these patients. Although Fisch[95] reported excellent results, others did not have the same success.[96] Paralytic ectropion, lagophthalmos, lip paresis, oral incompetence, blunted facial expression, and other complications from neurolysis have been reported.[97,98] Myectomy has been offered as a safer, more specific procedure for permanent resolution of synkinesis after facial paralysis.[96] Myectomy results in a more predictable result because the removed muscle does not regrow, a phenomenon that can be seen with neurolysis. In patients desiring no further treatment with botulinum toxin, or for whom botulinum toxin was ineffective, a myectomy may be performed. Selective myectomies can be performed on synkinetic facial muscles.

Summary

A variety of techniques are available for facial nerve rehabilitation after paralysis. The surgeon should know the advantages and disadvantages of the various techniques to apply them properly in each clinical situation. Thorough knowledge of neuromuscular pathophysiology also is important in the understanding of how time affects the available rehabilitative procedures. When properly informed of the limitations of these operative procedures, most patients can be rehabilitated and many of their symptoms can be alleviated.

SUGGESTED READINGS

Barrs DM. Facial nerve trauma: optimal timing for repair. *Laryngoscope.* 1991;101:835.

Bernstein L, Nelson RH. Surgical anatomy of the extraparotid distribution of the facial nerve. *Arch Otolaryngol.* 1984;110:177.

Borodic GE, Pearce LB, Cheney M, et al. Botulinum A toxin for treatment of aberrant facial nerve regeneration. *Plast Reconstr Surg.* 1993;91:1042.

Clark JM, Shockley W. Management of reanimation of the paralyzed face. In: Papel I, Larrabee W, Holt G, Park S, Sykes J, eds. *Facial Plastic and Reconstructive Surgery.* 2nd ed. New York: Thieme Medical Publishers; 2002:660.

Conley J, Baker DC. Myths and misconceptions in the rehabilitation of facial paralysis. *Plast Reconstr Surg.* 1983;71:538.

Conley J, Baker DC. The surgical treatment of extratemporal facial paralysis: an overview. *Head Neck Surg.* 1978;1:12.

Fisch U. Extracranial surgery for facial hyperkinesis. In: May M, ed. *The Facial Nerve.* New York: Thieme Medical Publishers; 1986:535.

Fisch U, ed. *Facial Nerve Surgery.* Birmingham, Ala: Aesculapius Publishing; 1977.

Fisher E, Frodel JL. Facial suspension with acellular human dermal allograft. *Arch Facial Plast Surg.* 1999;1:195.

Freeman MS, Thomas JR, Spector JG, et al. Surgical therapy of the eyelids in patients with facial paralysis. *Laryngoscope.* 1990;100:1086.

House JW, Brackmann DE. Facial nerve grading system. *Otolaryngol Head Neck Surg.* 1985;93:146.

Jelks GW, Smith B, Bosniak S. The evaluation and management of the eye in facial palsy. *Clin Plast Surg.* 1979;6:397.

Kazanjian VH, Converse JM. Facial palsy. In: Converse JM, ed. *Surgical Treatment of Facial Injuries.* Baltimore: Williams & Wilkins; 1974.

Kumar PA, Hassan KM. Cross-face nerve graft with free-muscle transfer for reanimation of the paralyzed face: a comparative study of the single-stage and two-stage procedures. *Plast Reconstr Surg.* 2002;109:451.

Levine R. Eyelid reanimation surgery. In: May M, ed. *The Facial Nerve.* New York: Thieme Medical Publishers; 1986.

May M, Sobol SM, Mester SJ. Hypoglossal-facial nerve interpositional-jump graft for facial reanimation without tongue atrophy. *Otolaryngol Head Neck Surg.* 1991;104:818.

Miehlke A, Stennert E, Chilla R. New aspects in facial nerve surgery. *Clin Plast Surg.* 1979;6:451.

Patel BCK, Anderson RL, May M. Selective myectomy. In: May M, Schaitkin BM, eds. *The Facial Nerve.* 2nd ed. New York: Thieme Medical Publishers; 2001:467.

Rubin LR: Reanimation of total unilateral facial paralysis by the contiguous facial muscle technique. In: Rubin LR, ed. *The Paralyzed Face.* St Louis: Mosby; 1991. pp 156-177.

Rubin LR, Lee GW, Simpson RI. Reanimation of the long-standing partial facial paralysis. *Plast Reconstr Surg.* 1986;77:41.

Shindo M. Facial reanimation with microneurovascular free flaps. *Facial Plast Surg.* 2000;16:357.

Smith JD, Crumley RL, Harker LA. Facial paralysis in the newborn. *Otolaryngol Head Neck Surg.* 1981;89:1021.

Wesley RE, Jackson CG. Facial palsy. In: Hornblass A, ed. *Oculoplastic, Orbital and Reconstructive Surgery. Vol I: Eyelids.* Baltimore: Williams & Wilkins; 1988.

For complete list of references log onto www.expertconsult.com.

Cranial Base

CHAPTER ONE HUNDRED AND SEVENTY-THREE

Surgical Anatomy of the Lateral Skull Base

Oswaldo Laércio M. Cruz

Key Points

- The temporal bone articulates with five other cranial bones and forms many sutures and foramina through which pass critical neural and vascular structures.
- Along with the greater wing of the sphenoid and a portion of the parietal bone, the temporal bone forms the lateral boundary of the middle cranial fossa.
- The petrous bone is a key element of the osseous anatomy of the middle and posterior cranial fossae.
- Medial and posterior to the foramen ovale the middle meningeal artery enters the middle cranial fossa through the foramen spinosum, and the greater superficial petrosal nerve is located medial to the middle meningeal artery.
- From superior to inferior, the greater superficial petrosal nerve, the tensor tympani muscle, and the eustachian tube all proceed in a similar anteroposterior plane.
- The greater petrosal nerve, the geniculate ganglion, and the labyrinthine segment of cranial nerve VII form an obtuse angle of approximately 120 degrees. The cochlea is embedded in the bone subtended by that angle.
- The cerebellopontine angle is traversed by the intracranial segments of cranial nerve V (superiorly) to cranial nerve IX (inferiorly) and by the premeatal, meatal, and postmeatal segments of the anterior inferior cerebellar artery (AICA).
- The medial aspect of the internal auditory canal is occupied by its four main neural components: the facial nerve (superior and anterior), the superior vestibular nerve (superior and posterior), the cochlear nerve (anterior and inferior), and the inferior vestibular nerve (posterior and inferior).
- The jugular foramen is located at the petro-occipital region and contains several vital neural and vascular components.
- The infratemporal fossa communicates with the orbit through the inferior orbital fissure, with the middle cranial fossa through the foramen spinosum, and with the pterygopalatine fossa through the pterygomaxillary fissure.

The lateral skull base presents a complex and conceptually challenging anatomy. The temporal bone, occupying a central and strategic position in supporting central nervous system (CNS) structures, articulates with five other cranial bones and forms many sutures and foramina through which pass critical neural and vascular structures. Familiarity with this complex anatomy is mandatory for an understanding of pathologic processes arising in the temporal bone and the middle and posterior cranial fossae, and for safe execution of skull base procedures.

This chapter is divided into four sections, on osseous anatomy of the lateral skull base, anatomy of the middle cranial fossa, anatomy of the posterior cranial fossa, and anatomy of the infratemporal fossa.

Osseous Anatomy of the Lateral Skull Base

The temporal bone occupies a central position at the lateral skull base, being the most important anatomic landmark in the lateral skull base anatomy.[1,2]

On lateral view, the squamosa presents a shape reminiscent of an open wing of a bird (Fig. 173-1). From its middle and caudal portions it contributes to the zygomatic arch and forms the superior wall of the external auditory canal. Its articulation with the tympanic bone in the anterosuperior external auditory canal forms the tympanosquamous suture. The zygomatic bone portion contributes to the roof of the glenoid fossa and the anterior part of the tympanic bone forms its posterior wall.

Along with the greater wing of the sphenoid and a portion of the parietal bone, the temporal bone forms the lateral boundary of the middle cranial fossa (Figs. 173-2 and 173-3). This medial aspect of the squamous bone forms the petrosquamous suture, which joins the caudal portion of the squamosa and the lateral superior portion of the petrosa. Anteriorly, at the articulation of the sphenoid with the squamous bone, is located the foramen spinosum, through which passes the middle meningeal artery into the cranium. The sulcus of this artery is easily identified on the medial surface of the squamosa (see Figs. 173-2 and 173-3).

The tympanic bone lies just inferior to the squamous portion and anterior to the mastoid and forms the tympanosquamous and tympanomastoid sutures with them (see Fig. 173-1). It is common for one edge of these suture lines (especially the tympanosquamous suture) to project as a spinous process exteding 1 to 3 mm into the lumen of the external auditory canal.[1,3,4]

The tympanic bone forms the anterior and inferior walls and a portion of the posterior wall of the external auditory meatus and is primarily responsible for the size and shape of the external auditory

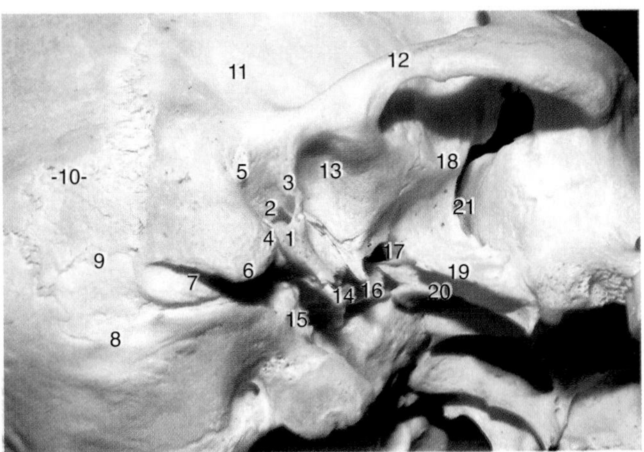

Figure 173-1. Cranium, lateral inferior view (right side): 1, tympanic bone; 2, external auditory canal; 3, tympanosquamous suture; 4, tympanomastoid suture; 5, suprameatal spine; 6, mastoid tip; 7, digastric sulcus; 8, occipital bone; 9, occipitomastoid suture; 10, parietomastoid suture; 11, squamous portion of the temporal bone; 12, zygoma; 13, glenoid fossa; 14, styloid process; 15, jugular foramen; 16, carotid canal; 17, sphenopalatine foramen; 18, greater wing of the sphenoid bone; 19, lateral pterygoid process; 20, medial pterygoid process; 21, pterygomaxillary fossa. *(Courtesy of Oswaldo Laércio M. Cruz, Helder Tedeschi, and Albert Rhoton.)*

canal. As mentioned, it also composes the posterior wall of the glenoid fossa (see Fig. 173-1).

At the medial extension of the external auditory canal, the tympanic bone ends at the tympanic sulcus or annular sulcus, into which the tympanic membrane inserts (Figs. 173-4 and 173-5; see also Fig. 173-1). On its inferior surface, the tympanic bone articulates with the petrous bone, forming the petrotympanic suture. It also contributes to the formation of the internal carotid artery canal (ascending portion) (see Figs. 173-4 and 173-5). Also, on its inferior aspect and lateral to the carotid canal, the tympanic bone forms the styloid process (see Fig. 173-1). Slightly posterior and medial to this process is the stylomastoid foramen, through which the seventh cranial nerve emerges (see Fig. 173-5).

The osseous anterior wall of the external auditory canal abuts the temporomandibular joint and is of variable thickness. The bony inferior wall is thick and related to the anterior aspect of the jugular bulb (posteriorly) and carotid canal (anteriorly) (Fig. 173-6; see also Figs. 173-1, 173-4, and 173-5). The posterior wall separates the external auditory canal from the mastoid cells and the descending portion of the facial nerve (see Fig. 173-6).[3,5]

The mastoid is a pneumatized bony process located at the most posterior and inferior part of the temporal bone that, in reality, can be considered an extension of the squamosa and a lateral projection of the petrous portion (see Figs. 173-1 and 173-2). It has a somewhat triangular form, with the vertex directed inferiorly and the base superiorly.

Anteriorly, the mastoid process forms the tympanomastoid suture as it joins the posterior portion of the tympanic bone. Above and lateral to the tympanomastoid suture is the suprameatal spine, an osseous elevation of variable size that anchors the nonosseous portion of the external auditory canal and auricle. Immediately posterior to this spine and inferior to the temporal line is a slightly depressed region called the cribriform plate, a multiperforated region that serves as a landmark for surgical access to the mastoid antrum (see Fig. 173-1).

Posteriorly, the mastoid portion presents a relationship with the parietal bone superiorly and the occipital bone inferiorly, forming the parietomastoid and occipitomastoid sutures. These two sutures join the occipitoparietal suture at a point called the asterion, an important surgical landmark for craniotomies to achieve posterior fossa access.

Medial to the mastoid tip, the posterior belly of the digastric muscle at its insertion forms an osseous depression or sulcus, running anterior to posterior. At its anterior termination, this sulcus is a land-

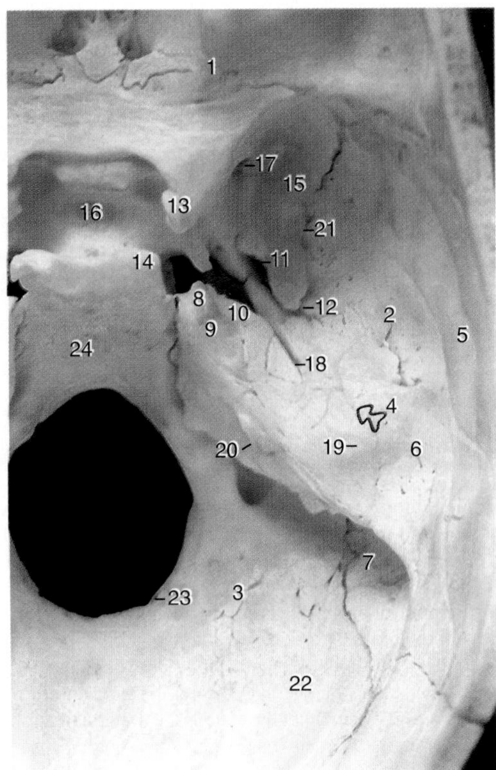

Figure 173-2. Superior view of anterior, middle, and posterior fossae, with the projection of petrous portion of temporal bone: 1, anterior fossa; 2, middle fossa; 3, posterior fossa; 4, petrous bone projection *(arrow)*; 5, squamous portion of the temporal bone; 6, mastoid tegmen; 7, sigmoid sinus impression; 8, petrous apex; 9, trigeminal depression (Meckel's cave); 10, foramen lacerum region; 11, foramen ovale; 12, foramen spinosum; 13, anterior clinoid process; 14, posterior clinoid process; 15, greater wing of sphenoid; 16, sphenoid bone and sella; 17, foramen rotundum; 18, greater petrosal nerve impression; 19, arcuate eminence; 20, internal auditory canal region; 21, petrosphenoid suture; 22, occipital bone; 23, foramen magnum; 24, clivus. *(Courtesy of Oswaldo Laércio M. Cruz, Helder Tedeschi, and Albert Rhoton.)*

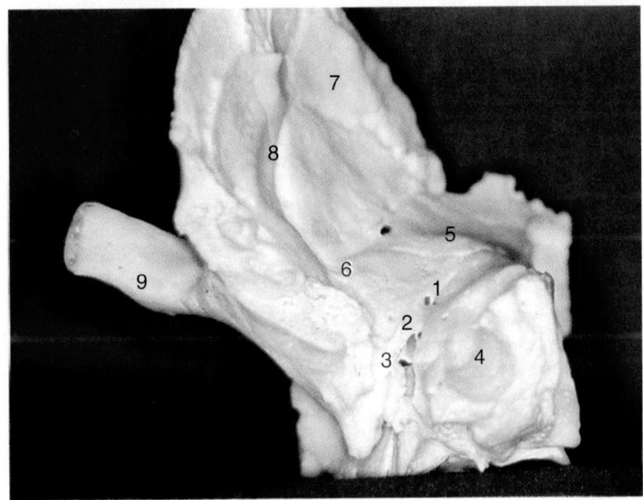

Figure 173-3. Anterior view of temporal bone (right side): 1, facial hiatus; 2, semicanal of the tensor tympani muscle; 3, osseous portion of the eustachian tube; 4, carotid artery canal (end of the horizontal portion); 5, arcuate eminence; 6, petrosquamous suture; 7, squamous portion of the temporal bone; 8, middle meningeal artery sulcus; 9, zygoma. *(Courtesy of Oswaldo Laércio M. Cruz, Helder Tedeschi, and Albert Rhoton.)*

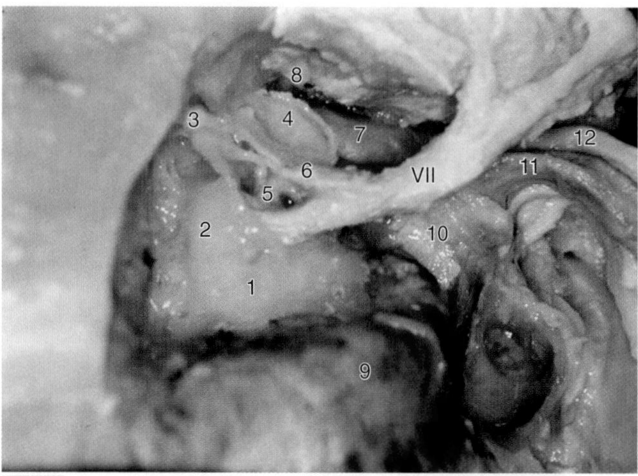

Figure 173-4. Lateral view of right temporal bone after resection of tympanic bone and mastoid and exposure of carotid artery and jugular foramen: 1, posterior semicircular canal; 2, lateral semicircular canal; 3, incus-malleus articulation; 4, tympanic membrane; 5, facial recess with view of round window niche, pyramidal eminence, stapes tendon, and incus-stapes articulation; 6, chorda tympani nerve; 7, carotid artery (ascending portion); 8, eustachian tube opening; 9, sigmoid sinus; 10, jugular bulb; 11, jugular vein (upper cervical portion); 12, cranial nerves X and XI emerging from neural intrajugular compartment of the jugular foramen; VII, facial nerve (seventh cranial nerve). *(Courtesy of Oswaldo Laércio M. Cruz, Helder Tedeschi, and Albert Rhoton.)*

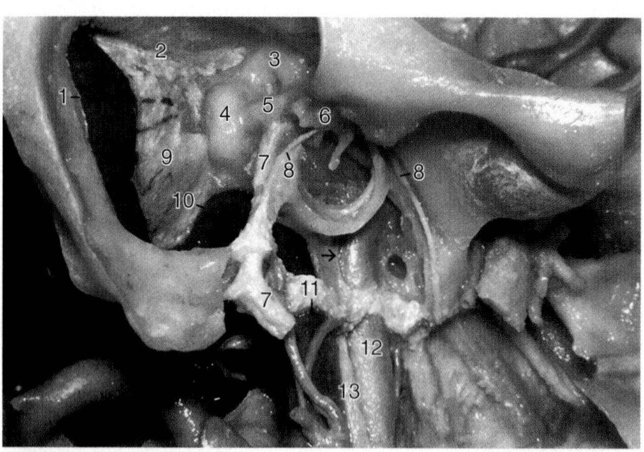

Figure 173-5. Lateral view of right temporal bone with mastoidectomy and resection of the tympanic bone, tympanic membrane, and glenoid process: 1, sigmoid sinus; 2, superior petrous sinus; 3, superior semicircular canal; 4, posterior semicircular canal; 5, lateral semicircular canal; 6, ossicular chain; 7, facial nerve; 8, chorda tympani nerve; 9, Trautmann's triangle—posterior fossa dura; 10, jugular foramen bulb; 11, jugular vein; 12, internal carotid artery: ascending portion and anterior turn or knee *(arrow)*; 13, cranial nerve IX. *(Courtesy of Oswaldo Laércio M. Cruz, Helder Tedeschi, and Albert Rhoton.)*

mark for the descending portion of the facial nerve and the stylomastoid foramen (see Figs. 173-1 and 173-6).

Viewed from above and from inside the cranium, the petrous bone is a key element in the osseous anatomy of the middle and posterior fossae. It has a configuration of a three-sided pyramid (see Fig. 173-2). The base of the pyramid constitutes its lateral surface and articulates with the squamous, tympanic, and mastoid portions of the temporal bone (Fig. 173-7; see also Fig. 173-2). Two sides of the pyramid are clearly recognized as medial projections: one superior, which forms much of the floor of the middle cranial fossa, and the medial surface,

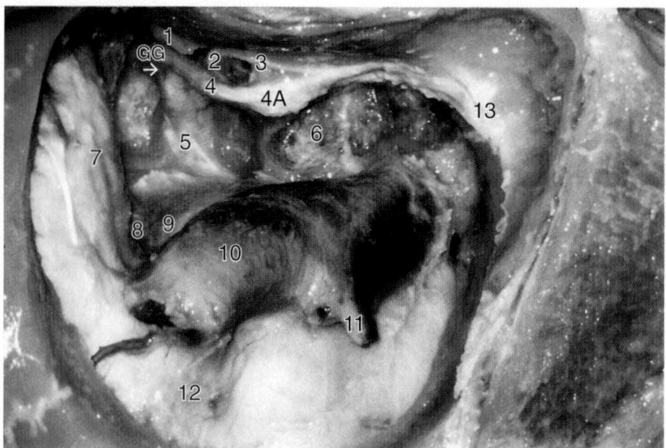

Figure 173-6. Lateral view of a right temporal bone with wide mastoidectomy, resection of the semicircular canals and exposition of the internal auditory canal: 1, incus; 2, stapes; 3, chorda tympani nerve; 4, tympanic portion of facial nerve continuing with mastoid segment (4A); 5, dura of the posterior wall of the internal auditory canal; 6, jugular foramen; 7, middle fossa dura; 8, superior petrosal sinus; 9, Trautmann's triangle (posterior fossa); 10, sigmoid sinus; 11, emissary vein; 12, transverse sinus; 13, digastric groove; GG, geniculate ganglion at the end of the labyrinthine segment of the facial nerve *(arrow)*. *(Courtesy of Oswaldo Laércio M. Cruz, Helder Tedeschi, and Albert Rhoton.)*

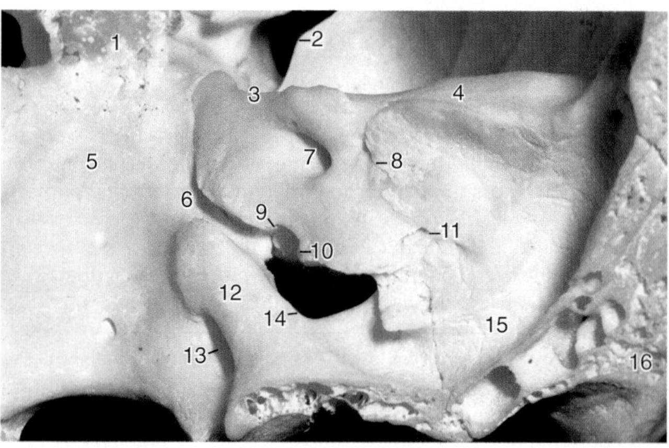

Figure 173-7. Medial view of lateral posterior fossa wall (right side): 1, sella; 2, superior orbital fissure; 3, trigeminal impression; 4, superior petrosal sinus impression; 5, clivus; 6, petro-occipital sulcus; 7, internal auditory canal; 8, subarcuate fossa; 9, cochlear aqueduct; 10, jugular process; 11, vestibular aqueduct; 12, jugular tuberculum; 13, hypoglossal nerve canal; 14, jugular foramen; 15, sigmoid sinus impression; 16, mastoid bone. *(Courtesy of Oswaldo Laércio M. Cruz, Helder Tedeschi, and Albert Rhoton.)*

which faces the posterior cranial fossa, forming most of its lateral wall. The third and inferior side articulates with the occipital bone (see Figs. 173-2 and 173-3). The anterior medial limit of the pyramid (petrous apex) reaches the greater sphenoid wing laterally, the body of the sphenoid medially and superiorly, and the clivus portion of the occipital bone medially and inferiorly (see Figs. 173-2 and 173-3). The petroclival sutures lie on either side of the midline within the circumference of the foramen magnum.

The superior surface of the petrosa forms the major portion of the middle fossa floor and presents key anatomic landmarks for otoneurologic surgery (Figs. 173-8 and 173-9; see also Figs. 173-2 and 173-3). At the most anterior medial portion (apex) is the foramen lacerum, through which passes the end of the horizontal portion of the carotid

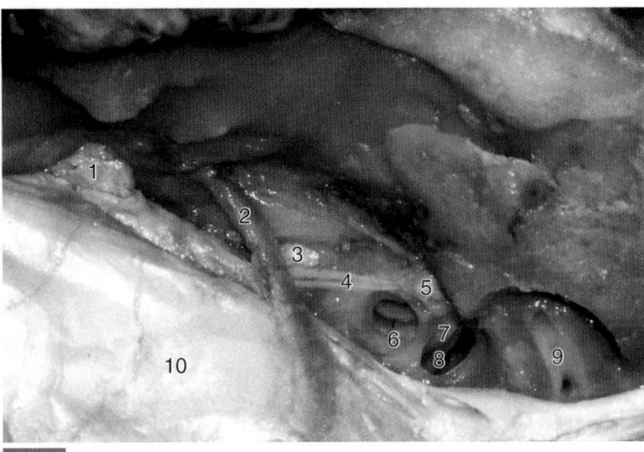

Figure 173-8. Right side view in middle cranial fossa surgical approach. The dura is detached from the temporal bone and the bone from the horizontal portion of carotid artery, cochlea, internal auditory canal, and the superior semicircular canal removed. 1, V_1 entering the foramen ovale; 2, middle meningeal artery coming from the foramen spinosum; 3, horizontal portion of the internal carotid artery; 4, greater superficial petrosal nerve; 5, geniculate ganglion; 6, cochlea; 7, facial nerve in the medial portion of the internal auditory canal; 8, superior vestibular nerve; 9, superior semicircular canal; 10, middle fossa dura. *(Courtesy of Oswaldo Laércio M. Cruz, Helder Tedeschi, and Albert Rhoton.)*

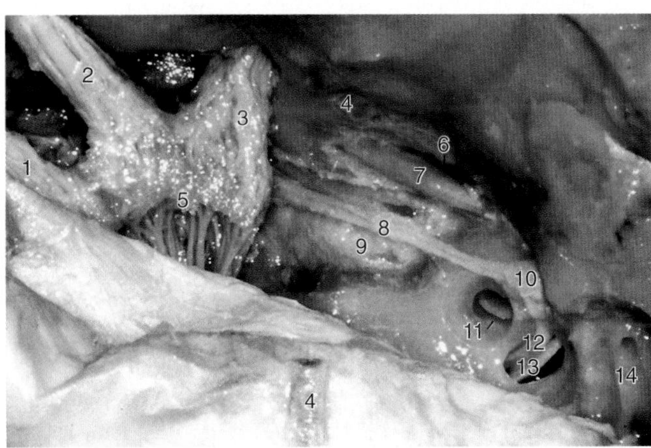

Figure 173-9. Surgical anatomy of the middle fossa approach after gasserian ganglion dissection, middle meningeal artery section, and eustachian tube and tensor tympani muscle exposure. 1, V_1: ophthalmic division of the trigeminal nerve; 2, V_2: maxillary division of the trigeminal nerve; 3, V_3: mandibular division of the trigeminal nerve; 4, middle meningeal artery; 5, gasserian ganglion; 6, eustachian tube; 7, tensor tympani muscle; 8, greater superficial petrosal nerve; 9, internal carotid artery; 10, geniculate ganglion; 11, cochlea; 12, facial nerve; 13, superior vestibular nerve; 14, superior semicircular canal. *(Courtesy of Oswaldo Laércio M. Cruz, Helder Tedeschi, and Albert Rhoton.)*

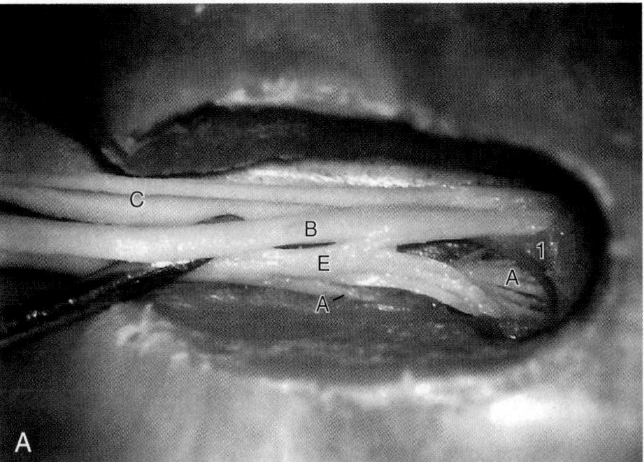

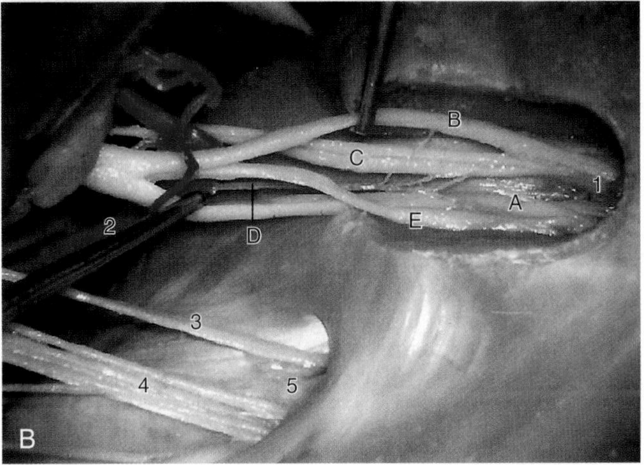

Figure 173-10. A, Closeup posterior view of the nerves in the internal auditory canal (right side). **B,** Close posterior view of the midface showing the petrous bone and internal auditory canal with nerve dissection. 1, transverse crest; 2, AICA (anterior inferior cerebellar artery); 3, cranial nerve IX (glossopharyngeal nerve); 4, cranial nerve X (vagus nerve); 5, dural septum; A, cochlear nerve; B, superior vestibular nerve; C, facial nerve and nervus intermedius (of Wrisberg); D, internal auditory artery; E, inferior vestibular nerve. *(Courtesy of Oswaldo Laércio M. Cruz, Helder Tedeschi, and Albert Rhoton.)*

artery on its way to the cavernous sinus. Medial to the foramen lacerum there is a depression in the bone border (trigeminal impression), where cranial nerve V fibers pass on their way to the Meckel's cave and gasserian ganglion. Lateral and slightly anterior to the ganglion and cave, at the junction to the sphenoid greater wing, is the foramen ovale, through which the third division of the trigeminal nerve (cranial nerve V_3) exits the cranium for the infratemporal fossa (see Figs. 173-2, 173-8, 173-9, and 173-15).

The foramen spinosum is lateral and posterior to the foramen ovale and transmits the middle meningeal artery. The facial hiatus is 10 to 15 mm medial to the foramen spinosum, a bony sulcus that receives the fibers of the greater petrosal nerve coming from the geniculate ganglion (see Figs. 173-2 and 173-3). Posterior and medial to the facial hiatus is the arcuate eminence, related to the most superior aspect of the superior semicircular canal. It is usually, but not always, elevated above the surrounding bone, and the mastoid and tympanic teguments are positioned laterally to it (see Figs. 173-2 and 173-3). The neural and vascular structures of this region are reviewed in the next section, "Anatomy of the Middle Cranial Fossa."

The medial or cerebellar surface of the temporal bone forms the anterolateral wall of the posterior fossa (see Figs. 173-2 and 173-7). Where the superior margin of the medial surface meets the medial margin of the superior surface, a bony sulcus accommodates the superior petrosal sinus on its course between the cavernous sinus and the transition zone between the lateral sinus to the sigmoid sinus. The inferior margin of the medial surface contains another sulcus at the petro-occipital junction for the inferior petrosal sinus, connecting the cavernous sinus and the jugular foramen.

The prominent structure of the petrosa's medial surface is the internal acoustic pore (porus acousticus), which represents the medial limit of the internal auditory meatus (see Fig. 173-7). The meatus ends laterally at the medial wall of the vestibule and the inferior surface of the modiolus and basal cochlear turn (Fig. 173-10; see also Figs. 173-6 and 173-7). A horizontal bony ridge located at the lateral limit divides the meatus into two compartments, superior and inferior. The upper compartment also is divided into anterior and posterior portions by a small vertical bony crest, commonly known as "Bill's bar" in honor of William House, who first drew attention to its presence and surgical importance. These bony ridges divide the fundus of the internal auditory canal into four quadrants, each carrying its own cranial nerve: an anterior-superior quadrant with the facial nerve, an anterior-inferior quadrant with the cochlear nerve, and posterior-superior and posterior-inferior quadrants occupied by the superior and the inferior vestibular nerves, respectively[6] (see Fig. 173-10A and B).

Posterior to the superior limit of the porus of the internal auditory canal and inferior to the arcuate eminence is the subarcuate fossa, which contains a channel to the subarcuate artery and veins (see Figs. 173-7 and 173-11). Posterior and caudal to the subarcuate fossa is a small bony fissure or depression that indicates the opening of the vestibular aqueduct and the position of the endolymphatic sac in the posterior fossa (see Fig. 173-7).

The inferior surface articulates with the occipital bone forming the petro-occipital suture which is in near continuity with the occipitomastoid suture and the sulcus of the sigmoid sinus. In this region lies the butterfly-shaped jugular foramen with its lateral margin formed by the petrous bone and its medial limits by the occipital bone (see Fig. 173-7). Immediately anterior to the jugular foramen is the petro-occipital sulcus, which contains the inferior petrosal sinus. The inferior petrosal sinus enters the jugular foramen in its anterior compartment.

Cranial nerves IX, X, and XI also exit the cranial cavity through the anterior compartment of the jugular foramen and are completely separated from the venous components by a dural septum and fibrous vascular tissue (as described later under "Anatomy of the Posterior Cranial Fossa") (see Figs. 173-4, 173-5, 173-13, and 173-14). The fossa of the jugular bulb lies superior to the posterior compartment and varies greatly in size (see Figs. 173-4, 173-5, and 173-13). The funnel-shaped opening of the cochlear canaliculus is at the superior border of the anterior compartment (see Fig. 173-7). Just inferior to the anterior compartment is the opening of the hypoglossal canal, through which cranial nerve XII leaves the cranium (see Fig. 173-7).

Lateral and anterior to the anterior component of the jugular foramen is the ascending portion of the carotid artery canal at the petrosa's junctions with the tympanic bone (see Figs. 173-4 and 173-5). Within it are the internal carotid artery and the venous and sympathetic nerve plexuses. Here the carotid artery pursues a cephalic course along the anterior wall of the tympanic cavity, parallel to the anterior portion of the tympanic bone and the glenoid fossa (see Figs. 173-4 and 173-5). Just medial to the tympanic ostium of the eustachian tube and immediately anterior to the cochlea, the carotid canal bends horizontally, forming the carotid "knee," and follows a horizontal course in the middle fossa toward the petrous apex and foramen lacerum (see Figs. 173-5, 173-9, and 173-15).

From an anterior perspective, two small openings are visible lateral to the carotid canal. The superior opening is the canal for the tensor tympanic muscle, and the inferior is the osseous portion of the eustachian tube (see Fig. 173-3).

When viewed from a lateral inferior perspective, the jugular foramen lies posterior and medial to the styloid process, and posterior and lateral to the carotid canal, formed by the medial-inferior aspect of the petrous bone and the occipital bone (see Fig. 173-1).

Anatomy of the Middle Cranial Fossa

This section describes relevant anatomy for the middle cranial fossa surgical approach. After a squamosal craniotomy, the temporal lobe dura is elevated, exposing the floor of the middle fossa (see Fig. 173-8).

The gasserian ganglion is located at the anterior aspect of the petrous apex (see Fig. 173-9). The mandibular division of the fifth cranial nerve (trigeminal nerve), V_1, passes anteriorly through the superior orbital fissure. The maxillary division, V_2, passes through the foramen rotundum, and the ophthalmic division, V_3, through the foramen ovale. Medial and posterior to the foramen ovale, the middle meningeal artery enters the middle cranial fossa through the foramen spinosum (see Figs. 173-2, 173-8, and 173-9). The greater superficial petrosal nerve is located medial to the middle meningeal artery. It is the principal surgical landmark for middle cranial fossa procedures because of its consistency and its intimate relationship with nearby structures[2] (see Figs. 173-2, 173-8, and 173-9).

Lateral to the greater petrosal nerve, semicanal to the tensor tympani muscle lies medial to the middle meningeal artery (see Figs. 173-3 and 173-9). The osseous portion of the eustachian tube parallels the course of the tensor tympani muscle laterally. Thus, from superior to inferior, the greater superficial petrosal nerve, the tensor tympani muscle, and the eustachian tube all proceed in a similar anteroposterior plane (see Fig. 173-3).

The horizontal portion of the carotid artery follows a course just inferior and medial to greater petrosal nerve and inferior to the gasserian ganglion on its way to the foramen lacerum and the cavernous sinus (see Figs. 173-8 and 173-9).

The posterior termination of the greater petrosal nerve is the geniculate ganglion. That ganglion is covered by a thin lamina of bone that is absent in 16% of cases. Medial and posterior to the geniculate ganglion is the labyrinthine segment of the facial nerve emerging from the internal auditory canal. After the superior wall of the internal auditory canal is removed, the facial nerve can be seen in the anterior superior portion of the canal and the superior vestibular nerve in the posterior superior portion (see Fig. 173-9). The greater petrosal nerve, geniculate ganglion, and labyrinthine segment of cranial nerve VII form an obtuse angle of approximately 120 degrees. The cochlea is embedded in the bone subtended by that angle (see Figs. 173-8 and 173-9).

The tegmen tympani and tegmen mastoideum are lateral to the geniculate ganglion. If they are partly removed, the epitympanum, the tympanic segment of the facial nerve, and the incudomalleolar joint are seen anteriorly and the mastoid antrum and the three semicircular canals are seen posteriorly. The groove for the superior petrosal sinus at the superior medial ridge of the petrosa marks the medial limit of the middle fossa approach. The opening of the superior petrosal sinus allows access to the posterior cranial fossa.

Anatomy of the Posterior Cranial Fossa

The cerebellopontine angle is traversed by the intracranial segments of cranial nerves VII and VIII. The posterior fossa also contains many other crucial neural and vascular structures, as shown in Figures 173-11 and 173-12. Also, the posteromedial aspect of the temporal bone contains the internal auditory canal and the jugular foramen, and familiarity with their relationships is essential.

Cerebellopontine Angle

The cerebellopontine angle is delimited as follows[2,6]:

- Anteriorly, by cranial nerve VI and the lateral aspect of the clivus
- Laterally, by the medial surface of the petrosa
- Medially, by the middle cerebellar peduncle, the pons, and the ventral surface of the cerebellum
- Superiorly, by cranial nerve V
- Inferiorly, by cranial nerves IX, X, and XI
- Posteriorly, by the cerebellar floccules

Contained within this space are cranial nerves VII and VIII; the premeatal, meatal, and postmeatal segments of the AICA; and the porus of the internal auditory canal. When cranial nerves VII and VIII leave the brainstem at the bulbopontine sulcus, cranial nerve VII lies 1 to 2 mm anterior to cranial nerve VIII. Both nerves follow a lateral and ascending course to enter the internal auditory canal (see Figs. 173-11 and 173-12). From its origin to the most lateral aspects of the internal auditory canal, cranial nerve VII occupies a more anterior and superior position in relation to cranial nerve VIII (see Fig. 173-10).

Internal Auditory Canal

The internal auditory canal develops a lateral and posterior path in relation to the medial surface of the temporal bone. Its length is 1.2 to

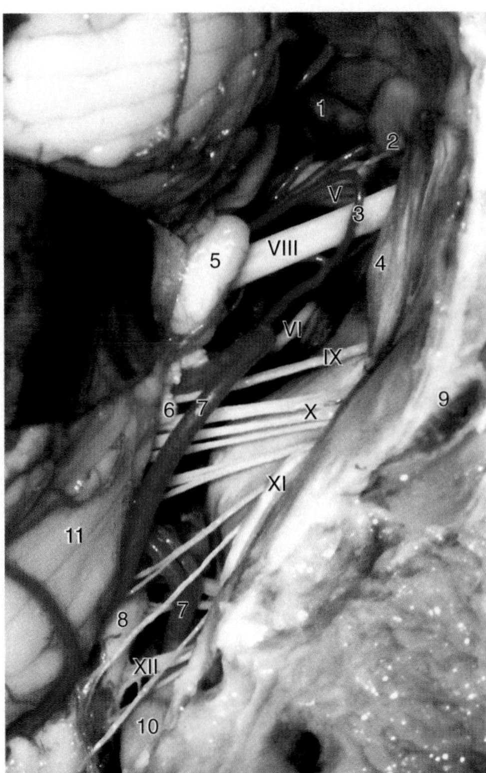

Figure 173-11. Posterior fossa and the middle surface of temporal bone relationships: posterior view as in the retrosigmoid approach (right side). 1, superior petrosal vein; 2, subarcuate artery; 3, anterior inferior cerebellar artery (AICA); 4, internal auditory artery; 5, cerebellar floccules; 6, choroid plexus; 7, posterior inferior cerebellar artery (PICA); 8, cerebellar olive; 9, sigmoid sinus; 10, vertebral artery; 11, cerebellar hemisphere. Roman numerals denote cranial nerves: V, trigeminal nerve; VI, abducens nerve; VIII, vestibulocochlear nerve; IX, glossopharyngeal nerve; X, vagus nerve; XI, spinal accessory nerve; XII, hypoglossal nerve. *(Courtesy of Oswaldo Laércio M. Cruz, Helder Tedeschi, and Albert Rhoton.)*

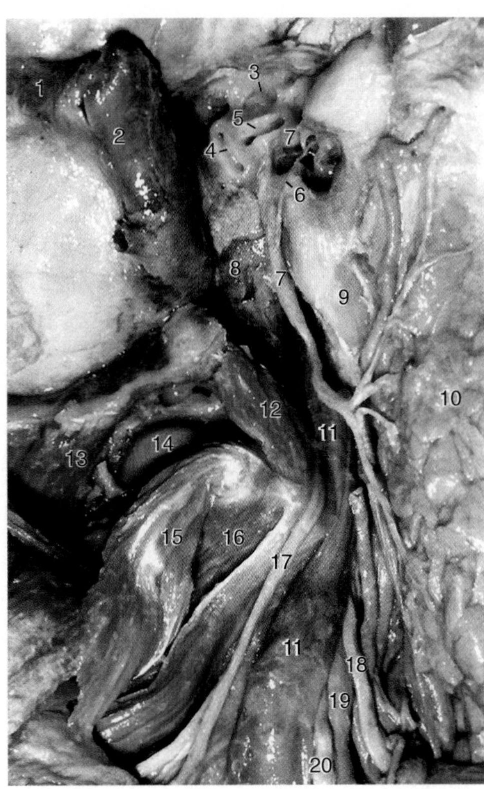

Figure 173-13. Lateral view of the lateral cranial base and the jugular foramen region. Posterior fossa and middle fossa craniotomies were performed, along with extensive mastoid resection and facial nerve exposure. 1, transverse sinus; 2, sigmoid sinus; 3, superior semicircular canal; 4, posterior semicircular canal; 5, lateral semicircular canal; 6, chorda tympani nerve; 7, cranial nerve VII (facial nerve); 8, jugular foramen; 9, tympanic bone; 10, parotid gland; 11, jugular vein; 12, rectus lateralis muscle; 13, rectus capitis major muscle; 14, vertebral artery; 15, superior oblique muscle; 16, inferior oblique muscle; 17, cranial nerve XI (accessory nerve); 18, cranial nerve XII (hypoglossal nerve); 19, internal carotid artery; 20, cranial nerve X (vagus nerve). *(Courtesy of Oswaldo Laércio M. Cruz, Helder Tedeschi, and Albert Rhoton.)*

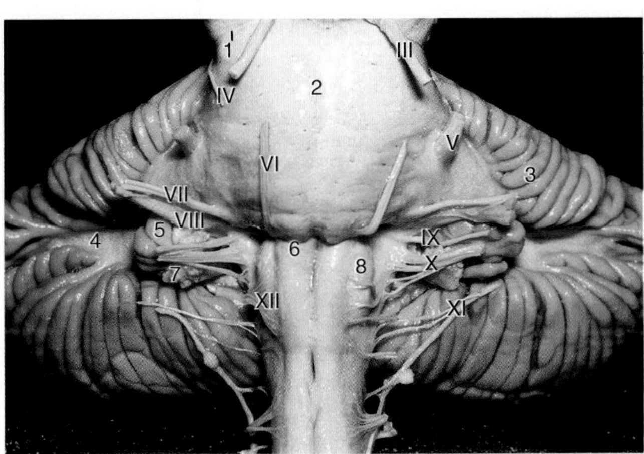

Figure 173-12. Anterior (rostral) view of the brainstem and the cerebellar hemispheres: 1, pontine-mesencephalic sulcus; 2, pons; 3, quadrangular cerebellar lobule; 4, cerebellar horizontal fissure; 5, cerebellar floccules; 6, bulbopontine sulcus; 7, choroid plexus of the IV ventricle; 8, cerebellar olive. Roman numerals denote cranial nerves. *(Courtesy of Oswaldo Laércio M. Cruz, Helder Tedeschi, and Albert Rhoton.)*

1.4 cm from the porus to the fundus, where it enters the inner ear[6] (see Figs. 173-6, 173-7, 173-9, and 173-10).

The lateral portion of the internal canal is divided into superior and inferior compartments by the falciform or transverse crest (see Fig. 173-10A and B). The superior compartment is further divided into anterior and posterior portions by the vertical crest (Bill's bar). Those four quadrants are occupied by the four main neural components of the internal auditory canal contents: the facial nerve (superior and anterior), the superior vestibular nerve (superior and posterior), the cochlear nerve (anterior and inferior), and the inferior vestibular nerve (posterior and inferior).

The inferior compartment does not have a bony division for the cochlear and inferior vestibular nerves, but the cochlear nerve leaves the internal auditory canal through a multiperforate osseous plate to enter the cochlear modiolus (see Fig. 173-10A). Posteroinferiorly, a small multiperforated region reflects the emergence of the inferior vestibular nerve fibers from the saccular macula, and a short distance away is the singular foramen that transmits the posterior ampullary nerve (singular nerve) from the ampulla of the posterior semicircular canal.

Jugular Foramen

The jugular foramen is located in the petro-occipital region and contains several vital neural and vascular structures (Fig. 173-13 and 173-14; see also Figs. 173-1, 173-3, 173-6, 173-7, and 173-11). The vascular structures include the sigmoid sinus, superior and inferior

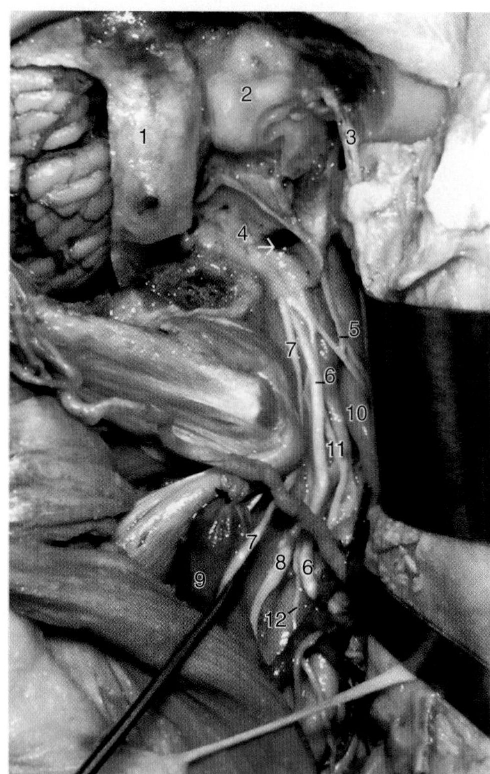

Figure 173-14. Lateral view of the posterior cranial base and the jugular foramen region. The dura of the posterior fossa has been opened, permitting an excellent view of sigmoid sinus position. The lateral aspect of jugular foramen (sigmoid portion) was removed after ligation of the jugular vein and section of the lateral wall of the sigmoid sinus. 1, sigmoid sinus; 2, semicircular canals; 3, facial nerve, anteriorly displaced; 4, medial wall of the jugular foramen with an opening for the inferior petrosal sinus *(arrow)*; 5, cranial nerve IX; 6, cranial nerve XII; 7, cranial nerve XI; 8, cranial nerve X; 9, jugular vein (with ligature); 10, internal carotid artery; 11, superior laryngeal nerve; 12, cervical branch of cranial nerve XII. *(Courtesy of Oswaldo Laércio M. Cruz, Helder Tedeschi, and Albert Rhoton.)*

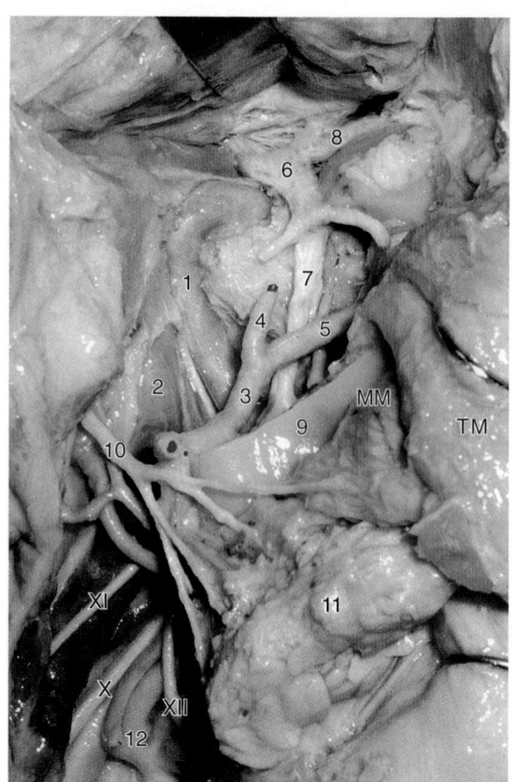

Figure 173-15. Lateral view of the infratemporal region after resection of the superior portion of the ascending ramus of the mandible. The parotid gland and the facial nerve were displaced inferiorly, as were the masseter and temporalis muscles. The lateral pterygoid muscle was resected to allow visualization of the mandibular nerve (V_3). 1, internal carotid artery; 2, jugular vein; 3, external carotid artery; 4, middle meningeal artery; 5, internal maxillary artery entering the pterygomaxillary fossa; 6, gasserian ganglion; 7, V_3 (mandibular nerve); 8, V_2 (maxillary nerve); 9, mandible (ascending ramus); 10, facial nerve, main trunk and divisions at parotid gland; 11, parotid gland; 12, inferior aspect of the external carotid artery; MM, masseter muscle; TM, temporalis muscle. Roman numerals denote cranial nerves. *(Courtesy of Oswaldo Laércio M. Cruz, Helder Tedeschi, and Albert Rhoton.)*

petrosal sinuses, jugular bulb, and meningeal branches from the ascending pharyngeal and occipital arteries. The neural components include cranial nerves IX (glossopharyngeal nerve), X (vagus nerve), and IX (spinal accessory nerve) and their respective ganglia. The jugular foramen also receives the opening of the cochlear aqueduct and is in close proximity to the hypoglossal canal and to cranial nerve XII (see Figs. 173-7, 173-11, and 173-14).

Traditionally, the jugular foramen has been divided into two parts: the larger posterior *pars venosa* and the smaller anterior *pars nervosa*. More recently, anatomic division into three compartments has been proposed[7]:

Sigmoid compartment: posterior and receiving the sigmoid sinus

Petrous compartment: anterior and receiving the inferior petrosal sinus

Neural intrajugular compartment: located between the two others and receiving the neural and arterial components

Cranial nerve IX penetrates a dural opening in the neural compartment and courses anteriorly and inferiorly near the opening of the cochlear aqueduct. Within the jugular foramen, cranial nerve IX forms two ganglia. The inferior ganglion gives rise to the auricular branch (Jacobson's nerve), which ascends across the promontory to form a sensory plexus and the lesser superficial petrosal nerve.

Cranial nerves X and XI penetrate the neural compartment inferior to cranial nerve IX and are separated from it by a dural septum. Cranial nerve X also forms a ganglion as it leaves the cranial cavity; the auricular branch of the vagus nerve (Arnold's nerve) arises from it. Arnold's nerve courses superiorly to emerge at the tympanomastoid fissure and provide sensory innervation to the posterior wall of the external auditory canal. Cranial nerve X leaves the jugular foramen and descends vertically posterior to the carotid artery and anterior to the jugular vein, parallel to and in close relationship with the cervical segment of cranial nerve XII immediately after it has left the cranial cavity (see Figs. 173-4, 173-5, 173-13, and 173-14).

Anatomy of the Infratemporal Fossa

The infratemporal fossa is a space delimited as follows (Fig. 173-15; see also Fig. 173-1):

- Anteriorly, by the posterior surface of the maxilla and the inferior orbital fissure
- Posteriorly, by the mastoid and tympanic portions of the temporal bone
- Superiorly, by the inferior surfaces of the greater wing of the sphenoid and the squamous portion of the temporal bone

- Medially, by the pterygoid process of the sphenoid, lateral portion of the clivus, first cervical vertebra, and inferior surface of the petrous portion of the temporal bone
- Laterally, by the zygomatic arch and ascending ramus of the mandible
- Inferiorly, by the the superior limit of the posterior belly of the digastric muscle and the angle of the mandible

The infratemporal fossa communicates with the orbit through the inferior orbital fissure, with the middle cranial fossa through the foramen spinosum, and with the pterygopalatine fossa through the pterygomaxillary fissure (see Figs. 173-1 and 173-15). The lateral and medial pterygoid muscles lie within the infratemporal fossa. The lateral pterygoid muscle is divided into superior and inferior parts. The superior portion arises from the roof of the infratemporal fossa, and the inferior arises from the lateral aspect of the lateral pterygoid process. Both portions insert onto the temporomandibular joint. The medial pterygoid muscle originates from the medial portion of the lateral pterygoid process and inserts on the medial surface of the angle of the mandible and the ascending ramus.

The infratemporal fossa also contains the mandibular division of the trigeminal nerve (V_3) and its branches (see Fig. 173-15), which provide motor innervation to the temporalis, masseter, and medial and lateral pterygoid muscles, as well as sensory innervation through the auriculotemporal, alveolar, lingual, and buccal nerves.

The chorda tympani nerve originates in the mastoid segment of the facial nerve (cranial nerve VII) midway in the descending portion, pursues a course anterior and superior to the posterior superior quadrant of the mesotympanum, passes through the tympanic cavity, and reaches the chorda tympani canaliculus in the petrotympanic fissure. It then passes forward and descends vertically and medially to the lateral pterygoid muscle to join the lingual nerve (see Figs. 173-4, 173-5, and 173-6).

The maxillary artery leaves the external carotid artery posterior to the ascending ramus of the mandible and enters the infratemporal fossa lateral to the lateral pterygoid muscle. It follows a trajectory anterior to the pterygomaxillary fissure and the pterygopalatine fossa (see Fig. 173-15). It divides within the infratemporal fossa. Its principal branches are the middle meningeal artery, the inferior alveolar artery, the deep temporal artery, branches to the pterygoid muscles, the auricular artery, and the anterior tympanic artery.

The venous drainage of the infratemporal fossa occurs by way of the pterygoid venous plexus, which drains posteriorly into the maxillary vein and anteriorly into the facial vein. The plexus also anastomoses with the cavernous sinus, ophthalmic veins, and pharyngeal venous plexus. Infection within the infratemporal fossa thus carries the risk of spread by hematogenous extension, especially to involve the contents of the orbit and cavernous sinus.

SUGGESTED READINGS

Costa SS, Cruz OLM. Exploratory tympanotomy: operative techniques in otolaryngology. *Head Neck Surg.* 1996;7:20-26.

Cruz OLM, Tedeschi H, Tzu WH, et al. Anatomia macroscópica do osso temporal. Section 1. In: Cruz OLM, Costa SS, eds. *Otologia Clínica e Cirúrgica.* Rio de Janeiro: Editora Revinter; 2000:2-33.

Duckert LG. Anatomy of the skull base, temporal bone, external ear, and middle ear. In: Cummings CW, Fredrickson JM, Harker LA, Krause CJ, Richardson MA, Schuller DE, eds. *Otolaryngology—Head and Neck Surgery.* 3rd ed. Vol 4. St Louis: Mosby–Year Book; 1988:2537-2547.

Katsuta T, Rhoton Jr AL, Matsushima T. The jugular foramen: microsurgical anatomy and operative approaches. *Neurosurgery.* 1997;41:149-202.

Pait TG, Harris FS, Paullus WS, et al. Microsurgical anatomy and dissection of the temporal bone. *Surg Neurol.* 1977;8:363-391.

Rhoton Jr AL, Tedeschi H. Microsurgical anatomy of acoustic neuroma. *Otolaryngol Clin North Am.* 1992;25:257-294.

Tedeschi H, et al. Anatomia microcirúrgica das fossas posterior e média relacionadas com o osso temporal. Section 3. In: Cruz OLM, Costa SS, eds. *Otologia Clínica e Cirúrgica.* Rio de Janeiro: Editora Revinter; 2000:7-33.

For complete list of references log onto www.expertconsult.com.

CHAPTER ONE HUNDRED AND SEVENTY-FOUR

Surgery of the Anterior and Middle Cranial Base

Colin D. Pero

Frank Culicchia

Rohan R. Walvekar

Bert W. O'Malley, Jr.

Daniel W. Nuss

Key Points

- Advances in oncologic and reconstructive surgery, anesthesiology, radiology, and other related fields have made surgery of the cranial base both technically feasible and therapeutically effective. As a result, surgical resection can be considered the primary management modality for many cranial base lesions previously considered inaccessible or inoperable.
- Symptoms from anterior and middle cranial base lesions may range from headache to impaired cranial nerve and central nervous system functions. These disorders are insidious in that they cause few symptoms until they have reached advanced stages and impinge on cranial nerves, major vessels, or the brain. This paucity of early symptoms makes early diagnosis difficult.
- Operative planning for the removal of lesions of this anatomically complex region requires that laboratory testing, imaging, and vascular interventional procedures be used to their fullest potential to guide the surgical and anesthetic teams, as well as the patient's expectations.
- Operative approaches should attempt to meet principal aims of (1) optimizing exposure, (2) preserving neurovascular structures, (3) implementing the use of image guidance and endoscope assistance to enhance the resection while limiting incision length and removal of normal tissue, and (4) planning surgical techniques that optimize functional and aesthetic reconstruction.
- Postoperative complications may entail serious morbidity and mortality; limiting postoperative neurologic and other complications requires anticipation of potential risks and an aggressive approach to their prevention and management.

The cranial base often is conceptually divided into three anatomic regions that are named for their intracranial relations to the overlying cranial fossae: anterior, middle, and posterior (Fig. 174-1). From a diagnostic and therapeutic point of view, it is useful to consider the anterior and middle cranial base regions together, for several reasons. They contribute to what is commonly referred to as the craniofacial junction, where the neurocranium and the viscerocranium meet (Fig. 174-2). Both share anatomic relationships with the orbits, the nasal airway, and the paranasal sinuses, and they are therefore affected by similar pathologic processes. The anterior and middle cranial base regions have traditionally been approached using craniofacial disassembly techniques, however, endoscopic approaches to the skull base have assumed a growing role in selected cases while minimizing surgical morbidity. Additionally, robotic-assisted surgery has been investigated and holds promise for the future of anterior and middle cranial base surgery. The posterior and lateral cranial base are clinically regarded as a separate region, often approached with combined neurotologic and neurosurgical approaches (Chapters 127, 173, 176, and 177). This chapter focuses on the surgical management of lesions that affect the anterior and middle cranial base.

Surgical Anatomy

Anterior Cranial Base

The anterior cranial base can be defined as that portion of the skull base adjacent to the anterior cranial fossa. It is bounded anteriorly by the frontal bone, which contains two surgically important structures: the frontal sinus and the supraorbital foramina (Fig. 174-3). The anatomy of the anterior cranial base is described in detail in Chapter 175, and briefly reviewed here. The supraorbital foramina, which may be incomplete (and therefore referred to as supraorbital notches), transmit the supraorbital nerves and vessels. These vessels supply the galea and the pericranium of the frontal region, and their preservation facilitates subsequent use in reconstructing anterior cranial base defects.

Superiorly, the anterior cranial base is formed by the frontal, ethmoid, and sphenoid bones (Fig. 174-4). An important visible land-

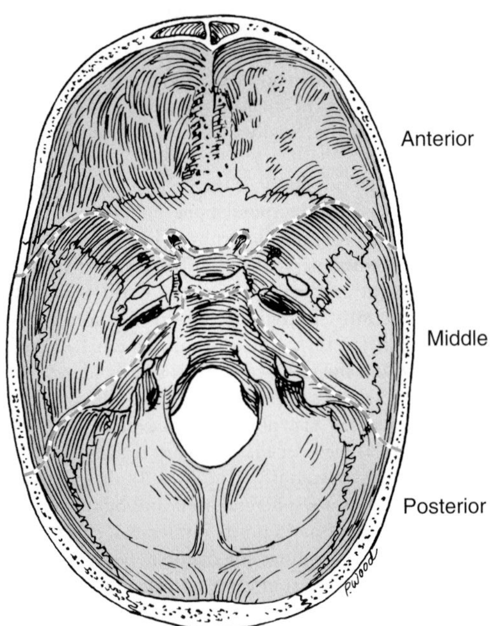

Figure 174-1. Intracranial view of cranial base showing boundaries of anterior, middle, and posterior divisions.

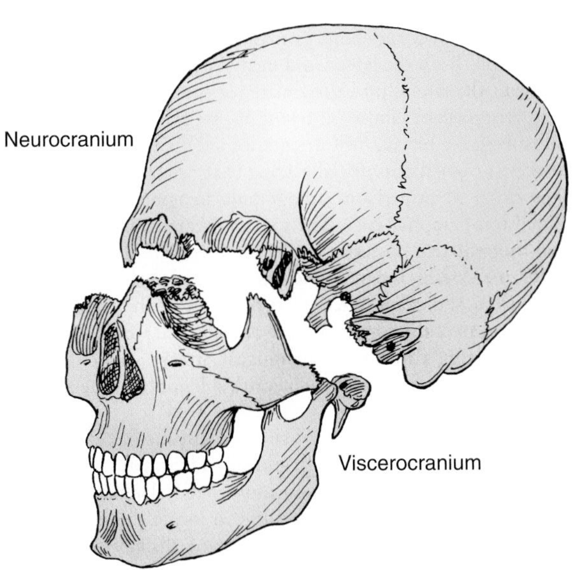

Figure 174-2. Disarticulated skull showing the junction of the neurocranium with the viscerocranium (craniofacial junction). The anterior cranial base forms the roof of the orbits and the nasal cavities, and the middle cranial base makes up the roof of the intratemporal fossa, the pterygopalatine fossa, and the nasopharynx. Operative approaches to the anterior and middle cranial base regions often traverse the viscerocranium.

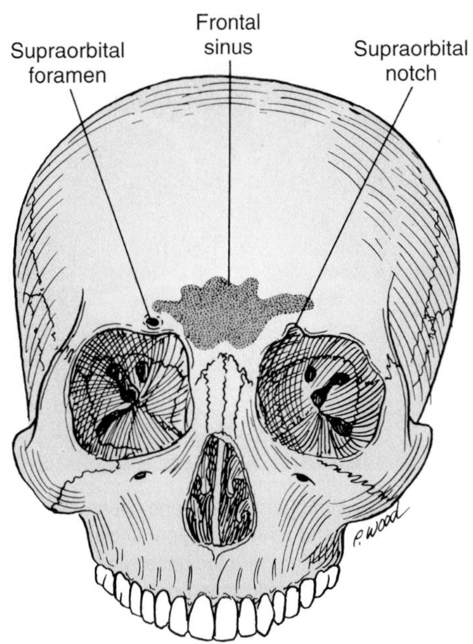

Figure 174-3. Anterior perspective of the anterior cranial base showing the outline of the frontal sinus *(shaded)* and the position of the supraorbital neurovascular pedicle exiting the supraorbital foramen *(left)* and the supraorbital notch *(right)*.

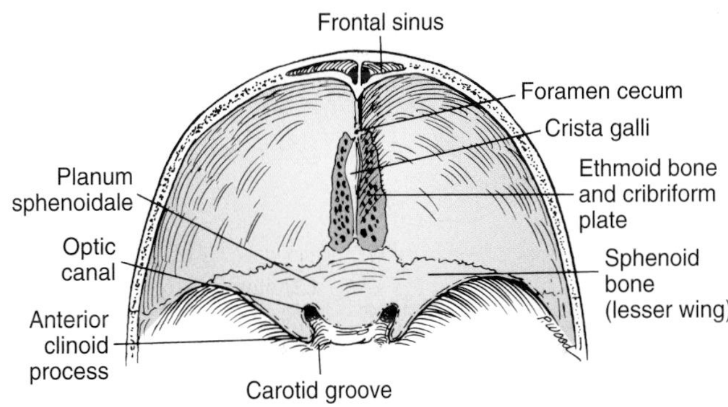

Figure 174-4. Intracranial view of the anterior cranial base and important landmarks.

mark is the foramen cecum, which is the site of a communication between veins of the nasal cavity and the origin of the superior sagittal sinus. The next landmark, the crista galli, protrudes upward from the midline to provide attachment for the falx cerebri. On either side of the crista are the openings of the cribriform plate, through which olfactory nerves are transmitted. Just posterior to the last of these olfactory foramina is a smooth-surfaced area known as the planum sphenoidale; it forms the roof of the sphenoid sinus when the sinus is well pneumatized. The anterior clinoid processes and lesser sphenoid wings delineate the most posterior limit of the anterior cranial base and delineate its boundary with the middle cranial base. Between and slightly below the clinoids are the optic canals and the internal carotid arteries (ICAs).

Extracranially, the anterior cranial base is related to the nasal cavity, the ethmoid and sphenoid sinuses, and the orbits (Fig. 174-5). The floor of the anterior cranial fossa is uneven, with the relatively flat orbital roofs sloping downward as they join the roof of the ethmoid sinuses medially. Thus, the ethmoid roof is lower than the orbital roof. The downward slope becomes even more exaggerated as the ethmoid roof joins the cribriform area (the roof of the nasal cavity), near the midline, which usually is the lowest point of the anterior skull base. The relative relationship of the height of the cribriform plate to the roof of the ethmoid is variable and has been classified by Keros into three categories: class 1, 1 to 3 mm; class 2, 4 to 7 mm; and class 3, 8 to 16 mm.[1]

This nonplanar arrangement of the cribriform area is important during transethmoid extracranial approaches to lesions of the anterior skull base. For example, an axial plane of dissection that is safe along the roof of the ethmoid may risk injury to the dura and frontal lobes if extended medially to encompass the cribriform plate territory.

The orbits contain several landmarks that can help surgical orientation during cranial base operations (Fig. 174-6). The superior orbital fissure transmits the oculomotor, trochlear, ophthalmic, and abducens

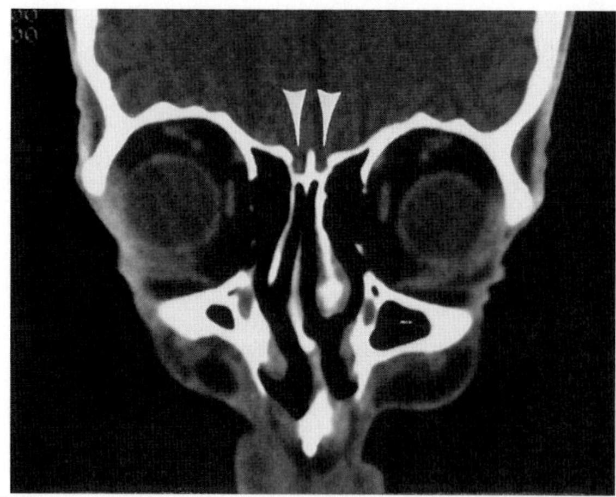

Figure 174-5. Coronal computed tomography scan through the anterior cranial fossa, orbits, and ethmoid region, showing the relationship of the anterior cranial fossa floor with the underlying orbits and sinuses. The cribriform area *(arrows)* is significantly lower than the ethmoid roof and the orbital roof. Extracranial approaches to this region should respect this anatomy to avoid injury to the dura and brain.

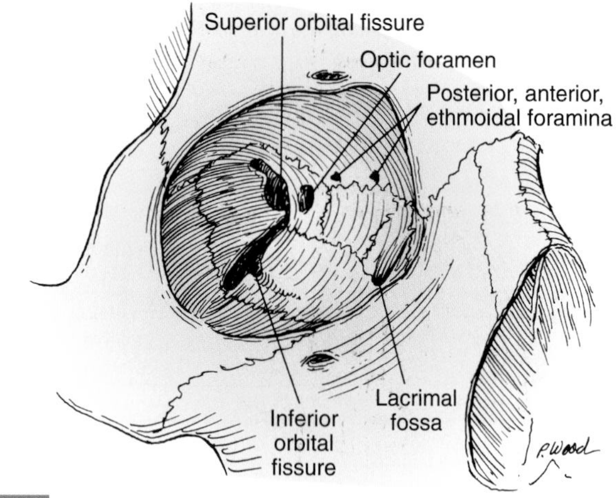

Figure 174-6. Important surgical landmarks of the orbital skeleton.

nerves (cranial nerves III, IV, V1, and VI) and the ophthalmic vein, and it communicates with the middle cranial fossa. The inferior orbital fissure contains the maxillary nerve (V2) and communicates primarily with the pterygopalatine fossa; the lateral end of this fissure is an important landmark for the placement of lateral orbital osteotomies. The optic canal transmits the optic nerve and the ophthalmic artery. The anterior and posterior arteries transmitted through ethmoid foramina should be controlled to reduce intraoperative bleeding in the nasal vault region. More important, these ethmoid foramina mark the position of the frontoethmoid suture line, a valuable guide to the level of the ethmoid roof and the anterior fossa floor. The posterior ethmoid foramen is of additional significance because of its consistent relationship with the optic canal, found 4 to 7 mm posteriorly.

Middle Cranial Base

The middle cranial base forms the floor of the middle cranial fossa. From the intracranial perspective (Fig. 174-7), the middle cranial base begins anteriorly at the posterior edge of the lesser sphenoid wing; posteriorly it ends at the posterosuperior edge of the petrous part of the temporal bone. The intracranial surface of the middle cranial base is formed by the greater wing and body of the sphenoid bone and the petrous and squamous portions of the temporal bone. As such, it forms the roof of the infratemporal fossa, middle ear, mastoid, and condylar fossa and the lateral wall of the sphenoid sinus.

Foramina along the floor of the middle fossa beginning anteriorly are the superior orbital fissure, optic canal, and foramen rotundum (representing the intracranial end of the inferior orbital fissure). Next, the foramen ovale delivers the mandibular nerve (V3) to the infratemporal fossa below, and the foramen spinosum transmits the middle meningeal artery.

The superomedial boundary of the middle cranial base is marked by the petrous part of the temporal bone containing the horizontal petrous ICA and the foramen lacerum. This foramen receives the greater superficial petrosal nerve (GSPN) (parasympathetic fibers from the facial nerve to the lacrimal gland) and conducts it to the pterygopalatine fossa inferiorly. Recognition of this relationship among the GSPN, the foramen lacerum, and the carotid canal often is helpful during surgery because the GSPN, which is readily identifiable, can be followed medially to the distal petrous ICA.

From an extracranial viewpoint, the middle cranial base extends from the posterolateral walls of the maxillary sinuses anteriorly to the petro-occipital sutures posteriorly (Fig. 174-8). It is formed by the greater wing and body of the sphenoid bone and by the temporal bone, including the condylar fossa. As on its intracranial surface, this region also contains numerous openings for major nerves and blood vessels, including the foramina ovale, spinosum, and lacerum and the stylomastoid foramen (cranial nerve VII), the jugular foramen (internal jugular vein, inferior petrosal sinus, cranial nerves IX, X, and XI), and the carotid canal (entrance of ICA into the temporal bone).

Operative approaches in this region often traverse the infratemporal fossa. Here, the muscles of mastication—the temporalis, masseter, and medial and lateral pterygoids—receive their blood supply from branches of the internal maxillary artery, which should be preserved if, for example, the versatile temporalis muscle is to be used as a flap for reconstruction. Both the lateral and medial pterygoid muscles originate in part from the lateral pterygoid plate (of the sphenoid bone), which serves as an excellent landmark owing to the following features: (1) it is a palpable guide for surgical orientation; (2) it can be easily exposed by dissection carried out medially along the greater sphenoid wing; and (3) it is easily identified on radiographic imaging studies, especially computed tomography (CT). The root of this lateral pterygoid plate is situated immediately posterior to the foramen rotundum and anterior to the foramen ovale. It can be used as an index to the positions of the maxillary (V2) and mandibular (V3) divisions of the trigeminal nerve (Fig. 174-9). After the foramen ovale is identified, the foramen spinosum (transmitting the middle meningeal artery) will be found just posterior to it. This leads to the next critical landmark: the spine of the sphenoid.

The sphenoid spine, which is situated just medial to the condylar fossa, serves as a palpable, radiographically identifiable landmark that is important because of its location immediately lateral to the carotid canal (see Fig. 174-8). It helps the surgeon locate the highest portion of the cervical ICA, which can be followed distally to expose and mobilize the petrous ICA. Because the sphenoid spine is just medial to the condylar fossa, the mandibular condyle often is displaced anteroinferiorly or resected to enhance exposure of the ICA as it enters the cranial base.

A thorough and detailed understanding of the regional anatomy of the cranial base is best achieved through the correlative study of dry skulls, cadaveric dissections, and radiographic images.

Preoperative Considerations

The principles of the clinical evaluation of presenting symptoms and physical findings (Chapter 175) and diagnostic imaging[2] (Chapter 135) are considered in detail elsewhere in this book.

Angiography

In many cases, it is important to have information about the vascularity of a given cranial base lesion and the possible involvement of major neighboring blood vessels. For this reason, cerebral angiography often is part of the diagnostic imaging sequence. This type of angiography permits the identification of the blood supply to the lesion and its own vascular pattern while simultaneously clarifying whether the ICA or other major vessels are compromised.

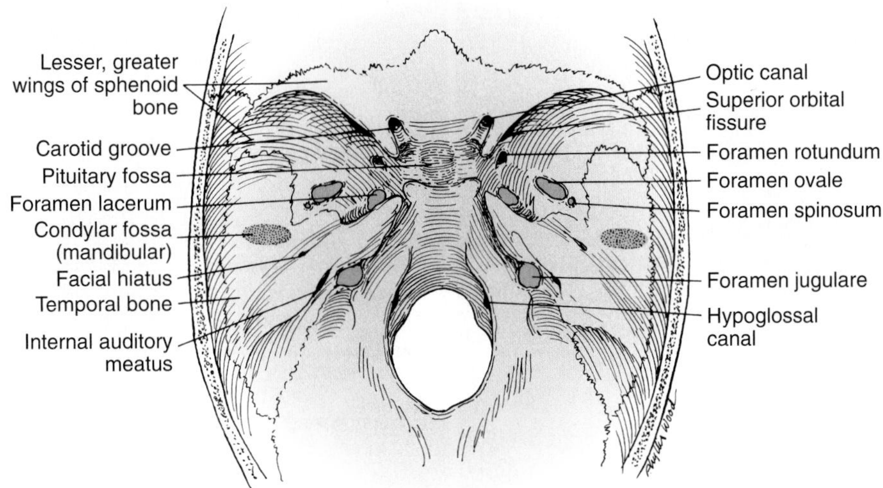

Figure 174-7. Intracranial view of the middle cranial base.

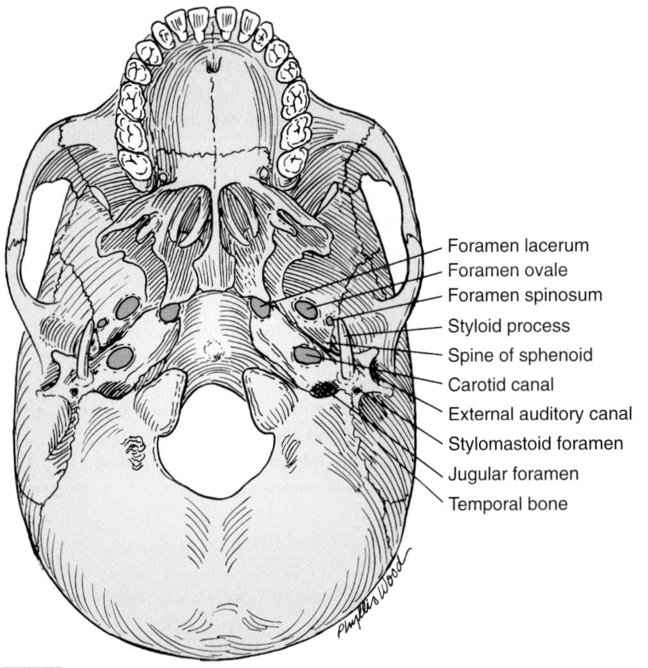

Figure 174-8. Extracranial aspect of the middle cranial base.

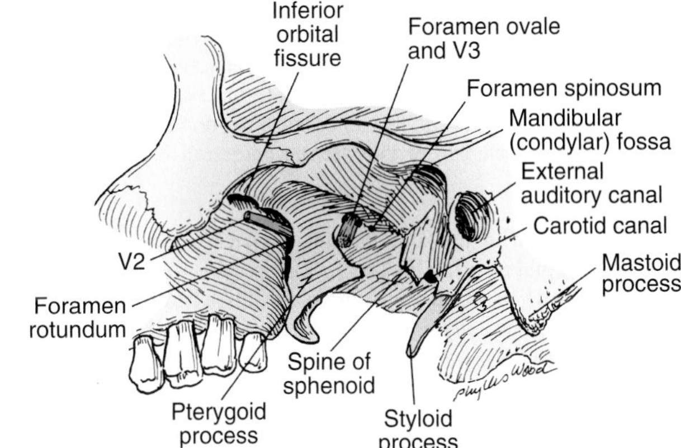

Figure 174-9. Lateral view of the pterygoid process of the sphenoid bone (pterygoid plate), showing the relationship of the foramina rotundum and ovale with associated structures. V2, maxillary nerve; V3, mandibular nerve.

Angiography also gives anatomic information about the integrity of the circle of Willis, existing collateral circulation to the cerebral hemispheres, and other possible anomalous blood supply patterns that may dictate the approach or prudent use of embolization.[3]

Angiography alone, however, does not give sufficient physiologic information about the adequacy of the circle of Willis or other collaterals with regard to supplying circulation to the brain.[4] To obtain detailed physiologic information, cerebral blood flow studies are performed.

Computed tomographic angiography (CTA), magnetic resonance angiography (MRA), and three-dimensional reconstructive technology have added relatively noninvasive options and adjuncts to conventional imaging and angiographic methods. One drawback to these modalities is the inability to incorporate interventional techniques including balloon occlusion and embolization as preoperative workup and adjunctive procedures (as discussed next).

Cerebral Blood Flow Evaluation

If a cranial base lesion involves or impinges on the ICA or if it will be necessary to manipulate the ICA during surgery, cerebral blood flow studies should be considered. These studies give a physiologic index of the adequacy of the circulation to the brain in a quantitative way and are useful for predicting whether a patient can tolerate occlusion of the ICA without major neurologic consequence.[5-8]

The test begins with a temporary occlusion of the ICA by means of a balloon-tipped catheter inflated within the vessel. The catheter is placed percutaneously through the femoral artery and guided into the cervical portion of the ICA under fluoroscopic control, just as is done for routine cerebral angiography. This is performed with the patient awake, and serial neurologic assessments are done during the 15-minute ICA occlusion. If a neurologic deficit develops during this part of the test, occlusion is immediately discontinued. A patient demonstrating such a deficit is considered to have failed the test and is presumed to be highly dependent on the flow in that ICA; thus, the risk for stroke is increased if the carotid is compromised at surgery. If the patient tolerates 15 minutes of ICA occlusion without the development of neurologic deficit, further study uses a quantitative test in which stable xenon gas is inhaled. The inhaled xenon is distributed throughout the circulation and into the brain, where it is visible on CT scanning; this gives a picture of cerebral blood flow distribution (Fig. 174-10). This xenon-enhanced CT scan is performed with the balloon inflated and deflated in the ICA. The uptake of xenon within both cerebral hemispheres is quantitated using the digitized data from the CT scan (when xenon CT is not available, single-photon emission computed tomography [SPECT] imaging can give similar blood flow imaging, although it is not quantitative).

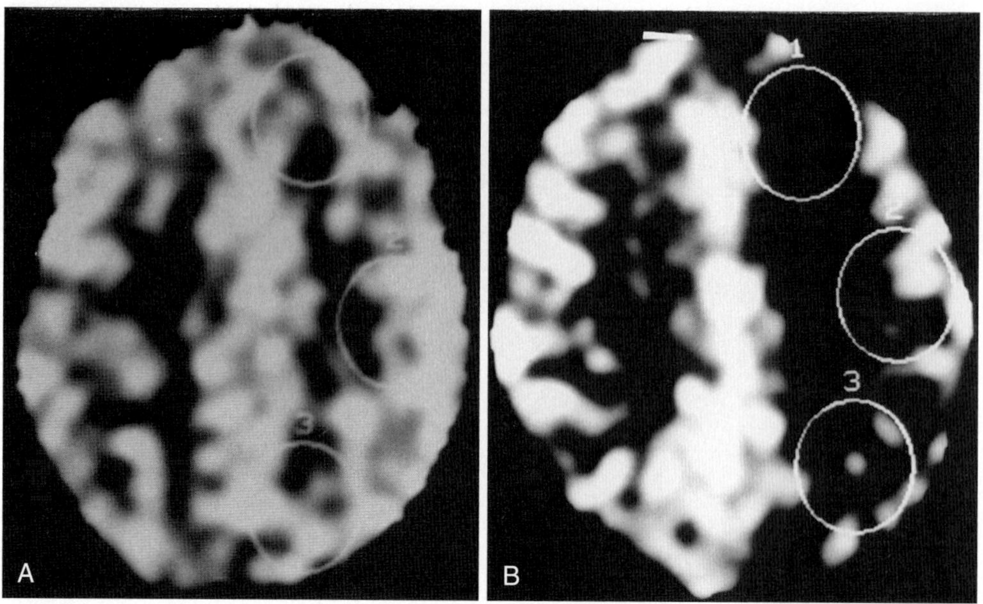

Figure 174-10. Axial slices, xenon-enhanced computed tomography scan through the level of the cerebral hemispheres. **A,** Normal cerebral blood flow distribution with symmetrical bilateral xenon uptake (*dark areas* within each hemisphere represent lateral ventricles). **B,** Significantly decreased hemispheric xenon uptake (on the right side of photograph) after inflation of a balloon within the ipsilateral internal carotid artery. From these xenon studies, cerebral blood flow in specific regions of interest *(circles)* can be quantitated. Such information is useful for predicting the patient's ability to tolerate occlusion of the internal carotid artery at surgery.

The patient who has a significant ipsilateral decrease in hemispheric xenon uptake during ICA occlusion (despite no clinically apparent neurologic deficit during the test) is considered to be at moderate risk for the development of neurologic sequelae should the ICA be occluded during surgery. Such patients would be candidates for extracranial-to-intracranial arterial bypass to enhance the intracranial circulation. Patients who have no drop in xenon uptake during balloon occlusion of the ICA are believed to be at low risk for postoperative stroke, even if the ICA is resected or permanently occluded.

Preoperative Embolization

Another advantage of preoperative angiography is the possibility for elective embolization of vascular tumor beds to help reduce intraoperative bleeding. In addition, the ICA may be electively embolized using detachable intra-arterial permanent balloons if the decision is made preoperatively that the ICA will have to be sacrificed. This is sometimes done to permit the resection of malignant tumors. These procedures are considered in more detail in Chapter 136.

Other Evaluations

For lesions near the orbits, visual acuity should be assessed quantitatively and measurements of the visual fields performed. For lesions near the temporal bone, audiologic and vestibular testing, electronystagmography, and facial electromyography (EMG) should be performed as indicated. These evaluations may help to uncover and quantify cranial nerve dysfunction in some patients. It may also help predict the degree of postoperative cranial nerve morbidity.

For lesions near the pituitary fossa, a complete endocrine evaluation should be performed. It is especially important to identify patients who preoperatively have syndrome of inappropriate antidiuretic hormone, diabetes insipidus, or hypothyroidism, because these conditions can lead to postoperative morbidity if not corrected. Also, abnormal levels of prolactin, growth hormone, or gonadotropins may be of diagnostic significance as indicators of tumors of the pituitary gland. Metastatic workup is conducted in patients with specific malignant tumors.

Pathology and Management Planning

Many disorders can affect the cranial base. Disorders in which surgery has played a significant therapeutic role include basicranial trauma; craniofacial anomalies; congenital syndromes (e.g., hypertelorism, Crouzon's syndrome); spontaneous cerebrospinal fluid fistulas; vascular problems (e.g., petrous carotid artery aneurysms); infectious diseases (e.g., petrositis, malignant external otitis); and neoplasms. Perhaps the widest acceptance and application of cranial base surgery has been in the management of neoplasms, in which the effectiveness of other modalities is limited.

Benign tumors and related lesions affecting the skull base have been reviewed by several authors and are summarized in Box 174-1.[9-11] In general, benign cranial base neoplasms are managed surgically. The surgical technique often involves "piecemeal" removal, with careful progression from one surgical landmark to the next, to permit the maximal preservation of functionally important structures. For larger tumors or those for which removal carries a high risk of damage to neighboring structures, incomplete resection with postoperative irradiation may be indicated.[12]

Malignant skull base lesions are listed in Box 174-2.[10] With some notable exceptions (i.e., leukemia, lymphoma, myeloma, metastases), malignant neoplasms are managed surgically, although in most cases surgery will not be used as the sole modality. Adjuvant management with radiation (by external beam, implantation, or brachytherapy) or chemotherapy is usually included in the therapeutic plan. Single-modality radiation therapy, including sterotactic radiotherapy, has been recommended by some investigators for certain smaller lesions.[13] Malignant lesions are surgically removed en bloc, with margins of uninvolved tissue after broad circumferential exposure whenever possible.[14]

When surgery is considered for tumors and tumor-like disorders of the cranial base, the first question that should be answered involves the biologic behavior of the lesion. As mentioned, an accurate clinical diagnosis often can be made on the basis of information obtained from the history, physical examination, and imaging studies. Whenever possible, this should be supplemented by a histologic diagnosis before definitive management is carried out.

When tumor is present within the nose, paranasal sinuses, middle ear, mastoid, oral cavity, pharynx, or neck, direct biopsy can be performed using standard techniques. When direct biopsy is not feasible, CT-guided needle biopsy may be done in selected cases (e.g., tumors of the infratemporal fossa). Occasionally a tumor may be inaccessible by either of these routes, or biopsy without adequate skull base exposure may be judged to be unsafe because of concerns about injury to nearby

Box 174-1

Benign Lesions of the Skull Base

Extracranial
Inverted papilloma
Angiofibroma
Salivary gland tumor
Paraganglioma (glomus)
Mucocele
Cholesteatoma

Intracranial
Pituitary adenoma
Craniopharyngioma
Meningioma
Schwannoma
Aneurysm
Arteriovenous malformation

Primary Basicranial
Fibrous dysplasia
Osteoma
Osteoblastoma
Chondroma
Chordoma*
Congenital
Cholesteatoma
Dermoid
Encephalocele

*Histologically benign but clinically malignant behavior.
Modified with permission from Dickins JRE. Approach to diagnosis of skull base lesions. *Am J Otol*. 1981;3:35.

Box 174-2

Malignant Lesions of the Skull Base

Extracranial
Squamous cell carcinoma
Adenoid cystic carcinoma
Mucoepidermoid carcinoma
Malignant mixed tumor
Leukemia
Lymphoma
Rhabdomyosarcoma
Neurogenic sarcoma
Undifferentiated carcinoma
Hemangiopericytoma
Synovial sarcoma
Adenocarcinoma
Basal cell carcinoma

Intracranial
Esthesioneuroblastoma
Malignant schwannoma

Primary Basicranial
Chondrosarcoma
Osteogenic sarcoma
Multiple myeloma
Histiocytosis X
Chordoma*

Metastatic
Breast
Lung
Kidney
Prostate
Melanoma

*Histologically benign but clinically malignant behavior.
Modified with permission from Dickins JRE. Approach to diagnosis of skull base lesions. *Am J Otol*. 1981;3:35.

critical structures or because of vascularity of the lesion. In these situations, the surgeon should proceed with an operative approach to the skull base that is designed to provide access to the tumor for safe biopsy before any irreversible ablative steps are taken. Then, if the frozen-section biopsy result contraindicates resection or is questionable, an alternative management plan may be made. On the basis of histologic criteria, extirpative surgery is usually not performed when one of the following conditions is present: (1) a malignant lesion is metastatic from a distant source; or (2) a malignancy is of a type that responds well to other management modalities (e.g., lymphoma).

Anesthesia

Anesthetic management is crucial for determining the outcome of cranial base operations. Techniques of neuroanesthesia are used, with the primary goals of maximal neuronal preservation and simultaneous facilitation of a controlled surgical environment.[15] Maintenance of hemodynamic factors is key in this scheme, because cerebral blood flow cannot be allowed to drop below critical levels for any significant length of time. Thus, close monitoring of arterial pressure, central venous pressure, cardiac function, and urine output is of paramount importance.

Electrophysiologic monitoring, including somatosensory-evoked potentials to assess cortical function and EMG to assess motor cranial nerve function, is another key element for the achievement of neuronal preservation. Appropriate selection of anesthetic agents and limited use of neuromuscular blocking drugs will enhance the reliability of such monitoring.

Cerebral edema, which is a common problem in intracranial surgery, can be minimized with the intraoperative use of colloids (albumin, plasma) rather than crystalloid fluids. It can be minimized by controlled hyperventilation, which, by virtue of decreasing arterial carbon dioxide tension ($P{CO_2}$), causes mild cerebral vasoconstriction and a corresponding reduction in intracranial volume. Generally, $P{CO_2}$ between 25 and 30 mm Hg is desirable for this purpose. Lower arterial CO_2 levels significantly reduce cerebral perfusion and are not recommended. Another technique that is helpful for reducing brain swelling is the preoperative placement of an indwelling lumbar drain, which decompresses the subarachnoid space by removing cerebrospinal fluid (CSF). Lumbar drains also are important postoperatively in selected cases, because short-term CSF decompression can decrease the possibility of CSF fistula formation. Such drains are not used in patients who have major intracranial space-occupying lesions because of the risk of brainstem herniation. Cerebral edema may be lessened with timely use of corticosteroids and diuretics, an especially helpful adjunct if edema is present preoperatively as a result of a mass lesion.

The anesthesia team also is responsible for the infusion of blood products to replenish surgical blood loss, which can be considerable in some cranial base procedures. Dilutional thrombocytopenia and other coagulopathies can occur after multiple transfusions of stored blood. These problems can be successfully managed with the replacement of clotting factors (in the form of fresh-frozen plasma) and platelets in proportion with erythrocyte transfusion. Related issues include the advance donation of autologous blood for transfusion and the use of "cell saver" devices to collect blood intraoperatively and reinfuse it. With concerns surrounding blood transfusion–related infectious diseases, these techniques are becoming increasingly important. One limitation of the cell salvage technique is that it should not be used when there is a risk of reinfusing tumor cells from the operative field.

The anesthesiologist is essential to the success of surgery for cranial base lesions. Optimal anesthetic management depends on close communication between the anesthesiologist and the surgeon before, during, and after the operation.

Operative Techniques

General Considerations

As the field of skull base surgery has evolved, more and more lesions previously thought to be unreachable or unresectable are now able to be addressed surgically. The contraindications to skull base surgery for malignancy as outlined by Donald[16] include anatomic, tumor, and patient factors. Absolute anatomic contraindications include involvement of the brain stem, portions of the cerebrum, superior sagittal sinus, both internal carotid arteries, both cavernous sinuses and certain vital bridging veins. Tumor factors representing contraindications to resection usually include distant metastic disease; although some authors advocate significantly prolonged survival in those with isolated distant metastases after resection of the primary tumor, this has not been well demonstrated in skull base tumors. Certain malignancies typically display aggressive behavior despite treatment, which must be considered before extensive resection. Patients should be well informed and motivated and without medical contraindications to the operation as well.[16]

Overview of Approaches

Surgical treatment of lesions involving the anterior skull base, nasal cavity, and paranasal sinuses has evolved into a single category of craniofacial approaches. A myriad of surgical approaches have been developed for exposure of the anterior and middle cranial base regions; these range from purely intracranial to purely extracranial. However, most approaches for dealing with lesions of the skull base use combined intracranial and extracranial methods. For anterior cranial base lesions, the most commonly used approaches combine frontal craniotomy with some form of transfacial (transnasal, transmaxillary, or transorbital) exposure. Most commonly, a team of neurosurgeons and otolaryngologists performs this procedure resulting in a bifrontal craniotomy from above and a transfacial approach from below. The transfacial approach often involves midfacial degloving, and facial disassembly, requiring facial incisions and facial osteotomies. Lateral rhinotomy, removal of the frontonasal unit, Le Fort I and II osteotomies, and splitting of the maxilla have been described as means of accessing lesions of the anterior cranial base. Janecka and coworkers[17] described the facial translocation approach, which also involves an extensive facial incision and facial disassembly for access to tumors in the anterior cranial base, cavernous sinus, clivus, and infratemporal fossa.

Since the 1990s, endoscopic sinus surgery has virtually replaced the conventional open techniques used by otolaryngologists in treating sinonasal disorders and is discussed in detail in Chapter 175. Use of the endoscope as a supplement to the surgical approaches can alleviate the need for some facial incisions by allowing the surgeon to observe areas hidden from the field of view of the microscope. For those tumors that invade the anterior cranial base, the endoscope may be utilized as an adjunct to the standard bifrontal craniotomy by allowing visualization of paranasal extension into the sphenoid, ethmoid, frontal, and maxillary sinuses. From nasal or maxillary portals, the endoscope allows visualization of all of the paranasal sinuses. As the technology of endoscope optics and video systems improves, the role of endoscopic cranial base surgery will augment and supplement current microsurgical techniques. Intraorbital lesions may be approached by frontal craniotomy or subcranial approaches, often combined with transfacial approaches.[18]

For middle cranial base lesions, access is most often provided by combining temporal or frontotemporal craniotomy with infratemporal fossa dissection, transfacial exposure, or transtemporal techniques. In addition, endoscope-assisted and image-guided navigational approaches are increasingly being applied (see Chapter 177). In anterior and middle cranial base approaches, craniofacial disassembly techniques have been widely used.

Implicit in the term *craniofacial disassembly* is the concept of the systematic, stepwise dissection of cranial and facial soft tissues on the basis of the knowledge of regional vascular territories and functional anatomy, followed by osteotomies and dismantling of the craniofacial skeleton. Some of these techniques, which were developed originally by plastic and reconstructive surgeons for the correction of congenital craniofacial deformities, are of major importance in cranial base surgery, because they allow wide exposure of the skull base through temporary displacement of the viscerocranium.[19,20] The enhanced exposure of the skull base from below the neuraxis significantly reduces the need for brain retraction and therefore helps minimize postoperative neurologic dysfunction. It also allows the surgeon greater oncologic precision during the extirpative phase, with preservation of the functional and aesthetic units of the face for reconstruction.[58]

Box 174-3
Goals of Cranial Base Surgery

1. Extirpation of disease
2. Protection of vital structures
3. Restoration of critical anatomic barriers
4. Functional and aesthetic reconstruction

Planning the Operative Approach

Whether the surgery is being performed for a benign tumor, a malignancy, or other indications (e.g., inflammatory or vascular lesions, CSF fistula), the approach should be planned and executed to accomplish the four specific goals that are applicable to all cranial base operations, summarized in Box 174-3.

GOAL 1. The approach should provide adequate exposure to allow extirpation of the disease process. To a large extent, the degree of needed exposure is based on information obtained from the physical examination and imaging studies.

GOAL 2. The approach should be designed to protect critical structures near the lesion. Traditionally, the safest way to protect critical structures has been to achieve surgical access beyond the boundaries of the lesion itself to allow for direct visualization and control over the structures of interest. For example, surgical exposure around a tumor would be broadened to identify, dissect, and perhaps displace nearby cranial nerves or the carotid artery. Although obtaining this additional exposure may increase the operative time, it can be a major factor in the reduction of postoperative morbidity.

More recently, the introduction and increased application of two major technical advances have given the surgeon additional options for the protection of critical structures, often without the need for increased surgical exposure: image-guided computer-assisted surgery and endoscopic surgery.

Image-guided (stereotactic) computer-assisted surgery has become a very useful alternative—or adjunct—to wide surgical exposure in selected cases.[21-26] Such "navigational surgery" employs one of a variety of referencing systems that can assimilate preoperative imaging studies into a computer-based algorithm that allows image reformatting in three dimensions (The preoperative reference images may be CT- or magnetic resonance imaging [MRI]-based, or they may be a "fusion study" that takes advantage of both types of studies). The reformatted images then serve as the basis for intraoperative navigation, which involves the use of an interactive probe that transmits spatial-orientation information back to the computer via transmitters; these can be either electromagnetic or optical. The computer screen then displays the appropriate preoperative images with the location of the probe superimposed, thus "targeting" the area of interest (Figure 174-11). With navigational systems, structures that are anatomically fixed (i.e., orbital walls, carotid canal, optic canal) can be precisely located, and the risk of injury can be minimized.

Reported uses of image-guided surgery include primary and revision endoscopic sinus surgery, osteoplastic frontal sinusotomy, transsphenoidal hypophysectomy, endoscopic cerebrospinal fluid leak and encephalocele or meningocele repair, endoscopic skull base tumor resection, orbital surgery, and endoscopic pterygomaxillary fossa biopsy.[27,28]

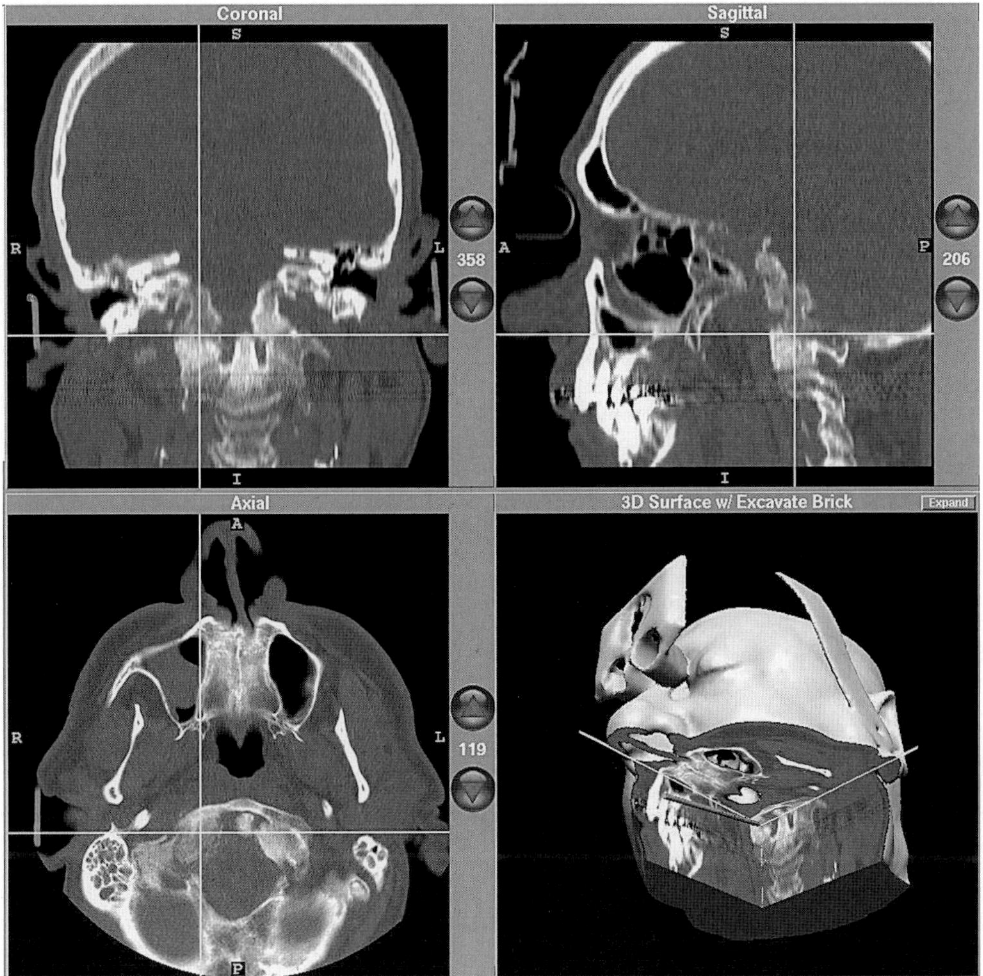

Figure 174-11. Navigational images as seen on intraoperative computer display. The patient's computed tomography images are displayed in the coronal *(top left)*, axial *(bottom left)*, and sagittal *(top right)* planes, and a three-dimensional cutaway view *(bottom right)* also is shown. On each image, the intersection of the crosshairs indicates the position of the navigational probe. As the probe is moved within the operative field, the images change to reflect the probe's precise location. In this case, a lesion that was both osteoblastic and osteolytic and that involved the occipital condyle was approached endoscopically through the nasal cavity without the need for an extensive disassembly approach. The lesion turned out to be a metastasis from a previous renal cell carcinoma.

The American Academy of Otolaryngology–Head and Neck Surgery endorses use of computer-aided surgery for the following specific procedures or conditions[29]:

- Revision sinus surgery
- Distorted sinus anatomy of development, postoperative, or traumatic origin
- Extensive sinonasal polyposis
- Pathology involving the frontal, posterior ethmoid, and sphenoid sinuses
- Disease abutting the skull base, orbit, optic nerve, or carotid artery
- CSF rhinorrhea or conditions that feature a skull base defect
- Benign and malignant sinonasal neoplasms

Intraoperative MRI or CT also has been proposed as a useful adjunct in skull base surgery. Proponents advocate the improved ability to detect residual tumor and evaluate for intraoperative complications, however, limitations of time and cost have prevented its widespread use outside of certain academic centers.[30]

Although large, multi-institutional prospective studies are yet to be accomplished, smaller studies and anecdotal reports demonstrate the efficacy of endoscope-assisted approaches for the treatment of selected skull base problems, most notably sinonasal neoplasms, pituitary tumors, and CSF leaks.[31-37]

Stamm[38] classifies endoscopic skull base approaches as follows:

1. Transnasal direct
2. Transethmoidal
3. Transseptal
4. Transplanum
5. Transsphenoidal-transpterygoid
6. Transsphenoidal-transclival
7. Transnasal-transpharyngeal (cranial-cervical junction)
8. Combined

The location and suspected pathology dictate the selection of approach.

Endoscopy-based approaches to the nasal cavity, olfactory groove, nasopharynx, ethmoid roof (anterior skull base), orbit and orbital apex, sphenoid sinus and sellar and parasellar areas, clivus, cavernous sinus, optic chiasm, pterygopalatine and infratemporal fossae, parapharyngeal space, craniocervical junction, petrous apex, and jugular foramen all have been described. In short, access to the central skull base from the frontal sinus to C2 and from the sella to the jugular foramen is now possible using the expanded endonasal approach.[39-43]

The endoscopic approach to the orbital apex and optic canal for orbital decompression in fibrous dysplasia, Graves' orbitopathy, compressive or traumatic optic neuropathy has been described. Of note, decompression is indicated only in patients with fibrous dysplasia with continuous deterioration of vision or undergoing removal of neighboring bone, but not as a prophylactic procedure.[44,45] This approach also is used in the management of clival lesions, anterior skull base tumors, and vascular malformations of the skull base.[46,47]

Kassam and associates described an approach to identify the petrous portion of the carotid artery following identification and retrograde dissection of the vidian artery. They found this to be a consistent landmark radiographically and intraoperatively.[48]

Endoscopic approaches to pituitary surgery offer benefits of improved cosmesis, decreased recovery time, and fewer complications. Three approaches exist: transnasal-transethmoid, transnasal-transseptal, and direct transnasal. The direct transnasal approach has been touted because of the advantages of avoiding the ethmoid complex, decreased operative time, and improved visualization.[2] Although endoscopic skull base surgery has been more extensively described for the anterior cranial base, endoscopic-assisted approaches to the middle cranial base also have been described.[49]

The protection of critical structures at the cranial base also is enhanced by the appropriate use of electrophysiologic monitoring, including intraoperative somatosensory evoked potentials, auditory brainstem evoked response, and EMG.[14] The injection of low-dose intrathecal fluorescein has been shown to be a useful adjunct intraoperatively to decrease the CSF leak rate and, when appropriate medication is provided, has been proven safe and without significant adverse effects.[50]

GOAL 3. The approach should be designed so that, at the completion of the extirpative phase, critical barriers between the neurocranium and viscerocranium can be reliably restored. These barriers, particularly the dura and subjacent soft tissues, normally serve to effectively insulate the intracranial contents and the ICA from exposure to the aerodigestive tract below, including the nasal cavity, sinuses, eustachian tube, and pneumatic spaces within the temporal bone. After they have been disturbed, the barriers should be restored to reduce the potential for such consequences as CSF fistula, meningitis, and septic carotid artery rupture. Also, an approach should respect the vascular territories of local tissues (i.e., the temporalis muscle, galea, and pericranium), which can then be used for the reconstruction.

Such vascularized local flaps are preferable to free flaps or nonvascularized grafts when available, however others have displayed excellent closure rates with materials ranging from acellular dermis to free microvascular transfers.[51,52] In general, smaller defects (less than 2 cm) are less likely to require vascularized tissue to achieve closure.[53,54]

Robotic endoscopic skull base surgery and transoral robotic surgery have been advocated by some researchers for the advantages of improved visualization, access, precise technique, and improved watertight closure following endoscopic skull base surgery. Although promising, more clinical investigation is needed before widespread acceptance of these techniques.[55,56]

GOAL 4. The choice of operative approach should reflect consideration for functional and aesthetic reconstruction, and it should include the placement of incisions within natural skin lines that respect aesthetic units of the face. The soft tissue closure should follow plastic surgery principles. Excellent skull base exposure usually can be achieved by elective osteotomies and the temporary removal of craniofacial bone segments, which are subsequently replaced, thereby preserving facial contour.[17,51,57-59] Even in cases in which aesthetically important segments should be removed for oncologic reasons, acceptable cosmesis can usually be accomplished through the judicious use of bone grafts and soft tissue flaps or through surgical closures designed to support alloplastic or prosthetic materials.

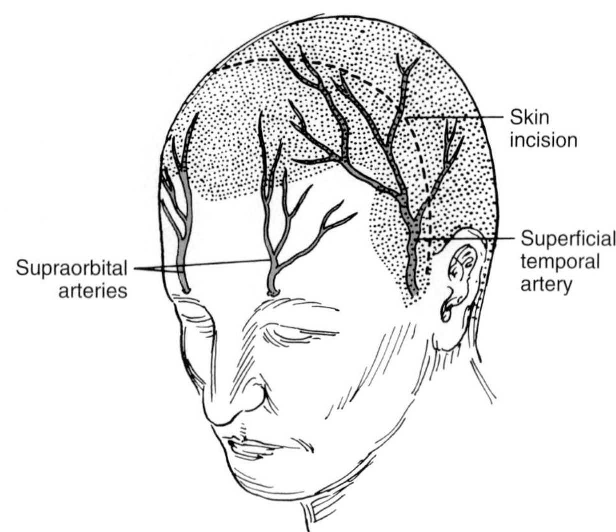

Figure 174-12. Bicoronal incision shown from the patient's left and demonstrating proper placement to allow for preservation of anterior branches of the superficial temporal artery. This incision design permits the use of a long pericranial or galeal flap (based on supraorbital vessels), which is important for the reconstruction of anterior cranial base defects.

Anterior Cranial Base Approaches

Surgical approaches to the anterior cranial base include methods that are purely extracranial and those that use combined extra- and intracranial exposures. The extracranial techniques—external ethmoidectomy, frontal sinusotomy, and intranasal ethmoidectomy—are suitable only for the management of discrete, well-localized lesions, such as CSF fistulas and some very limited benign anterior cranial base tumors. These procedures are well described elsewhere.[60,61]

Most of the remaining anterior cranial base lesions are best managed using the combined intracranial and extracranial techniques, of which there are basically two types: the classic anterior craniofacial resection and the basal subfrontal approach. Both of these approaches require bifrontal craniotomy for obtaining intracranial exposure. Except in special circumstances (e.g., in the presence of scars from previous-surgery or trauma), the most utilitarian incision for surgery of the anterior cranial base is the bicoronal incision.

Technical Note: The Bicoronal Incision

The bicoronal incision should be in the true coronal plane at the level of the top of the helix of the ear or slightly anterior to it (Fig. 174-12). A short, forward-directed, preauricular extension can be made on both sides to enhance scalp flap rotation. This coronal placement of the incision preserves the anterior branches of the superficial temporal artery, enhancing viability of the scalp flap. In addition, it substantially increases the length of vascularized galea and pericranium available for reconstruction as compared with incisions along the anterior hairline, the midforehead crease, or the brow. Additional length can be gained by back-elevating the scalp flap before division and elevation of the pericranial flap.

The central portion of the anterior scalp flap (i.e., the portion between the two superior temporal lines) is elevated in the subgaleal plane if a pericranial flap may be used and in the subperiosteal (subpericranial) plane if not. Lateral to the two superior temporal lines, it is elevated in the plane just above the deep temporal fascia. Therefore, at the temporal lines, the pericranium should be sharply incised to separate it from the origin of the deep temporal fascia (see Fig. 174-15). The pericranium is divided far enough posteriorly to provide sufficient

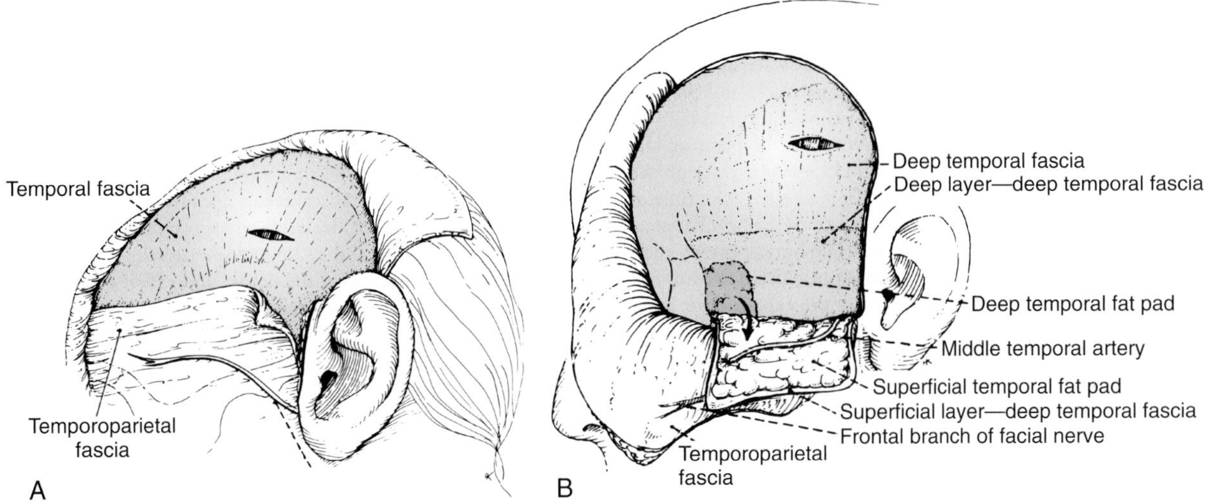

Figure 174-13. Relationship of the frontal branch of the facial nerve to layers of the temporal fascia. **A,** Anatomic dissection showing superficial temporal fascia (temporoparietal fascia), through which the nerve courses; attempts at surgery to elevate this relatively thin fascial layer alone may injure the nerve. **B,** Surgical dissection showing a deeper plane of fascial elevation that is less likely to cause injury to the frontal branch of the facial nerve. *(From Stuzin JM, Wagstrom L, Kawamoto HK, Wolfe SA. Anatomy of the frontal branch of the facial nerve: the significance of the temporal fat pad.* Plast Reconstr Surg. *1989;83:265-271.)*

length to the flap; then the dissection is carried forward in the subperiosteal plane as described earlier.

This deep temporal fascia begins to split into superficial and deep layers, beginning at approximately the level of the superior orbital rim.[62] These fascial layers diverge to envelop the lateral and medial surfaces of the zygomatic arch inferiorly; between the layers is the temporal fat pad. The frontal (temporal) branches of the facial nerve course just superficial to the zygoma along the superficial temporal fascia (temporoparietal fascia) and are prone to injury if the dissection is done at that level (Fig. 174-13A). Often these injuries can be avoided by maintaining the plane of dissection at the level of the deep layer of the deep temporal fascia (i.e., at the surface of the temporalis muscle itself). This deep plane of exposure essentially elevates the fat pad along with the superficial fascia and the superficial layer of the deep temporal fascia, thereby protecting the facial nerve branches (see Fig. 174-13B).[63,64] After the dissection reaches the level of the zygomatic arch, the arch is palpated, and its superior surface is directly exposed by sharply incising the fat pad and periosteum.

Further medially, flap elevation proceeds down the frontal area toward the supraorbital rims. Care should be taken to preserve the supraorbital supply of the galea and pericranium. This is best performed with elevation of the supraorbital rim periosteum that begins laterally and proceeds medially. A fine elevator is used first to palpate the supraorbital foramen (or notch) and then to expose its margins. If the pedicle is completely surrounded by bone, a 3-mm osteotome is used to fracture the inferior margin of the foramen, thereby liberating the pedicle and allowing it to be elevated intact, along with the remaining pericranium and underlying periorbita (Fig. 174-14). If the entire scalp flap is difficult to rotate inferiorly, the preauricular parts of the incision can be extended to as low as the tragus (without danger to the facial nerve trunk) or anteriorly (as far as the temporal hairline) to further enhance flap rotation.

Anterior Craniofacial Resection

Anterior craniofacial resection (Fig. 174-15) combines bifrontal craniotomy with transfacial exposure of the nasal cavity, ethmoid, maxillary, and orbital areas, usually by modifications of lateral rhinotomy, midfacial degloving, or other transfacial approaches.[65-67] Anterior craniofacial resection most often is used for removal of neoplasms that originate in the sinonasal tract and invade the anterior cranial fossa floor, such as squamous cell carcinoma, esthesioneuroblastoma, and adenocarcinoma. For cases in which tumor frankly invades the soft tissues of the orbit, the approach is extended to include orbital exenteration.[68]

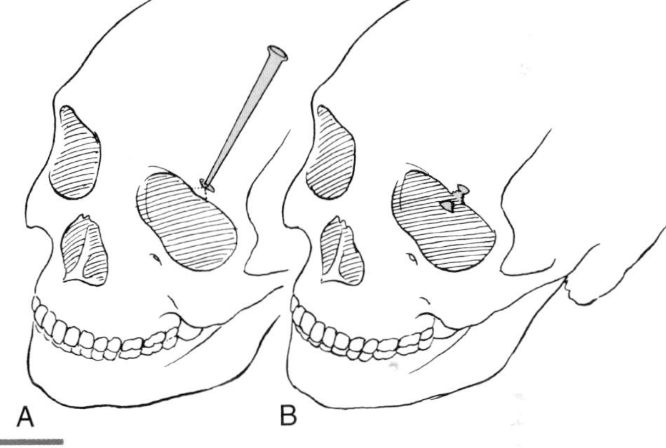

Figure 174-14. Technique for preserving the supraorbital neurovascular pedicle. **A,** After the foramen has been identified, a 3-mm osteotome is inserted along its lower border. **B,** A small segment of bone along the inferior rim of the foramen is fractured to liberate the nerve and vessels, which are reflected downward, along with soft tissues of the bicoronal flap.

The operation begins with transfacial exposure, which is followed by bifrontal craniotomy performed by the neurosurgeon. If the patient has a large frontal sinus, an osteoplastic flap may be elevated to avoid burr holes in the forehead area, which could later become aesthetically unsatisfactory. In such cases, the thin posterior table of the frontal sinus is opened with a diamond burr to expose the dura and then removed. If the frontal sinus is small, a frontal bone flap is developed using a guarded craniotome introduced through burr holes placed above the hairline or in the temporal areas. Near the midline, care is taken to separate the dural fold containing the sagittal sinus away from the bone to protect it before the craniotome is allowed to cross the sagittal plane. The lower horizontal bone cut should be kept low (within 1 cm of the superior orbital rims) to lessen the need for subsequent brain retraction. Withdrawing 25 to 50 mL of CSF from the lumbar subarachnoid catheter, lowering P_{CO_2} through controlled hyperventilation, and occasionally administering mannitol or corticosteroids will further reduce the need for mechanical frontal lobe retraction.

Next, the frontal lobes are elevated from the anterior cranial fossa floor by incising the dura and severing the olfactory nerves at the cribriform plate. This always results in some leakage of CSF, which is controlled by direct dural suture or a dural patch (from temporal fascia, fascia lata, or pericranium). The dural closure should be as watertight as possible. Dura is further elevated to expose the orbital roofs and planum sphenoidale and finally the base of the anterior clinoid processes.

If disease extirpation mandates the removal of the planum, the intracranial portions of the optic nerves should be exposed through the unroofing of the optic canal to protect them from injury at the time of sphenoid osteotomy.[14] If the disease is confined to the cribriform area, however, the planum may be entered with a cutting burr or osteotome[66] to establish the posterior bony margin without optic nerve decompression. This completes the intracranial portion of the exposure for anterior craniofacial resection.

The transfacial exposure often involves modifications of a lateral rhinotomy incision, which may transect the upper lip; this depends on whether a total maxillectomy will be done in conjunction with the resection. The periosteum is elevated from the nasal bone and from the medial and inferior surfaces of the orbit, and the nasolacrimal duct is identified and transected distally. The anterior and posterior ethmoid arteries are identified and cauterized or clipped. In most cases, it is necessary to perform a complete en bloc ethmoidectomy. For this purpose, a contralateral Lynch incision is made to elevate the contralateral periorbita, cauterize the anterior and posterior ethmoid vessels, and make the appropriate osteotomies using a sagittal saw. If preoperative imaging studies or intraoperative observations confirm the presence of tumor within the soft tissues of the orbit, then orbital exenteration may be performed after extending the skin incision laterally to include a portion of the eyelids. Depending on the nature and extent of the tumor, osteotomies also may be made to include part or all of the maxilla.

At this point, a reciprocating saw or cutting drill bit is used to create the osteotomies of the cranial floor. The frontal lobes are retracted or protected from the cutting instrument by inserting an appropriate malleable retractor. The reciprocating saw or cutting drill bit is introduced through the nasal and ethmoid exposures, and, under direct

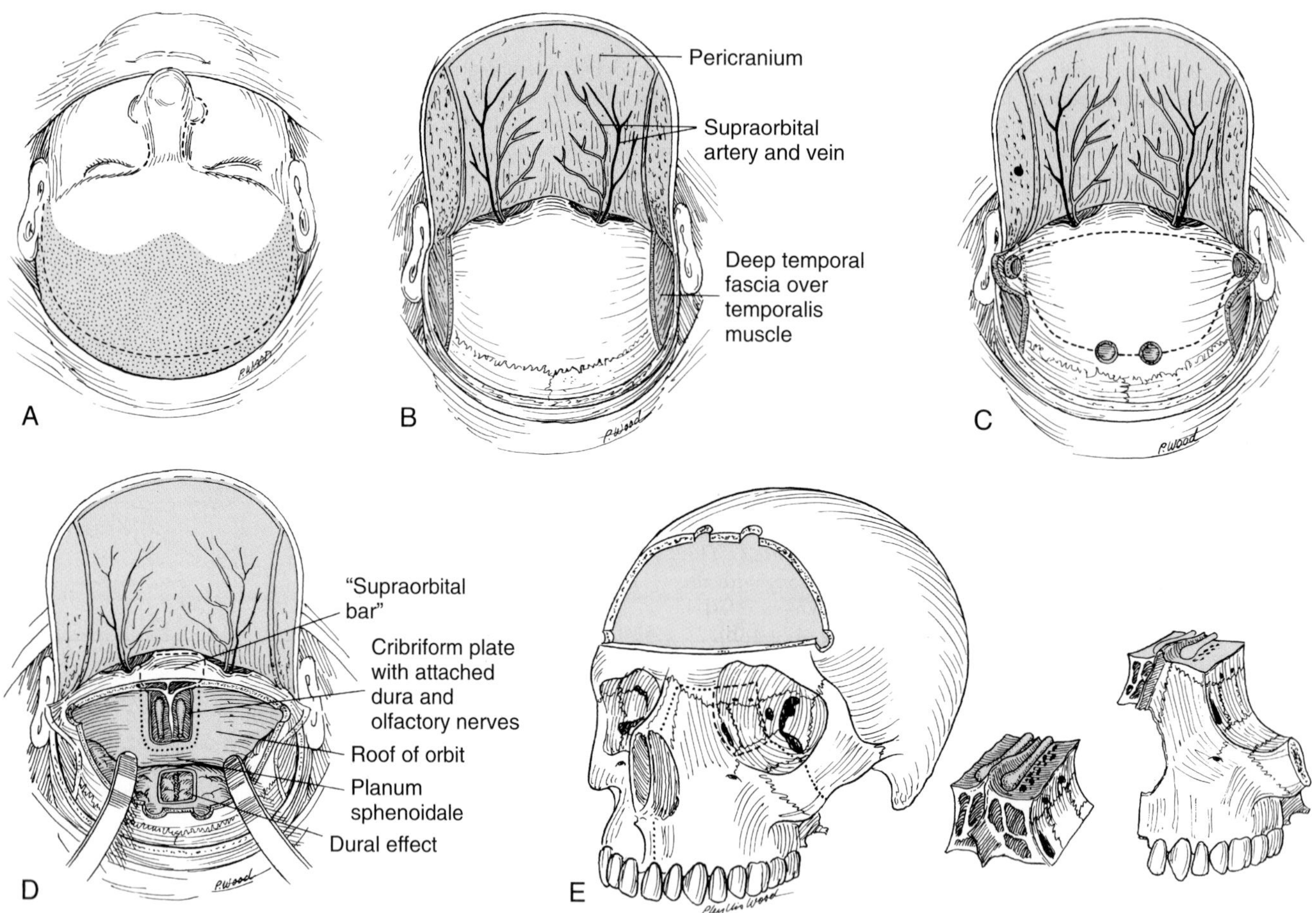

Figure 174-15. Anterior craniofacial resection. **A,** Incisions. High bicoronal incision preserves the optimal length of the galea and the pericranium for use as a reconstructive flap. Facial incisions usually include lateral rhinotomy and contralateral Lynch incisions, but these may be modified to suit the clinical situation. **B,** Elevation of the bicoronal scalp flap. The pericranium has been incised bilaterally at the superior temporal lines to separate it from the deep temporal fascia. Supraorbital vessels have been released from the supraorbital foramina to allow for the exposure of the superior orbital rims (zygomatic arches may be exposed using bicoronal incision by dissecting further laterally, as may be required for extended anterolateral craniofacial resections). **C,** Bifrontal craniotomy. *Dashed lines* represent the outline of the planned craniotomy. Temporalis muscles have been partially elevated so that burr holes may be placed below the temporal lines; superior burr holes are placed above the level of the frontal hairline. Such placement helps minimize postoperative cosmetic deformity. Paramedian positioning of superior burr holes aids in protection of superior sagittal (venous) sinus while the bone flap is being cut. **D,** Intracranial exposure. The frontal lobes have been retracted, and the dura has been incised, thereby leaving olfactory nerves and the margin of the dura to be resected en bloc, along with the cribriform plate and the ethmoid labyrinth (*dotted line*). The amount of dura and anterior cranial fossa floor resected will depend on the extent of tumor. To enhance exposure and direct visualization, the supraorbital bar *(dashed lines)* may be included in the resected specimen; after resection margins have been verified, this portion of bone is detached from the tumor-bearing part of the specimen and replaced. **E,** Osteotomies as seen from transfacial exposure. *Dashed lines* illustrate bone cuts used for en bloc ethmoidectomy, which result in the obtaining of a specimen *(left)*. *Dotted lines* indicate additional osteotomies to be used when total maxillectomy (with or without orbital exenteration) also is performed, thereby resulting in the obtaining of a specimen *(right)*. In both cases, resection encompasses part of the anterior cranial fossa floor. The extent of anterior fossa floor resection varies and should be modified as required by the extent of tumor.

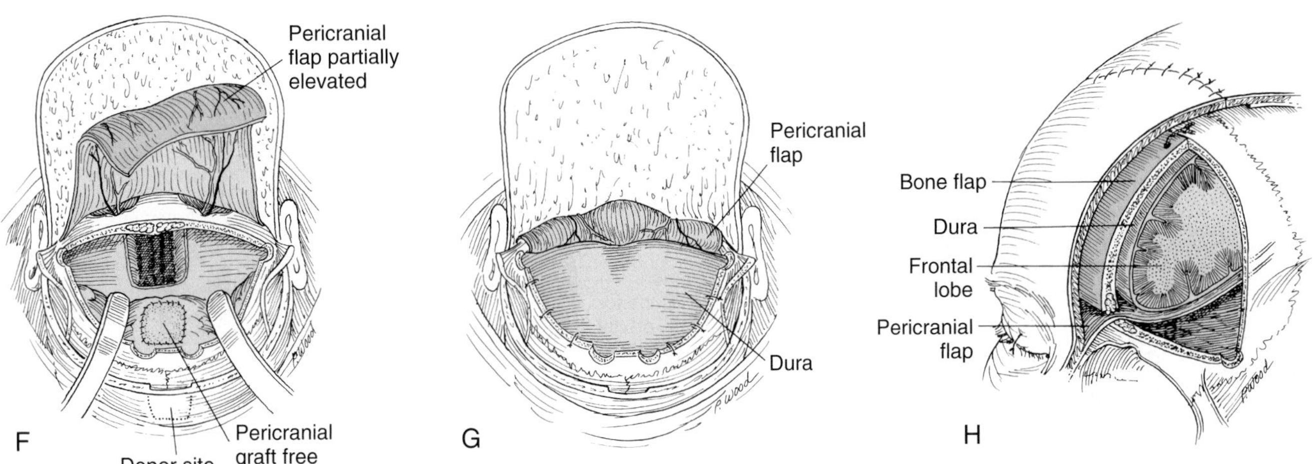

Figure 174-15, cont'd. **F,** Operative defect and preparation for closure. Large communication between the anterior cranial fossa and nasal cavity is closed by an inset of vascularized pericranial flap (shown here partially elevated from the galea). A dural defect created by resection of the olfactory nerves and surrounding dura has been closed with free graft of the pericranium taken from the posterior scalp *(dotted lines)*. Frontal sinuses have been stripped of mucosa and filled with autogenous fat after obliterating the frontonasal ducts. **G,** Cranial base defect repaired. A pericranial flap has been turned intracranially to line the anterior cranial fossa floor. Release of the frontal lobe retraction and clamping of the spinal drain have allowed for reexpansion of the brain and obliteration of the epidural dead space. The frontal bone flap is replaced and secured, with care taken to avoid compression of the pericranial flap. **H,** Cutaway view of final closure, showing the position of the pericranial flap relative to the brain and the cranial base. *(**A** to **G**, Adapted from Schramm VL. Craniofacial resection. In: Sasaki CT, McCabe BF, Kirchner JA, eds.* Surgery of the Skull Base. *Philadelphia: JB Lippincott; 1984.)*

vision, osteotomies are created from the planum sphenoidale, along the ethmoid roof, and forward to the front of the cribriform plate. These osteotomies may or may not include the supraorbital bar of bone, which is a portion of the frontal bone between the supraorbital rims (see Fig. 174-15D). If the tumor extends anteriorly to a significant degree, this supraorbital bar is removed with it as a single specimen, which can be closely inspected. If the supraorbital bar is not actually involved by tumor, it may be detached from the specimen and replaced for reconstruction at the completion of the operation.

After the resection margins have been verified by frozen section and are negative, reconstruction begins. As mentioned, it is critical that the dura be closed in a watertight fashion. This usually involves the placement of a patch of pericranium, temporal fascia, or fascia lata, followed by the placement of a vascularized pericranial flap over the defect in the floor of the anterior cranial fossa. The pericranial flap is developed by sharp dissection from the previously reflected scalp flap (see Fig. 174-15F).[69] Elevation of this flap of pericranium is continued down to the level of the glabella, with care taken to not injure its vascular pedicles. It is then rotated intracranially and positioned to form a bridge of soft tissue across the orbital roofs and back to the planum sphenoidale. If necessary, the distal end of the pericranial flap may be sutured to the dura over the planum for security; this provides a vascularized tissue barrier between the dura above and the nasal cavity below (see Fig. 174-15G and H). Unless a large amount of anterior cranial fossa bone has been resected and concern for brain herniation exists, it is usually not necessary to place a bone graft across the bony defect. Also, it is not necessary to place a skin graft on the undersurface of the pericranium (facing the nasal cavity), because this tissue mucosalizes readily on its nasal surface. After the pericranial flap is in place, the spinal drain is clamped so that no further intraoperative CSF decompression will take place. This will allow the gradual reexpansion of the brain to make contact with the pericranial flap, thereby obliterating any residual dead space. Because the pericranial flap traverses the frontal sinus, it is necessary to obliterate the frontonasal ducts and to remove all mucosa from within the sinus. A small amount of fat or free muscle may be packed into the ducts to obliterate any dead space inferiorly. The flap covers the frontonasal duct orifices and sinus floor. If the sinus is small, it may be obliterated by packing it with abdominal fat. If the sinus is large, however, removing the posterior table completely and allowing the brain and dura to expand and fill the space (cranialization of the frontal sinus) may be advisable.

In closing the facial incision, the medial canthal ligament is identified and secured to the remaining medial orbital wall. The upper and lower lid canaliculi may be intubated with a canalicular stent to prevent dacryostenosis. Before further closure, several tacking sutures are placed to secure the frontal dura to the margins of the craniotomy site; this will help in the prevention of postoperative epidural fluid and blood collections. The bifrontal craniotomy bone flap is then replaced and secured according to the surgeon's preference; this may be done with wires, plates, or sutures.

Basal Subfrontal Approach

The basal subfrontal approach or transbasal approach (Fig. 174-16)[14,70] is in many ways similar to the anterior craniofacial resection operation, except that the transfacial exposure is less extensive. Because the target area in this approach is more posterior (sphenoid and clivus) than that in the anterior craniofacial resection (ethmoids and cribriform), the craniotomy bone flap generally is somewhat larger and the orbital bone cuts are broader. This approach is used for lesions that primarily or secondarily involve the bony cranial base in the regions of the sphenoid body and upper clivus (e.g., meningiomas, fibrous dysplasia, chordomas, chondrosarcomas, ossifying fibromas).[63]

This approach also begins with a bicoronal incision. After exposing the orbital rims, periorbita is elevated from beneath the orbital roofs and medial walls in preparation for osteotomy. The anterior and posterior ethmoid arteries are identified bilaterally as landmarks, but they need not be divided because the axial ethmoid osteotomy can be made just above this level. Bifrontal craniotomy is then performed, and dura is elevated from above the orbital roofs and cribriform areas, as described. Using malleable retractors to protect the orbital contents and the brain, the reciprocating saw is used to create osteotomies that result in the temporary removal of both orbital roofs and the supraorbital bar (see Fig. 174-16A).

The coronal osteotomies along the posterior orbital roof should be made as far posteriorly as possible to simplify reconstruction, to conserve orbital contour, and to prevent postoperative pulsatile exophthalmos. These orbital cuts can be made as far back as the posterior ethmoid foramen but should be made only under direct vision from intra- and extracranial perspectives. With the use of these osteotomies, a very broad and basal exposure of the entire anterior cranial base is achieved (see Fig. 174-16B).

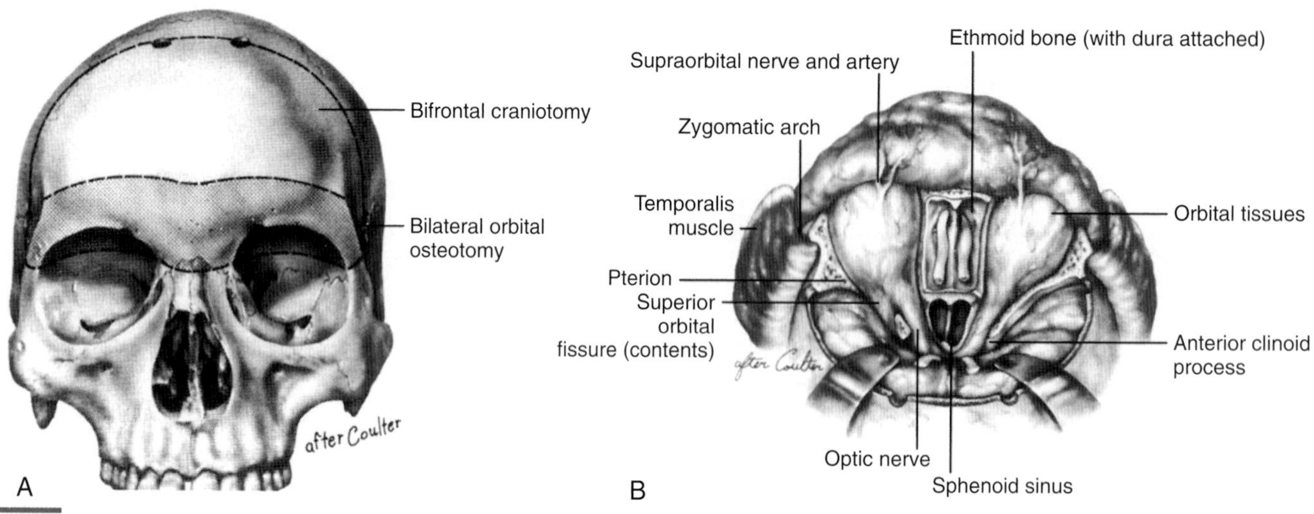

Figure 174-16. Basal subfrontal approach to the cranial base. **A,** Outlines of bifrontal craniotomy and bilateral orbital osteotomies. **B,** Surgeon's view from above after the removal of cranial and orbital bone segments. Olfactory nerves have been transected to allow sufficient brain retraction for exposure of the anterior fossa floor and decompression of the optic nerves. The sphenoid sinus has been widely opened. *(From Sekhar LN, Janecka IP. Intracranial extension of cranial base tumors and combined resection: the neurosurgical perspective. In: Jackson CG, ed.* Surgery of Skull Base Tumors. *New York: Churchill Livingstone; 1991.)*

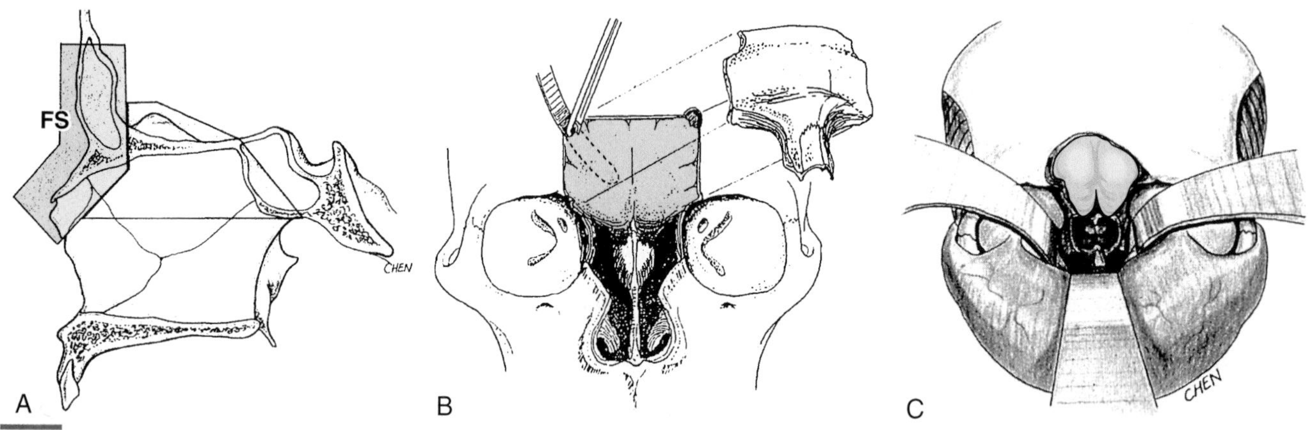

Figure 174-17. Subcranial approach to the anterior cranial base as described by Raveh.[71-73] **A,** Sagittal schematic showing the osteotomized frontonasal segment (FS), which is removed to allow access to deeper structures and then later replaced. **B,** Initial exposure afforded by the removal of the frontonasal bony segment; note the protection of the dura by a malleable retractor. **C,** Extent of exposure after lesion extirpation, with sphenoid sinus, sella, and orbital apices visible at the depth of the wound. Note that the bicoronal scalp flap has been elevated quite extensively along the lateral and medial orbital rims and nose to permt the frontonasal osteotomies and to compensate for the very low plane of access to the anterior cranial base while avoiding facial incisions *(see text)*. *(From Raveh J, Laedrach K, Ilzuka T, et al. Subcranial extended anterior approach for skull base tumors: surgical procedure and reconstruction. In: Donald PJ, ed.* Surgery of the Skull Base. *Philadelphia: Lippincott-Raven; 1998. With permission.)*

Working with the aid of the microscope, the approach is completed by rongeuring or drilling a small amount of bone remaining posteriorly to unroof the optic nerves, the superior orbital fissures, and the sphenoid sinus. Extirpation proceeds as required by the tumor and is followed by reconstruction, which is similar to that done for anterior craniofacial resection.

Raveh and colleagues[71-73] have described and refined an approach, now generally referred to as the subcranial approach, that offers significant advantages over the traditional anterior craniofacial resection and the basal subfrontal approach while combining elements of each. In the subcranial approach, facial incisions are not used; instead, the bicoronal scalp flap is reflected much further inferiorly to more completely expose both orbits and the nasomaxillary bony framework (Fig. 174-17). Extensive access along the entire anterior cranial base is possible as far back as the sella, the orbital apices, and the upper clivus. Advantages of the subcranial approach include minimal brain retraction, wide exposure, and the absence of facial scars.

Middle Cranial Base Approaches

In contrast with the anterior cranial base, surgical approaches to the middle cranial base are numerous and varied. This reflects the anatomic complexity of the region and the diversity of lesions found there. This discussion reviews several approaches and presents examples of those that have been found to be most useful.

Division into Central and Lateral Compartments

When considering surgical approaches to the middle cranial base, it is helpful to subdivide the region into a single central compartment and paired lateral compartments (Fig. 174-18).[74] When viewing the skull from the inferior perspective, the central compartment may be defined as that area between two parasagittal lines drawn from the medial pterygoid plate to the occipital condyle on each side. These lines correspond approximately to the pathways of the ICAs through the skull base. Thus, the central compartment consists of the pituitary fossa, the sphenoid rostrum and lower sphenoid sinus, the nasopharynx, the pterygopalatine fossa, and the lower portion of the clivus. (The lower

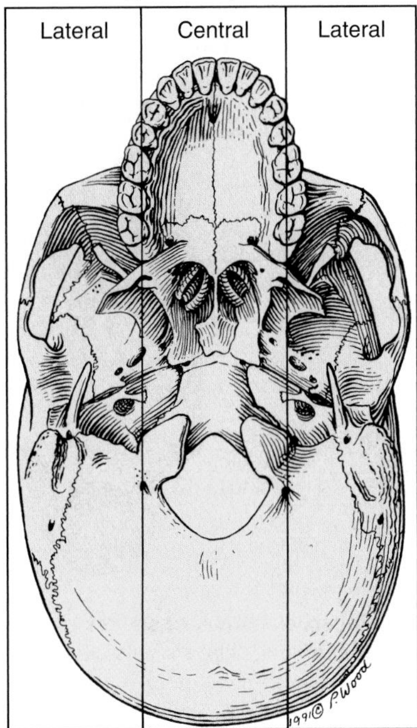

Figure 174-18. Compartments of the middle cranial base. The pathways of the internal carotid arteries as they traverse the middle cranial base region divide the region into one central and two lateral compartments. *(From Krespi YP, Sisson GA. Transmandibular exposure of the skull base. Am J Surg. 1984;148:534-538.)*

clivus actually is part of the occipital bone and not technically part of the middle cranial base. However, the surgical approaches to this area and also to the craniovertebral junction and upper cervical spine are essentially extensions of the approaches to the central compartment.)

The lateral compartment includes the entire infratemporal fossa, the parapharyngeal space, and the petrous portion of the temporal bone. This area is important because of the high density of neural and vascular structures within, including, extratemporally, the ICA; the internal jugular vein; the maxillary nerve (V2); the mandibular nerve (V3); the facial nerve (VII); cranial nerves IX, X, XI, and XII; the sympathetic nerves; and major branches of the external carotid artery, and, intratemporally, the cochlea, the vestibule, and cranial nerve VIII.

These distinctions between central and lateral compartments are valid in the sense that limited lesions within their respective boundaries will clearly be more amenable to resection using one type of approach vs another. However, it is not unusual for advanced lesions to extend beyond the line that separates the central from the lateral compartment; therefore, the surgical approach should be tailored to suit each clinical situation.

Approaches to the Central Compartment

The major surgical approaches to the central compartment of the middle cranial base are listed in Table 174-1, along with the anatomic areas for which they provide useful exposure. Except for pituitary surgery, these approaches are used primarily for the management of extradural lesions along the skull base.

Although most central compartment approaches in the literature can give access to the sphenoid sinus, not all are suitable for pituitary or parasellar surgery because of indirect exposure or oblique angle of entry into the sinus, which increases the risk of injury to adjacent neurovascular structures. When lesions are limited to the sphenoid sinus or the pituitary fossa, the transethmoidal sphenoidotomy (Fig. 174-19)[75,76] and the transseptal sphenoidotomy (Fig. 174-20)[77,78] are

Table 174-1

Surgical Approaches to the Middle Cranial Base: Central Compartment

	Anatomic Area(s) Exposed								
Approach	**SS**	**Sella**	**Clivus**	**NP**	**PPF**	**Maxilla**	**Ethmoid**	**C spine**	**ACB**
Transseptal sphenoid	+	+	–	–	–	–	–	–	–
Transethmoidal sphenoid	+	+	–	–	–	–	+	–	+
Lateral rhinotomy	+	NR	±	+	+	+	+	–	+
Transantral	+	+	±	+	+	+	+	–	–
Midfacial degloving	+	+	+	+	+	+	+	–	+
Le Fort I osteotomy	+	+	+	+	+	+	±	+	–
Transpalatal	+	–	+	+	–	–	–	+	–
Transoral	–	–	+	+	–	–	–	+	–
Mandibulotomy	–	–	+	+	–	–	–	+	–
Extended maxillotomy	+	±	+	+	+	+	+	+	–
Midfacial split	+	+	+	+	+	+	+	+	+
Intratemporal fossa	+	±	+	+	+	±	–	–	–
Facial translocation	+	+	+	+	+	+	+	–	+

ACB, anterior cranial base; C spine, cervical spine; NP, nasopharynx; NR, not recommended; PPF, pterygopalatine fossa; SS, sphenoid sinus; ±, exposure possible but limited.

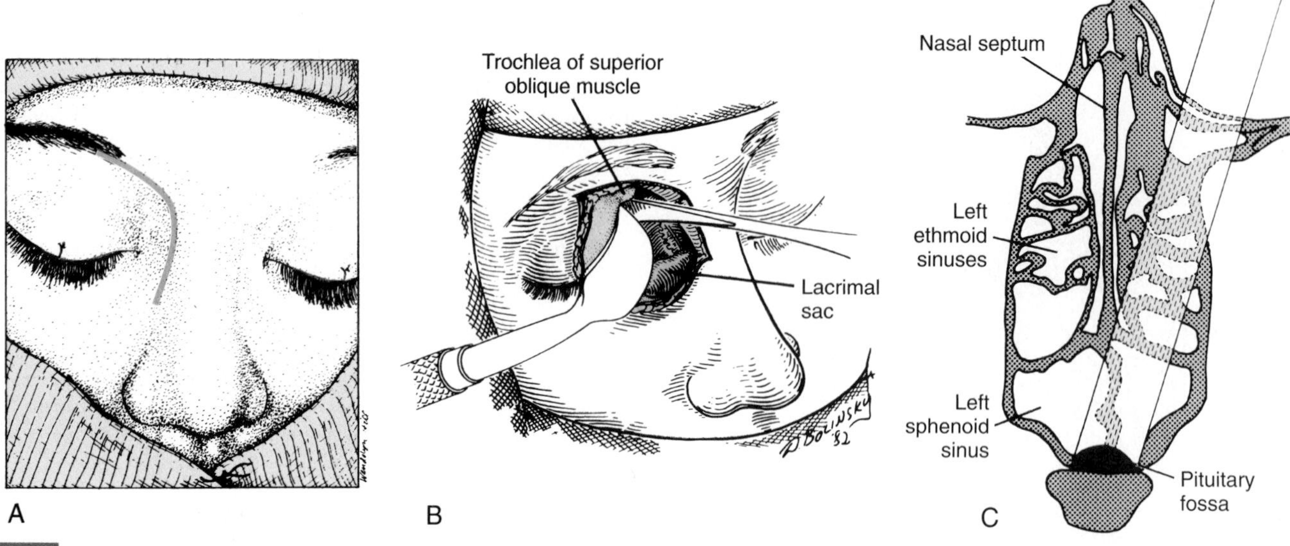

Figure 174-19. Transethmoidal-transsphenoidal approach to the cranial base. **A,** Incision. **B,** Retraction of orbital contents exposes the ethmoid labyrinth. **C,** Axial section at the level of the ethmoid and sphenoid sinuses. Progressive removal of ethmoidal air cells allows for entry into the sphenoid sinus and pituitary fossa. *(**A** and **C,** From Sasaki CT. Pituitary ablation for carcinoma of the breast: transethmoidal approach to the sella.* Otolaryngol Clin North Am. *1981;14:391; **B,** from Kirchner JA. Transethmoidal approach to the sella. In: Sasaki CT, McCabe BF, Kirchner JA, eds.* Surgery of the Skull Base. *Philadelphia: JB Lippincott; 1984.)*

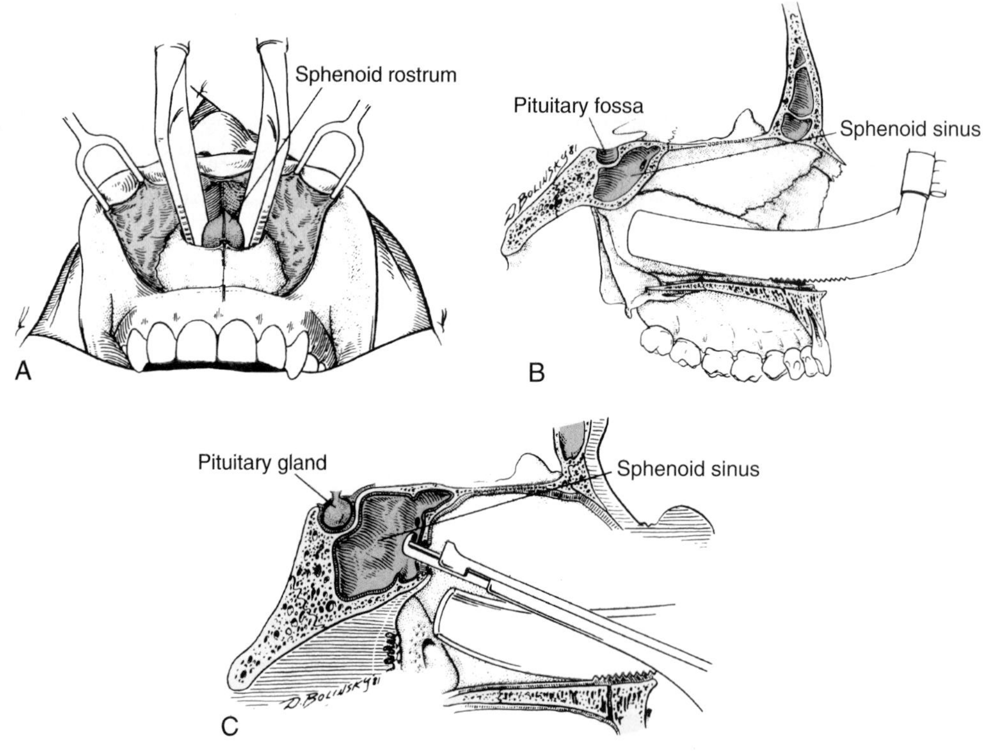

Figure 174-20. Transseptal-transsphenoidal approach to the cranial base. **A,** A sublabial incision is used to gain access to the premaxilla and to the nasal septum, which is exposed from the anterior nasal spine to the sphenoid rostrum in the subperichondrial-superiosteal plane. **B,** Lateral view of exposed area, showing a self-retaining speculum in position at the sphenoid rostrum. **C,** Sphenoid sinus is opened. A transseptal-transsphenoidal approach may be used for pituitary fossa surgery, for the removal of limited lesions of sphenoid region, or for the biopsy of tumors that involve the area. *(From Sasaki CT. Transseptal-transsphenoidal approach to the sella. In: Sasaki CT, McCabe BF, Kirchner JA, eds.* Surgery of the Skull Base. *Philadelphia: JB Lippincott; 1984.)*

usually satisfactory, safe, and effective. These approaches are useful for obtaining biopsy specimens of more extensive lesions that involve that region. For larger lesions that involve adjacent areas, however, the exposure is inadequate, because the operative field is deep and narrow, thus requiring the use of the operating microscope in most cases.

With trends toward less invasive surgical techniques, endoscopic procedures are gaining popularity as primary or adjuvant approaches in cranial base surgery. For tumors of the pituitary gland, endoscopic transnasal-transsphenoidal resection is another valuable option. Proponents of endoscopic pituitary surgery report fewer complications of facial swelling, septal perforations, nasal septal deviation or synechia formation, and numbness of the upper incisors; they also report a shorter hospital stay.[79,80] The surgery is performed with the patient under general anesthesia in the supine position with the head elevated 10 degrees. In most cases, the operation can be performed through one nostril, the choice of which depends on the width of the nasal cavity and the laterality of the pituitary tumor. The nose is decongested topically, and further vasoconstriction is achieved by infiltrating the mucosa over the rostrum of the sphenoid, the middle turbinate, and the posterior septum with lidocaine hydrochloride 1% with epinephrine 1 : 100,000.

Using a rigid zero-degree endoscope, the sphenoid ostium is identified, and its position may be confirmed by the use of C-arm fluoroscopy or image-guided navigation. The middle turbinate can be outfractured or removed to provide increased exposure to the sphenoid rostrum. The sphenoid ostia are identified and fractured inferomedially. Kerrison rongeurs or Hardy punches are used to widen the sphenoidotomy and to remove the sphenoid rostrum. The posterior septum may be rongeured to provide wide visualization, including that of the contralateral sphenoid sinus cavity. The 30-degree endoscope is inserted into both sides of the sphenoid sinus for identification of the optic and carotid protuberance, the opticocarotid recess, the clival indentation, and the anterior wall of the sella[81] (Fig. 174-21). After removal of the intersinus septum, the sella and dura are exposed and entered in the standard fashion. For resection of macroadenomas, insertion of the 30-degree endoscope allows the surgeon to follow intrasellar and extrasellar extension of the tumor and to identify and preserve the arachnoid membrane[81] (Fig. 174-22). The ability to directly visualize tumor and healthy pituitary gland through the endoscope is a major advantage over the operating microscope. This increased visualization may allow

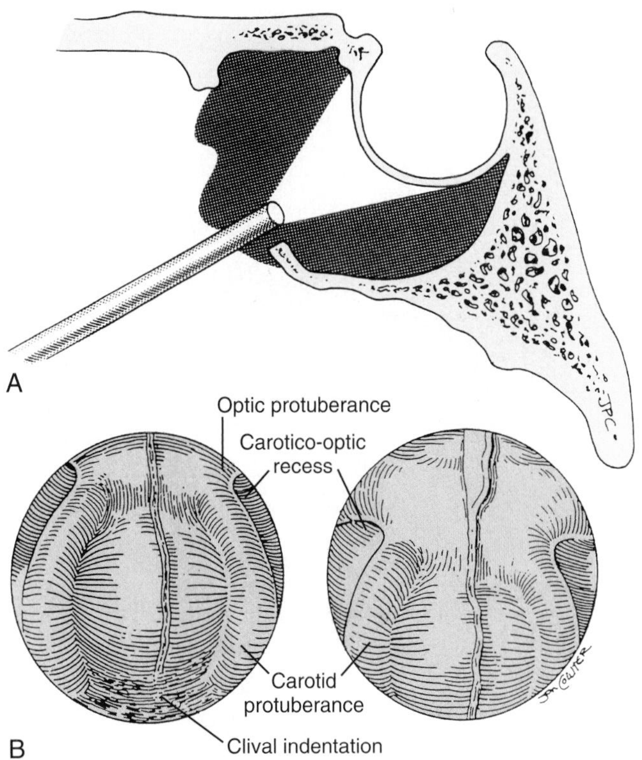

Figure 174-21. A, Endoscopic view of the sphenoid sinus after the completion of anterior sphenoidotomy and resection of the sphenoidal septum. **B,** *Left*: View with a zero-degree endoscope reveals the carotico-optic recesses, carotid protuberances, and clival indentation to the anterior wall of the sella. *Right*: A 30-degree endoscope provides a better panoramic view of the optic protuberances, the carotico-optic recesses, the carotid protuberances, and the upper portion of the anterior wall of the sella. *(From Jho HD, Carrau RL, Ko Y. Endoscopic pituitary surgery. In: Rengachary SS, Wilkins RH, eds.* Neurosurgical Operative Atlas. *Vol 5. Park Ridge, Ill: AANS; 1996. Copyright by the American Association of Neurological Surgeons.)*

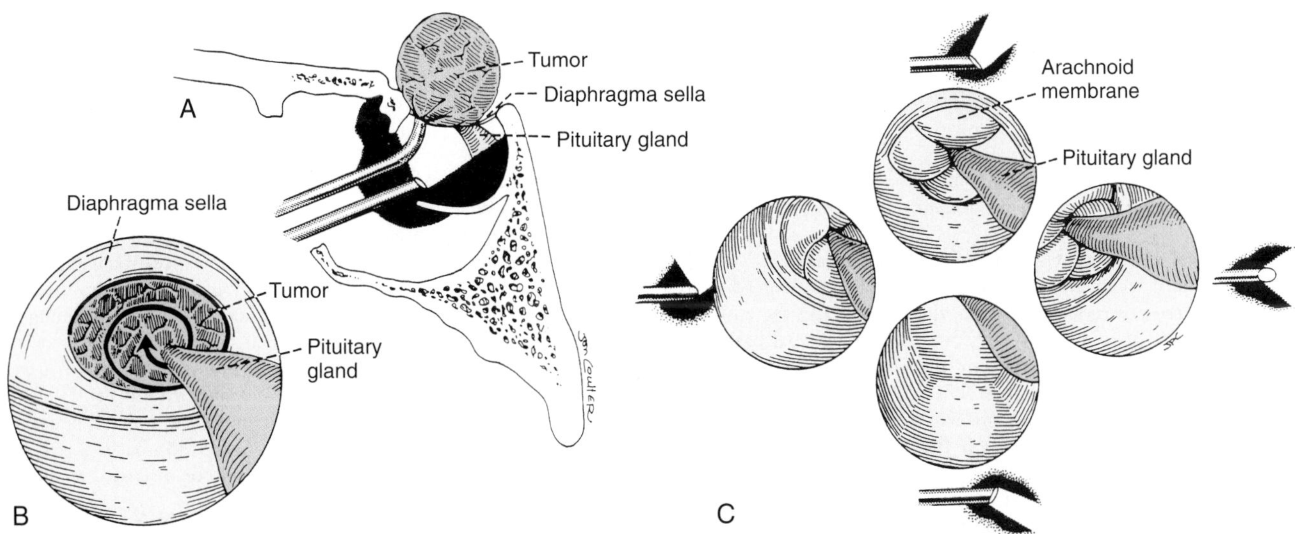

Figure 174-22. A, Sagittal view of the sella. **B,** 30-Degree endoscopic view of the suprasellar tumor. The suprasellar portion of the tumor is removed with a curved suction cannula beginning around the edge of the diaphragma sella circumferentially and heading toward the center of the tumor gradually. The healthy pituitary gland tissue is preserved, if possible. **C,** The arachnoid membrane will herniate down gradually when the suprasellar portion of the tumor has been completely removed. The center of the flower-shaped arachnoid membrane will be the pituitary stalk. Any healthy-looking pituitary gland tissue is preserved. When the 30-degree–angled endoscope placed inside the sella is rotated, it will reveal the suprasellar region superiorly, the lateral wall of the sella laterally, and the floor of the sella inferiorly. Residual tumor is removed from all corners by rotating the 30-degree endoscope. *(From Jho HD, Carrau RL, Ko Y. Endoscopic pituitary surgery. In: Rengachary SS, Wilkins RH, eds.* Neurosurgical Operative Atlas. *Vol 5. Park Ridge, Ill: AANS; 1996. Copyright by the American Association of Neurological Surgeons.)*

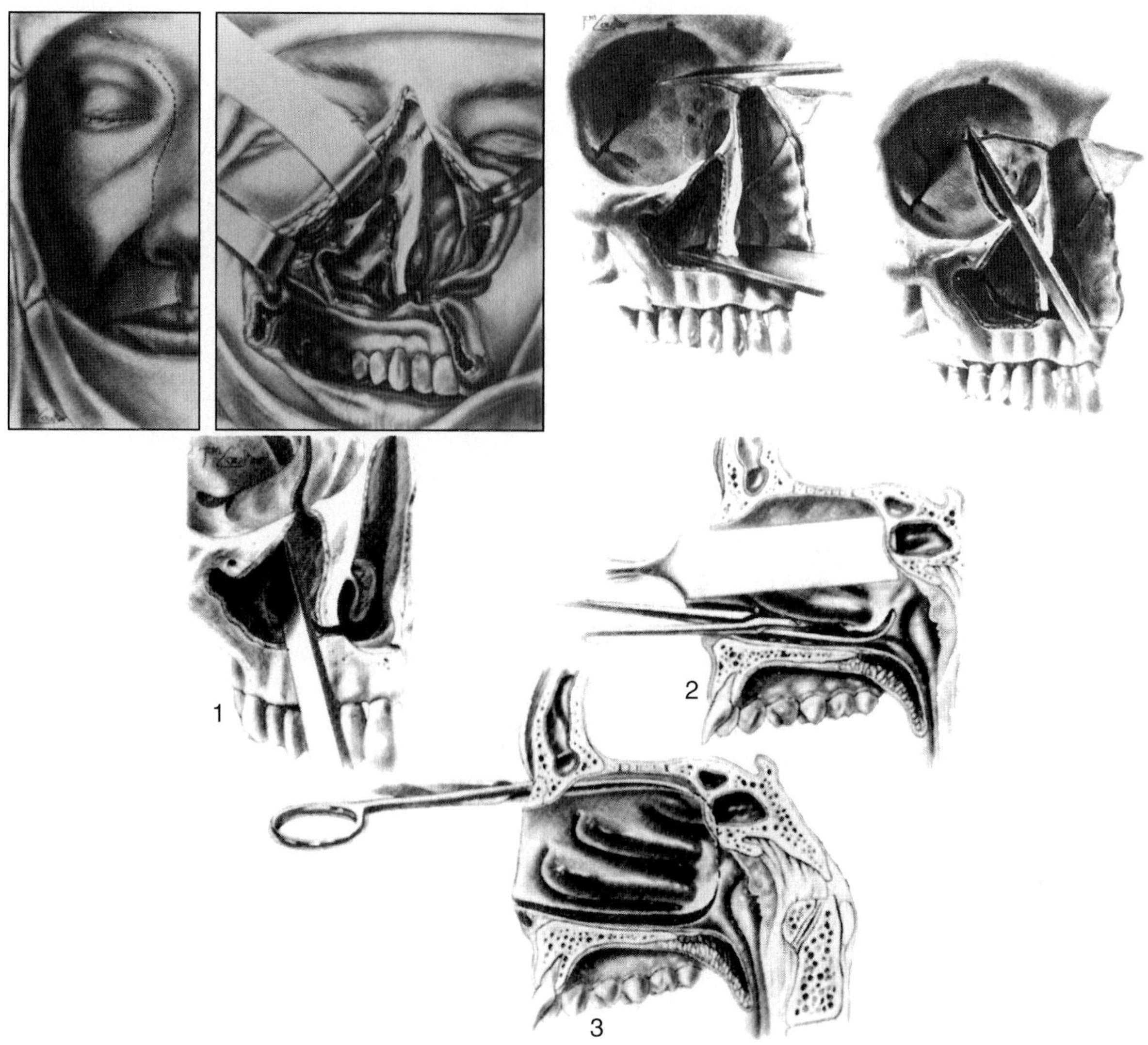

Figure 174-23. Lateral rhinotomy. *Top left,* Incision and soft tissue exposure followed by maxillary antrostomy. *Top right,* Osteotomies of the orbit and maxilla. *Bottom,* Anterior (1) and sagittal (2 and 3) views of posterior osteotomies and soft tissue cuts to remove medial portions of the orbit and maxilla. Such exposure can provide access to the face of the sphenoid, nasopharynx, pterygopalatine fossa, and ethmoid regions. *(From Schramm VL, Myers EN. "How I do it"—head and neck. A targeted problem and its solution. Lateral rhinotomy.* Laryngoscope. *1978;88:1042-1045.)*

for more complete tumor resection, while limiting the potential complications associated with blind curettage of the superior and lateral sella contents.

The lateral rhinotomy (Fig. 174-23)[82] and transantral (Fig. 174-24)[83] procedures afford wider access to the anterior sphenoid and adjacent nasopharynx, the pterygopalatine fossa, the maxilla, and the ethmoid regions. However, they generally are unsatisfactory for extirpation of any but the smallest lesions situated in the sphenoidal-clival area. The midfacial degloving approach (Fig. 174-25)[84] is more suitable for dealing with larger central compartment lesions, because it allows for improved midline access through the nose and both maxillary sinuses. Medial maxillectomy and resection of the ascending process of the palatine bone are included, if necessary, giving the surgeon good visualization of the nasopharynx and the adjacent skull base. The Le Fort I osteotomy (Fig. 174-26)[85,86] can be an alternative method for reaching these areas from a slightly more inferior angle, or it may be used as an adjunct to midface degloving, offering additional access to the oronasopharynx and clivus by displacing the hard and soft palate inferiorly.

For lesions of the clivus that also involve the upper cervical vertebrae (the craniovertebral junction), mandibulotomy (Fig. 174-27)[74,87,88] will afford a paramedian route to reach the lower areas of extension. The transpalatal (Fig. 174-28)[89,90] and transoral (Fig. 174-29)[91,92] approaches are also used for the management of lesions at the craniovertebral junction and may be used concomitantly with mandibulotomy, if necessary. A significant benefit of such a combined approach is that, with mandibulotomy, it is also possible to expose the parapharyngeal space and therefore to safely dissect along the ICA from the neck up to its entrance into the temporal bone.[74,87,88] This advantage is important when removing tumors that arise primarily in the central compartment but that have extended laterally. Conversely, for lesions that originate in the lateral compartment and extend centrally, the infratemporal fossa approach or one of its modifications can be used.[93] These approaches and the facial translocation approach,[17] which is suitable for lesions in both compartments, will be discussed in the following section.

An alternative approach for the removal of extensive lesions of the clivus and craniovertebral junction is the extended maxillotomy operation or its modification, the subtotal maxillectomy (Fig. 174-30).[94] In general, these innovative techniques combine the advantages of many approaches. They afford wide exposure of the central compartment by unilaterally displacing or resecting the hemimaxilla.

For very extensive clival and craniovertebral junction tumors, when bilateral transmaxillary access is needed, the midfacial split approach (Fig. 174-31) can be used.[51,57] This approach provides access to the entire central skull base in a unified surgical field that can extend

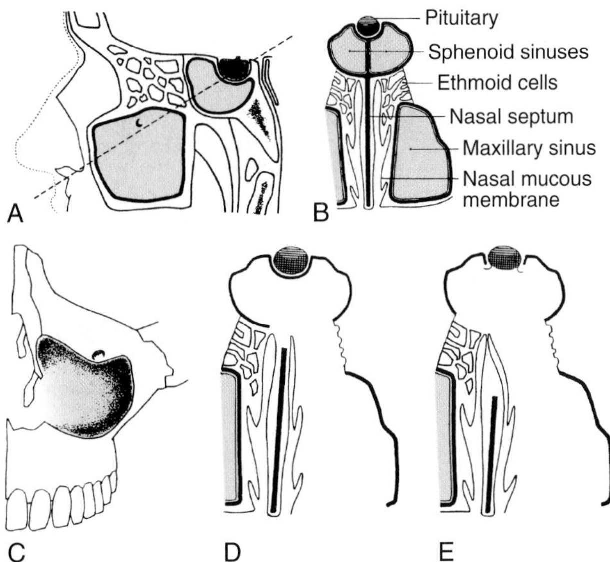

Figure 174-24. Transantral (transantrosphenoidal) approach to the cranial base as used for hypophysectomy. **A,** Near-sagittal section through the skull base and midface showing surgical route to the sphenoid region via the maxillary antrum. **B,** Oblique section in plane of the *dotted line* shown in **A** demonstrating the relationship among the maxillary sinus, the ethmoid air cells, and the sphenoid sinus. **C,** Partial medial maxillectomy performed to facilitate access. **D,** Ethmoidectomy and removal of the anterior wall of the sphenoid sinus. **E,** Exposure within the sphenoid sinus and pituitary fossa after partial submucous resection of the nasal septum. *(From Hamberger CA, Hammer G, Norlen G, Sjogren B. Transantrosphenoidal hypophysectomy.* Arch Otolaryngol. *1961;74:2-8.)*

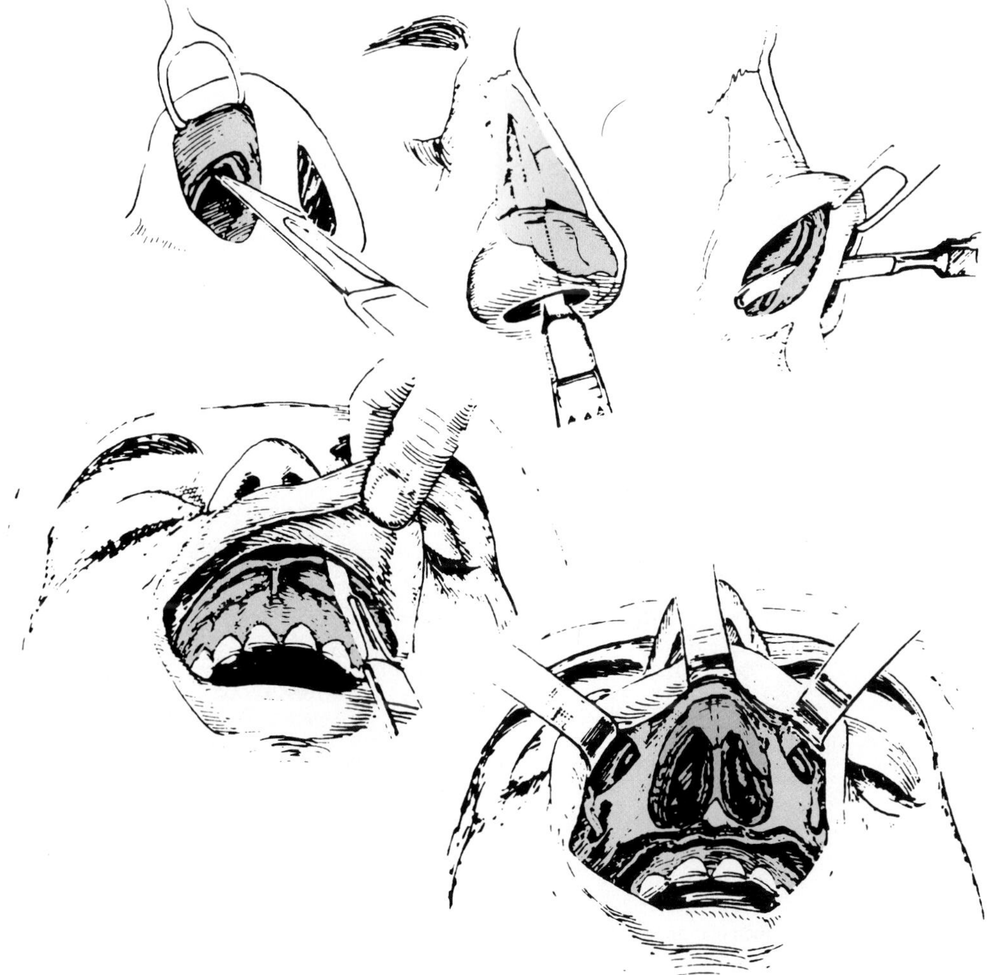

Figure 174-25. Midfacial degloving approach. Intranasal and sublabial incisions are used to elevate skin and soft tissues from the anterior facial skeleton (degloving). Subsequent bone removal and skull base exposure are similar to that shown for lateral rhinotomy, with an added benefit of bilateral access. *(From Casson PR, Bonanno PC, Converse JM. The midface degloving procedure.* Plast Reconstr Surg. *1974;53:102-103.)*

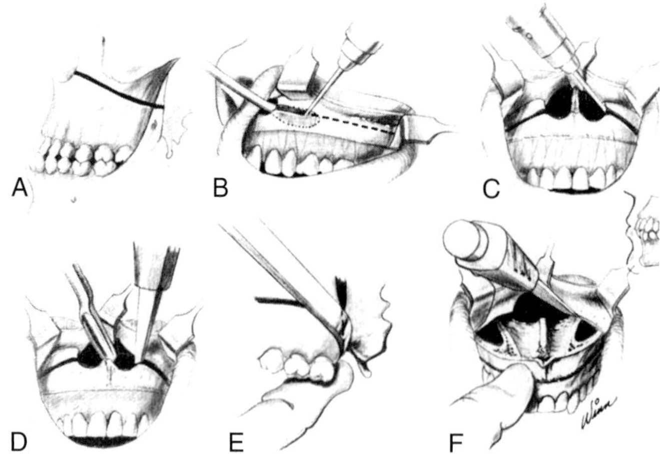

Figure 174-26. Le Fort I osteotomy approach. **A,** Lateral view of proposed osteotomy site just above the level of the nasal floor. **B** and **C,** Incisions and bone cuts along the anterolateral maxillary surface. **D,** Separation of the nasal septum with an osteotome. **E,** Separation of the maxilla from the pterygoid plate with a curved osteotome. **F,** Down-fracture of the maxilla to allow access to the maxillary sinuses, nasopharynx, and adjacent skull base. *(From Bell WH. Le Fort I osteotomy for correction of maxillary deformities.* J Oral Surg. *1975;33:412-426.)*

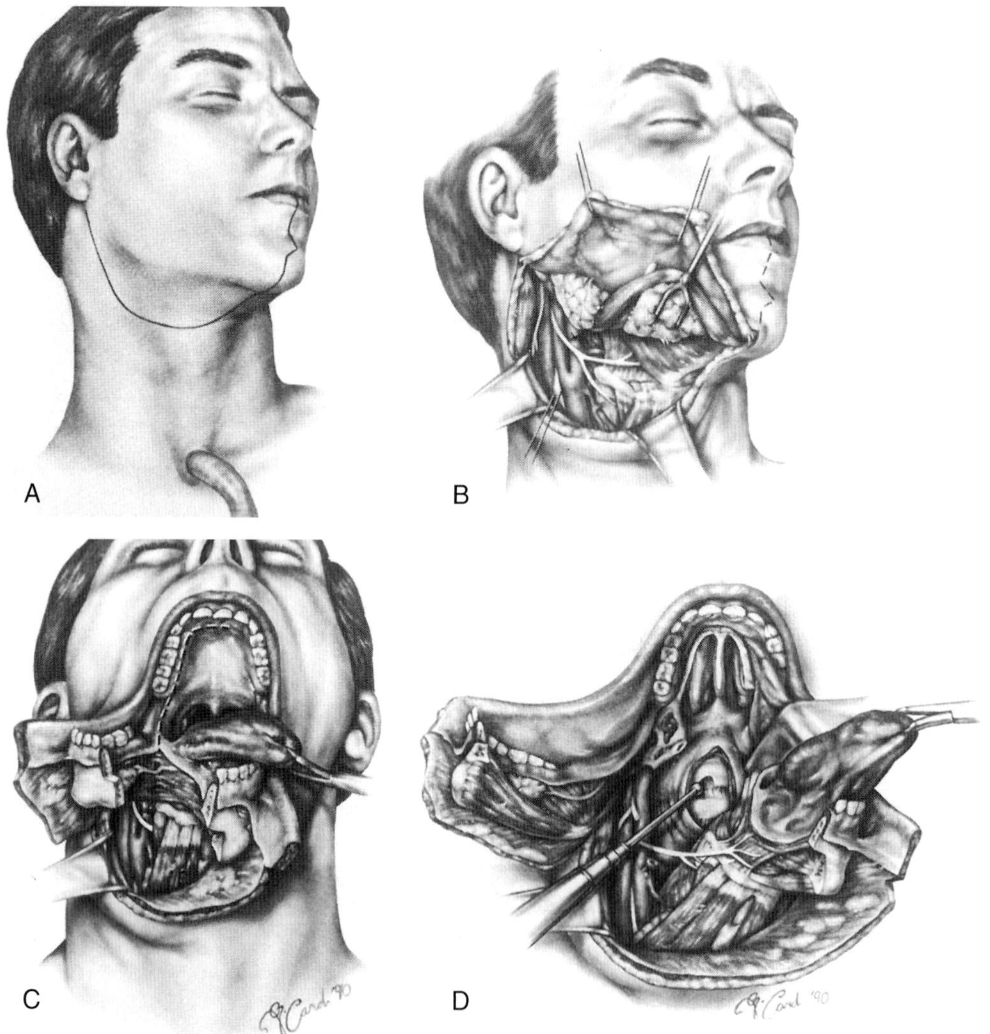

Figure 174-27. Mandibulotomy or transmandibular approach to the cranial base. **A,** Incision. **B,** Identification of major vessels and nerves in the neck. **C,** Paramedian mandibulotomy and intraoral incisions of the gingivolingual and palatal areas. **D,** After retraction of the mandible, tongue, and suprahyoid structures, major vessels may be dissected up to the skull base. Hard and soft palates are displaced to expose the nasopharynx and clivus, and upper cervical vertebrae are likewise accessible. Such an approach is useful for the management of tumors of the parapharyngeal space and the craniocervical junction. *(From Krespi YP, Cusumano RJ. Transpalatal and transmandibular approaches to the skull base. In: Jackson CG, ed.* Surgery of Skull Base Tumors. *New York: Churchill Livingstone; 1991:185-193.)*

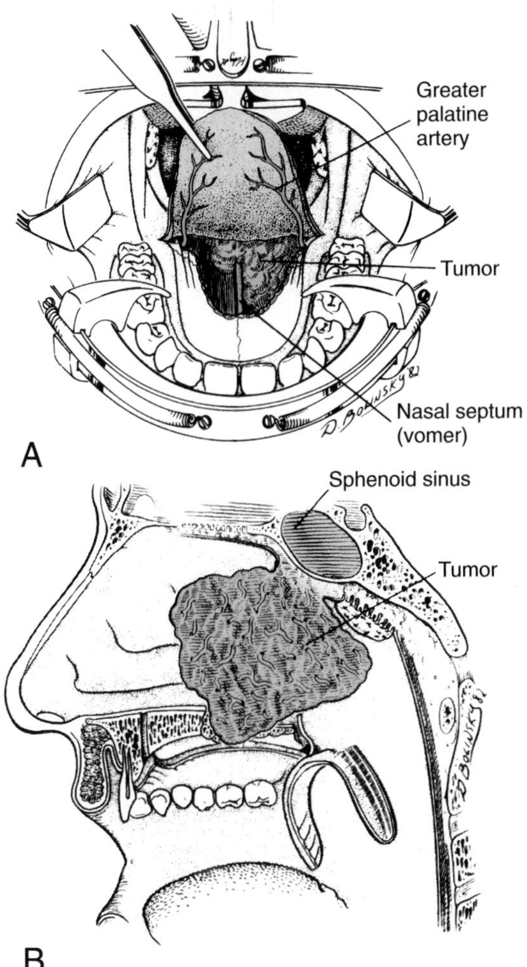

Figure 174-28. Transpalatal approach to the cranial base. **A,** A U-shaped incision has been made in the palatal mucoperiosteum, which has been elevated with care taken to preserve the greater palatine arteries bilaterally. The posterior portion of the bone of the hard palate has been removed to expose the nasal cavity and the tumor within. **B,** Sagittal view of the exposure obtained with a transpalatal approach. *(From Jenkins HA, Canalis RF. Transpalatal approach to the skull base. In: Sasaki CT, McCabe BF, Kirchner JA, eds.* Surgery of the Skull Base. *Philadelphia: JB Lippincott; 1984.)*

vertically from the anterior fossa floor to the level of the second cervical vertebra (and lower, if combined with mandibulotomy) and horizontally from jugular fossa to jugular fossa. This exposure is achieved using craniofacial disassembly to completely displace the midfacial skeleton, including both maxillae, the orbital floors, and the palate. It is especially useful for the management of large tumors that originate in the central compartment and that have also involved the adjacent anterior cranial base, the craniovertebral junction, or the lateral compartment.

Approaches to the Lateral Compartment

Numerous approaches have been developed and advocated for obtaining surgical access to the lateral compartment of the cranial base. Despite this apparent diversity of techniques and the sometimes confusing terminology by which they are described, considerable overlap exists. Most of the currently used approaches arrive at the cranial base through one (or more) of four main avenues: transtemporal, infratemporal, transfacial, or intracranial. These avenues refer to the primary direction or orientation from which the surgical exposure is ultimately achieved. In most cases, this orientation will influence the usefulness and morbidity of the operation. The cranial base surgeon should be

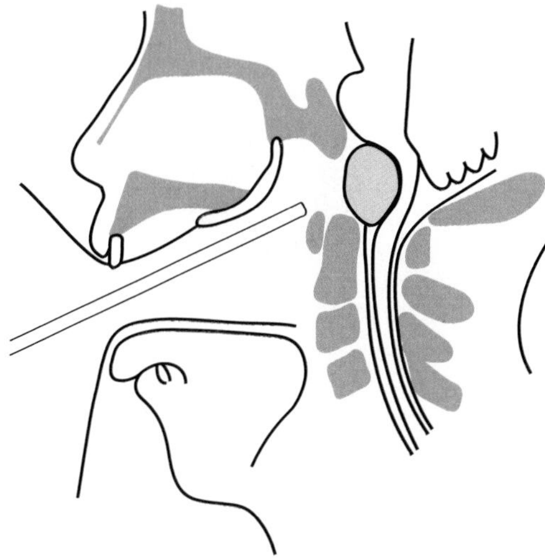

Figure 174-29. Transoral approach to the cranial base, showing access to the craniocervical junction through the open mouth, with retraction of the soft palate. *Light orange* represents a tumor of the clivus, with concomitant compression of the brainstem. *(From Crockard HA, Bradford R. Transoral transclival removal of a schwannoma anterior to the craniocervical junction. Case report.* J Neurosurg. *1985;62:293.)*

familiar with the advantages and limitations of each of these four routes. For extensive lesions, it often becomes necessary to combine approaches.

Transtemporal Approaches

The transtemporal routes include the transcochlear,[95] translabyrinthine,[15,96] presigmoid, retrolabyrinthine,[2] and combined[97] approaches. These are lateral, primarily extradural techniques that traverse the mastoid and petrous portions of the temporal bone to provide exposure of lesions of the petrous apex, the clivus, and the cerebellopontine angle. The anterior limit of purely transtemporal approaches is the intrapetrous course of the ICA, and these approaches therefore give only limited access to the middle cranial base. Accordingly, they more often are used for the management of tumors of the posterior cranial base (e.g., acoustic neuromas, petroclival meningiomas, aggressive cholesteatomas), and they will therefore be discussed in more detail in Chapter 177. With respect to the middle cranial base, the transtemporal approaches are useful mainly as adjunctive techniques in combination with craniotomy, infratemporal, or transfacial approaches. They can be used to enhance exposure of advanced lesions of the middle cranial base that have secondarily extended into or beyond the petroclival region and posterior to the course of the ICA. Postoperative consequences include permanent unilateral deafness with or without disequilibrium caused by functional loss of the middle or inner ear structures and facial paralysis of variable degree and duration caused by seventh nerve decompression or transposition.

Infratemporal Approaches

The infratemporal routes to the lateral compartment include the infratemporal fossa, lateral transparotid, extended rhytidectomy, lateral transtemporal-sphenoid, lateral facial, and subtemporal-infratemporal approaches.

The infratemporal fossa approach of Fisch and colleagues[93,98,99] encompasses three variations for use in specific clinical situations (Fig. 174-32). The type A approach provides exposure between the sigmoid sinus and the condylar fossa, and it is designed to reach to the petrous apex and infralabyrinthine areas. It is most useful for the management of cholesteatomas, meningiomas, and glomus tumors of those regions. The type B approach allows access from the sigmoid sinus to the petrous tip (including exposure of the horizontal ICA and foramen ovale) to reach lesions of the clivus, such as chordomas, meningiomas, and extensive apex cholesteatomas. The type C approach expands this access to include the parasellar region, the cavernous sinus, the foramen

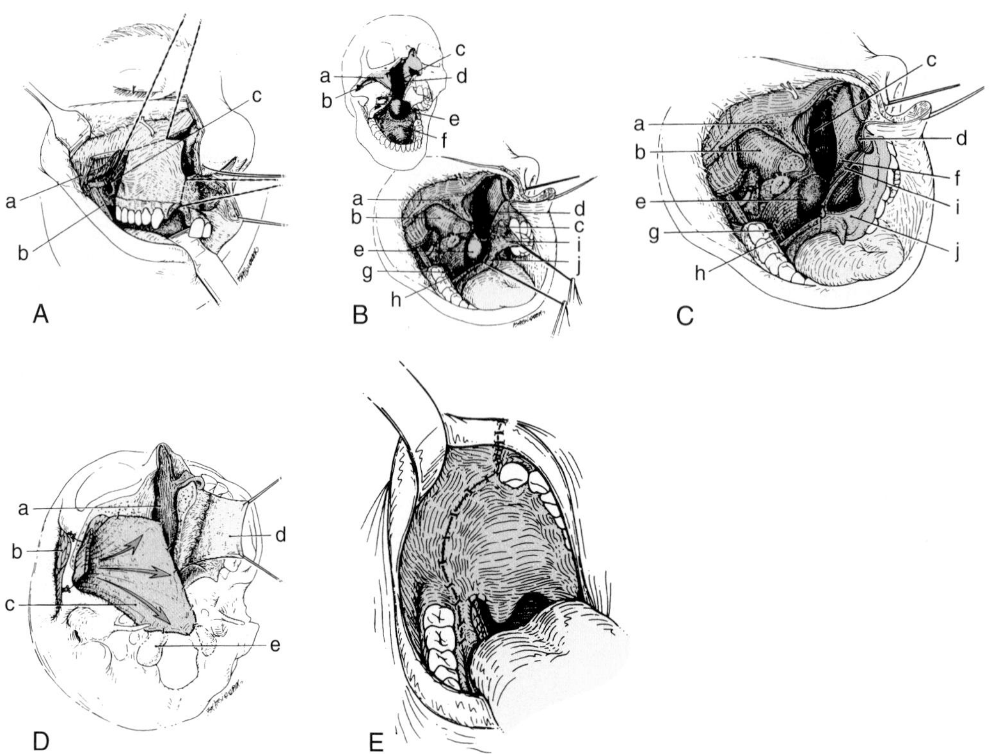

Figure 174-30. Extended maxillotomy; subtotal maxillectomy approach to the cranial base. **A,** Maxillectomy variation. Modified Weber-Fergusson incision followed by osteotomies to remove the hemimaxilla: a, masseter muscle divided; b, coronoidectomy defect; c, lateral pterygoid plate. **B,** Maxillectomy; defects: a, maxillary roof; b, infratemporal fossa; c, sinonasal defect; d, nasal septum; e, clivus tumor; f, C1 vertebra; g, lateral pharyngeal wall; h, pharyngeal wall incision; i, mucoperiosteum of hard palate; j, soft palate. **C,** Maxillotomy variation in which the hemimaxilla (j) is preserved but temporarily translocated, based on mucoperiosteum of the hard palate. See key in **B** for other lettered structures. Exposure is otherwise similar to that shown for maxillectomy. **D,** Temporalis muscle transferred into operative defect for reconstruction: a, sinonasal defect; b, fat graft; c, temporalis muscle flap; d, mucoperiosteum of hard palate; e, occipital condyle. **E,** Closure of the oral cavity and lip after subtotal maxillectomy. *(From Cocke EW Jr, Robertson JH, Robertson JT, Crook JP Jr. The extended maxillotomy and subtotal maxillectomy for excision of skull base tumors.* Arch Otolaryngol Head Neck Surg. *1992;116:92-104.)*

rotundum, and the foramen lacerum. Removal of the pterygoid plates in this approach also facilitates access to the nasopharynx. This approach is used in the resection of small nasopharyngeal carcinomas, adenoid cystic carcinomas, and angiofibromas. All three variations of the infratemporal fossa approach involve mastoidectomy, facial nerve dissection (and transposition), and obliteration of the eustachian tube, middle ear, and external auditory canal with resultant permanent conductive hearing deficit. Thus, types A, B, and C infratemporal fossa approaches share some features of the basic transtemporal approaches and yet extend the field of access anteriorly to reach the middle cranial base by virtue of exposing and controlling the petrous ICA (see Chapter 176).

For lesions of the middle cranial base that involve the infratemporal fossa, the upper pterygomaxillary space, the lateral orbit, and the orbital apex, the lateral facial approach[100] (Fig. 174-33) and the lateral transtemporal sphenoid approach[101] (Fig. 174-34) have been described. These procedures reach the infratemporal fossa from a slightly more superior direction by displacing the zygomatic arch inferiorly and reflecting the temporalis muscle. The greater wing of the sphenoid is followed to the lateral pterygoid plate, which is used as a surgical landmark, as outlined earlier. These approaches also incorporate partial removal of the greater wing of the sphenoid, which means that they include subtemporal craniectomy and extradural dissection. The advantages of these procedures are that they require no facial nerve dissection (the temporal branch of cranial nerve VII is retracted inferiorly with the skin flap), and they allow some access to the cranial base from both intracranial and extracranial perspectives.

The lateral facial approach is useful as a straightforward approach to a limited area of the middle cranial base that is technically simple to perform (after the anatomy is well understood) and that incurs relatively little morbidity. It is applicable in the management of small- to medium-sized benign tumors with limited intracranial extension, such as that which occurs with some angiofibromas. The similarly oriented lateral transtemporal sphenoid approach can be extended so that it is significantly more complex than the lateral facial approach but affords additional exposure, thus making it useful for the management of lesions in the clivus, the parasellar region, the nasopharynx, the petrous apex, and the infratemporal fossa. As the name implies, the lateral transtemporal sphenoid approach is a combination of techniques. It is similar to the infratemporal fossa approaches of Fisch except that it does not usually result in permanent conductive hearing loss, and it does not require rerouting of the facial nerve.

The subtemporal-preauricular infratemporal approach (Fig. 174-35)[14,102] is a combination of the transparotid and lateral transtemporal sphenoid procedures in addition to temporal craniotomy. It provides excellent exposure of much of the middle cranial base and allows for improved access for intracranial dissection when necessary. The orientation of the exposure begins laterally and progresses medially so that it is useful for the management of lesions of the greater sphenoid wing, the petrous apex, and the middle and lower clivus. This approach is used extensively for the resection of tumors such as meningiomas, chondrosarcomas, chordomas, and petrous apex cholesteatomas. It illustrates many important techniques used in surgery of the middle cranial base.

A hemicoronal or curved temporal incision is extended into the preauricular and cervical regions to expose the temporalis muscle, the zygomatic arch, the parotid gland, and the upper neck. (As discussed in the description of the bicoronal incision, the temporal fascia and fat

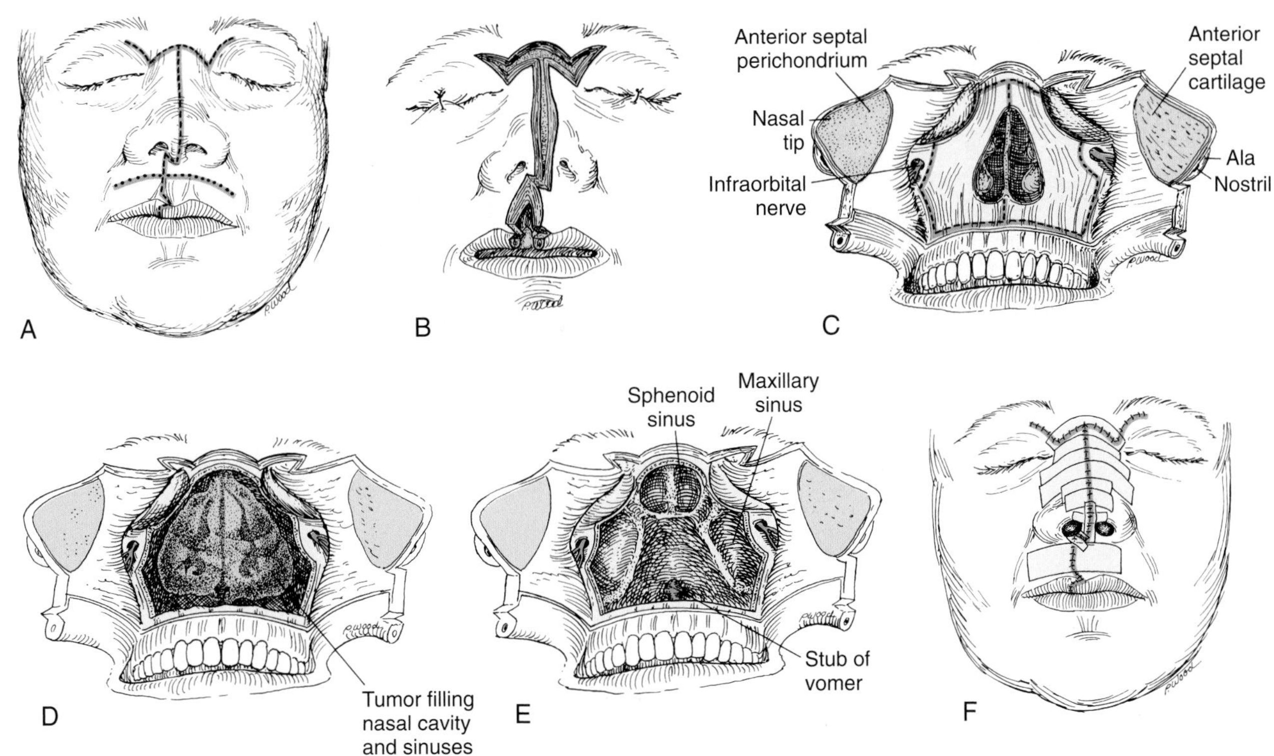

Figure 174-31. Midfacial split approach to the cranial base. **A,** Incisions. Horizontal incision across the nasion allows access to the upper orbits. Midline nasal incision divides skin and separates upper and lower lateral cartilage to expose septum; it is carried inferiorly along one side of the philtrum, splitting the upper lip. Gingivolabial incision *(dotted line)* facilitates exposure of the maxilla bilaterally. **B,** Partially developed facial soft tissue flaps, with attached nasal cartilages. **C,** Soft tissue flaps fully developed and reflected laterally to expose the orbitonasomaxillary skeleton. Proposed osteotomy sites are indicated by *dotted lines*. **D,** Midfacial exposure after osteotomies and temporary removal of bone segments, including portions of the medial and inferior orbital walls, the anterior maxilla, and the nasal bones. When necessary, osteotomies also may include the hard palate, which gives additional access to the oropharynx, the nasopharynx, and the clivus. In this example, tumor fills the posterior nasal cavity and nasopharynx and extends into the sphenoid sinus. **E,** After removal of the tumor, which included the nasal septum, the medial maxillae, and the sphenoid rostrum. **F,** Final closure. Orbitonasomaxillary bone segments are replaced and secured using microplates, and soft tissues are primarily repaired. Adhesive strips are applied, and silicone nasal stents are used for 1 week postoperatively.

pad are elevated with the skin flap, thereby protecting the frontal branch of the facial nerve). The cervical extension is used to gain access to the ICA, the internal jugular vein, and cranial nerves IX through XII, and to help identify the facial nerve extratemporally. The parotid gland is mobilized away from the sternocleidomastoid muscle, and the underlying styloid complex is divided, revealing the high cervical ICA, the internal jugular vein, and cranial nerves IX to XII. Next, the zygomatic arch is osteotomized with a reciprocating saw and removed temporarily, thereby allowing the temporalis muscle to be reflected inferiorly to expose the greater wing of the sphenoid and the underlying infratemporal fossa. In cases in which the lesion also involves the orbit (e.g., sphenoid wing meningiomas), the lateral orbital wall and rim may also be osteotomized and removed along with the zygoma. The condyle of the mandible may be retracted or resected to expose the spine of the sphenoid and its nearby structures, including the middle meningeal artery, cranial nerve division V3, and the ICA at its entrance into the carotid canal. More medially, V2 can be identified just anterior to the lateral pterygoid plate.

A low temporal craniotomy is performed, and, by extradural dissection, the temporal lobe is elevated off of the middle fossa floor, thereby revealing the intracranial landmarks: the GSPN, the middle meningeal artery, and cranial nerve divisions V2 and V3.

By progressive removal of the greater wing of the sphenoid, cranial nerve divisions V3 and V2 may be completely unroofed. If necessary, the sphenoid sinus may be opened by removing the bone between V2 and V3 and the base of the pterygoid plates. The superior orbital fissure may be unroofed in the same way.

The intrapetrous course of the ICA may be exposed, beginning at the infratemporal opening of the carotid canal and extending to just above the foramen lacerum (where the ICA enters the cavernous sinus). This is accomplished with a high-speed drill and a diamond burr using a technique analogous to that used for facial nerve decompression. To facilitate this exposure, the middle meningeal artery and the GSPN should first be divided, and the high cervical ICA with its fibrous periosteal sheath should be rendered accessible by removal of the styloid process and the surrounding bone. The ICA may be displaced forward out of its bony canal; this is useful whenever the lesion involves the clivus medial to the ICA or the petrous part of the temporal bone posterior to the ICA. The inferior aspect of the cavernous sinus may also be approached from this exposure.[7]

The sequence and extent of exposure at the skull base depend on the nature of the lesion to be extirpated. Certain steps in the procedure may be eliminated or modified to suit the needs of the particular case. For example, it is only necessary to dissect the neck if the procedure will benefit from proximal control of the ICA or from low exposure of the internal jugular vein or cranial nerves IX through XII. Otherwise, the cervical extension may be avoided.

After the lesion has been extirpated, the wound is irrigated with antibiotic solution and carefully inspected. Any dural openings are meticulously repaired primarily or by using grafts of pericranium, temporalis fascia, or fascia lata. In addition to repairing dura, every effort is made to reconstitute a functional barrier between the intracranial compartment and the visceral spaces of the head and neck. Usually this does not include any attempt to rebuild the bony basicranium. Instead,

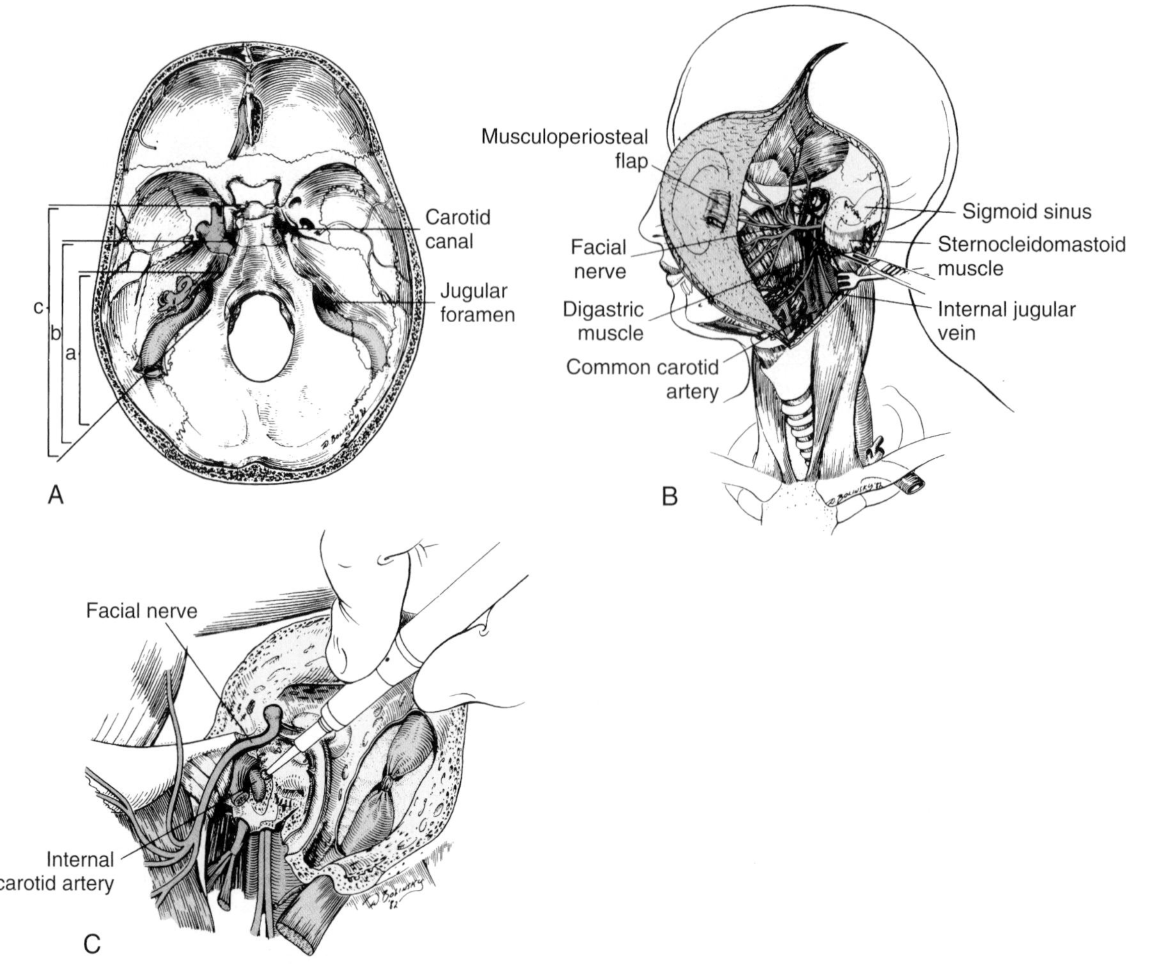

Figure 174-32. Infratemporal approach to the cranial base. **A,** Areas of the skull base accessible by each of the variations of the infratemporal approach: a, jugular foramen and petrous apex; b, clivus; c, parasellar and parasphenoid compartments. **B,** Postauricular incision with extensions into the scalp and neck. Sternocleidomastoid and digastric muscles have been divided at the mastoid tip, thereby allowing access to the carotid artery and the internal jugular vein. The facial nerve has been identified extratemporally. The external auditory canal has been closed by turning the musculoperiosteal flap. **C,** Radical mastoidectomy has exposed the sigmoid sinus (which has been ligated) and the middle fossa dura. The tympanic membrane and ossicles have been removed. The facial nerve has been unroofed and transposed anteriorly. By progressive drilling, the internal carotid artery can be traced distally through its petrous course to reach the cavernous sinus. Similarly, additional bone removal anteriorly will allow access to the parasellar region and the nasopharynx. *(From Fisch U, Pillsbury HC, Sasaki CT. Infratemporal approach to the skull base. In: Sasaki CT, McCabe BF, Kirchner JA, eds.* Surgery of the Skull Base. *Philadelphia: JB Lippincott; 1984.)*

efforts are focused on the interposition of reconstructive soft tissues—vascularized tissues, whenever possible—into the surgical defect.

Any communications with the aerodigestive tract are identified. These most often include the sphenoid sinus, the nasopharynx, and the eustachian tube. If the sphenoid sinus has been opened, its mucosa is removed, and it is obliterated with autogenous fat or by the transfer of vascularized temporalis muscle medially. If the eustachian tube has been entered, it is denuded of mucosa, packed with fat or muscle, sutured closed, and covered with vascularized temporalis muscle. If the nasopharynx has been violated, the opening is filled with a temporalis muscle flap or a free microvascular flap (e.g., rectus abdominis), depending on the size of the defect. Special care is taken to ensure that the ICA is covered with vascularized tissue throughout its course, particularly in cases in which the nasopharynx has been entered. Failure to protect the ICA in this way may result in continued exposure of the artery to bacterial contamination from the upper aerodigestive tract, with subsequent carotid rupture.

Finally, the zygomatic and craniotomy bone segments, which were previously displaced by osteotomy, are returned to their anatomic positions and secured appropriately. If the temporalis muscle has not been used as a reconstructive flap, it is returned to the temporal fossa. If a temporalis flap has been used, the temporal fossa may be filled with autologous fat from the abdomen or thigh to minimize the temporal fossa depression. Soft tissue closure then follows.

Transfacial Approaches

Transfacial exposure of the cranial base, particularly of the lateral compartment (middle cranial base region), is not a new concept. Operative procedures for the removal of neoplasms from this region were described by several authors in the 1960s.[103,104] These early procedures, which were used initially for the radical resection of malignant tumors, resulted in unacceptably high morbidity and mortality rates and considerable deformity, largely because methods to adequately reconstruct major cranial base defects were not yet available. With the introduction of craniofacial disassembly techniques and vascularized reconstructive flaps, it has become possible to dismantle the facial skeleton, to extirpate deep-seated lesions, and to perform functional reconstruction to a greater extent than ever. Accordingly, lesions of the lateral and central compartments are more amenable to surgery.

A transfacial approach to this region is desirable because it eliminates the viscerocranial skeleton as an obstacle to exposure, thereby opening up the entire infratemporal fossa and the nasal cavity, the

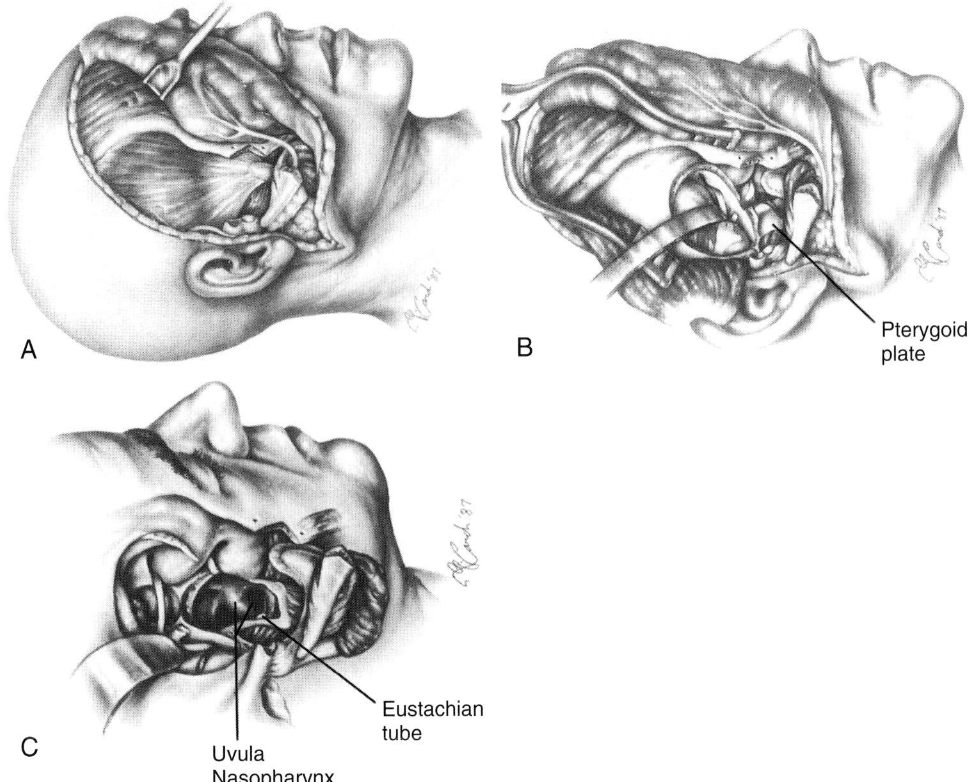

Figure 174-33. Lateral facial approach to the cranial base. **A,** A temporal and preauricular incision is used to expose the temporalis muscle and the zygomatic arch. The zygoma is sectioned to allow access to the insertion of the temporalis at the coronoid process. The frontal branch of the facial nerve is preserved within the skin flap. **B,** With the temporalis muscle retracted, the greater wing of the sphenoid is partially removed (subtemporal craniectomy). Retraction of the temporal lobe dura reveals branches of the trigeminal nerve and attachment of the pterygoid plate at the base of the sphenoid bone. **C,** Division of the maxillary nerve (V2) and resection of the pterygoid plate expose the nasopharynx. *(From Gates GA. The lateral facial approach to the nasopharynx and infratemporal fossa.* Otolaryngol Head Neck Surg. *1988;99:321-325.)*

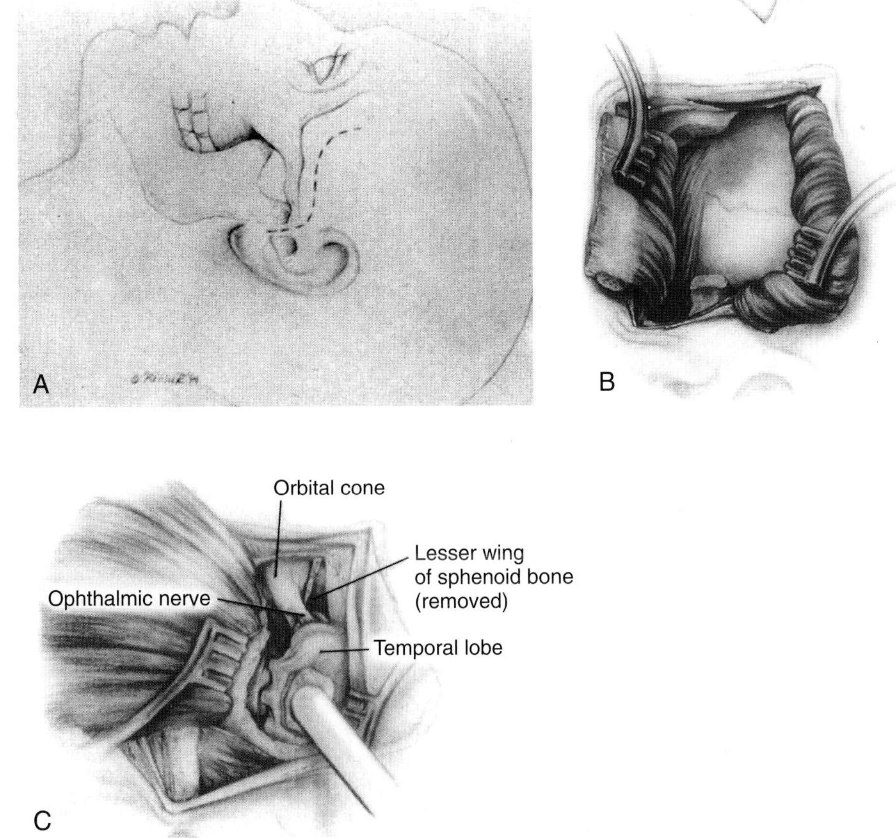

Figure 174-34. Lateral transtemporal sphenoid approach to the cranial base. **A,** Incision. **B,** Retraction of the temporalis muscle to expose the greater wing of the sphenoid. This muscle should be preserved intact and reflected inferiorly if muscle flap reconstruction of a skull base defect is anticipated. The zygomatic arch has been temporarily removed. **C,** Subtemporal craniectomy exposes the orbital apex and the floor of the middle cranial fossa. *(From Holliday MJ. Lateral transtemporal-sphenoid approach to the skull base.* Ear Nose Throat J. *1986;65:153-162.)*

Superficial temporal artery
VII
XII
Interior jugular vein
X
Carotid artery
A

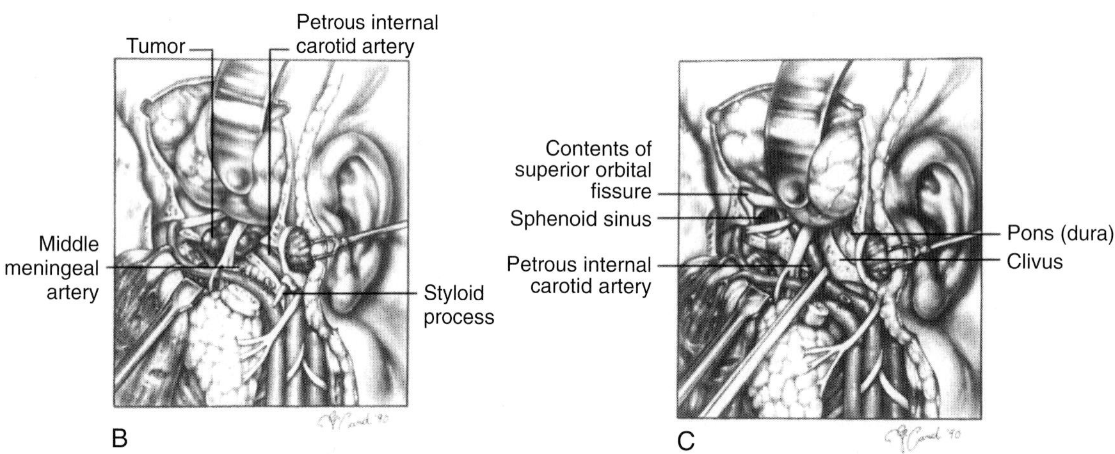

Figure 174-35. Subtemporal-preauricular and infratemporal approach to the cranial base. **A,** Initial exposure. Distal branches of the facial nerve are for demonstration only; in most cases they are not dissected. The frontal branch is included with the skin flap and retracted inferiorly. **B,** The temporalis muscle has been reflected inferiorly *(bottom left)* after temporarily removing the zygomatic arch, the mandibular condyle has been resected, and a subtemporal craniectomy has been performed. After dividing the styloid complex, the carotid artery is traced distally through part of its course within the temporal bone to separate it from the tumor. The facial nerve need not be transposed, and the conducting mechanism of the middle ear remains undisturbed in this approach. **C,** Progressive dissection exposes the clivus, the sphenoid sinus, the superior orbital fissure, and the adjacent neural and vascular structures. *(From Sekhar LN, Janecka IP. Intracranial extension of cranial base tumors and combined resection: the neurosurgical perspective. In: Jackson CG, ed.* Surgery of Skull Base Tumors. *New York: Churchill Livingstone; 1991.)*

nasopharynx, the pterygopalatine fossa, and the sphenoid region to direct access all at once. The facial translocation approach (Fig. 174-36)[17] is such a procedure.

Incisions are made in the face and scalp as shown in Figure 174-36A. The horizontal incision connects a lateral rhinotomy with a hemicoronal incision to create superior and inferior soft tissue flaps. (At this stage, the frontal branches of the facial nerve are identified using evoked EMG, tagged, and divided to be reconnected later on during the procedure. This horizontal incision is a key element in the exposure because it allows a single, unified surgical field that is unhampered by the need to work alternatively from separate cranial and facial incisions that limit the surgeon's ability to develop three-dimensional exposure at the cranial base.) The soft tissue flaps are then elevated in the subperiosteal plane from the zygoma and maxilla. Periorbita is likewise elevated from the lateral, inferior, and medial orbital rims and walls. A reciprocating saw is used to create osteotomies, and the orbitozygomaticomaxillary skeletal segment is temporarily removed.

After the temporalis muscle is reflected inferiorly, the subtemporal skull base is fully exposed, and further dissection proceeds as dictated by the lesion, using the same skull base landmarks as for other approaches. Intracranial exposure is readily obtained, if needed, by subtemporal craniectomy or by frontal or temporal craniotomy. Similarly, the pterygoid plates and muscles may be removed, thus revealing the nasopharynx, the sphenoid sinus, and the clivus. As mentioned previously, facial translocation may therefore be used as an approach to the central compartment of the middle cranial base; it provides a unified surgical field with access to both compartments.

At the completion of the extirpation, reconstruction follows the same principles as discussed. After dural repair, the temporalis muscle is used to fill the skull base defect. Because of its appreciable soft tissue bulk, the muscle also is useful for obliterating the maxillary sinus space. There it serves as a vascularized tissue bed for the orbitozygomaticomaxillary bone segment, which is replaced and secured as a free bone graft. Bony stabilization is achieved with sutures or miniplates. If it has not been resected for oncologic reasons, the infraorbital nerve (which was transected during the development of the lower facial soft tissue flap) is rerouted through its maxillary canal and reconnected to its distal trunk by suture neurorrhaphy. The frontal branches of the facial nerve also are repaired. The nasolacrimal system is stented to prevent dacryostenosis, and the medial canthal ligament is secured to the lacrimal

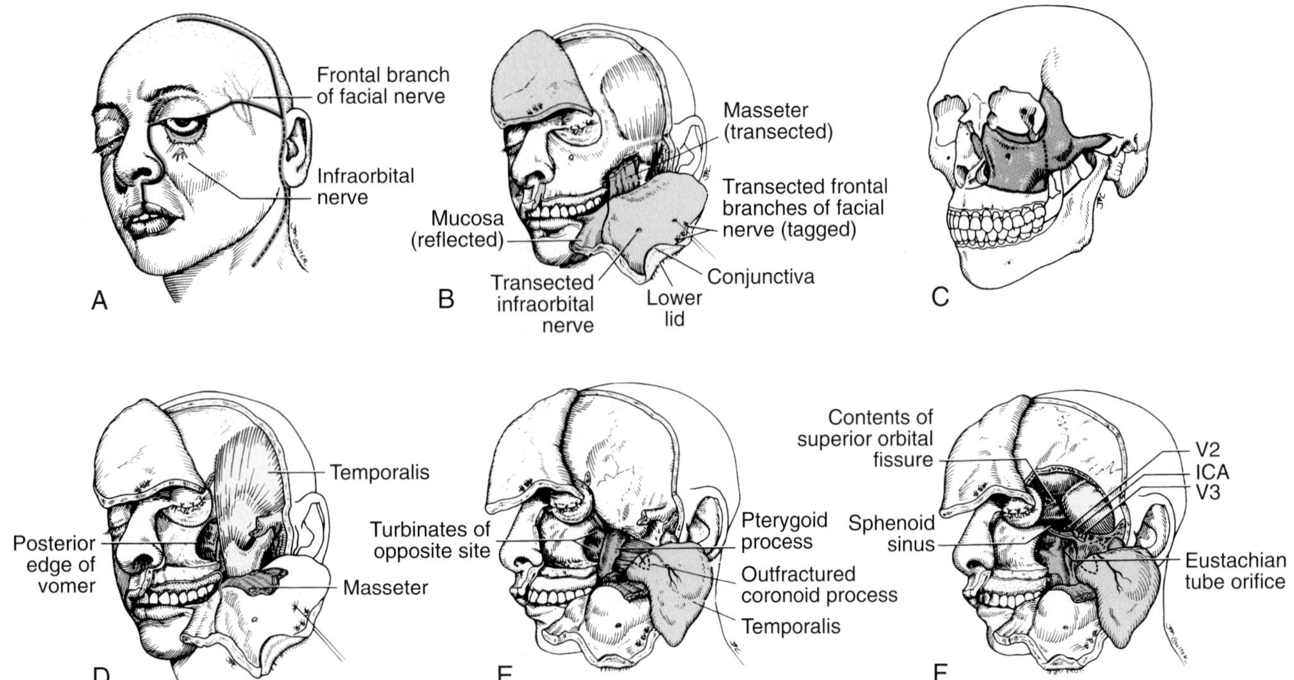

Figure 174-36. Facial translocation approach to the cranial base. **A,** Incisions. Infraorbital portion of an incision is made in the inferior fornix of the conjunctiva. The lip-splitting portion may be omitted in many cases in which low maxillary exposure is not needed. **B,** Facial soft tissue flaps fully developed and reflected to expose the craniofacial skeleton. **C,** Outline of osteotomies of the orbitozygomaticomaxillary skeleton. **D,** Exposure after temporary removal (translocation) of the orbitozygomaticomaxillary segment. **E,** Inferior reflection of the temporalis muscle—enhanced by outfracture of the coronoid process—gives access to the pterygoid region and the nasopharynx. **F,** Subtemporal craniectomy allows exposure of the middle fossa floor, the sphenoid sinus, and the adjacent neural and vascular structures. ICA, internal carotid artery. *(From Janecka IP, Sen CN, Sekhar LN, Arriaga M. Facial translocation: new approach to cranial base.* Otolaryngol Head Neck Surg. *1990;103:413-419.)*

crest. Temporary tarsorrhaphy helps support this repair during the early postoperative period. Closure of skin incisions completes the procedure.

Postoperatively, tarsorrhaphy sutures may be removed within 1 week; nasolacrimal stents remain in place for 6 to 8 weeks. In most patients, infraorbital sensation returns within 3 to 6 months, and frontalis muscle function resumes in 6 to 9 months.

The facial translocation technique is valuable for obtaining the broad exposure needed when managing large or advanced lesions of the lateral and central compartments of the middle cranial base, especially those in which much of the lesion is extracranial. Because of its modular nature, it also can be applied in various scaled-down versions that are tailored for dealing with smaller cranial base lesions.

Intracranial Approaches

Temporal craniotomy is the traditional, standard neurosurgical method for gaining access to the middle cranial fossa. For intradural lesions within the temporal lobe or for extradural lesions along the lateral convexity of the middle fossa, it is the most direct approach.[105] For lesions at the cranial base, however, temporal craniotomy alone is often less than ideal, because it requires (by virtue of its superolateral-to-inferomedial orientation) significant retraction or, in some cases, resection of the brain to reach a target area. Such brain manipulation can result in intraoperative and postoperative cerebral edema; temporal encephalomalacia; deficits of speech, memory, and cognition; and long-term risk of seizure disorder. These risks increase as the location of the lesion becomes more medial and more temporal lobe retraction is required.

Still, temporal craniotomy alone is useful for some limited lesions of the lateral compartment–middle cranial base region, such as meningiomas of the sphenoid wings. Risks of intracranial complications can be minimized by designing the craniotomy bone flap as low as possible, thereby giving a more basal and direct access to the skull base, with less need for brain retraction. The limiting factors are the petrous ridge of the temporal bone and the zygomatic arch. When preoperative imaging suggests that these structures will impede adequate exposure, a wider approach should be chosen, such as the subtemporal-infratemporal, lateral facial, or transtemporal sphenoid approach.

The middle fossa approach of House[106] involves the use of temporal craniotomy as a preliminary step to reach the IAC by the removal of bone from the superior surface of the petrous portion of the temporal bone. Because most lesions in these areas originate in relation to the seventh and eighth cranial nerves, this approach is considered in more detail in Chapters 171, 176, and 177.

When the skull base is involved only to a minimal extent and the lesion is mostly infracranial, a subtemporal craniectomy may be performed (see Figs. 174-33 and 174-36). In this procedure, only a limited area of cranial bone is removed, generally as a safe means of establishing a superior margin in resecting, for example, the base of the pterygoid plates and surrounding soft tissue. Subtemporal craniectomy may be performed by inserting a Kerrison or a similar rongeur extradurally inside the foramen ovale and gradually removing bone in the direction of the foramen rotundum. The resulting bone window allows for the protection of the middle fossa dura under direct vision while the subjacent lesion is removed.

For many lesions of the lateral compartment of the middle cranial base, temporal craniotomy and subtemporal craniectomy are used in combination with transtemporal, infratemporal, or transfacial exposure. These intracranial approaches provide added control over the neural and vascular structures in the region. As is true for all transcranial operations for cranial base lesions, close cooperation between the otolaryngologist and the neurosurgeon is essential.[107]

Reconstruction

As stated previously, use of locoregional vascularized flaps is the primary reconstructive method for skull base defects; however, support is growing for microvascular reconstruction of these defects, especially large ones, or in revision surgery, when locoregional flaps may be unavailable.[53,54,108]

In a retrospective study, Newman and associates found a 95% success rate in reconstructing anterior and middle skull base defects. Despite a 30% overall complication rate, no cases of intracranial complication or CSF leak or deaths were associated with this reconstruction.[109] Other authors have experienced higher rates of complications including flap failure and intracranial problems (cerebrovascular accident [CVA], syndrome of inappropriate antidiuretic hormone [SIADH], meningitis, seizure, pneumocephalus, CSF leak), although most reported series have been smaller with a retrospective study design.[110]

The progression of expanded endoscopic approaches has also necessitated the development of nonvascularized materials to repair skull base defects. Acellular dermis, hydroxyapatite cement, free abdominal fat, autologous cartilage and bone grafts may be used to match each defect. Of importance, hydroxyapatite cement must not be allowed to contact the sinonasal mucosa, to avoid infection and failure.[2,111]

Postoperative Concerns

Initial Postoperative Care

All patients initially are admitted to an intensive care unit that is staffed by nurses who are experienced in neurosurgical and head-and-neck surgical care. Consultants in critical care medicine, internal medicine, and other specialties actively participate in management, when appropriate. Typically, patients will have a continuous recording of the electrocardiogram, oxygenation status (monitored by pulse oximetry), and systemic blood pressure (monitored by arterial catheter). In specific circumstances, Swan-Ganz catheters or central venous lines are used to assess cardiovascular status and fluid balance. These parameters are crucial for maintaining optimal intravascular volume, cardiac output, and cerebral blood flow.

Given the complexity of intraoperative fluid and electrolyte management, close monitoring of hematologic and chemical parameters is essential (i.e., hemoglobin; hematocrit; platelets; prothrombin and partial thromboplastin times; sodium, potassium, calcium, magnesium, and phosphorus concentrations; and serum osmolality). The appropriate replacement of blood components maintains oxygen delivery (erythrocytes) and prevents coagulopathy (platelets, plasma). Electrolyte balance is especially important, because deviation from physiologic norms can lead to confusion, agitation, stupor, or seizure activity, which may be otherwise mistaken for surgery-related neurologic insults.

Pharmacologic therapy plays an important role in the prevention of complications. Antibiotics are routinely given, beginning just before surgery and for a duration of 24 to 48 hours afterward. Inhibitors of gastric acid secretion are given postoperatively to reduce the chance of stress ulceration and gastrointestinal bleeding, and they are continued until the patient is tolerating adequate enteral nutrition. Anticonvulsants are used to prevent seizures whenever significant frontal or temporal lobe manipulation is necessary. Once instituted, anticonvulsant therapy should be periodically monitored using serum drug levels and should be continued for at least 6 to 12 months after surgery. Analgesic therapy is limited in most cases to the judicious use of intramuscular codeine, which has a mild, predictable (and reversible) effect on mental status and respiratory drive. Stronger narcotics and benzodiazepines and related sedatives generally are avoided because of their more profound and less predictable influences on these functions, potentially confounding accurate neurologic assessment.

For most procedures in which the cranial vault has been opened, a CT scan is obtained on postoperative day 1. This scan serves as a baseline study for comparison with any subsequent studies performed to investigate neurologic complications if they arise.

Prophylaxis against deep vein thrombosis and pulmonary embolism includes the intraoperative and postoperative use of dynamic compression stockings. In addition, patients are mobilized as soon as feasible after surgery.

Complications

Many of the most serious complications of cranial base surgery are related to the brain,[14] and their prevention and management demand neurosurgical expertise. First, brain manipulation, especially by excessive retraction, can lead to cerebral edema, subdural hematoma, and acute brain dysfunction specific to the anatomic site involved. In the long term, it may cause encephalomalacia and deficits of speech, memory, and cognitive and intellectual functions. Brain injury (by contusion) also may predispose the patient to seizures, especially when the temporal lobe is affected. These problems are best prevented by obtaining adequate surgical exposure through basal bone removal and craniofacial disassembly (thereby limiting the need for significant brain manipulation) and by intraoperative brain relaxation through the use of subarachnoid CSF drainage, hyperventilation, and corticosteroids.

Pneumocephalus may occur as a sudden event during the early postoperative period, after a patient attempts (against advice to the contrary) to blow his or her nose, thereby inadvertently insufflating air through the dural closure. This rapid-onset pneumocephalus may cause intracranial mass effect (tension pneumocephalus), with confusion, obtundation, and progressive neurologic deterioration. Pneumocephalus also may develop more slowly as a result of the overdrainage of CSF from a lumbar spinal drain, which can cause a siphon effect, drawing air upward from the nasal cavity. Preventive measures therefore include the following: (1) keeping patients intubated or tracheotomized until they are alert enough to follow instructions; and (2) judiciously using spinal drainage at a conservative rate and for a short duration. In most patients after cranial base surgery, the lumbar catheter is allowed to drain 25 to 50 mL every 8 hours and is removed after 24 to 72 hours. When pneumocephalus is suspected, prompt CT assessment is necessary. Small collections of air may be observed, whereas larger ones may require decompression by needle aspiration (through an osteotomy site or burr hole) or by reexploration and reinforcement of the reconstruction. In cases of acute-onset pneumocephalus, the administration of 100% oxygen is a useful adjunctive measure to enhance resorption of the intracranial air. Lumbar subarachnoid CSF drainage should be discontinued in the presence of any significant pneumocephalus.

CSF fistula is another brain-related complication that is important because of its association with meningitis. It usually manifests as rhinorrhea, but it also may cause the patient to experience a salty taste in the throat. If the nature of nasal discharge is doubtful, the β_2-transferrin assay may be used to confirm or rule out the presence of CSF.[112] For small-volume leaks, which are the most common, observation and continued spinal drainage (or serial lumbar spinal taps) usually suffice. For high-volume leaks (grossly apparent rhinorrhea) or those that are persistent, careful sinonasal endoscopy or CT cisternography can be used to localize the fistula site (i.e., frontal, ethmoid, sphenoid, eustachian tube, temporal bone), after which operative repair frequently is needed. A CSF fistula may manifest as otorrhea or as wound discharge; the management principles are similar in either case. In some situations, the original repair simply needs to be revised; in others, additional vascularized tissue may be needed to obliterate the fistula site. Such tissues may include temporalis muscle, galeal, or free microvascular flaps (e.g., rectus abdominis, omentum). In selected cases, the closure may be augmented by the judicious use of free autogenous fat grafts or fibrin glue. The risk of reconstructive failure is substantially decreased if the original repair is performed using vascularized local tissue.[69]

CNS infections, including meningitis and brain abscess, also may occur. These complications can lead to extreme neurologic morbidity or death. Preventive measures include the use of perioperative antibiotics, strict adherence to sterile technique, the minimization of dural exposure to the aerodigestive tract, and meticulous attention to reconstruction, as outlined earlier. Management consists of antimicrobial drugs (given intravenously and sometimes intrathecally) and surgical exploration when necessary to drain abscesses or to obliterate sources of continued bacterial contamination.

Cerebrovascular complications are of major concern during the perioperative period. These events may have several causes. Carotid rupture may occur as a result of infection (and pseudoaneurysm) or excessive adventitial dissection. This complication is often sudden and fatal, but it may sometimes be preceded by a sentinel bleed, which, if recognized as such, can provide time for prompt intervention (i.e., reexploration and bypass or permanent ICA occlusion). Thrombotic

ICA occlusion or embolism into distal vessels can cause stroke and death. The strict maintenance of systemic blood pressure intraoperatively and postoperatively avoids hypotension, which can precipitate ICA thrombosis. Careful surgical technique when working in the vicinity of the ICA and cautious postoperative anticoagulation in high-risk patients may decrease embolic phenomena. Although the incidence of stroke in cranial base surgery is low, stroke is a source of considerable morbidity when it does occur; this morbidity can usually be lessened when the cranial base team adopts a vigorous approach to intervention and rehabilitation. Intervention after stroke should include the tight control of the hemodynamic factors that affect cerebral blood flow to prevent extension of the infarct. It also should include measures to ensure optimal homeostasis, such as control of the airway and oxygenation, maintenance of fluid and electrolyte balance, and nutritional support. Rehabilitation of stroke patients (and of patients with neurologic deficits from other causes) is greatly facilitated by input from professionals in rehabilitation medicine, physical and occupational therapy, and speech therapy.

Cranial nerve deficits deserve special consideration because of their profound impact on postoperative recovery and quality of life. The sacrifice of olfactory nerves (cranial nerve I) often is regarded as a minor disability, but it can contribute to significant malnutrition in some patients who, because of anosmia, no longer enjoy eating. Deficits of cranial nerves II, III, IV, and VI lead to visual disability of variable degree, depending on the extent of surgical trauma and nerve involvement by the disease process itself. Dense palsies of the extraocular muscles seldom recover completely. Patients in whom such deficits are predictable should therefore be prepared for the loss of binocular vision before surgery is undertaken. Extraocular muscle surgery by the ophthalmologist can sometimes help to compensate for such deficits. The loss of visual acuity is a potential complication of anterior cranial base surgery, but it is unusual unless the optic nerves are compromised preoperatively. In these patients, recovery of optic nerve function is difficult to predict.[63]

Deficits of the fifth and seventh nerves are dangerous, mainly because of loss of sensation (V1) or protection (VII) of the cornea. Tarsorrhaphy and careful attention to ocular lubrication are important means of preventing keratitis and visual loss in these cases. Fifth nerve dysfunction, in addition to the obvious sensory deficits, may also cause significant problems with mastication (and with nutrition) because of the loss of motor innervation to the pterygoid, temporalis, and masseter muscles (V3). Seventh nerve paralysis can be a tremendous social and emotional handicap and should be rehabilitated aggressively whenever possible. Eighth nerve deficits, although rarely reversible, usually can be compensated for (when unilateral) by audiologic and vestibular training.

Deficits of cranial nerves IX, X, and XII are potentially life-threatening, especially when they occur together, because of aspiration and dysphagia with subsequent pneumonia and malnutrition. Management of patients in whom these deficits are present preoperatively or expected postoperatively should include tracheostomy and gastrostomy at the time of the cranial base surgery or very soon thereafter, before complications compromise the patient's recovery. Laryngoplasty or injection of collagen or fat into the unilaterally paralyzed larynx also may be beneficial. Patients who have multiple bilateral deficits of cranial nerves IX, X, and XII are extremely difficult to rehabilitate. Management of these cases nearly always involves permanent tracheostomy and gastrostomy and, sometimes, laryngotracheal separation.

Many complications of cranial base surgery are not brain related (Table 174-2) and can affect any physiologic system. Despite the relatively less invasive appearance of endoscopic skull base surgery, these procedures carry many of the same risks of more traditional open skull base procedures. CSF leaks remain the most common complication, and additional serious complications including damage to cranial nerves, meninges, blood vessels, and venous sinuses can present in the immediate postoperative period. Delayed complications include meningitis, brain abscess, and tension pneumocephalus, anosmia, and synechia formation. Visual loss or changes may result from damage to the optic nerve or chiasm or orbital contents, including extraocular musculature. Damage to the pituitary stalk also may result with transsphenoidal approaches.[38] Postoperative diabetes insipidus rates are reported to be as much as 50% lower in endoscopic cases.[113]

Table 174-2

Non-neurologic Complications in Cranial Base Surgery

Type of Complication	Examples
Cardiovascular	Myocardial infarction Hypotension Congestive heart failure
Respiratory	Pulmonary embolism Pneumonia Aspiration Respiratory distress syndrome Pulmonary edema
Hematologic	Post-transfusion coagulopathy Anemia Deep venous thrombosis
Renal	Acute tubular necrosis Drug-induced nephropathies
Infectious	Pneumonia Sepsis Thrombophlebitis Wound infections Viral hepatitis Urinary tract infections
Gastrointestinal	Malnutrition Stress ulcer Gastrointestinal bleeding
Metabolic	Derangements of serum sodium, potassium, calcium, phosphorus, magnesium, and other minerals
Endocrine	Diabetes insipidus Syndrome of inappropriate antidiuretic hormone Hypopituitarism
Hepatic	Drug-induced hepatitis Cholestasis

Outcomes

Although the many technical advances and multispecialty approaches in cranial base surgery have expanded the ability to achieve complete and safe tumor resection, the question remains regarding the extent that patients benefit from these invasive procedures. A 1995 review of 40 years of cranial base surgery for carcinomas and sarcomas provided some insight into the answer to this question.[114] Three general eras of major advancement in the field were analyzed for survival outcomes and trends in morbidity.

From the 1960s to the 1970s, surgical pioneers achieved 3- and 5-year survival rates of 52% and 49%, respectively. The application of skull base approaches was limited, and tumors were designated as inoperable if they extended intracranially or into the pterygopalatine fossa. Morbidity rates were significant, with overall infection rates of 54% and CSF leaks occurring in 31% of cases. From the 1970s to the 1980s, the number of cranial base cases and the number of surgeons performing these cases increased. The major advancement was that patients with tumors previously designated as inoperable underwent attempts at complete tumor resection. Reports included tumors that extended intracranially and intracerebrally and into the pterygopalatine fossa. The 3-year survival rates rose slightly from 57% to 59%, with only limited reports of 5-year survival rates in the range of 49%. Infection rates ranged from 4% to 48%, but the incidence of CSF leaks dropped from 3% to 19%. From the 1980s to the 1990s, a multispecialty approach to cranial base surgery was introduced. Complications dropped significantly, with infection rates ranging from zero to 28% and CSF leaks diminishing from 2% to 4%. Another significant factor is that local disease control improved greatly. The 3-year survival rate increased from 67% to 74%, and the 5-year survival rate increased from 56% to 70%.[114] A recent multi-institutional study of patients undergoing craniofacial resection revealed 5-year overall, disease-specific, and recurrence-free survival rates of 48%, 53%, and 45%, respectively. Poor prognostic indicators included positive surgical margins and intracranial and orbital involvement. Melanoma and undifferentiated carcinoma carried the worst outcomes and esthesioneuroblastoma and low-grade sarcoma the best.[115]

In a large multi-institutional study of craniofacial resection patients, postoperative complications occurred in 36%. Increased risk of postoperative complications was found with the following factors; comorbid illness, previous radiation therapy, and tumor extension. Overall wound complication rates were less than 20%.[116]

Although reports in the literature are encouraging,[117-119] a need for controlled investigations and prospective clinical trials remains. This undertaking will prove to be very difficult. Unlike head and neck cancer, in which most cases are squamous cell carcinoma, cranial base tumors are less common and more varied in histologic type. Compounding the problem of broad histologic variation is the lack of uniformity of location and patterns of invasion of tumors in this complex anatomic region. When these factors are taken into consideration, investigations with adequate patient numbers to yield an accurate reflection of outcomes become nearly impossible. Multi-institutional studies may be required to circumvent these difficulties and to provide important information about the value of cranial base surgery. Such collaborative efforts may help establish the consistent use of primary and adjuvant therapies for tumors of the cranial base.

SUGGESTED READINGS

Anand VK, Schwartz TH. *Practical Endoscopic Skull Base Surgery.* San Diego: Plural Publishing; 2007.

Barnes L, ed. *Surgical Pathology of the Head and Neck.* 3rd ed. New York: Informa HealthCare; 2008.

Carrau RL, Snyderman CH, Vescan AD, et al. Cranial base surgery. In: Myers EN, Eibling DE, eds. *Operative Otolaryngology–Head and Neck Surgery.* 2nd ed. Section 11. Philadelphia: Elsevier; 2005.

Wenig BM. *Atlas of Head and Neck Pathology.* Philadelphia: WB Saunders; 1993.

For complete list of references log onto www.expertconsult.com.

CHAPTER ONE HUNDRED AND SEVENTY-FIVE

Transnasal Endoscopic-Assisted Surgery of the Anterior Skull Base

Aldo Cassol Stamm

Shirley S. N. Pignatari

Key Points

- Effective and safe treatment of lesions involving the anterior skull base and brain depends on several factors, including a careful clinical history, preoperative evaluation and imaging studies, familiarity with regional anatomy and cerebrovascular physiology, and refined surgical technique.
- Technologic advances such as image-guided systems and enhanced endoscopic surgical techniques and equipment have facilitated approaches to the anterior skull base and brain, optimizing the surgical exposure and reducing the risk of complications while avoiding extensive brain retraction and nerve damage.
- Use of a multidisciplinary team approach has increased survival and decreased complication rates from skull base surgery, and this type of surgery is contraindicated without such a team. The multidisciplinary team should include neurosurgery, otolaryngology, anesthesiology, pathology, endocrinology intensive care, and paramedical staff, familiar with the care of patients at risk for significant neurologic sequelae.
- The development of new reconstruction techniques for closing dural defects has been assisted by the use of pedicled nasal septal flaps and has enabled more extensive resections and reduced complication rates. However, infection, cerebrospinal fluid leakage, and difficulty controlling intradural bleeding still present a challenge, and a frank discussion of the risk of these problems is essential for the patient to give informed consent.

The past decade has brought about technologies and insights that have revolutionized our strategy in treating patients with lesions involving the skull base, orbit, and optic nerve. Our work developed from microscopic anterior skull base approaches that aimed to avoid nerve and brain retraction and were developed along two basic anterior midline routes, the transoral and the transnasal.[1-3] We have expanded the scope of the surgery we perform through these approaches and have expanded our armamentarium in achieving postresection reconstruction. Effective and safe treatment of lesions involving the skull base still presents significant challenges, however, because although we have improved postresection reconstruction, the expanded scope of surgery has added risks to the procedures.

Surgical Anatomy

Anterior Cranial Fossa

The anterior cranial fossa is composed of the orbital portion of the frontal bone anteriorly, the cribriform plate of the ethmoid bone centrally, and the lesser wing and body of the sphenoid bone posteriorly (Fig. 175-1A). The cribriform plate is located in a midline depression between the orbital roofs and separates the anterior cranial fossa from the nasal cavity. It has 15 to 20 small foramina that transmit the olfactory nerves from the superior nasal mucosa to the olfactory bulb. The crista galli projects upward at the median anterior portion of the cribriform plate and serves as the site of attachment of the falx cerebri. Between the crista galli and the frontal crest, the foramen cecum in the frontoethmoidal suture transmits an emissary vein to the superior sagittal sinus. The anterior and posterior ethmoidal branches of the ophthalmic artery exit the orbit by passing through the ethmoidal foramina to enter the cranium at the anterolateral and posterolateral edges of the cribriform plate, respectively (see Fig. 175-1B). Posteriorly, the cribriform plate articulates with the sphenoid body, which from anterior to posterior is the site of the planum sphenoidale, limbus sphenoidale, chiasmatic sulcus, tuberculum sella, pituitary fossa, and the dorsum sella. The planum sphenoidale forms the roof of the posterior ethmoid sinus and the anterior part of the sphenoid sinus and borders on the optic canals posterolaterally.[4]

Nasal Cavity

The nasal cavity is wider below than above and is bounded superiorly by the anterior cranial fossa, laterally by the orbits and the maxillary sinus, and inferiorly by the hard palate. This cavity is divided sagittally

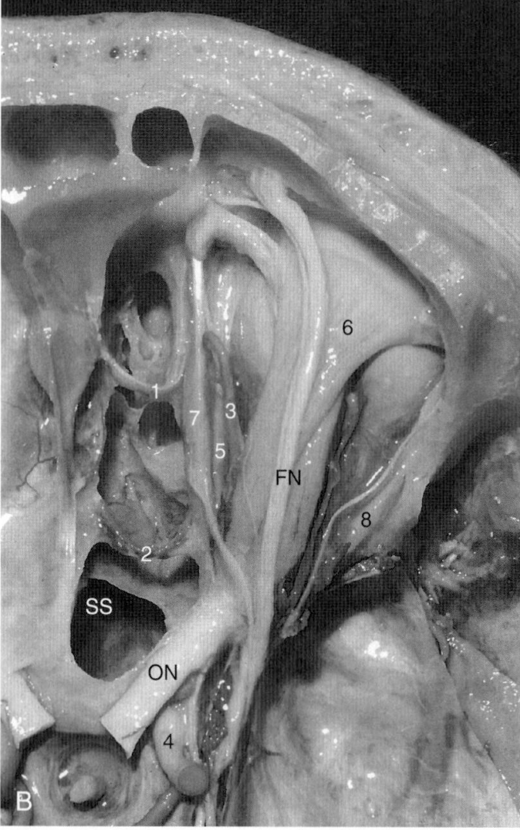

Figure 175-1. **A**, Cranial view of the skull base: 1, foramen cecum; 2, crista galli; 3, cribriform plate; 4, planum sphenoidale; 5, optic canal; 6, chiasmatic sulcus; 7, anterior clinoid process; 8, pituitary fossa; 9, dorsum sellae; 10, foramen ovale; 11, foramen lacerum. **B**, Cranial view of the skull base after removal of the floor of the anterior cranial fossa: 1, anterior ethmoidal artery; 2, posterior ethmoidal artery; 3, ophthalmic artery; 4, internal carotid artery; 5, medial rectus muscle; 6, superior rectus muscle; 7, oblique rectus muscle; 8, lateral rectus muscle. FN, frontal nerve; ON, optic nerve; SS, sphenoid sinus.

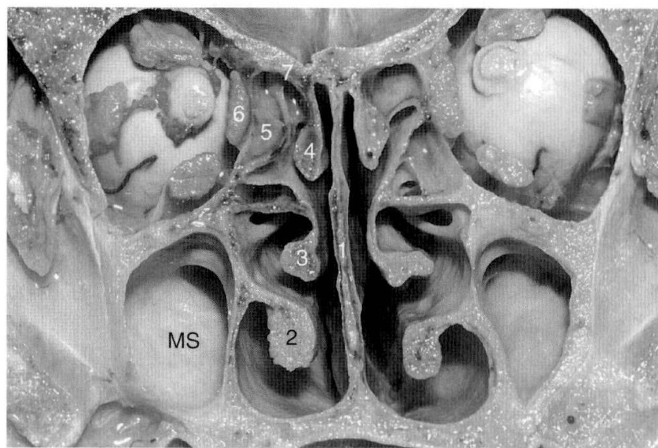

Figure 175-2. Posterior view of a coronal section of the nasal cavity and paranasal sinuses: 1, nasal septum; 2, inferior nasal turbinate; 3, middle turbinate; 4, superior turbinate; 5, ethmoid sinus; 6, medial rectus muscle; 7, fovea ethmoidalis. MS, maxillary sinus.

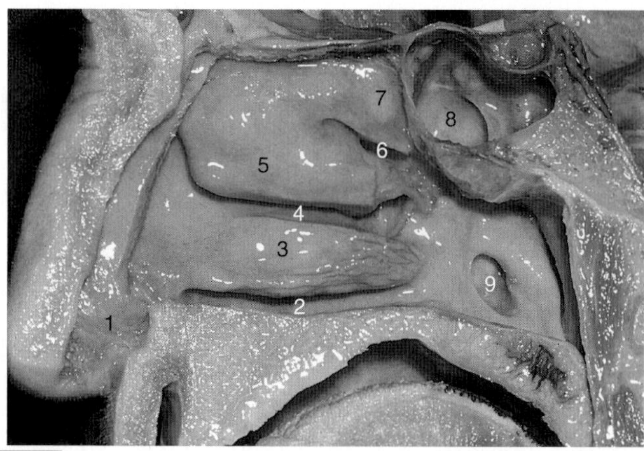

Figure 175-3. Lateral nasal wall, right side: 1, nostril; 2, inferior meatus; 3, inferior turbinate; 4, middle meatus; 5, middle turbinate; 6, superior meatus; 7, superior turbinate; 8, sphenoid sinus; 9, pharyngeal opening of the eustachian tube.

by the nasal septum, which is formed anteriorly and superiorly by the perpendicular plate of the ethmoid bone, posteriorly and inferiorly by the vomer, and anteroinferiorly by septal cartilage (Fig. 175-2). The nasal cavity opens anteriorly onto the face through the pyriform anterior nasal aperture and is continuous posteriorly with the nasopharynx at the posterior nasal apertures.

Each posterior nasal aperture measures approximately 25 mm vertically and 13 mm transversely and is bordered above by the anterior aspect of the sphenoid body that contains the sphenoid sinus, below by the posterior margin of the hard palate (horizontal plate of the palatine bone), medially by the nasal septum (vomer), and laterally by the medial pterygoid plate of the sphenoid.

The lateral nasal wall usually has three medially directed projections: the superior, middle, and inferior nasal turbinates or conchae (Fig. 175-3). The airway passages below these turbinates are termed the superior, middle, and inferior nasal meatuses, respectively. The paired sphenoethmoidal recesses are located above and behind the superior turbinate and in front of the upper anterior aspect of the sphenoid body. They are the sites of the paired sphenoid ostia that form the communication between the nasal cavity and the sphenoid sinus (Fig. 175-4). The upper half of the lateral nasal wall corresponds to the medial orbital wall. From anterior to posterior, it is composed of the frontal process of the maxilla, the lacrimal bone, and the orbital plate of the ethmoid bone (lamina papyracea), each separated from the next by a vertical suture. The extremely thin lacrimal and ethmoid bones contain the ethmoid air cells that separate the nasal cavity from the orbit. The nasolacrimal groove and canal (the site of the lacrimal sac and nasolacrimal duct, respectively) pass downward in front of the anterior end of the middle turbinate and open into the inferior nasal meatus. The frontoethmoidal suture is located at the level of the roof of the nasal cavity and the cribriform plate.

The anterior and posterior ethmoidal foramina transmit the anterior and posterior ethmoidal arteries and nerves and are located in, or just above, the frontal ethmoidal suture. These arteries and nerves exit the ethmoidal foramina and enter the anterior cranial fossa at the lateral

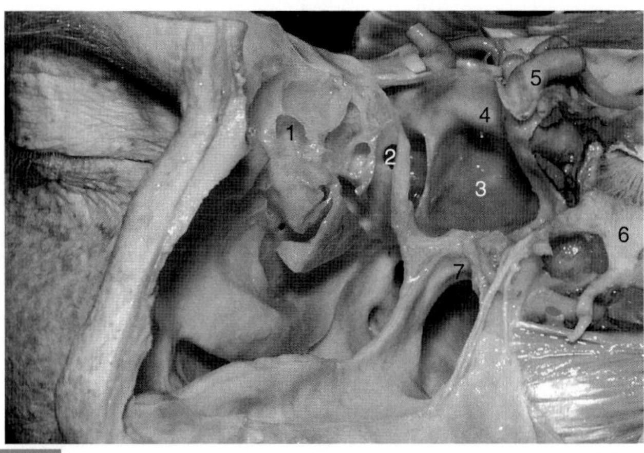

Figure 175-4. Oblique view of the right lateral nasal wall and sphenoid sinus region after removal of the nasal septum and the anterior wall of the sphenoid sinus: 1, ethmoid sinus; 2, sphenoid ostia; 3, sphenoid sinus; 4, anterior sella wall; 5, internal carotid artery; 6, trigeminal nerve; 7, superior arch of the choana.

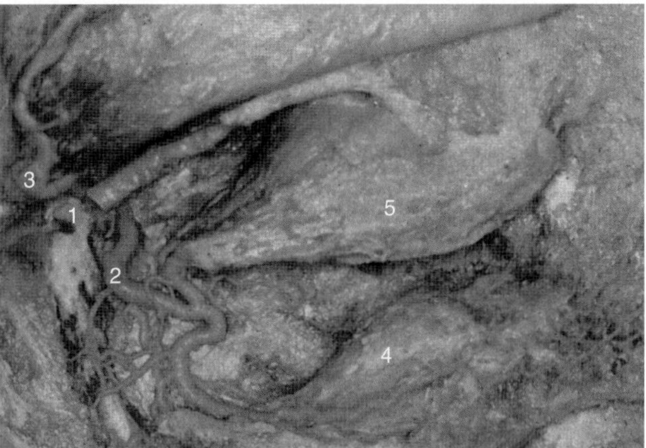

Figure 175-5. Lateral nasal wall demonstrating the terminal branches of the maxillary artery: 1, sphenopalatine foramen; 2, posterior lateral nasal artery; 3, septal artery; 4, inferior turbinate; 5, middle turbinate. *(Courtesy of Prof. Joao Navarro.)*

edge of the cribriform plate. The anterior ethmoidal artery is a terminal branch of the ophthalmic artery and supplies the mucosa of the anterior and middle ethmoid air cells and the dura covering the cribriform plate and the planum sphenoidale. The posterior ethmoidal artery usually is smaller than the anterior and is absent in nearly 30% of persons.[5] It supplies the mucosa of the posterior ethmoid cells and the dura of the planum sphenoidale. The distance from the anterior lacrimal crest of the maxilla's frontal process to the anterior ethmoidal foramen is 22 to 24 mm; the distance between the anterior and posterior ethmoidal foramina is 12 to 15 mm, and that between the posterior ethmoidal foramina and the optic canal usually is 3 to 7 mm. In the midline transfacial procedures, these ethmoidal arteries can be divided in a subperiorbital plane along the medial orbital wall. Care should be taken to prevent damaging the optic nerve, which sometimes is located immediately behind the posterior ethmoidal foramen (see Fig. 175-1B).

The inferior half of the lateral nasal wall comprises part of the medial wall of the maxillary sinus. It is formed anteriorly by the maxilla and posteriorly by the perpendicular plate of the palatine bone. The base of the middle turbinate attaches to the lateral nasal wall near the junction of the orbit and the maxillary sinus. Thus, the medial wall of the maxillary sinus is made up of the lateral wall of the middle and inferior nasal meati and the inferior turbinate. The maxillary sinus communicates with the middle nasal meatus through an opening located in the medial wall just below the roof of the sinus.[4]

The pterygopalatine fossa is situated between the posterior wall of the maxillary sinus anteriorly and the pterygoid process of the sphenoid posteriorly. The pterygopalatine fossa contains the pterygopalatine ganglion, which receives the nerve of the pterygoid canal (vidian nerve), the maxillary nerve just as it leaves the foramen rotundum, the internal maxillary artery (one of the two terminal branches of the external carotid artery), and the maxillary artery's two terminal branches, the posterior lateral nasal artery and the septal artery. Both of these terminal branches enter the nasal cavity through the sphenopalatine foramen just above the caudal aspect of the bony end (not the soft tissue end) of the middle turbinate. The septal artery courses along the roof of the nasal cavity toward the sphenoid rostrum and divides into a number of vessels that extend to the septum and the superior nasal walls. In the lateral wall of the nasal cavity, the posterior lateral nasal artery divides and provides nourishment to the turbinates and meatal spaces[6] (Fig. 175-5).

Paranasal Sinuses

The paranasal sinuses are the frontal, ethmoid, sphenoid, and maxillary. The frontal sinus consists of two large cells separated by an intersinus septum. The anatomic relationships of the sinus are mainly with the roof of the orbit, agger nasi cells, and the anterior cranial fossa. It drains through the frontal recess into the middle meatus. The ethmoid sinus is composed of two groups of air cells: The anterior air cells drain into the middle meatus and the posterior group into the superior meatus.

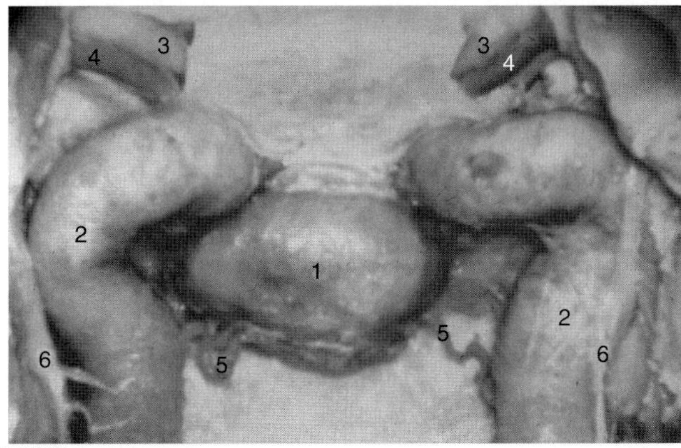

Figure 175-6. Frontal view of the central skull base after removal of the walls of the sphenoid sinus and the dura: 1, pituitary gland; 2, internal carotid artery; 3, optic nerves; 4, ophthalmic arteries; 5, inferior hypophyseal arteries; 6, sympathetic nerves. *(Courtesy of Drs. I. Inoue and A. Rhoton.)*

Posterior ethmoid cells can become pneumatized far laterally and to some degree superiorly to the sphenoid sinus, in which case they are called *sphenoethmoid cells* (Onodi cells). The optic nerve and carotid artery may project into these cells, where they can be damaged during a surgical procedure. The ethmoid sinus is in intimate relation with the medial orbital wall and the floor of the anterior skull base.

The sphenoid sinus varies in shape and size and is asymmetrically divided into two parts by an irregular septum. When the sphenoid sinus is well developed, its thin lateral wall is the medial wall of the cavernous sinus. The intracavernous portion of the internal carotid artery is the most medial structure within the cavernous sinus, and in well-developed sphenoid sinuses it produces a serpiginous bony elevation in the lateral wall of the sinus called the *carotid prominence*. The carotid prominence is divided into presellar, infrasellar, and retrosellar segments.[11] The presellar segment corresponds to the anterior vertical segment and the anterior bend of the intracavernous portion of the internal carotid artery. The infrasellar segment corresponds to the short horizontal portion of the carotid, and the retrosellar segment reflects the posterior bend and posterior vertical segment (Fig. 175-6).

The optic canal often is partially encircled by the sphenoid sinus and creates a bony bulge in the superoanterior portion of its lateral wall.

The bony depression between the optic canal and the presellar segment of the carotid prominence is called the *opticocarotid recess*; it extends a variable distance into the optic strut. The bony lateral sphenoid sinus wall over the internal carotid artery and the optic nerve usually is very thin and may be absent in some areas. Although Lang[7] observed that the canal of the optic nerve was dehiscent in 6% of cases, Seibert[8] found that 57% of the optic nerves bulged into the sphenoid sinus and 1% had no bony canal. Seibert[8] also noted that the horizontal portion of the intracavernous carotid artery extended prominently into the sphenoid sinus in 67% of cases and that its bony covering was dehiscent in 6%. In his series, the maxillary nerve was prominent in the sphenoid sinus in 48% of specimens and dehiscent in 5%, and the pterygoid nerve (vidian nerve) was prominent 18% of the time.

Just below the tuberculum sellae, where they are closest to each other, the average distance between the left and right internal carotid arteries is 13.9 mm (range, 10 to 17 mm). At the anterior wall of the sella, the carotid arteries are separated by 20 mm (range, 13 to 26.5 mm), and at the level of the clivus, the distance between them is 17.4 mm (range, 10.5 to 26.5 mm).[9]

The maxillary sinus has thin walls that face the lower nasal cavity medially, the orbit superiorly, the infratemporal fossa posterolaterally, the pterygopalatine fossa posteromedially, and the soft tissue of the cheek anterolaterally. The maxillary sinus provides a transantral avenue for extending a midline surgical approach for more extensive lateral exposures of the cavernous sinus and the infratemporal fossa.[4]

Nasopharynx

The nasopharynx is situated behind the posterior nasal apertures where the septum and the inferior turbinate end. It is partially separated from the oropharynx below by the soft palate. The roof of the nasopharynx is formed by the mucoperiosteum of the upper clivus. The posterior nasopharyngeal wall is formed in successive layers by the mucosa, the superior pharyngeal constrictor muscle, the prevertebral fascia, and the longus capitis muscle. It abuts the mid- to lower clivus, the anterior aspect of the foramen magnum, and the anterior arch of the atlas (see Fig. 175-3). The pharyngeal tubercle is a small bony elevation located in the midline at the junction of the middle and lower clivus approximately 1 cm above the foramen magnum and serves as the site of attachment of the pharyngeal raphe of the superior pharyngeal constrictor muscle. The longus capitis muscles are attached to the clivus lateral to the pharyngeal tubercle on each side.

The eustachian tube, also termed the pharyngotympanic or auditory tube, opens into the lateral wall of the nasopharynx immediately posterior to the medial pterygoid plate. The fossa of Rosenmüller (pharyngeal recess) is located at the junction of the lateral and the posterior walls of the nasopharynx and projects laterally just behind the orifice of the eustachian tube. At the posterolateral depths of the fossa of Rosenmüller, only a thin layer of fibroconnective tissue separates the mucosa from the cervical internal carotid artery. The horizontal segment of the internal carotid artery in the petrous portion of the temporal bone is located immediately medial and posterior to the eustachian tube.[4]

Clivus

The clivus separates the nasopharynx from the posterior cranial fossa. It is composed of the posterior portion of the sphenoid body (basisphenoid) and the basilar part of the occipital bone (basiocciput), and it is further subdivided into upper, middle, and lower thirds. The upper third of the clivus is at the level of the sphenoid sinus and is formed by the basisphenoid bone including the dorsum sella. The middle clivus corresponds to the rostral part of the basiocciput and is located above a line connecting the caudal ends of the petroclival fissures. The lower third of the clivus is formed by the caudal part of the basiocciput. The intracranial surface of the upper two thirds of the clivus faces the pons and is concave from side to side.

The extracranial surface of the clivus gives rise to the pharyngeal tubercle at the junction of the middle and lower clivus. The upper clivus faces the roof of the nasopharynx, which extends downward in the midline to the level of the pharyngeal tubercle (Fig. 175-7).

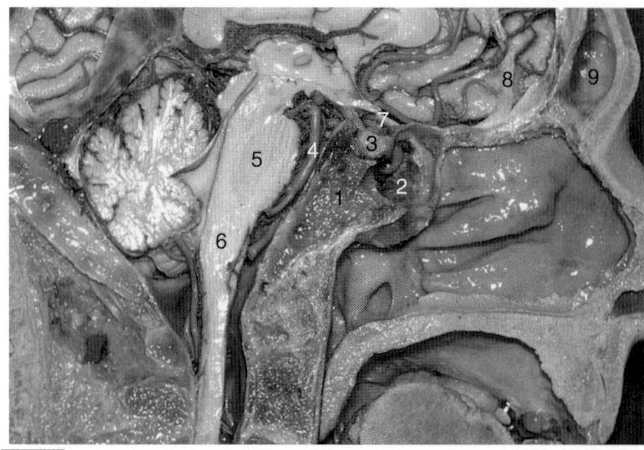

Figure 175-7. Midline sagittal section of the cranium: 1, clivus; 2, sphenoid sinus; 3, pituitary gland; 4, basilar artery; 5, pons; 6, medulla; 7, optic nerve; 8, frontal lobe; 9, frontal sinus.

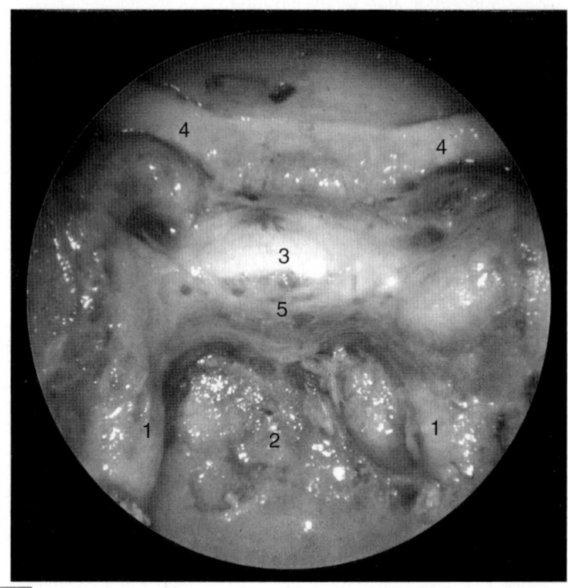

Figure 175-8. Endoscopic view of the posterior wall of the sphenoid sinus: 1, prominence of the internal carotid arteries; 2, clivus; 3, anterior sellar wall; 4, optic nerves; 5, intercavernous sinus.

The upper and middle clivus are separated from the petrous portion of the temporal bone on each side by the petroclival fissure. The basilar venous plexus is situated between the two layers of the dura of the upper clivus and is related to the dorsum sella and the posterior wall of the sphenoid sinus. It forms interconnecting venous channels between the inferior petrosal sinuses laterally, the cavernous sinuses superiorly, and the marginal sinus and epidural venous plexus inferiorly. The basilar sinus is the largest communicating channel between the paired cavernous sinuses.

Retroclival Region

When all the bone of the posterior and lateral walls of the sphenoid sinus has been removed, only periosteum covers the underlying anatomy (Fig. 175-8). The tectorial membrane protects the clival dura in the middle and lower clivus. When the external layer of the dura is opened, the basilar venous plexus and cranial nerve VI (the aducens nerve) on each side can be seen. The average distance between the two abducens nerves at the dural emergence is 19.8 mm.[10]

On opening the inner layer of the clival dura, the view through the 0-degree endoscope reveals the vertebral arteries, basilar artery and its branches (superior cerebellar arteries, anterior inferior cerebellar

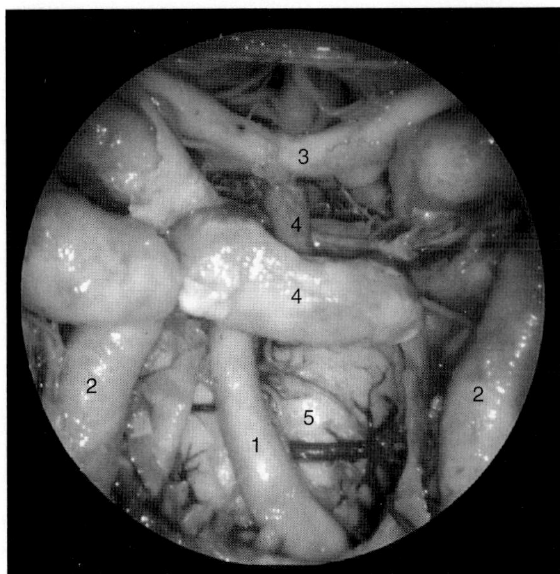

Figure 175-9. Endoscopic view of the posterior fossa after the removal of the posterior wall of sphenoid sinus and upper clivus: 1, basilar artery; 2, internal carotid arteries; 3, optic nerves and chiasm; 4, pituitary gland and pituitary stalk; 5, brainstem.

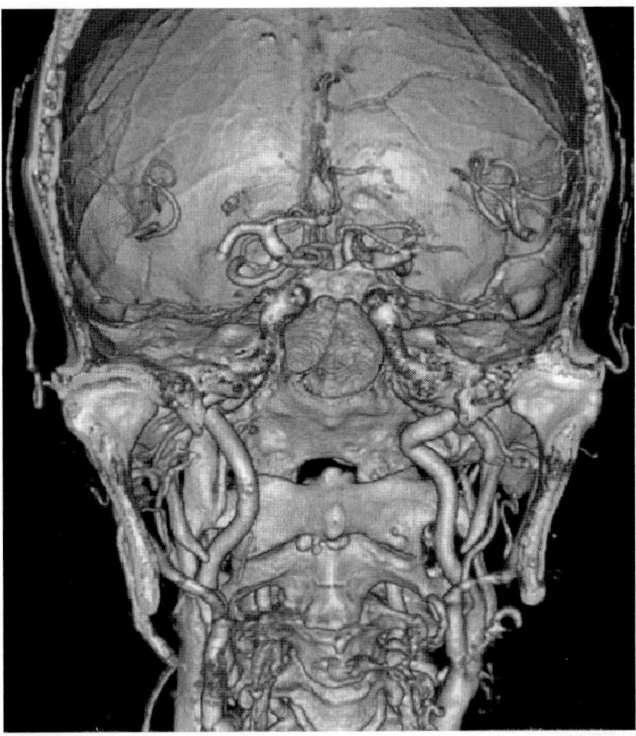

Figure 175-10. Coronal projection, computed tomographic angiography of the head and neck, showing the main vessels of the skull base region. Note the course of the internal carotid arteries and its division.

arteries), posterior cerebral arteries, brainstem, mammillary bodies, and the intradural pathway of cranial nerves III, IV, V, and VI. Just above the pituitary gland, the pituitary stalk, optic nerves, and optic chiasm can be seen. By introducing a 30-degree or 45-degree angled endoscope, it also is possible to view the cerebellopontine angle and cranial nerves VII and VIII, as well as the lower cranial nerves and the retrosellar region (Fig. 175-9).

Preoperative Assessment

The success of any skull base procedure depends on several factors, including a thorough clinical history, a careful preoperative evaluation, a well-developed surgical plan, and physician-patient conversations that include a frank discussion of the diagnosis, surgical plan, possible complications, and the roles of both the physician and the patient in the anticipated postoperative care plan.

Physical examination includes endoscopic assessment of the nasal cavity performed with the patient in a semisitting position. The nasal cavity is prepared with a topical anesthetic solution containing a vasoconstrictor. The examination is performed with rigid 4.0-mm 0-degree, 30-degree, and 70-degree endoscopes. In children, the flexible 3.2-mm endoscope is preferable, and occasionally a straight 2.7-mm endoscope is used.

Appropriate radiographic imaging studies always include diagnostic computed tomography (CT) and are essential in the assessment of all skull base lesions. CT permits assessment of critical anatomic information important during surgery including the presence and extent of erosions of the skull base; integrity of the medial orbital wall; position of the anterior skull base vessels; integrity and degree of aeration of the paranasal sinuses (particularly the sphenoid sinus); location and presence of intersinus septa; position of the internal carotid arteries, optic nerves, and cavernous sinuses; relationships between the ethmoid sinuses and the orbits and optic nerves; relationship between the roof of the ethmoid sinuses and the cribriform plate; and the presence of an Onodi cell. In assessing the frontal sinus, it is important to verify the presence of the intersinus septum and the relationship between the frontal sinus and the supraorbital ethmoid cells, the distance between the anterior and posterior sinus walls, and any bony erosions of the orbit, anterior wall, or posterior wall (anterior cranial fossa).

If the image-guided system is to be used, a multislice helical CT study is mandatory and should be performed as close as possible to the day of surgery. The images are stored on a compact disc and are used at surgery to provide a three-dimensional reconstruction of the patient's skull base region.

CT angiography is a robust technology that allows simultaneous visualization of bony and vascular structures. Venous and arterial structures can be visualized separately in the venous and arterial phases, or seen together. "Angio-CT" is especially useful in assessing the internal carotid and vertebrobasilar systems. Venous structures of particular interest include the cavernous sinus, the inferior aspect of the superior intercavernous sinuses, and the basilar venous plexus. This technology allows us to better plan surgical procedures[11] (Fig. 175-10).

Magnetic resonance imaging (MRI) is important to demonstrate the morphology of the soft tissues and the presence of liquid, but it is not helpful in assessing bony architecture. It helps to differentiate between neoplastic or inflammatory tissue and retained secretions, and to assist in clarifying the diagnosis of skull base malformations when meningoencephalocele, meningocele, or nasal glioma is suspected. MRI also is valuable to demonstrate erosion of the lateral sphenoid wall.

Magnetic resonance angiography (MRA) assesses the structure of medium-sized to large arteries and should be considered in patients with erosion of the lateral and posterior sphenoid walls to visualize the relationship between the basilar and internal carotid arteries.

Although conventional angiography is not routinely performed, it can provide essential information in some specific situations. If a lesion is suspected to involve, impinge on, or displace the internal carotid artery, the surgeon must have accurate preoperative knowledge of the position of the internal carotid artery and its relationship with the lesion, especially when the transnasal-transsphenoidal approach is contemplated (accessing the skull base through the posterior and lateral walls of the sphenoid sinus). Angiography also is helpful to verify the functional integrity of the circle of Willis and the extent of any carotid artery narrowing or occlusion, and to differentiate an aneurysm from tumor.

Operative Technique

The patient is prepared in the usual fashion for transnasal endoscopic-assisted surgery. The patient lies in a supine position on the operating

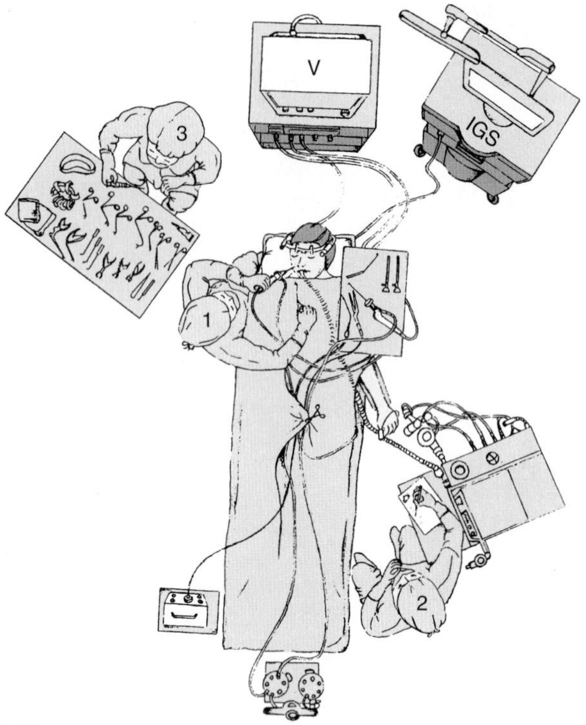

Figure 175-11. Surgical team setup in the operating room: 1, surgeon; 2, anesthesiologist; 3, nurse. IGS, image-guided system; V, video system.

table with the dorsum elevated 30 degrees, and with the head slightly extended and turned toward the surgeon. Head fixation is used when the navigation guidance system is required.

Transnasal endoscopic-assisted surgery of the skull base is performed with the patient under general controlled hypotensive anesthesia (Fig. 175-11). Compressed-rayon surgical sponges (Cottonoids) containing epinephrine, 1 : 2000 concentration, are placed in the nasal cavity, especially over the areas of surgical access. These Cottonoids are left in place for approximately 10 minutes before the surgical procedure is begun. If the surgical access is through the nasal septum, the septum is infiltrated with lidocaine and epinephrine, 1 : 100,000. When the surgery includes the pterygopalatine and zygomatic fossae and the sphenoid, the region of the sphenopalatine foramen is infiltrated with approximately 2.0 mL of the same concentration solution with an angulated 25-gauge spinal needle after first aspirating. If necessary, epinephrine-soaked Cottonoids are used for hemostasis during the surgery. If a CSF fistula is suspected, intrathecal fluorescein can be introduced at the beginning of the surgical procedure to facilitate its precise location.[12] If the use of the image-guided system is contemplated, the head frame is set up for calibration.

Instrumentation

Most skull base surgical procedures are performed with the endoscope attached to an endocamera and a video monitoring system. Endoscopes angled 0 degrees, 45 degrees, and 70 degrees can be used. In conjunction with KARL STORZ Endoscopy-America, Inc. (Culver City, California), we are developing a 5-mm wide-angle 0-degree telescope for these procedures to increase the field of view and illumination.

Although conventional surgical instrumentation also can be used, most of the microendoscopic surgical instruments for these cases are slightly longer and thinner, but just as strong or stronger. Most have an articulation located at the edge, allowing adequate visualization of the operative field. Extra-long handpieces for the surgical drill are essential and are used almost exclusively with diamond burrs of various sizes. Suction cannulas should have a blunted edge to avoid unnecessary trauma and mucosal bleeding. We recommend a micro-Kerrison punch to remove thin delicate bony plates such as those of the ethmoid air cells near the medial wall of the orbit and the bony canal of the optic nerve.

Monopolar and bipolar electrocautery can be used to control bleeding intraoperatively. Bleeding originating from branches of the anterior and posterior ethmoid arteries is more safely controlled by bipolar coagulation. Bleeding from the basilar venous plexus is not coagulated. Compression with oxidized cellulose (Surgicel) packing and obliteration of involved bony channels by diamond burrs are helpful measures.

Powered instrumentation was developed initially for soft tissue shaving and represents a major advance in transnasal endoscopic-assisted surgery. These instruments—microsurgical débriders, or "microdébriders"—have multiple functions, including suction, cutting, and irrigation. At present, newer instruments with curved blades and burrs are able to remove bone such as ethmoidal cells, drill out the frontal sinus, and debulk some tumors. The newer microsurgical débriders also produce a more precise cut of the diseased tissue, avoiding mucosal stripping, and are provided with continuous irrigation, which improves visualization and diminishes blood loss.

The new-generation image-guided systems are precise and have been very helpful in some cases of skull base surgery. These three-dimensional navigation systems provide important information about the location of anatomic structures in the operative field and create an individual anatomic map generated from a preoperative helical CT study. The advantage of this system lies in diminishing the chances of surgical complications, because it delineates the exact anatomic location of an instrument. On the basis of our experience in skull base surgery with such image-guided systems (Evolution computerized image-guided tracking system, Medtronic-Xomed, Jacksonville, Florida), we believe that they are very safe and precise and can be particularly helpful for surgery in patients who have unusual or high-risk anatomic variations, who have diseases involving the frontal sinus recess or sphenoid sinus that put the carotid artery and the optic nerves at risk, or who have recurrent or extensive disease.[13] The navigation system currently in use in our practice allows visualization of CT or magnetic resonance images or both simultaneously. This greatly improves the surgeon's ability to identify the extradural and intradural extent of the various lesions.

Transnasal Surgical Approaches to the Skull Base

Several transnasal approaches to the skull base have been described. The choice of the appropriate transnasal technique for each patient depends on the nature, location, and extent of the lesion. We currently are using the following extended transnasal surgical approaches:

- Transsphenoidal: transsellar and parasellar, transclival, and petrous apex
- Transcribriform
- Transtuberculum-transplanum
- Transmaxillary/transpterygoid/infratemporal
- Craniocervical junction

The transsphenoidal approaches (transsellar and parasellar, transclival, and petrous apex) require previous sphenoidectomy, which can be accomplished by several ways as briefly described below: direct transnasal access, transseptal access, transseptal transnasal access, and transethmoidal access. Regardless of the chosen expanded approach, the first step of the surgical procedure is the creation of a large pedicled septal flap originating at and based on the vascular pedicle of the sphenopalatine foramen. The extent of this flap is determined by the chosen approach. A vertical incision is made approximately 1 to 2 cm from the caudal edge of the nasal septum, followed by two horizontal incisions, one parallel to and just above the floor of the nasal cavity and the other approximately 0.8 cm to 1.0 cm beneath the upper limit of the nasal septum. The inferior incision borders the superior edge of the choana toward to the sphenopalatine foramen. The flap should be subperichondrial and subperiosteal, preserving the vascular pedicle. During the procedure, the flap can be safely placed into the maxillary sinus cavity through a large middle meatus antrostomy. This maneuver avoids any obstruction of the surgical field by the flap.[14]

Transsphenoidal Approach

The great majority of the transnasal endoscopic skull base operations directly involve the sphenoid sinus, which is the focal point for several of the surgical approaches. Although the operative lesion may involve the sella or parasellar region, the clival region, or the petrous apex, the specific nature and location of the lesion will determine the technique to access the sphenoid sinus. Choices include the direct transnasal, transseptal (anterior incision, posterior incision), transseptal-transnasal (binostril approach), and transnasal plus transethmoidal (middle turbinate removal) approaches. The direct transnasal approach is used for removal of lesions involving the roof of the nasal cavity without involvement of the ethmoid sinus, lesions of the nasopharynx, and some lesions involving the sphenoid sinus. The transseptal approach is used primarily for removal of lesions involving the sphenoid sinus and sella such as pituitary adenomas.[15] The transethmoidal approach is useful for disease localized to the ethmoid sinus, the roof of the ethmoid sinus, the orbits, or lesions involving both the ethmoid and sphenoid sinuses.

Direct Transnasal Access

With direct transnasal access, the procedure is carried out through one nostril. If the nasal cavity is very narrow and the passage of the endoscope and operating instruments is limited because of a septal deviation, septoplasty is done first. After identification of the middle and superior turbinates, the posterior region of the nasal septum, and the choanal arch, the ostium of the sphenoid sinus is probed with the seeker-palpator. If diseased tissue such as polyps obstructs the access to the sphenoid recess, a microsurgical débrider can be helpful. To improve access, the superior turbinate is identified and removed with a through-cutting forceps. When the surgical access is very narrow, the posterior portion of the middle turbinate also can be removed by means of microscissors.

The initial opening of the sphenoid sinus is made with a micro-Kerrison punch, beginning at the ostium. The sphenoidotomy is enlarged inferiorly, with care taken to avoid damaging or cauterizing the septal artery that crosses the anterior wall of the sphenoid sinus in that region. If both sphenoid sinuses are to be surgically exposed, the mucoperiosteum of the anterior wall and the sphenoid rostrun are displaced laterally. The anterior wall, rostrum, and all intersinus septa are resected by semicutting or diamond burrs, giving wide exposure of the sinus (Figs. 175-12 and 175-13).

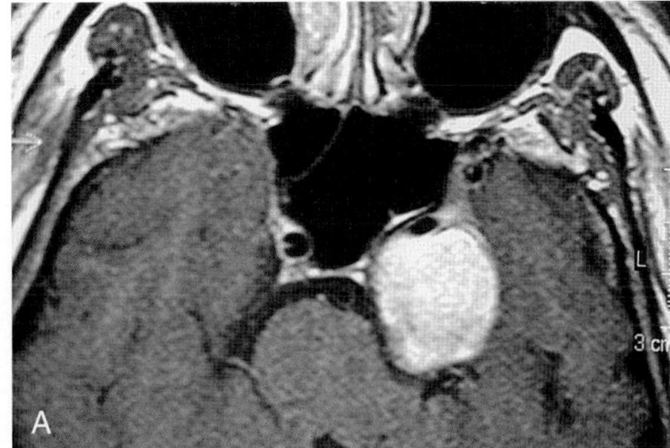

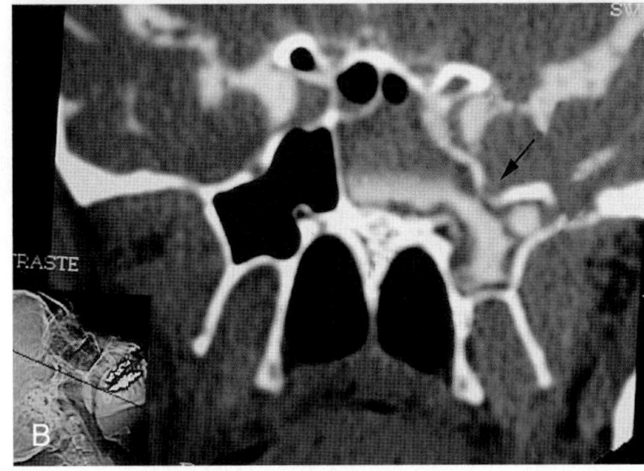

Figure 175-12. **A,** Axial view, magnetic resonance imaging, of a petrous apex cholesterol granuloma. **B,** computed tomography cisternogram showing a cerebrospinal fluid fistula at the lateral wall of the sphenoid sinus *(arrow)*.

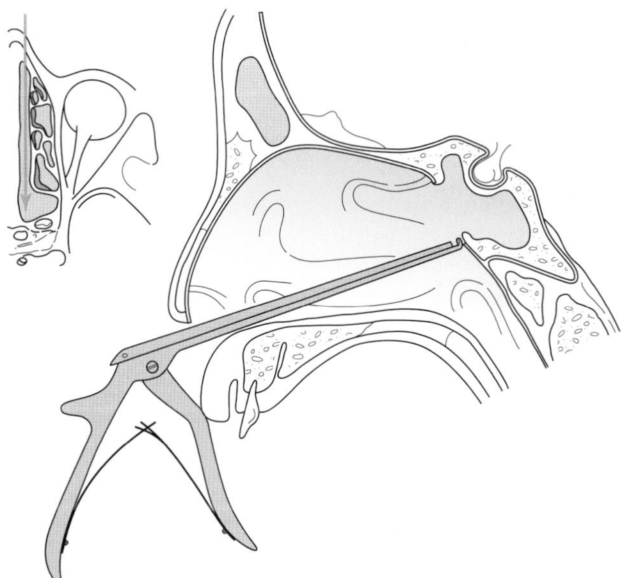

Figure 175-13. Opening of the sphenoid sinus anterior wall by means of a micro-Kerrison punch through a direct transnasal approach (*arrow* on *inset*).

Transseptal Access

Thetransseptal approach was conceived to provide a midline access to the sphenoid sinus region through the nasal septum, avoiding damage to the structures in the nasal cavity and avoiding the lateral wall of the sphenoid sinus and the nearby carotid artery and optic nerve. This approach has been particularly useful for obtaining access to the clivus, sella, and parasellar regions, because they are midline structures.

The surgeon first performs a submucoperichondrial and submucoperiosteal infiltration with lidocaine (2%) and epinephrine (1 : 100,000), producing a hydraulic dissection that facilitates surgical elevation. A vertical hemitransfixion incision is made at the caudal edge of the septal cartilage, and septal flaps are elevated as in performing a septoplasty. Disarticulation of the osseocartilaginous junction (septal cartilage, ethmoid plate, and vomer) is performed with the suction elevator, with preservation of the uppermost part of the osseocartilaginous junction to avoid postoperative dorsal nasal saddling. The posterior attachment of the septum to the perpendicular lamina of the ethmoid is fractured. The posterior part of the septal bone, which obstructs access to the sphenoid rostrum, is resected with a Jansen-Middleton forceps. The mucoperiosteum of the anterior wall of the sphenoid sinus is elevated until the sinus ostia on both sides are visualized. At this point, a self-retaining speculum is introduced between the two leaves of septal mucosa, and the anterior wall of the sphenoid sinus is entirely exposed. The anterior wall is then opened with a chisel and is enlarged with a micro-Kerrison punch (Fig. 175-14). The sphenoidotomy is made large enough to allow easy simultaneous introduction of a 4-mm endoscope and a surgical instrument. Once the septum is

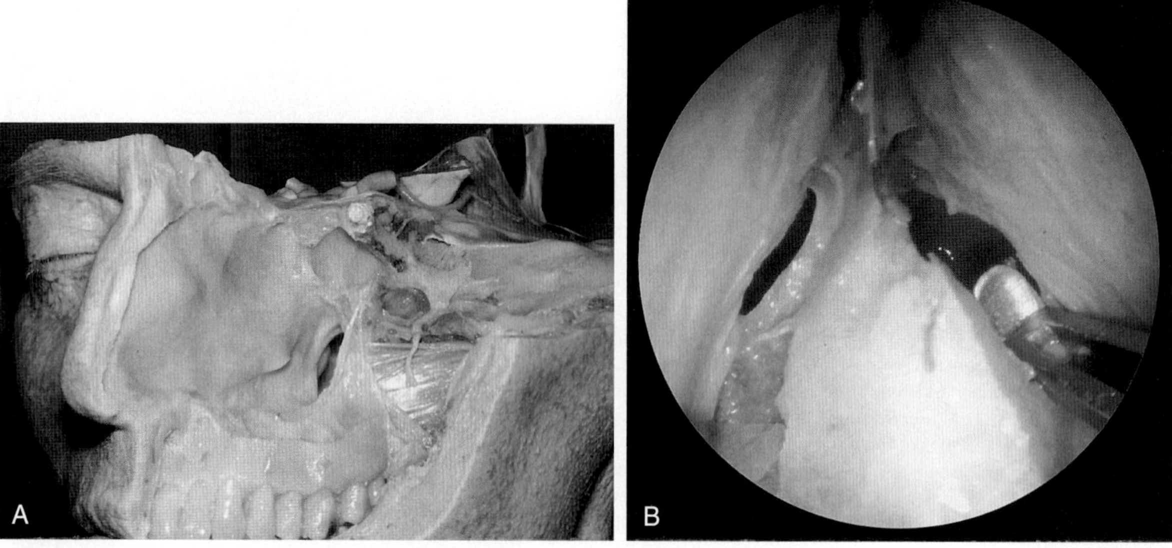

Figure 175-14. **A,** Anatomic oblique view of the nasal septum and its relation with the sphenoid sinus. **B,** Endoscopic view of the sphenoid rostrum being removed by a micro-Kerrison punch.

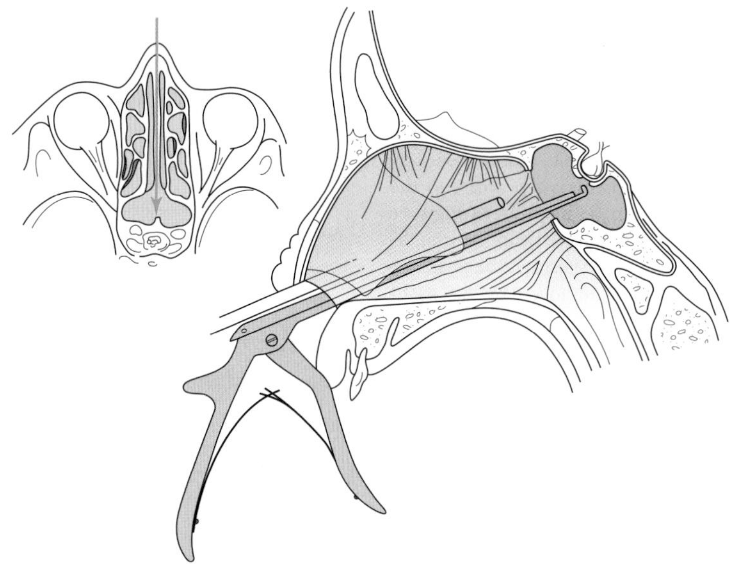

Figure 175-15. Schematic drawing of the transseptal approach (*arrow* on *inset*) to the sphenoid sinus and sellar region.

resected and the two septal flaps are displaced, the self-retaining speculum can be removed, and the surgeon can work exclusively with an endoscope and the instruments (Fig. 175-15).

Transseptal-Transnasal Access

For the transseptal-transnasal (binostril) approach (Fig. 175-16), a classic anterior septoplasty incision is made. A submucoperichondrial-mucoperiosteal dissection is performed on both sides. The posterior portion of the nasal septum is removed, with preservation of the inferior portion as a landmark for the midline. The sphenoid rostrum and anterior wall of the sphenoid sinus are exposed. The next step is the creation of a nasal septal mucosal flap on one side. Three incisions are made: vertical, superior horizontal, and inferior horizontal. These incisions can be completed with scissors or other sharp instruments as necessary, creating a mucosal flap that is displaced onto the nasal floor. This nasal septal flap preserves a posterolateral pedicle containing the sphenopalatine neurovascular bundle. Multiple modifications in length and width are possible, and the flap should be designed in accordance with the size and shape of the anticipated skull base defect. This approach has several advantages: It allows two surgeons to simultaneously manipulate surgical instruments using both nostrils; it has a very robust tissue pedicle to help in the closure of skull base defects; and it preserves the nasal septal mucosa on one side, avoiding nasal septal perforation (see Fig. 175-16).[16]

Transethmoidal Access

Transethmoidal surgical access usually is indicated for cases in which lesions extend into or involve the ethmoid and sphenoid sinuses. The most common of these lesions are hemangiopericytoma, inverted papilloma, schwannoma, meningoencephalocele, meningocele, and malignant tumors. CSF fistulas also commonly affect this area.[17]

First, an ethmoidectomy is performed beginning with the resection of the uncinate process and followed by resection of the ethmoid bulla and the remaining ethmoid cells. During the resection of the posterior ethmoid cells, the surgeon must correlate direct observation and intraoperative review of the CT scan to determine whether an Onodi cell is present, and, if so, to recognize its relationship to the optic nerve canal and the internal carotid artery.[18,19]

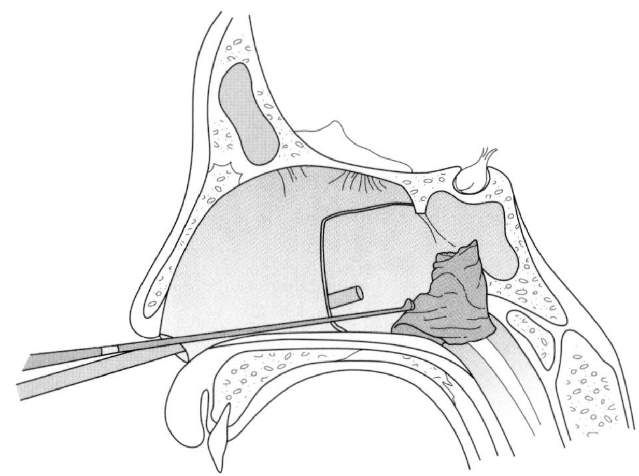

Figure 175-16. Nasal septum mucosal flap. Surgical instrument enters through one nostril and the endoscope through the septum; contralateral septal mucosa is intact and preserved.

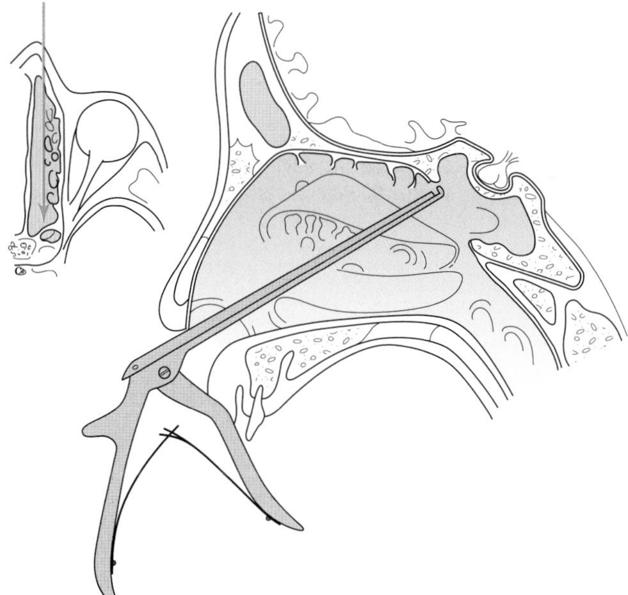

Figure 175-17. Transethmoidal approach (*arrow* on *inset*) to the sphenoid sinus.

Next, the posterior ethmoid artery is identified anterior to the front wall of the sphenoid sinus, which makes an angle of approximately 90 degrees with the roof of the ethmoid sinus. The initial opening of the sphenoid sinus is made with a delicate curette or with an atraumatic aspirator medially and inferiorly. The sphenoidotomy is then enlarged with a micro-Kerrison punch, incorporating the natural ostium into the opening (Fig. 175-17). Figure 175-18 shows a fracture of the optic nerve canals. Removal of the middle turbinate may be necessary when the lesion is located in the roof of the ethmoid sinus or the cribriform plate, as occurs in some cases of inverted papilloma, osteoma, or schwannoma. When the middle turbinate is removed, its mucoperiosteum can be used as a free graft to repair dural defects that were created by the lesion or its removal. Figure 175-19 shows removal of a schwannoma by this technique.

Transsellar and Parasellar Approaches

After the opening of the sphenoid sinus, the next step consists of opening the pituitary fossa. The anterior wall of the sphenoid sinus must be largely exposed, to facilitate the identification of the principal anatomic structures of this region, such as the prominence of the internal carotid artery canals, optic nerve canals, clivus, planum sphenoidale, and also the floor of the sella. Any intersinus and or intrasinus septa are resected by means of a strong through-cutting forceps. The mucoperiosteum of the sphenoid sinus covering the floor of the sella is displaced laterally and preserved for use in reconstruction. The next step consists of wide resection of the sellar bone, exposing the dura from one internal carotid artery to the opposite internal carotid artery and from the planum sphenoidale to the clivus. This usually is performed with a diamond burr and a micro-Kerrison punch. Thereafter, a quadrangular dural incision is made very carefully, with an attempt to visualize the precise localization of the cavernous sinus and the superior and inferior intercavernous sinuses, and of both internal carotid arteries through the exposed dura (Fig. 175-20).

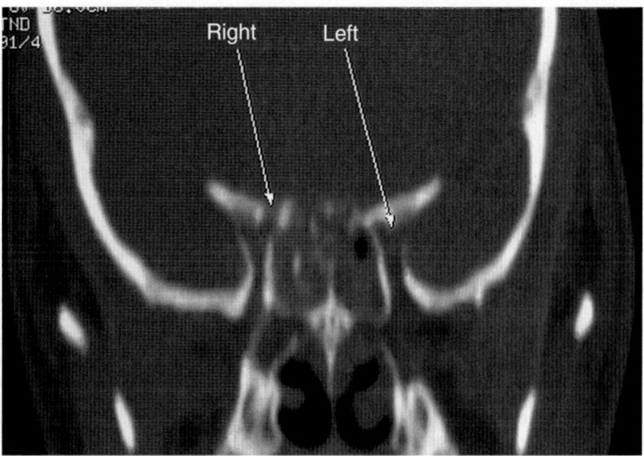

Figure 175-18. Coronal computed tomography scan showing bilateral fracture of the optic nerve canals.

These structures represent the anatomic limits of the dural opening. The dura mater, along with any attached fragments of tumor, is removed and sent for histopathologic examination. Resection of the tumor begins laterally with a 45-degree angled endoscope and curved suction tube, first identifying the angle between the arachnoid and the ICA. The arachnoid is the limit of the superior and posterior dissection (classically known as the diaphragma sella). When a complete removal is accomplished, the arachnoid frequently descends to fill the space occupied by the tumor. This can partially obstruct the surgical field of view and is one factor in incomplete tumor removal. In pituitary adenoma surgery, disection is more important than the use of the curette. Occasional bleeding is carefully controlled by application of warm saline solution, Surgicel packing, and other measures as appropriate.

If no fistula is present, the mucoperiosteum of the sphenoid sinus is replaced and secured with fibrin glue. In the presence of a CSF leak, the defect is sealed with fascia lata, fat, and mucoperiosteum of the sphenoid sinus. Fibrin glue completes the sealing process. In larger defects with high fluid flow, in addition to the previous steps, we use a pedicled flap originating from the mucoperiosteum of the posterior nasal septum to cover the region of the sella. Packing of the sphenoid sinus and nasal cavity for 5 to 7 days is recommended.

Transclival Approach

Approach to the Clivus and Cavernous Sinus

The transsphenoidal-transclival approach is used for lesions involving the clivus or retroclival region. Anterior approaches to the craniovertebral junction and clivus originally were proposed in the 1960s for the treatment of neoplasms and vertebrobasilar aneurysms.[20-23] Anterior procedures include the transseptal, transsphenoidal,[24,25] transmaxillary,[26,27] transpalatal and transoral-transpalatal,[28,29] transmandibular,[30] transmaxillary-transnasal,[31] and facial translocation approaches.[32]

Despite the fact that anterior approaches offer a more direct anatomic approach to the structures beyond the clivus, the risks of CSF leakage and infection limit most of the aforementioned approaches to extradural lesions, especially those approaches that traverse a nonsterile

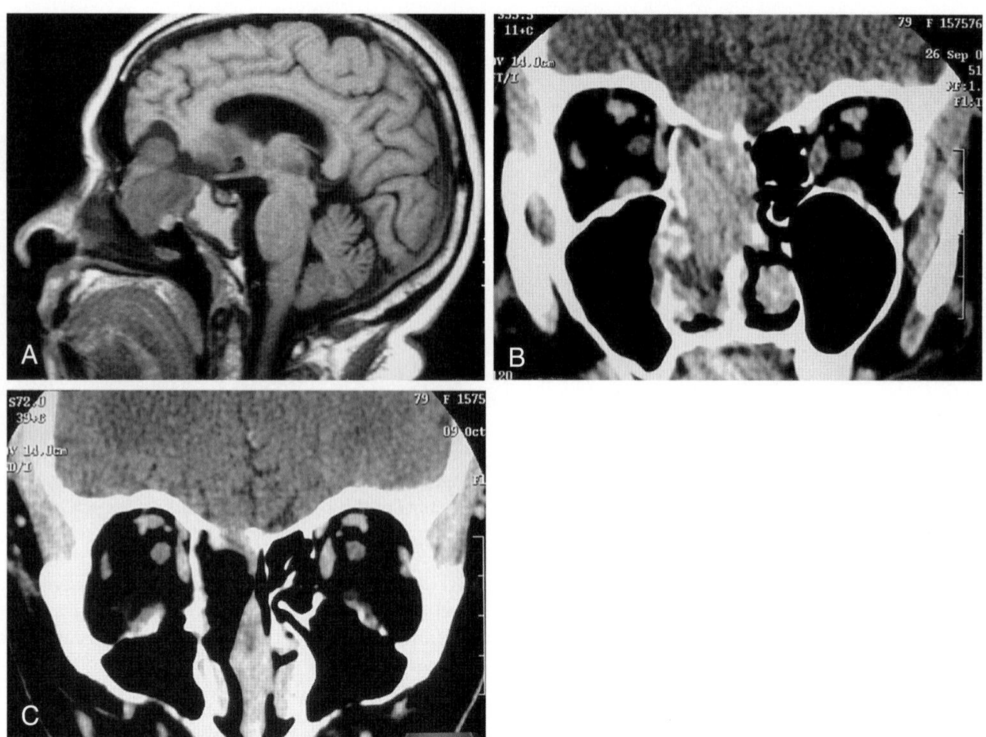

Figure 175-19. Schwannoma of the ethmoid region, with intradural extension, in a 68-year-old woman. **A,** Sagittal view, magnetic resonance imaging. **B,** Coronal reconstruction, computed tomography (CT), showing the extent of the lesion. **C,** Postoperative CT appearance, coronal reconstruction.

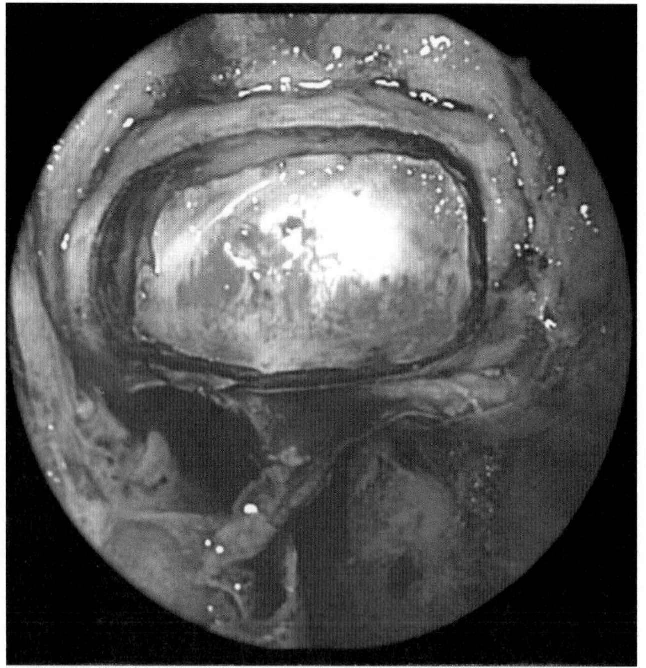

Figure 175-20. Quadrangular incision area in sellar dura.

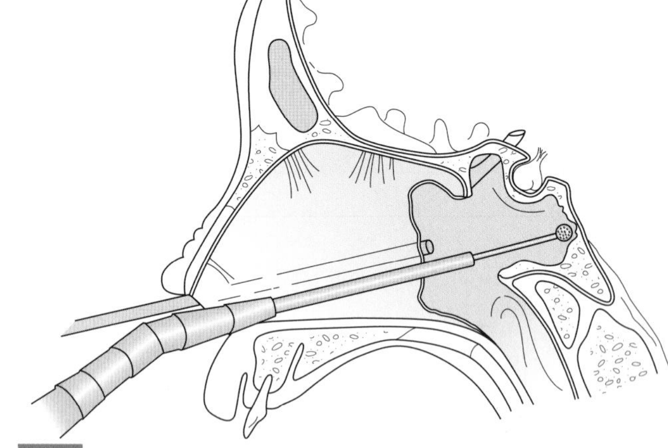

Figure 175-21. Schematic drawing showing a modified transseptal approach to the posterior sphenoid sinus wall (clivus). A surgical drill with a long handpiece and a diamond burr is used to remove the bone of the upper clivus.

operative field.[10] The major advantage of the midline transfacial approaches is the direct anterior surgical access through the large spaces of the nasal cavity, nasopharynx, oral cavity, and paranasal sinuses. However, these midline routes are restricted by critical neurovascular structures such as the internal carotid artery, optic nerve, cavernous sinus, cranial nerves, and the orbital contents.[4]

The transnasal endoscopic-assisted surgical technique begins with one of the surgical approaches to the sphenoid sinus (transnasal direct, transethmoidal, or transseptal). A wide opening of the anterior sphenoid sinus wall is obtained with a micro-Kerrison punch. The floor of the sella, the two carotid protuberances, the medial aspect of the optic canals, and the upper clivus are visualized. The sinus mucosa that lines the clival area is reflected carefully, exposing the clival bone. The bone removal initially is done with a drill system that uses a diamond burr and continued carefully with a micro-Kerrison punch if necessary (Fig. 175-21). The limits of clival bone removal are the floor of the sella superiorly, the foramen magnum inferiorly, and the bony canals of the sixth cranial nerves, the internal carotid arteries, and the occipital condyles laterally. To obtain an intradural exposure, the external layer of the dura is first incised, and the basilar venous plexus and cranial nerve VI are encountered. Bleeding in the plexus cannot be cauterized safely but usually can be controlled with small pieces of Surgicel. Large lesions

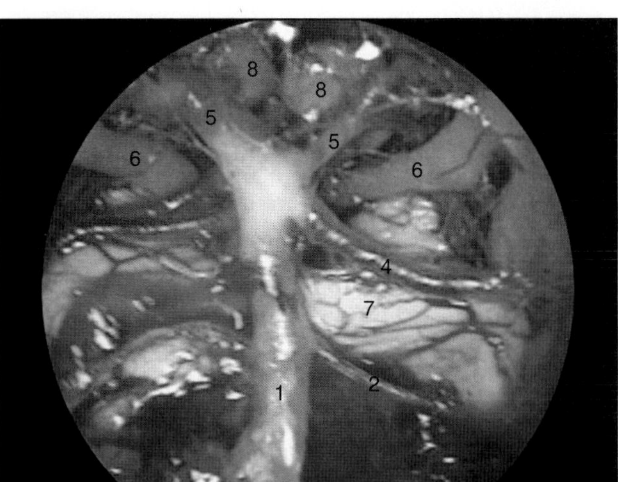

Figure 175-22. Surgical endoscopic view during a transseptal transclival approach: 1, basilar artery and branches; 2, anterior inferior cerebellar artery; 3, vertebral artery; 4, superior cerebellar artery; 5, posterior cerebral arteries; 6, intradural course of cranial nerve III; 7, brainstem; 8, mammillary bodies.

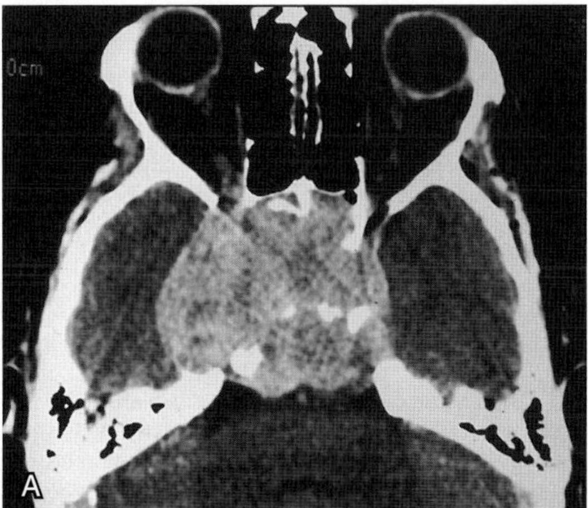

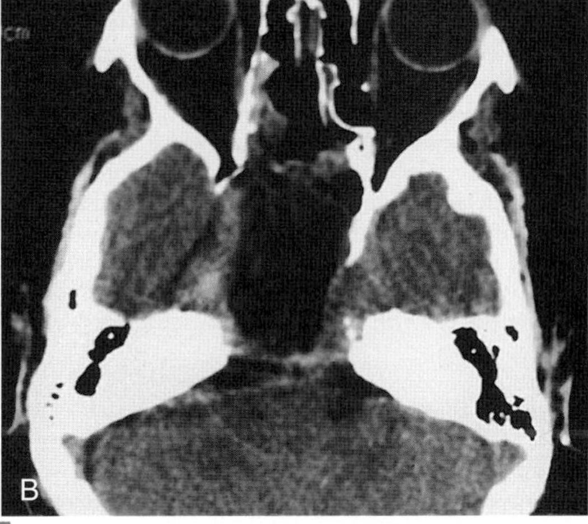

Figure 175-23. Preoperative **(A)** and, postoperative **(B)** axial computed tomography images of the operated region in a patient with clivus chordoma. An endoscopic-assisted combination transnasal, transsphenoidal, transclival surgical approach was used.

often encroach on and obliterate much of the plexus, but if the lesion is not large or if the plexus is not completely compressed, profuse and intense venous bleeding can occur. Judicious packing, time, patience, and experience are required to control such bleeding.

The opening of the internal layer of the dura at the level of the middle and superior clivus must be accomplished with great care to avoid injury to the underlying basilar artery. Once the dura is opened, minor bleeding is stopped with bipolar coagulation, and it is finally possible to introduce the endoscope carefully into the intradural space and to identify the major vessels of the posterior fossa (basilar artery and branches, anterior inferior cerebellar arteries, vertebral arteries, superior cerebellar arteries, and posterior cerebral arteries); the intradural course of cranial nerves III, IV, V, and VI; the brainstem; and the mammillary bodies. The cerebellopontine angle, cranial nerves VII through XII, and the retrosellar regions are best visualized by use of endoscopes angled 30 degrees, 45 degrees, or 70 degrees (Fig. 175-22).

Dural repair at the clivus region is difficult. If the defect is large, we occlude it with abdominal fat first and then cover the defect with grafts of fascia lata or synthetic dura (Duraform, Duragen). These grafts are covered by a large pedicled nasal septal flap, as described previously, secured in position with fibrin glue and pieces of surgical gel (Gelfoam). For small defects, the nasal cavity is packed with Merocel for 5 to 7 days, whereas for larger ones, the packing is made with gauze embedded in antibiotics for 10 to 14 days. Broad-spectrum antibiotics are given for 10 to 14 days.

The main advantages of the transsphenoidal-transclival approach with removal of the posterior nasal septum are the avoidance of cerebral retraction and a decreased incidence of injury to the lower cranial nerves. In addition, the approach is direct without external incisions, is relatively quick, and best preserves the anatomic structures. Even though endoscopes do not allow a three-dimensional perspective, they do provide a close view of the operative field from different angles. However, this technique requires working in a narrow operative field limited by critical neurovascular structures, such as internal carotid arteries, optic nerves, cavernous and basilar sinuses, and the pituitary gland. The risks of major intradural bleeding, CSF leakage, and meningitis are not to be taken lightly. Figure 175-23 illustrates this approach in a patient with a clivus chordoma.

Petrous Apex Access

This type of surgical access can be useful for biopsy and drainage purposes. It can be particularly helpful in selected cases of cholesterol granuloma of the petrous apex because complete excision is unnecessary (see Fig. 175-14). Although surgical drainage is usually accomplished through the temporal bone, the transsphenoidal endoscopic approach may be indicated when the lesion abuts against the posterior and lateral wall of the sphenoid sinus. In these cases, the use of an image-guided system can be very helpful, especially to precisely identify the internal carotid artery, optic nerve, and the lesion.

The clival region is completely exposed, and both carotid canals are identified. When the anatomy is clearly apparent, these canals are easily recognized. If the canals are difficult to identify, use of diamond burrs with suction-irrigation can help identify the vertical segment, particularly at the junction of the cavernous and petrous portions of the internal carotid artery.

The transmaxillary-transpterygoid access also permits approaching the petrous apex by exposing completely the pterygopalatine and infratemporal fossae. First, the vidian nerve canal, foramen rotundum and superior orbital fissure, and V_2 are dissected along their entire extradural extent. The early identification of the vidian canal is very important, because this can be an excellent guide to the identification of the canal of the internal carotid artery between its petrous and paraclival portions.[34] After exposure of the lateral recess of the sphenoid sinus and the lateral portion of the cavernous sinus, a diamond burr is used laterally and inferiorly, exposing the petrous apex. The petrous part of the internal carotid artery must be identified after careful dissection and resection of its bony canal. By mobilizing the artery laterally, a complete exposure of the petrous apex can be accomplished.

Transcribriform Approach

The transcribriform approach is indicated to remove lesions involving the olfactory groove, hypophysis, or crista galli; it can be performed unilaterally or bilaterally. Among the most common lesions treated using the transcribriform surgical approach are CSF leaks, meningoencephaloceles, encephaloceles, meningiomas, esthesioneuroblastomas, and malignancies.

Transcribriform Unilateral Access

The unilateral transcribriform approach is designed to remove the cribriform area and to preserve the crista galli, with or without resection of the dura mater. The procedure begins with a wide middle meatal antrostomy. The middle turbinate is removed to the level of the skull base and a complete sphenoethmoidectomy is performed, including removal of the lateral wall of the orbit, exposing the periorbita. Next, the frontal recess and frontal sinus are exposed. The anterior and posterior ethmoid arteries are then identified, coagulated, and divided. The bone of the roof of the ethmoid sinus is removed, completely exposing the dura. The medial dissection is accomplished by removing the posterior and superior portions of the ipsilateral nasal septum. Perichondrium and periosteum of the contralateral side are preserved to be used in the reconstruction.

Especially in cases of malignancy in which the lesion presents intradural extension, the dura is then removed. Reconstruction of the dural defect is achieved with one or two layers of fascia lata, covered by the contralateral septal flap. These layers are kept in place with fibrin glue and nasal packing. Lumbar drainage usually is not necessary. This endoscopic-assisted unilateral transnasal approach preserves the olfactory area on one side, which represents a great advantage over the classic craniofacial approach.

Transcribriform Bilateral Access

In cases with bilateral involvement, intradural extension of the lesion is very commom. The procedure is performed in the same way on both sides as decribed above. In such cases however, it is necessary to make a large aperture of the frontal sinus through a Draf III surgical access. Depending on the extent of the lesion, and especially in malignant tumors, the upper part of the nasal septum is also removed.

The limits of the dissection are as follows: laterally, the medial wall of the orbit; anteriorly, the frontal sinuses, and posteriorly, the sphenoid sinuses. The anterior and posterior ethmoid arteries of both sides are identified and coagulated with a bipolar cautery.

Next, complete removal of the skull base bone in this region is performed with a drill system and suction irrigation. The dura mater within the aforementioned limits is then resected. The opening of the dura is initiated with a surgical knife with a No. 11 blade after bipolar cauterization and is completed with microscissors on both sides of the falx. The falx is coagulated and the sagittal sinus packed with Surgicel, if necessary. The falx is transected and detached from the crista galli. When the lesion has a subpial extension, the dissection must be performed extremely carefully, with special attention directed at possible bleeding from branches of the anterior cerebral artery, such as the frontopolar artery. The dural defect may be large, necessitating meticulous reconstruction using two layers of fascia lata (one intradurally and another between the dura and the bone). The nasal flap, including mucoperiosteum-mucoperichondrium, is used to cover the grafts. If this flap is not available because the tissues are involved by a malignant lesion, a mucoperichondrial flap from the floor of the nasal cavity can be used (Fig. 175-24).

Transtuberculum-Transplanum Approach

We use the transtuberculum-transplanum approach for removal of lesions involving the planum sphenoidale and tuberculum sella, most typically meningiomas. It also is useful to remove lesions that compromise the suprasellar cistern region and pre– and post–optic chiasma lesions such as pituitary microadenomas, craniopharyngiomas, Rathke's pouch cysts, and even optic nerve gliomas.

The first step in the procedure is the development of a nasal mucoperichondrial flap pedicled on the sphenopalatine foramen to be used for reconstruction at the end of the procedure. The surgical access portion of the procedure consists of a wide sphenoidotomy with resection of the posterior part of the nasal septum and the intersinus septum. To obtain adequate exposure, it also is necessary to perform bilateral posterior ethmoidectomies and to resect both middle turbinates.

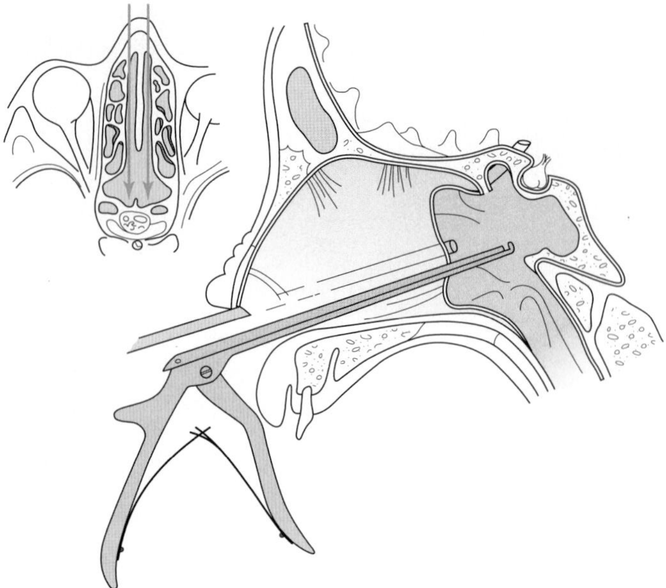

Figure 175-24. Schmatic drawing of a modified transseptal approach (*arrows* on *inset*) to the sphenoid and parasphenoid sinus regions.

The ethmoidectomies remove all cells laterally to both medial walls of the orbits and anteriorly to the level of the posterior ethmoid arteries, in order to avoid damaging the neuroepithelium. All bone in the region of the planum sphenoidale is exposed by using a high-speed drill with irrigation, continuing until the bone is as thin as an egg shell. The final layer is removed carefully with a micro-Kerrison punch.

We are especially careful not to damage the optic nerves by excessive heat generated by the use of the drill, and use shorter periods of drilling and copious irrigation. The eggshell bone over the internal carotid arteries in the parasellar region also is removed with a micro-Kerrison punch.

After the dura mater from the sellar region to the anterior portion of the planum and laterally to the lamina papyracea is exposed completely, the superior intercavernous sinus is cauterized using a bipolar system and transsected. The posterior ethmoidal arteries are coagulated and sectioned. Then the dura mater is opened carefully avoiding any damage to the attached vessels.

The intradural dissection is critical, and it is imperative to identify the internal carotid arteries in the paraclinoid region, the anterior cerebral arteries (A_1 and A_2), the anterior communicating artery, and the recurrent artery of Heubner. The optic nerve and chiasm must be identified more superiorly and also the pituitary stalk. Dissection in the arachnoidal plane is highly recommended whenever possible, as is the avoidance of excessive coagulation and traction, in order to reduce the possibility of minor surgical trauma to neurovascular structures.

Reconstruction is begun with a double layer of fascia lata, which is then covered with the pedicled nasal septal mucosal flap. We secure these with fibrin glue and place nasal packing, to remain for 7 to 10 days. We do not use external lumbar drainage.

Transmaxillary-Transpterygoidal-Infratemporal Approach

The transmaxillary approach is excellent for removing lesions that involve the medial portion of the maxillary sinus, and for larger lesions in the pterygopalatine, zygomatic, or infratemporal fossa such as angiofibromas. This approach also can be extended to gain exposure to the cavernous sinus.

The procedure begins with an anterior ethmoidectomy and continues with a wide middle meatus antrostomy to give maximal exposure

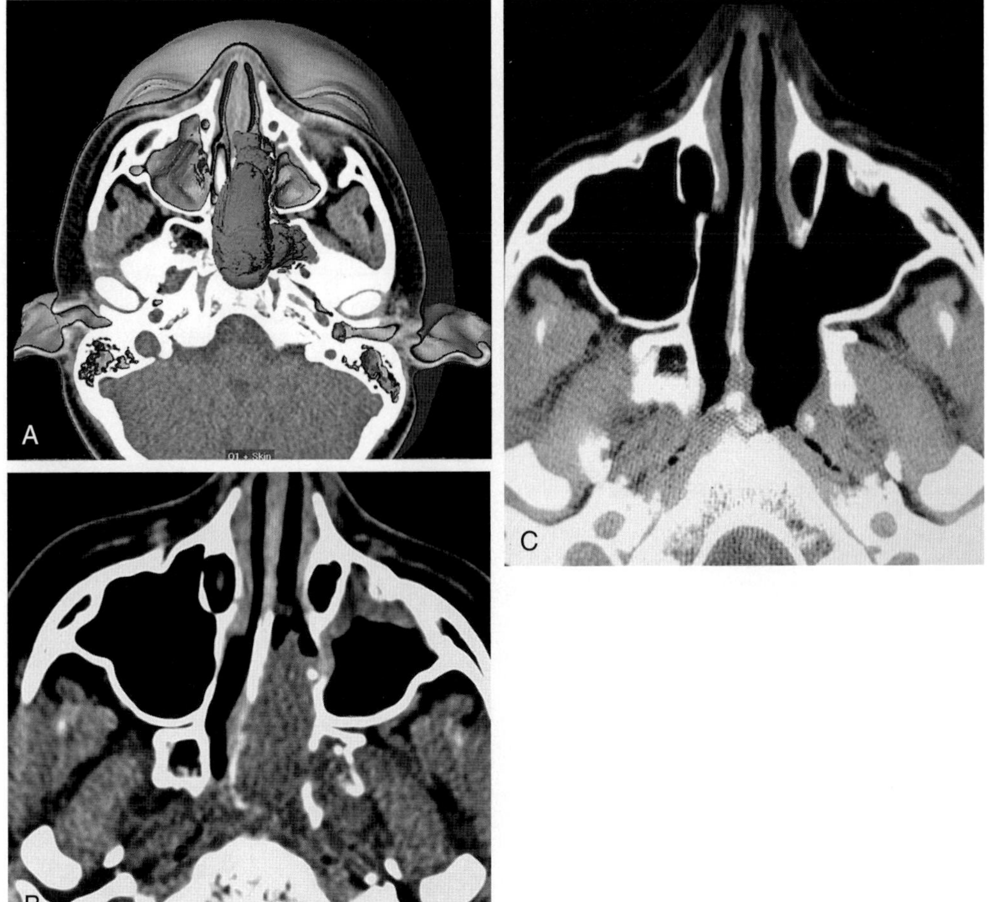

Figure 175-25. Angiofibroma in a 13-year-old boy. **A,** Axial three-dimensional computed tomography (CT) reconstruction. **B,** Preoperative axial CT scan. **C,** Postoperative axial CT scan.

of the posterior maxillary sinus wall. Sometimes it is necessary to remove the inferior turbinate, entirely resecting the medial wall of the maxillary sinus to obtain adequate exposure of the posterior and posterolateral portions of the wall of the sinus. During removal of the inferior turbinate, special care must be taken to avoid injuring the terminal branches of the maxillary artery at the sphenopalatine foramen and the second division of the trigeminal nerve.

The amount of posterior wall bone to be removed depends on the location and extent of the lesion as determined by preoperative image studies or by information from the image-guided system at the time of surgery. The posterior wall of the maxillary sinus can be opened by enlarging the sphenopalatine foramen with a micro-Kerrison punch and exposing the periosteum of the pterygopalatine, zygomatic, and infratemporal fossae. It is important to try to preserve the integrity of the periosteum and avoid fat protrusion into the operative field. If fat does protrude into the sinus, it is reduced by bipolar electrocoagulation, which also is used to control any bleeding. This technique is particularly useful in removing angiofibroma, when early identification of the feeding vessels is essential. Figure 175-25 illustrates removal of an angiofibroma using this technique.

The transpterygoid and infratemporal approaches are extensions of the transmaxillary access. In the transpterygoid approach, lateral extensions of the sphenoid sinus (pterygoid recess) and lesions involving the pterygopalatine fossa and zygomatic fossa can be accessed. This may require removal of the medial and sometimes lateral pterygoid processes in order to achieve access to the lateral and pterygoid regions of the sphenoid sinus. A wide sphenoidotomy is performed at the beginning or during the surgical operation. This access allows treatment of lesions involving the cavernous sinus that are lateral to the paraclival internal carotid artery.

The infratemporal access adds a medial endoscopic maxillectomy, including section of the nasolacrimal duct (a dacryocistorhinostomy is needed afterward). In this surgical access, we resect the posterior wall and sometimes the lateral wall of the maxillary sinus, particularly in situations with lateral expansion of the lesion.

Craniocervical Junction–Odontoid Approach

The most common indication for craniocervical junction–odontoid access is an extradural compressive lesion, the basilar invagination, which may be secondary to rheumatoid arthritis, exostosis, osteotoma, or other disorders (Fig. 175-26). Foramen magnum meningiomas, clivus chordomas with inferior extension, metastasis (especially in the odontoid process) also can be approached in this manner.

The procedure consists of the following sequence: general exposure, osseous exposure, removal of the lesion, and reconstruction. The otolaryngologic surgeon is responsible for the exposure of and access to the lesions. The surgery procedure usually is accomplished through both nostrils (four-hand technique), to permit use of multiple surgical instruments such as suction tubes, drills, and navigation system devices. The drill system must be thin, delicate, and long enough to allow its passage through the nose but without interfering with endoscopic vision. The image guide system is very helpful in these cases.

A panclival exposure creates a single cavity that extends from the sphenoid sinus to the level of the fossa of Rosenmüller. To expose the odontoid and the foramen magnum, additional soft tissue removal is required. The nasopharyngeal mucosa is cautherized with monopolar eletrocautery and then resected from the sphenoclival junction to the level of the soft palate. The longus capitis and longus colli muscles are exposed and partially resected to expose the ring of C1. Care should be taken to stay medial to the eustachian tube, especially during use of

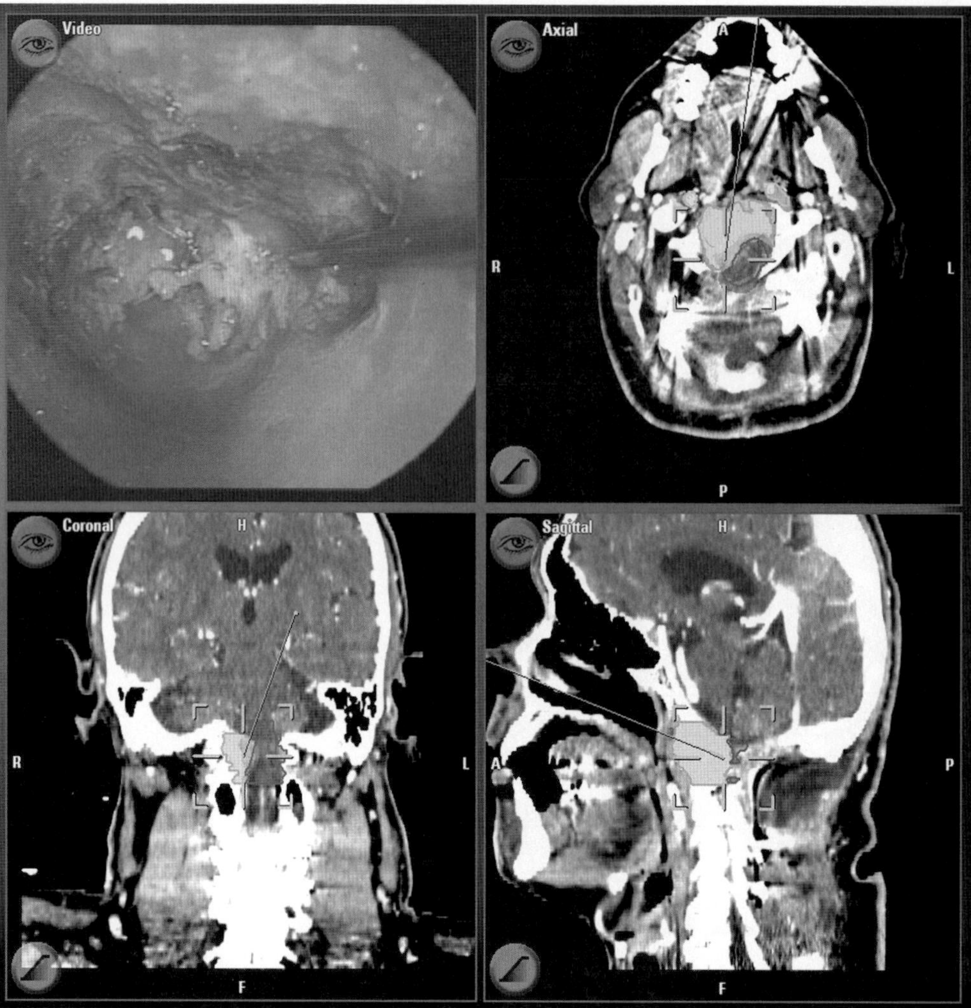

Figure 175-26. A surgical image-guided system was used to identify an osteoma located at the craniocervical junction.

electrocautery, because the parapharyngeal internal carotid artery is directly posterolateral to the eustachian tube. At the completion of the procedure, the nasopharyngeal tissues do not need reapproximation, and the surgical defect is covered with fibrin glue. The nasal passages are cleared of blood, and Silastic septal splints are inserted to minimize the risk of postoperative synechia formation.

Combined Approaches

Unfortunately, many lesions do not respect the anatomic boundaries for which the previously outlined approaches are ideal. In many instances, it is necessary to combine some of the previous approaches—for example, the transnasal direct with the transethmoidal or the transmaxillary with the transethmoidal.

Reconstruction

Reconstruction of the skull base after transnasal endoscopic surgery remains a major challenge, particularly when the dural defects are large and located at the posterior fossa.

The basic principle in sealing the dural defect is based on the use of several layers of tissue for the closure. We use fascia lata and free mucoperiosteum grafts from the floor of the nasal cavity or the middle or inferior turbinates. More recently we have used a septal flap pedicled at the region of the sphenopalatine foramen arteries. All of these layers are kept in position with fibrin glue.

If a large free space remains between the cerebral tissue and the dura, it is filled with fat (abdominal or from the thigh where the fascia was previously removed) before the first layer of fascia lata. The first layer of fascia lata is placed in a circumferential fashion, as an underlay graft between the dura and the nervous tissue. The second layer is then positioned between the dura and the bony skull base margins. The fascia lata can be substituted by artificial dura such as the collagen matrix graft (Duragen, Duraform). The third layer consists of vascularized mucoperiosteum-perichondrial flap pedicled at the region of the sphenopalatine foramen arteries. Fibrin glue is used to give support to these layers. When the septal flap is not large enough or is unavailable because of previous surgery, free mucosal grafts from the nasal floor, septum, and turbinates constitute an option. In this situation, they are ultimately covered by pieces of Gelfoam and supported by sponge packings (Merocel). When the dural defect is very large, gauze soaked in antibiotics is preferable to Merocel; over the gauze, a Foley catheter balloon is inflated to keep the tissues in position and to avoid displacement of the nasal packing into the nasopharynx. The balloon must be positioned under direct vision and inflated with no more than 10 mL of saline solution. It is left for approximately 5 days; the packing can remain for 10 to 14 days, depending on the extent of the reconstruction.

Postoperative Care

The goal of surgical treatment is to ensure the complete removal of the disease and the best possible functional result. A satisfactory postoperative result depends on both appropriate operative technique and meticulous postoperative care.

Wide-spectrum antibiotics are given during the operation and for 10 days postoperatively or until the nasal packing is removed. Adequate postoperative care of the operative site requires appropriate instrumentation, including 4-mm 0-degree, 45-degree, and 70-degree angled endoscopes, straight and curved atraumatic aspirators, and straight and curved microforceps.

For extended endoscopic skull base and brain surgery, the nasal cavity packing can remain in place as long as 2 weeks, depending on the type of procedure and dural reconstruction grade. The operative cavity is carefully suctioned, and any residual bone fragments are removed. The patient is instucted to peform frequent nasal irrigations with 0.9% or 3% saline solution. Nasal vasoconstriction with oxymetazoline is peformed by the patient until postoperative day 5. If the procedure includes repair of a dural defect, the patient is instructed to refrain from moderate or intense physical activity, straining, nose blowing, and sneezing for approximately 30 days. To prevent constipation, a high-fiber soft diet and laxatives are recommended.

The patient returns for postoperative visits every 2 weeks. At each visit, the operated nasal cavity is cleaned of crusts, granulation tissue, clots, and secretions. Imaging exams are performed when the cavity is well healed; the timing varies with the clinical course.

Complications

Every skull base surgical procedure has potential to cause complications. For example, a U.S. survey conducted in 1997 addressed complications of transsphenoidal surgery for pituitary gland lesions and documented carotid artery injury in 1.1% of cases, central nervous system injury in 1.3%, loss of vision in 1.8%, CSF fistula in 3.9%, and meningitis in 1.5%. The estimated mortality rate was 0.9%. These data were derived from several centers that used different transnasal approaches for only one surgical site but illustrate that serious complications do occur.[33] In the experience of Kassan and colleagues,[34] the incidence of neurovascular complications in 700 patients who underwent an expanded endonasal endoscopic approach was approximately 1.0%.

Prevention of the complications of transnasal endoscopic-assisted surgery of the skull base begins with an adequate preoperative evaluation of the patient, including history of the use of medications and previous operations. High-resolution CT in coronal and axial projections with sagittal reconstruction, MRI, and sometimes angiography are essential to plan the procedure and to execute it safely with the lowest possibility of complications.[35]

Complications can be classified by severity as minor or major and by time of appearance as immediate or delayed. Minor complications are associated with little morbidity and do not compromise the life of the patient, although they may be annoying and troublesome. Most resolve with time and conservative treatment. However, major complications are the cause of significant morbidity and increased risk of death. Most orbital complications stem from direct injury to the optic nerve or the extraocular muscles or from arterial or venous bleeding within the rigid bony orbit. These injuries can result in diplopia, hematoma, proptosis, and decreased visual acuity or blindness (which can be temporary or permanent). Blindness secondary to orbital hematoma can be reversible, mandating prompt hematoma evacuation to relieve the increased pressure compromising the blood supply to the retina or the optic nerve. Direct or indirect damage to the optic nerve usually occurs at the superolateral sphenoid sinus wall or in the posterior ethmoid cells.

Intracranial complications can result from direct injury to brain, cranial nerves, meninges, blood vessels, or venous sinuses. The resulting deficits reflect the loss of function of the damaged structures in the case of brain and cranial nerves, or the effects of loss of vascular supply to critical areas (stroke), or the mass effects of a resulting hematoma. Also, CSF leakage can cause symptoms directly, as well as predisposing the patient to the development of meningitis, and air entering the brain (pneumocephalus) can cause mass effect symptoms.

Bleeding is a risk in any surgical procedure, but seldom are so many important vessels susceptible to injury. The transnasal approaches outlined previously visualize and put at risk the anterior and posterior ethmoid arteries; the sphenopalatine and maxillary arteries and their branches; the internal carotid, anterior cerebral, basilar, and vertebral arteries and their branches; and the venous sinuses of the skull base: the cavernous sinus, basilar venous plexus, and the anterior intercavernous sinus.[36]

Immediate complications occur during surgery. The most frequent of these are CSF leakage, intraoperative bleeding, orbital hematoma, brain injury, and intrasellar complications, which can include injuries of the diaphragma sella, arachnoid membrane, pituitary stalk, intra-arachnoid vascular structures, and the hypothalamus, optic nerve, and chiasm and the vessels surrounding them. Injuries to cranial nerves III and VI are uncommon except in transsphenoidal-transclival approaches.

Delayed complications include progressive loss of vision or smell, meningitis, bleeding, synechia, and infection. The surgeon also must be aware of the possibility of transitory or permanent endocrinologic complications that can result from manipulation, compression, or traction of the pituitary stalk. The surgeon must be able to diagnose acute anterior pituitary insufficiency and be able to manage the condition or have available appropriate consultants who can do so.

Summary

Dramatic improvements in technology have made it possible to extend endoscopic surgical procedures well beyond the sinuses to all three cranial fossae, as well as to the orbit and pterygopalatine, zygomatic, and infratemporal fossae. Visualization is superior, morbidity is lower, and complications of endoscopic skull base and brain surgery, particularly vascular and neurologic lesions, CSF leak, and infection, are the same as after open procedures.

Despite all of the technologic and surgical advances, extensive dural defect repair remains a considerable challenge. Even with the dazzling technical advances, surgical success depends more on other factors: The surgeon must have a perfect knowledge of the involved anatomy, extensive endoscopic surgical training and experience, good surgical skills and judgment, and a highly skilled neurosurgical colleague. Only then can transnasal endoscopic-assisted surgery of the skull base reach its full potential.

SUGGESTED READINGS

Bouche J, Guiot G, Rougerie J, et al. [The trans-sphenoidal route in the surgical approach to chordoma of the clivus.] *Ann Otolaryngol Chir Cervicofac.* 1966;83:817.

Ciric I, Ragin A, Baumgartner C, et al. Complications of transsphenoidal surgery: results of a national survey, review of the literature, and personal experience. *Neurosurgery.* 1997;40:225.

Drake CG. The surgical treatment of vertebral-basilar aneurysms. *Clin Neurosurg.* 1969;16:114.

Ducasse A, DeLattre JF, Segal A, et al. Anatomical basis of the surgical approaches to the medial wall of the orbit. *Anat Clin.* 1985;7:15.

Fujii K, Chambers SM, Rhoton AL Jr. Neurovascular relationship of the sphenoid sinus. A microsurgical study. *J Neurosurg.* 1979;50:31.

Haddad G, Bassagasteguy L, Carrau RL, et al. A novel reconstructive technique following endoscopic expanded endonasal approaches vascular pedicle nasoseptal flap. *Laryngoscope.* 2006;116:1.

Harsh GR 4th, Joseph MP, Swearingen B, et al. Anterior midline approaches to the central skull base. *Clin Neurosurg.* 1996;43:15.

Hitotsumatsu T, Matsushima T, Rhoton AL. Surgical anatomy of the midface and the midline skull base. *Oper Tech Neurosurg.* 1999;2:160.

Janecka IP, Nuss DW, Sen CN. Facial translocation approach to the cranial base. *Acta Neurochir Suppl (Wien).* 1991;53:193.

Kassan AB, Snydermann CH, Carrau RL, et al. *The Expanded Endonasal Approach to the Ventral Skull Base: Sagittal Plane.* Tuttlingen, Germany: Endo-Press; 2007.

Kennedy DW, Keogh B, Senior B, Lanza D, et al. Endoscopic approach to tumors of the anterior skull base and orbit. *Oper Tech Otolaryngol Head Neck Surg.* 1996;7:257.

Lang J. *Clinical Anatomy of the Nose, Nasal Cavity and Paranasal Sinus.* New York: Thieme Medical Publishers; 1989.

Navarro JC. Surgical anatomy of the nose, paranasal sinuses, and pterygopalatine fossa. In: Stamm AC, Draf W, eds. *Micro-Endoscopic Surgery of the Paranasal Sinuses and the Skull Base.* Heidelberg: Springer; 2000.

Puxeddu R, Lui MWM, Chandrasekar K, et al. Endoscopic-assisted transcolumellar approach to the clivus: an anatomical study. *Laryngoscope.* 2002;112:1072.

Rabadan A, Conesa H. Transmaxillary-transnasal approach to the anterior clivus: a microsurgical anatomical model. *Neurosurgery.* 1992;30:473.

Sandor GK, Charles DA, Lawson VG, et al. Transoral approach to the nasopharynx and clivus using the Le Fort O osteotomy with midpalatal split. *Int J Oral Maxillofac Surg.* 1990;19:352.

Sano K, Jinbo M, Saito I. Vertebro-basilar aneurysms, with special reference to the transpharyngeal approach to basilar artery aneurysm. *No To Shinkei.* 1996;18:1197.

Sasaki CT, Lowlicht RA, Astrachan DI, et al. Le Fort I osteotomy approach to the skull base. *Laryngoscope.* 1990;100:1073.

Sethi DS, Pillay PK. Endoscopic management of lesions of the sella turcica. *J Laryngol Otol.* 1995;109:956.

Stamm AC. Transnasal endoscopic-assisted skull base surgery. *Ann Otol Rhinol Laryngol.* 2006;115(Suppl 196):45.

Stamm AC: Micro-endoscopic surgery of the paranasal sinuses. In: Stamm AC, Draf W, eds *Micro-Endoscopic Surgery of the Paranasal Sinuses and the Skull Base.* Heidelberg: Springer; 2000.

Stamm AC, Pignatari SNP. Transnasal endoscopic surgical approaches to the posterior fossa. In: Anand VK, Schwartz TH, eds. *Practical Endoscopic Skull Base Surgery.* San Diego: Plural Publishing; 2007.

Stamm AC, Pignatari SSN, Vellutini E. Transnasal endoscopic surgical approaches to the clivus. *Otolaryngol Clin North Am.* 2006;39:639.

Stamm AC, Pignatari SSN, Vellutini E, et al. A novel approach allowing binostril work to the sphenoid sinus. *Otolaryngol Head Neck Surg.* 2008;138:531.

Yasargil MG. *Anterior Approaches to the Clivus. Microsurgery Applied to Neurosurgery.* Stuttgart: Georg Thieme Verlag; 1969.

For complete list of references log onto www.expertconsult.com.

CHAPTER ONE HUNDRED AND SEVENTY-SIX

Temporal Bone Neoplasms and Lateral Cranial Base Surgery

Michael Marsh

Herman A. Jenkins

Key Points

- Patients with encasement of the internal carotid artery by tumor, contour irregularity on angiography, or anticipated internal carotid artery resection should undergo preoperative temporary balloon test occlusion (BTO) with neurologic monitoring with or without quantitative cerebral blood flow (CBF) assessment. When preoperative BTO reveals neurologic deficit or CBF is less than 30 mL/100 g per minute, definitive resection is not an option, unless extracranial-intracranial bypass can be accomplished beforehand. The decision regarding revascularization versus permanent balloon occlusion optimally is made preoperatively.
- The minimal procedure for treatment of carcinoma of the external auditory canal usually is a lateral temporal bone (LTB) resection. If radiation therapy is anticipated postoperatively, the cavity should be obliterated, in view of the high risk of osteoradionecrosis in irradiated open cavities.
- Carcinomas of the external auditory canal extending to the mesotympanum are optimally treated with a subtotal temporal bone resection and postoperative radiation therapy.
- High-grade malignancies of the temporal bone with extension outside the petrous bone to the petrous apex, extensive dural involvement, frank parenchymal involvement, gasserian ganglion involvement, or invasion along the skull base portend a poor outcome in nearly all cases. Palliation should be strongly considered.
- Aneurysms of the upper cervical and petrous internal carotid artery can be managed by endovascular stenting, balloon trapping, or surgical resection with or without revascularization or extracranial-intracranial bypass, as indicated by angiography and BTO assessment findings.
- Glomus tympanicum tumors whose borders are clearly seen through the tympanic membrane can be removed transtympanically; otherwise, an extended facial recess approach is indicated.
- Glomus jugulare tumors are best removed through a Fisch type A infratemporal approach. Staging may be necessary with significant intracranial extension. Preoperative embolization may greatly lessen intraoperative blood loss.
- Radiotherapy for glomus jugulare tumors may be indicated for recurrences or unresectable lesions, or in the presence of a medical contraindication to surgery.
- Jugular foramen schwannomas that are primarily intracranial are most easily approached suboccipitally. Jugular foramen schwannomas that are intraforaminal or combination tumors are removed in the safest manner using an infratemporal fossa approach with (Fisch type A) or without facial nerve transposition.
- The classic history of facial nerve schwannomas is one of a slowly progressive facial paralysis over months to years, not days to weeks, although sudden onset of paralysis, fluctuating paresis, and facial tic may occur. It is recommended to wait for facial function to deteriorate to House-Brackmann grade IV before surgical resection, because this may be the best expected outcome with facial nerve resection and reanastomosis.
- Drainage of cholesterol granulomas can be performed through the perilabyrinthine pathways or transsphenoidally using endoscopic image guidance techniques.
- Surgical management of a congenital cholesteatoma involving the petrous apex requires either complete removal of the cholesteatoma matrix or permanent exteriorization.
- Chordomas of the clivus can be resected using postauricular (Fisch type B) or preauricular lateral temporal bone techniques. Transnasal endoscopically assisted approaches also may result in complete extirpation, with greatly reduced morbidity compared with lateral skull base or facial translocation anterior techniques.

Lateral approaches to the skull base require numerous manipulations of intervening structures to gain access to the various regions of the skull in and around the posterior and middle cranial fossae. Advances in preoperative assessment, surgical techniques, and perioperative care have permitted removal of tumors previously regarded as unresectable. Concomitantly, the morbidity and mortality rates associated with these procedures have decreased significantly. A cohesive skull base team affords the patient the best possible preoperative assessment, planning, and surgical execution. The team requires the expertise of an otolaryngologist or neurotologist working with the neurosurgeon, neuroradiologist, interventional arteriographer, and anesthesiologist. The reconstructive surgeon may play a major role, especially if free flaps are required. This chapter reviews pertinent anatomy, various approaches to the lateral skull base, and selected pathologic entities.

Benign and malignant lesions (Box 176-1) involving the middle ear and temporal bone are located in one of the most inaccessible areas of the body. Although a variety of histologic types of tumor are found in these areas, each is uncommon, and clinical experience in their diagnosis and management is not easily acquired. Surgical approaches to the skull base are difficult, and the risks of neurologic deficit are significant. The major arteries and veins supplying the brain, intracranial structures, and all of the cranial nerves either exit through or are contiguous with the temporal bone. Modern surgical technique strongly stresses the minimization of cosmetic or neurologic loss in the management of benign and malignant lesions of the temporal bone. Through the years, collaborative approaches to the temporal bone have been developed for treatment of benign lesions and are being expanded to encompass malignant lesions as well. Nevertheless, considerable knowledge of temporal bone anatomy and adequate temporal bone-drilling laboratory experience are essential in adapting these approaches for each patient. Many histologic types are encountered only rarely, accounting for isolated case reports in the literature. Dividing tumors into benign and malignant categories, in combination with knowledge of the particular tumor biology and meticulous preoperative planning, greatly facilitates selection of the appropriate surgical approach and successful outcome.

Skull Base Anatomy

An overview of skull base anatomy may be found in Chapters 127 and 173. With lateral approaches to the skull base, anatomic structures are approached from a vantage point different from that presented in classic anatomic texts in terms of the course of dissection, in that such approaches are designed to enhance exposure while preserving neurovascular structures. The superior boundary of the infratemporal fossa as described by Grant[1] consists of the greater wing of the sphenoid the temporal fossa containing the temporalis muscle. The medial limit is

Box 176-1
Temporal Bone Neoplasms

Primary Benign Tumors
- Paraganglioma
- Neurofibroma/schwannoma
- Meningioma
- Adenomas
  - Ceruminous adenoma
  - Eccrine cylindroma
  - Pleomorphic adenoma
- Mesenchymal
  - Chondroma
  - Chondroblastoma
  - Chondromyxoid fibroma
  - Hemangiomas
  - Lipoma
  - Myxoma
  - Fibro-osseous tumors
    - Ossifying fibroma
    - Fibrous dysplasia
  - Giant cell granuloma
  - Aneurysmal bone cysts
  - Osteoblastoma
  - Osteoma/exostosis
  - Unicameral bone cyst
  - Teratoma
- Dysontogenic tissue
- Choristoma
- Glioma

Metastatic Tumors
- Prostate
- Breast
- Gastrointestinal
- Renal cell
- Lung
- Multiple myeloma
- Lymphoma
- Leukemia (chloroma)

Primary Malignant Tumors
- Epidermal carcinomas
  - Squamous cell carcinoma
  - Verrucous carcinoma
  - Basal cell carcinoma
  - Melanoma
- Adenocarcinomas
  - Ceruminous adenocarcinoma (low-grade and high-grade)
  - Adenoid cystic
  - Mucoepidermoid
  - Sebaceous cell
  - Papillary cystadenocarcinoma
- Mesenchymal
  - Rhabdomyosarcoma
  - Fibrosarcoma
  - Chondrosarcoma
  - Osteosarcoma
  - Liposarcoma
  - Dermatofibrosarcoma protuberans
  - Fibrohistiocytoma
  - Angiosarcoma
  - Osteoclastoma
  - Chordoma
- Plasmacytoma

Contiguous Tumor Invasion
- Neuronal structures
  - Meningioma
  - Gliomas
  - Neurofibroma/schwannoma
  - Choroid plexus papilloma
- Parotid gland neoplasm
- Pituitary tumors
- Craniopharyngioma
- Chordoma
- Scalp tumors
- Nasopharyngeal carcinoma

the lateral pterygoid plate, and the lateral limit is the mandibular ramus and condyle. The posterior wall of the maxillary sinus marks the anterior limit, and posteriorly and inferiorly, the infratemporal fossa opens into the parapharyngeal space, where fascial bands and ligaments subdivide the enclosed spaces.[2-4]

The facial nerve exits the stylomastoid foramen to enter the parotid gland and then emerges from the gland distally encased in the superficial muscular aponeurotic system fascia.[5] The glenoid fossa may limit superior exposure in lateral approaches.

As low-pressure, valveless channels, the venous system in the skull base is pivotal in lateral approaches. The torcular Herophili is the confluence of the transverse sinus (lateral sinus), superior longitudinal sinus, straight sinus, and occipital sinus. Bisaria[6] found that this confluence of sinuses was missing in 24.5% of 110 cadaver dissections. Ligation of the transverse sinus may lead to massive cerebral edema if the torcular Herophili is absent.[7] The vein of Labbé, or inferior anastomotic vein, connects the superficial middle cerebral vein with the transverse sinus, draining the superficial posterior temporal and inferior parietal lobes. It occurs on the right 66% of the time and on the left 77% of the time.[8] When present, it empties into the transverse sinus just proximal to the sigmoid sinus. Interruption of the vein of Labbé may lead to temporal lobe edema and infarction, unless good collateral drainage is present.[7,8] The superior petrosal sinus runs along the posterosuperior edge of the petrous bone from the cavernous sinus to the junction of transverse and sigmoid sinuses, receiving tributaries from the tympanic cavity and from the cerebellar and inferior cerebral veins.[9] The jugular bulb, averaging 15 mm in width, usually is separated from the tympanic cavity by bone but has been reported to be dehiscent in 6% of temporal bones.[10] The inferior petrosal sinus courses between the jugular bulb and cavernous sinus in the petro-occipital fissure, receiving tributaries from the internal auditory canal, pons, medulla, and inferior cerebellum.[9] The inferior petrosal sinus, occasionally the vein of the cochlear aqueduct, and the occipital sinus drain into the jugular bulb. Cranial nerves IX, X, and XI pass through the anterior medial portion of the jugular foramen and may be compressed during maneuvers to obtain hemostasis of the inferior petrosal sinus.[11]

The internal carotid artery ascends deep to the digastric and styloid muscles to enter the carotid siphon medial to the styloid process, ascending through vertical and horizontal segments. In the vertical segment near the genu, the artery is just deep to the eustachian tube orifice, posteromedial to the glenoid fossa. The osseous eustachian tube orifice is separated from the internal carotid by, on average, 1.5 mm of bone and may have dehiscences.[12,13] The midportion of the vertical arterial segment is anteromedial to the basal turn of the cochlea. The distance to the cochlea averages approximately 1.34 mm.[14] The average length of the vertical segment is approximately 10 mm (range, 5 to 15 mm).[12,15] The horizontal segment travels obliquely in a lateral to medial direction from the genu to the intracranial entry of this vessel at the superior aspect of the foramen lacerum. Its average length is 20 mm (range, 14.5 to 26 mm).[12,15] Relevant lymphatic anatomy includes the preauricular and parotid lymphatics that drain the external ear, with more medial aspects of the external auditory canal draining into deep jugular and postauricular nodes. The mucosa of the middle ear and mastoid drains into channels surrounding the eustachian tube, which then drains into the deep superior jugular and retropharyngeal nodes.[16]

Evaluation of Skull Base Lesions

Accurate diagnosis and evaluation of tumor extent of the middle ear space and temporal bone require appropriate physical examination and audiologic, vestibular, and radiologic assessment. Tumors of the middle ear space frequently can be seen on physical examination. The combination of the frequency of certain lesions and their classic presentations often suggest the tumor type. Tumors of the lateral skull base often manifest with cranial nerve deficits, including hearing loss, pulsatile tinnitus, and eustachian tube dysfunction. A thorough history and physical examination with special attention to the cranial nerves should be undertaken. Audiometry is useful in surgical planning, particularly when removal of the labyrinth will be necessary. Radiographic evaluation provides information regarding location, extensions, surrounding structural relationships, and probable histologic findings.[17-25]

Computed Tomography and Magnetic Resonance Imaging

Preoperative computed tomography (CT) and magnetic resonance imaging (MRI) are indispensable to modern skull base surgery (see Chapter 135). Hirsch and Curtin[26] noted that MRI and CT are "complementary and not competitive in the initial evaluation of skull base lesions." Modern CT affords exquisite bony detail and fairly good soft tissue information. The strength of CT lies in delineating the effect of the tumor on the bone of the skull base. Soft tissue–soft tissue discrimination is still limited because of the narrow range of electron densities in soft tissues of interest. More soft tissue discrimination is available with CT if iodinated contrast material is administered intravenously. The advent of MRI with its superb soft tissue sensitivity has resulted in fewer indications for use of iodinated contrast CT techniques. Although MRI is able to evaluate alterations in bony structure, it does so only indirectly, because cortical bone has few mobile water protons and hence nearly no intrinsic signal. For this reason, MRI is inferior to CT in the evaluation of subtle bony changes. Such features are important findings in temporal bone masses. The fine soft tissue discrimination of MRI is improved by the intravenous infusion of the MRI contrast medium gadolinium. Another advantage of MRI is its ability to display numerous imaging planes without repositioning the patient, which makes it easier to acquire coronal, sagittal, and even off-axis oblique images. For these reasons, MRI is superior to CT in defining brain or meningeal effects from temporal bone lesions. Because of potentially dangerous magnetic effects, MRI cannot be used in patients with certain cardiac pacemakers or valves, ferromagnetic cerebral aneurysm clips, some vena cava filters, and ferromagnetic intraocular foreign bodies.

The usual evaluation of a potential temporal bone mass begins with noncontrast temporal bone CT. This study will immediately show large lesions and usually suggests the presence of smaller lesions. Even though results of temporal bone CT may be negative, follow-up MRI may be indicated if clinical findings strongly suggest a mass. Like CT, MRI is focused to the region of interest instead of just providing thick-slice imaging of the entire head. Temporal bone MRI almost always is performed without and with gadolinium. Many practitioners choose to bypass CT if they believe the disease is retrocochlear. CT then can be added after the MRI study if precise bone detail is required.

Both CT and MRI are computerized imaging techniques. For this reason, either can be reformatted in any desired digital display. A popular type of reformatted display is a three-dimensional image. Three-dimensional displays may assist the surgeon by making it easier to understand the extent of the lesion, but they almost never provide diagnostic information that was not available on the standard axial or coronal slices. Moreover, three-dimensional displays are heavily post-processed. Significant image information can be lost in such processing. At present, three-dimensional images are used almost exclusively as supplemental displays, as dictated by the preference of the practitioner.

Preoperative Carotid Artery Assessment

In extirpation of skull base tumors, appropriate management of the internal carotid artery remains paramount (Fig. 176-1). The morbidity associated with carotid artery occlusion is well known. The first documented carotid ligation, for a sword injury, performed in 1585 by Paré, resulted in stroke.[27] Literature review reveals that unselected abrupt sacrifice of this vessel resulted in 26% (65 of 254) cerebral infarctions, with a 46% fatality rate (30 of 65).[28] Gradual occlusion, as with a Silverstone clamp, does not seem to alter morbidity. Berenstein and associates[29] noted that a significant reduction of blood flow or pressure does not occur until a cross-sectional area less than 2 mm^2 is attained, regardless of the diameter of the vessel. Late-onset complications from cervical internal carotid artery ligation may result after several hours, as a result of stasis with distal thrombosis and embolic phenomena.

Four-Vessel Arteriography

All patients considered for extensive lateral skull base surgery should undergo a four-vessel carotid angiogram with venous phase (see

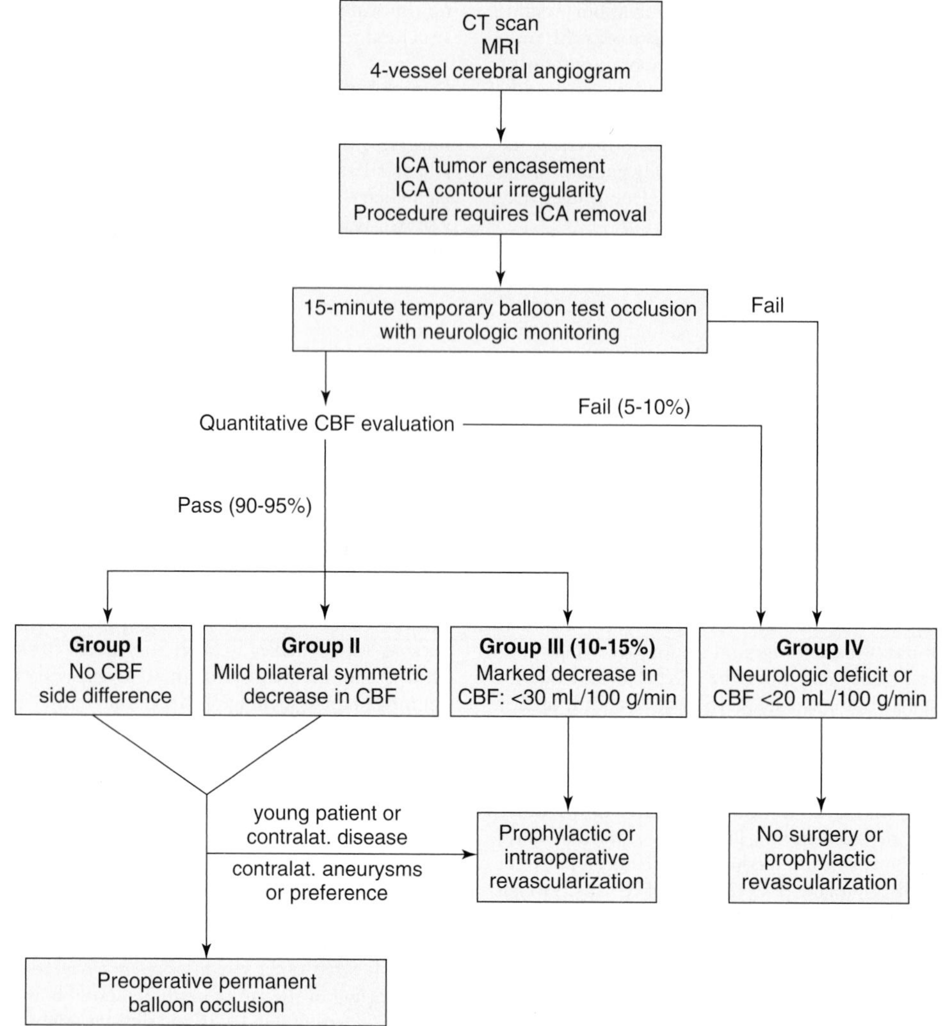

Figure 176-1. Algorithm for preoperative internal carotid artery (ICA)/cerebral blood flow (CBF) evaluation. CT, computed tomography; MRI, magnetic resonance imaging.

Chapters 135 and 136). Angiography is only qualitative but may provide critical information (Fig. 176-2).

According to Fisch and colleagues, angiographic evidence of ICA contour irregularity or stenosis at the level of lesion should prompt consideration of elective preoperative ipsilateral carotid balloon occlusion.[30] Intraoperative carotid occlusion is associated with a higher rate of permanent neurologic sequelae.

The venous phase provides critical information regarding collateral venous drainage, should ligation of the transverse sinus or the vein of Labbé be required.

Cerebral Blood Flow Assessment

Some understanding of cerebral blood flow (CBF) is essential to carotid artery management. Normal CBF approximates 50 mL/100 g per minute.[31] In alert humans, CBF less than 20 mL/100 g per minute produces failure of brain function, resulting in at least temporary hemiparesis or hemiplegia.[32] At this point, electroencephalography (EEG) usually reveals changes reflecting synaptic transmission failure.[31] As CBF decreases below 15 mL/100 g per minute, electrical activity is lost.[33] Jones and coworkers[34] found that long-lasting ischemia in monkeys from local CBF less than 17 to 18 mL/100 g per minute resulted in infarction. The time course of irreversible neuronal damage at various CBF levels in humans is unknown.

Functional assessment of CBF is required in the following clinical circumstances:

1. En bloc resection of a malignant tumor necessitating resection of the internal carotid artery
2. Tumor encasement of the internal carotid artery as seen on MRI or CT
3. Angiographic contour irregularity or stenosis at the level of the tumor

Qualitative Cerebral Blood Flow Evaluation

Various methods have been proposed to assess functional collateral circulation in the circle of Willis. Simplest is the Matas test, in which the ipsilateral carotid artery is compressed against a vertebral transverse process while the examiner observes for deterioration of neurologic function.[35] Cross-compression carotid arteriography will give a qualitative feel for ipsilateral CBF.[36] Direct intraoperative carotid stump pressures can estimate collateral circulation. A back-pressure of 50 mm Hg has been considered to be indicative of adequate CBF,[37] but stump pressures have been shown to be unreliable.[38,39] Ocular plethysmography and transcranial Doppler velocitometry of the middle cerebral artery[40] have similar theoretic limitations. In a series of patients undergoing carotid surgery, intraoperative EEG revealed no change in 18% to 56% of those with CBF levels less than 20 to 24 mL/100 g per minute, depending on the anesthetic used.[41] EEG, therefore, may be too insensitive for detection of CBF abnormality in patients who experience prolonged occlusions of the internal carotid artery.

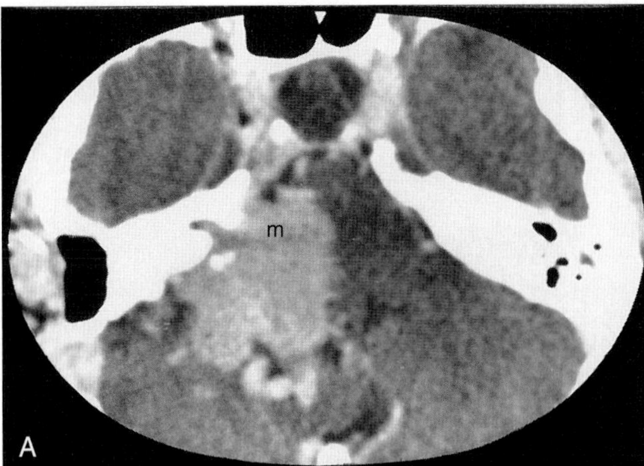

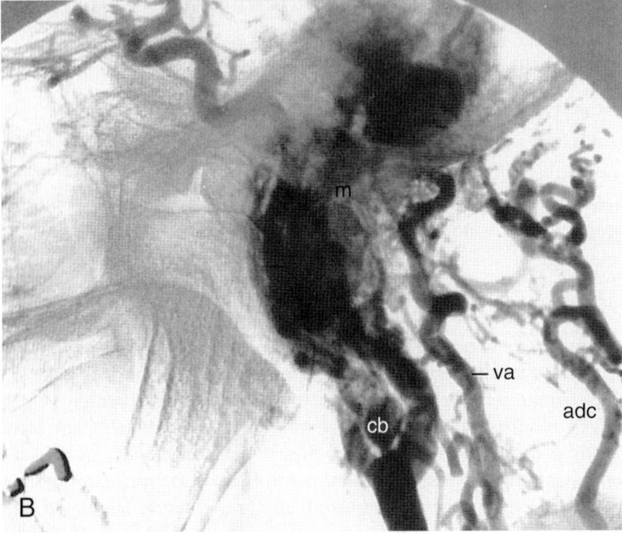

Figure 176-2. Two right-sided paragangliomas in a 61-year-old woman. **A,** Axial view, computed tomography after administration of intravenous contrast. A dense, pathologically contrast-enhancing mass (m) with tortuous dilated vessels is demonstrated. This lesion has ascended from the glomus jugulare up into the cerebellopontine angle cistern. It covers the internal auditory canal. **B,** Innominate artery angiogram, lateral subtraction view centered at the craniocervical junction. The wildly hypervascular nature of the paraganglioma is demonstrated. The tumor has parasitized the vertebral artery (va) and is ascending the deep cervical arteries (adc). These vessels have dilated and become tortuous because of the increased flow demanded from them. Besides the large glomus jugulare paraganglioma (m), the patient has a small carotid body paraganglioma (cb).

Generally accepted evaluations of CBF all involve the interventional radiologic technique of balloon test occlusion (BTO). The assessment of CBF will be either qualitative or quantitative with BTO with neurologic monitoring. Fisch uses qualitative BTO as the sole method to assess collateral CBF, with the neuroradiologist making an experienced, qualitative judgment regarding which patients should undergo permanent occlusion.[30] The collateral circulation may be stressed during BTO with pharmacologically induced hypotension or acetazolamide. Other qualitative techniques for CBF evaluation, such as single photon emission computed tomography (SPECT) and magnetoencephalography, attempt to "quantify" CBF.[42-45]

Quantitative Cerebral Blood Flow Evaluation

The impetus for quantitative evaluation of CBF is to identify the 10% to 25% subset of patients who "pass" BTO (as described next under "Carotid Management Algorithms") but are still at moderate to high risk of irreversible neurologic damage in the event of internal carotid artery occlusion. Quantitative methods of CBF evaluation during BTO include (1) positron emission tomography (PET), (2) MRI techniques, (3) cerebral perfusion CT, and (4) xenon CT or xenon 133 nuclear studies.

PET has the advantage of measuring CBF and metabolic parameters simultaneously.[46] Of the tests mentioned, PET provides the most accurate knowledge regarding cerebral hemodynamics, although it requires expensive infrastructure, is not widely available, and is time consuming.

New advances show that functional MRI (fMRI) has the potential to supplant xenon flow studies.[47-51] Such MRI studies have been used to evaluate CBF preoperatively and postoperatively for extracranial-intracranial bypass procedures.[52] The potential advantage of fMRI lies in that it requires only software upgrades to current MRI scanners. Disadvantages include the need for transport away from the vascular suite and for special equipment tolerant of the highly magnetic field.

Cerebral perfusion CT with or without acetazolamide challenge can be performed quickly on any standard helical (spiral) CT scanner with perfusion maps generated by software.[53,54] Further studies are needed to validate perfusion CT as a quantitative technique comparable to xenon CT.

Xenon 133 scintillation shows excellent correlation with quantitative assessments of CBF in a defined region with a scintillation counter on the scalp[41] and also may be used intraoperatively.

Xenon CT blood flow mapping is the best studied clinical, quantitative measure of CBF.[28,42,55-58] Inhaled xenon acts as a contrast agent, whose uptake and diffusion from cerebral tissue is proportional to blood flow. CBF distribution is estimated with specialized computer software before and after BTO of the internal carotid artery during serial CT scans and from which a blood flow map is calculated. An algorithm for carotid artery management has been proposed on the basis of preoperative xenon CT blood flow mapping with temporary carotid balloon occlusion (see Fig. 176-1). Group 3 patients (see Fig. 176-1), although "passing" BTO, have CBF values between 20 and 30 mL/100 g per minute and are thought to be in hemodynamic decompensation without neurologic deficit but entirely dependent on systemic blood pressure.[56] As is well recognized, intraoperative or postoperative blood pressure fluctuations after ICA occlusion may send these patients over the precipice. It is estimated that 90% of group 3 patients will have a major stroke after permanent occlusion of the internal carotid artery.[59]

Carotid Management Algorithms

A decision regarding management of the internal carotid artery is best made preoperatively. Intraoperative carotid occlusion usually is performed to control massive bleeding under suboptimal circumstances, resulting in a higher neurologic complication rate. Intraoperative balloon occlusion or intra-arterial shunt placement may be required if the carotid is lacerated and control is difficult.[60-62]

After preoperative functional evaluation of the internal carotid artery, either qualitative or quantitative, decisions about management of the carotid are dependent on the following factors:

- Results of the functional evaluation
- Young age
- Contralateral skull base tumor or vascular disease

Vein graft reconstruction, instead of sacrifice of the artery, may be a consideration regardless of the BTO result, especially in young patients and in cases in which contralateral involvement is a possibility, to restore physiologic circulation and reduce risk of late intracranial aneurysms.[33,42] The rationale for preservation of an ICA encased by benign tumor when this is possible, or revascularization when preservation is not possible, is valid.[63]

Opinion differs further regarding algorithms for management of the internal carotid artery based on functional evaluations, just as opinion differs regarding what constitutes an adequate evaluation in the first place. The results of temporary BTO can be classified as either "pass" or "fail," as follows:

Pass: no neurologic deficit and CBF greater than 30 mL/100 g per minute (if quantitative evaluation has been performed)

Fail: neurologic deficit or CBF less than 30 mL/100 g per minute (if quantitative evaluation has been performed), or both

For patients with BTO results in the "fail" category, definitive resection may not be possible; alternatively, extracranial-intracranial bypass antecedent to the resection procedure should be considered.[42,64-66]

Patients who "pass" are further subclassified depending on whether qualitative or quantitative testing has been done. Fisch[30] using qualitative BTO, recommends permanent occlusion of the internal carotid artery preoperatively if the neuroradiologist confirms adequate cross-circulation and no neurologic deterioration occurs during the test. In a series reported by Zane and colleagues, only 5% (2 of 46 patients, 1 preoperatively and 1 postoperatively) had permanent neurologic sequelae after occlusion when this algorithm was used.[30] If quantitative testing has been performed, transarterial permanent balloon occlusion may be considered for operative candidates in groups 1 and 2 (CBF greater than 30 mL/100 g per minute) (see Fig. 176-1) for the same indications as those that occasioned functional CBF testing. If the decision for occlusion of the internal carotid artery is reached preoperatively, permanent balloon occlusion should be performed 1 to 4 weeks before the resection to lessen thromboembolic sequelae. Placement proximally at the level of the carotid bifurcation and distally just before the ophthalmic artery minimizes late thromboembolic sequelae.[67] The long-term sequelae of carotid occlusion are unknown, although xenon CT blood flow mapping after BTO correlates well with medium-term neurologic outcome.[28] Direct vein graft reconstruction is indicated to allow complete tumor resection (see Fig. 176-1) in patients assigned to group 3 by quantitative CBF assessment (CBF less than 30 mL/100 g per minute), those with bilateral lesions, and young patients with benign tumors, according to Sen and Sekhar.[64] Intraoperative revascularization is associated with increased operative time, graft occlusion, need for transfusion, and potential for postoperative blowout.[30] Risk of graft occlusion is especially high among patients with long grafts.

Disregarding the surgeon's preference for revascularization or permanent balloon occlusion, the decision optimally is made under controlled circumstances preoperatively.

Surgical Approaches

Although the biologic behavior of tumors involving the skull base may vary, certain general principles should be followed in their extirpation. It is essential, if possible, to determine preoperatively whether the lesion is benign or malignant. Small, benign lesions in the middle ear space whose borders are clearly visible through the tympanic membrane can be removed through the external auditory canal. When removing the tumor, the surgeon should clearly differentiate it from vascular anomaly, because injury to the internal carotid artery in its intratemporal portion is hazardous and may require ligation of the artery for control of bleeding. Benign tumors limited to the mesotympanum whose borders are not visible through the tympanic membrane may be approached through a combined transcanal and facial recess or through an extended facial recess approach. Occasionally, the facial recess is narrow, necessitating removal of all or part of the bony posterior wall of the external auditory canal. Basic surgical approaches to the mastoid and mesotympanum are described in Chapters 127 and 142. Malignancies are best removed en bloc, whereas benign lesions may be extirpated piecemeal, although depending on biology, resection may require establishing a cuff of normal tissue. Surgical approaches to lesions deeper within the temporal bone should be chosen either to provide adequate exposure for complete excision or to allow easy access to an exteriorized cavity, to preserve useful residual hearing if possible, to preserve facial nerve and other cranial nerve functions when possible, to avoid injury to the brainstem and internal carotid artery, and to provide for wound closure without cerebrospinal fluid (CSF) leak.

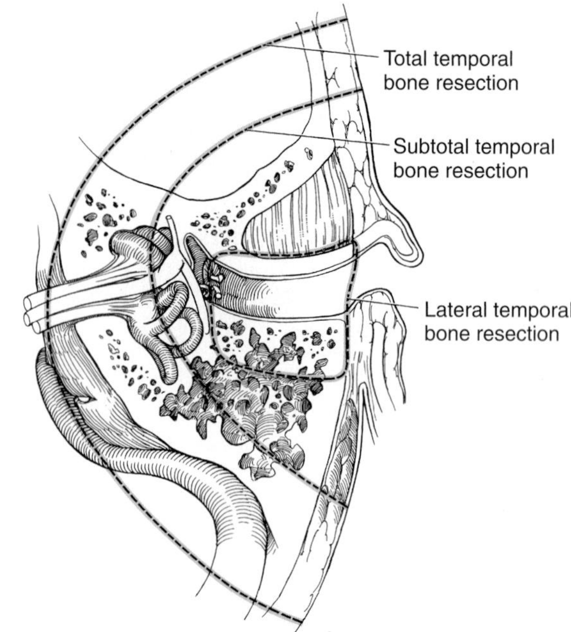

Figure 176-3. Margins of resection for lateral temporal bone, subtotal temporal bone, and total temporal bone resections.

The operative approach and intraoperative technique should maximize safe exposure and minimize morbidity. Surgeons should be well versed in all methods of exposure for various regions of the skull base. Circumferential exposure of tumor margins for benign tumors and en bloc technique for malignant lesions, minimization of blood loss by preoperative selective embolization and intraoperative selective vessel ligation, proximal and distal control of the internal carotid artery around the tumor, and preservation of cranial nerves facilitated with intraoperative monitoring by electromyography (EMG) (see Chapter 178) whenever necessary are essential to a successful outcome.

Sleeve Resection of External Auditory Canal

A sleeve resection of the external auditory canal removes the cartilaginous portion and some or all of the bony canal wall skin circumferentially without bone removal. Split-thickness skin grafts are used in the conchal bowl and external auditory canal. Some surgeons include the tympanic membrane as a medial margin to a sleeve resection, although this type of procedure generally is reserved for malignancies localized to the cartilaginous portion of the canal. Malignancies localized to or involving the osseous portion require at least a lateral temporal bone resection.

Lateral (Partial) Temporal Bone Resection

A lateral temporal bone resection[68-71] removes en bloc the entire osseous and cartilaginous portions of the external auditory canal and tympanic membrane using the extended facial recess approach (Fig. 176-3). This procedure is indicated for patients with malignant neoplasms localized to the osseous canal with no encroachment on the medial mesotympanum. Parotidectomy, neck dissection, and mandibular condylectomy are performed as adjunctive surgical procedures if indicated by preoperative radiologic or intraoperative findings. Intraoperative facial nerve monitoring is useful in this procedure.

Incisions

A soft tissue cylinder is designed to include the tragus and conchal bowl. The incision is taken vertically downward, posterior and superior to the temporal bone. The external auditory canal is sutured shut. A postauricular incision is created approximately a fingerbreadth behind the postauricular sulcus (Fig. 176-4A). It may be extended inferiorly into a neck crease for parotidectomy as required. Retractors then are placed.

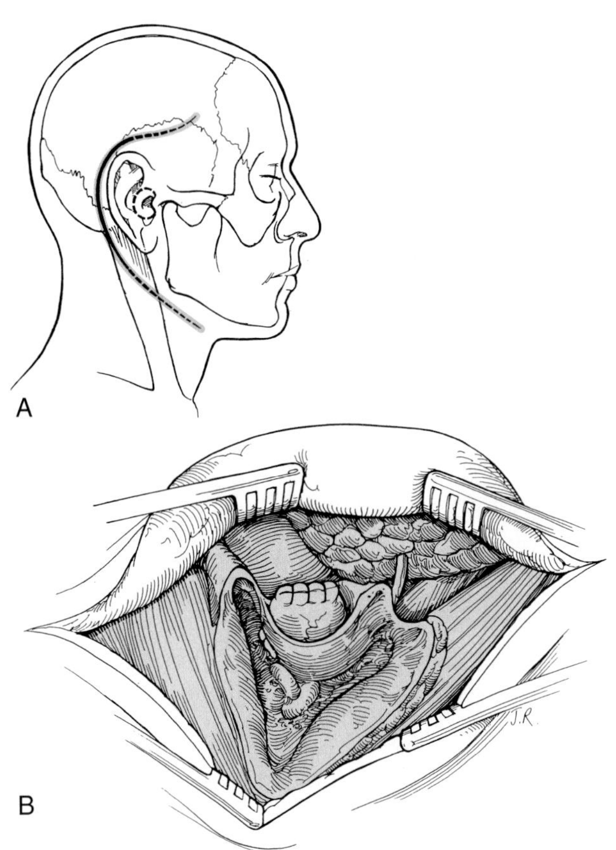

Figure 176-4. Lateral temporal bone resection: incision and initial exposure. **A,** Incisions include a central external auditory canal core, which is sutured closed. Extend incision as needed for neck dissection or temporal muscle rotation flap. Note that the tragus can be preserved for better cosmesis. **B,** Canal closure, mastoidectomy, and epitympanic dissection have been completed.

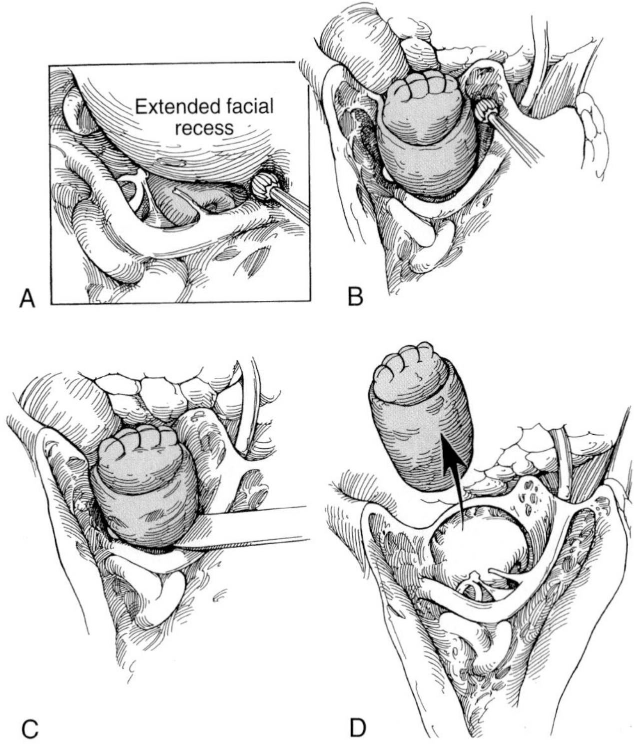

Figure 176-5. Lateral temporal bone resection: specimen delivery. **A,** Extended facial recess dissection. **B,** Hypotympanic dissection. **C,** Specimen fractured with osteotome. **D,** Specimen separated from soft tissue.

A modified neck dissection, total parotidectomy, and partial mandibulectomy may be performed if indicated by perioperative radiologic studies or intraoperative findings.

Mastoidectomy and Facial Recess Approach

A complete mastoidectomy is performed. The superior mastoid dissection is carried to the root of the zygoma, with care taken not to penetrate the osseous portion of the external auditory canal or the tegmen. Epitympanic dissection in an anterior direction should extend into the temporomandibular joint, as depicted in Figure 176-4B. An extended facial recess approach is then performed by "eggshelling" the vertical segment of the facial nerve from the second genu to the stylomastoid foramen (Fig. 176-5A). The incudostapedial joint is separated, and the pillar of bone between the facial recess approach and the fossa incudis also is removed. The tensor tympani tendon is cut with Bellucci scissors. Hypotympanic dissection is performed by extending the facial recess approach through the chorda tympani nerve. Drilling with either a diamond or cutting burr is continued along the inferior aspect of the hypotympanum medial to the annulus and lateral to the jugular bulb and carotid canal until soft tissue is reached, with care taken not to injure the intraparotid facial nerve (see Fig. 176-5B).

Removal of Specimen

Continuity between the hypotympanic dissection and the anterior epitympanic dissection is established by drilling along the anterior mesotympanum into the temporomandibular joint or by fracturing with a curved osteotome (see Fig. 176-5C). Either cautery or sharp dissection is used to separate the bony anterior canal wall from soft tissue of the temporomandibular joint and the superficial lobe of the parotid. The specimen then is sent en bloc for histopathological examination (see Fig. 176-5D).

Closure

If ancillary procedures such as parotidectomy or mandibular resection are not performed and if postoperative radiotherapy is not anticipated, creation of a large mastoid cavity is acceptable. The eustachian tube orifice should be obliterated with temporalis fascia as in a radical mastoidectomy. The mesotympanum and facial ridge may be covered with temporalis fascia graft to facilitate healing. Further conchal bowl cartilage may need to be removed to create a large meatoplasty. A split-thickness skin graft is then sutured to the edges of the conchal bowl and anterior facial skin or tragal skin and allowed to drape into the mastoid cavity and anterior cavity soft tissue. The skin graft then can be tacked into place with absorbable sutures along the soft tissue areas. Use of a graft will minimize postoperative meatal stenosis.[72] Absorbable gelatin then can be placed on the medial aspect of the mastoid cavity, followed by packing with gauze strips.

If postoperative irradiation is anticipated, the mastoid cavity should be obliterated to avoid osteoradionecrosis.[73] This may be achieved with use of abdominal fat and rotation of a temporalis graft to cover the defect. Alternately, a superiorly based sternocleidomastoid muscle flap based on the occipital artery may be rotated by incising the sternocleidomastoid muscle at the clavicle. A skin graft then is sutured to the conchal bowl margins and tacked down to underlying muscle.

Subtotal Temporal Bone and Total Temporal Bone Resections

A subtotal temporal bone resection[70,74-84] essentially allows en bloc resection of the medial surfaces of the mesotympanum, leaving the air cells of the petrous apex and portions of the bony labyrinth (see Fig. 176-3). This type of resection is indicated for patients with malignancies involving the middle ear.

A total temporal bone resection involves an en bloc resection of the temporal bone, including the petrous apex and the sigmoid sinus

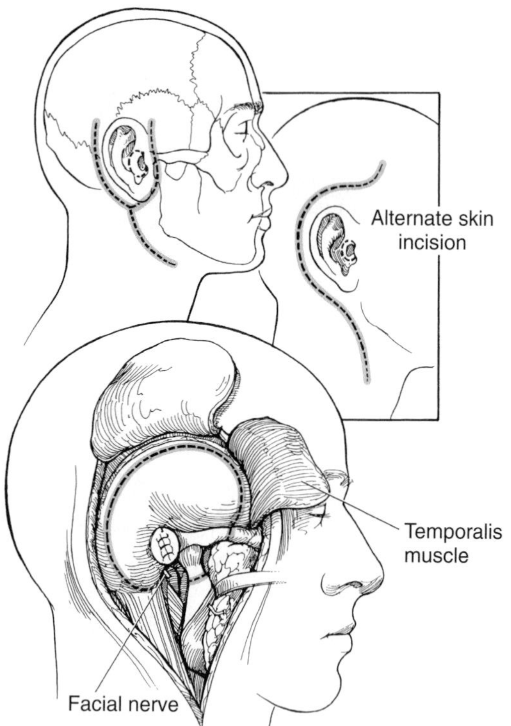

Figure 176-6. Subtotal temporal bone resection. Incisions include a central external auditory canal core, which is sutured closed. Note the tragus can be preserved for better cosmesis. Temporal craniotomy for subtotal temporal bone resection is smaller than for a total temporal bone resection. Parotid gland with main trunk of facial nerve has been elevated from masseter muscle.

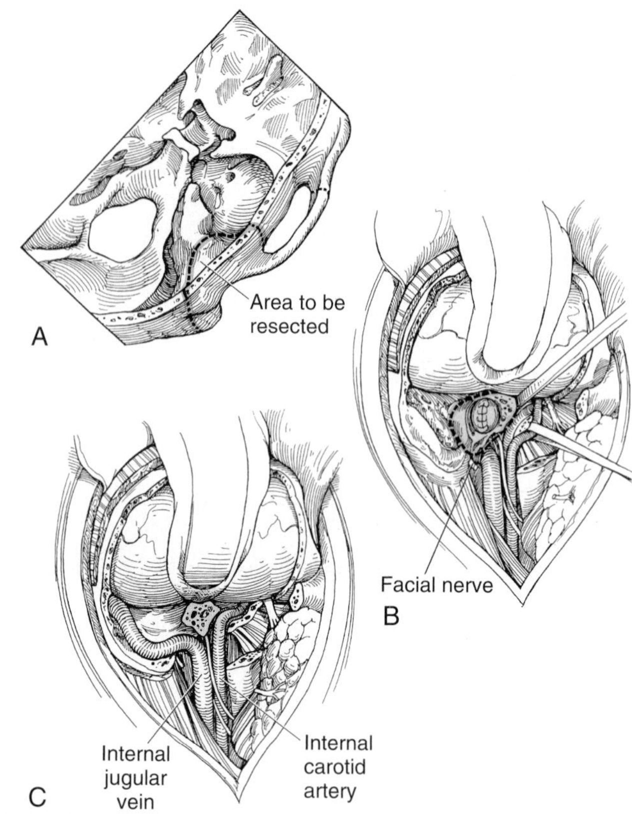

Figure 176-7. Subtotal temporal bone resection. **A,** Bird's-eye view of proposed resection. Note the facial nerve can be exposed for clean sectioning in the labyrinthine segment. **B,** Osteotome at carotid canal first genu directed at internal auditory canal fundus. **C,** Specimen removed showing remaining petrous apex and otic capsule. Roman numerals denote cranial nerves.

(see Fig. 176-3). The petrous internal carotid artery may be included in this resection. Total temporal bone resection is of questionable added benefit if a high-grade tumor involves the petrous apex or internal carotid artery or extends outside of the petrous bone intradurally or toward the cavernous sinus. Total resection may be indicated for low-grade malignancies.[83]

Incision

A large C-shaped postauricular incision or Y-shaped incision can be designed with a central island removed (Fig. 176-6). Alternately, a preauricular incision may be used for cases with involvement of the external auditory canal. In performing the incision, care should be taken to preserve the greater auricular nerve, because this nerve may be used for facial nerve interposition grafting. Also, care should be taken in elevating the flap off the zygoma, so as to not injure the peripheral frontal branch of the facial nerve.

Facial Nerve Management

With parotid involvement or involvement of the facial nerve, the distal branches or main trunks of the facial nerve may be identified and transected and marked for future interposition grafting. If no such involvement is present, the facial nerve is identified at the stylomastoid foramen and transected. The parotid is carefully dissected off the masseter. Proximal facial nerve management is considered later.

Proximal Vascular Control, Neck Dissection

If preoperative imaging indicates lymphadenopathy, a supraomohyoid modified neck dissection can be performed. Regardless of lymph node involvement, proximal vascular control of the carotid artery and internal jugular vein can be obtained, and vascular loops are placed around these vessels. The lower cranial nerve, internal carotid artery, and internal jugular vein can be followed superiorly. The sternocleidomastoid muscle is separated from the mastoid tip, as is the digastric muscle.

Infratemporal Fossa Dissection

The masseter attachment to the zygoma is detached. A mandibular osteotomy is performed from the mandibular notch to the angle of the mandible. The mandibular condyle is separated from the glenoid fossa, detaching the lateral and medial pterygoid musculature, with care taken not to injure the internal maxillary artery. Should the internal maxillary artery be injured, brisk back-bleeding would indicate good blood flow from the pterygoid plexus, presaging a viable temporalis muscle useful for reconstruction. The temporalis muscle is elevated off the skull in a subperiosteal fashion and reflected inferiorly, still attached to the coronoid process. A superior infratemporal fossa dissection should allow identification of the foramen spinosum and foramen ovale.

Temporal Craniotomy

A temporal craniotomy is performed to allow exposure of the superior surface of the petrous bone. A larger craniotomy is performed for a total temporal bone resection. The dura is elevated off the petrous bone, proceeding from posterior to anterior.

Subtotal Temporal Bone Resection

The vertical petrous portion of the internal carotid artery is identified (Fig. 176-7). This resection is performed by drilling with diamond burrs through the glenoid fossa and across the eustachian tube orifice. Mobilization of the carotid is just distal to the first genu. The distal eustachian tube orifice should be either sutured or closed with autologous tissue.

Delineation of the Sigmoid Sinus and Jugular Bulb

Presumably, if a subtotal temporal bone resection has been selected, the mastoid air system is not involved in patients with carcinoma. A mastoidectomy is performed, removing the mastoid cortex with cutting burrs. The sigmoid sinus and jugular bulb are carefully delineated with diamond burrs, and the jugular bulb is carefully dissected from the temporal bone, with recognition that the inferior petrosal veins enter it inferomedially. The sigmoid sinus may require ligation or extradural packing for vascular control later in the procedure.

Proximal Facial Nerve Management

Although an osteotomy may be performed at this point, with sectioning of the proximal facial nerve during an often bloody dissection, it probably would cause further stretch injury to the facial nerve. If grafting of the facial nerve is desired, further stretch injury is best avoided. The facial nerve may be delineated from the labyrinthine segment to the internal auditory canal as with routine middle cranial fossa nerve decompression or may be identified by a translabyrinthine approach (see Fig. 176-7A). Nonetheless, clean sectioning of the facial nerve facilitates interposition grafting and later facial nerve function.

Osteotomy

A groove may be drilled along the floor of the middle fossa connecting the glenoid fossa area, lateral internal auditory canal, and posterosuperior mastoid. An osteotome is inserted into the carotid canal just distal to the first genu and pointed toward the internal auditory canal (see Fig. 176-7B). The temporal bone specimen is brought out (see Fig. 176-7C), which often will result in inferior petrosal sinus bleeding, requiring intraluminal packing of the inferior petrosal sinus with oxidized cellulose or control of the jugular bulb and sigmoid sinus.

Total Temporal Bone Resection

The internal carotid artery is dissected to the foramen lacerum (Fig. 176-8). The vessel may have been permanently occluded perioperatively in accordance with the surgical plan. The internal jugular vein is ligated and cut. A suboccipital craniotomy is performed, extending over the transverse sinus and lateral posterior fossa. The dura is divided over the cerebellum, and the transverse sinus is ligated between the vein of Labbé and the superior petrosal sinus. The tentorium is divided from the lateral sinus across the superior petrosal sinus to the inferior edge of V_3 with continued dural incision along the floor of the middle cranial fossa laterally. Cranial nerves VII and VIII and the labyrinthine artery are divided at the internal carotid artery. Cranial nerves IX, X, and XI are divided intradurally. The inferior dural incision along the clivus extends from Meckel's cave caudal to the lower cranial nerve to the postsigmoid dural edge. An osteotome is inserted just posterior to the foramen ovale and directed slightly posteriorly to avoid entering the foramen lacerum. This will release the temporal bone specimen, with the occasional need for osteotomy just above the jugular bulb to separate the petro-occipital synchondrosis.[84,85] Alternatively, a groove is drilled under direct vision through the posterior fossa to connect to an externally drilled groove posterior to the petrous internal carotid artery.[83]

Reconstruction

The facial nerve and other appropriate cranial nerves can be cable grafted. Dural defects are closed as needed with fascia or pericranium. The temporalis muscle can be rotated and sutured to surrounding soft tissue. Alternately, regional or free flaps are used. Craniotomy bone and zygoma are secured with wire or miniplates. A closed suction drain then is placed before skin closure.

Infratemporal Fossa Approaches

Attacking various problems of the skull base through a lateral approach transgresses the temporal bone and infratemporal fossa. The postauricular infratemporal fossa approaches as described by Fisch[61,86-88] and the preauricular[89-92] approaches offer the best access to the jugular bulb, internal carotid artery, petrous apex, clivus, pterygomaxillary fossa, and nasopharynx. Proponents of these approaches have written extensively on the subject, and the techniques described here have been adapted from their work. Anatomic maneuvers may be added as needed to facilitate tumor exposure and extirpation.[93,94]

Postauricular Approaches to the Infratemporal Fossa

Fisch[61] has been the primary innovator of these techniques and should be credited for his work. He has divided these techniques into three basic approaches: *Type A* dissection entails radical mastoidectomy, anterior transposition of the facial nerve, exploration of the posterior infratemporal fossa, and cervical dissection permitting access to the jugular bulb, vertical petrous carotid, and posterior infratemporal fossa. *Type B* dissection explores the petrous apex, clivus, and superior infratemporal fossa. *Type C* allows exposure of the nasopharynx, peritubal space, rostral clivus, parasellar area, pterygopalatine fossa, and anterosuperior infratemporal fossa.

Incisions and Skin Flaps

The planned incision should allow for further extensions without devascularization of the elevated skin flap (Fig. 176-9A). Cervical exposure to a variable extent and anterior extension for dissection toward the clivus and parasellar area should be permitted. Keeping the inferior limb of the incision in a posterior location over the mastoid tip allows extension into the cervical area for dissection while protecting the marginal mandibular nerve. Similarly, extending the incision anterosuperiorly into the frontal area permits elevation over the zygoma to the orbital rim.

The flap should be elevated superficially to the temporalis and postauricular muscles, leaving a periosteal flap based on the external auditory canal (see Fig. 176-9B). The canal is transected with care to protect the branches of facial nerve anterior to the canal.

The plane of dissection in an anterior direction is in the subcuticular tissue over the temporal, parotid, and cervical areas. In the type A approach, the tertiary branches of the facial nerve are identified and protected, whereas in the type B and type C approaches, the frontal branch is exposed and protected near the lateral orbital rim.

Closure of the External Auditory Canal

The external auditory canal is closed in a watertight blind sac. The cartilaginous canal skin is undermined to approximately the level of the conchal bowl with tenotomy scissors. The cartilaginous canal skin then is everted and sutured with absorbable sutures and reinforced medially with the periosteal flap elevated off the mastoid cortex (see Fig. 176-9C to F).[96]

Removal of External Auditory Canal Wall Skin and Tympanic Membrane

The skin of the osseous portion of the external auditory canal wall is elevated circumferentially down to the annulus. With an operating microscope, the tympanic annulus is elevated, the incudostapedial joint is separated, the tensor tympani tendon is cut, and the neck of the malleus is nipped, allowing total removal of the canal wall skin, tympanic membrane, and attached manubrium (Fig. 176-10).

Cervical Dissection

Cervical dissection is done as needed to expose the inferior margins of the tumor. This part of the procedure is not required in most type B and type C approaches, except to gain cervical control of the vascular structures if needed. The greater auricular nerve should be sectioned as distally as possible in the parotid for potential use as an interposition graft if needed. Major structures, including the common, external, and internal carotid arteries, the internal jugular vein, and cranial nerves IX to XII, are identified (Fig. 176-11). Division of the posterior belly of the digastric near the mastoid facilitates identification of these structures up to their entrance in the skull base. Ligation of the occipital artery and ascending pharyngeal artery is indicated when these vessels prove to be the vascular supply to the tumor on arteriography. Transection of the glossopharyngeal nerve often is necessary to follow the carotid artery into the skull base. Vascular loops are placed around the internal carotid artery and jugular vein for quick identification and control in the event of bleeding (see Fig. 176-11).

Extratemporal Facial Nerve Dissection

The extratemporal facial nerve may be located deep to the midpoint of a line between the tragal pointer cartilage and the mastoid tip. After release of parotid tissue from the sternocleidomastoid muscle, the tragal cartilage is dissected medially, identifying the facial nerve just inferior to the pointer. The facial nerve is dissected out to tertiary branches by cutting overlying the parotid gland and freeing it from the underlying parotid tissues. This exposure is required for anterior transposition in the type A approach (see Fig. 176-11). In the type B and type C approaches, facial nerve transposition is not required; only the frontal branch is followed distally to allow its preservation when the zygoma is transected. The parotid gland is bluntly dissected off the masseteric fascia to reduce traction on the facial nerve when the mandible is retracted.

Radical Mastoidectomy

The radical mastoidectomy removes the air cell tracts lateral and adjacent to the otic capsule (Fig. 176-12A). Exenteration of all tracts is important to prevent long-term complications after cavity obliteration.[96] The stapes suprastructure is removed to prevent inner ear trauma. The facial nerve is skeletonized in preparation for transposition. The eustachian tube is obliterated with bone wax impregnated with bone dust and a muscle plug. Removal of the external auditory canal, tympanic membrane, ossicles, and air cells of the temporal bone lateral to the otic capsule constitute the radical mastoidectomy.

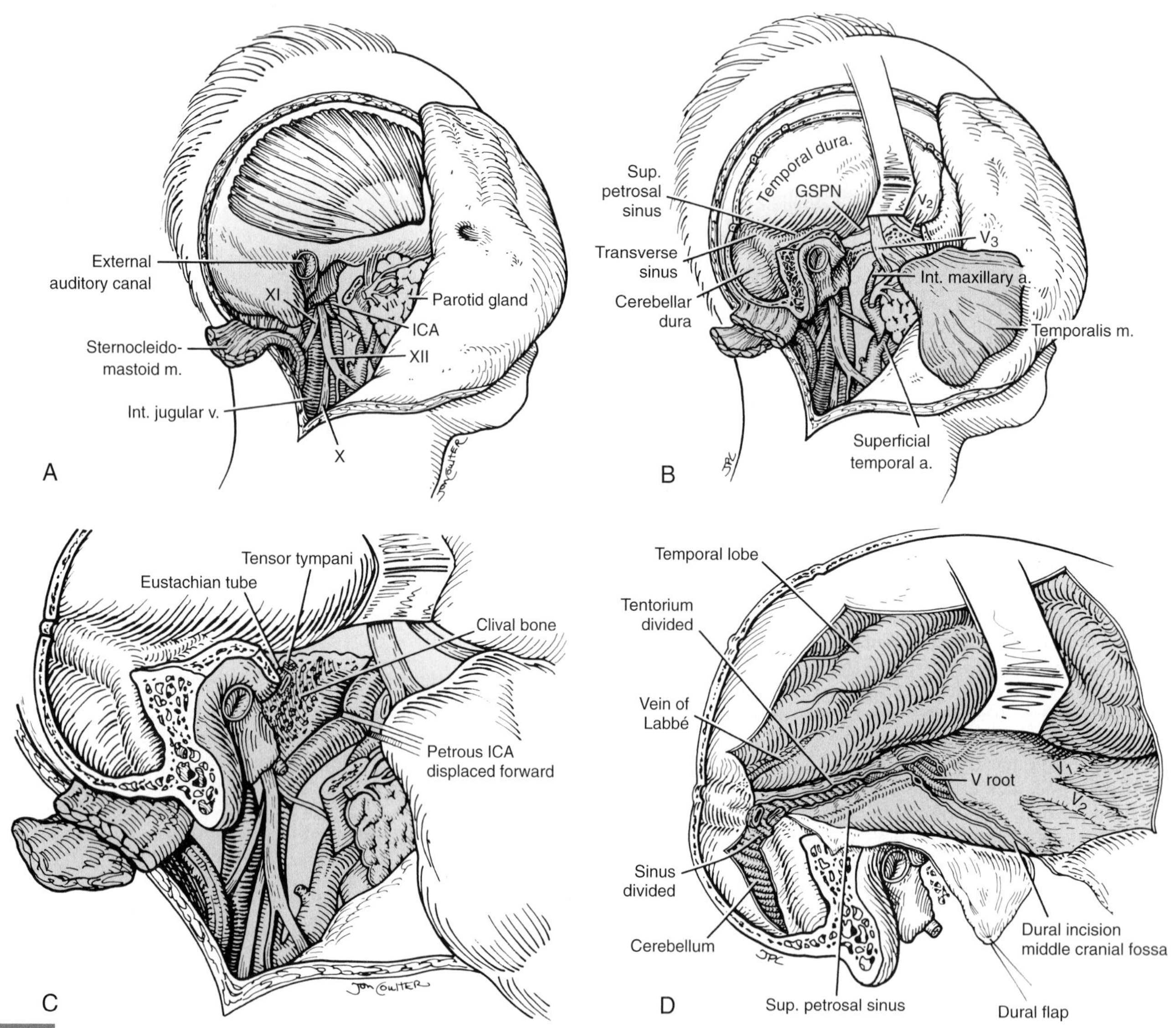

Figure 176-8. Schematic depiction of total temporal bone resection. Roman numerals denote cranial nerves. **A,** The frontotemporal-retroauricular-cervical skin flap is rotated forward. The external ear canal has been transected. The facial nerve has been transected just beyond the stylomastoid foramen. The temporomandibular joint has been opened and the mandibular ramus resected. Cranial nerves IX through XII and the jugular and carotid vessels are exposed to the neck. **B,** A temporal and suboccipital craniotomy has been extended over the transverse sinus and lateral posterior fossa. A zygomatic osteotomy and a partial mastoidectomy have been performed. The osseous middle fossa floor has been partially resected to expose second (V_2) and third (V_3) divisions of the cranial nerve V and the greater superficial petrosal nerve (GSPN). The middle meningeal artery has been transected. **C,** Continuing resection of the osseous middle fossa floor; the eustachian tube and the tensor tympani muscle have been transected. The ascending and transverse segments of the petrous ICA have been unroofed, and the ICA has become mobilized anteriorly. **D,** The temporal and retrosigmoid portions of the dura have been opened. The lateral sinus has been ligated at its junction with the sigmoid; the tentorium has been opened along the inferior edge of the mandibular nerve, trigeminal ganglion, and roof, with the interruption of the superior petrosal sinus. If the superior petrosal sinus is uninvolved, its drainage into the transverse sinus may be preserved by changing the dural incision lines. The dura has been cut over the cerebellum; the transverse sinus has been ligated and transected, and a dural flap has been brought down from over the temporal lobe. The tentorium has been divided from the transverse sinus transection, alongside and behind the petrous ridge, and anteromedially across the sinus. This cut has been connected to an incision in the dura on the middle cranial fossa floor anterior to the petrous base. The outline of the trigeminal ganglion and roots can be seen through the middle fossa dura.

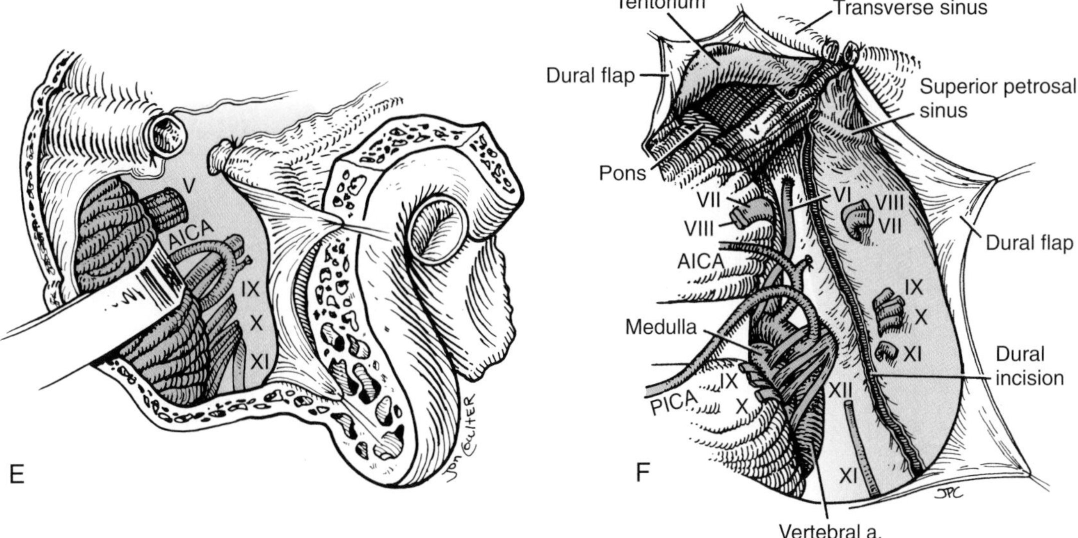

Figure 176-8, cont'd. **E,** With the cerebellum retracted medially, cranial nerves V and VII through XI can be seen. The labyrinthine (internal auditory) artery has been transected at its origin from the anterior inferior cerebellar artery (AICA). **F,** Cranial nerves VII through XI have been transected, and the underlying dura has been incised as the posterior border of the en bloc resection of the petrous bone. The petrous bone specimen then is disconnected from any remaining attachments and removed. ICA, internal carotid artery; PICA, posterior inferior cerebellar artery. *(Used with permission from Sekhar LN, Pomeranz S, Janecka IP, Hirsch B, Ramasastry S. Temporal bone neoplasms: a report on 20 surgically treated cases.* J Neurosurg. *1992;76:578-587.)*

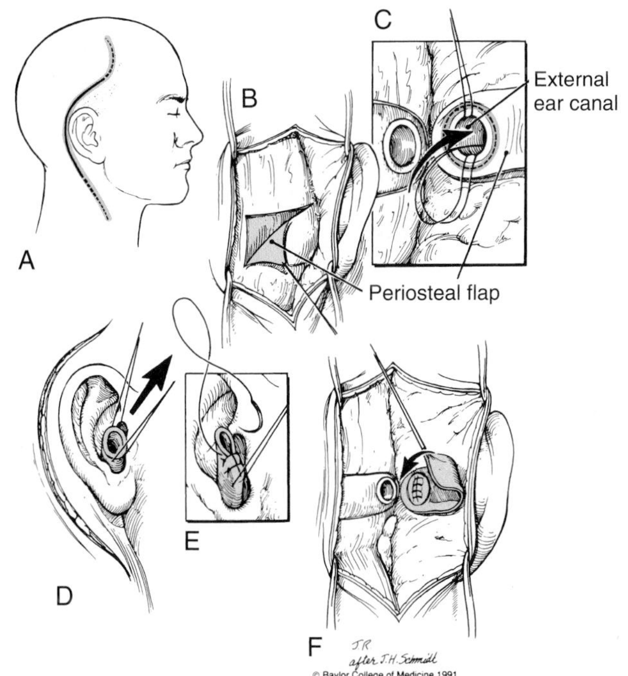

Figure 176-9. **A,** Skin incision for Fisch type A infratemporal fossa dissection. **B,** Anteriorly based periosteal flap elevation. **C** to **E,** Cartilaginous canal skin elevated, everted, and blind sac closure of external canal. **F,** Blind sac closure reinforced with periosteal flap.

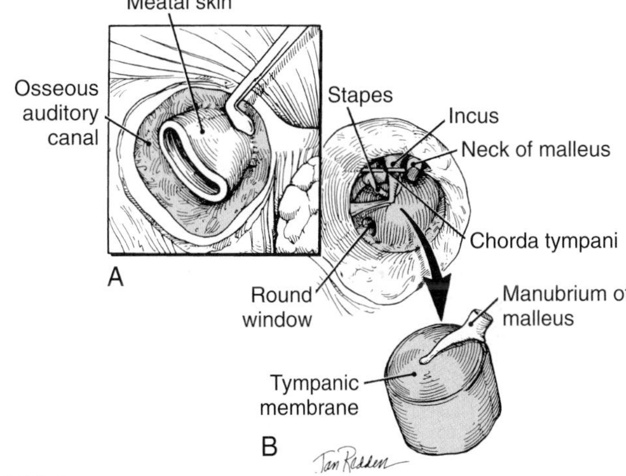

Figure 176-10. **A,** Skin of osseous external auditory canal elevated to annulus (note that lateral skin is already removed). **B,** Removal of canal skin, tympanic membrane, and attached manubrium.

Type A Approach

FACIAL NERVE TRANSPOSITION. The facial nerve should be skeletonized and freed of its bony canal 180 degrees circumferentially from the geniculate ganglion distal to the stylomastoid foramen. The horizontal semicircular canal is in jeopardy at the second genu, and bone should be removed only on the tympanic side of the facial nerve. The air cells of the mastoid tip are exenterated lateral to the digastric ridge; the cortical shell is removed with a rongeur after incising the attached digastric muscle. At the stylomastoid foramen, the facial nerve is densely adherent to the surrounding fibrous tissue, and these tissues are elevated as a unit to prevent devascularization and stretch injury to the nerve. A new bony canal is drilled in the anterior wall of the epitympanum to receive the nerve. The facial nerve is elevated carefully from the geniculate ganglion to the pes anserinus and is transposed into the new groove and secured within the parotid soft tissue (see Fig. 176-12B).

Meticulous handling of the facial nerve decreases the risk of permanent facial nerve dysfunction after transposition. Use of the operating microscope, diamond burr, and constant irrigation minimizes direct trauma. The epineurium is kept intact. The stapedius nerve, the soft tissue of the stylomastoid foramen including periosteum and enclosed facial nerve, and all medial attachments to the nerve should be sharply dissected to prevent stretch injury.

Intraoperative facial nerve monitoring with EMG is of great benefit during transposition in preventing injury (see Chapter 178).[80]

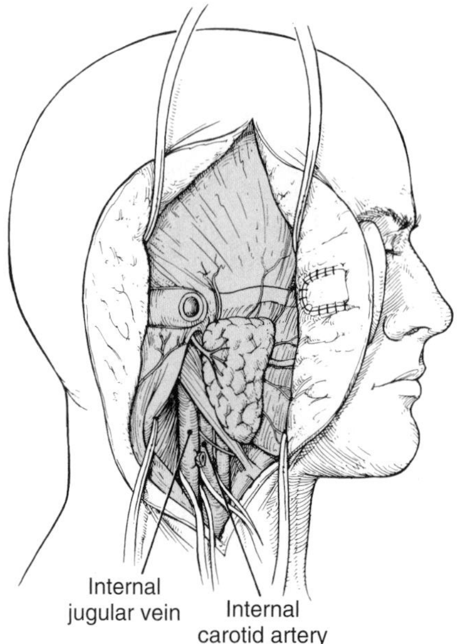

Figure 176-11. Preparatory dissection with flap elevation and proximal vascular control.

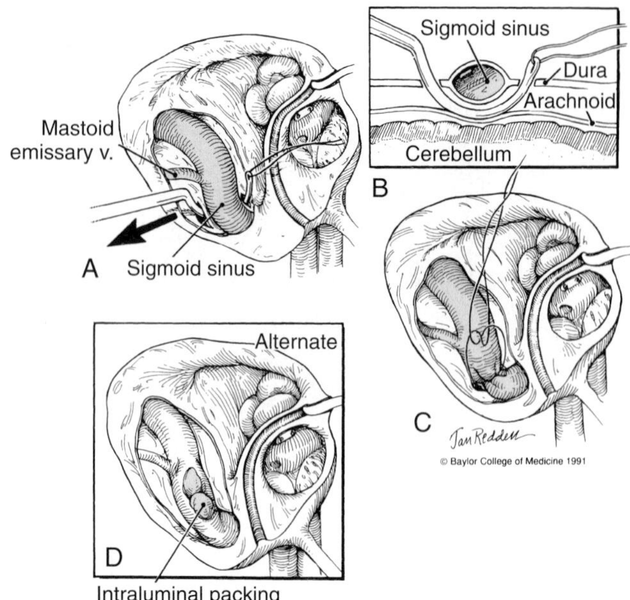

Figure 176-13. **A** to **C,** Ligation of the sigmoid sinus below the mastoid emissary vein. **D,** Alternate method of sigmoid sinus occlusion with intraluminal absorbable packing.

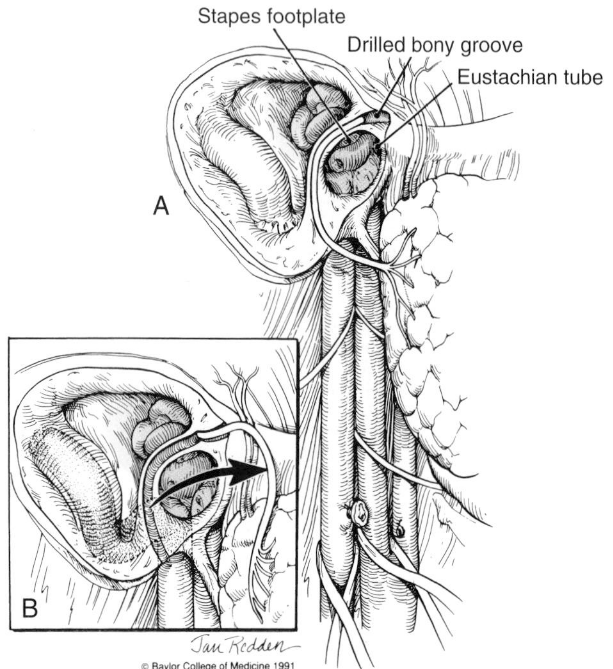

Figure 176-12. **A,** Radical mastoidectomy with facial nerve skeletonization. **B,** Anterior transposition of the facial nerve.

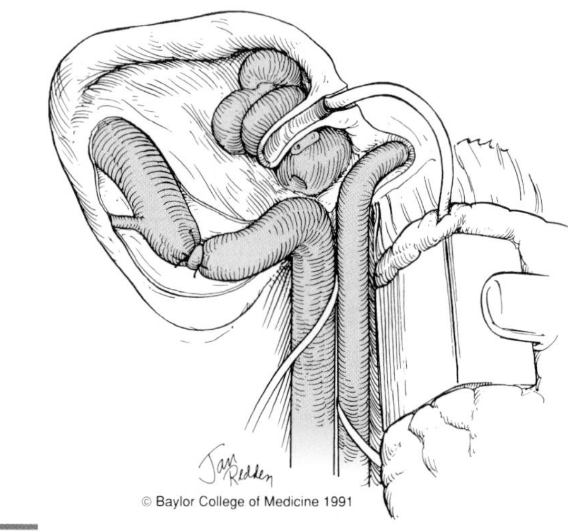

Figure 176-14. Fisch type A infratemporal fossa exposure and vascular control completed by removal of bone over carotid artery and jugular bulb.

Immediate feedback is available to the surgeon during manual manipulations, helping prevent direct trauma and stretch injury, the latter being the most common reason for postoperative dysfunction. With feedback monitoring, the surgeon can remove bone over the facial nerve more aggressively.

OCCLUSION OF THE SIGMOID SINUS. Bone is removed over the posterior fossa dura anterior and posterior to the sigmoid sinus to allow ligation. The mastoid emissary vein is left undisturbed, and ligation is performed below it if possible. Dural vessels are coagulated; the dura is elevated with dural hooks, incised in front of and behind the sigmoid sinus, and a blunt-tipped aneurysm needle is used to pass a double 2-0 silk ligature (Fig. 176-13A to C). A small CSF leak may occur and is easily controlled with a sutured muscle plug. Other methods of sigmoid sinus interruption, involving intraluminal absorbable packing (see Fig. 176-13D), are used by Jackson[97] and Holliday[98] and their coworkers.

EXPOSURE OF JUGULAR BULB AND INTERNAL CAROTID ARTERY. A clamp is passed medial to the styloid process to protect the internal carotid artery while the process is fractured and removed with the attached muscles. The parotid gland is dissected from the tympanic bone, and a modified self-retaining laminectomy retractor (Karl Storz, D-7200, Tuttlingen, Germany) is placed behind the ramus of the mandible to effect anterior subluxation. The facial nerve EMG activity is monitored to avoid stretch injury or compression of branches in the parotid gland. Exposure of the posterior infratemporal fossa now permits isolation of the vertical intrapetrous segment of the internal carotid artery. With removal of bone over the carotid artery and beneath the otic capsule, the jugular fossa is exposed for tumor removal (Figs. 176-14 and 176-15).

TUMOR REMOVAL. After exposure and distal control of the internal carotid artery are accomplished, the tumor may be carefully

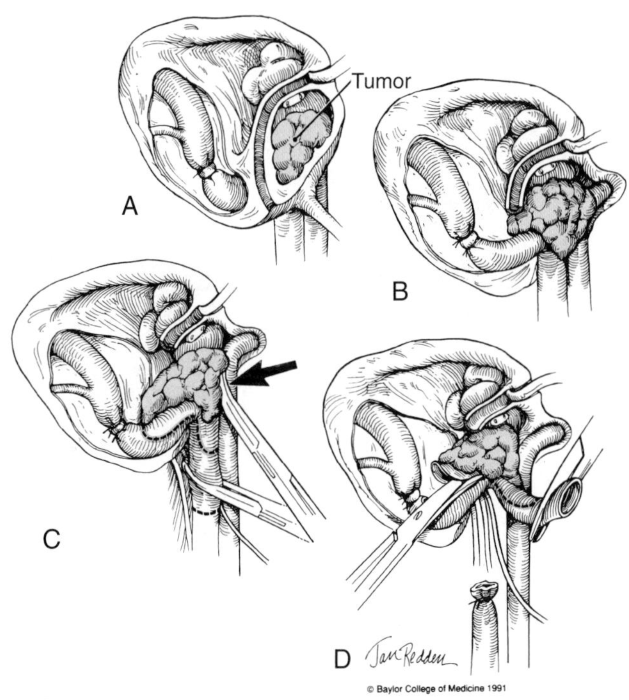

Figure 176-15. **A** to **D,** Removal of paraganglioma of the jugular bulb using the Fisch type A infratemporal fossa approach.

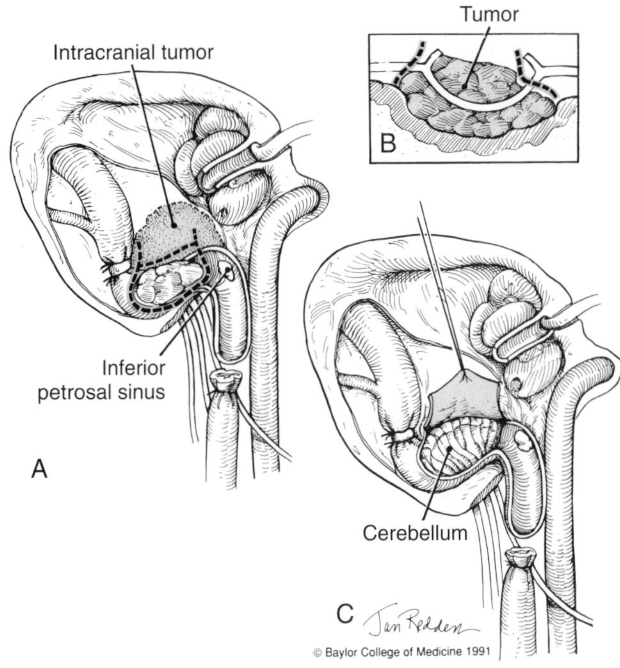

Figure 176-16. **A** and **B,** Intracranial paraganglioma extension into posterior fossa. **C,** Intracranial paraganglioma removed.

removed.[95,99] The jugular vein is ligated to prevent tumor and air embolism. Dissection begins by freeing the internal carotid artery and rotating the tumor posteriorly (see Fig. 176-15C). The lateral wall of the sigmoid sinus is removed along with intraluminal tumor (see Fig. 176-15D). The medial wall forms the barrier to the CSF. The inferior margin of the tumor is elevated, and the extracranial tumor is removed (see Fig. 176-15D). If the tumor extends intracranially, it is amputated sharply at this point. Profuse bleeding may occur from the entrances of the inferior petrosal sinus into the jugular bulb. Control is achieved by surgical packing.

After hemostasis is obtained, the posterior fossa dura is opened, and the intracranial portion of the tumor is excised (Fig. 176-16) at the same setting for intracranial tumors smaller than 2 cm. Larger tumors may be staged and removed at a later time.[100,101] Care should be taken to preserve the blood supply to the brainstem.

CLOSURE OF WOUND. The dura usually is left with a defect too large for primary closure. Fascia lata provides the best material for reconstruction, although lyophilized dura can be used to seal the defect. Abdominal fat is used to obliterate the dead space of the temporal bone, and the temporalis muscle is rotated inferiorly for reinforcement of the wound (Fig. 176-17). The skin is closed routinely, and a bulky pressure dressing is applied for a minimum of 5 days to prevent leakage of CSF.

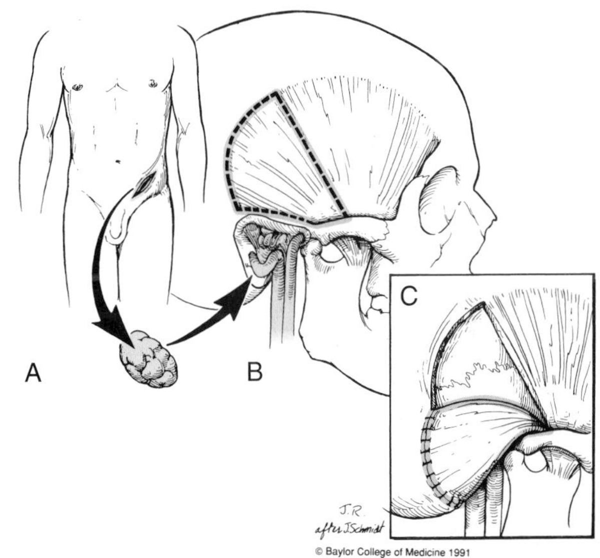

Figure 176-17. **A** to **C,** Obliteration of wound defect with abdominal fat and rotated temporalis muscle.

Type B Approach

The type B approach differs from the type A approach with respect to the facial nerve in that transposition of the nerve usually is not required. The steps up to transposition are identical to those for the type A approach. Reflection of the temporalis muscle still attached to the coronoid process and the zygoma allows the retractor to expose the superior infratemporal fossa (Fig. 176-18, A to C). Monitoring of facial nerve EMG activity during mandibular displacement helps prevent stretch injury. The limits of operative exposure in the type B approach are defined by the middle cranial fossa floor, mandibular condyle, and reflected temporalis muscle (see Fig. 176-18D).

Thinning bone under the MCF dura improves exposure. The middle meningeal artery and V_3 branch of the trigeminal nerve require bipolar cauterization and transection, respectively, thereby giving exposure to the superior 4 cm of the infratemporal fossa. The carotid artery may be uncovered from its vertical segment to its anterior limit at the foramen lacerum after separation from the soft tissues around the eustachian tube (Fig. 176-19A). The geniculate ganglion of the facial nerve and cochlea may be prone to injury if not properly recognized.

Petrous apex lesions, such as cholesteatoma or low-grade chondrosarcomas, may be removed at this point with careful anterolateral retraction of the internal carotid artery. The artery can be elevated from the foramen lacerum to the canalis caroticus to permit temporary transposition of the vessel (Fig. 176-20B). This maneuver may easily result in hemorrhage and should be performed with care. Extensive benign lesions involving the petrous apex and perilabyrinthine area may require a transotic approach combined with posterior facial nerve transposition, accomplished by cutting the greater superficial petrosal nerve and by liberating the facial nerve from the porus acusticus to the stylomastoid foramen (see Fig. 176-20).[102,103] In addition, the middle fossa

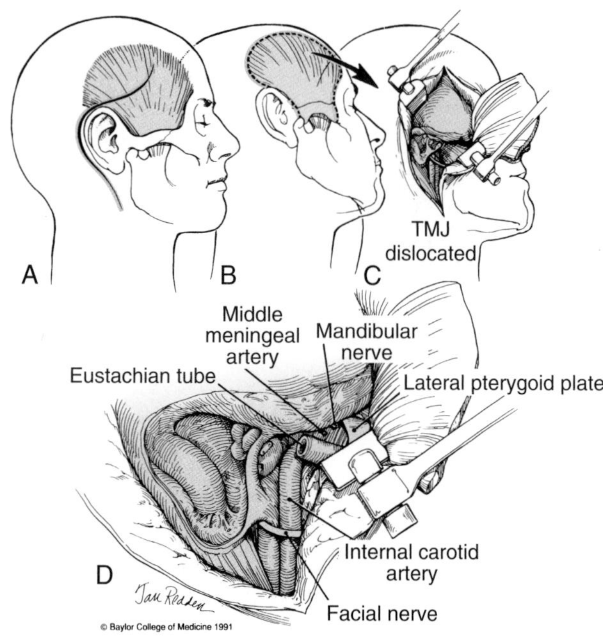

Figure 176-18. Fisch type B or C approach, incorporating the steps of the type A approach, as shown in Figures 176-9 through 176-12A. Note, however, that the intratemporal facial nerve is *not* skeletonized.) **A** to **C,** Dissection also includes transection of zygoma, elevation of the temporalis muscle and periosteum of skull base, and self-retaining retractor dislocation of the mandible inferiorly. **D,** Bone is removed to identify the middle meningeal artery and V_3 (transected here). TMJ, temporomandibular joint.

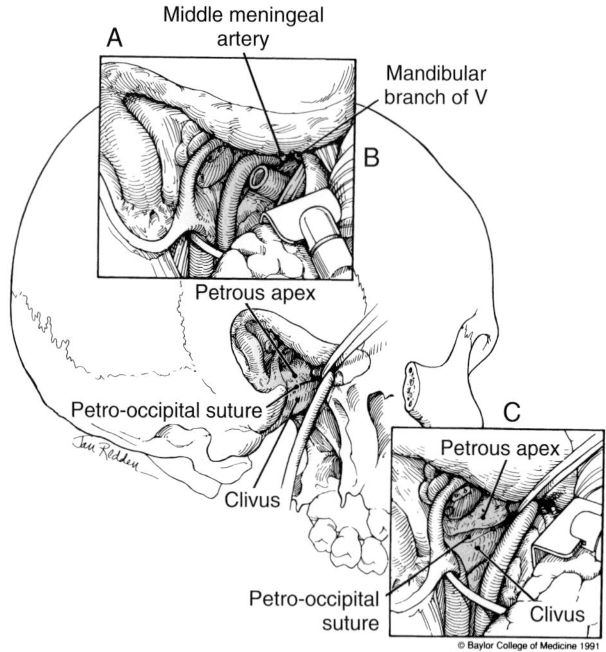

Figure 176-19. **A,** Removal of the eustachian tube permits access to the internal carotid artery up to the foramen lacerum. **B** and **C,** Elevation of the carotid artery permits additional access to the petrous apex and clivus.

may easily be accessed through a temporal craniotomy (see Chapter 174). Exposure of the clivus can be obtained by sharp incision of the fibrous attachments at the petro-occipital fissure. Tumors of the clivus, such as chordomas, up to the parasellar area may be removed through the type B approach (see Fig. 176-19C). Removal of the mandibular

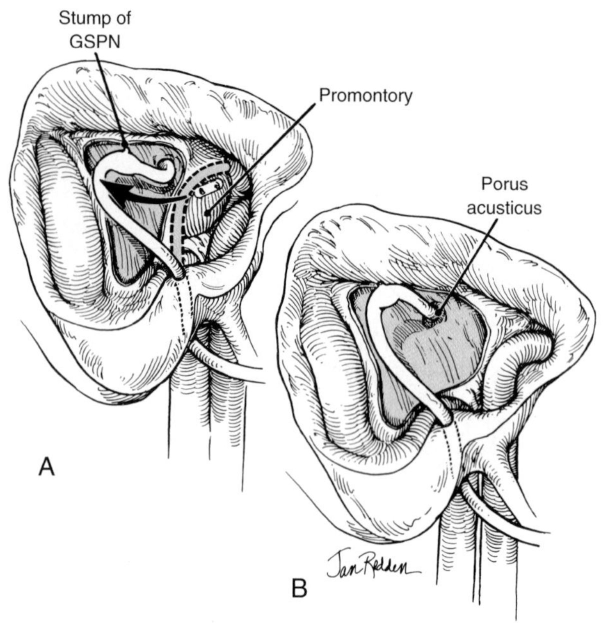

Figure 176-20. Transcochlear approach to the petrous apex. **A,** Posterior translocation of the facial nerve. GSPN, greater superficial petrosal nerve. **B,** Subtotal petrosectomy with removal of the otitic capsule.

condyle may give better exposure to the inferior clivus and upper cervical vertebrae. With inferior extension of the tumor, the facial nerve may be transposed as in a type A approach. Tumors located superior or medial to the horizontal portion of the internal carotid artery may require further mobilization of the cervical and vertical petrous carotid or the addition of a middle cranial fossa craniotomy. The superior and inferior petrosal sinuses may require removal in these extended dissections.

Type C Approach

The type C approach is an anterior extension of the type B approach. The type C infratemporal fossa approach permits posterolateral access to the rostral clivus, cavernous sinus, sphenoid sinus, peritubal space, pterygopalatine fossa, and nasopharynx and to the areas exposed by the type B approach. The type C infratemporal fossa approach, in essence, permits access anterior to the foramen lacerum up to the posterior aspect of the maxillary sinus and nasopharynx.

The base of the pterygoid process is removed to approach the sphenoid sinus and cavernous sinus (Fig. 176-21). Removal of the pterygoid base uncovers V_2 in the foramen rotundum and the inferior orbital fissure. Removal of bone from the pterygoid base permits better visualization of the sphenoid sinus; with the sinus exposed, the floor of the sella turcica can be visualized. The cavernous sinus is exposed by thinning the bone of the middle cranial fossa floor anterior to the V_2 stump. The middle cranial fossa dura may be retracted, giving an inferolateral view of the cavernous sinus.

To enter the lateral nasopharyngeal cavity, the lateral and medial pterygoid processes are removed, and the buccopharyngeal fascia and nasopharyngeal mucosa are incised. Separation of the pterygoid muscles from the mandible allows en bloc removal of the lateral nasopharyngeal wall, peritubal space, and superior infratemporal contents when needed for tumor extirpation (Fig. 176-22).

Tumors involving the pterygopalatine space require resection of the pterygoid process and a portion of the greater wing of the sphenoid with sacrifice of the maxillary branch of the trigeminal nerve. A portion of the posterior maxillary wall may be removed for further access.

Preauricular Infratemporal Approach

The preauricular approaches to the skull base described by various investigators, including Sen and Sekhar and colleagues,[90-92,104] can

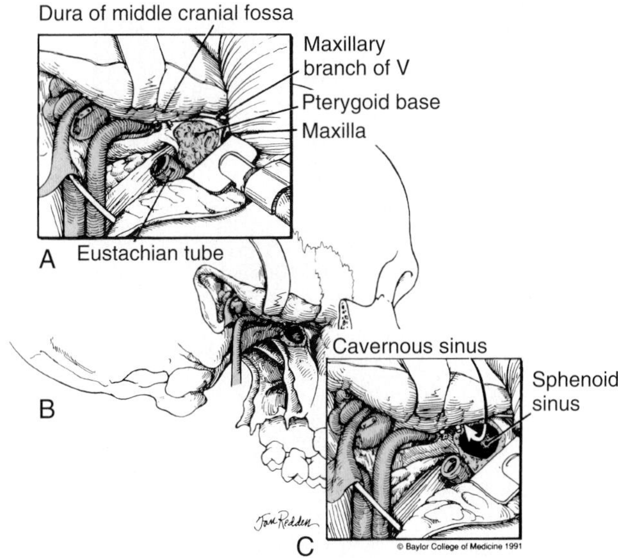

Figure 176-21. Fisch type C approach. **A,** Pterygoid base dissected with exposure of V_2. **B** and **C,** Sphenoid sinus entered.

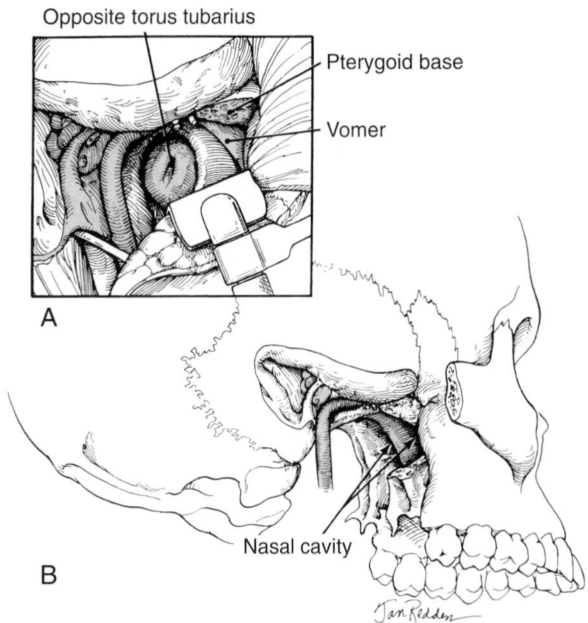

Figure 176-22. Fisch type C approach to nasopharyngeal exposure. **A** and **B,** Removal of pterygoid process and lateral wall of the nasopharynx exposing the opposite torus tubarius.

expose the upper cervical segment (without facial nerve transposition) and the intrapetrous segment of the internal carotid artery. These infratemporal dissections expose virtually the same areas as in the Fisch type B and type C approaches, albeit from a purely lateral vector of exposure. The preauricular approach permits access to the petrous apex, clivus, and superior infratemporal fossa and may be extended to include the nasopharynx, parasellar area, pterygopalatine fossa, and anterior infratemporal fossa. A frontotemporal craniotomy may be included for intracranial extension.[105] The petrous bone may be entered for access to the internal carotid artery, but the external auditory canal is not removed, and the tympanic cavity is not obliterated; therefore, the middle ear function is preserved, although the eustachian tube may be sacrificed, resulting in permanent serous otitis media. Although resecting the mandibular condyle in the preauricular approach facilitates the exposure of the internal carotid artery, such resection usually is not required in the postauricular approaches, because a posterior vector of orientation improves access.

The preauricular incision may be extended into the frontoparietal and upper cervical areas to expand exposure into the anterior infratemporal fossa (Fig. 176-23A). Identification and control of vascular structures in the neck are similar to those with the postauricular approaches. The superior cervical dissection is hindered by the facial nerve exiting the stylomastoid foramen to enter the parotid gland. Retraction of the mandible anteroinferiorly permits exposure of the upper cervical segment of the internal carotid artery (see Fig. 176-23B). Constant EMG monitoring during application of retractors greatly reduces the risk of facial nerve injury. Reflection of the temporalis muscles and zygoma as previously described for Fisch type B and type C approaches permits dissection of the anterior infratemporal fossa (see Fig. 176-23C).

The added time required for performance of a subtotal petrosectomy followed by obliteration is a disadvantage of the Fisch approach. Conductive hearing loss is inevitable, although transposition of the facial nerve, required in the type A approach, provides better access to the jugular fossa and the internal carotid artery at the skull base. The primary disadvantage of the preauricular approach is the inability to resect lesions extending into the temporal bone or posterior fossa.

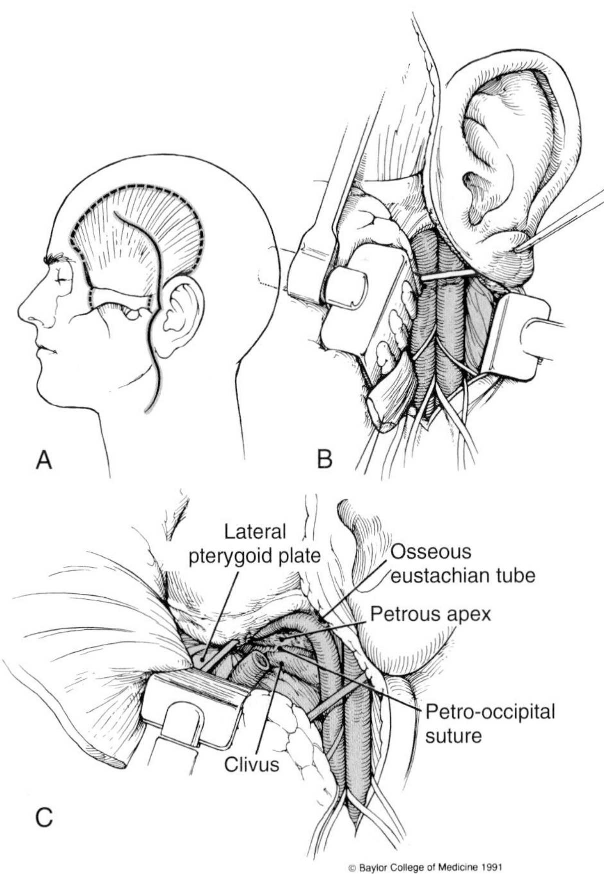

Figure 176-23. Preauricular lateral skull base approach. **A,** Incision for approach to infratemporal fossa. **B,** Exposure of major vessels to the skull base. **C,** Exposure of the infratemporal fossa.

Selected Problems

Rhabdomyosarcoma

A rhabdomyosarcoma is the most common childhood middle ear and mastoid malignancy. The recent spectacular improvement in 5-year survival rates in patients with this disease has been achieved by several continued refinements of combined therapy: more accurate staging of parameningeal disease, adjustments of chemotherapeutic agents and dosage schedules, and advances in radiotherapy techniques.[95,106,107] Although total tumor removal is the surgical goal when possible, surgical debulking is an important concept in this disease. Gross total removal with preservation of the dura, otic capsule, and neurologic and vascular structures is performed, followed by postoperative chemotherapy and radiotherapy.

Carcinomas of the External Auditory Canal and Temporal Bone

Carcinomas and benign tumors of the external auditory canal and temporal bone are uncommon. Squamous cell carcinoma is by far the most common malignant tumor of the external auditory canal, followed by basal cell carcinoma and adenoid cystic carcinoma.[35,108-123] Carcinomas of the external auditory canal usually occur in persons 40 to 60 years of age, with some reports of carcinomas originating from cerumen glands somewhat earlier.

Pertinent Anatomy

The outer third of the cartilaginous portion of the external auditory canal contains all cerumen glands, which are modified sweat glands and sebaceous glands. The cartilage of the cartilaginous canal is J-shaped, being absent posteriorly. Anteriorly, the cartilage has small dehiscences known as the fissures of Santorini. The junction of the cartilaginous and osseous canal also permits radial spread.[124] The cartilaginous canal thus facilitates radial tumor extension. The osseous or medial two thirds of the external auditory canal for the most part is devoid of glandular tissue. The epithelium has no underlying subcuticular tissue and is closely adherent to the periosteum. The bone provides resistance to radial spread, so longitudinal spread toward the tympanic membrane is an early phenomenon. Radial spread through Huschke's foramen, a developmental defect in the tympanic ring, may permit anterior extension into the parotid. The tympanic membrane is thought to act as a barrier to longitudinal spread, although McCabe[125] has warned that microscopic extension around the annulus into the mesotympanum may occur even when the tympanic membrane is intact or grossly uninvolved. Entry of tumor into the middle ear space permits a myriad of paths of least resistance through air cell tracts and the eustachian tube.[126]

Symptoms and Signs

Carcinoma of the external auditory canal and temporal bone often will masquerade as chronic external otitis or chronic otitis. The frequency of these complaints in "routine" clinic patients has led to an average 6-month delay in diagnosis. Persistence of external otitis, despite adequate management by routine treatment measures, should increase suspicion for carcinoma and inflammatory processes as potential etiologic disorders, leading to biopsy. Persistent pain that is inordinately severe for the abnormality or a change in pain pattern with a chronically painful ear should precipitate further investigation. Some adenoid cystic carcinomas have been preceded by ear pain for several months before any abnormality is noted; therefore, serial examinations are important.

Squamous cell carcinoma may appear as a meaty or polypoid lesion in the external auditory canal. Adenoid cystic carcinoma usually is epithelium-covered and may appear as a small pimple, accompanied by complaints of significant pain. Basal cell carcinoma may exhibit serpiginous ulceration, with absence of the typically pearly edges because of characteristics of the thin, adherent canal epithelium. Hearing loss usually is conductive, from obstruction of the canal. Cochlear hearing loss and vertigo indicate labyrinthine involvement and an aggressive, advanced lesion. A parotid mass, cranial nerve paresis, and cervical lymphadenopathy also are late signs portending a grave prognosis. It is important to assess the nasopharynx to ascertain that a tumor does not originate from this area. Carcinomas of the external auditory canal should prompt close evaluation of the parotid gland, because the tumor may have originated from the parotid gland.

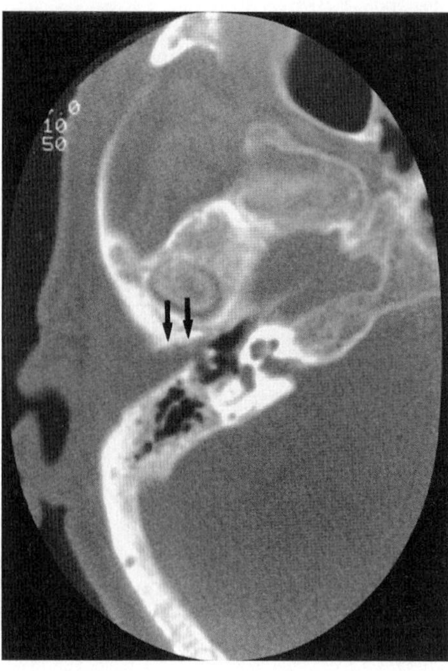

Figure 176-24. Squamous cell carcinoma of the right external acoustic canal in a 73-year-old woman: Axial view, computed tomography (CT) with bone algorithm. Only a focused bone algorithm CT scan would reveal the subtle bone erosion *(arrows)* associated with this carcinoma.

Staging

Planning management depends critically on preoperative evaluation. Thin-slice temporal bone CT, with soft tissue and bone protocols with intravenous contrast, will delineate the medial extent of disease and provide evidence of osseous erosion and some soft tissue detail[127] (Fig. 176-24). With extensive lesions or CT evidence of osseous erosions or soft tissue extension, MRI with gadolinium enhancement of the temporal bone, parotid gland, and upper neck will provide further soft tissue detail around the canal and intracranial involvement. Four-vessel carotid angiography and functional CBF assessment may be useful if extensive resections are indicated. An appropriate workup for metastatic disease also should be performed.

A system for staging carcinoma of the external auditory canal has been described by investigators from the University of Pittsburgh. Arriaga and Janecka[124] proposed a primary tumor–regional nodes–metastasis (TNM) staging system based on clinical examination, preoperative imaging studies, and intraoperative findings (Box 176-2). Of note, imaging may understage soft tissue extension seen intraoperatively. Other investigators have supported the clinical usefulness of this staging system.[128,129]

Management

In treating these carcinomas, the clinician should heed the admonition of Jesse and colleagues[130]: "One factor becomes painfully obvious, that the first treatment is the only one that has a chance of curing the patient, while subsequent treatment is simply palliative." For this reason, initial treatment by whatever modality chosen should be radical enough to eliminate the cancer. Consensus regarding management of carcinomas of the external auditory canal and temporal bone is not easily found in the literature, mainly because of the rarity of these lesions. Most series have one or two cases per year, extending over 2 decades or longer. Some of the larger series represent evolution of management philosophy, making critical analysis difficult. Authors often lump together all malignancies of the external auditory canal, regardless of histology, involvement of the middle ear, or other signs of advanced disease.

En bloc surgical resection of external auditory canal malignancies is considered by almost all investigators to be the primary therapy, with an adjunctive role for radiotherapy. Most recurrences are local. Positive

Box 176-2

University of Pittsburgh Tumor–Lymph Node–Metastasis Staging System Proposed for Neoplasms of the External Auditory Canal

T Status

T_1 Tumor limited to the external auditory canal without bony erosion or evidence of soft tissue extension

T_2 Tumor with limited external auditory canal bony erosion (not full-thickness) or radiographic finding consistent with limited (less than 0.5 cm) soft tissue involvement

T_3 Tumor eroding the osseous external auditory canal (full-thickness) with limited (less than 0.5 cm) soft tissue involvement, or tumor involving middle ear or mastoid, or patients presenting with facial paralysis

T_4 Tumor eroding the cochlea, petrous apex, medial wall of middle ear, carotid canal, jugular foramen or dura, or with extensive (greater than 0.5 cm) soft tissue involvement

N Status

Involvement of lymph nodes is a poor prognostic finding and automatically places the patient in an advanced stage (i.e., stage III [T_1, N_1] or stage IV [T_2, T_3, and T_4, N_1] disease).

M Status

Distant metastasis indicates a poor prognosis and immediately places the patient in the stage IV category.

margins, despite postoperative radiotherapy, have an almost uniform fatal result.[131] Advanced lesions involving the middle ear and medial structures can be handled with combined therapy or palliatively, depending on clinical factors.

An algorithm for the management of high-grade carcinomas of the external auditory canal and temporal bone is presented in Figure 176-25.

"Local" resections in rare circumstances may be appropriate but in general are to be condemned. T_1 tumors localized to the cartilaginous canal can be appropriately managed with sleeve resection of the external auditory canal with frozen section sampling of medial margins. Such cases are rare. Lateral temporal bone resection (or en bloc removal of the canal and tympanic membrane) is the minimum operation for patients with carcinoma of the osseous portion of the canal (T_1 and T_2 tumors) and with carcinomas abutting the chondro-osseous junction. Moore and coworkers[132] argue that "canal wall down" mastoidectomy technique with anterior canal drillout (i.e., not en bloc) is equal in efficacy to an en bloc lateral temporal bone resection. Spector[133] suggests that all patients should receive postoperative radiotherapy after en bloc resections. Other workers believe that postoperative radiotherapy should not be used unless aggressive clinical or pathologic features are noted, such as soft tissue extension, metastatic lymphadenopathy, or any osseous or cartilaginous invasion on pathologic examination. If postoperative radiotherapy is likely, the mastoid cavity should be obliterated at the time of the operation to prevent osteoradionecrosis.[73]

These operations yield complex surgical specimens, and it is incumbent on the surgeon to orient the pathologist and request information regarding osseous or soft tissue invasion to gain maximum benefit for the patient. Temporal bone laboratory techniques have been advocated.[134] However, temporal bone laboratory techniques may not provide clinically pertinent information in a timely manner.

Extension into the mesotympanum, stage T_3 disease, gives rise to several other therapeutic options. The least aggressive option includes a lateral temporal bone resection plus subtotal petrosectomy followed by postoperative radiotherapy (for a 28.6% 5-year survival rate),

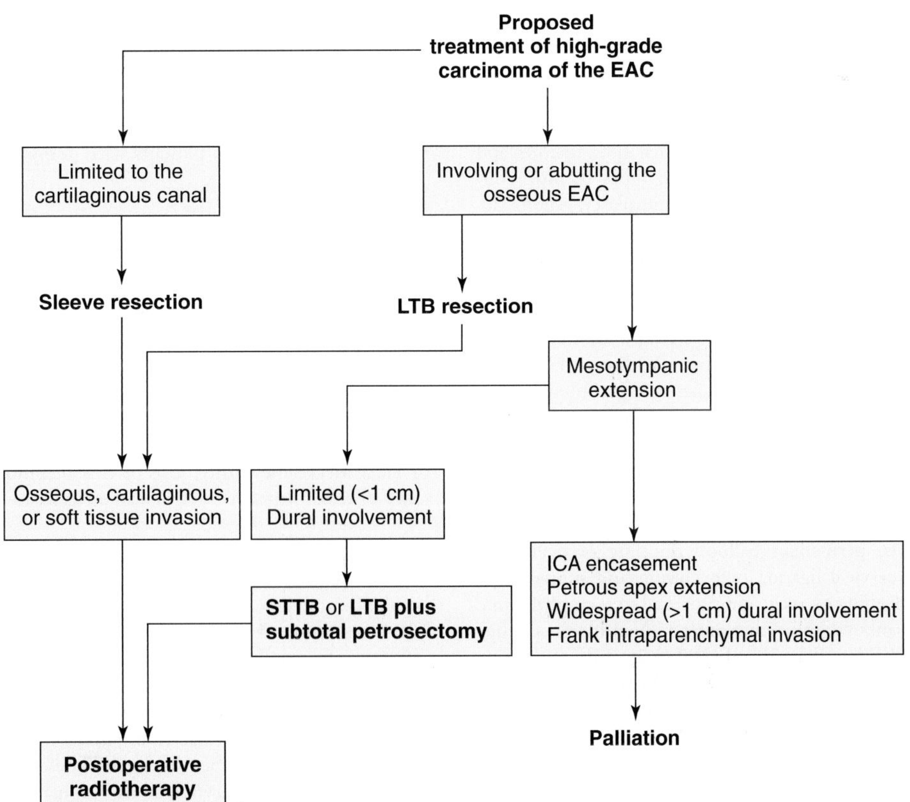

Figure 176-25. Algorithm for management of high-grade malignancies of the external auditory canal (EAC) and temporal bone. ICA, internal auditory canal; LTB, lateral temporal bone; STTB, subtotal temporal bone.

although this modality has been shown on literature analysis to be inferior to subtotal temporal bone resection (associated with a 41.7% 5-year survival rate).[84,85] Although it is uncertain whether postoperative radiotherapy provides added benefit after subtotal temporal bone resection,[84,85] we recommend subtotal temporal bone resection followed by postoperative radiotherapy. T_4 lesions with transdural extension generally have been thought to be inoperable. However, Moffat and associates[135] have successfully treated well to moderately differentiated T_4 tumors with limited temporal lobe involvement. A study by Ducic and colleagues,[136] supported by the International Study of Cranial Facial Surgery,[137] involving high-grade carcinomas of the anterior cranial fossa addressed issues of dural and intraparenchymal involvement. If dural involvement is limited (less than or equal to 1 cm) and frank intraparenchymal involvement is not apparent intraoperatively, the disease-free survivial or locoregional control shows no statistical difference with respect to dural involvement, but a dramatic decline in survival is associated with parenchymal invasion. Preoperative MRI may show dural or parenchymal involvement when none is found at surgery, possibly due to edema or inflammation. However, if overt intraparenchymal involvement is noted on frozen section, the procedure is abandoned, because as noted by Ganly and coworkers, "resection margin can still be achieved when either bone or dura is involved, but less likely when brain parechyma is involved."[137] The morbidity associated with subtotal temporal bone resection includes stroke, meningitis, and that due to sacrifice of the audiovestibular nerve and facial nerve, with a 5% perioperative mortality rate.

Total temporal bone resection also results in further morbidity from additional sacrifice of cranial nerves IX, X, and XI. Total temporal bone resection extends a subtotal resection by including the petrous apex and the entire mastoid air cell system. High-grade malignancies of the temporal bone with extension outside the petrous bone or to the petrous apex, extensive dural involvement, frank parenchymal involvement, gasserian ganglion involvement, or invasion along the skull base portend a poor outcome in nearly all cases. Palliation should be carefully and strongly considered. Patients with low- to medium-grade malignancies or extensive benign tumors, T_3 or T_4, may benefit from total temporal bone resection.[138]

Aneurysms of the Upper Cervical and Petrous Internal Carotid Artery

Primary lesions of the upper cervical and petrous segments of the internal carotid artery are decidedly rare. They include those lesions with a congenital aberrant course,[139,140] aneurysms, spontaneous and traumatic dissections, and lacerations. Aneurysm types include congenital, infectious (mycotic), pseudoaneurysms (traumatic), atherosclerotic, luetic, and fibromuscular dysplasia. Although upper cervical carotid aneurysms are associated with a high incidence of ischemic attacks and strokes, reports of rupture are unusual.[141-146] Petrous internal carotid artery aneurysms are associated with a high risk for cranial nerve dysfunction and aural hemorrhage.[147] In light of the natural history, observation is undesirable in most patients with internal carotid artery aneurysms unless other medical exigencies take precedence. Cervical carotid occlusion carries a high risk of cerebrovascular complications.

BTO aids in management decision-making (see Fig. 176-1).[148] CBF greater than 30 mL/100 g per minute carries a low risk for postocclusion infarction, thereby permitting surgical or endovascular trapping or occlusion. Surgical or permanent balloon trapping or occlusion, consisting of proximal cervical ligation or occlusion and supraclinoid internal carotid artery clipping or occlusion proximal to the ophthalmic artery, avoids late thromboembolic phenomena. Neurologic change observed on BTO or CBF less than 30 mL/100 g per minute necessitates some form of revascularization if the internal carotid artery is to be trapped or occluded. Transarterial detachable balloon trapping and cervical internal carotid artery occlusion preceded by extracranial-intracranial arterial bypass have been used.[29,149]

Preservation of internal carotid artery patency is desirable. Endovascular stenting has been performed for a petrous carotid pseudoaneurysm, preserving patency of the vessel and occluding the pseudoaneurysm with detachable coils,[150] as well as for extracranial

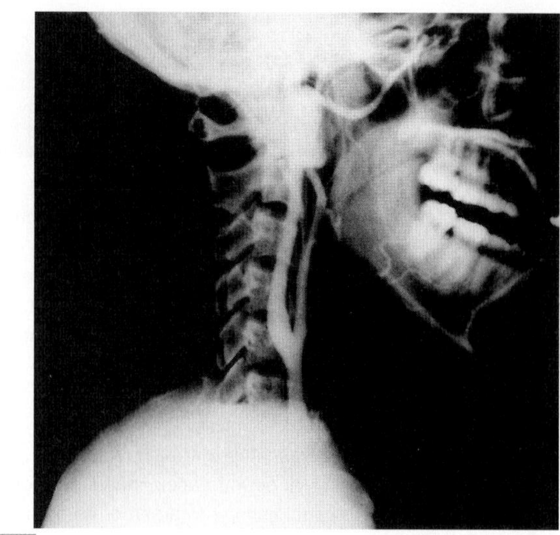

Figure 176-26. Preoperative angiogram of an upper cervical internal carotid aneurysm at the skull base.

aneurysms and dissections of the artery.[151,152] When surgical intervention is feasible or necessary, internal carotid artery reconstitution with direct reanastomosis or saphenous vein interposition grafting is preferable. A preauricular approach as described by several investigators[89,142,143,145,153] may be used to expose upper cervical carotid aneurysms, although these approaches are hindered by the facial nerve, mandible, styloid process, and tympanic bone. Lateral mandibulotomy may give access to upper cervical lesions.[154] For extension of the aneurysm to the skull base or vertical petrous internal carotid artery, the postauricular (Fisch type A or B) approach gives maximal vascular control with good distal exposure of the vessel[100,155] (Figs. 176-26 and 176-27) or routing a saphenous graft from the external carotid artery to the horizontal petrous internal carotid through a retroauricular groove.[153] Aneurysms involving the horizontal petrous segment may be approached through a Fisch type B or preauricular approach as described by Sekhar and coworkers.[91] Inadequate exposure and distal control of the horizontal petrous segment may lead to uncontrolled entry into these aneurysms. Some form of trapping with or without extracranial-intracranial bypass should be considered in patients with poorly accessible lesions.

Jugular Foramen Tumors

Tumors of the jugular foramen primarily include glomus jugulare (paraganglioma) and schwannomas of cranial nerves IX, X, and XI. The Fisch type A approach with transposition of the facial nerve and the Farrior approach[156] with limited mobilization of the vertical segment of the facial nerve both allow adequate exposure of the jugular bulb area. Donald and Chole[76] advocate a transcervical-transmastoid technique to gain access to the jugular fossa without transposing the facial nerve. This procedure, although technically feasible, provides less exposure and more limited vascular control but has the advantage of absence of facial nerve morbidity. Use of this technique is more desirable in cases in which extensive retrofacial air cells are present.

Schwannomas of the Jugular Foramen

Schwannomas originating from cranial nerves IX, X, and XI at the jugular foramen are decidedly uncommon, with only slightly more than 100 cases reported in the world's literature.[157] These tumors may be intracranial, intraforaminal, or cervical, or a combination thereof.[158] For removal of intracranial tumors, the suboccipital approach clearly is the most direct and effective route. Intraforaminal and combination tumors are removed in the safest manner through the infratemporal fossa approaches described by Fisch. These tumors originate anatomically from the pars nervosa of the jugular foramen and are situated anteromedial to the jugular bulb and internal jugular vein and posterior to the upper cervical and petrous internal carotid artery. Transposition of the facial nerve, as in the Fisch type A approach,[159] is helpful for

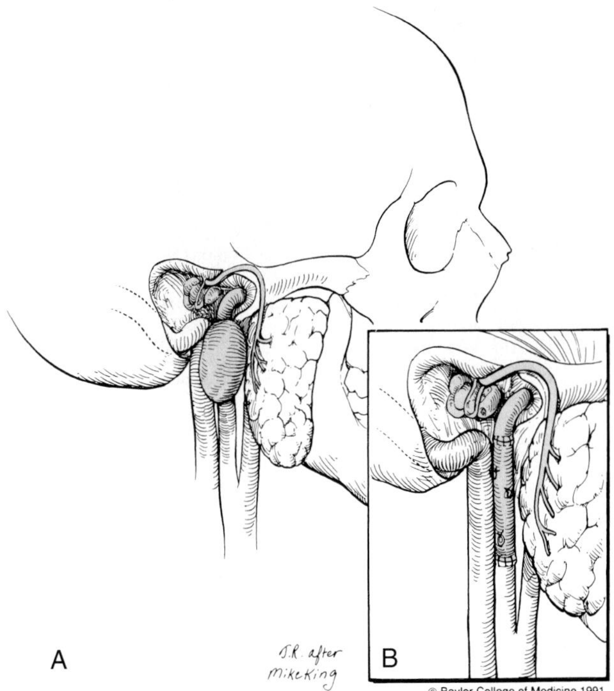

Figure 176-27. **A** and **B,** Saphenous vein repair of the aneurysm shown in Figure 176-26 with a Fisch type A infratemporal fossa approach.

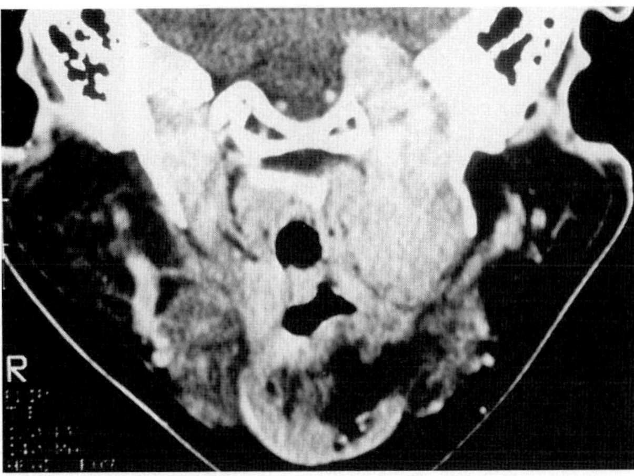

Figure 176-28. Coronal computed tomography scan revealing a jugular foramen schwannoma with a small intracranial extension removed by way of a Fisch type A infratemporal fossa approach.

control of these vascular structures and tumor exposure (Fig. 176-28). Farrior's limited approach also may have a role in small tumors.[160] Pellet[161] gave consideration to the use of an extended transcochlear route, in which a Fisch type A dissection is performed followed by sacrifice of the labyrinth to gain access to large tumors extending into the cerebellopontine angle. Oghalai and colleagues[162] describe a "transjugular craniotomy" whereby the facial nerve is not mobilized but left in a bridge of bone between an extended facial recess approach and a presigmoid craniotomy. These workers have used this technique for removal of intracranial glomus jugulare tumors.

Paragangliomas of the Temporal Bone

The glomus tumor of the temporal bone is the most frequently encountered neoplasm after the acoustic neuroma. Glomus tumors are divided into two broad categories on the basis of their site of origin: glomus tympanicum and glomus jugulare. Several classification systems have described paragangliomas of the temporal bone.[61,97,163,164] The classifications are similar and allow clinicians to communicate and compare findings and results.

Symptoms

Alford and Guilford[163] thoroughly described the signs, symptoms, and classification of glomus tumors of the temporal bone. The glomus tympanicum most frequently manifests with pulsatile tinnitus of insidious onset and a conductive hearing loss, although it also may be an incidental finding on routine physical examination.[165,166] The glomus jugulare tumor originates within the dome of the jugulare bulb and commonly appears late, after considerable growth and bony destruction. It may cause dysfunction of cranial nerves passing through the jugular bulb (cranial nerves IX to XII), facial nerve paresis caused by tumor extension into the mastoid, or sensorineural hearing loss caused by bony erosion of the labyrinth. Occasionally, either a glomus tympanicum or a glomus jugulare tumor may erode the tympanic membrane and appear as a bleeding mass in the external auditory canal.

Diagnostic Evaluation

Accurate diagnosis and evaluation of the extent of a glomus tumor of the temporal bone require appropriate physical examination and radiologic assessment.[167] The physical examination infrequently differentiates between the two kinds of glomus tumors. Only if all borders of the tumor are visible through the tympanic membrane can it be assumed that it is a glomus tympanicum tumor. If all of the borders are not visible behind the tympanic membrane, the tumor may be either a large glomus tympanicum tumor or a much larger glomus jugulare tumor that extends from the jugular bulb into the hypotympanum. If cranial nerve abnormalities are associated with a lesion, it is more likely to be a glomus jugulare tumor.

Although physical examination helps deduce the extent of a paraganglioma, radiologic evaluation is required to precisely define the lesion. CT and MRI usually are used for this evaluation (Fig. 176-29; see also Fig. 176-2). Glomus jugulare tumors require four-vessel angiography, for reasons previously discussed. Paragangliomas are vascular neoplasms. Arteriography is required if preoperative embolization of the lesions is desired. Such embolization takes place through specialized intra-arterial catheters and can lead to a marked reduction in vascularity of these masses, which reduces intraoperative blood loss and hemorrhage-related complications. The glomus jugulare paraganglioma, the most common of these tumors, causes somewhat selective erosion of the pars vasculosa portion of the jugular foramen. It also frequently destroys the bony septum between the internal carotid artery and the internal jugular vein. This bony septum is a distinctive structure whose absence is easily seen. Confounding lesions include schwannomas of cranial nerve IX, X, or XI, because these lesions also destroy the jugular foramen (Fig. 176-30). These lesions, however, usually destroy the more medial portion of the pars vasculosa or, if originating from cranial nerve IX, the pars nervosa.

At times, the paraganglioma manifest only after becoming large and eroding nearly all of the jugular foramen. Simple differentiation by the localization of bone erosion is not possible in such cases. MRI is helpful in defining these lesions, but results should be interpreted carefully. The complex flow characteristics of venous blood result in the presence of many signal artifacts in and about the jugular vein. Although experienced practitioners have become used to these artifacts, errors can still be made, and careful attention to the precontrast and postcontrast-enhanced MRI or fMRI is necessary so that the flow-related signal artifacts are not interpreted as a vascular lesion. Vasoactive peptides are produced by 1% to 3% of these tumors; therefore, patients should be screened with quantitative urine vanillylmandelic acid and hydroxyindoleacetic acid assays.

Surgical Approach

Only small glomus tympanicum tumors whose borders are clearly visible through the tympanic membrane can be removed through the external auditory canal. In radiologically proven glomus tympanicum tumors whose borders are not entirely visible through the tympanic

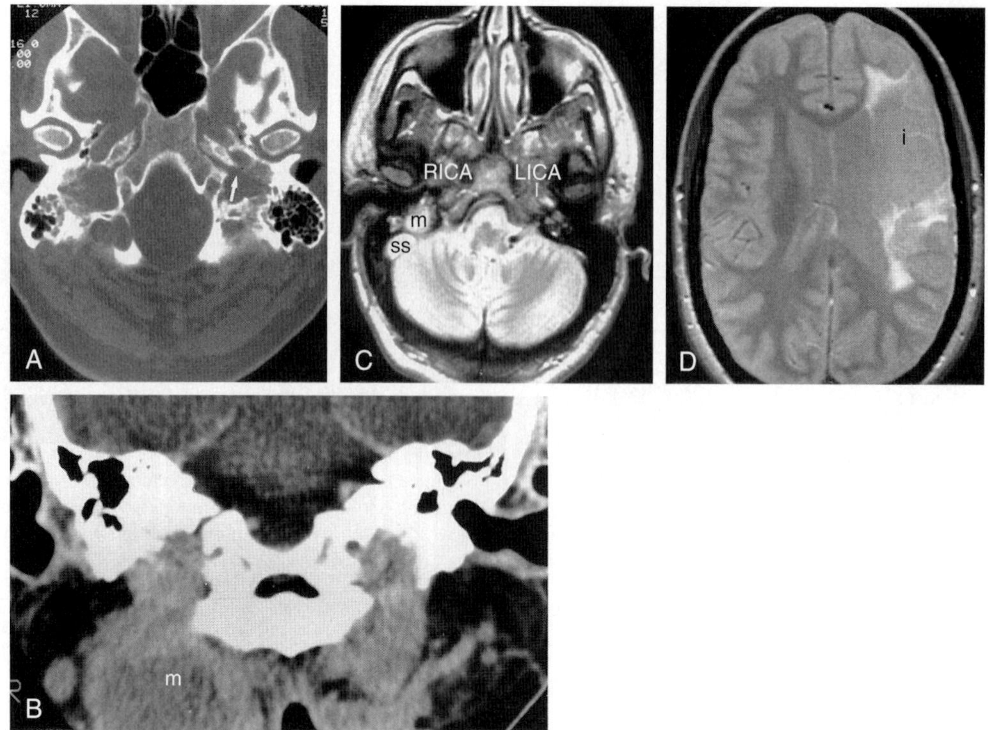

Figure 176-29. Familial paragangliomas in a 53-year-old woman.The tumors included bilateral glomus jugulare paragangliomas, a right-sided glomus vagale paraganglioma, and bilateral carotid body paragangliomas. **A,** Axial view, computed tomography (CT), bone algorithm. This CT study is performed with a small field of view and a bone algorithm to increase the resolution of bone edges. The bilateral glomus jugulare paragangliomas are destroying bone from the pars vasculosa laterally. On the left side, the lesion is destroying the septum between the internal carotid artery and the internal jugular vein. These are common findings in a glomus jugulare paraganglioma *(arrow)*. **B,** Coronal view, CT with intravenous contrast. Both glomus jugulare paragangliomas extend into the neck. However, another large mass can be seen on the right, a glomus vagale paraganglioma (m). **C,** Axial view, T2-weighted magnetic resonance imaging (MRI). The high-signal-intensity lesion, a glomus jugulare paraganglioma (m), has occluded the sigmoid sinus, which shows high-intensity signal (ss). The left internal carotid artery (LICA) shows signal of pathologic high intensity. This vessel has been occluded by a large paraganglioma in the neck *(not shown)*. Compare the signal intensity of this vessel with the normal dark black appearance of internal carotid artery flow on the right (RICA). Although MRI cannot provide the fine bony resolution of CT (see **B**), it gives more information about vascular patency. **D,** The LICA occlusion has resulted in a middle cerebral arterial distribution infarct (i).

membrane, the extended facial recess approach is recommended.[166] Occasionally, the facial recess is narrow, requiring removal of all or part of the bony posterior external auditory canal.

Glomus jugulare tumors are best approached by the Fisch type A route. Alternatively, Oghalai and colleagues[162] advocate a "transjugular craniotomy," which does not involve facial nerve transposition and its attendant morbidity. Staging may be necessary with those large tumors with extensive intracranial extension (Fig. 176-31). Bleeding intraoperatively remains a major problem in removal of glomus tumors. The efficacy of preoperative embolization of glomus tumors in reducing intraoperative blood loss is debated.[97] Some studies suggest major reduction in intraoperative blood loss and operative time after embolization.[50,67,168,169] Intraoperative ligation of the feeding vessels, such as the ascending pharyngeal, stylomastoid, caroticotympanic, internal maxillary, and superior tympanic arteries, before extirpation may lessen bleeding, although ancillary blood supply from various other sources may mitigate this result.[50] Piecemeal tumor removal, as in acoustic neuroma surgery, is impractical for management of these vascular tumors and often will result in hemorrhage, obscuring anatomic landmarks.

Lack of cranial nerve dysfunction is not a reliable indicator of intraoperative nerve integrity in patients with these tumors.[170] Cranial nerves VII and IX to XII may be involved at the skull base. In superficial involvement, segmental removal of involved epineurium may clear the tumor. Neural invasion requires segmental neurectomy. Paragangliomas often invade the periosteum of the carotid canal but rarely involve the adventitia itself.[60] Good preoperative angiographic assessment is of absolute necessity. A subperiosteal plane of dissection is developed intraoperatively. If the adventitia is involved, surgical manipulation may result in a large laceration of the carotid artery. Preoperative transarterial permanent balloon occlusion of the internal carotid artery should be considered in those tumors with infiltration of the wall of the horizontal petrous segment of the artery or with intracranial extension receiving significant blood supply from the artery and for reasons identified in Figure 176-1. If the status of the internal carotid artery is not appreciated preoperatively, several options are possible. Lacerations may be sutured directly. Saphenous vein interposition grafting may be performed with or without shunt placement.[48] The internal carotid artery may be transarterially balloon-occluded intraoperatively with or without angiographic confirmation, depending on the urgency of the situation.[60,61,169]

Radiotherapy

Although radiotherapy is not the modality of choice for treatment of surgically resectable glomus tumors of the temporal bone, tumor reductions after radiotherapy have been recorded.[171-173] Glomus tumors have been shown to have nonuniform responses, and tumor sterilization by radiotherapy is infrequent. Radiotherapy is useful for management of recurrences and unresectable lesions.

Facial Nerve Schwannomas

Schwannomas may involve the facial nerve along its intracranial, intratemporal, or extratemporal course. Altmann[174] presented the first comprehensive description of a facial nerve schwannoma and believed that its symptoms were sufficiently pathognomonic for the facial nerve schwannoma to be diagnosed clinically. These reported cases generally

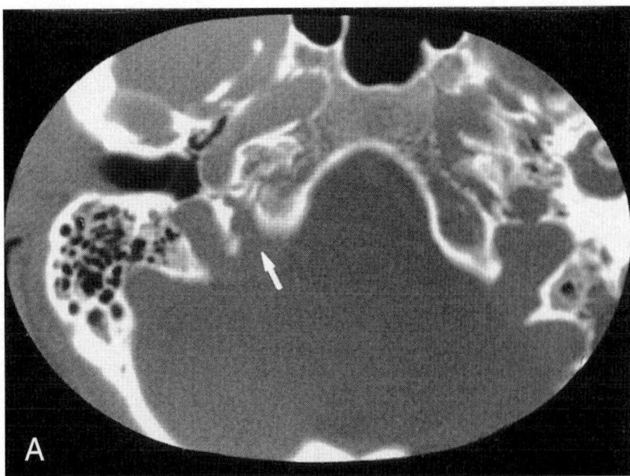

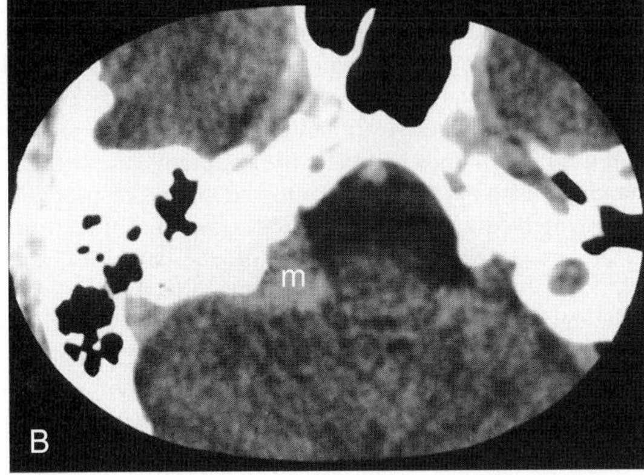

Figure 176-30. Right glossopharyngeal schwannoma in a 50-year-old woman **A,** Axial view, computed tomography bone algorithm. The neoplasm has focally expanded and destroyed the pars nervosa portion of the jugular foramen *(arrow)*. This is a helpful finding in this type of schwannoma. **B,** Axial view, computed tomography brain algorithm. This patient's neoplasm is large. It has ascended past the cochlear aqueduct toward the internal acoustic canal. If only this level were viewed, the mass (m) could simulate a vestibular schwannoma.

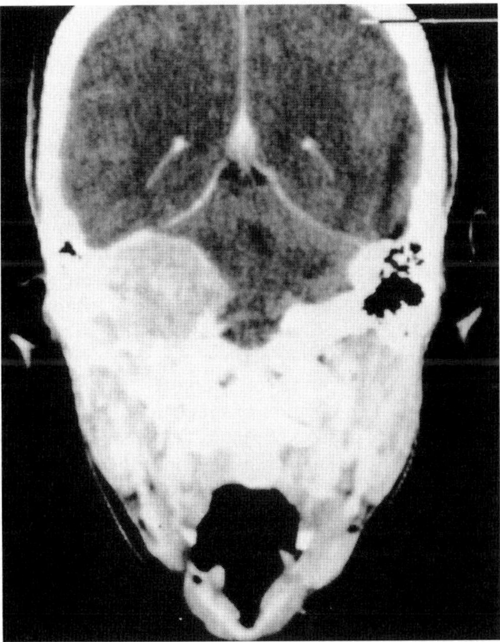

Figure 176-31. Paraganglioma of the jugular bulb with intracranial extension. The tumor was removed in one stage using a Fisch type A infratemporal fossa approach.

were diagnosed late; the patients presented with long-standing facial nerve paralysis and obstruction of the external auditory canal with tumor. More recently, with the increased awareness of this clinical entity and improved neurotologic diagnostic methods, earlier diagnosis is possible.

Diagnostic Evaluation

Facial weakness has been the most common presenting symptom in a number of series.[175,176] The classic history is one of slowly progressive facial paralysis over months to years, not days to weeks, although sudden onset of paralysis, fluctuating paresis, and facial tic may occur.[177] Hearing loss is the second most common presenting manifestation.[178] Conductive hearing loss may occur with middle ear involvement caused by tumor expansion and pressure on or disruption of the ossicular chain. In such cases, a gray-white polypoid mass frequently can be seen behind the posterosuperior tympanic membrane. Sensorineural hearing loss may result from erosion into the labyrinth or tumor compression on the cochlear nerve.

An intratemporal facial nerve schwannoma generally extends along the course of the facial nerve for a greater distance than that anticipated from the clinical or radiologic findings. The schwannoma visualized in the middle ear may extend intracranially into the internal auditory canal and cerebellopontine angle or extratemporally into the parotid gland. Preoperative radiologic assessment addresses this potential spread, but the surgeon should be prepared for more extensive nerve involvement than that suggested by clinical or radiologic testing. Topographic testing of facial nerve function, including tearing, stapedius reflex, taste, and salivation, may be helpful, but it is not definitive in the evaluation of the extent of facial nerve neuroma. Definitive assessment of facial canal alterations is made with axial and coronal temporal bone CT. The entire bony path of the facial nerve can be traced with certainty. In the normal structure, seldom is much variation observed in this path from side to side. Hence, it is simple to compare right and left to determine abnormality. The most common abnormality seen in patients with facial schwannomas is simple enlargement of the fallopian canal by a soft tissue mass. These lesions usually follow the exact path of the facial nerve. One great mimic of facial schwannomas is the facial nerve hemangioma. This uncommon lesion probably originates from arteriovenous plexus around the geniculate ganglion, internal auditory canal, or vertical segment of the facial nerve near the chorda tympani takeoff.[179] Differential diagnostic imaging characteristics include calcification-based higher CT attenuation in a hemangioma compared with a schwannoma. MRI is superior to CT in delineating a soft tissue mass along the facial nerve, especially when MRI contrast material is used. This material provides such sensitivity that the arteriovenous plexus along the fallopian portion of the facial nerve is visualized. This plexus normally can enhance in a spotty fashion, making it possible for inexperienced practitioners to identify this abnormality. In addition, inflammatory lesions of the facial nerve also will result in contrast enhancement. Accordingly, facial nerve enhancement on MRI should not be considered to be indicative of neoplasm unless a soft tissue mass is present. The clinical, CT, or MRI findings should be correlated before diagnosis of a facial nerve neoplasm. If this correlation is not definite, later follow-up imaging evaluation after a clinically appropriate amount of time has passed should resolve the issue.

In some patients with facial paralysis, radiologic evidence for tumor is lacking. Surgical exploration of all progressive facial palsies that occur over an extended period of time or facial palsies that show no return of tone or function after 6 to 12 months has been recommended, and facial schwannomas occasionally are discovered.

Management and Surgical Approach

Timing of intervention requires extensive discussion with the patient, especially if facial function is intact. McMonagle and coworkers advocate observation with serial scans until facial function deteriorates to House-Brackmann grade IV.[180] The management goals of facial nerve neuroma surgery are complete removal of the tumor with preservation of hearing and restoration of facial nerve function.[181,182] Most commonly, the transmastoid and middle cranial fossa approaches are

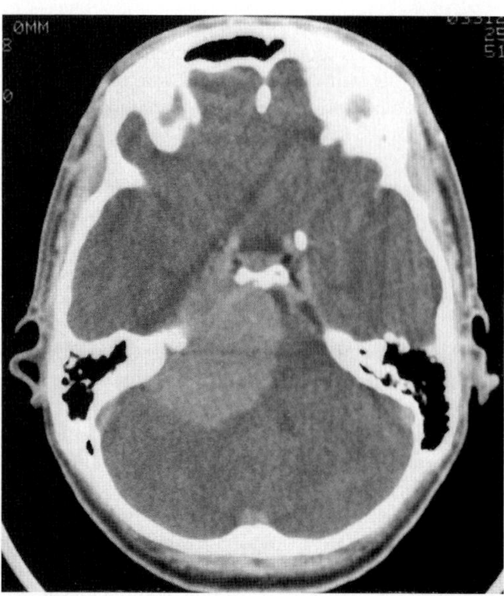

Figure 176-32. Computed tomography scan of a large posterior fossa meningioma with petrous apex involvement. The tumor was removed through a retrosigmoid craniotomy with petrosectomy, with posterior facial nerve transposition.

adequate for exposure of neuromas of the intralabyrinthine facial nerve segments. In patients with no serviceable hearing, a translabyrinthine exposure of the facial nerve may be indicated. Surgical removal and cable grafting of the facial nerve with frozen section histologic control is indicated in most patients. The nerve graft usually is placed in the fallopian canal, and its ends are approximated and stabilized with packing. Approximation of the cable graft to the facial nerve stump in the internal auditory canal is difficult. When the involved segment of nerve is limited to less than 1 cm, a facial nerve transposition and primary anastomosis sometimes can be performed. If primary anastomosis or cable grafting fail, hypoglossofacial anastomosis may be necessary (see Chapters 171 and 172).

Petrous Apex Lesions

Primary tumors of the petrous apex, either benign or low-grade neoplasms, such as cholesteatoma, schwannoma, chondroma, meningioma, chordoma, and low-grade sarcomas, are best removed totally to prevent recurrence.[183-185] The infratemporal fossa approaches to the petrous apex (i.e., Fisch type B or perhaps type A approach) give better exposure and control of the internal carotid artery and may be combined with the middle cranial fossa, retrosigmoid, transcochlear, or translabyrinthine routes as needed (Fig. 176-32). In patients with serviceable hearing, the petrous internal carotid artery may be temporarily transposed to gain access to the petrous apex with major risk of hemorrhage. The combination of the transcochlear or translabyrinthine route with posterior translocation of the facial nerve offers the best access to the petrous apex (see Figs. 176-20 and 176-32). Total temporal bone resection also is an option for low grade maligancies.

Benign cystic lesions such as cholesterol granulomas or cephaloceles are generally not extirpated. Drainage of cholesterol granulomas can be performed through the perilabyrinthine pathways[186] (see also Chapters 139 and 140) or transsphenoidally using endoscopic imaging guidance.[187-189] Symptomatic petrous apex cephaloceles can be either marsupialized intracranially using a posterior fossa approach or obliterated through a middle cranial foassa approach.[190]

Congenital Cholesteatoma

Congenital cholesteatomas of the temporal bone may be divided into four anatomic groups: middle ear, perigeniculate area, petrous apex, and cerebellopontine angle. These cholesteatomas originate from epithelial rests and should be distinguished from acquired cholesteatomas and from congenital auditory canal cholesteatomas associated with congenital atresia of the external auditory canal.

Diagnostic Evaluation

The clinical presentation of a congenital cholesteatoma varies, depending on its location. Middle ear cholesteatomas originally were described by House,[191] and clinical series have been reviewed by House and Sheehy[59] and Curtis.[192] Conductive hearing loss and a bulging whitish mass behind an intact tympanic membrane are common findings in patients with middle ear congenital cholesteatomas.[193] One half of all patients present with recurrent otitis media, and the lesions may fistulize through the tympanic membrane. The lesions also may be discovered incidentally at the time of a myringotomy or routine physical examination in children. Perigeniculate and petrous apex cholesteatomas usually present with insidious or rapidly progressive facial nerve paralysis.[194,195] Sensorineural hearing loss from labyrinthine or internal auditory canal erosion is common, but a conductive hearing loss also may result from cholesteatoma extension into the middle ear or blockage of the eustachian tube. Facial twitching may occur in the presence of congenital cholesteatomas and with facial nerve neuromas. Vestibular dysfunction may complete the symptom complex. On occasion, the cholesteatoma may erode into the middle or posterior fossa and expand markedly before producing symptoms. Preservation of hearing despite extensive destruction of the labyrinth has been reported.[45,74]

Radiologic evaluation of the temporal bone is essential in the evaluation of a congenital cholesteatoma (Fig. 176-33). Only the largest lesions will show on plain radiographs. High-resolution, focused CT of the temporal bone is ideal in this evaluation, because any alteration in normal bony structure can be seen. At times, the normal asymmetry in aeration, inflammatory, or passive effusion and bone marrow deposition in the petrous apices can cause diagnostic difficulties. These difficulties usually are resolved by clinical correlation; if the findings are problematic, MRI will provide further definition, because congenital cholesteatomas almost always will have a slightly higher signal intensity than that of spinal fluid on T1-weighted images, with moderately high signal intensity on T2-weighted images. By contrast, bone marrow fat will have a high signal intensity on T1-weighted images and then go on to fade dramatically on T2-weighted images. Typical effusions will have a low signal intensity on T1-weighted sequences, with high signal intensity on T2-weighted sequences. Giant cholesterol granulomas can be difficult to separate from congenital cholesteatomas of the petrous apex (Fig. 176-34), although giant cholesterol granulomas, but not congenital cholesteatomas, tend to show capsular enhancement.

Surgical Approach

Surgical management of a congenital cholesteatoma requires either complete removal of the cholesteatoma matrix or permanent exteriorization. The isolated middle ear cholesteatoma may be removed transtympanically. At surgery, it is essential to visualize clearly the complete extent of the cholesteatoma in the middle ear, particularly on the medial aspect of the tympanic membrane. Routine middle ear reconstructive techniques may be used if ossicles are eroded or removed or if the tympanic membrane is sacrificed. Removal of congenital cholesteatomas of the perigeniculate area or petrous apex may be accomplished by the transmastoid, middle cranial fossa approach,[196] the transsphenoidal approach,[197] or by a combination of these procedures.[94] Frequently, a cholesteatoma must be dissected from the facial nerve, and occasionally, the intralabyrinthine portion of the nerve must be mobilized to allow complete removal of a perigeniculate cholesteatoma. This maneuver may require sectioning of the greater superficial petrosal nerve and transposition of the facial nerve posteriorly at the geniculate ganglion. The cholesteatoma also may insinuate itself between the dura and the middle fossa floor and may extend for a considerable distance along this plane. Petrous apex cholesteatomas may act similarly and erode the bony labyrinth or internal auditory canal. Only by careful and often tedious dissection can injury to these structures be prevented. Cholesteatomas of the petrous apex may be exteriorized into the mastoid cavity or the sphenoid sinus, although frequent cleansing of debris from

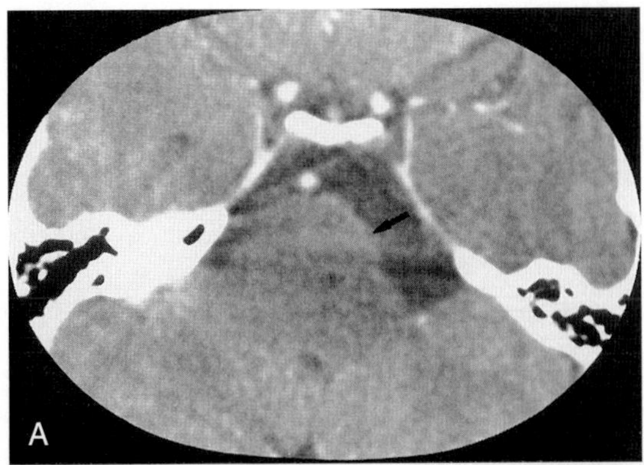

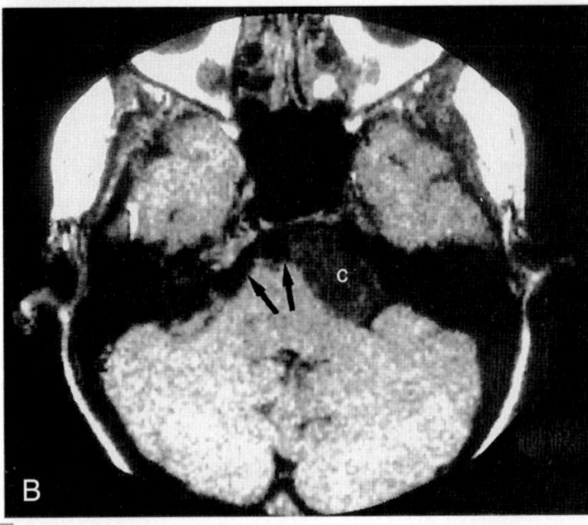

Figure 176-33. Left cerebellopontine cistern congenital epidermoid cyst in a 36-year-old man. **A,** Axial view, computed tomography (CT). Displacement of the pons to the right *(arrow)*. This displacement seems to be caused by cerebrospinal fluid (CSF) attenuation material. Accordingly, this could be an arachnoid cyst. **B,** Axial view, T1-weighted noncontrast magnetic resonance imaging. The cystic lesion (c) is now clearly seen to have higher-intensity signal than the CSF in the right cerebellopontine angle cistern *(arrows)*. This slightly higher signal intensity on T1-weighted images is helpful in separating epidermoid cysts from arachnoid cysts. This relative hyperintensity is caused by lipid, mostly cholesterin. The lipid is not seen on the CT scan as low attenuation because higher-attenuation keratin is mixed with the cholesterin. The sum of these two components balances out to nearly CSF attenuation.

the cholesteatoma cavity is required to prevent inspissations and subsequent infection.[198]

Encephalocele and Cerebrospinal Fluid Leaks

Postsurgical and postinfectious encephaloceles herniating through the tegmen tympani and tegmen mastoideum are well-recognized complications in otology.[199-201] Temporal bone herniation of the mastoid cavity is a result of loss of bony and dural support. Subsequent management should deal with CSF leakage, herniation of the brain into the mastoid cavity, and skin and cholesteatoma matrix in the middle ear and mastoid. Less frequently recognized is a spontaneous congenital encephalocele associated with CSF otorrhea or rhinorrhea.[202-207]

Diagnostic Evaluation

The appearance of postsurgical encephaloceles may occur early or late in the postoperative course. Early occurrences generally are associated with maceration of exposed brain and CSF leakage. Late occurrences are associated with pulsatile tinnitus and/or progressive prolapse of skin-covered brain into the mastoid cavity. Spontaneous congenital encephalocele may manifest as serous otitis media, CSF rhinorrhea, or CSF otorrhea through a tympanic membrane perforation or pressure-equalizing tube. Occasionally, prolapsed brain can be present as a mass behind the tympanic membrane. Because small and often multiple bony defects can be involved, carefully focused CT in the axial and coronal planes is needed to find these fenestrations. If necessary, the subarachnoid space can be opacified with myelographic contrast material, and the actual flow of the contrast-opacified spinal fluid through the fenestrations can be observed. Occasionally, encephaloceles also may be discovered as an intraoperative surprise.

Surgical Approach

Temporal bone encephaloceles and CSF leaks may be surgically approached either transmastoidally or through the middle cranial fossa intradurally or extradurally. Although transmastoid repair of the defect frequently is successful, repair through the middle cranial fossa allows greater visualization. Techniques for repair of the tegmen defect through the mastoid approach have included intracranial placement of reconstructive material (i.e., fascia, cartilage, or prosthetics) from the mastoid combined with obliteration of the mastoid with flaps or free tissue.[200,204,205,207,208] A fascia (banked)-bone-fascia technique incorporating use of a modified radical cavity, with neurosurgical consultation, followed by postoperative lumbar drainage, has been used successfully on several occasions by one of us (MM). A middle cranial fossa approach for repair provides greater visualization and can be either extradural or intradural.[209,210] A variety of closure techniques, including primary dural repair and fascia-bone-fascia, bone, cartilage, or synthetic supports, have been used. The bony and dural defects in spontaneous encephaloceles are routinely small and multiple.[211] Frequently, an encephalocele exists in the anterior epitympanum, where visualization may be inadequate and surgical repair through the transmastoid approach is difficult without ossicular disruption. Although transmastoid exposure defines the defect, repair may be better accomplished through the middle cranial fossa. The bony defects usually are small and do not require repair. The dural defects can be sealed by wide coverage of the middle cranial fossa with temporalis fascia and bone or cartilage as necessary.

Approaches to the Clivus

Clival tumor extirpation, both planning and execution, is perhaps the most difficult of skull base surgical procedures. Surrounding neurovascular structures of the brainstem and both internal carotid arteries are at risk during surgery. House and Hitselberger[103] reported use of a transcochlear route to the petrous tip and midclivus, sacrificing ipsilateral cochlear and vestibular function. This approach may be useful in removing tumors that are not intrinsic (primary) neoplasms of the clival bone itself, such as cholesteatoma and meningioma, because only the dorsal midclivus is exposed. The Fisch type B approach is useful for removal of tumors involving the midclivus with extension to the petrous apex.[61] Tumor extension medial and superior to the horizontal segment of the internal carotid artery in the petrous apex requires temporary transposition of the artery. Adding a middle cranial fossa subdural dissection may circumvent this problem.

A transcochlear dissection added to a Fisch type B approach also may improve access to the clivus. Tumor of the posterior clinoid (retrosellar) is not accessible through this route, but an intradural middle cranial fossa approach may be of benefit.[212]

With the preauricular approaches,[92,105] limitations are similar to those for techniques already discussed, but the transcochlear route cannot be used for further exposure in combination with the preauricular approach. Numerous anterior approaches to the clivus also have been described (see also Chapter 173).[124,213-217] Transnasal endoscopically assisted approaches also may result in complete extirpation with greatly reduced morbidity compared with lateral skull base or facial translocation anterior techniques (see also Chapter 174).[218] Hanna and colleagues have begun exploring robotic endoscopic surgery of the anterior and central skull base.[219]

Lesions Involving the Cavernous Sinus

The cavernous sinus is a small plexus of veins enclosed by leaves of dura on either side of the sella turcica.[220] In the cavernous sinus lie the internal carotid artery, sympathetic nerves, and cranial nerves III, IV,

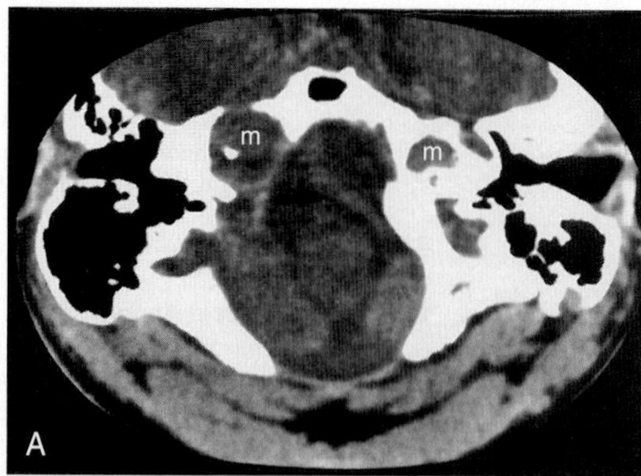

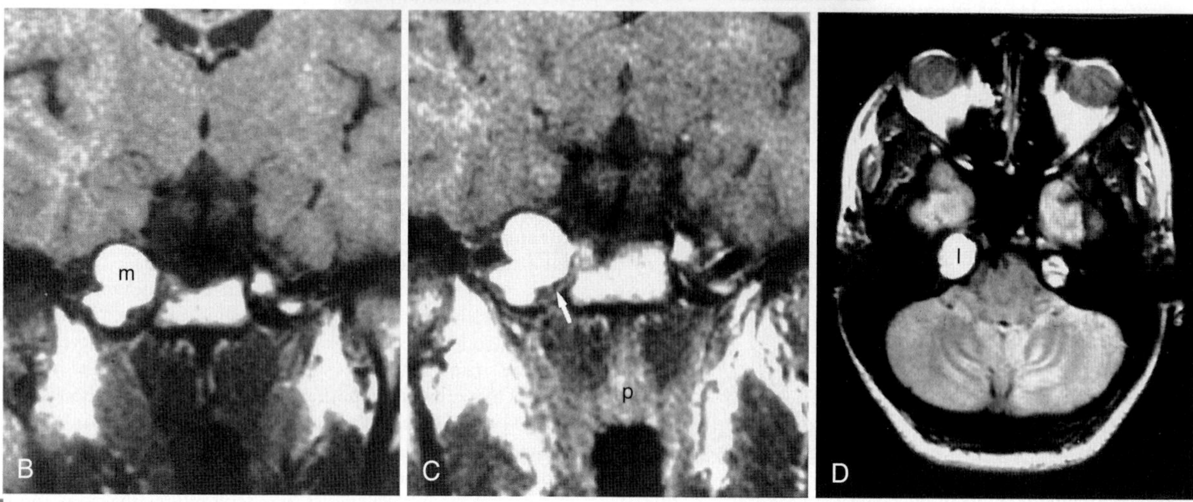

Figure 176-34. Cholesterol cysts in a 21-year-old woman. **A,** Axial view, computed tomography (CT) with intravenous contrast. Expansile, slightly low-attenuation masses (m) are seen in both petrous apices. **B,** Coronal view, T1-weighted sequence on noncontrast magnetic resonance imaging (MRI). High signal intensity is evident within both petrous apices, more pronounced in the larger, right-sided mass (m). **C,** Coronal view, T1-weighted sequence on MRI after administration of intravenous gadolinium contrast material. The edges of the lesion show enhancement *(arrow)*. The larger high-signal-intensity portion does not change. Notice the increased signal intensity in the pharyngeal mucosa (p). This is a normal finding after gadolinium administration. **D,** Axial view, T2-weighted MRI. The right-sided lesion (l) shows extremely high signal intensity. The left-sided lesion is similar but intensty increase is less marked. There is only slight inhomogeneity in this signal reflected by small patches of lower signal intensity. The combination of the CT appearance with extremely high signal intensity on T1- and T2-weighted sequences is distinctive for a cholesterol cyst. The slight inhomogeneity in the lesions is due to bone fragments, calcification, and small hemorrhages of varying ages.

VI, V_1, and sometimes V_2. Primary tumors of the cavernous sinus commonly include meningiomas or schwannomas,[89] but this region usually is invaded secondarily. Operations involving the cavernous sinus are fraught with potential complications, including bleeding, cranial nerve deficits, and carotid injury. Palliative therapy such as with conventional irradiation or gamma knife techniques may be warranted for patients with lesions in this location.

Chordoma

Cranial chordomas originate from the clivus and progressively destroy the skull base[202,204,206] (Figs. 176-35 and 176-36). They may extend ventrally into the nasopharynx, nose, or sinuses and cause obstruction. Headache, loss of vision, and cranial nerve deficits with involvement of the abducens, trigeminal, facial, and acoustic nerves are common presenting complaints. Because of the inaccessibility of the tumor site, surgical exposure and tumor removal may be difficult. Surgical debulking of the tumor followed by high-dose radiotherapy is historically the treatment of choice and may afford good palliative results. More recently, skull base surgeons have become more aggressive, tailoring surgical approaches to individual lesions to ensure complete removal. Because of the difficult accessibility, surgical control of chordoma is a unique challenge to the skull base surgeon and lends itself to creative surgical approaches (see Chapter 173). Anterior, endoscopic approaches rather than lateral skull base approaches are being pioneered to resect these difficult tumors, with great promise (see also Chapter 174).[218]

Tumors of the Parapharyngeal Space

Tumors involving the infratemporal fossa or parapharyngeal space at the skull base and extending into the temporal bone or middle cranial fossa require lateral skull base techniques. For tumors confined to the parapharyngeal space, a cervical approach, often with mandibular transection, may be indicated. Radical en bloc procedures for malignancy may require removal of the mandibular ramus and condyle.[221,222] A labiomandibulotomy[223,224] or extraoral mandibulotomy will give improved access to the tumor within the middle to upper infratemporal fossa. Reflection of the temporalis muscle and zygoma provides improved access to the superior infratemporal fossa. Retracting the mandibular condyle or resecting it may obtain further exposure. Middle cranial fossa approach may be added for superior extension (Fig. 176-37).

Approaches to the Nasopharynx

In patients with extensive benign tumors of the nasopharynx (e.g., juvenile angiofibromas), a lateral approach may be indicated. These approaches may be combined with any of the anterior approaches as the situation warrants. The Fisch type C (see Fig. 176-22) and Sekhar lateral approaches to the nasopharynx provide similar exposures, and either approach may be extended to include removal of tumor from the sphenoid sinus or pericavernous sinus area. Transmaxillary endoscopic approaches also may provide adequate exposure while minimizing operative morbidity (see Chapter 175).

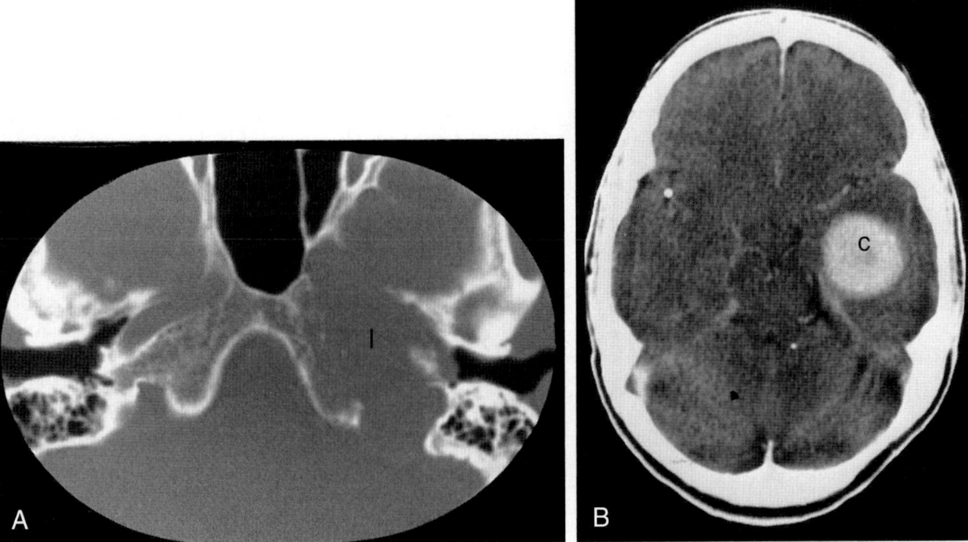

Figure 176-35. Massive petrous apex chordoma on the left in a 57-year-old man. **A,** Axial view, bone algorithm computed tomography (CT). Off-midline destructive changes characteristic of this lesion (I). Whereas most chordomas are midline, some can be quite far lateral. **B,** Axial view, brain CT with intravenous contrast. The chordoma (c) was so large that it extended up into the left temporal lobe.

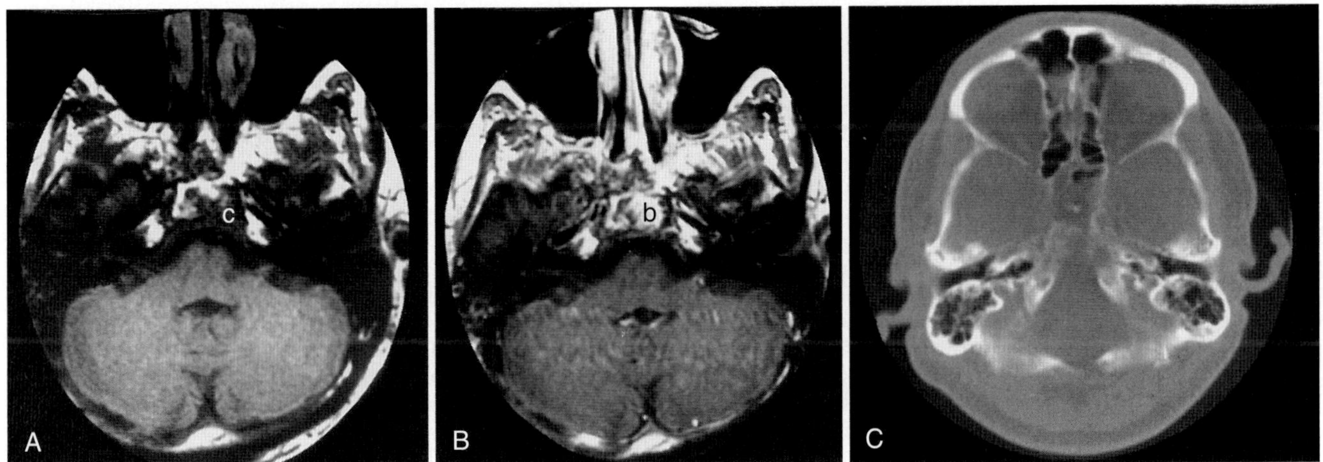

Figure 176-36. Clivus chordoma in a 59-year-old man. **A,** Axial view, T1-weighted magnetic resonance imaging (MRI). Subtle permeative changes can be seen extending into the clival bone marrow. The chordoma (c) is the darker area (of lower signal intensity) invading the brighter area (high-signal intensity) normal bone marrow fat. **B,** Axial view, T1-weighted MRI, after administration of intravenous gadolinium contrast material. The area of low signal intensity on the previous scan demonstrates markedly increased intensity (b). However, it is difficult to assess the degree of bone destruction with MRI. **C,** Standard computed tomography (CT), bone windows. Even on this nonfocused CT scan, the gross destructive changes associated with this clivus chordoma are visible. MRI is less sensitive than CT in showing bone destruction.

Excision of malignant lesions of the nasopharynx is fraught with controversy. Wang[225] has shown that patients with recurrent squamous cell carcinoma of the nasopharynx staged T_1 to T_3 may have improved survival rates if the lesions are excised. Fisch type C approach and Sekhar's approach permit en bloc removal of the lateral nasopharyngeal wall with the pterygoid and tubal musculature for persistent or recurrent tumor postradiation.

Complications

Intraoperative Complications

Intraoperative complications result mostly from lack of vascular control or coagulopathy. Management of unexpected blood loss from an internal carotid artery laceration is facilitated by proximal and distal control before repair. A lack of exposure may result in the need for emergency intraoperative balloon occlusion and ligation when hemorrhage occurs. Bleeding from the cavernous sinus can be massive, and an air embolus may occur, although this bleeding can be stopped with patient application of oxidized cellulose hemostatic strips (Surgicel). Carotid spasm may require termination of the procedure.[97]

Coagulopathy may occur as a result of massive transfusions of packed erythrocytes from citrate-induced hypocalcemia, depletion of clotting cascade proteins, hypothermia, thrombocytopenia, disseminated intravascular coagulopathy, or incompatible blood. When massive transfusion is necessary, 2 units of fresh frozen plasma and platelets should be given for every 10 units of packed erythrocytes.[226] Vasoactive glomus tumors or concomitant pheochromocytomas may lead to unexpected hypertension intraoperatively. For this reason, patients with glomus should be screened preoperatively with urine vanillylmandelic acid and hydroxyindoleacetic acid assays to rule out vasoactive tumors.

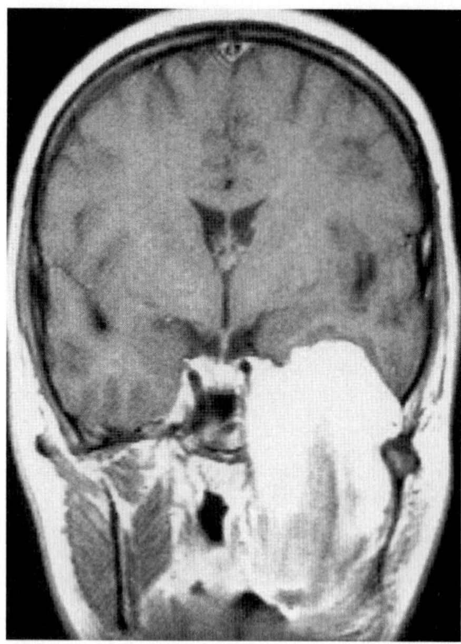

Figure 176-37. Intracranial-extracranial trigeminal schwannoma: Coronal view, magnetic resonance imaging. Excision through a preauricular approach with extraoral transection of mandible and temporal craniotomy.

Postoperative Complications

CSF leakage is one of the more common postoperative complications from infratemporal fossa surgery when the dural space must be entered. The risk of meningitis with high attendant morbidity rate is increased, as is length of hospital stay. Postoperative lower cranial nerve deficits leading to aspiration and subsequent coughing increases CSF pressure, adding another adverse variable to the management equation. Most CSF collections beneath flaps may be managed with compressive dressings, head elevation, and repeated aspirations. A lumbar subarachnoid drain best manages leakage of CSF through the wound or persistent otorhinorrhea.

In patients with large tumors and intracranial extension, the subarachnoid space should be entered for tumor exposure and extirpation. Jackson and associates[97] secured autogenous fascia to existing bone or dural margins for small to medium dural defects with temporalis muscle rotations for reinforcement. Obliteration with fat is not used. For larger defects, Gulya and coworkers[227] have used an infant-size ventriculocardiac shunt from the wound bed to the jugular stump to the right atrium, to allow continuous drainage. Lumbar subarachnoid drains combined with pressure dressings usually suffice to control leakage for large dural defects.

Cranial Nerve Deficits

The invasive nature of glomus tumors, especially those extending into the posterior fossa, has led historically to rather high rates of postoperative paralysis. Aside from intraoperative electrophysiologic monitoring,[80] the proximal identification of cranial nerves IX, X, XI, and XII in the posterior fossa and distal identification at the skull base should improve preservation of these nerves.[101] Unfortunately, these cranial nerves often are encased in tumor extending transdurally into the posterior fossa toward the root entry zones, making their preservation extremely difficult.

Most preoperative cranial nerve deficits persist postoperatively if they result from tumor invasion rather than compression. Creation of new cranial deficits, although necessary for complete tumor removal, can result in a prolonged rehabilitative phase and substantially reduce the quality of life. The patient's age and cardiopulmonary status should be carefully weighed against the tumor pathology, extent of disease, and natural course of the disease. Responses to other forms of therapy, such as radiotherapy or chemotherapy, should be considered before extensive skull base surgery is attempted. Younger, healthier patients, in general, tolerate new cranial deficits better than older patients do. Patients with marginal cardiac output are at high risk for myocardial infarction or congestive heart failure when subjected to prolonged surgery and recovery; those with compromised pulmonary function have poor tolerance for the problems created by lower cranial nerve deficiency (i.e., aspiration and decreased cough).

The oculomotor nerve can potentially be injured in cavernous sinus surgery or orbital apex. Neurapraxia or axonotmesis usually leads to a good functional recovery in 2 to 8 months, respectively. Functional recovery with reanastomosis after transection has been reported.[228] Loss of the trochlear nerve is reported to be associated with minimal functional disability. Good recovery with reanastomosis has been reported.[175] The abducens nerve has the longest intracranial course and is most prone to injury, especially in surgery for tumors of the clivus, petrous apex, or cavernous sinus. Good functional return should be expected with stretch injury, because this is a purely motor nerve.[228]

Prevention of facial nerve paresis already has been mentioned. If transection is required and the site optional, it is best to section the nerve at tertiary branches to limit synkinesis. In order of reconstructive preference for the facial nerve, options include direct reanastomosis, interposition grafting, and cranial nerve XII to VII crossover. Ocular care, with prevention of exposure keratitis, especially if the V_2 branch has been sacrificed, is of paramount importance postoperatively if the facial nerve has been injured. A lateral tarsorrhaphy affords the best protection to the eye for a combination deficit involving cranial nerves V and VII.

The approaches by Fisch to the infratemporal fossa by definition preserve cochleovestibular function. Inadvertent stapes subluxation or tumor invasion of the otic capsule may lead to sensorineural hearing loss. Exposure of the upper cervical internal carotid commonly entails loss of the glossopharyngeal nerve. Sequelae from its loss are infrequent, except when such loss is combined with other lower cranial nerve defects involving X and XII. Intraoperative reanastomosis of a vagal nerve is not indicated because of an association with paradoxic vocal cord motion. High vagal injuries can lead to a prolonged rehabilitative period. Not only are the quality of voice and protective sphincter function breached, but deglutition also is impaired through disruption of the pharyngeal plexus; when combined with losses of cranial nerves IX and XII, its loss may be debilitating. Persistent aspiration will lead to pneumonia. Tracheostomy is indicated if paresis of this combination of nerves is expected. Vocal cord medialization with endoscopic polytetrafluorethylene (Teflon) or surgical gel (Gelfoam) injection may be considered to protect the airway. Modified barium swallow may help in the decision regarding the need for a temporary feeding gastrostomy when aspiration persists.

Injury to the spinal accessory nerve usually is well tolerated in skull base procedures, because C2 and C3 ventral roots supply some motor innervation to the trapezius muscle. The suprascapular muscle also has a role in shoulder girdle stabilization. Nevertheless, reanastomosis or interposition grafting should be performed, if possible. Physical therapy and exercise instruction often are helpful in preventing persistent shoulder dysfunction.

The hypoglossal nerve often is involved with tumors of the clivus or jugular foramen. Because use of the hypoglossal nerve is an important reanimation option in facial nerve injury, its preservation is of added importance. Unilateral hypoglossal nerve loss usually is well tolerated unless combined with cranial nerve IX and X paralysis. Reconstruction of a transected hypoglossal nerve can lead to good functional recovery.[228]

Cerebrovascular Complications

The extensive manipulation of the internal carotid artery required by lateral skull base techniques understandably may lead to stroke. Preoperative angiographic evaluation and collateral circulation studies are mandatory. Anesthetic techniques such as increasing blood pressure, hypervolemia, pharmacologic vasodilation, calcium channel inhibitors, hemodilution, hyperosmolarity, and anticoagulation (when the carotid is occluded) theoretically reduce the risk.[229]

Cerebral edema or venous stroke is a concern, especially if a connection at the torcular Herophili is absent or if the vein of Labbé is interrupted.[7,8] Ligation of the sigmoid sinus is potentially more hazardous than extracranial jugular vein ligation. Collateral drainage through the superior and inferior petrosal sinuses may not be present. Presumably, the vertebral venous system compensates for posterior fossa outflow, and cerebral edema from venous occlusion is uncommon. At present, no good preoperative tests to predict this risk are available. Therefore, anastomotic veins, such as the superior petrosal sinus, inferior petrosal sinus, and mastoid emissary vein, should not be indiscriminately sacrificed.

SUGGESTED READINGS

Anand V. *Practical Endoscopic Skull Base Surgery.* Hong Kong: Plural Publishing; 2007.

Arriaga M, Curtin HD, Takahashi H, et al. The role of preoperative CT scans in staging external auditory meatus carcinoma: radiologic-pathologic correlation study. *Otolaryngol Head Neck Surg.* 1991;105:6-11.

Brackmann DE, Teufert KB. Chondrosarcoma of the skull base: long-term follow-up. *Otol Neurotol.* 2006;27:981-991.

Brackmann DE, Toh EH. Surgical management of petrous apex cholesterol granulomas. *Otol Neurotol.* 2002;23:529-533.

Coker NJ, Jenkins HA, Fisch U. Obliteration of the middle ear and mastoid cleft in subtotal petrosectomy: indications, technique, and results. *Ann Otol Rhinol Laryngol.* 1986;95(1 Pt 1):5-11.

DiNardo LJ, Pippin GW, Sismanis A. Image-guided endoscopic transsphenoidal drainage of select petrous apex cholesterol granulomas. *Otol Neurotol.* 2003;24:939-941.

Field M, Jungreis CA, Chengelis N, et al. Symptomatic cavernous sinus aneurysms: management and outcome after carotid occlusion and selective cerebral revascularization. *AJNR Am J Neuroradiol.* 2003;24:1200-1207.

Fisch U, Mattox D. *Microsurgery of the Skull Base.* New York: Thieme Medical Publishers; 1988.

Guthikonda M, Guyot LL, Diaz FG. Future of extracranial-intracranial bypass. *Neurol Res.* 2002;24(Suppl 1):S80-S83.

Hanna EY, Holsinger C, DeMonte F, et al. Robotic endoscopic surgery of the skull base: a novel surgical approach. *Arch Otolaryngol Head Neck Surg.* 2007;133:1209-1214.

Hoeffner EG, Case I, Jain R, et al. Cerebral perfusion CT: technique and clinical applications. *Radiology.* 2004;231:632-644.

For complete list of references log onto www.expertconsult.com.

House WF, De la Cruz A, Hitselberger WE. Surgery of the skull base: transcochlear approach to the petrous apex and clivus. *Otolaryngology.* 1978;86:ORL-770-ORL-779.

Isaacson B, Kutz JW, Roland PS. Lesions of the petrous apex: diagnosis and management. *Otolaryngol Clin North Am.* 2007;40(viii):479-519.

Jenkins HA, Canalis RF. Transpalatal approach to the skull base. In: McCabe BF, Kirchner JA, Sasaki CT, Lewis JS, eds. *Surgery of the Skull Base.* Philadelphia: Lippincott; 1984:254.

Jenkins HA, Fisch U. Glomus tumors of the temporal region. Technique of surgical resection. *Arch Otolaryngol.* 1981;107:209-214.

Jenkins HA, Franklin DJ. Infratemporal approaches to the skull base. In: Jackson CG, ed. *Surgery of Skull Base Tumors.* New York: Churchill Livingstone; 1991:291.

Leonetti JP, Anderson DE, Marzo SJ, et al. The preauricular subtemporal approach for transcranial petrous apex tumors. *Otol Neurotol.* 2008;29:380-383.

Leonetti JP, Smith PG, Kletzker GR, et al. Invasion patterns of advanced temporal bone malignancies. *Am J Otol.* 1996;17:438-442.

Moore MG, Deschler DG, McKenna MJ, et al. Management outcomes following lateral temporal bone resection for ear and temporal bone malignancies. *Otolaryngol Head Neck Surg.* 2007;137:893-898.

Mura J, Rojas-Zalazar D, de Oliveira E. Revascularization for complex skull base tumors. *Skull Base.* 2005;15:63-70.

Nadol Jr JB, Schuknecht HF. Obliteration of the mastoid in the treatment of tumors of the temporal bone. *Ann Otol Rhinol Laryngol.* 1984;93(1 Pt 1):6-12.

Neely JG, Forrester M. Anatomic considerations of the medial cuts in the subtotal temporal bone resection. *Otolaryngol Head Neck Surg.* 1982;90:641-645.

Oghalai JS, Leung MK, Jackler RK, et al. Transjugular craniotomy for the management of jugular foramen tumors with intracranial extension. *Otol Neurotol.* 2004;25:570-579.

Sekhar L. The exposure, preservation, and reconstruction of cerebral arteries and veins durig the resection of cranial base tumors. In: Sekhar L, Schramm VL, eds. *Tumors of the Cranial Base.* Mount Kisco, NY: Futura Publishing; 1987.

Sekhar LN, Schramm Jr VL, Jones NF. Subtemporal-preauricular infratemporal fossa approach to large lateral and posterior cranial base neoplasms. *J Neurosurg.* 1987;67:488-499.

CHAPTER ONE HUNDRED AND SEVENTY-SEVEN

Neoplasms of the Posterior Fossa

Derald E. Brackmann

Moisés A. Arriaga

Key Points

- Extra-axial neoplasms of the posterior cranial fossa have distinguishing imaging characteristics.
- Vestibular schwannomas and meningiomas are the most common lesions. Although both enhance with gadolinium on T1-weighted MRI, meningiomas tend to be eccentric to the porus acusticus, have enhancing dural "tails," and often demonstrate adjacent hyperostosis or intralesional calcifications on CT.
- Epidermoids and arachnoid cysts both are nonenhancing lesions hypointense to brain on T1-weighted and hyperintense on T2-weighted MRI studies. They are distinguished from one another on intermediate spin sequences and diffusion-weighted imaging (DWI) sequences, with arachnoid cysts exhibiting CSF characteristics and epidermoids demonstrating restricted diffusion (bright) on DWI.
- Vascular imaging studies including traditional angiography, magnetic resonance angiography (MRA), magnetic resonance venography (MRV), and CT angiography (CTA) are useful for demonstrating the proximity of these lesions to important vascular structures.
- Treatment of extra-axial neoplasms is individualized, with consideration of patient factors, tumor size, and tumor type. The treatment objectives are patient safety and functional preservation of cranial nerves.
- Treatment strategies include observation with serial imaging, stereotactic radiosurgery or radiotherapy, and surgical removal. Total surgical removal of these lesions usually is curative.
- Neuro-otologic surgical approaches are team therapies including the translabyrinthine approach, retrosigmoid approach, middle fossa approach, extended middle fossa approach, petrosal approach, and a series of petrous apex drainage approaches. Each strategy must be considered in the context of tumor size and location, patient symptoms and overall health, and short- and long-term outcomes.

With the evolution of advanced audiovestibular testing, sensitive imaging technologies, and modern skull base surgical teams, diagnosis and management of extra-axial posterior fossa neoplasms constitute a consideration in the daily practice of otolaryngology. This chapter reviews diagnostic issues and surgical management.

Approach to Diagnosis of Neoplasms of the Posterior Fossa

Cerebellopontine angle (CPA) lesions are the predominant skull base neoplasms that affect the posterior fossa. Although acoustic neuromas account for most primary neoplasms in this category, many other lesions should be considered in the differential diagnosis.

The diagnostic evaluation begins with a thorough neuro-otologic history and physical examination. Any suspicious neuro-otologic finding should be evaluated thoroughly, because these lesions produce minimal signs and symptoms until they are far advanced. As noted, acoustic neuromas are the most common posterior fossa skull base tumors; less common lesions usually can be diagnosed accurately with the application of modern audiologic and imaging modalities and a systematic approach to evaluation of their differing characteristics. Today's improved diagnostic capabilities facilitate routine detection of tumors smaller than those detectable previously.

Posterior fossa skull base neoplasms may be grouped into common CPA lesions, including lesions of the internal auditory canal; petrous apex lesions; rare CPA lesions; and intra-axial lesions. The signs, symptoms, and diagnostic procedures for tumors within the designated categories (Box 177-1) are described next.

Common Cerebellopontine Angle Neoplasms

In published series of CPA neoplasms, acoustic neuromas are the most common tumors, accounting for more than 90%. The remaining primary tumors were meningiomas (3%), primary cholesteatomas (2.5%), and facial nerve schwannomas (1%), with less common tumors composing the remaining lesions.[1] When secondary tumors also are considered, paragangliomas constitute up to 10% of CPA neoplasms.[2]

Acoustic Neuroma

Acoustic neuroma refers to a benign schwannoma of the eighth cranial nerve. These lesions are relatively common and account for 8% to 10% of all intracranial tumors. Acoustic neuromas arise principally from the vestibular division of the nerve. The superior and inferior divisions are equally affected; intraoperatively, the nerve of origin usually is difficult to determine. The 1992 National Institutes of Health Consensus Conference made *vestibular schwannoma* the official nomenclature term for these lesions. Acoustic neuromas are slowly growing neoplasms that

Box 177-1

Skull Base Neoplasms Involving the Posterior Fossa

Common Cerebellopontine Angle Lesions
Acoustic neuroma
Meningioma
Epidermoid
Nonacoustic neuroma
Paraganglioma
Arachnoid cyst
Hemangioma

Petrous Apex Lesions
Cholesterol granuloma
Epidermoid
Asymmetric pneumatization
Retained mucus or mucocele
Petrous carotid artery aneurysm

Uncommon Cerebellopontine Angle Lesions
Metastatic tumor
Lipoma
Dermoid
Teratoma
Chordoma
Chondrosarcoma
Giant cell tumor

Intra-axial Tumors
Hemangioblastoma
Medulloblastoma
Astrocytoma
Glioma
Fourth ventricle tumor

originate in the nerve sheath and consist of schwannoma cells in a collagenous matrix. They typically are circumscribed, grossly encroaching on and displacing neural structures without direct invasion. Consistency varies, ranging from firm and dense to soft with large cystic spaces.

In the past it was taught that acoustic neuromas usually arise near the myelin-glia junction near the porus acusticus. However, no published histopathologic study has confirmed this assertion. These lesions usually arise within the internal auditory canal; however, they occasionally develop in the CPA medial to the porus. Because acoustic neuromas produce symptoms by exerting pressure on surrounding neurovascular structures, auditory and vestibular symptoms develop earlier with tumors of the internal auditory canal than with tumors of the CPA.

Of the 2000 to 3000 acoustic neuromas diagnosed annually in the United States, more than 95% occur as unilateral and nonhereditary lesions. The remaining acoustic neuromas are manifestations of the neurofibromatoses, which consist of at least two distinct genetic disorders.

Neurofibromatosis type 1 (NF1), or von Recklinghausen's disease, is a relatively common disorder of autosomal dominant inheritance with variable penetrance and an incidence of 1 in 4000 live births. The gene responsible for NF1 has been localized to chromosome 17. NF1 neuromas occur throughout the body, arising both intracranially and extracranially from the Schwann cells of any nerve; however, acoustic neuromas develop in less than 5% of patients, and bilateral acoustic neuroma is not a part of the syndrome.

Type 2 neurofibromatosis, NF2, is the central form of the disease, characterized by bilateral acoustic neuromas in up to 96% of patients. Schwannomas of the other cranial nerves, meningiomas, and ependymomas also are observed much more commonly in patients with NF2.[3]

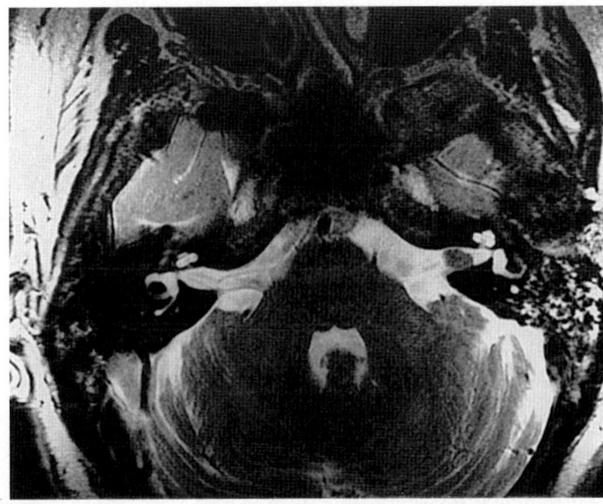

Figure 177-1. On T2-weighted fast spin echo magnetic resonance imaging, this axial reconstruction shows a 5-mm intracanalicular tumor on the *left*.

The precise frequency of NF2 is unknown, but it is far less frequent than NF1. The gene responsible for the condition encodes a membrane protein (merlin or schwannomin) and is located on chromosome 22. Acoustic neuromas in NF2 are characterized by an onset early in life, often before the age of 21 years, as opposed to unilateral lesions, most of which are diagnosed between the ages of 40 and 60 years. Thus, acoustic neuromas appearing before the age of 30 years mandate particularly close evaluation of the contralateral ear. Although the acoustic neuromas in NF1 and NF2 resemble the lesions in nonhereditary acoustic neuromas, they are technically more challenging to remove because of a tendency to adhere to nearby structures. The clinical presentation of acoustic neuroma in neurofibromatosis is identical to that of unilateral acoustic neuroma.

Malignant schwannomas may rarely occur. They often are associated with neurofibromatosis, but they also may occur with solitary schwannomas. Another very uncommon variant is a pigmented schwannoma.[4]

Natural History

The growth rate of acoustic neuromas is extremely variable. These tumors generally are slow-growing, with average reported growth rates of 0.2 cm per year; however, growth rates in excess of 2 cm per year have been documented. Acoustic neuromas that are not treated are potentially lethal. Gradual enlargement can lead to indentation of the brainstem, increased intracranial pressure, and death during a course of 5 to 15 years.[5]

Growth of acoustic neuromas generally occurs in three phases: internal auditory canal, cisternal, and brainstem compression (Figs. 177-1, 177-2, and 177-3). Growth within the internal auditory canal results in acoustic and facial nerve compression and attenuation. Displacement of the seventh cranial nerve, the acoustic (eighth) nerve, and the anterior inferior cerebellar artery occurs just medial to the porus acusticus (cisternal portion). Medial tumor growth augments the blood supply of the tumor with bridging vessels from the brainstem surface. Fourth ventricle shift often occurs when the CPA component reaches 2 to 3 cm and total ventricle obstruction with resulting hydrocephalus occurs with continued tumor growth. Trigeminal compression occurs at approximately the 3-cm stage, which permits the superior portion of the tumor to abut the fifth cranial nerve. Massive tumor growth with hydrocephalus, brainstem compression, and cerebellar tonsil herniation may occur even with modern imaging. The otolaryngologist should remain vigilant for signs and symptoms suggestive of retrocochlear pathology.

Signs and Symptoms

Sensorineural hearing loss (SNHL), tinnitus, dysequilibrium, and facial hypesthesia are, in descending order, the most common symptoms of

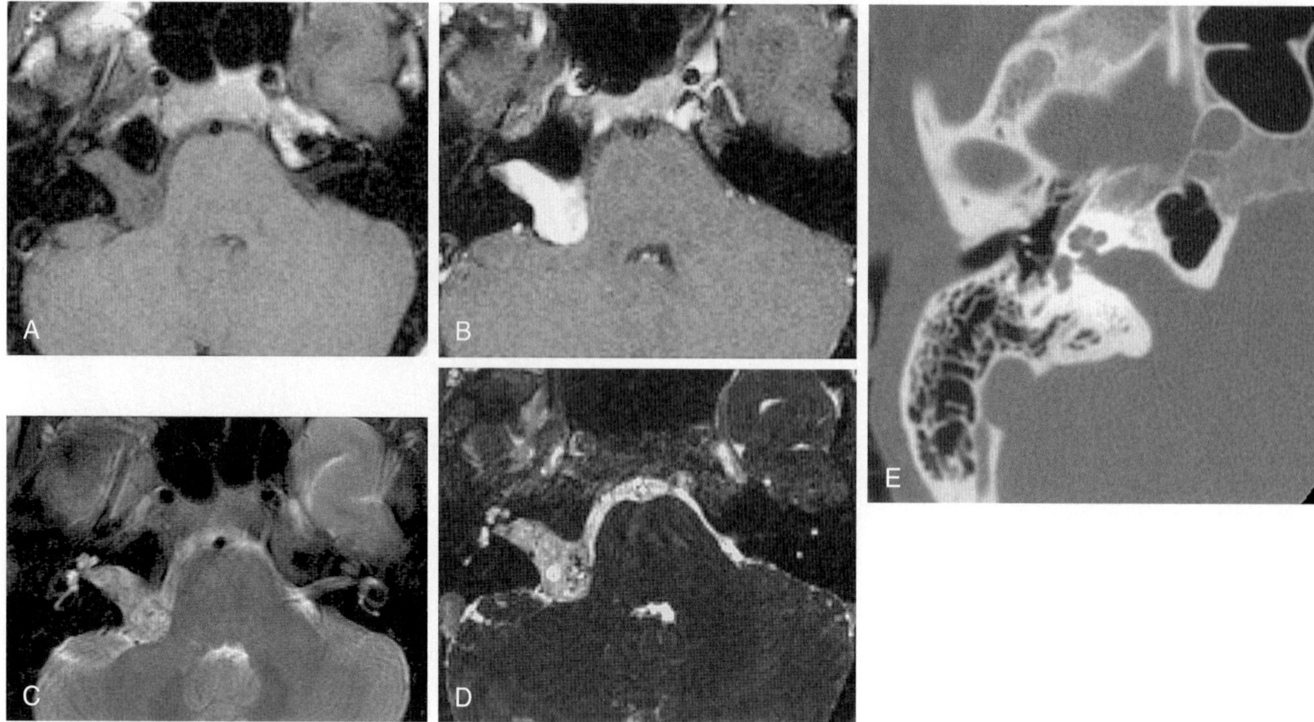

Figure 177-2. A medium-sized vestibular schwannoma, demonstrated by magnetic resonance imaging **(A** to **D)** and computed tomography **(E)**. **A** and **B,** T1-weighted images before and after intravenous administration of gadolinium contrast The tumor in the right internal auditory canal (IAC), which is mushrooming into the cerebellopontine angle and enlarging the canal, is isointense to mildly hypointense to the cerebellum and enhances markedly with contrast. **C** and **D,** T2-weighted and constructive interference in steady-state (CISS) images. The tumor is moderately hyperintense on the T2-weighted images. CISS images precisely demonstrate the cochlea, cystic, and calcified components of the tumor and surrounding vascular structures. **E,** CT bone windows. Note the enlargement of the IAC. *(Adapted from Maya MM, Lo WWM, Kovanlikaya I. Temporal bone tumors and cerebellopontine angle lesions. In: Som PM, Curtin HD, eds.* Head and Neck Imaging. *4th ed. Philadelphia: Mosby; 2003:245.)*

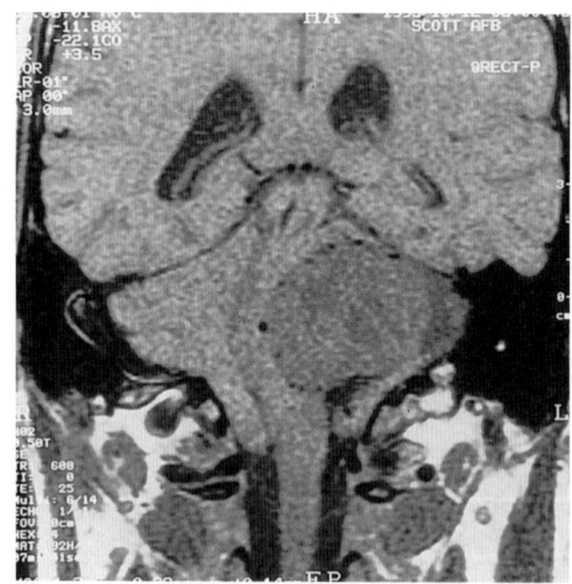

Figure 177-3. Noncontrast coronal T1 magnetic resonance image of a large acoustic neuroma with hydrocephalus, brainstem shift, and cerebellar tonsil herniation.

acoustic neuroma. Although progressive unilateral SNHL is the most common symptom, loss of speech discrimination is characteristic of retrocochlear dysfunction of the cochlear nerve presumably from pressure on the auditory nerve. The symptoms usually are slowly progressive, with a median duration of 2 years in one series.[6,7] However, up to 20% of affected patients experience sudden SNHL, although complete recovery of hearing has been reported.[8] Overall, only 1% of patients with sudden SNHL are found to have acoustic neuroma, whereas up to 5% of patients with acoustic neuroma have normal hearing.[9] Thus, any patient with asymmetric or sudden hearing loss (even after total recovery) should be considered for further evaluation for a possible retrocochlear lesion.

The dysequilibrium associated with acoustic nerve tumors usually is a mild balance disturbance, which often is so minor that the patient does not mention it and only careful questioning elicits it. Rotatory vertigo is far less common.

Diminished facial sensation or corneal reflex results from compression of the fifth cranial nerve, which is more likely with medium-sized and large tumors. As large acoustic neuromas compress the fourth ventricle and brainstem, long tract signs, ataxia, and findings of increased intracranial pressure (e.g., headaches, nausea) are produced.

Diagnostic Studies

Two categories of studies are performed in the diagnosis of acoustic neuroma. Auditory and vestibular studies assess the functional integrity of the audiovestibular system, whereas imaging studies are performed for the definitive anatomic diagnosis.

Audiometry

Routine air, bone, and speech discrimination studies may suggest the possibility of an acoustic neuroma. Asymmetric SNHL or impairment of speech discrimination disproportionate to the pure tone loss requires specific investigation for a retrocochlear lesion. In the past, an extensive audiometric test battery was necessary for timely tumor diagnosis.[6,10] In the magnetic resonance imaging (MRI) era, specialized audiometric tests are not sensitive or specific enough to detect small acoustic neuromas consistently.[11]

Auditory Brainstem Response Testing

Until recently, auditory brainstem (evoked) response (ABR) testing was considered the most sensitive modality for the detection of even small tumors, with detection rates of 95% to 100%.[12] The brainstem response to an 83-dB broadband click is recorded while the contralateral ear is masked by 78-dB white noise.[13] The latency for detection of wave V for the two ears is compared, and an adjusted interaural latency for wave V greater than 0.2 msec is considered abnormal. An approximately 10% false-positive rate has been reported for patients with SNHL who do not have a CPA tumor. Since the advent of gadolinium-enhanced MRI, however, the ABR false-negative rate (missing tumor diagnosis) has been 18% to 30% for intracanalicular tumors.[14] The possibility of false-negative results with intracanalicular acoustic neuromas has lessened the role of ABR testing for routine screening.[15] Stacked ABR testing is a modified ABR technique that offers improved sensitivity for detection of intracanalicular acoustic neuromas. It consists of testing the audiometric spectrum in a frequency-specific fashion followed by temporal alignment of the results; amplitude changes thus detected are much more sensitive for diagnosing small acoustic tumors than with routine ABR.[16,17] Nonetheless, the technique has not yet been verified in widespread clinical practice.

Vestibular Tests

Vestibular testing is not a useful screening test for acoustic neuroma. Electronystagmography (ENG) and infrared video caloric testing are helpful in defining whether the tumor arises from the superior or the inferior vestibular nerve.[18] Such information is valuable when hearing preservation surgery for acoustic neuromas is under consideration, because theoretically better results may be obtained with resection of tumors of the superior vestibular nerve.

Imaging

Computed tomography (CT) and MRI with the paramagnetic intravenous contrast agent gadopentetate (gadolinium-DTPA) are the principal imaging modalities for CPA lesions. Lo[19] proposed a scheme for the CT or MRI differential diagnosis of CPA lesions by anatomic location (extra-axial, extradural, or intra-axial) and by incidence (rare or common) (Table 177-1). In adults and teenagers acoustic neuromas, meningiomas, and epidermoids are the three most common lesions. Acoustic neuromas are very rare in children. Instead, brainstem gliomas (which can enlarge the internal auditory canal) are the most common CPA lesion in younger children.[20] Distinguishing among the three most common CPA lesions is based on specific imaging characteristics on CT and MRI (Table 177-2).

Although CT revolutionized the diagnosis of CPA tumors, gadolinium contrast MRI is sensitive and specific for detection of acoustic neuroma and is the diagnostic imaging technique of choice for the evaluation of acoustic neuroma and other CPA lesions (see Fig. 177-2).[21,22] Acoustic neuroma images on MRI are isointense or mildly hypointense to brain on T1-weighted images and mildly hyperintense to brain on T2-weighted images.[19] MRI for investigation of possible acoustic neuroma should be performed with intravenous contrast. Gadolinium increases the diagnostic sensitivity of MRI on T1-weighted images, and detection of lesions as small as 3 mm has been reported.[21] In addition to improving sensitivity in diagnosing acoustic neuromas, MRI is noninvasive, and the patient incurs no radiation exposure.

Before MRI, CT was the principal study for CPA lesions. Now the role of CT is to provide adjunctive information regarding the osseous structures surrounding a CPA lesion. It also can be the primary imaging modality in patients who cannot undergo MRI because of medical reasons (e.g., cardiac pacemaker or cochlear implant) or unmanageable phobic reactions. The CT finding characteristic of an acoustic tumor is an ovoid lesion centered on the internal auditory canal with moderate enhancing qualities. The tumor often is not homogeneous, exhibiting areas of lesser and greater enhancement. Approximately 85% of acoustic neuromas show acute angles at the bone-tumor interface, in contrast with meningiomas, in which the interface is obtuse in 75% of tumors.[19]

Intravenous contrast CT can fail to detect acoustic neuromas smaller than 1.5 cm in greatest dimension. Oxygen cisternography has been used to diagnose small, mainly intracanalicular lesions. In this technique, 4 mL of oxygen was introduced into the subarachnoid space through the opening afforded by a lumbar puncture, to highlight the structures of the internal auditory canal. This technique was very sensitive for detection of small lesions; however, it was limited by a false-positive rate of 5% and the need for a lumbar puncture.[23]

The improved availability of MRI has led to the development of MRI-based internal auditory canal screening protocols, which in many centers are comparable in cost to ABR-based internal auditory canal screening.[11] Special T2-weighted fast-spin echo sequences may achieve the accuracy of T1-weighted sequences with gadolinium without the need for contrast (see Fig. 177-1).[24] Although the software for these special sequences is not generally available, initial findings with this technique are very encouraging.

Table 177-1

Differential Diagnosis of Cerebellopontine Lesions by Imaging Location* and Incidence

Location	Incidence	Type
Extra-axial	Most common	Acoustic neuroma
	Common	Meningioma
	Common	Epidermoid (and other cysts: arachnoid, cysticercal, dermoid)
	Rare	Nonacoustic neuromas (cranial nerves V, VII, IX, X, XI, XII)
	Rare	Vascular lesions (loops, aneurysms, malformations)
Extradural	Common	Paraganglioma (glomus jugulare, glomus vagale)
	Rare	Bone lesions (benign or malignant; primary or metastatic)
Intra-axial	Rare	Astrocytoma, ependymoma, papilloma, hemangioblastoma, metastasis

*Computed tomography or magnetic resonance imaging.
Adapted from Lo WM. Tumors of the temporal bone and cerebellopontine angle. In: Som PM, Bergeron RT, eds. *Head and Neck Imaging*. St Louis: Mosby; 1991:420-445.

Meningiomas

Meningiomas represent up to 18% of all intracranial tumors and approximately 3% of CPA tumors.[25] The cells lining the arachnoid villi are the cells of origin. These cells are distributed throughout the intracranial space predominantly in relation to veins and dural sinuses. Meningiomas are benign but locally aggressive tumors, which occur at different anatomic sites in the following order of frequency: parasagittal region, falx, convexity, olfactory groove, tuberculum sellae, sphenoid ridge, petrous face (CPA), tentorium, lateral ventricle, clivus, and others.[26]

The gross appearance typically is that of a globular mass firmly adherent to the dura mater, with characteristic speckles scattered throughout the tumor that correspond to the microscopic psammoma bodies. The tumor displaces but does not invade adjacent neural tissue and has a thin investing capsule. Meningiomas can invade bone without destruction by extension along haversion canals. Adjacent bone is hyperostotic in 25% of cases.[26]

Many histopathologic classifications have been proposed, but a single, widely used system distinguishes among syncytial, transitional, fibrous, angioblastic, and sarcomatous types.[27] The specific histopathologic subtypes and growth characteristics are reviewed elsewhere.[28] In

Table 177-2

Imaging Features of the Three Most Common Cerebellopontine Angle Lesions

Feature	Acoustic Neuromas	Meningiomas	Epidermoids
Location	Centered on the internal auditory canal	Eccentric to the internal auditory canal	Anterolateral or posterolateral to brainstem
Bone changes	Most enlarge the internal auditory canal	Occasional hyperostosis	Occasional erosion
Shape	Spherical or ovoid, acute bone-tumor angle	Hemispherical, rarely plaquelike; may herniate through tentorium; obtuse bone-tumor angle	Variable—tends to dumbbell into middle fossa or contralateral cerebellopontine angle
Computed tomography density	Mostly isodense	Slightly hypodense; some calcified	Mostly hypodense; occasional peripheral calcium
Computed tomography enhancement	Moderate to marked; often inhomogeneous	Marked and homogeneous	Nonenhancing
T1-weighted magnetic resonance imaging	Isointense or hypointense	Isointense or hypointense	Hypointense
Gadolinium enhancement	Marked	Moderate	Nonenhancing
T2-weighted magnetic resonance imaging	Isointense or hypointense	Variable	Hyperintense

Adapted from Lo WM: Tumors of the temporal bone and cerebellopontine angle. In: Som PM, Bergeron RT, eds. *Head and Neck Imaging*. St Louis: Mosby; 1991:420-445.

the posterior fossa, meningiomas usually arise on the posterior surface of the petrous bone, away from or at the edge of the internal auditory canal, or along the sigmoid sinus. Because they usually arise outside of the canal, these tumors may become large before producing signs and symptoms of cranial nerve VIII compression. Most meningiomas eventually involve cranial nerve VIII.

Signs and Symptoms

Audiovestibular symptoms usually are the first indication of a posterior fossa meningioma. Among patients presenting to neurosurgeons, a higher proportion first experienced symptoms referable to the trigeminal nerve.[29] The signs and symptoms of meningiomas are similar to those of acoustic neuromas. Small tumors produce hearing loss, tinnitus, and imbalance. Larger tumors also produce signs and symptoms of involvement of other cranial nerves and hydrocephalus.

Diagnostic Studies

Audiovestibular Testing

It is impossible to distinguish acoustic neuromas from meningiomas on the basis of audiovestibular testing. Because meningiomas cause cranial nerve VIII compression, auditory and vestibular test findings become abnormal in a pattern similar to that with acoustic neuromas. Because meningiomas usually do not arise within the internal auditory canal, the sensitivity of audiometric and vestibular testing is lower with meningiomas than with acoustic neuromas. For instance, only 75% of patients with meningiomas exhibit an abnormal ABR.

Imaging

Table 177-2 summarizes features of meningiomas that assist in differentiating them from acoustic neuromas. Unlike acoustic neuromas, meningiomas usually are eccentric to the porus. Whereas acoustic neuromas seldom herniate into the middle fossa, approximately 60% of meningiomas extend to the middle fossa.[19] Meningiomas usually are hemispheric because of their broad-based attachment to the posterior petrous wall, accounting for the obtuse bone-tumor angles in 75% of meningiomas. Unlike the site of origin of acoustic neuromas, that of posterior fossa meningiomas is varied (Figs. 177-4 and 177-5).

On CT, approximately two thirds of meningiomas are hyperintense relative to the brain. Unlike acoustic neuromas, meningiomas are homogeneous and occasionally calcified. They show homogeneous enhancement with iodine infusion, which usually permits differentiation from acoustic neuromas. Hyperostosis of adjacent bone is infrequent but characteristic of meningiomas when present.

On MRI, meningiomas are of extremely variable intensity on T2-weighted images and isointense or slightly hypointense to brain on T1-weighted images. The different signal intensities among meningiomas correspond to different histopathologic subtypes.[27] Surface flow voids on MRI correspond to marginal pial blood vessels, and arborizing flow voids represent active feeders to the tumor. Calcification and cystic foci cause heterogeneity on MRI images of meningiomas.

Primary Cholesteatomas

Primary cholesteatomas (epidermoids) consist of a stratified squamous epithelial lining surrounding desquamated keratin, which originates from epithelial rests within the temporal bone or CPA. These lesions usually are slow-growing, and symptoms often do not become apparent until the second to fourth decades of life. As the lesions expand, compression and irritation of surrounding structures produce the signs and symptoms.

Primary cholesteatomas arise adjacent to the brainstem. Because they expand into the area of least resistance, primary cholesteatomas have variable shapes with irregular surfaces. They may burrow into crevices on the surface of the brain or extend in a dumbbell pattern into the middle fossa.

Signs and Symptoms

Although primary cholesteatomas produce pressure on cranial nerves VII and VIII with continued growth, these lesions can become quite large without producing any symptoms. Facial twitching is a distinguishing clinical manifestation of primary cholesteatomas. Progressive

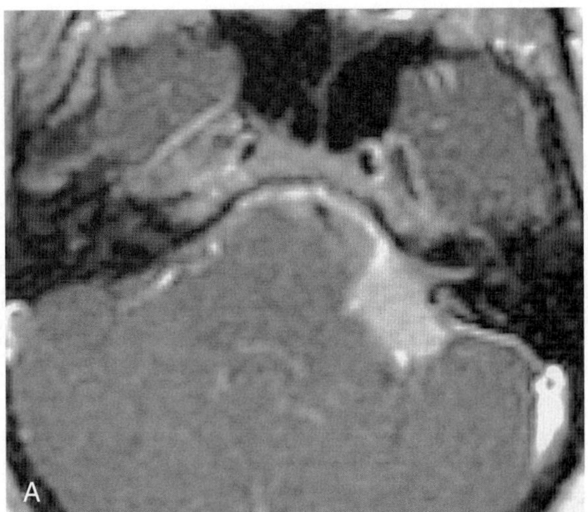

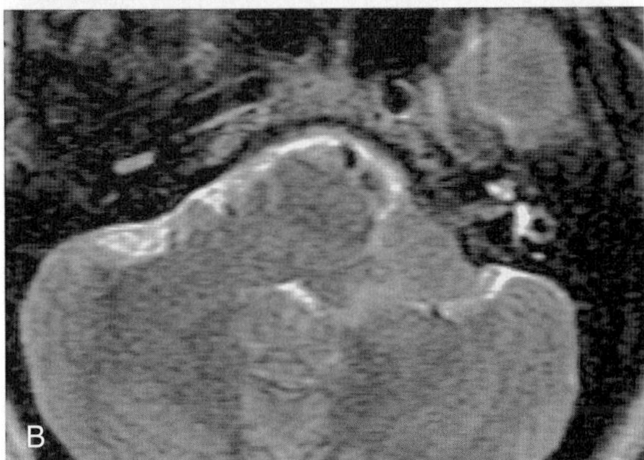

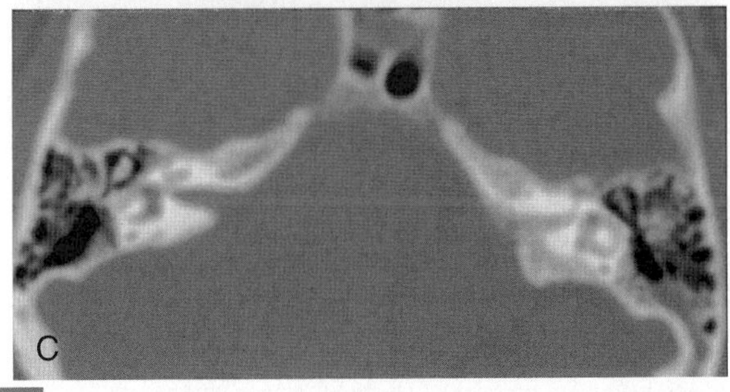

Figure 177-4. Cerebellopontine angle meningioma with classic features on magnetic resonance imaging (MRI) and computed tomography (CT). **A,** Post-gadolinium T1-weighted MRI: The tumor is eccentric to the internal auditory canal (IAC) and broadly dura-based, with obtuse angles at the bone-tumor interface. This hemispherical tumor shows uniform enhancement. Note the lack of IAC involvement. **B,** T2-weighted MRI: The tumor is homogeneously isointense to gray matter. **C,** CT bone windows. The tumor shows extensive hyperostosis underlying the dural base. *(From Maya MM, Lo WWM, Kovanlikaya I. Temporal bone tumors and cerebellopontine angle lesions. In: Som PM, Curtin HD, eds.* Head and Neck Imaging. *4th ed. Philadelphia: Mosby; 2003:245-250.)*

facial paralysis is more common with these lesions than with schwannomas.

Diagnostic Studies

Auditory Testing

Auditory testing does not show any distinguishing features. As with other retrocochlear lesions, speech discrimination is poorer than would be expected from the degree of pure-tone loss. ABR also is frequently abnormal in primary cholesteatomas.[30]

Imaging

CT and MRI are useful to differentiate primary cholesteatomas from other lesions. Epidermoids originating in the CPA should be distinguished from arachnoid cysts, and epidermoids in the petrous apex should be distinguished from the much more common cholesterol granulomas. This distinction affects therapy because adequate management for primary cholesteatoma requires excision, whereas drainage is sufficient for cholesterol granulomas and arachnoid cysts.

On CT, primary cholesteatomas are less dense than brain (having a density approximating that of cerebrospinal fluid [CSF]) and exhibit no enhancement with intravenous contrast. These lesions have irregular margins and are eccentric to the porus acusticus. Enhancing components suggest an associated malignancy.[31] With MRI, primary cholesteatomas are inhomogeneous and hypointense to brain on T1-weighted images, and homogeneous and isointense or hyperintense to brain on T2-weighted images (Fig. 177-6). Schwannomas, meningiomas, and chondromas are similar to primary cholesteatomas by intensity criteria; however, epidermoids are differentiated because they are nonenhancing.

Arachnoid cysts of the CPA are difficult to distinguish from epidermoids on CT and MRI. Both lesions are of CSF density and nonenhancing; compared with primary cholesteatomas, however, arachnoid cysts have smoother surfaces, and special MRI sequences such as diffusion-weighted images (DWIs) may differentiate the intensity of the epidermoid from the CSF intensity of the arachnoid cyst (Fig. 177-7).

Facial Nerve Neuroma

Facial nerve neuromas (schwannomas) are uncommon benign neoplasms of Schwann cells that may arise anywhere along the course of the facial nerve.

Signs and Symptoms

Symptoms associated with these tumors depend on the portion of the nerve affected by the neoplasm. Peripheral involvement can manifest as a parotid mass, middle ear involvement can produce conductive hearing losses, and internal auditory canal or CPA involvement may result in SNHL. Unlike hemangiomas of the facial nerve, schwannomas do not produce facial weakness until they become very large. Sometimes a facial nerve tic is evident, which helps distinguish facial neuromas from acoustic neuromas but not from primary cholesteatomas. Of note, intratemporal lesions, with the possibility of neural entrapment, are more likely than CPA lesions to result in facial paralysis.[32]

Diagnostic Studies

Auditory Testing

The mechanisms for conductive hearing impairment and SNHL have already been described earlier in this chapter. Impedance testing may reflect motor fiber impairment on ipsilateral reflex testing or cranial nerve VIII involvement on contralateral reflex testing. ABR testing of tumors arising in the internal auditory canal shows abnormalities similar to those seen with acoustic neuroma.[13]

Electroneurography

Electroneurography, also known as electroneuronography (ENoG), measures the muscle response to a maximal bipolar stimulation of the facial nerve near the stylomastoid foramen. ENoG potentials may be reduced in facial nerve neuroma even when no facial weakness or tic is present, whereas ENoG findings remain normal in acoustic neuroma until the tumor becomes very large. Some reports suggest that the value of preoperative ENoG in patients with acoustic neuroma lies in predicting whether the lesion actually represents a facial nerve tumor.[33,34]

Imaging

Intratemporal facial nerve lesions may produce bone destruction. Because the clinical presentation and audiometric study findings in facial neuroma are not distinct, CT and MRI constitute the mainstays of diagnosis.

Because facial nerve neuromas are histologically identical to acoustic neuromas, they have the same enhancement characteristics. It

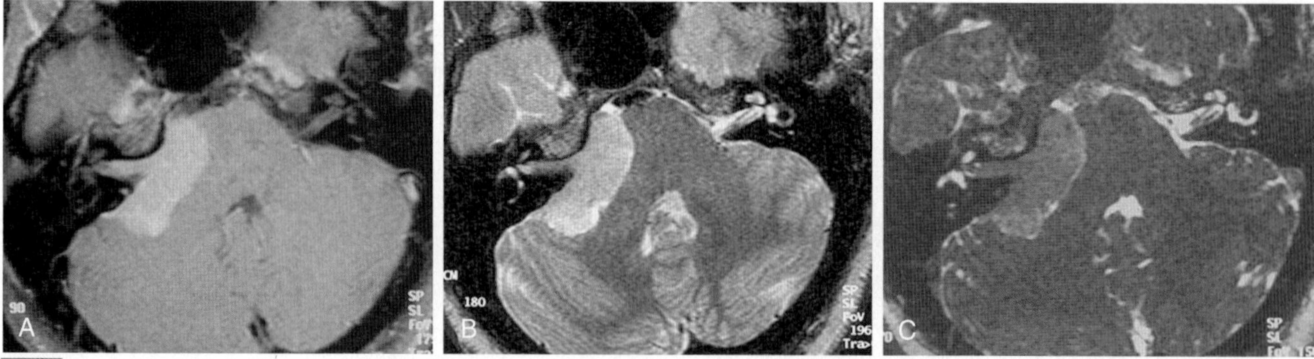

Figure 177-5. Cerebellopontine angle meningioma with intracanalicular extension, demonstrated by magnetic resonance imaging. **A,** Post-gadolinium T1-weighted image. Typical hemispherical tumor with intracanalicular extension. The dural tail of the tumor extending posteriorly is best seen on post-gadolinium images. **B,** T2-weighted image demonstrates the cerebrospinal fluid spaces and clefts surrounding the tumor. **C,** Constructive interference in steady-state (CISS) image. The internal auditory canal extension and margins of the tumor are better delineated on CISS images than on T2-weighted images. *(From Maya MM, Lo WWM, Kovanlikaya I. Temporal bone tumors and cerebellopontine angle lesions. In: Som PM, Curtin HD, eds.* Head and Neck Imaging. *4th ed. Philadelphia: Mosby; 2003:245-250.)*

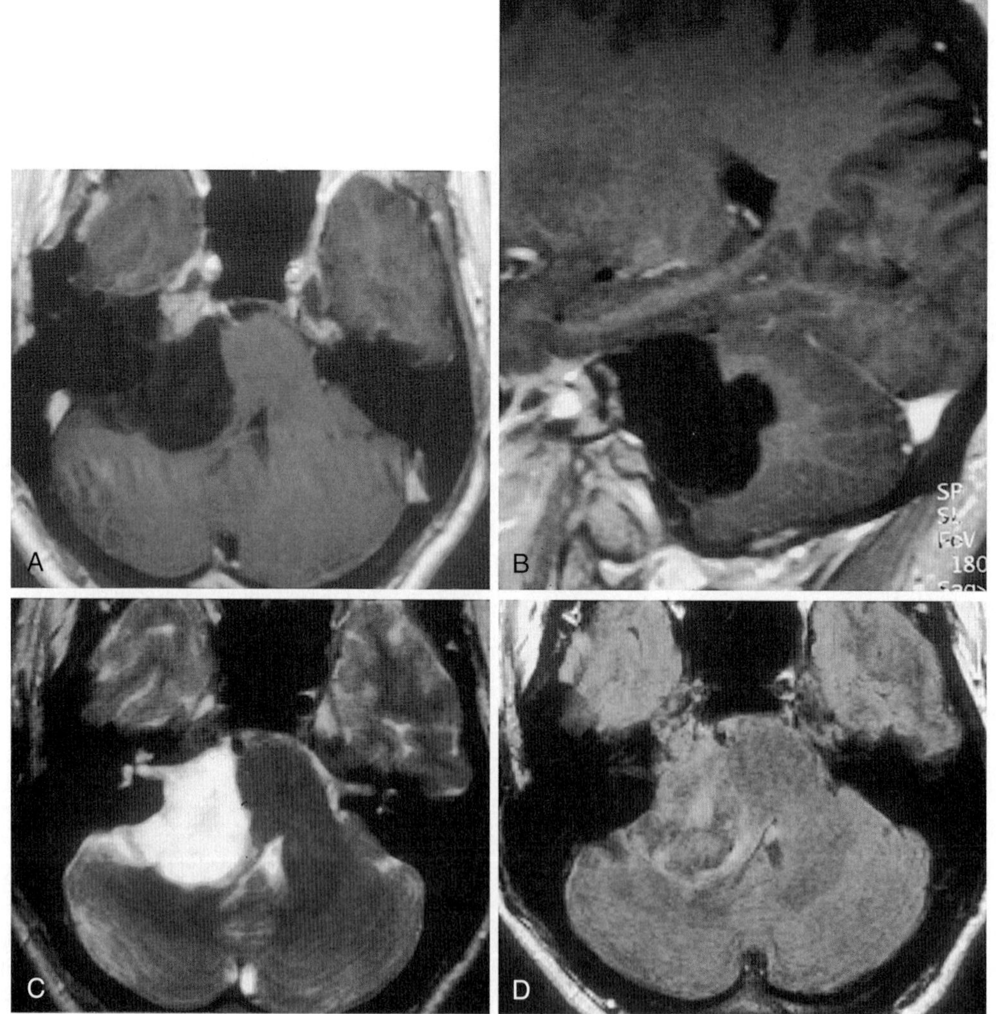

Figure 177-6. Cerebellopontine angle (CPA) epidermoid, demonstrated by magnetic resonance imaging. **A** and **B,** T1-weighted axial and sagittal images after gadolinium administration. The CPA mass extending to the prepontine cistern is isointense to cerebrospinal fluid (CSF) and shows no enhancement. **C,** T2-weighted image. The tumor, with irregular, cauliflower-like margins, is isointense to CSF, as in T1-weighted images, and is compressing the fourth ventricle. The internal auditory canal is normal. **D,** On this fluid-attenuated inversion recovery (FLAIR) sequence image, the epidermoid has heterogeneous hyperintense foci, enabling differentiation of an epidermoid from an arachnoid cyst in this case. *(From Maya MM, Lo WWM, Kovanlikaya I. Temporal bone tumors and cerebellopontine angle lesions. In: Som PM, Curtin HD, eds.* Head and Neck Imaging. *4th ed. Philadelphia: Mosby; 2003:245-250.)*

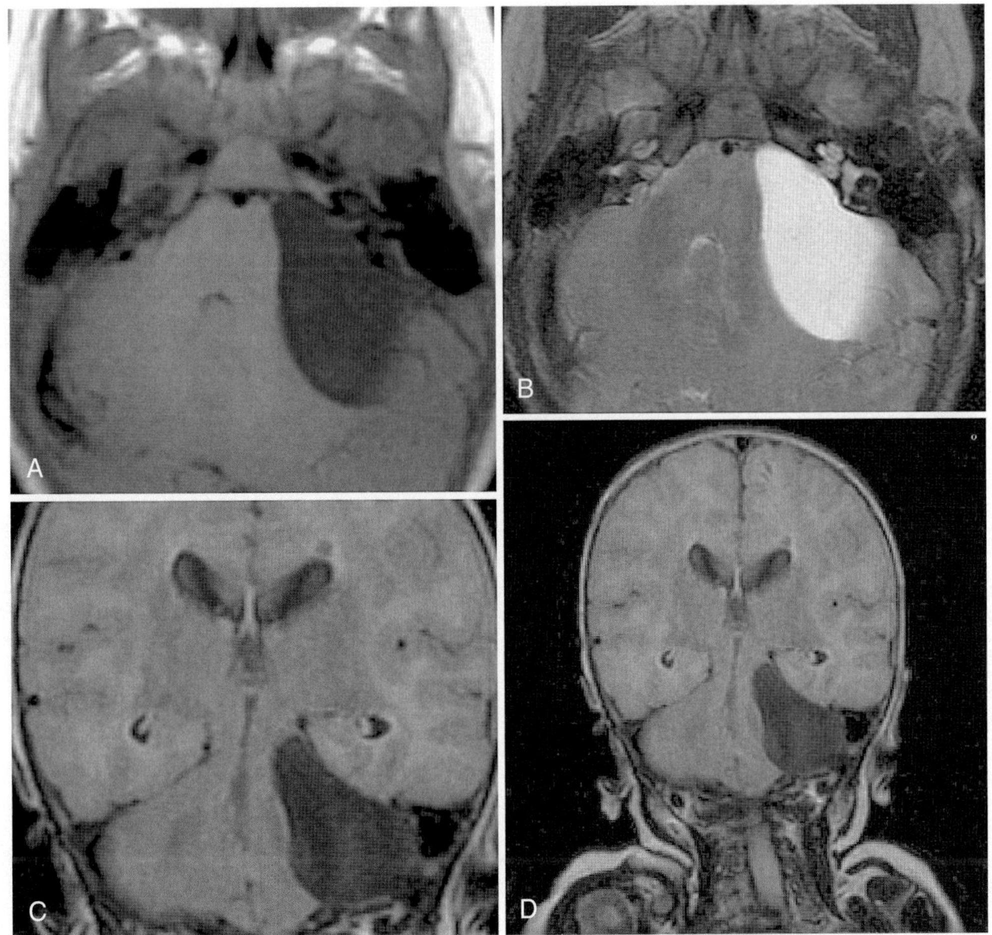

Figure 177-7. Cerebellopontine angle arachnoid cyst, demonstrated by magnetic resonance imaging. **A,** T1-weighted image. **B,** T2-weighted image. **C** and **D,** T1-weighted coronal and axial images, respectively. The cyst is isointense to CSF on all sequences. It is homogeneous, with a smooth surface, which can be helpful in differentiating it from an epidermoid. *(From Maya MM, Lo WWM, Kovanlikaya I. Temporal bone tumors and cerebellopontine angle lesions. In: Som PM, Curtin HD, eds.* Head and Neck Imaging. *4th ed. Philadelphia: Mosby; 2003:245-250.)*

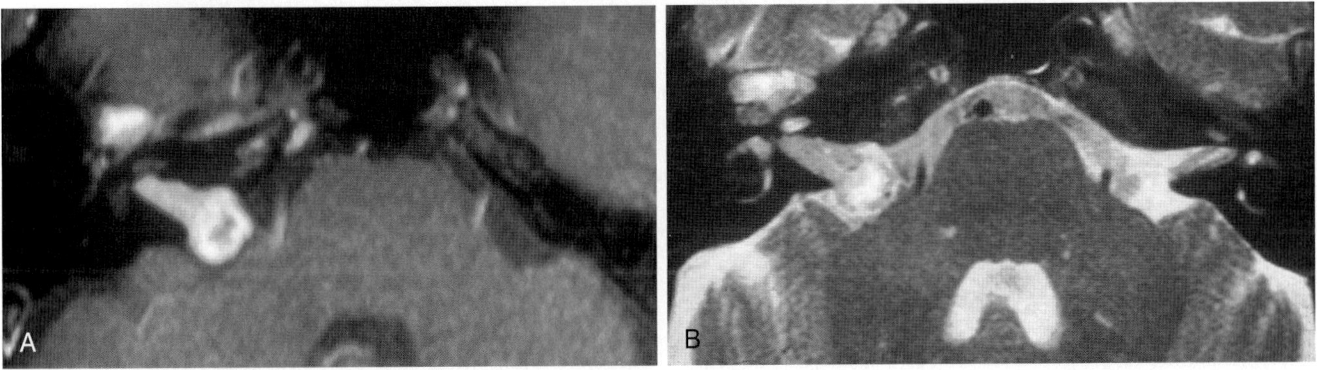

Figure 177-8. Facial schwannoma of internal auditory canal, demonstrated by magnetic resonance imaging. **A** and **B,** Post-gadolinium T1-weighted and T2-weighted images. The patient presented with progressive sensorineural hearing loss, with later development of facial palsy. The enhancing intracanalicular tumor is indistinguishable from an acoustic schwannoma. Note also the extension of the tumor to the geniculate ganglion. *(From Maya MM, Lo WWM, Kovanlikaya I. Temporal bone tumors and cerebellopontine angle lesions. In: Som PM, Curtin HD, eds.* Head and Neck Imaging. *4th ed. Philadelphia: Mosby; 2003:245-250.)*

usually is impossible to identify these lesions using CT. Anterosuperior erosion of the internal auditory canal or erosion of the labyrinthine facial nerve canal if present may be the only diagnostic clue.[19] More distal tumors enlarge the geniculate ganglion and fallopian canal.

As with CT, MRI of facial neuroma produces imaging characteristics identical to those of acoustic neuromas (Fig. 177-8). The preoperative diagnosis of intracranial facial neuroma is difficult. Early facial nerve symptoms are an obvious warning that a CPA lesion may rarely be a facial nerve neuroma. Patients diagnosed with CPA neuromas should be warned preoperatively of a 1% risk of facial nerve neuroma. This possibility is emphasized if findings on preoperative ENoG are abnormal on the tumor side. In some tumors, the lesion may extend

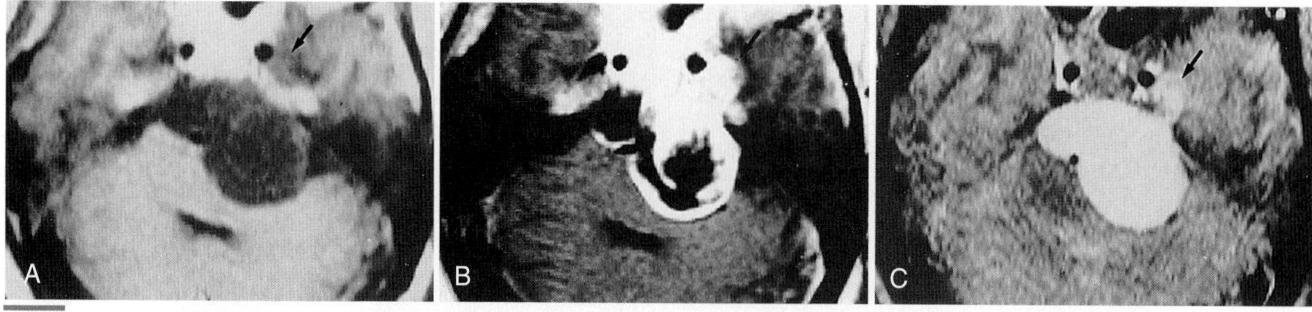

Figure 177-9. Cystic trigeminal schwannoma, demonstrated by magnetic resonance imaging. **A,** T1-weighted image. **B,** Gadolinium T1-weighted image. **C,** T2-weighted image. The bulk of the tumor lies in the posterior fossa, with a small middle cranial fossa component enlarging the left Meckel's cave *(arrow)*. Note the similarity of the tumor to an arachnoid cyst (see Figure 177-7) on the noncontrast images (**A** and **C**). The tumor is nearly of CSF intensity because of the predominance of the intratumoral cystic components. *(From Jackler RK, Brackmann DE, eds.* Neurotology. *St Louis: Mosby; 1994.)*

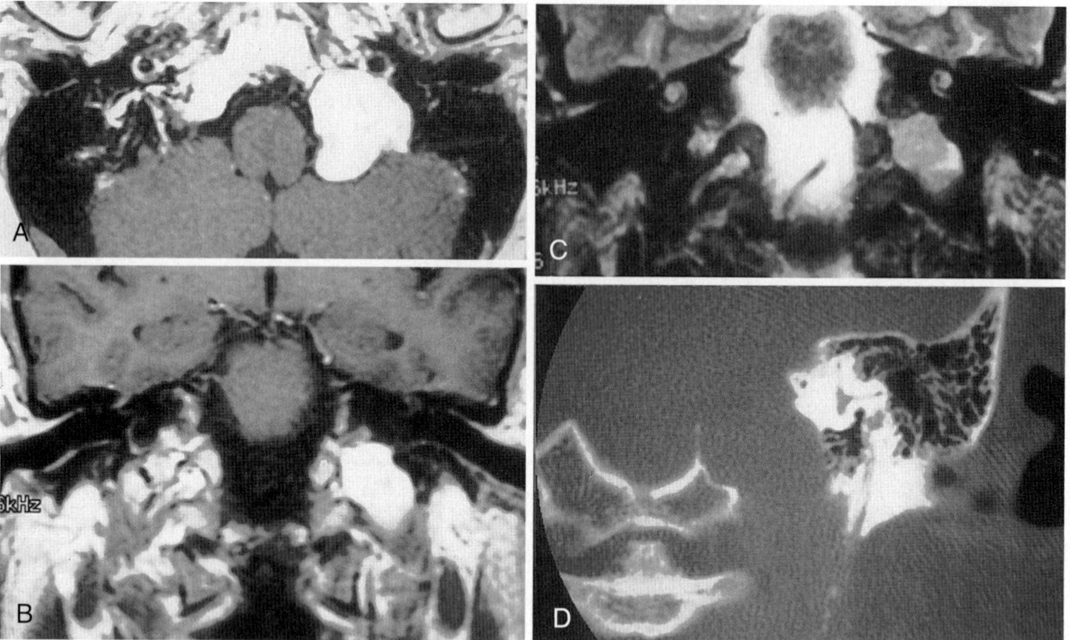

Figure 177-10. Jugular foramen schwannoma, demonstrated by magnetic resonance imaging (MRI) and computed tomography (CT). **A** and **B**, Axial and coronal T1-weighted post-gadolinium images. The large tumor in the left jugular fossa is extending inferiorly. It shows avid enhancement. **C,** Coronal T2-weighted image depicts the extracranial portion of the tumor, which is hyperintense to gray matter. **D,** CT bone windows, coronal image. Expansion of the jugular foramen is symmetric, and the margins are well defined. *(From Maya MM, Lo WWM, Kovanlikaya I. Temporal bone tumors and cerebellopontine angle lesions. In: Som PM, Curtin HD, eds.* Head and Neck Imaging. *4th ed. Philadelphia: Mosby; 2003:245-250.)*

from the CPA through the temporal bone course of the nerve to the extratemporal nerve in the parotid gland.

Other Cranial Nerve Neuromas

Neuromas may arise on any other cranial nerve in the posterior fossa. On imaging studies, nonacoustic neuromas have the same characteristics as those of acoustic neuromas except for their location. Overall, acoustic neuromas represent 95% of intracranial schwannomas, and trigeminal neuromas are the next most common; however, schwannomas also have been reported on cranial nerves IX, X, XI, and XII. These lesions are distinguished by their different location and by symptoms of dysfunction of the cranial nerve of origin.

Trigeminal neuromas arise intradurally, from the nerve root in the CPA and Meckel's cave, and extradurally, from the gasserian ganglion in the middle cranial fossa.[35] Typically these lesions enlarge Meckel's cave and produce hypesthesia of the face (Fig. 177-9).

Neuromas of cranial nerves IX, X, and XI produce smooth enlargement of the jugular foramen and classically cause hypesthesia and weakness of the palate, vocal cord, and shoulder, respectively (Fig. 177-10). If they arise in the posterior fossa, these tumors may grow to a large size before producing predominantly acoustic or cerebellar signs. Accurate preoperative differentiation of these tumors from acoustic neuromas is important because residual hearing is more likely to be preserved with lower cranial nerve neuromas. Hypoglossal neuromas produce motor hemiatrophy of the tongue and enlargement of the hypoglossal canal on radiography.

Glomus Tumors

Glomus tumors (paragangliomas) are discussed in detail in Chapter 176. Because glomus jugulare tumors and glomus vagale tumors may extend into the posterior fossa, they constitute an important consideration in the differential diagnosis of skull base neoplasms.

The first symptom often is pulsatile tinnitus, after which a conductive hearing loss develops. Involvement of the nerves of the jugular foramen and the hypoglossal nerve causes progressive neurologic deficits related to those nerves.

The characteristic appearance on CT with bone windows is irregular destruction of the jugular foramen, as compared with jugular

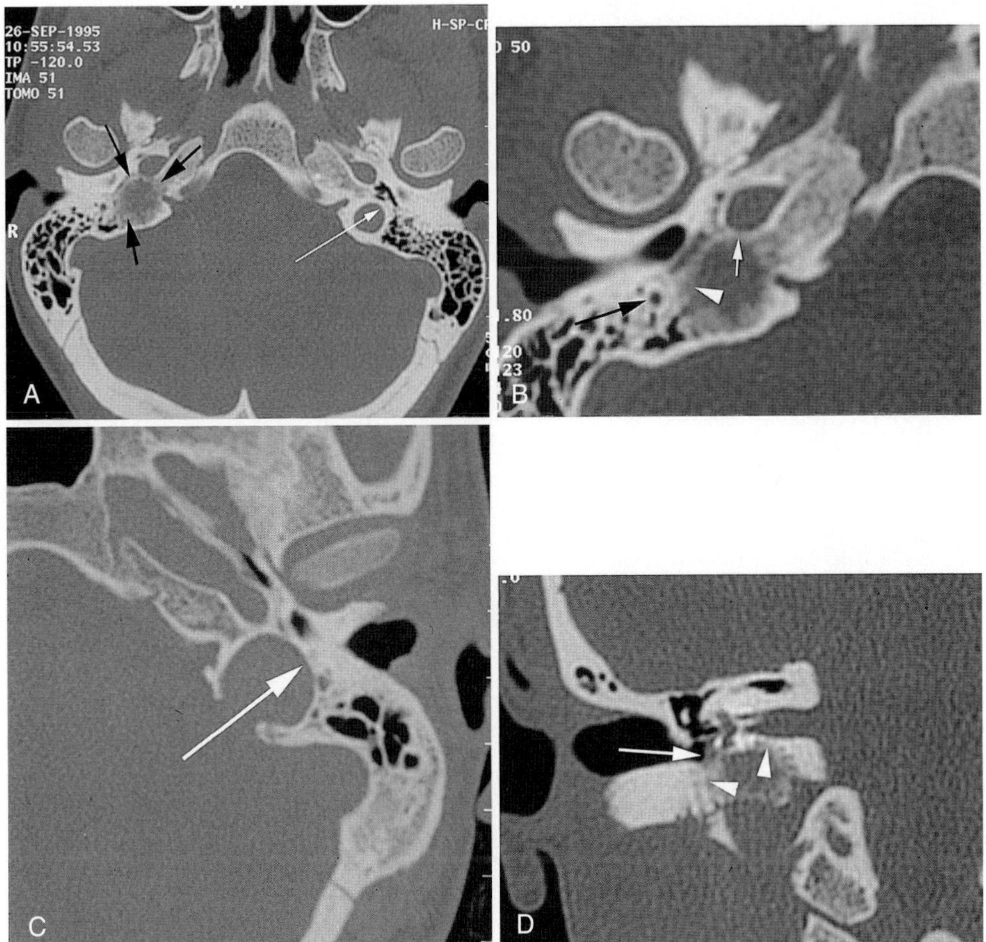

Figure 177-11. Glomus jugulare tumor, demonstrated by computed tomography. **A,** Axial image shows demineralization of the bony margins of the jugular foramen on the right side *(black arrows)*. There is demineralization of the fine cortical line usually demonstrated along the lateral aspect of the vascular portion of the jugular foramen. Compare with intact cortical plate on the opposite side *(white arrow)*. Note the demineralization of the bony wall separating the carotid canal from the jugular foramen. **B,** Enlarged axial image shows the demineralization of the lateral cortical plate *(arrowhead)*, as well as slight demineralization of the bony plate between the carotid canal and the jugular foramen *(white arrow)*. Note the proximity of the demineralized bone to the vertical section of the facial nerve canal *(black arrow)*. **C,** Axial image enlarged through the normal side shows the intact white cortical line *(arrow)* along the lateral aspect of the jugular foramen. The integrity of this line essentially excludes a glomus jugulotympanic tumor. **D,** Coronal image shows demineralization of the margins *(arrowheads)*, as well as the soft tissue of the intratympanic portion of the tumor *(arrow)*. *(From Maya MM, Lo WWM, Kovanlikaya I. Temporal bone tumors and cerebellopontine angle lesions. In: Som PM, Curtin HD, eds.* Head and Neck Imaging. *4th ed. Philadelphia: Mosby; 2003.)*

foramen schwannomas, which produce smooth enlargement (Fig. 177-11). The vascular pattern of paragangliomas on angiography is characteristic (Fig. 177-12), and biopsy of these lesions is not indicated.[36] Diagnostic angiography should be performed concomitantly with preoperative embolization when surgical resection is planned.

MRI produces a unique salt-and-pepper mixture of intensities on T1- and T2-weighted images. Arborizing flow voids reveal the prominent tumor vessels of this lesion. Lo[19] described two limitations of MRI in evaluating paragangliomas: (1) bone changes and the relation of tumor to bone landmarks are not visualized; and (2) distinguishing tumor from bone marrow is difficult, especially on gadolinium-enhanced T1-weighted images. Thus, MRI may provide complementary information about infralabyrinthine and intracranial tumor extensions, but bone algorithm CT is the cornerstone of imaging evaluation in paragangliomas.

The combination of CT, MRI, and angiography can provide extensive information about involvement of the internal carotid artery. Magnetic resonance angiography (MRA) is an adjunct to intra-arterial catheterization and formal angiography (see Fig. 177-12). Angiography is a necessary step in preoperative embolization of glomus tumors; however, it is unlikely that MRA can replace direct intravascular angiography in glomus tumor management. For resection of skull base neoplasms involving the posterior fossa, if surgical resection requires manipulation of the artery, preoperative assessment of the adequacy of collateral flow by way of the circle of Willis is necessary. Temporary balloon occlusion of the carotid artery in combination with radioisotope imaging or xenon-enhanced CT can accurately quantify collateral blood flow.[37]

Arachnoid Cysts

Arachnoid cysts are thin-walled sacs that contain yellow, entrapped CSF. The current theory is that these lesions represent congenital developmental anomalies.[38] Symptoms are produced by the mass effect of the cyst on surrounding structures and may be similar to the symptoms of acoustic neuromas. These patients may experience mild to profound hearing loss with a retrocochlear pattern.[39]

These lesions have CT and MRI characteristics similar to those of epidermoids. Enlargement of the internal auditory canal often is noted but is not characteristic of these lesions. The typical appearance is that of a smooth-surfaced lesion, which on CT approximates CSF and is nonenhancing and on MRI exhibits isointensity or hypointensity to brain on T1-weighted images and hyperintensity to brain on T2-weighted images (see Fig. 177-7). In most patients, no direct inter-

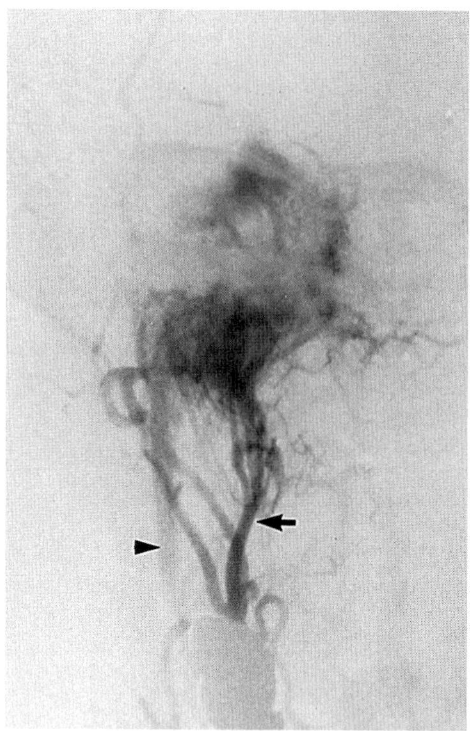

Figure 177-12. Glomus jugulare tumor. As seen on this selective external carotid angiogram, the characteristically hypervascular tumor is supplied by the hypertrophic ascending pharyngeal artery *(arrow)*. Note the early draining vein *(arrowhead)* seen during the midarterial phase. Considerations in the differential diagnosis include other hypervascular tumors such as metastatic hypernephroma, metastatic pheochromocytoma, and myeloma. *(From Maya MM, Lo WWM, Kovanlikaya I. Temporal bone tumors and cerebellopontine angle lesions. In: Som PM, Curtin HD, eds.* Head and Neck Imaging. *4th ed. Philadelphia: Mosby; 2003.)*

vention is necessary. When treatment is necessary to control symptoms, management of these lesions is not total resection. Instead, surgical drainage by way of retrolabyrinthine exposure is the usual recommended therapy; however, diuretic therapy provides symptomatic relief in a few patients.

Hemangiomas

Hemangiomas are hamartomatous neoplasms originating from blood vessels. Although benign, they produce symptoms by compression of adjacent structures. Hemangiomas are capillary or cavernous.

Capillary hemangiomas typically arise in the area of the geniculate ganglion in association with a perigeniculate capillary plexus.[40] The lesion is characterized by a progressive facial weakness despite being much smaller than facial nerve neuromas. The expanding lesion with the production of pulsatile tinnitus may expose the upper basal turn of the cochlea. CT shows a smooth enlargement of the geniculate ganglion and enlargement of the labyrinthine portion of the fallopian canal by a soft tissue mass. Although capillary hemangiomas are enhancing, they produce facial weakness at such an early stage that only subtle findings may be apparent on CT, and a very small enhancement in the area of the labyrinthine segment may be the only finding. Other CT findings include honeycomb bone, irregular and indistinct bone margins, and intratumoral bone spicules (Fig. 177-13). These findings contrast with those in facial nerve neuromas, which are larger, more obvious lesions with sharp bone margins.

Cavernous hemangiomas are the second type of hemangioma. These lesions arise in the internal auditory canal and produce symptoms typical for an acoustic neuroma. Although they tend to produce symptoms more rapidly than do acoustic neuromas, these two tumor types are identical on CT. However, on MRI, cavernous hemangiomas tend to be slightly more hyperintense than the typical acoustic neuroma.

Table 177-3

Imaging Features of Petrous Apex Cystic Lesions

Features	Cholesterol Granuloma	Epidermoid	Mucocele
Computed tomography density	Isodense	Hypodense	Hypodense
T1-weighted MRI appearance	Hyperintense	Hypointense	Hypointense
Gadolinium contrast MRI appearance	Nonenhancing	Nonenhancing	Rim enhances; mass is nonenhancing
T2-weighted MRI appearance	Hyperintense	Hyperintense	Hyperintense
Borders of lesion	Smooth	Scalloped	Smooth

MRI, magnetic resonance imaging.
Adapted from Lo WM: Tumors of the temporal bone and cerebellopontine angle. In: Som PM, Bergeron RT, eds. *Head and Neck Imaging*. St Louis: Mosby; 1991:420-445.

Petrous Apex Lesions

Petrous apex lesions constitute an important category of skull base neoplasms that may involve the posterior fossa. Some of the specific lesions have been described earlier under "Common Cerebellopontine Angle Neoplasms." The critical distinction in diagnosis of petrous apex lesions is between cholesterol granulomas, which require drainage procedures, and mass lesions, which generally require complete excision.

Cholesterol Granulomas

A cholesterol granuloma arises in the pneumatized spaces of the temporal bone presumably as a result of occlusion of the air cell system. Hemorrhage into the air cells results in a foreign body reaction and progressive granuloma formation. An expansile lesion of the temporal bone results, with extension into the CPA and resultant signs and symptoms of cranial nerve VIII dysfunction. A recent theory suggests that exposed bone marrow may hemorrhage into the pneumatized petrous apex air cells, producing the foreign body reaction and granuloma formation.[41] This newer concept more adequately explains the presence of cholesterol granuloma in well-pneumatized temporal bones.

The CT and MRI findings with this lesion are distinguishable from those with the other common lesions of the petrous apex (Table 177-3). On CT, the lesions result in a punched-out appearance of the temporal bone with an isodense mass of the petrous apex that does not enhance; however, rim enhancement is evident with intravenous contrast. On MRI, T1- and T2-weighted images are hyperintense with respect to brain (Fig. 177-14). Primary cholesteatomas are the main lesions from which cholesterol granulomas should be distinguished. Cholesterol granulomas are much more common and occur 20 times more frequently than epidermoids. Overall, cholesterol granulomas are relatively uncommon compared with acoustic neuromas. Only 1 cholesterol granuloma is identified for every 35 acoustic neuromas diagnosed. Imaging distinguishes petrous apex epidermoids from petrous apex cholesterol granulomas. On CT, epidermoids show rim enhancement. With MRI, cholesterol granulomas are hyperintense on T1- and T2-weighted images, whereas epidermoids are hyperintense only on T2-weighted images.

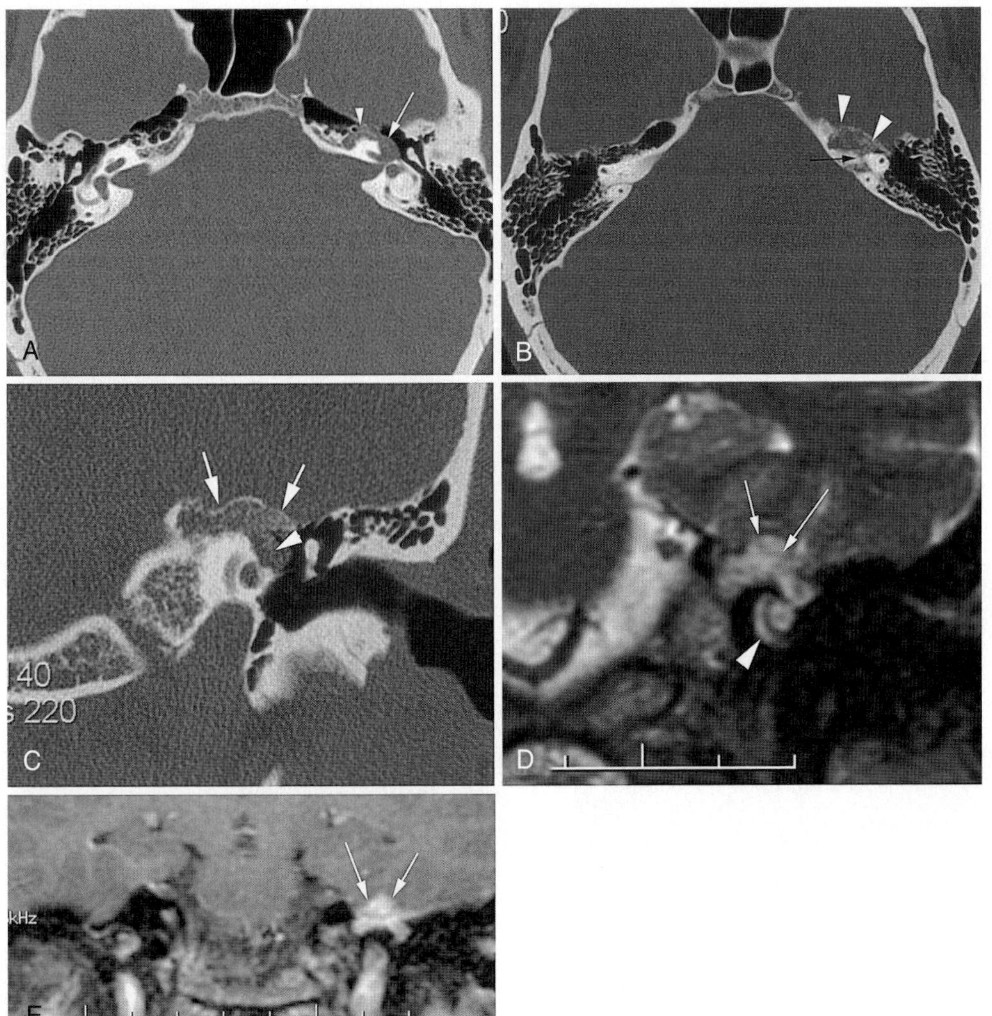

Figure 177-13. Intratemporal vascular tumor in the region of the geniculate ganglion, demonstrated by computed tomography (CT) and magnetic resonance imaging. **A,** CT image through the region of the geniculate ganglion shows expansion of the facial nerve *(arrow)*. Irregular bone is seen extending medially toward the petrous apex *(arrowhead)*. **B,** In this CT image, at a level slightly superior to **A,** demineralization is evident in the region of the labyrinthine segment of the canal *(black arrow)*. Note that the lesion *(arrowheads)* contains small spicules of bone. **C,** Coronal CT image shows the demineralized bone *(arrows)*. The abnormality extends inferiorly to enlarge the FNC *(arrowhead)* and involve the facial nerve. **D,** Coronal T2-weighted image shows the relatively high signal *(arrows)* of the vascular lesion. The fluid within the cochlea *(arrowhead)* is noted for comparison and orientation. **E,** Coronal postcontrast gadolinium T1-weighted magnetic resonance image shows the enhancement *(arrows)* of the lesion. *(From Maya MM, Lo WWM, Kovanlikaya I. Temporal bone tumors and cerebellopontine angle lesions. In: Som PM, Curtin HD, eds.* Head and Neck Imaging. *4th ed. Philadelphia: Mosby; 2003.)*

Total excision of cholesterol granulomas usually is unnecessary. Drainage may be achieved by a transmastoid or transcanal infralabyrinthine approach with preservation of cranial nerve function. The transcanal, infracochlear, hypotympanotomy approach is preferred because it affords dependent drainage and the possibility of revision, if necessary, through a myringotomy.[42] In cases with unfavorable anatomy for infracochlear or infralabyrinthine drainage, middle fossa drainage is an option. Suprisingly, long-term follow-up imaging has demonstrated that middle fossa catheter drainage to the mastoid remains patent.[43]

Asymmetric Petrous Apex Pneumatization

Although asymmetric pneumatization of the petrous apex does not represent a true neoplasm, this condition can be confused with and should be distinguished from true neoplasms. The fat content of bone marrow in a nonpneumatized petrous apex can produce a hyperintense appearance on T1-weighted noncontrast MRI (Fig. 177-15). The lack of bone destruction or expansion on CT, absence of contrast enhancement with gadolinium, and hypointensity on T2-weighted images distinguish this condition from a neoplasm.

Mucocele, Mucus Retention Cysts, and Petrous Apex Effusion

Petrous apex air cells may become obstructed, resulting in retained secretions as a mucus retention cyst in the petrous apex (Fig. 177-16) or an expansile mucocele (Fig. 177-17). CT reveals a nonenhancing lesion limited to the petrous apex air cell system. The MRI appearance is consistent with a mucus-filled lesion (hypointense on T1-weighted and hyperintense on T2-weighted images). A symptomatic mucocele behaves like chronic mastoiditis, with pressure symptoms that require drainage for relief. Occasionally, retained petrous apex fluid also can cause symptoms even without mucocele. Medical treatment as for a middle ear effusion or surgical drainage usually is therapeutic.[43]

Petrous Carotid Artery Aneurysms

Although aneurysms of the horizontal carotid artery are rare, they may appear as expansile, well-defined masses (Fig. 177-18). Their preoperative identification is critical for obvious reasons. Carotid aneurysms may be confused with chondrosarcomas on the basis of radiologic appearance.

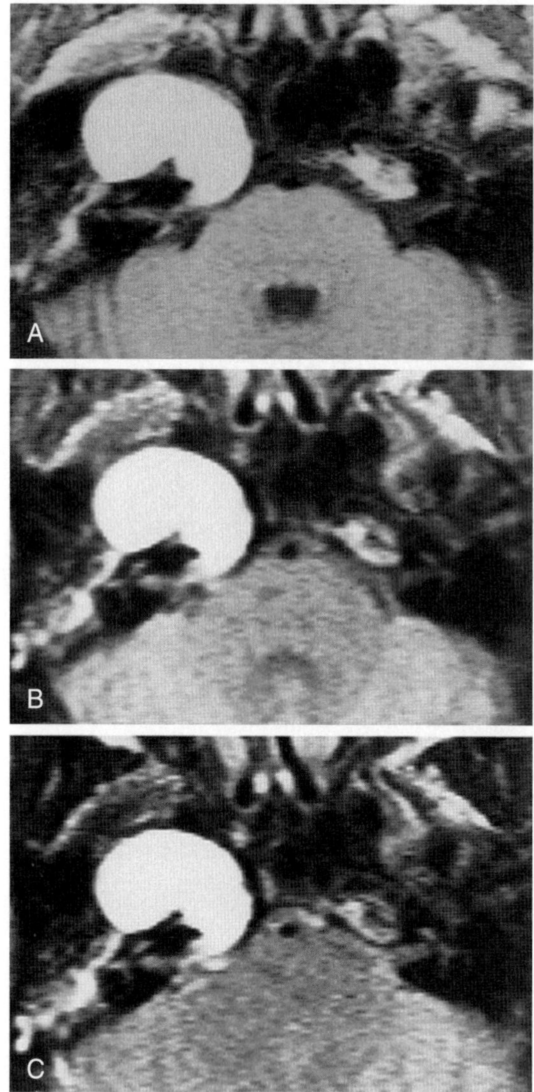

Figure 177-14. Petrous apex cholesterol granuloma, demonstrated by magnetic resonance imaging. **A** to **C,** T1-weighted, proton density, and T2-weighted images, respectively. The lesion is hyperintense on all three images. Note the hypointense rim medial to the lesion accentuated on **B** and **C**, attributable to a hemosiderin deposit or chemical shift artifact. *(From Maya MM, Lo WWM, Kovanlikaya I. Temporal bone tumors and cerebellopontine angle lesions. In: Som PM, Curtin HD, eds.* Head and Neck Imaging. *4th ed. Philadelphia: Mosby; 2003.)*

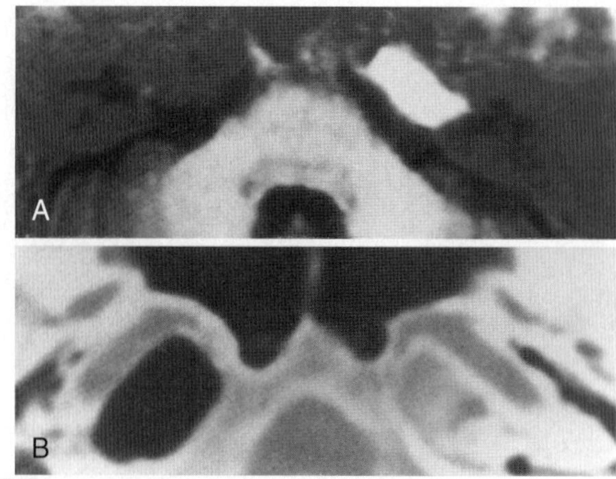

Figure 177-15. Asymmetric pneumatization of the petrous apex, demonstrated on an axial T1-weighted image **(A)** and an axial computed tomography (CT) scan **(B)**. Note that the area of hyperintensity on the T1-weighted image could be confused with a neoplasm. The CT scan reveals extensive pneumatization on the contralateral side and limited pneumatization on the side with hyperintense signal on magnetic resonance imaging.

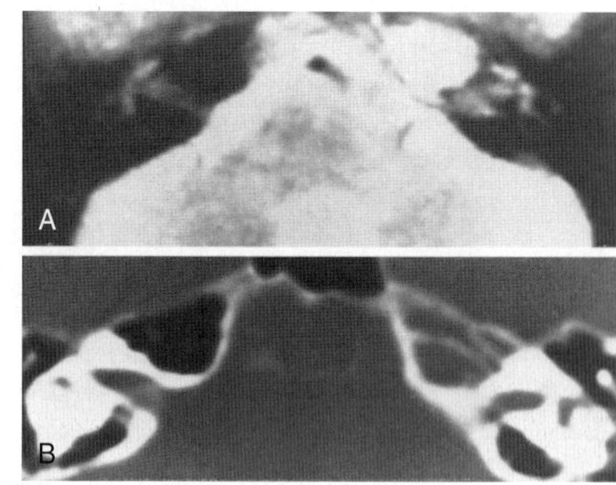

Figure 177-16. Retained mucus in petrous apex air cells, demonstrated on an axial T2-weighted magnetic resonance image **(A)** and an axial computed tomography (CT) scan **(B)**. Note that the mucus is hyperintense on the T2-weighted image, and the CT scan identifies fluid density within the petrous apex air cells.

Giant Cell Tumors

Giant cell tumors are extremely rare primary neoplasms of the temporal bone. They originate from undifferentiated cells of the supporting connective tissue and consist of multinucleated giant cells in a background of spindle-shaped stromal cells. Patients with this unusual condition demonstrate retrocochlear signs and symptoms. CT typically shows a diffuse lesion of the temporal bone compressing the contents of the internal auditory canal.

Miscellaneous Cerebellopontine Angle Lesions

Metastatic Tumors

Tumors may metastasize to the CPA from other sites, including lung, breast, prostate, oropharynx, and skin (i.e., cutaneous melanomas).[44] Tumors from these sites are distinguished by their rapid progression of symptoms and associated neurologic signs, in addition to hearing loss and dizziness. Associated lytic lesions in the petrous apex constitute another distinguishing feature of metastatic tumors. Rapid impairment of hearing, other cranial neuropathies, and brainstem dysfunction suggest malignant neoplasms of the posterior fossa, especially in a patient with a history of another malignancy.

Chordomas

Chordomas are dysontogenetic neoplasms that arise in remnants of the embryonic notochord. Although more than one half of these tumors arise in the sacrococcygeal region, more than one third occur at the skull base in the region of the clivus or, less commonly, the upper cervical vertebrae.[45] The prominent clinical characteristics are extensive bone destruction and progressive cranial nerve palsies. Extension of clivus chordomas to the petrous apex, sphenoid, or CPA is not unusual. Although fronto-orbital headache and vision complaints (e.g., limited visual fields, diplopia, loss of acuity) are more common, occasionally the initial symptoms reflect extension into the CPA. On CT, the bone destruction is readily apparent, and the masses are homogeneous with moderate enhancement and a greater density than that of bone

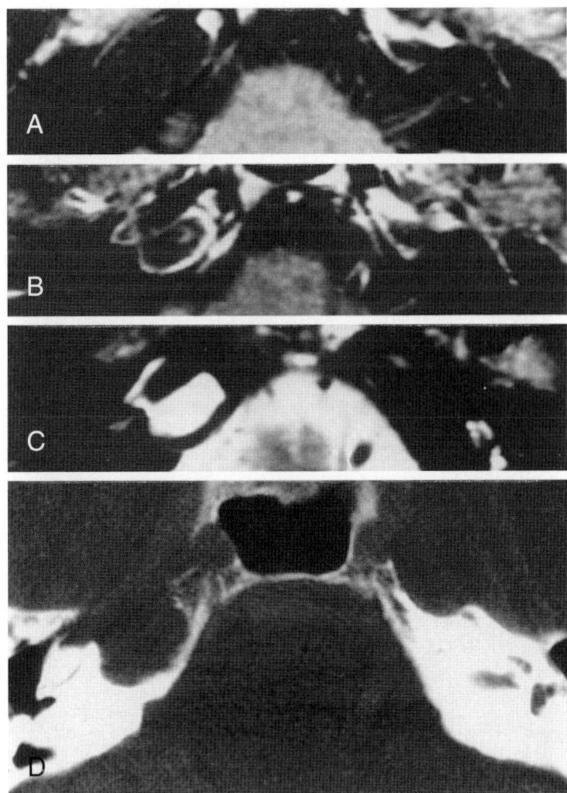

Figure 177-17. **A** to **C,** Axial magnetic resonance images of a petrous apex mucocele: T1-weighted without gadolinium **(A),** T1-weighted with gadolinium **(B),** and T2-weighted **(C).** The lesion is hypointense on the T1-weighted image and shows only rim enhancement with the addition of gadolinium. Note the hyperintensity of the mucocele on the T2-weighted image. **D,** Axial computed tomography scan of the same lesion. Note that the expansile lesion has eroded the petrous apex.

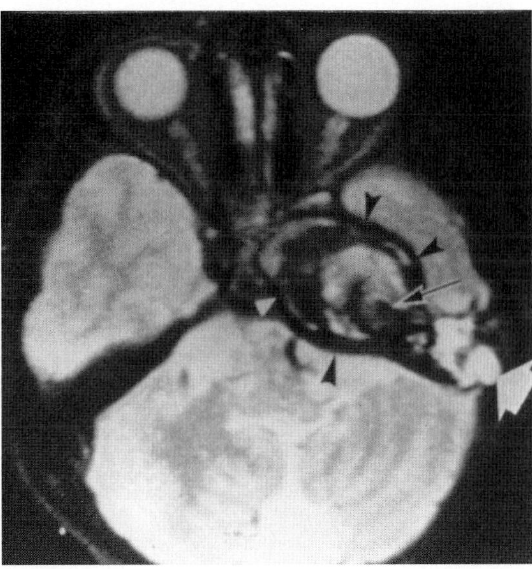

Figure 177-18. Axial T2-weighted magnetic resonance image of a petrous carotid aneurysm. The lesion is heterogeneous and shows decreased signal intensity within the thrombus. The circumscribing areas of low signal intensity *(arrowheads)* probably represents hemosiderin. The lumen *(long thin arrow)* has intermediate signal intensity as a result of slow flow as noted on the arteriogram *(not shown)* and is difficult to distinguish from thrombus. High-signal-intensity fluid is seen in multiple mastoid air cells *(short wide arrow). (From Tsuruda JS, Halbach VV, Higashida RT, Mark AS, Hieshima GB, Norman D. MRI evaluation of large intracranial aneurysms using cine low flip angle gradient-refocused imaging.* Am J Neuroradiol. *1988;9:418.)*

(Fig. 177-19). MRI reveals isointensity on T1-weighted images and hyperintensity on T2-weighted images (Fig. 177-20).

Chondrosarcomas

Chondrosarcomas of the skull base also may arise in the CPA. They are clinically indistinguishable from chordomas except that they are centered more laterally. CT shows characteristic bone destruction and invasiveness. MRI shows this lesion well, which is hyperintense on T2-weighted images in the area of bone destruction in the skull base (Figs. 177-21 and 177-22).

Lipomas

Lipomas are hamartomas that are thinly encapsulated and poorly delineated. They appear as soft, multilobular masses of typical adult adipose tissue. Lipomas within the internal auditory canal can produce symptoms typical of an acoustic neuroma. Although on CT these lesions are less dense than neuromas, MRI is diagnostic. The lesions are hyperintense on T1-weighted images, nonenhancing with gadolinium, and hypointense on T2-weighted images (Fig. 177-23). Fat-suppression techniques with T1-weighted sequences are confirmatory because the previously identified lesion that was hyperintense on nonenhanced T1-weighted images is rendered hypointense with fat suppression (Fig. 177-24).

Dermoid Tumors

A dermoid is a skin-lined cystic tumor containing dermal and adnexal structures. The lining of the cyst is mature, stratified squamous epithelium. A dermoid is a slowly expanding lesion that produces symptoms similar to those of a primary cholesteatoma. It may be differentiated

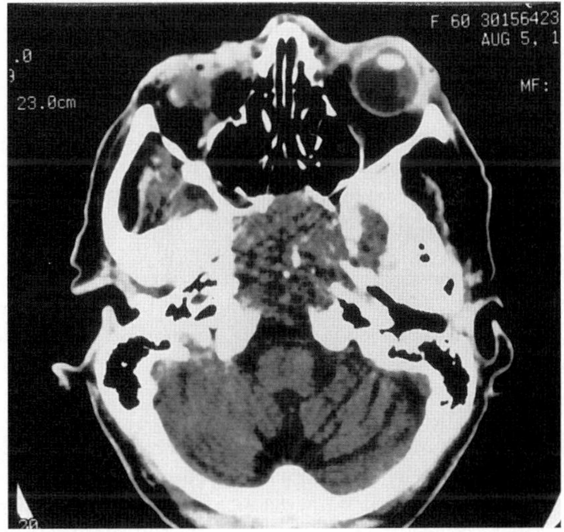

Figure 177-19. Axial computed tomography scan shows a large midline chordoma involving the petrous apex bilaterally.

on CT as a nonhomogeneous cystic mass that contains calcium but that is otherwise less dense than brain.

Teratomas

Teratomas arise from multipotential cells that differentiate into various tissues, representing more than one germ layer. They contain ectodermal, mesodermal, and endodermal tissues. Carcinomatous or sarcomatous changes occur in 10% to 35% of these tumors. When malignant degeneration occurs, symptoms progress rapidly; otherwise, slow progression is the rule, making the lesions indistinguishable from other benign CPA tumors. CT shows a nonhomogeneous lesion of less density than brain without enhancing characteristics.

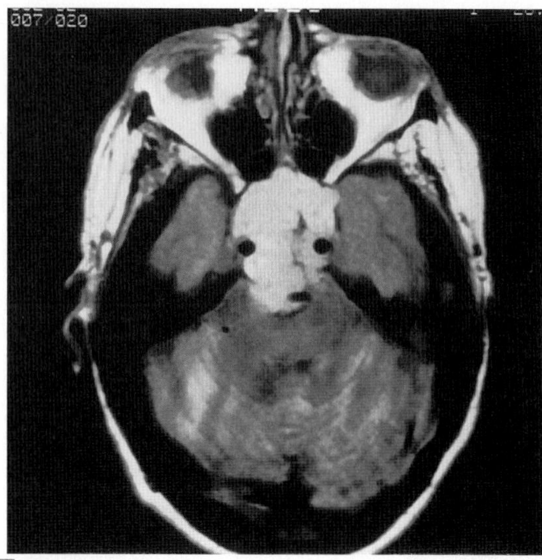

Figure 177-20. Noncontrast T1-weighted axial magnetic resonance image of the same chordoma as in Figure 177-19.

Intra-axial Tumors

Intra-axial tumors may occasionally be confused with CPA tumors as a result of extension to the CPA or compression of CPA structures. Intra-axial tumors may arise from the brainstem (gliomas), the cerebellum (medulloblastomas from the vermis or astrocytomas from the peduncles), or the fourth ventricle (choroid plexus papillomas and ependymomas). Although such lesions are highly unusual, the possibility cannot be ignored. In children, brainstem gliomas are reportedly the most common CPA neoplasms. Intra-axial tumors usually are isointense on T1-weighted MRI and hyperintense on T2-weighted images.[20,21]

Hemangioblastomas

Hemangioblastomas are tumors of blood vessel origin occurring primarily in the cerebellum. They also may occur in the cerebral hemispheres and in association with a similar retinal tumor and may be multicentric. Although histologically benign, hemangioblastomas may produce major neurologic dysfunction by compression of the brainstem.

Rapidly progressive signs and symptoms of cerebellar dysfunction are characteristic of this tumor. Hearing and balance are likely to remain normal. Imaging studies identify a tumor intrinsic to the cerebellum that may extend into the CPA.

Medulloblastomas

Medulloblastomas arise from the cells of the external granular layer of the cerebellar folia. They may appear as exophytic masses on the cerebellum with extension into the CPA. Symptoms are produced by destruction of cerebellar tissue and mass effect of the tumor on the CPA's adjacent structures.

Medulloblastomas are characterized by a rapid development of symptoms. In addition to hearing loss and dizziness, associated neurologic findings include facial weakness, dysmetria of speech and hand motion, perverted nystagmus, and abnormal peripheral reflexes. Temporal bone imaging findings are normal, but CT and MRI show a lesion intrinsic to the cerebellum.

Brainstem Gliomas

Exophytic gliomas may arise on the surface of the pons and grow into the CPA. Gliomas also may be intrinsic to the brainstem. Exophytic gliomas may produce signs and symptoms similar to those of acoustic neuromas, whereas the intrinsic variety produces predominantly long tract signs.

Patients with exophytic lesions may be diagnosed preoperatively to have acoustic neuromas. Long tract signs in association with characteristic brainstem distortion on imaging make preoperative diagnosis possible in the patients with intrinsic lesions.

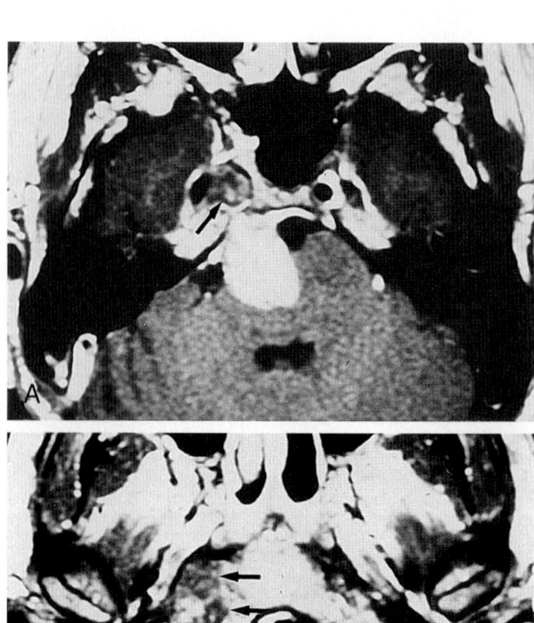

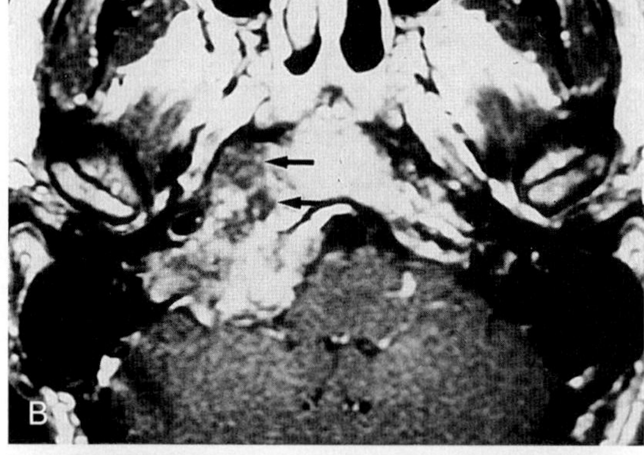

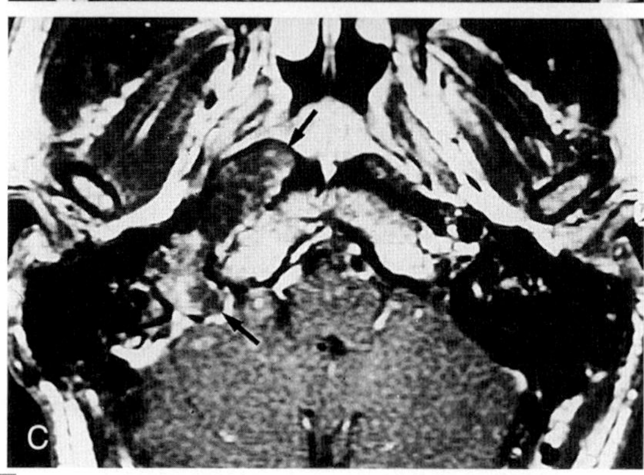

Figure 177-21. Right petrous apex chondrosarcoma. **A** to **C,** On gadolinium T1-weighted magnetic resonance imaging, the mass is markedly but inhomogeneously enhancing, with components containing small, poorly enhancing or nonenhancing foci in Meckel's cave (*arrow* in **A**) and in the petrous apex (*arrows* in **B**), as well as involvement of the longus colli muscle and jugular fossa (*arrows* in **C**). Note the markedly enhancing transdural components in the posterior fossa and the dural "tail" in **A** and **B**. *(From Maya MM, Lo WWM, Kovanlikaya I. Temporal bone tumors and cerebellopontine angle lesions. In: Som PM, Curtin HD, eds.* Head and Neck Imaging. *4th ed. Philadelphia: Mosby; 2003.)*

Tumors of the Fourth Ventricle

Malignant Choroid Plexus Papillomas and Ependymomas

Choroid plexus papillomas and ependymomas arise from the fourth ventricle and cause CPA symptoms by growing through the foramen of Luschka. In this location, they produce early signs of cranial nerve VIII dysfunction. In malignant choroid plexus papillomas, CT shows a mass with enhancing characteristics of a schwannoma (Fig. 177-25). These tumors are distinguishable from an acoustic schwannoma by being separate from the internal auditory canal. Ependymomas may

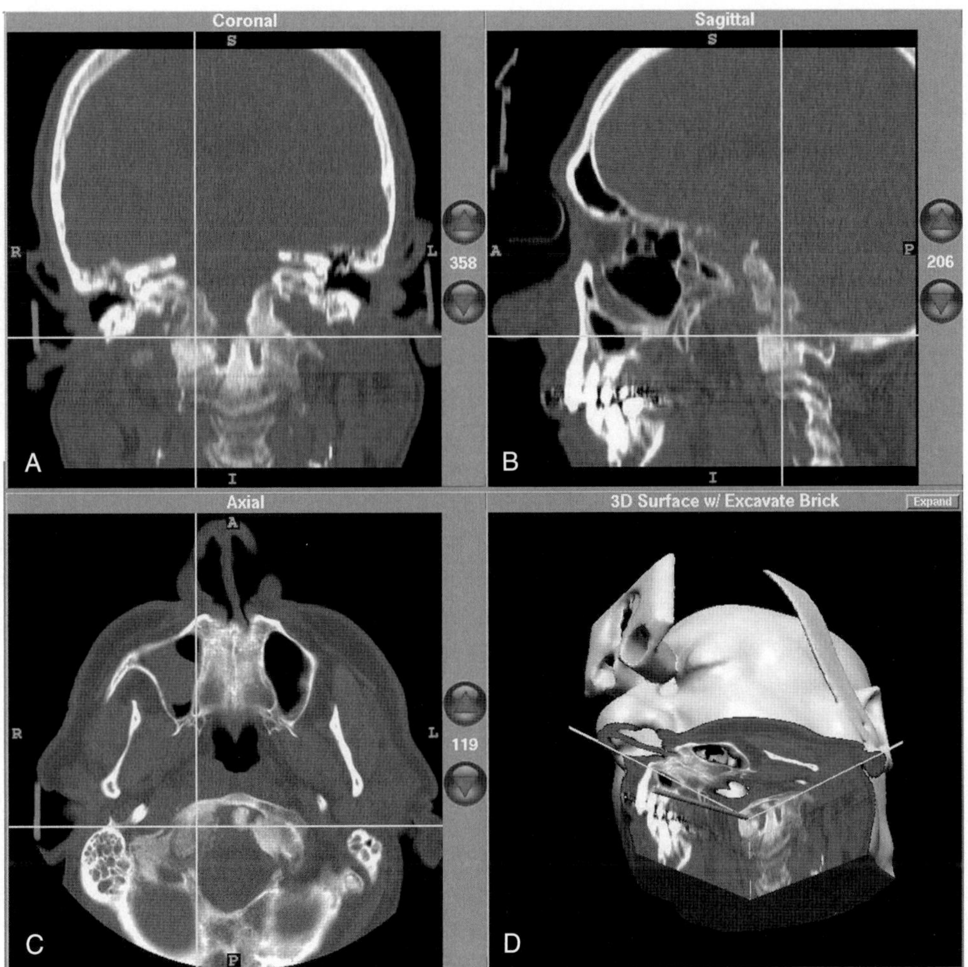

Figure 177-22. Skull base chondrosarcoma, demonstrated by magnetic resonance imaging. **A** and **B,** Axial T1-weighted pre- and postgadolinium images. **C,** Axial T2-weighted images. **D,** Coronal T1-weighted image after gadolinium enhancement. *(From Maya MM, Lo WWM, Kovanlikaya I. Temporal bone tumors and cerebellopontine angle lesions. In: Som PM, Curtin HD, eds.* Head and Neck Imaging. *4th ed. Philadelphia: Mosby; 2003.)*

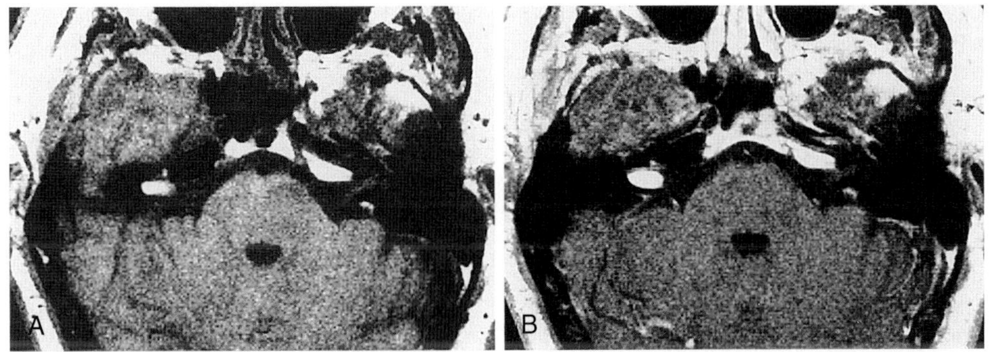

Figure 177-23. Lipoma of the right internal auditory canal, demonstrated by magnetic resonance imaging. **A,** T1-weighted image without gadolinium enhancement. **B,** Postgadolinium T1-weighted image. The lipoma has high signal intensity without gadolinium, which does not change after administration of contrast. *(From Maya MM, Lo WWM, Kovanlikaya I. Temporal bone tumors and cerebellopontine angle lesions. In: Som PM, Curtin HD, eds.* Head and Neck Imaging. *4th ed. Philadelphia: Mosby; 2003.)*

calcify, and those portions have variable imaging characteristics. At MRI, both lesions are isointense to brain on T1-weighted images and mildly hyperintense to brain on T2-weighted images (Fig. 177-26). Malignant ependymomas require multimodality therapy. The role of surgery is for biopsy, brainstem decompression, and management of hydrocephalus.

Surgery of the Posterior Cranial Fossa

This section addresses surgical management of extra-axial lesions of the posterior cranial fossa and internal auditory canal. Adequate exposure for skull base neoplasms involving the posterior fossa requires precise management of the temporal bone. The modern era for skull base surgery and transtemporal techniques began in 1961, when House

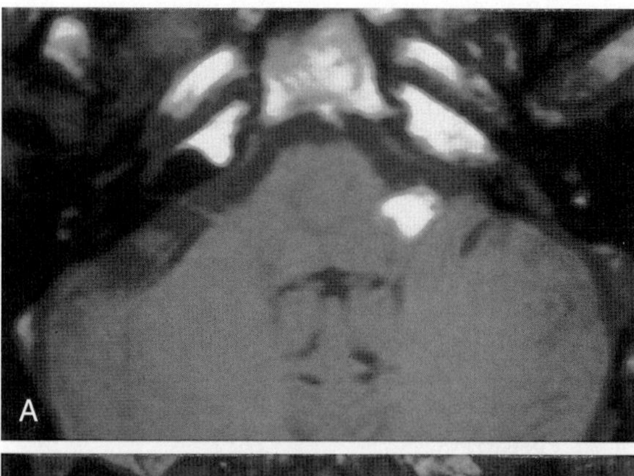

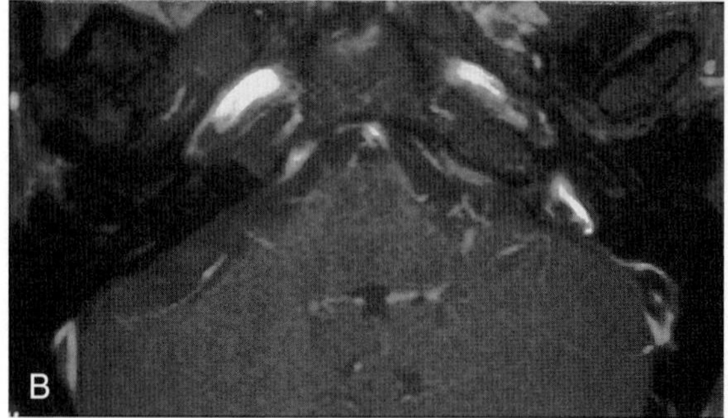

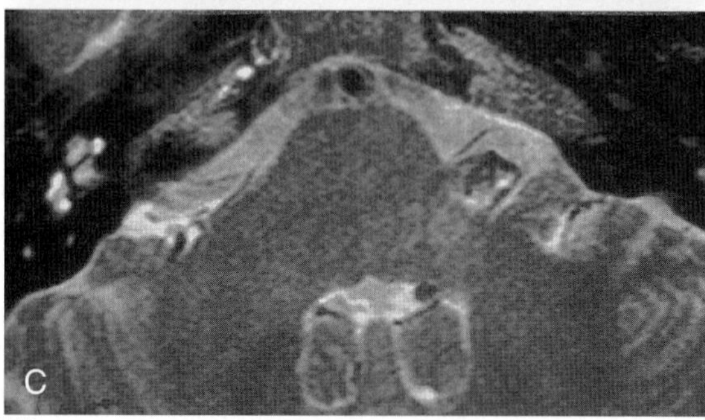

Figure 177-24. Cerebellopontine angle lipoma, demonstrated by magnetic resonance imaging. **A** and **B,** T1-weighted and fat-saturated postgadolinium images. The signal intensity of the tumor is similar to that of bone marrow. Note the signal loss of the tumor and fatty bone marrow on the fat-saturated images. No enhancement of the lesion is seen. **C,** T2-weighted image. The lipoma typically is moderately hypointense and is seen with surrounding signal void vessels. *(From Maya MM, Lo WWM, Kovanlikaya I. Temporal bone tumors and cerebellopontine angle lesions. In: Som PM, Curtin HD, eds.* Head and Neck Imaging. *4th ed. Philadelphia: Mosby; 2003.)*

introduced the operating microscope and multidisciplinary team surgery for removal of acoustic neuromas. With the vastly reduced mortality and excellent facial nerve preservation rates of the translabyrinthine approach for acoustic neuromas, House established the translabyrinthine approach as the procedure with which all other microsurgical approaches to the CPA are compared.[46] Subsequently, multiple approaches to the CPA have been developed, each with its own advantages and indications.

Thus, the modern skull base surgical team can choose from among various approaches for resection of posterior fossa neoplasms. The procedure should be tailored to the individual patient's pathology and physiologic status. Realistic counseling of patients is critical for informed decisions concerning surgical approaches and possible cranial nerve sequelae. Skull base surgery is a team endeavor, and the full array of experts familiar with the specific needs of these patients is necessary for a successful outcome.

This section details the basic approach, specific indications, techniques, and special features of the translabyrinthine, retrosigmoid, suboccipital, retrolabyrinthine, transcochlear, transotic, middle fossa, extended middle fossa, and petrosal approaches for skull base neoplasms involving the posterior fossa. Table 177-4 summarizes the basic indications for and drawbacks of the various approaches for resection of these tumors.

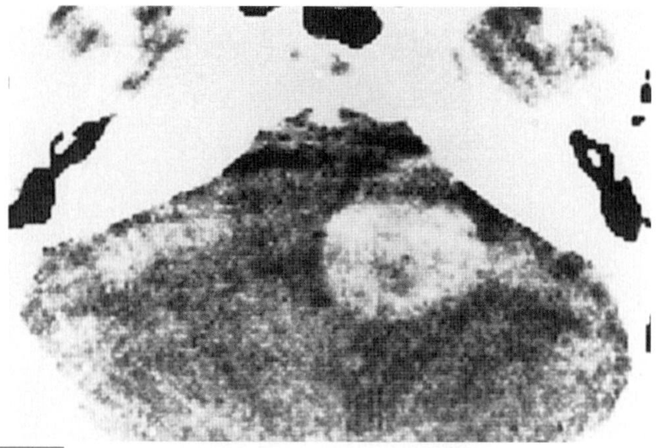

Figure 177-25. CPA choroid plexus papilloma, demonstrated by contrast computed tomography. The tumor is located at the foramen of Luschka. It is more sharply defined than an ependymoma. Like a giant aneurysm, it is detached from the petrous bone, in contrast with schwannomas and meningiomas. *(From Maya MM, Lo WWM, Kovanlikaya I. Temporal bone tumors and cerebellopontine angle lesions. In: Som PM, Curtin HD, eds.* Head and Neck Imaging. *4th ed. Philadelphia: Mosby; 2003.)*

In addition, the surgical approaches for skull base lesions that are adequately managed by drainage also are reviewed. A method for selecting the surgical approaches for removal of acoustic neuromas suitable for hearing preservation is presented, and general principles of patient management and management of complications of posterior fossa tumor surgery are outlined.

Translabyrinthine Approach

Basic Approach

A transmastoid labyrinthectomy and skeletonization of the sigmoid sinus and posterior fossa dura permit identification of the facial nerve with wide exposure of the internal auditory canal and CPA (Fig. 177-27).

Indications

The translabyrinthine approach is the principal neuro-otologic approach for all lesions of the CPA and internal auditory canal. This technique is ideal for removal of medium-sized and large acoustic neuromas, because hearing preservation is unlikely by any approach in tumors larger than 2 cm and because this approach carries the highest rate of preservation of facial nerve function. Small acoustic neuromas in patients without serviceable hearing also are removed by the translabyrinthine approach.

The approach is suited for removal of any neoplasms requiring exposure of the CPA, including meningiomas, nonacoustic neuromas, gliomas, chordomas, and skull base chondrosarcomas. In addition, if serviceable hearing is not present, the translabyrinthine approach is useful for complete facial nerve decompression and vestibular neurectomy.

Technique

The following discussion details patient positioning, preparation, monitoring, and tumor removal for the translabyrinthine approach. The same techniques are used for the other approaches except when otherwise specified.

The patient is positioned supine with the head turned to the opposite side. Head-holding pins or supports are not used. Electromy-

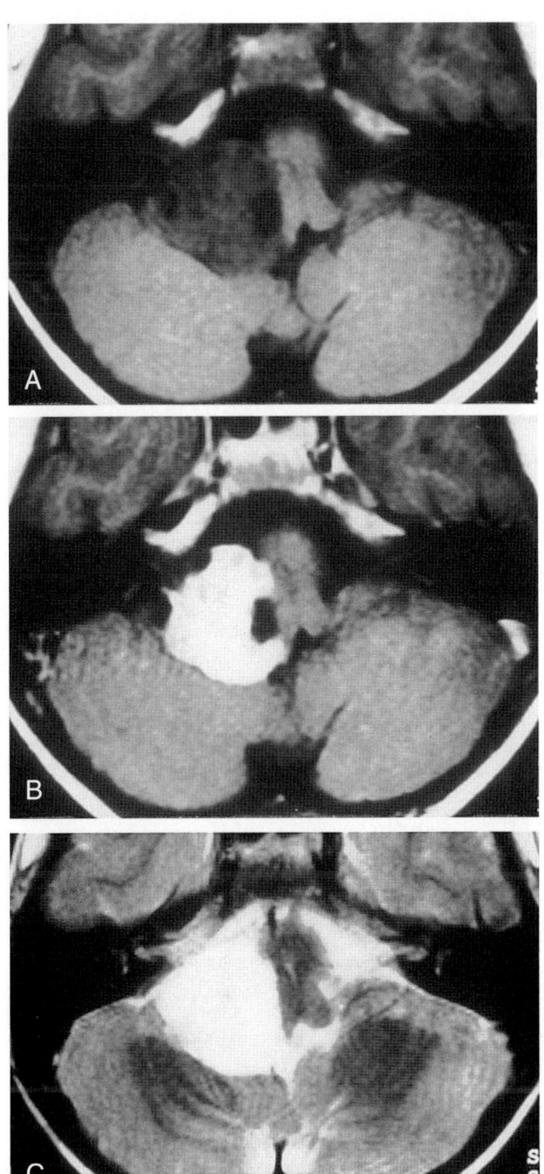

Figure 177-26. CPA ependymoma, demonstrated by magnetic resonance imaging. **A** and **B,** Pre- and postgadolinium images. The mass protruding into the right CPA from the foramen of Luschka shows clear demarcation and strong enhancement. **C,** T2-weighted image. The tumor is hyperintense and does not extend into the IAC. *(From Maya MM, Lo WWM, Kovanlikaya I. Temporal bone tumors and cerebellopontine angle lesions. In: Som PM, Curtin HD, eds.* Head and Neck Imaging. *4th ed. Philadelphia: Mosby; 2003:240-250.)*

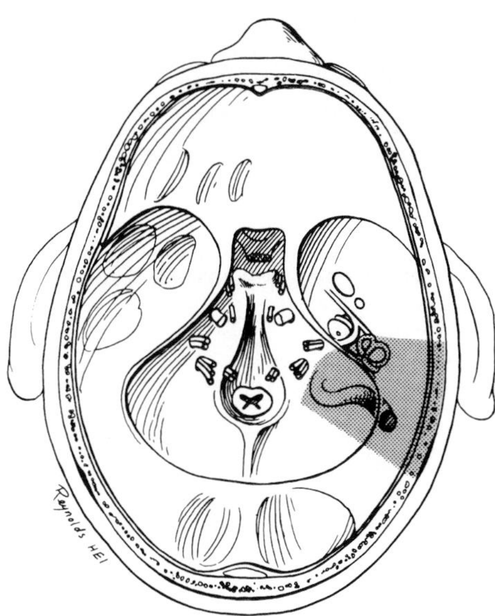

Figure 177-27. Surgical exposure in the translabyrinthine approach to the cerebellopontine angle (CPA). This approach permits direct access to the CPA without retraction of the cerebellum.

ography (EMG) electrodes for intraoperative facial nerve monitoring are inserted into the orbicularis oris and orbicularis oculi. Intravenous antibiotic is administered when the patient arrives in the operating room. Antibiotic also is used in the irrigation solution. Hyperventilation usually is sufficient for brain relaxation.

The curved postauricular incision is made with the apex 3 cm posterior to the postauricular crease. The soft tissue and periosteum are elevated from the mastoid and adjacent occipital bone, and self-retaining retractors are inserted.

The bone removal is accomplished in four stages and is performed using the operating microscope, a high-speed drill, and continuous suction-irrigation.[5] Most of the drilling is performed with cutting burrs; however, diamond burrs are used when drilling is performed on the dura or venous sinuses. The *first stage* is a complete mastoidectomy. Posteriorly, the bone is removed beyond the sigmoid sinus, and the sinus is skeletonized. The extent of bone removal posterior to the sinus and decompression of the posterior fossa depends on the size of the tumor. Greater posterior removal provides greater exposure of the CPA. Superiorly, the middle fossa plate is identified and thinned. Anteriorly, the facial nerve is identified in its vertical segment but left covered with bone for protection against inadvertent burr trauma.

The *second stage* is complete labyrinthectomy. The horizontal, superior, and posterior semicircular canals are systematically removed. Particular care is required in working along the inferior border of the horizontal canal because of the proximity of the facial nerve, and along the ampulated end of the posterior canal because this end lies medial to the facial nerve.

The *third stage* of bone removal consists of actual decompression of the middle and posterior fossa dura and removal of bone around the internal auditory canal. The bone overlying the posterior fossa is removed with cutting and diamond burrs, except for an island of bone over the sigmoid sinus ("Bill's island"). The mastoid emissary vein should be transected to permit retraction of the sinus and posterior fossa dura. Accordingly, bleeding from the emissary should be controlled with sutures, cautery, or bone wax. The petrous ridge, which is the junction between the middle fossa dura and the posterior fossa dura, should be removed. The superior petrosal sinus, which lies under the petrous ridge, is sometimes adherent to the bone. The resulting bleeding is controlled with bipolar cautery or extradural packing with oxidized cellulose strips (Surgicel). The entire middle fossa dura and posterior fossa dura adjacent to the mastoid are exposed.

The *final stage* of bone removal consists of skeletonization of the internal auditory canal. The orientation of this structure is roughly parallel to the external auditory canal. Thus, the fundus of the canal is just medial to the floor of the vestibule, which was exposed during the labyrinthectomy. By contrast, identification of the porus requires extensive bone removal as the internal auditory canal is dissected medially. The basic principle of exposing the internal auditory canal is that all bone removal should be accomplished before the dura is opened, and complete bone removal requires decompression of 270 degrees around the circumference of the canal to avoid obscuring any ledges of bone. By completing bone removal before opening the dura, the risk of accidental injury to the nerves of the internal auditory canal is minimized. The inferior border of the canal is skeletonized first. This edge of the canal is identified by gradually enlarging a trough between the inferior edge of the vestibule and the jugular bulb. The cochlear aqueduct

Table 177-4

Surgical Approaches for Resection of Posterior Fossa Skull Base Neoplasms: Indications, Advantages, and Disadvantages

Approach	Indications	Advantages	Disadvantages
Translabyrinthine	Large, medium-sized, or small cerebellopontine angle tumor	Wide exposure not limited by tumor size; facial nerve identified at the cerebellopontine angle and fundus of the internal auditory canal; immediate repair of facial nerve is possible; bone removal is extradural; limited cerebellar retraction	Total hearing loss
Retrosigmoid (suboccipital)	Cerebellopontine angle tumors without extensive internal auditory canal involvement	Hearing preservation possible; wide exposure; familiarity to most neurosurgeons	Internal auditory canal fundus not exposed in hearing preservation cases; cerebellar retraction may produce hydrocephalus; intradural drilling may result in severe headaches
Retrolabyrinthine	Selected cerebellopontine angle lesions without internal auditory canal involvement, biopsy of cerebellopontine angle lesions	Hearing preservation possible; bone removal is extradural; no cerebellar retraction	Limited exposure
Transcochlear	Extensive lesions of petrous apex and clivus	Wide exposure of skull base with access to clivus and vertebral and basilar arteries and full exposure of petrous carotid artery	Temporary facial nerve paralysis; total hearing loss
Transotic	Same as for transcochlear; some advocate use in acoustic neuromas with unfavorable venous anatomy	Same as for transcochlear; no facial nerve transposition	Facial nerve in the internal auditory canal and mastoid segments limits exposure; total hearing loss
Middle fossa	Intracanalicular tumors with minimal cerebellopontine angle involvement and good hearing	Hearing preservation possible	Small tumors only; temporal lobe retraction
Extended middle fossa	Petroclival lesions involving posterior and middle fossa with good hearing	Hearing preservation possible	Extensive temporal lobe retraction
Petrosal	Large petroclival lesions with good residual hearing	Widest posterior and middle fossa exposure available	Cerebellar and temporal lobe retraction

usually is identified as the dissection proceeds anteromedially. This structure becomes the inferior limit of the dissection, thereby protecting the lower cranial nerves from injury. After the inferior border of the internal auditory canal has been identified, the bone overlying the porus acusticus is thinned with cutting and diamond burrs. The superior border of the canal is identified last, because the facial nerve is more susceptible to injury in this area. A burr size that will fit between the middle fossa dura and the superior border of the internal auditory canal is used to expose the superior border. The entrance of the facial nerve into the canal can be positively identified just medial to a vertical crest of bone, "Bill's bar," along the superior aspect of the fundus. At this point, the bony exposure has been completed, and tumor removal can begin (Fig. 177-28).

Tumor Removal

With small lesions, opening the dura of the internal auditory canal exposes the tumor. Attention is focused on the fundus of the canal, and an angled hook placed lateral to Bill's bar is used to reflect the superior vestibular nerve inferiorly and then transect it. This maneuver protects the facial nerve and identifies the lateral plane between the facial nerve and the tumor. Sharp and blunt dissection can proceed with scissors and angled hooks from lateral to medial, but without actually placing traction on the facial nerve. With some small tumors, the dissection can be completed entirely without debulking.

With large tumors, CPA exposure is necessary. Intracapsular tumor debulking is completed before the tumor is dissected directly from the facial nerve. In essence, a large tumor is reduced to a small tumor. The dural flaps are developed carefully to avoid injury to the underlying petrosal vein or even branches of the anterior inferior cerebellar artery that can reach the dura. The incision is placed midway between the sigmoid sinus and the porus acusticus. The incision is carried directly to the porus and then continued in a curve around the porus.

Debulking should be accomplished to allow positive identification of the facial nerve medial to the tumor and to complete dissection of the tumor from the brainstem. Vessels that do not actually enter the tumor are reflected away, and the posterior aspect of the tumor is incised. Intracapsular debulking is accomplished with small dissection

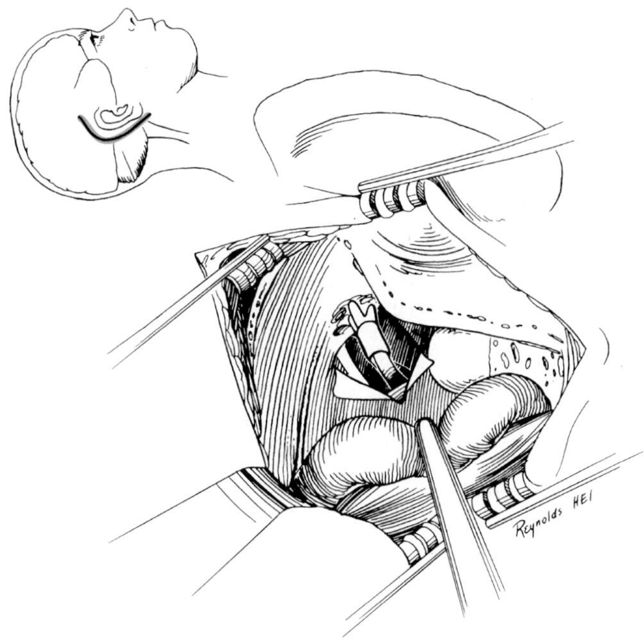

Figure 177-28. Surgical exposure in the translabyrinthine approach to the cerebellopontine angle (CPA). This approach permits positive identification of the facial nerve in its bony canal at the fundus of the internal auditory canal and at the brainstem. *Inset* shows skin incision in relation to the CPA.

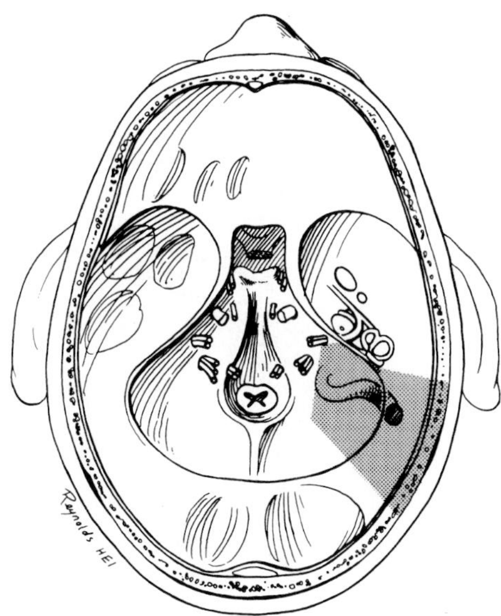

Figure 177-29. Surgical exposure in the retrosigmoid approach to the cerebellopontine angle (CPA). This approach permits wide access to the CPA; however, the cerebellum is between the surgeon and the CPA. Thus, cerebellar support (retraction) is required to permit complete visualization of the CPA.

forceps, scissors, or a rotatory dissector (e.g., House-Urban dissector) or one of the power dissectors used in endoscopic sinus surgery. Some surgeons prefer to use the laser or ultrasonic aspirator for debulking. Such intracapsular debulking permits the tumor to collapse onto itself for easier manipulation during its dissection from the facial nerve. The arachnoid sheath that binds the tumor to the nerve anteriorly is released with small hooks.

In tumor dissection, it is important to avoid pushing the tumor medially into the CPA, because this maneuver stretches the nerve at its lateral fixed bony attachment. The tumor and capsule are removed by separating them completely from the facial nerve. Once tumor debulking is completed and the facial nerve is identified medially, attention is focused on the fundus of the internal auditory canal. Final tumor dissection proceeds as for a small tumor. In this manner, most of the tumor has been removed, while the facial nerve has been protected in the dura of the internal auditory canal.

After tumor removal, eustachian tube closure is achieved by removing the incus, transecting the tensor tympani tendon, and filling the eustachian tube with Surgicel. The temporalis muscle closes the eustachian tube. By opening the facial recess during drilling, the surgeon obtains wide exposure for eustachian tube occlusion. The edges of the dura are approximated with sutures, and the mastoidectomy defect is filled with strips of abdominal fat. The ends of the strips are placed through the dural defect to plug the dural opening. Cranioplasty with use of hydroxyapatite cement or titanium mesh is a useful technique to reduce the incidence of CSF fistula postoperatively and to enhance long-term wound healing and the cosmetic result.[47,48] The wound is closed in layers, and a compressive dressing is applied.

Special Features

The translabyrinthine approach provides wide and direct access to CPA tumors with minimal cerebellar retraction. The versatility of this approach for large and small tumors makes it the most common approach for resection of acoustic neuromas.

The fundamental advantage of the translabyrinthine approach, particularly in medium-sized and large tumors, is that it permits positive identification of the facial nerve, laterally at the fundus and medially at the brainstem. Thus, the tumor can be dissected from either direction with optimal control of the facial nerve. Such medial and lateral identification of the nerve has permitted anatomic preservation of the facial nerve in greater than 98.5% of 759 acoustic neuromas removed in one large surgical series.[49] Furthermore, if the facial nerve is transected, as occurs in cases of CPA facial nerve neuroma, the tympanic and mastoid portions of the nerve are available for rerouting and reanastomosis or grafting.

Properly performed, with wide exposure of the middle and posterior fossae, the translabyrinthine approach provides exposure of the CPA as good as with any other neurosurgical approach; however, the direct route of exposure of the CPA eliminates the need for cerebellar support (retraction).

The disadvantage of this approach is that hearing cannot be preserved. In a series of 300 consecutive cases of acoustic neuromas diagnosed before the advent of gadolinium-enhanced MRI, only 5% of patients, using the broadest criteria, could be considered candidates for hearing conservation surgery.[50] The advent of gadolinium-enhanced MRI resulted in an increased percentage of acoustic neuromas among those detected, which are diagnosed at a small size before hearing is affected. Thus, hearing conservation procedures are becoming a more frequent consideration.

Retrosigmoid (Suboccipital) Approach

Basic Approach

Transmastoid decompression of the sigmoid sinus and a retrosigmoid craniotomy permit access to CPA tumors without disturbing the labyrinth. Intradural removal of the posterior wall of the internal auditory canal permits direct access to the medial two thirds of the canal (Fig. 177-29).

Indications

Because the principal advantage of this approach is hearing preservation, this technique is excellent for removal of acoustic neuromas of the CPA in patients with serviceable hearing and limited involvement of the internal auditory canal. Nonacoustic neoplasms of the CPA that do not involve the internal auditory canal, such as meningiomas, can be approached in this fashion with an opportunity for hearing preservation.

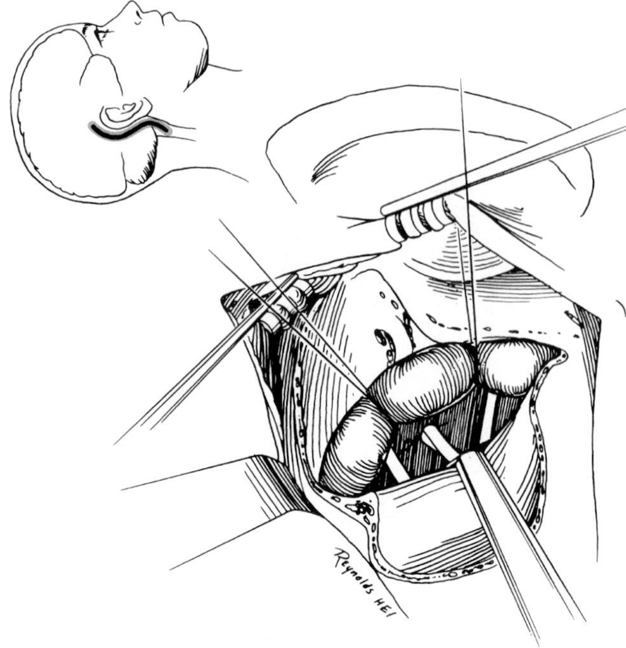

Figure 177-30. Surgical exposure in the retrosigmoid approach to the cerebellopontine angle (CPA). The mastoidectomy in conjunction with the retrosigmoid exposure permits anterior retraction of the sigmoid sinus, which improves anterior exposure. The mastoidectomy also allows positive identification of the posterior semicircular canal, which facilitates removal of the posterior lip of the internal auditory canal. *Inset* shows skin incision in relation to the CPA.

Technique

The soft tissues of the ear are reflected anteriorly and the muscles are widely reflected from the retromastoid region. Complete mastoidectomy is performed, and the sigmoid sinus is skeletonized and decompressed. The posterior semicircular canal also is skeletonized, and the posterior fossa dura up to the posterior semicircular canal is exposed. This area of exposed dura identifies the location of the posterior semicircular canal if the posterior lip of the internal auditory canal needs to be removed later in the procedure. A bone flap is removed posterior to the sigmoid sinus with the otologic drill. This flap can be preserved for replacement at the conclusion of the procedure. Alternatively, in cases with favorable venous anatomy, a craniectomy with skeletonization of the dura and sinus can be performed without entering the presigmoid mastoid air cells.

The dura is incised posterior to the sigmoid sinus, with care taken to avoid injury to the underlying vessels that may be adherent to the dura. Adequate drainage of CSF is necessary to minimize the need for cerebellar retraction. The cerebellum is exposed and supported with retractors to allow visualization of the tumor in the CPA. The neurosurgical techniques for tumor removal at the brainstem are the same regardless of the approach chosen. If the tumor is too large to permit proximal identification of the facial nerve, debulking of the tumor is performed. Once the debulking has been accomplished, the tumor is dissected from the facial nerve toward the porus acusticus (Fig. 177-30).

If the tumor extends into the internal auditory canal, the posterior lip of the canal is removed with diamond burrs. A dural flap is created lateral to the porus and reflected medially. Drilling of the posterior lip of the canal is continued until the lateral extent of the tumor is visualized. The anatomic limit for exposure of this posterior lip that will preserve hearing is the posterior semicircular canal. Attention to the area of dura previously exposed just posterior to the posterior semicircular canal will direct the surgeon to the precise location of the posterior canal when the posterior lip of the internal auditory canal is removed. Once the lateral limit of the tumor has been identified, tumor removal is accomplished in the same manner as with the translabyrinthine approach.

Unlike in the translabyrinthine approach, in which Bill's bar permits definitive identification of the facial nerve at the fundus, in the retrosigmoid approach the surgeon relies primarily on the facial nerve monitor for identifying the nerve laterally in the internal auditory canal. Once the location of the nerves is known medially and laterally, the tumor usually can be removed with preservation of the facial nerve. With surgery attempting hearing preservation, the cochlear nerve also should be preserved. Particular care is taken to preserve the blood supply to the internal auditory canal, because hearing preservation depends on an intact blood supply.

After tumor removal, the edges of the dura are reapproximated, and the mastoid and the internal auditory canal are obliterated with abdominal fat. The bone flap is replaced and the wound is closed in separate layers. A compressive dressing is applied. Alternatively, fat with hydroxyapatite cement or titanium can be used.

Special Features

The retrosigmoid approach, in selected cases, offers an opportunity for hearing preservation, with success rates ranging from 30% to 65%, depending on the selection criteria used for hearing preservation surgery.[51-53] This approach is particularly useful for removal of CPA tumors smaller than 2 cm in patients with good hearing and limited involvement of the internal auditory canal. The principal limitation of this approach is that the fundus of the canal is not directly visualized. This approach is being used more frequently as small tumors of the CPA are diagnosed with enhanced MRI and minimal auditory symptoms.

Extension of tumor to the fundus is a relative contraindication to use of the retrosigmoid approach for hearing preservation. With the retrosigmoid approach, tumor removal in the fundus is accomplished by "feel" with hooks or indirect visualization with mirrors and endoscopes. This approach risks leaving residual tumor.

Bill's bar in the fundus of the internal auditory canal cannot be used to identify the facial nerve laterally in the retrosigmoid approach. Thus, this step is more difficult in the retrosigmoid approach and relies more heavily on the nerve monitor. Although the rates of facial nerve preservation are comparable for the translabyrinthine and the retrosigmoid techniques, in our experience, facial nerve preservation rates are better with the translabyrinthine approach because it allows positive identification of the facial nerve in medial and lateral directions.[52,54,55]

A 10% incidence of severe postoperative headaches has been reported with this approach.[56] This symptom may be related to the intradural spread of bone dust, which occurs as a result of drilling the posterior lip of the internal auditory canal. Unlike in the translabyrinthine approach, drilling should be intradural in the retrosigmoid approach. Replacing the retrosigmoid bone flap with microplates or cranioplasty with synthetic materials has reduced the incidence of headaches with retrosigmoid surgery, suggesting that scar and muscle adherence to the dura also is an important factor.

Another objection to use of this approach has been the need for cerebellar retraction. Skeletonizing the sigmoid sinus and reflecting it anteriorly can minimize cerebellar retraction. However, medium-sized and large lesions require significantly more cerebellar retraction than is necessary with the translabyrinthine approach. Nonetheless, the retrosigmoid approach offers the most panoramic view of the posterior fossa.

Middle Fossa Approach

Basic Approach

A temporal craniotomy permits exposure of the internal auditory canal after identification of the superior semicircular canal and geniculate ganglion (Fig. 177-31).

Indications

The middle fossa approach is ideally suited for resection of intracanalicular acoustic neuromas. It provides limited exposure for surgery of lesions involving the CPA. CPA involvement beyond 1 cm is a relative contraindication to this approach. Decompression of the internal audi-

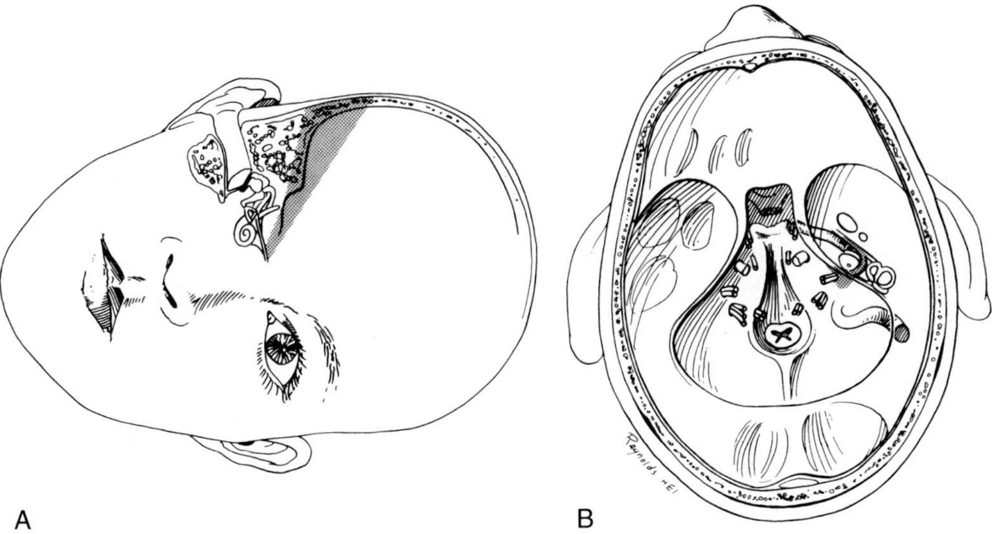

Figure 177-31. **A,** Coronal view: surgical exposure in the middle fossa approach to the cerebellopontine angle (CPA). A temporal craniotomy permits retraction of the temporal lobe and access to the floor of the middle fossa and internal auditory canal (IAC). **B,** Axial view: surgical exposure in the middle fossa approach to the CPA. The *shaded area* indicates the area of bone removal on the floor of the middle fossa. Note that although wider exposure is possible at the porus, limited space is available between the cochlea and the superior semicircular canal as the surgeon approaches the fundus of the IAC.

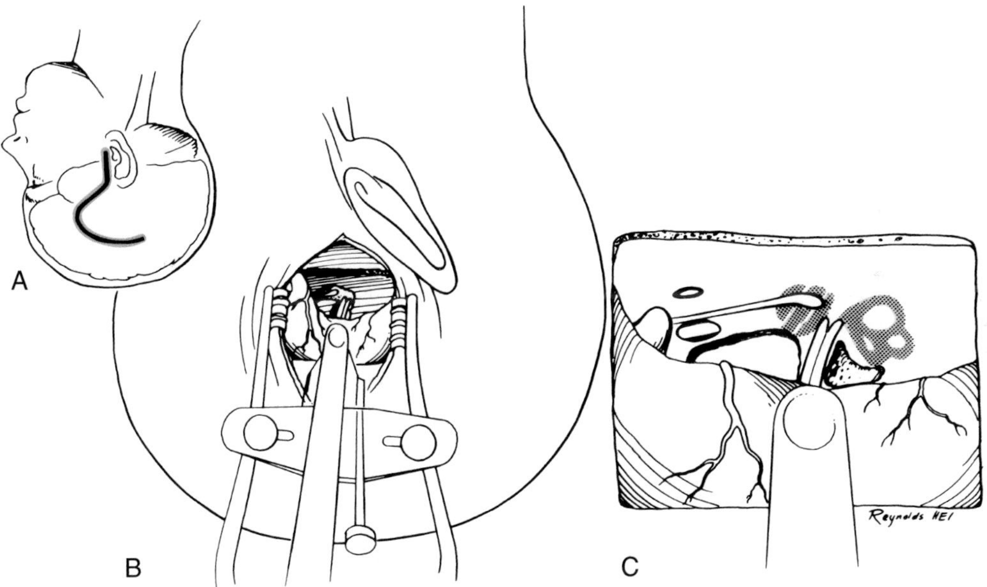

Figure 177-32. **A,** Skin incision for the middle fossa approach. Although the traditional vertical incision is used in middle fossa facial nerve decompression, the larger flap facilitates bony exposure for tumor removal. **B,** Surgeon's view of the internal auditory canal (IAC) via the middle fossa approach. Note the temporal lobe retractor in position. The proximity of the cochlea, labyrinth, and labyrinthine portion of the facial nerve at the fundus of the IAC requires precise identification of anatomic landmarks in this approach. **C,** Surgeon's view of the extended middle fossa approach. The anterior limit of bone removal is the carotid artery and the posterior limit is the labyrinth. In the illustration, the middle meningeal artery at the level of the foramen spinosum has been transected, and the horizontal carotid artery is identified coursing parallel to the greater superficial petrosal nerve and medial to the foramen ovale. Continued dissection anteromedially permits access to the cavernous sinus.

tory canal in cases of acoustic nerve tumors in only hearing ears can be accomplished in this fashion.[57]

Technique

The basic surgical exposure is illustrated in Figure 177-32A and B. Mannitol and furosemide are used in addition to hyperventilation for brain relaxation. A lumbar drain placed at the beginning of the procedure can facilitate dural elevation before open drainage of the cerebrospinal fluid. A preauricular incision is extended along the temporal region. The temporalis muscle may be reflected inferiorly or split and retracted to expose the squamosa of the temporal bone. A 5 cm × 5 cm craniotomy is centered over the zygomatic root.

The floor of the middle fossa is exposed by dissecting and elevating the dura from posterior to anterior to avoid injury to the geniculate ganglion, which can be dehiscent in up to 15% of patients. The principal landmarks for orientation are the greater superficial petrosal nerve

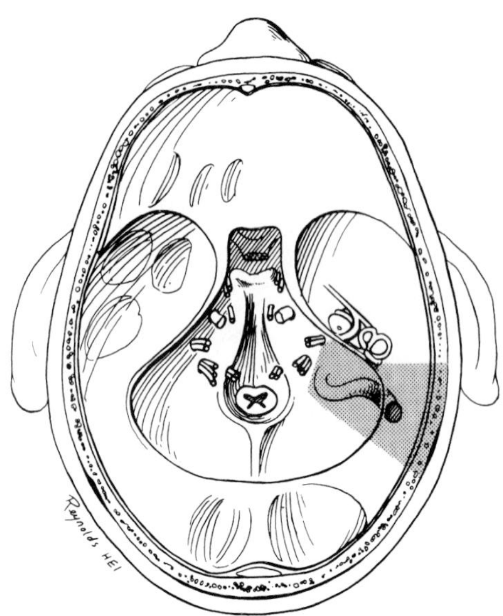

Figure 177-33. The retrolabyrinthine approach to the cerebellopontine angle (CPA). Although the exposure is limited anteriorly, removal of the bone posterior to the sigmoid sinus permits wide access to the CPA.

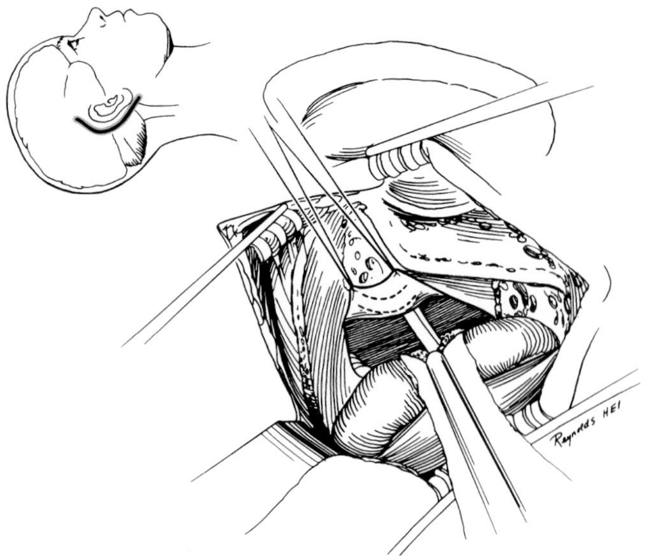

Figure 177-34. Surgeon's view of the cerebellopontine angle (CPA) with the retrolabyrinthine approach to the internal auditory canal. The dura is incised around the endolymphatic sac and reflected anteriorly. Wide posterior bone removal permits access to the CPA without a brain retractor, although suction is used to maintain the exposure. *Inset* shows skin incision in relation to the CPA.

and the arcuate eminence; however, these can be deceptive. Antidromic stimulation of the greater superficial petrosal nerve with the facial nerve stimulator can be helpful for orientation.[58] In addition, preoperative coronal CT can reveal the extent of pneumatization over the internal auditory canal and labyrinth.

Surgeons should be familiar with all techniques for identifying the internal auditory canal in middle fossa surgery, but some prefer to begin drilling medially near the porus acusticus. In this fashion, the cochlea and superior semicircular canal are not approached until the internal auditory canal has been identified. Wide skeletonization of this canal can be performed medially; however, the proximity of the cochlea and superior semicircular canal only permit unroofing the internal auditory canal laterally.

The dura is opened along the posterior aspect of the internal auditory canal. The facial nerve is freed from the tumor, and dissection proceeds in a medial to lateral direction. The canal is sealed with abdominal fat or temporalis muscle and the bone flap is replaced.

Special Features

Intracanalicular tumors, particularly those in the lateral portion of the internal auditory canal, are amenable to removal using the middle fossa approach in cases suitable for attempted hearing preservation. Because use of the approach has been limited to small lesions, the theoretic problem of limited access to the posterior fossa in case of bleeding has not been an issue.

The success of hearing preservation in selected patients is more than 70%; however, the limiting factor is the cochlear blood supply.[59] Just as in retrosigmoid hearing preservation cases, the rate of cochlear nerve preservation is substantially higher than that of actual hearing preservation. The approach is not usually recommended in patients older than 65 years because in this age group, the dura is more adherent and fragile.

Retrolabyrinthine Approach

Basic Approach

A wide mastoidectomy with skeletonization of the posterior semicircular canal permits access to the CPA with preservation of the seventh and eighth cranial nerves (Fig. 177-33).

Indications

The principal indication for the retrolabyrinthine approach is vestibular nerve section for intractable vertigo or for neurotomy in tic douloureux.[60] With posterior fossa neoplasms, the retrolabyrinthine approach affords adequate exposure and hearing preservation in selected cases of arachnoid cysts, meningiomas, and metastatic lesions of the CPA. In situations in which tissue diagnosis is required before proceeding with definitive surgery, the retrolabyrinthine approach permits wide exposure with minimal morbidity for exploration of lesions of the CPA.

Technique

The incision and soft tissue exposure for the retrolabyrinthine approach are identical to those for the translabyrinthine approach. Mannitol and furosemide are used for brain relaxation. A complete mastoidectomy is performed. The fossa incudis and the lateral and posterior semicircular canals are identified. The facial nerve is skeletonized but kept covered with bone.

Because exposure with this approach depends on collapsing the sigmoid sinus posteriorly, bone is completely removed from the sigmoid sinus and the subocciput posterior to the sinus. Extensive exposure of the retrosigmoid dura is necessary for adequate exposure with this approach. The middle fossa dura is exposed and the petrous ridge is removed to increase the exposure.

The dura is opened as a flap that begins just medial to the sigmoid sinus and preserves the endolymphatic sac. The flap is held anteriorly with sutures and tumor dissection can be performed in the posterior fossa (Fig. 177-34). Once the CPA is entered and CSF is released, the cerebellum falls away. Accordingly, cerebellar retractors are not necessary to expose the cranial nerves in the CPA. Instead, the sigmoid is collapsed posteriorly with fenestrated suction.

When tumor removal is completed, the dura is closed with sutures. The defect is obliterated with abdominal fat with the optional use of hydroxyapatite cement or titanium mesh. Closure is performed in layers, and a compressive dressing is applied.

Special Features

The indications for the retrolabyrinthine approach in tumor removal are limited. If exposure of the internal auditory canal is not needed for a small neoplasm of the CPA, however, this approach can preserve hearing and avoids the greater degree of cerebellar retraction required for the retrosigmoid approach.

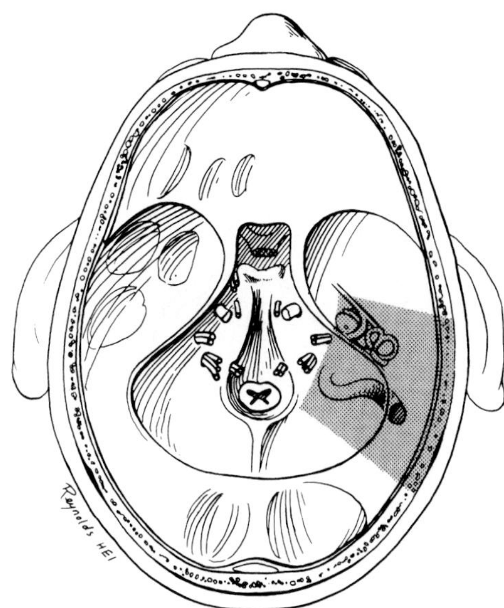

Figure 177-35. The transcochlear approach to the cerebellopontine angle petrous tip and clivus. Removal of the cochlea and anterior portion of the petrous bone permits wide visualization of the clivus and skull base.

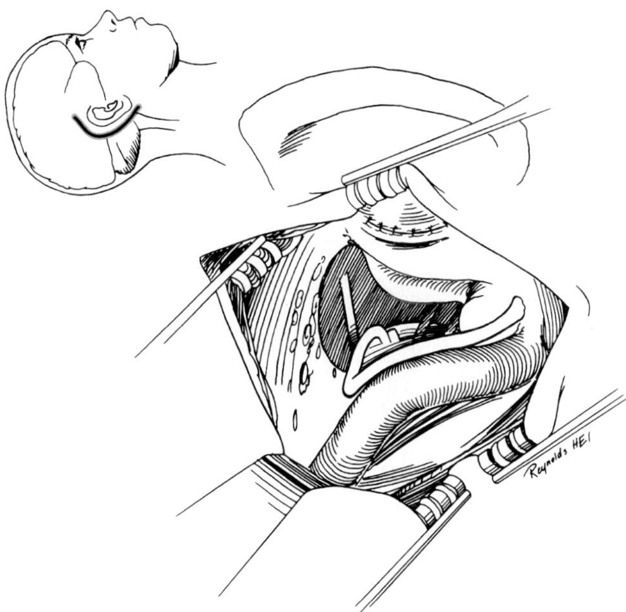

Figure 177-36. Surgeon's view of the skull base with the transcochlear approach. The external auditory canal is transected and sutured closed. Posterior transposition of the facial nerve permits unobstructed visualization from the superior petrosal sinus to the inferior petrosal sinus, anteriorly to the carotid artery, and medially to the clivus. *Inset* shows skin incision in relation to the cerebellopontine angle.

Transcochlear Approach

Basic Approach

As an extension of the translabyrinthine approach, the transcochlear approach affords additional exposure of the skull base. This is obtained by displacement of the facial nerve and removal of the cochlea to provide surgical access to lesions of the petrous tip and clivus (Fig. 177-35).

Indications

Petroclival meningiomas and epidermoids of the petrous tip are the principal lesions for which the transcochlear approach has been applied.[61] However, extensions of this approach have been used with glomus jugulare tumors, temporal bone carcinomas, and extensive nonacoustic neuromas of the CPA.

Technique

The incision, soft tissue exposure, complete mastoidectomy, labyrinthectomy, posterior and middle fossa dura decompression, and skeletonization of the internal auditory canal are performed as in the translabyrinthine approach.

The facial nerve is decompressed from the stylomastoid foramen to the geniculate ganglion. After sectioning of the chorda tympani nerve using an extended facial recess approach and transection of the greater superficial petrosal nerve, the facial nerve can be transposed posteriorly. Transposition of the nerve removes the obstacle to extending the exposure anteriorly. The transcochlear approach has been modified to include transection of the external auditory canal and two-layered closure of the meatus. This modification permits removal of the posterior wall of the external auditory canal, thus allowing wider anterior exposure in the areas of the jugular bulb and internal carotid artery. Next, the incus and stapes are removed. The cochlea is removed, thereby exposing the carotid artery anteriorly, the jugular bulb and inferior petrosal sinus inferiorly, and the superior petrosal sinus superiorly. The bony exposure leaves a dura-covered window extending from the superior petrosal sinus to the inferior petrosal sinus and reaching the clivus medially (Fig. 177-36).

The same principles of tumor removal are used as with the other approaches to the CPA. However, the position of the facial nerve in relation to the tumor and the proximity of the basilar artery make certain aspects of tumor removal with the transcochlear approach different from other approaches to the CPA. Unlike acoustic neuromas, tumors of the petrous apex and clivus often have the facial nerve on their posterior surface. Thus, the nerve should be dissected free of the tumor and protected. The position of the vertebrobasilar arterial system should be considered. As tumor dissection proceeds medially, the basilar artery will be anterosuperior and the vertebral artery will be posteroinferior. Extensive tumors that cross the midline are removed by reflecting the vessels posteriorly from the tumor capsule. Particular care is taken to preseve small perforating vessels that supply the brainstem, because their damage could be fatal. The surgical defect is filled with abdominal fat (often with hydroxyapatite or titanium mesh, or both), the wound is closed in layers, and a compressive dressing is applied.

Special Features

The transcochlear approach provides direct access to the base of implantation and blood supply of tumors arising from the petrous tip and petroclival junction. Temporary facial nerve paralysis occurs uniformly with the posterior transposition of the facial nerve required by this approach. Such paralysis is most likely to be the consequence of devascularization of the perigeniculate segments of the nerve caused by transection of the greater superficial petrosal nerve and its accompanying vessels. Because partial recovery of facial nerve function is the rule (to House-Brackmann grade 3/6 or 4/6), the approach has limited application except for removal of the most extensive life-threatening lateral skull base lesions such as malignancies or vertebrobasilar aneurysms.

Transotic Approach

Basic Approach

The transotic approach is similar to the modified transcochlear approach, in which the external auditory canal is closed and the posterior wall of the external auditory canal is removed. The distinction is that with the transotic approach, the facial nerve is skeletonized but left in its bony canal in the surgical field.

Indications

The transotic approach is indicated for removal of lesions of the CPA extending inferiorly into the jugular foramen or anteriorly into the

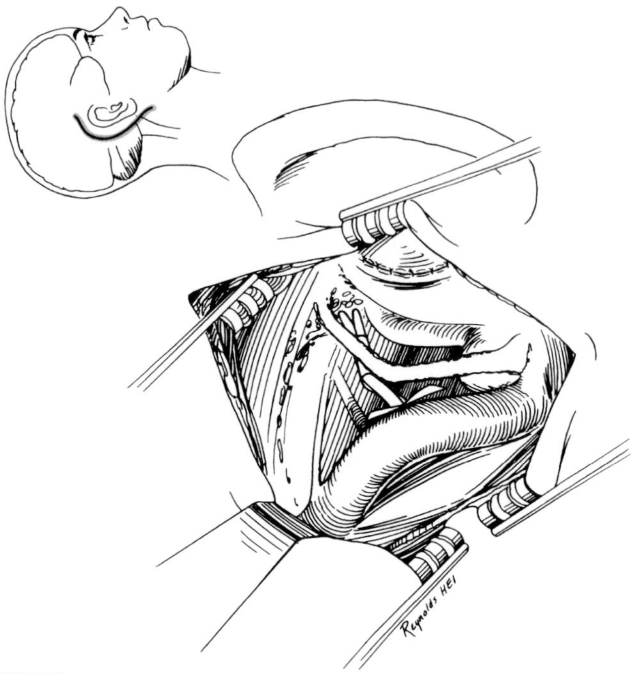

Figure 177-37. Surgeon's view of the transotic approach to the skull base. Note that the approach is identical to the transcochlear approach except that the facial nerve is not transposed. Instead, the nerve is left in its bony canal suspended across the surgical field. The in situ facial nerve limits the exposure in its internal auditory canal and mastoid segments (compare with Fig. 177-36). *Inset* shows skin incision in relation to the cerebellopontine angle.

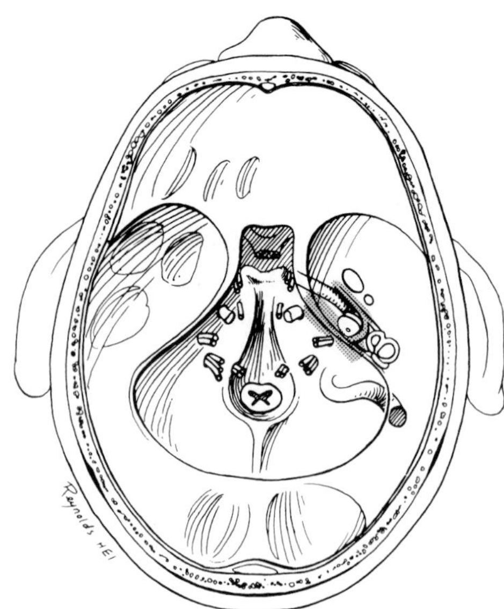

Figure 177-38. Schematic view (axial) of the extended middle fossa approach to the skull base. By removing the bone posterior and medial to the labyrinth and medial to the carotid artery, the exposure of the middle fossa approach is extended to lesions of the cerebellopontine angle that have spread beyond the tentorium or even into the cavernous sinus.

clivus. Some proponents of this approach use the additional exposure anteriorly in cases of high jugular bulbs or anteriorly placed sigmoid sinuses in small to medium-sized acoustic neuromas.[62] The translabyrinthine approach with wide decompression of the sigmoid sinus and posterior fossa dura provides adequate exposure of the internal auditory canal and CPA, even with large acoustic neuromas with unfavorable venous anatomy.

Technique

Through a postauricular incision, the ear is reflected anteriorly, and the external auditory meatus is transected and closed in two layers. Essentially the same procedure as that described for the transcochlear approach is performed, with the exception that the facial nerve is not completely freed from the fallopian canal. Rather, the nerve is skeletonized and left in its canal. At the conclusion of the exposure, the facial nerve is suspended, traversing the surgical field with a bony cover. The tympanic ring is removed, with systematic exposure of the jugular bulb, jugular foramen, and carotid canal. By working around the facial nerve, the surgeon has access to lesions of the internal auditory canal, CPA, clivus, and jugular foramen (Fig. 177-37). Closure is performed with obliteration of the defect with abdominal fat and optional placement of hydroxyapatite cement or titanium mesh.

Special Features

The transotic approach combines the added exposure provided by removal of the tympanic ring and access medial to the facial nerve with the added safety of the avoidance of transposing the facial nerve. This approach also offers an alternative strategy for management of the anterior sigmoid or high jugular bulb in cases of CPA tumor removal in which hearing preservation will not be attempted. Leaving the facial nerve in situ is an attractive means of avoiding excessive manipulation of the facial nerve; however, leaving the nerve without transposition requires added vigilance by the surgeon as dissection proceeds medial to the plane of the facial nerve. Furthermore, exposure is limited at the brainstem because the labyrinthine segment of the facial nerve and the contents of the internal auditory canal are not transposed.

Extended Middle Fossa Approach

Basic Approach

For the extended middle fossa approach, the skull base surrounding the otic capsule is carefully removed through a wide temporal craniotomy. This approach exposes lesions extending from the posterior fossa through the tentorium and incisura and anteriorly up to the region of foramen lacerum and the posterolateral aspect of the cavernous sinus (Fig. 177-38).

Indications

The extended middle fossa approach is indicated in extensive petrous ridge and petroclival lesions involving the temporal bone that have serviceable hearing. Petrous ridge lesions with extension through the tentorium into the middle fossa are especially amenable to removal using this approach.

Technique

The patient is positioned in the supine position with the head turned to the side. Mannitol, furosemide, and hyperventilation are used for brain relaxation. After performing a wide temporal craniotomy, the temporal lobe is progressively retracted to permit identification of the middle meningeal artery anteriorly, the petrous ridge posteriorly, and the petroclival junction medially. The internal auditory canal is uncovered using the standard middle fossa technique as described. The extension in the exposure is accomplished by removing the petrous ridge and posterior aspects of the temporal bone up to the labyrinth. Anteriorly, the temporal bone is removed up to the foramen lacerum and the internal carotid artery (see Fig. 177-32C). The area of Meckel's cave is clearly identified, and the posterolateral portions of the cavernous sinus are accessible.

Special Features

The extended middle fossa approach permits safe removal of extensive lesions (especially meningiomas) of the middle and posterior fossa that have not directly involved the otic capsule or internal auditory canal. Preservation of hearing and the facial nerve is possible with this technique despite wide access to the lesion.

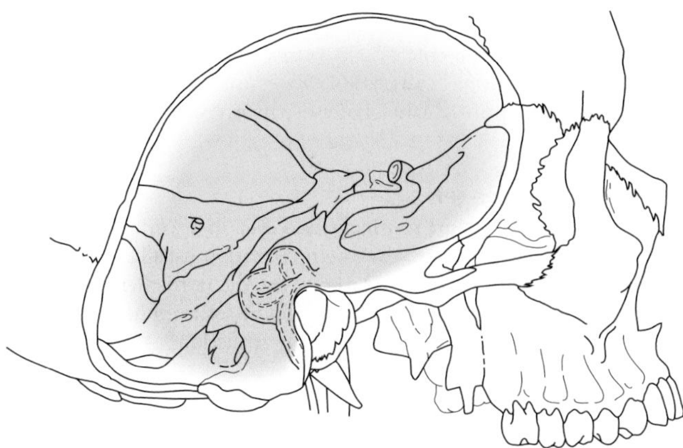

Figure 177-39. Combined petrosal approach uses the extended middle fossa, retrolabyrinthine, and retrosigmoid exposure while preserving the labyrinth.

Combined Techniques (Petrosal Approach)

Basic Technique

The previously described techniques for access to posterior fossa lesions may be combined to provide superior and posterior exposure.

Indications

Lesions involving the posterior and middle fossae or extensive lesions of the clivus are amenable to removal using combined approaches, especially if the patient retains serviceable hearing.

Technique

The usual procedures in the petrosal approach combine extended middle fossa exposure with full retrosigmoid and retrolabyrinthine exposure[63] (Fig. 177-39). The middle cranial fossa, internal auditory canal, posterior fossa, and clivus all are exposed while the otic capsule is preserved. By contrast, the translabyrinthine or transcochlear approach also can be combined with the extended medial fossa approach to provide the widest possible exposure.

Special Features

The petrosal approach provides wide exposure of the skull base from foramen magnum to the cavernous sinus while retaining the possibility for hearing preservation. The wide bone removal maximizes surgical exposure and minimizes the need for brain retraction. If hearing preservation is not a realistic expectation, the addition of otic capsule removal provides even wider surgical exposure.

Experimental Approaches

Attempted hearing preservation with partial or complete labyrinthine resection has been reported. McElveen[64] and Molony[65] and their colleagues reported systematic sealing of the vestibule during labyrinthectomy with successful hearing preservation after translabyrinthine tumor removal. To expose the lateral internal auditory canal with the retrosigmoid approach, Arriaga and Gorum[66] reported posterior semicircular canal resection with successful hearing preservation and total tumor removal in two of three enhanced retrosigmoid procedures. In extensive skull base lesions, labyrinthine procedures can be converted to partial labyrinthine resection procedures with concomitant opportunity for preserved hearing.[67]

Although these findings are promising, such techniques are currently experimental, and further investigation is necessary for such approaches to be offered routinely in clinical practice.

Approaches for Skull Base Lesions Requiring Drainage

As described earlier in this chapter, cholesterol granulomas are nonneoplastic lesions that may expand the petrous apex and produce symptoms related to the nerves of the posterior fossa. Similarly, mucoceles of the petrous apex may produce symptoms by their expansion. Both lesions are adequately managed by surgical drainage.

Translabyrinthine Approach

If hearing and vestibular function are absent, the translabyrinthine approach provides the most direct route for aeration from the mastoid through the surgical defect to the petrous apex.[68] Usually, however, this approach is inappropriate because patients often have excellent hearing despite large cholesterol granulomas.

Middle Cranial Fossa Approach

The middle cranial fossa approach permits hearing preservation but requires temporal lobe retraction for exposure. Placing a catheter from the mastoid tegmen to the apex facilitates drainage, and despite its relatively long course, the catheter remains patent, with radiologic follow-up confirmation of aeration.[43]

Infralabyrinthine Approach

After a complete mastoidectomy, the sigmoid sinus is decompressed, the posterior semicircular canal and jugular bulb are identified, and the infralabyrinthine air cells are followed into the petrous apex. The cyst is incised, drained, and stented open into the mastoid[68] (Fig. 177-40). This approach may be technically impossible in a patient with a high jugular bulb. Furthermore, although reexploration is possible in the face of an occluded stent, revision surgery requires formal reexploration of the transmastoid approach.

Transcanal Infracochlear Approach

The external auditory canal is transected and a superiorly based tympanomeatal flap is elevated. The bony external meatus is widened, and the air cell tract between the jugular bulb and carotid artery is followed into the petrous apex (Fig. 177-41). This approach permits dependent drainage of the petrous apex into the middle ear (see Fig. 177-14). If the drainage tube becomes obstructed, it may be revised through an office myringotomy. The principal disadvantages are the prolonged healing time required for the external auditory canal and the need for direct exposure of the petrous carotid artery.[42]

Selection of Surgical Approach

The rationale for selecting a particular surgical approach for acoustic neuromas is similar to that for other posterior fossa neoplasms. The principal goal is tumor removal with minimal postoperative morbidity. Accordingly, the surgical approach should be tailored to the patient's specific pathology and functional status. The notion that a single approach should be used with all lesions of the posterior fossa is counterintuitive and subjects patients to unnecessary morbidity. In patients without serviceable hearing, the translabyrinthine approach provides wide and direct access to the CPA, with maximal facial nerve safety, minimal cerebellar retraction, and a low incidence of severe postoperative headache.

Patients with small tumors and good hearing have three options for surgical removal: the translabyrinthine approach, which destroys hearing; the middle fossa approach in young patients with small, mainly intracanalicular tumors; and the retrosigmoid approach in small tumors of the CPA that do not extend to the fundus of the internal auditory canal. In general, the best hearing and functional outcomes result from individualizing the surgical approach to patient and tumor characteristics.[69]

Realistic patient counseling is necessary regarding hearing conservation procedures. Gardner and Robertson[51] rigorously reviewed the literature on hearing preservation in acoustic neuroma surgery. Of 621 reported cases of attempted hearing preservation, the success rate was 33%. Reported successful hearing preservation rates often refer only to measurable hearing. The rate is far lower if useful hearing (speech reception threshold [SRT] greater than 30 dB and speech discrimination less than 70%) or serviceable hearing (SRT greater than 50 dB and speech discrimination less than 50%) is considered. Furthermore, long-term follow-up studies reveal that 56% of patients experience significant loss of the preserved hearing over time.[59]

After a discussion of the risks and benefits of the various surgical approaches, many potential candidates for hearing preservation choose

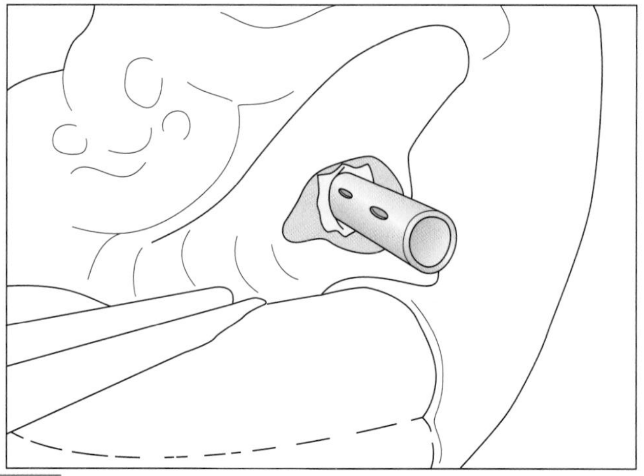

Figure 177-40. Surgeon's view of the completed transmastoid infralabyrinthine drainage of a cholesterol granuloma. The dissection is performed medial to the facial nerve and inferior to the level of the labyrinth. The drainage tube permits aeration of the cholesterol granuloma.

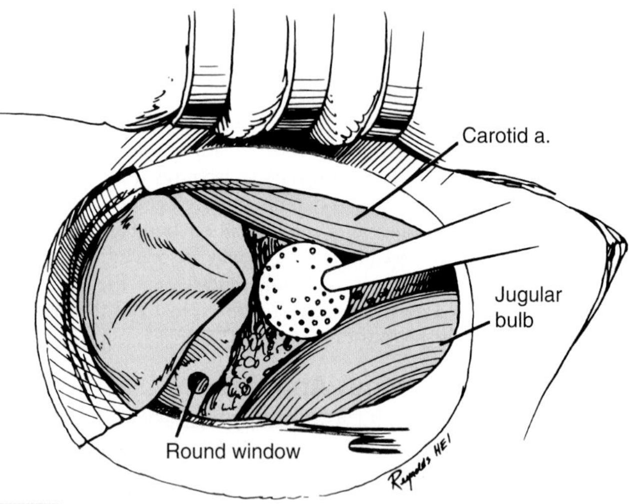

Figure 177-41. Surgeon's view of the transcanal infracochlear approach to the petrous apex. After transection of the ear canal, a superiorly based tympanomeatal flap is elevated. Diamond burrs are used to expose widely the hypotympanum, jugular bulb, and petrous carotid artery. The infracochlear cell tract is followed between the carotid artery and jugular bulb. *(From Giddings NA, Brackmann DE, Kwartler JA. Transcanal infracochlear approach to the petrous apex.* Otolaryngol Head Neck Surg. *1991;104:29.)*

the translabyrinthine approach, with its slightly higher rate of facial nerve preservation, rather than hearing conservation procedures.

With meningiomas and tumors that do not affect the internal auditory canal and have not impaired hearing, the extended middle fossa approach is used if posterior and middle fossa exposure is necessary. The retrolabyrinthine approach is used for removal of limited lesions of the CPA only, whereas the retrosigmoid approach would be applicable for resection of more extensive lesions of the posterior fossa. Extensive anteromedial exposure is needed with lesions of the clivus. Hearing preservation usually is not feasible in treatment of such lesions, and the transcochlear or transotic approach may be used.

Patient Management and Surgical Complications

Comprehensive management of patients with skull base neoplasms of the posterior fossa requires a team of specialists familiar with the particular needs of this patient group. In addition to neuro-otologists and neurosurgeons, designated internists, anesthesiologists, radiologists, ophthalmologists,[70] and critical care nurses are essential members of the team for optimal care of these patients with very specialized needs.

Preoperative Management

Preoperative antibiotics are routinely used even in uncomplicated cases. Osmotic agents and diuretics for brain relaxation usually are not used in the translabyrinthine approach; however, the retrolabyrinthine, retrosigmoid, middle fossa, and extended middle fossa approaches require such techniques to minimize the need for retraction.

Intraoperative Monitoring

Facial nerve monitoring is used routinely in all cases of posterior fossa neoplasm surgery. Continuous monitoring is performed with EMG electrodes and monitoring equipment with instantaneous visual and loudspeaker output. An audiologist assists with interpreting monitoring signals and stimulating the facial nerve when required to identify nerves intraoperatively.

Although ABR monitoring often is used in hearing preservation cases, this modality provides only delayed feedback to the surgeon and cannot affect intraoperative decision-making or tissue manipulation in a meaningful way. The advent of direct eighth nerve recording systems and electrocochleography (ECoG) modifications may make a practical real-time feedback system available to the surgeon in hearing preservation cases.[71]

Postoperative Care

The compression mastoid dressing applied in the operating room is left in place until the fourth postoperative morning if hydroxyapatite or titanium mesh was not employed. The patient is observed in the neurologic intensive care unit for 1 day and then transferred to the general ward. Limited activity is begun on the first postoperative morning, and ambulation usually resumes on the second postoperative day, with discharge home on postoperative day 3 or 4.

Complications

Anteroinferior Cerebellar Artery

Tumor manipulation at the brainstem may result in changes in vital signs. Such changes are related to ischemia, which usually is in the distribution of the anterior inferior cerebellar artery. Manipulation is stopped temporarily until vital sign changes have resolved. Vital sign alterations that do not resolve or that recur with any tumor manipulation constitute an indication to terminate the procedure. Complete interruption of this vessel may result in Atkinson's syndrome, infarction of the lateral tegmental pons, which often is fatal.[72] This complication can occur in a nonfatal form if branches of the anterior inferior cerebellar artery are transected.

Cerebrospinal Fluid Leaks

In the translabyrinthine approach, CSF leakage through the wound is rare with meticulous closure. The incidence of CSF rhinorrhea is less than 5%, and the leak usually responds to replacement of the compression mastoid dressing. The routine obliteration of the eustachian tube has nearly eliminated this problem. In the rare case of persistent leakage, spontaneous sealing of the leak can be expected after 3 days of lumbar CSF drainage. However, surgical closure of the ear canal with direct obliteration of the eustachian tube is promptly effective. Hydroxyapatite cement and titanium mesh cranioplasty techniques have been highly effective in reducing the leakage rate.

In the retrosigmoid approach, the mastoidectomy defect also is obliterated with fat. In some institutions, the mastoid is not routinely entered, and fluid communication is possible through exposed air cells, which ultimately permit fluid leakage through the eustachian tube. Aggressive application of bone wax over mastoid air cells is necessary to avoid leaks. In cases of persistent leakage, additional fat obliteration of the mastoid plus waxing of air cells usually is successful.

Meningitis

Any procedure that exposes the subarachnoid space can be complicated by postoperative meningitis. The diagnosis is suspected in a patient with a toxic appearance including stiff neck, recent headache, and fever. Appropriate CSF studies will confirm the diagnosis. The mean time to onset of meningitis in patients with acoustic neuroma is 8 days postoperatively. Aggressive medical management of this complication successfully avoids any serious complications from meningitis, other than a delayed hospital discharge.[73]

Facial Nerve Injury

Facial nerve transection ideally is managed by immediate repair or with an interposition graft.[74] In the translabyrinthine approach, access to the middle ear and mastoid portions of the nerve can provide a longer distal segment to ensure a tension-free anastomosis.[75] In cases in which direct repair is impossible or in which an intact nerve does not resume function within 1 year, the facial hypoglossal anastomosis provides reliable facial reanimation.[76] Temporalis muscle transfer is an alternative technique for reanimation of the paralyzed face that offers the benefit of immediate effects.

Ophthalmologic Considerations

The combination of facial paralysis and corneal insensitivity, which is more likely with surgery of large tumors, predisposes the cornea to significant trauma. Patients who are expected to have prolonged facial paralysis (6 months) are managed with a brow lift and placement of eyelid springs or gold weights. In cases of partial facial weakness or when the paralysis is expected to be short term, aggressive medical management including a regimen of lubricating drops or ointments, use of contact lenses, moisture chamber protection, and nightly taping of the affected eye is undertaken.[26] In some centers, gold weight implantation in the upper lid is the preferred technique for managing corneal exposure.

SUGGESTED READINGS

Arriaga MA, Chen DA. Hydroxyapatite cement cranioplasty in translabyrinthine acoustic neuroma surgery. *Otolaryngol Head Neck Surg.* 2002;126:512.

Arriaga MA, Luxford WM, Atkins Jr JS, et al. Predicting long-term facial nerve outcome following acoustic neuroma surgery. *Otolaryngol Head Neck Surg.* 1993;108:220.

Arriaga MA. Petrous apex effusion: a clinical disoder. *Laryngoscope.* 2007;116:1349.

Atkinson WJ. The anterior inferior cerebellar artery: its variations, pontine distribution and significance in the surgery of cerebellopontine angle tumors. *J Neurol Neurosurg Psychiatry.* 1949;12:137.

Brackmann DE, Anderson RG. Cholesteatomas of the cerebellopontine angle. In: Silverstein H, Norrell H, eds. *Neurological Surgery of the Ear.* Birmingham, Ala: Aesculapius Publishing; 1979:54-63.

Brackmann DE, Bartels LJ. Rare tumors of the cerebellopontine angle. *Otolaryngol Head Neck Surg.* 1980;88:555.

Brackmann DE, Hitselberger WE. Retrolabyrinthine approach: technique and newer indications. *Laryngoscope.* 1978;88:286.

For complete list of references log onto www.expertconsult.com.

Brackmann DE, Kwartler JA. A review of acoustic tumors: 1983-1988. *Am J Otol.* 1990;11:216.

Carrier D, Arriaga MA. Cost-effective evaluation of asymmetric sensorineural hearing loss with focused magnetic resonance imaging. *Otolaryngol Head Neck Surg.* 1997;116:567.

Daspit P, Spetzler R. The petrosal approach in otologic surgery. In: Brackmann DE, Shelton C, Arriaga MA, eds. *Otologic Surgery.* Philadelphia: WB Saunders; 1994:677-690.

Don M, Masuda A, Nelson R, et al. Successful detection of small acoustic tumors using the stacked derived-band auditory brainstem response amplitude. *Am J Otol.* 1997;18:608.

Gardner G, Robertson JH. Hearing preservation in unilateral acoustic neuroma surgery. *Ann Otol Rhinol Laryngol.* 1988;97:55.

Giddings NA, Brackmann DE, Kwartler JA. Transcanal infracochlear approach to the petrous apex. *Otolaryngol Head Neck Surg.* 1991;104:29.

Glasscock ME, Steenerson RL. A history of acoustic tumor surgery 1961-present. In: House WF, Leutje CM, eds. *Acoustic Tumors.* Baltimore: University Park Press; 1979:33-44.

House WF. Translabyrinthine approach. In: House WF, Leutje CM, eds. *Acoustic Tumors.* Baltimore: University Park Press; 1979:43-88.

House WF, De la Cruz A, Hitselberger WE. Surgery of the skull base: transcochlear approach to the petrous apex and clivus. *Otolaryngology.* 1978; 86:770.

Jackler RK, Cho M. A new theory to explain the genesis of petrous apex cholesterol granuluma. *Otol Neurotol.* 2003;24:94.

Janecka IP, Sekhar LN, Horton JA, et al. General blood flow evaluation. In: Cummings CW, Frederickson JM, Harker JM, et al, eds. *Otolaryngology—Head and Neck Surgery.* Update II, St Louis: Mosby; 1990:54-63.

Kevanishvili Z. The detection of small acoustic tumors: the stacked derived-band ABR procedure. [Comment on *Am J Otol.* 1997;18:608.] *Am J Otol.* 2000;21:148.

Lo WM. Tumors of the temporal bone and cerebellopontine angle. In: Som PM, Bergeron RT, eds. *Head and Neck Imaging.* St Louis, Mosby; 1991:420-445.

McElveen Jr JT, Wilkins RH, Erwin AC, et al. Modifying the translabyrinthine approach to preserve hearing during acoustic tumor surgery. *J Laryngol Otol.* 1991;105:34.

Samii M, Turel KE, Penkert G. Management of seventh and eighth nerve involvement by cerebellopontine angle tumors. *Clin Neurosurg.* 1985;32:242.

Sekhar LN, Jannetta PJ. Cerebellopontine angle meningiomas: microsurgical excision and follow-up results. *J Neurosurg.* 1984;60:500.

Selters WA, Brackmann DE. Acoustic tumor detection with brainstem electric response audiometry. *Arch Otolaryngol Head Neck Surg.* 1977;103:181.

Shelton C, Hitselberger WE, House WF, et al. Hearing preservation after acoustic tumor removal: long-term results. *Laryngoscope.* 1990;100:115.

Thomsen J, Tos M, Harmsen A. Acoustic neuroma surgery: results of translabyrinthine removal in 300 patients. Discussion of choice of approach in relation to overall results and possibility of hearing preservation. *Br J Neurosurg.* 1989;3:349.

CHAPTER ONE HUNDRED AND SEVENTY-EIGHT

Intraoperative Monitoring of Cranial Nerves in Neuro-otologic Surgery

Yasmine A. Ashram

Charles D. Yingling

Key Points

- Effective neurophysiologic recordings to guide the neurotologic surgeon rely on consistent protocols of neural stimulation and arrangement of the recording montage.
- In particular, a well-developed literature now demonstrates the effectiveness of monitoring facial nerve activity during vestibular schwannoma surgery by recording spontaneous and mechanically evoked activity. Recorded electrophysiologic activity reflects both nerve integrity and nerve responsivity.
- Similar methods are applicable to monitoring cranial nerves during other types of procedures, including resection of glomus jugulare tumors and prepontine tumors, microvascular decompression, parotidectomy, and tympanomastoidectomy.
- Other motor nerves—the third, fourth, motor portion of fifth, sixth, tenth, eleventh, and twelfth nerves—also can be monitored by placement of electrodes in appropriate target muscles.
- The cochlear nerve can be monitored by use of auditory brainstem response (ABR) or direct nerve action potential recordings.
- Numerous studies have confirmed that cranial nerve monitoring both reduces the incidence of postoperative deficits and can provide valuable prognostic information.
- Anticipated future developments, including the use of transcranial motor evoked potentials for continuous facial nerve stimulation, are expected to further enhance the utility of monitoring techniques.

The advent of sensitive diagnostic techniques and the refinement of microsurgical procedures have brought about a marked reduction in mortality rates for posterior fossa surgery; accordingly, increasing emphasis has been placed on preservation of cranial nerve function. This goal has in turn stimulated the development of techniques for monitoring cranial nerves during surgery. Seventh nerve monitoring during acoustic neuroma surgery has now become routine at most major medical centers, and anatomic preservation of the facial nerve has been achieved in more than 95% of the cases in some series.[1] Although facial motility often is compromised in the immediate postoperative period, the long-term prognosis is good if the nerve can be electrically stimulated after tumor removal. Preservation of hearing has been more difficult to achieve because of the more intimate relationship of such tumors with the cochleovestibular nerve but is now often achieved in smaller tumors with the aid of eighth nerve monitoring. Furthermore, the techniques developed for facial nerve monitoring are now readily adapted for monitoring other cranial motor nerves. We have reviewed these topics in greater detail elsewhere.[2]

The emphasis in this chapter is on the practical aspects of instrumentation, electrode placement, different neurophysiologic techniques used, artifact identification, types of responses encountered, and the relationship between intraoperative recordings and clinical outcome. Somatosensory evoked potential (SEP) recording[3] is not treated here, although SEP monitoring can be useful in monitoring large posterior fossa tumors with significant brainstem compression; discussions of SEP monitoring can be found in textbooks by Nuwer[4] and Møller.[5] This chapter is based primarily on the experience of the senior author with more than 700 posterior fossa procedures, as well as a review of the literature through 2007; also described are the methods currently available for cranial nerve monitoring, emphasizing facial and cochlear nerve monitoring during acoustic neuroma surgery but also including extension of these techniques to other nerves encountered in a variety of skull base procedures.

Neurophysiology in the Operating Room

Personnel

Successful intraoperative monitoring requires more than simply bringing another piece of equipment into the operating room (OR). The OR, unlike the typical clinical neurophysiology laboratory, presents a time-pressured and electrically hostile environment. Providing technically adequate recordings in the OR requires the services of professional personnel with specialized skills and experience despite the additional costs incurred. Attempts to monitor without such personnel may result in failure, or, even worse, inadequate monitoring, with inaccurate and misleading feedback to the surgeon. Accordingly, a new specialty field of intraoperative neurophysiologic monitoring has evolved, with its own professional organization, the American Society of Neurophysiological Monitoring (ASNM).

Professional certification for surgical neurophysiologists is now offered by two national organizations in the United States. At the technologist level, the American Board of Registered Electrodiagnostic Technologists (ABRET) offers a Certification in Neuro-physiological Intraoperative Monitoring (CNIM). The American Board of Neurophysiologic Monitoring (ABNM) offers board certification to monitoring professionals holding advanced degrees and with a minimum of 3 years' experience and 300 cases monitored. Because the demand for monitoring services is growing rapidly, there is a growing need for training programs to ensure an adequate supply of qualified personnel.

Technical Considerations

Instrumentation

The basic instrumentation requirements for cranial nerve electromyography (EMG) monitoring are an isolated electrical stimulator that can be precisely controlled at low levels; several low-noise EMG amplifiers; a multichannel display; and an audio monitor with a squelch circuit to mute the output during electrocautery. A system that provides multiple channels is recommended to allow simultaneous monitoring of multiple divisions of the facial nerve independently as well as other cranial nerves.

Auditory brainstem response (ABR) monitoring requires a system that includes high-gain (100 to 500,000 K) differential amplification with multiple band-pass filtering capabilities, acoustic stimulus intensity ranging from threshold to at least 70- to 80-dB hearing level (HL), signal averaging with real-time display of the evolving averages and the input signal, and permanent disk storage with hard copy printout capability.

For complex surgical cases requiring additional EMG monitoring channels or increased ABR averaging capability, or both, several commercial multichannel systems have been developed for intraoperative use. Currently available systems allow multiple independent time bases and functions to operate simultaneously; for example, some channels may be devoted to free-running EMG at slow sweep speeds and others to stimulus-triggered EMG at a faster sweep, and still others can be used for collection of averaged ABRs.

Recording Electrodes: Type and Placement

The most commonly used recording electrodes are the platinum or stainless steel subdermal needles designed for EEG; these have a larger uninsulated surface than that of electrodes designed for single-fiber EMG and thus are more likely to detect activity arising anywhere in the monitored muscle. Disposable, presterilized electrodes are available from several sources, and their use is highly recommended.

Intramuscular hook wire electrodes, which are inserted with a hypodermic needle, also have been used.[6] These are more delicate and have higher impedance, so the simpler needle electrodes are preferred, except in situations in which the electrodes cannot be easily fastened with tape, as in procedures involving the tongue, or when the use of insulated needles is desirable to avoid crosstalk from overlying muscles. An example of the latter case is recording from extraocular muscles, for which the electrodes must pass through the orbicularis oculi muscle and will therefore respond to facial nerve activity as well.

For monitoring the facial nerve, it is desirable to place the electrodes in at least two different muscles supplied by the nerve. Mechanical trauma to the seventh nerve often causes sustained EMG activity that can make identification of the facial nerve with electrical stimulation difficult. With two or more close-spaced bipolar channels, at least one often will be quiet enough to allow responses to stimulation to be identified without signal averaging even with high tonic EMG activity.

For recording the ABR in hearing conservation procedures, one electrode is placed in the ipsilateral ear canal and another on the forehead or vertex. The placement of the second electrode is not critical so long as it is near the midline. The best electrode option for the ear canal is the Nicolet Tiptrode, which is a compressible foam insert covered with gold foil. The acoustic signal is delivered through a tube in the center of the foam, which provides an acoustic seal, and the foil provides the electrical contact for recording.

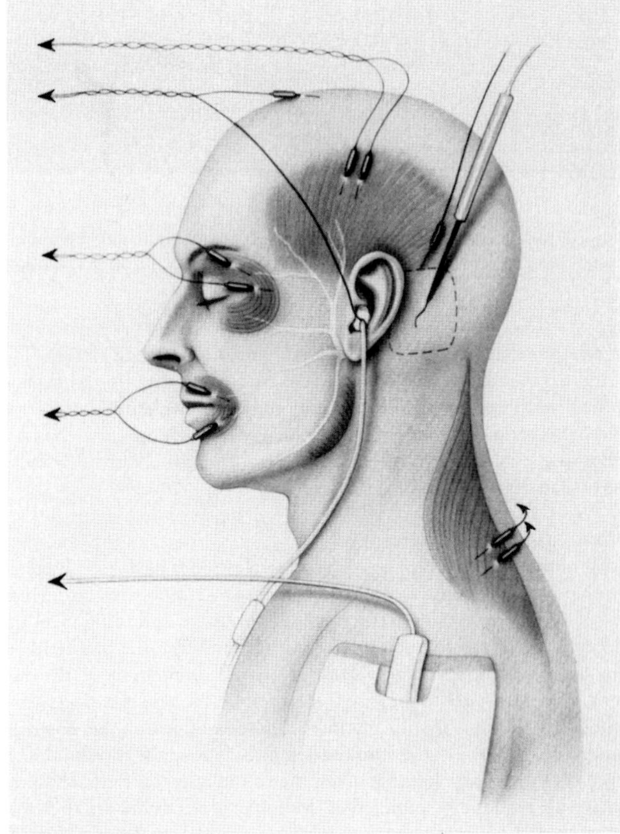

Figure 178-1. Diagrammatic representation of electrode placement for monitoring acoustic neuroma surgery with attempted hearing conservation. Pairs of needle electrodes are placed in the following muscles: temporalis (supplied by V3m), orbicularis oculi and orbicularis oris (supplied by the seventh nerve), and trapezius (by the eleventh nerve). Note that wires are twisted together to reduce 60-Hz pickup. Broadband click stimuli from a small transducer on the chest are fed through plastic tubing into the ipsilateral ear through a foil-covered sponge insert that also serves as a recording electrode and referred to a needle electrode on the forehead or vertex. An electrocautery ground pad is placed on the arm or shoulder as a signal ground. A flexible-tipped probe is used to stimulate cranial motor nerves, with a needle electrode as the stimulator ground placed in the margin of the craniotomy. *(From Yingling CD. Intraoperative monitoring of cranial nerves in skull base surgery. In: Jackler RK, Brackmann DE, eds.* Neurotology. *St Louis: Mosby; 1994:967).*

Figure 178-1 shows the positioning of recording electrodes for a middle fossa or retrosigmoid craniotomy for acoustic neuroma resection with a goal of hearing preservation. For a translabyrinthine approach, the same configuration is used, with the exception of the earphone and electrodes for ABR recording, because hearing conservation is not possible with this approach. Two channels are devoted to the facial nerve itself, with electrode pairs placed in orbicularis oculi and orbicularis oris muscles. One of the electrodes in the orbicularis oculi pair is placed at the lateral canthus, where it also will record volume-conducted activity in the lateral rectus muscle (from the sixth cranial nerve). One channel is used to record from the masseter or temporalis muscle (V3m) using hookwire electrodes, rather than subdermal needles, to reduce crosstalk, and the fourth channel is connected

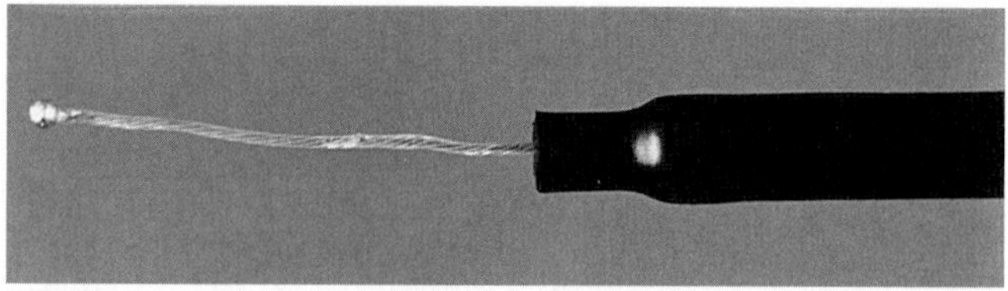

Figure 178-2. Close-up view of flexible-tipped probe used for intracranial stimulation. The entire probe and the flexible wire are insulated, except for the 0.5-mm ball on the end, to achieve localized stimulation.

to electrodes in the ipsilateral trapezius muscle (eleventh nerve). The latter two channels serve two functions: First, larger tumors may expand to involve these nerves, so monitoring may help in their identification and preservation. Second, even with smaller tumors, the extra channels serve as a control for nonsurgical causes of increased EMG activity, particularly light anesthesia.

Stimulating Electrodes

Both monopolar and bipolar stimulating electrodes have been used for intraoperative electrical stimulation. In theory, a bipolar electrode can provide more precise localization, with less current spreading from the electrode to adjacent structures. In practice, however, the threshold for bipolar stimulation depends strongly on the orientation of the two contacts with respect to the axis of the nerve.[7] Maintenance of a specific bipolar orientation is difficult in the close confines of the posterior fossa. Furthermore, if the stimulus intensity is near the threshold level (see later), a spatial resolution of less than a millimeter is easily obtained even with monopolar stimulation. Monopolar electrodes are therefore more commonly used; however, Schekutiev and Schmid[8] and Dankle and Wiegand[9] have described coaxial bipolar electrodes that may eliminate the problem of orientation.

The monopolar electrode should be connected to the cathode of the stimulator; the anodal return usually is a needle inserted into the periphery of the wound, preferably on the posterior margin of the incision to minimize stimulus artifact. This is particularly important in recording from extraocular muscles, which yield small-amplitude and short-latency responses that can easily be swamped by electrical artifacts. Several types of monopolar electrodes are available. Prass and Lüders[10] developed a malleable electrode, with the insulation continuous to a flush-tip that could be bent so that only the central portion of the tip contacted the desired tissue. They showed that this design minimized the spread of current to adjacent structures. Yingling and Gardi[11] developed a probe with a flexible platinum-iridium tip, insulated except for a 0.5-mm ball on the end (Fig. 178-2). This electrode can be used to stimulate within dissection planes or even behind the tumor, out of the surgeon's view, without concern for inadvertently damaging unseen neural or vascular structures (Fig. 178-3). With this probe, the facial nerve frequently can be located electrically even before it can be seen; dissection can then proceed in the most advantageous manner to avoid neural damage. Kartush and coworkers[7] developed a set of Rhoton-type dissecting instruments that are insulated except at the cutting surface, allowing simultaneous dissection with constant stimulation. These "stimulus dissectors" are particularly useful for removing the last portions of tumor capsule that are closely adherent to a nerve.

Stimulation Criteria

Little agreement has been achieved regarding the appropriate stimulation parameters to be used in cranial nerve monitoring, which vary considerably from one center to another. Our preference is to use a monopolar constant-voltage stimulator delivering pulses 0.2 ms in duration at a rate of 5 to 10 per second. In our experience, this is an effective and reliable choice that usually evokes a response from normal nerves at a threshold ranging between 0.05 and 0.2 V and averaging approximately 0.1 V.

Although the issue of whether constant-current or constant-voltage stimulators should be used has been a source of continuing controversy, there is no clear advantage of one method over the other. In many cases, however, the features of available equipment will limit the type of stimulation. Whether constant current or constant voltage is used, the more important issue is what actual level of stimulation is most appropriate. Rather than adhering to a simple "set it and forget it" approach, more useful information can be gained by varying the stimulation intensity in different surgical contexts, such as locating a nerve in relation to a tumor or testing the responsiveness of an already identified nerve.

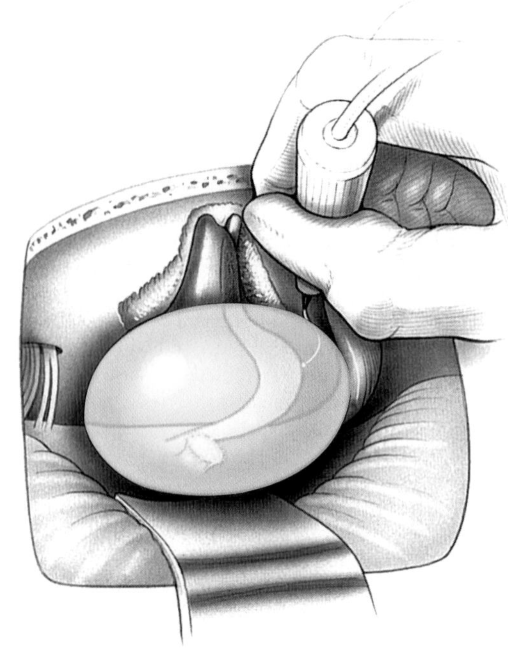

Figure 178-3. Surgical view of large acoustic neuroma (retrosigmoid approach) showing use of flexible-tipped probe to locate the facial nerve on the medial surface of the tumor out of direct view. Early identification of the facial nerve "around the corner" on the ventral surface of the tumor helps speed the procedure by allowing rapid removal of the remaining capsule. Tumor is drawn as if transparent to show details of anatomy on the hidden surface. *(Adapted from Yingling CD, Gardi JG. Intraoperative monitoring of facial and cochlear nerves during acoustic neuroma surgery.* Otolaryngol Clin North Am. *1992;25:413.)*

Anesthesia

Cortical evoked potentials are notoriously sensitive to many anesthetic agents, so careful adjustment of anesthesia levels is necessary in applications such as spinal cord monitoring with SEPs. Fortunately, the ABR and EMG responses that are used for cranial nerve monitoring are essentially unaffected by any commonly used anesthetics. The major anesthetic consideration is a contraindication to the use of muscle relaxants, because blockade of the neuromuscular junction interferes with monitoring of EMG activity. A few reports[12-14] have suggested that partial blockade can be used to prevent patient movement without blocking the ability to elicit EMG responses with facial nerve stimulation. However, in our experience, although electrically evoked EMG is relatively preserved, both spontaneous and mechanically elicited EMG activity tends to be suppressed by these agents. Therefore, *no paralytic agents should be used during surgery with cranial nerve monitoring*, other than short-acting agents such as succinylcholine given to facilitate intubation. Because the ABR and EMG are not significantly affected by routine concentrations of common anesthetics, no other constraints on anesthetic technique generally are necessary.

Finally, if local anesthetic is used at the incision site, care must be taken to avoid injection near the stylomastoid foramen to avoid anesthetizing the facial nerve. Alternatively, epinephrine 1 : 100,000 without any local anesthetic may be used to aid hemostasis.[15]

Facial Nerve (Seventh Nerve) Monitoring

Acoustic Neuroma and Other Cerebellopontine Angle Tumors

Facial nerve (seventh nerve) monitoring is routinely used in procedures to remove acoustic neuromas and other cerebellopontine angle tumors. Several techniques for facial nerve monitoring have been developed, including the use of sensitive detectors mounted on the face to detect facial nerve activity,[16-19] intraoperative EMG, recording of compound nerve action potentials (CNAPs) from the facial nerve,[20-22] intraoperative recording of nasal muscle F-wave,[23,24] and video analysis to detect facial movements.[25,26]

Electromyography

Because of its higher sensitivity[6,7,11,16,27-46] and easy application, EMG has by far overshadowed the other aforementioned methods and has become the most widely used modality for routine facial nerve monitoring. EMG recordings are used for monitoring cranial motor nerve activity in two distinct ways. First, intracranial electrical stimulation is used to identify and map the course of the nerves with evoked EMG activity and to determine the functional integrity of a nerve. Second, spontaneous EMG activity is continuously monitored to detect changes related to mechanical, thermal, or electrical irritation of the nerves by intraoperative maneuvers such as retraction,[47] tumor dissection, use of electrocautery or lasers,[48,49] or ultrasonic aspiration.

Activity Evoked by Electrical Stimulation

Use of Stimulation to Identify and Map Nerves in Relation to Tumor

Electrical stimulation is used in two main ways: (1) to rule out the presence of a nerve in a region to be dissected (using suprathreshold stimulation levels, i.e., 1 V) and (2) to map the precise locations of cranial nerves and determine their functional integrity, using stimulation levels at or just above threshold (i.e., 0.05 to 0.3 V).

Before electrical stimulation begins, correct functioning of the stimulating and recording system must be confirmed as soon as possible to avoid potentially catastrophic false-negative results. The presence of a stimulus artifact is not an unequivocal test; it is possible to have a stimulus artifact with only one lead (either the anodal return or the cathodal stimulator) connected. However, the absence of any artifact usually indicates an open circuit somewhere in the system. To avoid any ambiguity, it is preferable to confirm the operation of the entire system before beginning tumor dissection. In a retrosigmoid approach, the eleventh nerve usually can be stimulated at the jugular foramen as soon as the dura has been opened and the cerebellum retracted; an EMG response in the trapezius muscle confirms that the system is operating correctly. This confirmatory maneuver usually is possible before tumor resection begins, except in operations involving very large acoustic tumors. If the eleventh nerve is not visible at the outset, the stimulating electrode can be placed directly on a muscle and a direct muscular response obtained, although muscle requires higher stimulation levels than those effective in nerve. In translabyrinthine procedures, the facial nerve can be stimulated within the mastoid bone in the course of the labyrinthine dissection (before the tumor is exposed), although the threshold will be higher (usually 0.6 to 1.0 V, although up to 2 V may be needed), depending on the thickness of the overlying bone.

Once system function has been verified, an attempt is made to locate and stimulate the facial nerve. In smaller tumors (cerebellopontine angle component of 1 cm or less), the nerve usually can be located at its brainstem entry and an electrical response confirmed before dissection begins. Once a threshold has been established, the voltage is increased to at least three times the threshold value, and the stimulator is swept across the exposed surface of the tumor to confirm the absence of facial nerve fibers before dissection is begun. With larger tumors, the location of the facial nerve may not be immediately apparent. In such cases, we start with 0.3 V and map the accessible region, and if no response is obtained, we repeat the search at 0.5 and 1.0 V. If no response is obtained at 1.0 V, it can be safely assumed that the facial nerve is not on the exposed surface, and dissection can proceed.

During dissection, the stimulator is used repeatedly to scan the operative field for the presence of facial nerve fibers as the tumor is mobilized, using suprathreshold stimulus intensities as described previously. Once a response is obtained, stimulus intensity is reduced to 0.1 to 0.2 V, and the responsive region is narrowed. When the nerve is in sight, the electrode is placed directly on the nerve, and a threshold is obtained by slowly increasing the stimulus level from zero until a response is obtained. Further stimulation for mapping the location of the nerve is carried out at approximately three to five times this threshold, which should be periodically rechecked as dissection proceeds.

The spatial resolution of electrical mapping with monopolar stimulation is determined by stimulus intensity. For the most accurate localization, the stimulus is kept at a low level. At just suprathreshold levels, the spatial resolution is less than 1 mm, allowing the facial nerve to be easily distinguished from the adjacent vestibulocochlear complex. Conversely, to confirm that the nerve is not in an area about to be cut or cauterized, higher levels of stimulation (up to 1.0 V) are used to reduce the likelihood of false-negative results. As more and more tumor is removed, the course of the facial nerve can be mapped from brainstem to internal auditory canal. Although the nerve may be relatively cylindrical at each end, it frequently is compressed by the tumor in the cerebellopontine angle and may be seen as a broad, flat expanse of fibers splayed across the surface of the tumor. Frequently, the only way to identify the nerve and distinguish it from arachnoid tissue is with electrical stimulation; the nerve may be literally invisible to photons and visible only with electrons!

Assessment of Functional Status of Nerves after Tumor Removal

The primary use of intraoperative stimulation is in localizing and mapping the course of cranial nerves in relation to cerebellopontine angle tumors. However, electrical stimulation also is used to determine changes in the functional status of these nerves and is a useful predictor of postoperative function. In general, facial EMG responses elicited by low-threshold stimulation of the seventh nerve at the brainstem after total tumor resection constitute a good but not infallible predictor of postoperative function, because transient or delayed-onset facial palsies may be seen even when a low threshold is obtained at the end of the operation.[50-53] Conversely, a substantially elevated threshold or the inability to elicit a response with stimulation up to 1 V carries a significant likelihood of postoperative facial dysfunction, particularly in the short run.[51]

Methods based on measurement of the compound muscle action potential (CMAP) amplitude after tumor removal also have been used to quantify the functional status of the seventh nerve.[32,54] Absolute amplitude is quite variable between patients, however, and may be partially determined by nonspecific factors such as precise electrode placement, amount of subcutaneous fat,[29] facial nerve dimensions, and muscle mass.[55] These variations have led some investigators to use ratios rather than absolute values for assessment of postoperative facial nerve function. Taha and associates[56] measured the ratio of CMAP amplitudes to stimulation at the brainstem proximally and at the internal auditory meatus distally after tumor excision and found that proximal-to-distal amplitude ratios greater than 2 : 3 were associated with excellent outcome. Similarly, Isaacson and colleagues[57] analyzed proximal-to-distal amplitude ratios and reported that a higher ratio reflected good immediate postoperative facial nerve function. Lin and coworkers[55] used the ratio between proximal amplitude measurement after tumor dissection and supramaximal amplitude measurement in response to transcutaneous facial nerve stimulation and found that a CMAP ratio greater than 50% of maximum had a 93% positive predictive value when measured at 0.3 mA.

Prediction of long-term rather than short-term facial nerve function is the surgeon's major concern, because this would allow for better patient counseling and planning of rehabilitative treatment.[58] It has been suggested that low threshold recorded at the brainstem after tumor resection is a good predictor of long-term facial nerve function[50,59-61]; however, the ability of threshold to accurately predict long-term function has been questioned by some.[62,63] Neff and colleagues[64] evaluated a combination of threshold and amplitude and found that a minimum threshold of 0.05 mA together with a CMAP amplitude greater than

240 μV predicts a good postoperative outcome 1 year postoperatively. Fenton and associates[65] concluded that a more reliable predictor of long-term facial nerve is the clinical grade of early postoperative facial function. They also demonstrated that all patients with a recordable EMG response to proximal stimulation after tumor dissection, irrespective of the threshold or amplitude, recovered to a follow-up grade III or better facial nerve function. Although this correlation has been previously reported,[53,54,61,66,67] its importance has gone unnoticed. Therefore, it is now accepted that whenever a recordable response to electrical stimulation of whatever amplitude or threshold can be demonstrated, the facial nerve is most likely to show signs of improvement with follow-up, and intervention is therefore not recommended within the first year.[65] On the other hand, the absence of response to stimulation at the end of surgery does not doom the patient to a bad outcome. If the nerve is anatomically preserved, even with an immediate postoperative palsy, there is still a good possibility of eventual return of function as functional nerve fibers regenerate. Partial recovery of function in patients with unrecordable responses after surgery has been previously reported.[68] The earlier the onset of recovery, the better its quality; however, ifevidence of recovery is lacking at 12 months, then it is unlikely to occur.[69]

Intraoperative Identification of the Nervus Intermedius

Anatomic identification of the nervus intermedius during cerebellopontine angle surgery is important in order to prevent confusing this nerve with the facial nerve itself. Electrical stimulation of the nervus intermedius during cerebellopontine angle surgery was found to produce a characteristic response in the orbicularis oris channel only: long latency, low amplitude, and higher in threshold than the facial nerve response[70] (Fig. 178-4). Initial confusion between the nervus intermedius and a facial nerve strand at the time of stimulation is possible, because the entire course of the facial nerve may not be visually apparent to the surgeon as it passes anterior to the tumor—most common surgical approaches are from the posterior. Furthermore, tumor growth causes the facial nerve to be stretched and widened, so it often cannot be identified as a solitary trunk but rather is seen as a wide ribbon. The surgeon must recognize that stimulation of the nervus intermedius can cause EMG activity in the facial nerve monitoring channels (at least the orbicularis oris) but that the main trunk of the facial nerve may lie in an entirely different location within the cerebellopontine angle (Fig. 178-5). To protect this critical structure, it is imperative for the surgeon to locate the facial nerve itself by stimulation.

Spontaneous and Mechanically Evoked Activity

EMG responses to intracranial stimulation are the most specific indicators of cranial nerve localization and functional status. However, spontaneous EMG activity and EMG responses related to intraoperative events also are useful in preserving neural function. Some patients, particularly those with significant preoperative facial deficits,

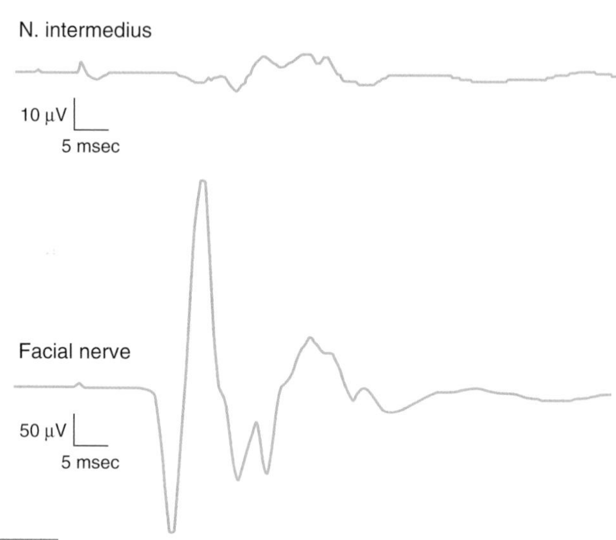

Figure 178-4. Responses in orbicularis oris to stimulation of nervus intermedius *(top)* and facial nerve *(bottom)*. Note smaller scale in nervus intermedius response, which is smaller, of longer latency, and seen only in the lower facial nerve channel. *(From Ashram YA, Jackler RK, Pitts LH, Yingling CD. Intraoperative electrophysiological identification of the nervus intermedius.* Otol Neurotol. *2005;26:274.)*

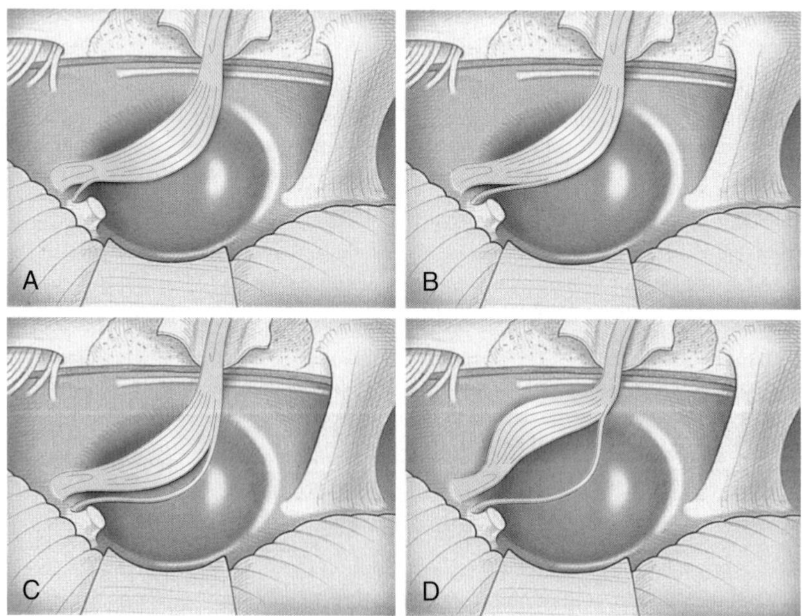

Figure 178-5. Anatomic variants in relationship between the nervus intermedius and the facial and vestibulocochlear nerves. **A,** Nervus intermedius joining nerve VII-VIII complex near brainstem root entry zone. **B,** Nervus intermedius joining nerve VII-VIII in mid-cerebellopontine angle. **C,** Nervus intermedius joining nerve VII-VIII near the porus acusticus. **D,** Nervus intermedius taking a separate course through cerebellopontine angle, where it can be misidentified as the facial nerve unless its unique response characteristics are recognized. *(From Ashram YA, Jackler RK, Pitts LH, Yingling CD. Intraoperative electrophysiological identification of the nervus intermedius.* Otol Neurotol. *2005;26:274.)*

demonstrate baseline tonic facial EMG activity; this often decreases as the nerve is decompressed with opening of the dura and draining of CSF. Virtually all patients exhibit some mechanically evoked facial EMG activity during tumor dissection, retraction, irrigation, or other intraoperative maneuvers. An increase in EMG activity associated with a particular surgical maneuver often is the earliest indicator of the location of the facial nerve. When such activity is elicited, the stimulator should then be used to search the area in question to positively identify the nerve if possible. Frequently, operative manipulations elicit EMG activity, even if the nerve is not in the immediate area, because of transmission of traction or pressure from the tumor to the nerve. In such cases, a negative response to electrical stimulation indicates that dissection can proceed. In other cases, stimulation after mechanically elicited activity results in identification of the nerve, which can then be precisely localized as described previously.

Finally, ongoing EMG activity often is an indirect indicator of depth of anesthesia, which is of particular concern when no muscle relaxants can be used. A simultaneous increase in spontaneous EMG activity on all channels is unlikely to result from localized dissection. When such a generalized increase occurs, the anesthesiologist should be notified immediately, because overt patient movement often occurs within a few seconds.

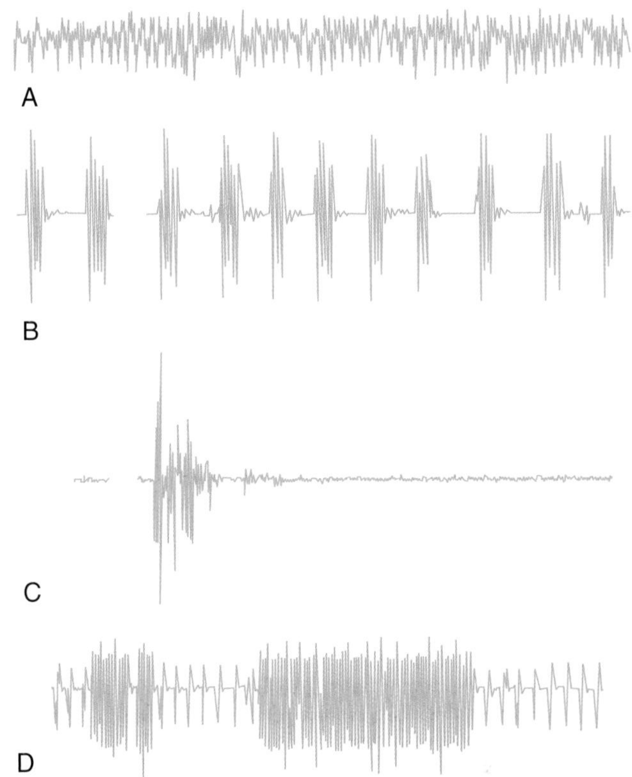

Figure 178-6. Illustrative examples of three types of electromyographic activity often seen during vestibular schwannoma surgery. **A,** Dense tonic (sustained) activity, often associated with nerve stretch and demonstrating a sinusoidal pattern. **B,** Lower tonic activity, called popcorn activity. **C,** Phasic (transient) burst activity typically associated with direct contact with the nerve. Such events are not of major significance unless they involve large-amplitude trains and occur during critical stages of dissection. **D,** Burst activity superimposed on ongoing small-amplitude train; it is important not to overlook such events overlapping on background activity, because they may pass unnoticed despite their significance. *(From Yingling CD, Ashram YA. Intraoperative monitoring of cranial nerves in skull base surgery. In: Jackler R, Brackmann DE, eds. Neurotology. 2nd ed. Philadelphia: Elsevier; 2005:958.)*

Patterns of Mechanically Evoked Electromyographic Activity

Prass and Lüders[6] distinguished two types of EMG activity associated with intraoperative events: *burst* and *train* activity. These investigators suggested that the phasic "burst" pattern, characterized by short, relatively synchronous bursts of motor unit potentials, corresponded to a single discharge of multiple facial nerve axons, and was associated with direct mechanical nerve trauma, free irrigation, application of pledgets soaked with lactated Ringer's solution over the facial nerve, or electrocautery. When burst activity occurs, it usually indicates that the facial nerve is being stimulated enough to result in depolarization and production of EMG response but not necessarily to the point of injury.[71] It generally is accepted that the occurrence of burst activity of small amplitude (less than 500 μV in amplitude) is not of major concern, and accordingly, the surgeon need not be warned each time such activity occurs.[72,73] On the other hand, the occurrence of large-amplitude burst activity (greater than 500 μV in amplitude) during the critical stages of dissection or final stages of drilling usually indicates a degree of facial nerve injury, the extent of which differs with the force and number of impacts.

As described by Prass and Lüders,[6] the second pattern, tonic or "train" activity, consisted of episodes of prolonged asynchronous grouped motor unit discharges that lasted up to several minutes. These episodes were most commonly associated with facial nerve traction, usually in the lateral to medial direction. The investigators further divided such train activity into higher-frequency trains (50 to 100 Hz), dubbed "bomber potentials" because of their sonic characteristics, and lower-frequency discharges (1 to 50 Hz), which were more irregular and had a sound resembling popping popcorn. The onset and decline of "popcorn" activity were more gradual than the more abrupt onset and decline of "bomber" activity.

Subsequently, Romstock and coworkers[72] classified train activity into three distinct patterns: A, B, and C trains. *A trains* are characterized by a sinusoidal symmetrical sequence of high-frequency and low-amplitude signals that have a sudden onset; *B trains* are regular or irregular sequences of repeated spikes or bursts with maximum intervals of 500 msec; and *C trains* are characterized by continuous irregular EMG responses that have many overlapping components. Although B and C trains did not correlate with postoperative function, the authors suggested a relation between the occurrence of A trains and poor postoperative facial nerve function.

Nakao and colleagues[74] classified train activity that occurred during the last stage of tumor resection into an *irritable* pattern with frequent EMG responses to the slightest stimuli, a *silent* pattern with few or no EMG responses, a *stray* pattern with persistent train responses up to 20 minutes despite temporary discontinuance of surgical manipulation, and an *ordinary* pattern related to mechanical stimulation of the nerve but not easily elicited. These workers found an association between the occurrence of silent or stray EMG patterns and poor postoperative outcome. The occurrence of train activity does not always imply an impending nerve injury but indicates the proximity of the facial nerve to the region of dissection and thus should be considered a reassuring sign denoting an intact and responsive nerve.[71] However, train activity of large amplitude (greater than 500 μV in amplitude) has been linked to postoperative nerve injury of variable degree,[75,76] and such events require prompt warning to the surgeon. The absence of large-amplitude train activity, on the other hand, does not always mean safe dissection, especially with large tumors producing significant facial nerve compression. The nerve axons become stretched, partially damaged, and less responsive than healthy ones, generating little EMG activity despite significant manipulation.[77] Therefore, spontaneous EMG activity may not be a reliable warning sign in large tumors, and the frequent use of electrical stimulation is important to map the tumor surface and measure any change of threshold from baseline to assess the condition of the nerve. Figure 178-6 shows representative samples of different types of EMG activity often encountered in vestibular schwannoma removal.

Limitations of Electromyographic Monitoring

Despite the wide use of intraoperative EMG monitoring, it still has its limitations. A major problem with EMG monitoring is its relatively low specificity. EMG channels can easily pick up artifacts, and the distinction between them and true EMG activity may sometimes be difficult. An example is artifacts produced by bimetallic potentials as a result of contact between surgical instruments made of different metals; because these may be associated with intraoperative events similar to those producing true EMG responses, they can be difficult to recognize. Some useful criteria include the fact that artifacts typically are higher in frequency content than EMG activity and thus sound more "crackly" than true EMG activity, which has more of a "popping" sound; and the tendency for artifacts to appear simultaneously on several channels, which is unlikely for EMG activity (Fig. 178-7). Experienced monitoring personnel are in an optimal position to make such decisions, rather than surgeons, who are focused on the operative field. Another limitation of EMG monitoring is that it is virtually useless during electrocautery, when the facial nerve is potentially at high risk. Attempts to reduce the artifact from bipolar cautery have met with limited success, because such devices generate high-amplitude, broadband noise that is difficult to filter out. Techniques based on detection of motion, which are not subject to electrical interference, such as video monitoring, may provide an important adjunct to EMG monitoring despite their relatively lower sensitivity. In our experience, the practical way to deal with this problem is to use electrical stimulation before bipolar electrocoagulation to confirm that the area to be cauterized is free from facial nerve fibers. The absence of a response to higher levels of electrical stimulation (up to 1 V) in an area about to be cauterized is an indication that electrocautery can proceed safely.

Another problem with EMG monitoring is that facial nerve integrity with stimulation cannot be assessed unless the nerve is accessible in the surgical field. However, with large tumors, the facial nerve is at risk of being traumatized before it is visually apparent to the surgeon and may not be responsive to mechanical manipulation. In this situation, the facial nerve location can be anticipated by use of a flexible-tipped probe to stimulate within dissection planes or even behind the tumor, out of the surgeon's view, without concern for damaging unseen vascular or neural structures. However, the development of continuous facial nerve monitoring methods that do not rely on visual identification of the nerve remains one of the major challenges for future research.

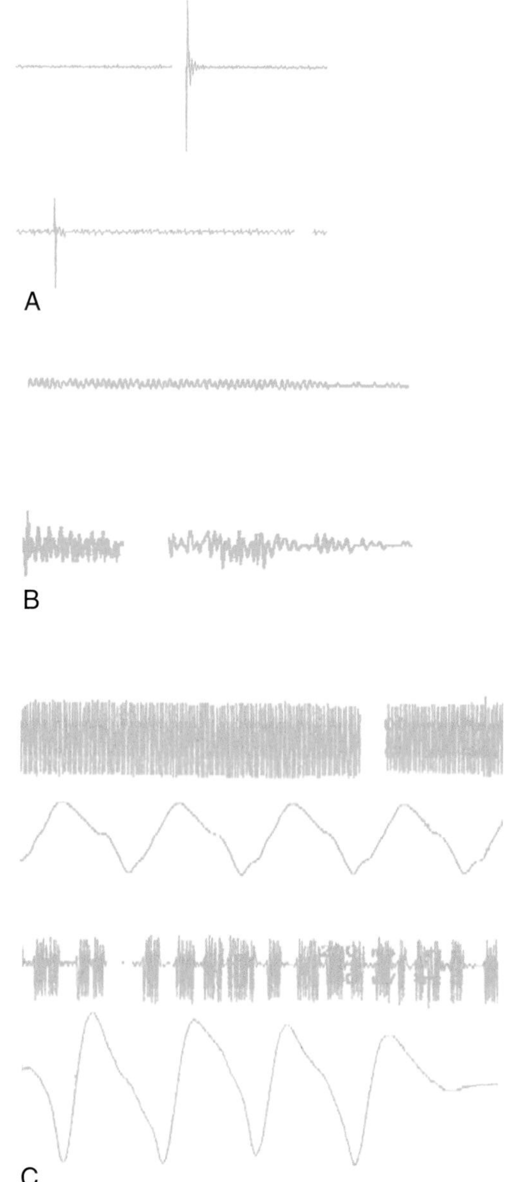

Figure 178-7. Electromyography (EMG) activity versus artifacts. **A,** *Upper trace*: Artifact produced by contact of different metallic instruments in surgical field. Note sharp edges on waveforms with exponential decay (may be confused with spike activity). *Lower trace*: Single electromyographic spike with a low-amplitude EMG background and no exponential decay. **B,** *Upper trace*: Regular sinusoidal artifact produced during drilling of the internal auditory canal (IAC). *Lower trace*: Irregular EMG activity while drilling IAC. **C,** *Upper two traces*: Regular artifact with two time scales, 200 msec/cm and 5 msec/cm. *Lower two traces*: EMG activity on the same two time scales. At 200 msec/cm, it may be difficult to differentiate between true EMG and artifact. However, with the faster 5 msec/cm time base, trace 2 shows that the artifact waveform is regular and synchronized, whereas trace 4 reveals the irregularities that characterize true EMG activity. *(From Yingling CD, Ashram YA. Intraoperative monitoring of cranial nerves in skull base surgery. In: Jackler R, Brackmann DE, eds.* Neurotology. *2nd ed. Philadelphia: Elsevier; 2005:958.)*

Microvascular Decompression

Microvascular decompression procedures for treatment of trigeminal neuralgia and hemifacial spasm involve potential damage to cranial nerves in the posterior fossa; therefore, EMG and ABR monitoring frequently are used with such procedures,[78] with the same techniques described elsewhere in this chapter.

In the specific case of microvascular decompression for hemifacial spasm, however, Møller and Jannetta[40] described a different technique. This method is based on the finding of abnormal muscle response in patients with hemifacial spasm, in whom muscles innervated by one branch of the facial nerve respond when another branch is stimulated. This response is due to abnormal spread of activity from one branch of the facial nerve to another on the affected side. Because it is not suppressed by anesthesia, it can be recorded intraoperatively so long as the patient is not paralyzed.

For a typical procedure, recording electrodes are inserted into the mentalis muscle (innervated by the marginal mandibular branch of the seventh nerve) and the orbicularis oculi (temporal branch). Subdermal needle electrodes also are inserted adjacent to the marginal mandibular and temporal branches of the seventh nerve for stimulation. Of note, the stimulation voltage required will be higher (4 to 20 V) than for direct stimulation of the nerve intracranially. Intracranial stimulation as described previously can, of course, also be used to ensure the integrity of the facial nerve in decompression procedures for hemifacial spasm. Figure 178-8 shows typical results with such a procedure.

If the abnormal response is not seen at the outset, it generally can be triggered by a brief train of stimuli at a high frequency (50 Hz). The amplitude of the abnormal response typically is lower than that of the normal response and may drop even further after the dura is opened, presumably because of a shift in the relation of the vessel to the nerve. Nevertheless, an abnormal response at some amplitude generally can be seen until the nerve is decompressed. Møller and Jannetta[40] recommend that the decompression be carried out until no abnormal response can be elicited. They state that the abnormal response disappears immediately when the offending vessel is removed from the nerve, a finding also reported by Halnes and Torres,[30] although in our experience, it may take a few minutes for the abnormal response to disappear completely. Debate continues over the association between the persistence or disappearance of the abnormal muscle response and ultimate clinical outcome. Kong and associates[79] found that long-term outcomes were

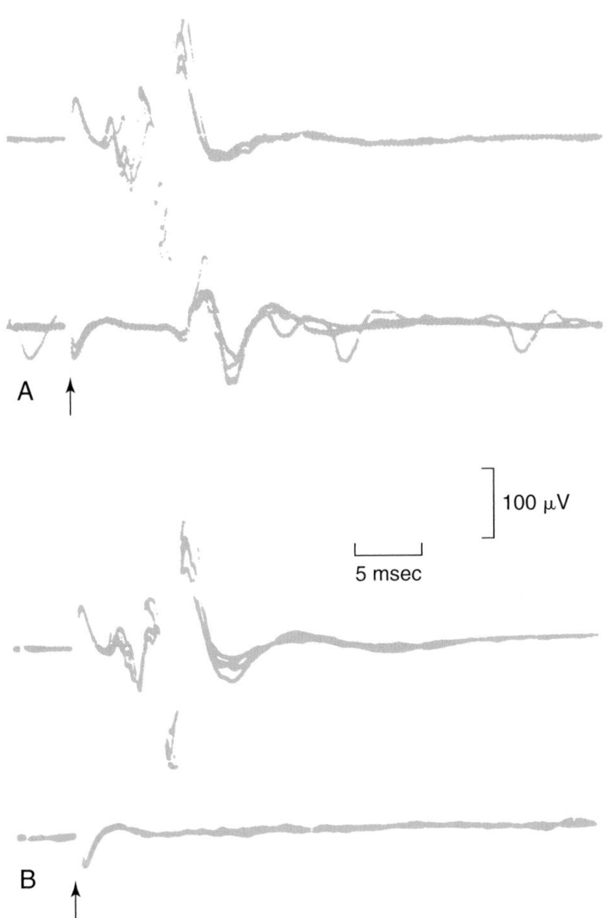

Figure 178-8. Responses during intraoperative monitoring of microvascular decompression for hemifacial spasm. Stimulating electrodes in temporal branch of facial nerve; recording channels orbicularis oculi *(top)* and mentalis *(bottom)*. **A,** *Before decompression*: The normal response in the orbicularis oculi to stimulation of the temporal branch is seen in the upper channel. The lower channel shows the abnormal response at prolonged latency in mentalis to stimulation (at time indicated by *arrow*) of temporal branch. **B,** *After decompression*: Abnormal response in mentalis no longer seen, normal response in orbicularis oculi unchanged. *(From Yingling CD. Intraoperative monitoring of cranial nerves in skull base surgery. In: Jackler RK, Brackmann DE, eds.* Neurotology. *St Louis: Mosby; 1994:967.)*

significantly better in patients whose abnormal response disappeared completely after decompression than in those with a persistent abnormal response; however, other investigators failed to prove this association.[80] More work is still necessary to elucidate the prognostic significance of the abnormal muscle response.

Parotid Surgery

Facial nerve monitoring during parotidectomy is similar to facial nerve monitoring in cerebellopontine angle surgery, except that the seventh nerve generally is the only nerve at risk. Thus, rather than using multiple EMG channels to monitor several nerves, all available channels can be used to monitor different branches of the facial nerve, which divides within the parotid gland (pes anserinus). Our typical four-channel montage includes closely spaced bipolar electrode pairs in the frontalis muscle (temporal branch of the seventh nerve), lower orbicularis oculi (zygomatic), upper orbicularis oris (buccal), and mentalis (marginal mandibular). The pattern of responses obtained with electrical stimulation can be used to determine which branch is being stimulated. EMG activity in a single channel indicates activation of a single branch of the nerve distal to the pes, activity in two or three channels generally indicates a location within the pes, and a response on all channels indicates activation of the main trunk of the nerve between the pes and the stylomastoid foramen. This is true both for mechanically elicited activity and for responses to electrical stimulation. The methods for recording both mechanically elicited activity and responses to electrical stimulation are similar to those used intracranially; of note, however, because the intracranial portion of the facial nerve lacks the thick epineurium found distally, thresholds for direct stimulation of the nerve within the parotid gland will typically be somewhat higher than those in the posterior fossa.

Other Otologic Surgery

Facial nerve monitoring also may be useful in many otologic procedures. For example, congenital aural atresia may be associated with an anomalous course of the facial nerve or may require rerouting of the nerve to expose the oval window. Surgery for chronic otitis media and cholesteatoma also may benefit from facial nerve monitoring, particularly when preoperative findings include preexisting facial dysfunction or computer tomographic (CT) evidence of fallopian canal erosion. Revision tympanomastoidectomies carry a higher risk of facial nerve injury because landmarks may be obscured by scar tissue. However, monitoring is not necessarily indicated in every routine case. There is no simple rule for determining when monitoring is indicated; a number of factors must be taken into consideration, including preexisting deficits, size and location of lesions, previous surgery, and the surgeon's experience. Besides serving as a guide to drilling, dissection, and verifying the integrity of the nerve, monitoring also is useful in detecting facial nerve dehiscence.[81,82] Noss and associates[81] suggested that the electrical stimulation threshold of the facial nerve is more reliable than surgical observation alone in identifying risk for injury secondary to dehiscence. These workers found that a facial nerve stimulation threshold less than 1 V identifies a nerve that is electrophysiologically dehiscent and thus should be considered at increased risk for injury.

Other Motor Nerve Monitoring

Third, Fourth, and Sixth Nerve Monitoring: Extraocular Muscles

Monitoring of the oculomotor (third), trochlear (fourth), and abducens (sixth) nerves, which innervate the various extraocular muscles, frequently is necessary in surgery for more anterior skull base lesions. These may include, for example, cavernous sinus tumors, prepontine tumors, and petrous apex lesions with significant anterior or medial extension. Although the basic principles are the same as for facial nerve monitoring, the relative inaccessibility of the target muscles causes special difficulties.

Paired hookwire electrodes are now preferred for monitoring of extraocular muscles, because they are flexible and thus less likely to traumatize the eye. The hookwire electrodes are inserted through the eyelids into proximity with the tendons of the target muscles, where they pick up volume-conducted activity from the muscles themselves (Fig. 178-9).

The oculomotor nerve (third nerve) is the easiest from which to obtain specific responses, because it innervates all of the extraocular muscles except for the lateral rectus and superior oblique. Placement of an electrode at the infraorbital margin, roughly one third of the distance out from the inner canthus, will result in pickup of activity from the inferior oblique or inferior rectus muscle, both of which are innervated by the third nerve (see Fig. 178-9). Similarly, activity in the lateral rectus muscle, innervated by the abducens (sixth) nerve, can be detected by an electrode inserted from the lateral canthus. The trochlear nerve (fourth nerve) is the most difficult to monitor, because the superior oblique muscle does not connect to the eyeball in the same straightforward fashion as for the other extraocular muscles. We have described these procedures in greater detail elsewhere.[2]

The latency of responses in the extraocular muscles to stimulation of the third, fourth, or sixth nerve typically is 2 to 3 msec, much shorter than that of responses to seventh nerve stimulation. This short latency helps prevent confusion of true third, fourth, or sixth nerve responses with seventh nerve activity, which is a common contaminant of recordings from these muscles (Fig. 178-10).

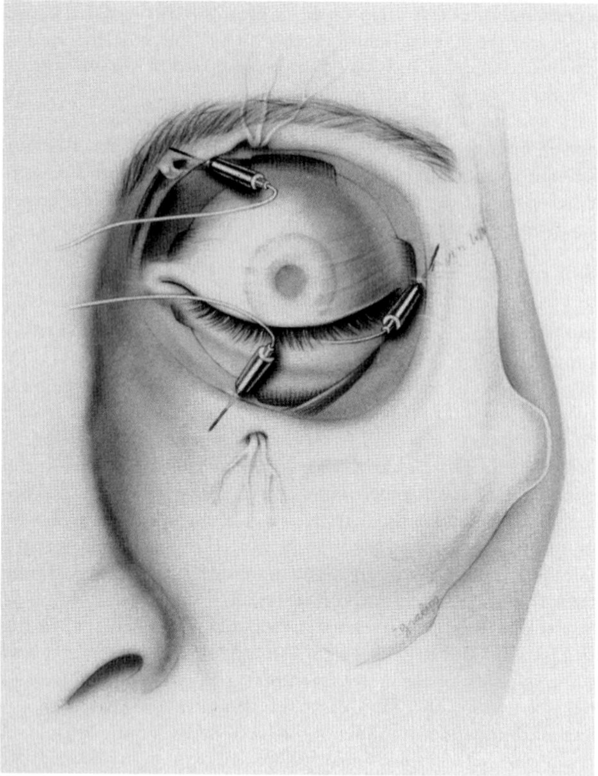

Figure 178-9. Placement of electrodes in extraocular muscles for monitoring cranial nerves III, IV, and VI. Electrodes are inserted through closed eyelids (drawn as if transparent), against inner surface of bony orbit, to record from inferior rectus/inferior oblique (third nerve), superior oblique (fourth nerve), and lateral rectus (sixth nerve). The illustration shows monopolar needle electrodes; flexible bipolar hookwire electrodes are now preferred for recording from extraocular muscles (see text for details). *(From Yingling CD. Intraoperative monitoring of cranial nerves in skull base surgery. In: Jackler RK, Brackmann DE, eds.* Neurotology. *St Louis: Mosby; 1994:967.)*

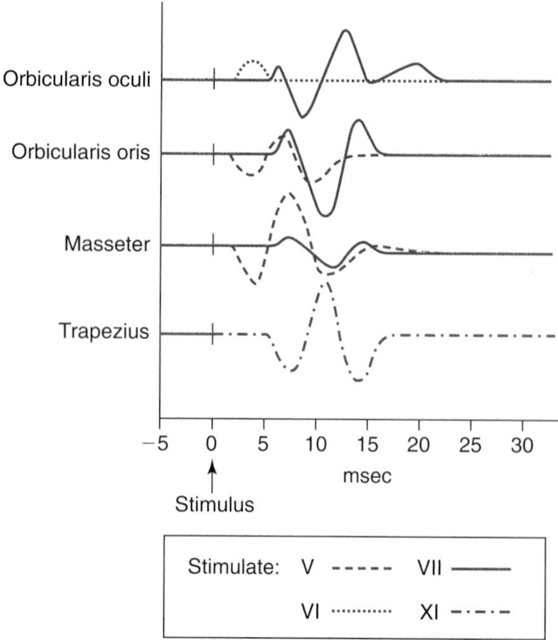

Figure 178-10. Schematic representation of responses obtained in four-channel montage (see Fig. 178-1) with intracranial stimulation of different motor nerves. Despite crosstalk in fifth and seventh nerve channels, these nerves can be clearly distinguished by the shorter latency of the responses to fifth nerve stimulation. Stimulation of the sixth nerve produces a short latency response localized to the orbicularis oculi channel because of volume conduction from the lateral rectus to the electrode at the outer canthus; stimulation of the eleventh nerve produces response restricted to the trapezius (see text for details). *(From Jackler RK, Pitts LH. Acoustic neuroma.* Neurosurg Clin N Am. *1990;1:199.)*

Complications (other than transient bruising) from monitoring of extraocular muscles are fortunately rare. It should be kept in mind, however, that the placement of electrodes near the globe is not without risk. In one of our patients, placement of an electrode near the superior oblique muscle resulted in bleeding and increased intraocular pressure, complicated by obstructed venous drainage due to compression of the posterior orbit by a neoplasm. Fortunately, this was detected before draping; the surgery was aborted and a lateral canthotomy was performed to relieve the excessive intraocular pressure. The tumor was removed a few days later, without further attempt to monitor fourth nerve function. Furthermore, diagnostic ocular EMG has been associated with rare occurrences of ecchymoses of the conjunctiva, subcapsular hemorrhage, and exposure keratitis, all of which clear without sequelae. Of greater concern is inadvertent perforation of the globe, which is more likely to occur in the presence of undetected glaucoma.[83]

Trigeminal Motor Branch Monitoring

Most efforts at intraoperative monitoring of the fifth nerve have concentrated on the motor portion (V3m), which is a branch of the third division of the nerve. There have been very few attempts to monitor the sensory branches, largely because of the technical problems encountered in overcoming stimulus artifact in trigeminal SEP recording, which is due both to the short latency of trigeminal SEPs and the proximity of the stimulation and recording sites.[84,85] However, Soustiel and coworkers[86] obtained good results with use of alternating-polarity stimuli to cancel the stimulus artifact.

The principles of monitoring V3m are the same as for seventh nerve monitoring. In practice, however, crosstalk between channels complicates the situation. Stimulation of V3m can produce large-amplitude CMAP responses that will be recorded by electrodes in masseter or temporalis and transmitted to facial muscles. Similarly, activity in facial muscles may be seen in the masseter or temporalis channels, creating the possibility of crosstalk in both directions. This overlap may pose a problem in interpreting the origin of mechanically elicited EMG activity. To minimize crosstalk, the V3m recording electrodes should be located where they will be minimally affected by facial muscle activity. We currently use hookwire electrodes placed in the temporalis muscle underneath the zygomatic arch, unless this is not possible because of the surgical approach (i.e., subtemporal or middle fossa); in such cases, the electrodes must be placed in the masseter.

Crosstalk presents less of a problem with the use of electrical stimulation because it is possible to distinguish between V3m and the seventh nerve by the latency of responses. Stimulation of the seventh nerve produces CMAP with an onset latency that typically ranges between 6 and 8 msec, depending on the exact site of stimulation, although it may be as short as 5 msec with stimulation in the far lateral internal auditory canal or delayed to as long as 20 msec if the nerve has been severely compromised by the tumor. On the other hand, stimulation of V3m produces responses of significantly shorter latency, ranging from approximately 3.5 to 5 msec. (Taken together, these findings suggest a useful mnemonic: "fifth nerve less than 5, seventh nerve approximately 7.") The differential pattern of responses seen in a typical acoustic neuroma case is shown in Figure 178-10.

Monitoring of Lower Cranial Nerves: Ninth, Tenth, Eleventh, and Twelfth Nerves

Larger acoustic neuromas with a significant inferior extension may involve the lower cranial nerves, and intraoperative monitoring of these nerves will be beneficial. More commonly, cranial nerves IX and XII are involved by tumors of the posterolateral cranial base, such as glomus jugulare tumors, meningiomas, or schwannomas of the ninth, tenth, or eleventh nerve. The morbidity associated with removal of tumors in this region is due primarily to neural damage, which may result in deterioration of voice, swallowing difficulties, or weakness and pain in the shoulder. These nerves can be monitored with EMG techniques analogous to those already described, with appropriate placement of recording electrodes.[87-89]

The glossopharyngeal (ninth nerve) nerve primarily mediates sensation to the upper pharynx and taste to the posterior third of the tongue. The only muscle innervated by this nerve is the stylopharyngeus, which is not easily accessible for insertion of EMG recording electrodes. However, electrodes in the posterior part of the soft palate ipsilateral to the tumor will pick up volume-conducted activity from the stylopharyngeus (Fig. 178-11; see also Fig. 178-13). The electrodes are inserted intraorally after intubation and are best sutured in place to prevent accidental dislodgement.

In contrast with other lower cranial nerves, mechanical stimulation of the ninth nerve during dissection typically produces little EMG activity, so it is the nerve for which function most commonly is lost. Fortunately, the deficits produced by isolated ninth nerve damage are relatively minor. Electrical stimulation of this nerve produces EMG responses at a latency of approximately 5 to 7 msec, which generally are of low amplitude, because recording electrodes are not placed directly in the stylopharyngeus. Similar responses often are seen with stimulation of the tenth nerve; however, it is easy to distinguish between the ninth and tenth nerves with multichannel recordings, because stimulation of the tenth nerve, but not the ninth nerve, also produces responses in the vocalis muscle (see later).

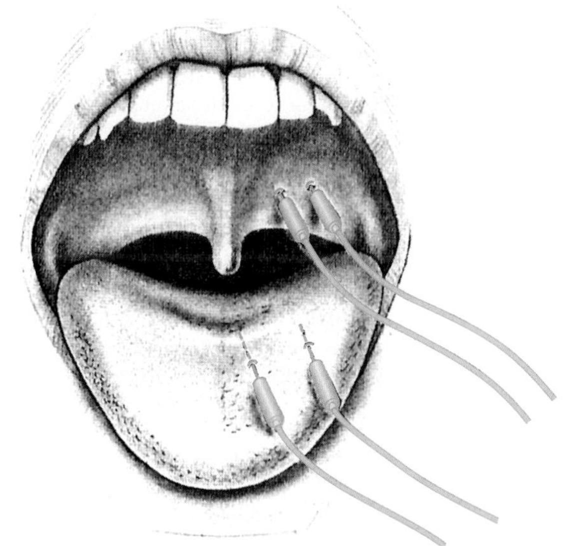

Figure 178-11. Placement of paired needle electrodes in the soft palate for monitoring the ninth cranial nerve and in the tongue for monitoring the twelfth cranial nerve *(From Lanser M, Jackler R, Yingling C. Regional monitoring of the lower (ninth through twelfth) cranial nerves. In: Kartush J, Bouchard K, eds.* Neuromonitoring in Otology and Head and Neck Surgery. *New York: Raven Press; 1992.)*

The vagus (tenth) nerve is one of the most complex cranial nerves, with myriad functions affecting the cardiac, respiratory, and gastrointestinal systems, as well as providing motor innervation to pharyngeal and laryngeal musculature. The vagus nerve commonly is monitored using an endotracheal tube with integral EMG electrodes (Medtronic-Xomed, Jacksonville, Florida), so that bipolar recordings can be obtained from both left and right vocalis muscles without additional electrodes (Fig. 178-12A).

Laryngeal surface electrodes (RLN Systems, Jefferson City, Missouri), which are inserted intraorally, posterior to the larynx, after intubation with a standard endotracheal tube also have been used (see Fig. 178-12B). They have a flat contact surface that records from the posterior cricoarytenoid muscle. The large contact surface may provide more stable recordings and greater reliability than are achievable with other methods.[90] Another laryngeal surface electrode is the bipolar electrode, which wraps around and adheres to a standard endotracheal tube and is positioned between the vocal cords as the tube is inserted (Neurovision Medical, Ventura, California). Finally, Leonetti and coworkers[91] have described a method for transcricothyroid membrane placement of bipolar hookwire electrodes in the vocalis muscle.

The latency of EMG responses to electrical stimulation of the tenth nerve varies with the site of stimulation. Intracranial stimulation in the posterior fossa or jugular foramen produces response latencies ranging from roughly 4 to 6 msec. Stimulation of the recurrent laryngeal nerve in the neck, as during thyroid surgery, produces a much faster response (2 to 3 msec latency). Another important consideration with stimulation of the vagus nerve is cardiac effects; bradycardia and even asystole have been documented with traction on the tenth nerve in both the posterior fossa and jugular foramen regions. (In such circumstances, however, the total heart rate in the OR generally remains constant, because that of the anesthesiologist rises in compensation!) Fortunately, this effect generally is not seen with threshold-level electrical stimulation; however, during surgery in this region, the anesthesiologist should be prepared to administer anticholinergic agents on short notice if necessary.

Monitoring of the eleventh nerve with electrodes in the trapezius muscle (Fig. 178-13) has already been briefly considered earlier, because activity of this muscle is the most readily observable marker for identifying the nerves of the jugular foramen in removal of large acoustic neuromas or other cerebellopontine angle tumors. During monitoring for tumors of the jugular foramen region itself, it also may be useful to place electrodes in the sternocleidomastoid muscle if extra channels are

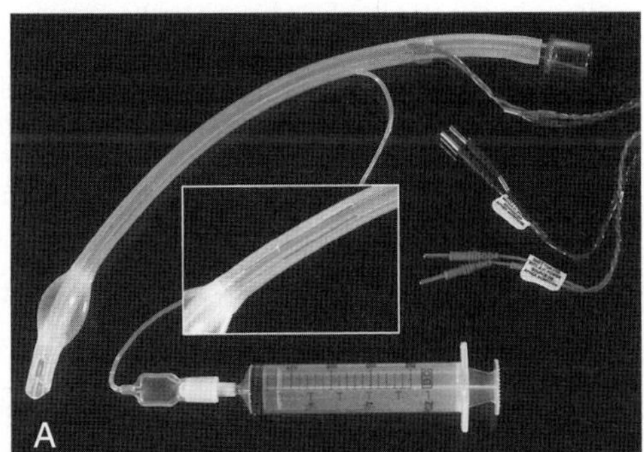

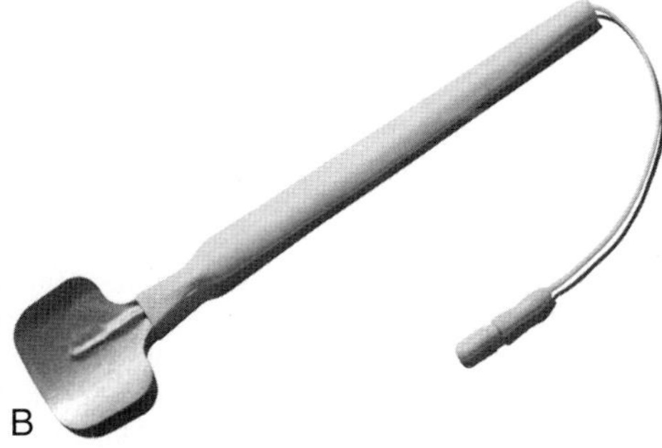

Figure 178-12. **A,** Electromyography (EMG) endotracheal tube. Two pairs of wires contact vocalis muscles bilaterally to record EMG activity resulting from activation of the recurrent laryngeal nerve, a component of the tenth cranial nerve **B,** Laryngeal surface electrode. The electrode is inserted into the postcricoid space after intubation with a standard endotracheal tube to record from the posterior cricoarytenoid muscles (tenth cranial nerve). *(**A,** Courtesy of Xomed-Treace, Jacksonville, Florida; **B,** courtesy of RLN Systems, Jefferson City, Missouri.)*

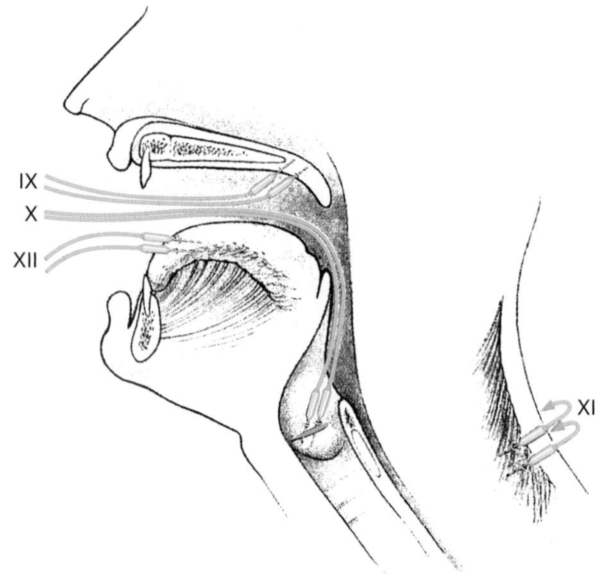

Figure 178-13. Sagittal view of placement of needle electrodes into the muscles used for lower cranial nerve monitoring. Needle electrode pairs are placed into the soft palate (ninth nerve), false vocal cord (tenth nerve), trapezius (eleventh nerve), and tongue (twelfth nerve). The electrodes placed in the false cord are unnecessary if one of the electrodes shown in Figure 178-12 is used instead. *(From Lanser M, Jackler R, Yingling C. Regional monitoring of the lower (ninth through twelfth) cranial nerves. In: Kartush J, Bouchard K, eds.* Neuromonitoring in Otology and Head and Neck Surgery. *New York: Raven Press; 1992.)*

available, especially if preoperative findings include preexisting eleventh nerve deficits and wasting of the trapezius. Because excessive movement from activation of trapezius muscles can be dangerous during surgery, stimulation of the eleventh nerve should be carried out at as low an intensity as feasible.

Finally, the twelfth cranial nerve provides motor innervation to the muscles of the tongue. Damage to this nerve produces the well-known sign of ipsilateral deviation seen on protrusion of the tongue, because of the predominance of the genioglossus muscle on the intact side, but in isolation does not usually produce major functional problems. However, damage to this nerve can lead to problems with chewing and swallowing, particularly in combination with deficits involving the eleventh and tenth nerves. This should be taken into account when facial reanimation with twelfth to seventh nerve anastomoses is under consideration in patients with lower cranial nerve deficits. The twelfth nerve can be monitored readily by insertion of electrodes into the lateral aspect of the anterior third of the ipsilateral tongue, with the electrodes sutured into place to prevent accidental dislodgement (see Figs. 178-11 and 178-13).

Cochlear Nerve (Eighth Nerve) Monitoring

The cochlear nerve is one of the most fragile of the cranial nerves and usually is much more intimately involved with acoustic tumors than the facial nerve. Thus, preservation of hearing generally is more difficult and less likely to be achieved than preservation of facial nerve function. However, recent advances in surgical and monitoring techniques have made preservation of hearing an attainable goal in removal of many smaller acoustic neuromas. Furthermore, the cochlear nerve is at risk in many other posterior fossa procedures, including resection of meningiomas and other nonacoustic tumors, vestibular neurectomies, and microvascular decompression of the fifth or seventh nerve. The most commonly used method for cochlear nerve monitoring has been intraoperative recording of the ABR.[2,11,38,55,93-110] ABR recording from the contralateral ear may be useful in cases with brainstem compression from large tumors, even if there is no hearing on the operated side.[92] More recently, direct eighth nerve action potentials,[11,38,45,49,77,111-114] electrocochleography (ECoG),[11,38,45,112,115-117] and recordings from the surface of the cochlear nucleus[118] also have been used. Finally, the use of evoked otoacoustic emissions, a more recently developed diagnostic technique, has been proposed as a potential method for monitoring cochlear nerve function.[119,120]

Auditory Brainstem Response Recording in the Operating Room

Since the ABR was first described in 1971,[121] ABR testing has become one of the most common neurophysiologic diagnostic modalities because of its ease of administration, relatively low cost, and ability to localize lesions in the peripheral auditory pathway.[122] The methods used in the OR are similar to those used clinically, with slight modifications.

Stimulus and Recording Parameters, Electrodes, and Placement

In clinical settings, stimuli for eliciting the ABR typically are delivered at rates of approximately 10 to 15 per second. For OR use, higher rates of 20 to 30 per second may be desirable to reduce averaging time. Stimulus intensity is maintained at a high level, usually at 95-dB peak sound pressure level (SPL) or higher, to obtain the best possible signal-to-noise ratio (SNR) (this is at least 60 dB above subjective click threshold levels). Although this is a high level for continuous stimulation, it does not seem to pose a problem; we are not aware of any reports of compromised hearing traceable to ABR recording over extended periods. Nevertheless, it is prudent to set the stimulus intensity at the lowest level that produces consistent waveforms.

It is necessary to use miniature earphones that do not compromise the surgical field. Møller[123] has successfully used small in-the-ear transducers designed for use with portable audio cassette players. Higher-quality transducers such as Etymotic Tubephones (Etymotic Research, Elk Grove Village, Illinois), which duplicate the frequency response of standard audiometric earphones, offer a more consistent, although expensive, alternative. For OR use, the main concern is obtaining clear definition of wave I, which often is the only useful ABR component in patients with acoustic neuroma. Any earphones that meet this criterion can be used with good success.

To minimize stimulus artifact, plastic tubing is used to conduct sound into the ear from a transducer placed a few inches away. The tube is terminated with a foam plug covered with a conductive gold foil (Tiptrode, Nicolet, Madison, Wisconsin), which also serves as one of the recording electrodes. In addition to providing acoustic isolation, this electrode provides improved definition of wave I over that obtainable with an earlobe or mastoid placement because of its closer proximity to the distal eighth nerve, the generator of wave I. The other electrode is placed at the vertex (Cz) or any point along the midsagittal plane between midforehead (Fpz) and vertex.

Because most of the power in the ABR is concentrated between 400 and 1400 Hz,[124] relatively narrow filter settings (i.e., 300 to 1500 Hz) produce more stable waveforms than wider settings (10 to 3000 Hz) typically used in the clinic, thereby facilitating rapid data collection. It also is desirable to collect a control ABR from the contralateral ear at the same time as that from the operated ear. This can be done by delivering stimuli alternately to each ear and separately averaging the left and right ear trials. Immediate comparison of the ABR from the operated side with that obtained from the contralateral ear provides a useful control for detection of nonspecific effects from factors such as anesthesia or temperature change. Of note, both ears must not be stimulated *simultaneously*, because the response from the contralateral ear could mask the loss of a response on the operative side.

Reducing Electrical and Acoustic Interference

It is imperative to take whatever steps are possible to minimize both electrical and acoustic artifacts. Electrical artifacts, which are of concern in both EMG and ABR monitoring, have already been covered. In addition, acoustic interference becomes a significant problem when either ABR or direct eighth nerve CNAPs are recorded. Drilling of the temporal bone to open the internal auditory canal can pose serious obstacles to auditory nerve monitoring because of acoustic masking, which can degrade or even obliterate the ABR or CNAP.

Unfortunately, the cochlear nerve, as well as the inner ear itself, is at great risk during this period in typical retrosigmoid approaches. It may therefore be necessary to deliberately halt drilling periodically to obtain valid readings. Alternately, the neurophysiologist can manually start and stop the averaging process to collect data during intervals in the drilling—for example, when changing drill burrs.

Because time is a major concern, efforts have been made to develop monitoring techniques that greatly reduce data collection times. The two major approaches that have been advocated are (1) emphasizing near-field recording techniques obtained from an electrode placed directly on the cochlear nerve and (2) the use of digital in addition to analog filtering.[123-125]

Interpretation of Responses in Surgical Context

ABRs are relatively unaffected by the level of anesthesia or the type of anesthetic agents used, provided normal brain temperature is maintained. Above 32° C, ABR absolute and interpeak latencies increase as a function of decreasing temperature at a rate of approximately 0.17 to 0.2 msec/° C.[126,127] Even though core temperature is maintained at near-normal values, brainstem temperature may still decrease, especially in tissue bordering the exposed cerebellopontine angle, and especially if it is irrigated with saline that is cooler than body temperature. If core temperature is not maintained, recording ABRs from the contralateral ear can help determine whether any changes are systemic or localized.

Another factor that typically affects the ABR is the craniotomy itself. New pathways for current flow caused by the craniotomy, changes in the local environment of the cochlear nerve with removal of CSF, and exposure of the nerve to air or insertion of metallic retractors into the opening all create differences in the relationship between the sites of ABR generation in the eighth nerve and brainstem and the recording electrodes. These changes are of no clinical significance but can lead to shifts in ABR amplitude, latency, and waveform that may be as large as those associated with intraoperative events that significantly affect auditory pathways. Fortunately, most of these changes occur in the early stages of the procedure before the cochlear nerve is in serious jeopardy; it is, however, important to obtain a new intraoperative baseline after opening and placement of retractors, rather than relying on the pre-incision baseline.

In most acoustic neuroma surgeries, ABR recordings from the operated side progressively deteriorate over the course of surgery, Cerebellar retraction, trauma from dissection, acoustic trauma, decreased local temperature, and disruption of cochlear perfusion may all affect ABR peak I, III, and V amplitude and latency values.[93,106] Retraction of the cerebellum, particularly in the medial to lateral direction,[102] is thought to be one of the principal maneuvers responsible for significant ABR deterioration.[93,94] Every effort should be made to reverse such effects by adjustment of the cerebellar retractor, by temporarily halting dissection, or by attempting dissection from a different angle or direction.[100] Occasionally, wave I amplitude will be acutely enhanced, possibly because of mechanical trauma to auditory efferent (inhibitory) fibers, which travel with the vestibular nerve. This enhancement often is followed by a rapid decrease in amplitude, suggesting disruption of the blood supply to the cochlea. Figure 178-14 shows typical ABR results from three patients undergoing surgical removal of acoustic neuroma.

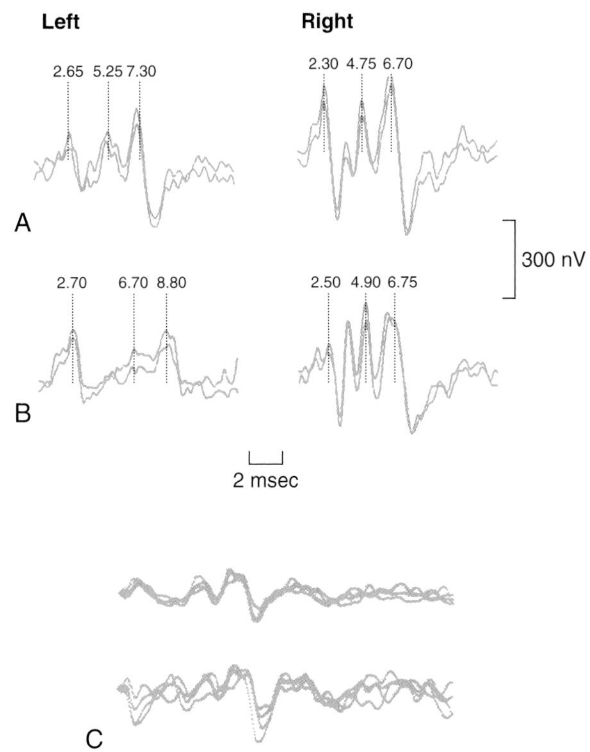

Figure 178-14. Representative examples of intraoperatively recorded auditory brainstem responses (ABRs) from three patients undergoing surgery for removal of acoustic neuroma. **A,** A 0.8-cm left-sided tumor in a 38-year-old woman with mild high-frequency hearing loss and speech discrimination scores of 92% for the left ear and 100% for the right ear. Pre-incision baseline shows well-defined ABRs on both sides. Note differences in interpeak latencies between left and right ears. **B,** A 1.8-cm tumor in a 52-year-old woman with moderate to moderate-severe sloping hearing loss and speech discrimination scores of 56% for the left ear and 90% for the right ear. Note that wave V is desynchronized and reduced in amplitude and that wave III is absent on the left side. Stimuli were alternating-polarity 100-msec clicks, presented at 80 dB above normal hearing level (nHL), 33.3/sec; 0.9-msec acoustic delay; averaged responses (N = 4000) were recorded from ipsilateral ear canal to vertex. Duplicate averages are overlaid. **C,** Intracanalicular right-sided tumor in a 48-year-old woman with nearly normal hearing, operated on by means of the middle fossa approach. *Top traces* are pre-incision baseline; *bottom traces* show preservation of auditory brainstem response after total removal of tumor, although a slight increase in latencies of waves IIII and V can be seen. Alternating-polarity 100-msec clicks, 80 dB above nHL, 21/sec; 0.9-msec acoustic delay; averaged responses (N = 1024) recorded from ipsilateral ear canal to midforehead. Four consecutive averages are overlaid. *(**A** and **B**, From Yingling CD, Gardi JG. Intraoperative monitoring of facial and cochlear nerves during acoustic neuroma surgery.* Otolaryngol Clin North Am. *1992;25:413;* ***C**, from Yingling CD. Intraoperative monitoring of cranial nerves in skull base surgery. In: Jackler RK, Brackmann DE, eds.* Neurotology. *St. Louis: Mosby; 1994:967.)*

Correlation of Intraoperative Auditory Brainstem Response with Postoperative Auditory Function

If ABR wave V is found to be intact after the tumor has been completely removed, preservation of useful hearing usually is achieved.[128] However, even with such favorable intraoperative findings, hearing may still be lost. Sometimes, hearing is present in the immediate postoperative period but disappears within 2 or 3 days. The mechanism of this delayed loss is unclear, but it may involve vasospasm of the cochlear artery.[129] If only wave I of the ABR is intact, preservation of useful hearing is much less likely. In several cases, we have recorded an intact wave I for more than an hour after the cochlear nerve was transected at the brainstem, an event that is unlikely to be compatible with hearing preservation! Furthermore, transient changes in wave I and the cochlear microphonic potential, even if the response returns over the course of surgery, may reflect pathogenic changes to the nerve with poor long-term prognosis.[38,112]

Most studies with intraoperative ABR recording agree that if waves I and V are preserved, the chances of hearing preservation are excellent,[109,130,131] although exceptions have been noted.[95,109] Conversely, if waves I and V are lost, there is little or no chance of hearing preservation,[42,109,128,131] although rare exceptions have been reported.[94,132] Therefore, the surgical decision to transect the cochlear nerve, even to facilitate tumor removal, should not be based solely on ABR findings.

Matthies and Samii[133] reported that loss of wave V, although the most definite sign of postoperative hearing loss, is the least helpful in hearing preservation, because its occurrence is a late indication of compromise of hearing. Relying on earlier warning criteria would seem to be more practical, such as a wave V latency increase by 0.5 msec[134] and observation of wave III for change. Wave III is the earliest and most sensitive sign of cochlear nerve affection; change or loss of wave III is an early sign that usually is followed by wave V loss. Wave III changes therefore warrant special attention to permit prompt warning to the surgeon.

Direct Eighth Nerve Action Potentials

Placement of Electrodes

To provide more rapid feedback on the functional status of the cochlear nerve, the rate of data acquisition can be enormously speeded up by recording near-field auditory CNAPs with an electrode placed directly on the cochlear nerve near the brainstem root entry zone.[11,45,111,135,136] With this configuration, clear averages can be obtained with 64 to 128 trials or less, compared with the 1000 or more usually required to record a reproducible ABR. The averaging time is thereby reduced from nearly 1 minute to approximately 5 seconds, permitting virtually on-line feedback to the surgeon, provided that the averaging computer can be programmed to automatically collect sequential averages and display the results so that changes can be readily identified. We have described this technique in detail elsewhere.[2]

Stimulus and Recording Parameters

The same stimuli used to elicit the ABR (brief clicks of fixed or alternating polarity) also are suitable for CNAP recording. Because the direct signal from the nerve is of higher amplitude than that of the ABR, however, the amplifier gain should be 5 to 10 times lower than for ABR recording; filter settings can remain the same. Usually 64 to 128 trials per average will produce an adequate waveform; at a stimulus rate of 20 per second, a new average can thus be obtained in approximately 5 seconds. An automated protocol for collecting sequential averages becomes important in this context to reduce the time to begin a new average after the previous one finishes.

Detection and Interpretation of Changes

It is important to determine the inherent amplitude and latency variability of the CNAP before operative manipulations that may potentially affect the cochlear nerve are undertaken, because this variability forms the background against which meaningful changes must be assessed. With an accurate and stable placement of the recording electrode on the nerve, the response can be quite repeatable from one average to the next. However, if the electrode position changes slightly, the variance may increase substantially. Unfortunately, some of the manipulations that may jeopardize the cochlear nerve (e.g., movement of a retractor) also are among the most likely to move the electrode. Figure 178-15 shows an example of a typical reversible change in CNAP amplitude.

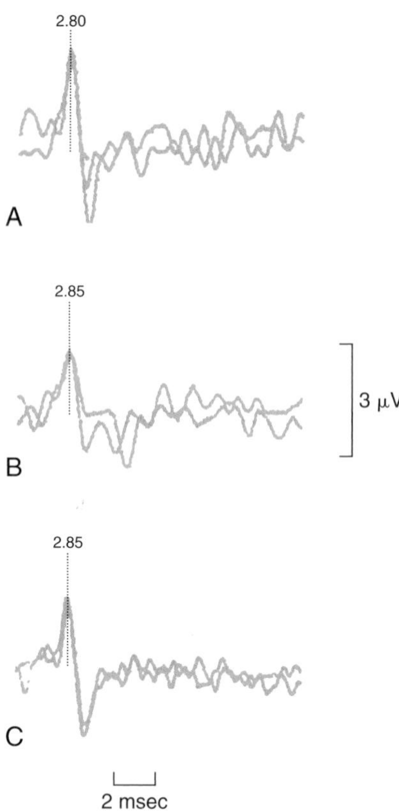

Figure 178-15. Representative changes in cochlear nerve compound action potentials during removal of a 0.6-cm intracanalicular acoustic neuroma. **A,** Just before mobilization of tissue adherent to cochlear nerve. **B,** Mobilization of tumor caused a sharp reduction (approximately 50%) in compound nerve action potential amplitude. **C,** Partial recovery of response after release of traction on nerve. Stimuli as described for Figure 178-14; 100 trials/average, duplicate averages are overlaid. *(**A** to **C**, From Yingling CD, Gardi JG. Intraoperative monitoring of facial and cochlear nerves during acoustic neuroma surgery.* Otolaryngol Clin North Am. *1992;25:413.)*

Relation of Monitoring to Outcome

Facial and Other Motor Cranial Nerve Preservation

Several studies have evaluated postoperative facial nerve function in series of cases with and without facial nerve monitoring.[31,32,36,37,43,51,137-139] As a result of these studies, it can now be generally accepted that although monitoring results in a small increase in the proportion of subjects with good outcomes (grade I or II), the main effect of monitoring has been to greatly decrease the incidence of poor outcomes (grade V or VI). This finding undoubtedly reflects the relative ease of locating and preserving the facial nerve in smaller tumors, coupled with a greater impact of monitoring with resection of larger tumors, when the nerve is more likely to be stretched and distorted and thus more difficult to identify by anatomic criteria alone.

The National Institutes of Health (NIH) consensus conference on vestibular schwannoma[140] concluded: "The benefits of routine intraoperative monitoring of the facial nerve have been clearly established. This technique should be included in surgical therapy for vestibular schwannoma." Facial nerve monitoring for vestibular schwannoma surgery is therefore now clearly established as the standard of care. Although less formal data are available concerning monitoring of other cranial motor nerves, the techniques and applications are virtually identical and should achieve similar benefits. The same NIH consensus panel concluded: "Routine monitoring of other cranial nerves should be considered." Accordingly, it is unequivocally recommended that EMG monitoring with as many simultaneously recorded channels as necessary be used during any skull base surgery in which cranial motor nerves are at risk.

Cochlear Nerve Preservation

No such unequivocal consensus has emerged concerning the usefulness of cochlear nerve monitoring. In studies in which tumor size was restricted to less than 2.0 cm, useful to adequate hearing preservation was maintained in approximately 30% to 45% of patients, as determined by preoperative and postoperative pure tone audiometry and speech discrimination testing.[42,109,131,141-144] At present, conservation of hearing is more a function of diagnostic (gadolinium-enhanced magnetic resonance imaging [MRI] detection of smaller tumors) and surgical (increased use of middle fossa approach) factors than of intraoperative monitoring. It is hoped that improved methods for rapid detection of intraoperative changes in cochlear and cochlear nerve function will help eighth nerve monitoring to contribute more substantially to improving clinical outcome.

Attempts to compare CNAP and ABR monitoring techniques during vestibular schwannoma surgery have revealed that although both

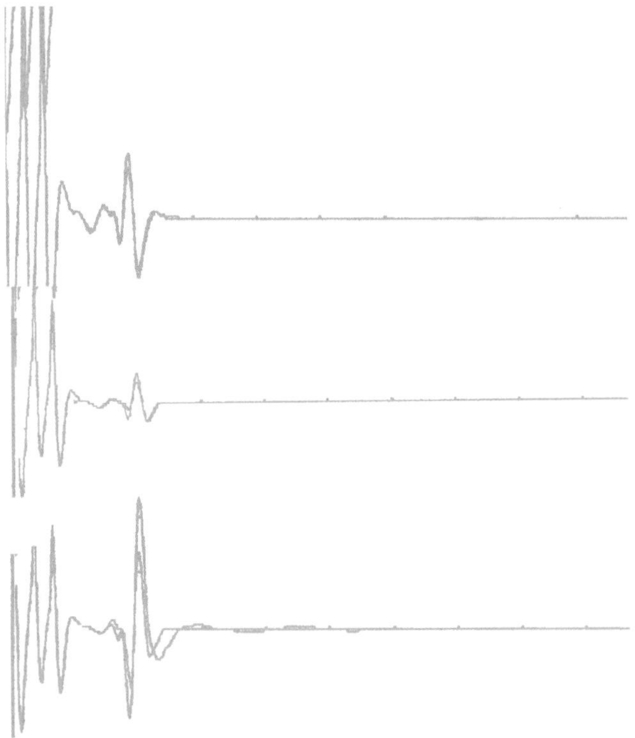

Figure 178-16. *Top*, Blink reflex recorded intraoperatively. *Middle*, Ipsilateral (R1) response recorded from orbicularis oculi after three-pulse train stimulus to supraorbital nerve. *Bottom*, Habituation of reflex response after repeated train stimulation. Restoration of reflex amplitude (dishabituation) after train stimulation of contralateral supraorbital nerve. *(From Yingling CD, Ashram YA. Intraoperative monitoring of cranial nerves in skull base surgery. In: Jackler R, Brackmann DE, eds.* Neurotology. *2nd ed. Philadelphia: Elsevier; 2005:958.)*

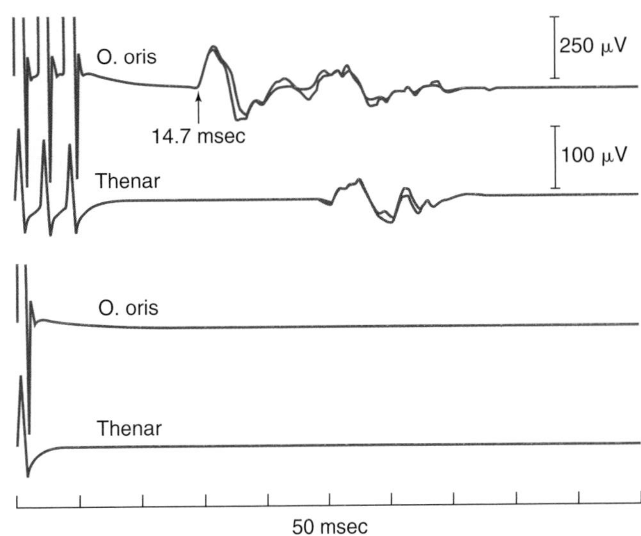

Figure 178-17. Intraoperative recordings of transcranial motor evoked potentials (tcMEPs). An example of facial MEP recorded from the left orbicularis oris (O. oris) muscle. The facial MEP response *(top trace)* is 300 mV in amplitude, generated by transcranial electrical stimulation of 3 pulses, 2-msec interstimulus interval, and 150 V. During stimulation, the anode was at M4 and the cathode at Mz. A simultaneous thenar muscle response also is shown *(second trace)*. Note the absence of same-intensity single-pulse responses *(third and fourth traces)* and the facial MEP onset latency of 14.7 msec, which indicate a central origin. Whether the apparent dispersion of the facial MEP relative to the expected duration of standard facial compound muscle action potentials (CMAPs) reflects preoperative facial nerve damage or normal temporal dispersion of facial motor neuron depolarization with pulse trains cannot be clearly determined without comparable normative data. *(From Dong CCJ, Macdonald DB, Akagami R, et al. Intraoperative facial motor evoked potential monitoring with transcranial electrical stimulation during skull base surgery.* Clin Neurophysiol. *2005;116:588.)*

ABR and CNAP are useful for predicting postoperative hearing, CNAP is more frequently obtainable, and CNAP monitoring is associated with a higher chance of hearing preservation.[145] Furthermore, CNAP monitoring is possible in patients with unrecordable ABR waveforms and may minimize cochlear nerve trauma.[146]

Colletti and associates[134] compared the value of ABR, ECoG, and directly recorded CNAPs in detecting damage to auditory structures during acoustic neuroma surgery. These investigators found that CNAPs had the highest predictive score for postoperative hearing. In particular, when a permanent loss of CNAPs occurred, sensitivity and specificity were 100%. These workers noted that ECoG activity was recorded in patients with lost CNAPs. This discrepancy was attributed to disconnection of the ear from the central auditory pathways associated with cochlear nerve damage,, with persistence of peripheral auditory function without propagation of the neural input. ABR monitoring was highly sensitive in detecting auditory damage, but its prognostic usefulness was marred by its poor specificity.

Future Directions and Conclusions

It is clear that facial nerve monitoring has had a marked impact on preservation of function in acoustic neuroma surgery. Although published data for other cranial motor nerves are more limited, the benefits are likely to be similar, because the principles are identical. The impact of monitoring on hearing preservation is less clear-cut, although the results thus far are improving and promising.

Equally clear is that much room for improvement remains. It is hopeful that the next decade will see improved techniques in a variety of areas, including better methods for automatic identification and rejection of artifacts; procedures for quantification of ongoing EMG activity; development of more sensitive non–EMG-based methods; and, perhaps most important, development of a technique for continuous assessment facial nerve integrity without direct electrical stimulation, analogous to continuous ABR recordings for assessing cochlear nerve function. This would be especially important with larger tumors, in which the nerve may be inaccessible for stimulation until extensive dissection has been done.

A possibility is to use the well-studied blink reflex,[83] which is elicited by stimulation of the supraorbital nerve (trigeminal afferents) and consists of an early ipsilateral EMG response (R1) and a later bilateral response (R2), both mediated by the facial nerve; it is the R1 response that can be recorded intraoperatively. Despite the usefulness of the blink reflex in clinical testing, it has not yet been reliably elicited in surgery because of the suppression of reflex activity by general anesthetics. It may become possible to overcome this problem by greater reliance on intravenous anesthetics, such as propofol, together with repetitive train stimulation (Fig. 178-16).

Another potentially valuable development is adapting the transcranial motor evoked potential (tcMEP) technique, now commonly used in spinal surgery, to facial nerve monitoring.[147-149] This technique entails placing a pair of stimulating needle electrodes on the scalp over the face motor area with the anode placed contralateral to the side of surgery.[150] The cortex is stimulated by multipulse constant-voltage stimulation, and EMG responses are recorded from appropriate facial muscles. The technique has some limitations, including the potential for excessive patient movement, which may not be appropriate for delicate intracranial surgery, generation of large stimulus artifact, and the possibility of extracranial current spread with peripheral facial nerve excitation; however, these limitations can be reduced by use of suitable electrode configuration and stimulation parameters.[148] Figure 178-17 shows intraoperative MEP recording from the orbicularis oris channel after multipulse transcranial electrical stimulation.

Finally, much is still to be learned about the relationship between intraoperative recordings and long-term clinical outcome. More controlled studies, with carefully characterized patient populations and standardized monitoring techniques with quantification of response parameters, are needed to address many of the issues discussed previously. The only certainty is that improvements in monitoring techniques and routine inclusion of professional monitoring personnel in the surgical team, coupled with advances in early diagnosis and microsurgical techniques, will continue to improve the prognosis for preservation of cranial nerve function in patients undergoing skull base surgery.

SUGGESTED READINGS

Ashram Y, Yingling C. Intraoperative facial nerve monitoring. In: Nuwer M, ed. *Intraoperative Monitoring of Neural Function*. vol 8. St. Louis: Elsevier; 2008:371-383.

Colletti V, Fiorino FG, Mocella S, et al. ECochG, CNAP and ABR monitoring during vestibular schwannoma surgery. *Audiology*. 1998;37:27.

Cueva RA, Morris GF, Prioleau GR. Direct cochlear nerve monitoring: first report on a new atraumatic, self-retaining electrode. *Am J Otol*. 1998;19:202.

Daube JR, Harper CM. Surgical monitoring of cranial and peripheral nerves. In: Desmedt JE, ed. *Neuromonitoring in Surgery*. Amsterdam: Elsevier; 1989.

Dong CC, Macdonald DB, Akagami R, et al. Intraoperative facial motor evoked potential monitoring with transcranial electrical stimulation during skull base surgery. *Clin Neurophysiol*. 2005;116:588.

Fenton JE, Chin RY, Fagan PA, et al. Predictive factors of long-term facial nerve function after vestibular schwannoma surgery. *Otol Neurol*. 2002;23:388.

Harner SG, Daube JR, Beatty CW, et al. Intraoperative monitoring of the facial nerve. *Laryngoscope*. 1988;98:209.

Jackler RK, Selesnick SH. Indications for cranial nerve monitoring during otologic and neurotologic surgery. *Am J Otol*. 1994;15:611.

Kartush J, Bouchard K, eds. *Neuromonitoring in Otology and Head and Neck Surgery*. New York: Raven Press; 1992.

Kartush J, Lundy L. Facial nerve outcome in acoustic neuroma surgery. *Otolaryngol Clin North Am*. 1992;25:623.

Kartush JM, Niparko JK, Bledsoe SC, et al. Intraoperative facial nerve monitoring: a comparison of stimulating electrodes. *Laryngoscope*. 1985;95:1536.

Lalwani AK, Butt FY, Jackler RK, et al. Delayed onset facial nerve dysfunction following acoustic neuroma surgery. *Am J Otol*. 1995;16:758.

Mandpe AH, Mikulec A, Jackler RK, et al. Comparison of response amplitude versus stimulation threshold in predicting early postoperative facial nerve function after acoustic neuroma resection. *Am J Otol*. 1998;19:112.

Møller AR. Monitoring auditory function during operations to remove acoustic tumors. *Am J Otol*. 1996;17:452.

Møller AR. *Intraoperative Neurophysiological Monitoring*. Clifton, NJ: Humana Press; 2006.

Møller AR, Jannetta PJ. Preservation of facial function during removal of acoustic neuromas. Use of monopolar constant-voltage stimulation and EMG. *J Neurosurg*. 1984;61:757.

Møller A, Jannetta PJ. Monitoring facial EMG during microvascular decompression operations for hemifacial spasm. *J Neurosurg*. 1987;66:681.

Nakao Y, Piccirillo E, Falcioni M, et al. Prediction of facial nerve outcome using electromyographic responses in acoustic neuroma surgery. *Otol Neurotol*. 2002;23:93.

Neu M, Strauss C, Romstöck J, et al. The prognostic value of intraoperative BAEP patterns in acoustic neurinoma surgery. *Clin Neurophysiol*. 1999;110:1935.

Noss RS, Lalwani AK, Yingling CD. Facial nerve monitoring in middle ear and mastoid surgery. *Laryngoscope*. 2001;111:831.

Nuwer M. *Evoked Potential Monitoring in the Operating Room*. New York: Raven Press; 1986.

Prass RL, Lüders H. Acoustic (loudspeaker) facial electromyographic monitoring: Part 1. Evoked electromyographic activity during acoustic neuroma resection. *Neurosurgery*. 1986;19:392.

Richmond IL, Mahla M. Use of antidromic recording to monitor facial nerve function intraoperatively. *Neurosurgery*. 1985;16:458.

Romstock J, Strauss C, Fahlbusch R. Continuous electromyography monitoring of motor cranial nerves during cerebellopontine angle surgery. *J Neurosurg*. 2000;93:586.

Silverstein H, Smouha EE, Jones R. Routine intraoperative facial nerve monitoring during otologic surgery. *Am J Otol*. 1988;9:269.

Yingling CD, Ashram YA. Intraoperative monitoring of cranial nerves in skull base surgery. In: Jackler R, Brackmann DE, eds. *Neurotology*. 2nd ed. Philadelphia: Elsevier; 2005.

Yingling CD, Gardi JG. Intraoperative monitoring of facial and cochlear nerves during acoustic neuroma surgery. *Neurosurg Clin N Am*. 2008;19:289.

For complete list of references log onto www.expertconsult.com.

CHAPTER ONE HUNDRED AND SEVENTY-NINE

Stereotactic Radiation Treatment of Benign Tumors of the Cranial Base

D. Bradley Welling

Mark D. Packer

Key Points

- Stereotactic radiation therapy demonstrates good short-term control for many benign cranial base tumors.
- Short-term quality of life outcomes favor stereotactic radiation therapy over conventional surgical management.
- Radiation-induced cranial nerve injury has been reduced as lower doses of radiation have come into use.
- Long-term control and radiation-induced malignancy risk will be known in the next decade with further study.

Stereotactic radiation therapy is an option for the treatment of most benign cranial base tumors including vestibular schwannomas. The literature to date, however, consists of retrospective studies, with their inherent biases. The same also is true of the alternative treatments, including surgical and observational protocols. Long-term prospective outcome studies with blinded independent observations are needed as a strong supplement on which to base clinical treatment.

Since the late 1990s, stereotactic radiation therapy has become an increasingly popular treatment for benign tumors of the cranial base, including vestibular schwannomas. After its introduction for clinical use in 1967 by Lars Leksell, the initial acceptance of this modality waned as early complications included brainstem radiation damage, hydrocephalus, and cranial neuropathies.[1] However, as delivery has become more precise through improved stereotactic guidance, and as the tolerance levels of cranial nerves for radiation have become better elucidated, the technique has gained popularity and now offers an alternative to surgical intervention or observation for many cranial base tumors. Additionally, the combined use of radiation and surgical treatment may be considered for tumors for which incomplete excision may be planned to reduce the danger to adjacent cranial nerves. The goal of stereotactic irradiation for the treatment of benign tumors generally is considered to be growth arrest.

This chapter summarizes the principal advantages, disadvantages, and areas needing further research related to this technique. When possible, standardized definitions of tumor control and hearing preservation are specified, but this is not possible for all studies reviewed.

Principles of Stereotactic Radiation Therapy

In general, *stereotactic radiation therapy* denotes the application of any kind of ionizing radiation in a precise dosing mechanism to a target while limiting radiation exposure and damage to the adjacent surrounding tissues. Several delivery techniques for stereotactic irradiation have been developed.

With gamma knife radiotherapy techniques, well-collimated beams of radiation from 201 cobalt-60 sources are directed through ports in a semispherical helmet, allowing the beams to converge and deliver a much higher dose to the target than to the surrounding structures. The precise delivery of the beam is increased by direct fixation of a head frame attached with surgical pins to the cranium (Fig. 179-1). Although the procedure commonly is referred to as stereotactic "radiosurgery," this is a misnomer, because the therapy is accomplished by the delivery of external radiation without a surgical incision. Today most teams are composed of neurosurgeons or neuro-otologic surgeons, a radiation oncologist, and a radiation biologist. The advantage of gamma knife techniques at present is the capability for highly controlled delivery of radiation by way of multiple isopoints to the tumor target. Additionally, newer units have more fully automated coordinate adjustments, allowing more rapid dosing. A disadvantage is that tumors located much below the level of the cranial base are not readily accessible for stereotactic radiation delivery by the gamma knife. Rigid fixation of the skull to a metal frame that locks into the radiation chamber allows precise, submillimeter stereotactic radiation delivery, but the gamma knife does not lend itself to multiple fractionated treatments.[2]

An alternative to the gamma knife was developed through the application of linear accelerators (LINACs). Instead of multiple sources aimed at a central designated target, the LINACs rotate the treatment beam of the unit around the target in a variable number of rotational arcs.[3] Although the tumor margin doses are similar to those achieved with the gamma knife, LINAC delivery typically uses fewer isocenters, and the dose to the tumor may be less precisely applied. Thermoplastic molded mask systems to limit positional variation in the radiation delivery allow for the potential of fractionated schedules without the placement of pins into the skull but may not restrict movement of the target as surely as rigid fixation. Controversy exists regarding the potential benefit of fractionated stereotactic radiation protocols. Some inves-

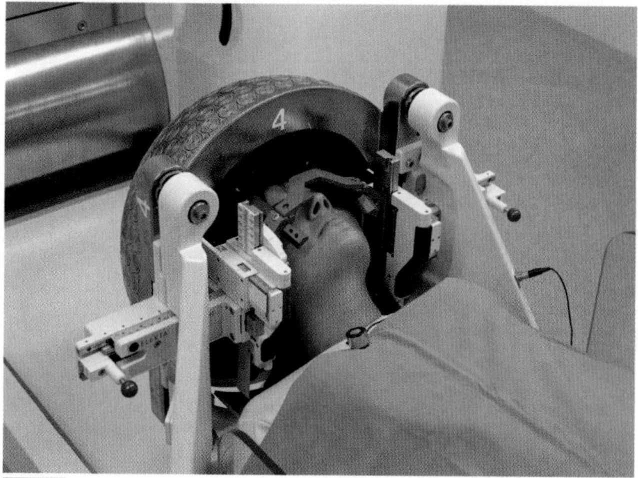

Figure 179-1. The gamma knife helmet. *(Courtesy of Elekta, Inc.)*

tigators maintain that a fractionated regimen, given over days or weeks, takes advantage of radiobiologic principles to reduce late toxicity while maintaining tumor control. However, in the case of vestibular schwannomas, both the tumor and the surrounding cranial nerves are late-reacting tissues; therefore, fractionating theoretically reduces the post-irradiation complications to the surrounding cranial nerves but also reduces the likelihood of desired tumor damage, DNA disruption, and apoptotic cell death.

Radiobiology

The therapeutic role of ionizing x-rays and gamma rays lies in their ability to alter and compromise DNA and other important biologic molecules of the cells targeted. Specifically, ionizing radiation excites electrons, which cause free radical damage of the involved cell structures. DNA damage prevents entering into the cell cycle and can lead to programmed cell death (apoptosis). Radiation damage to the phospholipids of the cell membrane also may lead to cell death. Ionizing radiation comes in two general varieties—electromagnetic, which consists of photons or packets of energy, and particulate radiation. X-rays and gamma rays are forms of electromagnetic radiation resulting when a photon indirectly transfers its energy to a target tissue. In an x-ray, a collision between an electron and the target tissue occurs, whereas gamma rays are produced when the contents of the nucleus of an atom return to their initial energy state from an excited level, a process known as gamma decay. As the electromagnetic waves pass through the tissues, they are absorbed, producing electron recoil and tissue damage as they lose their strength.

Protons are heavy charged particles that cause damage directly. They are positively charged and of a much higher mass than electrons. When a proton beam strikes its target, it delivers almost all of its energy at its delivery range, which results in a rapid dropoff of energy level, thereby limiting tissue damage past the target of interest. This characteristic is exploited to deliver a high dose of radiation directly to the target tissues with sparing of tissues deep to the delivery area. Dose inhomogeneity may increase the risks of complications for large target volumes treated with stereotactic radiation when the target area is less than a perfect match for the radiation delivery field. Complications were fewer with conformal multiple-isocenter gamma knife treatment plans than with less elaborate two-isocenter LINAC stereotactic radiation plans, which were associated with a higher risk of complications, with possible high-dose overlap regions extending into normal tissues.[4] The newer, more precise delivery systems are less likely to expose tissues out of the target regions to high doses of radiation.

Imaging

Typically, a lesion is diagnosed and confirmed by magnetic resonance imaging (MRI). On the day of the planned radiation treatment, a second MRI study is performed to precisely plan the radiation delivery after the patient's head has been fixed in the head frame. Post-irradiation MRI scans are obtained at 6 months and then yearly thereafter to observe the effect of the stereotactic radiation. Because of the long-term potential for delayed growth of the tumors and also because of the potential for malignant change, at present we recommend that yearly follow-up MRI scans be obtained.

Dose Selection

Dose selection in stereotactic radiotherapy has been evolving over the past decade as experience has been gained. Early animal studies by Kondziolka and associates[4a] demonstrated that xenograft vestibular schwannomas in the renal capsule of athymic mice showed significant reductions in tumor volume following stereotactic radiation with 40 Gy at 2 weeks and after 1 month in a 20-Gy group. Tumor vascularity was reduced in the 20- and 40-Gy groups respectively, but not in the 10-Gy group at 3-month follow-up evaluation. In humans today, however, in order to decrease facial nerve neuropathies, 17 Gy or less is delivered to the 50% isodose line (Fig. 179-2). Also, the auditory portion of the eighth cranial nerve appears to have a tolerance for approximately 11 Gy, with an 50% hearing preservation rate.[4b] Simply put, the lower the dose, the lower the complication rate—but the lower the likelihood of tumor control over the long-term follow-up period of observation.

Benign Tumors of the Cranial Base: Vestibular Schwannoma

Vestibular schwannomas have increasingly been treated with stereotactic radiation. Some centers favor this therapy over conventional surgical techniques or observation. In reporting the outcomes with gamma knife, LINAC, and fractionated stereotactic irradiation, "tumor control" has been defined in two ways. Some investigators define tumor control as no growth, whereas others report the percentage of tumors that required no further treatment. The latter definition may overestimate the true control rate, because cases in which tumors may have been growing but not requiring surgical intervention would be counted as those with successful outcomes. The most useful information that can be gleaned from the literature at this time is a compilation of reported outcomes. The lack of well-controlled studies has been duly noted. The longer the follow-up, the more valuable the study. Outcomes data extracted from the recent literature, including reports on tumor control, facial nerve function, hearing preservation, and trigeminal neuralgia, are summarized in Tables 179-1 to 179-3.

Fractionation versus Nonfractionation

Considerable debate is ongoing regarding whether or not fractionated stereotactic radiation is more favorable than single-dose stereotactic radiation for cranial nerve functional preservation in vestibular schwannoma treatment. Although fractionated radiation may give less immediate damage to the surrounding cranial nerves, damage to the slowly growing schwannoma cells also is less likely, thereby increasing the likelihood of growth. Flickinger[4c] argues that the available data in the literature are simply inadequate to allow definitive conclusions regarding which of the two delivery plans is better for cranial nerve preservation and tumor control; carefully planned, prospective controlled longitudinal studies are needed to address this concern. Indeed, the data shown in Tables 179-1 to 179-3 seem to confirm his opinion.

Traditionally, in our own practice, stereotactic radiation has been reserved for a select patient subset for the treatment of vestibular schwannoma. Elderly patients with small to medium-sized tumors with proven growth or those not fit for a surgical resection have been recommended to receive stereotactic radiation treatment. Chen, reporting data for three 5-year periods between 1990 and 2005, noted that vestibular schwannomas were being diagnosed at statistically higher ages, at smaller sizes, and in a greater proportion of patients older than 65 years of age.[5] During these periods, the frequency of observation as a treatment choice for vestibular schwannoma rose from 12% to 37%, microsurgery was performed in 59% of patients, and frequency of use of stereotactic radiation therapy rose to 4% of cases. As life expectancy

Table 179-1

Gamma Knife–Based Irradiation Protocols and Outcomes

Study	No. of Patients	Follow-up	Tumor size (cm^3)	Marginal Dose (Gy)	Isodose (mean)	Post-irradiation Tumor Control	Post-irradiation Hearing Preserved	FN Weakness	TrN Toxicity	Other
Mathieu et al, 2007[18]*	62 NF2 (74 tumors)	53 mo	5.7	14	50%	5 yr: 85% 10 yr: 81% 15 yr: 81%	1 yr: 73% 2 yr: 59% 5 yr: 48%	8%	4%	Volume/ dose-related†
Hempel et al, 2006[20]*	123	8.2 yr	1.0	13	40-85% (55%)	97%	47% 18% drop 73% audio	0	5.8	Tinn 4% Vert 13% hc 2.4%
Chung et al, 2005[14]	187	31 mo	4.1	13 11-18	50-94% (57%)	7 ya: 95%	60%	1.4%	1.1%	Blood-brain barrier disruption in 45% at <6 mo‡
Hasegawa et al, 2005[11]	317	7.8 yr 77: >10 yr	5.6	13.2	40-80% (51%)	5 ya: 93% 10 ya: 92%	68% audio/tele	1%	2%	Malignancy: 7% hc§
Huang et al, 2005[21]	45	25 mo	4.5	11.5		96%	77%	0	2%	
Paek et al, 2005[22]	25/pros	45 mo	3.0	12	50%	92%	52% 36% no loss	0	5%	Cochlear dose‖
Wowra et al, 2005[23]*	111 10 NF2	7 yr	1.6	13	45-85%	6 ya: 95%	Mean loss 10 dB (range +20 to −75)	0	12%	Tumor expansion¶
Lunsford et al, 2005[9]*	829 62 NF2	252: >10 yr	2.5	13 10-20	50%	97%	70%, 5 ya	<1%	<3%	
Landy et al, 2004[25]	34	43.4 mo		10-14	45-70%	97%	100% subjective	0	0	Arachnoid cyst
Inoue et al, 2005[26]	13	>6 yr	15.2	10-12		100%	4/5 tele	0	0	
Total	1758	>25 mo	>1.6	10-14	40-85%	81-97%	47-100%	0-8%	0-4%	

*Some studies used the same subject population: The series of Mathieu et al was the same as the NF2 subpopulation in the series of Lunsford et al; Hempel et al and Wowra et al also studied the same patients.
†Dose and volume were predictive of hearing deficit.
‡14.5% of irradiated tumors showed high signal intensity on T2-weighted sequences in peritumoral regions, consistent with disruption of the blood-brain barrier.
§One malignant transformation occurred at 48 months, resulting in death. Tumor volumes greater than 15 cm^3 were significant for treatment failure.
‖Higher doses to cochlear nucleus were deemed significant for hearing loss.
¶39% showed transient tumor expansion. Hearing loss associated with increased age and tumor expansion.
audio, audiometric data; FN, facial nerve; hc, hydrocephalus; NF2, neurofibromatosis type 2; pros, prospective; tele, telephone data; Tinn, tinnitus; TrN, trigeminal nerve; Vert, vertigo; ya, years of actuarial data.

is increasing, it seems likely that vestibular schwannomas under expectant management will be more likely to show growth when observed over longer periods of time, as demonstrated by Charabi and associates.[6] Smouha and colleagues, in a retrospective meta-analysis of patients managed without intervention, demonstrated that 43% of 1244 vestibular schwannomas showed growth over a mean follow-up period of 3.2 years.[7] Hearing loss occurred in 51% of 347 patients. Only 20% of 1001 patients from 15 studies eventually failed observation, showing growth sufficient to warrant active treatment. Smouha's data are similar to our own prospective findings, which demonstrated that 66% of tumors grew more than 15% when measured volumetrically after a mean follow-up period of 3.8 years.[8]

Outcome Assessment

Advocates of the use of stereotactic irradiation as a primary treatment for vestibular schwannomas without first documenting growth must bear in mind that over the short term, many tumors do not demonstrate growth. This calls into question whether or not post-irradiation stability of a nongrowing tumor should be considered to represent treatment success. In fairness, many patients in whom tumors are removed surgically are not followed to determine growth before treatment either. However, a fundamental difference remains between outcome assessments of the different treatment modalities. The key anatomic measure of outcome in surgery—absence of tumor or a residual of a small portion of the original tumor—typically

Table 179-2

LINAC-Based Stereotactic Irradiation Protocols and Outcomes

Study	No. of Patients	Follow-up	Tumor size (cm^3)	Marginal Dose (Gy)	Isodose (mean)	Post-irradiation Tumor Control	Post-irradiation Hearing Preserved	FN Weakness	TrN Toxicity	Other
Radu et al, 2007[27]	22	18 mo	1.85	12		100%	71% (grades I, II)	4.5%	9%	
Rutten et al, 2007[28]	26	49 mo		10-14	80%	5 yr: 95%	96%	0	8%	Volume/ dose-related
Roos et al, 2006[13]	65 4 NF2	48 mo	22 (mm)	12	85% 70-90%	95%	47%	6.1%	10.8%	Enlarging tumor: 17%* hc 1.8%
Combs et al, 2006[29]	26 2 NF2	110 mo	15 (mm)	13 11-20	80%	5 ya: 96% 10 ya: 91%	9 yr: 55%	5.2%	8%	
Chung et al, 2004[65]	27 3 NF2	27 mo 26 mo	2.6 2.4	12	80%	5 ya: 87%	1 yr: 85% 2 yr: 57%	11.8%	9.5%	SRT changes†
Friedman et al, 2006[30]	390/ pros	40 mo 63 >5 yr	2.2	12.5 10-22.5	70-80%	1 ya: 98% 2 ya: 98% 5 ya: 90%	Not reported	4.4%	3.6%	
Total	556	18-49 mo	1.9-2.6	10-14	70-90%	87-96%	47-96%	0-12%	4-11%	

*17% enlarge an average of 4 mm within the first year.
†Pre-reatment SRT was 20 dB; post-treatment SRT increased to 38 dB in 59%.
FN, facial nerve; hc, hydrocephalus; NF2, neurofibromatosis type 2; SRT, speech reception threshold; TrN, trigeminal nerve; ya, years of actuarial data.

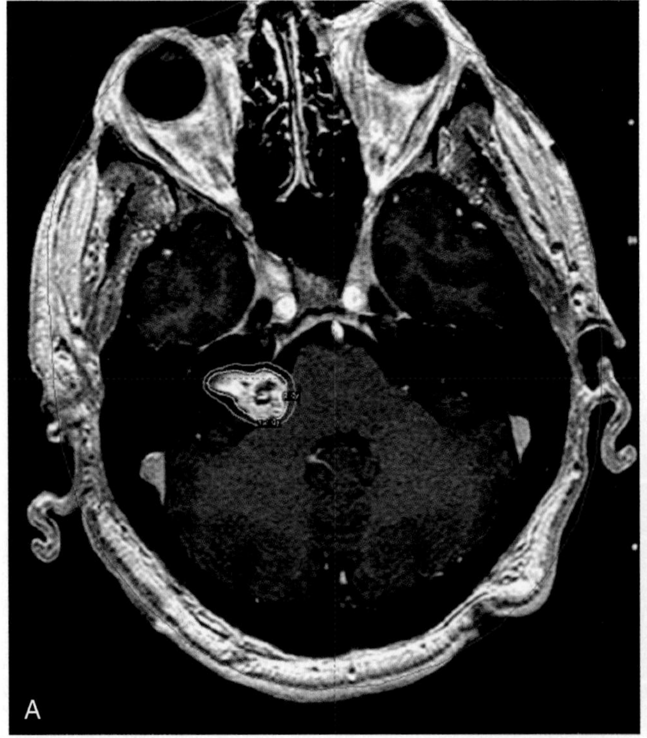

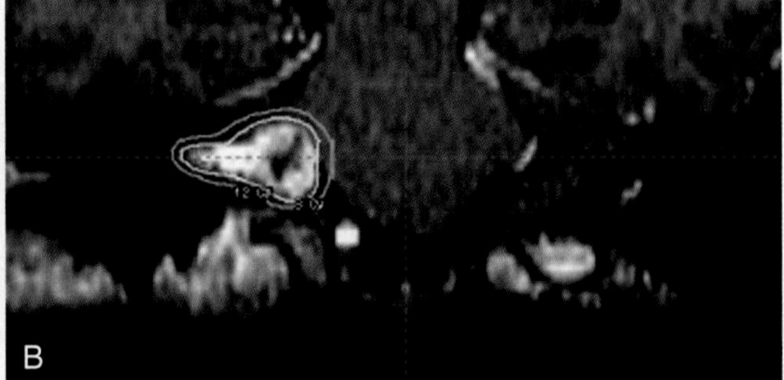

Figure 179-2. Axial (**A**) and coronal (**B**) images of radiation dose plan for a vestibular schwannoma. Multiple shots can be arranged within the tumor at various radiation doses to give homogeneous exposure to the tumor while avoiding unnecessarily high levels of radiation to adjacent structures.

Table 179-3

Fractionated Irradiation Protocols and Outcomes

						Post-irradiation				
Study*	No. of Patients	Follow-up (mo)	Tumor Size	Total Dose (Gy)	Fraction/ Isodose	Tumor Control	Hearing Preserved	FN Weakness	TrN Toxicity	Other
Thomas et al, 2007[33]	34/pros	37	1.1 cm^3	45	25 90%	2 ya: 100% 4 ya: 96%	2 yr: 63% 3 yr: 63%	6%	0	Cochlear dose†
Horan et al, 2007[34]	42 5 NF2	19	21.5 mm	50	30	2-5 ya: 97%	100% useful 73% drop**	3.2%	0	
Koh et al, 2007[35]	60	32	4.9 cm^3	50	25 95-100%	5 ya: 96% 5 y: 93%	77.3%	0	0	GBM‡
McClelland et al, 2008[67]	20	22	2.1 cm^3	54	30 90%	100%	100% useful 44% drop**	0%	10%	
Maire et al, 2006[32]	45	80	31 mm	51	28	5 ya: 86%	77.8%	0	0	MPNST§
Combs et al, 2005[36]	106/pros 14 NF2	49	3.9 cm^3	57.6	32 90%	3 ya: 94% 5 ya: 93%	5 yr: 94%	2.3%	3.4%	29/65 audio††
Chan et al, 2005[31] XKnife‡‡	70 11 NF2	45	2.4 cm^3	54	30 95%	3 ya: 100% 5 ya: 98%	3/5 yr: 84%, tele	1%	4%	>8 cm^3 significant‖
Chang et al, 2005[66] Cyberknife	61	48	18.5 mm	18-21	NR	98%	74%	3.3%	ND	
Selch et al, 2004[37]	50	36	2.51 cm^3	54	30 90%	100%	5 ya: 92% tele	2.1%	2.1%	Vertigo¶
Dhanachai et al, 2004[38]	5 NF2	19	5.4 cm^3	44-60 (8 pts) 30 (2 pts)	25-33	90%	40%	0	0	
Total	493	19-48	1.1-5.4 cm^3	54	25-32 >90%	86-100%	63-100%	0-6%	0-4%	

*Radiation source stated if known.
†Cochlear doses predicted hearing losses.
‡One malignant transformation occurred at 5.8 years after fractionated radiotherapy, resulting in death. 45% treated without tumor progression.
§One malignant transformation occurred at 18 years after fractionated radiotherapy, resulting in death.
‖Tumor volume larger than 8 cm^3 was predictive of hearing loss. No differences were noted in the patients with NF2.
¶Post-treatment ataxia and vertigo developed in 30%.
**100% reported having retained useful hearing, although hearing level or speech discrimination (function) dropped in 27% (73% retained current level). McClelland showed 100% retained useful functional hearing, even though 44% dropped some function.
††29 of 65 patients received audiograms.
‡‡XKnife (Integra Radionics, Burlington, MA) is a software package for 3D radiation therapy planning using LINAC = based radiotherapy units.
audio, audiometric data; FN, facial nerve; GBM, glioblastoma multiforme; hc, hydrocephalus; MPNST, malignant peripheral nerve sheath tumor; NF2, neurofibromatosis type 2; NR, not reported; pros, prospective; pts, patients; tele, telephone data; TrN, trigeminal nerve; y, years of progression-free control; ya, years of actuarial data.

differs from the growth of persistent tumor after stereotactic irradiation.

Information on outcomes pertaining to the therapeutic use of stereotactic radiation treatment is expanding. Moreover, although debate continues regarding the optimal treatment of vestibular schwannomas, a growing consensus is that focal radiation therapy, delivered in single- or fractionated-dose regimens, has an important role in the treatment of selected skull base tumors.

Because stereotactic radiation treatment of vestibular schwannomas is still evolving, results are not easily comparable on a study-to-study basis, nor are they easily grouped to add power to institutional reporting by meta-analysis. Dosing parameters have changed over time and differ among patients, among doctors, and among institutions within studies.[9-11] This variability in retrospective studies is problematic, making optimal dosing parameters difficult to discern. Dose planning is enhanced with improved imaging shot selection, and blocking strategies that safeguard neural structures. Automation in delivery systems and better understanding of the biologic effect of radiation also should result in improved outcomes.[10,11]

Because the goal of stereotactic irradiation differs from that of microsurgery and with observation, outcomes are difficult to compare. In most cases, microsurgery results in complete tumor removal. Imaging assessment gives an immediate quantifiable result. Imaging assessment of stereotactic radiation outcomes is subject to the inherent variability of the tumor response to treatment, the quality and resolution of the imaging, the examiner's judgment, the accuracy of post-imaging software, and interobserver comparison of imaging at different time points. The definition of success is not standardized at present but appears to be moving toward a crterion of progression-free survival. Since the objective of stereotactic radiation is tumor control rather than eradication of disease, criteria for success should be objectively compared to the natural progression of these slow-growing benign tumors.

After irradiation, tumors show signs of treatment effect by loss of central enhancement within the first 6 to 12 months.[12,13] Approximately one fourth (23%) will show *expansion*, or transient tumor swelling (on average 2 to 4 mm but as much as 10 mm) generally 6 to 24 months after treatment, but swelling can be seen up to 5 years after treatment. This temporary expansion may take 6 months to 5 years to resolve.[2] Fifty percent of these tumors will undergo a loss of central contrast enhancement that may correlate histopathologically with tumor necrosis.[14] Eventually, residual tumors show return of enhancement and possibly further shrinkage. Few show peritumoral edema. More recent studies recognize these signs of radiation effect, and continued observation often validates eventual stability or regression.[2] This understanding alone has prevented surgery for what was thought to be tumor progression in earlier studies and is manifested in improved control rates in newer data. Tumors that were excised, possibly for mistaken post-irradiation progression, have shown histopathologic evidence of radiation-induced vascular changes, including intimal thickening, perivascular inflammation, and focal hemorrhage.[14] Profuse interstitial fibrin deposits also were seen. Schwannomas surgically removed after stereotactic radiation failure also have shown typical and viable schwannoma cells with increased vascularity, as well as other foci showing delayed radiation changes such as nucleolar and cytoplasmic enlargement, proliferation of endothelial cells, and necrosis.[15-17]

In 2006, Weil and colleagues published a thorough review of the English language literature regarding single-fraction stereotactic radiation.[10] Similarly, Backous and Pham and Likhterov and associates reviewed the current literature and summarized the stereotactic irradiation data, including outcomes of fractionated stereotactic radiation protocols, through 2005.[2,3] Tables 179-2 and 179-3 present outcomes data from these reviews, along with those from the most recent studies on stereotactic irradiation.[10,12,14,15,18-39] Studies with fewer than 15 patients or less than 12 months of follow-up were excluded.

Tumor Control

Current data show that after irradiation, 1% to 2% of vestibular schwannomas resolve completely; however, tumor control is achieved in 74% to 100% over varied durations of follow-up. The definition of tumor control has not been consistent. Control in some series is considered no radiographic enlargement over some set parameter (e.g., 2 mm in tumor diameter or 10% change in tumor volume). Failure in others is considered progression requiring microsurgical resection. Some centers do not consider repeat stereotactic irradiation or neurosurgical relief of radiation-induced or tumor-related hydrocephalus by ventriculoperitoneal shunting to represent treatment failure, whereas other centers do. Outcomes in patients in earlier series may have been counted as failures before recognition of the phenomenon of transient tumor expansion, thereby falsely lowering control rates in those studies. A more recent trend in reporting tumor control is to provide actuarial data. Few studies have data to report beyond a median follow-up period of 48 months. To make up for this shortcoming, probable data are generated from the few leading patients in each study to provide Kaplan-Meier survival curves with confidence intervals predicting progression-free statistics. Considering the foregoing caveats, for the studies reviewed, the weighted summary of the 5-year-progression-free tumor control was 95% for single-dose stereotactic irradiation and 94% for fractionated regimens.

Hearing Outcomes

Hearing outcomes have steadily improved since the early 1980s as a result of decreasing marginal doses, improved conformality and shielding of important structures, or better patient selection, or a combination of these factors. Dose tolerances of the cochlea, cochlear nerve, and cochlear nucleus are still under investigation.[2,22,33] In a prospective follow-up study of 34 patients, Thomas and colleagues found the cochlear dose to be the only variable that was statistically predictive of hearing preservation.[33] These investigators showed that if the percentage volume of the cochlea exposed to 90% of the total treatment dose was less than 73.3%, the median hearing loss was 10 dB, compared with 25 dB for the cochleas exposed more than 73.3%. Paek and coworkers found that treatment doses to the cochlear nucleus below 10 Gy were the only statistically significant prognostic indicator for hearing preservation in their study of primary gamma knife therapy in a select group of 25 patients with pretreatment Gardner-Robertson hearing of grade I or II.[22] Chopra and colleagues have shown that hearing outcomes improve when the marginal dose to the tumor is reduced to 13 Gy or less. Increased age, tumor swelling, radiation exposure to greater lengths of the cochlear nerve, and increased dose to the cochlear nucleus also have been associated with poorer hearing outcomes.[40] Massager and colleagues analyzed the radiation doses delivered to the cochlea during gamma knife stereotactic irradiation and concluded that the cochlea received significantly higher radiation doses in patients with worsening of hearing after treatment. The cochlear dose was significantly associated with the intracanalicular dose of radiation delivered.[41,42]

Table 179-4

Gardner-Robertson Scale*

Hearing Grade		Pure Tone Average (dB)	Speech Discrimination (%)
Grade I	(good to excellent)	0-30	70-100
Grade II	(serviceable)	31-50	50-71
Grade III	(nonserviceable)	51-90	5-49
Grade IV	(poor)	91-max	1-4

*If pure tone average and speech do not correlate, the lower grade is assigned.

Hearing status and hearing outcomes are not universally evaluated and have not been examined in a standardized fashion if included, causing difficulty in comparing data.[10,31] Because fewer patients have serviceable hearing than the already low number of patients in some series, the power of reporting hearing outcomes in these studies is compromised. The timing of audiometric follow-up testing is not always clear and does not necessarily match the duration of tumor control surveillance. Few studies offer serial data on the hearing data they collect. Thomas and colleagues reported the only prospective series of outcomes encountered.[33] Not all studies rely on objective audiometric data for reporting, and some include the use of telephone or survey information with the hearing outcomes. When audiometric data are used, the definition of serviceable hearing has varied, using either hearing levels or speech discrimination, or a combination. The Gardner-Robertson classification of hearing is most commonly used today as a scale to gauge useful hearing (Table 179-4). Class I or II hearing, or speech reception thresholds better than 50 dB and speech discrimination better than 50%, is considered to be serviceable hearing for a majority of studies (see Table 179-4). That being said, preservation of any sound perception is important and useful for lip reading and voice modulation when the contralateral hearing is compromised, as in cases of neurofibromatosis type 2 (NF2).

After stereotactic irradiation, hearing loss becomes evident over the ensuing 6 to 24 months. Hearing levels decline by 15 to 20 dB on average after treatment. Hearing continues to decline with the duration of follow-up.[2,20] A profile of progressive loss is similar to that in natural history trends derived from tumor observation data but presumably is related to radiation effect. Tumor size may impede attempts at hearing preservation. Prasad and associates showed that useful hearing was retained in 75% of patients with tumors smaller than 1 cm^3, whereas 57% of those with tumors larger than 1 cm^3 demonstrated a hearing level of Gardner-Robertson class I or II.[43]

Hempel and coworkers documented an average drop of 18 dB with treatment.[20] These workers reported standardized follow-up data for 123 patients for a mean of 8.2 years after stereotactic gamma knife irradiation of median 1.6-cm^3 vestibular schwannomas treated with a mean marginal dose of 13 Gy. Pre- and post-treatment audiometric data were available for analysis in 63 patients. Post-treatment audiograms were obtained 1 to 24 months after treatment; in 46 of the patients (73%), audiometry was not performed until more than 5 months after treatment. Hearing declined an average of 18 dB, moving the group from a 42% pretreatment slight to moderate hearing difficulty level, on average, to 60% post-treatment moderate to high-grade hearing loss. No audiometric hearing loss occurred in 17 of 63 patients (29%), and subjectively, 53 patients (47.3%) reported that their hearing had not changed with treatment.

Thomas and colleagues, using fractionated stereotactic irradiation, conducted a prospective follow-up study in a select group of 34 patients with small tumors and good hearing and reported standardized hearing results at a median of 36.5 months.[33] Patients received doses of 50 Gy in 25 fractions to the 90% isodose line, treating median tumor volumes of 1.06 cm^3. As assessed using the Gardner-Robertson grading scale (see Table 179-4), 28 patients had grade I hearing levels before treatment, 5 had grade II hearing, and 1 had grade III hearing but was included in this select group because he felt subjectively that his hearing was serviceable. Speech reception thresholds were 20 dB on average before treatment and 40 dB after. Twenty patients (59%) retained serviceable hearing and 12 (35%) retained their pre–irradiation course Gardner-Robertson grade. Actuarial hearing preservation rates at 2, 3, and 5 years were 63%, 63%, and 56%, respectively.

Overall, reported hearing preservation rates range from 33% to 100% with gamma knife irradiation, from 47% to 96% with LINAC-based irradiation, and from 46% to 100% with fractionated protocols. The weighted average of pooled gamma knife data for more than 100 patients over more than 36 months showed a hearing preservation rate of 68%. No studies with single-dose LINAC-based protocols with more than 100 patients reported hearing outcomes; however, fractionated protocols showed a weighted hearing preservation rate of 69%.

Facial Nerve Outcomes

Stereotactic irradiation continues to offer excellent results in regard to function of the facial nerve. Improved outcomes were achieved by reducing the marginal tumor dose to less than 16 Gy, which decreased the rate of facial neuropathies to 15%. At 13 Gy or less, persistently improved facial nerve outcomes are achieved. Today, facial nerve injury is rare and usually transient. Improved outcomes are further enhanced by better conformality of treatment planning and limiting the irradiation field to the minimum length of nerve necessary for adequate tumor treatment. Tumor volume is debatable as a predictive factor for cranial neuropathy.[31,44] Reported rates of facial nerve injury in the low-dose era of treatment (12 to 14 Gy) range from 0% to 10.3% after gamma knife irradiation with up to 5.2% permanent injury, 0% to 11.8% with up to 8% permanent with LINAC-based radiotherapy, and 0% to 6% with up to 6% permanent for fractionated protocols. Facial synkinesis and spasm are sometimes discussed separately; according to the available evidence, they occur at similar rates.

Trigeminal Nerve Outcomes

Trigeminal nerve toxicity is seen in a low number of patients treated by stereotactic irradiation. Reported symptoms range in severity from trigeminal neuralgia to mild hypesthesia. The incidence ranges from 0% to 16% after gamma knife irradiation but more consistently falls between 2% and 5%. Single-dose LINAC protocols produce injury in 0.7% to 18% but more commonly in 7.5% to 10.8%. Fractionated protocols show trigeminal nerve injury in up to 14%, and routinely in up to 5% (see Tables 179-1 to 179-3).

Neurofibromatosis 2–Related Vestibular Schwannoma

In patients with the burden of multiple intracranial and spinal tumors, an effective method of treatment less invasive than surgical removal would be of great value. Concern arises, however, over irradiating benign tumors in young patients who have an inherited predisposition to tumor formation from loss of the NF2 tumor suppressor gene. In a retrospective study by Vachhani and Friedmann[45] of stereotactic radiation treatment of 14 NF2-related schwannomas, with a mean follow-up period of 38 months, no growth was noted in the radiation-treated tumors in 92% at 2 years and in 92% at 5 years. In the untreated tumors, 78% showed no growth at 2 years and 21% at 5 years.[45] Mathieu and colleagues reported the University of Pittsburgh experience, which included stereotactic radiation treatment of 74 schwannomas in 62 patients with NF2. These workers found tumor volume to be a significant predictor of local control. Actuarial control rates were 85%, 81%, and 81% at 5, 10, and 15 years, respectively. The actuarial serviceable hearing preservation rate for the 35% of patients presenting with serviceable hearing was 73% at 1 year, 59% at 2 years, and 48% at 5 years after gamma knife radiation treatment.[18]

Cystic Schwannomas

Debate is ongoing regarding the effectiveness of stereotactic radiation control of cystic vestibular schwannoma. Pendl and colleagues initially advised caution in recommending stereotactic irradiation to patients with cystic vestibular schwannoma.[46] These recommendations were based on a series of treatment failures that manifested as progressive neurologic symptoms after treatment with a mean dose of 13.8 Gy to the tumor margins. Surgical intervention was required in five of the six patients. Shirato and colleagues also claim that patients with cystic vestibular schwannomas are at significant risk for experiencing subacute expansion of the cyst after fractionated-dose stereotactic irradiation and reported that 45% showed growth in the 3-year actuarial follow-up period.[47]

In an effort to characterize the phenomenon of tumor expansion, Hasegawa and colleagues reported that of 254 vestibular schwannomas treated with high-dose irradiation between 1991 and 1998, 42 tumors (17%) continued to grow.[12] Of the 42 expanding tumors, 14 were characterized by central necrosis, 16 were solid tumors, and 12 demonstrated cystic formation or expansion. Of the 14 patients whose tumors demonstrated central necrosis, 3 required further salvage treatment. Of the 16 patients with solid tumors, 7 required additional treatment (including treatment for the malignant transformation of one tumor). All of the 12 patients in whom cysts developed or expanded eventually required craniotomy. The investigators concluded that patients shown to have cyst enlargement with neurologic deterioration after irradiation or those with new cyst formation will require surgery.

Delsanti and Régis showed only a 6.4% treatment failure rate for stereotactic irradiation of these tumors.[48] It is possible that these discrepancies are due to the low proportions of vestibular schwannoma that are cystic, or to the selection bias inherent in retrospective analysis. It is likely that truly cystic vestibular schwannomas do not respond as well as solid vestibular schwannoma to treatment by stereotactic irradiation. Further prospective studies of this variety of vestibular schwannoma are necessary before firm recommendations can be made.

Hydrocephalus

Hydrocephalus occurs in a low percentage of patients after stereotactic irradiation. Theoretically, this problem could be due to post-irradiation tumor or tissue swelling, or to new cyst formation with consequent obstructive hydrocephalus, radiation-induced fibrosis, or hemorrhage resulting in cerebrospinal fluid malabsorption and communicating hydrocephalus. Treatment by ventriculoperitoneal shunting resolves this problem in most situations, but salvage microsurgery for failed tumor control or to remove new cyst formation sometimes is necessary. Hydrocephalus occurs in 0.8% to 8% of cases with gamma knife treatment, 0% to 7.5% of LINAC single-dose protocols, and 0% to 12% of fractionated protocols, although more commonly 0% to 4%. See Tables 179-1 to 179-3.

Treatment of Stereotactic Radiation Failures

Fortunately, in most patients treated by stereotactic irradiation for vestibular schwannoma, tumor control is achieved, and follow-up with careful observation constitutes adequate management. Surveillance protocols vary, but follow-up imaging should be carried out indefinitely, or until longer-term follow-up studies in adequate numbers of patients treated at current dosing levels show this to be unnecessary. Stereotactic irradiation failure is defined as progression of tumor volume or diameter beyond the expected post-treatment expansion, progressive neurologic symptoms from active growth, or threatened brainstem compression. Although most failures manifest within 3 years of treatment, reports of failures beyond 5 years also are seen.[11,32,35,42]

Tumor volume has been shown to be a predictor of treatment failure. Hasegawa and colleagues showed actuarial 10-year progression-free control rates of 57% for tumors larger than 15 cm^3 and 95% for those smaller than 15 cm^3.[11] These workers also reported two occurrences of failures more than 5 years after stereotactic irradiation. One case involved new cyst formation, presumably secondary to intratumoral hemorrhage at 69 months, and the other involved malignant transformation of a vestibular schwannoma at 51 months. Chan and colleagues saw a similar statistical difference in progression-free survival. The 5-year actuarial rates of freedom from any neurosurgical intervention was 97% for patients with tumor volume less than 8 cm^3 and 47% for patients with tumor volume of at least 8 cm^3.[31]

The outcomes with microsurgical treatment of radiosurgical failures are unclear. Friedman and associates compared data for resection of 38 tumors after radiosurgical failure with those for resection of 38 matched primary tumors.[15] The mean follow-up period was 3.3 years. These workers noted moderate to severe adherence to the facial nerve in 89% of radiation failures, compared with 63% of primary resections. House-Brackmann grade I or II facial nerve outcomes were obtained in 37% of irradiated cases, compared with 70% of primary treatment cases. Limb and colleagues found similar difficulty for resection of radiosurgical failures compared with matched controls.[49] They also described increased operative time and uncertainty about the completeness of tumor removal. Shuto and colleagues reported data for 12 patients operated on after failed stereotactic irradiation.[50] Four also had had a previous microsurgical dissection. These investigators described difficult identification and dissection of the facial nerve and resorted to subtotal resections in order to preserve its integrity. They also found difficulty dissecting the tumor from the brainstem owing to adhesions. Hearing was sacrificed in all cases. Bleeding was scant, possibly as a result of the irradiation. Shuto's group recommend subtotal excision in revision cases and showed that growth of the residual tumor was rare.

The ultimate failure of stereotactic irradiation would be the transformation of a benign process into a malignant disease. The risk at present appears to be on the order of 0.01% to 0.3% for non–NF2-associated vestibular schwannomas.[35,51] Malignant change of a schwannoma has been reported up to 18 years after radiation treatment. Such extensive follow-up has been achieved in only a few patients.[30,52] Malignant transformation usually is a fatal event and may take more than 30 years to develop, as indicated by data on the treatment of other benign disease processes and from occupational exposure to radiation sources. The peak occurrence takes place approximately 15 years after low-dose radiation exposure, but the relative risk remains elevated well past 40 years.

The current literature does not have adequate numbers of procedures to be predictive of long-term risk. Actuarial data, although often quoted, are of no value in predicting malignant changes. Evans and colleagues as well as Ron and colleagues note an 18.8-fold increased relative risk of schwannoma induction and a 9.5-fold increased relative rate of meningioma induction after radiation doses of 2.5 Gy for the treatment of tinea capitis, adenotonsillar disease, and capillary hemangiomas.[53,54] The radiobiologic effect was dose-dependent, similar to the tissue effect and tumor growth response observed in post–World War II Japan.[55] Preston and colleagues showed that vestibular schwannomas were the most abundant intracranial tumors encountered, with a high propensity for Schwann cell mutation in response to radiation damage.[55] Overall, the risk of radiation-induced tumors appears to be approximately 0.1% to 3% after 30 years.[51,53] In light of the 33% to 40% lifetime risk of malignancy in the general population, Evans and colleagues feel that the benefits of single-dose radiation treatment for vestibular schwannoma is justified for patients with documented tumor growth who refuse surgery, or for the elderly or infirm. However, patients with NF2 in particular are the disproportionate recipients of radiation-induced malignant tumors. In a series of 829 subjects with vestibular schwannomas, 62 (7%) had NF2; yet in a review of the documented cases of malignant changes induced by stereotactic irradiation of vestibular schwannomas, 50% occurred in NF2 patients. Evans and colleagues strongly caution against the use of radiation treatment for benign tumors in childhood and in tumor-prone conditions such as neurofibromatosis.[53] We concur.

Quality of Life

In treatment of a benign disease with a natural history of general slow progression, the patient's satisfaction with the treatment outcomes is highly relevant. Quality of life measurements are useful tools for obtaining such information. Pollock and colleagues have reported the only prospective quality of life assessment to date.[56] They matched 36 microsurgical (suboccipital 69%, middle cranial fossa 6%, or translabyrinthine 25%) patients with 46 patients that underwent stereotactic irradiation. The surgical therapy group was composed of statistically older patients and showed a trend to larger tumor size when compared with the radiation therapy group. Outcomes were measured by a health status questionnaire, dizziness handicap inventory (DHI), and a tinnitus and headache survey. The questionnaires were evaluated at 3 months, 1 year, and the last follow-up. The mean follow-up period was 48 months. Responses showed statistically significant decline in the health status questionnaire parameters for the microsurgical group that resolved with follow-up. The parameters of bodily pain and mental health remained significantly different from the stereotactic irradiation group, although scores for both groups were elevated from baseline. The stereotactic irradiation group had lower DHI scores than those for the microsurgery group at last follow-up evaluation.

Myrseth and coworkers retrospectively looked at 168 patients, using the SF-36 questionnaire and the Glascow Benefit Inventory (GBI) as a measure of subjective quality of life.[57] Patients in the microsurgical therapy group (retrosigmoid 38%, translabyrinthine 62%) were significantly younger (mean age of 48.2 years, vs. 53.9 years). A larger group was lost to follow-up because of death in the stereotactic therapy group (16 vs. 8). Data were obtained by subject response for 83.3% of the patients over a 1-year follow-up period. The investigators concluded that the SF-36 did not bring out the differences between the two cohorts as well as the GBI, which showed that at 1 year, the score for the "general" category was significantly lower in the microsurgery group, although the two cohorts did not differ significantly on the "physical" and "social" scales.

Sandooram and associates also used the GBI as a quality of life measure.[58] This retrospective study, based on an 80% response from 165 subjects, included 102 patients managed with microsurgery and 10 with stereotactic irradiation. No significant age or tumor size difference was found between patients choosing microsurgery (49% retrosigmoid, 51% translabyrinthine) or stereotactic irradiation. The patients in the microsurgery group were followed for a median period of 4.8 years, whereas those in the stereotactic irradiation group were followed for a median 1.8 years. Patients in both groups showed decline in their GBI scores, although the decrease in the stereotactic irradiation group did not reach significance. A minimum follow-up period of 3 years should be sought for quality of life studies.[9] Longer follow-up is recommended for the following clinical reasons: (1) the natural progression of vestibular schwannoma shows nonlinear growth; (2) the progression of vestibular schwannoma growth in observed patients in our series was 66% at 3.8 years; and (3) the long-term failure rate for stereotactic radiation therapy is yet unknown. These considerations reinforce the need to standardize surveillance protocols and reporting definitions and measures so that future recommendations can be based on actual evidence.

No truly prospective randomized study with sufficient power or duration of follow-up that would give sufficient power has been conducted to compare the results of stereotactic irradiation. Meta-analysis

Table 179-5

Stereotactic Irradiation Protocols and Outcomes for Treatment of Glomus Jugulare Tumors

Study with Radiation Source	No. of Tumors	Local Control Rate	Hearing Preservation	Cranial Neuropathy: Facial Nerve	Cranial Neuropathy: Cranial Nerves IX, X, XI	Dose*
Sharma et al, 2008[61] Gamma knife	15 primary, 9 secondary; 10 patients with follow-up	100% at 24 mo in 10 patients	NR	NR	15/24 (62%)	16.4 Gy
Lim et al, 2004[62] Cyberknife plus LINAC	16	100% at 41 mo	1 transient loss	NR	1/16 (6%)	14-27 Gy
Eustacchio et al, 1999[63] Gamma knife	10 primary, 9 recurrent	95% at 46 mo	NA	NA	NA	13.5 Gy in a 91-year-old patient who died 9 months later
Liscak et al, 1999[64] Gamma knife	30 primary, 24 recurrent	100% at 24 mo	11/14	NA	5%	16.5 Gy
Pollock, 2004[60] Gamma knife	19 primary, 23 recurrent	98% at 44 mo	81% at 4 yr	11% 43%	3%	14.9 Gy

*Mean marginal dose of 16.4 Gy.
LINAC, linear accelerator (stereotactic irradiation); NR, not reported; NA, not available.

of retrospective data can be helpful, but a meta-analysis by Weil and colleagues in 2006 concluded that current studies are subject to a number of confounding factors, are not sufficiently statistically powered, and present limited long-term actuarial outcome data.[10] These investigators did not provide sufficient confidence to support the claim that low-dose stereotactic radiation is as effective as higher doses. Hearing results also are shown to decline over time. This also is true in patients with untreated tumors under observation. Weil's group noted that the small size of patient cohorts and the small proportion of patients at 5 years provide for large confidence intervals with considerable uncertainty. Furthermore, a recent study with longer follow-up suggests worse actuarial tumor control in patients treated with a marginal dose less than 12 Gy, compared with doses of 12 Gy or higher.[14]

Despite these difficulties in comparing reports, the short-term efficacy of stereotactic irradiation for treatment of vestibular schwannoma is impressive. Stereotactic irradiation is a valuable option for treatment of sporadic vestibular schwannomas in elderly patients. It may be useful in limiting the morbidity of microsurgery or stereotactic irradiation alone when used as an adjunct to subtotal resection of tumors with large volumes. Caution is still warranted in considering its application for tumors with undocumented growth, or in younger or tumor-prone patients.

Jugular Foramen Schwannomas

Martin and associates reported results of stereotactic irradiation in 34 patients with 35 jugular foramen schwannomas treated with gamma knife protocols between 1990 and 2005.[59] Twenty-two patients had undergone previous surgical resection, and 13 patients, in whom the diagnosis was based on imaging studies, underwent primary stereotactic irradiation. One or more cranial nerve deficits were present before stereotactic irradiation in all 34 patients. The marginal dose ranged from 12 to 18 Gy, and the dose to the maximum range was 21 to 36 Gy. Follow-up periods ranged from 1.5 to 14 years, with a mean or median of 7 years. These workers reported that 33 of 35 lesions decreased in volume or were stable at 5 years. When the lower motor cranial nerves (glossopharyngeal, vagus, spinal accessory, and hypoglossal) were considered as a group, a total of 105 ipsilateral nerves were affected at the time of stereotactic irradiation; 35 were intact, with no associated symptoms. Improvement of the affected cranial nerves was noted in 22 (20%), whereas 81 (77%) remained stable and only 2 were worse. All 35 unaffected cranial nerves remained unaffected.

Paraganglioma

Paraganglioma treatment reports in the literature have fewer numbers and shorter follow-up than those for vestibular schwannomas, but reported control rates are similarly encouraging (see Table 179-5).[60-64] A summary of five representative studies in the recent literature follows. In a report by Pollock, 42 patients underwent gamma knife surgery as the primary management (19 patients) or for recurrent glomus jugulare tumors (23 patients).[60] Facial weakness and deafness were more common in patients with recurrent tumors than in those in whom primary gamma knife stereotactic irradiation was performed (48% compared with 11%). The mean tumor volume was 13.2 cm^3; the mean tumor margin dose was 14.9 Gy. The mean follow-up period for the 39 patients in whom evaluation was possible was 44 months (range, 6 to 149 months). After gamma knife surgery, 12 tumors (31%) decreased in size, 26 (67%) were unchanged, and one (2%) grew. The patient whose tumor grew underwent another course of stereotactic irradiation. Progression-free survival after gamma knife surgery was 100% at 3 and 7 years and 75% at 10 years. Six patients (15%) experienced new deficits (hearing loss alone in three, facial numbness and hearing loss in one, vocal cord paralysis and hearing loss in one, and temporary imbalance or vertigo in one). In 26 patients in whom hearing could be tested before stereotactic radiation therapy, hearing preservation was achieved in 86% and 81% at 1 and 4 years after treatment, respectively. No patient suffered a new lower cranial nerve deficit after one stereotactic radiotherapy session.

Other studies evaluating stereotactic irradiation for paragangliomas similar to Pollock's are summarized in Table 179-5. The difficulty in preserving the lower cranial nerves with the excision of glomus jugulare tumors makes stereotactic irradiation an attractive alternative if the long-term results are as good as the reported short-term results, and if the cranial nerve preservation rates with these irradiation protocols are better than the surgical salvage rates.

Conclusions

Stereotactic radiation therapy is a useful addition to the armamentarium for the treatment of benign cranial base tumors. Good short-term and mid-term outcomes with quick recovery times have been shown in largely retrospective studies. The literature to date, on both the surgical and radiation treatments for these lesions, is marked by the biases inherent in the retrospective study design, and the evidence presented is at best level 4—not strong enough on which to base dogmatic opinions regarding critical clinical decisions. Therefore, the patient's personal preference often is the deciding factor, after a thorough discussion of the advantages and disadvantages of all the possible treatment options. Long-term prospective outcome studies with blinded independent observations are necessary to obtain high-quality of data to advance clinical care in this area.

SUGGESTED READINGS

Backous DD, Pham HT. Guiding patients through the choices for treating vestibular schwannomas: balancing options and ensuring informed consent. *Otolaryngol Clin North Am.* 2007;40:521-540.

Chen DA. Acoustic neuroma in a private neurotology practice: trends in demographics and practice patterns. *Laryngoscope.* 2007;117:2003-2012.

Chopra R, Kondziolka D, Niranjan A, et al. Long-term follow-up of acoustic schwannoma radiosurgery with marginal tumor doses of 12 to 13 Gy. *Int J Radiat Oncol Biol Phys.* 2007;68:845-851.

Evans DG, Birch JM, Ramsden RT, et al. Malignant transformation and new primary tumours after therapeutic radiation for benign disease: substantial risks in certain tumour prone syndromes. *J Med Genet.* 2006;43:289-294.

For complete list of references log onto www.expertconsult.com.

Friedman RA, Brackmann DE, Hitselberger WE, et al. Surgical salvage after failed irradiation for vestibular schwannoma. *Laryngoscope.* 2005;115:1827-1832.

Hasegawa T, Kida Y, Yoshimoto M, et al. Evaluation of tumor expansion after stereotactic radiosurgery in patients harboring vestibular schwannomas. *Neurosurgery.* 2006;58:1119-1128.

Lunsford LD, Niranjan A, Flickinger JC, et al. Radiosurgery of vestibular schwannomas: summary of experience in 829 cases. *J Neurosurg.* 2005;102(Suppl):195-199.

Massager N, Nissim O, Delbrouck C, et al. Irradiation of cochlear structures during vestibular schwannoma radiosurgery and associated hearing outcome. *J Neurosurg.* 2007;107:733-739.

Mathieu D, Kondziolka D, Flickinger JC, et al. Stereotactic radiosurgery for vestibular schwannomas in patients with neurofibromatosis type 2: an analysis of tumor control, complications, and hearing preservation rates. *Neurosurgery.* 2007;60:460-468.

Pollock BE, Driscoll CL, Foote RL, et al. Patient outcomes after vestibular schwannoma management: a prospective comparison of microsurgical resection and stereotactic radiosurgery. *Neurosurgery.* 2006;59:77-85.

Smouha EE, Yoo M, Mohr K, et al. Conservative management of acoustic neuroma: a meta-analysis and proposed treatment algorithm. *Laryngoscope.* 2005;115:450-454.

Thomas C, Di Maio S, Ma R, et al. Hearing preservation following fractionated stereotactic radiotherapy for vestibular schwannomas: prognostic implications of cochlear dose. *J Neurosurg.* 2007;107:917-926.

Weil RS, Cohen JM, Portarena I, et al. Optimal dose of stereotactic radiosurgery for acoustic neuromas: a systematic review. *Br J Neurosurg.* 2006;20:195-202.

PART EIGHT

Pediatric Otolaryngology

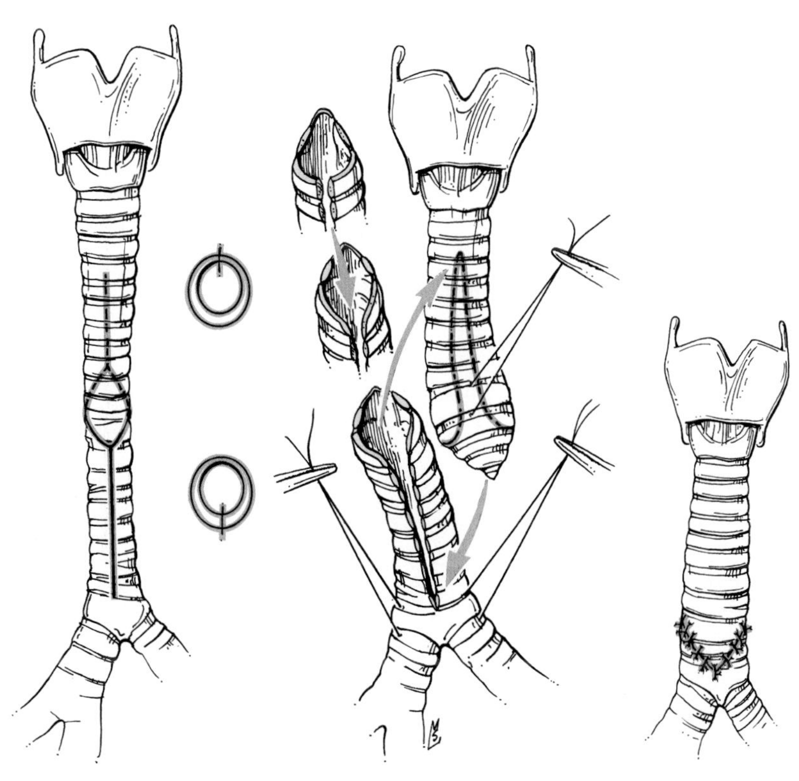

CHAPTER ONE HUNDRED AND EIGHTY

General Considerations in Pediatric Otolaryngology

J. Scott McMurray

Key Points

- Children are physiologically different from adults. Familiarity with these differences is required for safe management of their medical and surgical problems.
- Providing optimal pediatric care requires attention to the child as patient and the adult guardians.
- Involving the child in play may alleviate anxiety regarding procedures in the physical examination.
- With practice, physical examination can be conducted in expedient fashion and will be relatively painless for the child, yet complete for the surgeon.
- Management of the pediatric otolaryngology patient often requires a multidisciplinary team approach.

For many practitioners, there is no greater reward than helping children afflicted with illness. Pediatric otolaryngology has developed as a subspecialty within otolaryngology as a bridge between the surgical discipline and pediatric medicine. Nearly every otolaryngologist will treat children during his or her professional career. An estimated 25% to 50% of a general otolaryngologist's practice may be related to pediatric problems. Pediatric otolaryngology has therefore become an important part of all training programs in this field.

As the saying goes, children are not simply little adults. Often unique approaches are required for their evaluation, diagnosis, and management. Although the child is of prime concern, the parents—as the child's guardians, who must make decisions regarding the ultimate treatment options—also must be kept informed and must be approached with compassion. This is obvious to nearly all persons who have had to make medical decisions for a loved one but may not be as obvious to those who have not. The love for and emotional bond with a child may make even the most calm and rational person unable to comprehend events and medical explanations. It is up to the surgeon to monitor and modify his or her approach and explanations to both the child and the parent. This is not always an easy task but one that is highly rewarding.

Smaller and more premature neonates are surviving and sicker children are recovering from significant illnesses as neonatal and pediatric intensive care units, as well as the skills of the physicians who care for them, continue to advance. This development has led to a demand for practitioners well versed in the management of disorders encountered in this population—namely, intubation trauma, bronchoesophageal processes, infectious disease, tumors, and congenital malformations. A multidisciplinary approach often is required. Agreement among the pediatric specialists and with the general pediatrician is important, raising a third layer of communication that is required for successful treatment of the child and family.

Physiologic differences among infants, children, and adults have occupied major research efforts and constitute the subject of complete textbooks. This chapter outlines basic differences relevant to the practice of otolaryngology, along with some related considerations. In the following discussion, the material presented for each of the major body systems is intended as a general introduction, to be used as a starting point for further investigation.

Respiratory System

Control of Ventilation

Emergence from an underwater world, in which the child relied on placental exchange of gases and nutrition, induces tremendous changes in the neonate's physiology and anatomy. Some of these changes occur rapidly at birth; others proceed more slowly. These significant changes can complicate interpretation of the neonate's problems. In particular, the assessment of the control of ventilation in the neonate may be difficult. Interventions used to obtain measurements, such as placement of a facemask or insertion of a laryngotracheal tube, may induce significant changes in ventilation. Measurements of ventilation to assess respiratory drive also depend on the assumption that the respiratory muscles are capable of converting this drive into work—which is not always the case in infants and neonates.

Muscle fibers have been found to fall into two categories. *Type I* fibers are slow twitch, highly oxidative, and fatigue resistant. *Type II* fibers are fast twitch and are easily fatigable. Newborns have a paucity of type I muscle fibers but develop them shortly after birth. The muscle fibers in the diaphragm of a preterm infant are composed of less than 10% of type I fibers. The muscle fibers of a full-term infant may be 30% type I fibers. The percentage of type I fibers increases to 55%, the expected adult level, during the first year of life. Preterm infants are more prone to respiratory fatigue; this predilection disappears as they reach maturity.

Other subtle differences in sleep patterns also affect control of ventilation. Preterm infants spend as much as 50% to 60% of their sleep state in the rapid eye movement (REM) state. During REM sleep, the intercostal muscles are inhibited, as are most of the other skeletal muscles. This places a greater burden on the diaphragmatic activity. Much of this activity may be wasted, because the chest wall can move paradoxically in the very young. This purposeless movement readily leads to hypoventilation, increased respiratory drive, and diaphragmatic fatigue.

Biochemical and reflex controls of ventilation are similar but incompletely developed in full-term neonates when compared with adults. Neonates have a higher basal metabolic rate than that in adults. This is reflected in higher ventilatory rates relative to body mass at any given partial pressure of carbon dioxide. Increases in ventilation are proportionately similar, however, in infants and adults with an increased partial pressure of carbon dioxide. This concordance in response is not seen in preterm infants. Their response to increases in partial pressure of carbon dioxide is blunted when compared with that in full-term infants and adults. Differences also are seen in the response to partial pressure of oxygen between premature infants and full-term infants and adults. The administration of 100% oxygen decreases ventilation in the very young, suggesting the existence of chemoreceptor activity not generally seen in adults.

Gestational age, postnatal age, body temperature, and sleep state modify the ventilatory response of newborns to hypoxia. Preterm and full-term infants less than a week old who are awake and euthermic usually demonstrate biphasic breathing patterns. They often experience tachypnea followed by hypoventilation. Hypothermic infants demonstrate a blunted response to hypoxia with respiratory depression, but they do not have the initial hyperpnea. The central effects of hypoxia on the respiratory center may cause depression of ventilation. Active peripheral chemoreceptors are unable to maintain a significant influence over this response. REM sleep also may decrease the response to hypoxia in these infants. Sleep states other than REM are associated with an increase in the ventilatory response to hypoxia. Arousal from sleep during hypoxia is not seen in newborns but develops during the first few weeks of life. In these slightly older infants, further maturation of the chemoreceptors increases their ventilatory drive to hypoxia. Of interest, a decreased response to hypercarbia associated with hypoxia also occurs in newborns but not in older infants and adults.

Reflexes arising from the lung and chest wall probably are more important in maintaining ventilation in newborns and in determining the respiratory tidal volume. Periodic breathing is common in preterm and full-term infants. These periods of alternating rapid ventilation followed by apnea may be common and can be considered normal. Periodic breathing is thought to result from dyscoordination of the feedback loops controlling ventilation. During the apneic part of periodic breathing, partial pressure of carbon dioxide may increase, but changes in heart rate do not. Generally, no serious physiologic consequences are seen. This response often ceases by the age of 6 years. Some preterm infants, however, may demonstrate serious and potentially life-threatening episodes of apnea. These episodes may last longer than 20 seconds and are accompanied by bradycardia. Apneic episodes may represent a failed response to hypoxia. Because these episodes are more commonly seen during REM sleep, ventilatory fatigue, as well as impaired chemoreceptor response to hypoxia, may be the cause. Usually, stimulation is all that is required to terminate the apneic event. Aminophylline treatment generally decreases the apneic episodes through central stimulation. Continuous positive airway pressure (CPAP) also may be helpful to decrease apneic episodes by modifying the lung and chest wall reflexes.

Laryngospasm

The primary function of the larynx is to protect the lungs from aspiration. Hence, the laryngeal adductor response is a very strong reflex. The robustness of the reflex has been shown to change with age and maturity in animal models. It is strong enough to be lethal in some instances. When laryngeal adduction is coupled with tachycardia, hypertension, and apnea, it is termed the *laryngeal chemoreflex* (LCR). The LCR can be induced by laryngeal exposure to acid, base, and pressure, but it is most sensitive to water and is ablated by saline. This may have implications for sudden infant death syndrome (SIDS). Evolving responses with age to hypoxia, hypercarbia, and the laryngeal stimulation that causes the LCR may explain the age pattern seen with SIDS. Deaths attributed to SIDS have dramatically decreased as a result of a change in the recommended sleep position of children—from prone to supine. Elimination of hypercarbia from rebreathing may be the mechanism behind the decrease in SIDS deaths. Hypercarbia is a known potentiator of the LCR. An increased awareness of and more aggressive stance toward the treatment of infant reflux also may have decreased a potential stimulus for the LCR. Decreased bolus size, increased feeding frequency, frequent burping, and positioning to discourage regurgitation have been helpful to decrease the incidence of reflux in infants and perhaps the incidence of apneic spells and infant breathing issues.

Lung Volumes

In proportion to body size, the total lung capacity, functional residual capacity, and tidal volume are roughly equivalent in adults and in infants. In the full-term infant the total lung volume is approximately 160 mL, with functional residual capacity at one half of this volume. Tidal volume is approximately 16 mL and dead space is approximately 5 mL. In comparison with adults, however, any increase in dead space is much more significant in infants, related to their small lung volumes. In contrast with static lung volumes, however, alveolar ventilation is proportionately much greater in newborns (100 to 150 mL/kg of body weight) than in adults (60 mL/kg of body weight). This higher alveolar ventilation in infants results in a higher alveolar–functional residual capacity ratio, 5 : 1, compared with 1.5 : 1 in adults. Consequently, the functional residual capacity is much less of a buffer in infants, so that changes in the concentration of inspired gases are much more rapidly reflected in alveolar and arterial levels. This explains why induction of anesthesia using inhalational techniques is easier in infants than in adults. Along with the higher metabolic rate for body weight seen in infants, this differnce also explains why the ventilatory reserve in infants is not as great as in adults. The time from apnea to oxygen desaturation is much shorter in infants than in adults. Accordingly, surgical maneuvers that require short apneic periods may pose more of a challenge in infants than in adults.

The total surface area of the air-tissue interface of the alveoli in infants is small (2.8 m^2). When this relatively small gas exchange area is combined with the higher relative metabolic rate, infants have a reduced reserve capacity for gas exchange. This difference is of increased importance when congenital defects interfere with lung growth and development or if the lung parenchyma becomes damaged. The remaining healthy lung may not be adequate to sustain life.

Respiratory Rate

The most efficient respiratory rate for newborns has been calculated to be around 37 breaths per minute. This rate is close to that observed for average newborns. Full-term infants are similar to adults in requiring approximately 1% of their metabolic energy to maintain ventilation. The cost of breathing is then 0.5 mL/0.5 L of ventilation. In preterm infants, this nearly doubles to 0.9 mL/0.5 L of ventilation. The cost of respiration also dramatically increases if the lung parenchyma is diseased or damaged by processes other than prematurity. In either case, the result is higher caloric and nutritional demands. Respiratory rate can directly affect the infant's ability to complete the suck-swallow-breathe cycle as well. If gas exchange is poor, ventilation rates may increase. This increase in respiratory rate may not allow adequate time for the suck-swallow portion of feeding. Caloric intake decreases precipitously as the infant chooses breathing over feeding. This vicious circle can eventuate in failure to thrive.

Ventilation-Perfusion Relationships

Ventilation and perfusion are imperfectly matched in the neonatal lungs. Some persistent anatomic shunts in the newborn circulatory system, as well as a relatively high closing volume in the lungs, cause this mismatch. The normal arterial oxygen tension in a newborn breathing room air is 50 mm Hg. This increases dramatically during the first 24 hours of life with changes in fetal circulation and maturation of lung parenchyma. It continues to change slowly during the ensuing months and years (Table 180-1).

Table 180-1

Arterial Oxygen Tension (Pa_{O_2}) in Healthy Infants and Children

Age	Pa_{O_2} in Room Air (mm Hg)
0-1 week	70
1-10 months	85
4-8 years	90
12-16 years	96

Table 180-2

Normal Heart Rate for Children by Age

	Heart Rate (beats/minute)	
Age	Average	Range
Newborn	120	100-170
1-11 months	120	80-160
2 years	120	80-160
4 years	100	80-120
6 years	100	75-115
10 years	90	70-110

Cardiovascular System

Newborn Heart and Cardiac Output

The heart of a healthy neonate is much different from that of an adult. The thickness of the right ventricle exceeds that of the left, as seen by the normal right axis deviation on the neonatal electrocardiogram. Shortly after birth and with closure of the fetal circulation, the left ventricle enlarges disproportionately. By the age of 6 months, the adult right-left ventricular size ratio is established.

The newborn myocardium is significantly different from the adult myocardium as well. The newborn myocardium contains fewer contractile fibers and more connective tissue. Consequently, neonatal ventricles are less compliant at rest and generate less tension during contraction. The usual Starling curves of contractility for adult cardiovascular physiology do not hold true for the neonatal heart. Cardiac output is rate-dependent in the neonatal heart. Bradycardia invariably equates with reduced cardiac output. Because of the differences in compliance and contractility in the neonatal heart, the increased contractility necessary to maintain cardiac output during bradycardia is not possible. The low compliance of the relaxed ventricle limits the size of the stroke volume; therefore, increases in preload are not as important in neonatal physiology as is heart rate. This distinction is extremely important to recognize during surgical and anesthetic procedures, which may induce bradycardia. Autonomic innervation also is incomplete in the neonatal heart, with a relative lack of sympathetic elements. This relative underdevelopment may further compromise the ability of the less contractile neonatal myocardium to respond to stress.

Heart rate is crucially important in the very young. The normal range for the newborn is 100 to 170 beats per minute. The rhythm is regular. As the child grows, the heart rate decreases (Table 180-2). Sinus arrhythmia is common in children, but all other irregular rhythms should be considered abnormal. The average newborn systolic blood pressure is 60 mm Hg; the diastolic pressure is 35 mm Hg.

Blood Volume

Intravascular blood volumes vary tremendously during the immediate postnatal period, related to the amount of blood transferred from the placenta to the child. "Stripping" the cord after birth or delays in clamping the umbilical cord may increase the blood volume by more than 20%, resulting in transient fluid overload and respiratory distress. Conversely, fetal hypoxia during labor causes vasoconstriction and a shift of blood to the placenta. Thus, fetal hypoxia may lead to hypovolemia after birth.

Because the total blood volume of an infant is small, significant blood loss can accompany relatively minor surgical blood loss. It has been observed during exchange transfusions that withdrawal of blood parallels a decline in systolic blood pressure and cardiac output. This decline is reversible to normal parameters with replacement of the same blood volume that was removed. Changes in arterial blood pressure with normal heart rates are thus proportional to the degree of hypovolemia. A newborn's ability to adapt the intravascular volume to the available blood volume is limited because of less efficient control of capacitance vessels and to immature or ineffective baroreceptors.

In the infant, systolic arterial blood pressure is closely related to circulating blood volume. Blood pressure is then an excellent guide to the adequacy of blood or fluid replacement during anesthesia, a fact that has been confirmed by extensive clinical experience.

Response to Hypoxia

Because of the relatively high metabolic rate typical of neonates and the relatively low reserve for gas exchange as described earlier in this chapter, hypoxemia can develop rapidly in neonates, in whom the first sign is bradycardia. During surgery, any unexplained episode of bradycardia should be initially treated with oxygen and increased ventilation. During hypoxemia, pulmonary vasoconstriction and hypertension occur more dramatically in the neonate than in the adult. Such changes can shift the infant back into fetal circulation, compounding the problem. Changes in cardiac output and systemic vascular resistance also differ from those in older children and adults. During hypoxemia in adults, the principal response is systemic vasodilation that, together with an increase in cardiac output, helps to maintain oxygen transport to the tissues. Fetuses and some neonates respond to hypoxemia with systemic vasoconstriction. In the fetus, hypoxemia shifts blood to the placenta to improve gas exchange and oxygenation. After birth, however, hypoxemia may lead to decreased cardiac output, thereby further limiting oxygen delivery and increasing cardiac work. In infants, early and pronounced bradycardia may result from myocardial hypoxia and acidosis.

Neonates exposed to hypoxemia suffer pulmonary and systemic vasoconstriction, decreased cardiac output, and bradycardia. Rapid recognition and intervention are necessary to prevent cardiopulmonary collapse, cardiac arrest, and death.

Blood Volume and Oxygen Transport

Neonatal blood volume is approximately 80 mL/kg at term and 20% higher in preterm infants. The hematocrit is 60% and the hemoglobin content is 18 g/100 mL. The values vary by infant, depending on when the umbilical cord is clamped. Little change in these values occurs during the first week of life, after which the hemoglobin level declines. The hemoglobin level change occurs more rapidly in preterm infants.

Approximately 70% to 90% of the hemoglobin in a full-term infant is the fetal type. Fetal hemoglobin has a higher affinity for oxygen than that of adult hemoglobin. It combines with oxygen more readily but also releases oxygen less efficiently at the tissue level than does adult hemoglobin. The increase in hemoglobin content in neonates is required to overcome this higher affinity of fetal hemoglobin for oxygen. A concentration less than 12 g/100 mL constitutes anemia. Correction of anemia by blood transfusion is indicated if the infant requires oxygen or is experiencing apnea.

Table 180-3

Ideal Electrolyte Composition for Infants

	Na^+ (mEq/L)	K^+ (mEq/L)
Intracellular	10	150
Extracellular	140	4.5

Table 180-4

Expected Fluid Losses in Children

System	Fluid Loss (mL/100 cal/day)
Sensible Losses	
Kidneys	55
Insensible Losses	
Lung	15
Skin	30
Total	100

During the first weeks of life, the hematocrit drops as a result of early suppression of erythropoiesis. The fetal type of hemoglobin is replaced with the adult type of hemoglobin with more optimal oxygen-carrying capacity. This physiologic anemia reaches its nadir at 2 to 3 months with a hemoglobin content of 9 to 11 g/100 mL. Provided that nutrition is adequate, the hemoglobin level will then gradually rise over several weeks to 12 to 13 g/100 mL, which is maintained throughout childhood.

Fluids and Fluid Management

As in adults, preoperative, intraoperative, and postoperative fluid management is extremely important in children. Some of the physiologic differences outlined earlier in this chapter make fluid administration even more critical. Because of their small intravascular volume (70 to 80 mL/kg), infants who experience small changes in fluid balance can easily become either dehydrated or overloaded with fluid. Extreme vigilance, early recognition, and tight control are required in managing fluid balance in children. Compartmentalization of total body water changes with age, but intracellular and extracellular electrolyte composition remains stable (Table 180-3). Calculating the maintenance fluid requirements for a child can be based on relatively simple formulas that vary according to metabolic and physical activity. The calculation of water loss per calorie is described in Table 180-4. The correspondence of necessary fluid intake proportional to weight is described in Table 180-5.

Complex fluid and electrolyte deficits are beyond the scope of this discussion. In most such cases, consultation with pediatric medical specialists is advised.

Pain Management

The management of pain in infants and children has undergone tremendous advances in recent years. It had been commonly believed that infants and newborns did not perceive pain because of their immature nervous system and that they do not have memory of pain if it occurs. Direct physiologic consequences have been observed in infants as a response to pain. Changes in heart rate, blood pressure, and respiration rate have been documented in infants experiencing painful stimuli. These changes can be physiologically as well as emotionally deleterious to the child.

The perception of pain depends on both sensory and emotional experiences that may be altered by various psychological factors. These

Table 180-5

Children's Maintenance Fluid Intake Calculated by Weight

Weight (kg)	Estimated Fluid Intake (mL/hour)
0-10	4 mL/kg/hour
11-20	40 mL/hour (2 mL/kg/hour)
>20	60 mL/hour (1 mL/kg/hour)

factors may be specific for each individual patient, based on his or her expectations and past experiences. Efforts to reduce stress, anxiety, and fear will help decrease the apprehension and perception of pain during procedures in the office or in the operating room. In patients of the appropriate age, relaxation techniques such as guided imagery, deep breathing, and hypnosis may diminish the emotional component of pain. An adequate and age-appropriate explanation of expectations also will reduce anxiety, increase cooperation, and decrease perceived pain. The caregiver or parent also should be coached regarding expectations, because children often look to the psychological state of their parent for cues. An anxious parent often increases the anxiety of the child. Conversely, a calm and collected parent can help calm the child during uncomfortable procedures.

Non-narcotic analgesics are helpful for pain management. Acetaminophen in doses ranging from 10 to 15 mg/kg every 4 hours is useful. Other nonsteroidal anti-inflammatory medications also are excellent for pain management. They often inhibit platelet function, however, and should be used only at the discretion of the surgeon.

Narcotic analgesics are indicated for moderate to severe pain in all age groups. Optimal use requires consideration of the needs of the individual patient. Neonates require special observation during the administration of narcotics. As noted previously, ventilatory responses to hypoxia and hypercarbia are diminished in this age group. Narcotics may further decrease these responses to potentially life-threatening levels. The metabolism and half-life of narcotics are different in neonates from those in older children and adults. The permeability of the blood-brain barrier also may be increased in neonates. The use of intravenous, intramuscular, and oral narcotics is safe in the appropriately monitored setting and with the proper dose. Unlike adults, who usually self-administer and therefore self-regulate narcotic analgesics, pediatric patients often rely on caregivers to administer pain medication, which can lead to underdosing, as well as overdosing.

Sedation

More often today, professional certification and credentialing for pediatric sedation are required at institutions caring for children. The development of sedation teams, often staffed by pediatric intensivists, has increased safety and monitoring for these patients. Otolaryngologists can participate in the team effort by assessing the airway of the patient referred for sedation. Occasionally, a general anesthetic procedure with a secured airway is required for the proper level of safety for a sedated patient. Although the otolaryngologist can accomplish assessments of airway safety, the professionals on the sedation team have the final word on whether they are willing to sedate a child. The requirements for certification, the makeup of the sedation team, and the success of the interaction as measured by family satisfaction and patient outcome are dependent on the institution involved. It is important to adhere to the guidelines of the institution and to work together as a team.

Referral Sources

Unlike adults, most pediatric patients have a primary caregiver—the pediatrician or family practice physician. School-aged children require vaccinations and usually will have a physician who provides this level of care. In turn, most pediatric patients seeking help for problems related to the ears, nose, and throat will be referred to the specialist by their primary care physician. Pediatric medicine is a specialty that legitimately considers its practitioners to be advocates for their patients. The child's primary care physician is responsible for his or her overall health and well-being. This physician can serve as a tremendous ally to help identify and refer problems early on, as well as to help translate the complex problems related to surgical management when adequate communication lines have not been established. Although every patient encounter requires an element of trust building and rapport development, a long-term relationship usually has already developed between the child's doctor and the family.

Pediatric medicine and its interface with surgery have a slightly different culture from its counterpart in the typical adult world. Often a multidisciplinary approach is used in the perioperative period. Although this approach can enhance the care of the patient, clear delineation of duties and responsibilities and open lines of communication are essential.

Although all parties involved must understand that the surgeon is ultimately responsible for the care of any patient undergoing surgery, a decision to proceed should always be accepted by the parents, as well as the referral source. Occasionally, expectations for surgery are initiated before the evaluation by the otolaryngologist. In such cases, how a decision is made must be explained clearly and logically. The surgeon makes the final recommendations for or against surgical management of a problem. All parties must clearly understand the steps leading to a logical decision.

Finally, pediatric otolaryngologists often direct their educational efforts directly to the families of the patients they treat. Education of their colleagues, specifically the primary care physicians caring for these patients, also is very important. Keeping these practitioners up to date through small education forums will maximize their ability to help with perioperative management, as well as increasing the visibility of the otolarygologist's contributions.

Patients

Although the entire family is involved in the care of a child, the child is the patient. Children experience the same fears of pain and discomfort as in adults but may lack the maturity and skills to overcome these fears. Delayed gratification is not often a concept familiar to a child. Whereas adults often bring themselves to the doctor and therefore have made the first hurdle toward obtaining medical care, children are brought by their parents and often have no idea why they are there. Establishing rapport with the child is important for myriad reasons. Not only will this put the child at ease, but it will often put the parents at ease when they see that the physician has a genuine interest in the well-being of their child. Children take cues from their parents. If the parent is apprehensive, the child will often be as well. It is important to explain not only to the parent what is to be expected during the history and physical examination but also to the child—on a level he or she may understand. Procedures that may be uncomfortable are best left to the end of the examination and are performed quickly but thoroughly.

Quickness and experience allow for a brief, but relatively complete, physical examination without undue stress on the child or the parent. Restraining an older child who may have been traumatized by a previous forceful examination is wrong and could be dangerous. In these cases, sedation or a general anesthetic is appropriate to complete the required examination.

Parents

Parents can find themselves in an uncomfortable position. They must make decisions for their sick child, decisions that may include treatment that may carry some discomfort and risk. It is important for the surgeon to be open and honest regarding the options and risks involved. Alternative treatment plans often are possible, and all of the options, with their set of risks and benefits, as well as expected outcomes, should be explained to the family. Finally, a single best option may exist, and the reasons that a surgeon considers one option better than others should be explained. Parents often have questions that may be biased by previous experiences or the advice of other family members or friends, or by exposure to the media. Time must be allotted to answer these questions.

Often, families have been referred by the primary care physician, who usually has answered many of the relevant questions. Having been referred to a specialist, the parents often identify the otolaryngologist as a person with expertise and added ability. It is important not to be placed in the situation of persuading parents to proceed with surgery. If they continue to have difficulties deciding after all of their questions have been answered, it may be suggested that they contact their primary care physician for another view. Finally, it may be more comfortable for families to make decisions regarding surgery at home with the understanding that they can call if more questions arise and will schedule an appointment if they wish to proceed.

Congenital Anomalies

Children with developmental or hereditary abnormalities often require a health care professional team approach for optimal treatment. As an example, for children with craniofacial anomalies, a craniofacial team consisting of at least an otolaryngologist, a craniofacial surgeon, dentist, geneticist, audiologist, speech-language pathologist, and social worker will bring the greatest benefit. It is important that a unified voice come from the specialists at hand. Conflicting information will only confuse the often devastated parents. Guilt regarding inheritable defects may be overwhelming to the parents. Counseling should be available from specialists in genetics when needed.

The goal of caring for children with congenital anomalies or developmental delays is to maximize their individual potential. It is important to know what difficulties a child may have from a particular disorder and then to offer advice or techniques proven to help such families cope with or manage the disability. This will be different for each child, family, and situation.

At one time, genetic counseling was routinely advised for families of all children with congenital abnormalities. The feeling today is that genetic counseling should be offered only to parents who desire it. Other than speaking in general terms of the inheritable nature of sensorineural deafness, cleft palate, or other problems, the clinician should not force the parents to face information they do not wish to acknowledge. The denial phase is related to their eventual acceptance of their child's problem. Once they have adapted to the child's abnormality, the parents are much more receptive to genetic counseling.

History

In treating children, several sources are available for historical data. A referral letter from the primary care physician often will accompany the child. This aspect of the history is important but does not replace the history taken from the parents or the child. Historical data from the primary physician give the added advantage of allowing the specialist physician to verify that the information provided by others and the data gathered during the examination are in agreement. The parents often give the history. They usually are very astute regarding their child's behaviors or symptoms and should therefore be listened to carefully. The child can be questioned as well, although he or she may not understand or be able to identify a problem. Often, chronic symptoms are not seen as problems to the child because such symptoms have been lifelong. The child, not ever having experienced life any other way, does not recognize his or her symptoms as abnormal. The difficult part for the pediatric otolaryngologist is to synthesize sometimes conflicting data into a coherent story.

Occasionally, admission to the hospital for observation is required. This allows for further collection of historical data. Symptoms described by the caregiver can be documented and perhaps better understood. Further testing also may document whether the child's safety is compromised because of symptoms or the severity of potential problems.

It also is very important to obtain a general family history, as well as a history of any diseases or illnesses affecting the child's siblings. Information regarding the pregnancy and delivery of the child also is important. Insight into any family stresses or school problems that may influence the child's psychosocial development also is helpful.

Physical Examination

Physical examination of a child can be done in a nonthreatening and calm manner. Rapport and trust are the key elements. Engaging the child as an active participant often leads to more cooperation. One technique is to let the child hold or examine the instruments before they are used. This often reduces the child's anxiety. Because many well child examinations are accompanied by vaccinations, children unfortunately often equate any visit to the doctor with a shot. The resulting apprehension and perhaps an attempt at maintaining independence or control of the self may underlie seemingly irrational behavior during an examination.

Most of the head and neck examination should be painless. Otoscopy generally is managed without difficulty. Pneumatic otoscopy can be performed but should be explained before proceeding so as not to surprise the child. Explanations build a child's trust in the examining physician. The use of a head mirror or headlamp light during the examination is the surgeon's choice. Things that cover the examiner's face often frighten children, which may decrease cooperation. Nasal endoscopy can be performed with the otoscope and a larger speculum, thereby eliminating the need to introduce a new instrument to the child. Oral examination often can be accomplished without a tongue depressor, although occasionally use of a depressor may be required to view the posterior pharynx. Palpation of the neck can be accomplished without any significant discomfort to the child, and masses or tenderness can be documented.

During the examination, further observations of the child's facial features can be made. It is important to ensure that the ears look normal, without pits or fistulas. The eyes also should be symmetrical in shape and alignment, without apparent hypertelorism or heterochromia. The nasal airway should be assessed for chronic mouth breathing and to help identify any abnormality of the palate. Listening to the child breathe, for the sounds of stridor or stertor, can help identify the level or site of potential airway obstruction. Auscultation of the neck and chest also generally is performed. The otolaryngologist will concentrate the physical examination on the particular area of interest, which is the head and neck. A general physical examination should be performed in a brief but complete manner, however.

Special Considerations

Microscopic Examination of the Ear

Otomicroscopy is an invaluable tool for assessing the ears. Children can have anxiety about this portion of the examination, however. Often, allowing the child to look through the microscope at the examiner's thumb will show that the microscope is simply a tool to obtain a magnified view of the ear. The parent can assist in reminding the child to hold still for the examination while cerumen or debris is removed from the ear canal. With the parent reclined on the examination chair or table, the child may lie on the parent like a table. The parent can then hug the child, to hold the arms and body still, while an assistant helps steady the head. Use of a papoose is possible in smaller children but often is not successful in older children. Sedation usually is not necessary but may be used in certain cases, in accordance with the sedation policies of the institution. Occasionally a general anesthetic is required to permit a complete and thorough examination.

Although usually not painful, suctioning is loud and can be frightening. The suction device is a very useful tool to quickly clean away debris and drainage. Some clinicians prefer to use cotton-tipped applicators instead. It is important to have a number of techniques in reserve and to use the one that will quickly and effectively accomplish the required task without undue stress and discomfort to the child.

Flexible Endoscopy

Nasopharyngoscopy is an invaluable tool for the otolaryngologist. With advances in technology, smaller-caliber endoscopes are being developed with improving optics. Although the mirror examination is useful, the fiberoptic endoscope allows for a dynamic examination of the nose, vellum, pharynx, hypopharynx, and larynx. When combined with videotaping, slow-motion replay is possible—an important option if only brief glimpses are obtained in a child who is not able to cooperate fully with the examination.

As in adults, topical anesthesia and nasal decongestion, with lidocaine gel or Pontocaine (tetracaine) spray and oxymetazoline, is very useful. Use of cocaine in young children is not advisable because of variable absorption rates. In infants, cocaine can produce unwanted irritability and nervousness. The parents should be counseled that after the topical anesthetic, the child should not eat or drink for approximately 30 minutes. Sedation generally is not necessary for this examination.

Complications from nasopharyngoscopy are rare. An emergency cart for airway management and the skills to use it are important to have on hand. Nasal bleeding, if it occurs, often is self-limiting or requires little intervention.

Needle Biopsy

Fine-needle aspiration (FNA) can be performed in children to obtain a biopsy specimen for histopathologic examination. Ideally, a cytopathologist should be available for interpretation of results. Many of the typical masses of the head and neck are very different from those encountered in adults and may be more difficult to characterize. This does not make FNA less useful, however. Children usually are very frightened of needles or sharp objects. EMLA cream (Astra Pharmaceuticals, Westborough, Massachusetts) or other anesthetic creams that are topically applied can render the introduction of the needle painless.

The site is prepared in a sterile manner. The 22- or 23-gauge needle, attached to a 10-mL syringe, is then placed into the mass while suction is applied. The sample obtained within the needle core is then applied to a glass slide and is placed in a fixative. It is optimal if the cytopathologist can attend or perform the procedure to provide immediate feedback regarding the adequacy of the specimen. If the specimen is inadequate and the child appears able to tolerate another attempt, FNA may be repeated using the same anesthetic. An adhesive bandage is applied when the procedure is done. FNA should be no more traumatic than obtaining a blood sample and should be explained in those terms to the parent.

Audiology

Every child can be tested for hearing loss. Pediatric otolaryngologists can help to accomplish this goal by educating the families and especially the primary care physicians of their patients. It has been shown that in children with hearing loss, early detection and treatment lead to dramatic increase in language ability later in life. Audiologists interested in pediatric screening generally are able to test children as young as 6 months of age with visual response audiometry. Visual response audiometry in experienced hands can be very reliable. Other techniques for younger children or children who are unable to conform to the demands of the task include otoacoustic emissions and auditory brainstem response (ABR) testing.

Early detection of hearing loss is extremely important to the speech and language development of the child. Currently, newborn hearing screening programs with automated ABR testing are being set up nationwide. If a screening test identifies the infant as requiring further investigation, it is essential for the otolaryngologist to provide any necessary referrals and follow-up evaluations. If no action is taken once a child has been diagnosed with hearing impairment, the test is useless and does not benefit the child or the family.

Preparation for Hospitalization and Surgery

Once the decision to proceed with hospitalization or surgery has been made, the child and parents should be readied emotionally to achieve a successful outcome. The details and expectations should be reviewed with the family by persons familiar with the process. Some institutions and most children's hospitals have programs to introduce the family to the hospital, operating room, and operating room procedures. A sense of familiarity and an understanding of what to expect will be helpful to all involved. Children can then role-play before hospital admission or surgery. With a clear understanding of what is expected, parents also are less apprehensive and help calm the child.

It is important to clarify arrival times and nothing-by-mouth requirements to the family. Special films and booklets are valuable tools for education. The parents must be encouraged to be truthful, to the best of their ability, about preparation for the upcoming surgery. It also is important that the surgeon communicate directly with both parents and child so that all questions are answered completely.

Hospital

A dedicated children's hospital is the preferred venue for pediatric otolaryngologic surgery, providing a team of physicians, nurses, and other professionals who can best handle a hospital stay or surgical procedurefor the pediatric patient. Children's hospitals constitute an important medical resource, and every surgeon involved in the care of children should support them. Unfortunately, not every community has one. In such instances, it is important to identify the best facilities in the community in which the physical plant, physicians, nurses, and support staff are capable of and enjoy caring for children. Ensuring an optimal environment for pediatric treatment will encourage the best outcomes and lead to the greatest satisfaction among patients and their families.

The concept of a team of professionals who deal strictly with pediatrics is not new; moreover, a team approach is becoming increasingly accepted as the standard of care. When complications arise, as they inevitably do in the course of even the best medical care, having the support facilities and the personnel available to handle any need promptly is vital for the best outcome possible.

Selecting Anesthesia

Pediatric anesthesia is a subspecialty in itself. Reaching a degree of proficiency to deliver an anesthetic to children of all ages requires considerable training and experience. The younger the patient, the more complex the problems encountered. As in all aspects of medicine, this subspecialty includes practitioners with special interests and expertise in particular fields. Those with expertise in safely delivering anesthesia to children should be sought when their assistance is required. Reliance on these specialists benefits both the patient and the surgeon.

With practice and special expertise, the interested clinician can devise techniques to safely and effectively perform nearly any technique. Local anesthesia as a primary anesthetic technique for pediatric surgery is possible but requires a cooperative child and an adept surgeon. Generally, local anesthetics are used for immediate postoperative pain management after surgery performed with the patient under general anesthesia. Young children generally do not understand the need for painful injections and have short attention spans, making it difficult for them to sit still for the procedure. The use of sedation for extended periods is not recommended unless support personnel are available to monitor the child during the sedation process. Many institutions have strict guidelines and require a certification process for the use of conscious sedation in children. Most invasive or painful procedures require a general anesthetic.

Postoperative Management

Probably the most important part of postoperative management is preoperative teaching. If the parent and the child are adequately prepared about the effects of surgery, they are more capable of handling the postoperative period in terms of decreased stress and optimal adherence to the postoperative regimen. Detailed teaching about the expected clinical course and unexpected possibilities is important. Providing written instructions, along with contact telephone numbers if the parents should have questions, also is very helpful. Knowing what to expect is the single most important factor in uneventful recovery from a surgical procedure without multiple phone calls and excessive concern from both patient and physician.

If a child must be hospitalized, it has been shown that the presence of a parent makes the stay less fearsome and stressful for the child. Whenever possible, parents should be encouraged to stay with the child while in the hospital. Arrangements should be made for this to be possible if it is not the norm at the hospital where the child will stay.

More often, short-stay and outpatient procedures are being performed. It is helpful for the child to return to the home setting as soon as possible. Safety is the main concern, however, and monitoring in the hospital should be done as long as necessary.

An awareness that modifications in surgical technique may be required in the management of pediatric problems is important. Dressing changes, suture removal, and postoperative manipulations should be kept to the required minimum so as not to provoke fear and discomfort in children who must undergo minor procedures. Sometimes sedation or a general anesthetic for packing or suture removal, not often required for adults, may be necessary in children. It is reasonable to plan ahead at the time of surgery to use absorbable suture material and dressings that need infrequent changing.

A Rewarding Experience

The care of children is an extremely rewarding experience. Children may become ill quickly but often recover just as quickly if put on the right pathway. Watching children grow and develop makes for lasting memories and personal satisfaction. For many clinicians, helping children with chronic illness to overcome disabilities and difficulties and watching them reach their full potential as they grow to adulthood have no match for reward.

SUGGESTED READINGS

Ashcraft KW, Murphy JP, eds. *Pediatric Surgery.* 3rd ed. Philadelphia: Saunders; 2000

Avery ME, Chernick V, Dutton RE, et al. Ventilatory response to inspired carbon dioxide in infants and adults. *J Appl Physiol.* 1963;18:89.

Bodegård G, Schwieler GH, Skoglund S, et al. Control of respiration in newborn babies. I. The development of Hering-Breuer inflation reflex. *Acta Pediatr.* 1969;58:567.

Bryan AC, Bryan MH. Control of respiration in the newborn. *Clin Perinatol.* 1978;5:269.

Children's Hospital and Medical Center. *Selected Handouts for Housestaff.* 14th ed. Seattle: Children's Hospital and Medical Center; 1990-1991.

Cook CD, Sutherland JM, Segal S, et al. Studies of respiratory physiology in the newborn infant. III. Measurements of mechanics of respiration. *J Clin Invest.* 1957;36:440.

Filston HC. *Surgical Problems in Children: Recognition and Referral.* St Louis: Mosby; 1982.

Gans S, ed. *Surgical Pediatrics: Non-operative Care.* New York: Grune & Stratton; 1980.

Graff TD, Sewall K, Lim HS, Kantt O, Morris RE Jr, Benson DW. The ventilatory response of infants to airway resistance. *Anesthesiology.* 1966;27:168.

Graham GR. Circulatory and respiratory physiology of infancy and childhood. *Br J Anaesth.* 1960;32:97.

Gregory GA, ed. *Pediatric Anesthesia.* New York: Churchill Livingstone; 2002.

James LS, Rowe RD. The pattern of response of pulmonary and systemic arterial pressures in newborn and older infants to short periods of hypoxia. *J Pediatr.* 1957;51:5.

Ledbetter MK, Homma T, Farhi LE. Readjustment in distribution of alveolar ventilation and lung perfusion in the newborn. *Pediatrics.* 1967; 40:940.

Nelson NM. Neonatal pulmonary function. *Pediatr Clin North Am.* 1966; 13:769.

O'Brien RT, Pearson HA. Physiologic anemia of the newborn infant. *J Pediatr.* 1971;79:132.

Raffensperger J, ed. *Swenson's Pediatric Surgery.* 5th ed. New York: Appleton-Century-Croft; 1990.

Ravitch MM, Welch KJ, Benson CD, Aberdeen E, Randolph JR, eds. *Pediatric Surgery*. 3rd ed. Chicago: Mosby–Year Book; 1979

Rigatto H. Apnea. *Pediatr Clin North Am*. 29:1105, 1982.

Rowe MI, Marchildon MB. Physiologic considerations in the newborn surgical patient. *Surg Clin North Am*. 1976;56:245.

Steward DJ, ed. *Manual of Pediatric Anesthesia*. 4th ed. New York: Churchill Livingstone; 1995.

Wallgren G, Barr M, Rudhe U. Hemodynamic studies of induced acute hypo- and hypervolemia in the newborn infant. *Acta Paediatr Scand*. 1964;53:1.

Wallgren G, Hansen JS, Lind J. Quantitative studies of the human neonatal circulation. Observations on the newborn infant's central circulatory response to moderate hypovolemia. *Acta Paediatr Suppl*. 1967;179: 43.

CHAPTER ONE HUNDRED AND EIGHTY-ONE

Anatomy and Developmental Embryology of the Neck

Daniel O. Graney

Kathleen C. Y. Sie

Key Points

- Anatomy of the neck is predictable. A detailed understanding of neck anatomy is critical for the otolaryngologist–head and neck surgeon.
- Congenital anomalies of the neck are related to the embryology of the neck.

Most descriptions of the neck divide the anatomy, for discussion purposes, into triangles. The use of triangles is simply an organizational approach to manage the volume of anatomic detail in the neck by parceling it into reasonable study units. When an incision is made over the carotid triangle, surgeons can thereby predict the structures they will encounter in precise order. Similarly, the embryologic correlates of the triangles are important in understanding the development and differential diagnosis of masses in the various triangles of the neck.

This chapter begins with descriptions of the posterior triangle and the subdivisions of the anterior triangle. Also presented is a description of the root of the neck that relates the anatomy of the two major triangles to the radical neck procedure. The chapter concludes with a discussion of the embryology of the branchial arches and the pharyngeal pouches and their contribution to various masses in the neck.

Strictly speaking, the term *triangle* connotes a planar form (i.e., a flat structure). The "triangles" in the neck, however, are three-dimensional spaces that should be visualized as shallow triangular boxes. These boxes have not only three sides but also a roof (top) and a floor (bottom). Most of the triangles are three-dimensional spaces bounded by bone and muscles, with distinct fascial layers forming the roof and floor of the space. In general terms, the triangular space contains blood vessels, nerves, lymphatic vessels, and lymph nodes. Using this somewhat contrived schema, the organization of the neck can be greatly simplified.

Posterior Triangle of Neck

The posterior triangle is bordered by the sternocleidomastoid muscle, the anterior border of the trapezius muscle, and the middle third of the clavicle (Fig. 181-1). Specific layers of deep fascia form the floor (medial wall) and roof (lateral wall) of the triangular box. An understanding of the fascial relationships in the neck is important not only because of the boundary relationships but also because fasciae form planes that provide routes of surgical access or pathways for hemorrhage and infection. For this reason, a brief discussion of the fascial planes is necessary before proceeding with the anatomy of the posterior triangle.

Fascia of Neck

One of the earliest lessons in anatomy is that there are two types of fascia in the body: the superficial and the deep. In the region of the abdominal wall, superficial fascia consists of two layers—a fatty layer (Camper's fascia) and a deeper, membranous layer (Scarpa's fascia). The deep fascial layer of the abdominal wall is not subdivided but simply envelops the abdominal muscles. In the neck the superficial fascia is very thin and is not divided into layers, whereas the deep fascia is divided into three layers.[1] The names of these layers vary with different authors, resulting in a somewhat chaotic terminology. Regardless of the terminology used, the divisions are arbitrary at best. A simple approach can provide a workable solution for either the anatomist or the surgeon.

Superficial Layer of Cervical Fascia

As just noted, the superficial layer of cervical fascia is a single layer of fascia underlying the skin. It usually is thin, except in the obese person, in which case it is thickened by adipose tissue. Its primary surgical significance is that it provides a fascial pad that protects underlying structures when a skin incision is made. In exceptionally lean people, however, the paucity of this layer may not protect underlying structures, such as the accessory nerve, so the surgeon should be wary when operating on such patients.

Deep Fascia

The deep fascia is divided into three layers, demonstrated best when the neck is viewed in cross section (Fig. 181-2). These are the external, middle, and internal layers of the deep cervical fascia. The external layer of deep fascia underlies the platysma muscle and completely invests or encircles all of the superficial neck structures. For these reasons, the external layer is also known as the superficial layer, or investing layer, of deep fascia. In the region of the sternocleidomastoid and trapezius muscles, it splits and envelopes the individual muscles. A middle layer of the deep cervical fascia encloses the visceral structures of the neck (the trachea and esophagus). Hence the synonym for the middle layer is the *visceral fascia*.

The third, or internal, layer of the deep cervical fascia surrounds the deep muscles of the neck and cervical vertebrae (Fig. 181-3). This

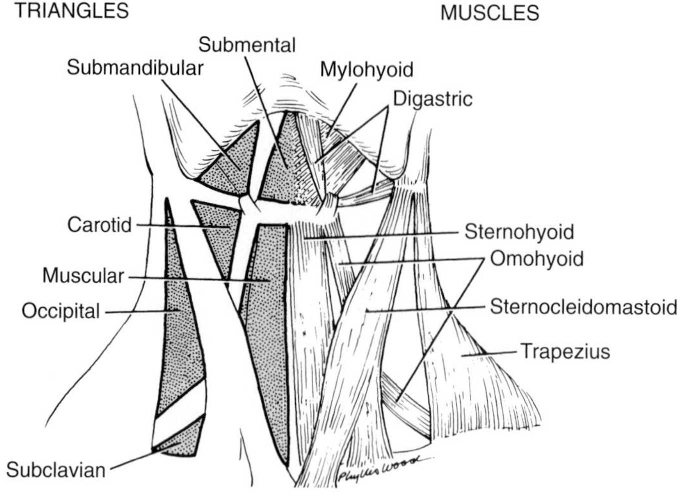

Figure 181-1. The triangles of the neck and their boundaries.

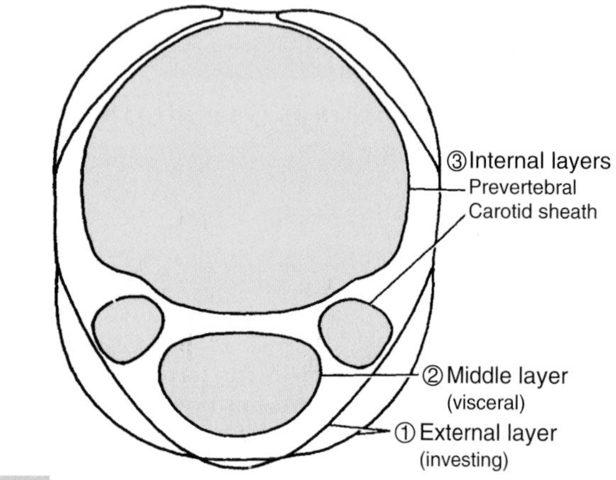

Figure 181-2. Divisions of the deep cervical fascia seen in transverse section at the level of cranial nerve VII.

layer also is known by its descriptive term *prevertebral fascia* (although "paravertebral fascia" would have been more appropriate). The muscles enclosed by the prevertebral fascia include the deep muscles of the neck (the cervical part of the erector spinae); the levator scapulae; the scalenus anterior, middle, and posterior muscles; and the longus colli and longus capitis muscles, which lie on the anterior aspect of the cervical vertebrae. The last-named pair of muscles serve as flexors of the vertebrae; the longus capitis also assists in flexion of the skull. The scalenus group underlies the prevertebral fascia in the region of transverse processes of the cervical vertebrae. The anterior tubercles of the transverse processes provide origin for the scalenus anterior muscle, whereas the posterior tubercles provide the origin for the scalenus medius and posterior muscles. Continuing posteriorly, in order, are the levator scapulae and deep cervical muscles already noted.

The internal layer of deep fascia is described by some authors as enveloping the carotid and jugular vessels. Hence, the carotid sheaths are included as part of the definition of the internal layer of deep fascia. An effective means of visualizing the spatial relationships of these layers of fascia is to examine a cross section of the neck. This view not only is informative in defining the three layers of deep fascia but also serves to relate them to the posterior triangle of the neck (see Fig. 181-2). Placing a finger over the middle of the posterior triangle (i.e., between the trapezius and sternocleidomastoid muscles) will clarify that the roof (lateral wall) of the triangle is formed by the superficial layer of deep fascia. Palpation deeper into the triangle will bring the tip of the finger into contact with the prevertebral fascia that forms the floor of the posterior triangle and invests the prevertebral muscles. If the superficial layer of the deep fascia is incised, a finger inserted into the space, exploring anteriorly between the sternocleidomastoid and prevertebral muscles, will encounter the carotid sheath. This is a surgical approach to the retropharyngeal area or to the carotid vessels for vascular surgery.

Contents of Posterior Triangle

The major contents of the posterior triangle are the cutaneous branches of the cervical plexus, the accessory nerve (cranial nerve XI), two arterial branches of the thyrocervical trunk, and an abundant number of lymph nodes associated with the veins of the region.

Cutaneous Branches of Cervical Plexus

The sensory branches of the cervical plexus contained within the posterior triangle are four cutaneous nerves, which supply the skin of the head and neck from the area of the posterior scalp to the supraclavicular region. These cutaneous nerves are the (1) lesser occipital, (2) great auricular, (3) anterior, and (4) supraclavicular (Fig. 181-4). The first three of these nerves contain cervical segments C2 and C3 and the supraclavicular nerves C3 and C4. The topographic relations of these nerves and their distribution to the skin are illustrated in Figure 181-5. The important landmark for the cervical nerves is the accessory nerve at the point where it enters the posterior triangle from under cover of the sternocleidomastoid muscle. If this point is viewed as the center of a clock face, the cervical nerves mimic the hands pointing in different directions (see Fig. 181-4, inset). For instance, on the right side, the lesser occipital nerve is approximately at the 11 o'clock position, the great auricular is at the 12 o'clock position, and the anterior cutaneous nerve of the neck can be found at the 3 o'clock position. The supraclavicular nerves consist of three or four bundles of filaments scattered between the 5 and 7 o'clock positions on the clock's face. Continuing this analogy, the accessory nerve can be seen to traverse the posterior triangle along the line of the 8 o'clock position until it enters the deep surface of the trapezius muscle. Viewed in this manner, the accessory nerve serves as a focus for organizing the pathways of the cutaneous nerves, as well as for emphasizing cranial nerve XI as a motor nerve in the posterior triangle.

Accessory Nerve

The accessory nerve supplies both the sternocleidomastoid and trapezius muscles; however, in the posterior triangle, the only fibers remaining in the nerve are those destined for the trapezius. The accessory nerve should be preserved whenever possible because paralysis of the trapezius muscle produces devastating effects on shoulder joint function. The range of shoulder abduction is diminished by at least 50 degrees when scapular rotation is impaired because of a trapezius palsy.

The accessory nerve is the only motor nerve in the posterior triangle as just defined. However, if the prevertebral fascia is incised, it is possible to encounter the motor nerves of the deep cervical muscles,

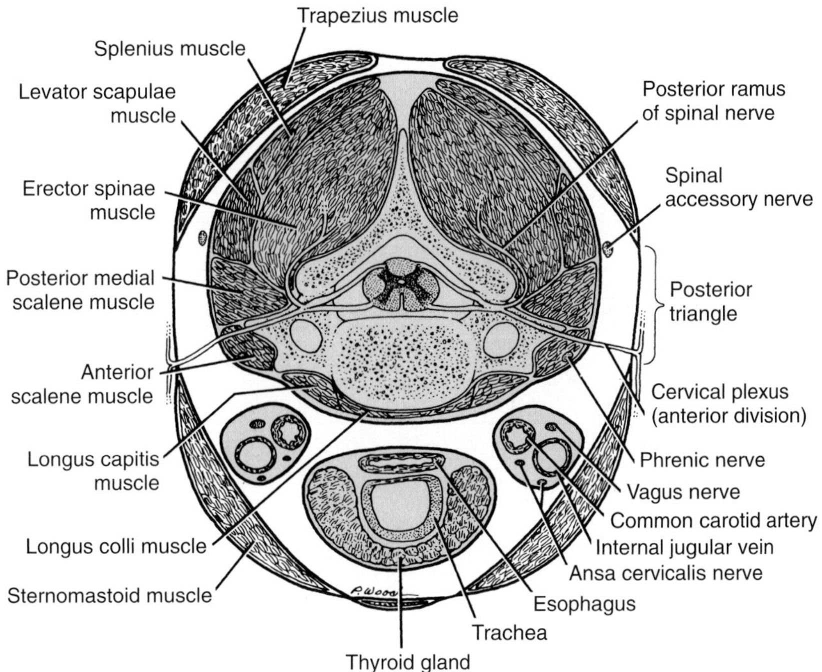

Figure 181-3. Structures contained by the deep cervical fascia seen in transverse section at the level of the cranial nerve.

the phrenic nerve, or the brachial plexus. With regard to its innervation of the sternocleidomastoid and trapezius muscles, cranial nerve XI is in fact a spinal nerve. Cell bodies of motor neurons innervating these muscles lie near the ventral horn in the upper cervical spinal cord, in the region of segments C2 through C4. The axonal fibers exit the anterior lateral portion of the cord as a series of fine filaments before becoming bundled as a nerve fiber within the subarachnoid space of the vertebral canal. The nerve ascends in the subarachnoid space, enters the posterior fossa through the foramen magnum, and joins with the cranial root of the accessory nerve before exiting the skull through the jugular foramen on the deep surface of the internal jugular vein. As the nerve descends the neck adjacent to the carotid sheath, motor or sensory filaments may join the nerve directly from segments C2 through C4.[2] After crossing the deep surface of the sternocleidomastoid muscle, the nerve enters the posterior triangle, as already described.

Arterial Branches

The major arteries of the posterior triangle are the suprascapular and transverse cervical arteries, located in the supraclavicular fossa near the base of the triangle. The arteries are derived from the thyrocervical trunk of the subclavian artery at the medial border of the scalenus anterior muscle. These arteries cross the muscle and the fossa transversely to course deep to the sternocleidomastoid muscle. Ascending and descending branches of the transverse cervical artery are usually described. The descending branch is of interest because it divides into a superficial branch that parallels the accessory nerve and a deep branch that parallels the nerve to the rhomboid muscle. The suprascapular artery, after crossing the fossa, is directed toward the suprascapular notch, where it supplies the posterior scapular muscle.

In addition to transverse cervical and suprascapular veins that parallel the course of the arteries, the posterior triangle contains the external jugular vein. It enters the triangle after crossing the superficial aspect of the sternocleidomastoid muscle in company with the great auricular nerve. The vein courses inferior to the base of the supraclavicular fossa, where it may anastomose with small vessels before entering the subclavian vein near the junction with the internal jugular vein.

Anterior Triangle of Neck

The anterior triangle of the neck is complementary to the posterior triangle and is bounded by the sternocleidomastoid muscle, the body of the mandible, and the midline of the neck. This space can be further subdivided into smaller triangular units, such as the submandibular triangle, and carotid and muscular triangles, which are included in this discussion (see Fig. 181-1).

Carotid Triangle

The carotid triangle is bordered by the posterior belly of the digastric muscle, the superior belly of the omohyoid muscle, and the midportion of the sternocleidomastoid muscle. The roof (lateral wall) of the carotid triangle is bounded by the superficial layer of deep fascia, whereas the floor (medial wall) is formed by the prevertebral fascia of the vertebral column and the visceral fascia covering the pharynx and larynx.

The contents of the carotid triangle are the carotid sheath structures. These include the common carotid with its internal and external branches, the last four cranial nerves (cranial nerves IX, X, XI, and XII), and the ansa cervicalis. In the carotid triangle, only a small branch of cranial nerve IX is left to supply the carotid sinus, because its main portion exits the sheath to enter the posterior third of the tongue. Cranial nerve XI, which also is in the upper portion of the carotid sheath, enters the sternocleidomastoid muscle at the apex of the carotid triangle, where the posterior belly of the digastric crosses the sternocleidomastoid muscle. The vagus nerve travels the entire length of the carotid sheath between the internal jugular vein and the carotid artery. Whereas the cranial nerves just mentioned lie in the posterior aspect of the carotid sheath, cranial nerve XII lies on the lateral and anterior aspect of the carotid sheath. At the level of the hyoid bone, cranial nerve XII courses anteroinferiorly to pass deep to the posterior belly of the digastric onto the surface of the hyoglossus muscle before entering the substance of the tongue.

The major focal point of the triangle is the bifurcation of the common carotid artery (Fig. 181-6). The internal carotid artery ascends the neck without branching. The external carotid artery provides several branches, many of which are important landmarks. The external carotid artery has anterior, posterior, and terminal branches.

Three anterior branches are common. In ascending order, they are the superior thyroid, lingual, and facial arteries. In some persons, the lingual and facial arteries form a common linguofacial trunk. Another important variation is the origin of the superior thyroid from the common carotid rather than the external carotid. The latter variation is important, because the external carotid occasionally is ligated (for

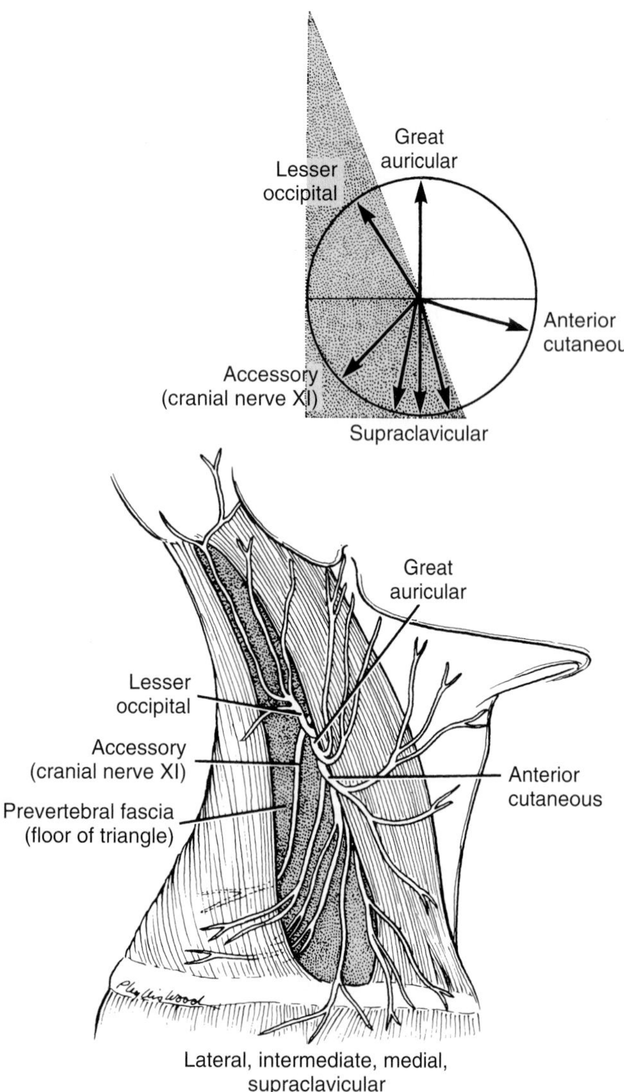

Figure 181-4. Nerves of the posterior triangle seen on the right side of the neck.

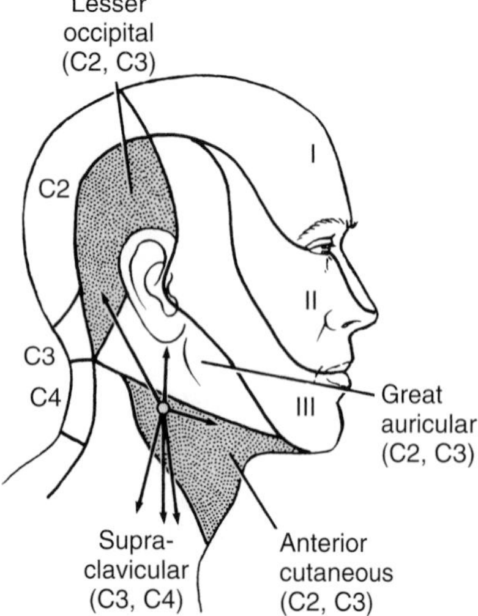

Figure 181-5. Distribution of the cutaneous branches of the cervical plexus.

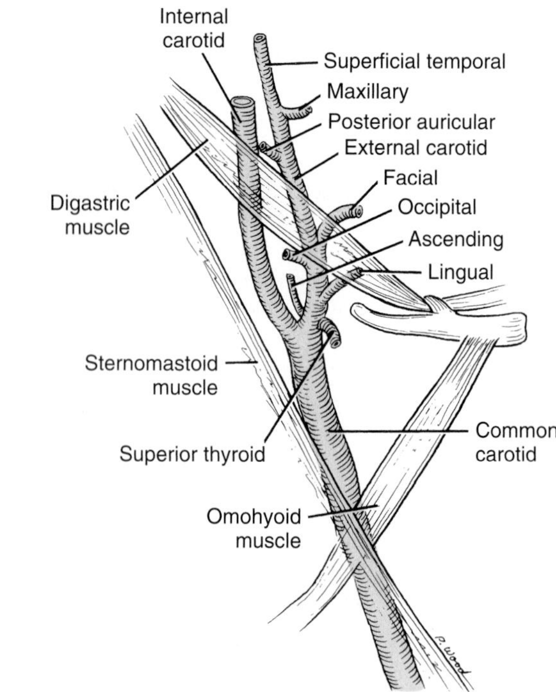

Figure 181-6. Arterial branches of the carotid triangle.

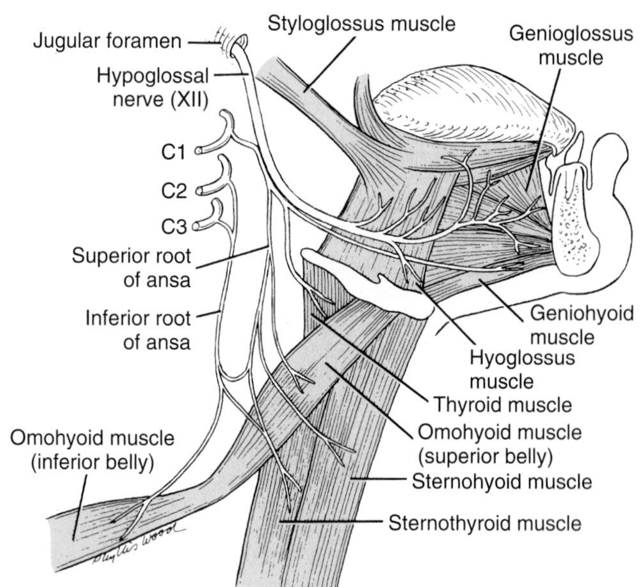

Figure 181-7. Distribution of the ansa cervicalis and the hypoglossal nerve (cranial nerve XII).

chronic epistaxis) at its origin from the common carotid. If the superior thyroid artery is used as a landmark in patients with this particular anatomic variation, it is possible to ligate the common carotid inadvertently instead of the external carotid.

The posterior branches of the external carotid are the occipital and the posterior auricular. The occipital is noteworthy for its small sternocleidomastoid branch, which supplies the sternocleidomastoid muscle. The origin of this small artery hooks cranial nerve XII as it courses anteroinferiorly and prevents it from ascending further in the neck. Thus, the sternocleidomastoid artery can be used to trace the position of cranial nerve XII. Similarly, the sternocleidomastoid artery enters its muscle near the point of cranial nerve XI, thereby also providing a means of locating the accessory nerve.

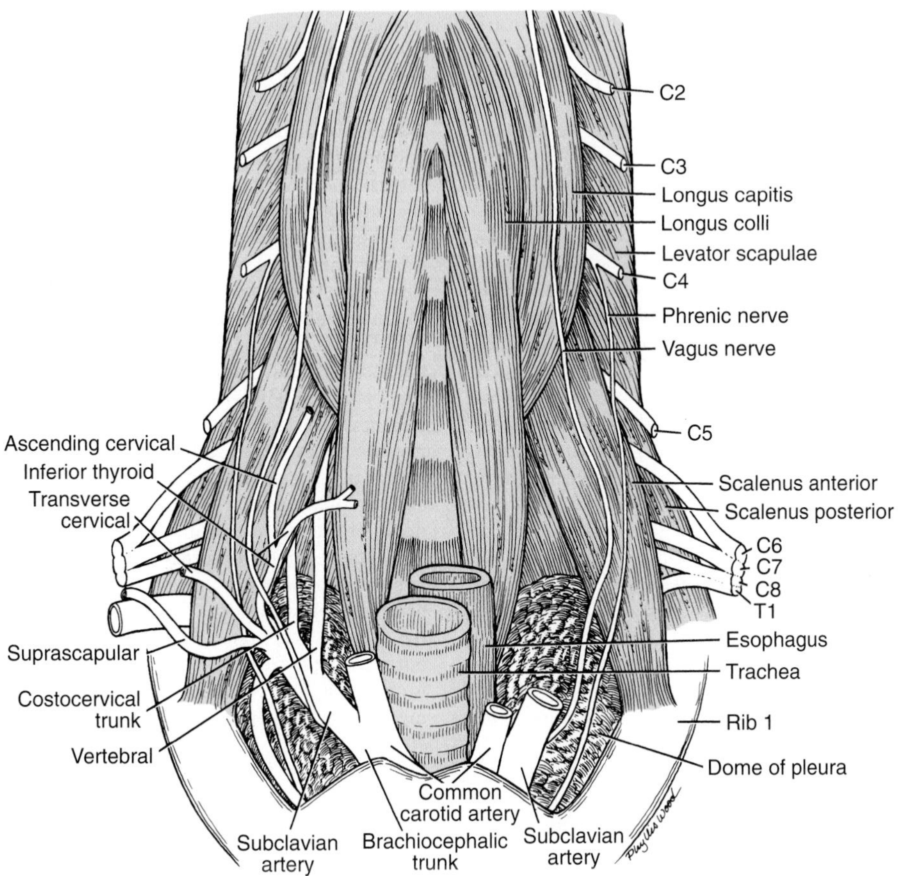

Figure 181-8. Root of the neck and subclavian artery. T1, first thoracic root; Rib 1, first rib.

Ansa Cervicalis

The ansa cervicalis is part of the cervical plexus. Its essential role is to supply the infrahyoid muscles: the sternohyoid, sternothyroid, and omohyoid muscles (Fig. 181-7). C1 fibers, which descend the neck, enter the hypoglossal nerve and travel as far as the occipital artery. At this point the hypoglossal nerve curves anteroinferiorly, but C1 fibers descend the neck to form the branch of cranial nerve XII, termed the superior root of the ansa. Fibers from C2 and C3 form an inferior root, which descends the carotid sheath on the surface of the internal jugular vein before turning anteroinferiorly to join the superior root. The ansa cervicalis is thus formed by the union of the two roots of the ansa. Three muscles are supplied directly by the ansa: the sternohyoid, sternothyroid, and omohyoid. At the origin of the superior root of the ansa, some C1 fibers do not follow the superior root but rather continue in the hypoglossal nerve transversely across the neck, before leaving cranial nerve XII to supply either the thyrohyoid muscle or the geniohyoid muscle (see Fig. 181-7). In summary, all four of the infrahyoid muscles are supplied by the ansa. In addition, one suprahyoid muscle, the geniohyoid muscle, also is supplied by the C1 fibers that have continued en route with the hypoglossal nerve. Except for proprioceptive fibers carried within the ansa, it is a motor nerve.

Thus far, two major groups of nerves of the cervical plexus have been discussed: the ansa cervicalis (principally motor) and the sensory (or cutaneous) branches of the posterior triangle. The cervical plexus comprises two other groups of fibers. One group of fibers is composed of motor filaments from cervical roots 3 and 4, supplying the levator scapulae muscle and located deep to the prevertebral fascia. The other group of fibers constitutes the phrenic nerve, derived from cervical segments C3, C4, and occasionally C5. This nerve not only is motor to the diaphragm but also supplies sensory fibers to the region of the central tendon of the diaphragm.

Root of Neck

The boundaries of the root of the neck are somewhat ill defined. The base of it is the plane of the thoracic inlet and can be traced from the manubrium laterally along the first ribs and then posterosuperiorly to the transverse process of C6 (Fig. 181-8). It contains the neck viscera and vessels. For the purposes of this discussion, it is divided unilaterally by the midline into a pyramidal space—bounded laterally by the scalenus anterior muscle, inferiorly by the first rib, and medially by the tracheoesophageal tract and midline.

The contents of the root of the neck include the great vessels emerging from the mediastinum, principally subclavian and common carotid arteries, brachiocephalic vein, vagus nerve, sympathetic trunk, and thoracic duct. As the great vessels traverse the thoracic inlet from the mediastinum, their course is divided by the scalenus anterior muscle. The subclavian vein crosses anterior to the muscle, whereas the subclavian artery courses between the cleavage plane of the scalenus anterior and scalenus medius muscles. In this region the subclavian vessels usually divide into three parts: the first part proximal to the scalenus, the second part posterior to the scalenus anterior muscle, and the third part between the lateral border of the scalenus and the lateral edge of the first rib.

A majority of the vascular branches arise from the first portion of the subclavian artery. The first branch of the subclavian artery normally is the vertebral artery, which ascends the root of the neck between the scalenus anterior and longus colli muscles to enter the foramen processus transversus of C6. The next is the thyrocervical trunk, which normally has four described branches. The first is a small ascending cervical, which supplies the prevertebral muscle region. The second branch of the thyrocervical trunk is the inferior thyroid artery coursing to the inferior pole of the thyroid gland. The inferior thyroid artery commonly supplies both the superior and inferior parathyroid glands. The third and fourth branches are the transverse cervical artery and the suprascapular artery, already described in relation to the posterior triangle of the neck. Two branches arise from the inferior surface of the subclavian artery: the costocervical trunk and the internal thoracic artery, which descends over the suprapleural fascia into the mediastinum and anterior chest wall. Multiple variations of these vessels have been described, as detailed by Daseler and Anson.[3]

The thoracic duct ascends into the root of the neck on the left side, anterior to the thyrocervical trunk. The thoracic duct empties chyle into the venous system at the junction of the left internal jugular and subclavian veins.

Other important relationships of this region are those involving the major nerves. On the right side, the vagus nerve lies in the posterior aspect of the carotid sheath and gives off its recurrent laryngeal branch at the level of the first rib. The recurrent branch circles the lateral aspect of the subclavian artery to cross medially and enter the tracheoesophageal groove. On the left side, the recurrent nerve arises from the vagus at the aortic arch and hooks posteriorly around the ligamentum arteriosum. It enters the tracheoesophageal groove, ascending the mediastinum and neck until it enters the larynx at the level of the cricothyroid membrane.

In the most posterior part of the root of the neck, against the longus colli muscle, the sympathetic trunk ascends from the mediastinum, following the prevertebral space to the level of C2, where the superior cervical sympathetic ganglion is located. The inferior cervical ganglion lies close to the level of C7, and sometimes a middle sympathetic ganglion is described at approximately the level of C4. Injury to the cervical sympathetic chain may result in Horner's syndrome, consisting of ptosis, miosis, and anhydrosis.

This region is of particular importance during radical neck surgery, because the deep dissection usually is begun by detaching the sternocleidomastoid muscle from its attachments to the manubrium and clavicle. This exposes the carotid sheath and its contents and opens up the posterior and anterior triangles. As the dissection proceeds, the internal jugular vein is mobilized, exposing the carotid and its branches, which have been left in place. Because the en bloc mass of the internal jugular vein and sternocleidomastoid muscle is mobilized superiorly, it is important to leave the prevertebral fascia intact. With this precaution, the fascia willprovide a protective veil over the brachial plexus, phrenic nerve, sympathetic trunk, and motor nerves to the deep cervical muscles. When the prevertebral fascia is exposed, two muscles—the scalenus anterior and the longus capitis—serve as important landmarks for the spinal nerves. As the nerves emerge from the intervertebral foramina, they lie in a groove on the transverse process of the cervical vertebrae. If the vertebrae and prevertebral muscles are envisioned as being enclosed in a cylinder of prevertebral fascia, the logical conclusion is that the spinal nerves must penetrate this fascia to reach superficial structures in the neck (see Fig. 181-3). With these guidelines it is possible to identify cervical nerves C1 through C4 at the lateral border of the longus capitis, and the roots of C5 through T1 can be identified at the lateral edge of the scalenus anterior (see Fig. 181-8).

At this point in the radical neck dissection, the cutaneous nerves of the posterior triangle are encountered at their origin from the spinal nerves, and the surgeon has returned to the anatomic relationships of the posterior triangle, as discussed at the beginning of this chapter.

Lymphatic Drainage of Head and Neck

Earlier in this chapter the deep cervical fascia was described as having external, middle, and internal layers. This same rule can be applied to the lymphatic drainage of the head and neck. This plan is similar to one described by Last.[4] The external layer can be thought of as an outer circle of superficial or regional lymph nodes, the middle layer as a visceral layer of nodes draining the viscera of the neck such as the larynx and pharynx, and the internal circle of nodes composed of the paired carotid sheaths containing the internal jugular vein and deep cervical lymph nodes. The deep cervical lymph nodes are tributaries for both the superficial and visceral circles of lymph nodes.

Superficial Lymph Nodes

The superficial nodes may be thought of as a circle of nodes beginning on the face and extending posteriorly to the occipital area of the scalp. The efferent lymphatics of these nodes drain inferiorly along the major veins of the face and scalp. On the anterior face, buccal nodes in the cheek and facial nodes along the path of the facial vein drain inferiorly across the mandible, into the submandibular triangle, and to submandibular nodes. Inferior to the mandible, the superficial circle is composed of submandibular and anterior cervical lymph nodes. Sublingual nodes adjacent to the tongue receive afferent lymphatics from the anterior part of the face, particularly the lower lip and tip of tongue, and then drain superficially on the neck to deep cervical nodes approximately at the level of the omohyoid. The lymphatics from these nodes then enter the plexus of lymphatics in the carotid sheath, follow the internal jugular vein, and connect with other deep cervical nodes.

In the more posterior portion of the face (in the region of the parotid), afferent lymphatics begin in the scalp along the path of the superficial temporal vessels and drain inferiorly to parotid nodes in the superficial aspect of the parotid gland. Efferent lymphatics from parotid nodes course inferiorly along the common facial vein and thence to deep cervical nodes. Posterior to the ear, retroauricular nodes and occipital nodes follow their major channels to the deep cervical nodes of the internal jugular vein.

The general rule is that in the more anterior regions of the face, lymphatic drainage to the lower portion of the neck is more rapid, because it occurs along a sparser chain of nodes before proceeding to the deep cervical nodes. By contrast, in the deeper and more posterior portions of the face, the chain of lymphatic nodes and channels usually is more complicated, so that drainage requires more time before reaching the jugular lymph chain.

Deep Cervical Lymph Nodes

The deep cervical lymph nodes are a series of nodes that parallel the course of the internal jugular vein from the base of the skull to its terminus at the brachiocephalic junction. Most of the nodes are closely associated with the vein within the carotid sheath and lie deep to the sternocleidomastoid muscle. Two particular areas are notable. One is the region in which the posterior belly of the digastric crosses the internal jugular. This region usually is the site of one or more palpable lymph nodes termed the jugulodigastric nodes. Similarly, another large node or series of small nodes exists at the junction of the superior belly of the omohyoid and sternocleidomastoid muscles, which are termed the jugulo-omohyoid nodes. Efferent lymphatics from the deep nodes drain into the internal jugular trunks, which ultimately enter the venous system at the jugulosubclavian angle.

Lymphatic Drainage of Pharynx and Larynx

The upper portion of the pharynx, the nasopharynx, drains directly to the upper deep cervical lymph nodes along the jugular chain. The oropharynx and, particularly, the tonsil drain through the parapharyngeal spaces to the region of the midportion of the jugular and particularly the jugulodigastric nodes. In some descriptions, the jugulodigastric nodes are referred to collectively as the tonsillar node. The region of the hypopharynx and larynx drains principally along the vascular pedicles of the hypopharynx and larynx. The upper portion of the larynx from the false cord drains along the superior laryngeal vessels to deep cervical nodes on the internal jugular vein near the bifurcation of the common carotid artery. The lower half of the larynx (from the true cords proceeding inferiorly) drains along the interior laryngeal vessels to nodes about the pretracheal region and eventually to deep nodes near the base of the internal jugular vein.

Classification of Cervical Lymphatics

Nomenclature of the cervical lymphatics historically has been inconsistent. As the focus of oncologic surgery has shifted from radical extirpation to functional preservation, it has become more important to standardize the classification system for the cervical nodes. The American Academy of Otolaryngology–Head and Neck Surgery, along with the American Society of Head and Neck Surgery, has developed a standardized classification system for the cervical lymphatic system and for neck dissections.

The groups of lymph nodes are designated as levels I to VI. *Level I* includes nodes in the submental and submandibular triangles. *Level*

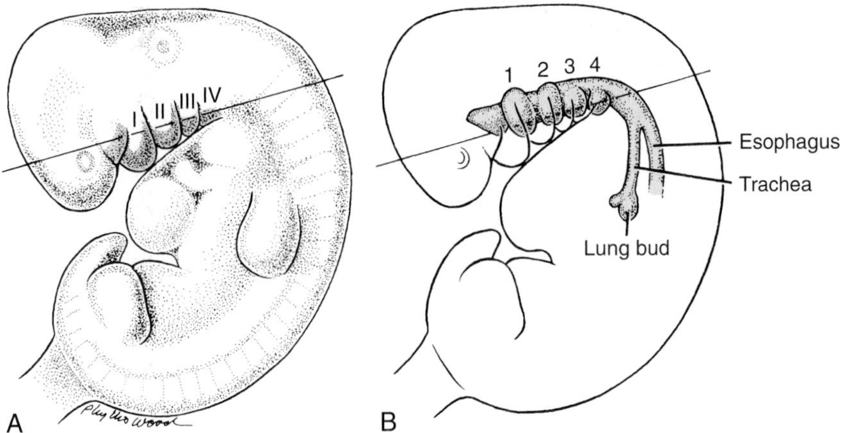

Figure 181-9. **A,** Branchial arches. **B,** Pharyngeal pouches.

II includes the upper jugular nodes located around the superior one third of the jugular vein and spinal accessory nerve extending from the carotid bifurcation or hyoid, inferiorly, to the skull base, superiorly. The anterior and posterior boundaries of this nodal group are the lateral border of the sternohyoid and the posterior border of the sternocleidomastoid muscle, respectively. *Level III* includes the middle jugular nodes around the middle third of the jugular vein, extending from the carotid bifurcation, superiorly, to the omohyoid (or cricothyroid notch, inferiorly). The anterior and posterior boundaries are the same as for level II. *Level IV* includes the lower jugular group surrounding the jugular vein from the omohyoid to the clavicle. The anterior and posterior borders are the same as in levels II and III. *Level V* is the posterior triangle group, consisting of the nodes surrounding the lower half of the spinal accessory nerve and the transverse cervical artery, including the supraclavicular nodes. The anterior boundary of level V is the posterior border of the sternocleidomastoid muscle and the posterior boundary is the anterior border of the trapezius muscle. *Level VI* includes the anterior compartment group surrounding the visceral structures of the neck from the hyoid, superiorly, to the sternal notch, inferiorly. The lateral boundary on either side of level VI is the medial aspect of the carotid sheath. This space crosses the midline and includes the perithyroidal, paratracheal, and precricoid nodes, as well as the nodes along the recurrent laryngeal nerve.[5] The terminology for neck dissection is discussed in Chapter 116.

Embryology of Head and Neck

The development of many structures in the head and neck is intimately related to either the branchial arches or the pharyngeal pouches (Fig. 181-9). These are transient embryonic structures that undergo substantial remodeling so that their original embryonic form is essentially unrecognizable by the time the infant is born. The derivatives of these structures nevertheless are important to adult morphology: Aberrations in branchial arch development may produce significant malformations.

Embryology of Branchial Arches

At 5 weeks of gestation, the area of the future face and neck of the embryo consists of five or six pairs of fingerlike masses of tissue named the *branchial arches*. Prominent in lateral profile (see Fig. 181-9), these masses are aligned in transverse orientation to the plane of the neck and are separated by clefts, termed the *branchial clefts*. The surface of the arches and clefts is lined by ectoderm, with mesodermally defined tissues contained within the branchial arches. The tissues underlying the region of the clefts are thin because of the close approximation of outpouchings from the foregut region called *pharyngeal pouches* (see Fig. 181-9). The derivatives of the arches and pouches are different because of the embryonic germ layers contained within the branchial arch (the mesoderm), whereas the pharyngeal pouches are composed of endoderm. Because of the differences in the embryonic germ layers, the following generalization can be made: In the adult, the derivatives of the branchial arch will be structures composed of muscle,

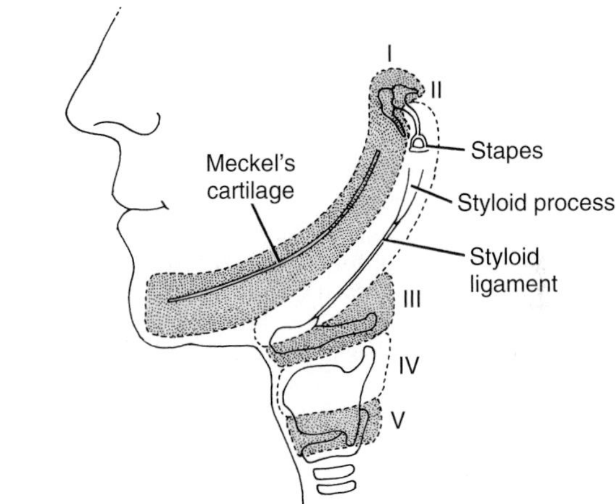

Figure 181-10. Skeletal derivatives of the branchial arches.

bone, or similar mesodermal derivatives; the derivatives of the endodermal pharyngeal pouch will be glandular or associated with the digestive tract.

Derivatives of Branchial Arches

In the early phase of branchial arch development, the mesodermal mass of the arch forms a bar of cartilage, which remodels into bone, cartilage, or other connective tissue elements in the adult. Similarly, the adult musculature of the face and neck also develops from the mesoderm of the arches. The development of these structures is considered separately.

Skeletal Derivatives

The first branchial arch is the proximal part of the first arch cartilage (Meckel's cartilage), which is remodeled and contributes to the formation of the ramus of the mandible (Fig. 181-10). The distal part of the cartilage withers, and the body of the mandible is formed from intramembranous bone. Other structures formed by the proximal part of the cartilage are the sphenomandibular ligament, anterior malleolar ligament, malleus (except for the manubrium, which is from the second arch), and incus (except for its long process, which is from the second arch).

The second branchial arch is the cartilage of the second branchial arch (Reichert's cartilage), which forms bony structures proximally and distally. Its central portion withers, leaving a fibrous band—the stylohyoid ligament. Proximally, it forms the styloid process, the manubrium of the malleus, the long process of the incus, and the stapes suprastructure. The stapes footplate is mostly derived from the otic capsule.[6,7] Distally (anteroinferiorly), the second arch cartilage forms a portion of the body of the hyoid and the lesser cornu of the hyoid bone.

In the adult, it is possible to trace the path of the embryonic second arch cartilage from the styloid process, to the stylohyoid ligament, ending at the lesser cornu of the hyoid bone (see Fig. 181-10).

The third branchial arch composes the remaining portions of the hyoid bone (i.e., the body and greater cornu).

The fourth through sixth branchial arches comprise the cartilaginous elements. These arches contribute to the formation of the thyroid, cricoid, arytenoid, corniculate, and cuneiform laryngeal cartilages.

Muscular Derivatives

In the first branchial arch, the muscles formed by mesodermal elements include the muscles of mastication: the temporalis, masseter, and medial and lateral pterygoid muscles. In addition, the tensor tympani, tensor veli palatini, anterior belly of the digastric, and mylohyoid muscles also are derived from first arch mesoderm.

In the second branchial arch, the muscles formed from mesoderm include all of the muscles of facial expression from the region of the scalp, inferiorly, to the platysma muscle in the neck. In addition to those muscles, grouped as the muscles of facial expression, the posterior belly of the digastric, the stylohyoid, and the stapedius muscles also are derived from second arch mesoderm.

In the third branchial arch, only one muscle is formed from mesoderm—the stylopharyngeus muscle, a small muscle that aids in elevating the pharynx during swallowing.

In the fourth through sixth branchial arches, the muscles include the muscles that form the pharynx and larynx. Pharyngeal muscles include the superior, middle, and inferior constrictor muscles. In addition, the mesodermal elements from these branchial arches also form the striated muscle composing the upper half of the esophagus. The inferior part of the esophagus usually is composed of smooth muscle derived from the splanchnic mesoderm of the primitive foregut.

The laryngeal muscles are also formed from mesodermal elements in the fourth, fifth, and sixth arches. These include the extrinsic muscle of the larynx and the cricothyroid, as well as all of the intrinsic muscles associated with movement of the arytenoid cartilage and true and false vocal folds.

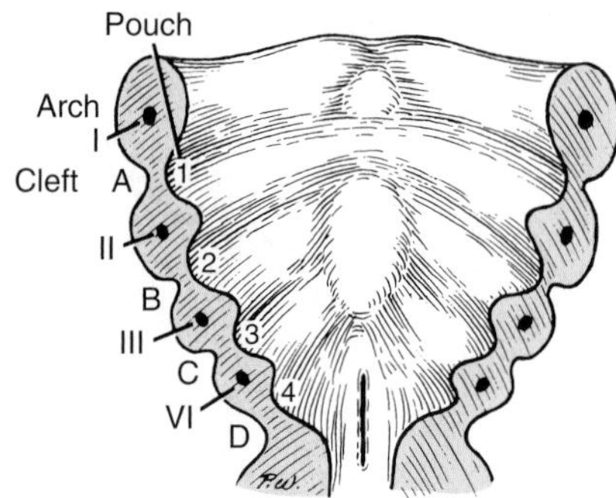

Figure 181-11. Relationships of the pharyngeal arches, clefts, and pouches in the floor of the mouth: stage I.

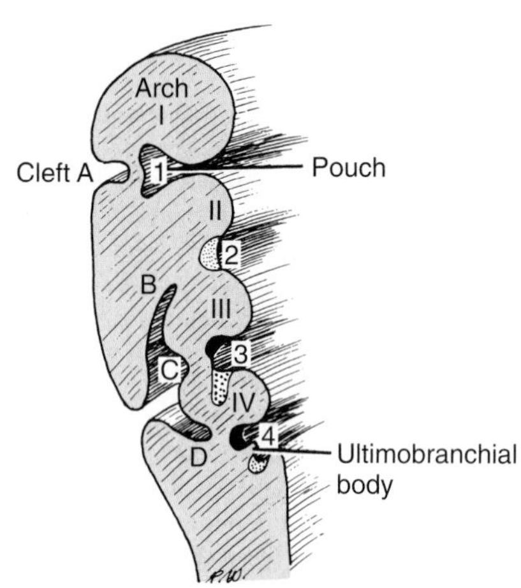

Figure 181-12. Derivatives of the pharyngeal pouches and formation of the cervical sinus: stage II.

Innervation

Because of the proximity of the developing branchial arches to the brainstem, each branchial arch receives motor or sensory innervation from an adjacent cranial nerve. A comparable parallel to this pattern occurs in the trunk, where a muscle is derived from the myotome region of a somite and receives its innervation from the adjacent segmental spinal nerve. In both cases, regardless of where the primordial muscle cell migrates, it retains its primary embryonic innervation. After each arch receives its cranial nerve innervation, then the adult pattern is established, regardless of its future migration onto the back of the head or base of the neck.

The nerve of the first branchial arch is the trigeminal nerve, which supplies motor innervation to all of the muscles derived from the first arch. In addition, sensory innervation is provided not only over the region of the mandible by the third division of the trigeminal but also over the maxillary process of the first arch and the frontal nasal process by the second and first divisions of the trigeminal nerve.

The nerve of the second branchial arch is the facial nerve, which supplies motor innervation to all of the muscles derived from this mesoderm. Other than a small sensory branch of cranial nerve VII, which may supply part of the external auditory meatus, sensory distribution of cranial nerve VII to ectoderm is absent.

Cranial nerve IX supplies the single muscle derived from the third arch—the stylopharyngeus muscle. As described later on, however, it also supplies sensory innervation to parts of the pharynx associated with this region.

The vagus nerve and the cranial part of the accessory nerve supply the muscles derived from branchial arches 3 through 6. Originating in the nucleus ambiguus of the medulla, the axonal processes of these nerves descend in the vagus nerve after exiting the skull through the jugular foramen. Specifically, the pharyngeal constrictors are supplied by the pharyngeal branch of the vagus and the transitional portion of the pharynx and esophagus by its recurrent laryngeal branch. The superior laryngeal nerve supplies sensation to the larynx by its internal branch and motor innervation to the cricothyroid muscle by the external branch. The recurrent laryngeal nerve supplies the intrinsic muscles of the larynx.

Embryology of the Pharyngeal Pouches

The pharyngeal pouches are lateral outpouchings of the foregut or region of the primitive pharynx (see Fig. 181-9). At the extreme lateral wall of each pharyngeal pouch, the endodermal lining contacts the ectodermal epithelium of a branchial cleft (Fig. 181-11). Thus, the branchial clefts are named in relation to the pharyngeal pouch with which they are apposed. The endodermal epithelium lining of either the branchial arch or the pharyngeal pouch contributes to the formation of specific elements of the pharynx in the adult.[8]

First Pharyngeal Pouch

The first pharyngeal pouch becomes elongated and incorporated into the temporal bone and forms the epithelial lining of the middle ear (Fig. 181-12). The most lateral portion of the pouch, along with the first closing plate of the first branchial cleft, forms the tympanic membrane (see Fig. 181-12). From this relationship, it is clear that the external auditory canal is nothing more than a remodeling of the first branchial cleft (Fig. 181-13).

Second Pharyngeal Pouch

The endodermal layer of the second pharyngeal pouch forms the epithelial lining of the palatine tonsil, whereas underlying mesenchymal elements contribute to the formation of the tonsil itself (see Figs. 181-12 and 181-13).

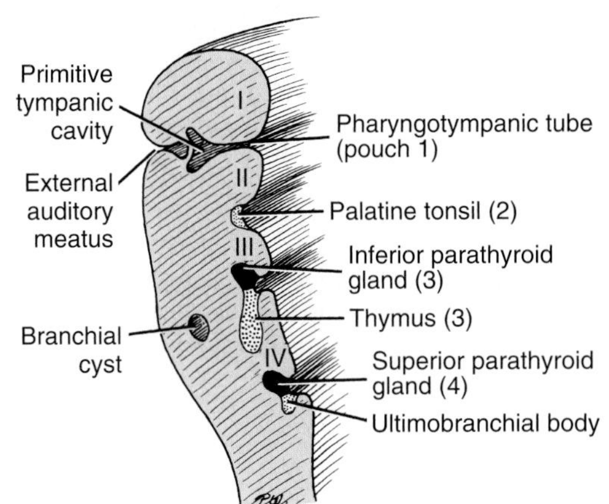

Figure 181-13. Maturation of the pharyngeal pouches: stage III.

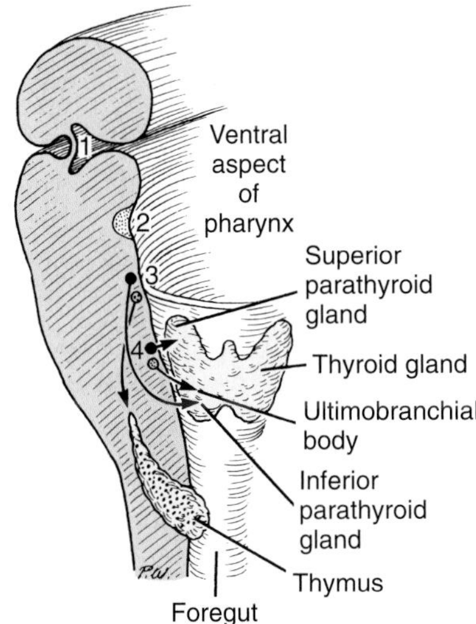

Figure 181-14. Migration of the pharyngeal derivatives into the neck: stage IV.

Third Pharyngeal Pouch

The region of the third pharyngeal pouch is subdivided into superior and inferior portions. The superior portion forms cells that eventually differentiate into the inferior parathyroid (see Fig. 181-12). The inferior portion of the third pouch becomes thymic tissue, which eventually migrates in the neck and mediastinum to form the thymus (Fig. 181-14).

Fourth through Sixth Pharyngeal Pouches

The endoderm of the fourth pouch forms the superior parathyroid gland. The adjacent area is variably named as the fifth or sixth pouch or the ultimobranchial body (see Fig. 181-13). Subsequently, the ultimobranchial body is infiltrated by cells migrating from the neural crest region. These cells eventually are incorporated into the thyroid gland and become the parafollicular cells (C cells) responsible for the secretion of calcitonin.[9,10]

Craniofacial Syndromes Related to Branchial Arch Structures

Hemifacial microsomia is thought to be related to a vascular injury in the region of the stapedial artery, resulting in microtia and mandibular hypoplasia.[11] Patients with this defect often have associated aural atresia. Mandibulofacial dysostosis, or Treacher Collins syndrome, is related to abnormalities of the first and second branchial arches. This syndrome is characterized by lid colobomata, down-slanting palpebral fissures, hypoplastic zygoma and mandible, and malformations of the external ear.[12] Other syndromes related to dysmorphogenesis of the first and second branchial arches include oculoauricular vertebral dysplasia (i.e., Goldenhar's syndrome) and branchio-oto-renal syndrome.

Branchial Cleft Remnants

The first branchial cleft becomes part of the external auditory canal, but the remaining branchial clefts are remodeled and normally do not form derivatives identifiable in the adult. However, the complicated morphodynamics of the branchial arch region seem to predispose this area to abnormalities, ranging from minor cysts to major orofacial malformations. The clinical terminology of the various branchial abnormalities is confusing. Part of the confusion results from the clinical spectrum of these anomalies—they may manifest as cysts, sinuses, or fistulae. A *cyst* has no communication with the body surface; a *sinus* communicates with a single body surface, either the skin or pharynx; and a *fistula* communicates with two body surfaces. A cystic dilation of the tract may be associated with either a sinus or a fistula. The terms *branchial cleft* and *branchial pouch* often are used interchangeably, although they refer to distinct structures. Occasionally, *groove* is used instead of *pouch* or *cleft*.

Abnormalities of First Branchial Cleft

Aberrant development of the first branchial cleft may lead to the formation of a cervical cyst or sinus in the region of the ear. Work[13] and Aronsohn and colleagues[14] emphasized the difference in the embryogenesis of preauricular cysts versus cysts of the first branchial cleft. Preauricular cysts or pits occur anterior to the external auditory canal, usually superior to the region of the tragus. In essence, they are inclusion cysts related to fusion of the ectodermal hillocks from the first and second branchial arches during formation of the auricle.[15]

By contrast, true first branchial cleft abnormalities are duplications of the membranous part of the external auditory canal, and they manifest clinically as cysts, sinuses, or fistulas. Work[13] has classified these into two types: type I, of ectodermal origin, involving only the membranous part of the canal; and type II, involving both ectoderm and mesoderm, in which duplication of cartilage also is a feature. As cystic masses or sinus tracts they may involve the parotid gland and cranial nerve VII (this particularly true of type II) or lie inferior to the ear, in the superior neck.

Abnormalities of Second through Fourth Branchial Clefts and Pouches

During closure of the cervical sinus lying between the second branchial arch and the epipericardial ridge, ectoderm may become trapped, resulting in an inclusion cyst at a later time (see Figs. 181-12 and 181-13). These are the more familiar branchial cleft cysts or sinuses, which lie on the lateral neck anterior to the sternocleidomastoid muscle. As such, they may overlie the carotid or muscular triangles of the neck. The fistulous forms of these abnormalities are surgically challenging because they may extend from the superficial area of the neck near the clavicle, superiorly, to the bed of the palatine tonsil. The course of the tract through the deep part of the neck usually lies between the internal and external carotid arteries. The pathway of this tract is easily explained on an embryologic basis. The medial wall of the cervical sinus is the region of closing plates 2 to 4 (see Fig. 181-12). A fistulous pathway breaking through into the pharynx will penetrate one of these closing plates and thereby enter either into the tonsillar bed (the second), the thyrohyoid membrane (third), or pyriform sinus or cricothyroid membrane (fourth).

Third branchial cleft sinuses, which communicate with the pharynx, travel deep to the carotid artery system in their superior extent. Thymopharyngeal cysts represent third branchial cleft remnants. As congenital cystic lesions of the neck, these are easily confused with lymphatic malformations. Remnants of the fourth branchial pouch, or pyriform sinus fistulas, may manifest as recurrent suppurative thyroiditis and usually are located on the left side.[16,17] These lesions may be associated with parathyroid, thymic, or thyroid tissue.

Isolated branchial arch remnants may manifest as subcutaneous cartilaginous tags along the anterior border of the sternocleidomastoid muscle.

Midline Lesions of the Neck

Thyroglossal duct cysts and dermoids are the most common midline lesions of the neck in children. These often are difficult to recognize clinically. The thyroglossal duct cyst derives from persistence of the embryonic thyroglossal duct, anywhere between the foramen cecum and the thyroid gland. Because of the attachments to the base of tongue, thyroglossal duct remnants will move superiorly in the neck when the patient protrudes the tongue. The thyroglossal duct remnant may contain ectopic thyroid tissue. Occasionally the cyst contains all of the functioning thyroid tissue. Because of the potential for permanent hypothyroidism after surgical excision, many investigators advocate routine preoperative assessment of the thyroid.[18,19] Ultrasound examination of the neck provides information regarding consistency of the cystic lesion and also can be used to assess for the presence of thyroid tissue in its normal position lower in the neck. Ultrasound examination is easily tolerated by children but does not give functional information. Radionuclide thyroid scans provide functional information regarding thyroid tissue (e.g., the possibility of malignancy within these lesions). Surgical excision is the treatment of choice. Thyroglossal duct remnants often involve the central part of the hyoid, necessitating removal of the midportion of the hyoid to minimize the risk of recurrence.[20]

Another midline developmental abnormality of the neck is the midline cleft. The clinical presentation varies, ranging from an area of subcutaneous absence of midline tissue, manifesting as a bluish area in the midline of the neck, to a midline vertical band. The vertical band becomes more restrictive with growth of the child and may interfere with mandibular excursion. Treatment involves excision of the band and Z-plasty.

Summary

The otolaryngologist–head and neck surgeon must be familiar with the developmental anatomy of the neck. A working knowledge of neck anatomy and embryology is critical in diagnosing and treating patients effectively.

SUGGESTED READINGS

Acierno SP, Waldhausen JH. Congenital cervical cysts, sinuses and fistulae. *Otolaryngol Clin North Am.* 2007;40:161.

Robbins KT, Clayman G, Levine PA, et al, and the Committee for Head and Neck Surgery. Standardizing neck dissection terminology: official report of the Academy's Committee for Head and Neck Surgery and Oncology. *Arch Otolaryngol Head Neck Surg.* 1991;117:601.

For complete list of references log onto www.expertconsult.com.

CHAPTER ONE HUNDRED AND EIGHTY-TWO

Anesthesia in Pediatric Otolaryngology

Veronica C. Swanson

Heike Gries

Jeffrey Koh

Key Points

- When anesthetic risk is correlated with age, children younger than 1 month of age are at the highest risk for adverse events during the procedure. The greatest improvements in patient safety have been in reducing the frequency of respiratory events. Elective procedures should be deferred until after the age of 6 months, when appropriate.
- The anesthetic plan is tailored to the patient's age—for physiologic differences as well as differences in psychological development.
- Preoperative preparation that includes patient education leads to greater satisfaction with the overall hospital experience for both child and parent.
- Routes of premedication and induction of anesthesia include oral, intranasal, intramuscular, intravenous, and inhalational.
- Decisions regarding deep versus awake extubation require careful consideration of clinical factors: Awake extubation is always the appropriate choice in patients who have difficult airway anatomy or full stomach physiology.
- Postoperative nausea and vomiting are best treated with multimodal therapy; a second dose of antiemetic agent in the same class of drug already given is rarely effective.
- Effective pain assessment and management are mandated by The Joint Commission for institutions to receive accreditation.
- Multimodal therapy for pain relief, with or without opioids, is now accepted as a more balanced approach to pain management in surgical patients. Such therapy aims to decrease the dose of any single agent, thereby improving antinociception and reducing side effects.
- Anesthetizing patients in locations outside the operating room minimizes interference with surgical needs and contributes to efficient delivery of care.
- Medical conditions with particular impact on aesthetic implications include upper respiratory infections, asthma, cystic fibrosis, diabetes mellitus, and congenital heart disease.
- The 2007 American Heart Association guidelines for the prevention of infective endocarditis in patients with congenital heart disease seek to minimize unnecessary exposure to antibiotics using evidence-based practices.
- Management of patients for bronchoscopy, adenotonsillectomy, and laryngeal surgery requires careful planning preoperatively and clear communication between surgeon and anesthesiologist throughout the procedure.

Because of the inherent complexity of the structure-function relationship in otolaryngology, pediatric otolaryngologists and anesthesiologists must work together closely in the operating room to provide optimal care to the patient. This chapter focuses on anesthesia topics that are relevant for the pediatric otolaryngologist, beginning with the safety of anesthesia for children, followed by preoperative assessment of pediatric patients. Perioperative management, including choice of drug and technique to match the situational demands, is described next. Finally, the anesthetic implications of specific diseases and the anesthetic considerations in commonly performed pediatric otolaryngology procedures are reviewed.

Anesthesia for Children

Anesthesia carries increased risk in children as compared with adults, as reported more than 50 years ago.[1] Work from the 1960s correlated this increased risk with age less than 1 year.[2] Nowadays children younger than 1 month of age are recognized as being at the highest risk,[3] which suggests that the risk of adverse events with anesthesia induction in infants is inversely proportional to age. In view of the physiologic changes that occur during the first year of life, this is not surprising. Respiratory control is immature in infants; carbon dioxide (CO_2) response curve is lower than it is in older children and adults, and hypoxia may induce apnea rather than hyperventilation.

Box 182-1

Intraoperative Monitoring Standards

Continuous presence of qualified anesthesia personnel in the operating room

Continuous evaluation of the following:

- Oxygenation
- Inspired oxygen concentration with an oxygen analyzer
- Blood oxygenation with a pulse oximeter
- Ventilation

Qualitative assessment, including chest excursion, observation of the reservoir bag, and auscultation of breath sounds

Quantitative assessment with end-tidal CO_2 analysis

A low-pressure disconnect alarm when mechanical ventilation is used

Circulation

Continuous electrocardiogram

Arterial blood pressure at least every 5 minutes

At least one of the following:

- Palpation of pulse
- Auscultation of heart sounds
- Intra-arterial blood pressure monitoring
- Ultrasound peripheral pulse monitoring
- Pulse plethysmography

Body temperature

Cardiovascular responses also are immature: The myocardium is poorly compliant, so cardiac output is rate dependent. Similarly, responses to anesthetic agents differ in accordance with patient age. Preterm and full-term newborns require lower concentrations of inhaled anesthetics than those needed in older children or adults. Inhalational agents may cause more depression of cardiac output in infants and may have a more profound effect on baroreflexes. Pharmacokinetic parameters of volume of distribution, hepatic clearance, and renal clearance differ profoundly from those in older children, affecting the dose of nearly every drug.

These differences in physiology and pharmacology are reflected in the types of anesthetic mishaps that tend to occur in newborns and infants. Inadequate ventilation and anesthetic overdose have been the most frequent sources of anesthetic morbidity and mortality in the 1980s.[4] Changes in anesthetic practice, such as improvement in monitoring (e.g., pulse oximeters and CO_2 monitors) and use of different drugs (e.g., sevoflurane instead of halothane) have decreased respiratory events and shifted the number of anesthesia-related cardiac arrests in infants toward cardiovascular causes of cardiac arrest.[5,6]

Adherence to the American Society of Anesthesiologists (ASA) monitoring standards[7] is basic to all anesthesia care performed by an anesthetist and has reduced the incidence of intraoperative complications.[8] The components of these standards are presented in Box 182-1. Most anesthesiologists consider pulse oximetry to be an indispensable part of the intraoperative monitoring armamentarium, although it has been difficult to document improvement in outcome as a result of this technique, even in a very large series.[9,10] The use of pulse oximetry alone or in combination with capnography has reduced the relative frequency of adverse respiratory events as compared with adverse cardiovascular events, perhaps because pulse oximetry and capnography are more effective for preventing respiratory events than cardiovascular events.[11]

Elective procedures should be deferred until the infant is at least 6 months to 1 year old, when anesthetic risk is likely to be lower. This is particularly true in infants who were born prematurely, because they have an increased risk of postoperative apnea until approximately 55 weeks of postconceptual age (see following). The use of trained subspecialty pediatric anesthesiologists for the care of infants and children has been suggested to be associated with improved outcomes,[12] although this contentious claim is difficult to prove.[13] More recent concern has been raised about the potential for neuronal damage in the developing brain caused by anesthetic agents. The available data are still preliminary, and no definitive human studies proving this concept have been performed. The United States Food and Drug Administration (FDA) recently launched the first phase of SAFEKIDS (Safety of Key Inhaled and Intravenous Drugs in Pediatrics), an initiative to provide seed funding for several clinical projects.[13a] Pediatric practitioners should be aware that more information probably will be presented in the coming years and may influence decisions about what age is safe to perform elective procedures.[14]

Current estimates of anesthetic mortality vary widely, depending on the definition of anesthetic death. However, mortality in healthy pediatric outpatients as the result of an anesthetic-related cause is very rare, with rates perhaps as low as 0.36 in 10,000 cases.[6,15] Accordingly, parents of otherwise healthy children can be reassured that outcomes in modern-day pediatric anesthesia are excellent.

Preoperative Assessment

Today's emphasis on cost containment has forced many changes in the practice of pediatric anesthesia. More and more patients with complex medical problems are having procedures as outpatients, which forces the preoperative contact between the anesthesiologist and the patients and family into a very few minutes. In addition, efficiency pressures have forced institutions to search for ways to maximize patient flow in surgery areas and to minimize unexpected delays or cancellations. Preoperative anesthesia clinics have developed in response to these changes.

A visit to the preanesthesia clinic before the day of surgery affords the opportunity for taking an anesthetic history; performing a physical examination; obtaining necessary laboratory tests; and informing the family about the anticipated procedures, including times for restriction of oral intake to nothing by mouth (i.e., NPO [*nil per os*]) status), premedication, anesthetic induction and maintenance, and postoperative pain management techniques. It also allows confirmation that all necessary paperwork, such as consent and surgical history and physical, is present in the medical record. An attending anesthesiologist is available for consultation for more complicated cases or to address specific clinical questions. Anesthetic risk can be discussed with patients and their families, with ample time allowed for them to ask questions. In addition, the clinic nurse can take this opportunity to educate the patient and family about the impending surgical visit and to identify fears and concerns of the parents and child.

A preoperative medical assessment includes a review of body systems and the patient's response to previous anesthetics, current medications, allergies, recent illnesses (including upper respiratory infections), and family history of problems with anesthesia. The physical examination concentrates on airway anatomy, including the mouth, jaw, teeth, and neck, and includes chest and heart auscultation to confirm the absence of significant cardiorespiratory disease. Laboratory tests are obtained as indicated by the child's condition and type of surgery planned, rather than as a routine component of the assessment.[16] Identification of clinical problems at a preanesthesia visit also allows appropriate evaluation or referral before surgery, thereby avoiding delay or cancellation on the day of surgery.

Preparation for Anesthesia

Behavioral Preparation

The days and hours leading up to surgery can be an anxious time for both children and parents. Fears about hospitalization are common among children, including fear of separation, pain, loss of control, and even death. Many of these fears are dependent on the child's age[17] (Table 182-1). Awareness of these developmental stages allows the anesthesiologist to better anticipate the needs of most children. In addition, understanding the impact of parental anxiety on a child's anxiety can help in the selection of interventions that will be helpful to both the child and the parents.

Details of the anesthetic and surgical experience should be presented in age-specific language for children of appropriate age.[18] Children who are given specific information before surgery have been shown to be less anxious than children who are given only general information.[19] Movies or videotapes can help children and parents cope with

Table 182-1

Age-Specific Concerns of Children

Age	Specific Concerns
Infant (6-18 months)	Separation anxiety
Toddler (1-2 years)	Fear of strangers, loss of mastery of the environment
Preschool (2-5 years)	Separation anxiety; difficulty distinguishing reality from fantasy; fear of pain, mutilation
School age (6-12 years)	Fear of the unknown, pain, mutilation, loss of control, autonomy
Adolescent (13-18 years)	Precarious sense of self; fear of pain, mutilation, loss of control, autonomy

From Orr RJ, Lynn AM. *Curr Rev Clin Anesth*. 1991;12:29.

the mysteries of hospital routines.[20] Comprehensive preoperative preparation programs have been shown to be helpful for reducing preoperative anxiety and enhancing coping behavior in children.[21] This may be especially important for children who will require repeated procedures, allowing them to learn coping strategies and to develop a better understanding of the environment in which they will receive their care. Parents also should be involved in these programs, because decreasing their anxiety is likely to provide the added benefit of decreasing the child's anxiety further.[22] These efforts are important even if pharmacologic agents will be used to decrease anxiety, because the combination of psychological and pharmacologic interventions can produce synergistic effects.[23]

Premedication

The choice of premedication is based on the age and specific needs of the patient. The usual goals of premedication are to reduce anxiety and to ease separation from parents. Because most children fear needles, the oral administration of sedatives has become the standard of care at many institutions. Children who are younger than 8 months of age generally do not need premedication and separate easily from their parents. Children between 8 months and 8 years of age often experience enough preoperative anxiety that preoperative medication may be helpful. Midazolam (0.5 to 1.0 mg/kg up to a maximum of 20 mg), mixed in flavored syrup and administered orally 10 to 20 minutes beforehand, usually smoothes the separation from the parents and induction of anesthesia, and has become the most popular agent for preoperative sedation for children.[24] Midazolam usually is well tolerated, although a rare decrease in oxygen saturation or blood pressure may be observed. In addition, intravenous flumazenil (10 µg/kg, administered over 1 minute, repeated as needed for a total of 5 doses; maximum 0.2 mg/dose, and 1 mg total dose) can be administered to reverse adverse effects such as oversedation, paradoxical effect, or emergence delirium.

Older children may be willing to have an intravenous line started preoperatively, especially if a topical anesthetic cream such as EMLA (eutectic mixture of local anesthetics) or ELA-Max (Ferndale Laboratories, Ferndale, Michigan) is used. EMLA cream is a mixture of lidocaine and prilocaine that penetrates intact skin and, when applied for 60 minutes or more, significantly decreases the pain associated with an intravenous insertion.[25,26] EMLA should be used with caution in children younger than 3 months of age or in children who are receiving other medications that may induce methemoglobin because of the risk of methemoglobinemia.[27] Plasma concentrations of lidocaine and prilocaine achieved with topical application are well below the toxic level,[27] but they may be higher in children with traumatized or inflamed skin. Another effect of EMLA that may be problematic is vasoconstrictive blanching, which makes the identification of potential intravenous insertion sites difficult for some practitioners. ELA-Max is an alternative to EMLA, and it contains only lidocaine in a liposomal matrix that allows for effective absorption across intact skin.[28] ELA-Max has been shown to provide equal topical anesthesia to EMLA, and it has a quicker onset of 30 minutes.[8,29] ELA-Max also produces less blanching than that seen with EMLA. If an intravenous line is placed, midazolam or another sedative can be titrated intravenously until the desired effect is achieved. Although the topical anesthetic creams are the most frequently used, alternative methods for providing topical anesthesia may be standard in some institutions.

Younger children may not accept oral premedication well, making this method of administration as anxiety-provoking as separating the child from his or her parents without any premedication. Alternative methods do exist. Intranasal administration of midazolam (0.2 to 0.3 mg/kg) using either an atomizer or simply a needle-less tuberculin syringe is easy in a patient small enough to be held or restrained.[30] This agent begins acting immediately after dosing and reaches peak concentrations by 14 minutes, having the advantage of increased bioavailability with minimal first-pass metabolism in the liver.[31] Intramuscular administration of premedication becomes necessary in larger children with behavioral issues that limit patient cooperation—autism, for instance. Because intramuscular injection is technically easier than intravenous line placement, this technique can be achieved quickly, and the child then be allowed some time with the parent, to minimize the trauma from the encounter. Intramuscular ketamine at a dose of 2 to 5 mg/kg or a combination of intramuscular ketamine and midazolam causes sedation and dissociation from the environment, making the patient more approachable for procedures, anesthesia induction, and so on. Larger doses of ketamine administered intramuscularly (up to 10 mg/kg) can induce general anesthesia (see following discussion). Anticholinergic agents may be desirable when copious airway secretions (commonly seen with ketamine) are a concern, or when vagal tone from airway manipulation produces decreases in heart rate and cardiac output. Halothane, an inhalation agent used only in a few countries outside of the United States, is more likely to cause bradycardia and a significant reduction in cardiac output in children younger than 6 months of age, than in in older children. The routine use of anticholinergic agents with halothane in these younger patients can prevent these changes.[32] Atropine (0.02 mg/kg) or glycopyrrolate (0.01 mg/kg) given intravenously at the time of induction can obviate the pain of an intramuscular injection.

Nothing-by-Mouth Orders

To minimize the risk of the aspiration of gastric contents during the induction of anesthesia, an adequate period of fasting must be maintained. Traditionally, both food and fluids have been withheld after the midnight before surgery. However, a prolonged period of fasting is uncomfortable for children, is unpleasant for the family, and risks hypovolemia. It has recently been recognized that the administration of clear liquids to children up to 2 to 3 hours before induction does not increase gastric residual volume or acidity as compared with a more prolonged fast.[33,34] In addition, morbidity and mortality rates for aspiration of gastric contents in children are exceedingly low.[35] Thus, fasting guidelines have been liberalized in recent years, and they are shown in Table 182-2. There is some debate about whether breast milk should be considered a solid or clear liquid, with many institutions allowing breastfeeding within the same guidelines as clear liquids. Nevertheless, in giving these instructions to parents, it is important to emphasize the safety issues involved to maximize compliance and avoid unnecessary delays in the start of the procedure.

Anesthetic Induction

Anesthesia can be induced by mask inhalation of a potent anesthetic agent in oxygen with or without nitrous oxide (inhalation induction), by injection of a sedative-hypnotic agent through an intravenous catheter (intravenous induction), or by intramuscular injection. As much as possible, the choice of technique is given to children; younger children tend to fear needles and prefer an inhalation induction, whereas

Table 182-2

Recommended Preoperative Fasting Guidelines for Children

Ingested Material	Minimum Fasting Period (hours)
Clear liquids	2
Breast milk	4
Infant formula	6
Light meal*	6

*A light meal typically consists of toast and clear liquids. Meals that include fried or fatty foods or meat may prolong gastric emptying time.
Adapted from Practice guidelines for preoperative fasting and the use of pharmacologic agents to reduce the risk of pulmonary aspiration: application to healthy patients undergoing elective procedures: a report by the American Society of Anesthesiologists Task Force on Preoperative Fasting. *Anesthesiology*. 1999;90:896-905.

older children and teenagers usually accept an intravenous induction. Inhalation induction will take longer in teen aged and older patients than in younger patients because of age-related physiologic differences. This prolonged time to effect must be taken into consideration if an inhalation induction is selected in this age group but does not preclude such an induction. Certain clinical factors (e.g., obesity, severe gastroesophageal reflux, full stomach) also may influence the choice of induction technique toward intravenous.

Parental Presence

With increasing frequency, parents are expressing a desire to be present at the time of their child's anesthetic induction.[36] Although parents' motives vary, most hope that the child's anxiety will be lessened by the emotional comfort of their presence. Some hospitals have induction areas outside of the sterile envelope of the operating room. If not, parents can be dressed in cover gowns and escorted into and out of the operating room for the induction.

Studies examining the impact of parental presence have had variable results, with some showing no significant impact,[37] some showing a decrease in patient anxiety,[38,39] and others showing an increase in patient anxiety.[40] Parents with a high anxiety level seem to have a negative impact on their child, whereas calm parents seem to have a positive impact on their anxious child during induction.[41] One survey reported that a majority of anesthesiologists are in favor of the practice of having parents present during induction,[42] and many hospitals tend to support this request as a mechanism to improve patient and parent satisfaction. Thus, it is likely that the trend will continue. Parents should be thoroughly educated about what to expect and how they can best help their child. They must agree to leave the induction area immediately when instructed to do so, and one member of the care team must be identified to help them during the induction. Highly anxious parents should be encouraged not to participate.

Inhalation Induction

For many years, halothane was the agent of choice for inhalation induction because of its lack of pungency relative to other agents. A more recently developed alternative, sevoflurane, is even less pungent than halothane and has fewer cardiovascular side effects, making it the current pediatric inhalational induction agent of choice. A small amount of favorably scented liquid (e.g., bubble gum flavor, for instance) applied to the inside of the mask disguises the odor of the anesthetic agent and improves the patient's acceptance of the technique.

Many anesthesiologists will begin the induction with the patient breathing 50% to 70% nitrous oxide (which is odorless) before introducing sevoflurane, thus making the addition of the sevoflurane less distressing. Noise in the room should be kept to a minimum during anesthesia induction, and the anesthesiologist often tells the child an entertaining story to direct the child's thoughts away from the reality of the situation. As the concentration of the anesthetic agent is increased, most children lose consciousness in less than 1 minute. The parents, if present, can be ushered out at this point, and an intravenous catheter can then be placed.

Intravenous Induction

Intravenous induction requires the presence of an intravenous catheter and thus is reserved for older children or teenagers, children with a preexisting intravenous catheter, children who need a rapid-sequence induction because of a full stomach, or children who object to an inhalation induction. Owing to slower uptake of inhaled anesthetic agents, inhalational induction takes much longer in older, heavier children, with consequently higher risk for laryngospasm and bronchospasm. An intavenous induction is therefore also the preferable method in this patient group.

The most common agent for intravenous induction is propofol, an alkylphenol that is formulated as a 1% solution in a white soybean oil, egg lecithin, and glycerol emulsion. Propofol is highly lipophilic and rapidly redistributes throughout body compartments, with a distribution half-life of approximately 2 minutes and an elimination half-life of approximately 30 minutes. The dose for the induction of anesthesia varies with age[43]: Infants 1 to 6 months of age require approximately 3 mg/kg, whereas older children require approximately 2.5 mg/kg. The major advantages of propofol are a rapid, clear-headed recovery with minimal associated nausea and vomiting. This has made it the intravenous induction agent of choice for outpatient procedures. The major disadvantage is pain on injection, particularly into small veins.[44] Lidocaine (0.5 to 1.0 mg/kg) administered intravenously before or during propofol injection may decrease the incidence of pain. Propofol may cause hypotension, apnea, and desaturation. Propofol also can be used for anesthesia maintenance as an intravenous infusion of 100 to 200 μg/kg per minute. This technique can be very useful for patients who have a history of severe postoperative nausea or who are undergoing procedures in which postoperative nausea is especially common (e.g., tympanoplasty). Many pediatric anesthesiologists use a propofol infusion to provide anesthesia during bronchoscopy, because it provides a reliable, stable method of administering anesthesia with spontaneous ventilation while sharing the airway and decreases the exposure of the surgeon to unscavenged anesthetic gases.

An alternative intravenous agent for induction is thiopental, an ultrashort-acting barbiturate that produces sleep in healthy, unpremedicated children; a dose of 4 to 6 mg/kg induces sedation within 1 minute of administration.[45] This drug can produce hypotension through both vasodilating effects and direct myocardial depression and must be used with caution in hypovolemic patients or patients with poor myocardial contractility. It also can produce prolonged sedation as a consequence of accumulation in fat stores if higher doses or repeated doses are given.

Rapid-Sequence Induction

Patients with a full stomach are at increased risk for the aspiration of stomach contents during the induction of anesthesia. Patients who require full stomach precautions include those who have not fasted for an adequate period, those with gastrointestinal obstruction, trauma patients whose gastric motility is depressed, or those who are at a mechanical predisposition for aspiration (e.g., patients with ascites). It is mandatory that these patients have an intravenous induction. Patients are preoxygenated with 100% oxygen by mask and then given an induction dose of a hypnotic and a rapid-acting muscle relaxant—either succinylcholine (2 mg/kg) or rocuronium (1.2 mg/kg). Application of manual pressure over the cricoid (known as the Sellick maneuver) can be performed in an attempt to seal the esophagus and to prevent passive regurgitation.[46] Pressure is not released until the endotracheal tube is in place, proper position is confirmed, and the cuff, if necessary, is inflated. At the end of the procedure, these patients should be allowed to emerge completely before extubation, to ensure adequate airway protection.

Intramuscular Induction

Ketamine is a derivative of phencyclidine with potent analgesic and amnestic properties. Anesthetic induction can be achieved with the recommended dose of 1 to 3 mg/kg intravenously or 5 to 10 mg/kg intramuscularly. As noted previously, ketamine is very useful as an intramuscular induction agent in children who are combative or unable to cooperate with a standard inhalation or intravenous induction, often because of intellectual disabilities and behavioral disorders. Ketamine is an excellent choice for anesthetic induction in hypovolemic patients because of its sympathomimetic properties; it rarely causes hypotension in these patients. Ketamine may be the intravenous induction agent of choice in patients with reactive airways[47] because it increases circulating catecholamines and causes the relaxation of tracheal, bronchial, and alveolar smooth muscle.

Ketamine tends to produce copious secretions and should be accompanied by the administration of atropine or glycopyrrolate. Nystagmus and diplopia are common side effects and will resolve as the drug is cleared from the patient's circulation. Intraoperative and postoperative dreams and hallucinations have been reported,[48] more often in older than in younger children, and less often when other sedative-hypnotic agents are used in conjunction with ketamine. If this agent is given preoperatively with the parents still present, they should be informed to expect these side effects.

Anesthesia Maintenance

Inhalational Agents

Nitrous Oxide

Nitrous oxide is a widely used inhalational induction agent in children. Its popularity is a result of its low solubility, which results in rapid uptake and distribution. Nitrous oxide also is odorless and does not cause cardiovascular depression. Although nitrous oxide allows the delivery of lower concentrations of other anesthetic agents, nitrous oxide itself is not a very potent anesthetic agent. Consequently, it must be delivered in high concentration to have an analgesic and hypnotic effect, thereby limiting the concentration of oxygen that can be delivered; it is not useful for patients who require high concentrations of oxygen and should be avoided in patients with pulmonary hypertension as it may aggravate it. Because of the lack of potency and the controversial increased incidence of postoperative nausea and vomiting (PONV), it has been used less and less for anesthesia maintenance. A 34-fold difference has been noted in the blood-gas coefficients of nitrogen (0.013) and nitrous oxide (0.46); thus, nitrous oxide will enter air-filled cavities faster than nitrogen can leave. In a fixed cavity such as the middle ear, the result is an increase in pressure. During tympanoplasty, the middle ear pressure generated by nitrous oxide can lift off the tympanic membrane graft. Therefore, nitrous oxide usually is avoided entirely during those procedures.[49] Nitrous oxide use also may present a hazard for patients with previous reconstructive middle ear surgery.[50]

Sevoflurane

Sevoflurane has completely taken the place of halothane in pediatric institutions in the United States. It is a valuable addition to the anesthesiologist's armamentarium for several reasons. First, it is less pungent than halothane, and it is even better tolerated during inhalation induction. Second, it has a blood-gas partition coefficient similar to that of nitrous oxide, so induction and emergence times are shorter than with halothane. Third, it has fewer cardiovascular effects than halothane.

Sevoflurane has several disadvantages: Its offset is so rapid that without adjunctive administration of narcotics, the perception of and response to pain may be accentuated.[51] There are reports in the literature of a significant incidence of emergence excitement associated with cases in which sevoflurane was used.[52] For these reasons, sevoflurane has assumed a role as an induction agent and a maintenance agent for very short procedures, but it often is replaced by isoflurane or desflurane after induction, depending on case type and anesthesiologist preference. Like all halogenated inhalational agents, it is a potential trigger agent for malignant hyperthermia and should be avoided in susceptible patients.

Isoflurane

Isoflurane has been used for many years as a standard maintenance inhalational agent for children and adults. In practice, it offers no clear advantage for the pediatric otolaryngology patient. It is more pungent and not nearly as well accepted by children during inhalation induction as sevoflurane. Isoflurane does increase rather than decrease heart rate. It also causes decreases in blood pressure, but unlike with halothane, the mechanism is peripheral vasodilation rather than direct myocardial depression.[53]

Desflurane

Desflurane is the newest inhalational agent to be introduced into clinical practice. Its principal advantage is its quicker time to recovery as compared with sevoflurane.[51] It appears to be well tolerated as a maintenance anesthetic, because it provides stable hemodynamics and respiratory parameters during its use. Similar to sevoflurane, desflurane has been associated with increased agitation and emergence delirium.[44] However, this effect does not seem to occur frequently enough to avoid its use in children.

Desflurane does have an irritant effect on the airway, making it contraindicated for inhalational induction or for use during airway procedures such as bronchoscopy. However, many centers have adopted a practice of inducing anesthesia with sevoflurane and then switching to desflurane to take advantage of its quick recovery time while avoiding its airway effects during induction. It also has been suggested that this agent may be particularly useful in neonates and formerly premature babies, in whom residual anesthesia effects may increase the risk of apnea postoperatively.[54]

Intravenous Agents

Opioids

Fentanyl

Fentanyl is the most commonly used supplement to anesthesia in children. Although the usual intravenous dose is 1 to 2 µg/kg, doses in excess of 100 µg/kg have been given to cardiac surgery patients with minimal cardiovascular depression.[55] An initial peripheral vasodilation occurs, but tachyphylaxis to this side effect occurs with additional dosing. Preterm and full-term newborns have variable and prolonged clearance, probably related to reduced hepatic blood flow.[56] In addition, they are extremely sensitive to the effects of fentanyl on chest wall rigidity. In neonatal patients who are not intubated, fentanyl should be given only in small increments.

The effect of low-dose fentanyl is terminated largely by redistribution, thereby resulting in a rapid reduction in clinical effect. Because fentanyl is highly lipophilic, however, higher or repeated doses result in drug accumulation. Clearance then becomes dependent on metabolism,[57] and the clinical effect, including respiratory depression, may last for hours. Chest wall rigidity has been reported after rapid fentanyl administration, although the etiology of this problem is unclear. Bradycardia may occur as a result of increased vagal tone, especially when given with other agents that may have a similar effect.

Morphine Sulfate

Overall, morphine is the most frequently used opioid in children. It can be used in the operating room to supplement inhalational agents and to provide postoperative analgesia. The usual intravenous dose is 0.05 to 0.1 mg/kg as part of a balanced anesthetic technique, although higher doses may be used for a narcotic-based technique. The dose may need to be reduced in critically ill children or young infants. The half-life after intravenous administration is approximately 3 hours in older children but is significantly longer in infants as a result of diminished clearance.[58] The major side effect is respiratory depression, which results in diminished minute ventilation, with a greater effect on respiratory rate than tidal volume. Many believe that newborns are at higher risk than older children for respiratory depression, although it is unclear whether this reflects a difference in pharmacokinetics or pharmacodynamics. Infusions of morphine at rates of 10 to 30 µg/kg per hour have been described in small infants without significant respiratory depression.[59] Appropriate monitoring for apnea should occur in premature infants and those neonates with a history of apnea and bradycardia. Histamine release is also common with the administration of morphine, and it most commonly results in a localized or generalized rash. Bronchospasm and hypotension have been reported, but they are much less common.

Hydromorphone

Hydromorphone has become a commonly used alternative to morphine. It is approximately five to seven times more potent than morphine, with the usual intravenous dose ranging from 0.015 to 0.02 mg/kg. Its half-life is similar to that of morphine, and it has a similar duration of action. Hydromorphone may be useful in patients with renal failure, because its metabolic by-products are less active than morphine's are. In addition, hydromorphone may be a good alternative for those patients who suffer side effects (e.g., itching, nausea, hallucinations) with morphine. As with other opioids, respiratory depression is the most concerning side effect, but it is rare with appropriate dosing.

Meperidine

The use of meperidine has dramatically decreased due to its unique side effect profile and the availability of equianalgesic alternatives. The principal metabolite of meperidine is normeperidine, a compound that can cause neurologic excitation manifested as tremors, irritability, or seizures. This side effect is especially pronounced with prolonged use or in patients with hepatic or renal dysfunction. Meperidine's superiority over other opioid agonists in the treatment of postoperative shivering probably is related to its kappa receptor activity and the one reason that it has not become entirely obsolete.

Alfentanil

As a short-acting analog of fentanyl, alfentanil commonly is used for short outpatient procedures. It is approximately one-fourth as potent as fentanyl and has one-third the duration of action. It has a very fast onset of action (1 minute) and a short elimination half-time (1.5 hours). It is less lipophilic than fentanyl, and the dose range is 10 to 20 μg/kg, given intravenously. Renal failure does not alter the clearance of alfentanil. Besides the opioid-related side effects, thorax rigidity and bradycardia may be seen.

Remifentanil

Remifentanil has the same analgesic potency as that of fentanyl. The key feature of remifentanil is the ester side chain hydrolysis by blood and tissue esterases, resulting in rapid metabolism (elimination half-time is 10 to 20 minutes). This results in zero order kinetics, meaning that its offset of action is 10 to 20 minutes after discontinuation of the infusion, regardless of the duration of the infusion. Said differently, it does not accumulate. It does have a rapid onset, and because of its short duration of action, it usually needs to be administered as an continuous intravenous infusion at the rate of 0.05 to 1 μg/kg/min for neonates and up to 2 μg/kg/min for older children. Pharmacokinetic parameters of remifentanil are unchanged by hepatic or renal disease. Disadvantages are the high cost and the lack of postoperative analgesia, which can be overcome with application of longer-acting opioids at the end of surgery.

Muscle Relaxants

Succinylcholine

Succinylcholine is the only depolarizing muscle relaxant. With the advent of intermediate-acting nondepolarizing relaxants, the use of succinylcholine for routine surgical procedures is declining, primarily as a result of side effects that relate to its depolarizing mode of action (see later). However, it remains the most rapid-acting of all muscle relaxants, and it is still indicated for use in rapid-sequence inductions and in the treatment of laryngospasm. Intravenous administration of 1.5 to 2.0 mg/kg achieves 95% twitch depression in 40 seconds,[60] resulting in excellent intubating conditions. Succinylcholine also can be given intramuscularly (4 to 5 mg/kg) if the intravenous route is unavailable, although the clinical effect is delayed in onset, depending on perfusion to the area of deposition.

The side effects of succinylcholine are numerous. Some degree of increase in masseter muscle tone is common and, in some cases, is extreme enough to mimic true trismus.[61] This is an important distinction to make, because as many as 50% of patients with trismus after succinylcholine are biopsy positive for susceptibility to malignant hyperthermia.[62] Succinylcholine can also cause bradycardia as a result of an increase in vagal tone; this effect is especially prominent in younger children and infants. The decline in heart rate usually is transient and, if not, is responsive to intravenous atropine; occasionally, asystole is seen. Hyperkalemia can be seen as a result of depolarization of the myoneural junction; increases of serum potassium of 0.5 mEq/L occur even in normal children.[63] Life-threatening hyperkalemia after succinylcholine administration can occur in children with burns, tetanus, paraplegia, encephalitis, crush injuries, and neuromuscular disease.[63] Myoglobinemia occurs in approximately 40% of children anesthetized with halothane who are given succinylcholine; this effect can be partially attenuated with a previous dose of a nondepolarizing agent to prevent fasciculations. A series of cardiac arrests were reported in boys who were given succinylcholine, with subsequent development of massive muscle breakdown and potassium release. The presumed etiology was previously undiagnosed muscular dystrophies.[64] In 1994, in response to these reports, the manufacturer placed a warning on the package insert cautioning the practitioner about the routine use of succinylcholine. As a result, many pediatric anesthesiologists have abandoned the routine use of succinylcholine except for rapid-sequence inductions and to treat laryngospasm. Succinylcholine may soon be replaced in that role by rocuronium, which has an onset of action of less than a minute, making it suitable for a rapid sequence induction. The disadvantage of rocuronium has been the long time to reversal after an intubating dose has been given. This makes it suboptimal and perhaps contraindicated for patients with a difficult airway. Sugammadex, a selective relaxant-binding agent, is in phase 3 trials. If approved, it would make rocuronium rapidly reversible and thereby make the risks of succinylcholine unnecessary. Sugammadex is not yet available for use in the United States.

Of note, 90% of an intravenous dose of succinylcholine is rapidly hydrolyzed in the plasma by pseudocholinesterase. Patients with deficient or reduced levels of pseudocholinesterase exhibit a prolonged effect from succinylcholine.

Nondepolarizing Muscle Relaxants

A variety of nondepolarizing muscle relaxants are available. These agents vary in dose, speed of onset, and duration of action. As shown in Table 182-3, the pharmacologic properties of these drugs may be different in infants from those in older children. The choice generally is based on the duration of the surgical procedure. As noted, rocuronium has been shown to produce good intubating conditions, but with a slightly longer onset of action (less than 1 minute) than with succinylcholine (less than 30 seconds).

Total intravenous anesthesia (TIVA) is a continuous titration of intravenous drugs for maintenance of anesthesia. Drugs used often are a propofol-remifentanyl or propofol-alfentanil combination. This technique provides malignant hyperthermia–safe anesthesia in the malignant hyperthermia–susceptible patient; it often is used in patients with severe postoperative nausea and vomiting and is also the technique of choice in some airway cases (see later on).

Emergence from Anesthesia

The decision of whether to extubate a patient while he or she is awake or under surgical planes of anesthesia (deep extubation) depends on a number of factors. Deep extubations are smoother and facilitate rapid turnover. Considerations in making this decision include the patient's age, airway anatomy, underlying disease, the presence of blood or secretions in the airway at the time of extubation, the presence of a full stomach preoperatively, the ability of the postanesthesia care unit staff to manage an obstructed airway, and the immediate availability of an individual skilled in reintubation should it be required. Deep extubation is preferred in patients with asthma or in those for whom coughing would be contraindicated. Factors that favor awake extubation include a full stomach at the start of the procedure, age younger than

Table 182-3

Intubation Doses, Onset Times, and Recovery Times for Commonly Used Muscle Relaxants

	Intubating Dose (mg/kg)			
	Adults	Children	Onset Times* (min)	Recovery Times in Infants (min)
Mivacurium	0.3	0.2-0.3	1.5-2	15-20
Atracurium	0.5	0.5	2	40-60
Cisatracurium	0.1	0.1-0.2	2.5	53
Vecuronium	0.07-0.1	0.1	2.4	35
Rocuronium	0.5-1.0	0.6-1.2	1.3	42
Pancuronium	0.1	0.1	2.5	50

*Time to maximal blockade.

6 months, difficult airway anatomy for either masking or intubating, copious blood or secretions in the airway, and a predisposition to apnea. Systematic comparisons of awake versus deep extubation have revealed that patients extubated while awake have lower oxygen saturations (probably because of coughing during emergence), but there is no difference in overall morbidity or mortality.[65,66] Either technique can be performed safely; the anesthesiologist should have both approaches in his or her armamentarium and, using clinical judgment, choose the one that best fits the situation.

Postoperative Management

Nausea and Vomiting

Nausea and vomiting can result in an unpleasant recovery from surgery and anesthesia as well as a delayed discharge from the postanesthesia recovery unit and an increase in overall cost. In the pediatric population, the incidence is variable and depends on the type of surgery, the type of anesthetic used, gender, age, history of motion sickness, and adequacy of hydration.[67] Although the overall incidence is lower in children younger than 2 years of age, children older than 3 years have an average vomiting incidence of more than 40%. Procedures such as tonsillectomy and middle ear surgery may be associated with an incidence of vomiting as high as 70%. The use of narcotics, halogenated inhalational agents, and perhaps nitrous oxide increases the risk of nausea and vomiting. By contrast, propofol reduces the incidence of vomiting as compared with that with halothane in children undergoing adenotonsillectomy.[17]

Therefore, antiemetics often are given prophylactically for children at risk for PONV and a multimodal approach has been shown to be the most effective one.[68] The use of intravenous ondansetron (50 to 100 μg/kg up to 4 mg), intravenous dexamethasone (150 to 500 μg/kg up to 8 mg), and intravenous droperidol (50 to 75 μg/kg up to 1.25 mg) is evidence-based for prophylaxis for patients at risk for PONV and for treatment of patients with PONV.

Serotonin (5-hydroxytryptamine$_3$)-receptor antagonists, such as ondansetron, have shown efficacy and safety in prophylaxis and therapy of PONV, having a greater antivomiting than antinausea effect.[69] When prophylaxis with serotonin receptor antagonist fails, a rescue therapy with serotonin receptor antagonists is not recommended within the first 6 hours of surgery because it confers no additional benefit.[70]

Another drug that has been shown to help control PONV during the 24 hours after surgery is dexamethasone. Children who receive a single intraoperative dose of dexamethasone were two times less likely to vomit during the first 24 hours than children who received placebo. Routine use in four children would be expected to result in posttonsillectomy emesis experienced by one fewer patient. Additionally, children receiving dexamethasone were more likely to advance to a soft to solid diet on posttonsillectomy day 1 than were those children receiving placebo.[71]

Droperidol is an antidopaminergic antiemetic. While effective in the treatment of PONV, its sedating and extrapyramidal side effects should be considered when choosing it.[72] In 2001, the U.S. FDA issued a black box warning against the use of this drug due to concerns of serious cardiac arrhythmias secondary to QT prolongation. Since that time, the restriction has been lifted. However, it has never returned to the prevalent use that was seen prior to the ban. An overwhelming majority of anesthesiologists surveyed (92%) did not consider the ban warranted, as torsades de pointes was seen mostly when the drug was administered in very high doses or when there were confounding factors. Still, prudence would limit its use to cases in which patients do not have underlying cardiac disease, other classes of antiemetics have been exhausted, and the maximum total pediatric dose is less than 100 μg/kg or 2.5 mg total.[73]

Finally, an inexpensive but effective method of reducing the incidence of nausea and vomiting is to withhold oral fluids during the postoperative period until the child asks for them, because forced oral fluids increase the incidence of vomiting and delay discharge.[67,74,75] This can be safely done by generously hydrating the patient with intravenous fluids intraoperatively. Nontraditional treatment methods such as acupressure are being studied and thus far confirm their effectiveness in the prevention of PONV; they are useful adjuncts, especially in view of the total absence of side effects.[76]

Postintubation Croup

In children up to approximately 8 years of age, the subglottis is the narrowest portion of the airway, and it may be the source of postoperative airway obstruction secondary to mucosal swelling. A reduction in the reported incidence of postintubation croup from 1%[77] to 0.1%[78] may be obtained with use of proper-sized, non–tissue-reactive tubes that allow an air leak around the tube at 25 cm H_2O or less.

Racemic epinephrine (0.5 mL of 2.25% in 2.5 to 3.0 mL of normal saline for children weighing 15 kg or more) nebulized in oxygen is the management of choice for postintubation croup; the effect is thought to result from the vasoconstriction of the subglottic mucosa. (The dose varies, ranging from 0.2 mL for infants weighing less than 5 kg, 0.3 mL for 5- to 10-kg infants, and 0.4 mL for 10- to 15-kg infants.) Because symptoms can recur within 2 to 4 hours, the child should be observed for 4 hours after treatment before being sent home. If frequent and repeated treatments are necessary, hospital admission should be considered. Dexamethasone (0.3 to 0.5 mg/kg) also may be tried,[79] although its effect is slow in onset if it occurs at all.

Pain Management

The theory that children, particularly neonates, perceive pain less acutely and therefore do not need pain medication is no longer accepted.[80] As a result, since the early 1990s there has been a significant change in how pediatric pain is approached. Perhaps the most powerful sign of this change was that the Joint Commission (formerly the Joint Commission on Accreditation of Healthcare Organizations [JCAHO]) added pain management to its accreditation review in 2000. Areas that now must be addressed by accredited institutions include pain assessment, pain treatment, and education about pain management.[81]

Pain assessment can be challenging in children. Assessing the degree of pain in preverbal children is problematic, although several observational scales have been developed to assist with this population.[82] Children 4 to 8 years of age have been shown to be capable of giving a self-report with simplified tools, and older children can use the same scales as those for adults.[83] Patients in the intensive care unit setting (immediately postoperatively) and cognitively impaired children remain populations to be studied in the area of pain assessment.

Intravenous opioids—whether given by bolus, infusion, or patient-controlled analgesia—are the mainstay of therapy for severe pain.[84] Children 8 years of age and older (and some mature 6- to 7-year-old children) do well with patient-controlled analgesia, tend to use less total drug, and have a better feeling of control than with traditional methods of administration. Younger children requiring intravenous opioids may benefit from administration accomplished using parent- or nurse-controlled analgesia. Appropriate parent education is a necessary prerequisite to parent-controlled analgesia.

Milder degrees of pain can be handled with nonopioid analgesics. Acetaminophen (10 to 15 mg/kg every 4 to 6 hours to a maximum of 4 g every 24 hours), alone or with oxycodone (0.1 to 0.15 mg/kg), is useful for children who can take oral medications. Rectal acetaminophen can also be given, although doses of 20 to 40 mg/kg are necessary to achieve serum levels equivalent to those obtained with 10 to 15 mg/kg given orally.[85] Ketorolac (0.5 mg/kg IM or IV every 6 hours for up to 48 hours) is a nonsteroidal anti-inflammatory agent that has potent analgesic properties; these may be equivalent to those of morphine[86] but without the respiratory depression or nausea associated with opioids. However, ketorolac requires 30 to 45 minutes for onset, has a 12% incidence of nausea, and may be associated with a higher incidence of bleeding because of effects on platelet function.[87] Nonopioid analgesics also are a good adjunct to opioid and other pain medications: multimodal therapy has been shown to be most effective in the treatment of pain, especially in difficult-to-treat cases.

Codeine, often used as a first-line oral opioid, seems to be a weak analgesic. Essentially a prodrug of morphine, it needs to be converted to its active form in the liver. Approximately 10% of the population lack the enzyme CYP2D6 and will not achieve pain relief from codeine. Accordingly, a more rational approach is to use a stronger oral analgesic as a first-line agent, especially after significantly painful procedures. As with all opioids, nausea and vomiting are potential side effects and may be more prevalent with use of codeine.

Sedation and Anesthesia Outside of the Operating Room

Over the past 10 years, an increasing number of procedures have been performed outside of the operating room. Reasons for this development include physician time constraints, reimbursement changes, new technology for procedures that cannot be done in the operating room, and the development of new anesthetic agents. This practice has been recognized to be accompanied by a risk of adverse events potentially greater than that for operating room procedures, as a result of monitoring variation, poor presedation evaluation, inadequate training, and lack of adequate recovery procedures.[88] More recently, a greater degree of scrutiny has been given to the practice of sedation for children outside of the operating room. In an effort to improve safety, the Joint Commission has been instrumental in forcing institutions to develop policies to improve the care of children and adults who are receiving sedation, as part of overall accreditation efforts. In addition, specialty organizations have developed policy statements about this topic.[89-91] In many institutions, this has meant that pediatric anesthesiologists are more directly involved with this activity than in the past.

A large number of procedures that are performed in hospitals may require use of sedation or analgesia, especially in children. Painful procedures (e.g., lumbar puncture, bone marrow biopsy, chest tube placement) are obvious examples. Other procedures, such as magnetic resonance imaging or gastrointestinal endoscopy, also may require sedation or anesthesia because of the distressing nature of one or more aspects of the examination or the need for immobility. In the context of otolaryngology, the most common candidates for out-of-the-operating-room or clinic procedures may be patients requiring the removal of pressure equalization tubes, nasal ciliary biopsy, fine-needle aspiration, or the removal of sutures. One report suggests that these procedures can be performed in the clinic safely and with less cost using intravenous sedation as compared with general anesthesia in the operating room.[92]

In general, a pediatric sedation service oversees sedation or anesthesia for a majority of out-of-the-operating-room procedures performed at our institution. All children scheduled for procedures receive a phone call before their appointment to identify any significant medical problems and to provide NPO instructions. On the day of the procedure, the patient arrives approximately 30 minutes before the planned time of the procedure for application of topical anesthesia cream. A sedation nurse then starts an intravenous line, after which the pediatric anesthesiologist provides intravenous sedation or anesthesia. After the procedure is completed, the sedation nurse oversees the patient's recovery until he or she is ready for discharge. For less invasive procedures in cooperative patients, the sedation nurse may provide conscious sedation with oral, intravenous, or intranasal medications rather than use the method described previously.

Another option is for the otolaryngologist to provide the sedation, often with oral or intravenous midazolam, possibly combined with fentanyl. Even with this type of conscious sedation, practitioners should be aware of their institution's policy about sedation. A preprocedure evaluation should be documented, monitoring should be performed during the procedure and documented, and appropriate recovery procedures should be followed. Documentation of NPO status also may be relevant, depending on the depth of sedation planned.

Medical Conditions with Anesthetic Implications

A number of medical conditions may modify preoperative preparation and intraanesthetic or postanesthetic management.

Upper Respiratory Infection

The decision of whether to anesthetize a child with an upper respiratory infection (URI) is recurrent in pediatric anesthesia. In making this decision, it is helpful to know the risks involved. Deterioration in pulmonary function is typical during a URI, including a decrease in flow rates such as forced expiratory volume in 1 second (FEV_1),[93] a decrease in mucociliary clearance,[94] and an increase in airway reactivity.[95] Resolution of these abnormalities can take up to 6 weeks after the resolution of symptoms.

These changes in pulmonary function have other clinical correlates. McGill and colleagues[96] reported on 11 cases (no denominator) of intraoperative atelectasis identified by chest radiography in children anesthetized within 4 weeks after a URI. Children with a URI may be at increased risk for postoperative desaturation,[97] croup, laryngospasm, airway obstruction, and reactive airway disease. Another prospective study evaluated adverse respiratory events in 1078 children with URIs undergoing elective surgical procedures. This study identified a significantly higher incidence of respiratory events among children with URIs, although none of these events was associated with long-term sequelae. Risk factors associated with adverse events included a history of prematurity, a history of reactive airway disease, parental smoking, and surgery involving the airway.[98,99] Conversely, a prospective study of a series of nonintubated children undergoing myringotomy failed to show a difference in perioperative complications between asymptomatic children and children with URI symptoms.[100]

Other factors also must be considered. Do the symptoms result from allergy rather than infection? How severe is the URI? A child with fever, cough, malaise, and myalgias may be at higher risk than a child with mild rhinorrhea. How elective is the surgery? How much inconvenience would result for the family from cancellation or postponement? Is an escalation in care likely from proceeding with the surgery at that time? How often is the child symptom-free? In view of the frequency of URIs in some children and the time required for the resolution of pulmonary function abnormalities, it may be difficult to find a disease-free interval.

Frequently, the decision seems to involve more art than science. In equivocal cases, a leukocyte count and a chest radiograph may be helpful.[98] Measurement of hemoglobin saturation in a patient breathing room air may identify some at-risk children, but it is not very sensitive. Unfortunately, no combination of historical features, physical findings, or laboratory tests can identify the child at risk. A discussion of the potential risks and benefits with the parents will allow them to participate in the decision-making process. Good communication between the anesthesiologist and the otolaryngologist is essential for establishing some consistency in approach.

Premature Infants

In the early 1980s, a high incidence of apnea was reported after the administration of general anesthesia during the first few months of life to children who had been born prematurely (at 37 weeks of gestational age or before).[101,102] The risk probably extends to approximately 55 weeks of postconceptual age, with the curve approaching but never reaching a zero percent risk, and is inversely related to both postconceptual and postgestational age and hematocrit.[45]

Although the etiology of apnea is unknown, most episodes are central in origin; however, nearly one third are associated with airway obstruction.[103] Halogenated inhalation anesthetics blunt the ventilatory response to CO_2 and hypoxia, even in subanesthetic concentrations,[29] thereby accentuating preexisting abnormalities of respiratory control that may result in an apneic event. Although apnea has been reported after general, spinal,[104] and caudal[105] anesthesia, one prospective series has suggested that the incidence is lower after regional techniques without adjunctive sedation than after either general or regional anesthesia with intravenous sedation.[106] Administration of caffeine intraoperatively also may lessen the incidence of postoperative apnea.[107]

Elective procedures should be postponed until premature infants reach 55 weeks' postconceptual age, at which time the incidence of apnea is less than 1%.[45] Children at risk for postoperative apnea should have cardiorespiratory and pulse oximetry monitoring for a period of time after surgery. There is some institutional variability in the exact duration of monitoring; however, most will monitor for a period of 4 to 24 hours, depending on the infant's actual postconceptual age, history of apnea, and overall health status.

Asthma

A history of asthma in a child is important to the anesthesiologist, because good preoperative preparation and careful intraoperative anesthetic management can usually prevent serious episodes of bronchospasm. History of severity (e.g., current medication, recent wheezing history, past need for emergency department visits or hospitalization) correlates well with intraoperative risk. For children with a history of frequent asthma attacks, consultation with the child's primary care provider can help ensure that treatment is maximized before surgery. A thorough physical examination that includes chest auscultation is necessary to rule out active bronchospasm. Elective surgery should not be performed in the presence of active wheezing. In a child with active wheezing, pulmonary function testing (especially FEV_1) may be useful for documenting the extent of obstructive disease and the potential for reversal with bronchodilators. Improvement in expiratory flow rates after a trial of bronchodilators suggests that adjustments in bronchodilator therapy before elective surgery may be beneficial.[108] A variety of bronchodilator compounds are available for preoperative and intraoperative use, including β_2-agonists, corticosteroids, and anticholinergics.[108] Nebulized β_2-agonists such as albuterol are the most commonly used agents during the perioperative period because of ease of administration, good efficacy, and low incidence of side effects. Preoperative administration of albuterol may be helpful for decreasing the incidence of intraoperative bronchospasm.

The most common cause of bronchospasm in susceptible patients is instrumentation of the airway under light planes of anesthesia.[109] Both general and regional anesthetic agents can be used to obtund airway reflexes. Lidocaine (1 to 2 mg/kg) can be sprayed into the trachea or given intravenously to prevent reflex-induced bronchospasm.[110] All inhaled halogenated anesthetics prevent or ameliorate bronchospasm by increasing bronchial caliber and pulmonary compliance, decreasing pulmonary resistance, and improving gas exchange during active bronchospasm.[111,112] Ketamine also acts as a bronchodilator and may be useful as an induction agent in patients with active wheezing. Extubation of the trachea while the patient is under surgical planes of anesthesia, followed by a slow, smooth emergence, minimizes the risk of bronchospasm. However, careful attention must be paid to airway patency until the child is awake.

Cystic Fibrosis

Early diagnosis and antibiotic treatment, management of chronic pulmonary disease and malabsorption have improved the health and survival of children with cystic fibrosis (CF); currently, nearly 50% of affected patients are older than 18 years of age.[112a] Pansinusitis develops in more than 90% of children with CF, and nasal polyps in 20%; the latter may require surgery. The child with CF presents a significant challenge to the pediatric anesthesiologist; malnutrition, dehydration, and pulmonary insufficiency are all potential concerns. One series reported that 13% of patients with CF had some anesthetic complication.[113]

Preoperative evaluation of patients with CF is important for minimizing postanesthetic morbidity. The severity of pulmonary disease can be quantitated with historical features (e.g., degree of exercise intolerance, amount of sputum production) and a thorough physical examination (e.g., respiratory rate, work of breathing, quality of breath sounds, skin color). Patients with evidence of significant disease should have oximetry and perhaps arterial blood gas analysis. Electrocardiogram and echocardiogram also should be considered to screen for right ventricular dysfunction (cor pulmonale). If the patient is cooperative, pulmonary function tests may help to quantitate the degree of pulmonary compromise and serve as a baseline to assess the impact of preoperative therapy. Consultation with the pulmonologist caring for the patient also may provide important information about baseline condition and medical therapy.

In patients with significant pulmonary disease, a preoperative "tune-up" may help prevent perioperative complications. A regular program of chest physiotherapy includes chest percussion and postural drainage. Sputum samples are sent for culture and sensitivity, and antibiotic therapy may be indicated. The patient should be well hydrated to avoid inspissation of secretions. Patients not taking oral vitamin K supplements are given enteral vitamin K. If premedication is required, a benzodiazepine can be given with minimal risk of respiratory depression. An anticholinergic can be given if desired; the concern about excessive drying of secretions has not been a significant clinical problem. General anesthesia can be maintained with inhalational agents, because they are potent enough to allow for the administration of high-concentration oxygen, and they provide bronchodilation. The shorter-acting inhalational agents (e.g., sevoflurane) may be of particular benefit because of their shorter recovery time. An endotracheal tube usually is placed to deal with the most commonly reported complications, which include copious secretions, airway irritability, and compromised oxygenation.[103] Ventilation usually is assisted or controlled, to prevent intraoperative loss of lung volume and subsequent atelectasis. All delivered gases are humidified, and intravenous hydration is maintained to facilitate the clearance of secretions. Tracheal suctioning is performed as necessary, with emphasis on maximal pulmonary toilet before extubation. At the end of the procedure, the trachea is extubated after the patient is awake and breathing spontaneously.

Diabetes Mellitus

The key to the successful anesthetic management of a child with diabetes mellitus is careful administration of dextrose and insulin and frequent monitoring of blood glucose. Knowledge of the patient's daily insulin type and amount and the resulting blood glucose is important to the development of an anesthetic plan. A normal diet and insulin regimen should be maintained up to the day of surgery. Diabetic children should be scheduled for the first surgical procedure of the day when possible, because this timing usually simplifies their glucose management.

One of several approaches to the management of glucose and insulin can be taken[114]:

1. On the morning of surgery, half of the usual morning insulin dose is given as regular insulin (onset in 30 minutes; peak effect in 2 to 4 hours; duration of action of 6 to 8 hours) after an intravenous infusion of 5% dextrose in 0.45% normal saline is established at 1500 mL/m^2 per day. Serum glucose levels are monitored frequently before and after surgery and are maintained between 100 and 200 mg/dL, with a sliding scale of regular insulin given until the patient is eating and can resume the usual insulin regimen.

2. On the morning of surgery, a continuous infusion of insulin and glucose is initiated (1 or 2 units of insulin per 100 mL of 5% dextrose). Adjustments can be made in the ratio to maintain blood glucose in the desired range.

3. For procedures that are brief and will allow oral intake in the recovery room (e.g., myringotomy), no insulin and no glucose are given. These cases should be scheduled as the first of the day. When oral intake is reinitiated, 40% to 60% of the usual daily insulin dose is given subcutaneously, and blood glucose is monitored carefully.

The appropriate use of short-acting anesthetic agents and nonsedating antiemetics will allow this group of patients to return to oral intake as soon as possible. Preoperative endocrinology consultation may be helpful for patients with poorly controlled blood glucose.

Congenital Heart Disease

Patients with congenital heart disease are seen by many other surgical specialists for management of congenital abnormalities associated with a specific syndrome, as well as for treatment of other diseases found in children without heart disease. Some will have had their defect already repaired (e.g., neonatal coarctation of the aorta). Some will have received surgical palliation and thus have achieved a state that is physiologically better tolerated but does not represent series circulation (e.g., hypoplastic left-sided heart syndrome in a patient who has had a stage 1 Norwood procedure). Some will not yet have had the defect repaired because it is of secondary priority to more urgent problem (e.g., a patient with an atrial septal defect who has a foreign body in the airway). In each of these situations, an in-depth understanding of the patient's anatomy and physiology will dictate anesthetic goals.

The first issue is whether the patient requires antibiotics for subacute bacterial endocarditis (SBE) prophylaxis. In 2007, the American Heart Association, in collaboration with a number of interested medical organizations, published revised evidence-based guidelines for the prevention of infective endocarditis. Of the underlying principles from which the previous (1997) guidelines had been formed, whether antimicrobial prophylaxis was effective in humans was called into question by the committee. The new guidelines pointed toward use of infective endocarditis prophylaxis in significantly fewer patients[115] (Tables 182-4 and 182-5). If given orally, the antibiotics should be administered 1 hour before the procedure. If given intravenously or intramuscularly, they should be administered within 30 minutes before the start of the procedure (Table 182-6). For recommendations outside the scope of otorhinolaryngology, appropriate practice guidelines should be consulted.

Premedication is the next consideration in this group of patients. In general, cardiac patients tolerate premedications well. We routinely give 0.7 to 1.0 mg/kg of oral midazolam 10 to 30 minutes before taking the patient to the operating room. In patients for whom this premedication has been insufficient in the past, we may add 5 to 10 mg/kg of oral ketamine, with the recognition that this will prolong recovery time. If an intravenous line has already been established, the usual doses of intravenous premedication agent is given. The relative exceptions are the patient with pulmonary hypertension and the patient in whom an increase in pulmonary vascular resistance (PVR) will cause right-to-left shunting—specifically cyanotic patients. Elevation in CO_2 as a result of hypoventilation from premedication causes this shift. With this patient population, an anesthesiologist should be in close proximity should the premedication not be well tolerated and control of the airway and ventilation becomes necessary. Monitoring is always indicated in these patients for administration of premedication.

For patients with a pacemaker, the child's electrophysiology cardiologist should be consulted about intraoperative recommendations, because all pacemakers are different. In most cases, the recommendation will be to have a magnet available that, when placed over the pacemaker, puts it into an asynchronous mode. In this case, it will fire

Table 182-4

Cardiac Conditions Associated with the Highest Risk of Adverse Outcome from Endocarditis for which Prophylaxis Is Recommended

Prosthetic cardiac valve
Previous infective endocarditis
Congenital heart disease (CHD)* • Unrepaired cyanotic CHD, including cases in which palliative shunts or conduits have been placed • Completely repaired congenital heart defect with prosthetic material or device, whether placed by surgery or by catheter intervention, during the first 6 months afte the procedure† • Repaired CHD with residual defects at the site or adjacent to the site of a prosthetic patch or prosthetic device (which inhibits endothelialization)
Cardiac transplant recipients in whom cardiac valvulopathy develops

*Except for the conditions listed above, antibiotic prophylaxis is no longer recommended for any other form of CHD.
†Prophylaxis is recommended because endothelialization of prosthetic material occurs within 6 months after the procedure.[114]

Table 182-5

Ear, Nose, and Throat Procedures and Subacute Bacterial Endocarditis Prophylaxis

Prophylaxis	Procedures
Recommended	Tonsillectomy, adenoidectomy Surgical procedures that involve respiratory mucosa Rigid bronchoscopy
Not recommended	Endotracheal intubation Flexible bronchoscopy Tympanostomy tube insertion

Table 182-6

Prophylactic Regimens for Oral and Respiratory Tract Procedures[115]

Regimen/ Patient Factors	Drug	Dosage
Standard		
Oral dosing	Amoxicillin	50 mg/kg PO up to 2.0 g
No oral dosing	Ampicillin *or*	50 mg/kg IM or IV up to 2.0 g
	Cefazolin *or*	50 mg/kg IM or IV up to 1.0 g
	Ceftriaxone	50 mg/kg IM or IV up to 1.0 g
Penicillin-allergic		
Oral dosing	Cephalexin *or*	50 mg/kg PO up to 2.0 g
	Clindamycin *or*	20 mg/kg PO up to 600 mg
	Azithromycin *or*	15 mg/kg PO up to 500 mg
	Clarithromycin	15 mg/kg PO up to 500 mg
No oral dosing	Cefazolin *or*	50 mg/kg IM or IV up to 1.0 g
	Ceftriaxone *or*	50 mg/kg IM or IV up to 1.0 g
	Clindamycin	20 mg/kg IV up to 600 mg

Table 182-7

Factors Influencing Pulmonary Vascular Resistance and Systemic Vascular Resistance

Vascular Resistance	Increases	Decreases
Pulmonary	PEEP, high airway pressure	Low airway pressure
	Low FiO_2	High FiO_2
	Acidosis, high $PaCO_2$	Alkalosis, low $PaCO_2$
	High hematocrit	Low hematocrit
	Sympathetic stimulation	Anesthesia
	Hypoxia	Drugs (e.g., NO, sildenafil)
	Atelectasis	
Systemic	Vasoconstrictors	Vasodilators
	Direct manipulation	Potent inhalation agents

FiO_2, inspired oxygen concentration; NO, nitric oxide; $PaCO_2$, arterial carbon dioxide concentration; PEEP, positive end-expiratory pressure.

without sensing (VOO mode). This is rarely necessary, because most (but not all) implanted pacemakers will do this automatically when faced with prolonged periods of electromagnetic interference. Finally, the grounding pad for the electrocautery should be placed as far away from the pulse generator as possible so that the path from electrocautery to grounding pad does not cross the mediastinum.

In managing the anesthetic procedure, it is important to prevent the administration of air bubbles in the intravenous fluids. Many of these patients have shunts that may allow air to pass from venous to systemic circulations, thereby increasing the risk for stroke, myocardial ischemia, renal ischemia, and so on.

For classification of the anatomy and circulation, the clearest view of the anatomy is obtained by visualizing a red blood cell traveling through the circulation, including all points at which a shunt may exist.

Table 182-8

Diagnosed Disorders by Age Group in Children Undergoing Bronchoscopy for Airway Obstruction

	Frequency (%) by Age Group		
Diagnosis	Younger than 1 Year	1 to 3 Years	Older than 3 Years
Congenital defects*	43	8	3
Acquired defects†	12	13	15
Normal findings	4	1	1
Total	69	22	19

*Laryngomalacia, tracheomalacia, bronchomalacia, vocal cord paralysis, vascular ring, hemangioma, cysts.

†Subglottic stenosis, papillomatosis, infection (e.g., tracheitis, epiglottitis).

Modified from Wiseman NE, Sanchez I, Powell RE. Rigid bronchoscopy in the pediatric age group: diagnostic effectiveness. *J Pediatr Surg*. 1992;27:1294.

Adopting this scheme makes it easier to sort out the anesthetic goals. Regardless of how the anatomy is arranged, it features a pulmonary circulation and a systemic circulation. With an understanding of their relationship to each other, the clinician can manipulate the resistances of the respective circulations and, in so doing, influence the degree and direction of shunting within the boundaries of what the anatomy will allow (Table 182-7). Poor ventricular function will dictate choice of an anesthetic that relies more on narcotics and less on inhalation agents.

In patients with cyanotic heart disease, polycythemia develops as a compensatory state to improve oxygen delivery in the long term. Hematocrit should therefore be measured early as a baseline and should be kept near 40 to support oxygen delivery. However, blood flow becomes sluggish when the hematocrit rises above 60. In these patients, phlebotomy may be considered to prevent ischemia resulting from stasis. The patient's cardiologist should be consulted if phlebotomy is considered as a therapeutic option.

Patients with congenital heart disease have very special needs. Except for the most severely ill of them, they tolerate noncardiac surgery quite well. However, their care needs to be optimized by an anesthesiologist who is familiar with the care of this patient population; understanding their physiology and anatomy is critical.

Anesthetic Considerations for Specific Procedures

Rigid Bronchoscopy

Anesthesia for rigid bronchoscopy presents a significant challenge for the pediatric anesthesiologist, for several reasons. First, bronchoscopy most often is indicated for the diagnosis and management of children younger than 1 year of age, predominantly because of congenital defects[116] (Table 182-8); this is relevant because anesthetic risk appears to be highest in this age group.[2,3] Second, patients who require bronchoscopy often present with difficult airway anatomy or with compromised oxygenation and ventilation; these factors may predispose them to intraoperative problems. Finally, the need to share the airway with the endoscopist demands effective two-way communication and coordination to ensure a smooth anesthetic and to prevent complications. Thus, the importance of communication between anesthesiologist and endoscopist during preoperative planning and intraoperative management cannot be overstated. Preparation should include assessment of the bronchoscope to facilitate a connection between the bronchoscope and the anesthesia circuit.

Anesthetic technique may be modified in accordance with the child's age and the suspected diagnosis, the underlying impairment of oxygenation and ventilation, the estimated duration of the procedure, and the training and experience of both the endoscopist and the anesthesiologist. The choice of anesthetic agents and techniques often is driven by the diagnosis. In evaluating a patient with stridor or other evidence of a compromised lumen, spontaneous breathing allows for the dynamic assessment of the pathophysiology that is critical for appropriate diagnosis. Anesthesia can be induced with either intravenous (sodium thiopental, ketamine, or propofol) or inhalation (sevoflurane) agents with oxygen. Inhaled rather than fixed agents are preferred when high-grade obstruction of the upper airway is suspected, because their effect is more readily reversed, and they more reliably preserve spontaneous ventilation during induction. In either case, after induction of anesthesia, total intravenous anesthesia (as with an infusion of propofol and alfentanil, for instance) avoids the disadvantageous situation of nonscavenging of inhaled anesthetics, with exposure of inhaled anesthetics to the health care team. Nitrous oxide must be used with caution in patients with compromised oxygenation, and it is contraindicated in patients with air trapping because of the risk of lung overinflation. Heliox, a low-density gas mixture that contains 70% helium and 30% oxygen, seems to be effective for improving the respiratory condition of infants with acute bronchiolitis or croup by increasing laminar gas flow through the narrowed bronchioles, thereby improving gas delivery and reducing accompanying tachycardia and tachypnea.[117]

After the patient is adequately anesthetized, the airway can be sprayed with 4% lidocaine, which provides local anesthesia to the larynx and trachea and reduces the total requirement of anesthetic agents. Lidocaine doses up to 7 mg/kg have been proved to be safe if they are administered over 15 minutes.[118] Intravenous lidocaine (1 to 2 mg/kg) is helpful,[119] but it is not as effective as the properly administered topical agent.

Use of a pediatric bronchoscope and rod lens telescope permits good visualization of the airway while oxygen with or without an inhaled anesthetic is delivered by way of the side-arm attachment. Use of the 2.5-, 3.0-, and 3.5-mm internal-diameter bronchoscopes, however, is associated with increased resistance to breathing. In combination with anesthetic agents that depress respiration, this increased resistance may result in compromised ventilation and oxygenation during spontaneous breathing.[120] The telescope should be removed periodically to allow the child to breathe without the resistive load. Constant communication between the anesthesiologist and the endoscopist is essential.

When spontaneous ventilation is not necessary, the adjunctive administration of short-acting muscle relaxants can allow the use of lighter planes of anesthesia. Propofol can be used adjunctively with airway topical anesthesia and a muscle relaxant or narcotic. Propofol has the advantage that it can be given continuously during the procedure, thereby resulting in a more constant level of anesthesia than can be achieved with inhalational agents, the delivery of which may be interrupted repeatedly. The choice of muscle relaxant can be made on the basis of the anticipated duration of the procedure. In practice, most bronchoscopic procedures are performed without any muscle relaxant; paralysis is the exception rather than the rule. Infusion of a short-acting narcotic (e.g., alfentanil, remifentanil) may be an alternative to a muscle relaxant, thereby allowing for adequate depth of anesthesia without muscle relaxation. Another advantage of total intravenous anesthetic is that the health care professionals in the room are not exposed to the inhalational gases that cannot be scavenged effectively using the side arm of a bronchoscope.

During the removal of a foreign body, close communication between the anesthesiologist and the endoscopist is essential. A joint decision should be made about maintaining spontaneous ventilation versus using positive-pressure ventilation. Adequate relaxation of the upper airway and glottis reduces the risk that the foreign body will be lost when it is pulled out of the airway with the grasping forceps and the bronchoscope.

In 1967, Sanders described a system in which oxygen at 50 to 60 psi was directed down the bronchoscope in intermittent bursts.[121] With this system, duration of bursts is determined by balancing chest rise with estimated airway pressures. Exhalation is then passive and depends on the recoil of the chest wall musculature. Although the device usually is successful for both oxygenating and ventilating patients, a number of potential problems exist. Because room air is entrained by the Venturi effect, hypoxemia may be seen in some patients. Peak inflation pressures and flow rates are influenced by the driving pressure, the diameter and shape of the bronchoscope, the diameter and length of the injector, and the angle from the axial line of the bronchoscope. Because of the smaller diameter of pediatric bronchoscopes, flow rates tend to be lower and inflation pressures to be higher than with use of adult bronchoscopes. Tidal volumes may be low in patients with poor lung compliance. Because of the higher inflation pressures, pneumothorax or pneumomediastinum may occur.[122] Finally, blood, infectious, or particulate matter in the airway may be forced distally by high-pressure bursts.

Hypoxemia and CO_2 retention are the most frequent complications of bronchoscopy. Early detection and prompt intervention usually result in resolution without incident. Pulse oximetry monitoring is mandatory. Monitoring of ventilation with capnography is impossible during bronchoscopy because of dilution of expired gas with high fresh gas flows, making observation of chest wall movement essential. A precordial stethoscope also is useful to auscultate breath sounds. Pneumothorax, although rare, must be kept in mind if acute deterioration of ventilation and oxygenation occurs, particularly if accompanied by a decrease in lung compliance and blood pressure. A portable chest radiograph should be obtained if the index of suspicion is high. Ventricular premature beats can occur in the presence of hypercarbia and light levels of anesthesia. Normal sinus rhythm usually returns promptly with a reduction in the CO_2 tension, an increase in the anesthetic depth, the administration of intravenous lidocaine (1 mg/kg), or a change to another anesthetic agent.

Bronchospasm can also occur during bronchoscopy, particularly in patients with a history of reactive airway disease or active inflammation of the airway. Frequently, bronchospasm results from instrumentation of an inadequately anesthetized airway, particularly if the bronchoscope is in contact with the carina. Removal of the instrument and deepening the anesthetic topically or systemically usually will resolve the problem. If these measures do not, administration of a β-sympathomimetic agent such as aerosolized albuterol (0.05 to 0.15 mg/kg in 5% solution) is indicated.

When the examination is complete, the bronchoscope is removed, and bag-and-mask ventilation with 100% oxygen is instituted. An endotracheal tube may be inserted if the patient is apneic; if bleeding, presence of secretions, or difficult anatomy makes the airway tenuous; or if the patient has a full stomach. Otherwise, the patient may be awakened without an endotracheal tube so long as close observation by qualified personnel can be provided until airway reflexes have returned.

Adenotonsillectomy

Adenotonsillectomy has become a less common procedure during the past decades, because the indications for this surgery have changed. With more effective antimicrobial therapy, the percentage of patients with recurrent infection as the indication for surgery has declined, and the percentage of patients with obstructive symptoms has increased; today, 75% of tonsillectomies are performed to remove obstructions.[123] With this change has come a greater appreciation that adenotonsillar hypertrophy may lead to obstructive sleep apnea (OSA) (Box 182-2) and, in the extreme, to cor pulmonale (see Chapter 183, Obstructive Sleep Apnea Syndrome). Because of the need to prevent cor pulmonale in patients with OSA, the adenotonsillectomy population has become younger; 60% of children operated on for obstruction are younger than 8 years of age.[124] Of children younger than 3 years who require tonsillectomy, 81% have an obstruction.[124] A careful history of coagulation disturbance in either the patient or a family member should be elicited preoperatively, with appropriate laboratory workup performed only for positive histories.

Box 182-2

ICSD-2 Criteria for Pediatric Obstructive Sleep Apnea

1. Parent or caregiver report of snoring, labored breathing, or other obstructive symptoms during sleep
2. Parent or caregiver report of at least one associated symptom:
   Paradoxical chest wall motion during inspiration
   Movement arousals
   Excessive perspiration
   Unusual sleeping positions (e.g., neck hyperextension)
   Daytime symptoms: hyperactivity, aggressive behavior, or sleepiness
   Impaired growth
   Headache on waking
   Secondary enuresis
3. Polysomnograph (PSG) documents at least one scoreable respiratory event lasting at least two respiratory cycles in duration per hour of sleep (criteria subject to revision as additional data become available)
4. PSG demonstrates either—
   At least one of the following findings:
   i. Frequent arousals associated with increased respiratory effort
   ii. Oxygen desaturation with apneic events
   iii. Hypercapnia in sleep
   iv. Excessively negative esophageal pressure fluctuations
   Periods of abnormal gas exchange during sleep (hypoxemia, hypercapnia, or both) with snoring, paradoxical chest wall motion, and at least one of the following:
   i. Frequent arousals during sleep
   ii. Excessively negative esophageal pressures swings
5. The disorder is not better explained by other sleep disorders, medical or neurologic conditions, or by medication or substance use

From American Academy of Sleep Medicine. *The International Classification of Sleep Disorders*. 2nd ed. Westchester, Ill: American Academy of Sleep Medicine; 2005.

Sedative premedication should be used with caution in children with OSA, because these patients are sensitive to both the sedative and the ventilatory depressant effects of sedative-hypnotic drugs. An inhalation induction is most commonly used, with careful monitoring and attention to airway patency, which often can be improved with jaw thrust, insertion of an oral airway, or the addition of continuous positive airway pressure during spontaneous breathing.

Intubation can be accomplished either with the patient under deep inhalational anesthesia or after the administration of a short- or intermediate-acting nondepolarizing muscle relaxant. An oral Ring-Adair-Elwyn (RAE) tube generally is used because of the low profile it provides under the self-retaining mouth gag. Careful monitoring of breath sounds is necessary, because the tube can become obstructed or dislodged during placement, insertion of and removal of the mouth gag.

Recently, the flexible laryngeal mask airway (LMA) has begun to be used as an alternative to intubation for adenotonsillectomy.[125] The flexible LMA has tubing that is much more flexible than that of the original LMA, thereby allowing use of the mouth gag without fear of dislodging the LMA from its proper position. Reports thus far suggest that the LMA is safe and reliable for managing the airway during this procedure,[113,126] and its use has become more common. Factors that may contraindicate the use of the LMA include full stomach, inability to ventilate adequately through the LMA, and surgeon preference. One study has directly compared LMA with the endotracheal tube for tonsillectomy, with results suggesting that the use of the LMA resulted in inferior surgical access.[127]

Anesthesia usually is provided with a volatile agent, most often sevoflurane, combined with nitrous oxide and oxygen. Delivered oxygen concentration should be measured at less than 50% before the initiation of electrocautery to prevent airway fires. Muscle relaxants may be used, but they generally are not necessary. Titration of supplemental narcotics helps provide a smooth anesthetic and emergence, but this must be done cautiously in patients with OSA. Because these patients have down-regulation of their mu receptors, their increased sensitivity dictates the use of short-acting narcotics, and in lower-than-usual doses. Once the child awakens, postoperative pain should be appropriately treated, but the total dose of narcotic usually is lower than in patients without OSA for reasons of this down-regulation. The decision regarding timing of extubation is left to clinical judgment, as previously discussed. Patients with OSA usually are extubated while awake, whereas patients without OSA can be extubated deep. If a deep extubation is chosen, thorough pharyngeal suctioning, placement of an oral airway, and lateral head-down positioning allows blood and secretions to drain cephalad.

Occasionally, reoperation is required for persistent hemorrhage; this occurs most commonly during the first 24 hours after the operation or at 7 to 10 days after the operation. Careful assessment of volume status and hematocrit are mandatory, and so is intravenous rehydration before anesthesia induction. Patients requiring reoperation have full stomachs and are candidates for rapid-sequence induction. Awake intubation should be considered if airway anatomy is distorted.

Most adenotonsillectomies can be performed on an outpatient basis, so long as the patient is monitored closely for at least 6 hours postoperatively.[128] Historically, most anesthesiologists have recommended overnight hospitalization after adenotonsillectomy in patients with OSA. However, a study that found improvements in polysomnograms in patients with mild OSA the night after adenotonsillectomy suggests that hospitalization is necessary only for high-risk patients.[129] At particular risk are children with OSA who are younger than 3 years of age, because the incidence of airway complications and delayed oral intake is higher in this age group. Other conditions that increase risk include cerebral palsy, seizure disorders, congenital heart disease, definitive syndromes, and prematurity.

Laryngeal Surgery

Like bronchoscopy, laryngeal surgery is challenging for the anesthesiologist, because the airway is shared with the surgeon and because the surgery often is performed on infants with congenital laryngomalacia, laryngeal clefts or webs, vocal cord disorders, or laryngeal tumors. Other common indications are acquired subglottic stenosis and recurrent laryngeal papillomatosis.

Several techniques allow the surgeon and the anesthesiologist to occupy the airway simultaneously. One such technique is the spontaneous ventilation technique, which is useful when the surgeon needs to assess airway dynamics.[130-132] If inhalation technique is used, the delivered concentration of agent must be high enough to prevent coughing or laryngospasm but not so high as to cause significant cardiovascular depression or apnea. Because this balance is difficult to achieve, especially with short-acting inhalation agents, adjunctive agents (e.g., propofol, narcotics) may be used to reduce the need for high concentrations of inhalational agent. Thorough topical anesthesia with 4% lidocaine (delivered either by atomizer or by syringe with a metal or plastic introducer needle) provides additional anesthesia and also may reduce systemic anesthetic requirements. As noted previously, a continuous infusion of propofol may be used instead of an inhalational agent to reduce operating room pollution and to provide a stable anesthetic level.

The spontaneous ventilation technique has been very useful for children with recurrent papillomatosis. The anesthetic technique for these children is basically the same as that described for bronchoscopy. Many of these children become psychologically sensitized by frequent needs for laser surgery, making good behavioral support important.

Premedication usually can be used in this population, unless the airway is particularly marginal. Child life or similar services have behavioral support programs that can also be especially helpful for these children. Often just the sight or smell of the anesthesia mask or inhalational agent can be quite anxiety-provoking for these children. An acceptable alternative to mask induction may be EMLA cream application followed by an intravenous start (sometimes with a butterfly needle) and then a propofol induction.

The apnea technique may be preferred if spontaneous ventilation is not necessary and if the anesthesiologist is uncomfortable with the unprotected airway. Anesthesia is provided with a combination of a muscle relaxant, high-concentration oxygen, and halothane or propofol. Topical anesthesia of the airway is accomplished before intubation. After the suspension laryngoscope is set up, the tube is removed, and the surgeon proceeds while the patient is apneic. The tube is replaced when the pulse oximeter indicates decreasing saturation, with a threshold established by the team. Repeated reintubation and ventilation are performed until the procedure is completed. The potential for CO_2 retention is high, particularly if only short periods of ventilation are used between periods of extubation and apnea.

Supraglottic jet ventilation incorporates the use of an intravenous anesthetic such as propofol with a muscle relaxant. After topical anesthesia is provided to the airway, the suspension laryngoscope is introduced, and a jet-ventilating device is attached. The characteristics and potential risks of this technique are the same as those for rigid bronchoscopy.

Finally, it is possible to place a small endotracheal tube around which the surgeon works, although this frequently proves to be awkward. With the availability of small-cuffed endotracheal tubes, older children can be more effectively ventilated with these smaller-diameter tubes.

SUGGESTED READINGS

General Guidelines and Articles

American Academy of Pediatrics. Guidelines for monitoring and management of pediatric patients during and after sedation for diagnostic and therapeutic procedures. *Pediatrics.* 1992;89:1110.

American Society of Anesthesiologists. Practice guidelines for sedation and analgesia by non-anesthesiologists. *Anesthesiology.* 1996;84:459.

American Society of Anesthesiologists. *Standards for Basic Anesthesia Monitoring: 2001 Directory of Members.* Park Ridge, Ill: American Society of Anesthesiologists; 2001.

American Society of Anesthesiologists. Practice advisory for preanesthesia evaluation. *Anesthesiology.* 2003;96:485.

Bhananker SM, Ramamoorthy C, Geiduschek JM, et al. Anesthesia-related cardiac arrest in children: update from the Pediatric Perioperative Cardiac Arrest Registry. *Anesth Anal.* 2007;105:344.

Coté CJ, Goudsouzian NG, Liu LM, et al. The dose response of intravenous thiopental for the induction of general anesthesia in unpremedicated children. *Anesthesiology.* 1981;55:703.

Ferrari LR, Donlon JV. Metoclopramide reduces the incidence of vomiting after tonsillectomy in children. *Anesth Analg.* 1992;75:351.

Habib AS, Gan TJ. Combination antiemetics: what is the evidence? *Int Anesthesiol Clin.* 2003;41:119.

Kurth CD, LeBard SE. Association of postoperative apnea, airway obstruction, and hypoxemia in former premature infants. *Anesthesiology.* 1991; 75:22.

Liu LMP, Goudsouzian NG, Liu PL. Rectal methohexital premedication on children: a dose comparison study. *Anesthesiology.* 1980;53:343.

Practice guidelines for preoperative fasting and the use of pharmacologic agents to reduce the risk of pulmonary aspiration: application to healthy patients undergoing elective procedures: a report by the American Society of Anesthesiologists Task Force on Preoperative Fasting. *Anesthesiology.* 1999;90:896.

Roy WL, Lerman J, McIntyre BG. Is preoperative hemoglobin testing justified in children undergoing minor elective surgery? *Can J Anaesth.* 1991;38:700.

Saint-Maurice C, Estève C, Holzer J, et al. [Better acceptance of measures of induction of anesthesia after rectal premedication with midazolam in children. Comparison of a placebo-controlled study.] *Anaesthesist.* 1987;36:629.

Sennaraj B. Management of post-strabismus nausea and vomiting in children using ondansetron: a value-based comparison of outcomes. *Br J Anaesth.* 2002;89:473.

Splinter WM, Rhine EJ, Roberts DW, et al. Ondansetron is a better prophylactic antiemetic than droperidol for tonsillectomy in children. *Can J Anaesth.* 1995;42:848.

Ved SA, Walden TL, Montana J, et al. Vomiting and recovery after outpatient tonsillectomy and adenoidectomy in children. *Anesthesiology.* 1996;85:4.

Watcha MF, Bras PJ, Cieslak GD, et al. The dose-response relationship of ondansetron in preventing postoperative emesis in pediatric patients undergoing ambulatory surgery. *Anesthesiology.* 1995;82:47.

Welborn LG, Hannallah RS, Norden JM, et al. Comparison of emergence and recovery characteristics of sevoflurane, desflurane, and halothane in pediatric ambulatory patients. *Anesth Analg.* 1996;83:917.

Williams AR, Conroy JM. The anesthetic management of the pediatric strabismus patient. *J AAPOS.* 1998;2:113.

Anesthesia in the Neonate

McGowan FX Jr. Anesthetic-related neurotoxicity in the developing infant: of mice, rats, monkeys and, possibly, humans. *Anesth Anal.* 2008;106:1599.

Behavioral Preparation and Premedication

Coté CJ. Preoperative preparation and premedication. *Br J Anaesth.* 1999;83:16.

Kain ZN, Caldwell-Andrews AA, Maranets I, et al. Predicting which child-parent pair will benefit from parenteral presence during induction of anesthesia. *Anesth Analg.* 2006;102:81.

Maxwell LG. Age associated issues in preoperative evaluation, testing and planning: pediatrics. *Anesth Clin North Am.* 2004;22:27.

McMillan CO, Spahr-Schopfer IA, Sikich N, et al. Premedication of children with oral midazolam. *Can J Anaesth.* 1992;39:545.

Postoperative Nausea and Vomiting

Gan TJ, Meyer T, Apfel CC, et al. Consensus guidelines for managing postoperative nausea and vomiting. *Anesth Analg.* 2003;97:62.

Habib AS, Gan TJ. Combination antiemetics: what is the evidence? *Int Anesthesiol Clin.* 2003;41:119.

Pain

Anand KJ, Hickey PR. Pain and its effects in the human neonate and fetus. *N Engl J Med.* 1987;317:1321.

Joint Commission on Accreditation of Healthcare Organizations. *Pain Assessment and Management: An Organizational Approach.* Oakbrook Terrace, Ill: Joint Commission on Accreditation of Healthcare Organizations; 2000.

McGrath PJ. Behavioral measures of pain. In: Finley GA, McGrath PJ, eds. *Measurement of Pain in Infants and Children.* Seattle: IASP Press; 1998.

Yaster M, Deshpande JK. Management of pediatric pain with opioid analgesics. *J Pediatr.* 1988;113:421.

Articles about Other Medical Conditions

Kretz FJ, Reimann B, Stelzner J, et al. [The laryngeal mask in pediatric adenotonsillectomy. A meta-analysis of medical studies.] *Anaesthesist.* 2000; 49:706.

Presland AH, Evans AH, Bailey PM, et al. The laryngeal mask airway in tonsillectomy: the surgeon's perspective. *Clin Otolaryngol.* 2000;25:240.

Stevens A, Roizen MF. Patients with diabetes mellitus and disorders of glucose metabolism. *Anesth Clin North Am.* 1987;5:339.

Tait AR, Malviya S, Voepel-Lewis T, et al. Risk factors for perioperative adverse respiratory events in children with upper respiratory tract infections. *Anesthesiology.* 2001;95:299.

Endocarditis Prophylaxis

Wilson W, Taubert KA, Gewitz M, et al. Prevention of infective endocarditis: guidelines from the American Heart Association: a guideline from the American Heart Association Rheumatic Fever, Endocarditis and Kawasaki Disease Committee, Council on Cardiovascular Disease in the Young, and the Council on Clinical Cardiology, Council on Cardiovascular Surgery and Anesthesia, and the Quality of Care and Outcomes Research Interdisciplinary Working Group. *J Am Dent Assoc.* 2008;139(suppl):3S-24S.

For complete list of references log onto www.expertconsult.com.

CHAPTER ONE HUNDRED AND EIGHTY-THREE

Obstructive Sleep Apnea Syndrome

Laura M. Sterni

David E. Tunkel

Key Points

- Obstructive sleep apnea syndrome (OSAS) is a common medical condition that can lead to significant morbidity in children.
- Sequelae of OSAS in children include poor growth, learning and behavior problems, and cardiovascular complications, with potential long-term consequences.
- The definitive diagnosis of OSAS in children is made using overnight polysomnography. Adult criteria for the scoring and interpretation of polysomnographic data cannot be applied to children.
- First-line therapy for OSAS in most children is adenotonsillectomy, with improvement expected in many. Children with severe OSAS or with significant risk factors for OSAS beyond adenotonsillectomy may require further evaluation and therapy.
- Children with OSAS at risk for postoperative respiratory compromise may be identified preoperatively. Risk factors include age younger than 3 years, severe OSAS documented by polysomnography, and abnormalities of upper airway tone or structure, as may be seen in children with neuromuscular disease, craniofacial anomalies, or obesity.
- Continuous positive airway pressure (CPAP) and bilevel positive airway pressure (BPAP) are the most commonly used nonsurgical modalities for management of OSAS and can be applied safely and successfully in children.

The stupid-lazy child who frequently suffers from headaches at school, breathes through his mouth instead of his nose, snores and is restless at night, and wakes up with a dry mouth in the morning, is well worthy of the solicitous attention of the school medical officer.

—W. Hill, 1889[1]

More than 100 years ago, clinicians began to recognize the manifestations of sleep-related breathing obstruction in children. Today, the obstructive sleep apnea syndrome (OSAS) is recognized as a common and important pediatric health problem. Sleep-related upper airway obstruction can lead to a variety of nighttime and daytime symptoms in children. If diagnosis and treatment are delayed, the consequences of OSAS can be severe.

Classification of Sleep-Related Upper Airway Obstruction

Snoring is the common feature of three clinical syndromes of sleep-related upper airway obstruction in children. The diagnoses of primary snoring, upper airway resistance syndrome (UARS), and OSAS separate patients according to the severity of their sleep-related upper airway obstruction and resulting clinical complications.

Primary Snoring

Approximately 10% of children snore during sleep on most or all nights, and the majority of these children have primary snoring.[2-5] *Primary snoring* has been defined as snoring during sleep without associated apnea, gas exchange abnormalities, or excessive arousals.[6] The factors that predispose children to primary snoring are similar to those described for OSAS and are discussed in detail later in this chapter. Major risk factors for snoring in otherwise healthy children are obesity, decreased nasal patency (rhinitis, septal deviation, nasal obstruction), and adenotonsillar hypertrophy.[7,8] Snoring in 6- to 13-year-old children also has been strongly associated with parental cigarette smoking.[4,7]

Primary snoring does not appear to progress to OSAS in young children and may resolve over time. Investigators have performed polysomnography in children 1 to 3 years after their diagnosis of primary snoring and found no significant difference in the apnea index or nighttime gas exchange.[9,10] Ali and coworkers found that 50% of children who were described by their parents as habitual snorers at 4 years of age had stopped snoring without treatment at a 2-year follow-up evaluation.[2]

In the past, primary snoring was considered a benign condition; however, more recent studies have challenged this assumption. O'Brien and colleagues found that primary snoring was associated with an increased probability of neurobehavioral deficits in children.[11] Daytime symptoms such as sleepiness, inattention, aggressiveness, and hyperactivity are reported commonly in habitual snorers and children with OSAS.[3,12-15] Disrupted microsleep architecture has now been demonstrated in children with primary snoring, providing a possible link between neurocognitive dysfunction and habitual snoring in children.[16,17]

Upper Airway Resistance Syndrome

Children with UARS snore and have partial upper airway obstruction that leads to repetitive episodes of increased respiratory effort ending in arousals and sleep fragmentation. Daytime symptoms similar to those seen with OSAS may exist.[18-20] Children with UARS have no evidence

Table 183-1

Childhood versus Adult Obstructive Sleep Apnea Syndrome

Feature	Adults	Children
Presentation		
Excessive daytime sleepiness	Main presenting complaint	Infrequent complaint
Associated obesity	Majority of patients	Minority of patients
Underweight/failure to thrive	Not seen	Frequent finding
Daytime mouth-breathing	Not seen	Frequent finding
Gender	Male/female = 2:1	Male/female = 1:1
Enlarged tonsils and adenoids	Rarely seen	Frequent finding
Sleep Pattern		
Obstructive	Obstructive apnea	Obstructive apnea or obstructive hypoventilation
Arousal with obstruction	Common	May be less frequent
Disrupted	Common	Not often seen
Management		
Surgical	Minority of patients with inconsistent results	Definitive in many
Medical (positive pressure)	Most common management	Only in selected patients

Adapted from Carroll JL, Loughlin GM. Diagnostic criteria for obstructive sleep apnea syndrome in children. *Pediatr Pulmonol.* 1992;14:71.

of apnea, hypopnea, or gas exchange abnormalities on polysomnography. The diagnosis of UARS currently is made with the use of esophageal pressure monitoring to identify increased respiratory effort with related arousals. When polysomnography is performed without esophageal pressure monitoring, snoring with marked paradoxical breathing movements or repetitive arousals may be suggestive of UARS. Treatment options for UARS are identical to those for OSAS and are discussed later in the chapter. The incidence of UARS in children is unknown, but some centers believe it may be more common than OSAS.[19]

Obstructive Sleep Apnea Syndrome

Approximately 1% to 3% of all children will have OSAS, and as many as 40% of snoring children referred to a sleep clinic or otolaryngologist may have OSAS.[21-25] Childhood OSAS has been defined as episodes of upper airway obstruction during sleep that usually are associated with a reduction in oxyhemoglobin saturation or hypercarbia, or both. Sleep-related upper airway obstruction in children may manifest as obstructive apnea or obstructive hypoventilation.[26] Obstructive hypoventilation results from continuous partial airway obstruction, which leads to paradoxical respiratory efforts, hypercarbia, and often hypoxemia. This pattern may be more common in children, who are less prone than are adults to collapse of the upper airway.[27] Diagnosis of obstructive hypoventilation in children requires end-tidal CO_2 monitoring during polysomnography. Despite the absence of complete airway obstruction during sleep, children with obstructive hypoventilation are at risk for all of the reported complications of OSAS.

Obstructive hypoventilation generally is not seen in adults with OSAS. A number of other important differences between adults and children with OSAS are detailed in Table 183-1.

Symptoms and Signs of Childhood Obstructive Sleep Apnea Syndrome

Children with OSAS almost always present with a history of snoring and difficulty breathing during sleep.[23,28,29] Parents often report nighttime sweating, restlessness, and unusual sleeping positions in their affected children. Chest retraction, use of accessory muscles, and paradoxical rib cage motion during inspiration are seen during episodes of upper airway obstruction. Paradoxical breathing (inward movement of the thorax during inspiration) can be normal during sleep in infants and toddlers. During rapid eye movement (REM) sleep, the tonic and phasic activity of the intercostal muscles disappears, and the infant chest wall becomes more compliant. The negative intrathoracic pressures generated during inspiration result in the paradoxical inward movement of the thorax. Paradoxical breathing decreases with age and is rare in healthy children older than 3 years of age.[30] Paradoxical respirations in older children are almost always the result of upper airway obstruction.

Enuresis has been associated with OSAS in children but is not a consistent finding.[29,31,32] Enuresis associated with OSAS may be related to disrupted, restless sleep patterns that affect arousal. Several studies have reported resolution of nocturnal enuresis after adenotonsillectomy in children with symptoms of nocturnal upper airway obstruction or polysomnography that is diagnostic for OSAS.[33-35]

Daytime symptoms associated with OSAS include mouth breathing, nasal obstruction, and hyponasal speech. Morning headaches have been associated with nighttime breathing obstruction, but controlled studies comparing children with OSAS with children with normal polysomnography results have found no significant difference in the frequency of this symptom.[29,31,36] Adults with OSAS often present with excessive daytime sleepiness, but this complaint is less frequent among children with OSAS.[23,31,32,37] OSAS can lead to significant cardiopulmonary complications, poor growth, and problems with learning and behavior. These important sequelae are discussed next.

Complications of Childhood Obstructive Sleep Apnea Syndrome

Growth Impairment

Failure to thrive was commonly described in early reports of children with OSAS.[28,29,36] Although overt failure to thrive is now seen less frequently, as a result of earlier diagnosis and management of OSAS, children with OSAS often grow poorly. Improved growth has been reported in childhood OSAS after treatment with adenotonsillectomy.[38-40] Marcus and colleagues reported decreased growth in children with even mild OSAS that appeared to be related to the increased work of breathing during sleep. After adenotonsillectomy, the patients had improved growth and decreased energy expenditure during sleep.[38] Nocturnal growth hormone secretion also appears to be decreased in children with sleep-related upper airway obstruction.[41] OSAS should be considered in the differential diagnosis for failure to thrive or impaired growth that is unexplained by other conditions.

Behavior and Learning Problems

Sleep-related breathing obstruction in children can lead to significant neurocognitive and behavioral complications. A comprehensive review of available data shows that pediatric OSAS is associated with shortfalls in academic performance, deficits in behavior and emotional regulation leading to problems such as hyperactivity and aggressiveness, difficulty with sustained and selective attention, and decreased alertness.[42] It also has been suggested that childhood OSAS may lead to problems with memory, intelligence, and executive functioning, but findings are inconclusive to date. Although the exact cause-and-effect relationships are unknown, both sleep fragmentation and intermittent hypoxia are emerging as likely components in the pathophysiology of neurobehavioral morbidity associated with sleep-disordered breathing.[43-45] Gozal and associates found that a group of children with OSAS and neurocognitive abnormalities had significantly increased levels of morning C-reactive protein when compared with children with OSAS and no cognitive dysfunction and with control subjects (i.e., children without OSAS).[46] This finding suggests that the greater the inflammatory response elicited by OSAS, the greater the risk of neurocognitive dysfunction, possibly secondary to neuronal injury.

In an encouraging trend, several studies have documented posttreatment improvement in children with OSAS who exhibited preoperative disturbances in behavior and cognition.[39,47-50] In one study of 12 children with moderate to severe OSAS, a significant reduction in inattention, aggression, and hyperactivity was seen after treatment, as assessed by the Conners Parent Rating Scale. The study authors also noted an improvement in vigilance on a continuous performance task.[47] Owens and colleagues found modest improvement after treatment in a small group of children with mild to moderate OSAS who had behavioral problems and mild deficits in executive functioning, attention, and motor skills.[50] Gozal reported evidence of learning difficulties in children with OSAS by documenting an increased incidence of snoring and nocturnal gas exchange abnormalities in a group of 297 first-grade children who were in the lowest 10th percentile of their class.[48] Of perhaps greatest interest, the children with sleep-associated gas exchange abnormalities who received treatment showed an improvement in academic performance in the second grade, whereas no academic improvements were seen in the affected children whose parents did not seek therapy.

Mitchell and Kelly assessed behavioral abnormalities in children with OSAS using the Behavioral Assessment System for Children before adenotonsillectomy, and again within 6 months after surgery and 9 to 18 months after surgery.[51] These investigators found improvements in behavioral measures after adenotonsillectomy that seemed to persist during long-term follow-up, although to a lesser degree than seen shortly after surgery. Similarly, Chervin and coworkers found that children undergoing adenotonsillectomy for any clinical indication (most often, suspected sleep-disordered breathing in this study) had increased difficulty with hyperactivity, inattention, and daytime sleepiness and were more likely to be diagnosed with attention deficit–hyperactivity disorder than control children undergoing other surgical procedures.[49] At 1 year after adenotonsillectomy, improvements were seen in all measures.

Clearly, sleep-disordered breathing, even in the mild to moderate range, carries a risk for significant and at least partially reversible neurobehavioral morbidity. It is not clear, however, if the cognitive and behavioral complications of OSAS are completely reversible. Gozal and Pope reported that children with lower academic performance in middle school were more likely to have snored loudly and frequently and to have required an adenotonsillectomy for snoring during early childhood.[52] These investigators suggested that the neurocognitive effects of sleep-related upper airway obstruction in young children may be only partially reversible and lead to a "learning debt" that adversely influences subsequent school performance. The diagnosis of OSAS should be considered in children with learning and behavior disorders. Although the ultimate prognosis remains uncertain, early recognition and therapy may help reduce possible life-long neurobehavioral limitations.

Cardiopulmonary Complications

Severe untreated OSAS can lead to pulmonary hypertension and cor pulmonale (Fig. 183-1).[28,29] Pulmonary hypertension results from the recurrent, severe, nocturnal hypoxemia, hypercarbia, and acidosis that occur during obstructive hypoventilation and apnea. Cor pulmonale generally is reversible with treatment for OSAS, but perioperative precautions are required in these high-risk patients. Amin and colleagues found that OSAS in children led to structural changes and hypertrophy of both right and left ventricles.[53] Most notably, the left ventricular hypertrophy seen in their OSAS patients was related to the degree of severity of the OSAS. These workers noted that left ventricular hypertrophy is a known risk factor for future cardiovascular disease. A follow-up study in children demonstrated a "dose-dependent" decrease in left ventricular diastolic function with increasingly severe OSAS.[54] Systemic hypertension, a frequent complication of adult OSAS, also has been reported in children with OSAS.[29,55-57] Pediatric OSAS has been shown to be associated with an increased systemic inflammatory response thought to increase the risk for atherosclerotic disease, as demonstrated by elevated levels of C-reactive protein and changes in levels of proinflammatory and anti-inflammatory cytokines.[58-60] Improvement in these inflammation indicators was noted after adenotonsillectomy, supporting the importance of early diagnosis and treatment of OSAS to avoid long-term cardiovascular morbidity.[58,59]

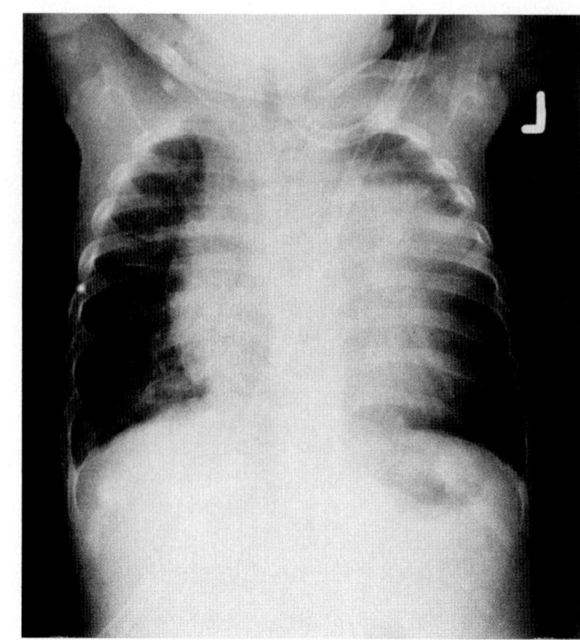

Figure 183-1. Chest radiograph of a child with cor pulmonale secondary to obstructive sleep apnea syndrome.

Pathophysiology of Obstructive Sleep Apnea

The upper airway is a collapsible muscular tube that includes the nasopharynx, oropharynx, and hypopharynx. Patency of the upper airway is determined by the tonic activity of the pharyngeal dilating muscles, as well as phasic contraction of these muscles in response to negative upper airway pressure (inspiration). Skeletal and soft tissue structures such as the tonsils and adenoids affect upper airway diameter and resistance and are important in determining airway patency. During sleep, reduced upper airway inspiratory muscle tone and diminished reflex dilation lead to airway narrowing. These effects are most pronounced in REM sleep, leading to increased obstructive events in predisposed patients.

In otherwise healthy children, adenotonsillar hypertrophy is a significant risk factor for OSAS.[36] However, no strict correlation has been found between size of the lymphoid tissues and the presence or severity of sleep-related breathing obstruction.[61-63] One child with significantly enlarged tonsils and adenoids may be asymptomatic (i.e., have no difficulty with sleep-related upper airway obstruction), whereas another with only moderate adenotonsillar hypertrophy will have severe OSAS. Furthermore, OSAS develops in only a small percentage of children with adenotonsillar hypertrophy. It is likely that a combination of structural factors and neuromotor abnormalities must be present for OSAS to occur.

Marcus and associates demonstrated that the pediatric upper airway behaves as a Starling resistor.[64] In the Starling resistor model, maximum inspiratory flow through the collapsible upper airway is determined by upstream (nasal) pressure and the pressure surrounding the collapsible segment. When airway collapse occurs, flow is independent of the downstream (tracheal) pressure. Airway collapse occurs when the pressure surrounding the airway becomes greater than the pressure within the collapsible segment. The pressure outside the airway is dictated by structural factors, as well as activity of the airway dilator muscles. These investigators found that children with OSAS had greater airway collapsibility than those with primary snoring. Although airway collapsibility was reduced after adenotonsillectomy in children with OSAS, it remained greater than in the patients with primary snoring.

Structural factors other than adenotonsillar hypertrophy may play a role in OSAS in otherwise healthy children. Arens and colleagues used magnetic resonance imaging to study the airway of children with OSAS and found a smaller upper airway volume than in control subjects.[65] In a second study, Arens' group found that the upper airway of children with OSAS was restricted along the upper two thirds, with greatest narrowing in the region of overlap of the tonsils and adenoids.[66]

Isono and associates studied children with OSAS who were given neuromuscular blockade under general anesthesia. These researchers found that the closing pressure of children with OSAS was positive and greater than that of normal children.[67] Collapsibility of the retropalatal and retroglossal segments was significantly increased in their OSAS subjects. They also determined that the cross-sectional area of the narrowest segment of the airway was significantly smaller in children with OSAS.

It appears that children with OSAS have subtle abnormalities in upper airway structure or neuromuscular control, in addition to adenotonsillar hypertrophy.

High-Risk Groups

Adenotonsillar hypertrophy is the leading cause of childhood OSAS. A number of other medical conditions also are strongly associated with OSAS in children, as listed in Table 183-2. Close follow-up is indicated in children in these high-risk groups to look for the development of signs and symptoms that may suggest sleep-related airway obstruction. Such signs and symptoms warrant polysomnographic testing to assess for the presence and severity of OSAS.

Table 183-2

Medical Conditions Associated with Obstructive Sleep Apnea Syndrome*

Achondroplasia and similar skeletal dysplasias
Apert's syndrome
Beckwith-Weidemann syndrome
Cerebral palsy
Choanal stenosis or atresia
Cleft palate after repair
Crouzon syndrome
Cystic hygroma
Down syndrome
Goldenhar syndrome/hemifacial microsomia
Hallermann-Streiff syndrome
Hypothyroidism
Klippel-Feil syndrome
Mucopolysaccharidosis
Obesity
Osteopetrosis
Papillomatosis (oropharyngeal)
Pierre Robin sequence
Pfeiffer's syndrome
Pharyngeal flap surgery
Prader-Willi syndrome
Sickle cell disease
Treacher Collins syndrome

*Other conditions not listed also may be associated with this syndrome.

Adapted from Marcus CL, Carroll JL. Obstructive sleep apnea syndrome. In: Loughlin GM, Eigen H, eds. *Respiratory Disease in Children: Diagnosis and Management*. Baltimore: Williams & Wilkins; 1994:475-499. Used with permission.

Obesity

Obese children are at risk for sleep-related breathing obstruction.[68,69] Deposition of adipose tissue within the muscles and soft tissues surrounding the upper airway in combination with external compression from the neck and jowls leads to upper airway narrowing in these patients.[70] Upward displacement of the diaphragm by the obese abdomen when the affected child is supine and decreased chest wall compliance lead to lower lung volumes during sleep, decreased oxygen stores, and increased risk of desaturation with obstructive events. Obese children are at increased risk for persistent OSAS after adenotonsillectomy. Mitchell and Kelly studied 30 obese children with OSAS and found a decrease in respiratory disturbance index (RDI) (see later under "Polysomnography") from a mean of 30 preoperatively to a mean of about 12 after adenotonsillectomy.[71] Although all children had an improved quality of life as defined by a validated questionnaire, OSAS was decreased in severity but not cured in these obese children.

Craniofacial Abnormalities

Children with craniofacial anomalies often have a multifactorial etiology for OSAS. Evaluation is directed toward examination of craniofacial issues such as skull base shape, maxillary size and shape, tongue size and support, and mandibular size and shape. Concomitant central nervous system abnormalities can affect pharyngeal tone, and any coexisting laryngotracheal anomalies should be evaluated. OSAS in such children may persist after adenotonsillectomy, and additional surgical and nonsurgical therapies may be necessary. Infants with craniofacial anomalies can be difficult to treat and may require tracheotomy.

Children with skeletal dysplasias such as achondroplasia may have mixed apnea syndromes. Compression of the brainstem at the craniocervical junction may cause abnormalities of ventilatory drive and central apnea. Cervicomedullary compression also can affect upper airway control, leading to airway obstruction during sleep. Adenotonsillar enlargement and the craniofacial features seen in these patients may also contribute to the development of OSAS.[72] Sisk and associates diagnosed OSAS in 38% of children with achondroplasia.[73] Adenotonsillectomy usually is effective, but additional therapy with continuous positive airway pressure (CPAP) or tracheotomy may be needed in such complicated cases.[74] Craniocervical decompression has been used in some patients with achondroplasia, but the effects on OSAS remain controversial.[75]

Neuromuscular Disease

Cerebral palsy in children is associated with decreased pharyngeal tone, resulting in OSAS. Adenotonsillectomy is a useful initial procedure for OSAS associated with pharyngeal hypotonia.[76] These children are at high risk for respiratory complications or persistent OSAS after adenotonsillectomy.[77-79] When pharyngeal hypotonia is marked, tracheotomy may be necessary to relieve OSAS. Aggressive craniofacial and pharyngeal surgical approaches have been used to avoid tracheotomy in neurologically impaired patients with OSAS.[80] Primary muscular diseases such as Duchenne muscular dystrophy also have been associated with the development of OSAS secondary to loss of upper airway muscle tone.[72]

Patients with Down syndrome have a high incidence of OSAS. A study of OSAS in these patients found that adenotonsillectomy alone was not adequate therapy for more than 60% of the patients.[81] It was concluded that the generalized hypotonia and anatomic abnormalities such as obesity, macroglossia, and midfacial and mandibular hypoplasia all contribute to nocturnal airway obstruction in these patients. Lefaivre and coworkers described a multilevel surgical approach to the management of OSAS in children with Down syndrome, using a combination of facial and mandibular bony advancement and pharyngeal soft tissue surgery to achieve improvement in sleep-related upper airway obstruction.[82] Merrell and Shott described the use of lateral pharyngoplasty (plication of the tonsillar pillars), along with adenotonsillectomy, in children with Down syndrome but found polysomnographic abnormalities in 75% of these children after adenotonsillectomy with or without this modification.[83]

Mucopolysaccharidoses

Mucopolysaccharidoses, such as the Hunter and Hurler syndromes, are associated with severe progressive OSAS in affected children. The head and neck manifestations in these syndromes include short neck, depressed nasal dorsum, macroglossia, adenotonsillar enlargement, and craniofacial abnormalities.[84] Bredenkamp and colleagues reported upper airway obstruction in 17 of 45 patients (38%) with mucopolysaccharidoses, 7 (16%) of whom required tracheotomy.[85] Leighton and associates found OSAS in more than 90% of patients with mucopolysaccharidoses, with the most severe OSAS found in the Hurler and Hurler-Scheie types.[86] Laryngeal tissues can be infiltrated and tracheal size decreased from mucopolysaccharide deposition, leading to airway obstruction at multiple levels.[87] Adenotonsillectomy and tracheotomy may be part of the surgical treatment of OSAS in such complicated cases.[88] Although its clinical applications are far from clear, enzyme replacement therapy may stabilize mild OSAS in children with Hurler syndrome and may improve upper airway size.[89]

Acute-Onset or Rapidly Progressive Obstructive Sleep Apnea Syndrome

Abrupt onset or rapid progression of OSAS in children suggests rapid enlargement of lymphoid tissue in the pharynx or other lesions rapidly growing near the airway. Viral syndromes can be associated with marked lymphoid hyperplasia and severe OSAS in children, the common example being infectious mononucleosis secondary to Epstein-Barr virus infection. Acute OSAS associated with Epstein-Barr virus infection is treated with a nasopharyngeal airway and steroids until the lymphoid hyperplasia resolves.[90]

Malignant and benign tumors of the head and neck may cause sleep-related upper airway obstruction, as discussed later on. A full head and neck examination should be directed at a search for intrinsic and extrinsic masses causing airway compromise. Biopsy, when clinically indicated, should be performed to direct additional therapy.

Diagnosis

Early diagnosis and treatment of OSAS in children will result in decreased morbidity. A study by Richards and Ferdman found that the mean period between onset of symptoms and treatment of OSAS in a group of 45 children was 3.3 years.[91] Delays in treatment were related to physician, parent, and third-party factors. Early diagnosis also may be cost-effective: Children with OSAS have been shown to have a 226% increase in health care utilization when compared with control subjects during the 1 year before they receive evaluation and treatment.[92] A clinical practice guideline on the diagnosis and management of OSAS in children released by the American Academy of Pediatrics has recommended that all children be screened for snoring as part of routine health care maintenance.[93] If snoring is reported, a more detailed evaluation is recommended.

History

Numerous studies have demonstrated that OSAS cannot be distinguished from primary snoring in children, based on clinical history and physical examination alone.[23,25,36,94-96] In one report, 89% of parents of children with OSAS observed the child struggling to breathe during sleep, as did 58% of parents of children with primary snoring.[23] A majority of parents of children with both disorders were frightened by their child's nighttime breathing, often staying up nights to watch the child breathe. Goldstein and associates evaluated 30 snoring children referred to a pediatric otolaryngology clinic using a focused history and physical examination in addition to a review of audiotaped breathing of the children during sleep.[25] In only one half of the 18 children believed to have definite OSAS clinically was polysomnography diagnostic for OSAS. In a systematic literature review, Brietzke and coworkers found that 11 of 12 articles in the literature concluded that clinical assessment is inaccurate in the diagnosis of childhood OSAS.[97] Although the clinical history may not be diagnostic, a thorough evaluation of daytime and nighttime symptoms is helpful in planning subsequent studies and interpreting the findings.

Physical Examination

The diagnosis of childhood OSAS is suggested by the patient's history and confirmed by polysomnography. The physical examination should note height and weight, because growth may be impaired by OSAS. Cardiopulmonary abnormalities associated with OSAS should be identified. A full otolaryngologic examination of the head and neck should establish the likely site or sites of dynamic or static airway obstruction.

Tonsil and adenoid size should be assessed in children with symptoms of nocturnal airway obstruction. Signs of adenoidal hypertrophy include decreased nasal airflow with an adequate nasal airway on rhinoscopy, a hyponasal speech pattern, and an open mouth breathing posture. Nasal examination should be focused to exclude obstructive septal deformity, intranasal masses, and mucosal or turbinate swelling within the nose. The oral examination should center on tonsil size and symmetry, pharyngeal dimensions, palate shape and size, and tongue size and motion.

Routine oral and nasal examination can be supplemented with fiberoptic nasal endoscopy to assess nasal patency, adenoid size, and effect of tonsil size and anatomy on awake respiration.[98] Croft and associates used fiberoptic endoscopy to evaluate the site of obstruction in children with polysomnogram-proven OSAS.[62] These workers identified distinct adenoidal, adenotonsillar, tongue base, and laryngeal sites of obstruction based on fiberoptic endoscopy and planned successful surgical therapy based on these findings.

The physical examination of children with craniofacial anomalies is directed at craniofacial structure, jaw size and position, and tongue size and position. Assessment of pharyngeal and laryngeal tone is necessary in children with neuromotor diseases such as cerebral palsy or muscular dystrophy. When sleep-disordered breathing is accompanied by daytime airway symptoms such as stridor or hoarseness, laryngotracheal examination with flexible or rigid endoscopy should be performed.

Polysomnography

Overnight polysomnography in a sleep laboratory is the "gold standard" method for diagnosing childhood OSAS. An accurate diagnosis of OSAS will ensure that appropriate treatment is provided when needed and will avoid unnecessary surgery in patients with primary snoring. The quantitative data obtained from polysomnography also can help predict which children are at risk for perioperative complications. Severe OSAS on polysomnography has been shown in several studies to be an important risk factor for postoperative respiratory compromise after adenotonsillectomy.[78,79]

Pediatric sleep laboratories should involve clinicians with expertise in pediatric respiratory disorders or sleep medicine to ensure that the studies are performed and the findings interpreted appropriately for this age group. Overnight polysomnography is recommended. Although a nap study that is positive for obstructive sleep apnea correlates well with the presence of obstructive apnea on an overnight study, a negative nap study result does not exclude the diagnosis of OSAS.[99] Nap studies are limited by the short recording time and the possible absence of REM sleep periods. The use of sedatives and sleep deprivation are not recommended because both may increase upper airway obstruction artifactually.[100,101]

In children, end-tidal CO_2 should be monitored to detect obstructive hypoventilation. The consensus statement adopted by the American Thoracic Society, Standards and Indications for Cardiopulmonary Sleep Studies in Children, also recommends measurement of (1) respiratory effort, as assessed by movement of the chest wall and abdomen; (2) airflow at the nose or mouth; (3) measurement of arterial oxygen saturation (Sao_2) by pulse oximetry; (4) electrocardiographic recording to monitor cardiac rate and rhythm; (5) electromyography performed

Table 183-3

Polysomnography for Obstructive Sleep Apnea Syndrome in Children

Sleep State
Electroencephalogram
Electro-oculogram (right and left)
Electromyogram (submental)
Respiratory Variables
Abdominal and chest wall movement (strain gauges, inductive plethysmography)
Oronasal airflow (thermistor)
End-tidal CO_2
Arterial oxygen saturation with pulse oximetry
Nonrespiratory Variables
Electrocardiogram
Electromyogram (tibial) to document movements and arousals
Recommended but Not Required
Audiovideo recording

in the anterior tibial region to monitor arousals; and (6) appropriate electroencephalography, electro-oculography, and electromyography measurements for sleep staging[102] (Table 183-3).

Sleep-related upper airway obstruction is diagnosed in children who have more than one obstructive apneic episode per hour or show evidence of significant obstructive hypoventilation. In adults, obstructive apnea is considered abnormal only if the episode lasts more than 10 seconds. Significant obstructive apneic episodes in children often are shorter than 10 seconds. Because of the higher oxygen consumption in children and the fall in functional residual capacity during sleep, Sao_2 may fall after only a few seconds of upper airway obstruction in the infant or toddler. Obstructive apneas or hypopneas lasting two or more consecutive breaths generally are considered abnormal in children. *Obstructive apnea* is defined as near-complete cessation of airflow despite ongoing respiratory effort. *Obstructive hypopnea* is diagnosed when partial upper airway obstruction results in a greater than 50% reduction in airflow associated with either an arousal or a desaturation of 3% or greater from baseline. Generally, obstructive apneas and hypopneas are combined to provide the apnea-hypopnea index (AHI), which reflects the number of discrete obstructive events per hour. Many laboratories may refer to this index as the respiratory disturbance index (RDI), whereas other laboratories will use the RDI to report the number of all scored respiratory events, including central apneas, per hour. Normal children have more frequent central apneas when compared with adults. Only an obstructive event index should be used to make the diagnosis of OSAS.[103]

Obstructive hypoventilation is diagnosed when peak end-tidal CO_2 is greater than 50 mm Hg for 25% or more of total sleep time in the presence of paradoxical respirations or snoring and in the absence of lung disease.[104] *Hypoxemia* is defined as an Spo_2 less than 92% and is correlated with the child's baseline readings and respiratory events. Sleep architecture is examined as well, because an adequate study should contain at least one REM period. Sleep efficiency and frequency of arousal from sleep in association with respiratory events also are analyzed.

Data correlating polysomnographic parameters with clinical outcomes in children are lacking, and no standard guidelines exist for classifying the severity of OSAS. OSAS and obstructive hypoventilation are diagnosed when polysomnographic parameters associated with upper airway obstruction fall outside the values that are currently accepted as normal.[105-107] In our laboratory, we classify children as having either mild, moderate, or severe OSAS based on the clinical picture, number of obstructive events per hour, peak end-tidal CO_2 pressure ($Petco_2$) or duration of elevated end-tidal CO_2 measurements, and frequency and severity of oxygen desaturation. We classify OSAS as severe if the patient has an obstructive event index of 10 or greater per hour because of the increased risk of respiratory compromise after adenotonsillectomy.[78] Representative polysomnographic tracings from pediatric patients are shown in Figure 183-2.

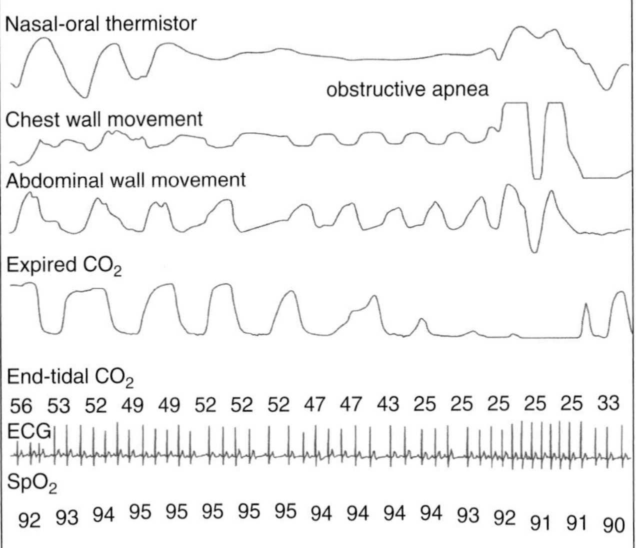

A

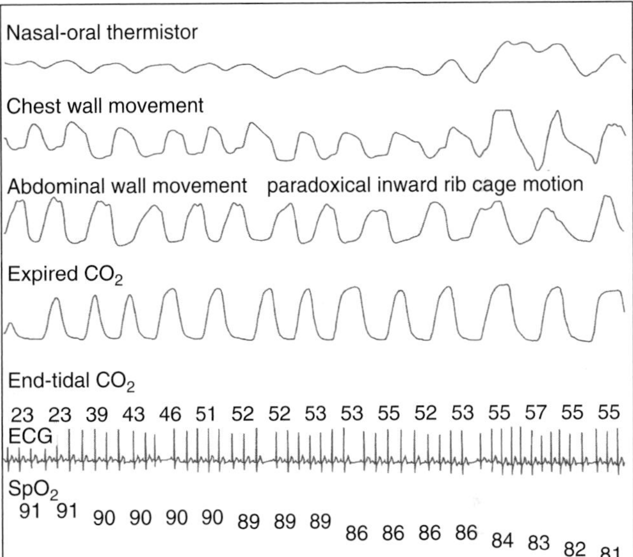

B

Figure 183-2. Typical polysomnographic recordings. **A,** Obstructive apnea. **B,** Obstructive hypoventilation. Evidence of paradoxical inward rib cage motion is seen in both tracings. In **A,** nasal-oral thermistor and expired CO_2 tracings flatten during the obstructive apneic episode, while respiratory efforts continue. Note the fall in arterial oxygen saturation (specifically, peripheral oxygen saturation [Spo_2]) measured by pulse oximetry that occurs shortly after the approximately 10-second event. In **B,** continuous partial airway obstruction results in elevated end-tidal CO_2 readings and a fall in Spo_2.

Other Studies

Because full polysomnography in children may be difficult to obtain, expensive, or inconvenient, screening methods to diagnose OSAS have been investigated. Having medical personnel directly observe a child experiencing apnea, retractions, and paradoxical respirations during sleep may allow the diagnosis of OSAS.[102] Making a diagnosis by observation, however, does not allow characterization of the severity of the OSAS, which may be important in determining management. Videotapes, audiotapes, and continuous pulse oximetry have been helpful in predicting OSAS when results are positive but unfortunately do not rule out OSAS when results are negative.[108-110] Therefore, children with negative results on screening studies should undergo a more comprehensive evaluation. Likewise, positive results on daytime nap studies have been shown to predict OSAS, whereas negative study results do not exclude the possibility of finding OSAS on an overnight study.[99,111] Questionnaires with emphasis on the symptoms and potential health outcomes of sleep-disordered breathing in children have not been shown to have sufficient sensitivity and specificity to diagnose OSAS in individual patients.[23,31,112,113] Reports from one center suggest that evaluation for sleep-disordered breathing may be accomplished with unattended home polysomnography.[114,115] The home test performed included measurement of oxygen saturation, ventilation, and video recordings. These tests are not widely available, and additional validation of unattended home sleep studies is needed.

Other diagnostic tests may be useful when evaluating a child for OSAS. A chest radiograph, electrocardiogram, and echocardiogram should be considered for any child with symptoms or signs of cardiovascular complications, such as congestive heart failure or hypertension. Children with multiple or lengthy episodes of hypoxemia or extremely severe hypoxemia on polysomnography may require formal cardiopulmonary evaluation as well. Children with these cardiovascular complications of OSAS should have repeat polysomnography after therapy to confirm resolution of OSAS.

Although airway radiographs, cephalometric studies, and computed tomography scans may assist in designing the treatment plan for high-risk children with OSAS caused by unusual anatomic abnormalities, these studies are of limited use in the diagnosis of OSAS in otherwise healthy children. Li and coworkers determined a ratio of tonsil size and pharyngeal depth on lateral radiographs that correlated with severity of OSAS, even though clinical measurements of tonsil size did not.[116] Jain and Sahni were able to predict OSAS based on a ratio of adenoid size to nasopharyngeal depth on lateral radiographs, although clinical tonsil size measurements were not helpful.[117] Sleep fluoroscopy has been described by Gibson and associates for evaluating children at risk for upper airway obstruction at multiple levels.[118] Although dynamic assessments of airway anatomy and function using endoscopy or imaging such as cine-magnetic resonance imaging during sleep have been used in adults with OSAS and in some children with OSAS within a complex clinical picture, these techniques require additional investigation before they can be recommended for widespread use in children.[119,120]

Indications for Polysomnography

Polysomnography remains the gold standard modality for diagnosing sleep apnea in children, because clinical assessment alone is sensitive but not specific for OSAS. The controversies regarding the use of polysomnography in otherwise healthy children with suspected OSAS are reviewed by Messner, who recognizes both the need for this test to diagnose childhood OSAS and the impracticalities of mandatory use before adenotonsillectomy.[121] Children who undergo adenotonsillectomy for recurrent pharyngeal infection may have obstructive symptoms as well. These children do not require polysomnography on a routine basis. Polysomnography is recommended to invetigate concerns that the patient also may have severe OSAS requiring intensive postoperative monitoring. The use of preoperative polysomnography is most controversial in healthy children with obstructive adenotonsillar hypertrophy and no other surgical indication. Historically, adenotonsillectomy has been used to manage obstructive symptoms in healthy children without preoperative polysomnography. In fact, in a recent survey of otolaryngologists and pediatric otolaryngologists by Kay and associates, history alone remains the most common method of establishing OSAS as a surgical indication for adenotonsillectomy in children.[122] Weatherly and colleagues estimated that less than 5% of children with sleep-disordered breathing undergo laboratory-based polysomnography before adenotonsillectomy.[123] An important point is that this practice will lead to potentially unnecessary tonsillectomy in some children with obstructive symptoms but without OSAS.

The use of polysomnography to both diagnose OSAS and assess perioperative risk is recommended in children with suspected sleep-related upper-airway obstruction prior to adenotonsillectomy by both the American Academy of Pediatrics and the American Thoracic Society. The use of preoperative polysomnography is especially important in high-risk patients, including those with craniofacial anomalies, neuromotor disease, or associated medical conditions that may complicate surgical management of OSAS. Baseline preoperative polysomnography is useful to assess postoperative improvement in such high-risk patients. Polysomnography also is useful in the evaluation of children for whom information from the history or physical examination may be inconsistent. Follow-up polysomnography is recommended for children who exhibit persistent snoring or other symptoms of sleep-related upper airway obstruction 4 to 6 weeks after surgery. A follow-up sleep study also should be considered for patients with significant complications from OSAS (e.g., cor pulmonale, failure to thrive), patients with severe OSAS on an initial sleep study, or patients who are very young (younger than 1 year of age) to ensure resolution of nighttime breathing abnormalities.[102]

Surgical Management

Tonsillectomy or Adenoidectomy

Tonsillectomy, adenoidectomy, or adenotonsillectomy is the most common surgical treatment for childhood OSAS. Adenoid and tonsillar hyperplasia appears to be a key element in the compromise of airway patency during sleep in otherwise healthy children with OSAS.[124,125] Brodsky and coworkers demonstrated that children undergoing adenotonsillectomy for obstruction had decreased lateral oropharyngeal dimensions compared with children undergoing adenotonsillectomy for chronic infection.[126] These investigators suggest that decreased oropharyngeal size, in addition to adenotonsillar hyperplasia, may contribute to OSAS in children. Removal of enlarged lymphoid tissue in Waldeyer's ring is curative for most of these children.[39,127-129] Adenotonsillectomy can be recommended for initial treatment of medically complicated children with complex OSAS as well, because this surgical procedure may be curative in appropriately selected children.[130]

Perioperative management of children undergoing adenotonsillectomy for OSAS should be individualized, with the recognition that these children have more frequent postoperative complications and the potential for serious respiratory compromise.[78,79] Children younger than 3 years of age, children with severe OSAS documented by polysomnography, and children with craniofacial anomalies or neuromotor impairment are at greatest risk for perioperative respiratory compromise.[77,78,131-133] Preoperative risk assessment centers on the severity of sleep disturbance as documented by polysomnography. A recent report noted the predictive value of polysomnography in identifying children at risk for respiratory compromise after adenotonsillectomy. The study investigators suggested that preoperative nocturnal oximetry may have similar value.[134] Patients with severe OSAS may be treated with CPAP before adenotonsillectomy if surgery is to be delayed or if significant cardiovascular complications are present. Children with OSAS should undergo routine assessment of hemostatic factors and anesthetic risk for adenotonsillectomy.[135,136]

Preoperative sedation should be used judiciously in children with documented or suspected severe OSAS. Cultrara and coworkers reported on a series of 65 children who were sedated with oral midazolam before adenotonsillectomy for OSAS, diagnosed either clinically or by polysomnography.[137] No adverse respiratory events were seen in any of these patients. In a similar prospective study of 70 children with OSAS, Francis and associates noted brief self-limited respiratory events in only two children after sedation with oral midazolam before adenotonsillectomy.[138] These results should be interpreted with some caution, owing to small numbers in these studies and heterogeneity of the sample population, including variability in the severity of OSAS.

Adenotonsillectomy is performed using standard techniques, with attention to minimizing edema in children at risk for postoperative obstruction. A majority of children who undergo adenotonsillectomy for mild OSAS experience immediate improvement as shown by sleep studies performed on the first postoperative night.[139] However, children with severe OSAS or complicating anatomic or neuromotor disorders often have a prolonged recovery or incomplete relief of OSAS.[77-79]

Radiofrequency tonsil reduction is a new technique that has been introduced as a potential treatment, in combination with surgical adenoidectomy, for OSAS in children. A pilot study of this technique demonstrated less pain when compared with conventional tonsillectomy and improvement in several clinical and polysomnographic parameters of OSAS.[140] Intracapsular subtotal tonsillectomy using several different surgical methods also has been introduced as a method of reducing perioperative morbidity in children being treated for OSAS.[141-143] Powered intracapsular tonsillectomy and adenoidectomy can reliably achieve at least short-term cure of moderate OSAS as documented by polysomnography in otherwise healthy children.[143a] The long-term efficacy of these techniques, as compared with conventional adenotonsillectomy, needs to be demonstrated in future studies.

Inpatient postoperative management, along with cardiorespiratory monitoring and pulse oximetry, is necessary for high-risk children who have moderate to severe OSAS.[78,133,144] Recovery should occur in an area in which signs of respiratory depression and airway swelling can be recognized and prompt intervention can be instituted.[136] Narcotics should be used judiciously, and postoperative oxygen supplementation should be used with careful monitoring for signs of depression of ventilatory drive. Several studies have demonstrated increased sensitivity to narcotics with regard to analgesic effects and respiratory depression in children with OSAS.[145,146] Steroids often are administered perioperatively, and nasopharyngeal airways are used in high-risk patients to support the airway after surgery. CPAP or bilevel positive airway pressure (BPAP) can be used for children with obstructive symptoms after adenotonsillectomy, including those necessitating airway support in the immediate postoperative period.[147-149]

Expected Results of Adenotonsillectomy for Obstructive Sleep Disorders in Children

Several authors have documented the clinical effectiveness of adenotonsillectomy for nocturnal upper airway obstruction in children.[128,150] Helfaer and colleagues performed polysomnography on otherwise healthy children with mild OSAS on the first night after adenotonsillectomy.[139] The number of apnea events decreased and oxygen saturation during sleep improved immediately after surgery in these children.

In some children, OSAS may persist after surgical treatment. Suen and coworkers reported that children with severe OSAS (RDI greater than 19.1) on preoperative polysomnography were likely to have residual OSAS after surgery.[95] Mitchell and Kelly found persistent OSAS in the majority of children with severe OSAS, as defined by a preoperative RDI 30 or greater, although most were improved by polysomnographic and quality of life measures.[151] In a large cohort of children diagnosed with OSAS by polysomnography, adenotonsillectomy resulted in significant relief of sleep and respiratory abnormalities found preoperatively but resulted in complete cure (defined as as obstructive apnea index of 1 or less) in only 25%.[152] In this study, 29% of the patients had an obstructive event index of 5 or higher after surgery. Children with high preoperative AHI and obese children were the least likely to be cured by surgery. Rapid relief of obstructive symptoms can be expected after adenotonsillectomy in children with mild OSAS, but OSAS may persist in severe cases or in children with significant risk factors for OSAS including obesity.

Brietzke and Gallagher performed a meta-analysis of available literature to try to determine the cure rate for adenotonsillectomy perfomed for childhood OSAS.[153] They identified 14 studies, all case series, and found a post-surgery reduction in AHI by approximately 14 events per hour. The summary success rate was 83%. Gozal and Kheirandish-Gozal reported a cure rate of 77% in a recent review but noted residual OSAS in up to 45% of children after adenotonsillectomy in their own prospective study.[154]

Of interest, more snoring and increased inspiratory effort during sleep were noted in teenagers studied 12 years after adenotonsillectomy.[155] This finding emphasizes the need for long-term study of both the natural history of and treatment outcomes for OSAS in children.

Quality of life improves for children after adenotonsillectomy for sleep apnea. De Serres and colleagues reported the results of a multicenter study of quality of life changes after adenotonsillectomy in children who had adenotonsillectomy for treatment of obstructive sleep disorders.[156] Large changes in quality of life were documented in almost 75% of children, with the most improved domains being sleep disturbance, caregiver concerns, and physical suffering. The OSA-18 is a well-validated quality of life instrument that has been useful in assessing the outcomes of patients treated for sleep-disordered breathing in several studies.[157] Using the OSA-18, Goldstein and associates found similar improvements in quality of life, again with the most significant improvements seen in the domains of sleep disturbance, caregiver concerns and physical discomfort, with concomitant improvements in behavior after adenotonsillectomy.[158] Mitchell and coworkers have documented more long-term quality of life improvements in children at 9 to 24 months after adenotonsillectomy.[159]

Other Pharyngeal Surgery

Resection of palatal and pharyngeal tissue in children as management of OSAS is almost always performed in combination with or subsequent to adenotonsillectomy. Uvulopalatopharyngoplasty (UPPP) is not widely used for the management of children with OSAS. It is used primarily for children at high risk for persistent obstruction because of neuromuscular dysfunction after adenotonsillectomy.[160] Seid and associates reported on the use of UPPP in combination with adenotonsillectomy in 10 children with obstructive apnea and mental retardation with neuromotor disease of diverse causes.[131] Only two patients required additional surgery to relieve OSAS, and one 15-month-old patient with cerebral palsy required subsequent tracheotomy. Tracheotomy was avoided in nine patients, but postoperative sleep studies were not performed.

Kosko and Derkay noted similar favorable results with UPPP combined with adenotonsillectomy in neurologically impaired children with OSAS, with 12 of 15 children showing improvement on pulse oximetry or formal polysomnography.[161] Donaldson and Redmond and also Strome have successfully used UPPP as part of the surgical management of OSAS in children with Down syndrome.[162,163] Kerschner and coworkers treated a diverse group of neurologically impaired children with OSAS with UPPP and adenotonsillectomy.[164] These workers noted long-term improvement in two thirds of their 15 patients but emphasized the need for close follow-up, because one third of their patients had recurrent or persistent upper airway obstruction severe enough to recommend tracheotomy. Potential postoperative velar dysfunction and voice alteration should be considered in the decision-making process for management of such high-risk children with OSAS. Fiberoptic endoscopy of velopharyngeal anatomy may be useful before UPPP is considered, especially in children with poor pharyngeal tone secondary to neuromotor disease.

Tongue reduction surgery has been proposed for the management of macroglossia in conjunction with OSAS, such as is seen in Beckwith-Wiedemann and Down syndromes.[165] Anterior tongue reduction probably improves cosmesis more than airway function, because the central and posterior tongue size may be more critical to airway patency. Rimell and colleagues noted that children with Beckwith-Wiedemann syndrome often required tracheotomy when airway obstruction occurred during the neonatal period.[166] These investigators also found that adenotonsillectomy probably was more beneficial than tongue reduction for managing OSAS in these children with macroglossia. Central tongue reduction has been reported to relieve symptoms of OSAS in children with Down syndrome and other craniofacial disorders.[167,168]

Obstructive sleep apnea has been described in children who have undergone pharyngeal flap surgery for correction of velopharyngeal incompetence.[169,170] Sleep-associated airway obstruction usually is most pronounced in the immediate postoperative period, and obstructive symptoms subside as the flap atrophies during the next several months. In a subset of these children, chronic OSAS may develop that may require flap revision or takedown. Predisposing anatomic factors may include tonsillar or adenoidal hypertrophy, micrognathia, or abnormalities of pharyngeal tone. OSAS after pharyngeal flap surgery appears to be more common in children born with the Pierre Robin

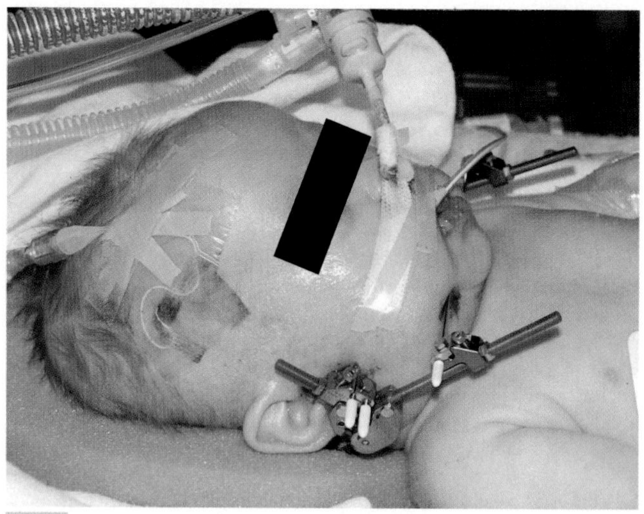

Figure 183-3. Neonate with mandibular distraction device to correct retrognathia.

sequence.[171,172] The need for close follow-up of children after pharyngeal flap surgery is emphasized by Liao and associates, who reported that 90% of children had abnormalities on polysomnograms done 6 months after flap surgery. This group used the strictest criteria for diagnosing OSAS in children: anRDI of 1 or greater.[173] Modifications of the pharyngeal flap technique, including the use of a shorter, more superiorly based flap in a procedure performed several months after planned first-stage adenoidectomy, can reduce the risk of OSAS in syndromic children.[174] Fortunately, when flap division is required for treatment of children with OSAS that persists, the speech and voice benefits of the flap surgery usually are preserved.[175]

Craniofacial Surgery

A variety of surgical procedures have been proposed to manage OSAS in children with complex craniofacial disorders or neuromotor disease. Burstein and associates successfully used mandibular advancement, tongue reduction, tongue-hyoid suspension, and other nasal and pharyngeal procedures to manage children with OSAS with abnormal craniofacial anatomy with or without neuromuscular disease.[167] Tracheotomy was avoided in 90% of this heterogeneous group of children with complex OSAS, including children with hemifacial microsomia, Down syndrome, and cerebral palsy.[176]

Children with severe OSAS and micrognathia may benefit from mandibular advancement or tongue suspension. Tracheotomy often is required in neonates and infants with these conditions to secure the airway until craniofacial growth and neuromotor maturation relieve the sleep-disordered breathing. Tomaski and coworkers have noted that children with isolated Pierre Robin sequence usually can be managed conservatively with nasopharyngeal tube placement and positioning, whereas syndromic children with associated anomalies often require tracheotomy for relief of airway obstruction.[177]

The principles of distraction osteogenesis have been used to treat children with OSAS from isolated mandibular hypoplasia.[178] Mandibular distraction has been used in children with more complex craniofacial conditions such as Treacher Collins syndrome or hemifacial microsomia, both to avoid tracheotomy and to achieve early decannulation.[179,180] A recent study documented dramatic improvement in polysomnographic measures in 10 syndromic children with upper airway obstruction after treatment with mandibular distraction.[181] Lin and associates documented the long-term benefits of mandibular distraction by performing polysomnography 4 years after surgery for neonatal upper airway obstruction[182] (Fig. 183-3). Four children had no evidence of residual or recurrent OSAS, whereas one child had severe OSAS requiring treatment. Midface distraction has been used to achieve decannulation in two patients with achondroplasia and OSAS.[183] Long-term follow-up of these children with complex OSAS-causing conditions is essential after such surgery, especially because relapse of upper airway obstruction after initial improvement has been observed in some children after mandibular distraction.[184]

Tracheotomy

Tracheotomy is indicated for the management of severe OSAS in children with complicated anatomic or neuromotor issues. A review of the literature on pediatric tracheotomy indicated that tracheotomy is now performed more often for dynamic airway issues such as severe OSAS than for fixed airway lesions.[185] Tracheotomy bypasses the areas of airway obstruction during sleep.

Tracheotomy should be considered for patients with severe OSAS associated with neuromotor disease. Tracheotomy can be avoided in some cases by UPPP, pharyngeal surgery, craniofacial surgery, or CPAP.[78,161,167] Although tracheotomy is almost always successful in relieving upper airway obstruction, the decision to perform tracheotomy must be made in the context of underlying medical conditions in the child with OSAS and the recognition of the detrimental effects of tracheotomy on the quality of life.[186]

Other Surgical Management

OSAS may be caused or worsened by nasal abnormalities or nasopharyngeal masses. Choanal atresia or stenosis can cause OSAS in neonates, and transnasal and transpalatal approaches for surgical repair are described earlier in this chapter. Nasal septal deviation as an isolated finding rarely causes childhood OSAS. Septoplasty and turbinate reduction have been used to relieve nasal obstruction and improve nocturnal breathing in adults.

Intranasal masses can cause snoring or OSAS in young infants, and removal usually is curative. Obstructive intranasal masses in children include foreign bodies, inflammatory polyps, mucoceles, and congenital masses such as nasolacrimal duct cysts.

Benign and malignant tumors of the head and neck can manifest with symptoms of OSAS. Supraglottic or parapharyngeal lymphangiomas (cystic hygroma) can cause symptoms of obstructive sleep apnea. Excision of such masses can relieve airway symptoms.[187] Nasopharyngeal carcinoma, juvenile nasopharyngeal angiofibroma, lymphoma, and rhabdomyosarcoma can manifest with obstructive symptoms when nasal or pharyngeal patency is affected. Appropriate oncologic treatment using combinations of surgery, chemotherapy, and radiotherapy can relieve airway symptoms, but airway support may be necessary until tumor regression occurs.

Nonsurgical Management

Children who fail to respond to or are not candidates for surgical intervention often can be managed successfully with nasal CPAP or BPAP.[148,149,188,189] Both modalities are safe, efficacious, and well tolerated by children. The level of positive pressure required to eliminate obstructive apneas and normalize ventilation and nighttime oxygen saturation must be determined in the sleep laboratory. Studies have demonstrated the need for serial evaluation and adjustment of CPAP in growing children, because their pressure requirements will change with time.[148,190]

Complications of CPAP or BPAP usually are minor. Local discomfort or irritation may result from poor mask fit. Regular follow-up to assess mask fit is important. Nasal symptoms such as congestion or rhinorrhea also are common. Nasal steroids or humidification of the delivered air can help relieve nasal obstruction. Hypoventilation and increased central apneas can be seen in children using CPAP or BPAP ventilators.[149] In these children, bilevel ventilation with a back-up rate can be employed. Potentially serious complications of CPAP and BPAP ventilation, including pneumothorax and clinically significant reductions in cardiac output, have not been reported in children treated for OSAS. One case report described the development of midface hypoplasia in a 15-year-old boy treated with nasal CPAP for 10 years for OSAS.[191] With long-term use of a nasal mask in children, regular evaluation of maxillomandibular growth and development is warranted.

Poor compliance is the greatest limitation to the use of CPAP and BPAP in the management of OSAS.[148,192] Pediatric centers have estimated compliance at 50% to 100%, with adolescents being the least compliant.[148] Rains improved compliance with CPAP therapy in four developmentally delayed children with OSAS by using intensive behavioral interventions including parent training, modeling, and desensitization.[193] In many cases, compliance problems are attributable primarily to the parent or caregiver rather than to the child.[148,192] With careful attention to training of caregivers and children, prompt and aggressive treatment of minor side effects, and close follow-up, the vast majority of families can be trained to successfully use CPAP or BPAP ventilation.

Nocturnal oxygen supplementation has been studied as a temporary treatment for hypoxemia associated with OSAS until definitive therapy can be provided.[194,195] Supplemental oxygen therapy in patients with OSAS may suppress hypoxic ventilatory drive, decrease upper airway tone, and worsen OSAS.[196] Aljadeff and coworkers administered supplemental oxygen to 16 children with OSAS secondary to adenotonsillar hypertrophy and found a decrease in apneic events, lessened paradoxical breathing, increased REM sleep, decreased arousals during sleep without hypoventilation, and increased central apneas.[194] Marcus and colleagues, however, noted significant hypercarbia in 2 of 23 children with OSAS when breathing supplemental oxygen.[195] In most cases, supplemental oxygen therapy will improve oxygenation during sleep without exacerbating sleep-disordered breathing. However, nocturnal oxygen therapy for children with OSAS should be initiated only under monitored conditions. Despite normalization of oxygen saturations, patients with OSAS treated with supplemental oxygen continue to have upper airway obstruction with resulting increased work of breathing, arousals and hypercapnia. Therefore, definitive therapy must still be pursued to prevent the long-term complications of OSAS.

Corticosteroids have been used with some success to treat obstructive symptoms in acute conditions that increase adenoid and tonsil size, such as infectious mononucleosis. A 5-day course of oral prednisone was not effective in treating children with OSAS from chronic adenotonsillar hypertrophy.[197] A few studies have demonstrated a beneficial response to topical intranasal steroids in pediatric patients with OSA. In one small trial, nasal fluticasone given for 6 weeks led to modest improvement in polysomnographic parameters in the treatment group.[198] Many patients, however, continued to have an abnormal apnea index after treatment and a significant number eventually had surgery. In a second study, a 4-week course of nasal budesonide led to an improvement in the mean AHI (from 5.2 to 3.2) and a mean symptom score. The improvement in the symptom score was sustained for several months after discontinuation of therapy.[199] Leukotriene receptor antagonists also have been examined in the treatment of children with OSAS. A small group of children with mild OSAS treated for 16 weeks with daily montelukast were found to have significant reductions in adenoid size and improved breathing during sleep documented by polysomnography.[200] Leukotriene receptor antagonists in combination with intranasal steroids were studied in 36 children with mild residual OSAS after adenotonsillectomy. After 12 weeks of therapy, children in the treatment group had improved AHI, higher nadir oxygen saturation, and decreased respiratory arousals compared with control subjects.[201] Both topical intranasal steroids and leukotriene receptor anatagonists may have promising roles in the management of OSAS, particularly mild OSAS, in children. However, further studies to evaluate effectiveness and appropriate dosing and duration of therapy are needed.

The use of orthodontic devices in the treatment of OSAS in children also appears encouraging in early studies. Rapid maxillary expansion (RME) is an orthodontic treatment that widens the palate and nasal orifices. The use of RME in children with OSAS described as having maxillary contraction has led to resolution of OSAS in this select group.[202,203] Use of orthodontic devices designed to advance the mandible also has led to improvements in sleep-related upper airway obstruction.[204,205] Again, further studies are needed to define the indications and candidates for and the effectiveness of orthodontic treatment in children with OSAS.

As in adults, weight loss is an important component of the management of OSAS in obese children.[206-209] Because weight loss will also lead to other significant health benefits, nutritional counseling with aggressive follow-up is necessary for these patients.

Summary

Obstructive sleep apnea in children is an important and common medical condition that can lead to significant morbidity. The diagnosis of obstructive sleep apnea in children requires clinical suspicion supplemented with the use of specific diagnostic tests. Polysomnography remains the key to diagnosis and helps assess the need for treatment, the risk for perioperative respiratory compromise, and the likelihood of persistent OSAS after treatment. Adenotonsillectomy is the mainstay of treatment, although children with complex medical conditions affecting upper airway anatomy and tone may require additional treatment.

SUGGESTED READINGS

American Thoracic Society. Standards and indications for cardiopulmonary sleep studies in children. *Am J Respir Crit Care Med.* 1996;153(2):866-878.

Beebe DW. Neurobehavioral morbidity associated with disordered breathing during sleep in children: a comprehensive review. *Sleep.* 2006;29(9):1115-1134.

Brietzke SE, Gallagher D. The effectiveness of tonsillectomy and adenoidectomy in the treatment of pediatric obstructive sleep apnea/hypopnea syndrome: a meta-analysis. *Otolaryngol Head Neck Surg.* 2006;134(6):979-984.

Brietzke SE, Katz ES, Roberson DW. Can history and physical examination reliably diagnose pediatric obstructive sleep apnea/hypopnea syndrome? A systematic review of the literature. *Otolaryngol Head Neck Surg.* 2004; 131(6):827-832.

Brown KA, Laferriere A, Lakheeram I, et al. Recurrent hypoxemia in children is associated with increased analgesic sensitivity to opiates. *Anesthesiology.* 2006;105(4):665-669.

Carroll JL, McColley SA, Marcus CL, et al. Inability of clinical history to distinguish primary snoring from obstructive sleep apnea syndrome in children. *Chest.* 1995;108(3):610-618.

Chervin RD, Archbold KH, Dillon JE, et al. Inattention, hyperactivity, and symptoms of sleep-disordered breathing. *Pediatrics.* 2002;109(3):449-456.

Chervin RD, Ruzicka DL, Giordani BJ, et al. Sleep-disordered breathing, behavior, and cognition in children before and after adenotonsillectomy. *Pediatrics.* 2006;117(4):e769-e778.

Cohen SR, Simms C, Burstein FD, et al. Alternatives to tracheostomy in infants and children with obstructive sleep apnea. *J Pediatr Surg.* 1999;34(1):182-186.

De Serres LM, Derkay C, Sie K, et al. Impact of adenotonsillectomy on quality of life in children with obstructive sleep disorders. *Arch Otolaryngol Head Neck Surg.* 2002;128(5):489-496.

Farber JM. Clinical practice guideline: diagnosis and management of childhood obstructive sleep apnea syndrome. *Pediatrics.* 2002;110(6):1255-1257.

Gozal D. Sleep-disordered breathing and school performance in children. *Pediatrics.* 1998;102(3 Pt 1):616-620.

Gozal D, Crabtree VM, Sans CO, et al. C-reactive protein, obstructive sleep apnea, and cognitive dysfunction in school-aged children. *Am J Respir Crit Care Med.* 2007;176(2):188-193.

Gozal D, Kheirandish-Gozal L. Sleep apnea in children—treatment considerations. *Paediatr Respir Rev.* 2006;7(Suppl 1):S58-S61.

Kheirandish L, Goldbart AD, Gozal D. Intranasal steroids and oral leukotriene modifier therapy in residual sleep-disordered breathing after tonsillectomy and adenoidectomy in children. *Pediatrics.* 2006;117:e61-e66.

Marcus CL. Pathophysiology of childhood obstructive sleep apnea: current concepts. *Respir Physiol.* 2000;119(2-3):143-154.

Marcus CL, Ward SL, Mallory GB, et al. Use of nasal continuous positive airway pressure as treatment of childhood obstructive sleep apnea. *J Pediatr.* 1995;127(1):88-94.

McColley SA, April MM, Carroll JL, et al. Respiratory compromise after adenotonsillectomy in children with obstructive sleep apnea. *Arch Otolaryngol Head Neck Surg.* 1992;118(9):940-943.

Monasterio FO, Drucker M, Molina F, et al. Distraction osteogenesis in Pierre Robin sequence and related respiratory problems in children. *J Craniofac Surg.* 2002;13(1):79-83.

Richards W, Ferdman RM. Prolonged morbidity due to delays in the diagnosis and treatment of obstructive sleep apnea in children. *Clin Pediatr (Phila).* 2000;39(2):103-108.

Rosen CL, D'Andrea L, Haddad GG. Adult criteria for obstructive sleep apnea do not identify children with serious obstruction. *Am Rev Respir Dis.* 1992;146(5 Pt 1):1231-1234.

Rosen GM, Muckle RP, Mahowald MW, et al. Postoperative respiratory compromise in children with obstructive sleep apnea syndrome: can it be anticipated? *Pediatrics.* 1994;93(5):784-788.

Tauman R, Gulliver TE, Krishna J, et al. Persistence of obstructive sleep apnea syndrome in children after adenotonsillectomy. *J Pediatr.* 2006;149(6):803-808.

Waters KA, Everett FM, Bruderer JW, et al. Obstructive sleep apnea: the use of nasal CPAP in 80 children. *Am J Respir Crit Care Med.* 1995;152(2):780-785.

For complete list of references log onto www.expertconsult.com.

Craniofacial

CHAPTER ONE HUNDRED AND EIGHTY-FOUR

Characteristics of Normal and Abnormal Postnatal Craniofacial Growth and Development

Frederick K. Kozak

Juan Camilo Ospina

Key Points

- All theories of facial growth control mechanisms are speculative, and none is fully satisfactory.
- In Moss's functional matrix hypothesis, regulation of growth of cartilage and bone is exerted by the functional matrix surrounding them.
- The craniofacial complex can be divided into three regions: neurocranium, nasomaxillary complex, and mandible.
- Asymmetry is recognized as an intrinsic facial characteristic.
- Ionizing radiation negatively affects developing bone and soft tissue, causing several side effects and facial alterations, both functional and cosmetic.
- The correlation between animal and human experiments regarding the effects of nasoseptal and sinus surgery on craniofacial growth remains unclear.
- Effects of functional endoscopic sinus surgery (FESS) on facial growth are yet to be consistently proven.
- The use of resorbable hardware systems is highly recommended in pediatric craniofacial surgery.
- Debate is ongoing regarding the correction of nasal septal deformity or deviation in neonates and older children. A conservative approach may be warranted until more definitive data are available.
- Controversy exists in the literature regarding the role that nasal or nasopharyngeal obstruction plays with regard to dentofacial growth and development.
- Robin sequence can appear as an isolated entity or as part of several craniofacial syndromes.
- Craniofacial surgery in patients with mandibulofacial dysostosis (Treacher Collins syndrome) using osteotomies and advancement techniques appears to assist in the orientation of subsequent growth in a more normal direction and to enlarge the airway at the same time.

Volumes of literature have been written on facial growth and development, and entire academic careers have been spent researching various concepts and theories. Searching through the published literature can be overwhelming. This chapter provides a place to begin the study of facial growth and development and reviews major changes in growth from birth to late adolescence. *Growth* refers to an increase in size, whereas *development* indicates an increase in complexity of structure and function.

An understanding of the abnormal first requires comprehension of the normal. Accordingly, this chapter is divided into two parts: A brief review of the main theories of postnatal craniofacial growth and the characteristics of normal postnatal facial growth and development is presented first. Subsequently, abnormal facial growth and development are examined through several clinical examples of relevance in pediatric otolaryngology. Embryology of the head and neck is covered in Chapter 181.

Theories of Craniofacial Growth

Postnatal facial growth appears to be a complex, multifactorial phenomenon. It is clear from the resemblance of children to their parents in both facial structure and soft tissue development that genetic factors play a significant role in basic facial pattern. However, "environmental" factors most certainly influence facial growth as well. These factors can range from intercellular influences to biomechanical forces (i.e., physical forces acting on bone). This essentially is Wolff's law (1870), which states that "changes in the function of a bone are attended by alterations in its structure."[1] Bone is a tissue that responds to the stresses placed on it. Bone remodels.

The genetic and environmental control mechanisms of postnatal facial growth and development are poorly understood. The three main theories of postnatal facial growth control are the genetic preprogrammed theory, the cartilage-mediated growth theory, and the functional matrix hypothesis. Following is a brief review of these theories, none of which is fully satisfactory.

Genetic Preprogrammed Theory (Growth Sites)

Early theorists believed that the sizes and shapes of bones were genetically determined within their cells and that sutural patterns were therefore predetermined. Because bone size and shape are defined by sutures in the head, these pioneers theorized that the position of sutures limits and controls the expansion of bones. Baume[2] described "growth centres" as places of endochondral ossification with tissue-separating force, resulting in an increase in skeletal mass, and "growth sites" as regions of periosteal or sutural bone formation and modeling resorption that are adaptive to environmental influences.[3] The cells of the sutures grew into the void left as the bone segments pulled apart from the tissue-separating force. In other words, growth sites are where growth literally takes place, and growth centers are areas in which genetically predetermined growth takes place. This theory was tested by experiments involving suture removal and transplantation, and the conclusion was that sutures are not primarily responsible for growth.[4] This theory is no longer accepted as correct.

Cartilage-Mediated Growth (Scott)

In 1953, Scott theorized that the cartilage of the nasal septum "is an extension of the cartilage of the cranial base."[5] In its growth, the cartilage of the nasal septum separates the facial bones from one another and from the cranial portion of the skull and allows growth to take place at the sutures by the ordinary mechanism of surface deposition. He held that the nasal septum and also the mandibular condyles and synchondroses (otherwise known as cephalic cartilages) are growth centers. As the nasal septum grows, it puts tension on the sutures of the nasomaxillary complex, thereby displacing it forward and downward, with resultant growth occurring at pressure-related growth sites. Tension occurring in the maxillary sutures causes new bone growth when the sutures are pulled apart. Therefore, suture growth is passive and secondary.

Latham[6] theorized that a septomaxillary ligament (connection between the septum and maxilla) in the fetus causes the maxilla to be pulled forward by the septum as the maxilla grows. It is unknown whether this ligament plays a role in postnatal growth, and experimentation related to the role of the nasal cartilage in this concept is unknown. Animal experimentation involving removal of septal cartilage shortly after birth[7] or secondary to trauma seems to result in midface hypoplasia, but such experiments cannot clearly prove that the cartilage removal causes the growth deficiency. Cartilage seems to play some role that has not yet been precisely determined.

The Functional Matrix Hypothesis (Moss)

The most fundamental dictum of the functional matrix hypothesis was stated by Moss,[8,9] as follows:

> The origin of all skeletal units, all of their subsequent changes in size, shape and location and their subsequent maintenance and being, are always, and without exception, secondary, compensatory and mechanical obligatory responses to the morphogenetically and temporally prior and primary alterations of the operational (functional) demands of their specifically related functional matrices. Put more succinctly, "Bones do not grow, they are grown."[10]

The basic premise of this theory is that bone and cartilage do not regulate their own growth. This theory proposes that craniofacial bony growth occurs as a reaction to—or in response to—the functional matrix surrounding it. A functional matrix consists of the cells that comprise muscle, soft tissue, teeth, glands, and nerves, as well as the functioning volumes of various cavities associated with the head and neck region (e.g., nasal, orbital, oral, pharyngeal, and neurocranial). A feedback system exists between the functional matrix and the bone and cartilage involved. Growth of cranial size occurs in response to growth of the brain, growth of the bony orbits occurs in response to the size of the orbit, and growth of the facial bones occurs in response to growth of the surrounding soft tissues. The resultant enlargement of the associated cavities of the head and neck occurs because of the functional demands of the airway, breathing, and eating "spaces." The craniofacial bones are in a dependent relationship with the surrounding soft tissues. Critics state that Moss's theory explains *what* happens during growth but does not explain *how* it happens. Moss's theory is quite useful in clinical practice because it allows separate assessment of each functional unit in the craniofacial skeleton (i.e., brain = cranium, eye = orbit, jaws (mandible) = mastication, nasomaxillary complex and associated airways = respiration, and the ear = temporal bone). The functional matrix operates within the genetic constraints of the cells and tissues involved.

Facial growth involves intimate morphogenic and biomechanical relationships among all of its component tissue parts, each influenced by and in turn influencing the other. A fundamental principle is that no part is developmentally independent or self-contained.[11]

At this time, all theories of growth control mechanisms are speculative, with strengths and faults in each. Further research is required before any definite conclusion can be made.

Bone Growth Concepts

Osteogenesis

A review of bone formation is required for a discussion of craniofacial growth. The initial step in osteogenesis is the laying down of primary or woven bone. *Primary bone* is immature bone defined by random orientation of collagen fibers and is temporary, except in a few locations such as the tooth sockets and sutures of the cranial bones. Primary bone generally either becomes secondary (lamellar) bone or is removed to leave bone marrow cavities. *Secondary bone* differs from primary bone in that its collagen has an orderly pattern and it has an increased number of osteoblasts. Osteogenesis occurs through intramembranous ossification in mesenchyme and endochondral ossification in preexisting cartilage.

Intramembranous Bone Formation

During intramembranous bone formation, mesenchymal cells differentiate into osteoblasts and accumulate in the area where bone is laid down. The osteoblasts begin to produce osteoid, which consists of collagenous fibers and a homogeneous matrix that is primary bone. Secondary bone replaces the primary bone through ossification of the osteoid.

Endochondral Bone Formation

In endochondral bone formation, simultaneous removal of cartilage and subsequent formation of bone occur. Endochondral bone formation is more complex than intramembranous bone formation. Various zones exist in active endochondral bone formation, including the zones of reserve cartilage, proliferating cartilage, hypertrophic cartilage, calcified matrix, and resorption. The hypertrophic cartilage cells enlarge, and the surrounding matrix becomes calcified. A separate collar of bone forms around the circumference of the center of this cartilage bar. This is periosteal or, more precisely, perichondral bone. A vascular bud migrates into the cartilage and a primary marrow cavity forms. Meanwhile, activity at the various zones continues. Erosion of the cartilage takes place at the two ends of the expanding primitive marrow cavity, and bone forms on the spicules of the cartilage at the erosion front. The epiphyseal plate of long bones allows simpler visualization of this process (Fig. 184-1).

This descriptive review of bone formation can be supplemented by a molecular view of bone formation.[12]

Remodeling and Displacement

Enlow and Hans[11] described the two basic types of growth movement: remodeling and displacement. This concept pertains to both bone and the surrounding soft tissues in the craniofacial complex. *Remodeling* involves changes in the size and shape of bone, the joining of separate bones and how they fit together, the adaptation intrinsically and extrinsically of these newly joined bones, and finally the relocation of these bones—each influenced by their overall enlargement. *Displacement* is the process whereby a space is created between bones as they enlarge. Resorption and deposition are ongoing in bones throughout the craniofacial complex during growth as part of the remodeling and displacement processes.

According to Rodan, "bone formation and bone resorption are finely regulated processes, controlled by local and systemic factors, carried out by a family of different interacting cells which communicate via cytokines, cell contacts, and elaboration of matrix which feeds back on cellular behavior."[13]

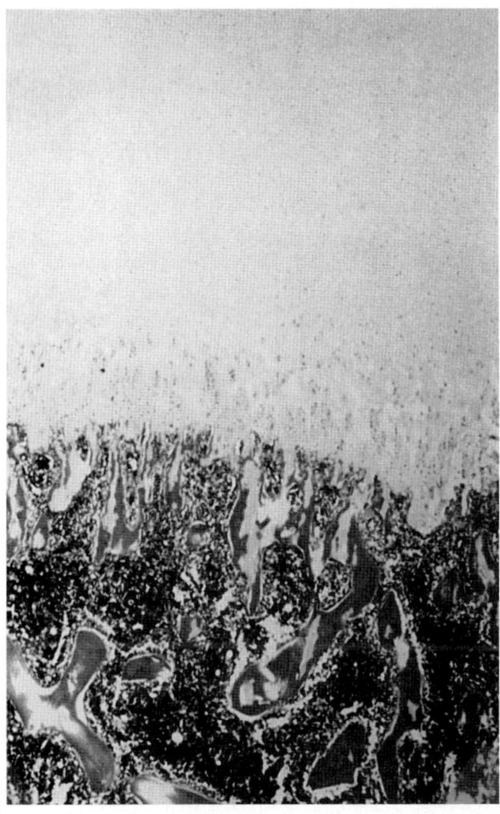

Figure 184-1. Endochondral bone formation at an epiphyseal plate.

Facial Changes during Normal Growth and Development

General

The faces of infants and children clearly differ from those of adults. Matching an infant's photograph with that of the corresponding adult photograph is challenging because of the changes that occur with growth and development of the craniofacial region. A baby's face is pudgy and round, relatively wide, and vertically short; the nose is small; the eyes appear relatively far apart; and there is a prominent forehead.

Infants have a large head relative to their body size. Their facial complex, which includes the nasomaxillary complex and mandible, is much smaller than the calvaria and basicranium (Figs. 184-2 through 184-4). With growth and development of the facial complex come changes in the size ratio of the cranium to the face. In infants the cranium-to-face ratio is approximately 3:1; whereas in adults it is approximately 2:1 (see Fig. 184-4).

With growth, increasing demands are made on the respiratory and masticatory systems. As part of the growth of the facial complex, the nose, mandible, and maxilla increase in size—resulting in the larger, coarser features of the adult face in comparison with the child's (see Fig. 184-3). The facial complex increases in size relative to the cranium. Similarly, body size increases relative to head size, to result in normal adult body and head proportions (Fig. 184-5).

Craniofacial Regions of Growth

The craniofacial complex can be divided into three regions: (1) the neurocranium, which is further divided into the calvaria and basicranium; (2) the nasomaxillary complex; and (3) the mandible. Figures 184-2 and 184-3 show the changes that occur in the craniofacial complex from birth to adulthood. The embryonic human skull has 110 ossification centers, many of which fuse, to result in 45 bones in the neonatal skull and ultimately 22 bones in the young adult skull.[1] Table 184-1 summarizes the changes in size of various anatomic sites that take place during growth and development from infancy to adulthood.[1,14-25]

Neurocranium (Calvaria = Roof and Basicranium = Floor)

Calvaria

The calvaria comprises the frontal, parietal, and parts of the temporal, occipital, and sphenoid bones. These bones are formed by intramembranous ossification, with the exception of noncalvarial parts of the occipital, temporal, and sphenoid bones, which are formed through endochondral ossification. These bones initially are separated by fontanelles, which develop into sutures early and then finally fuse in adult life (Fig. 184-6).

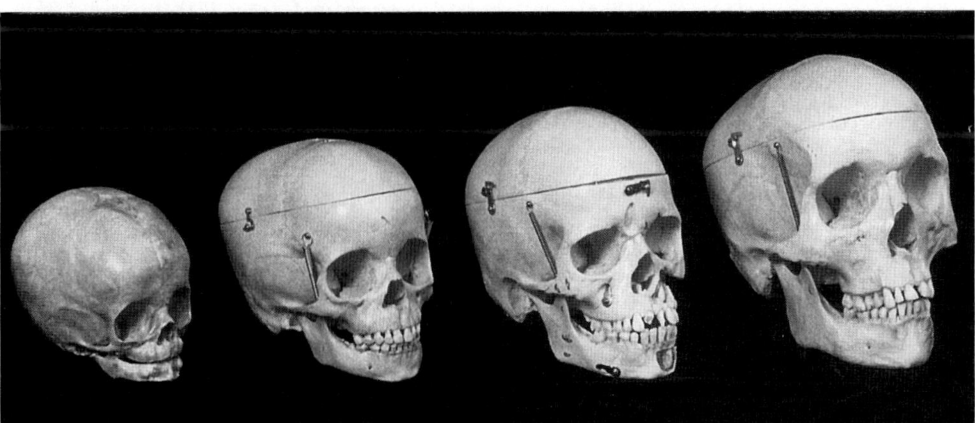

Figure 184-2. The skulls of an infant (approximately 8 months of age), a 5- to 6-year-old, a 10- to 12-year-old, and an adult. Note the bony craniofacial changes with increasing age.

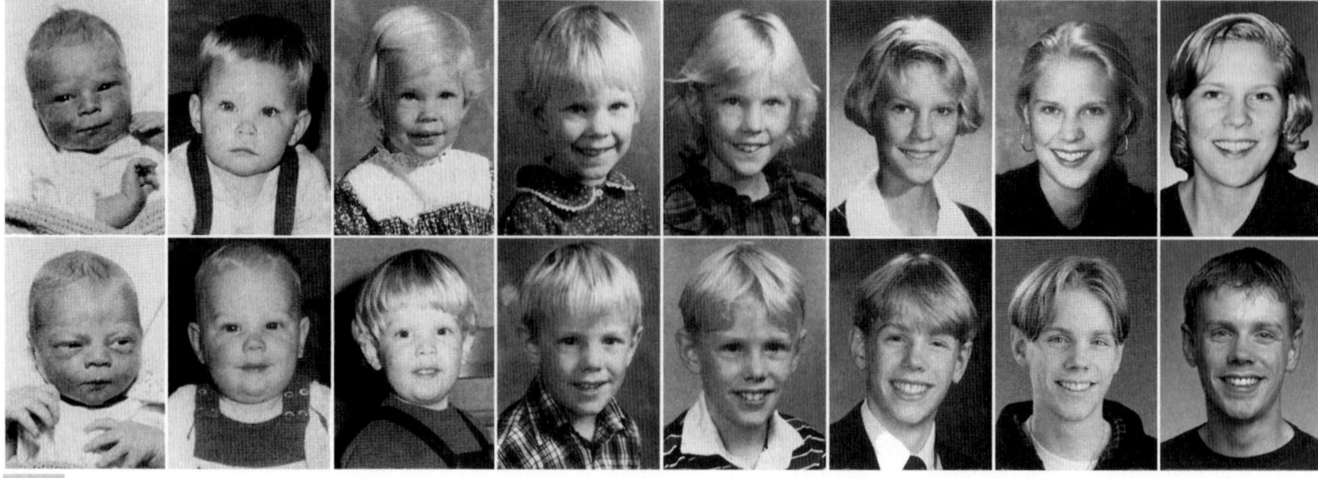

Figure 184-3. Photographs of two siblings from birth to adulthood, demonstrating changes in the craniofacial complex with growth and development. The girl is shown at birth, 10 months, 2.5 years, 6 years, 10 years, 14 years, and 18 years of age, with the last photo in adulthood at 25 years of age. Her brother male is shown at birth, 7 months, 2 years, 5 years, 9 years, 15 years, 19 years, and 25 years of age.

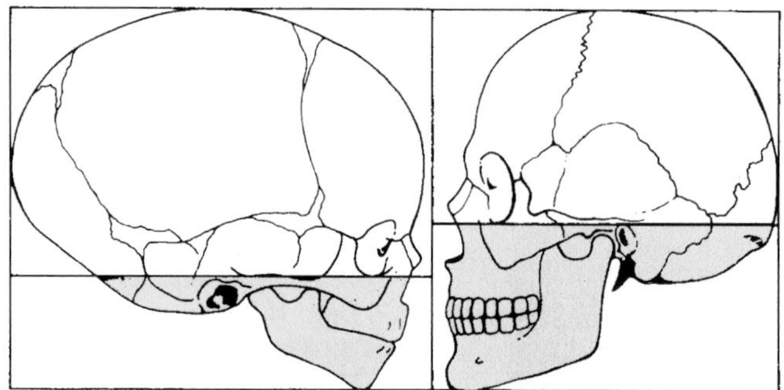

Figure 184-4. The size ratio of the cranium to the face changes considerably during growth and development. In the newborn, the cranium/face ratio is approximately 3:1, whereas in adults, this ratio is approximately 2:1. *(From Proffit WR.* Contemporary Orthodontics. *2nd ed. St Louis: Mosby; 1993.)*

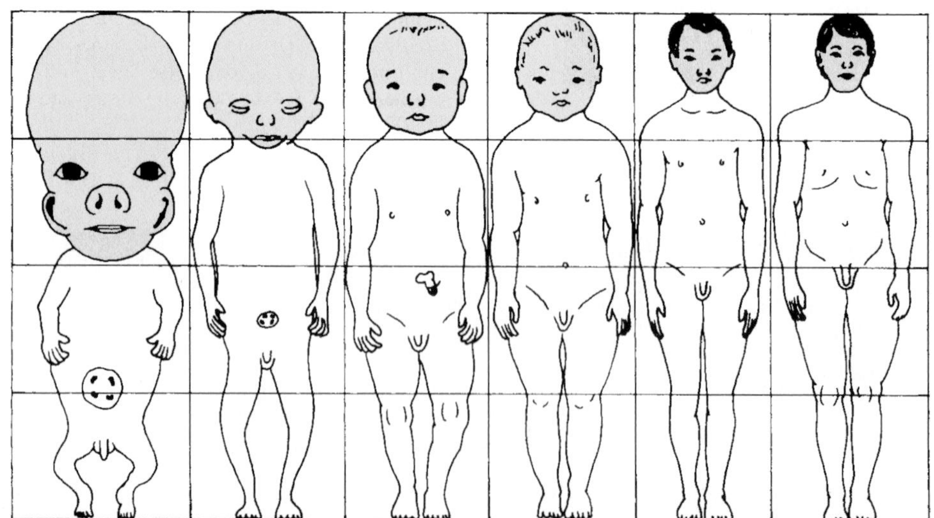

Figure 184-5. Schematic drawing showing the changes in body proportions during normal growth and development. *(From Proffit WR.* Contemporary Orthodontics. *2nd ed. St Louis: Mosby; 1993.)*

Table 184-1
Normal Craniofacial Growth and Development

Growth Aspect	Age/Development
Neurocranium growth	Birth/25% of ultimate growth 6 months/50% of ultimate growth 2 years/75% of ultimate growth 10 years/95% of ultimate growth
Facial skeletal growth	10 years/65% of ultimate growth
Neurocranium/face size ratio	Birth/8:1 2 years/6:1 5 years/4:1 Adult/2.1:1 to 2.5:1
Brain size	Birth to adulthood/3.5∞ increase
Fontanelle closure	3 months after birth/anterolateral Second year of life/posterolateral 2 months after birth/posterior Second year of life/anterior
Orbits	2 years/50% of ultimate growth 7 years/100% of ultimate growth
Inner ear	6 months of fetal life/full adult size
Brain weight	Full-term infant/25% of eventual weight 6 months/50% of eventual weight 2 years/80% of eventual weight 10 years/almost eventual weight
Postnatal brain growth	1 year/60% of ultimate growth 2 years/80% of ultimate growth 8 years/95% of ultimate growth Minimal growth continues to at least age 25 years
Facial height (males)	Birth/40% to 61% of ultimate growth
Upper facial height	1 year/63 to 86% of ultimate growth 3 years/72 to 90% of ultimate growth 5 years/82 to 100% of ultimate growth (mean, 89%)
Total facial height	Birth 38% to 45% of ultimate growth 1 year/50 to 66% of ultimate growth 3 years/66 to 78% of ultimate growth 5 years/68 to 82% of ultimate growth (mean, 77%)
Facial dimension	3 months/equivalent to 40% of adult size 2 years/equivalent of 70% of adult size 5 years/equivalent of 80% of adult size
Nasal height and nasal bridge length	Fully mature in boys at age 15, girls at age 12
Nasal tip protrusion	Boys age 15, females age 13
Upper and lower nasal dorsum	Males age 14, females age 12
Anterior and posterior nasal depth	Males age 14, females age 12
Foramen magnum	1 year/80% of transverse adult size 1 year/74% of sagittal adult size
Skull base (basion = nasion)	Birth/56% of adult length 2 years/70% of adult length 10 years/90% of adult length Prechordal part contributes 75% of the postnatal length and parachordal (basioccipital) contributes to 25%
Dentition eruption	8 months-2.5 years/primary teeth 6 years-20 years/permanent teeth
Maxillary antrum height	Birth/20% 7 years/50% 10 years/55%
Bizygomatic width	Birth/60% 3 years/80% 5 years/82% 10 years/85%
Cranial width	Birth/65% 3 years/85% 5 years/92% 10 years/95%
Cranial length	Birth/60% 3 years/85% 5 years/90% 10 years/95%

Data from references 1, 14-25.

As the child's brain grows, the calvarial bones are displaced. This displacement theoretically results in the deposition of new bone on the sutural edges. Growth of bone is seen on both the internal and external tables of the calvaria. This also results in an expanded medullary space. Significant thickening occurs from infancy to adulthood. The ascendancy (dominance) of the neurocranium over the facial complex during the early stages of life is clearly related to the inordinately early development of the brain.[21] The major portion of calvarial growth is completed by the age of 4 years (Fig. 184-7).

Basicranium

Growth of the cranial base creates space for the enlarging brain and oronasal structures with their associated airway. The basicranium grows more slowly than the neurocranium. At birth and at 10 years of age, the cranial base exhibits 63% and 95%, respectively, of its ultimate size.[21] The basicranium comprises parts of the occipital, temporal, sphenoid, and ethmoid bones. The occipital, temporal, and sphenoid portions form through endochondral ossification. The ethmoid and inferior nasal concha form solely by intramembranous bone formation.

In the midline, synchondroses are present (Fig. 184-8). These synchondroses remain after the chondrocranium (cartilage precursor of the basicranium) has ossified. During childhood, the spheno-occipital synchondrosis is the principal growth cartilage of the basicranium, and its growth persists into early adolescence.[3,11] Other synchondroses of the basicranium are the sphenoethmoidal, intersphenoidal, sphenofrontal, and frontoethmoidal synchondroses, all of which play a minimal

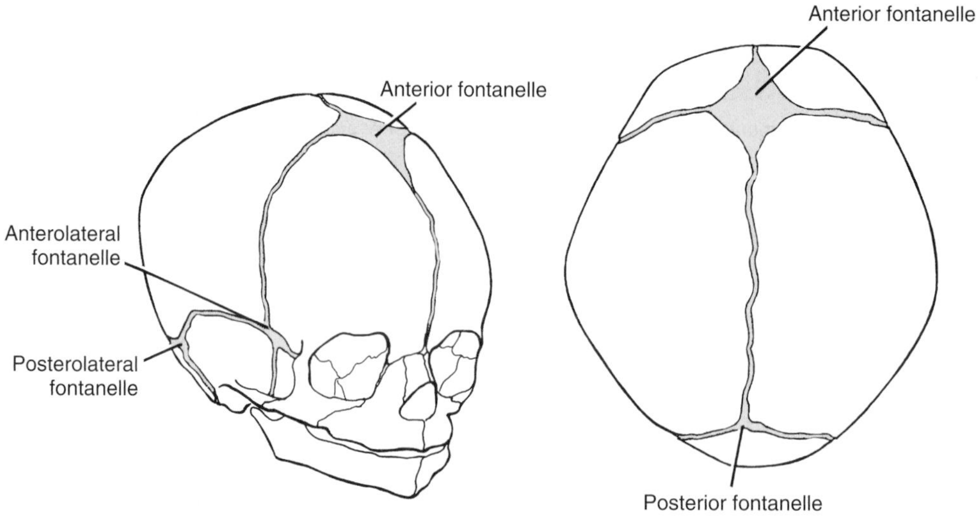

Figure 184-6. Newborn skull fontanelles.

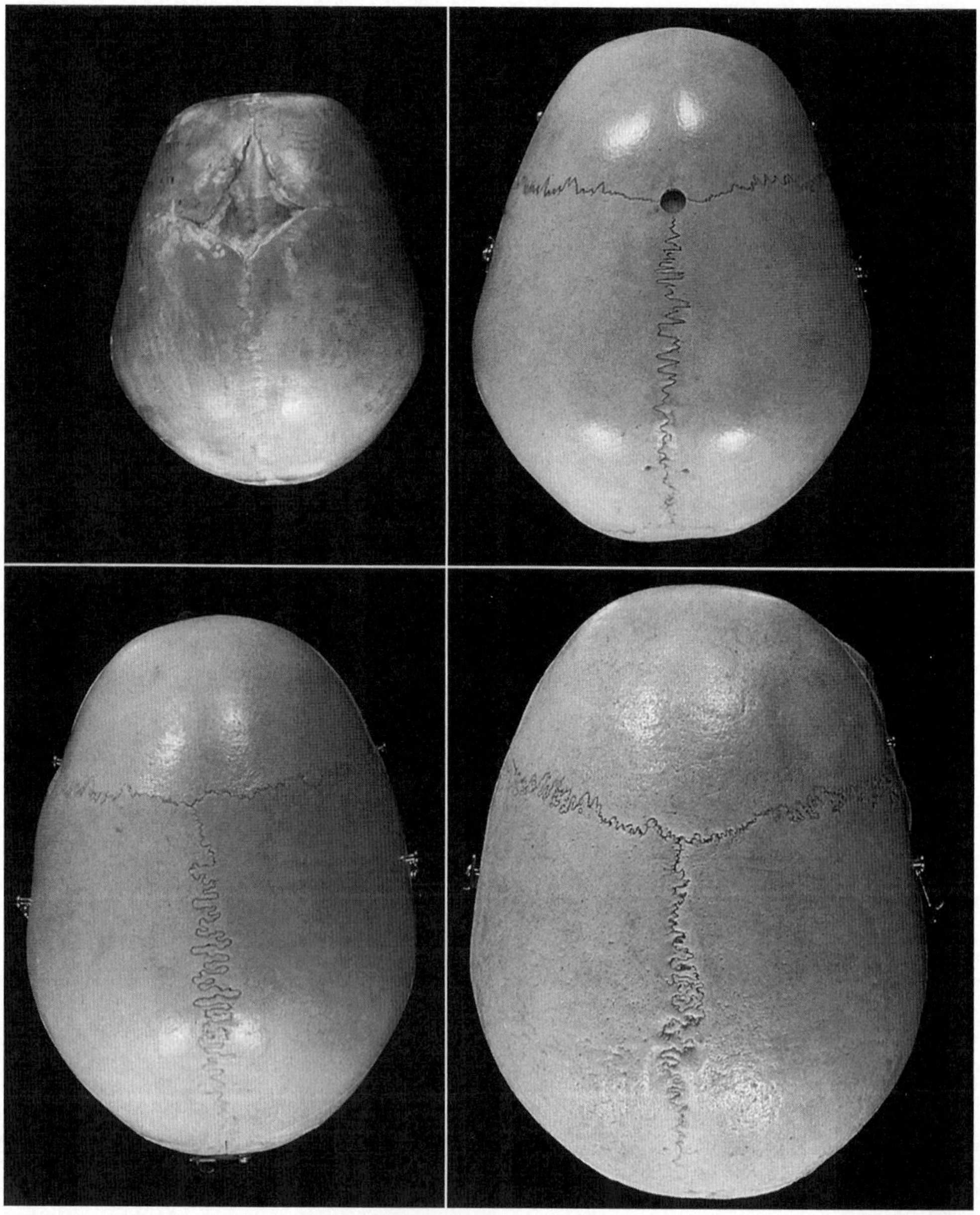

Figure 184-7. Top view of skulls showing the shape change that occurs from infancy to adulthood. Shown are infant (approximately 8 months of age), 5- to 6-year-old, 10- to 12-year-old, and adult skulls.

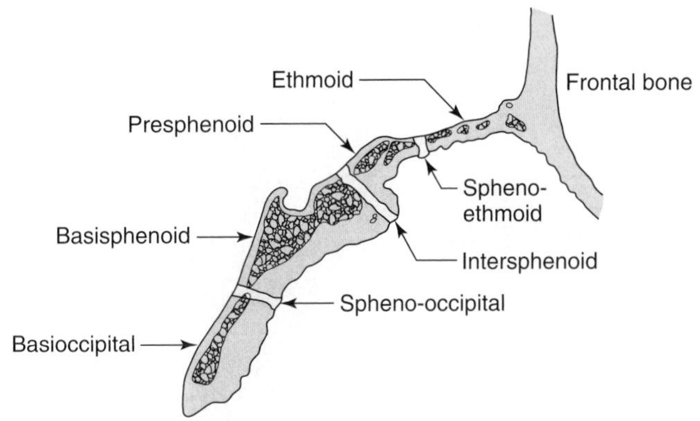

Figure 184-8. Diagrammatic representation of the synchondroses of the cranial base, showing the location of these important growth sites. *(From Proffit WR. Contemporary Orthodontics. 2nd ed. St Louis: Mosby; 1993.)*

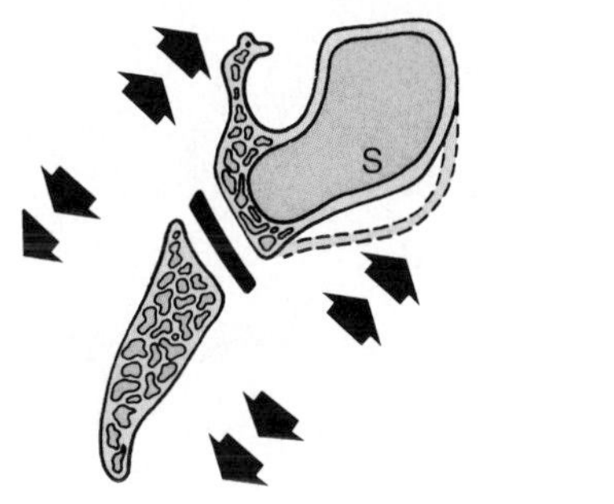

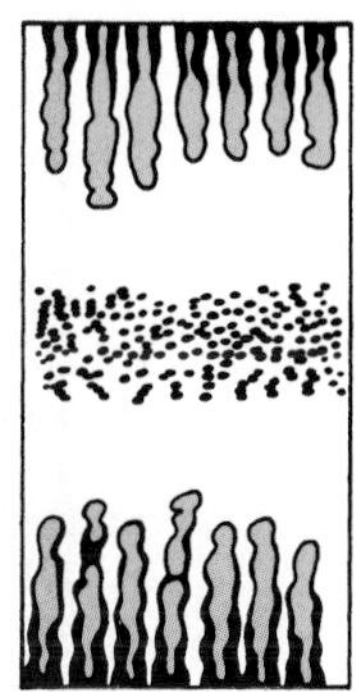

Figure 184-9. Diagrammatic representation of growth at the intersphenoid synchondrosis. A bank of immature proliferating cartilage cells is located at the center of the synchondrosis, whereas a band of maturing cartilage cells extends in both directions away from the center. Endochondral ossification occurs at both margins. Growth at the synchondrosis lengthens this area of the cranial base. S, sphenoid sinus. *(From Proffit WR. Contemporary Orthodontics. 2nd ed. St Louis: Mosby; 1993.)*

role in postnatal growth. The synchondroses have zones similar to those in the epiphyseal cartilage of long bones. However, growth occurs in two directions, resulting in elongation of the basicranium until its ultimate ossification is completed (Fig. 184-9).

The development of ossification center sutures and synchondroses in the chondrocranium throughout childhood hase been chronicled by means of computed tomography (CT). These data can provide standards for skull base maturity. In addition, postnatal normal CT variants and magnetic resonance imaging (MRI) assessment of the cranial base have been characterized.[26,27]

In newborns and infants, the cranial base is quite flat. With growth into childhood, a more convex superior or flexed appearance emerges, with further enlargement during adolescence and adulthood. The spheno-occipital synchondrosis becomes more flexed as the maxillary portion of the nasomaxillary complex moves toward the foramen magnum and moves under the anterior cranial fossa (Fig. 184-10). Components of the cranial base can be seen more clearly in older pediatric skulls than in infant skulls. The foramen magnum approaches adult size and the primary dentition has erupted by 3 years of age. By 8 years of age, the occipital bone has fused around the foramen magnum, and the secondary dentition is erupting. The major difference between the adolescent and adult skull is fusion of the spheno-occipital synchondrosis. Fusion of this synchondrosis begins at approximately 15 years of age for boys and at 12 or 13 years of age for girls on the cerebral surface. Ossification on the external aspect is complete by age 20[1] (Fig. 184-11). The chondrocranium-basicranium is a junction between both the neurocranial and facial complex bones. Its alteration affects not only neurocranial and skull growth but also facial morphology.[3]

Nasomaxillary Complex

The nasomaxillary complex develops through intramembranous ossification. It includes the nasal, lacrimal, maxillary, zygomatic, pterygoid, and vomer bones.

The nasomaxillary complex is displaced forward and downward from the cranial floor (basicranium) as a result of growth of the associated soft tissues. New bone growth occurs at sutural contact surfaces on both sides of the suture, with a resultant increase in the size of both bones involved (Fig. 184-12). Bone is added at the frontal maxillary, zygomaticotemporal, zygomaticosphenoidal, zygomaticomaxillary, ethmoidomaxillary, frontoethmoidal, nasomaxillary, nasofrontal, frontolacrimal, palatine, and vomerine sutures. Interaction between the basicranium and the nasomaxillary complex constantly occurs. Rotatory displacement is caused by the downward and forward growth of the middle cranial fossa, resulting in greater or lesser amounts of displacement and remodeling growth in the posterior and anterior parts of the maxilla, depending on the biomechanical forces involved.[11]

The anterior surface of the maxilla is an area of significant resorption (Fig. 184-13). Even though bone is being resorbed here, the

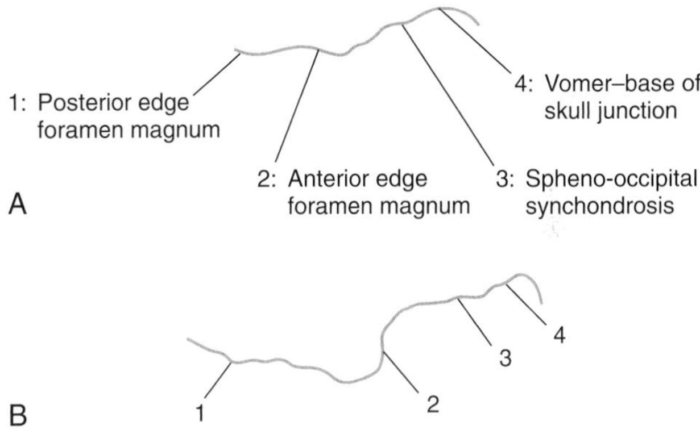

Figure 184-10. Flexion of the cranial base. With growth, a more convex superior or flexed appearance develops from infancy to adulthood. **A,** Infant. **B,** Adult.

maxilla is still growing forward. This is a good example of remodeling and displacement (Fig. 184-14). Growth and development of the nasomaxillary complex are shown in Figure 184-15. Vertical nasomaxillary growth occurs at the frontomaxillary, frontozygomatic, frontonasal, ethmoidomaxillary, and frontoethmoidal sutures as a result of orbital and nasal growth.

The orbits, which are linked to cranial growth, are quite large at birth because of their relationship with the globe. Orbital remodeling is quite complex—50% of postnatal orbital growth is achieved by the age of 2 years, and it is almost complete by age 7 years.[21] The superior aspect of the orbit in toddlers is similar to that in adults, although the inferior aspect differs. The floor of the nose is almost at the level of the inferior orbital rim in infants; then the distance progressively increases so that the floor is significantly lower in adults. The eyes in the adult face are not much farther apart than those in a child's. According to Enlow and Hans,[11] however, "because of the larger nose, higher nasal bridge, increase in the vertical facial dimension and the widening of the cheekbones, the eyes of the adult appear much closer together." The main contribution to the widening face is from the lateral expansion of the zygomaticomaxillary sutures and the intermaxillary suture growth. Eruption of the primary and secondary teeth results in an increase in the size of the maxilla. As the maxilla moves downward and forward and secondary teeth erupt, the maxillary sinuses increase in size as well.

Sinuses

At birth, the maxillary sinus is large enough to be seen radiologically. Relatively rapid growth occurs between ages of 1 and 4 years; by age

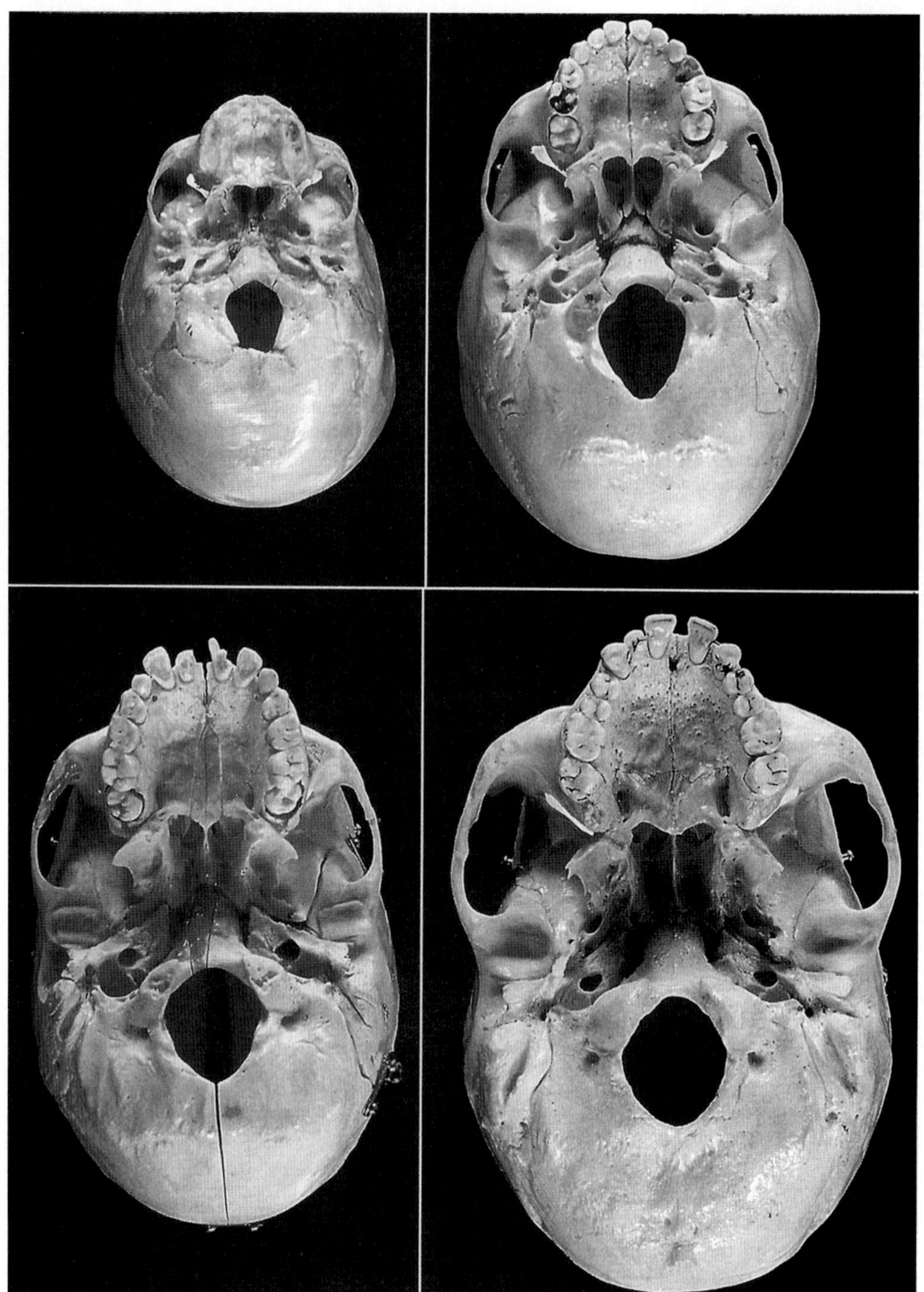

Figure 184-11. Basal extracranial views of the skulls of an infant (at 8 months of age), a 5- to 6-year-old, a 10- to 12-year-old, and an adult. Components of the cranial base are more clearly seen in the older skulls. Note the open spheno-occipital synchondrosis in the 5- to 6-year-old skull and that the most posterior molar on the right side of the photograph is not the patient's—it was inserted.

5, the sinus has started to expand laterally beyond the infraorbital foramen, although its floor does not extend below the nasal cavity. As the permanent dentition erupts, there is growth inferiorly of the floor of the sinus. By the age of 16 years, the maxillary sinus reaches full size (Fig. 184-16). The ethmoid sinuses are present at birth and have attained adult size by the early teens. The frontal sinus distinguishes itself from the ethmoids around age 5 and demonstrates a variable growth rate until reaching adult size in late puberty. The sphenoid sinus is the last to develop and is present radiologically at approximately age 6. Growth of the sphenoid sinus continues well past puberty into the early adult years.[28]

Shah and coworkers reviewed 91 CT scans in 66 patients (16 obtained serially over time) between the ages of 0 and 12 and demonstrated periods of significant growth in the paranasal sinuses in children. The ethmoid sinuses were the first to fully develop, followed by the maxillary, sphenoid and frontal sinuses.[29]

Mandible

The mandible forms in relation to the first branchial cartilage, otherwise known as Meckel's cartilage. Meckel's cartilage is interesting in that it is not replaced by bone. Instead, membranous bone forms lateral to Meckel's cartilage, and Meckel's cartilage then disappears[30] (Fig.

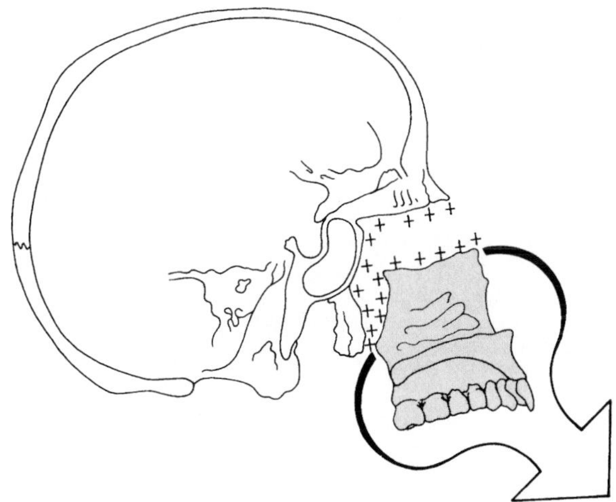

Figure 184-12. As growth of the surrounding soft tissues translates the maxilla downward and forward, opening space at its superior and posterior sutural attachments, new bone is added on both sides of the sutures. *(From Proffit WR.* Contemporary Orthodontics. *2nd ed. St Louis: Mosby; 1993.)*

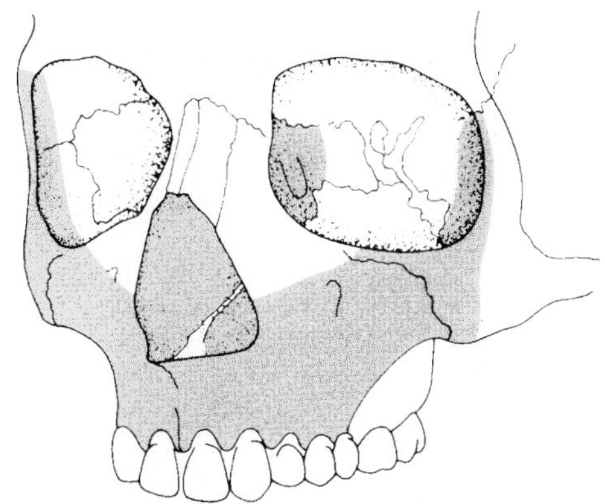

Figure 184-13. As the maxilla is carried downward and forward, its anterior surface tends to resorb. Resorption surfaces are shown in *gold.* Only a small area around the anterior nasal spine is not affected. *(From Proffit WR.* Contemporary Orthodontics. *2nd ed. St Louis: Mosby; 1993.)*

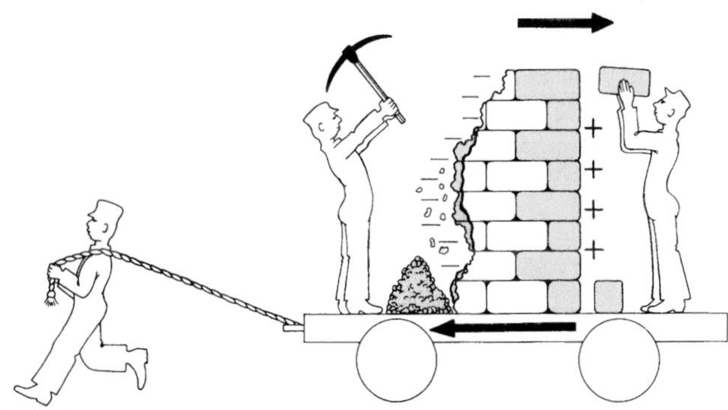

Figure 184-14. Surface remodeling of a bone—in the direction opposite that in which the bone is being translated by growth of adjacent structures—creates a situation analogous to that depicted in this cartoon. The wall is being rebuilt to move it backward at the same time the platform on which it is mounted is being moved forward. *(From Proffit WR.* Contemporary Orthodontics. *2nd ed. St Louis: Mosby; 1993.)*

184-17). At birth, the mandible comprises two bones with the symphysis menti between them. This suture closes by the age of 1 year, after which the major portion of mandibular growth occurs posteriorly.

Resorption occurring anteriorly and deposition occurring posteriorly result in the overall growth of the mandible (Fig. 184-18). Although the condyles are a major site of growth, they are not a master growth center, as was previously thought.

Variation of endochondral bone growth occurs at the articular contact portion of the condyle. The main contribution of condylar cartilage is to provide regional adaptive growth by maintaining the condylar area in a proper anatomic relationship with the temporal bone as the whole mandible is simultaneously being carried downward and forward.[11] The mandible grows by enlarging and widening in response to the increase in size of the muscles of mastication and an enlarging oropharynx, which accommodates the concomitant growth of the nasomaxillary complex. The ramus grows posteriorly and at the same time increases the inter-ramal dimension along with the laterally expanding cranial floor. The coronoid processes grow superiorly and buccally, with the anterior edges of the rami being continually resorbed in the process. The condyles grow posteriorly, superiorly, and laterally (Fig. 184-19). Even though it is a single bone, Sperber[1] described the mandible functionally as six skeletal subunits. These subunits are the alveolar, coronoid, and angular bones, the condylar process, and the chin, all of which are attached to the "body" of the mandible. Moss's concept of functional matrices then influences the growth of each subunit (teeth: alveolar unit; action of the temporalis muscle: coronoid process; masseter and medial pterygoids: angle and ramus; lateral pterygoid–condylar process, perioral muscles, tongue, and expanding oropharyngeal cavity: entire mandible).

The infant mandibular arch is U-shaped; whereas the adult arch is more V-shaped (Fig. 184-20). The gonial angle (the angle between the ramus and the body) is more obtuse in infants than in adults (Fig. 184-21). Mandibular growth takes place in two specific growth spurts, the first between the ages of 5 and 10 years and the second between ages 10 and 15 years.[31] Growth in mandibular width is completed during early adolescence. Growth in mandibular length is complete 2 to 3 years after menstruation in females and approximately 4 years after attainment of sexual maturity in males. Growth in mandibular height is complete in the late teens in females and early twenties in males (see Fig. 184-21).

Internal and external rotational changes of the mandible occur during growth and, of course, in conjunction with rotational changes in the maxilla (Fig. 184-22). Bjork and Skieller[32] described this in detail using metallic implants. Miller and Kerr[31] supported their findings but used a digitizer program for longitudinal follow-up with cephalograms in a number of patients. Overall mandibular growth is not uniform and steady, because corpus length and ramus height grow in an irregular pattern.[25,34] Jaw rotation influences the degree of tooth eruption.

Craniofacial cephalometric and anthropometric studies are abundant in the literature, and normative data are available. A review of these topics is beyond the scope of this chapter; however, these measurements may be used to assist in the interpretation of optimal growth and development in the clinical situation.[35-42]

Abnormal Facial Growth and Development

Asymmetry of the human face is well recognized as a normal finding and in fact is an intrinsic facial characteristic. According to Ferrario and colleagues, "the skeletal structures show a greater degree of asymmetry than their soft tissue drape."[43] Age is certainly one factor that influences asymmetry. Melnik[44] found that the left side of the face was larger at the age of 6 years, whereas the right side of the face was larger at age 16. Disagreement exists in the literature regarding the degree, side, and localization of normal facial asymmetry, although some researchers believe that this is because of methodologic differences.[43] Normal facial asymmetry involves many subtle differences that are not readily apparent to the viewer. Conversely, abnormal facial asymmetry typically is quite obvious.

Our culture is obsessed with physical attractiveness, which to a large extent is based on facial symmetry and what is perceived to be "normal." Langlois[45] found that the preference for attractive persons is

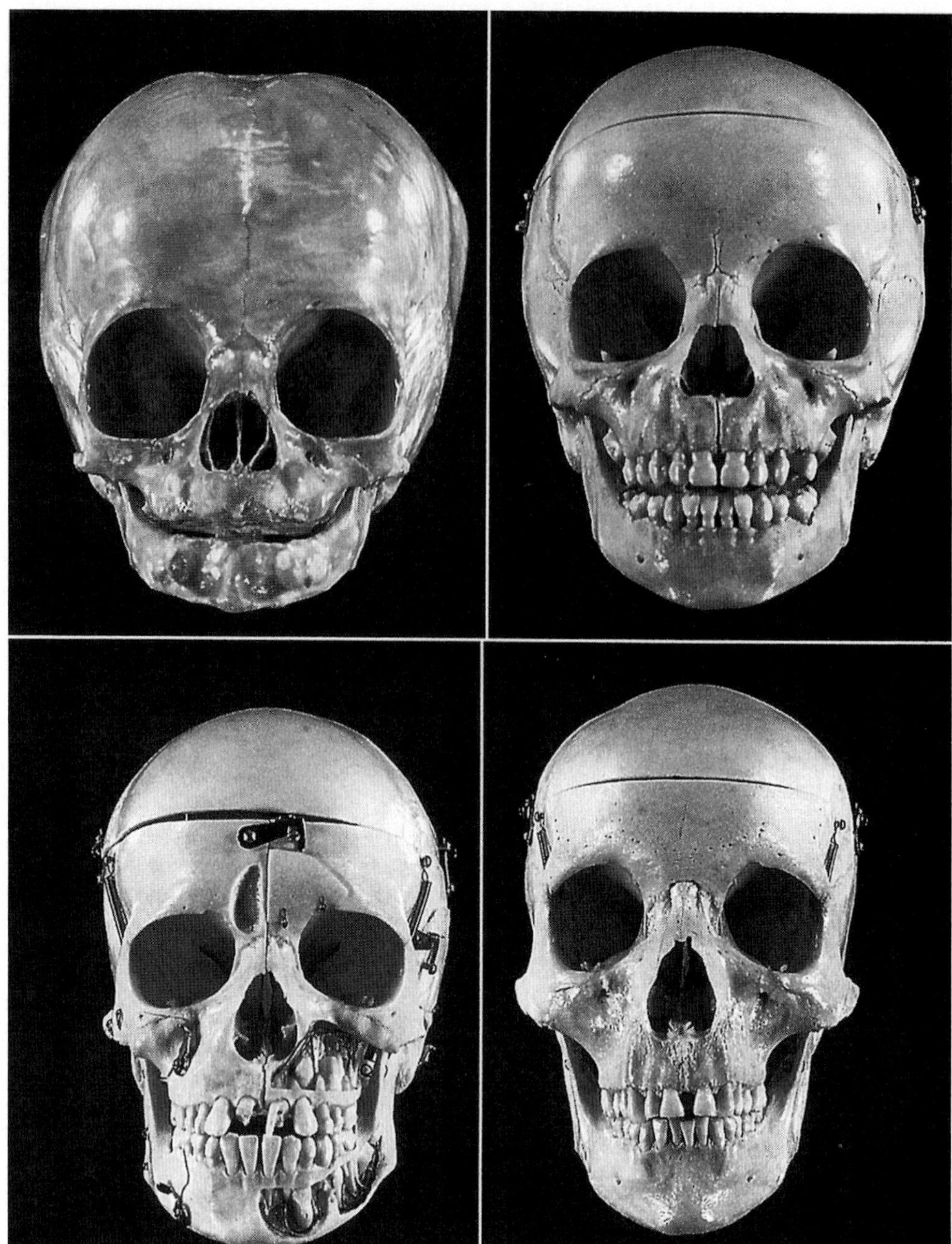

Figure 184-15. Anterior view of the skulls of an infant (8 months of age), a 5- to 6-year-old, a 10- to 12-year-old, and an adult. Note the overall change of skull shape and the facial complex/cranium ratio, the relationship of the orbits to the floor of the nose, nasomaxillary and mandibular growth, and dental changes.

evident early in life and involves all age groups and races. As a result, people whose appearance is divergent from the "norm," with or without intellectual impairment, are viewed differently in our society.

Abnormal facial growth and development may be of iatrogenic, traumatic, mechanical, or genetic etiology: Radiotherapy, functional endoscopic sinus surgery (FESS), internal fixation, nasoseptal trauma and surgery, and nasal obstruction related to dentofacial growth, as well as genetic conditions, all have been recognized as causes. Some etiologic categories relevant to pediatric otolaryngology are reviewed next.

Radiotherapy

Ionizing radiation is widely recognized as detrimental to the growth of developing tissue. In a majority of cases, this consequence is a result of the application of full doses to radiosensitive tumors.[46] Rhabdomyosarcoma and undifferentiated sarcomas constitute the most common type of malignant tumor of soft tissue of childhood. Of these sarcomas, 35% are found in the head and neck region. Retinoblastoma is the most frequent malignant ocular tumor in childhood and is a frequent indication for radiotherapy in the pediatric population.[47,48] Multimodal therapy (radiotherapy and chemotherapy) has been effective in the treatment of these tumors with a 3-year relapse-free survival rate of between 70% and 100%.[49-52] The value of radiotherapy has not been questioned given its success rate,[53] but as more children have been cured of cancer and the survival rates have increased, concerns about the long-term side effects of these therapeutic regimens (alone or in combination) have arisen.[50,51]

The effects of radiation therapy on facial growth, as well as radiation's collateral effects, are detailed in Table 184-2. Virtually 100% of children who have received radiotherapy suffer from alterations in the development of facial soft tissues, and in more than 60% of these

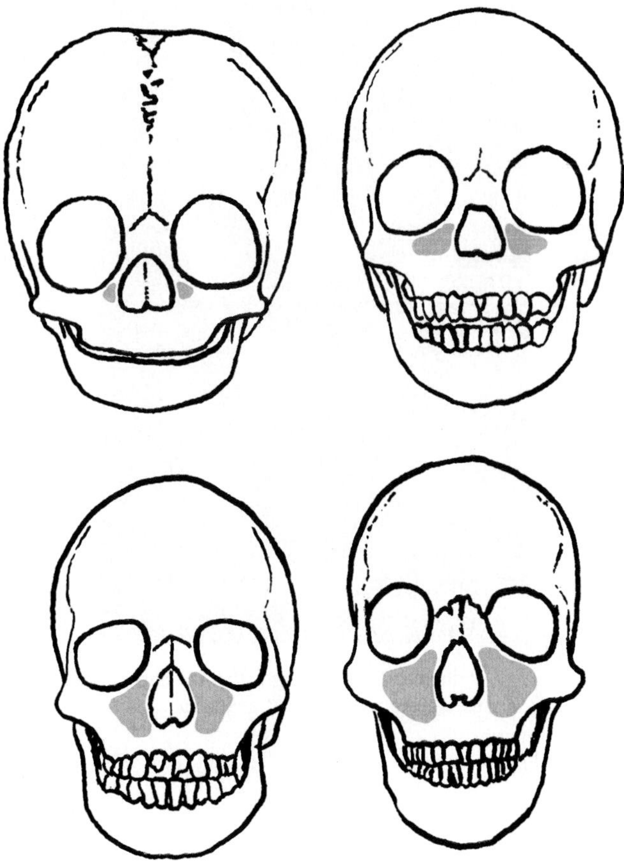

Figure 184-16. Maxillary sinus growth in an infant (8 months of age), a 5- to 6-year-old, a 10- to 12-year-old, and an adult. Drawings from x-ray images of skulls.

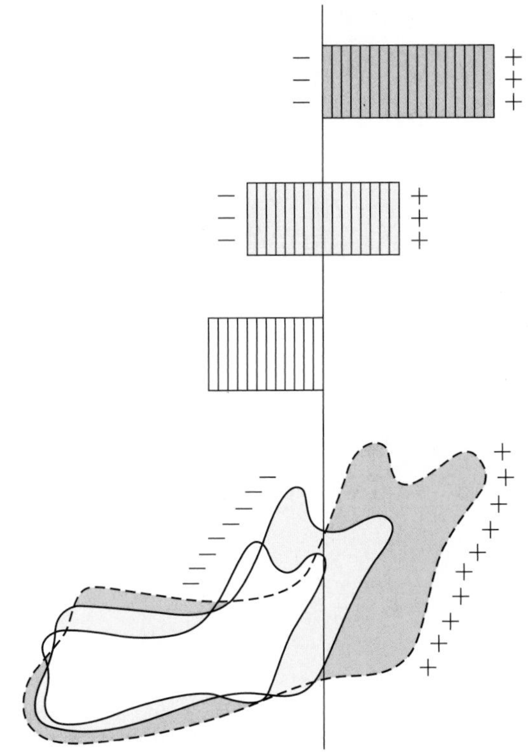

Figure 184-18. As the mandible lengthens, the ramus is extensively remodeled—so much so that the bone at the tip of the condylar process at an early age can be found at the anterior surface of the ramus some years later. Given the extent of surface remodeling changes that occur, it is an obvious area to emphasize endochondral bone formation at the condyle as the major mechanism for growth of the mandible. *(From Proffit WR.* Contemporary Orthodontics. *2nd ed. St Louis: Mosby; 1993.)*

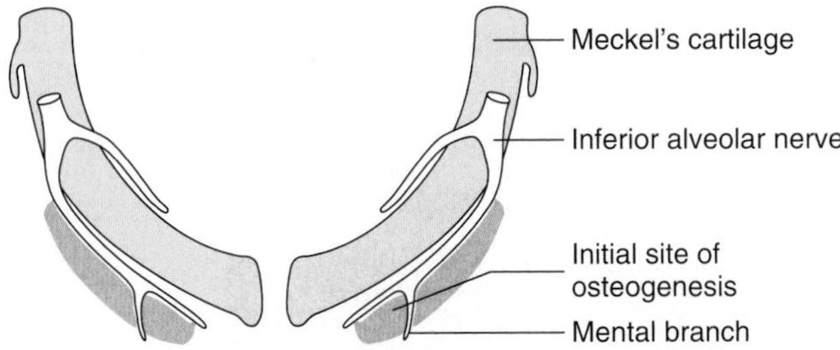

Figure 184-17. Diagrammatic representation of the relation of the site of initial bone formation in the mandible to Meckel's cartilage and the inferior alveolar nerve. Bone formation begins just lateral to Meckel's cartilage and spreads posteriorly along it without any direct replacement of the cartilage by the newly forming bone of the mandible. *(From Proffit WR.* Contemporary Orthodontics. *2nd ed. St Louis: Mosby; 1993.)*

children, the facial bones are affected.[47,54] The younger the patient at the time of irradiation, the greater the effects on craniofacial development.[51,55,56] These side effects are more frequent and more severe within the first 10 years after irradiation.[54]

It has been difficult to determine the safest dose of irradiation that keeps side effects on growing tissue to a minimum but at the same time is effective in eradicating the cancer.[46,53,54] Techniques for radiotherapy administration have changed during the past 20 years. The principal aim is to achieve a balance between cure and late toxicity of the treatment.[54] Changes to minimize undesirable effects include radiotherapy with megavoltage, hyperfractionation, three-dimensional therapy, intensity-modulation, and conformal radiation with multiple fields.[47,55]

In all children undergoing radiotherapy of the head and neck, it is mandatory that multidisciplinary follow-up be part of the ongoing management.

Functional Endoscopic Sinus Surgery

FESS has become the standard of care in the surgical management of chronic sinusitis and other sinus disorders in the pediatric population. Its effectiveness has been accepted when clear indications for surgery are established.[57,58] However, concerns have arisen regarding potential negative effects on the growth and development of paranasal sinuses and the nasomaxillary complex in the pediatric patient.[59]

A knowledge of sinus anatomy during different stages of development, as well as of pathologic circumstances such as chronic sinusitis, is imperative in decisions regarding FESS in the pediatric population.[28,60-62]

The absolute and relative indications for FESS in the pediatric population varied during the 1990s and into the millennium. These changes were related to the evolving definitions of sinus disorders and short- and long-term outcome measures.[60,63-68] This topic is covered in Chapter 195.

Although the relationship between nasal breathing and sinus development remains unclear, it is generally accepted that the development of the paranasal sinuses is linked to the growth of the nasomaxillary complex. A reasonable assumption, therefore, is that any intervention at this level, either an endoscopic technique or a Caldwell-Luc procedure, on a growing patient will have negative effects on the normal process of remodeling, expansion, and pneumatization.

Results of animal studies have varied depending on the species and the intervention. Kraut and Kronman examined 36-day-old New Zealand White rabbits and unilaterally filled their maxillary sinuses with polyhydroxyethylmethacrylate without adverse effect on

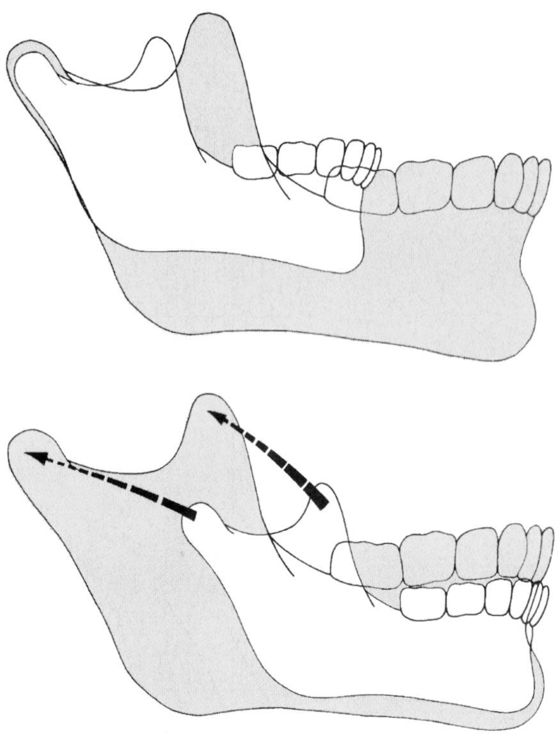

Figure 184-19. Mandibular growth as viewed from the perspective of vital staining dyes. Note the minimal changes in the body and chin area, whereas exceptional growth and remodeling occur in the ramus, moving it posteriorly. The correct concept of mandibular growth is that the mandible is translated downward and forward and grows upward and backward in response to this translation, maintaining its contact with the skull. *(From Proffit WR.* Contemporary Orthodontics. *2nd ed. St Louis: Mosby; 1993.)*

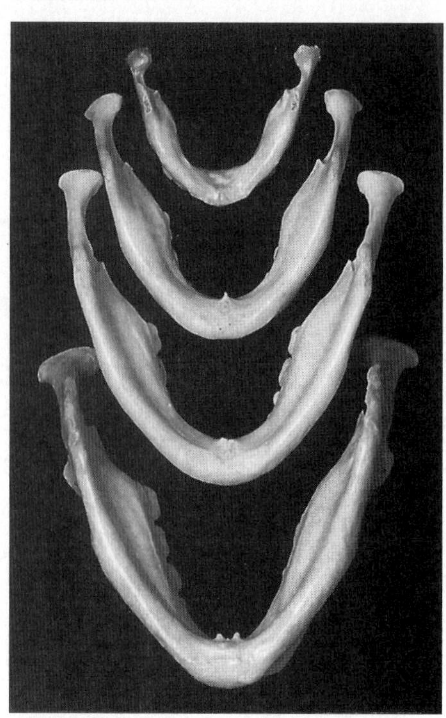

Figure 184-20. With mandibular growth, the U shape of the infant mandible *(top)* changes to more of a V shape, as seen in the adult *(bottom)*.

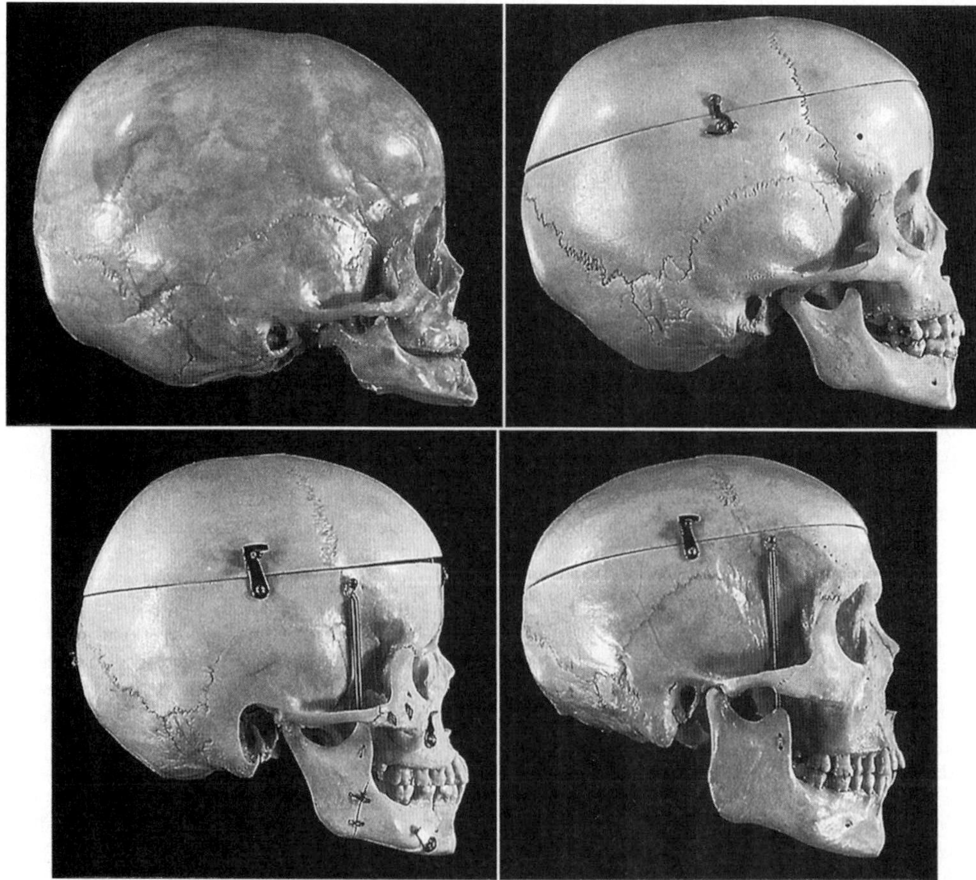

Figure 184-21. Lateral view of the skulls of an infant (at 8 months of age), a 5- to 6-year-old, a 10- to 12-year-old, and an adult. Note that the gonial angle of the mandible is more obtuse in the infant. The overall change in size of the mandible through time is dramatic.

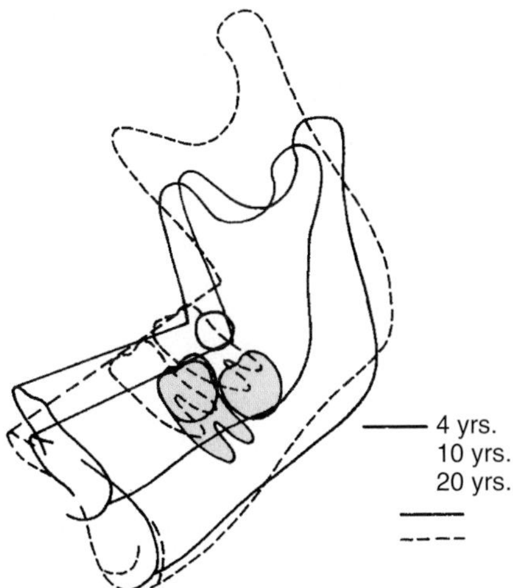

Figure 184-22. Superimposition on implants for a patient with a normal growth pattern showing surface changes in the mandible from ages 4 to 20 years. For this patient, there was a −19 degree internal rotation but only a −3 degree change in the mandibular plane angle. Note dramatic remodeling in the area of the gonial angle, with a net resorption during this period. This surface remodeling or external rotation compensates for, and conceals the extent of, the internal rotation. *(From Bjork A, Skiller V. Normal and abnormal growth of the mandible: a synthesis of longitudinal cephalometric implant studies over a period of 25 years.* Eur J Orthod. *1983;5:1.)*

craniofacial growth.[69] Mair and coworkers studied eight newly weaned piglets subjected to unilateral FESS. The researchers examined the piglets 6 months after surgery, noting significant reduction of the facial growth and maxillary-ethmoidal sinus development on the operated side.[70] Carpenter and associates found significant restrictive effects on piglet facial skeletal development after FESS.[71] Verwoerd-Verhoef and Verwoerd demonstrated that controlled resection of the bony sinonasal wall and partial resection of anterior ethmoid did not affect later development of nasal bones and maxilla on 20 young New Zealand White rabbits.[72]

Several studies in children have been undertaken. Mair and coworkers analyzed the uncinate processes and ethmoids of 84 children (mean age of 6 years; age range, 1 to 18 years) who previously had undergone FESS. In children younger than 9 years of age, woven and lamellar bone were present, in contrast with the presence of exclusively lamellar-mature bone in the children older than 9 years of age. These results suggest that the safest age at which a pediatric patient should be operated on is 9 or older.[70] Kosko and colleagues in 1996 presented five cases of children (mean age of 30 months) who had undergone bilateral FESS for refractory chronic sinusitis. At mean postoperative month 42, four children showed unilateral maxillary hypoplasia and one child showed bilateral hypoplasia without apparent changes in facial symmetry.[59] Sinus hypoplasia can be from primary causes related to individual development or secondary causes associated with a response to facial trauma, chronic sinusitis, or FESS, which has affected the activation of bone formation factors or the removal of growth centers.[59,61,73] In 2000, Senior and associates did not find long-term significant differences in sinus volumes in eight patients (age range, 2 to 14 years) who had required FESS after unilateral orbital complications of acute sinusitis, but the age range was so wide they could not determine any age-related association.[74] In a 2002 retrospective study, Bothwell and coworkers reported no evidence of facial growth disruption 10 years after FESS in 67 children between 2 and 4 years of age.[63]

Lusk and colleagues reported results of a 10-year retrospective follow-up study in children (aged 2 to 5 years) treated with FESS for chronic rhinosinusitis. Parental satisfaction regarding nasal symptoms was significantly higher in the surgically managed group than in the medically treated group. The study focused on six symptoms: day cough, night cough, irritability or crankiness, headaches, nasal airway obstruction, and purulent rhinorrhea. In comparisons of individual symptoms, no statistically significant difference was found between the two groups. However, when the mean was controlled for baseline symptom severity and CT severity, additional analysis noted a statistically significant decrease in nasal airway obstruction and in rhinorrhea in the surgical treatment group.[75]

In a small series of 14 patients with cystic fibrosis ranging in age from 9 to 28 years, Van Peteghem and Clement found no impact on the outcome of facial growth in comparison with their control group of 5 patients with cystic fibrosis who did not require surgery.[76]

In view of the small sample sizes in several studies and the lack of prospective studies, concerns still remain regarding FESS in the pediatric population. Unless the patient has an acute complication of sinus origin, FESS for chronic sinusitis should ideally be delayed until maximal medical therapy has been undertaken in order to avoid potential negative effects on facial growth.[58,77] It is recommended that one be prudent regarding the timing and extent of FESS in children and that clear indications for surgery be followed. If FESS is performed, conservative treatment preserving as much as possible of the normal mucosa, periosteum, and bone is recommended.[59,64,70,71] Further prospective studies in both animal and humans are required to clarify the role of FESS in the facial growth of children.

Internal Fixation and Facial Growth

Midface skeletal maturity is complete by approximately age 12 years. An important point is that any trauma or reconstructive surgery before this age may adversely effect facial growth.[78] However, according to Singh and Bartlett's review of data for surgically treated children for craniofacial fractures, a majority of cases had a favorable outcome with regard to facial growth and development on long-term follow-up, except for isolated condylar fractures and patients with complex centrofacial trauma.[79] There were significant limitations to this retrospective descriptive paper.

Some basic principles should be followed in planning the management of these patients. Complete clinical and image-guided assessment, early repair of fracture and soft tissue injury, minimal but sufficient surgical exposure, and correct technical application of fixation devices are required to achieve good bone stability without disrupting long-term facial growth.[78,80-83]

The direct effect of plates and screws on facial skeletal development has been studied. Lin and associates found significant growth retardation in a craniofacial segment in kittens that underwent osteotomies in conjunction with different fixation systems.[84] However, Mooney and coworkers did not find significant effects in rabbits.[85] These workers suggested, along with Carinci and colleagues, to avoid crossing sutures with plates and screws, because of the risk of synostosis.[86] Yaremchuk and coinvestigators found that osteotomy and fixation in the infant rhesus monkey affected craniofacial growth.[87] Growth deformity in selected craniometric parameters was greater when the complexity of fixation (longer plates and more screws) were used.[87,88] Courtemanche and associates found that the use of rigid internal fixation in the growing skull of piglets resulted in a contour deformity of the calvaria, and that the microplate and screw became completely incorporated into the bone. These workers suggested that this type of fixation not be used in the infant craniofacial skeleton.[89] Salyer and colleagues concluded that absorbable materials did not disrupt bone growth in canine puppies, but in this study, osteotomies were not performed.[90] In 1996, Canady and coworkers designed an animal model using conventional vitallium hardware after osteotomies without the restriction from routine rigid fixation. This system permitted more normal growth of the rabbit head compared with the rigid fixation system.[91,92] Laurenzo and associates concluded in 1995 that experimental osteotomies cause severe bony restriction in rabbits, regardless of the use of rigid plate fixation, supporting the theory that trauma itself affects growth and development.[93] However, the validity of studies using animal models has been criticized because of the lack of full applicability in humans.[87]

Imola and colleagues published a 2001 retrospective study of patients treated with resorbable plate fixation systems, concluding that this method is safe, with results comparable to those with use of metal

Table 184-2
Side Effects of Radiotherapy

Category	Manifestations
Skin	Dryness, abnormal pigmentation, telangiectasis, malignant degeneration, atrophy, alopecia, sebaceous cysts
Mucosa	Xerostomia, atrophy, fibrosis
Soft tissues	Atrophy, hypoplasia, sensitivity to infections
Facial bones	Growth retardation, hypoplasia, dysplasia, appositional growth restriction, weak resistance to infections, loss of cortical bone density, atrophy of alveolar process, micrognathia, facial asymmetry, condylar hypoplasia, "bird face," abnormal occlusion
Teeth	Failure to erupt, disturbed eruption, damage to tooth buds, anodontia, hypodontia, pseudoanodontia, mineralization, caries, root foreshortening, enamel dysplasia, atypical root morphology
Orbit	Bone and soft tissue hypoplasia, persistent infections.
Eyes	Cataracts, xerophthalmia, retinopathy, corneal lesions, loss of vision, keratoconjunctivitis, dryness of globe, enophthalmos, stenosis of lacrimal duct
Head and neck muscles	Atrophy, trismus, fibrosis
Risk of second malignancy	Osteogenic sarcoma, soft tissue sarcomas usually within radiation fields, thyroid, breast, acute myeloid leukemia, histiocytoma
Brain	Cerebral function damage
Middle ear	Serous otitis media, chronic otorrhea
Paranasal sinuses	Bone hypoplasia, chronic sinusitis
Audiology	Sensorineural or conductive hearing loss
Speech	Velopharyngeal incompetency
Hormonal	Growth retardation, growth hormone deficiency
Psychologic	Psychologic disorders
Cosmetic	Bone or soft tissue hypoplasia, facial asymmetry, severe neck fibrosis, nuchal asymmetry
Various	Nutritional and vitamin deficiency

Data from references 46-48, 50, 51, 53; and from Berkowitz RJ, Neuman P, Spalding P, Novak L, Strandjord S, Coccia PF. Developmental orofacial deficits associated with multimodal cancer therapy: case report. *Pediatr Dent*. 1989;11:227; Larson D, Kroll S, Jaffe N, Serure A, Goepfert H. Long-term effects of radiotherapy in childhood and adolescence. *Am J Surg*. 1990;160:349; Sklar CA. Overview of the effects of cancer therapies: the nature, scale and breadth of the problem. *Acta Paediatr Suppl*. 1999;88:1; and Sonis AL, Tarbell N, Valachovic RW, Gelber R, Schwenn M, Sallan S. Dentofacial development in long-term survivors of acute lymphoblastic leukemia. A comparison of three treatment modalities. *Cancer*. 1990;66:2645, 1990.

plates, but without the negative effect on the growth and development of the facial skeleton, because of its resorptive capacity once the fracture is healed.[94]

As more data over time are acquired regarding internal fixation and facial growth in the pediatric population, clarity regarding long-term outcome is sure to be achieved.

Nasoseptal Trauma and Surgery

It has long been suggested that nasal trauma or surgery has a detrimental effect on the nasofacial development of growing children. The literature notes that in adults with a deviated nasoseptal complex, up to 65% had sustained trauma in childhood.[95] It is important to recognize that nasoseptal deformities are a result of a complex interaction of factors, including trauma, surgery, inheritance, and individual growth patterns. Surgical correction of nasoseptal deformities during childhood remains very controversial because of potential adverse functional or aesthetic long-term sequelae.[96-98]

Animal Studies

Historically, various animal models of nasal septal trauma have been analyzed in attempts to find a valid correlation with humans. Sarnat and Wexler reported that in 1858 Flick removed septal cartilage from several different types of newly weaned animals and found significantly shortened hard palates on autopsy specimens suggesting that palatal growth depended on the growth of the nasal septum. They also reported that the degree of snout deformity was proportional to the amount of septum and perichondrium resected from rabbits.[99] Wexler confirmed these findings in a follow-up study.[100] Moss and colleagues wrote that the septum played a passive role in the development of the midface, acting only as a support structure in guinea pigs.[101] Hartshorn had similar findings after septectomies in puppies.[102] Stenstrom and Thilander studied guinea pigs, noting that in this species the septum is not the primary structure determining facial growth.[103]

Beginning in the 1970s, experimental models changed because the animal procedures to date frequently had been carried out in a destructive fashion and not as they would have been carried out in humans. Bernstein did not find growth retardation in dogs after conservative septoplasties in which the mucoperichondrium was preserved and the removed cartilage was reinserted but not sewn in.[104] Nordgaard and Kvinnsland noted severe deformities in rats after septoplasty, regardless of whether there was preservation of the mucoperichondrium.[105] Verwoerd and associates reported that the basal portion of cartilage, the perpendicular lamina, and the junction between cartilage and the premaxilla and cartilage with the sphenoid were the key areas in nasal development in rabbits.[106] Cupero and colleagues found that septal surgery preserving mucoperichondrium did not affect facial development in ferrets.[107] However, concerns persisted in the literature because of the lack of clear correlation between animals and humans.

Human Studies

In human studies it is difficult to differentiate the proportion of long-term sequelae on nasofacial growth and development attributable to trauma alone or in combination with surgery. A number of authors have theorized on the growth centers of the septum[106,108-111] (Fig. 184-23). Clinical cases such as that seen in Figure 184-24 invite researchers to question the role the septum plays in nasal growth. In the case depicted, a septal abscess developed at the age of 1 year. Serial photographs of the patient follow nasal growth at ages 1, 7, and 12 years. Nasal size appears to be smaller than expected; however, until the patient goes through a facial growth phase as an adolescent, it is difficult to comment on what the final proportion of his nose to the rest of his face will be. Clinically, he also has nasal obstruction secondary to a significantly deviated septum.

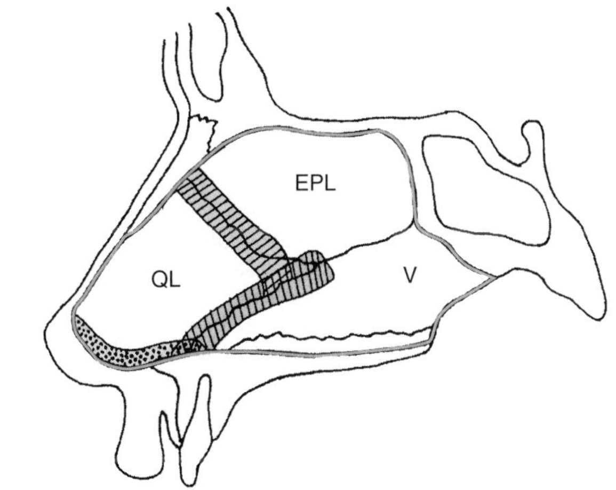

Figure 184-23. Proposed growth centers of the septum. EPL, ethmoid perpendicular lamina; QL, quadrangular lamina; V, vomer.

Alpini and colleagues examined 423 newborns, finding pyramid deformities with septal dislocation and columella deviation, assumed to be related to labor trauma with vaginal delivery. No infant delivered by cesarean section had a pyramid deformity. Septal deviation and subluxation were postulated to be related to developmental defects, and findings were essentially the same in the vaginally delivered and cesarean section–delivered infants.[112]

Traditionally, it has been accepted that nasoseptal surgery in children should be delayed until nasal maturity has been reached, at approximately the age of 15 years in boys and 12 years in girls. Parameters for the male and female such as facial maturity (15 and 12 years, respectively), near complete projection of the nasal tip (16 and 14 years, respectively), and the completion of growth spurts at ages 1 to 6 years and 12 to 16 years have been used to justify delay of surgical correction.[14,98,113] Akguner and coworkers, after analyzing anthropometric studies of 140 boys and 140 girls (age range, 11 to 17 years), concluded that the safest age for a septorhinoplasty in children was 15 years for boys and 13 for girls.[14] El-Hakim and associates compared 11 anthropometric variables in children who had undergone open rhinoplasty and found no long-term sequelae, although Béjar and colleagues previously had found a trend in growth retardation in the dorsum length (length from nasion to pronasale), which was not statistically significant.[96,114]

As noted by Pirsig, several clinical trials and studies with children were published during the early to mid-twentieth century: Krieg (1900), Freer (1902), Killian (1908), Metzembaum (1929), Cottle (1939, 1964). Those studies suggested that septoplasty be undertaken at the age of 16 years.[115] Farrior and Connolly postulated that a preadolescent could undergo conservative septoplasty in cases of severe deformity or impairment of nasal function.[116] In Pirsig's series of 261 children 4 to 14 years of age who underwent septoplasty, 80% achieved positive functional and aesthetic long-term outcomes, whereas 15% did not.[115] Pirsig, as well as other investigators, classified failures as the following anomalies found after trauma or surgery or both: mucosal atrophy, soft tissue scars, resorption or regeneration of cartilage (frequently ectopic) resulting in septal redeviation, bony resorption, fibrosis, hypoplasia (after septal hematoma or abscess), or hyperplastic changes (resulting in humps or crests).[95,115] Ortiz-Monasterio and

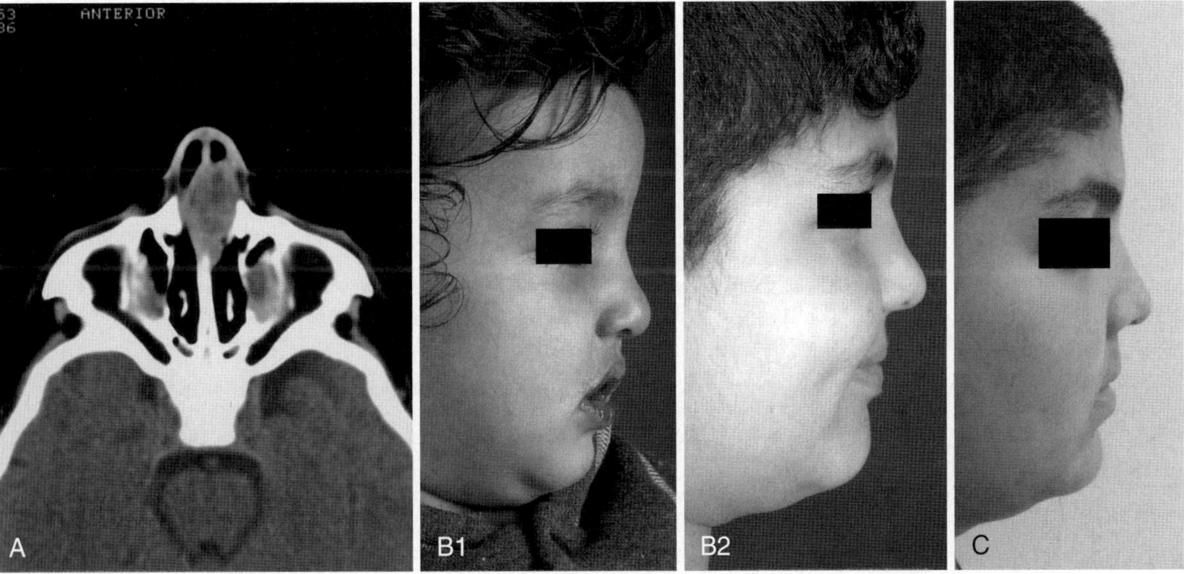

Figure 184-24. **A,** Septal abscess in a 1-year-old boy. **B1** and **B2,** Nasal profile in the same patient at ages 1 and 7 years, respectively. **C,** Nasal profile in the same patient at age 12.

Olmedo demonstrated no long-term negative outcomes in 44 children (8 to 12 years of age) after formal rhinoplasty including medial and lateral osteotomies. In this series, 65% of patients underwent septoplasty with limited dissection of mucoperichondrium and minimum cartilage excision and, when indicated, cartilage was crosshatched and replaced. Patients were followed up with preoperative and postoperative photographic and anthropometric studies.[117]

Surgical Timing and Approach

Timing of nasal surgery depends on when the injury or traumatic event has taken place and the amount of time to presentation to the surgeon. Some investigators have addressed the possibility of intervention in neonates with septal deviations secondary to delivery related injuries. Emami and Sooknundun and their coworkers advocate closed reposition or reduction of anterior septal nasal deformities and subluxations within the first few days of life in order to avoid future deformities.[118,119] However, many deviated noses of the newborn, both externally and internally do resolve on their own over several days to weeks. Kawalski and Spiewak concluded that anterior septal deviations caused by birth injuries are likely to resolve spontaneously within the first 3 days of life, suggesting that any intervention should be considered only for older children.[120]

Hippocrates (fifth century BC) described in detail the technique of nasal fracture reduction.[121] Pirsig suggested that the best time to correct nasal fractures in the pediatric population was between 6 and 10 days after injury.[95] He also felt that open reduction 2 to 3 weeks after injury was possible in cases of "massive pathologic signs." Many surgeons advocate waiting a period of 7 to 10 days after injury for the optimal time frame for fractures requiring closed reduction. Timing for surgery in patients presenting long after the traumatic event is more varied in the literature. Farrior and Connolly believed that it was wise to delay the procedure until achieving complete facial maturity, except in cases of severe functional impairment, in which it was important to do a limited resection, with proper reposition of cartilage. Alar or dorsum procedures were recommended to be delayed as long as possible.[116] It should be noted that much of the literature is anecdotal or lacks a scientific basis for the recommendations and opinions expressed.[122]

Different surgical approaches have been proposed. Loh and Chang described the basic septoplasty technique in children, with no noteworthy differences from adults, except for the conservative excision of cartilage and bone.[123] For severe deformities, Jugo proposed open rhinoseptoplasty, excising, and replacing the septum, without violating the K point (i.e., the junction between nasal bones and upper lateral cartilages on the nasal dorsum), neither cutting the septospinal ligament nor dissecting inferior tunnels. In less severe cases, a conventional Cottle's septoplasty is advised.[124] Koltai and colleagues agreed with this.[125] Crysdale's group proposed two approaches in children 6 years of age and older. When the deviation is located caudally and posterior to an imaginary line from the anterior nasal spine to the anterior aspect of the nasal bones, a hemitransfixion incision and limited excision of cartilage, maxillary crest, and vomer is indicated. If the deviation is anterior to this line, they suggested an open approach removing the whole quadrilateral cartilage and replacing it using its posterior edge, creating a "new" septal midline.[96,98,114,126,127]

In conclusion, rhinoseptoplasty in children remains a controversial topic.[127-130] It would appear impossible not to interfere to some degree with the growth pattern in operating on a developing nose. Farrior and Connolly in 1970 counseled prudence in this regard:

> There has not been adequate documentation by anatomic sections, embryologic study, and clinical verification of just what components of the nasal structure should not be disturbed or removed and what portions of these various structures should be either removed or preserved. The actual rates of growth of each component and what precisely located surgical trauma would do to future development have not been well studied. In any event, conservatism and repositioning without removal of tissue, or with minimal tissue disturbance, seems to be the wise approach.[116]

Although further study has taken place since Farrior and Connolly's delineation of the problem, questions remain regarding timing of and approach to this not uncommon reconstruction. Therefore, these procedures should be performed conservatively and, when possible, delayed until facial maturity is attained. However, should severe deformities be present, corrective procedures are indicated. A second surgical repair may be required once facial growth is completed or nearly completed, depending on the age of the child at the time of the initial procedure. Before proceeding to surgery, the child's functional, aesthetic, and psychologic parameters must be considered, and it is paramount that these considerations be discussed fully with the patient and the family.

Nasal Obstruction and Dentofacial Growth

Genetic factors clearly play a role in dentofacial growth in humans. Controversy exists in the literature regarding the role that nasopharyngeal obstruction plays with regard to dentofacial growth and development. Two schools of thought prevail: (1) that nasal obstruction plays a role and (2) that it does not.[131,132]

Nasal obstruction results in increases in both nasal flow resistance and nasal power (rate of energy required to move air through the nose), such that the child may be forced to switch to mouth breathing. When mouth breathing, the child has an open-mouth posture (OMP)—the mandible and tongue are displaced downward and backward and the head is tilted backward. It has been hypothesized that OMP affects the direction of jaw growth and the interaction of the teeth both horizontally and vertically. Stress from the suprahyoid muscles and the platysma is thought to influence growth on the lower aspect of the mandible. Sperber[1] makes reference to Moss's functional matrix hypothesis, noting that the nasal cavity also may influence growth of the face. Enlarged adenoids in young children are one of the most common causes of nasal obstruction, potentially resulting in the typical "adenoid facies" (narrow, increased facial height, protruding teeth, OMP, short upper lip and larger lower lip, small nose, high-vaulted palatal arch, and the appearance of a vacant or dull facial expression (Fig. 184-25). However, the cause-and-effect relationship of nasal obstruction and this facial morphology has not been substantiated. Heredity also may be involved to some degree.[1]

It should be noted that the term *mouth breathing* is in fact a misnomer, because most persons identified as using this mode of breathing are in fact oronasal breathers. Complete mouth breathing is unusual, and Ung and colleagues reported only 2 of the 49 children they studied to be 100% mouth breathers.[133] In fact, the accurate determination of respiratory mode (oral, nasal, or oronasal breathing) remains elusive, leading to significant difficulties in researching the effect of nasal obstruction on facial growth. The nasal valve area also may play a significant role in nasal obstruction. Ung's group found that the breathing modes of growing children varied on different days of testing. Hairfield and associates concluded that "the variation in respiratory mode we observed may make it impossible to identify clear cause-and-effect relationships regarding upper airway function on facial development."[134] The lack of normative data on nasorespiratory breathing and problematic measurement of respiratory mode must be kept in mind in reviewing the literature regarding implications of nasal obstruction on facial growth and development.

Open Mouth Posture

OMP in children may result from nasal obstruction secondary to enlarged adenoids, from significant allergic disease, from habit developed during previous nasal airway blockage, or from lack of encouragement from adult caregivers to maintain closed-mouth posture. However, oral respiration and OMP are quite common in children and may be unrelated to nasal airway obstruction. Indeed, it may be a normal part of development for some children. Warren and coworkers found that, before the age of 8 years, the proportion of nasal breathers and that of oral breathers were roughly equal. After 8 years of age, a majority of

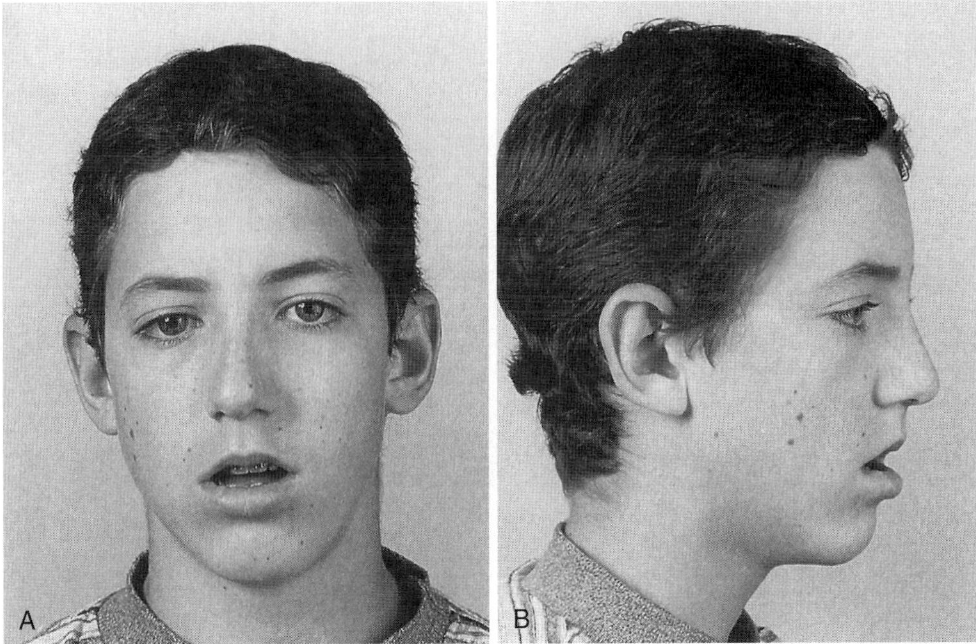

Figure 184-25. **A** and **B,** Typical "adenoid facies" in a 14-year-old boy. Note the long face, open mouth posture, short upper lip, larger lower lip, small nose, and dull facial expression.

children were nasal or predominantly nasal breathers.[135] Black children appear to abandon OMP more quickly over time at a faster rate than that noted in white children.[136] In evaluating children for chronic mouth breathing, OMP does not necessarily imply significant nasal obstruction, because some children will have OMP but are nasal breathers. In their study of children with severe nasopharyngeal obstruction, Woodside and colleagues found that 80% converted to nasal breathing after adenoidectomy.[137] The remaining 20% of their study population did not convert to nasal breathing following adenoidectomy. Soft tissue components of the oral cavity also may contribute to OMP (e.g., the tongue, by means of tongue thrusting).

Review of the Literature

Several studies have considered the specific effect of nasal airway obstruction on dentofacial growth. Complete nasal obstruction appears to alter dentofacial growth.[138] Paul and Nanda[139] and Gross and coworkers[136] found that children with OMP had less growth of the maxillary arches compared with children with closed-mouth posture. Brodie postulated that in some patients, the force of the buccinator muscle and its attachment may result in poor maxillary arch expansion.[140] A narrow maxillary arch frequently is associated with skeletal open bite and anterior crossbite.[22,141] Oulis and associates[142] found that the presence of posterior crossbite was high in children with severe upper-airway obstruction. Linder-Aronson summarized the conclusions of several studies[143-146]:

1. Monozygotic twins are more alike in mandibular growth direction than dizygotic twins, indicating some genetic influence.

2. Children with enlarged adenoids resulting in nasopharyngeal obstruction and subsequent mouth breathing have a longer total and longer lower anterior facial height. They also have an inclination toward a retrognathic mandible in comparison with unaffected children. Children with enlarged adenoids experience subsequent alteration of the dentofacial structures, resulting in an increase in the incidence of open bite, posterior crossbite, and narrower upper maxillary arches.

3. Children with enlarged adenoids and malocclusion, at 5-year follow-up after adenoidectomy, were found to have an increase in maxillary arch width and a decrease in lower facial height and mandibular plane angle. Affected girls demonstrated more horizontal mandibular growth.

4. Some children may undergo partial reversal of dental and skeletal anomalies after relief of nasal obstruction. Specifically, after adenoidectomy some children have shown evidence of a "partial recovery" from abnormal facial growth direction of the mandible and a decrease in lower facial height.

5. Changes in specific tooth positioning (incisors) after adenoidectomy have been noted.

In their study of 38 children observed over 5 years after adenoidectomy, Woodside and others[137] concluded that mandibular growth was greater in both males and females at the chin than in control subjects and that midface growth was greater in males, although no change in maxillary growth direction was observed for either gender.

Extended head posture is characteristic with mouth breathing and reverses when normal nasal breathing is resumed.[141] Studies in primates with obligatory oral breathing have shown that partial recovery of lower facial height and mandibular steepness occurred when normal respiration was resumed.[147,148] Extrapolation of primate studies on nasal obstruction and growth to humans is not clear. Houston[149] postulated that "growth in anterior face height is determined primarily by growth in the length of the cervical column and the associated stretch of the cranio-cervical fascia and musculature." Muscular influence in this area is supported by the primate studies noted previously.

In many of these studies the differences in measurements were statistically significant but not greatly so. In comparing "long face" and "normal face" adolescents, Fields and colleagues[150] showed data suggesting that decreased nasal respiration may add to a long face phenotype but is not the only cause. Although a large proportion of oral breathers are represented in the long face population, a significant number of long face persons do not have nasal obstruction.[22] Ung and coworkers[133] found a weak association of maxillary and mandibular incisors and class II malocclusion with retroclination. These workers questioned the clinical significance, even though the correlation was statistically significant. In addition, the association between dentofacial variables and respiratory pattern was weak in establishing generalizations about causal relationships when assessed subjectively and objectively. Mahony and associates, in their study of 80 children (45 with

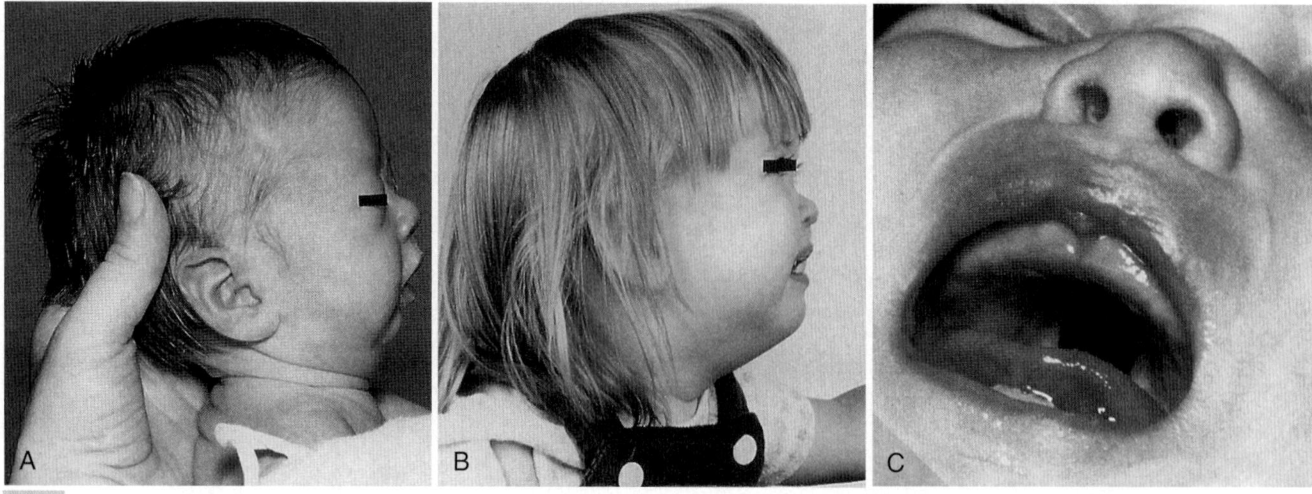

Figure 184-26. **A,** A newborn with Robin sequence. **B,** The same child at 2 years of age. Note the partial mandibular catch-up growth. **C,** U-shaped cleft palate in a patient with Robin sequence.

nasal obstruction who received an adenoidectomy and 35 age- and sex-matched controls), concluded that the changes in the dentoalveolar heights of the maxillary molars and the ratio of the upper and lower anterior face heights seem to be associated with the change in mode of breathing from mouth to nose breathing after adenoidectomy.[151] Hartgerink and Vig[152] could find no significant correlation between the respiratory and morphologic features studied, although they described associations among lip posture, lower anterior facial height, and nasal resistance.

Perhaps there is a period in facial growth and development during which a decrease in nasal breathing and an increase in oral breathing critically influence dentofacial growth. If so, then the timing of intervention would be important to alleviate or lessen the adverse aspects of the ultimate facial result.[133]

Rapid maxillary expansion (RME) with and without surgery has been shown to decrease nasal resistance and increase repiratory area. The study investigators advocate that the pubertal or prepubertal age period is the most suitable age for this intervention in patients with both maxillary constriction and a posterior cross-bite.[153] RME improved obstructive sleep apnea by changing the anatomic structure (widening of the nasal fossa and release of the septum) in 42 patients reported by Pirelli and colleagues; however, this study did not include a control group.[154]

Taking into account the research conducted in this area, the role that breathing patterns and modes play in dentofacial growth is still open to debate. Although the evidence is not entirely clear and the exact mechanisms remain unknown, it appears that craniofacial changes occur in persons with significant nasal obstruction secondary to adenoidal hypertrophy. This has led some researchers in the field to say that adults should watch for OMP in children and encourage them to "maintain appropriate lip seal posture" because of the high incidence of OMP in the orthodontic population. In the event that closed mouth posture cannot be maintained, the clinician should search for a treatable cause of OMP, such as an adenoidectomy.

Variations in response to the relief of nasal obstruction occur in patients, and it may be difficult to decide who would benefit from an adenoidectomy. Although the literature contains a growing body of data that nasal obstruction influences facial characteristics and that reversal may occur under certain conditions, this is still open to debate.

Hartgerink and Vig[152] concluded that "neither orthodontists nor otolaryngologists can predict or accurately diagnose nasal airway impairment from the patient's facial proportions or lip separation at rest." The prudent otolaryngologist should review in detail the findings in a specific case before embarking on a surgical procedure to possibly alter or reverse dentofacial growth.

Craniofacial Abnormalities

Robin Sequence (Pierre Robin Syndrome)

The combination of micrognathia, cleft palate, and glossoptosis is known as the Robin sequence (Fig. 184-26). Previously known as Pierre Robin syndrome, this entity is now recognized to demonstrate etiologic heterogeneity; thus, it does not meet the criteria for a syndrome, with a single identifiable etiology. Cohen[155] proposed that "etiologic heterogeneity suggests pathogenetic heterogeneity in Robin sequence."

There are various definitions of the Robin sequence, including the presence or absence of a cleft palate, glossoptosis, and airway difficulty. This variability has caused confusion in the literature. The Robin sequence can be classified as either isolated (nonsyndromic) or in association with a syndrome (syndromic). Shprintzen[156] found that approximately 20% of patients had isolated Robin sequence, with the remaining 80% of cases associated with various syndromes. The primary clinical implications of this condition are airway obstruction and feeding difficulty. Anatomically, the larynx is under the base of the tongue in patients with micrognathia and glossoptosis, making direct laryngoscopy or intubation difficult and occasionally impossible.[157] Cleft palate and respiratory difficulty can hamper feeding and contribute to failure to thrive.

Whether the Robin sequence is isolated or associated with a syndrome has very significant implications with respect to mandibular growth. A common error made by physicians is to convey to the family of a newborn with Robin sequence that the child's mandible will reach relatively normal size within a couple of years.[158] If the Robin sequence is associated with a known syndrome (primary error or nondeformational cause), such as Treacher Collins or Stickler syndrome, mandibular hypoplasia will persist throughout the patient's life unless surgical intervention is undertaken. In these cases, postnatal catch-up growth does not occur.

If the Robin sequence is isolated, however, with the etiologic pathogenesis related to deformation, then catch-up growth does occur. Pruzansky[159] believed that postnatal growth potential should be included in the analysis of differences between malformed mandibles and that "some mandibles are capable of considerable postnatal recuperations."

It was formerly thought that once affected patients were full-grown, their mandibles would be of essentially normal size. Pruzansky[159] noted that the mandible in such patients differed from the normal mandible in that "the gonial angle was more obtuse, the condyle extended distally from the ramus, and ramus-to-body proportions were deviant because of the greater reduction in body length." He also noted that these features persisted from infancy into adulthood. The mandible appears to grow faster than normal in such patients during the first few months of life, resulting in alleviation of breathing problems and feeding difficulty in many. Not all patients are so fortunate, however, and numerous measures have been advocated to address these issues: positioning, subperiosteal tongue release, and tracheostomy, among others.[156,157,160-163]

Even in the isolated Robin sequence, full or complete catch-up growth does not occur (see Fig. 184-26A and B). Figueroa and associates[164] performed a retrospective longitudinal cephalometric study analyzing size, growth, and the relation of the mandible, tongue, and airway in isolated nonsyndromic Robin sequence infants. These investigators found that the increased mandibular growth rate in these infants was significant but did not reach values seen in healthy infants. Craniofacial variables were significantly different between healthy patients and those with the Robin sequence. This study supported the concept of "partial mandibular catch-up growth." The investigators also discussed an unpublished study from their institution in which adolescent patients with Robin sequence were compared with healthy children. Results indicated that craniofacial dimensions, including the maxilla, mandible, and airway, were smaller in Robin sequence patients. Laitinen and Ranta[165] and Laitinen[166] found the dental arches at birth of patients with Robin sequence (isolated or possibly syndromic) and those of patients with isolated cleft lip and palate to be equal. By the age of 6 years, the dental arches in patients with Robin sequence were smaller than isolated cleft palate arches, which in turn were smaller than those in children without clefts.

The U-shaped cleft palate in Robin sequence and its mode of development are different from those of the usual V shape seen in primary defects (see Fig. 184-26C). Hanson and Smith[167] hypothesized that with micrognathia, the posteriorly displaced tongue is interposed between the palatal shelves. The palatal shelves do not close, resulting in less posterior growth of the soft palate and subsequently the U-shaped cleft palate. That is, the small mandible causes the tongue to be placed abnormally in the posterior portion of the oral cavity, in between the palatal shelves, and the subsequent lack of closure and growth of the palatal shelves and the lack of growth of the soft palate result in the U-shaped defect.

Robin sequence is relatively common, occurring in approximately 1 in 8500 births. Prevalence is confusing, however, because of the isolated versus syndromic differentiation. The most important issue in these patients is first to ensure an adequate airway and feeding; and then to determine whether there is an associated syndrome in order to communicate to the family the degree of intervention that is likely to be needed.

Down Syndrome (Trisomy 21)

Down syndrome (trisomy 21) is the most common malformation syndrome (Fig. 184-27). It occurs in approximately 1 in 650 live births, and the prevalence is greater with increasing maternal age. Affected persons, who have an extra copy of the genetic material on chromosome 21, have a highly characteristic appearance.[168,169] More than 100 different physical signs can be present with Down syndrome. The main features, in addition to intellectual deficit, are the craniofacial physical characteristics listed in Box 184-1. These characteristics make persons with Down syndrome appear significantly different from the rest of the population. Pueschel and Pueschel[170] extensively reviewed the biomedical concerns of Down syndrome patients, including growth and devel-

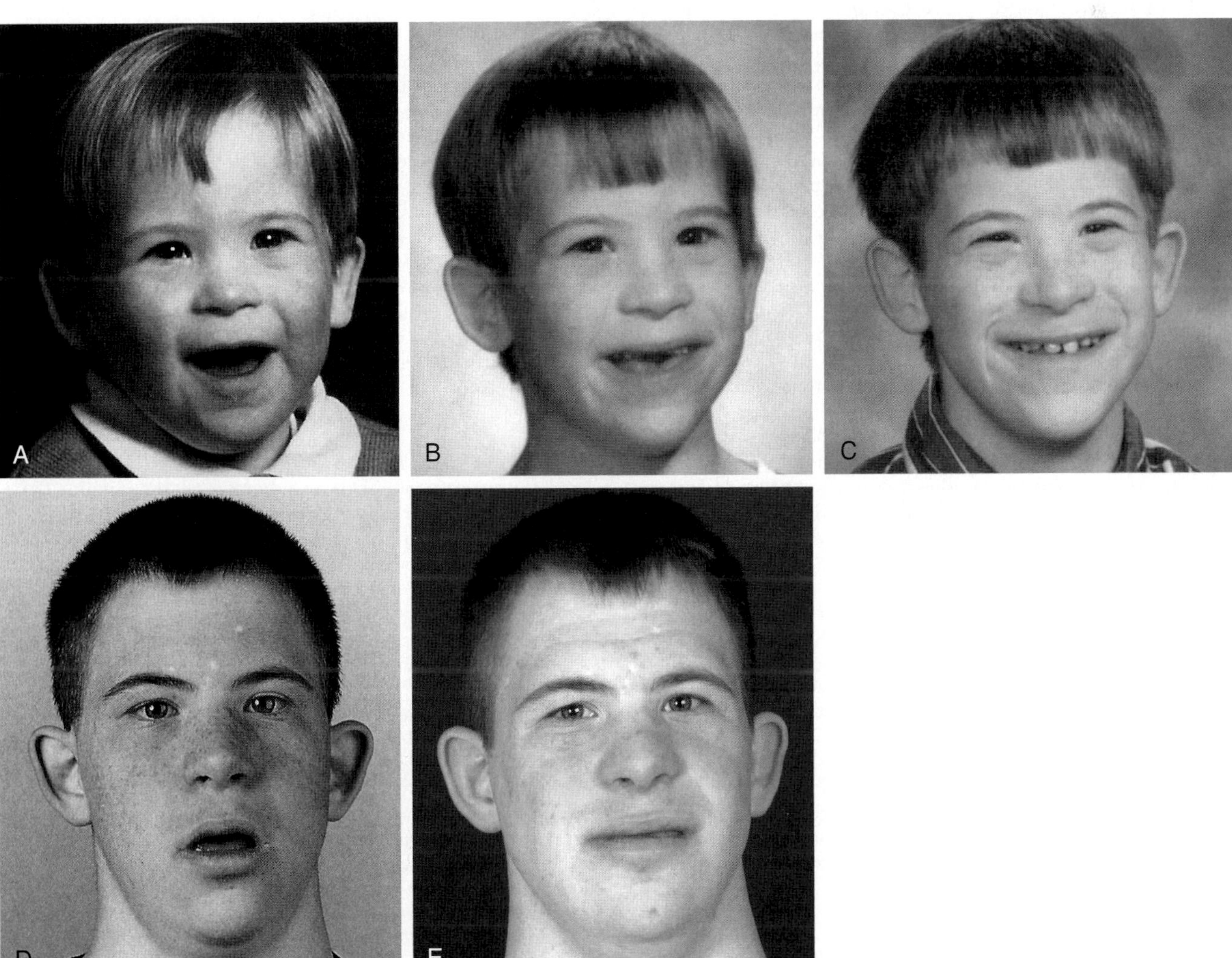

Figure 184-27. **A,** A 2-year-old boy with Down syndrome (trisomy 21). **B,** At age 5. **C,** At age 11. **D,** At age 14. **E,** The patient at age 20.

Box 184-1
Craniofacial Features of Down Syndrome

- Brachycephaly
- Flat occiput
- Upward-slanting palpebral fissures
- Epicanthic folds
- Short, small nose
- Abnormal small ears
- Short neck
- Midface hypoplasia
- Large fissured lips
- Large fissured tongue
- Dental abnormalities

opment. The specific dysmorphic facial features of Down syndrome, outlined in Box 184-1, can be further classified into five main regions: skull, midface, mandibular and oral, ears, and eyes. The growth changes in each of these regions are reviewed next.

Skull

A majority of patients with Down syndrome have brachycephaly. Head breadth (the largest lateral diameter of the head) and head length (measured from the nasion to the largest length across the occiput) were found to be essentially normal in the first 6 months of life when compared with healthy children.[171,172] At 6 months and 1 year, however, the mean values were less by 1 SD for head breadth and 2 to 3 SDs for head length. The greater difference in head length versus head breadth suggests that cranial growth is more reduced at the cranial base than in the area of the calvaria. In 1979, Hamill and associates[173] determined that head circumference is smaller in persons with trisomy 21; however, this reduction from the norm is thought to be a reflection of overall body size. When head circumference is plotted against body/length ratios, these values are found to be within normal range. Head circumference is related to intracranial or brain growth; whereas cranial base growth probably is under the same control as for total body growth. The occiput also is found to be flat, which is especially noticeable in the profile view. Allanson and colleagues[174] obtained 21 craniofacial anthropometric measurements from patients with trisomy 21 between the ages of 6 months and 61 years of age. Their data were compared with normal known standards and were in agreement with previous studies involving craniofacial findings in Down syndrome. These investigators specifically mention brachycephaly, round face, and small ears but add that underdevelopment of the maxilla in comparison with the mandible also occurs. More recently, computerized anthropometry has been used in patients with trisomy 21 and compared with normal reference data. Several differences have been noted, particularly related to midfacial hypoplasia, decreased nasal protrusion, and a lower facial third region (mandible).[175] Allanson's group found that as age increases, maxillary growth is reduced in comparison with mandibular growth, resulting in a change from the usual round face seen in infants to the more oval shape seen in older patients (see Fig. 184-27).

Sperber[1] indicated that the reduced cranial base results in an increased angulation because of the loss of the flattening effect of the growth of the spheno-occipital synchondrosis. In a skull of normal or reduced capacity, an increase in the basal angle is highly suggestive of Down syndrome.[176] This results in a "dish" deformity of the midface, accentuated by the large neurocranium. The anterior fontanelle is late to close, and the so-called third fontanelle, an open sagittal suture in the region of the parietal bone, is present.[177] A metopic suture is quite common in Down syndrome patients.

Midface

Benda[178,179] noted a deficiency in postnatal development of the nasal bones, the ethmoid, and the maxilla that results in continuance of the fetal proportions of the face in persons with Down syndrome. He also noted that hypoplastic or even absent paranasal sinuses also contribute to midface hypoplasia. Shapiro and associates[180] found that Down syndrome patients have narrower and shorter palates. The deficiency in palatal length, in comparison with that in healthy persons, was so great in the patients from their study (age range, 7 to 18 years) that they could distinguish between a Down syndrome patient and a healthy person on the basis of this dimension alone. Palatal vaults previously were thought to be abnormal (higher-arching) in patients with trisomy 21, but Shapiro's group confirmed that they are within the normal range.[180] Smaller nasal bones appear to contribute to the saddle nose–small nose of these patients.[1] Interorbital distance is reduced, and the mandible is more obtuse.[181] The angle between the base of the skull and the hard palate is less acute than normal in patients with trisomy 21, and the nasopharynx generally is small because of soft tissue encroachment. Although limited by a small sample size, another study compared rapid maxillary expansion in 13 children and no intervention in 13. Acoustic rhinometry measured nasal patency; those children undergoing expansion showed a significant increase in the total nasal volume. The investigators also noted that the widening of the maxillary bones also gives more space for the tongue in the oral cavity and that there is positive dental improvement. However, these two areas were not reviewed objectively in this article.[182]

Sperber[1] theorized that the neural crest tissues involved in facial bone formation, (including the nose) either "may be deficient in number, may not complete migration to their destination, or fail in their inductive capacity or cytodifferentiation." The generalized retardation in midface growth, along with the underdevelopment of the sinuses in patients with trisomy 21, results in the overall poor development and flat facial profile of the midface.

Ears

Persons with Down syndrome have long been recognized to have small ears. The ears are frequently small and boxlike and can be low-set with abnormal overlapping or folding of the helix. Aase and colleagues[183] noted that "of all the anthropomorphic measurements studied, the longitudinal dimensions of the pinna fell furthest below the expected norm at all age levels studied." This finding usually was greater than 2 SDs below the norm in newborns to 1-year-olds and 1 SD in patients older than 1 year of age. External ear canal narrowing is extremely common, and middle ear abnormalities exist.[184,185] The mastoid abnormalities in Down syndrome are mainly hypoplasia and sclerosis.[186] These abnormalities may have an inflammatory etiology from increased problems of middle ear pathology secondary to eustachian tube dysfunction. Generalized hypotonia in Down syndrome may affect the tensor veli palatini muscle, resulting in eustachian tube dysfunction.

Mandible and Oral Manifestations

The oral manifestations of Down syndrome are outlined in Box 184-1. Thickened and fissured lips as the patient advances in age, a large, fissured tongue (possibly related to a relatively small oral cavity), and various dental abnormalities are very common in these patients.[170,187-191] After the age of 16 to 18 years, progressive mandibular prognathism may occur and is believed to be related to the large tongue in a small oral cavity.[192]

Eyes

Using radiographic methods, Gerald and Silverman[181] described narrowing of the interorbital distance in patients with Down syndrome and concluded that this orbital hypotelorism is the skeletal substrate for the characteristic face in these patients. Cohen and associates[193] agreed that ocular hypotelorism is true when measured; however, they also noted that the hypertelorism may appear to be more pronounced in these patients because of the characteristic epicanthic folds and low nasal bridge. Other factors that contribute to the illusion of extreme hypertelorism include exotropia, narrow palpebral fissures, dystopia canthorum, and widely spaced eyebrows. In Down syndrome, epicanthic folds appear to result from underdevelopment of the nasion.[178] An alternative theory is that the epicanthic folds result from an abnormal distribution of the orbicularis oculi muscle, with some fibers passing circularly in front of the tendon rather than inserting wholly into the ligament.[23]

Abnormal and Poor Growth in Down Syndrome

No specific gene or genes on chromosome 21 have been identified to contribute to the current understanding of how the many phenotypic findings arise in Down syndrome. However, it is postulated that a dosage effect occurs because of the extra chromosome. No growth-regulating genes have been mapped on chromosome 21, but Pueschel and Pueschel[170] postulate that "gene coding for growth-regulating proteins may play a part in the growth retardation observed in individuals with Down syndrome." According to this theory, the extra chromosome 21 is responsible for the abnormal embryogenesis of the fetus with Down syndrome, and somehow the balance in the growth process is altered. Further studies in the molecular biology of growth and development will ultimately delineate this unknown.

Achondroplasia

Achondroplasia is the most common of the chondrodysplasias. A full description of this disorder of bone formation can be found in the works of Jones[169] and Gorlin and colleagues[168] and in the Online Mendelian Inheritance in Man (OMIM) database.[194]

Achondroplasia is an autosomal dominant disorder, with a majority of cases representing a new mutation. Bone formed from cartilage is abnormal because of a mutation in the fibroblast growth factor receptor-3 gene, *FGFR3*, which is located at 4p16.3.[195,196] Two different point mutations have been found in *FGFR3* in patients with achondroplasia, and both lead to the substitution of an arginine residue for a glycine at position 380 of the mature protein, which is in the transmembrane domain of *FGFR3*.[194] In addition to expression of the receptor in cartilage, *FGFR-3* transcripts are present in fetal and adult brains, which have the highest levels of any tissue. This finding may indicate that the effects of the gene involve calvarial content as well as skeletal cartilage, leading to true megalencephaly.[194,197] The exact process leading to the phenotypic appearance is unclear.

Persons affected by this disorder have short stature secondary to rhizomelic shortening of the limbs, as well as abnormalities of a number of other bones, including the lumbar spine, carpals, metacarpals, phalanges, and pelvis (Fig. 184-28A and C). The characteristic facial appearance of achondroplasia results from early spheno-occipital closure, a short cranial base, a small foramen magnum, and resultant megalocephaly with frontal bossing, sunken bridge of the nose, and midface hypoplasia (see Fig. 184-28B and D). In addition, the eustachian tube is shortened. Head growth normally is rapid in the first 6 months of life in patients with achondroplasia.[198]

It is postulated that the genetic defect in achondroplasia leads to reduced growth of the occipital bones, resulting in the small foramen magnum.[19] Premature fusion of the associated synchondroses could also explain the abnormal foramen magnum configuration. Measurement of the foramen magnum may identify affected persons at risk for possible neurologic complications in achondroplasia. Basilar kyphosis is present, with the angle between the ethmoidal plane and clivus reduced to 85 to 90 degrees (normal angle, 110 to 120 degrees).[199] The clivus is vertical, and the sphenoid sinus frequently extends into it.[200] The sella may be small and abnormally J-shaped.[201] The petrous portion of the temporal bone is very distorted, and the internal and external acoustic meatus and labyrinths are abnormally oriented. Of interest, balance is not affected in these patients. Mastoid development is minimal.[200] The chondrocranium is short and narrow, as noted earlier. Dorst[16] observed that the midface is recessed in profile because the facial bones "hang down" from the chondrocranium. Articulation is normal.[199] The mandible is not affected by the genetic mutation but appears disproportionately large. Class 3 dental occlusion is common. Surgical correction using standard craniofacial procedures and nasal bone grafting improves the cosmetic appearance if this is desired.[201,202]

Mandibulofacial Dysostosis (Treacher Collins Syndrome, Franceschetti-Klein Syndrome)

Mandibulofacial dysostosis (MFD), also known as Treacher Collins syndrome, is a rare malformation syndrome associated with a very characteristic appearance,[203] as shown in Figure 184-29. The craniofacial abnormalities in mandibulofacial dysostosis are outlined in Box 184-2,[168,169] and the syndrome is covered in detail elsewhere.[168,169,204]

Mandibulofacial dysostosis is a rare autosomal dominant condition with complete penetrance and variable expression. Sixty percent of cases are the result of spontaneous new mutations. The gene was first localized to 5q32-33.1 by linkage analysis and was subsequently identified by positional cloning.[205] The identification of mutations in the *TCOF1* gene (also referred to as the *TREACLE* gene) in five different families confirmed the causative nature of this gene in MFD. Its function is unknown. At present, linkage analysis or mutational analysis can be undertaken to identify affected family members who may exhibit only mild phenotypic features of this syndrome.

Marsh and colleagues[21,206] provide an exhaustive, outstanding review of the cranial dysmorphology in mandibulofacial dysostosis, deriving their data both from the literature and from three-dimensional reformation imaging from CT scans. From a clinical standpoint, pharyngeal hypoplasia in affected persons is significant because it makes these patients prone to airway difficulty both early in life and later in life. Pharyngeal hypoplasia existed in all 11 patients with mandibulofacial dysostosis reviewed by Shprintzen and coworkers.[207] In fact, patients with a mild or incomplete phenotype were equally at risk. Shprintzen's group recommended nasopharyngoscopy and anterior posterior roentgenography to aid in the diagnosis. With growth, there is an increase in basilar kyphosis exacerbating the problem. MFD patients reported in the literature have responded to craniofacial surgery to alleviate their apnea.[208,209]

Patients with MFD have an abnormal acute cranial base that is 2 to 3 SDs below normal.[156] Peterson-Falzone and Figueroa[210] reviewed the longitudinal measurements of cranial base angulation in 24 patients with mandibulofacial dysostosis. These investigators showed an increase

Box 184-2

Craniofacial Findings in Mandibulofacial Dysostosis (Treacher Collins Syndrome)

Eyes

Downward-slanting palpebral fissures
Lower lid coloboma
Partial to total absence of lower eyelashes

Ears

Auricular malformations with or without tags and preauricular blind fistulas
Stenosis or atresia of the external ear canals
Middle ear and ossicular abnormalities

Face

Malar hypoplasia (hypoplastic zygomatic bones) and nonfusion of the zygomatic arches
Flat frontal nasal angle
Hypoplastic supraorbital rims and ridges
Narrow nares and hypoplastic alar cartilages
Tongues of hair onto cheeks

Mandible and Oral Cavity

Mandibular hypoplasia and severe hypoplasia of the mandibular condyle
Microstomia
High-arched, narrow, or cleft palate
Dental abnormalities

Data from Gorlin RJ, Cohen MM Jr, Levin LS, eds. *Syndromes of the Head and Neck*. 3rd ed. New York: Oxford University Press; 1990; and Jones KL, ed. *Smith's Recognizable Patterns of Human Malformation*. 5th ed. Philadelphia: WB Saunders; 1997.

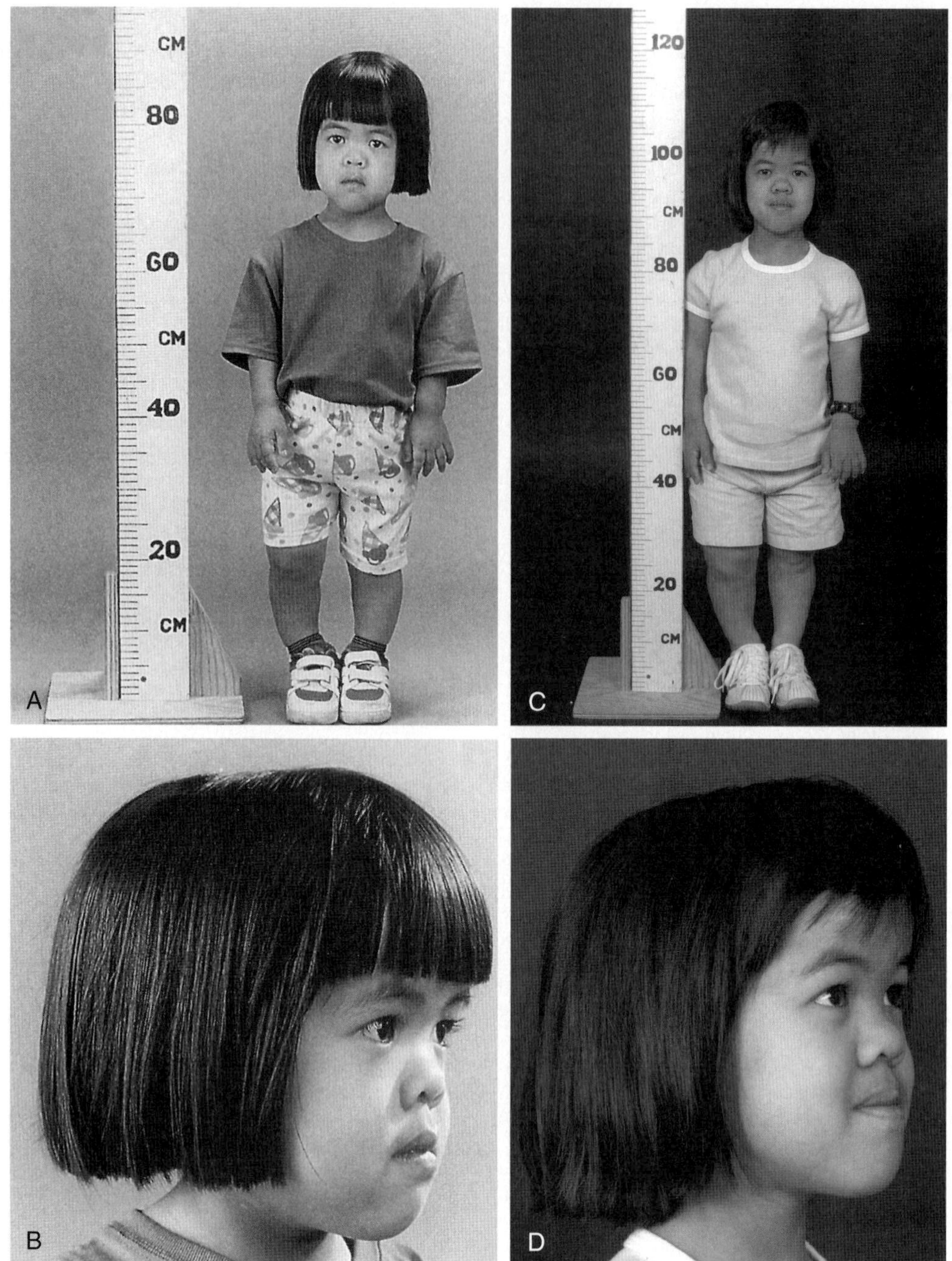

Figure 184-28. **A,** A 6-year-old girl with achondroplasia. **B,** The child manifests the characteristic facial appearance of achondroplasia: frontal bossing, sunken bridge of the nose, and midfacial hypoplasia. The normal mandible appears larger than usual. **C** and **D,** At age 12 years.

in the flexure of the cranial base angle over time, with more than 50% of cases falling into the kyphotic range, confirming previous reports of this finding in the literature. The investigators attribute the increasing flexion to intracranial resorption and extracranial bony apposition as described by Hans[11] and Enlow.[17] They speculate that the increased flexion may be greater in mandibulofacial dysostosis because the clivus resorbs to a greater degree during cranial base development. This may be because of a disproportion between normal brain mass in persons with mandibulofacial dysostosis and the reduction in facial height and the association with the anterior cranial base.

Deficient growth of the spheno-occipital and intersphenoidal synchondroses also plays a role in the formation of the abnormal cranial base. Kreiborg and Dahl[211] studied craniofacial growth in two children with MFD. Progressive basilar kyphosis occurred in both children, and the researchers hypothesized that bending took place at the sphenofrontal suture. They believed that this, along with abnormal growth of the mandible, led to impairment of the airway, that the calvaria appeared to rotate backward and downward in relation to the anterior cranial base, and that the sphenofrontal suture acted as a joint. Kreiborg and Dahl also concluded that the abnormal growth of the mandible occurred at the condyle, which is in agreement with Enlow and Hans' work.[11,17] This study also is consistent with previous findings of hypoplasia of the greater wings of the sphenoid and pterygoid plates.

The mandible in mandibulofacial dysostosis is hypoplastic. The gonial angle (ramus to body angle) is obtuse. The condyles are hypoplastic or completely absent. Antegonial notching (the concavity on the inferior border of the mandible anterior to the ramus-body junction) has been described as characteristic of mandibulofacial dysostosis, distinguishing it from other syndromes that involve the mandible. These features have been presented from studies of lateral cephalograms, longitudinal roentgen cephalometric analyses using metallic implants, and a review of dry skulls.[212-214] Grayson and coworkers[215] disputed this

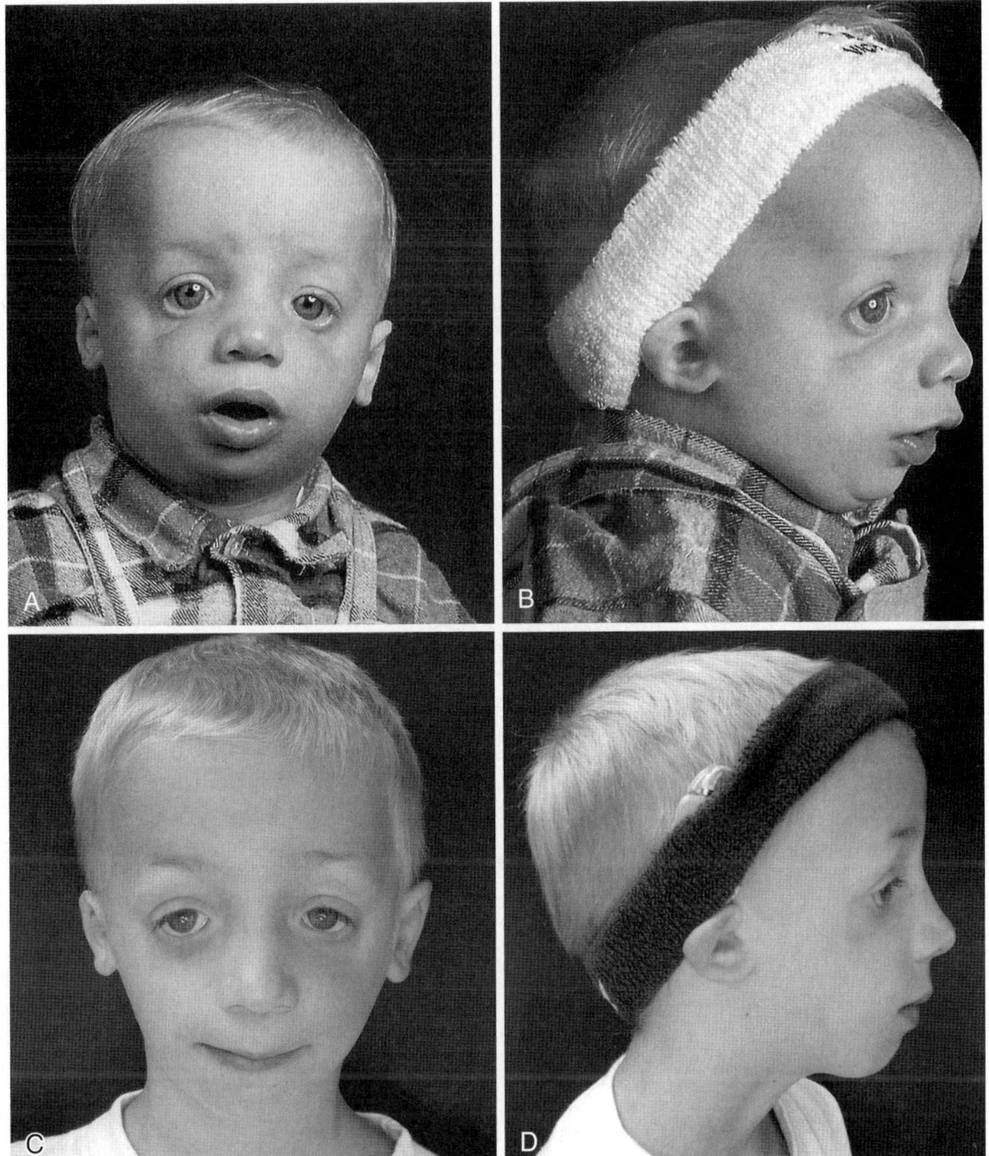

Figure 184-29. **A,** Characteristic facial appearance of a 10-month-old child with mandibulofacial dysostosis (Treacher Collins syndrome). **B,** Oblique view of same patient. Note the absent external ear canal, which is bilateral, and the headband, which holds bone conduction hearing aids. **C** and **D,** At age 6.

conclusion, although their methods did not employ classic cephalographic landmarks. They believed that complex craniofacial deformities require assessment from more than just conventional methods of measurement.[216]

Moss's functional matrix theory involves the concept that the mandible exhibits plasticity as it relates to the functional matrix with which it is involved, namely the anatomic features related to respiration and feeding. To know what the relationship is between the abnormal mandible—seen in mandibulofacial dysostosis and its functional matrix (respiration and feeding) in the context of Moss's functional matrix hypothesis in experimental form—would be helpful to better understand how the abnormal mandible functions in affected patients.[4,7-10]

Arvystas and Shprintzen[35] used 12 patients, ranging in age from 3 to 22 years (mean age, 10 years 4 months), as a sample population of mandibulofacial dysostosis. A number of cephalometric analyses were undertaken. These workers concluded that the characteristic appearance of the face in Treacher Collins syndrome (i.e., mandibulofacial dysostosis) is a product of the distinctive relationship among the abnormal basicranium, the dysmorphic mandible, and anomalous maxillary-malar complex. The anterior displacement of the temporomandibular joint, the short ramus, short mandibular body, synthesis distortion, and displaced maxilla all result in the characteristic appearance in this syndrome.[35]

Craniofacial surgery for patients with Treacher Collins syndrome is mandatory when problems with the airway become life threatening or are so severe as to compromise the individual. Previously, onlay techniques and soft tissue augmentation were used. However, craniofacial surgery using osteotomies and advancement techniques appears to assist in the orientation of subsequent growth in a more normal direction and to enlarge the airway at the same time. This results in both cosmetic and functional improvement.

As patients with MFD grow, their abnormally formed bones also grow, maintaining their original anatomy. "As they are malformed, so shall they grow."[217] Some researchers believe that the facial appearance of MFD individuals may improve during childhood growth.

Other Conditions and Syndromes

Numerous other syndromes and conditions may result in abnormalities of craniofacial growth and development. Cleft lip and palate and the craniosynostoses are two complex conditions resulting in abnormal craniofacial growth and development. These conditions cannot be given justice in a brief review, and the reader is directed to the significant body of literature covering these topics.

Conclusions

Craniofacial growth and development are extremely complex. Despite the voluminous amount of literature on this topic, little is known about the control mechanisms involved, even though the current understanding has increased because of the genetic revolution. The latter part of this chapter has described craniofacial growth in several genetic conditions from a primarily anatomic perspective, because at present this is all that is known.

Genetic predetermination is involved to a certain extent in facial growth and development, and many studying the field of craniofacial growth support the concept of Moss's functional matrix hypothesis and its interaction within the genetic constraints of the cells and tissues involved. As some critics have stated, however, Moss's theory explains *what* happens during growth but does not explain *how* it happens. The same can be said in describing abnormal facial growth and development. The cellular interaction within and between craniofacial regions remains unknown. It also seems likely that genes related to craniofacial growth and development are related to neurodevelopment. In the mid-1990s, an understanding of molecular genetics and craniofacial malformations began to emerge.[218,219] Although much progress has occurred in the study of genes for growth factors and signaling factors, much more is still to be learned.[220]

Acknowledgment

We thank Dr. Lorna E. Hruby for her expert editorial assistance and Dr. Doug Courtemanche for reviewing the first edition of this chapter.

SUGGESTED READINGS

Anderson PJ. Fractures of the facial skeleton in children. *Injury.* 1995;26:47.

Basciftci FA, Mutlu N, Karaman AI, et al. Does the timing and method of rapid maxillary expansion have an effect on the changes in nasal dimensions? *Angle Orthod.* 2002;72:118.

Baume LJ. Principles of cephalofacial development revealed by experimental biology. *Am J Orthod.* 1961;47:881.

Berkowitz RJ, Neuman P, Spalding P, et al. Developmental orofacial deficits associated with multimodal cancer therapy: case report. *Pediatr Dent.* 1989;11:227.

Berryhill WE, Rimell FL, Ness J, et al. Fate of rigid fixation in pediatric craniofacial surgery. *Otolaryngol Head Neck Surg.* 1999;121:269.

Bothwell MR, Piccirillo JF, Lusk RP, et al. Long-term outcome of facial growth after functional endoscopic sinus surgery. *Otolaryngol Head Neck Surg.* 2002;126:628.

Connelly SM, Smith RJH. Effects of rigid plate fixation and subsequent removal on craniofacial growth in rabbits. *Arch Otolaryngol Head Neck Surg.* 1998;124:444.

Demianczuk ANA, Verchere C, Phillips JH. The effect on facial growth of pediatric mandibular fractures. *J Craniofac Surg.* 1999;10:323.

Edwards RC, Kiely KD, Eppley BL. Resorbable PLLA-PGA screw fixation of mandibular sagittal split osteotomies. *J Craniofac Surg.* 1999;10:230.

Enlow DH, Hans MG. *Essentials of Facial Growth.* Philadelphia: WB Saunders; 1996.

Eppley BL, Sadove AM. Effects of resorbable fixation of craniofacial skeletal growth: a pilot experimental study. *J Craniofac Surg.* 1992;3:190.

Eppley BL, Sadove AM. Effects of resorbable fixation on craniofacial skeletal growth: modifications in plate size. *J Craniofac Surg.* 1994;5:110.

Eppley BL, Sadove AM. A comparison of resorbable and metallic fixation in healing of calvarial bone grafts. *Plast Reconstr Surg.* 1995;96:316.

Eppley BL, Sadove AM, Havlik RJ. Resorbable plate fixation in pediatric craniofacial surgery. *Plast Reconstr Surg.* 1997;100:1.

Ferrario VF, Sforza C, Poggio CE, et al. Distance from symmetry: a three-dimensional evaluation of facial asymmetry. *J Oral Maxillofac Surg.* 1994;52:1126.

Guyuron B, Dagys A, Munro I. Long-term effects of orbital irradiation. *Head Neck Surg.* 1987;10:85.

Hebert RL, Bent JP. Meta-analysis of pediatric functional endoscopic sinus surgery. *Laryngoscope.* 1998;108:796.

Klein JC. Nasal respiratory function and craniofacial growth. *Arch Otolaryngol Head Neck Surg.* 1986;112:843.

Koltai PJ, Rabkin D. Management of facial trauma in children. *Ped Clin North Am.* 1996;43:1253.

Kumar AV, Staffenberg DA, Petronio JA, et al. Bioabsorbable plates and screws in pediatric craniofacial surgery: A review of 22 cases. *J Craniofac Surg.* 1997;8:97.

Larson D, Kroll S, Jaffe N, et al. Long-term effects of radiotherapy in childhood and adolescence. *Am J Surg.* 1990;160:349.

Lin KY, Bartlett SP, Yaremchuk MJ, et al. An experimental study on the effect of rigid fixation on the developing craniofacial skeleton. *Plast Reconstr Surg.* 1991;87:229.

Linder-Aronson S. Adenoids: their effect on mode of breathing and nasal airflow and their relationship to characteristics of the facial skeleton and the dentition. *Acta Otolaryngol Suppl.* 1970;265:1.

Luhr HG. Indications for use of a microsystem for internal fixation in craniofacial surgery. *J Craniofac Surgery.* 1990;1:35.

Lusk RP, Bothwell MR, Piccirillo J. Long-term follow up for children treated with surgical intervention for chronic rhinosinusitis. *Laryngoscope.* 2006;116:2099.

Mair EA, Bolger WE, Breisch EA. Sinus and facial growth after pediatric endoscopic sinus surgery. *Arch Otolaryngol Head Neck Surg.* 1995;121: 547.

Marsh JL, Vannier MW, eds. *Comprehensive Care for Craniofacial Deformities.* St Louis: Mosby; 1985.

Moss ML. Growth and development of the craniofacial complex: an epigenetic viewpoint. In: Goodrich UT, Hall CD, eds. *Craniofacial Anomalies: Growth and Development from a Surgical Perspective.* New York: Thieme Medical Publishers; 1995:1-7.

Moss ML. The functional matrix. In: Kraus BS, Riedel RA, eds. *Vistas in Orthodontics.* Philadelphia: Lea & Febiger; 1962.

Moss ML. The primacy of functional matrices in orofacial growth. *Dent Pract.* 1968;19:65.

Orringer JS, Barcelona V, Buchman SR. Reasons for removal of rigid internal fixation devices in craniofacial surgery. *J Craniofac Surg.* 1998;9:40.

Paulino AC, Simon JH, Zhen W, et al. Long-term effects in children treated with radiotherapy for head and neck rhabdomyosarcoma. *Int J Radiat Oncology Biol Phys.* 2000;48:1489.

Pirsig W. Septal plasty in children: influence on nasal growth. *Rhinology.* 1977;15:193.

Posnick JC, Wells M, Pron GE. Pediatric facial fractures: evolving patterns of treatment. *J Oral Maxillofac Surg.* 1998;51:836.

Poswillo D. The aetiology and pathogenesis of craniofacial deformity. *Development.* 1988;103(suppl):207.

Pueschel SM, Pueschel JK. *Biomedical Concerns in Persons with Down Syndrome.* Baltimore: Paul H Brookes Publishing; 1992.

Scott JH. The cartilage of the nasal septum. *Br Dent J.* 1953;(July):37.

Shah RK, Dhingra JK, Carter BL, et al. Paranasal sinus development: a radiographic study. *Laryngoscope.* 2003;113:205.

Shprintzen RJ. Pierre Robin, micrognathia, and airway obstruction: the dependency of treatment on accurate diagnosis. *Int Anesthesiol Clin.* 1988;26:64.

Sklar CA. Overview of the effects of cancer therapies: the nature, scale and breadth of the problem. *Acta Paediatr Suppl.* 1999;88:1.

Sonis AL, Tarbell N, Valachovic RW, et al. Dentofacial development in long-term survivors of acute lymphoblastic leukemia. A comparison of three treatment modalities. *Cancer.* 1990;66:2645.

Tatum SA, Kellman RM, Freije JE. Maxillofacial fixation with absorbable miniplates: computed tomographic follow-up. *J Craniofac Surg.* 1997;8:135.

Thaller SR, Huang V, Tesluk H. Use of biodegradable plates and screws in a rabbit model. *J Craniofac Surg.* 1992;2:168.

Tourne LPM. The long face syndrome and impairment of the nasopharyngeal airway. *Angle Orthod.* 1990;60:167.

Winzenburg SM, Imola MJ. Internal fixation in pediatric maxillofacial fractures. *Facial Plast Surg.* 1998;14:45.

For complete list of references log onto www.expertconsult.com.

CHAPTER ONE HUNDRED AND EIGHTY-FIVE

Craniofacial Surgery for Congenital and Acquired Deformities

Jonathan Z. Baskin

Sherard A. Tatum, III

Key Points

- Craniofacial anomalies are relatively common deformities, many of which can treated by the otolaryngologist–head and neck surgeon with pediatric and/or facial plastic training.
- Craniofacial defects are often part of a larger syndrome affecting many functional systems.
- Appropriate care is best rendered by a clinically diverse team.
- The underlying pathology is etiologically diverse and heterogeneous.
- Craniofacial skeletal anomalies can be treated surgically with techniques that are reliable and reproducible.
- The application of craniofacial surgical principles, developed to treat congenital problems, also serves well for tumor extirpation and trauma repair.
- Several materials are currently available to reconstruct the craniofacial skeleton, but there is wide effort to develop more biomimetic bone substitutes.

Craniofacial surgery is a broad and continually growing field that addresses a wide array of congenital and acquired deformities. Much of the growth in this field has occurred in the last few decades, thus it is a relatively young discipline that is still actively evolving. This medical and surgical subspecialty includes a set of approaches and techniques developed in the last 50 years that allow for safe, reliable manipulation of the craniofacial skeleton. Although the field is focused primarily on congenital problems, the techniques can be broadly applied to trauma and tumor surgery of the craniofacial structures. *Craniofacial anomaly* refers to any malformation that involves the face, cranium, and cranial base. In the pediatric population the field is more commonly concerned with congenital anomalies, whereas in adults the more commonly encountered applications relate to trauma and neoplasm.

Congenital craniofacial deformities commonly occur as isolated defects and less often as part of a syndrome. The Committee on Nomenclature and Classification of Craniofacial Anomalies of the American Cleft Palate Association has organized craniofacial malformations into the following five categories: (1) facial clefts/encephaloceles and dysostoses; (2) atrophy/hypoplasia; (3) neoplasia/hyperplasia; (4) craniosynostosis; and (5) unclassified. Clinical entities such as orbital hypertelorism often exist with a syndrome that clearly fits into one of the aforementioned classifications.[1] Hypoplasia of the midface and micrognathia would be incorporated into the second category. In children, hematologic disorders and overly aggressive cerebrospinal fluid (CSF) shunting can result in secondary craniofacial disorders, which can be put into the third or fifth category. Acquired deformities of the craniofacial complex also include those inflicted by means of a traumatic event. Neoplasm (third category) and its treatment are classified as acquired deformities.

As is plainly evident, the field of craniofacial surgery is large with many and varied subfields. The objective of this chapter is to provide an overview of craniofacial surgery. The pathophysiology of major craniofacial anomalies is discussed in order to provide a framework for an understanding of the important clinical issues. The focus of the discussion is on cranial vault and craniofacial bony defects. Those disorders of first and second branchial arch derivatives that give rise to known craniofacial anomalies are briefly described. Trauma and neoplasm are important contributors to craniofacial disease and are examined briefly in this chapter but discussed in greater detail elsewhere in the text. Facial and palatal clefting is a very important subject in craniofacial surgery and is briefly discussed from a basic perspective. A clinical discussion of these defects, however, is the focus of another chapter.

Epidemiology

Craniofacial anomalies have been reported to constitute approximately one third of all congenital defects. The incidence of assorted individual deformities and syndromes varies. However, the overall incidence is considered to be 0.2 to 0.5 per 1000 births.[2] Interestingly, some craniofacial deformities occur at a uniform rate across racial and ethnic populations, whereas others occur at a frequency that varies as a function of race and ethnicity.

Several craniofacial malformations appear to have a genetic etiology. Several familial types have been well documented, and transmission can occur via autosomal dominant or recessive modes. With occasional exceptions males and females tend to have similar incidences for most anomalies. Craniofacial anomalies have been reported to occur as part of a genetic condition in about 20% of cases.[2] However, with the discovery of new syndromes and the recognition that "isolated defects" often have a genetic etiology, the 20% figure is probably an underestimate. Furthermore, as discussed here, the pathogenesis of craniofacial anomalies is complex, and generally it is most accurate to describe their etiology as multifactorial.

Mechanisms of Postnatal Facial Growth

It was once thought that craniofacial growth (like all other growth) was regulated, to a large extent, by the central nervous system. It is now understood to be much more complex. On a cellular level, the signal-sensitive membranes of the many types of cells respond to several different cues. On a developmental level, the functional needs of a particular structure and its relationship to adjoining structures strongly influence patterns of growth. Craniofacial bony growth is secondary to neural tissue growth and expansion. The brain as an organ mass develops early in embryogenesis. The developing brain highly influences the morphology of the basicranium, which in turn functions as a template for subsequent facial growth. The face can be viewed as a series of stratified vertical levels or fields that are strongly affected by growth of the brain and basicranium.[3]

Physiologically, there are two primary forces at play during the growth of individual craniofacial bones and structures, displacement and remodeling (Fig. 185-1). Growth does not indicate uniform enlargement of a structure; rather, it refers to a combination of displacement and remodeling. Displacement occurs when the bone is pushed away from its articulation with other bones (by the combined effects of growth of the surrounding soft tissue and growth center/sutural activity). Remodeling occurs by resorption and deposition of new bone that result in a net vector of growth. It is in this way that the correct tissue mass is achieved and that enlargement occurs proportionally and in the appropriate direction.

In the craniofacial complex the basicranium (along with the related soft tissues) influences the naso-orbito-maxillary complex and the ramus of the mandible, which conform through continual remodeling. Growth of the naso-orbito-maxillary complex displaces the maxillary dento-alveolus. This displacement together with growth of the mandibular ramus then affects growth of the corpus (body) of the mandible. The importance of soft tissues in growth is demonstrated in such clinical manifestations as the "adenoid face." The entire system is plastic and in flux throughout the growing period (even after periods of growth, albeit to a far lesser extent). It is for this reason that rigid nonbiologic implants such as those of titanium have the potential to interfere with normal growth if used during active development; they lack the plasticity that is so vital to dynamic growth.[4-6]

Throughout the period of craniofacial growth an overriding homeostasis exists among the different fields of growth. Small aberrations in one field can be counterbalanced by compensatory growth in another, resulting in constant equilibrium. This is very important for the physician to bear in mind when planning surgical or orthodontic intervention. Treatment failure or relapse is likely if that equilibrium is significantly disrupted.[7] Generally, interventions are more likely to succeed if the cause of the abnormality is addressed during periods of rapid growth. In contrast, the effect of the abnormality is more successfully treated during periods of slow growth.[3]

Craniofacial synostosis, or premature closure of a suture, is a good example of the morphologic consequence of defective skeletal growth. It also illustrates the importance of homeostasis in craniofacial development. The causes of craniosynostosis are likely multifactorial and the source of some controversy.[8,9] It has been shown to be associated with abnormalities in sutural biology, various biomechanical forces,[10] and defects in the primary growth centers of the involved bones. Sutural growth is also affected by surrounding tissue interactions. The contacting dura, for instance, influences the continued patency of sutures and helps regulate its closure.[11-14]

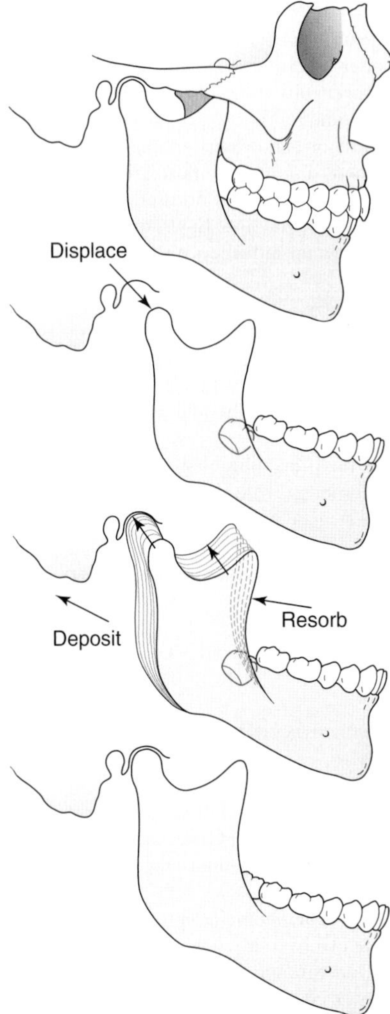

Figure 185-1. Schematic representation of displacement and remodeling in the mandible. Remodeling occurs through a combination of resorption and deposition. *(From The facial growth process. In Enlow: DH (ed).* Facial Growth. *3rd ed. Philadelphia: WB Saunders; 1990.)*

Regardless of the underlying etiology, the morphologic cause of the defect is premature closure of the suture, and this disruption in normal growth upsets the homeostasis inherent to the process. Consequently, compensatory growth occurs elsewhere as a means of achieving a new homeostasis. If the synostotic suture is treated early in life (while craniofacial growth is still quite active) the normal homeostasis can be restored by releasing the synostotic suture and thereby addressing the cause of the problem. If it is treated later in life, when active growth is largely complete, the morphologic results of the defect (including the anatomy associated with the compensation) have to be addressed because the sutural growth is no longer relevant.

Fusion of the facial processes during embryogenesis is another fundamental aspect of facial growth that is critical to normal development. Orofacial clefting results from a defect in this process. For opposing facial processes to fuse in the midline, the contacting epithelia must be eliminated so that the underlying mesenchymal tissue can become continuous. In the palate this elimination has been shown to occur through apoptosis, epithelial to mesenchymal cell transdifferentiation, or cell migration.[14-17] Underdevelopment of the mesenchyme of the involved subunits might preclude proper fusing, as can excessive apoptosis. Inadequate migration or proliferation of neural crest ectomesenchyme might have the same result. Facial clefting can also result from constricting anatomic defects. In the case of stunted mandibular growth, a Pierre Robin sequence can ensue whereby the palatal shelves are prevented from fusing in the midline.

Pathophysiology

As previously mentioned, the etiology of congenital craniofacial disorders is most often multifactorial and incompletely understood. A diverse and heterogeneous group of factors can contribute to abnormal craniofacial development. Various genetic defects have been implicated in the development of craniofacial anomalies. This field of study has yielded an enormous amount of information in the last few decades. In addition, numerous metabolic diseases are known to interfere with bone growth and suture function. Environmental factors have also been shown to exert important influences on embryologic craniofacial development.

Molecular Genetics

Several genetic defects have been identified that are directly associated with various craniofacial defects (Table 185-1). The products of these genes tend to fall into one of the following categories:

- Growth factor receptors: fibroblast growth factor receptors (FGFRs) 1, 2, and 3; tumor growth factor-β receptors (TGFβRs) 1 and 2; PTC and FGDY gene products
- Ephrins: membrane-anchored ligands for Eph receptor tyrosine kinases
- Transcription factors: MSX2, ALX4, GLI3, MITF, PAX3, RUNX2, TWIST
- Connective tissue structural proteins: type II and XI collagen, fibrillin-1 (FBN1)

These genetic defects have been linked to syndromes as well as isolated defects. For instance, defective FGFRs have been identified as the etiologic basis of some types of craniosynostosis as well as various syndromes (see Table 185-1).[18-45]

FGFRs are transmembrane receptors for fibroblast growth factors (FGFs). FGFs are involved in regulating cell proliferation, differentiation, and migration through a number of pathways. The receptor is made up of an extracellular domain (receptor-ligand binding), a transmembrane domain, and an intracellular tyrosine kinase enzymatic domain (Fig. 185-2A). There are several variations of the FGFR protein—all with important cell growth functions. Signaling via FGFR1, for instance, has been shown to facilitate neural crest migration, and a defective receptor has been linked to midline facial clefting in mice.[45] Defects in FGFR1 have been found to cause Kallmann's syndrome 2, which can include cleft lip and palate (see Fig. 185-2B).[46] Defects in FGFR1 and FGFR2 have been linked to syndromes such as Pfeiffer's syndrome (in which both receptors are defective) and to conditions of which craniosynostosis is a feature.[38,47] Defects in FGFR2 alone have been found in Apert's syndrome,[20,48] Jackson-Weiss syndrome,[28] Crouzon's syndrome,[29] and Beare-Stevenson cutis gyrata syndrome.[49] A defective FGFR3 protein is responsible for Crouzonodermoskeletal syndrome (Crouzon's syndrome with acanthosis nigricans),[30] for Muenke-type craniosynostosis,[32] and also for the disease process seen in achondroplasia.[50] In this disease the epiphyseal growth plates in long bones prematurely fuse. There are gross and histological similarities of long bone growth plates to the synchondroses of the calvaria. This work has led to the understanding that FGFR3 is involved in regulation of skeletal growth. In FGFR3 knockout mice (mice in which the gene that encodes this protein has been eliminated), there is severe retardation of skeletal maturation.[48,51-53]

The link between known syndromes or anomalies and genetic defects, however, can be complex and difficult to characterize. Defects in each of the three domains (in different FGFRs) have been discovered in association with craniofacial abnormalities, yet defects in the same domain of one FGFR type can cause two separate syndromes. For instance, identical mutations have been discovered in patients with Crouzon's, Pfeiffer's, and Jackson-Weiss syndromes, suggesting the involvement of other factors in the ultimate phenotypic expression.[38] Conversely, as is evident in Figure 185-2B, mutations in several distinct domains on one particular FGFR can result in the same phenotype.

As previously mentioned, defects in transcription factors and connective tissue proteins are also implicated in the pathogenesis of craniosynostosis. MSX2 is a homeobox gene that encodes a DNA binding transcription factor. It has been associated with nonsyndromic craniosynostosis (Boston type),[24,54] and ALX4, another homeobox gene, has been linked to parietal foramina.[34] Most cases of Saethre-Chotzen syndrome are caused by haplo-insufficiency of the TWIST gene, which appears to encode a transcription factor.[41] The GLI-3 gene and the transcription factor that it encodes are defective in Grieg's cephalopolysyndactyly (a rare syndrome that can include craniosynostosis).[31,55]

Genetic defects encoding several different extracellular matrix constituents can lead to anomalies of the craniofacial complex. Defective collagen, such as that seen in osteogenesis imperfecta, is clearly associated with bony abnormalities, although this disease only occasionally affects the craniofacial skeleton. Defective fibrillin (encoded by FBN1) results in Shprintzen-Goldberg syndrome with craniosynostosis and maxillary/mandibular hypoplasia.[43] The defective genes responsible for Stickler's syndrome are *COL2A1* and *COL11A2*, which encode types II and XI collagen, respectively.[56,57]

Metabolic Disorders

Several metabolic derangements are known to interfere with craniofacial development. The best known is the group of disorders known as the *mucopolysaccharidoses*. This group of disorders is characterized by a deficiency of lysosomal enzymes that results in a buildup of mucopolysaccharides. Although there are several clinical entities, patients with some of the more severe variations of the disease have large and dolichocephalic (long and narrow) skulls with premature closure of the sagittal suture and poorly developed mastoids and paranasal sinuses. Mucolipidosis, hyperthyroidism, and rickets are also known causes of craniosynostosis.[58,59]

Intrauterine Causes

In utero environmental contributors to craniofacial maldevelopment fit into the following four general categories: teratogenic, infectious, nutritional, and mechanical. Fetal alcohol syndrome can involve a wide range of defects, including holoprosencephaly. Tobacco use during critical periods of embryogenesis has also been shown to adversely affect craniofacial development. Medications such as hydantoin, phenytoin, valproic acid, and isotretinoin (a vitamin A derivative used in the treatment of acne) can exert deleterious effects on embryogenesis, as can toluene, the environmental contaminant dioxin, and ionizing radiation.[14,60,61]

Viral infections during pregnancy have been shown to cause cleft lip/palate via mutations in PVRL1 and IRF6.[62,63] Nutritional intake is also clearly linked to craniofacial development. Sonic hedgehog signaling, which is important in mediating parts of craniofacial development, is modulated by cholesterol. Therefore diets and medications that profoundly influence cholesterol levels can cause craniofacial malformations.[64,65] The link between a diet deficient in folic acid and neural tube defects has been well documented and has led to the widespread supplemental addition of folic acid to many processed foods throughout the developed world.

Finally, intrauterine constraint can cause deformation of the craniofacial skeleton. Factors that have been associated with intrauterine constraint include breech presentation, persistent fetal lie, early pelvic engagement of the head, oligohydramnios, prima gravidity, multiple gestations, uterine malformations, amniotic bands, and defects in fetal neuromuscular development.[66,67]

Acquired Craniofacial Deformities

Several postnatal conditions predispose an infant to disrupted craniofacial growth. Hematologic diseases such as thalassemias, sickle cell anemia, congenital hemolytic icterus, and polycythemia vera are known to cause craniosynostosis. Hyperplasia of the bone marrow leads to bony overgrowth in the skull. This in turn can cause the calvarial sutures to fuse prematurely.[68] Iatrogenic craniofacial anomalies can occur in patients who require ventricular shunts. If the shunt volumes in such patients are excessive, there is a lack of tension across the

Table 185-1

Craniofacial Anomalies with Phenotype and Known Gene Mutation

Condition	Craniofacial Phenotype	Gene*	OMIM Code†	Chapter Reference(s)
Aortic aneurysm, arterial tortuosity, hypertelorism, cleft palate/bifid uvula, craniosynostosis	Craniosynostosis, cleft palate, hypertelorism	TGFβR1 TGFβR2	190181 190182	19
Apert's syndrome	Craniosynostosis (brachycephaly); wide midline defect closes by coalescence of bony islands; midface malformations; dental crowding; cleft or narrow palate with swellings	FGFR2	101200	20-22
Beare-Stevenson cutis gyrata syndrome	Craniosynostosis (kleeblattschädel)	FGFR2	123790	23
Boston-type craniosynostosis	Craniosynostosis (kleeblattschädel), forehead retrusion, frontal bossing	MSX2	123101	24
Cleidocranial dysplasia	Delayed suture closure, frontal parietal bossing, wormian bone(s), hyperdontia, tooth eruption defects	RUNX2	119600	25
Craniofrontonasal syndrome	Craniosynostosis (brachycephaly), central defect between frontal bones, hypertelorism, divergent orbits	EFNB1	304110	26
Craniolacuna and pansynostosis	Multiple rounded calvarial bone defects, widespread craniosynostosis, hydrocephalus	FGFR2		27
Crouzon's syndrome	Craniosynostosis (brachycephaly), pronounced digital impressions of skull, midface hypoplasia, shallow orbits	FGFR2	123500	28, 29
Crouzonodermoskeletal syndrome	Craniosynostosis	FGFR3	134934	30
Grieg's cephalopolysyndactyly	Craniosynostosis in small percentage of cases, frontal bossing, sagittal ridging, hypertelorism	GLI3	175700	31
Muenke-type craniosynostosis (nonsyndromic)	Craniosynostosis (brachycephaly)	FGFR3	602849	32, 33
Parietal foramina	Symmetric parietal bone defects, cleft lip/palate	MSX2 ALX4	168500 605420	34-36
Parietal foramina with cleidocranial dysplasia	Symmetric parietal bone defects	MSX2	168550	37
Pfeiffer's syndrome	Craniosynostosis (brachycephaly)	FGFR1 FGFR2	101600	38-40
Saethre-Chotzen syndrome	Craniosynostosis (especially brachycephaly), flat forehead, low hairline	TWIST	101400	41, 42
Shprintzen-Goldberg (marfanoid) syndrome	Craniosynostosis (especially lambdoid and sagittal sutures), maxillary and mandibular hypoplasia, palatal abnormalities	FBN1	182212	43
Thanatophoric dysplasia II	Craniosynostosis (cloverleaf skull)	FGFR3	187601	44

*Gene abbreviations that have not been defined/spelled out are not acronyms or abbreviations.
†Online Mendelian Inheritance in Man database; available at www.ncbi.nlm.nih.gov/omim/
EFNB1, ephrin-B1; FBN, fibrillin; FGFR, fibroblast growth factor receptor; TGF-βR, tumor growth factor-β receptor
Adapted from Rice DP. Craniofacial anomalies: from development to molecular pathogenesis. *Curr Mol Med.* 2005;5:699-722.

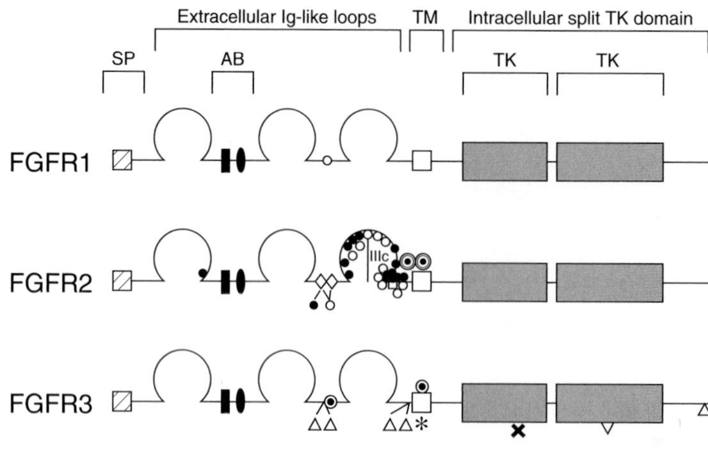

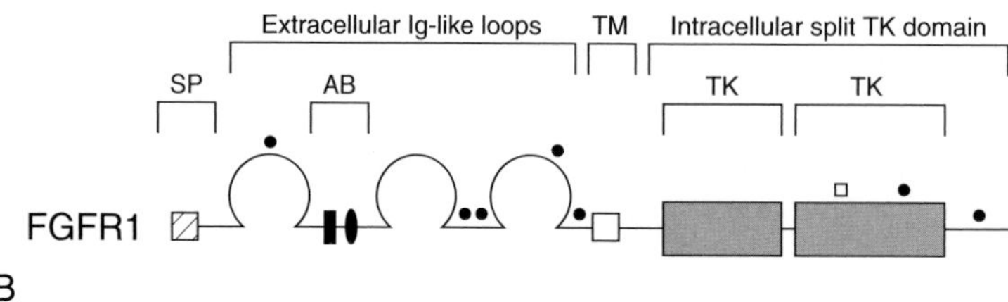

Figure 185-2. DNA mutations lead to several known defects in the fibroblastic growth factor receptor (FGFR) protein. **A,** Depicted are three receptors with defects involving different domains. Two phenotypically distinct syndromes can be caused by genetic mutations in the same functional domain of the same receptor type. **B,** Several different mutations of FGFR1 (*circles* refer to missense mutations, and *square* refers to a frameshift mutation) widely distributed along several distinct domains of the receptor that have been associated with one recognizable phenotype, Kallmann's syndrome. AB, acidic box; Ig, immunoglobulin; SP, signal peptide; TK, tyrosine kinase; TM, transmembrane domain. (**A** from Cohen MM Jr, Maclean RE. *Craniosynostosis: Diagnosis, Evaluation and Management.* 2nd ed. New York: Oxford Press; 2000. **B** adapted from Trarbach EB, Costa EM, Versiani B, et al. Novel fibroblast growth factor receptor 1 mutations in patients with congenital hypogonadotrophic hypogonadism with and without anosmia. *J Clin Endocrinol Metab.* 2006;91:4006-4012.)

sutures, which produces an environment that mechanistically resembles the one seen in microcephaly. In these conditions there is an increased risk of secondary craniosynostosis.[58] Etiologically, trauma and neoplasm can cause acquired craniofacial deformity, although they do so rarely.

Clinical Manifestations

Congenital Craniofacial Abnormalities

Craniofacial anomalies range from mild functionally asymptomatic defects (certain single-suture craniosynostoses) to severe anomalies that are not compatible with life (forms of holoprosencephaly). Typically, the pediatrician consults the craniofacial surgeon about a neonate who has an abnormally shaped head or unusual appearance. A fundamentally important point is to suspect the deformity to be part of a wider syndrome and to initiate a comprehensive examination in search of other abnormalities. However, the majority of cases of craniosynostosis are isolated with no associated anomalies.[69] Descriptions of some of the more common craniofacial abnormalities follow.

Craniosynostosis

Craniosynostosis refers to premature closure of the involved bony suture. The consequence is that growth is inhibited in the direction perpendicular to the suture line (Fig. 185-3). Ensuing developmental growth occurs in a compensatory pattern that permits, to the extent possible, continued expansion of the intracranial content in unrestricted directions. It must be stressed that the compensatory growth that occurs is the normal biologic response to sutural constraint. The functional and aesthetic imbalance that occurs is, in part, a byproduct of normal physiology. The various types of craniosynostosis are as follows.

Scaphocephaly

Scaphocephaly is the most common of cranial synostotic conditions. The sagittal suture, or part of it, prematurely fuses (Fig. 185-4). This anomaly prevents calvarial growth in the transverse dimension. The compensatory growth occurs in the anteroposterior (AP) direction, leaving the patient with decreased biparietal and bitemporal dimensions. The resulting head shape is long and narrow. There are several variations ("saddle deformity," "football deformity"), depending on the extent of premature sagittal fusion and also on whether the metopic suture is involved.

Trigonocephaly

Trigonocephaly refers to a triangular forehead (as viewed from above) and is associated with metopic suture synostosis. There is a decrease in bifrontal diameter. It is a mild form of craniosynostosis with rare func-

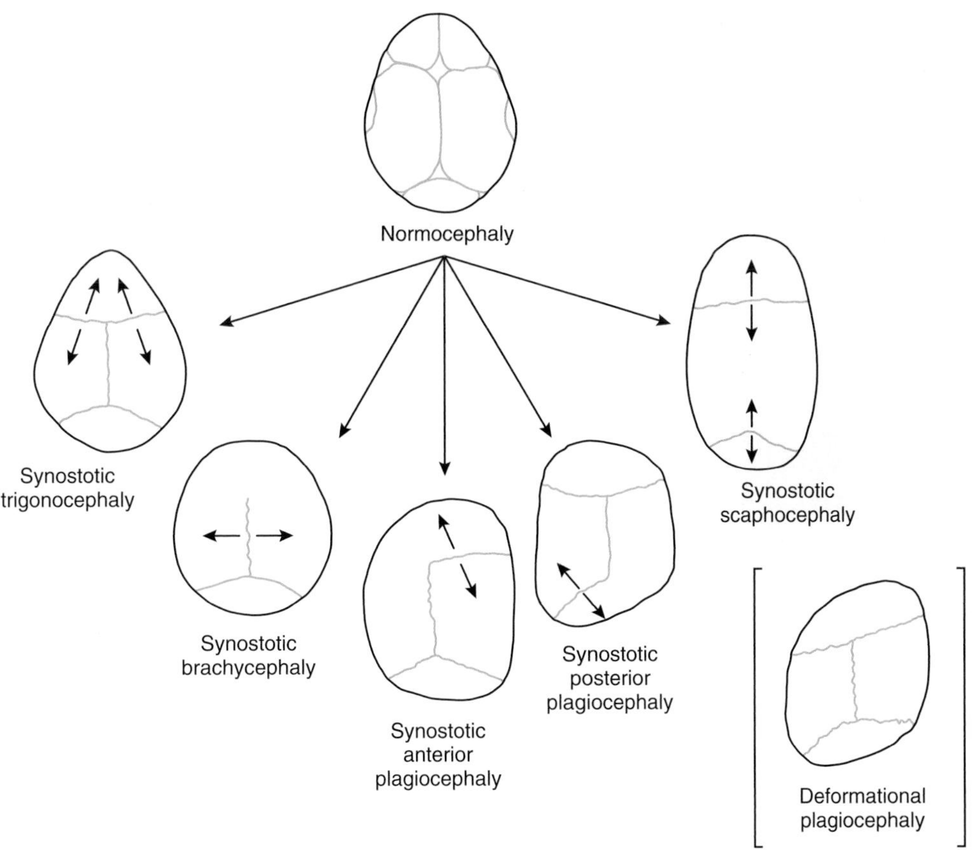

Figure 185-3. In craniosynostosis, growth is prevented from occurring across the fused suture. *Arrows* demonstrate compensatory growth that occurs across open sutures with continued intracranial expansion. (From Cohen MM Jr, Maclean RE. *Craniosynostosis: Diagnosis, Evaluation and Management.* 2nd ed. New York: Oxford Press; 2000:122.)

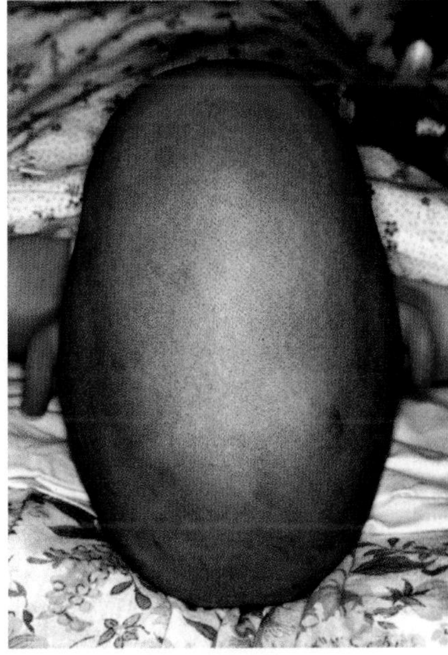

Figure 185-4. Sagittal suture synostosis without premature metopic closure resulting in scaphocephaly.

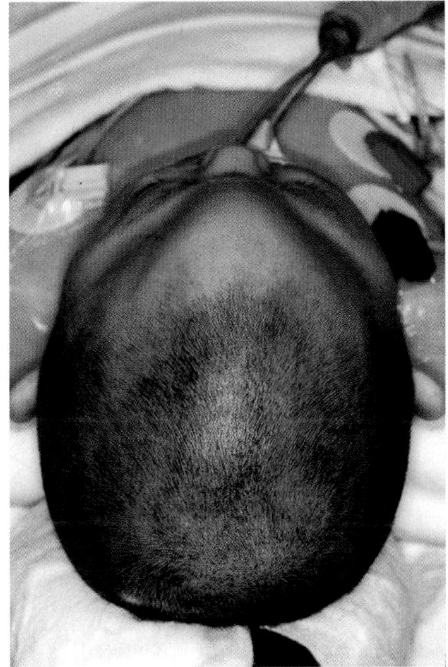

Figure 185-5. Metopic suture synostosis resulting in trigonocephaly.

tional consequences (Fig. 185-5). The suture area is thickened, resulting in an anterior midsagittal ridge. This appearance has been described as resembling the keel of a ship. There can be associated hypotelorism. In mild cases there may be only suture ridging without significant forehead deformity.

Plagiocephaly

In *plagiocephaly,* the head is asymmetric, flattened in one or more regions. It can be either synostotic or deformational and can be anterior or posterior. *Synostotic plagiocephaly* refers to either unilateral coronal (Fig. 185-6) or lambdoid synostosis. In coronal synostosis the forehead

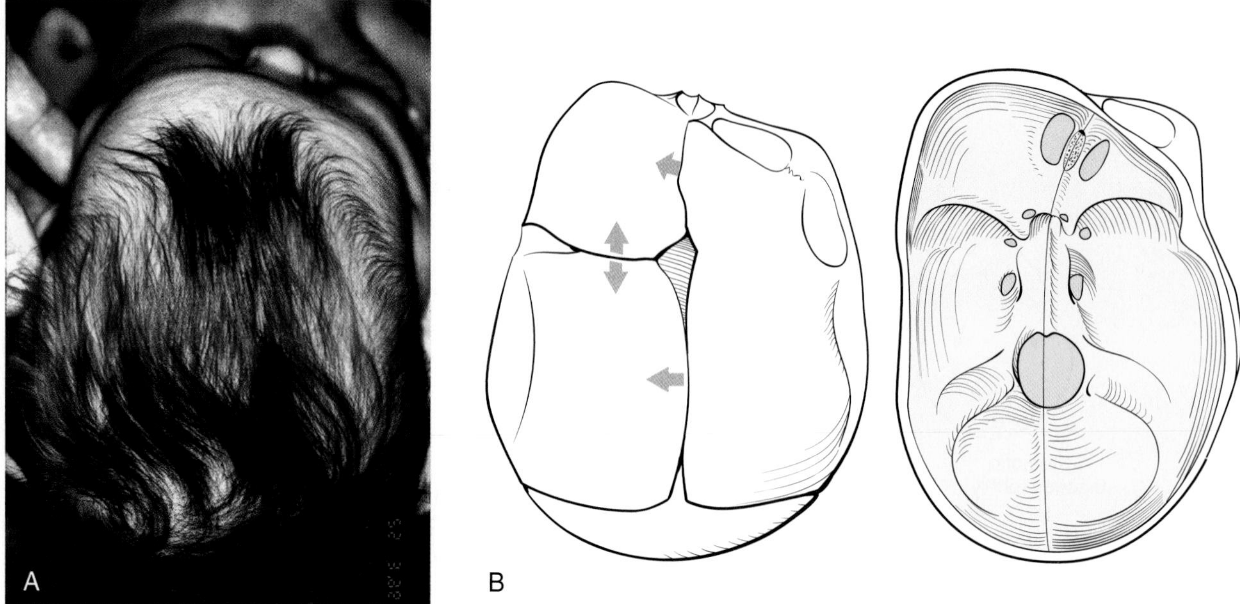

Figure 185-6. **A,** Unilateral coronal synostosis resulting in plagiocephaly. Note that the cranial vault irregularities are not confined to those ipsilateral to the defect. Compensatory growth has resulted in frontal bossing on the contralateral side. **B,** A schematic representation of plagiocephaly.

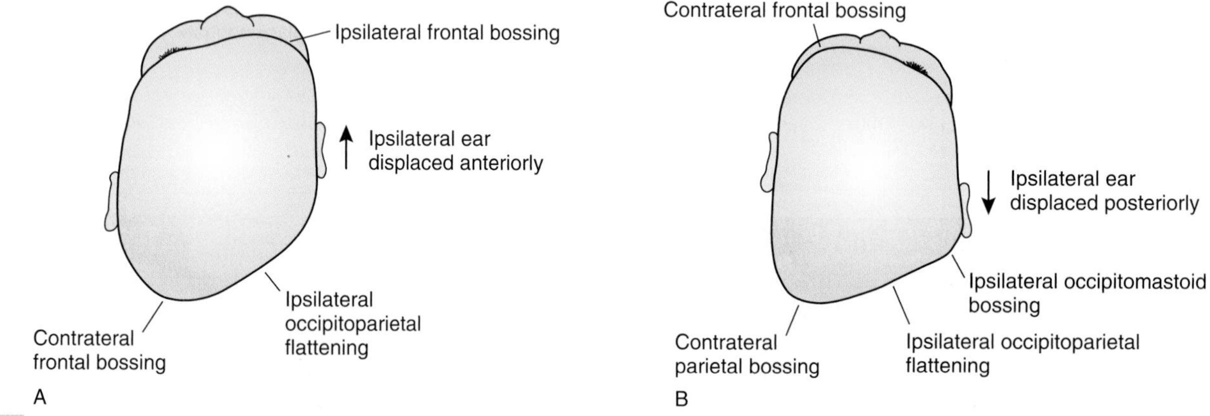

Figure 185-7. Deformational and synostotic plagiocephaly give rise to different characteristic head shapes. **A,** Posterior deformational plagiocephaly results in a parallelogram shape to the head with an anteriorly displaced ipsilateral ear. **B,** Unilateral lambdoid synostosis gives rise to contralateral posterior and occasional anterior bossing. The ipsilateral ear is displaced posteriorly. *(From Cohen MM Jr, Maclean RE.* Craniosynostosis: Diagnosis, Evaluation and Management. *2nd ed. New York: Oxford Press; 2000:128.)*

of the affected side is flat whereas the supraorbital rim is elevated and displaced posteriorly. The rim lies at or posterior to the plane of the cornea although it should normally be about 1 cm anterior to the cornea. The nasal root can be deviated to the side of the defect. The contralateral forehead is bossed, and the supraorbital rim can be pushed down. The ipsilateral auricle is anteriorly displaced but the occiput is minimally affected.

In unilateral lambdoid synostosis, there is an occipital flatness on the affected side. The ipsilateral auricle is posteriorly displaced, but the forehead is not typically affected. True lambdoid synostosis is a rare entity. Lambdoidal synostosis is frequently confused with posterior deformational plagiocephaly.

Deformational plagiocephaly is far more common and can be influenced by the previously noted intrauterine constraint factors, hypotonia, and prematurity. It is further compounded by sleeping in the supine positioning, with a predilection of the infant to sleep on one side owing to a prominent occiput and poor head control. This phenomenon has increased since the American Academy of Pediatrics, in an effort to reduce sudden infant death syndrome (SIDS), issued its recommendations to place sleeping infants in the supine position.[58,69] Additionally, persistent fetal lie, vertebral anomalies, muscular disorders, ocular abnormalities as well as assorted other conditions, can cause torticollis, further aggravating sleep position problems. The sutures in deformational plagiocephaly remain open so there is no ridging. The differences in head shape between synostotic and deformational plagiocephaly are illustrated in Figure 185-7.

Brachycephaly

Brachycephaly is the term used for bilateral coronal synostosis (Fig. 185-8). It is often accompanied by turricephaly (tall head) or acrocephaly (pointed head). As a result of this sutural synostosis, the skull is unable to expand in the AP dimension. In order to accommodate the expanding intracranial content, the skull grows in the lateral and superior dimensions. The neonate's cranium, therefore, has a smaller AP distance and greater lateral dimensions. The forehead comes right off the nose with a low hairline, and the glabellar depression is absent.

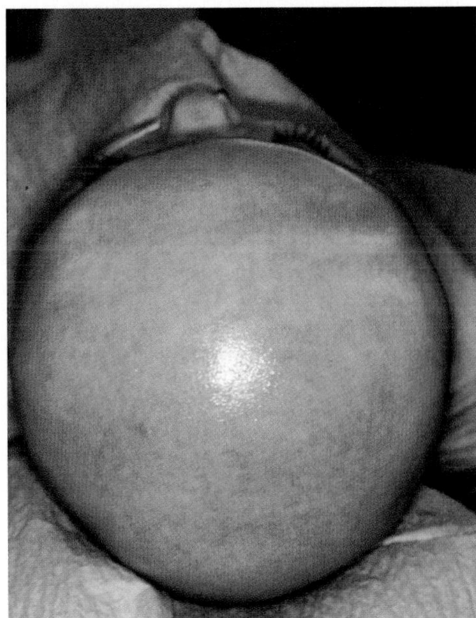

Figure 185-8. Bilateral coronal suture synostosis resulting in brachycephaly.

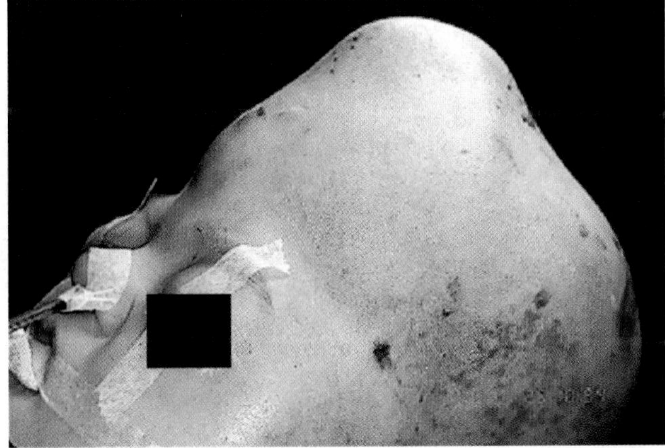

Figure 185-9. Coronal and sagittal suture synostosis in this child with Apert's syndrome resulted in acrocephaly.

Acrocephaly

Acrocephaly (also known as oxycephaly and turricephaly) consists of a skull that is high and conical (Fig. 185-9). This abnormality can develop as a result of progressive postnatal involvement of both the sagittal and coronal sutures. Compensatory growth occurs through the anterior fontanel.

Kleeblattschädel

Kleeblattschädel is also known as cloverleaf skull (Fig. 185-10). It results from synostosis of all the sutures previously discussed except for the metopic suture. The bone overlying the sutures is very thick but the intervening bone is thin. The expanding intracranial content tends to cause a ballooning of the thin bone between the sutures. This compensatory growth, in addition to expansion through the remaining open sutures, gives the characteristic lobular appearance of a cloverleaf. The skull growth falls drastically short of the needs of intracranial expansion, giving rise to neurologic impairment, increased intracranial pressure (ICP), and, often, secondary hydrocephalus. These patients exhibit exorbitism and therefore are at risk for globe exposure, and their optic nerves can also be at risk for damage. This anomaly requires prompt surgical attention to release the binding skull.

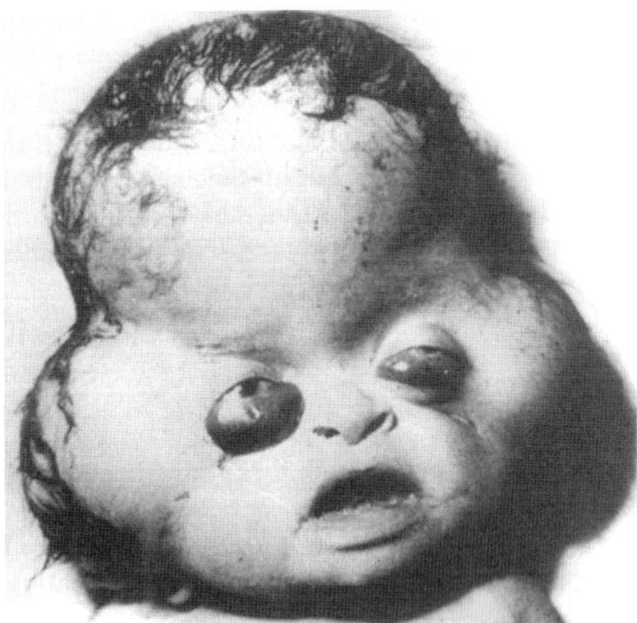

Figure 185-10. Premature fusion of all the cranial sutures except for the metopic and squamosal sutures results in kleeblattschädel or cloverleaf skull. (From Cohen MM Jr, Maclean RE. *Craniosynostosis: Diagnosis, Evaluation and Management.* 2nd ed. New York: Oxford Press; 2000.)

Facial Clefts

Facial clefts make up a large category of facial anomalies. A facial cleft is classified on the basis its position relative to the midsagittal plane. Although rare, facial clefts can present uniquely challenging problems to the surgeon. A further discussion of facial clefts is beyond the scope of this chapter.

Encephalocele

An *encephalocele* is a protrusion of intracranial content through a defect in the craniofacial skeleton (Fig. 185-11). It is classified according to its position in the skull. If the protruding content contains meninges, it is referred to as a *meningocele*. If it contains meninges and brain, it is called a *meningoencephalocele*, and if the protrusion additionally contains ventricle, it is known as a *meningoencephalocystocele*.[70]

Syndromes

The syndromes that cause craniofacial anomalies are quite varied in their clinical presentation. Because craniofacial anomalies frequently manifest as part of these syndromes, a familiarity with some of the well-described syndromes is important. This knowledge leads to more focused examination. Once a full survey is done, the proper consultations can be sought. Brief descriptions of several syndromes follow.

Crouzon's Syndrome

Crouzon's syndrome is an autosomal dominant condition that exhibits complete penetrance and variable expressivity. It often results in brachycephaly, but multiple sutures can also be affected. The calvarial suture defects can occur prenatally or throughout the first 5 years of life. There is associated midface (maxillary) hypoplasia, which leads to a class III malocclusion (the mandible is typically near normal). Exorbitism occurs as a result of decreased bony orbital volume (in contrast to exophthalmos, which results from greater intraorbital content). Intelligence is usually normal if patients are appropriately managed.

Apert's Syndrome

Apert's syndrome resembles Crouzon's syndrome in several ways. Most cases of Apert's syndrome arise sporadically through new mutations, although some familial cases with autosomal dominant transmission have been reported.[71] The disorder is characterized by brachycephaly

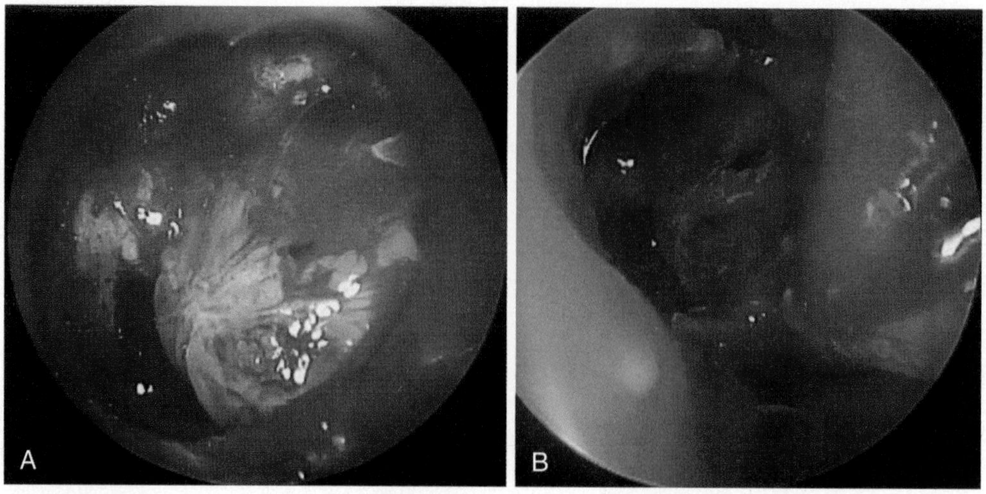

Figure 185-11. An endoscopic view of a meningoencephalocele protruding through the lateral wall of the sphenoid sinus. This was associated with a cerebrospinal fluid leak and a history of bacterial meningitis. **A,** An endoscopic view of the sphenoid ostium, which has been widened to allow sufficient access to the skull base defect. **B,** After mild (intrathecal) decompression but prior to endoscopic repair, the dural defect is clearly seen.

(with resultant turricephaly) and midfacial hypoplasia (with associated orbital and dental issues). Unlike patients affected with Crouzon's syndrome, patients with Apert's syndrome have symmetric syndactyly of the hands and feet as well as other axial skeletal abnormalities. The palate frequently has a high arch and may be cleft. The defects in Apert's syndrome are present at birth, and intelligence is often decreased.

Pfeiffer's Syndrome

Pfeiffer's syndrome is an autosomal dominant disorder that features craniosynostosis. The coronal sutures are frequently involved, giving rise to brachycephaly, but the sagittal and lambdoid sutures can also be involved. Affected patients can have midface hypoplasia (with associated orbital and dental issues) as well as enlarged thumbs and big toes.

Jackson-Weiss Syndrome

Jackson-Weiss syndrome is an autosomal dominant disorder with high penetrance and variable expressivity that resembles Pfeiffer's syndrome. Brachycephaly is common, the big toes are abnormally wide, but the thumbs are typically normal. Midfacial hypoplasia is more common than in Pfeiffer's syndrome. Jackson-Weiss syndrome was originally identified in an Amish population but can affect other individuals as well.

Saethre-Chotzen Syndrome

Saethre-Chotzen syndrome is an autosomal dominant disorder with full penetrance. Affected patients have craniosynostosis (often brachycephaly) with a low hairline, ptosis, brachydactyly, and a high arched palate with occasional palatal clefting. Midface hypoplasia is not common.

Carpenter's Syndrome

Carpenter's syndrome is a rare syndrome that is autosomal recessive. Patients affected by this syndrome usually suffer from craniosynostosis that can involve the sagittal, lambdoid, and coronal sutures. Midfacial hypoplasia can be a component but is usually mild. Other features are preaxial polysyndactyly of the feet and other syndactyly. Children with Carpenter's syndrome generally have developmental delays.

Stickler's Syndrome

Stickler's syndrome, also known as arthro-ophthalmopathy, is an autosomal dominant syndrome and is one of the more common syndromes, affecting about 1 in 10,000 people. It is caused by mutations in genes that encode type II collagen, type XI collagen, or both. This connective tissue disorder has ocular, orofacial, skeletal, cardiac, and auditory manifestations. The phenotypic orofacial expression is characterized by occasional midface underdevelopment, mandibular hypoplasia, and cleft palate. Stickler's syndrome is the most common syndrome to be associated with Pierre Robin sequence. It has been estimated that between 30% and 40% of patients diagnosed as having the Pierre Robin sequence (micrognathia, cleft palate, and glossoptosis) in fact have Stickler's syndrome. Given its variable expressivity, this syndrome, in its mild forms, often goes unrecognized.

Velocardiofacial Syndrome

Velocardiofacial syndrome is autosomal dominant with variable expressivity and penetrance and may be the most common syndrome after Down syndrome. There are numerous associated anomalies aside from the well-documented craniofacial, cardiac, and vascular malformations. The craniofacial anomaly broadly consists of a more open angle of flexion in the basicranium. This has an impact on the appearance of the midface and lower face (mandible). Clefting of the secondary palate can be overt or can take the form of an occult cleft that is apparent only on nasopharyngoscopy.[72] Velocardiofacial syndrome can easily be overlooked because affected patients are often not obviously abnormal in appearance.

Mandibulofacial Dysostosis

Mandibulofacial dysostosis, also known as Treacher Collins syndrome, is an autosomal dominant disorder with variable penetrance and expressivity. It involves numerous bilateral developmental abnormalities in structures that derive from the first and second branchial arches. Clinical features include zygomatic hypoplasia, micrognathia, dysplastic ears, antimongoloid slants to the eyes, colobomas of the lower eyelids, and deficient eyelashes in the medial two thirds of the lower eyelids. Mandibulofacial dysostosis is associated with Pierre Robin sequence and palatal clefting in 35% of cases. Severe obstructive apnea secondary to the micrognathia and glossoptosis often requires medical intervention.

Facio-Oculo-Auriculo-Vertebral Spectrum

Facio-oculo-auriculo-vertebral spectrum (FOAVS) refers to a group of anomalies that originate from unilateral defects in the first and second branchial arches. Most cases are sporadic, although familial cases have been reported. There is evidence that this syndrome results from a unilateral hemorrhagic event involving the stapedial artery during early craniofacial development.[73] FOAVS (also known as hemifacial microsomia), which includes Goldenhar's syndrome, can be quite diverse in terms of severity and scope. It is a rare disorder (1/5600 live births) that is present at birth. It involves the unilateral soft and skeletal tissues of the face and external and middle ear. It can manifest as temporal, zygomatic (malar), maxillary, and mandibular hypoplasia, hypoplastic facial musculature, and cleft lip and palate. It involves a wide variety of external and middle ear deformities related to structures that derive from the first and second branchial arch. Atresia of the external auditory canals and preauricular skin tags can all exist in FOAVS. The eye can be involved, with the occurrence of colobomas, epibulbar choristomas, blepharophimosis, and strabismus. Vertebral anomalies include fusion of vertebrae, spina bifida, and other more specific abnormalities. A variety of other, non-craniofacial abnormalities are associated with FOAVS.

Trauma

The basic concepts of craniomaxillofacial trauma and treatment are similar in the pediatric and adult populations. The differences mostly concern patterns of fracture in young children and how repair of fractures affect subsequent craniofacial growth. The pattern of facial fractures in children is influenced by several factors. The facial bones are not fully mineralized and are therefore more pliable and elastic, resulting in more "greenstick" fractures. Tooth buds replace much of the bone of the dental arches, creating a different stress-strain curve in the mandible and maxilla. Depending on the patient's age the sutures may not be fused, and there is a higher proportion of cancellous bone with thinner cortices. The face is also much smaller relative to the cranial cavity with minimal aeration of the sinuses, and the buttress system is not fully developed. In adolescence the face has matured sufficiently so that patterns of facial fractures more closely resemble those seen in the adult.

The incidence of facial fractures in the pediatric population has been estimated to range from 1% to 14.7%, and head injuries are frequently associated with them. The group least likely to suffer from facial trauma is children younger than 5 years. The preponderance of injuries in children has been reported to occur in boys, though some studies have found no gender predilection. According to some reports motor vehicle accidents are responsible for these injuries in up to 80% of cases. However, in the last 20 years, with the wider use of seatbelts and federally approved child-safe car seats, the incidence has significantly declined. Injuries that do result in pediatric maxillofacial trauma are usually quite severe and therefore are frequently accompanied by other systemic injuries.[74,75]

In general, fractures involving the forehead, frontal sinus, naso-orbital-ethmoid complex, and optic canals, as well as Le Fort fractures are managed through the craniofacial techniques similar to those developed for congenital anomalies. Facial trauma that is best managed via craniofacial techniques is usually severe but fortunately also rare. Complex midface fractures including Le Fort fractures are uncommon. (Although the Le Fort system is used to describe complex midface fractures in children, later classification systems tend to be functional and are based on the force of the impact and the resultant extent of bony disruption.) Fronto-orbital fractures and other fractures of the upper face occur with an even lower frequency.

Neoplasm

Craniofacial or skull base tumors are fortunately rare occurrences in the pediatric population. Head and neck tumors account for about 5% of all childhood cancers, and those involving the skull base are a small proportion of that figure. Of the solid nonhematologic lesions, brain tumors are the most common, followed by neuroblastoma and rhabdomyosarcoma, non-rhabdomyosarcoma sarcomas, salivary gland tumors, and teratomas. Benign tumors in the craniofacial region are also rare; they include fibrous dysplasia (Fig. 185-12), angiofibromas, granulomas, pituitary adenomas, and other unusual lesions.

Patient Evaluation

Craniofacial Team

Given the complexity of the problems found in the patient with a craniofacial disorder, the principle that care must be delivered by a clinically diverse and highly trained team has become the standard of care. Careful timing and coordination of procedures maximize benefits while minimizing trauma to the patient and family. In addition to the craniofacial surgeon, a typical team might consist of a pediatrician, neurosurgeon, ophthalmologist, dentist, orthodontist, oral surgeon, prosthodontist, geneticist, nurse, speech pathologist, audiologist, anthropologist, psychologist, and nutritionist. The emphasis is on taking a comprehensive approach to the health care of the individual. This approach is based on the recognition that these abnormalities, as well as their treatment, can affect many different functional systems. Open and unimpeded communication among the different members of the team is essential for full realization of the benefit of this approach.

History and Physical Examination

At the initial evaluation, a personal, family medical, and genetic history must be obtained. It is prudent to suspect that any defect of the craniofacial complex is part of a larger syndrome, so a full body survey is performed. All anomalies are noted, with an attempt to group them into a known syndrome. The head shape should be observed from front, rear, sides and vertex. The forms and positions of the eyes and ears are examined. The head is evaluated by palpation of the sutures and fontanelles to detect not only patency but also ICP. There should be no sutural ridging, and the fontanelles should not be bulging. The head circumference, the AP, bifrontal, bitemporal, and biparietal diameters, and the vertical height of the skull from the supraorbital border are all measured. In normal children the posterior and anterior fontanelles close at approximately 3 and 18 months, respectively, and the cephalic index (the ratio of the greatest width of the head to its greatest

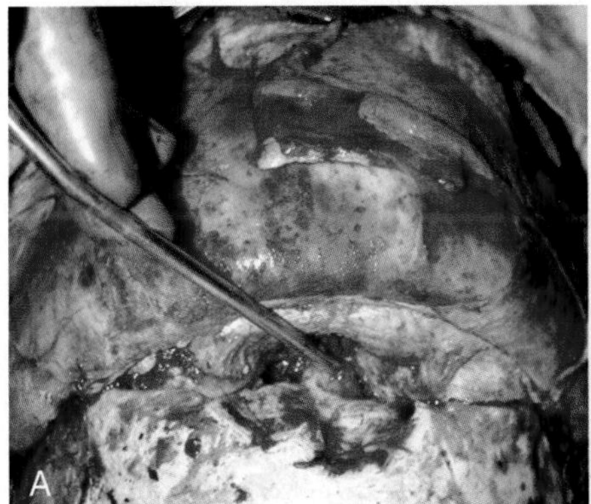

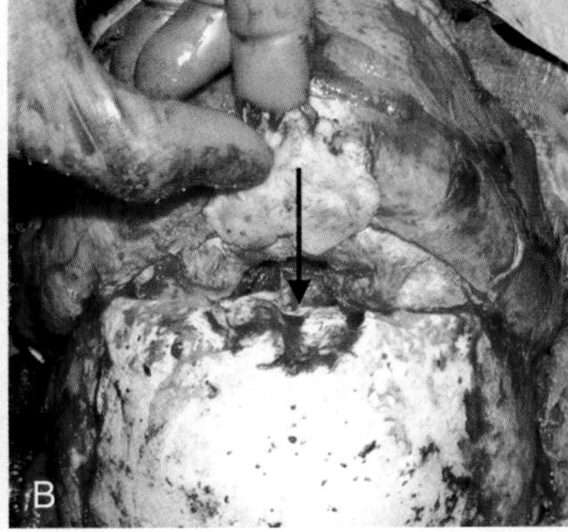

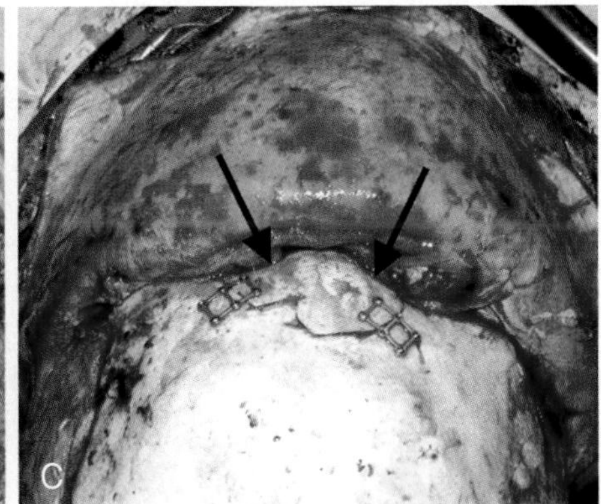

Figure 185-12. Operative images of a patient with fibrous dysplasia involving the anterior skull base who initially presented in her teenage years. Earlier endoscopic attempts at removal had failed and left the patient with strabismus, a mucocele of the frontal sinus, and exposed dura. **A,** A subcranial approach was utilized to remove the fibrous dysplasia. The suction tip is pointing to the lesion. **B,** The lesion has been removed, and the *arrow* is pointing to the area of dural exposure. The bone flap is shown. **C,** The bone flap has been replaced. *Arrows* are pointing to the pericranial flap that has been placed under the bone flap and used to seal the dural defect and obliterate the frontal sinus.

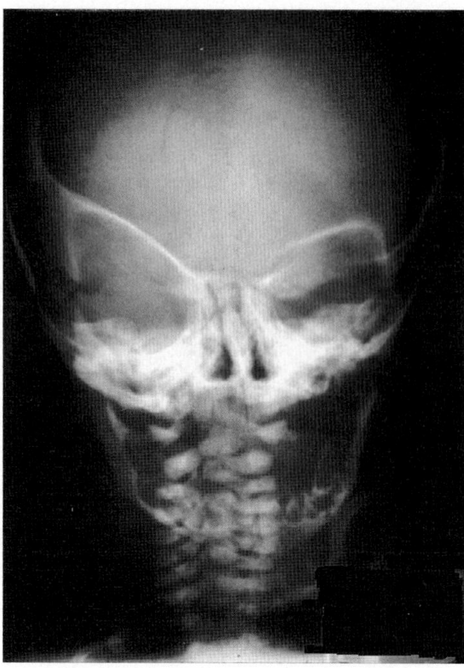

Figure 185-13. Skull film demonstrating the "harlequin mask" appearance seen in patients with unilateral coronal suture synostosis.

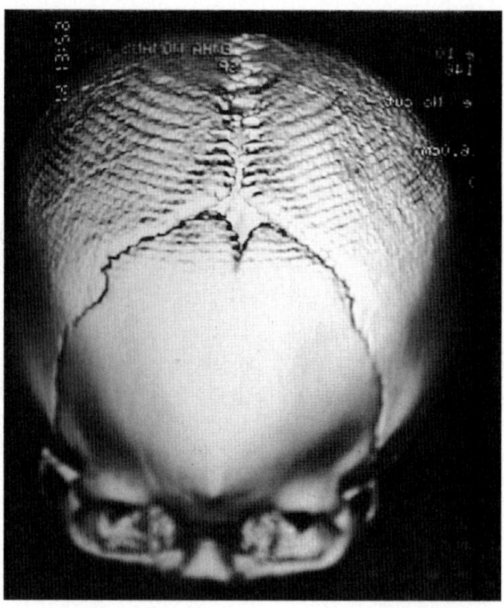

Figure 185-14. Three-dimensional computed tomography reconstruction demonstrating trigonocephaly.

length multiplied by 100) is 75 to 80. Although occlusion cannot be evaluated in the neonate, the relative dimensions of the mandible and midface are noted. The symmetry and range of motion of the neck must be examined as well.

Imaging

Plain radiographs can be useful in certain circumstances. The absence of normal sutural lucency may indicate synostosis. In plagiocephaly and brachycephaly, premature fusion of the frontoethmoid and frontosphenoid sutures causes elevation of the lesser wing of the sphenoid, producing the harlequin mask appearance (either unilateral or bilateral) on a plain AP film of the skull (Fig. 185-13). The hammered-copper or thumb-printing appearance of the inner table of the skull on cranial radiographs is associated with increased ICP and craniosynostosis; although its presence is easily detected, its clinical significance has been questioned.[76] Lateral and AP cephalometric radiographs continue to be useful, especially for evaluation of the progress of craniofacial growth.

However, for most defects computed tomography is the ideal modality for evaluation. Given its ubiquity and declining costs it has largely replaced plain radiography. Additionally, the software for three-dimensional reconstruction is widely accessible and provides detail of the bony anatomy that is unsurpassed (Fig. 185-14). Various cephalometric and volumetric analyses can be easily achieved. If necessary, a stereolithographic model based on three-dimensional studies can be built that provides an accurate template of the patient's craniofacial skeleton. Sophisticated software is also available to help in planning reconstruction (Fig. 185-15). Planning software is particularly helpful when one is preparing to reconstruct unilateral or some asymmetric defects. Although valuable information about the central nervous system can be obtained with computed tomography, magnetic resonance imaging is usually the modality of choice for evaluating the brain.

Indications for and Timing of Intervention

When one is considering treatment for craniofacial diseases and anomalies, it is helpful to stratify a patient into one of the following three categories based on the nature of the problem: life-threatening issues, functional impairments, and aesthetic issues. Issues classified as life-threatening include upper airway obstruction. An example is a neonate with severe Pierre Robin sequence. Another example is severe syndromic craniosynostosis affecting multiple sutures with dangerous ICP elevations. The second category, functional impairment, includes a broad spectrum of problems that range from visual impairment to neurocognitive problems as the child reaches school age. The third category is that of a mild deformity that results in what society might consider an abnormal aesthetic appearance.

The treatment algorithm for life-threatening problems is usually straightforward. The neonate with upper airway obstruction is treated either by distraction of the mandible (discussed in greater detail later) or a tracheotomy. The patient with kleeblattschädel requires urgent release of the binding skull by total cranial vault remodeling, and the child with dangerously high ICP is often treated with a ventriculoperitoneal shunt. The algorithm becomes more complex, however, for neonates with functional impairment.

The complexity arises because the consequences of not intervening or of the intervention itself are not always fully understood. Significant fronto-orbital retrusion is at the more severe end of the spectrum, as it may portend serious functional, neurologic, or ophthalmic problems. The presence of more than one synostosis is often associated with neurocognitive compromise. Anomalies of the maxilla and mandible not only affect appearance but also can impact the airway, dentition, and speech and therefore frequently require therapeutic intervention. Hypertelorism and other orbital dystopias can manifest as significant visual issues, in which case surgical reconstruction is necessary. Nonsyndromic single-suture craniosynostosis (SSC) is particularly difficult to classify because the association between the anomalies and functional sequelae is controversial. The incidence of increased ICP and neurocognitive deficiencies in nonsyndromic single-suture craniosynostosis is still debated, and further investigation of this issue is warranted.[77-79]

When the neonate has the mildest of craniosynostoses, such as some types of single-suture craniosynostosis or partial synostosis, positional plagiocephaly, mild FOAVS, and other mild craniofacial anomalies, the problem can be classified as aesthetic in nature. In such cases the craniofacial team and the involved family members must weigh the severity of aesthetic deformity against the risks of surgical intervention. The temptation to develop a strict algorithm based on the defect alone has to be resisted, as demonstrated by metopic suture synostosis. This deformity manifests with a wide range of severity in fronto-orbital malposition and hypotelorism, and the metopic suture closes earlier than previously thought.[80] The implication that prior standards used to guide the surgeon in deciding when to intervene surgically are not quite as relevant. In the case of positional plagiocephaly, the treatment does tend to be more clear-cut. Changing sleep position, treating causes

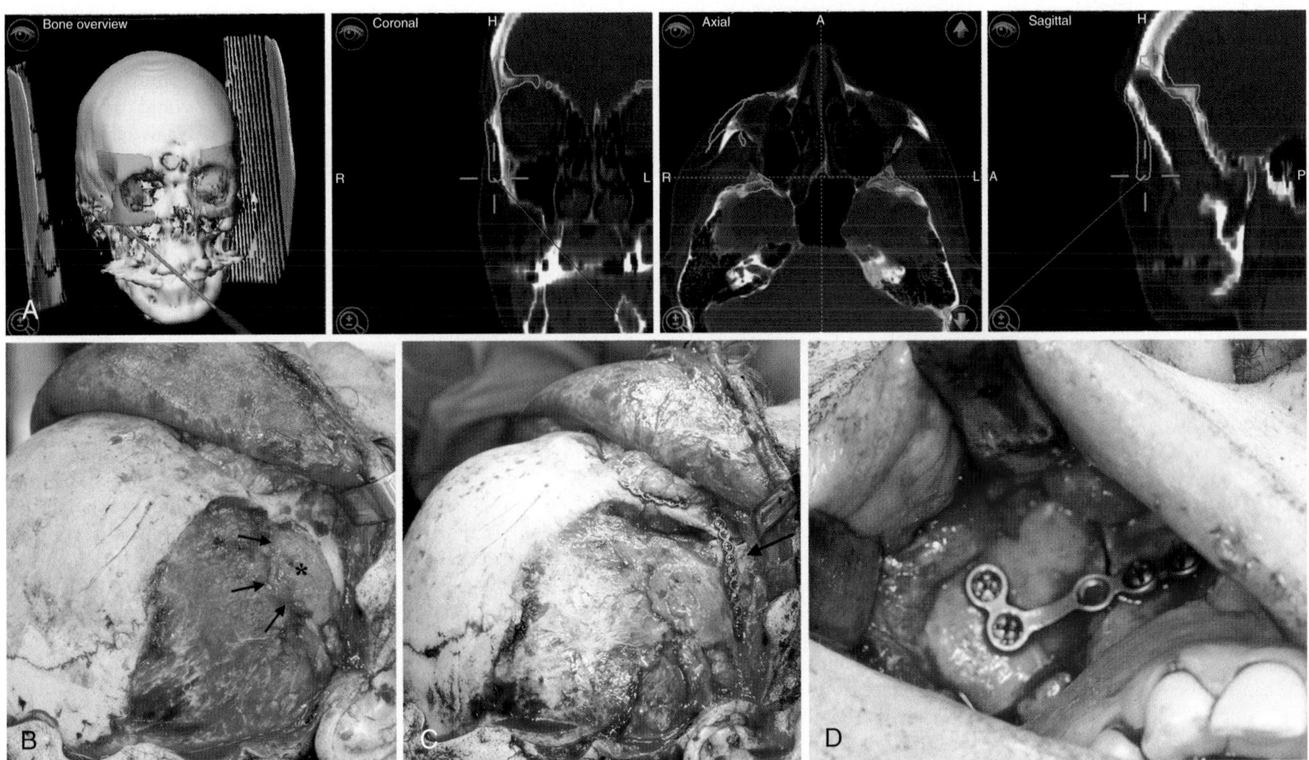

Figure 185-15. Images of a patient who had suffered from traumatically displaced fractures of the orbit and zygomatico-maxillary complex (ZMC) about a half year prior to presentation. Because of the delay in treatment, the skeletal segments healed in a malunion, resulting in a facial deformity as well as orbital dystopia. **A,** With the use of planning cranio-maxillo-facial software, the facial skeleton is displayed in the coronal, axial, and sagittal planes. The *green line* in the upper left image of the skull refers roughly to the planes in which the other three slides are shown. **B,** A bicoronal flap has been elevated to expose the orbit and ZMC. *Arrows* indicate where the superficial layer of the deep temporalis fascia has been incised at the temporal line of fusion and elevated to expose the temporal fat pad (indicated by *asterisk*). This is necessary to gain wide exposure to the zygomatic arch, which had been fractured in multiple places. **C,** Appropriate osteotomies have been made, and the displaced segment mobilized. Using the reconstructed image generated by the planning software the image guidance system helps in the proper placement of the osteotomized segment, which is fixed in place with titanium plates (this patient is old enough to allow for nonresorbable fixation). *Arrow* indicates calvarial bone grafting that was used to buttress the new construct (harvest not shown). **D,** A sublabial incision is necessary to make the inferior cut and apply the fixation.

of torticollis, and cranial molding orthotics can all be used quite effectively when appropriately applied.

The age at which surgical correction is appropriate depends on the particular anomaly, the extent of functional compromise, and the overall health of the patient. Pediatric anesthesia has greatly improved in the last several years, making surgery in infants significantly safer. This issue is particularly important in craniofacial surgery because many of the procedures are easier to conduct in young patients. Patients younger than 1 year have remarkable bony regenerative capacity. The bone is also thinner and more pliable, making it easier to cut and contour. Of course, with younger patients, there are risks that must be considered, such as intolerance to even mild blood loss.

Neonates suffering from airway obstruction are treated immediately if extubation fails. In the case of kleeblattschädel, multiple synostectomies must be performed within the first few weeks of life to prevent severe functional deficits and even death. Early intervention is also indicated for increased ICP and corneal exposure. Simple synostectomies (in treating scaphocephaly, for example) are often performed in patients 2 to 6 months old. The authors generally perform fronto-orbital advancement and cranial vault remodeling procedures in infants 6 to 9 months old. Monobloc surgery of the forehead, orbits, and midface is often done at 3 to 4 years, although with distraction osteogenesis, the tendency is toward earlier intervention. Whole orbit movements are typically done while patients are 2 to 4 years old. Surgery effecting change in the occlusal relationships is often delayed until the teenage years. Depending on the severity and scope of the deformities, multiple procedures may be required to maximize the correction.

Surgical Techniques

Congenital Craniofacial Abnormalities

Because much of the surgery for craniofacial anomalies is performed on very young patients, special attention needs to be given to tightly monitoring and regulating the patient's vital functions. Infants have such a small blood volume blood that transfusion is often required in lengthy craniofacial procedures. Young patients also have decreased thermoregulatory capacity, so the room temperature is kept relatively high, especially during induction of anesthesia. Venous and arterial lines are inserted, as is a bladder catheter, preferably with a core temperature sensor. In a combined extracranial-intracranial procedure, antibiotics and steroids are routinely given. Shaving of the scalp for the incision is optional and based on the surgeon's preference. The scalp is scrubbed with a soap solution and povidone-iodine solution, and the face is generally also prepared with antiseptic scrub. The oral and nasal cavities should be irrigated if there is a likelihood that they will be part of the surgical field.

The eyes are protected by gentle application of ophthalmic ointment followed by covering with a clear plastic dressing. If access to the eyes is necessary, no taping is applied. Corneal shields are avoided when a bicoronal flap is elevated because the flap, when turned on itself, can often exert a fair amount of pressure on the shields, which could lead to eye damage. If necessary, a tarsorrhaphy suture can be used to protect the eyes.

Given that the head position is frequently altered during these procedures, it is very important to properly secure the endotracheal tube to the patient and, if necessary, bring part of the tube into the field. If access to the maxilla is necessary, then the tube must be secured to the mandible. Although prone and sphinx positions are preferred by some surgeons, we prefer to perform most craniofacial procedures with the patient supine and the head flexed. In orthognathic procedures it is generally necessary to intubate the patient nasally. The tube must be draped in such a way so as to make it easily accessible to the anesthesia team if inspection of the ventilatory circuit is necessary. During draping of the patient, it is best to leave as much of the face (including the ears) in the field as possible. This exposure is helpful to maintain orientation. Prior to incision, a vasoconstricting agent can be injected into the skin, but doses must be carefully titrated in the young pediatric population. An epinephrine solution of 1 : 200,000 or 1 : 400,000 is recommended.

Although the coronal incision is the most widely used approach for gaining access to the craniofacial skeleton, other, smaller incisions are used for different applications. For cases of mild to moderate sagittal synostosis, an endoscopic approach can be used or a midsagittal (wavy) incision can be employed to gain access to the synostotic portion of the suture. However, whenever access to the supraorbital bar is necessary, the bicoronal incision is necessary.

Coronal Incision

The coronal incision can extend pre- or postauricularly. When extended into the postauricular area, the incision is hidden, and adequate exposure of the cranium and the upper and part of the middle thirds of the face can still be obtained. The incision is designed as a wavy line that extends across the vertex of the head (Fig. 185-16).[13,81] The overall incision can be rotated more anteriorly to allow more anterior/inferior retraction of the flap. Some surgeons sharply zigzag the incision so as to make multiple V-Y closures possible if the advancement is so significant as to preclude normal closure of the coronal flap. The flap can then be elevated in a subperiosteal or subgaleal plane over the calvarium. The dissection is continued to the deep temporalis fascia elevating the temporal-parietal fascia. Dissection in this plane enables the frontal branch of the facial nerve to be elevated in the flap. If access to the zygomatic arch is required, the superficial layer of the deep temporalis fascia is elevated starting at the temporal line of fusion (see Fig. 185-15). This maneuver has the added advantage of adding an extra layer of tissue in between the dissection and the facial nerve branch. In some types of cranial vault remodeling, it is necessary to elevate the temporalis muscle as well, but this step is performed independent of the scalp elevation.

Sagittal Synostosis

Sagittal synostosis requires that the skull be allowed to expand in the transverse dimension and reduced in the AP dimension. There is a spectrum of procedures for scaphocephalic correction. Mild cases treated before 3 months of age may be managed with strip craniectomy alone (Fig. 185-17). A strip craniectomy is performed by removing sagittal or parasagittal sections of bone. Severe cases and patients treated after 9 to 12 months may require total cranial vault remodeling. In these cases coronal and lambdoid osteotomies can be made, and the parietal bones out-fractured. In severe cases the frontal bone can be significantly bossed and often has to be reshaped or transposed to improve the contour of the forehead. This requires a coronal incision (Fig. 185-18).

Fronto-Orbital Advancement

Centrally, the dissection exposes the supraorbital bar in the subperiosteal plain (if the dissection was done in a subgaleal layer, the periosteum is incised 2 cm above the supraorbital rims). The supraorbital rims and frontonasal region are fully exposed, with preservation of the supraorbital neurovascular bundles, which can be quite small in the neonate. In the very young patient this structure rarely exits via a foramen; rather, it lies in a groove in the medial half of the supraorbital rim, generally over the pupil. If there is a foramen, the inferior rim must be osteotomized in order to dissect and mobilize the neurovascular bundle. Progressing medially, the lacrimal crests can be exposed, if necessary, after separation of the medial canthal ligaments from their bony attachments and elevation of the lacrimal sac. In the midline the

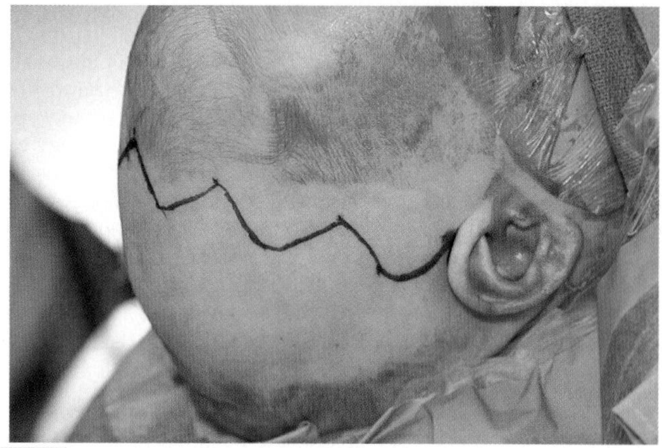

Figure 185-16. A wavy-line bicoronal incision that extends postauricularly is well concealed once the hair has grown in sufficiently.

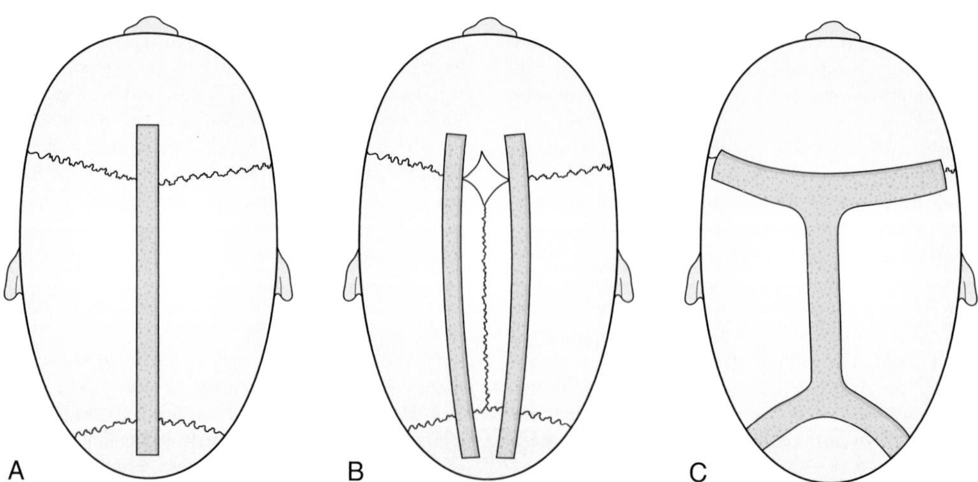

Figure 185-17. A range of surgical treatments can be employed for repair of scaphocephaly, depending on the severity. **A,** Removal of the suture. **B,** Strip craniectomies. **C,** Removal of the suture as well as coronal and lambdoid cuts. The latter is frequently combined with out-fracture of the parietal bones.

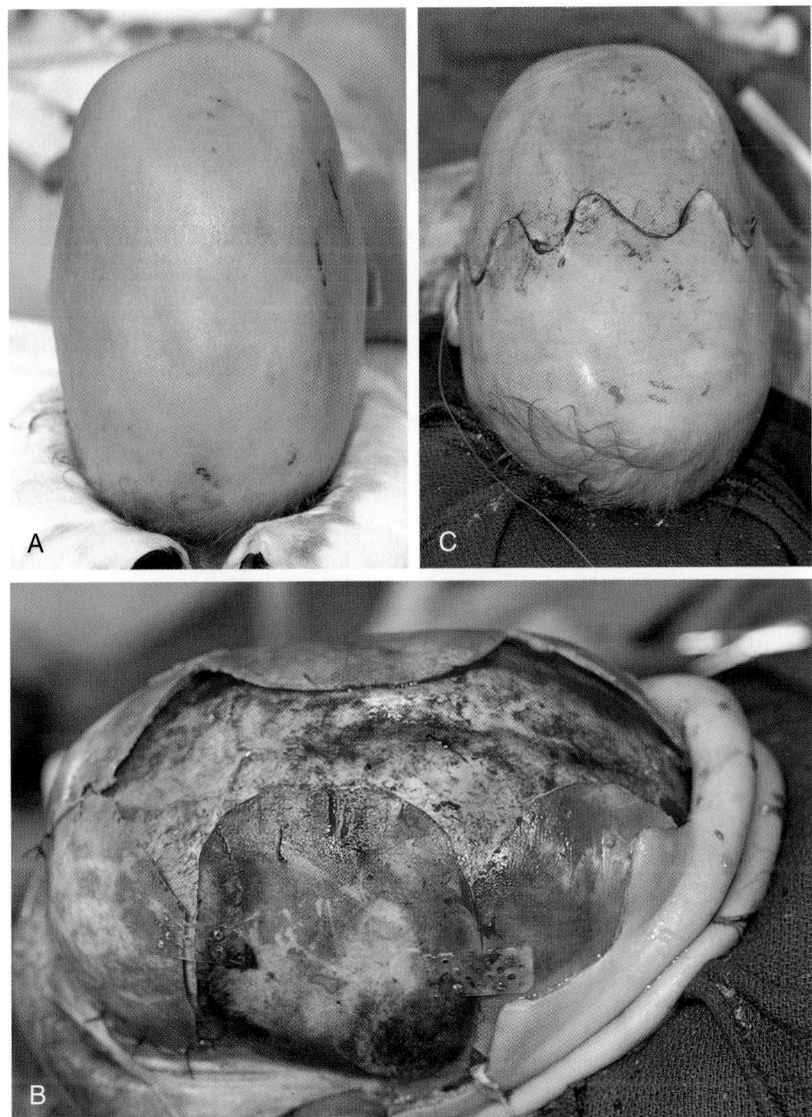

Figure 185-18. Scaphocephalic repair. **A,** Preoperative view of severe scaphocephaly. **B,** Repair required total cranial vault remodeling—the temporal-parietal complex was out-fractured on each side. Note the combined use of resorbable sutures and plates to achieve a stable construct. **C,** Postoperative view.

dissection is carried just past the nasofrontal suture. Laterally, exposure is extended from the zygomatic arch medially to the body of the zygoma. Fronto-orbital procedures generally require inferior exposure only to the level of the frontozygomatic suture. The lateral orbital rim is then exposed, and this dissection is connected to that of the supraorbital bar. The orbital roof is carefully dissected in the subperiosteal layer. The lateral orbital walls are exposed by elevation of the anterior aspect of the temporalis muscle from the temporal fossa.

Once the dissection is complete, intended osteotomy sites for both the supraorbital bar and the bifrontal craniotomy are marked. A side-cutting power craniotome is typically used once strategic bur holes have been drilled. The bifrontal craniotomy (Fig. 185-19) is done initially, with care taken to leave a transverse bar of bone above the supraorbital rims that is between 10 and 15 mm in width. The dura is freed from the anterior aspect of the anterior cranial fossa but left adherent over the cribriform plate. The supraorbital bar or bandeau is then marked for osteotomy. The superior osteotomy for the supraorbital bar was created by the bifrontal craniotomy. If a strip of bone was left over, the sagittal sinus it is cut from the bandeau. Laterally, the superior bandeau osteotomy is extended into the squamous portion of the temporal bone. Inferiorly, the central transverse osteotomy is made at or just above the

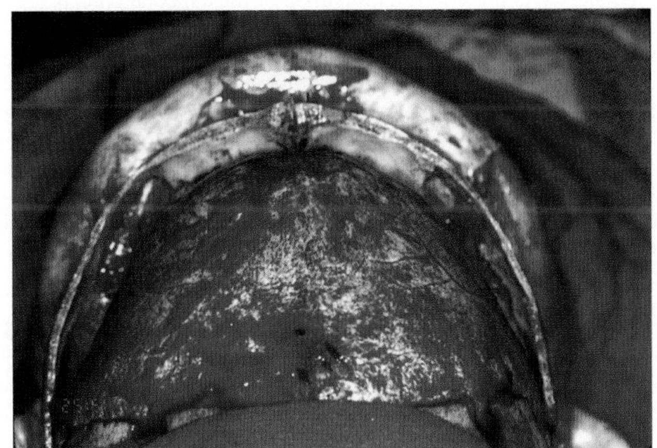

Figure 185-19. A bifrontal craniotomy has been performed. Note the elevation of the dura from the anterior cranial fossa in preparation for removal of the bandeau.

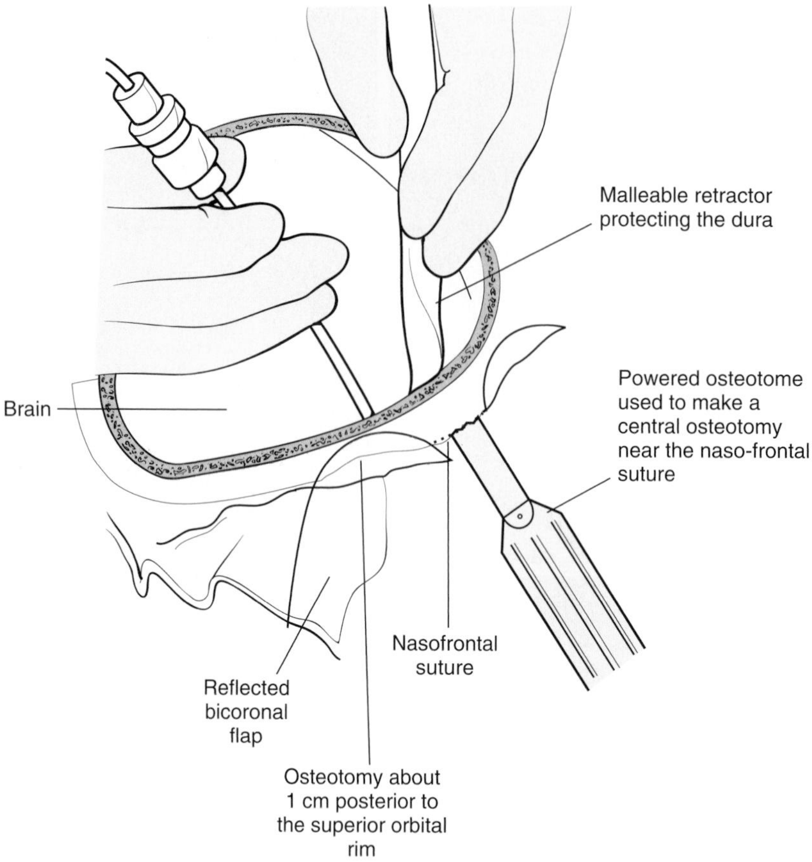

Figure 185-20. The central cut of the bandeau is illustrated. This cut is made above the nasofrontal suture. It is extended into the anterior cranial fossa anterior to the crista galli while protecting the brain with a malleable retractor. This way olfaction is preserved, and the barrier between the intracranial and nasal cavities is left intact. *(Adapted from Salyer K.* Techniques in Aesthetic Craniofacial Surgery. *New York; Gower Medical; 1989:35.)*

frontonasal suture (Fig. 185-20). This cut extends directly to the anterior cranial fossa at a point anterior to the crista galli. This location preserves olfaction as well as the barrier between the brain and the nasal cavity. The osteotomy is then carried into the medial orbit just above the lacrimal fossa. The osteotomy turns superiorly 5 to 10 mm inside the orbital rim, traverses the orbital roof around 10 mm posterior to the superior orbital rim, and extends down the lateral orbital wall to the level of the zygomaticofrontal suture. The lateral orbital rim is cut at the suture, and that cut extends posteriorly into the greater wing of the sphenoid and the squamous portion of the temporal bone parallel to and 10 to 15 mm inferior to the previous cut into this region. This site corresponds intracranially with the junction of the anterior and middle cranial fossae near the pterion. Enough length of the temporal portion of the bandeau will allow a tongue-and-groove action at this lateral point in order to increase the bony contact once the advancement has been completed. This maneuver facilitates bony stability. Removal of the bandeau is frequently hindered by incomplete osteotomy at the trifurcation (of the anterior extent) of the middle cranial fossa, the lateral orbital wall, and the greater wing of the sphenoid. The anterior tip of the temporal lobe must be protected while this cut is completed.

Once the bony segments are removed, they are reshaped on a separate table. The supraorbital bar can be reshaped to the extent required by the deformity (Fig. 185-21). Bone is removed as needed in thickened areas to facilitate bone bending. In unilateral synostosis (plagiocephaly) the central angle of the forehead is mildly affected, and only small alterations are necessary to increase the central angle to 150 to 170 degrees. Although only one side is affected in plagiocephaly, minor changes are required on the unaffected side because of compensatory frontal bossing. More drastic measures might be required for trigonocephaly, in which the central angle of the forehead can be as acute as 90 degrees. It is sometimes necessary to split the bandeau in the midline and add a bone graft in order to widen the central angle (Fig. 185-22). The components are then fixed to one another with absorbable plates, sutures, or both. Just above the lateral orbital rims, the angle between the supraorbital rim and the temporal fossa is adjusted to between 100 and 110 degrees. The orbital bar is then replaced in an advanced position.

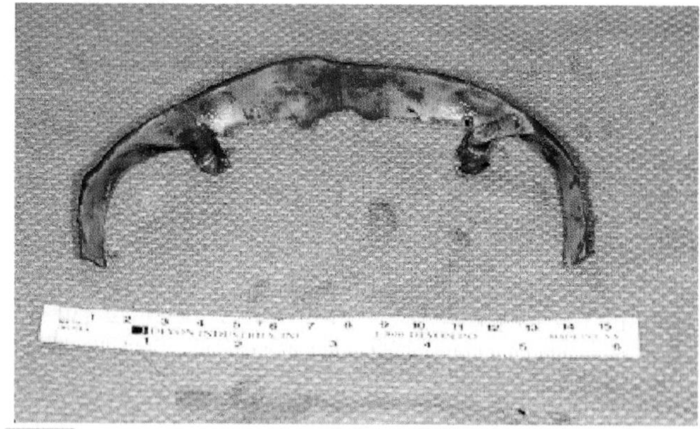

Figure 185-21. The bandeau following removal.

The extent of advancement obviously depends on the nature of the anomaly. In trigonocephaly and plagiocephaly, the orbital advancement is predominantly lateral, with the medial portion advancing little if any. In brachycephaly the entire bandeau is usually advanced, but the movement is still greater laterally than medially (Fig. 185-23). Maintaining contact between the supraorbital bar and the root of the

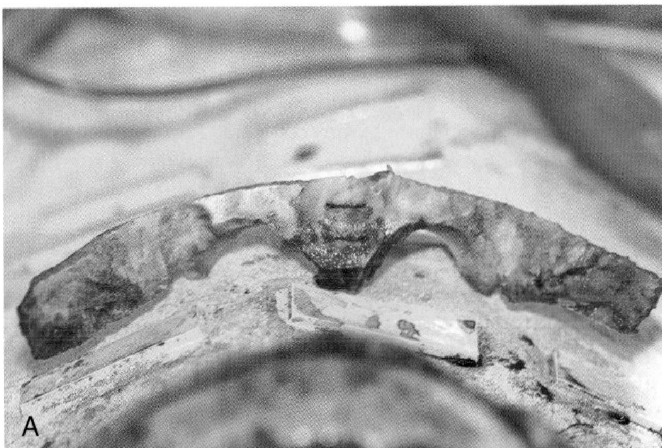

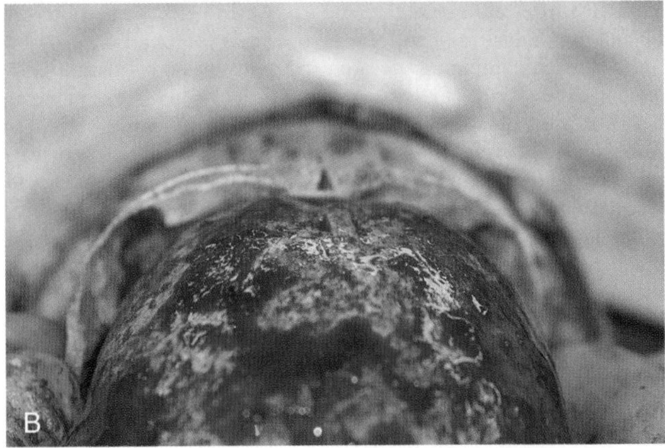

Figure 185-22. **A,** The bandeau can be split and a graft used to stabilize the new supraorbital construct. **B,** The bandeau is in place.

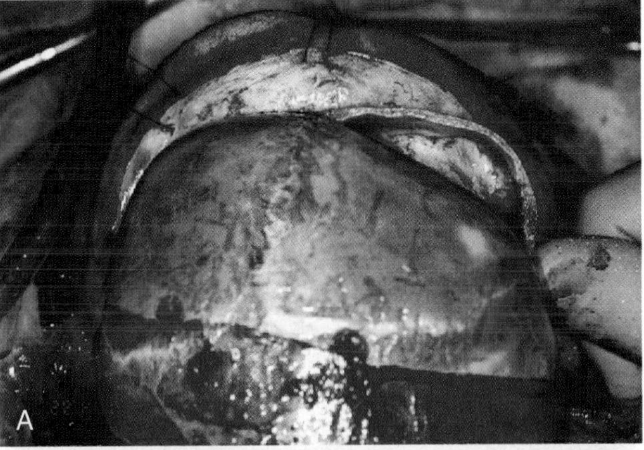

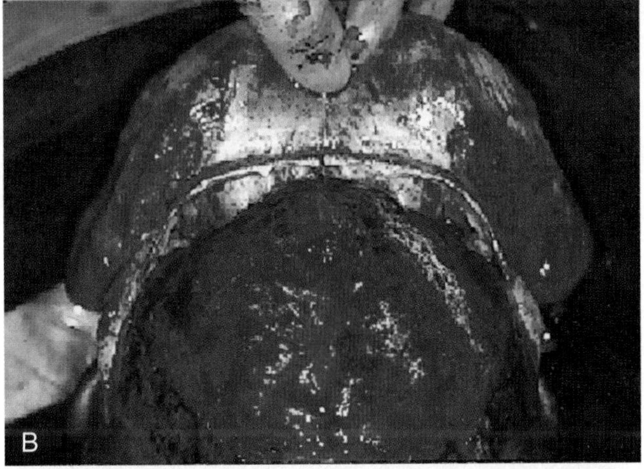

Figure 185-23. **A,** In this plagiocephalic repair, the lateral advancement of the bandeau is dramatic, whereas centrally little advancement was necessary. **B,** In this brachycephalic repair, there is more central advancement relative to the plagiocephaly repair but still far less than the lateral advancements.

nose is also important from the perspective of frontal sinus development, which later enhances central forehead projection.[82] It is important to establish symmetry with the advancement. Both rims should be about 1 cm anterior to the cornea. In severe cases the bandeau can be advanced as much as 2 cm, but bone grafting may be necessary. The supraorbital bar is fixed to the skull with absorbable plates, sutures, or both at the nasion and laterally (Fig. 185-24).

Lambdoid synostosis is repaired in much the same way as coronal synostosis. However, instead of removing and reshaping a supraorbital bar, the surgeon removes an occipital bar and advances it posteriorly and the occipitoparietal complex is reshaped to create posterior symmetry. Other types of cranial vault remodeling, including severe scaphocephaly, are also done via the coronal incision.

Resorbable plate technology represents a breakthrough in this treatment.[83] It offers dependable rigid fixation without the use of metallic plates.[84] Resorbable plates are less likely to interfere with craniofacial growth and development the way that titanium plates can, and they also rarely require removal.[85] The problem of intracranial plate migration with growth is avoided as well—typically the plates lose a large proportion of their strength within the first 6 months and are resorbed in less than 18 months. The calvarial bone flaps are then reshaped to provide normal contour to the head. Sometimes it is necessary to further osteotomize the flaps. The various components can be replaced in different positions to give the best contour. The bones are then fixed to the surrounding skull with absorbable plates or sutures. Maintaining large pieces of bone that are bent to the desired conformation, rather than creating small segments of bone with many osteotomies, provides for a more stable construct with less fixation than would be required if the bones were cut into smaller pieces.

Because of the advancement, there will be defects in the bone at various places. In patients younger than 1 year, bony defects are generally not of major concern because of bone regeneration. However, in older children and adults, large defects must be addressed. The orbital roofs represent a clear example. If there is a persistent communication between the orbit and the brain, pulsatile ophthalmopathy can develop. Therefore, these defects must be repaired with bone grafts (Fig. 185-25). Calvarial defects in the child or adult can be repaired with bone grafts or other bone replacement materials.

When the skeletal reconstruction is complete, attention is directed to a multilayer and precise closure. If the temporalis muscle has been elevated, it must be advanced to the lateral orbital rim and sutured. If this step is not performed, temporal hollowing occurs, creating an unaesthetic appearance. The muscle can be sutured to holes drilled in the lateral orbital rim or to one of the fixation plates. The galea aponeurosis is reapproximated with absorbable suture. The skin can then be closed with permanent or absorbable suture. We prefer to avoid suture removal in young children, so we perform a subcuticular closure with absorbable suture. In older children, skin staples can be used. If a sharp zigzag incision was used and the skin cannot be easily approximated (particularly in repair of severe brachycephaly), cutaneous closure can be performed, with use of the V-Y technique at each peak of the zigzag. We avoid using drains, especially in young patients. A gentle pressure and occlusive dressing is placed over the head.

Monobloc Advancement

Older children (>2-4 years) who present with fronto-orbital retrusion in conjunction with midface retrusion are potential candidates for a one-stage procedure. The (frontofacial) monobloc advancement originally described by Ortiz-Monasterio and colleagues[86] combines a fronto-orbital advancement with a Le Fort III level facial advancement (Fig. 185-26). The procedure is performed through the coronal inci-

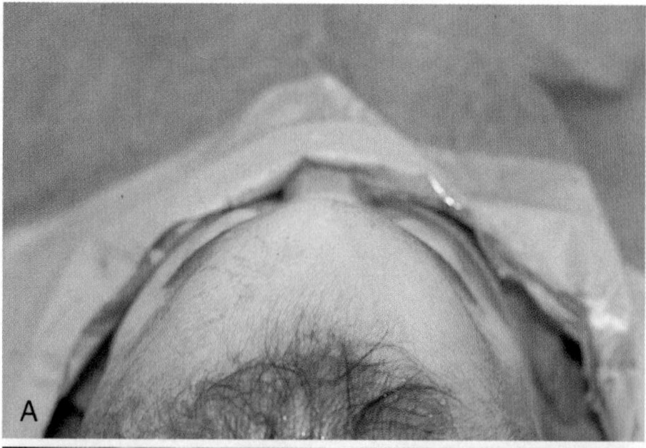

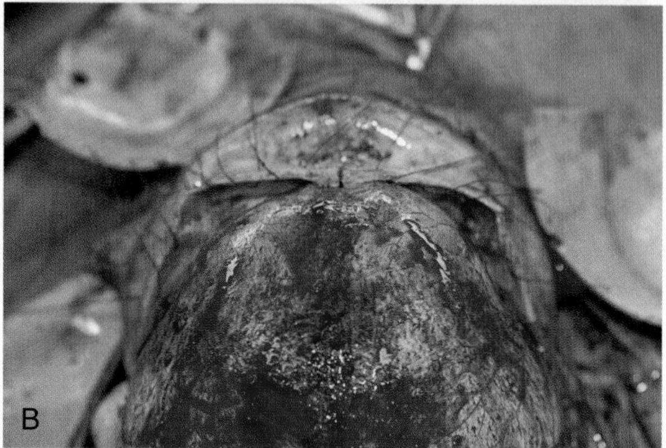

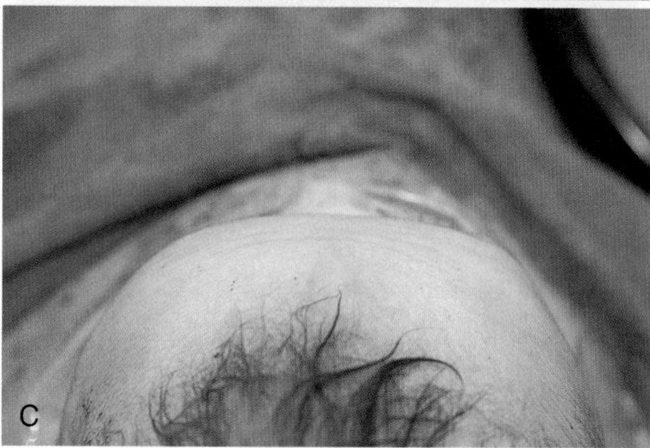

Figure 185-24. Trigonocephalic repair. **A,** Preoperative view. **B.** Intraoperative view. **C,** Postoperative view.

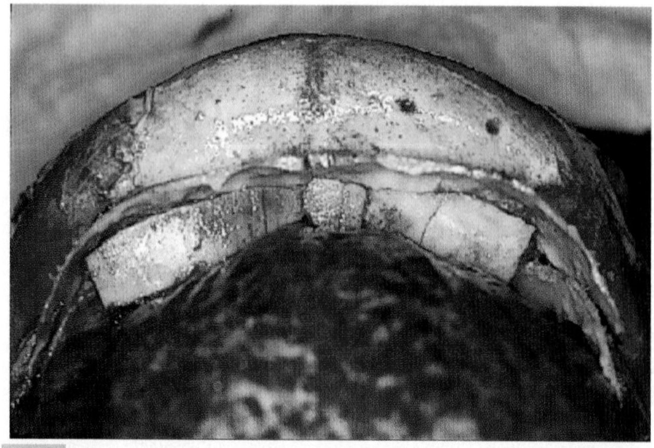

Figure 185-25. Bone grafts are placed between the orbit and the anterior cranial fossa in an effort to reconstitute the orbital roof.

sion. The craniotomy is similar to the one performed in a fronto-orbital advancement. The zygomatic arches are cut. The frontal bar is included with the Le Fort III segment. Circumferential orbital bony cuts are made with use of both extracranial and intracranial approaches. The lateral and inferior orbital walls are osteotomized starting in the inferior orbital fissure. The medial wall is cut just posterior to the posterior lacrimal crest. The orbital roof osteotomy is made intracranially. The nasal septum is cut via the frontoethmoid osteotomy. Finally, through the infratemporal fossa or the mouth, the maxilla is separated from the pterygomaxillary junction. The monobloc segment is then advanced and rigidly fixed with use of absorbable or titanium plates.

In some craniofacial deformities, such as those commonly seen in patients with Apert's syndrome, hypertelorism is present in association with maxillary deformities. Facial bipartition is a technique used to simultaneously correct hypertelorism and maxillary arch abnormalities (Fig. 185-27). Bone grafts are used to help maintain the advancement. Pericranial flaps and tissue glues are also used to create a seal between the anterior cranial fossa and the nasal cavities.

Although combining the two corrections into one procedure, has an obvious advantage, it is also associated with a higher rate of infection, presumably because of an incomplete seal of the central nervous system from the nasal cavities. It is for this reason that patients must be carefully selected for such a procedure. In situations in which the monobloc advancement is clearly the procedure of choice, distraction (in place of craniofacial advancement during the operation) may offer a safer way to achieve the desired results (see Fig. 185-26). The approach and the osteotomies are no different from the en bloc advancement just described.

Orbital Hypertelorism and Dystopia

In the correction of orbital hypertelorism, the approach is similar to that used in a fronto-orbital advancement, except that circumferential periorbital elevation is required. A bifrontal craniotomy is performed; however, a 1- to 1.5-cm strip of bone is left intact just above the orbital rims and below the bifrontal craniotomy. The anterior cranial fossa is exposed but the cribriform plate and crista galli are left intact to preserve olfaction. The periorbita is freed up to the infraorbital fissure. Four (box) osteotomies are made to encircle the entire bony orbit. The cuts outside the supraorbital, lateral, and medial rims can be made via the bicoronal exposure; however, the inferior cuts are facilitated by either a transconjunctival or subciliary incision. The bony orbits are mobilized by making a second set of circumferential osteotomies inside the orbit (using the inferior orbital fissure as a landmark) to separate the anterior part of the orbit from the posterior part. Upon mobilization of the orbits, a central bony block is osteotomized from the nasoethmoid complex. The anterior ethmoid fovea and air cells are often removed in this maneuver. The cribriform plate, along with the olfactory fibers and mucosa, are left intact. The bony orbits are then translocated to more medial positions. Vertical or rotational dystopia can be addressed at this point by addition or removal of bone in the appropriate areas to achieve proper orbital position. The bony segments are then fixed in their new positions with either resorbable or metallic plates. Closure proceeds as previously discussed. Because of instability of the mobilized orbit in the very young child, this type of correction is typically deferred until after age 2 years.

Distraction Osteogenesis

Distraction osteogenesis has been employed in the long bones for just under a century now. It was first applied to the craniofacial skeleton more than 80 years ago[87] but has come into widespread clinical use only in the last 25 years.[88] *Distraction osteogenesis* refers to creation of a controlled fracture in a bony structure followed by separation of the bony segments in a controlled and gradual manner. This process induces the formation of new bone in between the distracted segments. The advantages of using distraction osteogenesis in the craniofacial skeleton are numerous. It allows for skeletal lengthening and advancement in three dimensions. The process is a gradual one that allows the skin–soft tissue envelope to adapt to and accommodate skeletal movement.[89] It is also safer than many of the traditional skeletal techniques. Distraction osteogenesis is less involved and requires less operative time

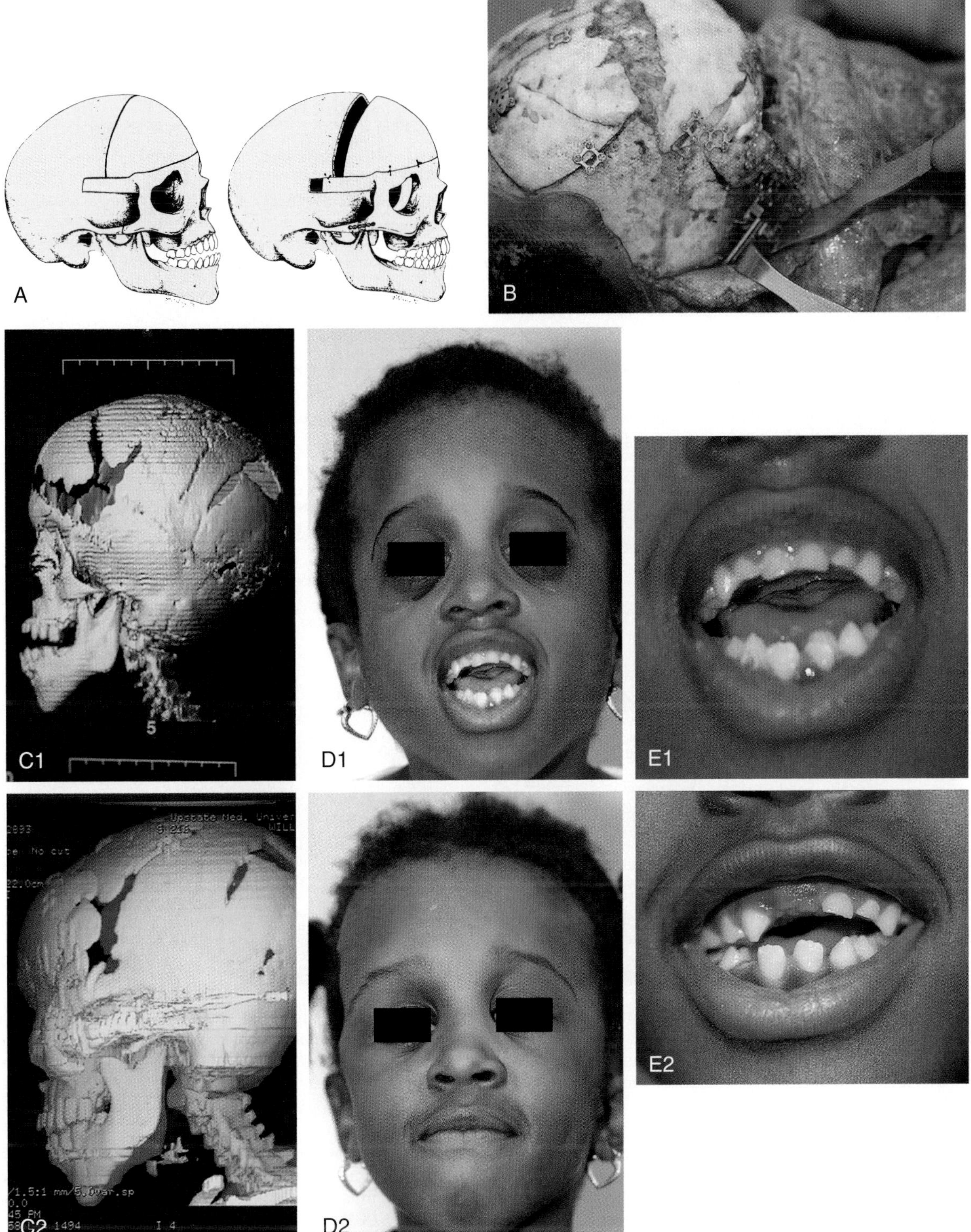

Figure 185-26. **A,** The monobloc advancement: Le Fort III osteotomies are performed in concert with a bifrontal craniotomy and mobilization of the bandeau. Fronto-orbital as well as midfacial advancements are then performed. **B,** Monobloc advancement with an internal distractor used to gradually advance the facial segment. (Note the right internal distractor device at the end of the retractors.) **C,** Preoperative (C1) and postoperative/postdistraction (C2) three-dimensional computed tomography scans. **D,** Preoperative (D1) and postoperative/post-distraction (D2) frontal photographs. **E,** Preoperative (E1) and postoperative/post-distraction (E2) dental/occlusal photographs.

(generating less blood loss) than the techniques it has replaced. As a result it is an attractive treatment alternative for children and infants with some craniofacial anomalies.

Distraction osteogenesis can be carried out with internal or external devices (Fig. 185-28). Internal devices have the advantage of not requiring big and bulky hardware protruding from the face and can, at times, be applied intraorally. The extent of control over the vectors of distraction is limited with internal devices. The external devices allow for three-dimensional distraction and better control of the vectors of distraction (see Fig. 185-28). The disadvantage lies in their bulkiness.

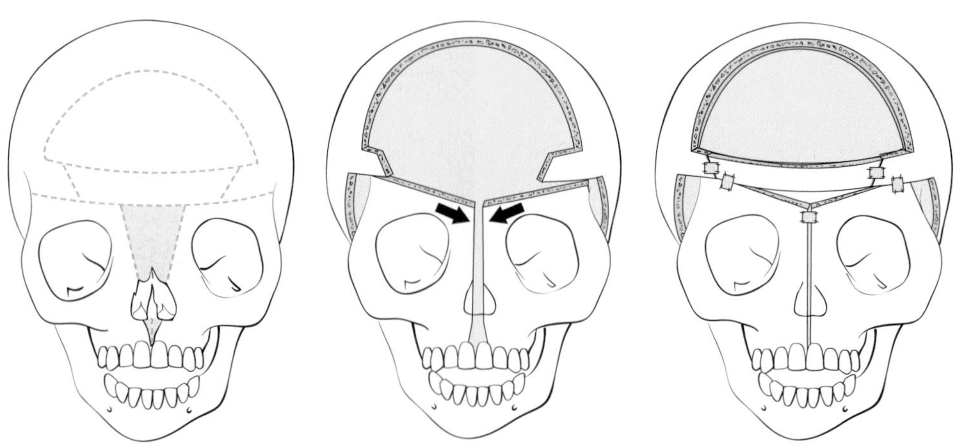

Figure 185-27. Facial bipartition can be used to move the orbits into more medial positions and narrow maxillary width as well. An inverted triangular wedge of bone is removed from the midline extending from the supraorbital ridge to the maxillary arch. The skeletal segments are then rotated, bringing the orbits into closer alignment and also reducing an open bite deformity. This procedure is also employed in the repair of some midfacial clefts. *(From Salyer K.* Aesthetic Craniofacial Surgery. *Philadelphia; Lippincott; 1989:67.)*

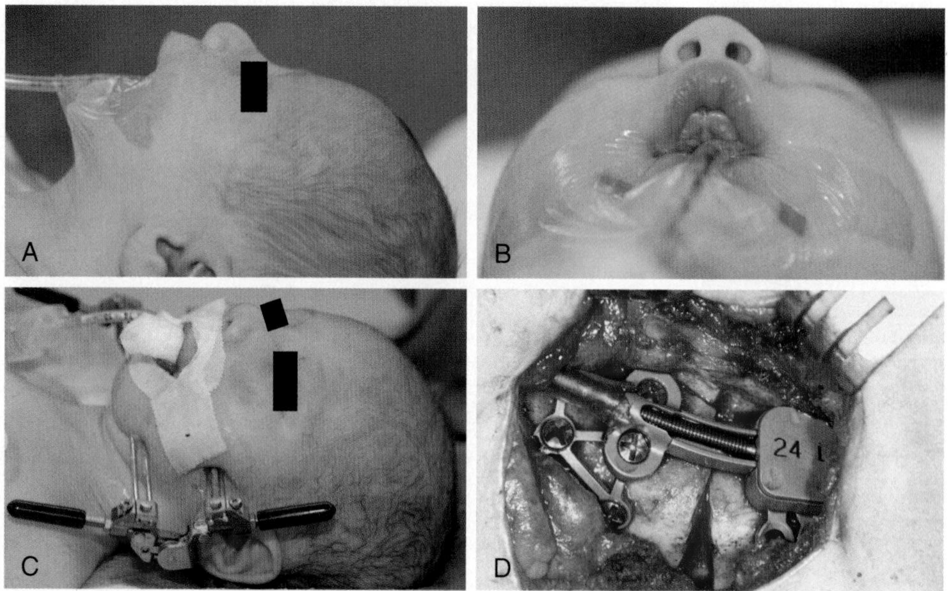

Figure 185-28. Distraction osteogenesis of the mandible. Profile view **(A)** and base view **(B)** of a neonate with Pierre Robin sequence. This patient could not achieve adequate ventilation without mechanical respiratory support. **C,** External distractors were placed after bilateral intra-oral osteotomies were created. The patient's mandible was ultimately distracted more than 1 cm, eliminating the need for any respiratory assistance. **D,** Internal distraction in a different patient. The distractors were applied after osteotomies were created through extra-oral incisions.

Pin migration scars can be significant as well. However, this is a rapidly evolving technique, and new devices are constantly being introduced. As the internal devices become more sophisticated, their roles will continue to expand.

The most common application of distraction osteogenesis in the craniofacial skeleton is the mandible. It is used for maxillary advancement and in the upper face and cranial vault as well. The process consists of several phases. At the time of surgery, the skin or mucosa and soft tissue are incised to expose the part of the facial skeleton that is to be distracted. The periosteum is incised directly over the intended site of osteotomy, which is marked out. The appropriate holes are drilled for fixation of the distraction device before the controlled osteotomy is made. In the mandible, the cortical cuts are made carefully to protect dental and neurovascular structures. Full mobility about the osteotomy sites must be confirmed to ensure total disunion of the bony segments; any bony continuity would hinder or prevent distraction. The distraction hardware is then put into place. Placement involves anchoring the device on both sides of the osteotomy with screws for an internal device or percutaneous pins for an external device. Some devices are borne by teeth or a dental implant. Distraction osteogenesis has a place in alveolar bone reconstruction and dental restoration as well.

A latency period is observed following osteotomy and placement of the device before actual distraction is begun. During this time the healing process commences with callus formation. The duration of the latency period depends on the age of the patient. In very young patients it can be as short as 24 hours, and in adults it can be as long as 1 week. It is more detrimental to wait too long than to begin too early, for premature fusion would render the distraction difficult or impossible. The beginning of distraction initiates what is termed the *distraction phase*. During this period, new immature bone is laid down between the osteotomized bony edges. The rate of distraction and the frequency with which it is done depend on the nature of the defect and the age of the patient. These variables are the subject of some debate, although the rate of distraction typically varies between 1 and 3 mm/day in one to three installments.

In the period subsequent to the distraction phase, the bone remodels and matures in what is known as the *consolidation phase*. The distraction hardware is left in place for a variable time. The rule of thumb we use is to allow consolidation to occur for a period that is at least twice the duration of distraction period. During the consolidation phase, the regenerate mineralizes and the soft tissue continues to change its shape and orientation so as to achieve balance with the new position of the bone. After several months the new bone is similar in volume to the native bone but with somewhat reduced mineral content and strength.

Trauma

The goal of treatment is the restoration of function and three-dimensional architecture. For severe and displaced fractures, internal fixation is often necessary.[90] The window of time in which fractures can be repaired is shorter in children as a result of the rapidity of their healing time. Many surgeons advocate using resorbable plates and screws for internal bony fixation, although others prefer using small titanium plates, arguing that complications from permanent (mini)plates are minimal.[75,85,91-93]

Neoplasm

Approaches to the skull base for tumor extirpation also require an intimate understanding of craniofacial anatomy because normal anatomy is often effaced. Several craniofacial approaches have been described in the pediatric population that can be used to gain access to tumors of the anterior and middle cranial fossae.[94] Historically, tumors of the anterior skull base were approached with a frontal craniotomy combined with a facial incision such as a lateral rhinotomy with or without a Weber-Ferguson facial incision. However, tumors of the anterior cranial fossa can be adequately exposed with a subcranial (subfrontal) approach without facial incisions (see Fig. 185-12). As previously mentioned, this latter exposure involves removal of the frontonasal complex. The extent of frontal and orbital rim bone removal is determined by the size, location, and nature of the lesion. In an extended subcranial approach, large sections of the bony orbit can be removed.[95]

The middle cranial fossa can be approached through a variety of techniques. The endoscopic transnasal-transsphenoidal approach can be effective in resection of midline tumors associated with the sella turcica, sphenoid cavity, and posterior nasal cavity. Figure 185-11 demonstrates repair of a sphenoid sinus encephalocele via this endoscopic approach. Even malignant or locally destructive lesions are occasionally accessible via this approach. Le Fort I, transpalatal, and midfacial degloving techniques can be used to gain limited access to lesions of the skull base.[96] More aggressive lesions that are off the midline (such as petroclival lesions) can be approached via the infratemporal fossa (or a modified version) or other transbasal approaches.[97] The cranio-orbito-zygomatic and transcondylar approaches provide excellent exposure of the infratemporal fossa. A frontotemporal craniotomy extends the exposure to the middle cranial fossa and the petrous internal carotid artery as well as other petroclival structures. When a lesion involves the middle cranial fossa, the infratemporal fossa, and the nasopharynx, a wider exposure is frequently necessary. The facial translocation procedure provides very wide exposure to lesions in this area and is well suited for malignancies, for which a margin of healthy tissue must be removed as well. It involves extended facial incisions as well as transection of facial nerve branches that are later reanastomosed. A maxillary-zygomatic bony segment is removed in order to gain access to the necessary extracranial lesion. A subtemporal craniotomy then provides intracranial exposure. In reconstruction of the bony framework, the same principles must be followed as for any other craniofacial procedure.

Biomaterials in Skeletal or Cartilaginous Defect Repair

When selecting materials for reconstituting craniofacial skeletal defects, the surgeon must recognize that no one material fills all needs. Several materials are available, reflecting the reality that there is no truly superior product in the field. The craniofacial surgeon starts the process of selecting a material by identifying a specific clinical need and a tissue substitute that will fill as much of that need as possible. Three types of factors are primarily responsible for outcomes of the use of bone substitute material, host factors, surgical technique, and the features of the material.

Host factors are of fundamental importance whenever a graft or implant is to be used. They include any systemic conditions, such as autoimmune illness, as well as the local environment. The local environment is profoundly influenced by anything that alters its vascularity, such as radiation therapy. The functional demands of the tissue being replaced are carefully considered. A calvarial defect, for instance, has different requirements from those of a mandibular defect, which has much greater load-bearing requirements. The extent of soft tissue coverage and mobility to which the implant is exposed are also key factors. Implants that work in the malar eminence might not work in the ear or nose.

Surgical technique can also play an important role in how well an implant is tolerated. Intra-oral approaches carry an increased risk of infection if closure is not executed with meticulous attention. For all approaches, appropriate handling of the soft tissues and the periosteum (when available) can be critical to success. Material preparation, such as pretreatment with an antimicrobial agent, can also be important in improving the likelihood of success.

The third factor is the material itself. On a general level a material that is nontoxic, noncarcinogenic, and nonimmunogenic to biologic systems is said to be *biocompatible*. Inflammation, which in previous discussions of the subject was considered a negative quality, can actually be advantageous as long as it is resolvable. The concept of biocompatibility, however, is more complex than even this definition implies. As previously discussed, a material that is biocompatible in one area may not be so in another. The use of expanded polytetrafluorethylene (ePTFE) is an excellent example. ePTFE has been successfully used for many years in vascular surgery,[98] but the use of Proplast, a closely related material, in reconstruction of the temporo-mandibular joint produced disastrous complications.[99] In some applications and locations, a material that causes a local but temporary reaction is desirable, whereas in others, a totally inert material is required. On the basis of this analysis, it is more precise to include application and local factors in the definition of biocompatibility.

Furthermore, it is most useful to think of biocompatibility as a broad spectrum with autogenous grafts on one end and alloplastic (synthetic) materials on the other. Allografts (homografts) and xenografts fall in the middle of that spectrum. Autogenous materials represent the "gold standard," but this category is not homogeneous. Cancellous bone grafts are quite different from cortical grafts. Cortical grafts can be further subclassified as endochondral or intramembraneous bone, with functional differences between the two.[100-102] Although there is a vast and successful experience with autogenous grafting,[103] this method still has its limitations. Donor site morbidity should not be taken lightly. In a prospective study evaluating iliac crest donor site pain, Sasso and colleagues[104] reported that a significant proportion of patients still had donor site pain 2 years after surgery. In addition, incomplete resorption and remodeling of cortical bone occurs in autogenous grafts, and unpredictable remodeling can be an issue as well.[105,106]

Allografts can be used in place of autogenous grafts. Demineralized bone matrix and irradiated cadaveric bone are examples of allografts currently used by some surgeons. Xenografts are also used; they include various collagen preparations that are employed as bone substitutes. The final category is synthetic biomaterials or alloplasts. This category consists of metals, ceramics, polymers, and biomimetic materials. This final subcategory refers to materials that mimic bone structurally or biologically and includes tissue-engineered constructs.

The metal most commonly used for craniofacial reconstruction is titanium. This metal not only has some osteoconductive properties but also has a modulus of elasticity that approaches that of bone. This feature results in less stress shielding than observed with stainless steel or Vitallium, both of which are rarely used today. Gold is inert, and its high density has made it useful in some applications, such as facial reanimation.

Polymers include a diverse set of materials some of which are nonresorbable and some resorbable. They have a successful track record for use in facial augmentation.[107] Methacrylates are nonresorbable and have been widely used for calvarial reconstruction since World War II. High-density porous polyethylene is a straight-chain aliphatic hydrocarbon that is inert and also nonresorbable. It has been used successfully in some craniofacial applications. The primary problem with these materials is associated with their risk for infection or extrusion during the life of the recipient. Implants fabricated from polylactic acid and polyglycolic acid are resorbable and have sufficient strength for some load-sharing applications. This material has been promising as a means of bony fixation without the use of a permanent material.

Ceramics include calcium phosphates such as hydroxyapatite and bioglass. Hydroxyapatite, which has the advantage of being closely related to the carbonated apatite found in bone, has been shown to be reasonably effective in animal models and has proven clinical efficacy in some applications.[108,109] However, in the sintered and cement forms, it is not entirely accessible to the remodeling activities of osteoclasts. Its osteoconductivity and osteoinductivity are often less than ideal.[106,110,111] Bioglasses are very osteoconductive, but some of their properties, such as stiffness and elasticity, render them inappropriate for many craniofacial applications.

The final subcategory is synthetic biomimetic materials. They are designed to replicate bone on a structural and biologic level. They are often composites and can include bioactive factors such as bone morphogenic proteins or cells in a tissue-engineered material. This field is very promising in offering the hope of an off-the-shelf material that can simulate bone and stimulate the bone remodeling cycle—so that it is resorbed via osteoclastic remodeling coupled with osteoblastic bone deposition. Biomimetic biomaterials are theoretically replaced with normal lamellar bone. Given the pace of research in this field, a true bone substitute material of this nature is certainly on the horizon.

Conclusion

The field of craniofacial surgery is a rapidly developing and complex field. Appropriate care can best be rendered by a multimember team with diverse and in-depth training. The craniofacial defects encountered are often part of a larger syndrome affecting many functional systems. The underlying pathology is etiologically diverse and heterogeneous. The application of craniofacial principles developed to treat congenital problems also serves well for tumor extirpation and trauma repair. Several materials are currently available to reconstruct the craniofacial skeleton, but there is also a wide effort to develop more biomimetic materials.

SUGGESTED READINGS

Bauer TW, Muschler GF. Bone graft materials: an overview of the basic science. *Clin Orthop Relat Res.* 2000:10-27.

Cohen MM Jr. Etiopathogenesis of craniosynostosis. *Neurosurg Clin North Am.* 1991;2:507-513.

Cohen M, Sutural pathology. In: Cohen M, MacLean R, eds. *Craniosynostosis: Diagnosis, Evaluation, and Management.* New York: Oxford University Press; 2000.

Hunt JA, Hobar PC. Common craniofacial anomalies: facial clefts and encephaloceles. *Plast Reconstr Surg.* 2003;112:606-615; quiz 616,722.

Imola MJ, Tatum SA. Craniofacial distraction osteogenesis. *Facial Plast Surg Clin North Am.* 2002;10:287-301.

McCarthy JG, Schreiber J, Karp N, et al. Lengthening the human mandible by gradual distraction. *Plast Reconstr Surg.* 1992;89(1):1-8; discussion 9-10.

Ortiz-Monasterio F, del Campo AF, Carrillo A. Advancement of the orbits and the midface in one piece, combined with frontal repositioning, for the correction of Crouzon's deformities. *Plast Reconstr Surg.* 1978;61:507-516.

Obwegeser JA. Maxillary and midface deformities: characteristics and treatment strategies. *Clin Plast Surg.* 2007;34:519-533.

Posnick J. *Craniofacial and Maxillofacial Surgery in Children and Young Adults.* Philadelphia: W.B. Saunders; 2000.

Slater BJ, et al. Cranial sutures: a brief review. *Plast Reconstr Surg.* 2008;121:170e-178e.

Tessier P, Kawamoto H, Matthews D, et al. Autogenous bone grafts and bone substitutes—tools and techniques: I: a 20,000-case experience in maxillofacial and craniofacial surgery. *Plast Reconstr Surg.* 2005;116(Suppl):6S-24S; discussion 92S-94S.

For complete list of references log onto www.expertconsult.com.

CHAPTER ONE HUNDRED AND EIGHTY-SIX

Cleft Lip and Palate

Oren Friedman

Tom D. Wang

Henry A. Milczuk

Key Points

- Cleft lip and palate deformities constitute the most common congenital defect of the head.
- The etiology of clefting is multifactorial. Its prevalence varies among ethnic groups and within families. Syndromes are common, especially among patients with cleft palate.
- Surgical decisions should be based on careful analysis of the defects. The goals are restoring function (e.g., lip closure, nasal airway, normal speech, eustachian tube function, useful dental occlusion) and maximizing lip, nose, and midface symmetry.
- Numerous surgical (and medical) approaches have been developed, and different teams use various management strategies for patients with clefting.
- Patients with cleft lip or cleft palate are best managed using a multidisciplinary approach. A coordinated medical and surgical care plan provides optimal long-term outcomes. The patient's medical and surgical needs change over time.

Cleft lip and cleft palate are among the more common congenital deformities. Patients with these deformities often may have associated problems including otologic disease, speech and language problems (delayed onset, articulation disorders, velopharyngeal incompetence or insufficiency), dental deformities (e.g., malocclusion; missing, malformed, or supernumerary teeth), facial growth deficiencies, and psychosocial issues. Some children have associated genetic syndromes or chromosomal abnormalities.

This chapter discusses some of these problems and their treatment strategies for the child with cleft lip or palate, or both, with emphasis on the need for a well-coordinated multidisciplinary approach to management.

Classification of Cleft Lip and Palate

A variety of classification systems have been proposed, but few have found wide acceptance. The embryologic development of the lip and palate serves as the foundation for a number of cleft classification systems. Some useful terms and concepts for cleft classifications are described in this section.

The incisive foramen divides the palate into the primary palate and the secondary palate. The secondary palate develops after completion of development of the primary palate, and extends from the incisive foramen anteriorly to the uvula posteriorly. The primary palate, which has the incisive foramen as its posterior border, consists of the premaxilla, lip, nasal tip, and columella.[1]

Cleft lip is classified as unilateral or bilateral, and its extent may be classified as complete or incomplete. A complete cleft involves the entire vertical thickness of the upper lip, and is often associated with an alveolar cleft, because the embryologic origins of the lip and primary palate are the same (Fig. 186-1). An incomplete cleft lip involves only a portion of the vertical height of the lip, with a variable segment of continuity across the cleft region. The variable continuous segment may present as a simple muscular diastasis with intact overlying skin or as a wide cleft with only a thin band of skin crossing the region of the cleft (Fig. 186-2). *Simonart's band* is the bridge or bar of lip tissue, of variable size, that bridges the cleft gap. Simonart's band usually consists of skin only, although some histologic studies have shown some muscle fibers to lie within the band.[2] Unilateral clefts of the lip should include a designation of whether the right or the left side is involved.

Palatal clefts also are described as being unilateral or bilateral, and their extent may be classified as complete or incomplete. In addition, cleft palates are classified according to their location relative to the incisive foramen. Clefts of the primary palate occur anterior to the incisive foramen, and clefts of the secondary palate involve the segment posterior to the incisive foramen. A unilateral cleft of the secondary palate is defined by a cleft in which the palatal process of the maxilla on one side is fused with the nasal septum (Fig. 186-3). A bilateral complete cleft of the secondary palate has no point of fusion between the maxilla and the nasal septum (Fig. 186-4). A complete cleft of the entire palate involves both the primary and secondary palate, including one or both sides of the premaxilla/alveolar arch, and frequently involves a cleft lip. An isolated cleft palate usually involves the secondary palate only, and has varying degrees of severity. The least severe incomplete cleft is the submucous cleft palate (SMCP) in which the underlying palatal musculature is deficient and inappropriately attached. Associated features include a bifid uvula, a zona pellucida (bluish midline region representing the muscle deficiency), and a notch in the posterior hard palate[3] (Fig. 186-5). All three elements are not required for the diagnosis of SMCP, however.

Embryology

For full appreciation of the variety of anatomic deformities that may be encountered in the patient with cleft lip and palate, an understanding of the normal embryologic development of the lip, palate, and nose

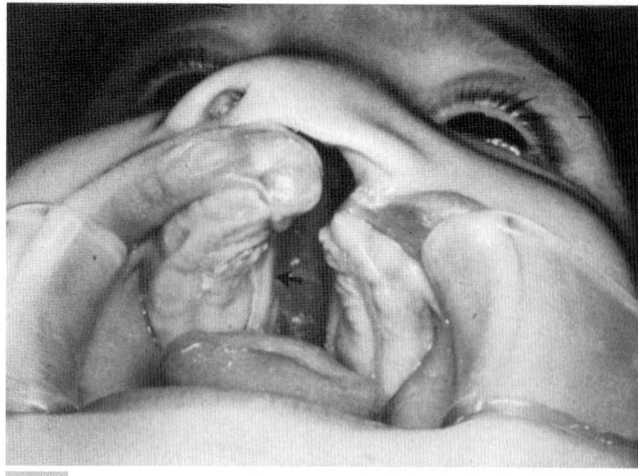

Figure 186-1. A patient with complete unilateral cleft of lip and palate. *Arrow* marks the junction of the nasal septum with the noncleft side of the palate.

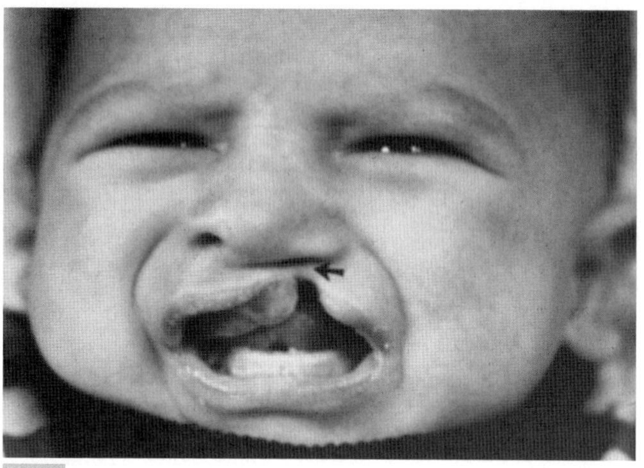

Figure 186-2. *Arrow* indicates Simonart's band connecting two sides in a patient with incomplete cleft lip.

is essential. At the end of the fourth embryonic week, the neural crest–derived facial prominences appear from the first pair of pharyngeal arches. The maxillary prominences are found laterally (Fig. 186-6). The frontonasal prominences, formed by the proliferation of mesenchyme ventral to the forebrain, form the upper border of the stomodeum. On either side of the frontonasal prominences are local thickenings of surface ectoderm which form the nasal placodes.[1]

During the fifth week of embryonic development, the nasal placodes invaginate to form the nasal pits. This invagination process creates a ridge of tissue around the pit, called the lateral nasal prominences laterally, and the medial nasal prominences medially (Fig. 186-7).

Over the next 2 weeks, the paired maxillary prominences grow medially and approximate the paired medial nasal prominences (Fig. 186-8). Over time, fusion of the paired medial nasal prominences and paired maxillary prominences occurs, thereby forming the upper lip. The medial nasal prominences fuse to form the philtrum, medial upper lip, nasal tip, and columella. The maxillary prominences form the lateral aspects of the upper lip. The lateral nasal prominences are not involved in the formation of the upper lip, but form the nose (Fig. 186-9).[1,3]

The nose is formed from five facial prominences: The frontonasal prominence forms the bridge, the fused medial nasal prominences form the tip and columella, and the lateral nasal prominences form the nasal alae (Table 186-1).

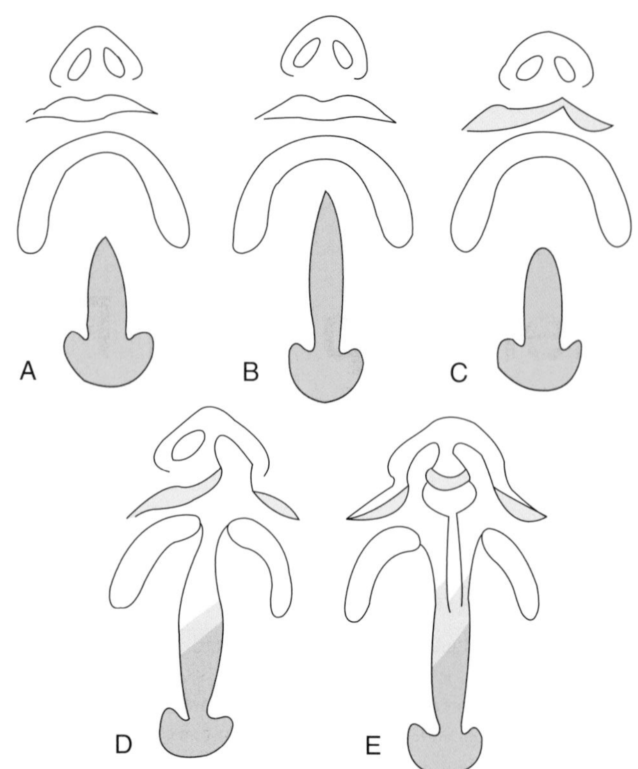

Figure 186-3. Classification of cleft palate. The division between primary palate (prolabium, premaxilla, and anterior septum) and secondary palate is the incisive foramen. **A,** Incomplete cleft of the secondary palate. **B,** Complete cleft of the secondary palate (extending as far as the incisive foramen). **C,** Incomplete cleft of the primary and secondary palates. **D,** Unilateral complete cleft of the primary and secondary palates. **E,** Bilateral complete cleft of the primary and secondary palates. *(After Kernahan and Stark, 1958. From McCarthy JG, Cutting CB, Hogan VM. Introduction to facial clefts. In: McCarthy JG, ed.* Plastic Surgery. *Vol 4. Philadelphia: WB Saunders; 1990:2443.)*

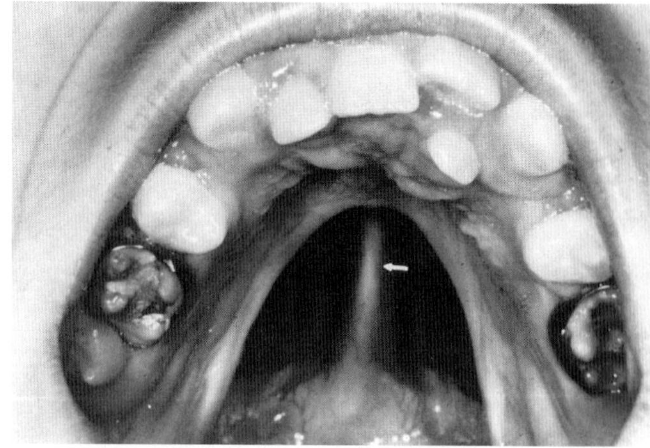

Figure 186-4. A patient with bilateral complete cleft palate. *Arrow* marks the nasal septum, which is not connected to either palatal shelf.

Palatogenesis begins at the end of the fifth week, with complete fusion occurring by 12 weeks of development. As the maxillary prominences grow and push the medial nasal prominences medially, the medial nasal prominences fuse not only at the surface but also at deeper levels (Fig. 186-10). Thus, the intermaxillary segment, or primary palate, which includes the central maxillary alveolar arch that houses the four incisor teeth and the hard palate anterior to the incisive foramen, is formed by the deeper levels of fusion of the two medial nasal prominences. Once the primary palate is completely developed, the secondary palate begins to develop.[1,3]

The secondary palate makes up the major portion of the palate. It is formed from the palatine shelves, which are two shelflike outgrowths of the maxillary prominences. In the sixth week of embryonic development, the palatine shelves are directed obliquely downward on either side of the tongue (Fig. 186-11). By the seventh week, the palatine shelves migrate inferomedially to lie horizontally above the tongue. It is in this horizontal position that the palatine shelves fuse in the midline to form the secondary palate (Fig. 186-12). The palatine shelves fuse with the previously formed primary palate anteriorly, and the nasal septum fuses with the newly formed secondary and primary palate. Palatal fusion occurs from anterior to posterior, beginning at the incisive foramen at 8 weeks of gestation and reaching completion by week 12 with uvular fusion (Fig. 186-13). The degree of clefting noted clinically is a consequence of the point in fetal development when the fusion process is interrupted.

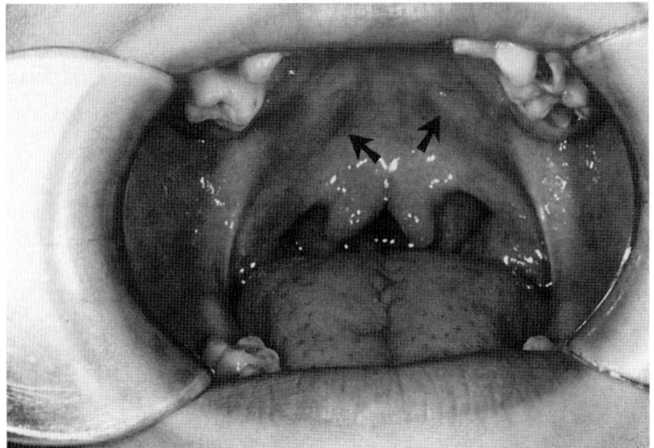

Figure 186-5. Submucous cleft palate with bifid uvula and muscular diastasis *(arrows)*.

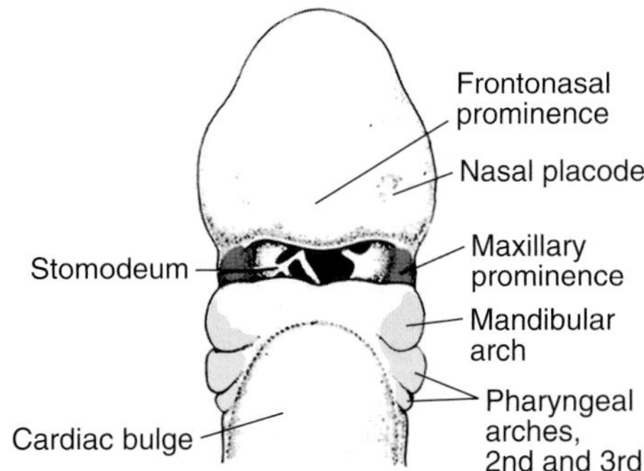

Figure 186-6. Lateral view of an embryo at the end of week 4, showing the position of the pharyngeal arches. *(From Sadler TW. Head and neck embryology. In: Sadler TW, ed.* Langman's Medical Embryology. *6th ed. Baltimore: Williams & Wilkins; 1990:315.)*

Diagnosis

Prenatal Diagnosis

The advent of ultrasonography for use in prenatal care and improvements in imaging now permits antepartum diagnosis of cleft lip and palate[4,5] (Fig. 186-14). Routine prenatal ultrasonography is now the standard practice in most communities. More reliable prenatal diagnosis can be made of cleft lip than of cleft palate.[6] Diagnostic accuracy is improved if two-dimensional ultrasonography is combined with three-

Table 186-1

Structures Contributing to the Formation of the Face

Prominence	Structures Formed
Frontonasal*	Forehead; bridge of the nose, medial and lateral nasal prominences
Maxillary	Cheeks, lateral portion of the upper lip
Medial nasal	Philtrum of the upper lip, crest and tip of the nose
Lateral nasal	Alae of the nose
Mandibular	Lower lip

*The frontonasal prominence represents a single unpaired structure, whereas the other prominences are paired.
From Sadler TW. Head and neck embryology. In: Sadler TW, ed. *Langman's Medical Embryology*. 6th ed. Baltimore: Williams & Wilkins; 1990:315.

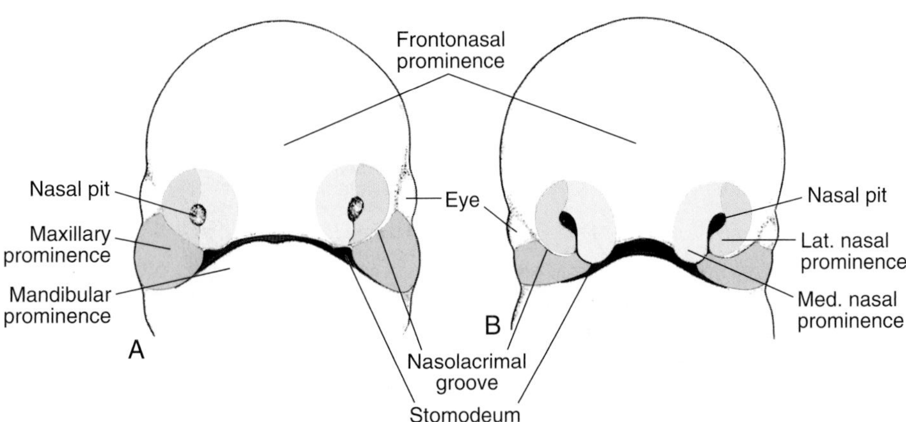

Figure 186-7. Frontal aspect of the face. **A**, Five-week embryo. **B**, Six-week embryo. The nasal prominences are gradually separated from the maxillary prominence by deep furrows. *(From Sadler TW. Head and neck embryology. In: Sadler TW, ed.* Langman's Medical Embryology. *6th ed. Baltimore: Williams & Wilkins; 1990:315.)*

dimensional ultrasonography.[7] The diagnosis can be made as early as 18 weeks, although the accuracy improves with the age of the fetus.[8] It is estimated that 12% of these fetuses will have other anomalies.[5] The parents frequently will want additional information and often are referred to cleft teams for counseling. Most families find antenatal counseling helpful in planning for care of the child with an orofacial cleft.[9]

Molecular Genetics of Orofacial Clefts

Clefts of the lip and/or palate are influenced by both genetic and environmental factors. Monozygotic twins demonstrate a concordance rate of 40% to 60% for clefting. Failure to reach 100% concordance in monozygotic twins suggests that genetics alone does not determine orofacial clefts. Embryology and genetics suggest that clefts of the primary palate, those that involve the lip with or without the remaining palate (CLP), arise from a different mechanism from that operative with clefts involving the secondary palate only (CP).[10] Currently, approximately 70% of CLP patients are thought to be nonsyndromic, whereas 50% of CP patients are nonsyndromic.[11] Syndromic clefts may be the result of a single gene transmission as occurs in autosomal dominant, autosomal recessive, or X-linked heredity. Facial clefting is a possible association in more than 200 syndromes.[12] The most common syndrome associated with cleft lip is van der Woude syndrome. Lower lip pits and CLP are the characteristics features of this syndrome, although CLP and isolated CP can be seen in the same

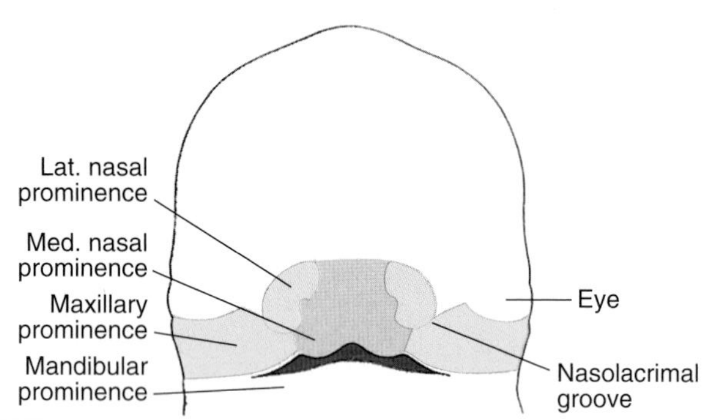

Figure 186-8. In a 7-week embryo, the maxillary prominences have fused with the medial nasal prominences. *(From Sadler TW. Head and neck embryology. In: Sadler TW, ed.* Langman's Medical Embryology. *6th ed. Baltimore: Williams & Wilkins; 1990:316.)*

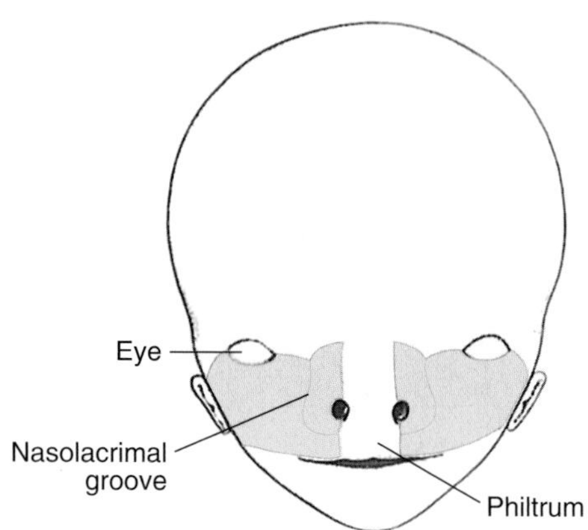

Figure 186-9. In a 10-week embryo, the maxillary prominences have formed the lateral lip and the medial nasal prominences have formed the philtrum. *(From Sadler TW. Head and neck embryology. In: Sadler TW, ed.* Langman's Medical Embryology. *6th ed. Baltimore: Williams & Wilkins; 1990:316.)*

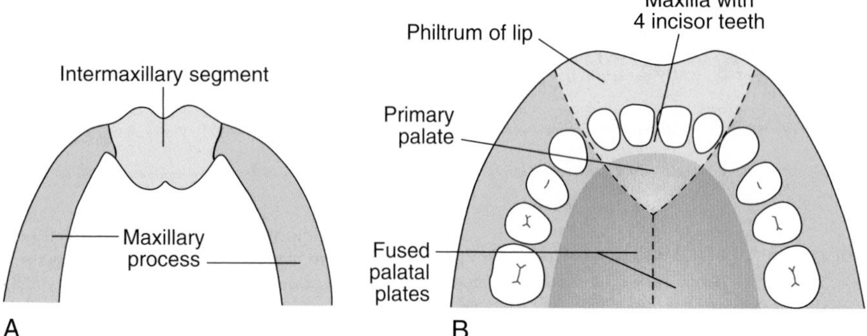

Figure 186-10. **A**, Schematic drawing of the intermaxillary segment and maxillary processes. **B**, The intermaxillary segment gives rise to the philtrum of the upper lip; the median part of the maxillary bone and its four incisor teeth; and the triangular primary palate. *(From Sadler TW. Head and neck embryology. In: Sadler TW, ed.* Langman's Medical Embryology. *6th ed. Baltimore: Williams & Wilkins; 1990:317.)*

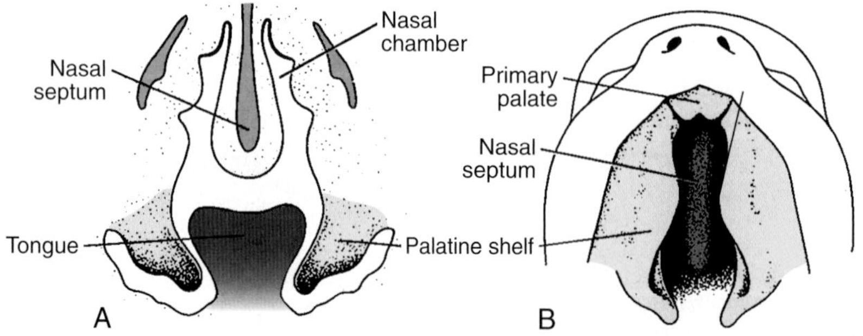

Figure 186-11. **A**, Frontal section through the head of a 6-week embryo. The palatine shelves are located in the vertical position on each side of the tongue. **B**, Ventral view of the palatine shelves after removal of the lower jaw and the tongue. Note the clefts between the primary triangular palate and the palatine shelves, which are still in a vertical position. *(From Sadler TW. Head and neck embryology. In: Sadler TW, ed.* Langman's Medical Embryology. *6th ed. Baltimore: Williams & Wilkins; 1990:317.)*

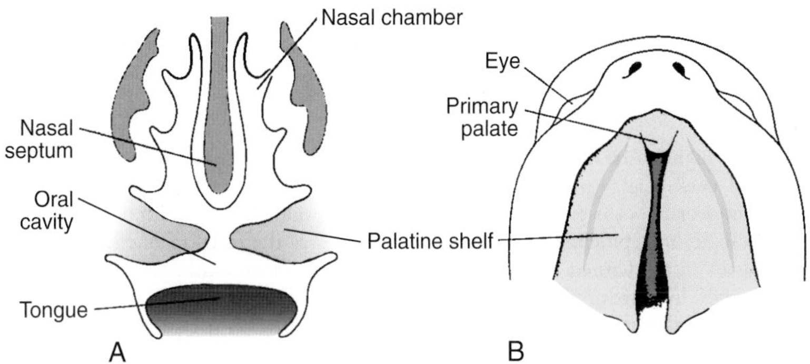

Figure 186-12. **A**, Frontal section through the head of a 7-week embryo. The tongue has moved downward, and the palatine shelves have reached a horizontal position. **B**, Ventral view of the palatine shelves after removal of the lower jaw and tongue. The shelves are in a horizontal position. Note the nasal septum. *(From Sadler TW. Head and neck embryology. In: Sadler TW, ed.* Langman's Medical Embryology. *6th ed. Baltimore: Williams & Wilkins; 1990:318.)*

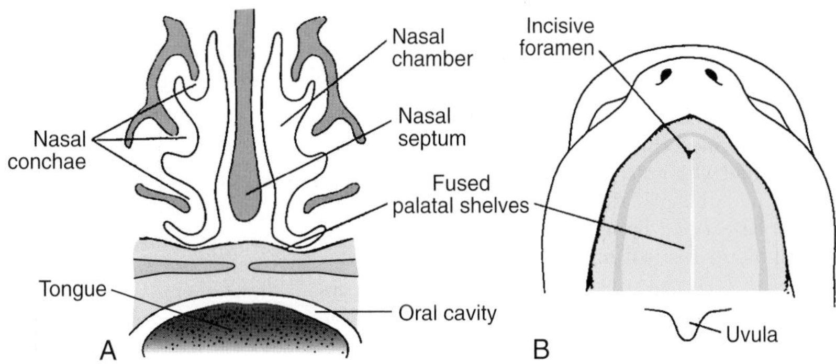

Figure 186-13. **A**, Frontal section through the head of a 10-week embryo. The two palatine shelves have fused with each other and with the nasal septum. **B**, Ventral view of the palate. The incisive foramen forms the midline landmark between the primary and the secondary palate. *(From Sadler TW. Head and neck embryology. In: Sadler TW, ed.* Langman's Medical Embryology. *6th ed. Baltimore: Williams & Wilkins; 1990:318.)*

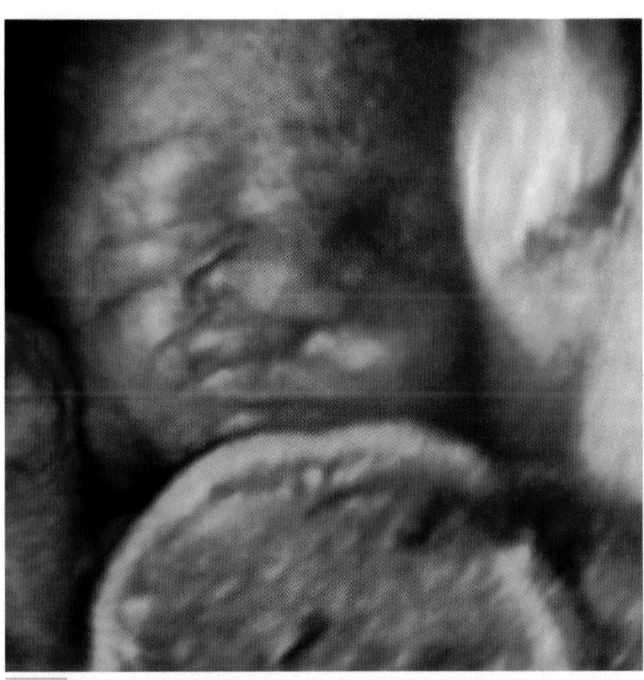

Figure 186-14. Surface-rendered three-dimensional ultrasound image of a 24-week fetus with isolated unilateral left cleft lip. *(Courtesy of Roya Sohaey, MD, Portland, Oregon.)*

family and lip pits are not found in 10%. Genetic studies indicate that the gene responsible for this autosomal dominant disorder is on chromosome 1.[13] A number of signaling molecules, transcription factors, and growth factors have been identified that are particularly important to the development of the lip and palate.[14] Mutations to the gene, delay in expression of the gene product, or exposure to an environmental factor affecting the gene or its product may result in a cleft.

Several teratogens have been implicated in cleft development. These include alcohol,[15] tobacco smoke,[16] phenytoin,[17] and retinoic acid.[18] Meta-analysis did not find maternal age to be a factor.[19] Multivitamin supplements lower risk for CLP and possibly isolated CP.[20] Whether preconceptual folic acid supplementation alone can reduce clefting is controversial.[21,22] Potential mechanisms of genetic, environmental, and biochemical interactions have been suggested and reviewed.[20,23] Human teratogen studies should be interpreted with caution due to the potential for confounding variables and recall bias.

Genetic linkage studies have suggested a number of potential loci for clefts,[24,25] though only loci on chromosome 6p have consistently demonstrated linkage to CLP.[26,27] Linkage studies are limited by small numbers of families available for study. Transgenic mouse models and mouse strains with spontaneous clefts have identified candidate genes that may also affect human clefting. Mice deficient in the *Msx1* gene, implicated in signaling between tissue layers during embryogenesis, all developed clefts of the secondary palate.[28] Another putative mediator of orofacial clefting is transforming growth factor beta-3 (TGF-β_3). Knockout of the TGF-β_3 gene in mice results in clefts, but the addition of TGF-β_3 to embryonic murine tissue culture stimulates palatal shelf adhesion.[29] Studies of South American children with CLP suggest and interaction between *Msx1* and TGF-β_3 loci increasing cleft susceptibility.[30] Transforming growth factor alpha also is considered to be a factor modulating CLP in humans.[31]

Epidemiology

Cleft lip and palate deformities are thought to be the most common congenital anomalies of the head and neck. Cleft lip with or without cleft palate must be distinguished from isolated cleft palate deformities because of different embryologic, etiologic, and epidemiologic factors.[32] Cleft lip occurs in 1 in 1000 live births in the United States, whereas cleft palate deformity occurs in 1 in 2000 live births. Cleft lip deformities occur with the highest incidence among Native Americans (3.6 in 1000 births), Asians (2.1 in 1000), and whites (1 in 1000) and with the lowest incidence among blacks (0.41 in 1,000).[12] By contrast, the incidence of cleft palate does not differ among ethnic groups, being reported as 0.5 in 1000 live births. Cleft lip occurs more commonly in boys than in girls, whereas cleft palate occurs more commonly in girls than in boys. Fusion of the palatine shelves 1 week later in girls than in boys is thought to be responsible for the higher frequency of cleft palate in girls.[1]

Recurrent risk rates for cleft lip with or without cleft palate and for isolated cleft palate have been determined and may be useful in counseling parents about the risk of cleft in future pregnancies.[32] Two unaffected parents with one child affected with a cleft have a 4.4% chance of having another child with a cleft lip and palate and a 2.5% chance of having a child with isolated cleft palate. One parent affected with a cleft has a 3.2% chance of having a child with cleft lip and palate and a 6.8% chance of having a child with isolated cleft palate. Presence of a cleft in one parent and in one sibling is associated with a 15.8% chance that the next child will have a cleft lip or palate, and a 14.9% chance that the next child will have a cleft palate.[32]

Multidisciplinary Cleft Team

Comprehensive care of the child with cleft palate is best done within a team of health care professionals trained in the care of various disorders that accompany and develop as a result of the cleft lip or palate.[33-35] This approach recognizes that no single discipline possesses all of the expertise needed for proper management of the many problems of these patients. The cleft team also will focus on the needs of the patient and family. Standards have been recommended by the American Cleft Palate–Craniofacial Association.[36] Specialties that often make up a cleft care team are listed in Box 186-1. Members should meet face to face to discuss patient care at least six times a year. Continuing education for the care of patients with cleft deformities should be an integral part of membership in a cleft team.

Team care begins when an infant is identified as having a cleft. The nursing staff or the pediatrician, within the context of a cleft care team approach, monitor feeding, growth, and development of the child. Parents are provided counseling, genetic information as needed, and verbal and written instructions regarding care plans. Most teams develop protocols for the management of children with cleft lip and palate deformities. These algorithms for care are based on the experience of the team members and assign care for anticipated needs of the child. A sample management protocol is outlined in Table 186-2. The otolaryngologist carries the roles of airway management, otologic care, and evaluation of velopharyngeal insufficiency and, in some teams, serves as the facial reconstructive surgeon.

Box 186-1

Specialty Members of a Cleft Care Team

- Reconstructive surgeon
- Otolaryngologist
- Plastic surgeon
- Oral maxillofacial surgeon
- Speech-language pathologist
- Orthodontist
- Pediatric or prosthodontic dentist
- Developmental or general pediatrician
- Genetics counselor
- Audiologist
- Nurse
- Social worker
- Psychologist

Adapted from the American Cleft Palate–Craniofacial Association.

Nursing Care

Special problems that are encountered in nursing care of the patient with a cleft deformity include initial feeding, postoperative airway and feeding management, and family care issues centered on frequent medical and surgical needs. Nurses often provide an additional and, for some parents, more secure source of information regarding treatment

Table 186-2

Example Protocol for Multidisciplinary Approach to Care of Patients with Cleft Lip and Palate

Age Range	Intervention
Prenatal	Refer to Cleft Palate Team Medical diagnosis Genetic counseling Address psychosocial issues
Neonatal (0-1 month)	Same as above Provide feeding instructions Monitor growth Hearing screening
1-4 months	Monitor feeding and growth Repair cleft lip Monitor ears and hearing
5-15 months	Monitor feeding, growth, and development Repair cleft palate Monitor ears and hearing; consider ear tubes Instructions in oral hygiene
16-24 months	Assess speech and language development Monitor ears and hearing; ear tubes if indicated Monitor development
2-5 years	Monitor speech and language development; manage velopharyngeal insufficiency Monitor ears and hearing; ear tubes if indicated Assess development and psychosocial needs Consider lip/nose revision before child reaches school age
6-11 years	Monitor speech and language; manage velopharyngeal insufficiency Orthodontic evaluation and treatment Alveolar bone graft Monitor school and psychosocial needs
12-21 years	Monitor school and psychosocial needs Orthodontics and restorative dentistry Genetic counseling Rhinoplasty (if needed) Orthognathic surgery (if needed)

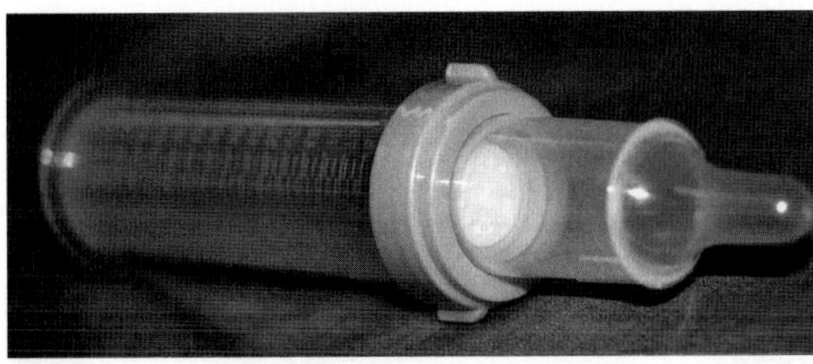

Figure 186-15. Haberman feeder.

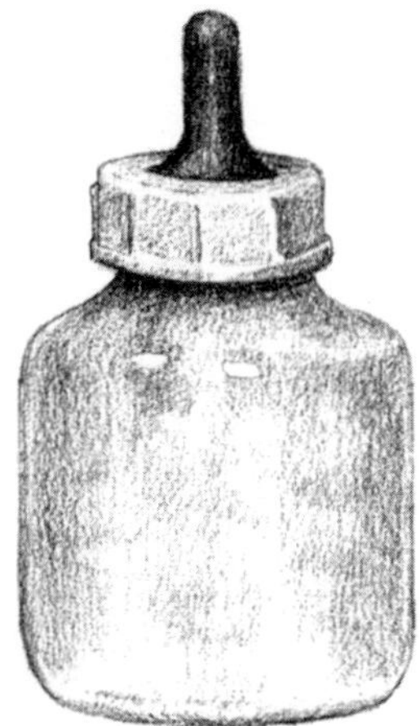

Figure 186-16. Mead-Johnson feeder.

plans. Parents may feel more comfortable revealing their concerns or frustrations related to their child to nursing staff. The participation of dedicated and skilled nurses is valuable within the cleft care team.

Infants with a cleft palate are limited in their ability to suck. The common cavity between the nose and the mouth permits air to leak as the infant tries to suck. Cleft lip alone usually does not cause feeding problems. Accordingly, a number of strategies have been devised and different feeders have been created for feeding the infant with a cleft palate. Generally, breast feeding is ineffective. Alternately, expressed (pumped) breast milk can be delivered using one of the specialized feeders. The three most commonly used cleft palate feeders are the Mead-Johnson, Haberman, and Pigeon bottles (Figs. 186-15 to 186-17). Each allows for parent-controlled delivery of the meal (expressed breast milk or formula). Parents and caregivers need to be taught how to properly use the feeder and observed for the first feed to insure proper use of the feeder.[37,38] Trial and error may be needed to discover the best technique and feeder for the infant. Children with cleft palate generally swallow much more air during feeds. Frequent burping often is necessary; this should be explained to parents. Attention should be paid to the child's growth. Following weight and length gains using standardized growth charts is very useful to ensure that the infant stays on the appropriate growth curves.

Nurses can help families find the best position and technique for feeding after surgery. Oral and facial wounds affect placement of a feeding nipple. Often, the same cleft feeder can be used as before surgery, although the feeding technique may need to be modified owing to pain and swelling. Wound care also can be taught by nursing staff. Fresh lip wounds should be kept clean (with soap and water) and moist with ointments. Often, padded elbow restraints that prevent flexion of the elbow but permit other arm and hand motion are placed after surgery. Children are discouraged from placing fingers or other things into the mouth that may potentially disrupt the suture line. Restraints also may be used after palatoplasty. The restraints are left on until the intraoral wounds have epithelialized. Close monitoring by nursing staff will facilitate return to normal activities after surgery.

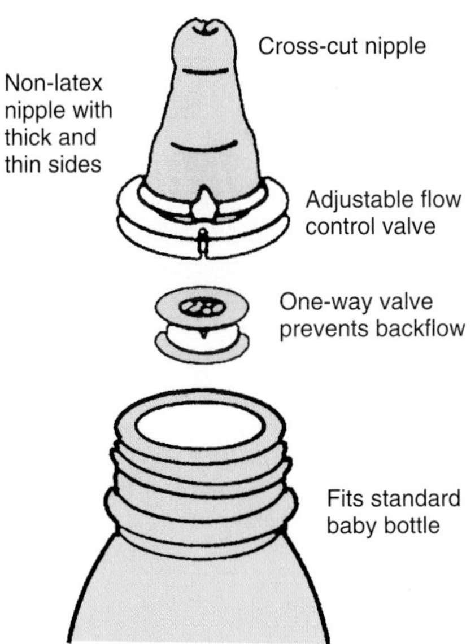

Figure 186-17. Pigeon feeder.

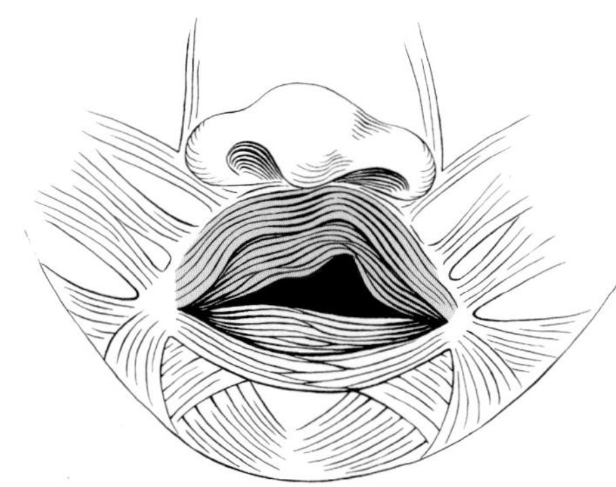

Figure 186-18. Muscle abnormality in an incomplete cleft lip that involves less than two thirds of the lip. Lower muscle fibers insert into tissue at the cleft margins; upper muscle fibers in the medial and lateral segment connect over the top of the incomplete cleft, forming a partial oral sphincter.

Anatomy

Anatomy of the Cleft Lip Deformity

The normal upper lip is divided into red and white components. The red lip is a mucous membrane, whereas the white lip is a cutaneous structure. The mucocutaneous junction at the vermilion border between the red and white lips is an important anatomic boundary that must be reconstructed meticulously in cleft lip repair for a natural-looking result. Failure to do so will draw attention to the irregularity at the vermilion border and create a poor cosmetic result.[3,39,]

In unaffected persons, the orbicularis oris muscle forms a complete sphincter around the oral cavity, providing the substrate for proper form and function of the lips and mouth. All patients with cleft lip deformities have muscular deficiencies and irregularities of varying degrees, leading to the abnormal appearance and function of the lip and mouth (Figs. 186-18 and 186-19). For proper correction of cleft lip deformities, it is essential not only to create symmetry of the lip superficially, at the skin level, but also to re-create the complete orbicularis muscular sling, for long-lasting cosmetic and functional results, and to re-establish complete mucosal coverage to ensure optimal healing and prevent distorting wound contracture. The muscle fibers in cleft lip deformities run in an inferior-to-superior direction along the margins of the cleft. They insert into the columella medially and along the nasal ala laterally. These fibers must be detached from their

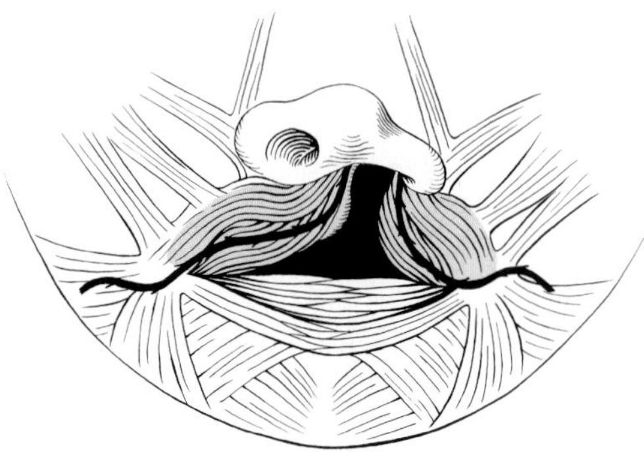

Figure 186-19. Abnormal direction and insertion of muscle fibers of medial and lateral segments of the cleft into the cleft margin, the area of the ala nasi (laterally), and the base of the columella (medially). *Dark line* indicates arterial supply.

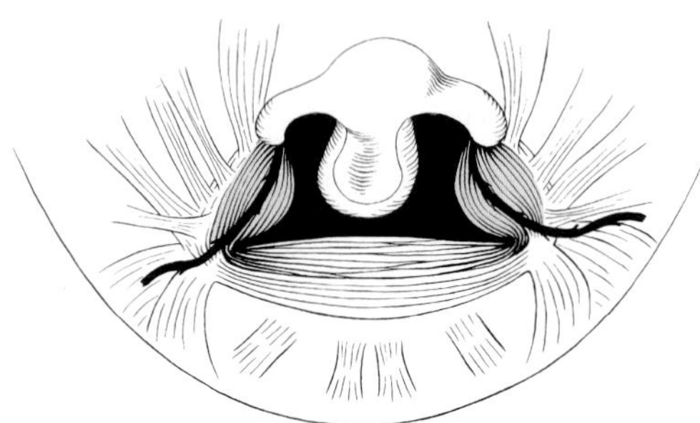

Figure 186-20. Abnormal muscle anatomy of a complete bilateral cleft. Both lateral muscle segments insert into the alae nasi, with the prolabium completely devoid of muscle tissue. Arterial supply is indicated by a *dark line*.

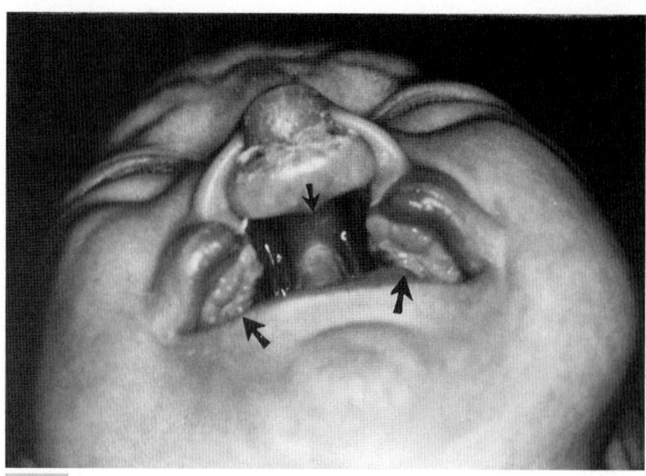

Figure 186-21. A patient with complete bilateral cleft lip and palate: *Top arrow*, protruding premaxilla; *bottom arrows*, collapse of alveolar arches.

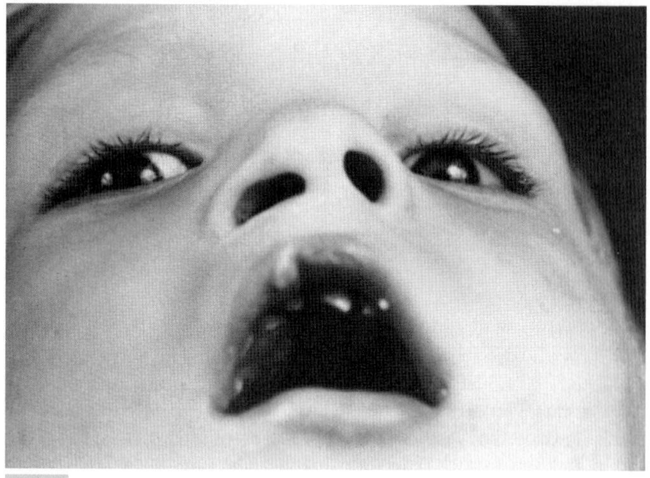

Figure 186-22. Classic nasal deformity associated with the unilateral cleft lip.

insertions and reoriented in a horizontal direction to bridge the cleft and create a complete muscular sling around the entire circumference of the oral cavity.[3,39]

Bilateral clefts also have abnormally oriented muscle fibers that run along the edges of the lateral aspect of the cleft (Fig. 186-20). Typically, the prolabial segment does not contain any useful muscle but is filled with connective tissue. In addition to the muscle and cutaneous irregularities, patients with bilateral cleft deformities have premaxillary and alveolar protrusion relative to the nasal septum. The premaxillary bony deformity may push the lip so far anteriorly and superiorly toward the nasal tip that the columella is severely diminished in strength and height and may even be obliterated completely (Fig. 186-21). There is often inadequate length to the medial crura; consequently, there is inadequate columellar skin. One of the major challenges in bilateral cleft repair is columellar reconstruction.[3,39]

The anatomic characteristics of the unilateral cleft lip nasal deformity include irregularities of the tip, columella, nostril, alar base, septum, and skeleton[40] (Fig. 186-22). The nasal tip is deflected toward the noncleft side, with a relatively short medial crus and long lateral crus on the cleft side. In addition, the lateral crus of the lower lateral cartilage is caudally displaced on the cleft side. The columella is shorter than normal on the cleft side, and the columella lies on the non-cleft side due to the unopposed action of the intact orbicularis oris muscle. The nostril on the cleft side is horizontally oriented rather than the normal vertical orientation.[17] Similarly, the nasal septum is deflected to the noncleft side. The alar base on the side of the cleft is displaced laterally, inferiorly, and posteriorly. Finally, there is a deficiency of maxillary bone on the cleft side, with the nasal floor often being absent.

The bilateral cleft lip nasal deformity differs from the unilateral deformity in several aspects other than laterality. The degree of nasal deformity relates to the severity of the cleft lip deformity—whether the cleft lip is complete or incomplete. It also is affected by the degree of premaxillary protrusion. Bilateral cleft lip nasal deformities are symmetrical, making the repair of the nose somewhat simpler with regard to gaining tip symmetry. The challenging aspect of the bilateral cleft lip nasal deformity is the lack of adequate columellar tissue. This lack of tissue includes deficiencies in the length of the lower lateral cartilages, as well as deficiency of skin overlying these shortened cartilages. The tip usually is broad and flat, and the alae are laterally displaced, with resultant horizontally oriented nostrils.[40]

Cleft Palate Deformity

Various degrees of deformity involving all tissue layers are seen in cleft palate. With soft palate cleft, deficiencies of the muscle and mucosal layers also are characteristic.

Five muscle pairs contribute to the soft palate. Normally, the levator veli palatini muscle has a transverse orientation, occupying the midportion of the soft palate, thereby creating a muscular sling for the velum.[41] This muscular sling is the principal structural component in closure of the nasopharynx during speech and swallowing. Other muscles that contribute to the velopharyngeal sphincter include the palatopharyngeus, superior constrictor, and musculus uvulae. The musculus uvulae runs beneath the nasopharyngeal musculus and extends from the tensor aponeurosis to the base of the uvula.[42] During speech, its contraction increases the midline bulk of the posterior edge of the soft palate. Deficiency of the musculus uvulae like that seen in

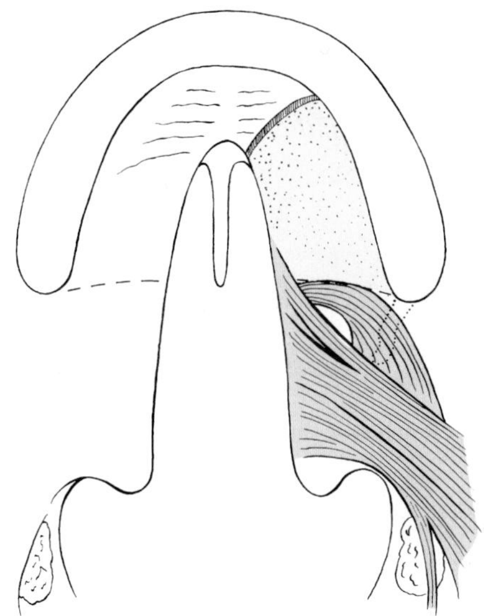

Figure 186-23. Abnormal muscle insertion into the posterior margin of the hard palate in a patient with clefting. Muscles are directed along the margins of the cleft, rather than across the soft palate as occurs normally.

submucous cleft palate may lead to velopharyngeal insufficiency and speech disorders (see Chapter 187, Velopharyngeal Dysfunction). The tensor veli palatini (TVP) muscle runs from its origins at the skull base and eustachian tube, wraps around the hamulus, and inserts into the posterior edge of the hard palate and forms an aponeurosis in the anterior midline of the soft palate.[43] Its functions are dilation of the eustachian tube and support for the soft palate during contraction.

In patients with cleft palate, the muscles of the soft palate may be hypoplastic,[44] in addition to exhibiting misdirection and abnormal insertions into the posterior hard palate (Fig. 186-23). Mucosa that envelops these muscles is deficient, except in the case of a submucous cleft palate. If the cleft involves the hard palate, then a midline bony deficiency of variable degree will extend toward the incisive foramen. The vomer usually is unattached in isolated cleft palate but may or may not be attached if there is a cleft lip. Abnormal muscle insertions combined with tissue absence or hypoplasia lead to palatal dysfunction. Palatoplasty aims to restore function by reorienting the muscles and reconstructing the continuity of the tissues.

Cleft Lip Repair and Cleft Rhinoplasty

The timing of cleft lip repair varies among surgeons. Some have suggested that lip repair be performed within 48 hours of the child's birth to prevent a separate hospitalization and to allow the parents to leave the hospital with a healthy-appearing newborn. Others prefer to delay surgery to allow for more tissue availability for the repair, more time for parent-child bonding, and more time for the parents to gain a better understanding and acceptance of the infant's congenital deformity. Commonly, the "rule of 10s" is applied, which suggests that surgery proceed when the infant is at least 10 weeks old, weighs 10 pounds, and has a hemoglobin level of 10 g/dL. We typically perform cleft repair during the child's second to third month of life, to gain the advantages just described.

Definitive Unilateral Lip Repair

Probably the most common technique for cleft lip repair is the Millard technique. Other techniques have been described, but this chapter focuses on only the Millard technique. The Millard rotation advancement closure for unilateral cleft lip repair entails the downward and lateral rotation of the medial segment of the cleft lip combined with the medial advancement of the lateral cleft segment into the defect. All cleft lips have a discrepancy between the vertical height of the lip from the Cupid's bow peak to the columellar base on the cleft and noncleft sides of the lip (philtral ridge height). The design and length of the rotation flap and the degree of back-cut required will depend on the difference in vertical height between the two sides. Advancement of tissue from the lateral segment of the cleft medially not only closes the tissue defect to bridge the gap but also serves to maintain the rotation flap in position and thus to maintain the amount of vertical height gained by the rotation flap and back-cut.[3,44]

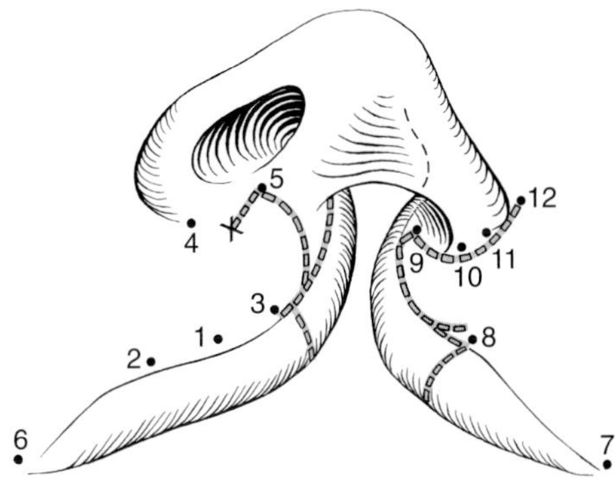

Figure 186-24. Rotation advancement technique: landmarks and incisions. See text for details.

The procedure begins with the skin markings, as shown in Figure 186-24. Skin markings are made with a 30-gauge needle and methylene blue dye. Extreme care should be paid to the measurements and placement of the skin markings, because these serve as the foundation for the surgical repair and provide stable anatomic landmarks in a changing surgical field.[31] The first marking, labeled 1 on the figure, is a point made at the mucocutaneous junction at the exact low point of Cupid's bow, which marks the central point of the upper lip. A second point (2) is placed at the height of Cupid's bow on the noncleft side of the upper lip. The distance between points 1 and 2 is measured—it normally is between 2 and 4 mm—and is used to establish the location of point 3, which represents the height of Cupid's bow on the cleft side of the upper lip. Thus, the distance from point 1 to point 2 is equal to the distance from point 1 to point 3. Point 4 marks the alar base on the noncleft side, and point 5 marks the columellar base on the noncleft side. Point 5 represents the superiormost extent of the vertical portion of the rotation flap, as discussed further later on. Point x, the back-cut point, is made at a variable distance from point 5 and is determined by estimating the amount of tissue needed to create symmetrical philtral ridges and to make up for the discrepancy in vertical height of the lip at the philtral ridge. Point x should never cross the philtral ridge on the noncleft side but should lie medial to it, so that the back-cut of the rotation flap runs parallel and medial to the normal philtral ridge on the noncleft side. This helps to maintain a scar-free philtral ridge on the noncleft side and improves the ultimate cosmetic result of cleft lip repair.

Point 6 marks the noncleft oral commissure, and point 7 marks the oral commissure on the cleft side. Point 8 marks the peak of Cupid's bow on the cleft side. It is placed at a distance from the commissure on the cleft side (distance from points 7 to 8) equal to that for the point placed at the peak of Cupid's bow on the noncleft side relative to the commissure on the noncleft side (distance from points 2 to 6). Point 9 is the medialmost point of the advancement flap and is placed at a distance from point 8 that is equivalent to the distance between point 3 and point 5 + x. Thus, the philtral ridge is formed by the union of the cleft edge on the side of the advancement flap (line 8-9) and the cut edges of the rotation flap on the non-cleft side (line 3-x). Point 10 is the cleft side alar base, point 11 is along the alar-facial crease, and point 12 is placed at the estimated lateralmost aspect of the advancement flap.

Surgical Technique—Rotation Flap

The normal philtral ridge height is 10 mm, and the rotation flap is designed to create a 10-mm-long segment for use in establishing philtral ridge symmetry. The rotation incision starts at point 3 and extends toward point 5, following a gentle curve and providing 4 to 5 mm of

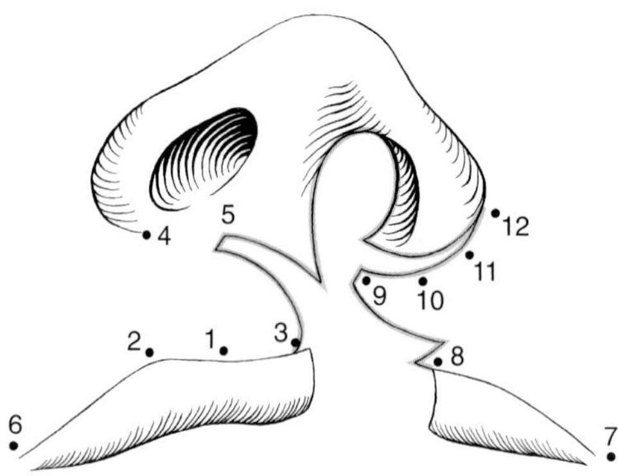

Figure 186-25. Rotation advancement technique: flaps incised and elevated. See text for details.

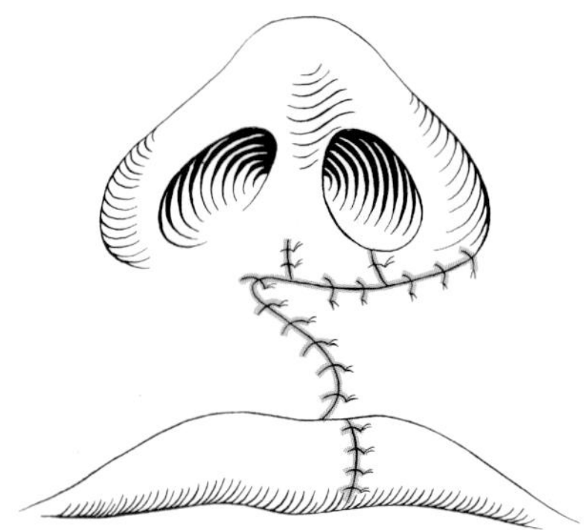

Figure 186-26. Rotation advancement technique: final suturing.

length toward the goal of 10 mm (Fig. 186-25). At the columellar base, the rotation flap incision follows a gentle curve and hugs the base of the columella, passing through point 5. This curve along the base of the columella adds an additional 3 mm of length toward the 10-mm goal. The final discrepancy in vertical height is compensated for with a back-cut to point x, using a stab incision with the No. 11 blade. The extension to the back-cut adds 2 to 3 mm of additional height that will be used to create philtral ridge symmetry. The back-cut is made at a 90-degree angle to the curved incision at the columellar base, to run parallel to rather than crossing the uninvolved philtral ridge. The rotation incisions are carried through the entire thickness of the orbicularis muscle and oral mucosa, to allow a complete release of the medial aspect of the cleft. Undermining along the edges of the rotation flap incision is continued for 1 to 2 mm on the cutaneous and mucosal surfaces, to permit eversion of the wound edges during skin closure.[32]

After completion of the rotation flap cuts, a "c" flap remains, which is a segment of skin that ran between the cut edge of the rotation flap and the edge of the cleft. The "c" flap may be used to add tissue length to the columella, which typically has a tissue deficiency.

Surgical Technique—Advancement Flap

The advancement flap starts with an incision from point 8 to point 9, creating the lateral edge of the new philtral ridge, which will be sutured to the edge of the previously created rotation flap (see Fig. 186-25). Thus, the length of line 8-9 is equal to the length of line 3-x. Release of the advancement flap is then achieved by continuing the incision horizontally along the alar base. Similarly, release of the gingivobuccal sulcus mucosa is performed with sharp dissection, to permit greater mobility. All incisions are carried down to the face of the maxilla, and blunt dissection along the face of the maxilla with scissors is performed, allowing the lateral lip segment freedom of mobility with minimal tension on the closure. Undermining the cutaneous and mucosal surfaces will allow eversion on wound closure.[3,32,45]

Closure—Rotation Advancement Flap

Once the rotation and advancement flaps are developed, approximation of the flaps is achieved with the help of skin hooks, followed by suturing of the flaps to one another to complete the lip reconstruction (Fig. 186-26). Four-0 Vicryl suture is used for all deep muscle stitches and oral mucosal stitches, and 6-0 fast-absorbing gut is used for the skin closure. The first key stitch attaches the muscle at the tip of the advancement flap to the muscle at the rotation flap back-cut point x. The next throw attaches the muscle layers of the advancement and rotation flaps at the level of the vermilion border. It is essential to align this stitch precisely in order to give a natural-appearing vermilion. Additional 4-0 Vicryl stitches are then used to reinforce the muscle layer of closure along the length of the philtral ridge. The mucosa is closed with 4-0 Vicryl suture placed in simple interrupted fashion. Skin closure is achieved with simple interrupted stitches of 6-0 fast-absorbing gut suture. The skin at the vermilion is closed with great precision to provide optimal cosmesis.[3,45]

Primary Rhinoplasty

The cleft lip deformity is always associated with nasal abnormalities. The extent of the nasal abnormality is related to the severity of the cleft lip. Nasal deformities associated with incomplete cleft lips are less severe than those associated with complete lip clefts. The goals of primary rhinoplasty include closure of the nasal floor, repositioning the lower lateral cartilages, and repositioning the alar base. These goals may be achieved through the same incisions that are used for the cleft lip repair, so that no additional incisions are required if the nasal deformity is addressed at the time of cleft lip repair.[40,46] Once the lip incisions are made, the muscle and soft tissue attachments of the ala are separated from the maxilla. Subsequently, through the same incisions, the lower lateral cartilages are freed from the overlying nasal skin along the entire nasal tip. Suturing of the lateral crura to the septum or to the ipsilateral dome helps to reposition the crura and alar base medially, increases tip projection, and creates greater symmetry between the two sides. Although secondary rhinoplasty frequently is still needed, the patient achieves greater social acceptance in the formative years when primary rhinoplasty is performed.

Bilateral Cleft Lip Deformities

The primary difference between the unilateral and bilateral cleft deformities lies in the position and characteristics of the premaxilla and prolabium. The lateral segments of the bilateral cleft lip deformity are similar to the lateral segments of the unilateral deformity. The difference lies in the medial segment of the cleft, the premaxilla. In bilateral deformities, the premaxilla is either partially or completely detached from both maxillae. The premaxilla and prolabium protrude anteriorly and superiorly and generally are unrelated to the maxilla itself. The columella is most often shorter than normal. Moreover, it may not be evident on surface inspection, though medial crura of the lower lateral cartilages are present. The prolabial soft tissue, though relatively scarce, should be used to form the full vertical length of the lip. The prolabial vermilion is used for the intraoral lining. The central vermilion is built up with vermilion-muscle flaps created from the lateral lip segments, and the vermilion ridge comes from the lateral lip segments. It may be helpful to use preoperative orthodontics to rotate the premaxillary segment posteriorly and rotate the lateral maxillary segments medially in order to increase the soft tissue available for closure and reduce the tension on the repair.[47] The repair we prefer for bilateral clefts is the single stage approach described by Millard, in which the orbicularis is advanced across the cleft, and straight vertical closure lines along the skin lie in the newly created philtral ridges[48] (Fig. 186-27A to F).

Cleft Palate Repair

All palatoplasty techniques share the same goals. These include separation of the nasal cavity from the oral cavity, creation of a competent velopharyngeal valve for both swallowing and speech, preservation of midface growth, and development of functional occlusion.

Controversy surrounds timing of cleft palate repair. Improved speech outcomes are seen when the soft palate is repaired early. Dorf and Curtin[49] demonstrated a 10% occurrence of articulation errors when palatoplasty was completed by 1 year and an 86% incidence of

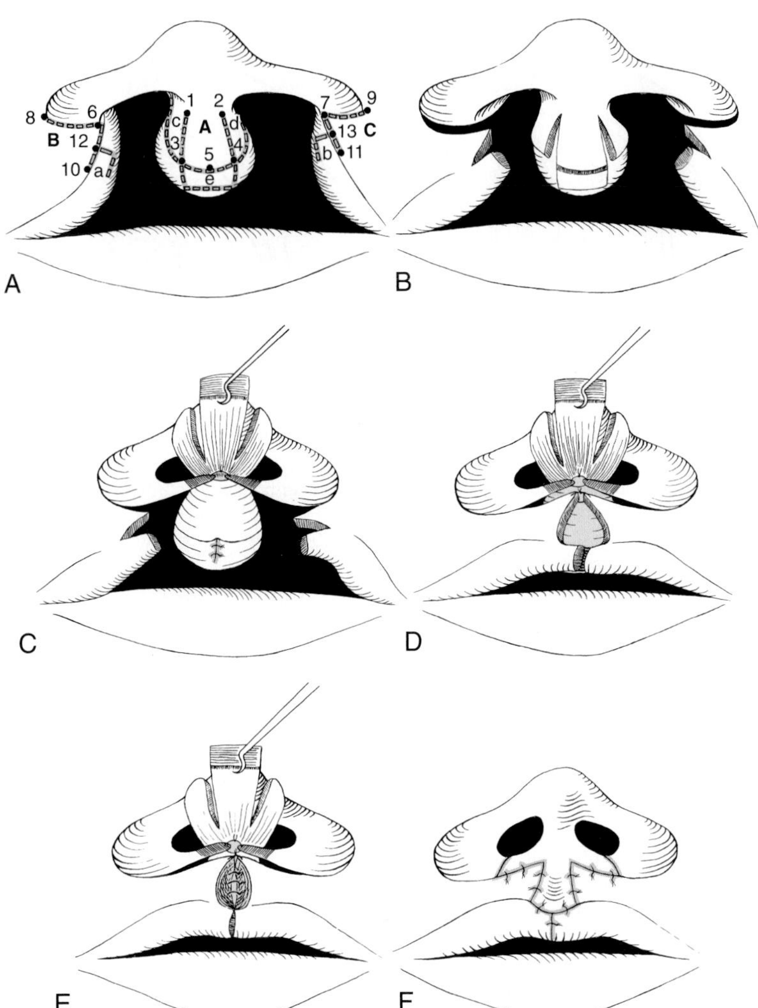

Figure 186-27. **A**, Bilateral cleft lip repair: landmarks and incisions. Prolabium provides philtral flap, A; forked flaps, c and d; and tubercle-reinforcing flap, e. Lateral lip provides flaps B and C and midline vermilion flaps a (within B) and b (within C). **B**, Bilateral cleft lip repair: flaps incised and elevated. **C**, Tips of the ala nasi de-epithelialized and sutured medially at the base of the prolabium. Excess prolabial mucosa provided the medial lining of the labial sulcus. **D**, Tips of the flaps sutured medially beneath the prolabium. **E**, Bilateral cleft lip repair: orbiuclaris oris muscle and mucosal approximation. **F**, Placement of forked flaps in the nasal sill and final suturing. Flap e (see **A**) may be used to reinforce the tubercle from behind.

articulation errors when repair was completed after 1 year. Similar results were found comparing early and late palatoplasty in isolated cleft palate. Haapanen and Rantala[50] compared three groups of children whose palatoplasty was done at mean ages of 12.9 months, 18.5 months, and 22.1 months. Significantly fewer children in the groups undergoing repair before 18 months had hypernasal speech or articulation errors or required secondary surgery to correct speech. Most surgeons and speech pathologists believe that soft palate repair should be done before the age of 12 months in order to minimize speech disorders.

Palate surgery during childhood may adversely affect facial growth. Case studies of adults with unrepaired clefts demonstrate normal midface development.[51,52] Animal studies suggest that disruption of the hard palate mucoperiosteum inhibits maxillary growth.[53] To preserve growth potential, some centers prefer a staged approach: early repair of the soft palate, obturation of the hard palate, then later surgical closure of the hard palate.[54,55] However, others have not found significant difference in maxillary development between patients who have single-stage palatoplasty versus two-stage repair.[56,57] Other factors that need to be considered are the type and severity of clefting. It appears that inherent growth deficiencies are associated with different cleft types.[58] More severe tissue deficiencies at birth in unilateral cleft lip and palate patients predict more growth retardation after cleft repair.[59] Given that this controversy over timing and staging of cleft palate repair has continued for several decades, prospective, multicenter clinical trials will be required to resolve many of the issues.

Palatoplasty Techniques

Preparation for palatoplasty requires analysis of abnormal anatomy. Knowledge of different techniques in palate repair will allow for an individualized surgical approach. The basic surgical techniques include primary veloplasty (Schweckendiek palatoplasty), bipedicled flap palatoplasty (von Langenbeck), V-Y pushback palatoplasty, unipedicled two-flap palatoplasty, and the double-opposing Z-plasty (Furlow) palatoplasty. Although credit is given to the original description of a palatoplasty technique by creating an eponym, it is important for the cleft surgeon to document the details of the technique used. Over time, many modifications have been advanced for each procedure. Important considerations for each technique are closure with minimal tension, layered closure, and reconstruction of the levator sling. The two most common techniques for palate closure are outlined next.

Two-Flap Palatoplasty

The two-flap palatoplasty is a commonly used technique for cleft palate repair and involves incisions that extend to the alveolar portion of the cleft or to the incisive foramen (Fig. 186-28). The nasal cavity can be

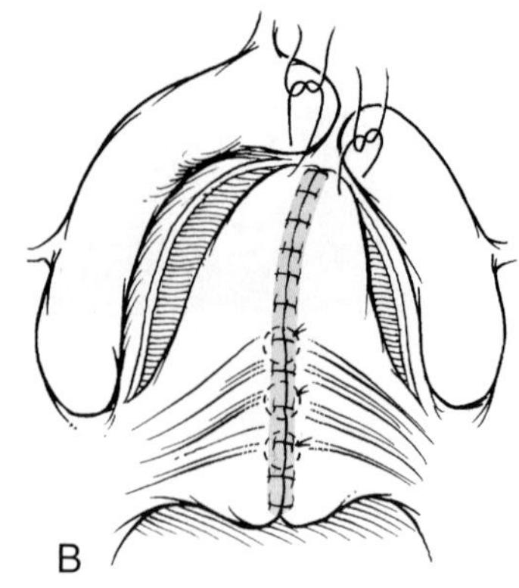

Figure 186-28. Two-flap palatoplasty. **A**, Incisions used to create unipedicled palate flaps. *Arrows* demonstrate rotation of bilateral flaps. **B**, The levator sling is reconstructed and closure is complete. In many cases, the hard palate mucoperiosteum can be reapproximated to the medial edge of the gingival incisions. This can minimize exposure of palate bone, which is believed to inhibit maxillary growth.

reconstructed by elevating vomer flaps, thereby creating four flaps used for reconstruction (not shown in Fig. 186-28). Vomer flaps are rotated laterally to unite with the mucosa at the medial edge of the nasal floor. The mucoperiosteal flaps are then rotated medially to close the cleft. The alveolar cleft is not closed using this method, nor is the palate lengthened unless a double-opposing Z-plasty (described next) is used to reconstruct the soft palate. This latter technique often is used for repair of complete primary and secondary cleft palate.

Furlow Palatoplasty (Double-Opposing Z-plasty)

The double-opposing Z-plasty palatoplasty was first described by Furlow in 1986.[60] This technique lengthens the soft palate and reconstructs the muscle sling. The two flaps containing muscle are rotated posteriorly and the two mucosa-only flaps are transposed anteriorly. It is more difficult to perform, especially in wide clefts. It can be combined with a unipedicled closure of the hard palate.[61] It also is commonly used to correct velopharyngeal insufficiency in patients with submucous cleft palate.[62] Speech outcomes are improved compared with those achieved with other palatoplasty techniques.[63,64]

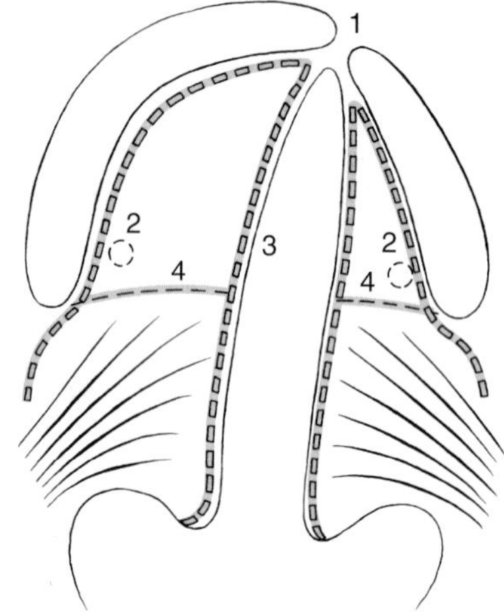

Figure 186-29. Two-flap palatoplasty. Landmarks are as follows: 1, alveolar cleft; 2, neurovascular bundle at the greater palatine foramen; 3, vomer; 4, posterior edge of hard palate. Incisions are indicated by the *dotted lines*.

Surgical Technique

Basic Principles

The patient should not have any active medical problems (other than otitis media). A family history of bleeding warrants an evaluation for a coagulopathy. Plans for airway management, especially for patients with Robin sequence, should be discussed with the anesthesiologist. A reinforced oral endotracheal tube should be used, to minimize kinking and ventilation problems while the mouth gag is in place. Most surgeons prefer the Dingman mouth gag for exposure of the oral cavity and pharynx. This mouth gag can exert significant pressure on the tongue.[65] If the mouth gag is then suspended from a Mayo stand, the exerted pressure may exceed arterial perfusion pressure to the tongue. Postoperative tongue edema risks airway obstruction and prolonged intubation. To minimize this risk, periodic release of the mouth gag during palatoplasty is recommended. Perioperative steroids (dexamethasone sodium phosphate 0.25 mg/kg) lower postoperative airway distress[66] and can reduce length of hospitalization[67] after primary palatoplasty. Perioperative antibiotics also may reduce the risk of infection. Injection of a topical anesthetic containing epinephrine into the planned incision and dissection sites and, if possible, into the greater palatine foramen helps reduce intraoperative blood loss.

Two-Flap Palatoplasty

Once general anesthesia has been achieved and the patient is in a supine position, the margins of the cleft at the junction of the nasal and oral epithelium are identified. The margins are incised sharply with a scalpel, separating the mucosa. Lateral releasing incisions are made medial to the alveolus and down to bone, and care is taken to avoid injury to the tooth buds and the neurovascular pedicle at the greater palatine foramen. This lateral incision is carried posteriorly just into the retromolar area and through mucosa only at this point (Fig. 186-29).

Dissection begins with the separation of the soft palate muscle from the nasal mucosa. At least 3 mm of mucosa is elevated sharply. To perform an intervelar veloplasty, the muscle should be freed from most of its nasal mucosa attachments laterally. This dissection is technically difficult, because the muscles adhere tightly to the nasal mucosa. In similar fashion, the oral mucosa is elevated from the soft palate muscles.

Next, the mucoperiosteum of the hard palate is elevated using a periosteal elevator. Anteriorly, this dissection is easy, but caution is taken posteriorly near the greater palatine foramen. Once the neurovascular bundle is identified, the surrounding fibrous attachments are carefully dissected from the bone. This maneuver will provide additional medial displacement of the flaps and minimize tension during repair. On the cleft side, the medial edge of the mucoperiosteal flap is released from the nasal mucosa. On the noncleft side, the mucoperiosteum is elevated from the vomer. Continuity is maintained between the vomerine mucoperiosteum and the nasal mucosa of the soft palate on this side. The soft palate muscles are then released from their abnormal attachments at the posterior edge of the hard palate (Fig. 186-30).

Rotating the flaps medially with forceps tests mobility of the flaps. If additional mobility is needed, then several other maneuvers can be used. A back-cut at the posterior edge of the vomer will allow easier closure of the nasal cavity. Extension of the relaxing incision posteriorly

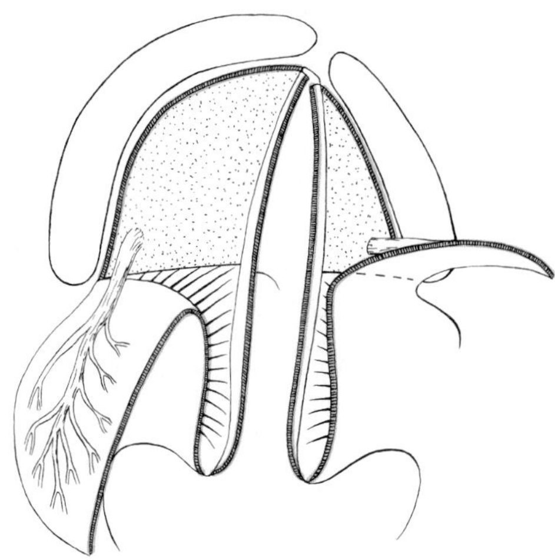

Figure 186-30. Two-flap palatoplasty: flaps incised and elevated.

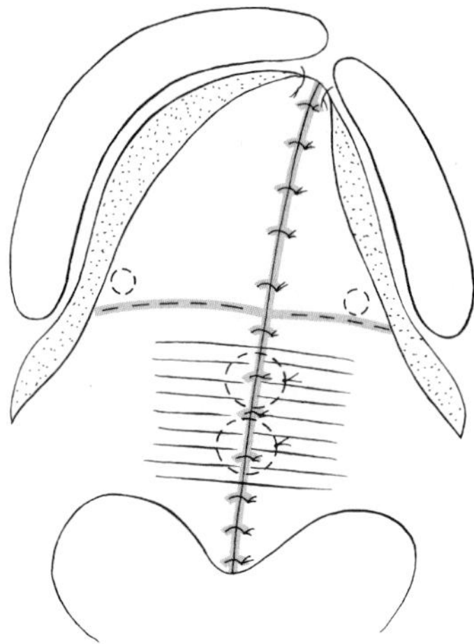

Figure 186-32. Two-flap palatoplasty: oral layer closed.

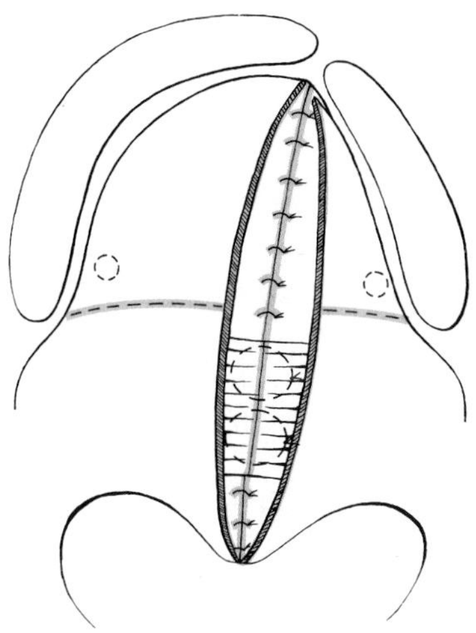

Figure 186-31. Two-flap palatoplasty: nasal mucosa and mucoperiosteum closed and levator reconstructed.

combined with blunt dissection between the pterygoid process and the superior constrictor muscle (space of Ernst) will further mobilize the anterior soft palate region. Wide clefts may require medial fracture of the hamulus, thereby releasing tension on the TVP, although concern about the potential adverse effect on eustachian tube function has been raised.[42]

Repair of the palate is done in three layers. Absorbable suture is used throughout. The nasal surface is closed with 4-0 or 5-0 suture. Tension usually is greatest at the junction of the hard and soft palate. In patients with wide clefts, primary closure of the nasal surface at this junction may not be possible. Clark and associates[68] report using acellular dermal grafts (LifeCell, Branchburg, New Jersey) placed between the nasal and oral surfaces to provide a biologic surface for healing by secondary intention. Several buried sutures placed using a horizontal mattress technique are used to repair the soft palate muscles and to reconstruct the levator sling (Fig. 186-31). The oral surface is closed first along the cleft edge. Mattress sutures help evert the edge of the mucoperiosteum. Simple sutures are used to close the oral mucosa. Laterally, closure is completed by reapproximating the mucoperiosteum to the medial alveolus; only sutures that do not increase tension along the cleft edge should be used (Fig. 186-32). If there is exposed bone or tissue (for example, the stippled area in Fig. 186-32), usually in the region of the hamulus and posterior hard palate, then microfibrillar collagen (Avitene; Bard, Salt Lake City, Utah) is packed into the open wounds to optimize hemostasis.

Double-Opposing Z-plasty Palatoplasty (Furlow Palatoplasty)

The double-opposing Z-plasty palatoplasty (Furlow palatoplasty) applies specifically to the repair of the soft palate and reconstruction of a levator sling. If the patient has a cleft involving the hard palate, closure of the hard palate is the same as for a two-flap palatoplasty. It is recommended that the soft palate dissection be completed before the incisions and elevation of flaps that are performed on the hard palate. By keeping the hard palate tissues intact, tension is provided to enable easier dissection of the soft palate needed for the Furlow palatoplasty. Elevation of the muscles from the nasal mucosa is technically challenging and is easier if the instruments are handled using a "forehand" grip and movements. For a right-handed surgeon, this means dissecting the muscles from the left aspect of the soft palate. Handedness then determines the types of flaps created elsewhere in the soft palate. A left-handed surgeon would perform the double-opposing Z-plasty in a mirror image of what is described next.

Incisions are first made sharply along the left cleft margin separating the oral and nasal mucosa. (If a double-opposing Z-plasty palatoplasty is being performed for repair of a submucous cleft palate, the midline incision should go only through the oral mucosa and leave the nasal mucosa intact until later.) A second incision is made from the apex of the cleft or 3 mm posterior to the junction of the hard and soft palate to just posterior to the hamulus. This incision parallels the posterior margin of the hard palate. It is important to leave at least 2 mm of mucosa posterior to the bony margin. Care must be taken not to tear or cut through the nasal surface. Dissection proceeds to the lateral pharyngeal wall from just superior to the tonsillar fossa to beneath the hamulus. The levator veli palatini muscle is released from the posterior edge of the hard palate using electrocautery (Fig. 186-33).

An anteriorly based oral mucosa flap is then created on the right soft palate. Incisions are made along the cleft margin and from the base of the uvula to just posterior to the hamulus. The mucosa and submucosa, a fatty layer that contains several unnamed feeder vessels, are elevated sharply from the muscle layer. This dissection plane is indistinct. By maintaining tension between the mucosa and muscle, thin muscle fibers are identified at the inferior edge of the muscle bundle. The oral mucosa flap is elevated to the posterior edge of the hard palate and over the hamulus (Fig. 186-34).

The right soft palate muscle is released from the posterior edge of the hard palate. Care must be taken to maintain at least 3 mm of nasal mucosa posterior to the edge of the hard palate. If this incision is too close to the bony edge, then suture closure becomes quite difficult once the left mucosa flap is transposed. The fourth flap is created from the left nasal mucosa. Scissors are used to incise from the base of the uvula to beneath the hamulus (Fig. 186-35). If a hard palate cleft repair is needed, the mucoperiosteal flaps are raised after creating the four flaps from the soft palate.

These four flaps are transposed so that the mucosa-only flaps are rotated anteriorly and the muscle-containing flaps are rotated posteriorly. Suturing is done with 4-0 or 5-0 absorbable suture. Use of a small needle with a high degree of curvature (P-2 needle; Ethicon, Somerville, New Jersey) often is necessary for closure along the posterior edge of the hard palate incisions. The nasal layer is closed before the oral layer (Fig. 186-36). It is helpful to first suture the apex of the flap into the recipient corner, thereby stretching the flap. Any length discrepancy between incisions can be accounted for during closure. The uvula should be reconstructed. Contracture of the oral mucosa-muscle flap may restrict its advancement during the oral closure. Occasionally, a short V-Y advancement can be done at the right anterior corner to facilitate watertight closure of the oral surface.

Complications

During palatoplasty, hemostasis should be secured with pressure and electrocautery. Typically, less than 50 mL of blood is lost if epinephrine is used during initial injections and careful hemostasis is maintained. Postoperative bleeding is rare unless open wounds exist. After removal of the mouth gag and before extubation, the floor of mouth and tongue should be inspected for signs of edema. Prolonged tongue ischemia may result in edema with the potential for airway obstruction. Periodic

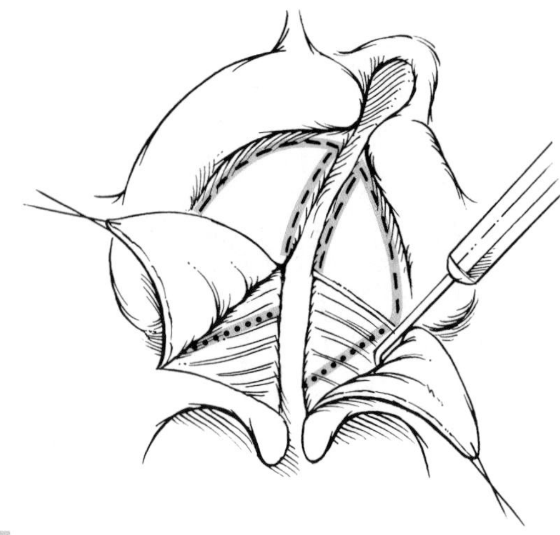

Figure 186-34. Oral mucosa flaps fully elevated. Soft palate muscles are seen on the right, and only the submucosa of the nasopharynx is exposed on the left. The *dotted lines* indicate where the incisions are planned for the next two flaps on the soft palate. *Dashed lines* on the hard palate indicate where incisions are to be made.

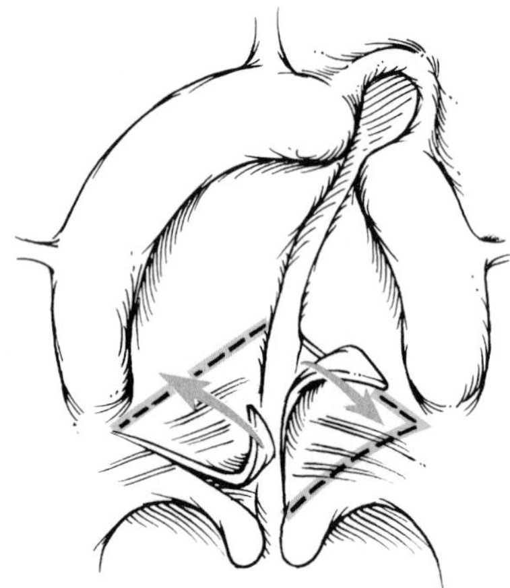

Figure 186-33. Double-opposing Z-plasty (Furlow) palatoplasty for a unilateral left complete cleft palate. Initial incisions and elevation of the first two flaps are indicated by the *arrows*. The left flap consists of oral mucosa and soft palate muscles. The right flap consists of oral mucosa and submucosa (perspective shown is that of a right-handed surgeon).

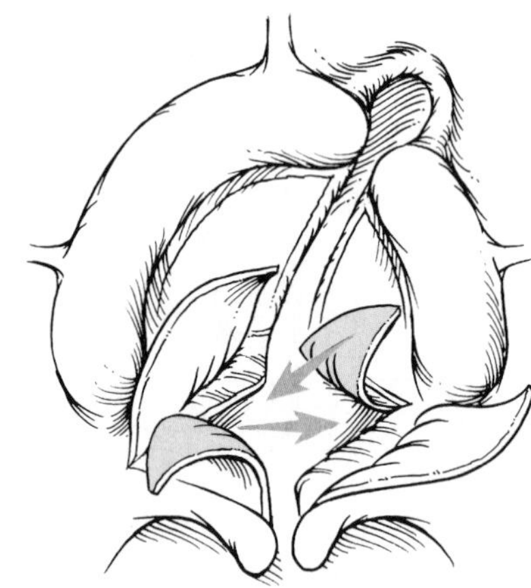

Figure 186-35. The nasopharyngeal mucosa flap from the left is transposed anteriorly. The flap containing soft palate muscle and nasopharyngeal mucosa from the right is transposed posteriorly.

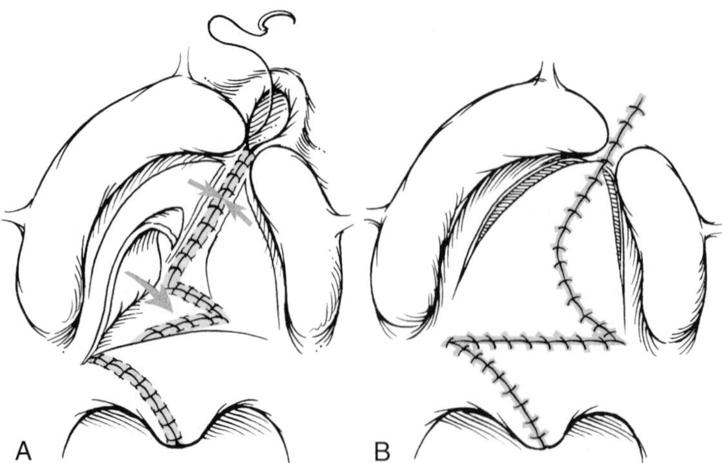

Figure 186-36. **A,** Closure of the oral surface of the soft palate. The muscle-mucosa flap from the right has been transposed and the oral mucosa is rotated anteriorly *(single large arrow)*. Nasal closure for double-opposing Z-plasty (Furlow) palatoplasty in a unilateral left complete cleft palate is also shown *(opposing smaller arrows)*. Nasal mucosa has been released along the cleft edge. Mucoperiosteal flaps were elevated bilaterally and pedicled from the greater palatine foramen *(not shown)*. **B,** Closure of the oral mucosa of both the hard and soft palate has been completed. If the incisions medial to the alveolus can be closed without substantially increasing tension, this is now performed.

release of the mouth gag during surgery should help prevent tongue ischemia.[65] Before extubation, a heavy silk suture typically is placed around the tongue tip. This "tongue stitch" may be used in lieu of an oral airway to aid postoperative airway management. This suture often is removed once the child is fully aware in the postanesthesia care unit but may be left until a safe airway is secure.

Historically, high rates of oronasal fistula formation have been reported after palatoplasty. When only fistulas that occur in the areas after primary repair (i.e., not intentional) are considered, the frequency of oronasal fistula is 8.7% to 23%.[69-71] Severity of clefting and type of cleft were the main risk factors identified. Recurrence rates after fistula repair range from 25% to 33%. Sites of fistulization typically are the anterior hard palate and the junction of the hard and soft palate.

The most common complication after palatoplasty is velopharyngeal insufficiency. Surgical technique may be a factor, with lower rates reported for double-opposing Z-plasty than for more traditional methods.[72] This topic is fully discussed in Chapter 187, Velopharyngeal Dysfunction.

Special Considerations in Patients with Cleft Palate

Robin Sequence

First described in 1923 in his native France and subsequently reported in the English literature in 1934, the Robin sequence is named for Dr. Pierre Robin, who highlighted the importance of the combination of micrognathia, glossoptosis, and cleft palate.[73,74] In the absence of other congenital abnormalities, the triad is considered a sequence because the micrognathia is the primary cause of the glossoptosis and cleft palate. However, the Robin sequence often is found associated with other abnormalities.[75,76] In such cases, the term "syndromic Robin sequence" has been used. Associated abnormalities are found in 52% to 83% of patients with Robin sequence. Stickler syndrome is the most common syndrome in children with Robin sequence, seen in 14% to 34% of cases. Sensorineural hearing loss and myopia are common findings in infants with Stickler syndrome. It is recommended that all children who present with features suggestive of Robin sequence have early hearing and vision screening. In nonsyndromic Robin sequence, it is unclear whether compensatory or "catch-up" growth occurs in the first years of life. The work of some investigators suggests that mandibular growth may be stimulated by tongue activity and oral motor development.[77,78] However, other work has shown that growth of the mandible in patients with Robin sequence is not significantly different from that in control subjects.[79-81]

Glossoptosis is an important factor that contributes to the upper airway obstruction commonly seen in Robin sequence. Retrodisplacement of the tongue into the oropharynx and inadequate support from the genioglossus muscle are the consequences of specific anatomic deficiencies of the mandible in these patients: a small body and short ramus. Negative pressure within the pharynx during inspiration and swallowing, combined with the anatomic and physiologic limitations imposed by micrognathia, frequently result in an unstable airway and dysphagia.[82-84] Severity of obstruction can be assessed by clinical evaluation, pulse oximetry, or polysomnography.[85]

Several strategies have been advocated for treating the airway obstruction in patients with Robin sequence.[82,83] These include prone positioning, which allows the tongue to fall away from the posterior pharyngeal wall.[82] If this strategy is ineffective in maintaining airway patency, a nasopharyngeal airway can help.[86] Maintenance of the nasopharyngeal airway can be challenging, as the tube requires suctioning and changing periodically. Oral feeding in this setting is made difficult owing to the frequent reflux of the meal through the tube. Gavage feeding may be needed in such cases.[87] Other centers will perform a glossopexy or lip-tongue adhesion in infants in whom positioning fails to maintain airway patency.[88-90] High success rates are reported when patients are selected on the basis of nasopharyngoscopy findings of an anterior-to-posterior collapse by the tongue, causing occlusion of the airway.[88] Complications of glossopexy include dehisence, which has been reported as high as 56%.[91]

Tracheostomy has traditionally been used for those patients with Robin sequence who also have severe airway obstruction or synchronous airway lesions, or in those infants in whom airway management by other methods has been unsuccessful.[82,83,92,93] Tracheostomy establishes an airway distal to the pharyngeal obstruction, and it has minimal impact on oropharyngeal swallowing mechanics. Another advantage of the tracheostomy is that it can be used during subsequent surgical procedures such as palatoplasty. A secure airway during palatoplasty is important, because airway problems occurring immediately after palatoplasty were most commonly seen in children with Robin sequence.[94] Nearly all patients with isolated Robin sequence who have tracheostomy performed to relieve airway obstruction can be decannulated after palatoplasty.[93] However, tracheostomy is not without difficulties in management and risks of serious complications.

Mandibular distraction osteogenesis is another method used to address the inadequate airway in infants with Robin sequence. First described in children in 1992,[95] the procedure is now advocated as primary treatment to relieve upper airway obstruction in these patients.[96,97] Bilateral mandibular osteotomies are performed and a distraction device is placed on either side of the osteotomy. Over the next several weeks, the distraction and subsequent consolidation across the osteotomy sites act to regenerate bone of the mandible, thereby lengthening the body or the ascending ramus. This in turn advances the tongue away from the posterior pharynx. In one series, all patients were successfully extubated or decannulated using this technique.[97] Selection criteria for mandibular distraction versus other airway management strategies have not been established.

Velocardiofacial or Microdeletion Chromosome 22 Syndrome

Velocardiofacial syndrome (VCFS) encompasses numerous phenotypic manifestations. It is the most common syndrome associated with isolated patients with isolated cleft palate.[98] It has become increasingly recognized in cleft palate patients and patients who present with velopharyngeal insufficiency (see Chapter 187, Velopharyngeal Dysfunction).[99,100] In one large series, 9% of patients had cleft palate and 32% had velopharyngeal insufficiency.[101] The palatal evaluation may reveal overt, submucous, or occult submucous clefting. Its phenotypic expression overlaps with DiGeorge syndrome and conotruncal anomaly face syndrome.[102] Because of the phenotypic overlap among these three syndromes, each a result of a deletion in the long arm of chromosome 22, the name "22q11 deletion syndrome" has been suggested.[103] More than 100 anatomic and functional abnormalities have been described in patients with VCFS.[101,104] The incidence of this deletion is estimated at 1 in 3000 to 1 in 4000 children.[105] Fluorescence in situ hybridization probes are available to identify patients with this deletion. The prevalence of patients with the phenotypic diagnosis of VCFS who test positive for the deletion is 68% to 81%.[102,106] Although its transmission is as an autosomal dominant trait, most cases represent a de novo deletion.[101,107]

The head and neck manifestations of VCFS are numerous. Facial dysmorphism can be subtle and several different findings are described. These include an elongated midface ("adenoid facies"), a shortened midface with malar hypoplasia, broad nasal base, low-set ears, thickened helical rims, mandibular micrognathia, and microcephaly.[108-110] Dysphagia is common and may present during infancy.[111] The dysphagia may be independent of cleft palate or cardiac involvement and may persist beyond infancy. Pharyngeal hypotonia and poor oral phase of swallowing are both felt to contribute to the dysphagia. Middle ear disease is common, with reports of 22% to 88% of patients affected.[108,109] Conductive hearing loss and chronic suppurative otitis media may result. These patients may require repeated tympanostomy tube placement. Adenoidectomy should be carefully considered in patients with VCFS, because a high incidence of postoperative velopharyngeal insufficiency has been described.[99] In addition to the high frequency of clefting seen in these patients, other factors may contribute to the eustachian tube dysfunction. An abnormally flattened basisphenoid has been described in patients with VCFS,[112] and palatal muscle dysplasia also is seen (Fig. 186-37). Medialized carotid arteries are found in some patients with VCFS, increasing risk for injury during pharyngeal

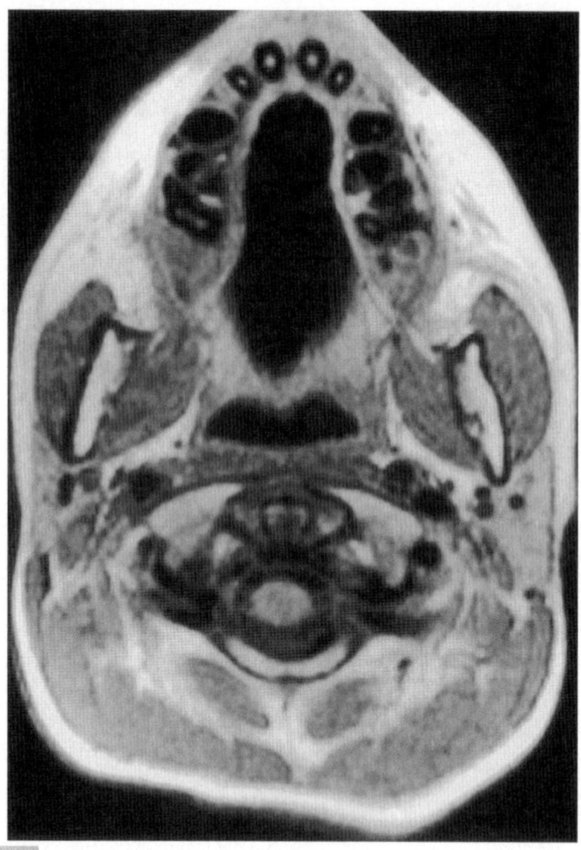

Figure 186-37. Magnetic resonance image of the soft palate in a patient with velocardiofacial syndrome. Note the increased signal intensity of this T1-weighted image, suggesting increased fat composition within the soft palate as compared with the surrounding facial and pharyngeal muscles.

surgery.[113] Imaging of the pharynx using magnetic resonance angiography is suggested,[114] although spontaneous resolution has been described.[115] Searching for pulsations along the posterior pharyngeal wall during nasendoscopy is recommended for this population. Velopharyngeal insufficiency is common in VCFS; the evaluation and management of this problem are covered elsewhere (see Chapter 187, Velopharyngeal Dysfunction). Vocal cord nodules may be found. Patients with velopharyngeal insufficiency may compensate by using glottal stops. Anterior laryngeal web also may be seen in these patients.[101]

Submucous Cleft Palate

A bifid uvula, a notch in the posterior hard palate due to the absence of the posterior vomerine spine, and a translucent zone in the midline of the soft palate constitute the classic findings with submucous cleft palate (SMCP) (see Fig. 186-5). Large population-based studies suggest a prevalence for SMCP of 1 in 1250.[116] An occult SMCP, not evident on oral examination, occurs when only the muscularis uvulae is dehiscent.[117] The diagnosis of occult SMCP is made during nasendoscopy for evaluation of velopharyngeal insufficiency[118] (see Chapter 187, Velopharyngeal Dysfunction).

The cause for the palatal dysfunction seen in patients with SMCP may involve several factors. Abnormal insertion of the levator palatini into the posterior margin of the hard palate and diathesis of the muscularis uvulae may result in the inability of the posterior margin of the soft palate to fully contact the pharyngeal wall. Histologic analysis of surgical specimens from patients with SMCP revealed increased fibrosis, especially within muscle fascicles; fascicular disorganization; and hypoplastic myocytes.[44] However, there does not appear to be differences in craniofacial morphology between symptomatic and asymptomatic children with SMCP.[119] Longitudinal studies indicate that more than 50% of patients with SMCP will develop speech disorders requiring surgery.[120,121] These studies were conducted in tertiary referral cleft clinics, thus the actual frequency of symptomatic patients with SMCP may be lower. SMCP appears more frequently in association with other craniofacial abnormalities. Occult SMCP is the most common palatal abnormality associated with VCFS, seen in 67% to 69% of affected patients. Overt SMCP may be found in another 24% of patients with this syndrome.[108,109] The soft palate should be diligently inspected and palpated prior to adenoidectomy because of the high prevalence of SMCP in cleft lip–only patients. The relationship between SMCP and otitis media is unclear. Higher rates of recurrent otitis media or need for tympanostomy tube placement in the first year of life were found in children with bifid uvula, but the difference was not significant. This difference was not seen at 3 years.[122] Similarly, no difference in effusions was found between surgical patients with and without bifid uvula.[123] Whether bifid uvula–only is an adequate marker for other deficiencies in SMCP is unknown. The discovery of SMCP in infancy or early childhood requires follow-up evaluation through adolescence. Because many children remain asymptomatic, surgical correction of the palatal deformity is indicated only when clinical problems are refractory to medical therapy.

Ear Disease

It has been recognized for some time that children with cleft palate have a very high frequency of middle ear disease compared with the noncleft population. Paradise and colleagues[124] first reported that all children with cleft palate examined by pneumatic otoscopy and otomicroscopy showed effusions. Muntz[125] reported that 96% of children with cleft palate required tympanostomy tube placement. Nearly 50% of these children required repeat tympanostomy tube placement. Complications in this group included chronic tympanic membrane perforation in 13%, chronic suppurative otitis media in 6%, and cholesteatoma in 1%. Dominguez and Harker[126] revealed the importance of routine follow-up care by an otolaryngologist to minimize complications of ear disease. The rates of cholesteatoma formation were reduced from 9% to 3% when a coordinated team approach to care of the CLP patient was instituted.

Otitis media with effusion develops within the first months of life in a child with cleft palate. In a prospective study, Dhillon[127] found middle ear effusions by aspiration in 97% of ears at 4 months of age. This study also demonstrated that eustachian tube function did not return within 2 years after palatoplasty in 80% of patients. Other prospective studies support poor eustachian tube function and otitis media as problems that persist during the first few years after palatoplasty.[128,129] It should be noted that in each of these studies, a "traditional" palatoplasty was performed. The potential effect that the type of palatoplasty has on otologic outcomes is unknown.

Frequency of otitis media decreases with increasing age of the child with cleft palate. Smith and colleagues[130] used audiology and tympanometry to determine that the average recovery time for eustachian tube function was 6 years after palatoplasty. Among children followed for at least 6 years, 70% of ears had normal eustachian tube function. More than 90% of the ears that recovered eustachian tube function were able to maintain normalcy. Tympanoplasty results were similar for patients with cleft palate (including SMCP) and children without cleft deformity with regard to postoperative air-bone gap, graft survival, and need for postoperative ventilation tube.[131]

Abnormalities of the cartilage and muscles surrounding the eustachian tube are responsible for the high prevalence of otitis media associated with cleft palate. Paratubal cartilage abnormalities have been described that may contribute to dysfunction in patients with cleft palate. Hypoplasia of the lateral cartilage relative to the medial cartilage was found in infants with cleft palate.[132,133] The curvature of the eustachian tube lumen, as determined by the shape of the surrounding cartilage, also was found to be abnormal when compared with noncleft specimens. Cephalometric data suggest that the width and angulation of the skull base with respect to the eustachian tube are different in patients with cleft palate.[134] Abnormal insertions of the TVP and levator veli palatini muscles into the cartilages and skull base also may adversely affect their role in eustachian tube function. Matsune and colleagues[135] studied temporal bone specimens from patients with cleft palate and compared them with those from non-cleft control subjects. No insertion of the TVP muscle to the lateral paratubal cartilage was found in 40% of CP specimens. All normal specimens demonstrated an insertion of the TVP to the lateral cartilage. Moreover, the length of TVP muscle inserted into the cartilage was reduced in CP specimens. Huang and coworkers[43] dissected fresh cadavers of normal adults. Their detailed analysis of the anatomy of the TVP and levator veli palatini muscles suggests that the TVP opens the eustachian tube directly by traction on the lateral cartilage. The levator veli palatini may open the eustachian tube by displacement of the medial cartilage. Some studies have identified the muscle fibers inserting into the lateral cartilage as a distinct muscle, the dilatator tubae.[136,137] It remains unclear to what degree the altered anatomy of the paratubal muscles directly affects eustachian tube dysfunction, because the levator veli palatini muscle is more severely affected by cleft palate.

Insertion of ventilation tubes is the standard treatment for otitis media in patients with cleft palate. Controversy surrounds the timing of ear tube placement. Otitis media with effusion is known to decrease hearing thresholds. Decreased hearing at a very young age may affect future speech and language development, especially in this high-risk group of patients. However, high rates of otorrhea from ears with ventilation tubes placed before palatoplasty have been reported; excessive compliance of the eustachian tube before palatoplasty has been suggested as the etiologic basis.[138] Chronic otorrhea resolved only after palatoplasty in four children who had early ear tube placement.[139] No long-term studies have been conducted to determine whether early placement of ventilation tubes, and correction of hearing loss, affect speech outcomes in patients born with cleft palate. Newborn hearing screening can provide an early indication of auditory function and help with treatment decisions such as when ear tubes should be placed.

SUGGESTED READINGS

Butts SC, Tatum SA 3rd, Mortelliti AJ, et al. Velo-cardio-facial syndrome: the pediatric otolaryngologist's perspective. *Curr Opin Otolaryngol Head Neck Surg.* 2005;13:371.

Huang MH, Lee ST, Rajendran K. Anatomic basis of cleft palate and velopharyngeal surgery: implications from a fresh cadaveric study. *Plast Reconstr Surg.* 1998;101:613.

Jones KL, ed. *Smith's Recognizable Patterns of Human Malformation.* 6th ed. Philadelphia: WB Saunders; 2005.

Mathes SJ. Pediatric plastic surgery. In: Mathes SJ, Hentz VR, eds. *Plastic Surgery.* 2nd ed. Philadelphia: Saunders; 2006.

McCarthy JG, Cutting CB, Hogan VM. Introduction to facial clefts. In: Mathes SJ, ed. *Plastic Surgery.* Philadelphia: WB Saunders; 1990.

Millard DR. *Cleft Craft: The Evolution of Its Surgery.* Boston: Little, Brown; 1980.

Muntz HR. An overview of middle ear disease in cleft palate children. *Facial Plast Surg.* 1993;9:177.

Myer, CM 3rd, Reed JM, Cotton RT, et al. Airway management in Pierre Robin sequence. *Otolaryngol Head Neck Surg.* 1998;118:630.

Sadler TW, ed. Head and neck embryology. In: *Langman's Medical Embryology.* 6th ed. Baltimore: Williams & Wilkins; 1990:315.

Sykes JM, Senders CW, eds. Surgery of cleft lip and palate deformities. *Facial Plast Surg Clin North Am.* 1996;4.

Zucchero TM, Cooper ME, Maher BS, et al. Interferon regulatory factor 6 (IRF6) gene variants and the risk of isolated cleft lip or palate. *N Engl J Med.* 2004;351:769.

For complete list of references log onto www.expertconsult.com.

CHAPTER ONE HUNDRED AND EIGHTY-SEVEN

Velopharyngeal Dysfunction

Harlan Muntz

Marshall E. Smith

Cara Sauder

Key Points

- Velopharyngeal inadequacy refers to any type of dysfunction and may be categorized as insufficiency, incompetence, and mislearning.
- "Phoneme-specific" velopharyngeal dysfunction (VPD) is diagnosed when one or more phonemes are abnormally produced with increased resonance while the rest of the speech is normal. The increased resonance most often is noted with /s/, /sh/, and /z/, and rarely, /f/ phonemes.
- Recommendations for management of VPD are best made jointly by a team that includes the surgeon, speech-language pathologist, and dentist or prosthodontist if needed.
- Compensatory articulation errors that are a result of VPD alone do not frequently occur with oral motor weakness. Therefore, oral motor exercises are not appropriate unless there is evidence of oral motor weakness in addition to VPD.
- The Furlow palatoplasty reorients the levator while also thickening and lengthening the palate.
- All surgical corrections of VPD may lead to airway obstruction.
- It is helpful for the otolaryngologist, speech-language pathologist, and other team members to take a "transdisciplinary" approach to the management of VPD.

In the English language, only three phonemes normally are produced with nasal air escape—/n/, /m/, and /ng/. All of the other sounds are produced with oral air flow. In speech production, the velopharynx is considered an articulator, as are the jaw, tongue, lips, pharynx, and larynx. These articulators work together to produce the various sounds of speech. Normal velopharyngeal function varies according to the sounds of speech produced. Factors that affect velopharyngeal valving include vowel height, consonant type, proximity of nasal sounds to oral sounds, utterance length, speaking rate, and tongue height. For vowels, velar position is higher for vowels with a high pharyngeal constriction such as /i/ and /u/ than for low-pharyngeal-constriction vowels such as /a/. The velar port generally is closed for vowels, except when the vowel is in proximity to a nasal consonant. The velopharyngeal port therefore changes its relatively open and closed states depending on the balance of oral versus nasal consonants occurring in the speech stimuli. Velar movement may vary widely in velocity and displacement with the tasks of the particular speech, particularly speaking rate.

If the velopharynx is not functioning correctly or if a defect in the palate allows the oral sound to resonate through the nose, speech may be perceived as abnormal. Incompetence of the velopharyngeal mechanism leads to increased hypernasality, nasal turbulence, or nasal emission. If an obstruction to nasal airflow is present, the resonance is hyponasal. Speech intelligibility is determined primarily by articulation; however, abnormal speech resonance distorts speech production, impairs overall speech quality, and can adversely affect intelligibility.

Functional Anatomy

The velopharyngeal port closes as the velum moves in a posterior-to-superior direction. The lateral pharyngeal walls may move medially. Occasionally, anterior movement of the posterior wall will be seen. The muscles of the velopharynx contribute to this closure (Table 187-1).

The elevation and posterior motion of the velum are attributed to the levator veli palatini (LVP). This is the main muscle mass of the velum.[1] Variation in the angle of insertion to the base of skull may change the elevation.[2] The palatoglossus and palatopharyngeus muscles pull the palate down, opposing the LVP. The palatopharyngeus muscle pull tends to stretch the velum laterally, thereby increasing the velar area and altering the shape of the contact.[2] This muscle can make subtle changes to velar height, especially when the velum is in the elevated position.[3] The musculus uvulae adds bulk to the dorsal side of the velum.

Lateral wall motion varies from person to person and depends on speech context. The greatest movement usually is below the levator eminence at the level of the full length of the velum and hard palate.[4] This movement is attributed to selective movement of the uppermost fibers of the superior constrictor. Because of the relationship between the lateral fibers of the superior constrictor and the palatopharyngeus, it has been suggested that this muscle is involved in the lateral wall motion as well.[5]

Passavant's ridge is a posterior wall feature seen in some persons during speech or swallow. It has been associated with lateral wall motion and is thought to be caused by a similar movement of the uppermost fibers of the superior constrictor and palatopharyngeus.[6] It may be involved in velopharyngeal closure in as many as one third of patients in whom Passavant's ridge is observed.[7,8] Its movement also can be seen below the level of the velopharyngeal port and therefore does not assist in the closure.

Table 187-1

Muscles of the Velopharynx

Muscle	Origination	Attachment	Function	Innervation
Tensor veli palatini	Vertical portion arises from the scaphoid fossa at the base of the internal pterygoid plate, from the spine of the sphenoid, and from the outer side of the cartilaginous portion of the eustachian tube	Terminates in a tendon that winds around the hamular process	Tenses the soft palate; opens the auditory tube during swallowing	Mandibular branch of the trigeminal nerve
Levator veli palatini	Arises from the undersurface of the apex of the petrous portion of the temporal bone and from the inner surface of the cartilaginous portion of the eustachian tube; found to occupy the intermediate 40% of the length of the soft palate*	Fibers spread out in the soft palate, where they blend with those of the opposite side	Acts as a sling when contracted to pull the velum in a posterosuperior direction[4]; major elevator of the velum[13]; positions the velum[†]	Pharyngeal plexus derived from the glossopharyngeal and vagus nerves and the facial nerve[‡]; course of the facial nerve is through the greater petrosal nerve[§]
Musculus uvulae	Palatal aponeurosis in a circumscribed area posterior to the hard palate[‖]	Inserts into the uvula	Adds bulk to the dorsal surface of the soft palate	Pharyngeal plexus; pharyngeal plexus derived from the glossopharyngeal and vagus nerves and the facial nerve[‡]
Palatoglossus	Has a fan-shaped attachment from the anterior surface of the soft palate[¶]	Courses through loose connective tissue within the anterior faucial pillar and has a tapering termination in the side of the tongue[¶]	Elevates the tongue upward and backward to constrict the pillars and probably lowers the velum**; positions the velum[†]	Pharyngeal plexus composed of branches from the glossopharyngeus and vagus cranial nerves and from the sympathetic trunk
Palatopharyngeal	Arises from the soft palate	Inserts with the stylopharyngeus into the posterior border of the thyroid cartilage	Adducts the posterior pillars, constricts the pharyngeal isthmus, narrows the velopharyngeal orifice, raises the larynx, and lowers the pharynx[††]; positions the velum[†]	Pharyngeal plexus
Superior constrictor	Arises from the lower third of the posterior margin of the internal pterygoid plate and its hamular process	Inserts into the median raphe	Medial movement of the lateral aspects of the pharyngeal walls[4]; high levels of activity are related to laughter[13]; may function to draw the velum posteriorly[13]; pulls the posterior wall and posterolateral angle	Pharyngeal plexus derived from the glossopharyngeal and vagus nerves and the facial nerve[‡]

*Data from Boorman JG, Sommerlad BC. Levator palati and palatal dimples: their anatomy, relationship and clinical significance. *Br J Plast Surg.* 1985;38:326.

†Data from Finkelstein Y, Shapiro-Feinberg M, Talmi YP, Nachmani A, DeRowe A, Ophir D. Axial configuration of the velopharyngeal valve and its valving mechanism. *Cleft Palate Craniofac J.* 1995;32:299.

‡Data from Nishio J, Matsuya T, Machida J, Miyazaki T. The motor nerve supply of the velopharyngeal muscles. *Cleft Palate J.* 1976;13:20.

§Data from Ibuki K, Matsuya T, Nishio J, Hamamura Y, Miyazaki T. The course of facial nerve innervation for the levator veli palatini muscle. *Cleft Palate Craniofac J.* 1978;15:209.

‖Data from Azzam NA, Kuehn DP. The morphology of musculus uvulae. *Cleft Palate J.* 1977;14:78.

¶Data from Kuehn DP, Azzam NA. Anatomical characteristics of palatoglossus and the anterior faucial pillar. *Cleft Palate Craniofac J.* 1978;15:349.

**Data from McWilliams BJ, Morris HL, Shelton RL. *Cleft Palate Speech*. Philadelphia: Mosby; 1990.

††Data from Meek MF, Coert JH, Hofer SO, Goorhuis-Brouwer SM, Nicolai JP. Short-term and long-term results of speech improvement after surgery for velopharyngeal insufficiency with pharyngeal flaps in patients younger and older than 6 years old: 10-year experience. *Ann Plast Surg.* 2003;50:13.

Approach to Diagnosis and Management of Velopharyngeal Dysfunction

Evaluation of velopharyngeal dysfunction (VPD) requires an understanding of the causes of the condition to make an appropriate diagnosis. Assessment includes an accurate study of the degree and nature of velopharyngeal function and its impact on speech production. This information is then used to formulate management recommendations, which generally include speech therapy, surgical intervention, or prosthetic obturation. These management options are reviewed later in the chapter.

Causes of Velopharyngeal Dysfunction

Velopharyngeal dysfunction refers to abnormal function of the velopharyngeal sphincter mechanism. However, it does not identify the cause. Perceptually, this dysfunction is considered a dysphonia because it affects the sound quality of the voice. The cause of the dysphonia needs to be identified. Campbell and associates[9] reported on 427 children referred to a pediatric voice and resonance clinic for voice problems. Of those children, 16% were actually found to have velopharyngeal, rather than laryngeal dysfunction. Different terminology has been used to describe the causes of VPD, and relevant terms and concepts are used inconsistently throughout the medical literature. In this chapter, we use the definitions summarized by D'Antonio and Crockett.[10] *Velopharyngeal inadequacy* refers to any type of VPD and can be divided into three etiologic categories: insufficiency, incompetence, and mislearning. Velopharyngeal *insufficiency* encompasses structural defects that result in insufficient tissue to accomplish closure—a well-known example being cleft palate. *Incompetence* describes impairment of motor control secondary to neurologic dysfunction, such as paresis or paralysis. Causes of incompetence include the sequelae of skull base surgery and tumors around the jugular foramen and vagus nerve, or central nervous system (CNS) impairment from brainstem stroke. *Mislearning* is the result of etiologic factors that are independent of structural defects or neuromotor pathology.

Congenital anatomic conditions affecting velopharyngeal function most commonly are attributable to clefting of the palate. VPD in the absence of an overt cleft palate also occurs. Affected children may have other anatomic abnormalities or functional disorders causing velopharyngeal insufficiency. These include congenital short palate, palatopharyngeal disproportion, a less overt palate deficiency called occult submucous cleft palate (absence of the musculus uvulae), and longitudinally oriented levators. Hypertrophic tonsils occasionally can cause insufficiency by impeding palate closure. Neurogenic causes of velopharyngeal incompetence include muscular dystrophies, myasthenia gravis, traumatic brain injury, Down syndrome, and velocardiofacial syndrome (22q11 deletion). An adenoidectomy can create or unmask VPD in any of these settings. In velopharyngeal insufficiency, a large adenoid can compensate for a short palate. In velopharyngeal incompetence, adenoidectomy can compensate for a poorly mobile palate. With removal of the adenoidal tissue, the mechanism of compensation is eliminated. Velopharyngeal inadequacy has been reported to occur after 1 in 1500 adenoidectomies.[11,12]

Assessment

Perceptual Speech Analysis

Most otolaryngologists will encounter children with VPD in their practice. In taking the history of a child referred for a voice or speech problem, the clinician should listen carefully to input from the parent or caregiver, who typically spends the most time hearing the child speak. Then, attention needs to be paid to the speech of the child, who often is shy and does not speak voluntarily. Playing games or asking direct questions can stimulate the child to begin spontaneous speech. This perceptual evaluation will provide the clinician with a sense of the language level, articulation, and the nasal resonance as the child is speaking. The possibility of a diagnosis of VPD should be considered even in children referred for other concerns.

If VPD is suspected, a few easy tests will further elucidate the problem. Many of these tests are quickly and easily performed in the office setting with a reasonably cooperative patient. These include nasal occlusion and mirror fogging tests during the child's production of various phonemes or phrases selected to provoke the symptoms.

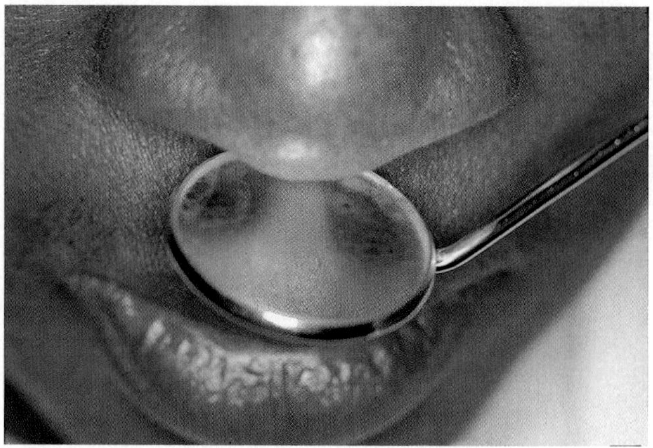

Figure 187-1. Mirror technique; note the fogging with nasal air escape.

Table 187-2

Examples of Tasks to Evaluate

Nasal Consonants	
Ma ma	Money
Na na	Monkey
Momma made lemon jam	Nancy is a nurse

Hyponasal resonance is most noted in the sounds /m/, /n/, and /ng/. These nasalized consonants will be altered with decreased nasal airflow. The /m/ will be changed to sound like /b/, the /n/ changed to sound like /d/, and the /ng/ to a hard /g/. Humming the /m/ sound will not change with nose plugging if the nose is already occluded. In addition, the examiner will not feel nasal vibrations. Normally, a mirror held under the nose should fog with voicing of the nasal consonants (Fig. 187-1). If the voice quality is the same with or without occlusion of the nose, then nasal or nasopharyngeal obstruction is present. Hyponasal resonance can be described as that quality of speech associated with the congestion of a common cold. Large adenoids or congested nasal turbinates also may be seen. Repetition of words or sentences that are loaded with nasal consonants will aid in documentation of this abnormality (Table 187-2). The velopharynx continues to be active during production of words and phrases with nasal consonant sounds but will be between a relaxed and a closed state.

Hypernasality or increased nasal resonance will be noted with production of non-nasal phonemes (Table 187-3). Because most sounds (vowels and consonants) in the English language are non-nasal, there are many phonemes to work with. The early phonologic repertoire usually includes the bilabial plosives /p, b/ and lingua-alveolar phonemes /t, d/. Using phonemes—words and sentences loaded with these sounds—allows the listener to assess speech resonance (normal or hypernasal). Plugging the nose while the child repeats the /p, b, t, d/ sounds or during sustained production of /s/ or /sh/ will result in noticeable change in resonance if there is hypernasality on these sounds. The use of a mirror beneath the nose during speech tasks also will assist in the detection of the nasal air escape (see Fig. 187-1). Fogging of the mirror typically is observed only for production of nasals and nasalized vowels. Increasing the complexity of the tasks (i.e., sounds to words to phrases to sentences) may document deterioration of the velopharyngeal competence. The degree of openness is determined by the phonetic environment. Some children will do less well if nasal and non-nasal phonemes are mixed. Repetition of tasks during a period of minutes

Table 187-3

Examples of Tasks to Evaluate

Non-Nasal Consonants		
Pa pa pa	Daddy did it	Sustain "s"
Baby	Too tight	Sustain "sh"
Puppy	Go get an egg	Count from "sixty to seventy"
Puffy	Forty-four fat fish	Baby bib
Daddy	Sissy saw it	Get it out

may unmask velopharyngeal fatigue, as seen in myasthenia gravis. Velar height or elevation is most pronounced during the "high" vowels of /i/ and /u/[13] and the fricative /s/.[14] Even if velopharyngeal function is improving, production of these sounds may remain difficult.

The clinician also may encounter "phoneme-specific" VPD, or mislearning. In this entity, one or more phonemes are produced abnormally with increased resonance, while the rest of the speech is normal.[15] It most often is noted with production of /s/, /sh/, /z/, and rarely, /f/ phonemes. A nasal fricative substitution is characteristic. Because these are predominant sounds in the English language, the patient often is believed to be globally hypernasal. Because other non-nasal sounds demonstrate no air escape, however, the velopharynx should be recognized to be otherwise functional. Appropriate articulation therapy usually will correct this abnormality.

The diagnosis of hypernasality may be confounded by concomitant dysphonia or hyponasality. Hoarseness will distort the sound enough that mild VPD may be overlooked. More than 40% of children with VPD also have dysphonia.[16] The use of the mirror test helps separate VPD from laryngeal pathology.

Children with VPD also may have nasal or pharyngeal airway obstruction that affects the nasal consonants. In such cases, both hyponasality and nasal air escape on production of non-nasal phonemes can occur. The abnormality is described as "mixed."

The presence of velopharyngeal insufficiency has a significant impact on the child's and the family's quality of life. Emotional and communication aspects are primarily affected. Parents seem to be an appropriate proxy in determining the impact of the altered speech on the child's quality of life.[17]

When VPD has been suspected on clinical examination, further testing is indicated. There are a number of techniques used for evaluation. Indirect measures to assess for VPD include nasometry and pressure-flow measurements. Imaging studies of the VP mechanism include lateral cephalometrics, speech videofluoroscopy, and speech endoscopy. Further specific resonance-related articulation assessment also is an important component in assessment of these patients.

Nasometry

Nasometry is an objective standardized assessment that measures the ratio of sound intensity between the nose and the mouth. This typically is done with voicing of standard phrases and passages. Standardized values exist for specific tasks. Calculation of the number of standard deviations from normative values for each phonemic set yields a measure of the severity of the resonance pattern. Nasometry can be used in the initial evaluation to document the degree of dysfunction. Perhaps more important, it is used in assessing progress during speech therapy or in following other interventions.[18] A discrepancy may exist between nasal scores and the perceived degree of hypernasality.[19] Figure 187-2 shows the Kay Elemetrics headgear used for this test.

Pressure Flow

Pressure and airflow measurement is another method of assessing velopharyngeal function during speech.[20-22] The nose is covered with a small mask to permit accurate measurement of nasal airflow. A probe is placed into the mouth to measure oral pressure. In the child with normal velopharyngeal function, no airflow will be detected during production of non-nasal phonemes. Oral pressure will be present if nasal air escape is detected during non-nasal sounds. An advantage to the pressure-flow technique is the ability to determine the timing of the air escape.[14] The pressure-flow technique also is used to calculate the cross-sectional nasopharyngeal airway area from the pressure-flow measures.

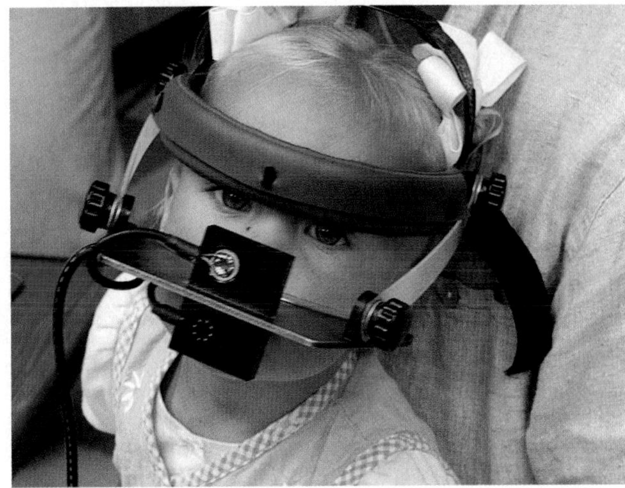

Figure 187-2. Nasometer apparatus in position.

Imaging Studies

An imaging study of the velopharyngeal mechanism is indicated when speech therapy is not progressing, if speech evaluation reveals significant hypernasality, if a diagnostic dilemma is present, or when surgery is under consideration. Lateral cephalometric x-ray studies were done in the past but are limited by a sagittal plane view and do not provide information on dynamic movement of the velopharyngeal mechanism. Current methods of imaging velopharyngeal function include speech videofluoroscopy and speech nasal endoscopy. Endoscopy has largely supplanted videofluoroscopy in most clinics today. Children older than 3 years of age most often will cooperate with the evaluation. The speech nasal examination may not be useful, however, in the child with significant developmental delays. If the child cannot produce appropriately articulated phonemes, the study will not give adequate speech information. The accuracy of articulation has a direct effect on the closure.[23] Velopharyngeal closure on swallow does not yield information regarding speech.[6] To be of value, the assessment requires appropriate articulation of phonemes.

Speech Videofluoroscopy

Videofluoroscopic evaluation has been a standard tool in assessment of the speech mechanism.[24] Generally, a speech-language pathologist attends this examination with a radiologist in the hospital imaging department, as is done for modified barium swallow studies. A small amount of barium is introduced through the nose to coat the velopharynx and improve visualization. While under fluoroscopy, the child repeats or reads a set of phoneme-specific speech tasks. Because the velopharyngeal sphincter functions in several planes of movement, accurate analysis will require at least two and preferably three views. The lateral view demonstrates the length, thickness, anterior-posterior, and superior motion of the palate, as well as the anterior movements of the posterior pharyngeal wall (Passavant's ridge). The anterior-posterior view assesses the lateral wall motion. An en face view (e.g., Towne's or submental vertex view) will look down the velopharynx and demonstrate lateral wall, velar, and posterior wall motion.

Videofluoroscopy has some limitations. Because of the radiation exposure, the speech sample may need to be shortened. Cooperation of the patient is still needed. Interpretation of the radiographs requires experience with analysis of the images. The examining team must include both a radiologist and a speech therapist with experience in this

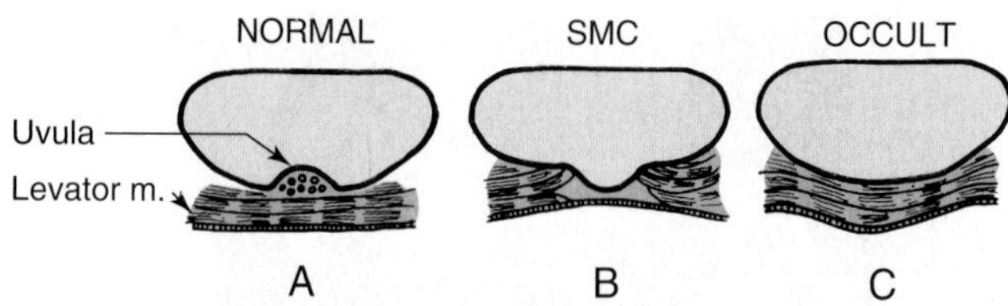

Figure 187-3. Muscle orientation of normal (**A**), submucous cleft (**B**), and occult submucous cleft (**C**). SMC, submucous cleft.

area of practice. With videofluoroscopy, closure patterns can be well defined and the level of Passavant's ridge and its participation in closure can best be assessed. Nevertheless, this assessment may still miss small fistulas and intermittent closure patterns. In addition, it is difficult to evaluate postsurgical changes. Many teams are moving toward the use of endoscopy as the standard first-line assessment tool.[25,26]

Speech Endoscopy

Speech endoscopy is now considered the most useful tool for evaluation.[27] Many otolaryngologists and some speech-language pathologists are experienced in the use of this minimally invasive diagnostic test. Ideally, the test is conducted with both the physician and speech-language pathologist in the room at the same time. If this is not possible, the examination can be video recorded for review. After topical anesthesia of the nose has been accomplished, a flexible nasopharyngoscope is introduced into the velopharynx.

The best image is obtained with the scope positioned higher in the nasopharynx to reduce parallax and fish-eye distortions. Passing the flexible scope in the middle meatus region (rather than along the floor) of the nose facilitates this optimal positioning. As with speech videofluoroscopy, a series of words, phrases, and sentences are spoken while the endoscopic images are recorded. It is important to use a microphone and record the voice, not just the video images. Endoscopy allows assessment of the static anatomy such as the nasal septum, eustachian tube orifice, adenoid pad, and structure of the musculus uvulae. Absence of the musculus uvulae is seen with occult submucous clefting (Fig. 187-3).

During speech tasks, the examiner observes velar and lateral wall motion and looks for Passavant's ridge. Incomplete closure can be documented by viewing the unclosed port or bubbling of mucus in the velopharynx. Contribution of the adenoid pad to closure, adenoid or posterior wall irregularities, and interference by the tonsils can be seen. There is no restriction on the duration of the speech sample, as constrained by the speech videofluroscopy. A clear and specific assessment can be made of both structure and function.

Four primary velopharyngeal closure patterns have been observed, as depicted in Figure 187-4.[28] These can be seen in both endoscopy and speech videofluoroscopy. These patterns are best understood in terms of the residual gap orientation on incomplete closure of the velopharynx.

The *coronal* closure pattern has a coronally oriented gap (seen in 55% of the population). The palate (velum) moves posteriorly without much contribution from the lateral walls or posterior wall. The *sagittal* closure pattern (seen in 10% to 15% of the population) leaves a gap oriented in a sagittal plane, because the major contribution to closure is from the lateral walls. The *circular* closure pattern has significant motion of the velum and the lateral walls, leaving a circular central gap (seen in 10% to 20% of the population). If the closure is *circular with Passavant's ridge*, then there is motion of the velum and lateral walls with additional presence of Passavant's ridge (seen in 15% to 20% of the population). Passavant's ridge may be present without contributing to closure.

The closure pattern may assist in prescribing surgical or prosthetic intervention. Knowing where the "gap" is should allow the clinician to decide how best to obturate that gap, as discussed next.[29-31]

Treatment

Management of VPD generally involves speech therapy or prosthetic or surgical treatment of the velopharyngeal defect, or combinations of

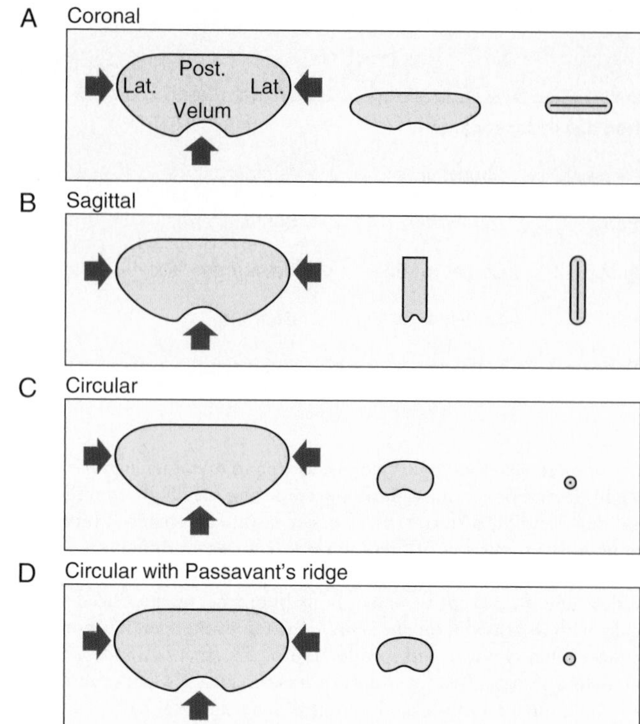

Figure 187-4. The closure patterns in the velopharynx. The pattern is based on the shape of the gap as it closes: **A,** coronal; **B,** sagittal; **C,** circular; **D,** circular with Passavant's ridge.

these approaches. Recommendations for each child generally are made jointly by a team that includes the surgeon, speech-language pathologist, and dentist or prosthodontist if needed.

Speech Therapy

Candidacy for and timing of speech therapy for children with VPD need to be examined closely by an experienced speech-language pathologist and the otolaryngologist. Speech therapy will not repair a deficiency in structure of the mechanism. Therefore, candidacy for therapy generally is limited to the following clinical circumstances: mild VPD in a child in whom appropriate stimulation yields improvement, inconsistent VPD, VPD occurring only when the child is fatigued, VPD with inappropriate articulation, VPD associated with oral-motor dysfunction, and failure of compensatory misarticulation to resolve spontaneously after surgical correction has been done. For patients who are candidates for speech therapy, the time of initiation of these services and the types of therapy recommended will depend on age, etiology, severity of VPD, cognition, hearing, phonetic inventory, expressive vocabulary, and the child and family's ability to participate in a therapeutic program.

Development of maladaptive articulations is common in children with VPD.[32,33] Excellent results from surgery can eliminate VPD, but impaired articulation may remain and greatly affect intelligibility. These abnormal articulation patterns include backing patterns, pharyngeal fricatives, glottal stops, and impaired sibilants. Speech intelligibility often is affected more by the presence of these articulation errors than by the resonance itself. If the maladaptive articulation is habituated, it may be difficult to reverse. Children who maintain articulation errors despite correction of VPD require speech therapy.[34] For children who receive surgical intervention of a structural deficit such as cleft palate, early intervention is recommended if stop oral consonants are not observed 6 to 8 weeks after surgery.[35] Phoneme-specific audible nasal air emissions can be present in children without VPD as well. Although appropriate referrals are important to rule out VPD, these children demonstrate an articulation disorder necessitating speech therapy as a primary means of treatment.

Articulation

Efficacy data regarding specific types of speech therapy techniques used to address articulation and resonance impairments in children with VPD are largely lacking. Correcting the placement and manner of articulation and adding additional phonemes to children's repertoires are primary goals of articulation therapy. Targets are selected on the basis of age appropriateness, impact on intelligibility, function, and stimulability. Careful evaluation of dentition to ensure that articulation errors are not a direct result of a structural problem also is required before initiation of therapy. The approach to articulation therapy does not vary significantly as a result of the presence or absence of VPD. However, glottal and nasal substitutions generally are considered atypical articulation disorders, so clinicians may have less experience in treating these types of substitutions. A generally recognized example of an articulation approach used to eliminate glottal stops involves repeating a stop plus vowel production first with a whisper and then gradually increase the voicing component.[36] Audible nasal air emissions that are phoneme-specific also are considered to be errors of articulation. Nasal air emissions generally occur during production of fricative, affricates, and sibilants. Clinicians frequently have the patient shape these sounds by increasing airflow during /t/ productions or use other voiceless stops with the same place of articulation as the targeted sound to establish correct productions. Nares-occluded oral productions of phonemes, syllables, words, and sentences also may be effective. Auditory, tactile, and visual training and feedback with respect to placement and manner of articulation as well as voicing components have demonstrated improvement in articulation of children with VPD as well.[37] Although some of the biofeedback techniques reported in the literature are not clinically relevant, they provide rationale for the use of auditory, visual, and tactile feedback during correct and incorrect productions of phonemes. Of note, compensatory articulation errors that are a result of VPD alone do not frequently occur with oral motor weakness. Therefore, oral motor exercises are not appropriate unless there is evidence of oral motor weakness in addition to VPD.

Resonance

It is unclear whether increasing strength or control of the muscles required for velopharyngeal closure by means of behavioral intervention is possible. Speech therapy generally is considered to be appropriate only when VPD is mild or inconsistently present, or if the affected child appears to fatigue throughout the day. Previous investigations of exercises to increase strength of the muscles needed for velopharyngeal closure have yielded poor results. Sucking, gagging, swallowing, and blowing exercises and electrical stimulation demonstrated no direct impact on improved velopharyngeal closure during speech tasks.[38-40] Attempts to train improved or more consistent velopharyngeal closure using speech therapy in children with mild hypernasality or intermittent closure rely heavily on auditory feedback. It is presumed that the ability to hear the difference between nasal and non-nasal productions is an important aspect of training production. Microphones, accelerometers, and tubing to assist with perception of airflow through the nose often are used. Resonance therapy and nasal occlusion with subsequent imitation of resonance without nares occluded are also commonly used to assist with auditory awareness and improve resonance. Visual feedback using the nasometer, which measures nasal and oral acoustic energy, is common instrumentation in many cleft palate and craniofacial settings. Some evidence supports its usefulness in reducing nasality with visual feedback.[14] However, long-term carryover has not been documented to the same degree.

Other forms of biofeedback, including Seescape, nasal stethoscope, and endoscopic feedback,[41,42] all have been used with some degree of success. Therapy techniques may include oral-motor awareness, continuous positive airway pressure (CPAP), and biofeedback techniques. Children with an inconsistent closure or those who on evaluation demonstrate minimal VPD may benefit from nasal CPAP. Nasal CPAP is used during speech tasks and resistance exercises performed to strengthen the velopharyngeal muscles. The exercises can be done at home. Although the reported results were variable, it may be helpful in some children for whom traditional therapy approaches do not result in significant improvement.[43]

Compensatory Strategies

Children who have undergone surgical repair of VPD but continue to demonstrate hypernasality often are referred for speech therapy to determine if altering speech production may improve speech to within socially acceptable limits. Strategies often include increasing breath support or loudness to increase sentence length, using increased jaw opening, and modifying pitch or breathiness of voice quality. Listener ratings of these changes either have not been studied in a systematic way or have yielded varied results.[44] Therefore, these therapy techniques generally are recommended on a trial basis.

Prosthetic Management

Prosthetic treatment has been used for many years and has been shown to be effective.[45] A palatal lift is created that pushes the palate up and back to contact the posterior pharyngeal wall (Fig. 187-5). If the palate is not too short, this maneuver will allow resolution of the VPD. Alternatively, an obturator (speech bulb prosthesis) is a round piece of acrylic that can be placed into the velopharynx so that with movement, the walls of the velopharynx will achieve closure as they contact the obturator (Fig. 187-6). "Weaning" from the obturator (bulb reduction therapy) subsequent to improved lateral wall and velar movement has been described.[46] Another study of clinical outcomes with the lift prosthesis did not seem to confirm this possibility.[47]

Prosthetic intervention is used in cases in which airway limitation is significant. The prosthesis can be removed at night to avoid obstructive apnea. It also is very useful in the case of stroke or central nervous system trauma[48] when there is a possibility of recovery. Older

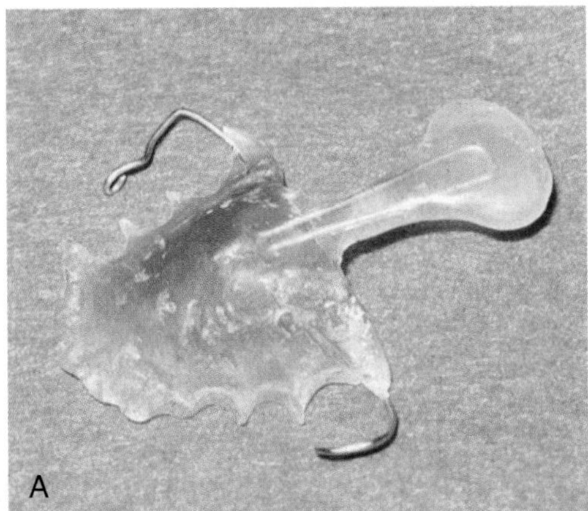

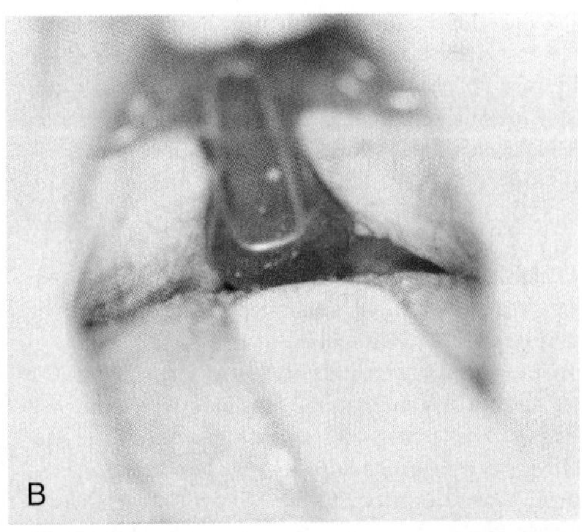

Figure 187-5. A palatal lift is shown out of the mouth **(A)** and in position **(B)**.

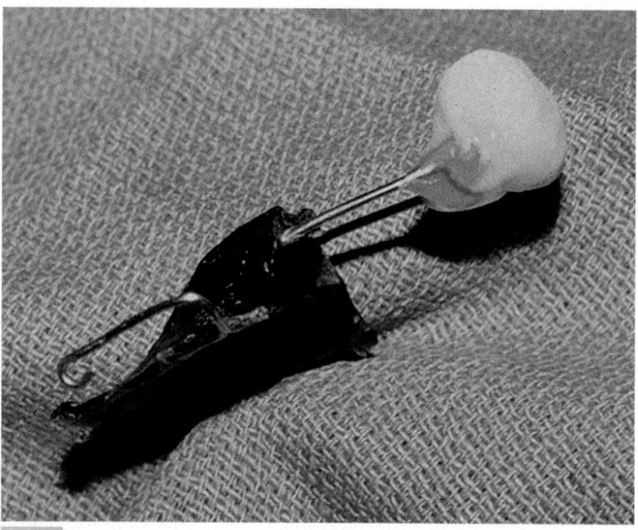

Figure 187-6. A palatal bulb obturator.

children and adults may be the most suitable candidates for this approach.

Prosthetic management has several limitations. First, an experienced prosthodontist is required for the fabrication, fitting, and maintenance of the appliance. Adequate maxillary dentition is mandatory, because the prosthesis is "hung" on the maxillary teeth. During the loss of deciduous teeth, keeping the prosthesis in place may not be possible. Similarly, during the rapid expansion of the maxilla in preparation for bone grafting, retention of the prosthesis is nearly impossible. The child must be cooperative with dental care. Finally, the prosthesis must be maintained with removal, cleaning, and repair. The inconvenience of this limits its widespread use and makes surgical options more desirable for long-term management in children.

Surgical Intervention

If a structural problem in velopharyngeal function exists, or speech therapy alone is ineffective, surgical intervention is a consideration. Options include intravelar veloplasty, Furlow double-opposing Z-plasty, sphincter pharyngoplasty, and superiorly based pharyngeal flap operations. The intravelar veloplasty and Furlow Z-plasty attempt to improve function by reorienting the levator sling. The (sphincter) pharyngoplasty borrows lateral wall tissue to obturate the lateral and posterior walls. The pharyngeal flap borrows tissue from the posterior wall to obturate the middle portion of the velopharynx.

Levator Repositioning

If the levator veli palatini muscle is oriented longitudinally, such as in a submucous cleft palate or after a palatoplasty, velar motion may be improved by reorienting the levator musculature. The traditional approach to this is an intravelar veloplasty. This operation dissects the levator muscles from their posterior attachment to the hard palate and nasal and oral mucosa to achieve a more anatomic transverse orientation. Although this is intuitively sensible, the results are not always satisfactory.[49] It has, however, been used with some success in "re-repair" of the palate if VPD follows a palatoplasty that did not include levator repositioning.[50]

The intravelar veloplasty can be done at the initial palate repair or as a secondary operation. An initial repair technique that can be slightly altered in revision surgery is described next.

After induction of general anesthesia and the securing of the endotracheal tube, a mouth gag is placed. This device secures the endotracheal tube against the tongue while retracting it out of the way with epinephrine. The greater palatine neurovascular bundle is injected with a small amount of local anesthetic. The palate will blanch, demonstrating a good local block. The soft palate is then additionally infiltrated to achieve further hemostasis.

The hard palatal flaps are elevated to the neurovascular bundle. Care is taken to dissect this without injury to the vascular supply. The lateral incision allows dissection around the hamulus. This maneuver will assist in freeing enough oral mucosa to allow closure.

The levator muscle inserts into the posterior border of the hard palate. This alignment makes the muscle nonfunctional. As the muscle is dissected from the posterior hard palate border, care is taken to avoid injuring the thinner nasal mucosa. The muscle is then freed from the oral mucosa and nasal mucosa. The dissection is best carried back to the hamulus and the levator followed toward the skull base. Debate is ongoing regarding the advantage of fracturing the hamulus to increase the mobility of the muscle bundle.

The palate is then closed in three layers. Nasal mucosa is closed with everting simple and mattress sutures from anterior to posterior. Absorbable sutures such as chromic are used. Uvular reapproximation, though not essential, is ideal. The muscle bundle often is attenuated. It is best closed with mattress sutures across the midline and may be tacked in this anatomic position. The oral mucosa is then closed as well.

Double-Opposing Z-plasty Palatoplasty

A current trend has been toward the use of the double-opposing Z-plasty originally described by Furlow (see Chapter 186).[38,51-54] This method reorients the levator while also thickening and lengthening the palate. The Furlow double-opposing Z-plasty also can be used as a primary closure, a repair of a submucous cleft palate, or a secondary procedure if the levators are longitudinally oriented. The Z-plasty is a well-known technique for lengthening a scar. The reorientation of the flaps also builds bulk in the posterior palate to aid contact of the posterior pharyngeal wall.

The Furlow double-opposing Z-plasty is done with the patient under general anesthesia. The mouth gag is used as well. After injection for hemostasis, as described earlier in the discussion of intravelar veloplasty, the four flaps are designed. The two myomucosal flaps are always posteriorly based and two mucosal flaps anteriorly based. A right-handed surgeon may find the elevation of the myomucosal flap on the patient's left more easily done, but this is not required.

If the palate is intact, it is divided in the midline. An incision is made on the left hemipalate, just posterior to the hard palate edge, leaving a small margin for ease of closure. This incision is carried through the muscle layer to the submucosal layer of the nasal mucosa. Care must be taken not to injure the thin nasal mucosa. The dissection is then carried posteriorly toward the free margin of the palate.

The oral mucosa is elevated from the muscle layer on the right hemipalate. This is based anteriorly. The incision is made just anterior to the free margin of the right hemipalate.

The right myomucosal flap is then developed by incising the muscle and nasal mucosa from the posterior edge of the right hard palate from medial to lateral. A cuff of tissue is left at the hard palate to facilitate closure.

The nasal mucosal flap on the left hemipalate is developed. An incision is made beneath the left myomucosal flap near the posterior edge of the soft palate toward the eustachian tube. This also creates a flap based anteriorly on the hard palate.

These four flaps are then repositioned to allow closure. The closure proceeds first with the nasal suture line repair, followed by the oral suture line closure. The left nasal mucosal flap is rotated across midline to the right hard palate margin. Everting sutures are tied with the knot toward the nose. The right myomucosal flap is then rotated to the left to insert into the left hemipalate. This maneuver brings the muscle bundle across the midline. The tension is not in the midline but lateral, reducing risk of fistula formation. The rotated flap is positioned so that the midline incision is now sewn to the posterior edge of the soft palate. The incision line that was at the hard palate is now sewn to the free edge of the nasal mucosal flap.

The oral mucosal flap from the right hemipalate is now rotated to the left, past the midline. The right oral mucosal flap is sutured to the incision at the posterior hard palate. The left myomucosal flap is then rotated to the right across the midline. The once-medial edge will be sutured to the posterior soft palate edge. The muscular flaps thus overlap each other, which thickens the soft palate. The lateral incision will be closed to the free margin of the oral mucosal flap. The uvula is reapproximated.

Pharyngeal Flap

For years, the pharyngeal flap operation has been the mainstay of management for VPD when performed as a secondary procedure in patients with cleft palate. Many surgeons have excellent success with this operation.[29,55-59] Although both inferiorly and superiorly based flaps can be designed, the superiorly based flap is in more common use.[60] This flap places posterior wall tissue in the center of the velopharynx, leaving a lateral port on either side. With use of lateral port control with an appropriately sized catheter, airway problems are reduced.[58] Because of the midline obturation, the pharyngeal flap is ideal for a sagittal or circular pattern with good lateral wall motion. It may be altered as a secondary procedure to improve results.[61,62] Lateral wall motion is necessary for closure, but some evidence suggests that the lateral wall motion will improve after the procedure.[57]

After induction of general anesthesia and endotracheal intubation, the Dingman mouth gag is introduced. Palatal injection is performed as described earlier. The posterior pharyngeal wall is injected as well.

The flap is designed based on previously obtained endoscopic or videofluoroscopic results. The width and length will be key. Care must be taken to avoid elevating the flap too far into the hypopharynx, to reduce scarring and postoperative dysphagia.

Lateral incisions are made to the prevertebral fascia. The flap is undermined. Division in the inferior aspect can be left until the palate is opened. It is important to recognize that the flap will shrink once the inferior cut is made. Adequate length is important, but little advantage accrues to creation of an exceptionally long flap.

This procedure may be done using a palatal split technique, with the nasal mucosa used to cover the raw surface of the flap. Alternatively, the flap may be introduced into a bivalved palate. Flap width can vary because of the vagaries of scarring.

If the bivalve or fish-mouth technique is chosen, the palate is retracted to expose the nasal surface. An incision is made just anterior to the free margin on the nasal side. The oral mucosa is then dissected from the muscle layer through this incision, creating a pocket. The width of the pocket is based on the preoperative assessment on the needed width of the flap.

The superiorly based flap is then released from its inferior connection. The flap is inserted into the pocket so that the raw surface is in contact with the raw surface of the pocket. Sutures are brought from the oral surface of the palate through the pocket. These are then placed from the raw surface of the flap through the mucosa about 1 cm from the tip. The suture is then placed back through the mucosa of the flap and brought through the pocket to come out on the oral mucosal surface. As these sutures are tied, the flap pulls itself into the pocket, with raw surface to raw surface and mucosa to mucosa. Lateral port control is helpful. The mucosa also can be removed from the distal end of the pharyngeal flap so that the sutures can be placed at the distal end of the flap. The denuded flap is inserted into the pocket. This technique, in one report, yielded inconsistent results when compared with others.[30]

If the surgeon prefers, a palatal split approach can be used. The palate is divided in the midline. The hemipalate sections are retracted laterally. Back-cuts are made through the nasal mucosa at the posterior margin of the hard palate to elevate a laterally based nasal mucosal flap from the soft palate. The pharyngeal flap is sutured to the midline at the soft-hard palate junction and laterally to the mucosal edge of the back-cut. Lateral port control is maintained by the placement of catheters. The size of the port is determined by how far laterally the flap is sewn to the back cut. The laterally based nasal mucosal flaps are then sewn over the pharyngeal flap, to reduce scar contracture and narrowing of the flap. The nasal mucosal incision is closed in the midline. The cut edges of the muscular layer are reapproximated. The oral mucosa is then closed.

The posterior wall defect can be partially closed to assist in the postoperative healing, but can also be left open to heal secondarily. Excessive closure narrows the pharynx, which can cause airway obstruction and consequent sleep apnea.

Pharyngoplasty

The sphincter pharyngoplasty is commonly used for treatment of VPD.[6,63-67] This procedure is a popular choice because of a perceived decrease in risk of postoperative airway obstruction and a high percentage of coronal and circular closure patterns. Bilateral myomucosal flaps are elevated from the lateral pharyngeal wall to be inserted into an incision on the posterior nasopharyngeal wall at the level of greatest closure. This obturates the posterior and lateral portions of the velopharynx. Movement of the palate to the flap accomplishes closure.[66,67] Sphincter pharyngoplasty is ideally suited for a coronal closure but also is useful in the circular closure if the palate has reasonable motion. This procedure is called a sphincter operation because it was felt that active movement of the myomucosal flap was possible. Although active motion of the flap occasionally is seen, it is not constant.[66,67] There seems to be improved palatal motion after this procedure.[67] The width, length, and degree of overlap of the myomucosal flaps determine the "tightness." Alterations in these three factors can compensate to some degree for limitation of palatal motion seen preoperatively.

The sphincter pharyngoplasty preparation is similar to the previously discussed palatal operations. Because no incisions are made in the palate, injection for hemostasis is only in the lateral pharyngeal wall and posterior nasopharynx.

The palate is retracted with a uvula retractor or red rubber catheters. Preoperative endoscopy or speech videofluoroscopy allows estimation of the amount of obturation needed and the level of maximal palatal excursion. The width of the lateral myomucosal flaps can be altered and the position of the incision for nasopharyngeal insertion decided, as needed. Adjustability is an advantage of this procedure. Even unilateral sphincter pharyngoplasty may be used on occasion.

A posterior incision is made at the level of the maximal palatal excursion. The flap placed at this level will allow the most closure during speech. The incision is carried bilaterally to the posterior limb of the outlined lateral flap. It is not carried through the deep fascia.

The lateral flaps are superiorly based myomucosal flaps. They may include the palatopharyngeal muscle (posterior tonsillar pillar) but can be taken directly from the constrictors.

Many variations are available on the placement of the flaps. Rotation into the velopharynx and suturing to the horizontal incision are necessary. The posterior border of the left flap can be sutured to the superior border of the horizontal incision in the nasopharynx. The right flap is rotated so that the anterior border is sutured to the inferior border of the horizontal incision. The two flaps are then sutured together at the remaining free edge.

The degree of overlap will determine the tightness of the sphincter, the degree of obturation, and obstruction. If vigorous movement of the palate is seen preoperatively, a narrow flap can be taken and secured with less overlap. If little preoperative palatal motion is possible, a wider flap is harvested and the overlap should be maximal.

In the postoperative period, all of these procedures warrant concern related to airway obstruction.[56,68-70] Close monitoring of the patient through the immediate postoperative period for acute obstruction is necessary. Chronic obstruction can manifest as obstructive sleep apnea. The use of CPAP can be helpful to allow resolution of edema and scar maturation. Some children can then "outgrow" the obstruction over time as the dimensions of the pharynx increase with growth.

Posterior Wall Augmentation

In the child who has a very small posterior midline "gap" that causes VPD, augmentation of the posterior pharyngeal wall may be tried. Although many materials have been used, including hyaluronic acid,[71] fat,[72] Teflon,[73] Proplast,[74] and cartilage,[75] most have achieved limited long-term success. A recent animal study looked at the duration of injectable micronized acellular dermal matrix in a submucosal area. Even after only 30 days, little of the injected material remained.[76] Gray and colleagues reported lasting improvement using a "rolled" posterior pharyngeal flap for autologous posterior wall augmentation.[77] In this procedure, a superiorly based pharyngeal flap is rolled or folded on itself and sutured to make a ridge in the posterior nasopharynx. Success may be variable, however: Durability of the obturation was not seen in a similar study using this technique.[78]

The autologous posterior wall augmentation uses the superiorly based pharyngeal flap. Lateral incisions are made, and the flap is elevated along the deep fascial plane. The flap is folded on itself. The distal end of the flap is secured at the base of the elevated flap into the deep fascia. This creates a mass effect on the posterior velopharyngeal wall. Preoperative endoscopy or speech videofluoroscopy can assist in determining the correct level for positioning the "rolled" flap. As in the pharyngeal flap operation, the posterior wall defect can be partially closed.

Choice of Surgical Intervention

Although basing selection of the surgical intervention on the gap seen at speech videofluoroscopy or endoscopy seems like a reasonable approach, alternative views have emerged. In one series, no difference was seen between superiorly and inferiorly based pharyngeal flaps.[79] A prospective multicenter study randomizing the patients to undergo either sphincter pharyngoplasty or a pharyngeal flap operation suggested no difference in outcomes.[63] Indeed, in centers that use pharyngeal flap operations as the mainstay of management for children with VPI, excellent results are obtained even though the most common closure pattern is coronal.[55] One protocol suggests that the initial decision be based on the orientation of the levators. A Furlow Z-plasty is done if they are suspected not to be horizontally placed. If that fails or if the orientation is normal in a child without a cleft deformity or if the cleft repair included this, a sphincter pharyngoplasty is used.[80]

Fortunately, most reported series do show very good results in the overwhelming majority of the patients. To that end, surgeons should consider maximizing competency in a particular technique and continuing to develop the skills for that technique. An important point is that although the velopharyngeal incompetence can be surgically eliminated, speech therapy may still be needed to correct the articulation errors, especially those that are maladaptive.

Conclusions

The diagnosis, assessment, and management of VPD involve a variety of diagnostic options, assessment tools, and management options. It is helpful for the otolaryngologist, speech-language pathologist, and other team members to take a "transdisciplinary" approach, in which each is thoroughly knowledgeable about the various disciplines involved in the care of children with these problems.[36] Identifying the need for speech therapy and the timely inclusion of surgical management, if needed, demand an understanding of the velopharyngeal mechanism and its relation to phonologic and articulation development, as well as awareness of the various surgical and prosthetic options and their short- and long-term consequences for the child.

SUGGESTED READINGS

Barr L, Thibeault SL, Muntz H, et al. Quality of life in children with velopharyngeal insufficiency. *Arch Otolaryngol Head Neck Surg.* 2007;133:224.

Croft CB, Shprintzen RJ, Rakoff SJ. Patterns of velopharyngeal valving in normal and cleft palate subjects: a multi-view videofluoroscopic and nasendoscopic study. *Laryngoscope.* 1981;91:265.

Dalston RM, Warren DW, Dalston ET. Use of nasometry as a diagnosis tool for identifying patients with velopharyngeal impairment. *Cleft Palate Craniofac J.* 1991;28:446.

D'Antonio LL, Muntz HR, Province MA, et al. Laryngeal/voice findings in patients with velopharyngeal dysfunction. *Laryngoscope.* 1988;98:432.

D'Antonio LL, Eichenberg BJ, Zimmerman GJ, et al. Radiographic and aerodynamic measures of velopharyngeal anatomy and function following Furlow Z-plasty. *Plast Reconstr Surg.* 2000;106:539.

Dejonckere PH, van Wijngaarden HA. Retropharyngeal autologous fat transplantation for congenital short palate: a nasometric assessment of functional results. *Ann Otol Rhinol Laryngol.* 2001;110:168.

Furlow LT Jr, Block AJ, Williams WN. Obstructive sleep apnea following treatment of velopharyngeal incompetence by Teflon injection. *Cleft Palate J.* 1986;23:153.

Furlow LT Jr, Williams WN, Eisenbach CR 2nd, et al. A long term study on treating velopharyngeal insufficiency by Teflon injection. *Cleft Palate J.* 1982;19:47.

Hallen L, Dahlqvist A. Cross-linked hyaluronan for augmentation of the posterior pharyngeal wall: an experimental study in rats. *Scand J Plast Reconstr Surg Hand Surg.* 2002;36:197.

Hardin-Jones MA, Chapman KL, Scherer NJ. Early intervention in children with cleft palate. *ASHA Leader.* 2006;32:8.

Kummer AW, ed. *Cleft Palate and Craniofacial Anomalies: The Effects on Speech and Resonance.* San Diego: Singular Publishing; 2001.

Levine PA, Goode RL. The lateral port control pharyngeal flap: a versatile approach to velopharyngeal insufficiency. *Otolaryngol Head Neck Surg.* 1982;90:310.

Liao YF, Chuang ML, Chen PK, et al. Incidence and severity of obstructive sleep apnea following pharyngeal flap surgery in patients with cleft palate. *Cleft Palate Craniofac J.* 2002;39:312.

Matsuya T, Miyazaki T, Yamaoka M. Fiberscopic examination of the velopharyngeal closure in normal individuals. *Cleft Palate J.* 1974;11:286.

Pamplona M, Ysunza A, Guerrero M, et al. Surgical correction of velopharyngeal insufficiency with and without compensatory articulation. *Int J Pediatr Otorhinolaryngol.* 1996;34:53.

Peat BG, Albery EH, Jones K, et al. Tailoring velopharyngeal surgery: the influence of etiology and type of operation. *Plast Reconstr Surg.* 1994;93:948.

Perkins JA, Lewis CW, Gruss JS, et al. Furlow palatoplasty for management of velopharyngeal insufficiency a prospective study of 148 consecutive patients. *Plast Reconstr Surg.* 2005;116:72-80.

Peterson-Falzone SJ, Graham MS. Phoneme-specific nasal emission in children with and without physical anomalies of the velopharyngeal mechanism. *J Speech Hear Disord.* 1990;55:132.

Pigott RW. An analysis of the strengths and weaknesses of endoscopic and radiological investigations of velopharyngeal incompetence based on a 20 year experience of simultaneous recording. *Br J Plast Surg.* 2002;55:32.

Powers G, Starr C. The effects of muscle exercises on velopharyngeal gap and nasality. *Cleft Palate J.* 1974;11:28-35.

Shprintzen RJ, Lencione RM, McCall GN, et al. A three dimensional cinefluoroscopic analysis of velopharyngeal closure during speech and nonspeech activities in normals. *Cleft Palate J.* 1974;11:412.

Sie KC, Tampakopoulou DA, de Serres LM, et al. Sphincter pharyngoplasty: speech outcome and complications. *Laryngoscope.* 1998;108:1211.

Sie KC, Tampakopoulou DA, Sorom J, et al. Results with Furlow palatoplasty in management of velopharyngeal insufficiency. *Plast Reconstr Surg.* 2001;108:17.

Sommerlad BC, Mehendale FV, Birch MJ, et al. Palate re-repair revisited. *Cleft Palate Craniofac J.* 2002;39:295.

Stringer DA, Witzel MA. Comparison of multi-view videofluoroscopy and nasopharyngoscopy in the assessment of velopharyngeal insufficiency. *Cleft Palate J.* 1989;26:88.

Ward PH, Stoudt R Jr, Goldman R. Improvement of velopharyngeal insufficiency by Teflon injection. *Trans Am Acad Ophthalmol Otolaryngol.* 1967;71:923.

Witt PD, O'Daniel TG, Marsh JL, et al. Surgical management of velopharyngeal dysfunction: outcome analysis of autogenous posterior pharyngeal wall augmentation. *Plast Reconstr Surg*. 1997;99:1287.

Witt PD, Rozelle AA, Marsh JL, et al. Do palatal lift protheses stimulate velopharyngeal neuromuscular activity? *Cleft Palate Craniofac J*. 1995;32:469.

Witzel MA, Rich RH, Margar-Bacal F, et al. Velopharyngeal insufficiency after adenoidectomy: an 8-year review. *Int J Pediatr Otorhinolaryngol*. 1986;11:15.

Ysunza A, Palmplona C, Toledo E. Change in velopharyngeal valving after speech therapy in cleft palate patients. A videonasopharyngoscopic and multi-view videofluoroscopic study. *Int J Pediatr Otorhinolaryngol*. 1992;24:45.

For complete list of references log onto www.expertconsult.com.

CHAPTER ONE HUNDRED AND EIGHTY-EIGHT

Congenital Malformations of the Nose

Ravindhra G. Elluru

Christopher T. Wootten

Key Points

- Most congenital nasal lesions relate to developmental errors in one of three embryologic zones: (1) anterior neuropore; (2) central midface; (3) nasobuccal membrane.
- Encephaloceles, gliomas, and dermoids share a common embryologic origin and frequently manifest as midline nasal masses that require surgical management.
- Appropriate preoperative imaging with CT or MRI, or both, and use of careful intraoperative dissection techniques are required to determine whether a dermoid extends intracranially. In such cases, optimal management consists of a combined approach involving otolaryngology and neurosurgery.
- The most common congenital nasal disorders of the central midface relate to cleft lip deformities. The typical appearance of the nose features a flattened, retracted nostril and a broad nasal tip.
- Congenital nasal pyriform aperture stenosis is associated with holoprosencephaly and a central maxillary megaincisor in a majority of cases. Pituitary abnormalities are also common.
- Up to 30% of infants are born with nasolacrimal duct obstruction, but only those with nasal obstruction and feeding difficulties secondary to nasolacrimal duct cysts require marsupialization.
- Choanal atresia is a relatively common cause of congenital nasal obstruction and more frequently is unilateral in presentation.
- Choanal atresia without a bony component does not exist. Transnasal approaches are the most popular technique. Mucosa-sparing techniques are associated with the best outcomes.

Overview

Congenital malformations of the nose and paranasal sinuses are rare manifestations of disordered development located at the origin of the aerodigestive tract. Clinical presentations range from subtle cosmetic deformities to life-threatening acute upper airway obstruction and feeding difficulties in neonates. This chapter focuses on the most common congenital lesions in the nose and paranasal sinuses. These lesions are considered within the framework of possible developmental errors in specific anatomic zones: (1) errors at the anterior neuropore, (2) errors of the central midface, and (3) errors of the nasobuccal membrane. Mesodermal and germline malformations not unique to the nose and paranasal sinuses also are discussed.

Developmental Errors of the Anterior Neuropore

The anterior neuropore persists medial to the optic recesses in the third week of life, and around it the skull base develops as the frontal, ethmoidal, and nasal bones. Behind the nasal bones but in front of the nasal and septal cartilages lies a potential space, the prenasal space. The foramen caecum forms a defect in the anterior skull base at the apex of the prenasal space, where the cribriform plate ultimately condenses. This structure is closed by its fusion with the fonticulus frontalis, a fontanelle between the inferior aspect of the frontal bones and the developing nasal bones. During the third through the eighth weeks of development, a projection of dura extends through the foramen caecum, traverses the prenasal space, and apposes ectoderm at the tip of the nasal bones (the future rhinion). As the foramen closes, the dural diverticulum detaches from the overlying ectoderm and retracts into the cranium. Irrevocably apposed ectoderm may be pulled posterosuperiorly toward and even through the foramen caecum, giving rise to a dermoid fistula, cyst, or sinus. Faulty or premature closure of the foramen may enable persistence of neural tissue in the nasal cavity as isolated heterotopic glial tissue (glioma) or as a patent central nervous system (CNS) communication (meningocele or encephalocele) (Fig. 188-1). The latter can occur in a paramedian position, as a nasoethmoidal encephalocele, or, more laterally through a medial orbital wall defect, as a naso-orbital encephalocele. Basal encephaloceles herniate posterior to the cribriform plate. Similar errors may occur above the developing nasal bones at the fonticulus frontalis. Intracranial contents may herniate through the patent fonticulus frontalis until the eighth week. If the fonticulus also closes abnormally, the result may be persistence of an extranasal path, leading to nasofrontal meningoceles or encephaloceles or gliomas[1] (Fig. 188-2).

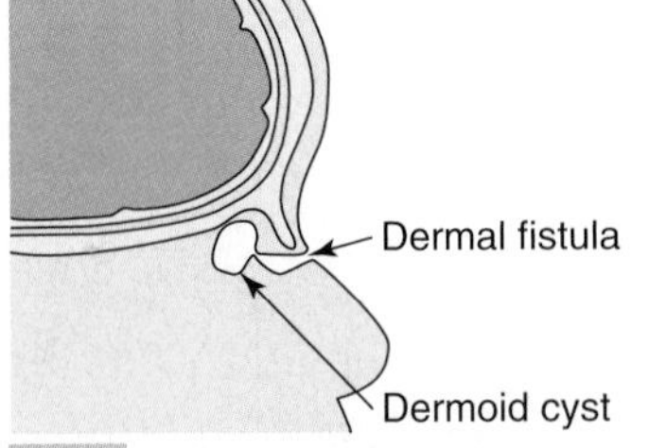

Figure 188-1. Schematic view of the common midline nasal masses.

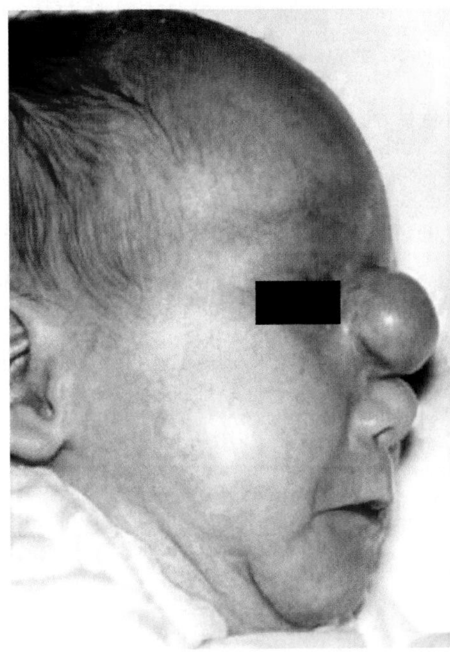

Figure 188-2. Sincipital encephalocoele. A soft, bluish compressible mass protruding from the glabellar region.

Encephaloceles

An *encephalocele* is an extracranial herniation of cranial contents through a defect in the skull. When the encephalocele includes meninges only, it is termed a *meningocele*; if it includes both brain and meninges, it is termed a *meningoencephalocele*. Estimates of the incidence of these lesions vary considerably, ranging from 1 in 3000 to 1 in 30,000 live births in North America and Europe. The incidence in Asian populations is higher, with a reported incidence of 1 in 6000 live births. Encephaloceles have no familial tendency or gender predilection. Approximately 40% of affected patients have other associated anomalies.[2-4]

Encephaloceles are divided into occipital, sincipital, and basal types (Tables 188-1 and 188-2). Occipital encephaloceles will not be discussed in this chapter as they occur outside the nose. *Sincipital* encephaloceles account for 25% of all encephaloceles, and they are further classified according to their location. Nasofrontal encephaloceles manifest as glabellar masses, causing telecanthus and inferior displacement of the nasal bones. Nasoethmoidal lesions manifest as dorsal nasal masses, causing superior displacement of the nasal bones and inferior displacement of the alar cartilages. Naso-orbital lesions manifest as orbital masses, causing proptosis and visual changes.[1] The anatomic course of each of these sincipital encephalocele presentations is shown in Table 188-1. *Basal* encephaloceles are less common, arising

Table 188-1

Sincipital Encephaloceles

Type	Course	Clinical Features
Nasofrontal	Through bone defect between orbits and forward between nasal and frontal bones to the area superficial to the nasal bones	Glabellar mass Telecanthus Inferior displacement of nasal bones
Nasoethmoidal	Through foramen caecum deep to the nasal bones, turning superficially at the cephalic end of the upper lateral cartilage to expand superficial to the upper lateral cartilage	Mass on the nasal dorsum Superior displacement of nasal bones Inferior displacement of the alar cartilages
Naso-orbital	Through the foramen caecum deep to the nasal and frontal bones through a lateral defect in the medial orbital wall	Orbital mass Proptosis Visual changes

Table 188-2

Basal Encephaloceles

Type	Course	Clinical Features
Transethmoidal	Through the cribriform plate into the superior meatus medial to the middle turbinate	Most common type Nasal obstruction Hypertelorism Broad nasal vault Unilateral nasal mass
Sphenoethmoidal	Passes through a bony defect between the posterior ethmoid cells and sphenoid	Nasal obstruction Hypertelorism Broad nasal vault Unilateral nasal mass
Transsphenoidal	Through a patent craniopharyngeal canal into the nasopharynx	Nasopharyngeal mass Nasal obstruction Associated with cleft palate
Spheno-orbital	Through the superior orbital fissure and out the inferior orbital fissure into the sphenopalatine fossa	Unilateral exophthalmos Visual changes Diplopia

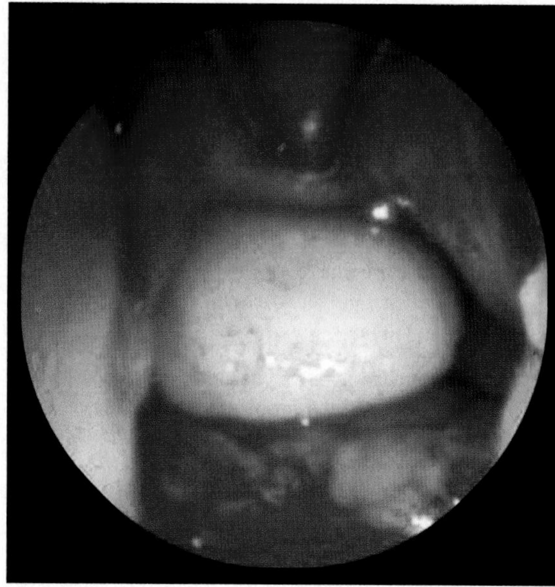

Figure 188-3. Basal encephalocele seen in nasopharynx with a 120-degree angled telescope.

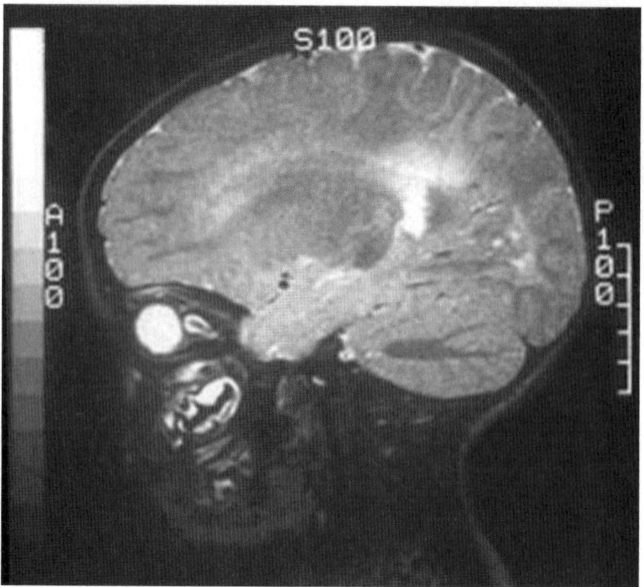

Figure 188-4. Sagittal magnetic resonance image of a basal meningoencephalocele protruding into the nasopharynx.

between the cribriform plate and the superior orbital fissure or posterior clinoid fissure and manifesting as an intranasal mass (Fig. 188-3). These masses may not manifest until later in childhood, when they cause nasal obstruction and drainage. Sincipital and basal encephaloceles appear as pulsatile, bluish compressible lesions that transilluminate. Classically, these lesions expand with crying, straining, or compression of the jugular veins.

On histopathologic analysis, sincipital and basal encephaloceles have a glial component, with astrocytes surrounded by collagen, submucosal glands, and sometimes nasal septal cartilage or calcification. When it is difficult to differentiate between gliomas and encephaloceles, the presence of ependymal tissue is consistent with an encephalocele.[5]

High-resolution computed tomography (CT) or magnetic resonance imaging (MRI) delineates encephaloceles and additionally helps to exclude associated anomalies such as agenesis of the corpus callosum and hydrocephalus.[5] CT outlines the bony cartilaginous defect, whereas MRI provides complementary information regarding the soft tissue characteristics of the mass (Fig. 188-4). MRI also differentiates meningoceles from meningoencephaloceles. Sagittal reconstructions and contrast enhancement are particularly advantageous for identifying an intracranial connection.

Once the diagnosis of encephalocele has been made, management is surgical. Most authorities advocate intervention in the first few months of life[2] to minimize the risk of meningitis and cosmetic deformity, but the risk of meningitis is not decreased with prophylactic antibiotics while surgery is being planned. Additionally, early intervention makes the identification of the intracranial connection technically easier and allows more complete repair of the dural defect.[2] Small lesions with minimal skull base defects may be managed endoscopically. Larger lesions require a combined approach with a craniotomy to resect condemned dura and cerebral tissue with concomitant endoscopic removal of the residual nasal tumor. The skull base defect can then be reconstructed using a pericranial flap or split-thickness calvarial bone graft.[5] The most commonly encountered postoperative complications are cerebrospinal fluid (CSF) leak, meningitis, and hydrocephalus. Postoperative neurologic function reflects the patient's preoperative performance. Encephalocele recurrence rates of 4% to10% have been reported.[6]

Gliomas

Gliomas consist of heterotopic glial tissue that lacks a patent CSF communication to the subarachnoid space; however, 5% to 20% of gliomas maintain a fibrous affiliation (see Fig. 188-1). Nasal gliomas are rare and show nonfamilial inheritance. They occur more commonly in males (in a ratio of 3:2). These benign masses manifest as extranasal (60%), intranasal (30%), or combined (10%) lesions.[7] *Extranasal* gliomas are smooth, firm, noncompressible masses that occur most commonly at the glabella, although they may arise along the side of the nose or the nasomaxillary suture line.[2] *Intranasal* gliomas are polypoid pale masses that may protrude from the nostril. The nasal fossa on the involved side may be obstructed. Intranasal gliomas most often arises from the lateral nasal wall near the middle turbinate and occasionally from the nasal septum.[7] Nasal gliomas rarely may extend into the orbit, frontal sinus, oral cavity, or nasopharynx. Because they lack a patent CSF connection, gliomas do not change in size with crying or straining and do not transilluminate.

Pathologically, gliomas are better termed nasal glial heterotopias, nasal cerebral heterotopias, or congenital nasal neuroectodermal tumors. Histologic analysis shows dysplastic, neuroglial, and fibrovascular tissue. Ependymal tissue is not found in gliomas, a distinction that allows differentiation from encephaloceles.

Diagnostic evaluation should include a CT scan to assess the bony anatomy of the skull base, an MRI study to accurately image soft tissue connections to the CNS, and nasal endoscopy to assess the location, origin, and extent of the nasal mass. As with encephaloceles, sagittal reconstructions and contrast enhancement are useful imaging adjuncts.

Proper management of gliomas requires surgical extirpation using a multidisciplinary approach involving otolaryngology and neurosurgery. Delaying intervention may lead to distortion of the septum or nasal bones, or infection. With cosmesis kept in mind, surgical access should provide exposure of the lesion and possible exploration of the skull base. For resection of extranasal gliomas, options include lateral rhinotomy, external rhinoplasty, transglabellar subcranial, bicoronal, and midline nasal approaches.[8] Except in the case of large glabellar lesions, the external rhinoplasty approach provides adequate surgical exposure while minimizing the use of facial incisions.[5] When a fibrous stalk is present that extends deep to the nasal bones toward the base of the skull, a nasal osteotomy is recommended to improve exposure. Following the stalk in its entirety is crucial in determining the possible presence of an intracranial extension. As a result of advancements in surgical instrumentation, image guidance, and surgical techniques, most intranasal gliomas can be removed endoscopically.[9,10] Reported recurrence rates are between 4% and 10%.[11]

Nasal Dermoids

Nasal dermoids are frontonasal inclusion cysts or tracts related to embryologic errors localized to the anterior neuropore. Congenital

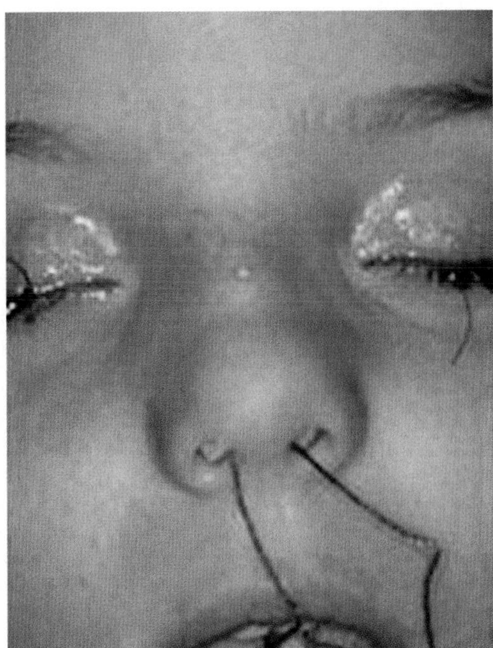

Figure 188-5. Nasal dermoid manifesting as a firm midline nasal swelling associated with a sinus opening.

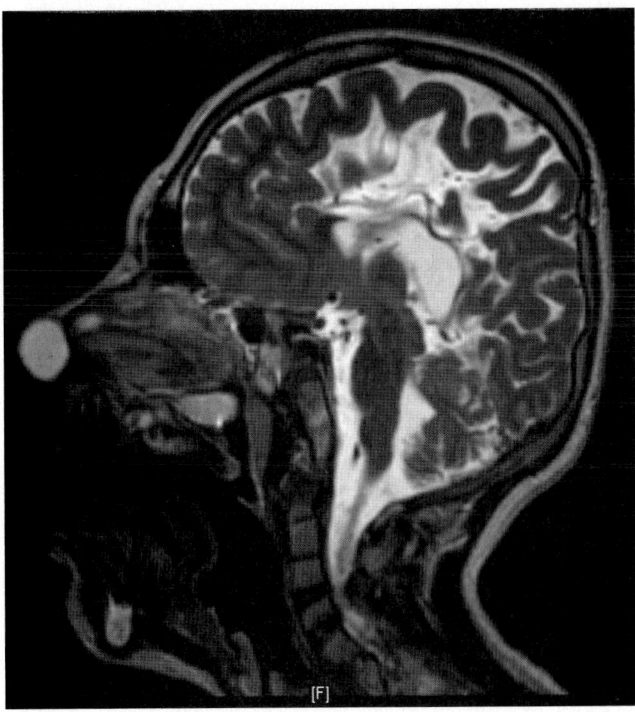

Figure 188-6. Sagittal magnetic resonance image of a nasal dermoid, evident as a region of signal hyperintensity in the anterior nasal septum as a hyperintense lesion.

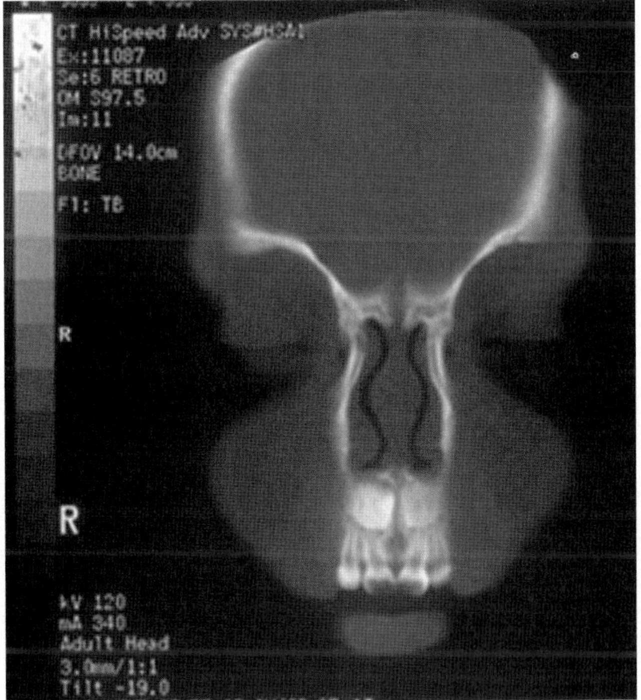

Figure 188-7. Coronal computed tomography scan showing a bifid crista galli and an enlarged foramen caecum.

midline nasal masses occur in 1 in 3000 to 1 in 40,000 live births, and dermoids are by far the most common.[12] Nasal dermoids account for 1% to 3% of all dermoids and approximately 10% to12% of head and neck dermoids. Most dermoid cysts occur sporadically, with a slight male preponderance,[13,14] although familial associations have been reported. Nasal dermoids may accompany aural atresia, pinna deformity, mental retardation, hydrocephalus, branchial arch anomalies, cleft lip and palate, hypertelorism, and hemifacial microsomia in 5% to 41% of presentations.[13]

Nasal dermoids usually manifest as a midline pit or mass. In approximately 50% of clinical presentations, a dimple is present at or near the rhinion, along with a widened nasal bridge; however, the true spectrum of disease includes cysts, sinuses, or fistulas that may occur anywhere along the embryologic line from the nasal tip into the cranial space. Mass lesions are firm, lobulated, and noncompressible and may be associated with a sinus opening (Fig. 188-5) with intermittent caseous discharge or infection. Although a protruding hair is seen in only a minority of patients, it is pathognomic for a nasal dermoid. A lesion within the nasal septum will cause nasal obstruction. Intracranial extension rates range from 4% to 45%.[13] Recurrent meningitis with typical skin flora may indicate an intracranial tract. Nasal dermoids do not enlarge with crying or straining and do not transilluminate.

Unlike teratomas, which contain all three embryonal germ layers, congenital dermoids contain only ectodermal and mesodermal embryonic elements. The latter include hair follicles, sebaceous glands, and sweat glands that are found in the wall of the cyst and thus differentiate these masses from simple epidermoid cysts. Keratin debris is another prominent feature on histologic examination, and dermoids also lack the glial features of encephaloceles and gliomas.

CT and MRI provide complementary information in the radiologic evaluation of nasal dermoids. Thin-slice (1 to 3 mm) CT scans with intravenous contrast are recommended to differentiate the dermoid from the surrounding nasal mucosa and to define the bony anatomy of the nose and anterior skull base (Fig. 188-6). Unique findings with intracranial dermoids include a bifid crista galli (Fig. 188-7) and an enlarged foramen caecum; a normal crista galli and foramen caecum may be used to exclude intracranial extension.[15] Multiplanar, thin-section contrast-enhanced MRI is used to depict the soft tissue anatomy of the anterior skull base, and contrast-enhanced MRI distinguishes the nonenhancing dermoid from enhancing lesions such as hemangiomas and teratomas. The neonatal crista galli does not contain marrow fat, so high signal intensity on T1-weighted images is suggestive of an intracranial dermoid.

As with other congenital anterior neuropore lesions, the management of nasal dermoids is surgical. Because aspiration, incision and drainage, curettage, and subtotal excision are associated with high recurrence rates, these management approaches generally are not advocated. Assessing the degree of intracranial extension is crucial, and in patients with features suggestive of intracranial extension, a combined intracranial-extracranial approach should be planned with the participating neurosurgeon. Extracranial access should fulfill four criteria: (1) excellent access to the midline; (2) access to the base of the skull; (3) adequate exposure for reconstruction of the nasal dorsum; and (4) an acceptable scar.[16] Several different extracranial approaches have been described. The external rhinoplasty incision generally gives the best cosmetic result and is therefore the most widely used approach. This approach also gives access to the skull base and allows for exposure of the nasal dorsum; nevertheless, it provides limited access to lesions in the glabellar region. Alternative approaches include lateral rhinotomy and midline vertical incisions, both of which provide excellent access.[13] For lesions in the glabellar area without a sinus tract, a transglabellar subcranial approach, a paracanthal incision, or a bicoronal approach is an acceptable alternative. Glabellar lesions with a sinus opening require an elliptic incision to excise the ostium, despite the possibility of a widened scar.

For lesions that extend into the cranial cavity, a multidisciplinary effort is required to perform a frontal craniotomy. This usually is carried out through a coronal incision using a combined intracranial-extracranial approach with a large frontal craniotomy; however, anterior small window craniotomies have been described.[17] Sessions[18] has suggested that craniotomy may be avoided altogether and the tract suture-ligated if it is devoid of epidermal and adnexal structures at the skull base. This information can be obtained by intraoperative frozen-section analysis of the tract. A number of investigators[13,15] agree with this approach. Other workers[19] have suggested that epidermal elements may be staggered along the tract and thus postulate that a single biopsy site may provide false-negative information regarding the presence of an intracranial extension of the dermoid tract. The overall recurrence rate after adequate excision is low; however, long-term follow-up is essential to diagnose the occasional late recurrence.

Developmental Errors of the Central Midface

Eruption of nasal pits into the choana, fusion of the palatal shelves, and growth of the nasal septum and soft palate coincide with the development of the lateral nasal wall and primitive sinus anatomy. For normal nasal and paranasal growth to occur, all of these rapid changes must take place with complete precision.[1]

Normal nasal development occurs between weeks 4 and 12 of life. During this time, neural crest cells migrate from their origin in the dorsal neural folds around the eye to form the first and second branchial arch–derived facial prominences surrounding the stomodeum. The stomodeum is surrounded by the frontonasal prominence superiorly, the maxillary processes laterally, and the mandibular processes inferiorly. The nasal placodes, which are two small thickenings in the frontonasal prominence, begin to burrow, forming nasal pits. This invagination process in the fifth week creates ridges of tissue around the pit; these are called the lateral nasal prominences laterally and the medial nasal prominences medially. Nasolacrimal duct development begins as a thickening of the ectoderm that becomes buried in the mesoderm of the nasal pits between the lateral nasal prominence and the maxillary process. This buried ectoderm canalizes from superiorly to inferiorly postnatally. The lateral and medial prominences finalize interaction with the developing maxillary process, creating the philtrum and medial lip (from the fused medial nasal prominences) and the lateral upper lip (from the maxillary prominences). The lateral nasal prominences form the nasal alae (Fig. 188-8).

Errors in central midface development underlie a host of congenital anomalies. Arhinia (congenital absence of the nose) may result from (1) abnormal migration of neural crest cells; (2) failure of fusion of the medial and lateral nasal processes; (3) overgrowth and premature fusion of the medial nasal processes; or (4) lack of resorption of the nasal epithelial plugs.[20] Similarly, polyrhinia probably results from incomplete development of the frontonasal process, which subsequently allows separation of the developing lateral portions of the nose.[1,21,22] The medial nasal processes and the septum continue to develop as scripted and are duplicated, thereby forming a "double nose."[1,2,11,23] Proboscis lateralis may result from mesodermal proliferation errors in the frontonasal and maxillary processes adjacent to the forming nasal pits. Epidermal breakdown then occurs, leaving the lateral nasal process sequestered as a tube arising in the frontonasal region. Also, because of this breakdown, the nasolacrimal duct is not formed.[1] Independent of proboscis lateralis, failure of the nasolacrimal ectodermal tract to canalize postnatally may result in formation of a nasolacrimal duct cyst in an otherwise normal patient.

Midline and paramedian fusion errors produce midfacial clefting. This may be isolated to the midface or occur as a part of cephalic clefting (Robert's syndrome) or holoprosencephaly. Errors in fusion of the medial nasal prominences with the medial aspect of the maxillary process produce a cleft lip, with its accompanying congenital nasal deformity. Finally, deficient development of the primary palate and bony overgrowth of the nasal process of the maxilla[24] are responsible for congenital nasal pyriform aperture stenosis. A developmental deficiency of the incisive os could explain the occurrence of a triangular plate, the narrow inferior portion of the nasal cavity, and the associated central maxillary mega-incisor, which is seen in 60% of cases[25] (Fig. 188-9). The term *holoprosencephaly* was introduced by DeMyer and coworkers to describe median facial anomalies and the brain morphology associated with these anomalies.[26] Holoprosencephaly is a failure of the embryonic forebrain to cleave sagittally into cerebral hemispheres, transversely into a diencephalon, and horizontally into olfactory and optic bulbs. This failure is associated with a spectrum of facial anomalies including (1) cyclopia (single eye and single orbit with arhinia and proboscis); (2) ethmocephaly (extreme hypertelorism, separate orbits, and arhinia; (3) cebocephaly (hypertelorism and proboscis-like nose without cleft lip); (4) median cleft lip (orbital hypertelorism and flat nose); and (5) median philtrum-premaxilla anlage (hypertelorism, bilateral cleft lip, and a median process representing the philtrum-maxilla anlage).

Complete Agenesis of the Nose (Arhinia)

Arhinia is part of the holoprosencephaly spectrum. This malformation is extremely rare, with approximately 30 cases described in the literature (Fig. 188-10). In the few reported cases, arhinia generally is sporadic in inheritance and may occur either as an isolated defect or in association with other facial and cerebral abnormalities.[27] Associations with genetic disorders such as trisomy 10, trisomy 13, and trisomy 21, as well as chromosome 9 inversion and translocation of chromosomes 3 and 12, also have been reported.[3,27,28]

The features of arhinia include absence of the external nose and nasal airways, hypoplasia of the maxilla, a small high-arched palate, and hypertelorism. Affected infants display respiratory distress and cyanosis associated with feeding. Older children may gulp food between breaths. Speech is characteristically hypernasal, and patients demonstrate evidence of hyposmia. Physical examination reveals an absence of the external nose, nasal septum, and sinuses. Rare associated abnormalities of the eye include anophthalmia and hypoplasia of the orbits.

Early management of arhinia focuses on nutrition. A cleft palate feeder or a gastrostomy tube is required. A prosthetic nose may be used until the child is older and can undergo definitive surgical repair. Vertical distraction osteogenesis of the midface has been reported to increase midfacial height, maximizing bone and soft tissue for later reconstruction.[29] Re-establishing the nasal passageway requires removing the incisors, creating an airway through the maxilla, and releasing the high-arched palate. The nasal passage is then lined with split-thickness skin grafts and maintained with long-term stenting. Restenosis is common, and serial dilations are required. Reconstruction of the external nose is a multistage procedure that requires the use of tissue expanders, bone, cartilage or prosthetic grafts, and local or regional skin flaps, with concomitant dacrocystorhinostomy to prevent recurrent conjunctivitis resulting from absence of the nasolacrimal ducts.[30]

Polyrhinia and Supernumerary Nostril

Polyrhinia (double nose) and supernumerary nostril (accessory nostril) are extremely rare anomalies, with only four reported cases of each.[21] These deformities may occur in isolation or in association with pseudohypertelorism. Patients with polyrhinia generally present with anterior (septal duplication, duplicated nasal passageways) and posterior (choanal atresia) nasal defects. The primary step in surgical

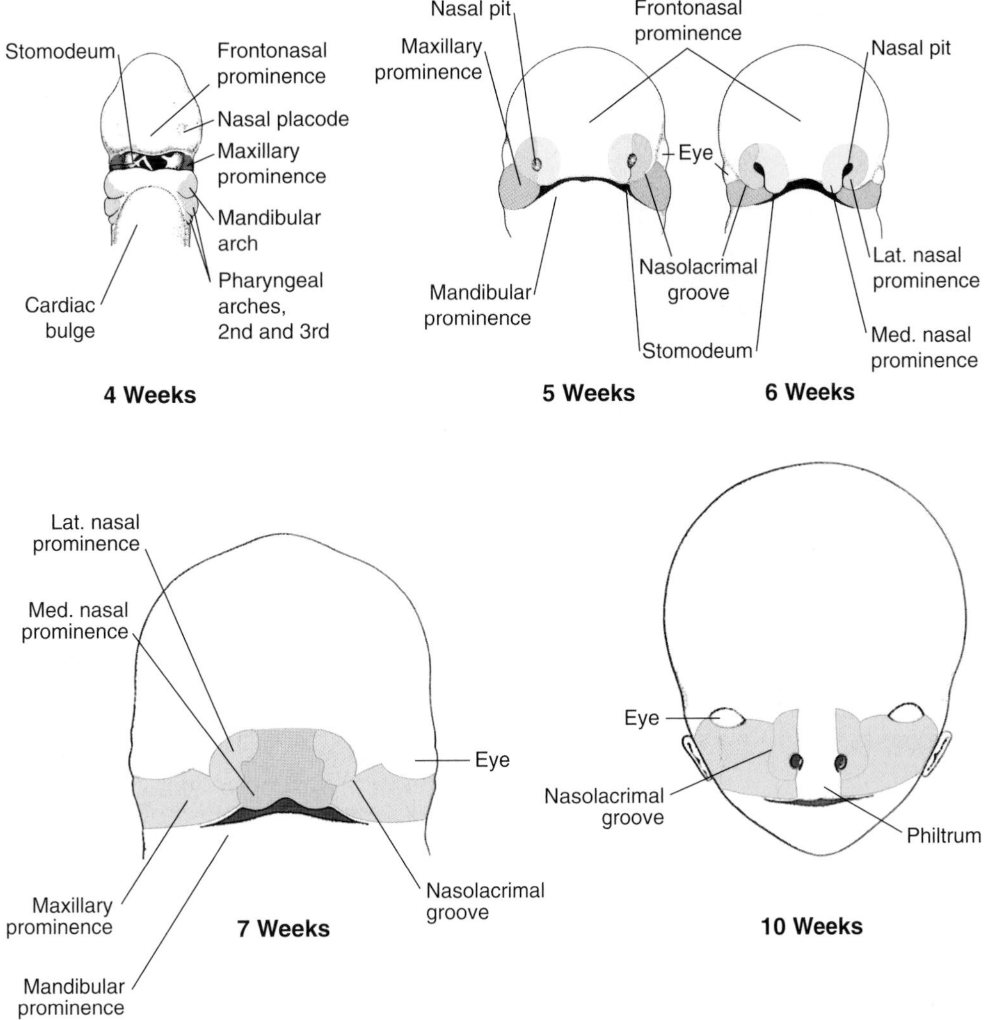

Figure 188-8. Embryo at weeks 4, 5, 6, 7, and 10, showing the developing nasal structures. *(From Sadler TW. Head and neck embryology. In Sadler TW, ed.* Langman's Medical Embryology. *6th ed. Baltimore: Williams & Wilkins; 1990:315-316.)*

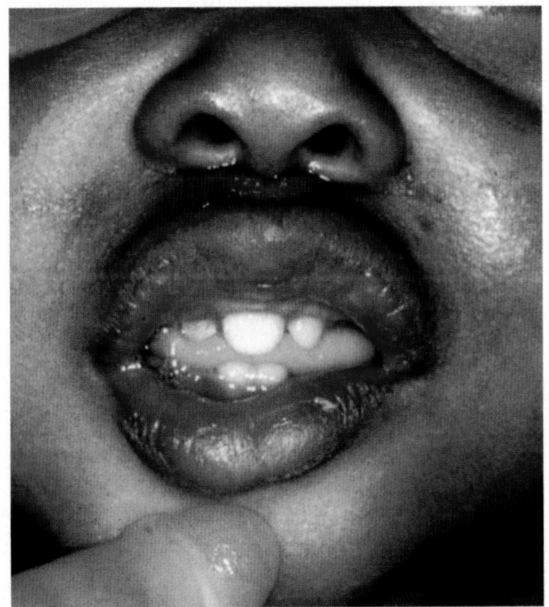

Figure 188-9. Maxillary mega-incisor in association with CNPAS.

Figure 188-10. Congenital arhinia.

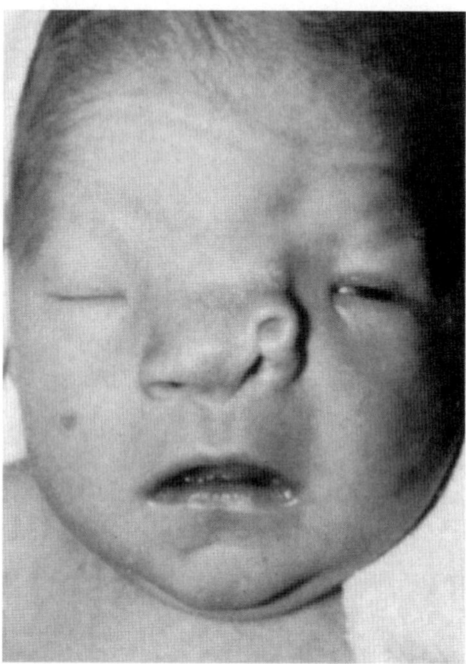

Figure 188-11. Proboscis lateralis. *(From Hengerer AS, Wein RO. Congenital abnormalities of the nose and paranasal sinuses. In: Bluestone CD, Stool SE, Alper CM, et al, eds.* Pediatric Otolaryngology. *4th ed. Philadelphia: Saunders; 2001:988.)*

management is correction of the choanal atresia. The nasal deformity is later corrected by removing the medial portions of each nasal passage and anastomosing the lateral portions in the midline.[2] The result is a broad flat nose with a depression in the midline, which can be corrected later on by medial in-fracture of the nasal bones and additional rhinoplasty techniques.

Supernumerary nostril manifests with the external appearance of a small accessory nasal orifice with surrounding redundant soft tissue. The orifice may be lateral, medial or superior to the nose. With a true fistula, a discharge from this orifice may occur. Treatment entails excision of the supernumerary nostril and primary closure of the defect or closure with the assistance of local flaps.[21]

Proboscis Lateralis

Proboscis lateralis is a rare disorder that manifests as a tubular sleeve of skin attached to the inner canthus of the orbit and heminasal aplasia on the affected side (Fig. 188-11). This deformity is thought to be secondary to fusion of the maxillary process on the affected side with the contralateral developing nasal process. Approximately 30 cases have been reported in the recent literature. Proboscis lateralis is associated with other CNS abnormalities and congenital ocular lesions, such as microphthalmus, coloboma, and arachnoid cysts. The diagnosis is made by physical examination, nasal endoscopy, and CT scanning. Treatment is delayed until facial growth is complete, and a prosthetic device is worn until reconstructive efforts begin. Reconstruction involves the use of bone and cartilage grafts and surrounding skin, including the tube of anomalous lateral nasal skin. Restenosis is common, and serial dilations with stenting often are required.[2]

Craniofacial Clefts

Craniofacial clefts are exceedingly rare and generally are not encountered in routine clinical practice. The hallmarks of this disorder are ocular hypertelorism; a broad nasal root; lack of formation of the nasal tip; anterior cranium bifidum occultum; median clefting of the nose, lip, and palate; and unilateral orbital clefting or notching of the nasal ala.[1,31] DeMyer[32] noted an association among hypertelorism, cephalic anomalies, and mental deficiency. The Tessier classification of cranial clefts[23] is the most widely used. This classification is based on specific axes (0 to 14) along the face and cranium. Because the orbit is common to the face and cranium, it distinguishes cranial clefts (9 to 14) from facial clefts (0 to 8).

There is a large degree of variability in the severity of median nasal clefts. This deformity, also known as bifid nose and internasal dysplasia, can range from a simple median scar at the cephalic end of the nasal dorsum to a completely split nose, forming separate halves with independent medial nasal walls. Disparate associations have been reported in the literature. A median cleft lip is a frequent associated anomaly.[33] The airway usually is adequate despite the cosmetic appearance. Before surgical reconstruction, it is important to rule out a possible dermoid cyst or encephalocele within the nasal-septal area. Surgical reconstruction requires the cooperative efforts of a multidisciplinary team, and treatment outcomes depend largely on the severity of the midline dysraphia.

Lateral nasal clefts are rare anomalies that involve defects of the lateral nasal wall or ala. They range from scarlike lines in the ala to triangular defects extending into the inner canthal fold and affecting the nasolacrimal apparatus. As with median nasal clefts, lateral nasal clefts require surgical reconstruction using a multidisciplinary approach.

Cleft Lip Nasal Deformity

Cleft lip deformity is among the most common congenital abnormalities of the head and neck. A complete cleft lip extends into the floor of the nose, whereas an incomplete cleft extends only partway through the upper lip. Cleft lip deformity shows a male predilection. Overall, the incidence of cleft lip and palate, singly or in combination, is between 1 in 1000 and 1 in 4000 live births. One half of these demonstrate cleft lip and palate, whereas 20% involve cleft lip alone. The distribution of left, right, and bilateral cleft lip deformities is approximately 6:3:1.

All complete clefts and many incomplete clefts involve the nose. The most severe defects are those associated with a bilateral complete cleft. Children with a bilateral deformity have a flattened nasal tip and a shortened columella. They also may have bilateral maxillary hypoplasia and relative prognathism. Less severe deformity is seen in children with unilateral clefting. In these children, the nasal ala on the side of the cleft is more laterally based, giving the appearance of a flat, retracted nostril. The caudal septum also is displaced to the cleft side. The maxilla on the cleft side is hypoplastic, and the nasal tip has a bifid appearance.

Treatment options for nasal deformities associated with cleft lip include both primary and secondary rhinoplasty. Many surgeons undertake redraping of the skin–soft tissue envelope over the lower lateral cartilages at the time of initial cleft lip repair within the first year of life. The flattened appearance of the nostril may be corrected by anchoring the skin–soft tissue envelope more medially on the lower lateral cartilage. This correction also adds definition to the tip subunit. Later, during a second procedure, a laterally based chondrocutaneous sliding flap procedure is performed to reposition the alar base; this often is combined with a columellar strut or shield graft placement to project the foreshortened columella. The secondary operation often is divided into stages. Stage 1, performed at the ages of 4 to 6 years, aims at providing cosmetic improvement. Stage 2, performed at ages 8 to 12 years, follows orthodontic correction and has the goal of making available an optimal skeletal framework. More definitive rhinoplasty is delayed until skeletal growth is completed. Accordingly, it is performed at the ages of approximately 16 to 18 years.[34] Both open and closed rhinoplasty techniques have been used.

Congenital Nasal Pyriform Aperture Stenosis

Congenital nasal pyriform aperture stenosis (CNPAS) is a rare anomaly that occurs secondary to bony overgrowth of the nasal process of the maxilla and typically manifests in the first few months of life. The stenosis may occur in isolation, or the patient may present with a central mega-incisor and the holoprosencephaly spectrum of congenital midline lesions. Hypertelorism, a flat nasal bridge, and the central mega-incisor are clinical features of the premaxillary dysgenesis associated with holoprosencephaly. Pituitary disorders and dental and facial anomalies also are part of this spectrum.

The pyriform aperture is the narrowest part of the nasal cavity, and small changes in the cross-sectional area significantly affect airflow by increasing nasal airway resistance. Newborns present with symptoms

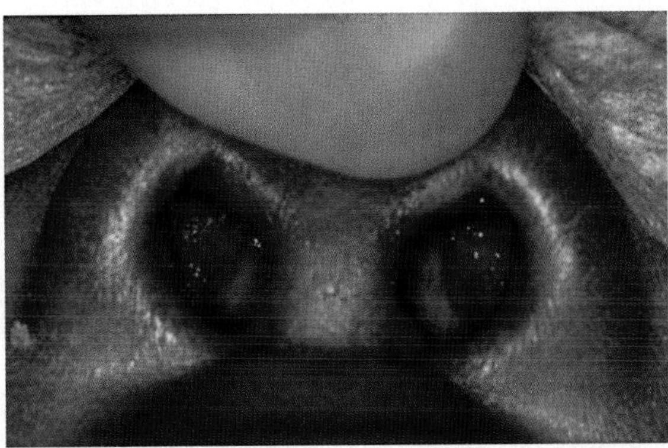

Figure 188-12. Congenital nasal pyriform aperture stenosis, as seen on anterior rhinoscopy.

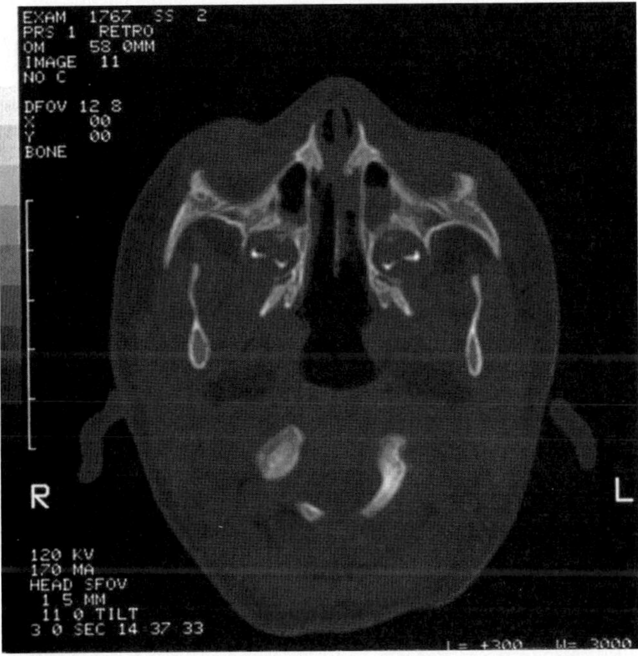

Figure 188-13. Axial computed tomography scan showing pyriform aperture stenosis secondary to overgrowth of the nasal process of the maxilla, causing reduction in the width of the piriform aperture.

similar to those of choanal atresia, and failure to pass a nasopharyngeal catheter may result in a misdiagnosis of choanal atresia. In older infants and children, nasal obstructive symptoms may be triggered by an upper respiratory infection, which further compromises the already narrow airway.

The diagnosis of CNPAS is established by physical examination and is best confirmed by CT, which shows that the width of the pyriform aperture, the cross-sectional area of the nasal cavity, and the width of the choana all are reduced. By contrast, the height of the nasal cavity and cross-sectional area of the choana are not altered (Figs. 188-12 and 188-13). Belden and colleagues[35] found the most helpful CT measurement to be the width of the pyriform aperture, defined as the distance between the medial aspects of the maxillae at the level of the inferior meatus, as measured on images in the axial plane. These workers reported that the width was never greater than 8 mm in their CNPAS group and never less than 11 mm in their control group. It is prudent for patients with a central maxillary incisor to undergo further investigation, to include central imaging for evaluation of CNS malformations, chromosomal analysis, and pituitary function testing.[36]

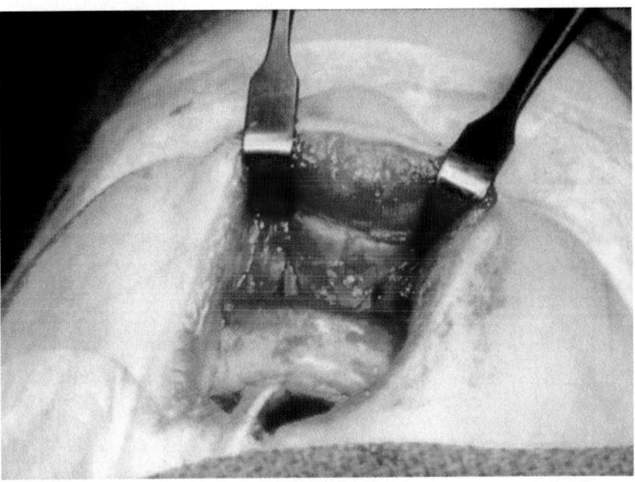

Figure 188-14. Sublabial approach to the piriform aperture. A gingivobuccal sulcus incision is made and a mucoperiosteal flap is raised to expose the piriform aperture.

Operative management is not always necessary for patients with CNPAS. Nonoperative management with nasal tubes and topical vasoconstrictive drops may be all that is required until growth results in increased nasal airway size. In patients who require surgery, repair is best accomplished through a sublabial approach, exposing the inferior and lateral pyriform aperture (Fig. 188-14). An otologic drill is used to widen the bony lateral and inferior margins. Brown and associates[24] recommend the use of nasal stents for up to 4 weeks.

Nasolacrimal Duct Cysts

Nasolacrimal duct cysts (dacrocystoceles) are uncommon abnormalities of the inferior meatus. These abnormalities may lead to nasal obstruction, respiratory distress, and epiphora. Although approximately 30% of all neonates have distal nasolacrimal duct obstruction at birth, formation of symptomatic cysts occurs only rarely in these children. The duct begins canalization at its lacrimal end and progresses inferiorly. In addition to producing nasal obstructive symptoms, the presence of a nasolacrimal duct cyst also makes neonates susceptible to aspiration and feeding difficulties. Infants with bilateral dacrocystoceles are the most severely affected. In most affected children, obstruction spontaneously resolves by 9 months of age.

The diagnosis of nasolacrimal duct cysts is made by anterior rhinoscopy or nasal endoscopy, which demonstrates a cystic mass in the inferior meatus (Fig. 188-15). This can be confirmed on a CT scan. The classic features evident on imaging are a dilated nasal lacrimal duct, an intranasal cyst, and cystic dilation of the lacrimal sac.[37]

Operative management is indicated for infants who have feeding problems, infection, or respiratory obstruction. The cyst is marsupialized endoscopically into the inferior meatus, opening the lesion with a curette or microsurgical débrider. This is best accomplished by a multidisciplinary team that includes an ophthalmologist, who may need to perform nasolacrimal duct probing and possible placement of nasolacrimal duct stents.

Developmental Errors of the Nasobuccal Membrane

During the third and fourth weeks of development, paramedian ectodermal nasal placodes appear. The nasal placodes, which are two small thickenings in the frontonasal process, begin to burrow, forming nasal pits. As these pits develop into the pouches of the nose and paranasal sinuses, the nasal pouches come to lie above the oral and buccal cavity. The nasobuccal membrane separates the nasal and oral or buccal spaces, and choanal atresia probably derives from failure of the nasobuccal membrane to rupture in the fifth and sixth weeks of development. An alternative theory suggests that abnormal migration of neural crest cells

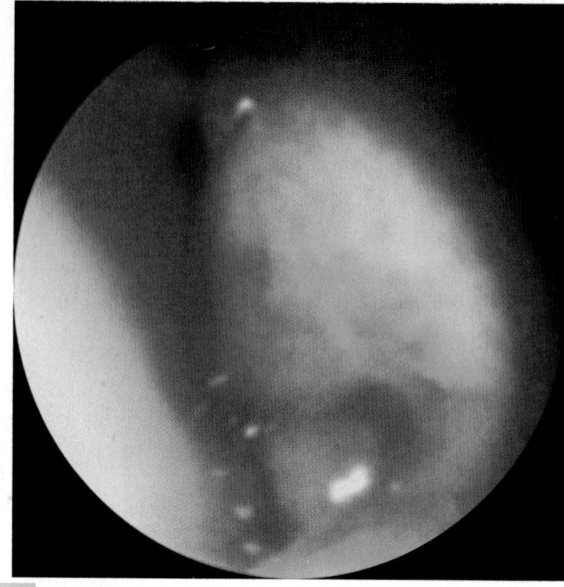

Figure 188-15. Left nasolacrimal duct cyst in the inferior meatus, as seen on anterior rhinoscopy.

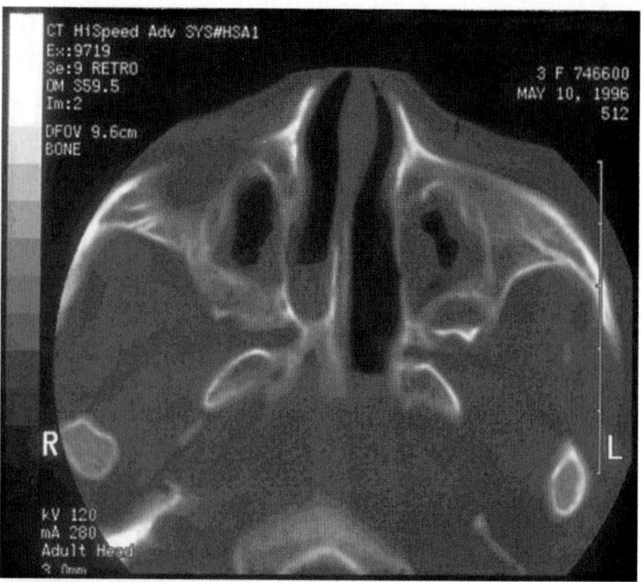

Figure 188-16. Axial computed tomography scan of unilateral choanal atresia, with a complete bony atretic plate and associated soft tissue.

results in choanal atresia. This theory is supported by the high incidence of choanal atresia in patients with mandibulofacial dysostosis (Treacher Collins syndrome), which is associated with abnormal neural crest migration.

Choanal Atresia

Choanal atresia occurs when the posterior nasal cavity fails to communicate with the nasopharynx.[1] This anomaly has a reported incidence ranging from 1 in 5000 to 1 in 8000 live births.[38] Up to two thirds of cases are unilateral, with atresia most commonly occurring on the right side.[1] Fifty percent of all patients with choanal atresia and up to 75% of patients with bilateral disease have other associated congenital anomalies.[2] These anomalies include CHARGE syndrome (*c*oloboma, *h*eart defects, *a*tretic choana, *r*etardation of growth and development, *g*enitourinary disorders, and *e*ar abnormalities); polydactyly; nasal, auricular, and palatal deformities; Crouzon's syndrome; craniosynostosis; microcephaly; hypoplasia of the orbit and midface; cleft palate; and hypertelorism.[39,40] The anatomic features that characterize choanal atresia include (1) a narrow nasal cavity; (2) lateral bony obstruction by the pterygoid plates; (3) medial obstruction caused by thickening of the vomer; and (4) membranous obstruction.[41-43] In a study conducted by Brown and associates,[41] the incidence of pure bony atresia was found to be 29%, whereas that of mixed bony-membranous atresia was 71%. No patients were found to have a purely membranous atresia.

The clinical presentation of choanal atresia varies between unilateral and bilateral disease. Patients with unilateral disease present later in life with rhinorrhea and nasal obstruction. On anterior rhinoscopy, the occluded nasal cavity is typically filled with thick, tenacious secretions. Patients with bilateral choanal atresia typically present as newborns with cyanotic events. An event begins with increasing efforts to breathe, tight mouth closure, and chest retractions followed by cyanosis. The cycle is broken by crying. A variant of bilateral choanal stenosis presents later in life with mouth breathing, recurrent sinusitis, chronic rhinorrhea, otitis media, failure to thrive, and defects of speech.

The diagnosis of choanal atresia is made clinically by failure to pass a 6F catheter through the nose into the nasopharynx (a distance of approximately 32 mm). CT is used to confirm the diagnosis and reveal the nature and thickness of the atresia.[44] Suctioning and pharmacologic vasoconstriction before imaging will improve resolution (Figs. 188-16 and 188-17). CT scanning also differentiates between complete atresia and stenosis. A diagnosis of choanal stenosis is made

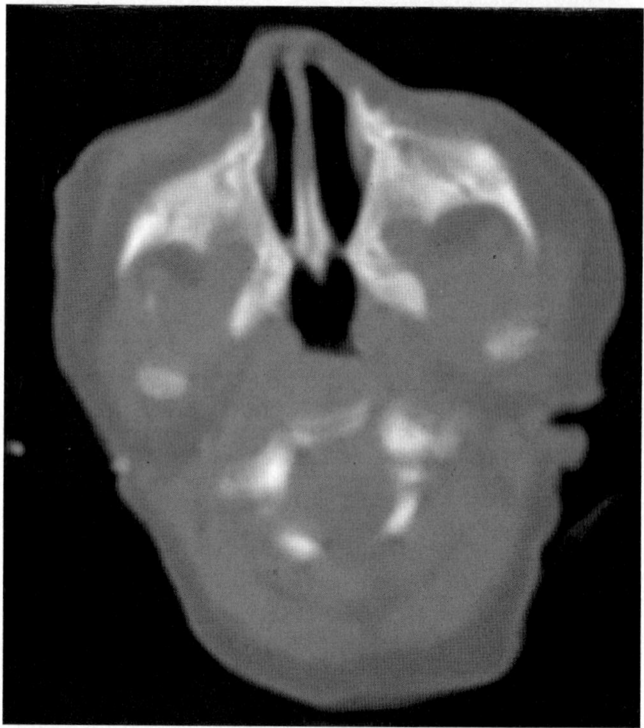

Figure 188-17. Axial computed tomography scan showing bilateral chonal atresia with soft tissue.

with recognition of a narrowed yet patent choana. Derkay and Grundfast[45] more specifically define this entity as a choanal space less than 6 mm across. This diagnosis should be confirmed by endoscopic evaluation (Fig. 188-18).

Unilateral atresia does not constitute an emergency. Treatment is delayed for several months, allowing for growth of the nose, which enhances the ease of surgery and reduces the risk of postoperative complications and restenosis. Bilateral atresia requires an initial intervention to establish an oropharyngeal or orotracheal airway and gastric feeding before definitive surgery. The timing of surgery is variable, and it may be preferable to wait several months until adequate facial growth has occurred (similar to the timing of cleft lip repair). In patients with

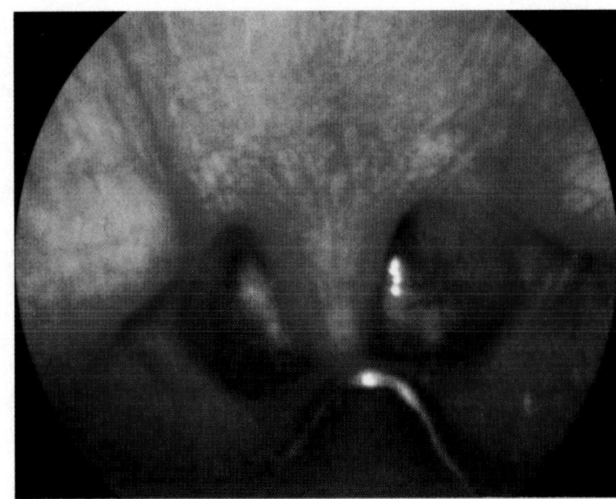

Figure 188-18. A view of bilateral choanal atresia through a 120-degree nasopharyngoscope.

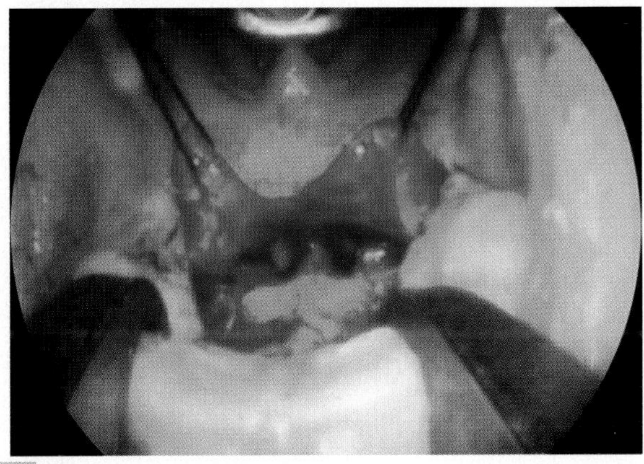

Figure 188-19. Transpalatal approach to choanal atresia repair. A pedicled hard palate mucoperiosteal flap based on the greater palatine artery is elevated to expose the choanae.

additional indications for tracheotomy, a surgical airway is obtained and definitive atresia repair is often delayed, allowing for facial growth. A shift has occurred in the surgical philosophy over the last few decades away from transpalatal (Fig. 188-19) and toward transnasal surgery. This shift can be attributed to reports citing a lower risk of dental and facial growth abnormalities associated with the latter approach. Most techniques begin the repair by perforating the atretic plate at its thinnest portion, using a urethral sound or suction instrument. A 0-degree transnasal endoscope or a 120-degree nasopharyngoscope is used for visualization (see Fig. 188-14). Subsequently, a backbiting forceps, a microsurgical débrider, a laser, and a drill are used as necessary to remove choanal soft tissue and bone. The posterior tip of the middle turbinate is a useful anatomic landmark. Restricting surgical maneuvers to remain inferior to this structure reduces the risk of intracranial injury.[46] The importance of stenting, as well as the use of fibroblast inhibitors (mitomycin C) and the preservation of mucosal flaps, remains controversial. Regardless of the techniques used, most studies[47,48] report significant recurrence rates, necessitating revision surgery. The lowest recurrence rates are seen in older children (with unilateral atresia), nonsyndromic patients, and patients who have undergone surgical procedures that minimize mucosal trauma.

Other Mesodermal and Germline Malformations

Mesodermally derived lesions such as hemangiomas and lipoblastomas may occur in the head and neck, although they rarely occur in the nose. These lesions present unique management challenges to the otolaryngologist or facial plastic surgeon. Similarly, germline malformations such as teratomas rarely localize to the nasopharynx. These foci may be remnants of normal embryologic structures that break off or fail to migrate along well-defined pathways to their normal destination.[49] The management of cutaneous hemangiomas follows principles detailed elsewhere in this text; the unique presentation and management of nasopharyngeal teratomas are described in this section.

Intranasal Hemangiomas

Infantile hemangiomas are discussed more fully elsewhere in this text. As suggested by Waner and colleagues, glucose transporter isoform 1 (GLUT1)-positive infantile hemangiomas have a predilection for embryonic fusion planes on the central face.[50] Thus, deep midface infantile hemangiomas may involve or distort the nasal lining. More typically, the intranasal hemangiomas described in the literature are lobular capillary hemangiomas and reparative cavernous hemangiomas. These noninfantile hemangiomas are GLUT1-negative and have been noted on the septum, the middle and inferior turbinates, and the lateral nasal wall.[51] These lesions frequently manifest with epistaxis and nasal obstruction. On examination, the hemangiomatous masses are friable, sessile or pedunculated, and reddish-purple in color. MRI shows high signal intensity on T2 sequences and enhancement with gadolinium on T1 sequences. CT may show associated bony remodeling. Whereas true infantile hemangiomas are amenable to both surgical and nonsurgical management, lobular capillary hemangiomas and cavernous lesions are treated by wide local excision of the lesion using endoscopic or open (midface degloving, open rhinoplasty, lateral rhinotomy) approaches.[51,52] Preoperative angioembolization has been described for larger lesions. The prognosis is excellent with complete excision.

Nasopharyngeal Teratomas

Teratomas are the most common germ cell tumors of childhood and are almost always benign. These lesions comprise representative tissues from each of the three embryonic germ layers (ectoderm, endoderm, and mesoderm) and generally contain tissues foreign to the anatomic site of origin. Teratomas occurring in infancy and early childhood generally are extragonadal, whereas those manifesting in older children more commonly occur in the ovary or testis.[53] Teratomas of the head and neck account for less than 5% of all teratomas. These rare neoplasms, which reportedly occur in 1 in 20,000 to 1 in 40,000 live births, may be located in the brain, orbit, oropharynx, nasopharynx, or cervical region.

Clinically, nasopharyngeal teratomas may be sessile or pedunculated and often protrude through the mouth. Anencephaly, hemicrania, and palatal fissures are associated with these lesions. The newborn usually presents with severe acute respiratory distress requiring endotracheal intubation or tracheotomy. In patients with smaller lesions, feeding difficulties may be the only presenting symptom.[54]

The diagnosis of congenital nasopharyngeal teratoma begins in utero. Maternal clinical characteristics may include polyhydramnios due to impaired swallowing and elevated α-fetoprotein levels. Larger lesions often are diagnosed by prenatal ultrasound examination. Such early detection enables planning for an EXIT (ex utero intrapartum treatment) procedure to secure the infant's airway before division of the maternal-fetal circulation. For lesions manifesting postnatally, fine needle aspiration may be used to assist in establishing the diagnosis.[54] Imaging is confirmatory. Lesions are seen as cystic and solid areas of fat density on CT and MRI (Fig. 188-20). Areas of bone and tooth formation may be present. Most nasopharyngeal teratomas are well encapsulated and demonstrate no intracranial connections.

The management of nasopharyngeal teratomas is surgical, and the approach depends greatly on the size of the lesion. Lesions can be excised through a transoral approach with or without endoscopic assistance. This approach may require splitting of the soft palate or palatal resection. Endoscopic assistance may obviate the need for palatal division or resection.[49] External approaches using a lateral rhinotomy incision or a transcervical incision also are used. If an intracranial component is present, a craniofacial approach is necessary. Outcomes generally are good, and α-fetoprotein levels are periodically measured to monitor for recurrence.

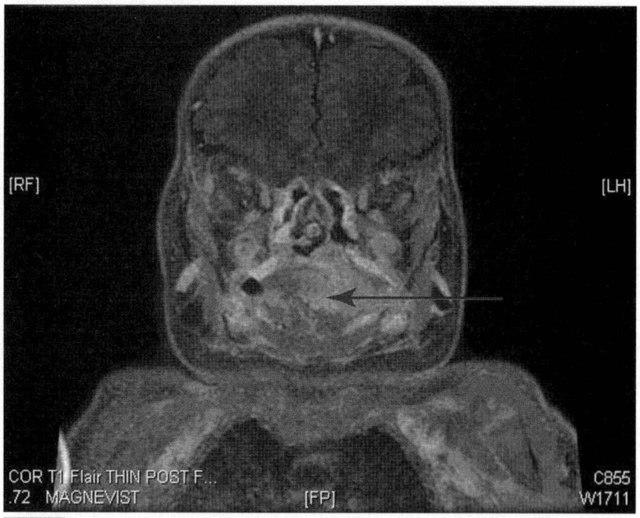

Figure 188-20. Nasopharyngeal teratoma on a coronal magnetic resonance image with characteristic heterogeneous signal intensity *(arrow)*.

SUGGESTED READINGS

April MM, Ward RF, Garelick JM. Diagnosis, management, and follow-up of congenital head and neck teratomas. *Laryngoscope.* 1998;108:1398-1401.

Belden CJ, Mancuso AA, Schmalfuss IM. CT features of congenital nasal piriform aperture stenosis: initial experience. *Radiology.* 1999;213:495-501.

Brown OE, Myer CM 3rd, Manning SC. Congenital nasal pyriform aperture stenosis. *Laryngoscope.* 1989;99:86-91.

Brown OE, Pownell P, Manning SC. Choanal atresia: a new anatomic classification and clinical management applications. *Laryngoscope.* 1996;106:97-101.

Derkay CS, Grundfast KM. Airway compromise from nasal obstruction in neonates and infants. *Int J Pediatr Otorhinolaryngol.* 1990;19:241-249.

Feledy JA, Goodman CM, Taylor T, et al. Vertical facial distraction in the treatment of arhinia. *Plast Reconstr Surg.* 2004;113:2061-2066.

Manning SC, Bloom DC, Perkins JA, et al. Diagnostic and surgical challenges in the pediatric skull base. *Otolaryngol Clin North Am.* 2005;38:773-794.

Rahbar R, Resto VA, Robson CD, et al. Nasal glioma and encephalocele: diagnosis and management. *Laryngoscope.* 2003;113:2069-2077.

Rahbar R, Shah P, Mulliken JB, et al. The presentation and management of nasal dermoid: a 30-year experience. *Arch Otolaryngol Head Neck Surg.* 2003;129:464-471.

Tessier P. Anatomical classification of facial, cranio-facial and latero-facial clefts. *J Maxillofac Surg.* 1976;4:69-92.

Van Den Abbeele T, Elmaleh M, Herman P, et al. Transnasal endoscopic repair of congenital defects of the skull base in children. *Arch Otolaryngol Head Neck Surg.* 1999;125:580-584.

For complete list of references log onto www.expertconsult.com.

CHAPTER ONE HUNDRED AND EIGHTY-NINE

Pediatric Facial Fractures

Paul R. Krakovitz

Peter J. Koltai

Key Points

- After the first month of life, trauma is the number one cause of pediatric deaths and a major contributor to long-term morbidity.
- Nasal fractures in children are the most common fractures of the facial bones in this age group. Mandible fractures are the most common facial fractures in children requiring hospitalization.
- Pediatric facial fractures often are complicated by associated neurocranial injury.
- Owing to rapid changes in facial dimensions with growth, patterns of fractures differ significantly among various pediatric age groups and between children and adults.
- Fractures to the developing body and ramus of the mandible are less likely to cause growth disturbance.
- Fractures to the developing mandibular condyles and the midface often lead to developmental deformities.
- Rigid fixation with plates and screws is avoided in the management of pediatric fractures unless the original features cannot be restored by simpler, less invasive means. These materials should be used in short segments so that crossing more than one osseous suture line is avoided. Use of resorbable plating systems is confined to non–load-bearing bone.
- After septal hematoma initially is ruled out in the evaluation of a child with a nasal injury, reexamination 3 to 5 days later is indicated to allow time for the resolution of edema. An accurate diagnosis can then be made in regard to a displaced nasal fracture, which if present necessitates reduction. Occult nasoethmoidal fracture is suspected when the clinical findings include marked flattening of the nasal dorsum.
- With internal fixation of fractures of the mandible or maxilla in children younger than 13 years, an understanding of the position of unerupted tooth buds is crucial. In regard to the mandible, monocortical miniplates are drilled in the lowermost margin.
- Maxillomandibular fixation is limited to 2 to 3 weeks and is followed by 6 to 8 weeks of use of guiding elastic bands.
- Delayed periorbital hematoma suggests fracture of the orbital roof.
- With extensive fractures of the orbital floor or demonstrable muscle entrapment, early surgery is appropriate. With more isolated injuries, waiting 7 to 10 days may prevent an unnecessary operation.

After the first month of life, trauma is the number one cause of pediatric deaths and a major contributor to long-term morbidity.[1,2] Nearly 15,000 children die and 100,000 others are disabled worldwide each year from trauma resulting from motor vehicle crashes, sports injuries, falls, altercations, and abuse.[2] More than $15 billion is spent annually in the United States for the treatment of childhood injuries.[1,3] Despite this epidemic of injuries, facial fractures in children remain uncommon.

Reconstruction of pediatric facial fractures requires an understanding of craniofacial development and of the consequences of injury for future growth. The patterns of facial fracture differ significantly not only between adults and children but also among pediatric age groups. Although some of the treatment strategies for facial fractures in adults and children are similar, children need to be considered in a different management algorithm because the repair of bony injuries is best accomplished by techniques that may adversely affect craniofacial development. This dilemma renders the treatment of facial fractures in children controversial. It is not possible to resolve all of the issues related to treatment; however, a rational approach to treatment that yields consistently excellent results can be formulated.

Epidemiology

Pediatric maxillofacial injuries account for approximately 5% of all facial fractures, although the incidence is reported as being between 1.5% and 15%.[4-18] Children younger than 5 years of age account for only 0.9% to 1.2%, whereas those 6 to 14 years of age account for 4% to 6% of all cases of maxillofacial trauma.[19,20] Bamjee and colleagues[19] found that 7% of pediatric traumatic injuries occur in children younger than 6 years, whereas 70% befall those between 13 and 18 years of age, indicating the increased vulnerability of the maturing face as well as the greater risk-taking behavior of a growing child.

In children, males are more prone to maxillofacial fractures than females, with an overall ratio of 1.5 : 1 to 2.3 : 1.[18,21-24] In children younger than 8 years, no difference between genders has been noted.[25] With approaching adolescence and greater involvement in sports and violence, the male-to-female ratio approaches 4.5 : 1.[25] In South Africa, male children are three times more likely to be involved in violence resulting in facial fractures; however, other types of injuries resulting in facial fractures are gender-neutral.[19] Nasal fractures are the most common fractures of the facial bones in children. Because most nasal fractures are treated in an office setting, precise statistics on their frequency are difficult to determine. Limited studies have reported the incidence to be between 45% and 60% of all facial fractures.[26,27]

Mandible fractures are the most common facial fractures in children requiring hospitalization. Depending on whether nasal fractures are included, mandible fractures account for between 5% and 50% of reported pediatric facial fractures.[1,16,21] The condyle is the most common site, accounting for 40% to 70% of mandibular fractures.[11,18,22,28] Mandibular body (0 to 20% of fractures, depending on the series), angle (3% to 17%), ramus (3% to 10%), and symphyseal fractures (2% to 30%) occur less frequently in young children.[9,12-14,22,25-27,29-37] As adolescence approaches, the incidence of fractures of the arch and body of the mandible reflects a more adult pattern.[38] Dentoalveolar fractures, like nasal fractures, often are treated in an office setting; hence, it is difficult to gauge their true frequency, which probably is higher than the 14% incidence reported in one large study.[29]

Complex facial fractures are rare in children. The literature shows a wide range of anatomic distribution. Reported incidence rates for orbital fractures range from 0.2% to 30%; for zygomatic complex fractures, 2.7% to 13.5%; and for Le Fort type fractures, 0 to 16%.[9,17,26,27,39,40] The sporadic distribution of midface injuries, especially among preadolescent children, highlights their uniqueness and emphasizes how limited a particular surgeon's experience can be with these complex injuries.

Associated injuries are a common feature of childhood maxillofacial trauma. In the pediatric age group, intracranial, intra-abdominal, and orthopedic injuries are associated with more severe types of facial fractures in 30% to 60% of the cases.[8,9,38,41] Temporal bone and soft tissue injuries also are commonly associated with facial fractures.[9] In young children, up to 86% of orbital roof fractures are associated with frontal skull fractures and concomitant intracranial injuries.[7,42] In 30% of orbital fractures, there are other associated facial injuries.[43] These statistics emphasize the importance of a complete initial assessment in children with facial trauma and highlight the dilemma of the timing of repair when medical instability conflicts with the limited period during which optimal reconstruction is best accomplished.

Etiology

In considering the cause of pediatric facial fractures, it is important to understand both the types of traumatic events that result in injury and the unique anatomic features of the child's face. These combined factors predispose children to patterns of injury that are different from those seen in adults.

Motor vehicle collisions constitute the main cause of serious pediatric facial trauma.[4-15,17,18] Fortunately, less than 1% of traffic accidents result in pediatric facial bone fractures.[44] The risk of injury is 1.6 times higher for children who are inappropriately restrained in the vehicle, and children seated in the front seat have nearly twice the risk of fracture as those sitting in the rear seat.[44] Air bags have been shown to decrease the mortality rate in the adult population; however, children younger than the age of 10 years have a 34% increased risk of dying in frontal crashes with air bag deployment.[45] The current recommendations for protection during motor vehicle travel by the American Academy of Pediatrics and the National Highway Traffic Safety Administration are use of child restraints for children weighing less than 40 lb, belt-positioning booster seats for children from 40 to 80 lb and up to 57 inches in height, and lap-shoulder belts for children weighing more than 80 lb and more than 57 inches tall, and placement of children younger than 13 years in the rear seat.[46-48]

Although a majority of serious pediatric facial fractures are incurred in motor vehicle collisions, childhood play is the most common cause of facial trauma (15% to 30%) when all forms of fractures are considered, including orbital, nasal, and dentoalveolar fractures.[49] Bicycle accidents remain an important cause of injury to children, and although wearing helmets has greatly reduced midfacial and intracranial injuries, the current designs of helmets do not protect against mandibular and dentoalveolar injury.[50-53] Other causes include falls (20% to 30%), aggravated assault (8% to 30%), and sports injuries (2% to 30%).* An uncommon cause of facial fracture is trauma from dog bites.[56,57] Isolated orbital fractures most commonly are seen in sports, with violence recognized as a significant risk among those 12 years and older.[43,58] Child abuse deserves special mention. Facial fractures, in particular, of the mandible, can be the result of child abuse.[8,14,33,59] It is important to consider the possibility of child abuse, especially in cases of facial injury among children younger than 5 years, because this is the age group at highest risk for battering.

Both social and anatomic differences account for the disparity in the incidence and in the nature of facial fractures between adults and children. Falls are frequent but generally occur from low heights and involve low speeds, so the likelihood of serious fractures is diminished. Children generally are in a more protected environment than adults that further reduces the risk of major injuries.

Understanding the difference in the patterns of fractures between children and adults requires familiarity with the development of the facial skeleton. At birth, the craniofacial ratio is 8 : 1, with the face located in a recessed position relative to a large skull. The cranium and forehead effectively shield the smaller lower and middle thirds of the face from injury. By the age of 2 years, the cranium has achieved 80% of its mature size. Facial growth also is rapid during this period, but it is only after the second year that facial growth outpaces cranial growth. Brain and ocular growth are near completion by age 7; however, facial growth continues into the second decade of life.[60,61] In adults, the craniofacial ratio is 2 : 1.[61,62] The consequence of the higher craniofacial ratio is that the cranium, especially the prominent forehead overhanging the face, absorbs the major portion of the impacting force. This accounts for the higher proportion of pediatric skull fractures relative to facial fractures and the rarity of serious midface fractures in young children, in whom the force necessary to cause major maxillary disruption often results in brain injury and death.[14,35]

Another resilient feature of young children is the makeup of the face with thick soft tissue, lack of sinus pneumatization, and elasticity of the bones. The greater proportion of cancellous to cortical bone explains the higher incidence of "greenstick" fractures in children.[63] The presence of unerupted and mixed dentition in the maxilla and mandible increases the resistance to fracture, although fractures can occur through developing tooth crypts. As the child enters adolescence and adulthood, the concomitant pneumatization of the paranasal sinuses, maturation of the dentition, hardening of bone, and thinning of the facial soft tissues, synchronized with higher-energy injuries associated with increased risk-taking behavior, all lead to a higher risk of fracture.[29,60,64-66]

Emergency Management

The first step in evaluating pediatric facial trauma is to follow the basic principles of trauma management. A primary survey must be made of the child's airway, breathing, and circulation. Airway-securing algorithms should be closely followed. In most cases of isolated facial trauma, careful posturing of the child is adequate. The oral cavity should be cleared of loose teeth and bone fragments, with suctioning of blood and secretions as necessary. In case of mandibular displacement, a midline traction suture on the tongue can help maintain a patent airway.

Orotracheal intubation is necessary in patients with concomitant cranial trauma, severe bleeding associated with midfacial fractures, or oropharyngeal obstruction and posterior retrusion of the mandible. Orotracheal intubation ideally is accomplished after the cervical spine is secured. Optimally, when oropharyngeal or laryngeal injuries are present, intubation is performed in the operating room with rigid instrumentation. "Crash" tracheotomy and particularly cricothyrotomy in the emergency department are ideally avoided in favor of orotracheal intubation. Once the airway is secured, elective controlled tracheotomy can be performed in the operating room when deemed necessary by the extent of injury. In one series of 73 patients with mandibular frac-

*References 12-14, 19, 21, 22, 25, 27, 32, 34, 36, 39, 54, 55.

tures, only one patient required airway control for obstruction; a tracheotomy was not necessary.[14] However, a controlled tracheotomy is a safe option in patients with panfacial fractures and associated major systemic trauma.[38]

Hypovolemic shock can result from the blood loss with injuries to the highly vascular face of a child. This blood loss may be a double threat if the bleeding is into the airway. Standard volume replacement practices should be implemented, along with transfusion of blood products as indicated.

The secondary survey of the head and neck is conducted in an orderly fashion, beginning with the neurologic assessment and proceeding to evaluation of the neck and cervical spine, inspection of the eyes, otoscopy, rhinoscopy, and finally, examination of the face and oral cavity.

Clinical and Physical Evaluation

If at all possible, an accurate history should be obtained, with the focus on the mechanism of injury as well as the energy and direction of the impact. An injury that appears inconsistent with the reported history should raise suspicion of child abuse.

Although cooperation may be limited in young children, the examination of the facial skeleton should begin with inspection followed by manual palpation in an orderly and systematic manner. Suggestive signs of facial fracture can include facial asymmetry, edema, ecchymosis, Battle's sign, "raccoon eyes," periorbital swelling, conjunctival chemosis, epistaxis, trismus, and malocclusion.

Bimanual examination of the facial skeleton begins over the zygomatic arches and systemically proceeds down the face. The examiner feels for asymmetry, tenderness, and crepitation. The forehead, malar eminences, orbital rims, and nasal bones are palpated. The premaxilla should be grasped with one hand and the head stabilized with the opposite hand to check midfacial stability. Further information can be obtained by intraoral digital examination of the maxillary buttresses.

The manual examination of the mandible begins with the palpation of the temporomandibular joints and the external auditory canals with opening and closing of the jaw. The entirety of the mandible is palpated both intraorally and extraorally. The oral examination includes inspection of the hard and soft palate, tongue, floor of the mouth, and dentition. The gingiva is closely examined for ecchymosis and lacerations; the occlusion is inspected.

A complete neurologic examination is important with evaluation of the level of consciousness (using the Glasgow Coma Scale) and of cranial nerve integrity. Particular attention to the sensory function of the fifth cranial nerve and the motor function of the seventh cranial nerve is essential. Ophthalmologic evaluation is important to rule out optic nerve injury, intraocular trauma, and ophthalmoplegia. This should include visual assessment (if possible), ophthalmoscopy, and tests for range of motion, diplopia, and pupillary reflexes. Forced duction testing should be performed with the patient under anesthesia whenever orbital trauma is suspected. The anterior external ear canal wall is inspected for lacerations from a condylar fracture; a hematotympanum may suggest a temporal bone fracture. Anterior rhinoscopy is valuable for evaluation for septal injury, septal hematoma, or cerebrospinal fluid (CSF) rhinorrhea.

Radiologic Examination

Computed tomography (CT) is invaluable in the evaluation of pediatric trauma. Axial and coronal cuts allow for a complete survey of the craniofacial, intracranial, orbital, and facial skeleton. Orbital injuries should be evaluated with 1.5- to 3.0-mm coronal and axial cuts. When the stability of the cervical spine is in question, and in the case of an uncooperative child, coronal cuts may be unobtainable. However, coronal reconstructions are universally available with the software of contemporary CT scanners, and these allow for appropriate preoperative assessment and surgical planning. Three-dimensional CT reconstructions also are routinely available to permit a more global understanding of the injury. Intraoperative findings generally correlate well with radiologic images.

The "gold standard" imaging study for displaying the mandible is the panoramic radiographic view (Panorex). This can be difficult to obtain in a multiply injured or uncooperative child. Alternatively, a plain film such as Towne's view is specific for the condyles. The lateral oblique view displays the condyle, coronoid, ramus, angle, and body. Intraoral projections can be helpful for symphyseal, parasymphyseal, and dentoalveolar fractures. In our experience, the axial CT scans of the mandible are the most useful for documenting mandible fractures in a multiply injured child and are best obtained when cranial and upper facial CT scanning is being performed.

Routine x-ray evaluation for isolated pediatric nasal trauma is rarely useful. Standard nasal radiographs frequently are inaccurate, especially in children whose nasal bones are not fully fused. However, when significant flattening or deformity of the nasal dorsum has occurred, both axial and coronal CT scans should be obtained.

Facial Growth and Trauma

Craniofacial bone growth is a complex process that is incompletely understood, and even less is known about the effects of trauma on this process.[67] See Chapter 184 for a detailed review of facial growth.

It is clear that facial growth is a complex process. What is unclear is the mechanism of control and coordination responsible for overall growth.[68] Practical concepts for the repair of facial fractures in children are based on the known effects of trauma in the growing face, as well as on an understanding of the operational mechanics of facial development (see Chapter 185, Craniofacial Surgery for Congenital and Acquired Deformities). The mandible appears to be generally resistant to abnormalities of growth as a result of trauma, unless its function is altered as a result of injury in or near the TMJ. Early return of mandibular mobility is desirable to facilitate the restorative bony changes that result from normal function.

The nose, nasoethmoidal complex, and maxilla are more prone to growth abnormalities resulting from trauma. This susceptibility probably stems from the minor restorative functional movement to which these bones are subject, the physiologic derangements that result from the fractures, the importance of the septum as a regional growth site, and the vulnerability of the multiple suture sites to scar formation. These factors suggest that basic tenets should be followed in the interfragmentary repair of pediatric fractures:

- Careful restoration of injured soft tissue, particularly the periosteum
- Close attention to septal injuries, with an emphasis on realignment rather than resection
- Reduction of fractures into their stable anatomic locations
- Correct realignment of suture lines
- Minimal periosteal elevation
- Three-dimensional, stable fixation of complex fractures
- Use of bone grafts in rigid fixation as a substrate for growth in areas of bone loss

Rigid Fixation

Controversy still exists over the use of rigid fixation in the developing face. See Chapter 184 for detailed discussion of rigid fixation in children.

With the current state of knowledge, plate fixation should be considered only for children with complex three-dimensional injuries that cannot be repaired by simpler means. Such caution is appropriate for several reasons: Access for plating often requires surgical trauma to facial soft tissues and extensive periosteal elevation, both important factors with potential for adverse alteration of facial growth. Bone is deposited at facial sutures as a result of tension fields across them. Plating across a suture line could potentially convert the sites to compressive fields, resulting in bony absorption. Plate and screw fixation also risks injury to maxillary tooth buds.

Nevertheless, with the recognition that each reconstructive technique has its strengths and its weaknesses, the use of rigid fixation is

Table 189-1

Physical Properties of the Common Monomeric Polymers Currently Used in Fabricating Bioresorbable Plates and Screws

Monomer	Glass Transition Temperature (° C)	Flexural Strength (MPa)	In Vivo Degradation Time	
			Strength	Mass
Polyglycolic acid	35-40	320	4-6 wk	6-12 mo
Poly L-lactic acid	60-65	190	6 mo	1-6+ yr
Poly DL-lactic acid	55-60	150	8-12 wk	12-16 mo
Polydioxanone	16	120	4-6 wk	6-12 mo

Adapted from Imola MJ, Hamlar DD, Shao W, Chowdhury K, Tatum S. Resorbable plate fixation in pediatric craniofacial surgery: long-term outcome. *Arch Facial Plast Surg*. 2001;3:79-90.

highly desirable in complex fractures in which the original features are difficult to restore. The alternative of no correction is unacceptable, and the use of interfragmentary wires requires tedious surgery and can lead to reconstruction of uncertain stability. As Rahn[69] has written, "Open reduction of a fracture may sometimes appear to be an aggressive approach. It can be justified when late reconstruction and secondary surgery is avoided. Thus an approach that appears initially to be more aggressive may be more conservative."

Permanent versus Resorbable Plating Systems

As noted, controversy is ongoing regarding the use of permanent plates and screws in the developing face. Although these techniques are excellent for fixation, leaving a metallic foreign body in a growing child has several drawbacks: Transcranial migration of metallic plates is a well-recognized problem.[70-72] Growth disturbances in both animal and human studies have been shown with use of permanent rigid fixation.[41,73-75] Metal hypersensitivity, potential for bone atrophy, interference with CT and MRI, allergy, and palpability all are potential problems with use of metallic plates. Accordingly, many surgeons routinely remove plates once the fracture line is well healed, especially in children.[76-80] However, others suggest that watchful waiting is appropriate and have found the need to remove plates for the aforementioned reasons in approxiamtely 8% of the pediatric population.[81] Of interest, in a rabbit study, Connelly and Smith[82] found that the removal of rigid plate fixation had a more deleterious effect on growth than if the rigid fixation was left in place. An alternative solution to this quandary is the use of absorbable plates and screws, the safety and efficacy of which have been shown by extensive animal research and subsequent use in craniofacial surgery and facial trauma reconstruction.[72,76,83-95] A study using resorbable copolymer in infant minipigs looked for local reaction as well as the complication of passive intraosseous translocation of plates. The investigators found the tissue reaction to be minimal and demonstrated that although the plates were embedded in the growing bone, this did not hinder degradation of the plates or screws.[95] Bioabsorbable plates are reasonable in cost and clinically safe. With experience in their application, resorbable systems are comparable in efficiency to metal plating systems.

The most commonly used craniofacial bioabsorbable materials are high-molecular-weight polyalphahydroxy acids: polylactic acid (PLA), polyglycolic acid (PGA), and polydioxanone (i.e., the suture material PDS) and their copolymers. Lactic acid has two enantiomeric forms: L-lactic acid (PLLA) and D-lactic acid (PDLLA). PLA and PGA are metabolized into carbon dioxide and water and are eliminated by respiration; the degradation products of PDS are excreted primarily in the urine.[93] The absorption occurs initially by hydrolysis and is completed by phagocytosis.[96] The physical properties of the polymers are outlined in Table 189-1.[90] Pure polymers have been shown to have disadvantages in strength, time to degradation, or local tissue reaction.[86,93,96] PGA has the best initial strength properties, equal to those of stainless steel.[97] PGA's mechanical properties are lost in 6 weeks, and resorption is complete within 1 year.[49,57] However, the use of pure PGA has resulted in adverse reactions in up to 60% of cases, including swelling, draining fistulas, and osteolysis.[98,99] In vivo sheep studies have shown that PLLA takes 5 years to resorb.[94] Reports on pure PLLA have demonstrated late tissue responses up to 4 years after implantation.[100]

Current resorbable plating systems take advantage of copolymers of PLA and PGA, which allow for variable duration of adequate mechanical strength and biodegradation time. LactoSorb was the first absorbable system approved by the U.S. Food and Drug Administration (FDA) in 1996, and at present there are five commercially available resorbable plating systems with different properties based on their individual polymer chemistry, as outlined in Table 189-2.[90] Because each plating manufacturer uses slightly different mixtures of copolymers, plate strength, absorption, and ease of handling will differ between the systems. Ideally, the plate used will retain full strength for 4 to 6 weeks, the time it takes for facial fractures to ossify.[101] The absorbable plates currently on the market maintain 60% to 90% of their strength through the 3-month mark.[96]

Complications with resorbable systems are comparable with results with metal plates, with the exception of the potential for long-term translocation with metal implants.[20,90,93,102-104] The most common adverse reactions are transient peri-implant edema and a high rate of temporary visibility or palpability of hardware, both of which resolve with time. Foreign body reaction in the surrounding tissue typically is minimal.[96] To date, the long-term studies on absorbable plating systems have exclusively used LactoSorb, which has a faster resorption time than some of the more recently released systems. Studies have shown that the available resorbable plating systems (1.5- and 2.0-mm screw diameters) provide flexural and tensile strength comparable with that of the microplate titanium systems (1.0- to 1.3-mm-diameter screws).[105] Definitive long-term studies in facial trauma have yet to conclude whether resorbable plates cause problems with growth restriction.

At this time, absorbable plates are not recommended for all types of pediatric facial fractures. As indicated by preliminary data on sagittal split osteotomy plated with absorbable systems, excellent results were obtained without the use of maxillomandibular fixation (MMF) in a 15-month follow-up study.[93] However, the use of absorbable plates in the mandible and "load-bearing" bone is still investigational in children, and long-term results are limited.[90,92] At this time, the indications for the use of absorbable systems in pediatric trauma are in non–load-bearing regions in the upper and middle thirds of the craniofacial skeleton.

From a practical point of view, the main difficulties we have found with use of resorbable plates are in complex midfacial fractures with

Table 189-2

Commercially Available Craniomaxillofacial Resorbable Plating Systems and Their Properties

System with Manufacturer and Date Introduced	Polymer Composition	In Vitro Time: Remaining Strength	In Vitro Time: Complete Resorption
LactoSorb W. Lorenz Surgical Inc., Jacksonville, Florida February 1996	PLLA 82%, PGA 18%	*8 wk*: 70% *12 wk*: 30%	6-12 mo
Macropore Medtronic, Minneapolis,Minnesota July 1998	PLLA (70%, PDLLA 30%	*6 mo*: 90% *12 mo*: 50%	1-3 yr
Bionx Bionx Implants Inc., Bluebell, Pennsylvania December 1998	PLLA 70%, PDLLA 30%	*8 wk*: 90% *6 mo*: 30%	1-2 yr
Resorbable Fixation System Synthes, Paoli, Pennsylvania February 2000	PLLA 70%, PDLLA 30%	*8 wk*: 68% *6 mo*: 30%	1-6 yr
DeltaSystem Stryker-Leibinger, Kalamazoo, Michigan March 2000	PLLA 85%, PDLLA 5%, PGA 10%	*8 wk*: 81% *6 mo*: 50%	1.5-3 yr

PDLLA, poly-DL-lactic acid; PGA, polyglycolic acid; PLLA, poly-L-lactic acid.
Adapted from Imola MJ, Hamlar DD, Shao W, Chowdhury K, Tatum S. Resorbable plate fixation in pediatric craniofacial surgery: long-term outcome. *Arch Facial Plast Surg*. 2001;3:79-90.

marked comminution or "cornflaking" of the bone. In such cases, the relatively large size of the resorbable instrumentation (especially the screws) makes fixation of multiple small fragments awkward and often impracticable. For similar reasons, problems with use of these devices also are on the infraorbital rim and in the nasoethmoidal area. Further evolution of resorbable plates and screws toward smaller, more refined sizes should improve their practicability for the rare highly comminuted midfacial injuries.

Maxillomandibular Fixation

In decisions regarding techniques to achieve MMF, primary considerations include the age and development of the teeth. In children who lack teeth or in whom the poor retentive shape of the deciduous teeth makes the use of arch bars and interdental wiring impractical, alternative methods of MMF need to be considered. Fortunately, 2 to 3 weeks of mandibular immobilization in children younger than 12 years is adequate.[38,106]

One approach is the use of an overlay acrylic mandibular splint held in place by circum-mandibular and transnasal wires. The splint's occlusal surface is placed in normocentric relation to the maxilla, and immobilization is accomplished by suspending a wire from the piriform aperture and tightening it around the mandibular midline wire that is holding the splint to the mandible (Fig. 189-1).

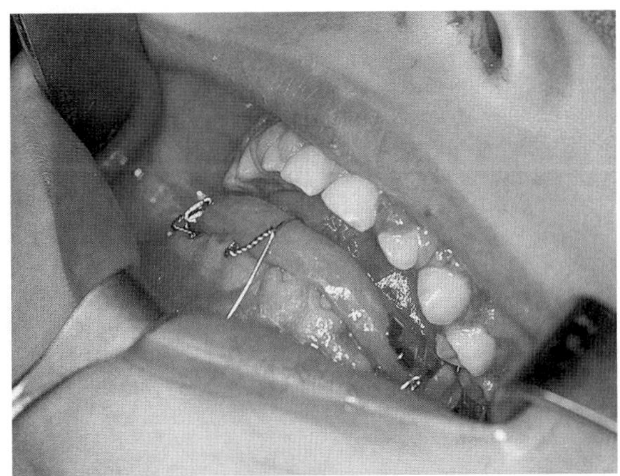

Figure 189-1. Circum-mandibular wires holding an acrylic splint in place in a 3-year-old child with a fracture of the body of the mandible, right side.

An alternative technique that adds more interocclusal stability is the placement of resorbable screws in the symphysis at the inferior border as well as that of the zygoma. The monofilament suture is tied between the two screws, thus avoiding the need for a circum-mandibular suture. The use of this MMF method in teenagers and adults is not advised, owing to the higher forces generated by the masticatory muscles.[107]

In children between the ages of 2 and 5 years, the deciduous incisors have firm roots, and if the deciduous molars have formed, they can be used for cap splints or arch bars. In general after age 10, the development of permanent teeth provides for safe anchors.[29] However, children develop at different rates, and the strength of the teeth should be carefully examined before the placement of any type of MMF instrumentation.

Surgical Approaches

Miniplate and microplate screw fixation systems have made open reduction with internal fixation (ORIF) the preferred method of treatment for midface fractures. The entire facial skeleton can be accessed and reconstructed using a combination of six incisions, which allows for rigid interfragmentary fixation of the entire midface[108] (Figs. 189-2 to 189-6). The *bicoronal* incision provides exposure of structures of the upper third of the face, including the zygomatic arches; lateral, medial, and superior orbital rims; and the nasoethmoidal region. The bicoronal

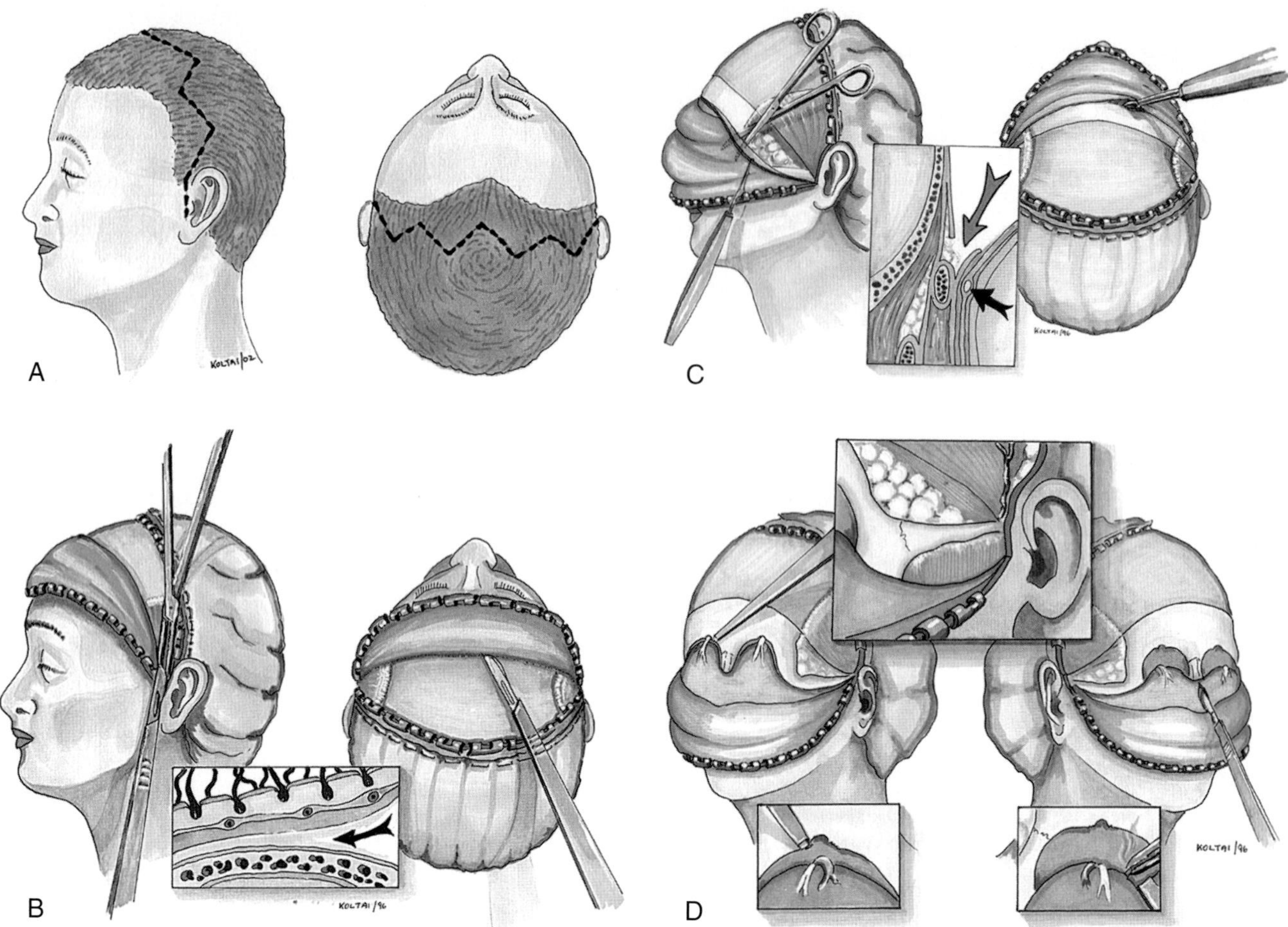

Figure 189-2. **A,** The incision line for coronal exposure begins in the preauricular crease above the tragus, enters the hairline above the attachment of the helix, and traverses the cranium 4 to 6 cm behind the hairline. The "stealth" modification of the traditional coronal incision leaves a broken-line, less visible scar. This technique also avoids parting of wetted hair along the incision line, a common postoperative complaint after repair using the traditional approach. **B,** The incision is carried down to the calvarial periosteum medially, which is contiguous with the deep temporal fascia laterally. The flap is elevated with a knife or blunt finger dissection in the subgaleal plane *(inset)*. Over the temporalis muscle, blunt dissection with a hemostat or scissor is used to develop the plane between the fascia and scalp. The scalp is incised over the instrument to prevent penetration of the deep temporal fascia, which will result in bleeding. **C,** Medially, the subgaleal dissection ends 2 cm above the supraorbital rims. The periosteum is incised, and dissection continues subperiosteally. Laterally, the temporal fat pad can be seen under the deep temporal fascia. The fascia is incised and dissection proceeds between the fascia and the fat pad, protecting the frontal branch of the facial nerve (*black arrow* on *inset*), which lies within the overlying temporoparietal fascia. **D,** The superior surface of the zygoma is exposed through sharp dissection of the periosteum, beginning at the temporal root of the arch *(upper inset)*. Medially, the supraorbital neurovascular bundle is released from its foramen using an osteotome or drill *(lower left inset)*. The medial orbit is exposed with blunt dissection and the anterior ethmoid neurovascular bundle, if still intact, is divided after bipolar cauterization *(lower right inset)*. A relaxing incision of the periosteum over the nasal dorsum allows for greater exposure. *(Reprinted with permission.)*

approach, which is subperiosteal over the cranium and subfascial over the temporalis muscle, permits access to the superior and medial orbital rims. Orbital roof and nasoethmoid exposure can be obtained by mobilizing the supraorbital neurovascular bundle. Detachment of the temporalis fascia from the lateral orbital rim and zygomatic arch reveals the bones of the entire upper face from the zygomatic root on one side completely around to the other. The exposure provides a means to realign and rigidly fix the frontozygomatic suture, the entire zygomatic arch, and the nasal bones. It also allows for harvesting of cranial bone grafts for orbital reconstruction and cantilever nasal reconstruction in complex nasoethmoid fractures. The inferior orbital rims and floor can be exposed by either a subciliary or transconjunctival incision. The medial orbit and apex can be exposed by a *transcaruncular* approach. The *gingivolabial sulcus* approach provides access to the entire maxilla, laterally to the malar bone and zygoma, anteriorly to the infraorbital nerve, and medially up to the lacrimal fossa. The exposure provides for the reestablishment of both the lateral zygomaticomaxillary buttress and the medial nasomaxillary buttress. The entire nasoethmoidal region can be exposed by a *midfacial degloving* incision.

The sequencing of procedures for repair of severe midfacial fractures, especially when the mandible is fractured, is important. Reestablishing occlusion by MMF and repair of the mandible establishes a solid base for upper face reconstruction. Different strategies with respect to the sequencing of maxillary fractures have evolved (Fig. 189-7). Traditionally, the external frame of the face is realigned, and then the work proceeds toward the central core. This approach emphasizes control of the facial width and projection, which is the function of the zygomatic arch.

Other reconstructive strategies emphasize the use of the anterior cranial base as a template for the midfacial reconstruction. This sequencing begins with reconstruction of the frontal bone to which the relations of the nasoethmoidal regions, orbit, and outer facial frame are reestablished. Reconstruction is then completed by connection of the midface to the occlusal unit at the Le Fort I level.

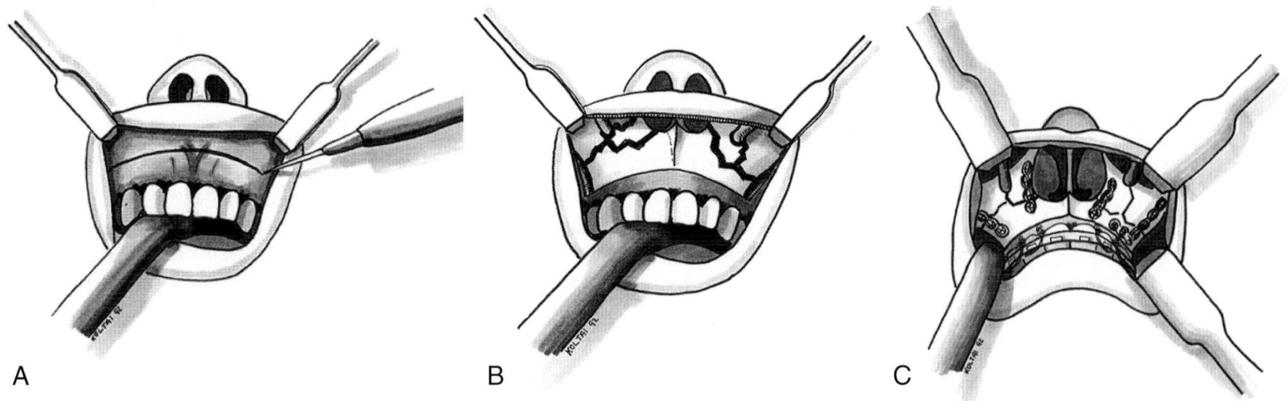

Figure 189-3. **A,** Using needle cautery, a maxillary gingivolabial sulcus incision is created, leaving a 3-mm cuff of tissue on the gingival side to facilitate closure. **B,** Fractures of the anterior and lateral buttresses have been exposed. **C,** The buttresses have been reduced and plated. *(Reprinted with permission.)*

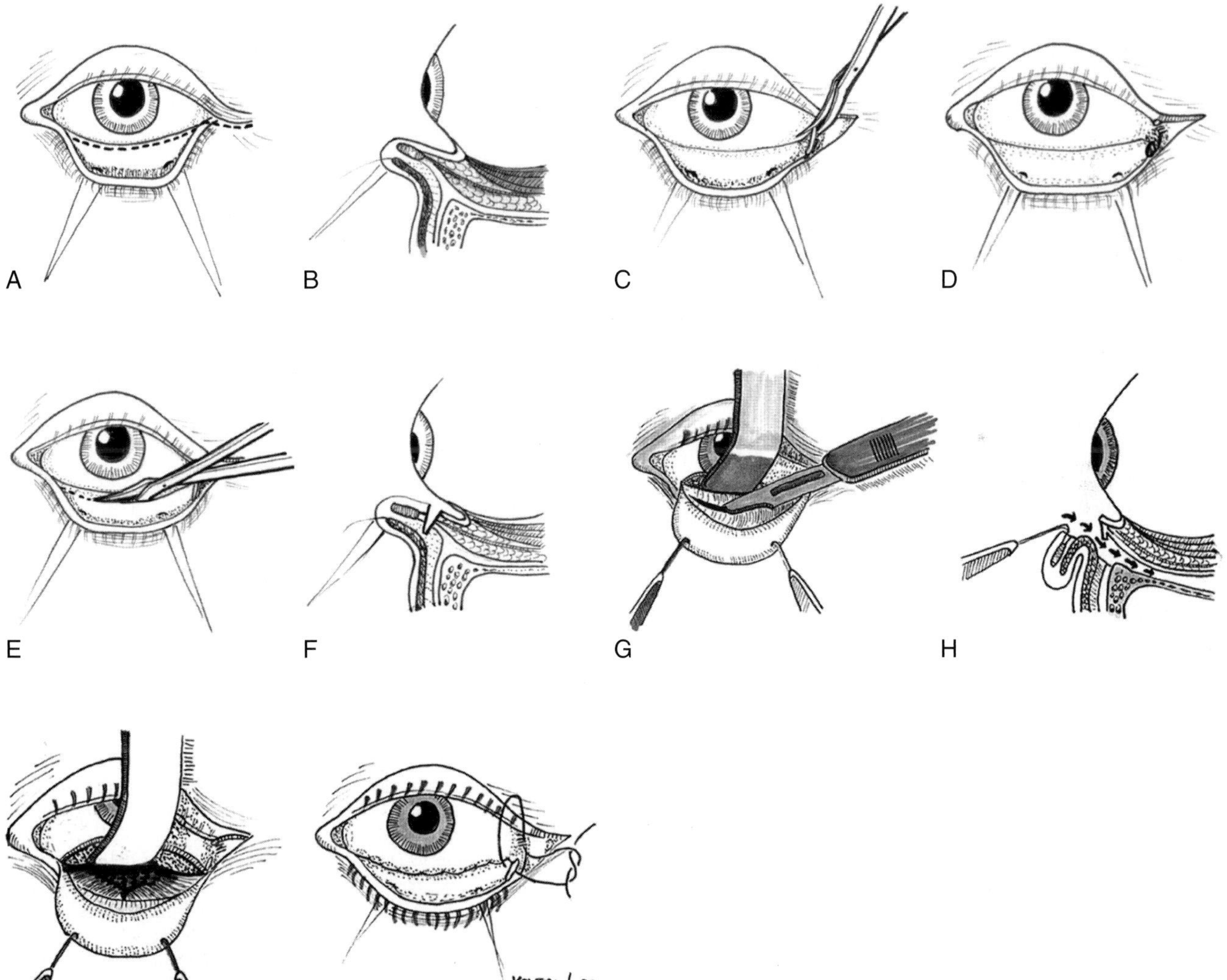

Figure 189-4. **A** to **F,** After traction, sutures are placed in the lower lid, and a lateral cantholysis is performed. Through the lateral canthotomy, sutures are introduced in the subconjunctival plane and blunt dissection proceeds inferior to the tarsal plate and medially up to, but not past, the lacrimal punctum. The conjunctiva is then incised below the tarsal plate **(E)**. The dissection can proceed in a preseptal or postseptal plane. **G** to **J,** The periosteum on the orbital rim is exposed and incised, allowing access to the floor. The procedure for closure consists of placement of running sutures of 6-0 chromic for the conjunctiva and 5-0 polydioxanone for repair of the cantholysis. *(Reprinted with permission.)*

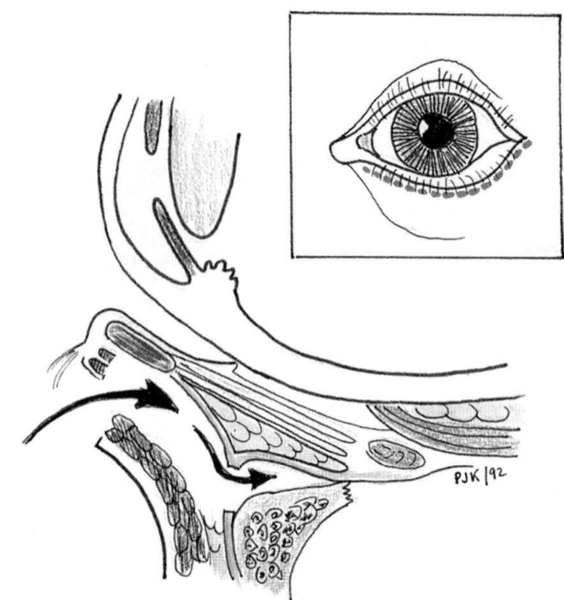

Figure 189-5. The subciliary incision is made 1 to 2 mm inferior to the lashes, through the skin and the orbicularis muscle. The plane of dissection is between the orbicularis muscle and the orbital septum. The periosteum is incised at the orbital rim, and the floor of the orbit is exposed. *(Reprinted with permission.)*

Our own approach to pediatric injuries is based on the recognition that the face is composed of component units connected by their associated buttresses and that the most prominent and most challenging aesthetic unit is the nasoethmoidal area. First, occlusion is established, and if necessary, the mandible is repaired. The central core is then reconstructed, followed by positioning of the orbits and the outer facial frame to the central core (Fig. 189-8).

Surgical Reconstruction

Fracture of the Mandible

Bicycle accidents, motor vehicle collisions, and falls are the most common source for mandibular fractures in children.[109] Greenstick injuries are more frequent in young children because of the presence of unerupted teeth, which increases density of bone, and a higher percentage of cancellous bone, which increases the elasticity.[110] Fractures through developing tooth crypts risk the maldevelopment as well as the devitalization of the respective teeth.[111]

The technical goal of repair in pediatric mandibular fractures is to restore the underlying bony architecture to its preinjury occlusion, tempered by the age-specific development of the mandible and the variable dentition. Before the age of 2 years, the eruption of the deciduous teeth is incomplete. From 2 to 5 years of age, the deciduous incisors and molars have firm roots. In children 5 and 9 years of age, resorption of the deciduous roots and incomplete eruption of the secondary dentition are characteristic. After 10 to 12 years of age, most children have a healthy complement of secondary dentition.

Complications of pediatric mandibular fractures include infection, nonunion, malunion, malocclusion, and TMJ dysfunction. Injuries to teeth in the fracture line account for 7% to 50% of all mandibular fractures.[18,112,113,] Post-traumatic ankylosis of the condyle is a rare but significant complication associated with injury in children younger than 3 years and those in whom MMF was prolonged.[122] One study showed a significant decrease in the vitality of teeth in proximity to fractures of the mandible treated by plates, which the investigators speculated was due to periosteal elevation and increased manipulation of bony fragments.[114] Several adult studies have shown an increased infection rate when teeth in the line of fracture are extracted during open repair.[115-119]

Condylar Fracture

Condylar fractures can be classified into three anatomic types. The first two are intracapsular and include crush-type fractures of the condylar head and high condylar fractures through the neck above the sigmoid notch. Before the age of 6 years, there is a preponderance of intracapsular fractures.[109] The third and most common type is a low or subcondylar fracture, often of the greenstick variety (Fig. 189-9). This fracture type is extracapsular and occurs from the sigmoid notch back toward the posterior ramus. The age discrepancy probably is related to anatomic development. When an injury occurs in a young child, the thickness of the condylar neck and the flexibility of the mandible direct the force toward the condylar head. Furthermore, children younger than 6 years are more likely to have other, systemic injuries concurrent with a mandible fracture.[14]

The condyle is an important site of mandibular growth, and controversy exists in the literature about the long-term issues surrounding preadolescent condylar fracture.[38] Lindahl and Hollender[120] showed that remodeling of the condyle after fracture resulted in normal anatomy in children aged 3 to 11 years but occurred to a lesser extent in adolescents and was minimal in adults. These findings have been the basis for the theory that younger children have fewer long-term problems.[10] However, more than one third of patients with arrested condylar development have a history of facial trauma.[121] Although most children heal without functional impairment,[122,124-126] multiple studies have demonstrated that between 5% and 20% of children with condylar fractures subsequently have some degree of functional or radiologic deformity.[13,16,32,122-124,127-129] Therefore, prolonged follow-up is mandatory, and orthodontia may be an important adjunct in the long-term management of condylar fractures.[38]

Clinical and experimental observations support a conservative, closed approach to the management of most pediatric condylar fractures. Although open surgical treatment is advocated by some experts, the primary decision is not whether to perform open reduction of the fracture but whether the child will need immobilization with MMF. Most unilateral and some bilateral condylar fractures will manifest with normal occlusion and mobility. A soft diet and movement exercises are all that is needed. Condylar fractures manifesting with an open bite, mandibular retrusion, or movement limitation are best treated with 2 to 3 weeks of immobilization. Early and persistent movement with an elastic jaw exerciser generally prevents the development of ankylosis and aids in restoring function (Fig. 189-10).

The indications for an open surgical approach to repair of pediatric condylar fractures are quite limited, and the procedure is reserved for the displacement of the condyle into the middle cranial fossa or interference with jaw mobility.[122] These circumstances are best approached with either a preauricular or submandibular approach, depending on the location of the fracture (Fig. 189-11).

Symphyseal and Parasymphyseal Fractures

Approximately one third of condylar fractures will have an associated symphyseal fracture.[109] With symphyseal and parasymphyseal fractures, the submental musculature exerts a downward and retrusive force, causing displacement of the fractured segments. These fractures with minimal to moderate displacement often can be realigned with careful manual manipulation of the patient under anesthesia and immobilized by the methods described for pediatric MMF.

The decision to treat with soft diet, MMF, or ORIF is best made on the basis of the degree of disruption in the fracture and the extent of occlusion change. The problem with MMF is that reducing the fracture on the side of the dentition (tension surface) often will result in distraction of the lower border (compression surface) of the mandible. To better reduce serious displacement, ORIF of the fragments is required. These midline areas are readily exposed using an intraoral approach. The lower border can then be reduced by wire fixation or by monocortical reconstruction with miniplates (Fig. 189-12). With both techniques, great care must be exercised in drill hole placement to prevent injury to the developing tooth buds (Fig. 189-13). Once preinjury occlusion has been established, a minor degree of osseous gap at the fracture site is of less consequence in the bony healing of pediatric mandibular fractures.[38] With both miniplate reconstruction and inter-

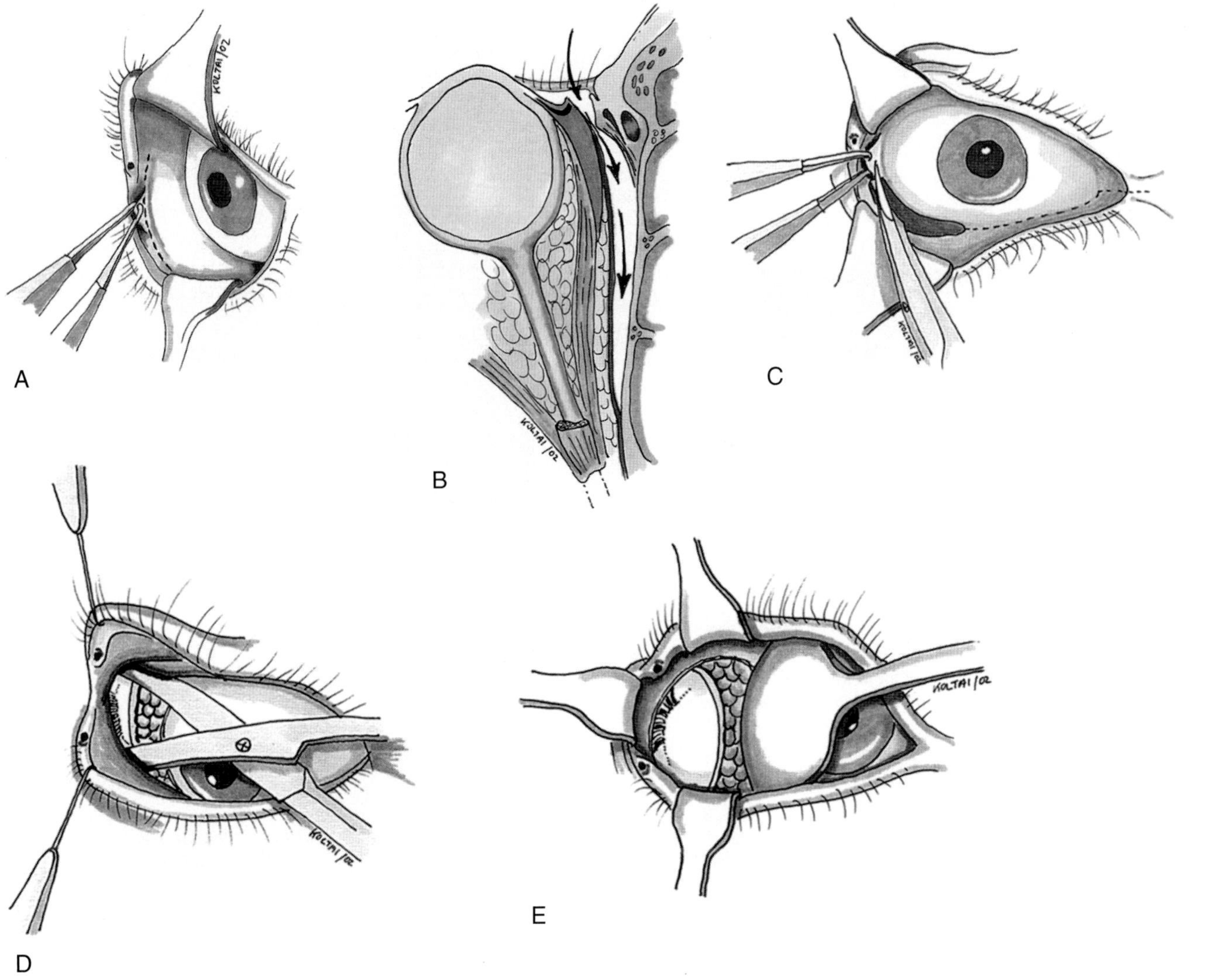

Figure 189-6. Transcaruncular approach. **A** and **B,** After retraction of the medial lid margins, the caruncle is incised along with the medial aspect of the superior and inferior conjunctival fornices. The incision can be continued into a transconjunctival approach with lateral canthotomy to expose the entire medial, inferior, and lateral orbit (*dotted line* in **A**). **C,** Blunt dissection in the plane between Horner's muscle medial and the orbital septum laterally is carried to the posterior lacrimal crest (*dotted line*). **D,** The periorbita is incised behind the posterior lacrimal crest; wide subperiosteal elevation exposed the medial orbital wall. **E,** Superior view of the orbit demonstrates the plane of dissection to gain wide exposure of the medial orbit to the apex. *(Reprinted with permission.)*

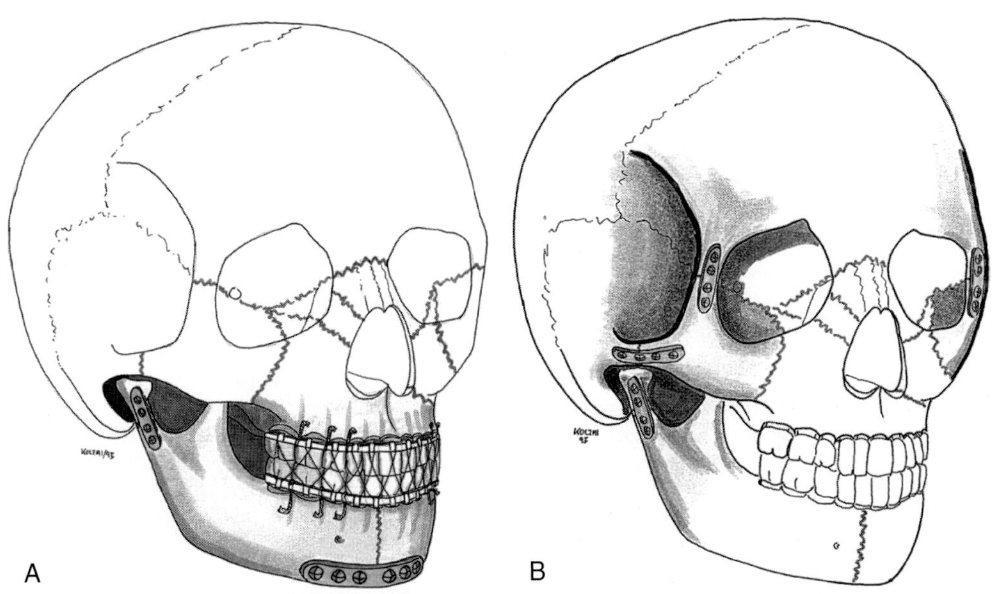

Figure 189-7. **A,** Bottom-up approach. Traditional sequencing begins with reconstruction of the occlusion and the mandible, which then serves as a template for the upper face. **B,** Outside-in approach. The outer facial frame is reconstructed with emphasis on the zygomatic arches, to narrow and project the face. *(Reprinted with permission.)*

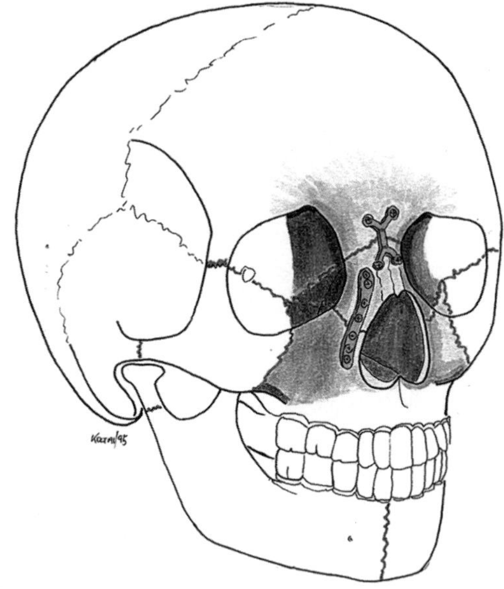

Figure 189-8. Inside-out approach. Reconstruction begins with the central core of the face, using the anterior skull base as the template, with the goal of improving the accuracy of the repair of the aesthetically most significant component of the face. *(Reprinted with permission.)*

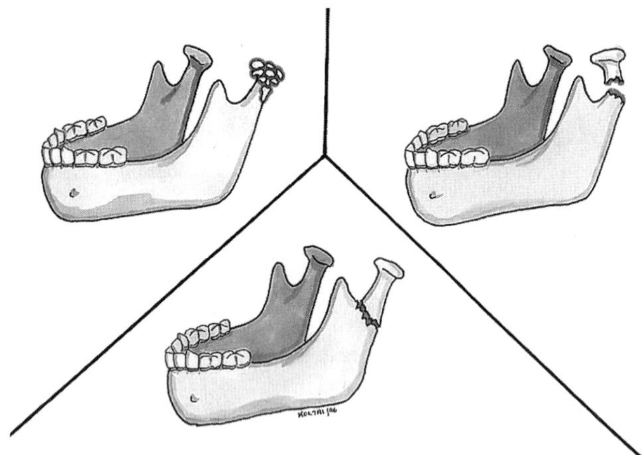

Figure 189-9. Three types of condylar fractures in children: crush injuries of the condylar head, high condylar fractures of the neck, and low subcondylar fractures. *(Reprinted with permission.)*

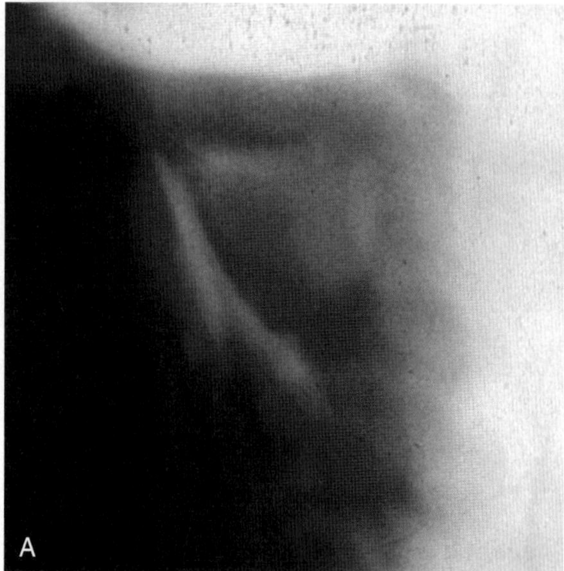

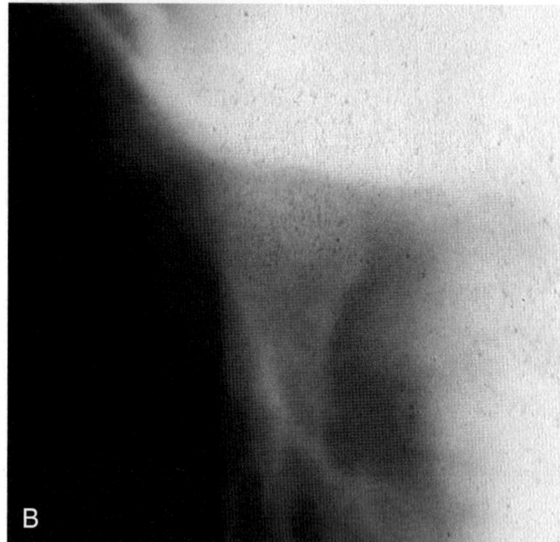

Figure 189-10. **A,** Polytomogram obtained in a 5-year-old child with a right subcondylar fracture, showing medial displacement of the condyle into the infratemporal fossa. The child was minimally symptomatic and treated only with analgesics, a soft diet, and range-of-motion exercises. **B,** Polytomogram obtained in the same child 6 months later, with the condyle restored to its normal position.

osseous wiring, a brief period of 2 to 3 weeks of MMF is required. In children with full, permanent dentition, the principles of bicortical, compression plate reduction are applicable.

Currently, absorbable plating systems in pediatric mandible fractures are not routinely used, nor are they FDA approved for this application.[90]

Angle and Body Fractures

Fractures of the body and angle frequently are monocortical greenstick fractures. Children with these injuries typically have normal occlusion and jaw movement. Treatment with soft diet, analgesics, and observation is appropriate. When the fracture components are displaced, treatment will depend on the availability of dentition, the directions of muscle pull, and the degree of distraction. For distracted body fractures, MMF with elastic traction usually is adequate. However, if misalignment of the lower border cannot be controlled in a conservative manner, then ORIF and the placement of monocortical miniplates will be necessary. The open reduction of posteriorly placed body fractures may require an external approach. However, the transcutaneous sleeve with improved plate holding instrumentation has made intraoral reduction technically simpler (Fig. 189-14).

Dentoalveolar Fracture

Falls and play accidents are the most common cause of dentoalveolar injury.[130,131] These fractures constitute dental emergencies because salvage of the traumatized bone segment and teeth requires prompt reimplantation. Isolated loss of the deciduous teeth without bone is not a problem; however, identification of tooth type, particularly during a period of mixed dentition, is difficult for practitioners unfamiliar with pediatric dentition. The maxillary incisors are the most commonly injured primary and permanent teeth, accounting for approximately 85% of dental injuries[130] (Fig. 189-15). Tooth luxation and concussion are more common in younger children, whereas crown fractures with dentin exposure are more common in children with permanent dentition.[131] Treatment is directed at arranging for immediate, definitive care of the child by a dentist. In the interim, the tooth is gently cleansed

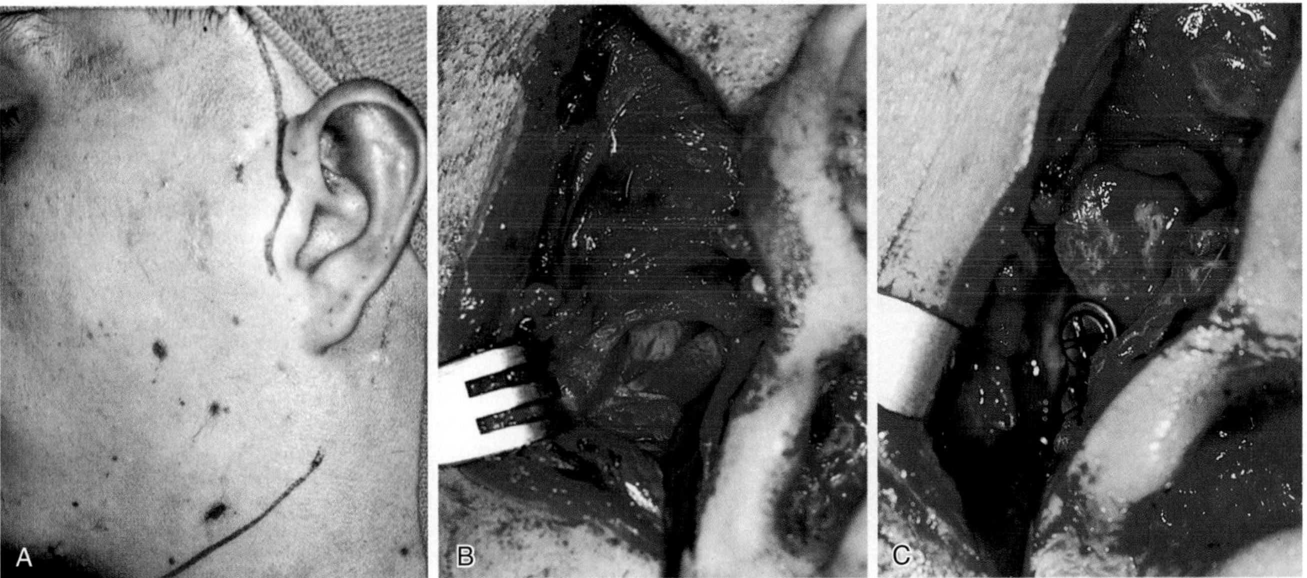

Figure 189-11. **A,** Surgical approach to a left subcondylar fracture in a 14-year-old adolescent male. **B,** Exposure of the temporomandibular joint with an empty glenoid fossa due to medial displacement of the condylar head. **C,** Open reduction and internal fixation of the condyle with titanium plates and screws.

with saline and handled by the crown. If possible, the tooth is replaced in the socket. However, if the child is uncooperative, then the tooth should be kept in saline-soaked gauze or a bowl of milk until a dentist can reimplant and stabilize the tooth. Every effort should be made to have the tooth reimplanted within 1 hour; beyond this time, tooth viability is less likely.

When an alveolar fracture is associated with a tooth fracture, treatment is more problematic. Tanaka and colleagues[15] found that dentoalveolar fractures were associated with the highest incidence of subsequent malocclusion among pediatric fractures. The problem often involves avulsed teeth, fractured roots, and displaced bone. Proper repositioning of the fragments can be very difficult, although reduction should be attempted. Prolonged periods of MMF often are required to maintain these fragments. Occasionally, stabilization with miniplates can be of some help if the bone is large enough to accept screw fixation and surgical space is adequate to avoid injuring healthy surrounding roots. A common outcome is loss of all of the components of a dentoalveolar fracture, despite aggressive measures.

Midface Fracture

Midface fractures in all age groups are described by the Le Fort classification. *Le Fort I fractures* separate the palate from the maxilla, extending through the floor of the nose, maxillary sinus, and the pterygoid plates. *Le Fort II fractures* separate the central midface from the cranium, extending through the pterygoid plates, along the lateral and anterior maxillary walls, the medial orbital wall, and the nasofrontal suture. *Le Fort III* fractures separate the entire face from the cranium extending through the zygomatic arch, frontozygomatic suture, lateral orbital wall, medial orbital wall, nasofrontal suture, septum, and the pterygoid plates.

Le Fort I fractures are rarely seen until approximately the age of 10 years, when the maxillary sinuses are well developed and the permanent teeth begin to descend.[132] In our experience, fractures in children rarely follow the typical Le Fort patterns of injury. Palatal fractures are more common in the pediatric midface injury due to incomplete fusion at the midline suture.[133] Manson[49] and Koltai[134] and their colleagues proposed a classification of midface fractures that is a simple and accurate preoperative tool. The classification, based on the energy of the impacting force, confirms that CT accurately defines the pattern of fracture and generally is the best guide for the extent and intensity of the reconstruction. Type I injuries are minimally displaced; type II fractures are moderately displaced, with some comminution; and type III fractures are severely displaced, with multiple comminution of the buttresses, resulting in a highly unstable injury that requires three-dimensional reconstruction and bone grafting.

Midface fractures in children are rare and manifest clinically with severe facial edema, prominent orbital ecchymosis, and malocclusion. Concomitant neurocranial injuries are frequent, because a force great enough to fracture the midface often will be transmitted intracranially. Axial and coronal CT scanning is indispensable for properly assessing the severity and degree of bony displacement and in developing a surgical plan. A team approach for care, including the expertise of pediatric intensivists, neurosurgeons, ophthalmologists, and anesthetists, is essential. Early operative intervention is ideal; however, this may not be possible owing to the medical condition of the child. Significant fracture displacement should be reduced within 10 days because of the high osteogenic potential of the periosteum and the growth centers; otherwise, rapid interfragmentary healing makes late correction difficult.[135] Acute reduction should be considered when fractures are accessible through open wounds.

The goals of therapy are to reestablish facial symmetry, appropriate occlusion, and normal three-dimensional proportions. Injuries with minimal or no displacement do not require correction. Active intervention is necessary when displacement has altered form or function (Fig. 189-16).

Zygomaticomalar Complex Fractures

Zygomaticomalar complex fractures correspond to the maxillary sinus pneumatization and are uncommon in children younger than 5 years. The frontozygomatic suture tends to be weak in children and easily displaced. Compared with those in adults, zygomaticomalar complex fractures in children tend to involve the lateral wall and orbital floor more extensively.[133,136] It is important to recognize orbital symptoms, including diplopia with ocular restriction and enophthalmos, signaling the possibility of an orbital floor fracture. Zygomaticomalar complex fractures can be classified by the patterns seen on CT scans, which generally correlate with the energy of the impacting force. Greenstick fracture with minimal displacement from the suture lines is typical with lower-force injuries. High-impact injuries lead to various degrees of disruption and comminution of the infraorbital rim, anterior

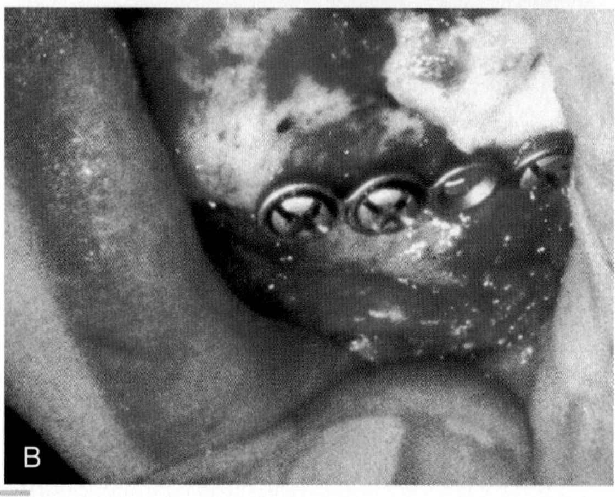

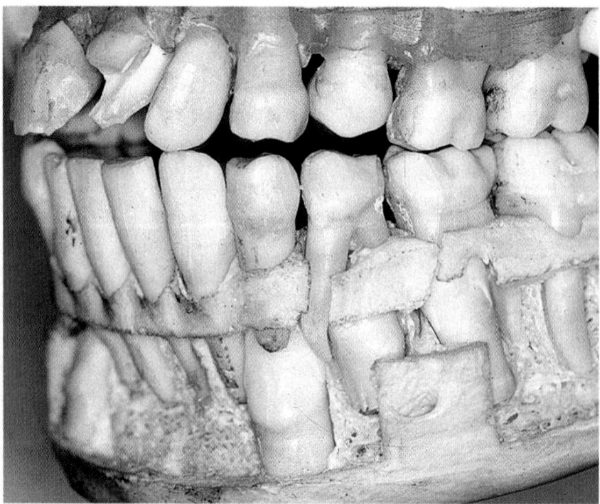

Figure 189-12. **A,** Basket-wire osteosynthesis of left parasymphyseal fracture in a 10-year-old boy. Note the proximity of the wire reduction to the lower mandibular margin. **B,** Monocortical miniplate osteosynthesis of a right parasymphyseal fracture in a 6-year-old boy. Note the proximity of the plate to the lower mandibular margin.

Figure 189-13. Cadaver preparation from an 11-year-old child. Note the proximity of the unerupted left lower canine tooth to the lower mandibular margin.

maxillary buttresses, and orbital wall and floor defects (Fig. 189-17). When the malar fragment has been laterally displaced, the fracture probably is unstable and will require fixation. The most severe injuries often are associated with Le Fort III fractures, again requiring rigid fixation.

The fracture typically involves the frontozygomatic suture, the infraorbital rim, the zygomaticomaxillary buttress, and the zygomatic arch, seen to be separated at the zygomaticotemporal suture. Minimally displaced fractures can be treated conservatively. A Gille's approach or transcutaneous bone hook can be used to reduce greenstick-type injuries, which frequently will not require internal fixation for stability. When simple reduction techniques result in unstable or nonanatomic reduction, ORIF is indicated.

Surgical correction involves adequate control of the frontozygomatic suture, the infraorbital rim, and the lateral buttresses. In most type I fractures, control of the infraorbital rim and the frontozygomatic suture can be accomplished with external palpation, and open visualization is necessary only for identification of the zygomaticomaxillary buttress through an intraoral gingivolabial sulcus incision. For type II fractures, open visualization can be accomplished through a brow, subciliary, or transconjunctival incision with lateral canthotomy, together with an upper buccal sulcus incision. For type III fractures for which significant reconstruction of the zygomatic arch also is required, a hemicoronal approach is necessary. Once exposure is achieved, most injuries can be reconstructed by one-point fixation of the zygomaticomaxillary buttress, or by two-point fixation with microplates at the frontozygomatic suture and infraorbital rim. Severe fractures will require three-point fixation of all of the buttresses. Zygomatic arch deformities usually can be repositioned by elevating through a brow or lateral canthotomy incision. When indicated, orbital floor exploration should be performed.

Nasal Fractures

The child's nose differs significantly from that of the adult. The soft, compliant cartilages that constitute the anterior projection of the nose bend easily during blunt trauma. The force causing the trauma is therefore dissipated across the maxilla and its buttresses, resulting in a broad area of edema. Rarely, the external cartilages can be dislocated from the bony framework. The septum is more rigid and thus likely to be fractured.

Several types of injury can affect the septum: Its perichondrial covering may become detached in response to the deformation of the cartilage during impact. This creates a potential space for the development of a septal hematoma. The septum also can be torn from its bony attachments or fractured in a vertical, horizontal, or stellate fashion. This can result in immediate or subsequent obstruction, delayed twisting deformities, and growth disturbances.

In young children, the nasal bones are rarely fractured because of minimal projection, but when they occur, fractures typically are of the greenstick type or occur along suture lines. When the blow is directly to the midline, an "open book" fracture can result, with central depression, lateral flaring, and splayed nasal bones over the frontal process (Fig. 189-18). With fractures of the nasal skeleton, a high index of suspicion should be maintained for more extensive but occult nasoethmoidal and orbital injuries. Fortunately, with isolated nasal fracture, growth retardation is rarely seen.[21,40]

The initial examination of a child with a suspected nasal fracture often is of limited value with regard to the external deformity because of edema. Several days may be required for the swelling to go down before the true extent of the deformity can be appreciated. However, immediate intranasal examination is essential to evaluate for septal injury, particularly septal hematoma. Nasal obstruction is the hallmark of septal hematoma and can be observed on anterior rhinoscopy as an obvious purple bulge on one side of the nose. The bulge is compressible but does not shrink with topical vasoconstriction. Septal hematoma is a serious complication and, left untreated, can result in a thick fibrotic and obstructive septum. The hematoma also can become infected, resulting in loss of cartilage and subsequent saddle nose deformity or septal perforation (Fig. 189-19). These injuries should be treated immediately with evacuation. In most cases this will require

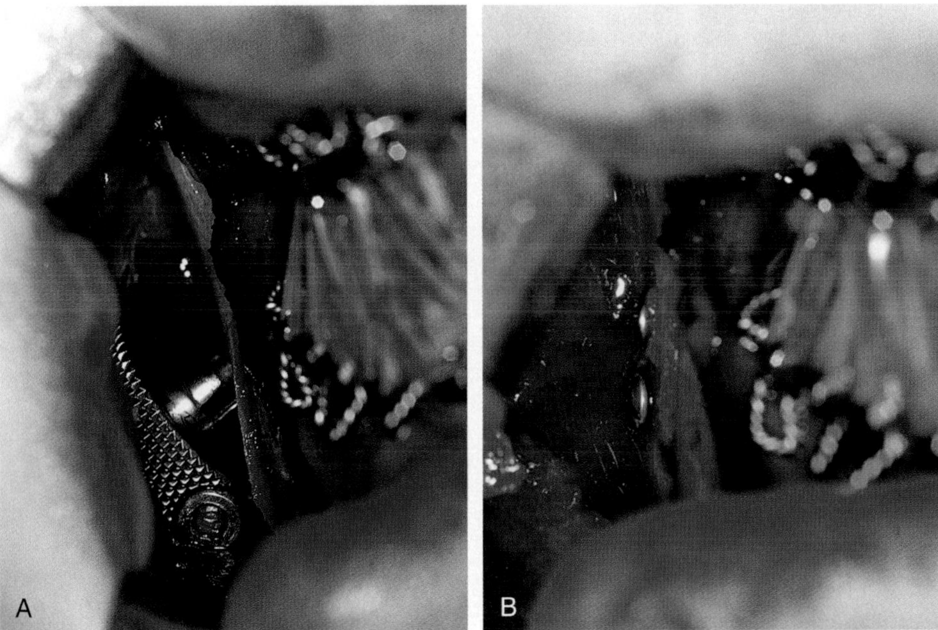

Figure 189-14. **A,** Transcutaneous instrumentation for intraoral reduction of a right-angle fracture in a 13-year-old girl. **B,** Open reduction and internal fixation of the fracture with lag screws.

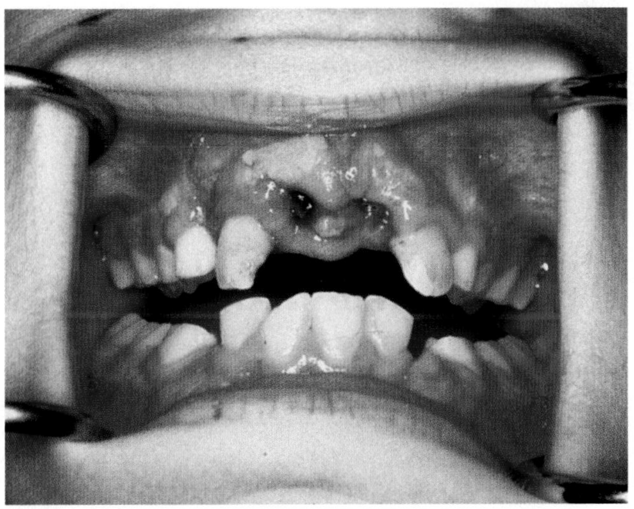

Figure 189-15. Avulsed central upper incisors in a 6-year-old boy.

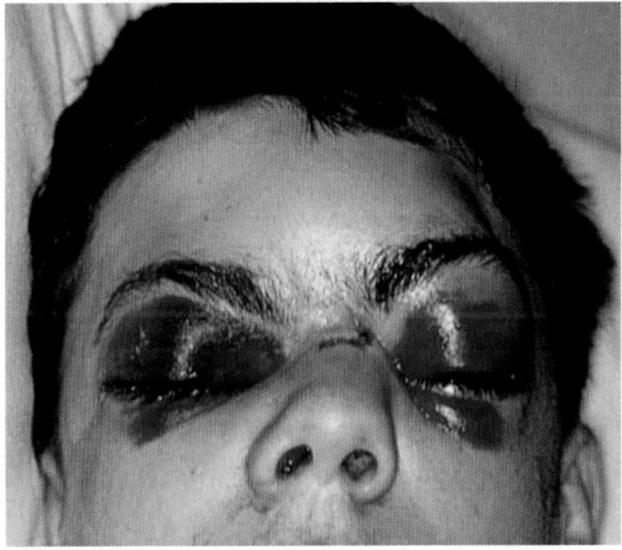

Figure 189-16. Clinical appearance of a 13-year-old boy with a nasoethmoidal fracture. Note the leftward displacement and upward rotation of the entire nasoethmoid complex.

general anesthesia. The use of a Killian septal incision allows for both drainage of the hematoma and investigation and suture reduction of any displaced septal fragments. After exploration has been completed, the mucoperichondrial leaflet is sewn back to the cartilage with a through-and-through suture. Septal splints and packing should be used for 2 to 3 days to prevent re-formation of the hematoma. Prophylactic oral antibiotics should be instituted. While the patient is under anesthesia, the bony nasal pyramid is examined, and if it is found to be dislocated, closed reduction can be accomplished.

If a septal hematoma has been ruled out and the possibility of nasal fracture is still a concern, the child is asked to return in 5 days, allowing time for the facial edema to subside. If a bony or septal fracture is present, resulting in a cosmetic deformity or a fixed nasal obstruction, then definitive surgical management is undertaken. Closed reduction of the bony fracture can be performed with intranasal instrumentation and bimanual external manipulation. Greenstick fractures may not always reduce into the desired position and sometimes require small osteotomies for proper alignment of the fragments. If significant dislocations are present or if the injury is more than 2 weeks old, open reduction may be necessary. The timing of open reduction is a subject of some debate; often, waiting is the best approach.

Newborn Nose

An occasional problem in newborn infants is an asymmetrical tip deformity. These infants typically have a flattened nasal tip off to one side, with the septum tilted in the same direction. The bony dorsum is invariably straight. Some controversy has arisen regarding whether this type of deformity is caused by birth trauma or by prolonged intrauterine positional pressure. Some surgeons advocate immediate surgical reduction of these deformities by straightening and relocating the septum.[137] In our experience, however, these deformities generally straighten over time despite lack of intervention, without late sequelae. The best approach with these children is to reassure the parents that the nose will straighten out in time. It is possible that such a displace-

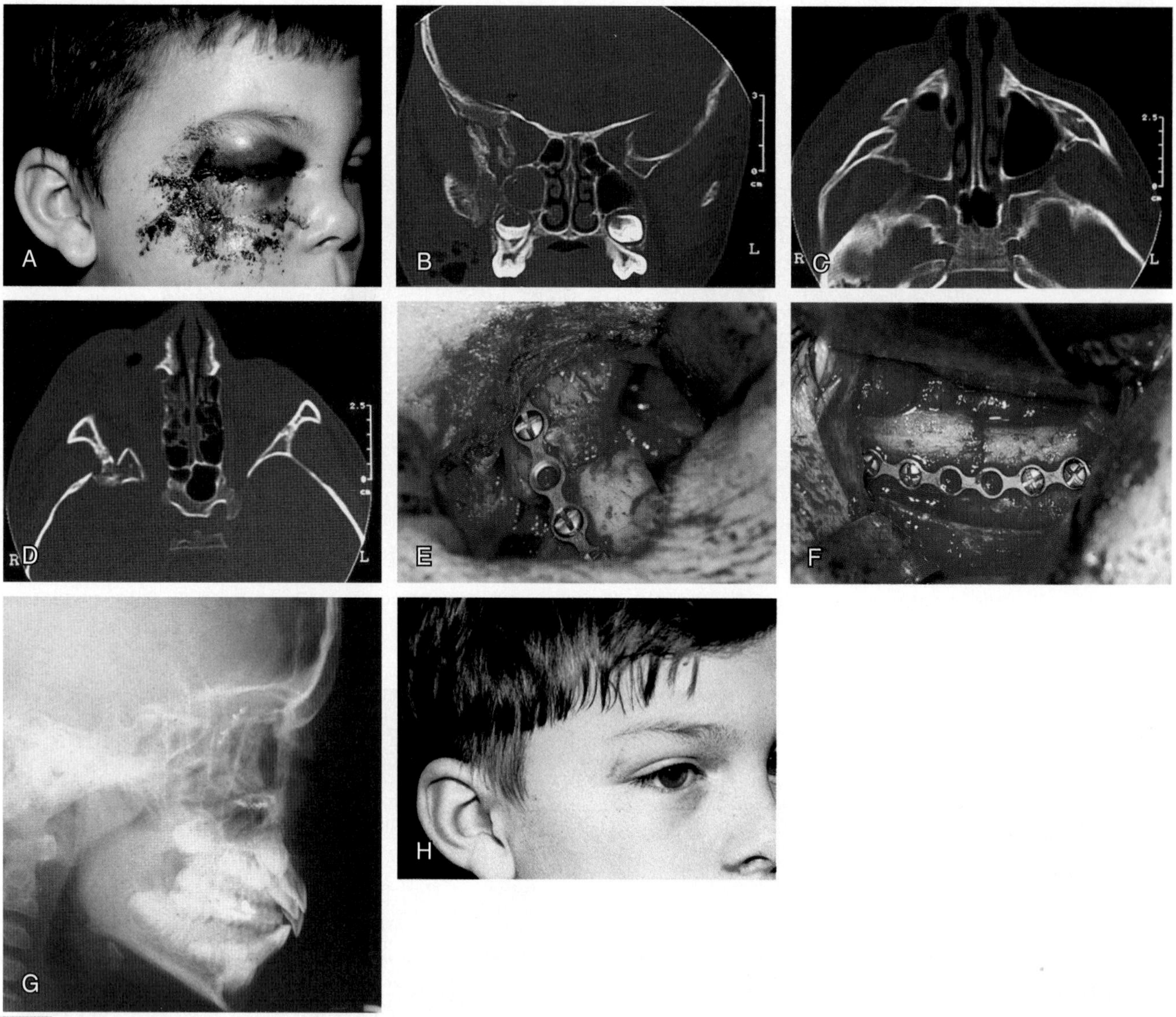

Figure 189-17. **A,** Clinical appearance of a 6-year-old boy with a right zygomaticomalar complex fracture. **B,** Coronal CT scan showing the medial rotation of the malar fragment. **C,** Axial CT scan showing the fractured zygomatic arch. **D,** Axial CT scan showing the buckling of the lateral orbital wall. **E,** Open reduction and internal fixation of a frontozygomatic fracture. **F,** Open reduction and internal fixation of an infraorbital rim fracture. **G,** Postoperative x-ray image of the reduction. **H,** Appearance at 1 year after reduction.

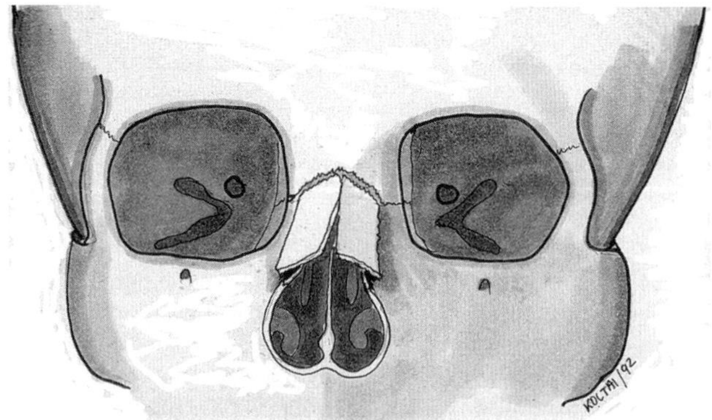

Figure 189-18. When the blow is directly to the midline, an "open-book" fracture can result, with central depression, lateral flaring, and splayed nasal bones over the frontal process.

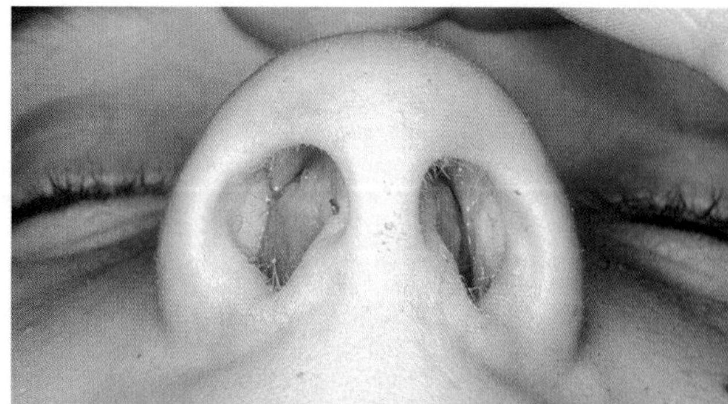

Figure 189-19. Bilateral septal hematoma in a 6-year-old child. Obstruction is present on both sides of the nose. There was no response to vasoconstriction.

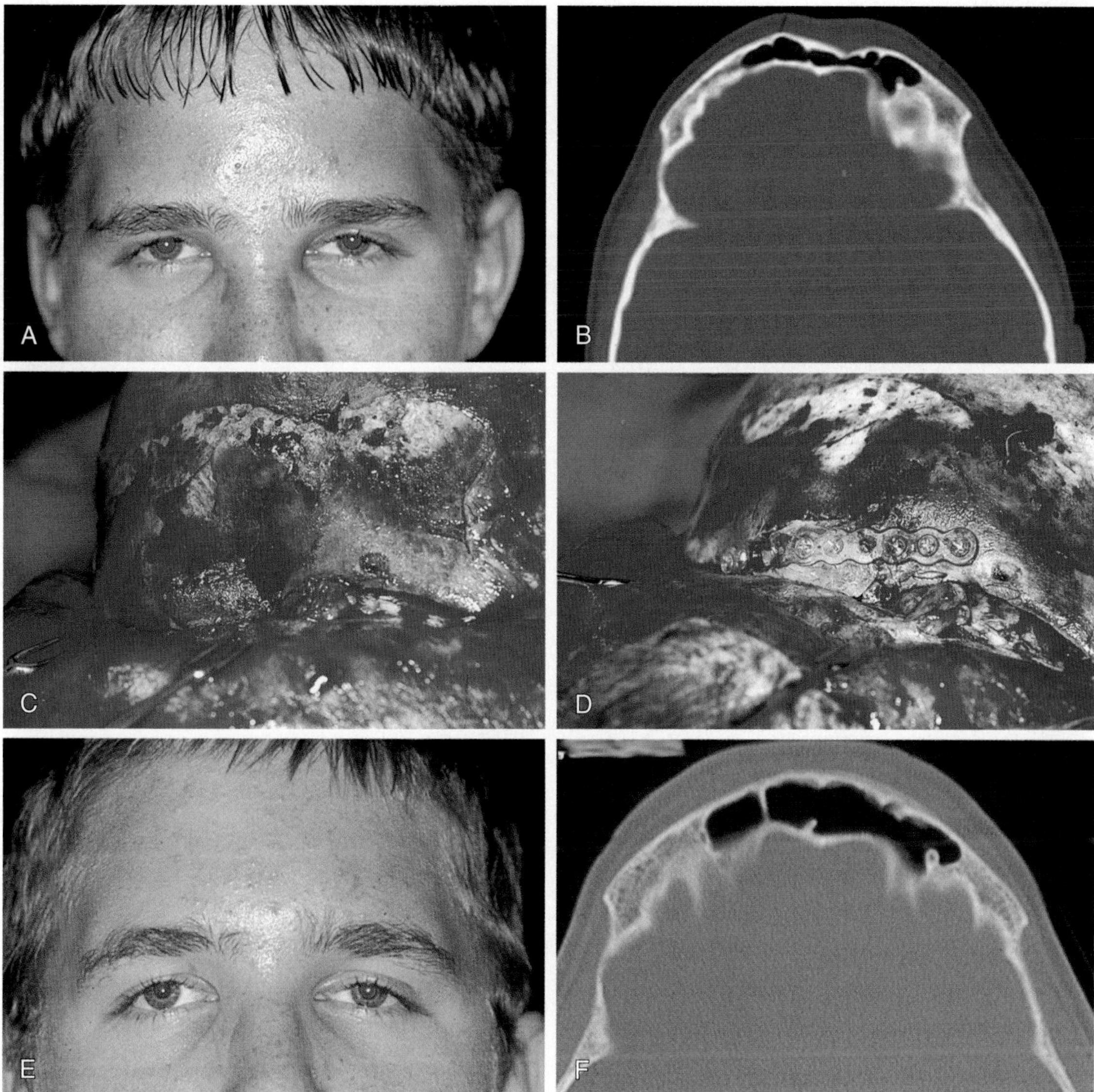

Figure 189-20. **A,** Clinical appearance of a 14-year-old boy with an anterior table frontal sinus fracture. Note the depression over the left brow. **B,** Axial CT scan demonstrates the left anterior table fracture. **C,** Surgical exposure of the depressed anterior table. **D,** Open reduction and internal fixation with resorbable plate. **E,** Postoperative view at 6 months shows resolution of the forehead depression. **F,** Axial CT scan at 6 months demonstrates normal anterior table contour.

ment can cause airway obstruction in a neonate who is an obligate nose breather, and in such cases, relocation of the septum is indicated.

Frontal Sinus Fracture

The frontal sinus is the last of the paranasal sinuses to develop in children and is therefore not prone to injury until adolescence. However, when fractures of the frontal sinus occur, 70% involve the posterior table, and the rate of CSF leak is 18%—nearly double that found in the adult population.[138] Management of pediatric frontal sinus fractures is similar to that of fractures in adults. When forehead deformity is present in a child with an anterior table fracture, it needs to be reduced (Fig. 189-20). The nasofrontal duct should be investigated both by direct visualization of the sinus floor and endoscopically. Posterior table fractures require open reconstruction, and severe comminution warrants neurosurgical consultation. Most posterior fractures are associated with anterior fractures, which can be repaired concurrently. The need for sinus obliteration is based on the same criteria as for adults. Long-term sequelae include CSF leak, intracranial abscess, and mucopyocele formation. It is important to maintain long-term follow-up with periodic imaging.

Fractures of the supraorbital rim can be treated as part of the neurosurgical repair and be approached either by extension of overlying laceration or through a coronal incision. Occasionally, a brow incision will be sufficient. Once frontal pneumatization has occurred, supraorbital rim fracture becomes more likely. Frontal sinus injury in this type of injury is common, and the approach is the same as for the adult.

Orbital Fracture

Injuries to the orbit and nasoethmoidal region can leave children with significant functional and cosmetic defects. The scope of these injuries is related to the magnitude of the force causing the injury and can vary, with injuries ranging from relatively minor fractures, such as "blowout" of the orbital floor, to complex fractures. Associated facial fractures occur in 30% of orbital fractures.[43]

Orbital fracture patterns in children tend to be age-specific. The two distinct factors in facial growth that affect the patterns of pediatric orbital fractures are craniofacial geometry and expansion and growth of the paranasal sinuses.[139] The ethmoid air cells steadily expand, reaching 70% of the interorbital width by the age of 7 years.[140] At birth, the maxillary sinus is medial to the globe, with the alveolar margin in close

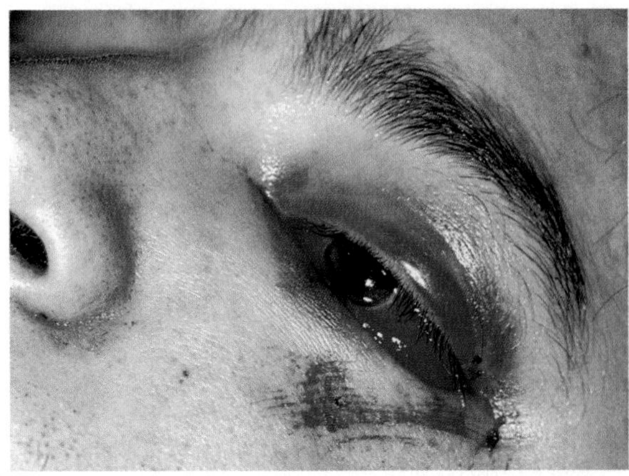

Figure 189-21. Periorbital edema, ecchymoses, and subconjunctival hemorrhage are indicative of orbital injury in this 13-year-old boy with lateral orbital wall and orbital floor fractures.

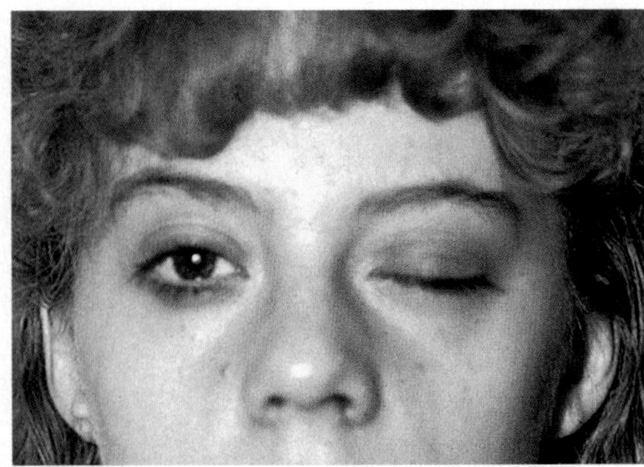

Figure 189-22. Left orbital apex fracture resulting in blindness, ophthalmoplegia, and ptosis in a 14-year-old girl.

proximity to the inferior orbital rim. By age 7, the maxillary sinus has widened past the midpupillary line to occupy one half of the lateral nasal wall. Also at this age, the slowly expanding frontal sinus begins to reside above the supraorbital rim.[141] Before the age of 7 years, the large cranium is more vulnerable to trauma than the face.

There are two proposed mechanisms of orbital wall fractures.[142] The first mechanism, called the *bone conduction process*, stipulates that force applied to the orbital rim is transmitted to the walls, which then fracture.[143] The second mechanism, called the *hydraulic process*, stipulates that the force applied to the globe causes an increase in intraorbital pressure, which then results in fracture of the walls. Both mechanisms probably are operational, although bone conduction accounts for most fractures.

Suspected orbital trauma warrants an ophthalmologic evaluation. Periorbital edema, ecchymoses, and subconjunctival hemorrhage are indicative of orbital injury. Propagation of the orbital wall buckling deformation can result in optic nerve injury without apex fracture; accordingly, the first priority is an assessment of visual acuity.[156] The position of the globe, often obscured by edema, is inspected for exophthalmos, enophthalmos, and vertical dystopia. Intraocular pressures are measured. The extraocular musculature is tested for voluntary range of motion and, if necessary, with forced duction with the patient under anesthesia. Intercanthal distance and the length of the palpebral fissures are measured, and the locations of the medial canthal ligaments are identified. The rims are palpated for disruption. Cranial nerve V is tested for sensitivity (Fig. 189-21).

The orbit has three anatomically distinct regions classified by fracture patterns.[144] The *anterior* component is the hard bone of the orbital rim and is divided into three subsections. The first is the supraorbital rim, a portion of the frontal bone. Second is the infraorbital rim, which is part of the zygomaticomalar complex. The third is the medial rim, to which the medial canthal tendons attach, and is part of the nasoethmoidal complex. The *middle* component consists of the thin lamellae of bone forming the roof, the floor, and the medial and lateral walls. The *posterior* component consists of the orbital apex, including the orbital fissures and the optic canal.

Some orbital fractures in children can be treated successfully by traditional closed or limited open techniques. However, for the severe injuries that require open reduction with rigid internal fixation, the development of hidden extended incisions for complete exposure has been a major advance.

Orbital roof fractures rarely require repair. However, if ocular mobility has not improved within 7 to 10 days of injury, repair should be performed. Permanent exophthalmos, vertical dystopia, and encephaloceles can result from unattended fractures. Reconstruction is best accomplished using basicranial exposure or a combined neurosurgical-maxillofacial approach, with intracranial exposure of the orbital roof. Timing of these repairs is based on implementation of any necessary neurosurgical intervention.

Orbital Apex Fracture

Orbital apex injuries in children are exceedingly rare in clinical practice, probably because the force required is lethal.[4,12,17,40,110] Fractures of the apex usually are due to posterior extensions of complex craniofacial injuries. Blindness is the greatest concern, potentially occurring as a result of optic nerve injury and vascular injury to the ophthalmic artery. Loss of visual acuity and afferent pupil defect are the hallmark findings for an optic neuropathy. Initial treatment is with high-dose steroids. If visual acuity does not improve, optic nerve decompression should be considered using either a transsphenoidal, intracranial, or endoscopic approach. Injury to the neurovascular structures entering the superior orbital fissure can result in ophthalmoplegia, ptosis, and fifth nerve hypesthesia. Treatment is expectant, and long-term deficits are common[144] (Fig. 189-22).

Orbital Floor Fracture

Orbital floor fractures are the most common injuries of the middle component of the orbit.[145-148] In children, the occurrence of these injuries parallels the pneumatization of the maxillary sinus, and they generally are not seen before the age of 5 years. They occur as isolated blowout fractures or in conjunction with zygomaticomalar or Le Fort–type fractures.

Isolated orbital floor fractures typically present with diplopia, infraorbital hypoesthesia, periorbital ecchymosis, and edema. "Trapdoor" and "saucer" fractures are the two major types of blowout or orbital floor fractures seen in the pediatric population. Serious ocular injury with blowout fractures occurs in less than 5% of cases.[149,150]

The *trapdoor fracture* is a pure orbital floor fracture, linear in form and hinged medially, that allows herniation of orbital contents through the fracture and then entraps these herniated contents.[149,150] It usually is a consequence of low-velocity blunt trauma and is seen most commonly in the pediatric population, probably as the result of a greenstick fracture phenomenon.[151-153] The trapdoor fracture, also known as the white-eyed fracture, can be subtle on presentation. The degree of orbital edema tends to be relatively minor in trapdoor cases and insufficient to explain the significant reduction in supraduction motility.[7,151,154-158] Furthermore, the trapdoor fracture frequently is associated with nausea and vomiting.[58,151] Trapdoor fractures are believed to cause tissue ischemia and necrosis, particularly of the inferior rectus and oblique muscles.[7,154-158] Failure to relieve the pressure on the muscle results in persistent diplopia.[153] With lid edema, the diagnosis can be difficult. It is therefore imperative to maintain a high index of suspicion for trapdoor fractures. CT scans classically show a trapdoor fracture along the canal of the infraorbital nerve.[153] However, entrapment is a clinical diagnosis, so CT scanning should be used to aid in the diagnosis. Severe limitation on forced duction testing is diagnostic for these fractures[155,157] (Fig. 189-23).

The second type of orbital floor rupture is the *saucer fracture*, characterized by a depressed crack in the orbital floor, resulting in enophthalmos. These fractures are more likely to cause enophthalmos

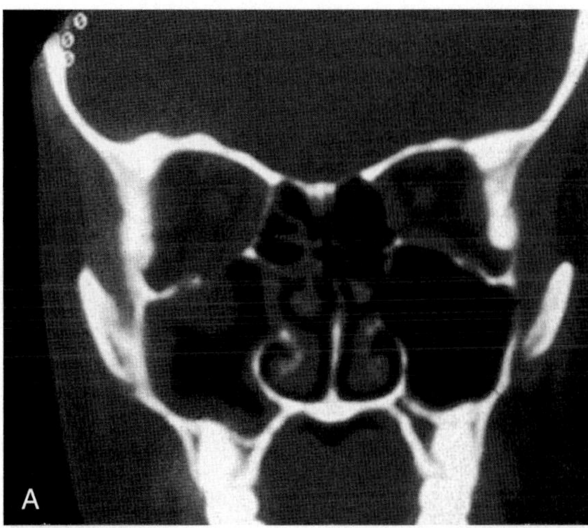

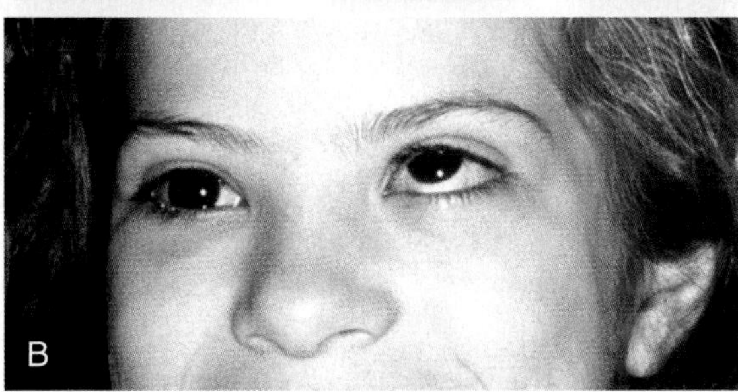

Figure 189-23. "Trapdoor" fracture of the right orbital floor in a 10-year-old child with entrapment of the inferior rectus muscle. **A,** CT scan demonstrating entrapment. **B,** Clinical photograph demonstrating the limitation of upward gaze on the right side. This problem resolved with exploration and freeing up of the entrapped muscle.

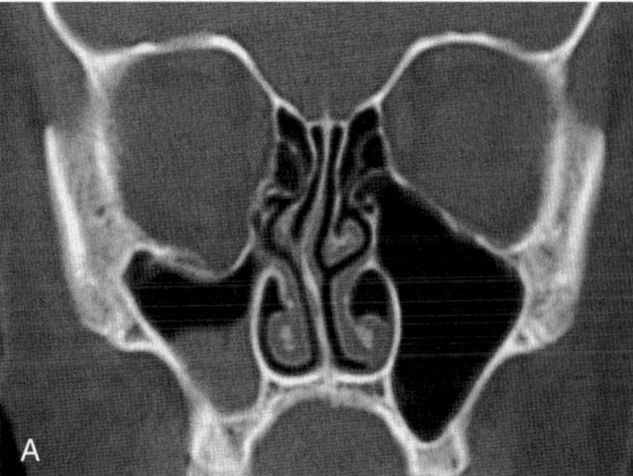

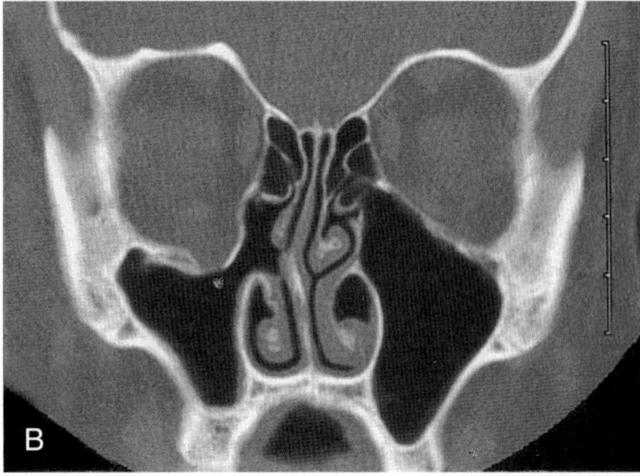

Figure 189-24. **A,** CT scan demonstrating unrecognized "saucer" fracture of the right orbital floor in a 15-year-old adolescent, causing obstruction of maxillary sinus outflow tract resulting in chronic maxillary sinusitis. **B,** Resolution of sinusitis after endoscopic maxillary antrostomy. Despite the obvious expansion of orbital volume noted on this coronal CT scan, the patient had only 1 mm of measurable enophthalmos and did not wish to have it repaired.

without significant duction deficits.[58] Because larger fractures tend not to impinge the muscle, they are less apt to cause muscle ischemia and can therefore be addressed after the resolution of edema (Fig. 189-24).

Differentiating between the two types of floor fractures is important, although management remains unnecessarily controversial. Relatively few studies evaluating the characteristics and management of internal orbital fractures in the pediatric population have been published. Putterman and colleagues popularized observation and a nonsurgical approach to all orbital blowout fractures, and for many years this was the trend in treatment.[159] However, failure to treat can lead to permanent gaze restriction, diplopia, and enophthalmos.[160,161] Accordingly, the practice of observation for all floor fractures has been challenged, with recognition of a role for surgery in some cases.

Indications for surgical intervention after an internal orbital fracture include significant (greater than 2 mm) enophthalmos, extraocular muscle restriction with positive results on forced duction testing (greater than 30 degrees), symptomatic diplopia, or CT findings of large orbital wall defect (involving more than 50% of the floor or orbital wall).[151,156,157,162,163] It is crucial that pseudoentrapment conditions such as orbital soft tissue swelling, extraocular muscle contusion, and cranial nerve injuries be distinguished from true muscular entrapment, because patients with the former conditions can be managed with observation only. The timing of surgery also is controversial. Patients with minimal diplopia, good ocular motility, absence of evidence of significant fracture or herniation on CT scans, and no significant enophthalmos can be managed by close observation over weeks.[164] However, some studies have demonstrated tight restriction of extraocular muscles. Patients with true muscle incarceration have an increased chance of ocular motility recovery with early intervention, preferably within 48 hours.[7,151,153-158,165,166]

The orbital floor can be exposed through a transconjunctival or subciliary approach. The orbital contents are gently teased back into the orbit, and bony fragments are reduced if possible. If a small defect or weakness persist, an implant of absorbable gelatin film (Gel-film) usually is adequate in children. Larger defects in children can be grafted with split calvarial bone.

Orbital Roof Fracture

Orbital roof fractures occur primarily in younger children, as a consequence of the proportionally larger cranium and the lack of frontal sinus pneumatization.[129,167] With aging, the orbital floor thins as the maxillary sinus enlarges. Consistent with maturation, the pattern of orbital fractures changes from roof fractures to the lower orbit around the age of 7 years.[8]

A history of a blow to the brow from a fall or blunt object associated with a late-developing periorbital hematoma should alert the clinician to the possibility of a roof fracture. Proptosis or dystopia can occur but may not be immediately evident (Fig. 189-25). In older children, orbital roof fractures occur as a component of more extensive craniofacial fractures, usually the result of high-velocity injuries. Up to 86% of all orbital roof fractures are associated with intracranial injury.[42,168] The orbit and globe rarely sustain long-term damage, so surgical repair is rarely necessary.[8] Fracture fragments that are displaced into the orbit will require combined intracranial and extracranial exploration with cranial bone graft reconstruction of the deficit to correct dystopia and exophthalmos and to prevent development of encephaloceles. Orbital encephaloceles have been reported as late sequelae, manifesting with vertical dystopia, axial proptosis, and pulsation of the globe.[26] Therefore, long-term follow-up with periodic imaging is important.

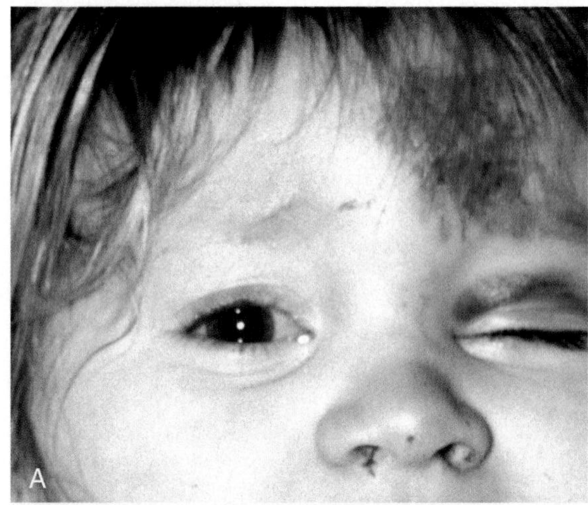

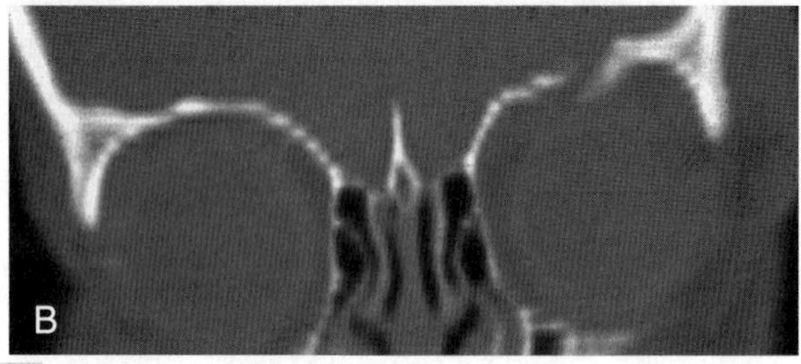

Figure 189-25. Left orbital roof fracture in a 3-year-old child from a blow to the left forehead. **A,** Note the upper eyelid hematoma. **B,** Coronal reconstruction CT scan shows the buckling of the orbital roof.

Lateral/Medial Orbital Wall

Pure fractures of the lateral and medial walls of the orbit are rare.[122,125,] When they do occur, orbital emphysema is commonly seen on CT scans. Surgical correction is necessary only for isolated injuries with nonresolving or fixed enophthalmos and entrapment within the ethmoid sinus. Surgical exposure can be accomplished using either a transcaruncular approach or through an external ethmoidectomy incision. The advantage of the transcaruncular approach is camouflage of the incision, with the small risk of medial fornix scarring[98,169,170] (Fig. 189-26).

Naso-orbitoethmoid Fractures

Fractures of the naso-orbitoethmoid (NOE) complex can vary in severity, ranging from minimal dislocations to highly comminuted compound fractures that extend into the surrounding frontal bone, orbits, and maxilla. The four-sided NOE fracture is anatomically defined by fractures of the nasofrontal suture, nasal bones, medial orbital rim, and infraorbital rim. This complex makes up the "central fragment" core of the midface.[144] Presence and degree of comminution of this core will determine the severity of the fracture and the complexity of surgery to achieve optimal cosmetic and functional results (Fig. 189-27).

CT scan is invaluable in the assessment of the NOE fracture. Evaluation of the medial canthal ligaments is mandatory and best performed with the patient under anesthesia by inserting a hemostat in the nose up toward the medial orbital rim (Fig. 189-28). Traumatic hypertelorism is evaluated by intercanthal distance, which is difficult owing to the lack of standard reference data and the great variation between males and females and among those of differing ethnic backgrounds. Nevertheless, the average intercanthal distance in children at the age of 3 years is approximately 25 mm; by age 12, it is 28 mm, and by adulthood, 30 mm.[140] An additional 5 mm of soft tissue widening above the age-adjusted average is suggestive of displaced fracture of the NOE complex, with 10 mm of displacement being diagnostic.

Most NOE fractures are best treated with ORIF. Although this is technically difficult, overcorrection of the NOE fracture is aesthetically superior to undercorrection.[171] Exposure is best obtained through preexisting lacerations or coronal incisions, with mobilization of the globes along the orbital roof to expose the nasal dorsum. The major fragments and the medial canthal ligaments are identified. Care is taken to preserve the attachment of the ligament to the bony insertion. To facilitate interfragmentary reduction and transnasal wiring, the central fragment is mobilized (Fig. 189-29).

Resetting the intercanthal distance is aesthetically the most important step for optimal results. Interorbital growth is nearly complete by the age of 8 years. It is crucial in children to set the intercanthal distance narrower than anticipated. In medial canthal reconstruction, a drill hole is made in the anterior lacrimal crest just above the insertion of the anterior limb of the tendon. A second drill hole is made in the posterior lacrimal crest just behind the insertion of the posterior limbs. Contralateral drill holes are made, and 28-gauge, stainless steel wire is passed transnasally between the two fragments and tightened in an effort to overcorrect the deformity. An alternative technique is to use a small screw as the anchor for the transnasal wires. Interfragmentary wiring is completed and, if the repair is unstable, further supported by plate fixation of the medial orbital rim[65,144] (Fig. 189-30).

The final step is reconstruction of the nasal dorsum, which often loses its support. A cantilever calvarial bone graft can be used to correct this deformity. It is best to place these grafts rigidly in hopes of limiting reabsorption. The tip of the graft should be deep to the upper border of the lower lateral cartilages (Fig. 189-31).

Direct injury to the lacrimal drainage system is uncommon in NOE fractures. Nevertheless, the lacrimal sac, duct, and canaliculi should be examined, and if injured, definitive repair with stents should be performed to prevent epiphora.

Conclusion

Children sustain severe maxillofacial injuries that require appropriate repair. The primary factor that distinguishes the management of pediatric fractures from that of adult fractures is facial growth. Trauma to the mandible is well compensated and growth disturbances are uncommon with appropriate treatment. Inadequate treatment of upper and midfacial injuries may result in serious alterations of facial growth. CT scanning, craniofacial exposure, bone grafting, and the advent of resorbable rigid fixation facilitate the reconstruction of the most complex three-dimensional disfigurements. These techniques have solid theoretic and practical applications in severe facial trauma.

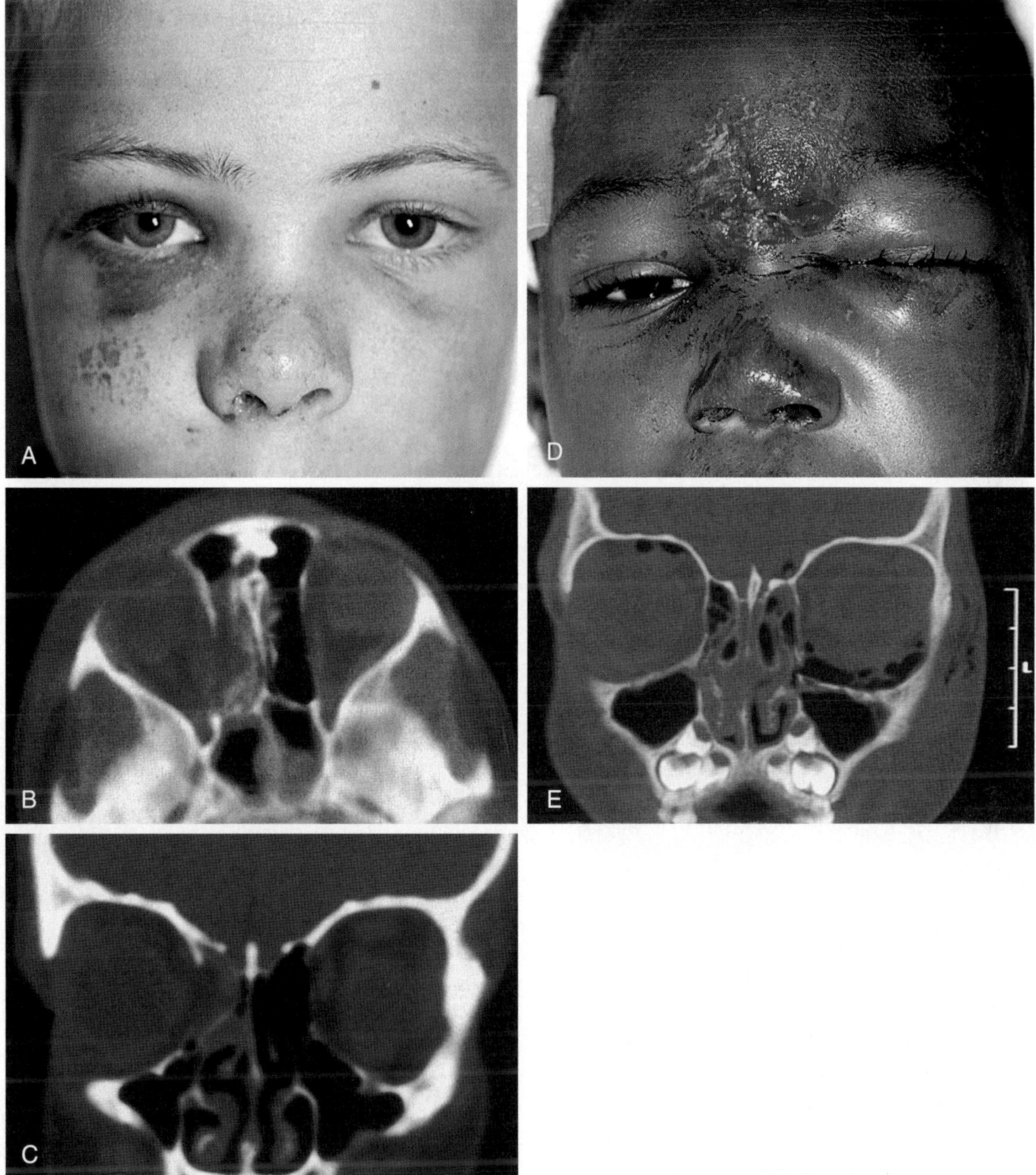

Figure 189-26. **A to C,** Right medial orbital wall fracture in a 9-year-old child. **A,** Note the lower eyelid and subconjunctival hematoma. **B** and **C,** Axial and coronal CT scans showing the medial displacement of the lamina papyracea. **D** and **E,** Nondisplaced bilateral medial orbital fractures in a 4-year-old child from a blow to the nasoethmoidal region and forehead. **D,** Clinical photograph. **E,** Coronal CT scan demonstrating orbital emphysema from the nondisplaced medial wall fractures. *(**B** and **C**, courtesy of Linda Brodsky, MD.)*

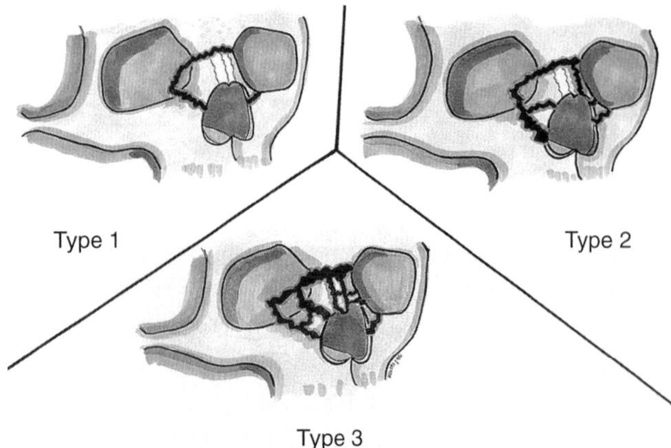

Figure 189-27. Classification of nasoethmoidal fractures. In type 1 fractures, the "central fragment" is intact as a single fragment of bone. In type 2 fractures, the central fragment is comminuted, but the fracture does not extend deep to the anterior lacrimal crest. In type 3 fractures, the comminution extends deep to the anterior lacrimal crest.

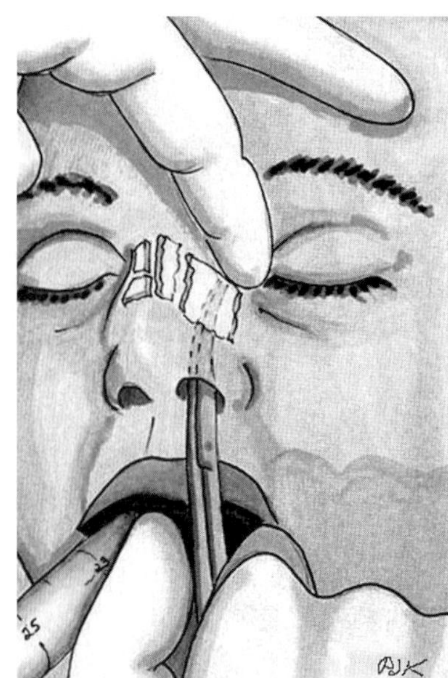

Figure 189-28. Bimanual test for medial canthal displacement. A hemostat is placed intranasally underneath the canthal bearing bone while the examiner's finger palpates the medial canthal tendon. The mobility of the canthal tendon-bearing fragment is an indication for medial canthopexy.

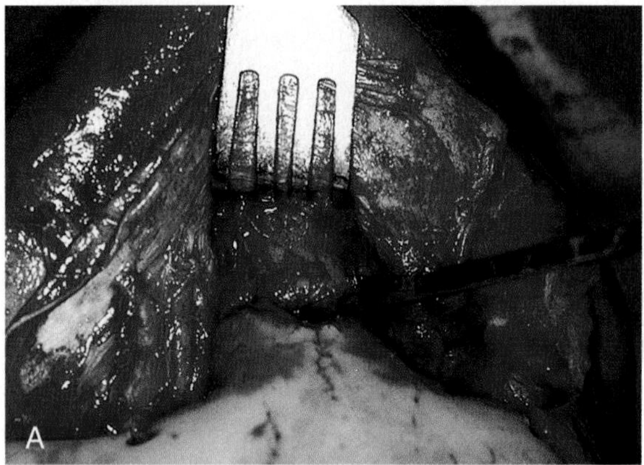

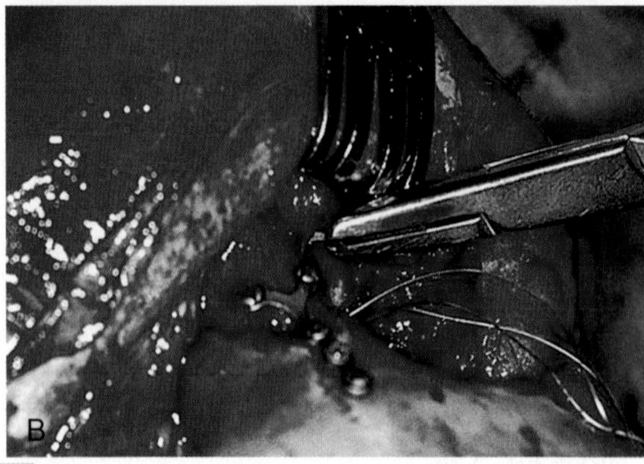

Figure 189-29. Repair of a nasoethmoidal fracture in a 3-year-old child was delayed for 3 weeks owing to concomitant neurocranial injuries, by which time the injury had begun to heal. **A,** At surgical repair, the fracture fragments required remobilization. **B,** Open reduction and internal fixation of the "central fragment" has been completed by suspension from the frontal bar by a "Y" plate. Medial canthopexy with transnasal wiring is demonstrated.

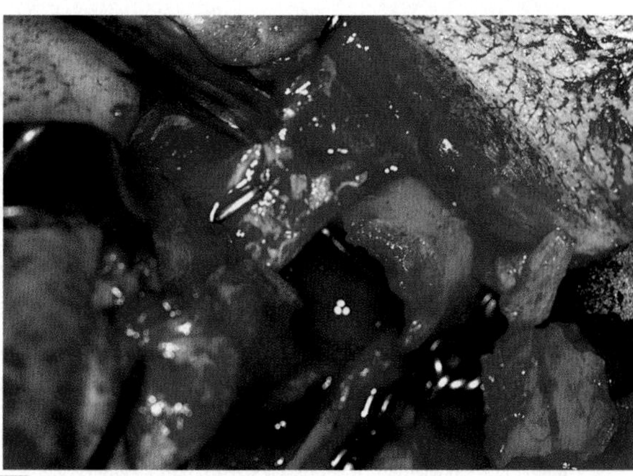

Figure 189-30. Repair of a comminuted compound type 3 nasoethmoidal fracture with bone loss in a 15-year-old adolescent. Medial canthopexy with transnasal wiring is shown.

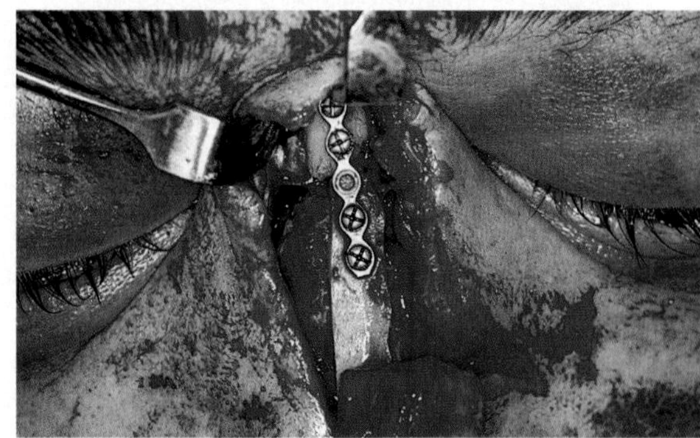

Figure 189-31. Cantilever calvarial bone graft has been used for reconstruction of the nasal dorsum.

SUGGESTED READINGS

Amaratunga NAS. The relation of age to the immobilization period required for healing of mandibular fractures. *Oromaxillofac Surg.* 1987;45:111-113.

Andersson L, Hultin M, Kjellman O, et al. Jaw fractures in the county of Stockholm (1978-1980). *Swed Dent J.* 1989;13:201-207.

Graham SM, Thomas RD, Carter KD, et al. The transcaruncular approach to the medial orbital wall. *Laryngoscope.* 2002;112:986-989.

Grant JH 3rd, Patrinely JR, Weiss AH, et al. Trapdoor fracture of the orbit in a pediatric population. *Plast Reconstr Surg.* 2002;109:482-489.

Hagan EH, Huelke DF. An analysis of 319 case reports of mandibular fractures. *J Oral Surg.* 1961;19:93-104.

Hirota Y, Takeuchi N, Ishio K, et al. Blowout fractures of the orbit—imaging modalities and therapeutic results. *Nippon Jibiinkoka Gakkai Kaiho.* 1991;94:1123-1135.

Hove C, Koltai PJ, Cacace A, Eames F. Age-related changes in the pattern of midfacial fractures in children: a chronographic analysis. *J Craniomaxillofac Trauma.* 2001;7:5-9.

Imola MJ, Hamlar DD, Shao W, et al. Resorbable plate fixation in pediatric craniofacial surgery: long-term outcome. *Arch Facial Plast Surg.* 2001;3:79-90.

Karlson TA. The incidence of facial injuries from dog bites. *JAMA.* 1984; 251:3265-3267.

Koltai PJ, Eames F, Selkin B. Midfacial fractures in children: a classification system based on CT findings to aid in surgical planning. *Facial Plast Surg Clin North Am.* 1999;7:169-173.

Koltai PJ, Rabkin D, Hoehn J. Rigid fixation of facial fractures in children. *J Craniomaxillofac Trauma.* 1995;1:32-42.

Lindqvist C, Sorsa S, Hyrkäs T, Santavirta S. Maxillofacial fractures sustained in bicycle accidents. *Int J Oral Maxillofac Surg.* 1986;15:12-18.

Marschall MA, Chidyllo SA, Figueroa AA, et al. Long-term effects of rigid fixation on the growing craniomaxillofacial skeleton. *J Craniofac Surg.* 1991;2:63-68.

McGuirt WF, Salisbury PL III. Mandibular fractures: their effect on growth and dentition. *Arch Otolaryngol Head Neck Surg.* 1987;113:257-261.

Messinger A, Radkowski MA, Greenwald MJ, et al. Orbital roof fractures in the pediatric population. *Plast Reconstr Surg.* 1989;84:213-216.

Moss ML, Bromberg BE, Song IC, et al. The passive role of nasal septal cartilage in mid-facial growth. *Plast Reconstr Surg.* 1968;41:536-542.

Moss ML, Rankow R. The role of the functional matrix in mandibular growth. *Angle Orthod.* 1968;38:95.

Moss ML, Salentijn L. The primary role of functional matrices in facial growth. *Am J Orthod.* 1969;55:566-577.

Moss ML, Young RW. A functional approach to craniology. *Am J Phys Anthropol.* 1960;18:281-292.

For complete list of references log onto www.expertconsult.com.

Munro IR. The effect of total maxillary advancement on facial growth. *Plast Reconstr Surg.* 1978;62:751-762.

Norholt S, Krishnan V, Pedersen S, et al. Pediatric condylar fractures: a long-term follow-up study of 55 patients. *J Craniomaxillofac Surg.* 1993;51:1302-1310.

Petrovic AG, Stutzman J, Gaxon N. The final length of the mandible: is it genetically predetermined? In: Carlson DS, ed. *Craniofacial Biology.* Ann Arbor: University of Michigan Center for Human Growth and Development; 1981.

Petrovic AG. Experimental and cybernetic approaches to the mechanism of action of functional appliances on mandibular growth. In: McNamara JA, Ribbeus KA, eds. *Malocclusion and the Peridontium. Monograph 15, Craniofacial Growth Series.* Ann Arbor: University of Michigan Center for Human Growth and Development; 1984.

Posnick JO. Management of facial fractures in children and adolescents. *Ann Plast Surg.* 1994;33:442-457.

Rowe IM, Fonkalsrud EW, O'Neill JA, et al. The injured child. In: Rowe MI, O'Neill JA, Grosfeld JL, et al, eds. *Essentials of Pediatric Surgery.* St Louis: Mosby; 1995.

Sarnat BG, Engel MB. A serial study of the mandibular growth after removal of the condyle in the *Macaca* rhesus monkey. *Plast Reconstr Surg.* 1951;7:364-380.

Sarnat BG, Greeley PW. Effect of injury upon growth and some comments on surgical treatment. *Plast Reconstr Surg.* 1953;11:39-48.

Sarnat BG. The face and jaws after surgical experimentation with the septovomeral region in growing and adult rabbits. *Acta Octolaryngol Suppl.* 1970;268:1-30.

Scott JH. Further studies on the growth of the human face. *Proc R Soc Med.* 1959;52:263-268.

Scott JH. Growth at facial sutures. *Am J Orthod.* 1956;42:381.

Scott JH. The analysis of facial growth from fetal life to adulthood. *Angle Orthod.* 1963;33:110.

Scott JH. The cartilage of the nasal septum. *Br Dent J.* 1953;95:37.

Shumrick KA, Kersten RC, Kulwin DR, et al. Extended access/internal approaches for the management of facial trauma. *Arch Otolaryngol Head Neck Surg.* 1992;118:1105-1112.

Thorén H, Iizuka T, Hallikainen D, et al. Different patterns of mandibular fractures in children: an analysis of 220 fractures in 157 patients. *J Craniomaxillofac Surg.* 1992;20:292-296.

Zimmermann CE, Troulis MJ, Kaban LB. Pediatric facial fractures: recent advances in prevention, diagnosis, and management. *Int J Oral Maxillofac Surg.* 2006;35:2-13.

CHAPTER ONE HUNDRED AND NINETY

Early Detection and Diagnosis of Infant Hearing Impairment

Susan J. Norton

Prabhat K. Bhama

Jonathan A. Perkins

Key Points

General

- Hearing loss may lead to delayed language development and poor school performance.
- Universal newborn hearing screening allows for earlier detection and intervention in infants with hearing loss, which may result in improved language development in affected children.
- Estimated rates of congenital sensorineural hearing loss (SNHL) range from 1 per 1000 to 3 per 1000 live births, depending on the degree of hearing loss.

Principles and Techniques of Newborn Hearing Assessment

- Screening outcomes are either "pass" (no further testing indicated) or "refer" (infant is at risk for hearing loss and requires diagnostic hearing evaluation).
- The auditory brainstem response (ABR) measures action potential responses of the eighth cranial nerve to an auditory stimulus.
- Evoked otoacoustic emissions (EOAEs) measure sound waves generated by the outer hair cells of the cochlea after an auditory stimulus.
- Most newborns with hearing loss do not have obvious abnormalities on physical examination, but ophthalmologic examination is warranted in these patients because of the high incidence of ocular defects in patients with severe to profound hearing loss.
- A strong association between hearing loss and impaired vestibular function in infants and children has been documented.
- Newborns who fail initial hearing screening tests should undergo careful otomicroscopic examination, because middle and external auditory canal problems are a frequent cause of such results.
- Diagnostic audiology (or visual reinforcement audiometry for infants unable to understand verbal instruction) is indicated by the age of 3 months for all infants not passing a newborn hearing screening test.
- Standardized laboratory tests in infants failing initial screening are not necessary or cost effective.

History of Infant Hearing Screening

The importance of early identification of hearing loss has been recognized for many years.[1-3] Undetected hearing loss present from an early age can impede acquisition of speech, language, cognitive, and social-emotional development.

Joint Committee on Infant Hearing

The Joint Committee on Infant Hearing (JCIH), of which the American Academy of Otolaryngology–Head and Neck Surgery is a founding member, was established in 1969 with the goal of developing more accurate and efficient methods of identifying neonatal hearing impairment. In 1972, the JCIH recommended the use of a High-Risk Registry (HRR) to identify neonates at higher-than-normal risk for hearing loss. It recommended these infants be referred for audiologic testing within the first 2 months of life. In 1982,[4] 1990,[5] and 1994[6] the JCIH issued updated high-risk criteria. The 1994 HRR included family history of hereditary childhood sensorineural hearing loss, in utero infection (e.g., toxoplasmosis, other viral infections, rubella, cytomegalovirus infection, and herpes simplex [TORCH]), craniofacial anomalies, birth weight less than 1500 g, hyperbilirubinemia severe enough to necessitate an exchange transfusion, ototoxic medications including but not limited to use of aminoglycosides in multiple courses or in combination with loop diuretics, bacterial meningitis, Apgar scores of 0 to 4 at 1 minute or 0 to 6 at 5 minutes, mechanical ventilation lasting 5 days or more, and presence of stigmata or other findings associated with a syndrome known to include sensorineural or conductive hearing loss. However, the JCIH recommended HRR use only if universal newborn hearing screening (UNHS) was unavailable. Only 2% to 5% of neonates with one or more risk factors exhibit a moderate to profound hearing loss. Conversely, 95% to 98% of neonates with one or more risk factors have normal hearing.[7] Furthermore, 50% of children with moderate to profound congenital hearing loss exhibit no risk factors for hearing loss.[8] This means that use of the HRR alone, as an indication for hearing testing, would leave at least 50% of infants with congenital hearing loss undiagnosed. In 2007, the JCIH recommended hearing screening for all newborns, with formal audiologic assessment in those who fail the initial screening test by 3 months of age, followed by intervention by 6 months of age for children with significant hearing loss.[9]

Delay in Identification

A significant delay exists in the identification and intervention of hearing impairment for infants without risk factors. For infants with mild to moderate hearing loss, a 1996 survey showed that parents of high-risk infants first suspected the loss when their infants were at a median age of 8 months. By contrast, the parents of infants without risk factors first suspected their infant had a hearing loss when the child was 15 months old.[10,11] Hearing loss was confirmed in infants without risk factors at 22 months of age, compared with 12 months of age for infants with risk factors, and infants were enrolled in intervention at 28 and 18 months, respectively. Ages of suspicion (7 to 8 months), diagnosis (12 to 13 months), and intervention (18 to 19 months) were essentially the same for infants with severe to profound hearing loss, regardless of whether risk factors were present. Recent retrospective studies indicate that infants with hearing loss enrolled in appropriate early intervention by 6 months of age incur significantly fewer delays than those who enroll after 6 months of age.[10,12] These findings are for children with all degrees of hearing loss, as well as for children with other handicapping conditions.

Universal Newborn Hearing Screening

In 1993, the National Institute for Deafness and Other Communicative Disorders (NIDCD) Consensus Conference on Early Identification of Hearing Loss recommended UNHS for infants within the first 3 months of life, preferably before hospital discharge.[13] Subsequently, several organizations and government agencies have endorsed UNHS as the best way to ensure early detection and habilitation of hearing loss. These groups include the Academy of Otolaryngology–Head and Neck Surgery, American Academy of Pediatrics, American Speech-Language-Hearing Association, American Academy of Audiology, and others. Despite considerable disagreement concerning the relative merits of specific measurement approaches for neonatal hearing screening and whether UNHS is even appropriate at this time,[14] universal newborn and infant hearing screening statutes have been passed in 41 states (legislation is pending in two states), and all states have implemented newborn hearing screening programs.[9] The goals of the U.S. Department of Health and Human Services' initiative Healthy People 2010 include UNHS by 1 month of age, diagnostic confirmation of hearing loss by 3 months of age, and enrollment in appropriate early intervention for children with hearing loss and their families by 6 months of age.[15] The Newborn Infant Hearing and Screening Intervention Act of 1999 provided funding to help states reach this goal. In 2008, the U.S. Preventive Services Task Force published a grade B recommendation to screen for hearing loss in all newborn infants.[16]

Prevalence of Sensorineural Hearing Loss in Children

Estimates of congenital sensorineural hearing loss (SNHL) vary, ranging from 1 per 1000 to 3 per 1000 live births, depending on the degree of hearing loss. Bilateral severe to profound hearing loss (70 dB HL or greater) occurs in 1 per 1000 live births. When the results of several studies are averaged, approximately 3 per 1000 infants have a hearing loss of 30 dB or greater.[17-21] The incidence of significant hearing loss is 10 times greater for infants with one or more risk factors than for those with no risk factors.

Progressive, late-onset, and acquired hearing loss in childhood is a continuing challenge. In its survey of deaf and hard-of-hearing school-aged children, Gallaudet Research Institute found a prevalence of significant hearing loss of 1.8% in children 3 to 17 years of age.[22] This figure is six times higher than the incidence of hearing loss in the neonatal period. Similarly, van Naarden and colleagues[23] reported that the average point prevalence of hearing losses 40 dB or greater increased with age from 0.67% at 3 years of age to 1.38% at 10 years of age. It is important that hearing, speech, and language development be monitored because of the occurrence of progressive, late-onset, and acquired hearing loss in early childhood.

Increase in Early Identification

In those states with UNHS, the average age of identification of congenital hearing loss has dramatically decreased. Rhode Island mandated UNHS in 1993. In 1998, Vohr and colleagues[24] reported that the average age at confirmation of permanent hearing loss in Rhode Island infants was 3 months. By contrast, in the absence of UNHS, the average age at diagnosis of permanent hearing loss in children was 31.25 months. In its 1999 Policy Statement, the American Academy of Pediatrics noted: "Reliance on physician observation and/or parental recognition has not been successful in the past in detecting significant hearing loss in the first year of life."[25] Long-term prospective studies of deaf and hard-of-hearing children identified through newborn hearing screening programs are needed to determine if in fact educational and vocational outcomes are significantly better for these children. A recently published controlled trial in the United Kingdom demonstrated that UNHS increased the proportion of 7- to 9-year-old children with permanent hearing loss who were identified before 6 months of age.[26] Strong data illustrating improved speech and language development from early interventions are lacking, but one controlled trial found that early detection of childhood hearing impairment leads to higher language scores (but not speech scores) in mid-childhood.[27]

Principles and Techniques of Newborn Hearing Assessment

Testing Protocols

The goal of newborn hearing screening is to identify those infants who need diagnostic hearing evaluations because they are at risk for significant hearing loss. With current technology, screening outcomes are either "pass" or "refer" (Fig. 190-1). "Pass" indicates the infant is not at risk for significant hearing loss and needs no further testing at this time. "Refer" indicates the infant is at risk for hearing loss and requires a diagnostic hearing evaluation. It is important to emphasize to parents and health care providers that "refer" does not mean that the baby has a hearing loss; this designation indicates only that the child has a greater risk of having hearing loss.

For many years, a primary barrier to UNHS was the lack of affordable, reliable, easy-to-use methodology. A hearing screening test has several requirements. First, the response being measured must be robust, specific to the peripheral auditory system, and present in all normal-hearing newborns. Second, the response criteria must be objective, based on scientific data, and applied consistently. Third, the measurement procedures must be noninvasive, rapid, reliable, and easy to use, with capability for separate testing of each ear. Behavioral methods do not meet these requirements. At present, one of two physiologic measures of auditory system status is used singly or in combination in most UNHS programs. Current technology uses automated protocols and pass-refer criteria. Such algorithms allow the use of less experienced testers, thereby reducing the cost of screening and removing some of the variability in test administration.

Auditory Brainstem Responses

The auditory brainstem response (ABR) is a series of scalp-recorded electrical potentials generated in the auditory nerve and brainstem during the first 10 to 20 ms after the onset of a transient stimulus. For the purposes of a hearing screening, responses typically are elicited by air-conducted clicks presented at a level that is thought to produce a response in ears with normal hearing and to produce no response in ears with

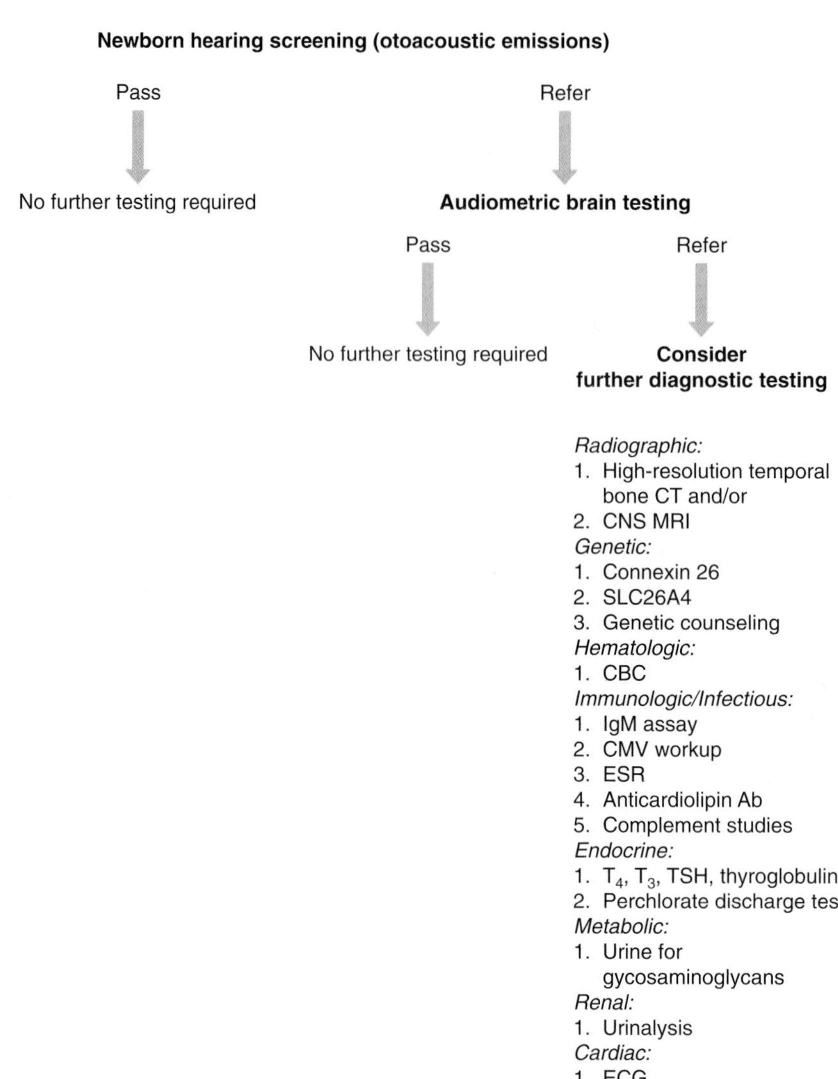

Figure 190-1. Algorithm for newborn hearing screening. Ab, antibody; CBC, complete blood count; CMV, cytomegalovirus; CNS, central nervous system; CT, computed tomography; ECG, electrocardiogram; ESR, erythrocyte sedimentation rate; IgM, immunoglobulin M; MRI, magnetic resonance imaging; T_3, triiodothyronine; T_4, thyroxine; TSH, thyroid-stimulating hormone.

hearing loss (30 to 35 dB normal hearing level [nHL]). Surface electrodes record the synchronized time-domain averaged response to the click.

In response to a click stimulus of known intensity, ABR latency and morphology are highly predictable for infants of a given age. This evoked potential is present in human neonates as early as 25 weeks of gestational age and is unaffected by sleep, attention, or sedation. ABR morphology changes rapidly with age during infancy because of maturation of the central nervous system (CNS). Therefore, it is important to use age-appropriate latency-intensity norms in judging the quality of ABR. ABR is affected by external and middle ear, cochlear, auditory nerve, and brainstem status. Middle ear disease or anomaly reduces the stimulus intensity, thus increasing the latency and decreasing the amplitude of the ABR. Cochlear abnormalities affect the quality and morphology of the ABR in many different ways. Response amplitude may be reduced, latency may be increased, or waveform morphology altered, depending on the degree and configuration of the hearing loss. Brief stimuli such as clicks have a broadband frequency spectrum. Click-evoked ABR is not frequency-specific. Any region of normal hearing can generate the response if there is sufficient energy in the stimulus at that frequency. ABR also is abnormal in the presence of eighth cranial nerve and lower brainstem abnormalities even if peripheral hearing loss is not present.

ABR has been used for many years to screen infants in the neonatal intensive care unit (NICU) before hospital discharge.[28-32] Recent advances have resulted in the development of automated ABR detection algorithms.[33-37] These systems replace the subjective impression of the tester as to the presence or absence of an ABR, with an objective statistical estimate of the likelihood or probability of a "response" distinct from the background "noise."

Evoked Otoacoustic Emissions

Evoked otoacoustic emissions (EOAEs) are also used widely for newborn hearing screening. EOAEs are acoustic signals generated by the cochlea in response to auditory stimulation. They are a physiologically vulnerable indicator of cochlear status, specifically outer hair cells. EOAE generation is independent of neural activity, so EOAE testing measures cochlear status independent of CNS status. Transient evoked otoacoustic emissions (TEOAEs) occur after a brief click stimulus.[38] TEOAEs provide information over a broad frequency range (approximately 500 to 6000 Hz). Distortion product otoacoustic emissions (DPOAEs) occur in response to simultaneous presentation of two pure tones with the appropriate frequency and amplitude ratios and provide frequency-specific information across a broad range of frequencies.[39]

Almost immediately after the first otoacoustic emissions (OAEs) reports by Kemp and Ryan[40] and Kemp, several investigators suggested that one of the potentially most useful clinical applications of OAE is assessment of cochlear status in infants.[41,42] In theory, OAEs were thought to (1) take less time to measure than an ABR, because OAEs do not require electrode attachment, (2) provide information over a broader frequency range than click-evoked ABR, and (3) provide cochlear-specific information unaffected by neurologic pathology.

Data from several groups of investigators indicate that robust, broadband TEOAEs can be measured in neonatal ears in the absence of external or middle ear pathology.[40,43,44] Likewise, data indicate that DPOAEs are robust in neonates and infants.[45-49]

Concerns about OAE-based neonatal hearing screening include difficulty testing in noisy environments, and the effects of vernix and other debris in the ear canal, as well as collapsing ear canals during the first 24 hours after birth.

Comparison of Otoacoustic Emissions and Auditory Brainstem Responses

In summary, technologic advances now make it possible to assess auditory function in neonates and infants. These electrophysiologic and acoustic responses can be safely applied without reliance on a behavioral response. However, neither OAE nor ABR tests evaluate hearing or describe how a particular person will use available hearing. OAE and ABR are physiologic responses related to peripheral hearing status but constitute indirect measures of hearing.

To predict hearing status in children 8 to 12 months of age, a multicenter longitudinal study compared the accuracy of click-evoked ABRs, TEOAEs, and DPOAEs. The results indicated no significant differences among the three measures.[48] However, a recent study comparing two-step TEOAEs and ABRs found that ABR was more effective for UNHS because it yields fewer false-positive results and a lower referral rate compared with TEOAE, resulting in a smaller percentage of infants lost during follow-up.[50]

Typically, a simple pass-refer criterion is chosen for a screening tool. Many studies and these programs assume a priori that all infants who "passed" the screen had normal hearing. To determine the true accuracy of neonatal tests, however, it is necessary to follow all infants evaluated during the neonatal period, regardless of neonatal test outcome.[48] Because the true hearing status of those infants who pass the screening test is not known, true sensitivity cannot be calculated. Errors made among infants with normal hearing can be known because these false-positive results are evaluated with additional testing. The fact that the "passes" may include infants with hearing loss will have little or no influence on the true-negative rate or specificity of the test, because the vast majority of infants have normal hearing. However, the errors among ears with hearing loss (false-negative results) cannot be known if only those infants failing the newborn hearing test are followed. This is because misses are not followed up. Assigning a "pass" to even a small number of babies with hearing loss can have a large effect on test sensitivity because of the small total number of those with hearing loss.

The sensitivity and specificity of ABR, TEOAE, and DPOAE testing alone or in combination depend on the target degree of hearing loss, the test parameters, and response criteria. For example, Hyde and associates[51] reported ABR sensitivity of 98% and specificity of 96% if the average target hearing loss is 40 dB nHL at 2 and 4 kHz. If the target degree of hearing loss is 30 dB nHL, sensitivity and specificity were 100% and 91%, respectively. Norton and coworkers held specificity at 80% and determined sensitivity for TEOAE, DPOAE, and ABR alone and in combination for a target loss of 30 dB nHL. Sensitivity ranged from 80% to 90%. If those infants with known progressive hearing loss were excluded, sensitivity improved.[48]

Because it is impossible for hospital-based screening UNHS programs to follow all infants screened regardless of test outcome, it is important to remember that no test is perfect. Click-evoked ABR often misses hearing losses in which hearing is normal at some frequencies. For example, a baby with a low-frequency hearing loss with normal thresholds at 2000 Hz and above will pass an ABR screening test. Likewise, a baby with high-frequency hearing loss with normal hearing at lower frequencies may pass an ABR screen. High-frequency hearing losses are relatively common and may have significant effects on speech and language development.

OAE testing may miss inner hair cell and eighth cranial nerve hearing losses. OAEs are generated by the outer hair cells and are independent of neural status. Recently, there are concerns about auditory dyssynchrony,[52] defined as robust OAEs and abnormal or absent ABR. This is an extremely heterogeneous population whose behavioral hearing status ranges from normal hearing to profound hearing loss. Good incidence data of this disorder in the neonatal population are scarce.

Physicians and parents must include regular monitoring of hearing, speech, and language milestones even for those infants who pass a newborn hearing screening test whether it is TEAOE, DPOAE, or ABR.

Common UNHS protocols include OAE testing before discharge followed by an outpatient OAE re-screen for inpatient referrals, OAE inpatient screen and ABR re-screen, OAE and ABR inpatient screens, and ABR inpatient and ABR re-screens. Outpatient re-screens help minimize the number of infants referred for diagnostic audiologic testing and hence costs. Persistent re-screening is inappropriate. Infants should be referred for diagnostic follow-up evaluation after two failed screenings.

Some hospitals implement two-stage screening, in which OAE is used as the preliminary screening test. Infants failing this test are then screened with the automated ABR (AABR). Those who fail the AABR undergo more diagnostic testing to evaluate for permanent hearing loss, but infants who pass the AABR are not tested further. A multicenter evaluation of the two-stage screening revealed that many infants with hearing loss may be missed, because infants who pass only the AABR are not referred for further testing.[53]

Diagnosis and Treatment of Hearing Loss in Infants

History

In infants who fail hearing screening tests, a directed history to identify potential sources of hearing loss is appropriate.[54] A careful family history looking for hearing loss, ocular abnormalities, congenital cardiac problems in first- and second-degree relatives, and any associated syndromes is essential. Prenatal history for possible maternal infection (i.e., TORCH), gestational diabetes, and hypothyroidism can help direct the evaluation. Maternal use of alcohol should be sought, because fetal alcohol syndrome is associated with auditory dysfunction. Other maternal illnesses and social habits (e.g., drug use and smoking) should be sought. Risk factors for hearing loss in the perinatal period are well known, as discussed earlier in this chapter.[6,55]

Physical Examination

A majority of newborns with hearing loss do not have abnormal physical features.[56] Nevertheless, a complete physical examination is essential. Presence of abnormal iris color, skin tags, anterior cervical neck pits, goiter, cleft palate, skull shape, abnormal numbers of digits, areas of hypopigmentation, and café au lait spots are potential signs of a syndromic disorder. Such a diagnosis, such as Wardenburg's or branchio-oto-renal syndrome, may explain hearing loss identified through infant hearing screening. Alternatively, these physical signs may prompt careful follow-up investigation and imaging to identify progressive sensorineural hearing loss or conductive hearing loss, which may occur in neurofibromatosis or craniosynostosis. Pendred's syndrome may be associated with goiter development. Stickler's syndrome has characteristic eye and facial features, along with cleft palate. Patients suspected of having possible branchio-oto-renal syndrome need a renal ultrasound examination. Those patients identified with severe to profound sensorineural hearing loss and neurologic and ocular abnormalities should have serial ophthalmologic evaluations to evaluate for retinitis pigmentosa. Electroretinography may uncover early forms of this abnormality, allowing early identification of Usher's syndrome. At this point the exact indications for this testing modality are unclear, but some investigators recommend electroretinography in all cases of undetermined bilateral severe to profound sensorineural hearing loss.[57] In any case, ophthalmologic examination is warranted, because up to one half of children with severe to profound hearing loss have ocular defects.[58]

Vestibular Function Assessment

When hearing loss is identified, careful attention to vestibular function is necessary.[59] A strong association exists between hearing loss and impaired vestibular function in infants and children. Neurologic and developmental milestones are important to record. Signs of peripheral vestibular dysfunction can occur with delayed motor development. Evaluation for the presence of nystagmus (i.e., spontaneous or head shaking type) can be done in infants. When nystagmus is present, further testing may be warranted.

Otomicroscopy

Infants who fail hearing screening tests should have careful middle and external auditory canal examinations with the otomicroscope, because a problem with the middle and external auditory canals is the most common source of failed initial hearing screening.[60] This type of examination allows careful cleaning of the ear canal and identification of external auditory canal stenosis or atresia.[61,62] Additionally, assessment of middle ear function may be possible with this method by assessing the thickness and character of the tympanic membrane, as well as its motion. In older children, tympanometry and pneumatic otoscopy by experienced examiners both measure middle ear status accurately, but in infancy (0 to 6 months of age) both measures can miss detection of middle ear effusions.[63]

Middle Ear Effusions

When persistent middle ear effusions are identified as a potential source of an abnormal hearing screening, observation is essential when there is no evidence of acute inflammation. The incidence of middle ear effusions in the first year of life is quite high and in infancy it is estimated to be as high 61%.[64] In our practice, we usually wait 2 to 3 months for spontaneous resolution of the middle ear effusion. If the effusion persists after that time, ABR testing is still performed to determine whether there is a response to sound. No clear guidelines for medical therapy have been developed for infants with persistent middle ear effusions. Oral steroid therapy can be given to clear the effusion, but in infancy the risks of this treatment must be weighed against its benefits.[65] If the child has acute otitis media, antibiotic therapy is necessary along with observation for effusion resolution. Tympanostomy tube insertion is done for persistent middle ear effusion. Usually the recommendations for treatment of persistent otitis media with effusion in children between 1 and 3 years of age as outlined in 1994 by the Agency for Health Care Policy and Research also are used in young infants.[66,67] However, no outcomes studies have been conducted to demonstrate the most effective therapy for middle ear effusions in children younger than 1 year of age.

Diagnostic Audiology

As mentioned earlier in this chapter, all infants not passing a newborn hearing screening should be referred for diagnostic audiology by 3 months of age. Diagnostic follow-up investigation for infants referred from newborn hearing screening programs should include threshold frequency–specific ABR and OAE testing. Frequency-specific ABR thresholds have good agreement with behavioral thresholds[68] and can be used to fit appropriate amplification and guide intervention. Air and bone conduction should both be evaluated using tone-pip ABR. A significant air-bone gap in ABR thresholds is indicative of external or middle ear pathology, just as with pure-tone audiometry. EOAE should always be obtained with ABR testing to rule out auditory neuropathy and other neural losses. Tympanometry using a probe-tone frequency of 1000 Hz or higher can provide information about middle ear status. In children younger than 4 months of corrected age, traditional tympanometry—using a 226-Hz probe tone—is invalid because of the characteristics of the neonatal ear canal.[69]

Visual Reinforcement Audiometry

Visual reinforcement audiometry (VRA) is a modification of standard audiometric testing, designed for infants who are unable to understand verbal instruction. In VRA, operant conditioning techniques are used to reward a natural orienting response of the infant by providing an enjoyable event to reinforce the likelihood of continued responses. An infant's natural response to sound is a head turn in the direction of the sound source. When that response is rewarded by the activation of a lighted, animated toy, the infant may continue to respond for a sufficient number of stimulus trials to obtain an audiogram.[70]

VRA thresholds for infants as young as 6 months of age have been shown to be within 10 dB of adult hearing thresholds. VRA thresholds have been shown to be comparable to thresholds obtained by play audiometry in children of preschool age.[71-74] Good agreement between VRA and tympanometry indicates that the method is sensitive enough to detect even slight threshold elevations, such as those due to middle ear effusion. VRA is not restricted to sound field testing. Numerous reports indicate that VRA testing can be done reliably under earphones. Infants born prematurely who have spent time in the NICU tend to perform better if testing is delayed until 6 to 8 months corrected age. By 12 months of age, infants have been shown to need fewer conditioning trials, be less variable in responses near threshold, and yield fewer false-positive responses in comparison with infants who are 6 months of age; however, older infants tend to reject earphones more frequently than younger ones.[73-76]

Ancillary Testing

Ancillary Laboratory Testing

No evidence shows that standardized batteries of laboratory tests in infants failing initial hearing screening are necessary or cost effective.[56] All testing in these infants should be directed by hearing testing results and patient age, history, and physical examination.[77] These tests usually exclude specific causes of hearing loss but on occasion can confirm a diagnosis. Routine blood chemistry and complete blood count are unhelpful in evaluating hearing loss in infancy. If there is a family history of hematologic disease, such as thalassemia or sickle cell disease, screening can be performed for these disorders.[78,79] Diseases with platelet abnormalities that usually appear later in life (e.g., Fechtner or Epstein-Barr syndrome) can be discovered.[80] Such diseases are associated with sensorineural hearing loss.[12,38] Similarly, Alport's syndrome can be suspected when laboratory evidence for renal dysfunction is present with hearing loss. Autoimmune-induced hearing loss can occur in children but is not routinely suspected in infants.[63] Metabolic disorders, such as mucopolysaccharidoses, are associated with both conductive and sensorineural hearing loss and should be tested for when assessment reveals a family history of metabolic disorders, with hearing loss or physical features consistent with this diagnosis.[81,82] When the family history includes syncopal episodes and hearing loss, an electrocardiogram should be obtained to look for evidence of Jervell and Lange-Nielsen syndrome.

Guidelines for Genetic Testing

Deafness in infancy is believed to be at least 50% genetic in origin, with the remaining 50% being acquired or of unknown etiology.[83] Of the cases of genetic deafness, 75% to 80% are autosomal recessive, 15% to 20% are autosomal dominant, and 1% to 2% are X-linked. A few patients acquire hearing loss through mitochondrial inheritance. Of note, newborn hearing screening does not identify progressive hearing loss, which does occur in preschool-aged children. It is estimated that 15% to 20% of young children identified with SNHL have progressive hearing loss. Among children with SNHL in infancy, chromosomal karyotyping is recommended for those with a maternal history of multiple miscarriages and an unrecognizable constellation of anomalies. Additionally, if there are any associated neurologic or cardiac defects, chromosomal karyotyping is essential. Rapid advances in molecular genetics ensure that many new diagnostic methods for detection of the genetic basis for hearing loss will become available by the next decade.

Screening for Connexin 26 Mutation

In the late 1990s and early in the millennium, the autosomal recessive inheritance of hearing loss was linked to mutations at *GJB2*.[84,85] This gene codes for connexin 26 and is believed to be responsible for up to one half of all cases of autosomal recessive congenital hearing loss. The 35delG deletion is responsible for 70% of all connexin 26 mutations. The autosomal recessive non-syndromic hearing loss mutation in connexin 26 is known as DFNB1 (in genetic notation, the prefix DFNB signifies autosomal recessive hearing loss).[86] DFNB1 is associated with prelingual nonprogressive bilateral sensorineural hearing loss without evidence of temporal bone computed tomography (CT) anomalies or vestibular abnormalities. The hearing loss associated with this deletion can range from mild deficits to profound deafness. Considerable interfamilial variation in degree of hearing loss is recognized among affected families. Because the 35delG mutation involves a single base pair, screening tests for this deletion are available. It is estimated that the connexin 26 deletion is responsible for 50% of the cases of autosomal recessive sensorineural hearing loss.[87] Within this family of connexins, however, 60 different allele variations exist and therefore the hearing loss may not always be simply a result of the 35delG mutation.[88] When a child is born homozygous for the 35delG mutation, the chance of recurrence is 25%. The same chance of occurrence is present in a heterozygous patient. Siblings of affected persons have a 66% chance of carrying the deletion while having normal hearing.[89] Therefore, when testing for the 35DelG mutation is performed, genetic counseling should also be available.

Testing for Pendred's Syndrome

Genetic testing can be performed when Pendred's syndrome is suspected.[86] Pendred's syndrome represents 10% of the cases of syndromic hearing loss and is the most common cause of syndromic hearing loss. It is associated with a dilated vestibular aqueduct on temporal CT scanning.[90] Screening for mutations at *SCL26A4* (*DFNB4*) is done in the research setting.[85] Results of thyroid function tests usually are normal, with the exception of thyroglobulin levels, which can be elevated. The perchlorate discharge test is nonspecific and difficult to perform in young children.

Temporal Bone Imaging

Noncontrast temporal bone CT scanning is the imaging test most commonly used for all children with SNHL. Increasingly, T2-weighted MRI is being used as new techniques have enhanced its capability to delineate anatomy. (See also Chapter 191 in this text.) The timing of the imaging is debated and is beyond the scope of this chapter to discuss. It should definitely be performed at any age in all patients with progressive SNHL or craniofacial anomalies. These clinical signs are the best predictive factors for abnormalities within the temporal bone.[91] As mentioned earlier, the dilated vestibular aqueduct is associated with Pendred's syndrome.[92] A dilated vestibular aqueduct is defined as one with a diameter greater than 1.5 mm at its middle third or greater than 2.0 mm anywhere along its length. When a dilated duct is discovered, testing for Pendred's syndrome should be initiated, along with serial audiologic examinations to detect progressive hearing loss. Mondini dysplasia reflects abnormal development of the cochlea and is associated with both Pendred's and branchio-oto-renal syndromes.[93] Abnormalities of the semicircular canals also are seen on temporal bone imaging and are associated with a well-recognized constellation of manifestations: coloboma, heart defects, atresia choanae, retardation of growth and development, genitourinary problems, and ear abnormalities—the CHARGE association.[94] Superior semicircular canal dehiscence also can be identified radiographically and has been associated with conductive hearing loss in children, albeit in rare cases.[95]

Identification of internal auditory canal stenosis and possible eighth cranial nerve aplasia is associated with hereditary deafness. This X-linked form of deafness (DFN3) is associated with conductive loss at birth, followed by SNHL at a later age. Magnetic resonance imaging (MRI) scanning can be used to visualize the acoustic nerve, exclude aplasia, and rule out inner ear destruction secondary to infectious causes.[96] In cases in which infection or neoplasia is suspected, MRI with contrast is favored.[97] Accurate imaging of the seventh and eighth cranial nerve complex may be necessary before consideration for cochlear implantation.[98] Functional MRI scanning may help elucidate the exact nature of SNHL found in infancy.[99,100] Additionally, central auditory processing may be further clarified with this modality.[101] Because of its soft tissue detail,[102] some investigators feel that MRI should be performed in cases of pediatric unilateral or asymmetrical SNHL in which CT findings are negative, to rule out a CNS cause of hearing loss.[103] MRI also is indicated in patients who may have neurofibromatosis type 2. If CT results are negative but hearing loss is progressive, or if audiologic testing reveals a possible retrocochlear pathology, MRI also may be warranted.[104]

Screening for Maternally Transmitted Infection

Other laboratory evaluations may include specific immunoglobulin M (IgM) testing for suspected intrauterine infection. IgM does not cross the placenta and, if present in the infant's blood, may suggest congenital cytomegalovirus (CMV), syphilis, or rubella infection. Further testing to elucidate these potential sources of hearing loss may include cultures for CMV in blood, urine, or saliva. Congenital CMV infection is a frequent congenital infection that can have significant neurologic sequelae.[12] Hearing loss can be the only manifestation.[105] The virus persists in infected infants and can be detected in the first 3 months of life. When the virus is detected, early treatment may lessen the severity of neurologic sequelae. With congenital syphilis, the fluorescent treponemal antibody absorption (FTA-ABS) test indicates intrauterine transmission of syphilis.[106] Congenital toxoplasmosis is present in 0.6% of newborns. Hearing loss is present in 10% to 15% of these newborns and usually is associated with other abnormalities (i.e., chorioretinitis, intracerebral calcification, and microcephaly). Early identification of the potential for this infection suggests that treatment may reduce the level of hearing impairment. Herpes simplex type 2 usually is transmitted through contact with vaginal lesions at the time of delivery and is associated with a low incidence of hearing loss. On the other hand, herpes simplex type 1 is associated with hearing loss in transplacental transmission.[107] Detection of IgM antibodies to this virus raises this infection as a possible source of hearing loss. Congenital rubella can be detected through serologic testing. Although the incidence of this infection has significantly decreased in recent times, it still is present, particularly in underdeveloped countries, and hearing loss is estimated to be the only sign of this infection in 50% of cases.[83]

Intervention Strategies

Surgical Therapy for Conductive Hearing Loss

Newborns with conductive hearing loss most commonly have middle ear effusions. If the actual hearing threshold needs to be established, then tympanostomy tube insertion is necessary. Other types of surgery to correct conductive hearing loss are beyond the scope of this discussion and are not usually attempted in infancy.

Bone Conduction Amplification

Hearing aids should be considered for any child who demonstrates a permanent bilateral hearing loss—both conductive and sensorineural—exceeding 20 dB HL between 1000 and 4000 Hz.[108] Even children with minimal hearing losses are at risk for experiencing educational difficulty.[109,110] A bone conduction hearing aid is fitted when the child is unable to wear air conduction hearing aids as a result of atresia, stenotic ear canals, or recurrent draining middle ears. Bone-anchored hearing aids are not approved by the U.S. Food and Drug Administration (FDA) for children younger than 5 years of age.

Amplification

Hearing aids should be fitted as soon as possible after confirmation of a hearing loss. As infants are identified earlier as a result of UNHS, audiologists face many challenges in fitting hearing aids, including size of the head and ear canal, poor head control, behavior, and rapid growth. Children younger than 7 years of age should be fitted with either behind the ear (BTE) hearing aids or bone conduction hearing aids.[108] Smaller styles of hearing aids, such as in the ear (ITE) and completely in canal (CIC) aids, are inappropriate for infants and young children whose ear canals are constantly increasing in size. Increasing ear canal size means that new ear molds must be made frequently to ensure proper amplification. ITE and CIC hearing aids would necessitate recasting, leaving the child without amplification during this process. Furthermore, ITE and CIC hearing aids pose a significant safety issue.

Hearing aid evaluation and selection involve determination of the appropriate circuitry and processing algorithm based on the child's degree, configuration, and type of hearing loss, plus the child's developmental needs and family resources. A selection and fitting technique designed for infants should be employed. The most widely used procedure involves measurement of the real-ear-to-coupler (RECD).[109-111] In addition, a technique such as the desired sensation level (DSL) method should be used to ensure audibility of the amplified speech, regardless of input level or vocal effort.[112,113]

Infants, particularly those with hearing losses of 55 dB and above, should be fitted with personal wireless frequency modulation (FM) systems to improve the speech-to-noise ratio. A receiver attaches to the child's hearing aid, and the caregiver wears a microphone and transmitter. Use of an FM system also reduces the feedback problems often encountered with infants, who have poor head control and mobility.

Regular follow-up appointments with the audiologist are critical for optimal fitting and usage of amplification devices for infants. Generally, infants are seen for follow-up appointments at least every 3 months during their first year. Ear molds may need to be remade even more frequently for some children. Other important considerations for children include tamper-resistant battery doors and controls, clips to secure the hearing aid to the child's clothing to prevent loss, listening tubes for parents, and extended warranties for loss and damage. Orientation for parents and other caregivers should include care and use of the hearing aid and FM system including wearing schedules, insertion, removal, storage, cleaning, and basic troubleshooting.

Sound field–aided testing often is used to confirm audibility. Aided testing provides information about how the child uses the signal provided by the hearing aid. That is, RECD and DSL are used to select, fit, and verify proper hearing aid function and audibility, whereas sound field testing provides information about how the child is using his or her hearing. Misleading information may be obtained in cases of severe to profound hearing loss or minimal hearing loss, or when nonlinear signal processing or digital noise reduction circuitry is used.[112]

Cochlear Implantation

A discussion of all aspects of cochlear implantation in children is beyond the scope of this chapter. Some general considerations are presented here.

When SNHL is identified and hearing aid amplification is applied with success, consideration for cochlear implantation is entertained. It is our practice to carefully evaluate each patient to establish candidacy for this procedure. As time has gone on, the indications for implantation have broadened and continue to evolve. Several studies indicate that the younger the age at which children with severe to profound hearing loss receive a cochlear implant, the better their auditory oral speech and language skills, and the more likely they are to be mainstreamed with their normal-hearing age peers. The FDA has approved cochlear implants for infants with profound hearing loss at 12 months of age and at 18 months of age for those with severe hearing loss. Increasingly, infants younger than 12 months of age are receiving cochlear implants. The key component of all treatment is identification of the type and extent of the hearing loss. Once this has been established, appropriate rehabilitative measures can be initiated, which eventually may include cochlear implantation. Several temporal bone abnormalities that may preclude this intervention are cochlear ossification and vestibular nerve aplasia. Enlarged vestibular aqueduct (EVA) syndrome has been thought to be a contraindication to implantation in the past, but not at present. Postmeningitic deafness is associated with cochlear ossification, and early implantation is recommended by some investigators to avoid the difficulties encountered when the cochlea is ossified. If the vestibular nerve is nonexistent, implantation will not help.

Early Intervention

Hearing loss in infants is primarily a communication problem, limiting the child's access to spoken language. Hearing loss happens to the family, not just the child. Providing the infant with full access to communication is the primary goal of early intervention. In addition to the use of assertive listening devices, parents learn to accommodate their baby's communication needs. The Individuals with Disabilities Education Act (IDEA) mandates early intervention services for children 0 to 3 years of age.[114] These programs are administered by individual states. Physicians should consult with local agencies to learn more about the services in their home state. Services for infants with hearing loss and families are generally home-based. There may be play groups and parent groups, but IDEA specifies that a majority of services be delivered in natural environments (i.e., where infants without disabilities are found). Because of the unique language and communication needs of deaf and hard of hearing (D/HOH) children, it is critical that services be provided by professionals with expertise in childhood hearing loss and early childhood education.

Historically, controversies in the education of D/HOH children have focused on communication methodology. Three broad categories exist: American Sign Language (ASL), simultaneous communication using spoken and signed English, and auditory-oral only. The history and nuances of this issue are beyond the scope of this discussion. Parents of children with hearing loss repeatedly stress that they want full unbiased access to information about their options, that they want to talk to other parents and not just to professionals, and that they are in charge of making decisions about their baby's communication needs.

SUGGESTED READINGS

Adcock LM, Freysdottir D. Screening the newborn for hearing loss. *UpToDate.* 2008; version 15.2.

American Academy of Audiology. *Pediatric Amplification Protocol.* Reston, Va: American Academy of Audiology; 2002.

Bamiou DE, MacArdle B, Bitner-Glindzicz M, et al. Aetiological investigations of hearing loss in childhood: a review. *Clin Otolaryngol.* 2000;25:98.

Bamiou DE, Phelps P, Sirimanna T. Temporal bone computed tomography findings in bilateral sensorineural hearing loss. *Arch Dis Child.* 2000;82:257.

Barsky-Firkser L, Sun S. Universal newborn hearing screenings: a three-year experience. *Pediatrics.* 1997;99:E4.

Denoyelle F, Weil D, Maw MA, et al. Prelingual deafness: high prevalence of a 30delG mutation in the connexin 26 gene. *Hum Mol Genet.* 1997;6:2173.

Early identification of hearing impairment in infants and young children. *NIH Consens Statement.* 1993;11:1.

Hone SW, Smith RJ. Medical evaluation of pediatric hearing loss. Laboratory, radiographic, and genetic testing. *Otolaryngol Clin North Am.* 2002;35:751.

Kennedy C, McCann D, Campbell MJ, et al. Universal newborn screening for permanent childhood hearing impairment: an 8-year follow-up of a controlled trial. *Lancet.* 2005;366:660.

Kennedy CR, McCann DC, Campbell MJ, et al. Language ability after early detection of permanent childhood hearing impairment. *N Engl J Med.* 2006;354:2131.

Lalwani AK, Castelein CM. Cracking the auditory genetic code: nonsyndromic hereditary hearing impairment. *Am J Otol.* 1999;20:115.

Prasad S, Cucci RA, Green GE, et al. Genetic testing for hereditary hearing loss: connexin 26 (GJB2) allele variants and two novel deafness-causing mutations (R32C and 645-648delTAGA). *Hum Mutat.* 2000;16:502.

Sanford B, Weber PC. Evaluation of hearing impairment in children. *UpToDate.* 2008; version 16.2.

Schrijver I. Hereditary non-syndromic sensorineural hearing loss. *J Mol Diagn.* 2004;6:4.

Universal screening for hearing loss in newborns: US Preventive Services Task Force recommendation statement. *Pediatrics.* 2008;122:1.

American Academy of Pediatrics, Joint Committee on Infant Hearing. Year 2007 position statement: principles and guidelines for early hearing detection and intervention programs. *Pediatrics.* 2007;120:898-921.

For complete list of references log onto www.expertconsult.com.

CHAPTER ONE HUNDRED AND NINETY-ONE

Congenital Malformations of the Inner Ear

Robert K. Jackler

Key Points

- In congenital SNHL, approximately 20% of inner ears demonstrate a radiographically detectable abnormality.
- Many patterns of deformity appear to result from disturbance in the embryogenesis of the inner ear during the first trimester.
- Enlargement of the vestibular aqueduct is most common, followed in frequency by semicircular canal and cochlear deformities.
- The imaging patterns of cochlear anomaly include aplasia, hypoplasia, incomplete partition, and common cavity.
- Semicircular canals may be absent (aplastic) or deformed (dysplastic).
- The eighth nerve may be aplastic or hypoplastic, especially when the internal auditory canal is narrow.
- Congenital ear malformations may be a feature of syndromes such as Pendred's and Usher's syndromes, the CHARGE association, and various trisomies.
- High-resolution T2-weighted MRI is superior to CT because it shows the endolymphatic sac and eighth nerve.
- Hearing in milder deformities is variable but tends to worsen over time.
- Pseudoconductive hearing loss may be present, with a high risk for dead ear and occurrence of CSF "gusher" at stapes surgery.
- Predilection for stapes gusher, due to modiolar defects, may be inherited in an X-linked pattern.
- Head trauma may cause sudden decrease in hearing.
- May be associated with transotic CSF leak and recurrent meningitis.
- Surgery on the endolymphatic sac or middle ear windows has not been shown to improve or stabilize hearing.
- Cochlear implantation usually is successful but carries a heightened risk for CSF leak, meningitis, and facial twitch.

Development of the inner ear begins early in embryogenesis. By the end of the eighth week, the membranous labyrinth has assumed its characteristic convoluted shape.[1] Gradual ossification of the otic capsule develops around the membranous labyrinth and is essentially complete by birth.[2] Maturation of the sensory epithelium occurs long after formation of the membranous labyrinth, during the late second and early third trimesters. By weeks 26 to 28 of gestation, hair cell and auditory neural development are largely complete. Thus, the normal human fetus may be able to hear 2.5 to 3 months before birth.

Most inner ear malformations arise when formation of the membranous labyrinth is interrupted during the first trimester of pregnancy.[2] This interruption may be either a result of inborn genetic error or a consequence of a teratogenic exposure during the period of inner ear organogenesis between the fourth and eighth weeks of gestation. Genetic errors may be either dominant or recessive and may manifest as sensorineural hearing loss (SNHL) alone or be associated with any of a number of syndromes.[4] A partial list of syndromes associated with radiologically detectable inner ear malformation includes Pendred's, Usher's, Waardenburg's, Wildervanck's (cervico-oculoacoustic), branchio-oto-renal, and Alagille's sundromes.[5-8] Nonsyndromic familial inner ear malformations have also been described.[9,10] Teratogenic influences known to affect inner ear organogenesis include in utero viral infection (e.g., rubella, cytomegalovirus infection), chemical teratogens (e.g., thalidomide), and radiation exposure.[11] Abnormalities in otic capsule structure and deficiencies in the organ of Corti appear to arise as secondary effects of the earlier error in development of the membranous labyrinth. Derangement of the otic capsule ossification process alone does not appear to be a major mechanism in congenital hearing loss. Ossification of the labyrinthine lumen, however, is a common finding in early acquired deafness, typically arising as a consequence of meningitis.

Developmental damage to cochlear structure and function is not restricted to agents that cause gross structural malformations. Even in doses below those that would be ototoxic in the adult, aminoglycoside antibiotics administered in the animal equivalent of the human first trimester of pregnancy cause severe hearing loss in several species.[12] This time frame corresponds to the maturation of the outer hair cells and initiation of the cochlear potentials. Human studies also document this. In 35 of the infants delivered by 72 women who received streptomycin prophylaxis for tuberculosis during the first 4 months of pregnancy, auditory deficits ranging from minor high-frequency threshold elevations to severe bilateral SNHL were noted.[13]

The risk is not restricted to the first trimester. Even at low doses, slighter hearing losses were noted when aminoglycoside antibiotics were administered during the human equivalent of the last two trimesters of pregnancy, which has obvious implications for use of these drugs in pregnant women and in premature infants who have not yet reached functional cochlear maturity.

Congenital anomalies of the inner ear may be considered in two broad categories: malformations with pathologic changes limited to the membranous labyrinth and malformations that involve both the osseous and membranous portions of the labyrinth. This division has been chosen because of its clinical relevance. Only patients with malformed otic capsules exhibit abnormalities on inner ear radiographs and therefore may be diagnosed during life. By inference, children with congenital SNHL and radiographically normal inner ears may be assumed to possess anomalies limited to the membranous labyrinth or neural pathways. Although several types of membranous deformities have been described, their classification is not yet of clinical use because differentiation requires histopathologic examination. Among the deformities that affect the otic capsule, a variety of morphologic patterns may be recognized radiographically, and classification may have prognostic and even therapeutic importance.

Incidence

Most children with congenital sensory hearing loss, with the possible exception of auditory neuropathy, would have detectable abnormalities in their inner ears if they could be examined histologically. Because most children with profound bilateral SNHL have radiographically normal inner ears, it can be inferred that malformations limited to the membranous labyrinth predominate. The incidence of malformations reported varies, depending on the hearing level of the study population, the sophistication of imaging used, and the definition of abnormality used by the observer. As a rule of thumb, approximately 20% of cases of congenital SNHL will demonstrate inner ear malformation with modern imaging technology. In a series of 234 children who had SNHL of varying degrees of severity, Reilly[14] found cochlear anomalies in only 4% of those evaluated by high-resolution computed tomography (CT). With improvements in CT imaging technology and greater awareness of inner ear deformities, Antonelli and colleagues found anomalies in 31% of 157 children with SNHL of variable degree.[15] In another CT study, anomalies were found in 17% of 185 ears of children with SNHL and none in the ears of 309 children without SNHL.[16] A large Korean study found 22% incidence of anomalies on radiologic imaging in 590 ears with profound SNHL.[17]

The incidence of deformities of the semicircular canals (SCCs) and inner ear aqueducts has been less well studied than that of cochlear deformities. In a series of patients with radiographically detectable malformations of the inner ear, the cochlea was involved in 76%, the semicircular canals were involved in 39%, and the vestibular aqueduct (VA) was affected in 32% of ears.[3] The total is more than 100%, because many cases demonstrate abnormalities of more than one portion of the inner ear. In recent years, a heightened awareness of VA enlargement, combined with the greater sensitivity of axial CT scans in demonstrating this deformity, has led to a substantial increase in its detection. The rapid accrual of cases by clinicians interested in inner ear malformations suggests that enlargement of the VA will ultimately prove to be the most common radiographically detectable inner ear anomaly.[6]

Among deaf children with radiographically normal inner ears, histopathologic studies indicate that cochleosaccular dysplasia (Scheibe's dysplasia) is by far the most common deformity.[18] Because of the paucity of pathologic specimens available for examination, it is impossible to estimate the relative frequency of the various membranous malformations.

Classification

The traditional nomenclature used to describe congenital anomalies of the inner ear involves a confusing array of eponyms that stem from the first reports of the various morphologic patterns, usually by 18th or 19th century authors. In this chapter, a descriptive classification system is used, along with the traditional eponymous terminology, to make this topic more logical, easier to learn, and more clinically relevant (Box 191-1). In membranous malformations, this classification is based on histopathologic changes in the inner ear; in combined osseous-membranous deformities, radiographic appearance is used to distinguish among the various entities.[3] Correct use of the terminology of pathoembryology is important, although these terms frequently are applied imprecisely in the earlier literature. Key terms are *aplasia* (complete lack of development), *hypoplasia* (incomplete development), and *dysplasia* (aberration in development). The classification scheme used in this chapter has proved to be of practical clinical use and has been employed in most published studies in recent years. Other classification schema that categorize observed anomalies have been proposed.[19]

Box 191-1

Classification of Congenital Inner Ear Malformations

Malformations Limited to the Membranous Labyrinth

- Complete membranous labyrinthine dysplasia
- Limited membranous labyrinthine dysplasia
  - Cochleosaccular dysplasia (Scheibe)
  - Cochlear basal turn dysplasia

Malformations of the Osseous and Membranous Labyrinth

- Complete labyrinthine aplasia (Michel)
- Cochlear anomalies
  - Cochlear aplasia
  - Cochlear hypoplasia
  - Incomplete partition (Mondini)
  - Common cavity
- Labyrinthine anomalies
  - Semicircular canal dysplasia
  - Semicircular canal aplasia
- Aqueductal anomalies
  - Enlargement of the vestibular aqueduct
  - Enlargement of the cochlear aqueduct
- Internal auditory canal anomalies
  - Narrow internal auditory canal
  - Wide internal auditory canal
- Eighth nerve anomalies
  - Hypoplasia
  - Aplasia

Malformations Limited to the Membranous Labyrinth

In malformations limited to the membranous labyrinth, which account for more than 90% of cases of congenital deafness, the bony labyrinth is normal.[20-23] In its most severe form, membranous dysplasia involves the entire labyrinth, including the cochlea, semicircular canals (SCCs), utricle, and saccule. A limited form of membranous labyrinthine dysplasia, involving only a portion of the inner ear, also has been described.

Complete Membranous Labyrinthine Dysplasia

Complete membranous labyrinthine dysplasia was first described by Siebenmann and Bing[24] and is extremely rare. It has been reported in association with cardioauditory (Jervell and Lange-Nielsen) and Usher syndromes.[25]

Limited Membranous Labyrinthine Dysplasia

Cochleosaccular Dysplasia (Scheibe's Dysplasia)

Incomplete development of the pars inferior is the most frequent histopathologic finding in congenital deafness. It was first described by Scheibe[26] and commonly is known as *cochleosaccular dysplasia*. The spectrum of pathologic findings in this anomaly, which is confined to the cochlea and the saccule, has been well described.[22,27-30] The organ of Corti is either partially or completely missing. The cochlear duct usually is collapsed, with Reissner's membrane adherent to the limbus. Less commonly, the duct is distended, presumably as a result of endolymphatic hydrops. The stria vascularis typically is degenerated and may contain colloidal inclusions. Schuknecht[31] described characteristic strial changes consisting of aplasia alternating with regions of hyperplasia and gross deformity. Cochlear changes may be severe in the base turn and gradually lessen in intensity toward the apex, or they may be severe throughout. The saccule usually is collapsed and has degenerated sensory epithelium. In cochleosaccular dysplasia, the SCCs and utricle are normal. Auditory neuronal survival is variable but may remain normal into adulthood, at least in some cases. Cochleosaccular dysplasia also has been demonstrated in a number of animal species, including the deaf white cat, Dalmatian dogs, and various mouse mutants.[32]

Cochlear Basal Turn Dysplasia

Dysplasia limited to the basal turn of the cochlea may be related to familial high-frequency SNHL. No description of membranous labyrinthine dysplasia limited to the pars superior was found in an extensive review of the literature. This outcome is not surprising, because affected persons probably are minimally symptomatic. They would have normal hearing and presumably would have compensated for their congenital vestibular deficit.

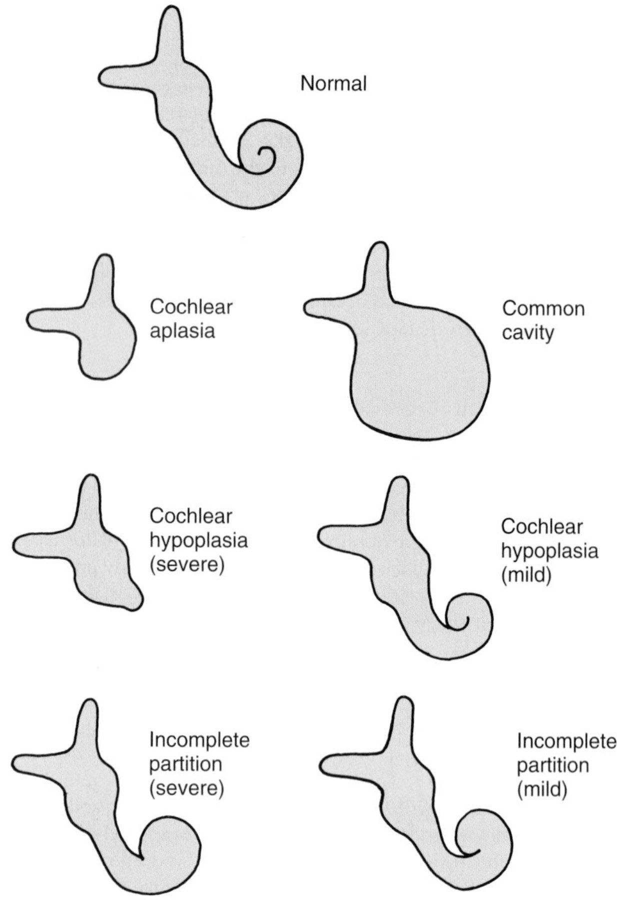

Figure 191-1. Cochlear malformations. Drawings were made from coronal computed tomography scans. *(From Jackler RK, Luxford WM, House WF. Congenital malformations of the inner ear: a classification based on embryogenesis. Laryngoscope. 1987;97[Suppl 40]:2.)*

Malformations of the Membranous and Osseous Labyrinth

Congenital anomalies of the inner ear that deform the otic capsule are of special interest to the clinician because they may be recognized and differentiated during life through radiographic imaging. As discussed previously, only approximately 20% of congenitally deaf people demonstrate radiographically anomalous inner ears. The clinical manifestations and natural history of these deformities are highly variable. Although some patients are deaf from birth, most maintain some residual hearing into adulthood. Slowly progressive deterioration of hearing during childhood, with eventual stabilization, is common. Sudden decrements in hearing are frequent and may appear to be spontaneous or may be triggered by head trauma, even minor in nature. Presumably, most of these cases are due either to internal fistulization secondary to membrane rupture within the cochlea, with admixture of perilymph and endolymph, or to external fistulization to the middle ear. Fluctuant hearing loss is unusual in these patients, and endolymphatic hydrops is an atypical finding. In some patients, hearing may be best preserved in very high frequencies (greater than 8000 Hz), which are not measured by conventional audiometry.[33] Residual ultra-audiometric hearing should be suspected in hearing-impaired children who manifest substantially better auditory function than would be predicted by pure tone results in the speech frequencies.[34] Occasionally, malformation of the inner ears may be associated with normal hearing.[35,36] This is especially the case for semicircular canal anomalies.[37] Vestibular symptoms, which occasionally are severe, are present in approximately 20% of patients.[3] Retardation of motor development has been documented in some children with malformed inner ears, particularly those in whom semicircular canals are absent.[38] A few patients experience vertigo when exposed to loud sounds—the so-called Tullio phenomenon.[39]

A wide variety of morphologic patterns of inner ear malformation has been observed radiographically and may involve the cochlea, SCCs, or vestibular aqueduct[3,40-45] (Fig. 191-1). Similar diversity has been observed on histologic analysis.[21,46-50] A majority of combined osseous and membranous malformations appears to arise from a premature arrest in the development of one or more components of the inner ear (Fig. 191-2). The strongest evidence for this theory comes from the resemblance of most malformed inner ears to the appearance of the inner ear during embryogenesis, particularly between the fourth and eighth weeks of gestation. As a general rule, the earlier the developmental arrest, the more severe the deformity and the worse the hearing will be.

Other anomalies cannot be explained by a premature arrest in development alone and appear to arise from an aberrant embryologic process. An example of this type of anomaly is a cochlea of normal length but abnormal size or coiling geometry.[46] In humans, the inner ear is of adult size at birth and shows strikingly little variation in size among individual patients. Pappas and colleagues[51] suggested that some children with congenital SNHL and apparently normal inner ear morphology on CT possess subtle abnormalities in the dimensions of inner ear structures. These investigators propose that such dimensional variations arise from a teratogenic insult during the second or third trimester, after the membranous labyrinth has formed but before it has reached adult size. Further study is needed to determine the clinical relevance of these observations.

Whereas some inner ear malformations involve only one portion of the inner ear, many patients have a combination of anomalies involving more than one component. Between the fourth and fifth weeks of development, the spheric otocyst develops three buds that ultimately form the cochlea, SCCs, and VA (see Fig. 191-2). An inner ear malformation may be limited to one of these anlages, may involve a combination of two, or may even affect all three.

The frequent coexistence of deformities involving the cochlea, SCCs, and VA has several possible explanations: (1) the anomaly is genetically predetermined; (2) an insult to the embryo occurred before the fifth week; or (3) each of the buds was susceptible to some teratogenic influence at a later stage of development. A majority of inner ear malformations are bilateral and symmetrical. In cases in which radiographs detect an anomaly on only one side, the opposite "normal" inner ear has a hearing loss in approximately 50% of cases.[3]

Before the evolution of high-resolution imaging technology, clinicians and histopathologists alike tended to lump these malformations together under the term *Mondini's dysplasia*, after the first report by Carlo Mondini. We are indebted to the late Dr. Peter Phelps and Latin scholar Gordon Hartley for an English translation of Mondini's original article.[52] Before the Academy of Sciences of the University of Bologna, Mondini described the inner ear findings in a deaf 8-year-old boy who was struck on the foot by a wagon and later died of gangrene.[53]

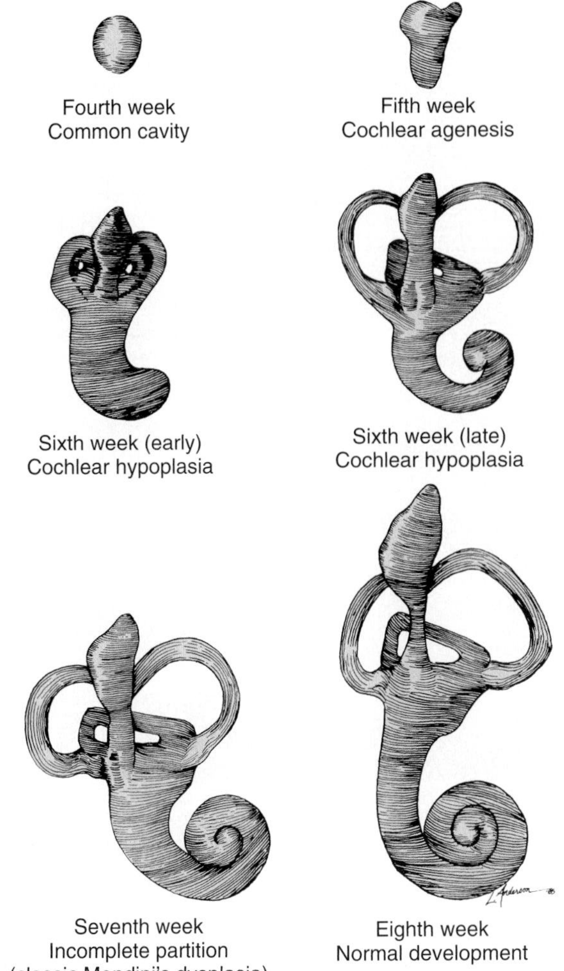

Figure 191-2. Embryogenesis of cochlear malformations. *(From Jackler RK, Luxford WM, House WF. Congenital malformations of the inner ear: a classification based on embryogenesis.* Laryngoscope. *1987;97(Suppl 40):2.)*

Table 191-1

Relative Incidence of Cochlear Malformations

Malformation	Incidence (%)
Incomplete partition (Mondini's dysplasia)	55
Common cavity	26
Cochlear hypoplasia	15
Cochlear aplasia	3
Complete labyrinthine aplasia (Michel's aplasia)	1

The cochlea possessed only 1.5 turns and had a hollow apical cavity. An enlarged vestibule and VA also were noted. This deformity is the most common form of cochlear anomaly (Table 191-1). Although numerous other distinct anatomic patterns of inner ear malformation are discernible radiographically and histologically, many workers continue to use the term Mondini's dysplasia to describe them all. To avoid a confusing and overly broad nomenclature system, this designation is best reserved for the particular subtype of cochlear malformation first described by Mondini, whether or not it is associated with other inner ear malformations.

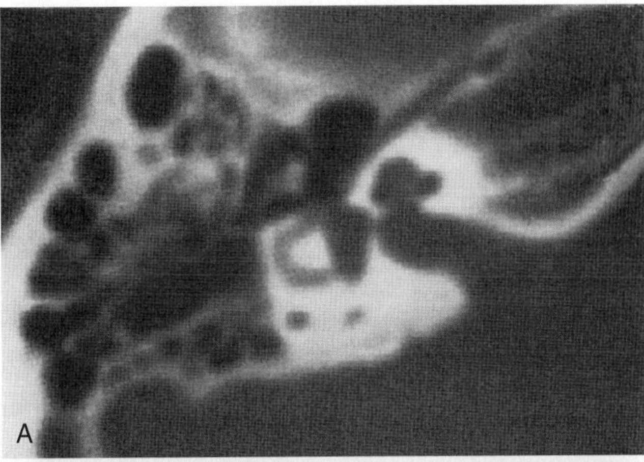

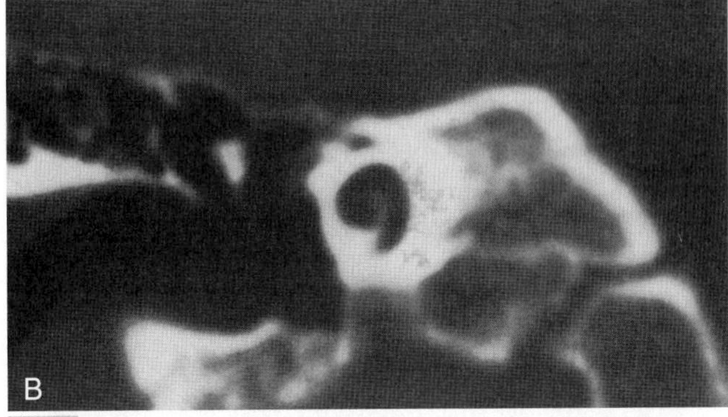

Figure 191-3. Radiographically normal inner ear as seen on axial (**A**) and coronal (**B**) high-resolution computed tomography scans. Note that the normal cochlea appears to have only 1.5 turns on the coronal scan, as a result of the oblique angle of section in relation to the axial scans of the modiolus.

Complete Labyrinthine Aplasia (Michel's Aplasia)

The most severe deformity of the membranous and osseous labyrinth, complete labyrinthine aplasia, was first described by Michel.[54] This malformation is exceedingly rare. Presumably, a developmental arrest occurs before the formation of an otic vesicle, resulting in a complete absence of inner ear structures. Complete labyrinthine aplasia has been reported in association with anencephaly and thalidomide exposure.[21,55] An association with external ear abnormalities also has been reported.[56] A purported case of Michel's aplasia actually described a cystic inner ear of the common cavity type.[57] This is but one example of the inaccurate use of traditional eponyms—a frequent occurrence in the literature. The incidence of complete labyrinthine aplasia is overestimated in the radiographic literature because it is confused with labyrinthine ossification. In the latter condition, which usually is acquired during life, a sizable and dense otic capsule is evident radiographically. In complete labyrinthine aplasia, the otic capsule is entirely absent[58] (Figs. 191-3 to 191-5). Such ears are, of course, uniformly deaf.

Cochlear Anomalies

Cochlear Aplasia

In cochlear aplasia the cochlea is completely absent, presumably as a result of an arrest in the development of the cochlear bud at the fifth week of gestation (see Fig. 191-1). This morphologic pattern is rare. Radiographically, only a vestibule and SCCs (usually deformed) are present. To differentiate this anomaly from labyrinthine ossification, it is necessary to assess the amount of otic capsule bone anterior to the internal auditory canal (IAC). In cochlear aplasia, the otic capsule is

Figure 191-4. Axial high-resolution T2-weighted magnetic resonance image (fast spin echo) of a normal inner ear at the level of the mid- and apical cochlea and lateral semicircular canal. Note the internal detail of the cochlea, which includes visualization of the scalar partitions and the modiolus. The seventh and eighth cranial nerves can be seen in the internal auditory canal outlined by cerebrospinal fluid.

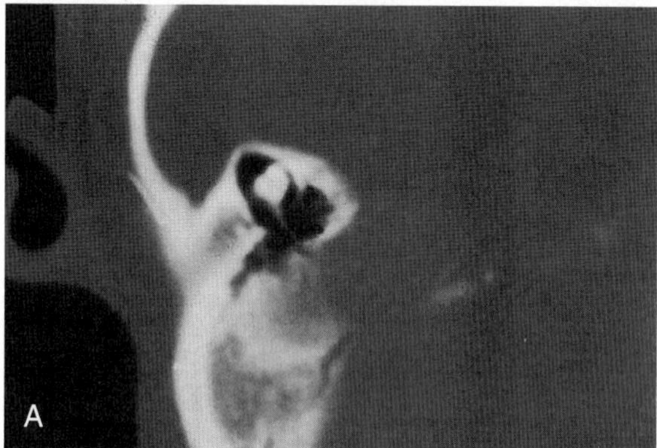

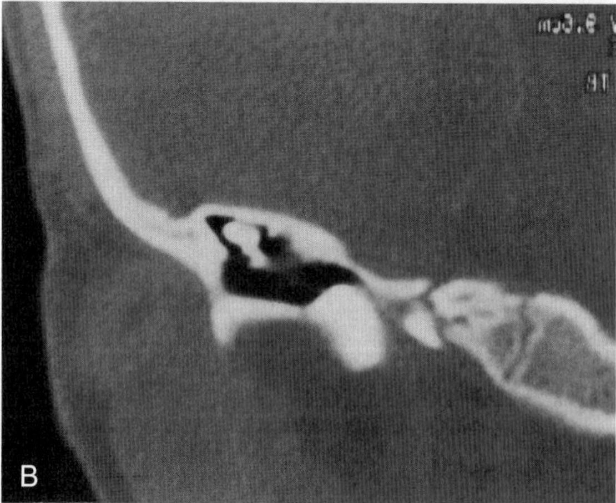

Figure 191-5. Complete labyrinthine aplasia as seen on axial (**A**) and coronal (**B**) computed tomography scans. Note the presence of an ear canal and middle ear but complete absence of the otic capsule. *(Courtesy of Joel Swartz, MD.)*

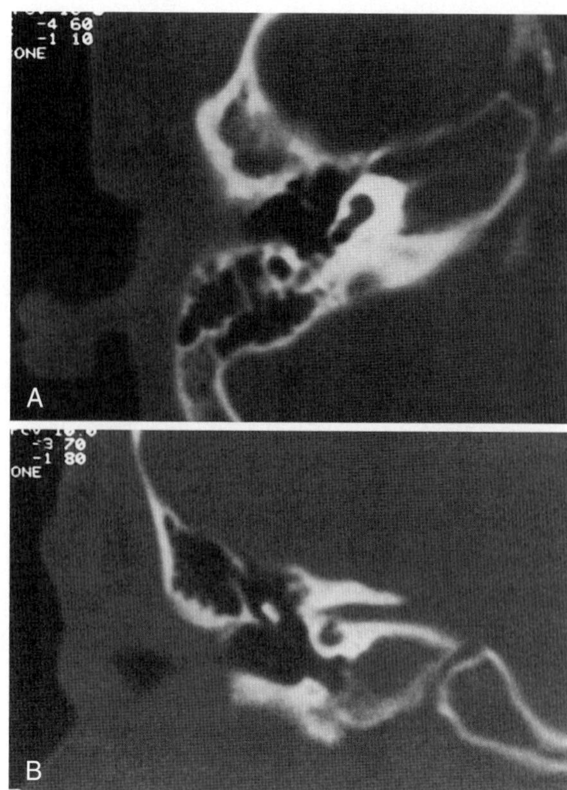

Figure 191-6. Cochlear hypoplasia as seen on axial (**A**) and coronal (**B**) computed tomography scans. The cochlea consists of only a small bud off the vestibule.

absent, whereas in osseous obliteration, it is dense and of normal dimensions. Ears with cochlear aplasia are devoid of auditory function.

Cochlear Hypoplasia

An arrest during the sixth week of gestation results in a hypoplastic cochlea consisting of a single turn or less. This deformity comprises approximately 15% of all cochlear anomalies. Radiographically, a small bud of variable length (usually 1 to 3 mm) protrudes from the vestibule (Fig. 191-6). The vestibule frequently is enlarged, with accompanying semicircular malformations in approximately one half of the cases. Small cochleas lacking a modiolus or other internal architecture have been described histologically.[27,50,59] Hearing is variable in these ears and may be remarkably good in view of the minute size of the cochlea. The variability of hearing presumably is accounted for by the degree of membranous labyrinthine development within the truncated cochlear lumen.

Incomplete Partition (Mondini)

Arrest at the seventh week of gestation yields a cochlea that has only 1.5 turns. This is the most common type of cochlear malformation, accounting for more than 50% of all such deformities. Radiographically, the cochlea is smaller than normal and partially or completely lacks an interscalar septum (Figs. 191-7 and 191-8). Although the cochlea usually measures 8 to 10 mm vertically, it is typically in the 5- to 6-mm range in incomplete partition deformity. Care must be exercised in counting the number of cochlear turns radiographically because this may be difficult to determine even using high-resolution CT. The radiographic diagnosis depends more on cochlear size and the absence of a scalar septum than on the number of cochlear turns perceived. Histologically, incomplete partition appears to be the radiographic correlate of classical Mondini's dysplasia (Fig. 191-9). In numerous reported cases, a small cochlea with 1.5 turns possessing an apical scala communis secondary to deficiency in the osseous spiral lamina has been described.[27,46,48] Sennaroglu and Saatci have subtyped the incomplete partition deformity into three variants[60] (Fig. 191-10).

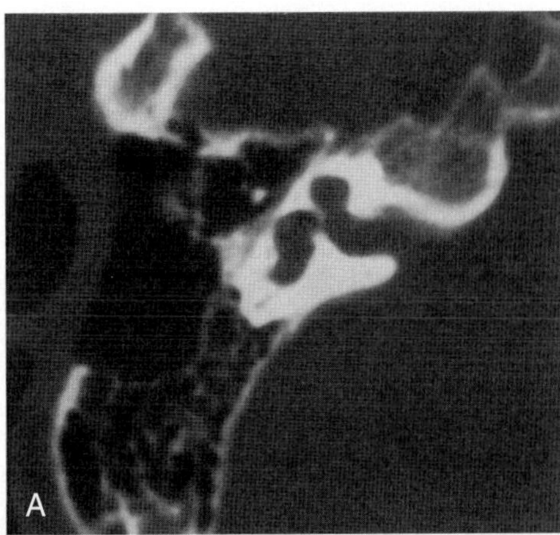

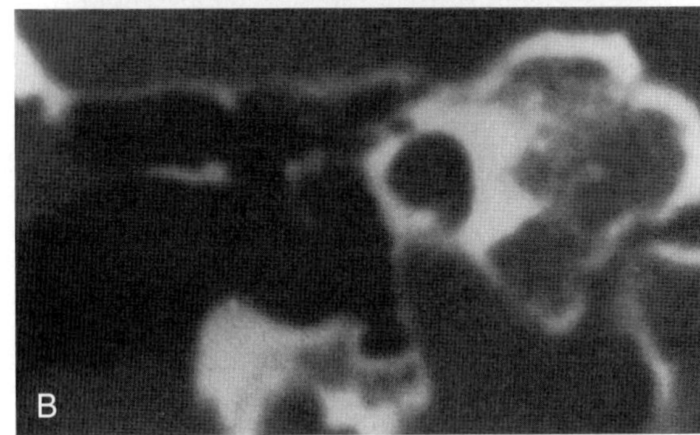

Figure 191-7. Incomplete partition as seen on axial (**A**) and coronal (**B**) computed tomography scans. Note the absence of an interscalar septum, which is more evident on the coronal scan.

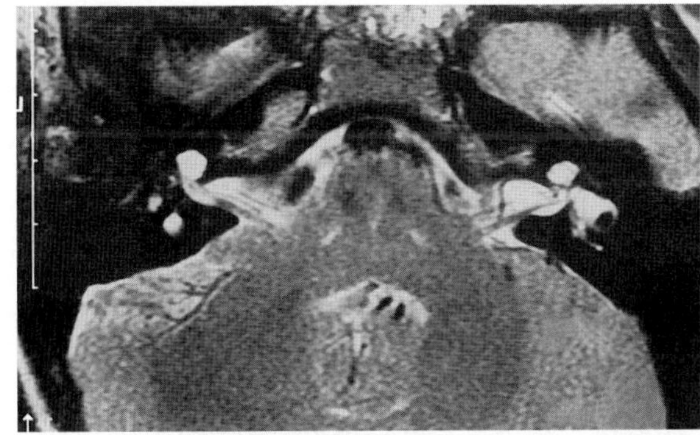

Figure 191-8. High-resolution T2-weighted magnetic resonance image (fast spin echo) of an incomplete partition deformity. Note the absence of intracochlear septation.

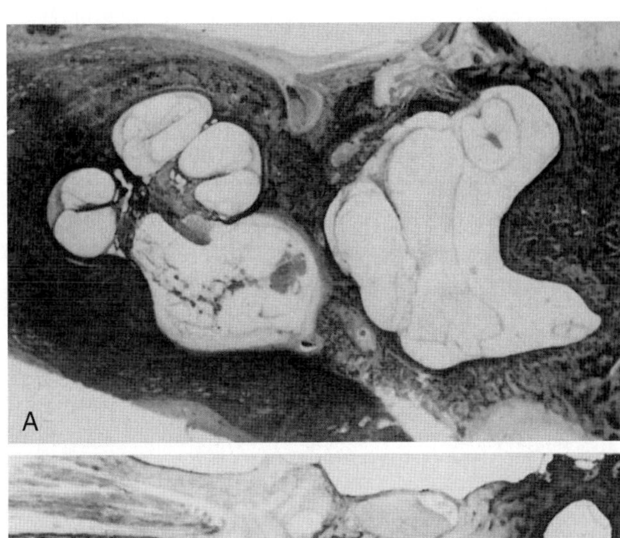

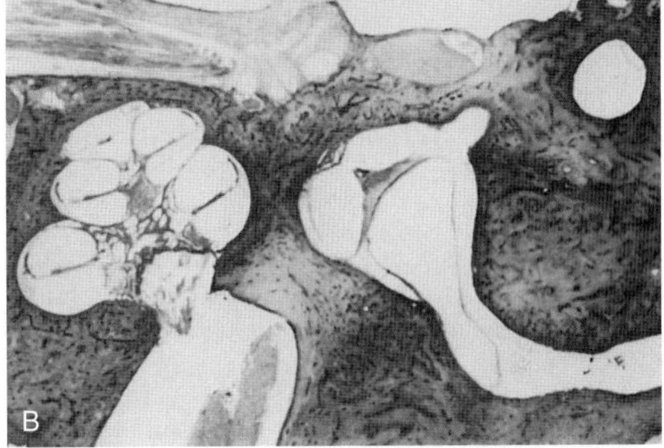

Figure 191-9. **A,** Photomicrograph of a malformed cochlea with the typical features of Mondini's dysplasia. The cochlea has 1.5 turns and an apical scala communis. **B,** Midmodiolar section through a normal cochlea for comparison. *(From Monsell EM, Jackler RK, Motta G, Linthicum FH Jr. Congenital malformations of the inner ear: histologic findings in five temporal bones.* Laryngoscope. *1987;97[Suppl 40]:18.)*

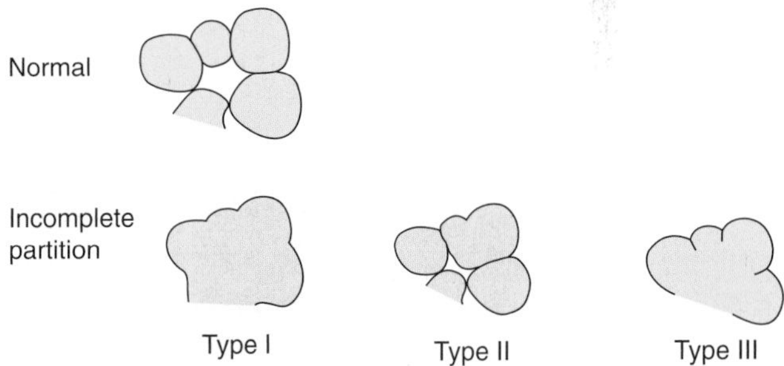

Figure 191-10. Subtypes of the incomplete partition deformity proposed by Sennaroglu and Saatci. *(From Sennaroglu L, Saatci I. Unpartitioned versus incompletely partitioned cochleae: radiologic differentiation.* Otol Neurotol. *2004;25:520.)*

Type I lacks the entire modiolus and interscalar septa and demonstrates a cystic appearance. Type II has a normal base turn but a cystic apex ("Mondini type"). Recently Sennaroglu has proposed a type III variant with deficient modiolus and partial interscalar septation at the cochlea's periphery (L. Sennaroglu, personal communication, 2007). Organ of Corti development is variable, as is the auditory neural population. As might be expected, auditory function also is variable, ranging from normal to profound SNHL. The mean hearing threshold (three-tone average) in a group of 41 ears with incomplete partition was 75 dB.[3] SCC deformities accompany incomplete partition of the cochlea in approximately 20% of cases.

Common Cavity

A deformed inner ear in which the cochlea and vestibule are confluent, forming an ovoid cystic space without internal architecture, may be explained by an arrest at the week 4 otocyst stage. Alternatively, this deformity may result from aberrant development at a later stage. An empty ovoid space typically longer in its horizontal dimension is seen radiographically. Although the size of the cyst may vary, it averages 7 mm vertically and 10 mm horizontally. It is quite easy to misdiagnose a dysplastic lateral SCC as a common cavity deformity. The key to differentiating between the two is that a common cavity cochlea lies predominantly anterior to the IAC on axial-plane CT, and a dysplastic vestibular system lies posterior to it. Histologically, an ovoid or spherical smooth-walled cystic cavity containing primordia of the membranous labyrinth has been described.[48,50,55] Sensory and supporting

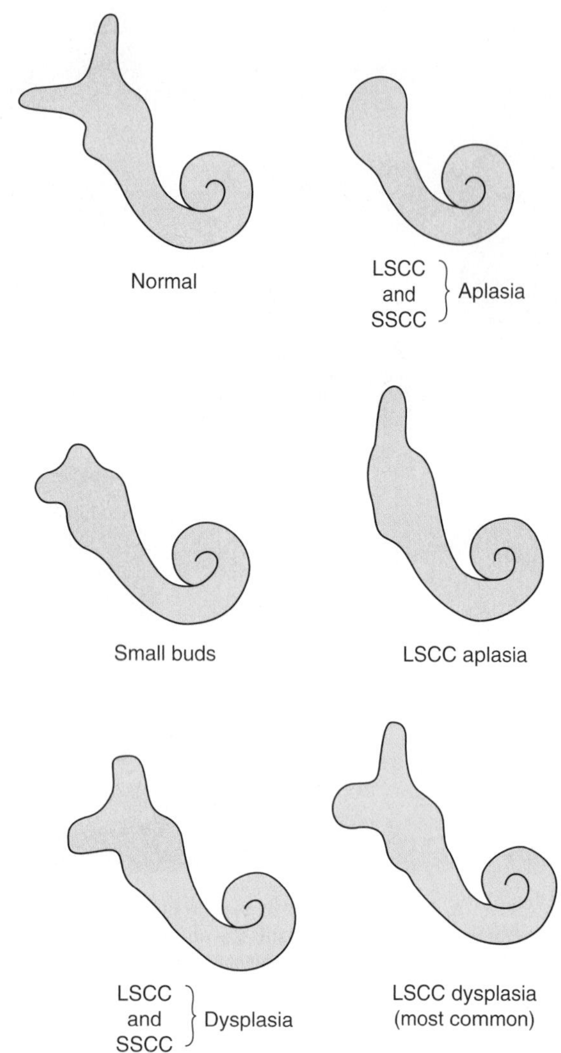

Figure 191-11. Semicircular canal malformations. LSCC, lateral semicircular canal; SSCC, superior semicircular canal. *(From Jackler RK, Luxford WM, House WF. Congenital malformations of the inner ear: a classification based on embryogenesis.* Laryngoscope. *1987;97[Suppl 40]:2.)*

cells may be differentiated into recognizable organs of Corti that are scattered peripherally around the walls of the cyst. Neural population usually is sparse or absent. Hearing is usually, but not invariably, poor.

Cochlear Hyperplasia

First reported in 2006, three temporal bones with a extra half apical turn have been described histologically.[61] Neither the clinical features nor the radiographic appearance of this anomaily has yet to be reported.

Labyrinthine Anomalies

Semicircular Canal Dysplasia

Dysplasia of the lateral SCC is a common type of inner ear malformation (Fig. 191-11). Approximately 40% of ears with a malformed cochlea will have an accompanying dysplasia of the lateral SCC.[3] Occasionally, dysplasia of the lateral SCC exists as the sole inner ear malformation. During the sixth week of development, the budding SCC normally forms a semicircular evagination from the vestibular anlage. The central portion of the pocket-shaped protrusion adheres, leaving a peripheral semicircular tube. When this central adhesion fails to occur, SCC dysplasia results (Fig. 191-12; see also Fig. 191-2). SCC dysplasia occasionally takes the form of a small bud, rather than the more common half-disk shape, presumably because of a slightly earlier timing of the developmental insult. The lateral SCC is deformed more often than the posterior or superior SCC, apparently because it forms earlier in embryogenesis. The typical radiographic appearance of SCC dysplasia is that of a short, broad cystic space confluent with the vestibule (Fig. 191-13).

Numerous histologic descriptions of SCC dysplasia exist in the literature.[46-50] The half-disk shaped cavity may contain a rudimentary crista ampullaris. The utricle and saccule may be distended, collapsed, or entirely absent. Caloric responses in SCC dysplasia are functionally absent or reduced in most cases, but a few may have normal responsiveness.[3] Ears with malformations limited to the vestibular system often have normal or near-normal hearing. When the cochlea also is abnormal, sensory hearing levels tend to be impaired, to a variable degree.[62] SCC dysplasia appears to have an association with conductive hearing loss, presumably because of inner ear micromechanical factors rather than stapes fixation.[63]

Semicircular Canal Aplasia

SCC aplasia is only one-fourth as common as SCC dysplasia.[3] It is usually associated with cochlear anomalies.[29] Presumably, SCC aplasia

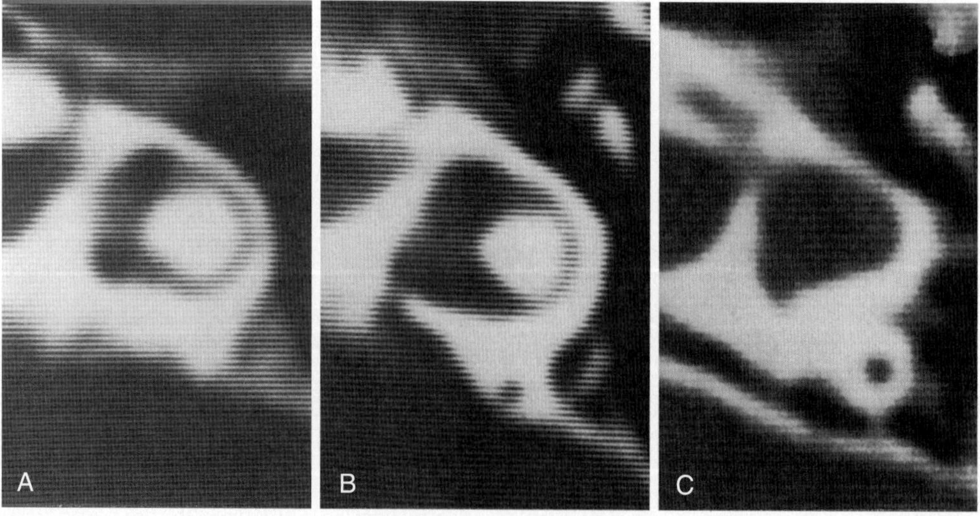

Figure 191-12. **A,** Lateral semicircular canal dysplasia as seen on an axial computed tomography scan. The normal appearance should be contrasted with that in mild, and severe dysplasia, in **B** and **C,** respectively. These images illustrate how semicircular canal dysplasia may arise from a failure of adhesion of the central region of the vestibular evagination during development. *(From Jackler RK, Luxford WM, House WF. Congenital malformations of the inner ear: a classification based on embryogenesis.* Laryngoscope. *1987;97[Suppl 40]:2.)*

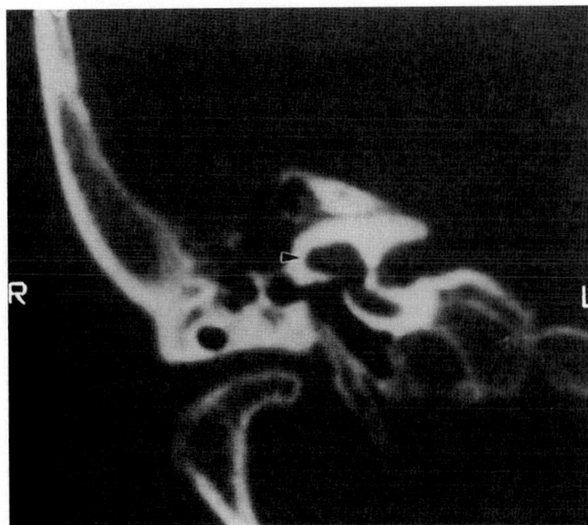

Figure 191-13. Lateral semicircular canal dysplasia *(arrowhead)* as seen on a coronal computed tomography scan. Note that the canal appears short, broad, and confluent with the vestibule.

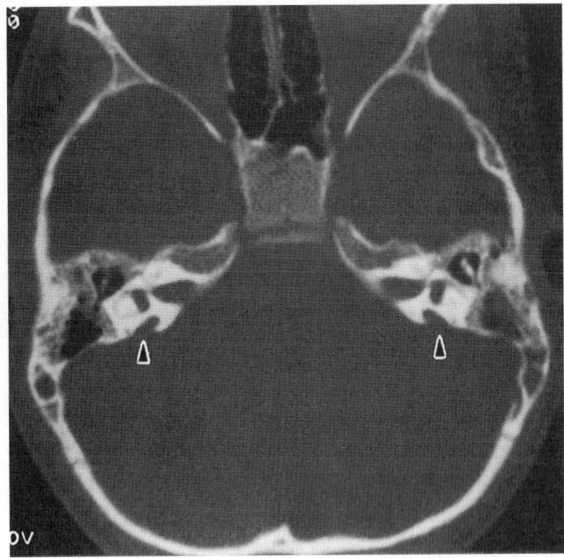

Figure 191-14. Bilateral enlargement of the vestibular aqueducts *(arrowheads)* as seen on an axial computed tomography scan.

arises from a failure in the development of the vestibular anlage before the sixth week of gestation. Most cases are syndromic, with a predominance of the CHARGE association (*c*oloboma, *h*eart defects, *a*tresia of the choanae, *r*etardation of growth and development, *g*enital, and *e*ar abnormalities or hearing loss).[64,65]

Malformations of the Vestibular and Cochlear Aqueducts

Enlargement of the Vestibular Aqueduct

Experience suggests that enlargement of the VA is the most common radiographically detectable malformation of the inner ear.[57,66-71] In earlier literature its incidence was underestimated, partly because of a lack of awareness but mostly because enlargement of the VA could be visualized only by lateral polytomography at a time when most studies were confined to the anteroposterior plane. The advent of high-resolution CT in the axial plane has made assessment of the VA much easier. The diameter of a normal VA, when measured halfway between the common crus and its external aperture, is between 0.4 and 1 mm. Enlargement of the VA is diagnosed when its diameter exceeds 2 mm, although enlarged VAs may exceed 6 mm in width. Whereas the VA is well visualized on axial CT (Fig. 191-14), the dilated endolymphatic sac is better seen with T2-weighted magnetic resonance imaging (MRI)[72,73] (Fig. 191-15). The sac often is seen to be enormously enlarged on MRI, sometimes measuring 2 cm or more in diameter.[74] In many cases, VA enlargement accompanies malformation of the cochlea or SCC. It also may be the sole radiographically detectable abnormality of the inner ear in a child with hearing loss. This condition is commonly referred to as the large VA syndrome, after Valvassori and Clemis's first descriptions.[75,76]

The VA derives from a diverticulum formed in the wall of the otocyst during the fifth week of gestation. It begins as a short, broad pouch but gradually elongates and thins until it achieves its characteristic J shape of adulthood (see Fig. 191-2). A premature arrest in development would be expected to produce a VA that is abnormally short and broad. However, an increasing body of evidence suggests that VA enlargement does not stem from an early arrest of sac development, but rather is an acquired deformity. Histologically, the sac and aqueduct are thin-walled and lack both vascularity and the rugose features thought to be important for physiologic function. Three observations suggest that a large VA stems from an abnormal communication between the subarachnoid space and the fluid chambers of the inner ear. The bone surrounding the VA may show signs of erosion, a finding that is inconsistent with a stable congenital deformity.[77] Serial MR images show variability in both the size and signal characteristics of the enlarged sac.[78] Presence of cerebrospinal fluid (CSF) under pressure,

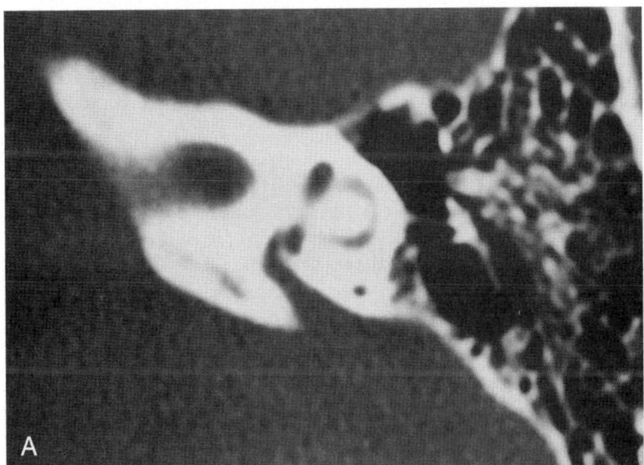

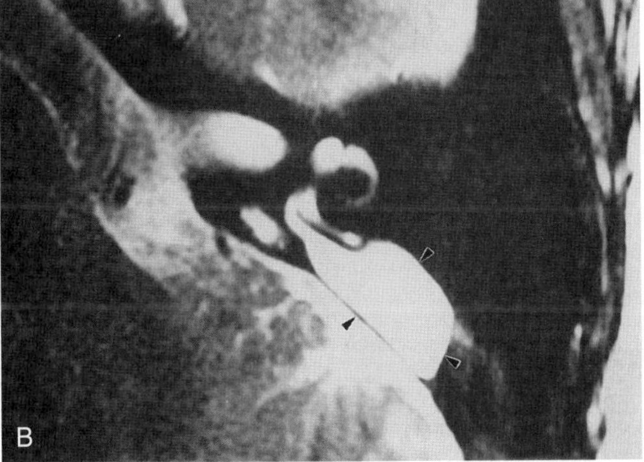

Figure 191-15. A comparison of computed tomography (**A**, axial scan), and magnetic resonance imaging (**B**), T2-weighted, fastspin echo sequence, of a large vestibular aqueduct deformity. Note that only the magnetic resonance image delineates the extent of the enormously enlarged endolymphatic sac *(arrowheads)*. *(Courtesy of Joel Swartz, MD.)*

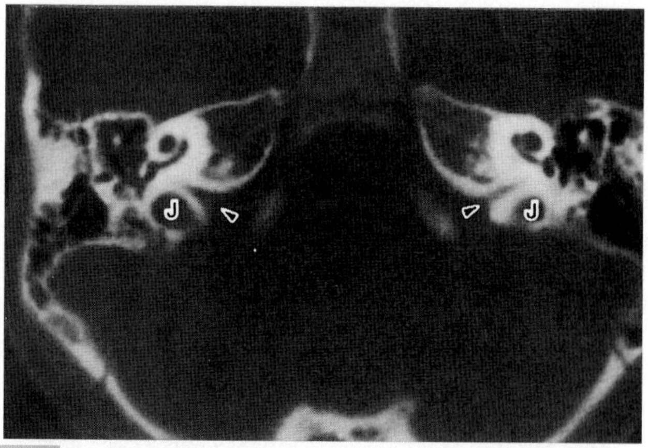

Figure 191-16. Axial computed tomography scan demonstrating a normal cochlear aqueduct bilaterally *(arrowheads)*. The external aperture typically lies inferior to the internal auditory canal and just above the jugular bulb (J).

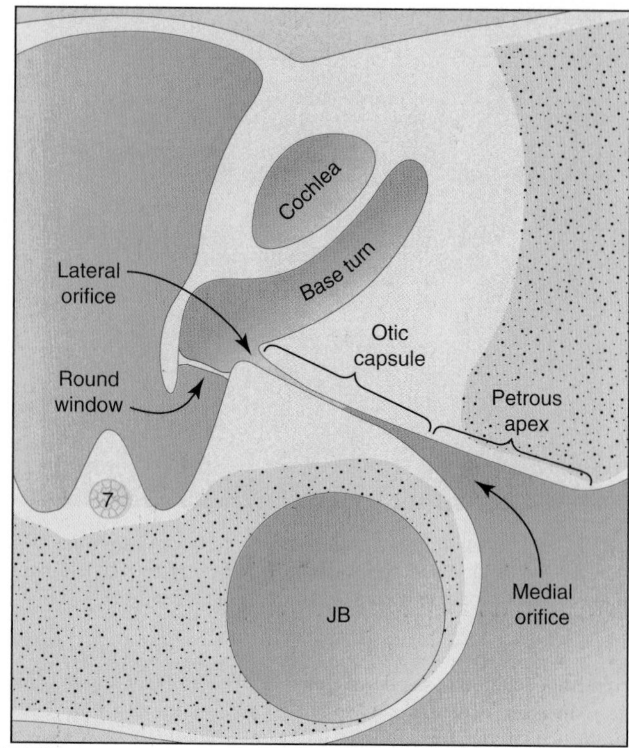

Figure 191-17. Illustration of the cochlear aqueduct in the axial plane. The diameter of the medial orifice is highly variable but often is wide (as depicted here) in normal-hearing persons. By contrast, the otic capsule portion typically is very narrow in both healthy and congenitally deaf persons. *(Adapted from Jackler RK, Hwang PH. Enlargement of the cochlear aqueduct: fact or fiction?* Otolaryngol Head Neck Surg. *1993;109:14.)*

with consequent "gusher," within the inner ear has been observed in ears with large VAs during both cochlear implantation and stapedectomy.[31,79] Furthermore, the existence of abnormal CSF in the inner ear pathway frequently has been observed with CT or MRI. This anomaly typically consists of a defect of the cochlear modiolus at the distal end of the IAC.[12,73] For CSF to become confluent with the endolymphatic space, the CSF fistula (subarachnoid space to perilymph compartment) must be accompanied by a second fistula joining the endolymph and perilymph spaces.

The large VA syndrome typically is bilateral. Affected children usually are born with normal or mildly impaired hearing that gradually deteriorates through childhood into adolescence and early adulthood. Hearing levels are variable, although at least 40% eventually develop profound SNHL.[80] As with other inner ear malformations, there is a tendency to suffer sudden decrements of hearing, particularly after head trauma. Conductive hearing loss may be present but is likely to be from intracochlear micromechanical disturbances rather than from impairment of ossicular mobility. Stapes surgery is best avoided because of the risk of CSF otorrhea.[79] Vestibular complaints in these patients have frequently been reported.[81,82] Large VA syndrome has been observed to occur in familial clusters.[10]

Surgical manipulation of the endolymphatic sac has been attempted in patients with large VAs. In a sizable series of shunt procedures, there was a high incidence of postoperative hearing loss.[67] Furthermore, a comparison of the operated and contralateral unoperated ears revealed no evidence of hearing stabilization after surgery. Recently, surgical obliteration of the enlarged endolymphatic sac with muscle and fascia has been advocated.[83] Results in a multicenter study indicated that the procedure not only lacks efficacy but actually injures one half of the operated ears.[84] Cochlear implantation has been quite successful in both adults and children with large VAs.[85,86]

Enlargement of the Cochlear Aqueduct

Enlargement of the cochlear aqueduct (CA) frequently is mentioned in the otologic literature because of its purported association with stapedectomy gusher and transotic CSF leak. Despite an active interest in the field and an extensive review of published radiographic images, I have never seen a radiograph that convincingly demonstrated CA enlargement.[87] Most cases presented as enlargement of the CA are misinterpretations of the wide internal funnel that opens into the posterior fossa.[88,89] In healthy subjects, the radiographic diameter of this aperture averages 3 to 4 mm but ranges from radiographically invisible to more than 10 mm[46,90-92] (Figs. 191-16 and 191-17). For enlargement of the CA to be diagnosed radiographically, the intraosseous portion coursing toward the vestibule must be enlarged beyond 1 mm, the practical resolution limit of contemporary CT scanners. If criteria analogous to those for enlargement of the VA are used, then an enlarged CA must have a diameter exceeding 2 mm throughout its course between the inner ear and the posterior fossa.

The preponderance of evidence suggests that the human CA usually is functionally patent.[92-94] In most persons, however, it can neither transmit sudden large pressure changes to the inner ear nor allow free flow of spinal fluid in any significant quantity (e.g., with outflow of perilymphatic fluid from perilymphatic fistula or an open vestibule). This observation reflects two anatomic features of the aqueduct: a narrow diameter of the bony channel and the presence of a fibrous tissue meshwork occupying and baffling the lumen. Schuknecht and Reisser[95] evaluated more than 1400 temporal bones in the Massachusetts Eye and Ear Infirmary collection and found no CA that exceeded 0.2 mm at its narrowest point. This series included 29 congenitally malformed inner ears. Of note, the CA was absent or nonpatent in 21 of these dysmorphic ears.

Some persons have less than normal or no fibrous tissue within the lumen, and the bony diameter is wider than normal. An opportunity may then exist for free flow of CSF from the oval window through the CA. According to Poiseuille's law, fluid flow through a tube varies with the fourth power of the radius, suggesting the possibility of free flow in an individual with a large-diameter unimpeded channel, as discussed by Allen.[96] Several histologic studies of congenital inner ear malformations have detected slightly larger CAs, particularly at their lateral orifice at the vestibule.[24,49] Even in these malformed inner ears, however, the aqueduct diameter remained well in the submillimeter range. From a clinical standpoint, a CA less than 1 mm in diameter is undetectable radiographically. Despite the theoretical possibility that a widely patent CA may cause a stapedectomy gusher, abnormal connections between the IAC and the vestibule appear to be etiologic in a majority of cases.[9,89,97,98]

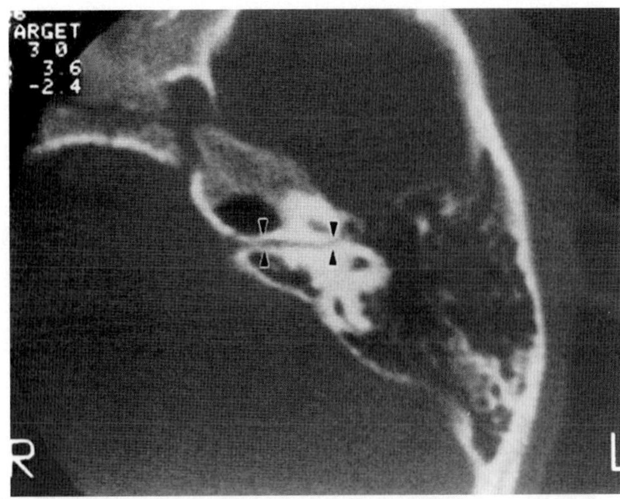

Figure 191-18. Axial computed tomography scan of a bulbous internal auditory canal (IAC). Note the minimal separation between the lateral end of the IAC from the vestibule *(arrowheads)*. Such an ear may be prone to spontaneous cerebrospinal fluid leakage and to "gusher" during stapes surgery.

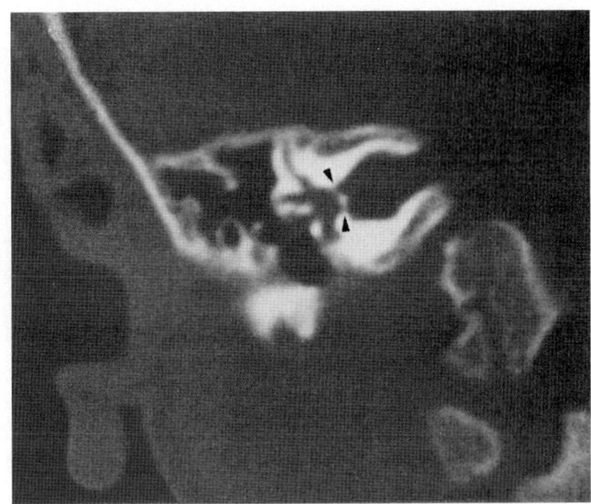

Figure 191-19. A pathologically narrow internal auditory canal (IAC) as seen on an axial computed tomography scan *(arrowheads)*. When the IAC is less than 3 mm in diameter, incomplete auditory nerve development is probable.

Developmental Anomalies of the Internal Auditory Canal

Wide Internal Auditory Canal

Unlike congenital narrowness of the IAC, a congenitally large canal may be an incidental finding in healthy individuals (Fig. 191-18). When a large IAC (larger than 10 mm in diameter) accompanies a malformation of the inner ear, it does not, as an independent variable, correlate with the level of hearing.[3] One report suggests that a wide IAC may be correlated with hearing loss.[99] The primary importance of detecting enlargement of the IAC is its association with spontaneous CSF leak and the occurrence of gusher during stapes surgery.[97] Because hearing after stapedectomy complicated by CSF gusher (often erroneously called "perilymph gusher") frequently is poor, a CT scan should be obtained before stapedectomy to address congenital fixation is undertaken. Dilation of the IAC, especially when the partition between the lateral end of the canal and inner ear appears deficient, should contraindicate stapedectomy.

Narrow Internal Auditory Canal

A narrow IAC may indicate a failure of eighth cranial nerve development. When a patient has normal facial function and an IAC less than 3 mm in diameter, it is likely that the bony canal transmits only the facial nerve (Fig. 191-19). A narrow IAC may accompany inner ear malformations or may be the sole radiographically detectable anomaly in a deaf child. A narrow IAC has been considered a relative contraindication to cochlear implantation, because it suggests that the eighth nerve may be insufficiently developed to conduct an auditory signal.[50] After cochlear implantation, some patients with narrow IACs have experienced facial pain and twitching without useful auditory sensation.

Anomalies of the Eighth Nerve

Hypoplasia and aplasia of the eighth nerve are often, but not inevitably, associated with congenital narrowness or even absence of the IAC. Similarly, although eighth nerve maldevelopment frequently accompanies malformation of the inner ear, the presence of a normal cochlea and semicircular canals does not guarantee normal development of the audiovestibular nerve.[100] High-resolution, thin-section MRI with T2-weighted sequences currently is the best means of assessing the fine anatomy of the eighth nerve in the IAC.[101,102] Such a study is warranted before cochlear implantation when the bony IAC is narrow on the CT scan, with severe types of inner ear malformation, and in syndromes known to be associated with maldevelopment of the eighth nerve (e.g., the CHARGE association, Möbius's syndrome).[103] Unilateral cochlear nerve aplasia, sometimes familial, is increasingly recognized as an important cause of congenital unilateral profound SNHL.[104,105] The internal auditory canal frequently is normal.[106] Increasingly refined MR techniques may reveal hypoplasia of the auditory nerve as more common than previously recognized.[107]

Syndromic Correlations and Familial Patterns

Inner ear malformations have been described in an increasing number of recognized syndromes associated with SNHL. Some of the more common examples are reviewed briefly next.

In Waardenburg's syndrome type I, absence of all three semicircular canals (17%) and cochlear hypoplasia (8%) have been reported.[108] In Waardenburg's syndrome type II, maldevelopment of the posterior semicircular canal has been described.[109] Semicircular canal agenesis or hypoplasia also has been noted in CHARGE syndrome.[110,111] In branchio-oto-renal syndrome, hypoplasia of the cochlea, sometimes accompanied by large VA, has been reported.[7,112,113] In Pendred's syndrome, large VA is a common feature, sometimes accompanied by modiolar deficiency.[114,115] Otic capsule anomalies also have been described in trisomy E and Usher's syndrome.[5,8] Down syndrome (trisomy 21) is associated with semicircular canal dysplasia and a variety of other inner ear malformations.[116]

Nonsyndromic familial patterns of inner ear malformation also have been identified.[9,10] An autosomal recessive pattern of Mondini's dysplasia has been reported.[117] In familial Mondini's dysplasia, genetic analysis has identified a deletion in locus DFN3.[118] Inherited complete labyrinthine aplasia (Michel's aplasia) has been described with a probable autosomal recessive inheritance pattern.[119] Familial lateral semicircular canal malformation has been described in association with anomalies of the external and middle ear.[120] Nonsyndromic familial occurrence of large VA has been associated with the Pendred gene.[121]

Cerebrospinal Fluid Leakage and Meningitis

Congenitally malformed inner ears may be a source of CSF otorhinorrhea.[122,123] For CSF leakage to occur, two abnormal connections must be present: one between the subarachnoid space and the inner ear and a second between the inner ear and middle ear. The most common pathologic interconnection between the subarachnoid space and the inner ear is through the fundus of the IAC. Histologically, large defects in the modiolar end of the IAC have been shown to exist in 10% of dysplastic ears.[95] Leakage may occur less often around the facial nerve at the lateral end of the IAC[124-126] (Fig. 191-20). The junction between the IAC and the inner ear may be evaluated with CT (Figs. 191-21 and 191-22). A well-defined bony plate normally partitions the distal IAC from the labyrinthine lumen. In a number of well-documented

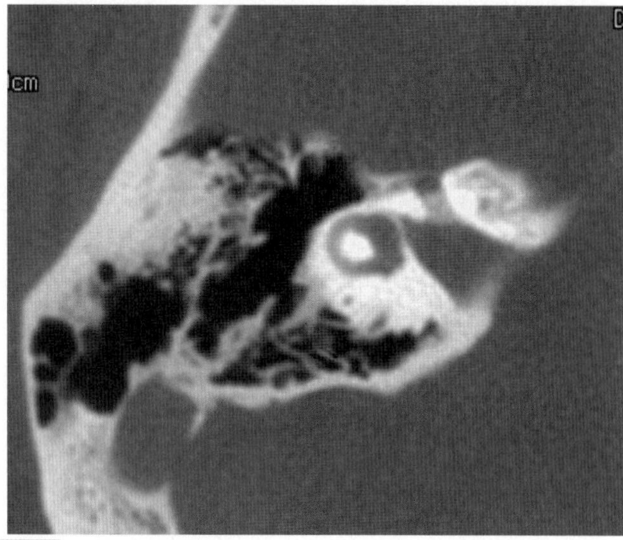

Figure 191-20. Dilated labyrinthine section of the fallopian canal associated with cochlear hypoplasia. This may serve as a conduit for cerebrospinal fluid leakage.

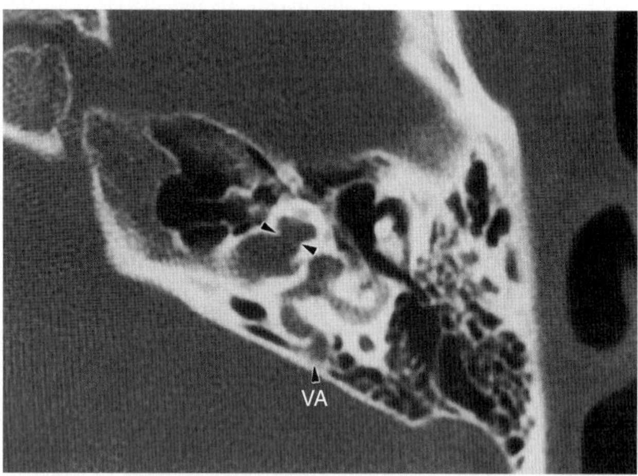

Figure 191-21. Axial computed tomography scan of an abnormal interconnection between the lateral end of the internal auditory canal and the cochlea. Note the absence of the modiolus *(arrowheads)* and the large vestibular aqueduct (VA).

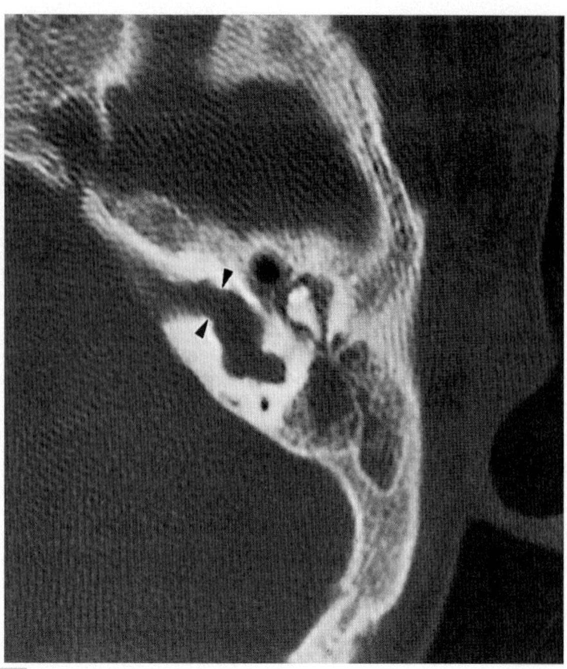

Figure 191-22. Axial computed tomography scan of an abnormal interconnection between the lateral end of the internal auditory canal (IAC) and a dysplastic vestibular system. Note the junction between the IAC and the dilated vestibule *(arrowheads)*.

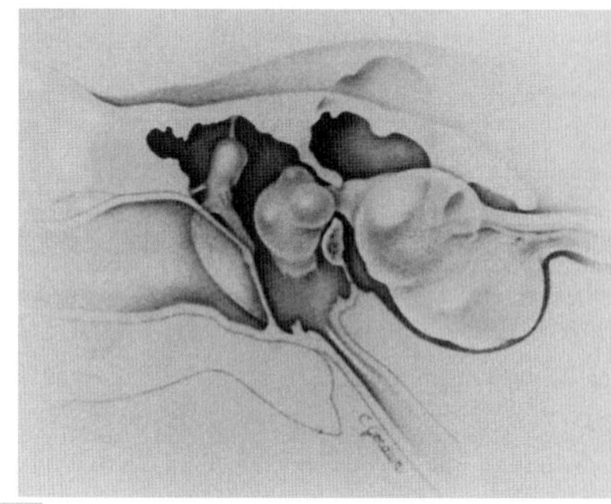

Figure 191-23. Drawing of a dural hernia protruding through the oval window in a child with cochlear hypoplasia, chronic cerebrospinal fluid leakage, and recurrent meningitis. *(From Herther C, Schindler RA. Mondini's dysplasia with recurrent meningitis.* Laryngoscope. *1985;95:655.)*

cases of CSF leakage, radiopaque contrast placed into the cerebellopontine angle cistern could be traced through the IAC into the inner ear.[122,124,127-129] The propensity of a dysplastic inner ear to leak CSF depends on its morphologic type. The common cavity deformity appears to be at particularly high risk. By contrast, Phelps and coworkers[130,131] maintain that the incomplete partition deformity (Mondini's dysplasia) is not associated with a heightened risk of CSF leakage. In ears with CSF fistulas, the SCCs usually are severely deformed. Although enlargement of the VA is a sign that CSF pressure is present within the inner ear, it does not necessarily imply the existence of an external leak into the middle ear. Rarely, transotic CSF leakage may be accompanied by a second congenital fistula in the anterior skull base.[132]

A second potential pathway between the subarachnoid space and the inner ear is the CA. As discussed previously in this chapter, there is little evidence to suggest that this pathway is a source of vigorous CSF leakage. In one published report, a CT metrizamide cisternogram was said to demonstrate a large CSF leak occurring through the CA; however, the published image showed the defect to be far anterior and superior to the region of the CA.[122]

A direct route between the subarachnoid space and middle ear, bypassing the inner ear, may exist in rare cases. Hyrtl's fissure, a congenital cleft that runs between the hypotympanum and posterior cranial fossa passing in proximity to the jugular bulb, has been reported to be a source of CSF leakage.[125] It is interesting that a diligent search of the historical literature has failed to find a publication on this subject by Hyrtl, despite his long eponymic association with this deformity.[133] In the interest of clarity, the descriptive term *tympanomeningeal fissure* is preferable.

The pathologic interconnection between the inner ear and middle ear most frequently is at the oval window. Numerous reports have described defects in the central portion of the footplate with a protruding membrane, most probably arachnoid[123,124,134-137] (Fig. 191-23). In other cases the defect is adjacent to the footplate, particularly just anterior to it. Much less frequently, leakage may occur through the round window or a fissure on the promontory.[123] Schuknecht and Reisser[95] evaluated the oval and round windows in 29 ears with congenital malformations of the inner ear. On histologic examination, the stapes were absent in 4, fixed in 6, and normal in 15 cases. In 4 cases the footplates were noted to have defects that were bridged by thin membranes only. The round windows were normal in 28 cases and abnormal in only 1 (bony closure). No deficiencies in the round window membranes were noted.

The primary clinical importance of CSF leakage is the risk of meningitis. There have been numerous reports of meningitis complicating congenital malformation of the inner ear.[122-124,134,136-138] Recurrent bouts of meningitis are typical, and recognition of the inner ear as the source frequently comes only after several episodes have occurred. Acute otitis media appears to be the bacterial source in most cases. All children with recurrent meningitis without an obvious cause should undergo CT of the inner ear to exclude inner ear malformation.[139] Even children with a single episode of meningitis should have a postrecovery audiogram followed by CT if unilateral or bilateral SNHL is discovered. The causative organisms in a review of 24 reported cases have been *Streptococcus pneumoniae* (in 71% of the cases), *Haemophilus influenzae* (in 33%), and β-hemolytic streptococci (in 8%). The total exceeds 100% because of the incidence of polymicrobial infection.

Surgical closure of transotic CSF leakage may be attempted at four anatomic levels: (1) the posterior cranial fossa; (2) the dysplastic inner ear; (3) the middle ear windows; and (4) the eustachian tube. In an ear with residual hearing, tympanotomy and overlay grafting of the site of leakage with a connective tissue graft is indicated as a first attempt. Unfortunately, recurrent leakage is common. When this technique fails and a useful amount of hearing persists, posterior fossa craniotomy with placement of a muscle plug in the IAC or connective tissue graft over the fistulous tract may prove to be successful and spare hearing.[122] When the hearing is poor, a direct approach to the dysplastic inner ear is indicated. After tympanotomy and removal of the footplate, an oversized piece of muscle may be used to obliterate the vestibule.[18,25,123,140] If the anatomy is unfavorable for this maneuver, a postauricular translabyrinthine approach to the IAC should prove to be effective. Farrior and Endicott[141] proposed a hypotympanic approach to ablation of the CA. However, this aqueduct has never been convincingly demonstrated to cause a high-volume CSF leak. The final option, closure of the eustachian tube, is not a good choice for children. After this procedure, the anomalous CSF pathway is still open to the middle ear—a disadvantageous situation at an age when acute otitis media is common. Subsequent to the repair of any CSF leakage, the patient is placed on bed rest with the head elevated 30 degrees for several days. Acetazolamide (Diamox) is administered to reduce CSF production, and fluids are restricted. Placement of a lumbar drain is a useful adjunctive measure, although it may be difficult to insert and maintain in young children.[90]

X-Linked Stapes Gusher Syndrome

A form of hereditary mixed conductive and sensory hearing loss associated with CSF gusher during stapes surgery has recently been described.[142] Inherited hearing loss follows an X-linked pattern.[143] The characteristic inner ear deformity may be seen radiographically.[144,145] On CT, the cochlear modiolus is deficient and the lateral portion of the IAC often is bulbous (see Fig. 191-21). These observations provide strong evidence that the abnormal interconnection between the subarachnoid space and the inner ear is by way of the lateral terminus of the IAC. The labyrinthine segment of the fallopian canal may be dilated. In the vestibular system, the posterior semicircular canal often is deformed, and the VA may be enlarged.

The occurrence of stapes fixation in X-linked gusher syndrome is questionable. It has been proposed that the observed air-bone gap may be accounted for by alteration in cochlear micromechanics rather than dysfunction of the conducting system.[146] Results of acoustic reflex testing and auditory evoked responses are more consistent with a pure sensory hearing loss than a mixed form. The outcome of stapes surgery in these patients usually is poor, with anacusis in the operated ear a frequent result. When surgery is contemplated for a congenital conductive hearing loss, preoperative imaging is advisable to screen for inner ear malformation.

Perilymphatic Fistula

In contrast with CSF leakage, a perilymphatic fistula requires only one abnormal pathway: an interconnection of the inner ear with the tympanic cavity. In all probability, perilymph fistula and CSF leak are part of a spectrum of related disturbances of inner ear fluid homeostasis. Although separation of the two topics may be artificial pathophysiologically, it can be justified by the different clinical settings of the two problems. With CSF leakage, the cardinal clinical issues are gross fluid leakage and recurrent meningitis; with perilymph fistulization, sudden or progressive hearing loss and vertigo are the primary manifestations.

Much controversy surrounds the diagnosis and management of perilymphatic fistula in children. The candidate group for exploratory tympanotomy consists of children with progressive or sudden SNHL. CT of the inner ear may demonstrate pneumolabyrinth, although this finding is rare (Fig. 191-24). Conservative surgeons have advocated exploration only in children with radiographically abnormal inner ears who have a clear antecedent event of head trauma or barometric pressure change.[147] Other workers have espoused the notion of surgical exploration in all children with unexplained SNHL.[14,148,149] Great variability exists in the number of fistulas "confirmed" at surgery. Pappas and colleagues[147] found only 4 fistulas in 36 ears (11%) explored for progressive SNHL during childhood. Of note, 50% of these ears had radiographically malformed inner ears. By contrast, Parnes and McCabe[148] found fistulas in 20 of 26 children's ears (77%), only 6 of whom had inner ear anomalies radiographically. A high incidence of fistulas among children with sensory hearing loss (64%), both with and without inner ear malformation, has been reported.[150,151] Furthermore, one group of investigators claim to have objective verification of the presence of perilymph in the middle ear through evaluation of β_2-transferrin levels in surgical aspirates.[152] An important point is that considerable doubt exists regarding whether this test is valid. A recent study in which perilymph samples were directly obtained during either stapedectomy or cochlear implant surgery failed to detect β_2-transferrin in this fluid.[153]

In exploration of a perilymph fistula, it is important to perform provocative maneuvers to render subtle perilymph flows more visible. Such maneuvers include performing a Valsalva maneuver, using the Trendelenburg position, and compressing the jugular veins. Many surgeons are either missing subtle or intermittent perilymphatic fistulas during explorations or overdiagnosing them by misinterpreting middle ear secretions or local anesthetic as perilymph. Attempts to make a

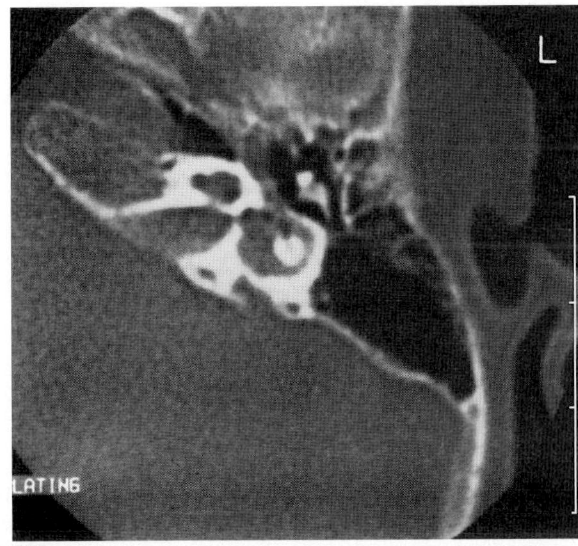

Figure 191-24. Air bubbles in the inner ear (pneumolabyrinth) in a congenitally deaf child with a perilymphatic fistula.

practical biochemical test for the presence of perilymph or CSF in the middle ear—through either assay of β_2-transferrin or intrathecal fluorescein administration—have not yet proved useful.[154,155] Most surgeons patch both oval and round windows with connective tissue whether or not a perilymphatic fistula was identified during exploration.

Rather than dwell on the controversy about how many fistulas are found, the critical observer should judge the effectiveness of the therapeutic intervention by analyzing its outcome relative to the natural history of the disease. In this regard, results of perilymphatic fistula exploration in children have been disappointing. In one series of 36 patients, hearing was better in 3, unchanged in 21, and worse in 12.[147] Similar results have been obtained in other childhood perilymphatic fistula series. It would be difficult to argue that these data represent a significant improvement over the natural history of the inner ear disease. Congenital progressive SNHL often is characterized by long periods of stability interspersed with periods of rapid deterioration. Even a relative improvement in hearing may occur after an episode of sudden loss. It is apparent that most children with sudden or progressive SNHL have suffered from cochlear diseases other than perilymphatic fistula. Examples are hereditary progressive loss, viral labyrinthitis (e.g., measles, mumps, cytomegalovirus), autoimmune inner ear disease (e.g., Cogan's syndrome), and endolymphatic hydrops. Even in the most suggestive clinical situation—sudden loss triggered by head trauma in a child with radiographically malformed inner ears—only a minority of patients demonstrate oval or round window fistulization. Many of these children probably lose hearing as a result of internal fistulization between the endolymphatic and perilymphatic space because of deficiencies of the osseous spiral lamina, rather than because of external fistulization to the middle ear. A minority of children with sudden or progressive SNHL have prominent vestibular symptoms. Results of perilymphatic fistula repair in the relief of vertigo have been quite good, although spontaneous recovery from vestibulopathy is common in this age group.

Inner Ear Malformations in Congenital Aural Atresia

Development of the external and middle ears is embryologically distinct from that of the inner ear. Anomalies of the lateral portion of the temporal bone typically result from derangement of the first or second branchial arches. Despite their embryologic separateness, congenital aural atresia may coexist with malformation of the inner ear.[156] In one study of patients with atresia, 12% (8 of 66) had a radiographically detectable inner ear abnormality.[157] In this group, SCC abnormalities were most common, including some ears with normal bone-conduction hearing. Cochlear anomalies were present in 5% (3 of 66) of these patients, all of whom had poor bone conduction hearing. It is an embryologic enigma that one patient with unilateral atresia had a malformed inner ear only on the contralateral side. In another polytomographic study of atretic ears, 8% (4 of 48) had SCC anomalies, and 2% (1 of 48) had a deformed cochlea.[158] As indicated by a comprehensive review of the relevant literature, approximately 5% of patients with atresia have cochlear deformities, whereas 10% have malformed SCCs. As a general rule, surgical reconstruction of atretic ears should not be attempted when they are associated with malformation of the inner ear. The deformed cochlea is more vulnerable to injury from vibratory trauma, and the risk of inducing a sensory hearing loss is increased. This surgery also carries a heightened risk of CSF leakage.

Imaging

During the 1980s and 1990s, CT was the gold standard imaging modality for investigation of patients suspected of having an inner ear malformation. In the early 21st century, new MRI techniques are capable of producing images superior to those obtained with CT. In contrast to CT, which depicts otic capsule bone, MRI displays inner ear morphology by imaging inner ear fluids. High-resolution, thin-section, T2-weighted sequences (e.g., fast-spin echo) provide exquisite detail of inner ear anatomy (see Fig. 191-4).[159] MRI is superior to CT in a number of ways. MRI can distinguish between a cochlea filled with fluid and one occluded by soft tissue. CT is unable to make this distinction—an observation of great importance in assessing scala tympani patency before cochlear implantation. MRI provides more information about large VAs than that provided by CT.[72,73,160] It displays not only the dilated osseous canal but also the dimensions of the often impressively expanded endolymphatic sac. Direct visualization of the eighth nerve in the IAC, where it appears as a linear filling defect outlined by CSF, is yet another advantage of MRI. This capability is important in certain severe deformities in which neural agenesis may be found. Three-dimensional renderings of inner ear malformations have been produced using both CT and MRI.[161,162]

In assessing images for possible inner ear malformation, it is important to measure the size of structures and not merely look for anomalous patterns. Normative data of inner ear dimension have been published to aid in this determination.[163] Quantitative measurement has been shown to increase diagnositc yield in cochlear hypoplasia (less than 4.4 mm cochlear height on coronal images) and semicircular canal dysplasia (bony island width on axial projection) even for experienced neuroradiologists.[164]

In addition to inner ear malformation, numerous causes of acute and chronic SNHL in children are recognized. Whereas either CT or MRI findings would be normal in the great majority of these, a few disorders can be visualized only by MRI. The obvious category is lesions of the cerebellopontine angle (e.g., tumors) and brainstem (e.g., adrenoleukodystrophy). On noncontrast T1-weighted MRI, acute hemorrhage results in hyperintensity of the inner ear. On gadolinium-enhanced studies, acute inflammation (e.g., viral infection) results in high signal intensity in the inner ear or along the course of the eighth nerve.

When selecting MRI as an imaging study to screen for inner ear malformation, it is important for the physician to be aware that standard MRI protocols designed to screen for central nervous system abnormalities provide only limited information concerning the inner ear. To be useful in screening for inner ear anomalies, specially designed protocols are needed.[159] One disadvantage of MRI is the difficulty young children have in tolerating the confined spaces of the magnet. In addition, fast-spin echo MRI requires considerably longer scan time than does CT. Whereas simple sedation usually is sufficient for CT, acquiring high-quality magnetic resonance images may require use of general anesthesia in pediatric patients. Accordingly, despite the numerous advantages of MRI (including the absence of ionizing radiation), CT is the pediatric examination of choice in many centers for this important practical reason.

Evaluation and Management

High-resolution CT or MRI of the inner ears is recommended for all children with suspected congenital malformation of the inner ear, including those with otherwise unexplained SNHL, regardless of whether it has existed from birth or occurred later. Scans usually are obtained when hearing impairment is first recognized. Use of thin slices of 1- or 1.5-mm thickness with 0.5-mm overlap will adequately image the minute inner ear structures.[59] If only one plane of view is to be obtained, the axial orientation is preferred because it provides superior images of the VA, a frequently malformed structure that is difficult to visualize on coronal scans. When possible, both axial and coronal views should be obtained, because certain subtle deformities, such as deficiency of the interscalar septum, are best seen in the coronal orientation. It is important to examine thoroughly all portions of the inner ear, because anomalies frequently are multiple (Fig. 191-25).

No medical or surgical therapy has been shown to prevent the progressive hearing loss associated with congenital malformation of the inner ear. After a sudden decrease in hearing, a short course of an oral corticosteroid (e.g., prednisone) is administered. Although no studies have assessed the efficacy of corticosteroids in children with inner ear deformities, studies of idiopathic sudden SNHL in adults suggest some benefit. Furthermore, autoimmune mechanisms may play a role in a few children with rapid hearing deterioration, a possibility that justifies a therapeutic trial. Of course, many patients experience spontaneous partial recovery after sudden losses, even without therapeutic intervention.

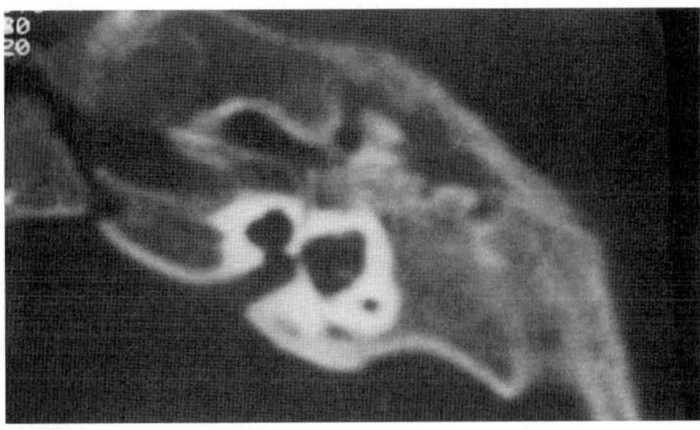

Figure 191-25. Axial computed tomography scan demonstrating a cochlear deformity (incomplete partition) as well as dysplasia of the lateral semicircular canal. Many congenitally malformed inner ears have abnormalities in more than one portion of the inner ear.

Few patients with congenitally malformed inner ears have a fluctuating pattern of hearing loss suggestive of endolymphatic hydrops. When fluctuations are encountered, however, a low-salt diet and diuretics are prescribed. Surgical intervention is indicated in a few well-defined circumstances. Obviously, CSF leakage and meningitis require intervention. Exploration for perilymphatic fistula is reserved for patients with radiographically abnormal inner ears who have suffered a sudden hearing deterioration temporally related to a precipitating event such as head trauma, rapid barometric pressure change, vigorous exercise, or sneezing. As discussed previously, even in these patients, only a minority have a fistula, and those who do frequently continue to lose hearing despite repair. House[165] and later others advocated endolymphatic sac surgery for congenital malformations of the inner ear[166-168]; however, a careful analysis of the outcome in a large series revealed no benefit of this surgery in terms of hearing stabilization.[169] In fact, nearly 30% of the patients suffered significant postoperative hearing deterioration. Patients with large VAs appear to be at particularly high risk for poor outcome after sac surgery. Surgical obliteration of the endolymphatic sac with muscle and fascia has been advocated in patients with enlargement of the VA.[83] Unfortunately, a multicenter study showed that this procedure not only fails to stabilize hearing but is associated with a 50% rate of sensorineural hearing deterioration.[84]

Preventive measures are important in the management of patients with congenitally malformed inner ears. The risk of CSF leakage may be estimated by CT or MRI of the inner ear. Anatomic features of concern include a wide IAC, deficient partitioning between the IAC and inner ear, and enlargement of the vestibule in the horizontal plane. Parents should be made aware of the risk of meningitis and instructed in recognizing its early symptoms and signs. Because most episodes of meningitis associated with inner ear malformation are pneumococcal, use of the pneumococcal vaccine is recommended.[170] Children with malformed inner ears should avoid head trauma and rapid barometric pressure changes, because these risk provoking a sudden hearing loss or even CSF leakage. Activities such as contact sports and scuba diving are discouraged. Finally, establishing a prognosis for future auditory function in a hearing-impaired child serves as a guide for educational and rehabilitative efforts. Recognizing an inner ear malformation on CT may be helpful, because certain morphologic patterns have more favorable prognoses than others.

Cochlear Implantation

Electrical stimulation of the auditory nerve has proved useful in many forms of sensory deafness, including those associated with congenital malformations of the inner ear. The fundamental premise of cochlear implantation is that some of the cochlear neural population survive despite the absence of hair cells. In congenital malformations of the inner ear, the auditory nerve population typically is less than with other forms of sensory deafness. The normal human spiral ganglion cell count usually is 25,000 to 35,000. In eight congenitally dysplastic ears, Schmidt[171] reported cell counts ranging from 7677 to 16,110, with an average of only 11,478. By contrast, ears with profound sensory hearing loss from ototoxicity, otosclerosis, or mechanisms of sudden loss have ganglion cell populations in the range of 18,000 to 22,000. This observation suggests that malformed inner ears could be electrically stimulated but that improvements in speech discrimination would fall below average for the deaf population at large. A narrow IAC on pre-implantation CT (less than 3 mm in diameter) is a strongly adverse predictor of neural survival.[23]

Cochlear implantation in deformities that involve both the membranous and osseous labyrinth raises several special considerations. Cochlear implantation in malformations limited to the membranous labyrinth is equivalent to implantation in the prelingually deaf child (see Chapter 159). Results of implantation with short, single-channel devices in patients with cochlear hypoplasia, common cavity, and incomplete partition deformities appear in the literature.[36,172,173] In successful cases, sound detection levels are similar to those in other prelingually deaf children.[174,175] Implantation of deformed cochleas with multichannel devices also has proved to be valuable in a majority of cases but is associated with a higher rate of complications.[31,176-179] Performance varies widely and appears, on average, to be somewhat below that realized in most other forms of deafness. The design of multichannel electrodes makes certain assumptions about the geometry of the scala tympani that affect the anticipated orientation of stimulating electrodes to neural elements. Although standard electrodes are not optimized for dysplastic cochleae, fabrication of custom electrodes for each malformed cochlea is not feasible with current technology. The degree of electrode insertion varies, in large part because of variability in size and geometry of the deformed cochlea.[180] Only partial insertion may be realized, particularly in hypoplastic cochleas, whereas complete insertion is more common with milder deformities such as incomplete partition.

One complication of unpredictable electrode positioning is stimulation of the facial nerve at current levels lower than the threshold for auditory perception. Cross-stimulation of the facial nerve has been reported with both single-channel and multichannel designs and has prevented some patients from using the device. Multichannel systems have a distinct advantage in this regard because the offending electrode pair or pairs may be programmed out of the stimulation map, thereby preserving the ability to provide auditory stimulation. The presence of a dysplastic inner ear may be a warning that the facial nerve is malpositioned.[181] An anomalous facial nerve course has been reported to occur in 16% of malformed inner ears.[176] In one patient with cochlear hypoplasia, an anomalous facial nerve was injured immediately above the round window niche, a highly vulnerable location during implant surgery.[31] Use of electrophysiologic facial nerve monitoring during implantation in patients with malformed inner ears is advisable. It also is possible for a persistent stapedial artery to traverse the round window region, thereby precluding implantation.[182]

Another complication of implantation in malformed cochleas is facial twitching consequent to inadvertent penetration of the IAC by the electrode.[179] When such a malpositioned electrode is activated, vigorous facial twitching may occur at an extremely low stimulation threshold. To avoid this complication, post-implantation CT is advisable before stimulation is undertaken to assess electrode position after implantation in a malformed cochlea.

CSF leak also has been a frequent complication during implantation of the malformed cochlea, occurring with an incidence of approximately 40%.[176] The leak typically is evident immediately on opening the round window and presumably occurs as a result of deficiencies in the partition between the modiolus and the dural envelope at the lateral end of the IAC. Leaks have been successfully handled by packing connective tissue around the electrode, but temporary CSF diversion may be required to obtain a lasting seal.[183] Multichannel cochlear implants, especially certain varieties designed to approximate the modiolus, have been associated with an increased long-term incidence of meningitis.[184] The incidence may well be higher in patients with malformed inner ears.[185]

SUGGESTED READINGS

Alexander G. Zur Pathologie und Pathologischen Anatomie der kongenitalen Taubheit. *Arch Otor Nas Kohlk Heilk.* 1904;61:183.

Anson BJ. The endolymphatic and perilymphatic aqueducts of the human ear: developmental and adult anatomy of their parietes and contents in relation to otological surgery. *Acta Otolaryngol (Stockh).* 1965;59:140.

Bamiou DE, Worth S, Phelps P, et al. Eighth nerve aplasia and hypoplasia in cochlear implant candidates: the clinical perspective. *Otol Neurotol.* 2001; 22:492.

Bluestone CB. Cochlear malformations, meningitis, and cochlear implants: what have we learned? *Otol Neurotol.* 2003;24:349.

Ceruti S, Stinckens C, Cremers CW, et al. Temporal bone anomalies in the branchio-oto-renal syndrome: detailed computed tomographic and magnetic resonance imaging findings. *Otol Neurotol.* 2002;23:200.

Collins WO, Buchman CA. Bilateral semicircular canal aplasia: a characteristic of the CHARGE association. *Otol Neurotol.* 2002;23:233.

Cremers WR, Bolder C, Admiraal RJ, et al. Progressive sensorineural hearing loss and a widened vestibular aqueduct in Pendred syndrome. *Arch Otolaryngol Head Neck Surg.* 1998;124:501.

Eisenman DJ, Ashbaugh C, Zwolan TA, et al. Implantation of the malformed cochlea. *Otol Neurotol.* 2001;22:834.

Govaerts PJ, Casselman J, Daemers K, et al. Audiological findings in large vestibular aqueduct syndrome. *Int J Pediatr Otorhinolaryngol.* 1999;51: 157.

Ishinaga H, Shimizu T, Yuta A, et al. Pendred's syndrome with goiter and enlarged vestibular aqueducts diagnosed by PDS gene mutation. *Head Neck.* 2002;24:710.

Ito K, Ishimoto S, Shotaro K. Isolated cochlear nerve hypoplasia with various internal auditory meatus deformities in children. *Ann Otol Rhinol Laryngol.* 2007;116:520.

Jackler RK, Hwang PH. Enlargement of the cochlear aqueduct: fact or fiction? *Otolaryngol Head Neck Surg.* 1993;109:14.

Jackler RK, Luxford WM, House WF. Congenital malformations of the inner ear: a classification based on embryogenesis. *Laryngoscope.* 97(Suppl 40):2.1987;

Johnson J, Lalwani AK. Sensorineural and conductive hearing loss associated with lateral semicircular canal malformation. *Laryngoscope.* 2000;110:1673.

Konigsmark BW, Gorlin RJ. *Genetic and Metabolic Deafness.* Philadelphia: WB Saunders; 1976.

Miyamoto RT, Robbins AJ, Myres WA, et al. Cochlear implantation in the Mondini inner ear malformation. *Am J Otol.* 1986;7:258.

Mondini C. Anatomia surdi nedi sectio. *De Bononiensi Scientiarum et Artium Instituto Arque Academia Commentarii, Bologna.* 1791;7:419.

Mondini C. The minor works of Carlo Mondini: the anatomical section of a boy born deaf. *Am J Otol.* 1997;18:288.

For complete list of references log onto www.expertconsult.com.

Nadol JB, Young YS, Glynn RJ. Survival of spiral ganglion cells in profound sensorineural deafness: its implications for cochlear implantation. *Ann Otol Rhinol Laryngol.* 1989;98:411.

Paparella MM. Mondini's deafness: a review of histopathology. *Ann Otol Rhinol Laryngol Suppl.* 1980;89:1.

Phelps PD. Imaging for congenital deformities of the ear. *Clin Radiol.* 1994;49:663.

Phelps PD, Coffey RA, Trembath RC, et al. Radiological malformations of the ear in Pendred syndrome. *Clin Radiol.* 1998;53:268.

Phelps PD, Proops D, Sellars S, et al. Congenital cerebrospinal fluid fistula through the inner ear and meningitis. *J Laryngol Otol.* 1993;107:492.

Phelps PD, Reardon W, Pembrey M, et al. X-linked deafness, stapes gushers and a distinctive defect of the inner ear. *Neuroradiology.* 1991;33:326.

Purcell DD, Fischbein N, Patel A, et al. Two temporal bone computed tomography measurements increase recognition of malformations and predict sensorineural hearing loss. *Laryngoscope.* 2006;116:1439.

Raphael Y, Fein A, Nebel L. Transplacental kanamycin ototoxicity in the guinea pig. *Arch Otorhinolaryngol.* 1983;238:45.

Rich PM, Graham J, Phelps PD. Hyrtl's fissure. *Otol Neurotol.* 2002;23:476.

Satar B, Mukherji SK, Telian SA. Congenital aplasia of the semicircular canals. *Otol Neurotol.* 2003;24:437.

Schuknecht HF. *Pathology of the Ear.* Cambridge: Harvard University Press; 1974.

Schuknecht HF, Reisser C. The morphologic basis for perilymphatic gushers and oozers. *Adv Otorhinolaryngol.* 1988;39:1.

Sennaroglu L, Saatci I. Unpartitioned versus incompletely partitioned cochleae: radiologic differentiation. *Otol Neurotol.* 2004;25:520.

Sennaroglu L, Saatci I. A new classification for cochleovestibular malformations. *Laryngoscope.* 2002;112:2230.

Streeter GL. On the development of the membranous labyrinth and the acoustic and facial nerves in the human embryo. *Am J Anat.* 1906;6:139.

Streeter GL. The histogenesis and growth of the otic capsule and its contained periotic tissue-spaces in the human embryo. *Carnegie Contrib Embryol.* 1918;7:5.

Usami S, Abe S, Weston MD, et al. Non-syndromic hearing loss associated with enlarged vestibular aqueduct is caused by PDS mutations. *Hum Genet.* 1999;104:188.

Wilson JT, Leivy SW, Sofferman RA, et al. Mondini dysplasia: spontaneous cerebrospinal fluid otorrhea. New perspectives in management. *Pediatr Neurosurg.* 1990-1991;16:260.

Wootten CT, Backous DD, Haynes DS. Management of cerebrospinal fluid leakage from cochleostomy during cochlear implant surgery. *Laryngoscope.* 2006;116:2055.

Zheng Y, Schachern PA, Djalilian HR, et al. Temporal bone histopathology related to cochlear implantation in congenital malformation of the bony cochlea. *Otol Neurotol.* 2002;23:181.

CHAPTER ONE HUNDRED AND NINETY-TWO

Microtia Reconstruction

Craig S. Murakami

Vito C. Quatela

Kathleen C. Y. Sie

Joseph Shvidler

Key Points

- The auricle is formed from the branchial arches starting at approximately 5 weeks of gestation.
- The auricle grows rapidly in the first 3 years of life and then grows more slowly until approximately 13 years of age for boys and 12 years of age for girls. Normal adult ear height ranges from 5.5 to 6.5 cm.
- The etiology of microtia most commonly is sporadic, possibly as the result of a vascular injury in the distribution of the stapedial artery. Other causes include teratogenic exposures and syndromic associations.
- Type I microtia is used to designate ears with mild deformity. Type II includes ears that have all major structures present to some degree. Type III deformities have few or no recognizable landmarks of the auricle, although the lobule usually is present and positioned anteriorly. Anotia is the complete absence of auricle and lobule.
- Options for microtia management include observation, prosthetic management, and reconstruction with autologous rib graft or Medpor implant with temporoparietal fascial flap.
- Observation is recommended until the child is at least 5 to 8 years old. This allows both growth of the donor rib cartilage and development of the contralateral normal ear. In general, microtia repair should precede atresia repair.

Microtia occurs with an overall frequency of approximately 1 to 3 cases per 10,000 population,[1] although certain ethnic groups, such as Navaho Indians in Mexico and the Japanese, may have higher incidence of microtia.[2] Microtia deformities appear to be more common on the right side and affect boys more often than girls at roughly a 2.5 : 1 ratio; unilateral cases outnumber bilateral cases by 4 : 1. Surgical management of microtia remains one of the greatest reconstructive challenges for an otolaryngologist.[3-6] Auricular reconstruction of the microtia deformity is a complex and labor-intensive process that requires careful preoperative planning, surgical skill, and artistry. This chapter provides a basic overview of clinical issues in children with microtia and reconstruction with autologus rib cartilage. Discussion of aural atresia is presented elsewhere.

Embryology

The inner ear begins as the otic placode at approximately the third week of gestation, and it then forms into the otic pit and otic cyst. The external ear begins to form in the fifth week of gestation. The auricle begins as six small buds of mesenchyme, classically known as the hillocks of His, surrounding the dorsal end of the first branchial cleft.[7-10] On either side of the first branchial cleft are the first (mandibular) and second (hyoid) branchial arches. Hillocks 1 through 3 arise from the first branchial arch, and hillocks 4 through 6 arise from the second branchial arch. Conventional teaching holds that the first hillock forms the tragus, the second and third form the helix, the fourth and fifth form the antihelix, and the sixth forms the antitragus. The majority of the central ear is derived from hillocks 4 and 5, and the lobule appears to be one of the last parts of the ear to develop (Fig. 192-1). It has been estimated that the hyoid arch forms about 85% of the auricle.[5] The exact embryology of each of these hillocks remains unclear. The position of the auricular complex begins at the anterior neck region. As the mandible develops during gestational weeks 8 through 12, the auricular complex moves in dorsal and cephalic directions. The etiology of microtia remains unknown in most cases, although the inciting event that arrests development of the ear must occur during the first trimester, and may be related to abnormal neural crest cell migration.

Known teratogens, such as the retinoic acid derivative isotretinoin (Accutane; Roche, Nutley, New Jersey), can produce forms of microtia in conjunction with craniofacial, cardiac, thymic, and CNS anomalies, a condition commonly known as retinoic embryopathy.[11] Thalidomide and mycophenolate mofetil also have been reported to be associated with microtia.[12,13] Microtia is associated with other anomalies about 50% of the time. Microtia is most commonly associated with other regional anomalies related to the first and second branchial arches, i.e., facioauriculovertebral syndrome. Within the facioauriculovertebral spectrum are malformations and syndromes that affect the first and second branchial arch derivatives, such as Goldenhar's syndrome (preauricular nodes, epibulbar dermoids, mandibular hypoplasia), hemifacial microsomia,[14] and oculoauricular vertebral dysplasia (microtia, cervical spine anomalies, and epibulbar dermoids).[15,16] It may be that Goldenhar's syndrome, hemifacial microsomia, oculoauriculovertebral dysplasia, and microtia are simply variants of the same entity.[4] Microtia also may be seen in syndromes such as Treacher Collins syndrome, which has an autosomal dominant inheritance pattern.

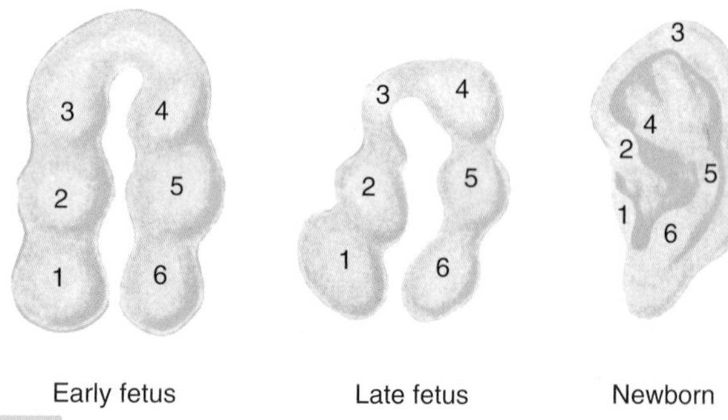

Figure 192-1. Embryonic development. The ear develops from six hillocks of His. Hillocks 1 through 3 are from the first branchial arch, and hillocks 4 to 6 are from the second branchial arch. Hillock 1 forms the tragus, hillock 2 forms the root of the helix, and hillock 6 forms the antitragus. Hillocks 2 through 5 appear to form the helix and antihelix.

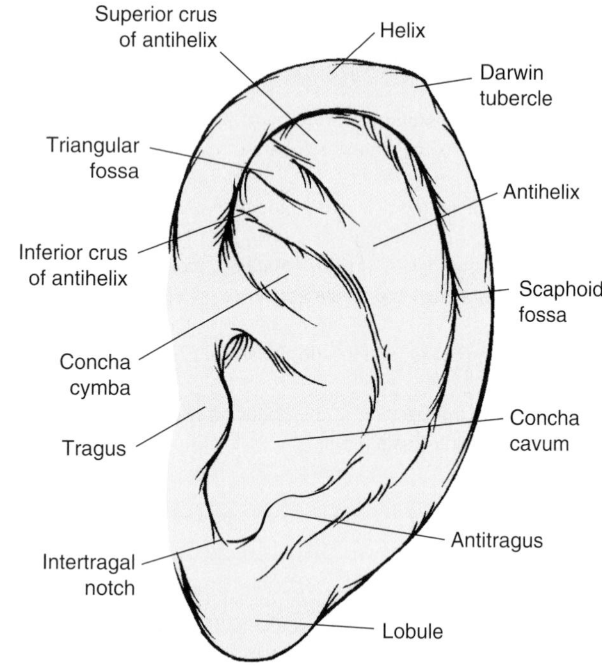

Figure 192-2. Normal anatomic landmarks of the ear.

Ear Anatomy

The anatomic contour of the normal ear must first be reviewed in order to understand the nature and extent of microtic ear deformities (Fig. 192-2). The auricle is an aesthetic sculpture of complex convexities, concavities, and curved lines such as the helix and the antihelix, which are smooth and uninterrupted. The elastic cartilage framework of the auricle is usually pliable yet structurally strong and extraordinarily resistant to trauma. The skin of the ear is fibrofatty and loose over the lobule and the margin of the helix but thin and fixed over the remaining cartilage framework.

Normal adult ear height ranges from 5.5 to 6.5 cm, which is typically attained by 13 years of age in boys and 12 years of age in girls. The ear goes through rapid growth between 2 and 3 years of age and reaches 95% of its adult size by about age 5. Thereafter it grows at a modest rate until it reaches its adult size during early teenage years. The horizontal width of the ear is achieved at a much earlier age. Protrusion of the ear from the surface of the mastoid should be 1.5 to 2.0 cm, thereby creating an angle between 15 and 20 degrees.[17] The superior margin of the helix is at the level of the tail of the eyebrow in 85% of people. Because the tail of the eyebrow is also quite variable, the level of the upper eyelid also may be used as a landmark if the patient has bilateral microtia.[18] The ear inclination is the angle formed by the vertical axis of the face and the longitudinal axis of the ear with the patient in the Frankfort horizontal position. This is approximately 24.8 degrees, with a standard deviation of 6.2 degrees.[19] Therefore, the longitudinal axis of the ear is not quite parallel with the dorsum of the nose (as is commonly thought), because the ear is in a slightly more vertical orientation.

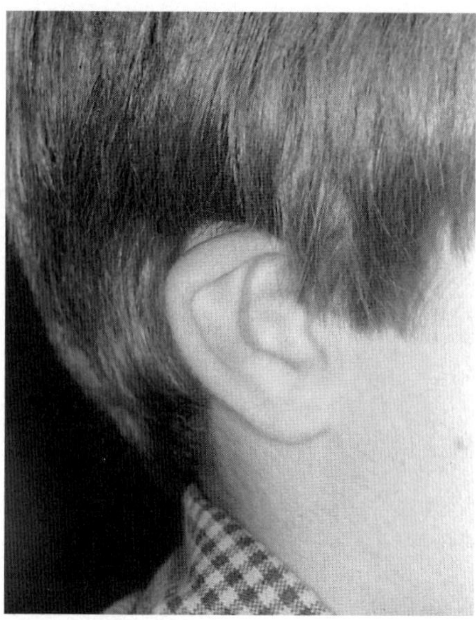

Figure 192-3. Type I microtia. A constricted ear with minimal tissue deficiency.

Microtia

Microtia deformities come in various shapes and sizes, and unfortunately, there is currently no universal, precise, and accurate classification scheme that is clinically useful. Classification schemes are further complicated if the status of the external auditory canal (EAC) and middle ear contents and the presence or absence of an associated syndrome are included.[5,20] Classification usually is simplified by evaluating the external auricular deformities alone. Perhaps *dysplasia* is a better term than *microtia* to use in describing ear deformities. Dysplasia deformities typically are divided into three broad and simple categories that have a great deal of overlap.[21] *Type I* (Fig. 192-3) is used to designate ears with mild deformity. All major structures are present to some degree, and reconstruction does not require additional tissue. *Type II* (atypical microtia) dysplasia (Fig. 192-4A to C) includes ears that have all major structures present to some degree. There is a deficiency of tissue, and surgical correction requires the addition of cartilage and skin. Mini-ear and severe cup-ear deformities are included in this category. The external auditory meatus is present, but it may demonstrate some degree of stenosis. *Type III* (classic microtia) dysplasia (Fig. 192-5A to C) deformities have few or no recognizable landmarks of the auricle, although the lobule usually is present and positioned anteriorly (see Fig. 192-16). *Anotia* is the complete absence of auricle and lobule. Reconstructive surgeons may find it more useful to simply note the status of the helix and antihelix, the conchal bowl, the lobule, the tragus, and the EAC, because these landmarks dictate the stages of ear reconstruction and the degree of surgical difficulty.

Evaluation

Children with microtia typically present to an otolaryngologist early during infancy because of the visible anomaly and parental concerns related to the child's hearing. The parents are usually concerned with the short- and long-term effects of monaural hearing on the child's speech development and the possibility of learning disabilities. Physical examination should focus on the mandibular shape and excursion, mouth, maxilla, eyes, and neck to rule out mandibular asym-

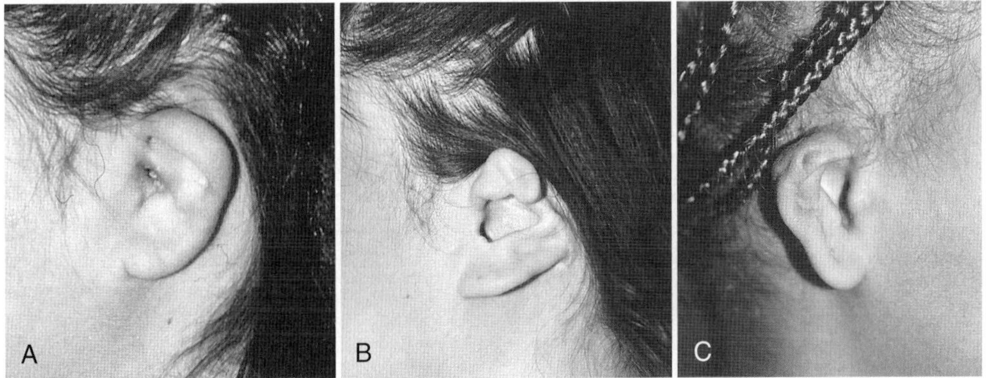

Figure 192-4. Type II microtia. **A,** A patient with type II microtia demonstrating a slight deformity with a small helix and missing antihelix. This patient also demonstrated canal stenosis. **B,** More extensive loss of the helix and antihelix, with a relatively normal canal and conchal cavum. **C,** A patient with loss of the superior crus of the antihelix and a constricted helix.

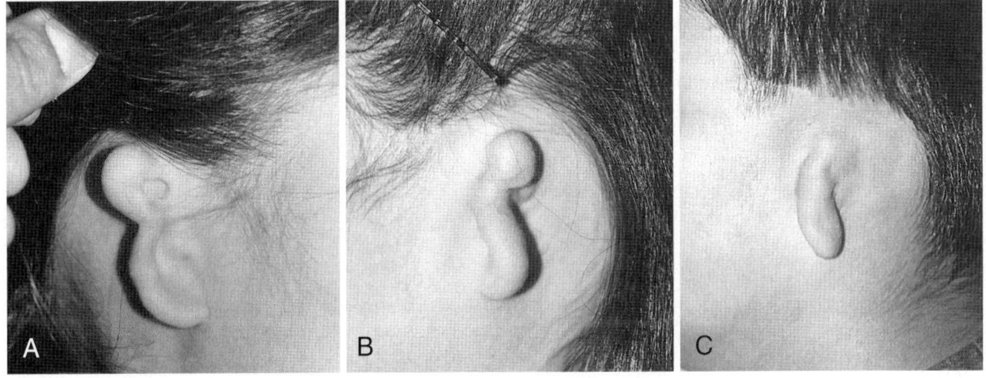

Figure 192-5. Type III microtia. **A** and **B,** Ears with moderate deformity and a few remaining visible landmarks of the helix. **C,** No recognizable landmarks of the auricle or canal are apparent, but the lobule is preserved.

metry, maxillary asymmetry, epibulbar dermoids, coloboma, and vertebral anomalies, which may indicate that the microtia is part of a syndrome.

Although patients with microtia typically have normal hearing in the contralateral ear, all patients with unilateral microtia should have age-appropriate hearing assessment. Hearing should continue to be monitored and eustachian tube dysfunction in the patent ear should be treated. Radiologic evaluation should include high-resolution computed tomography (CT) scan of the temporal bones to assess degree of atresia; cervical spine films to rule out vertebral anomalies; renal ultrasound to rule out congenital renal malformations; and panoramic (Panorex) films to assess the status of the mandible. If multiple anomalies are found, the child is referred to a multidisciplinary craniofacial team for more comprehensive evaluation.

Planning

Early evaluation by an otologist who is familiar with aural atresia is generally recommended. In most cases of unilateral microtia with aural atresia and a contralateral normal-hearing ear, canal reconstruction is controversial because speech development is expected to be normal. However, children with unilateral hearing loss predictably will have difficulties with sound localization and speech discrimination in a noisy setting. Careful review of the middle ear status, ossicular mass, position of the facial nerve, formation of the cochlea, and vestibular structures on CT scan helps the otologic surgeon determine candidacy for atresia repair.

If the patient is considered to be a favorable candidate, atresia repair should be performed after completion of microtia reconstruction. Patients with bilateral microtia and normal bone conduction thresholds may benefit from bone conduction hearing aids. Bone-anchored hearing aids may be considered in children older than 5 years of age.

With regard to the pinna, the patient and family are presented with three options: observation; prosthetic management, either adhesive- or implant-retained; and reconstructive options including staged reconstruction with autologous rib graft, and reconstruction with linear high-density polyethylene (Medpor) surgical implant material and temporoparietal fascial flap. Generally, observation is recommended until the child is at least 5 to 8 years old. This allows both growth of the donor rib cartilage and development of the contralateral normal ear, which will act as a template for the microtic side. Waiting until the child is older may reduce the risk of the development of a thoracic deformity as a result of harvesting of cartilaginous rib graft, although we feel this risk is minimal.[22] Finally, waiting until the child is school-aged allows the child to participate in these important decisions. We feel that it is important for the child to understand the options and participate in the decision making. The general health of the child is assessed, with particular attention paid to growth, maturation, and lung function. It is important to assess lung function, because the risk of pneumothorax and postoperative atelectasis and pneumonia is significant. This assessment usually is performed by the child's pediatrician. It is important to question the child about his or her personal concerns and to inquire about the effects of the microtia on social interaction with friends and classmates. Each child and parent will have different concerns that should be explored preoperatively.

During the planning stage of reconstruction, the surgical benefits, risks, and alternatives are discussed with the patient and the parents (Table 192-1). Complications such as infection, bleeding, scarring, graft loss, displacement or resorption, asymmetry, and pneumothorax should be discussed in detail. The possibility of a less-than-optimal aesthetic result also is discussed, and the expectations of the patient, parents, and surgeon must be realistic and clearly defined. Providing postoperative photographs of previous patients often is

Table 192-1
Overview of Treatment Options for Microtia

Treatment	Details	Advantage(s)	Disadvantages
Observation		No risk	Cosmesis Psychosocial issues
Prosthesis	Adhesive retained	Appearance	More difficult to incorporate atresia repair Requires removal of prosthesis at night and replacement in the morning Cost of prosthesis and maintenance
	Implant retained	Secure retention Appearance	Requires two surgical procedures that include removal of the microtic remnant Daily maintenance of implant site Appearance of implant site Cost of prosthesis and maintenance Eliminates possibility of reconstruction in the future
Reconstruction	Autogenous rib	Autogenous tissue Minimum maintenance More easily accommodates atresia repair	Appearance Donor site morbidity Multiple surgical procedures
	Medpor	Less donor site morbidity Less variability in carving	Foreign body More challenging to do atresia repair Increased risk of exposure of the framework

helpful to patients if the pictures depict a realistic result of a similar deformity.

One alternative for older children or adults may be the use of an auricular prosthesis. In some institutions, placement of a permanent auricular prosthesis with osseointegrated implants is recommended as the primary management modality. The aesthetic appearance often is excellent. However, most reconstructive surgeons discourage the use of osseointegrated implants for younger patients as a primary modality for several reasons: The implant sites will require daily care to maintain the health of the soft tissue surrounding the percutaneous osseointegrated implants. The prosthesis needs to be removed at night and replaced in the morning. The patient may unnecessarily avoid situations that may accidentally dislodge the ear and cause embarrassment. The placement of the osseointegrated implants requires removal of the soft tissue with skin grafting to bone to create nonmobile skin surrounding the posts. This eliminates the possibility of reconstructive surgery in the future. Furthermore, the prostheses are expensive and often not covered by third-party payers, leaving the patient at risk for having the osseointegrated implants in place without a prosthesis to wear in the future.

Finally, other materials for auricular reconstruction should be mentioned as part of a thorough informed consent, even if your institution may not offer these types of reconstructions. Implantable materials such as Medpor are used as alternatives to autogenous cartilage. Use of synthetic frameworks eliminates the need to harvest and carve the rib. However, the likelihood of extrusion and the lifelong risk of infections may outweigh their benefit. Stem cell technology is still emerging, and stem cell–derived implants may someday replace the need for rib graft harvesting. To date, no reliable cartilage implant created from stem cells is available.

Autogenous Costochondral Reconstruction

The use of rib cartilage in auricular reconstruction was pioneered by Tanzer[23] and refined by the meticulous work and accomplishments of Brent.[24,25] Reconstruction using the standard rib-grafting technique requires three to four stages, each separated by 2 to 6 months, beginning when the patient is approximately 6 to 8 years old.

The surgeon must develop carving and sculpting skills before undertaking a microtia reconstruction on a patient. For obvious reasons, fresh cadaveric rib cartilage is the best material with which to practice carving and harvesting grafts. If this cannot be obtained, carving the basic auricular framework can be practiced using soap or potatoes.

The surgical procedure described next is appropriate for reconstruction in patients with the most common class III dysplasia, or "peanut" ear.

Classic Microtia Reconstruction

Stage I: Cartilage Implantation

The first stage of microtia reconstruction is undoubtedly the most tedious and crucial of the entire process.[24] One of the most important objectives during the first stage is to place the auricular framework in a position that achieves the best symmetry for the patient's face. Placement of the reconstructed ear is determined by the position of the normal ear, and we do not alter this position to accommodate future reconstruction of the canal atresia or a low-lying hairline. If the hairline is low, the initial ear reconstruction is destined to have hair along the helix that will require depilation or excision at a later date. Preoperative tissue expansion to increase the amount of non–hair-bearing skin is not recommended, because the expanded skin capsule does not contour well over the implanted cartilaginous framework.

Three templates are made using radiographic film: a positioning template, a sizing template, and a carving template. The positioning template is made by carefully tracing the contour of the normal ear. It has the outline of the normal ear, with the landmarks of the lateral palpebral fissure and the lateral oral commissure for reference points. The landmarks are etched onto the radiographic film with an 18-gauge needle or scalpel to avoid losing these reference points (Fig. 192-6). The distance from the lateral palpebral fissure to the root of the helix is also measured on the template and should approximate 6.5 cm, or the length of the normal ear. The sizing template, which is a tracing of the entire ear, is used to test the size of the skin pocket in which the cartilaginous framework is placed. The carving template is drawn from the sizing template to include the landmarks of the antihelix, the triangular fossa, the scaphoid fossa, the medial aspect of the helix, and the antitragus. It is drawn 1 to 2 mm smaller than the sizing template to compensate for the thickness of the overlying skin. It is also used to determine the best donor site during rib harvesting and as a template for sculpting the cartilaginous framework. After the landmarks are permanently etched, the templates are autoclaved. The entire head and neck region is prepared so that the contralateral normal side can be easily visualized to evaluate symmetry. The eyes and mouth are covered with a transparent drape to allow visualization of the lateral palpebral fissure and the lateral commissure and to facilitate placement using the positioning template. The recipient ear site is injected with lidocaine

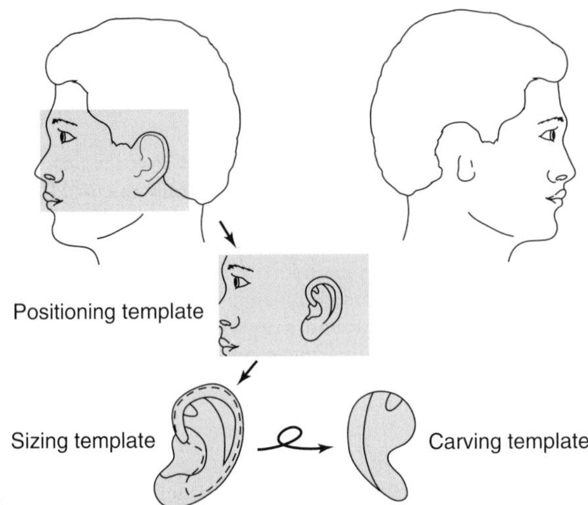

Figure 192-6. Templates for reconstruction. The positioning template, which is drawn with reference landmarks, is used to create the sizing and carving templates. The sizing template is drawn to match the exact size of the normal ear. The carving template is slightly smaller than the sizing template to compensate for the thickness of the skin flap.

with epinephrine to assist with hemostasis, and the incision is drawn along the anterior and superior margin of the rudimentary lobule. The contralateral side of the chest is prepared, because the contralateral rib graft has better contour characteristics. The chest incision is drawn just superior to the margin of the rib cage.

We generally use two surgical teams to reduce operating time. The donor site incision is made on the contralateral side of the chest, and the inferior margin of the rib cage is exposed. We have refined a minimally invasive technique, using a 2-cm skin incision (Fig. 192-7A). Two cartilaginous segments are required: a segment of free-floating cartilage to create the helical rim and a portion of synchondrosis to create the auricular framework.

The floating eighth rib is isolated, and dissection is continued posterolaterally to the bony-cartilaginous junction. Ideally this segment is 8 to 9 cm in length. Then the synchondrosis, usually between sixth and seventh ribs, is exposed. The carving template is used to determine the best donor site for the synchondrosis (see Fig. 192-7B to D). The rib cartilage is harvested with the superficial perichondrium intact. After removal of both segments, the donor site is checked for violation of the pleura. The chest wound is filled with saline and the anesthesiologist is asked to deliver positive-pressure ventilation to sustain a pressure of 40 cm H_2O. If a defect in the pleura is identified, a red rubber catheter is introduced into the pleural space and placed on continuous suction. The catheter is removed during positive-pressure ventilation, and the wound is closed with an airtight closure. A suction drain is placed in the subcutaneous space after closure of the rectus muscle. Intercostal bupivacaine blocks are placed at the end of the procedure to reduce postoperative pain.

All incision planning should take into consideration future stages of reconstruction. The recipient incision is made vertically along the anterosuperior margin of the lobule. This incision site will be used for the second-stage lobule transfer. The rudimentary cartilage segment is meticulously removed, with great care taken to avoid perforating or traumatizing the skin flap. The recipient pocket is elevated over the

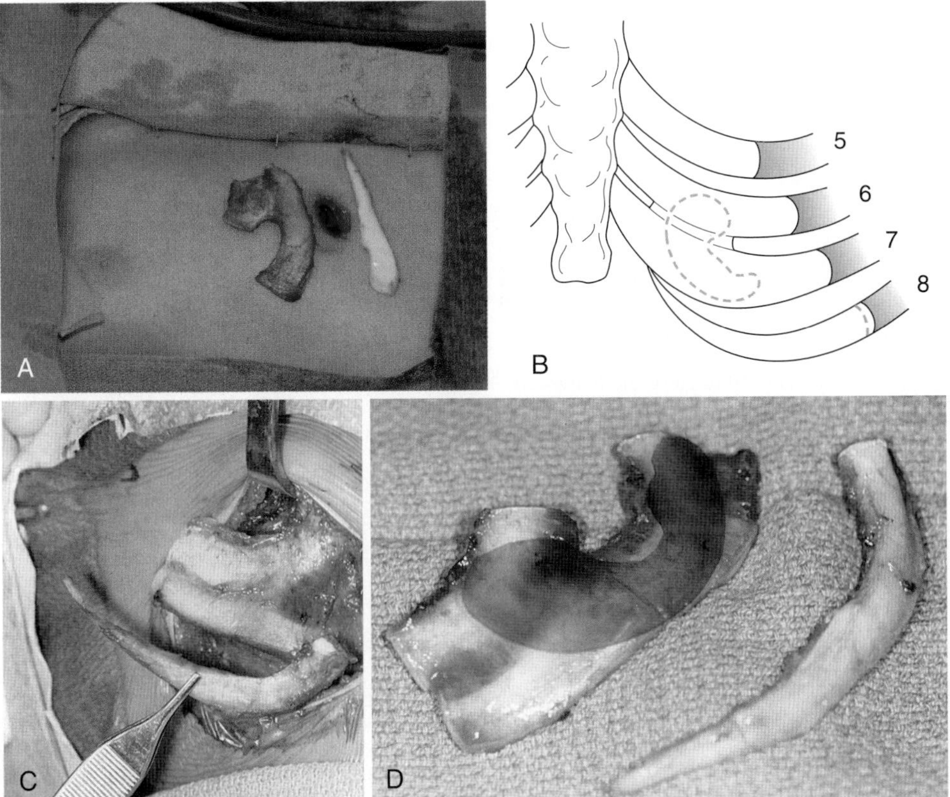

Figure 192-7. The donor site. **A,** A minimally invasive 2-cm incision is used to harvest rib segments. **B** to **D,** The contralateral chest is chosen for the donor site. The sixth, seventh, and eighth ribs and the synchondrosis between the sixth and seventh ribs are depicted. (The longer incision depicted in **C** is rarely necessary.) The donor sites of the auricular framework and the helical rim are indicated.

mastoid in a subcutaneous plane. The flap is thinned to a uniform thickness. In the hair-bearing region, the skin is thicker, because it becomes continuous with the scalp and contains a layer of galea. Dissection must be superficial to this layer of galea so that the flap remains uniformly thin and pliable. The sizing template is used to ensure that the pocket is large enough to accommodate the framework. The sizing template reduces the number of times that the reconstructed cartilage framework is transferred in and out of the pocket while adjustments are made; this helps reduce the amount of unnecessary handling and the risk of fracturing the framework.

The framework and helix are carved using Nos. 10, 11, and 15 scalpel blades. The 6700 Beaver blade can also be used (Fig. 192-8). As much perichondrium as possible is left intact over the lateral surface to enhance revascularization and tissue fixation. Suture or wire fixation is needed occasionally to reinforce the synchondrosis and to provide additional support to the framework. Additional cartilage grafts can be sutured to the posterior surface of the synchondrosis for more rigidity. The helix is carved from the eighth rib using the thicker part of the graft for the root of the helix and the thin distal tip of the graft for the caudal helix. The graft is carefully thinned until it is pliable enough to bend around the framework, and it is sutured into position with 4-0 clear nylon sutures. Additional thinning of the scaphoid and triangular fossa can be done after the helix is adequately fixated (Fig. 192-9A to C).

The reconstructed framework with attached helix is then placed into the pocket in a rotational manner, beginning with the root of the helix and then rotating the framework clockwise for the right side and counterclockwise for the left. If the pocket is excessively tight and the overlying skin remains blanched with poor vascular refill, the implant is removed and the pocket enlarged. After the graft is properly positioned, a small round suction drain is placed deep to the framework and brought out through the skin in the hairline. After the wound is sealed, the skin should conform to the framework, and the details of the helix and antihelix should be clearly visible (Fig. 192-10). The concavities of the ear are packed with petroleum gauze and secured with 4-0 chromic bolster sutures. A Glasscock dressing is applied using fluffed gauze to avoid unnecessary pressure. The drains are placed on intermediate suction. One of us (CSM) prefers continuous suction for 24 hours before placing the drains on bulb suction; another (VQ) recommends the continuous use of butterfly drains connected to vacuum-sealed red rubber–topped tubes.

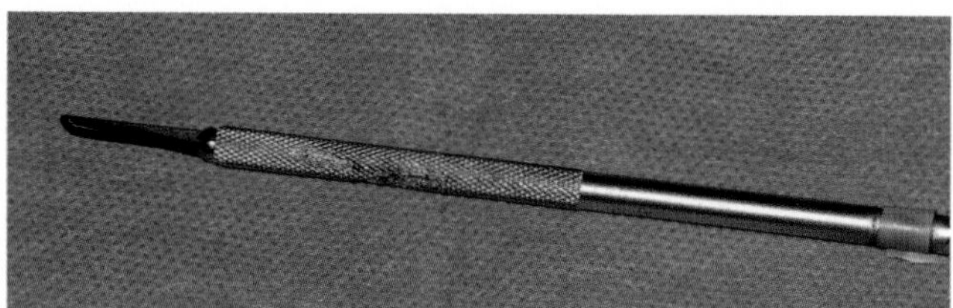

Figure 192-8. A 6700 Beaver blade is used to carve the framework.

A chest radiograph is obtained in the recovery room to rule out the possibility of pneumothorax. These patients are admitted for 48 hours for pain control, and intravenous antibiotics. The chest drain is removed on the first postoperative day, and the ear drain is removed after 2 to 3 days when there is little or no drainage. The vascularity of the skin overlying the helix is inspected on a regular basis, and the mastoid dressing is removed at 24 to 48 hours. A Glasscock dressing is then applied for the next 2 weeks to protect the ear. The patient must refrain from strenuous activity for 4 to 6 weeks, and the patient is not allowed to participate in contact sports for 1 month to avoid injuring the donor rib site.

Stage II: Lobule Transfer

The second surgery is performed 2 to 3 months after the first stage. A transposition flap is designed to move the vertically oriented lobule to the tail of the framework. After the incisions are made, a pocket is created within the lobule to accommodate the tail of the framework. The tail is elevated from the mastoid cortex so that the lobule can be wrapped around the posteroinferior margin of the cartilage framework. Care is taken to evert the wound margins in an attempt to avoid a stepoff at the junction of the lobule and framework. One to two Z-plasties are performed across the transverse portion of the incision (Fig. 192-11A to F).

Stage III: Creation of Postauricular Sulcus

This procedure is performed approximately 3 months after stage II (Fig. 192-12A to D). An incision is made around the helical rim. However, if there is hair on the helix, the incision is made slightly lower on its lateral surface to minimize the hair-bearing skin over the framework. The non–hair-bearing auricular skin is advanced 2 to 3 mm superiorly over the helical rim, and absorbable tacking sutures are placed between the subcutaneous tissue and the cartilaginous framework. The ear is released by dissecting into the postauricular sulcus and leaving the perichondrium intact to protect the cartilage graft. The postauricular skin over the mastoid is undermined and advanced into the postauricular sulcus, to help project the ear laterally away from the mastoid. After the postauricular skin is advanced and secured, the remaining defect is measured. It usually measures approximately $4 \times 8\,cm^2$. An elliptical thick split-thickness graft is harvested freehand from the left groin. The donor site is closed primarily. The graft is secured into the newly created postauricular sulcus with 5-0 chromic sutures. A bolster is secured into the sulcus with a 4-0 nylon. The ear is covered with a Glasscock dressing for protection for 1 to 2 weeks. The bolster is removed after 5 to 7 days, and the skin graft is kept moist for 2 to 3 weeks.

For some patients, the contralateral ear is prominent, contributing to the asymmetrical appearance of the ears. Otoplasty of the normally formed ear can be combined with this procedure, and the skin excised for the otoplasty can be used for grafting of the newly created postauricular sulcus of the microtic ear.

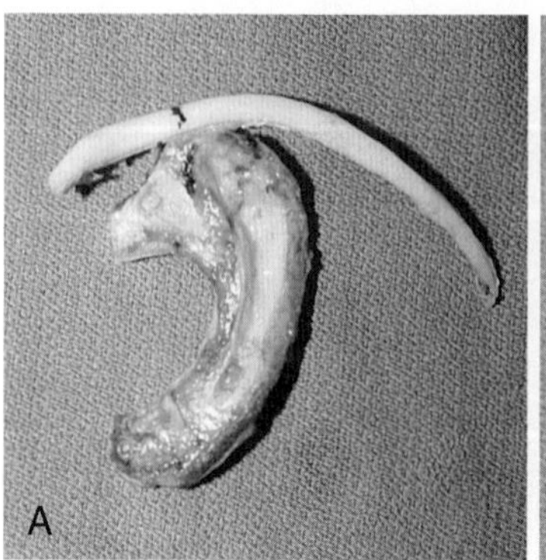

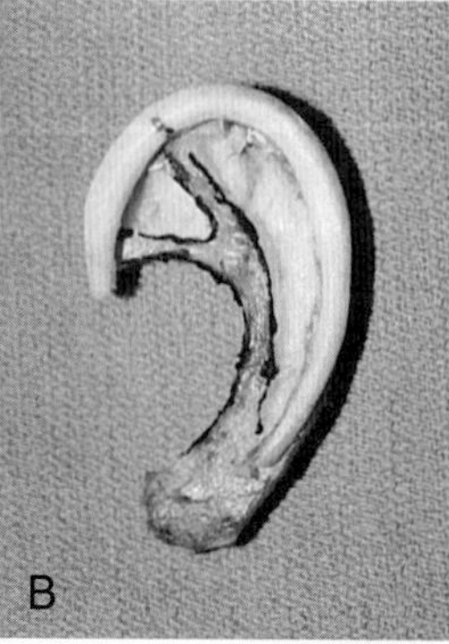

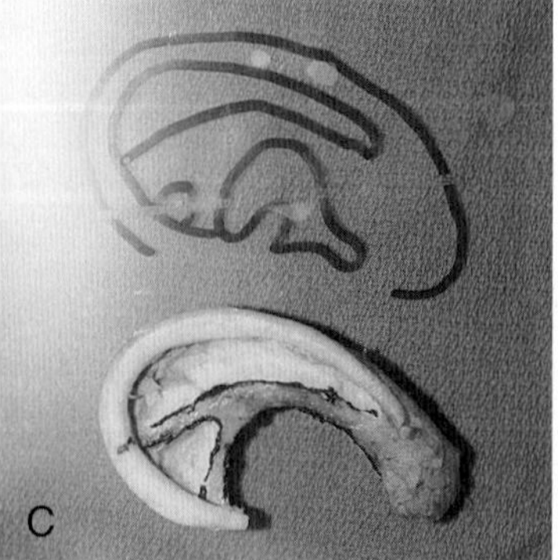

Figure 192-9. Construction of the implant. **A,** The framework is carved from the sixth and seventh ribs. The helix is carved from the eighth rib and is bent gently around the framework. **B,** The helix is secured with 4-0 clear nylon or wire. **C,** The implant is compared with the template.

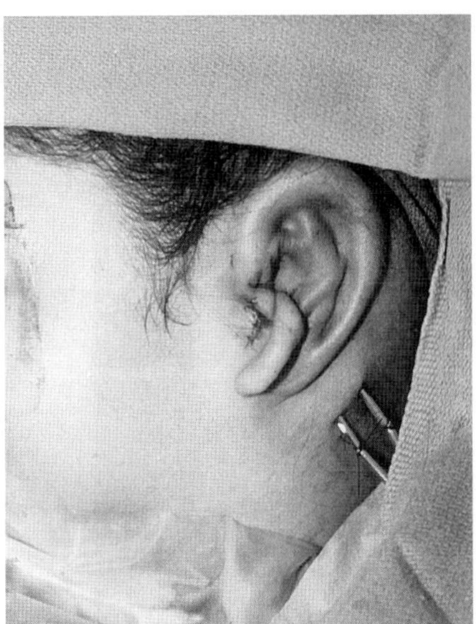

Figure 192-10. Placement of the implant. The implant is placed into the pocket and positioned using the positioning template. One drain is placed over the surface of the implant as one is placed deep to the implant. The drains are then placed on suction. Note the contouring of the skin over the cartilaginous framework, with the drain traversing over the antihelix and into the scaphoid fossa.

Stage IV: Tragus Reconstruction

The fourth stage of reconstruction is to form a tragus and conchal bowl. If the conchal bowl is well defined, a composite graft can be used to reconstruct the tragus. An elliptical composite graft is removed from the concha cymba of the contralateral ear. An incision is made along the posterior border of the future tragus, and the composite graft is placed on the posterior surface to give the tragus some projection. The shadowing effect gives the illusion of an external auditory meatus. If the conchal bowl is not defined, an incision is made along the posterior border of the future conchal bowl, and an anterior-based cutaneous circular flap is created. The conchal bowl is then debulked of scar tissue and any rudimentary skin and cartilage that might remain. Because of facial nerve anomalies, a facial nerve monitor is recommended. The flap is folded onto itself to create a tragus that is then reinforced with a small piece of auricular or rib cartilage, and the surface of the conchal bowl is covered with a small skin graft (Fig. 192-13A to C). The bolster is removed in 3 to 5 days. Occasionally, an additional operation is needed to further elevate the reconstructed ear away from the mastoid using grafts of cartilage implanted medial to the framework.

Atypical Microtia Repair

Second-degree dysplasia or atypical microtia presents a more difficult surgical challenge. As previously discussed, many components of the auricular structure are recognizable, but there is a distinct tissue deficiency that necessitates the transportation of cartilage and skin. The additional structure often eliminates the necessity for complete framework insertion. When the vertical height difference between the two ears is greater than 20 mm, consideration is given to using a rib framework. When the difference is less than 20 mm, the result is achieved by

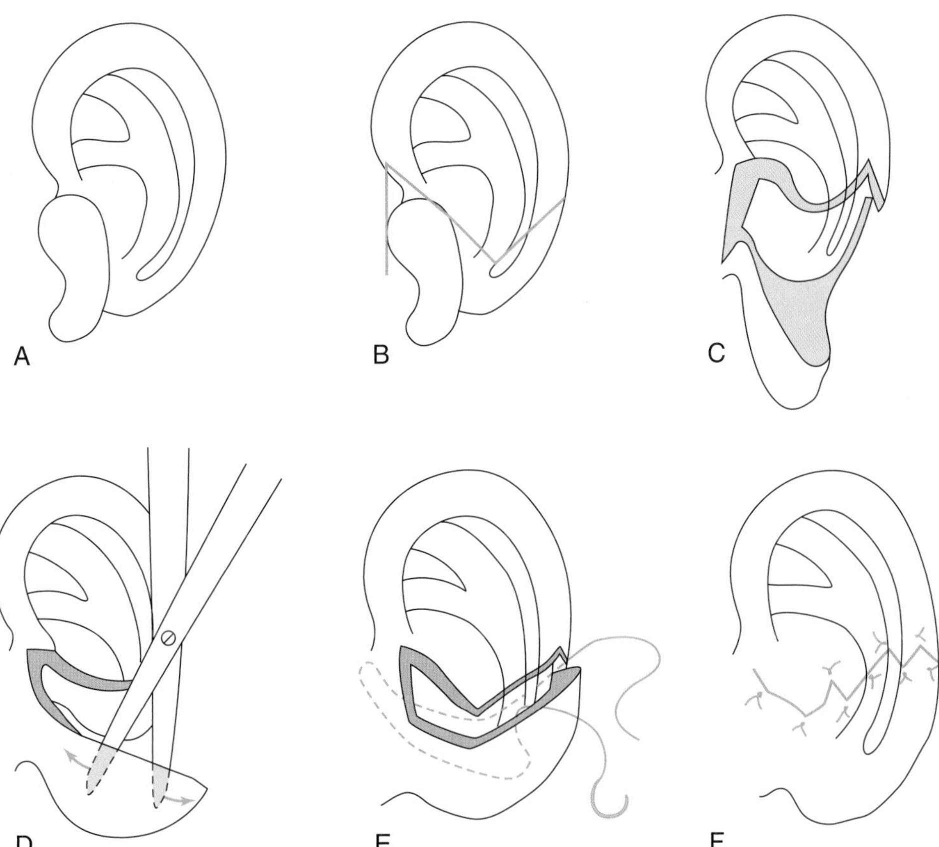

Figure 192-11. Stage II lobule transfer. **A,** Preoperatively, the lobule is noted to be malpositioned anteriorly. **B,** A lobule transposition flap incision is drawn. **C,** Lobule is elevated and posteroinferior margin of the framework is dissected out. **D,** A pocket is dissected within the lobule, and the lobule is transposed over the posteroinferior margin of the graft. **E,** Suture is placed from the pocket in the lobule to mastoid periosteum in order to reduce the flare of the lobule. **F,** Several mini Z-plasties are created along the incision to break up the scar and prevent contracture. Incisions are closed with mattress sutures.

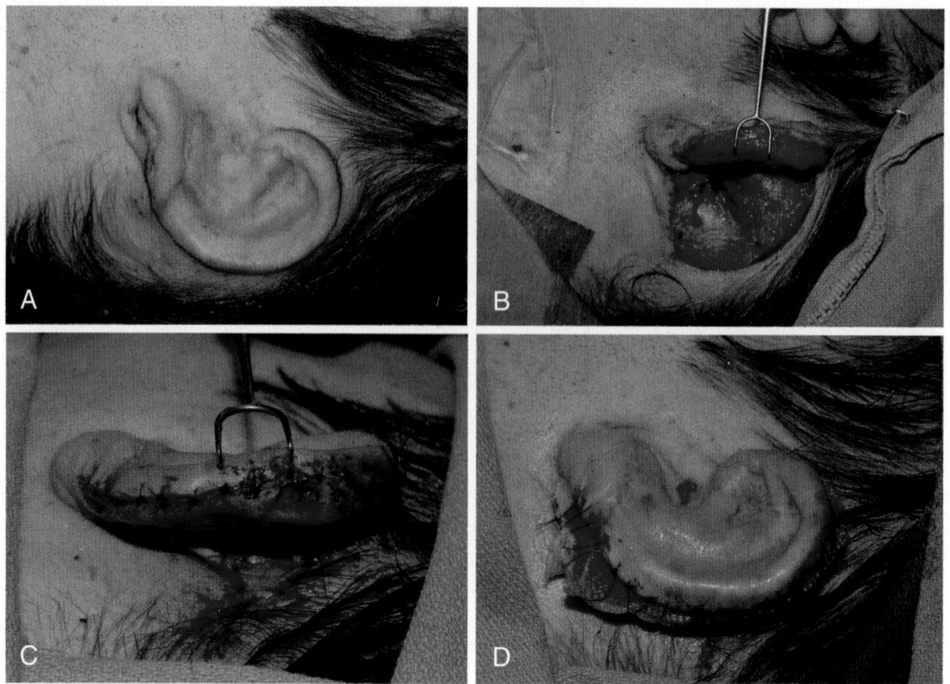

Figure 192-12. Stage III skin grafting. **A,** Before the procedure. **B,** Release of the skin, leaving the perichondrium intact. Dissection is carried into the postauricular sulcus, and postauricular skin is advanced. **C,** Skin graft in place. **D,** Skin graft secured with a soft bolster.

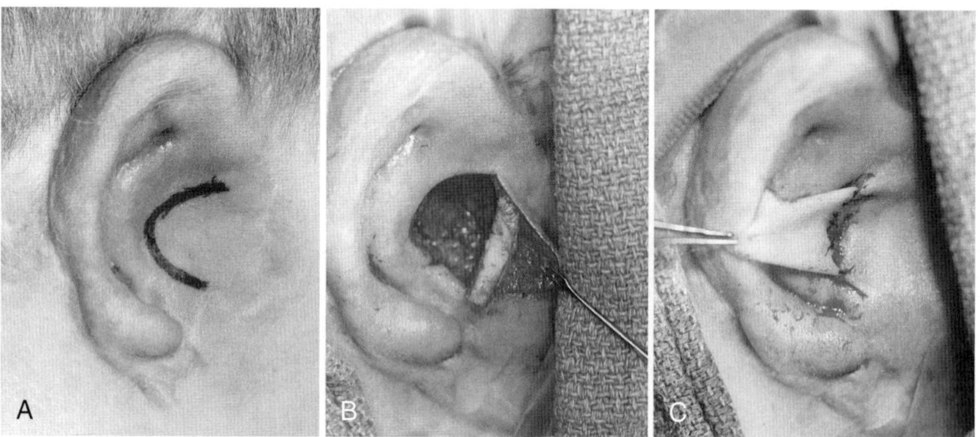

Figure 192-13. Stage IV tragus reconstruction. **A,** In bilateral microtia, tragal reconstruction is more difficult, because both ears are reconstructed; thus, normal concha cymba is not available for composite grafting. A longer flap must be elevated to provide both medial and lateral tragal lining. **B,** A free cartilage graft is placed to prevent contraction and is lined by the skin flap. **C,** The conchal bowl is deepened and lined with a skin graft. *(From Quatela VC, Goldman ND. Microtia repair.* Facial Plast Surg. 1995;11:257. Used with permission.)

expanding the existing structure; this is done by a combination of unfurling, uncupping, and increasing the vertical height with the use of cartilage composite grafts (Fig. 192-14A to H).[26] The helical root can also be advanced in a V-Y fashion into the helix to help augment the vertical height. Unlike classic microtia reconstruction, the use of vestigial remnants as a main framework does not lead to consistent results. Figure 192-15A to F shows a child with atypical microtia with an undeveloped lobule that was reconstructed by placing a cartilage implant that was harvested from the contralateral conchal bowl. This reconstruction was followed by a staged skin graft with an advancement flap of postauricular skin.

Complications

Major complications are rare. However, seemingly minor complications may lead to loss of the graft if they are not treated expeditiously. Immediate postoperative complications include pneumothorax and hematoma formation. Short-term complications include skin flap necrosis and infection. If a graft becomes exposed postoperatively secondary to breakdown of the overlying skin flap, the patient is placed on antibiotics that provide coverage for *Staphylococcus* and *Pseudomonas* infections, and the exposed site is covered with moist continuous dressings. If the exposure is small (1 to 2 mm) and the perichondrium is intact, the wound may granulate with local wound care. If the perichondrium is gone and the cartilage exposed, the framework may become devitalized, desiccated, and infected. Early coverage of the site with a local flap or a temporoparietal fascia flap with an overlying skin graft should be considered. Prolonged antibiotic therapy after flap coverage is necessary to avoid progression of the infection and eventual collapse and resorption of the graft.

Minor complications include malpositioning, scar contracture or hypertrophy, and poor contouring. Generally, problems with scar formation and poor contouring resolve with time if the cartilage has not

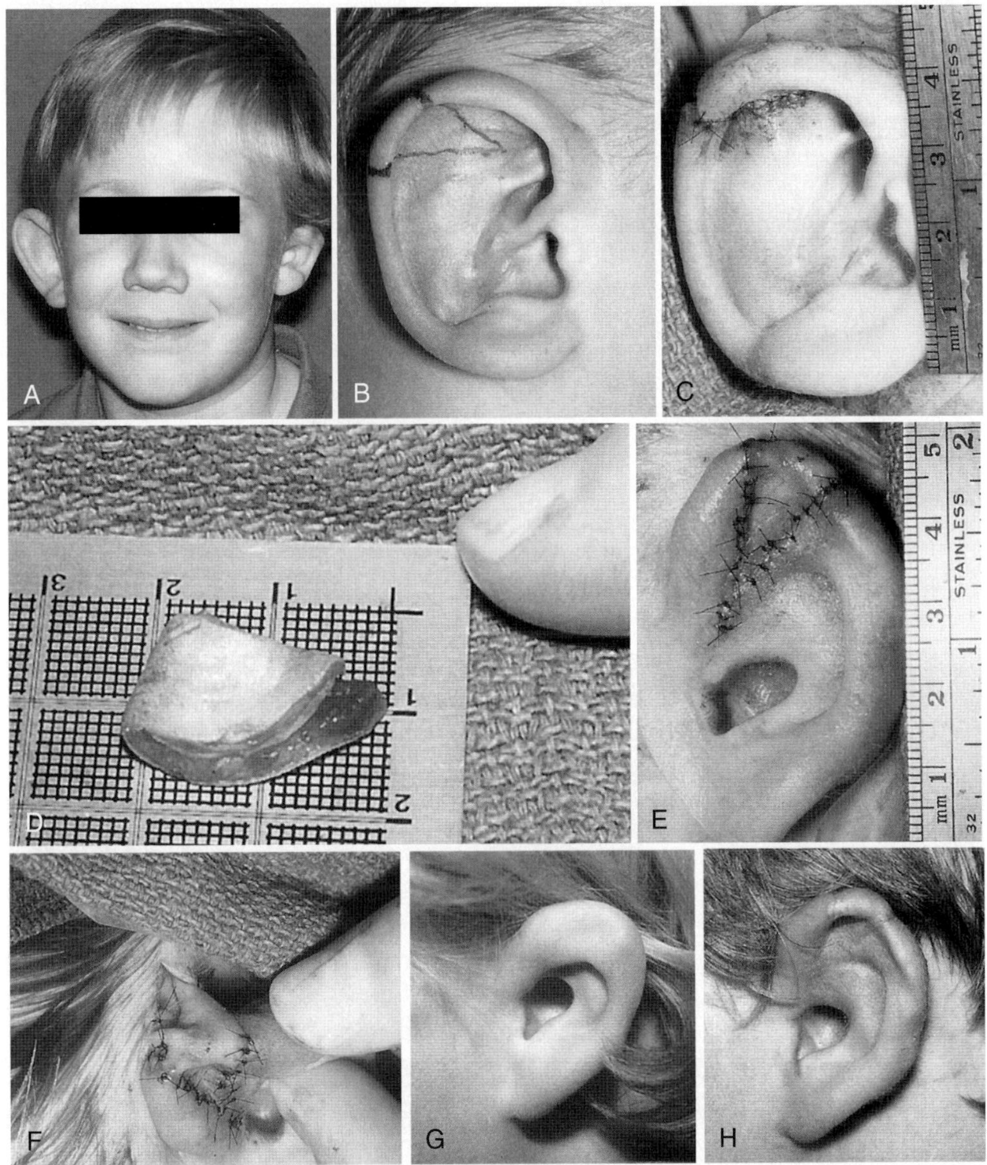

Figure 192-14. Atypical microtia reconstruction. **A,** A congenital defect of the ear with more than 20 mm of vertical height than in the contralateral healthy ear. **B,** The donor site composite graft is harvested to equal to one-half the size of the recipient defect, thereby reducing the disparity. The donor site is closed primarily, with the only resultant deformity being shortened vertical height, which is desirable in this patient's ear. **C,** The donor ear is shortened by 1 cm but retains good form. **D,** The composite graft. **E,** The composite graft sutured into position; vertical height is increased by approximately 1 cm. **F,** Epithelium is removed from the medial aspect of the composite graft, and the graft placed into a postauricular subcutaneous pocket. The medial skin is still attached at the rim as a hinge flap. The medial perichondrium is in contact with the retroauricular soft tissue; this will ensure maximum recipient contact for graft survival. Release is accomplished 2 weeks later, using the hinge flap skin for medial resurfacing. **G,** Before surgery. **H,** The final result at 1 year.

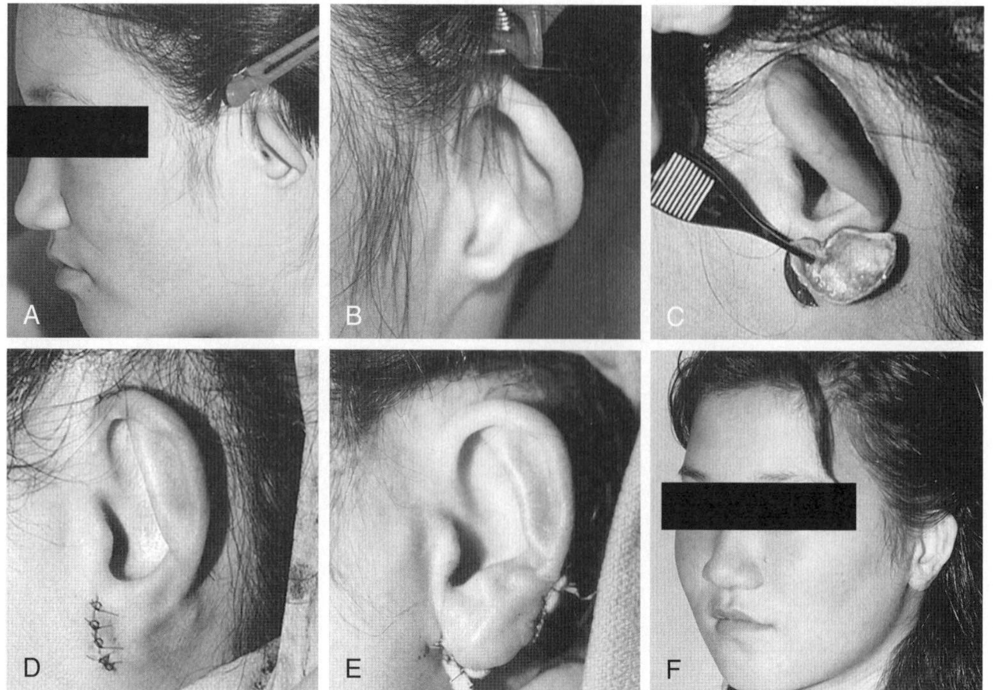

Figure 192-15. **A** and **B,** Type II atypical microtia with a missing lobule and a dysmorphic helix and antihelix. **C** to **E,** Two-stage reconstruction required placement of a conchal cartilage graft followed by delayed release of the lobule, advancement of postauricular skin, and placement of a full-thickness skin graft that was secured with a bolster dressing. **F,** Final postoperative result at 1 year.

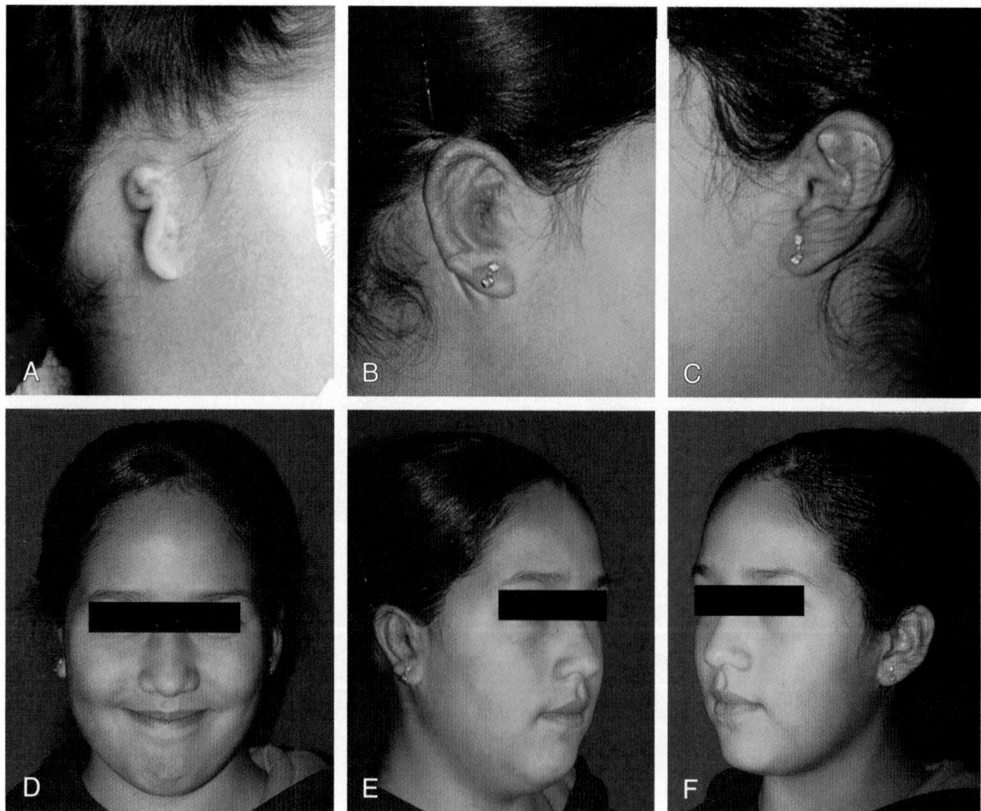

Figure 192-16. **A,** Type III microtia with anteriorly positioned lobule. **B** to **F,** At 2 years after completion of microtia reconstruction. Note the height symmetry and angle of the auricle in relation to Frankfurt horizontal plane.

become infected or undergone resorption. Minor scar revisions may be necessary when indicated, and the surgeon should be careful not to expose the cartilage graft. Problems with malposition are usually minor if proper template techniques were used, and they are commonly related to preexisting lobule asymmetry or generalized facial asymmetry caused by hemifacial microsomia. Major malposition problems are usually related to poor preoperative planning.

Conclusions

Managing patients with microtia can be a rewarding experience for both the patient and the surgeon if proper training, preparation, and planning are done. Each patient and each ear deformity are unique, thus making the management of these patients a humbling, challenging, and perpetually stimulating problem. In many respects, microtia surgery is similar to rhinoplasty, in which the surgeon continually strives to achieve the elusive "perfect" aesthetic and functional result through meticulous planning and attention to detail.

SUGGESTED READINGS

Aase JM, Tegtmeier RE. Microtia in New Mexico. *Birth Defects.* 1977;13:113.

Aguilar EA. Major congenital malformations of the auricle. In: Bailey BJ, Johnson JJ, Kohut RI, Pillsbury HC III, Tardy ME, eds. *Head and Neck Surgery–Otolaryngology.* Philadelphia: JB Lippincott; 1993.

Bennun RD, Mulliken JB, Kaban LB, et al. Microtia: a microform of hemifacial microsomia. *Plast Reconstr Surg.* 1985;76:859.

Brent B. Correction of microtia with autogenous cartilage grafts: I. Classic deformity. *Plast Reconstr Surg.* 1980;66:1.

Brent B. Correction of microtia with autogenous cartilage grafts: II. Atypical and complex deformities. *Plast Reconstr Surg.* 1980;66:13.

Brent B. *The Artistry of Reconstructive Surgery.* St Louis: Mosby; 1987.

Farkas LG. Anthropometry of the normal and defective ear. *Clin Plast Surg.* 1990;17:213.

Fukuda O. Long-term evaluation of modified Tanzer ear reconstruction. *Clin Plast Surg.* 1990;17:241.

Gorlin RJ, Pindborg JJ, Cohen MM Jr. Oculoauriculovertebral dysplasia. In: Gorlin RJ, Pindborg JJ, Cohen MM Jr, eds. *Syndromes of the Head and Neck.* New York: McGraw-Hill; 1976.

Granstrom G. Retinoid-induced ear malformations. *Otolaryngol Head Neck Surg.* 1990;103:702.

For complete list of references log onto www.expertconsult.com.

His W. Austellung von entwickelungsnormen zweiter monat. *Anat Mensch Embryonen.* 1883;55:Part II.

His W. Die Formentwickelung des ausseren Ohres. *Anat Mensch Embryonen.* 1885;3:211.

Jarvis BL, Johnson MC, Sulik KK. Congenital malformations of the external, middle, and inner ear produced by isotretinoin exposure in mouse embryos. *Otolaryngol Head Neck Surg.* 1990;102:391.

Jones KL. *Smith's Recognizable Patterns of Human Malformation.* Philadelphia: WB Saunders; 1988.

Karmody CS, Annino DJ. Embryology and anomalies of the external ear. *Facial Plast Surg.* 1995;11:251.

Kaye CI, Rollnick BR, Hauck WW, et al. Microtia and associated anomalies. *Am J Med Genet.* 1989;34:574.

Lammer E. Preliminary observations on isotretinoin-induced ear malformations and pattern formation of the external ear. *J Craniofac Genet Dev Biol.* 1991;11:292.

Lucente FE, Lawson W, Novick NL. *The External Ear.* Philadelphia: WB Saunders; 1995.

Marx H. Beitrag zur Morpholgie und Genese der Mittelohrmissbildungen mit Gehorgangsatresie. *Z Hals Nasan Ohrenheilkd.* 1922;2:230.

Mastroiacovo P, Corchia C, Botto LD. Epidemiology and genetics of microtia-anotia: a registry based study on over one million births. *J Med Genet.* 1995;32:453.

Melnick M, Myrianthopoulos NC. *External Ear Malformations: Epidemiology, Genetics and Natural History.* New York: Alan R Liss; 1979.

Moore KL. *The Developing Human.* Philadelphia: WB Saunders; 1977.

Posnick JC, Al-Qattan MM, Whitaker LA. Assessment of the preferred vertical position of the ear. *Plast Reconstr Surg.* 1993;91:1198.

Rosa FW. Teratogenicity of isotretinoin [letter]. *Lancet.* 1983;2:513.

Skiles MS, Randall P. The aesthetics of ear placement: an experimental study. *Plast Reconstr Surg.* 1983;72:133.

Streeter GL. Development of the auricle in the human embryo. *Control Embryol.* 1922;14:111.

Sulik KK, Dehart DB. Retinoic-acid-induced limb malformations resulting from apical ectodermal ridge cell death. *Teratology.* 1988;37:527.

Tanzer R. Total reconstruction of the external ear. *Plast Reconstr Surg.* 1959;23:1.

Westerman ST, Gilbert LM, Schondel L. Vestibular dysfunction in a child with embryonic exposure to Accutane. *Am J Otol.* 1994;15:400.

CHAPTER ONE HUNDRED AND NINETY-THREE

Reconstruction of the Auditory Canal and Tympanum

Antonio De la Cruz

Karen B. Teufert

Key Points

- Atresiaplasty aims to create a patent, skin-lined external auditory canal and to achieve a postoperative air-bone gap within 20 to 30 dB.
- In bilateral or unilateral cases of congenital atresia, auricular reconstruction and atresiaplasty are recommended at 6 years of age. Reconstruction with porous high-density polyethylene (Medpor) can be done at an earlier age. In unilateral cases, atresiaplasty is indicated only in minor deformities.
- The microtia repair is performed first because of the need for an excellent blood supply to cover the autologous rib graft, and the hearing restoration surgery is performed 2 months after the last step of the microtia repair.
- There are two requirements for planning surgery in congenital aural atresia: radiographic three-dimensional evaluation of the temporal bone and audiometric evidence of cochlear function.
- The following four anatomic parameters as seen radiographically are crucial for surgical planning: the status of the inner ear, the extent of pneumatization of the mastoid, the course of the facial nerve (both the relationship of the horizontal segment to the oval window and the location of the mastoid segment), and the presence of the oval window and stapes footplate.
- Ideal surgical candidates display a well-developed mastoid and a good oval window/footplate–facial nerve relationship.
- Ossicular reconstruction with the patient's own ossicular chain is preferred to the use of a prosthesis.
- Complications of atresiaplasty include lateralization of the tympanic membrane, stenosis of the meatus, sensorineural hearing loss, and facial nerve palsy.
- Graft lateralization is the most common delayed cause of a poor hearing outcome, usually occurring in the first 12 months after surgery.
- Polymeric silicone sheets, hydroxylated polyvinyl acetate wicks, absorbable gelatin film disks, and tabs in the fascia graft have helped lower the incidence of tympanic membrane lateralization by keeping the tympanic membrane graft in position.
- The incidence of stenosis has been significantly reduced with the use of one-piece split-thickness skin grafts covering all exposed bone, and polymeric silicone sheets and hydroxylated polyvinyl acetate wicks in the external auditory canal.
- It is important that drilling on the ossicular chain be minimized when it is dissected away from the atretic bone to reduce the risk of noise-induced sensorineural hearing loss.
- Intraoperative facial nerve monitoring is essential in all cases because there are often no clearly identifiable landmarks in atretic ears.
- Bone-anchored hearing aids are an alternative to atresiaplasty for rehabilitation of hearing loss resulting from congenital aural atresia, particularly in patients who are not good candidates for surgery.

Congenital aural atresia (CAA) represents aplasia or hypoplasia of the external auditory canal (EAC) resulting from failed or aborted development and is often associated with other malformations of the temporal bone, including external, middle, and inner ear deformities. CAA is unilateral more often than bilateral (occurring at a ratio of 3 : 1), preferentially affects males and the right side, and occurs in 1 in 10,000 to 1 in 20,000 live births.[1] Bony atresia occurs more frequently than membranous atresia. Fusion of the malleus and incus is the most common associated middle ear deformity, whereas the stapes footplate is usually normal.[2] Microtia is common in patients with CAA, and generally the severity of the external deformity correlates with the extent of middle ear deformity.[3-5] As opposed to middle ear malformations, the incidence of inner ear abnormalities in patients with CAA is relatively low, reflecting the earlier and independent embryonic development of the inner ear. The facial nerve typically lies in a normal position but may be displaced anteriorly and laterally in the vertical segment. Atresiaplasty aims to create a patent, skin-lined EAC and to achieve a postoperative air-bone gap within 20 to 30 dB. Surgical success depends on the appropriate selection of candidates for surgery and on proficient application of all modern tympanoplasty techniques, including meatoplasty, canalplasty, tympanic membrane grafting, and ossicular reconstruction.

Embryology

Knowledge of normal ear development aids understanding of the potential combinations of malformations possible in ears with CAA. This understanding helps physicians select appropriate surgical candidates and avoid complications during surgery. Because the inner ear, middle ear, and external ear develop independently, deformity of one does not necessitate deformity of another. Fortunately, inner ear structure and function are usually normal in ears with outer and middle ear abnormalities.[6]

The external auditory meatus develops from the first branchial groove. During the second month, a solid core of epithelium extends inward from the primary meatus to the primitive tympanic cavity forming the meatal plate.[7,8] During the 21st week, this core resorbs and canalizes, forming the precursor to the EAC. Failure of resorption and canalization accounts for most cases of CAA. Subsequent posterior and inferior development carries the middle ear and facial nerve to their normal locations. By the end of the third gestational month, the primitive auricle has formed from six hillocks derived from the first and second branchial arches.

The eustachian tube, tympanic cavity, and mastoid air cells derive from the first branchial pouch, and the tympanic membrane forms from the plaque of tissue where this pouch meets the epithelium of the EAC.[7,8] Pneumatization of the middle ear and mastoid occurs late in fetal development, is usually present by birth, and continues to expand postnatally. Meckel's cartilage (first branchial arch) gives rise to the neck and head of the malleus and the body of the incus, whereas Reichert's cartilage (second branchial arch) forms the long processes of the malleus and incus as well as the stapes superstructure. The stapes footplate has a dual embryologic origin, developing from the second arch and from the otic capsule. The ossicles achieve their final shape by the fourth month and are covered with a mucous membrane from the expanding tympanic cavity by the end of the seventh to eighth month.

The facial nerve is the nerve of the second branchial arch. Its general course is established by the end of the embryonic period; however, its ultimate intraosseous course depends on later bony expansion of the tympanic ring and cavity.[9] The auditory placode on the lateral surface of the hindbrain gives rise to the membranous inner ear during the third to the sixth week. The surrounding mesenchyme transforms into the bony otic capsule.

Classification Systems

In atresiaplasty, surgery classification systems that help in the identification of best candidates and in comparison of outcome and multiple schemes have been developed. The De la Cruz classification divides abnormalities into "minor" and "major" categories (Box 193-1).[2] The clinical importance of this classification is that surgery in cases of minor malformations has a good possibility of yielding serviceable hearing, whereas cases of major malformations are best treated with the bone-anchored hearing aid (BAHA) system.

The point-grading system for preoperative assessment of the best candidates for hearing improvement developed by Jahrsdoerfer and colleagues[10] assigns points on the basis of preoperative temporal bone CT scan findings of mastoid pneumatization, presence of the oval and round windows, facial nerve course, status of the ossicles and mesotympanum, and presence of the stapes, as well as on the external appearance (Table 193-1). Each parameter receives 1 point except for the presence of the stapes, which receives 2 points. A score of 8 or higher predicts the best chance of surgical success (greater than 80% success). A score of 7 implies a fair result, a score of 6, a marginal result; and a score less than 6 indicates that the patient would have poor results from atresiaplasty.

Ishimoto and colleagues[11] evaluated the relationship between hearing level and temporal bone abnormalities in patients with microtia, using the Jahrsdoerfer scoring system and high-resolution CT (HRCT) scans of the temporal bone.[11] The hearing level in microtic ears best correlated with the formation of oval/round windows and ossicular development but not with the degree of middle ear aeration, facial nerve aberration, or severity of microtia.

Box 193-1
De la Cruz Classification of Congenital Aural Atresia

Minor Malformations
- Normal mastoid pneumatization
- Normal oval window footplate
- Good facial nerve–footplate relationship
- Normal inner ear

Major Malformations
- Poor pneumatization
- Abnormality or absence of oval window/footplate
- Abnormal course of the facial nerve
- Abnormalities of the inner ear

Adapted from De la Cruz A, Linthicum FH Jr, Luxford WM. Congenital atresia of the external auditory canal. *Laryngoscope*. 1985;95:421-427.

Table 193-1
Jahrsdoerfer Grading System of Candidacy for Atresiaplasty

Parameter	Points
Stapes present	2
Oval window open	1
Middle ear space	1
Facial nerve normal	1
Malleus-incus complex present	1
Mastoid well pneumatized	1
Incus-stapes connection	1
Round window normal	1
Appearance of external ear	1
Total available points	10

Total Score	Type of Candidate
10	Excellent
9	Very good
8	Good
7	Fair
6	Marginal
≤5	Poor

Modified from Jahrsdoerfer RA, Yeakley JW, Aguilar EA, Cole RR, Gray LC. Grading system for the selection of patients with congenital aural atresia. *Am J Otol.* 1992;13:6-12.

Other classifications systems have been developed by Altmann,[12] Chiossone,[13] and Schuknecht.[14] Congenital cholesteatoma occurs in 14% of patients with CAA and is not included in any of the grading systems because these systems are used only for predicting hearing results in patients undergoing elective procedures.

Initial Evaluation

Several issues should be addressed in infants presented with CAA. In addition to the malformations of the temporal bone, other congenital abnormalities may be present and should be excluded. Evaluation of auditory function with auditory brainstem response (ABR) audiometry should be performed during the first few days of life in patients with either unilateral or bilateral atresia, because ipsilateral and contralateral inner ear abnormalities may be associated with CAA. Occasionally, a patient with unilateral atresia has a total sensorineural hearing loss (SNHL) on the side of the normal-looking ear. To maximize speech and language development, proper hearing amplification must begin promptly. For the patient with bilateral CAA, a bone conduction hearing aid should be applied as soon as possible, ideally at 3 or 4 weeks of age. Hearing amplification is not necessary in the patient with unilateral atresia if hearing is normal in the contralateral ear.

Parents of a child with sporadic, nonsyndromic CAA are counseled that the possibility of CAA in their subsequent children is no greater than that for the general population. Options regarding future auricular reconstruction are also reviewed with the parents, and the need for proper hearing rehabilitation is stressed. Early enrollment in special education enhances speech and language development. Children with CAA in association with other syndromes (e.g., hemifacial microsomia, Treacher Collins or Crouzon's syndrome, Pierre Robin sequence) are poor surgical candidates for whom long-term bone-conduction aids or BAHAs offer the best rehabilitation.

The two requirements for elective atresiaplasty are (1) audiometric evidence of cochlear function and (2) radiographic three-dimensional evaluation of the temporal bone. As noted, audiometric evaluation should occur within the first few days of life; however, radiologic evaluation with HRCT of the temporal bone is deferred until age 5 or 6 years. A patient with CAA may experience an infected or draining ear or acute facial palsy with or without a congenital cholesteatoma. In such a case, resolution of the infection and removal of the cholesteatoma, if present, take priority, and HRCT scanning may be indicated before age 5 or 6 years.

Timing of Ear Reconstructive Surgery

Auricular reconstruction precedes hearing restoration surgery by at least 2 months to optimize the blood supply for the autologous rib graft and complex flaps.[15] For patients with binaural or unilateral atresia, microtia repair and atresiaplasty are recommended at 6 years of age. By this age, mastoid pneumatization is complete and the costal cartilage has developed sufficiently for auricular reconstruction. Auricular defects can be rehabilitated with an osseointegrated percutaneous mastoid implant prosthesis, with or without bone-conduction aids such as a BAHA.[16] Alloplastic materials have been used for microtia repair in the past, but a high risk of extrusion is associated with their use. However, new materials, such as porous high-density polyethylene (Medpor), seem to be very well tolerated.[17,18] Medpor reconstruction can be done before or after atresiaplasty because intact blood supply is not indispensable to its success.

In unilateral cases, atresiaplasty surgery may be indicated in a patient who has "minor" unilateral atresia with normal middle ear, ossicles, and facial nerve and excellent pneumatization. In such a patient, atresiaplasty may be offered in childhood with the parents' consent. An adult with unilateral atresia commonly requests atresiaplasty when presbycusis develops in the normal ear.

Preoperative Evaluation and Patient Counseling

Palpation of the mastoid tip, suprameatal spine of Henle (if present), condyle, and zygomatic arch provides a reasonable clinical estimate of the size of the mastoid. This is a useful measure because the new ear canal will be created at the expense of the mastoid air-cell system. The preoperative imaging study is HRCT of the temporal bone in both axial and coronal planes (Fig. 193-1). The surgeon and the radiologist should both review the HRCT scans. Particular attention is given to the following elements, which are the most critical for surgical planning: (1) the status of the inner ear, (2) the extent of temporal bone pneumatization, (3) the course of the facial nerve, with emphasis on the relationship of the horizontal portion to the footplate and the location of the mastoid segment, and (4) the presence of the oval window and stapes footplate. The ideal surgical candidate displays a well-developed mastoid and a good oval window/footplate–facial nerve relationship. In addition to the elements mentioned, HRCT also delineates the thickness and form of the atretic bone, the soft tissue contribution to the atresia, the size and status of the middle ear cavity, and the presence or absence of congenital cholesteatoma. These factors are less critical for the repair.

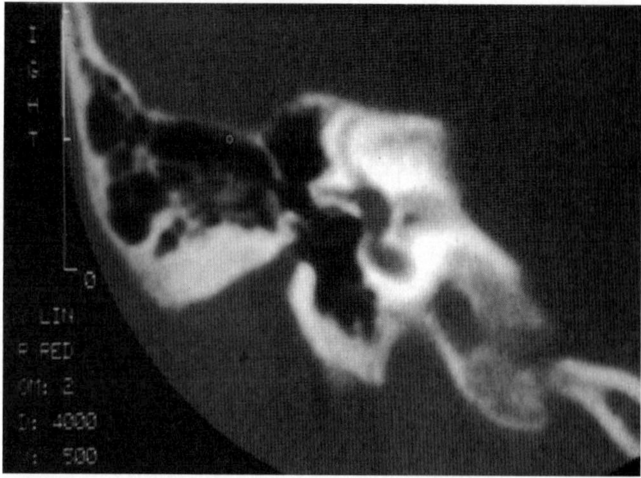

Figure 193-1. Congenital aural atresia, right ear. Coronal high-resolution computed tomography demonstrates atretic external auditory canal and normally developed mastoid system, with normal inner ear.

Poor pneumatization is the most common cause of inoperability in CAA. Fortunately, the majority of patients have normal pneumatization. A facial nerve overlying the oval window may prevent ossicular reconstruction and hearing improvement. If the oval window is absent, it is possible to fenestrate the lateral semicircular canal to improve hearing. However, hearing results are generally poorer in such cases and there is increased risk of SNHL. Patients with these findings are usually best rehabilitated with hearing amplification. Atresiaplasty carries potential for facial nerve injury. The nerve often lies more laterally than usual and may assume a more acute angle than its usual 90 to 120 degrees at the mastoid genu (Fig. 193-2). Even in patients in whom the facial nerve follows a normal course, the distances between the nerve and the temporomandibular joint and between the nerve and the posterior wall of the tympanic cavity are significantly reduced.

Preoperative patient and parent counseling carefully considers reasonably expected surgical results and the potential risks and complications.[19-25] Patients who have minor malformations or a score of 8 or better on the Jahrsdoerfer grading scale are given a greater than 80% chance of significant hearing improvement. Of surgical patients, we find that 50% achieve a long-term postoperative air-bone gap of 30 dB or less.[26] The risk of graft lateralization is less than 4%, the risk of high-tone SNHL is approximately 7%, and the risk of facial nerve palsy is less than 1%. Other risks and complications are comparable to those for other tympanomastoidectomy procedures. Patients and parents are reminded that frequent postoperative visits are critical in the early postoperative period and that a split-thickness skin graft will be taken from the low abdomen to line the new ear canal.

Surgical Approach

Although three approaches to drilling the new ear canal have been described, we have used only an anterior approach for the past 25 years,

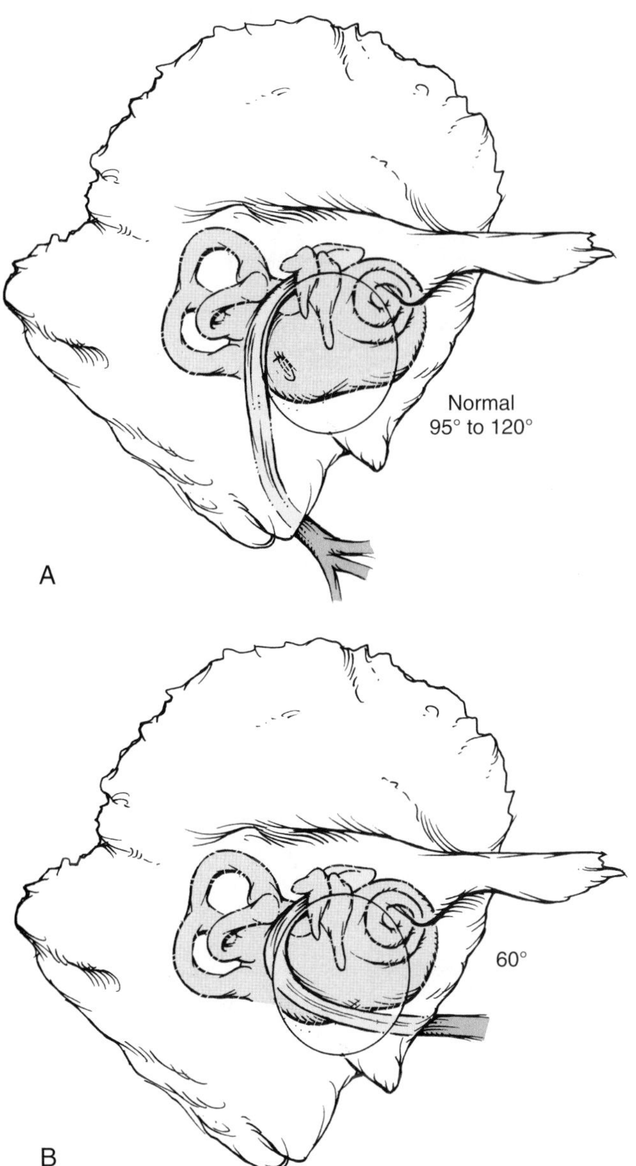

Figure 193-2. The facial nerve in congenital aural atresia. **A,** Normal intratemporal facial nerve anatomy. **B,** Intratemporal facial nerve anatomy in congenital aural atresia. *(© 2008 by Johns Hopkins University, Art as Applied to Medicine.)*

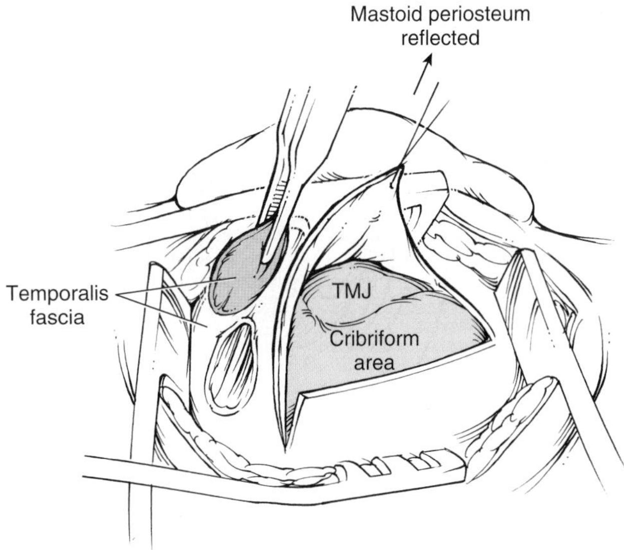

Figure 193-3. Incision, harvesting temporalis fascia, T incision, and elevation of periosteum. TMJ, temporomandibular joint. *(© 2008 by Johns Hopkins University, Art as Applied to Medicine.)*

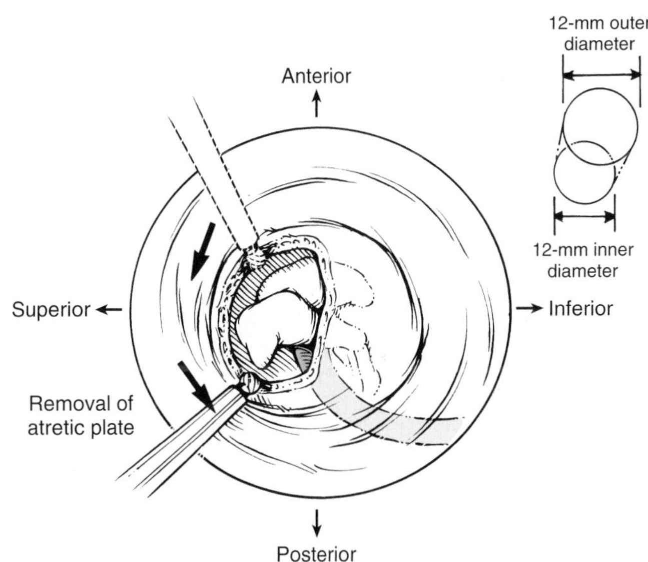

Figure 193-4. Anterior approach: Removal of atretic plate and adhesions, exposing the ossicles, and drilling for the new ear canal. *(© 2008 by Johns Hopkins University, Art as Applied to Medicine.)*

and only this standard approach is described here.[27] Under general endotracheal anesthesia, the patient is placed in the otologic position with the head turned away. Facial nerve monitoring electrodes are placed, and muscle relaxants are avoided. The postauricular area is shaved, and the auricle and postauricular area are prepared with povidone-iodine and then draped. The lower abdomen is similarly prepared for the skin graft donor site.

The approach in all cases is through a postauricular incision. In patients with prior auricular reconstruction, care is taken not to expose the grafted costal cartilage. A T-shaped incision is made in the periosteum, and the subcutaneous tissue and periosteum are elevated anteriorly to allow identification of the glenoid fossa (Fig. 193-3). The temporomandibular joint space is gently explored to ensure that an anomalous facial nerve or tympanic bone remnant is not lying within it. Temporalis fascia is harvested and dried.

If a remnant of tympanic bone is present, drilling for the new ear canal begins at the cribriform area. If no such remnant exists, drilling of a 12-mm cylindrical canal begins at the level of the linea temporalis, just posterior to the glenoid fossa. Dissection proceeds anteriorly and medially, taking into consideration the lack of landmarks in atretic bone. The middle fossa plate is identified and followed to the epitympanum, where the fused malleus head–incus body mass is identified (Fig. 193-4). Care is taken to avoid exposure of the temporomandibular joint space or to avoid opening an excessive number of mastoid air cells. A radical mastoidectomy–like approach is to be avoided. Once the ossicular mass is identified, the atretic bone is removed with diamond micro-drills and curettes to completely expose the ossicles (Fig. 193-5A). It is important to minimize drilling on the ossicular mass because transmission of high-speed drill energy to the inner ear may result in high-tone SNHL. An argon laser is used to free the malleus-incus complex from its soft tissue attachments to reduce potential drill trauma to the inner ear. The ossicular mass in the epitympanum is meticulously dissected free of the atresia plate and left intact. Although the temporomandibular joint often limits anterior dissection, particular effort is made to try to create a space of 2 mm or greater

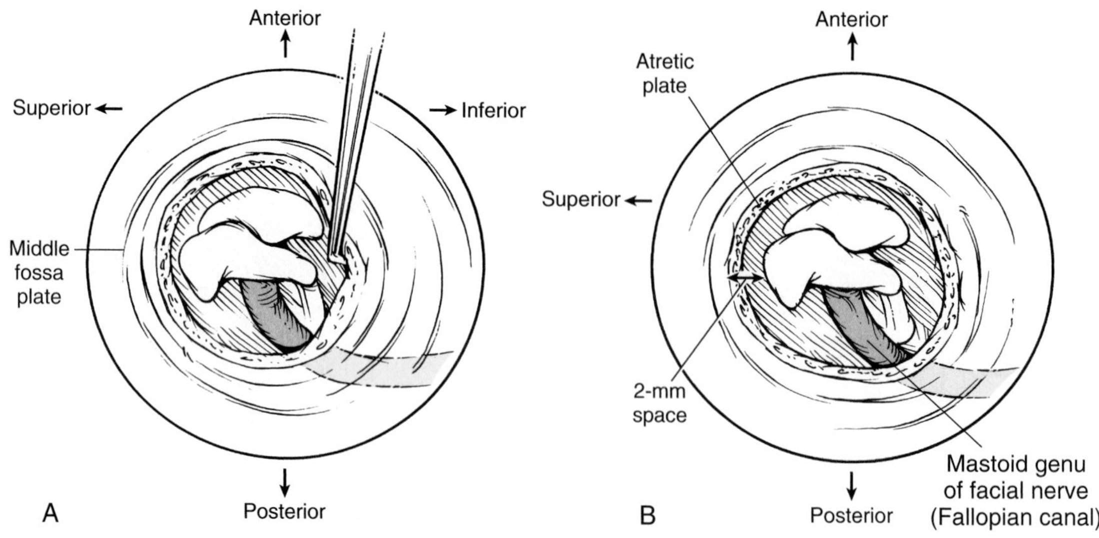

Figure 193-5. **A** and **B,** Anterior approach: The ossicular mass is dissected free of the atretic plate, and a 2-mm space is created around the ossicles. *(© 2008 by Johns Hopkins University, Art as Applied to Medicine.)*

anterior to the ossicular mass (Fig. 193-5B). The horizontal facial nerve always lies medial to the ossicular mass. During dissection of the inferior and posterior aspects of the canal, an aberrant facial nerve may be encountered as it passes laterally through the atretic bone. Drilling for the new ear canal continues until it measures about 12 mm. This circumference is most difficult to achieve medially, where the facial nerve, temporomandibular joint capsule, and middle fossa plate limit larger exposure.

Reconstruction with the patient's own ossicular chain is performed in almost all cases, even if the ossicular chain is deformed. Therefore, if the ossicular chain is intact, it is left in place and used for ossicular reconstruction. When this is not possible, a total or partial ossicular reconstruction prosthesis to either a mobile footplate or the stapes head is used for reconstruction. If access to the oval window footplate is impossible because a dehiscent facial nerve obliterates the window, hearing restoration can be accomplished with the use of a BAHA.[28-30]

Drilling continues to create an external auditory canal. It must be one-and-one-third times the size of a normal canal (12 mm vs. 9 mm) to allow for contracture healing in the postoperative period. During creation of the external auditory canal, care is taken not to enter the temporomandibular joint or unnecessarily open mastoid cells.

A dermatome is used to obtain a 0.008-inch thick, 6 × 6-cm split-thickness skin graft (STSG) from the hypogastrium. Pressure with a gauze sponge wet-soaked in 1% lidocaine with epinephrine 1 : 100,000 and thrombin solution aids hemostasis of the donor site. When dry, the donor site is dressed with a sterile wound dressing such as a Tegaderm dressing (3M, St. Paul, MN). This step reduces most of the pain associated with other methods of donor site care. One edge of the skin graft is cut in a zigzag fashion to create four or five triangular points (Fig. 193-6). To facilitate inspection of the skin graft in the final stages of the procedure, the tips of each point and the two corners on the opposite edge are colored with a skin marker.

The dried temporalis fascia is trimmed to size, ideally a 20 × 15-mm oval, and a small (4-mm) "tab" is cut into the anterior-inferior aspect of the graft in an attempt to prevent lateralization. (Lateralization is the most common delayed cause of a poor hearing outcome, usually occurring in the first 12 months after surgery. Once the graft starts lateralizing, it pulls away from the ossicles, and the original good hearing results slowly deteriorate.) Thirty minutes before grafting begins, nitrous oxide administration is discontinued. The fascia is placed over the ossicular chain medial to the malleus, if present, or over the cartilage that covers the prosthesis (Fig. 193-7). The tab of the graft is placed medially into the protympanum to help prevent lateralization of the new eardrum.

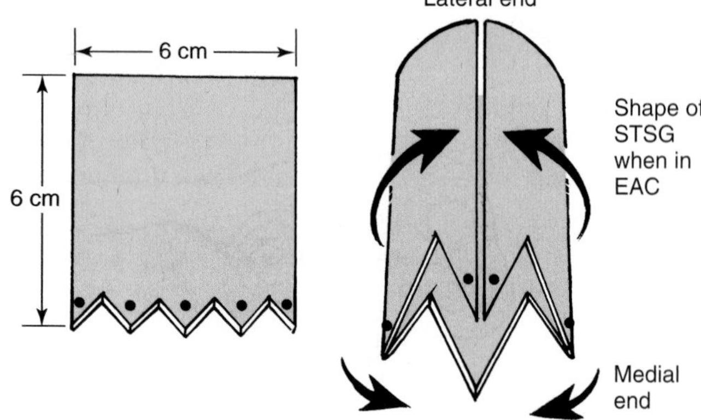

Figure 193-6. Split-thickness skin graft (STSG) used to line new external auditory canal (EAC). *(© 2008 by Johns Hopkins University, Art as Applied to Medicine.)*

Next, the new ear canal is circumferentially lined with the STSG so that all the bone is completely covered (Fig. 193-8). The triangular corners of the skin graft are placed medially and partially overlap the fascia. The previous coloring of the points helps ensure that no skin lies folded on itself and that the entire width of the graft is used. A single layer of antibiotic-soaked absorbable gelatin sponge (Gelfoam; Pfizer Inc, New York) holds the fascia and skin graft in place. To reproduce the anterior tympanomeatal angle, a disk of absorbable gelatin film (Gelfilm; Pfizer Inc) is placed over the fascia and skin graft. After the fascia and skin graft are in proper position, three 0.020-inch polymeric silicone (Silastic; Dow Corning Corporation, Midland, MI) strips are placed to line the skin (Fig. 193-9). This step helps prevent adhesions between the skin graft and the ear canal packing and ensures good contact between the skin graft and ear canal bone. A 9 × 15-mm hydroxylated polyvinyl acetate sponge wick (Merocel; Medtronic USA, Inc., Jacksonville, FL) is placed in the bony canal.

A 12-mm meatus is created, with the anticipation that a third of its diameter will diminish through normal healing. Before the meatoplasty is begun, the ear is turned back and the periosteum is brought back in place with one absorbable suture at the superior level of the new ear canal. This maneuver stabilizes the pinna and helps ensure that the meatus is at the same level as the new ear canal. Skin, subcutaneous tissue, and cartilage are removed in a 12-mm-diameter core over the new meatus. An attempt is made to avoid exposing the grafted cartilage or other materials used for auricular reconstruction. The lateral edge of the STSG is brought through the meatoplasty, and the lateral portion of the new ear canal and the meatus are packed with a large 15 × 25-mm Ambrus Merocel Ear Wick (Medtronic Xomed Surgical Products, Jacksonville, Fla.). This packing applies diffuse pressure over the entire lateral skin graft and widely packs the meatoplasty. Five tacking sutures

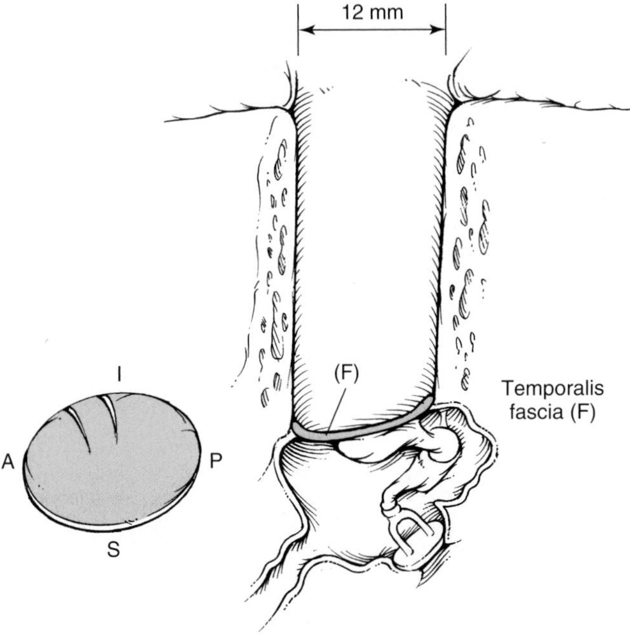

Figure 193-7. Temporalis fascia graft with tabs used over an ossicular mass or a partial ossicular replacement prosthesis and cartilage. A, anterior; I, inferior; P, posterior; S, superior. *(© 2008 by Johns Hopkins University, Art as Applied to Medicine.)*

of 5-0 Ti-Cron (Covidien, Mansfield, MA) attach the lateral edge of the skin graft circumferentially to the meatal skin. Finally, 6-0 fast-absorbing plain gut is used in a running manner between each Ti-Cron sutures (Fig. 193-10). The periosteum is sutured back into position. The postauricular incision is closed using absorbable sutures (3-0 polyglactin 910 [Vicryl; Ethicon, Inc, Somerville, NJ]). Steri-Strip surgical skin closures (3M) cover the incision, a mastoid dressing is applied, anesthesia is reversed, monitoring equipment is removed, and the patient leaves the operating room.

Silastic sheets and Merocel wicks have helped decrease both the incidence of TM lateralization by keeping the TM graft in position and the incidence of postoperative EAC stenosis by covering all exposed areas of bone that may cause granulation tissue formation.[26] The Merocel wicks that are now available in many sizes for canal stenting help prevent postoperative infection and granulation tissue by allowing administration of topical antibiotic medication to the entire external auditory canal.

Postoperative Care

The mastoid dressing is removed on the first postoperative day. The Tegaderm dressing remains over the STSG donor site for at least 3 weeks to allow epithelialization to occur under the plastic. The patient is seen 1 week after surgery, at which time the tacking Ti-Cron sutures at the meatus and the postauricular Steri-Strips are removed. Any dried blood or crusting on the lateral end of the meatus pack should be trimmed. The postauricular site can now be washed, but water precautions continue for the ear canal. We continue to see the patient on a weekly basis. At 2 weeks, the Merocel packs and Silastic sheet are removed, and the meatus is repacked with antibiotic-soaked Gelfoam. At this point, the patient or parent(s) should apply antibiotic suspension to the packing in the ear canal twice a day for 8 to 12 weeks. Usually by 3 weeks, the abdominal donor site has completed the initial re-epithelialization, and the Tegaderm dressing may be removed.

By 6 to 8 weeks postoperatively, nearly all of the Gelfoam is usually gone and the canal is healing well. The first postoperative

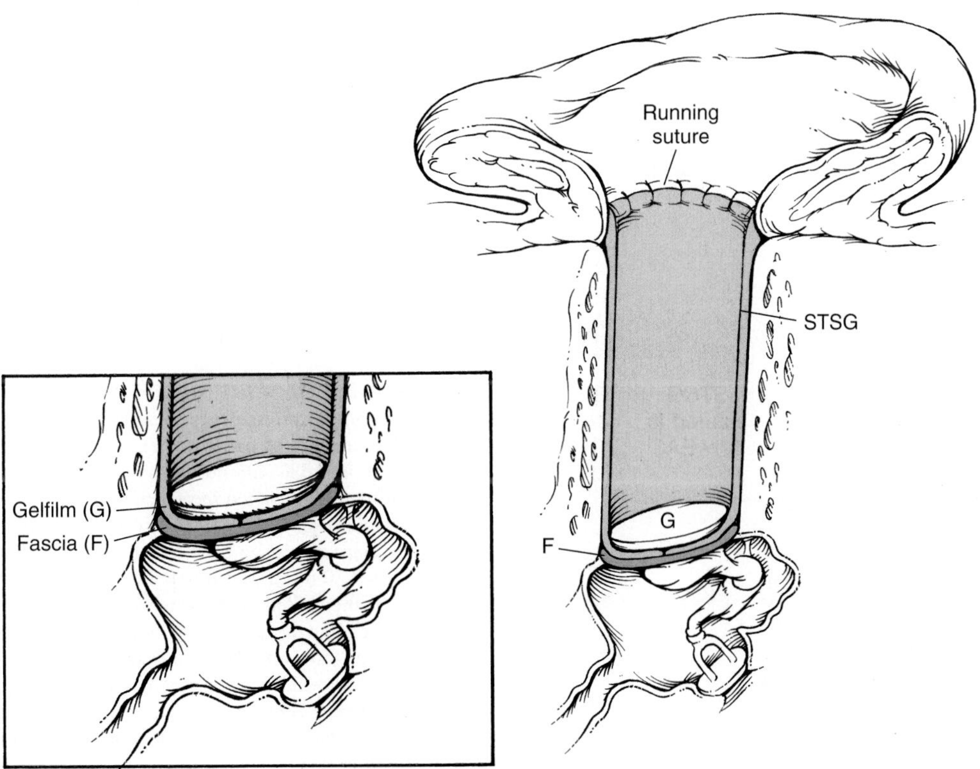

Figure 193-8. Two views of a split-thickness skin graft (STSG) in place over fascia, lining new external auditory canal, and disk of Gelfilm over fascia and skin graft. *(© 2008 by Johns Hopkins University, Art as Applied to Medicine.)*

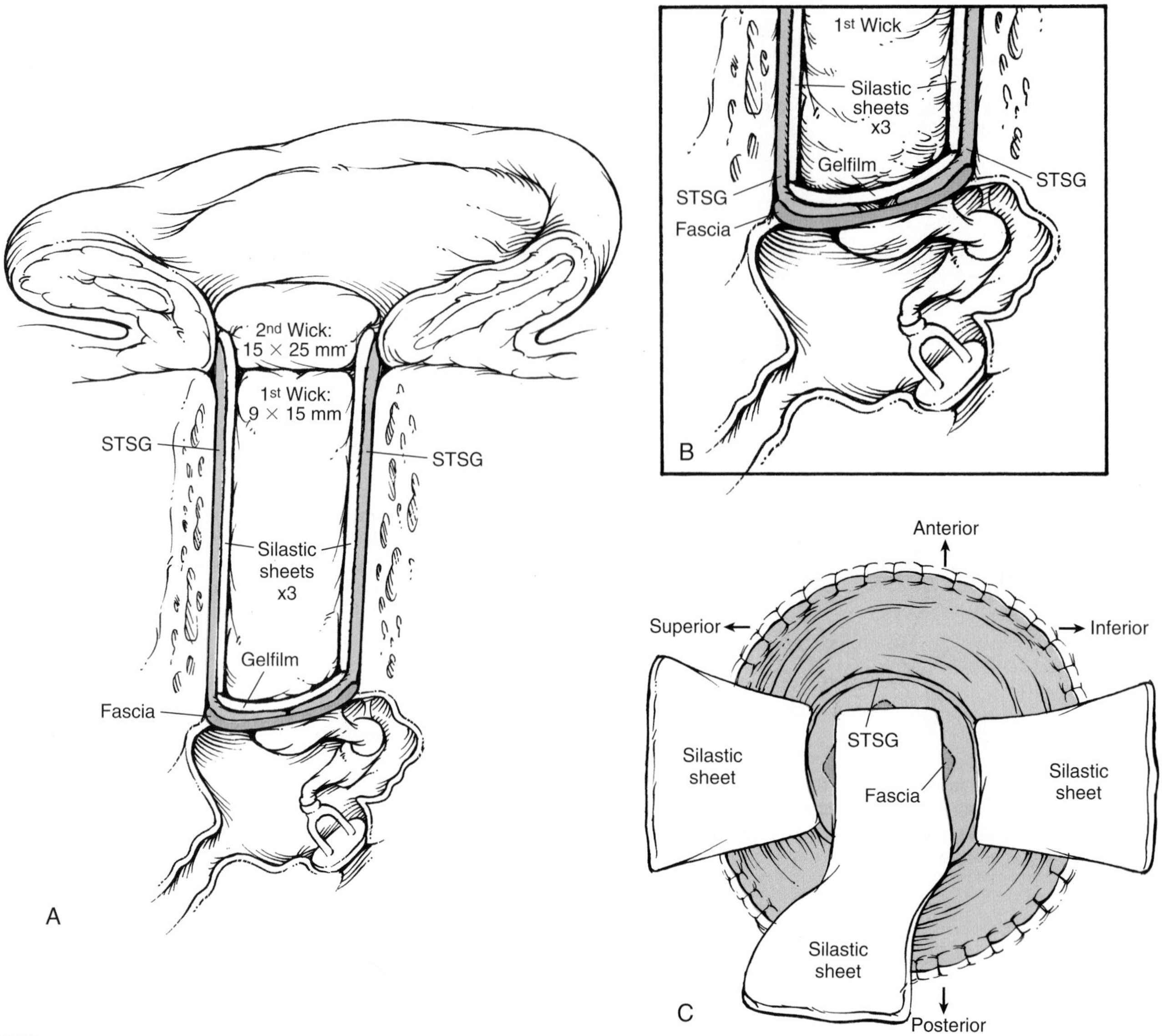

Figure 193-9. Split-thickness skin graft (STSG) and Silastic (polymeric silicone) strips with ear wicks to maintain contact with bony external auditory canal, and wide meatus. *(© 2008 by Johns Hopkins University, Art as Applied to Medicine.)*

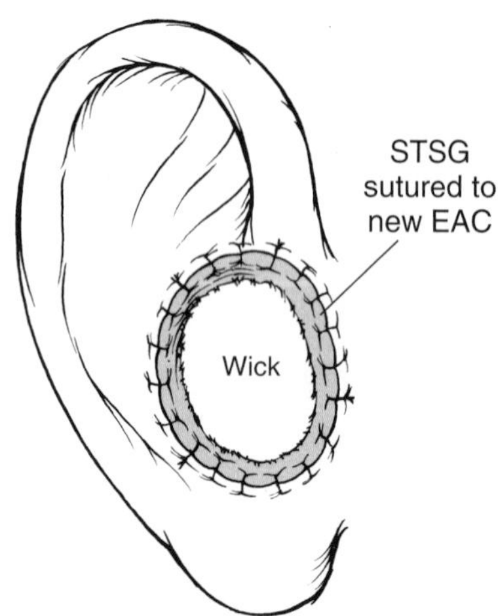

Figure 193-10. Split-thickness skin graft (STSG) sutured into place at meatus, to new external auditory canal (EAC). *(© 2008 by Johns Hopkins University, Art as Applied to Medicine.)*

audiogram is obtained at that time, and audiography is repeated in 6 months, in 1 year, and yearly thereafter.

Avoidance of Complications

Complications of atresiaplasty include lateralization of the tympanic membrane in 3.4% of patients, stenosis of the meatus in 3.8%, high-tone SNHL in 7.5%, and facial nerve palsy in less than 1%.[26,31] Other investigators have reported meatal stenosis in 7% and tympanic membrane lateralization in 18% of their cases.[32] Attention to intraoperative measures helps minimize graft lateralization: Nitrous oxide should be discontinued 30 minutes before grafting. The graft should be anchored medially to the malleus and the tab should be placed into the protympanum. Use of an accurately sized Gelfilm disk attempts to recreate an anterior tympanomeatal angle and keeps the graft in position. Silastic sheets and Merocel wicks placed in the EAC also help minimize the incidence of graft lateralization. The patient must be followed carefully for at least 24 months, because lateralization has been known to occur up to 12 months postoperatively.

The incidence of stenosis has been significantly reduced with the use of one-piece STSGs covering all exposed bone, and Silastic sheets and Merocel wicks in the EAC.[26] Of equal importance to surgical technique are consistent postoperative follow-up and office care. Patients or their parents should understand beforehand that they must strictly follow the postoperative instructions and that they must keep all scheduled postoperative visits. We check the circumference of the pack each week to ensure that there is no ingrowth of grafted skin into the pack. If the meatus appears to be narrowing, usually at the third month, it should be dilated every 2 weeks and restented with the large Merocel wick for several months to 2 years. This measure usually avoids the need for reoperation. Early identification and treatment of infection are also necessary to prevent graft failure and canal stenosis.

High-tone SNHL occurs in up to 7.5% of cases.[26,31] To reduce the risk of noise-induced hearing loss, it is critical to minimize drilling on the ossicular chain while it is being dissected away from the atretic bone, but noise transmission during creation of the ear canal cannot be completely avoided. Use of the laser helps minimize manipulation when the surgeon is trying to free the malleus-incus complex from the atretic plate. With better imaging techniques, oval window problems can be identified preoperatively, and problems of SNHL due to oval window drill-out are avoided. Likewise, patients with computed tomography evidence of severe malformations are likely to have poor surgical results and so are best fitted with conventional bone-conduction hearing aids or BAHAs instead.

Intraoperative facial nerve monitoring is essential in all cases because there are often no clearly identifiable landmarks in atretic ears. If the monitor is off transiently because of the use of electrocautery, the surgeon can monitor the facial nerve manually by placing a hand on the patient's face. It is also important to remember that in a poorly pneumatized temporal bone, the otic capsule may be difficult to distinguish, and care must be taken to avoid "blue lining" (or worse) of the semicircular canals.

Surgical Alternatives to Atresiaplasty

BAHAs provide a good alternative to atresiaplasty for rehabilitation of hearing loss resulting from CAA.[28,33] BAHAs are especially suitable for patients with bilateral CAA and who, because of the severity of the malformations, would have poor results with atresiaplasty. The BAHA is a better alternative than a conventional bone hearing aid. Conventional bone hearing aids have the following drawbacks: discomfort because of constant pressure from the steel spring, worse sound quality because of higher-frequency attenuation by the skin, and poor aesthetics and insecure positioning of the device. The BAHA works without pressure on the skin and provides direct bone transmission without air interface.

Surgery for the BAHA can be performed under local or general anesthesia and is a one-stage procedure. To implant the BAHA, a small titanium abutment is implanted behind the ear, where it osseointegrates to the mastoid bone. After a 3-month healing period the BAHA processor can then be connected.

Audiologic indications for the BAHA include a pure-tone average bone-conduction threshold better than or equal to a 45-dB hearing level (average of 500, 1000, 2000, and 3000 Hz). A maximum speech discrimination score better than 60% for use of the PB word lists is recommended. From an audiologic point of view, the side with the better cochlear function (the better bone-conduction threshold) should be used. Patients with a bone-conduction threshold of 25 to 45 dB hearing level will be expected to improve but may not achieve levels in the normal range. Patients with a bone-conduction threshold of less than 25 dB hearing level can be expected to experience hearing improvements that restore hearing levels to normal ranges. Patients must be able to maintain the abutment/skin interface of the BAHA. Careful consideration must be given to the patient's psychological, physical, emotional, and developmental capabilities to maintain hygiene. Titanium implants can be installed in most patients because allergy to titanium is extremely rare. Alternative treatments should be considered for patients with a disease state that might jeopardize osseointegration.

In general, we do not recommend implantable hearing aids in young children, because the surgical scars may preclude any future microtia repair. However, the BAHA titanium implant is ideally placed 5 to 6 cm behind and 3 cm above the ear canal in a hair-bearing area. This placement seems to allow for the possibility of future microtia repair that would transplant costal cartilage to an area with unscarred skin. On the other hand, the titanium implants for a bone-anchored ear epithesis are ideally placed 18 to 20 mm behind the (future) ear canal. This site would interfere with the skin of a future auricle, if reconstruction is contemplated.

Summary

The treatment of congenital aural atresia represents a challenging, complex problem. Early identification, appropriate hearing amplification, and speech and language therapy are crucial in patients with bilateral disease. Surgical coordination with the auricular reconstruction surgeon allows for the best aesthetic and functional success. Strict radiologic and clinical criteria are necessary to appropriately identify atresiaplasty candidates. Classification of patients into those with minor and major malformations provides prognosis for hearing improvement and potential risks of surgery. A thorough understanding of the embryologic development of the ear and adherence to the surgical principles of tympanoplasty, canalplasty, and facial nerve surgery enable optimal and safe hearing restoration. Maintenance of good initial surgical results and avoidance of late complications requires diligent postoperative office care. BAHAs provide a good alternative for patients in whom atresiaplasty results would be poor.

SUGGESTED READINGS

Altmann F. Congenital atresia of the ear in man and animals. *Ann Otol Rhinol Laryngol.* 1955;64:824-828.

Anson BJ, Davies J, Duckert LG. Embryology of the ear. In: Paparella MM, Shumrick DA, Gluckman JL, Meyerhoff WI, eds. *Otolaryngology.* 3rd ed. Philadelphia: WB Saunders; 1991.

Brent B. Microtia repair with rib cartilage grafts: a review of personal experience with 1000 cases. *Clin Plast Surg.* 2002;29:257-271.

Chandrasekhar SS, De la Cruz A, Garrido E. Surgery of congenital aural atresia. *Am J Otol.* 1995;16:713-717.

Chang SO, Choi BY, Hur DG. Analysis of the long-term hearing results after the surgical repair of aural atresia. *Laryngoscope.* 2006;116:1835-1841.

Chiossone E. Surgical management of major congenital malformations of the ear. *Am J Otol.* 1985;6:237-242.

De la Cruz A, Chandrasekhar SS. Congenital malformation of the temporal bone. In: Brackmann DE, Shelton C, Arriaga M, eds. *Otologic Surgery.* Philadelphia: WB Saunders; 2001.

De la Cruz A, Linthicum FH Jr, Luxford WM. Congenital atresia of the external auditory canal. *Laryngoscope.* 1985;95:421-427.

De la Cruz A, Teufert KB. Congenital aural atresia surgery: long-term results. *Otolaryngol Head Neck Surg.* 2003;129:121-127.

Digoy GP, Cueva RA. Congenital aural atresia: review of short- and long-term surgical results. *Otol Neurotol.* 2007;28:54-60.

Evans AK, Kazahaya K. Canal atresia: "surgery or implantable hearing devices? The expert's question is revisited." *Int J Pediatr Otorhinolaryngol.* 2007;71:367-374.

Federspil P, Delb W. Treatment of congenital malformations of the external and middle ear. In: Ars B, ed. *Congenital External and Middle Ear Malformations: Management.* Amsterdam: Kugler Publications; 1992.

Gasser RF, Shigihara S, Shimada K. Three-dimensional development of the facial nerve path through the ear region in human embryos. *Ann Otol Rhinol Laryngol.* 1994;103:395-403.

Ishimoto S, Ito K, Karino S, et al. Hearing levels in patients with microtia: correlation with temporal bone malformation. *Laryngoscope.* 2007;117:461-465.

Jahrsdoerfer RA, Yeakley JW, Aguilar EA, et al. Grading system for the selection of patients with congenital aural atresia. *Am J Otol.* 1992;13:6-12.

Kountakis SE, Helidonis E, Jahrsdoerfer RA. Microtia grade as an indicator of middle ear development in aural atresia. *Arch Otolaryngol Head Neck Surg.* 1995;121:885-886.

Melnick M. The etiology of external ear malformations and its relation to abnormalities of the middle ear, inner ear, and other organ systems. *Birth Defects Orig Artic Ser.* 1980;16:303-331.

Naumann A. Plastic surgery to correct deformities of the ear. *MMW Fortschr Med.* 2005;147:28-31.

Niparko JK, Langman AW, Cutler DS, et al. Tissue-integrated prostheses in the rehabilitation of auricular defects: results with percutaneous mastoid implants. *Am J Otol.* 1993;14:343-348.

Patel N, Shelton C. The surgical learning curve in aural atresia surgery. *Laryngoscope.* 2007;117:67-73.

Romo T 3rd, Presti PM, Yalamanchili HR. Medpor alternative for microtia repair. *Facial Plast Surg Clin North Am.* 2006;14:129-136.

Schuknecht HF. Congenital aural atresia and congenital middle ear cholesteatoma. In: Nadol JB, Schuknecht HF, eds. *Surgery of the Ear and Temporal Bone.* New York: Raven Press; 1993.

Shih L, Crabtree JA. Long-term surgical results for congenital aural atresia. *Laryngoscope.* 1993;103:1097-1102.

Teufert KB, De la Cruz A. Advances in congenital aural atresia surgery: effects on outcome. *Otolaryngol Head Neck Surg.* 2004;131:263-270.

Van de Water TR, Maderson PF, Jaskoll TF. The morphogenesis of the middle and external ear. *Birth Defects Orig Artic Ser.* 1980;16:147-180.

For complete list of references log onto www.expertconsult.com.

CHAPTER ONE HUNDRED AND NINETY-FOUR

Acute Otitis Media and Otitis Media with Effusion

Margaretha L. Casselbrant

Ellen M. Mandel

Key Points

- The presence or absence of signs and symptoms and findings on the otoscopic examination provide the basis for diagnosis of the different types of otitis media.
- Proper treatment depends on differentiation between acute otitis media and otitis media with effusion.
- The highest incidence of otitis media occurs between the ages of 6 and 11 months and decreases with age. Risk factors include both host and environmental factors.
- Prevention of disease through use of vaccines and risk factor reduction is desirable.
- For children 2 years of age or older with nonsevere acute otitis media, published guidelines have given the option of observing rather than treating with antibiotics immediately.
- Antihistamines and steroids are ineffective for the treatment of otitis media.
- Tympanostomy tube insertion is effective in reducing recurrent episodes of otitis media and persistent middle ear effusion.
- Adenoidectomy *is not* recommended for the initial surgical treatment of otitis media unless nasal obstruction is present but *is* recommended for children in whom a repeat surgical procedure is needed.
- Careful follow-up is needed to identify complications and sequelae of otitis media as well as of its treatment.

Otitis media is not only a disease of modern times. It has been a major health problem in many societies. In the 8th century, the most common approach to healing was water from wells named after various saints.[1] Otitis media is in general a childhood disease, and in most children it resolves with anatomic and physiologic changes with growth. Until the condition has resolved, it may affect balance, hearing, and speech and language development and cause poor school performance. This disease affects not only the child but the whole family, from an economic as well as a societal standpoint. It is more than the cost for medicine or visits to the doctors; passing sleepless nights due to a crying child, having to take off from work to stay home with the child, and taking the child to the doctors can be very stressful for the family. The cost for medical and surgical therapy for otitis media in children 5 years of age or younger is estimated at $5 billion annually in the United States.[2]

Diagnosis

Definition/Symptoms and Signs

Although considered to constitute a continuum of disease, otitis media can be subclassified into *acute otitis media* (AOM) and *otitis media with effusion* (OME) on the basis of signs and symptoms. Because the treatments for AOM and for OME differ, it is important to accurately diagnose the two conditions. AOM generally is characterized by rapid onset of signs and symptoms of inflammation in the middle ear accompanied by middle ear effusion (MEE). Signs of inflammation include bulging or fullness of the tympanic membrane (TM), erythema of the TM, and acute perforation of the TM with otorrhea. Symptoms include otalgia, irritability, and fever. OME, on the other hand, is defined as MEE without signs and symptoms of acute inflammation as found in AOM.

Physical Examination

In addition to the examination of the ears, a proper head and neck examination is invaluable, because it may identify conditions that may predispose the patient to otitis media. Facial features should be assessed for craniofacial anomalies such as those of Down syndrome and Treacher Collins syndrome, because they are associated with increased incidence of otitis media. Examination of the oropharynx may show a bifid uvula or a cleft palate. Hypernasality indicates velopharyngeal insufficiency, whereas hyponasality may be caused by obstructing adenoids or nasal obstruction due to nasal polyposis or deviated septum.

Pneumatic otoscopy is the primary diagnostic tool to evaluate the status of the middle ear, because it allows assessment of the TM and its mobility. The normal TM is translucent and concave and moves briskly with application of positive and negative pressure. A visible landmark is the handle (manubrium) of the malleus, which is attached to the TM, with the umbo in the center of the TM. To adequately visualize the TM, the external ear canal must be cleared of cerumen and debris. The assessment of the TM should note *position, color, degree of translucency,* and *mobility.* To ascertain the mobility of the TM, a good airtight seal must be obtained between the speculum and the ear canal. The largest speculum that fits comfortably should be used. A bulb through which air is puffed should be attached to the otoscope, allowing for visualization of TM mobility. Reduced or no mobility of the TM indicates loss of compliance of the TM, either as a result of effusion in the middle ear or from increased stiffness due to scarring or increased thickness of the TM. Total absence of mobility of the TM may also be due to an opening in the TM either as a perforation or a patent tympanostomy tube. Other features, such as fluid levels or bubbles, may be more easily discerned with movement of the TM. The position of the TM ranges from severely retracted to bulging. Mild to moderate retraction indicates negative pressure, MEE, or both, whereas a severely retracted TM usually is associated with effusion. Fullness and bulging of the TM are caused by increased pressure or fluid, or both, in the middle ear. Opacification of the TM may be caused by thickening or scarring or presence of MEE. A red but translucent TM is a typical finding in a crying or sneezing infant, secondary to engorgement of blood vessels in the TM. On the other hand, a "red" TM that is full or bulging often is a sign of AOM. A pink, gray, yellow, or blue retracted TM with reduced or no mobility usually is seen with OME. Myringitis is inflammation of the TM without fluid in the middle ear. Use of an operating microscope may clarify features seen on otoscopy, and visualization of scarring and atrophy of the TM may be enhanced.

Immittance Testing (Tympanometry)

Immittance testing is an excellent adjunct to the assessment of middle ear status and the management of otitis media. When otoscopic evaluation is inconclusive or difficult to perform, tympanometry can be very useful in evaluating ear disease in children older than 6 months of age. It is easy to perform and most often is well accepted by the patient. It has been used for school screening as well as in pediatricians' offices. It also is valuable for documentation of middle ear status over time with repeat testing. A small probe, which emits a tone, is placed in the ear canal with an airtight seal. The tympanogram is obtained by plotting the immittance (acoustic energy of the reflected tone) of the middle ear as a function of the pressure in the external ear canal, which varies, ranging from −400 to +200 daPa (decapascals). The instrument provides measures such as peak compensated (static) admittance, tympanometric peak pressure, acoustic reflex, and tympanometric width (TW) (a measure of gradient). The following set of criteria uses TW to categorize middle ear status[3]:

TW less than 150 daPa = no OME

TW greater than 350 daPa = OME

TW 150-350 daPa = presence or absence of OME is determined by otoscopy

A flat or rounded pattern (TW greater than 350 daPa) with a small ear canal volume indicates MEE, whereas a flat pattern with a large ear canal volume suggests a perforation or a patent tympanostomy tube. In a normal air-filled middle ear with equal pressure on both sides of the TM, the peak pressure of the tympanogram is 0 daPa. Algorithms have been developed to determine the presence or absence of MEE, some combining pneumatic otoscopy and tympanometry. Other methods of ascertaining middle ear status have been investigated, including spectral gradient acoustic reflectometry[4,5] and ultrasound evaluation,[6] but they have been found to have limitations, although they may be useful for screening.

Audiometry

MEE usually results in a mild to moderate conductive hearing loss. The assessment of hearing is essential to management, because hearing impairment can predispose the affected child to delays in speech and language development and may later affect school performance. Audiometry should be used to determine specific management strategies, with a more aggressive approach considered in children with significant hearing impairment.

Behavioral audiometry requires cooperation of the child with the examination and the test is adapted to the age of the child. *Visual reinforcement audiometry* is used for children 6 months to 2 years of age and involves presentation of a sound stimulus in the sound field with observation of the child's conditioned head turn response. This reaction is rewarded with a visual reinforcement such as an animated toy. *Play audiometry*, for children older than 2 years, is similar to *conventional audiometry* (for children over 5 years of age), but the child places toys in a bucket rather than raising a hand to acknowledge hearing the sound. Hearing thresholds in the sound field or ear-specific are determined at 0.25, 0.5, 1, 2, 4, and 8 kHz, depending on the age of the child.

Auditory brainstem audiometry (ABR) and *transitory otoacoustic emissions* (TOAE) are excellent methods for testing children who do not cooperate with behavioral hearing evaluation because of very young age or developmental delay. Except for infants, sedation or general anesthesia is usually necessary for ABR testing in younger children. Three electrodes are placed (forehead and each mastoid process) to record the response to clicks of 2000 to 4000 Hz or pure tone burst. The ABR consists of five to seven vertex-positive waves. Waves I to III presumably reflect activity of the auditory centers in the eighth nerve fibers and pons, waves IV and V reflect auditory centers in mid- to rostral pons and caudal midbrain, respectively; activity from waves VI and VII is less certain. The ABR reflects auditory neural electrical responses that are adequately correlated to behavioral hearing thresholds. However, a normal response on the ABR suggests only that the auditory system up to the midbrain level is responsive to the stimulus employed. Thus, it does not guarantee normal hearing.

Otoacoustic emissions (OAE) testing measures cochlear function (outer hair cells) and is a means of objective assessment of auditory function. It commonly is used for newborn hearing screening because it is fast and easy to perform. It is excellent for testing children who do not cooperate with behavioral testing. MEE may confound the results. Therefore, if the OAEs are absent, immittance testing should be performed to assess the middle ear. For children who "fail" OAE testing, follow-up audiologic testing must be done to assess type and degree of hearing loss.

Pathophysiology and Pathogenesis

The pathophysiology of otitis media is multifactorial, with various overlapping factors (Fig. 194-1).

Eustachian Tube Function

The eustachian tube in the infant is shorter, wider, and more horizontal than in the adult, which accounts for the high rate of otitis media in infants and children. By the age of 7 years, when the tube has a more

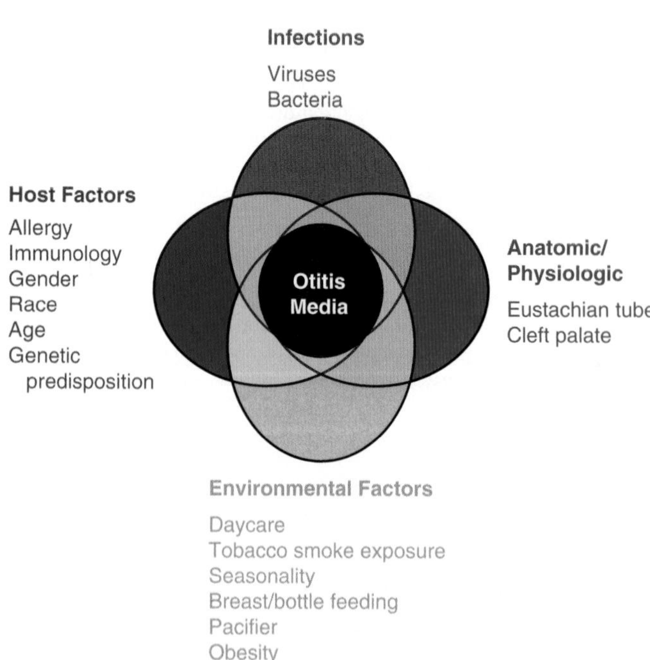

Figure 194-1. Various factors interact in the pathogenesis of otitis media.

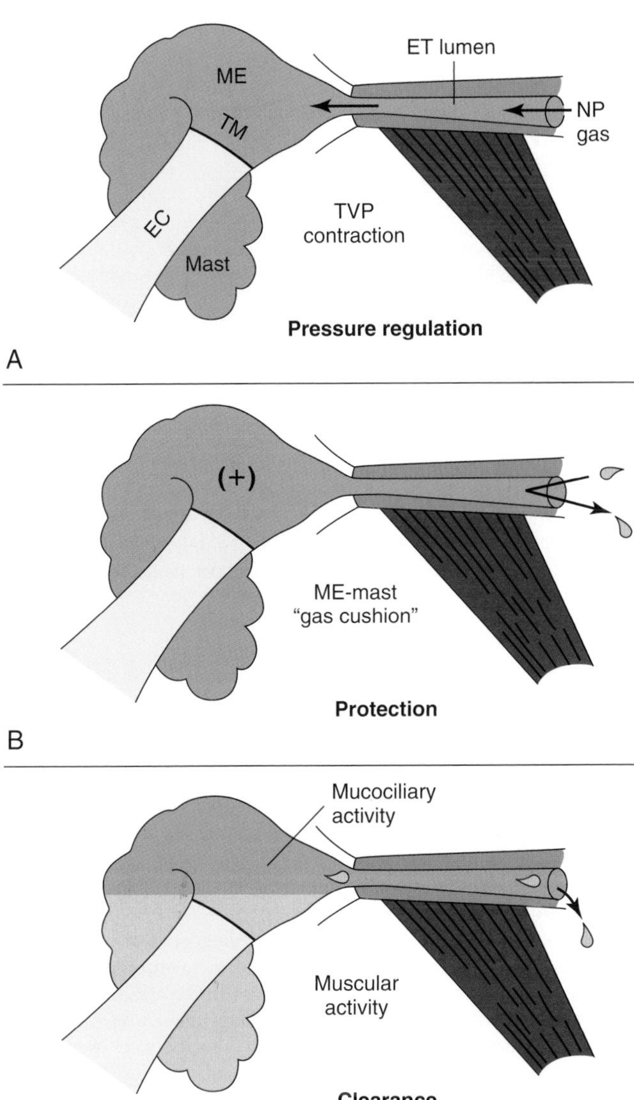

Figure 194-2. Functions of the eustachian tube (ET)-middle ear (ME)-mastoid (mast) gas cell system. **A,** Pressure regulation function is related to active dilation of the tube by contraction of the tensor veli palatini muscle (TVP). **B,** Protective function is dependent in part on an intact middle ear and mastoid gas cells to maintain a gas cushion. **C,** Clearance function is enhanced by mucociliary activity and muscular activity during tubal closing. EC, external canal; NP, nasopharynx; TM, tympanic membrane. *(Adapted from Bluestone CD.* Eustachian Tube: Structure, Function, Role in Otitis Media. *Hamilton, Ont: BC Decker; 2005:51.)*

adult configuration, the prevalence of otitis media is low.[7] The three physiologic functions of the eustachian tube are (1) *pressure regulation* (ventilation), (2) *protection*, and (3) *clearance* (drainage). Of these three functions, pressure regulation is the most important[8] (Fig. 194-2). Middle ear pressure is equilibrated to atmospheric pressure through active intermittent openings of the eustachian tube caused by contraction of the tensor veli palatini muscle during swallowing, jaw movements, and yawning. If active function is impaired, negative pressure will develop in the middle ear. Pressure regulation can be impaired by failure of the opening mechanism (*functional obstruction*) or anatomic (*mechanical*) obstruction. Using a pressure chamber, Bylander and associates evaluated eustachian tube function in children and adults who were considered otologically normal with intact TMs.[9] Although only 5% of the adults were not able to equilibrate negative middle ear pressure, as many as 35.8% of the children could not equilibrate negative pressure. Children 3 to 6 years of age performed worse than children 7 to 12 years of age. These studies indicate that in even apparently otologically normal children eustachian tube function is worse than in adults, but it does improve with age. The improvement in the eustachian tube function parallels the decrease in the incidence of otitis media. Stenström and colleagues tested eustachian tube function in 50 otitis-prone children and 49 children with no history of AOM (control group) using a pressure chamber.[10] The otitis-prone children had significantly poorer active tubal function than the normal control subjects, suggesting that recurrent AOM is the result of functional obstruction of the eustachian tube.

In ears with normal eustachian tube function, the eustachian tube is collapsed when at rest. This arrangement protects the middle ear from nasopharyngeal sound pressure and reflux of secretions from the nasopharynx.

The clearance of secretions produced within the middle ear into the nasopharynx is provided via the mucociliary system and through the "pumping action" of the eustachian tube during closing. The passive closing of the tube is initiated at the middle ear end of the eustachian tube and progresses toward the nasopharyngeal end, facilitating removal of the secretions.

Infection

Bacteriology

Before the year 2000, studies in the United States reported that *Streptococcus pneumoniae* was the single most common bacterial pathogen in AOM, followed by *Haemophilus influenzae* and *Moraxella catarrhalis*; *Streptococcus pyogenes* and other miscellaneous bacteria accounted for just a few cases. From ears with chronic OME, *H. influenzae* was the single most common pathogen, with *S. pneumoniae*, *M. catarrhalis*, and other bacteria accounting for a small percentage of cases each. Data obtained during the 1980s from a single institution is shown in Figure 194-3.[11] There was great hope that the introduction and subsequent use of the heptavalent conjugated pneumococcal vaccine (PCV7) for infants and young children, licensed in the United States in 2000, would lead to a substantial decrease in AOM. However, data from vaccine trials conducted in California[12] and Finland[13] revealed only a 7.8% and a 6% relative risk reduction, respectively, in AOM. Casey and Pichichero examined the experience of children in a suburban Rochester, New York, practice in the years 2001 to 2003 (after the introduction of PCV7) compared with the years 1995 to 2000 and reported a 24% decrease in persistent AOM and AOM treatment failures.[14] These investigators also reported a decrease in recovery of *S. pneumoniae* from the ears of such children and an increase in *H. influenzae*. McEllistrem and coworkers looked at middle ear cultures obtained between 1999 and 2002 at five institutions.[15] They reported that the percentage of AOM episodes due to non-PCV7 serogroups increased after 2000, from 12% in 1999 to 32% in 2002, and the nonvaccine serotypes were more frequent in those who received more than one dose of vaccine. The frequency of penicillin nonsusceptible strains in the vaccine and nonvaccine serotypes remained unchanged.

Nasopharyngeal carriage also was examined. Pelton and associates enrolled 275 infants and children 2 to 24 months of age in a surveillance study in which nasopharyngeal swabs or nasal washes were obtained at all well-child visits and at visits for AOM.[16] From 2000 to 2003, these workers noted a decrease in vaccine serotypes with an increase in nonvaccine serotypes. Tracking antimicrobial susceptibility, they found that the MIC50 and the MIC90 for amoxicillin were stable until the 6-month period from October 2002 to March 2003, when they both increased significantly. Jacobs and associates examined the nasopharyngeal flora in children undergoing tympanostomy tube placement in March 2004 to March 2005 and also found a decrease in vaccine serotypes with a concomitant increase in nonvaccine serotypes, many of which were antibiotic-resistant strains.[17]

These data point to a changing bacteriology and the need for continued surveillance. A remarkable decrease in serious disease has occurred with the use of the newer pneumococcal vaccines, but the impact on otitis media continues to evolve.

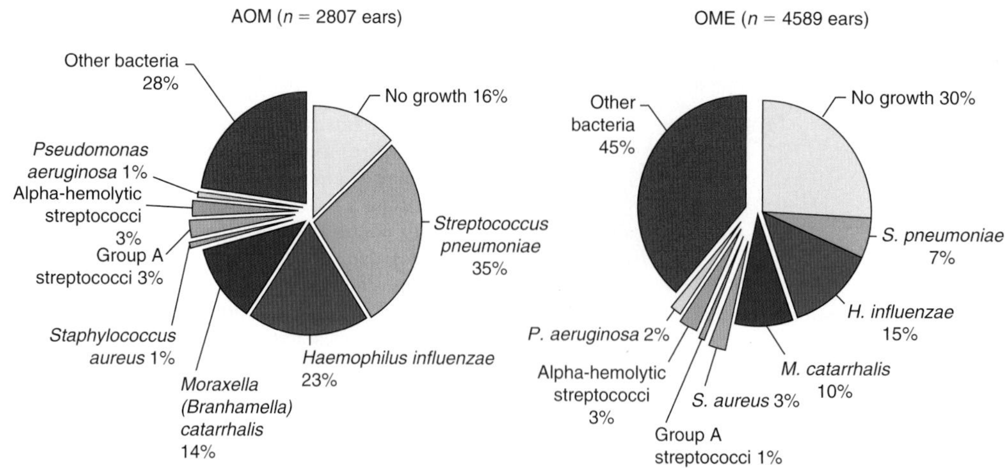

Figure 194-3. Comparison of distribution of isolates in 2807 effusions from patients with acute otitis media (AOM) and 4589 effusions from patients with otitis media with effusion (OME) at the Pittsburgh Otitis Media Research Center, 1980 to 1989. Total percentages are greater than 100% because of multiple organisms. *(Adapted from Bluestone CD, Klein JO. Otitis Media in Infants and Children. 4th ed. Hamilton, Ont: BC Decker; 2007:103.)*

Biofilms

Bacterial biofilms are sessile communities of interacting bacteria attached to a surface and encased in a protective matrix of exopolysaccharides rather than living in a motile "planktonic" or free-floating state. The exopolysaccharide matrix provides protection from phagocytosis and other host defense mechanisms due to lack of accessibility by immunoglobulins and complement. The reduced metabolic rate of bacteria in the biofilm renders them resistant to antimicrobial treatment. The bacterial community relies on a complex intracellular communication system that provides for organized growth characteristics known as "quorum sensing." Biofilms have been known to exist on hard surfaces such as metal pipes or teeth. However, recent animal and human studies have suggested that biofilms can also be isolated from the middle ear. Post and coworkers, using polymerase chain reaction (PCR) methodology, found evidence of bacteria in 48% of culture-negative MEE specimens from children undergoing tympanostomy tube insertion for chronic OME.[18] Hall-Stoodley and colleagues obtained confocal laser scanning microscopy images from the middle ear mucosa of 26 children scheduled for tympanostomy tube insertion for recurrent or persistent otitis media and 8 control subjects (3 children and 5 adults) who underwent cochlear implantation.[19] Generic stains and species-specific probes for *H. influenzae*, *S. pneumoniae*, and *M. catarrhalis* were used to evaluate biofilm morphology. Mucosal biofilms were visualized in 92% of the mucosa from children with chronic and recurrent otitis media but were not observed in any of the 8 control subjects. The investigators suggested that the findings supported the hypothesis that chronic middle ear disease is biofilm-related. Biofilms also have been identified in the nasopharynx of children with otitis media, and it was suggested that the biofilm may act as a reservoir for bacterial pathogens resistant to antibiotics. The mechanical débridement of the nasopharyngeal biofilms may explain the observed clinical benefit associated with adenoidectomy in subsets of pediatric patients.[20]

Viruses

Until the introduction of PCR, viruses were not considered a major factor in the etiology of otitis media, probably because of the technical difficulties in isolating the viruses. Using PCR techniques, however, it has been possible to identify respiratory syncytial virus (RSV), influenzavirus, adenovirus, parainfluenza virus, and rhinoviruses in MEE.[21,22] There is strong evidence that viruses have a crucial role in the development of AOM.[22] In a majority of children, viral infection of the upper respiratory tract mucosa initiates the whole cascade of events that finally leads to the development of AOM, and AOM may be regarded as a complication of a preceding or concomitant viral infection. In a study of 60 children (in 24 families) who were followed from October 2003 through April 2004 by daily parental recording of illness signs, weekly pneumatic otoscopy and viral PCR analysis of nasal secretions collected during "colds" or when MEE was noted, or from enrolled siblings without these conditions, one or more viruses were identified from 73% of secretions collected during a cold but only 18% collected at a time without a cold.[23] Of 93 episodes of otitis media, 70% occurred during a cold, and nasal secretions from 77% of children at the time of these episodes were positive for virus.

Allergy and Immunology

Even though allergy is considered in the pathogenesis of otitis media, the causal mechanism is not understood, and well-controlled studies to prove the efficacy of anti-allergic medication in the treatment of OM are lacking. Several mechanisms by which allergy may cause otitis media have been suggested: (1) the middle ear is a "shock organ" (target); (2) allergy may induce inflammatory swelling of the eustachian tube mucosa; (3) allergies produce inflammatory obstruction of the nose; and (4) bacteria-laden allergic nasopharyngeal secretions may be aspirated into the middle ear. The last three mechanisms involve an association between allergy and abnormal eustachian tube function. Prospective studies have reported a relationship between upper respiratory tract allergy and eustachian tube obstruction in a series of provocative, intranasal allergen–inhalation challenge studies.[24]

Recent studies focus on the analysis of the inflammatory markers in MEE to determine the role of allergy. Both TH1 and TH2 inflammatory patterns in helper T cells have been found in OME. TH1 cytokines antagonize allergic inflammation and play a key part in the defense against viruses and intracellular pathogens, whereas TH2 cytokines promote IgE production, eosinophil growth, and mucus production.[25] The chemoattractant cytokine RANTES (*r*egulated upon *a*ctivation, normal *T* cell–*e*xpressed and *s*ecreted) and eosinophilic cationic protein (ECP), signs of a TH2 process, were assessed in MEE samples from 25 children with allergy and 20 nonallergic children who were 5 to 11 years old at the time of tympanostomy tube insertion.[26] RANTES and ECP levels were significantly higher in the MEE samples from children with allergy than in children without allergy ($P < 0.01$ and < 0.05, respectively). A positive correlation also was found between RANTES and ECP in MEE ($P < 0.01$) in children with allergy, which suggests that allergy is a contributing factor in the pathogenesis of otitis media.

Children with major immune deficiencies may have recurrent otitis media as part of their overall clinical picture, but most otitis-prone children may have only a subtle immunologic abnormality that predisposes them to recurrent infections.[27] The three major pathogens of otitis media—*S. pneumoniae*, *H. influenzae*, and *M. catarrhalis*—frequently colonize the nasopharynx. There are many strains of these organisms, and among the different strains are heterologous surface (strain specific) antigens and conserved antigens. Conserved antigens induce broadly protective antibodies while strain-specific antigens induce limited protection. Otitis-prone children may display strain-specific immunity but fail to develop a broadly protective antibody response, which makes them susceptible to recurrent and persistent otitis media.[28]

Recurrence of bilateral OME after tympanostomy tube insertion was more likely in children with poor eustachian tube function and low IgA or low IgG2 and decreased levels of mannose-binding lectin than in children with poor tubal function and high IgA and IgG2 measured at the time of tube insertion.[29] This suggests that an interaction between various immune factors may increase the risk for the development of otitis media.

Gastroesophageal Reflux

In 2002 Tasker and associates reported finding pepsin/pepsinogen, using enzyme-linked immunosorbent assays, in 90.8% of 65 MEE samples obtained at the time of myringotomy in children.[30] The pepsin-pepsinogen levels ranged from 0.8 to 213.9 µg/mL, which is 1000 times higher than serum levels. He and colleagues, using a sensitive and specific pepsin assay, detected pepsin activity in 14.4% of 152 subjects undergoing tympanostomy tube insertion.[31] The levels of pepsin ranged from 13 to 687 ng/mL. Crapko and associates also identified pepsin activity in the middle ear fluid in 60% of 20 subjects also undergoing tympanostomy tube insertion.[32] In this group of children the pepsin levels ranged from 80 to 1000 ng/mL. The latter studies have shown that pepsin is identified less frequently and at lower levels of pepsin, which may be due to differences in methodology. However, it may be concluded from these studies that gastroesophageal reflux may be a causative factor in otitis media, with a potential role for antireflux therapy in the treatment of otitis media in some children, but adequate controlled trials have not been done.

Epidemiology

Incidence and Prevalence

Otitis media is considered a worldwide pediatric health care problem. The Early Childhood Study—Birth Cohort (ECLS—B), a nationally representative longitudinal study of more than 8000 children born in 2001, showed that otitis media was diagnosed in 39% of children by 9 months and 62% of children by 2 years of age.[33] Although the highest incidence of otitis media is in young children, it also occurs in older children, adolescents, and adults. The Oslo Birth Cohort enrolling infants born in a 15-month period in 1992 to 1993 found that 13% of 10-year-olds had at least one episode of otitis media in the previous 12 months.[34] Approximately 3% to 15% of patients with otitis media referred to otolaryngology clinics are adults.[35]

Acute Otitis Media

Most children experience at least one episode of AOM during their childhood. The cumulative incidence of the first episode of AOM based on studies from various countries ranges from 19% to 62% by age 1 year and 50% to 84% by 3 years of age[36-42] (Fig. 194-4). In a majority of these studies, the peak incidence of AOM was during the first 6 to 12 months of life.[39] The incidence decreases with age, and by the age of 7 years, few children experience episodes of AOM. Recurrent episodes of AOM are common in young children. By 6 months of age, 20% have had two or more episodes.[43] Occurrence of three or more episodes of AOM by the ages of 1, 3, 5, and 7 years has been documented in 10% to 19%, 50%, 65%, and 75% of children, respectively.[39] Occurrence of six or more episodes of AOM was documented in 39% of children by the age of 7 years.

Otitis Media with Effusion

It may be difficult to determine the "true" incidence of OME because, by definition, OME is asymptomatic. Furthermore, most screening studies determine the presence of MEE without differentiating between AOM and OME. Also, a short time between observations is needed for precise assessment of the onset and time to resolution of each new

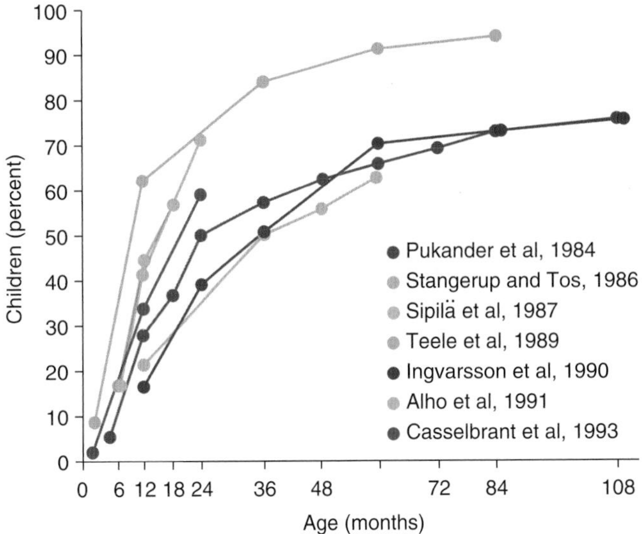

Figure 194-4. Cumulative incidence of first episode of acute otitis media. *(Reproduced from Casselbrant ML, Mandel EM. Epidemiology. In: Rosenfeld RM, Bluestone CD, eds.* Evidence-Based Otitis Media. *2nd ed. Hamilton, Ont: BC Decker; 2003:147.)*

episode of OME, because approximately 65% of OME episodes in children 2 to 7 years of age resolve within 1 month.[44] Monthly examinations with otoscopy and tympanometry in 2- to 6-year-old children in a day care center in Pittsburgh revealed MEE at least once in 53% to 61% of the children. Lous and Fiellau-Nikolajsen found an incidence of MEE of 26% in 7-year-old children followed monthly for 1 year using tympanometry.[45]

The point prevalence of MEE from different countries shows a wide variation, depending on the age of the child, season of the year, and type of assessment. Thus, it must be emphasized that comparison of outcomes between studies will require careful evaluation of study methodology, as well as caution in drawing conclusions. However, nearly all children had experienced at least one episode by the age of 3 years.[46]

Trend over Time

Even though otitis media remains a major problem in the United States, several recent studies point to a trend toward reduction in the burden of otitis media. Grijalva and associates compared the national rates of outpatient visits for pneumonia and otitis media in children in 1994 to 1999 to those in 2002 to 2003 using the National Ambulatory Medical Care Survey and the National Hospital Ambulatory Medical Care Survey.[47] The results showed that otitis media visit rates declined by 20% in children younger than 2 years of age while there was no significant decrease in outpatient visit rates for pneumonia or other respiratory infections in children in this same age group. The second study compared the risk of developing frequent otitis media or having tympanostomy tubes inserted in four birth cohorts (1998 to 1999, 1999 to 2000, 2000 to 2001, and 2001 to 2002).[48] The study population included all children at birth in TennCare or selected upstate New York commercial insurance plans as of July 1998 and followed them for 5 years. When comparing the 2000-2001 cohort to the 1998-1999 cohort frequent otitis media declined by 17% and 28% and tympanostomy tube insertion declined by 16% and 23% for Tennessee and New York cohorts, respectively. The decline may be the result of infant immunization, catch-up doses in older children, and herd immunity after introduction of the heptavalent pneumococcal conjugate vaccine in the United States in 2000. In a comparison of the 2000 to 2001 and 2001 to 2002 birth cohorts, frequent otitis media and tympanostomy tubes remained stable in New York but increased in Tennessee. The investigators attributed this to several possible factors including increase in disease due to nonvaccine serotypes and change in medical care utilization.

A decline in the incidence of otitis media also has been reported from several European countries. Kvaerner conducted a study in Norway of hospital admissions for AOM from 1999 to 2005 among children aged 7 years or younger.[49] Hospitalization for AOM was less frequent but the incidence of acute mastoiditis remained stable at approximately 6 per 100,000 children over time. The consultation rates to the general physicians in the Netherlands for otitis media during 1995 to 2003 in children from birth to 13 years of age were assessed using the research database of the Netherlands University Medical Center Utrecht Primary Care Network.[50] The overall consultation rates decreased by 9% for AOM and 34% for OME. In children aged 2 to 6 years and those aged 6 to 13 years, the rate of AOM declined by 15% and 40%, respectively; the rates of OME declined by 41% and 48%, respectively. In children younger than 2 years of age, however, the rates of AOM and OME increased by 46% and 66%.

Data from the General Practitioner Database in the United Kingdom were analyzed for events classified as AOM or "glue ear" in the years 1991 to 2001.[51] Total consultations for AOM and glue ear in children aged 2 to 13 years had changed from 105.3 to 34.7 and 15.2 to 16.7 per 1000 per year, respectively.

Further surveillance is needed. As noted previously, disease rates must continue to be monitored to determine the effects of vaccines and changes in treatment on the epidemiology of otitis media.

Risk Factors

Risk factors can be host-related (age, gender, race, prematurity, allergy, immunocompetence, cleft palate and craniofacial abnormalities, genetic predisposition) as well as environmental (upper respiratory infections, seasonality, day care, siblings, tobacco smoke exposure, breastfeeding, socioeconomic status, pacifier use, and obesity) and are considered important in the occurrence, recurrence, and persistence of middle ear disease.

Host-Related Factors

Age

The highest incidence of AOM is between 6 and 11 months of age,[39] and onset of the first episode of AOM before 6 months[39] or 12 months of age is a powerful predictor of recurrence.[52] The risk of persistent MEE after an episode of AOM is inversely correlated with age,[39] and children who experience their first episode of MEE before 2 months of age are at a higher risk for persistent fluid during their first year of life than are children who have their first episode later.[53]

Sex

Most investigators have reported no apparent sex-based difference in the incidence of OME.[46] Paradise and coworkers, in a study involving more than 2000 infants, found males had more time with MEE, although the difference was not large.[54] Some studies have found a significantly higher incidence of AOM in males as well as more recurrent episodes than in females, but others have not found this.[46]

Race

Earlier studies have suggested a lower incidence of otitis media in African-American children than in white children. More recent studies in which the children were followed prospectively from infancy to age 2 years with routine examinations of the ears every 6 weeks showed no difference between the African-American and white children in their experience with otitis media.[54,55] A third study, part of an American population-based sample survey evaluating schoolchildren 6 to 10 years of age with tympanometry, reported no difference between African-American and white children. However, the prevalence of OME was significantly higher in Hispanic children compared with white children.[56] In another study of more than 11,000 infants followed only from the ages of 1 through 6 months at two urban and one suburban location in the United States, non-Hispanic white children had significantly higher rates of otitis media after multivariant adjustment than non-Hispanic black or Asian children. There was no difference between Hispanic and non-Hispanic children.[57]

Prematurity

Some studies have shown a possible association between low birth weight and prematurity and otitis media, but others have not. In many of these studies, however, the sample sizes have been relatively small. A recent study analyzing data from more than 10,000 births showed some relationship between very low birth weight (less than 1500 g) and frequent otitis media, but no increased risk was found for recurrent otitis media and moderately low birth weight (1500 to 2499 g). In a prospective cohort study of 136 children treated with tympanostomy tubes, a positive but nonsignificant association was documented between low birth weight or low gestational age or history of incubator care and recurrent OME.[58]

Allergy

There is still controversy regarding the role of allergy in the pathogenesis of otitis media. Allergy is a common problem in children, occurring at a time when respiratory infections and otitis media are common. Most, but not all, of the epidemiologic studies have supported an association. Pukander and Karma followed 707 children with AOM and found that in children with atopic manifestations, persistence of MEE for 2 months or longer was more common than in children without allergy.[59] In another study, however, atopic diathesis was not found to predispose affected children to the development of AOM.[60] The Japanese investigators Tomonaga and associates determined that allergic rhinitis was present in 50% of 259 patients (mean age of 6 years) in whom OME had been diagnosed, and OME was present in 21% of 605 patients (mean age of 9 years) in whom allergic rhinitis had been diagnosed.[61] Among 108 children 5 to 8 years of age (mean age of 6 years) in whom neither condition had been diagnosed, the occurrence rates for allergic rhinitis, OME, and both of these conditions were 17%, 6%, and 2%, respectively. Another investigative group (Kraemer and coworkers) compared risk factors for persistent MEE among 76 children hospitalized for bilateral myringotomy with tube insertion (M&T) and 76 control subjects matched by age, gender, and season of admission for a general surgical procedure.[62] Results showed a nearly fourfold increase in the risk of persistent MEE in children who had atopic symptoms for more than 15 days per month. In another study, Bernstein and Reisman determined the allergy status of a group of 200 children who had undergone one or more M&T procedures.[63] These workers diagnosed allergy in 23% of the entire group but found that the frequency was 35% among the 88 children with multiple myringotomies with tube insertions. The frequency of allergy in these patients was higher than that reported for children of similar age in the general population. The foregoing studies generally found a higher frequency of OME in allergic children than in age-matched nonallergic children, as well as higher frequencies of allergy in children with OME than in children without OME.

Immunocompetence

Children with recurrent otitis media as well as other recurrent infections may have a defect in the immune system such as a defect in phagocyte function, humoral immunity, local immunity, or other immune defects.[8] Children infected with the human immunodeficiency virus (HIV) demonstrate a significantly higher recurrence rate than in normal children or children who have seroconverted.[64]

Cleft Palate/Craniofacial Abnormality

Otitis media is considered "universal" in infants younger than 2 years of age with unrepaired cleft palate.[65] After surgical repair of the palate, the occurrence of otitis media is reduced, probably because of improvement in eustachian tube function. However, many children continue to have problems up into the teens. Otitis media also is common in children with other craniofacial abnormalities or Down syndrome, also due to anatomic or functional eustachian tube abnormalities.[66] In children with Down syndrome, low resistance of the tube, in addition to poor active eustachian tube function, predisposes them to reflux of nasal secretions into the middle ear.[67]

Genetic Predisposition

The frequency of the occurrence of one episode of otitis media is so high that a genetic predisposition is highly unlikely. However, a predisposition to recurrent episodes of otitis media and chronic MEE may have a significant genetic component. The etiology of otitis media is multifactorial, involving environmental as well as genetic factors. A large number of genes may be involved, each contributing to a particular increase in disease risk.

Twin and triplet studies have been used to assess the heritability of otitis media. Two retrospective studies using questionnaires have been published. The first study, using 2750 Norwegian twin pairs, estimated the heritability at 0.74 in females and 0.45 in males.[68] In the second study, the estimated heritability was, on average, 0.57 at the ages of 2, 3, and 4 years.[69] In a prospective twin-triplet study from Pittsburgh with monthly assessments of middle ear status, the heritability estimate for otitis media at age 2 years was 0.79 in females and 0.64 in males.[70] Heritability is a population statistic used to ascertain if a trait is heritable, and linkage and association studies may identify genetic regions or specific genes influencing the particular trait or disease. Daly and coworkers, using genome-wide linkage analysis, have suggested that chromosomal regions on 19q and 10q contain genes contributing to the susceptibility to chronic OME or recurrent AOM.[71] Subsequent fine mapping of both regions further strengthened the evidence for this linkage.[72] In addition, evidence for an association between polymorphisms in *FBXO11*, the human homolog of a mouse model gene for chronic otitis media, and chronic OME/recurrent AOM (COME/ROM) has been reported.[73]

Environmental Factors

A study was conducted to assess the variation in environmental risk factors for otitis media across Western countries, including European countries, the United States, Canada, and Australia.[74] The main risk factors for otitis media were day care atendance, number of siblings, tobacco smoke exposure, breastfeeding, birth weight, socioeconomic status, and air pollution. However, the results indicated large variations in rates across the various countries: day care at ages 1 to 3 years: Sweden 75% versus Italy 6%; breastfed at 6 months: Norway 80% versus Poland 6%; and women smoking: Germany, France, and Norway 30% to 40% versus Portugal less than 10%.

Upper Respiratory Infection/Seasonality

Both epidemiologic evidence and clinical experience strongly suggest that otitis media frequently is a complication of an upper respiratory infection (URI). The incidence of AOM is highest during the fall and winter months and lowest during spring and summer months, which parallels the incidence of URI.[44] This correlation supports the hypothesis that an episode of URI plays an important role in the etiology of otitis media. Rhinovirus, RSV, adenovirus, and coronavirus have been detected in MEE during episodes of AOM.[21,75] Upper respiratory tract infections with RSV, influenzavirus, and adenovirus often precede an episode of AOM.[22] In a prospective study of Finnish children, 54% of ensuing AOM episodes were diagnosed by day 4 after the onset of URI symptoms.[76]

Day Care/Home Care/Siblings

Almost universally, day care center attendance remains a very important risk factor for development of otitis media. For example, prevalence of high negative ME pressure and flat tympanograms (type B), indicative of MEE, have been shown to be highest in children cared for in day care centers with many children, intermediate in children in family day care with fewer children, and lowest in children cared for at home.[77] Children attending day care centers also have been shown to be more likely to have tympanostomy tubes inserted than children cared for at home.[78]

Birth order has been shown to be associated with episodes of otitis media and percentage of time with MEE.[55] First-born children had a lower rate of episodes of AOM and less time with MEE during the first 2 years of life than children with older siblings. Also, having more than one sibling was significantly related to early onset of otitis media.[59]

The increased morbidity among children in day care centers and in children with older siblings may be related to the greater opportunity for exposure to viral URI, which may cause eustachian tube dysfunction, leading to the development of otitis media.

Tobacco Smoke Exposure

An association between otitis media and passive exposure to smoking has been reported by many investigators while others have not been able to demonstrate such an association. In most studies the information regarding smoke exposure has been obtained from the parents. A few recent studies have measured cotinine, a metabolite of nicotine, in blood, urine, or saliva of the child and have been able to more accurately determine the association between otitis media and smoke exposure.[43,79] More information about the pathogenesis and duration and intensity of exposure is needed to clarify this association. Two recent studies have shown an association between middle ear status and parental smoking. In children exposed to parental smoking, tympanostomy tubes stayed in place for 59 weeks, compared with 86 weeks in children who were not exposed to smoking.[80] Also, myringosclerosis was more prevalent in children with two smoking parents compared with those with no smoking parents (64% versus 20%) and maternal smoking was associated with a highly increased risk of recurrent otitis media after insertion of tympanostomy tubes.[81]

Breastfeeding/Bottle Feeding

Currently, most national and international authorities, including the American Academy of Pediatrics and the American Academy of Family Physicians, the World Health Organization (WHO), and the United Nations Children's Fund, recommend 6 months of exclusive breastfeeding. In 2004, Kramer and Kakuma published a comprehensive review of the world literature to determine health benefits of exclusive breastfeeding for 6 months compared with 3 to 4 months.[82] They reported a decrease in the risk for gastrointestinal infection even in developed areas. It had not been shown previously that exclusive breastfeeding for 6 months or longer compared with 4 to less than 6 months in the United States provided greater protection against respiratory infections. Therefore, a secondary analysis of data from the National Health and Nutrition Examination Survey III, a population-based cross-sectional home survey conducted from 1988 to 1994, was undertaken.[83] After adjustment for demographic variables, child care, and smoke exposure, the data revealed statistically significant increased risk for both pneumonia (odds ratio [OR]: 4.27; 95% confidence interval [CI]: 1.27-14.35) and three or more episodes of otitis media (OR: 1.95; 95% CI: 1.06-3.59) in those children breastfed 4 to less than 6 months. These findings further support the current recommendations that infants receive breast milk exclusively during the first 6 months of life.

Socioeconomic Status

Socioeconomic status and access to health care are factors that may affect the incidence of otitis media. It has been generally thought that otitis media is more common among persons in the lower socioeconomic strata as a result of poor sanitary conditions and crowding. Paradise and colleagues followed 2253 infants for 2 years in the United States and found an inverse relationship between the cumulative proportion of days with MEE and socioeconomic status.[84] However, many studies have not revealed any correlation between socioeconomic status of the child's family and the incidence of MEE.

Pacifier Use

Niemelä and associates reported that pacifier use increased the annual incidence of AOM and calculated that pacifier use was responsible for 25% of AOM episodes in children younger than 3 years.[85] They reported the results of an intervention trial in which parents in various well-baby clinics were taught that pacifier use was harmful and should be limited, and parents in other clinics were not provided with this information. This led to a 29% decrease in AOM in the group provided with pacifier information. Pacifier use has been theorized to contribute to the development of otitis media, possibly due to the sucking action of the child propelling nasopharyngeal secretions into the middle ear or by the pacifier acting as a fomite. However, Brook and Gober cultured the surface of pacifiers from children with AOM but found no pathogens typical of AOM.[86] The role of pacifier use in AOM remains unclear.

Obesity

Recent studies have indicated a possible association between otitis media and body mass index (BMI). Tympanostomy tube insertion and overweight were studied in two cohorts of children followed from birth to 2 years of age.[87] Weight-for-length and BMI-for-age were calculated using well-child visit data. In the cohort of predominantly white children, a history of tympanostomy tube insertion significantly predicted risk of BMI index beyond the 85th percentile at the age of 2 years. In the other cohort of American Indian children, a history of recurrent AOM increased the likelihood of weight-for-length index beyond the 95th percentile. Further studies are needed to clarify the association.

Prevention of Disease

Prevention and modification of risk factors and vaccine development are two recommended strategies for the prevention of disease.

Management of Environmental Factors

Promotion of breastfeeding in the first 6 months of life, avoidance of supine bottle feeding and pacifier use, and elimination of passive tobacco smoke may be helpful in reducing the risk of development of otitis media. Alteration of child care arrangements such that the child is exposed to fewer children may also be of benefit.

Vaccines

The three most common bacteria isolated from the middle ear are *S. pneumoniae*, *H. influenzae* and *M. catarrhalis*. At present, the *S. pneumoniae* vaccines (Pneumovax and Prevnar) are the only bacterial vaccines available for otitis media. Although respiratory viruses, such as RSV, influenzavirus, adenovirus, parainfluenza virus, and rhinovirus, have been isolated in MEE using PCR, influenza vaccine is the only available recommended viral vaccine today that may have an impact on otitis media.

Bacterial Vaccines

Streptococcus pneumoniae *Vaccine*

Pneumovax is a 23-valent polysaccharide vaccine that is not efficacious in children 2 years or younger because of poor antigen production in this age group. Prevnar is a conjugated vaccine in which pneumococcal polysaccharides are conjugated to a nontoxic mutant of diphtheria toxin. The 7-valent vaccine (PCV7), which includes serotypes 4, 6B, 9V, 14,18C, 19F, and 23F, was licensed for use in the United States in 2000 and recommended for use in children younger than 6 years of age by the American Academy of Pediatrics.[88] Infants are immunized at the ages of 2, 4, 6, and 12 to 15 months. For previously unimmunized children 7 to 23 months of age, a reduced number of doses is recommended, and for children 24 to 59 months of age and children at high risk at any age, two doses of PCV7 and one dose of the 23-valent vaccine are recommended.

The efficacy for AOM of the conjugated vaccine has been evaluated in several randomized clinical trials. The trial from Northern California Kaiser Permanente enrolling 37,868 children randomly assigned to either pneumococcal conjugate vaccine or a meningococcal type C conjugate vaccine and followed prospectively, reported an overall reduction of episodes of otitis media of 7%.[12] However, children with recurrent otitis media benefited from the vaccine with a reduction in otitis media episodes ranging from 9.3% to 22.8%, increasing as the frequency of episodes of AOM increased. In addition, immunized children were 20.1% less likely to require tube placement than control subjects. The PCV7 vaccine demonstrated a much higher efficacy (greater than 80%) in reducing invasive pneumococcal disease than in reducing the burden of otitis media. Additional follow-up of the study subjects continued to demonstrate a modest amount of protection against episodes of AOM and need for tympanostomy tube insertion.[89] In a Finnish study of 1662 children randomized to receive either PCV7 vaccine or a hepatitis B vaccine, with follow-up to the age of 24 months, a bacterial diagnosis was made based on a culture of the middle ear fluid, in addition to the clinical assessment of episodes of AOM.[13] The vaccine reduced the number of AOM episodes from any cause by 6%, the number of culture-confirmed pneumococcal episodes by 34%, and the number of episodes due to the vaccine serotypes by 57%. The number of episodes attributed to serotypes that were cross-reactive with those in the vaccine was reduced by 51%, whereas the number of episodes due to all other serotypes increased by 33%. The modest response in reducing number of episodes of AOM was due to a decrease in vaccine efficacy against serotype-specific infections as well as an increase in AOM episodes due to nonvaccine serotypes. A second trial was conducted in Finland using a 7-valent pneumococcal polysaccharide–meningococcal outer membrane protein complex conjugate vaccine (PncOMPC) in 1666 children who were followed for 24 months.[90] This trial showed no reduction in overall number of AOM episodes. The reduction in number of AOM episodes due to any culture-confirmed pneumococci was 25% and to vaccine serotype pneumococci, 56%—results similar to those with the PCV7. This vaccine failed to show protection against cross-reactive serotypes. An increased rate of carriage of nonvaccine serotypes was noted among infants vaccinated with the pneumococcal conjugate vaccine.

With use of the vaccine, pneumococcal colonization in the nasopharynx has changed as the vaccine has caused a reduction in the carriage rate of vaccine serotypes and replacement with nonvaccine serotypes.[17,91] It should be noted that a reduction in nasopharyngeal carriage of vaccine serotypes and an increase in nonvaccine serotypes has also been seen in children younger than 7 months of age.[16]

In the United States and Finland, the initial immunization with PCV7 is at age 2 months based on the results from the clinical trials. However, the question of whether or not the results obtained in the Finnish and U.S. trials could be extrapolated to older children who already had a history of recurrent episodes of AOM was addressed by Dutch and Belgian trials.[92,93] Seventy-eight and 383 children with documented histories of recurrent AOM were enrolled in the Belgian and Dutch studies, respectively. In both trials children between 1 and 7 years old were immunized at entry with PCV7 followed by a booster immunization with a 23-valent pneumococcal polysaccharide vaccine 7 months later and followed up for a total of 18 months in the Dutch trial and 26 months in the Belgian trial. The results from these two studies did not lend any support to the use of pneumococcal conjugate vaccine to prevent AOM in previously unvaccinated toddlers and children with a history of recurrent AOM. The differences in outcome between the studies in older children and those in healthy infants may be caused by differences in age at immunization. In the infant studies the PCV7 immunization may prevent or delay nasopharyngeal colonization of the most frequent pneumococcal serotypes and consequently delay pneumococcal episodes of AOM until a later age. In older children, who already are carriers of pneumococci, there is rapid replacement of pneumococcal vaccine serotypes with nonvaccine serotypes.

An 11-valent polysaccharide pneumococcal serotype vaccine conjugated to *H. influenzae*–derived protein D was evaluated in a clinical trial conducted in the Czech Republic enrolling a total of 4968 children, who were followed to the end of the second year of life.[94] Middle ear fluid was cultured when episodes of AOM were diagnosed. The vaccine reduced the overall incidence of AOM episodes by 33.6%. Vaccine efficacy was 57.6% for episodes of AOM caused by pneumococcal serotypes included in the vaccine and 66% for vaccine-related cross-reactive pneumococcal serotypes. There was no significant change in number of AOM episodes due to other nonvaccine serotypes. Of great interest is that there was 35.3% efficacy against AOM episodes caused by nontypeable *H. influenzae*. These results indicate that using the *H. influenzae*–derived protein D as a protein for conjugation of pneumococcal polysaccharides not only allowed for protection against pneumococcal otitis, but also against otitis media due to nontypeable *H. influenzae*. The use of the *H. influenzae*–derived protein D and the two additional pneumococcal serotypes probably explains the 33.6% reduction in numbers of all types of AOM episodes by the vaccine, which is significantly better than in the previously mentioned trials.[12,13]

Maternal Immunization

Infants immunized with PCV7 are unlikely to elicit protective serum antibody concentrations during the first 4 to 6 months of life, when recurrent AOM begins. Maternal immunization with pneumococcal vaccine is another approach that is currently being studied in animals as well as in humans.[95,96] A randomized clinical trial was conducted to evaluate the immunogenocity and reactogenicity of the 23-valent pneumococcal polysaccharide vaccine among pregnant women in the Philippines. A significant rise in antibody to polysaccharides varying from 3.3- to 9.1-fold for individual serotypes between pre- and postvaccination was seen in the immunized mothers relative to that in the control subjects. The level of polysaccharide-specific antibody in cord blood was also significantly higher in the immunized group, indicating transfer from mother to infant to provide enhanced protection. Adverse reactions were mild and required no treatment. Healy and Baker, reviewing the subject of maternal vaccination, found strong evidence that maternal immunization would be a feasible approach, particularly for providing early protection to children at high risk.[97] The main concerns with maternal immunization appear to be the fear of risk of birth defects.

Haemophilus influenzae *Vaccine*

Because nontypeable *H. influenzae* is the second most common bacterial pathogen isolated from middle ear fluid in AOM, much effort has been channeled into developing an effective vaccine. Many different approaches using animal models have been used to develop vaccine antigens for nontypeable *H. influenzae*–induced otitis media, including the following proteins: outer membrane protein (OMP) P5, 26, P2, P6, Htr protein, protein D, phosphorylcholine (ChoP), detoxified lipo-oligosaccharides (dLOSs), and type 1V Pili. For the first time, however, it was possible to demonstrate an effective *H. influenzae* antigen for otitis media in a clinical trial using an 11-valent vaccine with the pneumococcal capsular polysaccharides conjugated to protein D, an outer membrane protein of *H. influenzae*, as previously mentioned.[94] Although the efficacy was only 35.3%, the results indicate that it would be feasible to develop an effective vaccine for *H. influenzae*.

Moraxella catarrhalis *Vaccine*

Moraxella catarrhalis is considered the third most common bacterial pathogen isolated from the middle ear. Although the frequency of *M. catarrhalis* infections has previously been rather modest, recent studies have indicated that the frequency of nasopharyngeal colonization with *M. catarrhalis* in children with otitis media increased with the widespread use of the pneumococcal conjugate vaccine.[98] Therefore, for the greatest impact on reducing otitis media episodes, the development of a vaccine that contains *M. catarrhalis*, as well as *S. pneumoniae* and *H. influenzae* antigens, is necessary. Very little progress has been made in defining the protective immune response in *M. catarrhalis*. However, recently, protective immune responses to *M. catarrhalis* in adults with chronic obstructive pulmonary disease have been identified.[99,100] Candidate *M. catarrhalis* vaccine antigens that have been shown to induce potentially protective responses include outer membrane protein OlpA, CopB, filamentous hemagglutinin (FHA-like protein), and lipo-oligosaccharides (LOSs).

Viral Vaccines

Based on evidence regarding the role of viruses in the pathogenesis of AOM, the development of viral vaccines should be strongly promoted.[22] It should be recognized that bacterial vaccines only prevent the bacterial complications of a viral infection, while viral vaccines act at an earlier stage in the pathogenesis of AOM. Thus, viral vaccines have the potential to prevent viral upper respiratory infections, thereby potentially preventing the development of AOM as a complication of bacterial colonization of the nasopharynx.

Influenza Vaccine

The only commercially available viral vaccine today used for prevention of otitis media is the influenza vaccine, which is recommended for all children 6 to 59 months of age and older children with high-risk conditions by the American Academy of Pediatrics.[101] Currently, two types of influenza vaccine are available. Trivalent inactivated influenza vaccine (TIV) contains killed viruses and is given intramuscularly to children 6 months and older and adults. Live-attenuated influenza vaccine (LAIV) contains live virus, is given intranasally, and currently is licensed by the U.S. Food and Drug Administration (FDA) for healthy persons 2 through 49 years of age.

A prospective study in children 13 years or younger was conducted during two respiratory seasons in Finland.[102] The average annual rate of influenza was highest (179 cases/1000 children) among children younger than 3 years of age. AOM developed as a complication of influenza in 39.7% of children younger than 3 years. For every 100 influenza-infected children younger than 3 years, there were 195 days of parental loss of work (mean 3.2 days). The investigators concluded that vaccination of children younger than 3 years of age may be beneficial for reducing the direct and indirect costs of childhood AOM.

Two recent clinical trials have addressed the efficacy of inactivated influenza vaccine in preventing otitis media. Hoberman and coworkers conducted a randomized double-blind, placebo controlled 2-year clinical trial in 786 children 6 to 24 months of age in Pittsburgh, Pennsylvania.[103] The investigators did not identify any significant reduction in the burden of AOM from administration of inactivated trivalent influenza vaccine. However, in the first year of the study, the efficacy of the vaccine against culture-confirmed influenza was 66%, whereas in the second year of the study the efficacy was −7%. The low efficacy rate in the second year may be explained by the fact that the attack rate of influenza virus in the second year did not reach epidemic proportions, in contrast with the first year (3.3% versus 15.9% in the placebo group). The second study was single-blinded and evaluated the efficacy of inactivated influenza vaccine in preventing otitis media. The study was carried out in 119 children 6 to 60 months of age attending day care in Turkey. Efficacy rates for the vaccine against AOM, OME, and otitis media were 51%, 18%, and 18%, respectively.[104]

A multicenter study enrolled and randomly assigned 8475 children 6 to 59 months of age in a double-blind fashion to intranasal trivalent live-attenuated influenza vaccine or trivalent inactivated influenza vaccine intramuscularly to assess the efficacy and safety of the vaccines.[105] The live-attenuated vaccine was overall superior to the inactivated vaccine in preventing influenza episodes. There were 54.9% fewer cases of culture-confirmed influenza episodes in the group that received the live-attenuated vaccine ($P < 0.001$). The superior efficacy of the live-attenuated vaccine was observed for both antigenically well-matched and drifted viruses. Rates of wheezing and hospitalization were higher in the youngest children who received the live-attenuated vaccine than in those given the inactivated vaccine. In 2007 the FDA approved the use of this vaccine for children 2 years of age and older without a history of recurrent wheezing or asthma. Additional studies to assess the safety of the vaccine in the youngest children need to be done.

Respiratory Syncytial Virus Vaccine

The seriousness of RSV infection in infants and children and the need for an RSV vaccine are widely recognized. In addition to causing lower airway infections, the RSV virus is one of the major viruses contributing to the development of AOM.[75] Only live-attenuated vaccines have been investigated. Karron and associates developed a recombinant live-attenuated RSV vaccine that was attenuated in RSV-seropositive children and was well tolerated and immunogenic in RSV-seronegative children.[106] Further studies are needed to assess the clinical efficacy.

An alternative approach to preventing RSV infection is maternal immunization. Munoz and colleagues conducted a study to assess safety and immunogenicity of an RSV purified fusion protein 2 (PFP-2) subunit vaccine in 35 pregnant women in their third trimester and the effect on the offspring.[107] The infants were followed during their first RSV season. Seventy-five percent of the immunized infants had a response to the PFP-2 by Western blot analysis, compared with none of the control subjects. The transplacental transfer of vaccine-induced maternal antibodies was efficient, and no increase in frequency or severity of respiratory tract infections was observed in the immunized infants. The infants were born healthy, and no adverse events related to maternal immunization were documented.

Treatment

The treatment of otitis media involves medical and surgical therapies.

Acute Otitis Media

Observation

In an effort to reduce antibiotic use and stem increasing bacterial resistance, observation without use of antibiotics is listed as an option for selected children with AOM in the guidelines document published by the American Academy of Pediatrics and American Academy of Family Physicians in 2004.[108] Children for whom this is an option are to be selected on the basis of diagnostic certainty, age, illness severity, and access to medical care. Severe disease is defined as moderate to severe otalgia, fever with temperatures higher than 39° C (102° F) orally or 39.5° C rectally, or a toxic-appearing child. Children younger than 6 months of age should be treated with antibiotics regardless; children 6 to 23 months, if the illness is nonsevere, may be observed if the diagnosis is uncertain, but if AOM is certain or severe, the child should be treated with antibiotics; children 24 months or older may be watched if the diagnosis is uncertain or disease is nonsevere but treated if AOM is severe.

Already a popular method of management in several countries outside the United States, observation, or "watchful waiting," is predicated on the results of several earlier studies showing a high spontaneous cure rate for AOM.[109-114] Wald, however, cited problems with the earlier studies: The definition of AOM used in the various studies may have allowed for the inclusion of subjects with asymptomatic OME; children younger than 2 years of age were not included in some studies and were underrepresented in others; the sickest children often were not selected for these studies; and the antibiotic selected may have been inappropriate and the doses used were often insufficient, all of which would make the efficacy of antimicrobial treatment appear lower.[115] A meta-analysis of studies of AOM with an observation group found that children younger than 2 years of age and those with bilateral AOM were more likely to have prolonged symptoms when not given antimicrobial treatment.[116]

Nonetheless, the practice of not treating AOM immediately with antibiotics, often giving a "backup" prescription in case of persistence of symptoms, is undergoing further scrutiny in this country and elsewhere. McCormick and associates reported their randomized trial of immediate antibiotics plus symptom medication versus symptom medication only in 223 subjects with "nonsevere" AOM, of whom 57% were younger than 2 years of age.[117] At day 12, 69% of TMs and 25% of tympanograms were considered to be normal in the antibiotic group, compared with 51% of TMs and 10% of the tympanograms in the nontreated group; 66% of the watchful-waiting group completed the study without antibiotics. Nasopharyngeal cultures at day 12 of the study revealed that *S. pneumoniae* was eradicated in most of the antibiotic-treated subjects, but the strains that were cultured were more likely to be antibiotic-resistant. Parental satisfaction with the assigned "treatment" was the same in both groups. Spiro and associates randomly assigned children 6 months to 12 years of age diagnosed with AOM (definition left to discretion of physician) to receive either immediate antibiotic treatment or a "wait-and-see" prescription, to be filled if the child was not improving or was worse at 48 hours.[118] In this study, performed in an emergency department population, the mean age of subjects was 3.2 years; approximately 84% had unilateral AOM. The investigators found that 62% of the group given instructions to delay filling the prescription did not fill the prescription, compared with 13% given the instructions to start the medication immediately ($P < 0.001$). The presence of fever or otalgia was associated with filling the prescription.

Vernacchio and coworkers surveyed physicians in a national practice-based pediatric research network regarding their preferred management of AOM.[119] Despite the studies showing that the use of observation or delayed prescribing may allow for spontaneous recovery in many children and the option of observation was offered in the AOM guidelines, they found that although 83% considered observation a "reasonable option," it was used only in a median of 15% of cases.

Medical Treatment

Antibiotics

Many antibiotics are available, but according to American Academy of Pediatrics–American Academy of Family Physicians guidelines,[108] amoxicillin is still the first-line antibiotic for non-severe episodes of AOM and, at 90 mg/kg per day in two divided doses, is recommended to provide coverage for *S. pneumoniae*, including resistant strains. For severe episodes of AOM, amoxicillin–clavulanic acid (amoxicillin 90 mg/kg per day and clavulanic acid 6.4 mg/kg per day in two divided doses) is recommended and will provide coverage for beta-lactamase–producing *H. influenzae* and *M. catarrhalis*. According to these guidelines, cephalosporins should be considered as accepted first-line treatment only for patients with penicillin allergy. Macrolides should be prescribed for patients with penicillin and cephalosporin allergies. Treatment failure is defined as persistence or recurrence of symptoms and signs 48 to 72 hours after institution of initial treatment. In such cases, the diagnosis should then be reassessed and antibiotics started if not given previously or changed to a broader-spectrum agent if antibiotics were previously prescribed (amoxicillin–clavulanic acid if amoxicillin failed to produce improvement and ceftriaxone for 3 days if amoxicillin–clavulanic acid was not effective). Tympanocentesis should always be considered if the child does not respond to the antibiotic treatment, in order to identify the bacteria in the MEE and to select an appropriate antibiotic.

Duration of Treatment

Ten days of antibiotic treatment has been the standard, but in an effort to reduce cost and the incidence of antibiotic resistance, the efficacy of shorter courses has been investigated. Studies have found the 10-day course has resulted in fewer early treatment failures in younger children,[8] in children recently treated for AOM,[120] and in those presenting with spontaneous perforation of the TM,[121] compared with a 5-day course. The recent U.S. guidelines recommend the standard 10-day course of therapy for younger children and for children with severe disease, and for those 6 years of age and older with mild to moderate disease, a 5- to 7-day course may be used.[108] Several short courses of antibiotics have been approved by the FDA for use in AOM. Cefpodoxime proxetil and cefdinir have been approved for a 5-day course; azithromycin may be given for 1-, 3-, and 5-day courses; one dose of IM ceftriaxone may be given, although results for penicillin-resistant *S. pneumoniae* are better with a 3-day course.[122]

Longer courses of antibiotics have also been proposed. In a randomized, double-blind trial of 10 days of amoxicillin versus 20 days of amoxicillin or 10 days of amoxicillin with an additional 10 days of amoxicillin-clavulanate, no advantage in treatment failure or duration of MEE was found with the longer courses.[123]

Decongestants/Antihistamines

A meta-analysis of studies of decongestant-antihistamine preparations for AOM found no benefit of these agents for early cure, symptom resolution, or prevention of surgery or complications. Although some benefit of the combination was found in number of subjects with persistent AOM at the 2-week endpoint, the 5- to 8-fold risk of side effects, along with the fact that finding benefit was inversely correlated with study quality, led the authors to not recommend the routine use of decongestant-antihistamine agents for AOM.[124] In 1994, Chonmaitree and associates reported increased levels of histamine in middle ear fluid from children with AOM and speculated that antihistamine may be clinically beneficial in reducing inflammation.[125] However, in a recent trial for AOM, antihistamine administered with an antibiotic did not result in improved clinical outcome and prolonged the duration of effusion.[126] At this point, neither decongestants or antihistamines, nor their combinations, are recommended for the treatment of AOM.

Steroids

Studies in rats suggested that steroid given with antibiotic reduced inflammatory changes in the middle ear mucosa to a greater extent than treatment with antibiotic alone.[127] McCormick and coworkers found no reduction in histamine or leukotriene B4 in children treated with oral antibiotic and steroid compared with children receiving antibiotic alone but did find a lower rate of treatment failure during the first 2 weeks and a shorter duration for MEE in those treated with steroids.[128] When a larger sample of subjects was studied, however, the same group of workers found that corticosteroid (2 mg/kg given for 5 days) administered with antibiotic did not provide any improvement in clinical outcome.[126]

Recurrent Acute Otitis Media

Antibiotic Prophylaxis

Many studies have examined the efficacy of antibiotics in preventing AOM in children with frequently recurrent episodes. Many antibiotics have been studied, particularly amoxicillin and sulfisoxazole, used at one-half of their recommended daily dose and given once per day for months. Studies generally have concluded that antimicrobials are effective in preventing disease.[129] This method of managing children with recurrent AOM is not recommended, however, because of the potential for increasing resistant organisms. Rather than daily medicine given for months at a time, treating intermittently at the time of upper respiratory tract symptoms has been tried, but efficacy is less than with continuous medication.[130]

Surgical Treatment

Myringotomy/Tympanocentesis

For episodes of AOM, a myringotomy or tympanocentesis is helpful for relief of pain and allows samples to be obtained for culture to identify the pathogen and to guide in the selection of antibiotics, but provides no advantage in duration of effusion or recurrence of episodes of AOM.[111]

Myringotomy with Tympanostomy Tube Insertion

When preventive and medical treatments for recurrent AOM have failed, tympanostomy tube insertion is recommended. Two recent randomized studies have assessed the efficacy of tympanostomy tube insertion for recurrent AOM. A randomized clinical trial to evaluate the efficacy of myringotomy with tympanostomy tube insertion (M&T) versus sulfisoxazole prophylaxis versus placebo enrolled 65 children 4 years or younger with recurrent AOM and followed them for 6 months or longer.[131] Treatment failure was defined as two episodes of AOM or otorrhea in less than 3 months. Five of 22 children in the M&T group experienced treatment failure, compared with 12 of 20 children in the placebo group ($P = 0.02$) and 8 of 21 children in the prophylaxis group. In a similar study to determine the efficacy of amoxicillin prophylaxis versus M&T versus placebo, 264 children 7 to 35 months of age with recurrent AOM were randomized to one of the three treatment arms and followed for 2 years.[132] The average proportion of time with OM (AOM or otorrhea) was 10% in the amoxicillin, 15% in the placebo, and 6.6% in the tube groups (placebo versus tube; $P < 0.001$). Rates of new episodes of any type per child was 0.6 in the amoxicillin, 1.08 in the placebo, and 1.02 in the tube groups (amoxicillin versus placebo; $P < 0.001$). The low rate of new episodes must be viewed in light of the fact that the study subjects proved not to be at as high risk for AOM as had been anticipated. However, in comparison with children who received placebo, children with tympanostomy tubes spent less time with OM. It should be kept in mind that episodes of otorrhea with tympanostomy tubes usually are less severe, without fever and otalgia, and in most cases resolve with ototopical drops and do not require oral antibiotics.

For children with recurrent episodes of AOM, usually defined as three or more episodes of AOM in 6 months or four or more episodes in 12 months, insertion of tympanostomy tubes is an option.

Adenoidectomy with and without Tonsillectomy

Two parallel randomized clinical trials compared the efficacy of adenoidectomy and adenotonsillectomy in 461 children 3 to 15 years of age with persistent or recurrent otitis media who had not previously undergone tympanostomy tube placement.[133] Children without recurrent throat infections were randomized to undergo adenoidectomy, adenotonsillectomy, or no surgery (no adenoidectomy or adenotonsillectomy), and children with recurrent throat infections, to undergo adenotonsillectomy or no surgery. A majority of children (91%) had a history of recurrent AOM. The benefit of surgery in both trials was modest and limited mainly to the first follow-up year. The largest difference was in the three-way trial between adenotonsillectomy and no surgery, with a mean annual AOM rate of 1.4 versus 2.1 ($P < 0.001$) and mean estimated percentage of time with otitis media of 18.6% versus 29.9% ($P = 0.002$). Based on the short-term efficacy of adenoidectomy and adenotonsillectomy as well as the morbidity rate and cost of these procedures, it was suggested that neither should be considered as the initial surgical procedure.

In a randomized clinical trial assessing the efficacy of adenoidectomy versus placebo versus long-term antimicrobial prophylaxis in preventing episodes of recurrent AOM, 180 children 10 to 24 months of age were enrolled and followed for 24 months. No significant difference was observed between the groups in the numbers of episodes of AOM, visits to doctors, antibiotic prescriptions, and days with symptoms of respiratory infection. The investigators concluded that adenoidectomy cannot be recommended as the primary treatment in this age group.[134]

Hammarén-Malmi and colleagues conducted a clinical trial in children 12 to 48 months of age with recurrent AOM (three or more episodes in 6 months or five or more episodes in 12 months) to evaluate the efficacy of adenoidectomy in children receiving tympanostomy tubes.[81] The children were randomized to undergo tympanostomy tube insertion (i.e., bilateral myringotomy with tube insertion) with or without adenoidectomy. During the follow-up period of 12 months, the mean number of AOM episodes was 1.7 for children in the adenoidectomy plus tube insertion group, compared with 1.4 in children in the tube insertion–only group. Adenoidectomy at time of tympanostomy tube insertion does not significantly reduce the incidence of AOM in otitis-prone children younger than 4 years of age.

Adenoidectomy may provide modest improvement in children with recurrent AOM but is not recommended as a first-line procedure unless indicated for airway obstruction. Tonsillectomy, in conjunction with adenoidectomy, provides no significant advantage over adenoidectomy alone, and the risks outweigh the benefits.

Otitis Media with Effusion

Observation

For children not at risk for speech and language or learning disabilities, "watchful waiting" may be appropriate. Hearing testing should be done if MEE persists for 3 months or longer or at any time that language delay, learning difficulties or significant hearing loss is suspected. If the average hearing level is below 20 dB, watchful waiting is suggested, but if it is greater than 40 dB in the better ear, surgery is recommended. For children with hearing levels in the better ear between 21 and 39 dB, management is based on the duration of effusion and severity of symptoms. For children not at risk, examination at 3- to 6-month intervals until the fluid has resolved, hearing loss, language, or learning delays are identified or there are suspected structural abnormalities of the ear drum, is recommended.[108]

Medical Treatment

Decongestant/Antihistamine

Decongestant with or without antihistamine was a popular treatment for OME, but clinical trials found no efficacy of these medications.[135-138] In studies of OME at the Children's Hospital of Pittsburgh, no efficacy was found for an oral decongestant-antihistamine combination given either alone[139] or with an antimicrobial agent.[140]

Antibiotics

Antibiotics came into prominence as treatment for OME toward the end of the 1970s and beginning of the 1980s, when studies showed the ineffectiveness of decongestant-antihistamine combinations. In addition, although effusions were thought to be sterile, studies showed that specimens from asymptomatic children with MEE contained bacteria.[11,141] Mandel and associates reported the results of their double-blind, randomized trial in which 518 children with OME of varying durations were divided into three treatment groups: (1) amoxicillin (40 mg/kg/day) for 14 days plus a decongestant/antihistamine combination for 28 days; (2) amoxicillin for 14 days plus placebo for decongestant/antihistamine for 28 days, or (3) placebo for both amoxicillin and decongestant/antihistamine.[140] At 4 weeks, the rate of resolution of MEE was twice as high in those treated with amoxicillin, with or without a decongestant-antihistamine agent, as those who received placebo (percentages of effusion-free: 31.6%, 28.8%, and 14.1% in the amoxicillin plus decongestant-antihistamine, amoxicillin alone, and placebo groups, respectively); the addition of the decongestant-antihistamine made no difference. Recurrence of effusion occurred in most subjects within 3 months after completion of treatment. Other antibiotics, including amoxicillin-clavulanate, ceftibuten, and penicillin, have been tested in clinical trials to determine whether all antibiotics had the same efficacy, but none has been clearly shown to have any long-term advantage over the others.[142-144] Mandel and associates compared the efficacies of cefaclor and erythromycin-sulfisoxazole to that of amoxicillin.[145] Besides not being better than placebo, cefaclor and erythromycin-sulfisoxazole showed no increased efficacy at 2 and 4 weeks after starting treatment compared with amoxicillin. Antibiotic used in prophylactic doses (generally half the total daily dose used for AOM, given once daily for months) has also been examined in the treatment of OME, but its efficacy is linked more to preventing AOM than treating OME.[146] Despite short-term efficacy, antibiotics are not recommended for routine treatment of OME, due to lack of long-term efficacy, the high spontaneous cure rate, and concern about overuse of antibiotics.[129,147]

Steroids

Theoretically, glucocorticoids should be efficacious in the treatment of OME: Anti-inflammatory properties are due to inhibition of phospholipase A_2, which then inhibits formation of arachidonic acid and the subsequent synthesis of inflammatory mediators; up-regulation of transepithelial sodium transport promotes fluid removal from the middle ear; and decreasing mucin production by suppressing MUC5AC.[148] In clinical trials, systemic steroids have demonstrated an advantage over placebo in resolving MEE, but owing to the high recurrence rate after treatment, steroids are not recommended for long-term management.[149]

Because of the side effects with use of systemic steroid, especially for prolonged courses of treatment, other routes of administration have been investigated. Tracy and colleagues used prophylactic antibiotics with and without (both an untreated group and a placebo group) intranasal beclomethasone to treat 59 children with chronic OME and recurrent AOM.[150] Although all groups improved initially, no difference in OME resolution was observed by the 12-week visit. Cengel and Akyol found, in a nonblinded, randomized (every other subject assigned to active treatment with nasal mometasone spray for 6 weeks, with the remaining subjects assigned to no treatment) study of patients with documented MEE of at least 3 months' duration, 42.2% of treated subjects resolved at 6 weeks, compared with 14.5% of untreated subjects ($P < 0.001$); no long-term follow-up was reported.[151]

Autoinflation

Popularized by Politzer more than 100 years ago, devices to insufflate air through the eustachian tube have been tried for the treatment of OME. However, studies using a number of devices have failed to show consistent efficacy,[152-155] so autoinflation is not recommended for routine use at this time. In their meta-analysis, Perera and associates concluded that because of its low cost and absence of adverse effects, autoinflation might be considered for use while awaiting spontaneous resolution of the effusion.[155]

Surgical Treatment

Myringotomy

Myringotomy alone has been shown to be ineffective for long-term management and is not recommended for chronic OME.[156,157] Laser-assisted myringotomy has been described as an alternative to the standard myringotomy in children with chronic OME, and the procedure can be done using local anesthesia and is considered safe. However, the mean time to closure of the perforation is only 2 to 3 weeks.[158,159]

Myringotomy with Tympanostomy Tube Insertion

In children with persistent MEE, the decision of whether to insert tympanostomy tubes is based on the child's hearing status and risk for developmental problems. Several randomized clinical trials have demonstrated evidence-based indications for the use of tympanostomy tube insertion for chronic OME.

The efficacy of M&T for the management of OME has been the subject of many studies. Mandel and coworkers reported the results of a 3-year clinical trial of 109 children, 7 months to 12 years of age, with OME of 2 months' duration or longer who were unresponsive to medical management and who were randomly assigned to receive myringotomy alone, M&T, or no surgery.[160] During the first year, over 50% of subjects in the myringotomy-only and the no surgery groups met preset treatment failure criteria and underwent M&T. A second study designed to correct some of the design flaws of the first study and to extend the time until treatment failure involved 111 children with OME for at least 2 months and whose pure-tone averages bilaterally were 35 dB or less.[157] This study also found high rates of treatment failure in children in the myringotomy-only group (70%) and the no surgery group (56%). The percentages of time with MEE during the first year in the myringotomy-only, M&T, and no surgery groups were 61%, 17%, and 64%, respectively ($P < 0.001$). From these studies, it was concluded that myringotomy offered no advantage over no surgery in regard to percentage of time with effusion, number of AOM episodes, and number of repeat surgical procedures, and M&T provided more disease-free time and better hearing than myringotomy only or no surgery.

Gates and associates studied the effects of various surgical treatments in children 4 to 8 years of age with chronic OME; 127 children were randomly assigned to undergo myringotomy and 150 were assigned to undergo M&T.[156] Compared with myringotomy only, M&T provided less time with effusion and more time with better hearing, and necessitated fewer surgical retreatments.

The previously mentioned studies[157,160] were performed at a time when it was considered "unethical" to allow a child to have MEE for more than 2 to 3 months because of the associated hearing loss and the possible detrimental effects on speech and language development. A more recent study by Paradise and colleagues randomly assigned 429 children younger than 3 years of age with persistent or recurrent OME either to prompt M&T or to M&T up to 9 months later.[84] Eighty-five percent of children in the promptly treated group and 41% of children in the late treatment group had undergone M&T by 6 years of age. On developmental testing at 6 years, there were no significant differences between the groups on 30 measures. Of interest, in both the randomized clinical trial and in children randomly selected from those followed in the study but who did not meet criteria for randomization, sociodemographic variables seemed to be the most important factors influencing developmental outcomes.

Adenoidectomy

A study by Maw enrolling children 2 to 11 years of age with chronic OME showed that adenoidectomy alone and M&T alone provided better results than no surgery, but the combination of the two surgical procedures provided better results than either alone.[161] The addition of tonsillectomy to adenoidectomy provided no additional benefit for middle ear fluid resolution. In the previously discussed study by Gates and associates,[156] the children randomly assigned to the adenoidectomy-myringotomy and the adenoidectomy-M&T groups both had a lower percentage of time with effusion than those who received M&T alone. Thus, on the basis of these results, Gates and associates recommended adenoidectomy-myringotomy as the first-line procedure.[156]

Paradise and colleagues studied 213 children 1 to 15 years old with recurrent AOM or OME who had previously had M&T.[162] Children were randomly assigned to undergo adenoidectomy or no adenoidectomy; M&T was also performed at the same time for specific indications. Among the 99 subjects who were randomized, a significant reduction in time with otitis media during the first 2 years was observed in the children who underwent adenoidectomy, in comparison with those who did not. For the remaining children, whose parents chose not to allow random assignment, the results favored adenoidectomy over no adenoidectomy.

A clinical trial enrolling 98 children ranging in age from 24 to 47 months who had bilateral OME for 3 months or longer, or unilateral OME for 6 months or longer, or recurrence of effusion after extrusion of previously placed tympanostomy tubes, randomized the subjects to undergo M&T versus adenoidectomy and myringotomy with and without insertion of tubes.[163] Adenoidectomy with M&T provided no advantage over M&T alone (11.9% versus 18.1%; $P = 0.12$) in regard to mean percentage of time with MEE during the 18-month follow-up period. However, the mean percentage of time with MEE in the adenoidectomy-myringotomy alone group (35.7%) was significantly higher than in both the M&T and the adenoidectomy-M&T groups ($P < 0.001$ and $P = 0.003$, respectively). Also, in the adenoidectomy plus myringotomy group, 25% of the children subsequently needed an additional procedure (M&T), compared with less than 10% in the two groups with initial M&T.

Several retrospective studies have looked at the efficacy of adenoidectomy in addition to M&T. Boston and associates evaluated risk factors for additional tube insertion in 2121 patients undergoing bilateral M&T.[164] In 19.9% of the children, two or more tube insertions were performed. After the initial tube insertion, as many as 45.1% of the patients needed an additional surgical procedure (tube insertion, adenoidectomy, or tonsillectomy with or without adenoidectomy). Patients younger than 18 months at the initial procedure were significantly more likely to have a second procedure (26.3% versus 15.9%; $P < 0.001$). Adenoidectomy was performed at the time of the initial tube insertion in 527 patients (24.5%). This reduced the probability of needing a second set of tubes (0.08 versus 0.24; $P < 0.001$). Also, the probability of needing a third set of tubes was reduced when adenoidectomy was performed at or before placement of the second set of tubes (0.15 versus 0.40; $P < 0.001$). The presence of craniofacial abnormalities and a family history of adenoidectomy, tonsillectomy, or tube insertion increased the likelihood of need for subsequent tube insertions ($P < 0.001$). Sex and race were not risk factors for subsequent tube insertion.[164]

Another retrospective study evaluated the effect of adjuvant adenoidectomy or adenotonsillectomy at time of tympanostomy tube insertion on the rate of reinsertion of tubes and re-hospitalization for otitis media–related conditions in 37,316 Canadian children (≤19 years) for whom tube insertion was their first surgical procedure.[165] Compared with tube insertion alone, adenoidectomy was associated with a reduction in the likelihood of reinsertion of tubes (relative risk [RR]: 0.5; 95% CI: 0.5-0.6; $P < 0.001$), as was adenotonsillectomy (RR: 0.5; 95% CI: 0.5-0.6; $P < 0.001$). Performing adenoidectomy or adenotonsillectomy at the time of the initial tympanostomy tube insertion substantially reduced the likelihood of additional hospitalization and operations related to otitis media among children 2 years of age or older.

A third large retrospective study assessing the benefits of adjuvant pharyngeal surgery (adenoidectomy, adenotonsillectomy and tonsillectomy) at the time of tympanostomy tube insertion examined the records of 51,373 children less than 10 years of age.[166] Twenty-nine percent of the children had pharyngeal surgery at the time of the first tube insertion. The study authors concluded that having adenoidectomy or adenotonsillectomy at the time of first or subsequent tube insertion was associated with reduced risk of further tube insertion.

Guidelines

In 2004 a revised Clinical Practical Guidelines for OME was published jointly by the American Academy of Family Physicians, the American Academy of Otolaryngology–Head and Neck Surgery, and the American Academy of Pediatrics.[108] The guidelines were evidence-based, and the quality of the evidence was assessed. The recommendations reflected the quality of the evidence and the balance between benefit and harm that is anticipated when recommendations are followed. The guidelines apply to children 2 months through 12 years of age with and without developmental disabilities or underlying conditions that predispose to OME and its sequelae. The decision regarding surgery for OME depends largely on hearing status, associated symptoms, the child's developmental risk, and the anticipated chance of timely spontaneous resolution of the effusion. Surgical candidates are children with (1) OME lasting 4 months or longer with persistent hearing loss or other signs or symptoms; (2) recurrent or persistent OME associated with increased risk of developmental problems regardless of hearing status; and (3) OME and structural damage to the TM or middle ear.

Tympanostomy tube insertion is the initial preferred procedure. Adenoidectomy should not be performed except for a specific indication (i.e., nasal obstruction, chronic adenoiditis). Repeat surgery consists of adenoidectomy plus myringotomy with or without tympanostomy tube insertion. Tonsillectomy alone or myringotomy alone should not be used to treat OME.

Quality of Life Assessment

The first validated quality of life (QOL) outcome study for otitis media used the OM-6 instrument developed by Rosenfeld and associates, representing six domains: physical stress, hearing loss, speech impairment, emotional distress, activity limitation, and caregivers' concerns.[167] Large, moderate, and small improvements after tympanostomy tube insertion were documented in 56%, 15%, and 8% of children, respectively, using this instrument.[168] Trivial changes were noticed in 17% of children and 4% of children had a poor outcome after tube insertion. The results indicate that tympanostomy tube insertion produces large short-term improvement in QOL for most children.

A QOL outcome study assessed the parents' appreciation of their child's general condition using the OM-6 scale before, after, and retrospectively before tube insertion in a group of Dutch children 12 to 36 months of age.[169] The results from the retrospective assessment of the child's general condition prior to tube insertion indicated that the parents underestimated the effects of otitis media before surgery. In particular, after tube insertion, parents were able to appreciate the extent of presurgical hearing loss.

Surgical Issues

Tympanostomy Tube Placement

Rationale

Myringotomy and tympanostomy tube insertion is currently the most common surgical procedure in children that requires general anesthesia. Insertion of a tympanostomy tube promotes ventilation of the middle ear and drainage through both the eustachian tube and the tympanostomy tube. Also the aeration of the middle ear may promote normalization of the middle ear mucosa. The removal of MEE restores the conductive hearing loss. However, reflux of nasopharyngeal secretions may occur in an ear with a tympanostomy tube, causing otorrhea due to loss of the middle ear air cushion effect.

Procedure

In most children insertion of tympanostomy tubes is performed under general mask anesthesia. In older children who are cooperative tympanostomy tube insertion could be performed using topical anesthesia such as phenol or lidocaine delivered by iontophoresis.

The procedure should be performed using a binocular operating microscope. After satisfactory removal of cerumen and debris the entire TM should be inspected to rule out any abnormalities. The myringotomy incision is performed in the anterior-superior or anterior-inferior quadrant of the pars tensa. A radial incision is made small enough to prevent premature tube extrusion but large enough that the tube can be easily inserted using an alligator forceps. If MEE is present, it should be aspirated. When the effusion is purulent or mucopurulent, it should be aspirated into a Juhn trap or Alden-Senturia trap and sent for culture (Fig. 194-5). If the MEE is too thick to be aspirated through the myringotomy incision with a large suction tip, a counterincision is

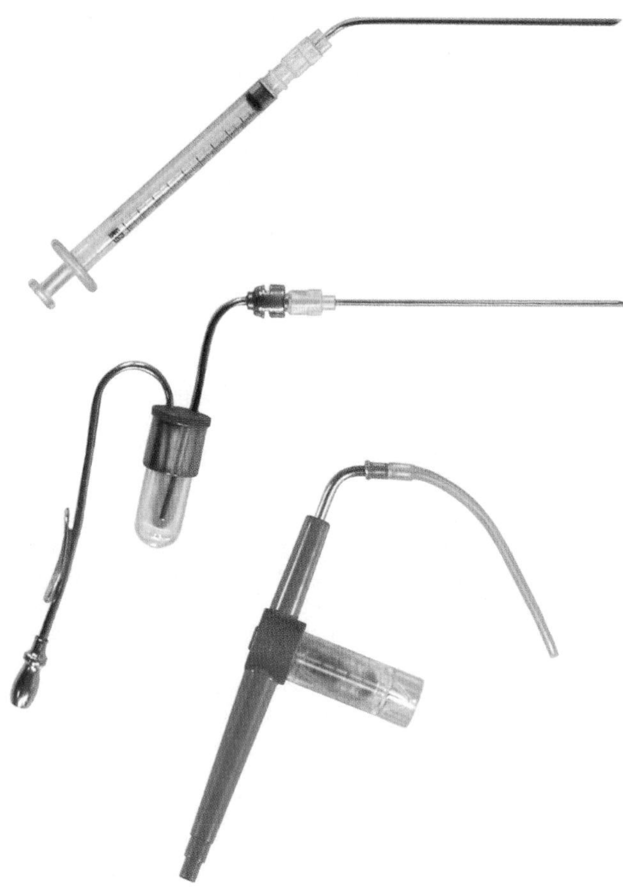

Figure 194-5. Collection vehicles for aspiration of middle ear effusions. *Top to bottom*: Syringe with spinal needle; Alden Senturia trap; Juhn Tym-Tap.

made in the inferior part of the tympanic membrane or sterile saline is placed in the canal or through the myringotomy to enhance the aspiration of the viscous fluid. There is still controversy regarding the best place to insert the tympanostomy tube. The anterosuperior quadrant is associated with a longer clincial tube life; however, a persistent perforation in that area is somewhat more difficult to repair.

Selection of Tympanostomy Tubes and Indications

Many different tympanostomy tubes have been developed, but most tympanostomy tubes are variations of the grommet or the T-tube. The duration of time before extrusion is shorter for grommet tubes than for T-tubes. Weigel and associates performed a randomized prospective trial of four different types of tympanostomy tubes in 75 children.[170] During the first 2 years, 93% of Shepard tubes, 80% of Armstrong tubes, 66% of Reuter-Bobbin tubes, and 31% of Goode T-tubes had extruded. In studies from Pittsburgh, the clinical life of the Armstrong-type tube was approximately 1 year; 50% had extruded by 12 months, and 75% by 18 months.[157] The time to extrusion is a function of the size, shape of the medial flange, absence of a lateral flange, and the material of the tube. Also, the coating of the tube may affect the time to extrusion, because it may prevent infections.[171,172]

In a young child with a history of recurrent or persistent otitis media, a tympanostomy tube that remains in place for at least a year is preferable. If the child has recurrent otitis media after the tubes have become nonfunctional or extruded, a similar type of tube should be recommended. Grommets with shorter duration are recommended in older children, who may not continue to have problems after the then current season. T-tubes or long-term tubes are recommended for older children with persistent problems due to poor eustachian tube function. These tubes also are recommended for children who have an atrophic TM after going through multiple sets of tympanostomy tubes, because a regular grommet tube may be very quickly extruded.

Perioperative and Postoperative Ototopical Drops

In an effort to reduce early postoperative otorrhea and tube blockage, use of ototopical antimicrobial drops at the time of surgery has been recommended, especially if MEE is present.[173,174] Only FDA-approved ototopical agents such as ofloxacin (Floxin) and ciprofloxacin (Ciprodex) should be considered.

Postsurgical Follow-up

All patients should return for a follow-up visit a few weeks after the surgery for an otoscopic examination to assess the status of the tympanostomy tube. Patients with a hearing loss documented preoperatively should have a repeat hearing evaluation postoperatively. Patients who did not have a preoperative hearing test should be examined postoperatively to document that the hearing is normal. Patients usually are evaluated 6 to 12 months after the insertion of the tubes and every 6 months thereafter, or when problems occur, to assess the status of the tubes and the TM.

Complications and Sequelae

Otorrhea

Otorrhea through a tube or perforation is a common problem after tympanostomy tube insertion and has been recorded in as many as 50% of children with tympanostomy tubes.[175] Transient otorrhea occurred in the postoperative period in 16% (range, 8.8 to 42.0) and later in 26% (range, 4.3 to 68.2) of patients; recurrent otorrhea occurred in 7.4% (range, 0.7 to 19.6), and chronic otorrhea in 3.4% (range, 1.4 to 9.9) of patients.[176] If untreated, acute otorrhea can develop into chronic suppurative otitis media. Pathogens typical of AOM (*S. pneumoniae, H. influenzae, M. catarrhalis,* and *S. pyogenes*) were found in 42% and *P. aeruginosa* and *S. aureus* in 44% of all episodes of acute otorrhea in 246 children with tympanostomy tubes followed prospectively.[175] The typical AOM pathogens were more common in children under 6 years of age than in older children (50% versus 4.4%; $P < 0.001$). *P. aeruginosa* was more common in children 6 years of age or older than in the younger children (43.5% versus 20.5%; $P = 0.052$). Roland and colleagues obtained 1309 isolates from 956 acutely draining ears and identified *S. pneumoniae* in 17%, *H. influenzae* in 18%, *S. aureus* in 13%, *P. aeruginosa* in 12%, and fungus in 5%.[177] Several clinical trials have demonstrated that ototopical agents such as ofloxacin otic solution and ciprofloxacin-dexamethasone otic suspension are effective when acute otorrhea occurs through a tympanostomy tube or perforation, even when no systemic antibiotic is given.[178] In a child who has severe systemic symptoms, a systemic antibiotic should be added. The ciprofloxacin-dexamethasone combination has been shown to be superior to ofloxacin in resolving granulation tissue.[179] The use of other ototopical agents in ears with a nonintact TM has not been approved by the FDA, because they can be ototoxic, especially those that contain aminoglycoside. If the drainage does not resolve in 7 to 10 days, suctioning of the ear canal should be performed and a culture specimen from the opening of the tube should be obtained to determine the causative pathogen. If yeast is the predominant organism, treatment with a topical antifungal drop such as clotrimazole should be initiated. Repeated aural toilet is a very important part of the treatment. Compliance with a regimen of frequent suctioning may be difficult for both the child and the parent, however. If aural toilet and topical treatment fail to produce improvement and the organisms are not sensitive to oral antibiotics, then intravenous antibiotics, removal of the tube(s), or simple mastoidectomy should be considered. CT scan of the temporal bones should be obtained before possible mastoidectomy, to look for complications such as coalescent mastoiditis. In older children with recurrent episodes of otorrhea, removal of the tubes is the treatment of choice, because in these children the eustachian tube may have matured and secretion from the nasopharynx may be refluxing into the middle ear. Also, the tube occasionally may act as a foreign body, causing a foreign body reaction with granulation tissue formation and infections.

Recently, biofilms were identified on a tympanostomy tube removed from a child with a chronic draining ear.[180]

Tympanosclerosis, Atrophy, and Retraction Pockets

A meta-analysis reviewing 134 articles estimated the incidence of TM sequelae after tube extrusion and reported that tympanosclerosis occurred in 32% (range, 7.2 to 64.3), focal atrophy in 25% (range, 1.6 to 75.0), and retraction pockets in 3.1% (range, 0 to 22.7) of ears.[176] The type of tube (short-term versus long-term) had no significant impact on these rates.

The sequelae of tympanostomy tube insertion in children with chronic OME followed for 8 years was reported by Daly and associates.[181] One hundred thirty-eight children (275 ears) followed for 3 years and 84 of these children (167 ears) followed for 8 years were evaluated in regard to TM myringosclerosis, atrophy, retraction pockets or perforations, hearing loss, and static admittance. In general, the annual incidence of sequelae was greater at the 4- to 5-year follow-up than at the 6- to 8-year follow-up. Although atrophy developed in 67% of the ears, myringosclerosis in 40%, and perforation in 3% between the 3- and 8-year follow-up evaluations, the annual risk of new sequelae declined considerably throughout the 3- to 8-year follow-up period for most sequelae studied. However, atrophy and pars tensa or pars flaccida retraction were present in 55% of ears at the 8-year follow-up evaluation, which may put children at risk for continuing middle ear problems during adolescence and adulthood. These results support the need for long-term follow-up in selected patients.

In reporting the incidence of TM abnormalities in children in the previously cited trial[84] of prompt versus delayed tube insertion, Johnston and associates noted that in children who underwent intubation, segmental atrophy and tympanosclerosis at age 5 years were more common than in children who did not receive tubes.[182] These workers found no significant relationship between hearing levels at 6 years of age and the presence or type of TM abnormalities.

Persistent Perforation

The incidence of persistent perforation after extrusion of tympanostomy tubes has been estimated at 4.8% (for short-term tubes, 2.2% [range, 0 to 12.3%]; for long-term tubes, 16.6% [range, 0 to 47.0%]).[176] Also, long-term tubes increased the relative risk of perforation by 3.5 (95% CI: 2.6 to 4.9) over that for short-term tubes. The perforations caused by tympanostomy tubes usually are small; consequently, hearing loss is very mild. The perforations are easily managed with a simple fat graft or surgical gel (Gelfoam), paper patch, or Steri-strip myringoplasty. Sckolnick and associates recently found that the success rate with Gelfoam myringoplasty was higher than with fat graft or paper patch.[183] Before closing the perforation, it is important to ensure that eustachian tube function is good; otherwise, there is a risk of nonclosure or reaccumulation of fluid in the middle ear. As a rule, the TM in the opposite ear should be intact and free of infection for 1 year.

Cholesteatoma

For all types of tubes, the combined incidence of cholesteatoma is 0.7%, but for short-term tubes, the incidence is 0.8% (range, 0 to 6.5) and for long-term tubes 1.4% (range, 0 to 3.0).[176] Any of several mechanisms may be responsible for the development of cholesteatomas. Tympanostomy tubes may be inserted to prevent the development of cholesteatoma in a retraction pocket. However, cholest atoma may result from ingrowth or transplantation of keratinized epithelium into the middle ear cleft around a tympanostomy tube. Also, an intratympanic cholesteatoma may develop after surgical manipulation of the TM. Patients with tympanostomy tubes require regular follow-up during the time the tubes are in place and after extrusion to assess the TM and middle ear for cholesteatoma development.

Early Extrusion

Premature extrusion of tubes occurs in approximately 3.9% of ears.[176] This is most likely due to infection in the middle ear that pushes the tube into the external ear canal. The tube may not have been properly inserted, especially if the TM is thickened owing to an infection at the time of tube insertion. An atrophic TM also may allow early tube extrusion.

Tube Blockage

The lumen of the tympanostomy tube may become obstructed from dried blood or mucus, granulation tissue or a polyp caused by infections in the middle ear. The incidence of plugging of the tube is 6.9% (range, 0 to 37.3) of ears.[176] The tube sometimes can be unplugged using a pick, suction, a Rosen needle or ototopical drops for 10 to 14 days. If the blockage cannot be resolved but the middle ear is effusion-free with normal middle ear pressure, the tube can be left in place and watched until extrusion. On the other hand, if fluid has accumulated in the middle ear or recurrent infections continue, replacement of the tube may be indicated.

Tube Displacement into the Middle Ear

The incidence of displacement of a tympanostomy tube into the middle ear is 0.5% (range, 0 to 1.3).[176] It occurs most commonly at the time of surgery, but it can also be seen later due to infection or trauma, which is very rare. If the tube is displaced into the middle ear during surgery, attempts should be made to retrieve the tube at the time of surgery. However, if a tube is visualized behind an intact TM, risks versus benefits have to be assessed, because a child would require general anesthesia and an incision of the TM to retrieve the tube. A tympanostomy tube displaced behind an intact TM rarely causes problems.

Retained Tympanostomy Tubes

A tympanostomy tube usually is not removed surgically, because most tubes extrude spontaneously. In some children, however, the tube remains in place in the TM and has to be removed surgically. Indications for removing a tympanostomy tube include the following clinical scenarios:

- Retention of one tube after extrusion of the other tube if the middle ear has been free of disease for 1 year or longer in a child 5 to 6 years old or older
- Bilateral retained tubes in an older child with good eustachian tube function
- Chronic or recurrent episodes of otorrhea that are not able to be managed medically, especially in an older child who previously has not had recurrent episodes of otorrhea, because this could be a sign of reflux of secretions from the nasopharynx due to maturation of the eustachian tube
- Blockage of a tympanostomy tube that has become embedded in granulation tissue

In children, most retained grommet, short-term tubes usually are removed with the patient under general anesthesia. After the tube has been removed, a paper patch or Gelfoam myringoplasty is performed. Soft long-term T-tubes may be removed in the office in older cooperative children. In these children, follow-up is esssential to see if the perforation closes spontaneously or requires myringoplasty.

Water Precautions

Several studies have been published, including two meta-analyses[184,185] demonstrating no increase in episodes of otorrhea in patients with tympanostomy tubes not using water precautions over the number of episodes of otorrhea in those using water precautions. In a clinical trial to assess the need for water precautions after insertion of tympanostomy tubes, 201 children, 6 months to 6 years of age, were randomized to swimming and bathing with and without ear plugs and evaluated monthly for 1 year and whenever an episode of otorrhea occurred.[186] At least one episode of otorrhea was documented in 47% of children who used ear plugs, compared with 56% in children with no ear plugs ($P = 0.21$). The mean rate of otorrhea per month for children who used ear plugs was 0.07, versus 0.10 for children not using ear plugs ($P = 0.05$). Although children who do not use ear plugs have a higher incidence of episodes of otorrhea, the clinical impact of using ear plugs is small, and their use should be individualized, rather than recommended on a routine basis.

A clinical survey was conducted in the Pacific Northwest to determine the recommendations given to parents and patients regarding water precautions for swimming with tympanostomy tubes.[187] A total of 263 physicians returned the survey (23.5% response rate). As indicated by the survey findings, most primary care physicians (83%) and approximately one half of the otolaryngologists (47%) still recommend water precautions for swimming with tympanostomy tubes.

Adenoidectomy

Rationale for Adenoidectomy

The rationale for removal of the adenoids in children with otitis media is that the enlargement of the adenoids may cause obstruction of the nasopharynx and blockage of the eustachian tube, preventing ventilation of the middle ear–mastoid system.[188] Also, the adenoid tissue in children with otitis media has been found to have increased bacterial colonization, which may predispose to recurrent infections.[189] Coticchia and associates have demonstrated that the adenoids are covered with biofilm, which may act as a reservoir for bacteria causing middle ear disease.[20] This may explain the clinical improvement obtained after mechanical débridement of the adenoids. The effect of adenoidectomy for children with otitis media is independent of the size of the adenoids.[156,162]

Procedure

Adenoidectomy requires general anesthesia accomplished by either endotracheal intubation or laryngeal mask anesthesia (LMA) and is performed using many different techniques, including curettage, electocautery, microsurgical débridement, or coblation to remove the midline adenoid tissue. The adenoidectomy is completed when the choanae are completely opened and the nasopharynx has a smooth, level contour. Care should be taken to avoid injury to the torus tubarius, which may potentially result in stenosis and eustachian tube dysfunction. In children with submucous cleft palate without airway obstruction, adenoidectomy is not recommended for otitis media because of the risk of velopharyngeal insufficiency. If obstruction exists, partial superior adenoidectomy should be performed, leaving an inferior strip of adenoid tissue for palate closure. Other complications include bleeding, respiratory distress, and atlantoaxial subluxation, which are rare.

Complications and Sequelae of Otitis Media

Complications and sequelae of otitis media are *intratemporal* (extracranial, i.e., temporal bone or neck) or *intracranial* (within the cranial cavity). The intracranial complications are rare in developed countries but are still common in developing nations.

A judicious approach to the use of antimicrobial therapy, including observation without antimicrobials for AOM, has been promoted by guidelines in many different countries owing to the development of increased bacterial resistance to the most common antibiotics. However, delaying antimicrobial therapy may increase the risk for development of complications. Schilder and coworkers compared the national prescription rate of antibiotics for AOM and the national incidence rate of acute mastoiditis across countries.[190] The study showed a slightly higher incidence rate of acute mastoiditis in children (i.e., approximately 4 per 100,000 person–years) in the Netherlands, where only 31% of patients with AOM receive antibiotics, as compared with 2 per 100,000 person-years in the United States, where almost all cases of AOM are treated with antibiotics. More recent studies have shown that use of antibiotics to treat AOM in children may not influence the subsequent development of acute mastoiditis.[191] Also, there is no difference in the proportion of pediatric mastoiditis caused by *S. pneumoniae* in the preconjugated pneumococcal vaccine era versus the postvaccine era.[192]

Intratemporal Complications

The intratemporal complications of otitis media include hearing loss, vestibular and balance problems, acute perforation of the TM, mastoiditis, petrositis, labyrinthitis, and facial paralysis. The intratemporal sequelae include chronic suppurative otitis media, atelectatsis of the middle ear, adhesive otitis media, cholesteatoma, cholesterol granuloma, tympanosclerosis, and ossicular discontinuity and fixation with hearing loss.

Hearing Loss and Balance Problems

Most children with MEE have hearing loss that can be fluctuating or persistent. It usually is a mild to moderate conductive loss averaging between 20 and 30 dB.[193] Rarely, a permanent sensorineural hearing loss may result from AOM or OME, possibly as a result of spread of the infection through the round or oval window or a suppurative complication. Behavioral hearing thresholds in the high frequencies (12 to 20 kHz) are significantly higher in children with a history of otitis media when the middle ear was effusion free.[194]

During an episode with MEE, balance and vestibular function seem to deteriorate, and when the effusion resolves or tympanostomy tubes are inserted, these functions improve.[55] Also, children with otitis media may be more visually dependent as a result of the deterioration of vestibular function causing excessive reliance on other nonvestibular sensory cues to maintain balance.[195] Children may have delayed development of motor coordination skills, such as walking or manipulating their environment; the resultant "clumsiness" may make them more accident-prone. Stenström and Ingvarsson reported that Swedish otitis-prone children were seen more often in the orthopedic and general surgery departments compared with children who were not otitis-prone.[196]

Speech-Language and Child Development

Many studies have investigated the association between otitis media and child development. Some studies have found an association, whereas others have failed to do so. In a recent article, Paradise and coworkers reported that there was no difference between children with otitis media with early versus late tympanostomy tube insertion with regard to hearing, speech-language, and developmental testing.[197] As indicated in the OME Guidelines,[108] however, it is recommended that children with OME undergo hearing testing every 3 to 6 months and be assessed for tympanostomy tube placement if they are at risk for any developmental difficulties due to otitis media, such as significant speech delay.

Mastoiditis

Mastoiditis remains the most common suppurative complication of AOM. Mastoiditis without periosteitis or osteitis most likely represents a continuation of the middle ear inflammation as the mastoid air cell system is in continuity with the middle ear. In acute mastoiditis with periosteitis the infection has spread to the periosteum covering the mastoid process. The spread from the mastoid cells to the periosteum usually is through the mastoid emissary veins. In acute mastoiditis with osteitis with and without subperiosteal abscess the infection can cause destruction of the mastoid cells, leading to "coalescence" of the cells (i.e., mastoid empyema), and present as a subperiosteal abscess. The infection also may spread medially to the petrous bone (petrositis), the labyrinth (labyrinthitis), and neck (Bezold's abscess) and involve the facial nerve or extend into the intracranial cavity.

The diagnosis is made by physical examination and imaging studies such as CT scans and MRI. In the early stage, there are no specific signs and symptoms of mastoid infection with later progression to erythema and tenderness over the mastoid area, to edema or a subperiosteal abscess with displacement of the pinna inferiorly and anteriorly and obliteration of the postauricular crease. The CT scan in the early stage most frequently shows a cloudy mastoid; the inflammatory process may progress and develop into osteitis, with destruction of mastoid bone. Mastoiditis with and without periosteitis often responds to medical treatment and tympanocentesis or tympanostomy tube insertion, whereas mastoiditis with osteitis and bone destruction usually requires cortical mastoidectomy.

Intracranial Complications

The middle ear and the mastoid air cell system are close to the intracranial cavity, and infection can spread to the intracranial structures. Suppurative intracranial complications due to AOM include meningitis, epidural abscess, subdural empyema, focal otitic encephalitis, brain abscess, lateral sinus thrombosis, and otic hydrocephalus. These are serious conditions and potentially life-threatening. The signs and symptoms are persistent headache, lethargy, malaise, irritability, severe otalgia, fever, and nausea and vomiting, as well as signs of intracranial complications including stiff neck, focal seizures, ataxia, blurred vision, papilledema, diplopia, hemiplegia, aphasia, dysdiadochokinesia, intention tremor, cranial nerve deficits other than of the facial nerve, dysmetria, and hemianopia. Any child with an intracranial infection such as meningitis or brain abscess should be evaluated for middle ear disease.

Meningitis

Hematogenous spread is the most common route of spread of infection from the middle ear to the meninges. It also may occur by direct extension through a preformed pathway or retrograde thrombophlebitis. Meningitis as a complication of otitis media is treated with high doses of broad-spectrum antibiotics; the dose is then adjusted according to the cerebrospinal fluid (CSF) culture results. Tympanocentesis or tympanostomy tube insertion should be done urgently to obtain material for culture to identify the causative agent of the otitis media. Surgery such as cortical mastoidectomy or tympanomastoidectomy may be necessary when the patient is stabilized.

Subdural Abscess and Subdural Empyema

Subdural abscess usually results when cholesteatoma or infection destroys bone next to the dura and there is an accumulation of granulation tissue and purulent material. A subdural empyema is an accumulation of purulent material between the dura and the arachnoid membrane. Treatment consists of broad-spectum antibiotics as well as surgical drainage by a neurosurgeon and otolaryngologist.

Brain Abscess

An otogenic brain abscess can develop directly from an acute or chronic middle ear infection or from the development of an adjacent infection such as a lateral sinus thrombophlebitis, petrositis or meningitis. The diagnosis is based on presence of clinical signs and symptoms and on CT and MRI findings. The CSF may be culture-negative if the abscess is deep. Treatment includes broad-spectrum antimicrobial agents and surgical treatment of the primary focus. Treatment for the brain abscess may consist of only long-term parenteral antibiotic therapy.

Lateral Sinus Thrombosis

Lateral and sigmoid sinus thrombophlebitis arises from an adjacent mastoid infection in contact with the sinus wall through inflammation of the adventitia and is followed by penetration of the venous wall. A thrombus is formed after the infection has spread to the intima; the mural thrombus may become infected and may occlude the lumen. Embolization of the thrombus may cause additional disease. Treatment includes parenteral broad-spectrum antimicrobial agents; anticoagulants are recommended by some experts, but consensus is lacking on this issue. Surgical treatment may include tympanostomy tube insertion alone or with tympanomastoidectomy. There is also controversy regarding opening the lateral sinus and removing the thrombus or ligating the jugular vein in the neck if the patient experiences repeated episodes of formation of septic emboli.

SUGGESTED READINGS

American Academy of Family Physicians; American Academy of Otolaryngology–Head and Neck Surgery; American Academy of Pediatrics Subcommittee on Otitis Media with Effusion. *Pediatrics.* 2004;113(5):1412-1429.

For complete list of references log onto www.expertconsult.com.

American Academy of Pediatrics Committee on Infectious Diseases. Policy statement: recommendations for the prevention of pneumococcal infections, including the use of pneumococcal conjugate vaccine (Prevnar), pneumococcal polysaccharide vaccine, and antibiotic prophylaxis. *Pediatrics.* 2000;106(2 Pt 1):362-366.

American Academy of Pediatrics Committee on Infectious Diseases. Prevention of influenza: recommendations for influenza immunization of children, 2007-2008. *Pediatrics.* 2008;121(4):e1016-e1031.

American Academy of Pediatrics Subcommittee on Management of Acute Otitis Media. Diagnosis and management of acute otitis media. *Pediatrics.* 2004;113(5):1451-1465.

Auinger P, Lanphear BP, Kalkwarf HJ, et al. Trends in otitis media among children in the United States. *Pediatrics.* 2003;112(3):514-520.

Berman S, Lee B, Nuss R, et al. Immunoglobulin G, total and subclass, in children with or without recurrent otitis media. *J Pediatr.* 1992;121(2):249-251.

Bluestone CD. *Eustachian Tube: Structure, Function, Role in Otitis Media.* Hamilton, Ont: BC Decker; 2005.

Bluestone CD, Klein JO. *Otitis Media in Infants and Children.* 4th ed. Hamilton, Ont: BC Decker; 2007.

Bluestone CD, Rosenfeld RM, eds. *Surgical Atlas of Pediatric Otolaryngology.* Hamilton, Ont: BC Decker; 2002.

Bluestone CD, Stool SE, Alper CM, et al, eds. *Pediatric Otolaryngology.* 4th ed. Philadelphia: Saunders; 2003.

Casselbrant ML, Mandel EM, Kurs-Lasky M, et al. Otitis media in a population of black American and white American infants, 0-2 years of age. *Int J Pediatr Otorhinolaryngol.* 1995; 33(1):1-16.

Derkay CS, Carron JD, Wiatrak BJ, et al. Postsurgical follow-up of children with tympanostomy tubes: results of the American Academy of Otolaryngology–Head and Neck Surgery Pediatric Otolaryngology Committee National Survey. *Otolaryngol Head Neck Surg.* 2000;122(3):313-318.

Healy CM, Baker CJ. Prospects for prevention of childhood infections by maternal immunization. *Curr Opin Infect Dis.* 2006;19(3):271-276.

Kaiser Permanente Vaccine Study Center Group. *Pediatr Infect Dis J.* 2000;19(3):187-195.

Mandel EM, Casselbrant ML. Recent developments in the treatment of otitis media with effusion. *Drugs.* 2006;66(12):1565-1576.

Mandel EM, Rockette HE, Bluestone CD, et al. Efficacy of amoxicillin with and without decongestant-antihistamine for otitis media with effusion in children. *N Engl J Med.* 1987;316:432-437.

Post JC, Hiller NL, Nistico L, et al. The role of biofilms in otolaryngologic infections: update 2007. *Curr Opin Otolaryngol Head Neck Surg.* 2007;15:347-351.

Rosenfeld RM, Bluestone CD, eds. *Evidence-Based Otitis Media.* 2nd ed. Hamilton, Ont: BC Decker; 2003.

Infections and Inflammation

CHAPTER ONE HUNDRED AND NINETY-FIVE

Pediatric Chronic Sinusitis

Rodney P. Lusk

Key Points

- Pediatric sinusitis is of primarily infectious origin secondary to immaturity of the immune system and small developing sinuses.
- Allergy, immunodeficiency, and GERD may be important associated diseases.
- Imaging is not required for medical management in children. Plain films are not useful in children. CT scans should be obtained only if ethmoidectomy is being contemplated.
- Medical management consists primarily of parental education regarding the frequency of upper respiratory tract infections and medical management but also may include broad-spectrum oral antibiotics as indicated, topical nasal steroid sprays if the patient is allergic, and appropriate management of GERD.
- Surgical management is considered in patients in whom medical management has failed and who have infections outside the norm. Options include endoscopic anterior ethmoidectomy and conservative maxillary antrostomy, adenoidectomy (to rid the nasopharynx of possible contamination secondary to biofilms), and rarely, sphenoidotomy.
- Surgical intervention has not been shown to interrupt facial growth in children and, in appropriately selected patients, is very successful.

The diagnosis of acute and chronic sinusitis is a common primarily clinical diagnosis. It is associated with significant morbidity. In a quality of life assessment, Cunningham[1] and colleagues found that sinusitis had a more significant impact on children and their families than asthma, juvenile rheumatoid arthritis, and other chronic disorders.

Pediatric sinusitis is estimated to complicate approximately 5% to 10% of upper respiratory infections in early childhood.[2] Because children average six to eight upper respiratory illnesses per year, sinusitis is a very common problem.

Etiology

Age is clearly one of the most significant etiologic factors in pediatric sinusitis.[3] Because of their immature immune system, children are more likely to develop upper respiratory tract viral infections and associated acute sinusitis. A strong association has been recognized between sinusitis and respiratory viral infections. Viral infections are thought to cause significant ciliary dysfunction by decreasing the ciliary beat frequency or destroying the ciliary blanket.[4] These changes result in inflammation and edema that obstructs the ostium and increases the chance of establishing a bacterial infection of the sinuses. The ciliary dysfunction and edema will interrupt the drainage in the osteomeatal complex, predisposing the patient to the development of acute and possibly chronic sinusitis. As the ciliary function improves, the sinuses clear and the infection resolves in 80% of patients. The role of allergy in chronic sinusitis remains controversial. Rachelefsky[5] and coworkers[6] were the first to point out an association between allergic symptoms and sinusitis in children. The allergic reaction also will be associated with edema, and the same pathophysiology may be present. Huang[7] studied this issue for 5 years in children with perennial allergic rhinitis (PAR) and seasonal allergic rhinitis (SAR). Huang found that the prevalence of sinusitis was significantly higher among patients with PAR than among those with SAR, regardless of age or season. The patients with mold allergy PAR had a higher risk than those with nonmold allergies. Huang concluded that mold allergy is an important risk factor for sinusitis.

According to Ponikau and colleagues,[8] allergic fungal sinusitis may be an important factor in polypoid disease in adults. A strong correlation does appear to exist between the allergic response and fungal infections in some patients. The presentation of pediatric patients with allergic fungal sinusitis is different from that of adults. Children have more malleable bones and therefore incur a higher incidence of obvious abnormalities of their facial skeletons. Obstruction and the disease appear to be more unilateral.

The incidence of sinusitis and that of seasonal allergic symptoms do not, however, show a high degree of correlation. Numerous studies show that approximately 50% of children with sinusitis also have allergies; however, cause and effect have not been definitively demonstrated. A long-standing association among asthma, allergies, and chronic sinusitis is recognized. Dixon and associates[9] found a strong correlation between asthmatics and patients with rhinitis or sinusitis. In a recent study, Riccio and coworkers[10] found that allergic asthmatic children with chronic rhinosinusitis have a typical Th2 cytokine pattern. Nonallergic asthmatic children share a similar pattern. Riccio's group postulated that these findings suggest the existence of a common pathophysiologic mechanism shared by upper and lower airways, consistent with the concept of unified airway disease. This concept of unified airway disease has been increasingly recognized.[11]

Gastroesophageal reflux disease (GERD) may be associated with chronic sinusitis.[9] The incidence of GERD in children is not known, but Bothwell and associates are convinced that GERD is present in a majority of children with chronic sinusitis and effective treatment of the reflux can prevent sinus surgery.[12] Chambers and colleagues[13] found that GERD was the only reliable historical symptom that predicted a bad outcome in adults. There is, however, conflicting information in the literature. Suskind and coworkers[14] studied patients undergoing antireflux surgery and who had failed medical management. In this very young group of patients (younger than 2 years), only two patients (14%) had severe chronic sinusitis and otitis media. Yellon and colleagues[15] also found an incidence of sinusitis in only 10% of patients with esophagitis proved by biopsy. These two studies lead one to conclude that sinusitis is not associated with GERD. Without a doubt, some children have sinusitis associated with GERD. Reflux may be intermittent and cannot be identified with a 24-hour pH probe study. If present, the GERD should be treated with a proton pump inhibitor, which could possibly prevent the need for surgery. Some investigators have recommended empirical therapy with a proton pump inhibitor before proceeding with surgical management.[16]

Without a doubt, the bacteria causing sinusitis are becoming more resistant to antibiotics, especially *Streptococcus pneumoniae*, which has made medical management of chronic sinusitis more difficult. The aerobic pathogens in pediatric chronic sinusitis include bacteria typical of acute sinusitis and organisms more characteristic of chronic disease, such as *Staphylococcus aureus*. These resistant strains have a significant effect on the usefulness of available antibiotic regimens for medical management.

Imaging

It is now clear that plain films do not adequately image the pediatric sinuses.[17] In the setting of acute sinusitis, Gwaltney and associates[18] showed a high incidence of opacification of the anterior ethmoid and maxillary sinuses with acute rhinovirus infections. For assessing the status of sinuses, the coronal CT study remains the imaging method of choice. Plain films do not reveal the true status of sinusitis in children.[19] In general, sinusitis is a clinical diagnosis, and radiographic imaging is not necessary in children for confirmation. This is in contrast with adults, for whom most otolaryngologists (73%) feel that a CT scan is required to confirm the diagnosis.[20] CT scans should be obtained when both the parents and the surgeon feel that surgical intervention is warranted. The CT scan is used primarily to look for anatomic abnormalities that would increase the risk of surgical complications and to help document the presence of disease. The CT scan should be obtained after a trial of maximum medical management that would include broad-spectrum antibiotics and topical nasal steroid sprays for at least 3 to 4 weeks. The CT scan should be obtained at the end of this course of management. It is difficult to assess the meaning of positive findings on a CT scan that has been obtained without prior medical management. It also is important to avoid being forced by an anxious or frustrated parent into operating on a child whose CT scan shows minimal disease. The best way to prevent this is to warn the parents, before obtaining the CT scan, that a small amount of disease does not necessarily require surgical intervention.

Treatment

Irrigation of the nose has been found to be efficatious; however, in the child, compliance can be a significant issue. Irrigation with saline has been found to be as effective as use of topical vasoconstrictors.[21] If the child can cooperate, irrigations should be included as a primary modality.

In general, cultures of the nasal cavity have not been readily used in the pediatric population. In fact, many laboratories will not run routine cultures of the nose. The literature is mixed regarding the efficacy of directed cultures. Jiang and coworkers[22,23] have shown that the bacteriology of the middle meatus was different from that found in the ethmoid bulla. They therefore concluded that the bacteriologic findings in the middle meatus may not reflect the real bacteriology in chronic sinusitis. Other studies have shown that bacteriologic findings in the middle meatus have a high correlation with antral punctures.[24] In the cooperative patient, endoscopically directed cultures of the middle meatus may be very useful, particularly in communities with increased resistance. If the patient is uncooperative, then broad-spectrum antibiotics would be appropriate.

Medical Management

Because antibacterial therapy most often is empirically chosen to treat the disorder, knowledge of the typical etiologic agents, as well as awareness of the antibacterial susceptibility profiles in a given community, is of paramount importance.

Much is unknown about antibiotic therapy and chronic sinusitis. Recent advances, however, include recognition of the importance of nontypable *Haemophilus influenzae* unresponsive to first-generation cephalosporins and of tetracycline-resistant gram-positive cocci and the increasing emergence of beta-lactamase–positive respiratory pathogens such as *H. influenzae* and *Moraxella catarrhalis*. These realities now mandate the more conservative use of antibiotics in upper respiratory tract infections and the use of newer therapeutic agents for acute and chronic sinusitis.

One subject on which most authors have agreed in recent publications on pediatric sinusitis is that patient expectations for antibotic usage need to be altered. Currently, antibiotics often are used to treat viral upper respiratory tract infections, even though they usually are ineffective. This frequent inappropriate antibiotic use contributes to the emergence of drug-resistant bacterial pathogens. It is frequently difficult to assess whether the infection is viral or has been complicated by a bacterial infection and would subsequently improve with antibiotic therapy. Reviews in the literature emphasize the need for primary medical, not surgical, management of sinusitis. In the most resistant cases, however, surgery can have a significant therapeutic role, as outlined later in this chapter.

Chronic sinusitis is best treated with broader spectrum antibiotics. For the most resistant strains of pneumococci, File and colleagues[25] found the newer form of amoxicillin-clavulanate (2000 mg-125 mg) and the fluoroquinolones[26] to be highly active against these cultured isolates from patients with community-acquired respiratory tract infection. These drugs, however, should be saved for the most resistant infections.

There are proponents of the use of long-term, low-dose therapy with erythromycin in patients who do not respond to aggressive medical management.[27] Don and associates have recommended intravenous antibiotic therapy as an alternative to endoscopic sinus surgery.[28] They believed this was warranted because of the risk of interference with facial skeletal growth and complications of endoscopic sinus surgery. Conclusive evidence now shows that endoscopic sinus surgery does not interfere with facial growth,[29] and the risks of endoscopic sinus surgery are small. Don and associates[28] found that 89% of the patients had complete resolution of symptoms after intravenous therapy with selective adenoidectomy; the remaining 11% failed to respond to intravenous therapy and required endoscopic surgery. In this study, the criteria for performing selective adenoidectomy are not clear, and significant complications were reported with intravenous therapy as well. Intravenous therapy is, however, a potential modality of therapy in resistant cases and can be used for complications of acute or chronic sinusitis.

Some investigators have recommended topical aerosolized antibiotics, but others have found them to be ineffective.[12] At this time, a firm recommendation about the use of topical aerosolized antibiotics cannot be made.

Prospective studies are lacking in the use of antihistamines and decongestants. In theory, decongestants would decrease the amount of edema and open the ostia. Topical steroids have been shown to decrease edema within 2 weeks and may be of modest benefit. Topical steroids have been shown to be safe and not to interrupt growth.[30]

Some investigators have used intravenous immune globulin (IVIG) to treat patients who do not have immune deficiencies but have chronic sinusitis.[31] They concluded that IVIG was successful in improving the medical management of chronic sinusitis. They also thought the mechanisms by which IVIG may be helpful are probably not based on the concept of immune replacement therapy, but more likely as an immune or inflammatory modulating agent.

Surgical Management

There is little doubt that chronic sinusitis–like symptoms occur in children with large obstructive adenoid pads (Fig. 195-1). If the obstructive adenoid pad is not removed, the nasal cavity cannot become healthy. Several studies indicate that adenoidectomy improves the signs and symptoms of sinusitis.[32,33] The efficacy of the treatment

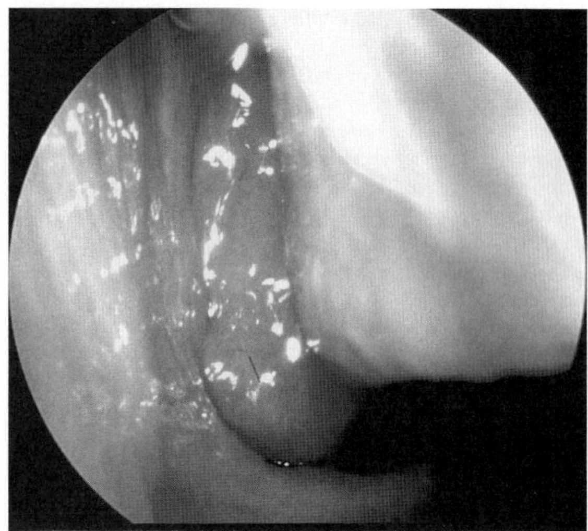

Figure 195-1. Endoscopic view of enlarged adenoid pad causing nasal obstruction and symptoms compatible with obstructive sleep apnea (OSA).

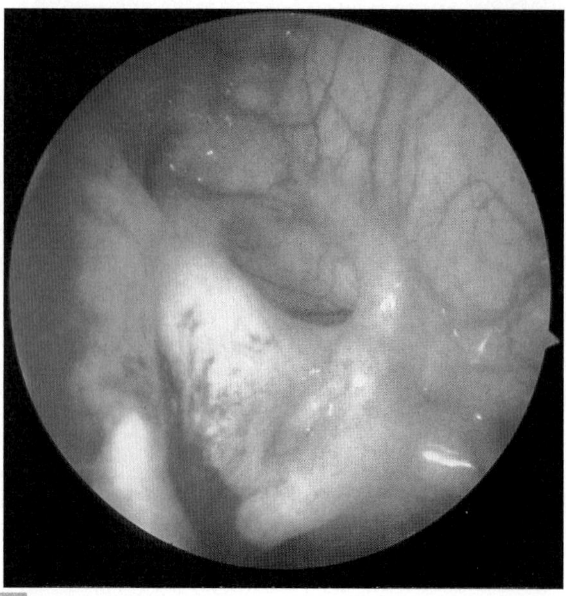

Figure 195-2. Endoscopic view of mucosa intact over the lamina papyracea and basal lamella.

appears to be independent of the size of the adenoid pad. Recently, biofilms have been discovered covering the adenoid tissue in children with chronic sinusitis.[34,35] Such biofilms may constitute a repository for bacterial seeding of the middle meatus; this theory is supported by the efficacy of adenoidectomy regardless of the size of the adenoid pad. Certainly more work needs to be performed in this area before a firm correlation can be established. Good prospective studies assessing the efficacy of adenoidectomy in well-documented cases of sinusitis have yet to be performed. Overall, adenoidectomy can be expected to help relieve the symptoms of chronic sinusitis in approximately 50% of patients. A majority of pediatric otolaryngologists perform an adenoidectomy as the initial step in surgical management of chronic sinusitis.[36]

Some investigators believe that endoscopic surgery is rarely indicated. Endoscopic sinus surgery has become, however, a primary method of surgical therapy for chronic sinusitis after adenoidectomy. The indications for endoscopic sinus surgery remain controversial. The Consensus Panel[37] preferred to divide its indications into absolute and possible indications:

Absolute indications include (1) complete nasal airway obstruction in cystic fibrosis due to massive polyposis or closure of the nose by medialization of the lateral nasal wall; (2) antrochoanal polyp; (3) intracranial complications; (4) mucoceles and mucopyoceles; (5) orbital abscess; (6) traumatic injury to the optic canal; (7) dacryocystorhinitis due to sinusitis and resistant to medical treatment; (8) fungal sinusitis; (9) some meningoencephaloceles; and (10) some neoplasms.

Relative or possible indications, which are present in the vast majority of patients, include chronic rhinosinusitis that persists despite optimal medical management and after the exclusion of any systemic disease. Optimal management includes 4 to 6 weeks of adequate broad-spectrum antibiotics and treatment of any concomitant diseases.

According to the Consensus Panel,[37] only a small fraction of all children suffering from chronic sinusitis will require functional endoscopic sinus surgery (FESS), but these children account for a majority of surgical patients, and the procedure has gained popularity. Reported success rates, defined mainly on the basis of improvement over preoperative symptoms, have been encouraging and ranged between 71% and 93%. Hebert and Bent[38] performed a meta-analysis that revealed a success rate of 88.4% with surgical management in children in whom medical management had failed to effect improvement. With more experience, many surgeons have modified their techniques to be less aggressive, with the aim of preservation of mucosa. Advances in instrumentation, including the advent of the microsurgical débrider and sharp through-biting instruments, also have contributed to realization of this goal. It is now possible to preserve mucosa over the lamina papyracea, middle turbinate, and basal lamella (Fig. 195-2). Extensive sphenoethmoidectomy usually is not justified in children unless they have symptomatic polyps secondary to cystic fibrosis or allergic fungal sinusitis (Fig. 195-3).

Most surgeons perform a limited procedure that involves an anterior ethmoidectomy and maxillary antrostomy.[36] The size of the maxillary antrostomy continues to be controversial. Many surgeons have become more conservative in the size of their antrostomy. The mucosa in the area of the root of the middle turbinate should not be removed. It is important to leave mucosa in this area to prevent scarring in the frontal recess. If the ostium can be seen with a 30-degree telescope, then it does not need to be enlarged. If, however, there is evidence of a polypoid mucosa in the ostium or if it is edematous and can only be identified with a seeker, then it may be enlarged posteriorly into the fontanelle, with through-biting instruments. On occasion, usually less than 30% of the time, the posterior ethmoid sinuses will need to be entered. In unusual circumstances, less than 10% of the time, the sphenoid sinus or frontal sinuses will need to be entered. The frontal recess in children is the source of the frontal sinuses, and frontal sinuses are not developed in children. Therefore, instrumentation of this area should be performed very carefully.

When the procedure was originally performed, a second-look operation that included cleaning of the cavity was believed to be necessary. In the pediatric population, this meant a second general anesthetic procedure. Ramadan[39] found that treatment with intravenous dexamethasone during endoscopic sinus surgery was safe and was helpful in reducing scarring and swelling noted during the second-look procedure. Use of corticosteroids was particularly helpful in children with asthma, lower CT scores, no exposure to smoking, and older than 6 years of age. Walner and associates[40] found that avoiding a second look did not increase the incidence of revision surgery. Fakhri and coworkers[41] concluded that second-look endoscopy did not decrease the incidence of revision surgery; therefore, the second look was of no benefit after routine FESS. It has now become more common practice to use some type of absorbable stenting material in children, to omit the second look. Most surgeons do not perform a second-look operation.[36]

Many areas of surgical management of sinusitis need further investigation but none is more important than the impact on facial growth. In two studies in animal models, piglets showed interruption of facial growth on the side of endoscopic surgery, but the animals clinically did not show evidence of abnormal growth.[42,43] Lund and associates[44] have

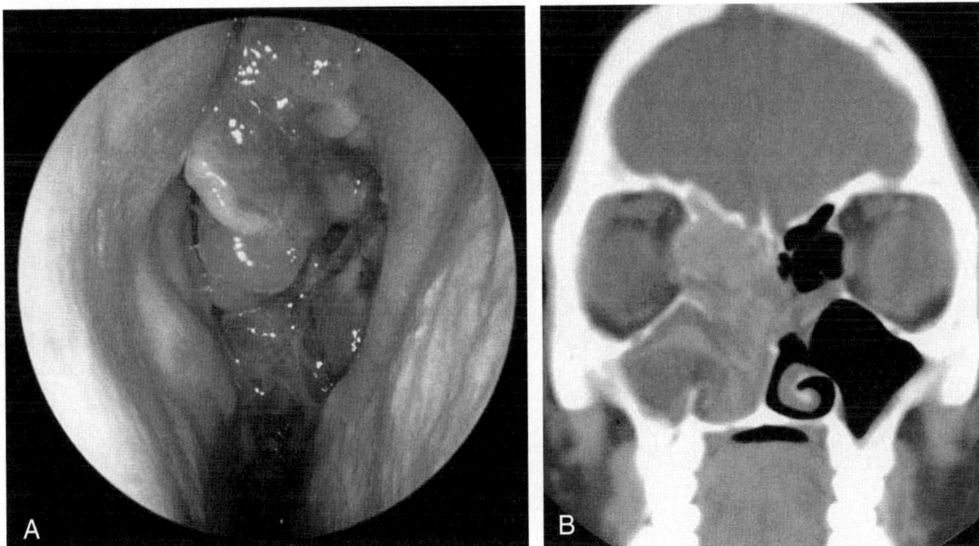

Figure 195-3. **A,** Endoscopic view of polyps secondary to fungal sinusitis. **B,** Computed tomography scan of a patient with fungal sinusitis.

evidence that very aggressive surgical management of midface lesions is not associated with interruption of facial growth. Wolf and colleagues[45] did not note any evidence of interruption of facial growth. However, these two studies did not perform accurate measurements of the facial skeleton.

Bothwell and associatess[29] sought to determine whether FESS performed in children with chronic rhinosinusitis alters facial growth. They evaluated 67 children with a mean age of 3.1 years at presentation. The patients were evaluated for facial growth 10 years later, at a mean age of 13.2 years. In this series, 46 children underwent FESS and 21 children did not undergo FESS and acted as a control group. Quantitative anthropomorphic analysis was performed using 12 standard facial measurements on both groups. A facial plastic surgery expert performed blinded qualitative facial analysis on standardized photographs. Both quantitative and qualitative analyses showed no trends or statistical significance in changes of facial growth between children who underwent FESS and those who had chronic sinusitis but did not undergo FESS. The data also showed no deviations, or trends toward deviation, from the standard norms in children. Bothwell's investigators concluded that evidence for an adverse effect of FESS on facial growth in children was lacking.

Large clinical studies are necessary to further elucidate the pathophysiology and medical and surgical management of chronic sinusitis. These studies will be difficult to perform because of the large numbers required.

SUGGESTED READINGS

Bothwell MR, Parsons DS, Talbot A, et al. Outcome of reflux therapy on pediatric chronic sinusitis. *Otolaryngol Head Neck Surg.* 1999;121(3):255-262.

Bothwell MR, Piccirillo JF, Lusk RP, et al. Long-term outcome of facial growth after functional endoscopic sinus surgery. *Otolaryngol Head Neck Surg.* 2002;126(6):628-634.

Coticchia J, Zuliani G, Coleman C, et al. Biofilm surface area in the pediatric nasopharynx: chronic rhinosinusitis vs obstructive sleep apnea. *Arch Otolaryngol Head Neck Surg.* 2007;133(2):110-114.

Hebert RL, Bent JP 3rd. Meta-analysis of outcomes of pediatric functional endoscopic sinus surgery. *Laryngoscope.* 1998;108(6):796-799.

Huang SW. The risk of sinusitis in children with allergic rhinitis. *Allergy Asthma Proc.* 2000;21(2):85-88.

McAlister WH, Lusk RP, Muntz HR. Comparison of plain radiographs and coronal CT scans in infants and children with recurrent sinusitis. *AJR Am J Roentgenol.* 1989;153:1259-1264.

Sobol SE, Samadi DS, Kazahaya K, et al. Trends in the management of pediatric chronic sinusitis: survey of the American Society of Pediatric Otolaryngology. *Laryngoscope.* 2005;115(1):78-80.

For complete list of references log onto www.expertconsult.com.

Pharyngitis and Adenotonsillar Disease

W. Peyton Shirley

Audie L. Woolley

Brian J. Wiatrak

Key Points

- An understanding of the anatomy, embryology, and physiology of Waldeyer's ring is important to learning how to diagnose and treat disease in this region.
- The physician must be familiar with and be able to diagnose a wide range of infections that may be seen in Waldeyer's ring. Once the diagnosis is made, the physician needs to know the treatment options and the potential complications that may result from pharyngitis and adenotonsillar disease.
- Adenotonsillar hypertrophy is a common cause of upper airway obstruction in children that has a wide range of clinical manifestations and complications. Newer research suggests that upper airway obstruction potentially leads not only to harmful physiologic alterations but also to pathologic changes in behavior and neurocognitive development.
- Proper preoperative assessment is crucial. A good history and thorough physical examination are the most important part of appropriate treatment of adenotonsillar disease. The physician must be familiar with and know how to optimally use all the available diagnostic tests and procedures. Finally, the surgeon must have a thorough understanding of the proper indications for adenotonsillectomy.
- Many techniques have been and continue to be used to perform adenotonsillectomy. The physician must have knowledge of all the surgical options available and must make an informed choice about the method. Whatever technique is chosen, careful surgical technique is important as well as an awareness of potential complications. The surgeon must be able to handle the potential complications but, more important, know how to avoid them.

Infectious and inflammatory diseases involving the pharynx, tonsils, and adenoids account for a significant proportion of childhood illnesses and pediatric health care expenditures. They often result in two of the most common surgical procedures of childhood, tonsillectomy and adenoidectomy (Fig. 196-1). Clinical research has now helped illuminate this vast area of pediatric otolaryngology, including the effects of adenotonsillar hypertrophy on obstructive sleep apnea and the many possible sequelae of obstructive sleep apnea, the microbiologic flora of the tonsils and adenoids and their role in chronic adenotonsillar hypertrophy, the relationship between adenotonsillar hypertrophy and craniofacial growth, and new techniques for adenotonsillectomy with improved management of perioperative morbidity. This chapter reviews the current understanding of pharyngitis and adenotonsillar disease processes.

History

Celsus was the first to report removal of the tonsils.[1] Describing his surgical technique, Celsus indicated that "the tonsils are loosened by scraping around them and then torn out."[1] Hemostasis was obtained using a vinegar mouthwash and painting the tonsillar fossa with a medication to reduce bleeding.[2] Aëtius of Amida on the Tigris described a technique for tonsillectomy in the first half of the sixth century, in which a hook was used to snare the tonsil and a knife was used for amputation. He warned of the severe dangers of hemorrhage when excision was too deep.[3] Subsequent surgical techniques were described by Paul of Aegina in 625, and Physick described a forceps to facilitate extirpation of the tonsil, which became the forerunner of the modern tonsil guillotine.[1,4] Mackenzie improved on the Physick tonsillotome and popularized its use for surgery of the tonsils in the late nineteenth century.[5]

The adenoids were first described by the Danish physician Meyer. In his 1868 paper "Adenoid vegetations in the nasopharyngeal cavity," Meyer described in detail his technique of posterior rhinoscopy to diagnose adenoid hypertrophy and recommended removal of adenoid tissue with the aid of a ring knife.[6] In 1885, Gottstein described the first adenoid curette.[6]

Crowe and colleagues[7] reviewed 1000 consecutive tonsillectomies performed between 1911 and 1917. In the study "Relation of tonsillar and nasopharyngeal infection to general systemic disorders," they provided a detailed description of a meticulous surgical technique by sharp dissection and described using the Crowe-Davis mouth gag. The low complication rate they described compares favorably with rates in modern reports of tonsillectomy.

Anatomy

Waldeyer's Ring

Together, the lingual tonsils anteriorly, the palatine tonsils laterally, and the pharyngeal tonsils (adenoids) posterosuperiorly form a ring of lymphoid or adenoid tissue around the upper end of the pharynx known as Waldeyer's tonsillar ring. All the structures of Waldeyer's ring have similar histology and, presumably, similar functions.

Palatine Tonsil

The palatine tonsil represents the largest accumulation of lymphoid tissue in Waldeyer's ring and, in contrast to the lingual and pharyngeal tonsils, constitutes a compact body with a definite thin capsule on its deep surface.[8] Tonsillar crypts, blind tubules from the epithelium on the surface of the tonsil that are lined with stratified squamous epithelium, extend deep into this tissue.

The tonsillar capsule is a specialized portion of the pharyngobasilar fascia that covers the surface of the tonsil and extends into it to form septa that conduct the nerves and vessels.[8] The tonsil is not, therefore, easily separated from its capsule, but the capsule is united largely by loose connective tissue to the pharyngeal muscles. One can easily dissect the tonsil from its normal position by separating the capsule from the muscle through this loose connective tissue.

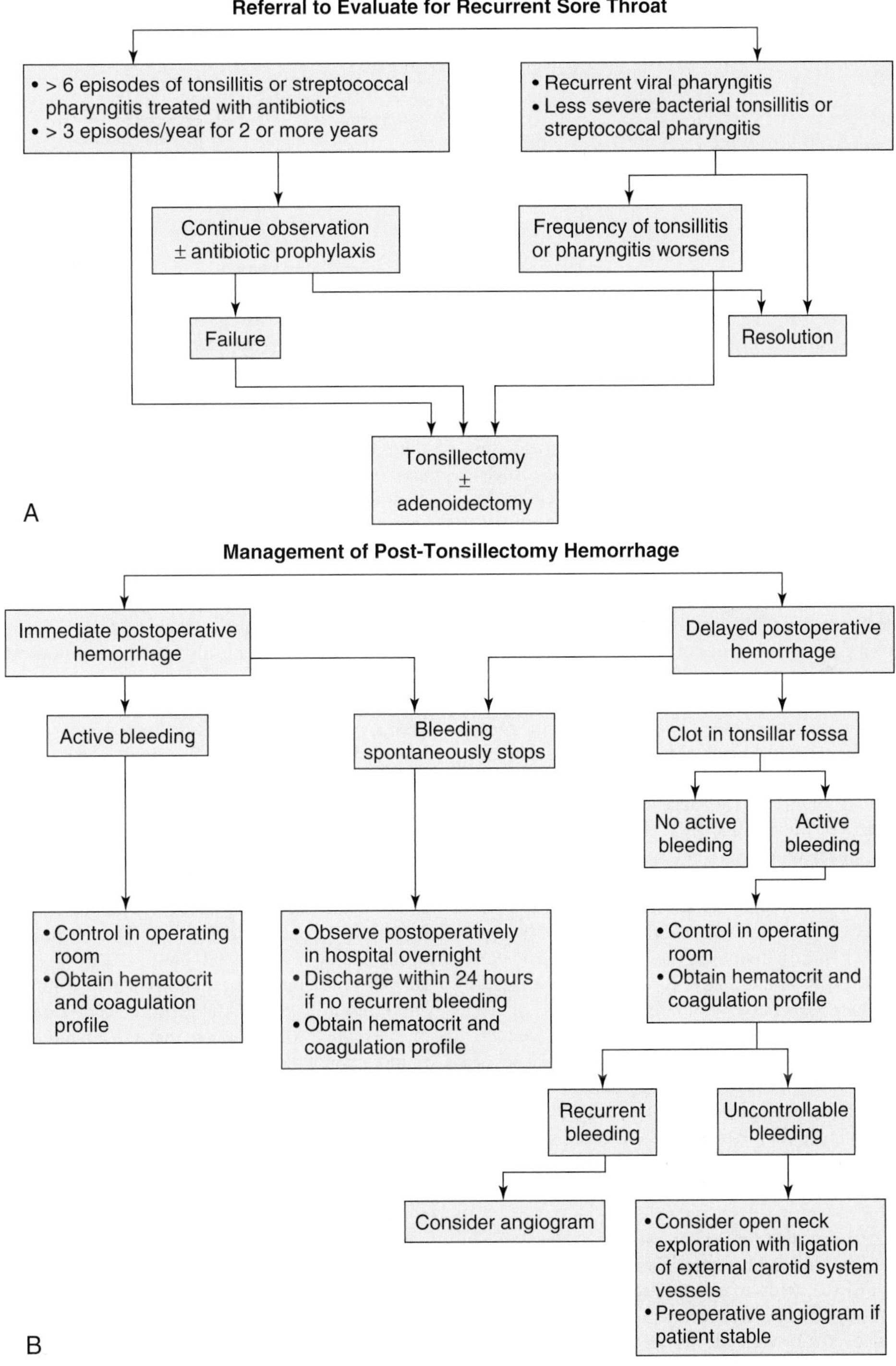

Figure 196-1. Management algorithms for pediatric pharyngitis and adenotonsillar disease. **A,** Algorithm for evaluation of a patient referred for recurrent sore throat. **B,** Algorithm for management of post-tonsillectomy hemorrhage. *Continued*

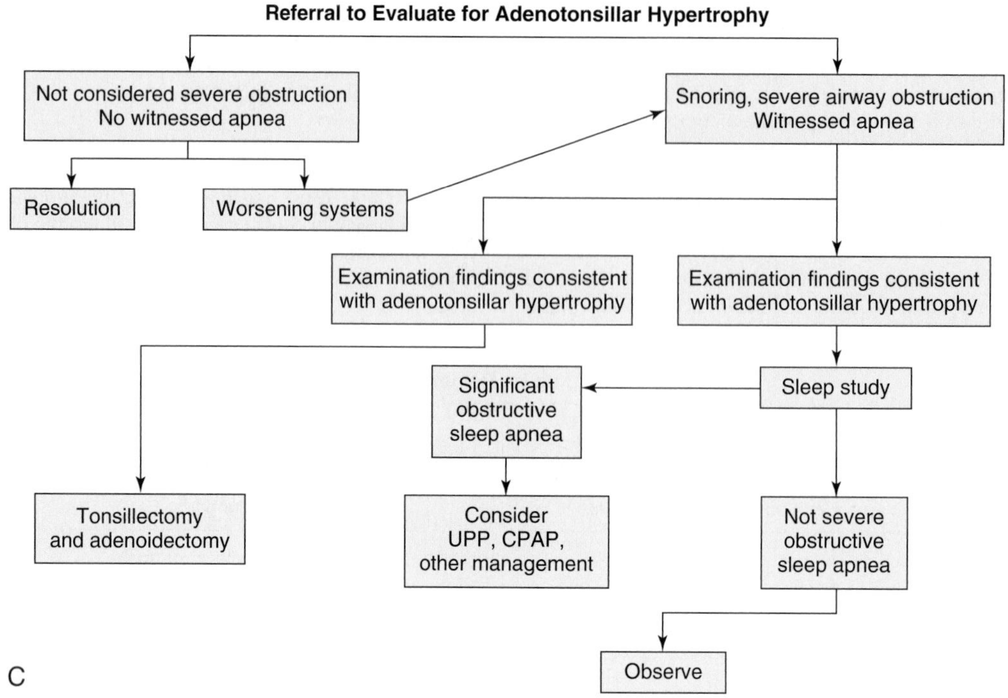

Figure 196-1, cont'd. **C,** Algorithm for evaluation of a patient referred for adenotonsillar hypertrophy.

The tonsillar fossa is composed of three muscles: the palatoglossus muscle, which forms the anterior pillar; the palatopharyngeal muscle, which is the posterior pillar; and the superior constrictor muscle of the pharynx, which forms the larger part of the tonsillar bed.[8] The muscular wall is thin, and immediately against it on the outer wall of the pharynx is the glossopharyngeal nerve. This nerve can be easily injured if the tonsillar bed is violated, and not uncommonly the nerve is temporarily affected by edema after tonsillectomy, which produces both a transitory loss of taste over the posterior third of the tongue and referred otalgia.

The arterial blood supply of the tonsil enters primarily at the lower pole, with branches also at the upper pole. There are typically three arteries at the lower pole: the tonsillar branch of the dorsal lingual artery anteriorly, the ascending palatine artery (a branch of the facial artery) posteriorly, and the tonsillar branch of the facial artery between them that enters the lower aspect of the tonsillar bed.[8] At the upper pole of the tonsil, the ascending pharyngeal artery enters posteriorly, and the lesser palatine artery enters on the anterior surface. The tonsillar branch of the facial artery is the largest. Venous blood drains through a peritonsillar plexus about the capsule.[8] The plexus drains into the lingual and pharyngeal veins, which in turn drain into the internal jugular vein.

The nerve supply of the tonsillar region is through the tonsillar branches of the glossopharyngeal nerve about the lower pole of the tonsil and through the descending branches of the lesser palatine nerves, which course through the pterygopalatine ganglion.[8] The cause of referred otalgia with tonsillitis is through the tympanic branch of the glossopharyngeal nerve. Efferent lymphatic drainage courses through the upper deep cervical lymph nodes, especially the jugulodigastric or tonsillar node located behind the angle of the mandible.[8]

Adenoids

The adenoid or pharyngeal tonsils form the central part of the ring of lymphoid tissue surrounding the oropharyngeal isthmus. The adenoid is composed of lymphoid tissue, with its apex pointed toward the nasal septum and its base toward the roof and posterior wall of the nasopharynx. The adenoid is covered by a pseudostratified ciliated columnar epithelium that is plicated to form numerous surface folds. The adenoid develops as a midline structure by the fusion of two lateral primordia that become visible during early fetal life, are fully developed during the seventh month of gestation, and continue to grow until the fifth year of life, often causing some airway obstruction.[6,9] Thereafter, the adenoid gradually atrophies, the nasopharynx grows, and the airway improves.[10]

The blood supply and drainage are from the ascending pharyngeal artery, the ascending palatine artery, the pharyngeal branch of the maxillary artery, the artery of the pterygoid canal, and contributing branches from the tonsillar branch of the facial artery.[9] Venous drainage is to the pharyngeal plexus, which communicates with the pterygoid plexus and then drains into the internal jugular and facial veins. The nerve supply is from the pharyngeal plexus. The efferent lymphatic drainage of the adenoids is to the retropharyngeal and pharyngomaxillary space lymph nodes.[9]

Immunology of the Adenoids and Tonsils

The adenoids and tonsils are predominantly B-cell organs; B cells account for 50% to 65% of all adenoid and tonsillar lymphocytes.[11] Approximately 40% of adenoid and tonsillar lymphocytes are T cells, and 3% are mature plasma cells. Conversely, 70% of the lymphocytes in peripheral blood are T cells.[12] The immunoreactive lymphoid cells of the adenoids and tonsils are found in four distinct areas: the reticular cell epithelium, the extrafollicular area, the mantle zone of the lymphoid follicle, and the germinal center of the lymphoid follicle.[11]

Ample evidence shows that the adenoids and tonsils are involved in inducing secretory immunity and regulating secretory immunoglobulin production. They contain a system of channels covered by specialized endothelium that can mediate antigen uptake much like Peyer's patches of epithelium in the bowel.[13] Both the adenoids and tonsils are favorably located to mediate immunologic protection of the upper aerodigestive tract as they are exposed to airborne antigens. Both organs, specifically the tonsils, are particularly designed for direct transport of foreign material from the exterior to the lymphoid cells.[11] This is in contrast to lymph nodes, which depend on antigenic delivery through afferent lymphatics. The tonsillar crypts are covered by stratified squamous epithelium. There are 10 to 30 of these crypts in the tonsils, and they are ideally suited to trapping foreign material and transporting it to the lymphoid follicles.[11]

The tonsils and adenoids rank among the secondary lymphatic organs. Intratonsillar defense mechanisms eliminate weak antigenic signals. Only when additional higher antigenic concentrations are presented does proliferation of antigen-sensitive B cells occur in the germinal centers.[11] Low antigen doses effect the differentiation of lymphocytes to plasma cells, whereas high antigen doses produce B-cell proliferation. The generation of B cells in the germinal centers of the tonsils is considered by Siegel to be one of the most essential tonsillar functions.[14]

Immunoglobulins (Igs) produced by the adenoid include IgG, IgA, IgM, and IgD.[11] IgG appears to pass into the nasopharyngeal lumen by passive diffusion.[11] The tonsil produces antibodies locally as well as B cells, which migrate to other sites around the pharynx and periglandular lymphoid tissues to produce antibodies.

T-cell functions, such as interferon-γ production and, presumably, production of other important lymphokines, have been shown to be present in tonsils and adenoids.[11] The role played by tonsillar and adenoid T cells in tumor response is still unknown.

The human tonsils are immunologically most active between ages 4 and 10 years. Involution of the tonsils begins after puberty, resulting in a decrease of the B-cell population and a relative increase in the ratio of T to B cells.[11,15] Although the overall Ig-producing function is affected, considerable B-cell activity is still seen in clinically healthy tonsils even at age 80 years.[16] The situation is different in disease-associated changes, such as when recurrent tonsillitis and adenoid hyperplasia are observed. Inflammation of the reticular crypt epithelium results in shedding of immunologically active cells and decreasing antigen transport function with subsequent replacement by stratified squamous epithelium.[17] These changes lead to reduced activation of the local B-cell system, decreased antibody production, and an overall reduction in density of the B-cell and germinal centers in extrafollicular areas.[17] In contrast to recurrent tonsillitis, the changes are less pronounced in adenoid hyperplasia, in which the immunoregulatory conditions necessary for maintenance of the B-cell population are well preserved. The reason is most likely that the reticular epithelium is less affected in inflammation of adenoids than of tonsils.

Reports conflict regarding the immunologic consequences of tonsillectomy and adenoidectomy, yet it is clear that no major immunologic deficiencies result from these procedures.[16,18] Ogra[19] showed a three- to fourfold drop in titers in children previously immunized with live poliovirus vaccine. Attempts to vaccinate seronegative children subjected to tonsillectomy and adenoidectomy have resulted in delayed and lowered nasopharyngeal secretory immune responses as measured by IgA antibodies to the poliovirus.[19] Fortunately, poliovirus epidemics are no longer an annual threat. Serum IgA levels in patients who had undergone tonsillectomy were lower than in age-matched controls, but this immunologic change did not appear to be clinically significant. Some studies actually point to improved immunologic activity after tonsillectomy. One study showed better neutrophil chemotaxis after tonsillectomy, and another demonstrated increased IgG and IgM production, possibly as a result of unblocking of the suppression that the immune system was subject to before tonsillectomy.[20,21] One large study, with a cohort of 1328 children, showed no higher incidence of atopic disease (asthma, allergic rhinitis, and eczema) in children who had adenotonsillectomy prior to age 8 than in those who had not undergone surgery.[22]

It is clear that the adenoids and tonsils are active immunologic organs that generally reinforce the mucosal immunity of the entire upper aerodigestive tract. The immunologic role of these organs should be considered before a patient undergoes adenoidectomy or tonsillectomy; nonetheless, clinical consideration still forms the actual basis of surgery.

Bacteriology

Establishment of normal flora in the upper respiratory tract begins at birth. *Actinomyces*, *Fusobacterium*, and *Nocardia* are acquired by age 6 to 8 months.[23] Subsequently, *Bacteroides*, *Leptotrichia*, *Propionibacterium*, and *Candida* are also established as part of the oral flora.[24] *Fusobacterium* populations reach high numbers after dentition and reach maximal numbers at 1 year of age.[23] The ratio of anaerobic to aerobic bacteria in saliva is approximately 10 : 1,[24] because of variations in oxygen concentration throughout the oral cavity.

Healthy children up to 5 years of age can harbor known aerobic pathogens. Ingvarsson and colleagues[24] reported that *Streptococcus pneumoniae* was recovered in 19% of healthy children, *Haemophilus influenzae* in 13%, group A *Streptococcus* in 5%, and *Moraxella (Branhamella) catarrhalis* in 36%. The frequency of pathogens decreases with age, possibly because of greater immunity. Changes in the pharyngeal bacteria flora noted during viral illnesses are thought to be a result of the increased adherence of *Staphylococcus aureus* as well as gram-negative enteric organisms.[25] Oral pharyngeal colonization during illness-free periods was found to vary from 12% to 18% for gram-negative enteric organisms and from 5% to 14% for *S. aureus*.[26] During an episode of viral upper respiratory tract infection, the colonization rates for gram-negative organisms and *S. aureus* increased to 60% and 43%, respectively.

Brodsky and Koch[27] found substantive differences between the types and numbers of aerobic bacteria found in nondiseased and diseased adenoids. The core samples of normal adenoids showed that 75% of children who were relatively free of upper respiratory disease, otitis media, and symptoms of adenoid obstruction had either no bacterial growth on culture or bacteria that are considered part of the normal flora and not pathogenic. Core samples in adenoids of only 45% of children who had chronic adenoid infection and 39% who had obstructive adenoid hypertrophy had no bacteria growth or only normal flora; the bacteria found in these children were more likely to be β-lactamase producers.

Infections of Waldeyer's Ring

Many organisms can induce inflammation of Waldeyer's ring. These include aerobic as well as anaerobic bacteria, viruses, yeasts, and parasites. Some of the infectious organisms are part of the normal oral pharyngeal flora, and others are external pathogens. Because the oropharynx is colonized by many organisms, most infections of Waldeyer's ring are polymicrobial. These organisms work synergistically and can be demonstrated in mixed aerobic and anaerobic infections.[28]

Another feature of mixed infections is the ability of organisms resistant to an antimicrobial agent to protect an organism susceptible to that agent by the production of an antibiotic-degrading enzyme that is secreted into the tissues.[29] Because of the polymicrobial nature of most infections around Waldeyer's ring, it is often difficult to interpret data derived from clinical samples obtained from mucosal surfaces and to differentiate between organisms that are colonized and those that are invaders.

Viruses

The classic "common cold" is the most frequent cause of otolaryngologic infection in children. A multitude of offending viral pathogens have been implicated in causing pharyngitis, including rhinovirus, influenzavirus, parainfluenza virus, adenovirus, coxsackievirus, echovirus, reovirus, and respiratory syncytial virus. Viral pharyngitis is usually mild in manifestations, with patients complaining of a sore throat and dysphagia. Most patients have a fever with erythema of the pharyngeal mucosa. The tonsils may be enlarged but frequently there is no associated exudate.

Herpangina caused by coxsackievirus is characterized by small vesicles with erythematous bases that become ulcers and are spread over the anterior pillar tonsils, palate, and posterior pharynx (Fig. 196-2). Herpes simplex virus commonly causes the well-known "cold sore." This virus can also cause exudative or nonexudative pharyngitis, mainly in older children and young adults. In younger children, the herpesvirus may induce gingivostomatitis.

Management of viral infections is nonspecific and symptomatic. Antibiotics are helpful in cases of secondary bacterial infection.[30]

Epstein-Barr Virus

One particular type of viral infection that deserves special attention is the Epstein-Barr virus (EBV). EBV induces the mononucleosis syndrome, which consists of high fever; general malaise; large, swollen, dirty-gray tonsils (Fig. 196-3); sore throat; dysphagia; and odynophagia. Petechiae located at the junction of the hard and soft palate are highly

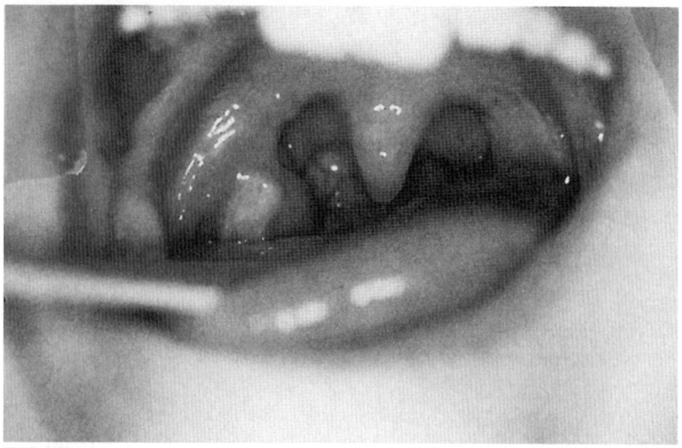

Figure 196-2. Viral ulcer on the right tonsil consistent with coxsackievirus infection.

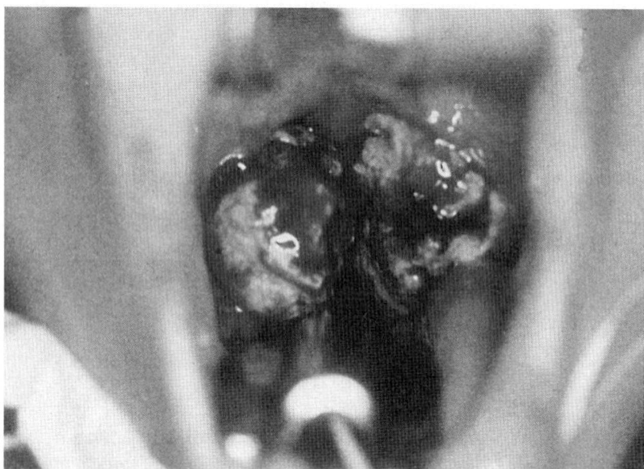

Figure 196-3. Tonsillar hypertrophy and mononucleosis with significant airway obstruction.

suggestive of EBV infection, although not pathognomonic. Often patients with EBV infection have hepatosplenomegaly with resultant liver damage. The most common method of transmission is oral contact.

Diagnosis of EBV is confirmed by laboratory studies. A differential blood count showing 50% lymphocytosis with 10% atypical lymphocytes is characteristic of EBV infection. Serologic studies include monospot and other serum heterophil antibody titer measurements. Results of these tests may be negative initially, and repeat testing in 1 to 2 weeks is warranted if clinical suspicion of EBV infection is strong. The heterophil antibody titers are detected by the Paul-Bunnell-Davidsohn or ox-cell hemolysis test. If the heterophil antibody agglutination test result is negative, the disease may still be present. Only 60% of patients with infectious mononucleosis have a positive result within the first 2 weeks after onset of the illness; 90% have a positive result 1 month after onset.[31] EBV-specific serologic assays have become the method of choice for confirmation of acute or convalescent EBV infection. Figure 196-4 shows the serologic response time. Management of this condition is symptomatic. Recovery may take weeks, and antibiotics are used to treat secondary bacterial infections. Ampicillin should be avoided because a rash may occur despite previous intake without similar reactions. Upper airway obstruction from severely enlarged tonsils can be life-threatening and should be managed promptly with the insertion of a nasopharyngeal airway and short-term high-dose steroid therapy. If the obstruction is severe and unrelieved by these measures, a tonsillectomy or tracheotomy may be necessary.

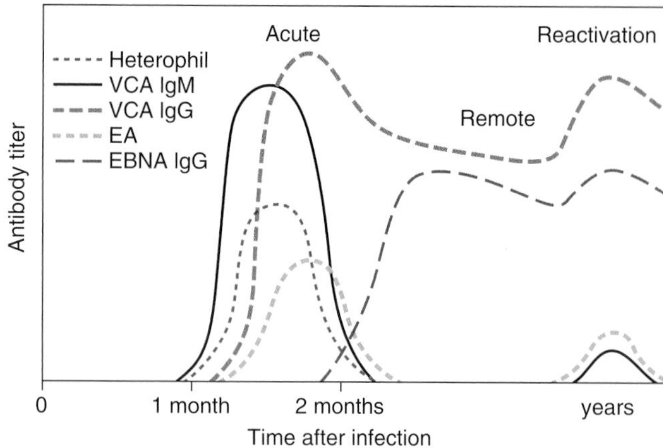

Figure 196-4. Serologic response time in diagnosis of EBV infection. EA, early antigen; EBNA, EBV nuclear antigen; Ig, immunoglobulin; VCA, viral capsid antigen. *(From Gulley ML. Molecular diagnosis of Epstein-Barr virus-related diseases.* J Mol Diagn. *2001;3:1-10.)*

Candida

Candidiasis can result in severe pharyngitis, particularly in patients who are immunocompromised or who have been undergoing treatment with antimicrobial agents. It is a fairly unmistakable syndrome consisting of coherent white plaques on the oral pharyngeal mucosa. Removal of these plaques may reveal a raw, bleeding surface. Management is with nystatin or, in refractory cases, fluconazole.

Neisseria

Pharyngitis as a result of *Neisseria gonorrhoeae* is common in homosexual men. It has been detected in 6% of adolescents with acute pharyngitis.[32] Although the infection is often asymptomatic, it can result and persist after treatment. Acute exudative tonsillitis is a manifestation of gonococcal pharyngitis. The clinical syndrome may range from an asymptomatic to an exudative pharyngitis, but most cases tend to fall toward the exudative pharyngitis end of the spectrum. Nonetheless, disseminated gonococcemia can result even from mild or asymptomatic infection. Penicillin and tetracycline are the most effective therapeutic agents.

Vincent's Angina

Vincent's angina is secondary to *Spirochaeta denticulata* and Vincent's fusiform bacillus *Borrelia vincentii* (*Treponema vincentii*). This condition arises slowly, manifesting both mild local and systemic symptoms. The infection arises most commonly in overcrowded conditions. Patients present with complaints of high fever, headache, sore throat, and physical findings of cervical lymphadenopathy and a membrane on the tonsil that, when removed, reveals an ulcer that remains confined to the surrounding tissue and usually heals in 7 to 10 days.[33] Management consists of penicillin therapy. Local treatment in the form of oral hygiene is helpful. This condition may be confused with trench mouth, which is caused by the same organisms but in which oral cavity ulcers include the gums and oral mucous membranes.[34]

Syphilis

Treponema pallidum infections in both the primary and secondary stages of syphilis can be associated with oral pharyngeal lesions. In primary syphilis, oral chancres appear about 3 weeks after exposure. Grayish superficial mucous membrane patches surrounded by an erythematous border are generally found in patients with secondary syphilis.

Corynebacterium diphtheriae

The incidence of *Corynebacterium diphtheriae* infection has declined markedly since the introduction of diphtheria vaccination. This organism causes an early exudative pharyngotonsillitis with a thick pharyngeal membrane. Infection can then spread to the throat, tonsils, palate, and larynx.[35] *C. diphtheriae* organisms also produce a lethal exotoxin that can damage cells in distant organs. Today only 200 to 300 cases of diphtheria occur in the United States each year, usually—but not exclusively—in people who have not been immunized.[36] The organism is a gram-positive pleomorphic aerobic bacillus that can be identified in a routine throat culture, particularly when the microbiologist is made aware of a clinical suspicion of this diagnosis. Only toxigenic strains infected with a bacteriophage can cause diphtheria.[30] Laryngeal inflammation combined with an exudative, necrotic, gray pharyngeal membrane may result in airway obstruction. Removal of this membrane causes bleeding. Early diagnosis is critical, and the goal of therapy is neutralization of unbound toxin with antitoxin. Myocarditis and neurologic sequelae resembling features of Guillain-Barré syndrome or poliomyelitis may result.[35,36] The organism is identified by fluorescent antibody studies. The presence of Klebs-Löffler bacillus in the membrane can be diagnosed with Gram staining.[34] Because diphtheria is an emergency condition, antitoxin must be given in the first 48 hours of onset to be effective. Airway obstruction should be managed with tracheotomy. Penicillin in high doses should be administered.

Streptococcal Tonsillitis-Pharyngitis

Group A *Streptococcus* is the most common bacterial cause of acute pharyngitis.[37] The public health importance of this infection lies not only in its frequency but also on the fact that it is a precursor of two serious sequelae, acute rheumatic fever and poststreptococcal glomerulonephritis. Although the incidence of rheumatic fever has decreased, all groups of β-hemolytic streptococci have been associated with rheumatic fever.[23]

Acute streptococcal tonsillitis is a disease of childhood, with a peak incidence at about 5 to 6 years of age, but can occur in children younger than 3 years and in adults older than 50 years.[34] Outbreaks may arise in epidemic forms in institutional settings such as recruit camps and daycare facilities. Acute tonsillitis manifests as a dry throat, malaise, fever, fullness of the throat, odynophagia, dysphagia, otalgia, headache, limb and back pain, cervical adenopathy, and shivering. Examination reveals a dry tongue, erythematous, enlarged tonsils, and yellowish white spots on the tonsils. In severe cases, a tonsillar or pharyngeal membrane or purulent exudate may exist along with jugulodigastric lymph node enlargement.[34]

The diagnosis of acute tonsillitis is made mainly on clinical grounds. The clinical manifestations of streptococcal and nonstreptococcal pharyngitis overlap so broadly that it is often impossible to make the diagnosis with certainty. For this reason, most authorities recommend that the diagnosis of group A β-hemolytic streptococcal (GABHS) pharyngitis be verified or ruled out by microbiologic tests in patients who appear likely, on the basis of clinical and epidemiologic considerations, to have this illness.[37,38] The time-honored method of diagnostic confirmation is the throat culture. This is a simple and extremely useful test but sampling must be skillfully performed by swabbing the posterior pharynx and tonsillar areas.[37] The specimen must also be appropriately processed and read. Such selective use of throat cultures represents good medical practice.

One of the major problems in the use of throat cultures in everyday medical practice has been the delay in obtaining results. The delay can range from 18 to 48 hours, which holds up the start of appropriate management but does not increase the likelihood of development of rheumatic fever. Nevertheless, it can be difficult for physicians to persuade parents of the wisdom of withholding antibiotics until results are known, especially if their children are cranky and febrile. If group A streptococcal pharyngitis is treated early in the clinical course, the period of communicability is reduced.[39] Management is thus initiated before culture results are available and unfortunately may not be terminated even when negative results are obtained. Development of rapid strep detection tests for the detection of the group A streptococcal antigen has therefore represented a useful advance.

Several rapid tests to detect group A streptococcal antigen in the pharynx have been developed. They employ either latex agglutination or enzyme-linked immunosorbent assay (ELISA) methods to extract the antigen from a swab. The streptococcal group A carbohydrate may be detected within a matter of minutes. The test kits are suitable for use in a physician's office. Although the rapid detection tests are highly specific, they are unfortunately not as sensitive as routine throat culture.[37,40,41] A negative rapid detection test result may prompt the practitioner to withhold antibiotic therapy while awaiting culture results. Most guidelines suggest that throat cultures should be performed when the body temperature is greater than 38.3° C or when the illness is characterized exclusively by a sore throat.[42] The most accurate and cost-effective method to diagnose acute GABHS infection is the use of the rapid strep test. This is followed by standard throat culture in patients with a negative rapid strep test result and a strong suspicion of streptococcal tonsillitis.

Even optimally obtained and processed, throat cultures are not without flaws. Throat culture cannot reliably differentiate acute from chronic infection. The treatment of all patients who have positive culture results leads to over-management. There are occasional false-negative results (approximately 10% of cases), although one report has found that patients with false-negative results are most likely carriers who do not require treatment.[37] Studies have reported that a single throat culture is 90% to 97% sensitive and 90% specific for GABHS growth.[43] The carrier state can be elucidated by serologic testing. A true infection is demonstrated by a positive throat culture result and at least a two-dilutional rise in the antistreptolysin-O titer.[44] A GABHS carrier without acute infection has a positive culture result with no change in dilution titer.[45] Excluding the diagnosis of group A streptococcal pharyngitis is quite important because the majority of patients with acute pharyngitis do not have "strep" throat.

Therapy has usually been directed at the aerobic pathogens traditionally associated with tonsillitis (e.g., GABHS). Penicillin is still the agent of choice in most cases. However, anaerobic bacteria play a major role in the complications associated with tonsillitis, so they are probably also involved in recurrent tonsillitis. One study has documented the prevalence of *Bacteroides* cultured from chronically inflamed tonsils.[46] Anaerobes also have been implicated in acute tonsillitis.[23] Clinical failure of penicillin should lead to the suspicion of β-lactamase–producing organisms. The reason for the treatment failure could be that these organisms either act as pathogens themselves, so-called direct pathogens, or protect susceptible pathogens from the effects of β-lactamase antibiotics, making them so-called indirect pathogens. In such cases, the patient complains of sore throat that never resolves completely despite penicillin management. An alternative to the use of penicillin is to use a penicillin plus a β-lactamase inhibitor such as clavulanic acid (e.g., amoxicillin/clavulanic acid). Other alternatives are clindamycin and a combination of erythromycin and metronidazole. Institution of antibiotic therapy within 24 to 48 hours of symptom onset will result in decreased symptoms associated with sore throat, fever, and adenopathy 12 to 24 hours sooner than without antibiotic administration. The use of antibiotics also minimizes the chance of suppurative complications and diminishes the likelihood of acute rheumatic fever.[47,48] Ten full days of therapy is necessary, as eloquently demonstrated by Schwartz and colleagues,[49] who showed that children receiving 10 days of therapy have lower clinical and bacteriologic recurrence rates than children receiving only 7 days of therapy.

There appears to be no need for further management for asymptomatic carriers because the carrier state does not lead to suppurative or nonsuppurative complications nor is the patient likely to spread the disease to others.[50] Although asymptomatic patients need neither culture nor management if results of follow-up culture are positive, certain high-risk situations should be approached differently. For example, if a family member had rheumatic fever or if a family has been experiencing recurrent streptococcal illness, another course of antibiotics would be recommended for the carrier. Patients who become symptomatic after an appropriate course of therapy may indeed represent true management failures for which a second course of therapy would also be justified.[50]

Tonsillar Concretions/Tonsilloliths

Tonsillar concretions or tonsilloliths (Fig. 196-5) arise from retained material and bacterial growth in the tonsillar or adenoid crypts and may exist in patients with or without a history of inflammatory disorders in either the tonsils or adenoids.[51] The clinical presentation of fetor oris (halitosis) and sore throat as well as the presence of whitish, expressible,

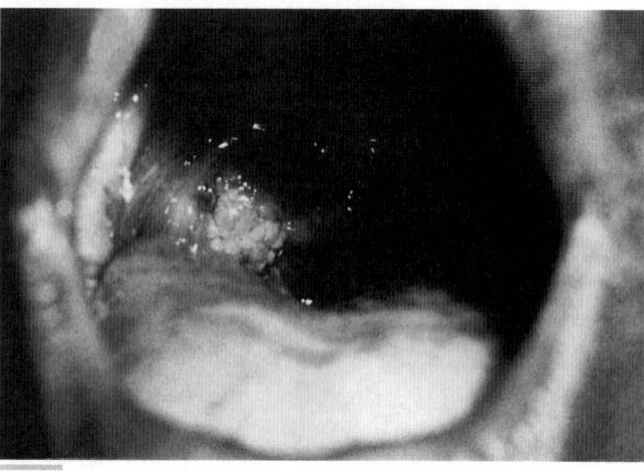

Figure 196-5. Tonsillolith of the right tonsil.

foul-tasting, and foul-smelling cheesy lumps from the tonsils characterizes the tonsillar concretions in many patients. Local management involves simple expression of the concretions by the patient, the use of pulsating jets of water to clean the pockets of debris mechanically, or application of topical silver nitrate to the tonsillar crypts in an effort to chemically cauterize and obliterate them. Persistent problems with pain, halitosis, foreign body sensation, or otalgia may require surgical removal of the tonsils as definitive therapy.

Complications of Tonsillitis

The complications of tonsillitis can be broken down into nonsuppurative and suppurative complications. Nonsuppurative complications include scarlet fever, acute rheumatic fever, and poststreptococcal glomerulonephritis. Suppurative complications are the result of abscess formation and include peritonsillar and parapharyngeal abscess development.

Nonsuppurative Complications

Scarlet fever is secondary to acute streptococcal tonsillitis or pharyngitis with production of endotoxins by the bacteria.[33] Manifestations include an erythematous rash; severe lymphadenopathy with a sore throat; vomiting; headache; fever; erythematous tonsils and pharynx; tachycardia; and a yellow exudate over the tonsils, pharynx, and nasopharynx. The membrane that is present over the tonsils is usually more friable than that seen with diphtheria. A strawberry tongue with a rash and large glossal papillae is a good diagnostic sign. Diagnosis of scarlet fever is made by culture and positive result of the Dick test, which is an intradermal injection of dilute streptococcal toxin.[34] Management of this condition involves intravenous administration of penicillin G. Otologic complications may include necrotizing otitis media with complete loss of the tympanic membrane and ossicles.

Fortunately, acute rheumatic fever is an uncommon illness in the United States today. The incidence of rheumatic fever following sporadic streptococcal infection is approximately 0.3%.[50] A patient with rheumatic fever who does not comply with penicillin prophylaxis should have a tonsillectomy and adenoidectomy because patients who have undergone surgery have a lower infection rate with β-hemolytic streptococcus.[52]

Poststreptococcal glomerulonephritis may be seen after both pharyngeal and skin infections. The incidence is approximately 24% after exposure to nephrogenic strains, but these strains account for less than 1% of the total pharyngeal strains.[50] Typically, an acute nephritic syndrome develops 1 to 2 weeks after a streptococcal infection. The infection is secondary to the presence of a common antigen of the glomerulus with the streptococcus. Penicillin management may not decrease the attack rate, and there is no evidence that antibiotic therapy affects the natural history of glomerulonephritis. A tonsillectomy may be necessary to eliminate the source of infection.

Suppurative Complications

Peritonsillar Infections

Peritonsillar abscess most commonly occurs in patients with recurrent tonsillitis or in those with chronic tonsillitis that has been inadequately treated. The spread of infection is from the superior pole of the tonsil with pus formation between the tonsil bed and the tonsillar capsule.[33] This infection usually occurs unilaterally and the pain is quite severe, with referred otalgia to the ipsilateral ear a few days after the onset of tonsillitis. Drooling is caused by odynophagia and dysphagia. Trismus is frequently present as a result of irritation of the pterygoid musculature by the pus and inflammation. There is gross unilateral swelling of the palate and anterior pillar with displacement of the tonsil downward and medially with reflection of the uvula toward the opposite side. Cultures of the peritonsillar abscess usually show a polymicrobial infection, both aerobic and anaerobic.[53]

Needle aspiration may be used to obtain a test aspirate and identify the site of the abscess. If pus is found on needle aspiration, the abscess may be opened with a long-handled scalpel to incise the mucosa over the abscess and a blunt-tip hemostat to spread and break up the loculi, draining as much pus as possible. If there has been a previous history of tonsillitis, a Quinsy tonsillectomy may be quite effective. This removes the possibility of recurrent infections and allows swift improvement of the patient's condition. This procedure is particularly favored in younger patients in whom further tonsillar infections are more likely and because of the difficulty of needle aspiration or surgical drainage in children under local anesthesia. Care must be taken to avoid abscess rupture and pus inhalation during the induction of anesthesia and endotracheal intubation.

Cellulitis should be differentiated from abscess in the management of peritonsillar infections. Some abscesses may be clinically obvious, whereas others are less obvious. When there is extension of infection of the peritonsillar abscess, computed tomography (CT) with contrast enhancement may be indicated (Fig. 196-6).

The choice between needle aspiration and incision and drainage in the management of peritonsillar abscesses is controversial. Traditional management has consisted of incision and drainage, with tonsillectomy 4 to 12 weeks later. Some surgeons advocate immediate tonsillectomy or Quinsy tonsillectomy as definitive management to ensure complete drainage of the abscess and to alleviate the need for a second hospitalization for an interval tonsillectomy.[54] Each therapeutic modality has advantages in certain situations. If incision and drainage or needle aspiration fails to drain an abscess adequately, a Quinsy tonsillectomy is indicated. In patients with a prior history of recurrent peritonsillar abscess or recurrent tonsillitis severe enough to warrant tonsillectomy, a Quinsy tonsillectomy should be considered. Quinsy tonsillectomy is particularly favored in children because they are likely to experience further episodes of tonsillitis, and needle aspiration or incision and drainage with a child under local anesthesia is often difficult or impossible.

Parapharyngeal Space Abscess

An abscess can develop in the parapharyngeal space if infection or pus drains from either the tonsils or from a peritonsillar abscess through the superior constrictor muscle.[33] The abscess is located between the superior constrictor muscle and the deep cervical fascia and causes displacement of the tonsil on the lateral pharyngeal wall toward the midline. Involvement of the adjacent pterygoid and paraspinal muscle with the inflammatory process results in trismus and a stiff neck. The thickness of the overlying sternocleidomastoid muscle often prevents the detection of fluctuance by palpation.

Patients with parapharyngeal space infections characteristically exhibit fever, leukocytosis, and pain. Progression of the infectious process of the abscess may spread down the carotid sheath into the mediastinum. As with most soft-tissue infections of the neck, lateral pharyngeal space infections are polymicrobial and usually reflect oropharyngeal flora. Intraoral examination reveals swelling of the lateral pharyngeal wall, especially behind the posterior tonsillar pillar. Anteromedial tonsil displacement is present. Clinically this may be confused with a peritonsillar abscess, so if indicated, a CT scan with contrast

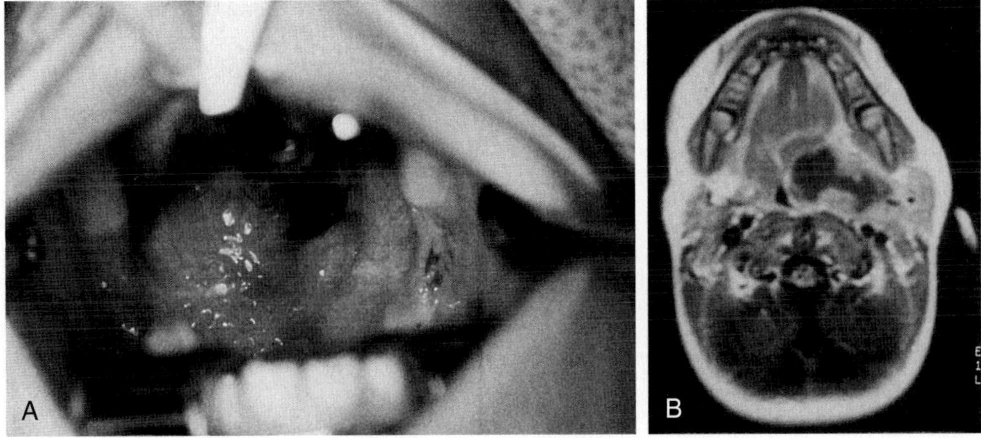

Figure 196-6. **A,** Left peritonsillar abscess in an 18-month-old child. **B,** Magnetic resonance image of the peritonsillar abscess in the same patient, showing extension of the abscess into the retropharyngeal space.

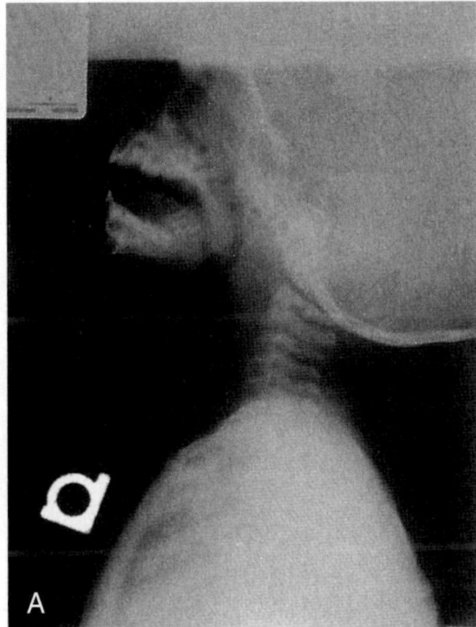

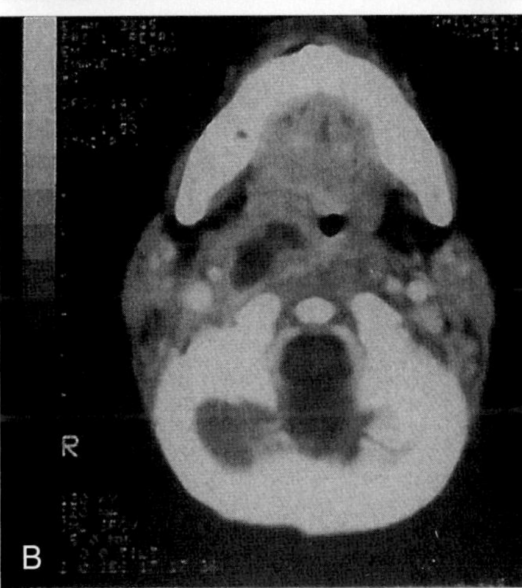

Figure 196-7. **A,** Lateral neck radiograph showing a retropharyngeal abscess. **B,** Computed tomography scan of the same patient.

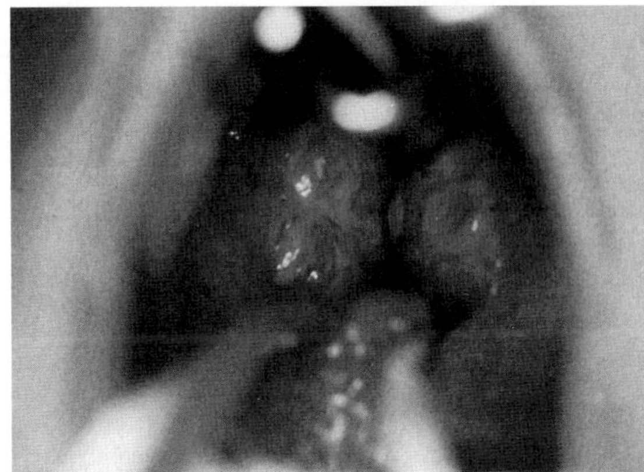

Figure 196-8. Tonsillar hypertrophy with significant pharyngeal obstruction.

enhancement should be obtained. Neurologic deficits involving cranial nerves IX, X, and XII may occur.

Initially, lateral pharyngeal space infections should be managed with aggressive antibiotic therapy, fluid replacement, and close observation. Surgical intervention is often required to bring about resolution of these infections. Intraoral approaches should be confined to management of peritonsillar abscesses and should not be used in true lateral pharyngeal space abscesses because of inadequate exposure if severe bleeding arises. An external approach to the parapharyngeal space usually consists of a transverse submandibular excision approximately 2 cm inferior to the mandibular margin, which extends from the anterior limits of the submandibular gland just past the angle of the mandible. The submandibular gland is freed inferiorly and posteriorly by sharp, blunt dissection, and access to the space is achieved by dissection between the tail of the submandibular gland and the anterior aspect of the sternocleidomastoid muscle. With this approach, the skull base can easily be explored.

Retropharyngeal Space Infections

The superior limit of the retropharyngeal space is the cranial base. Inferiorly, the retrovisceral space extends into the mediastinum to approximately the level of the tracheal bifurcation. The buccal pharyngeal fascia is adherent to the prevertebral fascia in the midline, so that infection in the retropharyngeal space is unilateral. Lateral neck radiography, CT, or ultrasonography may help ascertain whether there is cellulitis or a true abscess (Fig. 196-7). The source of the retropharyngeal abscess is a chain of lymph nodes present on either side of the midline in the retropharyngeal space. These lymph nodes receive drainage from the nose, paranasal sinuses, pharynx, and eustachian tube.

Retropharyngeal space infections occur most commonly in children younger than 2 years. Children with infection in the retropharyngeal space usually present with irritability, fever, dysphagia, muffled speech, noisy breathing, stiff neck, and cervical lymphadenopathy. Physical examination usually shows unilateral posterior pharyngeal swelling, which is visualized on inspection of the child's pharynx.

A transoral approach is recommended for incision and drainage of retropharyngeal space abscesses. If the abscess extends inferiorly below the hyoid bone (shown on the CT scan), an external approach should be used. The patient must undergo oral intubation, which can be done safely by introduction of the tube on the side opposite the abscess to avoid aspiration of purulent material. The patient must be positioned in the head-down Trendelenburg position, and packing should be placed around the endotracheal tube inferiorly. Gram staining, culture, and antimicrobial sensitivity staining should be performed on the purulent material. A small vertical incision is made in the lateral aspect of the posterior pharyngeal wall at a point between the junction of the lateral one third and medial two thirds of the distance between the midline of the pharynx and the medial aspect of the retromolar trigone.[55] The space is gently probed with a hemostat to break up the loculations and drain the abscess. A drain is not used because of the possibility of aspiration if swallowed postoperatively. If the abscess extends laterally to involve the parapharyngeal space, it should be drained through an external approach.

Chronic Adenotonsillar Hypertrophy

Etiology

Chronic adenotonsillar hypertrophy—manifesting as various degrees of airway obstruction in children—has become the most common indication for adenotonsillectomy in the United States.[56] Typically, the tonsils and adenoids are very small at birth and progressively enlarge over the first four years of life as a result of increased immunologic activity (Figs. 196-8 and 196-9). Brodsky and colleagues[27,57] reported that hypertrophied and chronically infected tonsils and adenoids had greater loads of pathogenic bacteria, especially β-lactamase producers, than nondiseased tonsils and adenoids.[57,58] These studies were based on core samples that were believed to be more accurate than surface cultures of the tonsils and adenoids. It is possible that equilibrium exists between the normal flora of the adenotonsillar tissue and their local immunologic response and that this equilibrium can become disrupted with recurrent acute viral or bacterial infections or colonization with pathogenic bacteria, resulting in hypertrophied lymphoid tissue.[27]

In addition to chronic bacterial infection, exposure to secondhand smoke has been implicated as a cause of adenotonsillar hypertrophy in children.[8]

Airway Obstruction

Obstructive sleep apnea is the most common indication for tonsillectomy in the pediatric population. Pediatric obstructive sleep apnea, confirmed by polysomnography, is reported to have an incidence of 1% to 3%.[59-61] The obstructive apnea is almost always associated with hypertrophy of the tonsils and adenoids. The tonsil and adenoid tissue, when large, fills the area of the oropharynx and nasopharynx, obstructing airflow. This obstruction is worse when the patient is supine and asleep owing to the effects of gravity and the relaxation of surrounding nasopharyngeal and oropharyngeal soft tissue. The obstruction can result in a mildly compromised airway, which leads to snoring, and most children with airway obstruction related to adenotonsillar hypertrophy have a history of significant snoring at night.[28,31,59,62,63] The obstruction may lead to intermittent complete airway obstruction with subsequent apnea and oxygen desaturation. The apnea typically is short and usually associated with a brief arousal wherein the patient repositions himself or herself and opens the airway. However, if the apnea is prolonged, oxygen desaturation can occur. Such desaturation episodes put stress on the cardiovascular system.

Before the syndrome of obstructive sleep apnea was widely recognized, children sometimes presented with pulmonary hypertension and

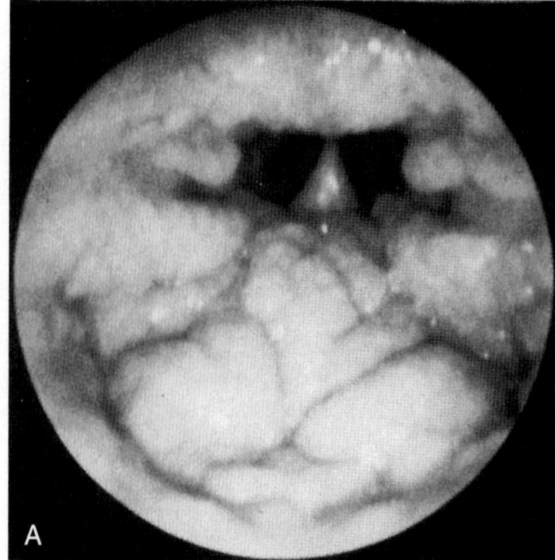

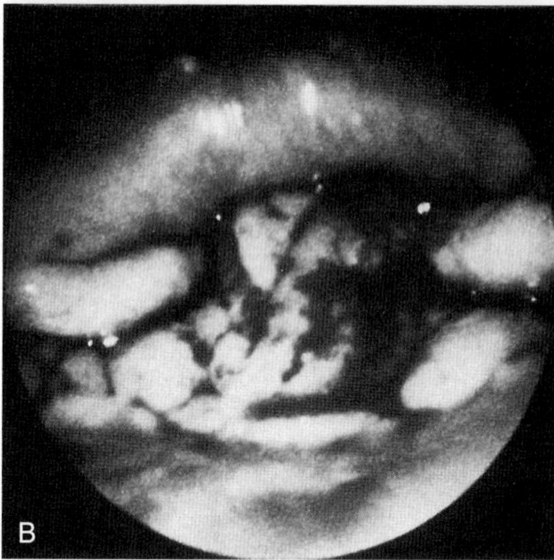

Figure 196-9. **A,** Endoscopic view of mild adenoid hypertrophy. **B,** Severe adenoid hypertrophy with total choanal obstruction.

cor pulmonale, failure to thrive, and developmental delay.[64] Such severe consequences rarely occur now, but the sleep disturbance manifests as multiple clinical symptoms that are commonly seen. Some of the more common symptoms that occur during the sleep of affected children are loud "heroic" breathing, diaphoresis, apnea, gasping, mouth-breathing, restless sleep, enuresis, drooling, night terrors, and sleepwalking. During the day affected children may suffer from daytime sleepiness, morning headache, dry mouth, halitosis, swallowing difficulty, behavioral difficulties and hyponasal speech, or, rarely, hypernasal speech (rhinolalia aperta) caused by enlarged tonsils impinging on normal palatal movement.[63] Behavioral difficulties include hyperactivity, inattentiveness in the classroom, problems with academic performance, and rebellious or aggressive behavior. The aforementioned behavioral difficulties are also clinical manifestations of the most commonly diagnosed psychiatric diagnosis in children—attention deficit–hyperactivity disorder (ADHD).

Today obstructive sleep apnea and its consequences are widely recognized, and for that reason it is the primary indication for tonsillectomy in this country.[65] There is no debate about the existence of the obstructive sleep apnea syndrome or that adenotonsillectomy is the treatment of choice. However, there is considerable debate about the methods of diagnosis and therefore considerable discussion about exactly how large a group of children is affected by the syndrome (see Chapter 183 for a full discussion).

Attention Deficit–Hyperactivity Disorder

As previously noted, inattention and hyperactivity are some of the daytime symptoms shown to have a relationship to pediatric sleep-disordered breathing (SDB). This relationship has been demonstrated in studies of children in whom obstructive sleep apnea syndrome has been documented by formal sleep study. However, an increased incidence of inattention and hyperactivity has also been found in children with significant snoring but with negative sleep study results, as well as in groups of snoring children without any formal sleep testing.

Numerous articles in the literature have shown a significant relationship between sleep-disordered breathing and the symptoms of ADHD. One study investigated 996 children aged 4 to 5 years seen consecutively in a community health clinic. Of the 782 for whom the questionnaires were completed, 95 or 12% of the children were found to snore on most nights. A group of 66 children considered at high risk for sleep disturbance was selected from these 95 children and compared with a control group who had no symptoms of sleep disturbance. The study used a modified version of the Conner's behavioral scale to assess symptoms of hyperactivity. These 66 children were studied with overnight oximetry and video monitoring. According to results of the overnight study, only 7 of the 66 children in the high-risk group had documented obstructive sleep apnea syndrome, but all the children in this high-risk group had significantly higher scores on parental and teacher reports of hyperactive behavior.[60]

Another study looked at the relationship between the symptoms of sleep-disordered breathing and problem behavior including hyperactivity and inattention. The study enrolled 3019 5-year-old children. The researchers used a questionnaire to evaluate for symptoms of sleep-disordered breathing as well as problems with behavior, and had a subset of 219 children's families complete the Revised Conners' Parent Rating Scale as a means of validating the results obtained with limited initial questioning. Symptoms of sleep-disordered breathing were present in 25% of the children. A strong association was found between parent-reported sleep problems and the parent-reported incidence of inattention, hyperactivity, and aggressiveness. Interestingly, a dose-response effect on problem behaviors was seen for both snoring frequency and snoring loudness. These results remained significant even when data were adjusted for sex, race, maternal education level, maternal marital status, household income, and respiratory history. Such adjustments had not been made in previous reports on the link between SDB and ADHD.[66]

A different study evaluated 2076 children and found 71 with behavioral or academic problems. These children had significantly more problems with snoring and difficulty breathing. This association was found to be strongest with children who had academic problems or in children whose specific behavioral problem was consistent with ADHD.[67]

Other studies have examined this issue from the opposite direction, evaluating a group of children diagnosed with neuropsychological problems and searching for signs and symptoms of SDB. These studies show that children with neuropsychological problems have a higher percentage of sleep problems than normal controls. Marcotte and associates looked at 200 children referred for psychiatric evaluation for possible ADHD; 79 children were diagnosed with ADHD, learning disability, or combined ADHD–learning disability. Through parent questionnaires, the investigators found a high incidence of reported sleep problems at night in comparison with the incidence in a control group of children. They did not find any difference in the reported length of sleep. Thus, the effect seems to depend on quality, not quantity, of sleep.[68]

Another study surveyed a group of parents at a child psychiatry unit and a group of patients at a general pediatric clinic. Children at the psychiatry clinic with the diagnosis of ADHD had a 33% incidence of habitual snoring, compared with 11% of the other children at the psychiatry clinic and 9% in those at the general pediatric clinic. Higher snoring scores derived from the validated pediatric sleep questionnaires were associated with higher levels of inattention and hyperactivity, again pointing to an apparent dose-response relationship.[69]

The pathophysiology of ADHD is unknown, but there are suggestions that an abnormal sleep pattern may be one causal factor. It has long been known that stimulants improve behavior in patients with ADHD. Stimulants are believed to work because ADHD is a disorder caused by hypovigilance rather than hypervigilance.[70] If hypovigilance is indeed the mechanism, it makes sense that a child with decreased or poor sleep secondary to obstructive sleep apnea syndrome would be much more likely to suffer from symptoms of ADHD. Consequently, if the sleep obstruction was removed, it should follow that the quality of sleep would improve and therefore symptoms of ADHD would diminish.

One small article in the European literature did show that symptoms of ADHD diminished after adenotonsillectomy.[71] At this point, however, no large prospective studies have looked carefully at this issue. This is an area of active research in the literature and one that receives a lot of attention, but still more work must be done to better clarify the cause-and-effect relationships.

Neurocognitive Development

Sleep is an important part of a child's growth and development, particularly during periods of brain maturation. Among different species, greater sleep requirements have been seen in maturing as opposed to fully mature individuals. Sleep, particularly in children, can be a very active process and may play a key role in proper brain maturation.

Multiple studies have indicated that children with a childhood history of snoring and SDB may have alteration in normal neurocognitive development. One study evaluated 297 first-grade children whose school performance was in the lowest 10th percentile in their class ranking. With both a parental questionnaire and overnight pulse oximetry monitoring and transcutaneous monitoring of partial pressure of carbon dioxide, the group was screened for signs and symptoms of a sleep disorder. The researchers found that 54 (18.1%) of these children had sleep-associated gas exchange abnormalities. Parents of these children were all offered surgical treatment, and 24 underwent tonsillectomy and adenoidectomy; parents of the remaining 30 refused surgical treatment. The group undergoing surgical treatment had a significant improvement in school scores the following year, whereas, the group refused treatment and a control group had no change in year-to year scores.[72]

In another study, the author sent questionnaires to the parents of seventh and eighth graders whose test scores placed them in either the top 25% or bottom 25% of the class. These students were matched for age, gender, race, address, and schools. The parents were sent questions related to their child's sleeping habits from age 2 to 6 years, in which the primary indicators of sleep disturbance were snoring frequency and loudness. Only those with reported loud frequent snoring during childhood years were included in the group with suspected sleep disorder. The few children with current snoring were excluded. The investigators ultimately had 800 students in each group and found that frequent and loud snoring was reported in 12.9% of the low-performing students, but in 5.1% of the high-performing children.[73] To the investigators, these results indicated that a significant sleep disturbance during the early important years of neurocognitive development may create deficits that cannot be overcome later in life, after the sleep disturbance has resolved.

One study compared the results of neurocognitive testing between 16 snoring children and 13 normal controls aged 5 to 10 years. Of the snoring children, 13 completed polysomnograms and none had clinically defined obstructive sleep apnea. The researchers found that the snoring children had lower attention, memory, and intelligence scores. They concluded that the impact of clinically mild SDB may be greater than suspected and may significantly affect future development of the child.[74]

Another study looked at a large community sample of 5-year-old children. The investigators screened the children for SDB and found that those with symptoms of SDB had significantly lower scores on a wide range of neurocognitive studies. These studies included assessments of executive function, memory, and general intellectual ability. All the test results were adjusted for any potentially confounding sociodemographic or health issues.[66] This study found that the differences in cognitive function were present even if the children with polysomnography-confirmed obstructive sleep apnea were excluded. Thus, even in children with what has been referred to as "primary snoring" were shown in this study to have measurable neurocognitive deficits.

The mechanism underlying possible cognitive deficits remains unclear. Three major processes occur during the sleep of children with upper airway obstruction—episodic hypoxia, repeated arousal leading to sleep deprivation or sleep fragmentation, and periodic or continuous alveolar hypoventilation combined with intermittent hypercapnia. Which of these sequelae or in what proportion they may be responsible for cognitive impairment is not known.[73] Central nervous system development is an ongoing process from infancy to adolescence, and developing neural elements are most likely more susceptible to injury. Neurocognitive deficits in children affected with SDB may be more prominent in the area of the prefrontal cortex because these areas do not finish development until adolescence.[75]

The National Institutes of Health–sponsored 2003 National Sleep Disorders Research Plan states, "In recent years it has become apparent that SDB and snoring are not as innocuous as previously thought." The report continues that failure to diagnose and treat such disorders in a timely manner may lead to long-lasting residual consequences. "However, the point of transition between what constitutes pathology and what is normal has yet to be defined."[76] In an editorial, one researcher active in this area discussed the accumulating evidence of a causal relationship between pediatric SDB and neurocognitive deficits. He concluded his thoughts, "The remaining but complex challenge will be to define at what age, and by what means, intervention will be required to prevent long-term neurocognitive dysfunction."[77]

An article by Garetz[78] offers a good review of the literature surrounding the issues of behavior and cognition associated with SDB. She discusses the need for further research while pointing out that none of the studies in this area has been randomized, and few studies have addressed well how ethnicity and obesity may play a role in these areas. Clearly, many questions are left unanswered at this point. First, we do not know what the dose-response relationship is between SDB and neurocognitive impairment. How long should a child be allowed to snore before treatment is recommended? We know snoring resolves spontaneously in many children, so how long do we allow a child's snoring to persist before we have concern that cognitive function will be affected? Is the tolerable length of time related to the age of the child—is a child more sensitive to the effects of sleep disturbance at 3 years or 7 years, and thus should we wait less time in a 3- year-old with significant SDB? These are all questions that further research must address.

Enuresis

Enuresis is another indicator of severe underlying airway obstruction in children. Weider and associates[79] described enuresis related to chronic adenotonsillar hypertrophy and significant airway obstruction that was relieved by adenotonsillectomy. In this study, all patients with secondary enuresis (developed later during childhood) showed response to adenotonsillectomy, whereas 24 patients with primary enuresis (congenitally present) showed no response to surgery, possibly as a result of other neurologic factors. A proposed cause of enuresis is poor nocturnal regulation of antidiuretic hormone release that is related to disorders of rapid eye movement (REM) sleep.

Growth Problems

Children with chronic adenotonsillar hypertrophy and airway obstruction may also present with failure to thrive.[64,80] A review of the literature further confirmed this apparent relationship between SDB secondary to adenotonsillar hypertrophy and the risk of growth failure in children.[81] This relationship may be related to abnormal regulation of growth hormone. During rapid eye movement sleep, growth hormone may be severely disrupted in children with obstructive sleep apnea.[80] Several studies have confirmed a postoperative increase in circulating insulin-like growth factor and its binding proteins in children with obstructive sleep apnea secondary to adenotonsillar hypertrophy.[82,83]

Cardiopulmonary Complication

Severe cases of sleep obstruction may result in cor pulmonale, pulmonary vascular hypertension, and alveolar hypoventilation, all of which may be reversed by adenotonsillectomy (Fig. 196-10).[19,84,85] The etiology of cor pulmonale is related to chronic upper airway obstruction, which leads to pulmonary ventilation-perfusion abnormalities and chronic alveolar hypoventilation. The result is chronic hypercapnia and hypoxia with respiratory acidemia, pulmonary artery vasoconstriction, and right ventricular dilation. Eventual cardiac failure may occur.[31,86,87] Relief of upper airway obstruction by adenotonsillectomy will eventually reverse this condition. However, increased partial pressure of carbon dioxide (P_{CO_2}) values may persist after relief of the obstruction, occasionally requiring prolonged endotracheal intubation and mechanical ventilation until P_{CO_2} values return to normal.

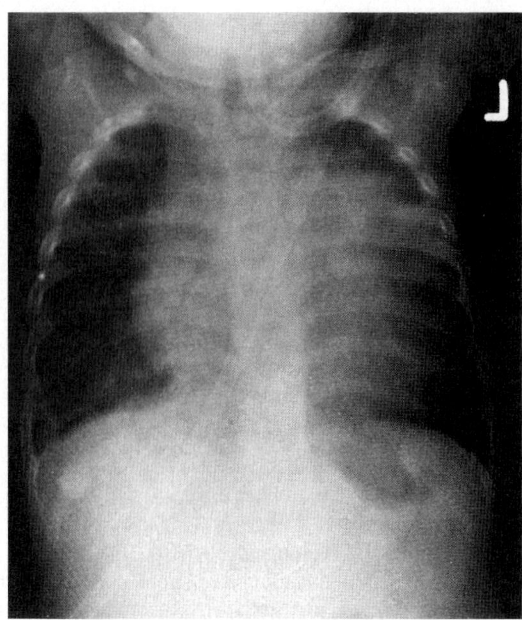

Figure 196-10. Posteroanterior chest radiograph of a patient with adenotonsillar hypertrophy, severe airway obstruction, pulmonary vascular hypertension, and cor pulmonale.

Craniofacial Growth and Adenotonsillar Hypertrophy

Chronic mouth-breathing secondary to adenotonsillar hypertrophy and upper airway obstruction has been shown to affect craniofacial growth patterns in children. As early as 1872, Tomes[88] reported that children who were chronic mouth-breathers secondary to adenoid hypertrophy displayed evidence of malocclusion and maxillofacial growth abnormalities. Mouth-breathing leads to downward and backward displacement of the mandible and tongue and potential postural changes of the head and neck that may secondarily affect dental occlusion and jaw growth.[89] Numerous animal and human studies have demonstrated the effect of chronic nasal obstruction on maxillofacial growth patterns. Harvold[90] showed that chronic nasal obstruction may lead to narrow maxillary dental arches in rhesus monkeys. Linder-Aronson and colleagues[91] demonstrated the classic stigmata of adenoid facies in children with chronic nasopharyngeal obstruction from adenoid hypertrophy. These consisted of longer total anterior face height with a tendency toward a retrognathic mandible in comparison with controls.

Adenotonsillectomy has been shown to reverse some of these findings.[91,92] Other investigators have confirmed the relationship between chronic nasal obstruction, adenotonsillar hypertrophy, and increased facial height.[93,94] A later study showed a significant correlation between adverse cephalometric data and adenotonsillar hypertrophy in a group of children 4 to 12 years old.[95] Although there is significant support in the literature for the effect of upper airway obstruction and adenotonsillar hypertrophy on craniofacial growth, other studies have been less conclusive about this relationship.[94,96,97] Maxillofacial growth disturbances in children who are mouth-breathers may also be multifactorial in etiology.[98] As a result of this apparent relationship among upper airway obstruction, adenotonsillar hypertrophy, and craniofacial

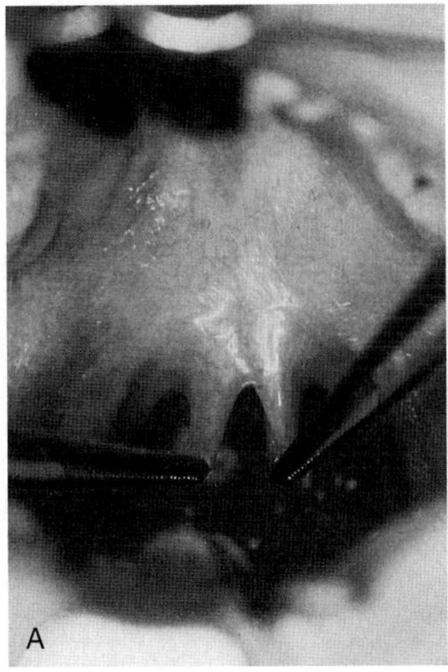

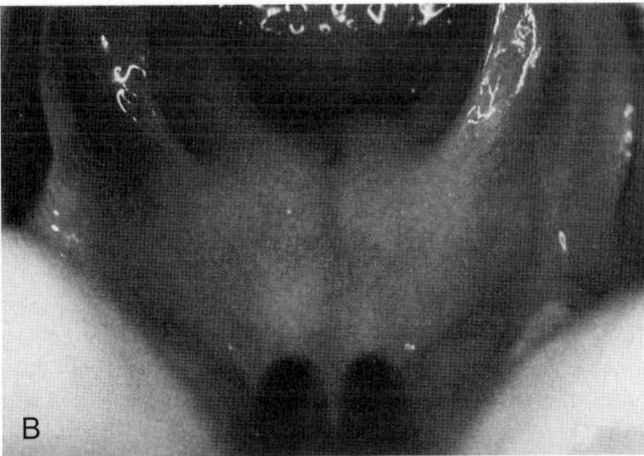

Figure 196-11. **A,** Bifid uvula in a patient with a submucous cleft palate. **B,** Submucous cleft palate.

growth disturbance, an otolaryngologic evaluation may be warranted in children undergoing orthodontic procedures for malocclusion who show evidence of adenotonsillar hypertrophy and mouth-breathing.

Diagnostic Assessment of the Tonsils and Adenoids

The physical examination of patients with suspected adenotonsillar disease should include a thorough head and neck examination to rule out manifestations of chronic adenotonsillar hypertrophy (i.e., the craniofacial stigmata of chronic nasal obstruction, which includes open-mouth breathing, an elongated face, dark circles under the eyes, and evidence of dental malocclusion). Other possible causes of nasal obstruction and these findings (e.g., turbinate hypertrophy secondary to allergic rhinitis) should also be evaluated. It is important to listen to the patient's speech to assess the presence of hyponasality. Having the child repeat words such as "Mickey Mouse," which emphasize nasal emission, and "baseball," which does not, better illuminates the presence of hyponasality.[4]

Brodsky and coworkers[57] described an assessment scale for tonsillar hypertrophy. In this scale, 0 indicates that the tonsils do not impinge on the airway; 1+ indicates less than 25% airway obstruction; 2+ indicates 25% to 50% airway obstruction; 3+ indicates 50% to 75% airway obstruction; and 4+ indicates more than 75% airway obstruction. It is also important to assess the palate on oral examination. Patients with evidence of overt or submucous cleft palate are at increased risk for the development of velopharyngeal insufficiency (VPI) after adenoidectomy. Submucous cleft palate may manifest only as a bifid uvula. However, notching of the posterior hard palate may be palpable, and an obvious translucent line through the mid–soft palate may be evident (Fig. 196-11). Although diagnostic assessment of the tonsils is apparent with oral examination, evaluation of adenoid tissue is much more difficult because it is not easily accessible on physical examination.

Lateral neck radiography may be helpful in assessing adenoid hypertrophy (Fig. 196-12). Fujioka and associates[99] determined that the adenoid-nasopharyngeal ratio, measured by lateral neck radiography, closely correlated with clinical symptomatology related to adenoid hypertrophy. This conclusion has been confirmed by other reports.[100] However, physiologic variations during nasal and oral breathing may affect these nasopharyngeal dimensions as measured by lateral neck radiography.[101] Furthermore, during an upper respiratory or sinonasal infection, significant nasopharyngeal secretions and purulence can obscure the nasopharynx and give the false impression of adenoid obstruction.

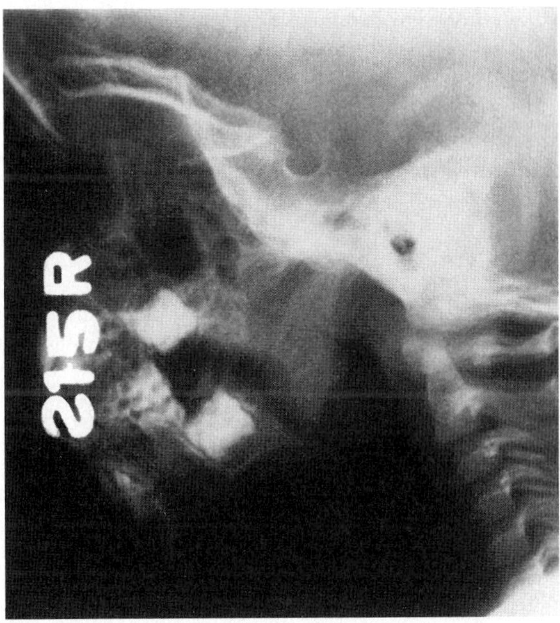

Figure 196-12. Lateral neck radiograph demonstrating significant adenoid hypertrophy and nasopharyngeal obstruction.

Lateral neck radiography is not necessary for the evaluation of all patients with suspected adenoid hypertrophy. Patients with significant obstructive symptomatology and obvious tonsillar hypertrophy most likely require surgical intervention, and findings on lateral neck radiography would not alter the decision to proceed with surgery. Patients with significant nasal obstruction and insignificant tonsillar hypertrophy should undergo radiographic assessment of the nasopharynx. Patients with significant nasal obstruction and evidence of allergic rhinitis may have concurrent underlying adenoid hypertrophy and would benefit from lateral neck radiography.

Flexible endoscopic nasopharyngoscopy may also be valuable in the assessment of adenotonsillar disease. With appropriate topical anesthesia, pediatric endoscopes, and reassurance from the physician, children generally tolerate this procedure well. The presence of adenoid tissue obstructing the posterior nasal choana will be apparent with this technique. The degree of hypopharyngeal extension of tonsillar hypertrophy may also be apparent. Sometimes tonsils that do not appear significantly large on oral examination can be seen to impinge upon and actually push back the epiglottis when viewed from above with the flexible laryngoscope. VPI secondary to tonsillar hypertrophy limiting palatal movement will be apparent on nasopharyngoscopy. The presence of adenoiditis may also be diagnosed from the presence of purulent secretions covering the adenoid pad. Wormald and Prescott[102] and Wang and others[103] demonstrated the greater efficacy of flexible nasopharyngoscopy in comparison with lateral neck radiography and clinical symptomatology in the assessment of adenoid hypertrophy in children. Rhinomanometry has also been demonstrated to correlate with the presence of nasal obstruction secondary to adenoid hypertrophy; however, this test is not well tolerated by children, is difficult and time-consuming to administer, and is probably not of clinical benefit in its current form.[104]

The role of polysomnographic testing in children has been previously reported.[64,80,105] Because of the high cost of polysomnography, it is important for the otolaryngologist to be selective in referring patients for this diagnostic modality. Furthermore there are few dedicated pediatric sleep laboratories and the wait for a study can often be very long. Patients with obvious symptoms related to adenotonsillar hypertrophy confirmed by physical examination most likely do not require polysomnographic testing. Patients with significant symptomatology—suggesting sleep apnea or a significant sleep disturbance without evidence of significant adenotonsillar hypertrophy on examination—should undergo polysomnographic testing to determine the severity of the sleep disturbance. Children with significant comorbidities that may increase surgical risk are also candidates for a polysomnogram to help in the preoperative risk-benefit assessment of surgical intervention. A polysomnogram may also help in the evaluation of the neurologically compromised child, in order to differentiate between obstructive and central apnea, because surgery is not likely to improve the latter. Screening chest radiography and electrocardiography are also recommended in the preoperative assessment of severe cases.

Preoperative Assessment

Preoperative assessment in patients undergoing adenotonsillectomy is crucial and may reveal problems that could complicate either surgery or the patient's postoperative course. It is crucial to detect the existence of any coagulation abnormalities. A family history of coagulation disorders or easy bruising may be a warning sign of an underlying bleeding disorder that warrants further hematologic evaluation. Routine evaluation of coagulation parameters before surgery in patients undergoing adenotonsillectomy is controversial. Manning and colleagues,[106] examining the records of 994 of 1050 consecutive patients undergoing tonsillectomy, adenoidectomy, or adenotonsillectomy, determined that evidence of coagulation disorders in patients with no clinical history of or findings consistent with a hematologic disorder was extremely low, thereby not justifying routine preoperative coagulation studies. This conclusion was confirmed by Close and associates,[100] who suggested that excessive bleeding associated with tonsillectomy was usually not the result of an identifiable coagulation disorder.

Conversely, Kang and coworkers[107] studied the risk of postoperative hemorrhage in 1061 children undergoing adenotonsillectomy. In this study, 2.5% of the children had at least one abnormality on preoperative coagulation screening, which consisted of determinations of prothrombin time, partial thromboplastin time, bleeding time, and platelet count. These researchers suggested that, although hematologic disorders were diagnosed infrequently by preoperative coagulation screening, the coagulation profile may detect patients who are more likely to bleed postoperatively.[107] This suggestion is consistent with the findings of Bolger and colleagues,[108] who demonstrated abnormal initial coagulation screening results in 11.5% of patients undergoing adenotonsillectomy. It is apparent that patients who have an obvious family or clinical history of excessive bleeding or an underlying hematologic disorder require close monitoring of coagulation profiles and consultation with a hematologist. Use of preoperative coagulation screening should be left to the discretion of the surgeon until its role is better clarified by further study.

Box 196-1

Surgical Indications for Tonsillectomy

Infection

Recurrent, acute tonsillitis (more than 6 episodes per year or 3 episodes per year for 2 years or longer)
Recurrent acute tonsillitis associated with other conditions:
- Cardiac valvular disease associated with recurrent streptococcal tonsillitis
- Recurrent febrile seizures

Chronic tonsillitis that is unresponsive to medical therapy and is associated with:
- Halitosis
- Persistent sore throat
- Tender cervical adenitis

Streptococcal carrier state unresponsive to medical therapy
Peritonsillar abscess
Tonsillitis associated with abscessed cervical nodes
Mononucleosis with severely obstructing tonsils that is unresponsive to medical therapy

Obstruction

Excessive snoring and chronic mouth-breathing
Obstructive sleep apnea or sleep disturbances
Adenotonsillar hypertrophy associated with:
- Cor pulmonale
- Failure to thrive
- Dysphagia
- Speech abnormalities
- Craniofacial growth abnormalities
- Occlusion abnormalities

Other

Suspected neoplasia–asymmetric tonsillar hypertrophy

Patients with obvious severe airway obstruction secondary to adenotonsillar hypertrophy may require polysomnography, chest radiography, electrocardiography, and, possibly, cardiology consultation. Patients with cor pulmonale and hypercapnia may need postoperative intensive care monitoring with mechanical ventilation to avoid postobstructive pulmonary edema. If the severity of airway obstruction is not clear from history supplied by the parents, polysomnography may be warranted.

Patients with other medical conditions may require further testing or preoperative consultation. Patients with a history of significant bronchospasm may require pulmonary medicine evaluation and management in the perioperative period. Black patients should be screened for sickle cell disease preoperatively, and girls of reproductive age should undergo a preoperative serum β-human chorionic gonadotropin test to rule out pregnancy. Velocardiofacial syndrome may require preoperative angiography to determine the presence of abnormally medially displaced carotid arteries, which may be at risk during tonsillectomy.[109]

Adenotonsillectomy

The technique of adenotonsillectomy has evolved significantly over the past 2000 years, and various techniques are used today for extirpation of the tonsils and adenoids. Multiple tonsillectomy techniques exist, including the sharp dissection initially described by Crowe and associates[7]; various electrocauterization techniques; lasers (including potassium-titanyl–phosphate [KTP][110] and CO_2[52]); the tonsil guillotine; as well as newer technologies and techniques such as Coblation (ArthroCare Corporation, Austin, TX), the Harmonic Scalpel (Ethicon Endo-Surgery, Inc., Cincinnati, OH), and the Microdebrider (Medtronic Xomed, Inc., Jacksonville, FL). The number of adenotonsillectomies

Box 196-2

Surgical Indications for Adenoidectomy

Infection

Purulent adenoiditis

Adenoid hypertrophy associated with:

- Chronic otitis media with effusion
- Chronic recurrent acute otitis media
- Chronic otitis media with perforation
- Otorrhea or chronic tube otorrhea

Obstruction

Adenoid hypertrophy associated with excessive snoring and chronic mouth-breathing

Sleep apnea or sleep disturbances

Adenoid hypertrophy associated with:

- Cor pulmonale
- Failure to thrive
- Dysphagia
- Speech abnormalities
- Craniofacial growth abnormalities
- Occlusion abnormalities
- Speech abnormalities

Other

Suspected neoplasia

Adenoid hypertrophy associated with chronic sinusitis

performed in the United States appears to have peaked in the 1940s and 1950s.[56] In 1959, 1.4 million tonsillectomies were performed. This number decreased to 500,000 in 1979 and fell even further to 340,000 in 1985.[50,56] In the past 30 years there has been a significant decrease in the number of adenotonsillectomies performed in the United States, as well as a change in the preoperative indications for surgery. Whereas chronic infection was the primary surgical indication for adenotonsillectomy in the 1950s and 1960s, airway obstruction and obstructive sleep apnea have now become the most common preoperative indications for surgery.[56] Apparent drops in the number of adenotonsillectomies performed in the United States reflect a higher degree of selectivity by otolaryngologists and referring primary care physicians.

Indications

The current indications for tonsillectomy and adenoidectomy are shown in Boxes 196-1 and 196-2. Generally, the indications for adenotonsillectomy can be related primarily to chronic upper airway obstruction in conjunction with adenotonsillar hypertrophy, which manifests as snoring, obstructive sleep apnea, or chronic infectious conditions such as chronic recurrent tonsillitis.

Upper Airway Obstruction

Patients with airway obstruction related to adenotonsillar hypertrophy typically present with excessive snoring and sometimes with witnessed brief apneic events. The severity of the condition can often be elicited with a history supplied by the parents. However, there may often be no indications of airway obstruction other than loud snoring. It has been demonstrated that patients who snore loudly at night may manifest significant sleep apnea on polysomnographic testing when no significant parental history of witnessed apnea has been noted.[111] Patients who have obvious adenotonsillar hypertrophy on physical examination, a significant history of loud snoring with the associated symptoms of restless, disturbed sleep, or daytime somnolence do not necessarily need preoperative polysomnographic testing. If the parent is unclear about the severity of airway obstruction or if the physical findings and history are not consistent, preoperative polysomnographic testing is warranted to demonstrate the severity of airway obstruction.

Chronic Infections

Patients with chronic recurrent tonsillitis or chronic tonsillitis may benefit from tonsillectomy and possibly adenoidectomy. In 1995, the American Academy of Otolaryngology–Head and Neck Surgery Clinical Indicators Compendium stated that patients who have three or more infections of the tonsils and/or adenoids per year despite adequate medical therapy are candidates for tonsillectomy and adenoidectomy.[112] Other indications are chronic tonsillitis unresponsive to medical therapy that results in a persistent foul taste or halitosis and recurrent tonsillitis associated with the streptococcal state that has not responded to β-lactamase–resistant antimicrobial therapy.[112] The efficacy of elective tonsillectomy for recurrent sore throats has been demonstrated by numerous investigators.[113,114] The efficacy of elective tonsillectomy has also been shown in children with recurrent throat infections, including GABHS.[114]

In a study by Paradise and associates,[114] 187 children participated in a randomized clinical trial. Inclusion criteria for the study were seven or more sore throat episodes in the preceding year that were treated with antibiotics; five or more sore throat episodes in the 2 preceding years; or three or more episodes in each of the 3 preceding years. Elective tonsillectomy or adenoidectomy resulted in better status than that in a control group of children who were managed nonsurgically. Factors that should be taken into account in the consideration of surgery for recurrent throat infections in children are (1) the severity of each episode, (2) how well infections have responded to medical therapy, and (3) quality of life issues (e.g., number of school days missed).

Tonsillectomy and adenoidectomy should be considered in patients with recurrent tonsillitis, as well as other medical conditions such as cardiac valvular disease with recurrent streptococcal tonsillitis, a history of febrile seizures, poorly controlled diabetes, and, possibly, ventricular peritoneal shunts. Systemic infections in these situations could become life-threatening.

Tonsillectomy is the management of choice for peritonsillar abscess in children who do not tolerate needle aspiration. Peritonsillar abscesses that have been successfully drained by needle aspiration are not necessarily absolute indications for tonsillectomy. However, tonsillectomy is definitely indicated in cases of recurrent peritonsillar abscess.[54,115-117]

Although diphtheria is currently unusual, tonsillectomy may be warranted in patients who are diphtheria carriers and have not shown response to antibiotic therapy. Finally, patients with chronic halitosis related to debris in the tonsillar crypts or secondary to chronic tonsillitis are candidates for tonsillectomy.

Adenoidectomy

Indications

Adenoid hypertrophy or chronic adenoiditis may cause significant problems requiring adenoidectomy in situations in which the tonsils themselves are not diseased and are not contributing to symptomatology. Patients with chronic adenoid hypertrophy causing craniofacial morphology problems, excessive snoring, or, possibly, quality of life issues (e.g., poor olfaction) are candidates for adenoidectomy.[118] Adenoid hypertrophy may be confirmed by flexible nasopharyngoscopy or lateral cervical radiography.

Patients with a history of chronic recurrent sinusitis may also benefit from adenoidectomy. Patients with chronic sinusitis and significant adenoid hypertrophy may initially benefit from adenoidectomy rather than undergoing more extensive sinus surgery.[119] In addition, patients with chronic purulent rhinitis secondary to chronic adenoiditis may also have response to adenoidectomy if their rhinitis has not responded well to appropriate medical therapy. Evidence now points to a possible reason for the efficacy of adenoidectomy in these situations. Coticchia and colleagues[120] showed that biofilms were prominent in the adenoids of children with chronic sinusitis. The group compared pediatric adenoids removed for chronic sinusitis with those removed for obstructive sleep apnea. In the sinusitis-related adenoids, 94.9% of the mucosal surface was covered with dense mature biofilms, compared with just 1.9% of the surface in the hypertrophy-only adenoids. This study suggests that the biofilms may be a natural reservoir for resistant bacteria and that their removal during adenoidectomy may be the reason for the observed benefit of the procedure.

Patients with hyponasal speech (rhinolalia clausa) are also candidates for adenoidectomy. Hypernasal speech (rhinolalia aperta) is a contraindication to adenoidectomy. However, in unusual cases, excessive tonsillar hypertrophy may impede palatal movement, which may improve after tonsillectomy.[121]

Although surgical intervention should be considered in cases of severe nasal obstruction related to adenoid hypertrophy, there is evidence that alternative medical therapy exists to manage adenoid hypertrophy. Demain and Goetz[122] demonstrated that aqueous nasal beclomethasone therapy led to significant improvement of nasal obstruction secondary to adenoid hypertrophy, which was confirmed by pre- and post-management flexible nasopharyngoscopy. In addition, patients with underlying inhalant allergies may benefit from antihistamine therapy and, possibly, from allergic immunologic desensitization therapy.

Conservative adenoidectomy should be performed in patients with a cleft palate or submucous cleft palate, leaving the lower portion of the adenoid pad intact to decrease the risk of postoperative VPI.

Adenoidectomy and Otitis Media

The role of the adenoids in the etiology of otitis media has been controversial. However, several investigations have demonstrated that appropriate management of the adenoids plays an important role in the diagnosis and management of chronic otitis media in children. Numerous reports have demonstrated that adenoidectomy alone or in conjunction with myringotomy tube placement may reduce the incidence of future episodes of otitis media and possibly reduce the necessity for future ventilation tubes.[123,124] Gates and colleagues[123] randomly assigned 578 children between the ages of 4 and 8 years to four management groups; group 1 underwent bilateral myringotomy and no ventilation tube placement; group 2 underwent placement of ventilation tubes; group 3 underwent adenoidectomy alone; and group 4 underwent adenoidectomy and placement of ventilation tubes. They demonstrated with statistical significance that patients who underwent adenoidectomy in conjunction with bilateral myringotomy had significantly lower postmanagement morbidity, as measured by hearing loss secondary to middle-ear effusion and the number of subsequent placements of ventilation tubes. Paradise and associates[124] randomly studied 213 children who had previously received ventilation tubes that had since extruded. These patients were randomized into two groups, those undergoing adenoidectomy and those who did not (control group). The adenoidectomy group had statistically significant less otitis media than control subjects. Another, large study further demonstrated the effectiveness of adenoidectomy in this regard. Kadhim and associates,[125] evaluating data on 50,000 children younger than 10 years who had undergone myringotomy tube placement, found that adenoidectomy at the time of tube placement decreased the odds of needing subsequent tube placement regardless of whether or not the child was having adenotonsillar disease. The actual mechanism by which adenoidectomy affects the course of otitis media in children is unclear. Surgical extirpation of the adenoids may remove a nasopharyngeal nidus of contaminated tissue that secondarily acts as a source of infection in the middle ear, or adenoidectomy may simply remove an anatomic obstruction of the eustachian tube. The actual size of the adenoid pad has not necessarily been implicated in the etiology of chronic otitis media with effusion. Many studies have been unable to determine the relationship between adenoid size and chronic otitis media with effusion.[126-129]

On the basis of current evidence, adenoidectomy should be considered in children undergoing primary ventilation tube placement who have symptomatology suggestive of chronic nasal obstruction or adenoid hypertrophy that is confirmed by nasopharyngoscopy or nasopharyngeal radiography. Patients who require subsequent sets of ventilation tubes also may be candidates for adenoidectomy, regardless of adenoid size or symptomatology. If surgery is elected, proper technique is important, as Bluestone[115] and McKee[130] reported that surgical manipulation of the eustachian tube during adenoidectomy may predispose children to eustachian tube malfunction and the subsequent development of otitis media with effusion.

Adenotonsillectomy: Surgical Technique

Many surgical techniques have been described for extirpation of the tonsils and adenoids. Crowe and associates[7] described the first meticulous surgical dissection technique with use of sharp instrumentation. More recently, however, dissection with electrocautery has become the most popular and common technique. Other current techniques are the Coblator (ArthroCare Corporation), the Microdebrider, the ultrasonic Harmonic Scalpel, bipolar electrocautery, and, less frequently, CO_2 or KTP laser tonsillectomy.[62,110,131-135] A 2007 survey of pediatric otolaryngologists showed monopolar cautery to be by far the most common method of tonsillectomy, favored by 53% of the respondents. Coblation at 16% was the second most common method, cold dissection combined with electrocautery was third at 10%, followed by bipolar electrocautery at 6%.[136] Evidence also suggests that sharp dissection may lead to slightly less postoperative pain. However, there may be less intraoperative blood loss with electrocautery techniques.[132,137,138] Guillotine tonsillectomy techniques are still used and have been shown to have a low complication rate.[140-141] In China, the technique of guillotine tonsillectomy in children without anesthesia has been described.[142]

Of the new technologies, Coblation tonsillectomy has received possibly the most attention and acceptance. Coblation technology utilizes a system of radiofrequency bipolar electrical current that passes through a medium of normal saline, which results in the production of a plasma field of sodium ions. These energized ions are able to break down intercellular bonds and effectively vaporize tissue at a temperature of only 60° C. This vaporization theoretically results in effective dissection with less postoperative pain from thermal injury.[143,144] The technique can be utilized for complete tonsillectomy or for intracapsular tonsillectomy, otherwise known as tonsillotomy, in which the tonsil is debulked, leaving a small amount of lymphoid tissue to cover the inferior constrictor muscle. Multiple newer studies suggest decreased pain and recovery time with Coblation than with electrocautery and the Harmonic Scalpel.[145-147] These studies report no higher incidence of postoperative hemorrhage with this technique. Some researchers, however, have found a higher bleeding rate with the Coblator, and this issue remains a concern for some writers.[148-150]

The Coblator consists of a hand piece with a suction irrigation tip that transmits the radiofrequency current and dissects tissue and also has a cautery capability for hemostasis. With the Coblation technique, a separate suction cautery device is theoretically not necessary, because adenoidectomy can be performed with the Coblator. The blade can be bent to allow placement into the nasopharynx to allow Coblation of adenoid tissue with use of mirror visualization. This technique may work adequately for small adenoid pads; however, it may not be as efficacious for large obstructive adenoid pads. Research is ongoing to improve the Coblator to enhance its capabilities to perform adenoidectomy.

The Harmonic Scalpel utilizes ultrasonic technology to cut and coagulate tissues, resulting in minimal tissue damage from thermal trauma. The device converts electrical energy from a generator into mechanical vibration through a transducer that consists of piezoelectric ceramics, generating a back-and-forth vibration of the blade at a frequency of approximately 55.5 kHz. The device can cut tissue on low- and high-power settings and can also coagulate bleeding tissue. Initially, the Harmonic Scalpel found its use in laparoscopic surgery in the field of pediatric and general surgery. However, its use in tonsillectomy has been reported to have encouraging results.[103,151] Wiatrak and Willging[151] reported on a prospective study consisting of 117 patients undergoing either traditional electrocautery technique or Harmonic Scalpel surgery. They found a trend toward decreased postoperative pain over the first 3 postoperative days and a significant increase in the ability to sleep comfortably through the first three postoperative nights in children undergoing Harmonic Scalpel surgery. The duration of the procedure was longer for the Harmonic Scalpel than for electrocautery. The complication rates were equivalent in the two groups. At this time the Harmonic Scalpel cannot be utilized for adenoidectomy, so other techniques must be used for that operation. A concern about its use is higher costs incurred for each blade utilized for tonsillectomy. Other studies have shown the Harmonic Scalpel to be an effective instrument for tonsillectomy but have not found it to have a significant advantage over electrocautery.[152]

Subtotal tonsillectomy has become a more popular technique over the last several years. The concept of partial intracapsular tonsillectomy or tonsillotomy is not new to otolaryngology.[153] This procedure can be performed using any of the described instruments but is now most commonly performed with powered instrumentation.[154,155] Ideally in this technique, the only tissue manipulated and dissected is the tonsil itself. No mucosal cuts are made, the peritonsillar capsule is not dissected, and there should not be any direct cauterization of the peritonsillar fascia and underlying pharyngeal musculature. All of the preceding features are thought to make the postoperative pain and discomfort much less with this technique. With use of a microsurgical debrider, the hypertrophied tonsils are sequentially shaved behind the levels of the anterior and posterior tonsillar pillars. Exposure is obtained by retraction of the anterior tonsillar pillar with a Herd retractor. Hemostasis is obtained with suction cautery. Multiple studies point to a reduced need for pain medicine and more rapid return to normal activity and normal diet with subtotal microsurgical debrider tonsillectomy.[156-158] The incidence of postoperative bleeding is not increased with this technique and may actually be slightly less than with traditional electrocautery.[159] However, at least one study did not show a significant difference in return to normal activity and pain resolution between these two methods.[160] The indications for this technique are controversial, with some advocating this technique as appropriate for all indications in all ages and others stating that it should be performed only in children without a history of tonsillitis, owing to the concern about persistent tonsillitis in the residual tonsil tissue. Cost is a factor in the use of disposable microsurgical debrider blades for partial intracapsular tonsillectomy. At this point there is little evidence that the residual tissue is associated with recurrent tonsillitis as the child ages, but more long-term data are needed for confirmation. The most significant concern with this technique is the possibility of regrowth and the subsequent recurrence of obstructive symptoms. In one series of 278 patients, the incidence of regrowth was 3.2%.[161] This event is rare but does occur, and the patient's parents must be made aware of this possibility during the informed consent discussion for this procedure.

The microsurgical debrider can be effective for performing adenoidectomy. Koltai and others have reported on and shown the safety and efficacy of this technique.[155,162-165] Koltai, Chan, and Younes[166] report that the utilization of power-assisted adenoidectomy allows more precise, rapid, and safe removal of adenoid tissue. This technique is especially useful in removing adenoid tissue that extends through the choanae and into the nasal cavity. However, the cost of microsurgical debrider blades continues to be an issue related to its use. Stanislaw and coworkers,[167] in a prospective evaluation of power-assisted adenoidectomy or curette adenoidectomy in 90 children, found that power-assisted adenoidectomy was 20% faster, involved 27% less blood loss, and provided a more complete resection and better control of depth of reception. It also had higher surgeon satisfaction.

Technique Description

Electrocautery tonsillectomy using a meticulous dissection technique and low electrocautery wattage results in very minimal intraoperative blood loss and acceptable postoperative discomfort. This technique is described in detail. Instrumentation is shown in Figure 196-13.

Patients should not eat solid foods for 8 hours before surgery. If the patient is closely supervised, he or she may drink clear liquids until 3 hours before surgery. Preoperative sedation with midazolam hydrochloride (0.5 to 1 mg/kg) approximately 30 minutes before surgery may be necessary for patients with excessive preoperative anxiety. Anesthesia is typically induced by mask ventilation, with subsequent intravenous access after the anesthetic has taken effect. Patients usually receive intravenous antibiotics such as ampicillin (20 mg/kg; maximum dose, 1 g). Telian and colleagues[168] demonstrated that intravenous antibiotics followed by a 1-week course of postoperative oral antibiotics significantly decreased morbidity after tonsillectomy.

Patients who have a significant history of obstructive sleep apnea or are younger than 3 years receive intraoperative corticosteroids, most commonly dexamethasone (0.5 mg/kg). Catlin and Grimes[169] reported that one dose of intraoperative intravenous corticosteroids improved

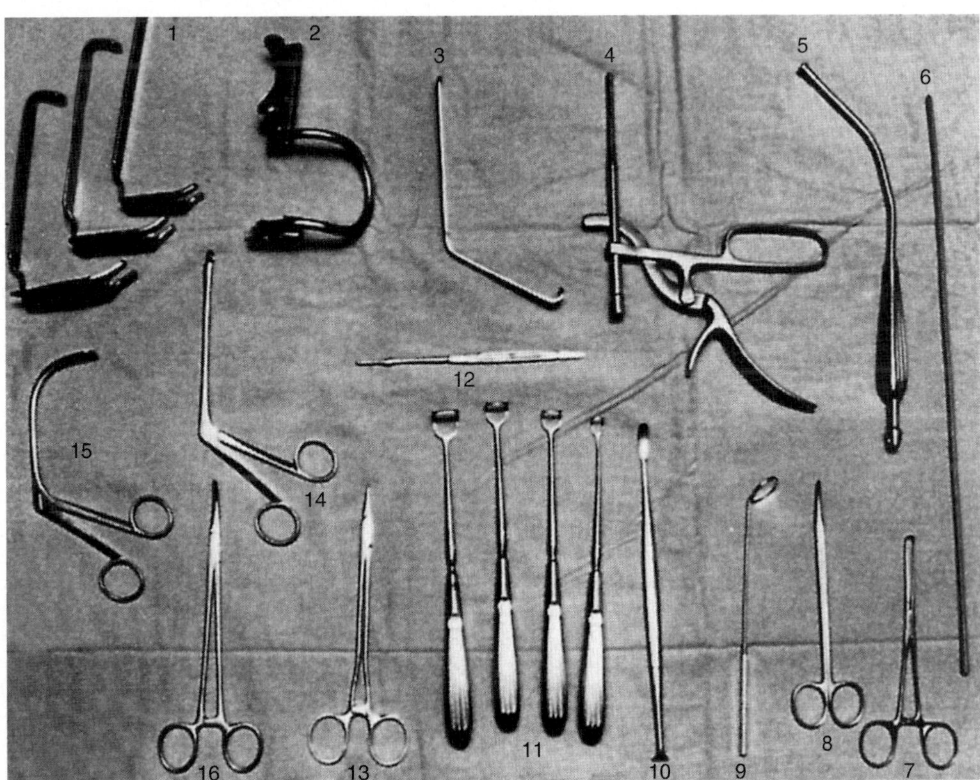

Figure 196-13. Instrumentation used in tonsillectomy and adenoidectomy procedures.

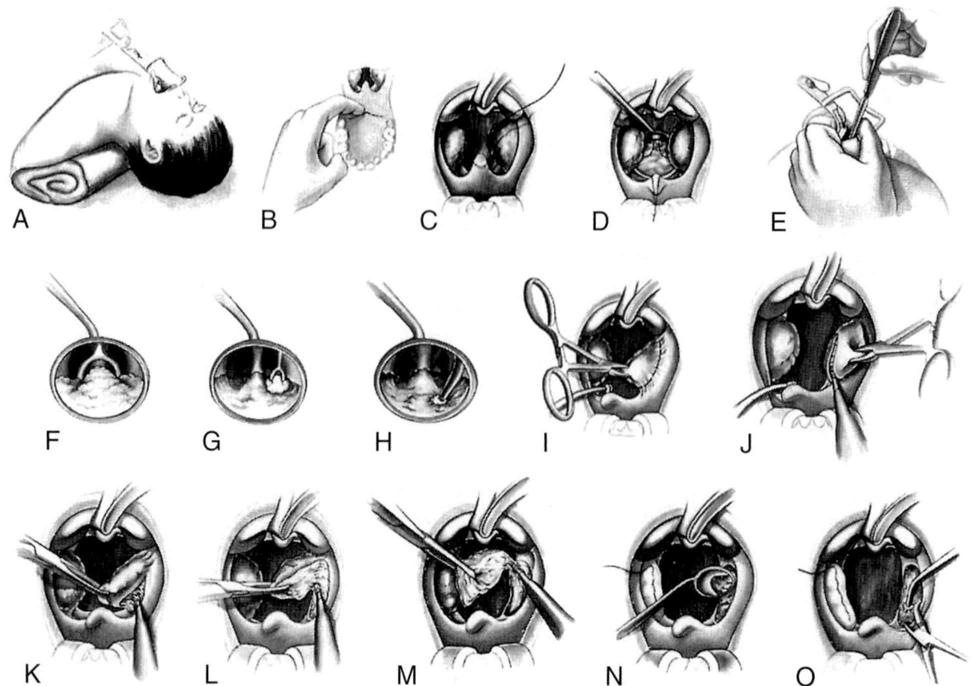

Figure 196-14. Adenotonsillectomy technique. **A,** Patient placed in Rose's position. **B,** Palate inspected for presence of submucous cleft. **C,** Nylon suture placed through uvula for retraction. **D,** Nasopharynx inspected with mirror. **E** and **F,** Positioning of curette for adenoid removal. **G,** Removal of adenoid remnants with small curette. **H,** Removal of adenoid remnants and control of bleeding with suction cautery. **I** and **J,** Grasping of right tonsil and incision of mucosa using cautery. **K** to **M,** Dissection of tonsil with cautery. **N,** Inspection of superior pole with mirror. **O,** Control of bleeding with suction cautery.

recovery time in children following tonsillectomy. However, Ohlms and associates[170] and Volk and coworkers[171] demonstrated no significant effects on recovery time of a single dose of intravenous steroids. We use corticosteroids to potentially reduce airway edema in patients who are more susceptible to airway complications after tonsillectomy. Although we do not routinely use peritonsillar infiltration with local anesthetic agents, numerous reports have described short-term benefit of this procedure with regard to postoperative pain in the immediate recovery period after tonsillectomy.[172-174] Peritonsillar infiltration with local anesthesia may also decrease intraoperative blood loss in patients undergoing sharp-dissection tonsillectomy.[172]

After induction of general anesthesia and placement of an endotracheal tube, the patient is placed in Rose's position (Fig. 196-14A) and a Crowe-Davis mouth gag is placed for exposure of the oropharynx. A red rubber catheter is placed through the right nares, brought back out through the oral cavity, and clamped with a Kelly clamp to retract the soft palate for better visualization of the nasopharynx. At this point the hard and soft palate are examined by visual inspection and palpation for evidence of a submucous cleft palate. Adenoidectomy should not be performed in the presence of an occult submucous cleft palate unless absolutely necessary. Conservative adenoidectomy should be considered in these situations. The Microdebrider is especially useful in this rare situation.

Adenoidectomy in the United States is still most commonly performed with adenoid curettes, which have either straight or curved handles.[175] The LaForce adenotome also has been described as an instrument for adenoid extirpation.[176] The nasopharynx is inspected with a nasopharyngeal mirror to assess the size of the adenoid pad and guide placement of the curette. The curette is placed high in the nasopharynx so it abuts the posterior aspect of the nasal septum. The adenoid pad is then carefully curetted, with care taken not to penetrate deeply into the prevertebral region. Care must also be taken during use of the curette not to extend too far laterally and thus potentially risking damage to the torus tubarius and eustachian tube orifice. Small curettes may be used to remove residual adenoid tissue in the posterior choanal region. This step entails removal of the superior portion of the adenoid pad and preservation of the inferior aspect with cautery or curettes. Packs are placed into the nasopharynx to obtain hemostasis.

With use of the Microdebrider, the exposure is the same. The instrument is set to oscillate at a maximum of 1500 rpm. With the nasopharyngeal mirror, the adenoids are débrided, with protection of the eustachian tube opening and care taken to not débride too deeply. When all the desired adenoid tissue has been removed, the nasopharynx is packed.

After tonsillectomy has been performed, the nasopharynx is reexamined, and hemostasis is obtained with suction electrocautery. It is important to remember that the mouth-gag tongue blade places pressure on the base of tongue and should be released intermittently to allow blood circulation in the tongue and possibly aid in reducing postoperative pain. A throat pack may be used to prevent blood and secretions from entering the esophagus. Swallowing of blood and secretions may lead to postoperative nausea and vomiting. In addition, blood oozing around the endotracheal tube may form a laryngeal clot, which may lead to postextubation airway obstruction. Children undergoing adenotonsillectomy typically have an uncuffed endotracheal tube, which may allow leakage of air around the tube with positive-pressure ventilation. Fires and endotracheal tube explosions have been reported during tonsillectomy, presumably related to oxygen leaking around uncuffed endotracheal tubes.[177]

At this point, the tonsillectomy is performed with electrocautery. The tonsil is grasped with an Allis clamp or tenaculum. It is then retracted medially, and the superior pole is incised with the electrocautery; the surgeon identifies the tonsillar capsule and carefully dissects the avascular plane between the capsule and the tonsillar bed. When sharp dissection is used, the superior mucosal incision may be made with a knife, and blunt dissection may be used to separate the tonsil from the tonsillar bed with a Thompson dissector or a Fischer knife. With the electrocautery, the tonsil is carefully dissected down to its inferior extent, where it is amputated. With sharp dissection, a tonsil snare can be used to amputate the tonsil at the inferior pole. If bleeding is noted at this point, a pack may be placed in the tonsillar fossa, and the other tonsil is then excised in the same manner. Care must be taken to preserve the mucosa and muscle in the posterior pillar, especially superiorly. Extensive cauterization and tissue loss of the posterior pillar may predispose the patient to postoperative nasopharyngeal stenosis. If electrocautery is being used, great care must be taken that other metal instrumentation in the oropharynx (e.g., the mouth gag or Yankauer suction) not touch the electrocautery blade, so as to avoid burning the oropharynx and lips. In addition, the electrocautery blade should be guarded with a nonconducting material.

After removal of the tonsillar fossa packs, residual bleeding may be controlled with electrocautery on a low-wattage setting. Significant bleeding vessels may have to be clamped and ligated. Great care should be taken in the use of suture ligatures in the tonsillar fossa. The external maxillary and lingual arteries may inadvertently be ligated in the region of the inferior tonsillar pole, thus leading to sloughing and severe hemorrhage. In addition, the internal carotid artery, which is in close proximity to the tonsillar fossa, may be damaged inadvertently, resulting in complications such as pseudoaneurysm formation and excessive hemorrhage.[52] After hemostasis has been obtained in the oropharynx and nasopharynx, the oral and nasal cavities are thoroughly irrigated. The hypopharynx is suctioned to evacuate all secretions and potential blood clots, and the stomach is also suctioned at this point. The patient is then awakened and extubated.

In general, accepted practice is to admit for overnight admission patients who have a significant history of obstructive sleep apnea, those younger than 3 years, and those with other medical problems or extenuating circumstances. If they are taking oral fluids adequately, all patients undergoing outpatient surgery are discharged after an observation period of approximately 2 to 4 hours. Intravenous fluids are administered according to deficit replacement and maintenance until oral intake resumes satisfactorily; lactated Ringer's solution or 0.5 normal saline is used. Acetaminophen with or without codeine is given for analgesia. A 1-week course of oral antibiotics is also prescribed. The patient's diet advances from clear liquids on the day of surgery to a soft diet the following day and then solid foods subsequently as tolerated. Soft foods are generally well tolerated. However, patients with unrestricted diets have not been shown to have significant complication rates postoperatively.[6,58,178] Patients or their parents are instructed to return immediately to the emergency room if there is any evidence of bright red bleeding from the nose or oral cavity.

Inpatient versus Outpatient Procedures

It has been clearly demonstrated in the literature that adenotonsillectomy in appropriately selected children may be performed on an outpatient basis.[14,25,105,179,180] It is important that patients are observed postoperatively and that they obtain significant postoperative intravenous rehydration. Postoperative observation times discussed in the literature vary from 136 minutes to 6 to 8 hours.[133,181] Although short-stay outpatient tonsillectomy has been demonstrated as a safe and cost-effective procedure, it is important preoperatively to identify outpatients who are at risk for postoperative complications and who may benefit from longer observation periods following surgery.

Numerous writers believe that children younger than 3 years should be admitted for observation after surgery because they are at increased risk for postoperative complications, most of which are airway-related.[94,180,182-185] The ultimate decision for postoperative admission lies with the surgeon. Other patients who may warrant admission after adenotonsillectomy include those with (1) a history of an abnormal bleeding disorder or abnormal preoperative coagulation profile, (2) evidence of severe obstructive sleep apnea, (3) underlying craniofacial abnormalities such as Down syndrome, and (4) systemic disorders such as cardiopulmonary disease or asthma. Postoperative admission also should be considered for patients undergoing tonsillectomy for peritonsillar abscess, for patients who live a long distance from the hospital (>60 miles or 1 hour driving time), or for patients whose home situation is not consistent with close postoperative observation.[116,117,186]

Complications

Serious postoperative complications secondary to surgery of the tonsils and adenoids are primarily related to pain, hemorrhage, airway obstruction, postoperative pulmonary edema, VPI, nasopharyngeal stenosis, and death.[187] Meticulous attention to surgical technique and technical advances in modern anesthesiology have significantly reduced the number of complications related to adenotonsillectomy. Paradise reported an overall complication rate of 14%; all of these complications were self-limiting.[124] Richmond described a series of 794 patients undergoing adenotonsillectomy, of whom 4.2% had variable degrees of postoperative bleeding and 1.3% had self-limiting postoperative airway obstruction. In 9409 pediatric patients undergoing adenotonsillectomy, Crysdale and Russel[188] reported an overall hemorrhage rate of 2.15%, with only 0.06% of patients requiring a second general anesthetic for hemostasis. For reasons other than the hemorrhage (including fever, airway distress, pneumonia, inadequate oral intake, vomiting, and pain), 0.6% of the patients required delayed hospitalization. The incidence of serious surgical complications has been reported to be approximately 15 cases per 1000.[189] Pulmonary abscess, although dreaded in the past, is now extremely rare. However, this complication may still be encountered, as may other rare complications, including Horner's syndrome, optic neuritis, meningitis, brain abscess, paralysis of the glossopharyngeal and recurrent laryngeal nerves, salivary fistulas from the submandibular gland to the tonsillar fossa, and mediastinal emphysema.[187,190,191]

Chronic postoperative pain related to fibrosis and calcification of the stylohyoid ligament (Eagle's syndrome) may be encountered occasionally. Pain referred to the ipsilateral ear may be diagnosed by palpation of the tonsillar fossa and from demonstration by radiographic studies of an elongated styloid process. Aspiration of foreign bodies (e.g., dislodged teeth, sponges, and lymphoid tissue) may also be encountered. If a tooth aspiration is suspected, a radiographic study should be obtained immediately. If a permanent tooth has been dislodged, a dental consultation should be obtained. A thorough investigation, including endoscopy, must be performed when a suspected foreign body has been aspirated.

Postoperative Hemorrhage

Postoperative hemorrhage is the most common serious complication of adenotonsillectomy. Reported postoperative hemorrhage rates range from 0.5% to 10%, although variable rates have been reported with different surgical techniques.[188,192-195] Meticulous attention to surgical technique and intraoperative hemostasis, regardless of the technique used, will lead to acceptable postoperative hemorrhage rates. Detection of underlying coagulation disorders by history and physical findings or through preoperative screening in appropriately selected patients will help avert significant intraoperative blood loss. Appropriate preoperative and intraoperative measures are taken in conjunction with a hematology consult. Certain analgesics (e.g., ketorolac tromethamine) have been associated with increased hemorrhage rates when given in the perioperative period and should be avoided in patients undergoing adenotonsillectomy.[63,196]

The extensive blood supply of the tonsillar fossa is composed of a complex network of anastomosing arteries primarily arising from the ipsilateral external carotid artery system. However, there are contributions from the internal carotid and vertebral arteries, and contralateral vessels circulate through the circle of Willis.[197] Therefore, extensive intraoperative or postoperative hemorrhage may not always cease after ligation of the external carotid artery. In rare, severe cases, ligation of other branches (e.g., the maxillary, facial, lingual, or superior thyroid artery) may be necessary.[192]

The arterial blood supply of the nasopharynx and adenoids arises from both the internal and external carotid arterial system. However, bleeding in this region can be controlled most commonly with compression and electrocautery. In severe cases, application of caustic agents (e.g., tannic acid, bismuth subgallate) or hemostatic agents (e.g., Avitene) may be beneficial. Aberrant arterial vessels in the oropharynx and nasopharynx may be damaged intraoperatively (Fig. 196-15). McKenzie and Wolfe[97] reported an aberrant carotid artery arising in Rosenmüller's fossa that was injured during adenoidectomy, necessitating subsequent ligation of the common carotid artery with resultant transient hemiplegia.

Bleeding can be intraoperative, immediately postoperative (within 24 hours), or delayed (after 24 hours). Intraoperative hemorrhage may

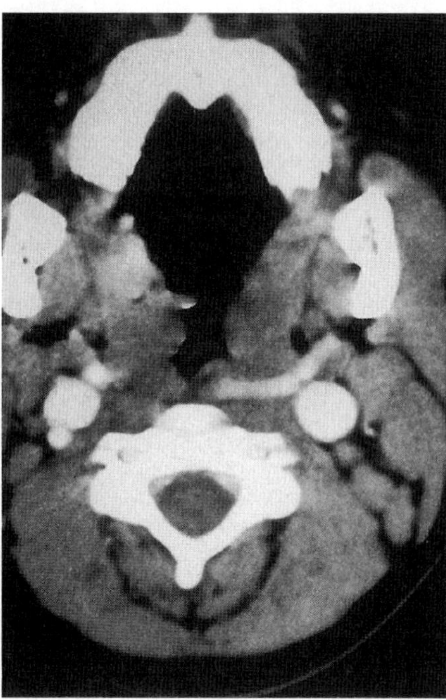

Figure 196-15. Computed tomography scan with contrast enhancement demonstrating an aberrant artery in the left retropharyngeal region.

be related to an underlying coagulopathy or possibly to major arterial damage in severe cases. Steps to control major intraoperative hemorrhage include use of suction cautery or ligation or, possibly, placement of a pack in the tonsillar fossa and over-suturing of the tonsillar pillars to provide constant compression of the fossa. Suture ligatures may damage underlying arterial vessels, thereby worsening the bleeding or possibly leading to delayed postoperative hemorrhage and should be placed with extreme care if they are used.[87,198] In severe cases, ligation of larger arteries through an open-neck exploration may be necessary. However, this should be an extremely uncommon step. Persistent hemorrhage from the nasopharynx after adenoidectomy is often related to residual remnants of adenoid tissue that should be completely removed to best obtain hemostasis.

Immediately postoperative bleeding after adenoidectomy may be controlled initially with topical decongestant nose drops. However, patients with severe bleeding should be taken back to the operating room for examination of the nasopharynx and definitive hemostasis, in which the clots are suctioned, adenoid remnants are removed, and the nasopharyngeal pad is definitively cauterized.

Delayed postoperative bleeding, although typically not as dangerous as intraoperative or immediately postoperative bleeding, may be fatal if not managed appropriately. Patients or parents should be well informed before discharge about the possibility of delayed postoperative hemorrhage and should be told to return for immediate evaluation if there is any evidence of bright red bleeding from the nose or mouth. The most common time for delayed postoperative bleeding is between the fifth and seventh postoperative days. When hemorrhage occurs, patients should be returned to the operating room for immediate hemostasis if active bleeding is confirmed on physical examination. If no active bleeding is apparent and a blood clot is evident in the tonsillar fossa, it should not be disturbed. However, if the surgeon cannot determine whether active bleeding is taking place, the clot should be suctioned to allow better examination. Blood clots often hide bleeding vessels and may prevent appropriate coagulation as a result of fibrinolysis.[199] Patients with delayed hemorrhage who are not actively bleeding and have a blood clot present in the tonsillar fossa should at least be admitted for overnight observation. A coagulation profile and hematocrit measurement should be obtained.

Airway Obstruction and Pulmonary Edema

Postoperative airway obstruction may occur after adenotonsillectomy, especially in children younger than 3 years.[58,182] Edema of the tongue, nasopharynx, and palate may necessitate temporary replacement of a nasal trumpet and also may require intravenous corticosteroid therapy. Dislodging of pharyngeal clots may obstruct the larynx postoperatively, resulting in death.[200] Therefore, all clots should be evacuated from the pharynx before termination of the procedure.

Postoperative pulmonary edema may arise in patients with long-term upper airway obstruction related to adenotonsillar hypertrophy, often necessitating prolonged mechanical ventilation. Patients with a prolonged history of obstructive sleep apnea—as documented by polysomnography and evidence of cor pulmonale—should be observed closely after surgery with pulse oximetry in a monitored setting. Patients with persistent hypercapnia may require planned postoperative mechanical ventilation until P_{CO_2} values return to normal.

Velopharyngeal Insufficiency

Velopharyngeal insufficiency (VPI), or hypernasality, is a relatively unusual complication primarily related to adenoidectomy. In patients with excessively large tonsils and preoperative VPI, the velopharyngeal insufficiency may actually improve after the obstructive tonsils have been removed. Patients with a history of cleft palate or evidence of an occult submucous cleft palate on physical examination (see Figure 196-11) should not undergo adenoidectomy unless it is absolutely necessary. In these situations conservative or partial adenoidectomy should be performed. The actual incidence of VPI after adenoidectomy in otherwise healthy children has been estimated to be between 1 in 750 and 1 in 1459.[189,201] It is important to determine preoperatively whether there is a family history of VPI or whether the patient had a prior history of hypernasal speech or nasal regurgitation as an infant. These signs may herald the development of postoperative VPI. If an underlying speech abnormality exists preoperatively, speech therapy evaluation should be performed. It also is important to determine whether reported hyponasal speech is truly related to a nasal obstruction or is actually related to hypernasal speech, which can be misinterpreted by parents.

Patients in whom postoperative VPI develops should be evaluated and managed initially by a speech pathologist. Most cases are transient and will resolve with time. However, severe cases may require surgical intervention, such as formation of a pharyngeal flap, sphincteroplasty, or, possibly, posterior pharyngeal wall augmentation. Reconstructive surgery should be considered in patients with persistent VPI that has not responded to speech therapy for at least 1 year. *Habit palsy* is transient postoperative VPI that develops secondary to pain when the patient has altered pharyngeal muscle control during speech and swallowing. If it is not resolved shortly after surgery, speech therapy is usually successful.

Nasopharyngeal Stenosis

Nasopharyngeal stenosis is an extremely difficult management problem that requires surgical intervention for satisfactory resolution. This situation may arise from excessive cauterization with extensive mucosal destruction involving the nasopharynx, lateral nasopharyngeal wall, and superior tonsillar pillar along with excessive resection of posterior tonsillar pillar tissue. Other predisposing factors are performance of surgery during an acute episode of pharyngitis or purulent sinusitis, revision adenoid surgery with removal of lateral pharyngeal bands, and keloid formation.[202] Figi[203] described 37 cases of nasopharyngeal stenosis, 22 of which were secondary to adenotonsillectomy.[109] Guggenheim[204] reported 18 cases of nasopharyngeal stenosis secondary to adenoidectomy caused by stripping of the lymphoid tissue from the torus tubarius, Rosenmüller's fossa, and the lateral nasopharynx.[205]

Numerous techniques have been described for surgical repair using a combination of skin flaps, local mucosal flaps, stents, skin grafts, and scar incisions.[206] Cotton[207] described a technique using incision of the stenosis with rotation of a laterally and inferiorly based pharyngeal flap to reline the nasopharynx. Occasionally, second-stage repair is necessary. Physical findings in patients with nasopharyngeal stenosis

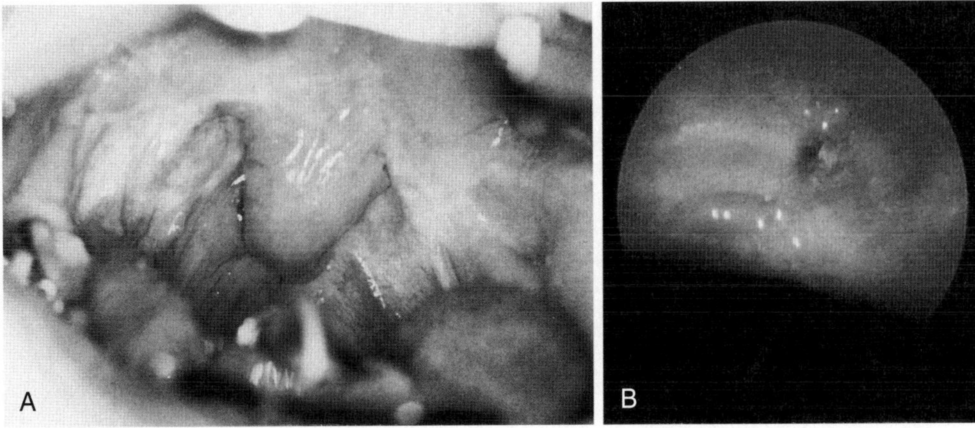

Figure 196-16. **A,** Oropharyngeal view of postadenotonsillectomy nasopharyngeal stenosis. **B,** Endoscopic view of nasopharyngeal stenosis by means of a 120-degree rod-lens telescope.

typically consist of scarring of the uvula down to the posterior pharyngeal wall with possibly a small opening visible on mirror examination or flexible nasopharyngoscopy (Fig. 196-16). The majority of the scarring is based laterally in the region of the posterior tonsillar pillars. This results in partial or complete obstruction of the nasopharyngeal airway and can be extremely debilitating.

Cervical Spine Complications

A rare complication of adenoidectomy or tonsillectomy is atlantoaxial subluxation (Grisel's syndrome). Although up to 10% of patients may report neck pain after adenoidectomy, patients with Grisel's syndrome have decalcification of the anterior arch of the atlas and laxity of the anterior transverse ligament between the atlas and axis.[63,208] This leads to complaints of stiff neck with spasm of the sternocleidomastoid or deep cervical muscle. The patient holds the head to one side with slight rotation toward the opposite side. Radiographic evaluation in suspected cases should include anteroposterior and lateral cervical spine radiography in addition to flexion-extension radiographs, which may detect mild subluxation. In severe cases, CT and possibly magnetic resonance imaging may demonstrate evidence of decalcification, which may be associated with cervical spine osteomyelitis. Most cases of atlantoaxial subluxation are related to infection or trauma and only rarely are secondary to adenotonsillectomy.[209] Patients with Down syndrome are more prone to traumatic atlantoaxial subluxation following adenotonsillectomy. Great care should be taken in cervical spine manipulation during surgery in patients with Down syndrome.[104]

Management of atlantoaxial subluxation after adenoidectomy or adenotonsillectomy should be individualized according to the duration and the symptoms present. Intravenous antimicrobial therapy and possibly cervical traction may be necessary. In the presence of cervical osteomyelitis, long-term (4-8 weeks) intravenous antimicrobial therapy, coupled with cervical stabilization, will be necessary.[209] Retropharyngeal abscess after adenoidectomy has also been reported.[190]

SUGGESTED READINGS

Ali NJ, Pitson DJ, Stradling JR. Snoring, sleep disturbance and behavior in 4-5 year olds. *Arch Dis Child.* 1993;68:360-366.

American Academy of Otolaryngology–Head and Neck Surgery. *1995 Clinical Indicators Compendium.* Alexandria, VA: American Academy of Otolaryngology–Head and Neck Surgery; 1995.

American Thoracic Society. Standards and indications for cardiopulmonary sleep studies in children. *Am J Respir Crit Care Med.* 1996;153:866-878.

Bluestone CD. Current indications for tonsillectomy and adenoidectomy. *Ann Otol Rhinol Laryngol Suppl.* 1992;155:58.

Bluestone CD, Wittel RA, Paradise JL, et al. Eustachian tube function as related to adenoidectomy for otitis media. *Trans Am Acad Ophthalmol Otolaryngol.* 1972;76:1325-1339.

Coticchia J, Zuliani G, Coleman C, et al. Biofilm surface area in the pediatric nasopharynx: chronic rhinosinusitis vs obstructive sleep apnea: *Arch Otolaryngol Head Neck Surg.* 2007;133:110-114.

Derkay CS, Darrow DH, Welch C, et al. Post-tonsillectomy morbidity and quality of life in pediatric patients with obstructive tonsils and adenoid: Microdebrider vs electrocautery. *Otolaryngol Head Neck Surg.* 2006;143:114-120.

Garetz SL. Behavior, cognition, and quality of life after adenotonsillectomy for pediatric sleep-disordered breathing: summary of the literature. *Otolaryngol-Head Neck Surg.* 2008;138(Suppl):S19-S26.

Gates GA, Avery CA, Cooper JC Jr, et al. Chronic secretory otitis media: effects of surgical management. *Ann Otol Rhinol Laryngol Suppl.* 1989;138:2-32.

Gates GA, Avery CA, Prihoda TJ. Effect of adenoidectomy upon children with chronic otitis media with effusion. *Laryngoscope.* 1988;98:58.

Gates GA, Avery CA, Prihoda TJ, et al. Effectiveness of adenoidectomy and tympanostomy tubes in the treatment of chronic otitis media with effusion. *N Engl J Med.* 1987;317:1444-1451.

Goldstein NA, Fatima M, Campbell TF, et al. Child behaviour and quality of life before and after tonsillectomy and adenoidectomy. *Arch Otolaryngol Head Neck Surg.* 2002;128:770-775.

Gottlieb DJ, Chase C, Vezina RM, et al. Sleep-disordered breathing symptoms are associated with poorer cognitive function in 5-year-old children. *J Pediatr.* 2004;145:458-464.

Gozal D. Sleep disordered breathing and school performance in children. *Pediatrics.* 1998;102:616-620.

Gozal D, Pope DW Jr. Snoring during early childhood and academic performance at ages thirteen to fourteen years. *Pediatrics,* 2001;107:1394-1399.

Javed F, Sadri M, Uddin J, et al. A completed audit cycle on post-tonsillectomy haemorrhage rate: Coblation versus standard tonsillectomy. *Acta Otolaryngol.* 2007;127(Mar):300-304.

Kay DJ, Mehta V, Goldsmith AJ. Perioperative adenotonsillectomy management in children: current practices. *Laryngoscope.* 2003;113;592-597.

Koltai PJ, Chan J, Younes A. Power-assisted adenoidectomy: total and partial resection. *Laryngoscope.* 2002;112:29.

Koltai PJ, Solares CA, Mascha EJ, et al. Intracapsular partial tonsillectomy for tonsillar hypertrophy in children: *Laryngoscope.* 2002;112(Suppl 100):17-19.

Littlefield PD, Hall DJ, Holtel MR. Radiofrequency excision versus monopolar electrosurgical excision for tonsillectomy. *Otolaryngol Head Neck Surg.* 2005;133;51-54.

Paradise JL, Bluestone CD, Bachman RZ, et al. Efficacy of tonsillectomy for recurrent throat infection in severely affected children: results of parallel randomized and nonrandomized clinical trials. *N Engl J Med.* 1984;310:674-683.

Paradise JL, Bluestone CD, Rogers KD, et al. Efficacy of adenoidectomy for recurrent otitis media in children previously treated with tympanostomy-tube placement: results of parallel randomized and nonrandomized trials. *JAMA.* 1990;263:2066-2073.

Telian SA. Sore throat and antibiotics. *Otolaryngol Clin North Am.* 1986;19:103.

For complete list of references log onto www.expertconsult.com.

CHAPTER ONE HUNDRED AND NINETY-SEVEN

Infections of the Airway in Children

Newton O. Duncan

Key Points

- The diagnosis of pediatric airway infections requires astute clinical acumen and judicious use of laboratory testing and imaging techniques.
- Prompt and evidence-based management of these potentially life-threatening infections provides reliable, successful outcomes.
- Viral croup, or laryngotracheitis, is the most common airway obstructive infection in children with well-defined diagnostic criteria and clinically documented management schemes.
- Supraglottitis or epiglottitis has become a rare clinical entity, but its diagnosis and management should not be forgotten.
- Bacterial tracheitis, or exudative tracheitis, is also uncommon, but prompt diagnosis and management may be lifesaving.
- Retropharyngeal cellulitis and abscesses are common airway infections in children and a high index of suspicion may be needed for diagnosis. Well-defined CT imaging results can help determine where surgical management is appropriate.

Children may experience a variety of infections involving the upper respiratory tract and surrounding structures. Some infections occur commonly, some may be self-limited, and some may be relatively inconsequential. However, other infections, some of which are more rare, may be life threatening. The astute clinician can often identify the various airway infections by an accurate clinical history and targeted physical examination. Radiologic imaging, laboratory studies, or airway endoscopy may also be helpful for accurate diagnosis. Nevertheless, a keen understanding of the various signs and symptoms of airway infections is important. The signs and symptoms of the various airway infections may have many similarities because the anatomic structures and tissues involved are close in proximity. These similar airway findings also can be present in children with acute tonsillitis, infectious mononucleosis, diphtheria, peritonsillar abscess, congenital airway anomalies, subglottic stenosis of any etiology, and in those with airway foreign bodies. Therefore great familiarity with the spectrum of childhood airway disease entities can be extremely important in their prompt diagnosis and management. This chapter emphasizes the current recognition and management of croup (laryngotracheitis), supraglottitis (epiglottitis), bacterial tracheitis, and retropharyngeal abscesses.

Croup (Laryngotracheitis)

The term *croup* is from the ancient Scottish language that refers to the harsh, barking cough that may be present in those with a number of different acquired or congenital disorders.[1,2] Several terms have been used synonymously with croup, leading to confusion about the exact nature of the disease. These terms include *croup, viral croup, laryngotracheitis, laryngotracheobronchitis, pseudomembranous croup, spasmodic croup,* and *postintubation croup.* This infectious disease primarily involves the vocal folds or glottis and the subglottis. Because viruses predominantly cause this entity, the most descriptive and widely used terms are either viral croup or, more properly, viral laryngotracheitis. Viral laryngotracheitis, or croup, is the most common form of infectious upper airway tract obstruction in children. It is estimated that this condition accounts for 90% of infectious airway obstructions and that 3% to 5% of children have at least one episode of croup. This condition can be recurrent in approximately 5% of children.[3] Most children with croup have mild-spectrum symptoms but some children (1.5% to 15%) with more severe spectrum croup require hospital admission for airway obstructive symptoms, and during hospitalization 1% to 5% may require intubation.[4] Parainfluenza viruses 1 and 2 primarily are implicated in this disease (up to 75%), but influenza A and B, respiratory syncytial virus, measles, adenovirus, varicella, and herpes simplex virus type 1 all have been isolated.[5] Measles involvement in those with croup historically leads to an aggressive form of the disease.[6] More recently, influenza viruses and herpes simplex viruses have both been implicated in more severe or prolonged courses of croup.[7,8]

Children are most commonly affected when they are between 6 months and 3 years of age, with a peak incidence at 18 to 24 months of age. Boys are more likely affected, by more than a 2 : 1 ratio. Although croup can occur at any time of the year, there is a strong seasonal occurrence in late autumn and winter. Croup may be called atypical if it occurs in infants younger than 6 months of age, lasts more than 7 days, or does not respond to appropriate treatment. Other etiologies besides acute viral laryngotracheitis should be considered in these atypical cases.

Viral croup transmission occurs by direct contact and exposure to nasopharyngeal secretions.[9] The incubation period before onset of clinical symptoms is 2 to 6 days for parainfluenza virus type 1, and children may continue to shed the virus for up to 2 weeks.[10] After acquisition, the viral infection involves the nasopharynx, producing nasal symptoms. Local spread to the larynx and trachea ensues. The mucosa of the vocal folds and subglottis become erythematous and swollen. Lymphocytes, histiocytes, and polymorphonuclear leukocytes infiltrate the lamina propria, submucosa, and adventitia. In addition, generalized mucosal edema is present. The duration of illness usually is from 3 to 5 days. The crucial factor in those with viral croup is the amount of swelling in the subglottic area. The subglottis is the narrowest portion of the upper respiratory tract and, because of the complete cartilaginous cricoid ring, any edema that occurs in the subglottis does so at the expense of the airway lumen. Because stridor does not occur until there is already significant airway obstruction and because any decrease in cross-sectional area is proportional to the square of the radius of the airway lumen, any further decrease in airway size caused

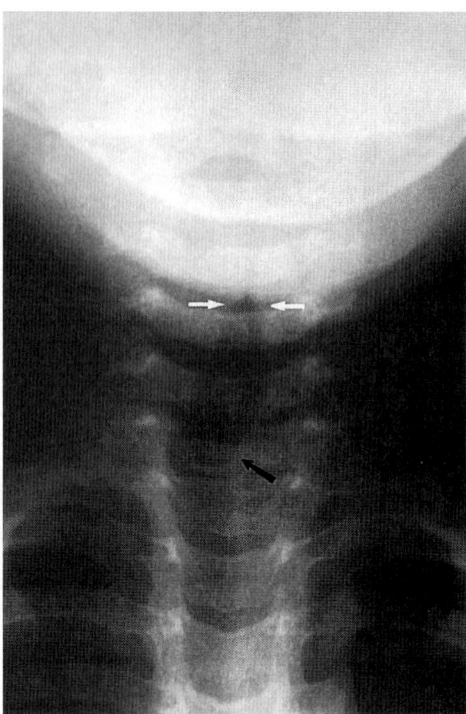

Figure 197-1. Normal anteroposterior radiographic view of the soft tissues of the neck demonstrating the normal shouldering contours of the proximal trachea *(white arrows)*. Many children will show slight angulation of the trachea, which is a normal variant *(black arrow)*.

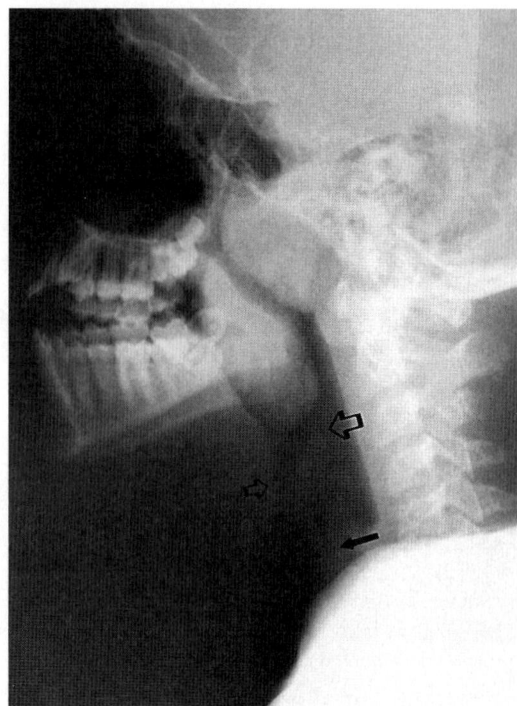

Figure 197-2. Normal lateral soft tissue radiograph of the airway with normal epiglottis *(large open arrow)* and well-defined vallecula *(small open arrow)*. The *black arrow* shows the laryngeal ventricle.

by mucous plugging or crusting may lead to rapid and complete airway obstruction.

Clinical Features

Characteristically, children with viral croup have a history of prodromal upper airway infection. Low-grade fever may be present. There also may be leukocytosis, although the leukocyte count in most patients is normal. Inspiratory stridor, hoarseness, and a barking cough are cardinal symptoms of viral croup. This cough is invariably present and may help distinguish croup from other illnesses. The presence of biphasic stridor, retractions, high respiratory rate, or oxygen desaturations indicates severe airway obstruction.

Viral croup may present with only mild symptoms of airway obstruction, but it also can be severe with life-threatening airway obstruction. Many different schemes have been developed to assess the spectrum and severity of croup in an effort to assist in determining how to best manage the different presentations of croup.[1,5,10] Regardless of the scheme used, it is important to consider the following parameters when evaluating children with croup or airway obstruction in general: (1) stridor—inspiratory versus expiratory; (2) respiratory rate; (3) chest retractions; (4) air entry into the chest by auscultation (decreased with severe obstruction); (5) anxiety or restlessness; (6) color or cyanosis; (7) oxygen desaturation by pulse oximetry; and (8) level of consciousness.

Diagnosis

The diagnosis of croup is highly suggested by history and physical examination alone. Detailed questioning about possible foreign body ingestion should be made, along with any previous intubation history. Radiographic imaging of the airway traditionally has been helpful in evaluating those with airway disorders (Figs. 197-1 and 197-2). The diagnosis can be confirmed radiographically by anteroposterior (AP) and lateral (high kilovoltage) films of the upper airway. The frontal AP view classically shows a "steeple sign" in the subglottic area, whereas the lateral view is characterized by haziness of the same area (Figs. 197-3 and 197-4). Flexible fiberoptic laryngoscopy occasionally may be helpful in establishing the correct diagnosis of viral croup. This procedure should be performed with utmost care if there are moderate-to-severe airway obstructive symptoms. In patients with severe airway obstruction, the diagnosis may be confirmed by direct laryngoscopy at the time of intubation (Figs. 197-5 and 197-6).

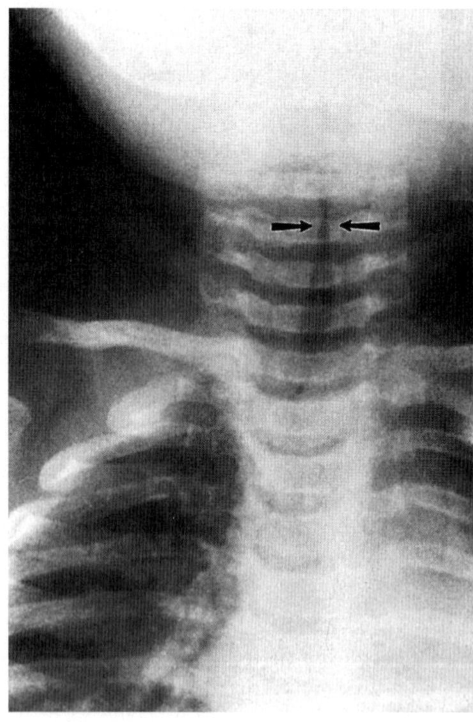

Figure 197-3. Narrowed subglottis in viral croup *(arrows)* in the anteroposterior radiographic view.

Differential Diagnosis

The most important differential diagnosis to consider in children with suspected croup is supraglottitis (Table 197-1). Thereafter, the possible

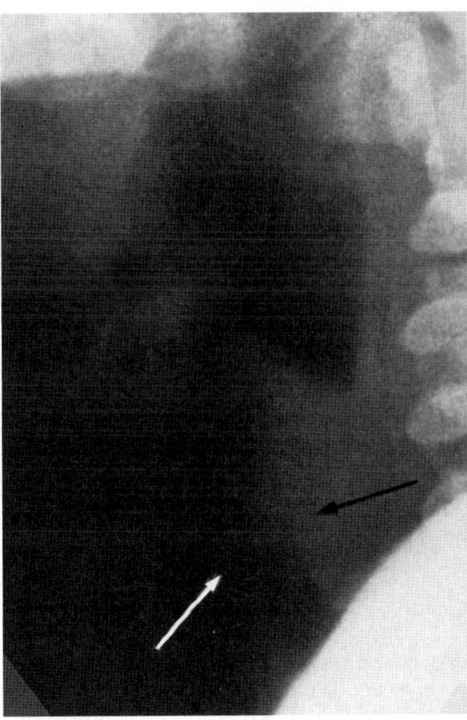

Figure 197-4. Hazy subglottis in the lateral radiographic view *(arrows)* seen in viral croup.

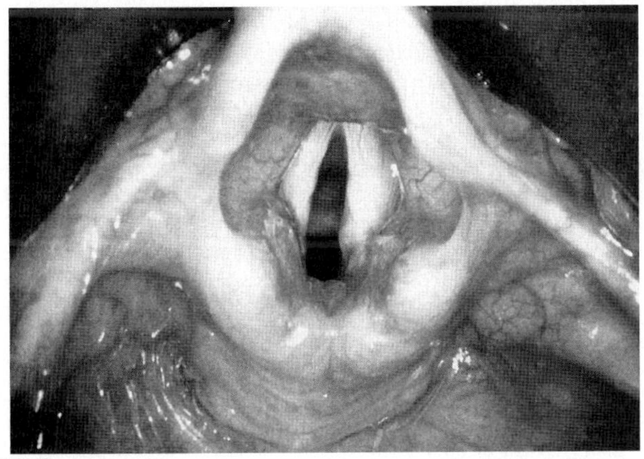

Figure 197-5. Normal child larynx with crisp vocal folds and widely patent subglottis visualized by a rigid rod telescope.

presence of any airway foreign body, particularly in the larynx or subglottis, must be considered. Subglottic hemangiomas may have similar symptoms in infants younger than 6 months of age. Recurrent episodes of a crouplike illness may occur not only in those with congenital subglottic narrowing, but also in children with acquired subglottic stenosis. Therefore a history of intubation may be important. Viral croup in the presence of any preexisting laryngeal or subglottic narrowing may lead to early or recurrent stridor and symptoms of croup. Atypical or recurrent symptoms of croup always demand close attention for other etiologies of airway compromise in addition to viral croup. Gastroesophageal reflux also may be a contributing cause of recurrent croup.[11] When viral croup is not responding to appropriate therapy and when children exhibit an increasingly febrile or toxic appearance, bacterial superinfection in the subglottis or trachea should be suspected. This may occur in 10% to 15% of patients hospitalized with more severe croup. Bacterial tracheitis actually may originate as a complication of viral croup.[12]

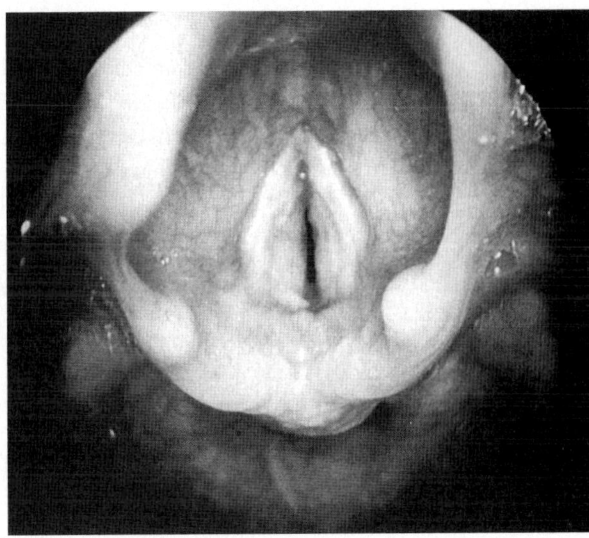

Figure 197-6. Viral croup with severe vocal fold and subglottic edema as seen with a rigid rod telescope.

Spasmodic Croup

Spasmodic croup is a poorly understood entity that is manifested by the sudden onset of stridor, usually at night, in a healthy child between 1 and 3 years of age with no concomitant upper respiratory tract infection. A barking cough and dyspnea accompany the stridor. These episodes may be recurrent in nature and usually resolve spontaneously or with cool humid air within several hours. The vocal folds may be involved with spasm, and mild, pale transient vocal fold and subglottic edema may be present. Some of the same viruses that cause viral croup may be involved with causing spasmodic croup. An increasing body of evidence suggests an association between spasmodic croup and recurrent croup with nonspecific bronchial hyperactivity, asthma, and allergic disease.[13-16] Spasmodic croup and viral croup also may well represent two ends of a broad spectrum in the clinical presentation of a single disease.[17]

Management

Most children with viral croup have symptoms within the mild spectrum of the illness and do not require a physician visit. The illness usually is self-limited, peaking in severity through 3 to 5 days with no specific treatment required at home. A quiet environment and parental comforting or support is universally important in the treatment of children with croup. Any stimulus or disturbance promotes crying and an increased respiratory rate. The airway is stabilized with less mucosal dryness when the child is quiet and when anxiety or crying is diminished.

Management strategies for viral croup have included glucocorticoids, racemic epinephrine, heliox, and mist. Although viral croup is the most common form of airway obstruction in young children, many controversies remain and there is no consensus regarding optimal treatment. Recently, croup clinical pathways have been devised to promote consistent, safe, and effective management that might result in reduced hospital admissions and earlier hospital discharge.[18]

Overwhelming evidence is present to support the use of glucocorticoids in both outpatient and inpatient settings in the management of moderate to severe decrease in croup.[19-22] Segal and others[23] have documented an 86% decrease in hospital admissions for treatment of croup when steroids were used. The exact mechanism of action of glucocorticoids in croup is unknown, but they probably decrease endothelial permeability, thus leading to decreased mucosal edema. This effect commonly takes at least 3 hours. In mild to moderate cases, oral prednisolone 2 mg/kg/day in two divided doses may be used in the outpatient setting or home for approximately 3 days. This regimen is particularly useful in milder, recurrent cases of croup, with parents keeping prednisolone at home to use when symptoms occur.

Table 197-1

Differential Diagnosis of Upper Airway Infections in Children

	Laryngotracheitis (Viral Croup)	Supraglottitis (Epiglottitis)	Bacterial Tracheitis	Retropharyngeal Abscess
Age	6mo to 3yr	1-8yr	6mo to 8yr	1-5yr
Onset	Slow	Rapid	Rapid	Slow
Prodrome	URI symptoms	None or mild URI	URI symptoms	URI symptoms
Fever	Variable or none	High	Usually high	Usually high
Hoarseness/barky cough	Yes	No	Yes	No
Dysphagia	No	Yes	Yes	Yes
Toxic appearance	No	Yes	Yes	Variable

URI, upper respiratory infection.

In the emergency center, dexamethasone has been extensively used in doses from 0.15 mg/kg to 0.60 mg/kg, with maximum doses of 1 mg/kg for moderate to severe croup.[22,24] Oral administration is as effective or better than intramuscular injection or nebulized therapy.[15,22] Nebulized budesonide has also been compared with dexamethasone but has had no clear clinical advantage.[24] If the symptoms of croup are severe enough to warrant the use of racemic epinephrine, then glucocorticoids are helpful in preventing any associated mucosal rebound edema 2 to 3 hours later. Glucocorticoids have had a significant impact in the outpatient setting but have also greatly decreased the severity of symptoms and the duration of hospitalization.[22,25,26] At this point it appears that an initial dexamethasone dose of 0.60 mg/kg orally is preferred because of its low dose and ease of administration.[27] Further doses of prednisolone (2 mg/kg/day) or dexamethasone (1 mg/kg/day) in divided doses may be used to sustain the glucocorticoid effect in either inpatients or outpatients. Intravenous administration is preferable in serious inpatient disease. Prolonged use of glucocorticoids should be monitored carefully, particularly when antibiotics may be used, to prevent candida overgrowth in the subglottis or trachea.[28] In the absence of clinical evidence of an emerging bacterial process, there is no support for the use of antibiotics in the management of viral croup.

Racemic epinephrine in an equal mixture of the d- and l-isomers of epinephrine has been used in the United States and Canada since 1971[29] but has become available and accepted in other countries as well. It has been shown that l-epinephrine is at least as effective as racemic epinephrine, is readily available worldwide, has no increased side effects, and is less expensive than d-epinephrine.[30] The α-adrenergic effects of epinephrine cause mucosal vasoconstriction, leading to decreased edema in the subglottic region. Using 0.5 mL of a 2.25% solution of racemic epinephrine diluted in 3 mL of saline delivered by a nebulizer results in rapid clinical improvement of moderate to severe respiratory distress within 10 to 30 minutes.[17,31] Alternatively, 5 mL of a 1:1000 solution of l-epinephrine produces equivalent results. This effect wanes and disappears by 2 hours after administration, with rebound mucosal edema in some patients. Because of this temporary effect and possible rebound, children should be observed closely after administering racemic epinephrine for 2 to 3 hours. Recent reports document the safe use of racemic epinephrine in an outpatient setting. These children were observed for at least 2 to 3 hours, were significantly improved, could easily return to the hospital if needed, and were closely followed as outpatients.[32-35] Racemic epinephrine has become widely used in outpatient settings for moderate to severe croup within similar observation criteria described in the studies. In an intensive care setting it can be used every 30 minutes, but it is usually spaced every 3 to 4 hours in a regular hospital unit. Glucocorticoid administration is important in any setting to prevent or diminish the mucosal rebound potential of racemic epinephrine. Racemic epinephrine should be used with great caution in patients with tachycardia or cardiac anomalies such as tetralogy of Fallot or idiopathic subaortic stenosis.

Heliox, a helium-oxygen mixture, may be helpful in severe croup. It decreases the work of breathing by promoting laminar flow through the partially obstructed airway. One study has shown similar improvement in croup scores with heliox administration when compared with patients given epinephrine.[36] Heliox may be used as an adjunct to all other medical therapy for croup.

Humidified air or mist has historically been used to treat croup before other medical therapy was available. Humidifiers or steam showers at home and mist tents or blow-by mist in hospital settings presumably moisten secretions, make for easier expectoration, and prevent drying or crusting that may further compromise a narrow airway. There may also be soothing of the involved mucosa, making children more comfortable and less likely to increase submucosal inflammation by vigorous coughing. However, only several studies have investigated the effectiveness of moist air in the management of croup and have demonstrated no benefit over control patients.[22,26,37,38] Furthermore, the issue of warm versus cool mist has not been settled. Despite the lack of objective benefit, strong anecdotal experience may support the continued use of mist, particularly in severe hospitalized cases of viral croup or in low-humidity environments. Mist tents should be avoided or used with caution because they may provoke more anxiety in children and therefore blow-by mist may be a better alternative. Well-designed studies are necessary to define the role of mist in the management of viral croup.

When medical therapy fails to alleviate respiratory distress, endotracheal intubation (nasotracheal or orotracheal) may be necessary. A tube at least a half size smaller than estimated for the child's size or age should be used. When possible, intubation should be done in a controlled situation in the operating room with an inhalation agent, while the child is spontaneously breathing. This also may allow for airway endoscopy at the same time. Optical rigid rod telescopes should be used to assess the airway, and rigid bronchoscopes should be avoided if possible to prevent further airway mucosal injury. Extubation can be performed when an air leak is detected. If no air leak is detected after 5 to 7 days, thorough airway endoscopy is indicated. Airway endoscopy also is important in recurrent, prolonged, or atypical cases of croup. Ideally, endoscopy should be performed 3 to 4 weeks after the acute episode has resolved so that acute inflammatory changes can be differentiated from previous existing anatomic abnormalities. A thorough evaluation of the larynx, subglottis, and trachea with rigid rod telescopes then should be performed.

Supraglottitis (Epiglottitis)

Since Michel's original description of "angina epiglottidea anterior" in 1878,[39] acute epiglottitis, or *supraglottitis* as it is more correctly called, has become recognized as a rapidly progressive, life-threatening airway

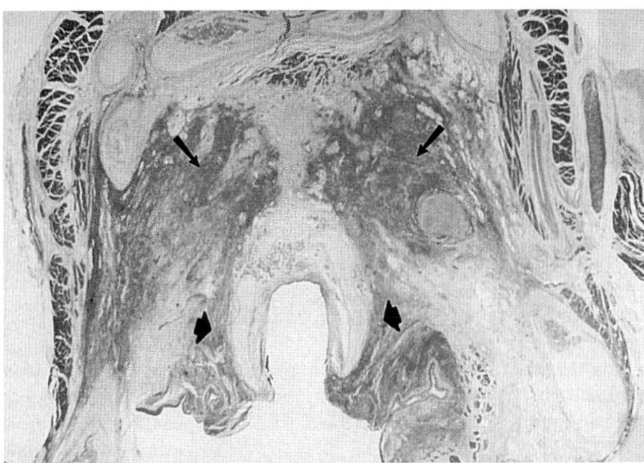

Figure 197-7. Histologic section of a larynx (postmortem) in supraglottitis showing posterior curling of the epiglottic cartilage *(arrowheads)* and severe inflammatory edema of the lingual surface of the epiglottis *(arrows)*.

emergency. Supraglottitis predominantly affected children in what may be termed the prevaccine era. A precipitous decline in supraglottitis in children has occurred since the introduction of the Haemophilus influenzae type b (HIB) vaccine.[40-42] Before widespread use of the HIB vaccination, the incidence of HIB among children ranged from 6 per 100,000 in Canada[43] to 34 per 100,000 in Switzerland.[44] In 1988 conjugated HIB vaccine was introduced with recommendations for universal use in children by 2 years of age in 1990 and immunized levels of at least 90% by 1995. Invasive HIB disease, primarily supraglottitis and meningitis, has declined nationally in the United States by 95%.[45] Immunization works by producing antibodies to the polysaccharide capsule of HIB. Supraglottitis may infrequently occur even when immunization has occurred because of failure of antibody production.[45] Acute supraglottitis remains a rare infection. Its importance lies in its high mortality if the diagnosis is not made promptly.

Supraglottitis is a cellulitis of all the supraglottic structures (not just the epiglottis) that may completely obstruct the airway. As the supraglottic edema increases, the epiglottis curls posteriorly and inferiorly as a result of diffuse inflammatory infiltration of the lingual surface of the epiglottis (Fig. 197-7). The aryepiglottic folds are also affected. With the airway partially occluded, mucus can easily complete obstruction of the airway. Diffuse infiltration of polymorphonuclear lymphocytes and inflammatory edema are seen histologically. Progress is rapid, in terms of hours rather than days. The disease classically occurred in children 2 to 6 years of age; however, it may occur at any age including in newborns.[28,46] A higher incidence may be seen in the winter or spring, although the disease may occur at any time of the year. Supraglottitis may be more commonly seen in older children and adults in today's HIB vaccine era.[23]

The causative organism most commonly identified in more than 90% of supraglottitis in the prevaccine era was *H. influenzae* type b (HIB).[40,47] This bacterial species may be part of the normal nasopharyngeal flora, or it may be acquired by respiratory transmission from other intimate contact. These bacteria may become blood borne and subsequently seed the epiglottis, meninges, facial skin, lungs, or joints. As the frequency of HIB disease has decreased in the HIB vaccine era, the epidemiology of supraglottitis has shifted.[48] Group A β-hemolytic streptococci comprise the majority of cases.[21,49] Other pathogens such as staphylococcus,[50] pneumococcus,[51] klebsiella,[52] Haemophilus parainfluenzae,[53] pseudomonas,[54] viruses,[53,55-57] and candida[58] have been isolated. Other rare causes including crack cocaine,[59] Kawasaki disease,[60] thermal epiglottitis caused by hot food or drink,[61,62] and post transplant lymphoproliferative disorder[63] have been reported. With the appearance of the human immunodeficiency virus (HIV), chronic epiglottitis associated with lymphoid hyperplasia within the epiglottis of an HIV-infected child has been reported.[64]

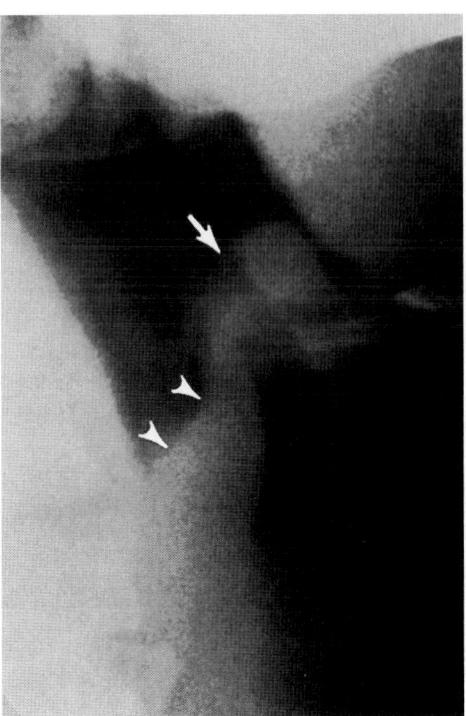

Figure 197-8. Supraglottitis seen on lateral soft tissue radiograph with a rounded epiglottis *(arrow)*, thickened aryepiglottic folds *(arrowheads)*, and distention of the hypopharynx.

Clinical Features

Due to the rarity of supraglottitis in the HIB vaccine era, the diagnosis may be more challenging. Regardless of the age at presentation, the three most common signs of supraglottitis are fever, difficulty breathing, and irritability. Children are toxic in appearance and have clinical evidence of major upper airway obstruction. The child exhibits shallow respiration, inspiratory stridor, retractions, and drooling. There is severe throat pain and dysphagia. Speech is limited because of pain. A cough or hoarseness is usually not present, but the voice may be muffled. Stridor occurs late when airway obstruction is almost complete. Activity is minimal, and the patient usually prefers sitting or leaning forward. The child may assume a "tripod" position (i.e., seated, with the hands braced against the bed and the head held in the sniffing position to maximize airflow through a narrowed laryngeal inlet). Sudden laryngospasm may occur with aspiration of secretions into an already compromised airway and produce respiratory arrest. Some of the atypical causes of supraglottitis may have a more protracted presentation.

Diagnosis

Prompt recognition of this acute airway emergency is essential to prevent airway obstruction. The diagnosis of acute epiglottitis is made by direct inspection of the supraglottic structures in a controlled environment, usually in the operating room. In a cooperative patient with no imminent complete airway obstruction, the pharynx may be visualized without a tongue blade to rule out acute tonsil or peritonsillar infection. Attempts to visualize the epiglottis in the office or emergency department without the ability or equipment to manage an obstructed airway are strongly discouraged.

The need for radiologic studies is controversial. Although there is no question that supraglottitis can be diagnosed on a lateral neck radiograph, the question arises whether this is a safe and necessary procedure. Most radiology suites lack the facilities to handle an obstructed pediatric airway. A child presenting with the previous signs and symptoms probably should forego radiologic testing and proceed directly to the operating room. If there is any question as to the correct diagnosis and if the child is not in respiratory distress, radiologic examination can confirm

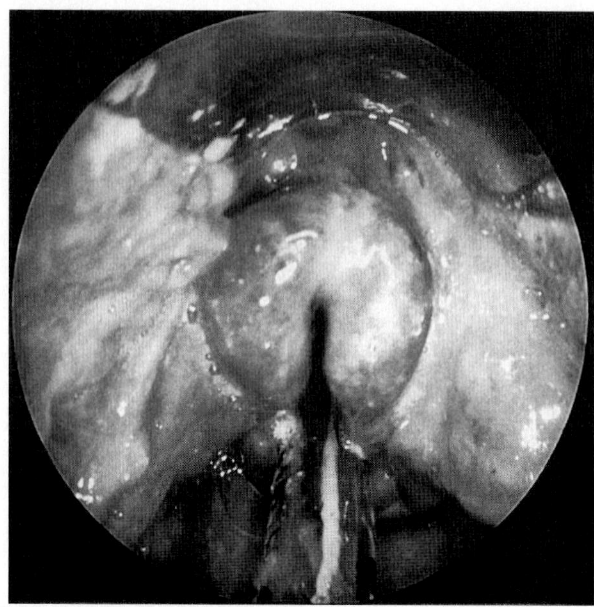

Figure 197-9. Supraglottitis just after intubation, visualized by a rigid rod telescope.

the diagnosis and exclude other causes of acute airway obstruction. Among the different diagnoses to be excluded are foreign bodies, retropharyngeal abscesses, and viral croup or laryngotracheitis.

Lateral neck radiographs in those with epiglottitis reveal swelling and rounding of the epiglottis with thickening and bulging of the aryepiglottic folds and distention of the hypopharynx (Fig. 197-8). In addition, the subglottic airway will appear normal on AP radiographs. In the operating room, examination of the supraglottis reveals an edematous, erythematous epiglottis with variable degrees of obstruction of the airway (Fig. 197-9). The cartilaginous landmarks are often obscured. Mucosal changes range from erythema to frank ulceration or sloughing. Rarely, an abscess can be found in the lingual surface of the epiglottis. The differential diagnosis of inpatients with possible supraglottitis includes viral croup or laryngotracheitis, bacterial tracheitis, uvulitis, acute tonsillitis, retropharyngeal or peritonsillar abscess, and diphtheria. Diphtheria is a rare infection seen only in certain areas with nonimmunized patients. A history of diphtheria immunization and the absence of pharyngeal membranes make the diagnosis unlikely. Foreign body aspiration in a child with an acute upper respiratory infection also may mimic supraglottitis.

Management

Close cooperation among the otolaryngologist, pediatrician, and anesthesiologist is paramount in the management of supraglottitis. If the diagnosis of acute supraglottitis is suspected, care should be taken to avoid stimulating the child. The child will naturally assume a posture and breathing pattern that maximizes ventilation. Any intervention may convert a functional—albeit unstable—airway into a nonfunctional, acutely obstructed airway. Anything that causes the child to cry may precipitate obstruction. Therefore drawing blood, throat examination, establishing an intravenous line, restraining for a radiograph, undressing the child, or even separating from a parent may cause distress and lead to airway obstruction. Any of these procedures should wait until a stable airway has been established.

Once the diagnosis of acute supraglottitis is made, survival is closely related to the establishment of an artificial airway. For many years, this meant a tracheotomy was performed when the diagnosis was made. Since the 1970s, the safety of intubation has been established, and now endotracheal intubation by nasal or oral routes has become the standard method of managing acute supraglottitis. The rationale for this change is based on the rapid response of the infectious process to appropriate antibiotic therapy. The edema of the supraglottic larynx usually subsides within 48 to 72 hours, allowing safe removal of the endotracheal tube.[65] Despite this observation, if personnel skilled in endotracheal intubation will not be available postoperatively or if the airway can only initially be secured with a rigid bronchoscope, then a tracheotomy still may be the most appropriate choice.

If supraglottitis is suspected, the patient should be taken to the operating room, accompanied by personnel experienced in the establishment of an emergency airway including tracheotomy. Once in the operating room, the patient undergoes gentle, slow, inhalational induction of general anesthesia with a nonirritating inhalation agent. Muscle relaxants should be avoided until an airway is established. Only after adequate anesthesia is obtained should blood samples be taken or intravenous lines be established. A small rigid rod telescope with an endotracheal tube threaded over it may also be useful in patients in whom the glottic airway cannot be visualized. The telescope is advanced through the larynx, and then the endotracheal tube is advanced over the telescope into the trachea. A rigid bronchoscope of the appropriate size and one size smaller should be available. In addition, equipment for a tracheotomy should be at hand. The larynx is examined by the otolaryngologist, and the diagnosis is confirmed. Temporary orotracheal intubation is performed. Cultures are taken from the surface of the epiglottis, and simultaneous blood cultures are drawn. Blood cultures are almost always positive for HIB when this is the causative organism. Orderly nasotracheal intubation can be performed in most patients with removal of the orotracheal tube. Nasotracheal intubation is preferred because there is less motion and resultant irritation of the subglottis. Adequate sedation or restraint is essential to prevent accidental self-extubation.

Appropriate antibiotic therapy is begun with the first dose given in the operating room. Ceftriaxone, cefotaxime, or ampicillin-sulbactam are all appropriate choices even in the HIB-vaccine era. Vancomycin may be used if the child is sensitive to cephalosporins. Adjustments in antibiotics can be made on the basis of culture results. The duration of antibiotic therapy depends on the clinical response of the child. Oral antibiotics indicated by culture results can be used to complete a 7- to 10-day course of therapy as soon as extubation has been accomplished and adequate oral intake is present. Adjunctive treatment with corticosteroids is controversial. Antibody levels to HIB should be measured if there is a history of HIB vaccine administration.

Extubation generally can be accomplished within 48 hours.[65] Criteria for extubation include decreased erythema and swelling of the epiglottis on laryngoscopy and the development of an air leak around the endotracheal tube or after an empirical 48 hours of intubation. Visualization of the supraglottis offers the best guide to extubation. When there is no air leak at 48 hours, flexible fiberoptic laryngoscopy or even direct laryngoscopy can be performed safely and quickly in the intensive care unit in an effort to determine when extubation is safe and to shorten the duration of intubation.

Complications

Although the airway compromise in supraglottitis itself is a life-threatening illness, other infections may occur simultaneously, which may have an equally deleterious effect. In the era of HIB supraglottitis, there was a 90% to 95% rate of positive blood culture for HIB.[66] Therefore it was not surprising that hematogenous dissemination of the disease occurred. The most common infectious complication was pneumonia. Other concomitant HIB infections included meningitis, cervical adenitis, pericarditis, septic arthritis, and otitis media.[66-68] Meningitis may be difficult to diagnose in a sedated patient, and therefore one must be cognizant of this manifestation of HIB disease. The dose of antimicrobial agent ordinarily given may be below that which is recommended for managing meningitis.

Noninfectious complications may also occur in patients with supraglottitis. Any patient with complete airway obstruction and respiratory arrest can suffer hypoxic damage of the central nervous system and other organ systems. Even patients who have had appropriate management of their airway obstruction can become hypoxic. The sudden relief of upper airway obstruction can result in postobstructive pulmonary edema with subsequent hypoxia.[69] This potential complication should be anticipated before the placement of an artificial airway, especially in those patients exhibiting a high degree of airway obstruction. Appropriate levels of positive end-expiratory pressure after endotracheal intubation can provide a protective mechanism against the development of pulmonary edema.

Bacterial Tracheitis (Exudative Tracheitis)

Bacterial tracheitis, perhaps better known as *exudative tracheitis,* has also been termed bacterial laryngotracheobronchitis, membranous laryngotracheobronchitis, and pseudo-membranous croup. It is a rare but potentially life-threatening disease. The disease was certainly described by C. L. Jackson in 1945, but it was not until 1979 that it was redescribed in detail.[70-72] Since then, there has been a growing consensus of opinion that bacterial tracheitis represents a secondary or complicating bacterial infection of viral croup or laryngotracheitis.[12,73] The secondary bacterial pathogen most often described is *Staphylococcus aureus,* but a more recent report found *Moraxella catarrhalis* to be the most frequently implicated pathogen followed by *S. aureus.* This series and others also suggested an epidemiologic change to a slightly less morbid condition.[74,75] Other pathogens include *Streptococcus pyogenes, H. influenzae,* and more rarely gram-negative enteric bacteria.[3]

Bacterial tracheitis primarily occurs during the respiratory virus seasons of autumn and winter, similar to viral croup. It may be seen in a wider range of ages than typical croup, with a mean age of 7.9 years.[72] The infectious inflammatory process involves the subglottis and trachea with marked edema in the subglottis as in those with viral croup. Diffuse mucosal ulceration and pseudo-membrane formation follow, with sloughing of these membranes into the tracheal lumen further contributing to airway obstruction. A purulent exudate is commonly present in copious amounts throughout the trachea and main bronchi as well. Blood cultures are usually negative, but tracheal cultures reliably reveal the bacterial pathogen.[3]

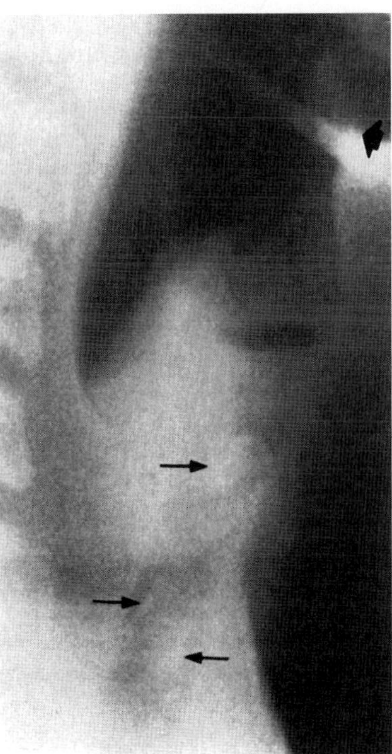

Figure 197-10. Bacterial tracheitis in a lateral soft tissue radiograph with obscured tracheal airway caused by sloughed mucosa *(arrows).* The epiglottis *(arrowhead)* is normal.

Clinical Features

The onset of bacterial tracheitis is variable. Some children become acutely ill and have severe respiratory distress within hours of the onset of illness. In other children there is a several-day prodromal period of stridor, barky cough, and hoarseness typical of viral croup that precedes the rapid, dramatic onset of higher fever, increasing respiratory distress, and toxic appearance. These patients often do not respond to racemic epinephrine because the disease rapidly progresses. High fever, cough, and stridor occur almost simultaneously over several hours. The rapid onset of the illness is similar to supraglottitis, but there usually is no dysphagia or drooling. Leukocytosis often is prominent in those with bacterial tracheitis.

Diagnosis

The diagnosis may be suspected on the basis of signs and symptoms, but it is confirmed by endoscopic examination of the airway. Plain radiographic imaging of the upper airway will show a "steeple" sign of the upper trachea or subglottis in anterior views, similar to viral croup, but it is the lateral view that can be most helpful. Diffuse haziness is present in the tracheal air column, along with soft tissue irregularities within the lumen, indicating pseudo-membrane detachment (Fig. 197-10).

No clinical, radiologic, or laboratory feature alone or in combination is a reliable predictor of bacterial tracheitis. The only diagnostic procedure that distinguishes bacterial tracheitis promptly and accurately from other acute upper airway disease is airway endoscopy.[76]

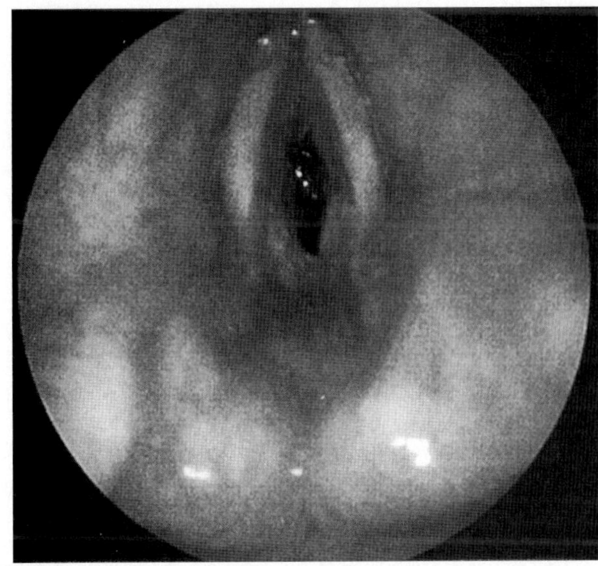

Figure 197-11. Bacterial tracheitis with severe glottic and subglottic edema with sloughed mucosa in the lumen.

Management

Airway endoscopy is not only diagnostic of bacterial tracheitis but also is therapeutic at the same time. Children should be taken to the operating room, where induction of anesthesia with spontaneous ventilation is similar to that in children with supraglottitis. Direct laryngoscopy then is performed with careful examination of the larynx, subglottis, trachea, and main bronchi with a rigid rod telescope (Fig. 197-11). A rigid bronchoscope may be necessary along with the rigid rod telescope to adequately suction and remove the copious secretions and pseudo-membranes. Cultures and a Gram stain should be obtained from the tracheal secretions. Orotracheal or nasotracheal intubation then can be performed to secure the airway, if necessary. When rigid bronchoscopy is performed, this may induce further mucosal injury and edema in the subglottis, requiring a longer period of intubation. Tracheotomy is rarely necessary.

Historically, the majority of patients (up to 80%) with bacterial tracheitis required intubation and ventilatory support.[44,72] More recent reports again suggest a milder illness with only 53% needing intubation.[75] While intubated, meticulous airway care with frequent saline administration and suctioning of the trachea should be performed to evacuate the thick and copious secretions. Occasionally, repeat rigid bronchoscopy may be necessary to handle unusually tenacious secretions. Initial parenteral antibiotic therapy should include vancomycin—because of the rise in resistant *S. aureus* organisms—along with cefotaxime or ceftriaxone for gram-negative organisms or mixed flora.

Gram's stain, culture results, and sensitivity results will direct ultimate antibiotic choices. Nafcillin, ampicillin-sulbactam, and cefuroxime may be good secondary antibiotic choices when culture and sensitivity results are known. Parenteral antibiotics should be continued beyond extubation when the child has undergone major clinical improvement. Extubation can be safely performed when the child's temperature has returned to normal, when a leak is present around the endotracheal tube, and when the secretions have markedly decreased. Oral antibiotics then can be used to complete a 10- to 14-day course of therapy. Intubation may be necessary for 6 to 7 days in more severe cases with a mean hospitalization of 10 days, which usually is longer than that of those with viral croup.[3]

The most common complication of bacterial tracheitis is pneumonia, occurring in about 50% of children. Severe hypoxia with death has occurred after respiratory arrest in severe cases of airway obstruction.[77]

Retropharyngeal Abscess

Retropharyngeal abscesses occur primarily in children, but they can be seen in adults where it is an entirely different disease associated with direct extension from adjacent structures, penetrating trauma, granulomatous disease, and cervical spine osteomyelitis. In children, retropharyngeal abscesses have been described since antiquity, but they have become less common as a result of antibiotic use since the 1950s.[78] However, Kirse and Roberson,[79] in a large review, reported a dramatic increase in the incidence of retropharyngeal abscess in 2001. Because of its anatomic location, a retropharyngeal abscess can still be a life-threatening illness that requires prompt diagnosis and treatment.

The retropharyngeal space extends from the skull base into the mediastinum as far as T6. It is limited posteriorly by the prevertebral fascia; anteriorly by the buccopharyngeal fascia, pharyngobasilar fascia over the three pharyngeal constrictor muscles, and the esophagus; and laterally by the carotid sheath. The space communicates directly with the parapharyngeal space anterolaterally. Within the retropharyngeal space are two vertical paramedian chains of lymph nodes that drain potential infections in the nasopharynx, oropharynx, paranasal sinuses, and possibly middle ear.[3] These lymph nodes are common in childhood, but they undergo atrophy by puberty. Suppuration of these nodes leads to abscess formation within the retropharyngeal space. Other sources of infection in this space include penetrating foreign bodies, endoscopy or intubation trauma, pharyngitis, pyogenic or mycobacterial vertebral body osteomyelitis, petrositis, and dental procedures.[80]

Retropharyngeal abscesses are most common in early childhood, with 70% of patients younger than 6 years of age and 50% younger than 3 years of age.[79,81] Coulthard and Isaacs[82] reported that 55% of their cases were younger than 1 year of age, and 10% presented in the neonatal period. Boys are more likely to be affected than girls by a 2:1 margin.[79]

Clinical Features

The symptoms of retropharyngeal abscess often, but not always, begin insidiously after an antecedent mild upper respiratory infection. Children usually present with fever, sore throat, progressive dysphagia, and drooling. Neck stiffness and mild torticollis may be present and may be suggestive of the diagnosis, distinguishing it from supraglottitis. Stridor is more prominent in younger children and increases as the abscess increases in size. Examination of the pharynx may reveal asymmetric swelling of the posterolateral oropharyngeal wall, but this may be difficult to assess in an uncooperative child with pooling of pharyngeal secretions. Cervical adenopathy also is common. Because of the presence of nonspecific signs and symptoms, a high degree of suspicion is required to ultimately make the diagnosis of retropharyngeal abscess.

Diagnosis

When there is clinical suspicion of retropharyngeal abscess, a complete blood count with differential and a lateral soft tissue radiograph of the neck should be obtained. The neck should be extended, and the radiograph should be taken on inspiration. The diagnosis of retropharyngeal cellulitis or abscess is suggested when the retropharyngeal space at the level of C2 is twice the diameter of the vertebral body (Fig. 197-12).[10]

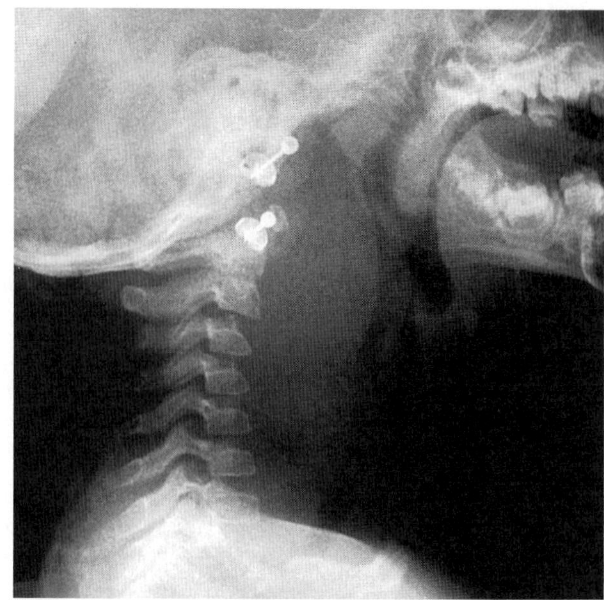

Figure 197-12. Retropharyngeal cellulitis and abscess seen on a lateral radiographic view with widened soft tissue in the retropharynx compared with the adjacent vertebral bodies.

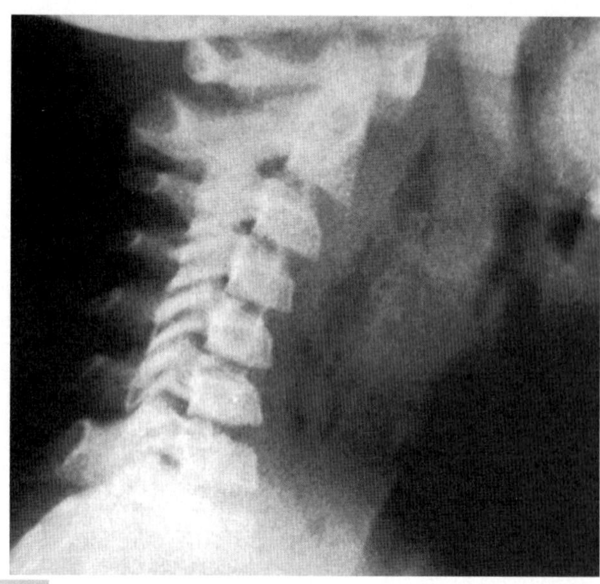

Figure 197-13. Retropharyngeal abscess in a lateral view with gas production within the soft tissues of the retropharynx.

This criterion has a sensitivity of nearly 90%.[82] The lateral radiograph also may reveal gas caused by gas-producing bacteria within the widened retropharyngeal tissues (Fig. 197-13). The normal cervical spine lordosis may be lost or even reversed, and the radiograph should be examined carefully for vertebral or intervertebral disease. The radiographic technique is extremely important because retropharyngeal thickening may be seen when the neck is flexed or when the view is taken on expiration. A chest radiograph should also be performed to exclude mediastinitis or aspiration pneumonia.

When the lateral neck radiograph reveals widened retropharyngeal soft tissues or there are equivocal findings with a strong clinical suspicion of retropharyngeal abscess, computed tomography (CT) of the neck with contrast is extremely helpful in differentiating an abscess from retropharyngeal cellulitis or phlegmon (Fig. 197-14). If there is no airway compromise, the child may be sedated for the CT scan, but, when significant obstruction is present, intubation may be necessary

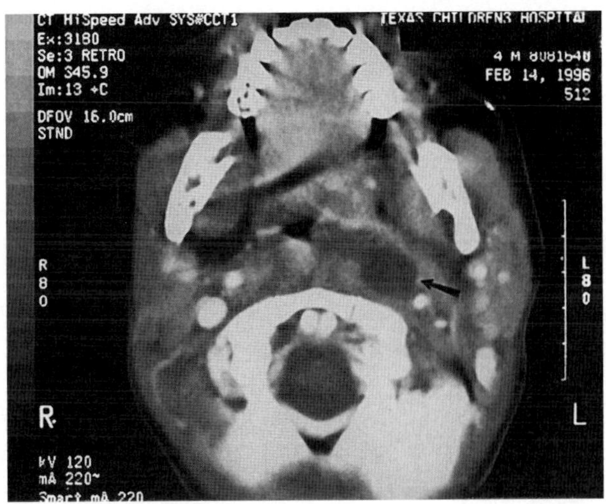

Figure 197-14. Axial computed tomography showing a hypodense area in the left retropharynx with early ring enhancement, indicating a retropharyngeal abscess *(arrow)*.

with the involvement of anesthesia and otolaryngology specialists. Scans should be obtained from the skull base to the thoracic inlet with delayed imaging at least midway through the intravenous contrast injection. Round, central hypodense nodes without clear ring enhancement suggest edematous nodes or phlegmon. When central hypodensity is associated with clear ring enhancement and irregular or scalloped walls, this is most suggestive of an abscess.[79] Using these criteria, CT imaging should accurately delineate abscess from cellulitis in more than 75% of cases. Roberson and colleagues[83] described a comprehensive practice guideline for diagnosis and management of retropharyngeal abscesses with standardized care and good outcomes. The CT scan also defines the exact abscess location and any possible extension into other anatomic areas such as the parapharyngeal space. This is most valuable information when incision and drainage of the abscess is performed.

Management

As in other airway infections, the airway should be secured in severe cases of respiratory distress before ever performing diagnostic procedures. Once the diagnosis is confirmed, initial antibiotic therapy is directed empirically toward aerobic and anaerobic flora of the nasopharynx. Aerobic species include Streptococcus, S. aureus, and Haemophilus. Group A β-hemolytic streptococci have emerged as important organisms either alone or in polymicrobial infections. Bacteroides, Peptostreptococcus, and fusobacteria are the most commonly encountered anaerobes.[79,80] Initial antimicrobial therapy should include clindamycin or ampicillin-sulbactam. An aminoglycoside or third-generation cephalosporin may also be necessary in neonates to provide management for gram-negative enterics.

When CT suggests only a phlegmon or cellulitis, a trial of intravenous antibiotics is warranted. If after 48 hours the child is clinically well, then outpatient antibiotic therapy is appropriate. If the clinical course is worrisome, however, a repeat CT scan or surgical intervention should be considered.

With the availability of CT imaging to distinguish retropharyngeal cellulitis from abscess formation, the surgeon can best determine those children who will require abscess incision and drainage. When an abscess is found or suspected, incision and drainage should be performed in most cases because this may greatly expedite resolution of this disease. Very small abscesses in children who are clinically improving may be treated medically. The transoral approach is indicated in almost all children, except in those rare cases when there is extension or involvement lateral to the great vessels. The vessels should be well examined on the imaging study to rule out the rare possibility of vascular wall compromise. Careful oral intubation should be performed to avoid abscess rupture and possible aspiration of purulent material. The pharyngeal incision is made over the most prominent bulging area, which is almost always located on one side of the posterior pharynx near the lateral pharyngeal wall. Blunt dissection may reveal thin secretions in early abscess formation but thicker mucopurulent secretions in a more defined abscess. Needle aspiration may be helpful in localizing a purulent collection. A drain is not required. When a child presents with a major inflammatory lateral neck mass and a large parapharyngeal space abscess, in addition to retropharyngeal involvement, a lateral cervical incision and drainage procedure is indicated with drain placement. Cultures of the purulent drainage from either approach will help direct antibiotic therapy. When the child is afebrile, asymptomatic, and swallowing well, appropriate oral antibiotics (e.g., amoxicillin–clavulanic acid or clindamycin) can be used to complete a 10- to 14-day course of therapy.

Complications

Complications that should be considered in children with retropharyngeal abscesses include airway obstruction, spontaneous abscess perforation, aspiration pneumonia, mediastinitis, and sepsis. More rarely, retropharyngeal abscess can result in chest empyema, thrombosis of the internal jugular vein, erosion of the carotid artery, and atlantoaxial dislocation.[10,80] With early suspicion of the clinical possibility of a retropharyngeal abscess, along with CT imaging, good anesthesia, and prompt surgical drainage, complications should be extremely low with near zero mortality.

Acknowledgments

I want to gratefully acknowledge the support of my mentor Dr. Bruce N. P. Benjamin, Sydney, Australia, in collecting the endoscopic airway photographs in this chapter; Dr. Lynn Trautwein, Texas Children's Hospital, Houston, for helping assemble the radiographs and imaging views; and Ms. Nancy Turner for manuscript editorial assistance.

SUGGESTED READINGS

Ausejo M, Saenz A, Pham B, et al. The effectiveness of glucocorticoids in treating croup: meta-analysis. *BMJ*. 1999;319:595.

DeBoeck K. Croup: a review. *Eur J Pediatr*. 1995;154:432.

Donnelly B, McMillan J, Win L. Bacterial tracheitis: a report of eight new cases and review. *Rev Infect Dis*. 1990;12:729.

Eckel H, Widemann B, Damm M, Roth B. Airway endoscopy in the diagnosis and treatment of bacterial tracheitis in children. *Int J Pediatr Otorhinolaryngol*. 1993;27:147.

Fitzgerald D, Kilhaven H. Croup: assessment and evidence-based management. *Med J Aust*. 2003;179:372.

Kirse D, Robertson D. Surgical management of retropharyngeal space infections in children. *Laryngoscope*. 2001;111:1413.

Klasser T. Croup—a current perspective. *Pediatr Clin North Am*. 1999;46:1167.

Loftis L. Acute infections upper airway obstructions in children. *PMID*. 2006;17:5.

Rafei K, Lichtenstein R. Airway infectious disease emergencies. *Pediatr Clin North Am*. 2006;53:215.

Rotta A, Wiryawan B. Respiratory emergencies in children. *Respiratory Care*. 2003;48:248.

Salamone F, Bobbitt DB, Myer CM, et al : Bacterial tracheitis re-examined: Is thee a less severe manifestation? *Otolaryngol Head Neck Surg*. 2004;131:871.

Shah R, Roberson DW, Jones DT. Epiglottitis in the *Hemophilus influenzae* type B vaccine era: changing trends. *Laryngoscope*. 2004;114:557.

Stroud R, Friedman N. An update on inflammatory disorders of the pediatric airway; epiglottitis, croup, and tracheitis. *Am J Otolaryngol*. 2001;22:268.

Wright R, Pomerantz W, Luria J. New approaches to respiratory infection in children. *Emerg Med Clin North Am*. 2002;20:93.

For complete list of references log onto www.expertconsult.com.

SECTION FIVE

Head and Neck

CHAPTER ONE HUNDRED AND NINETY-EIGHT

Differential Diagnosis of Neck Masses

Ralph F. Wetmore

William P. Potsic

Key Points

- The two major categories of neck masses in children are congenital and acquired lesions. Congenital cysts make up the majority of the congenital lesions, whereas infectious masses comprise a majority of the acquired ones.
- A good history and physical are essential to narrow the differential diagnosis of a pediatric neck mass. Computed tomography (CT), magnetic resonance imaging (MRI), and neck ultrasound are the major radiologic studies that help in the evaluation of a neck mass.
- Most branchial cleft cysts are either second or third branchial derivatives. Thyroglossal duct cysts develop within the embryonic thyroid descent tract.
- Hemangiomas are proliferative lesions, rather than neoplastic, and typically begin to involute at 18 to 24 months of age. Vascular and lymphatic malformations are also congenital lesions but do not involute.
- Most infectious lymphadenopathy is viral, but streptococcal or staphylococcal organisms may cause suppurative lymphadenopathy.
- Lymphoma is the most common neck malignancy in children and presents as an enlarging neck mass with or without systemic symptoms of fever, weight loss, night sweats, or fatigue. Malignant neck lesions tend to occur most commonly in either the posterior cervical or supraclavicular regions.

The presentation of a neck mass in a pediatric patient has many diagnostic possibilities not normally encountered in an adult (Fig. 198-1). Neoplastic disease, especially malignant, is the primary consideration in the evaluation of a neck mass in an adult. In contrast, diagnosis of a pediatric neck mass can be categorized, depending on the location, growth factors, and the child's age. The possibility of malignancy should always be considered in the differential diagnosis in pediatric patients; however, it is not as overriding a concern as in adults.

The two major categories of pediatric neck masses include congenital and acquired lesions. Congenital masses have a high incidence (>50% in some series),[1] which initially differentiates them from acquired masses. The primary type of acquired masses is inflammatory (acute and chronic), which further narrows the differential diagnosis. Benign and malignant lesions are rare in the pediatric patient.

The approach to the child with a neck mass depends on the history and physical examination. Radiographic and laboratory studies may prove helpful, but some masses require surgical biopsy to establish the diagnosis. Thus the pediatric neck mass often poses a challenge to the surgeon.

History

In the evaluation of a pediatric patient with a neck mass, a detailed history alone can often exclude many lesions in the differential diagnosis. Consideration of temporal relationships can often prove helpful. A history of infection elsewhere in the patient or recent travel or exposure to farm animals may suggest an infectious origin. Preceding trauma may signal a hematoma, whereas an increase in the size of the mass or pain with eating may point to a salivary gland problem. Exposure to drugs such as phenytoin may also be contributory.

The growth characteristics of the neck mass are important. Slow growth suggests a benign process, whereas rapid enlargement occurs with infectious or malignant lesions. Some masses fluctuate in size (e.g., hemangiomas increase in size with straining and crying). Fever, weight loss, night sweats, or fatigue suggest a malignant process.

Physical Examination

In the evaluation of a child with a neck mass, comprehensive head and neck examination is essential. Clues to the pathogenesis of the neck mass may be found anywhere in the head. Likewise, a total physical examination should be performed with special attention to other lymph node groups such as the axillae and groin. Palpation for an enlarged spleen should always be attempted.

Infants frequently have small palpable lymph nodes in the posterior cervical region, whereas older children have palpable nodes in the anterior cervical, posterior cervical, and submandibular regions. Any node greater than 2 cm in diameter falls outside the range of these normal hyperplastic nodes and should be evaluated further.

In examination of abnormal lymph nodes or a neck mass, the location is important for determining the site of the precipitating infection or the primary source of a malignant neoplasm. For example, infection in the nasopharynx tends to drain into the posterior cervical

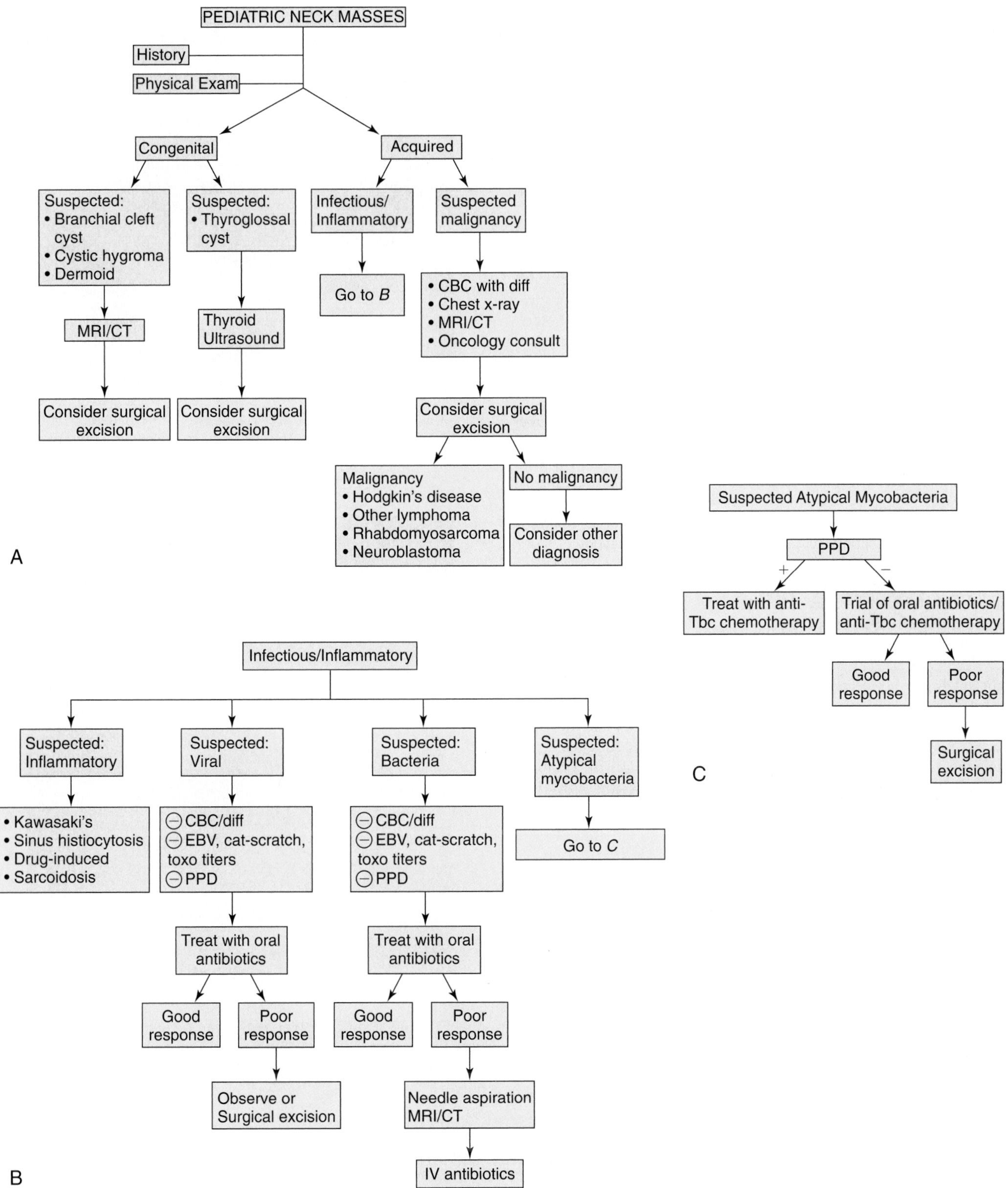

Figure 198-1. **A** to **C**, Algorithms for the differential diagnosis of neck masses.

region, whereas tonsillitis may cause enlargement in the anterior cervical region. Moussatos[2] and Putney[3] noted an increased incidence of malignancy in the posterior cervical triangle; in contrast, Torsiglieri and colleagues[1] reported an increased incidence in the supraclavicular region.

The consistency of a neck mass is frequently helpful in categorizing the mass. For example, hard masses tend to occur with infection or a malignant process. Fixation of a mass to the skin or deeper structures of the neck suggests a malignancy. A fluctuant mass tends to occur with abscess formation or a cyst.

Radiologic Studies

Depending on the clinical impression of a neck mass from the history and physical examination, selected radiographic studies may help narrow the differential diagnosis. Chest radiography is helpful if a malignancy, sarcoidosis, or pulmonary tuberculosis is suspected. In the evaluation of the nasopharynx, cervical spine, or retropharyngeal region, lateral neck radiography may show an abnormality. Likewise, a sinus series may show evidence of an infection or neoplasm in the paranasal sinuses.

In cases of infection in the neck, computed tomography (CT) with contrast may differentiate cellulitis that may respond solely to antibiotic therapy from an abscess with rim enhancement that may necessitate surgery. CT with contrast also helps identify vascular masses such as hemangiomas. Magnetic resonance imaging (MRI) provides even better detail of soft tissue. When combined with contrast, MRI is also useful in the evaluation of vascular lesions.

Ultrasound of the neck is most helpful in differentiating a cystic structure from a solid mass. It should be included as part of the evaluation of any thyroid mass. Before excision of a thyroglossal duct cyst, ultrasound can confirm the presence of a thyroid gland in its normal position, ruling out the possibility of ectopic thyroid. Use of ultrasound in these cases is easier and more economical. Thyroid scanning remains essential in the evaluation of any thyroid mass.

Laboratory Studies

As with radiography, selected laboratory studies may be useful in the evaluation of the pediatric neck mass. A complete blood count with differential is indicated if a malignancy or systemic infection is suspected. Serologic testing for Epstein-Barr virus (EBV), cytomegalovirus, toxoplasmosis, syphilis, or cat-scratch disease may be diagnostic. An elevated serum calcium level is highly suggestive of sarcoidosis, whereas thyroid function studies are necessary in the evaluation of most thyroid masses. Urinary collection for vanillylmandelic acid (VMA) is helpful when neuroblastoma is suspected. Although not as accurate as a culture of infected tissue, skin tests, if available, remain a reliable indicator of mycobacterial disease.

Surgical Diagnosis

Although fine-needle aspiration of a suspected malignancy is not as reliable in children as in adults, fine-needle aspiration of a neck infection decompresses the mass and provides material for culture. In some cases, especially when the diagnosis of malignancy is considered, an incisional or excisional biopsy is indicated. Advantages of a biopsy include inspection of the lesion, providing a cuff of healthy surrounding tissue and tissue for frozen and permanent section, electron microscopy, and tumor markers.

Congenital Masses

Branchial Cleft Cysts

Although the definitive mechanism for the development of branchial cleft cysts is unclear, it is suspected that these congenital masses result from the cervical sinus of His becoming entrapped without an external or internal opening. An epithelium-lined cyst results. Others suggest that these cysts develop from epithelial rests of tissue from Waldeyer's ring.[4] Branchial cleft cysts are relatively common; in one series, they comprise one third of congenital neck masses.[1]

Branchial cleft cysts typically are seen as nontender, fluctuant masses that may become inflamed and abscess during an upper respiratory infection (Fig. 198-2). First branchial cleft cysts, although rare, typically present near the angle of the mandible (Fig. 198-3). Second branchial cysts are found high in the neck and deep to the anterior border of the sternocleidomastoid muscle. Third branchial cleft cysts, also rare, are seen near the upper pole of the thyroid gland. Other symptoms, depending on the size of the cyst, include dysphagia, dyspnea, and stridor.

Radiologic evaluation of a branchial cleft cyst may include ultrasound, CT, and MRI. Ultrasound shows a fluid-filled cyst and can differentiate cystic lesions from solid masses. CT and MRI also confirm the cystic characteristics of the mass and, more importantly, delineate the relationship of the cyst to surrounding structures (Fig. 198-4).

Management of branchial cleft cysts is surgical excision. It is advisable, if possible, to manage an infected cyst with antibiotics, allowing the inflammation to resolve before excision is attempted.

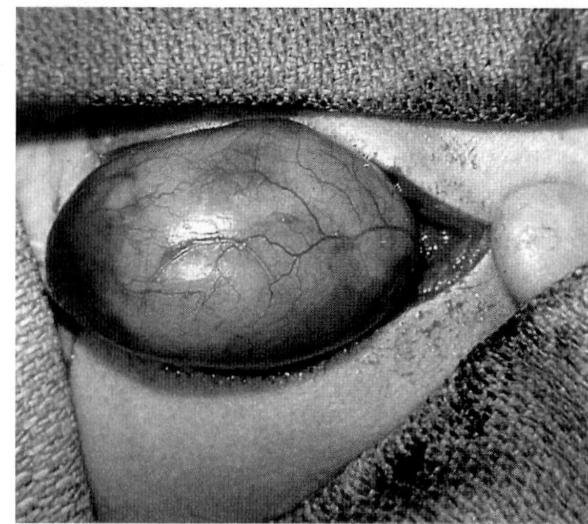

Figure 198-2. A typical branchial cleft cyst is an epithelium-lined cyst filled with mucoid material. This cyst presents along the anterior border of the sternocleidomastoid muscle.

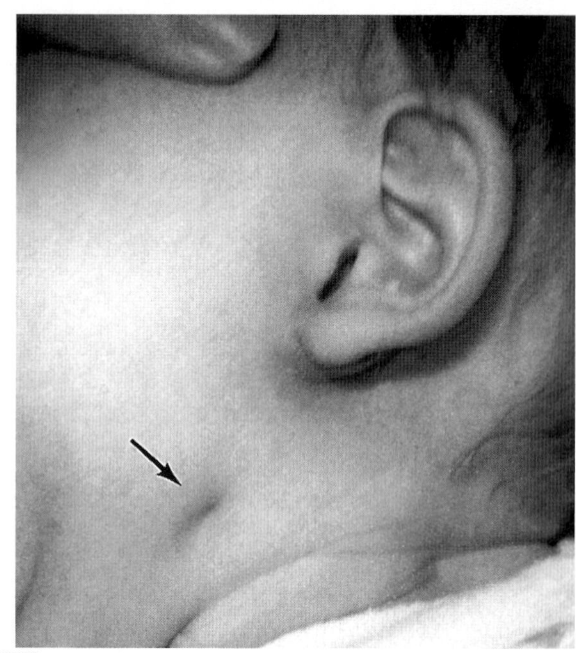

Figure 198-3. First branchial derivatives present as a pit or a mass near the angle of the mandible *(arrow)*. They frequently originate in or near the external canal and, during their course, involve the facial nerve.

Thyroglossal Duct Cysts

Thyroglossal duct cysts form in a persistent thyroid descent tract that begins as an elongation of the thyroid diverticulum. Beginning at the foramen caecum of the tongue, this tract may extend to the thyroid gland itself, where some tissue may persist in the region of a pyramidal lobe. These remnants are cysts and are not associated with a cutaneous sinus or fistula tract unless surgically drained and inadequately excised. They comprise approximately one third of congenital neck masses in children.[1]

Most thyroglossal duct cysts are seen in the midline near the level of the hyoid bone because the tract passes just anterior to the hyoid bone (Fig. 198-5). Some cysts may present laterally and are not infrequently found superior to the hyoid or as low as the level of the thyroid gland. Thyroglossal duct cysts that occur off the midline may be

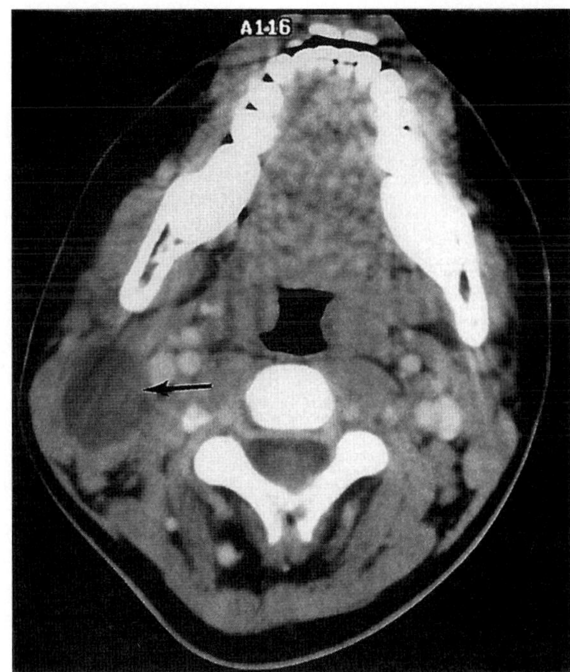

Figure 198-4. Axial computed tomography of the neck shows a branchial cleft cyst in the hypolucent area *(arrow)*.

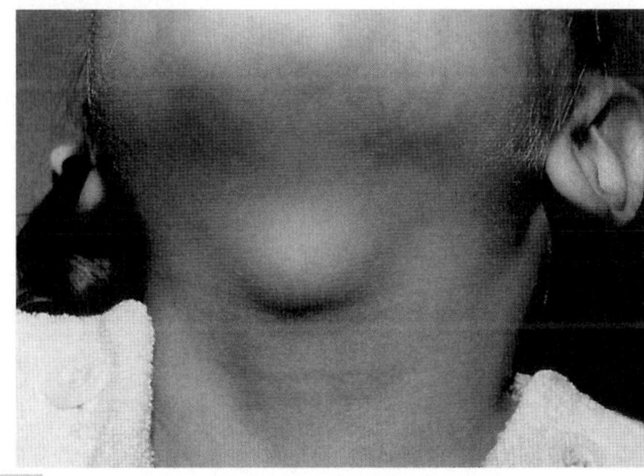

Figure 198-5. Thyroglossal duct cysts are often found in the midline of the neck at or near the hyoid bone.

difficult to differentiate from branchial cleft cysts, an important factor in their surgical excision. Other unusual presentations of thyroglossal duct cysts include formation on either side of the hyoid bone as dumbbell-shaped lesions and, rarely, as cystic lesions in the larynx. Thyroid tissue is found in surgical specimens in up to 45% of cases.[5]

A thyroglossal duct cyst usually presents as an asymptomatic mass but may be associated with mild dysphagia. Not infrequently, presentation of these cysts may be accompanied by infection, causing rapid enlargement that may produce significant dysphagia and choking.

In cases in which a thyroglossal duct cyst is suspected, it is important to differentiate ectopic thyroid from a cyst. Although only 10% of ectopic thyroid is found in the neck, it may represent the only thyroid tissue in 75% of patients.[6] Children with ectopic thyroid may be mildly hypothyroid; however, excision of this tissue necessitates hormone replacement for the remainder of the patient's life. Thyroid ultrasound and radionucleotide scanning can differentiate ectopic thyroid from a thyroglossal duct cyst; ultrasound is easier to perform, less expensive, and does not use radioisotopes.

The Sistrunk operation is the standard method of thyroglossal duct cyst excision. The cyst is excised along with a cuff of tissue including the center portion of the hyoid bone. Incision and drainage of an infected cyst should be avoided because violation of the cyst capsule may invite recurrence. Recurrence rates of nearly 10% have been reported in children who have undergone uncomplicated Sistrunk operations.[1]

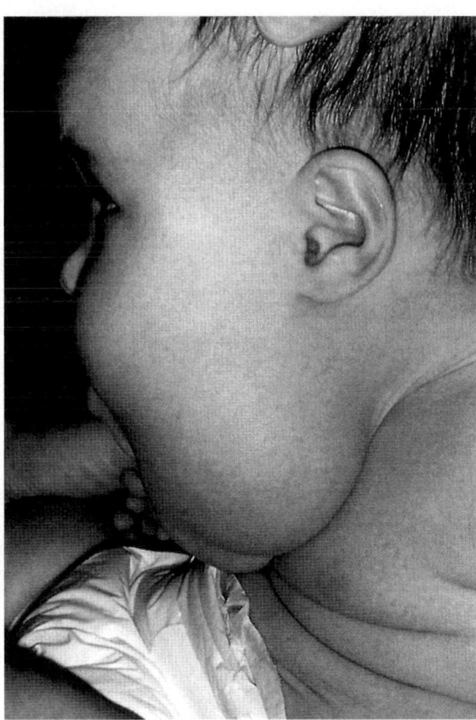

Figure 198-6. Lymphangiomas of the neck may cause significant cosmetic deformity and may impair respiration or alimentation.

Lymphatic Malformations (Lymphangiomas)

The term *lymphatic malformation* is a better definition of the lesion that was previously termed *lymphangioma.* Lymphatic malformations are congenital malformations of lymph tissue that result from the failure of lymph spaces to connect to the rest of the lymphatic system. Lesions containing both lymphatic and venous components may be labeled combined venolymphatic malformations. Macrocystic lymphatic malformations (previously termed *cystic hygroma*) contain large thick-walled cysts that have less infiltration of surrounding tissue. Microcystic lymphatic malformations have more extensive infiltration of the soft tissue structures of the head and neck, especially in the tongue and floor of mouth, making their excision difficult.

A lymphatic malformation presents as a soft, smooth, nontender mass that is compressible and can be transilluminated (Fig. 198-6). Typically, lymphatic malformations fluctuate in size as a result of infection or hemorrhage. They mostly impact the cosmetic appearance of the child. Depending on the size and location of the mass, there may be respiratory compromise and difficulty in feeding.

Radiographic evaluation with MRI or CT is invaluable for diagnosis and determination of the extent of the lesion. Radiography shows fluid-filled spaces with surrounding connective tissue. Because these malformations lack a capsule and extend along the lymphatic channels, MRI or CT is essential in defining normal anatomic structures that should be preserved when surgical excision is performed.

The goals of surgery are to improve cosmetic appearance and to counter impaired breathing or eating. Because of the infiltrative nature of these malformations, complete surgical excision is often difficult; debulking of the mass often accomplishes these goals.

Some experts recommend staging of surgical excision in extensive cases.[7] Management with radiotherapy has not been effective.[8] Macrocystic lesions can be treated with sclerotherapy using alcohol. An experimental lyophilized streptococcal compound, OK-432, has been used successfully to sclerose macrocystic lesions.[9]

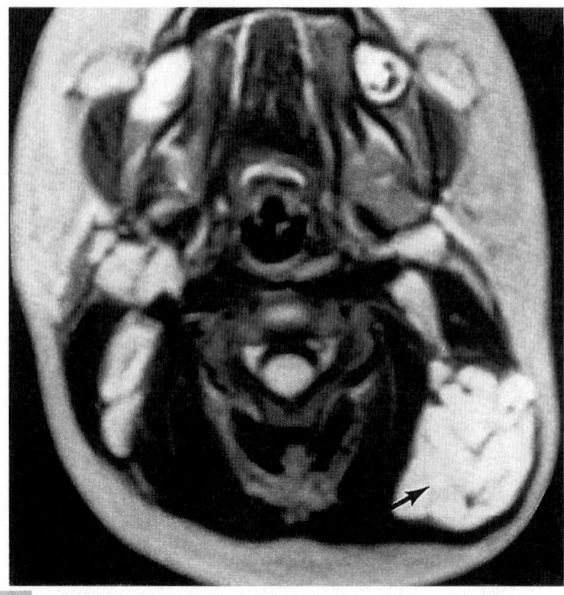

Figure 198-7. Magnetic resonance imaging with contrast shows an enhancing vascular lesion in the posterior neck consistent with a hemangioma *(arrow)*.

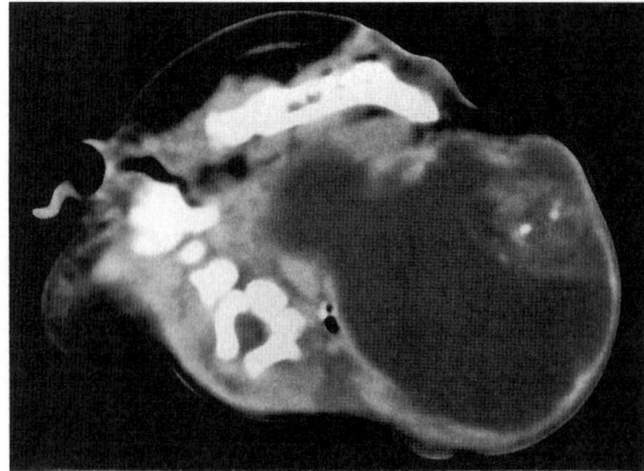

Figure 198-8. Computed tomography shows a large teratoma cyst in a newborn that severely compromised the respiratory tract and required a tracheostomy.

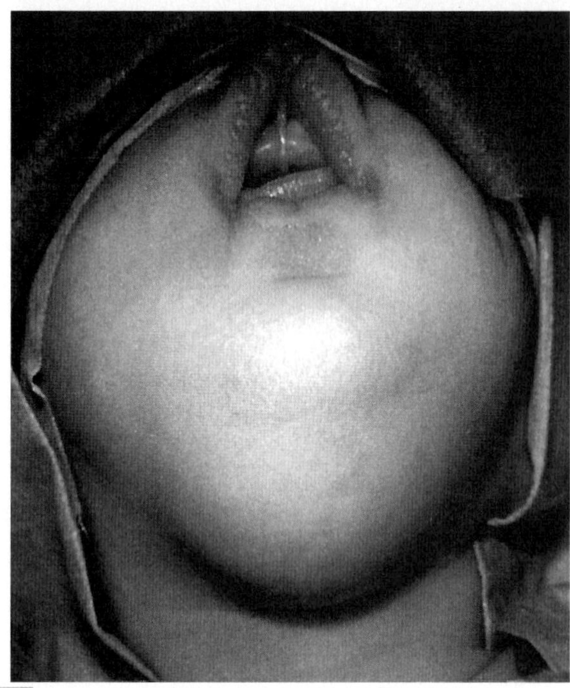

Figure 198-9. A large dermoid cyst presents in the midline of the submental region.

Hemangiomas

Hemangiomas are proliferative endothelial lesions rather than true neoplasms. Hemangiomas present at birth, grow rapidly during the first year of life, and begin to slowly involute at 18 to 24 months of age. Hemangiomas occur in up to 10% of children with a female-to-male ratio of 2 : 1.[10]

Hemangiomas are seen as red or bluish soft masses that frequently have a skin component. Typically, these masses are compressible and increase with straining or crying. With large hemangiomas, a bruit may be heard over the lesion. CT or MRI with contrast often confirms the diagnosis of a vascular lesion (Fig. 198-7).

Because hemangiomas typically involute after several years, the usual management is observation, unless there is functional impairment, bleeding, skin necrosis, or a coagulopathy caused by thrombocytopenia. Use of systemic corticosteroids may be helpful in the management of complications such as skin ulceration, dysphagia, dyspnea, thrombocytopenia, or cardiac failure.[11-14] Surgical excision or laser therapy may be helpful in cases of incomplete involution or when mild functional or cosmetic abnormalities remain. Management with radiotherapy may lead to malignant transformation, and the use of sclerosing agents and cryotherapy has produced poor results.[8,15]

Teratomas

Teratomas in the head and neck are rare, comprising only 3.5% of all teratomas in one series.[16] Although there is a female-to-male preponderance of 6 : 1 in other body regions, the female-to-male ratio is equal in the head and neck.[17] Teratomas arise from pluripotential cells and consist of tissues foreign to the site from which they arise. A history of maternal polyhydramnios has been noted in up to 18% of neonates who have a cervical teratoma (Fig. 198-8).

Most teratomas present as firm neck masses. With large teratomas, there may be symptoms of respiratory compromise caused by tracheal compression. Intrinsic calcifications may be seen on CT or MRI, a finding that may assist diagnosis. Management is by surgical excision; failure of complete excision may result in recurrence.

Dermoid Cysts

Similar to teratomas, to which they are pathologically related, dermoid cysts arise from epithelium that has been entrapped in tissue during embryogenesis or by traumatic implantation. Dermoid cysts consist of epithelium-lined cavities filled with skin appendages (e.g., hair, hair follicles, sebaceous glands). They are found at other sites in the head and neck including the orbit, nose, nasopharynx, and oral cavity.

Typically, dermoid cysts are seen in the midline of the neck, usually in the submental region (Figs. 198-9 and 198-10). They are attached to and move with the overlying skin and are painless unless infected. Management is by complete surgical excision.

Laryngoceles

A laryngocele is an abnormal dilation or herniation of the saccule of the larynx. If this dilation lies within the limits of the thyroid cartilage, the laryngocele is internal. If it extends beyond the thyroid cartilage in a cephalad direction to protrude through the thyrohyoid membrane, the laryngocele is external. Some laryngoceles present with internal and external components. Laryngoceles are rare in infants and children but may present congenitally in newborns. Clinical differentiation of air-filled laryngoceles from fluid-filled saccular cysts may be impossible.[18]

Hoarseness, cough, dyspnea, and dysphagia suggest a laryngocele. CT may be helpful in diagnosis, especially in delineating the extent of the lesion and differentiating the laryngocele's air-filled space from the

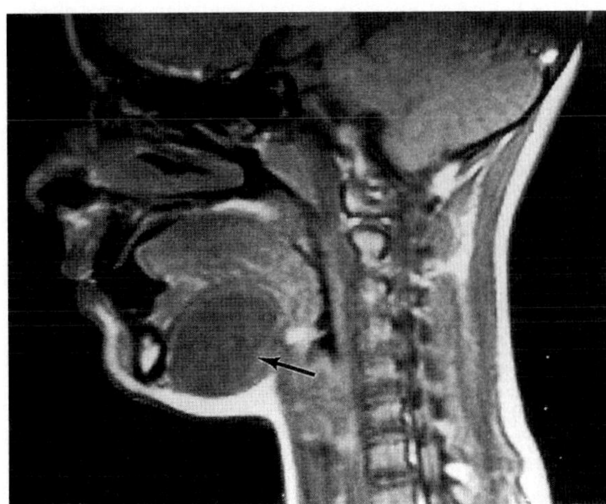

Figure 198-10. Magnetic resonance imaging (sagittal view) shows a large dermoid cyst in the submental region just deep to the tongue *(arrow).*

fluid of a saccular cyst. Surgical excision through an external approach is the management of choice.

Thymic Cysts

The thymus develops from the third pharyngeal pouch and descends into the chest. An implant of thymic tissue along this descent tract anywhere in the neck may result in a thymic cyst. Thymic cysts may be more common than suggested by several reports in the literature.[19] Almost all are unilateral (most commonly on the left side of the neck), and 90% are cystic.[20]

Typically, a thymic cyst presents as an asymptomatic mass, but it may be painful if infected or if there is a rapid increase in its size. CT or MRI may help differentiate a thymic cyst comprising a single cystic lesion from a cystic hygroma that has multiple large cysts within the mass. The preferred management is surgical excision. Diagnosis is confirmed by histologic identification of Hassall's corpuscles.

Vascular Malformations

Vascular malformations can be divided into two groups depending on blood flow. Slow-flow lesions include capillary malformations and venous malformations, whereas arterial and arteriovenous malformations are typically fast-flow lesions. Vascular malformations represent congenital structural anomalies, grow at the same rate as the child, and do not involute.

Venous anomalies of the external jugular vein may occasionally present as a neck mass.[21] Typically, the external jugular vein empties into the subclavian vein, but it may empty into the internal jugular vein outside the carotid sheath, forming a venous plexus. Jugular malformations present as soft, compressible masses along the anterior border of the sternocleidomastoid muscle. Management is by ligation or excision of the anomaly.

Sternocleidomastoid Tumors of Infancy

Neonates with sternocleidomastoid tumors present with neck masses that are usually not apparent at birth but appear at 1 to 8 weeks of age. Pathologically, the mass is characterized by dense fibrous tissue and the absence of normal striated muscle (Fig. 198-11). As the mass resolves, the remaining muscle continues to degenerate into fibrous tissue. The etiology of this disorder, also known as *congenital torticollis,* is unclear; however, birth trauma, ischemia of the muscle, and intrauterine positioning have been implicated.

Most patients are firstborn[22]; siblings are rarely affected.[1] Congenital torticollis presents as a firm, painless, discrete, fusiform mass within the sternocleidomastoid muscle that slowly increases in size for 2 to 3 months and then slowly regresses for 4 to 8 months (Fig. 198-12). Because the mass disappears in more than 80% of cases,[23] conservative management with physiotherapy (passive and active motion) prevents the development of restrictive torticollis. In resistant cases, surgical section of the sternocleidomastoid muscle may be required.

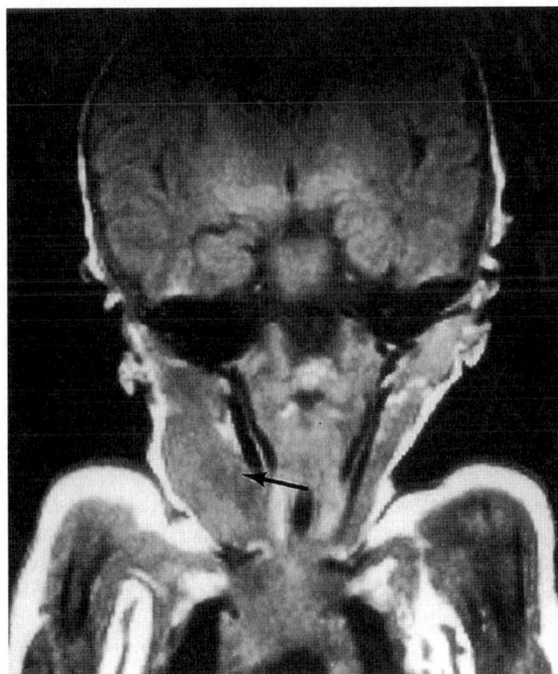

Figure 198-11. Magnetic resonance imaging of an infant with congenital torticollis shows enlargement of the sternocleidomastoid muscle *(arrow).*

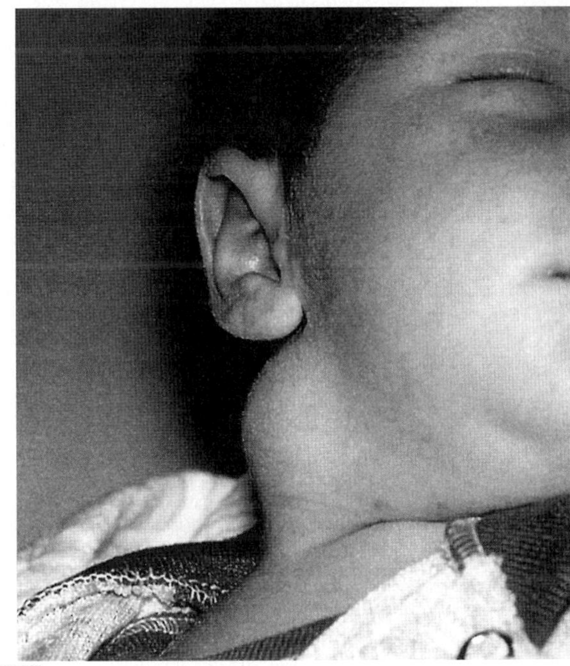

Figure 198-12. A firm mass in the midportion of the sternocleidomastoid muscle is seen in an infant with congenital torticollis.

Acquired Masses

Viral Lymphadenopathy

Reactive lymph nodes result from viral upper respiratory tract infections such as adenovirus, rhinovirus, or enterovirus (coxsackievirus A and B). EBV often presents with massive lymphadenopathy in addition to enlargement of other lymphoid tissue (e.g., tonsils, spleen). On pathologic examination, there is a proliferation of normal cells; however, in contrast to neoplastic disease, the nodal architecture is intact.

Reactive lymphadenopathy is frequently bilateral and is associated with symptoms of the underlying respiratory infection. Management is observation, although not infrequently these nodes are biopsied because their consistency mimics lymphoma and their regression in size is often slow.

Unlike most cases of viral lymphadenopathy, human immunodeficiency virus (HIV) infection may result in acquired immunodeficiency syndrome (AIDS) whose associated findings, aside from generalized lymphadenopathy, include hepatosplenomegaly; weight loss; susceptibility to viral, bacterial, and fungal infections; and fevers. Pediatric AIDS should be suspected in cases in which multiple neck nodes are involved with bacterial infection and in cases that fail to respond to adequate antibiotic therapy.

Cervical lymphadenopathy is also a manifestation of posttransplantation lymphoproliferative disease (PTLD). PTLD is associated with an Epstein-Barr infection in patients who have undergone either solid organ or bone marrow transplantation. Histologic examination of a biopsied node and Epstein-Barr titers are essential in the diagnosis of this disorder.[7,24]

Bacterial Lymphadenopathy

Suppurative Lymphadenopathy

Staphylococcus aureus and group A β-*Streptococcus* are the most common causative organisms of suppuration in the neck, although other bacteria such as *Haemophilus* and *Moraxella* species have been implicated. Brodsky and colleagues[25] found a 19% incidence for anaerobic bacteria versus 67% for aerobic bacteria. Brook[26] reported a similar anaerobic incidence and β-lactamase-positive organisms in 34%. In neonates the offending organisms may be *Staphylococcus* or *Streptococcus,* but *Pseudomonas* and other gram-negative bacteria have also been reported.[27,28] Several studies have documented a rising incidence of methicillin-resistant *S. aureus* (MRSA) as the pathogen in community-acquired pediatric cervical neck infections.

No major differences between the *Staphylococcus* and *Streptococcus* groups are evident when demographic factors and occurrence of symptoms are compared. Frequently, the neck mass develops in the submandibular region, but it may occur in the anterior and posterior cervical triangles (Fig. 198-13).[29] Associated symptoms include a history of upper respiratory infection, sore throat, earache, and skin lesions.[29] Initial management is with antibiotic therapy, either orally or intravenously, depending on the severity of the infection. Failure to respond to medication may indicate the need for fine-needle aspiration or incision and drainage.

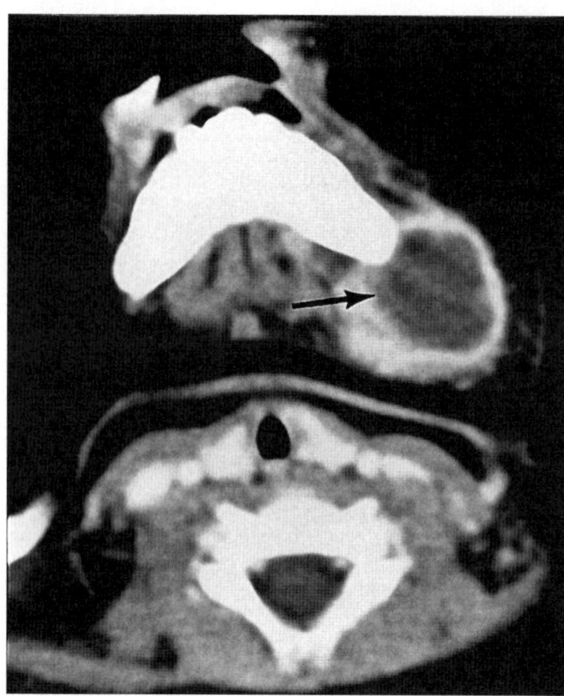

Figure 198-13. Computed tomography with contrast shows a neck abscess in the submandibular triangle *(arrow).* Abscess formation is characterized by hypolucency and rim enhancement.

Cat-Scratch Disease

Most cases of cat-scratch disease occur in patients younger than 20 years,[30] and males are affected more frequently than females.[31] More than 90% of patients have a history of feline contact, and there is a fall and winter prevalence. Although the symptom complex of cat-scratch disease has been recognized for almost 50 years, only recently has the bacterium *Bartonella henselae* been implicated as the etiologic agent.[32] Serologic testing by indirect fluorescent antibodies for *Bartonella* DNA has a high sensitivity and specificity. Typically, affected children are seen with lymphadenopathy associated with mild fever and other symptoms of malaise. Antibiotic therapy with azithromycin, an aminoglycoside, or ciprofloxacin is usually curative.[32] Rarely is the infection severe enough to require surgery.

Toxoplasmosis

Infection with *Toxoplasma gondii* is usually contracted through the consumption of poorly cooked meat or ingestion of oocytes excreted in cat feces. Symptoms include fever, malaise, sore throat, and myalgias. Cervical adenitis occurs in greater than 90% of cases.[33] Complications of toxoplasmosis include myocarditis and pneumonitis. The diagnosis is confirmed by serologic testing, and management is with pyrimethamine or sulfonamides.

Mycobacterial Infection

Most atypical mycobacterial infections are caused by a variety of mycobacteria including *Mycobacterium avium-intracellulare, Mycobacterium scrofulaceum, Mycobacterium kansasii, Mycobacterium fortuitum,* and *Mycobacterium haemophilum.* In the past few years, the reemergence of *Mycobacterium tuberculosis* has been noted; *M. tuberculosis* as a cause of cervical adenopathy is associated with pulmonary tuberculosis in endemic areas of the United States. In a series on the cause of mycobacterial neck infections, Hawkins and colleagues[35] showed a 59% incidence for atypical mycobacteria compared with 29% for *M. tuberculosis.*

Skin tests for *M. tuberculosis* and atypical mycobacteria are available[34] and were positive in 95% of cases in the series by Hawkins and colleagues.[35] Mycobacterial infection is definitively diagnosed by culture, which frequently takes weeks.

The most common site of mycobacterial infection in the neck is the anterior superior cervical region, followed by the posterior cervical, middle cervical, supraclavicular, and submental regions. Atypical mycobacterial infection is not infrequently found in the preauricular region (Fig. 198-14). It tends to occur unilaterally, whereas *M. tuberculosis* is more diffuse and frequently bilateral.[35] A painless, firm, enlarging mass in the face of antibiotic therapy suggests the diagnosis. The overlying skin is frequently discolored with atypical mycobacterial infection. In patients with *M. tuberculosis* infection, weight loss, fever, and anorexia may also be present.

The current management of *M. tuberculosis* infection is with antituberculous chemotherapy, usually including two drugs, although lymph nodes infected with atypical mycobacteria are best managed by surgical excision or incision and curettage. Hawkins and colleagues[35] showed resolution of neck masses in 4 of 18 cases of atypical mycobacterial infection with chemotherapy alone.

Fungal Infections

Fungal infections of the neck typically present in immunocompromised patients with symptoms and signs that suggest viral or bacterial infection. The usual pathogens include *Candida, Histoplasma,* and *Aspergillus.* The diagnosis is made by serology or fungal smear and culture.

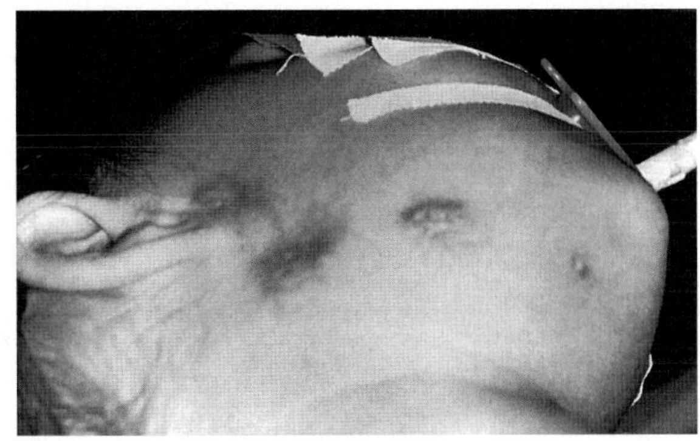

Figure 198-14. Atypical mycobacterial infection frequently involves the submandibular triangle and preauricular regions.

Management of fungal lymphadenopathy requires intravenous amphotericin B.

Sialadenitis

The salivary glands are susceptible to viral and bacterial infection and, at times, may resemble infection of surrounding lymph nodes. Although rare since the development of a vaccine, mumps is a paramyxoviral infection that may cause orchitis, meningitis, or sensorineural hearing loss. One or both parotid or submandibular glands may be involved. Management includes supportive measures such as analgesics and hydration.

In addition to viral infection, dehydration and generalized disability of patients often predispose to bacterial infection of the salivary glands. The causative organisms include *S. aureus, Streptococcus* species, and *Haemophilus influenzae.*

Children with sialadenitis have a rapid onset of pain and swelling of the affected glands. Fever, chills, and malaise may also occur. Examination of the oral cavity may reveal purulent discharge from the ducts of the involved glands (Stensen's or Wharton's). Management of bacterial sialadenitis is hydration and oral or intravenous broad-spectrum antibiotic therapy.

Noninfectious Inflammatory Disorders

Kawasaki Disease (Mucocutaneous Lymph Node Syndrome)

Kawasaki disease is an acute multisystem vasculitis of unknown etiology that tends to affect children younger than 5 years of age.[36] To confirm this diagnosis, the patient should have fever persisting for 5 days and four of the following features: (1) acute, nonpurulent cervical lymphadenopathy that is usually unilateral; (2) erythema, edema, and desquamation of the hands and feet; (3) polymorphous exanthem; (4) bilateral painless conjunctival infection; and (5) erythema and infection of the lips and oral cavity.

Associated findings in the acute stage include thrombocytosis and cardiac signs of pericardial effusion.[37] In the subacute stage, coronary artery aneurysms may develop in 15% to 20% of cases.[36] The goal of management is to reduce the inflammatory response with aspirin and γ-globulin therapy.

Sinus Histiocytosis (Rosai-Dorfman Disease)

Children with sinus histiocytosis have massive nontender cervical lymphadenopathy that is similar to infectious mononucleosis or lymphoma. The disease is thought to represent an abnormal histiocytic response to some precipitating cause, possibly either a herpesvirus or EBV.[38] Biopsy shows dilated sinuses, many plasma cells, and marked proliferation of histiocytes. In addition to massive adenopathy, fever and skin nodules may be present. Management of this disorder is expectant.

Drug-Induced Lymphadenopathy

Although phenytoin is the most well-known cause of drug-induced lymphadenopathy, pyrimethamine, allopurinol, and phenylbutazone have also been implicated.[39] Typically, the adenopathy resolves when drug therapy is discontinued; however, long-term use of phenytoin has been reported to progress to a premalignant pseudolymphomatous state.

Sarcoidosis

The etiology of sarcoidosis is unknown, but clusters of cases tend to suggest an infectious or toxic origin. It is found most commonly in the second decade of life, and men and women are affected equally. Patients typically have lymph node enlargement, fatigue, and weight loss. Depending on the sites of involvement, there may also be cough, dyspnea, hoarseness, bone and joint pain, visual symptoms, headaches, fever, and skin rash. Abnormalities on chest radiography help suggest the diagnosis, which is confirmed by finding noncaseating granulomas on biopsy of involved tissue. Management is expectant, although corticosteroids may be helpful in acute settings.

Benign Neoplasms

Lipomas

Lipomas are benign encapsulated fatty tumors found in subcutaneous tissue. In general, they rarely occur in the head and neck. The usual management is surgical excision.

Thyroid Adenomas

A thyroid adenoma presents as an isolated mass that is palpable within the thyroid gland. On ultrasound, an adenoma appears as a solid mass in contrast to a thyroid cyst. On thyroid scanning, an adenoma appears as a cold nodule; however, some adenomas take up radionucleotide and show function, although not as much as that seen with typical hyperfunctioning nodules. Thyroid adenomas usually require excision to differentiate them from thyroid carcinomas.

Neurofibromas

Neurofibromas are circumscribed tumors that arise from small cutaneous nerves and are composed of Schwann cells, nerve fibers, and fibroblasts. They may be solitary or more rarely occur as multiple neurofibromas (e.g., in von Recklinghausen's disease). Management is excision, taking care not to injure nearby anatomic structures.

Pleomorphic Adenomas

Pleomorphic adenomas are salivary gland tumors that typically arise in the lateral portion of the parotid gland. They present as slow-growing painless masses that show no evidence of nerve or skin involvement. A superficial parotidectomy is necessary for surgical excision.

Malignant Neoplasms

Lymphomas

Lymphomas are the most common neck malignancy in large pediatric series.[1,40] They may be divided into two histologic categories, Hodgkin's and non-Hodgkin's, which have different clinical courses and prognoses.

Rye classified Hodgkin's disease into four histologic types: nodular sclerosing, mixed cellularity, lymphocyte predominant, and lymphocyte depleted. Males of any age are more commonly afflicted with Hodgkin's disease than females, although the incidence is nearly equal during the teenage years.[41] Hodgkin's disease often presents as an asymptomatic cervical or supraclavicular mass (Fig. 198-15). Fever is commonly associated with cough, night sweats, and weight loss. After confirmation of cell type by biopsy, management consists of chemotherapy or radiotherapy, depending on the histologic findings and staging.

Non-Hodgkin's lymphoma is more likely to be disseminated and extranodal. Histologic types include lymphoblastic, large cell, and undifferentiated. The liver, lung, and bone marrow are the most common sites of extralymphatic involvement. In the neck, non-Hodgkin's lymphoma is less common than Hodgkin's disease.[42] Weight

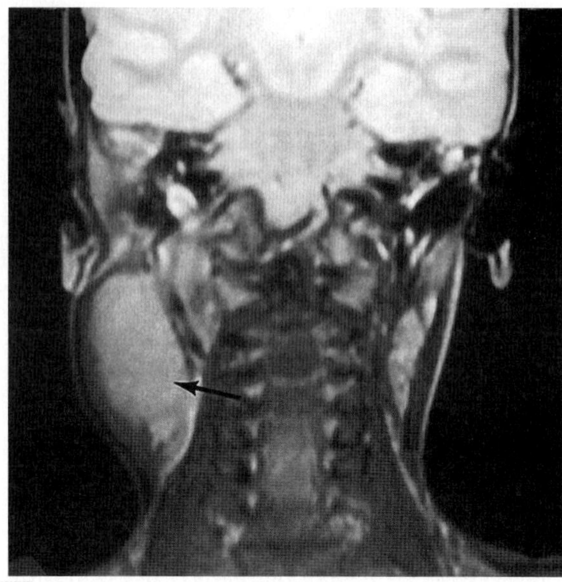

Figure 198-15. Magnetic resonance imaging of the neck shows Hodgkin's disease presenting in the posterior cervical region *(arrow)*.

loss, night sweats, and fever are common, especially when disease is more disseminated. Chemotherapy is the mainstay of management of non-Hodgkin's lymphoma.

Rhabdomyosarcomas

Soft tissue sarcomas comprise a small percentage of all childhood malignancies. Rhabdomyosarcoma is the most common soft tissue sarcoma; because it occurs most commonly in the head and neck, it comprises a significant percentage of malignant neck masses in series of pediatric patients.[43] The peak incidence of rhabdomyosarcoma occurs at 2 to 5 years, with another peak between 15 and 19 years of age.[44] White children are affected more often than children of other races, and there is a slight male predominance.[44] Embryonal rhabdomyosarcoma is the most common cell type, followed by alveolar and pleomorphic.[45]

Predominant sites of rhabdomyosarcoma in the head and neck include the orbit, nasopharynx, paranasal sinuses, ears, and oral cavity. Primary involvement of the neck occurred in 89% of cases in one series.[46] Metastatic disease from one area of the head to the neck is rare.[47]

Management of rhabdomyosarcoma includes a combination of surgery, radiotherapy, and chemotherapy. The role of surgery, biopsy, debulking, or radical excision depends on the site, extent, and presence of recurrence. Radiotherapy to the primary site is given at 5000 to 6000 cGy in children older than 3 years of age and lesser doses in younger children. Two thirds of patients experience long-term survival or cure.[43,9]

Thyroid Carcinoma

Thyroid carcinoma is uncommon in the pediatric age group but has been associated with exposure to low-dose ionizing radiation.[48] Female children are more commonly affected but less so than female adults. The usual histology is papillary or mixed papillary-follicular. Involved patients have a solitary mass in the anterior neck. More worrisome signs include rapid growth of the mass, hoarseness, dysphagia, and fixation of the mass to the surrounding structures. Metastases, when present, are found in regional lymph nodes and the lungs or bones. Ultrasound or thyroid scanning is helpful in diagnosis, although frozen section at the time of surgical excision is definitive. Because almost all thyroid carcinoma in children is papillary, management should be subtotal or total thyroidectomy with neck dissection if there is nodal involvement. Thyroid suppression is often used to prevent recurrence, and radioactive iodine helps eliminate unresectable tumor.

Salivary Gland Malignancies

Mucoepidermoid and acinic cell carcinomas of the salivary glands account for approximately 60% of malignant epithelial neoplasms in children.[49] With mucoepidermoid carcinoma, local invasiveness, regional metastasis, and prognosis depend on histologic differentiation; the behavior of acinic cell carcinoma does not correlate with histology. Mucoepidermoid and acinic cell carcinomas present as solitary firm masses that grow painlessly, usually in the parotid gland. Both tumors tend to be low grade and are seldom fatal.[49] Depending on which gland is involved, initial management is by superficial parotidectomy or submandibular gland excision. The use of adjuvant therapy including neck dissection or radiotherapy depends on cell type and tumor growth characteristics.

Nasopharyngeal Carcinoma

Nasopharyngeal carcinoma may present with a mass in the neck associated with a nasopharyngeal mass, unilateral otitis media, rhinorrhea, and nasal obstruction. In advanced cases, there may be one or more cranial nerve palsies. There is an increased incidence of nasopharyngeal carcinoma in black and Asian teenagers.[50,51] Titers of EBV types 2 and 3 have been elevated in patients with nasopharyngeal carcinoma.[6] Although the diagnosis is confirmed by biopsy, CT and MRI may help determine the extent of tumor involvement. Bone or liver metastasis may be identified with a bone scan or CT of the abdomen. Management depends on clinical staging and includes radiotherapy with or without chemotherapy.

Neuroblastomas

Neuroblastomas are malignant neoplasms that originate from primitive neuroblasts and neural crest cells. Only 2% to 4% of neuroblastomas originate in the neck.[52] In the neck, these masses may be associated with an ipsilateral Homer's syndrome.[53] Because systemic involvement is common, evaluation of the patient should include MRI and CT of the neck, chest, and abdomen, looking for metastatic spread. Elevated urinary VMA found on 24-hour collection strongly suggests neuroblastoma. Management depends on the extent of involvement and may include surgical excision, radiotherapy, and chemotherapy.

Summary

A neck mass may provide a diagnostic challenge to the clinician and a source of anxiety to the parents. Systematic evaluation, paying particular attention to important details in the history and physical examination, can narrow the differential diagnosis and allow selection of appropriate radiologic and laboratory studies when indicated. In children, congenital and inflammatory masses are most common, but malignancy should be considered, especially if the mass continues to grow after appropriate therapy.

SUGGESTED READINGS

Brodsky L, Belles W, Brody A, et al. Needle aspiration of neck abscesses in children. *Clin Pediatr (Phila)*. 1992;31:71.

Brook I. Aerobic and anaerobic bacteriology of cervical adenitis in children. *Clin Pediatr (Phila)*. 1980;19:693.

Civantos FJ, Holinger LD. Laryngoceles and saccular cysts in infants and children. *Arch Otolaryngol Head Neck Surg*. 1992;118:296.

Cunningham MJ, Myers EN, Bluestone CD. Malignant tumors of the head and neck in children: a twenty-year review. *Int J Pediatr Otorhinolaryngol*. 1987;13:279.

Edgerton MT. The treatment of hemangiomas: with special reference to the role of steroid therapy. *Ann Surg*. 1976;183:517.

Garfinkle TJ, Handler SD. Hemangiomas of the head and neck in children: a guide to management. *J Otolaryngol*. 1980;9:5.

Handler SD, Raney RB. Management of neoplasms of the head and neck in children. I. Benign tumors. *Head Neck Surg*. 1981;3:395.

Luna MA, Batsakis JG, El-Naggar AK. Pathology consultation: salivary gland tumors in children. *Ann Otol Rhinol Laryngol.* 1991;100:869.

Ossowski K, Chun RH, Suskind D, et al. Increased Isolation of methicillin-resistant *Staphylococcus aureus* in pediatric head and neck abscesses. *Arch Otolaryngol Head Neck Surg.* 2006;132:1176.

Raney RB, Handler SD. Management of neoplasms of the head and neck in children. II. Malignant tumors. *Head Neck.* 1981;3:500.

Torsiglieri AJ Jr, Tom LW, Ross AJ 3rd, et al. Pediatric neck masses: guidelines for evaluation. *Int J Pediatr Otorhinolaryngol.* 1988;16:199.

For complete list of references log onto www.expertconsult.com.

CHAPTER ONE HUNDRED AND NINETY-NINE

Vascular Anomalies of the Head and Neck

Jonathan A. Perkins

Eunice Y. Chen

Key Points

- The most common types of head and neck vascular tumors are hemangioma of infancy (HOI), whereas the most common head and neck vascular malformations are lymphatic malformations.
- HOIs are absent at birth, occur in infancy, proliferate up to the age of 9 to 10 months, and variably involute or shrink over years.
- HOIs and lymphatic malformations each have unique endothelium that distinguishes them from other types of vascular tumors and malformations.
- Periocular hemangiomas of infancy can cause deprivation amblyopia and astigmatic amblyopia.
- Superficial HOIs and other red, cutaneous vascular lesions can be treated with a pulsed dye laser.
- Surgical excision of focal hemangiomas can be done to both prevent complications and improve treatment outcomes.
- Lymphatic malformations are classified by stage and radiographic appearance as macrocystic or microcystic or a combination of both.
- Lymphatic malformations occur in utero and manifest at birth or in association with an infection or trauma later in life. Most malformations manifesting at birth or later in life are associated with a normal karyotype.
- Macrocystic lymphatic malformations can resolve spontaneously or be treated with either surgery or sclerotherapy. Microcystic suprahyoid lymphatic malformations are difficult to treat with any modality and frequently cause macroglossia.
- Venous malformations are associated with tyrosine-kinase type 2 receptor dysfunction, which causes abnormal venous structure. Histologically, venous malformations are a combination of both blood vasculature as well as lymphatic vasculature.
- Kasabach-Merritt phenomenon is most commonly associated with the vascular tumors kaposiform hemangioendothelioma and tufted angioma.
- Arteriovenous malformations are high-flow venous malformations that occur in any area of the head and neck and frequently require a combination of embolization and surgical therapy for treatment. Medical therapy is ineffective.

Vascular anomalies encompass vascular tumors and malformations and involve the head and neck 70% to 80% of the time. Clinical and radiographic findings, and occasionally histologic evidence, are used to distinguish among various vascular anomaly subtypes. A vascular anomaly classification system has been developed based on these factors[1,2] (Table 199-1). Hemangiomas of infancy (HOIs) were the first vascular lesions to be distinguished from other vascular anomalies, based on their natural history.[3] HOIs, unlike other vascular anomalies, are absent at birth, appear during infancy, grow rapidly within the first year of life, and then undergo a variable period of involution. Numerous recent discoveries have further solidified the distinction between vascular tumors and vascular malformations.[4-6]

Vascular tumors usually are benign, have neoplastic characteristics, and represent disordered angiogenesis.[4] Radiographically these tumors can be characterized by describing lesion size, blood flow, and location.[7,8] Certain clinical conditions, such as Kasabach-Merritt phenomenon and PHACES syndrome (*p*osterior fossa abnormalities, *h*emangiomas, *a*rterial anomalies, *c*ardiac anomalies, *e*ye abnormalities, *s*ternal or abdominal clefting), are associated with vascular tumors and not vascular malformations.[9-11] Vascular malformations often contain all vessel types—arterial, venous, and lymphatic—and seem to represent disordered vasculogenesis. Most vascular malformations are present at birth and demonstrate growth parallel to the child's growth. These lesions have a distinct radiographic appearance in their location, size, and blood flow—in particular, that through the lesion. Additionally, certain types of vascular malformations are characterized on the basis of the radiologic architecture of the lesion. This characterization has been most useful in identifying lymphatic malformations. These malformations also are associated with either local tissue or bony overgrowth (Fig. 199-1). Since the original distinction of hemangiomas from other types of vascular tumors and malformations, molecular characteristics as well as radiographic features of individual vascular anomaly subtypes have allowed further distinction between various types of vascular anomalies. This chapter outlines these distinctions and explains how these distinctions have led to treatment improvements, potentially leading to better clinical outcomes.

A genetic and molecular basis for some vascular anomalies is being investigated.[12-14] The most apparent link between genetic defect and disease is seen in inherited venous malformations, in which a mutation in the protein receptor for tyrosine kinase (Tie2), which normally allows endothelial–smooth muscle communication essential for venous morphogenesis.[15] Defects in the smooth muscle layer of vessels with venous malformations result from this mutation. Similarly, vascular malformations in hereditary hemorrhagic telangiectasia types 1 to 3 are associated with gene mutations that adversely affect endothelial function.[16] Familial HOIs are linked to defects in the fifth chromosome.[17] Sporadic HOI endothelium is clonal.[18,19] Glomangiomas have defective "glomulin" function, distinguishing them from other venous malformations.[20] Ateriovenous malformations occurring with atypical capillary malformations have been linked to a gene *RASA1*.[21] Hypertrophy of tissues near vascular malformations has been linked in certain syndromes to a mutation in the *PTEN* tumor suppressor gene.[22,23] This information creates a basis for understanding the mechanisms behind the pathogenesis of vascular anomalies.

Table 199-1

Vascular Anomaly Classification*

Vascular Malformation	Vascular Tumor
Single-Vessel Type	Hemangioma
Capillary	Hemangioma of infancy
Venous	Congenital hemangioma
Lymphatic	Rapidly involuting congenital hemangioma (RICH)
Combined/Complex	Noninvoluting congenital hemangioma (NICH)
Malformations	Lobular hemangioma (pyogenic granuloma)
Arteriovenous	Vascular Neoplasm
Lymphaticovenous	Kaposiform hemangioendothelioma
Capillary-venous	Angiosarcoma
Capillary-lymphaticovenous	Hemangiopericytoma
Capillary-arteriovenous	Miscellaneous
	Tufted angioma

*Binary classification system adopted by the International Society for the Study of Vascular Anomalies (ISSVA) in 1996.

Vascular Tumors

Hemangiomas of Infancy

HOIs are absent at birth and appear in infancy; they proliferate for 6 to 9 months and then involute partially or completely over several years[24-26] (Fig. 199-2). Vascular lesions not following this pattern should be considered for alternative diagnoses.[6] In addition to clinical diagnosis, HOI diagnosis can be further confirmed through molecular staining and imaging.[27,28] HOI endothelium has several unique surface markers detected by immunohistochemistry. The first marker for HOI described was glucose transporter-1 (GLUT-1); others have since been described. GLUT-1 detection separates HOIs from other vascular anomalies and congenital hemangioma.[28] Improvements in image acquisition with both computed tomography (CT) scanning and magnetic resonance imaging (MRI) allow differentiation between HOIs and other vascular anomalies[8,29,30] (Fig. 199-3).

Clinical Presentation

At birth, HOI can be completely absent or may be present as a slight redness or pallor in the area in which a HOI subsequently appears.[24] In the first several months of life, HOIs grow rapidly and can involve any area of the head and neck. Often multiple hemangiomas are present in areas outside the head and neck. Two thirds of HOIs occur in girls. HOIs are more prevalent in premature infants and infants born to mothers of advanced maternal age, with a history of chorionic villus sampling. Terminology to describe types of HOIs and their appearances and locations[31] are illustrated in Figure 199-4. Segmental HOIs usually are superficial, variably involve cutaneous dermatomes, and have more associated morbidity than focal HOIs. These lesions are thought to occur in embryologic prominences that are related to neural crest cells, which influence vascular patterning.[32] In the head and neck, focal HOIs occur in identifiable patterns that are thought to be associated with lines of embryonic tissue fusion.[31,32] Building on the concept of embryonic fusion planes, several groups of investigators have observed that midface HOIs do not predictably involute.

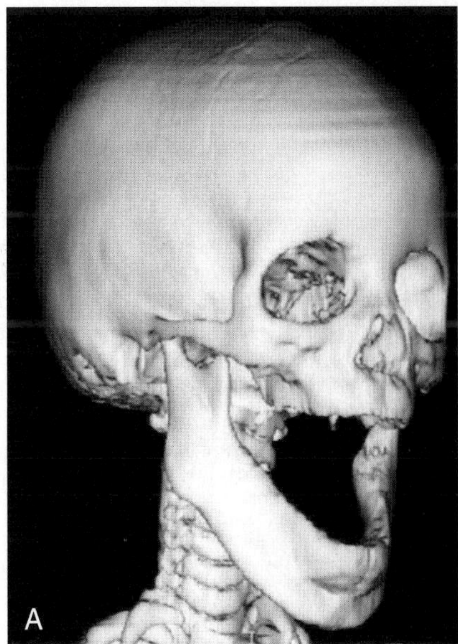

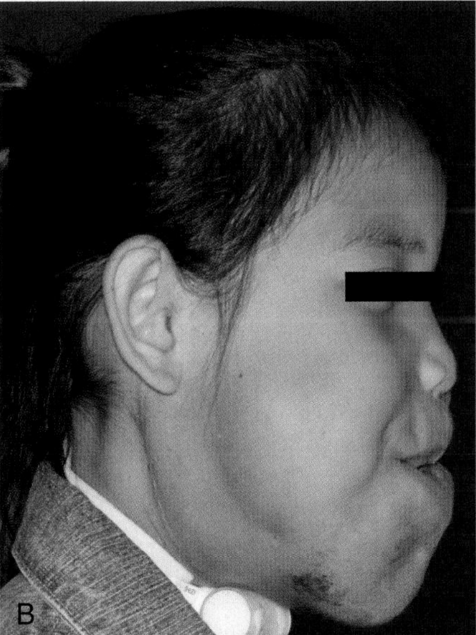

Figure 199-1. Mandibular overgrowth associated with lymphatic malformation. **A,** Three-dimensional computed tomography reconstruction in infancy. **B,** Clinical photograph of same patient at a later age.

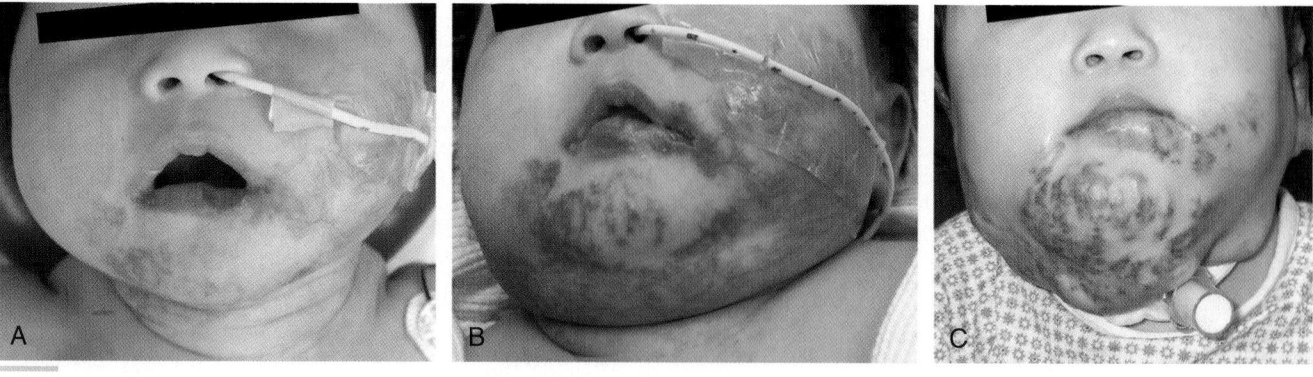

Figure 199-2. Segmental hemangioma appearance. **A,** Initial appearance in infancy. **B,** Late proliferative stage. **C,** Beginning involutional phase.

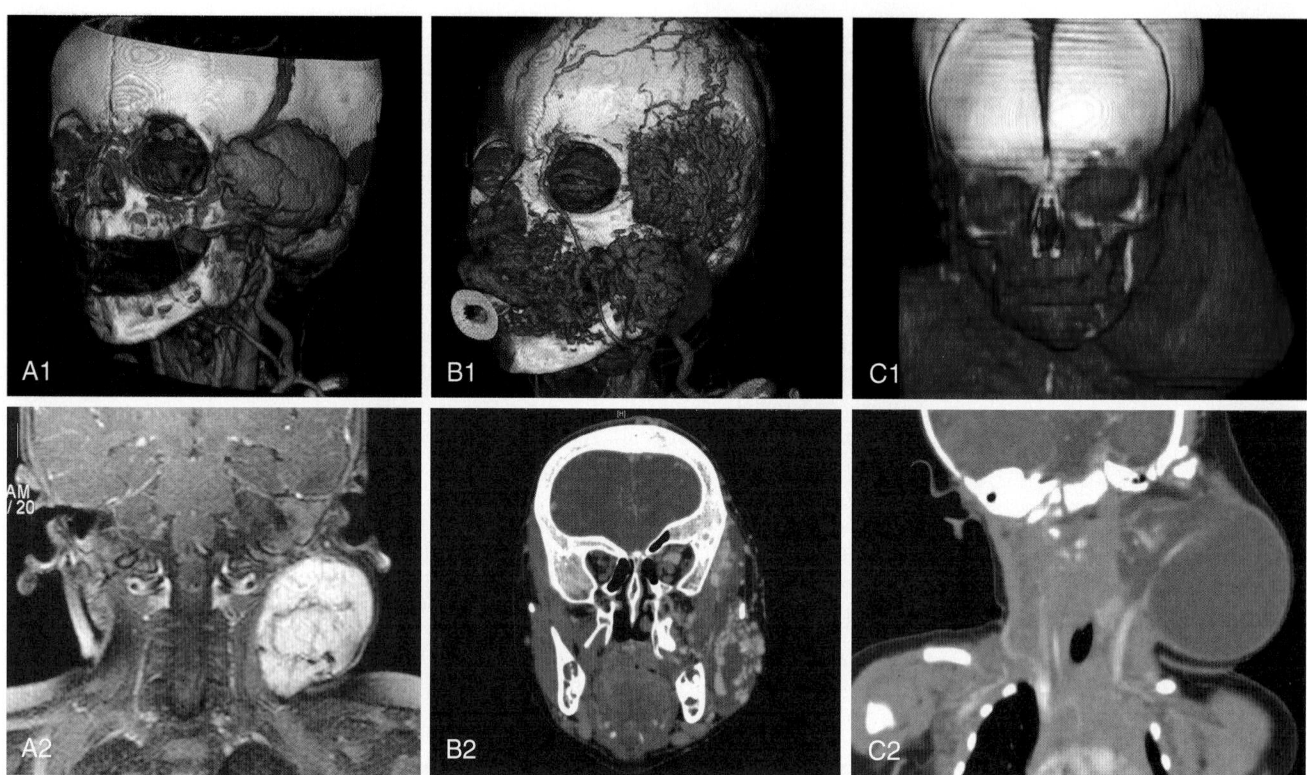

Figure 199-3. Vascular anomaly imaging. **A,** Three-dimensional CT angiography (A1) and coronal CT scan (A2) of deep hemangioma of infancy. **B,** Three-dimensional CT angiography and coronal CT scan of venous malformation. **C,** Three-dimensional CT angiography and coronal CT scan of lymphatic malformation.

PHACES Syndrome

An association between some HOIs and ventral clefting, congenital cardiac malformations, intracranial malformations, and ocular abnormalities has been described; the specific manifestations collectively make up the PHACES syndrome[11] (Fig. 199-5). Central nervous system symptoms include developmental delays, seizures, and congenital stroke. Patients suspected to have PHACES syndrome should undergo head imaging, ophthalmologic examination, and cardiac evaluation. Some clinicians recommend antiplatelet therapy for patients with abnormal cerebral vasculature, to prevent congenital stroke.[33,34] Further analysis of HOI biology is necessary to elucidate these associations.

Other Types of Vascular Tumors

Congenital Hemangioma

High-flow vascular tumors manifesting at birth that are histologically identical to HOIs except for positive GLUT-1 staining are called *congenital hemangiomas*.[73,74] There are two types of congenital hemangiomas—those that rapidly resolve over the span of a year and those that persist. Accordingly, they are named *rapidly involuting congenital hemangioma* (RICH) and *non-involuting congenital hemangioma* (NICH), respectively. These lesions often are difficult to distinguish from HOIs unless a careful history is taken and histologic analysis is performed. Often the diagnosis remains uncertain until the clinical behavior of a given lesion is observed (Fig. 199-6). Medical therapy is ineffective for congenital hemangiomas. Treatment for RICH usually is limited to observation, whereas NICH may require laser or surgical therapy.

Kaposiform Hemangioendothelioma and Tufted Angioma

Most nonhemangioma vascular tumors are benign. These tumors occur rarely in the head and neck. The two most common tumors are kaposiform hemangioendothelioma (KHE) and tufted angioma (TA). KHEs occur anywhere in the head and neck and have a significant lymphatic component in addition to blood vascular endothelium.[75] Clinically,

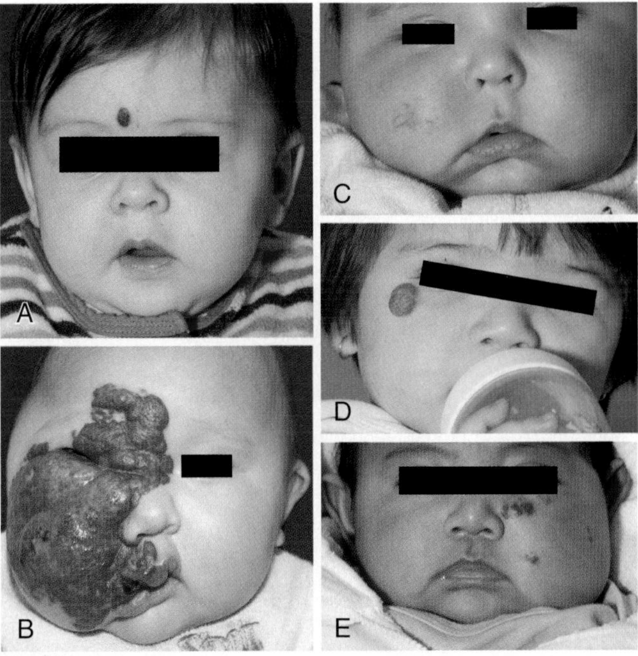

Figure 199-4. Hemangioma of infancy, types. **A,** Superficial focal hemangioma; forehead. **B,** Mixed segmental hemangioma; midface, lip, forehead. **C,** Deep focal hemangioma; malar region. **D,** Mixed focal hemangioma; malar lower eyelid. **E,** Mixed segmental hemangioma; cheek, malar region.

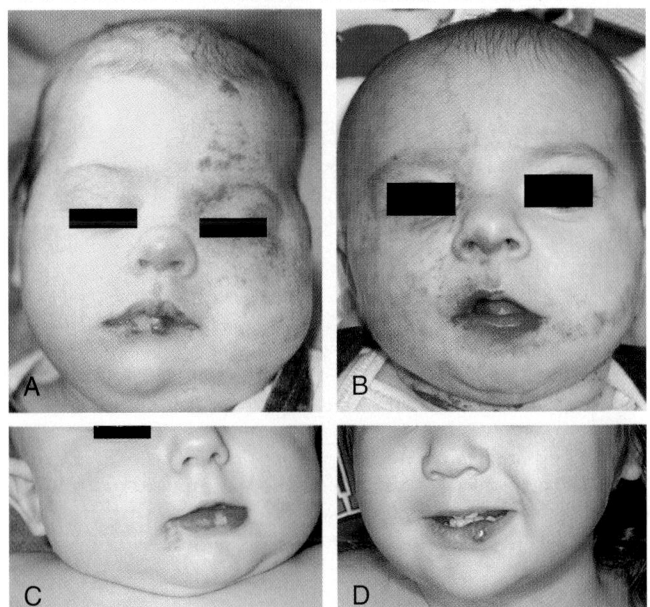

Figure 199-5. Clinical appearance in PHACES syndrome. **A,** Segmental hemangioma involving the lips, nose, left upper and lower face. **B,** Segmental hemangioma involving the lips, nose, left upper and bilateral lower face. **C,** Segmental lower lip hemangioma with sternal cleft. **D,** Focal lower lip hemangioma with sternal cleft.

KHEs appear as violaceous cutaneous nodules extending into deep tissues locally (Fig. 199-7). Their radiographic appearance is one of diffuse infiltrative vascular process (see Fig. 199-7). Careful assessment through imaging and diagnostic biopsy should guide KHE therapy. TAs are more localized and may or may not involve the skin. Treatment for both KHE and TA is centered on proper diagnosis, prevention of

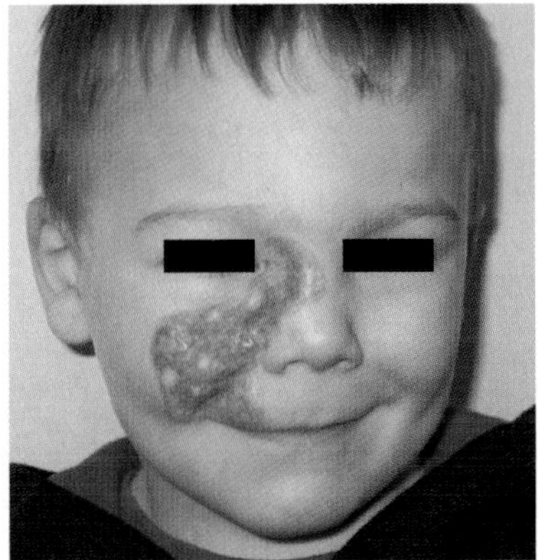

Figure 199-6. Appearance of noninvoluting congenital hemangioma.

complications, and tumor control. Diagnosis requires an incisional biopsy with possible immunohistochemical staining. Curative surgical resection is possible and advisable for some localized tumors, but for large lesions, surgery may not be curative. With extensive KHEs or TAs that are causing pain, loss of function, or significant disfigurement, antiangiogenic chemotherapy may be necessary. The natural history of these lesions in the head and neck often is unclear; therefore, treatment needs to be individualized.

Common Complications of Vascular Tumors

Because most vascular tumors are HOIs, which proliferate rapidly, complications occur most frequently with these lesions. HOI complications occur primarily from lesion-induced functional compromise and cutaneous ulceration. Breathing can become compromised and obstructed from airway HOI. HOI can cause biphasic stridor by narrowing the infant's subglottic airway[35] (Fig. 199-8). Obstruction of the visual axis by a proliferating HOI occurs with eyelid lesions, inducing deprivation amblyopia[36] (Fig. 199-9). Deformation of the eye from lesion compression or periocular tissue distortion before the age of 6 months induces astigmatic amblyopia.[37] Proliferating HOI located in places of repetitive skin trauma such as the lips and neck skinfolds can ulcerate, resulting in scarring. The reasons for ulceration are unclear, but when present, ulcerations begin as brown crusts, become painful, bleed, and require local wound care for healing. Extensive ulcerations of the hemangioma can become infected and result in tissue loss, further complicating healing and treatment[38] (Fig. 199-10). Ulceration involving the lip often makes oral feeding challenging because of pain and hemangioma-induced lip distortion. Large, deep head and neck HOIs involving the parapharyngeal and scalp regions often are associated with high-output cardiac failure, due to the increased blood flow in these vascular lesions.[39] The psychosocial consequences of HOI for the family and patient are important to consider in treatment planning.[40]

Unusual Conditions Associated with Vascular Tumors

Kasabach-Merritt Phenomenon

Kasabach-Merritt phenomenon is the occurrence of profound thrombocytopenia in association with vascular tumors. For unknown reasons, KHE and TA, not HOI, are the vascular tumors most frequently associated with Kasabach-Merritt phenomenon.[9,10,76] This occurs in infancy and requires extensive chemotherapy to reduce the risk of bleeding associated with thrombocytopenia. The mechanisms leading to thrombocytopenia are unknown. Before the capability of histologic distinction between the endothelium of KHE, TA, and HOI, many vascular tumors were called simply "hemangiomas," and Kasabach-Merritt phenomenon was associated erroneously with HOI. Newly described vascular entities, not classified as vascular tumors, also are associated with thrombocytopenia. The spectrum of this phenomenon as it relates to vascular anomalies is still being defined.[77]

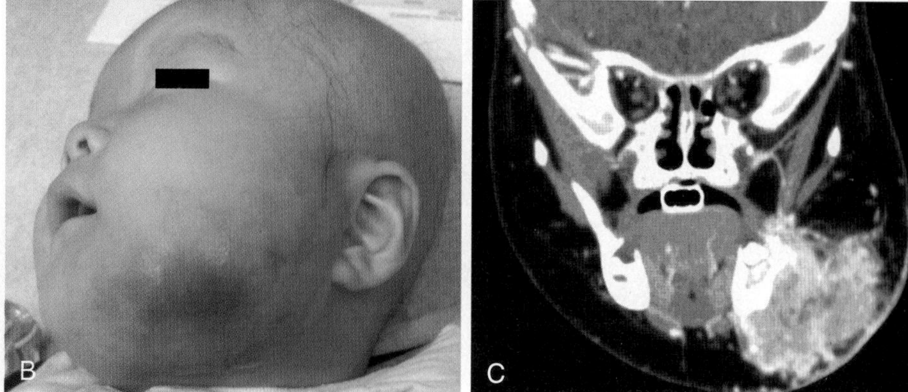

Figure 199-7. Kaposiform hemangioendothelioma, clinical and radiographic appearance. **A,** Cutaneous nodules. **B,** Deep lesion extending to the skin. **C,** Coronal computed tomography scan of lesion shown in **B.**

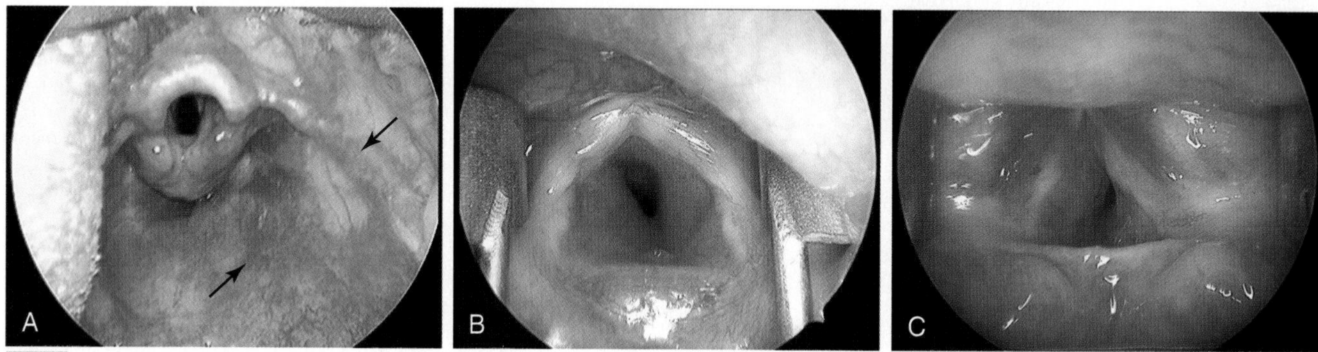

Figure 199-8. Endoscopic appearance of airway hemangioma of infancy. **A,** Diffuse hypopharyngeal mucosal involvement *(arrows)*. **B,** Unilateral posterior focal hemangioma; left subglottis (see also Fig. 199-16A and B). **C,** Circumferential, segmental hemangioma; subglottis (see also Fig. 199-16C and D).

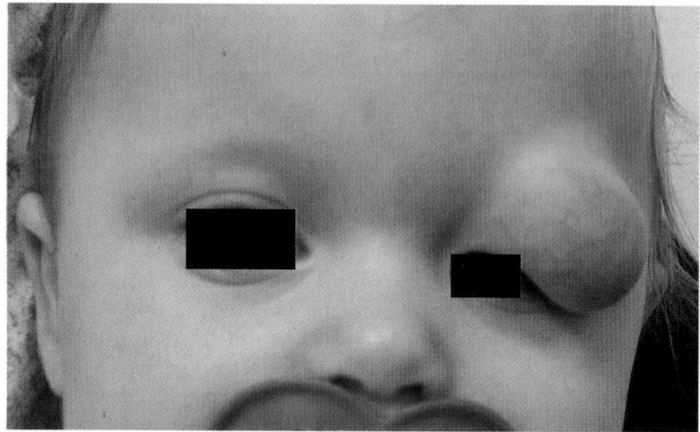

Figure 199-9. Deep focal hemangioma of infancy, upper eyelid, impinging visual axis.

Bone Resorption

Bone resorption can occur in association with KHE, resulting in localized osteopenia. The mechanisms for bone resorption are unknown. When bone loss occurs, chemotherapy has not been shown to change outcome.

Treatment Overview

Analysis and Treatment of Facial Hemangiomas

A complete discussion of all aspects of facial hemangioma treatment is beyond the scope of this chapter.[72] Some general concepts and principles useful in management decisions follow:

1. Societal attitudes and recognition of treatment possibilities for HOIs that involve the face are changing. Lesions that formerly were allowed to "involute," followed by delayed treatment of residual skin changes, are being managed more aggressively in early childhood (Fig. 199-11).

2. HOIs in certain areas of the face are prone to complications and noninvolution. This is especially true of midface lesions. Recognition of the varied natural history of facial HOI is essential to treatment planning and family counseling.

3. HOIs distort involved tissue by creating tissue excess and sometimes inducing adjacent bone and soft tissue hypertrophy (Fig. 199-12). This hypertrophy creates surgical and reconstructive challenges that differ from usual tissue deficits associated with facial tumor resection.

4. Large facial HOIs require more intensive monitoring and treatment planning than smaller lesions. Often the treatment of these lesions requires combined modalities and occurs in multiple stages over several years (Figs. 199-13 and 199-14).

5. An understanding of the medical, laser, and surgical treatment implications and options associated with HOI type and facial location is essential in planning treatment of these lesions.

Medical Therapy

Medical therapy for proliferating HOI is directed at stopping angiogenesis and decreasing peritumoral inflammation; in contrast, medical therapy for nonproliferating HOI is ineffective.[4,41,42] Although controversial, the mainstay of medical therapy has been systemic corticosteroid administration, which is antiangiogenic and anti-inflammatory.

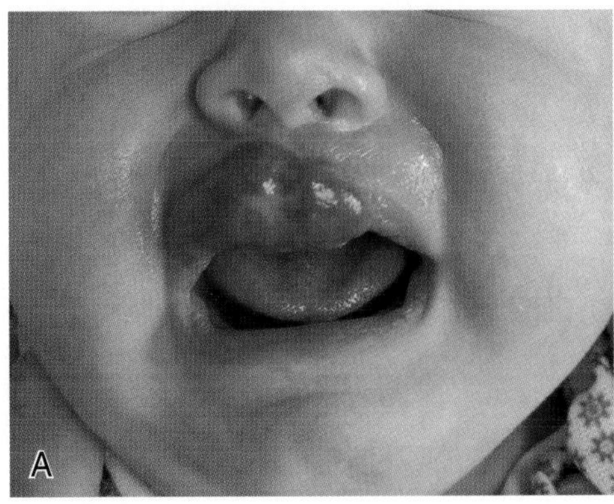

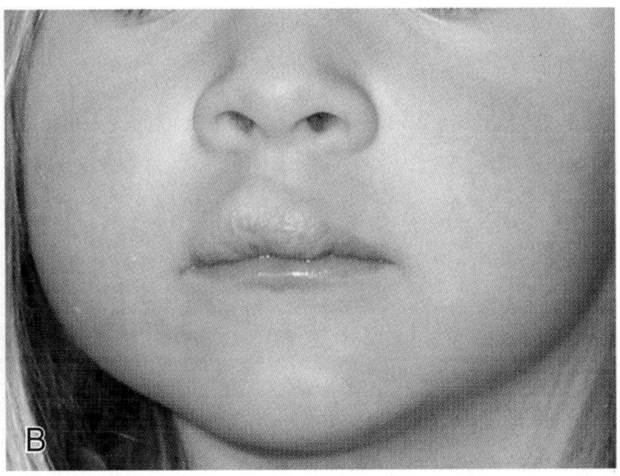

Figure 199-10. Hemangioma of infancy, lip. **A,** Ulcerated hemangioma during proliferation. **B,** Lip appearance after several pulsed dye laser treatments and ulcer healing.

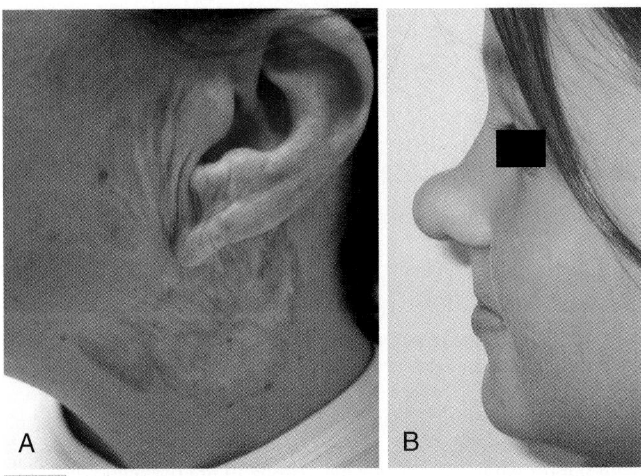

Figure 199-11. Persistent tissue changes from hemangioma of infancy. **A,** Fibrofatty skin changes from involuted mixed parotid hemangioma of infancy in adult. **B,** Enlargement of nasal tip from persistent deep focal hemangioma of infancy in adolescent.

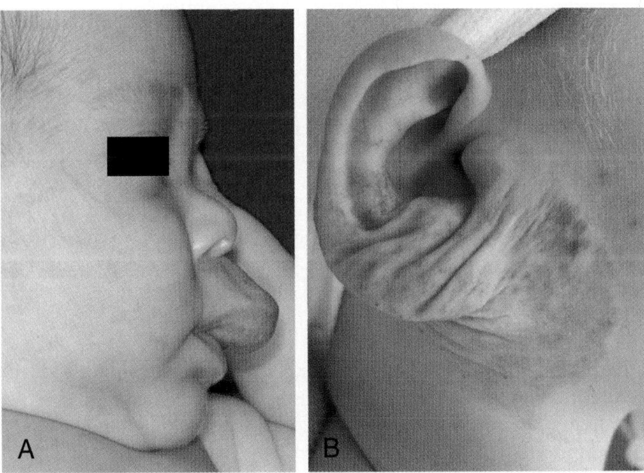

Figure 199-12. Tissue expansion and hypertrophy associated with hemangioma of infancy. **A,** Focal upper lip hemangioma: Lateral view demonstrating increased lip height and width. **B,** Mixed parotid-ear hemangioma: Lateral view demonstrating enlargement of lower third of the auricle.

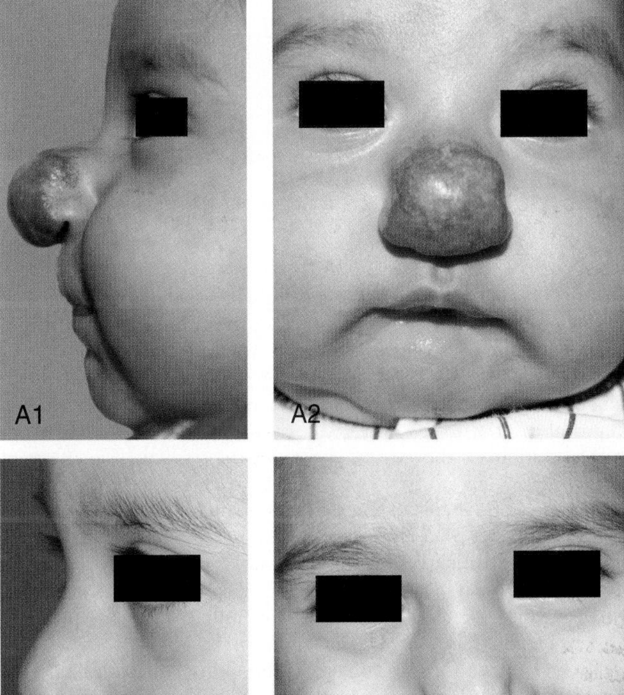

Figure 199-13. Combined laser and surgical treatment of large nasal tip mixed focal hemangioma of infancy. **A,** Before treatment. **B,** After residual deep hemangioma excision via external rhinoplasty approach.

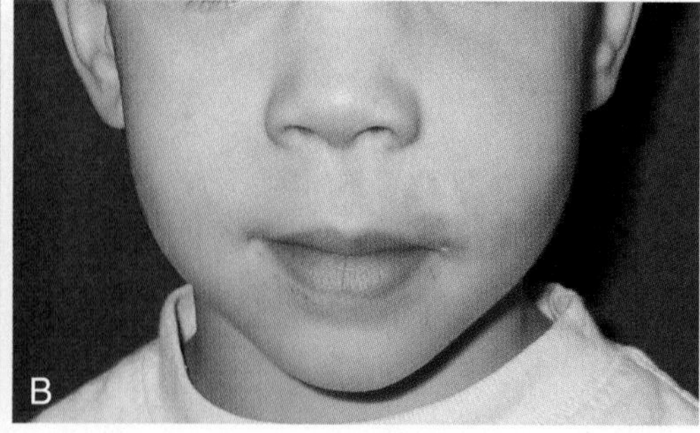

Figure 199-14. Combined laser and surgical treatment of large upper lip–cheek mixed segmental hemangioma of infancy. **A,** Before treatment. **B,** After laser treatment and deep hemangioma excision.

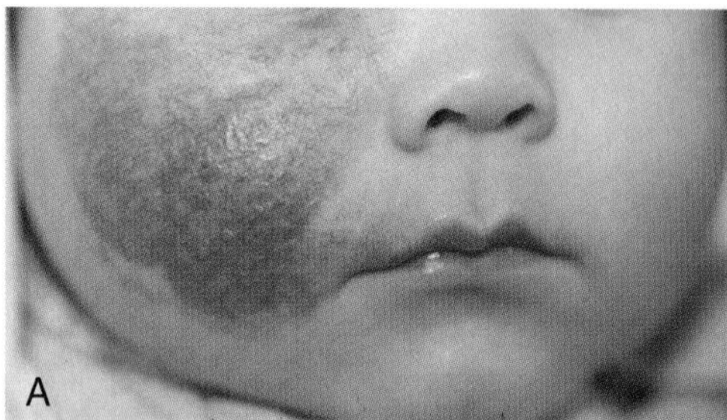

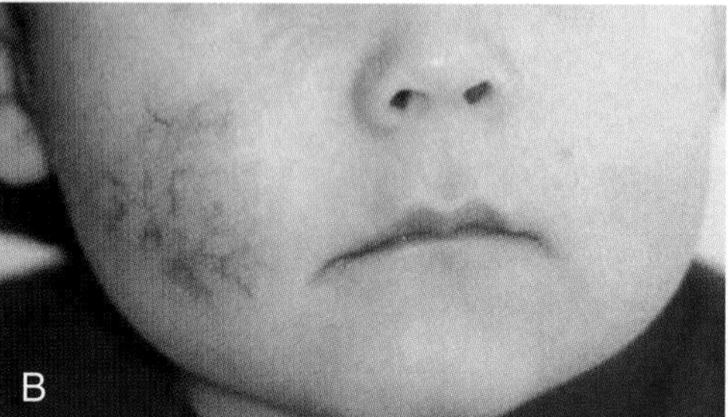

Figure 199-15. Laser treatment of superficial hemangioma. **A,** Pretreatment appearance. **B,** Appearance after three pulsed dye laser treatments.

The major indication for corticosteroid use depends on the presence of HOI complications or the attempt to prevent such complications, which occur more frequently with extensive segmental lesions.[26] For extensive proliferating HOI, prednisolone is given orally with doses ranging from 1 to 5 mg/kg/day in treatment courses that begin with an empirical burst at a high dose and then a slow 4- to 6-week taper off the medication. In theory, this minimizes the systemic side effects of steroid usage, but no long-term efficacy studies have been done.[43] Effectiveness of therapy is monitored throughout therapy; live vaccine administration is avoided, and blood pressure is monitored. Focal HOI of the head and neck can be injected with corticosteroids to localize drug delivery.[44,45] This practice is controversial and specialty specific, owing to the risk of blindness, training differences, and uncertain efficacy. Despite this, it is frequently done under general anesthesia for eyelid HOI while directly visualizing the retina.[36,46] In this location steroids are very effective in reducing HOI size, thereby decreasing the risk of HOI-induced visual impairment, but intralesional steroid injections can induce measurable adrenal suppression.[46] The role of topical medications to treat hemangiomas is being defined.[47] Other forms of antiangiogenic chemotherapy, such as interferon, have been used to treat HOIs.[48,49] The initial optimism for interferon as an effective agent for treatment of extensive HOI was subdued by the realization that before the age of 1 year, the central nervous system appears to be sensitive to this medication; neurologic complications such as spastic dysplegia were frequent.[50] For this reason, interferon is not used without serious consideration. However, it is still used in selected patients during times of rapid HOI proliferation. The proper dose of interferon is controversial, because previously reported complications were attributed to inappropriately high interferon dosing. More recently, vincristine has been investigated as a medication that can be used safely for treatment of extensive HOI.[51,52] Trials are under way to determine its efficacy in comparison with corticosteroids. Most recently, propranolol has been found to have an effect on reduction of HOI size. Further study is necessary to refine its use in the treatment of HOI.[78]

Laser Therapy

Superficial HOIs are red; the pulsed dye laser with a cooling device can reduce and even remove this skin redness, while the epidermis overlying the HOI is preserved.[53,54] The pulsed dye laser does not reduce HOI volume. This device is advantageous because it spares the superficial epidermis and allows for treatment of cutaneous redness without scarring (Fig. 199-15). However, when this device is used in patients younger than 6 months of age, when the HOI is actively proliferating, it can induce epithelial disruption, ulceration, and scarring.[55] For this reason, most clinicians recommend waiting to use the pulsed dye laser until after the age of 6 months. Often, reducing HOI redness is the only therapy necessary, because the deep portion of the lesion resolves with involution.

Surgical Therapy

When HOIs cause functional compromise of vision or breathing and are unresponsive to medical therapy, surgical excision may be necessary to preserve function.[56-58] HOIs that partially involute may leave significantly abnormal fibrofatty skin changes, requiring surgical resection.[59] A variety of techniques for HOI removal and reconstruction have been described. In most cases, waiting until the HOI has stopped proliferating is advisable.[60,61] When the HOI is causing airway or visual compromise, surgery during proliferation may be necessary. HOI occurring on the face can be significantly disfiguring and may be best treated with surgical excision.[62] When this type of lesion is mixed, with a larger superficial component, staged treatment with pulsed dye laser induces skin and dermal thickening, allowing HOI excision with minimal skin loss and tension-free closure of the defect (see Fig. 199-13).[63]

Assessment and Treatment of Airway Hemangiomas

One of the conditions associated with HOI that warrant the direct involvement of the otolaryngologist is an airway hemangioma. HOIs can occur anywhere in the upper and lower airways.[35] Usually the lesion is asymptomatic, involving the superficial mucosa. When a parapharyngeal HOI is large and abuts the pharynx, extrinsic compression of the airway can occur, particularly during sleep. Symptoms of sleep-disturbed breathing may arise during HOI proliferation or inflammation. Laryngeal involvement with HOI frequently manifests during infancy in the proliferative phase in association with an upper respiratory infection, or later in life with recurrent croup.[64] This clinical

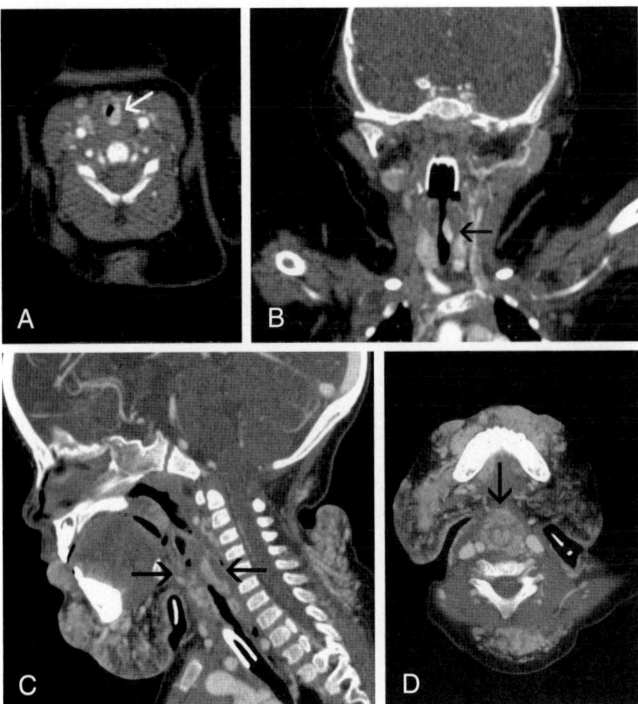

Figure 199-16. Computed tomography (CT) assessment of airway hemangioma of infancy. **A** and **B**, CT appearance of focal airway hemangioma of infancy. **A**, Axial scan; **B**, coronal scan. Compare endoscopic photograph of the same patient in Figure 199-8B. **C** and **D**, CT appearance of segmental airway hemangioma of infancy. **C**, Sagittal scan; **D**, axial scan. Compare endoscopic photograph of the same patient in Figure 199-8C.

feature is different from those of other types of hemangiomas, such as a lobular hemangioma (also known as a pyogenic granuloma).[65] Because the subglottic airway is the narrowest portion of the pediatric airway, HOIs in this area induce the greatest degree of respiratory embarrassment. Assessment of a stridorous infant must include the possibility of an airway hemangioma, especially if a cutaneous HOI is present. Segmental HOIs in the lower face are associated with airway lesions in at least 50% of cases.[66] Stridor in association with this type of HOI should prompt hospital admission, fiberoptic laryngoscopy, and even operative endoscopy if the initial evaluation is nondiagnostic. Advances in CT imaging techniques enable accurate assessment of HOI extent, to include evaluation of airway lesions (Fig. 199-16). Along with careful endoscopy, such imaging will reveal a pattern of HOI in the airway that can be described as similar to cutaneous HOI. In other words, there can be focal HOIs located only in the subglottis or segmental HOIs that are transglottic and extend into the soft tissues surrounding the airway.

Treatment of airway HOI is aimed at preventing the need for a tracheotomy. Initial treatment with high-dose oral corticosteroids usually improves the respiratory status within 24 hours. Empirical use of steroids in any patient with cutaneous HOI and new-onset stridor can be used as a diagnostic assessment. If rapid improvement occurs, then presence of an airway HOI is likely. If no improvement is obtained, some other problem exists. Airway protection, when necessary, can be accomplished with endotracheal intubation using a small uncuffed endotracheal tube. This option allows safe transfer to a facility capable of comprehensive HOI care and avoids using a tracheotomy for immediate airway protection. Chemotherapy has been used to treat these lesions, but safety of this management method is controversial.[67] Numerous methods of operative interventiont have been used successfully for many airway hemangiomas.[56,57,68-70] Several themes have emerged from analysis of airway hemangiomas over several decades. "Focal" lesions that involve one side of the subglottis are successfully treated with steroid injection, laser ablation, or surgical excision. Larger circumferential "segmental" lesions are more difficult to treat and may necessitate tracheotomy management. Frequently, these lesions respond temporarily to steroid treatment. Laser use for circumferential lesions is done only on one side of the larynx at a time, necessitating multiple treatments that can result in airway scarring and stenosis.[71] Surgical excision as initial treatment for extensive airway HOI is being done more routinely and successfully, but careful case selection is imperative.[56] In all airway hemangiomas, use of oral corticosteroids, intermittently and long-term, usually is necessary until the HOI stops proliferating. Analysis of treatment outcomes for airway hemangiomas is in its infancy, owing to ongoing changes in the current understanding of HOI biology.[35]

Vascular Malformations

Lymphatic Malformations

In our experience, lymphatic malformations are the most common vascular malformation affecting the head and neck in children.[79,80] Seventy-five percent of all lymphatic malformations occur in the head and neck. The etiology of lymphatic malformations remains unknown. Histologically, they consist of abnormally dilated lymphatic channels. Most lymphatic malformations are present at birth, although some appear later in childhood when they enlarge in response to infection or trauma. Unlike the detection of nuchal thickening and lucency in utero, the postnatal presence of these malformations is not associated with chromosomal abnormalities.[81-83] Up to 60% of all lymphatic malformations are detected by ultrasound examination in utero.[84] It has been suggested that the sporadic occurrence of lymphatic malformations is due to de novo somatic mutations.

Diagnostic Evaluation

Diagnosis and characterization of lymphatic malformations can be accomplished with either MRI or CT scanning.[7] On MRI, T1-weighted images show nonenhancing muscle signal intensity, whereas T2-weighted images demonstrate nonenhanced high signal intensity without any feeding or draining vessels. CT scans show nonenhancing fluid density areas.[8] Either modality is useful for classifying the lesion as macrocystic (cystic spaces measuring 2 cm or larger), microcystic, or mixed.[85] Additionally, the prominent venous component of microcystic suprahyoid malformations is demonstrated with CT. Prenatal ultrasound examination can be used not only to detect the malformation but also to determine if there is a possibility of airway compromise at birth.[86] If further information regarding the lesion is required, a prenatal MRI study also can be used. With this information, delivery procedures that protect the infant airway while maintaining maternal-fetal circulation can be planned.[87]

Clinical Assessment and Behavior of Lesions

Clinical understanding of lymphatic malformation behavior and treatment outcome has improved through better diagnostic imaging and head and neck staging systems[88] (Fig. 199-17). Macrocystic malformations in the posterior neck, without septations, that are infrahyoid can resolve without treatment.[89] In general, macrocystic malformations in any location in the neck can be obliterated with sclerotherapy or surgery.[90-92] By contrast, bilateral suprahyoid lesions, which tend to be microcystic or mixed, respond poorly to any treatment and are more often associated with complications.[92-94] These lesions frequently involve the oral and pharyngeal mucosa, with consequent recurrent tongue swelling, persistent tongue hypertrophy, mucosal bleeding, speech difficulty, and airway compromise. In general, lymphatic malformations lateral to the lateral canthal line tend to be macrocystic, whereas medial midfacial lesions tend to be more mixed. Midface involvement is uncommon and usually is completely microcystic[95,96] (Fig. 199-18). The larger and more extensive suprahyoid malformations have the most unpredictable clinical behavior and cause the most problematic dysfunction of the upper aerodigestive tract.

Associated Conditions

Lymphatic malformations are associated with unique problems that complicate treatment. Repeated episodes of malformation swelling

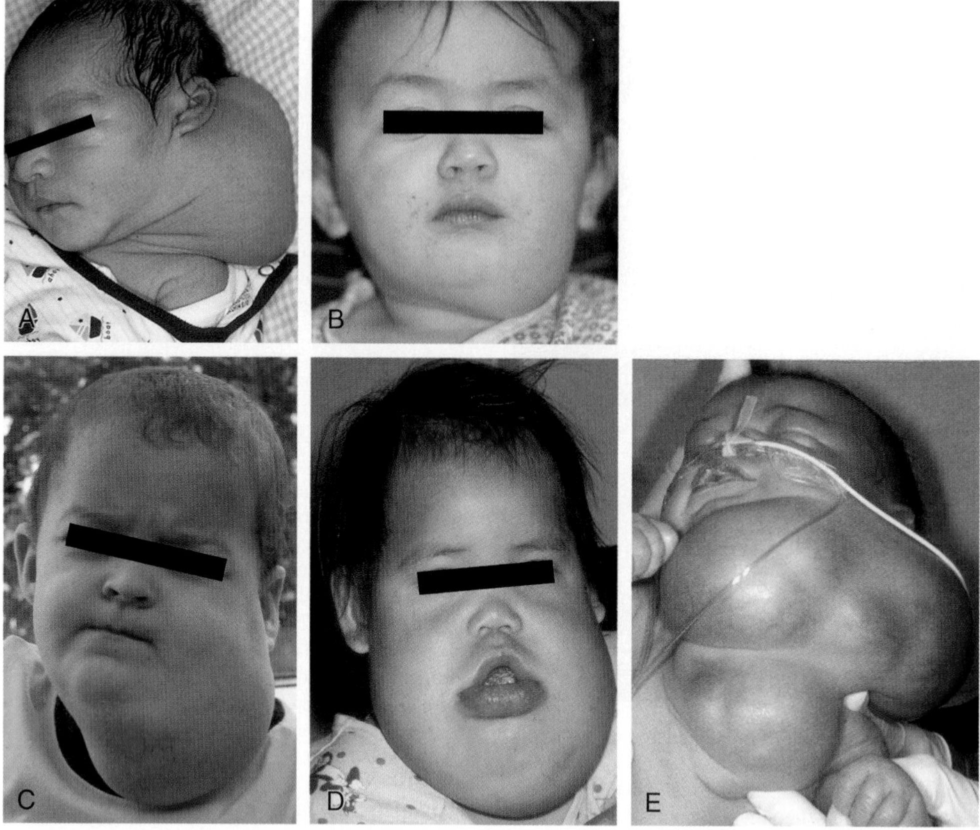

Figure 199-17. Head and neck lymphatic malformation stages. **A,** Stage 1, unilateral infrahyoid. **B,** Stage 2, unilateral suprahyoid. **C,** Stage 3, unilateral supra- and infrahyoid. **D,** Stage 4, bilateral suprahyoid. **E,** Stage 5, bilateral supra- and infrahyoid.

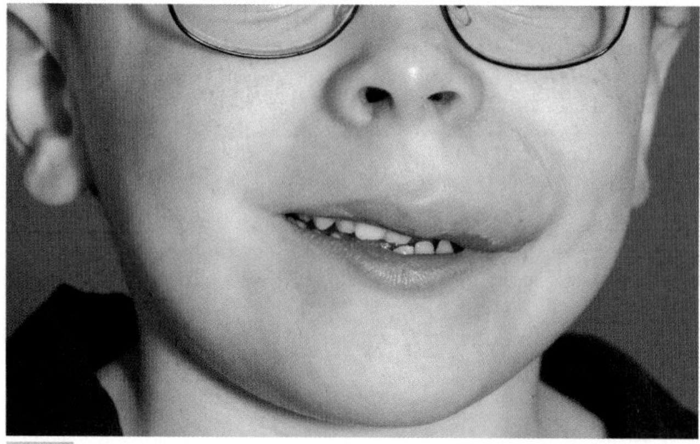

Figure 199-18. Microcystic lymphatic malformation involving left upper lip.

in association with presumed infection or trauma frequently occur, especially in suprahyoid microcystic or mixed lymphatic-venous malformations with oral mucosal involvement.[97] Mucosal inflammation can trigger intermittent aggravation of airway and feeding issues. These inflammatory-infectious episodes are treated effectively with appropriate broad-spectrum antibiotics with or without systemic corticosteroids.[80] Patients with transmural tongue involvement by malformation benefit significantly from this treatment both acutely as well as prophylactically. What triggers inflammation of lymphatic malformations is unknown, but in some cases recurrent or persistent inflammation may be related to immune dysfunction. Patients with large bilateral or microcystic lymphatic malformations can have significant lymphocytopenia involving T, B, and natural killer (NK) cell subsets.[98] This lymphocytopenia is not related to lymphocyte sequestration within the malformation, as was previously thought. Large bilateral or microcystic lesions involving the oral mucosa require more intensive treatment in lymphopenic patients than in patients without lymphocytopenia.[99]

Lymphatic malformations frequently involve and can distort the facial skeleton. This distortion is most evident in the mandible in association with large bilateral suprahyoid lesions[93] (Fig. 199-19; see also Fig. 199-1). The reasons for skeletal overgrowth are unknown. Early surgical excision of the soft tissue lymphatic malformation does not appear to change the rate or incidence of bony involvement. When the mandible is enlarged by malformation, mandibular reduction surgery may be indicated. In rare cases, large lymphatic malformations near the skull and skull base may be associated with bone resorption and more widely disseminated lymphatic growth, which can be fatal.[78] Bone loss also occurs with some lymphatic malformations. Gorham syndrome (disappearing bone disease) is the most striking manifestation of lymphatic vessels overtaking bony structures.[99a]

Treatment Options: Sclerotherapy versus Surgery

Favorably staged lymphatic malformations, such as unilocular macrocystic posterior lateral malformations, can be observed over time. If problems such as infection do not occur during observation, the lesion may regress spontaneously[89] (Fig. 199-20). A decision for intervention usually is triggered by concerns for airway, feeding, speech, infection, and appearance.

Sclerotherapy

Sclerotherapy for macrocystic (cysts larger than 2 cm in diameter) malformations is no longer new, but popularity for this intervention appears to be on the rise, even though it is infrequenly used according to some reports.[100,101] Sclerotherapy with all reported agents is usually ineffective for microcystic lesions.[102] Sclerotherapy involves percutaneous needle aspiration of macrocystic spaces under fluoroscopic guidance

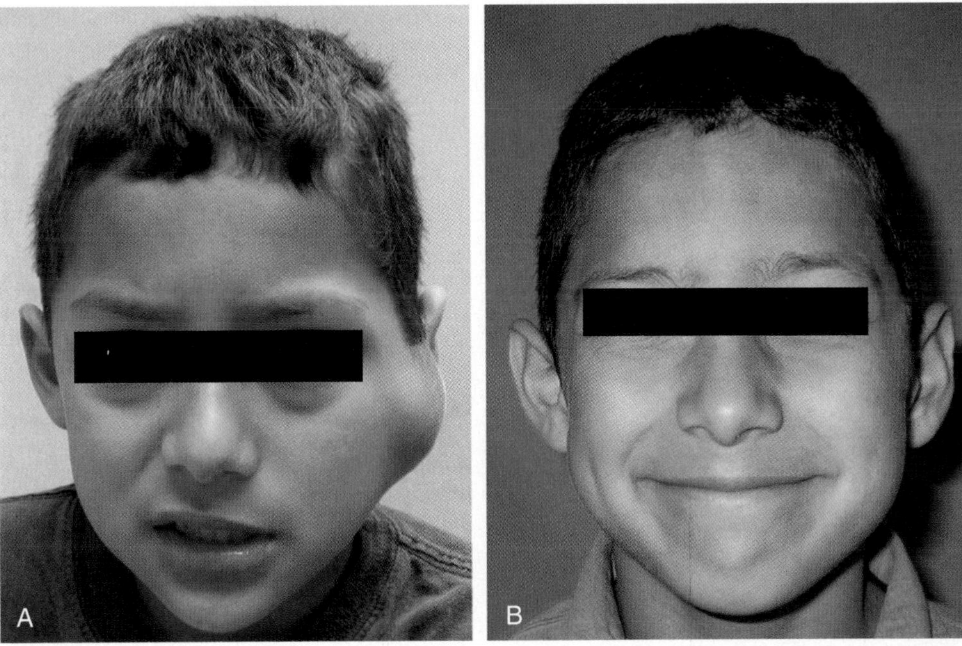

Figure 199-19. Facial asymmetry in parotid lymphatic malformation. **A,** Swollen lymphatic malformation before treatment. **B,** Persistent facial asymmetry after treatment; asymmetry involves both soft tissue and bone.

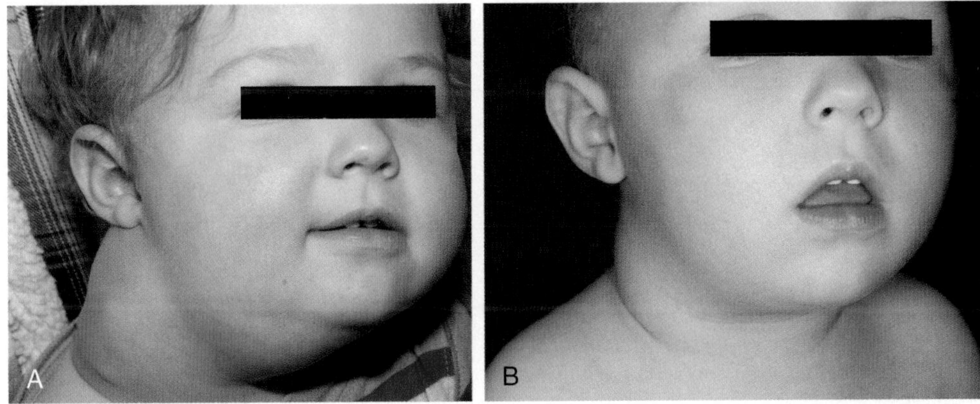

Figure 199-20. Spontaneous resolution of macrocystic posterior cervical lymphatic malformation. **A,** Initial appearance, before the age of 6 months. **B,** Complete resolution by the age of 1 year.

with subsequent injection of the sclerosing agent. Use of OK-432 (Picibanil, Chugai Pharmaceutical Company, Tokyo) as a sclerosant, because of its decreased toxicity and scarring risks, has led to increased interest in sclerotherapy. OK-432 is not commercially available in the United States, but published reports show promising results for macrocystic lesions after multiple treatments.[102,103] Similar efficacy for treatment of macrocystic lesions has been reported for doxycycline, bleomycin, ethanol, and sodium tetradecyl sulfate.[104,105] Major toxicity issues, including pulmonary fibrosis with bleomycin and permanent nerve injury with ethanol, are rare. Other rare complications include sepsis, shock, stroke, and seizures. Minor issues such as skin blistering and loss, fever, and erythema and pain at the injection site are more common.

Surgery

Surgical excision, the traditional treatment of choice for most types of lymphatic malformations, is still the most common treatment modality.[100] Excision of localized macrocystic lesions in the posteroinferior neck and parotid and submandibular regions generally has a high rate of complication-free surgical success.[80] However, in some reports, the complication rate, especially for large mixed suprahyoid lesions, is high.[93] Complications include cranial nerve or great vessel injury, tongue edema requiring tracheotomy, bleeding, and infection.

Surgical goals should be total excision with preservation of vital structures, when possible. Subtotal excision, not surprisingly, results in more postoperative persistent problems but may be necessary to preserve vital structures.[95] Lymphatic malformations are infiltrative and involve nerves, vessels, and muscles. It is common in large facial malformations to have facial nerve branches weave back and forth in the cyst walls and within the lesion, resulting in unusual nerve location and greater nerve length.[106] Intraoperative electromyographic nerve mapping can aid in these difficult dissections (Fig. 199-21). For bilateral suprahyoid lesions with mucosal involvement, waiting as long as possible before surgery and doing one side at a time (staged excision) may reduce the potential for permanent tongue enlargement. When the tongue becomes enlarged, surgical reduction may be indicated[107] (Fig. 199-22). Postoperative drainage of the surgical site is essential after resection, because significant lymphorrhea can occur.[108]

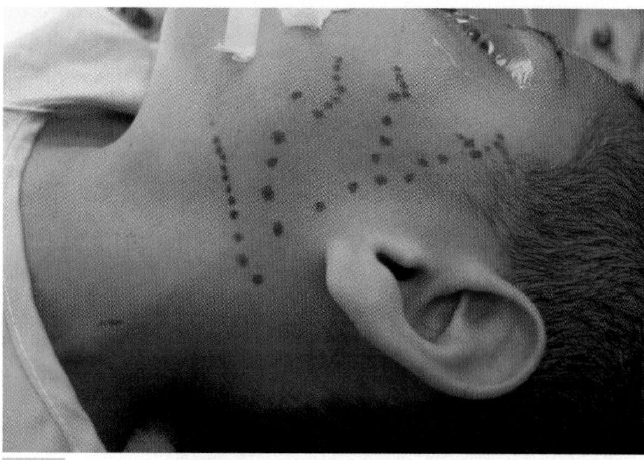

Figure 199-21. Preoperative facial nerve mapping before lymphatic malformation excision.

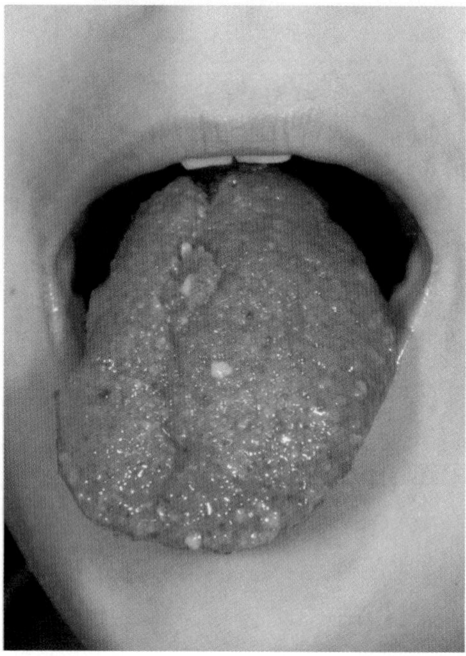

Figure 199-22. Microcystic lymphatic malformation, mucosa and deep tongue involvement.

Treatment Option Conclusions

New consensus views regarding treatment of lymphatic malformations appear to be emerging. The practice of waiting for the possibility of spontaneous resolution for unilocular or nearly unilocular lesions, especially if they are located in the posteroinferior neck, is becoming more common. Most vascular anomaly centers are treating macrocystic disease with either sclerotherapy or surgery. Systemic steroids, in addition to antibiotics, are used to treat severe acute inflammation and infection, although controlled studies are lacking and immune surveillance is necessary. Anecdotal evidence has led many clinicians to delay surgery, if necessary, as long as possible and to perform surgery for large suprahyoid lesions in stages to reduce complications (e.g., tongue edema). Little consensus exists regarding treatment to reduce mandibular and other facial overgrowth.

Venous Malformations

Venous malformations consist of tangled abnormal blood vessels filled with slow flow blood. Some of these lesions have been associated with a receptor tyrosine kinase (Tie2) dysfunction.[13] Other molecular mechanisms may be involved in the disordered vasculogenesis associated with these lesions.[109] These lesions frequently are present in muscle tissue, are compressible, enlarge with Valsalva maneuver or dependent positioning, and give a bluish hue under involved skin or mucosa[110] (Fig. 199-23). Occasionally, intracranial and skull base extension can occur, particularly with periorbital lesions.[111] Histologically, many of these lesions comprise blood and lymphatic vascular elements.[112] They usually are present at birth, slowly enlarge over time, and may become inflamed and painful during puberty and with trauma.[113] Diagnosis can be made clinically with radiographic confirmation. Duplex scanning shows slow blood flow, and lesions have a bright signal on T2-weighted sequences on MRI.[7] CT scans frequently demonstrate calcified phleboliths. Treatment consists of symptom management and malformation ablation or excision in selected lesions. Pain from enlargement is thought to be due to adjacent nerve irritation from the malformation and may be related to the intralesional consumptive coagulopathy present in some patients.[112,113] This coagulopathy can be detected through elevated D-dimers and low fibrinogen. Antiplatelet and anti-inflammatory agents can help control symptoms. In extreme situations, low-dose heparin may be necessary in conjunction with hematology consultation. Venous malformation ablation can be achieved with complete surgical excision if possible. Careful preoperative assessment is essential to detect any evidence of a subclinical coagulopathy. Combined therapy with sclerosis and surgery usually is necessary to minimize blood loss and morbidity.[110,114] When excessive intraoperative bleeding occurs, novel hemostatic measures have been used effectively.[115] For lesions that are amenable to sclerotherapy, intralesional sclerosants or laser can be utilized[116-118] (Fig. 199-24). Often, periodic treatments are necessary.

Arteriovenous Malformations

Arteriovenous malformations are high-flow vascular malformations that can manifest as enlarging masses throughout the head and neck, most frequently involving the cheek or auricle.[119] Some arteriovenous malformations are found with cutaneous capillary malformations and are associated with gene abnormalities.[21] Functionally, these congenital lesions arise from a nidus of blood vessels that have abnormal precapillary communication from arteries to veins. This creates the arteriographic diagnostic finding for arteriovenous malformations of "early venous filling." By contrast, arteriovenous fistulas are a solitary abnormal communication between arteries and veins that usually are acquired secondary to trauma. Diagnosis of arteriovenous malformations requires imaging with MR or CT angiography[29,120] (Fig. 199-25). Occasionally, interventional angiography also is necessary, but usually this can be done in conjunction with embolization, immediately before surgical treatment. The natural history of these malformations often is unclear, but four clinical stages—dormancy, expansion, destruction, and heart failure—have been described and correlated with treatment outcome.[119] In the dormancy stage, these malformations can be mistaken for other vascular anomalies. In some patients, enlargement and growth can occur during adolescence. Treatment of arteriovenous malformations includes nonintervention or intervention with a combination of preoperative embolization followed by surgical excision of the nidus.[121] Lesions contained within bone can be managed with embolization alone, but once the lesion involves adjacent soft tissue, surgery may be necessary.[122] These lesions recur commonly, so treatment decisions must be carefully planned.

Capillary Malformations

Skin capillaries that are persistently dilated form malformations commonly known as *port-wine stains.*[123] These capillary malformations frequently are seen in the mid- and upper face. In the upper face and eyelid region, they are associated with Sturge-Weber syndrome.[124] This condition is characterized by capillary malformations involving the eye, skin, and leptomeninges. Capillary malformations in the upper face warrant concomitant evaluation with brain MRI and ophthalmologic examination to rule out this syndrome. These lesions progressively darken and thicken throughout life and are associated with local tissue hypertrophy and hamartomatous nodule formation that may require

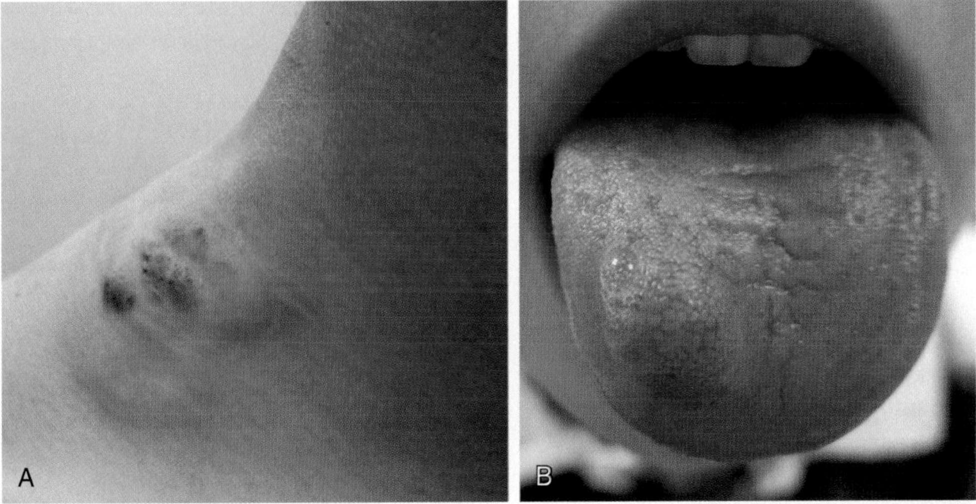

Figure 199-23. Venous malformation appearance. **A,** Skin. **B,** Tongue.

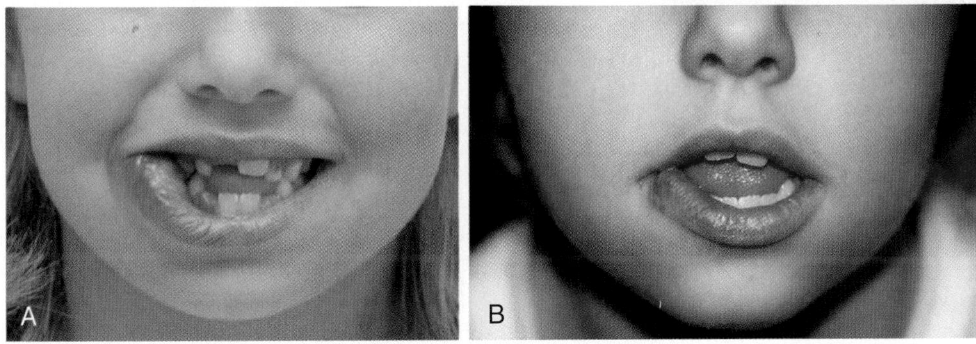

Figure 199-24. Venous malformation treatment with interstitial laser. **A,** Lip before treatment. **B,** Lip after two laser treatments.

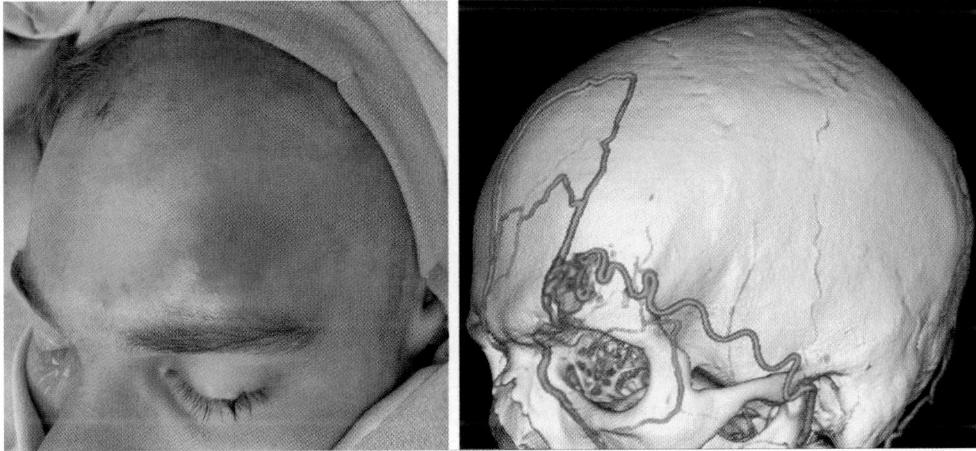

Figure 199-25. Computed tomography angiography and clinical appearance of quiescent arteriovenous malformation nidus, left brow.

treatment[125] (Fig. 199-26). The superficial component of these lesions can be managed with serial pulsed-dye laser treatments.[126] Some malformations are resistant to this therapy, and other laser modalities can be used.[127] No therapy is curative.

Summary

Current understanding of vascular anomalies is evolving with new advances in molecular, genetic, diagnostic, disease staging, and therapeutic outcomes research. As a field of clinical medicine, the management of these anomalies crosses traditional boundaries between medical and surgical disciplines. This overlap necessitates a multidisciplinary approach, in order to optimize patient care and treatment outcomes. It is anticipated that future diagnostic and treatment modalities will be more effective in predicting the clinical course and preventing complications of these common and benign yet problematic lesions.

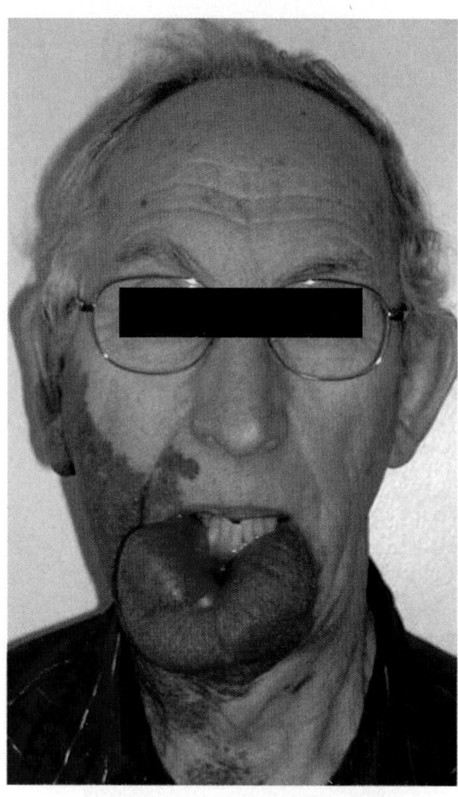

Figure 199-26. Capillary malformation of lower face and lip. The lip hypertrophy was related to the capillary malformation. *(Courtesy of Dr. J. Gruss.)*

SUGGESTED READINGS

Hemangioma of Infancy

Barlow CF, Priebe CJ, Mulliken JB, et al. Spastic diplegia as a complication of interferon alfa-2a treatment of hemangiomas of infancy. *J Pediatr.* 1998;132:527-530.

Bitar MA, Moukarbel RV, Zalzal GH. Management of congenital subglottic hemangioma: trends and success over the past 17 years. *Otolaryngol Head Neck Surg.* 2005;132:226-231.

Ceisler EJ, Santos L, Blei F. Periocular hemangiomas: what every physician should know. *Pediatr Dermatol.* 2004;21:1-9.

Greene AK, Rogers GF, Mulliken JB. Management of parotid hemangioma. *Plast Reconstr Surg.* 2005;116:676-677.

Metry DW, Haggstrom AN, Drolet BA, et al. A prospective study of PHACE syndrome in infantile hemangiomas: demographic features, clinical findings, and complications. *Am J Med Genet A.* 2006;140:975-986.

Mulliken JB, Glowacki J. Hemangiomas and vascular malformations in infants and children: a classification based on endothelial characteristics. *Plast Reconstr Surg.* 1982;69:412-422.

North PE, Waner M, Buckmiller L, et al. Vascular tumors of infancy and childhood: beyond capillary hemangioma. *Cardiovasc Pathol.* 2006;15:303-317.

For complete list of references log onto www.expertconsult.com.

North PE, Waner M, Mizeracki A, et al. A unique microvascular phenotype shared by juvenile hemangiomas and human placenta. *Arch Dermatol.* 2001;137:559-570.

Phung TL, Hochman M, Mihm MC. Current knowledge of the pathogenesis of infantile hemangiomas. *Arch Facial Plast Surg.* 2005;7:319-321.

Vijayasekaran S, White DR, Hartley BE, et al. Open excision of subglottic hemangiomas to avoid tracheostomy. *Arch Otolaryngol Head Neck Surg.* 2006;132:159-163.

Waner M, Buckmiller L, Suen J. Surgical management of hemangiomas of the head and neck. *Operative Tech Otolaryngol Head Neck Surg.* 2002; 13:77-84.

Waner M, North PE, Scherer KA, et al. The nonrandom distribution of facial hemangiomas. *Arch Dermatol.* 2003;139:869-875.

Weiss AH, Kelly JP. Reappraisal of astigmatism induced by periocular capillary hemangioma and treatment with intralesional corticosteroid injection. *Ophthalmology.* 2008;115:390-397.

Vascular Tumors

Enjolras O, Wassef M, Mazoyer E, et al. Infants with Kasabach-Merritt syndrome do not have "true" hemangiomas. *J Pediatr.* 1997;130:631-640.

North PE, Waner M, James CA, et al. Congenital nonprogressive hemangioma: a distinct clinicopathologic entity unlike infantile hemangioma. *Arch Dermatol.* 2001;137:1607-1620.

Vascular Malformations

Azuma H. Genetic and molecular pathogenesis of hereditary hemorrhagic telangiectasia. *J Med Invest.* 2000;47:81-90.

de Serres LM, Sie KC, Richardson MA. Lymphatic malformations of the head and neck. A proposal for staging. *Arch Otolaryngol Head Neck Surg.* 1995;121:577-582.

Forrester MB, Merz RD. Descriptive epidemiology of cystic hygroma: Hawaii, 1986 to 1999. *South Med J.* 2004;97:631-636.

Giguère CM, Bauman NM, Sato Y, et al. Treatment of lymphangiomas with OK-432 (Picibanil) sclerotherapy: a prospective multi-institutional trial. *Arch Otolaryngol Head Neck Surg.* 2002;128:1137-1144.

Kennedy TL, Whitaker M, Pellitteri P, et al. Cystic hygroma/lymphangioma: a rational approach to management. *Laryngoscope.* 2001;111:1929-1937.

Kohout MP, Hansen M, Pribaz JJ, et al. Arteriovenous malformations of the head and neck: natural history and management. *Plast Reconstr Surg.* 1998;102:643-654.

Perkins J, Maniglia C, Magit A, et al. Clinical and radiographic findings in children with spontaneous lymphatic malformation regression. *Otolaryngol Head Neck Surg.* 2008;138:772-777.

Persky MS, Yoo HJ, Berenstein A. Management of vascular malformations of the mandible and maxilla. *Laryngoscope.* 2003;113:1885-1892.

Raveh E, de Jong AL, Taylor GP, et al. Prognostic factors in the treatment of lymphatic malformations. *Arch Otolaryngol Head Neck Surg.* 1997;123:1061-1065.

Tempero RM, Hannibal M, Finn LS, et al. Lymphocytopenia in children with lymphatic malformation. *Arch Otolaryngol Head Neck Surg.* 2006;132: 93-97.

CHAPTER TWO HUNDRED

Pediatric Head and Neck Malignancies

Carol J. MacArthur

Richard J. H. Smith

Key Points

- Each year in the United States, cancer is diagnosed in 1 of every 7000 children 0 to 14 years of age.
- Although accidents are the leading cause of death in children, malignancies remain the most common cause of death from disease in the 1- to 14-year-old age group.
- Unlike adults, most childhood tumors are mesenchymal or neuroectodermal in origin.
- Nearly one third of pediatric malignancies are leukemias, and an additional 12% are lymphomas. Nonhematologic solid tumors account for the remaining 55%.
- Every child with suspected leukemia-lymphoma or neuroblastoma should have a workup to evaluate for gene translocations, antigen expression, and gene amplification. Critical to this histopathologic workup is the delivery of fresh tissue to the pathologist for proper handling.
- Pediatric head and neck cancer treatment is guided by the guidelines developed in accordance with collaborative, multimodality therapeutic protocols, such as the Intergroup Rhabdomyosarcoma Study Groups Committee (IRSC).
- Because of the high rate of metastatic disease in pediatric cancers, combined therapy usually is required (surgical biopsy or excision, chemotherapy, radiation therapy if needed for local control).
- With increasing numbers of long-term survivors of pediatric head and neck cancer, ongoing management of sequelae from treatment is essential, including attention to development of secondary malignancies 1 to 2 decades after treatment.

Each year in the United States, cancer is diagnosed in 1 of every 7000 children 0 to 14 years of age. In 1998, the diagnosis of cancer was given to 8700 children before their 15th birthday and to 3700 young adults between 15 and 20 years of age in the United States.[1] Data collected by the Surveillance, Epidemiology, and End Results (SEER) Program of the National Cancer Institute (NCI) between 1972 and 1990 suggested that these numbers were on the rise. In 1972, 12 cancers were diagnosed per 100,000 children under the age of 15 years; by 1990, that number had increased to nearly 14 per 100,000.[2,3] However, the rates have been stable since 1990.[4] Among malignancies of the head and neck, the incidence rate increased from 1.1 to 1.49 per 100,000 person–years.[5] During this same period, cancer-related mortality rate decreased. Therefore, the changes in incidence probably coincided with earlier diagnosis because of advances in central nervous system (CNS) diagnostic imaging such as computed tomography (CT) scanning and magnetic resonance imaging (MRI), and not a true increase in rates of disease.[4] However, malignancies remain the most common cause of death from disease in the 1- to 14-year-old age group. Childhood cancers are exceeded only by accidents as the leading cause of death in children older than 1 year of age.

Certain populations of children are at a higher risk for developing childhood malignancies. Down syndrome (DS) patients have a 20-fold increased chance of developing leukemia over the normal population. Post-transplantation pediatric patients and children who have received chemotherapy or radiotherapy are at increased risk for development of a second malignancy, most commonly non-Hodgkin's lymphoma or leukemia. Beckwith-Wiedemann syndrome and hemihyperplasia (previously termed hemihypertrophy) is linked with an increased risk of Wilms' tumor and hepatoblastoma. Patients with Bloom's syndrome, ataxia-telangiectasia, X-linked hypogammaglobulinemia, Wiskott-Aldrich syndrome, common variable immunodeficiency syndrome, severe combined immunodeficiency syndrome, X-linked lymphoproliferative disorder, selective IgA deficiency syndrome, and autoimmune diseases are all at increased risk for development of lymphoma, leukemia, and solid tumors.

The types and relative frequencies of childhood cancers are vastly different from those of cancers in adults. Most childhood tumors are mesenchymal or neuroectodermal in origin, whereas adult tumors are usually epithelial in origin. Nearly one third of pediatric malignancies are leukemias, most commonly acute lymphocytic leukemia, and an additional 12% are either Hodgkin's lymphoma or non-Hodgkin's lymphoma. Nonhematologic solid tumors comprise the remaining 55%. Of all solid tumors in children younger than 15 years of age, brain tumors are most common, followed in frequency by neuroblastoma, Wilms' tumor, non-Hodgkin's lymphoma, Hodgkin's disease, and rhabdomyosarcoma.

Impressive gains have been made in survival rates for some childhood cancers. In children younger than 15 years of age who are

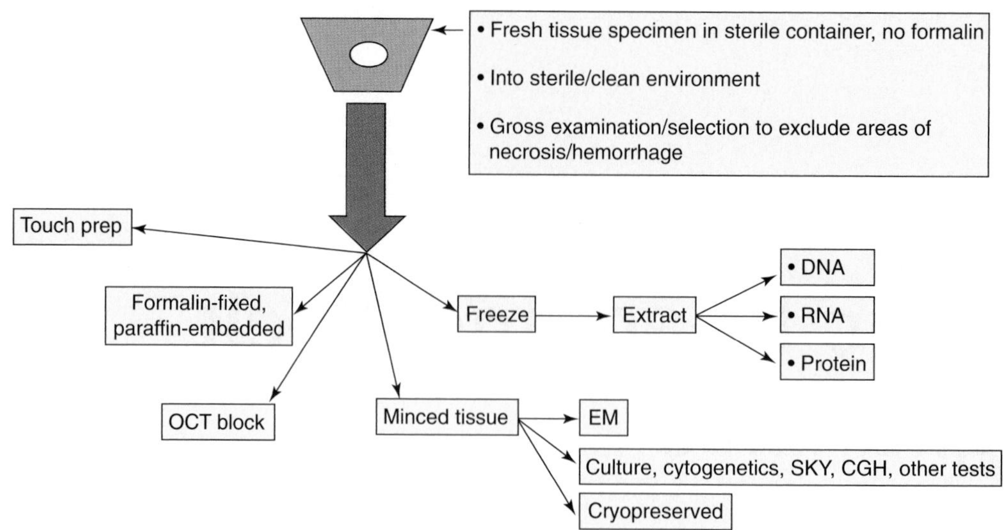

Figure 200-1. Tissue-handling algorithm for histopathologic workup. CGH, comparative genomic hybridization; EM, electron microscopy; FISH, fluorescence in situ hybridization; SKY, spectral karyotyping.

diagnosed with solid tumors, the survival rate has more than doubled—from 28% in 1960 to a more than 75% 5-year survival rate in 1993 and an 80% 3-year survival rate in 1995.[6] Particularly impressive survival gains have been achieved with Wilms' tumor and Hodgkin's lymphoma, both of which now have cure rates exceeding 90%.[2] Outcome data during this 30-year period show that the slopes of curves describing survival over time have remained fairly constant for all types of tumors. Advances in treatment and gains in survival have been achieved in a slow, incremental manner based on results of multicenter clinical trials. In spite of these advances, approximately 25% of children diagnosed with cancer will die of their disease.

The progress in survival rates for childhood cancer largely reflects the impact of clinical trials. Initiated first in 1948 to enable Farber and colleagues[7] to document the efficacy of methotrexate in inducing remission in some children with acute lymphocytic leukemia, most clinical trials today are conducted by the Children's Cancer Group or the Pediatric Oncology Group. In these trials, standard therapy is compared with a modification of that therapy, and if the modified protocol is superior, it then becomes the new standard. Progress is tedious, but from the perspective of time, it has been tremendously rewarding.

The possibility of more rapid advances in diagnosis and management is becoming increasingly real as studies of the molecular biology of childhood malignancies elucidate several requisite steps for tumorigenesis. Two important cytogenetic events, translocation and amplification, are important in tumor development and can act synergistically to generate potent oncogenic activity.[8] Nonrandom chromosomal translocations typically activate oncogenes by one of two mechanisms.[9] The first mechanism, frequently found in lymphoid malignancies, places the coding sequence of one gene under the regulatory control of a second gene. This juxtaposition results in increased or inappropriate expression of the first gene. The second mechanism generates a new gene, which is a chimera of two other genes that is formed by joining their coding regions. For amplification events, additional copies of a cellular gene are generated in the form of double-minute chromosomes or homogeneously staining regions.[10]

The pathologic evaluation of childhood tumors is very different from that of adult tumors. Because of the large numbers of mesenchymal tumors that can look very primitive and similar on light microscopy—small round blue cell (SRBC) tumors—use of newer techniques such as immunochemical, molecular, or ultrastructural analysis is necessary for accurate diagnosis. Proper diagnosis is crucial to developing a treatment plan and for prediction of clinical behavior. Every child with suspected leukemia-lymphoma or neuroblastoma should have a workup to evaluate gene translocations, antigen expression, and gene amplification. Critical to this pathologic workup is the delivery of fresh tissue to the pathologist for proper handling. Figure 200-1 shows proper tissue handling to ensure the availability of tissue for all types of analysis. Fresh tissue has the messenger ribonucleic acid (mRNA) necessary to carry out cell cultures for molecular genetic analysis and for growth of a permanent cell line. Because tissue often is not handled properly and is fixed in formalin before arriving at the pathologist's laboratory, techniques have been developed to obtain molecular genetic information from fixed or frozen tissue by such means as reverse transcriptase–polymerase chain reaction (RT-PCR) analysis, flow cytometry, fluorescence-activated cell sorting (FACS), and fluorescence in situ hybridization (FISH). However, RT-PCR analysis requires intact RNA, which can be obtained only by snap-frozen tissue stored at −70° C from viable tumor areas without tumor necrosis. Some success has been achieved with use of fixed, paraffin-embedded tissue for RT-PCR assays, but further work is needed in this effort.

Because resources are limited, a practical way to handle biopsy tissue must be adopted (see Fig. 200-1). After delivery of fresh tissue to the pathologist, the tissue is examined by routine hematoxylin and eosin (H&E) stains. If the diagnosis is not clear, additional methods are brought into play to establish a diagnosis such as immunohistochemistry, molecular genetic analysis, electron microscopy, cytogenetic studies, and deoxyribonucleic acid (DNA) sequencing (Table 200-1). These evolving techniques are used judiciously and are rarely all needed. The most common secondary procedure after examination of H&E stains is immunohistochemistry, followed by special stains, electron microscopy, and molecular studies. Immunohistochemistry is used to confirm the histogenesis of a tumor. Approximately 35 antibodies are commonly used in pediatric tumor workups in the categories of general (vimentin), hematopoietic, neural, myogenic, epithelial, and miscellaneous. Immunohistochemistry and electron microscopy have largely replaced the use of special stains, but a few are still useful, such as trichrome, pentachrome, reticulin, myeloperoxidase, and periodic acid–Schiff (PAS) stains. Electron microscopy is used primarily to clarify conflicting results from other studies such as immunohistochemistry. Molecular genetic techniques include five major methods: polymerase chain reaction (PCR) analysis, cytogenetic studies, FISH, spectral karyotyping (SKY), and comparative genomic hybridization (CGH). These techniques are used to detect genomic alterations (translocations, amplifications, or deletions) from chromosomal analysis. Many protocols require the use of special studies for ploidy and molecular genetics to enter a patient into a protocol treatment arm. The availability of molecular genetics has revolutionized childhood cancer diagnosis, providing accurate diagnoses that help guide therapy and predict clinical aggressiveness. Molecular genetic analysis of childhood tumors should not be taken with blind faith because two problems can be encountered: certain tumor-specific translocations only occur in a percentage of tumors, and in some cases, the same translocation can occur in a phenotypically different tumor. Still, molecular genetics has enormous value in the diagnostic workup of the difficult, primitive pediatric tumors.

Head and neck tumors of childhood are reviewed in this chapter. This subset of malignancies accounts for approximately 12% of all childhood cancers and, in order of relative prevalence, includes lymphomas (27%: Hodgkin's lymphoma 17%, non-Hodgkin's lymphoma 10%), neural tumors (23%: retinoblastoma and neuroblastoma), thyroid malignancies (21%, with papillary carcinoma the most common pathologic diagnosis), and soft tissue sarcomas (12%: rhabdomyosarcoma; 8%, nonrhabdomyosarcoma soft tissue sarcomas [NRSTSs]).[5] Age has a marked effect on tumor type and modifies this order of prevalence considerably. The age factor is obviously pertinent to a directed evaluation and diagnostic workup (Table 200-2).

Discussion in this chapter is limited to lymphomas, rhabdomyosarcomas, neuroblastomas, NRSTSs, salivary gland malignancies, thyroglossal duct carcinomas, post-transplantation lymphoproliferative disorders, malignant teratomas, and the histiocytoses. Thyroid and nasopharyngeal carcinomas are adequately covered elsewhere in this book.

Table 200-1

Diagnostic Methods for Tumor Diagnosis

Method	Comment
Light microscopy	Used in all cases
Immunohistochemistry	Widely used ancillary diagnostic
Molecular genetic: reverse transcriptase–polymerase chain reaction (RT-PCR)	Common molecular diagnostic method
Molecular genetic: FISH	Replacing cytogenetics in many cases
Molecular genetic: in situ hybridization	Specialized use
Special stains	Still useful in some cases, inexpensive
Electron microscopy	Used to augment light microscopy
Cytogenetics	Used when no suitable FISH probes available
Molecular genetic: SKY, CGH	Newer diagnostic methods
Molecular genetic: DNA sequencing	For rare cases

CGH, comparative genomic hybridization; FISH, fluorescence in situ hybridization; SKY, spectral karyotyping.

Lymphomas

Non-Hodgkin's Lymphomas

Acute lymphoblastic leukemia, defined as leukemic involvement of greater than 25% of the bone marrow, is the most common pediatric malignancy. *Lymphomas*, defined as leukemic tumor cells extending beyond bone marrow sites and involving less than 25% of the bone marrow, are the third most common cancers in children in the United States,[11] and non-Hodgkin's lymphomas represent 60% of these diagnoses. The annual incidence in children younger than 15 years of age is 7 to 8 per 1 million, with peak ages between 7 and 11 years. Boys are preferentially affected in a 3 : 1 ratio,[12,13] and the disease is twice as common in whites as in blacks.[14] Although adult lymphomas are primarily nodal, childhood lymphomas are predominantly extranodal. Since 1973, the annual incidence of non-Hodgkin's lymphoma has risen by approximately 30%. Although the reasons for this increase remain unclear, specific populations of children who are at greater risk for non-Hodgkin's lymphoma have been identified. These groups include children with congenital immunodeficiency syndrome (Wiskott-Aldrich syndrome, ataxia-telangiectasia, and X-linked lymphoproliferative disease), children with acquired immunodeficiency syndrome (AIDS), and children who have received immunosuppressive therapy for organ or bone marrow transplantation. Patients treated for Hodgkin's lymphoma and solid tumors with chemotherapy are at an increased risk for non-Hodgkin's lymphoma as well. Common to all these patients is deficient or impaired T-cell function.

Geographic differences in the incidence rates and subtypes of non-Hodgkin's lymphoma are striking. For example, non-Hodgkin's lymphoma is rare in Japan, whereas in equatorial Africa and northeastern Brazil, Burkitt's lymphoma is endemic and accounts for approximately 50% of all cancers.[11] An association with Epstein-Barr virus (EBV) and BL has been demonstrated in these areas.[15] Even in cases of sporadic Burkitt's lymphoma in the United States for which standard screening yields a negative result,[16] EBV genomic DNA can be detected with molecular biology.

Presentation and Evaluation

Characterized by an acute onset with rapid progression, prompt diagnosis and initiation of therapy are important to reduce morbidity and ensure long-term survival.[17] In 23% to 46% of affected children, primary disease occurs within the abdominal cavity and involves, in decreasing order of frequency, the distal ileum, cecum, and appendix.[18,19] Mediastinal primary tumors are slightly less common and are

Table 200-2

Age-Incidence Ranking for Head and Neck Tumors in Children

Ranking of Tumors by Age (years)			
0-1	1-5	6-10	11-20
Neuroblastoma	Rhabdomyosarcoma	Lymphoma	Lymphoma
Rhabdomyosarcoma	Lymphoma	Rhabdomyosarcoma	Thyroid malignancies
Lymphoma	Neuroblastoma	Nonrhabdomyosarcoma soft tissue sarcoma (NRSTS)	Nasopharyngeal malignancies
NRSTS	NRSTS	Thyroid malignancies	Salivary gland neoplasms

Table 200-3
Diagnostic and Staging Evaluation for Non-Hodgkin's Lymphoma

Essential	Useful	Occasionally Indicated
History	Intravenous urography	Contrast studies of the gastrointestinal tract
Physical examination	Special radiologic views (airway)	CT, MRI of the brain
Specimens for histology, cytology, immunophenotyping, genotyping	CT, MRI of primary site	CT, MRI of spinal cord
Complete blood count		Creatinine clearance
Serum chemistries (electrolytes, liver, renal serum chemistries, LDH, uric acid)	Epstein-Barr virus studies	Urinary uric acid Serum lactic acid
Bone marrow aspiration and biopsy	Protein electrophoresis	
Cerebrospinal fluid analysis	Acid-base studies	Liver biopsy
Urinalysis		Bone scan
Chest radiography		
Gallium-67 scanning		
Abdominal imaging		

CT, computed tomography; LDH, lactate dehydrogenase; MRI, magnetic resonance imaging.

diagnosed in 15% to 45% of cases.[20] Primary head and neck involvement occurs in 5% to 10% of children and originates in the salivary glands, larynx, paranasal sinuses, orbit, scalp, and Waldeyer's ring.[19] Proximity to the CNS makes direct extension possible.

The rapid progression of disease mandates prompt referral to a specialized management center before biopsy so that a pediatric oncologist can expedite the diagnostic and staging evaluation (Table 200-3) and determine the site and procedure to obtain tissue for histologic, cytologic, immunophenotyping, and genotyping analyses, with consultation from the surgeon and pathologist if necessary. Definitive diagnosis requires biopsy, sometimes by excision of a cervical node. Mediastinal involvement should be assessed by neck and chest CT before any procedure under general anesthesia. Disseminated disease is the rule, however, and often adequate numbers of malignant cells are found in the bone marrow, spinal fluid, or pleural or ascites fluid, obviating surgical intervention entirely. The presence of pancytopenia suggests bone marrow involvement, and when more than 25% of the marrow is replaced with tumor, children are assigned a diagnosis of acute lymphoblastic leukemia.

Management

Dramatic improvement in overall cure rates among children with non-Hodgkin's lymphoma reflects the incremental development of effective multimodal chemotherapeutic regimens through well-planned clinical trials. Systemic therapy is imperative because occult micrometastases affect more than 80% of children with non-Hodgkin's lymphoma and cure rates are less than 20% when only local therapy is used.[17] Management protocols are based on the extent of disease as determined by the staging workup and the histologic subtype.

The most widely used staging classification is the St. Jude Children's Research Hospital classification, based on the Ann Arbor staging system for Hodgkin's lymphoma, modified for non-Hodgkin's lymphoma (Table 200-4). Chemotherapy with combination drug therapy is the backbone of management, traditionally with agents used for acute lymphoblastic leukemia (i.e., cyclophosphamide, doxorubicin, vincristine, and prednisone, and for extensive or recurrent disease, methotrexate, Ara-C, etoposide, and ifosfamide). Overall cure rates are in the range of 70% to 90%, depending on tumor subtype. Radiotherapy has no routine role in the treatment of non-Hodgkin's lymphoma. Its use is reserved for massive disease, and surgery is used only occasionally in children with life-threatening tracheal compression. Response to therapy is assessed by monitoring tumor size and activity using a variety of imaging modalities or invasive techniques.

Histopathology and Molecular Biology

The histopathology of non-Hodgkin's lymphoma is extremely variable and has been categorized in various ways. The traditional and widely adopted Rappaport classification uses histologic pattern, cell type, and degree of differentiation to categorize tumors. In children, the categories seen with the most frequency are B-cell phenotype (Burkitt's lymphoma, Burkitt's-like lymphoma, large B-cell lymphoma), pre-T-cell origin (lymphoblastic lymphoma), and T-cell origin (anaplastic large-cell lymphomas and peripheral T-cell lymphomas). The diffuse histologic pattern is almost universal within these categories.[17]

The development of immunologic markers has added refinement to categorization and contributed to the identification of molecular mechanisms in pathogenesis. Best studied are the small, noncleaved-cell lymphomas, particularly Burkitt's lymphoma (Fig. 200-2). In Burkitt's lymphoma, EBV, a B-cell mitogen, probably fosters the establishment of a premalignant state by expanding the pool of lymphocytes in which chromosomal transformations can occur. Classic to Burkitt's lymphoma is the translocation of the *myc* gene from chromosome 8 to a position juxtaposed to an immunoglobulin receptor subunit gene on chromosomes 14 (80%), and less commonly to chromosomes 2 or 22 [t(8;14), t(8;2), t(8;22), respectively].[21,22] Unregulated expression of the *myc* gene disrupts regulation of the expression of target genes that are required for the normal progression of the cell cycle.[23-25]

Approximately 80% of large-cell lymphomas have a t(2;5) chromosomal rearrangement.[26] The precursor RNA can be detected by a RT-PCR assay, which has become an important diagnostic tool.[27] Although the impact of molecular biology has yet to revolutionize clinical practice, it will inevitably refine our diagnostic capabilities and permit the development of target tumor–specific therapy.

Hodgkin's Lymphoma

In 1832, Thomas Hodgkin described the disease that now bears his name. Although characterized by the presence of mononuclear cells (Hodgkin's cells) and binucleated or multinucleated tumor cells (Reed-

Table 200-4
Staging Systems for Non-Hodgkin's Lymphoma

Stage	Staging System: Ann Arbor	St. Jude Children's Research Hospital
I	Involvement of a single lymph node region (I) or of a single extralymphatic organ or site (IE)	Single tumor (extranodal) or single anatomic area (nodal) excluding the mediastinum or abdomen
II	Involvement of two or more lymph node regions on the same side of the diaphragm (II) or localized involvement of extralymphatic organ or site and of one or more lymph node regions on the same side of the diaphragm (IIE)	Single extranodal site with regional lymph node involvement; two or more nodal areas on the same side of the diaphragm; two single extranodal tumors ± regional node disease on the same side of the diaphragm; primary gastrointestinal tract tumor, usually in the ileocecal area ± involvement of associated mesenteric nodes
III	Involvement of lymph node regions on both sides of the diaphragm (III) ± extranodal involvement (IIIE) ± splenic involvement (IIIS), or both (IIISE)	Two single extranodal tumors ± regional node disease on opposite sides of the diaphragm; two or more nodal areas on opposite sides of the diaphragm; all extensive primary intra-abdominal disease; unresectable; all primary intrathoracic tumors (mediastinal, pleural, thymic); all primary paraspinal or epidural tumors regardless of other sites
IV	Diffuse involvement of one or more extralymphatic organs; organs or tissues ± associated lymph node enlargement	Any of the above + initial CNS or bone marrow involvement (<25%)

CNS, central nervous system.

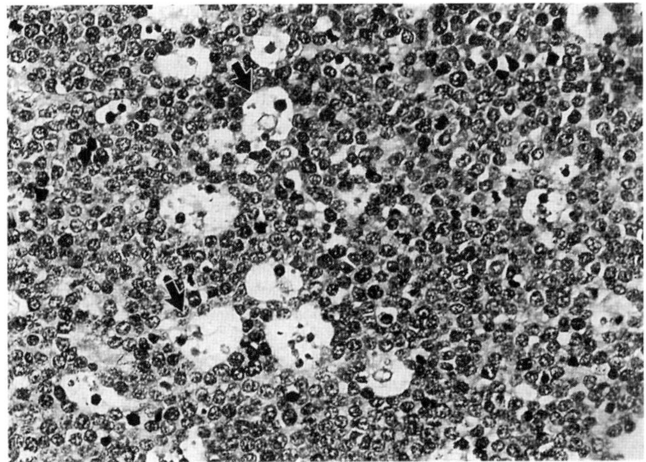

Figure 200-2. Non-Hodgkin's lymphoma categorized as malignant lymphoma with diffuse, small, noncleaved cells (Burkitt's lymphoma EBL7). Small non-cleaved lymphocytes diffusely replace this lymph node. The size is monotonous, differentiating it from non–Burkitt's lymphoma BL, which exhibits more variation in nuclei size and shape. Histiocytes *(arrows)* with their abundant pale cytoplasm and engulfed cellular material are scattered among the malignant lymphocytes, giving a "starry-sky" appearance. (Original magnification, 400×.)

Sternberg cells) in a background of variable and often abundant reactive cells, a single unifying principle of the biologic nature of Hodgkin's lymphoma and of the origin of the Reed-Sternberg cell has remained elusive.[28] Current data suggest that Hodgkin's lymphoma represents a group of diseases with an uncertain relationship to each other.[29] Age at diagnosis follows a bimodal distribution, with the first peak occurring between 15 and 40 years of age and the second peak occurring after age 50. Approximately 4% of cases occur in children younger than 10 years of age, and 11% are found in children between 10 and 16 years of age.[30]

Presentation and Evaluation

In more than 90% of childhood and adult cases, Hodgkin's lymphoma arises in the lymph nodes, typically causing an asymmetrical adenopathy that is firm, rubbery, and nontender. Particularly common is the combination of mediastinal and right supraclavicular nodal disease. The spleen is the most common extranodal site of involvement. Constitutional symptoms (B symptoms) may be present and include fever of 38° C or higher, drenching night sweats, or unexplained loss of 10% or more of body weight. Diagnosis is made by lymph node biopsy, and the disease is then staged using the classification developed in 1971 by the Ann Arbor workshop[31] and modified 18 years later to incorporate newer procedures such as CT (see Table 200-4, Ann Arbor staging system).[32] Substage classifications include A for asymptomatic disease, B for B symptoms (as described earlier in the chapter), and E for extension to an adjacent extranodal site. The staging system is based on the premise that Hodgkin's lymphoma spreads through the lymphatics to contiguous nodal groups and through the circulation to extranodal sites, although these modes of spreading have not been clearly established and multifocal involvement may represent multicentric disease.[29]

Clinical staging procedures include history, physical examination with measurement of lymph nodes, chest radiograph, CT scan of neck and chest, CT or MRI of abdomen, and laboratory tests (complete blood count with differential, erythrocyte sedimentation rate determination, renal and hepatic function tests, alkaline phosphatase assay). CT has limited sensitivity for detection of abdominal adenopathy in children because of their lack of retroperitoneal fat.[33] Therefore, abdominal MRI may be a better study for determining extent of abdominal and pelvic disease. Pathologic staging includes excisional lymph node biopsy. Bone marrow aspiration and biopsy is reserved for patients with stage III or IV disease or B symptoms. Routine use of surgical staging with splenectomy and lymph node sampling is no longer in use because of improved imaging techniques, routine use of systemic therapy, and the knowledge that splenectomy is associated with increased infectious and neoplastic complications. Stage at presentation is similar among children and adults, with approximately 60% of patients presenting with stage I or II disease and 40% of those presenting with stage II or IV disease, regardless of age.[30] In children younger than 10 years of age, however, stage I disease is more common (18%) and stage IV disease is less common (3%) than in adolescents

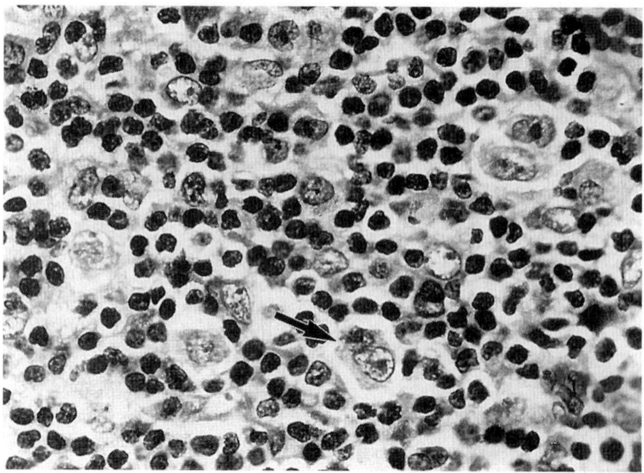

Figure 200-3. Hodgkin's lymphoma of the nodular sclerosing subtype. A mixed population of lymphocytes, histiocytes, and plasma cells along with binucleated Reed-Sternberg cells *(arrow)* are present. (Original magnification, 480×.)

(8% and 15%, respectively) and adults (11% and 11%, respectively). Systemic B symptoms also are less likely in younger patients (19%) than in adolescents (30%) and adults (32%).

Management

Management of Hodgkin's lymphoma varies according to stage. In most centers, radiation therapy is recommended for stage IA and stage IIA disease. Because of the high relapse rate among children with stage IIA disease of the mediastinum, chemotherapy also may be given.[34] For more advanced disease, chemotherapy either alone or as part of a combined regimen including radiotherapy is used.[35]

Long-term results for pediatric patients with early-stage Hodgkin's lymphoma suggest a prognosis similar to that in adults, with cure rates of approximately 90%.[36] With use of combined-modality therapy for stage IV disease, overall survival rates are slightly lower (approximately 80%).[35] When patients who have received only chemotherapy demonstrate relapse at nodal sites, salvage radiotherapy should be considered.[37]

Histopathology and Molecular Biology

The major histologic types of Hodgkin's lymphoma recognized by the Lukes, Butler, and Rye classifications include lymphocytic predominance, mixed cellularity, nodular sclerosis, and lymphocytic depletion (Fig. 200-3).[29] Further subclassification probably is unncessary, because current management protocols have eliminated differences in survival rates between the most common types (mixed cellularity and nodular sclerosis).

Micromanipulation of histologic sections to isolate and analyze individual Hodgkin's and Reed-Sternberg cells has verified an origin from B-lineage cells at various stages of development.[38] Ig heavy chain rearrangements have also been detected by PCR amplification in approximately 25% of cases.[39] These studies suggest that Hodgkin's lymphoma represents a clonal lymphocyte population and that different chromosomal rearrangements may be associated with different subclasses of disease.

Post-Transplantation Lymphoproliferative Disorder

As solid organ transplantation success rates have improved, diseases related to chronic immunosuppression have increased in prevalence. Post-transplantation lymphoproliferative disorder (PTLD) is the term for all abnormal proliferations of lymphoid tissue in the transplant recipient, ranging from lymphoid hyperplasia to malignant non-Hodgkin's lymphoma. Risk factors for the development of PTLD are the degree of immunosuppression, use of potent immunosuppressive agents such as tacrolimus, EBV seronegative status at time of transplantation, young age, donor-recipient mismatch, severe graft-versus-host disease (GVHD), T-cell depletion of donor marrow, use of anti–T-cell monoclonal antibodies, and high-dose antithymocyte globulin for GVHD prophylaxis. The rate of PTLD ranges from 8% to 28%,[40] depending on the immunosuppressive agents used. The rate of PTLD is higher in liver, heart, and heart-lung transplant recipients. The rate of PTLD is lower for renal transplant recipients, probably because of the higher level of immunosuppression needed in the former group.[41] Most PTLDs are of B-cell origin, but early PTLD can manifest as plasmacytic hyperplasia or as a polymorphic lymphoid process.[42] When PTLD affects the tonsils and adenoids, it often is of the plasmacytic hyperplasia type. When PTLD is seen in the lymph nodes, it is often a polymorphic lymphoid lesion. Treatment of PTLD includes decreasing the immunosuppression, to which most patients respond. When a transplant recipient presents with enlargement of the tonsils and adenoids, removal of the affected tissue (i.e., by tonsillectomy and adenoidectomy) is indicated to evaluate the tissue for PTLD. Removal of the affected tissue often is curative. Other therapies for PTLD include intravenous immunoglobulin, interferon alfa, antiviral therapy (with acyclovir or ganciclovir), and immunotherapy with donor T-lymphocyte infusion.

A correlation between EBV infection and PTLD is well documented.[43] In immunosuppressed patients, the T-lymphocyte response to the EBV infection is suppressed and the B-cell proliferation turned on by the virus infecting the B-lymphocytes is allowed to proceed unchecked. Thus, EBV seronegativity at the time of transplantation is a risk factor for the development of PTLD, because active EBV infection after transplantation can initiate this polyclonal response from the B lymphocytes infected with the Epstein-Barr virus.

Sarcomas

Rhabdomyosarcoma

Rhabdomyosarcoma is the most common soft tissue sarcoma of childhood, representing 13% of all pediatric malignancies. Rhabdomyosarcoma is the third most common neoplasm in childhood after neuroblastoma and Wilms' tumor. The annual incidence of this tumor in children younger than 20 years of age is 4.3 cases per 1 million children, affecting approximately 350 children in the United States each year.[44] Approximately 35% of these children present with disease in the head and neck. Sites of involvement include the orbit, nose and paranasal sinuses, oropharynx, soft tissues, nasopharynx, and external ear or mastoid. Because of the high possibility of contiguous spread to the CNS, the paranasal sinuses, infratemporal fossa, middle ear, and nasopharynx are classified as parameningeal sites.

In the 1960s, fewer than one third of children with rhabdomyosarcoma survived, but cure rates now approximate 70%, largely reflecting advances made by the Intergroup Rhabdomyosarcoma Study Committee (IRSC).[45,46] Before the formation of the IRSC in 1972, the relatively small numbers of patients, short follow-up times, and the confounding effects of varied treatments limited univariate and multivariate analyses, especially for small subgroups of patients. However, when three pediatric centers agreed to pool patients and investigate resources, it became possible to identify prognostic variables of crucial importance for stratifying patients in clinical trials. Valid comparisons of alternative therapies were developed, and therapies were tailored according to the risk of relapse. The data obtained through the collaborative, multimodality therapeutic protocols developed and studied by the IRSC have allowed a steady improvement in the curability of rhabdomyosarcoma, especially the locally extensive tumors.

Presentation and Evaluation

A majority of affected children are younger than 6 years of age when the diagnosis of rhabdomyosarcoma is made.[47] The spectrum of presenting signs and symptoms varies greatly depending on the site of the primary tumor, the age of the child, and the presence or absence of metastatic disease. Presentation in the head and neck most frequently is heralded by a local swelling. Fewer than one half of these children have pain. Nasal discharge or obstruction, signs of cranial nerve involvement, otorrhea, hearing loss, fetor, and proptosis are even less frequent.[48]

The orbit is involved in nearly one third of rhabdomyosarcomas of the head and neck,[48] with the typical presentation being that of a rapidly developing, unexplained proptosis. In decreasing order of frequency, rhabdomyosarcoma also affects the oral cavity and pharynx (29%), the face and neck region (24%), and the ears and sinuses (9%). Nasopharyngeal and paranasal sinus involvement can cause nasal obstruction or epistaxis, and otitis media, facial nerve palsy, or tumor filling the ear canal is often the presenting symptom of temporal bone disease.[49]

The diagnostic workup of children with suspected rhabdomyosarcoma must address two complementary issues: the nature and extent of the primary disease and the presence or absence of locoregional or metastatic disease. To assess the former, CT and MRI are essential. To assess the latter, common sites for metastases must be evaluated, including the lungs, bone, and bone marrow. A minimal test battery consists of complete blood count, serum electrolyte panel, liver and renal function tests, baseline coagulation studies, CT scan of the chest, a ^{99m}Tc-diphosphonate bone scan, and bilateral aspiration and biopsy of iliac bone marrow.

Surgery is a necessary part of the diagnostic and staging evaluation and is an essential component in the Intergroup Rhabdomyosarcoma Study Clinical Grouping Classification (IRSCGC) (Table 200-5). Although this staging system is widely used, it was revised in 1991 and the primary tumor, regional lymph nodes, and distant metastasis (TNM) classification is now used for Intergroup Rhabdomyosarcoma Study (IRS) patients in IRS groups IV and beyond. For instance, patients in IRSCGC group III represent a heterogeneous collection of patients who have resectable and unresectable tumors, depending on the experience of the institution. As surgery techniques have advanced, especially in the skull base, and reconstructive techniques such as microvascular reconstruction are more widely available, complete extirpation often is feasible for rhabdomyosarcoma in the head and neck.[48] In some centers, however, surgery may be limited to partial removal or excisional biopsy to establish the diagnosis. Additional important variables that were not considered in the IRSCGC were the degree of local extension and the status of the primary echelon nodes. To address these shortcomings, the IRSC now uses the TNM classification, similar to that used to characterize disease extent in adults with solid tumors (Table 200-6).

Table 200-5

Intergroup Rhabdomyosarcoma Study Clinical Grouping Classification*

Group	Definition
I	Localized disease, completely resected
II	Compromised or regional resections with microscopic residual disease
III	Incomplete resection or biopsy with gross residual disease
IV	Distant metastatic disease present at onset

*Used in Intergroup Rhabdomyosarcoma Studies I through III.

Management

Multimodal, multiagent therapy is the mainstay of management of rhabdomyosarcoma, along with surgical removal or biopsy and radiotherapy for local control. Several different chemotherapeutic agents are used, with appropriate selections based on the initial extent of disease and its site of origin. During the 1980s and 1990s, cisplatin, etoposide, and dacarbazine have been used in combination for rhabdomyosarcoma. Other agents used include ifosfamide and either etoposide or doxorubicin for new and recurrent rhabdomyosarcoma. IRS IV looked at combinations of these drugs; for metastatic rhabdomyosarcoma, it found that the combination of ifosfamide and doxorubicin improved outcome.[50] Some children, such as those with orbital rhabdomyosarcoma, require less intensive, two- or three-drug therapy and do well. By contrast, children with metastatic disease require extremely intensive therapy and still do poorly. Although they respond to initial chemotherapy, 75% relapse within 18 to 24 months.[51] To improve this outcome, efforts are ongoing to develop new active chemotherapeutic agents and to use dose-intensifying regimens with hematopoietic growth factors or autologous hematopoietic progenitor cells.

Radiotherapy is required to eradicate residual tumor cells at the primary site or to treat gross persistent disease. Guidelines for dosage and radiation fields evolved during the IRS I, II, and III. Local control is achieved in 80% to 90% of children using 4000 to 4500 cGy for microscopic residual disease and 4500 to 5000 cGy for tumors larger than 5 cm.[52] Prophylactic irradiation of clinically uninvolved regional nodes is unnecessary. With parameningeal tumors, 4500 to 5500 cGy is required. With overt parenchymal, meningeal, or cerebrospinal fluid involvement, whole-brain irradiation and intrathecal chemotherapy are indicated.[53,52] Hyperfractionation was evaluated in IRS IV as an approach to maintain local control rates and to reduce late side effects. Hyperfractionation did not result in significant improvement in local disease control over conventional radiation therapy.[54] Radiation therapy guidelines in IRS V have been simplified, with the basic emphasis placed on reducing the dose of radiation for most patients. This is being

Table 200-6

TNM Pretreatment Staging Classification for IRS Study IV

Stage	Sites	T*	Size	Nodes†	Metastases‡
1	Orbit, head and neck (excluding parameningeal), genitourinary (excluding bladder/prostate)	T1 or T2	A or B	N0, N1, or Nx	M0
2	Bladder/prostate, extremity, cranial parameningeal sites, other (includes trunk, retroperitoneum)	T1 or T2	A	N0 or Nx	M0
3	Bladder/prostate, extremity, cranial parameningeal	T1 or T2	B	N0, N1, or Nx	M0
4	All	T1 or T2	A or B	N0 or Nx	M1

*Tumor: T1, confined to anatomic site of origin; T2, extension or infiltration into surrounding tissue (A ≤5 cm in diameter; B >5 cm in diameter).
†Nodes: N0, no distant metastases; Nx, clinical status unknown; N1, clinically involved.
‡Metastases: M0, no distant metastases; M1, distant metastases present.
IRS, Intergroup Rhabdomyosarcoma Study; TNM, tumor-node-metastases.

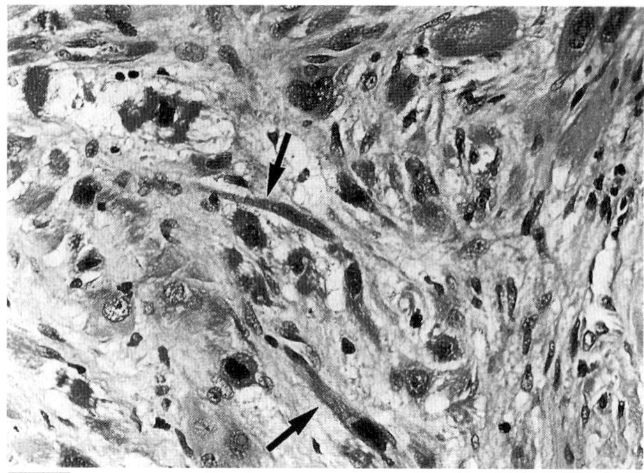

Figure 200-4. Embryonal rhabdomyosarcoma. The cells show a mixture of shapes but a spindled or elongated morphology is evident overall. Strap cells *(arrows)*, which resemble primitive muscle cells and are classically described in rhabdomyosarcomas, are easily seen in this example but may be difficult to identify in some cases. Immunohistochemical staining for muscle-specific markers can be useful in these instances. (Original magnification, 350×.)

accomplished in conjunction with delayed surgical resection of alveolar type tumors or initially unresectable tumors in anatomically unfavorable sites. With the refinement of aggressive craniofacial and intracranial surgical techniques that minimize postoperative morbidity, surgery is playing a more important role in selected patients with head and neck rhabdomyosarcoma. Specifically, if the tumor can be completely resected, the patient can avoid radiotherapy and its long-term complications, with no compromise in survival. Patients who are able to have complete removal of their tumors fare much better than those in whom gross residual tumor is left behind. Complete resection of skull base–parameningeal rhabdomyosarcoma is now more often a reality with advances of skull base surgery techniques and use of free-tissue transfer techniques for reconstruction.[55] In addition, salvage surgery after cytoreductive combination chemotherapy and radiotherapy can be offered to convert a partial response (PR) or stable disease (SD) to a complete response (CR).[56] For most children in group III, intensification of therapy using a risk-based study design has significantly improved management outcome. The largest gains have been realized in children with gross residual tumor after biopsy. In selected patient subsets, it also has been possible to decrease therapy.[57]

Histopathology and Molecular Biology

The histologic classification of rhabdomyosarcoma is based on the resemblance of these tumors to normal fetal skeletal muscle before innervation. The first formal classification was proposed by Horn and Enterline[58] in 1958 and subsequently was adopted by the IRSC and the World Health Organization. Subtypes include embryonal, botryoid (a subtype of embryonal), alveolar, and pleomorphic. Embryonal rhabdomyosarcoma of the botryoid subtype is the most common variant, accounting for 60% of tumors. It is characterized by variable amounts of spindle and primitive cells that are either tightly packed or loosely dispersed in a myxoid background. Rhabdomyoblasts are present in a variety of shapes, leading to unusual designations like tadpole, racquet, or strap cells (Fig. 200-4). The botryoid subtype accounts for 5% of cases and tends to arise in the mucosa-lined organs of the nasopharynx, external auditory canal, and genitourinary tracts. It is characterized grossly by the presence of polypoid masses and microscopically by the presence of subepithelial aggregates of tumor cells known as the cambium layer. Metastases are rare and the prognosis is excellent. Alveolar rhabdomyosarcomas are diagnosed in 20% of affected children and are characterized by the presence of fibrovascular septa that form alveolus-like spaces that contain freely floating monomorphous round malignant cells with abundant eosinophilic cytoplasm. Pleomorphic rhabdomyosarcomas show features of both embryonal and alveolar subtypes but are uncommon in children.[46] Cytogenetic studies of alveolar rhabdomyosarcoma have identified frequent chromosomal rearrangements and amplification. The most commonly recognized translocation events, t(2;13) and t(1;13), are found in 64% and 18% of cases, respectively.[59] The result is fusion of the *PAX3* gene on chromosome 2 or the *PAX7* gene on chromosome 1 with the *FKHR* gene on chromosome 13. In the case of *PAX3*, the new chimeric transcription factor excessively activates transcription from binding targets of wild-type *PAX3*. Molecular assays for *PAX3-PAX7* fusion genes have identified additional cases that do not have cytogenetically detectable rearrangements. On the basis of these more sensitive studies, the overall frequency of *PAX3-PAX7-FKHR* chimera appears to be higher than 90%.[8] Also, the presence of the *PAX3-FKHR* and *PAX7-FKHR* gene fusions correlate with poor clinical outcome. The prevalence and presumed importance of these fusion genes in tumorigenesis suggest that drugs designed to block their intracellular activity may be effective chemotherapeutic agents.

Nonrhabdomyosarcoma Soft Tissue Sarcomas

NRSTSs of childhood have a combined annual incidence of approximately 2 to 3 cases per 1 million and comprise a large number of uncommon tumors, including fibrosarcoma, dermatofibrosarcoma protuberans (DFSP), epithelioid sarcoma, synovial sarcoma, malignant fibrous histiocytoma, hemangiopericytoma, chondrosarcoma, osteosarcoma, leiomyosarcoma, liposarcoma, and soft tissue clear cell sarcoma.[47] Although rhabdomyosarcoma accounts for 60% of soft tissue sarcomas in children younger than 5 years of age, NRSTSs account for approximately 75% of all soft tissue sarcomas in teenaged patients (15 to 19 years of age).[44] The diagnostic evaluation for a child with a suspected NRSTS is identical to that for a child with rhabdomyosarcoma because tumor distinction is impossible on clinical grounds alone. This limitation makes it imperative to obtain enough tissue to establish a diagnosis without compromising the possibility of future surgical extirpation.

The rarity of these tumors has made the IRSCGC the most commonly used staging system (see Table 200-6), although the TNM system for soft tissue sarcomas in adults also has been applied by modifying the histologic grading classification.[60,61] The pathologic evaluation of these tumors typically takes into consideration factors such as necrosis, mitotic activity, cellularity, matrix formation, and pleomorphism. Because specific chromosome translocations define many of the soft tissue sarcomas, measures of ploidy and the demonstration of certain molecular genetic abnormalities will undoubtedly prove valuable in guiding prognostically based management protocols in the future.

Currently, the most important factors determining the likelihood of cure are histologic grade and tumor resectability.[62] The latter is particularly important for high-grade malignancies. Unfortunately, tumor size and invasiveness preclude complete resection in 30% to 50% of cases, and long-term locoregional control with adjuvant chemoradiotherapy usually is unsuccessful in the presence of either gross residual or metastatic disease (1 of 26 survivors with gross residual or metastatic disease versus 29 of 36 survivors with completely resected tumors or microscopic residual disease). Although the roles of radiotherapy and chemotherapy have not yet been standardized, data from the NCI Pediatric Branch indicate that a substantial number of children may benefit from appropriate intense multimodality therapy. Management of these children should be based on selected clinical protocols designed to assess responsiveness and long-term outcome.

Fibrosarcoma

Fibrosarcoma is a rare malignancy of the head and neck, with only 7 of 53 cases (13%) reported by the Armed Forces Institute of Pathology and 22 of 110 cases (20%) reported by Soule and Pritchard.[63] Neck disease occurs most commonly, followed in descending order of frequency by involvement of the oral cavity, scalp, auriculoparotid region, and face.[64] Hematogenous and lymphatic spread are extremely rare.[65]

Children of all ages are affected and typically present with an asymptomatic, slowly enlarging mass.[66] In infants, a unique form of

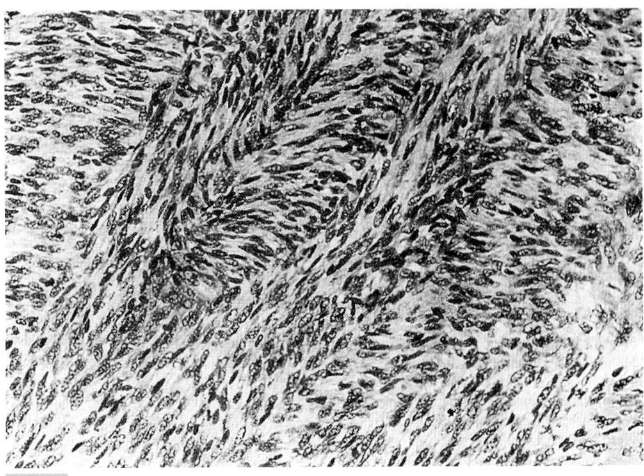

Figure 200-5. Fibrosarcoma. Discrete fascicles of spindle cells form intersecting patterns, sometimes producing a herringbone effect. (Original magnification, 200×.)

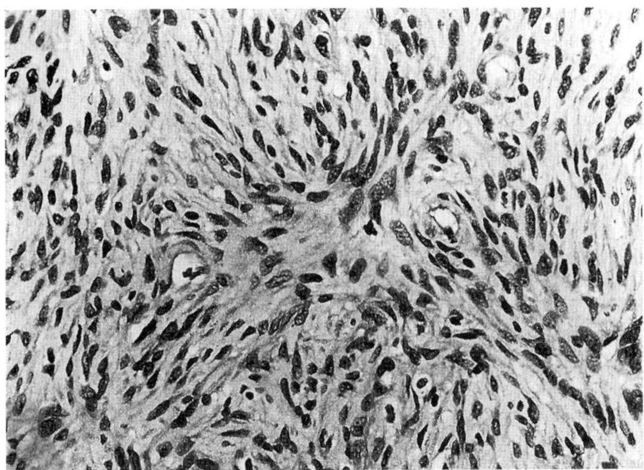

Figure 200-6. Dermatofibrosarcoma protuberans. This intermediate-grade malignancy is in the group of fibrohistiocytic tumors. Many of the tumors in this group have plump spindle cells arranged in patterns frequently described as cartwheel, whorling, or storiform (from the Latin *storea*—a rush mat) because of its woven appearance. (Original magnification, 275×.)

congenital fibrosarcoma occurs that is considered a histologically low-grade fibrosarcoma.[67] Although these tumors can be large, the long-term outlook is quite good, perhaps reflecting an enhanced sensitivity to chemotherapeutic agents. Some unresectable congenital fibrosarcomas respond to preoperative chemotherapy, permitting a later, less mutilating surgical procedure with clear margins.[68,69] By contrast, fibrosarcoma is more aggressive in older children, survival rate is lower, and the impact of multimodal therapy is not obvious. Management requires wide local excision to optimize the chances of survival. The absence of a true capsule makes intraoperative assessment of the degree of tumor spread difficult.

The excised mass typically is gray-tan with hemorrhagic and necrotic areas.[70] Composed mostly of spindle-shaped fibroblasts or myofibroblasts with scanty cytoplasm, histologic grading is possible and is based on degree of cellularity, cellular maturity, and amount of collagen production (Fig. 200-5). Cytogenetic studies have shown an association with trisomies of chromosomes 8, 11, 17, and 20.[71,72] Karyotyping studies show a recurring t(12;15) translocation.

Dermatofibrosarcoma Protuberans

Dermatofibrosarcoma protuberans is a nodular cutaneous tumor with a high propensity for local recurrence after simple excision. It usually appears as a firm, solitary, flesh-colored nodule, although multiple masses or an area of induration can occur. The trunk is the favored site of involvement, followed by the extremities and the head and neck, especially the scalp and supraclavicular fossa.[73]

Approximately 12% of affected persons are older children,[73] but dermatofibrosarcoma protuberans has been diagnosed in patients younger than 10 years of age. Time to diagnosis may exceed 2 years, with size at diagnosis up to 2 cm. Management requires wide excision for a successful long-term outcome, reflecting the "pseudocapsule" and finger-like extensions of this tumor. With surgical margins less than 2 cm, recurrence rates approximate 40%; with margins wider than 2 cm, recurrence rates drop to 25%; and with margins wider than 3 cm, few recurrences are reported.[74,75] However, given the regional anatomy of the head and neck, achieving a 2.5- to 3-cm margin can be difficult. Even with Mohs' technique, extensive surgery may be required.[76] Although local recurrence rates of 50% to 70% are reported, with repeated procedures, 90% of affected patients can be rendered free of disease.[77] Consensus is lacking regarding the cell of origin of dermatofibrosarcoma protuberans. The primary mass usually is grossly encapsulated and well circumscribed, although it can send multiple pseudopod-like projections laterally and deeply (3 cm or more).[78] These extensions are easily missed on histologic sectioning. Histologic examination shows elongated cells with a storiform organization (Fig. 200-6).

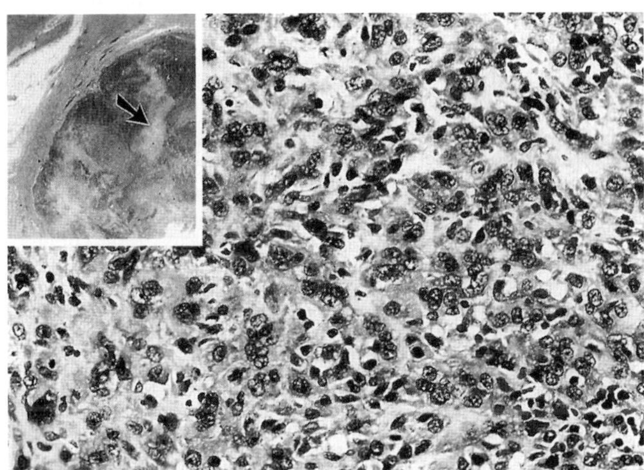

Figure 200-7. Epithelioid sarcoma. This unusual tumor is composed of epithelial-like cells that have polygonal-shaped cytoplasm. The lower-power view *(inset)* reveals a distinct nodular appearance. Necrosis *(arrow)* in the center of the nodules is characteristic. (Original magnification, 400×; low-power inset: original magnification, 5×.)

Epithelioid Sarcoma

Epithelioid sarcoma can easily be confused with a variety of benign and malignant conditions such as necrobiotic granuloma, rhabdoid tumor, rhabdomyosarcoma, and Ki-1 lymphoma.[79-82] It occurs throughout infancy and early childhood, although most individuals are not diagnosed until the second to fourth decades of life.[83] Approximately 10% of cases involve the head and neck, produce nontender, nonulcerated swelling, and follow a protracted course of repeated local recurrences with eventual distant metastases. More aggressive tumors that metastasize early are uncommon. Once the diagnosis has been made, complete surgical resection should always be attempted because the role and efficacy of chemotherapy and radiotherapy have not been clearly established.

The characteristic histologic pattern is one of nodules separated by fibrous septa (Fig. 200-7). The cells inside the nodules are polygonal, are variable in size, and may cluster, suggesting squamous differentiation. Areas of necrosis and an inflammatory infiltrate are common. The molecular biology of epithelioid sarcoma has shown multiple structural changes, most frequently the deletion of 1p21-22.[83]

Neuroectodermal Tumors

Neuroblastomas

Neuroblastomas are the most common extracerebral solid tumors of infancy and childhood.[84] Their annual incidences in white and nonwhite children under 15 years of age are 10.4 and 8.3 per 1 million, respectively.[85] Arising from primitive neuroectodermal cells of neural crest origin as embryonal tumors of the sympathetic nervous system, neuroblastomas can develop wherever sympathetic nervous tissue is found. Primary tumors occur paravertebrally along the sympathetic chain from the neck to the pelvis and from paraganglia from the adrenal medulla, the organ of Zuckerkändl, or the retroperitoneal, inguinal, paratesticular, testicular, oviductal, or ovarian paraganglia. The most unusual aspect of this tumor is the frequent occurrence of spontaneous regression, typically in infants with a small primary tumor, liver involvement, subcutaneous nodules, and patchy bone marrow infiltration without major replacement of hematopoietic cells.[86]

Presentation and Evaluation

Primarily a tumor of infancy and early childhood, as many as 50% of cases are diagnosed in infants younger than 1 year of age and 80% are detected in children younger than 5 years of age.[87] Presenting signs and symptoms depend on the site of the primary lesion, the presence and site of metastases, and the secretion of hormones and vasoactive substances. The most common site of origin is the adrenal medulla or adjacent retroperitoneum, but 2% to 5% of neuroblastomas develop in the head and neck region.

Primary cervical tumors generally are detected at an earlier age and at a lower stage than tumors detected elsewhere, reflecting the greater facility with which abnormalities in the neck are recognized. Laryngotracheal or pharyngeal compression can lead to airway obstruction, dysphagia, or aspiration. Ipsilateral ptosis occurs if the superior cervical ganglion is involved. Primary neuroblastoma of the orbit may cause proptosis, periorbital ecchymoses (panda eyes), and ocular muscle paresis. However, more subtle findings such as edema of the conjunctivae or eyelids, papilledema, and retinal hemorrhage may be noted. Because the sympathetic nervous system is intimately associated with the development and maintenance of eye color, heterochromia irides is possible.[88] Another finding peculiar to the head and neck is the cardiofacial syndrome, or "asymmetrical crying face." This type of congenital facial weakness becomes most apparent with crying and reflects disease involvement of the motor cortex, the nucleus or peripheral root of cranial nerve VII, or the muscles of facial expression.[89]

Paraspinal neuroblastoma may extend through adjacent intervertebral foramina into the spinal cord (*en sablier* tumors) to produce paraplegia. Although this finding is most commonly associated with mediastinal and retroperitoneal tumors, it can occur with cervical disease.[90,91] Neuroblastoma also is a noteworthy cause of congenital paraparesis; clinical features of neurologic dysfunction in neonates are difficult to recognize, however, and diagnosis may be delayed.

The diagnostic and metastatic evaluation of children with neuroblastoma of the head and neck requires multiple imaging studies, immunocytochemistry studies, routine histologic examination, and cytogenetic analysis. For suspected cervical disease, CT and MRI to evaluate the neck should be complemented by abdominal CT and MRI, chest radiograph, bone scans, and bone marrow aspirates and biopsies to appropriately stage the tumor. The International Neuroblastoma Staging System (INSS) was developed in 1991 to help stage patients uniformly for clinical trials and biologic studies. The staging system is based on clinical experience with neuroblastoma, reflecting the degree of tumor burden, surgical resectability, and the pattern of metastatic spread (Table 200-7).

Several genetic markers have been identified in neuroblastoma tumors correlating with clinical course, but determination of the best predictors awaits further study in large numbers of patients. These markers include tumor cell DNA index, *MYCN* gene copy number, allelic loss of 1p, and unbalanced gain of 17q. *MYCN* amplification occurs in approximately 25% of primary neuroblastomas and amplification is associated with advanced stage and poor prognosis. Tumor markers such as catecholamine metabolites, ferritin, neuron-specific enolase, lactate dehydrogenase, and the disialoganglioside G_{D2} are helpful in diagnosis and disease monitoring but have largely been replaced by genetic markers (e.g., *MYCN* amplification) for risk stratification.[86] The frequency of abnormal elevations depends on disease burden and therefore hampers detection of neuroblastoma at an early stage. Catecholamines and their metabolites (vanillylmandelic acid, homovanillic acid, and dopamine) are elevated in 90% to 95% of children with neuroblastoma and have been very successfully developed by the Japanese for use in urine screening programs despite high false-negative rates.[92] Tests on 115,000 infants suggest that a majority of neuroblastomas can be discovered before the age of 1 year, when prognosis is most favorable.[92]

Table 200-7

International Neuroblastoma Staging System

Stage	Description
1	Localized tumor with complete gross resection, with or without microscopic residual disease; representative ipsilateral lymph nodes negative for tumor microscopically (nodes attached to and removed with the primary tumor may be positive)
2A	Localized tumor with incomplete gross excision; representative ipsilateral nonadherent lymph nodes negative for tumor microscopically
2B	Localized tumor with or without complete gross excision, with ipsilateral nonadherent lymph nodes positive for tumor (enlarged contralateral lymph nodes must be negative microscopically)
3	Unresectable unilateral tumor infiltrating across the midline, with or without regional lymph node involvement; or localized unilateral tumor with contralateral regional lymph node involvement; or midline tumor with bilateral extension by infiltration (unresectable) or by lymph node involvement
4	Any primary tumor with dissemination to distant lymph nodes, bone, bone marrow, liver, skin, or other organs (except as defined for stage 4S)
4S	Localized primary tumor (as defined for stages 1, 2A, or 2B), with dissemination limited to skin, liver, or bone marrow (limited to infants younger than 1 year of age)

Management

Management of neuroblastoma is determined by the stage of disease and sites of involvement. Patients are stratified into low-, intermediate-, and high-risk groups based on the various prognostic variables available (age at diagnosis, INSS stage, tumor histopathology, DNA content of the tumor, and *MYCN* amplification). Treatment of stage I neuroblastomas consists of surgical removal. Chemotherapy is the main modality of treatment in intermediate- and high-risk patients. Radiation therapy is also used, but by itself is not curative due to the high rate of metastatic disease. In the head and neck, surgical intervention most commonly implies excisional biopsy for stages II, III, and IV. A cervical sympathetic ganglion is usually involved and is resected. Adjacent, enlarged nodes should also be removed, although a formal radical neck dissection is not required.[93] In cases in which complete resection would cause unacceptable morbidity, a second surgical procedure can be planned

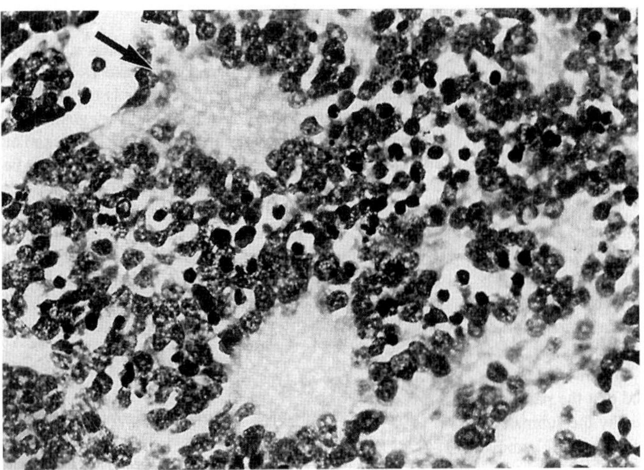

Figure 200-8. Neuroblastoma. Small blue cells characterize this neoplasm. The differential diagnosis of "small blue cell" tumors in children also includes lymphoma and peripheral neuroectodermal tumor/Ewing's sarcoma. Other tumors can also be considered in this group. Neuroblastoma can be differentiated by its relatively uniform cell appearance and neurofibrillary material between the cells. Pseudorosettes (Homer-Wright rosettes) are illustrated *(arrow)* but often are not seen. Immunohistochemical marking and electron microscopy can be useful to demonstrate neural-associated proteins or neural-associated structures (e.g., neurosecretory granules). (Original magnification, 425×.)

12 to 24 weeks after completion of chemotherapy.[94] Unfortunately, despite the large number of chemotherapeutic agents that are active in newly diagnosed patients, long-term remission remains elusive for children older than 1 year of age with INSS stage IV disease (approximately 45% of all children with neuroblastoma).

Histopathology and Molecular Biology

Grossly, neuroblastoma is a discrete solid mass with well-circumscribed contours. Coagulative necrosis may develop in nonviable areas, sometimes with dystrophic calcification. Microscopically, the tumor represents one of the "small blue cell" neoplasms of childhood that is exquisitely susceptible to smear or crush artifact. Iatrogenic damage may obscure cytologic details, making it difficult to make an unequivocal histologic diagnosis.[95] The prototype neuroblastoma is composed of small uniform cells that are 7 to 10 mm in diameter and have dense hyperchromatic nuclei with minimal perinuclear cytoplasm (Fig. 200-8). Immunohistochemistry has revolutionized diagnostic histopathology, and a battery of selected antibodies is used to evaluate specific cellular and subcellular aspects of these neoplasms.

Elucidation of molecular biology also has affected diagnosis and management protocols. Deletions in the short arm of chromosome 1 (1p36) are the most common structural aberration and identify children with a poor prognosis.[84] A less frequent abnormality is amplification of the N-*myc* oncogene.[96,97] This event is associated with advanced stages of disease and rapid tumor progression, perhaps because amplification usually accompanies 1p deletions.

The clinical implication of these studies is that infants with 1p deletions, N-*myc* amplification, and diploidy or tetraploidy are at high risk for recurrence and require aggressive therapy at diagnosis. Management failures appear to be a result of the development of multidrug resistance associated with overexpression of multidrug resistance–associated protein, even when a diverse range of structurally and functionally unrelated chemotherapeutic agents is used.[98]

Based on advances in the molecular biology of neuroblastoma, priorities for future trials will include defining subsets of children who do not require therapy, improving durability of remissions for disseminated disease by exploiting cytokines for dose intensification, defining the place of autologous bone marrow transplantation, exploring means for reversing drug resistance, evaluating tumor-targeted radiotherapy, and identifying new active chemotherapeutic agents.

Ewing's Sarcoma Family of Tumors

Ewing's Sarcoma and Peripheral Primitive Neuroectodermal Tumor

Ewing's sarcoma (ES) and peripheral primitive neuroectodermal tumor (PPNET) are now considered to be in the same spectrum of malignancy—the Ewing's sarcoma family of tumors (ESFTs). Based on molecular genetic and cytogenetic information, both of these tumors are now known to be of neural crest origin. The chromosomal translocation [t(11;22)(q24;q12)] is present in 85% of ESFTs.[99] This reciprocal translocation results in the formation of an *ews*-fli1 fusion gene. ES is a neuroectodermal tumor primarily affecting the long bones and pelvis. Extraosseous ES can occur in soft tissue. A more differentiated form of ES, PPNET (or neuroepithelioma) also can occur in bone or soft tissue. Both ES and PPNET appear similar on histochemical staining and share a unique nonrandom translocation. ESFTs occur primarily in the second decade of life and are seen in whites but rarely in blacks in the United States and in Africa. Although these tumors are primarily found in the extremities, pelvis, chest wall, and spine-paravertebral region, they can manifest in the head and neck as a primary or metastatic tumor. Cure can be expected in up to two thirds of patients with localized disease.

Evaluation of patients with ESFT should include plain films and MRI studies of the primary site, CT scan of the chest, bone scans, bone marrow aspiration and biopsy, complete blood count, baseline blood chemistry studies, and serum lactate dehydrogenase determination. Surgery, radiation therapy, and chemotherapy all are important modalities in treatment. Virtually all patients will have metastases or microscopic metastatic disease at presentation; therefore, chemotherapy is always needed.

Salivary Gland Malignancies

Childhood malignancies of the salivary glands are rare. In a review of 2135 children under 16 years of age who developed salivary gland tumors, only 17 (0.79%) malignancies were recorded (15 [0.7%] mucoepidermoid and 2 [0.09%] acinar cell carcinomas).[100] Most of these malignancies involved the parotid gland. Other authors have confirmed this bias, and from an overview of nine different studies, Rasp and Permanetter[101] concluded that the parotid gland is the favored site (88.5%), followed by the submandibular gland (7.7%), the minor salivary glands (3.3%), and the sublingual gland (0.5%). A unique feature of these tumors is that most appear to be induced by radiation.[102]

Presentation and Evaluation

Children with salivary gland malignancies usually are in their second decade of life at diagnosis. The majority also are survivors of another malignancy, most frequently acute lymphoblastic leukemia diagnosed 10 years earlier for which cranial radiotherapy was required.[103] Chemotherapy, age at the time of therapy, and genetic susceptibility are additional risk factors that may contribute to the development of secondary salivary gland malignancies.[102]

Regardless of location, the most common presentation is as an asymptomatic mass, although facial nerve involvement occasionally accompanies parotid gland disease.[103] The presence of cervical adenopathy does not imply metastatic disease. It more likely reflects common childhood reactive hyperplasia seen as a sequela of repeated upper respiratory infections. Evaluation by CT and MRI is helpful to delineate tumor boundaries and for planning surgical resection.

Management

Salivary gland malignancies in children should be excised. Although the primary principle of surgical excision is accepted, the extent of the procedure and the value of multimodal therapy are not as clearly defined. For parotid gland disease, superficial or total parotidectomy is required, and unless tumor invasion dictates otherwise, the facial nerve should be spared. Complete excision should also be the goal for tumors

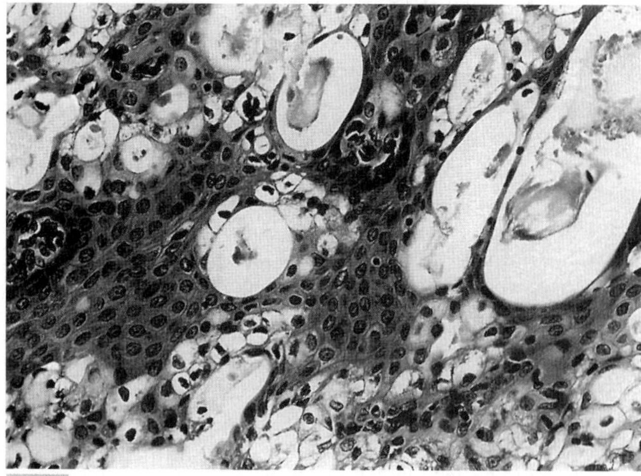

Figure 200-9. Mucoepidermoid carcinoma. Mucus-producing and squamous tumor cells are the prime histologic components of mucoepidermoid carcinomas. Mucous cells containing rounded intracytoplasmic mucous droplets are evident along with pavement-like squamous cells with distinct cellular boundaries. Larger cysts containing mucus also are present. (Original magnification, 320×.)

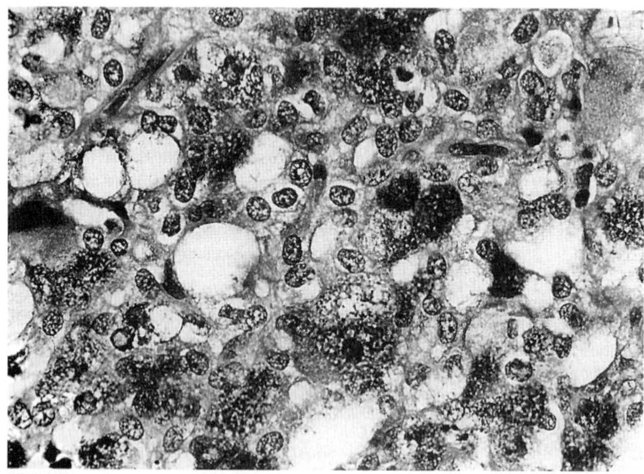

Figure 200-10. Acinic cell carcinoma. Tumor cells appear similar histologically to normal acinar unit cells, but their lack of arrangement of organization into functional units helps in differentiation. These cells have a granular appearance, and some show large basophilic granules. Microcystic changes are seen in this case. (Original magnification, 420×.)

of the submandibular, sublingual, and minor salivary glands. Radiotherapy is reserved for children with high- or intermediate-grade malignancies of the major salivary glands and high-grade malignancies of the minor salivary glands. The value of radiotherapy as adjuvant therapy in intermediate-grade tumors of the soft palate is debatable. Routine use of elective neck dissection for patients with clinically negative necks is not recommended or beneficial for children with malignant salivary gland disease. Chemotherapy with cisplatin-based drugs is reserved for palliation or metastatic disease.

Histopathology and Molecular Biology

Mucoepidermoid and acinic cell carcinomas account for 60% of childhood salivary gland malignancies (45% and 15%, respectively),[104] although the former is the only type that has been diagnosed in the intraoral salivary glands.[105,106] Mucoepidermoid carcinomas are usually low grade and are seldom fatal (Fig. 200-9), whereas acinic cell carcinomas behave like their adult counterparts (Fig. 200-10). Probably the only epithelial salivary gland tumor unique to children is the embryoma, or sialoblastoma.[107] Recognized only in newborns or during the first year of life, this malignancy is morphologically similar to stages in the development of the embryonic anlage of salivary gland tissue. Fewer than one quarter of such tumors show either biologic or histologic signs of malignancy, and complete surgical excision is curative.[107]

Table 200-8

Teratoma Types

Type*	Distribution of Cases (%)	Frquency of Hydramnios (%)	Mortality Rate (%)
I	12.4	56	100
II	45.6	23	43.4
III	17.1	8.1	2.7
IV	14.3		3.2
V	10.6		43.5

*I, moribund neonate or stillborn infant; II, neonate with respiratory distress; III, neonate without respiratory distress; IV, child 1 month to 18 years of age; V, adult.

Teratomas

Teratomas are the most common extragonadal germ cell tumors of childhood. They arise most commonly in a midline or paraxial location from the brain to the sacral area and involve the head and neck in 1 of every 40,000 births.[108] In this region, sites of involvement include the soft tissues of the neck (cervical teratomas), superficial facial structures in and about the temporal fossa and zygomatic area, oral cavity, oronasopharynx, and orbit.[109]

Presentation and Evaluation

More than 75% of cervical teratomas are diagnosed in neonates, two thirds of whom have respiratory distress significant enough to cause stridor.[62] Hydramnios, stillbirth, and premature labor are other frequent accompaniments.[109] This information, in addition to age at diagnosis and respiratory ability, was used by Jordan and Gauderer[110] to define five different disease types (Table 200-8). The high mortality rate in the adult group (type V) reflects the correspondingly high rate of malignant transformation. By contrast, death in neonates usually results from respiratory obstruction as a result of lesion bulk and location. Malignant degeneration is much less common, although it does occur.

Rothschild and associates[111] described seven neonates with teratomas that metastasized to the cervical nodes, lungs, and liver. The metastatic deposits were composed of either mature glial tissue or a mixture of mature and immature elements. Differentiation suggests that the presence of metastases does not necessarily portend a bleak prognosis.[112] This impression was supported by the findings of Rothschild's group,[111]: Death was secondary to metastatic disease in only one patient with metastases. Benign teratomas arising in the paranasal sinuses are extremely rare, and all of the malignant lesions of the sinonasal tract have occurred in adults.[109]

Management

The recommended treatment for head and neck teratomas is surgical excision. When a neonate is experiencing respiratory difficulty, the first priority should be stabilization of the airway. In utero diagnosis of a large cervicofacial teratoma will allow time for perinatal planning of the ex utero intrapartum treatment (EXIT procedure), to secure the infant's airway before the maternal-fetal circulation is divided.[113]

Histopathology and Molecular Biology

Teratomas in neonates and infants contain tridermic tissue elements: ectoderm, endoderm, and mesoderm. Although the preponderant tissue is most often neuroepithelium, other tissues that can be involved include fetal cartilage, myogenic tissue, and epithelium (squamous, ciliated, columnar, enteric, and endocrine). In type II and type III teratomas, malignancy is not equated with the degree of immaturity of the tissue elements and instead reflects immaturity of the host (Fig. 200-11).[109]

Thyroglossal Duct Carcinomas

Thyroglossal duct carcinoma may arise in a thyroglossal duct cyst, although this is a rare occurrence. It may be an incidental finding on removal of the benign-appearing cyst or may manifest as a midline enlarging mass with features suggestive of malignancy, especially if the cyst has a largely solid character. Treatment consists of complete removal along with the midline portion of the hyoid bone, as is done in the Sistrunk procedure. Close follow-up is necessary along with thyroid suppression.[114] Prophylactic total thyroidectomy is necessary if metastasis to the thyroid gland is detected. Incidence of papillary carcinoma in the remaining thyroid gland is 25%. Therefore, some workers recommend prophylactic total thyroid gland removal.[115]

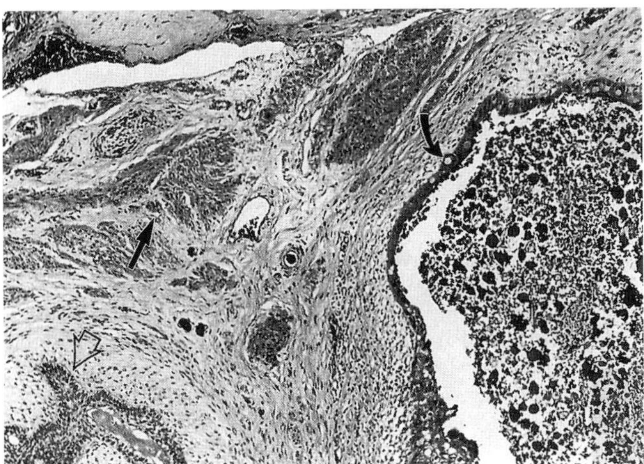

Figure 200-11. Teratoma. Multiple cell types in a haphazard arrangement are evident in this low-power view showing squamous cells *(open arrow)*, mucus-containing goblet cells *(curved arrow)* lining a cyst, and smooth muscle cells *(solid straight arrow)*. (Original magnification, 50×.)

Histiocytoses

The histiocytoses are a family of disorders of histiocytes that can range in clinical importance from focal and easily controlled to fatal. The histiocytoses are diseases of histiocytes. Accordingly, infiltration or accumulation of cells of the monocyte-macrophage series is seen in the involved tissues. A majority of the histiocytoses are not malignant but proliferative lesions, possibly disorders of immunoregulation. It is thought that perhaps the initiating event for the histiocytoses is immunologic stimulation of a Langerhans cell, an antigen-presenting cell, which then continues proliferating in an uncontrolled manner. The International Histiocyte Society has proposed the classification system shown in Table 200-9.[116] Class I histiocytosis, formerly known as histiocytosis X, is now known as *Langerhans cell histiocytosis*, which includes the diseases formerly classified under the histiocytosis X label: eosinophilic granuloma, Hand-Schüller-Christian disease, and Letterer-Siwe disease.

Pathology

Grossly, the lesions of Langerhans cell histiocytosis are granulomatous. By light microscopy, Langerhans cells are seen. By electron microscopy, Birbeck granules are seen. The lesions may be purely histiocytic or may be a mixture of histiocytes and eosinophils.

Clinical Presentation and Evaluation

The clinical presentation varies from an asymptomatic lytic bone lesion, found incidentally on radiographs, to generalized manifestations such as diabetes insipidus, fever, or weight loss. The first step in the evaluation and management of a patient with such a lesion must include a biopsy of the involved tissue. Care must be taken with the biopsy, because Langerhans cells with Birbeck granules can be found in normal skin. Pathologically, the diagnosis can be confirmed by Birbeck granules on electron microscopy, or by CD1a-positive staining in lesional cells. S100 immunostaining also is present in Langerhans cell histiocytosis cells and not on normal histiocytes. Once the lesion is identified

Table 200-9

Classification of Childhood Histiocytoses

Class I	Class II	Class III
Dieases included: Langerhans cell histiocytosis	IAHS; FEL; grouped together as the hemophagocytic lymphohistiocytoses (HLH)	Malignant histiocytosis; acute monocytic leukemia; true histiocytic lymphoma
Cellular characteristics of the lesions: Langerhans cells with cleaved nuclei and Birbeck granules seen on electron microscopy; cell surface antigens include S100 and CD1a; cells mixed with varying proportions of eosinophils; multinucleated giant cells sometimes seen	Morphologically normal, reactive macrophages with prominent erythrophagocytosis; process involves entire reticuloendothelial system	Neoplastic cellular proliferation of cells exhibiting characteristics of macrophages or dendritic cells or their precursors; localized or systemic
Proposed pathophysiologic mechanisms of the histiocytoses: Immunologic stimulation of a normal antigen-presenting cell—the Langerhans cell—in an uncontrolled manner	Histiocytic reaction secondary to an unknown antigenic stimulation (FEL) or to an infectious agent (IAHS), with erythrophagocytosis possibly reflecting foreign antigens adsorbed on erythrocytes or activation of macrophages by excess lymphokine production because of abnormal immunoregulation	Neoplasm; clonal autonomous uncontrolled proliferative process

FEL, familial erythrophagocytic lymphohistiocytosis; IAHS, infection-associated hemophagocytic syndrome.

as being in the histiocytosis family, the workup should include a complete blood count, skeletal survey, a CT scan of the head, liver function tests, coagulation studies, and determination of urine osmolality after water deprivation. Monostotic bone disease (formerly known as eosinophilic granuloma) clearly carries a better prognosis than polyostotic bone disease (formerly known as Hand-Schüller-Christian disease). The fulminant presentation, formerly known as Letterer-Siwe disease, is most commonly seen in infants younger than 2 years of age.

Treatment

Class I histiocytoses can be treated with curettage, excision, intralesional steroids, systemic steroids, or low-dose radiotherapy. Curiously, single monostotic lesions often regress spontaneously after biopsy, curettage, or steroid injection. If a single lesion is not resolving and is threatening a vital structure, low-dose radiotherapy, in the range of 500 to 800 cGy, can be curative,. The role of chemotherapy is reserved for multisystem involvement and widespread disease. The agents used are vinblastine and etoposide, with or without steroids. In general, the poor-prognosis groups are those comprising children younger than 2 years of age and children with organ dysfunction (liver, bone marrow, lungs). Unfortunately, little gain has been obtained in the treatment of the 15% of cases of Langerhans cell histiocytosis that are resistant to treatment or progress in a fulminant fashion. In an effort to optimize therapy for disseminated Langerhans cell histiocytosis, the Histiocyte Society opened a prospective, randomized treatment study in 1991, LCH-1. LCH-1 showed that vinblastine and etoposide are equivalent drugs in terms of response, toxicity, survival probability, probability of disease reactivation, and sequelae.[117] LCH-1 also identified lack of rapid response to treatment (less than 6 weeks) as another poor prognostic indicator. Other experimental treatment approaches include bone marrow transplantation, and 2-chlorodeoxyadenosine (an antimetabolite) for severe cases.

Class II histiocytoses, infection-associated hemophagocytic syndrome and familial erythrophagocytic lymphohistiocytosis (FEL), are diseases of the mononuclear phagocytic cell series, excluding Langerhans cells (see Table 200-9). The histiocytic reaction in these disorders is presumed to be from an underlying pathogenic process. FEL is usually rapidly fulminant and fatal, despite chemotherapy. Because the cells causing this disease are benign, it is not surprising that chemotherapy is usually not successful. Bone marrow transplantation is currently being studied in a controlled study and the initial results have been encouraging.

Class III histiocytoses are the only malignant histiocytoses (see Table 200-9). Three types are recognized: acute monocytic leukemia, malignant histiocytosis, and true histiocytic sarcoma. These diseases are treated with systemic chemotherapy.

Sequelae of Management

More than 12,000 children and adolescents under 20 years of age are diagnosed with cancer each year in the United States.[118] The overall survival rate is nearly 80%. A growing population of survivors requires long-term follow-up. The morbidity of managing head and neck cancers in children must be measured not during a 5- to 10-year interval but throughout a lifetime of more than 70 years. As cure rates improve, therapy must be refined to optimize growth potential and fertility and minimize the risk of second malignancies without sacrificing the primary goal of tumor eradication. The immediate sequelae of radiotherapy to the head and neck are similar in both children and adults. Acutely, mucositis, otitis externa, and alopecia are common. Subacutely, somnolence develops in approximately one third of children who receive whole-brain irradiation. Transient demyelination also can occur, leading to a sensation of electrical shocks at various levels below the neck elicited by flexion of the head or torso (Lhermitte's syndrome). Late effects include problems with transverse myelopathy, sensorineural hearing loss, endocrinopathies, and abnormal development of irradiated structures.[119]

Most disheartening of all is the possibility of a second malignancy. This risk is not insubstantial: Children who have survived one malignancy are three to six times more likely to develop another cancer than is the general population.[120] Thus, the risk of a second malignancy in long-term survivors (5 years) of all forms of childhood cancer appears to be 2% to 3%.[121] Contributing factors include radiotherapy, chemotherapy, age at treatment, and genetic susceptibility. Especially vulnerable are children previously treated for retinoblastoma and survivors of Hodgkin's lymphoma who receive mantle irradiation. Reported tumors include acute leukemias; bone and soft tissue sarcomas; and carcinomas of the skin, breast, thyroid, and salivary glands.[102]

Because children can tolerate greater doses or greater dose intensities of irradiation than adults, they also are at higher risk for delayed or chronic toxicities that become evident years after treatment. Growth retardation is found in approximately one third of pediatric brain tumor survivors, and in approximately 10% of pediatric leukemia survivors. Children treated at an age younger than 5 years with irradiation for brain tumors are especially susceptible to the linear growth retardation. Musculoskeletal problems such as scoliosis, avascular necrosis of bone, and osteoporosis are seen in approximately one third of pediatric cancer survivors, secondary to irradiation or steroid use, especially dexamethasone. Dental problems such as arrested tooth development or malocclusion and caries are common with radiotherapy to the facial or pharyngeal areas. Learning problems and neuropsychological problems are seen with cranial irradiation, especially in children younger than 36 months of age. Radiation to the neck also can cause thyroid dysfunction as a late effect.

Most radiation-induced second neoplasms occur more than 15 years after treatment of the first. Unfortunately, as duration of follow-up increases, so does risk.[122] Among chemotherapeutic agents, cyclophosphamide has been implicated in the development of solid tumors. Etoposide, an epipodophyllotoxin that acts by inhibiting the enzyme topoisomerase II, has been implicated in the development of second leukemias. The sobering reality is that the treatment of primary malignancies of the head and neck in children is extremely toxic, and the burden of a successful outcome can be immense. Addressing these issues remains a challenge for the 21st century.

SUGGESTED READINGS

Albright JT, Topham AK, Reilly JS. Pediatric head and neck malignancies. *Arch Otolaryngol Head Neck Surg.* 2002;128:655.

Bown N, Cotterill S, Lastowska M, et al. Gain of chromosome arm 17q and adverse outcome in patients with neuroblastoma. *N Engl J Med.* 1999; 340:1954.

Caron H, van Sluis P, de Kraker J, et al. Allelic loss of chromosome 1p as a predictor of unfavorable outcome in patients with neuroblastoma. *N Engl J Med.* 1996;334:225.

Charache H. Hodgkin's disease in children. *N Y State J Med.* 1946;46:507.

Chilcote RR, Brown E, Rowley JD. Lymphoblastic leukemia with lymphomatous features associated with abnormalities of the short arm of chromosome 9. *N Engl J Med.* 1985;313:286.

Coene IJ, Schouwenburg PF, Voûte PA, et al. Rhabdomyosarcoma of the head and neck in children. *Clin Otolaryngol.* 1992;17:291.

Crist WM, Kelly DR, Radab AH. Predictive ability of Lukes-Collins classification for immunologic phenotypes of childhood non-Hodgkin's lymphoma: an institutional series and literature review. *Cancer.* 1981;48:2070.

Cunningham MJ, Myers EN, Bluestone CD. Malignant tumors of the head and neck in children: a twenty-year review. *Int J Pediatr Otorhinolaryngol.* 1987;13:279.

Daya H, Chan HS, Sirkin W, et al. Pediatric rhabdomyosarcoma of the head and neck: is there a place for surgical management? *Arch Otolaryngol Head Neck Surg.* 2000;126:468.

Donaldson SS, Meza J, Breneman JC, et al. Results from the IRS-IV randomized trial of hyperfractionated radiotherapy in children with rhabdomyosarcoma—a report from the IRSG. *Int J Rad Oncol Biol Physics.* 2001;51:718.

Donaldson SS, Link MP. Childhood lymphomas: Hodgkin's disease and non-Hodgkin's lymphoma. In: Mossa AR, Robson MC, Schimpff SC, eds.

Comprehensive Textbook of Oncology. 2nd ed. Baltimore: Williams & Wilkins; 1991.

Evans AE, et al. Factors influencing survival of children with nonmetastatic neuroblastoma. *Cancer*. 1976;38:661.

Evans AE, D'Angio GJ, Randolph J. A proposed staging for children with neuroblastoma. *Cancer*. 1971;27:374.

Gadner H, Grois N, Arico M, et al. A randomized trial of treatment for multisystem Langerhans' cell histiocytosis. *J Pediatrics*. 2001;138:728.

Gurney JG, Young JL, Roffers SD, Smith MA, Bunin GR. Soft tissue sarcomas. In: Gloeckler Ries LAG, Smith MA, Gurney JG, Linet M, Tamva T, Young JL, Bunin GR, eds. *SEER Pediatric Monograph: Cancer Incidence and Survival among Children and Adolescents, United States SEER Program 1975-1995*. Bethesda, Md: National Cancer Institute; 1999.

Halperin EC, Kun LE, Constine LS, Jarbell NJ. Hodgkin's disease. In: Halperin EC, Kun LE, Constine LS, et al, eds. *Pediatric Radiation Oncology*. New York: Raven Press; 1989.

Harmer MH, ed. *International Union Against Cancer: TNM Classification of Malignant Tumors*. 3rd ed. Geneva: International Union Against Cancer; 1982.

Healy GB, Upton J, Black PM, et al. The role of surgery in rhabdomyosarcoma of the head and neck in children. *Arch Otolaryngol Head Neck Surg*. 1991;117:1185.

Hudson MM, Jones D, Boyett J, et al. Late mortality of long-term survivors of childhood cancer. *J Clin Oncol*. 1997;15:2205.

Jenkin RDT, Peters MV, Darte JMM. Hodgkin's disease in children. *Am J Roentgenol*. 1967;100:222.

Kao GD, Willi SM, Goldwein J. The sequelae of chemo-radiation therapy for head and neck cancer in children: managing impaired growth, development, and other side effects. *Med Pediatr Oncol*. 1993;21:60.

Kramer S, Meadows AT, Jarrett P, et al. Incidence of childhood cancer: experience of a decade in a population-based registry. *J Natl Cancer Inst*. 1983;70:49.

Linet MS, Ries LA, Smith MA, et al. Cancer surveillance series: recent trends in childhood cancer incidence and mortality in the United States. *J Natl Cancer Inst*. 1999;91:1051.

Lukens JN. Progress resulting from clinical trials. Solid tumors in childhood cancer. *Cancer*. 1994;74:2710.

Mark RJ, Bailet JW, Tran LM, et al. Dermatofibrosarcoma protuberans of the head and neck. *Arch Otolaryngol Head Neck Surg*. 1993;119:891.

Mecucci C, Van Den Berghe H. OKT8-Positive T-cell lymphoma associated with a chromosome rearrangement t(2;17) possibly involving the T8 locus. *N Engl J Med*. 1985;313:185.

Michaelis J, Kaatsch P. Cooperative documentation of childhood malignancies in the FRG: system design and five-year results. *Mongr Paediatr*. 1986;18:56.

Morris SW, Kirstein MN, Valentine MB, et al. Fusion of a kinase gene, ALK, to a nucleolar protein gene, NPM in non-Hodgkin's lymphoma. *Science*. 1995;267:316.

Nag S, Grecula J, Ruymann FB. Aggressive chemotherapy, organ-preserving surgery, and high-dose-rate remote brachytherapy in the treatment of rhabdomyosarcoma in infants and young children. *Cancer*. 1993;72:2769.

National Cancer Institute. *Surveillance, Epidemiology, and End Results (SEER) Program*. Public Use CD-ROM (1973-96). Bethesda, Md: National Cancer Institute, Division of Cancer Prevention and Control, Surveillance Program, Cancer Statistics Branch; April 1999.

Newell KA, Alonso EM, Whitington PF, et al. Posttransplant lymphoproliferative disease in pediatric liver transplantation. Interplay between primary Epstein-Barr virus infection and immunosuppression. *Transplantation*. 1996;62:370.

Pappo AS, Shapiro DN, Crist WM, et al. Biology and therapy of pediatric rhabdomyosarcoma. *J Clin Oncol*. 1995;13:2123.

Rabbitts TH. Chromosomal translocations in human cancer. *Nature*. 1994;372:143.

Reis LAG, Eisner MP, Kusary CL, et al. *SEER Cancer Statistics Review, 1973-1998*. Bethesda, Md: National Cancer Institute; 2001.

Robison LL. General principles of the epidemiology of childhood cancer. In: Pizzo PA, Poplack DG, eds. *Principles and Practice of Pediatric Oncology*. 2nd ed. Philadelphia: JB Lippincott; 1993.

Rutigliano DN, Meyers P, Ghossein RA, et al. Mucoepidermoid carcinoma as a sedondary malgnancy in pediatric sarcoma. *J Pediatr Surg*. 2007;42(7):E9.

Sandlund JT, Pui CH, Roberts WM, et al. Clinicopathologic features and treatment outcome of children with large-cell lymphoma and the t(2;5)(p23;q35). *Blood*. 1994;84:2467.

Schneider AB, Lubin J, Ron E, et al. Salivary gland tumors after childhood radiation treatment for benign conditions of the head and neck: dose-response relationships. *Radiat Res*. 1998;149(6):625.

Smith MA, Gloeckler Ries LA. Childhood cancer incidence, survival, and mortality. In: Pizzo PA, Poplack DG, eds. *Principles and Practice of Pediatric Oncology*. 4th ed. Philadelphia: JB Lippincott; 2002.

Smith RJH, Katz CD. Neuroblastoma of the head and neck. In: Pochedly C, ed. *Neuroblastoma: Tumor Biology and Therapy*. Boca Raton, Fla: CRC Press; 1990.

Sokal EM, Antunes H, Beguin C, et al. Early signs and risk factors for the increased incidence of Epstein-Barr virus-related posttransplant lymphoproliferative diseases in pediatric liver transplant recipients treated with tacrolimus. *Transplantation*. 1997;64:1438.

Straus DJ. Treatment of early stage Hodgkin's disease. *Blood Rev*. 1993;7:34.

Ward VM, Langford K, Morrison G. Prenatal diagnosis of airway compromise: EXIT and fetal airway surgery. *Int J Pediatr Otorhinolaryngol*. 2000;53:137.

White L, Meyer PR, Benedict WF. Establishment and characterization of human T-cell leukemia line (LALW-2) in nude mice. *J Natl Cancer Inst*. 1984;72:1029.

White L, Siegel SE. Non-Hodgkin's lymphoma in childhood. In: Sutow WW, Fernbach DF, Vietti TJ, eds. *Clinical Pediatric Oncology*. St Louis: Mosby; 1984.

Writing Group of the Histiocyte Society: Histiocytosis syndromes in children. *Lancet*. 1987;1:209.

Xia Y, et al. TAL2, a helix-hoop-helix gene activated by the (7;9)(p34;q32) translocation in human T-cell leukemia. *Proc Natl Acad Sci U S A*. 1991;88:11416.

For complete list of references log onto www.expertconsult.com.

CHAPTER TWO HUNDRED AND ONE

Salivary Gland Disease in Children

Gresham T. Richter

David L. Walner

Charles M. Myer, III

Key Points

- A good history and physical examination is the best tool in diagnosing salivary gland problems in children.
- Ultrasound with or without fine-needle aspiration is useful for diagnosis of most parotid and submandibular gland diseases in children who are tolerant of the procedure.
- For complete evaluation of the nature and extent of salivary gland masses, cross-sectional imaging with CT or MRI with contrast is necessary.
- Inflammatory conditions are the most frequently encountered salivary entities in young children.
- Salivary neoplasms are uncommon in children, mostly occur in the second decade, and are malignant in more than 50% of cases.
- The incidence of mumps virus parotitis is waning since the advent of the mumps vaccine. Beyond mumps, common viral etiologies of parotitis include Epstein-Barr virus, parainfluenza viruses, and adenovirus.
- A solid, firm, and fixed salivary mass that persists for greater than 6 weeks is an appropriate candidate for open surgical biopsy.
- Hemangiomas are the most frequently encountered benign tumors of the parotid gland. Pleomorphic adenomas are the most common benign epithelial tumors.
- Mucoepidermoid carcinoma is the most common malignancy of the parotid and most common tumor secondary to radiation exposure.
- Persistent sialorrhea beyond 4 years of age is considered abnormal and should be investigated for treatment including medical (glycopyrrolate) and surgical (submandibular gland excision and parotid duct ligation) options.

Salivary gland disease is an uncommon but manageable condition in the pediatric population. Inflammatory conditions of the salivary glands are more frequently encountered because salivary tumors account for only 1% of all childhood neoplasms. Infections can be either acute (bacterial and viral) or chronic (ductal obstruction, mycobacterial, and granulomatous disease) with the parotid being the most frequently affected gland. When a persistent salivary gland mass is present, possible neoplastic and congenital processes should be explored with an understanding that the risk of malignancy for salivary tumors is greater in young children. A complete differential diagnosis includes inflammatory, neoplastic, vascular, congenital, traumatic, and a myriad of less common diseases (Table 201-1). Clues gleaned from a thorough history and physical examination can help identify the disease in each pediatric patient. Ultrasound, computed tomography, magnetic resonance imaging, and fine-needle aspiration (FNA) have proven to be safe and valuable diagnostic tools for delineating inflammatory from benign and malignant salivary gland conditions (Figs. 201-1 to 201-3). Chronic sialorrhea (drooling) is a frequent and chronic problem, especially in neurologically impaired children, that can be addressed with both medical and surgical therapy.

Anatomy

The salivary system consists of the major paired parotid, submandibular, and sublingual glands and the minor salivary glands. All salivary glands are derivatives of ectoderm. During their development, they pierce the surrounding mesenchyme and arborize before terminating into multiple acini. The parotid gland lies between the external auditory canal, mandibular ramus, and mastoid tip. It is separated, by the stylomandibular ligament, from the submandibular gland, which rests between the anterior and posterior digastric tendons just below the body of the mandible. Both glands are covered by the superficial portion of the deep cervical fascia that either envelops (parotid) or separates (submandibular) the gland from adjacent lymph nodes. The largest salivary gland is the parotid, which is located in the parotid space harboring the facial nerve, external carotid artery, and retromandibular vein. It is artificially divided into two lobes, the deep and superficial, by the facial nerve. Accessory parotid glands with a connection to the parotid duct can be identified along the masseteric muscle in 20% of people. Although rare, agenesis of the parotid gland has also been reported.

An arborized draining system leads to a single and final secretory duct for both the parotid and submandibular glands known as Stensen's

Table 201-1

Differential Diagnosis of Pediatric Salivary Gland Disease

Inflammatory		Congenital	Neoplastic				
Acute	**Chronic**	**Cysts**	**Benign**	**Malignant**	**Traumatic**	**Autoimmune**	**Other**
Bacterial	*Obstructive*	Dermoid	*Vascular Anomaly*	*Epithelial*	Penetrating cheek	Benign lymphoepithelial disease	Allergy
Suppurative	Sialectasis	Branchial cleft	Hemangioma	Mucoepidermoid carcinoma	Blunt gland trauma	Sjögren's syndrome	Medication induced
Lymphadenitis	Sialolithiasis	Branchial pouch	Lymphatic malformation	Acinic cell carcinoma	Radiation injury		Chronic sialorrhea
Viral	Mucocele cyst	Congenital ductal	Arteriovenous malformation	Adenocarcinoma			Systemic conditions
Mumps	*Granulomatous*		Venous malformation	Adenocystic carcinoma			Obesity
EBV	Mycobacterial		*Epithelial*	*Nonepithelial*			Prader-Willi
Parainfluenza	Actinomycosis		Pleomorphic adenoma	Rhabdomyosarcoma			Cystic fibrosis
HIV	Sarcoid		Cystadenoma lymphomatosum	Lymphoma			
			Monomorphic adenomas				

EBV, Epstein-Barr virus; HIV, human immunodeficiency virus.

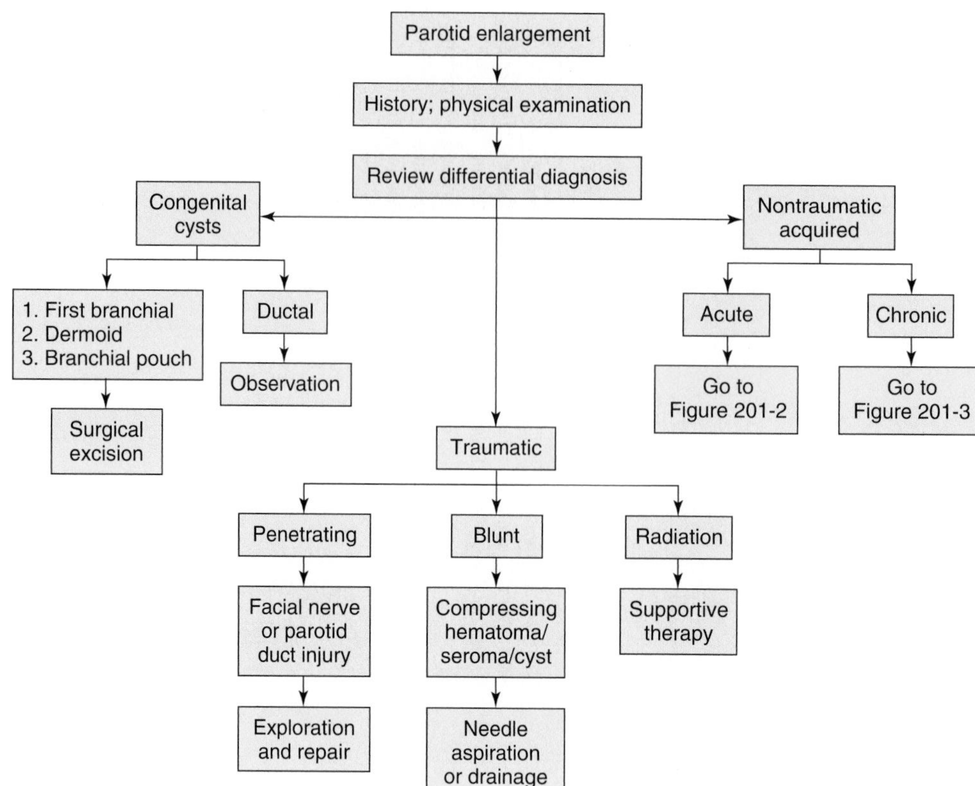

Figure 201-1. Parotid enlargement.

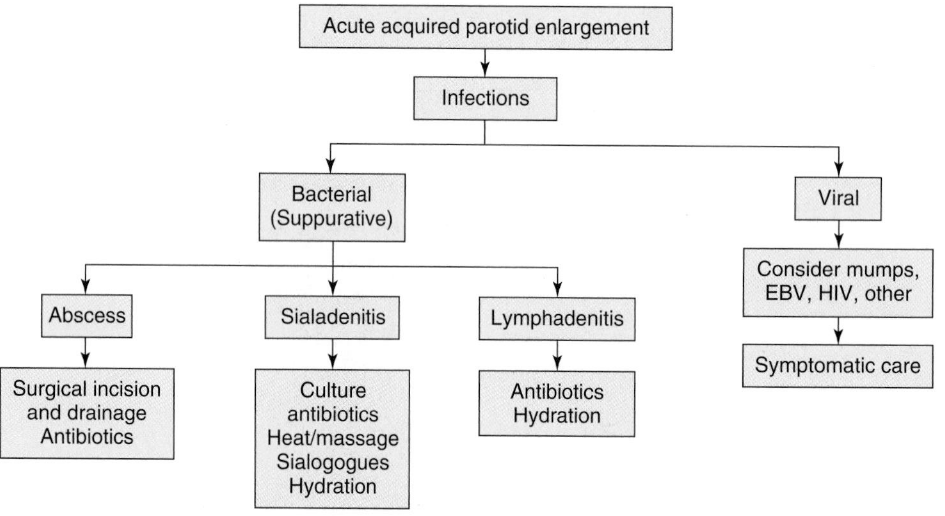

Figure 201-2. Acute acquired parotid enlargement. EBV, Epstein-Barr virus; HIV, human immunodeficiency virus.

and Wharton's ducts, respectively. The sublingual glands are located in the floor of the mouth immediately below the mucosa and drain at its medial surface via 10 to 12 small ducts (ducts of Rivinus). They are the source of mucoid cysts, otherwise known as *ranulas,* which are frequently discovered in young children. The remaining upper aerodigestive tract is lined by literally hundreds of minor salivary glands that lie just deep to the mucosa. The highest concentration of minor glands are in the buccal, lingual, labial, and palatal regions. Each minor gland uses only one draining duct. Occlusion of these ducts can lead to small mucoceles. Frequently found along the lower lip of young children, treatment involves excision or marsupialization.

A few salient differences exist in the anatomy of the salivary system and its adjoining structures in children and adults. In infants the parotid gland is lighter and rounder. It lies wedged between the masseter muscle and the ear and gradually grows during childhood over the surface of the parotid duct. The facial nerve exits the skull base just deep to the subcutaneous tissue to enter the parotid gland in children younger than 2 years of age, making it particularly prone to traumatic injury. Thereafter, formation of the tympanic ring and mastoid tip allows the facial nerve to take a deeper and more protected position behind the mastoid bone and tragal cartilage. Similarly, after exiting the stylomastoid foramen, the nerve takes a more abrupt and lateral course in children than in adults, with the marginal mandibular nerve often riding in a superficial course over the mandible. These variations in facial nerve anatomy contribute to parotid and mastoid surgery as common iatrogenic causes of facial paralysis in children. Familiarity

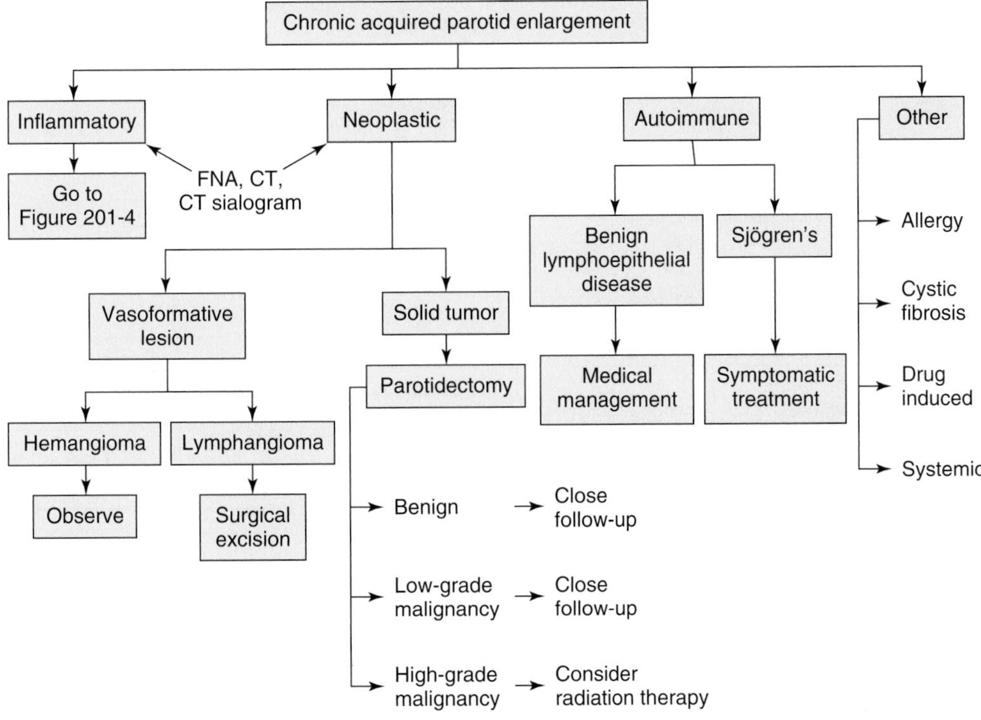

Figure 201-3. Chronic acquired parotid enlargement. CT, computed tomography; FNA, fine-needle aspiration.

with pediatric anatomy is thereby recommended before operating in a young patient.

In addition, the submandibular and sublingual glands are small in infants. Rapid growth of up to five times their initial size occurs during the first 2 years of life. Surgeons should be aware that, in very young children, the sublingual and submandibular glands are often anatomically contiguous.

Physiology of the salivary glands is thoroughly addressed in Chapter 84. Briefly, salivary flow is controlled by the superior salivatory nuclei (submandibular and sublingual glands) and inferior salivatory nuclei (parotid gland) via the autonomic nervous system. Only a small amount of saliva is secreted during the night because resting salivary flow increases during the day and peaks in the late afternoon. Resting salivary secretions are produced predominantly by the submandibular (60%) and sublingual (10%) glands with the submandibular glands creating the bulk of the fluid. The production of parotid secretions, which are serous in nature, is increased during eating. Saliva produced from all glands is critical for deglutition and acts as an infectious barrier for the mucosa and dentition by creating a surface coat of mucoid secretions, enzymes (e.g.. lysosyme), and immunoglobulins (IgA). In select children, excessive saliva and drooling (sialorrhea) can lead to aspiration, pulmonary compromise, mouth and skin maceration, and social isolation.[1] These patients often require medical or surgical therapy, or both, to reduce salivary flow from the major glands.

History and Physical Examination

A thorough history is the most important tool in diagnosing salivary gland problems in children. The onset, duration, and severity of symptoms provide valuable clues to the pathologic nature of the problem and allow the practitioner to quickly delineate among neoplastic, congenital, and inflammatory processes. Congenital disorders such as hemangiomas and cysts will often become evident shortly after birth. Neoplastic processes are more frequently seen in children older than 10 years.[2-4] In contrast, an inflammatory condition is the most common salivary pathology in toddlers and is marked by acute onset, brief duration, and painful swelling. Chronic conditions may be more difficult to differentiate by history alone, but gradual and painless growth at or near salivary tissue is suspicious for neoplasm until proven otherwise. Intermittent swelling associated with eating will signify salivary duct obstruction by stones or strictures, whereas recurrent and diffuse bilateral cheek swelling may indicate recurrent parotitis or chronic sialectasis.

The location and number of glands involved should be elicited in the history. Diffuse edema of the involved gland suggests inflammatory disease while focal and palpable lesions are the hallmark of neoplasm (Fig. 201-4). Bilateral involvement suggests systemic conditions. The character, quality, and quantity of the salivary secretions are also important. Serous secretions suggest a viral etiology, whereas malodorous purulent material indicates bacterial disease. The presence of fever, chills, or a recent upper respiratory infection should also be ascertained. An immunization history for mumps vaccine should be obtained. Questioning should elicit any history of trauma including injury from blunt or sharp objects, animal scratches, or recent dental procedures. The presence of congenital anomalies or cysts should be identified. Awareness of any underlying systemic diseases, which may include immune deficiency, allergy, or autoimmune disease, can be helpful.

The physical examination should include bimanual palpation of all major salivary glands. This consists of simultaneous palpation of the salivary gland structures in both intraoral and extraoral manners. This will also help distinguish salivary gland enlargement from cervical lymphadenopathy. It is important to identify whether the mass is cystic or solid, tender or nontender, and mobile or fixed. Facial movement (CN VII) should be assessed for subtle asymmetry or weakness. Symmetry and mobility of the tongue (CN XII) and sensation of the tongue (CN V) should be checked. Fixed nodules, cervical lymphadenopathy, and facial nerve involvement suggest malignant disease. Floor-of-mouth masses with enlarged perifacial lymph nodes need to be assessed for submandibular malignancy. Careful inspection of the salivary gland orifices should be performed with attention focused on the quantity (minimal, adequate, or excessive) and consistency (serous or suppurative) of the salivary content during palpation or "milking" the gland. Repeat examination may be helpful and necessary to follow the natural history of the disease.

Laboratory Studies

Laboratory studies are helpful in diagnosing and following salivary gland disease in children. If an infectious etiology is present, the leukocyte count will assist in determining whether adequate therapy is

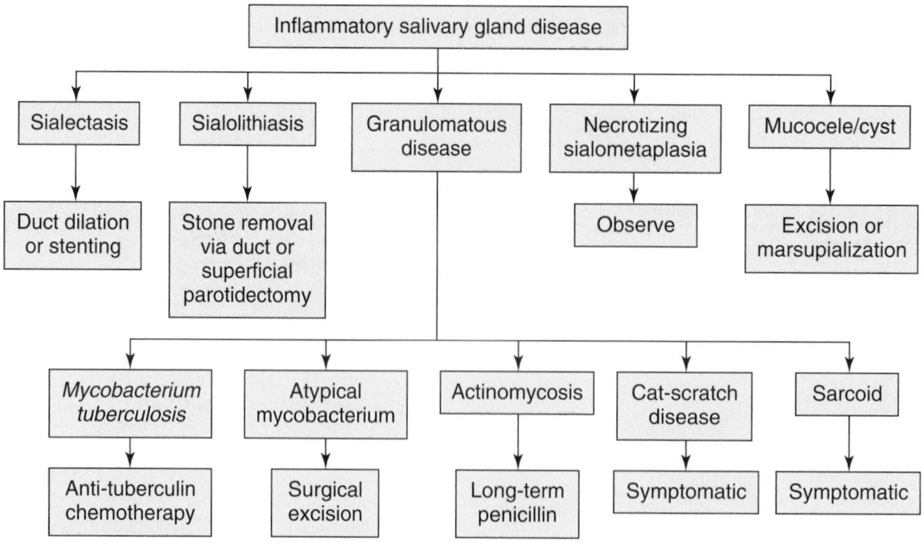

- Inflammatory salivary gland disease
  - Sialectasis → Duct dilation or stenting
  - Sialolithiasis → Stone removal via duct or superficial parotidectomy
  - Granulomatous disease
    - *Mycobacterium tuberculosis* → Anti-tuberculin chemotherapy
    - Atypical mycobacterium → Surgical excision
    - Actinomycosis → Long-term penicillin
    - Cat-scratch disease → Symptomatic
    - Sarcoid → Symptomatic
  - Necrotizing sialometaplasia → Observe
  - Mucocele/cyst → Excision or marsupialization

Figure 201-4. Inflammatory salivary gland disease.

being used. C-reactive protein is another nonspecific marker for bacterial infections and can be followed for treatment progress. Patients with risk factors or suspicion for human immunodeficiency virus (HIV) must be tested appropriately. A purified protein derivative (PPD) skin test and chest radiograph are employed in the pediatric population with salivary disease when mycobacterial infections (tuberculosis and atypical) are considered. Aerobic and anaerobic cultures of purulent material draining from duct orifices may help direct antibiotic coverage.

FNA is an easy and relatively safe technique for the diagnosis of palpable or deep-lying salivary masses. This can often be employed as an adjunct to diagnostic ultrasonography during the evaluation of pediatric salivary masses. With a well-trained cytopathologist, FNA can be an effective tool in diagnosing difficult lesions. In adults, up to 93% of benign and malignant lesions of the salivary glands can be differentiated.[5] Unfortunately, FNA is not commonly employed in the pediatric population because sedation or general anesthesia is often required. Moreover, pediatric pathologists are not universally versed in identification of salivary tumors due to the rarity of neoplasms in this population. Nonetheless, the unique architecture of pleomorphic adenoma and Warthin's tumor often makes it easy to diagnose them by FNA. Cytologic evaluation of sialadenitis shows polymorphonuclear leukocytes in a background of necrotic cellular debris. Cultures may also be obtained from aspirated contents at the time of FNA. Cystic lesions and poorly differentiated carcinomas are more difficult to assess by FNA and should undergo excisional biopsy for definitive answers.

In general, unusual and longstanding salivary masses should undergo FNA in tolerant pediatric patients before a surgical plan is developed. Surgical resection of discovered malignancies by FNA can be designed more appropriately. Misdiagnoses and nondiagnostic results are rare in FNA of pediatric head and neck masses. Regardless, most fine-needle aspirates lead to the diagnosis of a chronic inflammatory condition and can offset the use of open procedures in pediatric patients.[6,7]

Radiology

Radiographic imaging has played an increasing role in the diagnosis and perioperative decision making for salivary gland lesions. Improved radiographic instruments have allowed practitioners to delineate inflammatory and benign disease from malignant processes. Commonly employed techniques include plain film radiography, ultrasonography, sialography, radionucleotide scanning, computed tomography (CT), and magnetic resonance imaging (MRI). New MR technologies such as dynamic contrast-enhanced MRI, diffusion-weighted MRI, and MR spectrscopy have proven helpful in better differentiating benign from malignant salivary gland tumors.[8]

In children, ultrasonography is the most useful tool in evaluating salivary gland pathology and can be employed as a primary radiographic modality in nearly all cases. Ultrasound is an expedient, safe, and relatively painless technique that is ideal for examining pediatric patients. Ultrasonography can identify and assess adjacent vascular structures, distinguish focal from diffuse disease, clarify cystic from solid masses, and guide FNA. Lesions can be measured and easily followed with repeat examinations. The location of obstructing calculi within salivary ducts, despite their radiolucency, can be identified clearly with ultrasound. Nearly all sialoliths greater than 2 mm in size can be detected. Additional advantages to ultrasonography include low cost, avoidance of radiation, and avoidance of anesthesia.

Simple plain film radiography has become a less frequently used imaging tool for pediatric salivary masses as imaging speed and quality has improved in more informative radiographic tools such as CT and MRI. However, plain films remain easy to perform and detect the presence of radiopaque ductal stones within the major salivary glands. Unfortunately, up to 20% of submandibular calculi and 80% of parotid calculi are radiolucent and not well visualized with this technique.

Sialography involves the injection of contrast medium into the salivary duct during radiographic imaging in order to outline the salivary ductal system. Similar to plain film radiographs, this technique is gradually being replaced by CT sialography, MRI, and salivary duct endoscopy.[9,10] CT sialography can be valuable for detecting sialolithiasis, ductal dilatation, and strictures of the major salivary glands and has been used to evaluate obstructive disease, inflammatory lesions, penetrating trauma, and mass lesions. A filling defect and dilation of the main duct or intraglandular ducts will be seen when calculi are present. Chronic sialadenitis may show sialectasis or ductal ectasia. Salivary fistula or sialoceles can be picked up using this technique following trauma to a salivary gland.[11] Regardless, in the face of acute sialadenitis, sialography should not be performed because this can exacerbate disease and injure the involved gland.

For complete evaluation of the nature and extent of salivary gland masses, cross-sectional imaging with CT or MRI is necessary. Contrast-enhanced CT is best fitted for evaluating inflammatory conditions such as abscesses, obstructing sialoadenitis, cystic disease, sialolithiasis, and acute inflammation. Imaging should be performed both before and after administration of intravenous contrast. CT is an excellent tool to study both intrinsic and extrinsic masses of the parotid gland, and the relationship of the mass to critical anatomic structures such as the facial nerve are well illustrated with coronal and sagittal reconstructions.[8] The main benefits of CT scans in children are its speed and quietness relative to the slow, claustrophobic, and loud nature of MRI machines.

Bony architecture is better defined by CT and can provide information on the integrity of adjacent bone in malignant processes.

However, in patients with suspected neoplastic disease, MRI provides the best information on the exact location and degree of disease penetration.[11] In malignant processes, tumor infiltration of adjacent structures, soft tissue destruction, perineural spread, and meningeal penetration is best detected by MRI. This provides more information for operative planning. Standard axial T1- and T2-weighted MRI illustrate tumor margins and growth patterns. Coronal images, fat suppression, and gadolinium enhancement help identify perineural spread. Moreover, newer MR techniques have the ability to delineate benign from malignant processes with reported sensitivities and specificities above 90% using dynamic contrast or diffusion weighted methodology.[8] The drawback of MRI is that it can be difficult for children to tolerate and thereby be subject to the risks of sedation or general anesthesia required to perform the procedure.

Sialendoscopy

Sialendoscopy is a novel technique that has gained acceptance as a tool for diagnosing and treating a variety of salivary gland lesions in adults.[12] Since its development in the early 1990s, improvements in instruments and technique have allowed its application in the pediatric population. Semirigid sialendoscopes with external diameters between 1.1 mm and 1.6 mm are now available and can accommodate the pediatric salivary duct orifices. The endoscope includes two channels, one for irrigation and the other for instrumentation. Following routine dilation of the salivary duct, sialendoscopy is performed with continuous irrigation to maintain patency during exploration. This tool is best designed, and has proven applicable, to diagnose and treat obstructive pathology of pediatric unilateral salivary diseases. Diagnosis of salivary duct stenosis can be achieved with this technique, while wire baskets, lithotripsy, and YAG lasers can be simultaneously deployed to address small obstructing sialoliths.[13]

Biopsy

When diagnosis of a salivary mass has proven difficult with other modalities, open surgical biopsy is the next best approach. A solid, firm mass that persists for more than 6 weeks is a good candidate for open surgical biopsy. An incisional biopsy is inappropriate unless lymphoma is present; the cell type must be determined to direct management. An excisional biopsy should be performed following nondiagnostic FNA in a mass with a high index of suspicion for malignancy. Also, when confidence in cytopathology is low or an FNA cannot be performed, excisional biopsy is warranted. For masses within the superficial lobe of the parotid gland, an excisional biopsy will include the whole lobe with identification and preservation of the facial nerve. Occasionally, an isolated parotid tail lesion can be excised without the need for a superficial parotidectomy or facial nerve dissection. Tumors of the submandibular gland require complete excision of the gland and removal of adjacent lymph nodes (perifacial) for appropriate oncologic workup. Local excision with wide margins should be performed with minor salivary gland lesions. Examination of the draining lymphatic beds should be performed both prior and during excisional biopsies. Radiographic imaging with CT or MRI will help assess the extent of deep tissue penetration before elective biopsy.

Inflammatory Diseases of the Salivary Glands

Inflammatory conditions of the salivary glands are rare in children. Acute processes occur in the majority of cases that involve either viral or bacterial disease. The peak incidence is during puberty with most cases occurring between 12 and 18 years of age (>40%).[14] Submandibular disease is most commonly associated with proximal sialolithiasis and should be investigated appropriately. Granulomatous disease is a cause for a significant bulk of cases (primarily in toddlers) due to inflamed periglandular lymph nodes. Similar to adults, immunocompromised children are particularly prone to salivary gland infections and ductal stasis and obstruction and should be monitored closely. The most common clinical manifestation of salivary gland involvement is xerostomia and bilateral painless enlargement of the parotid glands.[15] Autoimmune disorders in children are rare but often manifest as inflammation of the major salivary glands.

Viral

Once the most common cause of viral sialadenitis, the mumps virus has virtually been eliminated as a cause of parotitis in the United States since the institution of the mumps vaccine in 1982. However, a few cases emerge annually in local and migrating patients who are without prior vaccination. The reader is directed to review the current guidelines and contraindications for mumps vaccination, which is beyond the scope of this chapter. However, other viruses can mimic mumps sialadenitis and should be included in the differential of vaccinated children with diffuse bilateral salivary gland disease. Beyond mumps, the most common viral sources of childhood sialadenitis are Epstein-Barr virus (EBV, incidence = 14%), parainfluenza viruses (4%, types 1, 2 and 3), adenovirus, (3%), HHV-6, human immunodeficiency virus, coxsackievirus, and influenza.[16] Most cases of viral sialadenitis are self-limited with conservative management of warm compresses, sialogogues, analgesics, anti-inflammatories, and hydration as the mainstay of therapy. The disease course of a few viral processes deserves special mention.

Mumps

Mumps parotitis is characterized by self-limiting bilateral diffuse parotid and submandibular gland enlargement. The gonads, meninges, and pancreas can also be involved and should be examined in these patients. The disease more frequently occurs during the winter and spring months, with 85% of cases occurring in the pediatric age group. The incubation period is 14 to 21 days, but the contagious period lasts from 2 to 3 days before the development of swelling and lasts until the swelling remits. During the incubation period, the patient develops a prodrome of symptoms including malaise, loss of appetite, chills, fever, and sore throat. The major salivary glands become tender and swollen, and the patient reports trismus and difficulty chewing. Although the duct orifice may be swollen, the saliva is clear. The temperature is elevated to 100° F to 103° F, and the leukocyte count is normal or slightly elevated with lymphocytosis. Although the diagnosis is clinical, amylase levels, complement fixation, and hemagglutination tests can be used for confirmation. Histologic examination reveals extensive cytoplasmic vacuolization of acinar cells. Management is symptomatic, and the swelling usually resolves over several weeks. Complications include sialectasis, exacerbation of diabetes, orchitis, meningoencephalitis, and sensorineural hearing loss (especially unilateral).

Epstein-Barr Virus

EBV is the cause of heterophil-positive infectious mononucleosis and has been implicated as a major cause of acute inflammation of the salivary glands in pubescent children.[16] Disease symptoms range from an asymptomatic infection to fulminant lymphoproliferative disease. EBV is emitted in the saliva and has been colloquially termed the "kissing" disease due to its oral transmission. In fact, 10% to 20% of healthy seropositive persons can shed EBV into their oropharynx.

The long incubation period of EBV ranges from 30 to 50 days. A triad of fever, sore throat, and posterior cervical adenopathy occurs in more than 80% of patients. Lethargy can persist for months in infected patients. The cervical adenopathy can involve the periparotid or perifacial (submandibular) lymph nodes with subsequent involvement of adjacent glands. Again, there is no specific therapy for EBV infection, but improvements in serologic detection have helped practitioners identify disease early and accurately. Children often need weeks of isolation and rest before returning to normal daily activity. Corticosteroids can be used for life-threatening complications but are unlikely necessary in isolated salivary gland cases. Recently, nearly 50% of salivary gland tumors and oral malignancies of nonodontogenic origin have been associated with EBV. Thus in children with rare oropharyngeal or salivary malignancies, isolation of EBV genome by polymerase chain reaction may help families come to terms with the source of such rare tumors.[17]

Human Immunodeficiency Virus

Salivary gland disease is a common manifestation of HIV in infected children. More than 50% of cases of pediatric HIV present with head and neck masses with the majority of patients having major salivary gland enlargement.[18] The enlargement can be lymphoproliferative, cystic, or both, with the parotid glands being the most frequently affected salivary entity. Parotid swelling of various degrees has been found in more than 10% of HIV-positive children.[19] The submandibular and sublingual glands can be involved as well. The incidence of ranula has been shown to be increased in HIV pediatric patients.[20] The high rate of salivary gland involvement is probably related to the presence of HIV within the saliva. Quantitative changes to the saliva can contribute to glandular hypertrophy, reduced salivary flow, stasis of secretions, and xerostomia.[21] Slow continuous enlargement is the hallmark disease in pediatric AIDS patients. The pathophysiology remains elusive. However, in children, bilateral lymphoepithelial cystic enlargement or intraglandular lymph node enlargement of the parotid glands is common. Cystic disease can often be seen in combination with lymphocytic interstitial pneumonitis.[22] Latent manifestation of EBV and cytomegalovirus in these patients may also contribute to salivary gland pathology.

Management of an HIV salivary lesion is generally conservative. Acute symptoms should be managed similarly to other salivary gland disease in healthy pediatric patients with techniques such as sialogogues and warm compresses. Imaging (CT or MRI) will help identify occult pathology. Antibiotic coverage for potential bacterial processes and fluoride treatment to prevent dental caries from xerostomia should also be employed. Consultation with an infectious diseases specialist is appropriate in these complex patients. Needle aspiration is indicated if a salivary lesion in an HIV-positive child grows to an uncomfortable or deforming size. Patients with HIV are particularly susceptible to lymphoma and Kaposi's sarcoma and can present with isolated salivary gland masses. Open biopsy is indicated only for lesions suspected of malignancy (lymphoma, Kaposi's sarcoma) that cannot be identified by FNA.

Bacterial

Primary bacterial salivary gland infections are rare in the pediatric population. Dental infections, periglandular lymphadenitis, and floor of mouth and submandibular triangle processes need to be considered in the differential of acute bacterial sialadenitis because these may be the source of inflamed salivary tissues. When suppurative sialadenitis does present, it most commonly occurs acutely and within the parotid gland. The normally serous saliva of these glands contains limited bacteriostatic activity (lysozymes) compared with the mucinous secretions of the submandibular and sublingual glands and likely contributes to the predominance of bacterial disease occurring in the parotid. Submandibular gland infections are associated with proximal sialolithiasis more than 40% of the time.[14] This is rare for the parotid gland.[23] The primary cause of submandibular infections appears to be salivary stasis of dependent and viscous mucous secretions of the submandibular duct. Predisposing factors include congential Wharton's duct stricture, ductal trauma, dehydration, autoimmune disorders, and congenital sialectasis. Similarly, recurrent sialadenitis has been associated with traumatic injury to the ductal orifices by repetitive biting of the buccal mucosa, dental appliances, and tooth eruption.[24] Retrograde oral bacteria transmission via the salivary ducts is thought be a culprit in disease.

Signs and symptoms of acute bacterial sialadenitis include rapid onset of focal pain, edema, and erythema of the soft tissues overlying the affected gland. Disease is predominantly unilateral. Spiking fevers are often present with symptoms worsening during deglutition. Purulent discharge found draining from the involved gland's duct is pathognomonic for disease. Most children remain nontoxic during acute episodes but, as the acute phase passes, residual induration and enlargement of the gland may persist for several months. Facial nerve paresis is extremely rare. The most common pathogens associated with bacterial sialadenitis are coagulase-positive *Staphylococcus aureus, Streptococcus viridans,* and *Haemophilus influenzae.* Less frequently identified bacteria include *Streptococcus pneumoniae, Escherichia coli, Bacteroides melaninogenicus,* and *Streptococcus micros* (Table 201-2).[25,26] Cultures of aspirated material or swabs of the purulent ductal secretions will help guide antibiotic coverage.

Table 201-2
Acute Suppurative Sialadenitis

Most common	*Staphylococcus aureus* (coagulase-positive) *Streptococcus viridans* *Haemophilus influenzae* *Peptostreptococcus* spp.
Less common	*Streptococcus pneumoniae* *Escherichia coli* *Bacteroides melaninogenicus*

Management includes the use of systemic antibiotics, local heat and massage, fluids, and sialogogues (lemon juice, sour candy). Penicillinase-resistant antistaphylococcal antibiotics are recommended to cover gram-positive and anaerobic organisms until culture results return. Rarely, patients not responding to initial therapy may require intravenous antibiotics and hospitalization. Screening for immunocompromised states is thereby recommended. Bacterial disease not responding to standard therapy should also be evaluated for underlying granulomatous or neoplastic processes including mycobacterial infections, cat-scratch disease, and lymphoma.

Abscess

Persistent inflammation, hyperpyrexia, and progressive edema overlying the parotid gland suggest the possibility of an abscess. The gland will not be fluctuant until late in abscess formation because of the numerous fascial investments within the gland. Ultrasonography can help diagnose and potentially guide FNA of a parotid abscess, so it should be employed initially in these cases. Significant involvement of adjacent structures or evidence of deep soft tissue disease warrants a CT examination of the head and neck. If an abscess is identified, surgical incision and drainage is appropriate. Drainage is accomplished through a standard parotid incision along the preauricular crease, raising a skin flap, and then opening the superficial glandular fascia parallel to the branches of the facial nerve. Drains should be placed, and the wound closed loosely to heal by secondary intention. One must observe for spread of disease into the contiguous fascial spaces of the neck and mediastinum.

Submandibular abscesses are frequently associated with proximal ductal sialolithiasis. Rapid enlargement of the submandibular triangle suggests diffuse disease within this confined space. Patients will complain of submandibular and floor-of-mouth pain shortly after a meal. Extension beyond the submandibular space can lead to Ludwig's angina and airway obstruction and should be treated urgently. Removal of the involved gland is recommended therapy with drainage of the overlying abscess within the submandibular and sublingual fascial compartments. Airway status and the need for temporary tracheotomy should be evaluated when managing patients with Ludwig's angina.

Recurrent Sialadenitis

Repeated infections of the salivary glands have been shown to cause ductal metaplasia, parenchymal restructuring, and an increase in mucin production and quantity of viscous secretions that can lead to recurrent salivary stasis. Patients with recurrent disease present with low-grade edema and tenderness of the gland with slightly purulent secretions. Unfortunately, once the glandular architecture is altered, opportunistic oral flora are more likely to cause recurrent disease. These patients are frequently chronically infected with various organisms, and immunologic dysfunction such as IgA deficiency appears to play a role in its development.[27,28] Broad-spectrum antibiotics should be used and measures to increase salivary flow and reduce viscosity need to be instituted. Ductal dilatation may improve cases of recalcitrant disease. Gland excision remains the last resort for treatment. Although the most effective and reliable mode of therapy is parotidectomy, many surgeons delay definitive surgery for fear of injuring the facial nerve during surgical dissection. A total parotidectomy with facial nerve preservation is appropriate for recurrent parotitis because superficial parotidectomy alone is thought to increase the risk of recurrent disease.

Neonatal Sialadenitis

Neonatal sialadenitis is more common in the parotid gland than in the submandibular gland. Possible causes of neonatal sialadenitis are anatomic deformities of the oral cavity, dehydration, sialolithiasis, and prematurity. Approximately 40% of neonates with parotitis are premature. The most common organism in neonatal sialadenitis is *S. aureus.* Other organisms identified are *E. coli, Pseudomonas aeruginosa, Moraxella catarrhalis,* and various streptococci. The salivary secretions should be cultured and a Gram stain obtained. The disease is usually limited to a single gland and signs and symptoms of systemic disease may not be seen. Diagnosis is confirmed by physical examination when a warm, tender, erythematous mass is palpated and pus is expressed from the accompanying salivary duct. Appropriate antimicrobial therapy and adequate hydration result in resolution of the disease in less than 1 week. Recurrence is uncommon.[29] Lymphadenitis of nodes surrounding the parotid or submandibular gland, or both, can mimic sialadenitis. This may be difficult to determine on physical examination. Ultrasonography is helpful in cases not responding to conservative medical management (hydration, antibiotics). Infections involving the scalp, face, or nasopharynx need to be considered.

Viral sialadenitis is seen infrequently during the perinatal period but may occur when there is maternal transmission of virus. This is influenced by the onset of maternal disease, the mode of transmission (transplacental or at delivery), the type of virus, and the host's defenses. A mumps infection in the newborn can range from mild to severe and careful observation is necessary. Cytomegalovirus is another potential viral source of sialadenitis in newborns. Diagnosis can be determined by urine examination. However, its course may be devastating and should be considered early in infants with salivary inflammation. Clearly, infants with suspected viral sialadenitis should be isolated from other newborns.

Necrotizing Sialometaplasia

Necrotizing sialometaplasia is a benign, self-healing (reactive) inflammatory process of salivary gland tissue that clinically and histologically mimics a malignant neoplasm. It most commonly affects adults but has been reported in adolescents. It arises in mucus-secreting cells and can be found in the parotid gland, sublingual gland, hard and soft palates, and lower lip. Its clinical appearance ranges from minor submucosal edema with overlying erythema to an erosive ulcer. It usually presents as a painless ulcerated lesion or a nodular swelling. Most cases involving the extrapalatal minor salivary glands and major salivary glands are iatrogenically induced after surgery, trauma, or radiotherapy, with a mean duration of 18 days from the insult to the development of the lesion. In the major salivary glands, necrotizing sialometaplasia occurs secondary to focal lobular sialadenitis and prior surgical manipulation.[25,30] Typically, the process appears as a 1- to 3-cm crater-like ulcerative lesion. Histologically, lobular necrosis is present with pools of mucin that elicit a granulation tissue reaction with associated acute and chronic inflammation. In addition, extensive squamous cell metaplasia is present. The lesion heals spontaneously in 6 to 12 weeks. Although total excision of the lesion may be carried out as definitive therapy, it is not necessary or indicated.[30]

Granulomatous Disease

Granulomatous diseases are characterized by intense inflammatory reactions, sponsored by the host, around a central pathogen or antigen within one or more organ systems. Granulomatous processes, despite the etiology, rarely involve the salivary system. However, several pathogens causing granulomatous inflammation of the major salivary glands have been identified. In particular, actinomycosis, tuberculosis, atypical mycobacterial infections, and sarcoidosis have all been implicated. Their incidence in children remains unknown, but they are considered unusual. In these conditions, salivary gland involvement is often the result of inflamed periglandular lymph nodes. Regardless, granulomatous diseases should be included in the differential of pediatric patients with atypical and chronic salivary gland inflammation.

Mycobacterial

Nontuberculous mycobacterial infections of the salivary glands are most frequently seen in children. The average age at presentation is 16 to 36 months. Cervicofacial lymphadenitis is the most common manifestation. *Mycobacterium avium-intracellulare* accounts for 70% to 90% of cases. Involvement caused by *Mycobacterium bovis* has become less common since the widespread pasteurization of milk. Infection may occur by *Mycobacterium kansasii* and *Mycobacterium scrofulaceum.*[31] Periparotid and submandibular lymph nodes are frequently involved with the formation of cutaneous sinus tracts (Fig. 201-5). The Mantoux test will likely be weakly positive, whereas chest radiography is generally normal. Diagnosis is based on clinical judgment and exclusion of other diseases. FNA may help to rule out an abscess; however, culture results can take 6 weeks until an organism is seen. Management of nontuberculous mycobacterial infections may be conservative but usually requires surgical removal of the disease process. If the parotid gland is affected,

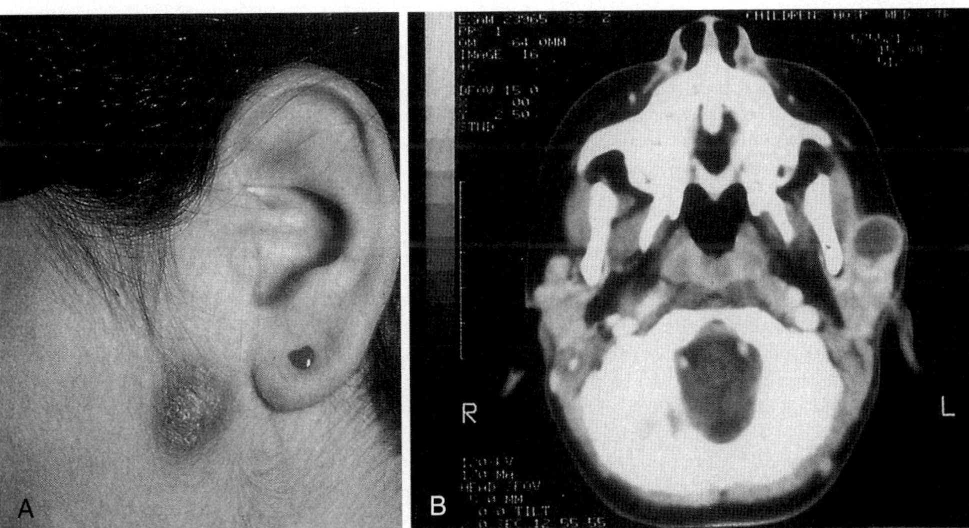

Figure 201-5. **A,** Patient with an atypical mycobacterial infection involving the parotid gland. **B,** Computed tomography with contrast of the same patient. Notice the rim-enhancing parotid lesion.

a superficial parotidectomy with facial nerve preservation is necessary. Removal of involved skin is often necessary during excision. Antituberculous drugs have not been effective in managing this condition. Use of a macrolide (e.g., clarithromycin) as an adjunct to surgery, especially in cases of incomplete excision, appears to be effective in some cases.

Primary tuberculosis of the salivary system is uncommon. No more than 100 cases affecting the salivary glands have been reported, but this disease entity should always be considered in patients with a slow-growing firm to hard nodular mass.[32] The parotid gland is most frequently involved and the disease generally stays unilateral. Primary tuberculosis parotitis is thought to develop from disease spreading via fascial communication with infected tonsils or teeth. Diagnosis may occur by FNA with aspirated material of the involved gland revealing *Mycobacterium tuberculosis* var. *hominis*. Polymerase chain reaction (PCR) testing of FNA contents has proven useful in difficult-to-diagnose cases. Treatment usually involves typical systemic antituberculosis drugs, but excision is frequently curative.

Actinomycosis

Actinomycosis is an infectious disease caused by a gram-positive anaerobic organism. Occurrence is usually in the cervicofacial region and frequently involves the salivary glands. Infections often follow dental extraction or oral trauma. The precipitating event allows mucosal invasion of the organism and a slowly progressive inflammatory reaction. Typically, patients have a painless, indurated enlargement of the gland that mimics a neoplasm. Lymph node necrosis characteristically leads to multiple draining cutaneous fistulae. FNA or fistulous tract drainage culture will reveal characteristic sulfur granules and gram-positive rods. Biopsy specimens are often multiloculated abscesses with whitish-yellow pus. Anaerobic cultures are positive. Management is with penicillin and consists of a 6-week parenteral course followed by 6 months of oral administration.[33] Cure rates approach 90%.

Sarcoid

Sarcoidosis is an idiopathic granulomatous disease. Sarcoidosis is less common in children but, when present, occurs in the second decade of life. It presents with bilateral diffuse enlargement of the parotid glands. Uveoparotid fever (Heerfordt's syndrome) is a form of sarcoidosis characterized by uveitis, parotid enlargement, and facial paralysis. Symptoms may include fever, malaise, weakness, nausea, and night sweats. Chest radiography looking for hilar adenopathy and an acetylcholinesterase level will assist with the diagnosis. A biopsy from the lip or tail of the parotid will confirm the diagnosis. The disease is self-limited, so no specific management is necessary with regard to salivary gland disease. Systemic involvement or complications may necessitate corticosteroid use.

Autoimmune Disease

Benign Lymphoepithelial Disease

Benign lymphoepithelial disease is typically seen in children older than 5 years of age. Although the cause is unknown, an autoimmune mechanism is suspected. It is characterized by unilateral or bilateral enlargement of the major or minor salivary glands or lacrimal glands.[34] Salivary gland enlargement in children with benign lymphoepithelial disease is usually sudden and is characterized by a tender gland accompanied by a fever. It persists for a variable length of time. In some cases, episodes of swelling are recurrent and the gland can remain enlarged. The condition usually resolves spontaneously during adolescence.

Benign lymphoepithelial disease is managed in an identical fashion to acute sialadenitis when purulent secretions are present. With recurrent disease, sialectasis and, rarely, cavitary changes can be shown on CT sialography or MRI. Medical therapy is appropriate unless cavitary changes occur, whereby the gland should then be removed. If an affected gland develops nodularity, distinction from a neoplasm is necessary. If FNA cannot differentiate the two, surgical excision is required.

Sjögren's Syndrome

Primary Sjögren's syndrome in children is uncommon. Sjögren's syndrome is characterized by lymphocyte-mediated destruction of the exocrine glands leading to xerostomia and keratoconjunctivitis sicca. Symptoms include burning oral discomfort and a sandy sensation in the eye. Patients with Sjögren's syndrome have a greater incidence of recurrent parotitis. If a child has recurrent parotitis and a history of dry eyes or xerostomia, further evaluation is indicated. Immunologic tests for antinuclear antibodies and antibodies to Sjögren's syndrome antigens A and B (SS-A and SS-B) are present in 50% to 80% of infected individuals. The sialographic abnormalities show varying degrees of sialectasis. This entity involves the minor salivary glands in 70% of patients and a diagnosis can be obtained with a labial, palatal, or tail of parotid biopsy. Management is symptomatic. In adults, this lesion is associated with an increased incidence of lymphoma.

Chronic Sialadenitis

Chronic inflammatory disease of the salivary glands, also known as *sialectasis,* is associated with repeated episodes of acute sialadenitis and subsequent obstruction of the glandular drainage pathway. The primary causative event is considered to be lowered secretion rate and salivary stasis. Chronic obstructive sialadenitis is associated frequently with salivary duct strictures or sialolithiasis. The strictures may have several causes including recurrent infection, trauma, neoplasms, or congenital abnormalities. Regardless of the cause, progressive dilation and sacculation of the salivary ductal system can lead to chronic uniglandular enlargement. This condition can lead to permanent damage to the gland with ductal ectasia, progressive acinar destruction, and lymphocytic infiltrate.[35]

A child with chronic sialadenitis usually presents with diffuse enlargement of a salivary gland. Massage of the gland will usually produce only small amounts of saliva at the duct orifice. Recurrent swelling will occur during eating, which is followed by gradual relief as emptying of the gland occurs over a 2-hour period. Over time, xerostomia becomes a complaint in up to 80% of patients. A stricture may sometimes be identified by sialography showing ductal dilation proximal to the stricture and delayed emptying of the ducts. Simple dilation or incision may correct the stricture. Repair of the parotid duct requires more elaborate surgery with a higher risk of failure. If a stricture is not found, chronic conservative therapy (sialogogues, massage, and antibiotics) will frequently control disease and prevent progression. When conservative measures fail, excision of the submandibular or parotid gland with facial nerve preservation is occasionally required. Chronic recurrent parotitis may lead to development of a benign lymphoepithelial lesion that may need removal for cosmetic reasons.

Juvenile Recurrent Parotitis

Although rare, juvenile recurrent parotitis (JRP) is the second most common inflammatory condition of the parotid gland next to mumps. It is marked by recurrent pain and swelling of one (60%) or both (40%) parotid glands that can have associated systemic features of fever and malaise. Xerostomia may be present as well. Nonpurulent secretions can be elicited from the parotid duct and set this disease apart from recurrent bacterial parotitis. The age of onset appears bimodal, with peak incidence around 3 to 6 and 10 years of age.[36] A decrease in the frequency of infections is observed during adolescent years.

Thought to be associated with nonobstructive sialectasis within the gland, JRP should be managed nonsurgically with conservative therapy such as analgesics, sialogogues, oral rinses, warm compresses, parotid massage, and antibiotics directed toward oral flora. JRP is an international phenomenon, but no consensus of etiology has been established. Causative factors may be congenital aberrations of the ductal architecture, autoimmune disease, genetic predisposition, allergy, or occult viral and bacterial infections. Regardless, ultrasound and sialography have been shown to help delineate JRP from other parotid entities. The heterogeneous echoes of JRP identified by ultrasound differ from the homogeneous echogenicity of parotid glands infected by mumps. Sialectasis identified by sialography or MRI supports the diagnosis.

Sialolithiasis

Salivary gland ductal calculi are unusual in children but should be considered in patients with chronic or recurrent salivary gland inflammation. Retrospective reviews suggest that only 3% to 13% of cases of sialolithiasis occur in the pediatric population. The average age of onset in this group is 12 years, with only rare presentations in children younger than 10 years old. As in adults, more than 90% of cases involve Wharton's duct of the submandibular glands, whereas calculi within Stensen's duct or the parotid gland are extremely unusual.[37] Salivary gland calculi form by deposition of calcium salts, predominantly calcium phosphate, around a central organic nidus (e.g., desquamated epithelial cells, bacteria, foreign body). Bacterial infection may initiate the process due to changes in pH, fluid composition, and ductal morphology. The submandibular glands release alkaline and viscous secretions that must traverse a long, tortuous, and narrow duct against gravity before entering the oral cavity. This leads to increased fluid stasis and susceptibility to calculi formation in contrast to the parotid gland, which expels serous material from a relatively short, broad, and dependent cannula.

Signs and symptoms of sialolithiasis in children are of shorter duration but more common than that seen in adults. Glandular pain and postprandial swelling are significant indicators of disease. In contrast to bacterial sialadenitis, purulent discharge is uncommon (2% to 12% of cases). Ductal obstruction leads to tenderness and inflammation of the involved gland. Symptoms increase with enlargement of the stone, ultimately requiring medical attention. Fevers may be present, too. In children younger than 10 years of age, tenderness is more often intraoral. A single calculus less than 1 cm in diameter within the distal aspect of the involved duct is generally the rule in children.[37] Often this can be palpated by bimanual examination and makes extraction easier. If necessary, dental occlusal radiographs and ultrasonography allow visualization and confirm the presence of calculi along the submandibular duct or parenchyma.

Management of a calculus near the orifice of the submandibular duct can be performed by probing the duct or through a small intraoral incision. If the calculus is positioned in the parenchyma of the submandibular gland, gland removal is required. During excision, the duct should be ligated as close to the mouth as possible to prevent infection of the ductal remnant. Parotid calculi near the orifice of the duct can be removed intraorally, but the duct should be repaired and stented to prevent postoperative stricture. If a calculus within the parenchyma of the parotid gland causes persistent symptoms, a parotidectomy, with facial nerve preservation, may be required.

Sialendoscopy is a novel option in addressing pediatric salivary gland stones. Endoscopes approaching 1.1 mm in size are now available. The endoscope constitutes two channels, one for the irrigation and the other for endoscopy. Continuous irrigation during endoscopy is required to maintain duct patency following standard dilatation. Wire baskets, YAG laser, and lithotripsy have proven effective in treating small obstructing stones from the salivary duct orifice of adult patients.[12] Some evidence suggest the applicability of sialendoscopy in children.[13,38]

Cysts and Mucoceles

Acquired

Acquired salivary cysts may be associated with neoplasms, benign lymphoepithelial lesions, trauma, parotitis, calculi, duct obstruction, or mucus extravasation. Mucous retention cysts usually involve the minor salivary glands and are commonly seen on the lips, buccal mucosa, and tongue. These true cysts with an epithelial lining result from duct obstruction. A ranula is a mucous retention cyst of the sublingual gland and is described as plunging when it extends from the floor of the mouth through the mylohyoid musculature into the neck. Mucoceles, in contrast, are not true cysts and do not contain an epithelial lining. Mucoceles represent mucous extravasation into the surrounding soft tissue. If necessary, management of mucous retention cysts and mucoceles is by excision or marsupialization.

Congenital

Congenital salivary gland cysts can be classified into dermoid cysts, congenital ductal cysts, and branchial cleft anomalies. Dermoid cysts characteristically contain white keratinizing squamous epithelium that is apparent on excision. These cysts are composed of elements from all three germinal layers. Dermoid cysts usually appear as isolated masses within the substance of the parotid gland. Total removal is necessary to prevent recurrence. This is best accomplished by a subtotal parotidectomy with facial nerve preservation. Congenital ductal cysts most commonly occur within the parotid gland and are rare at other salivary locations. In contrast to dermoids, congenital ductal cysts generally manifest in infancy as enlargement of the parotid gland. The diagnosis can be confirmed with sialography and observation is advised unless recurrent infections occur.

Derivatives of embryologic branchial clefts can also emerge within or adjacent to major salivary glands. The parotid gland is often involved when a first branchial cleft anomaly is present. These can be either type 1 or type 2 first branchial cleft anomalies, which are defined by their location and presence of ectoderm, with or without mesoderm, within the cyst parenchyma (see Fig. 201-8). Type 2 anomalies are more frequently associated with the parotid gland as they course anterior and inferior to the auricle into the gland parenchyma along their path toward the neck. The tract always passes close to the facial nerve and often ends inferior to the angle of the mandible. Infections or drainage of these anomalies often lead to their diagnosis. Safe removal of these anomalies requires preoperative CT or MR imaging and intraoperative facial nerve dissection.

Type 1 branchial defects are duplication anomalies of the membranous external auditory canal. These defects are composed only of ectoderm. Located within the periauricular soft tissues and the parotid gland, they commonly present as sinus tracts or areas of localized swelling near the postauricular sulcus, concha, or anterior tragus. The tympanic membrane and middle ear space are rarely involved. Complete surgical removal is curative. Histologic examination reveals a squamous epithelial lining without skin appendages. When the lesion extends into the parotid gland, the facial nerve should be identified and preserved.

Vascular Anomalies

Vascular anomalies of the head and neck commonly involve one or more salivary entities. On the basis of the histologic classification derived by Mulliken and Glowacki,[39] and agreed on by the International Society for the Study of Vascular Anomalies in 1996, vascular anomalies are classified as either vascular tumors or vascular malformations. Hemangiomas are the most frequently encountered representative of the former. They are composed of aberrant and rapidly proliferating endothelial cells often confined within the substance of the cutaneous and subcutaneous tissue. Extension into deeper structures may occur as seen in the parotid gland. Most will present within the first 6 weeks of life and, unlike other tumors, will characteristically involute over time. This has led to a benign neglect approach to hemangiomas because most will resolve without sequelae. Other vascular tumors include Kaposi-like infantile hemangioendotheliomas and glomus tumors that develop from aberrant proliferation of vascular cells but do not follow the natural course of hemangiomas. In contrast, vascular malformations consist of ectatic development of vascular channels of one or more elements of the normal circulatory system. On the basis of their source vessels, they are subclassified into venous, lymphatic, arterial-venous, and lymphatic-venous malformations. They grow by expansion and vascular recruitment and, without intervention, can eventually invade normal structural architecture including muscle and bone. Although rare, vascular malformations can be notoriously difficult to cure because recurrence is common depending on their type.

Hemangiomas

Hemangiomas are the most common benign tumor of the parotid gland. Of salivary gland hemangiomas, 80% occur in the parotid gland, 18% in the submandibular gland, and 2% in the minor salivary glands. This parotid tumor is generally contained within the subcutaneous and intracapsular portion of the gland with rare extension into the submucosa, mucosa, or dermis (Fig. 201-6). They are usually discovered shortly after birth (3 to 6 weeks). After it appears, the hemangioma grows rapidly over months and plateaus for a period of time before its slow but progressive involution. Of affected children, 50% have com-

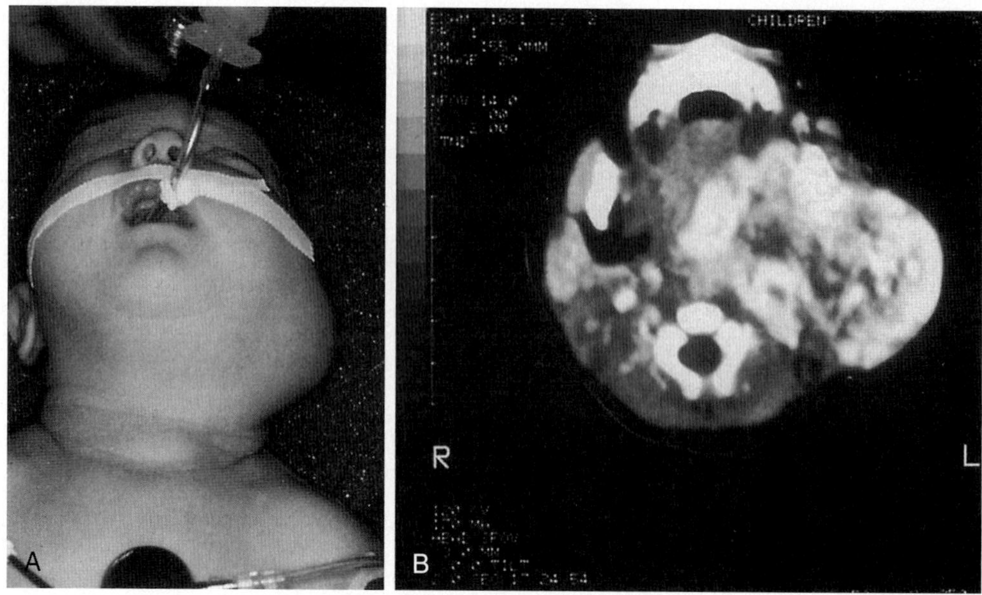

Figure 201-6. **A,** Patient with a hemangioma of the parotid gland. **B,** Computed tomography with contrast shows a parotid gland mass consistent with a hemangioma and extension into the retropharyngeal space.

plete involution of the lesion by age 5 years, 70% have involution by 7 years of age, and 90% by 9 years of age.[40]

Infants with parotid hemangiomas typically present with asymptomatic facial asymmetry and a fluctuant cheek mass that is soft to rubbery on palpation. Vascular staining may indicate disease. Bright red macules or bluish discoloration will indicate either superficial or deep (subcutaneous) disease, respectively. Parotid hemangiomas can be either segmental or focal with the former often engaged in other locations of the face either in a random or more frequently encountered "beard" distribution with involvement of both parotid glands. Hemangiomas can cause the parotid gland to increase up to five times its normal size. Focal disease frequently undergoes a defined proliferative phase up to 1 year of life that is followed by gradual involution. The proliferative phase of segmental disease is less clear because these lesions generally grow larger, take longer to involute, and are more difficult to eradicate than their focal counterparts. Regardless, the general lobular architecture of the native gland is typically preserved with limited or no impact on the acini and ductal structures.

Diagnosis is usually by history and physical examination. If necessary, ultrasound, CT, or MRI will confirm the diagnosis. Biopsy is unnecessary; however, if the mass is firm, painful, or rapidly grows, histologic sampling may be necessary to rule out a malignancy. Most of these tumors undergo spontaneous involution, which requires the use of observation to follow up most of these lesions. Potential complications of hemangiomas may include a localized consumptive coagulopathy known as the *Kasabach-Merritt syndrome.*

Excision of a salivary gland hemangioma is indicated when there is excessively rapid growth of the mass, severe facial deformity, functional impairment, infection, hemorrhage, or ulceration. Laser therapy has not proven completely effective over natural involution to reduce vascular staining or speed involution of these tumors.[41] However, use of the flash pump dye laser is appropriate for ulcerative and bleeding lesions because this can lead to rapid epithelialization and repair of these sites.[42] If necessary, subtotal parotidectomy, with facial nerve preservation, or total submandibular gland excision can be performed and only after the end of the proliferative phase of these lesions. Bipolar cautery is recommended because it eases dissection of these highly vascular tumors. Segmental disease is likely better managed with either systemic or intralesional injections (triamcinolone acetonide/betamethasone [Kenalog/Celestone] mixture) of corticosteroids because resection of these multiple lesions and sites can be difficult. Steroids should be instituted only during the proliferative phase. Although controversial, recent investigation into these treatment modalities has illustrated improved functional and cosmetic results.[43,44] Nonetheless, the risk of systemic side effects of corticosteroids including hypertension, irritability, Cushing's syndrome, and adrenal insufficiency should be respected and frequently monitored during their use. Tapering systemic doses to therapeutic response is advocated.[44] Interferon is no longer recommended for fear of spastic diplegia and has been circumvented by the use of vincristine for complicated disease. Of final note, patients with segmental facial hemangiomas involving the parotid should be screened for associated anomalies of PHACES syndrome including Posterior fossa abnormalities, Arterial anomalies, Cardiac anomalies, Eye abnormalities, and Sternal defects, with MRI, echocardiogram and ophthalmologic referral.

Lymphatic Malformations

Of the vascular malformations, lymphatic malformations are those that most commonly affect the salivary structures, making them the second most common vascular anomaly found in the salivary glands. Before the recent classification of vascular anomalies, these lesions have been previously named cystic hygromas and lymphangiomas. A venous component to these lesions is also common (lymphatic-venous malformations) and should be considered at initial evaluation and when surgical resection is considered.

Lymphatic malformations are soft, painless, and compressible benign masses that represent areas of regional lymphatic dilation. Lymphatic malformations have been divided into two categories on the basis of the size of their lymphatic channel aberrations. Lesions consisting predominantly of small lymphatic spaces, less than 2 cm in diameter, are considered microcystic. Those with spaces greater than 2 cm are known as *macrocystic lymphatic malformations* and have been known as cystic hygromas in the past. Mixed lesions of these two types are also common.

Lymphatic malformations involve the head and neck in more than 50% of cases. Infiltration of the salivary glands is common but not frequently the source of disease.[45] These malformations can involve any of the major salivary glands and usually present as an asymptomatic fluctuant mass (Fig. 201-7). They are present at birth and grow at unpredictable rates. However, rapid growth and ectasia can occur with upper respiratory tract infections. Approximately 50% to 60% of patients present with these tumors before age 1 and about 90% of the tumors occur before the end of the second year of life. The diagnosis can be confirmed when cystic areas, septations, and air fluid levels are found on imaging with ultrasound, CT, or MRI. Gadolinium-enhanced MRI will provide clarity of all soft tissues involved and is recommended

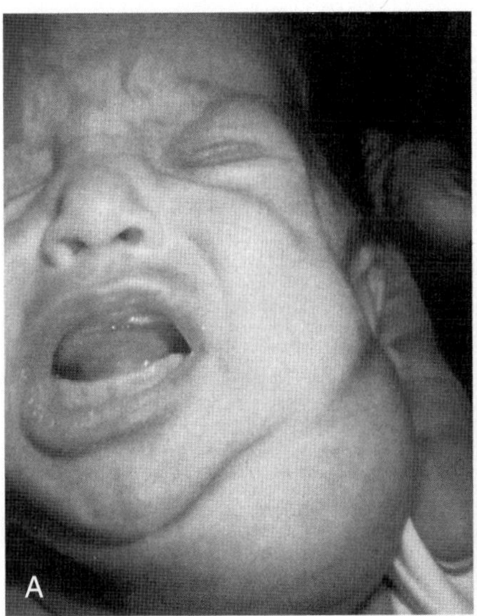

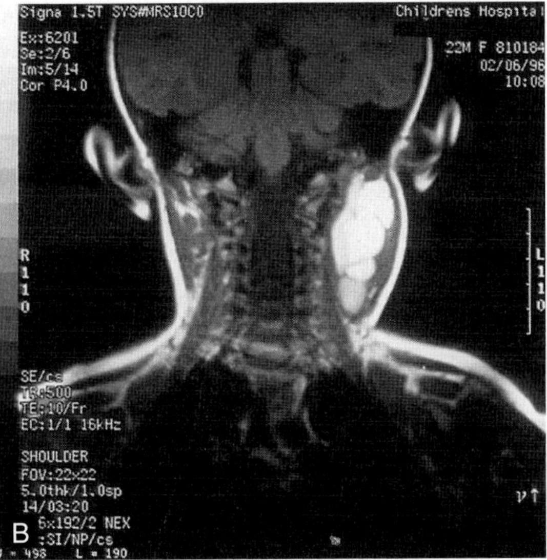

Figure 201-7. **A,** Lymphangioma with involvement of the submandibular and parotid glands. **B,** Magnetic resonance imaging (T1-weighted) shows multiple loculated spaces consistent with a lymphangioma.

as a primary imaging modality. Examination of the chest, mediastinum, and airway is recommended in larger lesions that are seen in approximately the lower third of the neck.

Unlike hemangiomas, lymphatic malformations rarely undergo spontaneous resolution. Although it has been reported in small lesions, resolution is thought to occur as a result of autosclerosis of the cystic space. More frequently, infiltration of local tissue, especially with microcystic disease, can lead to destruction and deformation of normal bone and muscle leading to significant functional and cosmetic consequences. Macrocystic disease (cystic hygroma) can be approached with either sclerotherapy or surgical resection. Sclerotherapy is recommended for deep lesions not surrounding prominent vascular or nervous structures because various agents (e.g., ethanol, bleomycin) have a small risk of associated nerve and vessel injury. Sclerosis of superficial lesions can also lead to skin ulceration. Consultation with the interventional radiologist is paramount for these vascular malformations.

Surgical removal of macrocystic disease is often curative. OK-432 (Picibanil) sclerotherapy, although not currently FDA approved, has been reported as a successful treatment of these lesions.[46] Definitive therapy potentially can be delayed until the child is several years old to make surgical dissection less difficult. Prompt removal of lymphatic malformations is necessary when the potential for airway obstruction exists. This potential is highest in tumors of the sublingual glands, submandibular glands, or minor salivary glands. A tracheotomy may be necessary if the malformation cannot be removed completely. Recurrence of macrocystic lymphatic malformation is uncommon when all evidence of gross tumor is removed. If residual disease remains, recurrence is estimated to occur in up to 35% of cases.[47] Microcystic disease is difficult to erradicate and often requires staged surgical resections with bony recontouring. Infiltration of muscle and nerve is common. Perioperative systemic steroids reduced postoperative edema often encountered following partial resection of these lesions. Use of systemic steroids is also recommended during upper respiratory infection in children with lymphatic malformations to prevent lymphatic edema and growth.

Neoplasms

Salivary gland neoplasms in children are uncommon, with an annual incidence of 1 to 2 cases per 100,000 juveniles. Salivary gland tumors account for 8% of all pediatric head and neck tumors with less than 5% of these occurring in patients 16 years of age or younger.[47] Pediatric salivary gland neoplasms are classified into three histologic groups: benign, low-grade malignant, and high-grade malignant. Sometimes intermediate-grade classification is also used. Management choices inherently depend on histologic type because more aggressive therapy (resection with radiation) is advocated for high-grade lesions.

As mentioned previously, the majority of benign salivary lesions are of vascular origin. The second most common are epithelial tumors. These are predominantly benign and occur most frequently in children in the second decade of life.[2,4,48] Overall, the most common epithelial tumor in children is the pleomorphic adenoma (Table 201-3). Others include Warthin's tumor, oncocytoma, and various adenomas. In contrast to adults, the incidence of malignant tumors is inversely proportional to the age of the patient. Several reports suggest that 23% to 50% of all salivary gland tumors in children are malignant.[3] Fortunately, most of these are of low-grade histology. The most common are mucoepidermoid and acinic cell carcinomas, which account for 60% of the malignant epithelial salivary neoplasms in children.[4] Rare but most frequently encountered nonepithelial malignancies are rhabdomyosarcoma and lymphoma.[2]

The parotid gland is the primary location for salivary gland neoplasms (85% to 90%).[4] These frequently present as a slow-growing mass with average time of onset to ultimate diagnosis approximating 1 to 2 years.[48] Thus it is safe practice to consider all deep, painless, and noninflammatory parotid masses as neoplasms until proven otherwise. Submandibular gland lesions also present as painless swellings but are harbored within the submandibular triangle. A rare minor salivary gland lesion will tend to occur as an oral mass or ulceration. In general, submandibular and minor salivary gland neoplasms have a higher rate of malignancy. Perineural involvement with symptomatic paresthesias (lingual nerve) or weakness (facial nerve or hypoglossal nerve) is suggestive of high-grade processes. Fixation and pain are also indicative of aggressive malignant disease. Pain (30%) and facial paralysis (15%) often accompany malignant parotid tumors.

Benign

Pleomorphic Adenoma (Benign Mixed Tumor)

The most common nonvascular or epithelial salivary gland tumor in children is the pleomorphic adenoma.[49] The highest incidence of pleomorphic adenoma in children is in the pubertal and prepubescent child.[3] These adenomas consist of both mesenchymal and epithelial cell lines derived from the intercalated duct reserve cell. The tumor most often presents as a slow-growing, firm, discrete nodule that is freely mobile and about 1 cm in diameter. Facial paralysis is atypical and should alert the physician that a malignant process is present. Although pleomorphic adenomas appear encapsulated, they have a highly lobular

Table 201-3

Salivary Gland Neoplasms in Children

Benign*		Malignant†	
Hemangioma	111	Mucoepidermoid carcinoma	122
Mixed tumor (pleomorphic adenoma)	94	Acinic cell carcinoma	30
Vascular proliferative tumor	40	Undifferentiated carcinoma	22
Lymphangioma	18	Adenocarcinoma	19
Lymphoepithelial tumor	3	Adenoid cystic carcinoma	16
Cystadenoma	3	Malignant mixed tumor	10
Warthin's tumor	3	Rhabdomyosarcoma	6
Plexiform neurofibroma	2	Undifferentiated sarcoma	5
Xanthoma	2	Mesenchymal sarcoma	5
Neurolemmoma	1	Unclassified carcinoma	4
Adenoma	1	Squamous cell carcinoma	3
Lipoma	1	Lymphoma	3
TOTAL	279	Ganglioneuroblastoma	1
		TOTAL	246

*Adapted from Schuller DE, McCabe BF. Salivary gland neoplasms in children. *Otolaryngol Clin North Am.* 1977;10:399.
†Adapted from Shikhani AH, Johns ME. Tumors of the major salivary glands in children. *Head Neck Surg.* 1988;10:257.

architecture with microscopic pseudopod extensions that prohibit enucleation as a therapeutic alternative. Recurrence rates approach 40% with this surgical technique. Multiglandular involvement in children is unusual. Most of these tumors are 1 to 3 cm in size and located within the superficial lobe or tail of the parotid gland.

The diagnosis of a pleomorphic adenoma, as is the case for most salivary neoplasms, is best confirmed by FNA with ultrasound guidance as needed. Incisional biopsies are contraindicated. MRI will provide better clarity of soft tissue extension in unusual cases. If FNA is inadequate or unavailable, excisional biopsy consisting of a lateral (superficial) parotid lobectomy with facial nerve preservation is appropriate. Total excision of the submandibular gland is necessary when pleomorphic adenomas are found in this gland. Rarely, a mixed tumor abutting the parotid gland, but not infiltrating it, can be removed with a completely intact capsule-sparing parotid tissue and facial nerve dissection. Recurrence after superficial parotidectomy for pleomorphic adenoma in the pediatric population is reported by Shikhani and Johns[50] to be as high as 19.5%, which is considerably greater than that seen in adults (1%). The reasons for this remain unclear but may be related to the misdiagnosis and drainage of previously presumed lymph node infections.

Other Benign

Several rare benign neoplasms have been described in the pediatric population. These include plexiform neurofibroma, Warthin's tumor (papillary cystadenolymphomatosum), embryoma, monomorphic adenoma (basal cell, clear cell, glycogen-rich adenoma), lipoma, and teratoma in descending frequency.[51]

Warthin's tumors theoretically arise from trapped ductal epithelium (striated ducts) within intraparotid lymph nodes and are histologically characterized by oncocytes lying among dense stoma of lymphatic origin. These are typically well-circumscribed lesions that are rare in children and occur in less than 2% of all benign epithelial salivary gland tumors. CT, MRI, and FNA will help diagnose these solid tumors that are often nestled within the tail of the parotid gland. Surgical excision with superficial parotidectomy is often curative, although small secondary lesions may arise later in the same gland. The remaining benign processes are managed similarly to Warthin's tumor both diagnostically and surgically with imaging and resection of the tumor with a wide cuff of adjacent normal gland. The exception is the plexiform neurofibroma that may involve numerous head and neck sites beyond the primary gland. Controversy on treatment, timing, and extent of resection is prevalent in the literature and beyond the scope of this chapter.

Malignant

Mucoepidermoid Carcinoma

Mucoepidermoid carcinoma is the most common malignant epithelial salivary gland neoplasm in children, accounting for approximately 50% of salivary gland malignancies. Most are low-grade lesions that tend to have a good prognosis.[2,49,52] These are also the most frequently encountered radiation-induced salivary gland tumors in children.[53,54] Mucoepidermoid carcinomas are composed of cells with squamous differentiation and cells with mucinous differentiation. Lower-grade neoplasms are commonly cystic, showing predominant mucinous differentiation. Higher-grade neoplasms show greater squamous differentiation and resemble squamous cell carcinoma. Again, histologic grade correlates well with prognosis.

Management is essentially the same in children and adults. Low-grade malignancies of the parotid gland are managed by an appropriate parotidectomy sufficient to remove the tumor with a generous cuff of normal parotid and preserving the facial nerve. The lymph nodes around the digastric triangle should be evaluated at the time of surgery and, if involved, a neck dissection should be done. High-grade malignancies are managed with total parotidectomy. Recurrence rates for superficial versus total parotidectomy for mucoepidermoid carcinoma of the parotid are 30.7% and 0%, respectively.[55] This underscores the implementation of more extensive resection for this disease. This is offset by the risks to the facial nerve. Temporary facial nerve paralysis has been reported to occur in 25% and 16% of total and superficial parotidectomies, respectively, after removal of parotid lesions and facial nerve preservation in children. Permanent loss is rare but more common in malignant tumors.

The facial nerve is preserved in all cases unless gross tumor invasion into the nerve is present. Radical surgery with nerve sacrifice should not be performed on the basis of the results of frozen section alone. However, once confirmed by permanent histologic evaluation, invasion of the nerve should be managed with resection until final sections reveal no further disease. Surgeons need to be prepared for mastoidectomy and temporal bone dissection in suspected cases. In this scenario, immediate facial nerve grafting is performed. Postoperative radiotherapy often is given to patients with high-grade malignancies.[52]

Submandibular gland malignancies are managed with submandibular gland excision and submandibular triangle nodal dissection. High-grade tumors often are given postoperative radiotherapy. Ten-year survival rates for low-grade mucoepidermoid carcinoma have approached 95%.[4]

Acinic Cell Carcinoma

Acinic cell carcinoma is the second most common malignancy and accounts for approximately 12% of the total number of epithelial malignancies of the salivary gland in children.[38] Most acinic cell carcinomas are low-grade malignancies and are diagnosed in pubescent adolescents. They are characterized by cells with bland nuclei and an abundant basophilic cytoplasm. The behavior of acinic cell neoplasms is similar to mucoepidermoid carcinoma because patients present with a slow-growing solitary mass with or without associated pain. Management is the same as low-grade mucoepidermoid carcinoma: an appropriate parotidectomy sufficient to remove the tumor with a generous cuff of normal parotid tissue, preserving the facial nerve.

Other Malignant

Adenocarcinoma and undifferentiated carcinoma, adenoid cystic carcinoma, and malignant mixed tumors are rare but can occur in the pediatric population. Primary sarcomas of the salivary glands in children are also uncommon. When present, rhabdomyosarcoma is the most common. All of these malignancies demonstrate high recurrence rates and poor prognosis. Undifferentiated carcinomas tend to occur in children younger than 10 years of age.[48] Epithelial salivary gland tumors identified in the first month of life are termed *embryomas* or *sialoblastomas* and are malignant in 25% of cases.

Surgery remains the mainstay for the more aggressive lesions with the goal of complete removal. Total parotidectomy is advocated because it may affect local control. Lymph node disease in the neck is estimated to occur in less than 15% of cases, oncologically warranting cervical lymphadenectomy in cases of gross nodal involvement or poorly differentiated lesions. In particular, elective neck dissection without clear involvement should be done only for high-grade malignancies where occult disease is estimated to be greater than 15% (high-grade mucoepidermoid, rhabdomyosarcoma, undifferentiated, and rare squamous cell carcinoma).

Minor salivary gland neoplasms are rare in the pediatric population. Most are pleomorphic adenomas or low-grade mucoepidermoid carcinomas. Regardless of etiology, wide local excision with a cuff of normal adjacent tissue is recommended for both diagnosis and therapy. This is usually curative for these and other malignant neoplasms of these glands.

Role of Irradiation

Irradiation of the major and minor salivary glands in children is generally reserved for high-grade lesions in which significant risk of recurrence and mortality is evident. Other indications include those seen in adults and include remaining gross or microscopic disease, inadequate margins, nodal involvement, perineural spread, and adjacent soft tissue extension. The risk of postradiation sequelae is high in young patients and includes limitations in facial growth, development of secondary tumors, dental caries and trismus.[56]

Trauma

Most salivary gland injuries are seen in association with penetrating wounds of the cheek. Few cause serious injury to the facial nerve or salivary duct system. Any penetrating wound deep to the parotideomasseteric fascia can injure these structures. If the laceration extends anterior to a line dropped from the lateral canthus of the eye, the facial nerve does not need to be explored. Satisfactory reinnervation will occur through peripheral nerve branches. When a laceration is posterior to this line and the facial nerve is paralyzed, exploration of the wound and reapproximation of the proximal and distal segments of the nerve are obligatory.

Exploration of the facial nerve should occur within 72 hours of the injury so that electrical stimulation of the distal segment is possible. Epineural repair of the severed branches can be accomplished with the aid of an operating microscope. A 6-0 to 8-0 nylon suture is ideal for this purpose. If tension exists on the suture line, a cable graft is preferable. The best results are obtained when the anastomosis is accomplished with fresh, sharp nerve ends. Recovery of facial nerve function after transection and repair requires 6 to 12 months.

The parotid duct (Stensen's duct) is located on a line drawn from the tragus to the midpoint between the upper lip margin and the columella. The parotid duct is likely to be injured if a laceration courses through the masseter muscle. Pooling of saliva in the wound is a frequent finding. Lacerations involving Stensen's duct should be repaired when they are detected because the resultant inflammatory response leads to a high probability of a salivary fistula, sinus tract, or an obstructive cyst. This repair should occur as early as the patient is medically stable and staff are available. The preferable method is to perform the ductal repair using 6-0 or 7-0 nylon suture over a small stent (polyethylene tubing). The tubing remains in place approximately 10 days. When the orifice of Stensen's or Wharton's duct has undergone significant injury, surgical rerouting of the remaining duct through the buccal mucosa may be necessary. If this is not possible, ligation at this site is also a reasonable option.

Blunt trauma to the salivary glands may cause less obvious injury than penetrating trauma. Injury to the parotid duct can result in a salivary pseudocyst with associated swelling and recurrence after FNA. Repeat aspiration and a pressure dressing may be necessary. Children who require dental appliances can develop chronic irritation of the salivary ducts resulting in stasis. Salivary gland swelling has been described in neonates resulting from a compression-type birth injury from a forceps delivery.

Sialorrhea

Sialorrhea (drooling) is defined by the unintentional loss of saliva beyond the lip margin. This usually results from an inability to coordinate oral control and swallowing and is a natural phenomenon in infants as they gradually gain function of their oral-motor skills. Drooling normally subsides in these children during neuromuscular maturity and should resolve around 18 months of age. Persistent sialorrhea beyond 4 years of age is thereby considered abnormal and should be investigated for treatment options. This most frequently occurs in neurologically impaired children with the highest incidence in patients diagnosed with cerebral palsy (10% to 25%). Specific delay in oral motor function in these patients can last up to 6 years of age and should be kept in mind when considering sialorrhea therapy.

The submandibular and sublingual glands produce the most saliva (70%) during the normal, unstimulated basal state. The role of saliva is to maintain oral homeostasis with respect to pH, dental health, control of bacterial growth, lubrication, and digestion of food (amylase). On sympathetic stimulation (eating and preparation to eat) the parotid gland produces the preponderance of saliva with dramatic increase in flow.[57] Excessive production or ineffective dissolution (voluntary swallowing) can lead to persistent drooling and its consequences including maceration of the lips and chin, chapping, dehydration, infection, foul odor, and aspiration. This can lead to significant hygienic issues, costs, and social isolation as patients continuously soil their clothes, furniture, and caregivers. Assessment of sialorrhea is often determined by subjective scales answered by the patient's caregivers with specific rating of the severity and frequency of drooling. The results thereby help guide management.

Medical Management

A multidisciplinary approach is appropriate for these patients because management decisions often include otolaryngologists, speech therapists, physical therapists, social workers, and pediatric dentists.[1] In otherwise healthy children with sialorrhea, nasal obstruction and dental disease are common sources and should be assessed carefully because management may be directed at this problem. Adenoidectomy, turbinectomy, allergic desensitization, and management of dental hygiene can be performed. In neurologically impaired children the approach is not as simple. In such patients with associated malocclusion, macroglossia, and orthodontic problems, surgical correction of these deformities or the application of orthodontic appliances can improve mild cases of sialorrhea.

However, neurologic dysfunction is the primary culprit for disease in sialorrhea patients. An initial attempt at speech therapy or physical therapy is appropriate before beginning extensive medical or surgical management. This method provides a physiologic approach to the problem using oral-motor and behavior modification. Conservative management includes correcting posture to more upright positions and techniques to improve oral competence (closing mouth) and reducing tongue thrust. Biofeedback has been used in higher-functioning patients and shown to be effective in mild to moderate cases of sialorrhea. This is aimed to elicit a swallow or mouth wiping by the patient on hearing a repeated tone. Unfortunately, habituation to the stimulus occurs in most patients over time.[58] Indications for delay in therapy include normally developing children up to 6 years of age with a sole complaint of sialorrhea, cerebral palsy patients with mild to moderate sialorrhea before 6 years of age, and sialorrhea following acute neurologic deficits (wait 6 to 12 months).[1]

Medical regimens have involved the use of oral (glycopyrrolate) and topical (scopolamine) anticholinergics. Unfortunately, these have generally been unsuccessful due to the broad side-effect profile, making their use unattractive. Even more selective agents with limited blood-brain barrier penetration such as glycopyrrolate have nearly 60% of patients experiencing various side effects such as hyperactivity, irritability, xerostomia, constipation, and urinary retention. Regardless, in patients without side effects, glycopyrrolate at dose 0.10 mg/kg has proven effective in maintaining reduction of sialorrhea. This is thereby often used before contemplating surgical intervention. Botulinum injection is also used in some cases and has been successful in temporarily reducing sialorrhea.

Surgical Management

Surgical management of sialorrhea is generally reserved for patients in whom nonsurgical measures have not been effective, those with moderate to profuse sialorrhea and older than 6 years of age, dramatically developmentally delayed children with moderate to profuse drooling, sialorrhea with more than one documented episode of aspiration pneumonia annually, and patients requiring chronic and frequent maintenance of secretions by their caregivers. Although less clear, patients who require several bib or clothing changes daily or hourly suctioning are considered appropriate candidates. Botox injections of the major salivary glands have proven effective in reducing sialorrhea and seems appropriate in patients with poor neurologic prognosis, surgical risk factors, and determining those in whom surgery may be effective.[1] However, repeated injections will be necessary, thus limiting its use in the general population of sialorrhea patients.

Bilateral submandibular gland excision with parotid duct ligation has most consistently controlled drooling. It has supplanted other surgical options including submandibular duct rerouting, submandibular duct rerouting with bilateral tympanic neurectomies and chorda tympani nerve sections, and tympanic neurectomies with chorda tympani nerve sections alone. This procedure is safe and reliable and results in few complications.[59] Another less invasive option is that of four-duct ligation, which includes ligation of both parotid ducts and both submandibular ducts all via transoral approach. No conclusive studies have determined the overall benefit from this less invasive procedure.

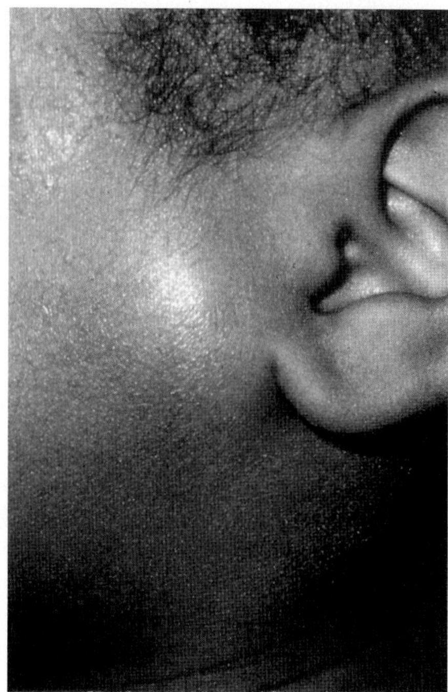

Figure 201-8. A first branchial cleft anomaly that has become an infected cyst.

Rare Disorders

Allergy

Allergic reactions can cause bilateral parotid enlargement. The enlargement is usually of rapid onset and transient nature. Resolution is usually spontaneous when the offending allergen is eliminated. Certain foods (seafood, strawberries) may precipitate this reaction. Investigation of the saliva or leukocyte differential may reveal a relative eosinophilia.

Cystic Fibrosis

Patients with cystic fibrosis can develop salivary gland enlargement. The submandibular gland is involved more frequently than the parotid gland. When a child younger than 2 years of age presents with diffuse parotid enlargement without an associated infection, a sweat chloride test should be performed to rule out cystic fibrosis. The mechanism of the swelling is unknown, but increased concentrations of calcium and phosphorus are found in the saliva.

Aberrant Salivary Glands

Heterotopic salivary gland tissue is defined as the existence of salivary tissue in locations external to the major and minor salivary glands. This is a rare entity and when present usually presents as a sinus tract in the right side of the lower neck along the anterior border of the sternocleidomastoid muscle with close proximity to the sternoclavicular joint. Most are noticed at birth or shortly thereafter. The tracts may drain saliva-like fluid related to meals. Excision is the treatment of choice. The sinus tracts are generally short in comparison with that of branchial cleft fistulas.[39]

Agenesis of the major salivary glands can occur. Diagnosis can be confirmed with pertechnetate nuclear medicine imaging. The scan may be diagnostic in a child with idiopathic xerostomia. Early identification is important so that proper oral hygiene can be started. The oral sequelae include dental carries and candidiasis.

Systemic Conditions and Medications

Systemic conditions in which bilateral diffuse salivary enlargement can occur include obesity, alcoholism, portal cirrhosis, malnutrition (kwashiorkor, hypovitaminosis A), gastrointestinal absorption disease (celiac disease, Chagas' disease), chronic pancreatitis, uremia, thyroid disease (hypothyroidism), diabetes, bulimia, and abnormalities of the pituitary-adrenal axis. Salivary gland enlargement has been associated with several drugs including phenytoin, thiourea, isoproterenol, methimazole, phenothiazine, thiocyanate, iodine compounds, and heavy metals.

SUGGESTED READINGS

Adams DM. The nonsurgical management of vascular lesions. *Facial Plast Surg Clin North Am.* 2001;9(4):601-608.

Banks WW, Handler SD, Glade GB, et al. Neonatal submandibular sialadenitis. *Am J Otolaryngol.* 1980;1(3):261-263.

Bradley P, McClelland L, Mehta D. Paediatric salivary gland epithelial neoplasms. *Orl J Otorhinolaryngol Relat Spec.* 2007;69(3):137-145.

Brannon RB, Fowler CB, Hartman KS. Necrotizing sialometaplasia. A clinicopathologic study of sixty-nine cases and review of the literature. *Oral Surg Oral Med Oral Pathol.* 1991;72(3):317-325.

Brook I. Aerobic and anaerobic microbiology of suppurative sialadenitis. *J Med Microbiol.* 2002;51(6):526-529.

Chung MK, Jeong HS, Ko MH, et al. Pediatric sialolithiasis: what is different from adult sialolithiasis? *Int J Pediatr Otorhinolaryngol.* 2007;71(5):787-791.

Crysdale WS, McCann C, Roske L, et al. Saliva control issues in the neurologically challenged. A 30 year experience in team management. *Int J Pediatr Otorhinolaryngol.* 2006;70(3):519-527.

da Cruz Perez DE, Pires FR, Alves FA, et al. Salivary gland tumors in children and adolescents: a clinicopathologic and immunohistochemical study of fifty-three cases. *Int J Pediatr Otorhinolaryngol.* 2004;68(7):895-902.

Davidkin I, Jokinen S, Paananen A, et al. Etiology of mumps-like illnesses in children and adolescents vaccinated for measles, mumps, and rubella. *J Infect Dis.* 2005;191(5):719-723.

Elluru RG, Azizkhan RG. Cervicofacial vascular anomalies. II. Vascular malformations. *Semin Pediatr Surg.* 2006;15(2):133-139.

Hockstein NG, Samadi DS, Gendron K, et al. Pediatric submandibular triangle masses: a fifteen-year experience. *Head Neck.* 2004;26(8):675-680.

For complete list of references log onto www.expertconsult.com.

Kim YH, Jeong WJ, Jung KY, et al. Diagnosis of major salivary gland tuberculosis: experience of eight cases and review of the literature. *Acta Otolaryngol.* 2005;125(12):1318-1322.

Laskawi R, Schaffranietz F, Arglebe C, et al. Inflammatory diseases of the salivary glands in infants and adolescents. *Int J Pediatr Otorhinolaryngol.* 2006; 70(1):129-136.

Leerdam CM, Martin HC, Isaacs D. Recurrent parotitis of childhood. *J Paediatr Child Health.* 2005;41(12):631-634.

Nahlieli O, Baruchin AM. Endoscopic technique for the diagnosis and treatment of obstructive salivary gland diseases. *J Oral Maxillofac Surg.* 1999;57(12):1394-1401; discussion 1401-1392.

Pinto A, De Rossi SS. Salivary gland disease in pediatric HIV patients: an update. *J Dent Child (Chic).* 2004;71(1):33-37.

Rice DH. Chronic inflammatory disorders of the salivary glands. *Otolaryngol Clin North Am.* 1999;32(5):813-818.

Shah GV. MR imaging of salivary glands. *Neuroimaging Clin N Am.* 2004;14(4):777-808.

Shapiro NL, Bhattacharyya N. Clinical characteristics and survival for major salivary gland malignancies in children. *Otolaryngol Head Neck Surg.* 2006;134(4):631-634.

Shikhani AH, Johns ME. Tumors of the major salivary glands in children. *Head Neck Surg.* 1988;10(4):257-263.

Shott SR, Myer CM 3rd, Cotton RT. Surgical management of sialorrhea. *Otolaryngol Head Neck Surg.* 1989;101(1):47-50.

Stong BC, Sipp JA, Sobol SE. Pediatric parotitis: a 5-year review at a tertiary care pediatric institution. *Int J Pediatr Otorhinolaryngol.* 2006;70(3):541-544.

Thoeny HC. Imaging of salivary gland tumours. *Cancer Imaging.* 2007;7:52-62.

Wolinsky E. Mycobacterial lymphadenitis in children: a prospective study of 105 nontuberculous cases with long-term follow-up. *Clin Infect Dis.* 1995;20(4):954-963.

Yu GY, Li ZL, Ma DQ, et al. Diagnosis and treatment of epithelial salivary gland tumours in children and adolescents. *Br J Oral Maxillofac Surg.* 2002;40(5):389-392.

CHAPTER TWO HUNDRED AND TWO

Congenital Disorders of the Larynx

Anna H. Messner

Key Points

- The most common cause of stridor in infants is laryngomalacia—but not all stridor can be assumed to be due to laryngomalacia.
- Laryngomalacia is most likely due to altered laryngeal tone and sensorimotor integrative function, which improves with increasing age.
- Infants with laryngomalacia are likely to have gastropharyngeal reflux requiring evaluation and treatment.
- Supraglottoplasty is a highly successful treatment for severe laryngomalacia with a low complication rate.
- Noniatrogenic neonatal unilateral and bilateral vocal cord paralysis will resolve spontaneously in greater than 50% of patients.
- Posterior glottic stenosis and arytenoid fixation can mimic neurologic vocal cord paralysis.
- All children with anterior laryngeal webs should undergo genetic testing for abnormalities of chromosome 22q11.
- Patients with subglottic hemangiomas often present with a history of "recurrent croup" because the lesion mimics the subglottic swelling of croup, and the symptoms improve with steroid treatment.
- Laryngeal cysts, including vallecular thyroglossal duct cysts, saccular cysts, and subglottic cysts, are a source of potentially severe airway obstruction.
- In the patient with feeding problems, recurrent aspiration, and stridor, the otolaryngologist must maintain a high index of suspicion that a laryngeal cleft may be present, as well as a low threshold to perform direct laryngoscopy in the operating room to rule out potential clefts.

Stridor is the hallmark of any laryngeal obstruction. Much can be learned about the nature of the laryngeal problem by closely observing the infant and listening to the noise produced as air passes through the obstruction. Stridor resulting from supraglottic or glottic obstruction is typically present on inspiration, whereas biphasic stridor originates from obstruction at or below the level of the glottis in the upper trachea. Expiratory stridor is the result of lesions in the distal trachea or mainstem bronchi.

Dynamic evaluation of the larynx by flexible laryngoscopy is best performed in the patient who is awake. Although at least a 2.5-mm diameter fiberoptic laryngoscope is recommended for optimal viewing, fiberoptic laryngoscopes with diameters as small as 1.9 mm allow the neonatal larynx to be viewed with a minimum of trauma to the young patient. Direct laryngoscopy of the neonatal larynx with a telescope or microscope provides the best optics (Fig. 202-1). To fully evaluate the larynx, the endoscopist should note findings in the vallecula, piriform fossae, postcricoid region, arytenoids, interarytenoid area, aryepiglottic folds, epiglottis, false vocal cords, ventricles, true vocal cords, and the subglottis.

Laryngomalacia

Without question, the most common cause of stridor in infants is laryngomalacia, a disease more commonly found in term infants, and in males more than females.[1] The newborn with laryngomalacia typically develops intermittent, inspiratory stridor within the first 2 weeks of life, which resolves slowly over several months. Many authors describe the stridor as high-pitched, but compared to the stridor of vocal cord paralysis it is relatively low-pitched and does not have a musical quality. The stridor nearly always worsens with feeding, and often the baby will need to take breaks while feeding in order to breathe. The stridor of mild laryngomalacia often improves with crying as tone in the pharynx is increased. Conversely, in moderate-to-severe laryngomalacia, the stridor typically will worsen with crying because of the increased airflow through the severely collapsed larynx. Laryngomalacia may be an isolated finding in the otherwise healthy infant or may be associated with other neurologic disorders such as cerebral palsy.

The median time to spontaneous resolution of stridor is 9 months of age, and 75% will have no stridor by 18 months of age.[2] Infrequently, the laryngomalacia is severe, resulting in feeding difficulties, failure to thrive, apnea, pectus excavatum, or cyanosis. In these cases, surgical intervention is recommended to prevent worsening failure to thrive, cor pulmonale, and cardiac failure.[1-3]

The inspiratory stridor of laryngomalacia results from collapse of the supraglotttic larynx, creating a narrow airway and turbulent airflow (Fig. 202-2). The etiology of this collapse has been elusive but it appears to be related to neuromuscular hypotonia. Sensorimotor integration of peripheral sensory afferent reflexes, brainstem function, and the motor efferent response are responsible for laryngeal function and tone.[1] The laryngeal adductor reflex (LAR) is a vagal nerve-mediated reflex activated by sensory stimulation of the mechanoreceptors and chemoreceptors of the superior laryngeal nerve located in the region of the aryepiglottic fold. Dysfunction anywhere along the afferent, brainstem,

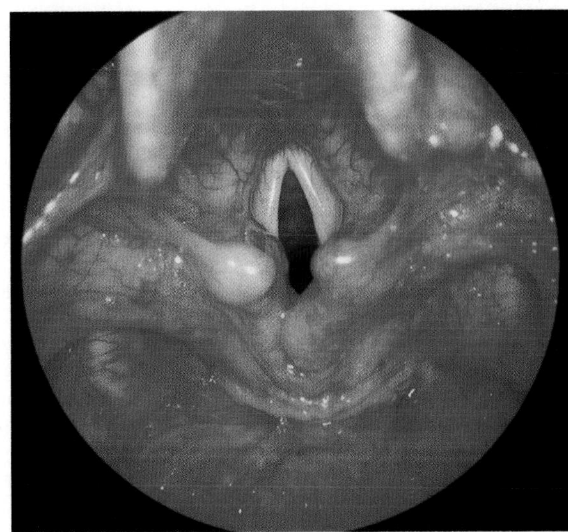

Figure 202-1. Normal infant larynx. Anatomic areas to be examined include epiglottis, vallecula, piriform sinuses, arytenoid cartilages, interarytenoid area, aryepiglottic folds, false vocal cords, ventricles, true vocal cords, anterior commissure, and subglottis. *(From Benjamin B. The pediatric airway, slide #2, Slide Lecture Series. American Academy of Otolaryngology–Head and Neck Surgery, 1992.)*

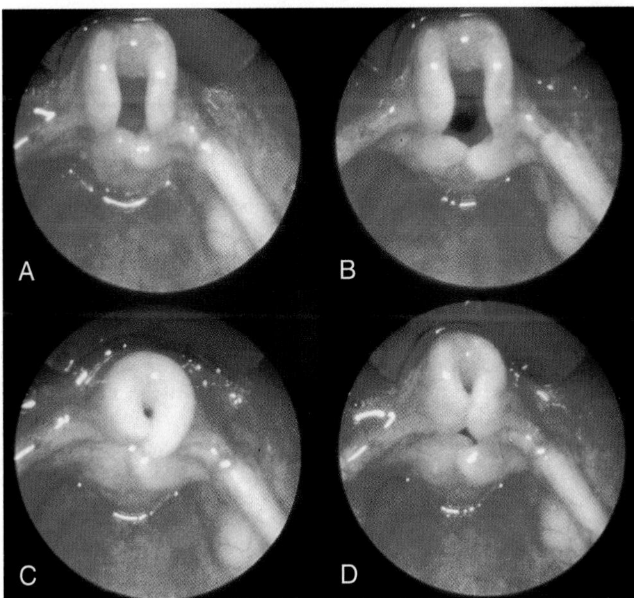

Figure 202-2. Laryngomalacia. Progressive airway obstruction on inspiration. Note omega-shaped epiglottis. *(From Benjamin B. The pediatric airway, slide #2, Slide Lecture Series. American Academy of Otolaryngology–Head and Neck Surgery, 1992.)*

or efferent pathway of the LAR can result in altered laryngeal tone and function. Infants with laryngomalacia have been found to have elevated laryngopharyngeal sensory testing thresholds, showing that the sensorimotor integrative function of the larynx is altered, likely leading to the weak laryngeal tone seen in infants with laryngomalacia.[1]

In several series, a high prevalence of gastroesophageal reflux disease (GERD) has been reported in patients with laryngomalacia (50% to 100%).[1,4-6] When present, GERD can cause airway edema and thus contribute to the airway compromise. Children with laryngomalacia should be evaluated for GERD and if airway surgery is needed, care should be taken to control GERD before surgery to avoid GERD-induced delayed healing.[6] Mild GERD may improve with the treatment of laryngomalacia when the negative intrathoracic intraesophageal pressures decrease. Conversely, treatment of GERD may improve laryngomalacia as acid ceases to irritate the larynx and edema resolves.[5] In the child with GERD related to airway obstruction, the GERD can be expected to improve significantly after aryepiglottoplasty.[7]

The diagnosis of laryngomalacia requires an endoscopic examination; however, the optimal type of endoscopic examination is somewhat controversial. If the patient is sedated and undergoes fiberoptic flexible laryngoscopy (FFL), the topical lidocaine typically used can cause increased collapse of the arytenoids and folding of the epiglottis during inspiration—possibly leading to overestimation of the severity of laryngomalacia.[8] These findings suggest that the optimal way to diagnose laryngomalacia is with FFL in the awake patient. Conversely, the awake technique has been found to miss mild laryngomalacia or lead to overdiagnosis in the patient with a normal airway.[9] The advantages of awake FFL compared to FFL under general anesthesia include the ability to perform the examination expediently in the clinic setting with the parents present, without the need for sedation, leading to less medical expense. The primary disadvantage of the awake FFL is that in nearly all cases the infant is crying during the examination, which can alter the appearance of the supraglottic structures. An omega-shaped epiglottis is often associated with laryngomalacia but can also be found in otherwise normal infants with no airway obstruction. If fluoroscopy is performed, downward anterior displacement and bowing of the aryepiglottic folds, horizontal infolding of the epiglottis, and in some cases, narrowing of the trachea are seen on inspiration, all of which reverse on expiration.[10]

Approximately 17% of infants with laryngomalacia have a second synchronous lesion that may lead to airway difficulties.[11] The decision to perform a bronchoscopy in patients who present with typical laryngomalacia is also controversial. Some contend that bronchoscopy need be done only in select infants with laryngomalacia who present with "apnea, failure to thrive, or features inconsistent with isolated laryngomalacia."[2,12] Others strongly recommend a complete evaluation of the tracheobronchial tree in all symptomatic infants to avoid missing life-threatening lesions.[13]

The anatomic abnormality causing the supraglotttic obstruction of laryngomalacia varies among infants. Most have anterior prolapse of the mucosa overlying the arytenoid cartilages (57%); others have short aryepiglottic folds that tether the epiglottis posteriorly (15%), posterior collapse of the epiglottis (12%), or some combination of these findings (15%).[2] Several classification systems have been proposed with none being predominant at this time.[2,14,15]

Approximately 10% to 31% of infants seen by a pediatric otolaryngologist require surgical intervention for their laryngomalacia.[1] Surgery is indicated if there is feeding difficulty with failure to thrive, cyanosis, apnea, respiratory distress, or hypoxia. The current standard treatment is supraglottoplasty (aryepiglottoplasty) (Fig. 202-3). The surgical resection can be performed using the carbon dioxide (CO_2) laser, laryngeal microscissors, or microdébrider.[1-3,5,16] Various types of supraglottoplasty have been described based on what portion of the prolapsing supraglottis is removed: the tissue overlying the arytenoids (with care taken to preserve the interarytenoid mucosa), the aryepiglottic folds, or the posterior portion of the epiglottis.[5] Unilateral supraglottoplasty has been advocated by some authors to relieve the airway obstruction while reducing the risk of postoperative supraglottic stenosis.[17,18]

Short aryepiglottic folds that tether the supraglotttic structures in close anterior and posterior approximation can be divided or excised.[19] If the epiglottis is displaced posteriorly, an epiglottopexy can be performed.[20] In this procedure the mucosa of the lingual surface of the epiglottis and the corresponding mucosa of the base of the tongue are removed with the CO_2 laser, then the epiglottis is sutured to the tongue base. These procedures are well tolerated by the infants, typically requiring only a short 1- to 3-day hospital stay. The success of the various forms of supraglottoplasty-epiglottopexy are high, with the vast majority of children obtaining relief from their obstruction.[3,16,19-23] Those children who do not improve with supraglottoplasty usually have underlying neurologic or syndromal abnormalities or associated tracheomalacia and may require a tracheotomy.[22,23] Complications are

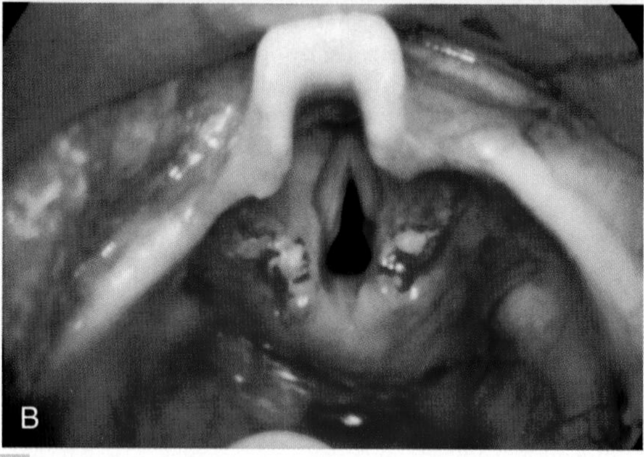

Figure 202-3. Laryngomalacia. Infant larynx before and after supraglottoplasty.

rare, with the most feared being supraglottic stenosis, which may occur in up to 4% of cases.[22] More frequently, transient dysphagia and aspiration can occur in approximately 10% to 15% of patients.[1]

Although laryngomalacia is typically thought of as occurring only in infants, it is occasionally observed in older children and adults. Neurologically impaired children (i.e., those with cerebral palsy) with poor pharyngeal control can develop laryngomalacia. Exercise-induced laryngomalacia results when enough inspiratory force occurs during exercise to draw the aryepiglottic folds into the larynx, partially obstructing the glottis.[24,25] In severe cases with redundant aryepiglottic folds, supraglottoplasty can be beneficial. Similarly, if the epiglottis is elongated and flaccid, a partial epiglottidectomy can be effective.[26]

Vocal Fold Paralysis

Vocal fold paralysis (VFP) is another common cause of neonatal stridor. The stridor is inspiratory or biphasic, with a high-pitched musical quality. VFP in a newborn may be idiopathic or can result from birth trauma, central or peripheral neurologic diseases, or thoracic diseases or procedures.[27,28] The diagnosis is best made by FFL in the awake patient so that the effect of anesthesia on vocal fold function is minimized.

Iatrogenic left VFP may be present following thoracic surgery, particularly patent ductus arteriosus (PDA) ligation or repair of an interrupted aortic arch. In these infants, the left recurrent laryngeal nerve is damaged at the point that it passes around the ductus arteriosus (unless a right aortic arch is present). The incidence of recurrent laryngeal nerve injury is estimated at 1% to 7.4% of PDA ligation cases.[29,30] Most infants with a unilateral VFP are brought to the attention of the otolaryngologist for evaluation of a weak cry or stridor or for inability to wean the infant off ventilatory support if thoracic surgery was performed.[30,31] Of those children evaluated by a pediatric otolaryngologist with a unilateral vocal fold paralysis after cardiac surgery approximately 35% will recover vocal fold function.[31] At least half of these patients will have swallowing dysfunction, usually aspiration or laryngeal penetration with modified barium swallow.[31,32] Although many of the patients with a unilateral vocal fold paralysis will be able to feed orally, many will initially require a gastrostomy tube.[31,32]

The more difficult problem is bilateral VFP. The degree of airway obstruction is often severe, requiring a tracheotomy in up to 73% of children.[33-35] The diagnosis of vocal fold paralysis can be made on FFL, but differentiation between bilateral vocal fold fixation and neurogenic VFP cannot be made unless direct laryngoscopy is performed and the glottis palpated. Laryngeal electromyography in the pediatric patient under a light plane of anesthesia can also be helpful to differentiate fixation vs paralysis and assist with prognosis.[36,37]

Workup of patients with idiopathic VFP should include a magnetic resonance imaging (MRI) scan of the brain to rule out an Arnold-Chiari malformation or other intracranial cause of brainstem compression.[38-40] If such a malformation is identified, then early decompression is recommended to obtain a better outcome.[40] If idiopathic congenital bilateral VFP is present, a genetics consultation is recommended to evaluate the patient for chromosome abnormalities.[41]

Approximately 70% of noniatrogenic unilateral vocal fold paralyses will resolve spontaneously, most within the first 6 months of life.[27] The patient with unilateral VFP is often able to compensate for purposes of feeding without medical intervention. Sometimes an infant will require nasogastric feeds on a short-term basis or a gastrostomy tube. An occupational or speech pathology feeding consult is helpful with these infants to rule out aspiration (as seen on modified barium swallow) and to counsel the parents on how to feed the patient. Most often, these infants should start with a slow-flow nipple, then work up to a regular nipple. The voice of most infants with a unilateral VFP is quiet but audible and gains strength with time.

Occasionally, the child with unilateral VFP has problems with severe aspiration and dysphonia. In these children, injection of the vocal fold can be helpful. Most commonly, injection materials used include cadaveric dermis (Cymetra), calcium hydroxyapatite (Radiesse or Radiesse Voice Gel), hydrated porcine gelatin powder (Surgifoam), or absorbable gelatin sponge (Gelfoam), or autologous fat.[42,43] Alternatively, in the older child a medialization laryngoplasty (thyroplasty) can be performed.[42-45] The retrospective review by Link and others of 12 type I thyroplasty procedures in eight pediatric patients ages 2 to 17 years demonstrated that the anatomically lower position of the vocal fold (compared with that in adults) must be taken into consideration if optimum outcomes are to be obtained in children.[45]

The vocal folds spontaneously become mobile in up to 65% of patients with bilateral VFP.[27,46] Prognosis is better if there are no associated anomalies.[33] Most recovery of vocal fold function occurs within 24 to 36 months, although it has been reported in patients up to 11 years of age.[33,34] If recovery occurs after 2 to 3 years, it is often incomplete because of laryngeal muscle atrophy, cricoarytenoid fixation, and synkinesis.[33] The timing of possible surgical intervention is debated. Some authors recommend intervention at a young age. Others suggest waiting until adolescence when the patient is able to decide.[33,34,47]

Many surgical options are possible to improve the airway of a patient with bilateral vocal cord paralysis.[48] The plethora of surgical options indicates that none is uniformly successful—particularly in the young patient. Endoscopically, a lateral cordotomy can be performed to increase the glottic area.[49,50] An arytenoidectomy can be performed via an endoscopic or external cervical approach or using the Woodman approach.[33,51] Alternatively, an arytenoidopexy can be performed using a laterocervical approach.[27,52,47] Triglia and colleagues performed an arytenoidopexy on 34 children with bilateral vocal cord paralysis who had a mean age of 20 months.[47] Of the 15 children who had a tracheotomy or endotracheal tube (ETT) before the procedure, 14 were successfully decannulated postoperatively. Another option is to expand the cricoid cartilage by placing a costal cartilage graft posteriorly, thereby separating the arytenoids and increasing the area between the vocal folds. This procedure can be performed with a laryngofissure or endoscopic approach.[53,54] Finally, lateralization of the paralyzed cord has been described as a potentially reversible approach to vocal cord paralysis.[55]

Hartnick and colleagues described 52 children who underwent surgery for bilateral VFP.[56] The procedures most successful in realizing tracheotomy decannulation were those that included vocal cord

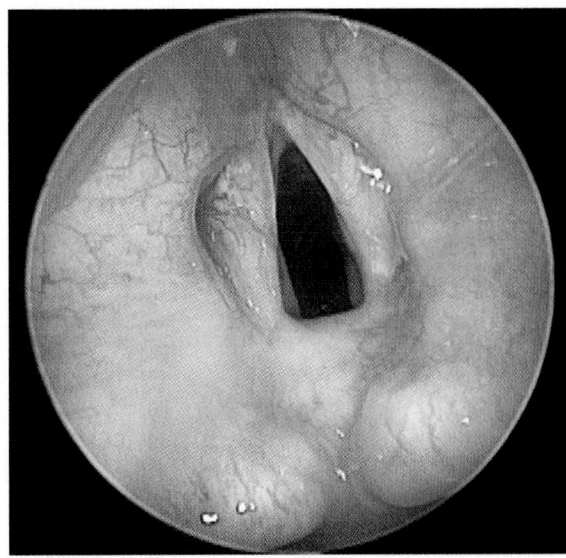

Figure 202-4. Interarytenoid web. *(Copyright Peter Koltai, MD.)*

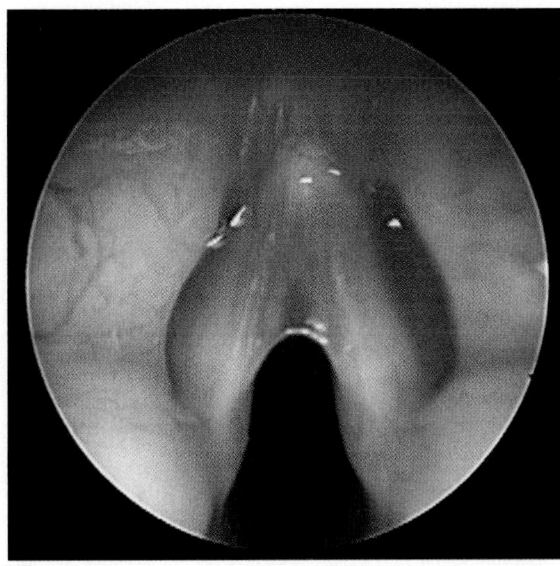

Figure 202-5. Anterior glottic web. Patient presented with chronic hoarseness and mild stridor. *(Copyright Peter Koltai, MD.)*

lateralization procedures combined with a partial arytenoidectomy (71% decannulation rate). These procedures were more successful than CO_2 laser cordotomy or arytenoidectomy procedures (29% decannulation), for isolated arytenoidopexy procedures (25% decannulation) or for posterior costal cartilage graft procedures (60% decannulation). No prospective randomized studies have been performed to evaluate the outcomes of these different surgical options, although meta-analysis has suggested that external arytenoidopexy and external arytenoidectomy are more effective than carbon dioxide ablation procedures.[57]

Laryngeal Web/Atresia

Posterior Webs

Apparent bilateral vocal cord paralysis may occur if an interarytenoid web is present in the posterior larynx causing limited vocal fold abduction (Fig. 202-4). This type of congenital web is rare and often necessitates a tracheotomy in the early years of life.[58] Stridor is the major presenting clinical feature, but patients can also present with obstructive cyanosis at birth or with episodes of apnea.

Diagnosis is made at the time of microscopic laryngoscopy with palpation of the interarytenoid area. Posterior webs may be associated with subglottic stenosis, and bulky arytenoids and abnormal laryngeal position are often present. Management options include long-term tracheotomy with probable decannulation after 3 to 5 years, division of the web (frequently unsuccessful), arytenoidectomy, or open airway reconstruction with a posterior cartilage graft.[58]

Anterior Webs

Anterior congenital laryngeal webs are also rare anomalies typically diagnosed in the neonatal period after an investigation for the source of aphonia and stridor (Fig. 202-5). Occasionally a minor web will not be diagnosed until the child is older and undergoes an evaluation for chronic hoarseness. Most commonly, a web will cause partial obstruction of the anterior glottis and will extend into the subglottic area, causing congenital subglottic stenosis.[59]

The most severe form of a laryngeal web is total atresia of the larynx (Fig. 202-6). A fetus with laryngeal atresia or a web obstructing nearly all of the larynx will develop congenital high airway obstruction syndrome (CHAOS). Magnetic resonance imaging of the affected fetus will show enlarged echogenic lungs, inverted diaphragms, massive ascites, and dilated airways (Fig. 202-7).[60,61] Death results in these infants unless a tracheotomy is performed at the time of birth, therefore delivery by ex utero intrapartum treatment (EXIT procedure) is recommended. The EXIT procedure establishes an airway before completion of birth, while the neonate remains on placental support.

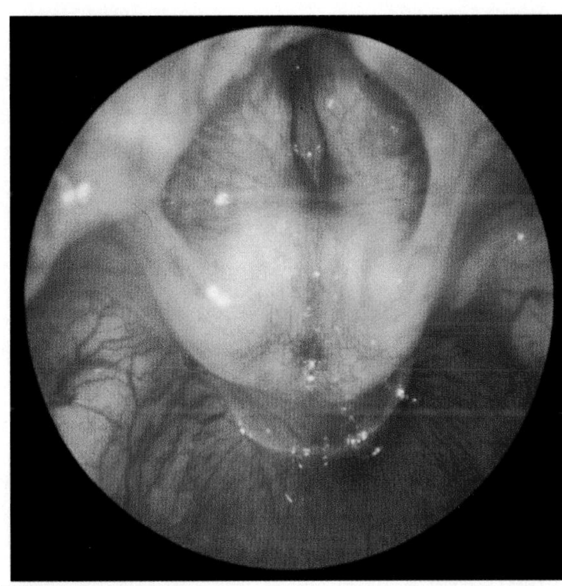

Figure 202-6. Laryngeal atresia. *(From Benjamin B. The pediatric airway, slide #33, Slide Lecture Series. American Academy of Otolaryngology–Head and Neck Surgery, 1992.)*

Many anterior laryngeal webs are associated with deletions of chromosome 22q11.[63] In a review of 17 patients with anterior glottic webs, 11 (65%) were found to be positive for chromosome 22q11.2 deletion.[63] These same microscopic and submicroscopic deletions cause a wide range of phenotypes including DiGeorge's syndrome, velocardiofacial (Shprintzen) syndrome, conotruncal anomaly face syndrome, and sporadic or familial heart defects (Table 202-1). The acronym CATCH 22 (cardiac defect, abnormal facies, thymus hypoplasia, cleft palate, hypocalcemia, and chromosome 22 deletion) has been used to describe the various phenotypes. For this reason, all patients with a diagnosis of laryngeal web should undergo genetic screening and a thorough cardiovascular evaluation, with particular attention being paid to the aortic arch. Delayed diagnosis of a vascular ring can occur in the patient with a laryngeal web whose stridor and dysphagia are attributed only to the presence of the web.[62]

Successful treatment of an anterior laryngeal web most often demands that an open approach be used so that the subglottic narrow-

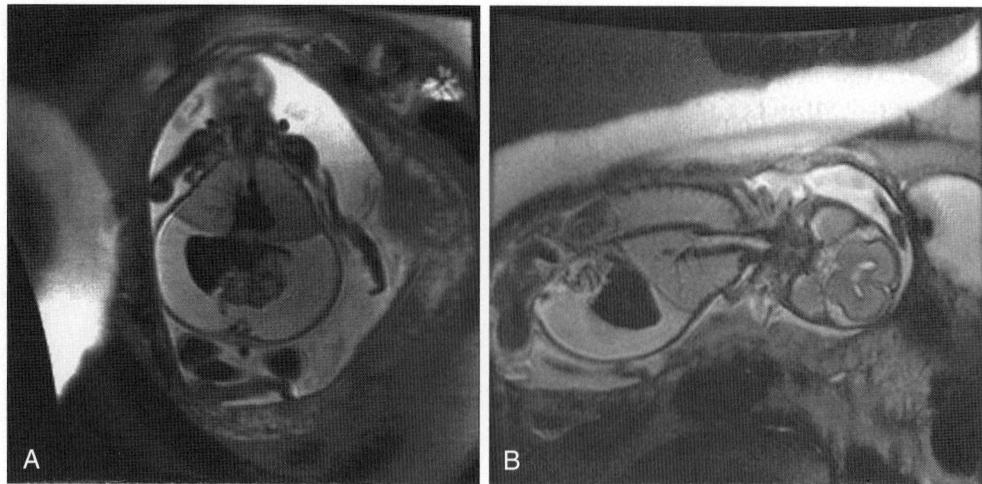

Figure 202-7. **A,** Fetus with congenital high airway obstruction syndrome due to laryngeal atresia. Magnetic resonance imaging (MRI) scan of the fetus in utero shows abnormally large, echogenic lungs and massively enlarged fluid-filled fetal lungs with associated chest deformation and fetal heart compression by the enlarged lungs. **B,** MRI shows an abrupt, V-shaped termination of the trachea with the apex pointing superiorly. *(From Erickson V, Messner A. Radiology quiz case 2. Congenital high airway obstruction syndrome (CHAOS).* Arch Otolaryngol Head Neck Surg. *2007;133:299-301.)*

Table 202-1

Syndromes Associated with Congenital Laryngeal Anomalies

Laryngeal Anomaly	Chromosome Affected	Associated Syndromes	Other Associated Anomalies
Laryngeal web	22q11	Velocardiofacial DiGeorge Conotruncal face	Cardiac anomalies Cleft palate–velopharyngeal insufficiency Hypocalcemia Abnormal facies
Laryngotracheal cleft or bifid epiglottis	GLI3	Pallister-Hall (congenital hypothalamic hamartoblastoma)	Polydactyly Pituitary dysfunction Imperforate anus Hamartoblastomas
Laryngotracheal cleft or hypoplastic epiglottis		Opitz-Frias	Hypertelorism Cleft palate–cleft lip Intracranial anomalies Hypospadias Bifid scrotum, uvula, tongue

ing can be corrected.[64,65] Laryngotracheal reconstruction or laryngofissure and silastic keel are used to correct the defect. If laryngotracheal reconstruction is performed, the approach can sometimes be single-staged. In rare cases in which the web is limited, endoscopic treatment may be successful.

Congenital Subglottic Stenosis

Subglottic stenosis in a term newborn is defined as a cricoid diameter of less than 3.5 mm.[66] Congenital, as opposed to acquired, stenosis is typically the result of malformation of the cricoid cartilage. Normally, at the inferior margin of the cricoid cartilage the transverse and anteroposterior diameters of the normal infant larynx are equal, resulting in a ring configuration. In some infants with congenital subglottic stenosis, an elliptical cricoid is present with a transverse diameter that is significantly smaller than the anteroposterior diameter, which may cause respiratory distress and predispose the larynx to injury from endotracheal tube intubation.[66,67] The elliptical cricoid may be found in association with a laryngeal cleft. An "occult" or submucous posterior laryngeal cleft may be associated with subglottic stenosis. This type of cleft is difficult to identify, however, because the soft tissue overlying the posterior cricoid appears normal.

In comparison with the elliptical cricoid, the transverse diameter may be greater than the anteroposterior diameter, causing a flattened cricoid, which again may lead to respiratory distress and intubation trauma. The flattened cricoid may be associated with a trapped first tracheal ring, where the first tracheal ring is inside the cricoid cartilage, thereby reducing the size of the lumen. A narrowed subglottic space can also be caused by a generalized thickening of the cricoid.

The stridor of subglottic stenosis may be inspiratory or biphasic and worsens with patient agitation (increased airflow). A mild stenosis may be asymptomatic until an upper respiratory tract infection causes subglottic edema and the child presents to medical personnel with symptoms consistent with croup. Prolonged or recurrent croup may be caused by mild subglottic stenosis.

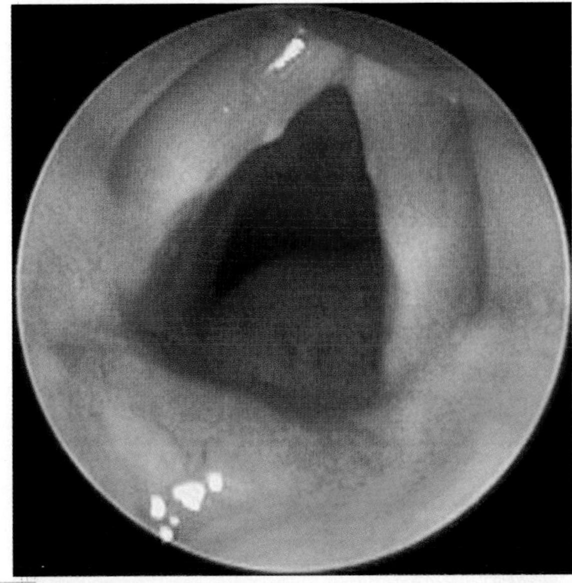

Figure 202-8. Right posterior subglottic hemangioma.

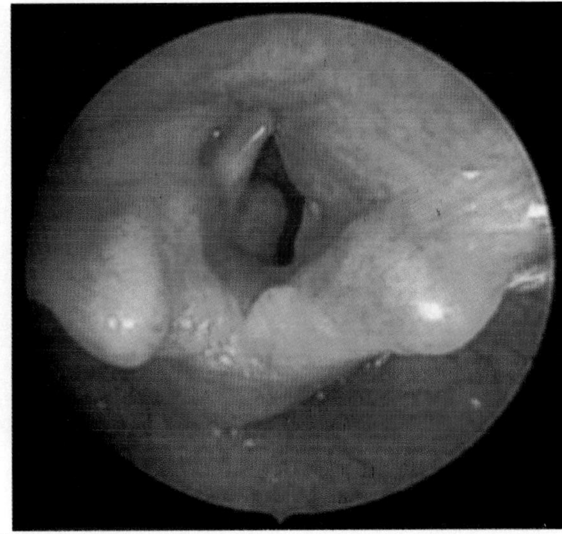

Figure 202-9. Left subglottic cyst.

Direct laryngoscopy and bronchoscopy are needed to fully evaluate subglottic narrowing. Objective measurement at the time of laryngoscopy by sequential gentle placement of endotracheal tubes of various sizes is recommended.[68] The stenosis is then graded: grade I, less than 50% obstruction; grade II, 52% to 70% obstruction; grade III, 71% to 99% obstruction; grade IV, no detectable lumen.[68]

In patients with grade I stenosis, a watchful waiting approach can be taken and the child will likely grow out of the problem as the cricoid cartilage grows. In the child with a more significant stenosis, surgical intervention is usually needed. Because it is primarily a cartilaginous problem, congenital subglottic stenosis does not typically respond to dilation or laser treatment, which is sometimes effective in soft tissue acquired stenoses. If the stenosis is grade II or III, a tracheotomy will likely be needed until the cricoid grows to a sufficient size to allow decannulation, or a laryngotracheal reconstruction performed to expand the cricoid ring. For further details of surgical management, see Chapters 71 and 206 on subglottic stenosis.

Hemangiomas and Subglottic Cysts

Mass lesions in the subglottic area can mimic the symptoms of subglottic stenosis. Subglottic hemangiomas are benign vascular malformations characterized by endothelial hyperplasia. They are twice as common in females as in males, and the patients typically present to medical caregivers in the first 6 months of life with inspiratory or biphasic stridor.[69,70] Often these patients are thought to have nonresolving croup, because they have a barking cough that responds temporarily to oral steroids. Hemangiomas grow rapidly in the first 6 months of life, stabilize for approximately a year, then slowly involute until they are gone, usually by the age of 3 years. To avoid total airway obstruction, medical or surgical intervention is usually needed.

Diagnosis is made at the time of direct laryngoscopy, with viewing of the subglottic area via telescope or microscope (Fig. 202-8). Narrowing of the subglottis can sometimes be seen on x-ray examination of the neck, and computed tomography (CT) or MRI scan can assist in the diagnosis.

The traditional medical treatment used for management of the patient with a subglottic hemangioma is systemic steroids. In most children, systemic steroids result in at least partial regression of the hemangiomas. Steroid therapy alone has been advocated as the primary method of management.[71] Long-term therapy lasting several months is needed if the hemangioma is to be controlled, leading to possible severe side effects such as Cushing's syndrome, hypertension, diabetes, and growth retardation. Intralesional steroids and short-term intubation also have been recommended as a method to control the subglottic hemangioma. Using a protocol of steroid injection followed by 1 week of intubation has resulted in patent airways at a mean of 9.5 months of age in 82% of the 15 patients treated at one institution.[72] Propanolol, a beta-blocking agent, has been used successfully to treat infantile hemangiomas. The conditions under which it will be most successful have not yet been identified.

The traditional surgical option to relieve the airway obstruction associated with subglottic hemangioma is a tracheotomy. The tracheotomy tube bypasses the lesion. Once the lesion involutes, the patient can be decannulated, on average 27 months after the tracheotomy was placed.[69] Accidental decannulation and tracheostomy tube obstruction are the major drawbacks of this approach. The mortality rate of a tracheostomy in an infant is generally accepted to be between 1% and 2%.[73] In addition, the care required to keep an infant with a tracheostomy tube safe is tremendous, causing a severe strain on the patient's family.

The carbon dioxide and potassium titanyl phosphate (KTP) lasers have been used to control hemangiomas.[69,74] Using a CO_2 laser has been reported to be successful,[70,75] but others have reported that the laser did not result in earlier tracheotomy decannulation.[69] It has been proposed that the KTP laser may be the superior instrument for treatment of the hemangiomas because the KTP beam is preferentially absorbed by hemoglobin, making it more applicable to the treatment of vascular lesions.[74] The most significant complication associated with the laser is subglottic stenosis, which has been reported in up to 18% of cases.[75,76] At least one report did not find any advantage of the tracheostomy and laser compared with the tracheostomy alone.[69]

Open surgical resection via a laryngofissure has been reported to be successful in several cases.[69,77,78] This approach seems to be particularly useful in the patients with circumferential or bilateral subglottic hemangiomas.

Another lesion that can mimic the symptoms of a subglottic hemangioma is the subglottic cyst (Fig. 202-9). In one review, 55 patients with subglottic cysts were identified.[79] All had been intubated in the neonatal period and 94% were born prematurely at 24 to 31 weeks of gestation. Intubation trauma is believed to be the cause of these lesions.[80] The cysts can be unroofed with either a laser or microlaryngeal instruments, but recurrence is common.[81,82]

Thyroglossal Duct Cyst

Cysts at the base of tongue in the vallecula are a rare but potentially lethal source of airway obstruction in a neonate (Fig. 202-10). Cases of acute airway obstruction with sudden death have been reported.[83-85] The obstructing cysts are of thyroglossal duct origin and have pseudostratified ciliated or squamous epithelium, with mucous glands and thyroid follicles in the subjacent stroma.[86] If thyroid follicles are not

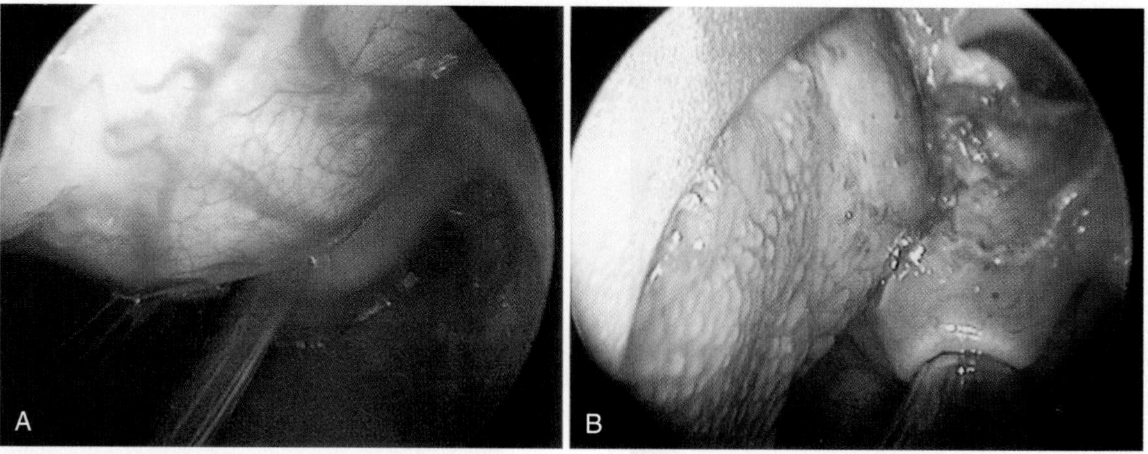

Figure 202-10. Vallecular thyroglossal duct cyst before and after marsupialization.

seen, the pathologist sometimes will call it a vallecular cyst instead of a thyroglossal duct cyst, but the origin is the same. In addition, cysts that occur on the epiglottis or in the vallecula and originate from obstruction of the submucosal glands are sometimes are called "ductal cysts."[87] Infants with thyroglossal duct cysts at the foramen cecum typically develop symptoms within the first few weeks of life. Most commonly the baby will present with stridor but feeding difficulties, coughing, cyanotic episodes, failure to thrive, and breath-holding spells may be present.[87-90] The voice may be normal or may have a muffled quality.

Diagnosis is made at the time of flexible or direct laryngoscopy. A lateral neck x-ray film, CT scan, or MRI scan may be helpful in the diagnosis, but endoscopy is the major diagnostic tool. Definitive treatment should not be delayed for these other investigations in the infant with airway obstruction.[88] The differential diagnosis of a vallecular mass in children also includes a dermoid, teratoma, lingual thyroid, lymphatic malformation, or hemangioma.[85] If a thyroglossal duct cyst or lingual thyroid is identified, then a thyroid scan or ultrasound should be performed to identify other functioning thyroid tissue.

Treatment of all types of vallecular cysts is by endoscopic surgical removal or marsupialization. Aspiration of the cysts for definitive treatment is not advocated because they will recur. In an emergency situation with a tenuous airway, the cyst can be aspirated, with definitive surgical treatment following.

Laryngeal Cysts

Saccular cysts and laryngoceles are unusual causes of respiratory obstruction in children. The anterior-superior portion of the laryngeal ventricle leads to a pouch of mucous membrane called the saccule. The saccule rises superiorly between the false vocal fold, the base of the epiglottis, and the inner surface of the thyroid cartilage. Scant muscle surrounds the saccule, compressing it to express its secretions on the vocal folds. Laryngoceles (abnormal dilation or herniation of the saccule) can be internal, confined to the interior of the larynx and extending posterosuperiorly into the area of the false vocal fold and aryepiglottic fold, or laryngoceles can be external, passing through the thyrohyoid membrane and presenting as a mass in the neck. If both an internal and external component are present, the laryngocele is termed a *combined laryngocele.* The radiographic finding of an air-containing rounded mass in the neck or supraglottic region, sometimes with air-fluid levels, confirms the presence of a laryngocele.[10]

Saccular cysts result from the obstruction of the laryngeal saccule orifice, or the collecting ducts of the submucosal glands located around the ventricle produce the saccular cysts. Saccular cysts may be anterior, protruding between the anterior and posterior vocal cords, or lateral, extending into the false vocal cord and aryepiglottic fold (Figs. 202-11 and 202-12). Laryngoceles produce intermittent upper airway obstruction and hoarseness because of episodic filling with air, whereas saccular cysts produce constant symptoms because of mucoid fluid within the cyst. Diagnosis is made at the time of flexible or direct laryngoscopy.

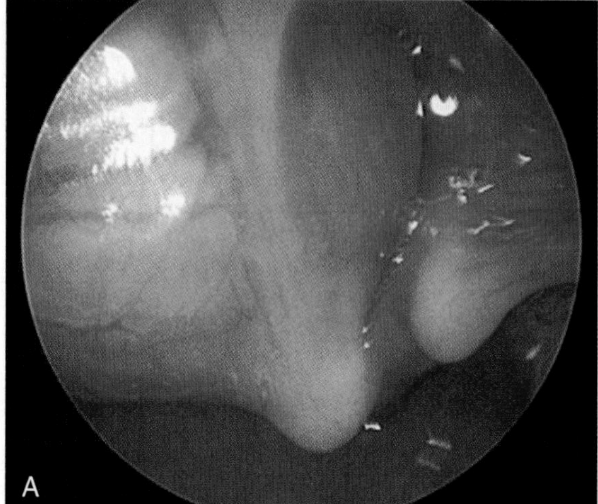

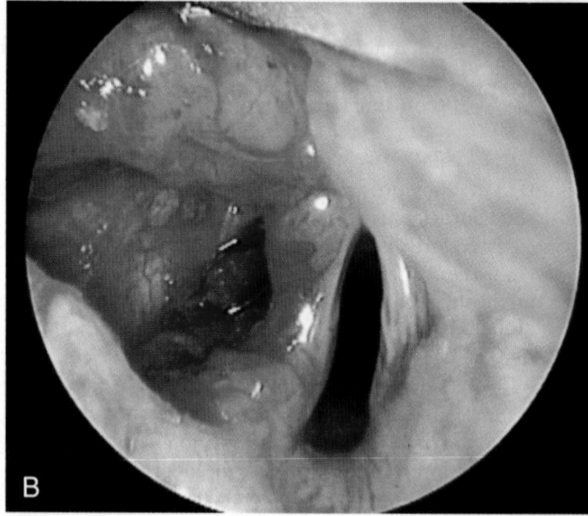

Figure 202-11. **A,** Left lateral saccular cyst. The 17-month-old female presented with a muffled cry and history of stridor when younger. **B,** Area of saccular cyst following endoscopic resection.

Other laryngeal lesions, such as hemangiomas, laryngeal duplication cysts, hamartomas, choristomas, and teratomas, can present with similar symptoms and appearance.[91-94]

Typically, treatment of the cysts involves endoscopic marsupialization of the cyst, most commonly with the CO_2 laser so that the back wall of the cyst can be ablated.[95] Recurrence after marsupialization of a posterior saccular cyst is common, often necessitating several

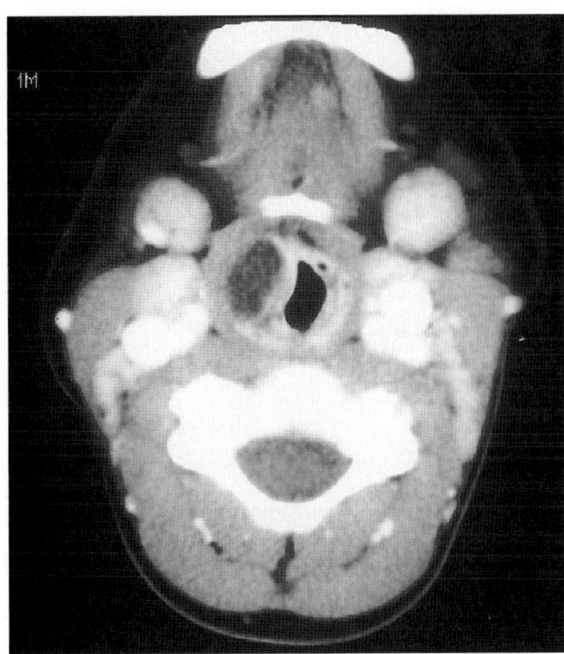

Figure 202-12. Computed tomography scan of child with a lateral saccular cyst.

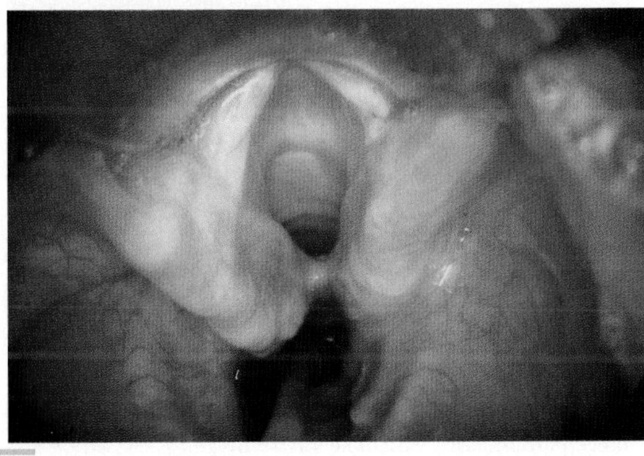

Figure 202-13. Laryngotracheal cleft—Benjamin-Inglis type 3. *(From Benjamin B: The pediatric airway, slide #34, Slide Lecture Series. American Academy of Otolaryngology–Head and Neck Surgery, 1992).*

endoscopic procedures.[96] Tracheotomy may be required and subglottic stenosis is a potential complication of the treatment. Alternatively, removal of the cyst can be achieved via a lateral cervical approach through the thyrohyoid membrane.[97]

Laryngeal-Laryngotracheoesophageal Cleft

Laryngeal cleft (LC) and laryngotracheoesophageal clefts (LTECs) are rare congenital anomalies caused by failure of the posterior cricoid lamina to fuse and incomplete development of the tracheoesophageal septum (Fig. 202-13). This developmental failure leads to an abnormal communication between the posterior portion of the larynx and esophagus.

Presenting symptoms depend on the extent of the cleft. Small clefts involving only the interarytenoid musculature (type 1) are difficult to diagnose and the need for a high index of suspicion cannot be overemphasized. There are wide variations in the reported incidence of presenting symptoms suggesting that the diagnosis of mild LCs is an inexact science. Feeding difficulties and aspiration have been reported to occur in 40% to 90% of patients, and stridor in 15% to 94% of patients.[98-100] Recurrent pneumonia and chronic cough are also commonly seen with this diagnosis. The severity of symptoms typically increases with the extent of the cleft. Patients with LTECs that extend into the trachea present with signs and symptoms of severe aspiration, respiratory distress, and cyanosis.[101]

Most patients with LC and LTECs have other congenital abnormalities, most commonly including tracheoesophageal fistula (TEF), esophageal atresia, congenital heart disease, cleft lip and palate, micrognathia, glossoptosis, laryngomalacia, and Opitz-Frias syndrome (see Table 202-1).[102] A tracheoesophageal fistula is present in approximately 25% of patients with an LC or LTEC and is an important prognostic indicator of possible failure of the surgical repair.[100-104]

Diagnosis is made at the time of microdirect laryngoscopy where the interarytenoid mucosa is spread laterally to reveal the cleft larynx. Care must be taken to look at and palpate the interarytenoid area, because the cleft may be missed if only a flexible bronchoscopy or direct laryngoscopy without palpation is performed. In a group of 20 children, the average interarytenoid notch height relative to the vocal folds has been found to be approximately 3 mm.[105] In this study, a low interarytenoid notch height was found to be significantly correlated with laryngeal incompetence and aspiration. In the patient with a laryngeal cleft, bronchoscopy and esophagoscopy should also be performed and a biopsy of the esophagus considered if there is any evidence of gastroesophageal reflux. Other diagnostic tests often performed include barium swallow, functional endoscopic evaluation of swallow (FEES), and chest x-ray study to evaluate the extent of aspiration.[98] Barium swallow shows spillover of barium from the esophagus into the trachea. High small clefts may be difficult to differentiate from high H-type tracheoesophageal fistulas.[10]

Multiple classification schemes have been described, all based on the vertical length of the cleft (Table 202-2), with the Benjamin-Inglis system being used most commonly (Fig. 202-14).[103,106-109] In addition, submucous "occult" laryngeal clefts have been described.[66,110,111] The submucous laryngeal cleft consists of a posterior midline cartilage defect, with intact soft tissue including mucosa and interarytenoid muscle. It is associated with subglottic stenosis and typically is not identified unless a postmortem examination is performed.

Early repair of LCs and LTECs are recommended to avoid irreversible pulmonary damage from continued aspiration.[108] The method of surgical repair for LCs and LTECs depends on the type of cleft present. For clefts that extend only through the interarytenoid musculature, antireflux therapy may be enough to control symptoms. At some centers, conservative treatment with temporary nasogastric tube feedings is recommended.[99] If a Benjamin-Inglis type I or II cleft is symptomatic, endoscopic or open surgical repair is possible.[100] If the significance of the cleft for a particular patient is unknown, Gelfoam can be injected into the interarytenoid area to determine whether symptoms are alleviated and to provide clarification of the contribution of the posterior laryngeal cleft to the clinical status of the patient.[112]

For some clefts that extend into the cricoid and all clefts that extend below the cricoid (Benjamin-Inglis type II-IV), an open procedure is required. These clefts are best repaired using an anterior laryngofissure to avoid injury to the vascular and neural structures.[113,114] If the cleft extends to the carina (type IV), an anterior laryngofissure and median sternotomy are recommended.[115] Most patients require a tracheotomy in at least the perioperative period. If the median sternotomy approach is used, then the intrathoracic part of the repair is performed with the patient on cardiopulmonary bypass or extracorporeal membrane oxygenation.[102,115] The prognosis is grim for patients with a type IV LTEC that extends all the way to the carina.[115]

Most commonly, a two-layer closure of the cleft is performed with absorbable sutures. If possible, the two layers should not directly oppose each other to minimize the chance for breakdown and recurrent clefting. Tracheoesophagoplasty with two overlapping flaps via an anterior approach has also been used with good results.[113] An interposition graft may be placed between the two suture lines. Possible grafts include a sternocleidomastoid or strap muscle flap (inferiorly based), tibial periosteum, auricular cartilage, or temporalis fascia.[101,104,114,115]

Outcomes of surgical repair vary.[101,113,114] A higher rate of suture line breakdown occurs in the more extensive clefts and after surgical repair of an LC or an LTEC in any child who also has a tracheoesopha-

Table 202-2
Laryngeal and Laryngotracheoesophageal Cleft Classification

Cleft Location	Petterson	Armitage	Evans	Benjamin/Inglis*	Myer/Cotton*
Laryngeal					
Interarytenoid	Type I	Type IA	Type I	Type I	LI
Partial cricoid	Type I	Type IB	Type II	Type II	LII
Complete cricoid	Type I	Type IC	Type II	Type II	LIII
Laryngotracheoesophageal					
Into cervical trachea	Type II	Type II	Type II	Type III	LTEI
To intrathoracic trachea/carina	Type III	Type III	Type III	Type IV	LTEII

*Most useful classification systems.

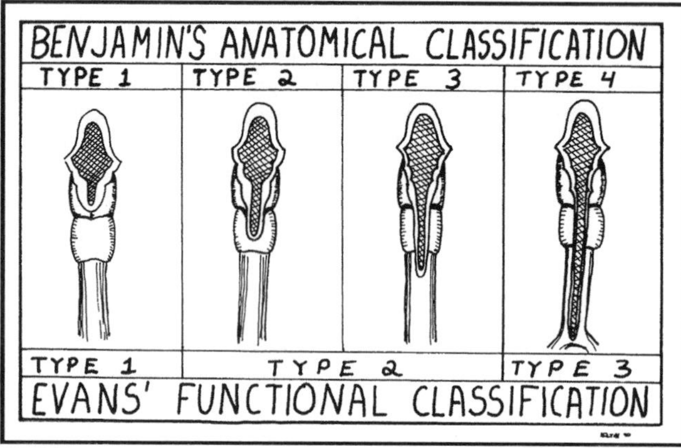

Figure 202-14. Benjamin-Inglis classification system for laryngeal clefts. *(Copyright Peter Koltai, MD.)*

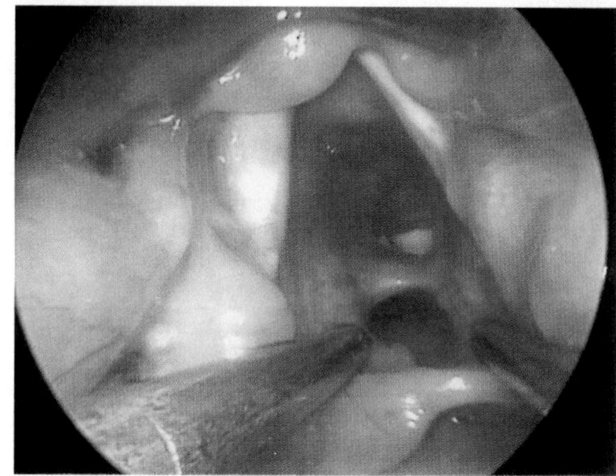

Figure 202-15. Benjamin/Inglis stage 3, Myer/Cotton Stage LTEI recurrent laryngotracheal cleft after two open attempts at repair. Note small mucosal bridge at proximal end of cleft and tracheotomy tube within the trachea.

geal fistula (see Fig. 202-14). In a retrospective review of 25 children who underwent a Myer-Cotton classification type LII, LIII, or LTEI cleft repair, 12 of 14 (86%) who had a previously repaired TEF subsequently developed a recurrent LC or LTEC (Fig. 202-15).[104] Of the remaining 11 patients who did not have a TEF, only one experienced a suture line breakdown. Gastroesophageal reflux and eosinophil gastroenteritis can also negatively affect the surgical repair and thus should be treated aggressively.[116-118]

Bifid Epiglottis

A bifid epiglottis is a rare anomaly defined as a cleft of the epiglottis encompassing at least two thirds of its length.[119] The infants typically present with stridor or aspiration, although they also can be asymptomatic. The diagnosis is made on laryngoscopy, and if the epiglottis is lax, prolapsing into the laryngeal inlet, supraglottoplasty can be performed.

Associated congenital anomalies are common and tend to be midline.[120] In the head and neck these anomalies include cleft palate, cleft uvula, micrognathia, and microglossia (see Table 202-1). Polydactyly has been reported in approximately 75% of patients with a bifid epiglottis.[121] The hypothalamic-pituitary axis is often disrupted in children with a bifid epiglottis. Congenital hamartomas or the absence of the pituitary gland can lead to growth hormone insufficiency with resultant growth retardation, secondary hypothyroidism with resultant cretinism, or secondary hypoadrenalism resulting in salt wasting and hypoglycemia.

Pallister-Hall syndrome (PHS), or congenital hypothalamic hamartoblastoma syndrome, is commonly associated with a bifid epiglottis.[122] Laryngoscopic examination of 26 subjects with PHS showed that 15 had a bifid or cleft epiglottis (58%). Other associated features of the syndrome include polydactyly, pituitary dysfunction, imperforate anus, and laryngotracheal cleft. It has an autosomal dominant inheritance pattern, with variable expressivity and is caused by a mutation in the GLI3 gene.[122] Because of the high incidence of hypothalamic-pituitary problems, all infants with a congenitally bifid epiglottis should undergo an MRI of the brain, an endocrine evaluation, and a genetics consultation.

Summary

Congenital laryngeal anomalies cause a spectrum of airway difficulties. In laryngomalacia, the stridor is transient and in most cases resolves spontaneously without intervention. Conversely, laryngeal atresia or obstructing vallecular cysts can lead to neonatal death. Although nearly all anomalies present with stridor, they can cause a host of other problems for the young child, including dysphagia, aspiration, failure to thrive, and dysphonia. Laryngoscopy, either direct or flexible, is the procedure most likely to diagnose the problem, although complete laryngotracheobronchial endoscopy may be needed to rule out a laryngeal cleft or other synchronous airway lesions.

SUGGESTED READINGS

Chien W, Ashland J, Haver K, et al. Type 1 laryngeal cleft: establishing a functional diagnostic and management algorithm. *Int J Pediatr Otorhinolaryngol.* 2006;70(12):2073-2079.

Daya H, Hosni A, Bejar-Solar I, et al. Pediatric vocal fold paralysis: a long-term retrospective study. *Arch Otolaryngol Head Neck Surg.* 2000;126:21-25.

Denoyelle F, Mondain M, Gresillon N, et al. Failures and complications of supraglottoplasty in children. *Arch Otolaryngol Head Neck Surg.* 2003; 129(10):1077-1080.

Hadfield PJ, Albert DM, Bailey CM, et al. The effect of aryepiglottoplasty for laryngomalacia on gastroesophageal reflux. *Int J Pediatr Otorhinolaryngol.* 2003;67:11-14.

Hartnick CJ, Brigger MT, Willging JP, et al. Surgery for pediatric vocal cord paralysis: a retrospective review. *Ann Otol Rhinol Laryngol.* 2003;112(1):1-6.

Hoeve LJ, Kuppers GL, Verwoerd CD. Management of infantile subglottic hemangioma: laser vaporization, submucous resection, intubation, or intralesional steroids? *Int J Pediatr Otorhinolaryngol.* 1997;42:179-186.

Holinger LD. Histopathology of congenital subglottic stenosis. *Ann Otol Rhinol Laryngol.* 1999;108:101-111.

Kirse DJ, Rees CJ, Celmer AW, et al. Endoscopic extended ventriculotomy for congenital saccular cysts of the larynx in infants. *Arch Otolaryngol Head Neck Surg.* 2006;132(7):724-728.

Kubba H, Gibson D, Bailey M, et al. Techniques and outcomes of laryngeal cleft repair: an update to the Great Ormond Street Hospital series. *Ann Otol Rhinol Laryngol.* 2005;114(4):309-313.

Lim FY, Crombleholme TM, Hedrick HL, et al. Congenital high airway obstruction syndrome: natural history and management. *J Pediatr Surg.* 2003;38(6):940-945.

Lim J, Hellier W, Harcourt J, et al. Subglottic cysts: the Great Ormond Street experience. *Int J Pediatr Otorhinolaryngol.* 2003;67:461-465.

Mathur NN, Peek GJ, Bailey CM, et al. Strategies for managing Type IV laryngotracheoesophageal clefts at Great Ormond Street Hospital for Children. *Int J Pediatr Otorhinolaryngol.* 2006;70(11):1901-1910.

Miyamoto RC, Parikh SR, Gellad W, et al. Bilateral congenital vocal cord paralysis: a 16-year institutional review. *Otolaryngol Head Neck Surg.* 2005;133(2):241-245.

Miyamoto RC, Cotton RT, Rope AF, et al. Association of anterior glottic webs with velocardiofacial syndrome (chromosome 22q11.2 deletion). *Otolaryngol Head Neck Surg.* 2004;130(4):415-417.

For complete list of references log onto www.expertconsult.com.

Nicollas R, Sudre-Levillain I, Roman S, et al. Surgical repair of laryngotracheoesophageal clefts by tracheoesophagoplasty with two overlapping flaps. *Ann Otol Rhinol Laryngol.* 2006;115(5):346-349.

O-Lee TJ, Messner AH. Open excision of subglottic hemangioma with microscopic dissection. *Int J Pediatr Otorhinolaryngol.* 2007;71(9):1371-1376.

Rahbar R, Rouillon I, Roger G, et al. The presentation and management of laryngeal cleft: a 10-year experience. *Arch Otolaryngol Head Neck Surg.* 2006;132(12):1335-1341.

Roger G, Denoyelle F, Triglia JM, et al. Severe laryngomalacia: surgical indications and results in 115 patients. *Laryngoscope.* 1995;105:1111-1117.

Scott AR, Chong PS, Randolph GW, et al. Intraoperative laryngeal electromyography in children with vocal fold immobility: A simplified technique. *Int J Pediatr Otorhinolaryngol.* 2008;72(1):31-40.

Sipp JA, Kerschner JE, Braune N, et al. Vocal fold medialization in children: injection laryngoplasty, thyroplasty, or nerve reinnervation? *Arch Otolaryngol Head Neck Surg.* 2007;133(8):767-771.

Sivan Y, Ben-Ari J, Soferman R, et al. Diagnosis of laryngomalacia by fiberoptic endoscopy: awake compared with anesthesia-aided technique. *Chest.* 2006;130(5):1412-1418.

Stevens CA, Ledbetter JC. Significance of bifid epiglottis. *Am J Med Genet A.* 2005 May 1;134(4):447-449.

Thompson DM. Abnormal sensorimotor integrative function of the larynx in congenital laryngomalacia: a new theory of etiology. *Laryngoscope.* 2007;117(6 Pt 2 Suppl 114):1-33.

Truong MT, Messner AH, Kerschner JE, et al. Pediatric vocal fold paralysis after cardiac surgery: rate of recovery and sequelae. *Otolaryngol Head Neck Surg.* 2007;137(5):780-784.

Van der Doef HP, Yntema JB, van den Hoogen FJ, et al. Clinical aspects of type 1 posterior laryngeal clefts: literature review and a report of 31 patients. *Laryngoscope.* 2007 117(5):859-863.

CHAPTER TWO HUNDRED AND THREE

Voice Disorders

Sukgi S. Choi

George H. Zalzal

Key Points

- Evaluation and management of voice disorders in children can be more challenging because of their inability to cooperate, lack of awareness of the problem, and lack of motivation to change.
- Otolaryngologic evaluation of a child with voice disorder begins with detailed history, physical examination, flexible laryngoscopy, and videostroboscopy.
- Voice evaluation by a speech pathologist should include perceptual, acoustic, and aerodynamic analyses.
- Voice therapy plays an essential role in management of pediatric voice disorders and should be used liberally both preoperatively and postoperatively.
- Voice disorders can be due to functional and organic etiologies. Organic voice disorders requiring primarily surgical management include vocal fold paralysis, laryngeal web, posterior glottic stenosis, recurrent respiratory papillomatosis (RRP), and malignant tumors. Vocal fold granulomas typically require medical management. Vocal nodules, cysts, polyps, and sulcus are initially managed with voice therapy but may require surgery.
- Surgery, especially in very young children, should be undertaken with caution.

Voice production starts with the expiration phase of respiration, which provides the air pressure to vibrate the vocal folds. The lowest periodic component of vocal fold vibration is termed *fundamental frequency* and is perceived as pitch.[1] Harmonics are integer multiples of fundamental frequency in voiced sounds. The energy or intensity in the harmonic components decreases as frequency increases.

Sound waves generated by vocal fold vibration are modified by the size, shape, and tenseness of the resonating chamber, which consists of the oropharynx, the nasopharynx, and the nasal cavities. The resonance of the vocal tract is termed *formant*.[1] Although an infinite number of formants exist, only the first four formants (F1, F2, F3, and F4) are of clinical interest; the lowest frequency formant is F1. Each formant is characterized by its center frequency and bandwidth. Constriction of the vocal tract near a volume velocity maximum or minimum can respectively lower or raise the formant frequency. The resulting sound wave is further modified by the articulators (lips, teeth, tongue), resulting in voice and speech production. A normal voice should be pleasing in quality and have appropriate balance of oral and nasal resonance, intensity, fundamental frequency level, and prosody. Voice disorder can result in a voice that is unpleasant for the listener or can interfere with effective communication.

The underlying cause of a voice disorder can be organic or functional. Organic voice disorders result from congenital or acquired anatomic abnormalities. Functional disorders are caused by emotional or psychological problems but can lead to anatomic alterations. However, even when a voice disorder results primarily from an organic cause, there is often a psychological overlay.[2]

Although the reported incidence of voice disorders in children varies greatly, most voice surveys of children show a 6% to 9% incidence of voice disorders.[3] Voice disorders are categorized depending on the area of problem: voice quality, resonance, loudness, and pitch. This classification is arbitrary, and a voice disorder often has several problem areas. Any anatomic abnormality involving the free edge of the vocal fold can affect voice quality and result in harshness, breathiness, or hoarseness. Disturbances in resonance can be caused by hypernasality or hyponasality. Loudness or intensity problems occur when a child speaks too loudly or too softly. Deviations in pitch occur with inappropriate speaking fundamental frequency, narrow pitch range, or excessive pitch breaks. An algorithm for the evaluation and management of voice disorders is outlined in Fig. 203-1.

Evaluation

The evaluation of a voice disorder in a child requires a systematic approach. Additional evaluation by specialists from a variety of disciplines including a pediatrician, pulmonologist, gastroenterologist, psychologist, and social worker may be necessary. A detailed history, including medical, birth, growth and development, and speech and language history is obtained, followed by detailed voice history to determine the cause of the voice disorder and its contributing factors, potentially including any pulmonary disease. Typically, voice history should include a description of the disorder, time of onset, any known causes, severity of the disorder, exacerbating or alleviating factors, voice use history, and any previous history of voice or speech therapy.

Social and functional impact of voice impairment can be evaluated using rating scales such as Pediatric Voice Outcomes survey (PVOS), Pediatric Voice-Related Quality-of-Life Survey (PVRQOL), and Pediatric Voice Handicap Index (pVHI).[4-6] These rating scales are designed to provide physicians with the parents' perception of the severity of the child's voice disorder and its impact on the child's daily life; they are used to follow the child's progress before and after therapy and surgical intervention.

Physical examination should concentrate on the head and neck areas. The ears are examined for evidence of previous and current ear disease. A nasal examination should reveal any deviation of the septum

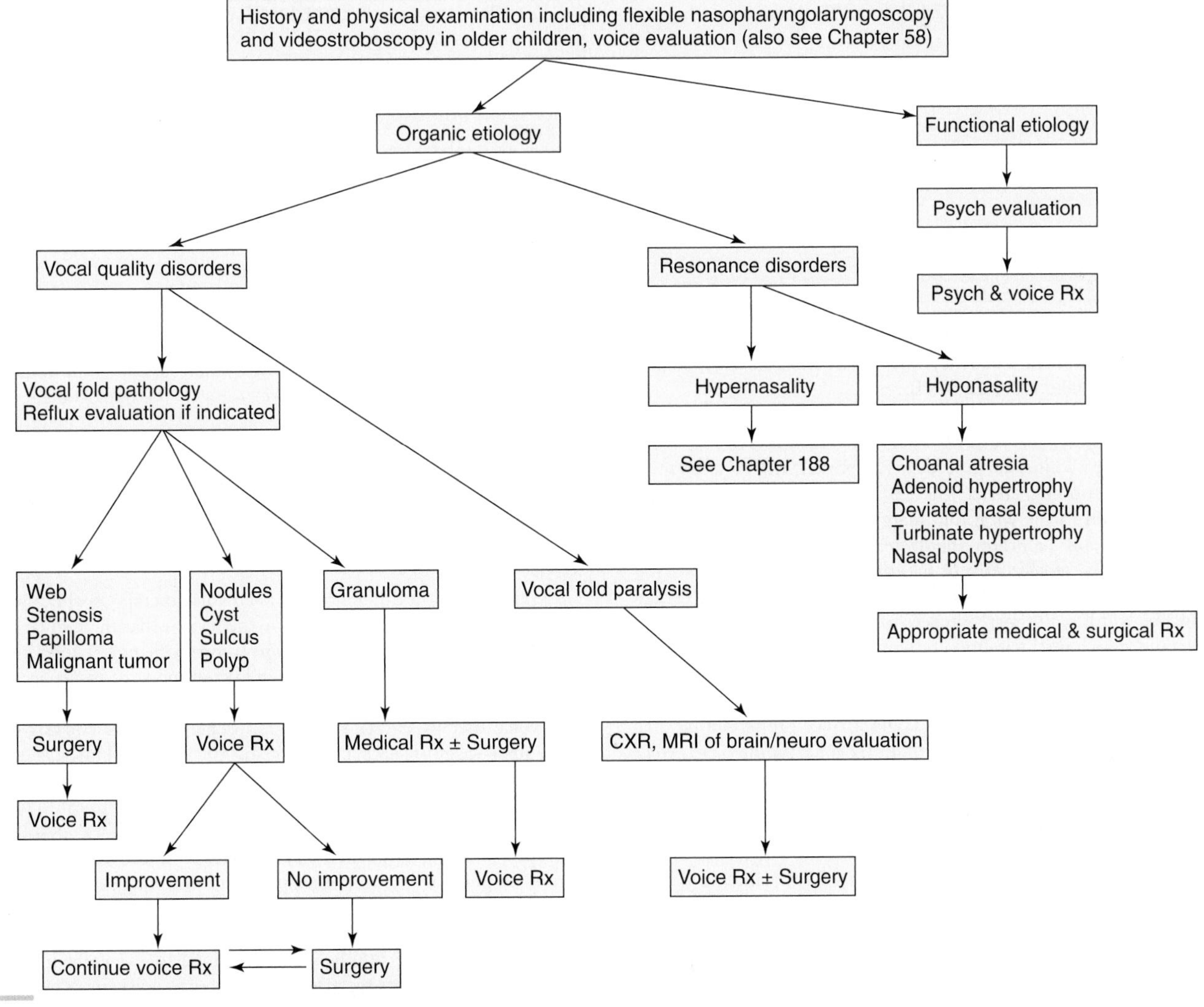

Figure 203-1. Evaluation and management of voice disorders in children.

and turbinate abnormalities. An oropharyngeal examination should focus on the structural integrity and mobility of the soft palate and is followed by flexible fiberoptic nasopharyngolaryngoscopy. Flexible fiberoptic scopes determine the size of the adenoid, velopharyngeal function, and any pathology in the supraglottic and glottic areas.

Stroboscopic examination, which uses a short burst of light in synchrony with vocal fold motion, can seemingly slow down the movement of the vocal folds and allow more careful examination of the vocal folds and their motion.[7] It is particularly useful in differentiating superficial from deep lesions. Laryngeal stroboscopy can delineate vocal fold symmetry, periodicity, vibratory amplitude, mucosal wave, glottal closure, and rigidity,[7] but it is not possible in many children. Bouchayer and Cornut[8] found that stroboscopic examination in children often had to be quick; therefore their results tended to be inconclusive. Hirschberg and colleagues[9] found that stroboscopy was possible only in children older than 6 or 7 years. McAllister and others[10] completed stroboscopic examination in only half of 60 patients age 10 years and older. The newer digital flexible endoscopes may allow stroboscopic examination in younger children.[11] In our voice clinic, digital flexible stroboscopy has been used successfully in children as young as age 3 years. Although stroboscopic examination can be instrumental in accurate diagnosis of a voice disorder, rigid endoscopy under anesthesia may be necessary in some children to establish diagnosis and for therapeutic intervention.

The child's voice is evaluated by a speech-language pathologist, usually in a voice laboratory. A typical voice evaluation consists of perceptual, acoustic, and aerodynamic analyses carried out as the child performs several speaking tasks. There are no universally accepted standards for speech and voice evaluation, and the speaking tasks, the speech parameters measured, and the method of measurement vary greatly.

There are several commonly used speaking tasks.[3] The first is oral reading, which is possible only in older children. Children who can read at third grade level or better are given a specific passage to read; younger children are allowed to select the reading material. The second task is conversational speech or connected speech at least 1 minute long. The child is asked to tell a story about a picture or talk about a specific topic (e.g., pets, a vacation, a hobby). Based on these two tasks, the speech-language pathologist can perceptually and acoustically analyze the child's speech for most voice parameters, including prosody.

The remaining speaking tasks are designed to evaluate more isolated aspects of the child's voice. The third task consists of counting from 1 to 10, 60 to 70, and 90 to 100.[3] The counting is done carefully, once slowly and then as rapidly as possible. This is repeated for three levels of loudness (soft, average, loud) and pitch (low, modal, high). This task reveals any problems with laryngeal tone, resonance, pitch, and loudness.

The fourth speaking task is the production of isolated speech sounds. This consists of sustaining certain vowel sounds (e.g., /a/, /i/) for at least 5 seconds and repeating them three times to determine laryngeal tone, resonance, and fundamental frequency. The child should then sustain /a/ at a comfortable pitch and loudness for as long as possible after a deep inspiration and repeat this three times with a break in between each attempt to determine the maximal phonation time and whether the child had adequate respiratory drive to maintain

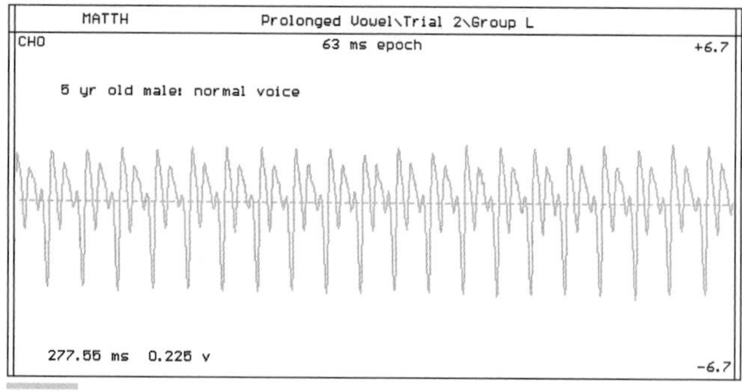

Figure 203-2. Voice tracing of a normal voice sustaining a prolonged vowel: mean fundamental frequency, 332.53 Hz; jitter, 0.36%; shimmer, 1.9%; harmonic/noise ratio, 12.37 dB.

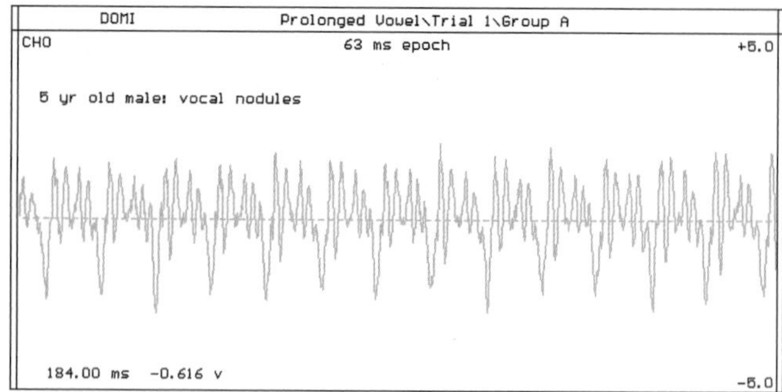

Figure 203-3. Voice tracing of a hoarse voice (caused by vocal nodules) sustaining a prolonged vowel: mean fundamental frequency, 220.60 Hz; jitter, 2.26%; shimmer, 4.34%; harmonic/noise ratio, 7.84 dB.

continuous voice.[3] This same procedure is repeated with /s/ and /z/. In a normally functioning larynx, the s:z ratio should be close to 1. However, a lesion in the vocal fold margins (e.g., vocal fold nodules) increases the amount of airflow and decreases the time on /z/, resulting in a ratio of 1.4 or greater 95% of the time.[12]

Finally, the examiner should instruct the child to repeat certain consonants, words, and short sentences to assess the child's articulation abilities and speech intelligibility. The words and sentences are typically chosen to bring out specific problems such as velopharyngeal insufficiency.

The speech samples are analyzed, and a voice profile can be then developed using scales such as the Buffalo III voice profile.[3] This voice profile classifies voice abnormalities as follows: 1, normal; 2, mild; 3, moderate; 4, severe; or 5, very severe. It evaluates laryngeal tone, pitch, loudness, nasal resonance, oral resonance, breath supply, muscles, voice abuse, rate, speech anxiety, speech intelligibility, and overall voice rating. Other perceptual scales such as GRBAS and Consensus Auditory-Perceptual Evaluation-Voice (CAPE-V) are also used in the evaluation of pediatric voice.[13,14]

Aerodynamic analysis provides objective measures of the velopharyngeal and vocal fold functions. The oral-nasal acoustic ratio and palatal efficiency rating computed instantaneously have been used to evaluate velopharyngeal function.[15,16] Laryngeal airway resistance can be measured to assess the effective closure of the vocal folds to airflow. This is measured noninvasively using an anesthesia mask, a pressure-sensing catheter, and a flow-sensing pneumotachometer. Values less than 30 cm H_2O/L/sec indicate inadequate closure, whereas values greater than 60 cm H_2O/L/sec are associated with hyperkinetic voice disorders.[17] Normative aerodynamic measures for children age 6 to 10 are available.[18] These techniques of aerodynamic analysis are being replaced by computer-assisted voice analysis programs.

Computer-assisted analysis of voice disorder was introduced in 1990 and is being used with increasing frequency.[19] This technology presents the opportunity to supplement perceptual evaluation of voice disorders and has replaced many traditional methods of evaluation. Evaluation of naturalness and intelligibility of speech still requires the human ear.

Computer-assisted voice analysis can provide the mean fundamental frequency, intensity, and amplitude of voice based on a small voice sample (0.5 second) for comparison with existing normative values for age and sex (Figs. 203-2 and 203-3).[19] Until recently, no normative data for children in these analyses was available and normative data from adult studies in the literature were used[20]; however, in 2002, Campisi and colleagues[21] published a pediatric normative database for computer-assisted voice analysis.

Other information provided by computerized voice analysis includes harmonics-noise ratio, amplitude perturbation (shimmer), frequency perturbation (jitter), and electroglottography. Aerodynamic measures can be obtained in less than 60 seconds using the pneumotachographic mask. Parameters that can be measured include subglottal pressure; transglottal airflow; oral pressure; nasal flow; airflow; resistance and efficiency; inspiratory, expiratory, and pause aerodynamics; and nasal and velopharyngeal resistance. Voice analysis is also discussed in Chapter 58.

Voice Therapy

There are important differences between voice therapy in children and in adults. Children often do not have the insight that their voice needs to be modified and they lack the motivation to change. Therefore, the therapist must work to increase the child's awareness of his or her vocal behaviors and awareness of behaviors that require change.

Voice therapy entails two stages.[22] The first stage consists of 10 exploratory sessions, each lasting 35 to 40 minutes. This stage helps determine the goals and specific procedures to be used in stage 2, which consists of regular voice therapy sessions for 2 to 5 months. The frequency of therapy is determined by the severity of the dysphonia. Therapy should be supplemented by practice at home to hasten resolution of dysphonia. The total therapy duration is approximately 4 to 5 months; improvement or resolution of dysphonia should be significant.

During the initial phase of voice therapy, the mechanisms of voice production and voice problems are explained to the child in simple terms, and a list of rules regarding good and bad voice are provided.[3,22] A main goal of therapy is to eliminate vocal abuse by decreasing the total amount of talking; however, even in highly motivated children, total voice rest may not be feasible. Listening training and auditory feedback are essential in voice therapy because, to correct a voice disorder, the patient should learn to differentiate normal and abnormal voices for comparison with his or her own voice.[3]

Problematic muscular tonus, loudness, pitch, and rate require therapy. These areas are often closely interrelated and should be managed simultaneously. The child is taught the following steps to correct a problematic voice parameter[3]: correct rules of specific voice parameters; identification of incorrect and correct voice habits in others; recognition of personal use of incorrect voice and modification of this habit; recognition of personal use of correct voice; recognition of situations that cause personal use of poor voice habits and good voice habits; and an increase in the amount of time that correct habits are used. These steps can be applied to any problematic voice parameter.

Voice production depends on well-coordinated movement of muscles involved in phonation. Hyperfunction or excessive muscular tonus frequently occurs in children with benign laryngeal pathology, whereas hypofunction with flaccid muscular tonus occurs in those with functional dysphonia. For both problems, control of muscular tonus and proper positioning of the laryngeal, pharyngeal, and oral structure should be taught. To correct hyperfunctional states, posture instruction, breathing exercises, relaxation procedures, muscle tension reduction technique, chewing method, muscle stretching exercises, and biofeedback can be used.[23-25] Wilson[3] found that the chewing method and progressive relaxation are particularly useful in reducing muscular tension. For hypofunctional states, the pushing method increases muscular tension.[26]

Excessive loudness of voice is accompanied by high pitch, rapid rate of speaking, and hyperfunctional state. Therefore it is often necessary to manage these problems simultaneously. Eliminating loud speaking is particularly important in children with vocal nodules. Correct training for loudness, pitch, and rate involves teaching the child to listen and to monitor various voice parameters. Often, modifying loudness lowers pitch, and attention to loudness and pitch normalize the rate of speaking.

Functional Etiology

Functional voice disorder is diagnosed when no anatomic or organic cause can be found. Functional dysphonia is categorized as disturbed mutation, psychological dysphonia, imitation, and faulty learning.[3] Mutation is the change of voice that occurs during puberty. Pitch lowers in males and, to a lesser extent, in females. Mutation can be delayed, prolonged, or incomplete. High pitch, hoarseness, and voice breaks are characteristic. Mutational voice disorder can result from endocrine pathology.[3]

Functional dysphonia resulting from psychological causes seldom occurs in children; only isolated case reports can be found in the literature.[27] The underlying psychological problems are related to or are part of tensional symptoms, adjustment, anxiety, or personality disorders.[28] Functional dysphonia may be a form of conversion hysteria. The disorder may be complete aphonia or partial loss of voice. The dysphonia is often variable, with effortful voice production and easy fatigue. Laryngeal examination may show ventricular band approximation, bowed vocal folds, or hypoadducted vocal folds (hysterical aphonia). Vocal fold movement is normal with inhalation and cough.

Faulty learning[29] occurs when a child imitates cleft palate or hearing-impaired speech or learns to talk louder than normal because of the presence of hearing-impaired persons in the household.

In adults, several approaches have been used to manage functional dysphonia, including behavior therapy, hypnosis, speech therapy, psychotherapy, and a combination of speech therapy and psychotherapy. In children, the optimal management is unknown but psychotherapy or psychological counseling is often carried out in conjunction with voice therapy.

Organic Etiology

Resonance Disorders

Resonance disorders include hypernasality and hyponasality. Hypernasality is usually caused by velopharyngeal insufficiency from underlying palatal abnormalities. Hyponasality can result from any underlying condition that causes nasal or nasopharyngeal obstruction. The underlying pathology may be choanal atresia, deviated nasal septum, turbinate hypertrophy, nasal polyps, or, most frequently, adenoid hypertrophy. In performing adenoidectomy, particular attention should be paid to the structural integrity of the palate to decrease the incidence of postoperative velopharyngeal incompetence. Accurate diagnosis and appropriate medical and surgical management of these underlying conditions are further discussed in Chapter 188.

Vocal Quality Disorders: Surgical Management

Vocal Fold Paralysis

Vocal fold paralysis in children results from birth trauma and congenital anomalies of the central nervous system and the heart and great vessels. Any infant or child with vocal fold paralysis should be evaluated with chest radiograph and imaging of the central nervous system.[30-33] Vocal fold paralysis is the second most common cause of congenital stridor in children and represents 10% of congenital anomalies of the larynx.[34] Prognosis for spontaneous recovery is better for acquired, right-sided, and unilateral paralysis.[35-37]

More than 50% of vocal fold paralysis in children is bilateral.[32,38] Because arytenoid fixation can be mistaken for bilateral vocal fold paralysis, the cricoarytenoid joint should be palpated at rigid endoscopy. Laryngeal electromyography may be the most specific and sensitive test to determine the presence of vocal fold paralysis. More than 50% of the time, bilateral vocal fold paralysis requires tracheotomy for the establishment of an airway; however, the voice is often normal. Although spontaneous recovery of vocal fold function is possible after 2 to 3 years, late recovery is often incomplete because of laryngeal muscle atrophy, synkinesis, and cricoid fixation.[39] If vocal fold function does not return spontaneously after 10 to 12 months, surgery to decannulate the child should be considered.[31,40]

Surgical options to correct bilateral vocal fold paralysis consist of reinnervation with a nerve-muscle flap, cordotomy, lateralization procedures (e.g., arytenoidopexy), arytenoidectomy through a posterolateral external approach, arytenoidectomy through laryngofissure, or endoscopic arytenoidectomy.[31,40-44] Reinnervation of the posterior cricoarytenoid muscle is not universally successful,[38] although Tucker[45] reported it to be the management of choice in children. Because of the small size of the laryngeal structure, endoscopic techniques can be more difficult and less successful in children.[31,46] Cordotomy, a procedure in which the membranous vocal fold is sectioned from the vocal process of arytenoid, has limited use in children and may be useful as an adjunct to other procedures.[41,47] Narcy and colleagues[40] found Woodman's procedure to have a higher failure rate and recommended arytenoidopexy by an external posterolateral approach. However, Bower and colleagues[31] recommended arytenoidectomy through a laryngofissure because it provided better exposure, better control over the final fold position, and a high rate of success (84%). Although most patients have adequate voice postoperatively, breathiness, hoarseness, and pitch change are seen, and patients may require voice therapy. The resulting voice disorder is inversely proportional to the adequacy of the airway.

Unilateral vocal fold paralysis rarely requires airway intervention and often goes unrecognized until the child is older. The voice in unilateral vocal fold paralysis is hoarse, weak, and breathy. It usually improves spontaneously over 6 to 12 months by contralateral vocal fold compensation; recovery may be hastened by the use of voice therapy. However, in a few patients, persistent problems with dysphonia or aspiration require surgical intervention.[48] Surgical options include vocal fold injection, surgical medialization, and reinnervation. Surgical interventions should be done in conjunction with preoperative and postoperative voice therapy.

Polytef injection immediately improves voice; however, it is irreversible and changes vocal fold vibratory characteristics and thus results in poor vocal quality. Furthermore, in children, determining the amount of polytef to inject is difficult because general anesthesia is often necessary and airway obstruction is possible because of the small size of the larynx.[45] Levine and colleagues[48] recommended injection of an absorbable gelatin sponge, which is similar to polytef injection except that its effects are temporary. Fat injection appears to be well tolerated by the body, does not cause the vocal fold to become stiff, and is not absorbed extensively.[49] Recently, other injection materials such as AlloDerm and calcium hydroxyapatite have become available[50] but they have not yet been widely used in children.

Several surgical techniques are available for medialization of the vocal fold.[45,51-53] Isshiki type I thyroplasty is theoretically reversible and does not change the vibratory characteristics of the vocal fold; however, it does not restore tensioning capability of the vocal folds and requires external incision and a temporary tracheotomy in most cases. In children, this procedure is technically more difficult and may cause airway compromise. Experience with thyroplasty in children has been limited because of a lack of knowledge about the effect of this technique on thyroid cartilage growth.[48] Gray and colleagues[47] recommended thyroplastic operations only in patients with mature larynx because they believed that the operation may fix the distance between the arytenoid and thyroid cartilage. Link and others[54] have reported their experience with thyroplasty in children ages 2 to 17 years and have recommended modified surgical approach in children to compensate for their lower position of vocal folds. Although voice quality improves using objective measurement, the resulting voice is not ideal.[55]

Selective reinnervation of the adductors of the larynx does not compromise potential spontaneous recovery, necessitate tracheotomy, or preclude eventual use of other techniques; it restores tensioning capability, thereby providing better pitch control. However, it is an open procedure, and motion may not be observed for up to 6 months.[45]

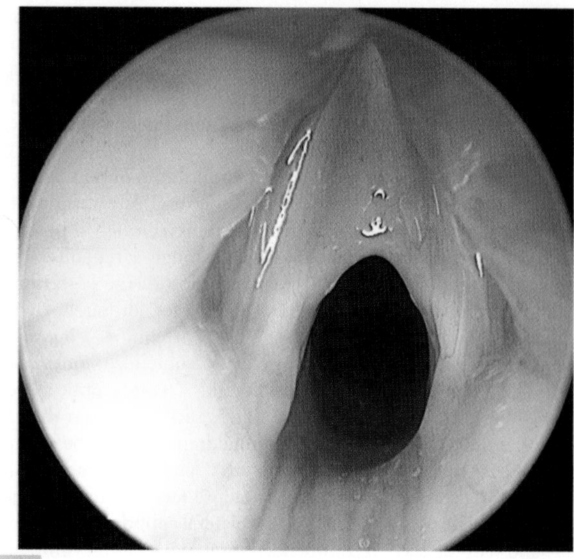

Figure 203-4. Type 2 laryngeal web.

Excellent results have been reported by Crumley[56] and Tucker.[45] Tucker advocated it to be the procedure of choice in children.[45]

Laryngeal Web

Smith and Caitlin[57] reported that glottic web and atresia account for 5% of congenital anomalies; however, some consider the true incidence of congenital web of larynx to be more common, whereas others consider it more rare. Web occurs because of failure of the epithelium, which temporarily obliterates the developing laryngotracheal lumen, to reabsorb during the eighth week of embryogenesis. Glottic web is classified depending on its severity.[58] Type 1 is an anterior web involving 35% or less of the glottis. True folds are visible within the web, and there is little or no subglottic extension. Although there is usually no airway obstruction, voice dysfunction is common. Type 2 is an anterior web involving up to 50% of the glottis (Fig. 203-4). True folds are usually visible within the web, and subglottic involvement is minimal. Voice disorder is the common presenting symptom. However, airway compromise can be seen with upper respiratory tract infections. Type 3 involves up to 75% of the glottis, and the anterior portion of the web is solid and extends into the subglottis. Most of the true folds are visible within the web. Airway obstruction and voice disorder are moderately severe. Type 4 involves up to 90% of the glottis, and the web is uniformly thick and extends into the subglottic area with resulting subglottic stenosis. Infants with this type of web are aphonic with severe airway compromise.

In 1985, Cohen and others[58] reviewed 51 cases of children with laryngeal web and recommended that surgery be tailored according to web severity. A type 2 web was divided with a knife, microsurgical scissors, or laser followed by dilations. Types 3 and 4 were managed by tracheotomy and insertion of a laryngeal keel through a laryngofissure. The anterior commissure is not adequately reconstructed by any surgical procedure, and the resulting voice continues to be abnormal and requires vocal rehabilitation.

Recommended management of a thin laryngeal web involves endolaryngeal division of the web with a knife or CO_2 laser with temporary placement of a keel to prevent readhesion. Thick glottic webs are approached through precise midline thyrotomy, a laryngofissure with removal of excess tissue under direct vision using a fiberoptic laryngoscope, and placement of a mucosal graft fixated with fibrin glue or stenting.[59] The use of CO_2 laser in cases of thick web is not recommended. The resulting voice is reportedly satisfactory, but objective postoperative analysis of voice is unavailable.

Posterior Glottic Stenosis and Cricoarytenoid Joint Fixation

Posterior glottic stenosis in children can be congenital (e.g., caused by interarytenoid web or cricoarytenoid fixation). More commonly, posterior glottic stenosis results from airway trauma from intubation. Bogdasarian and Olson[60] classified posterior glottic stenosis into four types. This classification was later modified for the pediatric population by Irving and associates.[61] Type I is vocal process adhesion, type II is posterior commissure or interarytenoid scar, type III is congenital or acquired unilateral cricoarytenoid fixation with or without interarytenoid scar, and type IV is congenital or acquired bilateral cricoarytenoid fixation with or without interarytenoid scar.

With interarytenoid web and scarring, there is bilaterally impaired abduction but normal adduction; these patients tend to have a normal voice.[62] The main presenting symptom in these cases is airway compromise. In cricoarytenoid joint fixation, adduction and abduction of the vocal fold are limited, which may also cause dysphonia. To distinguish cricoarytenoid joint fixation from vocal fold paralysis, palpation of the cricoarytenoid joint at rigid endoscopy is necessary. Laryngeal electromyography may be necessary for definitive diagnosis.

Benjamin and Mair[62] noted that interarytenoid webs are often associated with other airway abnormalities. They recommend that interarytenoid web be managed by long-term watchful waiting or by tracheotomy if associated abnormalities of the airway exist. In the case of pediatric posterior glottic stenosis, arytenoidectomy should be avoided to prevent the possibility of aspiration, deterioration of voice, and difficulty with future airway repair.[63] Although many techniques have been tried, anterior and posterior cricoidotomy with posterior graft appears to give the most consistent results and is considered the procedure of choice in children.[61,63] Improved vocal fold mobility has been observed postoperatively with this technique.[63,64]

The postoperative voice is considered to be functional in most children; a voice disorder consisting of hoarseness and breathiness often persists.[63] Bogdasarian and Olson[60] noted in adult patients that final voice results depended on the severity of stenosis; the same applies to children.

Recurrent Respiratory Papillomatosis

RRP is the most common benign neoplasm of the larynx. Papilloma patients present with hoarseness or airway obstruction. Papillomas have a predilection for anatomic sites where ciliated and squamous epithelia are juxtaposed. Common sites in the larynx are the mid zone of the laryngeal surface of the epiglottis, the upper and lower margins of the ventricles, and the undersurface of the vocal folds.[65] Recurrent respiratory papillomatosis is often diagnosed in patients between the ages of 2 and 3 years. Juvenile and adult-onset forms of the disease are possible; the juvenile form has a more aggressive clinical course. The need for tracheotomy in juvenile RRP is reportedly 14% to 21%.[66,67]

An association between cervical human papillomavirus (HPV) types 6 and 11 in the mother and RRP in the child has been established.[68-70] HPV is found in the genital tract of approximately 25% of women of child-bearing age and is clinically apparent in 2% to 5%. Shah and others[71] estimate the risk of HPV transmission to be 1 in 400 vaginal births in mothers with active condylomata.

Surgery is the management of choice, although it is only palliative because the natural history of RRP is one of recurrence. The goal of surgery is to establish a stable airway and a serviceable voice. Surgical options are CO_2 laser ablation and microlaryngoscopy with forceps removal; CO_2 laser ablation is generally accepted as the procedure of choice.[67] More recent reports indicate that removal of papillomas with microdébrider can be more efficient and atraumatic.[72] Papillomas are removed to the level of the mucosa or submucosa, avoiding the deeper muscular and ligamentous levels. Caution should be exercised in removing papillomas from the anterior and posterior commissure areas because irreversible scarring can result. Although removal of RRP temporarily improves the voice, the increasing number of required procedures results in scarring of the vocal folds and deterioration of the voice.

Leventhal and others[73] recommended the use of interferon in any patient requiring surgery every 2 to 3 months. The duration of management should be 6 months. If there is neither a response nor a complete response, management should be discontinued, but if there is a partial response management should be continued. However, the results of interferon management of RRP have been disappointing. After the cessation of interferon therapy, there is a rebound effect and papillomas recur at an increased rate.[74] Intralesional administration of cidofovir, an acyclic nucleoside phosphate, has shown promise in treating severe cases of RRP in pediatric patients.[75] Other adjuvant therapies (e.g., photodynamic therapy, acyclovir, ribavirin, isotretinoin, indole 3-carbinol) are infrequently used.[67]

Malignant Tumors

Malignant tumors of the pediatric larynx are rare. Isolated case reports are seen in the literature, but more extensive experience is lacking. A 15-year review of malignant laryngeal tumors at a tertiary pediatric referral center revealed only four cases.[76] These laryngeal tumors are usually in the sarcoma group, most commonly rhabdomyosarcoma. Other malignancies include squamous cell carcinoma, lymphoma, mucoepidermoid carcinoma, neuroectodermal tumor, and metastatic carcinoma.[77-80] Spontaneous malignant degeneration of longstanding RRP has an incidence of 2% to 3%.[81] In addition, squamous cell carcinoma may be seen in patients who have RRP and a history of radiotherapy.

Patients with laryngeal tumors present with voice change (often hoarseness), stridor, and progressive airway obstruction. Delay in diagnosis is common because of a low suspicion for malignancy. Any child with persistent hoarseness should thus be fully evaluated. Management goals are patient survival and preservation of laryngeal function, when possible. Management depends on the tumor histology and consists of combination surgery, radiotherapy, and chemotherapy.

Radiotherapy of a prepubescent larynx can result in a fibrotic infantile larynx with no useful voice, airway, or swallowing function.[76] This should be considered when deciding on a management protocol. Ohlms and associates[76] provide an example of a prepubescent child with a laryngeal rhabdomyosarcoma. Although radiotherapy may have provided adequate local control, total laryngectomy was chosen to improve local control. Total laryngectomy was justified because it provided a better chance of cure, whereas the larynx may have been useless after undergoing radiotherapy.

Vocal Quality Disorders: Medical Management

Granuloma

Patients with vocal fold granuloma commonly exhibit hoarseness. Granuloma often results from intubation trauma. Habitual throat clearing, excessive glottal attacks, and reflux esophagitis are also important causal factors.[82] Inflammation over the vocal process of arytenoid progresses to infection involving the perichondrium and formation of granuloma. Histologically, the granulomas are nonspecific reparative granulation tissue covered by hyperplastic squamous epithelium.[83]

Children with vocal fold granuloma should be evaluated for gastroesophageal reflux disease (GERD). The most reliable means of diagnosing GERD is prolonged (24 hours) pH manometry study.[84] A reflux event is defined as a drop in the pH to less than 4. Normally, the time that pH is less than 4 is approximately 6.3% upright, 1.2% supine, and 4.2% total.[85] Other less specific and less sensitive methods are barium esophagography, radionuclide scanning, and lipid-laden macrophage testing for aspiration.

The primary management of vocal fold granuloma is management of the underlying GERD. Most granulomas resolve with medical management. Management of GERD involves[86] (1) dietary and lifestyle modifications and the use of antacids; (2) H_2 blockers (cimetidine, ranitidine, famotidine), prokinetic agents (bethanechol, metoclopramide, cisapride), and mucosal cytoprotectants (sucralfate) in combination; and (3) proton pump inhibitors (omeprazole, lansoprazole) combined with surgical repair of hiatal hernia and the reestablishment of lower esophageal sphincter function.

Surgical removal (CO_2 laser or sharp incision with microlaryngeal instruments) of the vocal fold granuloma is reserved for lesions causing airway obstruction (Fig. 203-5).[83,84] Regardless of the surgical technique used, recurrence is frequent. Although voice therapy has been recommended, it does not appear to be an effective primary management modality for vocal fold granulomas.

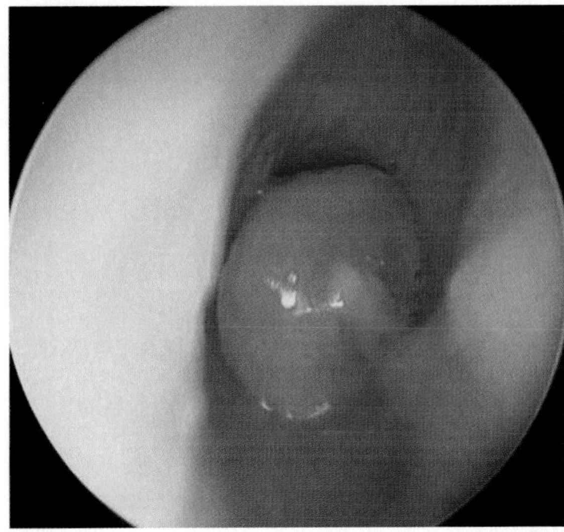

Figure 203-5. Large granuloma with laryngeal obstruction requiring surgery.

Vocal Quality Disorders: Voice Therapy with or without Surgery

Opinions about the management of cysts, polyps, sulcus vocalis, and nodules differ widely. Traditionally, surgery was discouraged in children because of the small size of the larynx, difficulty in reinforcing voice rest postoperatively, and high recurrence when underlying vocal behavior is not modified. Surgery was recommended for only the most recalcitrant and severe dysphonia. However, some surgeons have reported that surgery of the pediatric larynx is safe and technically feasible with good results, as seen in a series by Bouchayer and Cornut[8] of 191 children who underwent microsurgery. Advocates of surgery recommend waiting until the child is 8 to 9 years old.[8,87] This recommendation is in agreement with the recent report describing the development of the three-layered vocal fold in children approximating that of adult vocal folds by age 7.[88] In addition to the age, a highly motivated patient and involved parents are prerequisites to surgery.

Preoperative and postoperative voice therapy is essential. Surgical intervention is most often performed by microsurgical technique, although CO_2 laser is infrequently used. The principles of surgery are to remove the pathology with maximal preservation of normal mucosa and to avoid injury to the anterior commissure and vocal ligament.

Nodules

Most voice disorders in children result from vocal nodules. Vocal nodules occur frequently, often as a result of misuse or overuse of the larynx (hyperfunctional state). Other conditions that can lead to predisposition for vocal nodules include gastroesophageal reflux and velopharyngeal insufficiency.[47] The incidence of hoarseness, a symptom of dysphonia, in schoolchildren is estimated to be approximately 5%.[89] Of children evaluated by an otolaryngologist for chronic hoarseness, 38% to 78% have vocal nodules. Thus more than 1 million children in the United States have vocal nodules. Vocal nodules are most often seen as a child enters a group activity. They occur more commonly in boys. Patients with vocal nodules exhibit hoarseness and breathiness. A stroboscopic examination shows decreased mucosal waves and incomplete approximation of the free edges.[89]

Vocal nodules result from mechanical trauma and occur at the free edge of the anterior and middle third of the vocal fold (Fig. 203-6). Often, vocal nodules are bilateral, although unilateral nodules can occur. Vocal nodules develop in three stages[90]: (1) an inflammatory phase with increased vascularity and protein accumulation; (2) localized

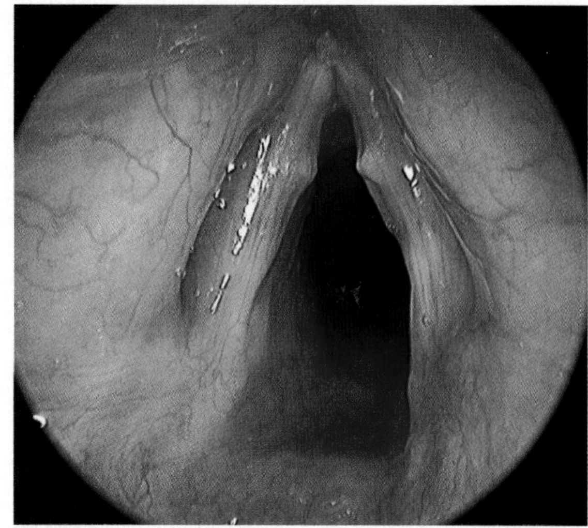

Figure 203-6. Vocal nodules.

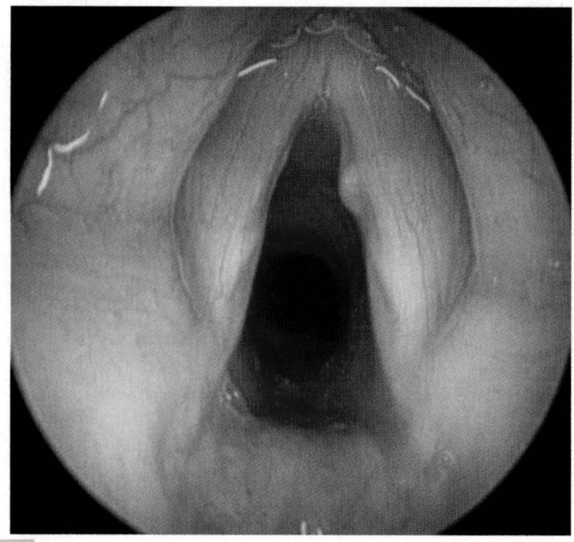

Figure 203-7. Right vocal fold cyst.

swelling on the edge of the vocal fold that appears as grayish, translucent thickening (nodules are reversible within 24 to 48 hours if trauma is eliminated); and (3) replacement of thickening by fibrotic tissue that appears gray or white. Histologically, circumscribed hyperplasia or hyperkeratinization and secondary hyaline degeneration in the lamina propria are seen.[91]

Management options include voice therapy, surgery, voice therapy plus surgery, and no intervention.[8,87,89,92-94] It is difficult to determine the success of differing modes of management because follow-up of control groups (no management) is rare. Because of the benign nature of nodules, patients who undergo medical or surgical management are often lost to follow-up evaluation. The fact that vocal nodules in children often resolve spontaneously by puberty may also influence management. The most widely accepted management option for vocal fold nodules in children is voice therapy. According to von Leden,[89] most nodules resolve or show significant improvement within 3 to 6 months of initiating voice therapy. Surgery is considered in children who fail to show improvement with voice therapy and in whom severe hoarseness interferes with daily functioning.[87,89]

The surgical management of choice is microsurgical excision, although CO_2 laser has been used. The nodule is stretched medially and removed at its base with microscissors without excessive mucosal removal. Bilateral nodules can usually be removed in one sitting; however, care should be taken to avoid injuring the anterior commissure. Some surgeons recommend removing bilateral nodules in stages that are 4 weeks apart.[87] Voice rest is recommended for 7 to 10 days. Long-term results depend on the quality of voice therapy, but they are generally good. Recurrences are frequent without voice therapy.

Cysts and Sulcus Vocalis

It is unclear whether epidermoid cysts and sulcus of the vocal folds are congenital or acquired lesions. Some authors[95,96] support the view that these lesions are acquired, whereas Bouchayer and colleagues[97] theorize that they are congenital. In a series of 2334 patients, Bouchayer and Cornut[8] found that congenital lesions of the vocal folds were the most frequently seen benign lesions requiring surgical intervention; they believe these congenital lesions are often overlooked or misdiagnosed.

Patients with either lesion often present with hoarseness, voice breaks, and vocal fatigue. With epidermoid cysts, unilateral submucosal swelling of the superior mid-third surface often occurs with associated edema of the contralateral vocal fold (Fig. 203-7). Reduced mucosal waves are seen on stroboscopy. Epidermoid cysts are lined with stratified keratinizing squamous epithelium and contain keratin debris. With sulcus vocalis, the surface epithelium invaginates into Reinke's space and adheres to the vocal ligament, resulting in a longitudinal furrow parallel to the edge of the vocal fold and an oval glottic chink. Stroboscopy shows incomplete closure of the free edges of the vocal folds.

Cysts and sulcus vocalis usually do not resolve spontaneously although voice can improve with therapy.[8,98] Epidermoid cysts are often mistaken for vocal nodules, and patients are thus referred for voice therapy. Referral to an otolaryngologist occurs when the voice disorder does not resolve after several months of voice therapy. Sulcus vocalis is often difficult to diagnose in children because careful examination of the larynx with a stroboscope is often impossible. These children are referred for voice abnormality that fails to improve with voice therapy.

Epidermoid cyst and sulcus vocalis are managed by microsurgery. For cysts, a mucosal incision is made on the superior surface of the vocal fold, parallel to the free edge, and the cyst is dissected. Bouchayer and Cornut[8] recommend intrafoldal injection of the surgical site with corticosteroid to decrease the inflammation. Woo and colleagues[99] reported improved laryngeal microsurgery results using 6-0 chronic Endoknot sutures to close the microflaps of the vocal fold. Sulci are resected by making incisions in the superior and inferior edges of the pocket and dissecting the pocket from the vocal ligament. A slicing mucosa surgical technique that detaches the mucosa of the sulcus and interrupts the longitudinal fibrotic tension line has been used with good results.[100] Although the resulting voice is improved compared with the preoperative state, it is not perfect. Postoperative voice therapy is important and has significant effect on voice results. Therapy is recommended for at least 3 to 6 months.

Polyps

Vocal fold polyps occur infrequently in children and adolescents.[101,102] They arise from chronic abuse of the larynx or from a single traumatic episode. Hoarseness is the most common presenting symptom. The polyps occur at the junction of the anterior and middle third of the vocal fold and may be fusiform, pedunculated, or generalized.[103] A recent study showed that polyps are caused by circulation impediment, thrombosis, exudation, and edema of the lamina propria. Inflammation and secondary atrophy of the vocal fold epithelium occur.[91]

Vocal fold polyps can improve with voice therapy but may require surgical removal.[8,90,98,103] Pedunculated polyps are removed at the base using CO_2 laser or microscissors. For generalized polyps, an incision is made over the superior surface of the vocal fold, and the fibrous exudate is suctioned out or vaporized.[8] The resulting voice quality depends on the degree of irreversible damage to the superficial layer of the lamina propria by fibrous or hyaline infiltration. Voice therapy is recommended before and after surgery to prevent recurrences.[8,22]

Summary

Voice disorders are commonly seen in children. Evaluation and treatment of voice disorders are more complicated in children than in adults because of their inability to cooperate, lack of awareness of the problem, and lack of motivation for change. There have been significant recent advances in technology and establishment of normative data for pediatric voice parameters. Surgery should be undertaken cautiously, especially in very young children because the larynx is not mature and surgery is more difficult. Voice therapy should be used extensively both preoperatively and postoperatively.

SUGGESTED READINGS

Benjamin B, Mair EA. Congenital interarytenoid web. *Arch Otolaryngol Head Neck Surg.* 1991;117:1118.

Benjamin B, Croxson G. Vocal cord granulomas. *Ann Otol Rhinol Laryngol.* 1985;94:538.

Benjamin B, Croxson G. Vocal nodules in children. *Ann Otol Rhinol Laryngol.* 1987;96:530.

Bogdasarian RS, Olson NR. Posterior glottic laryngeal stenosis. *Otolaryngol Head Neck Surg.* 1980;88:765.

Boseley ME, Hartnick CJ. Development of the human true vocal fold: depth of cell layers and quantifying cell types within the lamina propria. *Ann Otol Rhinol Laryngol.* 2006;115:784.

Bouchayer M, Cornut G, Witzig E, Loire R, Roch JB, Bastian RW. Epidermoid cysts, sulci and mucosal bridges of the true vocal cord: a report of 157 cases. *Laryngoscope.* 1985;95:1087.

Bouchayer M, Cornut G. Microsurgical treatment of benign vocal fold lesions: indications, technique, results. *Folia Phoniatr (Basel).* 1992;44:155.

Bower CM, Choi SS, Cotton RT. Arytenoidectomy in children. *Ann Otol Rhinol Laryngol.* 1994;103:271.

Cohen SR. Congenital glottic webs in children: a retrospective review of 51 patients. *Ann Otol Rhinol Laryngol.* 1985;14:2.

Cohen SM, Garrett CG. Utility of voice therapy in the management of vocal fold polyps and cysts. *Otolaryngol Head Neck Surg.* 2007;136:742.

Crumley RL. Teflon versus thyroplasty versus nerve transfer: a comparison. *Ann Otol Rhinol Laryngol.* 1990;99:759.

For complete list of references log onto www.expertconsult.com.

Derkay CS. Task force on recurrent respiratory papillomas. *Arch Otolaryngol Head Neck Surg.* 1995;121:1386.

Healy GB, Gelber RD, Trowbridge AL, Grundfast KM, Ruben RJ, Price KN. Treatment of recurrent respiratory papillomatosis with human leukocyte interferon: results of a multicenter randomized clinical trial. *N Engl J Med.* 1988;319:401.

Hirano M. *Clinical Examination of Voice.* New York: Springer-Verlag; 1981.

Holinger LD, Holinger PC, Holinger PH. Etiology of bilateral abductor vocal cord paralysis: a review of 389 cases. *Ann Otol Rhinol Laryngol.* 1976; 85:428.

Isshiki N, Morita H, Okamura H, Hiramoto M. Thyroplasty as a new phonosurgical technique. *Acta Otolaryngol (Stockh).* 1974;78:451.

King JM, Simpson CB. Modern injection augmentation for glottic insufficiency. *Curr Opin Otolaryngol Head Neck Surg.* 2007;15:153.

Kleinsasser O. Pathogenesis of vocal cord polyps. *Ann Otol Rhinol Laryngol.* 1982;91:378.

Levine BA, Jacobs IN, Wetmore RF, Handler SD. Vocal cord injection in children with unilateral vocal cord paralysis. *Arch Otolaryngol Head Neck Surg.* 1995;121:116.

Narcy P, Contencin P, Viala P. Surgical treatment for laryngeal paralysis in infants and children. *Ann Otol Rhinol Laryngol.* 1990;99:124.

Pransky SM, Brewster DF, Magit AE, Kearns DB. Clinical update on 10 children treated with intralesional cidofovir injections for severe recurrent respiratory papillomatosis. *Arch Otolaryngol Head Neck Surg.* 2000;126:1239.

Wilson DK. Management of voice disorders in children and adolescents. *Semin Speech Lang.* 1983;4:245.

Zalzal GH. Posterior glottic fixation in children. *Ann Otol Rhinol Laryngol.* 1993;102:680.

Zalzal GH, Loomis SR, Derkay CS, Murray SL, Thomsen J. Vocal quality of decannulated children following laryngeal reconstruction. *Laryngoscope.* 1991;101:425.

Zalzal GH, Loomis SR, Fischer M. Laryngeal reconstruction in children: assessment of vocal quality. *Arch Otolaryngol Head Neck Surg.* 1993;119:504.

CHAPTER TWO HUNDRED AND FOUR

Recurrent Respiratory Papillomatosis

Craig S. Derkay

Russell A. Faust

Key Points

- Recurrent respiratory papillomatosis (RRP) is a devastating, rare disease in which papillomas of the airway cause hoarseness and airway obstruction.
- The disease is caused by human papillomavirus (HPV) 6 or 11, the same subtypes responsible for the development of genital warts and low-risk cervical intraepithelial neoplasias of the genitourinary tract.
- The age of disease onset and clinical course are highly variable.
- Surgical therapy for RRP requires a team approach with otolaryngologists, anesthesia providers, and operating room personnel working together in a facility properly equipped to manage difficult airways.
- In addition to surgical débridement accomplished with the use of microdébriders, pulsed dye and carbon dioxide (CO_2) lasers and microlaryngoscopy "cold-steel" techniques, multiple medical modalities have been used without consistently effective results.
- Parental support and education are invaluable adjuncts to the safe care of children with RRP.
- The recent introduction of a quadrivalent HPV vaccine offers hope for prevention of transmission of the virus to neonates and may significantly reduce the future incidence of RRP and oropharyngeal cancers.

Recurrent respiratory papillomatosis (RRP) is the most common benign neoplasm of the larynx in children. Despite its benign histology, RRP has potentially fatal consequences and is often difficult to treat because of its tendency to recur and spread throughout the respiratory tract. Long neglected from an epidemiologic standpoint, initiatives to better understand this disease process have been launched in the United States through coordination between the Centers for Disease Control and Prevention (CDC) and the American Society of Pediatric Otolaryngology (ASPO) and internationally through the British Association of Paediatric Otolaryngology (BAPO) and by Canadian Paediatric Otolaryngology physicians.

This chapter discusses the etiology, immunology, epidemiology, and transmission of RRP. Clinical features including pertinent aspects of the history, physical examination, airway endoscopy, and other considerations are highlighted. Management principles for performing surgical and nonsurgical treatments, the indications and results for employing adjuvant therapies, and their results are discussed. Ongoing research initiatives, promising strategies, the potential for a quadrivalent human papilloma vaccine (HPV) to reduce its incidence and the RRP Task Force's contributions to understanding this frustrating disease are also reviewed.

Epidemiology

Recurrent respiratory papillomatosis is a disease of viral etiology, caused by human papillomavirus (HPV) types 6 and 11, and is characterized by the proliferation of benign squamous papillomas within the aerodigestive tract.[1-3] Although it is a benign disease, RRP has potentially fatal consequences because of its involvement of the airway and because of the risk, albeit low, of malignant conversion.[4] In addition to the emotional burden to the patients and their families associated with the need for repeated surgery,[5] the economic cost of this relatively rare chronic disease is high, having been estimated at $150 million annually.[6]

RRP is both the most common benign neoplasm of the larynx among children and the second most frequent cause of childhood hoarseness.[7] The disease is often difficult to treat because of its tendency to recur and spread throughout the aerodigestive tract. Although it most often involves the larynx, RRP may involve the entire aerodigestive tract. The course of the disease is variable, with some patients experiencing spontaneous remission, whereas others may suffer from aggressive papillomatous growth and respiratory compromise, requiring multiple surgical procedures through many years.

RRP may have its clinical onset during either childhood or adulthood. It may affect people of any age, with the youngest patient identified at 1 day of life and the oldest at 84 years.[6] Two distinct forms of RRP are generally recognized: a juvenile or aggressive form and an adult or less aggressive form. The aggressive form, although most prevalent in children, can also occur in adults. Children whose RRP was diagnosed at younger ages (younger than 3 years) have been found to be 3.6 times more likely to have more than four surgical procedures per year and almost two times more likely to have two or more anatomic sites affected than children whose RRP was diagnosed at older ages (older than 3 years).[6] Similarly, children with disease progression are generally diagnosed at younger ages than those who remain stable or become disease-free.[8-10] In most pediatric series, the delay in diagnosis from the time of onset of symptoms averages about 1 year.[6,11] In 75% of children with RRP, diagnosis was made before the fifth birthday.[12]

The true incidence and prevalence of RRP are uncertain. It is estimated that between 80 and 1500 new cases of childhood-onset RRP occur in the United States each year.[6,13] While the incidence among children in the United States is estimated at 4.3 per 100,000 children, the incidence among adults is 1.8 per 100,000.[6,14] These figures are comparable with those found in a Danish survey. In a subpopulation incorporating 50% of the population of that country, the rate among children was 3.62 per 100,000, whereas adult-onset cases occurred at a rate of 3.94 per 100,000.[15] The National Registry of children with RRP, composed of the clinical practices at 22 pediatric otolaryngology sites, calculates a mean number of procedures at 19.7 per child with an average of 4.4 procedures per year.[6,14] Based on the incidence data, this translates into more than 10,000 surgical procedures annually for children with RRP in the United States.

Virology of Human Papillomavirus

HPV, belonging to the Papovaviridae family, is a small deoxyribonucleic acid (DNA)-containing, nonenveloped, icosahedral (20-sided), capsid virus with a double-stranded circular DNA of 7900 base-pairs long. HPV is epitheliotropic (infects epithelial cells). The HPVs have been grouped on the basis of shared genetic code homology, with viruses that share less than 90% identity in specific regions of the virus being defined as separate types. On this basis, the HPVs are numbered to distinguish them. Nearly 100 different HPV types have been identified. Grouping HPV types based on their DNA homology has allowed us to identify closely related types. Functionally, these groupings correlate with their tissue preference as well as similar pathophysiology.[16] The HPVs are members of a large family of papillomaviruses that infect vertebrates ranging from birds to humans, causing epithelial neoplasms that can be benign or malignant. These viruses are designated by their natural host species (e.g., bovine papillomavirus, murine papillomavirus, and human papillomavirus). Each papillomavirus is specific for its host species, and this specificity is thought to be absolute. Within each species, similar types of papillomavirus exhibit specificity for epithelial tissues of different sites (e.g., oral mucosa, genital mucosa, or skin). In humans, this tissue specificity is less absolute, and some HPV types exhibit more of a preference for certain tissues.

Until the 1990s, HPV had been suspected but not confirmed as the causative agent in RRP. This uncertainty resulted from an inability to culture the virus in vitro and from the failure to demonstrate viral particles consistently in papilloma lesions using electron microscopy or HPV antibodies. With the advent of molecular probes, HPV DNA has been identified in virtually every papilloma lesion studied. The most common types identified in the airway are HPV 6 and HPV 11—the same types responsible for more than 90% of genital condylomata. Specific viral subtypes may be correlated with disease severity and clinical course. Children infected with HPV 11 appear to have a more obstructive airway course early in the disease and a greater likelihood of undergoing tracheotomy to maintain a safe airway.[10,17]

In addition to the HPV group that includes HPV 6 and 11, two other major groups of HPV are associated with mucosal lesions in the aerodigestive and genital tracts. HPV 6 and 11, responsible for the majority of RRP, are members of a group believed to have a low malignant potential compared with some other groups. In contrast, the group that contains HPV 16 and HPV 18 is associated with malignancies in the genital and aerodigestive tracts.[16] The group that contains HPV 31 and HPV 33 exhibits malignant potential that lies somewhere in between.

HPV is thought to infect stem cells within the basal layer of mucosa.[18,19] After infection of the stem cells, the viral DNA can either be actively expressed or it can exist as a latent infection in mucosa that remains clinically and histologically normal. To produce viral proteins or to replicate the virus, the viral DNA must somehow reactivate the host replication genes. The viral genome consists of three regions: an upstream regulatory region and the two regions named according to the phase of infection in which they are expressed—early (E) and late (L) regions. The E-region genes are involved in the replication of the viral genome, interaction with the host cell intermediate filaments, and transforming activities, and are potential oncogenes, depending on the HPV type. The L-region genes encode the viral structural proteins.[20-22]

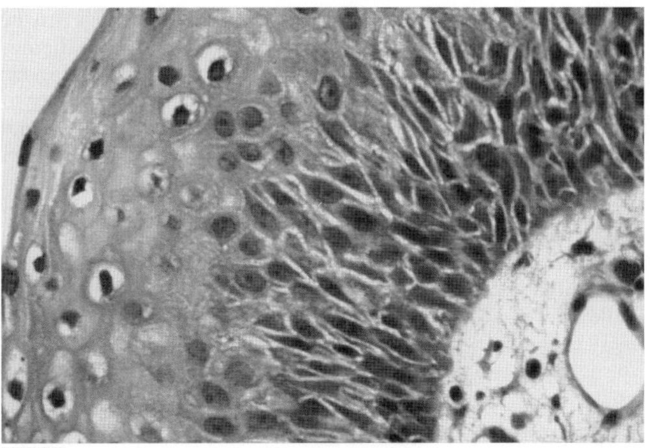

Figure 204-1. Histopathology of human recurrent respiratory papillomatosis. Micrograph of laryngeal mucosa infected with human papillomavirus.

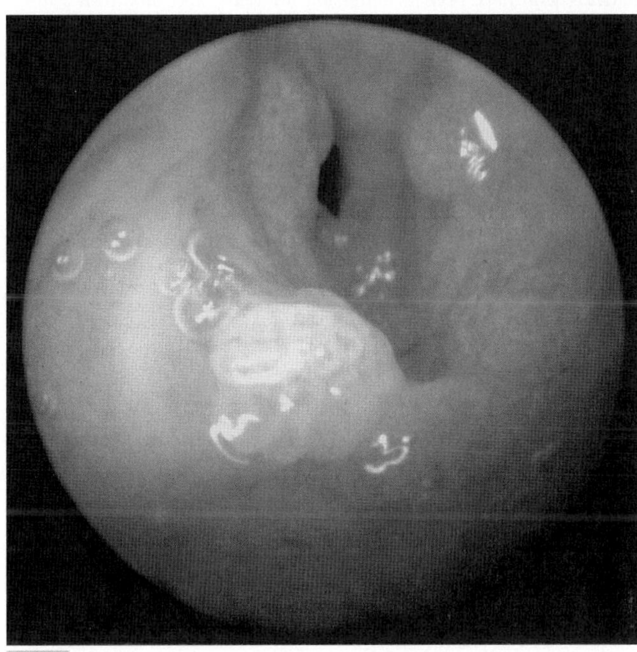

Figure 204-2. Gross appearance of respiratory papillomas during laryngoscopy. Appearance of massive, exophytic papillomatosis of the larynx.

The induction of cellular proliferation is a fundamental property of HPV, although the mechanism of action remains unclear. We are slowly gathering information regarding the interaction of viral gene products with cellular proteins. For example, several of the viral E-region gene products have been shown to bind and inactivate certain cellular tumor-suppressor proteins.[21,23] Conversely, HPV has been shown to activate the epidermal growth factor (EGF) receptor pathway, known to be associated with proliferation of epithelial cells.[3] Thus there are likely several mechanisms by which HPV induces cellular proliferation in the aerodigestive mucosa.

Histologically, this mucosal proliferation results in multiple "fronds" or finger-like projections with a central fibrovascular core, covered by stratified squamous epithelium (Fig. 204-1).[18] When papillomas are microscopic, they may assume a superficial-spreading configuration, with a velvety appearance (Fig. 204-2). When they exhibit a more macroscopic or exophytic growth pattern, they appear grossly as "cauliflower" projections (see Fig. 204-2). Papilloma lesions may be sessile or pedunculated and often occur in irregular exophytic clusters. Typically, the lesions are pinkish to white in coloration. Iatrogenic implantation of papilloma may be preventable by avoiding injury to nondiseased squamous or ciliated epithelium adjacent to areas of frank papilloma. Ciliated epithelium undergoes squamous metaplasia when exposed to repeated trauma and is replaced with nonciliated epithelium that creates an iatrogenic squamocellularly junction. This may also explain the observation that RRP flourishes in the presence of uncontrolled gastroesophageal reflux. Most RRPs do not exhibit dysplasia, abnormal mitoses, or hyperkeratosis.[18] Without exception, RRP exhibits delayed maturation of the epithelium, resulting in significantly thickened basal cell layer and nucleated cells in the superficial layers.[24] This is thought to be in part because of the interaction of HPV gene products with the EGF receptor pathway.[3] The sum result of these cellular effects is that, although HPV-infected cells do not rapidly divide, there is a disproportionate increase in the number of dividing basal cells. Thus expansion of the RRP tissue mass may occur very rapidly, because of the large number of dividing cells.[19]

During viral latency there is very little viral RNA expressed. Even so, HPV DNA can be detected in normal-appearing mucosa in RRP patients who have been in remission for years, and unknown stimuli can result in reactivation and clinical recurrence following years of remission.[25,26] Thus activation of viral expression can occur any time after the establishment of latent infection. Gene products of early region gene E6, E7, and possibly E5 are required for papilloma induction, but the details of the mechanism of HPV activation are unknown. To "cure" RRP, it is necessary to modulate the host response to the virus and, ideally, eliminate latent infection.

It is likely that the host immune system plays an important role in the pathogenesis of HPV-induced lesions. Both the humoral and the cellular immune responses may be compromised in children with RRP, and the patient's immunocompetence may be associated with the clinical course of the disease. The role of cytokines, such as interleukin-2, interleukin-4, and interleukin-10, and expression of the major histocompatibility complex (MHC) antigens in the dysfunction of the cell-mediated immune response in children with RRP has been demonstrated.[27,28]

Transmission

An association between cervical HPV infection in the mother and the incidence of RRP has been well established. However, the precise mode of transmission is still not clear.[18] The universality of HPV in the lower genital tract rivals that of any other sexually transmitted disease in humans. It is estimated that at least one million cases of genital papillomas occur per year in the United States.[29] These are most commonly manifested as condylomata acuminata involving the cervix, vulva, or other anogenital sites in women or the penis of male sexual partners of affected women. Colposcopic (subclinical) changes are seen in about 4% of women, whereas DNA positive biopsies without a visible lesion are seen in 10% of women. HPV antibody positivity (without DNA or a clinical lesion) is estimated in 60% of women (81 million). HPV has been estimated to be present in the genital tract of as many as 25% of all women of child-bearing age worldwide. One study reported that the incidence of HPV infections in sexually active young college women is highest, with a cumulative incidence of 43% during a 36-month period.[30] Clinically apparent HPV infection has been noted in 1.5% to 5% of pregnant women in the United States.[31] More than 30% of American women are currently infected with HPV with 7.5 million 14- to 24-year-olds currently infected and one fourth of women younger than 60 years of age infected at any given time.[32] Up to 90% of lesions are undetectable clinically at 2 years. The highest prevalence is in women 20 to 24 years of age. More than 50% of women will initially acquire HPV within 4 years of their first sexual intercourse. As in RRP, HPV 6 and HPV 11 are the most common subtypes identified in cervical condylomata.

Vertical transmission occurring during delivery through an infected birth canal is presumed to be the major mode of transmitting the infection in children whereas in utero and transplacental transfer of HPV, sexual abuse, and direct contact are thought to play a minor role. The support for vertical transmission lies in the fact that overt maternal condyloma are seen in more than 50% of mothers who give birth to children with RRP.[33] The same subtypes (HPV 6 and 11) are involved, and cesarean delivery of children seems to be preventive to some extent.[34]

Patients with childhood-onset RRP are more likely to be first born and vaginally delivered than are control patients of similar age.[35,36] Kashima and others hypothesized that primigravid mothers are more likely to have a long second stage of labor and that the prolonged exposure to the virus leads to a higher risk of infection in the first-born child. They also suggested that newly acquired genital HPV lesions are more likely to shed virus than longstanding lesions, accounting for the higher incidence of papilloma disease observed among the offspring of young mothers of low socioeconomic status—the same group that is most likely to acquire sexually transmitted diseases such as HPV.[35,36]

Despite the close association between maternal condylomata and the development of RRP, only a small portion of children exposed to genital condylomata at birth actually go on to development of clinical RRP.[37] Although HPV could be recovered from the nasopharyngeal secretions of 30% of infants exposed to HPV in the birth canal, the number of infants expected to manifest evidence of RRP is only a small fraction of this population.[37] Clearly, other factors (patient immunity, timing, length and volume of virus exposure, local trauma) must be important determinants in the development of RRP. Even though cesarean section delivery would seem to reduce the risk of transmission of the disease, this procedure is associated with a higher morbidity and mortality for the mother and a much higher economic cost than elective vaginal delivery. Furthermore, reports of neonatal papillomatosis suggest that, in at least some cases, transmission may occur in utero.[1] However, with such a high rate of subclinical maternal HPV infection and such a low rate of actual new cases of childhood RRP, elective cesarean delivery as a means of preventing RRP is currently not practical or recommended.[1] The risk of a child contracting the disease from a mother who has an active genital condyloma lesion during vaginal delivery is only approximately 1 in 231 to 400.[22,34,36] The characteristics that distinguish this one child from the other 230 to 399 remain elusive. In summary, a better understanding of the risk factors associated with RRP is needed before the efficacy of cesarean delivery or other preventive measures can be fully assessed.

Prevention

The new quadrivalent HPV vaccine (Gardasil, Merck and Co., Inc.), is licensed and indicated for the prevention of cervical cancer, adenocarcinoma in situ, and intraepithelial neoplasia grades 1-3; vulvar and vaginal intraepithelial neoplasias grades 2-3; and genital warts associated with HPV 6, 11, 16, and 18. The CDC Advisory Committee on Immunization Practices (ACIP)[32] has recommended vaccination for all girls ages 11 to 12, girls and women ages 13 to 26 who have not yet been vaccinated, and girls as young as age 9, in whom the physician believes it would be appropriate. Based upon the pivotal clinical studies, the vaccine is predicted to reduce the incidence, morbidity, and mortality of cervicovaginal HPV disease. An added and often overlooked benefit may be a concomitant decrease in the incidence of RRP and HPV-associated head and neck cancers.

The ability of the quadrivalent vaccine to prevent HPV 6/11/16/18-associated cervical and genital disease was established in the phase 3 FUTURE I and II trials, and their immunogenicity in the target group of vaccinees was established in immunogenicity bridging trials.[38] In FUTURE I, the quadrivalent vaccine was 100% effective in preventing cervical intraepithelial neoplasia (CIN) or worse, genital warts, and vulvovaginal neoplasia. In FUTURE II, the vaccine was 100% effective in preventing HPV 16/18-associated CIN. Both Future I and II were conducted in women in the age range at highest risk for HPV acquisition.[38,39] However, it appears that the vaccine will be most effective if administered to individuals who have not yet become sexually active. Immunogenicity bridging studies were conducted to assess the immunogenicity of the vaccine in this population, and established that immunogenicity among younger girls was equal to if not superior to the response among 16- to 23-year-old women, suggesting that the quadrivalent HPV vaccine is immunogenic in this population and thus likely to be effective in preventing disease.[40] A separate study in 9- to

15-year-olds established that in this younger population immunogenicity lasts at least 18 months.[41]

There is also a bivalent HPV vaccine currently in phase 3 trials. This vaccine provides protection against HPV 16 and 18, but not 6 and 11.[38] Early phase 2 data for this vaccine suggest that it is 100% effective in preventing incident and persistent cervical HPV 16 and 18 infections in the according-to-protocol (ATP) sample, and 93% effective in preventing HPV 16- or 18-related disease in the intention-to-treat analysis; efficacy against disease was not presented for the ATP cohort. This vaccine's efficacy against HPV 16 and 18 suggests that, like the quadrivalent vaccine, it may reduce the incidence of HPV-associated head and neck cancers. However, because the bivalent vaccine does not protect against HPV 6 and 11, it will not likely affect the vertical transmission of HPV 6 or 11 from mother to child.

Widespread use of the quadrivalent HPV vaccine promises to dramatically reduce the morbidity and mortality of cervical cancer and drastically reduce the incidence of genital warts. If the vaccine is as effective in preventing HPV infection of the oral cavity as of the cervix and genital tract, then, vaccination could be expected to reduce the incidence of HPV-associated oropharyngeal cancers by as much as 30%. In addition, a near-universal vaccination program providing the quadrivalent vaccine should all but eradicate RRP in future generations. Thus vaccination against HPV offers additional benefits above and beyond prevention of cervical cancers, some of which are unique to the quadrivalent vaccine.

Clinical Features

Inasmuch as the vocal fold is usually the first and predominant site of papilloma lesions, hoarseness is the principal presenting symptom in RRP.[42] The child's voice may be described as hoarse or weak from the time of birth. Particularly in very young children, changes in voice may go unnoticed. Stridor is often the second clinical symptom to develop, beginning as an inspiratory noise and becoming biphasic with progression of the disease. Less commonly, chronic cough, recurrent pneumonia, failure to thrive, dyspnea, dysphagia, or acute life-threatening events may be the presenting symptoms. The duration of symptoms before diagnosis varies. Not uncommonly, a mistaken diagnosis of asthma, croup, allergies, vocal nodules, or bronchitis is entertained before a definitive diagnosis is made. However, the initial presentation in infants, whose airway dimensions are small, may be with acute respiratory distress during an otherwise routine upper respiratory tract infection. The natural history of RRP is highly variable. After presentation, the disease may undergo spontaneous remission or persist in a stable state requiring only periodic surgical treatment. At the other extreme, RRP may become extremely aggressive, requiring frequent surgical treatment (every few days to weeks), prompting early institution of medical adjuvant therapy. A waxing-waning clinical course of remissions and exacerbations is common for RRP.

Because of the rarity of RRP and the slowly progressive nature of the disease, some cases may go unrecognized until respiratory distress results from papillomas obstructing the airway. The result is a relatively high need for tracheotomy to be performed in these children. Shapiro and others noted that RRP tracheotomy patients presented at a younger age and with more widespread disease, often involving the distal airway before tracheotomy.[43] In their experience with 13 patients, they did not believe that the tracheotomy itself led to spread of disease outside the larynx. In the CDC National RRP Registry, children with tracheotomy were initially diagnosed with RRP at a younger age (2.7 years) than those without a tracheotomy (3.9 years).[14] Others have suggested that tracheotomy may activate or contribute to the spread of disease lower in the respiratory tract.[44] Cole and colleagues reported that tracheal papillomas developed in half of their tracheotomy patients and that, despite attempts to avoid this procedure, 21% of their patients still required a long-term tracheotomy.[45] Prolonged tracheotomy and the presence of subglottic papillomata at the time of tracheotomy have been associated with an increased risk of distal tracheal spread. Most authors agree that tracheotomy is a procedure to be avoided unless absolutely necessary. Interestingly, Boston and colleagues from Cincinnati noted successful laryngotracheal reconstruction in a series of children with subglottic stenosis and RRP.[46] When a tracheotomy is unavoidable, decannulation should be considered as soon as the disease is managed effectively with endoscopic techniques. Children with bronchopulmonary dysplasia who require prolonged endotracheal intubation may also be at increased risk for development of RRP.[47] Through interruption of the continuous respiratory mucosal surface, an endotracheal tube may have the same role in the mechanical dissemination-implantation of RRP as tracheotomy, as a risk for distal spread of disease. Several authors have noted an association between RRP caused by HPV 11 (as opposed to HPV 6) and distal spread of papilloma.[10]

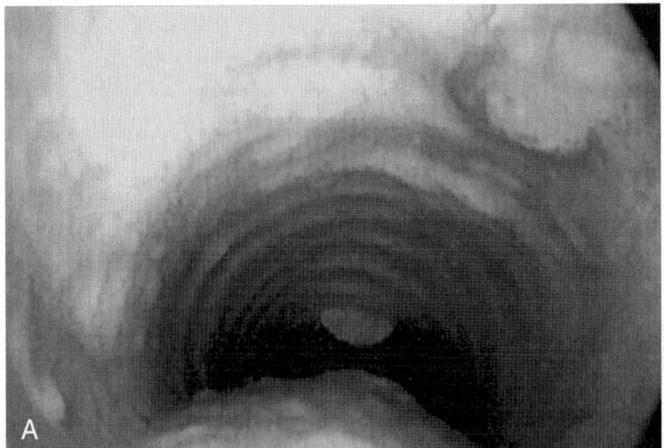

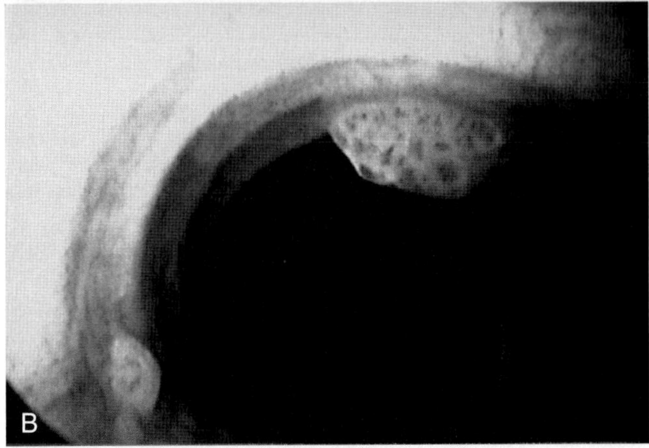

Figure 204-3. Tracheal spread of recurrent respiratory papillomatosis. Note nodular, exophytic lesions in distal trachea.

Extralaryngeal spread of respiratory papillomata has been identified in approximately 30% of children and in 16% of adults with RRP.[6] The most frequent sites of extralaryngeal spread were, in decreasing order of frequency, the oral cavity, trachea, and bronchi (Fig. 204-3).[6,42] Pulmonary papilloma lesions begin as asymptomatic noncalcified peripheral nodules.[48] These lesions eventually enlarge to undergo central cavitation and central liquefactive necrosis with air-fluid levels on a computed tomography scan (Fig. 204-4). These patients present clinically with recurrent bronchiectasis, pneumonia, and declining pulmonary status. The clinical course of the pulmonary spread of RRP is insidious and may progress through the years, but eventually manifests in respiratory failure because of destruction of lung parenchyma. For this reason, the finding of pulmonary lesions in a patient with RRP is a grave development with no currently available treatment modality that has shown more than anecdotal promise. Furthermore, pulmonary dissemination is anecdotally associated with a higher risk of malignant transformation of RRP.

Malignant transformation of RRP into squamous cell carcinoma has been documented in several case reports. A total of 26 patients was identified as having progressed to squamous cell carcinoma in the task force survey.[6] Dedo and Yu reported malignant transformation in 4 of 244 (1.6%) RRP patients treated during 2 decades.[49] When death occurs in a patient with RRP, it is usually as a complication of frequent

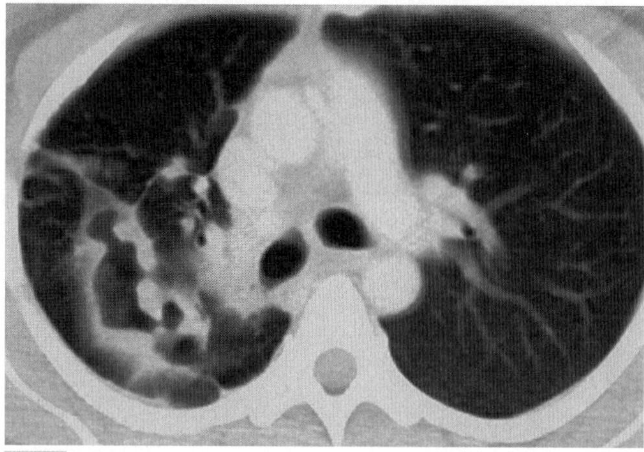

Figure 204-4. Pulmonary spread of recurrent respiratory papillomatosis. Note lytic, cavitary lesions on computed tomography.

surgical procedures or caused by respiratory failure because of distal disease progression. RRP presenting in the neonatal period is thought to be a negative prognostic factor, with a greater likelihood for mortality and need for tracheotomy.[8,9]

Patient Assessment

History

Persistent or progressive stridor and dysphonia, with the possible development of respiratory distress, are the most consistent signs and symptoms of RRP in children (see the Practice Pathway Flow Chart, Fig. 204-5). In the absence of severe respiratory distress, a careful history should be obtained. Information regarding the time of onset of symptoms, possible airway trauma including a history of previous intubation, and characteristics of the cry are obviously important. Hoarseness, although a common and often benign clinical complaint in young children, always indicates some abnormality of structure or function. Because of the precision of laryngeal mechanics, hoarseness may result from a remarkably small lesion and thus be an early sign in the course of a disease process. On the other hand, if the lesion's origin is remote from the vocal cords, hoarseness may present as a late sign. Although histologically the same lesion, a papilloma that produces hoarseness in one patient may produce stridor and obstruction in another, depending on the size and location of the lesion. The quality of the voice change may give only limited clues to its etiology, whereas other characteristics such as age of onset, rate of progression, associated infection, history of trauma or surgery, and the presence of respiratory or cardiac distress may be of much greater significance. A low-pitched, coarse, fluttering voice suggests a subglottic lesion, whereas a high-pitched, cracking voice; aphonia; or breathy voice suggests a glottic lesion. Associated high-pitched stridor also suggests a glottic or subglottic lesion. Although stridor that has been present since birth is more often associated with laryngomalacia, subglottic stenosis, vocal cord paralysis, or a vascular ring, it should be realized that neonates can also present with papillomatosis. Associated symptoms such as feeding difficulties, allergic symptoms, vocal abuse, and the presence of hereditary congenital anomalies may help distinguish RRP from alternative diagnoses, including vocal fold nodules, vocal fold paralysis, subglottic cysts, subglottic hemangioma, and subglottic stenosis. In the absence of any history suggesting these lesions, review of the perinatal period may reveal a history of maternal or paternal condylomata. If the onset of stridor and dysphonia is gradual and progressive through weeks or months, then neoplastic growth compromising the airway must be considered and investigated.

Certainly not every child with a hoarse voice or cry merits investigation beyond an assessment of symptoms. However, in the presence of hoarseness with respiratory distress, tachypnea, decreased air entry, tachycardia, cyanosis, dysphagia, chronic cough, failure to thrive, recurrent pneumonia, or dysphagia, the larynx must be visualized and a firm diagnosis of the cause of hoarseness must be made. Any child with slowly progressive hoarseness merits investigation and the clinician should not wait until total aphonia or airway problems occur.[50]

Physical Examination

Children presenting with symptoms consistent with RRP must undergo a thorough and organized physical examination. The child's respiratory rate and degree of distress must first be assessed. The physician should observe the child for tachypnea or the onset of fatigue that may indicate impending respiratory collapse. The child should be observed for flaring of the nasal ala and the use of accessory neck or chest muscles. Increasing cyanosis and air hunger may cause the child to sit with the neck hyperextended in an attempt to improve airflow. If a child is gravely ill, additional examination should not be undertaken outside the operating room (OR), the emergency department, or the intensive care unit, where resuscitation equipment for intubation of the airway, endoscopic evaluation, and possible tracheotomy are readily available. In the stable, well-oxygenated child, additional examination can proceed. The most important part of the examination is auscultation with the aid of a stethoscope. The physician should listen over the nose, open mouth, neck, and chest to help localize the probable site of the respiratory obstruction. The authors prefer to pull the bell off the stethoscope and listen over these areas with the open tube. The respiratory cycle, which is normally composed of a shorter inspiratory phase and a longer expiratory phase, should then be observed. Stridor of a laryngeal origin is most often musical and may begin as inspiratory, but will progress to biphasic as airway obstruction worsens. Infants with stridor should be placed in various positions to elicit any changes in the stridor. A child with RRP would not be expected to demonstrate much change in the stridor with position change in contrast to infants with laryngomalacia, a vascular ring, or a mediastinal mass. Pulse oximetry can add objective information on the child's respiratory status. In the stable patient in whom asthma is a likely diagnosis, pulmonary function testing may also be helpful.

Airway Endoscopy

The preoperative diagnosis of RRP is best made with a flexible fiberoptic nasopharyngoscope. Careful, sequential inspection of the pharynx, hypopharynx, larynx, and subglottis provides the critical information necessary to make the diagnosis of RRP and allows estimation of lumen size, vocal cord mobility, and the urgency of operative intervention. Advances in instrumentation of flexible nasopharyngoscopes have resulted in instruments as small as 1.8 mm in diameter, which when combined with the newest low-light, three-chip endoscopic cameras, allow passage in even the smallest newborns. Even the smallest diameter scopes provide excellent images that can be viewed on a video monitor and recorded for later review. Topical decongestant and local anesthesia can be applied by spray, dropper, or pledget. Oxymetazoline is the decongestant of choice because of its lack of cardiac side effects. Topical Pontocaine may be used to enhance patient cooperation, but the dosage must be critically monitored in the small infant to avoid cardiotoxicity.

Most clinicians find that visualization with the flexible nasopharyngoscope is far superior to that obtained with indirect mirror laryngoscopy in young children. Patient cooperation, however, is required even with good topical anesthesia. In infants, this is not a large issue because they can easily be restrained in an upright, sitting position in the parent's or nurse's lap for evaluation. Likewise, most children older than 6 or 7 years of age can be "talked into" cooperating for the examination. It is the intermediate age group, between 1 and 6 years of age, who may be the most difficult to examine, taxing the patience and skill of even the most experienced clinicians. Although dynamic evaluation can be appreciated when children are spontaneously breathing, endoscopy in the OR under anesthesia is warranted in any child suspected to have RRP who cannot be fully examined in the outpatient setting.[50]

Surgical Management

Classic Management

At present, there is no "cure" for RRP, and no single modality has consistently been shown to be effective in eradication of RRP. The

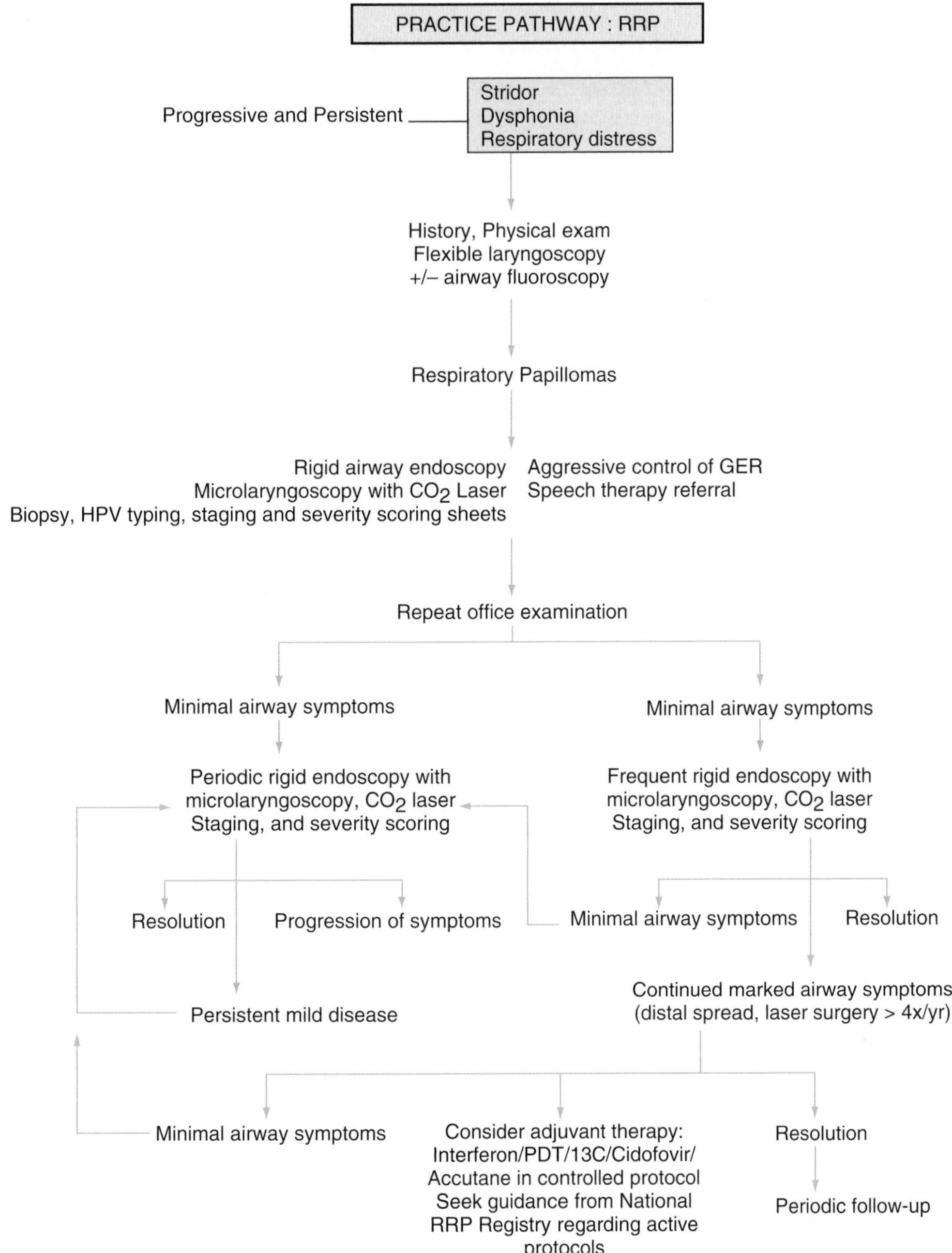

Figure 204-5. Practice pathway for recurrent respiratory papillomatosis. GER, gastroesophageal reflux; HPV, human papillomavirus; PDT, photodynamic therapy; RRP, recurrent respiratory papillomatosis.

current standard of care is surgical therapy with a goal of complete removal of papillomas and preservation of normal structures. In patients in whom anterior or posterior commissure disease or highly aggressive papillomas are present, the goal may be subtotal removal with clearing of the airway. It is advisable to debulk as much disease as possible while preserving normal morphology and anatomy and preventing the complications of subglottic and glottic stenosis, web formation, and resulting airway stenosis. Table 204-1 lists treatment options for RRP.

Until recently, the CO_2 laser has been favored over cold instruments in the treatment of RRP involving the larynx, pharynx, upper trachea, and nasal and oral cavities.[6] When coupled to an operating microscope, the laser vaporizes the lesions with precision, causing minimal bleeding. When used with a no-touch technique, it minimizes damage to the vocal cords and limits scarring. Dedo reported on a series of 244 patients with RRP treated with the CO_2 laser used every 2 months and achieved "remission" in 37%, "clearance" in 6%, and "cure" in 17%.[49] The CO_2 laser has an emission wave length of 10,600 nm and converts light to thermal energy. The CO_2 laser delivers energy that is absorbed by intracellular water, effectively vaporizing the cells.[51] It provides a controlled destruction of tissues with vaporization of water, and it cauterizes tissue surfaces. The smoke plume contains water vapor and destroyed tissue material. Its drawbacks relate to safety of the operating room personnel, patient, and surgeon. The laser may glance off metal used in the suspension of the larynx and injure eyes or skin that it hits. A misfire may also hit areas on the patient that are not protected by a wet towel to absorb the laser energy. In addition, the laser smoke or "plume" has been found to contain active viral DNA, a potential source of infection.[52-54] Smoke evacuators are necessary for safety of exposed individuals. Most importantly, since the laser generates heat, ignition of the endotracheal tube may occur with an inadvertent laser strike. In the oxygen-rich environment provided by anesthetic gases, this can lead to explosion or fire in the airway. The surgeon who

Table 204-1

Treatment Options in RRP

Treatment	Number of Patients Reported
Laser therapy The standard for papilloma removal.	**Hundreds**
Microdébrider removal An evolving standard for papilloma removal.	**Hundreds**
Acyclovir Inhibits thymidine kinase, an enzyme not encoded by HPV. 4 patients treated with postoperative acyclovir, with "no recurrence in 3 cases"[105] 4 patients treated with acyclovir as adjuvant therapy to routine surgical/laser treatment. One of the 4 patients exhibited "less aggressive disease during the treatment period." The authors conclude that acyclovir "is not recommended in the treatment of juvenile respiratory papillomatosis."[106]	**8**
Cidofovir First member of group of antiviral agents known as acyclic phosphonate nucleotide analogs; they inhibit viral DNA polymerase. Cidofovir is directly injected into laryngeal sites of RRP. Large-scale trials are ongoing. 14 of 17 patients with "severe" RRP who underwent cidofovir injections experienced a "complete response."[71] 10 of 10 children with RRP who underwent cidofovir injections showed a response with short-term follow-up.[72] 14 of 14 adults with RRP exhibited disease remission after 1 to 6 injections of cidofovir.[107] Similarly, percutaneous injections of cidofovir resulted in clinical improvement in 5 of 5 adults and 5 of 5 children undergoing intralesional injections.[108,109] A larger study of 26 adults and children receiving intralesional injections found that one third exhibited complete remission; two thirds of the patients exhibited reduction in disease; none exhibited worsening of disease.[75,76] A report of a single patient with pulmonary spread of RRP suggests that systemic cidofovir may be effective in some instances. A patient had documented regression of lung RRP lesions in response to systemic cidofovir.[78]	**>50**
Indole-3-carbinol (I-3-C) I-3-C affects the ratio of estradiol hydroxylation. 18 patients, Phase I trial: one third (6 patients) exhibited "cessation of their papilloma growth"; one third exhibited "reduced papilloma growth rate"; one third exhibited "no clinical response."[84]	**18**
Interferon-alpha This most widely used adjuvant therapy appears to modulate host immune response to virus. Most common adverse side effects include flulike symptoms, but can include severe central nervous system effects such as coma.[67,68]	**>100**
Mumps vaccine 11 children with RRP were treated with regular laser excision; 9 of 11 patients (82%) had "remission induced by 1 to 10 injections, with follow-up at 5 to 19 months." In subsequent series, remission was induced in 29 of 38 patients (76%) by 4 to 26 injections, with follow-up at 2 to 5 years.[95]	**49**
Retinoids ANY in RRP trials?	**?**
Photodynamic therapy (PDT-DHE)	**>100**
Photodynamic therapy (PDT-Foscan)	**Ongoing Clinical Trials**
Vaccines A fusion protein composed of heat shock protein and the E7 gene product of human papillomavirus (HSP-E7) has been used successfully as a novel vaccine in patients with anogenital warts, where 13 of 14 adult patients had resolution of warts at week 24.[110] This novel approach had been in clinical trials as potential therapy for RRP; however, the pharmaceutical company responsible was financially insolvent and clinical trials have been halted. The quadrivalent HPV vaccine indicated for the prevention of cervical cancer[32] promises to dramatically reduce the morbidity and mortality of cervical cancer, but also has the potential to reduce aerodigestive squamous cell carcinoma as well as to eradicate RRP in future generations.[32]	**Ongoing Clinical Trials**

is not aware of injury to deeper tissue layers with injudicious laser usage may cause unacceptable scarring and subsequent abnormal vocal fold function. Inappropriate and aggressive use of the laser may also cause injury to tissues that are not affected and create an environment suitable for implantation of viral particles. Use of the CO_2 laser can also result in delayed local tissue damage, which may be related to the total number of laser surgeries and the severity of RRP disease.

Although the CO_2 laser allows for precision of surgery and excellent hemostasis, multiple procedures are often necessary. Frequent interval laser laryngoscopies are recommended in an attempt to avoid tracheotomy and permit the child to develop good phonation with preservation of normal vocal cord anatomy. The latest generation of laser microspot micromanipulator enables the surgeon to use a spot size of 250 mm at 400-mm focal length and 160 mm at 250-mm focal length.

Although the CO_2 laser is the most commonly used laser for RRP in the larynx, the potassium titanium phosphate (KTP), 585-nm flash dye, and argon laser could also be used. Papillomata that have extended down the tracheobronchial tree often require use of the KTP or pulse dye laser coupled with a ventilating bronchoscope for removal. Occasionally, the ventilating resectoscope can also be used in these circumstances.

Emerging Technologies

The use of the CO_2 laser on the true vocal folds must be judicious given the potential for significant postoperative scar tissue formation from unrecognized heat transfer. To minimize the risk of scar formation in the true vocal folds, cold steel excision can be used successfully following the principles of phono-microsurgery, submucosal dissection, and microinstrumentation. This approach may have treatment advantages over CO_2 laser surgery, especially in the adult RRP patient.[55-57] In their initial series, Zeitels and Sataloff report recurrence of papilloma in none of the six adults at 2 years follow-up after resection for primary disease. Of those who presented with recurrent papillomatosis, 6 of 16 (38%) continued to recur after their microflap procedure.[57]

Publications have highlighted the potential benefits of other surgical technologies in managing RRP. Bower and others evaluated the feasibility and safety of the flash pump dye laser in nine children and found good early results.[58] McMillan and others published preliminary results regarding their positive experience with the 585-nm pulsed dye laser in three patients.[59] Zeitels reported on office-based use of the 532-nm pulsed KTP laser for treatment of recurrent glottal papillomatosis and dysplasias, noting at least 75% regression of disease in two thirds of patients who could tolerate the procedure.[60] Rees and Koufman also demonstrated tolerance for in-office pulsed dye laser treatments involving 328 procedures in 131 adult patients, with patients overwhelmingly preferring the in-office pulsed dye laser over surgeries under general anesthesia.[61] Zeitels and others currently favor use of a solid-state fiber-based thulium laser that functions similarly to a CO_2 laser with the benefit of being delivered through a small glass fiber.[62]

A number of investigators are now replacing their use of the CO_2 laser with the endoscopic microdébrider as a means of quickly debulking laryngeal disease. In a small, randomized study, Pasquale and others observed improved voice quality, less OR time, less mucosal injury, and a cost benefit in direct comparison of the microdébrider and the CO_2 laser.[63] El-Bitar and Zalzal, and Patel and others, have observed similar improved outcomes with the use of the endoscopic microdébrider.[64,65] A web-based survey of members of the American Society of Pediatric Otolaryngologists (ASPO) found the majority of respondents now favoring the use of "shaver" technology.[4]

Because no therapeutic regimen reliably eradicates the HPV, when there is a question about whether papilloma in an area needs to be removed, it is prudent to accept some residual papilloma rather than risk damage to normal tissue and produce excessive scarring. Even with the removal of all clinically evident papilloma, latent virus remains in adjacent tissue. Therefore the aim of therapy in extensive disease should be to reduce the tumor burden, decrease the spread of disease, create a safe and patent airway, optimize voice quality, and increase the time interval between surgical procedures. Staged papilloma removal for disease in the anterior commissure is appropriate to prevent the apposition of two raw mucosal surfaces.

Anesthetic Techniques

Several different anesthetic techniques have been advocated in endoscopic procedures to remove papillomas in children. With all methods, the airway must be handled with the utmost delicacy to minimize iatrogenic microtrauma to the mucosa.

Spontaneous Ventilation

In spontaneous ventilation, intravenous agents such as propofol are used along with oxygen and anesthetic gases such as sevoflurane that are entrained through a side port of the laryngoscope or through an endotracheal tube or nasal trumpet placed in the pharynx. The patient's own efforts are responsible for maintenance of anesthesia. Advantages are the unobstructed surgical field, but the technique is hard to master and requires an anesthesiologist who is well attuned to his or her patient. Laryngospasm, awakening, and other movement can take place with disastrous results.

Intermittent Apnea-Reintubation

Intermittent apnea-reintubation allows for the widest range of anesthetic types and provides for an unobstructed surgical view. The patient is anesthetized, intubated, suspended, and examined. The microscope is used to visualize the larynx and the tube is withdrawn while the laser or microdébrider is used. The tube is then replaced under direct visualization if the patient's oxygenation diminishes and/or the carbon dioxide level rises. Although the time for operative intervention is limited, this method is simple and effective. It does have the drawback of potentially spreading the virus through the repeated placement of the tube, however.

Wrapped or "Laser-Safe" Endotracheal Tube

Use of a wrapped or "laser-safe" endotracheal tube to protect the tube from accidental ignition by the laser can be effective and permits no significant alteration in anesthetic or surgical management. The tube remains in the surgical field, potentially obscuring the posterior glottis and subglottis. A wrapped tube must be protected (usually with electromagnetic tape or foil) to reduce risk of airway fire. There are commercially available "laser safe" tubes. Cuffs must also be protected with moist surgical cottonoids to prevent their rupture.

Jet Ventilation

Another anesthetic alternative is the use of jet ventilation for microsurgery of the larynx. Jet ventilation eliminates the potential fire hazard inherent in the use of the endotracheal tube when used with the CO_2 laser and allows good visualization of the vocal cords. A limitation of this technique is the possibility of transmission of HPV particles into the distal airway. The jet cannula can be placed either above or below the vocal cords and each approach has its own particular benefit. It is preferable to place the cannula proximal to the end of the laryngoscope to decrease the risk of possible pneumothorax or pneumomediastinum. With large laryngeal lesions, narrowed airways, and ball-valve lesions, there may develop a high degree of outflow obstruction that could lead to increased intrathoracic pressure and a subsequent pneumothorax. This may also result if there is inadequate muscle relaxation. Jet ventilation also requires constant communication between the operating surgeon and the anesthesiologist. Excessive mucosal drying and damage can occur, as can insufflation of air into the stomach with gastric distention. As mentioned earlier in this chapter, there is also the potential risk of disseminating papilloma or blood into the tracheobronchial tree.

Although not appropriate for most children with RRP, office endoscopy using light or topical anesthesia can be used along with the pulsed dye laser in selected adults.

Adjuvant Treatment Modalities

Although surgical management remains the mainstay therapy for RRP, ultimately as many as 20% of patients with the disease will require some form of adjuvant therapy. The most widely adopted criteria for initiating adjuvant therapy are a requirement for more than four surgical procedures per year, rapid regrowth of papilloma disease with airway compromise, or distal multisite spread of disease. Some of these adjuvant treatment options are summarized in Table 204-1.

Antiviral Modalities

Interferon

The first widely employed adjuvant therapy was alpha-interferon.[6,66,67] The exact mechanism by which interferon elicits its response is unknown. It appears to modulate host immune response by increasing production of a protein kinase and endonuclease, which inhibits viral protein synthesis.[68] Interferons are a class of proteins that are manufactured by cells in response to a variety of stimuli including viral infection. The enzymes that are produced block the viral replication of RNA and DNA and alter cell membranes to make them less susceptible to viral penetration.

Common interferon side effects fall into two categories: acute reactions (fever and generalized flulike symptoms, chills, headache, myalgias, and nausea that seem to decrease with prolonged therapy) and chronic reactions (decrease in the growth rate of the child, elevation of liver transaminase levels, leukopenia spastic diplegia, and febrile seizures). Thrombocytopenia has been reported, as have rashes, dry skin, alopecia, generalized pruritus, and fatigue. Acetaminophen has been found to effectively relieve fever, and interferon injections are best tolerated at bedtime. Interferon produced by recombinant DNA techniques appears to have fewer side effects and better efficacy than blood bank-harvested interferon. If the side effects can be tolerated then therapy is initiated at 5 million units/m^2 body surface area administered by subcutaneous injection on a daily basis for 28 days, then 3 days per week for at least a 6-month trial. After 6 months in children with excellent responses and no severe side effects, the dosage can be decreased to 3 million units/m^2 for 3 days a week with further slow weaning as tolerated.

Ribavirin

Ribavirin is an antiviral drug used to treat respiratory syncytial virus pneumonia in infants that has also shown some promise in the treatment of aggressive laryngeal papillomatosis. Ostrow and others at the University of Minnesota have completed a small trial in eight patients using ribavirin in an oral form at 23 mg/kg/day divided four times daily after an initial intravenous loading dose, showing an increase in surgical interval in those treated.[69]

Acyclovir

Another antiviral treatment that has been advocated in the treatment of RRP is acyclovir. Although the activity of acyclovir is dependent on the presence of virally encoded thymidine kinase, an enzyme that is not known to be encoded by papillomavirus, conflicting clinical results have been obtained in several small series. Theoretically, it would not be expected to have a positive effect. However, it has been postulated that perhaps acyclovir is most effective when there are simultaneous disease factors such as infection with herpes simplex virus. Such viral co-infections with herpes simplex virus 1, cytomegalovirus, and Epstein-Barr virus (HSV-1, CMV, and EBV) have been demonstrated in RRP patients, and these patients with viral co-infections appear to have a more aggressive clinical course.[70]

Cidofovir

Recent reports have stimulated interest in the intralesional injection of cidofovir (Vistide)—(S)-1-[3-hydroxy-2-(phosphonylmethoxyethyl)-propyl]-cytosine (HPMPC)—a drug approved by the U.S. Food and Drug Administration for use in human immunodeficiency virus (HIV) patients with cytomegalovirus under expedited, fast-track guidelines. Despite a lack of controlled, randomized, blinded clinical trials in children with RRP, cidofovir is currently the most frequently used adjuvant drug.[4] Snoeck and others reported a series of 17 patients with severe RRP treated with cidofovir at 2.5 mg/mL injected directly into the papilloma bed after laser surgery experienced a complete response in 14 days.[71] Pranksy and coworkets have used this therapy in 10 children with severe RRP with short-term follow-up showing a response in all 10 patients,[72] and long-term follow-up has been encouraging.[73,74] Similarly encouraging results have been reported by Naiman and others in a small cohort of adults and children treated with a protocol-driven approach using a high dose of cidofovir at 2-week intervals.[75,76] Co and Woo have also demonstrated efficacy in a small cohort of adults with RRP treated with serial office-based intralesional injections of cidofovir.[77] Finally, there has been one encouraging successful treatment of pulmonary multicystic papillomatosis using systemic cidofovir.[78]

Based on animal studies that demonstrated a high level of carcinogenicity, and on case reports of progressive dysplasia in patients with RRP,[79] the RRP Task Force has published guidelines for clinicians interested in using cidofovir in their RRP patients.[80] Despite the anecdotal nature of most of the cidofovir studies and reports, the preliminary results are encouraging enough to consider this a treatment option in severely affected RRP patients.

Photodynamic Therapy

Photodynamic therapy (PDT) applied to the treatment of RRP has been studied extensively at Long Island Jewish Hospital by Shikowitz and associates.[81] PDT is based on the transfer of energy to a photosensitive drug. The original drug used was dihematoporphyrin ether (DHE), which has a tendency to concentrate within papillomas more so than in surrounding normal tissue. Patients are typically treated intravenously with 4.25 mg/kg of DHE before photoactivation with an argon pump dye laser. A small but statistically significant decrease in RRP growth, especially in patients whose disease was worse, was seen with the use of PDT and DHE. The drawback of this therapy is that patients become markedly photosensitive for periods lasting 2 to 8 weeks. A new drug, m-tetra(hydroxyphenyl)chlorine (Foscan), has shown efficacy in HPV-induced tumors in rabbits with minimal tissue damage and less photosensitivity. A clinical trial using this drug in a parallel-arm, randomized trial of 23 severely affected patients ages 4 to 60 resulted in improvement in laryngeal disease; however, remissions failed to be maintained over 3 to 5 years and the therapy was poorly tolerated by a quarter of the patients.[82]

Indole-3-Carbinol

There has been recent interest in the dietary supplement, indole-3-carbinol, a compound that is found in high concentration in cruciferous vegetables such as cabbage, cauliflower, and broccoli. Results in an open label, multicenter study coordinated by Rosen of treating RRP with indole-3-carbinol were encouraging. During the short follow-up of the study (a minimum of 8 months), one third of the patients had a cessation of their papilloma growth and did not require further surgery, one third of the patients exhibited reduced papilloma growth rate, and one third did not show a clinical response.[83,84] The role of estrogens on the growth of RRP has been conjectured since the discovery that RRP exhibits increased binding of estrogen.[85] Subsequent to that report, inhibition of estrogen metabolism using indole-3-carbinol has been shown to reduce the formation of HPV-induced papilloma tumors in immunocompromised mice by nearly 75%.[86] Most recently, the clinical response to indole-3-carbinol in children with RRP was closely correlated with the ratio of hydroxylated estradiol in urine.[84] Longer follow-up of a larger, blinded, controlled trial seems warranted before universally recommending this therapy.

Celecoxib

Celecoxib (Celebrex) is a selective inhibitor of the enzyme COX-2, which is overexpressed in RRPs and stimulates their growth.[87] Preliminary encouraging results in a small cohort of adults with Celebrex has led to an NIH-funded multicenter trial led by investigators at Long Island Jewish Hospital that is currently active (no longer enrolling) for adults with RRP.

Retinoids

Retinoids, which are metabolites and analogues of vitamin A, are known modulators of cellular proliferation and differentiation of diverse histologic cell types. In the aerodigestive tract, excess vitamin A has been found to suppress squamous differentiation, and may result in mucous metaplasia.[88] In contrast, vitamin A deficiency may result in hyperkeratinization and squamous metaplasia.[89] However, there are a variety of retinoids with opposing effects on epithelial cell metabolism.[90-93] Thus to state that retinoids as a class of agents have a beneficial or deleterious effect on mucosal differentiation would be an oversimplification. With this caveat, 13-cis-retinoic acid (Accutane) has gained some popularity as a systemic treatment for RRP.[94] The dosage for retinoic acid is 1 to 2 mg/kg/day. This therapy is maintained for 6 months or until the patient develops side effects he cannot tolerate. Care has to be taken in sexually active patients because Accutane has well-known teratogenic effects.

Mumps Vaccine

Intralesional injection of mumps vaccine and MMR vaccine has been investigated in an open-label single-center trial with moderate success.[95]

STAGING ASSESSMENT FOR RECURRENT LARYNGEAL PAPILLOMATOSIS

PATIENT INITIALS : ___ DATE OF SURGERY:___ SURGEON:___
PATIENT ID #: ___ INSTITUTION:___

1. How long since the last papilloma surgery? ___days, ___weeks,___months,___years, ___ don't know, ___1st surgery
2. Counting today's surgery, how many papilloma surgeries in the past 12 months?___
3. Describe the patient's voice today: ___aphonic, ___abnormal, ___normal,___other
4. Describe the patient's stridor today: ___absent, ___present with activity, ___present at rest, ___ don't know
5. Describe the urgency of today's intervention: ___scheduled, ___urgent, ___ emergent

FOR EACH SITE, SCORE AS: 0 = NONE, 1 = SURFACE LESION, 2 = RAISED LESION, 3 = BULKY LESION

LARYNX
Epiglottis
Lingual surface _____ Laryngeal surface ____
Aryepiglottic folds: Right___ Left___
False vocal cords: Right___ Left___
True vocal cords: Right___ Left___
Arytenoids: Right___ Left___
Anterior commissure_____ Posterior commissure_____
Subglottis_____

TRACHEA:
Upper one-third _____
Middle one-third_____
Lower one-third_____
Bronchi: Right_____ Left_____
Tracheotomy stoma_____

OTHER:
Nose_____
Palate_____
Pharynx_____
Esophagus_____
Lungs_____
Other_____

TOTAL SCORE ALL SITES: __________

Figure 204-6. Staging assessment sheet for recurrent respiratory papillomatosis. *(From Derkay CS, Malis DJ, Zalzal G, et al. A staging system for assessing severity of disease and response to therapy in recurrent respiratory papillomatosis.* Laryngoscope. *1998;108:935-937.)*

These positive results, however, have not been reproduced by other investigators.[96]

Antireflux Therapy

The role of gastroesophageal reflux in exacerbation of RRP deserves special mention. Recent case reports have shown that the rate of recurrence of respiratory papillomatosis in children may decrease significantly after antireflux therapy.[97,98] The H_2-antihistamine Cimetidine (ranitidine) has been shown to have immunomodulatory effects.[99,100] This has resulted in several reports of its use against various virally based diseases, including RRP.[98,101] A recent small case series from Buffalo demonstrated efficacy in previously resistant children with RRP.[102] It is for these reasons that optimal control of extraesophageal reflux disease has been advocated as a means of improving outcomes, along with surgical therapy. The authors routinely place their RRP patients on an antireflux regimen.

Staging Severity

It is helpful when tracking the progression of a child's disease, communicating with other surgeons, and treating patients in a protocol format to have a surgical scoring system to assess severity and clinical course of RRP disease. Although several scoring and staging systems have been proposed, clinicians and researchers have not yet adopted a uniformly acceptable nomenclature for describing RRP lesions that is simple yet comprehensive. This has created confusion in the RRP literature and in physician-to-physician communications regarding patients' response to therapies. In addition, the absence of a universally accepted staging system has hampered our abilities to accurately report the results of adjuvant therapies or document the natural course of the disease. We have introduced a severity-staging system for RRP in a format that incorporates the best qualities of the existing systems by numerically grading the extent of papillomatosis at defined aerodigestive subsites, assessing functional parameters, diagrammatically catalogs subsite involvement, and assigning a final numeric score to the patient's current extent of disease (Figs. 204-5 through 204-7).[47,103,104] Using software designed at the University of Washington (Seattle) and licensed to the ASPO, this staging system is now computerized and available to pediatric otolaryngologists and bronchoesophagologists to allow them to objectively and subjectively measure an individual patient's clinical course and response to therapy through time. Health Insurance Portability and Accountability Act–compliant encryption technology with this software offers promise to allow clinicians from

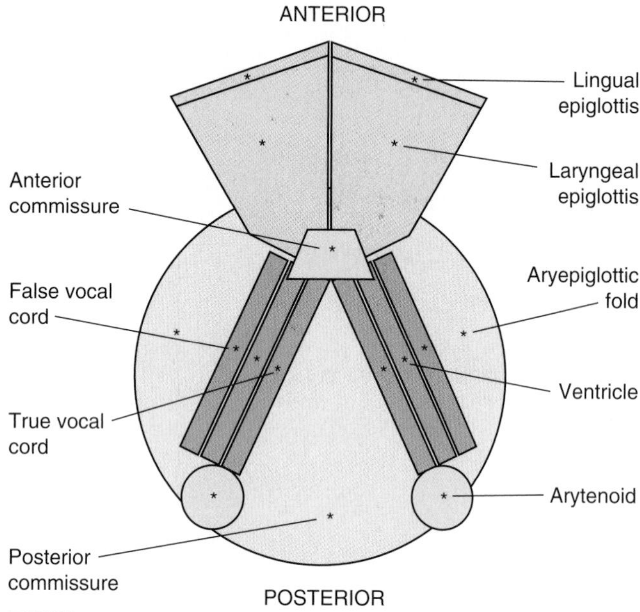

Figure 204-7. Diagram of laryngeal sites that may be scored. *(From Hester RP, Derkay CS, Burke BL, Lawson ML. Reliability of a staging assessment system for recurrent respiratory papillomatosis.* Int J Pediatr Otorhinolaryngol. *2003;67:505-509.)*

around the world to anonymously share some of their patient data to enhance our knowledge of this disease and promote multi-institutional investigations.

Registry and Task Force Initiatives

It should be stressed that participation in national and regional protocols of adjuvant treatment modalities is essential for the scientific community to learn more about RRP. A national registry of patients with RRP has been formed through the cooperation of the ASPO and the CDC.[14] The registry tracked nearly 600 children at 22 sites with data on more than 11,000 surgical procedures. Data from the national registry aided in the identification of patients suitable for enrollment in multi-institutional studies of adjuvant therapies and better defined the risk factors for transmission of HPV and the cofactors that may determine the aggressiveness of RRP. An RRP task force, made up of the principal investigators at each of the registry sites as well as representatives from the adult RRP research community and patient/parent advocacy groups, meets twice yearly to facilitate research initiatives. The RRP task force has completed a set of Practice Guidelines (RRP Task Force, 2000) to help guide the clinician in the diagnosis and management of children with RRP, and has authored public health guidelines regarding RRP and statements on the use of cidofovir. The Task Force is engaged in providing a statement on the value of viral typing and is facilitating an investigation of the genes responsible for aggressive RRP. They have also facilitated the development of similar groups of RRP investigators in Canada and Europe and are currently working with their colleagues outside of the United States to study the benefits of the quadrivalent HPV vaccine for treatment and prevention of RRP.

Other Considerations

Children with newly diagnosed RRP warrant a substantial time commitment on the part of the otolaryngologist to engage the family in a frank and open discussion of the disease and its management. Support groups such as the Recurrent Respiratory Papilloma Foundation (www.rrpf.org) and the International (www.rrpwebsite.org) can be a vital resource for information and support. RRP patients require frequent office visits and endoscopic procedures at the outset to establish the aggressiveness of their disease. The patients are encouraged to return to the office or call as often as necessary while family members and the health care team become familiar with the child's symptoms and level of distress. While infant home intercom-type monitors are often recommended, apnea-bradycardia monitors and pulse oximetry are generally not necessary. Repeat flexible fiberoptic laryngoscopy may be used in the office, and speech and language therapy is offered early in the course of the disease. Control of other medical factors such as reflux and asthma is also aggressively pursued.

Summary

RRP is a frustrating, capricious disease with the potential for morbid consequences because of its involvement of the airway and the risk of malignant degeneration. The goals of surgical therapy are to maintain a safe airway with a serviceable voice while avoiding excessive scarring. No single modality of therapy has been consistently shown effective in eradicating RRP. When children require surgical therapy more frequently than four times in 12 months or have evidence of distal spread of RRP outside of the larynx, adjuvant medical therapy should be considered. Many adjuvant therapies have been investigated to supplement surgical therapy. These range from dietary supplements and control of extraesophageal reflux disease to potent antiviral and chemotherapeutic agents and photodynamic therapies. Although several of these modalities have shown promise, no adjuvant therapy to date has "cured" RRP.

Strides are being made in learning more about the natural history of the disease. A registry of RRP patients, and software to help clinicians share information on and accurately follow their RRP patients, has been developed. Future research is needed regarding prevention of transmission of HPV from mother to child. Specifically, the roles of cesarean section and gynecologic surgery during pregnancy need to be elucidated. Universal or near-universal use of an HPV vaccine that provides protection against HPV 6 and 11 may do for RRP what the Hib vaccine has done for *H. influenzae* type B epiglottitis—virtually eliminating new cases in less than a decade. Further refinements in surgical techniques, including the use of new office-based lasers to minimize laryngeal scarring, also need to be studied. Surgical therapy for RRP requires a skilled team consisting of otolaryngologists, anesthesia providers, and operating room personnel working together in a facility properly equipped to manage difficult pediatric airways. Because of the recurrent nature of RRP and the potential for airway obstruction, parental support and education can be invaluable to the safety of the child with RRP.

SUGGESTED READINGS

Armstrong LR, Derkay CS, Reeves WC. Initial results from the National Registry for juvenile-onset recurrent respiratory papillomatosis. *Arch Otolaryngol Head Neck Surg.* 1999;125:743-748.

Dedo HH, Yu KC. CO_2 laser treatment in 244 patients with respiratory papillomatosis. *Laryngoscope.* 2001;111:1639-1644.

Derkay CS, Malis DJ, Zalzal G, et al. A staging system for assessing severity of disease and response to therapy in recurrent respiratory papillomatosis. *Laryngoscope.* 1998;108:935-937.

Derkay CS. Task force on recurrent respiratory papillomas: a preliminary report. *Arch Otolaryngol Head Neck Surg.* 1995;121:1386-1391.

Derkay CS, Smith RJ, McClay J, et al. HspE7 treatment of pediatric P: final results of an open-label trial. *Ann Otol Rhinol Laryngol.* 2005;114;730-737.

Derkay CS. Cidofovir for recurrent respiratory papillomatosis (RRP): a re-assessment of risks. *International Journal Pediatric Otolaryngology.* 2005; 11:1465-1467. Epub 2005 Sep19.

Freed G, Derkay CS. HPV vaccines and RRP. *International Journal of Pediatric Otorhinolaryngology.* 2006;70(November (11)):1-5.

Healy GB, Gelber RD, Trowbridge AL, et al. Treatment of recurrent respiratory papillomatosis with human leukocyte interferon. *N Engl J Med.* 1988; 319:401-407,

Kashima HK, Mounts P, Leventhal B, Hruban RH. Sites of predilection in recurrent respiratory papillomatosis. *Ann Otol Rhinol Laryngol.* 1993;102:580-583.

Kosko J, Derkay CS. Role of cesarean section in the prevention of recurrent respiratory papillomatosis: is there one? *Int J Pediatr Otorhinolaryngol.* 1:31-38, 1996.

Leventhal BG, Kashima HK, Weck PW, et al. Randomized surgical adjuvant trial of interferon alpha-n1 in recurrent papillomatosis. *Arch Otolaryngol Head Neck Surg.* 1988;114:1163-1169.

Maloney EM, Unger ER, Reeves RA, et al. Longitudinal measures of HPV 6 and 11 viral loads and antibody response in children with RRP. *Arch OTOHNS.* 2006;132:711-715.

Mounts P, Shah KV, Kashima H. Viral etiology of juvenile- and adult-onset squamous papilloma of the larynx. *Proc Natl Acad Sci U S A.* 1982;79:5425-5429.

Pasquale K, Wiatrak KB, Wooley A, et al. Microdébrider versus CO_2 laser for RRP: a comparative study. *Laryngoscope.* 2003;113(1):139-143.

Pransky SM, Magit AE, Kearns DB, et al. Intralesional Cidofovir for recurrent respiratory papillomatosis in children. *Arch Otolaryngol Head Neck Surg.* 1999;125:1143-1148.

Reeves WC, Ruparelia SS, Swanson KI, et al. National registry for juvenile-onset recurrent respiratory papillomatosis. *Arch Otolaryngol Head Neck Surg.* 2003;129(9):976-982.

Rimmel FL, Shoemaker DL, Pou AM, et al. Pediatric respiratory papillomatosis: prognostic role of viral typing and cofactors. *Laryngoscope.* 1997;107:915-918.

Schraff S, Derkay CS. Survey of ASPO membership regarding management of RRP distal spread and the use of adjuvant therapies. *Arch Otolaryngol Head Neck Surg.* 2004;130:1039.

Shah K, Kashima HK, Polk BF, et al. Rarity of cesarean delivery in cases of juvenile-onset respiratory papillomatosis. *Obstet Gynecol.* 1986;68:795-799.

Shah KV, Stern WF, Shah FK, et al. Risk factors for juvenile-onset recurrent respiratory papillomatosis. *Pediatr Infect Dis J.* 1998;17:372-376.

Shapiro AM, Rimell FL, Shoemaker D, et al. Tracheotomy in children with juvenile-onset recurrent respiratory papillomatosis: the Children's Hospital of Pittsburgh experience, *Ann Otol Rhinol Laryngol.* 1996;105:1-5.

Shikowitz MJ, Abramson AL, Steinberg BM, et al. Clinical Trial of photodynamic therapy with meso-tetra (hydroxyphenyl) chlorin for respiratory papillomatosis. *Arch Otolaryngol Head Neck Surg* 2005;131;99-105.

Wiatrak BJ, Wiatrak DW, Broker TR, et al. Recurrent respiratory papillomatosis: a longitudinal study comparing severity associated with human papilloma viral types 6 and 11 and other risk factors in a large pediatric population. *Laryngoscope* 2004;114(November (11 Pt 2 Suppl 104)):1-23.

Zeitels SM, Sataloff RT. Phonomicrosurgical resection of glottal papillomatosis. *J Voice.* 1999;13:123-127.

Zeitels SM, Akst LM, Burns JA, et al. Office-based 532 nm pulsed KTP laser treatment of glottal papillomatosis and dysplasia. *Ann Otol Rhinol Laryngol* 2006;115:679-685.

For complete list of references log onto www.expertconsult.com.

CHAPTER TWO HUNDRED AND FIVE

Evaluation and Management of the Stridulous Child

David Albert

Simone Boardman

Marlene Soma

Key Points

- The quality of stridor may be *characteristic* of a particular pathology but is never *diagnostic*; the diagnosis can only be confirmed with certainty after endoscopy.
- Improvement in stridor can paradoxically be due to worsening airway obstruction and reduced airflow.
- Laryngotracheobronchoscopy is the gold standard in the assessment of the stridulous child. It is now a highly technical procedure and the whole team (surgeon, anesthetist, and nursing assistant) needs to work closely together to perform the examination safely and to optimize the assessment.
- Children with croup who demonstrate increased work of breathing in the clinics or emergency departments should be treated with glucocorticoids.
- The risk with low tracheobronchial obstruction is that neither intubation nor tracheostomy will relieve the obstruction, although positive pressure will tend to improve malacia and to a lesser extent stenosis.
- A difficult and potentially dangerous situation occurs if a tracheotomy is attempted for tapering long segment tracheal stenosis. Not only is it not possible to insert a normal neonatal size tracheotomy tube but the tracheotomy itself severely limits the therapeutic options for surgical reconstruction of the stenosis.
- Medical therapy with steroids, antireflux treatment, nebulized adrenaline (epinephrine), heliox, and antibiotics in some cases may avert the need for more invasive measures such as tracheotomy.
- Therapeutic surgical options to manage the stridulous child include tracheotomy, endoscopic and open laryngeal surgery. Treatment is individualized depending on the underlying pathology, associated comorbidity, and social circumstances.

A stridulous child with airway obstruction demands prompt attention from parents and clinicians alike. There are many good reasons to treat pediatric patients with great respect; they have less respiratory reserve and their smaller airways are more easily compromised. In the acute situation, the infant airway can deteriorate rapidly and provide significant clinical challenges. The history and examination are rarely sufficient for a firm diagnosis; however, deciding which patients require further investigation may be difficult. Even after appropriate noninvasive investigations (e.g., imaging), there may still be a number of possible diagnoses. Flexible endoscopy in the office is useful but gives limited information beyond the glottis. The definitive diagnostic tool of laryngotracheobronchoscopy requires highly specialized equipment and an experienced surgical, anesthetic, and nursing team.

Advances in medical technology impact the likely underlying diagnoses of modern-day stridor and its management.[1] Developments in neonatal intensive care have seen improved neonatal survival and the associated challenges of the airway pathology seen in these children. Routine childhood immunization with the *Haemophilus influenzae* type B (HiB) vaccine has led to a precipitous decline in epiglottitis, making it a rarity. Improvements in endoscopic equipment have revolutionized the quality of optical images obtainable and captured for digital recording. It has also allowed for the development of endoscopic interventions in the compromised pediatric airway, many of which may now be used in combination to avoid tracheotomy or open airway surgery.

This chapter describes a current and safe approach to assessing and treating the airway of the stridulous child. The diagnostic workup is reviewed in detail and the medical and surgical management of acute and chronic airway obstruction is reviewed, with special attention given to the situations of postextubation stridor and postpartum neonatal airway obstruction. The principles of tracheotomy, endoscopic, and open laryngeal surgery are discussed.

Definition and Physical Principles

Stridor is an audible respiratory noise derived from turbulent airflow due to narrowing or obstruction of the upper airway. Stridor may be inspiratory, biphasic, or expiratory in nature. It is classically a harsh sound, which can vary in quality from a squeak to a whistling noise. Stertor describes the snoring-like noise, which typically originates from nasopharyngeal or oropharyngeal obstruction. Clinically, however, the supraglottic larynx can occasionally produce this quality of noise.

Table 205-1

Differential Diagnosis of Airway Obstruction

	Supralaryngeal	Laryngeal	Tracheobronchial
Congenital	Choanal atresia	Laryngomalacia	Tracheomalacia/bronchomalacia
	Choanal/midnasal/piriform aperture stenosis	Vocal cord palsy	Tracheal stenosis
	Benign tumor	Laryngeal atresia	Extrinsic compression
	Nasal glioma	Laryngotracheal stenosis	Vascular compression (e.g., aberrant brachiocephalic, double aortic arch, vascular ring, pulmonary artery sling)
	Encephalocele	Laryngeal web	Mediastinal tumor
	Meningocele	Posterior laryngeal cleft	Tracheal atresia
	Nasopharyngeal mass (e.g., hairy polyp, teratoma)	Cysts	Complete tracheal rings
	Structural	Vallecular cyst	Tracheal cysts
	Midface hypoplasia (e.g., Apert's, Crouzon's, Down syndrome)	Laryngeal cyst	
	Micrognathia (e.g., Pierre Robin, Treacher Collins)		
	Macroglossia (e.g., Down syndrome, cystic hygroma, lingual thyroid)		
	Cysts		
	Dermoid		
	Thyroglossal duct cyst		
	Neurological dysfunction		
Acquired	Adenotonsillar hypertrophy	Trauma	Postintubation/instrumentation
	Infection	Intubation trauma (e.g., subglottic stenosis)	Tracheal stenosis
	Tonsillitis	Cricoarytenoid joint fixation	Foreign body
	Adenoiditis	Surgical trauma (e.g., laser)	Reflux
	Infectious mononucleosis	Thermal and caustic burns	Infection
	Retropharyngeal abscess	Infection	Croup
	Ludwig's angina	Croup	Bacterial tracheitis
	Rhinitis	Epiglottitis	Postsurgical malacia (e.g., tracheostomy, tracheoesophageal fistula repair)
	Foreign body	Reflux laryngitis	Extrinsic compression
	Thermal and caustic burns	Benign tumor	Mediastinal tumor (e.g., hemangioma, cystic hygroma, lymphadenopathy, thyroid mass)
		Papillomatosis	
		Hemangioma	
		Cystic hygroma	
		Malignant tumor (e.g., rhabdomyosarcoma)	
		Foreign body	

Obstruction from all levels of the airway should thus be considered when approaching the differential diagnoses of airway obstruction (Table 205-1).

It is helpful to review the physical principles of tubular flow according to Poiseuille's law, which states that $Q = [\pi r^4(P_1\text{-}P_2)]/8\eta L$; where Q is flow, r is radius, P is pressure, η is viscosity, and L is length of tube. From this law, resistance is inversely proportional to the radius to the fourth power. From a practical viewpoint, this explains why minor narrowing in a child's airway is of much greater consequence than in an adult. For example, 1 mm of edema in a 4-mm diameter pediatric airway will reduce the cross-sectional area by 75% (16-fold increase in resistance), whereas in a 12-mm adult airway, the same 1 mm of edema reduces the airway area by just 30% (twofold increase in resistance) as demonstrated in Fig. 205-1.[2]

Assessment

It is important to perform a rapid initial evaluation of the stridulous child to assess their degree of respiratory distress and thus the urgency of their clinical presentation. If the patient has acute airway obstruction with significant respiratory distress, particularly if the patient is tiring, then the history, examination, and initial resuscitation must take place simultaneously. A comprehensive history and exhaustive examination can be completed once the situation is controlled. If the child's condition is stable, then a thorough assessment can be conducted.

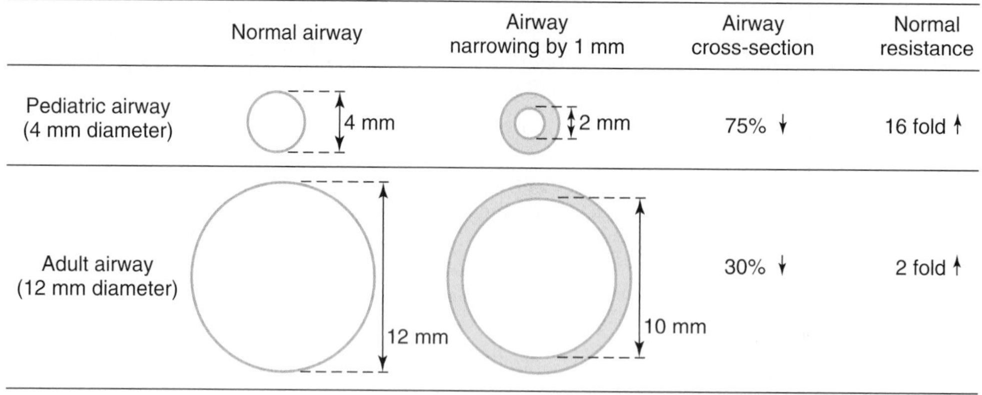

Figure 205-1. Effect of airway narrowing upon airway cross-section and resistance in the pediatric and adult airway.[2]

Stridor may be *characteristic* of a particular pathology but is never *diagnostic*. The diagnosis can be confirmed with certainty only after endoscopy. However, the combination of a thorough history, examination, and investigation can in some conditions (e.g., mild laryngomalacia) provide sufficient diagnostic probability to avoid initial rigid endoscopy. Seventeen percent of infants with laryngomalacia have a synchronous lesion that may be contributing to their airway compromise.[3] This may be missed without assessment via rigid endoscopy.

History

In an acutely stridulous child, even a brief history may aid in determining the source of the airway obstruction. Particular note should be taken of any possible foreign body ingestion or concurrent illness. A careful and thorough history will aid in formulating the differential diagnosis as long as the child has a stable airway.

Features of the stridor, including the timing of onset, progression, variability, and presence of exacerbating or relieving factors should be carefully established. Stridor present from birth suggests an underlying anatomic cause. This generally denotes a fixed congenital narrowing such as a laryngeal web, subglottic stenosis, or tracheal narrowing.[4] Dynamic conditions such as laryngomalacia typically become evident in the first few weeks of life, while congenital vocal cord palsy is also a common cause of neonatal stridor. A gradual increase in severity of stridor or airway compromise implies progressive obstruction. The obstruction may be luminal (as in a subglottic hemangioma) or extrinsic (as with a mediastinal mass or vascular anomaly). Alternatively over a longer period of time, increasing stridor may coincide with increased respiratory demands as the child becomes more active. Typically, laryngomalacia improves during rest or sleep but is worsened by crying, feeding, or physical activity. Airway obstruction associated with supine positioning may occur with supralaryngeal obstruction, such as micrognathia wherein there is associated airway obstruction by the tongue base. More rarely a pedunculated laryngeal mass, for example, a vallecular cyst, can give positional variation in the stridor as it is displaced in and out of the airway (Fig. 205-2). Improved airway obstruction with crying may occur in gross nasal obstruction such as bilateral choanal atresia.

Airway obstruction produces a number of associated symptoms (Table 205-2) that may be useful in formulating a differential diagnosis. Parents have often observed signs of increased respiratory work, including tracheal tug, subcostal recession, and suprasternal or sternal indrawing. Apneas with cyanosis may occur and parents often attempt resuscitation if these are severe. These episodes are typical of severe tracheobronchomalacia and are sometimes termed *dying spells*. The differential diagnosis includes underlying congenital cardiac disease, hence these episodes should be investigated further. Cough is typical of tracheoesophageal fistula and tracheomalacia, and raises the possibility of aspiration. Hoarseness suggests laryngeal pathology such as laryngeal papillomatosis (Fig. 205-3), whereas supralaryngeal pathology may give a muffled voice. Voice change may also occur in vocal cord palsy, although these children can also present with airway compromise and a normal voice.[5,6] Tachypnea and dyspnea are not limited to upper airway obstruction, but a clear description of exertional dyspnea in an older child may provide a useful functional assessment of severity.

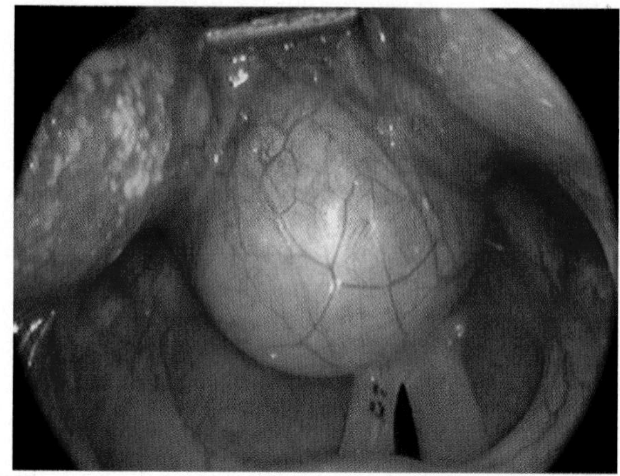

Figure 205-2. Endoscopic view of supraglottic larynx demonstrating a vallecular cyst.

The baby may feed slowly due to airway obstruction and "run out of breath" or "come up for air" during feeds. Bottle-fed babies may require thickened feeds or a "slow teat" (i.e., one with small holes). Uncomplicated slow feeding, although often a source of significant maternal anxiety, is not necessarily of concern in isolation. However, if there is failure to thrive and documented poor weight gain on the centile growth chart, further investigation and possible intervention should be considered. Laryngomalacia commonly gives rise to feeding difficulties but it is important to consider other causes. Choking episodes, documented aspiration, or recurrent chest infections may occur with vocal cord palsy, tracheoesophageal fistula, or rarely a laryngeal cleft (see Fig. 205-21). Gastroesophageal reflux is also common in infants with stridor and may exacerbate airway obstruction via edema.

The possibility of foreign body aspiration should always be raised with the parents although it is an unusual cause of isolated stridor. The clinician must however maintain a high index of suspicion to avoid missing this diagnosis, particularly if there is a history of a choking episode. The parent or caregiver may not necessarily witness events of foreign body aspiration and so the likelihood of this should be assessed. Caustic ingestion or thermal injury to the hypopharynx or supraglottis sustained by the infant drinking from microwave-heated bottles can also cause upper airway obstruction.

The clinician should determine whether the child has been systemically unwell, possibly with high temperatures. Acute episodes of airway infection will cause acute inflammation and obstruction. Viral laryngotracheitis (croup) classically has a barking cough with low-grade

Table 205-2

Features of History and Examination in the Stridulous Child

Symptoms	Signs
Stridor	Characteristics of stridor
Timing of onset	Quality, duration, timing
Progression	General appearance/syndromic features
Variability	
Exacerbating/relieving factors	Work of respiration:
Features of systemic infection	Respiratory rate, distress,
Apneas/cyanosis (dying spells)	fatigue, accessory muscle
Parental observation of recession	use, recession, nasal flaring, tracheal tug
Shortness of breath, respiratory rate	Positioning for optimal airway
	Drooling
Cough	Quality of cry
Feeding difficulties	Observation chart: temperature,
Aspiration/reflux	pulse rate
Cry/hoarseness	Nasal patency
Specific questioning regarding foreign body aspiration	Oropharynx—mandible, tongue, tonsils
Past history:	Neck—fullness/masses,
Perinatal	torticollis
Intubation history	Auscultation of upper airway
Recurrent/persisting croup or	and chest
bronchiolitis	Remainder of earn, nose,
Comorbidities (e.g.,	throat assessment (e.g.,
neurologic—Arnold-Chiari,	ears)
vascular malformation,	
cardiac disease/surgery,	
"birth marks"	

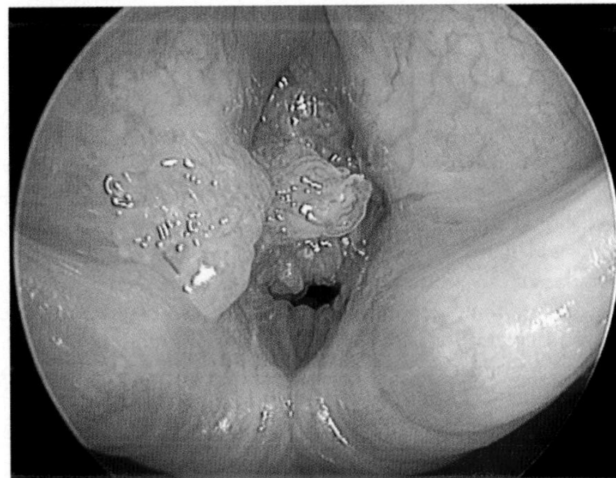

Figure 205-3. Laryngeal papillomata involving the vocal cords and extending onto the right false cord with significant airway obstruction and dysphonia.

fever and a preceding prodromal upper respiratory tract infection. Epiglottitis typically produces rapidly progressive upper airway obstruction in association with drooling, marked odynophagia, and a "muffled" voice. It is now very rare due to a dramatic reduction in incidence since implementation of Hib immunizations. Bacterial tracheitis has a variable onset with a toxic appearance, high fevers, cough, and stridor.

The obstetric and perinatal histories are often relevant, especially if the child was born prematurely and required ventilation. Parents should be specifically asked about neonatal intubation. This history must be taken carefully because the passage of nasogastric tubes for feeding or nasal/oral mucous suctioning may be mistaken for intubation. Previous intubation places the child at an increased risk of acquired subglottic stenosis (see Fig. 205-13). If the child was recently intubated or is being assessed due to failed extubation, it is worthwhile to obtain details, including size of the endotracheal tube used in comparison to the predicted age-appropriate tube, presence of a leak during intubation, use of steroids at the time of extubation, and any previous history of failed extubations.

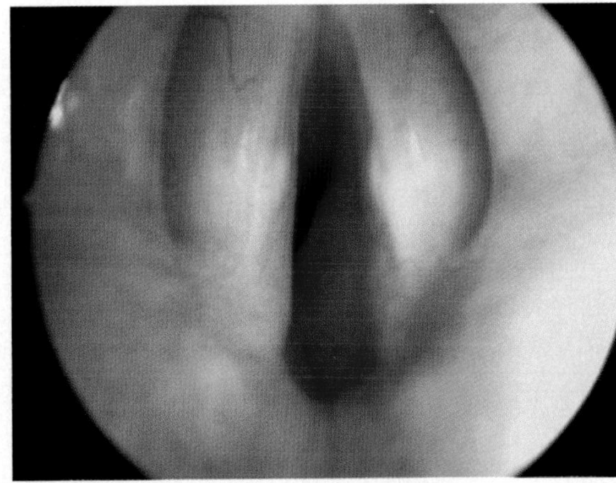

Figure 205-4. Endoscopic view of subglottic hemangioma presenting with increasing stridor.

Other comorbidities may predispose to airway obstruction, for example, vocal cord palsy in Arnold-Chiari malformation or birth injury, neurologic disease giving rise to hypotonia, or iatrogenic injury following cardiac surgery. A previously diagnosed syndrome may alert the clinician to potential pathology that is recognized as a component of the syndrome, for example, laryngeal webs in velocardiofacial syndrome. Vascular malformations, congenital cardiac disease, or vascular anomalies may give extrinsic compression of the airway and subsequent tracheomalacia. Parents should be asked about the presence of any "birthmarks," in that 50% of children with a subglottic hemangioma have a cutaneous lesion at the time of diagnosis (Fig. 205-4).[7] There is a markedly increased risk for children with cutaneous hemangiomas in a "beard" distribution, with 63% having significant airway involvement (Fig. 205-5).[8] The clinician should be particularly vigilant in assessing children with a history of recurrent episodes of laryngotracheitis or bronchiolitis that has been slow to settle. These children ought to be thoroughly assessed for an underlying source of airway obstruction that is being exacerbated by superimposed upper respiratory tract infection (Fig. 205-6).

Examination

An overall assessment of the degree of respiratory distress and airway compromise should be expedited in the acute situation and a full examination completed if the child's condition is stable (see Table 205-2). Observation of the child at rest in the parent's arms provides an initial assessment of the degree of respiratory distress, the characteristics of any stridor, and whether the child appears systemically unwell. It also allows time to gain the child's confidence before any further examination. A careful general examination is necessary to avoid missing subtle features of related syndromes or of other general pediatric disease. Syndromic features, if present, may suggest likely sources of airway obstruction associated with the particular syndrome, for example, micrognathia in Pierre Robin sequence, macroglossia in Beckwith-Wiedemann syndrome, or anterior glottic webs in velocardiofacial syndrome (Fig. 205-7).

Simple inspection of the child reveals valuable information regarding the work of breathing and degree of obstruction. Potential findings of increased respiratory work include suprasternal or sternal recession, subcostal indrawing, "see-saw" or paradoxical abdominal movement

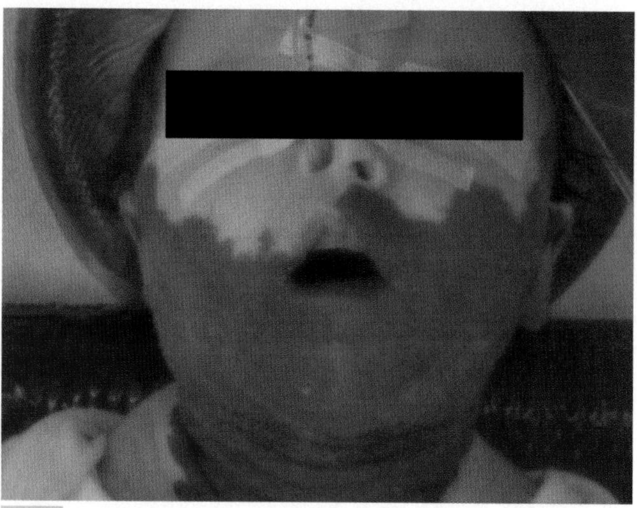

Figure 205-5. Extensive cutaneous cervicofacial hemangioma in a "beard" distribution in an infant with transglottic, tracheal, and mediastinal hemangioma.

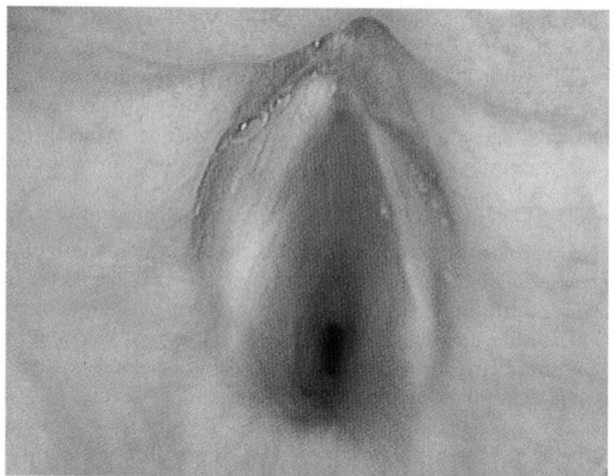

Figure 205-6. Severe congenital (grade III) subglottic stenosis presenting for rigid laryngobronchoscopy on a background of recurrent episodes of croup.

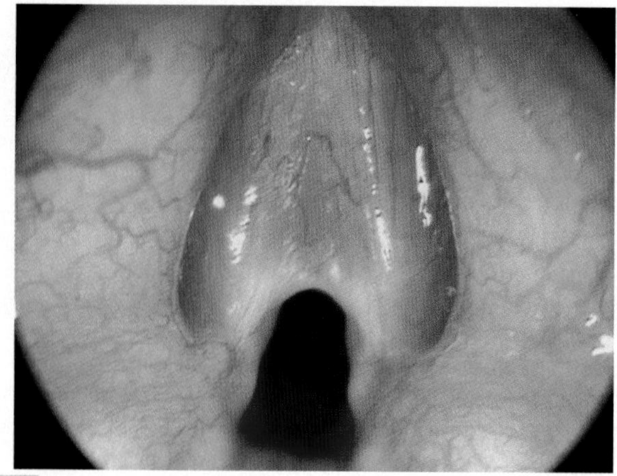

Figure 205-7. Anterior glottic web presenting with stridor in a child with velocardiofacial syndrome.

during respiration, nasal flaring, tracheal tug, anxiety, irritability, or evidence of fatigue. The amount of recession is a better indicator of the severity of airway compromise than the degree of stridor. Stridor can paradoxically become quieter and less apparent as the obstruction worsens due to the diminishing airflow and may be a sign of impending respiratory arrest. Pallor and subsequent cyanosis are late events in pediatric patients and no comfort should be taken from the fact that a child still appears pink. Children may position themselves to optimize their own airway as is classically described in epiglottitis, where children prefer to sit upright with their head in a "sniffing" position. Pectus excavatum may be seen in children with chronic airway obstruction due to negative intrathoracic pressure in their highly compliant rib cage.[2]

The observation chart should be checked for elevated temperatures, tachycardia, or tachypnea. Drooling may occur in epiglottitis, severe oropharyngeal inflammation, or deep neck space infection. Any cough or change in voice or cry should be noted. The clinician should listen carefully to the audible respiratory noise to differentiate between inspiratory stridor, biphasic stridor, expiratory stridor or wheeze, and stertor. This can be useful in determining the likely anatomic site of the pathology, although this is not absolute and is only useful as a guide.

Inspiratory stridor typically occurs due to obstruction at the level of the supraglottis or glottis. Obstruction arising in the bronchi or lower trachea classically produces an expiratory stridor or prolongation of the expiratory phase. Biphasic stridor can occur with obstruction anywhere in the laryngotracheobronchial tree but is classically associated with either upper tracheal or subglottic pathology where it is attributed to the fixed luminal diameter of the cricoid. The characteristic sound of stridor, even in a common condition such as laryngomalacia,[9] is so variable as to be of little diagnostic use in isolation. Laryngomalacia has been traditionally described as having stridor that is of a musical quality, while stridor in vocal cord palsy has a breathy quality, viral laryngotracheitis has a barking cough and tracheomalacia has a brassy cough. It is important to recognize that these descriptions are highly subjective and their assessment is not reliably reproducible.

Nasal patency is assessed via fogging of a mirror or metal tongue depressor. Nasal airflow may also be detected via a wisp of cotton wool or using the bell end of a stethoscope. This is particularly relevant if supralaryngeal obstruction is suspected. The clinician should also make a conscious assessment of jaw and tongue size. Stridor and recession vary as the child rests, cries, and sleeps. It can be useful to observe the child while the child feeds, particularly if poor feeding or aspiration has been reported. Auscultation may be used to aid in localizing the site of maximal obstruction but the transmission of sound through the thorax is variable, often making this technique difficult. Auscultation is useful to detect heart murmurs and wheeze.

The nose, throat, neck, and ears should also be examined. The oropharynx is examined to assess the size and appearance of tonsils and palate, and to check for oropharyngeal swelling or fullness. The neck is also inspected and palpated to identify swelling or masses. The usual caution should be used in examining a child with possible epiglottitis wherein sudden airway obstruction may be precipitated. In this situation, equipment for immediate intubation must be present if examination is to be attempted. It is also acceptable to make a provisional diagnosis of epiglottitis based on history and appearance of the child, with formal examination performed in the safety of the operating room under endoscopic control.

Nonendoscopic Investigations

Investigations should not be routinely conducted but judicious use may be helpful. Selection of investigations should be tailored to the clinical presentation on the basis of the history and examination findings and are not necessary in every patient.

O_2 Saturation Monitoring

O_2 saturation monitoring is noninvasive and readily accessible, although considerable airway obstruction may occur without desaturation, as long as the child is not tiring and continues to have the energy to overcome the obstruction. Care should be taken in administering supplemental oxygen because this can maintain O_2 saturations while masking raised levels of CO_2. Arterial blood gases are useful in this situation. From a clinical viewpoint, cyanosis occurs very late in pediatric respiratory distress.

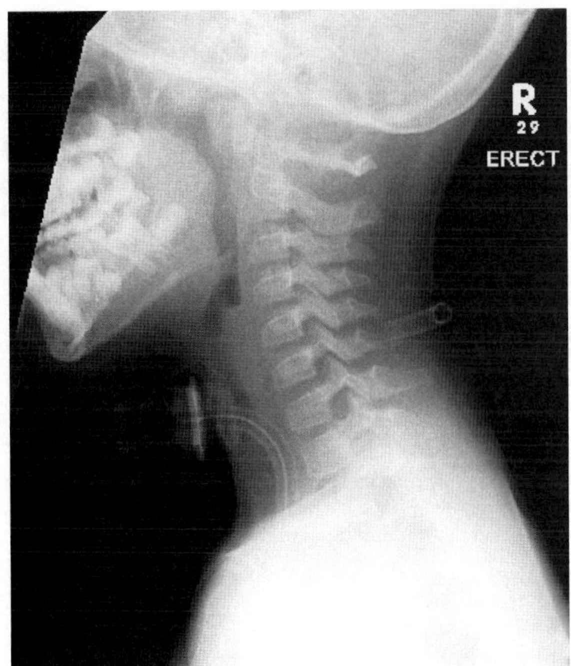

Figure 205-8. Lateral neck x-ray study with enhancement of the tracheal air column demonstrating a stenotic segment with obliteration of the airway for 7 mm craniocaudally from the glottic level.

Radiology

Soft tissue lateral neck x-ray examination demonstrates the airway outline from the nasopharynx to the subglottis. Posterior-anterior chest x-ray study shows the lung fields and mediastinum. Persistent air trapping may be demonstrated on the side of a bronchial foreign body in inspiratory/expiratory views. A decubitus view may be useful in young children, where normally the dependent lung deflates.[10] A Cincinnati (high-kilovoltage filter) view enhances the tracheal air column while de-emphasizing bony cervical spine to demonstrate the major airways. These x-ray techniques may be useful as screening investigations (Fig. 205-8).[11,12] Careful consideration of the stability of the child's airway is mandatory and radiology should not be undertaken if there is any potential for acute airway deterioration. Policy for suspected epiglottitis differs between centers; however, the result of the x-ray study may not influence management[13] and may be associated with significant risk to the child. Further imaging should be performed according to the endoscopy findings.

Videofluoroscopy is an excellent way of demonstrating tracheomalacia and can be combined with a contrast swallow to exclude vascular compression,[14,15] tracheoesophageal fistula, or aspiration. It may demonstrate diaphragmatic immobility on the side of a foreign body airway obstruction. Bronchograms using safe nonionic contrast media are useful for outlining the luminal surface of the lower airway, demonstrating tracheobronchial stenosis and malacia. Opening pressures of the collapsed bronchi and lower trachea can also be measured to determine the level of airway support needed. Computed tomography (CT) and magnetic resonance imaging (MRI)[12,16,17] continue to lack sensitivity in assessing airway stenoses and cannot replace endoscopic assessment. They are useful in demonstrating vascular anomalies and extrinsic compression of the airway (Fig. 205-9). Virtual endoscopy uses radiologic data to create computer simulations that may be viewed as one would conventional endoscopy. Helical CT with multiplanar reconstruction provides three-dimensional images, which are used in real time to simulate endoscopy views. It is noninvasive and allows retrograde luminal airway views. Although it demonstrates some fixed airway stenoses, it is not helpful in detecting obstruction during dynamic movement as occurs in tracheomalacia or vocal cord palsy. There is also a lack of detail, with airway pathology such as glottic webs being poorly demonstrated.[18]

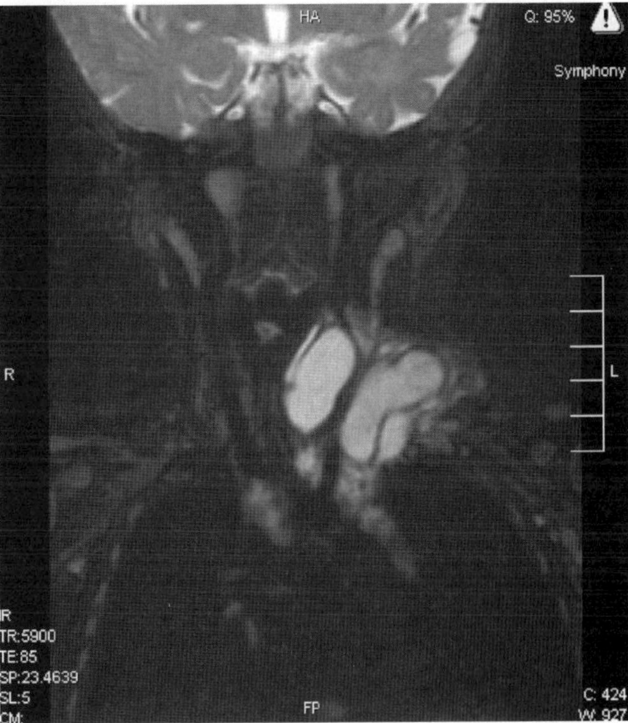

Figure 205-9. Magnetic resonance imaging study of head and neck demonstrating cystic hygroma in the left cervical region with airway compression, tracheal displacement to the right, and mediastinal extension.

Other Investigations

Vocal cord ultrasound can be used, with experience, to demonstrate vocal cord palsy to complement the endoscopic findings.[19] The role of *laryngeal EMG* in the management of vocal cord immobility is yet to be fully defined.[20] Airway obstruction that worsens during sleep is usually a feature of pharyngeal obstruction, such as adenotonsillar obstruction or craniofacial anomaly. Laryngotracheal pathology at any level including laryngomalacia may, however, occasionally worsen during sleep, thus requiring *sleep study* investigation.[21] *Pediatric lung function tests* are seldom used because of compliance and cooperation issues. Flow volume loops[22] may help localize the site of obstruction and other tests such as peak flows or ventilation-perfusion scans may be used upon the advice of a pulmonologist. Gastroesophageal reflux[23-26] is not discussed in detail in this chapter but can be investigated via double probe pH studies, contrast studies, milk scan, or esophagoscopy with lower esophageal biopsy. Echocardiography detects congenital heart disease but does not demonstrate all abnormal vasculature, thus it cannot be used to exclude vascular anomalies.

Endoscopy

Pediatric airway endoscopy requires a full range of specialized pediatric endoscopy equipment and an experienced team. An inadequate evaluation needs to be repeated, and referral to an experienced center should be made as required to ensure a single comprehensive and definitive evaluation. A systematic approach provides a diagnosis in most cases.[27]

Flexible Endoscopy in the Office or Ward

The introduction of ultrathin endoscopes[28] in a range of diameters with good optics has allowed even neonates to undergo endoscopy without the need for a general anesthetic. This is usually considered a screening procedure, in that the view of the larynx may be suboptimal. Rigid endoscopy of the airway is superior in examining the airway for structural abnormalities. Flexible endoscopy is useful in assessing the dynamic airway for vocal cord movement or features of laryngomalacia. A systematic approach must be adopted, observing first the nasal cavity followed by the postnasal space, oropharynx, supraglottis, and glottis during dynamic respiration and phonation. It is difficult to obtain good views of the subglottis. This is purely a diagnostic procedure, with no opportunity for therapeutic procedures, in contrast to a rigid laryngotracheobronchoscopy. Flexible endoscopy under sedation in an endoscopy suite is widely practiced by pediatricians and pulmonologists[29-31] and is used by otolaryngologists as an adjunct to rigid endoscopy.[32] Rigid endoscopy is helpful if the diagnosis remains unclear despite flexible endoscopy, if there is clinical suspicion of a second airway lesion, or if subglottic/tracheal or bronchial pathology is suspected.

Laryngotracheobronchoscopy

Laryngotracheobronchoscopy[33] is the gold standard in the evaluation of the stridulous child. It enables a thorough assessment to be performed while the airway is maintained and allows findings to be visually recorded for future reference. The airway may be formally sized to grade any narrowing. It also may incorporate therapeutic procedures, including foreign body removal or the endoscopic management of airway pathology. It requires an experienced team skilled in airway assessment, including the surgeon, anesthetist, and nursing assistant, who work closely to ensure an optimal and safe examination. The use of a video is essential to facilitate training and allows the anesthetist and nurse to follow the procedure and status of the airway on the monitor.

It is vital that accurate records are kept in a standardized form within a department.[34] Digital prints provide a valid record of static conditions while video clips record dynamic findings. Digital images and video recordings should be saved and archived. This provides an invaluable source of information for sequential clinical comparisons, teaching, and medicolegal purposes.

Anesthetic Considerations

This procedure requires a cooperative approach to airway management with both the anesthetic team and surgeon sharing the control of the airway. The use of atropine premedication provides a dry surgical field and improves the efficacy of topical anesthesia. It is most effective via intramuscular injection. Anesthesia is often induced using slow masked inhalational anaesthesia. Halothane is a volatile agent that has been traditionally used and is nonirritating to the airway, allowing for smooth maintenance of anesthesia during instrumentation of the airway. Halothane is now difficult to obtain and other inhalational agents such as isoflurane, sevoflurane, and intravenous agents are being used. Sevoflurane[35] is also nonirritating, rapid in onset, and allows rapid delivery of high concentrations. Topical lidocaine is applied to the airway to minimize airway stimulation during the procedure and helps avoid laryngospasm. Lidocaine dose needs to be carefully measured to avoid overdosage.[36,37]

Anesthetic practice varies between centers but most units use spontaneous respiration for pediatric patients rather than paralysis and jet ventilation simulating normal respiration. Jet ventilation prevents coughing or gagging[38-40] but requires pressures above physiologic levels[38,41] with an associated risk of pneumothorax in neonates and smaller children. Dynamic conditions such as malacia and cord palsy cannot be identified. Apneic endoscopy is also possible after initial hyperventilation with 100% oxygen, although progressive hypoxemia and hypercarbia limit the operating time and condition of the patient.[42]

After induction, the child is ventilated down to a level of anesthesia that allows the rigid endoscope to be passed without gagging but maintains spontaneous respiration. The child may be intubated before the endoscopy or alternatively the airway may be controlled via a mask. Ideally the endoscopist has a view of an airway that is not altered by the passage of an endotracheal tube and, if the child is intubated, the tube is withdrawn during the procedure. A transnasal endotracheal tube may be positioned with the tip in the hypopharynx to optimize delivery of anesthetic gases and oxygen without obstructing the view of the airway. Airway control can be regained at any stage via intubation or through the use of a bronchoscope.

A laryngeal mask[43] may be useful for fiberoptic bronchoscopy particularly if the patient is difficult to intubate due to mandibular hypoplasia.

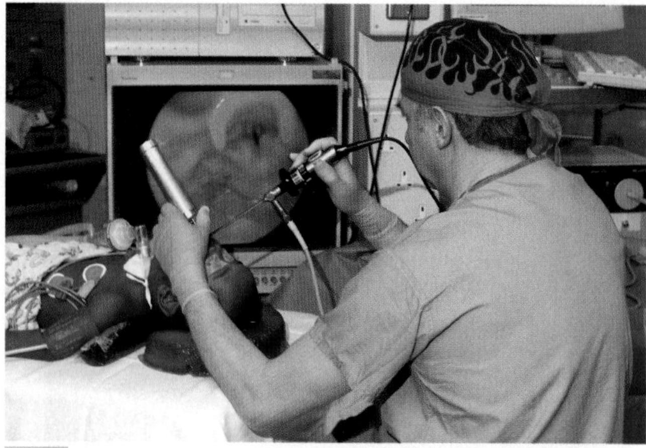

Figure 205-10. Rigid laryngobronchoscopy using a zero degree telescope demonstrating optimal positioning of the child and operating room set-up to allow accurate airway assessment.

Operative Technique

A suspension laryngoscope and microscope are traditionally used to examine the larynx, with a ventilating bronchoscope to examine the tracheobronchial tree (Fig. 205-10). Rigid telescopes provide excellent images and many centers now perform the assessment using a telescope, with digital images recorded at each anatomic level. High-quality images may be captured via the use of a wide Storz photographic telescope. A 4-mm rigid telescope should provide adequate images for data records, provided there is careful focusing and appropriate camera settings to ensure optimal captured images. For routine examination, the telescope and camera can be held in the left hand with a probe used in the right while the laryngoscope is in suspension. The microscope is used if there is to be manipulation of the airway requiring both hands of the operating surgeon. Differing techniques are adopted, according to individual departmental preferences. The procedure may be combined with rigid esophagoscopy, according to departmental protocols.

Preparation and Positioning

It is essential to anticipate equipment requirements so all equipment can be checked and prepared before commencement. A range of Hopkins rod telescopes should be available, which includes all lengths and diameters that may be required, so the endoscopist is fully prepared for all eventualities. Charts that predict age-appropriate sizes of bronchoscopes should be consulted and be readily available in the operating room.[44] The appropriate bronchoscope needs to be checked and assembled and at least one size smaller must be on hand. A 30-degree telescope may be used to enable assessment of the supraglottis without splinting. It may also assist assessment of an anteriorly placed larynx. A microscope should be available with the 400-mm lens to be used with standard laryngeal instruments. A 350-mm lens may be useful in small neonates by "bringing the patient closer" to allow easier manipulation of larynx.

A small sandbag is placed under the shoulders, with supporting lateral sandbags placed for children with long thin heads, as is typically seen in ex-premature neonates. A Mayo table supports the laryngostat clear of the chest.

Microlaryngoscopy Technique

A suspension straight-blade laryngoscope is gently inserted while assessing the overall appearance of the laryngopharynx, taking care to protect the teeth, lips, and oral mucosa while keeping the tongue midline to provide a well-centered view. The laryngoscope is placed in the vallecula and the epiglottis is carefully lifted forward. An overall assessment of the larynx can be made while an endotracheal tube is in situ and while providing a degree of stability, particularly in a compromised pediatric airway. Removal of the endotracheal tube allows a superior view and a probe may be used to independently palpate the arytenoids

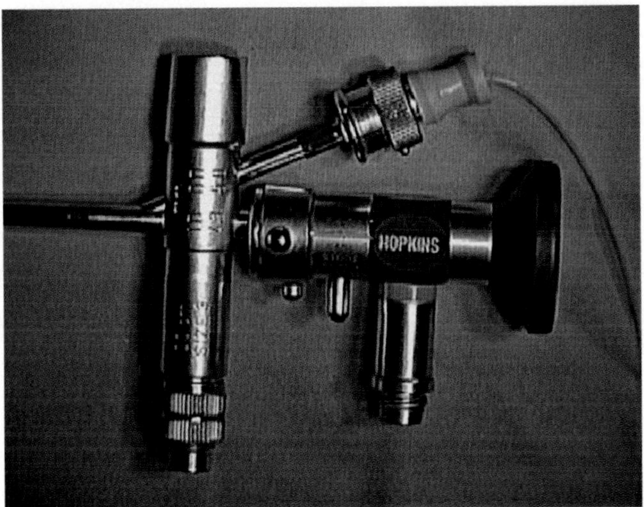

Figure 205-11. Ventilating bronchoscope.

to assess the mobility of the cricoarytenoid joints and any limitation in joint movement. Absence of independent arytenoid movement on palpation is indicative of interarytenoid scarring. A posterior laryngeal cleft should be excluded by passing the probe between the arytenoids to allow comparison of the inferior limit of the interarytenoid groove with the posterior commissure. The subglottis should also be inspected from above. Topical decongestion and vasoconstriction of the airway may be helpful, particularly in the presence of low-grade inflammation or edema. Any airway narrowing should be formally sized. The largest endotracheal tube that permits a leak at less than 30 cm H_2O of pressure provides a measure of the airway diameter. Subglottic stenosis may then be graded using the Cotton-Myer grading system,[45] thus allowing reproducible assessment of the stenosis and aiding in treatment selection. If there is airway compromise or instability, assessment time may be limited. It is thus essential to be prepared to move ahead with bronchoscopy at any stage.

Bronchoscopy Technique

Traditionally, a ventilating bronchoscope (Fig. 205-11) has been used to assess the distal airway, which provides a means of actively ventilating the patient during the procedure, if required. An age-appropriate sized bronchoscope is used unless stenosis is suspected. A smaller-diameter rigid Hopkins rod telescope can be used as an alternative to examine the airway in a spontaneously breathing child, particularly if there is significant subglottic stenosis. The rigid telescope may reduce local airway trauma and lessen airway splinting, while allowing the distal airway to be visualized.

An anesthetic laryngoscope is placed in the vallecula while passing the bevel of the bronchoscope through the vocal cords under vision or via the monitor. The subglottis, trachea, carina, and main bronchi are systematically examined and findings recorded via digital images and/or videos. Evidence of tracheomalacia should be sought in the absence of positive airway pressure to avoid splinting of the airway and using a small bronchoscope withdrawn from the area being assessed. The ratio of cartilage to trachealis is significant in recording the type of malacia. The presence of complete tracheal rings is of importance when considering slide tracheoplasty for the treatment of long segment tracheal stenosis.[46] Extrinsic compression and prominent transmitted pulsation may be evident where there is an underlying vascular anomaly, which can be confirmed with imaging.

Dynamic Airway Assessment

A dynamic assessment of the larynx may be performed as the child lightens and is observed while the child recovers from the anesthesia. Dynamic views can be achieved by withdrawing the bronchoscope so that it is positioned just posterior to the tip of the epiglottis. This allows a good view of the vocal cords to exclude vocal cord immobility. It is useful if the anesthetist calls the phase of respiration, thus allowing the endoscopist to check for paradoxical cord movement. The arytenoids and adjacent mucosa can also be visualized to check for evidence of laryngomalacia. Anterior collapse of the epiglottis may be masked, however. A 30- or 70-degree telescope may offer improved views for dynamic assessment.

An excellent technique for dynamic assessment of vocal cord movement utilizes a laryngeal mask with a fiberoptic bronchoscope passed through to visualize the airway. The flexible endoscope is positioned just proximal to the laryngeal inlet to observe airway dynamics.[47]

Complications

Complications are unusual in rigid laryngobronchoscopy with a reported overall complication rate of 1.9%.[48] Possible complications include oral injury, subglottic injury, pneumothorax, cardiac complications, loss of control of the airway, and bleeding. Blood in the airway impairs oxygenation and ventilation, rather than giving rise to difficulties due to volume of blood loss.[42] Risks associated with procedural complication include cardiac anomalies, airway foreign body, tracheal stenosis, and biopsy or abscess drainage,[48] and particular care should be taken in these cases.

Postoperative Care and Planning

Airway obstruction may increase following the procedure due to underlying pathology, edema, blood, secretions, or postintubation croup. Edema is usually maximal within 4 hours and settles by 24 hours. Humidified oxygen by mask is initially tried. Nebulized epinephrine (1:1000) may be tried but the child must be kept under observation and reviewed within an hour for recurrence due to its limited duration of action.[42] The patient may be given intraoperative dexamethasone if there is a potential for edema from instrumentation of the airway. Steroids may be continued in the postoperative period depending on the endoscopy findings and underlying airway pathology. The patient must be recovered by nursing staff experienced in the care of pediatric airways and remain as an inpatient for close observation until the airway is adequately stable for discharge.

The operative record should clearly record the endoscopy findings, ideally with a photographic record of the findings. Using the endoscopic assessment, a plan of management can then be decided upon and discussed with the parents postoperatively.

Treatment of Acute Airway Obstruction

Medical Treatment

The child who arrives in the emergency department with acute airway obstruction should undergo rapid evaluation. Assessment, history, and active resuscitation should proceed while measures are taken to stabilize the airway. The physician should determine the degree of airway obstruction by observing the child for recession and work of respiration while taking a brief history from the accompanying adult. Details will be obtained regarding the length of history, recent systemic illness, and possibility of foreign body inhalation. The nursing staff should check the oxygen saturation and set up humidified oxygen. Another team member should contact the operating room and anesthesiologist to advise that the child may require intubation. The otolaryngologist may also be contacted and asked to attend the intubation,[49] depending on the unit's protocol. This situation clearly benefits from careful planning, with most units having a protocol for how to deal with the stridulous child.

Supplemental oxygen reduces the ventilatory requirement to maintain adequate oxygen saturation in cases of airway obstruction with normal alveolar function. The potential for CO_2 retention should be kept in mind. Heliox (helium-oxygen gas mixture) may be used to relieve respiratory distress, decrease the work of breathing, and improve gas exchange.[50] It does this due to its low density, which results in a lower resistance to gas flow.[51,52] It has no direct effect on the underlying pathology and thus must be viewed only as a "therapeutic bridge," allowing time for definitive treatment to be commenced.[50] Steroids and nebulized epinephrine may also be used to help optimize the airway in the acute situation.

Laryngotracheitis (viral croup) can be treated with intravenous, oral, or nebulized steroids. There is no objective evidence that raising the humidity of the inspired air is beneficial.[53] Nebulized budesonide[54] is used in the home environment for children with recurrent croup. Corticosteroids are beneficial and are routinely recommended for the treatment of croup.[55] Klassen[56] recommends that children with croup symptoms and increased work of breathing should be treated with either nebulized budesonide (2 mg) or oral/intramuscular dexamethasone (0.15 to 0.6 mg/kg). Oral dexamethasone is easily administered, widely available, and low in cost. L-epinephrine (5 mL of 1 : 1000) or racemic epinephrine (0.5 mL) should be considered if there is moderate or severe distress because it has been found to give clinical improvement and reduce the need for intubation.[57]

Other infective causes of airway obstruction respond promptly to antibiotic therapy. This includes bacterial tracheitis or epiglottitis, which is rare, although vaccine failure[58,59] has been documented. Appropriate intravenous antibiotic therapy should be commenced while the airway is stabilized via short-term intubation if required.

Therapeutic Intubation

Intubation is increasingly used as an alternative to tracheotomy in acute airway obstruction. Pediatric tracheotomy is avoided if possible due to the potential for morbidity, even with short-term usage. Intubation may not be possible, for example, in severe subglottic stenosis, impacted foreign bodies, or advanced epiglottitis. As this situation may be unexpectedly encountered even by skilled, experienced pediatric anesthesiologists, most hospitals require an otolaryngologist to be informed if a child with airway obstruction is to be intubated. It may be necessary to have an emergency tracheotomy set open with the correct size tube already selected.

The child is "gassed down" slowly and the larynx is inspected to exclude epiglottitis. The child may then be manageable on a nasal pharyngeal airway with continuous positive airway pressure (CPAP). If intubation is required, it is important to minimize any damage to the inflamed subglottic mucosa. This is achieved by gentle intubation with a small, soft tube that is adequate for ventilation and suction of secretions. A nasotracheal tube is preferable to an oral intubation to help minimize tube movement. The secure nasotracheal tube ought to be placed and assessed by suctioning the secretions and testing for a leak. Any persisting element of airway obstruction or tenacious secretions should be further investigated by passing a ventilating bronchoscope. This helps exclude bacterial tracheitis[60,61] or a foreign body. Endoscopic suctioning and clearance of debris from the airway may be performed and is particularly beneficial in bacterial tracheitis. Significant tracheobronchomalacia may also give persisting obstruction after intubation and will usually respond to CPAP.

Emergency Tracheotomy

Emergency tracheotomy is a rare occurrence in departments with experienced pediatric anesthesiologists.[49,62] Otolaryngologists are often asked to attend a potentially difficult intubation but are rarely needed. If emergent tracheotomy is required, however, the surgical set and appropriate tube must be immediately available. The neonate needs to be in a straight supine position with the neck extended over a roll. A long, vertical, strictly midline incision is made through skin and down to the trachea, guided by palpation of the trachea. The main danger lies in drifting off the midline and a finger on either side of the larynx is helpful. If a pediatric tracheotomy tube is not available, a pediatric endotracheal tube can be used, ensuring it remains above the carina.

Endoscopic Removal of Foreign Bodies

Foreign body removal has been greatly facilitated by the introduction of foreign body optical extraction forceps that have a central channel for an extra-long Hopkins rod telescope. Different forceps are available for the removal of various types of foreign bodies. The foreign body and adjacent airway can be carefully examined while the removal is planned using a fine suction catheter in the bronchoscope alongside the rigid telescope. The use of topical adrenaline before any attempt at removal optimizes local conditions by vasoconstricting the mucosa and reducing bleeding.[63]

Table 205-3

Management Options for the Difficult to Extubate Neonate

Treat reflux
Leave tube in place for at least 1 week between trials of extubation
Steroids to cover extubation
Nasal prong ± CPAP postextubation to support airway
Endoscopic optimization of airway—removal of small granulations, cysts
Cricoid split
Single-stage laryngeal reconstruction
Tracheotomy ± stent to maintain airway

Approach to Postextubation Stridor

Extubation should not be attempted until the child has an optimal chance of success. Failed extubation requiring subsequent reintubation predisposes to further deterioration of the airway with additional edema, ulceration, and perichondritis. There should be no active respiratory infection, minimal pressure support, and a normal oxygen requirement at the time of extubation. Reflux should be adequately treated and steroids commenced if indicated. Extubation should proceed once sedation has worn off and the child is awake to maximize the likelihood of success. If postextubation stridor and obstruction occur, the airway can be further optimized with nebulized epinephrine,[64] intravenous dexamethasone[65] before and after extubation, and continuous positive airway pressure via nasal cannula. Therapeutic reintubation for laryngeal rest has been demonstrated to be beneficial,[66-68] allowing any reversible component of the airway inflammation to settle.

If extubation fails, despite appropriate medical measures and laryngeal rest, endoscopic procedures are being increasingly used to optimize the airway (Table 205-3). Alternatively, a cricoid split may be performed. Single-stage laryngotracheal reconstruction can be used in patients who fail cricoid split or who have a mature stenosis. Tracheotomy is reserved for those who are not suitable for an alternative approach. These surgical options are discussed later.

Expected Airway Obstruction in the Postpartum Neonate

Antenatal diagnosis of airway obstruction enables a definitive plan of management to be formulated before delivery. Routine prenatal ultrasonography may diagnose large masses, including cervical teratoma,[69,70] cystic hygroma,[71] or rhabdomyosarcoma[72] with associated airway obstruction. Further details of the anatomy can then be defined using MRI.[73,74] Airway obstruction may be detected on ultrasound, even in the absence of a mass. Antenatally diagnosed congenital high airway obstruction syndrome (CHAOS) exhibits features including tracheal dilation and lung hypertrophy, as seen in laryngeal atresia.[75] Polyhydramnios may also occur if an obstructing lesion is compressing the esophagus and impairing fetal swallowing.[76] Other ultrasound features may include diaphragmatic eversion, ascites, and ultimately fetal hydrops.[77] Holinger and others first described the successful airway management of an antenatally diagnosed cervical teratoma in 1985.[70] The technique of securing the neonatal airway while the uteroplacental blood flow was maintained was subsequently described in the early 1990s.[73,78] This procedure has become known as the ex utero intrapartum treatment (EXIT)[79,80] or OOPS (operation on placental support)[71] and should be considered when perinatal airway obstruction is anticipated. The multidisciplinary team usually includes pediatricians, obstetricians, anesthetists, and ENT surgeons. Other specialties may be involved, depending on the underlying pathology. At planned cesarean section, adequate uteroplacental flow is maintained while the airway is established. The placenta allows continued gas exchange while the airway is stabilized. Direct laryngoscopy and intubation is then

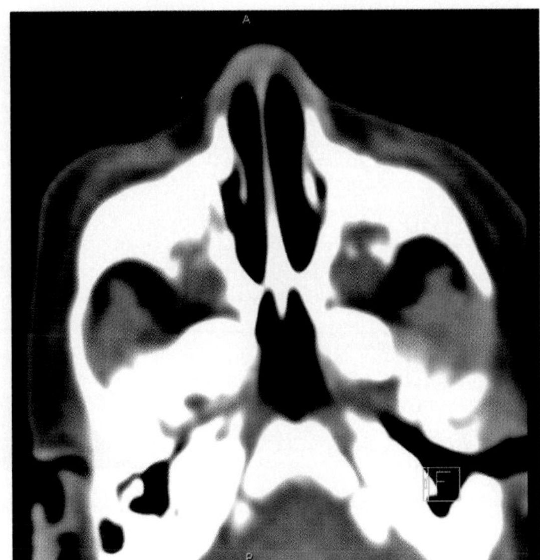

Figure 205-12. Computed tomography scan (axial view) demonstrating bilateral choanal atresia.

performed. Rigid laryngobronchoscopy may be used to define the anatomy and possibly place a guidewire for intubation guidance if there is marked distortion or poor visualization of the airway. If intubation is not possible, the trachea is exposed and a tracheotomy performed. The surgeon should be mindful that a large neck mass will hyperextend the neck and anteriorly displace the trachea. This may mean that the tracheotomy is placed more distally than planned. Once the airway is secured the umbilical cord is clamped and the delivery is completed.[76] Extracorporeal membranous oxygenation can be used particularly in the presence of severe congenital cardiac disease.[81] Resection of an obstructing mass is usually delayed until the child's condition is stabilized.[81]

Unexpected Airway Obstruction in the Postpartum Neonate

Airway obstruction may not always be antenatally diagnosed. The delivery team may be presented with a neonate with unexpected airway obstruction. An anatomic approach to the differential diagnoses and management of these infants is helpful.

Supralaryngeal

Nasal or nasopharyngeal obstruction can be highly significant in the newborn who is an obligate nasal breather. Nasal suction removes secretions and allows assessment of the patency of the nasal airway. Choanal atresia is the most common diagnosis in complete nasal obstruction and can be investigated via CT scan (Fig. 205-12). It may be difficult to pass a nasal suction catheter in a neonate with prominent turbinates or, less commonly, piriform aperture stenosis, midnasal stenosis, or choanal stenosis. Nasopharyngeal masses such as teratomas may also obstruct the airway. Nasal or nasopharyngeal airway obstruction is relieved by an oral airway. Oropharyngeal sources of obstruction (such as micrognathia with a retroposed tongue) may also be improved by positioning and oral airway placement.

Laryngeal

Laryngeal obstruction shows no improvement with an oral airway but is relieved by intubation. Airway obstruction associated with severe laryngomalacia, vocal cord palsy, laryngeal cysts, or polyps will improve with intubation. A small-shouldered tube may be temporarily positioned through a laryngeal stenosis to secure the airway. Some units now advocate using a laryngeal mask for neonatal resuscitation[82] to avoid exacerbation of the stenosis by attempts at intubation. It may be possible to ventilate a neonate with laryngeal atresia and a low tracheoesophageal fistula although this is rare. In these cases, there will be none of the characteristic findings of congenital upper airway obstruction on antenatal ultrasound. On closer examination in this instance, the tube is found in the esophagus with ventilation occurring via the fistula.[83]

If intubation is not possible and there is inadequate ventilation via a laryngeal mask or very fine endotracheal tube, the trachea must be opened to ventilate the neonate. In the emergency situation, needle puncture of the cricothyroid membrane or trachea is possible but not easy, while emergency open tracheotomy is also difficult unless the surgeon has current experience of neonatal tracheotomy. It may be difficult to palpate the laryngeal cartilage in a neonate. It is of greater importance to remain in the midline when locating the airway, rather than focusing on the level of entry. The principles of emergency tracheotomy are discussed earlier. In tracheal puncture, the first and second fingers of the left hand are placed either side of the trachea and the needle inserted vertically, strictly in the midline until air can be aspirated. Larger needles can be inserted above or below the first if necessary. A tracheotomy will bypass laryngeal lesions such as congenital webs or subglottic stenosis.

Tracheobronchial

Obstruction due to distal tracheal or bronchial pathology, including tracheobronchomalacia, may not improve with either intubation or tracheotomy. Positive pressure will aid in splinting the airway and improve malacia. It is less helpful for distal airway stenosis. Use of an extended (long) tracheotomy tube will physically support tracheomalacia but will not assist in carinal malacia or bronchomalacia. A tapering long-segment tracheal stenosis presents a difficult clinical situation, because it is often possible to insert only a very small tracheotomy tube. In addition the tracheotomy severely limits the therapeutic options for surgical reconstruction of the stenosis. The patient with a long-segment tracheal stenosis requires referral for consideration of slide tracheoplasty, which is recognized as the best treatment for this condition in the current era.[46]

Treatment of Chronic Airway Obstruction

The evaluation of a child with chronic airway obstruction is not dissimilar to the acute situation; however, one has the luxury of time to perform a thorough clinical assessment and systematic investigations as required. The management options are more complex as the emphasis shifts from acute resuscitation and relieving the obstruction to addressing the underlying condition and preventing complications. The choice of treatment is influenced by the severity of the symptoms and signs, coexisting morbidity, the patient's social situation, surgeon's preference, availability of equipment, and other pediatric services, particularly intensive care.

Conservative options include watchful waiting and the use of medical treatments to address general and specific conditions. Tracheotomy may be chosen to "buy time" until the child grows and the condition resolves, or in some situations it may be definitive. Other surgical treatments include a vast spectrum of endoscopic techniques available to open laryngeal framework surgery.

Medical Management

There are several conditions presenting with chronic airway compromise that may be managed expectantly with regular clinical review and supportive therapy only (e.g., mild to moderate laryngomalacia, unilateral vocal cord palsy, grade I subglottic stenosis). The input of allied health departments such as speech and language therapy and dietetics is beneficial with regard to concurrent feeding, swallowing, and aspiration issues. Respiratory review to manage underlying lung disease and the consideration of CPAP may be appropriate in some situations. The use of a nasopharyngeal airway to bypass supralaryngeal airway obstruction is highly effective and relatively noninvasive.[84] It may be used to avoid surgery in certain cases of midface hypoplasia, neuromuscular disorders, glossoptosis, and micrognathia/retrognathia. It is also a valuable postoperative adjunct following adenotonsillectomy in the child with severe obstructive sleep apnea.

Gastroesophageal reflux is thought to aggravate airway conditions and possibly contribute to apnea, recurrent upper respiratory tract infections, laryngomalacia, and subglottic stenosis, although consistent

Table 205-4

Indications for Pediatric Tracheotomy

- Upper airway obstruction
  - Anatomic, e.g., craniofacial abnormality, laryngeal pathology
  - Functional, e.g., vocal cord palsy
- Prolonged ventilatory support
- Neurologic dysfunction
- Facilitation of major head and neck surgery
- Management of secretions

evidence to support the hypothesis is limited.[85,86] Adjuvant antireflux treatment is generally well tolerated and effective in the pediatric population. Its use, although empirical at times, may improve airway symptoms, circumvent the need for surgery, and enhance surgical outcomes.

Systemic steroids are often used intermittently to treat acute deterioration in the setting of chronic airway obstruction. Long-term doses require careful monitoring for side effects but have been successfully used as an adjuvant treatment for conditions such as subglottic hemangioma in many series.[87-89] Airway edema from croup responds well to steroids and some children with this condition benefit from having dexamethasone available for recurrent attacks at home.[57]

Antibiotics are useful to treat acute infective exacerbations in the setting of chronic airway obstruction. The prophylactic use of antibiotics is also recommended in the setting of open laryngeal surgery to reduce the chance of postoperative wound infection from direct exposure to the respiratory tract.

Tracheotomy

The indications for insertion of a pediatric tracheotomy have changed over the past decades.[90] Tracheotomy is more commonly requested to bypass chronic airway obstruction from craniofacial or upper airway abnormalities, or to support prolonged ventilation than for acute infective conditions such as laryngotracheobronchitis and epiglottitis (Table 205-4). Tracheotomy may be a temporary treatment while waiting for the child to outgrow the underlying condition (e.g., subglottic hemangioma or severe laryngomalacia), or until the child is old enough to undergo other definitive procedures. Its insertion may be permanent but is generally not undertaken without consideration of care requirements and the potential morbidity associated with it. The overall complication rate is up to 44% and tracheotomy-related death as high as 3.6% in some series.[91,92]

Techniques to avoid tracheotomy include the use of maximal medical treatments to reduce edema and inflammation while surgical alternatives are directed toward addressing the site of obstruction and minimizing resistance to airflow. For example, in developing subglottic stenosis, the options of laryngeal rest,[67] cricoid split,[93-95] endoscopic balloon dilatation with mitomycin C,[96] and single-stage laryngotracheal reconstruction[97,98] may avoid the need for tracheotomy. A case of early subglottic stenosis and its response to balloon dilatation is shown in Figs. 205-13 and 205-14.

Once the decision has been made to proceed with a pediatric tracheotomy, a comprehensive discussion should take place with the primary care clinicians before surgery. Informed consent encompasses not only details of the operative procedure and possible complications, but also a full brief on the long-term implications of caring for a child with a tracheotomy, preferably meeting another family of a child with a tracheotomy. The family circumstances need to be assessed, home suctioning equipment arranged, basic life support training given, and other support offered if needed.

Surgical Procedure

The operation is usually conducted under general anesthesia with the child intubated or a laryngeal mask in place. The position is supine with a small shoulder roll to provide slight neck extension. An adhesive tape under the chin retracts any dewlap and anchors the head (Fig.

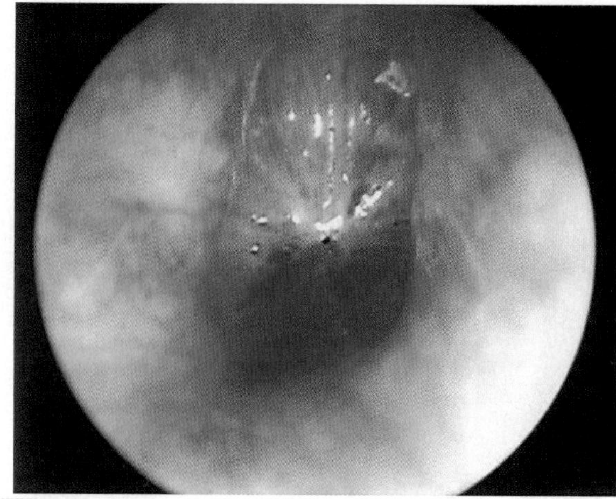

Figure 205-13. Balloon dilatation of early subglottic stenosis—before dilatation.

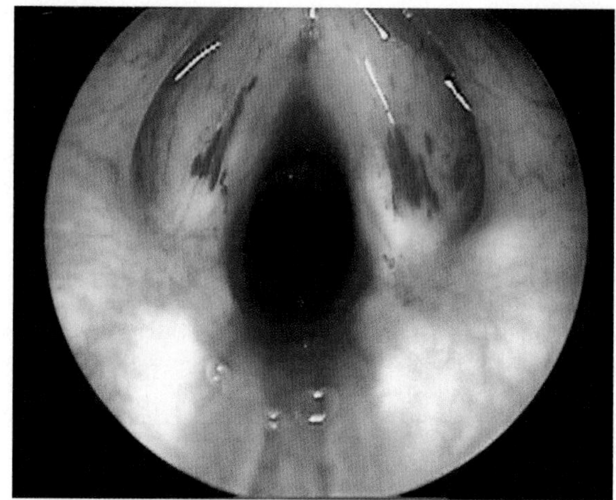

Figure 205-14. Balloon dilatation of early subglottic stenosis—after dilatation.

205-15). Skin marking of the cricoid and sternal notch is useful although may be difficult to palpate in a small infant. Either a horizontal or short vertical skin incision can be used. In children, removal of a subcutaneous fat plug is helpful and the thyroid isthmus can be simply divided using bipolar diathermy. It is crucial to stay midline in a pediatric tracheotomy and one should frequently pause to check the dissection plane. A vertical incision is made through the third and fourth tracheal rings without removal of cartilage and nonabsorbable stay sutures placed on either side of the incision (Fig. 205-16). These sutures assist in replacement of a tube ,which is dislodged before the tract is established. The sutures are removed with the first tube change at 1 week. If a future laryngotracheal reconstruction (LTR) or open laryngeal cleft repair is planned, the tracheal opening may be placed lower, being mindful of the innominate (brachiocephalic) vessels and lung apices. Occasionally, a high innominate vein needs to be protected from the tracheotomy tube by a small inferiorly based flap instead of the vertical incision. Vicryl maturation sutures from the tracheal opening to the skin reduce the chance of false passage creation and assist in establishment of the stomal tract. They have not been shown to increase the rate of tracheocutaneous fistula.[99,100]

Local policy will dictate tracheotomy tube type but beware inserting one that is too long, particularly in neonates, for whom special short tubes are available. Consideration of the underlying condition, patient anatomy, and frequency for tube change influences the choice of tracheotomy tube.[101] An extended length tube may be required if the neck and chest wall are bulky, or length may be required internally to

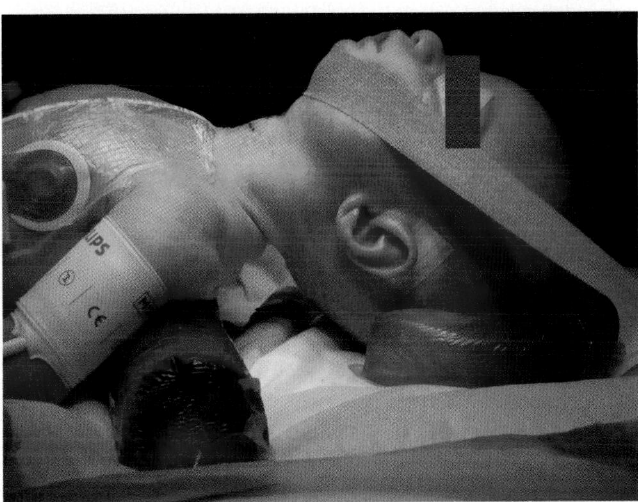

Figure 205-15. Ideal positioning for pediatric airway surgery using shoulder roll, head ring, and chin strap to stabilize the head.

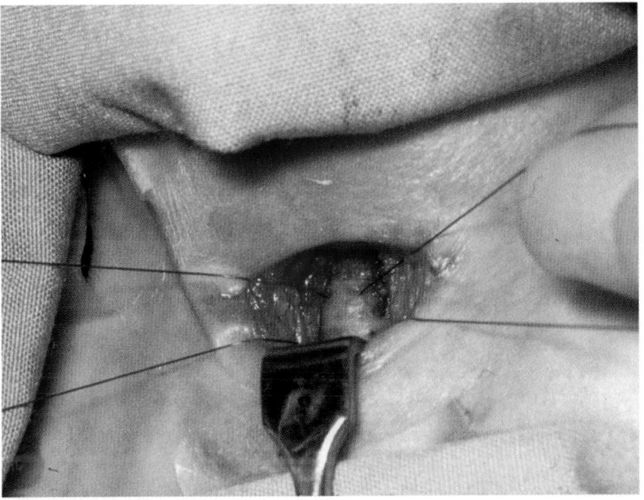

Figure 205-16. Nonabsorbable stay sutures placed on either side of the tracheotomy opening as a safety measure to assist in replacement of a dislodged tube.

support tracheomalacia or a tracheal stenosis. Cuffed tracheotomy tubes are placed infrequently in the pediatric population except to protect the airway in the presence of aspiration. The use of a cuffed tube is usually unnecessary and avoided if possible in that the pediatric airway is particularly sensitive to ischemic insult and prone to ulceration, granulation, and ultimately stenosis.[102] Lateral skin sutures to close the tracheotomy neck wound should not be applied tightly because this predisposes to surgical emphysema.

The percutaneous technique of tracheotomy is not suitable for children because the landmarks may be hard to distinguish, the trachea is soft, pliable, and mobile, the lumen is small, and one may easily drift from the midline.

Tracheotomy Complications

Early complications such as accidental tube dislodgment may be a life-threatening emergency in a small child. This can be prevented by adjusting the tapes carefully to only allow one fingerbreadth between the skin and the tapes, and by providing stay sutures through the trachea on either side of the incision (see Fig. 205-16). These sutures are pulled apart in the event of tube dislodgment to open the incision, bring the trachea to the surface, and guide tube reinsertion into the tracheal lumen. Conventional adult tracheal dilators are usually too large, but a small, curved artery clamp may help. The technique of using a cut suction catheter through the lumen of an appropriate sized tracheotomy tube to guide its insertion has the advantage of confirming tracheal position by successful suctioning of secretions and the opportunity for jet ventilation to maintain oxygenation if required.[103] An emergency box should always be at the child's bedside containing two spare tracheotomy tubes (one a size smaller), suction catheters, lubricant, scissors, and spare tapes. Tube blockage is avoided by humidification, frequent suctioning, and an awareness of the problem.

Postoperatively, a chest x-ray study is imperative to check the tube length and exclude a rare pneumothorax, which can occur from puncturing the lung apex or from positive-pressure ventilation. Hemorrhage is rarely a complication in children if the thyroid isthmus has been divided with electrocautery rather than ligated after division between clamps. Subcutaneous emphysema may be prevented by having a snug fit of the tube in the trachea and avoiding tight wound closure and excessively high-pressure ventilation. Tube dislodgment and blockage remain the most important late complications and are responsible for tracheotomy-related mortality. Stomal and tracheal granulations are the result of physical factors such as movement and plasticizers in the tube, combined with infective factors from the skin and airway. The use of antibiotic ointment around the tube may improve but never remove the granulations. Longstanding suprastomal granulations within the tracheal lumen are associated with the development of suprastomal collapse, which is commonly responsible for difficult decannulation that requires further surgery. Tracheal erosion may occur because of a poor-fitting tracheotomy tube, particularly if metal. Erosion can involve the mediastinum, esophagus, or major vessel. An acquired tracheoesophageal fistula requires closure with an open operation and interposition of muscle. Small bleeds around or from the tracheotomy tube may herald the dramatic erosion of a major vessel.[104] Although suprastomal and tracheal granulations can give rise to small hemorrhages, any tracheotomy bleeding should be taken seriously and investigated radiologically or endoscopically. In very longstanding tracheotomy, the tube may migrate and require surgical repositioning.

Tracheotomy Decannulation

Adults and children with a short-duration tracheotomy (less than 1 month) can be decannulated after appropriate assessment by simply having the tube removed and the stoma covered with an occlusive dressing.[105] Most children, however, are more difficult to decannulate because of multiple factors including suprastomal collapse and granulation, the relatively small size of the airway, and, possibly, psychological dependence or attachment to their tracheotomy tube. A more controlled process for decannulation is used in these children. A recent formal endoscopic examination of the airway, ideally within 1 month, is required before any attempt is made to try decannulation.[106] The most common causes of failed decannulation are significant suprastomal collapse and granulation, and this should be addressed at the time of surgery.

The child is admitted to hospital for a supervised trial of "ward decannulation." The tracheotomy tube is downsized in a stepwise manner, usually one to two sizes smaller each day until the smallest tube has been tolerated. The tracheotomy tube is then blocked for 24 hours and the child is kept on the ward for careful observation at night. If the trial of capping is uneventful, the tube is completely removed and the stoma covered with an occlusive dressing. A further 48-hour period of observation is recommended in that failure may occur at any stage. In the case of failed decannulation, the smallest tube is simply reinserted in the stoma and gradually upsized. Time may be required to allow the airway to grow; however, a repeat endoscopy should be performed before any further trials of decannulation to exclude concurrent pathology such as cord fixation or palsy, suprastomal granuloma or collapse, and tracheomalacia.[107]

Surgical Decannulation

If significant suprastomal collapse is identified that is not responsive to endoscopic measures, a "surgical decannulation" will be required. In principle, the stoma is formally closed, sometimes with additional support from a cartilage graft and period of intubation. At the beginning of the operation, the child is intubated nasally with an age-appropriate tube. The tracheocutaneous fistula is excised, preserving the tracheal wall, unless a cartilage graft is required. If cartilage is not required (mild to moderate collapse only), the stoma is closed primarily and sutures are taken laterally to the sternomastoid to prevent collapse of the repair. If cartilage is required, it is harvested from a rib and carved to a boat shape as for laryngotracheal reconstruction (see open surgical techniques section). The malacic wall is excised until firmer cartilage is exposed. The cartilage graft is sutured to strengthen the anterior tracheal wall with minimal or no air leak. If the trachea is very malacic, an oversize graft can be supported on the sternomastoids, lifting the graft and anterior tracheal wall forward. Postoperatively, the patient remains nasally intubated for 5 to 7 days with the endotracheal tube acting as a stent for the reconstruction.

Endoscopic Treatment of the Larynx and Tracheobronchial Tree

The microsurgical techniques and equipment that are needed in pediatric laryngology are much closer to those of adult phonosurgery than general adult laryngology. Skill, patience and special instrumentation are required. Any damage to the delicate vocal fold may produce lifelong dysphonia that could prove difficult to correct. Optimal anesthetic conditions with the child breathing spontaneously without laryngeal intubation are crucial in this setting. Endoscopic treatment provides the opportunity for therapeutic intervention at the time of a diagnostic procedure, thus avoiding further general anesthesia and open surgery. Many techniques are minimally invasive with reduced trauma and risk to adjacent tissues than in open techniques. The opportunity for photo and video documentation is also extremely useful. Pledgets soaked in 1:10,000 adrenaline (epinephrine) help prepare the operative site before any procedure. Suspension laryngoscopy allows two-handed surgery; however, some may prefer the magnification, distal access, and range of movement afforded by newer generation telescopes and cameras. The surgeon's armamentarium includes the use of "cold steel" microinstrumentation, lasers (CO_2, KTP, thulium), balloons, microdébriders, indwelling stents, grafts, and sutures. Topical medical treatments such as steroids, cidofovir, and mitomycin C can also be administered endoscopically.

Microinstrumentation

Sharp dissection using cupped forceps and microscissors is precise and causes minimal damage to surrounding structures, and the mucosal injury is generally quick to heal. Cystic lesions and nodules may be successfully marsupialized or resected with less trauma than with a laser. Indeed, in inexperienced hands the laser probably has greater potential for damage. Aryepiglottic trimming for laryngomalacia[108] was originally described using sharp dissection. The aryepiglottic folds may simply be released or a small wedge of bulky arytenoid mucosa removed to prevent the forward prolapse of the posterior larynx and arytenoids, which is typical of the condition. Microinstrumentation with the sickle knife and sharp blades can be used to perform other procedures such as an endoscopic cricoid split (Fig. 205-17). In these cases, decompression of the cricoid ring followed by short-term stenting with an endotracheal tube may allow sufficient expansion of the subglottis to enable extubation and avert the need for a tracheostomy in early subglottic stenosis.[109]

Laser

The CO_2 laser for the larynx, and more recently the KTP laser for the trachea and bronchi, have been considered an essential part of the equipment needed to manage the pediatric airway. Other lasers such as the Nd:YAG and thulium laser have also been used in the respiratory tract. Newer techniques and instrumentation, however, may supersede use of the laser due to the delicate nature of the pediatric airway and its sensitivity to thermal injury. A number of improvements, including super pulsing, have reduced the collateral damage that occurs around the intended area of vaporization, making the laser relatively safe and effective in experienced hands. One should always err on the side of conservatism when using the laser in the pediatric airway (Fig. 205-18). Great care must be taken not to damage normal tissues and produce a

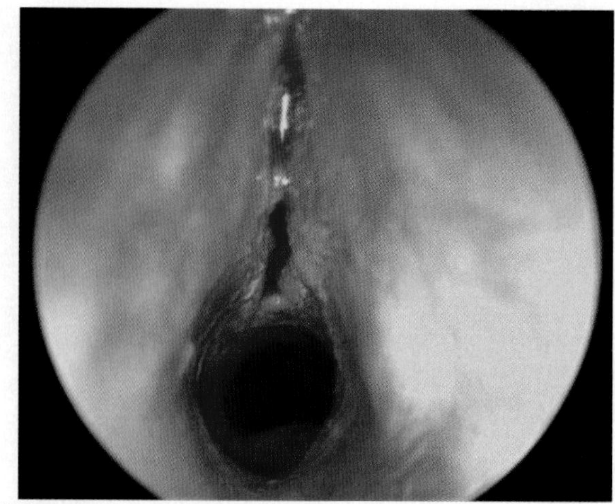

Figure 205-17. Endoscopic cricoid split performed in anterior midline using a sickle knife followed by balloon dilatation for subglottic stenosis.

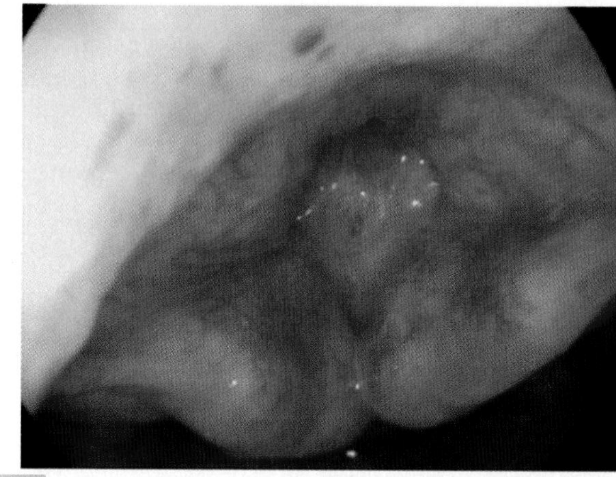

Figure 205-18. Acquired complete glottic stenosis following excessive laser treatment for subglottic hemangioma.

secondary stenosis. A laser-safe tube must be used to provide anesthesia in all these cases; it is withdrawn into the pharynx and the inspired oxygen concentration is reduced to allow safe lasering of an unobstructed field.

The radiant energy produced by the CO_2 laser with a wavelength of 10.2 μm is strongly absorbed by tissues with a high water content with minimal penetration of surrounding tissues. It is useful for supraglottic and laryngeal pathology when attached to the operating microscope. CO_2 laser bronchoscopes have been developed, however, the optics are vastly inferior to normal telescopes, the technique is different, and its use is limited.

The KTP laser emits light at 532 nm (similar to the argon laser) that is preferentially absorbed by hemoglobin and has a greater penetration depth. It may be delivered via fiberoptic fibers to the lower airway, allowing precise access to distal lesions that cannot easily be reached with the CO_2 laser. The KTP laser fibers are sufficiently thin to be passed alongside a suction catheter of a conventional ventilating bronchoscope, providing an excellent view, hemostasis, and controlled vaporization.

The thulium laser is a continuous wave laser with a wavelength of 2013 nm. It has the advantage of being deliverable down a glass fiber with precise cutting and coagulation characteristics, and limited deep tissue penetration. Its use in the pediatric airway for laryngomalacia, laryngeal cysts, vocal cord palsy, tracheal hemangioma, and papillomatosis has recently been described.[110]

Techniques employed with the laser include excision of a wide variety of lesions,[111] vaporization of tissue, the encouragement of controlled scarring, and its use as a precise dissection tool. Postintubation granulomas can be accurately excised or vaporized, and cystic lesions marsupialized or debulked with good hemostasis and minimal postoperative edema. Subglottic hemangioma can be controlled with regular treatments, although the time to resolution is unchanged and there is a potential risk of subglottic scarring and stenosis especially with the CO_2 laser.[87-89] Propanolol is a recent therapy that can cause hemangiomas to regress.

Laser arytenoidectomy may be used for vocal cord palsy to remove the arytenoid and posterior vocal cord. This provides a posterior airway while preserving the function of the anterior vocal cord for phonation. Laryngeal papillomatosis responds well to vaporization with the laser, with potential reduction of viable viral particles that may seed down the trachea. Laser epiglottoplasty and supraglottoplasty for laryngomalacia is quick and bloodless,[112] and when used in the vallecula, scarring is promoted with elevation of a prolapsing epiglottis. Similarly, KTP laser to suprastomal granulomas secondary to tracheostomy tube placement may improve the airway lumen and stiffen up the anterior tracheal wall, facilitating subsequent decannulation.[113,114] Attempts to use the laser to divide anterior webs or subglottic stenosis, however, have generally been unsuccessful due to the tendency for recurrent and sometimes more severe stenoses.

Balloons

Endoscopic treatment of the pediatric airway using vascular-type balloons has become more popular in the last decade. They may be positioned under direct vision using the Hopkins rod or operating microscope and gradually inflated until the desired diameter and pressure are reached. The radial force generated is gentle and there is little mucosal injury. When using a spontaneous inhalational anesthetic technique, the anesthetist must be prepared for a period of total airway occlusion and apnea. One should avoid exceeding the burst pressure of the balloon or overstretching the airway, which potentially risks the development of cartilaginous injury and malacia. There are several situations in which endoscopic balloon dilatation is used for the stridulous child: in the case of early evolving stenosis following airway surgery or intubation, after division of posterior glottic scar bands, with endoscopic cricoid split, and to assist or maintain expansion of tracheal and bronchial stents.[96,115-117]

Microdébrider

The powered microdébrider was initially introduced to otolaryngologists as an additional tool in the treatment of nasal polyps and endoscopic sinus surgery. The development of longer blades with smaller angled cutting surfaces has seen its use migrate to the airway, including the pediatric airway. The concurrent suction attached to the handpiece allows abnormal tissue to be drawn into the blade and precise excision follows. This has been particularly suitable for cases of recurrent respiratory papillomatosis in which preservation of the submucosal tissues is crucial to avoid damage to the vocal ligament and scarring. In fact, a recent survey of members of the American Society of Pediatric Otolaryngology has noted that the microdébrider is now favored for the treatment of laryngeal papillomatosis over the CO_2 laser.[118] The technique is relatively fast, safe, and well tolerated. It has also been shown to cause equivalent immediate postoperative pain, greater improvement in voice quality and the overall procedure cost is lower in some centers.[119-121] The blade may be passed into the subglottis and upper trachea but access may be limited distally. The microdébrider has also been used to remove granulations and even subglottic hemangioma in some centers.[88,122]

Stents, Keels, and Grafts

Maintenance of the pediatric airway occasionally requires techniques of anatomic augmentation or the use of foreign materials to prevent collapse and to discourage stenosis. Many of these procedures can be performed endoscopically, thus avoiding an open operation and related potential morbidity. Glottic and subglottic stents may be positioned, secured, and later removed endoscopically. Expandable metallic stents used for tracheal and bronchial pathology can be placed endoscopically under radiologic guidance. Silastic sheeting used as a keel at the anterior commissure in cases of anterior webbing may be temporarily sutured into place through the neck. The use of the Montgomery T-tube in specialized circumstances of laryngotracheal disease can be inserted endoscopically using a heavy Prolene suture to guide the proximal limb toward the larynx. Recent reports of insertion of cartilage expansion grafts into the posterior larynx following endoscopic posterior cricoid split are also promising.[123]

Endoscopic Sutures

The development of endoscopic instrumentation such as the Lichtenberger needle holder has expanded the options available to the endoscopic airway surgeon. Type I and II laryngotracheoesophageal clefts may be sutured closed after endoscopic trimming of the common mucosal cleft wall. Interrupted sutures are used to close the defect on the tracheal and esophageal aspects with particular attention given to repairing the distal-most point where a fistula may persist. Two-layered repairs of type III laryngeal clefts have also been described, although the technique remains challenging.[124] In cases of vocal cord paralysis, endoscopic arytenoidopexy using a lateralizing suture has been performed with some success.[125,126] This may be temporizing or permanent.

Endoscopic Administration of Topical Treatments

Certain topical treatments can be applied endoscopically to the pediatric airway to assist in the management of the chronically stridulous child. Direct intralesional injection of papillomas with the antiviral cidofovir after debulking of the lesions is effective in reducing recurrence in approximately 60% of severe cases.[127] Its mechanism of action is via inhibition of the HPV viral DNA polymerization process; however, its use is reserved for those patients with aggressively progressing disease as the long-term side effects and potential for malignant transformation have yet to be documented.[128] Corticosteroids may be injected into evolving stenoses and into subglottic hemangiomas followed by a short period of postoperative intubation. The results have been encouraging so far.[87] Mitomycin C is an antineoplastic agent that has been used against solid tumors in the breast, lung, pancreas, and bladder. It was first used in the airway in 1998[129] and has since been applied topically to inhibit fibroblast growth, granulation tissue formation, and cicatricial scarring in many sites including the airway. The optimal dosage has yet to be agreed upon, although most centers tend to prefer 0.2 to 0.4 mg/mL applied on cotton pledgets for up to 5 minutes.[130]

Principles of Open Laryngeal Surgery

Open laryngeal framework surgery allows access to the upper respiratory tract from the supraglottis to the cervical trachea. These procedures are generally performed in the elective setting with careful consideration of the nature of the airway problem and its etiology, the patient's comorbidity and healing tendencies. As for tracheotomy, a meticulous dissection technique is essential, with attention paid to midline anatomic landmarks. The oblique fibers of the cricothyroid muscles are a useful guide to the cricoid cartilage. Anesthesia and ventilation may be maintained via endotracheal intubation or a temporary tracheotomy distal to the operative site depending on the circumstances. If a full laryngofissure is required, the position of the anterior commissure at the vertical midpoint of the thyroid cartilage is marked to allow accurate apposition on closure. Failure to do this may result in suboptimal voice outcomes. Placement of a surgical drain is strongly advised when postoperative air leak is likely to occur to reduce the chance of wound infection and surgical emphysema.

Open procedures may definitively address anatomic narrowing by allowing removal of tissue (stenoses, granulomas and other pathology), decompression of the lumen (cricoid split; Fig. 205-19), or expansion and augmentation with cartilage grafting (laryngotracheal reconstruction (Fig. 205-20), surgical decannulation and stomal reconstruction). Complete resection of a severe stenosis with end-to-end anastomosis is appropriate in some settings (cricotracheal resection). Subglottic hemangiomata may be definitively excised with a single stage open

Figure 205-19. Principles of the anterior cricoid split operation: the cricoid and upper tracheal ring are opened in the midline to decompress the airway.

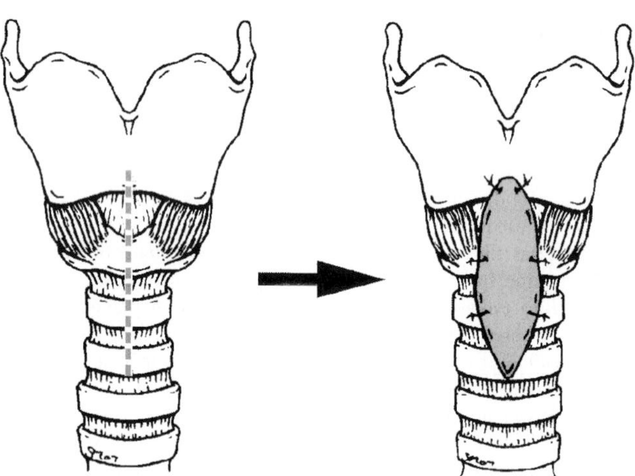

Figure 205-20. Principles of laryngotracheal reconstruction: an anterior cartilage graft is used to augment the subglottic lumen; this may be combined with a posterior cricoid split with or without posterior cartilage graft.

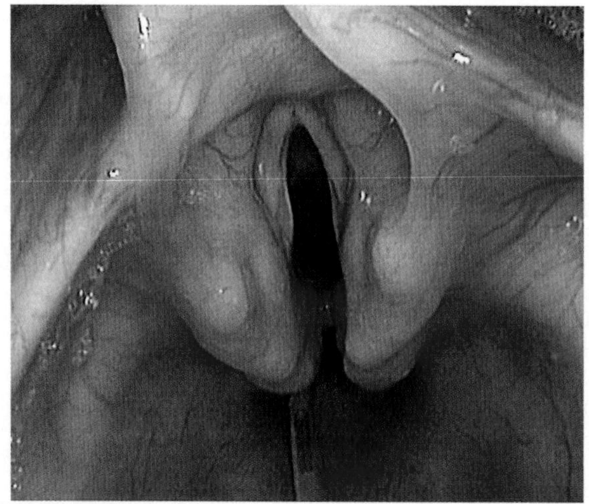

Figure 205-21. Endoscopic view of type 3 laryngeal cleft[131] (total cricoid cleft extending completely through the cricoid cartilage).

resection incorporating the techniques of cartilage augmentation into the repair. Laryngotracheoesophageal clefts can be repaired in two layers using a temporalis fascia or tibial periosteum graft as a reinforcing layer (Fig. 205-21). Maximal supportive medical therapy in the perioperative period with nutritional support, steroids, antibiotics, and antireflux treatment are important adjuncts to open surgery. Endoscopic follow-up is essential to monitor outcomes, granulations, and tendency to restenosis. This may need to be frequent in the early postoperative stages. (See Chapters 202 and 206 for further coverage of laryngeal surgery.)

The Future

The evaluation and management of the stridulous child can be a challenge for the general and pediatric otolaryngologist. Improved neonatal care and a greater understanding of the effects of intubation has led to a decline in iatrogenic airway disease in the last few decades. A systematic approach is essential with direct rigid endoscopic assessment remaining the gold standard investigation over other modalities. Medical management of the compromised airway is preferable if it can be achieved without jeopardizing patient safety. Minimally invasive therapeutic endoscopic measures are gaining popularity and may avert the need for a tracheotomy or open surgery in certain circumstances. The provision of optimal anesthetic conditions is pivotal to success of many pediatric airway procedures. Reconstructive airway techniques continue to be applied to a range of conditions with great success.

SUGGESTED READINGS

Axon PR, Hartley C, Rothera MP. Endoscopic balloon dilatation of subglottic stenosis. *J Laryngol Otol.* 1995;109:876.

Benjamin B. Prolonged intubation injuries of the larynx: endoscopic diagnosis, classification, and treatment. *Ann Otol Rhinol Laryngol Suppl.* 1993;160:1.

Bitar MA, Moukarbel RV, Zalzal GH. Management of congenital subglottic hemangioma: trends and success over the past 17 years. *Otolaryngol Head Neck Surg.* 2005;132:226.

Cherry JD. Clinical practice. Croup. *N Engl J Med.* 2008;358:384.

Craig MF, Bajaj Y, Hartley BE. Maturation sutures for the paediatric tracheostomy—an extra safety measure. *J Laryngol Otol.* 2005;119:985.

de Jong AL, Kuppersmith RB, Sulek M, et al. Vocal cord paralysis in infants and children. *Otolaryngol Clin North Am.* 2000;33:131.

Durden F, Sobol SE. Balloon laryngoplasty as a primary treatment for subglottic stenosis. *Arch Otolaryngol Head Neck Surg.* 2007;133:772.

Eze NN, Wyatt ME, Hartley BE. The role of the anterior cricoid split in facilitating extubation in infants. *Int J Pediatr Otorhinolaryngol.* 2005;69:843.

Gupta VK, Cheifetz IM. Heliox administration in the pediatric intensive care unit: an evidence-based review. *Pediatr Crit Care Med.* 2005;6:2041.

Hartley BE, Cotton RT. Paediatric airway stenosis: laryngotracheal reconstruction or cricotracheal resection? *Clin Otolaryngol Allied Sci.* 2000;25:342.

Inglis AF Jr, Perkins JA, Manning SC, et al. Endoscopic posterior cricoid split and rib grafting in 10 children. *Laryngoscope.* 2003;113:2004.

Jaquet Y, Lang F, Pilloud R, et al. Partial cricotracheal resection for pediatric subglottic stenosis: long-term outcome in 57 patients. *J Thorac Cardiovasc Surg.* 2005;130:726.

Lichtenberger G. Reversible immediate and definitive lateralization of paralyzed vocal cords. *Eur Arch Otorhinolaryngol.* 1999;256:407.

MacKenzie TC, Crombleholme TM, Flake AW. The ex-utero intrapartum treatment. *Curr Opin Pediatr.* 2002;14:453.

Mathur NN, Peek GJ, Bailey CM, et al. Strategies for managing type IV laryngotracheoesophageal clefts at Great Ormond Street Hospital for Children. *Int J Pediatr Otorhinolaryngol.* 2006;70:1901.

Pasquale K, Wiatrak B, Woolley A, et al. Microdebrider versus CO2 laser removal of recurrent respiratory papillomas: a prospective analysis. *Laryngoscope.* 2003;113:139.

Rahbar R, Nicollas R, Roger G, et al. The biology and management of subglottic hemangioma: past, present, future. *Laryngoscope.* 2004;114:1880.

Rahbar R, Rouillon I, Roger G, et al. The presentation and management of laryngeal cleft: a 10-year experience. *Arch Otolaryngol Head Neck Surg.* 2006;132:1335.

Sharp HR, Hartley BE. KTP laser treatment of suprastomal obstruction prior to decannulation in paediatric tracheostomy. *Int J Pediatr Otorhinolaryngol.* 2002;66:125.

Senders CW. Use of mitomycin C in the pediatric airway. *Curr Opin Otolaryngol Head Neck Surg.* 2004;12:473.

Soma MA, Albert DM. Cidofovir: to use or not to use? *Curr Opin Otolaryngol Head Neck Surg.* 2008;16:86.

Tweedie DJ, Skilbeck CJ, Cochrane LA, et al. Choosing a paediatric tracheostomy tube: an update on current practice. *J Laryngol Otol.* 2008;122:161.

Vijayasekaran S, White DR, Hartley BE, et al. Open excision of subglottic hemangiomas to avoid tracheostomy. *Arch Otolaryngol Head Neck Surg.* 2006;132:159.

Wyatt ME, Bailey CM, Whiteside JC. Update on paediatric tracheostomy tubes. *J Laryngol Otol.* 1999;113:35.

Wyatt ME, Hartley BE. Laryngotracheal reconstruction in congenital laryngeal webs and atresias. *Otolaryngol Head Neck Surg.* 2005;132:232.

For complete list of references log onto www.expertconsult.com.

CHAPTER TWO HUNDRED AND SIX

Glottic and Subglottic Stenosis

George H. Zalzal

Robin T. Cotton

Key Points

Majority are caused by trauma:

- Iatrogenic
    - Prolonged intubation
    - Laryngeal surgery
- External neck trauma to a lesser extent
- Congenital (usually less severe and less frequent) even more infrequently
- Burns, ingestions
- Infection
- Inflammation (gastroesophageal reflux or Wegener's)
- Types:
- Anterior, posterior, circumferential, complete: all may be associated with movement disorders
- Prevention:
    - Repair of laryngeal fractures and lacerations
    - Proper tracheotomy techniques
    - Appropriate endolaryngeal surgery
    - Avoidance of intubation trauma
- Diagnosis:
- History and Physical
- Radiology
    - Soft tissue AP and lateral
    - CT
    - MRI
- Endoscopy (flexible and rigid)
- Others
- Pulmonary functions, voice assessment, pH probe, FEES, PFTs
- Management is through (1) expansion or (2) resection. Specifically:
- Endoscopic
- Anterior cricoid split
- Expansion surgery
    - Grafting and stenting
    - Single stage laryngotracheoplasty
- Resection
- Cricotracheal

Chronic laryngeal stenosis is a partial or complete cicatricial narrowing of the endolarynx and may be congenital or acquired. The condition is rare and presents multiple problems affecting soft tissue and cartilage. Iatrogenic injuries and external neck trauma account for most cases. Chronic laryngeal stenosis in pediatric patients may be managed differently from that in adult patients, but the principles of expansion versus resection surgery remain the same. Of all laryngeal stenoses, chronic subglottic stenosis is the most common and presents significant challenges in management (Fig. 206-1).

Etiology and Pathophysiology

Congenital Laryngeal Stenosis

Congenital stenosis is secondary to inadequate recanalization of the laryngeal lumen after completion of normal epithelial fusion at the end of the third month of gestation.[1] The final pathologic findings depend on the degree of recanalization. Thus if the laryngeal lumen is not recanalized and remains completely obliterated, it will result in complete laryngeal atresia; if it is partially recanalized, incomplete atresia,

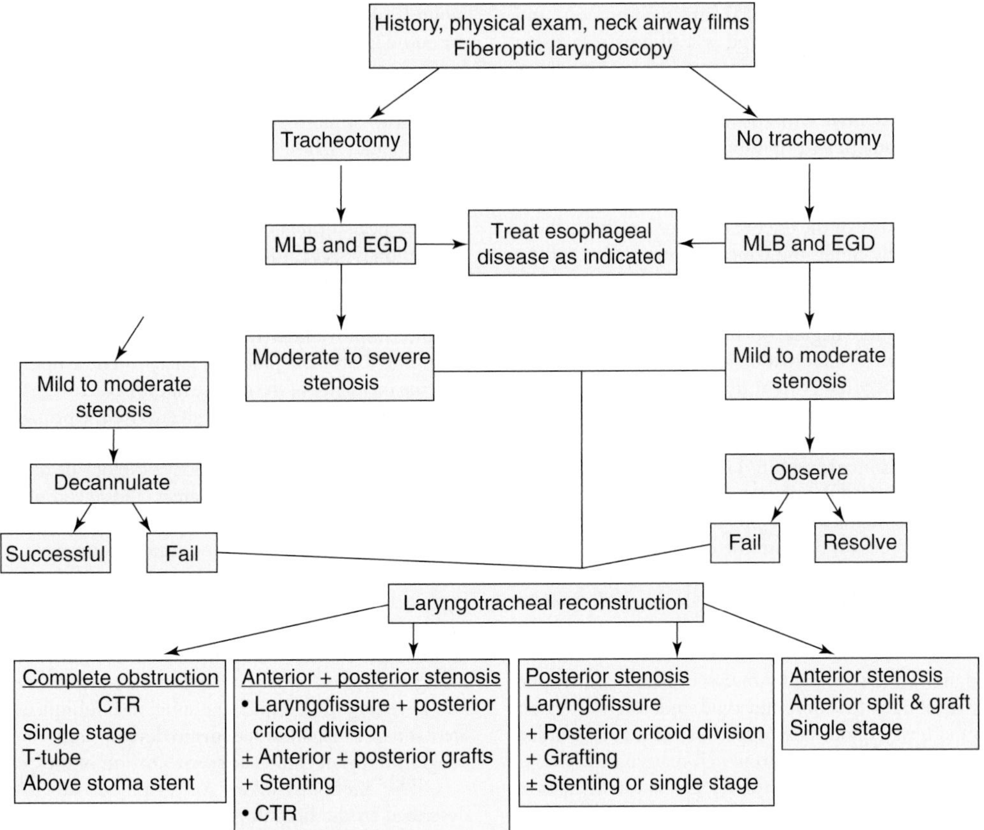

Figure 206-1. Algorithm for management of laryngeal stenosis.

stenosis, or webbing will occur. The cricoid cartilage is usually abnormally developed.

Congenital Laryngeal Atresia and Web

Laryngeal atresia can occur at any laryngeal level or combination of levels. The clinical picture depends on the severity of the lesion. In complete atresia, the glottis is closed at or above the vocal cords by a firm fibrous membrane. The neonate is aphonic, tries vigorously to breathe, undergoes rapid deterioration, becomes cyanotic despite continued respiratory efforts, and soon dies of asphyxia unless immediate tracheotomy is performed.[2,3] The condition is incompatible with life unless an emergency tracheotomy is performed or there is an associated tracheoesophageal or bronchoesophageal fistula. The most severe type of congenital laryngeal atresia presents as stillbirth and may not be recognized.

Congenital laryngeal webs account for about 5% of congenital anomalies of the larynx.[4] About 75% occur at the glottic level, and the rest are supraglottic or subglottic.[5] An association between anterior glottic web, the chromosome 22q11.2 deletion, and velocardiofacial syndrome has been established.[6-8] All patients with anterior glottic web should have their chromosome 22q11.2 deletion status determined by standard fluorescent in situ hybridization (FISH) analysis. Most webs present at birth or in the first few months of life. The severity of the web varies. Only a few are severe enough to require airway support by intubation or tracheotomy. A laryngeal web is often an abnormality of the glottis and the subglottic cricoid region (Fig. 206-2). The differential diagnosis includes bilateral vocal cord paralysis and congenital interarytenoid joint fixation. It is important to detect associated anomalies of the larynx, the respiratory tract, and other organ systems.

Treatment of congenital laryngeal atresia and web is presented later in this chapter under treatment of specific disorders.

Congenital Subglottic Stenosis

The normal subglottic lumen diameter in the full-term neonate is 4.5 to 5.5 mm and in premature babies is about 3.5 mm. A subglottic

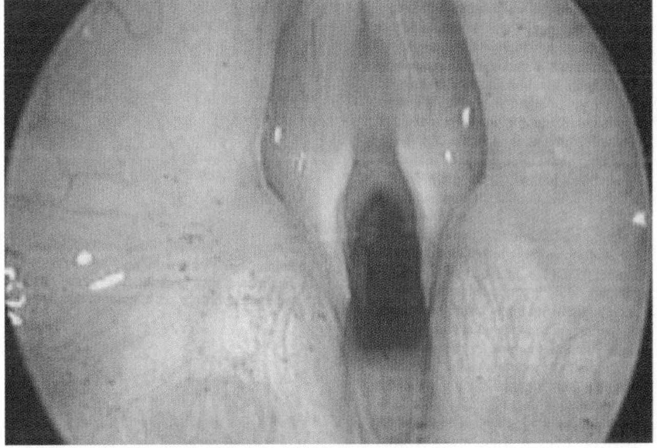

Figure 206-2. Endoscopic view of a congenital glottic web with subglottic extension.

diameter of 4 mm or less in a full-term neonate is considered to be narrowed.

Congenital subglottic stenosis (SGS) is considered to be congenital in the absence of a history of endotracheal intubation or other apparent acquired causes of stenosis. The diagnosis may be difficult to confirm, and it is unknown how many intubated premature infants who fail extubation have underlying congenital stenosis. Thus, by best approximation, congenital subglottic stenosis is the third most common congenital disorder of the larynx after laryngomalacia and recurrent laryngeal nerve paralysis. Acquired subglottic stenosis is more common than congenital stenosis because of the use of prolonged endotracheal intubation for respiratory support.

Congenital SGS is a clinical endoscopic diagnosis describing various histopathologic conditions that produce narrowing of the subglottic airway. Congenital SGS can be divided into membranous and cartilaginous types.[9-11] The membranous type is a fibrous soft tissue thickening of the subglottic area caused by increased fibrous connective tissue or hyperplastic dilated mucous glands with no inflammatory reaction. It is usually circumferential, with the narrowest area 2 to 3 mm below the true vocal cords, sometimes extending upward to include the true vocal cords.[12]

The cartilaginous types are more variable, but the most common type is a thickening or deformity of the cricoid cartilage causing a shelf-like plate of cartilage, partially filling the concave inner surface of the cricoid ring and extending posteriorly as a solid rigid sheet, leaving only a small posterior opening.[13]

Symptoms depend on the degree of subglottic narrowing. In severe cases, respiratory distress and stridor are present at birth; in milder cases, the symptoms become evident during the first few weeks or months of life, presenting as prolonged or recurrent croup. Differential diagnosis includes subglottic hemangioma and subglottic cysts. Infants usually become symptomatic within 3 months of birth because of increased activity and increased ventilation requirements.[2,9]

Minimal laryngeal swelling secondary to infection or endoscopy may precipitate airway obstruction because the cricoid cartilage limits the swelling of tissue in any direction except toward the laryngeal lumen at the expense of the airway. Therefore great care is needed when endoscopy is performed on these children to prevent trauma to the subglottic mucosa.

Endoscopic diagnosis is essentially by means of flexible fiberoptic endoscopy to assess vocal cord function and rigid endoscopy to assess the degree of anatomic obstruction. Postendoscopic edema is avoided by operating on a quiet, relaxed infant who is well-oxygenated. Cooperation between the endoscopist and anesthesiologist is essential, as is gentle instrumentation, preferably with the rigid rod lens system telescope alone without the sheath. If postoperative edema occurs, aggressive management should be started with cool mist racemic epinephrine by aerosol or intermittent positive-pressure breathing, and a short course of high-dose intravenous corticosteroids.

Congenital subglottic stenosis is most often less severe than acquired stenosis and may therefore be managed more conservatively. Some patients outgrow the condition.[12-14] Management depends on the degree and severity of stenosis, shape (whether the cricoid cartilage is normal or abnormal), and whether there are associated congenital anomalies.

Mild cases of stenosis are managed conservatively by watchful waiting and regular follow-up because many children outgrow the problem. During observation, vigorous medical management of viral infection is recommended. More severe cases requiring airway support may be managed by tracheotomy and reconstructive repair, or by single-stage laryngotracheal reconstruction using costal cartilage grafting for expansion of the subglottic airway.

Acquired Laryngeal Stenosis

Trauma is the most common cause of acquired laryngeal stenosis in children and adults and may be external or internal.

External Laryngeal Trauma

Blunt trauma to the neck sustained during motor vehicle accidents injures the larynx when the anterior surface of the extended neck strikes the dashboard or steering wheel, causing a laryngeal framework fracture. This is more common in adults than in children, in whom the prominent mandible and relatively high position of the larynx protect the latter from injury. Fractures of the larynx occur secondary to in-home accidents when the neck is injured by striking furniture such as a coffee table. Chronic acquired laryngeal stenosis is a sequela of severe laryngeal trauma with fracture of the cricoid and thyroid cartilages with or without displacement, or of inadequately managed early stages of laryngeal trauma.

Another mechanism of blunt laryngeal trauma, the so-called clothesline injury, occurs when a person riding a bicycle hits the anterior neck on a branch or clothesline, sustaining laryngeal fracture, and thyrotracheal or cricotracheal separation. A patient may have a separation of the cricoid and trachea and still survive the injury. Penetrating wounds of the larynx are usually less common than blunt trauma and are more common in adults than in children.

Internal Laryngeal Trauma

Most cases of internal laryngeal injury are iatrogenic, secondary to prolonged endotracheal intubation, which is the most common cause of chronic laryngeal stenosis. Approximately 90% of cases of acquired chronic subglottic stenosis in infants and children occur secondary to endotracheal intubation.[12,14] The reported incidence of stenosis after intubation ranges from less than 1% to 8.3%.[15-19] This rate is much lower than the 12% to 20% reported in the late 1960s and early 1970s because of recognition of the problem and institution of preventive methods. Despite improvement in neonatal care, the incidence has stabilized at around 1% over the past 10 years.[19,20] These figures may underestimate the true incidence of the disease in the pediatric population because many infants who are intubated do not survive the primary illness. In addition, some acquired subglottic stenosis may not be recognized unless an infection of the upper respiratory tract develops or the patient requires reintubation later in life. The areas most commonly injured are the subglottic region in children and the posterior endolarynx in adults.[21]

In children, the subglottic region is especially prone to injury from endotracheal tube intubation for various reasons. First, the cricoid cartilage is the only area in the upper airway that has a complete circular cartilaginous ring, preventing the outward extension of traumatic edema. Second, the pseudostratified, ciliated, columnar respiratory epithelium lining this region is delicate and tends to deteriorate under the stress of an indwelling tube. Third, the subglottic submucosa is made up of loose areolar tissue that allows edema to develop easily and quickly. Fourth, the subglottic region is the narrowest portion of the pediatric airway.[12]

The pathophysiology of acquired subglottic stenosis is well described in the literature.[3,22-24] The endotracheal tube causes pressure necrosis at the point of interface with tissue, leading to mucosal edema and ulceration. As ulceration deepens, normal ciliary flow is interrupted, with mucociliary stasis leading to secondary infection and perichondritis. With further infection, chondritis and cartilaginous necrosis occur, especially with collapse of the airway during inspiration. Healing occurs by secondary intention with granulation tissue proliferation in the areas of ulceration and deposition of fibrous tissue in the submucosa. Primary healing of the laryngeal injury is hindered by the presence of loose and mobile subglottic mucosa, poor blood supply to the cartilage, and constant motion of the larynx associated with swallowing and head movement.[23,25] Study of intubated larynges from infants of 22 to 40 weeks' gestation who survived a few hours to 300 days showed acute injury was almost invariable and up to 100% of the subglottic epithelium was lost within a few hours of intubation, but progression of injury was relatively short lived. Ulcer healing started after a few days, rapidly progressed from day 10, and, in most cases, was complete after 30 days. This study suggests that longstanding acute injury of the subglottis is the exception rather than the rule, even with the endotracheal tube remaining in place.[23]

Duration of intubation and the size of the endotracheal tube are the most important factors in the development of laryngeal stenosis. No definite safe time limit for endotracheal intubation has been established. Severe injury has been reported after 17 hours of intubation in adults[22] and 1 week after intubation in neonates.[26] Several studies in adults have shown that a 7- to 10-day period is acceptable, after which prolongation of intubation is accompanied by an increased incidence of laryngotracheal complications.[21] Premature infants tolerate more prolonged intubation (weeks rather than days). Explanations include relative immaturity of the laryngeal cartilage in the neonates (more hypercellular with scant gel-like matrix) rendering it more pliable, thus yielding to pressure,[27] and the high location of the neonatal larynx in the neck with its posterior tilt and funnel shape.[25]

Insertion of an oversized endotracheal tube increases the risk of laryngeal injury. In children, the tube size should allow an air leak at 20 cm H_2O pressure if possible. Polymeric silicone and polyvinyl chloride are considered the safest materials for prolonged intubation.

Shearing motion of the tube causes abrasive traumatic action on the mucosa, especially in patients who are restless, those on respirators, and those with orotracheal intubation. Superimposed bacterial infec-

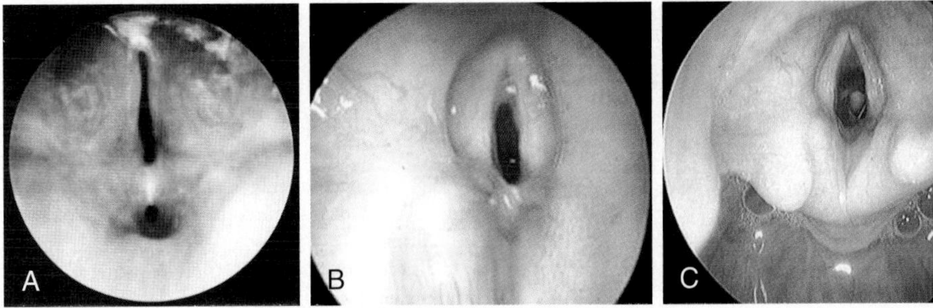

Figure 206-3. **A,** Endoscopic view of interarytenoid adhesion shows a posterior fistular tract resulting from a scar tissue band between the vocal process of the arytenoids cartilages. **B,** Endoscopic view of posterior glottic stenosis with vocal cord fixation. **C,** Same lesion as in **B,** after repair with posterior cartilage grafting and stenting, achieving full vocal cord mobility.

tion compounds the mechanical mucosal trauma by increasing the inflammatory response and scar tissue formation. Repeated intubations cause increased trauma and increase the risk of sequelae. Nasogastric tubes can cause pressure necrosis and cricoid chondritis if placed in the midline. Coexistence of endotracheal and nasogastric tubes may increase laryngeal complications.

When inexperienced personnel care for intubated patients, intubation complications may increase. Education of physician and nursing personnel caring for intubated patients markedly increases the expertise of that care. Systemic factors including chronic illness, general disability, immunosuppression, anemia, neutropenia, toxicity, dehydration, hypoxemia, poor perfusion, radiotherapy, and the presence of gastric acid reflux encourage the vulnerability of laryngeal mucosa to injury by decreasing tissue resistance and increasing infection rate.

Other Causes of Laryngeal Stenosis

Laryngeal stenosis may occur secondary to laryngeal injury resulting from laryngeal surgery. Emergency cricothyroidotomy through the cricothyroid membrane[28] and high tracheotomy can produce severe stenosis, particularly in children. Supraglottic stenosis and collapse may be related to prior laryngeal or tracheal injury. Acquired anterior glottic web can occur after excision of a laryngeal polyp or papilloma in the anterior commissure area if the anterior portions of both vocal cords are denuded simultaneously.[29] Laryngeal stenosis also is described after endoscopic microsurgery with modalities such as electrocautery or laser.[30]

Chondroradionecrosis can lead to scarring and stenosis shortly after radiotherapy or as long as 20 years later.[31] Intralaryngeal burns from fumes, smoke inhalation, or caustic lye ingestion can give rise to chronic laryngeal stenosis.[32]

Chronic Infection

Laryngeal stenosis secondary to chronic infection is rare except in isolated endemic geographic areas. It has been described in tuberculosis, syphilis, leprosy, glanders, typhoid fever, scarlet fever, diphtheria, mycosis, and laryngeal scleroma.

Chronic Inflammatory Disease

Laryngeal stenosis has been described secondary to sarcoidosis, lupus erythematosus, Behçet's syndrome, Wegener's granulomatosis, relapsing polychondritis, pemphigoid, epidermolysis bullosa, amyloidosis, and major aphthous ulceration. Management of laryngotracheal stenosis in Wegener's granulomatosis is complex, requiring individualized and often multimodality interventions to achieve satisfactory results.

Chronic inflammation secondary to gastroesophageal reflux (GER) may cause laryngeal stenosis. GER in children can be classified as physiologic, functional, pathologic, or secondary.[33] Many airway manifestations have been attributed to GER including stridor, recurrent croup, exacerbation of subglottic stenosis, and chronic cough. Diagnosis is difficult unless the index of suspicion is high.[34] The role of GER on the outcome of pediatric laryngotracheal reconstruction remains unknown.[35] Until this is clear, the authors recommend that GER is investigated and treated in patients undergoing laryngeal reconstruction during the perioperative period.

Laryngeal Neoplasm

Chondroma, fibroma, hemangioma, and carcinoma can cause laryngeal stenosis because of tumor infiltration or secondary to infective perichondritis, postradiation perichondritis, or postsurgical scarring and stenosis.

Types of Stenosis

Acquired glottic stenosis may be anterior, posterior, circumferential, or complete. Anterior glottic stenosis can be a thin glottic web, which is a bridge of scar tissue covered by epithelium located between the vocal cords involving the anterior commissure. This usually results from enthusiastic endoscopic surgery involving both true cords simultaneously. Thick, anterior glottic scarring is usually more extensive and results in true vocal cords, false cords, and laryngeal ventricles adhering to one another without any intervening web. The cause is often unmanaged severe external laryngeal trauma. Posterior glottic stenosis usually results from prolonged endotracheal tube intubation.

Pressure necrosis of the mucosa overlying the vocal process of the arytenoid occurs, followed by ulceration and granulation tissue formation on the medial surface of the body of the arytenoid cartilage. A similar process occurs to a variable degree in the interarytenoid area with involvement of the interarytenoid muscle, causing fibrous ankylosis of one or both cricoarytenoid joints.[36] Posterior glottic scar frequently extends downward to the subglottic region. It is important to differentiate between a complete posterior glottic stenosis, in which the scar is located in the interarytenoid space and posterior commissure, and an interarytenoid adhesion, in which the scar is between the vocal processes of the arytenoids with a small posterior, mucosally lined sinus tract in the posterior commissure area (Figs. 206-3 and 206-4A). The scarring of the posterior commissure may be confined to the submucosa (see Fig. 206-4B) or extend into one (see Fig. 206-4C) or both (see Fig. 206-4D) cricoarytenoid joints.

The voice is generally good because of the adducted position of the vocal cords. The major symptoms are referable to the airway. In mild or moderate cases, the patient may be able to ventilate without a tracheotomy and may experience only exercise intolerance. Patients who have a more severe stenosis may need a tracheotomy for adequate respiratory exchange. Diagnosis by indirect laryngoscopy is difficult and may be confused with bilateral vocal cord paralysis.[37] Diagnosis at direct laryngoscopy is made by careful observation of the posterior commissure. The true vocal cords are closely approximated because the vocal processes, and occasionally the arytenoid bodies, are tethered together by heavy scar. A posterior sinus tract should be carefully sought and is particularly difficult to see in the pediatric larynx. Unlike vocal cord paralysis, in posterior glottic stenosis the cricoarytenoid joints are partially or completely immobile on a passive motion test. Palpation of the arytenoids shows that they may be rocked in an anteroposterior direction but will not slide from side to side. Complete total glottic stenosis rarely occurs in isolation and is usually accompanied by supraglottic or subglottic stenosis. In children, it is a sequela of endotracheal intubation, lye ingestion, and thermal burn.

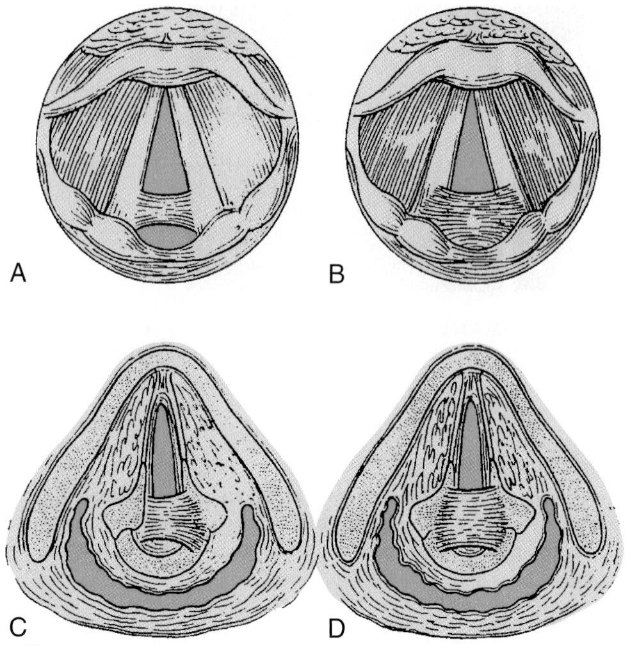

Figure 206-4. Posterior subglottic stenosis. **A,** Interarytenoid adhesion with a mucosally lined tract posteriorly. **B,** Posterior commissure and interarytenoid scar without a mucosally lined tract posteriorly. **C,** Posterior commissure scar extending into the right cricoarytenoid joint. **D,** Posterior commissure scar extending into both cricoarytenoid joints.

Prevention

Factors important in reducing the incidence of laryngotracheal stenosis include:

1. Early exploration of laryngeal fractures to minimize serious sequelae.
2. High tracheotomy and cricothyroidotomy should be avoided except in extreme emergencies. If it is suspected that a high tracheotomy or cricothyroidotomy has been performed, endoscopy is indicated. If the suspicion is confirmed, the neck should be explored, and the tracheotomy site should be relocated to a lower position to prevent chronic subglottic stenosis. However, if the repair of a cricotracheal resection is planned, a high tracheotomy rather than a lower one is advantageous because it reduces the length of the resection.
3. When performing a tracheotomy, the surgeon should avoid extensive resection of the tracheal wall and use the smallest size tracheotomy tube compatible with ventilation and suctioning.
4. Aggressive endoscopy for benign laryngeal lesions should be avoided, especially for those in the anterior commissure area, to prevent formation of an anterior glottic web. The procedures should be staged 2 weeks apart for each side. Different principles may be appropriate for malignant lesions.
5. Intubation and endoscopy should be performed gently on relaxed patients.
6. Circumstances contributing to laryngeal trauma secondary to prolonged intubation should be recognized and avoided whenever possible.

Diagnosis of Congenital and Acquired Laryngeal Stenosis

Laryngeal stenosis is diagnosed by a thorough history and physical examination, radiologic evaluation, and endoscopic examination of the airway and esophagus.[38] Other investigations such as pulmonary function tests also may be helpful.

History and Physical Examination

Mild to moderate laryngeal stenosis is usually asymptomatic until an infection of the upper respiratory tract causes additional narrowing of the airway, resulting in respiratory distress. These patients usually have a tendency toward prolonged courses of upper respiratory tract infections.

In acquired stenosis, there is a history of laryngeal insult. Symptoms usually occur 2 to 4 weeks after the original insult, although the latent period can occasionally be longer. In congenital stenosis, symptoms usually appear at or shortly after birth, suggesting the possibility of a laryngeal anomaly.

The main symptoms of laryngeal stenosis relate to airway, voice, and feeding. Progressive respiratory difficulty is the prime symptom of airway obstruction with biphasic stridor, dyspnea, air hunger, and vigorous efforts of breathing with suprasternal, intercostal, and diaphragmatic retraction. Abnormal cry, aphonia, or hoarseness occurs when the vocal cords are affected. Dysphagia and feeding abnormality with recurrent aspiration and pneumonia can occur.

Complete physical examination of the upper aerodigestive tract should be performed to rule out associated congenital anomalies or acquired injuries.

Radiologic Evaluation

Radiologic evaluation is performed after stabilization of the airway. Radiography helps assess the exact site and length of the stenotic segment, especially for totally obliterated airways. The soft tissue radiograph is the single most important view in children. The anteroposterior high-kilovoltage technique increases visibility of the upper airway by enhancing the tracheal air column while deemphasizing the bony cervical spine. In acquired stenosis, small areas of calcification may be seen, denoting the site of previous injury. Fluoroscopy is helpful in studying tracheal dynamics.

Computed tomography (CT) and magnetic resonance imaging (MRI) are useful. High-speed CT has reduced imaging time and is becoming more popular in the assessment of airway lesions. MRI still requires a significant amount of time, necessitating sedation in younger patients.

Evaluation of swallowing is important before airway reconstruction because dysfunctional feeding may complicate airway reconstruction by increasing the risk of aspiration postoperatively. Patients undergoing surgical correction of airway anomalies should have a historical screen for feeding problems. Patients with marginal feeding skills may be unable to compensate for the altered anatomy created by the reconstruction.

Videofluoroscopic swallowing studies (VSS) provide radiographic reviews of the bolus during swallowing. The presence of laryngeal penetration and aspiration can be documented and assessment of the ability of the child to protect the airway can be made. Many children with congenital anomalies of the airway, however, cannot tolerate the volume of contrast necessary to visualize the swallowing mechanism, and have significant oral aversion behaviors that preclude the introduction of any material into the mouth because of lack of exposure to nutritional stimuli at developmentally sensitive periods of their development. This makes the assessment of swallowing safety impossible by this method and an endoscopic evaluation of swallowing should be performed.

Endoscopic Examination

Indirect laryngoscopy alone is inadequate for diagnosis. Direct endoscopic visualization of the larynx is essential to study the stenosis carefully. Flexible fiberoptic endoscopy assesses the dynamics of vocal cord function and the upper airway, including the trachea.[39] In patients with severe burns with neck contractures, flexible endoscopy may be the only method to visualize the larynx. Flexible retrograde tracheoscopy through the tracheotomy site may provide useful information in some cases.

Rigid and flexible endoscopy of the airway and esophagus should be performed in the operating room with the patient under general anesthesia. The rigid telescope is especially important in the examination of children because it better visualizes the small larynx. However, it is important to recognize that the airway lumen should be measured by passing bronchoscopes or endotracheal tubes of known sizes and cannot be gauged by the use of telescopes alone.[40]

Flexible endoscopy and spiral CT with mutiplanar resolutions have to be considered complementary techniques to rigid endoscopy in the preoperative evaluation and follow-up of children with laryngotracheal stenosis.[41]

Evaluation of Gastroesophageal and Gastrolaryngopharyngeal Reflux

GER is a common occurrence in children and adults. Many infants have no pathologic symptoms related to GER (the happy spitters). The current prevailing, although not universal, opinion is that GER and gastrolaryngopharyngeal reflux (GLPR) are likely to play a role in the development and exacerbation of SGS and may affect adversely the successful outcome of laryngotracheal reconstruction (LTR). GER and GLPR are defined as involuntary passage of gastric contents into the esophagus and pharynx, and are commonly occurring physiologic phenomena. It is not the presence of reflux that determines gastroesophageal reflux disease (GERD) or gastrolaryngopharyngeal reflux disease (GLPRD), but rather the frequency, intensity, and associated symptoms of reflux that distinguishes GERD and GLPRD from GER and LPR. Unfortunately, there is no gold standard for recognizing or excluding GERD and GLPRD, and differentiation between physiologic and pathologic reflux can be difficult. All diagnostic tests available for GER and GLPR have significant limitations. Generally, they tend to have high specificity but low sensitivity. Of the tests available today, 24-hour esophageal pH probe using a dual probe technique is believed to be the most reliable. This test, when used in conjunction with history, esophagoscopy, and esophageal biopsy, yields the best information in determining the likelihood of GERD and GLPRD.

Esophagogastroduodenoscopy with Biopsy

Esophagogastroduodenoscopy (EGD) allows direct visualization of the esophageal, gastric, and duodenal mucosa, as well as facilitating biopsy of any suspicious lesions. Any esophageal mucosal irritation, erosion, ulceration, epithelial metaplasia as in Barrett's esophagitis, or stricture should be noted and biopsied. Histologic findings of esophagitis are confirmed. EGD is a surgical procedure, with its own potential risks of bleeding, infection, intestinal perforation, mediastinitis, or peritonitis. This test is recommended when esophagitis is suspected, but not required for every patient undergoing reflux evaluation. When esophagitis is detected, EGD with biopsy may be repeated to determine treatment efficacy.

It is important to recognize eosinophilic esophagitis as a separate entity from GER. Control of this is important prior to surgical reconstruction of the airway.

Treatment of GER and GLPR starts with dietary and lifestyle modifications and can be supplemented by pharmacologic agents. If control of GER and GLPR is not achieved with maximum medical therapy, a surgical consultation should be obtained. Proper communication between the otolaryngologist, the gastroenterologist, and the surgeon based on the previous investigations leads to instituting the most appropriate therapeutic program for the individual patient.

Functional Endoscopic Evaluation of Swallowing

The functional endoscopic evaluation of the swallow (FEES) study requires the passage of a flexible endoscope transnasally into the hypopharynx. The hypopharynx can be visualized and parameters similar to those rated in VSS related to airway protection can be determined. In addition, secretions spilling from the oral cavity that pool in the hypopharynx may be visualized and their aspiration risk assessed. An assessment of hypopharyngeal sensation also can be made by demonstrating the laryngeal closure response elicited from a calibrated air stimulus to the larynx. Decreased sensation is correlated with an increased aspiration potential. If VSS is precluded because of oral aversion, then a FEES study is performed.

Table 206-1
Grading of Laryngeal Stenosis

Grade	Percentage of Laryngeal Lumen Obstruction
I	Less than 70%
II	70% to 90%
III	More than 90%; identifiable lumen is present (no matter how narrow)
IV	Complete obstruction; no lumen

Voice Assessment

Psychoacoustic evaluation and acoustic analysis of the voice may be used to establish the degree of vocal abnormality before surgery and compare it with voice analysis after surgery.[42,43]

Although assessment of pre- and postoperative vocal quality in young children may be frustrating, improvement in technology has made the task easier and several reports have been published regarding specific voice issues. In general, the voice results are unsatisfactory, with the vocal parameters suggesting a pattern of lower than optimum pitch and a restricted pitch range. Vocal quality appears to be disturbed in most patients; however, laryngeal reconstruction makes oral communication possible.[43-46]

Pulmonary Function Test

Pulmonary function tests with the spirometric maximum inspiration and expiration flow rates, flow volume loops, or pressure flow loops show characteristic changes in upper airway stenosis and can be used to compare the postoperative results with preoperative values.[47]

Management

Management should be individualized according to pathologic findings, patient age, degree and consistency of stenosis (hard or soft and percentage of stenosis), and general condition of the patient. Management of adults differs from that of children, and some operations useful in children are not applicable to adults.

All cases of moderate or severe laryngeal stenosis require a tracheotomy at or below the third tracheal ring to establish a safe airway. Stenosis that does not require a tracheotomy constitutes a mild case. A four-stage grading system has been widely adopted (Table 206-1).[40,48]

The first thing to do is to secure the airway if immediate repair cannot be performed. Severe cases of congenital subglottic stenosis or marked cartilaginous cricoid deformity need a tracheotomy to maintain an adequate airway. When a tracheotomy is performed, the smallest tube that permits adequate ventilation should be used. The tube should allow air leakage to occur to avoid injury to the tracheal mucosa and simultaneously preserve phonatory potential.

Tracheotomy was required in congenital subglottic stenosis in less than half of a large series of patients.[12] Once the airway is secured, two basic management modalities are considered: endoscopic or external. Endoscopic methods include traditional dilation including balloon dilation and techniques that use laser excision of stenotic areas. Open surgical methods include expansion and resection surgery. The morbidity of open reconstruction is higher, but this is balanced against the multiplicity and futility of endoscopic procedures when inappropriately used. In general, less severe cases respond to endoscopic methods, and more severe cases require external reconstruction. If the cartilaginous framework of the larynx is significantly deficient, endoscopy is unlikely to be successful.

The best chance for the patient lies in the first operation.[49] Endoscopic techniques for isolated subglottic stenosis may be successful in grade I and occasionally grade II subglottic stenosis. Expansion laryngotracheal surgery is very successful in grades II, III, and some grade IV. Partial cricotracheal resection is successful in some grade III and

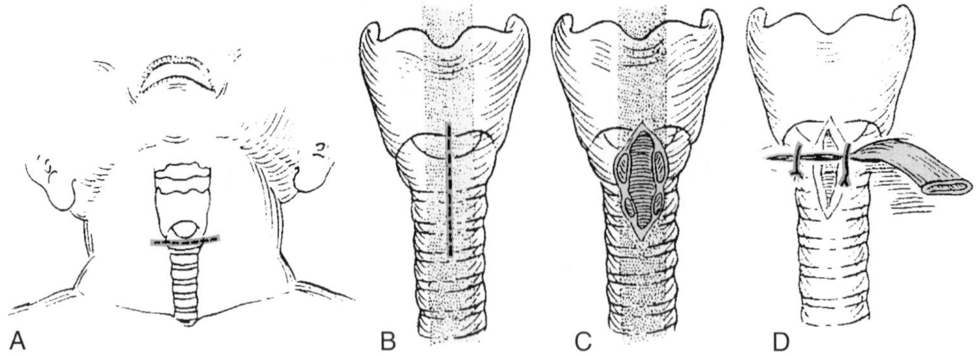

Figure 206-5. Anterior cricoid split. **A,** Skin incision. **B,** Midline laryngeal incision through cartilage and mucosa. **C,** With the cricoid cartilage decompressed, the endotracheal tube is ghosted in **B** and **C.** **D,** Loose skin closure with a drain inserted.

IV stenosis where there is a clear margin between the stenosis and the vocal cords.

Endoscopic Management

Dilation is sometimes useful early in the development of stenosis. It is not recommended for mature, firm stenosis or cartilaginous stenosis. Dilation is usually performed alone or supplemented with local or systemic corticosteroids or intralaryngeal stenting. The use of corticosteroids in all stages of acquired SGS is controversial. Corticosteroids tend to decrease scar formation by their anti-inflammatory action of delaying synthesis of collagen in early stages of wound healing and increasing collagen lysis in the later phases. Corticosteroids also delay wound healing by delaying the epithelial migration necessary to resurface the denuded area, thus increasing scar formation and predisposing to infection. Corticosteroids may be used systemically or locally. Local injection into subglottic scar is technically difficult and may be ineffective if a pressure injection system is not used. Resorption of cartilage secondary to the presence of local corticosteroids is a serious complication. Inhalation corticosteroids are believed to reduce granulation tissue formation after stent removal or early after endotracheal tube injury.

Mitomycin C is an antineoplastic antibiotic that acts as an alkylating agent by inhibiting deoxyribonucleic acid and protein synthesis. Experimental animal studies[50] and postendoscopic application[51,52] seem promising; however, there seems to be no advantage to its use after open surgical repair.[53] There is a risk of acute airway obstruction from excessive accumulation of fibrinous debris at the operative site in humans and animals after applying mitomycin to sites treated with CO_2 laser and dilatation.[54,55]

Endoscopic scar excision using the carbon dioxide (CO_2) laser is popular because it allows the surgeon to vaporize scar tissue with precision, producing minimal damage to healthy areas. Tissue destruction is directly related to the amount of energy delivered by the laser and the duration of exposure. If minimal energy of short duration is delivered, damage to the underlying and normal surrounding structures is minimal. However, if the laser is used at high energy levels for long times, it acts similar to any other uncontrolled method of tissue excision. The laser is useful for managing early stenosis with granulation tissue and may improve the airway without causing significant bleeding or edema, thus avoiding the need for a tracheotomy. Many authors have reported adequate results in managing early or mild SGS using the CO_2 laser,[56,57] generally with multiple procedures. CO_2 laser treatment was found to be effective in 92% of grade I subglottic stenosis but declined to 46% in grade II and to 13% in grade III. In order to avoid worsening of the airway it is recommended that CO_2 laser treatment be used only once if the airway lumen does not improve.[58] Endoscopic management has not been successful in the presence of the following conditions:

1. Circumferential cicatricial scarring
2. Abundant scar tissue greater than 1 cm in vertical dimension
3. Fibrotic scar tissue in the interarytenoid area of the posterior commissure
4. Severe bacterial infection of the trachea after tracheotomy
5. Exposure of perichondrium or cartilage during CO_2 excision, predisposing to perichondritis and chondritis
6. Combined laryngotracheal stenosis
7. Failure of previous endoscopic procedures
8. Significant loss of cartilaginous framework

Anterior Cricoid Split Operation

The anterior cricoid split operation (Fig. 206-5) was described in 1980 as an alternative to tracheotomy in the management of acquired SGS in premature infants.[59] The procedure has subsequently been used in the management of congenital SGS.[60] The concept is to split the cricoid and upper first and second tracheal rings in the midline anteriorly, thus allowing expansion of the cricoid ring. It is indicated in cases of congenital SGS caused by a small cricoid ring (i.e., not otherwise seriously deformed) or extensive submucosal fibrosis with healthy cricoid cartilage. It should be used only in patients whose condition is severe enough to require airway support and in whom lung function is adequate to permit decannulation. Use of auricular,[61] thyroid alar cartilage,[62] and hyoid[63] grafts has been reported to improve the success rate of the cricoid split operation. There are many factors that determine the success of the cricoid split procedure and hence the variability of its success from a low of 35% to a high of 88%.[64,65] Performing a cricoid split on a healthy infant with isolated subglottic stenosis yields the best results. Poor results occur when patients are generally sick and the airway lesion is not restricted to the subglottis.

With the patient under general endotracheal anesthesia, a horizontal skin incision is made over the cricoid to expose the cricoid and upper two tracheal rings. A single vertical incision is made through the anterior cartilaginous ring of the cricoid and through the mucosa to expose the endotracheal tube. The incision is extended inferiorly to divide the upper two tracheal rings in the midline. When the incision is made through the cricoid, the cricoid springs open, and the endotracheal tube is readily visible in the lumen. The incision in the larynx is extended superiorly in the midline to include the lower third of the thyroid cartilage to a level just inferior to the anterior commissure, but it can be extended to within 2 mm of the thyroid notch (Fig. 206-6).[66] Stay sutures of 3-0 Prolene are placed on each side of the incised cricoid. These can be used as retractors in the postoperative period if the endotracheal tube becomes dislodged and cannot be reinserted. The skin is loosely approximated around an elastic band drain. The endotracheal tube is left in place for about 7 days and acts as a stent while the mucosal swelling subsides and the split cricoid and tracheal rings heal.

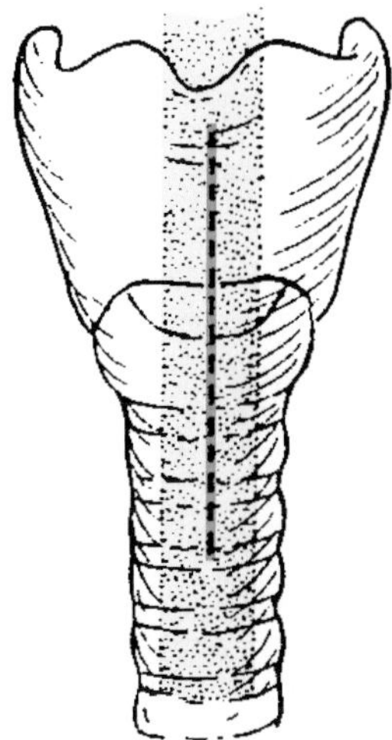

Figure 206-6. Incision for an anterior cricoid split in the management of SGS in infants (compare with Fig. 206-7.)

Endoscopy is not performed at extubation. Corticosteroids are administered before extubation and continued for 5 days.

External Expansion Surgery

Surgical reconstruction is recommended when conservative efforts to establish a satisfactory airway are inappropriate or have failed. In weighing the advantages of open reconstruction versus endoscopic management, the surgeon should consider his or her personal expertise and the severity of the lesion. In general, SGS grades III and IV lesions require external methods. Grade II may be amenable to either method. Occasionally, open surgery is required when the stenosis is of such a degree that tracheotomy has not been required.

Before surgery is performed, vocal cord paralysis should be ruled out. There should be no reason for the patient to continue to be tracheotomy-dependent despite adequate patency of the airway (e.g., presence of neurologic deficit or chronic pulmonary disease). The goal and rationale of open reconstructive surgery are to achieve early decannulation with minimal detrimental effect on the voice.

External surgical repair should be directed at the site and severity. Each case should be individualized. The two main methods of repair are resection and expansion surgery.[67-71] Expansion surgery is a collection of techniques that aim to widen the glottic and subglottic lumen. These techniques combine the use of laryngeal and cricoid splits, cartilage grafts, and stenting with success rates of higher than 90%.[72-75] Many techniques for correction of stenosis are available, but choosing the most appropriate procedure and achieving a successful outcome are problematic. Surgical repair at the youngest age possible is important for a child's speech and language development, as well as for eliminating the morbidity and mortality associated with a tracheotomy.

Combined Laryngofissure and Posterior Cricoid Division

Division of the posterior cricoid lamina through a partial laryngofissure is the method of choice for combined posterior glottic and SGS for grade II and moderate grade III. The operation is effective in patients of all ages. Cartilage grafts can augment the lumen. Scar removal is unnecessary in this procedure.

With the patient under general anesthesia administered via the tracheotomy, a horizontal skin incision is made incorporating the upper portion of the stoma (Fig. 206-7). Subplatysmal flaps are elevated superiorly and inferiorly, and the strap muscles are retracted laterally, exposing the thyroid, cricoid, and upper tracheal rings. A midline anterior incision is made in the larynx and upper trachea, extending from the superior thyroid notch to the tracheotomy site. After injection of 1% lidocaine with epinephrine 1 : 100,000 into the posterior larynx, the posterior scar and full length of the posterior lamina of the cricoid are divided, taking care to cut strictly in the midline, down to the level of the hypopharyngeal mucosa. The laryngeal scar should not be

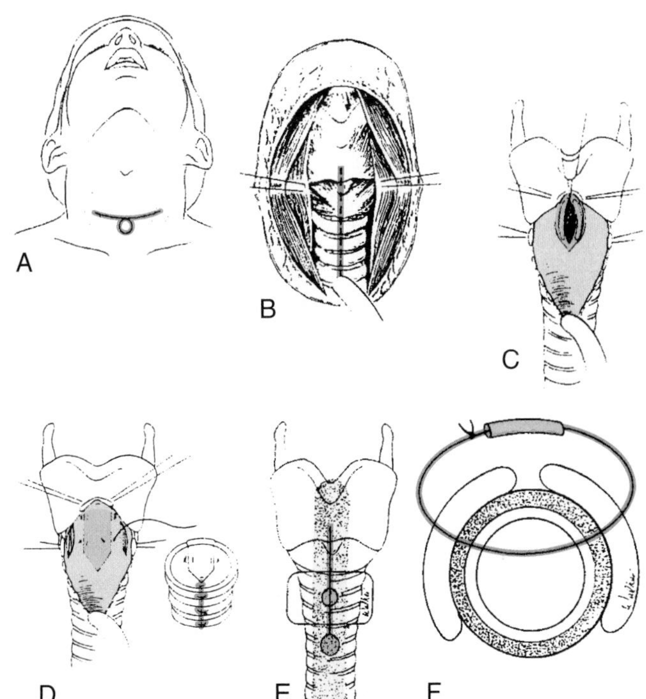

Figure 206-7. Anterior laryngofissure with division of the posterior and lateral lamina of cricoid, together with posterior cricoid cartilage graft insertion. **A,** Horizontal skin incision incorporates the superior aspect of tracheotomy. **B,** Skin flap elevated in the neck and laryngofissure. **C,** Division of the posterior lamina of the cricoid. **D,** Autogenous cartilage graft interposed posteriorly between divided ends of the cricoid lamina and sutured in place. **E,** Laryngofissure closed anteriorly with a suprastomal stent in place. **F,** Anchoring suture through suprastomal stent.

excised. The incision is carried superiorly into the interarytenoid area through the interarytenoid muscle (when fibrosed) and inferiorly for about 1 cm into the membranous tracheoesophageal septum. The divided halves of the posterior cricoid lamina are distracted laterally and an autogenous costal cartilage (see Fig. 206-7) is used to maintain separation of the divided halves of the cricoid lamina. A stent is inserted suprastomally for 2 to 6 weeks. A variety of stents is advocated and each has its own specific application. The use of stents is being replaced more and more by the use of single stage laryngoplasty. It is also advisable to avoid a complete laryngofissure so as not to disrupt the anterior commissure, which could lead to deleterious voice results.

Grafts

In children, autogenous costal cartilage is the graft material of choice, especially when there is little identifiable cricoid cartilage remaining anteriorly.[12,76,77] Because of the abundance of available costal cartilage, any length of cartilage can be obtained to graft the subglottis and trachea. Ear cartilage[75] and free thyroid cartilage graft are alternatives in special circumstances. The use of vascularized hyoid interposition techniques should be discouraged in children because the hyoid is too small to augment effectively the subglottic lumen, the bone is too hard to sculpture, and the muscle pedicle tends to ossify, causing secondary compression of the larynx. Cartilage graft survival has been proven experimentally and clinically in children and adults.[78]

Thyroid alar cartilage is excellent for use in the anterior subglottic region but is limited to grade II and few grade III lesions[79] because of its limited thickness compared to costal cartilage and inability to use it in the posterior cricoid area. Removal of the alar cartilage does not seem to cause a laryngeal deformity but no long-term follow-up is available.[80,81]

Autogenous Costal Cartilage Reconstruction

The patient is positioned in an extended neck position. The tracheotomy tube is replaced with an endotracheal tube to allow easy access to

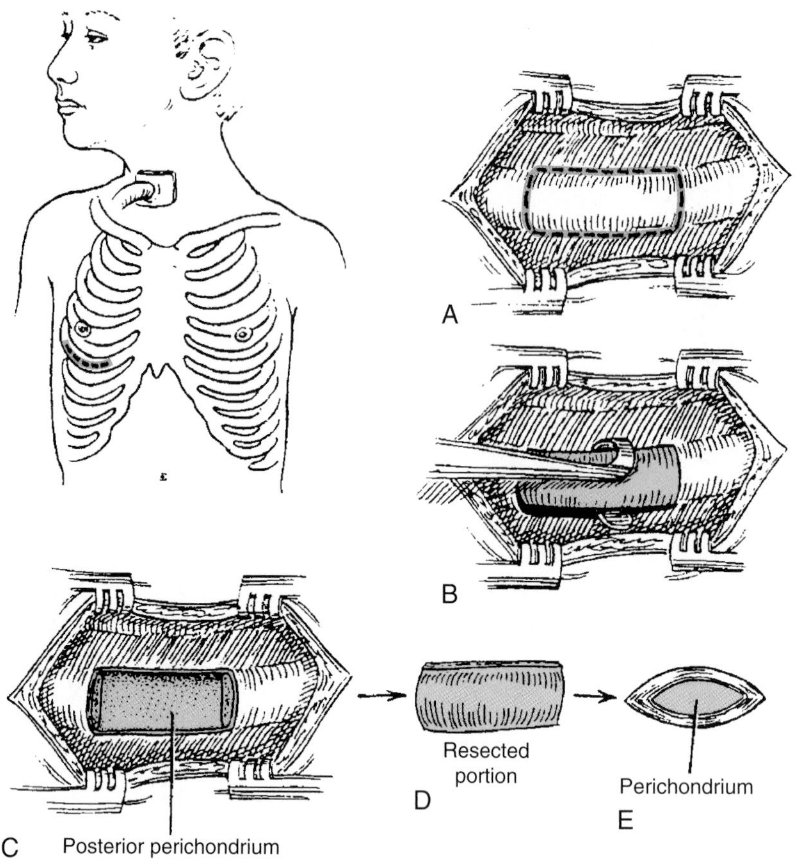

Figure 206-8. Donor site of a costal cartilage graft used for anterior augmentation of stenotic cricotracheal area. **A,** Incision over the fifth costal cartilage to obtain a costal cartilage graft. **B,** Perichondrial incisions are made along the inferior and superior borders of the rib, with care taken not to injure underlying cartilage. **C,** Dissection in the subperichondrial plane is accomplished so that the pericardium on the posterior part of the rib remains in situ on the chest wall of the patient. **D,** A 4-cm length of costal cartilage is removed and placed in physiologic saline solution. Lining perichondrium remains only on the anterior aspect of the graft. **E,** Costal cartilage graft is shaped into an ellipse and beveled to prevent the graft from settling into the lumen.

the neck and adequate anesthesia. The lower face, neck, and chest are scrubbed and draped. A 3-cm horizontal skin incision is made just inferior to the right mammary gland and is deepened to include the subcutaneous tissue and muscle. Costal cartilage is identified (Fig. 206-8), and the longest straight segment is removed with overlying lateral perichondrium, leaving the medial perichondrium in situ. The cartilage is fashioned to fit the intended site of transplantation. If the stenosis is anterior, cartilage is trimmed to a modified boat shape (see Fig. 206-8).[82] Flanges at the edges of the cartilage graft prevent prolapse into the lumen and allow maximum use of the width of the graft for distraction of the cricoid and upper trachea (Fig. 206-9). The regular boat-shaped graft is used for distraction of posteriorly cut cricoid segments in the management of posterior glottic and subglottic stenosis.[83] Indications for use of a cartilage graft in the posterior glottis and subglottis are: (1) posterior glottic or subglottic stenosis; (2) isolated subglottic shelves; and (3) circumferential SGS, when the posterior cricoid lamina has been divided. Despite suturing, creation of flanges, or both, the graft is not stable enough to remain in place and stenting is needed for several days.

A large series of posterior cartilage grafting with animal study documentation of survival of posteriorly placed cartilage grafts has been reported.[84] In cases of severe SGS, anterior and posterior grafts have yielded success rates greater than 90% after a single procedure within a short time after removal of the stent.[85,86]

Stents

Stents are used to counteract scar contractures and promote a scaffold for epithelium to cover the lumen of the airway. Stents also hold the reconstructed area in place and prevent mechanical disruption secondary to movement of the laryngotracheal complex during breathing, swallowing, and attempts at phonation. Stenting is necessary when using grafts to expand stenosed areas of the airway. Grafts provide rigidity and support and fill gaps in the incised and distracted segments to avoid the formation of fibrous tissue with subsequent contraction. If the grafts are dislodged, failure to correct the stenosis will follow.

When choosing stents, the physician should focus on the material, size, location, and duration of stenting. Many types of stents have been used and each has its own application. T-tubes continue to be used successfully in children and adults, special care is needed to avoid tube blockage.[87] Repair of laryngotracheal stenosis in almost all cases, except the anterior subglottis, requires brief stenting to keep the grafts in place and lend support to reconstructed areas. Long-term stenting is occasionally indicated.

Single-Stage Laryngotracheal Reconstruction

Single-stage laryngotracheal reconstruction (SSLTR) implies the use of cartilage grafts to obtain stability of the reconstructed airway and compress the prolonged stenting period of traditional LTR methods into a briefer period of endotracheal intubation. SSLTR may include an anterior cartilage graft, a posterior cartilage graft, or both, and often includes a cartilage graft of the former stoma site. The grafts are supported temporarily by a full-length endotracheal tube fixed in position through the nasal route. The optimal time for intubation has not been established definitively. In general, approximately 2 to 4 days of intubation are necessary for anterior cartilage grafts alone, and about 7 days are recommended if a posterior graft is used as well. A tendency exists to decrease the time of intubation with increasing age through childhood. SSLTR demands comprehensive knowledge of the principles of LTR

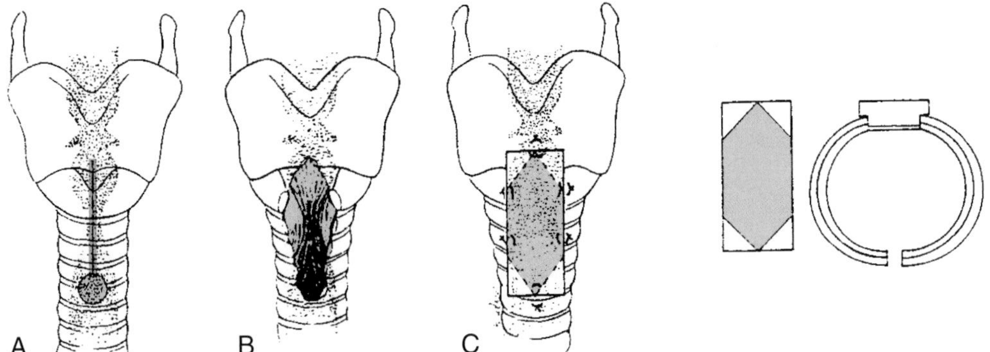

Figure 206-9. Anterior cartilage graft. **A,** Vertical incision is made into the thyroid cartilage from a point immediately below the anterior commissure through the upper tracheal rings, with care taken to remain in the midline. **B,** Intraluminal scar and lining mucosa are incised along the length of the stenotic segment. **C,** Costal cartilage is shaped into a modified boat (*inset*) and placed in position with the lining of the perichondrium facing internally.

and significant experience in the techniques. In addition, the otolaryngologist must have complete confidence in the nursing, anesthesia, and intensive care resources available at his or her institution.

SSLTR is indicated primarily in SGS without significant obstructions in the trachea or significant tracheomalacia. SSLTR may include all variations of the cricoid cartilage division and, in most cases, these divisions are stabilized by the use of a cartilage graft.

The concept of SSLTR is appealing because of the advantage of immediate decannulation or even the avoidance of tracheotomy altogether in a child who does not have a tracheotomy in place. Long-term stenting with its potential complications is also unnecessary. These advantages must be weighed against the potential for airway complications in the perioperative period, possible replacement of the tracheotomy, and complications that may arise during the intensive care required by these patients intubated for a prolonged period of time.

Certainly one requirement of SSLTR is meticulous management of the patient's condition in the ICU postoperatively. The nasotracheal airway must be maintained securely during the time of stenting without accidental extubation. Toddlers are prone to self-extubation unless carefully managed and sedated as appropriate. Older children and adults often can tolerate endotracheal intubation without any sedation.[88] Some centers use titration sedation to prevent agitation and accidental self-extubation, avoiding pharmacologic paralysis. One argument for using paralysis is that even if the patient is not accidentally extubated, motion of a nasotracheal tube in a surgical site results in poor healing. Although many variables determine success in the expansion of SGS, including preoperative grade, PR, underlying medical conditions, airway, and surgical technique, it has not been possible to quantify this particular effect. Further argument against the use of heavy sedation is the withdrawal symptoms that many children experience after cessation of the sedation drugs. The argument against pharmacologic paralysis is the necessity for immediate reintubation, should accidental extubation occur, and that postoperative pulmonary morbidity is high. These children develop migratory atelectasis, often with exacerbation of reactive airway disease or pulmonary infiltrates despite intensive pulmonary toilet, bronchodilator therapy, broad-spectrum antibiotics, and chest physiotherapy. The success of SSLTR is dependent on not only the surgical technique but also on intensive careful postoperative management.

Most surgeons exclude patients with notable craniofacial or vertebral anomalies from SSLTR to avoid a potentially difficult emergent reintubation.

SSLTR remains an excellent treatment modality for the repair of SGS in infants. It is reported that infants weighing more than 4 kg and those with a gestational age greater than 30 weeks have a greater chance for successful extubation and eventual airway patency. It appears that infants weighing fewer than 4 kg have more complications surrounding extubation. This may be because of the other underlying disease states often present in these neonates.

Cricoid Resection with Thyrotracheal Anastomosis

Surgical resection of the anterior arch of the cricoid cartilage, together with a portion of the posterior cricoid lamina below the cricothyroid articulation with thyrotracheal anastomosis, was first suggested in 1953[89] and resurgence of this procedure in adults[90-93] encouraged use in children. Several authors report good results.[60,88,109] In children with isolated tracheal stenosis, repair with resection and end-to-end anastomosis yields excellent results.[94] When the stenosis involves the subglottis, the resection becomes technically difficult, but excellent results have been reported by several authors.[67,95-100] The procedure is applicable to the few patients in grades III and IV SGS. Arytenoid prolapse has been described as a complication in children[101] but not in adults.[102] Several reports favor CTR over LTR for grade 4 stenosis.[68,69] The current recommended strategy is to perform partial cricotracheal resection (PCTR) as a primary or salvage procedure in patients with grades III and grade IV stenosis.[102] Risk factors for failure are presence of unilateral or bilateral vocal cord paralysis.[103] Cricotracheal resection has been reported in children weighing less than 10 kg with excellent results.[104] No deleterious effects on laryngeal growth or function have been observed in humans.[105] In cases where the margins for resection are close to the vocal cords especially posteriorly, PCTR with grafting is indicated. It is very important not to resect a significant portion of the posterior cricoid plate, since animal studies have shown airway impairment in such cases. Vertical posterior cricoid laminotomy is safe.[106] The partial cricotracheal resection procedure has eliminated the need for four-quadrant cricoid division which still is an excellent procedure with good results in some cases.[107]

With the patient under general anesthesia through the tracheotomy, the larynx and upper airway are dissected and identified. The dissection is performed on the cricoid in a subperichondrial plane to avoid injury to the recurrent laryngeal nerve. The superior resection line starts at the inferior border of the thyroid cartilage and passes obliquely posteroinferiorly to cross the lower margin of the cricoid plate below the level of the cricothyroid joints (Fig. 206-10). The distal resection line is made immediately below the inferior border of the stenosis. To compensate for the disparity in the diameters between the tracheal and subglottic lumen, the superior cut of the tracheal lumen is beveled, and the membranous trachea may need to be plicated. Primary thyrotracheal anastomosis is accomplished by advancement of the distal segment superanteriorly to the residual posterior shell of the cricoid cartilage and suturing a tongue of mucosa from the posterior trachea to the remaining laryngeal mucosa. Cartilage sutures are then placed at the anastomosis, which should be kept free of tension. This is best accomplished by suprahyoid laryngeal mobilization and tension-relieving sutures in the cartilage. After surgery, extension of the neck is to be avoided for 10 days by placing three sutures from the chin to the upper chest area. Stenting is generally used either with an endotracheal tube (single-stage technique), a T-tube, or a suprastomal stent.

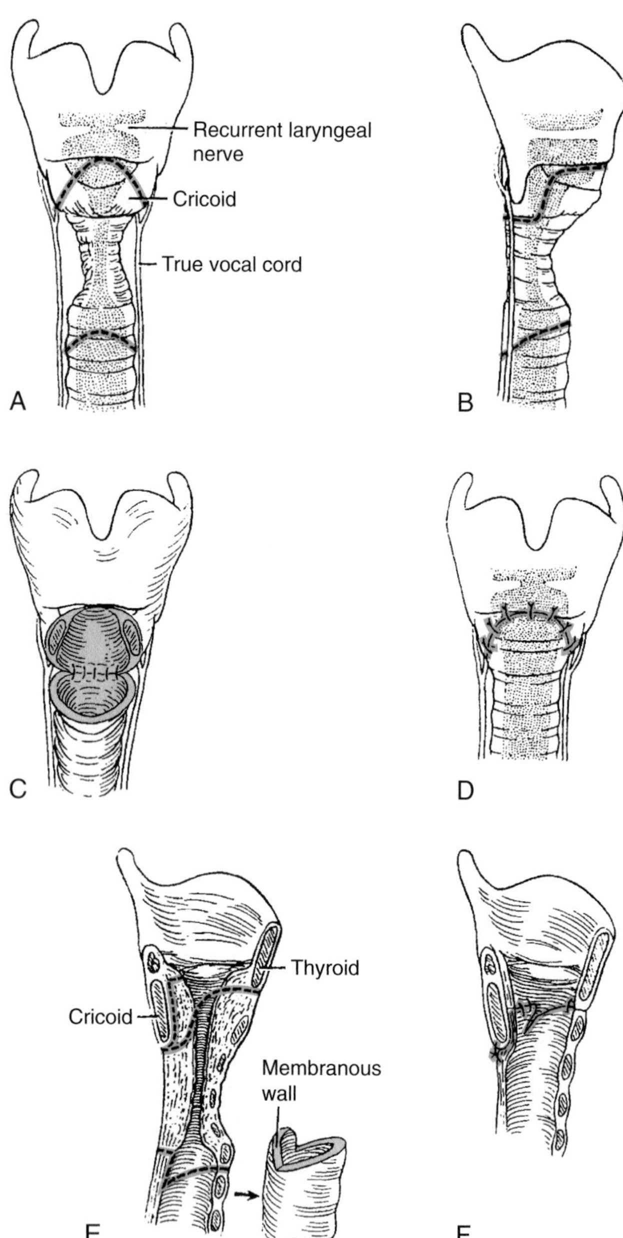

Figure 206-10. Partial cricoid resection with thyrotracheal anastomosis. **A,** Anterior view of the stenotic area to be resected, including the anterior cricoid lamina. **B,** Lateral view of the same area. Note the preservation of the posterior cricoid lamina and the location of the recurrent laryngeal nerve. **C,** After resection. The trachea is beveled and approximated to the subglottis. **D,** Suturing is completed (3-0 polyglactin 910). **E,** If a posterior subglottic thick scar is present, it is resected with preservation of the posterior cricoid cartilage, and a mucosal flap is developed from the posterior tracheal wall. **F,** Suturing of the mucosal flap is performed, and coverage of raw areas is achieved.

Management of Specific Disorders

Congenital

Atresia and Webs

The immediate management of laryngeal atresia is by establishing an airway at birth through an emergency tracheotomy. Rarely, it may be possible to pass a small bronchoscope through an incomplete atresia into the trachea, followed by a tracheotomy. It is extremely difficult to insert a large-bore needle into the highly mobile trachea of infants, and a neck incision with tracheotomy is the preferable method of establishing an emergency airway. Occasionally, tracheal agenesis coexists. After adequate airway is maintained, the elective surgical correction of laryngeal atresia generally restores respiratory function, but the phonatory and protective functions may remain significantly impaired after surgery.

Treatment of laryngeal webs depends on the thickness of the web.[3] A thin web may be broken down by passage of the bronchoscope or incised with a surgical knife, scissors, or the CO_2 laser. An attempt should be made to incise the web along one vocal cord, followed 2 weeks later by incision along the opposite side (to prevent further web formation). However, the smaller the larynx, the more difficult this is to achieve.

The less common thick glottic webs are more difficult to manage, and may be difficult or impossible to incise or dilate because of the associated subglottic-cricoid abnormality.

Tracheotomy may be required to establish the airway. Surgical excision of the glottic web and cartilaginous abnormality via a laryngofissure approach, followed by stenting and placement of an anterior autogenous costal cartilage graft, can be performed in a single or double stage.[108,109] The optimum age for surgery is unknown, and the possibility of aggravating the situation with an ill-judged operation should be considered. However, infants with severe obstruction above the tracheotomy are at greater risk of dying of cannula obstruction because of their decreased reserve airway above the tracheotomy. In such cases, earlier reconstruction should be considered. Endoscopic placement of a keel in children is difficult, and the external approach is recommended for best results.

Anterior Glottic Stenosis

Small anterior webs less than 2- to 3-mm wide produce minimal or no symptoms, and surgery is usually unnecessary. Thin anterior webs can be managed by microendoscopic incision of the web with a microsurgical knife or CO_2 laser. A keel may be placed endoscopically[110]; however, if this technique fails or if longer, thick anterior glottic scars are present, an external approach is needed. Tracheotomy is performed, followed by laryngofissure and incision of the stenotic area or web with the surgical knife. Resection of scar tissue should be minimized because this creates further mucosal loss. The umbrella keel gives reliable results and should be inserted for 2 weeks. The keel prevents restenosis in the anterior commissure during reepithelialization. If the keel is used for 2 weeks or fewer, granulation tissue formation is minimal. The design of the keel is such that contact with the posterior glottis is avoided, thus minimizing scarring secondary to the keel itself.

Stenosis and Vocal Cord Paralysis

Vocal cord paralysis can accompany anterior, posterior, or complete glottic stenosis. Bilateral vocal cord paralysis, associated with acquired glottic stenosis, needs a partial arytenoidectomy with lateralization of the true cord in addition to the operation discussed earlier in this chapter for correction of glottic stenosis. This is generally required unilaterally and occasionally bilaterally. Arytenoidectomy is reliably performed through the anterior thyrotomy approach. If done as a separate and later operation, an endoscopic laser arytenoidectomy is a valid alternative.[111] Arytenoid separation has been reported to be helpful.[112]

Posterior Glottic Stenosis

Management of posterior glottic stenosis varies with the degree of pathologic findings.[113] A simple interarytenoid adhesion requires a different approach from scarring involving both cricoarytenoid joints (see Fig. 206-4). It is a major challenge because the voice is generally excellent. Children with Down syndrome have a higher rate of posterior glottic stenosis than the general population.[114] Endoscopic division of the adhesion is sufficient if a mucosally lined sinus tract is present posteriorly. This is easily accomplished with a microsurgical knife while the posterior surface of the mucosally lined sinus is protected by inserting a microsuction tip. In the absence of a mucosally lined sinus tract, simple endoscopic incision of the scar results in restenosis. Partial laryngofissure, however, is the most common approach for such cases and is required for more advanced cases with cricoarytenoid joint fixation. Endoscopic posterior cricoid split with grafting is another approach for repair.[115]

In children with severe posterior glottic scarring with cricoarytenoid joint fixation or subglottic extension, a division of the posterior cricoid lamina in the midline with insertion of a free autogenous costal cartilage graft (see Fig. 206-7) is recommended.[83,116] Complete glottic stenosis is difficult to manage, and voice results are usually poor because of severe scarring involving the vocal cords. Also, it may be associated with a decrease in the anteroposterior diameter of the larynx secondary to external trauma. Management involves incising the scar in an anteroposterior manner, posterior cartilage grafting, and placing a stent. Cartilage grafts should not be used in the anterior commissure area.

Anterior Subglottic Stenosis

Anterior subglottic stenosis is managed by incising the scar anteriorly and placing a modified boat-shaped cartilage graft[82] (see Fig. 206-9) to keep the segments of the cricoid distracted. The perichondrium of the graft should be at the level of the mucosa. At the end of the procedure, endoscopic examination of the subglottic airway is recommended to check for possible poor placement or partial collapse of the graft. The cartilage graft can usually be extended inferiorly to cover the tracheostomy if a single stage is planned.

Endotracheal intubation after a single-stage laryngotracheoplasty can range from 2 days for simple anterior cartilage[117] grafting to 2 weeks for moderately severe stenosis repaired with anterior and posterior grafts.[118]

Postoperative Management

Postoperative management[119] is affected by whether a stent was used. In patients in whom stents were not used, antibiotics for 2 weeks after the surgery are recommended and endoscopy is indicated once the patient is ready for decannulation. When stenting has been used, long-term, low-dose antibiotics are recommended for the duration of stenting to prevent infection. Appropriate tracheotomy care is extremely important. The caregiver should be proficient and knowledgeable about routine and emergency care because the control of GER is important.

Decannulation

The tracheotomy tube is gradually downsized and eventually plugged. Children should always be under adult supervision.[120] Once a child is ready for decannulation, endoscopy should be performed to ensure the airway is clear and the factors that influence successful decannulation after surgery have been well described. Occasionally suprastomal granulomas are seen. If the child is being considered for decannulation, these granulomas should be removed; however, if the child is not ready for decannulation, removal of suprastomal granulomas is not indicated unless they are completely obstructing the airway.[121]

The presence of suprastomal collapse can prevent decannulation, and further management may be needed.[122] When the child can tolerate the tracheotomy plugging for as long as he or she is awake, the decision for decannulation is made and the child is admitted to the hospital where the tracheotomy is plugged overnight with continuous monitoring. If there is no oxygen desaturation or apnea, the tracheotomy tube is removed the following morning, the stoma is covered with an occlusive dressing, and the child is kept for an additional night, again with continuous monitoring. Tracheotomy tube fenestration is not performed. A residual tracheocutaneous fistula may need to be surgically closed.

Summary

Glottic and subglottic stenosis, although rare, are difficult to manage. Surgical goals are to produce as early as possible[123] an adequate airway, an acceptable voice, and a competent larynx to avoid aspiration. The keys to successful outcome depend on (1) accurate preoperative and intraoperative assessment; (2) correct choice of surgical procedure; (3) meticulous surgery directed at the site of the lesion; and (4) close postoperative care and monitoring.

SUGGESTED READINGS

Bailey M, Hoeve H, Monnier P. Pediatric laryngatracheal stenosis: a consensus paper from three European centres. *Eur Arch Otorhinolaryngol.* 2003; 260(3):118-123.

Choi SS, Zalzal GH. Changing trends in neonatal subglottic stenosis. *Otolaryngol Head Neck Surg.* 2000;122:61.

Choi SS, Zalzal GH. Pitfalls in laryngotracheal reconstruction. *Arch Otolaryngol Head Neck Surg.* 1999;125:650.

Cotton RT. The problem of pediatric laryngotracheal stenosis: a clinical and experimental study on the efficacy of autogenous cartilaginous grafts placed between the vertically divided halves of the posterior lamina of the cricoid cartilage. *Laryngoscope.* 1991;12:1.

Forte V, Chang MB, Papsin BC. Thyroid alar cartilage reconstruction in neonatal subglottic stenosis as a replacement for the anterior cricoid split. *Int J Pediatr Otorhinolaryngol.* 2001;59:181.

Garabedian EN, Nicollas R, Roger G, et al. Cricotracheal resection in children weighing less than 10 kg. *Arch Otolayngol Head Neck Surg.* 2005;131(6):505-508.

Hartley BE, Gustafson LM, Liu JH, et al. Duration of stenting in single-stage laryngotracheal reconstruction with anterior costal cartilage grafts. *Ann Otol Rhinol Laryngol.* 2001;110:413.

Hueman GM, Simpson CB. Airway complications from topical mitomycin C. *Otolaryngol Head Neck Surg.* 2005;133:831.

Jacobs BR, Salman BA, Cotton RT, et al. Postoperative management of children after single-stage laryngotracheal reconstruction. *Critical Care Med.* 2001; 29(1):164-168.

Jauet Y, Lang F, Pulloud R, et al. Partial cricotracheal resection for pediatric subglottic stenosis: long-term outcome in 57 patients. *J Thorac Cardiovasc Surg.* 2005;130(3):726-732.

McArthur CJ, Kearns GH, Healy GD. Voice quality after laryngotracheal reconstruction. *Arch Otolaryngol Head Neck Surg.* 1994;120:641.

Monnier P, George M, Monod ML, et al. The role of the CO_2 laser in the management of laryngotracheal stenosis: a survey of 100 cases. *Eur Arch Otorhinolaryngol.* 2005;262:602-608.

Myer CM III, O'Connor DM, Cotton RT. Proposed grading system for subglottic stenosis based on endotracheal tube sizes. *Ann Otol Rhinol Laryngol.* 1994;103:319.

Richardson MA, Inglis AF Jr. A comparison of anterior cricoid split with and without costal cartilage graft for acquired subglottic stenosis. *Int J Pediatr Otolaryngol.* 1991;22:187.

Rutter MJ, Cotton RT. The use of posterior cricoid grafting in managing isolated posterior glottic stenosis in children. *Arch Otolaryngol Head Neck Surg.* 2004;130(6):737-739.

Rutter MJ, Hartley BE, Cotton RT. Cricotracheal resection in children. *Arch Otolaryngol Head Neck Surg.* 2001;127:382.

Seid AB, Pransky SM, Kearns DB. One stage laryngotracheoplasty. *Arch Otolaryngol Head Neck Surg.* 1991;117:408.

Silva AB, Lusk RP, Muntz HR. Update on the use of auricular cartilage in laryngotracheal reconstruction. *Ann Otol Rhinol Laryngol.* 2000;109:343.

Triglia J, Nicollas R, Roman S, et al. Cricotracheal resection in children: indications, technique and results. *Ann Otolaryngol Chir Cervicofac.* 2000;117:155.

Wyatt ME, Hartley BE. Laryngotracheal reconstruction in congenital laryngeal webs and atresias. *Otolaryngol Head Neck Surg.* 2005;132(2):232-238.

Zalzal GH. Stenting for pediatric laryngotracheal stenosis. *Ann Otol Rhinol Laryngol.* 1992;101:651.

Zalzal GH. Treatment of laryngotracheal stenosis with anterior and posterior cartilage grafts: a report of 41 children. *Arch Otolaryngol Head Neck Surg.* 1993;119:82.

Zalzal GH, Choi SS, Patel KM. The effect of gastroesophageal reflux on laryngotracheal reconstruction. *Arch Otolaryngol Head Neck Surg.* 1996;122:297.

Zalzal GH, Loomis SR, Fischer M. Laryngeal reconstruction in children: assessment of vocal quality. *Arch Otolaryngol Head Neck Surg.* 1993;119:504.

Zalzal GH. Rib cartilage grafts for the treatment of posterior glottic and subglottic stenosis in children. *Ann Otol Rhinol Laryngol.* 1988;97:506.

For complete list of references log onto www.expertconsult.com.

CHAPTER TWO HUNDRED AND SEVEN

Diagnosis and Management of Tracheal Anomalies and Tracheal Stenosis

Greg R. Licameli

Mark A. Richardson

Key Points

- The management and diagnosis of tracheomalacia and tracheal stenosis is complex and has evolved over the last two decades as experience grows with this condition.
- This chapter addresses tracheomalacia, congenital tracheal stenosis, and the management of tracheal stenosis with various surgical techniques.

The diagnosis and surgical management of tracheal stenosis, whether acquired or congenital, remains a challenge. In infants and children, tracheal stenosis has a high morbidity and mortality, particularly for those with severe disease, and is often associated with other congenital anomalies that require concomitant repair. Over the past 2 decades, certain principles of management have been developed that have improved patient outcomes. The evaluation and development of a logical management plan for these complex cases often requires the involvement of multiple medical specialties.

Embryology

The trachea develops as an evagination of foregut mesenchyme in the fourth week of gestation. This gradually expands caudally to form the developing lungs and joins together posteriorly to form the common membranous wall of the esophagus and trachea. Initially, this evagination has an extensive communication with the ventrocaudal part of the pharynx. From this primordial outgrowth, the trachea extends caudad ventral to and roughly parallel with the esophagus. Only the epithelial lining and the glands of the trachea are derived from the original entodermal outgrowth from the pharynx. The cartilage, connective tissue, and muscle of its wall are formed by mesenchymal cells that migrate to become massed around the growing entodermal tube. Usually by the ninth week, developing cartilaginous rings can be identified.

Tracheomalacia

Tracheomalacia, which is the absence or deformity of the tracheal cartilage, can present with inspiratory and expiratory stridor, wheezing (which may be mistaken for asthma), chronic cough, and recurrent respiratory infections. It may be subdivided into two categories: primary tracheomalacia, which is an intrinsic deformity of the tracheal cartilage in the absence of any other pathology, and secondary tracheomalacia, which is due to extrinsic compression, most commonly related to cardiac or vascular anomalies, as well as tracheoesophageal fistula.[1,2]

The symptoms of primary tracheomalacia tend to improve as the child's tracheobronchial tree grows in caliber, and surgical intervention is often not required. This condition occurs in both premature and mature infants. In contrast, the causes of secondary tracheomalacia usually require surgical correction to remove the cause of the compression and subsequently to assess the residual tracheal wall integrity.

Vascular Anomalies—Vascular Rings

Vascular rings are the result of abnormal development of the aortic arch complex. The most common complete vascular ring is a double aortic arch, in which the ascending aorta bifurcates to encase both the trachea and esophagus as it joins the descending aorta. Symptoms begin early in childhood and are related to both respiration and feeding. A barium swallow study shows a posterior compression of the esophagus.

A second but less common vascular ring arises from the persistence of the right aortic arch, with a left ligamentum arteriosum usually associated with a retroesophageal left subclavian artery, or less commonly, mirror branching of the right and left subclavian and common carotid arteries, and may present with similar symptoms as a double aortic arch.[3]

Surgical division of the ring immediately improves symptoms related to swallowing; however, symptoms related to the associated tracheal deformity may take some time to resolve as the patient grows.

Vascular Anomalies—Arterial Compression

The most common cause of vascular compression of the trachea is from an anomalous innominate artery compression. A more distal origin of the innominate artery from the aorta causes compression of the right anterior trachea that endoscopically demonstrates a triangular-shaped

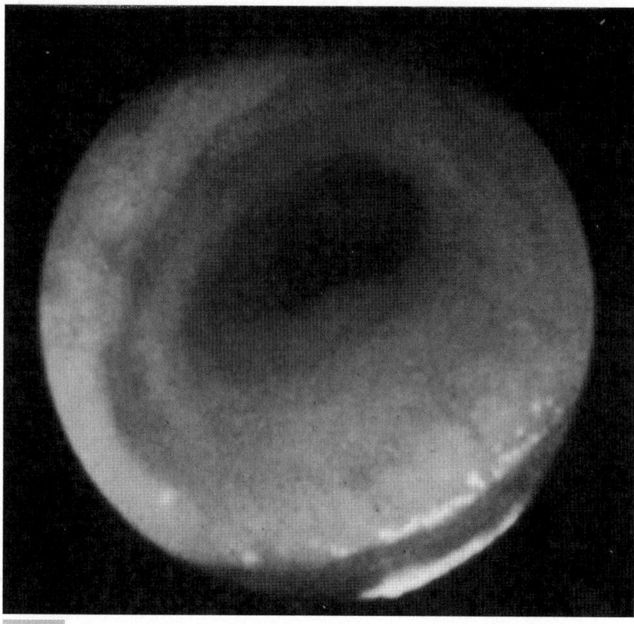

Figure 207-1. Long-segment tracheal stenosis (complete rings).

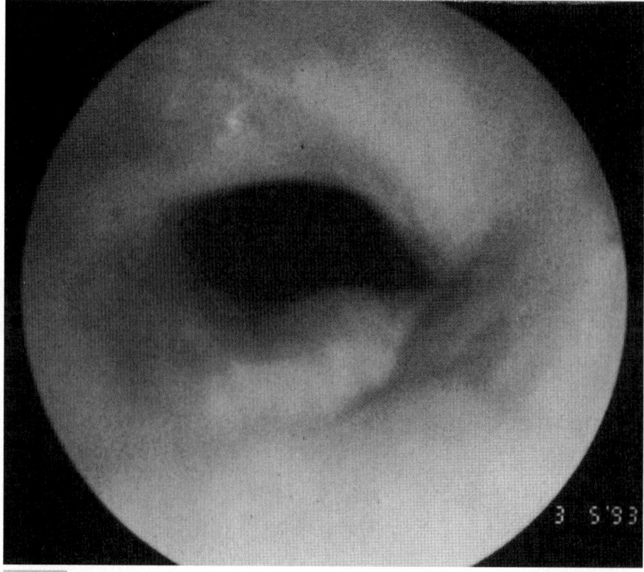

Figure 207-2. Short-segment tracheal stenosis.

deformity. Lifting the tip of the bronchoscope against the artery diminishes the right brachial pulse. Chest radiographs show anterior tracheal compression but no esophageal deformity.[3] Often these patients present with inspiratory or biphasic stridor, cough, recurrent respiratory infections and reflex apnea, with the latter often referred to as "dying spells."[4]

Pulmonary artery anomalies can also cause tracheal compression. In this situation, the aberrant left pulmonary artery arises on the right and passes between the esophagus and trachea, causing compression of the trachea and right bronchus, which is seen on endoscopy. Division of the artery with reanastomosis improves symptoms of stridor and wheezing.[5]

Other tracheal pathologies (e.g., congenital tracheal enlargement, cysts, abnormal tracheal bifurcation) are also in the differential diagnosis for congenital anomalies of the tracheobronchial tree.

Tracheoesophageal Fistula

Tracheoesophageal fistula is a common congenital abnormality, presenting at birth with respiratory distress, excessive mucus, feeding difficulties, and aspiration. It is often associated with tracheomalacia.[6] Five types have been described, with the most common abnormality occurring with the proximal esophagus ending in a blind pouch and the lower esophagus connected to the trachea via a fistula. The majority of cases are diagnosed by the inability to pass a catheter orally into the stomach.[7] Severe aspiration can occur with the use of radiologic contrast studies; therefore its use is controversial. Endoscopic examination is critical in the evaluation and planning of surgical intervention.[8] One half of all patients have congenital anomalies of other organ systems, including cardiac, genitourinary, and gastrointestinal abnormalities. A small percentage of patients have an intact esophageal lumen with a small connection to the trachea, known as an *H-type fistula.* These patients are usually less dramatically affected and diagnosis may be defied for months. Careful investigation with both contrast radiography and endoscopy is required to identify the small connection from the upper posterior trachea to the esophagus.[9]

Diagnosis

The severity of tracheal stenosis usually determines the age of presentation, which can be quite variable, ranging from days to weeks or even months. A long-segment stenosis with a markedly limited tracheal diameter would ordinarily present in early infancy with evidence of respiratory obstruction, especially when the airway may be compromised by secretions or infection, which produce additional incremental difficulties in adequate respiration (Fig. 207-1). Shorter segments, with a more moderate degree of obstruction in terms of tracheal diameter, may appear later in infancy or early childhood when the increasing respiratory demands of growing infants outstrip the capacity of the narrow airway to provide adequate levels of air and gas exchange (Fig. 207-2).

Any child who is being considered for bronchoscopy and who has atypical asthma, inspiratory and expiratory stridor, and recurrent respiratory disease should also have a potential diagnosis of tracheal stenosis. Poor weight gain and sometimes poor feeding are also associated with tracheal stenosis. Chest radiography may be helpful but is often nondiagnostic due to the dynamic aspects of the pediatric trachea. In some cases, however, a suggestion of the stenosis can be evident on close examination of the radiograph. A minority of patients with congenital tracheal stenosis present without any associated malformations and a careful assessment of particularly the cardiac vasculature is required.[10]

Endoscopy

Endoscopic evaluation with a rigid bronchoscope is clearly the most accurate means of diagnosing tracheal stenosis and assessing its length, degree, and character. Due to the limited diameter of the trachea, however, endoscopy must be approached expertly and with full availability of the smallest equipment possible. In some cases, placement of an endotracheal tube through the larynx to the level of the stenosis may cause a loss of ventilatory capability as a result of obstruction of the tube at the site of the stenosis. Additionally, even the smallest bronchoscope (4-mm outer diameter) might not pass through the stenosis and, in some cases, placement of a rigid bronchoscope for ventilation and the use of the longer rigid telescope (2.5-mm outer diameter) or ultra-thin flexible bronchoscope (2-mm outer diameter) might be the only means of visualization of the length of the stenosis and identification of any distal abnormalities in the tracheobronchial tree.

Endoscopic evaluation of the airway performed with rigid instrumentation and with the patient under general anesthesia is, however, accompanied by the greatest risk and requires skill in performing anesthesia, expert endoscopic skills, and a full complement of pediatric endoscopic instruments and photographic documentation capability. Minor trauma to the mucosa could precipitate an obstructive event. Once the patient has been given general anesthesia, additional anesthesia can be administered by applying lidocaine topically to the tracheal mucosa. Ideally the patient can maintain spontaneous ventilation, so that the adequacy of neuromuscular movement in the larynx can be assessed. It is generally wise to use the telescope as an initial form of evaluation without the accompanying bronchoscope for tracheoscopy to determine whether there is a significant stenosis and to identify its approximate location and the nature of the tracheal rings (i.e., whether they are complete or incomplete). In some cases, even the smallest 2.5-mm pediatric bronchoscope (4-mm outer diameter) will not pass through the stricture, and again, the bronchoscopic telescope might be the only instrument able to pass through the stenosis to visualize the carina and distal bronchi. The patient must be hyperventilated for such an examination to be possible, but in so doing the length of the trachea affected can be gauged and a potential surgical procedure designed.

The length of the stenotic segment should always be estimated during the course of endoscopy as well as the degree of involvement of the trachea and the main bronchi, and is frequently underestimated. The determination whether a tracheal stenosis is congenital or acquired is an important one. Commonly, the congenital stenotic tracheal segment is associated with a somewhat longer trachea than the native and normal trachea of newborns. Congenital problems are often associated with other abnormalities of vascular structure and genetic defects. Acquired stenoses are accompanied by irregular scarring, perichondritis, and loss of cartilaginous support, which complicate surgical resection and reanastomosis.

Radiology

Computed tomography (CT) and magnetic resonance imaging (MRI) provide accurate evaluations of the airway, with MR images having a slight edge in depicting finer detail and the actual nature of the stenosis. There is an inherent risk for infants and children, who may require sedation or general anesthesia before examination.

Because some cases of congenital tracheal stenosis are often associated with a vascular ring or pulmonary artery sling, some means of determining whether there are abnormalities in the great vessels of the heart should be performed. Echocardiography or MRI might be satisfactory in some cases, although arteriography or heart catheterization may be necessary to fully identify or rule out the possibility of aberrant vasculature.

If additional information must be obtained, contrast bronchography can be performed with a thin solution of contrast material to outline the tracheal dimensions and bronchial branchings. This contrast material must be thinned because the secretions themselves and inflammation—which is sometimes stimulated by the contrast—can cause significant problems in ventilation for the patient. Despite the inherent danger in contrast bronchography, it does provide a measurable evaluation of long-segment tracheal stenosis and any accompanying bronchial abnormalities, which are often seen in congenital stenoses. There is increasing evidence that bronchography and angiography is being supplanted by spiral CT with multiplanar reconstruction and MRI.[11]

Advances in CT/MRI have allowed for fine detail three-dimensional reconstructions to provide a virtual endoscopy of the airway. It is limited by not being able to provide a dynamic assessment of either tracheomalacia or bronchomalacia, may not provide enough resolution to define subtle anatomic abnormalities, and can underestimate the degree and extent of the narrowing.[12] It has the advantages of being able to evaluate the airway distal to a stenosis that cannot be traversed by bronchoscopy and can be used in the measurement of the airway caliber over time. It should be considered as a complementary technique to formal rigid or flexible endoscopy in selected patients.[13]

Associated Anomalies

Congenital tracheal stenosis is often associated with other developmental anomalies. Cardiovascular anomalies are the most common, occurring in up to one half of cases, and include patent ductus arteriosus, ventricular septal defects, left pulmonary artery sling, aberrant subclavian artery, and double aortic arch.[10] Anomalies of the bronchopulmonary, gastrointestinal, renal, or skeletal systems should also be sought. Several authors believe that the simultaneous repair of both tracheal and cardiac defects provides better postoperative management and long-term outcomes.[14,15]

Louksnov and colleagues thought that a key element to achieving a 97% survival rate in 37 patients who underwent surgical repair was the use of cardiopulmonary bypass, which allowed them extensive mobilization of the tracheobronchial tree and a tension-free anastomosis,[14] as well as better exposure of the operative field.[16]

Table 207-1

Cantrell and Guild Structural Classification

Type 1	Generalized hypoplasia of the entire trachea
Type 2	Funnel stenosis—normal proximal trachea with distal narrowing to carina
Type 3	Segmental stenosis with up to three rings involved

Data from Cantrell JR, Guild H. Congenital stenosis of the trachea. *Am J Surg.* 1964;108:297-305.

Table 207-2

Anton-Pacheco Functional Classification

Type: Mild	None or occasional symptoms
Type: Moderate	Respiratory symptoms without respiratory compromise
Type: Severe	Respiratory compromise
Subtype A	No other associated malformations
Subtype B	Associated malformations

Data from Anton-Pacheco J, et al. Patterns of management of congenital tracheal stenosis. *J Pediatr Surg.* 2003;38:1452-1458.

Classification

Congenital tracheal stenosis was originally classified based on anatomic morphologies as described by Cantrell and Guild,[17] and was augmented by the development of a clinical symptom classification by Anton-Pacheco.[11] These complementary approaches allow better correlation of anatomic findings with patient symptoms, important for surgical planning and outcome (Tables 207-1 and 207-2).

Surgery

Surgery for tracheal stenosis can be categorized generally in the following ways: (1) conservative management; (2) endoscopic, using laser or dilation; (3) resection and reanastomosis, including slide tracheoplasty; or (4) augmentative procedures using cartilage, perichondrium, or vascularized tissue.

Conservative Management

The role of conservative or nonsurgical management of congenital tracheal stenosis has recently been better defined. Historically, patients were treated conservatively because of poor surgical outcomes. There is increasing evidence that a carefully selected group of patients with congenital tracheal stenosis will resolve their difficulties with growth of the airway. This is largely due to the fact that tracheal airflow is proportional to the fourth power of the radius of the trachea. Patients with mild stenosis and occasional symptoms can be managed with respiratory physiotherapy, antibiotics in case of infection, supplemental oxygen, and close observation.[11,18] Rutter and colleagues described seven patients with complete tracheal rings who did not require surgical intervention.[19]

Cheng and colleagues reported their experience with 22 consecutive patients, 11 who underwent surgery and 11 who were followed nonsurgically. Initial diagnosis was made with bronchoscopy and supported by radiologic and clinical findings. The patients who were observed later (1.5 vs 0.4 years), were less symptomatic, had less severe tracheal narrowing (58% vs 30% of normal tracheal diameter), and had a lower mortality than the surgical group. Six of the 11 patients in the observation group underwent serial CT measurements of the tracheal diameter. These data showed that five of six patients experienced an increased rate of tracheal growth compared with normal pediatric tracheal growth until approximately 7.5 years of age, when it then grew at a normal rate. The researchers suggested conservative management if the stenosis was not long segment and if the most stenotic segment was less than 60% of the normal trachea.[18]

Surgical management broadly involves two modalities: endoscopic tracheoplasty and open tracheal reconstruction. Endoscopic options include tracheal dilation, intraluminal stent placement, and laser ablation. Biopsies can be performed if there is suspicion of systemic disease such as amyloidosis or sarcoidosis. Open tracheal reconstruction can include the use of autologous, homologous, or inert stenting material to enlarge the airway diameter or to remove stenotic segments. The morbidity of an endoscopic approach is less than that of an open procedure but often involves repeated surgery. Selection of a therapeutic approach depends on the type of airway anomaly and can involve a variety of endoscopic modalities either alone or combined with an open approach to the trachea.

Dilation

Dilation of strictures has traditionally been performed with Jackson or Maloney rigid dilators. This method involves serial dilation with progressively larger-diameter bougies but has a tendency to shear tissue, which may create more scarring and further stricture formation.[20] In comparison, balloon tracheoplasty imparts only radial forces to the lesion and is less traumatic to the surrounding tissues. Balloon devices range from catheters developed for percutaneous transluminal angioplasty to specially designed balloons that fit over the tip of a rigid bronchoscope. Balloon-tipped catheters are connected to an inline pressure gauge and a water-filled syringe that delivers a steady, constant dilation. Serial dilation is performed with increasingly larger balloons. Balloon-tipped catheters can also be placed under radiologic guidance to confirm placement (Fig. 207-3).[21]

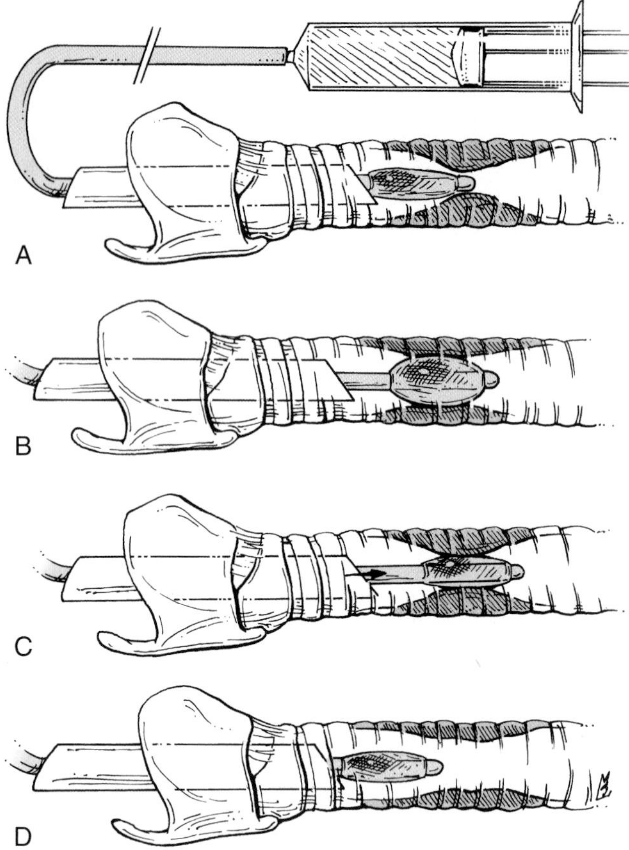

Figure 207-3. Pneumatic dilation of short-segment, acquired stenosis. Balloon insertion **(A)** and inflation **(B)**, reduction of stenosis **(C)**, and balloon deflation and removal **(D)**.

A 15-year experience of balloon tracheoplasty in 37 patients was reported by Hebra and associates.[20] Short-term improvement for both congenital and acquired lesions was seen in 90% of patients, with long-term improvement in 54%. Complications were infrequent and included tracheitis, atelectasis, and pneumomediastinum. This method appears to be most useful in the management of soft granulation tissue or to aid in delaying open reconstruction in premature or medically unstable infants.

Messino and colleagues[22] and Bag and associates[23] have described aggressive balloon dilation of complete tracheal rings with endotracheal stenting in children younger than 2 years of age. The posterior wall of a complete ring is the weakest point, as demonstrated by their postmortem studies, and allows disruption of the trachea with subsequent fibrotic healing. This method should be reserved for critically ill patients because complications can be life threatening.

Laser Therapy

Laser therapy is often combined with dilation procedures in the endoscopic management of tracheal strictures or obstructing masses. Use of the laser allows precise tissue ablation with less trauma to the surrounding tissue compared with cryosurgery and electrocautery.[24] Early reports described the use of the carbon dioxide laser with a bronchoscopic coupler and a rigid bronchoscope to manage tracheal lesions.[25] With the development of improved optics and laser micromanipulators mounted directly to the microscope, visualization and precision have improved. Lesions most amenable to this technique are soft granulation and short segments of mature fibrosis. Simpson and others[24] and Ossoff and associates[26,27] listed the following factors as contributing to laser therapy failure: circumferential scarring, fibrosis greater than 1 cm in vertical length, tracheomalacia, and severe bacterial infection in the presence of a tracheostomy.

A method using radial incisions and dilation with a rigid bronchoscope for moderate to severe subglottic and tracheal stenosis was described by Shapshay and coworkers.[28] Success was attributed to the preservation of islands of epithelium between the radial incisions. Results were good at 1-year follow-up (Fig. 207-4). Mucosal preservation was also advocated by Dedo and Sooy,[29] who described the use of the carbon dioxide laser in the elevation of mucosal flaps. An incision is made into the superior surface of the scar, creating a trapdoor flap, and the underlying fibrous tissue is ablated with the laser with replacement of the mucosal flap (Fig. 207-5). Success with these techniques appears to be dependent on reepithelialization before scar formation, avoidance of extensive tissue damage, preservation of mucosa, and careful patient selection.

Intralesional and systemic corticosteroids have been suggested by some authors to aid in the prevention of scar formation and stenosis at the site of mucosal injury. However, corticosteroids may reduce epithelial migration, increase scar formation, or weaken existing cartilaginous support.[30] Other adjunctive measures include the use of antibiotics and antireflux medications. Mitomycin C is an antitumor antibiotic that inhibits fibroblastic proliferation and has been used in airway reconstruction to help prevent scar formation, with varied success.[31-33]

The combination of endoscopic laser division of tracheal stenosis or complete tracheal rings with balloon dilatation has been successfully reported.[34-36] Advantages purported by Andrew and associates include the ability to perform this technique with spontaneous respiration in a patient with a suboptimal airway, and the avoidance of endotracheal intubation after the procedure, which could incite further stenosis.[36]

Stents

Stents are important in the management of tracheal stenosis and can be used in either endoscopic or open approaches. Montgomery[37] first described the use of a polymeric silicone (Silastic T tube; Boston Medical Products) in 1965. This type of stent allows ventilation, support for soft tissue grafts and cartilage, and tracheal lumen suctioning. This tube is used in conjunction with a tracheostomy and is placed under endoscopic guidance. Maniglia[38] reported on the use of the T-tube stent in 53 adult patients with tracheal stenosis, subglottic stenosis, or both, with good results in 85%. Problems associated with

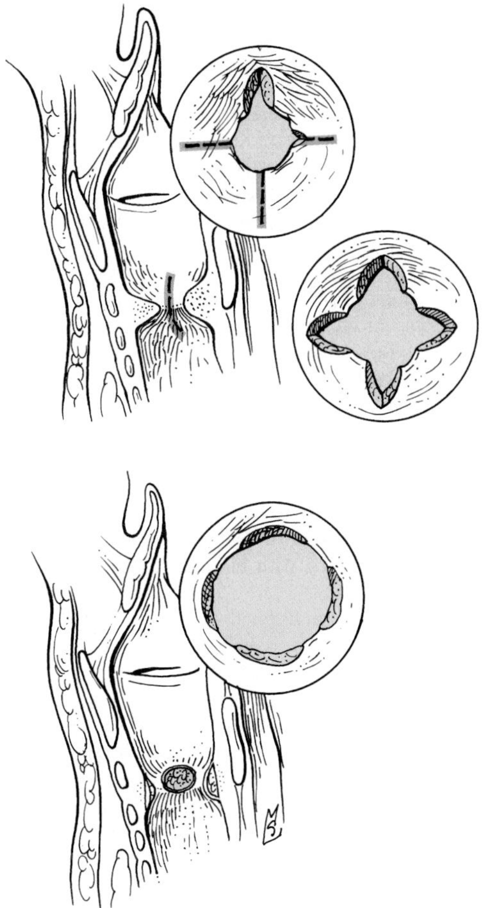

Figure 207-4. Star-shaped laser incision and dilation (Shapshay).

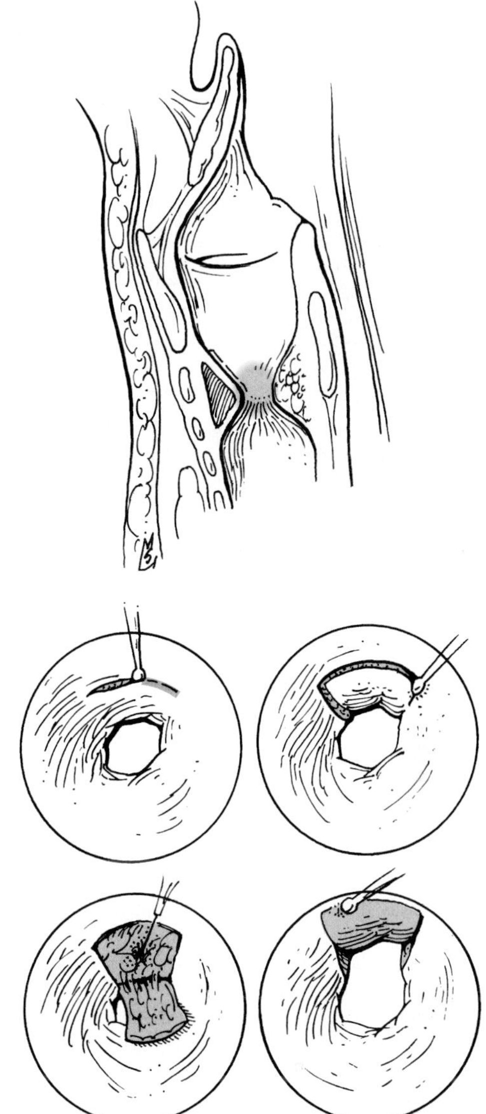

Figure 207-5. Laser trapdoor flap.

stents include obstruction, granulation tissue formation, infection, and malposition. Phillips reported use of this tube in 10 children with complex airway stenosis, the majority requiring stenting due to difficulties with severe granulation and stenosis of the subglottis after laryngotracheal reconstruction. This author and others emphasized the need for meticulous postoperative care to prevent luminal obstruction with secretions.[39]

The use of solid stents in children is limited. One version is the Dumon stent, modified from the Montgomery T-tube stent. It is a cylindrical solid silicone stent with external studs to hold it in place. Its main advantage is ease of removal, but its use in children has been limited because wall thickness itself can cause luminal obstruction in relatively small-caliber airways. Migration and occlusion from secretions, due to impairment of mucociliary clearance, are more problematic than expandable stents.

Experience with indwelling expandable stents in children has been limited, and initially these devices were used primarily in adults with advanced tracheobronchial malignancies.[40] Materials currently in use include self-expanding woven polymers and stainless steel wire, which are placed bronchoscopically. Mair and colleagues[41] demonstrated faster mucosalization and improved tracheal patency with polymer stents versus stainless steel stents both in a piglet model and in children. Bugmann and associates[42] reported on the successful use of an expandable Z-shaped wire stent in a 6-month-old patient with severe tracheomalacia. No complications were reported at 2-year follow-up. In adults, Nashef and colleagues,[43] among others,[23] found that the most common complication of stent placement was the formation of granulation tissue. Concerns raised by the authors regarding their use in children include the uncertainty of long-term tolerance of these stents, mucosal hypersecretion, and the risk of perforation and migration (Fig. 207-6).

Over the past decade, experience with expandable metal stents has increased. Filler and colleagues[44] reported on 16 children who required 30 balloon expandable metallic stents (Palmaz) over a 5-year period. All patients had improvement of their respiratory status, and three died of underlying cardiac disease. Obstruction in these patients was due to tracheomalacia, bronchomalacia, prior surgery, or vascular compression. Vinograd outlined his experience with metallic stents in 32 pediatric patients retrospectively reviewed. Initial stent insertion was uncomplicated, but the degree to which the stent needed to be expanded within the airway was much more difficult to gauge. Underexpansion could potentially cause stent displacement and overexpansion could cause mucosal injury and excessive granulation tissue formation. Although most patients had immediate relief of their airway obstruction, repeated endoscopies for removal of granulation tissue was required in 20 patients, and excessive granulation tissue occurred in another six patients who subsequently required stent removal. The authors also raised the question of the optimal period of time to leave the stent in place. Periodic expansion of the stent with patient growth needs to be balanced with the unknown effects on tracheal growth. In addition, stent removal was considered difficult with the potential development of life-threatening airway obstruction during extraction.[45]

A potential advantage to this type of stent is the ability to reexpand the stent as the child grows to accommodate a larger airway caliber.

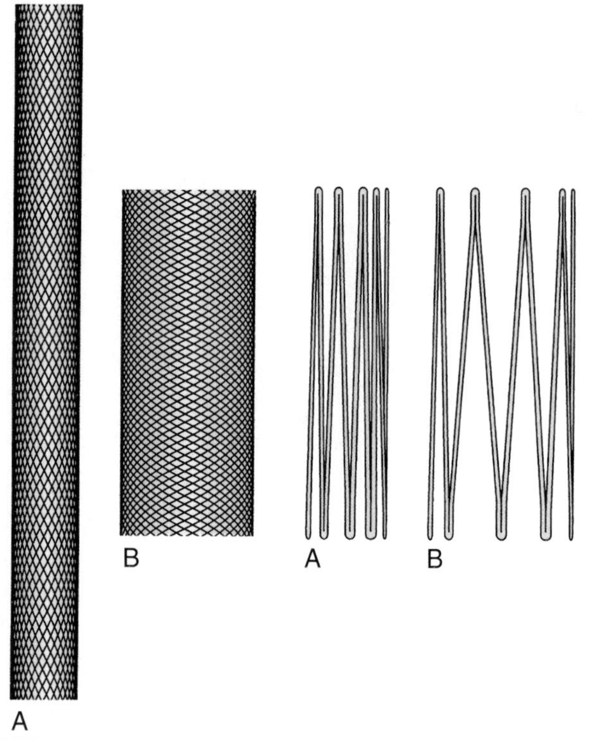

Figure 207-6. Polymer and wire stents in unexpanded **(A)** and expanded **(B)** forms.

Another advantage is that the stent is balloon expandable and can be removed more easily than a self-expanding stent such as the Gianturco stent, which is primarily used in adults. Furthermore, the wire mesh design preserves mucociliary clearance and hinders migration of the stent, unlike solid silicone stents.

The most common complication with the Palmaz stent was development of obstructing granulation tissue that necessitated early removal of the stent in three patients in the Filler[22] series. Because of the inability to remove the stent in a patient who underwent laser resection of stent granulation tissue, the authors advocate balloon compression or endoscopic scraping to address this problem. Furman and colleagues[46] reported on six patients requiring 12 Palmaz stents over a 3-year period with similar results and believed that stenting should be used in patients for whom conventional therapy had failed.

In a group of five infants ranging in age from 7 days to 12 months, Maeda and colleagues[47] reported on their success in treating congenital tracheal stenosis with stenting over a 3-year period. At follow-up bronchoscopy, the stents were found to be covered with respiratory mucosa. Granulation tissue developed at the site of the stent in all children, and one child died of intractable pneumonia related to recurrent granulation tissue.

A multicenter review by Jacobs and colleagues discussed the use of stenting in 33 children and highlighted the need to adapt the various stents available to the patient and their particular pathology, as evidenced by their use of custom carinal stents fashioned from cardiopulmonary bypass venous cannulas. They emphasized the need for accurate diagnosis before the surgical treatment of any extrinsic and intrinsic airway obstruction. In this series, stents were used as a primary modality to stabilize the airway or to support reconstruction after a variety of reconstructive procedures, with complications similar to earlier published reports.[48]

Experience with Nitinol stents in two children with tracheal stenosis was favorable.[49] Nitinol stents are formed from the metal alloy of nickel and titanium and are less reactive in the airway than stainless steel stents, potentially avoiding difficulties with granulation tissue formation. Another property of this alloy is its ability to reduce in size with temperature cooling, potentially facilitating its removal from the airway. Another promising area is the use of extraluminal microplates to support tracheal expansion[50] and the use of stainless steel wire to act as a scaffolding for pericardial patch tracheoplasty.[51]

In summary, stents can be useful as a primary modality for treatment, allowing time for very small children or children in unstable condition to grow and tolerate more complex open repairs if necessary. They can also be used in the postoperative period to support the repair or to salvage the airway in the case of stenosis. Experience in this area continues to grow in this small group of complex patients.

Open Repair

Acquired stenoses are often further complicated by scarring, poor vascular supply, and chronic infection. Tracheal resection and reanastomosis have been widely used in hundreds of adult patients for tracheal stenosis since the 1960s; however, Halsband[52] found only 26 reports of these procedures in children between 1969 and 1984. In general, surgical therapy should be pursued when conservative or nonsurgical therapy fails or is deemed inappropriate. A variety of techniques are available for the surgical management of tracheal stenosis, including tracheoplasty with autologous material, wedge resection, slide tracheoplasty, total resection with end-to-end anastomosis, tracheal homograft reconstruction, and stenting with bioinert materials. Often, multiple techniques must be used.

Tracheoplasty can be performed with rib cartilage as described by Kimura and others.[53] Cartilage is a rigid autologous tissue that derives its nutritional support through diffusion and can survive without a direct vascular supply. Because of this, cartilage has been widely used as a tracheal graft material. The surgical technique involves securing the airway either by a previously placed tracheostomy or by endotracheal intubation, which is performed orally and then converted to a transtracheal site once the trachea is exposed. The area of stenosis is exposed anteriorly and the extent of the stenosis is outlined bronchoscopically, either by palpation with the bronchoscope or using the light of the telescope. The external appearance of the trachea can underestimate the extent of the stenosis.[54] Intraluminal granulation tissue is removed and the scar is incised. A rib graft is harvested (usually a fifth or sixth rib on the right is used) and fashioned as described previously. Perichondrium is preserved on the anterior surface of the rib graft and becomes the luminal surface of the airway. The graft is held in place by interrupted suture material and, depending on the extent of the stenosis, is supported with an endotracheal tube for 5 to 7 days (Fig. 207-7). For longer-term stenting, an Aboulker or T-tube stent can be used. The decision of whether to use cardiopulmonary bypass, extracorporeal membrane oxygenation, or distal tracheal intubation during the procedure is controversial and depends on the site of the lesion and the surgeon's personal preference. Pericardium is the most commonly used alternative to rib augmentation and also has good long-term survival rates (Fig. 207-8).[55-58] Other autologous materials that can be used include periosteum,[59] pedicled muscle flaps,[60,61] composite grafts,[62] the esophagus,[63,64] omentum,[65] and solvent-preserved dura.[66]

Kimura and others[53] were the first to report successful repair of a 1-year-old with complete stenosis of the trachea using costal cartilage. Their experience was updated with an additional four patients in 1988.[67] Long-term survival was 80%, with one death due to respiratory distress 10 months after repair. Complications related to this procedure include anastomotic breakdown, stenosis, and granulation tissue formation at the suture line. Jaquiss and colleagues,[54] among others,[68] described six patients who underwent rib tracheoplasty (mean age, 14 weeks) with an average stenosis of 70% of the total length of the trachea. All patients had survived at a follow-up of 6 months to 7.6 years. Bronchoscopy was performed three times or fewer postoperatively in all but one patient. These authors advocated cardiopulmonary bypass to obtain an unobstructed view of the airway during repair. Lobe and others[66] reported on seven infants with congenital tracheal stenosis, four of whom underwent repair with costal cartilage.[69] One death caused by pneumonia occurred 5 weeks postoperatively.

The experience with costal cartilage tracheoplasty continues to grow. Forsen and colleagues[70] reported on 10 patients with congenital long-segment tracheal stenosis repaired at an average age of 18 weeks with costal cartilage tracheoplasty. They were followed up for an

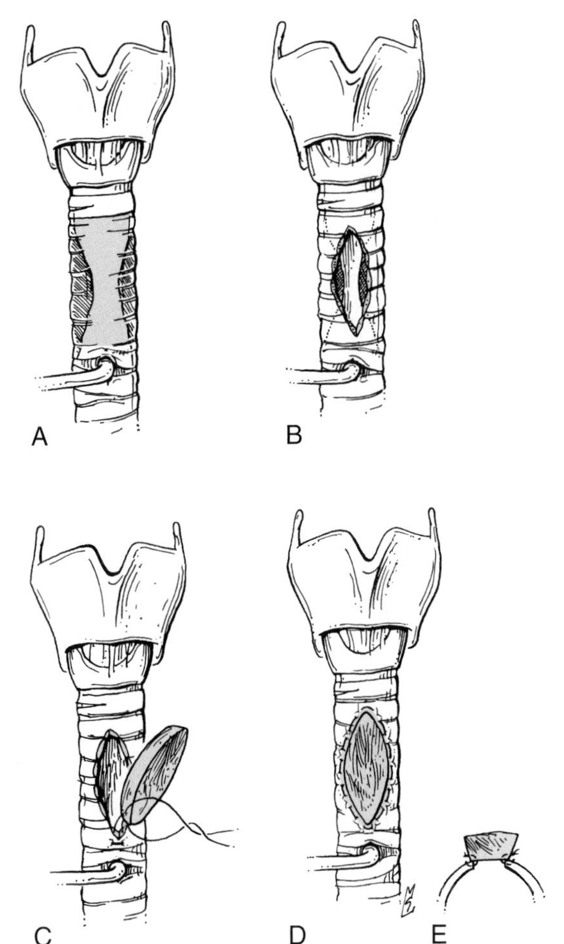

Figure 207-7. Cartilage graft placement for augmentation of tracheal stenosis. **A**, Area of stenosis. **B**, Stenosis excised. **C** and **D**, Placement of graft. **E**, Surgical result. Note the graft placement in lumen **E**.

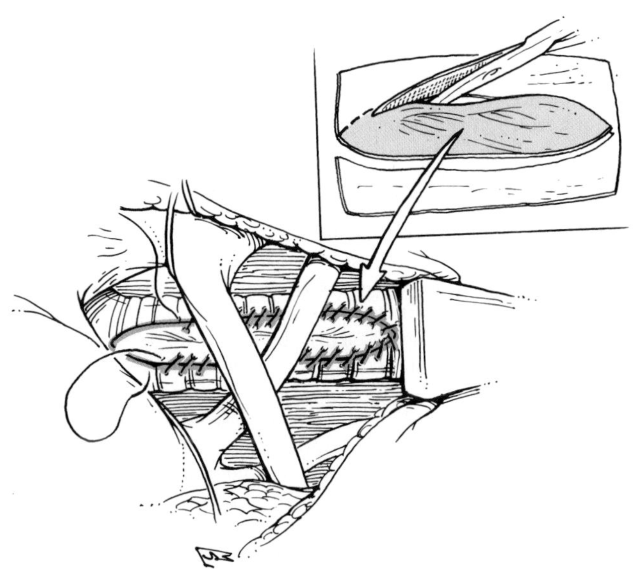

Figure 207-8. Pericardial patch sewn in position.

average of 8 years, and 70% of patients were active without tracheostomy. Kamata and colleagues[71] detailed their experience with 11 infants who underwent tracheobronchial reconstruction with costal cartilage grafts. Similar to other studies, frequent postoperative bronchoscopies were needed, and the use of extracorporeal membrane oxygenation

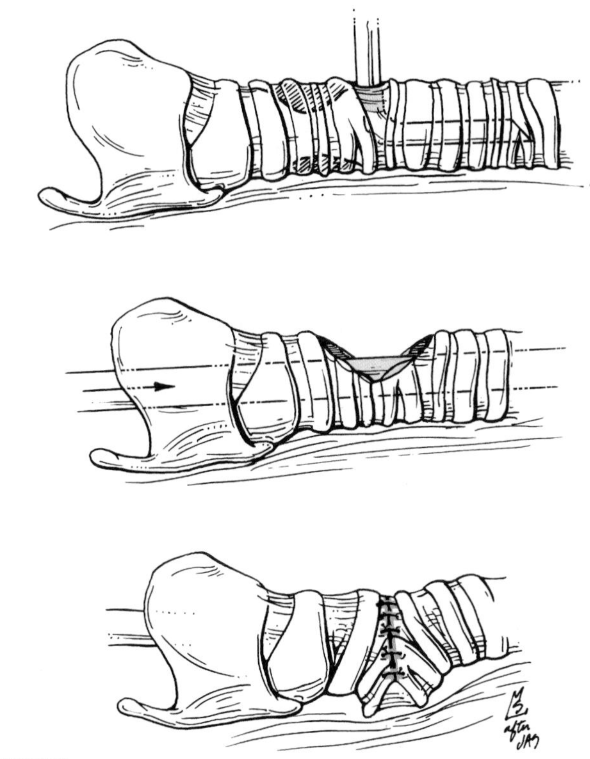

Figure 207-9. Wedge section and closure.

(ECMO) facilitated repair. A common finding in all these series was a high incidence of associated cardiovascular and pulmonary anomalies.

Troublesome to repair is the formation of granulation tissue at the graft site. One advantage of rib graft in contrast to pericardial grafts is that the endotracheal tube does not need to be beyond the proximal edge of the graft for stenting purposes and subsequently decreases granulation tissue formation.[54] DeLorimier and others[72] have suggested that the formation of granulation tissue is more likely if the graft involves 30% or more of the luminal surface. Epithelialization of costal cartilage grafts in the trachea has been demonstrated in both animals and humans.[73] Grillo and colleagues[74] have stated that the use of absorbable (polyglycolic acid polymer) versus nonabsorbable suture material reduces the amount of granulation seen at the anastomotic site.

The technique of wedge resection is most useful for a localized stenosis involving one or two tracheal rings. This method may be useful in small infants in whom the recurrent laryngeal nerve can be difficult to identify. After oral intubation, the lesion is defined and an anterior wedge of trachea is removed. The defect is closed primarily with interrupted sutures. Weber and colleagues[75] used this procedure successfully in four patients with localized stenosis (Fig. 207-9).

Segmental resection is successful for repair of long-segment tracheal stenosis comprising less than 50% of the tracheal length. In children, this operation uses the principles of tracheal repair that were developed for adults.[76] Following endoscopy to outline the extent of the lesion, the stenotic segment is excised. Dissection beyond the stenosis is kept to a minimum to preserve the vascular supply to the trachea. Sutures are placed submucosally and tied extraluminally. Important to the success of the repair is the ability to achieve a tension-free anastomotic suture line. Various techniques can be applied, including suprahyoid release, infrahyoid release, peritracheal mobilization, intercartilaginous incisions, perihilar release, dissection of the pulmonary vasculature, transplantation of the left mainstem bronchus, and neck flexion with chin-to-chest suturing (Fig. 207-10).[77-79]

The results of several authors have been encouraging.[75,78,80,81] Nakayama and others[82] reported on 10 patients, four of whom underwent tracheal resection. They emphasized the association of multiple tracheobronchial and vascular anomalies in these patients and the need for a detailed preoperative evaluation. Healy[69] reported on three chil-

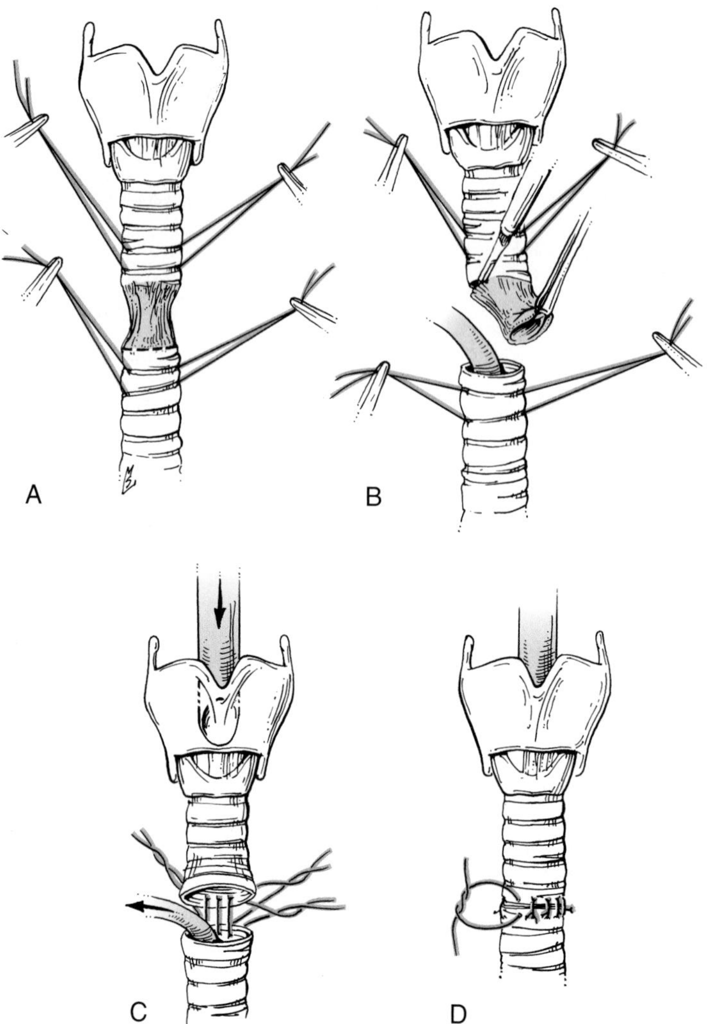

Figure 207-10. **A**, Area of stenosis. **B**, Resection of stenosis with intubation of trachea distally. **C**, Interrupted absorbable sutures placed circumferentially and reintubated from above **(D)**.

dren, ages 4 weeks to 3 years, who were successfully resected. The author thought that three to five tracheal rings could be resected in children without a laryngeal release. He also commented that postoperative endotracheal intubation can often be avoided in adults, but in children the cartilage is still very pliable and may not offer sufficient resistance to tracheal collapse at the anastomotic site. Two patients who required postoperative nasotracheal intubation were not mechanically ventilated but were allowed to breathe spontaneously in an intensive care unit setting and were successfully extubated several days later. DeLorimier and others[72] detailed their experience with 45 patients with tracheobronchial stenoses. Seventeen patients underwent segmental resection, with three anastomotic strictures developing postoperatively. These strictures were resected with success in two patients. In their series of 52 patients ranging in age from 7 weeks to 15 years, Grillo and Zannini[83] undertook segmental resection in 20. Good results were obtained in 17 patients. The remaining 32 patients were treated conservatively, with 24 requiring either a T tube or tracheotomy. In their series of 21 patients with congenital tracheal stenosis, Benjamin and colleagues[84] also treated 12 patients without surgery. This experience lends support to the individualized treatment options and the nonsurgical management of selected patients.

Segmental resection is often not possible due to the length of trachea to be resected. First described by Tsang and others,[85] slide tracheoplasty involves dividing the stenosis transversely in the midportion and then incising the upper segment vertically posteriorly and the lower segment vertically anteriorly. The two ends are then placed over each other, effectively halving the stenotic segment while doubling the circumference. The distance that the tracheal ends need to move is half that of a resection and primary reanastomosis. This fact aids in reducing tension along the suture line, which may be more critical in children than in adults.[51] Grillo[86] described two children (ages 3 months and 3 years) and two young adults, all of whom had complete cartilaginous rings. The stenotic areas were 36% and 50% of the total tracheal length for each group, respectively. Short-term results were deemed good. An advantage to this technique is decreased granulation tissue that is often seen at the site of the cartilage graft reconstruction. Other advantages to this procedure are the avoidance of graft materials, decreased tracheal mobilization, and a good success rate (Fig. 207-11).

Cotter and colleagues[87] reported on 17 patients with congenital tracheal stenosis who underwent tracheoplasty over a 10-year period; 11 underwent augmentation with pericardial grafts or costal cartilage. Five of six patients who had resection and reanastomosis did well for 2 to 9 years after surgery, seven of eight patients with tracheoplasty did well for 2 to 4 years after surgery. This study found that the former group had fewer postoperative bronchoscopies and fewer difficulties with the development of granulation tissue at the suture line. Important in the management of these patients was frequent postoperative bronchoscopy, and the use of cardiopulmonary bypass for some made the operation technically easier. No complications were related to the use of cardiopulmonary bypass. The authors advised segmental resection, when possible, with early extubation to reduce mucosal injury.

Recent reports favor the use of slide tracheoplasty over augmentation with cartilage or pericardial patch grafts for long-segment tracheal

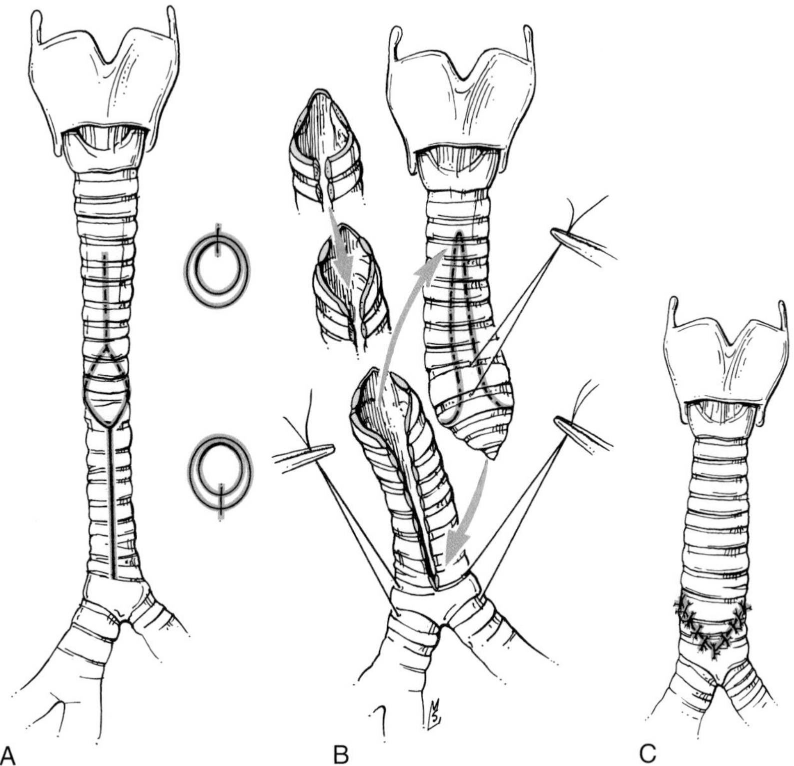

Figure 207-11. Slide tracheoplasty. **A**, Area of stenosis. **B**, The trachea is divided on an angle and then vertically anteriorly and posteriorly. **C**, Surgical result.

stenosis. According to Grillo and colleagues,[88] "Patch tracheoplasty met a previously urgent need but should perhaps be largely reserved for unusual problems." In all juvenile patients, the repaired tracheal segment continues to grow, with complications related to suture line granulomas (two of seven slide tracheoplasty patients) that resolve with a single bronchoscopy without recurrence. Others have reported similar experience with long-term growth of the reconstructed airway and few complications.[88-92]

In the series by Acosta,[93] six patients were treated with resection and reanastomosis and three with slide tracheoplasty. The latter group had favorable outcomes with regard to anastomosis complications such as leaks, mediastinitis, fibrosis, or stenosis. Kim compared eight patients between 12 days and 6 months with congenital tracheal stenosis, four who underwent slide tracheoplasty, three had pericardial patch, and one had resection and end-to-end reanastomosis. Bothersome granulation tissue formation was seen in the pericardial patch subset. Tsugawa compared 17 pediatric patients who underwent slide tracheoplasty with 12 pediatric patients who underwent costal cartilage tracheoplasty and concluded that slide tracheoplasty was the preferred method[94] with similar findings in a group of 10 patients described by Matute.[95] These findings have prompted these authors to recommend slide tracheoplasty as the procedure of choice.

Tracheal homograft transplantation with cadaveric human tracheal homograft is an exciting new modality for the repair of severe long-segment tracheal stenosis in children. Initially described in 1980 in adult patients,[96] 24 children were recently reported by Jacobs and others.[97] An 83% survival rate was achieved, with follow-up ranging from 5 months to 10 years. Tracheal homograft banks exist in Europe, and specimens are fixed in formalin, washed in thimerosal (sodium ethylmercurithiosalicylate), and stored in acetone. The trachea is exposed through a neck incision, a median sternotomy, or both. Cardiopulmonary bypass is used to facilitate the operative field. The anterior part of the trachea is removed, leaving only a posterior tracheal wall intact. Dumon stents are then sutured into the native trachea to provide support for the homograft for 10 to 12 weeks until the graft hardens and reepithelialization occurs. The endotracheal tube is positioned to lie within the lumen of the Dumon stent. The homograft is fashioned to the defect and sutured in place with interrupted sutures (Fig. 207-12).

Postoperative care includes 2 weeks of intravenous antibiotics followed by 4 weeks of oral trimethoprim as well as inhaled albuterol and corticosteroids. No immunosuppression is needed because the thimerosal used in the preparation of the homograft destroys antigenicity. Frequent bronchoscopy is required to remove granulation tissue at the site of the stents.

Advantages to the tracheal homograft include an adequate supply of tissue, which can be placed without suture-line tension, and the presence of a carina, which is needed for distal reconstruction. Ciliated columnar epithelium has been shown to coat the homograft. Tracheal homograft reconstruction is an exciting new approach to severe or recurrent tracheal stenosis.

In 1999, Jacobs and colleagues[98] updated the worldwide experience with tracheal autografts in 31 children. Twenty-one of these patients underwent previous surgical attempts at airway reconstruction, and results were encouraging for both the short and medium terms. Mortality overall was 16%; however, three of the five patients who died had functional airways. Twenty-six patients survived, with 22 patients deemed asymptomatic on follow-up bronchoscopy that showed epithelialization of the grafts. Continued follow-up of these patients is planned in an established database.

Backer and colleagues[99] described six patients with tracheal stenosis resulting from complete tracheal rings that were constructed with partial tracheal resection, posterior end-to-end anastomosis, and anterior repair with the patients' own resected trachea. In four patients, the anterior repair was augmented with pericardial patch. The use of a free tracheal autograft was based on the senior author's observation that the trachea in children with complete tracheal rings was usually longer than average. This technique is more appealing than performing tracheal homografts because the autograft is lined with respiratory epithelium, will not reject from its donor, and has the potential to grow. Intermediate-term results were reported with an additional four patients added to the study in 2000.[100] Nine of ten children were reported on 2 to 44 months postoperatively. One child had dehiscence of the autograft requiring repair within the aortic homograft, and two patients were

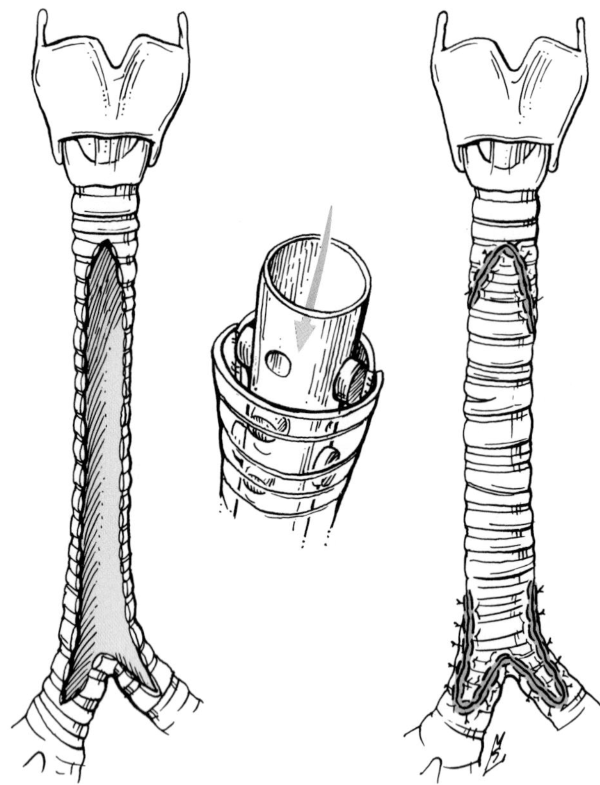

Figure 207-12. Homograft transplant with a Dumon stent.

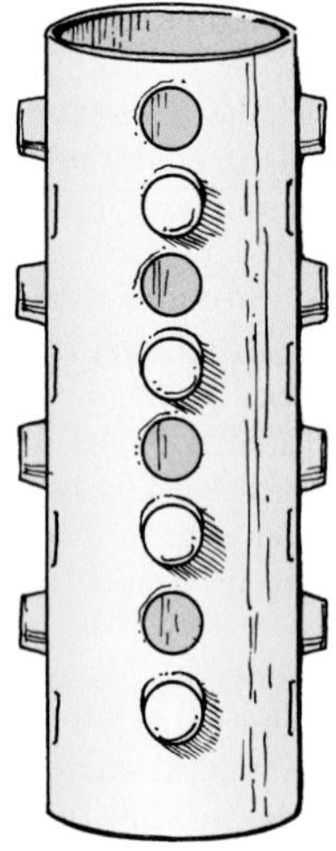

Figure 207-13. Silastic Dumon stent.

trachea dependent. One child died of sepsis and multisystem organ failure, and subsequent autopsy showed that the autograft was well healed. Autografts on serial bronchoscopy appeared to grow with the patient and are difficult to distinguish from the surrounding trachea.

Synthetic tracheal prostheses have not enjoyed the same success as prosthetic devices used elsewhere in the head and neck because the trachea is much more susceptible to infection. Synthetic devices that have been used include ceramic rings, Marlex mesh, and silicone stents.[101] These are complicated by dense granulation tissue reaction, migration of the prosthesis, recurrent stenosis, and the risk of vascular erosion (Fig. 207-13).

Fortunately, over the last few years, several papers have been published looking at these multiple surgical techniques. In a study by Anton-Pacheco and colleagues involving 19 patients from 3 days to 7 years, 14 underwent surgery over a 13-year period. For symptomatic cases with short segment stenosis, defined as less than 30% of total tracheal length, tracheal resection with anastomosis was preferred, and in long-segment stenosis (greater than 70%), slide tracheoplasty was recommended.[102] Backer reviewed a single institution's experience with four surgical techniques over 18 years involving 50 patients. Current management included resection/anastomosis for short stenosis (up to eight rings), and for long-segment stenosis, a tracheal autograft technique later supplanted by the pericardial tracheoplasty procedure in use until 1996.[103] Chui performed a retrospective analysis of 68 patients treated at six centers to determine prognostic factors that influence mortality after repair with either cartilage patch or slide tracheoplasty. No difference was seen between the two techniques, but a higher mortality was seen in two groups of patients: those younger than 1 month of age and those with intracardiac anomalies.[104] These findings were also corroborated by Herrera in 2007 in an excellent review of the literature. In reviewing the literature over a 42-year period, the researcher concluded that short segment stenosis was best treated with resection and long-segment stenosis was best treated with tracheoplasty, with cardiopulmonary bypass as part of the standard of care for these operations.[105]

Complications related to open surgical resection have been addressed by several authors.[52,67,74,106] The most common complication of tracheal reconstruction is the formation of granulation tissue at the anastomotic site or around the stent. This problem is usually managed with bronchoscopic-guided laser removal and with intravenous or intralesional injection of corticosteroid. Anastomotic leak or separation is often caused by excessive tension at the site of resection. Several techniques have been described to lessen the tension, including the supralaryngeal-, tracheal-, and hilar-releasing maneuvers mentioned earlier. Recurrent laryngeal nerve injury is rare and is usually managed conservatively if it is unilateral. Aspiration can also complicate recurrent laryngeal nerve injury and may be seen after thyrohyoid or suprahyoid release.

Complications can be avoided by ensuring several factors before surgery.[107] Ideally, the surgical resection candidate should not be mechanically ventilated, should not be taking steroids, and should not have prior radiotherapy to the area. Muscle flaps between the esophagus and trachea can reduce the incidence of fistula formation. Glottic competence should be evaluated, especially in neurologically compromised patients.

Conclusion

Evaluation and management of tracheal stenosis is a complex undertaking, as evidenced by the numerous methods available for reconstruction. In general, limited tracheal stenoses can be managed endoscopically, whereas longer stenoses are better corrected through an open approach. The trend over the last decade is for segmental resection and reanastomosis for short-segment stenosis and use of slide tracheoplasty or augmentation of long-segment stenosis. The experience with both tracheal homografts and autografts continues to grow. No one surgical method is appropriate for every setting, and often the surgeon must use several therapeutic options. Furthermore, the surgeon must recognize the limitations and complications of each of the various management options to ensure a successful outcome.

SUGGESTED READINGS

Backer CL, et al. Tracheal surgery in children: an 18 year review of four techniques. *Eur J Cardiothorac Surg.* 2001;19:777-784.

Elliot M, et al. The management of congenital tracheal stenosis. *Int J Pediatr Otorhinolaryn.* 2003;67:183-192.

Herrera P, Caldarone C, et al. The current state of congenital tracheal stenosis. *Pediatr Surg Int.* 2007;(11):1033-1044.

For complete list of references log onto www.expertconsult.com.

CHAPTER TWO HUNDRED AND EIGHT

Foreign Bodies of the Airway and Esophagus

Lauren D. Holinger

Sheri A. Poznanovic

Key Points

- The highest incidence occurs in children 1 to 3 years old.
- Most airway foreign bodies are located in the bronchi.
- Most esophageal foreign body impactions occur in the cervical esophagus, just below the cricopharyngeus muscle.
- An aerodigestive tract foreign body frequently mimics other conditions and is often the result of an unwitnessed episode; the diagnosis must be considered in any patient with prolonged or unusual pulmonary symptoms.
- Complete airway obstruction resulting from a foreign body and esophageal impaction with a battery are emergencies. Delayed diagnosis may lead to complications.
- Esophageal foreign body impaction is frequently associated with vomiting and dysphagia, but may also manifest with respiratory distress.
- There is a high rate of spontaneous passage of esophageal coins into the stomach.
- Negative radiographic findings do not rule out the presence of a foreign body. Generally, chest radiography is an adjunctive procedure to a thorough history and physical examination.
- Communication with the anesthesiologist regarding the anesthetic and endoscopy plan is essential before any surgical intervention.
- Endoscopic instrumentation revolutionized the field of bronchoesophagography, and reduced the mortality associated with aerodigestive tract foreign bodies.
- Careful endoscopic removal of foreign objects under direct vision is the safest management for patients with foreign bodies of the airway and esophagus.
- Stricter industry standards for toy part sizes and increased public awareness have helped to decrease fatalities from choking.

Foreign bodies in the airway, pharynx, and esophagus continue to be a diagnostic and therapeutic challenge for practicing otolaryngologists. Despite improvement in public awareness and emergency care, foreign bodies result in approximately 150 deaths per year in children secondary to asphyxiation.[1] Most deaths occur before hospital intervention.

Although the role of the otolaryngologist begins after the child is evaluated initially by emergency department or primary care physicians, otolaryngologists and primary care physicians should have a high index of suspicion for foreign body aspiration or ingestion. Because a foreign body can mimic other conditions, particularly without a witnessed event, there can be a delay in management that may lead to complications.

Before the 20th century, bronchotomy was the method of choice for airway foreign body removal. Most patients with foreign body aspiration died from the initial event, the attempt at removal, or complications thereof. Although intubation of the airway was suggested at the time of Hippocrates, Killian in 1895 was the first to use a hollow tube to evaluate the tracheobronchial airway.[2] He used this technique to remove a bone from the right main bronchus in 1897, becoming the first to perform endoscopic removal of an airway foreign body.

Endoscopic illumination was initially used in esophagoscopy and was incorporated into a bronchoscope by Jackson,[2] who revolutionized the field of bronchoesophagography with the development of instruments and techniques for foreign body removal. The principles he and his son developed[3] were paramount in reducing the mortality associated with airway foreign bodies and are still the basis of foreign body removal today.

The introduction of the rod-lens telescope in the 1970s greatly improved the visualization of bronchoscopic removal of foreign bodies. Foreign body removal has been performed with topical anesthesia and sedation. With new, safer anesthetic agents and improved anesthesia techniques and monitoring, however, general anesthesia is now routine.

Children frequently swallow objects that pass through the gastrointestinal tract without problems. This also may occur in adults. Foreign bodies occasionally become lodged in the esophagus because of the object's size or shape, narrowing of the esophageal lumen, extrinsic compression, or anatomic abnormalities.

Before the mid-1850s, the most common management for suspected esophageal foreign body impaction was to attempt to push the object into the stomach. Various instruments, including curved hooks, forceps, and even a walking cane, were used. Dupuytren was reported to pinch the neck of patients vigorously to crush a food impaction in the cervical esophagus, allowing it to pass to the stomach.[2] The first esophagoscope used in 1890 by Mackenzie was later improved by Jackson, Ingals, and Mosher. The earliest rigid esophagoscopies for foreign body extraction by Jackson and Ingals were performed on awake patients in a sitting position. Because anesthesia risks have decreased, and instrumentation for endoscopic removal of esophageal foreign bodies has improved, these procedures are now performed with the patient supine and under general endotracheal anesthesia.

Epidemiology

The incidence of airway and esophageal foreign bodies has not changed significantly, but the safety in removal has increased dramatically. Most aerodigestive foreign bodies are esophageal—85% as reported by Hsu and colleagues.[4] Most airway foreign body aspirations occur in patients younger than 15 years old. In this age group, choking-related episodes treated in the emergency department number approximately 29.9 per 100,000 population.[1] The highest incidence occurs between 1 and 3 years of age; 25% of patients are younger than 1 year.[5-9] The reasons toddlers are most susceptible are (1) they lack molars necessary for proper grinding of food; (2) they have less-controlled coordination of swallowing, and immaturity in laryngeal elevation and glottic closure; (3) there is an age-related tendency to explore the environment by placing objects in the mouth; and (4) they are often running or playing at the time of ingestion.[10] Older children and adolescents may have an anatomic abnormality[11] or a neurologic impairment.[12] Accidental aspiration or ingestion of objects tends to be twice as common in boys. Vegetable matter is seen in approximately 70% to 80% of airway foreign body ingestions; the most common are peanuts in the United States, watermelon seeds in Egypt,[13] and pumpkin seeds in Greece.[14] The percentage of aspirated and ingested metallic foreign bodies, especially safety pins, has decreased, primarily because of the widespread use of disposable diapers. Plastic pieces constitute approximately 5% to 15% of airway foreign bodies; plastic pieces tend to remain longer because they are inert and radiolucent.

The most common esophageal foreign bodies are coins (75% of cases).[5-9] Meat and vegetable matter impactions are less common in children. Round objects, trinkets, disk batteries, and sharp objects constitute less than 20% of impacted esophageal foreign bodies. The duration of impaction before endoscopic removal is less than 24 hours in most patients, more than 1 week in 6%, and of unknown duration in 10%.[6,7]

Of patients with multiple esophageal foreign body impactions, 80% have an esophageal anomaly on further evaluation.[6] Of patients with recurrent esophageal foreign bodies, 19% have esophageal anomalies that previously required surgical repair.

Location

Most airway foreign bodies become lodged in the bronchi because their size and configuration allow passage through the larynx and trachea (Fig. 208-1). Larger objects become impacted in the larynx or trachea, sometimes causing complete obstruction, which is an acute emergency. Bronchial foreign bodies are more common in the right main bronchus in adults, which is thought to be caused by the position of the carina to the left of the midline and its lesser angle of divergence from the tracheal axis.[15] Several authors report airway foreign bodies in children with equal frequency in the right and left main bronchi, with no clear explanation for this occurrence.[2,16,17]

Most esophageal foreign body impactions occur in the cervical esophagus just below the cricopharyngeus muscle (Fig. 208-2).[5,6,8] Another 4% to 5% of esophageal foreign bodies become lodged at the midesophagus or distal esophagus, often caused by extraluminal compression by the aortic arch or left main bronchus (Fig. 208-3). Esophageal foreign body impactions also can occur above an esophageal stricture.[6]

Acute Airway Obstruction

Complete airway obstruction resulting from a foreign body is an absolute emergency. Food (e.g., hot dogs, candies) and nonfood objects (e.g., toys, balloons) commonly become lodged in the larynx and trachea. Increased public awareness, availability of emergency personnel, and the widespread use of the Heimlich maneuver have greatly reduced the mortality of acute obstruction.[18] The most important factor in reducing mortality is recognition of the person in acute airway distress. Coughing and gagging indicate partial obstruction. Older children and adults may signal choking by grasping the neck.

The Committee on Accident and Poison Prevention of the American Academy of Pediatrics developed guidelines in accord with the American Red Cross and the American Heart Association for manage-

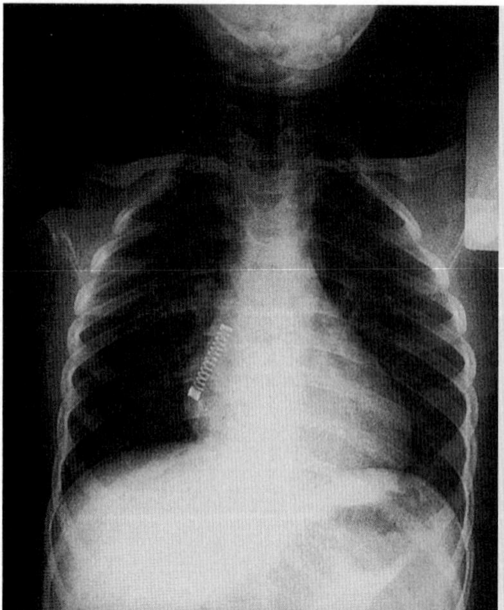

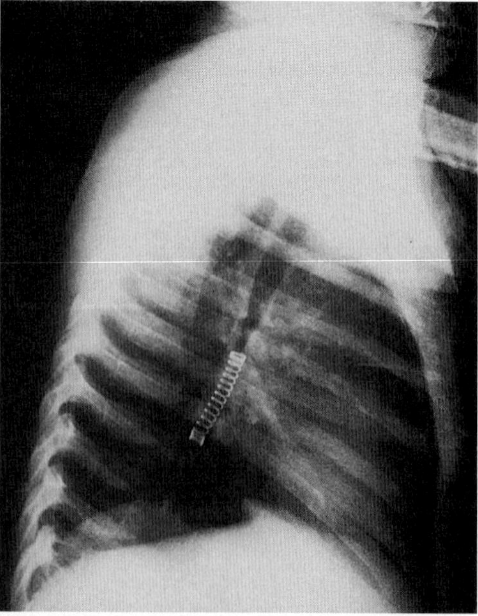

Figure 208-1. Posteroanterior and lateral views of a pen spring in right main bronchus.

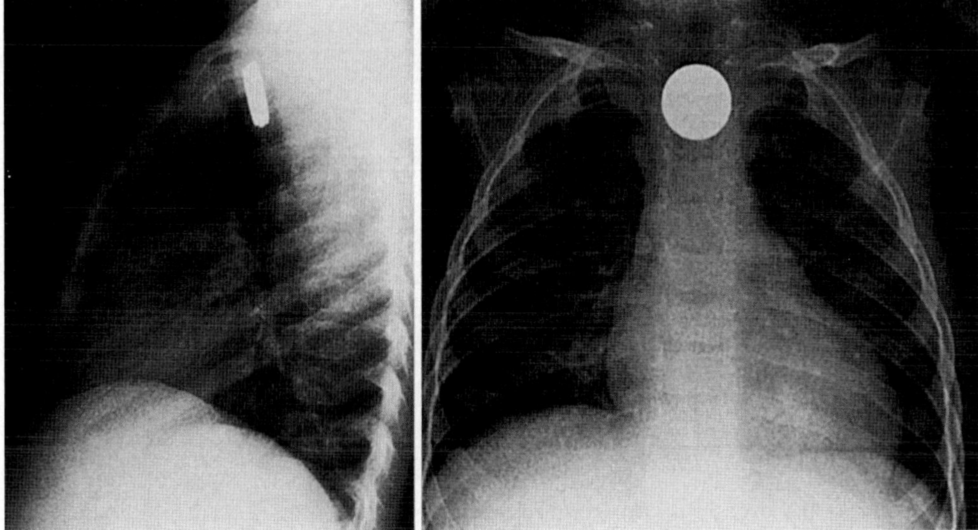

Figure 208-2. Posteroanterior and lateral films of two pennies and a nickel in a typical esophageal location immediately below the cricopharyngeus.

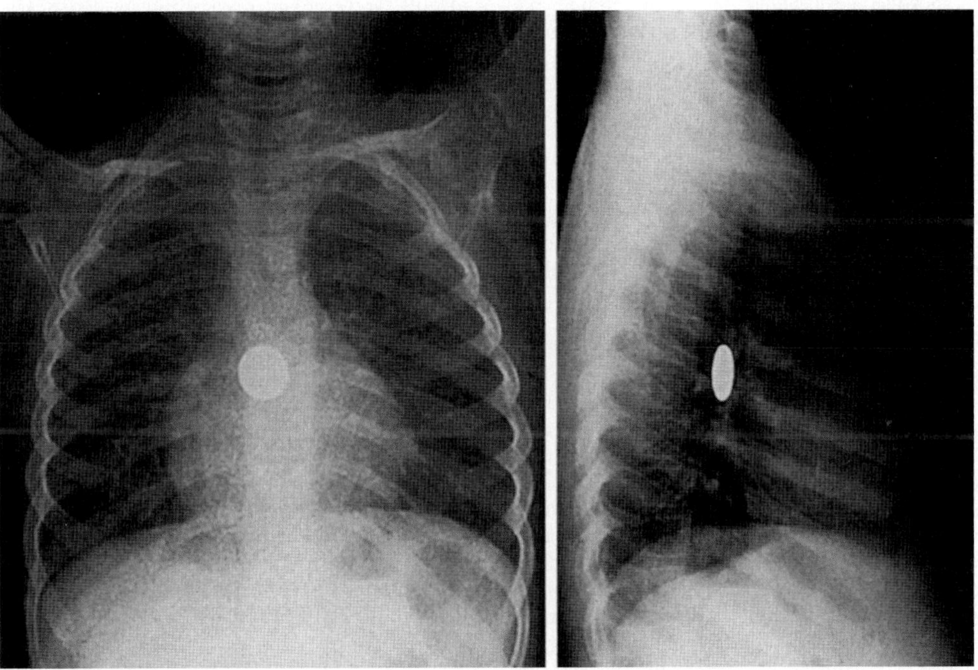

Figure 208-3. Posteroanterior and lateral chest films of a coin in the midesophagus.

ment of choking victims.[19] For infants, rescue breaths and chest compressions are recommended. Children older than 1 year require gentle abdominal thrusts while supine. Older children and adults are positioned standing, sitting, or recumbent for the Heimlich maneuver. Back blows or abdominal thrusts in individuals with only partial obstructions could lead to complete obstruction and are not recommended.

Symptoms

Foreign body aspiration is suspected when a victim has acute choking or severe coughing with respiratory distress. The diagnosis sometimes is obscured if the event is unwitnessed in a young child. Some children do not admit to aspiration because of fear of punishment. Symptoms of foreign body aspiration can mimic conditions such as asthma, croup, and pneumonia. Onset of wheezing in an otherwise healthy child should prompt suspicion of foreign body aspiration.

There are three clinical phases of foreign body aspiration.[15] The initial phase consists of choking, gagging, and paroxysms of coughing or airway obstruction that occur at the moment of aspiration. The choking, gagging, and coughing subside during the asymptomatic phase when the foreign body becomes lodged, and the reflexes fatigue. The asymptomatic phase can last hours to weeks. Complications occur in the third phase, when obstruction, erosion, or infection causes hemoptysis, pneumonia, atelectasis, abscess, or fever.

A careful history and physical examination are most important in diagnosing foreign body aspiration. Determining the site of the obstruction is important in the management of the problem.

Laryngeal Foreign Bodies

A foreign body in the larynx may constitute an airway emergency that requires lifesaving first aid before transport to the hospital. Irregular foreign bodies or orientation in the sagittal plane may produce only

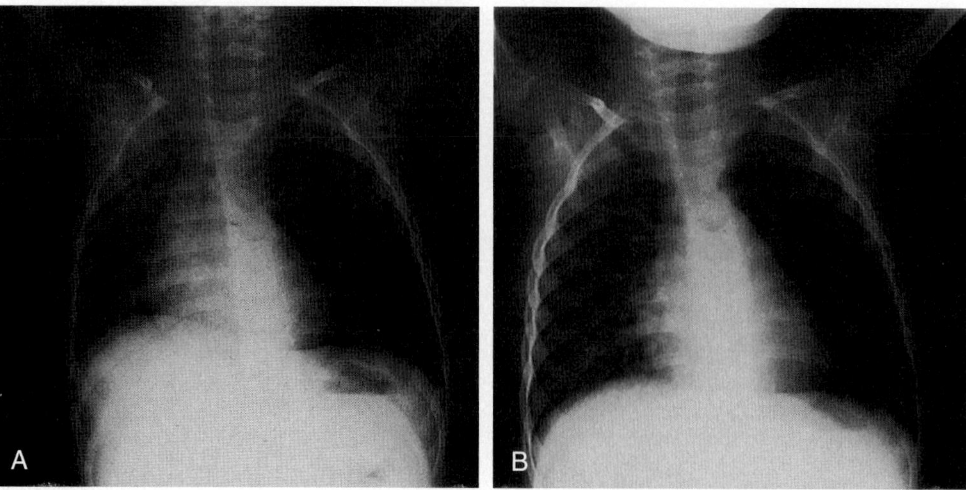

Figure 208-4. **A** and **B,** Expiratory **(A)** and inspiratory **(B)** chest films show hyperinflation on side of left bronchial foreign body (a peanut fragment). This is a typical early finding.

partial obstruction, allowing adequate air movement around the obstruction. Resulting laryngeal edema can lead to complete obstruction. Typically, these patients have symptoms of obstruction and hoarseness. Some symptoms can mimic croup.[3] Delayed diagnosis may lead to complications.

Tracheal Foreign Bodies

Patients with tracheal foreign bodies are seen in similar fashion, but typically do not have hoarseness. Jackson and Jackson[3] described three signs associated with tracheal foreign bodies: the "asthmatoid wheeze," the "audible slap" produced from foreign body contact with the trachea, and the "palpable thud" over the trachea. As with laryngeal foreign bodies, edema can progress to complete obstruction.

Bronchial Foreign Bodies

Of airway foreign bodies, 80% to 90% are found in the bronchi.[20] These patients typically have a triad of cough, wheezing, and decreased breath sounds. One large series reported that 65% have the classic triad,[17] but 95% have at least one finding.[16]

The asymptomatic phase may give a false sense of security that the problem has resolved and lead to a delay in diagnosis. Chest auscultation may reveal decreased breath sounds or wheezing. Sudden onset of wheezing is particularly suggestive of a bronchial foreign body, especially if unilateral, but may be a subtle finding.[21] Occasionally, bronchial foreign bodies can cause respiratory compromise as a result of swelling of dried vegetable matter (e.g., dried beans and peas) or edema around the object, producing complete obstruction and lobar collapse. Movement of the foreign body from one main bronchus to the other produces respiratory distress, resulting from obstruction of the previously normally ventilating lung.

Esophageal foreign body impaction is most frequently associated with vomiting, odynophagia, dysphagia, and ptyalism.[5-8] If the ingestion is witnessed, gagging or choking may be reported. A large foreign body may cause symptoms of airway obstruction and cough caused by compression or irritation of the upper airway. In long-standing esophageal foreign body impaction, fever and other symptoms of respiratory infection may be present.[6]

A careful history and physical examination are the first steps necessary to diagnose esophageal foreign body impaction. Appropriate radiographic evaluation further aids diagnosis and management.

Radiographic Evaluation

Laryngotracheal Foreign Bodies

Airway films—high-kilovolt posteroanterior and lateral soft tissue radiographs of the neck—are the radiographic examination of choice to identify laryngeal and tracheal foreign bodies. Chest radiographs are ordered before intervention. Neck films may show subglottic narrowing. Esclamado and Richardson[20] reported that 92% of patients with tracheal foreign bodies had abnormal neck radiographs, whereas 50% had normal chest films. When such children do not respond rapidly to medical management, foreign body aspiration must be ruled out.

Bronchial Foreign Bodies

Children with bronchial foreign bodies can be radiographically normal or may show obstructive emphysema (air trapping or hyperinflation—an early finding) and atelectasis or consolidation (late findings). Even if the diagnosis is strongly suspected by history and physical examination, posteroanterior and lateral chest radiographs are performed. Chest radiography generally is an adjunctive procedure because the history and physical examination are sufficient to suspect a bronchial foreign body.

During normal respiration, the airway dilates with inspiration and contracts on expiration. This respiratory cycle can be altered by the presence of bronchial foreign bodies.[22] Small objects may cause no radiographic abnormalities. Foreign bodies that obstruct mainly on expiration generate a check-valve effect, resulting in hyperinflation of the affected side and mediastinal shift to the opposite side (Fig. 208-4). This is a typical early finding. A ball-valve effect is produced later when foreign bodies obstruct on inspiration and open on expiration, producing atelectasis on the affected side and a mediastinal shift toward the affected side (Fig. 208-5). When the object completely obstructs the bronchus, a stop-valve effect occurs, leading to consolidation of the lobe involved.

Inspiratory and expiratory chest films can aid in the diagnosis, showing hyperinflation on expiratory films or atelectasis on inspiratory films. In younger children who cannot cooperate, lateral decubitus films may help. The dependent lung should collapse normally, but remains inflated in bronchial obstruction. Fluoroscopic evaluation is of little benefit; decreased diaphragmatic movement on the side of the obstruction is helpful in only 50% of cases.[16] Simultaneous biplane fluoroscopy is used for extraction of radiopaque foreign bodies in the lung periphery.

Radiographic findings often suggest but do not diagnose foreign body aspiration. Asthma and mucous plugging can simulate foreign body aspiration. Mu and associates[23] reported that 35% of patients having normal radiographic studies were later found to have bronchial foreign bodies. Other studies show the lack of sensitivity or specificity of radiographs in diagnosing airway foreign bodies.[24,25] In cases of suspected foreign bodies, endoscopic evaluation is important because negative radiographs are not enough to rule out the presence of a foreign body.[24]

Esophageal Foreign Bodies

When an esophageal foreign body is suspected by history and physical examination, a radiologic evaluation is performed to assess its location and size, and to anticipate the possibility of multiple foreign bodies. Posteroanterior and lateral airway films and posteroanterior and lateral chest films, including the abdomen, are performed. Foreign bodies rotate to the greatest diameter of the lumen; flat objects in the esophagus usually are oriented in the coronal plane.[26] It is imperative to obtain a lateral airway and chest film to evaluate for possible battery ingestion because a battery can easily mimic a coin on posteroanterior view.

There is a high rate of spontaneous passage of esophageal coins into the stomach.[27] Predictors for a high rate of spontaneous passage include location in the distal esophagus, male gender, and age older than 5 years.[28] An observation period of 8 to 16 hours is considered appropriate management in otherwise healthy children with asymptomatic esophageal coins.[29] A repeat radiograph is warranted before attempted removal to confirm the location of the coin. A handheld metal detector may improve the timing and ease of confirming the location of blunt metallic foreign objects within the esophagus just before administration of general anesthesia.[30]

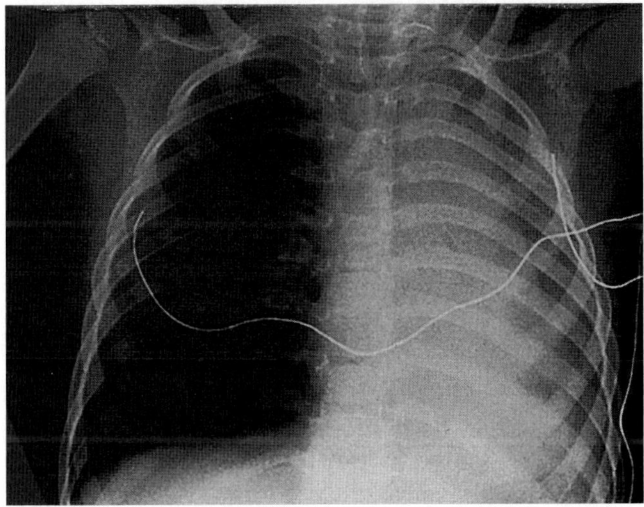

Figure 208-5. Anteroposterior chest film of left lobar collapse secondary to candy corn in the left main bronchus.

In rare cases in which an esophageal foreign body was not found on initial endoscopy and migrated extraluminally, fluoroscopy with contrast material may aid in preoperative location of the object. Open surgical exploration is rarely required to retrieve a foreign body.[26]

Management

Most patients who arrive at the hospital with airway foreign bodies have passed the acute phase and are no longer in respiratory distress. Patients in respiratory distress are given support until the endoscopy team can safely attempt removal. This support may include oxygen, heliox,[31] or intubation. With rare exceptions, esophageal foreign body impactions are not dire emergencies. There is time to obtain a history regarding the ingestion and a pertinent medical history. An inadequate diagnostic workup and hasty preparation of the operating suite likely lead to a poor outcome. Other associated conditions, such as tetanus immunization status or blood lead levels,[32] should be appropriately ascertained and treated.

The standard radiographic posteroanterior and lateral airway and chest films may give adequate information for foreign body removal. If the foreign body is sharp or irregularly shaped, a radiograph in the plane of the greatest dimension of the foreign body may help plan removal. If a suspected esophageal foreign body is radiolucent, a barium contrast study should be avoided because it would delay endoscopy in that the patient can no longer take anything by mouth, and the foreign object may be obscured by the material swallowed. Generally, the patient should take nothing by mouth for 6 hours, and then be adequately hydrated.

The basic principles of endoscopic foreign body removal have not changed since Jackson's time.[3,8] The type and size of endoscope depend on the age of the patient and the location of the object. Foreign body forceps are selected on the basis of practice with a similar object, preferably a duplicate brought in by the patient's family. It is important that the operating room personnel be familiar with the planned procedure, and that communication with the anesthesiologist regarding the anesthetic and endoscopy plan has occurred.

Equipment

Age-appropriate equipment for endoscopic foreign body removal is carefully selected before the patient is brought to the operating room (Table 208-1). Equipment should be in good working order and checked before the procedure. All members of the endoscopy team should be familiar with the location, setup, and use of the instrumentation. If there is inadequate equipment or a lack of trained personnel, transfer of the patient to an adequately equipped center with an experienced endoscopy team should be considered.

Table 208-1

Guidelines for Selection of Bronchoscope, Esophagoscope, and Laryngoscope for Diagnostic Endoscopy by Age

Mean Age (Range)	Bronchoscope Size*	mm*	Laryngoscope Size*	Esophagoscope Size*
Premature infant	2.5	3.7	8	4
Term newborn (newborn to 3 mo)	3	5.8	8	4-5
6 mo (3-18 mo)	3.5	5.7	9	5-6
18 mo (1-3 yr)	3.7	6.3	10.5	6
3 yr (2-6 yr)	4	6.7	10.5-12	6-7
7 yr (5-10 yr)	5	7.8	12	7
10 yr (>10 yr to adolescent)	6	8.2	16	8

*Outside diameter given in millimeters.

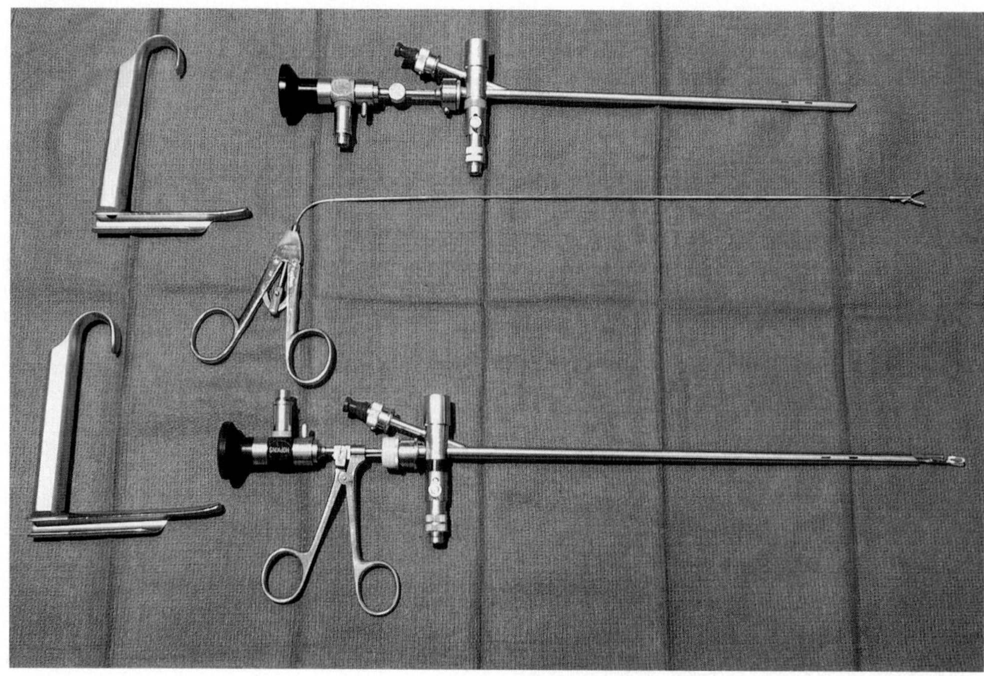

Figure 208-6. Instruments for endoscopic removal of an airway foreign body.

Laryngoscopy visualizes laryngeal foreign bodies and facilitates passage of a bronchoscope. Preferred bronchoscopes with a rod-lens telescope are the Doesel-Huzly bronchoscopes (Karl Storz) (Fig. 208-6). Age-appropriate sizes minimize laryngeal edema. For airway foreign bodies, two bronchoscopes are prepared so that if one fails, another is immediately available. For esophageal foreign bodies, an esophageal speculum and appropriate-sized esophagoscope for the patient's age and size are chosen. Suctions and forceps should be checked to ensure they are of adequate length to be used with the endoscopy equipment. Active or passive action forceps may be used; in most situations, the improved visualization achieved with optical forceps is preferable. Because of their size, optical forceps may impair the ability to ventilate a patient adequately through the bronchoscope; alternate forceps should be readily available.[3,7,8] With all endoscopic foreign body procedures, safety glasses should be worn by the endoscopy team, and a dental guard should be placed before introduction of the endoscope.

Anesthesia

Unless the patient is in extremis, foreign body removal is performed under general anesthesia to provide optimal airway control and patient comfort. The plan for induction and maintenance of anesthesia, and the method of evaluation and removal of the foreign body should be communicated preoperatively between the anesthesiologist and endoscopist. Patients are given nothing by mouth for an adequate time to reduce the risk of aspiration. Patients are placed supine for mask induction using volatile inhalational agents for children. Eye protection prevents corneal abrasions. Spontaneous respiration is maintained. The larynx is topically anesthetized with 1% to 4% lidocaine to inhibit laryngeal reflexes and to reduce the incidence of laryngospasm.

For a suspected laryngeal foreign body, patients are preoxygenated. After mask induction, anesthesia is maintained with an insufflation catheter through the nares into the hypopharynx. For tracheobronchial foreign body removal, the laryngoscope tip is placed in the vallecula to expose the larynx for passage of the bronchoscope. The patient breathes through the bronchoscope until the conclusion of the procedure. For esophageal foreign bodies, the patient undergoes endotracheal intubation. The endotracheal tube prevents inadvertent aspiration of the foreign body into the airway during attempted removal, and minimizes any tracheal compression caused by a rigid esophagoscope.

Technique

For bronchial foreign bodies, the healthy bronchus is examined first. The bronchoscope is positioned above the foreign body, and secretions are gently suctioned to expose the object fully. Before and during the attempt at removal, 100% oxygen is given. The forceps are placed through the bronchoscope, and the foreign body is engaged. The bronchoscope, forceps, and foreign body are removed as a unit, and the bronchoscope is returned immediately to the airway for ventilation and assessment for other foreign bodies. As previously mentioned, simultaneous biplane fluoroscopy can be used for extraction of radiopaque foreign bodies in the lung periphery.[33]

Occasionally, attempts at endoscopic retrieval fail, and thoracotomy is required. If the foreign body is too large to be extracted through the larynx, the foreign body may be broken into small fragments and removed through the bronchoscope. Alternatively, a tracheotomy is performed, and the foreign body is removed through the neck, maintaining the airway and delivering the object with bronchoscopic guidance.[34,35]

For esophageal foreign body removal, an esophageal speculum or esophagoscope is passed through the right side of the mouth and directed toward the pyriform sinus. The scope is angled toward the sternal notch. The esophageal lumen is kept in view at all times while the esophagoscope is gently advanced until the foreign body is visualized. The foreign body is engaged with the forceps; the esophagoscope is advanced toward the object; and the foreign body, forceps, and esophagoscope are removed as a single unit. If multiple foreign bodies are suspected, the esophagoscope is reinserted to assess the condition of the esophageal mucosa, and to identify additional foreign bodies below the primary one. Multiple foreign bodies are found in 5% of patients (Fig. 208-7).[6]

Removal of Sharp Objects

Extraction of sharp, pointed, or unusually shaped objects can be extremely challenging.[7,36] Locating the point is crucial. Usually, the tip of a pointed object engages the mucosa, causing the object to tumble and proceed with the point trailing. Pointed objects may be bendable or breakable; analysis of a duplicate may aid in this determination. The endoscope is aligned parallel to the long axis of the airway or esophagus to minimize the likelihood of damage to the surrounding mucosa. During the extraction, the object first is moved distally to disengage the point.

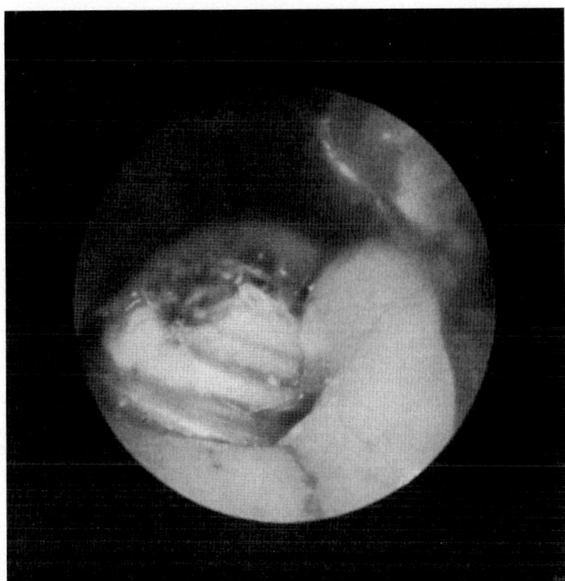

Figure 208-7. Multiple coins in the esophagus of a patient with a history of tracheoesophageal fistula.

Pin-bending forceps may be used for bendable objects; this reconfigures the object's point to trail on removal. Safety pins are uniquely challenging; pins that become lodged are invariably open. The incidence of safety pins as foreign bodies has decreased with the introduction of disposable diapers. Two methods of removal are suggested: (1) sheathing the point within the endoscope while locking the forceps closed to hold the keeper against the outside of the tube particularly during extraction through the larynx, and (2) gastric version (under fluoroscopic guidance) of esophageal safety pins, using rotation forceps to flip the safety pin point down within the stomach. The Clerf-Arrowsmith pin-closing forceps risk entanglement with the safety pin, which becomes virtually impossible to remove. This dangerous tool is not recommended. If a sharp object is severely impacted or embedded, an open surgical approach may be the safest method of foreign body removal.[5,7]

Long or large objects in children younger than 2 years may not pass through the duodenum. It is preferable to remove these objects from the stomach endoscopically before they migrate further or perforate a bowel wall. If a disk battery traverses beyond the esophagus, and the patient remains asymptomatic, parents are advised to check the patient's stools for passage and to return immediately to the hospital if fever or abdominal pain occurs.[7,37] An abdominal film should be obtained for delayed passage. Children younger than 6 years who have swallowed a battery 15 mm in diameter or larger that has not passed out of the stomach within 48 hours should undergo endoscopic removal. Many batteries 15 mm or greater do not pass out of the stomach and cause corrosive injury in an acidic environment.

Disk Battery Ingestions

Disk batteries are commonly used in hearing aids, calculators, watches, and other portable electronic devices. The peak incidence of ingestion occurs at age 1 to 2 years. In 33% of cases, the ingested battery is from the child's hearing aid.[38] A patient with a history of ingestion and esophageal lodging of disk batteries (also known as button batteries) requires immediate action.[7,37,38] In 1 hour, the esophageal mucosa may be damaged; in 4 hours, leakage of caustic battery contents may cause erosion through the muscular wall of the esophagus; and within 6 or more hours, an esophageal perforation leading to mediastinitis, tracheoesophageal fistula, or death may occur.[7,37,38] If esophageal lodging of a disk battery is suspected, radiography localizes the battery. An immediate esophagoscopy is performed to remove the battery and assess the patient's esophageal mucosa. Most batteries of this type are of a smaller diameter (<15 mm) and usually traverse the gastrointestinal tract with only minor injury. Larger button batteries (≥15 mm in diameter) are more likely to lodge in the esophagus or stomach, causing serious corrosive injury. Mercuric oxide–containing batteries can cause systemic mercury poisoning if they open in the gastrointestinal tract. The imprint code of a duplicate battery should be conveyed to a Poison Control Center or Button Battery Ingestion Hotline for specific information.[38]

Pill Ingestions

Medications in pill form may lodge within the esophagus because of delayed esophageal transit, dry swallow (i.e., swallowing without liquids), adherent tablets, or a supine swallow. The pill may cause caustic injury through various mechanisms because of prolonged contact with the esophageal mucosa.[39] More than 70 different medications in pill form have been reported to cause caustic injury. Antibiotics and antivirals account for 60% of cases. Most heal without significant injury. Anti-inflammatory medications have been reported in fewer cases, but a third of these patients have had significant hemorrhage or had strictures develop.[39]

Most injured patients have no predisposing factor other than improper swallowing of pills; however, any functional or anatomic abnormality of the esophagus may give rise to this condition. Patients usually are seen with sudden onset of retrosternal pain, dysphagia, and odynophagia.[39] Fever, hematemesis, and dehydration are less common presenting symptoms. Often, patients recall the sensation of a pill sticking in the esophagus before the onset of symptoms, or have swallowed a pill without water or at bedtime.[39] Most symptoms resolve over days to weeks.

Endoscopy should be considered if the symptoms are severe, persistent, or atypical, or if hematemesis or a stricture is suspected.[39] Esophagoscopy can differentiate other potential causes, such as infection, malignancy, or gastroesophageal reflux disease. In addition, any pill remnants may be removed, and an accurate assessment may be made of the degree of mucosal injury. The most common findings on esophagoscopy are small, shallow, discrete ulcers that may be single or multiple. Large, circumferential lesions several centimeters in length have been reported.[39] Most shallow ulcers heal spontaneously. Deep injuries may lead to stricture formation and perforation. Education of the public and health care personnel in methods of proper pill swallowing is important to prevent pill-induced esophageal injuries.

Esophageal Perforation

Perforation of the esophagus in a patient with an impacted esophageal foreign body may be caused by the object itself, by the length of time that the object has been lodged, or by attempts to retrieve the object.[8,26,38,40-42] If perforation is suspected preoperatively, esophageal perforation may be diagnosed on preoperative radiographic evaluation. Cervical subcutaneous emphysema, retroesophageal abscess, or an obvious extraluminal portion of the esophageal foreign body may be apparent.[5] Fever with tachycardia, tachypnea, and increased pain all may be early signs of a perforation.[5,43] With early recognition and management, the mortality rate for esophageal perforation has decreased from 60% to 9%.[42] After esophagography has been performed to locate and evaluate the extent of the injury, early institution of nothing by mouth and broad-spectrum antibiotics may be all that is necessary in pharyngoesophageal perforations,[41,43] the most common area injured in endoscopic removal of esophageal foreign bodies. In more severe injuries, drainage, closure, or more complex surgical repairs may be necessary.

Postoperative Management

After esophagoscopy for foreign body extraction, children are observed and given nothing by mouth for 4 hours. Patients are monitored for fever, tachycardia, and tachypnea, all signs of possible perforation. Antibiotics are not routinely given unless significant esophageal injury is evident.

When appropriate-sized bronchoscopes are used for brief procedures, racemic epinephrine or corticosteroids are not given. Chest physiotherapy may help to clear inspissated secretions. A routine postoperative radiograph is unnecessary unless the patient's symptoms

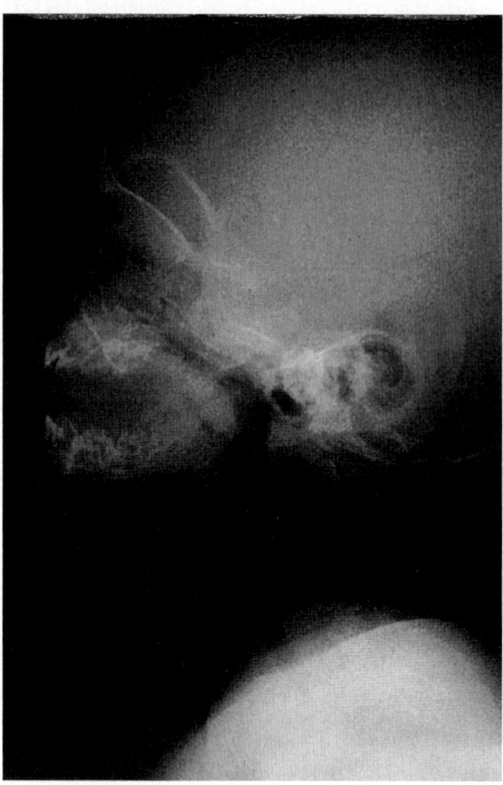

Figure 208-8. Lateral neck film reveals retroesophageal abscess.

persist or progress. When extraction attempts fail or are incomplete, patients are rested for several days, and then returned to the operating room for repeat endoscopy. One more recent study examined factors associated with increased pulmonary recovery time after foreign body removal. A recovery time of more than 1 week was associated with preoperative inflammatory findings by radiologic study, procedure time greater than 50 minutes, and worsening postoperative radiologic findings.[44]

Complications

Before the 20th century, the mortality rate caused by foreign body aspiration was high, with most patients dying of complications. In 1882, Weiss reported 937 cases for which bronchotomy was performed, with a 27% mortality rate; however, 23% died without management.[2] Jackson's techniques reduced the mortality rate to about 2%.[22] The present rate is 2% or less.[4,11,16,17,45,46]

Most complications are the result of delayed diagnosis and treatment.[17,21,47,48] Earlier diagnosis correlates with fewer complications.[48] Of laryngotracheal foreign bodies, 45% were associated with major complications, and 67% were associated with major complications when the delay was longer than 24 hours.[20] The introduction of rod-lens telescopes has reduced the incidence of missed or incomplete removal of foreign bodies, reducing complications further.

Pneumonia and atelectasis are the most common complications after bronchial foreign body removal. Patients usually respond to intravenous antibiotics and chest physiotherapy. Bleeding can occur because of granulation tissue or erosion into a major vessel. Pneumothorax and pneumomediastinum can result from an airway tear. Small perforations typically heal spontaneously, and do not require specific management. Impaction of the foreign body can cause airway obstruction, converting a controlled situation into an emergency. Laryngeal inflammation and edema have decreased significantly with the use of appropriate-sized endoscopic equipment.

Long-term complications (e.g., granulation tissue, stricture formation) can occur at the site where the foreign body is lodged. Certain foreign bodies are more likely to cause more complications.[48] The oils of nuts may contribute to edema and granulation tissue.[3]

The most frequent complications of endoscopic esophageal foreign body removal are categorized as those occurring before endoscopy, during endoscopy, and after endoscopy.[39] Vomiting and respiratory distress are most common preoperatively. During esophagoscopy, the endotracheal tube may be dislodged, and the patient may have cricopharyngeal spasm, esophageal mucosal injury, or perforation. After esophagoscopy, vomiting, aspiration, a second missed foreign body, and fever are the most common complications. Esophageal perforation, retroesophageal abscess, mediastinitis, and death are rare (Fig. 208-8). In several large series of endoscopic esophageal foreign body removal, there were no life-threatening complications.[5,6,41,42]

Controversies in Management

Nonendoscopic means of foreign body extraction have been suggested. These methods have been detrimental in some cases, causing emergent situations and even death. Although chest physiotherapy and bronchodilators have been suggested as a management for airway foreign bodies, this proposal has been retracted.[49]

Flexible bronchoscopic removal of airway foreign bodies seems attractive, with more recent literature advocating its use in adults and increasing experience in pediatrics as a diagnostic tool.[9] Unless the endoscopist also is skilled at rigid bronchoscopy, flexible bronchoscopic foreign body removal in children is not recommended,[25] especially in small children. The main problems are poor control of the airway and of the foreign body itself.[9,25]

For impacted esophageal foreign bodies, bougienage with esophageal dilators or a nasogastric tube has been proposed to push foreign bodies into the stomach.[2,49] This blind technique may cause esophageal injury and is not universally accepted. Foley catheter removal with fluoroscopic control of blunt radiopaque esophageal foreign bodies has been recommended for a single object lodged below the cricopharyngeus for a short duration.[23,42,50] Advantages include reduced cost and avoidance of general anesthesia. Few serious complications have been reported when this technique was used in healthy children. Other authors[6,26,49] point out that the risks of general anesthesia in these patients are small. This technique does not allow a postretrieval assessment of the esophageal mucosa or identification of a nonradiopaque second foreign body. Because the coin is not grasped using this technique, loss of control of the coin at the level of the posterior pharynx can result in an airway emergency. In addition, there is a risk of vomiting and aspiration with an unprotected airway, and young patients who have this procedure while awake and restrained in a steep head-down position may experience emotional trauma.

Use of various pharmacologic agents in the management of esophageal foreign bodies has also been proposed. Papain (meat tenderizer) has been used in patients with impacted esophageal meat boluses.[49] Papain was given as a 5% solution to adult patients, with the meat passing in most instances. However, there were at least two cases of mediastinitis and death in these patients caused by necrosis of the esophagus and perforation. Glucagon produces relaxation of the smooth muscle of the esophagus, promoting passage into the stomach. One open-label study in pediatric patients failed to show a higher incidence of passage in patients who received glucagon versus placebo.[51] Sumatriptan prolongs fundic relaxation and delays gastric emptying. Studies conducted so far have revealed an increase in the rate of gastroesophageal reflux and the number of esophageal mother waves.[52,53]

Flexible esophagoscopy has been used for removal of blunt objects or meat impaction. Sharp objects pose a greater risk, however, because of the inability to sheath the object as with a rigid esophagoscope.[36]

Careful endoscopic removal of foreign objects under direct vision is the safest management for patients with foreign bodies of the airway and esophagus. Prevention is ideal, with increased education of the public, especially individuals who supervise children—parents, teachers, and other care providers—on age-appropriate foods and household objects. Stricter government and industry standards for toy part sizes and appropriately sized containers have helped to decrease fatalities from choking, but have come about only through the cooperation of physicians, consumer advocacy groups, and governmental public health agencies.[54,55]

SUGGESTED READINGS

Assefa D, Amin N, Stringel G, et al. Use of decubitus radiographs in the diagnosis of foreign body aspiration in young children. *Pediatr Emerg Care.* 2007;23:154.

Aydogan LB, Tuncer U, Soylu L, et al. Rigid bronchoscopy for the suspicion of foreign body in the airway. *Int J Pediatr Otorhinolaryngol.* 2006;70:823.

Bloom DC, Christenson TE, Manning SC, et al. Plastic laryngeal foreign bodies in children: a diagnostic challenge. *Int J Pediatr Otorhinolaryngol.* 2005; 69:657.

Centers for Disease Control and Prevention (CDC). Nonfatal choking-related episodes among children—United States, 2001. *MMWR Morbid Mortal Wkly Rep.* 2002;51:945.

Chatterji S, Chatterji P. The management of foreign bodies in air passages. *Anesthesia.* 1972;27:390.

Chung MK, Jeong HS, Ahn KM, et al. Pulmonary recovery after rigid bronchoscopic retrieval of airway foreign bodies. *Laryngoscope.* 2007;117:303.

Clerf LH. Historical aspects of foreign bodies in the air and food passages. *South Med J.* 1975;68:1449.

Committee on Accident and Poison Prevention. First aid for the choking child. *Pediatrics.* 1988;81:740.

Darrow DH, Holinger LD. Foreign bodies of the larynx, trachea and bronchi. In: Bluestone C, Stool S, eds. *Pediatric Otolaryngology.* Philadelphia: Saunders; 1996.

Deutsch ES, Dixit D, Curry J, et al. Management of aerodigestive tract foreign bodies: innovative teaching concepts. *Ann Otol Rhinol Laryngol.* 2007; 116:319.

Gaafar H, Abdel-Dayem M, Talaat M, et al. The value of x-ray examination in the diagnosis of tracheobronchial foreign bodies in infants and children. *ORL J Otorhinolaryngol Relat Spec.* 1982;44:340.

For complete list of references log onto www.expertconsult.com.

Heimlich HJ. A life-saving maneuver to prevent food-choking. *JAMA.* 1975;234:398.

Holinger LD. Management of sharp and penetrating foreign bodies of the upper aerodigestive tract. *Ann Otol Rhinol Laryngol.* 1990;99:684.

Inglis AF, Wagner DB. Lower complication rates associated with bronchial foreign bodies over the last 20 years. *Ann Otol Rhinol Laryngol.* 1992;101:61.

Kikendall JW. Pill-induced esophageal injury. *Gastroenterol Clin North Am.* 1991;20:835.

Lemberg PS, Darrow DH, Holinger LD. Aerodigestive tract foreign bodies in the older child and adolescent. *Ann Otol Rhinol Laryngol.* 1996;105:267.

Litovitz T, Schmitz B. Ingestion of cylindrical and button batteries: an analysis of 2382 cases. *Pediatrics.* 1992;89:747.

Maves MD, Carithers JS, Birck HG. Esophageal burns secondary to disc battery ingestion. *Ann Otol Rhinol Laryngol.* 1984;93:364.

Reilly JS, Cook SP, Stool D, et al. Prevention and management of aerodigestive foreign body injuries in childhood. *Pediatr Clin North Am.* 1996;43:1403.

Rimell FL, Thome A Jr, Stool S, et al. Characteristics of objects that cause choking in children. *JAMA.* 1995;274:1763.

Silva AB, Muntz HR, Clary R. Utility of conventional radiography in the diagnosis and management of pediatric airway foreign bodies. *Ann Otol Rhinol Laryngol.* 1998;107:834.

Singh B, Kantu M, Har-El G, et al. Complications associated with 327 foreign bodies of the pharynx, larynx, and esophagus. *Ann Otol Rhinol Laryngol.* 1997;106:301.

Soprano JV, Fleisher GR, Mandl KD. The spontaneous passage of esophageal coins in children. *Arch Pediatr Adolesc Med.* 1999;153:1073.

Tomaske M, Gerber AC, Stocker S, et al. Tracheobronchial foreign body aspiration in children—diagnostic value of symptoms and signs. *Swiss Med Wkly.* 2006;136:533.

Waltzman M. Management of esophageal coins. *Curr Opin Pediatr.* 2006;18:571.

CHAPTER TWO HUNDRED AND NINE

Gastroesophageal Reflux and Laryngeal Disease

Philippe Contencin

Thierry Van den Abbeele

Natacha Teissier

Key Points

- Other than gastroesophageal reflux (GER) disease, with its digestive and general signs and symptoms and valid tests, the definition of GER-related laryngeal disorders remains unclear.
- No true specific features of GER-related laryngeal disorders have been found, and the role of refluxed acid (or nonacid) gastric content in their occurrence is still unknown.
- Only a statistical correlation between GER and some inflammatory processes of the pediatric larynx has been found.
- Several possible mechanisms have been described, including direct epithelial injury, and indirect harm via vague mediated reflexes with or without vocal misuse.
- In addition to classic signs and symptoms of GER, the diagnosis is based on therapeutic trials, esophageal pH, and, for the future, impedance monitoring.
- Although most controlled studies (in adults) show no efficacy, anti-GER treatment or proton pump inhibitors or both are advised in selected cases of apnea with laryngospasm, associations with regional neuromuscular disorders (including laryngomalacia), recurrent croup, and laryngeal surgery.

First reported in the 19th century for bronchitis, the involvement of gastroesophageal reflux (GER) in the respiratory tract is still a controversial topic. Most pulmonologists consider GER as a possible aggravating factor for asthma. The involved mechanism of it is unknown, however.

The pediatric larynx is a sensitive organ subject to spasm and edema in case of minor harm. Evidence of the association of GER and laryngeal disorders in newborns to adults has been found. Data suggesting a cause-and-effect relationship are still missing, however.

History

Internists and otolaryngologists have reported possible airway involvement in adult patients with upper digestive disorders. By the end of the 19th century, Osler mentioned the occurrence of dyspnea in the postprandial period when the gastric cavity is full. From the early 1970s, with the description of "hiatal hernia" in adults, to more recent pediatric studies, it has become obvious that some laryngeal inflammatory processes develop in conjunction with upper digestive malfunctions, including GER.

The first modern clinical demonstration of GER-related laryngeal harm was made by Ward and colleagues[1] in glottic granulomas and contact ulcers in adults, and by Little and colleagues[2] in subglottic stenosis in an animal model. In infants and children, GER was initially shown through barium studies to be responsible for recurrent croup.[3] Similarly, apnea in premature newborns and various forms of laryngitis were linked to GER by means of esophageal and pharyngeal pH monitoring.[4,5] Finding decreases in pharyngeal pH to 2 at the laryngeal inlet or above in cases of pediatric chronic rhinitis/laryngitis raises a high index of suspicion of the role of acid reflux in these disorders of the airway. There was a statistically significant difference in upper and lower pH monitoring data between these patients and controls.[6] Some control patients and even gastroenterology patients might have pH variations that were close to each other, however, without any rhinolaryngologic symptoms. Since those studies were performed, control infants and children could not ethically be tested. Many studies focused on in vitro tests and on the efficacy of anti-GER treatments in patients.

Definition

GER is an abnormal and repeated ascent of gastric content into the esophagus (and possibly above it). There is a physiologic GER that occurs mainly in the postprandial period. Small amounts of refluxed material may cause burping at any age and a small degree of emesis in the infant. Sometimes it is also called "functional" GER because esophageal pH monitoring may show a few acid periods (<5% of recorded time at pH less than 4 on a 20-hour basis) that are considered unharmful to the esophagus. In this case, no other digestive symptom is noted, and upper digestive endoscopy is normal.

GER disease (GERD) is believed to have gastrointestinal or extra-gastrointestinal signs. Gastrointestinal signs include emesis, dysphagia, choking, gagging, and failure to thrive in children. Extragastrointestinal signs include chronic coughing, wheezing, hoarseness, sore throat, stridor, recurrent croup, and obstructive apnea. Heartburn is extremely rare.

GERD was defined using gastrointestinal criteria; normal values for GER tests were established according to this definition. These criteria are not entirely appropriate in cases of a laryngeal disorder (also improperly called "laryngopharyngeal reflux" in adults). An extensive assessment for GER with "normal" results may be associated with chronic laryngeal inflammation; however, abnormal results indicating GERD may be found in cases of asymptomatic and endoscopically normal larynges. Many authors emphasized the particular pH profile of "airway-linked" GER. In a cohort of 90 children with pH monitoring, Zalesska-Krecicka and coworkers[7] found a high prevalence of daytime refluxes when patients with laryngeal disorders were in the upright position.

Physiopathology

The anatomic proximity and the neurofunctional collusion of the human larynx to the hypopharynx and upper esophagus lead to its unique vulnerability.[8] In no other mammal species is the larynx so caudal compared with the digestive tract organs. This positioning can explain the diffusion of the gastric juice up to the laryngeal mucosa.[9] Although many patients have GER, why do so few have true laryngeal disorders? It seems that a mechanism peculiar to the larynx is involved, and this can be due to direct contact with the gastric juice or to a vague mediated reflex.

Studies by Willging and Thompson[10] emphasized the role of laryngeal sensitivity in the development of pediatric anomalies such as laryngomalacia and GER-induced laryngeal reflexes. Paradoxical vocal cord motion, laryngospasm, and saliva and food aspiration are associated with abnormal thresholds of local chemoreceptors and mechanoreceptors. It has been shown that premature infants develop progressive swallowing ability and control of the lower esophageal sphincter postnatally, depending on the status of their respiratory and neurologic systems. GER and laryngeal sensitivity are intimately related and involved in cases of prematurity.[11]

Lipan and associates[9] discussed possible mechanisms of potential harm of the larynx by GER. They stated that, compared with classic intraesophageal reflux, cranial involvement by GER may be the result of four failing "barriers" including upper esophageal sphincter and pharyngolaryngeal mucosal resistance. These two domains warrant specialized interest and involvement of gastroenterologists, pathologists, and immunologists to know what exactly differentiates patients with gastrointestinal symptoms from patients with head and neck symptoms affected by GER. In 1998, an experimental rabbit model–based study emphasized the role of hydrogen chloride and pepsin inducing a chemical trauma and the individual laryngeal chemosensitivity.[12] In 2003, Altman and colleagues[13] found expression of a proton pump in the laryngeal mucosa. These mechanisms are held responsible for inflammatory laryngeal pediatric processes and for adult laryngeal carcinomas.[14] Eventually, in an "in vitro" model of laryngeal cultures, Ylitalo and Thibeault[15] showed more changes in gene expression of postcricoidal fibroblasts after 60 seconds of exposure to pepsin at low pH. Some authors denied the role of acid secretions in this domain, however, considering the inefficacy of gastric acid suppressors (i.e., proton pump inhibitors) in healing chronic laryngitis in adults.[16]

Diagnosis

A patient history of combined digestive and respiratory symptoms may help suggest the diagnosis of GERD. In infants, feeding difficulties with tears, apparent life-threatening events with hypotonia, and rise of refluxed food while supine are useful signs that may lead to empirical treatment. Radiographic studies with barium swallow, a search for lipid-laden macrophages at bronchial lavage, and a thoracic scintiscan with ingestion of nuclide elements are not routinely performed. Esophagoscopy with a flexible fiberscope may show esophagitis and large hiatal hernia. These abnormalities are rare, however, in cases with no gastrointestinal symptoms. It is unclear whether laryngoscopy and bronchoscopy can point to marks of GER because no specific features are described other than cobblestoning of the posterior supraglottic or subglottic area.[17,18]

Esophageal pH monitoring is considered by gastroenterologists to be the gold standard for diagnosing GER. Acid periods recorded over 18 to 24 hours can be correlated with airway manifestations (e.g., cough, stridor). An abnormal percentage of the recorded time at a pH less than 4 allows the physician to manage the GER. The question is what percentage should be considered abnormal in the absence of gastrointestinal signs and symptoms. It is unknown whether nonacid or weakly acid reflux may also play a role in the pathogenesis of GER-related laryngeal disorders.[19,20] A negative test does not rule out GER without esophageal lesion, however. Combined pharyngeal and esophageal pH records showed that brief refluxes can reach the laryngeal inlet and cause problems, whereas classic standards for this pH test are considered normal with a poor total acid time. Pharyngeal pH recordings are subject to drifts by dryness, however, and are not used routinely. Many studies have shown that brief diurnal refluxes are usual features of airway-disordered GER. Brief, pharyngeal and nonacid refluxes may be diagnosed easily by a promising test: esophageal impedance recording. This technique, which includes pH monitoring, allows recording of any refluxate, and is expected to enter routine practice.[21]

In adults with laryngeal symptoms and suspicion of GER, a therapeutic trial with a proton pump inhibitor is sometimes recommended, although more recent studies denied any efficacy of these treatments compared with placebo.[16,22] A therapeutic trial with a proton pump inhibitor would not be recommended as a diagnostic test in infants and children.

McMurray and coworkers[23] summarized the optimal assessment in cases of suspected esophagopharyngolaryngeal reflux: endoscopy with mucosal biopsy and dual probe pH monitoring are advocated.[23] This assessment underlies the principle of a mandatory abnormal GER (under gastrointestinal specifications) to start a specific treatment that is still subject of doubt.[9,24]

Disorders

The most frequent GER-related disorders in the airway of children of any age are classically the laryngeal diseases listed in Box 209-1. In older children and adults, dysphonia is the most frequently reported pathologic sign, along with pharyngeal symptoms (e.g., pain, globus sensation). Recurrent subglottic laryngitis with dyspnea (croup) is the most common consequence of GER on the airway in children. A statistically significant correlation with GER was found in patients with recurrent croup using two-channel pH monitoring.[5] Successful anti-GER therapeutic trials and recurrences after stopping management also were noted in patients with recurrent croup.[25]

GER has been shown to have an important role in the development of subglottic stenosis. Long-term endotracheal intubation leads to increased acid pharyngeal reflux. Animal studies have shown that acid placed on the subglottic mucosa after local trauma leads to granulation tissue and fibrous scarring with subsequent stenosis.[2] Some authors believe that successful surgical management of subglottic stenoses in children depends on the control of GER.[26]

Box 209-1

Gastroesophageal Reflux–Related Laryngeal Disorders in Infants and Children

- Apnea, laryngospasm
- Paradoxical vocal cord motion
- Laryngomalacia
- Recurrent croup
- Laryngeal granulations
- Acquired glottic web
- Hoarseness, chronic cough
- Aspiration
- Subglottic stenosis (and laryngeal surgery)

The most important GER-associated laryngeal phenomena in infants are motor disorders. GER is found in more than 90% of cases of laryngomalacia.[27] GER may cause edema at the laryngeal inlet. GER also may be induced by the negative endothoracic pressure resulting from the airway obstruction. GER is probably associated only with pharyngoesophageal motor anomalies that are caused by the neurologic dysfunction that determines laryngomalacia.[27] Glottic and pharyngoesophageal dysfunctions that occur simultaneously with GER lead to aspiration. In return, laryngeal adductor responses seem to coincide with reflux in premature newborns, with subsequent obstructive reflex apnea.[4]

Apnea in neonates and obstructive sleep apnea in adults have been reported as linked to GER. The concomitant time with GER episodes has been shown in premature infants by Orenstein and colleagues.[4] Senior and associates[28] described a decline of obstructive sleep apnea scores at polysomnography with anti-GER treatment. Dyce and coworkers[29] stated that GER is associated with many congenital disorders, including Pierre Robin sequence and 22q11 deletion syndrome.

Hoarseness and vocal fold nodules are sometimes described as a result of GER. Mandell and colleagues[30] compared the results of esophageal biopsy with endoscopic findings and bronchioalveolar lavage in a series of 127 hoarse children including 104 with nodules. There was no correlation between biopsy and bronchioalveolar lavage results, and endoscopy was more contributory than any other test. In a study of 254 pediatric patients, Shah and associates[31] found only one quarter of GER-positive cases. It seems that the incidence of GER in hoarse children may vary depending on the criteria used and the type of assessment made. Vocal cord dysfunction or laryngeal dyskinesia are strongly associated with psychiatric illness and GER.[32]

A link between GER and recurrent respiratory papillomatosis has been suggested by McKenna and Brodsky[33] from a series of four children whose noncompliance with anti-GER treatment determined occurrence of laryngeal symptoms and reappearance of papillomas at endoscopy. All these studies widely favor the close relationship between GER and inflammatory features of the larynx. They do not carry any direct evidence of the role of GER, however, owing to nonspecific aspects of the described features (except for contact ulcers, which are very rare in children).

Possible Role of Gastroesophageal Reflux

Because no direct role of GER has been shown by GER tests, endoscopy, and biopsy, therapeutic trials were used to search for indirect evidence. Besides acid and pepsin, many other components of refluxed material may be harmful, according to experimental animal or in vitro studies. Even powerful antagonists of gastric H^+ ion secretion may be useless in cases of documented GER with laryngeal involvement without esophagitis.

A retrospective study examined the impact of anti-GER treatments on the development of subglottic stenosis after surgery, and found there were fewer tracheostomies remaining in the treated group.[34] This study's method may be biased, however, and the same suspicion arose in other small series.[26,35] Of five published randomized controlled trials on the efficacy of GER treatments versus placebo in adult laryngeal disorders, four were negative, and the positive trial was considered weak because it included only 11 patients in each group.[16]

The implication of GER in laryngeal pathologies remains a controversial topic. It is still unclear how refluxed material ascending from the stomach may be harmful to the laryngeal mucosa, and which mechanisms, common muscular or immune or both, lead to GER and laryngeal inflammation. In the first hypothesis, we may wonder why many patients with GERD have no laryngeal disorder (even while vomiting and aspirating). In the latter, is the common digestive mechanism the cause or the consequence of laryngeal diseases? If it is not the consequence, further studies are necessary to find out if different types of reflux exist, or, more likely, if different types of laryngeal sensitivity could explain the controversial results in the described series. This laryngeal sensitivity may be related to other particular laryngeal descriptions, such as apnea encountered in preterm infants,[36] and laryngeal dysfunctions such as laryngomalacia[10,37] and paradoxical vocal fold motion.[38]

Management

The first step in antireflux management is to ensure that the patient has an age-appropriate diet and lifestyle. Foods that relax the lower esophageal sphincter should be avoided. Small meals at regular times and avoidance of any food or drink 1 hour before bedtime are common recommendations. Infants should be given milk thickened with rice, and fruit juice should be avoided. The posture of the patient at rest also is extremely important. Gravity reduces the frequency and strength of reflux episodes. Raising the head of the bed by 10 to 15 degrees is recommended for children, whereas infants who weigh up to 10 kg can be placed on a special mattress with a 30- to 45-degree slope. Pillows should be avoided. When not in bed, infants should be as upright as possible, even when physiotherapy is applied.

Recommended antireflux drugs (prokinetics) stimulate esophageal and gastric motility, while reinforcing the tonicity of the lower esophageal sphincter. Domperidone and metoclopramide can be prescribed despite their risk of adverse side effects (extrapyramidal syndrome with high dosage). Alginates coat the gastric contents and prevent its reascension. H_2 blockers inhibit gastric acid secretion and have been successfully used in some difficult cases, but some pediatric patients are nonresponders. Proton pump inhibitors (e.g., omeprazole, lansoprazole, esomeprazole) are now widely used in adult and pediatric patients. They prevent the release of hydrogen ions and are useful in severe forms resistant to other management. Management usually continues for years. Drugs can be limited to 2- to 3-month cycles, however, because the spontaneous course of the disease is typically episodic except in infants, in whom management may be continued for longer periods. Surgery (mainly Nissen fundoplication) is appropriate in cases in which severe disorders recur as soon as drugs are withdrawn, or in which medical control is impossible to achieve.

Conclusion

GER is strongly associated with many laryngeal disorders in infants and children, although evidence of a causal relationship is still lacking. This phenomenon is probably explained by different local sensitivities among subjects. The significant association is a strong argument, however, in favor of an anti-GER treatment in the absence of another obvious cause, or when critical surgery involving the airway is planned. Based on their experience, most laryngologists recommend that GER should be sought and managed in cases of recurrent laryngitis and of surgery for subglottic stenosis and other laryngeal abnormalities, such as nodules, cysts, and posterior cleft.[39] Whether prokinetic or anti-H^+ agents are most efficacious is still unknown.

SUGGESTED READINGS

Altman KW, Haines GK 3rd, Hammer ND, et al. The H+/K+-ATPase (proton) pump is expressed in human laryngeal submucosal glands. *Laryngoscope.* 2003;113:1927-1930.

Berkowitz RG. Failed paediatric laryngotracheoplasty. *Aust N Z J Surg.* 2001;71:292-296.

Carr MM, Nagy ML, Pizzuto MP, et al. Correlation of findings at direct laryngoscopy and bronchoscopy with gastroesophageal reflux disease in children: a prospective study. *Arch Otolaryngol Head Neck Surg.* 2001;127:369-374.

Contencin P, Maurage C, Ployet MJ, et al. Gastroesophageal reflux and ENT disorders in childhood. *Int J Pediatr Otorhinolaryngol.* 1995;32(Suppl):S135-S144.

Ford CN. Evaluation and management of laryngopharyngeal reflux. *JAMA.* 2005;294:1534-1540.

Halstead LA. Gastroesophageal reflux: a critical factor in pediatric subglottic stenosis. *Otolaryngol Head Neck Surg.* 1999;120:683-688.

Karkos PD, Wilson JA. Empiric treatment of laryngopharyngeal reflux with proton pump inhibitors: a systematic review. *Laryngoscope.* 2006;116:144-148.

Lipan MJ, Reidenberg JS, Laitman JT. Anatomy of reflux: a growing health problem affecting structures of the head and neck. *Anat Rec B New Anat.* 2006;289:261-270.

Manning SC, Inglis AF, Mouzakes J, et al. Laryngeal anatomic differences in pediatric patients with severe laryngomalacia. *Arch Otolaryngol Head Neck Surg.* 2005;131:340-343.

McKenna M, Brodsky L. Extraesophageal acid reflux and recurrent respiratory papilloma in children. *Int J Pediatr Otorhinolaryngol.* 2005;69:597-605.

McMurray JS, Gerber M, Stern Y, et al. Role of laryngoscopy, dual pH probe monitoring, and laryngeal mucosal biopsy in the diagnosis of pharyngoesophageal reflux. *Ann Otol Rhinol Laryngol.* 2001;110:299-304.

Miller CK, Willging JP. Advances in the evaluation and management of pediatric dysphagia. *Curr Opin Otolaryngol Head Neck Surg.* 2003;11:442-446.

Senior BA, Khan M, Schwimmer C, et al. Gastroesophageal reflux and obstructive sleep apnea. *Laryngoscope.* 2001;111:2144-2146.

Thach BT. Reflux associated apnea in infants: evidence for a laryngeal chemoreflex. *Am J Med.* 1997;103:120S-124S.

Tilles SA. Vocal cord dysfunction in children and adolescents. *Curr Allergy Asthma Rep.* 2003;3:467-472.

Vaezi MF, Richter JE, Stasney CR, et al. Treatment of chronic posterior laryngitis with esomeprazole. *Laryngoscope.* 2006;116:254-260.

Vandenplas Y, Salvatore S, Vieira MC, et al. Will esophageal impedance replace pH monitoring? *Pediatrics.* 2007;119:118-122.

Willging JP, Thompson DM. Pediatric FEESST: fiberoptic endoscopic evaluation of swallowing with sensory testing. *Curr Gastroenterol Rep.* 2005;7:240-243.

Wilson JA, White A, von Haacke NP, et al. Gastroesophageal reflux and posterior laryngitis. *Ann Otol Rhinol Laryngol.* 1989;98:405-410.

Ylitalo R, Thibeault SL. Relationship between time of exposure of laryngopharyngeal reflux and gene expression in laryngeal fibroblasts. *Ann Otol Rhinol Laryngol.* 2006;115:775-783.

Zalesska-Krecicka M, Krecicki T, Iwanczak B, et al. Laryngeal manifestations of gastroesophageal reflux disease in children. *Acta Otolaryngol.* 2002;122:306-310.

Zoumalan R, Maddalozzo J, Holinger LD. Etiology of stridor in infants. *Ann Otol Rhinol Laryngol.* 2007;11:329-334.

For complete list of references log onto www.expertconsult.com.

CHAPTER TWO HUNDRED AND TEN

Aspiration and Swallowing Disorders

David J. Brown

Maureen A. Lefton-Greif

Stacey L. Ishman

Key Points

- In evaluating children with aerodigestive disorders, the first priority is securing a safe airway.
- The coordination of breathing and swallowing is crucial to survival because both functions share the pharynx as a common conduit.
- The four phases of swallowing are the oral preparatory, oral, pharyngeal, and esophageal phases.
- The characteristics of dysphagia are defined by the anatomic site of impairment: nose and nasopharynx, oral cavity and oral pharynx, hypopharynx and larynx, and trachea and esophagus.
- Swallowing must provide sufficient nutrition and fluid for optimal growth and development.
- Videofluoroscopic swallow studies and flexible endoscopic evaluation of swallowing are commonly used evaluation tools to assess the pharyngeal phase of swallowing deficits.
- Dysphagia management may include feeding modifications, supplemental nutrition, oral motor and swallowing therapies, and alternative feeding routes.

Swallowing involves multiple, highly integrated, and partially overlapping actions; however, for discussion purposes, it is frequently separated into three phases—*oral, pharyngeal,* and *esophageal.* During the *oral phase,* food is processed into a "swallow-ready ball" (bolus), and then transported to the back of the mouth. This phase is limited to sucking fluid from a nipple during infancy. After approximately 6 months of age, this phase is sometimes subdivided to include the *oral preparatory phase,* which conditions solid foods requiring chewing. The *pharyngeal phase* comprises a series of complex and interrelated events that direct and propel boluses through the pharynx into the esophagus while the airway is protected. During this phase of swallowing, the velum rises and approximates the pharyngeal walls, breathing stops, the larynx rises, the vocal folds adduct, and the base of tongue and pharyngeal muscles propel the bolus through a relaxed upper esophageal sphincter. The act of swallowing results in mechanical closure of the airway and cessation of breathing. The *esophageal phase* begins when the bolus enters the esophagus and ends when it passes into the stomach.

Typical swallowing maturation involves transformation from the primitive sucking and swallowing reflexes used during infancy into the mature and volitional functions of biting, chewing, and bolus formation necessary for the safe and adequate delivery of nutrients in older children and adults. Appropriate adjustments to growth and developmental changes of the aerodigestive system and changes in airway protective responses are essential to competent postnatal maturation processes. Changes in the anatomic relationships of the oral cavity, pharynx, and larynx occur throughout the first few years of life and are well described. In addition, neurodevelopmental, cognitive, and sensory inputs modulate deglutitive function, and consequently may influence the maturation process.

Competent deglutition (the act of swallowing) is crucial to survival. Two primary functions of swallowing are to direct oral secretions, liquids, and food from the mouth to the stomach while protecting the airway, and to provide sufficient amounts of nutrients and fluids for children to grow and develop optimally. Appropriate adjustments to growth and increases in nutritional needs are crucial to successful postnatal deglutition. Because breathing and swallowing share common conduits, such as the oral cavity and pharynx, their functions are intertwined.

Dysphagia (swallowing dysfunction) may be caused by any condition that interferes with structural integrity of the structures comprising the aerodigestive tract or their coordination. Congenital or acquired structural or anatomic anomalies may cause airway and swallowing defects. This chapter focuses on the evaluation of infants and children with suspected dysphagia and the associated primary aerodigestive tract anomalies. Management approaches to swallowing and airway-related problems are reviewed.

Evaluation of Infants and Young Children with Suspected Dysphagia

Clinical or Bedside Evaluation

Evaluation of all children with feeding and swallowing difficulties begins with taking a thorough history and performing a physical examination. Children with anatomic anomalies are at increased risk for dysphagia when the underlying conditions interfere with the structural integrity of the oropharynx or the complex coordination of neuromuscular and airway processes involved in deglutition; consequently, the focus of the clinical evaluation is the identification of diagnostic tests that determine the nature and extent of the swallowing impairments, and assist with management decisions. Children who present with structural anomalies as one component of a complex medical history or syndrome (e.g., bronchopulmonary dysplasia or Smith-Lemli-Opitz syndrome) may require other specialized evaluations (e.g., direct laryngoscopy and bronchoscopy) to determine the impact of the associated comorbidities on swallowing.

Instrumental Evaluation

When the clinical evaluation identifies problems that may be caused by or reflect problems that are invisible, an instrumental evaluation is typically recommended. Common examinations that allow for direct visualization of the structures involved in swallowing include radiologic (e.g., upper gastrointestinal series [UGI] and videofluoroscopic swallow studies [VFSS]) and endoscopic (e.g., flexible endoscopic evaluation of swallowing [FEES]) procedures. Clinicians need to be cautious about the interpretation of negative findings of aspiration during UGI, VFSS, and FEES. Each of these evaluations may establish a diagnosis of dysphagia by identifying specific aspects of the pathophysiology of the dysfunction; however, they may fail to detect aspiration even in children who aspirate, particularly when aspiration is episodic.

Upper Gastrointestinal Series

UGI may provide important information for children with anatomic anomalies, particularly when the anomaly is distal to the oropharynx. UGI provides information that allows for assessment of the anatomy and physiology of the esophagus, stomach, and duodenum; defines gastrointestinal obstructions; and identifies malrotation. In addition, it serves as a screen of the oropharyngeal structures and their functions. Decisions about whether liquid barium should be administered orally or by nasogastric tube are determined by the specific diagnostic questions, and whether children are at risk for aspiration secondary to swallowing dysfunction.

Videofluoroscopic Swallow Study

VFSS, sometimes referred to as a modified barium swallow study, may be useful in children suspected to have oropharyngeal dysphagia because it images the structures of the oral cavity, pharynx, and cervical esophagus during deglutition.[1] VFSS may screen gastrointestinal structures distal to the cervical esophagus. The goals of VFSS are to provide information that helps determine whether anatomic or structural abnormalities are present; ascertain if coordination of the structures and functions of the upper aerodigestive tract supports safe and efficient bolus passage; and identify strategies that enhance the safety and efficiency of feeding, while minimizing the dysphagic problems. During VFSS, children ingest liquids or foods or both impregnated with barium contrast material to simulate functional feeding as closely as possible. Consequently, children must be ready, willing, and able to cooperate with VFSS.[2,3]

Flexible Endoscopic Evaluation of Swallowing

FEES is an extension of the routine flexible fiberoptic nasopharyngolaryngoscopy examination, and may be used to evaluate the structures and functions of the nasopharynx, oropharynx, and larynx during phonation, spontaneous swallows, and swallows of liquids and foods.[4,5] FEES may be particularly useful in children who are nonoral feeders, who are unable to cooperate with VFSS, who have vocal fold dysfunction, or in whom their ability to handle their secretions is questionable.

FEES may provide sensory information when the endoscope touches adjacent mucosa or structures. To standardize evaluations of responses to sensory input, calibrated air pulses have been administered endoscopically.[6] The utility of FEES plus sensory air pulse testing (FEES-ST) has been shown during the evaluation and treatment of children with specific diagnostic conditions (e.g., type I laryngeal clefts) and during preoperative evaluations for pediatric airway reconstruction.[7,8] Elevated laryngopharyngeal sensory thresholds have been documented in children with clinical diagnoses of recurrent pneumonia, neurologic disorders, and gastroesophageal reflux disease (GERD).[6] Table 210-1 outlines the utility of using VFSS and FEES based on the anatomic or structural condition.

Other Diagnostic Evaluations

Other diagnostic tests may be needed to determine the cause of the swallowing dysfunction. Imaging of the brainstem may be needed to diagnose abnormalities of the skull base or spine as potential underlying conditions. Specialized evaluations may be needed for children with refractory respiratory conditions. Chest radiographs, pulmonary function tests, high-resolution computed tomography (CT), and bronchoscopy provide information regarding the extent of lung injury. Endoscopy of the gastrointestinal tract may be beneficial for patients with histories or presentations suggestive of gastrointestinal conditions.

Four Anatomic Sites of Dysphagia

The four primary anatomic sites with anomalies of the aerodigestive tract that may adversely affect swallowing and contribute to dysphagia are the nose and nasopharynx, oral cavity and oral pharynx, hypopharynx and larynx, and trachea and esophagus (Fig. 210-1).

Nose and Nasopharynx

Anomalies of the nose and nasopharynx affect the oral and pharyngeal phases of swallowing. Dysphagia from anomalies of the nose and nasopharynx is secondary to upper airway obstruction and the caliber of the upper airway and the child's ability to compensate while swallowing (Fig. 210-2). Bilateral disease has a more significant impact on airway patency and swallowing than unilateral disease.

Any cause of nasal airway obstruction can lead to feeding difficulties, particularly during infancy when nasal airflow is an important component of breathing and feeding. Nasal obstruction can result from myriad conditions, including midface hypoplasia, congenital nasal pyriform aperture stenosis, septal deviation or hematoma, chronic or acute rhinitis, congenital midline nasal masses (including dermoids, encephaloceles, and gliomas), nasal or nasopharyngeal tumors, choanal atresia, and adenoidal hypertrophy. These children frequently have difficulty coordinating feeding and breathing, and may have failure to thrive or recurrent aspiration.[9]

Unilateral nasal disease may not be detected for years and is often associated with unilateral nasal congestion or rhinorrhea. Bilateral disease has a more significant impact on airway patency and swallowing than unilateral disease and is usually recognized soon after birth because the child commonly has severe respiratory difficulties with cyclical cyanosis relieved by crying.[10] These children are also unable to feed effectively, and may have coughing and choking with cyanotic spells when attempting to eat. Diagnostic evaluation often starts with attempted passage of a 6F feeding tube through the nares. A thorough evaluation with flexible fiberoptic endoscopy and imaging should be carried out if nasal obstruction is suspected. Figure 210-2 outlines the evaluation for children with dysphagia that is suspected to originate from the nose and nasopharynx.

Oral Cavity and Oral Pharynx

Anomalies of the oral cavity and oral pharynx may affect the oral and pharyngeal phases of swallowing, and many have the potential for upper airway obstruction. The respiratory issues should be evaluated and stabilized before initiating the feeding efforts or evaluations for suspected dysphagia (Fig. 210-3).

Functional swallowing depends on efficient bolus formation and movement of the bolus from the mouth to the stomach, and coordination of breathing with bolus passage to protect the airway. Successful bottle-feeding and breastfeeding requires compression of the nipple and the generation of sufficient negative intraoral pressure for suction. Anatomic abnormalities that compromise either the compression or the suction actions of nipple feeding may create feeding difficulties by decreasing the efficiency of feeding. Although abnormalities of the oral

Table 210-1

Anatomic Locations, Conditions, Phases of Swallowing Dysfunction, and Utility of Videofluoroscopic Swallow Studies and Flexible Endoscopic Evaluation of Swallowing

Anatomic Location	Anatomic or Structural Condition	Potential Phase of Swallowing Impairment			Indication for VFSS	Indication for FEES
		Oral	Pharyngeal	Esophageal		
Nose and nasopharynx	Midface hypoplasia	+	+		Sometimes	Sometimes
	Pyriform aperture stenosis	+	+		Sometimes	Sometimes
	Deviated septum	+	+		No	No
	Encephalocele	+	+		No	No
	Tumor	+	+		No	No
	Choanal atresia	+	+		No	No
	Adenoid hypertrophy	+	+		No	No
Oral cavity and oropharynx	Cleft lip/palate	+			No	No
	Micrognathia or retrognathia	+	+		Sometimes	Sometimes
	Macroglossia	+	+		Sometimes	Sometimes
	Tumor	+	+		Sometimes	Sometimes
Hypopharynx and larynx	Vallecular cyst		+		No	No
	Laryngomalacia		+		Sometimes	Sometimes
	Vocal fold paralysis/paresis		+		Yes	Yes
	Laryngeal web		+		Sometimes	Sometimes
	Posterior laryngeal cleft		+	+	Yes	Yes
	Subglottic stenosis		+	±	Sometimes	Sometimes
	Subglottic hemangioma		+	±	Sometimes	Sometimes
Trachea and esophagus	GERD		±	+	Sometimes	No
	Eosinophilic esophagitis		±	+	Sometimes	No
	Vascular ring			+	Sometimes	No
	Tracheal stenosis			+	Sometimes	No
	Tracheomalacia			+	Sometimes	No
	Tracheoesophageal fistula			+	Sometimes	No

+, yes; ±, sometimes; FEES, flexible endoscopic evaluation of swallowing; GERD, gastroesophageal reflux disease; VFSS, videofluoroscopic swallow studies.

cavity and oropharynx may occur in isolation, they frequently co-occur with defects in other portions of the aerodigestive tract, and may also compromise airway function. As always, airway concerns are the first priority and are addressed before attention is focused on feeding and swallowing. This section reviews common conditions affecting the oral cavity and oropharynx, including cleft lip and palate, micrognathia or retrognathia, and macroglossia.

Cleft lip may affect infant feeding by interfering with the lips and tongue creating a seal around the nipple. This interference may compromise the compression phase of sucking and cause excessive fluid loss. Palatal clefts may compromise the suction phase of nipple feeding by interfering with the generation of the negative intraoral pressure needed to extrude fluid from the nipple. The extent of the impact of any anatomic defect depends on multiple factors (e.g., location and extent of impairment, the presence of other anomalies or comorbidities). Some children with isolated small cleft lips or submucous clefts feed without problems or have mild problems that are amenable to feeding routine adaptations.[11] Special feeders, such as the Haberman feeder or Mead-Johnson nurser, allow infants to compensate when there are problems with the compression phase of nipple feeding. Caregivers squeeze the bottles to deliver fluids. Additionally, a cross-cut nipple can be used to facilitate fluid flow. These adaptations are often used before surgical repair of the cleft lip or palate. Clinicians must be cautious about airway protective mechanisms (i.e., aspiration potential) before recommending any feeding routine adaptation that increases the rate of fluid flow.

Common craniofacial syndromes associated with cleft lip and palate are Apert's, Stickler's, and Treacher Collins syndromes; Pierre Robin sequence; CHARGE (coloboma, heart disease, atresia choanae, retardation, genital hypoplasia, and ear anomalies) association; and 22q11 deletion syndromes including velocardiofacial syndrome and DiGeorge syndrome.[12] These conditions may interfere with aspects of feeding and swallowing beyond those localized to the oral cavity or oropharyngeal structures.

Micrognathia and retrognathia can occur in isolation; however, they also occur in association with Pierre Robin sequence and genetic syndromes such as Goldenhar's, Treacher Collins, Smith-Lemli-Opitz, and cri du chat syndromes. Retrognathia and micrognathia may compromise airway patency and feeding secondary to retrodisplacement of the tongue. In Pierre Robin sequence, airway obstructive patterns are caused by pharyngeal collapse and velum elongation leading to palatal and base of tongue obstruction.[13] In addition to the interference with the compression and suction phases of nipple feeding, the combination of a relatively small oropharynx and nasopharyngeal reflux secondary to a cleft palate may compromise breathing and swallowing coordination. The diagnosis is made by clinical evaluation and confirmed by instrumental assessment, if warranted. The prognosis for successful oral feeding depends on the degree of respiratory distress and the presence

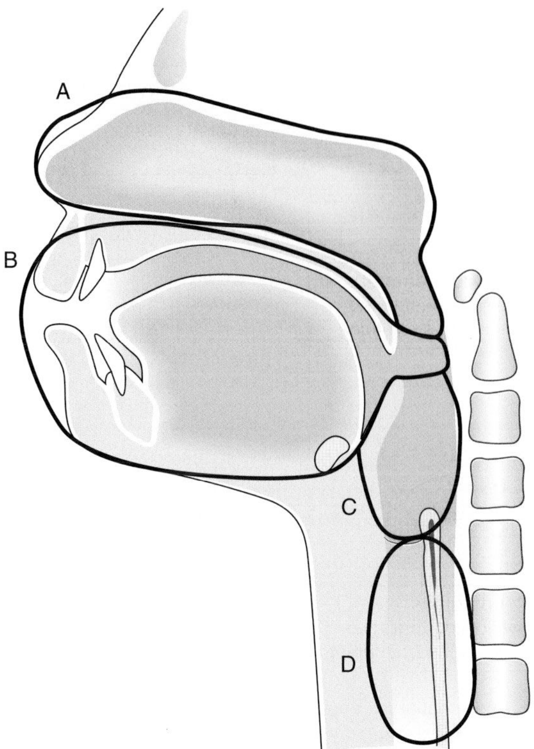

Figure 210-1. Four anatomic sites of dysphagia. **A,** Nose and nasopharynx. **B,** Oral cavity and oral pharynx. **C,** Hypopharynx and larynx. **D,** Trachea and esophagus. *(© 2008 by Johns Hopkins University, Art as Applied to Medicine.)*

of associated issues or diagnoses. Patients with Pierre Robin sequence–associated syndromes generally require gastrostomy tube placement despite successful airway intervention.[14]

Macroglossia often leads to feeding difficulty because tongue enlargement may interfere with the creation and maintenance of an adequate lip-tongue and nipple seal. Additionally, tongue movement may be restricted, leading to difficulty controlling food in the oral cavity. Macroglossia is associated with Down syndrome and Beckwith-Wiedemann syndrome. Feeding problems are reported in 50% to 80% of children with Down syndrome; specific dysphagia characteristics include delayed and aberrant oral-motor function, abnormal tongue and mandibular function, and delayed initiation with difficulty of the oral phase of swallowing.[15,16] Hypotonia may also compound feeding and swallowing problems in children with Down syndrome.

Pharyngeal diverticula or tumors are less commonly seen in children. The effects of these conditions depend on the size and location of the defect, and there may be no impact on feeding unless these are significantly enlarged.

Hypopharynx and Larynx

Anomalies of the hypopharynx and larynx may affect the pharyngeal and esophageal phases of swallowing. Initial evaluation usually involves performing a flexible fiberoptic laryngoscopy (Fig. 210-4).

Vallecular cysts are rare mucous retention cysts that manifest with stridor, respiratory distress, dysphagia, and failure to thrive. These cysts sit in the vallecular space and can cause significant retroflexion of the epiglottis, which leads to respiratory distress and dysphagia. Dysphagia can result from interference with base of tongue and epiglottic movement and from obstruction of the natural lateral flow of food around the epiglottis during swallowing. Vallecular cysts can be diagnosed by flexible fiberoptic laryngoscopy, direct laryngoscopy, or a swallow study. They can be seen on CT and magnetic resonance imaging (MRI), but are difficult to see on plain films of the neck.

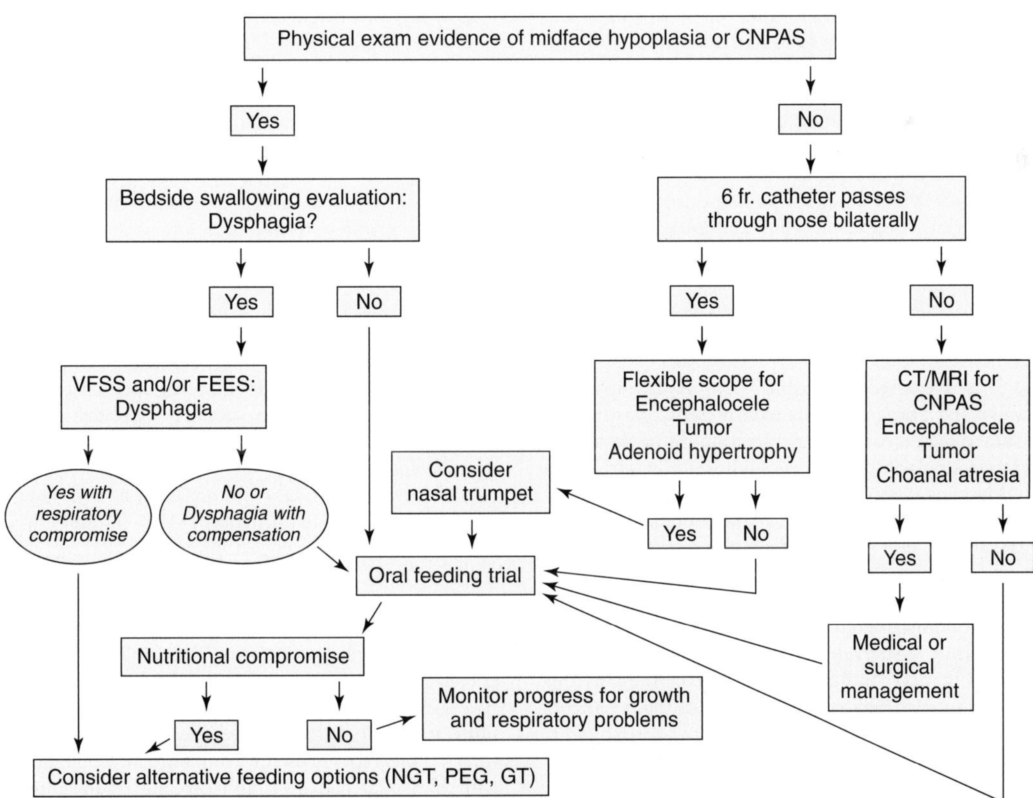

Figure 210-2. Evaluation and management of dysphagia with suspected nose and nasopharynx anomaly. CNPAS, congenital nasal pyriform aperture stenosis; FEES, flexible endoscopic evaluation of swallowing; GT, gastrostomy tube; NGT, nasogastric tube; PEG, percutaneous endoscopic gastrostomy; VFSS, videofluoroscopic swallow studies.

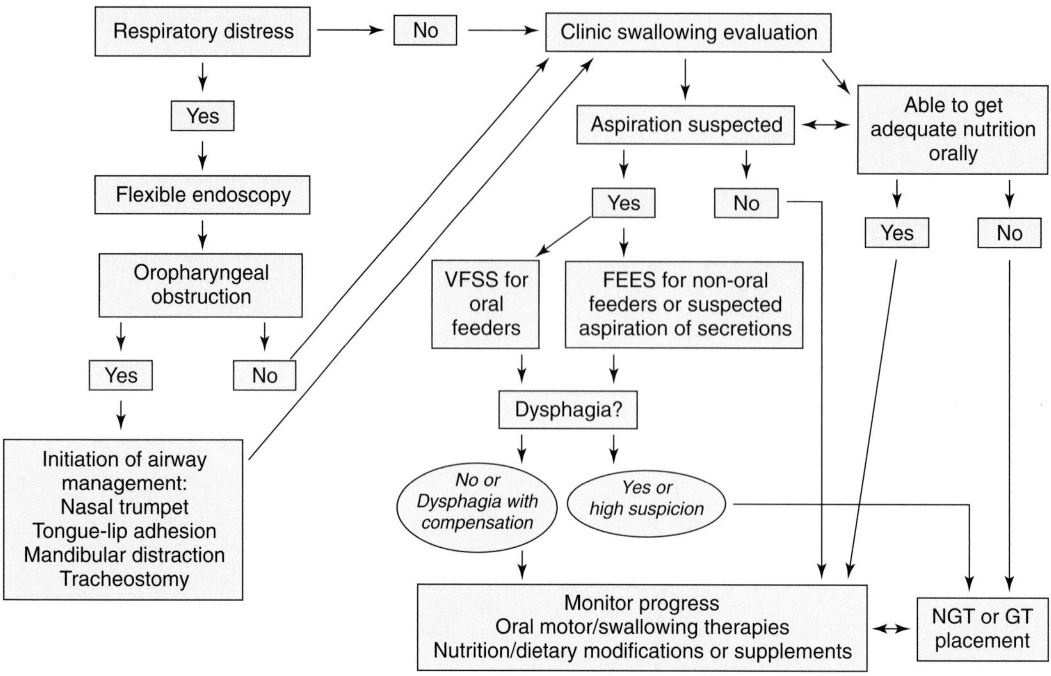

Figure 210-3. Evaluation and management of dysphagia with suspected oral cavity and oropharynx anomaly. FEES, flexible endoscopic evaluation of swallowing; GT, gastrostomy tube; NGT, nasogastric tube; VFSS, videofluoroscopic swallow studies.

Surgical management of vallecular cysts is recommended by marsupialization of the cyst and removal of the mucosal lining, which can be performed with a carbon-dioxide laser, cold knife, or a microdébrider. Yao and colleagues[17] described an 11-week-old infant with a vallecular cyst, choking with feeds, failure to thrive, stridor, laryngomalacia, and gastroesophageal reflux.[17] After surgical removal of the cyst, the aerodigestive symptoms resolved within days, as is often the case. This patient showed improvement in weight percentiles from less than 10th percentile at the time of surgery to the 50th percentile 12 weeks later.

Laryngomalacia is the most common cause of stridor in infants, representing more than 70% of cases. These children present with inspiratory stridor secondary to collapse of the epiglottis or arytenoids or both during inspiration. Many studies have found that laryngomalacia is associated with gastroesophageal reflux and underlying neurologic conditions.[18-20] Respiratory distress can be seen in more severe cases with cyanosis, obstructive sleep apnea, supraclavicular retractions, and subcostal retractions. Severe laryngomalacia can also contribute to feeding difficulties heralded by choking while feeding, failure to thrive, and emesis.

Laryngomalacia is diagnosed by flexible fiberoptic laryngoscopy with the infant awake and upright. Infants with presentations suggestive of dysphagia should have a swallowing evaluation. More than 90% of patients with laryngomalacia are treated nonsurgically with close clinical follow-up. Matthews and coworkers[21] found that of 24 infants diagnosed with laryngomalacia who had 24-hour double-probe pH monitoring, all had at least one episode of pharyngeal refluxate, and greater than 90% had three episodes. Because GERD and laryngomalacia seem to coexist, many clinicians manage laryngomalacia patients with antacids or proton pump inhibitors. For patients with respiratory distress or failure to thrive, a supraglottoplasty is recommended. Lee and associates[22] showed that carbon-dioxide laser supraglottoplasty can improve substernal and suprasternal retractions, but that many patients continued to have choking and feeding problems postoperatively. This condition warrants a postoperative swallowing evaluation and close clinical follow-up.

Vocal fold paralysis represents 10% of congenital laryngeal anomalies. Infants may have unilateral or bilateral vocal fold paralysis, and can present with stridor, recurrent aspiration, and dysphagia from the inability to protect the airway. The diagnosis is best made by flexible fiberoptic laryngoscopy in an awake patient. Management of vocal fold paralysis in children should focus first on establishing a safe airway. After the airway is stable, the nutritional needs should be assessed.

Swallowing difficulties can be evaluated by VFSS or FEES or both. These evaluations can identify penetration, aspiration, the patient's ability to protect the airway adequately, and the effect of changes in feeding utensils (e.g., fast vs. slow flow nipples) or different liquid viscosities (e.g., thin vs. thick liquids). Some infants benefit from a slower swallowing transit time, which can be accomplished by decreasing the flow from the bottle's nipple or by thickening the formula or breast milk. Other infants require a feeding tube to obtain adequate nutrition and hydration.

Laryngeal webs can be congenital, secondary to incomplete resorption of the laryngeal lumen epithelium during embryologic development, or acquired from vocal fold trauma secondary to laryngeal surgery or endotracheal intubation. Infants may present with stridor, a weak cry, hoarseness, respiratory distress, and aphonia, and some may have dysphagia. Laryngeal webs are associated with cardiac and 22q11 anomalies. The diagnosis is made by flexible fiberoptic laryngoscopy or direct laryngoscopy. Thin webs can be managed by endoscopic lysis, whereas thicker webs require an open laryngeal fissure and placement of a laryngeal keel or stent. For patients with preoperative dysphagia, a follow-up swallowing evaluation should be performed postoperatively.

Posterior laryngeal clefts are uncommon congenital anomalies caused by incomplete formation of the septum between the esophagus and the airway. This laryngeal anomaly is associated with tracheoesophageal fistulas in one third of cases. The Benjamin-Inglis classification system describes four types of posterior laryngeal clefts: Type 1 clefts are interarytenoid and lie above the level of the true vocal folds, type 2 clefts extend below the true vocal folds and partially through the cricoid cartilage, type 3 clefts extend into the extrathoracic trachea, and type 4 clefts extend into the intrathoracic trachea.[23] Common presentations are stridor, choking, aspiration, chronic cough, and failure to thrive. Direct laryngoscopy and bronchoscopy should be performed with bimanual palpation and probing of the interarytenoid area to confirm the diagnosis. Microaspiration and penetration can be seen on FEES or VFSS.

The management of posterior laryngeal clefts depends on the extent of the cleft. Chien and colleagues[7] found type 1 posterior

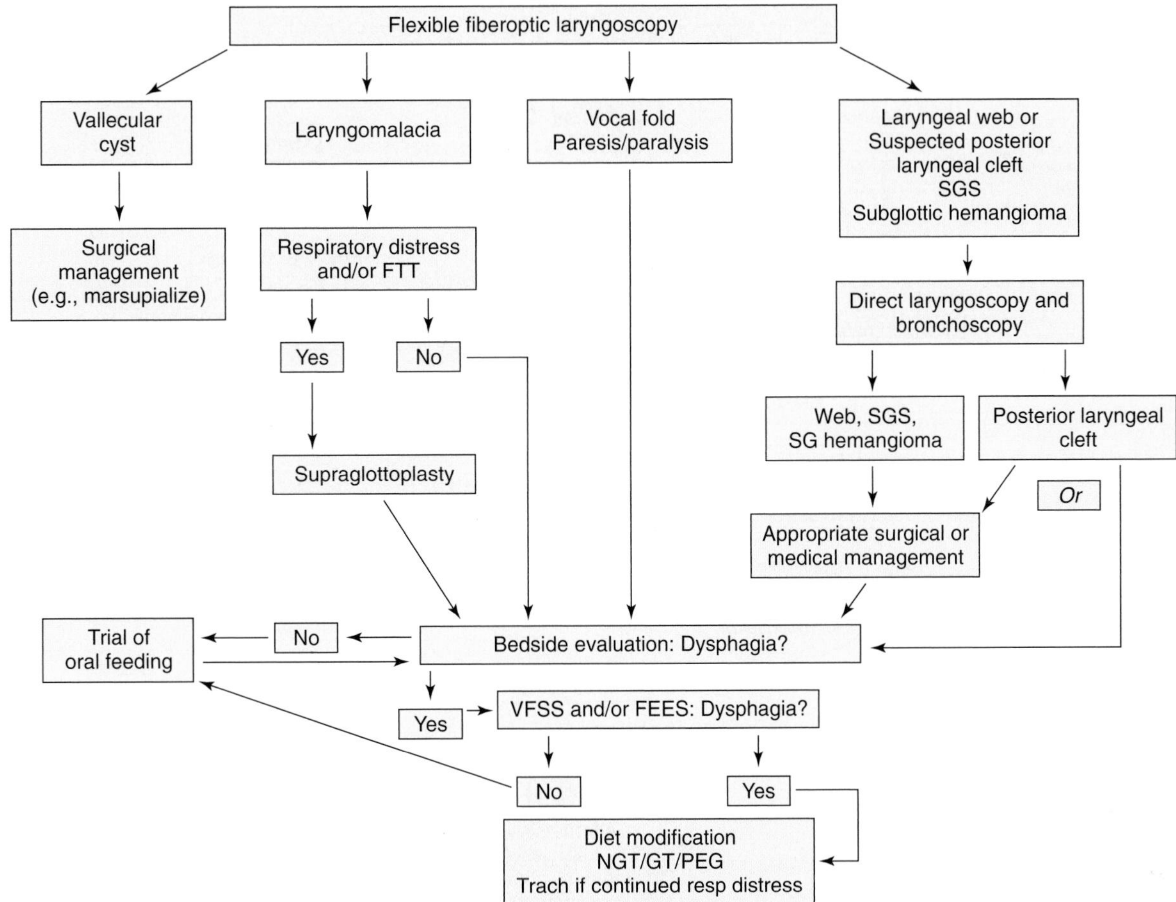

Figure 210-4. Evaluation and management of dysphagia with suspected hypopharynx and larynx anomaly. FEES, flexible endoscopic evaluation of swallowing; FTT, failure to thrive; GT, gastrostomy tube; NGT, nasogastric tube; PEG, percutaneous endoscopic gastrostomy; SG, subglottic; SGS, subglottic stenosis; VFSS, videofluoroscopic swallow studies.

laryngeal clefts in 1 of 13 patients presenting to their institution with symptoms of chronic cough or aspiration over a 3-year period. They recommend that type 1 clefts have a trial of nonsurgical management first with a proton pump inhibitor to treat GERD, upright feedings, and thickened feedings. Children who fail conservative treatment should have surgical repair. Types 1 and 2 posterior laryngeal clefts can be repaired endoscopically, whereas type 3 and 4 clefts require an open surgical repair. A postoperative swallowing study should be performed.

Subglottic pathologies such as stenosis and hemangiomas affect swallowing in similar ways. Subglottic anomalies manifest with inspiratory or biphasic stridor, and the best evaluation method is by direct laryngoscopy and bronchoscopy. MRI or three-dimensional CT may be useful in delineating the extent of subglottic narrowing. The increased work of breathing can lead to increased laryngeal refluxate, penetration, and aspiration. The acidic refluxate into the subglottis can lead to further airway edema and narrowing. The first priority for these patients is to ensure a stable airway. When that has been achieved, swallowing function can be assessed by a bedside swallowing evaluation, and VFSS or FEES if indicated.

Trachea and Esophagus

Dysphagia of the trachea and esophagus may affect the pharyngeal and esophageal phases of swallowing. In addition to structural anomalies, inflammatory conditions such as GERD and eosinophilic esophagitis can affect these areas. The initial evaluation depends on the specific condition suspected. Figure 210-5 outlines a working algorithm for evaluating these patients.

GERD symptoms such as regurgitation and emesis occur in 50% to 67% of normal children, with most having symptom resolution by 1 to 2 years of age.[24,25] Children younger than 2 years old present with airway symptoms (stertor, stridor, or cyanosis) and feeding abnormalities (vomiting, dysphagia, and failure to thrive).[26] GERD can affect all of the major aerodigestive anatomic areas (see Fig. 210-1), and has been implicated in stertor, lingual tonsil hypertrophy, arytenoid edema, vocal fold edema, subglottic edema, cobblestoning of the trachea, and blunting of the carina.[27,28]

GERD is also associated with other known conditions that affect the aerodigestive tract. Giannoni and colleagues[20] prospectively evaluated 33 consecutive infants diagnosed with laryngomalacia and noted that 64% had GERD. Additionally, GERD was associated with more severe cases of laryngomalacia and cases with complicated clinical courses. Animal studies have linked gastric acid and pepsin to subglottic stenosis and vocal fold granulomas.[29,30]

When GERD affects the upper aerodigestive tract, it is referred to as *laryngopharyngeal reflux*. The diagnostic workup for LPR in infants lacks consensus and includes symptom assessment questionnaires, flexible fiberoptic laryngopharyngoscopy, single-lumen or double-lumen pH probe, barium esophagogram, scintigraphy, impedance, and laryngeal biopsy. Often a trial of antireflux medication is given to see if symptoms resolve.

GERD can affect the sensation of the larynx and blunt protective reflex mechanisms. Suskind and coworkers[31] retrospectively reviewed 28 infants with GERD and found altered laryngeal sensation by FEES and FEES-ST and dysphagia by VFSS and FEES. GERD was managed medically or surgically, and repeat VFSS and FEES-ST testing showed improved laryngeal sensation and swallowing function. These authors hypothesize that the refluxate causes laryngeal edema and decreased sensation, which alters the laryngeal adductor reflex, and then disrupts the suck-swallow-breathe sequence and causes dysphagia.

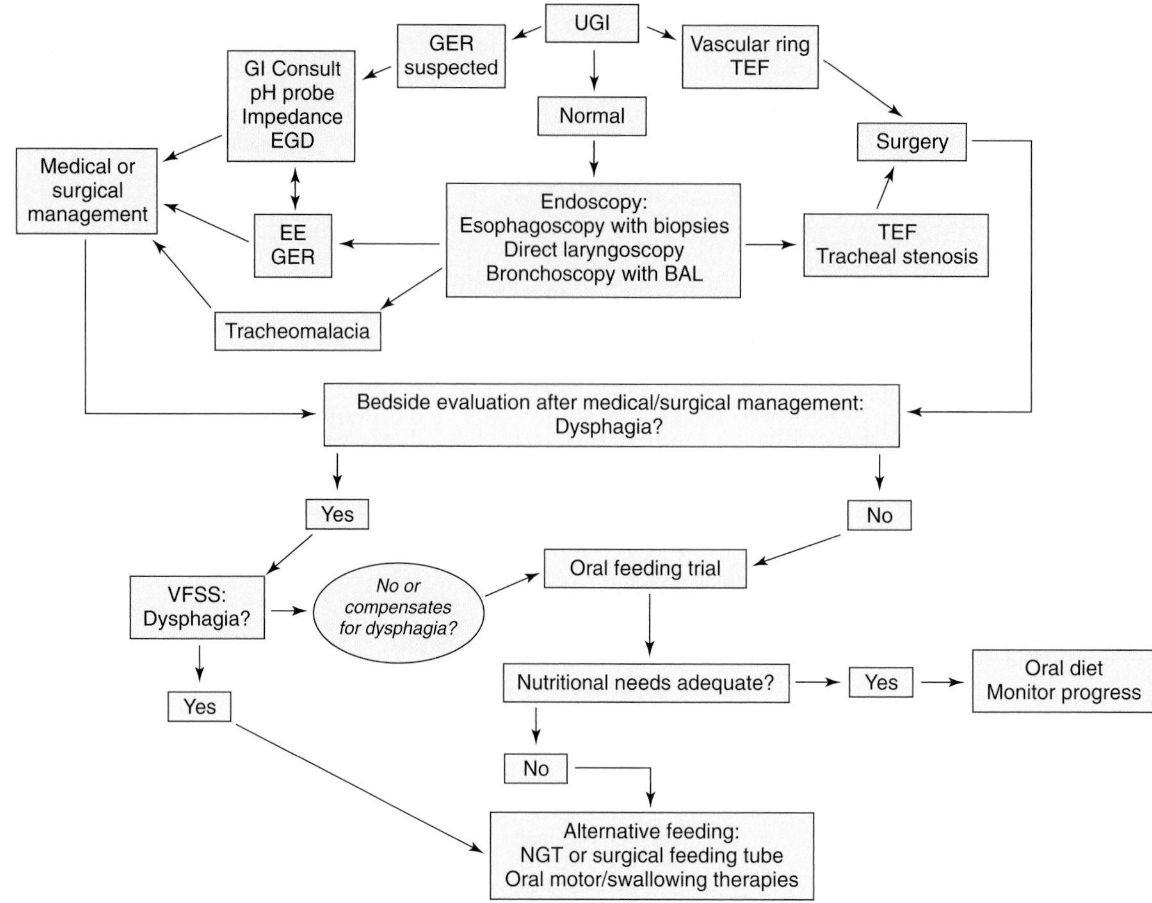

Figure 210-5. Evaluation and management of dysphagia with suspected trachea and esophagus anomaly. BAL, bronchoalveolar lavage; EE, eosinophilic esophagitis; EGD, esophagogastroduodenoscopy; GER, gastroesophageal reflux; GI, gastrointestinal; NGT, nasogastric tube; TEF, tracheoesophageal fistula; UGI, upper gastrointestinal series; VFSS, videofluoroscopic swallow studies.

Eosinophilic esophagitis is an inflammatory process of the mucosal and submucosal layers of the esophagus.[32] Symptoms often mimic the symptoms of GERD with feeding difficulties predominating in infants and toddlers; vomiting and abdominal pain are common in school-age children, and dysphagia is evident in preadolescents.[33] Food impaction may occur in older children and adults. Diagnosis of eosinophilic esophagitis is made by a combination of the clinical symptoms listed previously and histologic confirmation of 15 eosinophils or more per high-powered field along with normal gastric and duodenal biopsy specimens. In addition, biopsies must be performed after 6 to 8 weeks of regular proton pump inhibitor therapy or have a documented negative pH probe study.[34,35] Eosinophilic esophagitis may be patchy, and the diagnosis requires multiple biopsies; often four or five are recommended.

In contrast to GERD, treatment with acid-blocking therapies is ineffective in alleviating symptoms. Dietary changes, such as implementation of an elemental diet, suggest that food allergies play an important part in the pathogenesis of this disease.[36] Elemental diets have been shown to be effective greater than 95% of the time; other approaches include directed elimination diets (>75% effective) and empirical elimination diets (>70% effective).[37] Systemic steroids have also been advocated. Histologic remission has been documented after 4 weeks of corticosteroid use, although recurrence is common within 6 months of the cessation of treatment.[38] Topical corticosteroids, swallowed instead of inhaled, have also been advocated to treat acute eosinophilic esophagitis, and are known to reverse the associated clinical symptoms and histologic changes.[37]

Congenital tracheal stenosis is a rare congenital anomaly consisting of complete, circular tracheal rings. More than one third are associated with pulmonary slings or other cardiovascular anomalies. The dysphagia can be secondary to increased work of breathing or the associated vascular anomalies. CT, three-dimensional CT, and MRI are useful in determining the stenotic length and the presence of associated vascular anomalies. Bronchoscopy confirms the presence of complete tracheal rings and the length of the stenosis. Although many of these children require surgical correction, Rutter and associates[39] estimated 10% can be managed without surgery. Adequate nutrition and growth are crucial for these children. Oral feeders should have evaluation by FEES or VFSS or both because aspiration can result in significant respiratory compromise in these children with small airway caliber.

Tracheomalacia is anterior-to-posterior collapse of the trachea. Children with tracheomalacia present with expiratory stridor, wheezing, coughing, and sometimes dysphagia. Conditions that affect the structural integrity of the trachea such as tracheoesophageal fistulas, esophageal anomalies, vascular rings and slings, and innominate artery anomalies can cause tracheomalacia. The dysphagia can be a result of increased work of breathing, from the associated esophageal anomaly, or from vascular anomalies compressing the esophagus.

The diagnosis can be made by either airway fluoroscopy or bronchoscopy. Esophagograms are useful to identify esophageal anomalies and vascular anomalies compressing the esophagus. MRI can evaluate the extent of vascular anomalies further.

Tracheomalacia related to weak tracheal cartilage often resolves spontaneously in 2 to 3 years, as the child and the tracheal airway grow. Infants who are symptomatic with respiratory distress may require continuous positive airway pressure. Infants with tracheal collapse from esophageal or vascular anomalies benefit from surgical correction of the offending anomaly. Assessment of swallowing function may include VFSS and UGI after surgical correction.

Conclusion

Functional swallowing involves a complex orchestration of events throughout the aerodigestive tract. We have outlined four anatomic areas of the aerodigestive tract that contribute to dysphagia if anomalies are present: nose and nasopharynx, oral cavity and oral pharynx, hypopharynx and larynx, and trachea and esophagus. These four anatomic areas provide a framework for the evaluation and management of dysphagia. When managing children with dysphagia, the first priority is to provide a safe airway for breathing. After the airway is stabilized, swallowing function should be assessed and managed with the ultimate goal of providing sufficient nutrition and fluid for optimal growth and development. The care for children with dysphagia is complex, and a team approach including members from speech-language pathology, nutrition, gastroenterology, and otolaryngology is ideal.

SUGGESTED READINGS

Arvedson JC, Lefton-Greif MA. *Pediatric Videofluoroscopic Swallow Studies: A Professional Manual with Caregiver Handouts.* San Antonio: Communication Skill Builders; 1998.

Langmore SE. *Endoscopic Evaluation and Treatment of Swallowing Disorder.* New York: Thieme; 2001.

Langmore SE, Schatz K, Olsen N. Fiberoptic endoscopic examination of swallowing safety: a new procedure. *Dysphagia.* 1988;2:216-219.

Logemann JA. *Manual for the Videofluorographic Study of Swallowing.* Austin: Pro-Ed; 1993.

Logemann JA. *Evaluation and Treatment of Swallowing Disorders.* San Diego: College Hill Press; 1983.

For complete list of references log onto www.expertconsult.com.

CHAPTER TWO HUNDRED AND ELEVEN

Caustic Ingestion

Glenn B. Williams

Rose Mary S. Stocks

J. Dale Browne

James N. Thompson

Key Points

- Injuries from caustic ingestion are rare in the United States; 5000 to 15,000 occur per year.
- The current strict public policy on solution labeling and concentration was spearheaded by Jackson in the early 20th century.
- In developing nations without such policies, caustic injuries are more common.
- Acid ingestion leads to coagulative necrosis; alkali ingestion leads to liquefactive necrosis.
- The antrum of the stomach is the most vulnerable to acid ingestion; areas of anatomic narrowing are at greatest risk after alkali ingestion.
- Because of their resemblance to disk-shaped batteries, all coin-shaped foreign bodies should be removed expeditiously.
- Endoscopy is the most useful tool in assessing injury to the upper gastrointestinal tract.
- Typically, infant and toddler caustic ingestions are accidental, whereas adolescent and adult ingestions are suicide attempts.

"Those who cannot remember the past are condemned to repeat it."

—George Santayana

The preceding quote comes to mind when reviewing more recent caustic ingestion literature, most of which is from developing countries. Over the last decade, numerous articles have been published from various institutions in the developing world.[1-10] The fundamental problem is "uncontrolled and cheaper domestic cleaners have been introduced through common informal or open markets."[6] More recent reports estimate the incidence of caustic injuries in the United States to be 5000 to 15,000 per year; this low incidence has not always been the case.[5] During the early 1900s, in concert with the ready availability of cleaning solutions composed of strong alkalis or acids, reports of caustic ingestions filled the medical literature. These early cleaning solutions were packaged in inconspicuous containers that concealed the potential danger of the content. This public health issue was highlighted in a landmark article in 1921 by Jackson,[10] developer of the first distal lighted esophagoscope. Supported by extensive lobbying efforts by Jackson, the U.S. Congress passed legislation that controlled the sale of these potential toxins in 1927. Legislation led to the 1953 creation of the first National Poison Control Center in Chicago. In 1971, the U.S. Federal Hazardous Substance and Poison Prevention Packaging Act passed, mandating childproof container caps and banning excessively hazardous products and concentrations.

Despite these measures, extensive medical literature, and a century's experience, serious injuries secondary to caustic ingestion persist in the United States and abroad. Pediatric caustic ingestions are typically accidental and involve common household items. In adolescents and adults, ingestions are more likely intentional and represent suicide attempts.

Pathophysiology

Acid and alkali solutions are the two main categories of caustic products. Commonly ingested substances include cleaning agents, bleach, concentrated laundry detergent, concentrated ammonia, dishwashing detergent, alkali hair straighteners, nail-decorating liquids, sodium hydroxide–containing glucose testing tablets, and disk batteries.[11-15] Extensive local damage can occur after ingestion of sodium hydroxide–containing glucose test tablets and disk-shaped batteries if they lodge in the esophagus. Disk-shaped batteries are easily swallowed, and if they become lodged cause injury by several mechanisms: leakage of alkali causing direct caustic injury; absorption of toxic substances; pressure necrosis; and electrical discharge, which can cause mucosal burns.[16] Subsequently, the following types of esophageal injuries may occur: esophageal burn with or without perforation, tracheoesophageal fistula, and aortoesophageal fistula. Caustic substances present in farming homes used as disinfectants, pipeline clearance, and cattle horn removal are not subject to U.S. protective packaging legislation.[17]

Acid ingestion leads to coagulative necrosis with eschar formation that subsequently prevents further tissue penetration. Esophageal damage secondary to acid ingestion is less likely because of the protection afforded by the slightly alkaline pH of the esophagus, and because of the resistance of the squamous epithelium to acids. The antrum of the stomach is the most vulnerable region of the upper digestive tract to acidic substances owing to pooling and prolonged contact with the compound.[18]

Alkalis are responsible for more severe caustic ingestion sequelae; multiple factors contribute to the extensive damage. Direct contact with cell membranes leads to their disruption secondary to saponification and proteinate formation as the alkali reacts with membrane components. Solubility of alkalis allows for deeper penetration of the caustic agents typically in areas of anatomic narrowing (e.g., cricopharyngeus,

Box 211-1

Signs and Symptoms of Caustic Ingestion

Oral mucosal erythema, ulceration
Drooling
Tongue edema
Stridor
Hoarseness
Dysphagia
Odynophagia
Chest or back pain
Epigastric pain or tenderness
Vomiting
Hematemesis

aortic arch, left main stem bronchus, and diaphragmatic hiatus).[18] Damage ceases only when the alkali is neutralized by its reaction with tissue. The histopathologic events that occur after a 10% sodium hydroxide burn of esophageal mucosa include edema of the submucosa, inflammation of the submucosa with thrombosis, sloughing of the superficial layers, necrosis of the muscular layer, fibrosis of the deep layers, and delayed re-epithelialization.[19]

Initial Assessment and Diagnosis

Patients with caustic ingestion present with many symptoms, ranging from asymptomatic to overt stridor with severe dysphagia secondary to laryngeal edema and hypopharyngeal or esophageal injury (Box 211-1). As with all injured patients, the primary survey focuses on airway, breathing, and circulation (ABCs). A rapid assessment of the patient's airway and determination of the need for intervention is of primary importance. Simultaneously, patients suspected to have a severe injury should have large-bore intravenous catheters for early fluid resuscitation and medication. Patients with significant oral mucosal burns, tongue edema, hoarseness, stridor, and dyspnea should be monitored closely for possible airway obstruction.

Fiberoptic laryngoscopy is an invaluable tool in the assessment of hypopharyngeal damage and the risk of airway compromise. In a patient with an injured but stable airway, dexamethasone (20 to 30 mg intravenous bolus in adults; 0.5 to 1 mg/kg in children) can help prevent further deterioration. Direct visualization of the larynx is necessary for a successful and safe intubation; blind nasotracheal intubation should be avoided for fear of destabilizing a tenuous airway. If orotracheal intubation cannot be performed safely because of edema or exudate or both, a surgical airway (cricothyrotomy or tracheotomy) is the safer choice. Dyspnea associated with rales and rhonchi may indicate aspiration of caustic material or pulmonary edema. Chest and abdominal radiography should be obtained to rule out pulmonary infiltrates or free air. Patient complaints of epigastric pain and examination findings of peritonitis (e.g., abdominal wall rigidity, tenderness) are highly correlated with gastric injury.[20]

Vital information necessary for appropriate care of a patient with a caustic ingestion includes identification of the ingested agent and its characteristics (pH, concentration, physical form [i.e., granular, liquid]), time and setting of ingestion, and volume swallowed. The social setting of the ingestion may provide clues to the amount of caustic involved in the injury and should be explored in the history. Children ingest caustic substances accidentally while exploring their surroundings or because of lack of parental education or parental neglect.[9,21] Adult ingestions are generally suicide attempts, and large volumes are ingested. In the laboratory, the amount of titratable base is a more accurate predictor of a strong alkaline substance.[22] Vancura and colleagues[23] showed esophageal ulceration at a pH 12.5 or greater and significant mucosal damage with sodium hydroxide concentrations of 0.4% in mongrel cats. pH is clinically a more practical, rapid method of estimating the risk of mucosal injury.

Large volumes of strong acids are generally required to create esophageal injury, whereas a few milliliters of strong alkali can cause extensive damage instantaneously. Injury to the upper gastrointestinal mucosa after acid ingestion is more prolonged and is aided by reflex pylorospasm. Entry of acid into the stomach and contact with the pylorus results in a reflex spasm, leading to increased length of exposure and a predominance of gastric mucosal injuries in these patients. Measures such as emetics or buffering attempts are not recommended because they do not lessen the injury, and they increase the risk of aspiration. Conservative measures are encouraged, such as cleaning oral mucosa burns with water to dilute any remaining caustic, and manually removing any visible lye granules to lessen continuing injury.

Although the acute crises of esophageal perforation and upper airway obstruction are more dramatic, the most common complications from strong alkaline burns result from the more protracted courses of fibrosis and delayed epithelialization. Superficial burns generally heal without sequelae; however, deeper injuries involving the muscular layer and submucosa are associated with a more extensive loss of mucosa with subsequent fibrosis. A characteristic esophageal stricture develops in four stages: (1) An intense inflammatory response with associated dysmotility occurs in the area of the burned mucosa and deeper layers. (2) Granulation tissue with fibroblasts brings a matrix of collagen fibers to the newly formed connective tissue. (3) These collagen fibers begin to contract 3 or 4 weeks after the initial injury, with irregular formation of this collagen matrix, which enables the formation of adhesive bands. (4) Pseudodiverticula form between these adhesions as the contracting process continues until a dense inflexible fibrous scar replaces the destroyed submucosa and muscular layers. Circumferential burns are much more likely to lead to a symptomatic stricture than are noncircumferential injuries.[24]

Endoscopy

The clinician's principal diagnostic challenge lies in accurately predicting which ingestion injuries are prone to rapid, inconsequential healing, and which are prone to stricture formation or perforation. Endoscopy is the most useful method of assessing whether esophageal injury has occurred. Traditional adjunctive studies, such as barium esophagogram, are inadequate because of the reliance on motility disturbance and mucosal irregularities to detect injury[25] and significant false-negative rates (30% to 60%).[26,27] The usefulness of technetium 99m–labeled sucralfate has been shown; it has high sensitivity and specificity in determining the presence of an esophageal injury after pediatric caustic ingestion.[28] The high sensitivity and specificity allow this nuclear medicine study to serve as a screen for injury; however, it does not determine severity of injury or enable intervention. Depending on radiography alone for guidance may lead the clinician to underestimate the degree of injury in some patients.

The timing and necessity of endoscopy remains a topic of debate. Proponents of endoscopy within 24 hours in all cases of caustic ingestions are supported by retrospective reviews detailing instances of significant esophageal injury despite the absence of symptoms or signs of mucosal burns.[3,4,6,29-32] In citing the poor correlation of signs, symptoms, and esophageal injury, such studies frequently do not differentiate the form of the ingested substance (liquid vs. granular), and whether the asymptomatic burns were from more potent liquid alkalis. This association may lead to the conclusion that any form of an ingested caustic may cause significant distal injury even in the absence of signs or symptoms of mucosal burns. Although conservative and cautious, this approach may subject patients (and parents) occasionally to unneeded procedures, worry, and expense. In a retrospective study of 41 ingestions that noted the type of lye ingested, the granular form did not cause significant mucosal injury, whereas all strictures resulted from liquid alkalis.[30]

An alternative view of when to perform endoscopy considers several factors, including form and strength of the caustic, presence or absence of multiple signs and symptoms, and age of the patient. Most adult patients ingest caustic agents as a suicide attempt—this is a more straightforward diagnostic assessment. The volume of agent swallowed is usually great, commonly causing dysphagia, stridor, or oropharyngeal burns. Suicidal adults may be unreliable historians, which forces the clinician to rely on physical findings to direct therapy, especially because oral mucosal injury may be absent when a strong alkali is quickly swallowed. Consequently, endoscopy is advisable for any adult having ingested a strong alkali or acid (e.g., sodium hydroxide, potassium hydroxide, hydrochloric acid, sulfuric acid), regardless of the lack of presenting symptoms or signs. In suicidal ingestions, the physician should examine the stomach for necrosis with endoscopy, laparoscopy, or laparotomy because a large volume of caustic may have been swallowed.

In contrast, toxic agents are accidentally swallowed in children as a result of innocent curiosity and confusion with food and drink. Just as children do not swallow a great deal of any distasteful food or medicine, they would not swallow any noxious, bitter acid or unpalatable granular lye. These compounds are rarely associated with significant esophageal burns because the volume ingested is generally very small.[30,33,34] Exceptions have been reported, but these cases are associated with presenting combinations of oral burns, drooling, and dysphagia that easily raise suspicion that a significant amount of the compound has been swallowed. In cases of pediatric ingestion of acids or granular lye, endoscopy can be reserved for children with significant oral burns, dysphagia, or stridor. A glucose test tablet or disk-shaped watch battery needs to be endoscopically removed as quickly as possible because these items cause localized transmural necrosis and esophageal perforation. This recommendation can be extended to any coin-shaped object lodged in a child's esophagus because some disk batteries may resemble a coin on chest radiographs (Fig. 211-1).

Most severe pediatric esophageal injuries are the result of just a few milliliters of a strong liquid alkali, usually sodium hydroxide. Some investigators have found that the presence of two or more signs and symptoms (e.g., oral burns, drooling, dysphagia, vomiting, stridor) reliably indicates esophageal injury significant enough to lead to stricture formation or perforation, requiring endoscopy.[33-35] Based on evidence from a retrospective study, one series concluded that unless a pediatric patient is symptomatic (e.g., vomiting, drooling, oral lesions, respiratory distress, hemostasis), endoscopy is unnecessary because asymptomatic children were not found to develop sequelae. The authors of the series confined this recommendation to developed countries with a more controlled, lower concentration of alkalis and acids.[36]

Although such criteria can be helpful in evaluating a child with a questionable history of liquid alkali ingestion, prudent evaluation of a pediatric patient with known ingestion of a strong liquid alkali should consider reported cases of an otherwise silent, significant injury appreciated only through endoscopy. In cases of known pediatric liquid alkali ingestion, endoscopy offers a direct assessment with low morbidity for the presence or absence of significant injury. In borderline patients, a technetium 99m–labeled sucralfate study can be useful. In children without a strong history and with only one presenting sign or symptom, the risk of significant injury is low, and endoscopy can be deferred or held, pending the results of a nuclear medicine study. Otherwise, it is safer to perform endoscopy in all children with known ingestion of a strong liquid alkali or who have positive findings on a technetium 99m–labeled sucralfate study.

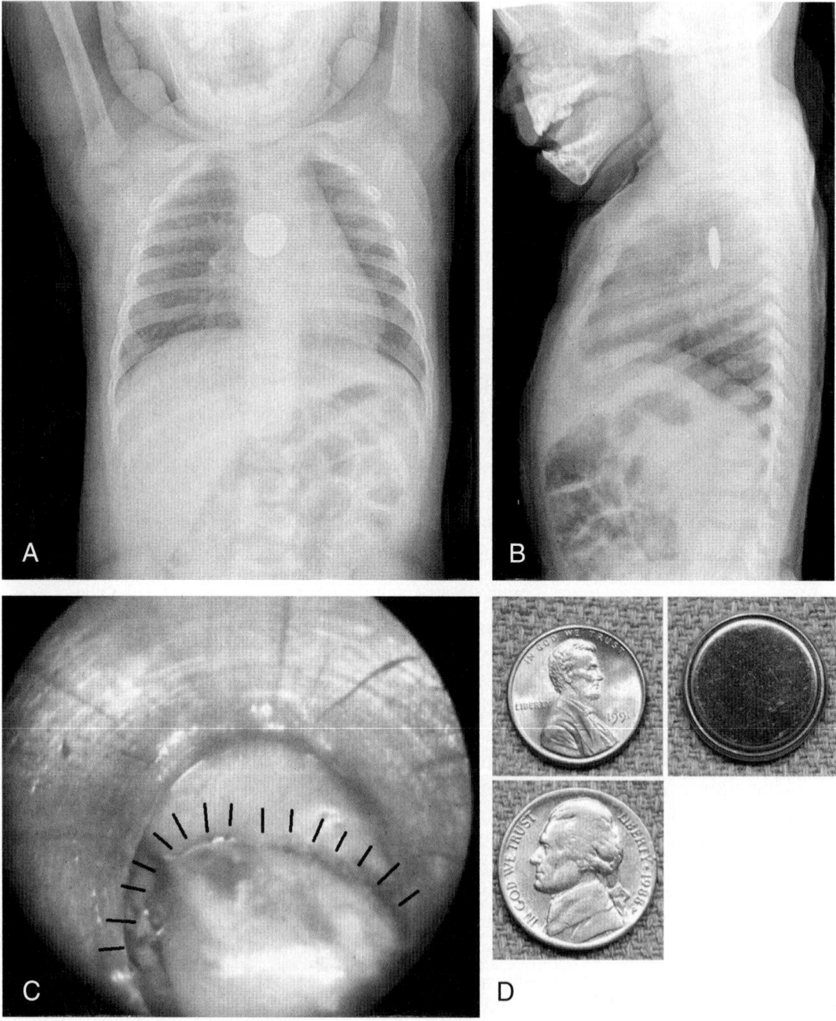

Figure 211-1. **A,** Anterior view of a chest radiograph of a child who has ingested a coin-shaped battery. Note its resemblance to a coin. **B,** Lateral view of battery within the chest. **C,** Endoscopic view of mucosal injury caused by the battery; lines mark circular burn at battery edge. **D,** Visual size comparison of a similar battery, a penny, and a nickel.

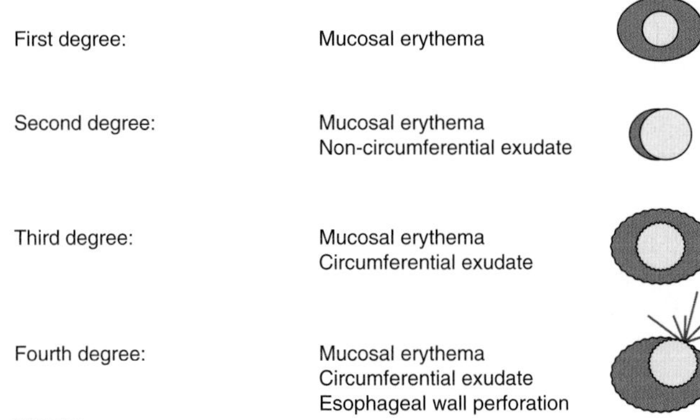

Figure 211-2. Four stages of esophageal burns.

Although any portion of the esophageal wall may be involved with the burn, the areas with the greatest extrinsic compression are most prone to injury. These are the cricopharyngeus, the aortic arch and left main stem bronchus compression sites, and the distal esophagus at the esophagogastric junction. As for other foreign bodies, this site is where solid caustics or batteries may lodge, causing severe localized injuries. When evaluating a significant burn of the esophagus, the endoscopist should be aware of the potential for a tracheoesophageal fistula resulting from the injury, especially at the upper esophageal and midesophageal narrowings. Tracheoscopy should be included when extensive burns are seen in these areas to examine the posterior tracheal wall for injury.

Staging

Methods of endoscopically staging and reporting esophageal burns vary. Historically, a classification borrowed from thermal burns has been used with references to first-degree, second-degree, and third-degree injuries that range from mild mucosal edema, to partial-thickness necrosis, to transmural necrosis.[37] Variations on this method have noted whether the lesion was circumferential. Recurrent difficulties in accurately and consistently applying this method include a failure to appreciate the true burn depth through the endoscope because of a necrotic exudate. Further contributing to endoscopic inaccuracy is difficulty in assessing the true amount of surface area burned because of mucosal edema. Such edema can prevent a complete, circumferential examination and obscure the sometimes subtle changes of an evolving submucosal necrosis, leading to an underestimation of injury in marginally burned areas.

Using modified classifications, four stages can provide the endoscopist with a consistent format for describing caustic injury to the esophageal lumen: first degree, mucosal erythema; second degree, erythema plus noncircumferential exudate; third degree, circumferential exudate; and fourth degree, circumferential exudate with esophageal wall perforation (Fig. 211-2).[38] Additional references to the site and length of the burn can be documented. In this staging system, only first-degree burns consistently heal uneventfully. Second-degree injuries occasionally form strictures, and all third-degree burns generally form strictures. Fourth-degree burns carry the additional risk of sepsis and mediastinitis. Because it is difficult to predict the true depth accurately, there is the potential for a third-degree burn eventually to extend into a fourth-degree burn—hence the need for close follow-up.

Several days after a caustic esophageal injury, any necrotic mucosa, submucosa, and muscular layer will have sloughed. At this point, the esophageal wall is at its weakest and may be prone to perforation, either spontaneously or secondary to an endoscope or nasogastric tube. The same is true for a transmural injury to the gastric wall. Close observation in all patients with third-degree esophageal burns is mandatory in a hospital for several days. Although antibiotics have not been shown to prevent strictures, broad-spectrum antibiotics are prudent in extensive third-degree burns that may lead to perforation.[30]

Additionally, endoscopy in the first 24 hours is safer to minimize the risk of perforation and for early identification of patients at risk for a fourth-degree injury. Although traditionally endoscopy has been aborted at the first significant burn,[10,17] the value and safety of full-length, careful esophagoscopy has been shown, especially in identifying patients with significant distal injury extending into the stomach.[30,37,39-42] With this in mind, endoscopy should be aborted when there is no definable lumen, rather than ceasing at the first severe burn. Although rigid and flexible endoscopes have been used to examine the full length of the esophagus successfully, the flexible model is necessary for adequate visualization of the stomach. If necrosis is identified extending into the gastric mucosa, direct visualization of the outer gastric wall should be strongly considered to rule out a transmural necrosis. Visualization may be by laparoscopy or laparotomy, depending on the surgeon's preference.

Therapy

When esophagogastric mucosal injury is diagnosed, the choice of therapy depends on the degree of injury. Injuries limited to first-degree burns of the esophageal mucosa require no further therapy. Blunt esophagectomy after identification of fourth-degree and selected extensive third-degree esophageal burns reduces the expected mortality from leaving a necrotic esophagus in place.[39,43] Identifying a perforation makes the decision for esophagectomy straightforward. For extensive third-degree burns, a thoracotomy or thoracoscopy for direct examination of the esophageal wall may be indicated to assess for transmural necrosis. Such decisions may be difficult, and may require the judgment and experience of the endoscopist. Débridement at the time of laparotomy or laparoscopy is dictated by the injury. In cases of gastric perforation, débridement of omentum, small bowel, and other intra-abdominal structures may be necessary.

The major controversy in therapeutic choices involves intermediate esophageal burns (i.e., second-degree and localized third-degree injuries). The goals of therapy are to maintain the esophageal lumen by the pharmacologic reduction or prevention of stricture formation and to maintain a conduit from the hypopharynx to the stomach by esophageal dilation, stenting, or reconstruction.

Pharmacologic Therapy

In 1950, Howes[44] and Spain[45] documented the retarding effect of corticosteroids on wound healing in separate laboratory studies. The following year, Rosenberg and coworkers[27] noted decreased stricture formation with corticosteroid therapy after alkali burns of rabbit esophageal mucosa. Although infection led to a high mortality rate, the supposed benefit from corticosteroids seemed clear. The addition of antibiotics reduced mortality, and the subsequent regimen of corticosteroids and antibiotics reduced esophageal strictures in the laboratory setting.[46-48] These findings led to the empirical therapeutic combination of corticosteroids and broad-spectrum antibiotics for significant second-degree and third-degree esophageal injuries. Retrospective analyses produce conflicting results. Some studies have shown benefit in reducing strictures, whereas others have not.[49,50]

In an attempt to resolve this controversy, Anderson and associates[51] reported on a prospective analysis through 18 years of 60 children with esophageal burns secondary to strong caustics (80% alkali). Patients were randomly assigned to receive 21 days of corticosteroids or no therapy, with the degrees of injury stratified equally in both groups. Of 21 patients identified as having circumferential burns, 20 developed strictures. Only 1 of 20 patients with a noncircumferential burn developed a stricture. Corticosteroids had no effect in the patients with circumferential burns. Ironically, the only stricture in the noncircumferential injury occurred in a child who received corticosteroids.

Lathyrogenic drugs that reduce collagen cross bonding have been used in attempts to decrease stricture formation.[52] Compounds such as β-aminopropionitrile, *N*-acetylcysteine, and penicillamine decrease stricture formation in laboratory settings, but their benefit in humans is unproven. Of these medications, penicillamine is the least toxic, and potentially may play a limited role.

Contact with acid and pepsin retards the healing of lye-induced esophageal burns in rabbits.[53] Clinically, the increase of gastroesophageal reflux has been documented in pediatric caustic strictures and subsequent loss of lower esophageal sphincter integrity.[54] With this information, it follows that efforts to decrease the effects of stomach acid on injured esophageal mucosa may be useful clinically. Sucralfate therapy for caustic esophageal burns has shown promise in the healing of ulcers without stricture formation.[55,56] Although unproven clinically in prospective caustic injury series, the low toxicity of pharmacologically reducing gastroesophageal reflux provides an attractive adjunctive measure in controlling strictures that is worthy of such a study.

Experience has been positive in the use of topical mitomycin in the management of pediatric tracheoesophageal strictures.[57-59] Mitomycin is an antibiotic used as an antineoplastic agent. Its usefulness stems from its behavior as an alkylating agent that inhibits deoxyribonucleic acid and protein synthesis, and fibroblast formation. Although experience in the use of this medication in caustic esophageal injuries is minimal, the successful use of this agent in selected aerodigestive tract lesions may herald some usefulness in caustic injuries.

Mechanical Therapy

The simplest mechanical method for maintaining a lumen in a third-degree esophageal burn is to place a nasogastric tube at the time of initial endoscopy. The true benefit of nasogastric tube stenting varies, with results ranging from spectacular to no benefit.[60,61] In a patient with a third-degree burn and dysphagia, a nasogastric tube provides a convenient stent and a means of nutritional support. Other types of stents have used polymeric silicone tubes in the esophagus with mixed success. Any clear benefit over serial dilations has not been shown.[62] Ideally, if this philosophy is used in guiding therapy, stents should remain in place long enough to allow re-epithelialization (2 to 3 weeks) with some reporting use for 9 to 14 months.[2]

Mild strictures can be serially dilated in a prograde fashion through an esophagoscope with filiform dilators. Cooperative patients (generally adults) may tolerate the periodic swallowing of weighted dilators in the office. Fluoroscopic guided balloon catheter dilation for acquired strictures has shown little success.[63] When identified, multiple strictures are managed most safely with retrograde dilators, popularized by Tucker[64] in the 1920s. A gastrostomy is necessary for the passage of an endless loop of silk exiting the mouth to allow slow, serial increases in caliber, while maintaining a secure position within the narrowed lumen and minimizing the risks of perforation (Fig. 211-3). If a significant, lengthy third-degree burn is identified at initial endoscopy, strong consideration should be given to the placement of a gastrostomy tube and

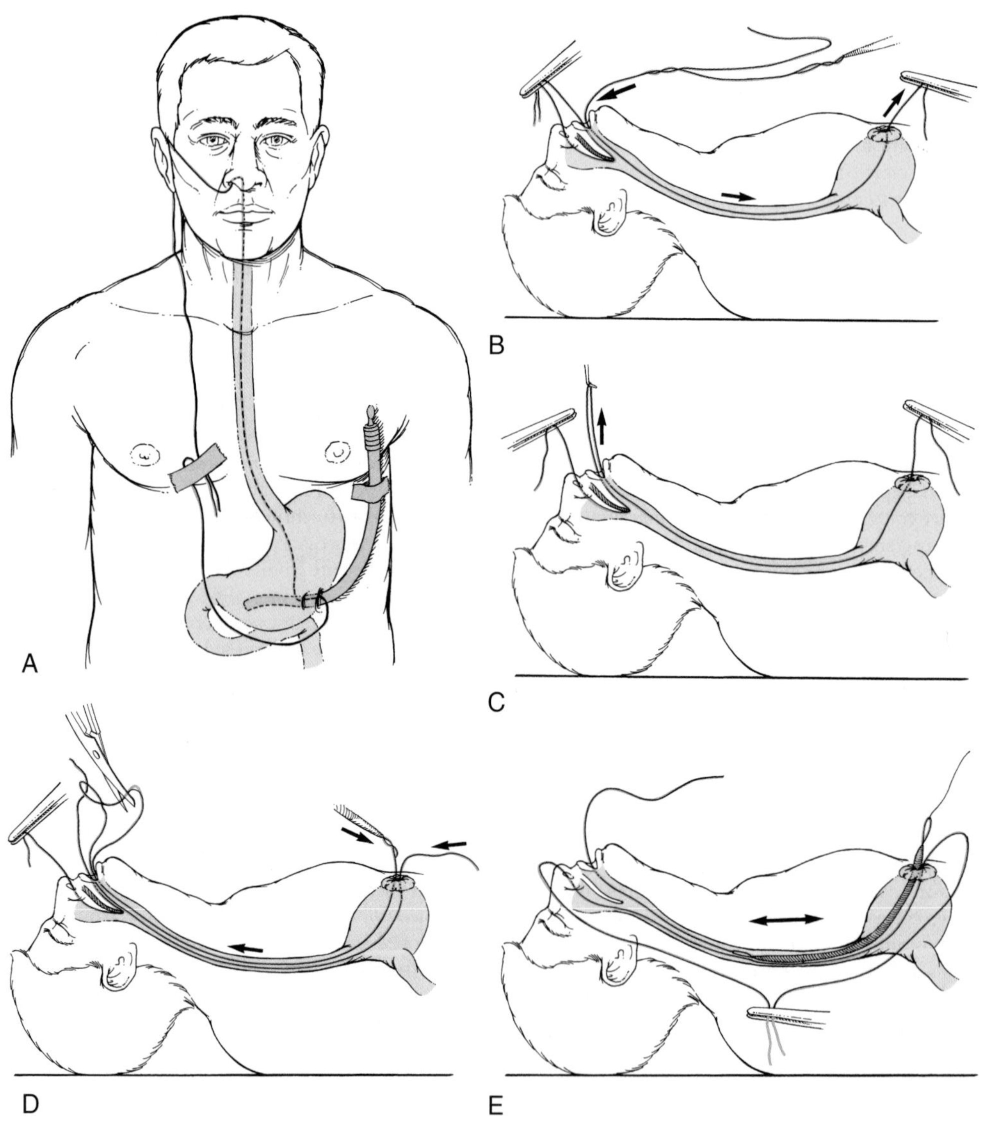

Figure 211-3. **A,** Appearance of a typical patient undergoing chronic retrograde dilations via gastrostomy. A guide string enters the nasal cavity, loops behind the ear, and enters alongside the gastrostomy tube. **B,** String (heavy silk) is retrieved from the posterior pharynx. **C,** A dilator is secured to silk exiting the mouth for gentle progressive prograde dilation. Care is taken to clamp the loop exiting the mouth and nose. **D,** A dilator is secured to silk exiting the gastrostomy tube for gentle progressive retrograde dilations. **E,** When dilator is within the lumen of the strictures, a gentle to-and-fro prograde or retrograde dilation may be accomplished. For security, a second heavy silk loop can be passed before any dilation in case the dilator string breaks.[64]

retrograde silk during the same anesthesia or before discharge to avoid a delay in safe dilation in the outpatient setting.

The timing of stricture dilation depends on the severity of the injury. In second-degree injuries, prophylactic dilation is not recommended, although periodic follow-up is important. Stricture formation may occur 6 weeks from the time of injury, and may become evident only when obstructed with food. Generally, a barium swallow at 3 weeks serves as a baseline in asymptomatic patients and as an initial study before prophylactic dilations in patients with lengthy third-degree injuries that are at high risk for stricture development. Routine barium esophagography is useful for 1 year to monitor progress of a managed stricture, and to rule out the development of an occult stricture. For symptomatic patients, the frequency of dilations depends on patient response. Weekly dilations may be necessary to maintain a viable lumen in severe injuries (Fig. 211-4).

When repetitive dilations fail to relieve symptoms, or when severe esophageal strictures render dilation impossible or fruitless, more aggressive techniques are indicated to reconstruct the conduit from hypopharynx to stomach. Esophageal replacement with gastric tubes, right colon, transverse colon, or descending colon has been described. The right colon has been reported to be the most useful conduit (Fig. 211-5).[65,66] When possible, blunt esophagectomy is preferable to thoracotomy. For isolated strictures, local resection with end-to-end reanastomosis, colon patch esophagoplasty, and esophageal stricture bypass with a colonic conduit have been reported in successful attempts to preserve an injured esophagus.[67-69]

Gastric outlet obstruction as a complication of acid ingestion is well known but uncommon, with an incidence 3.8% to 8.2% in pediatric series.[7,70] Less common is outlet obstruction secondary to alkali ingestion, with 5.3% (9 of 168) of patients developing gastric outlet obstruction in addition to esophageal strictures in the series reported by Ciftci and colleagues.[70] Presenting symptoms include frequent nonbilious emesis and secondary marked weight loss.[7] Treatment is surgical and includes gastrojejunostomy[7] or Billroth I[70] for complete obstruction and the Finney or Heineke-Mikulicz pyloroplasty for patients with partial obstruction.[70]

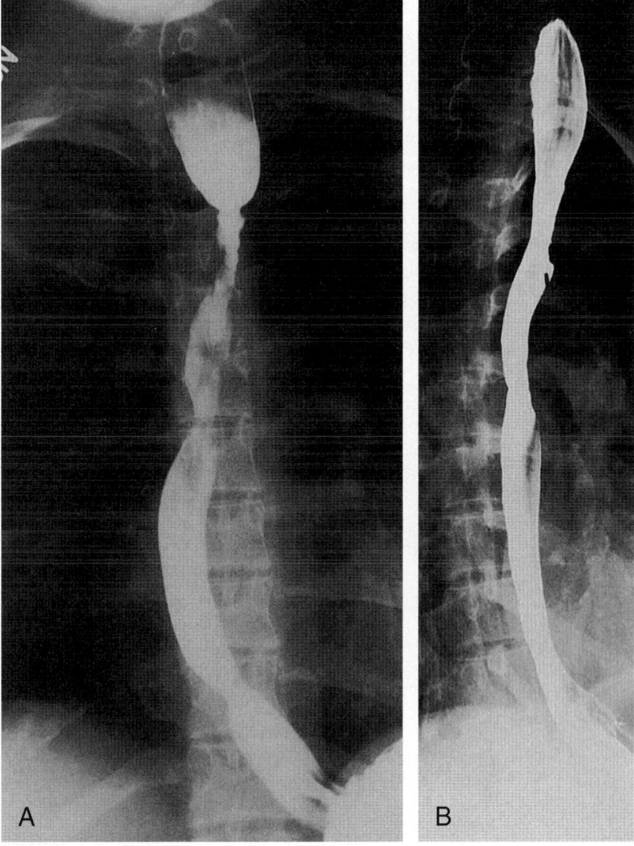

Figure 211-4. **A,** Barium swallow shows midesophageal stricture after lye ingestion in an adolescent 4 weeks after ingestion and at the beginning of retrograde dilations. **B,** Same patient 5 years later, after 4 years of repetitive dilations; the patient has a stable stricture and is generally nonsymptomatic.

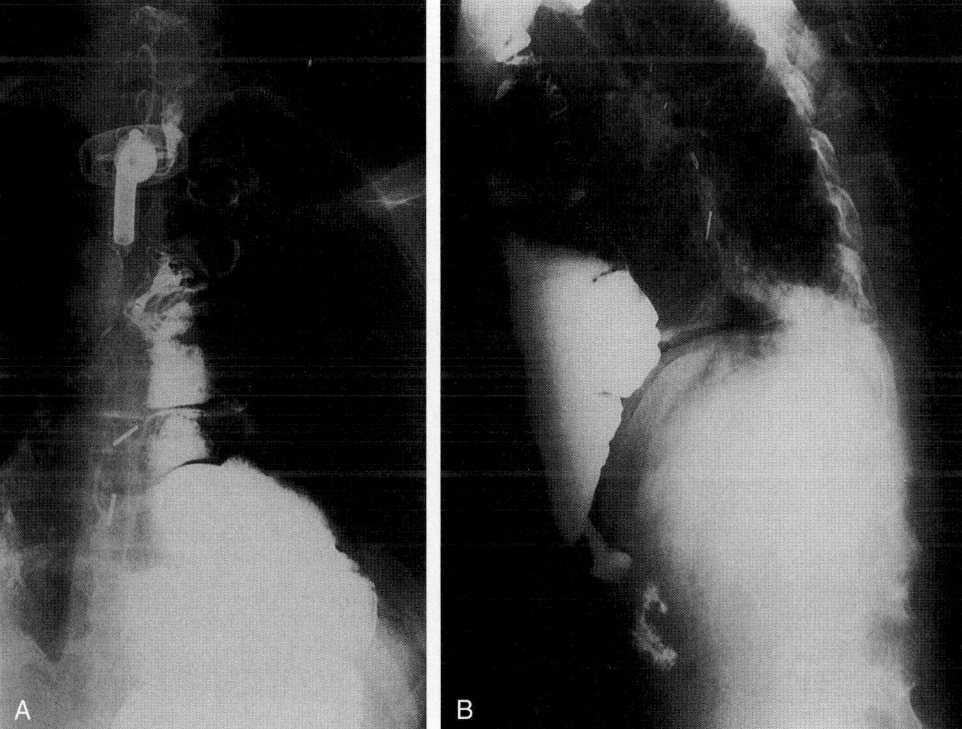

Figure 211-5. **A,** Anterior view of a barium swallow of a patient with a fourth-degree burn necessitating a total blunt esophagectomy with subsequent reconstruction using the right descending colon. The tracheotomy was originally placed emergently because of laryngeal obstruction secondary to supraglottic necrosis or edema. **B,** Lateral view of the same patient. Note the position of colon transfer in the anterior mediastinum.

The benefits from esophagectomy are not limited to the reconstruction of a swallowing conduit. In large series of esophageal carcinomas, a 1% to 4% incidence of caustic ingestion is typical. Although the true increased risk of carcinoma is unknown, it has been estimated at 1000-fold. The tendency for local extension of these malignancies is lower than expected with a higher potential rate of cure because they develop in the fibrotic, stenotic scar.[71] With this in mind, long-term follow-up is essential in any patient with a caustic esophageal stricture. The redevelopment of dysphagia after years of minimal difficulties should prompt an investigation with at least barium esophagography and, if abnormal, esophagoscopy with appropriate biopsy specimens.

In selected patients with a severely strictured esophagus requiring a lifetime of repetitive dilations necessary to maintain any useful lumen, elective esophagectomy with subsequent reconstruction may be reasonable. Additionally, a hiatal hernia, esophagitis, and peptic stricture may develop decades after a severe caustic injury, with resultant progressive fibrosis and dysfunction of the gastroesophageal sphincter. In this setting, the use of traditional dilation techniques as primary long-term therapy actually worsens the situation and the reflux.[72] Aggressive prophylactic antireflux measures with proton pump inhibitors may improve the outlook for these patients by increasing the long-term success of dilation, avoiding the need for aggressive surgery.

Conclusion

Caustic ingestion is an uncommon injury in the United States that varies widely in severity, ranging from minimal mucosal erythema to frank transmural necrosis of the esophagus and stomach with viscous perforation (Fig. 211-6). After appropriate identification of concentra-

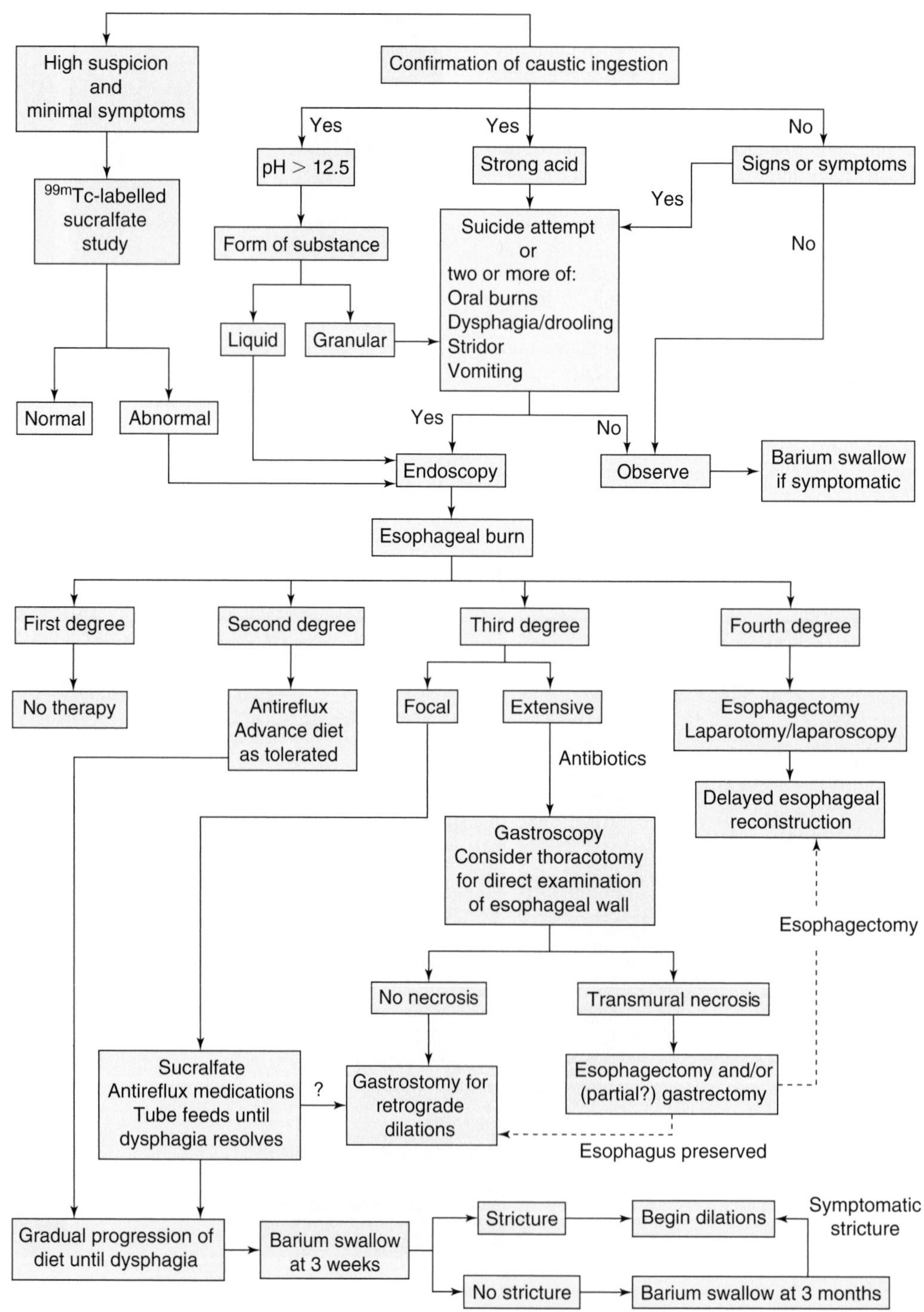

Figure 211-6. Evaluation and treatment of caustic ingestion.

tion, pH, and form of the ingested substance, the clinician should decide whether to evaluate the upper aerodigestive tract further. Full-length esophageal endoscopy is the most accurate initial method of examination, and is indicated after any ingestion of a strong liquid alkali. The need for endoscopy in other settings depends on the strength, volume, and form of the ingested caustic and associated signs and symptoms. Esophageal stricture formation is the chief long-term complication with a potential devastating impact on quality of life. Although repetitive stricture dilations are the mainstay of management, prevention or reduction in the severity of this complication is promising. Extensive necrotic esophageal injuries are doomed to fibrosis, but protocols emphasizing mucosal protectants with aggressive antireflux management may provide a means to minimize stricture formation in second-degree and localized third-degree injuries.

SUGGESTED READINGS

Anderson KD, Rouse TM, Randolph JG. A controlled trial of corticosteroids in children with corrosive injury of the esophagus. *N Engl J Med.* 1990;323:637.

Arevalo-Silva C, Eliashar R, Wohlgelernter J, et al. Ingestion of caustic substances: a 15-year experience. *Laryngoscope.* 2006;116:1422.

Bosher LH Jr, Burford TH, Ackerman L. The pathology of experimentally produced lye burns and strictures of the esophagus. *J Thorac Surg.* 1951; 21:483.

Brown JD, Thompson JN. Caustic ingestion. In: Cummings CW, Flint PW, Harker LA, et al., eds. *Cummings Otolaryngology Head and Neck Surgery.* 4th ed. St Louis: Mosby; 2005.

Christesen HBT. Prediction of complications following unintentional caustic ingestion in children: is endoscopy always necessary? *Acta Paediatr.* 1995; 84:1177.

Ciftci AO, Senocak ME, Buyukpamukcu N, et al. Gastric outlet obstruction due to corrosive ingestion: incidence and outcome. *Pediatr Surg Int.* 1999; 15:88.

Crain EF, Gershel JC, Mezey AP. Caustic ingestions: symptoms as predictors of esophageal injury. *Am J Dis Child.* 1984;138:863.

For complete list of references log onto www.expertconsult.com.

Dogan Y, Erkan T, Cokugras FC, et al. Caustic gastroesophageal lesions in childhood: an analysis of 473 cases. *Clin Pediatr (Phila).* 2006;45:435.

Gasset D, Sarfati E, Celerier M. Early blunt esophagectomy in severe caustic burns of the upper digestive tract: report of 29 cases. *J Thorac Cardiovasc Surg.* 1987;94:188.

Gun F, Abbasoglu L, Celik A, et al. Early and late term management in caustic ingestion in children: a 16-year experience. *Acta Chir Belg.* 2007;107:49.

Hollinger PH. Management of esophageal lesions caused by chemical burns. *Ann Otol Rhinol Laryngol.* 1968;77:819.

Howes EL, Plotz CM, Blunt JW, et al. Retardation of wound healing by cortisone. *Surgery.* 1950;28:177.

Jackson C. Esophageal stenosis following the swallowing of caustic alkalis. *JAMA.* 1921;77:22.

Kennedy AP, Cameron BH, McGill CW. Colon patch esophagoplasty for caustic esophageal stricture. *J Pediatr Surg.* 1995;30:1242.

Lamireau T, Rebouissoux L, Denis D, et al. Accidental caustic ingestion in children: is endoscopy always mandatory? *J Pediatr Gastroenterol Nutr.* 2001;33:81.

Moore WR. Caustic ingestions: pathophysiology, diagnosis, and treatment. *Clin Pediatr.* 1986;25:192.

Postlewhait RW, Sealy WC, Dillon ML, et al. Colon interposition for esophageal substitution. *Ann Thorac Surg.* 1971;12:89.

Rosenberg N, Kunderman PJ, Vroman L, et al. Prevention of experimental esophageal strictures by cortisone, II: control of suppurative complications by penicillin. *Arch Surg.* 1953;66:593.

Thompson JN. Corrosive esophageal injuries, II: an investigation of treatment methods and histochemical analysis of esophageal strictures in a new animal model. *Laryngoscope.* 1987;97:1191.

Tiryaki T, Livanelioglu Z, Atayurt H. Early bougienage for relief of stricture formation following caustic esophageal burns. *Pediatr Surg Int.* 2005;21:78.

Weisskopf A. Effects of cortisone on experimental lye burns of the esophagus. *Ann Otol Rhinol Laryngol.* 1952;61:681.

Index

Note: Page numbers followed by b, f, or t indicate boxes, figures, or tables, respectively.

A

A ring, 967
A trains, in electromyography, 2547
AABR (automated auditory brainstem response), 2721
AAMC (Association of American Medical Colleges), 84t-87t
AAV (adeno-associated virus) vectors, for gene therapy, 18, 18t
  of inner ear, 2191t, 2192
Abbé flap, 352
  in cleft-lip nose repair, 563f-564f
Abbreviated Profile of Hearing Aid Benefit (APHAB), 57
Abducens nerve
  intraoperative monitoring of, 2549-2550, 2550f
  in surgical anatomy of anterior cranial base, 2474
  in surgical anatomy of lateral skull base, 2439f
Abductor spasmodic dysphonia, botulinum toxin therapy for, 839, 841f
ABI. *See* Auditory brainstem implant (ABI).
Ablative vestibular surgery
  labyrinthectomy as, 2366-2368, 2367f
  patient selection for, 2364-2366
    clinical history in, 2364-2365
    consideration of other potential treatments in, 2366
    identification of intracranial pathology in, 2366
    identification of offending labyrinth in, 2365-2366
    poor compensation *vs.* unstable labyrinthine disease in, 2364, 2365t
    residual hearing and selection of procedure in, 2366
    therapeutic trial of vestibular rehabilitation in, 2365
    vestibular testing in, 2365, 2365b
  vestibular compensation after, 2370
  vestibular nerve section as, 2368-2370, 2368f-2369f
ABMS (American Board of Medical Specialties), 80, 84t-87t
  core competencies of, 80, 80b
ABOto (American Board of Otolaryngology), 80b, 84t-87t
ABR. *See* Auditory brainstem response (ABR).
Abrasions, 306
Abrasive surgery, for skin lesions, 294
ABRS (acute bacterial rhinosinusitis), 703-705, 704f
Abscess
  Bezold, 1985-1986, 1986f-1987f
    due to temporal bone infection, 1980t
  brain, 1994
    due to cranial base surgery, 2468
    epidemiology of, 1980t-1981t, 1994
    imaging of, 1994f-1995f
    otitis media and, 2777
    pathogenesis of, 1994
    symptoms of, 1994
    treatment of, 1994
  dentoalveolar, 1252
  epidural, 1995-1996
    epidemiology of, 1980t-1981t
  of infrahyoid prevertebral space, 162f
  of masticator space, 151-152, 152f
  of neck, imaging of, 1407, 1407f
  odontogenic (*See* Odontogenic infections)
  of oral cavity, 156f
  of parapharyngeal space, in children, 2788-2789
  parotid gland, 1152f-1153f
Abscess *(Continued)*
  peritonsillar, 1407, 1407f
    in children, 2788, 2789f
  postauricular, 1985, 1985f-1986f
  retropharyngeal, 1407, 1465-1466
    in children, 2789-2790, 2789f, 2810-2811
      anatomy of, 2810
      clinical features of, 2810
      complications of, 2811
      diagnosis of, 2810-2811, 2810f-2811f
      differential diagnosis of, 2806t
      epidemiology of, 2810
      historical background of, 2810
      imaging of, 2810-2811, 2810f-2811f
      management of, 2811
    imaging of, 1465-1466, 1466f
    infrahyoid, 134
    suprahyoid, 153, 155f
  of salivary gland, in children, 2856
  septal, 2627, 2627f
  subdural, otitis media and, 2777
  of sublingual space, 156, 157f
  temporal root, 1986
  tonsillar, 148, 148f
Absolute alcohol, for embolization, 1933
Absolute ethanol, for embolization, 1933
Absorption
  of laser energy, 28-29, 29f
  of photon, 26, 26f
Abutments, in prosthetic maxillary obturation, 1338-1339
AC (atypical carcinoid), of larynx, 1507
Acantholytic squamous cell carcinoma (ASCC), of larynx, 1506
ACC. *See* Adenoid cystic carcinoma (ACC).
Accelerated fractionation, 1040
Accessible population, 68, 68t
Accessory cartilages, of nose, 496-497, 497f
Accessory nerve. *See* Spinal accessory nerve (SAN).
Accreditation Council for Continuing Medical Education (ACCME), 79, 84t-87t
Accreditation Council for Graduate Medical Education (ACGME), 84t-87t
  core competencies of, 80, 80b
Accuracy, 65
Accutane (13-*cis* retinoic acid)
  for cancer chemoprevention, 1018, 1061-1062
    laryngeal, 1491
ACE (Advanced Combination Encoder), for cochlear implants, 2230, 2231f
ACE-27 (Adult Comorbidity Evaluation 27), 53
Acetaminophen, in children, for pain, 2572
  postoperative, 2594
Acetazolamide (Diamox)
  for Meniere's disease, 2337
  for migraine, 2350
Acetic acid, for cerumen removal, 1958t
Acetic acid with aluminum acetate (Domeboro Otic), 1959t-1960t
  for ear hygiene or chronic ear drainage, 1958
  for otitis externa
    bacterial, 1946, 1953
    fungal, 1954
Acetyl-L-carnitine, for noise-induced hearing loss, 2145
Achalasia, 963-965
  cricopharyngeal, 1398-1399, 1400f
  defined, 963
  differential diagnosis of, 1400
Achalasia *(Continued)*
  endoscopy of, 964, 964f
  esophageal manometry for, 964, 964f
  etiology and pathogenesis of, 963
  imaging of, 1399-1400, 1400f-1401f
    esophogram for, 963-964, 963f-964f
  management of, 964-965
  manometric findings with, 959t
  symptoms of, 963
  vigorous, 1399-1400, 1401f
Achondroplasia, craniofacial abnormalities in, 2633, 2634f
Acid(s), caustic ingestion of, 2956-2957
Acid reflux. *See* Gastroesophageal reflux disease (GERD).
Acid reflux laryngopharyngitis, 863, 863f
Acid taste, transduction of, 1209
Acidifying agents, ototopical, 1959t-1960t
  for ear hygiene or chronic ear drainage, 1958
  for otitis externa
    acute bacterial, 1953
    fungal, 1954
Acid-sensing channels, in sour taste, 1209
Acinic cell carcinoma, of salivary glands, 1185-1186, 1187f
  in children, 2820, 2846, 2846f, 2863
Acinic cell tumor, of parotid gland, 151f
Acinus(i), of salivary gland
  anatomy of, 1133-1134, 1134f, 1162, 1163f
  classification of, 1134, 1134t
  in secretory process, 1134-1135
Acne, after dermabrasion, 399
Acoustic analysis, for voice evaluation, 829t, 834-835
  cepstral peak prominence in, 829t, 830
  combined frequency and intensity in, 829, 829f, 829t
  Fast Fourier Transform in, 829t, 830, 830f
  frequency in, 829, 829t
  intensity (sound pressure level) in, 829, 829t
  linear predictive coding in, 829t, 830, 830f
  long-term average spectrum in, 829t, 830
  nasalance in, 829t, 830
  phonetogram (voice range profile) in, 829, 829f, 829t
  of professional voice, 849
  spectral displays in, 829t, 830, 830f
    with professional voice, 849
  variability in, 829-830, 829t
  of velopharyngeal function, 829t, 830
Acoustic changes, in geriatric patients, 236
Acoustic coupling, 1839-1840, 2000
  with hearing aids, 2205f
Acoustic desensitization protocol, for tinnitus, 2135
Acoustic feedback, with traditional hearing aid, 2204
Acoustic immittance testing, 1890-1891, 1890f, 2020
Acoustic impedance, 1839, 2000, 2017-2018
Acoustic meatus
  anatomy of, 1824f
  external, 320f, 2010f
Acoustic neuroma(s), 2514-2517
  of cerebellopontine angle, 1929t, 2514-2517
    diagnostic studies of, 2516-2517
    imaging of, 2517, 2517t-2518t
    natural history of, 2515, 2515f-2516f
    signs and symptoms of, 2515-2516
  cystic, stereotactic radiation therapy for, 2563
  defined, 2514-2515

Acoustic neuroma(s) *(Continued)*
diagnosis of, 2516-2517
audiometry for, 1897, 1898f, 2516
auditory brainstem response in, 1896-1899, 1898f-1899f, 1911, 2517
errors in, 1901, 1902f
imaging in, 2517, 2517t-2518t
vestibular tests in, 2517
facial nerve involvement in, 2413-2414
vs. facial nerve neuroma, 2414, 2519-2522
imaging of, 173, 175f, 2517, 2517t-2518t
of internal auditory canal, 173, 1928, 1928f
intraoperative monitoring for
of auditory brainstem response, 2553, 2553f
of cranial nerve function, 2543-2545, 2543f-2544f
of direct cochlear nerve action potentials, 2554f
intravestibular, 1921, 1924f
malignant, 2515
natural history of, 2515, 2515f-2516f
in neurofibromatosis type 1, 2515
in neurofibromatosis type 2, 2515
pathogenesis of, 2514-2515
sensorineural hearing loss due to, 2124-2125, 2125f, 2515-2516
sudden, 2128
signs and symptoms of, 2515-2516
stereotactic radiation therapy for, 2558, 2560f
cystic, 2563
fractionation *vs.* nonfractionation of, 2558-2559, 2561t
gamma knife–based, 2559t
hydrocephalus due to, 2563
LINAC-based, 2560t
neurofibromatosis 2–related, 2563
outcome assessment with, 2559-2563
facial nerve outcomes with, 2563
hearing outcomes with, 2562-2563, 2562t
trigeminal nerve outcomes in, 2563
tumor control in, 2562
quality of life with, 2564-2565
radiation dose plan for, 2560f
treatment of failures of, 2564
tumor control with, 2562
unilateral and nonhereditary, 2515
vertigo due to, 2353
Acoustic reflex decay, 1891
Acoustic reflex evoked potentials, to assess facial nerve function, 2388
Acoustic reflex testing
for conductive hearing loss, 2020
for otosclerosis, 2030, 2030f
for sensorineural hearing loss, 2117
Acoustic reflex threshold test, 1891
Acoustic rhinometry, 486-487, 644-645
in allergic rhinitis, 651
to assess effect of treatment, 651-652
equipment for, 486-487, 486f, 644
interpretation of results of, 645
intranasal sites assessed by, 644
reporting results of, 645
rhinogram generated by, 486-487, 487f, 645
vs. rhinomanometry, 644
for snoring and sleep apnea, 651
sources of variability in, 651
technical concerns and testing pitfalls with, 645
technique of, 644-645
Acoustic schwannoma. *See* Acoustic neuroma(s).
Acoustic trauma, 2121-2122, 2121f-2122f, 2141
Acoustic-based treatment strategies
for hyperacusis, 2139
for tinnitus, 2133
acoustic desensitization protocol as, 2135
ambient stimulation as, 2133-2134
combined with education and counseling, 2134-2135
Acoustic-based treatment strategies *(Continued)*
personal listening devices as, 2134
total masking therapy as, 2134
Acousticofacial ganglion, 1851-1852, 1851f
Acquired immunodeficiency syndrome (AIDS), 2114-2115. *See also* Human immunodeficiency virus (HIV)/HIV infection.
nasal manifestations of, 660
otologic manifestations of, 2114-2115
sensorineural hearing loss due to, 2124, 2161-2162
sudden, 2128
Acquired immunodeficiency syndrome (AIDS)-defining conditions, 210-211, 211t
Acquired immunodeficiency syndrome (AIDS) dementia complex, 223
Acquired immunodeficiency syndrome (AIDS)-related parotid cysts, imaging of, 1146, 1146f
Acrivastine (Semprex D), for nonallergic rhinitis, 701t
Acrobot, 39
Acrocephaly, synostotic, 2645, 2645f
Acrochordon, 291
Acromegaly, oral manifestations of, 1251
Acrylic mandibular splint, for pediatric facial fractures, 2701, 2701f
ACS (American College of Surgeons), 84t-87t
Actin filaments, in stereocilia, 2074, 2075f-2076f
Actin $\gamma 1$ *(ACTG1)* gene, in deafness, 2051t-2058t, 2074-2075
Actinic cheilitis, 283
Actinic keratoses, 283, 284f
Actinic lentigo, 288
Actinomyces israelii, otitis externa due to, 2194-2195
Actinomycosis
deep neck space infections due to, 201
laryngeal and tracheal manifestations of, 893
of salivary glands, 1159
in children, 2858
Action potential (AP), in electrocochleography, 1892-1894, 1907
in Meniere's disease, 2337
Active head movement analysis techniques, 2323-2324, 2324f
Actors, voice disorders in. *See* Professional voice disorders.
Acute bacterial rhinosinusitis (ABRS), 703-705, 704f
Acute chemical labyrinthine upset, due to intratympanic gentamicin, 2189
Acute exacerbation of chronic rhinosinusitis (AECRS), 705, 707, 707f
surgical management of, 741
Acute lymphocytic leukemia, otologic manifestations of, 2108f
Acute myelogenous leukemia, otologic manifestations of, 2108f
otorrhea as, 2197
Acute otitis media (AOM), 1979-1981
in children, 2761-2777
complications and sequelae of, 2776-2777
intracranial, 2776-2777
intratemporal, 2776
diagnosis of, 2761-2762
audiometry in, 2762
immittance testing (tympanometry) in, 2762
physical examination in, 2761-2762
symptoms and signs in, 2761
epidemiology of, 2765-2768
incidence and prevalence of, 2765-2766, 2765f
risk factors in, 2766-2768
trend over time in, 2765-2766
pathophysiology and pathogenesis of, 2762-2765, 2762f
Acute otitis media (AOM) *(Continued)*
allergy and immunology in, 2764-2765
eustachian tube function in, 2762-2763, 2763f
gastroesophageal reflux in, 2765
infection in, 2763-2764, 2764f
prevention of, 2768-2769
antibiotic prophylaxis for, 2771
management of environmental factors in, 2768
vaccines in, 2768-2769
quality of life assessment for, 2773
recurrent, 2771
treatment of, 2770-2771
medical, 2770-2771
observation in, 2770
for recurrent disease, 2771
surgical, 2771, 2773-2776
clinical features of, 1980
complications and sequelae of, 1963, 1979-1981 (*See also* Temporal bone infections, complications of)
in children, 2776-2777
intracranial, 2776-2777
intratemporal, 2776
otitis media with effusion as, 1963
tympanosclerosis as, 1974
diagnosis of, 2761-2762
audiometry in, 2762
immittance testing (tympanometry) in, 2762
physical examination in, 2761-2762
symptoms and signs in, 2761
epidemiology of, 1979-1980
in children, 2765-2768
incidence and prevalence of, 2765-2766, 2765f
risk factors in, 2766-2768
trend over time in, 2765-2766
immunosuppression and, 222-223
pathophysiology and pathogenesis of, 1980-1981, 2762-2765, 2762f
allergy and immunology in, 2764-2765
eustachian tube function in, 2762-2763, 2763f
gastroesophageal reflux in, 2765
infection in, 2763-2764, 2764f
prevention of, 2768-2769
antibiotic prophylaxis for, 2771
management of environmental factors in, 2768
vaccines in, 2768-2769
recurrent, 2771
treatment of, 1980-1981, 2770-2771
medical, 2770-2771
observation in, 2770
for recurrent disease, 2771
surgical, 2771, 2773-2776
Acute retroviral syndrome (ARS), 197
Acute rhinosinusitis (AR, ARS)
bacterial, 703-705, 704f, 732
endoscopic sinus surgery for, 761
frontal, 775
pathogenesis of, 703-705, 704f
radiologic appearance of, 672-673, 673f
recurrent, 705
surgical management of, 741
Acute vestibular deafferentation syndrome, due to intratympanic gentamicin, 2189
Acyclovir (Zovirax)
with chemical peels, 397
for herpes zoster, 2396
for recurrent respiratory papillomatosis, 2890t, 2892
AD (auditory dyssynchrony)
cochlear implant for, 2220, 2240
neurodiagnostic studies with, 1899-1901, 1900f
otoacoustic emissions as, 1907

Ad (adenoviral) vectors
conditionally replicating, 22
for gene therapy, 17-18, 17f, 18t
of inner ear, 2191t, 2192
Ad5CMV-p53 vector, in gene therapy, 21-22
Adams suspension wiring, 335-336
Adaptation
and olfactory testing, 633
in vestibular compensation, 2374-2375
Adaptation exercises, in vestibular rehabilitation, 2372-2373, 2375f, 2378
Adaptive immune system, 209, 599-605
B cells in, 603
development of, 603
responses by, 603
basophils and mast cells in, 605
eosinophils in, 604
innate *vs.*, 597-598
monocytes and macrophages in, 604
natural killer cells in, 603-604
neutrophils in, 604
overview of, 597-598
platelets and erythrocytes in, 605
stem cells in, 599-600, 600f
T cells in, 600-603
development of, 600-601
effector, 601-603
priming of, 601
Toll-like receptors and, 598
ADCC (antibody-dependent cellular cytotoxicity), 603-604, 606
Addax (ethylene oxide polyoxypropylene glycol), for cerumen removal, 1958t
Addison's disease
oral manifestations of, 1251
preoperative evaluation of, 105
Additive effect, of chemoradiation, 1041
Adductor breathing dystonia, 839
Adductor spasmodic dysphonia, botulinum toxin therapy for, 839, 840f
A-delta fibers, in dental pain, 1202-1203
Adeno-associated virus (AAV) vectors, for gene therapy, 18, 18t
of inner ear, 2191t, 2192
Adenocarcinoma(s)
breast
metastatic to ear, 2108f
skull base metastases of, 173f
esophageal, 973, 974f
cervical, 1425
GERD and, 899
of hypopharynx, 1425
of paranasal sinuses, 1131
of salivary glands
basal cell, 1191
NOS, 1191
polymorphous low-grade, 1184-1185, 1186f
Adenoid(s)
anatomy of, 2784
radiographic, 1399f, 1462-1463
bacteriology of, 2785-2788
diagnostic assessment of, 2793-2794, 2793f
hypertrophic, and otitis media, 1872, 1873f
in immune system, 605, 2784-2785
Adenoid cystic carcinoma (ACC)
of larynx, 1507
of masticator space, 155f
of nasopharynx, 1351
of oral cavity, 1299
of paranasal sinuses, 1131
of salivary glands
histopathology of, 1183-1184, 1185f
imaging of, 1146-1147, 1146f-1147f, 1180f
minor, 1362-1363
of trachea, 1614, 1614f
"Adenoid facies," 618, 2628, 2629f, 2639
Adenoid hypertrophy, rhinitis due to, 619b
Adenoid pads, 1869, 1869f
enlarged, and pediatric chronic sinusitis, 2779-2780, 2780f
Adenoid squamous cell carcinoma, of larynx, 1506
Adenoid tissue, 101
Adenoidectomy, 2795-2796
for chronic sinusitis in children, 2779-2780, 2780f
immunologic consequences of, 2785
indications for, 2795-2796, 2795b
Microdebrider for, 2797-2798
for obstructive sleep apnea, 2608-2609
for otitis media, 2796
acute, 2771
with effusion, 2772-2773, 2776
procedure for, 2776, 2798
rationale for, 2776
in vocal professional, 858
Adenolymphoma, of salivary glands, 1170-1171
imaging of, 1146, 1146f
Adenoma(s)
parathyroid (*See* Parathyroid adenoma)
pleomorphic (*See* Pleomorphic adenoma(s))
sebaceum, 292
thyroid, 1758-1759
autonomously functioning, 1759
in children, 2819
clinical presentation of, 1758
management and prognosis for, 1759
pathology of, 1758-1759
sestamibi–technetium 99m scintigraphy of, 1785f
toxic, 1744
Adenomatoid odontogenic tumor, 1277
microscopic features of, 1277
radiographic features of, 1277
treatment of, 1277
Adenopathy, physical examination of, 95-96
Adenosine triphosphatase (ATPase)-driven sodium-potassium (Na^+,K^+) pump, in salivary gland secretion, 1135
Adenosine triphosphate (ATP)–magnesium chloride complex, and skin flap viability, 1074
Adenosquamous carcinoma (ASC)
of hypopharynx and cervical esophagus, 1425
of larynx, 1506
Adenotonsillar disease, in children, 2782-2802
adenoidectomy for, 2795-2796
indications for, 2795-2796
and otitis media, 2796
adenotonsillectomy for (*See* Adenotonsillectomy)
anatomy of, 2783-2784
due to bacterial infections, 2785-2788
due to candidiasis, 2786
chronic adenotonsillar hypertrophy as, 2790-2793
airway obstruction due to, 2789f-2790f, 2790-2793, 2795
algorithm for evaluation of, 2783f-2784f
with attention deficit–hyperactivity disorder, 2791
cardiopulmonary complications of, 2792, 2792f
craniofacial growth and, 2792-2793
diagnostic assessment of, 2793-2794, 2793f
and enuresis, 2792
etiology of, 2789f-2790f, 2790
and growth problems, 2792
and neurocognitive development, 2791-2792
and obstructive sleep apnea, 2790-2793
complications of, 2788-2790
nonsuppurative, 2788
parapharyngeal space abscess as, 2788-2789
peritonsillar infections as, 2788, 2789f
retropharyngeal space infections as, 2789-2790, 2789f
suppurative, 2788-2790
due to *Corynebacterium diphtheriae*, 2786-2787
diagnostic assessment for, 2793-2794, 2793f
Adenotonsillar disease, in children *(Continued)*
history of, 2782
imaging of, 2793-2794, 2793f
immunology of, 2784-2785
due to infections of Waldeyer's ring, 2785
management algorithms for, 2782, 2783f-2784f
microbiology of, 2785-2788
due to *Neisseria gonorrhoeae*, 2786
preoperative assessment for, 2794
due to streptococcal infection, 2787
due to syphilis, 2786
due to tonsillar concretions/tonsilloliths, 2787-2788, 2788f
due to Vincent's angina, 2786
due to viral infections, 2785-2786, 2786f
with Epstein-Barr virus, 2785-2786, 2786f
Adenotonsillar hypertrophy
chronic, in children, 2790-2793
with ADHD, 2791
airway obstruction due to, 2789f-2790f, 2790-2793, 2795
algorithm for evaluation of, 2783f-2784f
cardiopulmonary complications of, 2792, 2792f
craniofacial growth and, 2792-2793
diagnostic assessment of, 2793-2794, 2793f
and enuresis, 2792
etiology of, 2789f-2790f, 2790
and growth problems, 2792
and neurocognitive development, 2791-2792
and obstructive sleep apnea, 2790-2793
obstructive sleep apnea due to, 252
in children, 2604-2606, 2790-2793
Adenotonsillectomy, 2796-2801
anesthesia for, 2598-2599, 2599b, 2797
antibiotic prophylaxis with, 2797
complication(s) of, 2799-2801
airway obstruction and pulmonary edema as, 2800
atlantoaxial subluxation (Grisel's syndrome) as, 2801
nasopharyngeal stenosis as, 2800-2801, 2801f
postoperative hemorrhage as, 2799-2800, 2800f
velopharyngeal insufficiency as, 2800
historical background of, 2794-2795
indications for, 2794b-2795b, 2795
chronic infections as, 2794b-2795b, 2795
upper airway obstruction as, 2794b-2795b, 2795
inpatient *vs.* outpatient, 2799
intravenous corticosteroids during, 2797-2798
for obstructive sleep apnea, 2608-2609
patient discharge after, 2798
patient preparation for, 2797-2798
preoperative assessment for, 2794
preoperative sedation for, 2797
surgical technique for, 2796-2799, 2798f
adenoidectomy in, 2798
Coblator in, 2796
electrocautery tonsillectomy in, 2797-2799
Harmonic Scalpel in, 2796-2797
hemostasis in, 2798-2799
instrumentation in, 2797, 2797f
Microdebrider in, 2797
options for, 2796
patient positioning in, 2798, 2798f
subtotal tonsillectomy in, 2797
Adenoviral (Ad) vectors
conditionally replicating, 22
for gene therapy, 17-18, 17f, 18t
of inner ear, 2191t, 2192
Adenovirus, pharyngitis due to, 198
Adenylate cyclase system, in salivary gland secretion, 1137
ADHD (attention deficit–hyperactivity disorder), sleep-disordered breathing and, 2791
Adhesion molecules, in allergic rhinitis, 616, 617f
Adipocyte hyperplasia, 452

Adipose origin, neoplasms of, of larynx, 881
Aditus ad antrum
anatomy of, 1827, 1829, 1852
vulnerability to injury of, 1829
Adjuvant analgesics, 243-244
anticonvulsant agents as, 243-244, 244t
antidepressants as, 244-245, 245t
Adjuvant radiation therapy, for salivary gland neoplasms, 1197-1198, 1198t
Adjuvant therapy, concomitant chemoradiation as, 1056
Adoptive T-cell immunotherapy, for head and neck squamous cell carcinoma, 1024
Adrenal diseases, oral manifestations of, 1251
Adrenal gland, preoperative evaluation of, 104-105
Adrenal insufficiency, idiopathic primary, preoperative evaluation of, 105
Adrenergic receptors, in salivary gland secretion, 1136, 1137t
ADSNHL (autosomal dominant sensorineural hearing loss)
genetic testing for, 2098
nonsyndromic, 2090-2093, 2092t
syndromic, 2093-2096, 2094t
Adult Comorbidity Evaluation 27 (ACE-27), 53
Adult Emergency Airway Cart, 116
Advanced Combination Encoder (ACE), for cochlear implants, 2230, 2231f
Advanced sleep phase disorder, 264
Advancement flaps, 345-346
bilateral, 345, 346f
for cheek defects, 358
V-Y, 358, 361f
for cleft lip repair, 2668, 2668f
for forehead repair, 360-363, 362f
island, 345
for lip defects, 352-353
for nasal defects, 347-348, 347f, 349f
unipedicle, 345, 345f
V-Y, 345-346, 346f-347f
for cheek defects, 358, 361f
Y-V, 346
Advancement rotation flaps, for forehead repair, 360-362, 362f
Adynamic segments, laryngeal videostroboscopy of, 820
AECRS (acute exacerbation of chronic rhinosinusitis), 705, 707, 707f
surgical management of, 741
AERD (aspirin-exacerbated respiratory disease), 731-732, 732f
Aerodynamic assessment, in voice evaluation, 828-829, 828t, 835
of airflow, 828, 828t
of children, 2878
of laryngeal airway resistance, 828-829, 828t
of maximum phonation time, 828
of phonation threshold pressure, 828, 828t
of professional voice, 849
of subglottic air pressure, 828, 828t
of velopharyngeal function, 828t, 829
AESOP (automated endoscopic system for optimal positioning), 39, 40f
Aesthetic facial analysis. *See* Facial analysis.
Aesthetic units, in facial analysis, 269-270, 274f
African-American nose. *See* Noncaucasian rhinoplasty.
AFRS. *See* Allergic fungal rhinosinusitis (AFRS).
Afterhyperpolarizations (AHPs), in vestibular afferent nerve fibers, 2284-2285, 2284f
AGA (androgenetic alopecia), 374-376, 375f
Agency for Healthcare Research and Quality (AHRQ), 52, 82, 84t-87t
Age-related hearing loss (AHL), 2125-2126, 2126f
genetic basis for, 2074
with tinnitus, 2132
Age-related plasticity, 1877, 1879, 1882f
AGES classification, of thyroid cancer, 1754, 1756t
Agger nasi, surgical anatomy of, 740
Agger nasi cells
in endoscopic dacryocystorhinostomy, 799-800, 800f
in frontal sinusitis, 776
normal anatomy of, 665-666, 665f-666f
Aging patients. *See* Geriatric patients.
Aging skin, 390-404
appearance of, 440f
classification of, 391, 391t
esthetician's role in management of, 402
evaluation of, 391
and facial expression, 439, 440f
facial resurfacing for
chemical peels for, 391-397
agents for, 392-394
complications of, 396-397
contraindications to, 391, 392t
in dark-skinned individuals, 392
deep, 394-395
equipment tray for, 393f
histologic changes with, 390-391
indications for, 391, 392t
medium-depth, 393-394, 393f-394f
patient selection and education for, 391-392
and phenol toxicity, 395
postoperative care after, 396, 396f
prepeel preparations for, 392
superficial, 392-393, 403
contraindications to, 391, 392t
dermabrasion for, 397-399
complications of, 399
equipment for, 398, 398f
micro-, 402-403
patient selection and consultation for, 397-398
postoperative care after, 399, 399f
technique of, 398-399, 398f-399f
indications for, 391, 392t
laser, 399-402
CO_2, 400, 400f
Er:YAG, 400
nonablative, 402, 403t
postoperative care after, 401-402, 401f
nonablative, 402, 403t
laser, 402, 403t
microdermabrasion for, 402-403
superficial chemical peels for, 403
histologic changes of, 390-391
intrinsic and extrinsic factors in, 439
medical skin care regimens for, 403-404
melolabial fold in, 406, 406f
of midface, 444, 444f
Agranulocytosis, oral manifestations of, 1256
AHI (apnea-hypopnea index), 251, 251b
AHIP (America's Health Insurance Plans), 84t-87t
AHL (age-related hearing loss), 2125-2126, 2126f
genetic basis for, 2074
with tinnitus, 2132
AHPs (afterhyperpolarizations), in vestibular afferent nerve fibers, 2284-2285, 2284f
AHRQ (Agency for Healthcare Research and Quality), 52, 82, 84t-87t
AI (apnea index), 251b, 252
AICA. *See* Anterior inferior cerebellar artery (AICA).
AIDS. *See* Acquired immunodeficiency syndrome (AIDS).
AIED. *See* Autoimmune inner ear disease (AIED).
Air leaks, due to neck dissection, 1722-1723
Air pollution, and rhinosinusitis, 731
Air pressure, subglottic
in professional voice production, 846
in voice evaluation, 828, 828t
Air stream, through nose, tests that assess, 643
Air-bone gap, 1888, 1888f
with conductive hearing loss, 2020, 2020f
Air-conduction testing, in pure-tone audiometry, 1888
masking for, 1889-1890
errors in, 1901-1902
Air-contrast pharyngogram, 1394, 1395f
Airflow
in olfaction, 624-625, 625f
and stridor, 2897, 2898f
in voice evaluation, 828, 828t, 849
Airflow measurement, for velopharyngeal dysfunction, 2679
Airflow rhinometry, 487
Airway
anatomy of, and tracheobronchial endoscopy, 998-999, 999f
difficult (*See* Difficult airway)
fire in, 119
foreign bodies in, 975-976, 2935-2943
acute obstruction due to, 2936-2937
complications of, 2942
epidemiology of, 2936
imaging of, 1411, 1412f, 2938-2939
vs. tonsillar calcifications, 1411, 1412f
location of, 2936, 2936f
management of, 2939-2941
anesthesia for, 2940
controversies in, 2942
equipment for, 2939-2940, 2939t, 2940f
history of, 2935
postoperative, 2941-2942
for sharp objects, 2940-2941
technique for, 2940, 2941f
symptoms of, 2937-2938
"Airway Alert," identification of, 115
Airway establishment, for odontogenic infections, 188
Airway hemangioma
assessment and treatment of, 2828-2829, 2829f
complications of, 2825, 2826f
Airway infection(s), in children, 2803-2811
bacterial tracheitis (exudative tracheitis) as, 2809-2810
clinical features of, 2809
complications of, 2810
diagnosis of, 2809, 2809f
differential diagnosis of, 2806t
endoscopy of, 2809, 2809f
epidemiology of, 2809
imaging of, 2809, 2809f
management of, 2809-2810, 2809f
pathogenesis of, 2809
terminology for, 2809
croup (laryngotracheitis) as, 2803-2806
clinical features of, 2803-2804
defined, 2803
diagnosis of, 2804
differential diagnosis of, 2804-2805, 2806t
epidemiology of, 2803
etiology of, 2803
imaging of, 2804, 2804f-2805f
laryngoscopy of, 2804, 2805f
management of, 2805-2806
pathogenesis of, 2803-2804
spasmodic, 2805
terminology for, 2803
retropharyngeal abscess as, 2810-2811
anatomy of, 2810
clinical features of, 2810
complications of, 2811
diagnosis of, 2810-2811, 2810f-2811f
differential diagnosis of, 2806t
epidemiology of, 2810
historical background of, 2810
imaging of, 2810-2811, 2810f-2811f
management of, 2811

Airway infection(s), in children *(Continued)*
supraglottitis (epiglottitis) as, 2806-2809
clinical features of, 2807
complications of, 2808-2809
diagnosis of, 2807-2808, 2807f-2808f
differential diagnosis of, 2806t
endoscopy of, 2808, 2808f
epidemiology of, 2806-2807
etiology of, 2807
histology of, 2807, 2807f
historical background of, 2806-2807
imaging of, 2807f, 2808
management of, 2808
Airway management
for deep neck space infections, 205
for laryngeal trauma, 936
with tracheal neoplasms, 1617
for tracheobronchial endoscopy, 1000
Airway obstruction
after adenotonsillectomy, 2800
in children (*See* Stridulous child)
due to chronic adenotonsillar hypertrophy, 2789f-2790f, 2790-2793, 2795
decongestion for, 655
due to foreign body, 2936-2937
in neonate
expected, 2904-2905
unexpected, 2905
laryngeal, 2905
supralaryngeal, 2905, 2905f
tracheobronchial, 2905
posterior to valve area, 655-656
in Robin sequence, 2673
sleep-related, 2607
valve area stenting for, 655
Airway pressure, subglottic
in professional voice production, 846
in voice evaluation, 828, 828t
Airway protection, during pharyngeal swallow, 1216-1217
Airway resistance, laryngeal, in voice evaluation, 828-829, 828t
Airway restriction
identification of side of nose with greater, 655
threshold level at which patient feels, 655
Airway Service, 116-117
Airway Service resources, 116
Airway stenosis, 943-952
classification of, 944, 944t
local application of mitomycin C for, 946
pathophysiology of, 943-944, 944b
surgical management of, 943-952
for chronic disease, 947-952
anterior glottic, 948
due to anterior wall collapse, 951
cervical tracheal, 951, 951b, 951f
cicatricial membranous, 951
complete glottic, 949-950
complete tracheal, 951-952, 952f
laryngeal release procedures in, 952
posterior glottic, 948-949, 949f
subglottic, 945f, 950-951
supraglottic, 947-948
endoscopic *vs.* open, 945
goals and assessment in, 944, 945f
microsurgical débridement in, 946, 946b, 946f
planning for, 946-947
skin and mucosal grafts in, 946-947
stent placement in, 947, 947f
timing of, 945
Akt receptor, in oral cancer, 1295
Ala
lateral angle of, 509f
medial angle of, 509f
5-ALA (5-aminolevulinic acid)-induced fluorescence, for premalignant lesions of larynx, 1488-1489
Alar base, overly narrowed, revision rhinoplasty for, 593-594, 594f
Alar base modification, in noncaucasian patients, 577-578, 578f
Alar batten grafts, 550, 551f
in revision rhinoplasty, 586-587, 587f
Alar cartilage, 496-497, 497f
lateral crus (crura) of, 496-497, 497f, 509f
in cleft-lip nose repair, 562f
transposition of, 551
medial crus (crura) of, 496-497, 497f, 509f
in cleft-lip nose repair, 561f-562f
Alar defects
extending into facial sulcus, 348
cheek advancement flap for, 348, 349f
cheek pedicle transposition flap for, 348, 349f
full-thickness, 347
bipedicle mucosal advancement flap for, 347, 347f
free cartilage grafts for, 348
melolabial interpolated flap for, 348
due to septoplasty, 491, 491f
Alar layer, 202
Alar margin implant, retrograde, 548, 550f
Alar pinching, revision rhinoplasty for, 587, 587f-589f
Alar reduction, for noncaucasian nose
alar soft tissue sculpting in, 557, 561f
nasal base sculpting in, 556-557, 559f-560f
Alar retraction, 548, 549f
revision rhinoplasty for, 587, 587f-589f
Alar rim grafts, in revision rhinoplasty, 587, 588f-589f
Alar soft tissue sculpting, for noncaucasian nose, 557, 561f
Alar-columellar complex, aesthetic analysis of, 270f-271f, 274
Alar-facial junction, 509f
Alaryngeal voice and speech, 1459, 1594-1610
electrolarynx, 1596, 1596f
esophageal, 1596, 1596f
history of, 1594-1595, 1595f
after laryngopharyngectomy, 1458-1459
physiology of, 1595-1597, 1596f
after total laryngectomy, 1572
after total laryngopharyngectomy, 1575
tracheoesophageal, 1597, 1597f
voice prosthesis(es) for, 1597, 1597f
indwelling *vs.* nonindwelling, 1597-1598, 1598f
postoperative management of, 1600
alimentary care in, 1600
pulmonary care in, 1600, 1602f
and radiotherapy, 1600, 1602b
replacement of, 1601
indications for, 1601
nonindwelling, 1602
for valve discrepancy (periprosthetic leakage), 1602
for valve incompetence (transprosthetic leakage), 1601-1602
secondary, 1600
surgical aspects of, 1598-1600, 1599f-1600f
creation of optimally contoured stoma as, 1599-1600, 1600f
pharyngeal mucosa closure as, 1599-1600, 1601f
prevention of excessively deep stoma as, 1599-1600, 1600f
prevention of hypertonicity of PE segment as, 1599-1600, 1599f
timing of insertion of, 1597-1599
troubleshooting with, 1603-1605
types of, 1597-1598, 1598f
Albers-Schönberg disease, 2112
Albright's disease, oral manifestations of, 1257
Albright's syndrome, fibrous dysplasia in, 2110-2111
Albumin, in saliva, 1139
Alcohol
absolute, for embolization, 1933
dizziness due to, 2310t
for ear hygiene or chronic ear drainage, 1958
Alcohol block, for neuropathic pain, 245-246
Alcohol consumption, and squamous cell carcinoma
of head and neck, 1016
of larynx, 1491, 1512-1513
of oral cavity, 1293, 1365
Alcoholism, oral manifestations of, 1255
Alcohol-vinegar solution, for otitis externa, 1953, 1959t-1960t
ALD(s) (assistive listening devices), 2270-2271
Aldara (imiquimod), for aural papillomatosis, 1957
Aldosteronism, primary, preoperative evaluation of, 104-105
Alendronate, for hyperparathyroidism, 1804
Alexander's law, 2297, 2299f, 2312, 2312f
Alfentanil, for pediatric anesthesia, 2592
Alginic acid, for GERD, 970
Alkali(s), caustic ingestion of, 2956-2958
Alkaptonuria, 2114
Allegra (fexofenadine), for nonallergic rhinitis, 701t
Alleles, 2088
Allergic component, in nonallergic rhinitis, 696
Allergic fungal rhinosinusitis (AFRS), 707, 712-715
in children, 2778, 2780, 2781f
chronic, 707, 733
classification of, 709
diagnosis of, 707, 712-713
epidemiology of, 713-714
imaging of, 706f, 713, 714f
immunochemical staining for, 731, 731f
pathogenesis of, 712-714, 714b
prognosis for, 713
therapy for, 713-715, 715b
Allergic granulomatous angiitis, nasal manifestations of, 659
Allergic nasal mucin, 733
Allergic otitis externa, 1945-1946
Allergic reactions, 608-612
parotid enlargement due to, 2864
Allergic rhinitis (AR), 612-614
burden of disease for, 614
classification of, 617-618
epidemiology of, 612-613
episodic, 617-618
evaluation and diagnosis of, 617-619
acoustic rhinometry in, 651
diagnostic tests in, 619
differential diagnosis in, 618, 619b
history in, 617-618, 619b
physical examination in, 618-619
rhinomanometry in, 651
hygiene hypothesis of, 613-614
intermittent, 618
mild, 618
moderate to severe, 618
pathophysiology of, 614-617, 618f
adhesion molecules and cellular recruitment in, 616, 617f
cellular events in, 615-616
early response to antigen in, 614
hyperresponsiveness in, 616-617
nonspecific, 617
specific, 616-617
late response to antigen in, 615
neuronal contribution to, 614-615
sensitization and immunoglobulin E production in, 614
and pediatric chronic sinusitis, 2778
perennial, 617-618
and pediatric chronic sinusitis, 2778
persistent, 618
seasonal, 617-618
and pediatric chronic sinusitis, 2778

Allergic rhinitis (AR) *(Continued)*
severity of, 618
symptoms of, 617
treatment of, 619-622
anticholinergics in, 620
antihistamines in, 620
anti-IgE in, 622
avoidance in, 619-620
combination, 622
cromolyn sodium in, 620
decongestants in, 620
for eye symptoms, 622
general planning for, 622-623
immunotherapy in, 621-622
novel extracts in, 622
subcutaneous, 621
sublingual, 621-622
intranasal steroids in, 621
leukotriene modifiers in, 620-621
systemic glucocorticosteroids in, 621
Allergic rhinoconjunctivitis, 622
Allergic rhinosinusitis, imaging of, 675
"Allergic salute," 618
Allergy
and otitis media, 2764-2766
preoperative evaluation of, 102
and rhinosinusitis, 731
chronic, 706-707, 706f
pediatric, 2778
Allocation bias, *vs.* efficacy of treatment, 62t
AlloDerm Regenerative Tissue Matrix (Cymetra)
for nasal reconstruction, 368
for tympanoplasty, 2000
for vocal fold medialization
history of, 905
by injection, 905-906
complications of, 907
laryngoscopic, 906-907
percutaneous, 906
Allograft(s)
for craniofacial defect repair, 2657
for ossiculoplasty, 2006
Allograft transplantation, 1098
Alloplastic grafting materials, for nasal skeletal reconstruction, 368
Alloplastic implants, in noncaucasian rhinoplasty, 569-570, 570f
complications of, 578, 578f-579f
Allopurinol, and skin flap viability, 1074
Almond oil, for cerumen removal, 1958t
Alopecia. *See also* Hair loss.
androgenetic, 374-376, 375f
areata, 376
scarring, 375-376
Alpha error, 65, 66t
Alpha particles, 1031-1032
5-Alpha reductase, in hair loss, 375, 375f
5-Alpha reductase inhibitor, for hair loss, 377-378
α- and β-blocker, intraoperative, 112
α-adrenergic blocking agents, and skin flap viability, 1073
α-amylase, in saliva, 1139-1141
α-defensins, 599
α/β ratio, for radiation therapy, 1038-1039
Alpha-hydroxy acids, for aging skin, 404
Alport syndrome (AS), sensorineural hearing loss in, 2051t-2058t, 2094t, 2096-2097
adult-onset, 2118
ALS (amyotrophic lateral sclerosis), laryngeal hypofunction due to, 842
Alternaria spp, rhinosinusitis due to, 705, 732-733
Alternate cover test, 2312-2313
Alternative medicine, for rhinosinusitis, 731, 735t
Alternobaric vertigo, 2343
Aluminum acetate otic drops (Burow's solution), 1959t-1960t
for fungal otitis externa, 1954
Alveolar canal, of mandible, 1319-1320
Alveolar cyst of newborn, 1266, 1266f
microscopic features of, 1266
treatment of, 1266
Alveolar hypoventilation, central, 262t
Alveolar process, of mandible, 1319, 1320f
Alveolar ridge
anatomy of, 1297-1298
squamous cell carcinoma of, 1304-1305
clinical presentation of, 1304, 1304f
epidemiology of, 1304
mandibulectomy for, 1304, 1304f-1305f, 1307f
maxillary, 1304
neck dissection for, 1304
survival with, 1304-1305
Alveolar soft part sarcoma, of neck, 1668
Alveolar ventilation, in newborns, 2570
Alveolus, 998
Alzheimer's disease
olfactory dysfunction in, 635
oral manifestations of, 1254-1255
AMA(s) (antimicrosomal antibodies), 1740-1741
AMA (American Medical Association), 84t-87t
Amalgam tattoo, 1243
clinical features of, 1243, 1243f
defined, 1243
differential diagnosis of, 1243
etiology of, 1243
histopathologic features of, 1243, 1243f
treatment of, 1243
Ambient stimulation, for tinnitus, 2133-2134
Ambulatory Care Quality Alliance (AQA), 84t-87t, 87-88
Ameloblastic carcinoma, 1274
Ameloblastic fibroma, 1274-1275
microscopic findings in, 1274-1275, 1275f
radiographic features of, 1274
treatment of, 1275
Ameloblastic fibro-odontoma, 1275
microscopic findings in, 1275, 1275f
radiographic findings in, 1275
treatment of, 1275
Ameloblastoma
intraosseous type, 1273-1274
defined, 1273
mandibular, 1274
maxillary, 1274
microscopic features of, 1273, 1273f
natural history and treatment of, 1273-1274
radiographic findings in, 1273, 1273f
malignant, 1274-1275
odonto-, 1278
of oral cavity, 1291, 1291f
peripheral (extraosseous), 1274
unicystic, 1271-1272
definitions, clarifications, and treatment for, 1272, 1272f
microscopic features of, 1271, 1271f
vs. multicystic or multilocular, 1272
radiographic features of, 1271
"simple," 1272
American Board of Medical Specialties (ABMS), 80, 84t-87t
core competencies of, 80, 80b
American Board of Otolaryngology (ABOto), 80b, 84t-87t
American College of Surgeons (ACS), 84t-87t
American Medical Association (AMA), 84t-87t
America's Health Insurance Plans (AHIP), 84t-87t
AMES classification, of thyroid cancer, 1754, 1756t
Ames waltzer mouse, deafness in, 2074
AMI (auditory midbrain implant), penetrating, 2262-2263, 2263f
Amifostine, for xerostomia, 1103
Amino acid taste, transduction of, 1209
Aminoglycoside ototoxicity, 1953-1954, 2169
clinical manifestations of, 2170
delayed, 2170
histopathology of, 2170
mechanisms of, 2170-2171
monitoring for, 2170
in noise-induced hearing loss, 2147
pharmacokinetics of, 2169-2170
risk factors for, 2170
sensorineural hearing loss due to, 2119-2120, 2170
with topical preparations, 2119-2120
susceptibility to, 2097, 2170
vertigo due to, 2201, 2310t
vestibular, 2170
5-Aminolevulinic acid (5-ALA)-induced fluorescence, for premalignant lesions of larynx, 1488-1489
Amiodarone (Cordarone)
dizziness due to, 2310t
thyrotoxicosis due to, 1744
Amitriptyline, for neuropathic pain, 244, 245t
Amoxicillin
for endocarditis prophylaxis, 1249t
for otitis media with effusion, 2771-2772
for pediatric surgery prophylaxis, 2597t
Amoxicillin-clavulanate
for acute otitis media, 2770
for pediatric chronic sinusitis, 2779
for rhinosinusitis, 734t
AMP(s). *See* Antimicrobial peptides (AMPs).
Amphotericin B, for rhinosinusitis, 735-736, 735t
fungal, 712, 713t
nonallergic eosinophilic, 714t
Ampicillin
for adenotonsillectomy, 2797
for endocarditis prophylaxis, 1249t
for pediatric surgery prophylaxis, 2597t
Amplitude
of sound waves, 1838-1839, 1839f
of vibration, laryngeal videostroboscopy of, 820, 821f, 848, 848t
Ampullae, of semicircular ducts
anatomy of, 1851f, 1853f, 1854
embryogenesis of, 1852
in vestibular sensation, 2277
Ampullofugal rotation, of endolymph, 2289
Ampullopetal rotation, of endolymph, 2289
Amputation neuromas, due to neck surgery, 1731-1732
Amylase, in saliva, 1139-1141
Amyloidosis
esophageal manifestations of, 979
laryngeal and tracheal manifestations of, 891, 891f
of oral cavity, 1289-1290, 1290f
Amyotrophic lateral sclerosis (ALS), laryngeal hypofunction due to, 842
AN. *See* Auditory neuropathy (AN).
Anagen phase, 374, 374f
Analgesia
patient-controlled, 240, 241t
preemptive, 241
Analgesic ladder, 242-243
Analgesics
adjuvant, 243-244
anticonvulsant agents as, 243-244, 244t
antidepressants as, 244-245, 245t
for cancer pain, 1103
oral sequelae of, 1247t-1248t
ototoxicity of, 2175-2176
hydrocodone as, 2175
salicylates as, 2175-2176
Analog hearing aids, 2267
Analog stimulation, for cochlear implants, 2230, 2230f

Analysis of variance (ANOVA), 71
Anaphylactic reaction, tension pneumothorax *vs.*, 119
Anaphylaxis, preoperative evaluation of, 102
Anaplastic thyroid carcinoma, 1764
  clinical presentation of, 1764
  management and prognosis for, 1764
  pathology of, 1764
Anatomic landmarks and reference points, in facial analysis, 269
  cephalometric, 270b, 272f
  Frankfort horizontal plane as, 269, 272f
  soft tissue, 270b, 271f
ANCAs (antineutrophil cytoplasmic antibodies), in Wegener's granulomatosis, 658, 2103
Androgen metabolic pathway, within skin, 375, 375f
Androgenetic alopecia (AGA), 374-376, 375f
Androgenic factors, in hair loss, 375, 375f
Anechoic tissue, 1643
Anemia
  Fanconi's, tumor suppressor gene in, 1020
  oral manifestations of, 1256
  and radiotherapy, 1041
Anesthesia
  adjuncts to
    antihypertensives as, 112
    paralytic agents as, 111-112
  for anterior and middle cranial base surgery, 2447-2448
  for arytenoid adduction, 914-915
  in children, 2575, 2587-2601
    for adenotonsillectomy, 2598-2599, 2599b
    for airway and esophageal foreign body removal, 2940
    emergence from, 2592-2593
    induction of, 2589-2591
      inhalation, 2590
      intramuscular, 2591
      intravenous, 2590
      parental presence during, 2590
      rapid-sequence, 2590
    intraoperative monitoring standards for, 2588, 2588b
    for laryngeal surgery, 2599-2600
    maintenance of, 2591-2592
      inhalational agents for, 2591
      intravenous agents for, 2591, 2593t
    medical condition(s) affecting, 2594-2597
      asthma as, 2595
      congenital heart disease as, 2596-2597, 2596t-2597t
      cystic fibrosis as, 2595
      diabetes mellitus as, 2596
      prematurity as, 2595
      upper respiratory infection as, 2594-2595
    outside of operating room, 2594
    postoperative management of, 2593-2594
      for nausea and vomiting, 2593
      for pain, 2594
      for postintubation croup, 2593
    preoperative assessment for, 2588
    preparation for, 2588-2589
      behavioral, 2588-2589, 2589t
      nothing-by-mouth orders in, 2589, 2590t
      premedication in, 2589
    for rigid bronchoscopy, 2597-2598, 2597t
    risks of, 2587-2588
  and cranial nerve monitoring, 2544
  for endoscopic sinus surgery, 744-745
    general, 745
    local, 744-745
  for facial trauma, 304
  fasting prior to, 112
  induction of
    agents for, 111
    in children, 2589-2591
Anesthesia *(Continued)*
      inhalation, 2590
      intramuscular, 2591
      intravenous, 2590
      parental presence during, 2590
      rapid-sequence, 2590
    sedatives and opioid as adjuncts to, 111
    standard *vs.* rapid-sequence, 112-113, 113f
  for laryngotracheobronchoscopy, 2902
  for laser surgery, 36-37
  local, 112
    oral sequelae of, 1247t-1248t
  for parathyroidectomy, 1790
  perioperative regional, for postoperative pain control, 241-242
  with recurrent respiratory papillomatosis, 2891
    intermittent apnea-reintubation, 2891
    jet ventilation, 2891
    spontaneous ventilation, 2891
    wrapped or "laser-safe" endotracheal tube, 2891
  for rhinoplasty, 515-519, 518f
    and surgical planes, 516-517, 516f-517f
  routine, 110-111
  for small fenestra stapedotomy, 2030
  topical
    for awake fiberoptic nasotracheal intubation, 124
    for tracheobronchial endoscopy, 1000
  with tracheal neoplasms, 1617
  for tympanoplasty, 2001
  volatile agents for, 111
Anesthesia Fiberoptic Cart, 116
Anesthetics
  local, 112
    oral sequelae of, 1247t-1248t
  topical
    for awake fiberoptic nasotracheal intubation, 124
    for tracheobronchial endoscopy, 1000
Aneuploidy(ies), 4-5
  in thyroid carcinoma, 1752
Aneurysm(s), carotid artery
  of petrous apex, 2525, 2527f
  upper cervical and petrous, 2504, 2504f-2505f
"Angel's kiss," 290-291
Angiitis, allergic granulomatous, nasal manifestations of, 659
Angina
  Ludwig's
    airway establishment for, 188
    due to mandibular space infections, 184, 185f
  Vincent's, 2786
Angiofibroma, 292
  epistaxis due to, 686f
  juvenile
    endovascular treatment of, 1937-1938, 1943f
    nasopharyngeal, 152, 154f, 1349-1351
      clinical features of, 1349
      diagnosis of, 1349-1350, 1350f
      growth patterns of, 1349
      management of, 1350-1351
      pathologic features of, 1349
      recurrence of, 1351
      staging of, 1350, 1350t
    sinonasal, 721-722
      classification systems for, 722
      endoscopic appearance of, 721, 721f
      imaging of, 721
      natural history of, 721
      origin of, 721, 721f
      postoperative surveillance for, 722
      preoperative embolization for, 721-722
      surgical approach for, 718t, 722, 722f-723f, 763
      transnasal endoscopic-assisted surgery for, 2483, 2483f
Angiogenesis
  in acutely raised skin flaps, 1069, 1069f
  in formation of granulation tissue, 1077-1078
Angiography
  prior to anterior and middle cranial base surgery, 2444-2445
  of anterior skull base, 2475
  catheters for, 1932-1933
  computed tomography
    of anterior skull base, 2475, 2475f
    of neck masses, 1637, 1637t
  equipment for, 1932
  of glomus jugulare/vagale tumor, 1935f
  magnetic resonance, 137
    of anterior skull base, 2475
    of neck masses, 1637, 1637t
    of petrous apicitis, 1989f
  of multiple chemodectomas, 1935f
  of neck masses, 1637, 1637t
  of paranasal sinus tumors, 1124
  for penetrating neck trauma, 1630-1632, 1631t, 1632f-1633f
Angiokeratoma corporis diffusum universale, oral manifestations of, 1257
Angioma(s)
  cherry (senile), 290-291
  spider, 291
  strawberry, 290
  tufted, 2824-2825
    Kasabach-Merritt phenomenon with, 2825
Angiopathy, diabetic, presbycusis due to, 232
Angiosarcoma, of neck, 1668
Angiosomes, 1064
  in acutely raised skin flaps, 1069, 1069f
Angular cheilitis, 1230, 1230f
  in HIV, 225, 226f
Angular gyrus, in central auditory pathway, 1837
Angular vestibuloocular reflex (aVOR), 2306, 2307f
  after labyrinthectomy, 2291-2292, 2291f-2293f
Ankle strategy, 2308
Ankylosis, of temporomandibular joint, 1281t, 1282
Ann Arbor staging system, for lymphoma, 1676, 1677t
Annular ligament, of stylomastoid foramen, 1826f
Annulus of Zinn, 440
Anosmia, 633
  congenital, 636
  specific, 636
Anotia, 2742
ANOVA (analysis of variance), 71
Ansa cervicalis
  anatomy of, 2579f-2580f, 2581
  characteristics of, 918-919
  in neuromuscular pedicle procedure, 920, 921f
Ansa cervicalis–recurrent laryngeal nerve anastomosis, for laryngeal reinnervation, 922-923
  advantages of, 922
  clinical results of, 923
  disadvantage of, 922
  history of, 917-918
  surgical indications and contraindications for, 922
  surgical technique for, 922-923, 923f
Ansa hypoglossi nerve, for facial nerve paralysis, 2426-2427
Antacids
  for extraesophageal reflux, 901
  for GERD, 970
Anterior ampullary nerve, 1854f, 2278f
Anterior cerebral artery, 2351f
Anterior cervical lymph nodes, 2582
Anterior cervical space, imaging of, 158, 160f, 162f
Anterior cervical trauma, laryngeal injury due to, 933-934, 934f

Anterior clinoid process
in surgical anatomy of anterior cranial base, 2442-2443, 2443f, 2472f
in surgical anatomy of lateral skull base, 2435f
Anterior commissure
anatomy of, 1486
laryngeal carcinoma of, 1486
anatomic basis for, 1486
imaging of, 161, 1474, 1474f
treatment of, 1496-1497, 1523
transoral laser microsurgery for, 1531
Anterior commissure tendon, surgical anatomy of, 1541-1542
Anterior communicating artery, 2351f
Anterior compartment lymph nodes, in neck dissection, 1704, 1704f, 1706t
Anterior cranial base
anatomy of, 1697
boundaries of, 2442, 2443f
anterior, 2442, 2443f
superior, 2442-2443, 2443f
surgical anatomy of, 741, 2442-2444
craniofacial junction in, 2442, 2443f
extracranial structures related to, 2443, 2444f
and surgical landmarks of orbital skeleton, 2443-2444, 2444f
for transnasal endoscopic-assisted surgery, 2471-2475
anterior cranial fossa in, 2471, 2472f
clivus in, 2474, 2474f
nasal cavity in, 2471-2473, 2472f-2473f
nasopharynx in, 2474
paranasal sinuses in, 2473-2474, 2473f
retroclival region in, 2474-2475, 2474f-2475f
Anterior cranial base irradiation, 1697-1699
Anterior cranial base surgery
anesthesia for, 2447-2448
bicoronal incision in, 2450-2451, 2450f
complications of, 2468-2469, 2469t
electrophysiologic monitoring during, 2450
flap elevation in, 2450-2451, 2451f
goals of, 2448, 2448b
intraoperative imaging during, 2449
operative approaches for, 2450-2454
anterior craniofacial resection as, 2451-2453, 2452f-2453f
basal subfrontal, 2453-2454, 2454f
endoscopic, 2448-2450
functional and aesthetic considerations in choice of, 2450
general considerations with, 2448-2450
image-guided computer-assisted, 2448-2449, 2449f
overview of, 2448
planning of, 2448-2450
robotic, 2450
subcranial, 2454, 2454f
outcomes of, 2469-2470
pathology and management planning for, 2446-2447, 2447b
postoperative care after, 2468
preoperative embolization for, 2446
preoperative evaluation for, 2444-2448
angiography in, 2444-2445
of cerebral blood flow, 2445-2446, 2446f
other evaluations in, 2446-2447
reconstruction after, 2467-2468
transnasal endoscopic-assisted, 2471-2486
anesthesia for, 2476
combined approaches for, 2484
complications of, 2485
craniocervical junction–odontoid approach for, 2483-2484, 2484f
instrumentation for, 2476
patient preparation for, 2475-2476
pedicled septal flap in, 2476-2477
postoperative care after, 2484-2485
Anterior cranial base surgery *(Continued)*
preoperative assessment for, 2475, 2475f
reconstruction after, 2484
surgical anatomy for, 2471-2475
anterior cranial fossa in, 2471, 2472f
clivus in, 2474, 2474f
nasal cavity in, 2471-2473, 2472f-2473f
nasopharynx in, 2474
paranasal sinuses in, 2473-2474, 2473f
retroclival region in, 2474-2475, 2474f-2475f
surgical team setup for, 2476f
transcribriform approach for, 2482
with bilateral access, 2482, 2482f
with unilateral access, 2482
transmaxillary-transpterygoidal-infratemporal approach for, 2482-2483, 2483f
transsellar and parasellar approaches for, 2479, 2480f
transsphenoidal approach for, 2477-2481
with direct transnasal access, 2477, 2477f
with petrous apex access, 2481
with transclival approach, 2479-2481, 2480f-2481f
with transethmoidal access, 2478-2479, 2479f-2480f
with transseptal access, 2477-2478, 2477f-2478f
with transseptal-transnasal access, 2478, 2479f
transtuberculum-transplanum approach for, 2482
Anterior cranial base tumors
benign, 2446, 2447b
fibrous dysplasia as, 2647f
malignant, 1697-1699, 2446, 2447b
esthesioneuroblastoma as, 1697-1698, 1698f, 1698t
sinonasal undifferentiated carcinoma as, 1698-1699
preoperative planning for, 2446-2447
Anterior cranial fossa
in surgical anatomy of anterior skull base, 2471, 2472f
in surgical anatomy of lateral skull base, 2435f
Anterior cranial fossa floor, in surgical anatomy of anterior cranial base, 2442-2443, 2443f-2444f
Anterior craniofacial resection, 2451-2453, 2452f-2453f
Anterior cricoid split operation, 2910f, 2918-2919, 2918f-2919f
Anterior cutaneous nerve, anatomy of, 2578, 2580f
Anterior disk displacement, of temporomandibular joint
with reduction, 1280, 1282f
without reduction, 1279-1280, 1282f
Anterior ethmoidal air cells, in frontal sinusitis, 776
Anterior ethmoidal artery
anatomy of, 682, 684f, 1124f
bleeding from, 690-691, 691f-692f
prior to endoscopic sinus surgery, 764, 765f
septal branch of, 483f
in surgical anatomy of anterior cranial base, 2471-2473, 2472f
Anterior ethmoidal foramen, 322f, 439
Anterior ethmoidal nerve, 483f
external branch of, 497, 497f
Anterior ethmoidectomy, in endoscopic sinus surgery, 747, 748f
Anterior fontanelle, 2618f
Anterior glottic gap, laryngeal videostroboscopy of, 819, 820f
Anterior glottic web, 2869, 2869f
stridor due to, 2899, 2900f
and velocardiofacial syndrome, 2899, 2900f, 2913
Anterior inferior cerebellar artery (AICA)
anatomy of, 1856f, 2351f
surgical, 2403-2404, 2404f
in posterior fossa surgery, 2540
in surgical anatomy of anterior skull base, 2481f
in surgical anatomy of lateral skull base, 2437f, 2439f
Anterior inferior cerebellar artery (AICA) occlusion, sensorineural hearing loss due to, 2123
Anterior lacrimal crest, 439
Anterior lamella, of eyelid, 442-443, 443f
Anterior laryngeal wall stenosis, 951
Anterior laryngofissure, with posterior cricoid division, for laryngeal stenosis, 2919, 2919f
Anterior mallear fold, anatomy of, 1825f
Anterior malleolar fold, anatomy of, 1827f
Anterior malleolar ligament, anatomy of, 1827f
Anterior meningoencephaloceles, surgical management of, 742
Anterior nasal aperture, 320f
Anterior nasal depth, 2617t
Anterior nasal spine, 320f, 509f
Anterior neck dissection, 1719
defined, 1719, 1719f
technique for, 1719, 1720f
Anterior neuropore, congenital malformations of nose due to developmental errors of, 2686-2690, 2687f
Anterior ostiomeatal channels, 666f
Anterior ostiomeatal unit, 664, 665f
Anterior palatal artery, 483f
Anterior partial laryngectomy, for glottic cancer, 1517t
Anterior petrous apex (APA), 1975-1976, 1976f
pneumatic, 1976, 1977f
Anterior rhinoscopy, 100, 484
Anterior scalene muscle, anatomy of, 2579f
Anterior scalp flap, 2450-2451
Anterior semicircular duct, anatomy of, 1851f
Anterior septal angle, 509f
Anterior skull base. *See* Anterior cranial base.
Anterior spinal artery, 2351f
Anterior spiral vein, 1856f
Anterior tonsillar pillar, 1297-1298
Anterior tracheal wall stenosis, 951
Anterior transhyoid pharyngotomy, for hypopharyngeal cancer, 1427-1429, 1428f
Anterior triangle, of neck, 96, 96f, 2578f, 2579-2581
ansa cervicalis in, 2580f, 2581
carotid triangle in, 2578f, 2579-2580, 2580f
Anterior triangle dissection, 1709-1710
Anterior tympanic artery, 1828f
Anterior vestibular artery, 1854, 1856f
Anterior visceral space, anatomy of, 203
Anterolateral fontanelle, 2618f
Anterolateral thigh flap, 1082t, 1083
for hypopharyngeal and esophageal reconstruction, 1455
for oropharyngeal reconstruction, 1379
of tongue base, 1390-1391
of tonsils and pharyngeal wall, 1386
Anthropometry, 269
Antiaging products, 403
Antiangiogenesis, in gene therapy, 22
Antiangiogenic compounds, for head and neck squamous cell carcinoma, 1060
Antiarrhythmics, oral sequelae of, 1247t-1248t
Antiarthritics, oral sequelae of, 1247t-1248t
Antibacterial activity, of saliva, 1141
Antibiotic(s)
for deep neck space infections, 205-206, 206t
for odontogenic infections, 178, 188
oral sequelae of, 1247t-1248t
for otitis media
acute, 2770
with effusion, 2771-2772

Antibiotic(s) *(Continued)*
ototopical, 1959t-1960t
for acute bacterial otitis externa, 1951-1953
evidence-based data on, 1952
hypersensitivity reaction to, 1954
mechanism of action of, 1951
ototoxicity of, 1953-1954
resistance to, 1953
for pediatric chronic sinusitis, 2779
for rhinosinusitis, 733-735
intravenous, 733-734, 735t
issues with, 736
long-term macrolide, 733, 734t
oral, 733
short-term, 734t
topical, 734-735, 735t
for stridulous child, 2906
for vocal professionals, 855
Antibiotic prophylaxis
for acute otitis media, 2771
for burns, 315
for orthopedic joint patients, 1253, 1253t
for sinus surgery, 743, 773
for temporal bone fractures, 2044-2045
Antibody-dependent cellular cytotoxicity (ADCC), 603-604, 606
Antibody-mediated hypersensitivity reactions, 608-612
Anticholinergics
for allergic rhinitis, 620
for nonallergic rhinitis, 701
Anticoagulants
dizziness due to, 2310t
oral sequelae of, 1247t-1248t, 1248, 1250
preoperative evaluation of, 105
Anticonvulsants
for chronic pain, 243-244, 244t
dizziness due to, 2310t
oral sequelae of, 1247t-1248t
Antidepressants
for chronic pain, 244-245, 245t
for migraine, 2350
in palliative care, 1104
for tinnitus, 2137
Antidiarrheal agents, oral sequelae of, 1247t-1248t
Antidromic potentials, to assess facial nerve function, 2388
Antiemetics, for postoperative nausea and vomiting, in children, 2593
Antiepileptics
for chronic pain, 243-244, 244t
dizziness due to, 2310t
oral sequelae of, 1247t-1248t
Antifungal agents
for rhinosinusitis
nonallergic eosinophilic fungal, 715-716
systemic, 735, 735t
topical, 735-736, 735t
topical, 1959t-1960t
for fungal otitis externa, 1954-1955
ototoxicity of, 1955
for rhinosinusitis, 735-736, 735t
Antigen presentation, 602f, 606, 606f
Antigen-presenting cells (APCs), 602f, 606, 606f
Antihelix, of ear, 476-477, 476f, 1824f, 2742f
Antihistamines
oral sequelae of, 1247t-1248t
for otitis media
acute, 2770
with effusion, 2771
for rhinitis
allergic, 620
nonallergic, 700-701, 701t
for rhinosinusitis, 734t, 737
for vocal professionals, 854
Antihypertensives
dizziness due to, 2310t
intraoperative, 112
oral sequelae of, 1247t-1248t, 1248
Anti–immunoglobulin E (anti-IgE)
for allergic rhinitis, 622
for rhinosinusitis, 735t, 737
Anti-inflammatory medications
oral sequelae of, 1247t-1248t
ototopical
classes of, 1956, 1956t
for eczematoid otitis externa, 1956-1957
hypersensitivity reaction to, 1954
mechanism of action of, 1951
ototoxicity of, 1956
Antilipidemics, oral sequelae of, 1247t-1248t
Antimalarials, sensorineural hearing loss due to, 2120
Antimicrobial peptides (AMPs), 598-599
cathelicidins as, 599
defensins as, 599
tissue distribution of, 599
Antimicrobial substances, in saliva, 1140
Antimicrosomal antibodies (AMAs), 1740-1741
Antimycotics, oral sequelae of, 1247t-1248t
Antineoplastic agent(s)
oral sequelae of, 1247t-1248t
ototoxicity of, 2171-2174
carboplatin as, 2173-2174
cisplatin as, 2171-2173
clinical studies on, 2171-2172
delayed, 2171-2172
experimental studies on, 2172
genetic predisposition to, 2172
histopathology of, 2172
mechanics of, 2172-2173
pharmacokinetics of, 2171
risk factors for, 2172
vestibular, 2172
difluoromethylornithine as, 2174
animal studies on, 2174
clinical studies on, 2174
conclusions on, 2174
Antineutrophil cytoplasmic antibodies (ANCAs), in Wegener's granulomatosis, 658, 2103
Antioxidants
for cisplatin ototoxicity, 2173
for noise-induced hearing loss, 2145
oral sequelae of, 1247t-1248t
Anti-Parkinsonian medications, oral sequelae of, 1247t-1248t
Antiphospholipid antibody syndrome, inner ear disease in, 2166
Antiproliferatives, oral sequelae of, 1247t-1248t
Antipyretics, oral sequelae of, 1247t-1248t
Antireflux agents
for extraesophageal reflux in children, 2946
oral sequelae of, 1247t-1248t
for recurrent respiratory papillomatosis, 2893
for rhinosinusitis, 735t, 737
Antireflux surgery, for GERD, 970
Antiretroviral therapy, highly active, 211
Antiseptics, ototopical, 1959t-1960t
for fungal otitis externa, 1955
Antithyroglobulin antibodies (ATAs), 1740
Antithyroid agents, 1739, 1739t
adverse reactions to, 1742
for Graves' disease, 1742
for Graves' ophthalmopathy, 1810
oral sequelae of, 1247t-1248t
for thyroid storm, 1745
Antithyroid antibodies, 1740-1741
Anti-thyroperoxidase (anti-TPO), 1740
Antitragus, 476-477, 476f, 1824f, 2742f
Antitumoral immune response, direct in vivo stimulation of, 21
Antiviral agents
for Bell's palsy, 2395
for rhinosinusitis, 731, 734t
Antrostomy, in endoscopic sinus surgery, 747, 747f
failure of, 764-766, 766f
Antrum, in mastoidectomy, 2011-2012
Anxiety
palliative care for, 1103-1104
professional voice disorders due to, 853
Anxiolytics, oral sequelae of, 1247t-1248t
AOM. *See* Acute otitis media (AOM).
AP (action potential), in electrocochleography, 1892-1894, 1907
in Meniere's disease, 2337
APA (anterior petrous apex), 1975-1976, 1976f
pneumatic, 1976, 1977f
APCs (antigen-presenting cells), 602f, 606, 606f
Apert's syndrome, craniofacial anomalies in, 2641t, 2645-2646
APHAB (Abbreviated Profile of Hearing Aid Benefit), 57
Aphthous stomatitis, 1289, 1289f
in HIV, 227, 227f
recurrent, 1236-1239
clinical features of, 1237-1238
defined, 1236-1237
differential diagnosis of, 1238, 1238t
etiology and pathogenesis of, 1237, 1237t
herpetiform-type, 1238, 1238f
histopathologic features of, 1239
major, 1237-1238, 1238f
minor, 1237, 1238f
treatment of, 1239
Apnea
defined, 251b
obstructive
in children, 2607
sleep (*See* Obstructive sleep apnea (OSA))
Apnea index (AI), 251b, 252
Apnea technique, for pediatric anesthesia, 2600
Apnea-hypopnea index (AHI), 251, 251b
Apoptosis, in ototoxicity, 2171
prevention of, 2189-2190
Appearance
physical examination of, 95
in voice evaluation, 827
Appendix, laryngeal, 876
Apple green birefringence, with amyloidosis, 1289-1290
Apron incision, for neck dissection
radical, 1709, 1710f
selective
of oral cavity, 1714, 1716f
of oropharynx, hypopharynx, and larynx, 1717-1718, 1717f
AQA (Ambulatory Care Quality Alliance), 84t-87t, 87-88
AR. *See* Acute rhinosinusitis (AR, ARS).
AR (allergic rhinitis). *See* Allergic rhinitis (AR).
Ar (argon) laser, 30, 31t
Ar (argon) plasma coagulation, interventional bronchoscopy with, 1010t
Ar (argon) tunable dye laser, 30, 31t
Arachidonic acid metabolism, in rhinosinusitis, 731-732, 732f
Arachis oil
almond oil, rectified camphor oil (Otocerol, Earex), for cerumen removal, 1958t
chlorbutol, paradicholorobenzene, oil of turpentine (Cerumol), for cerumen removal, 1958t
Arachnoid cysts, of cerebellopontine angle, 2523-2524
vs. cholesteatoma, 2519, 2521f
imaging of, 1928, 1929t
Arcanobacterium haemolyticum, pharyngitis due to, 193

Arch bars, in maxillofacial fracture repair, 333, 333f, 337
Arch of Corti, 1840
ARCON treatment, with radiotherapy, 1041
Arcuate eminence
anatomy of, 1822, 1822f
in surgical anatomy of lateral skull base, 2436f, 2437
Arcuate fasciculus, in central auditory pathway, 1837
Area ratio, in auditory physiology, 1839-1840, 1840f, 2018-2019
L-Arginine, and skin flap viability, 1074
Argon (Ar) laser, 30, 31t
Argon (Ar) plasma coagulation, interventional bronchoscopy with, 1010t
Argon (Ar) tunable dye laser, 30, 31t
Arhinia, 2690, 2691f
Aromatase, in hair loss, 375, 375f
ARS (acute retroviral syndrome), 197
ARS (acute rhinosinusitis). *See* Acute rhinosinusitis (AR, ARS).
Arterial compression, of trachea, 2925-2926
Arterial cutaneous flaps, 1067, 1067f
Arterial embolization
for epistaxis, 690, 691f
for vascular repair, 1633
Arterial oxygen tension (Pao_2), in children, 2570, 2571t
Arteriography
cross-compression carotid, for cerebral blood flow evaluation, 2490
four-vessel, prior to lateral cranial base surgery, 2489-2490, 2491f
of neck masses, 1637, 1637t
parathyroid, 1788
for penetrating neck trauma, 1630-1632, 1631t, 1632f-1633f
Arteriovenous fistulas, embolization of
dural, 1940-1942, 1940f
facial, 1940, 1940f
Arteriovenous malformation (AVM), 2832, 2833f
embolization for, 1942, 1942f
of neck, 1662-1663
of salivary glands, 1172
Arthritis
infectious, of temporomandibular joint, 1281-1282, 1281t
osteo- (degenerative)
oral manifestations of, 1253
of temporomandibular joint, 1281-1282, 1281t
rheumatoid
laryngeal and tracheal manifestations of, 891, 891f
oral manifestations of, 1253, 1253t
of temporomandibular joint, 1281t, 1282
Arthrocentesis, of temporomandibular joint, 1283
Arthroscopy, of temporomandibular joint, 1283
Arthrotomy, of temporomandibular joint, 1283
Articular disk, of temporomandibular joint, 1279-1280
Articular tubercle, 2010f
Articulation
in speech, 810-812, 833
speech therapy for, with velopharyngeal dysfunction, 2681
Artifacts
in auditory brainstem response recording, 2552-2553
in electromyography, 2547-2548, 2548f
on MRI, 133-134, 134f
Artificial larynx. *See* Voice prosthesis(es).
Aryepiglottic folds
anatomy of, 1422
radiographic, 1398f-1399f, 1463f, 1471, 1471f
carcinoma of
imaging of, 1475, 1478f
supraglottic laryngectomy for, 1554-1555
Aryepiglottic muscle, 1542f-1543f
Aryepiglottoplasty, for laryngomalacia, 2867, 2868f
Arytenoid abduction, for bilateral paralysis, 916
Arytenoid adduction, 912-916
anesthesia for, 914-915
cricoarytenoid joint in, 913
cricoarytenoid muscle in, 913, 914f
future directions in, 916
for long-standing laryngeal paralysis, 914
membranous vocal fold in, 914
overview of, 912, 913f
postoperative care after, 916
surgical procedure for, 915-916, 915f-916f
vs. thyroplasty, 912-913
vs. vocal fold injection, 912-913
vocal process in, 913-914, 913f-914f
Arytenoid cartilage
anatomy of, 805-806, 1422f
radiographic, 1399f, 1471, 1473f
surgical, 1541, 1542f
laryngeal carcinoma of, 1541
movement of, 805, 806f
videoendoscopy of, 816
Arytenoid involvement, supraglottic laryngectomy with, 1554-1555
Arytenoid muscle, 1543f
Arytenoidectomy
laser, 2909
for posterior glottic stenosis, 949, 949f
AS (Alport syndrome), sensorineural hearing loss in, 2051t-2058t, 2094t, 2096-2097
adult-onset, 2118
ASC (adenosquamous carcinoma)
of hypopharynx and cervical esophagus, 1425
of larynx, 1506
A-scale, 2140
ASCC (acantholytic squamous cell carcinoma), of larynx, 1506
Ascending cervical artery, in root of neck, 2581-2582, 2581f
Ascending pharyngeal artery, 2580f
Ascending "w," in nasal breathing assessment, 644
Ascertainment bias, *vs.* efficacy of treatment, 62t
Asian nose. *See* Noncaucasian rhinoplasty.
ASIMO, 38, 39f
Asimov, Isaac, 38
Aspergillus fumigatus
otitis externa and otitis media due to, immunosuppression and, 222-223
rhinosinusitis due to, 220-221, 220f
Aspergillus niger, otitis externa due to, 2195
Aspergillus spp
otitis externa due to, 1944-1945, 1945f
rhinosinusitis due to, 705, 710-711, 712f
chronic, 732-733
in immunocompromised host, 220-221, 220f
Aspiration
due to abnormal swallow, 1217 (*See also* Dysphagia)
chronic, 925-3
defined, 925
etiology of, 925, 926b
evaluation of, 926
nonsurgical management of, 926-927
surgical management of, 927-932
endolaryngeal stents for, 928, 930f
epiglottic flap closure of larynx for, 928, 930f
glottic closure for, 929-931, 931f
"ideal" procedure for, 927, 927b
laryngectomy for, 927, 928f
laryngotracheal separation for, 931-932, 931f
partial cricoidectomy for, 928
subperichondrial cricoidectomy for, 927-928, 929f
tracheoesophageal diversion for, 931-932, 931f-932f
vertical laryngoplasty for, 928-929, 930f
Aspiration *(Continued)*
symptoms of, 925-926
tracheotomy for, 927
vocal cord medialization for, 927
foreign body, 975-976, 2935-2943
acute obstruction due to, 2936-2937
complications of, 2942
epidemiology of, 2936
imaging of, 1411, 1412f, 2938-2939
vs. tonsillar calcifications, 1411, 1412f
interventional bronchoscopy for, 1008
location of, 2936, 2936f
management of, 2939-2941
anesthesia for, 2940
controversies in, 2942
equipment for, 2939-2940, 2939t, 2940f
history of, 2935
postoperative, 2941-2942
for sharp objects, 2940-2941
technique for, 2940, 2941f
stridor due to, 2898
symptoms of, 2937-2938
Aspiration pneumonia, 1250
Aspirin
for chemoprevention of oral cancer, 1315
after free tissue transfer, 1096
for head and neck squamous cell carcinoma, 1018
preoperative use of, 105
sensorineural hearing loss due to, 2120
for vocal professionals, 855
Aspirin desensitization therapy, for rhinosinusitis, 734t, 737
Aspirin sensitivity, in rhinosinusitis, 731-732, 732f
Aspirin-exacerbated respiratory disease (AERD), 731-732, 732f
Assistive listening devices (ALDs), 2270-2271
Association auditory cortex, 1847
Association of American Medical Colleges (AAMC), 84t-87t
ASSR (auditory steady-state response), 1911-1912
clinical applications of, 1910f, 1912
for cochlear implants in children, 2234-2235
Astelin (azelastine)
for allergic rhinitis, 620
for nonallergic rhinitis, 701t
for rhinosinusitis, 734t, 737
Asterion, 320f
Asthenia, in voice evaluation, 827t
Asthma
exercise-induced, in professional singers, 853
and GERD, 971
oral manifestations of, 1250
pediatric anesthesia with, 2595
ASV (automatic speaking valve), 1599-1600
A-T procedure, for forehead repair, 362, 363f
ATA(s) (antithyroglobulin antibodies), 1740
Ataxia
cerebellar, 2356-2357
familial episodic, 2357
Friedreich's, 2357
ATB. *See* Audiologic test battery (ATB).
Atelectasis, middle ear, 1964, 1964f-1965f
tympanoplasty with, 2003-2004
Athletes, rhinosinusitis in, 737
Atlantoaxial dislocation, 2355-2356
Atlantoaxial instability, 2355-2356
Atlantoaxial subluxation, due to adenotonsillectomy, 2801
Atlas, assimilation (occipitalization) of, 2355
Atmospheric barotrauma, 2343
Atoh1
in hair cell regeneration and repair, 2144
in murine deafness, 2058t-2060t
ATP (adenosine triphosphate)–magnesium chloride complex, and skin flap viability, 1074
ATP2B2, in deafness, 2051t-2058t, 2080
ATP6B1, in deafness, 2051t-2058t

ATPase-driven sodium-potassium (Na^+,K^+) pump, in salivary gland secretion, 1135
Atracurium, for pediatric anesthesia, 2593t
Atresiaplasty, 2754-2757
  alternatives to, 2759
  avoidance of complications of, 2758-2759
  candidacy for, 2753, 2753t
  contraindications to, 2754
  creation of split-thickness skin graft in, 2756, 2756f
  dissection of ossicular mass in, 2755-2756, 2756f
  drilling for new ear canal in, 2755-2756
  ear wick packing in, 2756-2757
  facial nerve in, 2754, 2755f, 2759
  harvesting of temporalis fascia in, 2755, 2755f
  meatoplasty in, 2756-2757
  outcomes of, 2754
  placement of split-thickness skin graft in, 2756, 2757f-2758f
  postauricular incision in, 2755, 2755f
  postoperative care after, 2757-2758
  preoperative evaluation and patient counseling for, 2754, 2754f-2755f
  reconstruction of ossicular chain in, 2756
  removal of atretic plate in, 2755-2756, 2755f
  Silastic strips in, 2756-2757, 2758f
  suturing in, 2756-2757, 2758f
  temporal fascia graft in, 2755f, 2756, 2757f
  timing of, 2754
Atrophic rhinitis, 696-697
Atropine, for premedication in children, 2589
Attention deficit–hyperactivity disorder (ADHD), sleep-disordered breathing and, 2791
Attenuation, 1032-1033
Atticotomy, in ossiculoplasty, 2007-2008
Atypical carcinoid (AC), of larynx, 1507
Atypical mole syndrome, 1107
Atypical neuralgia, *vs.* myofascial pain dysfunction syndrome, 1284t
Audax (choline salicylate and glycerol), for cerumen removal, 1958t
Audibility, threshold of, 1888
Audimax Theraband, for tinnitus, 2136-2137
Audiogram, 1888
  with acoustic neuroma, 1897, 1898f
  of cochlear implant map, 2255
  for dizziness, 2326
  of hearing loss
    conductive, 1888f
    mixed, 1889f
    sensorineural, 1906f
      high-frequency, 1889f, 1907f
  in Meniere's disease, 1894, 1895f
  for nasopharyngeal carcinoma, 1354
  with normal hearing, 1906f-1907f
  and otoacoustic emissions
    distortion product, 1905, 1907f
    transient evoked, 1905, 1906f
Audiologic test battery (ATB), 1887-1903
  for cochlear implantation
    in adults, 2223
    in children, 2225
  to evaluate functional hearing loss, 1901
  to evaluate middle ear function, 1890-1891, 1890f
  historical background of, 1887-1890
  masking in, 1889-1890
  neurodiagnostic studies for auditory neuropathy or dyssynchrony in, 1899-1901, 1900f
  objective tests for differential diagnosis in, 1891-1892
    auditory brainstem response as, 1896, 1896f
      neurodiagnosis with, 1896-1899, 1898f-1899f
    electrocochleography as, 1892-1896, 1894f-1895f
    otoacoustic emissions as, 1891-1892, 1892f-1893f
Audiologic test battery (ATB) *(Continued)*
  sources of error in, 1901-1902
    in clinical judgment, 1901, 1902f
    technical, 1901-1902
  speech testing in, 1888-1889
  test for hearing sensitivity or acuity in, 1888, 1888f
    pure-tone air-conduction testing as, 1888
      masking for, 1889-1890
    pure-tone bone-conduction testing as, 1888, 1888f-1889f
Audiology
  in children, 2574
  effects of radiotherapy on, 2626t
  in infants, 2722
Audiometric correlates
  of ossicular discontinuity, 2005-2006
  of ossicular fixation, 2006
Audiometric thresholds, 1888
  based on auditory brainstem responses
    click-evoked, 1909
    using more frequency-specific stimuli, 1909-1910, 1910f
  based on auditory steady-state response, 1912
Audiometry, 2087
  with acoustic neuroma, 1897, 1898f, 2516
  for otitis media, 2762
  for otosclerosis, 2030, 2030f
  pure-tone (*See* Pure-tone audiometry)
  for sensorineural hearing loss, 2117
  visual reinforcement
    in infants, 2722
    for otitis media, 2762
Auditory brainstem, 1845-1846
Auditory brainstem implant (ABI), 2258-2264
  alternative strategies to, 2263
  anatomy and surgical approaches for, 2260, 2261f
  auditory performance with, 2262
  biocompatibility of, 2259
  with cochlear nerve aplasia, 2263-2264
  complications of, 2260-2261
  history of clinical approaches to, 2259-2260, 2259f
  indications for, 2260
  intraoperative monitoring of, 2260, 2261f
  in patients without neurofibromatosis type 2, 2262
  penetrating, 2262, 2262f
Auditory brainstem response (ABR), 1896, 1908-1911, 2087
  with acoustic neuroma, 1896, 1898f-1899f, 1910-1911, 2517
  advantage of, 1908
  artifacts with, 2552-2553
  audiometric thresholds based on
    click-evoked, 1909
    using more frequency-specific stimuli, 1909-1910, 1910f
  with auditory neuropathy or dyssynchrony, 1899-1901, 1900f
  automated, 2721
  in Bell's palsy, 2393-2394
  with central neural auditory prosthesis, 2260, 2262f
  click-evoked, 1909
  clinical applications of, 1896, 1908-1911
    to assess hearing sensitivity, 1909-1910, 1910f
    in CHAMP procedure, 1911
    for differential diagnosis, 1910-1911
    for intraoperative monitoring, 1899f, 1911
    for neurodiagnosis, 1896-1899, 1898f-1899f
    otoneurologic, 1910-1911
  for cochlear implant, 1913f
    in children, 2225, 2234-2235
  defined, 1896, 1908
  effect of intensity on, 1908, 1909f
  electrically evoked, 1912-1913, 1913f
Auditory brainstem response (ABR) *(Continued)*
  electrocochleography and, 1908
  in infants, 2719-2721
  instrumentation for, 2543
  interpretation of, 1896
  intraoperative monitoring of, 2552-2554
    interpretation of, 2553-2554, 2553f
    and postoperative auditory function, 2553-2554
    reducing electrical and acoustic interference in, 2552-2553
    stimulus and recording parameters, electrodes, and placement in, 2552
  maturational changes in, 1908
  with normal hearing, 1896, 1896f, 1908, 1909f, 1913f
  for otitis media, 2762
  and otoacoustic emissions, 1891-1892, 1893f
  procedure for, 1896, 1908
  for sensorineural hearing loss, 2117
  speech-evoked, 1911
  stacked, 1911
  tone burst–evoked, 1909-1910
Auditory cortex, in central auditory pathway, 1835f-1836f, 1836-1837, 1847
Auditory distortion, with migraine, 2349
Auditory dyssynchrony (AD)
  cochlear implant for, 2220, 2240
  neurodiagnostic studies with, 1899-1901, 1900f
    otoacoustic emissions as, 1907
Auditory evoked potentials, middle and long latency, 1912, 1913f
Auditory meatus
  anatomy of, 1824f
  external, 320f
Auditory midbrain, 1845-1846
Auditory midbrain implant (AMI), penetrating, 2262-2263, 2263f
Auditory nerve
  anatomy of, 1825f, 1834
  in auditory physiology, 1844-1845, 1845f
  in central auditory pathway, 1835f
Auditory neural plasticity. *See* Neural plasticity, in otology.
Auditory neuropathy (AN)
  cochlear implant for, 2220, 2240
  genetic basis of, 2081
  neurodiagnostic studies with, 1899-1901, 1900f
    otoacoustic emissions as, 1907
Auditory pathway(s)
  afferent, 1834, 1834f
  central, 1834-1837, 1835f
    auditory cortex in, 1835f-1836f, 1836-1837
    cochlear nerve in, 1834-1835
    cochlear nucleus in, 1835, 1835f
    inferior colliculus in, 1835f, 1836
    lateral lemniscus in, 1835-1836, 1835f
    medial geniculate body in, 1835f, 1836
    superior olivary complex in, 1835, 1835f
  efferent, 1834, 1834f, 1847-1849
    middle ear muscle reflex pathways as, 1847, 1848f
    olivocochlear reflex pathways as, 1848-1849, 1848f
  neural plasticity in (*See* Neural plasticity, in otology)
Auditory perceptual assessment, of voice, 826-831
  CAPE-V for, 826
  GRBAS for, 826, 827t
  other aspects of, 826-827
  for professional voice, 850
Auditory performance, with cochlear implants
  in adults, 2244-2245
  bilateral, 2247-2251
  in children, 2246
    early studies of, 2246
    measurement of, 2246
    more recent studies of, 2246-2247, 2247f

Auditory performance, with cochlear implants *(Continued)*
factors related to measurement of, 2244-2247
with hearing preservation, 2245-2246
in infants, 2247
predictors of, 2245, 2245f
tests of, 2244
Auditory physiology, 1838-1849
auditory cortex in, 1847
auditory nerve in, 1844-1845, 1845f
cochlear nucleus in, 1845-1846, 1846f
efferent auditory system in, 1847-1849
middle ear muscle reflex pathways in, 1847, 1848f
olivocochlear reflex pathways in, 1848-1849, 1848f
external ear in, 1839
impedance in, 1839
inferior colliculus in, 1846
inner ear in, 1840-1844
basilar membrane of, 1840-1842, 1841f-1842f
cochlea of, 1840, 1841f-1842f
cochlear partition of, 1840-1842, 1842f
endocochlear potential in, 1840, 1841f-1842f
endolymph of, 1841f-1842f
hair cells of
inner, 1841f, 1842, 1844f
outer, 1841f, 1844, 1844f
stereocilia of, 1841f, 1842, 1843f
tip links of, 1841f, 1842, 1843f
tonotopic tuning of, 1844, 1844f
organ of Corti of, 1841f
perilymph of, 1841f-1842f
Reissner's membrane of, 1841f
scala media of, 1840, 1841f-1842f
scala tympani of, 1841f-1842f
scala vestibuli of, 1841f-1842f
spiral ligament of, 1841f
spiral limbus of, 1841f
stapes footplate of, 1840, 1842f
stria vascularis of, 1840, 1841f
tectorial membrane of, 1841f
"third window" of, 1842, 1843f
lateral lemniscus in, 1846
medial geniculate body in, 1846-1847
middle ear in, 1839-1840, 1840f
sound and its measurement in, 1838-1839, 1839f
superior olivary complex in, 1846
Auditory potentials, electrically evoked, 1912-1914
auditory brainstem response as, 1912-1913, 1913f
clinical applications of, 1914
compound action potential as, 1912-1913
with cochlear implants, 1913f, 1914
middle and long latency response as, 1912-1914, 1913f
Auditory rehabilitation, after cochlear implantation, 2253-2257
in adults, 2254-2255
in children, 2254-2255
efficacy of, 2253-2254
Auditory signal, mechanoelectrical transduction of, 1840, 1841f
Auditory steady-state response (ASSR), 1911-1912
clinical applications of, 1910f, 1912
for cochlear implants in children, 2234-2235
Auditory symptoms, of migraine, 2348-2349
distortion as, 2349
hearing loss as, 2348-2349
phonophobia as, 2349
tinnitus as, 2349
Auditory training, after cochlear implantation, 2253-2257
in adults, 2254-2255
in children, 2254-2255
efficacy of, 2253-2254
Auditory tube. *See* Eustachian tube.
Auerbach's plexus, 953, 954f
Aura
migraine with, 247, 2347, 2347b
migraine without, 2347b
Aural atresia, congenital. *See* Congenital aural atresia (CAA).
Aural cholesteatoma. *See* Cholesteatoma.
Aural fullness, 2198
Aural papillomatosis, 1957, 1957f
management options for, 1957
Aural polyp, 1965
Auricle(s), 476-477, 476f
anatomy of, 1823, 1824f, 1944, 2742
physical examination of, 97
Auricular branch block, 242
Auricular cartilage, 476-477
burns of, 316
Auricular defects, prosthetic management of, 1345-1346, 1345t, 1346f
Auricular hematomas, 97, 310, 2038
Auricular muscle group, 442f
Auricular nerve injury, due to otoplasty, 479
Auricular prosthesis, 1345-1346, 1345t, 1346f
Auricular reconstruction. *See* Atresiaplasty.
Auriculocephalic angle, 477
Autofluorescence
in early glottic carcinoma, 1516
in premalignant lesions of larynx, 1488-1489
Autofluorescence bronchoscopy, 1009
Autogenous cartilage grafts
for nasal reconstruction, 368-369, 369f-370f
in noncaucasian rhinoplasty, 569, 570f
complications of, 578, 579f
Autogenous cartilage struts, for nasal tip projection, 535-536, 536f
Autogenous costal cartilage grafts, for laryngeal stenosis, 2919-2920, 2920f
Autogenous costochondral reconstruction, for microtia, 2744, 2744t
Autografts
for craniofacial defect repair, 2657
for ossiculoplasty, 2006, 2025
Autoimmune disorders
laryngeal involvement in, 887, 887f
otologic manifestations of, 2114
of salivary glands, 2858-2863
sensorineural hearing loss due to, 2123-2124
sudden, 2128
Autoimmune inner ear disease (AIED), 2164-2168
clinical presentation of, 2165-2166
cochlear implant for, 2221
defined, 2164
diagnosis of, 2166, 2167t
differential diagnosis of, 2166
epidemiology of, 2165
future directions for, 2167-2168
pathology and pathogenesis of, 2165
animal studies of, 2165
human temporal bone studies of, 2165
sensorineural hearing loss due to, 2124, 2165
fluctuating, 2199
rapidly progressive, 2199-2200
treatment of, 2166-2167
Autoimmune thyroiditis, 1747
oral manifestations of, 1251
ultrasound of, 1644
Autoinflation, for otitis media with effusion, 2772
Autologous fat, for vocal fold medialization, 905-906
Autologous temporalis fascia grafts, for medialization thyroplasty, 910
Autologous whole-cell vaccine, for head and neck squamous cell carcinoma, 1024
Automated auditory brainstem response (AABR), 2721
Automated endoscopic system for optimal positioning (AESOP), 39, 40f
Automatic speaking valve (ASV), 1599-1600
Autonomic control, in salivary gland secretion, 1136
Autonomic dysfunction, preoperative evaluation of, 106
Autonomic reflexes, of oral cavity, 1205-1206
Autoregulation, of capillary blood flow, 1066
Autosomal dominant disorder, 6, 6f, 2088, 2088f
Autosomal dominant sensorineural hearing loss (ADSNHL)
genetic testing for, 2098
nonsyndromic, 2090-2093, 2092t
syndromic, 2093-2096, 2094t
Autosomal recessive inheritance, 2088-2089, 2089f
Autosomal recessive sensorineural hearing loss
nonsyndromic, 2089-2090, 2090f, 2091t
syndromic, 2094t, 2096
Avita (tretinoin)
for aging skin, 403-404
with chemical peels, 392-393
for chemoprevention of oral cancer, 1315
Avitene (microfibrillar collagen), for embolization, 1933
AVM. *See* Arteriovenous malformation (AVM).
Avoidance
for allergic rhinitis, 619-620
for nonallergic rhinitis, 699-700
aVOR (angular vestibulo-ocular reflex), 2306, 2307f
after labyrinthectomy, 2291-2292, 2291f-2293f
Avulsions, soft tissue, 307, 308f
Awake fiberoptic nasotracheal intubation, 122-123
advantages of, 123
avoiding failure in, 125, 126b
bronchoscopy cart for, 123, 123f
conscious sedation for, 124
fiberoptic bronchoscope in, 123-125, 125f
historical perspective on, 122-123
indications for, 123, 123b
keys to successful, 124b
monitoring during, 124
nasal trumpet placement for, 124, 125f
optimal setup for, 125f
patient preparation for, 123-124
technique of, 124-125
topical anesthesia for, 124
Axial pattern flaps, 1067, 1067f
Axonotmesis, 2384-2385
of facial nerve, 2040
Azelastine (Astelin)
for allergic rhinitis, 620
for nonallergic rhinitis, 701t
for rhinosinusitis, 734t, 737
Azithromycin
for endocarditis prophylaxis, 1249t
ototoxicity of, 2176
for pediatric surgery prophylaxis, 2597t

B

B cells, 602f, 603
development of, 603
responses by, 603
T cell–dependent and T cell–independent, 606
B ring, 966f, 967, 968f
B trains, in electromyography, 2547
Bacterial biofilms
on adenoid pads, and pediatric chronic sinusitis, 2779-2780
for chemoprevention of oral cancer, 1315
in chronic rhinosinusitis, 706, 732
disruption of, 735
in chronic suppurative otitis media, 2221
in otitis media and cholesteatoma, 1974, 2764
Bacterial infections
oral manifestations of, 1252
otitis media due to, 2763, 2764f
pediatric chronic sinusitis due to, 2779
of salivary glands, 1151-1153
in children, 2851t, 2856-2857

Bacterial labyrinthitis, 2160
Bacterial laryngitis
acute, 884
chronic, 885
Bacterial laryngotracheobronchitis. *See* Bacterial tracheitis.
Bacterial lymphadenopathy, in children, 2818, 2818f-2819f
Bacterial meningitis, hearing loss due to, 2160-2161
Bacterial otitis externa, 1944
ear wick for, 1945-1946, 1951, 1951f
otorrhea due to, 2194-2195
systemic antibiotics for, 1953
topical therapies for, 1951-1953
acidifying agents for, 1953
failure to respond to, 1953, 1953t
options for, 1951-1953, 1951f
ototopic antibiotics for, 1951-1953
Bacterial pharyngitis, 191-196
due to *Arcanobacterium haemolyticum,* 193
due to *Chlamydia pneumoniae,* 194
due to *Corynebacterium diphtheriae,* 195-196
in children, 2786-2787
due to *Francisella tularensis,* 195
due to group A beta hemolytic *Streptococcus pyogenes,* 191-193
in children, 2787
due to *Mycobacterium tuberculosis,* 195
due to *Mycoplasma pneumoniae,* 194-195
due to *Neisseria gonorrhoeae,* 193-194, 194f
due to *Neisseria gonorrhoeae* (gonococcal), in children, 2786
due to non–group A beta hemolytic streptococcal infections, 193
in children, 2787
complications of, 2788
due to *Treponema pallidum,* 194
in children, 2786
due to *Yersinia enterocolitica,* 196
Bacterial rhinosinusitis
acute, 703-705, 704f, 732
chronic, 732, 733f
Bacterial tracheitis, 2809-2810
clinical features of, 2809
complications of, 2810
diagnosis of, 2809, 2809f
differential diagnosis of, 2806t
endoscopy of, 2809, 2809f
epidemiology of, 2809
imaging of, 2809, 2809f
management of, 2809-2810, 2809f
pathogenesis of, 2809
terminology for, 2809
Bacterial vaccines, to prevent otitis media, 2768-2769
BAFF (B-lymphocyte–activating factor belonging to the TNF family), 609t-610t
BAHA. *See* Bone-anchored hearing aid (BAHA).
Baker's solution, for deep chemical peels, 394-395
BAL (bronchoalveolar lavage), flexible fiberoptic bronchoscopy for, 1003-1004
Balance exercises, in vestibular rehabilitation, 2372-2373, 2378-2379
Balance function studies, in assessment of vestibular compensation, 2376-2377
Balance problems, due to otitis media, 2776
Balance rehabilitation. *See* Vestibular and balance rehabilitation therapy (VBRT).
Balanced carrier, 5
Balanced chromosome complement, 5
Balanced orbital decompression, for Graves' ophthalmopathy, 1814
Baldness. *See also* Hair loss.
male-pattern, 374-376, 375f
Ballenger swivel knife, for septoplasty, 489-490
Balloon(s), for embolization, 1933
Balloon bronchoplasty, interventional bronchoscopy for, 1009
Balloon catheter sinusotomy, 752-753, 753f
frontal, 782-783
Balloon dilatation
of esophageal strictures, 966
transnasal esophagoscopy in, 984, 984f
for stridulous child, 2906, 2906f, 2909
for subglottic stenosis, 2906, 2906f
for tracheal stenosis, 2928, 2928f
Balloon occlusion test (BOT), for embolization, 1934, 1934f
Balloon test occlusion (BTO), for cerebral blood flow evaluation, 2491
Balloon tracheoplasty, for tracheal stenosis, 2928, 2928f
Bamford-Koval-Bench (BKB) Sentences, for cochlear implants, 2223
Bandeau, in fronto-orbital advancement
removal of, 2651-2652, 2652f
reshaping of, 2652, 2652f-2653f
splitting of, 2652, 2653f
Bannwarth's syndrome. *See* Lyme disease.
BAPTA, and interstereociliary linkages, 2077
Barium swallow
for hypopharyngeal and cervical esophageal cancer, 1423-1424
modified, 1394, 1396
for swallowing disorders, 1217-1218, 1219f
in children, 2949, 2950t
for penetrating neck trauma, 1631t, 1633
Baroreflex failure syndrome, due to carotid paraganglioma surgery, 1661
Barotrauma
atmospheric, 2343
eustachian tube dysfunction due to, 1872
facial paralysis with, 2400
peripheral vestibular disorders due to, 2343
sensorineural hearing loss due to, 2122, 2199
Barrett's esophagus
endoscopic appearance of, 967f, 972, 972f
gastroesophageal junction in, 957f
GERD and, 972-973
grading of dysplasia in, 973, 973t
histologic appearance of, 972, 972f-973f
imaging of, 1403-1404, 1404f
long-segment, 972f
short-segment, 972f
surveillance for, 972-973, 973t
transnasal esophagoscopy in, 983, 983f
Bartonella henselae
deep neck space infections due to, 201
salivary gland infection due to, 1159
Bartter syndrome, deafness in, 2051t-2058t, 2083
Barttin, in deafness, 2051t-2058t
Basal cell(s)
of olfactory epithelium, 626f, 627
of taste buds, 1208
Basal cell adenocarcinoma, of salivary glands, 1191
Basal cell adenomas, of salivary glands, 1170
Basal cell carcinoma (BCC), 283-285
diagnosis of, 284-285
epidemiology of, 283
immunosuppression and, 213t, 215, 284
morpheaform, 284, 284f
nodular, 284f
noduloulcerative, 284f
pigmented, 284, 284f
recurrent, 284, 285f
risk factors for, 283-284
Basal cell hyperplasia theory, of cholesteatoma formation, 1966-1967, 1967f
Basal cell nevus syndrome, 1268
treatment of, 1268
Basal encephaloceles, of nose, 2687-2688, 2687t, 2688f
Basal lamella, 665f, 667f
Basal subfrontal approach, for anterior cranial base surgery, 2453-2454, 2454f
Basaloid carcinoma, of oral cavity, 1299
Basaloid squamous cell carcinoma (BSCC)
of hypopharynx and cervical esophagus, 1425
of larynx, 1506
Base(s)
cranial (*See* Cranial base)
nucleotide, 4
of tongue (*See* Tongue base)
Base view, of facial bones and sinuses, 130
Baseline, assessment of, 53
Basicranium, growth and development of, 2617-2619, 2617t, 2619f-2620f
Basilar artery, 2351f
in surgical anatomy of anterior cranial base, 2474-2475, 2474f-2475f, 2481f
Basilar impression, 2355
Basilar membrane (BM)
anatomy of, 1831-1832, 1832f, 1840
in auditory physiology, 1840-1842, 1841f-1842f
in cochlear transduction, 2061f-2062f, 2065f
physical dimensions of, 2060, 2063f
radial displacement patterns of, 2067, 2069f
radial shearing forces and displacement of, 2065-2067, 2069f
in traveling wave, 2061-2062, 2064f
tuning curves of, 1844, 1844f
Basilar migraine, 2349
Basilar sinus, in surgical anatomy of anterior cranial base, 2474
Basilar venous plexus, in surgical anatomy of anterior cranial base, 2474
Basion, growth and development of, 2617t
Basophil(s)
in adaptive immune system, 605
in allergic rhinitis, 616
Bassoon *(Bsn)* gene, in murine deafness, 2058t-2060t, 2080
Battery(ies)
for external speech processors, 2233
ingestion of, 2941, 2958, 2958f
Battle's sign, 97
BCC. *See* Basal cell carcinoma (BCC).
B-cell lymphoma, diffuse large. *See* Diffuse large B-cell lymphoma (DLBCL).
BDNF (brain-derived neurotrophic factor)
for facial nerve paralysis, 2427
in gene therapy, 2192
for prevention of ototoxicity, 2189-2191
B2E (Bridges to Excellence), 84t-87t
Beam pattern, of surgical laser, 27
Beam waist, of surgical laser, 27-28, 28f
Beamlets, in intensity-modulated radiation therapy, 1696-1697
Beare-Stevenson cutis gyrata syndrome, craniofacial anomalies in, 2641t
Beclomethasone, for otitis media with effusion, 2772
Beclomethasone nasal (Vancenase, Beconase), for nonallergic rhinitis, 700t
Becquerel, 1031-1032
Becquerel, Antoine, 1031
Becquerel, Henri, 1031
Bed rest, fluid utilization during, for children, 2572t
Behavior problems, obstructive sleep apnea and, 2603-2604
Behavioral audiometry, for otitis media, 2762
Behavioral modification, for extraesophageal reflux, 900-901
Behçet's disease
esophageal manifestations of, 979
imaging of, 1405
nasal manifestations of, 660-661
oral manifestations of, 1254
Behind-the-ear (BTE) external speech processors, 2229, 2232, 2232f

Behind-the-ear (BTE) hearing aids, 2269-2270, 2270f
in children, 2274
comparison of features of, 2206t
in infants, 2723-2724
selection of, 2266-2267, 2270
Bell stage, of enamel organ development, 1259
Bell's palsy, 2391
auditory symptoms of, 2393-2394
in children, 2397
CNS changes in, 2393-2394
corticosteroids for, 2409-2410, 2410t
defined, 2391
and diabetes, 2401
differential diagnosis of, 2391, 2392t
electromagnetic stimulation in, 2394-2395
electrophysiology and testing for, 2394
electromyography in, 2394
electroneurography in, 2394
interpretation of electrical tests in, 2394
maximal stimulation test in, 2394
nerve conduction velocity in, 2394
nerve excitability threshold in, 2394
etiology of, 2391-2393
facial nerve imaging in, 1924, 1927f, 2395
familial, 2397
histopathology of, 2393
incidence of, 2391-2396
management of, 2395-2396
middle cranial fossa decompression for, 2409-2410, 2409t
oral manifestations of, 1255
polyneuropathy in, 2391, 2398f
prognosis and statistics for, 2395
recurrent, 2397
Bell's phenomenon, 445-446
Benadryl (diphenhydramine)
for allergic rhinitis, 620
for nonallergic rhinitis, 701t
Benign intracranial hypertension (BIH)
CSF rhinorrhea due to, 787
facial paralysis due to, 2400-2401
sensorineural hearing loss due to, 2123
Benign lymphoepithelial cyst (BLEC), in HIV, 217-218, 218f
Benign lymphoepithelial disease, of salivary glands, 1154
in children, 2858
Benign mesenchymal neoplasms, of larynx, 878-882
chondroma as, 881-882
granular cell, 882
lipoma as, 881
mixed, 881
neurilemmoma as, 882
neurofibroma as, 882
oncocytic, 881
recurrent respiratory papillomatosis as, 868f-869f, 878-880
adult-onset, 879
epidemiology of, 878
etiology of, 878-879
juvenile form of, 879
treatment of, 879, 880f
rhabdomyoma as, 881
vascular, 880-881
laryngeal hemangiomas as, 880-881
polypoid granulation tissue as, 880
Benign mixed tumors. *See* Pleomorphic adenoma(s).
Benign paroxysmal positional vertigo (BPPV), 2330-2332
diagnosis of, 2330-2331
findings on examination in, 2330-2331, 2331f
history in, 2330
test results in, 2331
etiology of, 2330
Benign paroxysmal positional vertigo (BPPV) *(Continued)*
historical background of, 2329-2330
horizontal (lateral) canal
positional testing for, 2315-2316, 2331
repositioning maneuver for, 2332
incidence of, 2330
mechanism of, 2330-2332
and migraine, 2350
posterior canal
anatomic and physiologic basis for, 2288-2289, 2288f
conversion of, 2332
positional testing for, 2315, 2315f, 2331, 2331f
repositioning maneuver for, 2331-2332, 2332f
surgical treatment of, 2332
superior canal
positional testing for, 2331
repositioning maneuver for, 2332
treatment of
with repositioning, 2331-2332, 2332f
surgical, 2332, 2360-2361
posterior semicircular canal occlusion as, 2360-2361, 2361f
singular neurectomy as, 2360, 2360f
vestibular rehabilitation for, 2376, 2378t
Benign paroxysmal vertigo, of childhood, and migraine, 2350-2351
Benign vocal fold mucosal disorder(s), 859-882
anatomy and physiology relevant to, 860, 860f-861f
bilateral diffuse polyposis as, 872-873, 872f
diagnosis of, 872
history in, 872
laryngeal examination in, 872
vocal capability battery in, 872
epidemiology of, 872
management of, 872-873
behavioral, 872
medical, 872
surgical, 872-873, 873f
pathophysiology and pathology of, 872
capillary ectasia as, 866-867
diagnosis of, 866-867
history in, 866
laryngeal examination in, 866-867
vocal capability battery in, 866
epidemiology of, 866
epidermoid inclusion cyst with, 868f
hemorrhagic polyp with, 868f
management of, 867
behavioral, 867
medical, 867
surgical, 867
pathophysiology and pathology of, 866
vocal nodules with, 867f
contact ulcer or granuloma as, 874-875, 874f
diagnosis of, 875
history in, 875
laryngeal examination in, 875, 875f
vocal capability battery in, 875
epidemiology of, 874
due to extraesophageal reflux, 902, 902f-903f
management of, 875
pathophysiology and pathology of, 874
epidemiology of, 859
etiology of, 859
patient beliefs about, 861
systemic medications that may affect larynx in, 863
evaluation of, 860-862
direct laryngoscopy and biopsy in, 862
history in, 860-861
common symptom complexes in, 861
onset in, 860-861
other risk factors in, 861
patient beliefs about causes in, 861
Benign vocal fold mucosal disorder(s) *(Continued)*
patient perception of severity and vocal aspirations and consequent motivation for rehabilitation in, 861
talkativeness profile in, 861
vocal commitments in, 861
objective measures of vocal output in, 862
office examination of larynx in, 862, 862f
vocal capability battery in, 861-862
general management options for, 862-863
for acute mucosal swelling of overuse, 863
hydration as, 862
laryngeal instillations for mucosal inflammation as, 863
management of acid reflux laryngopharyngitis as, 863, 863f
sinonasal management as, 862-863
glottic sulcus as, 870-872, 871f
diagnosis of, 870-871
history in, 870
laryngeal examination in, 870-871
vocal capability battery in, 870
epidemiology of, 870
management of, 871-872
behavioral, 871
medical, 871
surgical, 871-872, 872f
mucosal bridge due to, 870, 871f
pathophysiology and pathology of, 869-870
with polypoid nodule, 871f
intracordal cysts as, 869-870
diagnosis of, 869
history in, 869
laryngeal examination in, 869
vocal capability battery in, 869
epidemiology of, 869
epidermoid inclusion, 868f-869f, 869
mucus retention (ductal), 869, 869f-870f
open, 869, 870f
pathophysiology and pathology of, 869
treatment of, 869-870
behavioral, 869-870
medical, 869
surgical, 870, 870f
intubation granuloma as, 875-876, 875f
diagnosis of, 875-876
history in, 875
vocal capability battery in, 875-876
epidemiology of, 875
management of, 876
pathophysiology and pathology of, 875
postoperative dysphonia as, 873-874, 873f
diagnosis of, 873-874
history in, 873
laryngeal examination in, 874
vocal capability battery in, 873-874
epidemiology of, 873
management of, 874
behavioral, 874
medical, 874
pathophysiology and pathology of, 873, 874f
surgery for, 863-865, 864f
symptoms of
in nonsingers, 859, 861
in singers, 859, 861
vocal fold hemorrhage and unilateral (hemorrhagic) vocal fold polyp as, 867-869
with capillary ectasia, 868f
diagnosis of, 868
history in, 868
laryngeal examination in, 868
vocal capability battery in, 868
epidemiology of, 867
pathophysiology and pathology of, 867-868

Benign vocal fold mucosal disorder(s) *(Continued)*
treatment of, 868-869
behavioral, 868
medical, 868
surgical, 868-869
vocal nodules as, 865-866
with capillary ectasia, 867f
defined, 865
diagnosis of, 865
history in, 865
laryngeal examination in, 865
vocal capability battery in, 865
epidemiology of, 865
management of, 865-866
behavioral, 865
medical, 865
surgical, 865-866, 866f, 867t
pathophysiology and pathology of, 865
voice therapy for, 863, 864f
Benzodiazepines, as adjuncts to induction of anesthesia, 111
Benzydamine hydrochloride, for mucositis, 1102
Bernoulli effect, in voice production, 846
Bernstein test, 962-963
Berry's ligament, anatomy of, 1751
Beta decay, 1032
Beta defensins, in middle ear protection, 1871
Beta error, 65, 66t
Beta particles, 1031-1032
Beta-adrenergic agents, for migraine, 2350
β_2-transferrin test, for CSF rhinorrhea, 789, 2044
β-all-*trans* retinoic acid, for cancer chemoprevention, 1061
β-blockers
for Graves' disease, 1743
intraoperative, 112
β-carotene
for cancer chemoprevention, 1061-1062
for chemoprevention of oral cancer, 1315
β-defensins, 599
β-lactamase inhibitors, for streptococcal pharyngitis, 2787
Betadine (povidone-iodine), for embolization, 1933
Betahistine, for Meniere's disease, 2337-2338
Beta-hydroxy acids, for aging skin, 404
Betamethasone valerate cream, for eczematoid otitis externa, 1955-1956
Beta-trace protein (βTP), in CSF rhinorrhea, 790
Betel nuts, and oral cancer, 1294, 1365
Bethanechol, for extraesophageal reflux, 901
Bevacizumab, for nasopharyngeal carcinoma, 1700
Bezold abscess, 1985-1986, 1986f-1987f
due to temporal bone infection, 1980t
BFU-E (burst-forming units–erythroid), 605
BFU-MEG (burst-forming units–megakaryocytes), 605
Bias, 53
allocation, 62t
ascertainment, 62t
detection, 62t
vs. efficacy of treatment, 62t
in outcomes research, 53
selection, 53, 68t
susceptibility, 62t
treatment, 53
Bias velocity, in rotatory chair testing, 2322
Bicarbonate (HCO_3)
in saliva, 1139
in salivary gland secretion, 1135
Bicellular reserve cell theory, of salivary gland tumorigenesis, 1163
Bicklemann, A. G., 251
Bicoronal incision, 2450-2451, 2450f
for nasal fracture repair, 505, 505f
for pediatric facial fracture, 2701-2702, 2703f
Bidirectional sensitivity, of vestibular system, 2278-2279
BIH (benign intracranial hypertension)
CSF rhinorrhea due to, 787
facial paralysis due to, 2400-2401
sensorineural hearing loss due to, 2123
Bilateral advancement flap, 345, 346f
Bilateral cochlear implantation, 2241
for adults, 2224
for children, 2226
results of, 2247-2251
Bilateral hockey stick incision, for neck dissection
radical, 1709, 1710f
selective, 1717-1718, 1717f
Bile, in reflux laryngitis, 886
Bile monitoring, ambulatory 24-hour, 960-961, 961f
Bilevel positive airway pressure (BiPAP), for obstructive sleep apnea
in children, 2610-2611
Bilitec 2000, 960-961, 961f
Bill's bar
anatomy of, 1822, 1823f
in surgical anatomy of lateral skull base, 2437-2439
Bilobed flap
for cheek defects, 357, 359f
for nasal defects, 365-366, 365f
Binaural cochlear implantation, 2241
for adults, 2224
for children, 2226
results of, 2247-2251
Binaural processing, 2248
Binaural squelch, 1846, 2248
Bing-Siebenmann dysplasia, 2727
Binostril approach, for transnasal endoscopic-assisted anterior skull base surgery, 2478, 2479f
Biochemical defects, in recessive disorders, 7
Biocompatibility, in skeletal or cartilaginous defect repair, 2657
Biofilms
on adenoid pads, and pediatric chronic sinusitis, 2779-2780
for chemoprevention of oral cancer, 1315
in chronic rhinosinusitis, 706, 732
disruption of, 735
in chronic suppurative otitis media, 2221
in otitis media and cholesteatoma, 1974, 2764
Bioinformatics, in head and neck squamous cell carcinoma, 1028-1029
Biologic agents, with radiotherapy, 1054, 1055f
Biomarkers
for head and neck squamous cell carcinoma, 1026-1027
epidermal growth factor receptor as, 1026
human papillomavirus as, 1026
loss of heterozygosity as, 1026
margin analysis for, 1027
in oral rinses and saliva, 1026
other, 1026-1027
polymorphisms in DNA repair enzymes as, 1027
serum analysis for, 1026-1027
for laryngeal squamous cell carcinoma, 1493, 1505
for oral cancer, 1295
for salivary gland neoplasms, 1163, 1194
Biomaterials, in skeletal or cartilaginous defect repair, 2657-2658
Biomimetic materials, for craniofacial defect repair, 2658
Bionx plating system, for pediatric facial fractures, 2701t
Biopsy
endobronchial and transbronchial, flexible fiberoptic bronchoscopy for, 1004-1005, 1004f-1005f
fine-needle aspiration
in children, 2574
of salivary glands, 2854
of lymphoma, 1675-1676
of neck masses, 1638
of oropharyngeal cancer, 1366
of salivary glands, 1149, 1149f, 1165-1166, 1180-1181
in children, 2854
of thyroid nodule, 1756-1758
repeat, 1759
ultrasound-guided, 1655f
ultrasound-guided, 1653-1654, 1655f
of glottic cancer, 1518
laryngeal, for benign vocal fold mucosal disorders, 862
of lymphoma
core-needle, 1676
corticosteroids prior to, 1676
fine-needle aspiration, 1675-1676
open, 1676
of melanoma, 1109
of neck masses, 1638
in children, 2814
of oropharyngeal cancer, 1366
fine-needle aspiration, 1366
of paranasal sinus tumors, 1124
of salivary glands, 1149, 1149f, 1165-1166, 1180-1181
in children, 2854-2855
sentinel lymph node (*See* Sentinel lymph node biopsy (SLNB))
of thyroid nodule, 1756-1758
repeat, 1759
ultrasound-guided, 1655f
Biotinidase deficiency, sensorineural hearing loss in, 2094t, 2096
BiPAP (bilevel positive airway pressure), for obstructive sleep apnea
in children, 2610-2611
Bipedicle flap, for nasal reconstruction, 371
Bipedicle mucosal advancement flap, for nasal defects, 347, 347f
Bipolaris, rhinosinusitis due to, 732-733
Birdshots, 1626, 1628t
Birth order, and otitis media, 2767
Bisphosphonates, for hyperparathyroidism, 1804
Bitter taste
individual differences in, 1211-1212
peripheral sensitivity to, 1211
transduction of, 1209
Bizygomatic width, 2617t
BK channel defects, and hearing, 2079
B-K mole syndrome, 288, 288f, 1107
BKB (Bamford-Koval-Bench) Sentences, for cochlear implants, 2223
Blair incision, modified, for parotidectomy, 1172, 1173f, 1195, 1195f
Blast trauma, peripheral vestibular disorders due to, 2343
Blastomycosis, laryngeal and tracheal manifestations of, 885, 892
BLEC (benign lymphoepithelial cyst), in HIV infection, 217-218, 218f
Bleeding
due to neck dissection, 1723
due to thyroid surgery, 1770
Bleeding disorders, oral manifestations of, 1256
Bleomycin, for induction chemotherapy, 1056-1057

Blepharoplasty, 439-451
adjunctive procedure(s) to, 451
Botox for, 451
injectable filler for, 451
skin resurfacing as, 451
aesthetic considerations and ideals and, 444-447
for brow position, 445, 445f
for eyelids, 445-447, 446f
and upper eyelid ptosis, 446-447, 447f
for midface, 447
complications of, 449-451
for facial paralysis, 2430
preoperative planning for, 447
surgical techniques for, 447-451
lid shortening procedure as, 449
of lower eyelid, 448-449
subciliary approach to, 449, 450f-451f
transconjunctival approach to, 448-449, 450f
with ptosis repair, 447-448
of upper eyelid, 447-448, 447f-449f
Blepharospasm, 2401
Blind nasal technique, for difficult airway, 114t
Blindness, due to neck dissection, 1723
Blink reflex, to assess facial nerve function, 2388
intraoperatively, 2555, 2555f
Blom-Singer duckbill prosthesis, 1598f
Blood clot, in wound healing, 1076
Blood dyscrasias, sensorineural hearing loss due to, 2123
Blood supply, to brain, 2351, 2351f
Blood viscosity, decreased, and skin flap viability, 1073-1074
Blood volume, in children, 2571
Blowout fracture, 170f, 321
Blue nevus, 286-287, 287f
Blunt neck trauma, 1634-1635
B-lymphocyte–activating factor belonging to the TNF family (BAFF), 609t-610t
BM. *See* Basilar membrane (BM).
B-mode sonography, 1643
BMPs (bone morphogenetic proteins), in mandibular reconstruction, 1327-1328, 1328f
Board certification, 79-80, 80b
Bode plot, in vestibular tests, 2302, 2303f
Body-cover concept, of phonation, 811
Body-worn (BW) external speech processors, 2229, 2232, 2232f
Boilermaker's deafness, 2121
Bolus fabrication, by maxillofacial prosthodontist, 1331, 1332f
Bone, primary *vs.* secondary, 2614
Bone conduction process, and orbital wall fractures, 2712
Bone disease
due to hyperparathyroidism, 1781
otologic manifestations of, 2108-2112
in fibrous dysplasia, 2110-2111, 2111f
in osteitis fibrosa cystica, 2112
in osteogenesis imperfecta, 2109-2110, 2110f
in osteopetroses, 2111-2112, 2112f-2113f
in Paget's disease, 2108-2109, 2109f
sensorineural hearing loss due to, 2124
Bone erosion
in cholesteatoma and chronic otitis media, 1971-1974, 1972f-1973f
of paranasal sinus walls, 672
Bone formation, 2614
endochondral, 2614, 2615f
intramembranous, 2614
Bone grafts
in cleft-lip nose repair, 559, 564f
for nasal fractures, 505, 505f
for nasal reconstruction, 369, 370f
Bone growth
osteogenesis in, 2614
endochondral, 2614, 2615f
intramembranous, 2614
Bone growth *(Continued)*
remodeling and displacement in, 2614-2615, 2639
of mandible, 2639f
of nasomaxillary complex, 2619, 2621f
Bone healing, 330-331
Bone morphogenetic proteins (BMPs), in mandibular reconstruction, 1327-1328, 1328f
Bone remodeling, 2614-2615, 2639
of mandible, 2639f
of nasomaxillary complex, 2619, 2621f
Bone resorption
in cholesteatoma and chronic otitis media, 1971-1974, 1972f-1973f
with vascular tumors, 2826
Bone sarcomas, of neck, 1666, 1667t
Bone scans, for nasopharyngeal carcinoma, 1354
Bone Source (hydroxyapatite), for chin implants, 465t
Bone-anchored hearing aid (BAHA), 2212-2216
background of, 2213
biology and histology of, 2213
biophysical principles of, 2213
comparison of features of, 2206t
complications of, 2215
components of, 2213f
for conductive hearing loss, 2027
for congenital aural atresia, 2759
design of, 2213
indications and contraindications for, 2212-2213, 2216t
location of, 2204f
materials for, 2213
operative technique for, 2213-2215, 2214f
radiologic implications of, 2213
results of, 2215-2216
sound transduction and coupling to auditory system with, 2205f
for unilateral sensorineural hearing loss, 2216
in young children, 2215
Bone-conduction implantable hearing aids, 2212-2216
background of, 2213
biology and histology of, 2213
biophysical principles of, 2213
comparison of features of, 2206t
complications of, 2215
components of, 2213f
design of, 2213
indications for and contraindications to, 2212-2213, 2216t
in infants, 2723-2724
location of, 2204f
materials for, 2213
operative technique for, 2213-2215, 2214f
radiologic implications of, 2213
results of, 2215-2216, 2216t
sound transduction and coupling to auditory system with, 2205f
for unilateral sensorineural hearing loss, 2216
in young children, 2215
Bone-conduction testing, in pure-tone audiometry, 1888, 1888f-1889f
Bony labyrinth
anatomy of, 1831, 1852, 1853f
embryogenesis of, 1852
Bony vault, rhinoplasty of, 540-542
for bony profile reduction, 540-541, 540f
for narrowing of nose, 541-542
double osteotomies in, 542, 542f-543f
lateral osteotomies in, 541, 542f
medial-oblique osteotomies in, 541, 541f
Boomerang incision, for neck dissection
radical, 1709, 1710f
selective, 1713-1714
BOR (branchio-oto-renal) syndrome
deafness in, 2051t-2058t, 2093-2095, 2094t
inheritance pattern of, 6, 2093-2095
inner ear anomalies in, 2735
Border cells of Held, 1832f
Bordetella pertussis, laryngeal and tracheal manifestations of, 892
Boric acid solution, for fungal otitis externa, 1954
Borrelia burgdorferi. See Lyme disease.
Borrelia vincentii, Vincent's angina due to, 2786
Boston-type craniosynostosis, 2641t
BOT (balloon occlusion test), for embolization, 1934, 1934f
Botryoid odontogenic cyst, 1265-1266
radiographic features of, 1266
treatment of, 1266
Bottle feeding, and otitis media, 2767
Bottom-up approach, for pediatric facial fracture repair, 2706f
Botulinum toxin (Botox)
for achalasia, 965
for alaryngeal speech, 1459
with blepharoplasty, 451
for depressor muscles, 432, 433f
for laryngeal hyperfunction, 839, 840f-841f
for synkinesis, 2432
Bouton vestibular afferent nerve fibers, 2283, 2283f
Bowen's disease, 286
Bowman-Bird protease inhibitor, for chemoprevention of oral cancer, 1315
Boyce's sign, 986-987
BPPV. *See* Benign paroxysmal positional vertigo (BPPV).
Brachiocephalic trunk, in root of neck, 2581f
Brachycephaly
in Down syndrome, 2632
synostotic, 2643f, 2644, 2645f
fronto-orbital advancement for, 2652-2653
Brachytherapy, 1036, 1047
interventional bronchoscopy with endobronchial, 1010t
maxillofacial prosthodontics in, 1332, 1335f
for oral cancer, 1314, 1314f
for unresectable tracheal tumor, 1621
Bradykinin, in skin blood flow, 1066
BRAF gene, in thyroid carcinoma, 1753
Bragg peak, 1034
Brain
blood supply to, 2351, 2351f
effects of radiotherapy on, 2626t
Brain abscess, 1994
due to cranial base surgery, 2468
epidemiology of, 1980t-1981t, 1994
imaging of, 1994f-1995f
otitis media and, 2777
pathogenesis of, 1994
symptoms of, 1994
treatment of, 1994
Brain fungus, due to otitis media, 1992-1993, 1993f
Brain growth, postnatal, 2617t
Brain hernia, due to otitis media, 1992-1993, 1993f
Brain injury, due to cranial base surgery, 2468
Brain size, 2617t
Brain weight, 2617t
Brain-derived neurotrophic factor (BDNF)
for facial nerve paralysis, 2427
in gene therapy, 2192
for prevention of ototoxicity, 2189-2191
Brain-evoked potentials, for olfaction, 632
Brainstem
efferent pathways from vestibular nuclei to, 1865
in surgical anatomy of anterior cranial base, 2475f, 2481f
in surgical anatomy of lateral skull base, 2439f
in vestibular function, 2308

Brainstem *(Continued)*
vestibular nerve terminations in, 1858f, 1859-1860
in vestibulo-ocular reflex, 2296-2297
anatomic and physiologic basis for, 2296
velocity storage in, 2296
velocity-to-position integration in, 2296, 2297f-2298f
clinical implications of, 2296-2297
for Alexander's law, 2297, 2299f
for head-shake nystagmus, 2296-2297
for interpreting rotary chair tests, 2297-2299
for pre- and post-rotatory nystagmus, 2296, 2298f
Brainstem gliomas, intra-axial, 2528
Brainstem lesions, laryngologic manifestations of, 837-838, 838t
Brainstem neoplasms, vestibular symptoms of, 2353-2354
Branchial arches, embryology of, 2583-2584, 2583f
craniofacial syndromes related to, 2585
innervation of, 2584
muscular derivatives of, 2584
skeletal derivatives of, 2583-2584, 2583f
Branchial cleft anomalies
embryology of, 2583
first, 2585
imaging of, 1410, 1410f
neck masses due to, 1639
second through fourth, 2585
Branchial cleft cyst, 2814-2817
in children, 2859
clinical presentation of, 2814, 2814f
embryology of, 2585, 2585f, 2814
imaging of, 131, 158f, 1410, 2814, 2815f
management of, 2814
otorrhea due to infection of, 2195
squamous cell carcinoma arising in, 1671
Branchial cleft fistula, 2585
imaging of, 1410, 1410f
Branchial cleft remnants, 2585
Branchial cleft sinus, 2585
imaging of, 1410
Branchio-otic syndrome, deafness in, 2051t-2058t
Branchio-oto-renal (BOR) syndrome
deafness in, 2051t-2058t, 2093-2095, 2094t
inheritance pattern of, 6, 2093-2095
inner ear anomalies in, 2735
Bravo wireless pH capsule, 961, 961f
Breast adenocarcinoma
metastatic to ear, 2108f
skull base metastases of, 173f
Breastfeeding, and otitis media, 2767
Breathiness, in voice evaluation, 827t
Breathing
laryngeal function in, 807-809, 808f-810f
oral (mouth), 809
pharyngeal function in, 809-810, 810f
in voice evaluation, 827
Bregma, 320f
Bremsstrahlung, 1032
Breslow microstaging, for melanoma, 1113f
Bridges to Excellence (B2E, BTE), 84t-87t
Brn3c, in deafness, 2051t-2058t
Brn4.0, in deafness, 2051t-2058t
Broca's area, in central auditory pathway, 1837
Bronchial foreign bodies
complications of, 2942
imaging of, 2938, 2938f-2939f
location of, 2936, 2936f
management of
anesthesia for, 2940
controversies in, 2942
technique for, 2940
symptoms of, 2938
Bronchial wash, flexible fiberoptic bronchoscopy for, 1003
Bronchioles, anatomy of, 998-999, 999f
Bronchitis, oral manifestations of, 1250
Bronchoalveolar lavage (BAL), flexible fiberoptic bronchoscopy for, 1003-1004
Bronchogenic duplication cyst, compression of pharynx and esophagus due to, 1409f
Bronchoplasty, balloon, interventional bronchoscopy for, 1009
Bronchoscope
fiberoptic, for awake fiberoptic nasotracheal intubation, 123-125, 125f
ventilating, 2903, 2903f
Bronchoscopic brush, flexible fiberoptic bronchoscopy for, 1007
Bronchoscopic lung volume reduction, 1011
Bronchoscopy
airway anatomy and nomenclature for, 998-999, 999f
autofluorescence, 1009
in children
anesthesia for, 2597-2598, 2597t
for foreign body removal, 2939t, 2940
for difficult airway
fiberoptic, 114t
rigid, 113f, 114t
flexible fiberoptic, 1001-1007
care of bronchoscopes for, 1001-1002
diagnostic, 999b, 1003-1007
for bronchial wash, 1003
for bronchoalveolar lavage, 1003-1004
for bronchoscopic brush sampling, 1007
for endobronchial and transbronchial biopsy, 1004-1005, 1004f-1005f
general approaches to, 1003
for transbronchial needle aspiration, 1005-1007, 1005f-1006f
for visual examination, 1003
range and special features of bronchoscopes for, 1001, 1002t, 1003f
imaging prior to, 999-1000
indications for, 999, 999b
innovations and future developments in, 1009-1011
autofluorescence bronchoscopy as, 1009
endobronchial ultrasonography as, 1011
endoscopic/bronchoscopic lung volume reduction as, 1011
interventional, 999b, 1007-1009
for balloon bronchoplasty, 1009
for endobronchial stent placement, 1009
for foreign body removal, 1008
in children, 2939t, 2940
general principles of, 1007-1008
patient preparation and instrument selection for, 1008
for tissue débridement, 1008-1009, 1010t
for laryngomalacia, 2867
patient discussion and informed consent for, 1000
patient positioning and route of entry for, 1000
for penetrating neck trauma, 1631t, 1634
rigid, 1000-1001
sedation and airway management for, 1000
for tracheal neoplasms
diagnostic, 1616-1617
therapeutic, 1619-1622
Bronchoscopy cart, for awake fiberoptic nasotracheal intubation, 123, 123f
Bronchospasm, during anesthesia, in children, 2595
Bronchus(i), anatomy and terminology for, 998-999, 999f
Brooke-Spiegler syndrome, 292
Brow
aesthetic proportions of, 428, 429f, 445, 445f
aging, 428-432, 429f, 445, 445f
Brow depressor muscles
botulinum toxin for, 432, 433f
release of, 434, 434f
Brow lift, 2430
direct, 430, 431t
endoscopic, 431, 431t
midforehead, 430, 431t
Brow muscles, 431, 433f
Brow position, ideal, 445, 445f
Brow ptosis, 445, 445f, 2430
Brow rejuvenation, 428-438
aesthetic proportions for, 428, 429f
brow muscles in, 431, 433f
and characteristics of aging brow, 428-432, 429f
patient selection for, 428-430
anatomic considerations in, 429-430
psychological considerations in, 428
postoperative care after, 434
results of, 434-438, 436f-438f
surgical goals of, 430
surgical technique for, 432-434
brow elevation and fixation in, 434, 435f
frontal and parietal bone dissection in, 432-433
incisions in, 432, 433f
local anesthesia in, 432
release of brow depressor muscles in, 434, 434f
temporal dissection in, 433-434, 433f-434f
technique(s) for, 430-432, 431t
browpexy for, 430, 431t, 432f
coronal forehead lift for, 430, 431t
direct brow lift for, 430, 431t
endoscopic brow lift for, 431, 431t
midforehead brow lift for, 430, 431t
midforehead lift for, 430, 431t
pretrichial forehead lift for, 430, 431t
temporal lift for, 431-432, 431t
treatment of depressor muscles with botulinum toxin for, 432, 433f
Brown-Guss provocation maneuvers, 500
Browpexy, 430, 431t, 432f
Brute force sample, 68, 69t
Bruxism, 262t
BSCC (basaloid squamous cell carcinoma)
of hypopharynx and cervical esophagus, 1425
of larynx, 1506
Bsn (bassoon) gene, in murine deafness, 2058t-2060t, 2080
BSND, in deafness, 2051t-2058t
BTE (Bridges to Excellence), 84t-87t
BTE (behind-the-ear). *See* Behind-the-ear (BTE).
BTO (balloon test occlusion), for cerebral blood flow evaluation, 2491
βTP (beta-trace protein), in CSF rhinorrhea, 790
Buccal bifurcation cysts, infected, 1264-1265
Buccal branch, of facial nerve, 1194f, 2418-2419, 2419f
Buccal carcinoma, 1308-1309
clinical appearance of, 1308f
epidemiology of, 1308
radiation and chemoradiation for, 1309
reconstruction for, 1308-1309, 1309f
squamous cell, 1308, 1308f
surgical treatment of, 1308-1309, 1309f
survival with, 1309
verrucous, 1308
Buccal fatpad, 321f
Buccal lymph nodes, 2582
Buccal membranes, physical examination of, 99
Buccal mucosa, 1295f, 1298
Buccal nerve, 321f
Buccal space involvement, in odontogenic infections, 181, 181f
Buccinator lymph nodes, 1360f
Buccinator musculomucosal flap, for soft palate reconstruction, 1381-1382, 1381f
Buckshots, 1626-1627, 1628t

Bud stage, of enamel organ development, 1259
Budesonide, for eczematoid otitis externa, 1955
Budesonide nasal spray (Rhinocort)
for nonallergic rhinitis, 700t
for rhinosinusitis, 734t, 736
Buffalo III voice profile, 2878
Buffering, saliva in, 1141
Buflomedil, and skin flap viability, 1073
Buildup region, in radiation, 1033
Bulb insufflator, for ear hygiene or chronic ear drainage, 1958, 1961f
Bulbar conjunctiva, 444
Bulbopontine sulcus, in surgical anatomy of lateral skull base, 2439f
Bulk flow, across interstitial space, 1066
Bulla frontalis, in frontal sinusitis, 776
Bullet(s)
expanding, 1626, 1627f
fragmenting, 1627f
high-velocity, 1626, 1626f
low-velocity, 1625
self-exploding, 1627f
tumbling, 1625-1626, 1627f
yaw of, 1625
Bullet injuries, of neck
due to handgun, 1625
due to rifle, 1626, 1626f-1627f
due to shotguns, 1626-1627, 1628t
Bullous myringitis, 1948, 1948f
Bullous oral mucosal lesions, 1231-1240
erythema multiforme as, 1239-1240, 1254
clinical features of, 1239, 1239f-1240f
defined, 1239
differential diagnosis of, 1239
etiology and pathogenesis of, 1239
histopathologic features of, 1239-1240
treatment of, 1240
herpes simplex infection as
primary, 1235, 1252
clinical features of, 1235, 1235f
defined, 1235
diagnosis of, 1235
differential diagnosis of, 1235
etiology and pathogenesis of, 1235
treatment of, 1235, 1252
recurrent, 1235-1236, 1252
clinical features of, 1236, 1236f
defined, 1235
differential diagnosis of, 1236
etiology and pathogenesis of, 1235-1236
histopathology of, 1236, 1237f
vs. recurrent aphthous stomatitis, 1238, 1238t
treatment of, 1236
mucous membrane (cicatricial) pemphigoid as, 1233-1235, 1254
clinical differential diagnosis of, 1234, 1234t
clinical features of, 1233-1234, 1233f-1234f
defined, 1233
etiology and pathogenesis of, 1233
histopathologic features of, 1234-1235, 1234f
treatment of, 1235
pemphigus vulgaris as, 1231-1233, 1254
clinical differential diagnosis of, 1232
clinical presentation of, 1232, 1232f
defined, 1231-1232
etiology/pathogenesis of, 1232
histopathologic features of, 1232-1233, 1232f-1233f
treatment of, 1233
recurrent aphthous stomatitis as, 1236-1239
clinical features of, 1237-1238
defined, 1236-1237
differential diagnosis of, 1238, 1238t
etiology and pathogenesis of, 1237, 1237t
herpetiform-type, 1238, 1238f
histopathologic features of, 1239
major, 1237-1238, 1238f
Bullous oral mucosal lesions *(Continued)*
minor, 1237, 1238f
treatment of, 1239
traumatic (eosinophilic) granuloma as, 1240
clinical features of, 1240, 1240f
defined, 1240
differential diagnosis of, 1240
etiology of, 1240
histopathologic features of, 1240, 1240f
treatment of, 1240
Bullous pemphigoid, esophageal manifestations of, 980
Bumetanide, sensorineural hearing loss due to, 2120, 2175
Bupivacaine, intraoperative, 112
Bupivacaine block, for neuropathic pain, 245
Bupropion, for neuropathic pain, 245, 245t
Burden, in psychometric validation, 55
Burkitt's lymphoma, 1679
in children, 2838, 2839f
clinical presentation of, 1674
treatment and prognosis for, 1679
Burns, 314-316
assessment and treatment of, 315-316
classification of, 314-315, 315f
of eyelids, 316
of lips and oral commissure, 316
of nasal and utricular cartilage, 316
Burow's solution (aluminum acetate otic drops), 1959t-1960t
for fungal otitis externa, 1954
Burow's triangles, with advancement flaps, 345, 346f
"Burst" activity, in facial nerve monitoring, 2387, 2547, 2547f
Burst-forming units–erythroid (BFU-E), 605
Burst-forming units–megakaryocytes (BFU-MEG), 605
Burstone analysis, for mentoplasty, 463, 463f
Burwell, C. S., 251
Bushy cells, in cochlear nucleus, 1835, 1845
Buttress(es), of facial skeleton, 331, 331f
repair of, 336
Buttress graft
in nasal tip refinement, 576
in revision rhinoplasty, 589
BW (body-worn) external speech processors, 2229, 2232, 2232f

C

C chemokines, 611t-612t
C fibers
in dental pain, 1202
in nonallergic rhinitis, 695
C trains, in electromyography, 2547
Ca^{++}. *See* Calcium (Ca^{++}).
CA (cochlear aqueduct). *See* Cochlear aqueduct (CA).
CA (compressed analog), for cochlear implants, 2230
CAA. *See* Congenital aural atresia (CAA).
Cachexia, palliative care for, 1104
Cacna1D, in murine deafness, 2058t-2060t, 2080
Cadherin 23 (CDH23), in tip links, 2074
Cadherin 23 *(CDH23)* gene, in deafness, 2051t-2058t, 2074
Cadherin expression, in oral cancer, 1301
CAHPS (Consumer Assessment of Health Providers and Services), 82, 84t-87t
Calcifications, tonsillar, 1411, 1412f
Calcifying epithelial odontogenic tumor, 1276
microscopic findings in, 1276
radiographic findings in, 1276, 1276f
Calcifying odontogenic cyst (COC), 1268-1269
microscopic features of, 1269, 1269f
radiographic features of, 1269
treatment of, 1269
Calcimimetic agents, for hyperparathyroidism, 1804
Calcitonin
in calcium homeostasis, 1775
serum levels of, with thyroid nodule, 1756
Calcitonin gene–related peptide (CGRP)
in salivary gland secretion, 1137
and skin flap viability, 1073
Calcitriol, in parathyroid hormone regulation, 1776
Calcium (Ca^{++})
in saliva, 1139
serum, 1782
Calcium (Ca^{++})-activated chloride (Cl$^-$) channels, in salivary gland secretion, 1135
Calcium (Ca^{++})-activated potassium (K$^+$) channels, in salivary gland secretion, 1135
Calcium channel blockers
for achalasia, 965
for migraine, 2350
Calcium channel defects, and hearing, 2080
Calcium deficiency, oral manifestations of, 1254
Calcium homeostasis, 1775-1777
Calcium hydroxyapatite (Radiesse dermal filler), for vocal fold medialization, 906
Calcium (Ca^{2+})-mediated adaptation, of mechanoelectrical transduction currents, 2078-2079, 2079f
Calcium phosphate cement, for nasal reconstruction, 368
Calcium (Ca^{2+})-transporting plasma membrane 2, in deafness, 2051t-2058t
Calcium–adenosine triphosphatase 2 (Ca^{2+}-ATPase 2), in deafness, 2051t-2058t, 2080
Calcium-sending receptor gene, in parathyroid neoplasm(s), 1775
Calculi, of parotid gland, 150
Calculous lesions, of salivary glands, 1647
Caldwell, George, 756
Caldwell view, 662, 663f
of facial bones and sinuses, 130
Caldwell-Luc procedure, 756, 756f
Calgary Sleep Apnea Quality of Life Index (SAQLI), 57
Caliber, of handgun, 1625
Caloric testing, 2319-2320
anatomic and physiologic basis for nystagmus during, 2290
convective component of, 2319, 2320f-2321f
nonconvective component of, 2319-2320
normative values for, 2320
protocol for, 2320
recording of eye movements in, 2320, 2321f
Calvaria, growth and development of, 2615-2617, 2617t, 2618f
Calyceal vestibular afferent nerve fibers, 2283, 2283f
Calyx ending, of hair cells, 1857, 1859f
CAMP (Clinical Assessment of Musical Perception), 57
cAMP (cyclic adenosine monophosphate)
in olfactory transduction, 629
in salivary gland secretion, 1137
Camper's fascia, 2577
Canal wall down mastoidectomy, 2010-2011
for chronic otitis media with cholesteatoma, 1969, 1970t
intact canal wall *vs.,* 2014
indications for, 2014-2015, 2015f
operative procedure for, 2013-2014, 2014f
Canal wall up mastoidectomy, 2010
vs. canal wall down procedure, 2014
for chronic otitis media with cholesteatoma, 1969, 1970t
indications for, 2014-2015
Canalicular cell adenomas, of salivary glands, 1170
Canalith repositioning, for benign paroxysmal positional vertigo, 2331-2332, 2332f

Canalithiasis, 2329-2330
of lateral semicircular canal, 2331
of posterior semicircular canal, 2331
Canalplasty, in tympanoplasty, 2002
with lateral graft technique, 2002-2003, 2002f
c-ANCAs (cytoplasmic antineutrophil cytoplasmic antibodies), in Wegener's granulomatosis, 658, 2103
Cancer, gene therapy for, 20-22, 21f
antiangiogenesis in, 22
conditionally replicating adenovirus therapy in, 22
cytotoxic or suicide gene strategies in, 21
direct in vivo stimulation of antitumor immune response in, 21
genetic modification of tumor-infiltrating lymphocytes in, 20-21
modifying oncogenes and tumor suppressor genes in, 21-22
Cancer pain, palliative care for, 1103
Cancer stem cell hypothesis, in head and neck squamous cell carcinoma, 1028
Candida albicans, otitis externa due to, 2195
Candida esophagitis, 976, 976f
imaging of, 1404, 1405f
Candida spp
otitis external due to, 1944-1945
pharyngitis due to, 199-200
Candida superinfections, in chronic suppurative otitis media, 2221
Candidal leukoplakia, 1231, 1231f
Candidiasis
laryngeal and tracheal, 884-885, 884f, 893
oropharyngeal, 199-200, 1229-1231, 1252
acute, 1230, 1230f, 1230t
angular cheilitis due to, 1230, 1230f
in children, 2786
chronic, 1230, 1230t
clinical features of, 1230-1231
defined, 1229
differential diagnosis of, 1231
erythematous, 1230, 1230f
etiology and pathogenesis of, 1229-1230
histopathologic/diagnostic features of, 1231, 1231f
in HIV, 225, 226f
hyperplastic, 1231, 1231f
pseudomembranous, 1230, 1230f
risk factors for, 1229, 1230t
treatment of, 1231
Canine smile, 2417-2418
Canine space involvement, in odontogenic infections, 180-181, 180f
Caninus, 321f
Cannulas, for liposuction, 453, 455f
Canthoplasty, 2420-2421
Cantilever bone graft, for nasal fractures, 505, 505f
CAP (compound action potential)
in Bell's palsy, 2394
electrically evoked, 1912-1913
with cochlear implants, 1913f, 1914
Cap graft
for nasal tip enhancement, 576, 577f
in revision rhinoplasty, 589
Cap stage, of enamel organ development, 1259
Capek, Joseph, 38
Capek, Karel, 38
CAPE-V (Consensus Auditory Perceptual Evaluation for Voice), 819, 826
Caphosol, for mucositis, 1102
Capillary ectasia, of larynx, 817, 866-867
diagnosis of, 866-867
history in, 866
laryngeal examination in, 866-867
vocal capability battery in, 866
epidemiology of, 866
epidermoid inclusion cyst with, 868f
Capillary ectasia, of larynx *(Continued)*
hemorrhagic polyp with, 868f
management of, 867
behavioral, 867
medical, 867
surgical, 867
pathophysiology and pathology of, 866
vocal nodules with, 867f
Capillary hemangioma, sinonasal lobular, 718t, 725, 725f
Capillary lake, 866-867
Capillary malformations, 2832-2833, 2834f
Capillary obstruction, in acutely raised skin flaps, 1070-1071
Capillary system, and skin flaps, 1065-1066, 1065f
acutely raised, 1068-1069
Capsaicin provocation test, in nonallergic rhinitis, 696
Capsid, in Epstein-Barr virus, 1352
Capsulopalpebral fascia, 444
Carbamathione, for noise-induced hearing loss, 2145
Carbamazepine, for neuropathic pain, 243, 244t
Carbamide peroxide (Debrox, Murine removal kit), for cerumen removal, 1958t
Carbogen, with radiotherapy, 1041
Carbon dioxide (CO_2) laser, 31t, 32-33
for airway stenosis, 945, 2918
for benign vocal fold mucosal disorders, 864
for glottic cancer, 1517t, 1519t
for laryngeal hemangiomas, 881
optical resonating chamber of, 26, 27f
for premalignant lesions of larynx, 1490
for recurrent respiratory papillomatosis, 879, 2889-2891
for stridulous child, 2908
for transoral laser microsurgery, 1528
Carbon dioxide (CO_2) laser endoscopic resection, for hypopharyngeal cancer, 1429-1430, 1442
outcomes of, 1436-1438
Carbon dioxide (CO_2) laser resurfacing
complications of, 402
equipment for, 400, 400f
postoperative care after, 401-402
results of, 401f-402f
technique of, 400, 400f
Carbon ion therapy, 1046
Carbon monoxide, in noise-induced hearing loss, 2147-2148
Carbonated apatite (Norian CRS), for chin implants, 465t
Carbonic anhydrase inhibitors, for Meniere's disease, 2337
Carboplatin
in combination chemotherapy, 1059-1060
ototoxicity of, 2173-2174
sensorineural hearing loss due to, 2120, 2173-2174
Carcinoembryonic antigen (CEA)-targeted vaccine, for head and neck squamous cell carcinoma, 1024
Carcinoid tumors
of larynx
atypical, 1507
typical, 1507
of trachea, 1615, 1615f
Carcinoma ex pleomorphic adenoma, of salivary glands, 1187-1189, 1188f
Carcinoma in situ (CIS)
of larynx, 1486-1491, 1489f-1490f, 1515
treatment of, 1489-1490, 1520-1521
oropharyngeal, 1361
Carcinosarcoma
of larynx, 1506
of salivary glands, 1187, 1188f
Cardiac bulge, 2661f, 2691f
Cardiac disease, oral manifestations of, 1246-1249, 1249t
Cardiac output, of newborn, 2571
Cardiac transplantation, oral sequelae of, 1248
Cardiopulmonary bypass, sensorineural hearing loss due to, 2120
Cardiopulmonary complications
of obstructive sleep apnea, in children, 2604, 2604f
of sleep-disordered breathing, in children, 2792, 2792f
Cardiovascular disease, oral manifestations of, 1246-1249, 1249t
Cardiovascular manifestations, of hyperparathyroidism, 1781
Cardiovascular system
in children, 2571-2572
and blood volume, 2571
and newborn heart and cardiac output, 2571, 2571t
and oxygen transport, 2571-2572
and response to hypoxia, 2571
preoperative evaluation of, 102
Caregiver Impact Questionnaire, 57
Carina fully implantable hearing system, 2210-2211
clinical results with, 2210-2211
components of, 2210, 2210f
history of, 2210
placement of, 2210, 2211f
Carinal resections, 1619, 1621f-1622f
reconstruction after, 1619, 1623f
Caroticotympanic arteries, 1870
Caroticotympanic canaliculus, 1824f
Carotid arteriography, cross-compression, for cerebral blood flow evaluation, 2490
Carotid artery
in surgical anatomy of lateral skull base, 2436f, 2438
preoperative management of, 2489
algorithm for, 2490f, 2491-2492
cerebral blood flow assessment in, 2490-2491, 2490f
four-vessel arteriography in, 2489-2490, 2491f
tinnitus-producing fibromuscular dysplasia of, endovascular treatment for, 1943
Carotid artery aneurysms
of petrous apex, 2525, 2527f
upper cervical and petrous, 2504, 2504f-2505f
Carotid artery canal
anatomy of, 1824f
inferior foramen of, 1822-1823
in surgical anatomy of lateral skull base, 2435f-2436f, 2438
in surgical anatomy of middle cranial base, 2445f
Carotid artery hemorrhage, due to neck surgery, 1728
Carotid artery injury, due to temporal bone trauma, 2039, 2040f, 2047
Carotid artery invasion, imaging of, 166-167
Carotid artery pseudoaneurysm, due to deep neck space infections, 207
Carotid artery rupture, 1479
due to cranial base surgery, 2468-2469
due to deep neck space infections, 207
due to neck dissection, 1723-1724
due to neck surgery, 1728
due to radiotherapy, 1048
Carotid artery stenosis, due to neck irradiation, 1695
Carotid blowout syndrome, 1479
due to neck surgery, 1728
due to radiotherapy, 1048
Carotid body, 1658-1659
Carotid body tumors, 1657-1658, 1934-1935, 1935f
endovascular treatment of, 1937, 1937f

Carotid cavernous fistula, due to temporal bone trauma, 2047
Carotid gland, 1657-1658
Carotid groove
  in surgical anatomy of anterior cranial base, 2443f
  in surgical anatomy of middle cranial base, 2445f
Carotid ligation, in extended neck dissection, 1719-1721, 1720f
Carotid paragangliomas, 1657-1658, 2506f
  anatomy and physiology of, 1658-1659
  classification of, 1660
  clinical presentation and diagnosis of, 1659-1660
  etiology of, 1659, 1659t
  history of, 1657-1658
  imaging of, 1658f, 1660-1661
  malignancy of, 1660
  multicentricity of, 1660-1661
  observation for, 1661-1662
  radiation therapy for, 1661
  surgical management of, 1660-1661
Carotid prominence, in surgical anatomy of anterior cranial base, 2473
Carotid sheath, anatomy of, 202
  in children, 2578-2579, 2578f
Carotid sinus syndrome syncope, due to carotid paraganglioma, 1659
Carotid space (CS)
  anatomy of, 203
  imaging of, 150-151, 151f-152f
  schwannoma of, 1663f
Carotid stump pressure, for cerebral blood flow evaluation, 2490
Carotid triangle, 96, 96f, 2578f, 2579-2580
  arterial branches of, 2579-2580, 2580f
Carpenter's syndrome, craniofacial anomalies in, 2646
Cartilage grafts
  for nasal reconstruction, 368-369, 369f-370f
  for nasal tip projection, 535-536, 537f, 549-550, 550f-551f
  for revision rhinoplasty, 583, 584f
  for saddle nose deformity, 555, 556f
Cartilage plumping grafts, for nasal tip projection, 535-536, 536f
Cartilage struts, autogenous, for nasal tip projection, 535-536, 536f
Cartilage tympanoplasty, 2004-2005
Cartilage-mediated growth, in craniofacial growth and development, 2614
Cartilage-splitting approaches, for nasal tip refinement, 522, 523f-526f
Cartilaginous defect repair, biomaterials in, 2657-2658
Cartilaginous glottis, 849
Cartilaginous neoplasms, of larynx, 881-882
Cartilaginous vault rhinoplasty, 536-540
  access to nasal skeleton in, 537-539, 539f
  aesthetic improvement after, 537, 538f
  factors to consider in, 537
  incremental cartilaginous profile alignment in, 539
  mucoperichondrium in, 539-540
  pollybeak deformity due to, 512, 512f, 539, 539f
  for reduction of overlong caudal quadrangular cartilage, 513f
  with traumatic or iatrogenic avulsion of upper lateral cartilage, 539-540, 540f
Carved polymeric silicone (Silastic) implants, for medialization thyroplasty, 908-910, 910f
Carving template, in microtia reconstruction, 2744-2745, 2745f
Case series, 54-55, 54t
  data interpretation with, 59-61
Case-control study, 54, 54t
Caspases, in cisplatin ototoxicity, 2173
Casts, for prosthetic maxillary obturation, 1338-1339, 1338f
Cat scratch disease (CSD)
  in children, 2818
  deep neck space infections due to, 201
  salivary gland involvement in, 1159
Catagen phase, 374, 374f
CATCH-22, 2869
Catenary lever, 2018
Cathelicidins, 599
Catheters, angiographic, 1932-1933
Cauda-conchal sutures, 476f
Caudal extension graft
  in noncaucasian rhinoplasty, 576, 576f
  in revision rhinoplasty, 593
Caudal helix, 476f
Caudal septal deviation, revision rhinoplasty for persistence of, 593
Caudal septal excision, excessive, revision rhinoplasty for, 591f, 593
Caudal septum
  repositioning of, 547, 547f
  in septoplasty, 491-492, 491f-492f
    overaggressive resection of, 492, 492f
  shortening of, 547-548, 547f-548f
"Cauliflower deformity," 310
Caustic esophageal injury, 942, 977-978
  in children, 2956-2964
    algorithm for, 2962f
    endoscopy for, 2957-2959, 2958f
    epidemiology of, 2956
    initial assessment and diagnosis of, 2957
    pathophysiology of, 2956-2957
    signs and symptoms of, 2957b
    staging of, 2959, 2959f
    therapy for, 2959
      mechanical, 2960-2962, 2960f-2961f
      pharmacologic, 2959-2960
  clinical features of, 977
  etiology of, 977
  grading of, 977, 978t
  imaging of, 1404-1405, 1405f
  prognosis for, 977-978
  squamous cell carcinoma due to, 978
  strictures due to, 977-978, 978f-979f
    imaging of, 1405, 1405f
Caustic laryngeal trauma, 939-941
  etiology of, 940-941
  incidence of, 939-940
  management of, 941
Cautery, for epistaxis, 687-688, 687f
Ca$_v$1.3, in murine deafness, 2058t-2060t, 2080
Ca$_v$1.3 channels, 2080-2081
Caval mucosa, in sensation of nasal obstruction, 641-642
Cavernous hemangioma, 290
  epistaxis due to, 684f
Cavernous sinus meningiomas, embolization of, 1938
Cavernous sinus thrombosis
  due to deep neck space infections, 207
  due to odontogenic infections, 181, 182f
  preseptal orbital, 676
Cavernous sinus tumors, surgical approach for, 2509-2510
Cavernous venous sinus, 1699
Cavity dumped lasers, 34
Cavum conchae, 476-477, 1824f
CBF evaluation. *See* Cerebral blood flow (CBF) evaluation.
CBT (cognitive-behavioral therapy), for tinnitus, 2135
CC chemokines, 611t-612t
CCDC50 (coiled-coil domain–containing protein 50/Ymer) gene, in deafness, 2051t-2058t
CCL chemokines, 611t-612t
CCR (cervicocollic reflex), 2307-2308
CD4$^+$ cells, 601
CD8$^+$ cells, 601
CDH23 (cadherin 23), in tip links, 2074
CDH23 (cadherin 23) gene, in deafness, 2051t-2058t, 2074
Cdkn2d (cyclin-dependent kinase inhibitor 2D) gene, in murine deafness, 2058t-2060t
CDP. *See* Computerized dynamic posturography (CDP).
CEA (carcinoembryonic antigen)-targeted vaccine, for head and neck squamous cell carcinoma, 1024
CECT. *See* Contrast-enhanced computed tomography (CECT).
Cefazolin
  for endocarditis prophylaxis, 1249t
  for pediatric surgery prophylaxis, 2597t
Ceftazidime, for rhinosinusitis, 734
Ceftriaxone
  for endocarditis prophylaxis, 1249t
  for pediatric surgery prophylaxis, 2597t
Cefuroxime, for rhinosinusitis, 734t-735t
Celecoxib (Celebrex), for recurrent respiratory papillomatosis, 2892
Celiac disease, oral manifestations of, 1254
Cell cycle, 12, 13f
Cell cycle arrest, due to radiation, 1037, 1037f
Cell division, 12, 13f
Cell membrane, 1066-1067
Cell surface receptors, in salivary gland secretion, 1136-1137, 1136f, 1137t
Cell survival curve, with radiation therapy, 1037-1039, 1038f
Cell-mediated immune response, 602f
Cellular immunodeficiency disorders, 2114
  otologic manifestations of, 2114
Cellular recruitment, in allergic rhinitis, 616, 617f
Cellular systems, and skin flaps, 1065-1067, 1065f
Cellulitis
  of external ear, 1946, 1948
  orbital, due to odontogenic infections, 181, 182f
  retropharyngeal, 2810-2811, 2810f
  of sublingual space, 156, 157f
Censored data, 63t, 64
Center of gravity, in vestibular function, 2308
Centers for Medicare and Medicaid Services (CMS), 84t-87t, 87
Centor scoring system, for GABHS pharyngitis, 193
Central adaptation, and olfactory testing, 633
Central alveolar hypoventilation, 262t
Central apnea index, 251b
Central compartment dissection, 1719
  defined, 1719, 1719f
  technique for, 1719, 1720f
"Central face," concept of, 322
Central facial paralysis, 2401
Central gustatory pathways, 1212-1213, 1212f
Central midface, congenital malformations of nose due to developmental errors of, 2690-2693, 2691f
Central nervous system (CNS) changes, in Bell's palsy, 2393-2394
Central nervous system (CNS) infections, due to cranial base surgery, 2468
Central neural auditory prosthesis, 2258-2264
  alternative strategies to, 2263
  anatomy and surgical approaches for, 2260, 2261f
  auditory performance with, 2262
  biocompatibility of, 2259
  in children with cochlear nerve aplasia, 2263-2264
  complications of, 2260-2261
  history of clinical approaches to, 2259-2260, 2259f
  indications for, 2260

Central neural auditory prosthesis *(Continued)*
intraoperative monitoring of, 2260, 2261f
in patients without neurofibromatosis type 2, 2262
penetrating
brainstem, 2262, 2262f
midbrain, 2262-2263, 2263f
"Central sensitization," 1203
Central sleep apnea, 251b, 256f, 263, 263b
Central tendency, 64t, 66t
Central vestibular disorder(s), 2346-3
cerebellar ataxia syndromes as, 2356-2357
cervical vertigo as, 2354
of craniovertebral junction, 2354-2356
assimilation of atlas as, 2355
atlantoaxial dissociation as, 2355-2356
basilar impression as, 2355
Chiari malformation as, 2356, 2356f
classification of, 2355-2356
pathophysiology of, 2355
focal seizure disorders as, 2357
intracranial complications of otitic infections as, 2347
migraine as, 2347-2350
auditory symptoms of, 2348-2349
distortion as, 2349
hearing loss as, 2348-2349
phonophobia as, 2349
tinnitus as, 2349
without aura, 2347b
aura with, 2347, 2347b
basilar, 2349
diagnosis and classification of, 2347, 2347b
epidemiology of, 2347
etiology of, 2349
without headache, 2349
management of, 2349-2350, 2350f
with neurotologic symptoms, 2349
vestibular disorders associated with, 2350
benign paroxysmal positional vertigo as, 2350
Meniere's disease as, 2350
vestibular disorders related to, 2350-2351
benign paroxysmal vertigo of childhood as, 2350-2351
paroxysmal torticollis as, 2351
vestibular symptoms of, 2347-2348
motion sickness as, 2348
nonspecific dizziness as, 2347
vertigo as, 2347-2348, 2348f
multiple sclerosis as, 2356, 2356f
neoplastic, 2353-2354
of brainstem, 2353-2354
cerebellar, 2354
vestibular schwannomas as, 2353
normal pressure hydrocephalus as, 2357
peripheral *vs.*, 2346, 2347t
physiologic dizziness as, 2357
in mal de débarquement syndrome, 2357
in motion sickness, 2357
vascular, 2351-2353, 2351f
cerebellar hemorrhage as, 2354f
cerebellar infarction as, 2353f
evaluation and management of, 2354f-2355f
lateral medullary syndrome as, 2352f, 2354f
lateral pontomedullary syndrome as, 2353f
vertebrobasilar insufficiency as, 2355f
Centric fusion translocation, 5
Cephalexin
for endocarditis prophylaxis, 1249t
for pediatric surgery prophylaxis, 2597t
Cephalic phase insulin release (CPIR), 1206
Cephalic phase responses, 1206
Cephalic rotation, in nasal tip refinement, 519, 536, 549-550, 551f
Cephalocele, 670, 671f
of petrous apex, 2508
Cephalometric radiography
lateral, for mentoplasty, 463, 463f
of obstructive sleep apnea, 255, 255f
Cephalometric reference points, in facial analysis, 270b, 272f
Cephalosporins
for acute otitis media, 2770
adverse reactions to, 102
Cepstral peak prominence (CPP), in acoustic analysis, for voice evaluation, 829t, 830
Ceramic allografts, for ossiculoplasty, 2006
Ceramics, for craniofacial defect repair, 2657-2658
Cerebellar ataxia syndromes, 2356-2357
Cerebellar atrophy, 2357
Cerebellar degeneration, paraneoplastic, 2357
Cerebellar floccules, in surgical anatomy of lateral skull base, 2439f
Cerebellar hemispheres, in surgical anatomy of lateral skull base, 2439f
Cerebellar hemorrhage, 2354f
Cerebellar horizontal fissure, in surgical anatomy of lateral skull base, 2439f
Cerebellar infarction, 2353f
Cerebellar lesions, laryngologic manifestations of, 837-838, 838t
Cerebellar neoplasm, vestibular symptoms of, 2354
Cerebellar olive, in surgical anatomy of lateral skull base, 2439f
Cerebellopontine angle (CPA)
imaging of, 1926-1928, 1929t
with acoustic schwannoma, 1929t
with arachnoid cyst, 1928, 1929t
with epidermoid tumor, 1928, 1928f, 1929t
with lipoma, 1928, 1929t
with meningioma, 1928, 1928f, 1929t
in surgical anatomy of lateral skull base, 2438
Cerebellopontine angle (CPA) neoplasm(s)
acoustic neuroma as, 2514-2517
diagnostic studies of, 2516-2517
imaging of, 2517, 2517t-2518t
natural history of, 2515, 2515f-2516f
signs and symptoms of, 2515-2516
arachnoid cysts as, 2523-2524
vs. cholesteatoma (epidermoid), 2519, 2521f
imaging of, 1928, 1929t
chondrosarcomas as, 2527, 2528f-2529f
chordomas as, 2526-2527, 2527f-2528f
choroid plexus papilloma as, 2528-2529, 2530f
common, 2514-2524, 2515b
dermoid tumors as, 2527
differential diagnosis of, 2517t-2518t
ependymoma as, 2528-2529, 2531f
facial nerve neuroma as, 2519-2522
diagnostic studies of, 2519-2522
imaging of, 2519-2522, 2521f
signs and symptoms of, 2519
glomus tumors as, 2522-2523, 2523f-2524f
hemangiomas as, 2524, 2525f
intraoperative cranial nerve monitoring with, 2545
lipoma as, 2527, 2529f-2530f
imaging of, 1928, 1929t
meningiomas as, 2517-2518
diagnostic studies of, 2518
imaging of, 1928, 1928f, 2518, 2519f
in differential diagnosis, 1929t, 2518t
with intracanalicular extension, 2520f
sensorineural hearing loss due to, 2125, 2125f
signs and symptoms of, 2518
metastatic, 2526
other cranial nerve neuromas as, 2522, 2522f
primary cholesteatomas (epidermoids) as, 2518-2519
diagnostic studies of, 2519
differential diagnosis of, 2518t, 2524t
imaging of, 2519, 2520f-2521f
signs and symptoms of, 2518-2519
Cerebellopontine angle (CPA) neoplasm(s) *(Continued)*
retrocochlear
hearing loss due to, 2199
vertigo due to, 2202
teratomas as, 2527
uncommon, 2515b, 2526-2527
Cerebellopontine cistern, congenital epidermoid cyst of, 2509f
Cerebellum
afferent pathways to vestibular nuclei from, 1864
efferent pathways from vestibular nuclei to, 1864-1865
in vestibular function, 2308
vestibular nerve projections to, 1860
Cerebral blood flow (CBF) evaluation
prior to anterior and middle cranial base surgery, 2445-2446, 2446f
prior to lateral cranial base surgery, 2490-2491, 2490f
qualitative, 2490-2491
quantitative, 2491
"Cerebral congestion," 2329
Cerebral edema
after lateral skull base surgery, 2513
due to neck dissection, 1723
Cerebral palsy, and obstructive sleep apnea, 2605
Cerebritis, due to temporal bone infection, 1980t
Cerebrospinal fluid (CSF)
in Bell's palsy, 2394
with enlarged cochlear aqueduct, 2734
with enlarged vestibular aqueduct, 2733-2734
physiology of, 786
volume of, 786
Cerebrospinal fluid (CSF) drainage, posturography and, 2326
Cerebrospinal fluid (CSF) fistula(s)
bacterial meningitis due to, 794
due to cranial base surgery, 2468
CT cisternogram of, 2477f
traumatic, 2044-2046
antibiotic prophylaxis for, 2044-2045
closure of, 2045-2046, 2045f
diagnosis of, 2044
infecting organisms with, 2045
meningitis due to, 2044-2045
pathogenesis of, 2044
signs and symptoms of, 2044
treatment algorithm for, 2045-2046, 2045f
Cerebrospinal fluid (CSF) gusher
with wide internal auditory canal, 2735, 2735f
X-linked syndrome of stapes, 2737
Cerebrospinal fluid (CSF) leakage
due to inner ear anomalies, 2735-2737, 2736f
treatment of, 2737, 2739
due to otitis media, 1992-1993, 1993f
due to posterior fossa surgery, 2540
temporal bone, 2509
diagnostic evaluation of, 2509
surgical approach to, 2509
traumatic, 2044
Cerebrospinal fluid (CSF) otorrhea, 788, 2197
Cerebrospinal fluid (CSF) pressure, 786
Cerebrospinal fluid (CSF) rhinorrhea, 785-2
classification of, 786, 786b
complications of, 785
diagnosis of, 788
chemical markers in, 789-791
CSF tracers in, 790-791, 790f
CT cisternography in, 790, 790f
CT in, 791, 791f-792f
diagnostic testing in, 789-791
differential, 788-789
localization studies in, 791, 791f-792f
MR cisternography in, 790-791, 790f
MRI in, 791, 791f
nasal endoscopy in, 791

Cerebrospinal fluid (CSF) rhinorrhea *(Continued)*
patient history in, 789
physical examination in, 789
radionuclide cisternography in, 790
epidemiology of, 786
etiology of, 786, 786b
due to intraoperative injury, with immediate recognition or onset, 795
nontraumatic, 786b, 795
traumatic, 786b, 794-795
after functional endoscopic sinus surgery, 679-680, 680f
historical perspective on, 786
and intracranial pressure, 786-787, 786b
management of, 791-795
comprehensive strategy for, 794-795
conservative, 791-792, 792b
extracranial techniques for, 792-794, 793f-794f
precautions in, 794
transcranial techniques for, 792
maxillofacial trauma with, 326, 334-339
due to nasal fracture, 507
pathophysiology of, 786-788, 787f-788f
patient education on, 794
surgical management of, 742
Cerebrospinal fluid (CSF) tracers, for CSF rhinorrhea, 790-791, 790f-793f
Cerebrovascular accident (CVA)
chronic aspiration due to, 926b
due to lateral skull base surgery, 2512
oral manifestations of, 1250
Cerebrovascular complications
of cranial base surgery, 2468-2469
of lateral skull base surgery, 2512-2513
Cerebrovascular diseases, oral manifestations of, 1250
Certification, 79-80, 80b
maintenance of, 80, 81b
Cerumen impaction, 1957
therapy options for, 1957, 1958t, 2021
Cerumenex (docusate sodium), for cerumen removal, 1958t
Cerumenex (trolamine polypeptide oleate-condensate), for cerumen removal, 1958t
Ceruminolytics, 1957, 1958t
Cerumol (arachis oil, chlorbutol, paradicholorobenzene, oil of turpentine), for cerumen removal, 1958t
Cervical adenopathy. *See* Cervical lymphadenopathy.
Cervical branch, of facial nerve, 1194f
Cervical dissection, in postauricular approach to infratemporal fossa, 2495, 2498f
Cervical epidural anesthesia, 242
Cervical esophageal cancer
advanced, 1439
chemotherapy for, 1439
quality of life with, 1439
approach to management of, 1426
chemoradiotherapy for, 1434
chemotherapy for, 1433-1434
clinical evaluation of, 1423
physical findings in, 1423
presenting symptoms in, 1423, 1423t
fasciocutaneous free flaps for, 1433
gastric pull-up for, 1432, 1432f
imaging of, 1423-1424
barium swallow for, 1423-1424
CT for, 1424, 1424f
MRI for, 1424
PET/CT for, 1424, 1424f
incidence of, 1423
lymph node metastasis of, 1434-1439
pathology of, 1424-1425
radiation therapy for, 1436
therapeutic outcome of, 1436
Cervical esophageal cancer *(Continued)*
reconstruction for
with circumferential defects, 1431-1432
fasciocutaneous free flaps for, 1433
gastric pull-up in, 1432, 1432f
jejunal free flap for, 1432-1433, 1433f
staging of, 1426-1434, 1426t-1427t
therapeutic outcomes for, 1435-1436
total pharyngo-laryngo-esophagectomy for, 1430-1431
Cervical esophagus, 1421-1422
Cervical exploration, for parathyroid adenoma, 1792-1793
Cervical fascia, 2577
deep, 202, 2577-2578, 2578f-2579f
superficial, 202, 2577
surgical anatomy of, 1543f
Cervical lymph node(s)
anatomy of, 1683, 1683f, 1684t
classification of, 1683, 1683f, 1684t, 2582-2583
deep, 2582
superficial, 2582
Cervical lymph node groups, in neck dissection, 1703-1705
levels of, 1703-1705, 1704f, 1706t
radiologic anatomic markers in, 1705, 1707t-1708t
sublevels of, 1704-1705, 1705f, 1706t
Cervical lymph node metastasis(es), 1682-1695
anatomic basis for, 1683, 1683f, 1684t
of cervical esophageal cancer, 1434-1439
chemoradiation therapy for
postoperative, 1693-1694, 1694t
primary, 1693, 1693t
classification of, 1684t
in contralateral neck, 1688, 1690
of hypopharyngeal cancer, 1434-1439
incidence and distribution of, 1686f, 1688t
radiation therapy for, 1689t
imaging of
contrast-enhanced CT for, 164-165, 167f
of laryngeal carcinoma, 1476, 1479f
MRI for, 165-166, 168f
incidence and distribution of, 1684-1688
from clinical and radiologic assessment, 1684-1687, 1685f-1686f
in contralateral neck, 1688
from hypopharyngeal tumors, 1686f, 1688t
from nasopharyngeal tumors, 1687f
from oral cavity tumors, 1685f, 1688t
from oropharyngeal tumors, 1685f, 1688t
pathologic, 1687, 1688t
from supraglottic laryngeal tumors, 1686f, 1688t
of laryngeal carcinoma, 1493-1494, 1493f
embryology and, 1482-1483
glottic, 1497-1498
imaging of, 1476, 1479f
radiation therapy for, 1690t
subglottic, 1501, 1501f
supraglottic, 1500-1501
incidence and distribution of, 1686f, 1688t
of nasopharyngeal carcinoma, 1352-1353, 1353f
incidence and distribution of, 1687f
radiation therapy for, 1690, 1690t
neck control for
with N0 status, 1688, 1690, 1692, 1692t
with N1-N3 status, 1692-1695
postoperative irradiation or chemo-irradiation for, 1693-1694, 1694t
after primary radiotherapy, 1692-1693, 1693t
neck dissection for (*See* Neck dissection)
of oral cavity tumors
incidence and distribution of, 1685f, 1688t
radiation therapy for, 1689t
Cervical lymph node metastasis(es) *(Continued)*
of oropharyngeal cancer, 1360f, 1361t
incidence and distribution of, 1685f, 1688t
radiation therapy for, 1689t
of paranasal sinus tumors, 1130
radiation therapy for
indications for neck node dissection after, 1694
late complications of, 1694-1695
with N0 status, 1688, 1690, 1692, 1692t
with N1-N3 status, 1692-1695
neck control after, 1692-1693, 1693t
postoperative, 1693-1694, 1694t
of retropharyngeal nodes, 1688
target volumes for, 1688-1690
delineation of, 1690-1691, 1691f
for hypopharyngeal tumors, 1689t
for laryngeal tumors, 1690t
for nasopharyngeal tumors, 1690, 1690t
for oral cavity tumors, 1689t
for oropharyngeal tumors, 1689t
techniques for, 1691, 1692f
recurrent, 1695
postoperative, 1693-1694, 1694t
after primary radiation therapy, 1695
retropharyngeal, 1687-1688
of salivary gland tumors, 1196-1197
staging of, 1683-1684, 1684t
of thyroid cancer, 1766
Cervical lymphadenectomy. *See* Neck dissection.
Cervical lymphadenopathy
in children
bacterial, 2818, 2818f-2819f
drug-induced, 2819
fungal, 2818-2819
reactive, 2818
suppurative, 2818, 2818f
viral, 2817-2818
imaging of, 1414-1415, 1415f
CT of, 139
with extracapsular spread, 164-166, 167f
inflammatory (reactive), 164
with invasion of carotid artery, 166-167
metastatic
contrast-enhanced CT of, 164-165, 167f
MRI of, 165-166, 168f
MRI of, 142
with non-Hodgkin's lymphoma, 165-166, 167f
ultrasound of, 143
in immunosuppressed patients, 218-219, 219t
neck masses due to, 1638
in children
bacterial, 2818, 2818f-2819f
fungal, 2818-2819
viral, 2817-2818
Cervical lymphatics, 1312-1313, 1313f
Cervical plexus, 2581
ansa cervicalis of (*See* Ansa cervicalis)
anterior division of, 2579f
cutaneous branches of, 2578, 2580f
for facial nerve grafting, 2422
Cervical plexus block, superficial, 242
Cervical sensory nerve injuries, due to neck surgery, 1731-1732
Cervical skin flaps, for hypopharyngeal and esophageal reconstruction, 1450-1451
Cervical space infections. *See* Deep neck space infections.
Cervical vertigo, 2354
Cervicocollic reflex (CCR), 2307-2308
Cervicofacial advancement flap, for buccal carcinoma, 1309f
Cervital, for ossiculoplasty, 2026t
Cetirizine (Zyrtec)
for nonallergic rhinitis, 701t
for rhinosinusitis, 734t

Cetuximab (Erbitux)
for metastatic squamous cell carcinoma, 1061
with radiotherapy, 1052, 1054
for laryngeal cancer, 1585
CF. *See* Cystic fibrosis (CF).
CFD (computational fluid dynamics), CT with, 643
CFU. *See* Colony-forming unit (CFU).
CGH (comparative genomic hybridization), for head and neck squamous cell carcinoma, 1019
CGRP (calcitonin gene–related peptide)
in salivary gland secretion, 1137
and skin flap viability, 1073
Chalasia, cricopharyngeal, 1399
CHAMP procedure, auditory brainstem response in, 1911
Chance, *vs.* efficacy of treatment, 62t
CHAOS (congenital high airway obstruction syndrome), 2869, 2870f, 2904-2905
Characteristic frequency, 1844-1845, 1845f
Charcot-Leyden crystal (CLC) protein, 604
Charcot-Marie-Tooth syndrome, deafness in, 2051t-2058t
CHARGE association
facial paralysis in, 2397
inner ear anomalies in, 2735
Charged particle beams, in radiotherapy, 1034-1035
Check ligament, 321f
Cheek advancement flap, for nasal defects, 348, 349f
Cheek defects, 355-359
advancement flaps for, 358
V-Y, 358, 361f
rotation flaps for, 357-358, 359f
sub-superficial musculoaponeurotic system dissection for, 357-358, 360f
transposition flaps for, 358-359, 361f
bilobed, 357, 359f
rhombus shaped, 355
Cheek pedicle transposition flap, for nasal defects, 348, 349f
Cheilitis
angular, 1230, 1230f
in HIV, 225, 226f
solar (actinic), 283
Cheiloplasty, 2431, 2431f
Chelating agents, oral sequelae of, 1247t-1248t
Chemesthesis, of oral cavity, 1202
Chemical labyrinthectomy, for Meniere's disease, 2185-2189, 2338-2339, 2338f
Chemical markers, for CSF rhinorrhea, 789-790
Chemical peels, 391-397
agents for, 392-394
complications of, 396-397
contraindications to, 391, 392t
in dark-skinned individuals, 392
deep, 394-395
equipment tray for, 393f
histologic changes with, 390-391
indications for, 391, 392t
medium-depth, 393-394, 393f-394f
patient selection and education for, 391-392
and phenol toxicity, 395
postoperative care after, 396, 396f
prepeel preparations for, 392
superficial, 392-393, 403
Chemical shift artifact, on MRI, 134
Chemical shift selective presaturation, for MRI, 135-136, 136f
Chemical surgery, for skin lesions, 294
Chemodectomas, 1657. *See also* Paragangliomas (PGLs).
multiple, 1934-1935, 1935f
Chemokine(s)
in humoral immune response, 608, 611t-612t
in wound healing, 1076
Chemokine connective tissue–activating peptide-III (CTAP-III), in wound healing, 1076
Chemokine receptor 2 (CXCR2), in wound healing, 1076
Chemokine receptor 4 (CXCR4), in head and neck squamous cell carcinoma, 1060
Chemoprevention
of head and neck squamous cell carcinoma, 1018, 1061-1062
clinical implications of, 1018
of laryngeal cancer, 1491
of oral cancer, 1315
Chemoradiation therapy (CRT), 1041-1043, 1052-1058
for cervical lymph node metastasis
postoperative, 1693-1694, 1694t
primary, 1693, 1693t
concomitant, 1052-1056, 1053t-1054t
as adjuvant therapy, 1056
induction chemotherapy with, 1041-1042, 1052-1053
with adjuvant therapy, 1056
for esophageal carcinoma
definitive, 1445-1447, 1446t-1447t
preoperative, 1444-1445, 1445t
for hypopharyngeal cancer, 1434, 1439, 1442-1444
RADPLAT technique for, 1592
for laryngeal carcinoma, 1501-1503, 1502f
glottic
in advanced stage, 1584-1585, 1584t
with nodal metastases, 1498
optimal dose-fractionation scheme for, 1585-1586
outcomes and prognostic factors with, 1586-1587, 1587t
RADPLAT technique for, 1592
supraglottic, in advanced stage, 1500, 1589
for maxillary sinus tumor, 1130
for nasopharyngeal carcinoma, 1355, 1699f
neck dissection after, 1724
for oral cancer, 1314-1315
RADPLAT technique for, 1054
for laryngeal and hypopharyngeal cancer, 1592
swallowing disorders due to, 1219
for thyroid cancer, 1772
Chemosomatosensory-evoked potentials, 632
Chemotherapy, 1015
adjuvant, for oral cancer, 1314-1315
combination, 1059-1060
for esophageal carcinoma
localized, 1444
metastatic, 1447
historical background of, 1051-1052
for hypopharyngeal cancer, 1433-1434, 1442
advanced, 1439
induction, 1443
for larynx preservation, 1443-1444
induction, 1056-1058, 1058f, 1058t-1059t
clinical trials of, 1056-1058
in concomitant chemoradiation, 1041-1042, 1052-1053
with adjuvant therapy, 1056
defined, 1056
for hypopharyngeal cancer, 1443
for laryngeal carcinoma, 1501-1503, 1502f
for oral cancer, 1314-1315
intra-arterial, 1939
for laryngeal carcinoma
early glottic, 1520
neoadjuvant, 1501-1503, 1502f
for melanoma, 1118
neoadjuvant, for laryngeal carcinoma, 1501-1503, 1502f
for oral cancer, 1314-1315
with radiation therapy (*See* Chemoradiation therapy (CRT))
Chemotherapy *(Continued)*
radiosensitizing, 1040-1043
for recurrent or metastatic disease, 1058-1061
combination, 1059-1060
prognostic factors with, 1058-1059
single agent, 1059
for rhabdomyosarcoma, 2841
for salivary gland neoplasms, 1199
single agent, 1059
for thyroid cancer, 1772
Chemotherapy resistance, gene therapy for, 24
CHEP. *See* Cricohyoidoepiglottopexy (CHEP).
Cherry angiomas, 290
Chest pain, due to esophageal disease states, 956, 971
Chest voice, 846-847, 851
Chest wall displacement, in voice evaluation, 828
Chest x-ray (CXR)
of early glottic carcinoma, 1516
for imaging of pharynx and esophagus, 1393
for neck masses, 1637
Chiari malformation, 2356, 2356f
Chiasmatic sulcus, in surgical anatomy of anterior cranial base, 2472f
Chief cell(s), 1778
Chief cell hyperplasia, of parathyroid glands, 1779
Chief complaint, 94, 94b
Child Health and Illness Profile–Child Edition (CHIP-CE), 57
Child Health Questionnaire (CHQ), 57
Childhood, benign paroxysmal vertigo of, and migraine, 2350-2351
Children
acute otitis media and otitis media with effusion in, 2761-2777
complications and sequelae of, 2776-2777
intracranial, 2776-2777
intratemporal, 2776
diagnosis of, 2761-2762
audiometry in, 2762
immittance testing (tympanometry) in, 2762
physical examination in, 2761-2762
symptoms and signs in, 2761
epidemiology of, 2765-2768
incidence and prevalence of, 2765-2766, 2765f
risk factors in, 2766-2768
trend over time in, 2765-2766
guidelines for, 2773
pathophysiology and pathogenesis of, 2762-2765, 2762f
allergy and immunology in, 2764-2765
eustachian tube function in, 2762-2763, 2763f
gastroesophageal reflux in, 2765
infection in, 2763-2764, 2764f
prevention of, 2768-2769
antibiotic prophylaxis for, 2771
management of environmental factors in, 2768
vaccines in, 2768-2769
quality of life assessment for, 2773
recurrent, 2771
treatment of, 2770-2773
medical, 2770-2772
observation in, 2770-2771
for recurrent disease, 2771
surgical, 2771-2776
adenotonsillar disease in, 2782-2802
adenoidectomy for, 2795-2796
indications for, 2795-2796
and otitis media, 2796
adenotonsillectomy for (*See* Adenotonsillectomy)
anatomy of, 2783-2784
due to bacterial infections, 2785-2788
due to candidiasis, 2786

Children *(Continued)*
chronic adenotonsillar hypertrophy as, 2790-2793
airway obstruction due to, 2789f-2790f, 2790-2793, 2795
algorithm for evaluation of, 2783f-2784f
with attention deficit–hyperactivity disorder, 2791
cardiopulmonary complications of, 2792, 2792f
craniofacial growth and, 2792-2793
diagnostic assessment of, 2793-2794, 2793f
and enuresis, 2792
etiology of, 2789f-2790f, 2790
and growth problems, 2792
and neurocognitive development, 2791-2792
and obstructive sleep apnea, 2790-2793
complications of, 2788-2790
nonsuppurative, 2788
parapharyngeal space abscess as, 2788-2789
peritonsillar infections as, 2788, 2789f
retropharyngeal space infections as, 2789-2790, 2789f
suppurative, 2788-2790
due to *Corynebacterium diphtheriae*, 2786-2787
diagnostic assessment for, 2793-2794, 2793f
history of, 2782
imaging of, 2793-2794, 2793f
immunology of, 2784-2785
due to infections of Waldeyer's ring, 2785
management algorithms for, 2782, 2783f-2784f
microbiology of, 2785-2788
due to *Neisseria gonorrhoeae*, 2786
preoperative assessment for, 2794
due to streptococcal infection, 2787
due to syphilis, 2786
due to tonsillar concretions/tonsilloliths, 2787-2788, 2788f
due to Vincent's angina, 2786
due to viral infections, 2785-2786, 2786f
with Epstein-Barr virus, 2785-2786, 2786f
airway infection(s) in, 2803-2811
bacterial tracheitis (exudative tracheitis) as, 2809-2810
clinical features of, 2809
complications of, 2810
diagnosis of, 2809, 2809f
differential diagnosis of, 2806t
endoscopy of, 2809, 2809f
epidemiology of, 2809
imaging of, 2809, 2809f
management of, 2809-2810, 2809f
pathogenesis of, 2809
terminology for, 2809
croup (laryngotracheitis) as, 2803-2806
clinical features of, 2803-2804
defined, 2803
diagnosis of, 2804
differential diagnosis of, 2804-2805, 2806t
epidemiology of, 2803
etiology of, 2803
imaging of, 2804, 2804f-2805f
laryngoscopy of, 2804, 2805f
management of, 2805-2806
pathogenesis of, 2803-2804
spasmodic, 2805
terminology for, 2803
retropharyngeal abscess as, 2810-2811
anatomy of, 2810
clinical features of, 2810
complications of, 2811
diagnosis of, 2810-2811, 2810f-2811f
differential diagnosis of, 2806t
epidemiology of, 2810
historical background of, 2810

Children *(Continued)*
imaging of, 2810-2811, 2810f-2811f
management of, 2811
supraglottitis (epiglottitis) as, 2806-2809
clinical features of, 2807
complications of, 2808-2809
diagnosis of, 2807-2808, 2807f-2808f
differential diagnosis of, 2806t
endoscopy of, 2808, 2808f
epidemiology of, 2806-2807
etiology of, 2807
histology of, 2807, 2807f
historical background of, 2806-2807
imaging of, 2807f, 2808
management of, 2808
anesthesia in, 2575, 2587-2601
for adenotonsillectomy, 2598-2599, 2599b
emergence from, 2592-2593
induction of, 2589-2591
inhalation, 2590
intramuscular, 2591
intravenous, 2590
parental presence during, 2590
rapid-sequence, 2590
intraoperative monitoring standards for, 2588, 2588b
for laryngeal surgery, 2599-2600
maintenance of, 2591-2592
inhalational agents for, 2591
intravenous agents for, 2591, 2593t
medical condition(s) affecting, 2594-2597
asthma as, 2595
congenital heart disease as, 2596-2597, 2596t-2597t
cystic fibrosis as, 2595
diabetes mellitus as, 2596
prematurity as, 2595
upper respiratory infection as, 2594-2595
outside of operating room, 2594
postoperative management of, 2593-2594
for nausea and vomiting, 2593
for pain, 2594
for postintubation croup, 2593
preoperative assessment for, 2588
preparation for, 2588-2589
behavioral, 2588-2589, 2589t
nothing-by-mouth orders in, 2589, 2590t
premedication in, 2589
for rigid bronchoscopy, 2597-2598, 2597t
risks of, 2587-2588
audiology in, 2574
Bell's palsy in, 2397
cardiovascular system in, 2571-2572
and blood volume, 2571
and newborn heart and cardiac output, 2571, 2571t
and oxygen transport, 2571-2572
and response to hypoxia, 2571
caustic ingestion in, 2956-2964
algorithm for, 2962f
endoscopy for, 2957-2959, 2958f
epidemiology of, 2956
initial assessment and diagnosis of, 2957
pathophysiology of, 2956-2957
signs and symptoms of, 2957b
staging of, 2959, 2959f
therapy for, 2959
mechanical, 2960-2962, 2960f-2961f
pharmacologic, 2959-2960
chronic sinusitis in, 2778-2781
cultures for, 2779
etiology of, 2778-2779
imaging of, 2779
irrigation for, 2779
medical management of, 2779
surgical management of, 2779-2781, 2780f-2781f

Children *(Continued)*
cochlear implants in, 2224-2226, 2239-2240
audiologic protocol for, 2225, 2234-2235
auditory rehabilitation with, 2254-2255
current trends that affect, 2226
ear selection in, 2226
factors that affect performance in, 2226
and language development, 2239-2240
other evaluations for, 2225
outcome expectations for, 2225-2226
recommendations for referral for, 2226
residual hearing and, 2240
results of, 2246
auditory performance assessments for, 2246
early studies of speech reception in, 2246
for educational placement and support, 2251-2253, 2251f, 2255-2256
for language acquisition, 2249-2251, 2250f
more recent studies of speech reception in, 2246-2247, 2247f
quality-of-life studies for, 2252-2253, 2253f
selection criteria for, 2225-2226
surgical techniques for, 2240
conductive hearing loss in, 2026-2027
with congenital anomalies, 2573
dysphagia in, 2948-2955
anatomic site(s) of, 2949-2954, 2951f
hypopharynx and larynx as, 2950t, 2951-2953, 2953f
nose and nasopharynx as, 2949, 2950t, 2951f
oral cavity and oral pharynx as, 2949-2951, 2950t, 2952f
trachea and esophagus as, 2950t, 2953-2954, 2954f
evaluation of, 2948-2949
clinical or bedside, 2948-2949
instrumental, 2949, 2950t
other diagnostic tests in, 2949
epistaxis in, 686
facial fractures in, 2647, 2697-2717
anesthesia for, 304
associated injuries with, 2698
clinical and physical evaluation of, 2699
complex, 2698
dentoalveolar, 2706-2707, 2710f
emergency management of, 2698-2699
epidemiology of, 2697-2698
etiology of, 2698
facial growth and, 2698-2699
front sinus, 2711, 2712f
mandibular, 2704-2706
arch and body, 2706, 2709f
complications of, 2704
condylar and subcondylar, 2704, 2706f-2708f
epidemiology of, 2698
symphyseal and parasymphyseal, 2704-2706, 2708f-2709f
mandibular immobilization for, 2701, 2701f
maxillomandibular fixation for, 2701
midface, 2707, 2710f
nasal, 2708-2711, 2711f-2712f
naso-orbitoethmoid, 2714
classification of, 2714, 2716f
evaluation of, 2714, 2716f
repair of, 2714, 2716f
open reduction with internal fixation for, 2701-2702
orbital, 2711-2714
evaluation of, 2712, 2713f
of lateral/medial orbital wall, 2712, 2714, 2716f
of orbital apex, 2712, 2713f
of orbital floor, 2712-2713, 2714f-2715f
of orbital roof, 2712-2713, 2716f
patterns of, 2711-2712
permanent *vs.* resorbable plating systems for, 2700-2701, 2700t-2701t

Children *(Continued)*
radiologic examination of, 2699
rigid fixation for, 2699-2700
sequencing of procedures for, 2702, 2704, 2706f
surgical approaches for, 2701-2704
bicoronal incision in, 2701-2702, 2703f
lateral cantholysis in, 2704f
maxillary gingivolabial sulcus approach in, 2701-2702, 2703f
midfacial degloving incision in, 2701-2702
subciliary incision in, 2705f
surgical approaches for, 2701-2704
transcaruncular approach in, 2701-2702, 2705f
surgical management of, 2648, 2649f, 2657
surgical reconstruction for, 2704-2714
zygomaticomalar complex, 2707-2708, 2710f
flexible endoscopy in, 2574
fluids and fluid management in, 2572
and expected fluid losses, 2572t
and fluid utilization during bed rest, 2572t
and ideal electrolyte composition for infants, 2572t
foreign bodies of airway and esophagus in, 2935-2943
acute airway obstruction due to, 2936-2937
complications of, 2942, 2942f
epidemiology of, 2936
esophageal perforation due to, 2941
imaging of, 2938-2939, 2938f-2939f
location of, 2936, 2936f-2937f
management of, 2939-2941
anesthesia for, 2940
controversies in, 2942
for disk batteries, 2941
equipment for, 2939-2940, 2939t, 2940f
historical background of, 2935-2936
for pills, 2941
postoperative, 2941-2942
for sharp objects, 2940-2941
technique for, 2940, 2941f
symptoms of, 2937-2938
general considerations with, 2569-2576
GERD-related laryngeal disease in, 2944-2947
diagnosis of, 2945
disorders due to, 2945-2946, 2945b
evidence of, 2946
history of, 2944
management of, 2946
physiopathology of, 2945
head and neck malignancies in, 2835-2849
vs. adults, 2835
age and, 2837, 2837t
clinical trials for, 2836
epidemiology of, 2835
histiocytoses as, 2847-2848, 2847t
lymphoma as
Hodgkin's, 2838-2840, 2840f
non-Hodgkin's, 2837, 2838t-2839t, 2839f
neuroectodermal, 2844-2845
neuroblastomas as, 2844-2845, 2844t, 2845f
peripheral primitive, 2845
pathologic evaluation of, 2836-2837, 2836f, 2837t
post-transplantation lymphoproliferative disorder as, 2840
risk factors for, 2835
salivary gland, 2845-2846, 2846f
sarcoma as, 2840-2843
dermatofibrosarcoma protuberans as, 2843, 2843f
epithelioid, 2843, 2843f
Ewing's, 2845
fibro-, 2842-2843, 2843f
nonrhabdomyosarcoma soft tissue, 2842
rhabdomyo-, 2840-2842, 2841t, 2842f

Children *(Continued)*
sequelae of management of, 2848
survival with, 2835-2836
teratomas as, 2846-2847
epidemiology of, 2846
histopathology and molecular biology of, 2847, 2847f
management of, 2846
presentation and evaluation of, 2846, 2846t
thyroglossal duct carcinomas as, 2847
tumorigenesis of, 2836
hearing aids in, 2274
bone-anchored, 2215
history taking with, 2573
hospital for, 2575
laryngeal stenosis in, 2912-2924
anterior glottic, 2922
anterior subglottic, 2923
due to atresia and webs, 2922
diagnosis of, 2916-2917
endoscopic examination in, 2916-2917
esophagogastroduodenoscopy and biopsy in, 2917
evaluation of GERD and GLPRD in, 2917
functional endoscopic evaluation of swallowing in, 2917
history and physical examination in, 2916
pulmonary function tests in, 2917
radiologic evaluation in, 2916
voice assessment in, 2917
etiology and pathophysiology of, 2912-2916
acquired, 2914-2915
congenital, 2912-2913, 2913f
grading of, 2917, 2917t
management of, 2917-2921
algorithm for, 2913f
anterior cricoid split operation for, 2918-2919, 2918f-2919f
autogenous costal cartilage reconstruction in, 2919-2920, 2920f-2921f
combined laryngofissure and posterior cricoid division for, 2919, 2919f
cricoid resection with thyrotracheal anastomosis for, 2921, 2922f
decannulation after, 2923
endoscopic, 2918
external expansion surgery for, 2919-2921
grafts in, 2919
postoperative, 2923
single-stage laryngotracheal reconstruction for, 2920-2921
stents in, 2920
posterior glottic, 2922-2923
prevention of, 2916
types of, 2915, 2915f-2916f
with vocal cord paralysis, 2922
laryngeal trauma in, 938
microscopic examination of ear in, 2574
nasal fractures in, 506-507
neck mass(es) in, 2812-2821
acquired, 2817-2819
bacterial lymphadenopathy as, 2818, 2818f-2819f
benign neoplasms as, 2819
drug-induced lymphadenopathy as, 2819
due to fungal infections, 2818-2819
in Kawasaki disease, 2819
malignant neoplasms as, 2819-2820, 2820f
in sarcoidosis, 2819
sialadenitis as, 2819
in sinus histiocytosis, 2819
viral lymphadenopathy as, 2817-2818
algorithm for differential diagnosis of, 2813f
biopsy of, 2814
congenital, 2814-2817
branchial cleft cysts as, 2814, 2814f-2815f
dermoid cysts as, 2816, 2816f-2817f

Children *(Continued)*
hemangiomas as, 2816, 2816f
laryngoceles as, 2816-2817
lymphatic malformations (lymphangiomas) as, 2815, 2817f
sternocleidomastoid tumors of infancy as, 2817, 2817f
teratomas as, 2816, 2816f
thymic cysts as, 2817
thyroglossal duct cysts as, 2814-2815, 2815f
vascular malformations as, 2817
history of, 2812
imaging of, 2813-2814
laboratory studies for, 2814
physical examination of, 2812-2813
needle biopsy in, 2574
obstructive sleep apnea in, 2602-2612
acute-onset or rapidly progressive, 2606
vs. adults, 2603, 2603t
anesthesia with, 2598, 2599b
complications of, 2603-2604
behavior and learning problems as, 2603-2604
cardiopulmonary, 2604, 2604f
growth impairment as, 2603
diagnosis of, 2606-2608
history in, 2606
other studies in, 2607-2608
physical examination in, 2606
polysomnography in, 2606-2607, 2607f, 2607t
epidemiology of, 2603
nonsurgical management of, 2610-2611
pathophysiology of, 2604-2605
polysomnography in, 2606-2607, 2607f, 2607t
indications for, 2608
risk factors for, 2605-2606, 2605t
craniofacial abnormalities as, 2605
mucopolysaccharidoses as, 2606
neuromuscular disease as, 2605-2606
obesity as, 2605
surgical management of, 2608-2610
craniofacial surgery in, 2610, 2610f
other pharyngeal surgery in, 2609-2610
other types of, 2610
tonsillectomy or adenoidectomy in, 2608-2609
tracheotomy in, 2610
olfactory testing in, 632-633
outcome scales for, 56t, 57
pain management in, 2572
paranasal sinus neoplasms in, 1132
parents of, 2573
as patients, 2573
pharyngitis in, 2782, 2783f-2784f
physical examination of, 2574
postoperative management of, 2575
preparation for hospitalization and surgery of, 2574-2575
primary snoring in, 2602-2603
referral sources for, 2572-2573
respiratory system of, 2569-2570
and control of ventilation, 2569-2570
and laryngospasm, 2570
and lung volumes, 2570
and respiratory rate, 2570
and ventilation-perfusion relationships, 2570, 2571t
rhinomanometry for, 645
rhinosinusitis in, 737
salivary gland disease in, 2850-2865
aberrant salivary glands as, 2864, 2864f
due to allergic reactions, 2864
anatomy and, 2850-2853
autoimmune, 2858-2863

Children *(Continued)*
benign lymphoepithelial, 2858
biopsy for, 2855
congenital, differential diagnosis of, 2851t
in cystic fibrosis, 2864
cysts and mucoceles as, 2859
acquired, 2859
congenital, 2859
differential diagnosis of, 2850, 2851t, 2852f-2853f
history and physical examination for, 2853
imaging of, 2854-2855
inflammatory, 2855-2858
abscess as, 2856
due to actinomycosis, 2858
bacterial, 2856-2857, 2856t
diagnostic algorithm for, 2853, 2854f
differential diagnosis of, 2851t
due to Epstein-Barr virus, 2855
granulomatous, 2857-2858, 2857f
due to HIV, 2856
due to mumps, 2855
mycobacterial, 2857-2858, 2857f
sarcoidosis as, 2858
viral, 2855
laboratory studies for, 2853-2854
due to medications, 2864-2865
necrotizing sialometaplasia as, 2857
neoplastic, 1192, 2861-2862, 2862t
benign, 2861-2862
differential diagnosis of, 2851t
malignant, 2862-2863
parotitis as, juvenile recurrent, 2858
sialadenitis as, 2819
acute suppurative, 2856, 2856t
bacterial, 2856-2857, 2856t
chronic, 2858
neonatal, 2857
recurrent, 2856-2857
viral, 2855
sialadenoscopy for, 2855
sialolithiasis as, 2858-2859
sialorrhea as, 2863-2864
in Sjögren's syndrome, 2858
in systemic conditions, 2864-2865
traumatic, 2863-2865
vascular anomalies as, 2859
hemangiomas as, 2859-2860, 2860f
lymphatic malformations as, 2860-2861, 2861f
sedation of, 2572, 2594
sleep-disordered breathing in, 2602-2612
and ADHD, 2791
cardiopulmonary complications of, 2792
classification of, 2602
and enuresis, 2792
and growth problems, 2792
and neurocognitive development, 2791-2792
primary snoring as, 2602-2603
upper airway resistance syndrome as, 2602-2603
stridulous (*See* Stridulous child)
thyroid neoplasms in, 1769-1770
tracheal stenosis in, 2925-2934
anomalies associated with, 2927
due to arterial compression, 2925-2926
classification of, 2927, 2927t
conservative management of, 2927-2928
diagnosis of, 2926-2927
dilation for, 2928, 2928f
embryology of, 2925-2926
endoscopic evaluation of, 2926-2927
imaging of, 2927
laser therapy for, 2928, 2929f
long-segment, 2926, 2926f
treatment of, 2934

Children *(Continued)*
open repair for, 2930-2934
complications of, 2934
costal cartilage tracheoplasty as, 2930-2931, 2931f
granulation at graft site with, 2931
long-segment, 2934
partial tracheal resection, posterior end-to-end anastomosis, and anterior repair with resected trachea in, 2933-2934
pericardial patch in, 2930, 2931f
segmental resection in, 2931-2932, 2932f
short-segment, 2934
slide tracheoplasty in, 2932-2933, 2933f
synthetic tracheal prostheses in, 2934, 2934f
tracheal homograft transplantation in, 2933, 2934f
wedge resection in, 2931, 2931f
short-segment, 2926, 2926f
treatment of, 2934
stents for, 2928-2930, 2930f
due to vascular rings, 2925
tympanoplasty in, 2005
upper airway resistance syndrome in, 2602-2603
voice disorder(s) in, 2876-2883
evaluation of, 2876-2878
aerodynamic analysis in, 2878
algorithm for, 2877f
computer-assisted voice analysis for, 2878, 2878f
history in, 2876
physical examination in, 2876-2877
for social and functional impact, 2876
speaking tasks in, 2877-2878
stroboscopic examination in, 2877
voice profile in, 2878
functional, 2876, 2879
incidence of, 2876
organic, 2876, 2879
of resonance, 2879
of vocal quality
due to cricoarytenoid joint fixation, 2880
due to epidermoid cysts, 2882, 2882f
due to granuloma, 2881, 2881f
due to laryngeal web, 2880, 2880f
due to malignant tumors, 2881
medical management of, 2881
due to posterior glottic stenosis, 2880
due to recurrent respiratory papillomatosis, 2880-2881
due to sulcus vocalis, 2882
surgical management of, 2879-2881
due to vocal fold paralysis, 2879-2880
due to vocal fold polyps, 2882
due to vocal nodules, 2881-2882, 2882f
voice therapy for, 2881-2882
voice therapy for, 2878-2879, 2881-2882
Chin
aesthetic analysis of, 275, 278f
double, liposuction for (*See* Liposuction)
senile ptosis of, 465, 466f
witch's, 465, 466f
Chin deformities
mentoplasty for (*See* Mentoplasty)
senile, 465, 466f
types of, 465, 466f
Chin implants, 465-467
anesthesia for, 465
clinical example of, 470, 471f
complications after, 470
dissection planes for, 465-467, 467f
incision and approach for, 465-467, 467f
intraoral approach for, 467
subperiosteal *vs.* supraperiosteal placement of, 465-467, 467f
surgical procedure for, 465-467
types of, 465, 465t, 467

CHIP-CE (Child Health and Illness Profile–Child Edition), 57
Chlamydia pneumoniae, pharyngitis due to, 194
Chlorbutol, for cerumen removal, 1958t
Chloride (Cl^-), in saliva, 1139
Chloride/bicarbonate (Cl^-/HCO_3^-) exchanger, in salivary gland secretion, 1135
Chloroma, 2107
Chloroquine
ototoxicity of, 2176
sensorineural hearing loss due to, 2120
Chlorpheniramine (Chlor-Trimeton), for nonallergic rhinitis, 701t
Choanal atresia, 2694-2695
bilateral, 2694-2695, 2694f-2695f
clinical presentation of, 2694
endoscopic evaluation of, 2694, 2695f
epidemiology of, 2694
imaging of, 2694, 2694f, 2905f
rhinitis due to, 619b
sinus surgery for, 742
treatment of, 2694-2695, 2695f, 2905
unilateral, 2694-2695, 2694f
Choanal stenosis, rhinitis due to, 619b
Choking, due to abnormal swallow, 1217
Cholesteatoma, 97
acquired, 1964-1965
diagnosis of, 1965, 1965f-1966f
otorrhea due to, 2196
pathogenesis of, 1966
anterior epitympanic, 1968, 1969f
of cerebellopontine angle, 2518-2519
diagnostic studies of, 2519
differential diagnosis of, 1929t, 2518t, 2519, 2524t
imaging of, 2519, 2520f-2521f
signs and symptoms of, 2518-2519
chronic otitis media with, 1964-1969
acquired, 1964-1966, 1965f-1966f
anterior epitympanic, 1968, 1969f
bone erosion in, 1971-1974, 1972f-1973f
complications of, 1968, 1969b
congenital, 1964-1966, 1966f
diagnosis of, 1965, 1965f-1966f
epidemiology of, 1965
management of, 1968-1969, 1969t, 1970b
pathogenesis of, 1965-1968, 1967f
posterior mesotympanic, 1968, 1968f
sensorineural hearing loss due to, 1974
chronic otitis media without, 1969-1971
diagnosis of, 1969, 1970f
management of, 1971
pathogenesis of, 1970-1971, 1971f, 1971t
congenital, 1964-1965
and congenital aural atresia, 2754
diagnosis of, 1965, 1966f
pathogenesis of, 1965-1966
of temporal bone, 2508-2509
diagnostic evaluation of, 2508, 2509f-2510f
surgical approach to, 2508-2509
defined, 1964-1965
diagnosis of, 1965, 1965f-1966f
of external auditory canal, 1949
imaging of, 1917, 1918f
labyrinthine fistula due to, 1989-1990, 1990f
mastoidectomy for, 1969, 1970t, 2014-2015
of middle ear, imaging of
acquired, 1919, 1920f
congenital, 1918-1919, 1919f-1920f
with CT, 174f, 1919f-1920f
with MRI, 1919, 1920f-1921f
pathogenesis of, 1965-1968, 1967f
acquired, 1966
basal cell hyperplasia theory of, 1966-1967, 1967f
congenital, 1965-1966
epithelial invasion theory of, 1967f, 1968

Cholesteatoma *(Continued)*
invagination theory of, 1966, 1967f
squamous metaplasia theory of, 1967f, 1968
of petrous apex, 1924t
drainage of, 2508
posterior mesotympanic, 1968, 1968f
properties of, 1968
retraction pocket, 1965-1966, 1965f, 1967f
of temporal bone
congenital, 2508-2509
diagnostic evaluation of, 2508, 2509f-2510f
surgical approach to, 2508-2509
traumatic, 2038, 2047
with tympanostomy tubes, 2775
Cholesterol, serum
and presbycusis, 232
subclinical hypothyroidism and, 1747
Cholesterol cysts, 2508, 2510f
Cholesterol granuloma
vs. cholesteatoma, 2508, 2510f
of petrous apex, 2524-2525
differential diagnosis of, 1924t, 2515, 2524t
imaging of, 1923, 1925f-1926f, 2477f, 2526f
of skull base, 171, 172f
transmastoid infralabyrinthine drainage of, 2540f
Cholestyramine
for Graves' disease, 1742-1743
for hyperthyroidism, 1739t
Choline salicylate and glycerol (Earex Plus, Audax), for cerumen removal, 1958t
Cholinergic receptors, in salivary gland secretion, 1136-1137
Chondritis, of external ear, 1946, 1948
Chondrocranium-basicranium, 2619
Chondrodermatitis nodularis helicis, 285, 285f
Chondroma
of larynx, 881-882
of trachea, 1612-1613
Chondrosarcoma(s)
of cerebellopontine angle, 2527, 2528f-2529f
of larynx, 1508
of neck, 1669-1670
of paranasal sinuses, 1131
of petrous apex, 2528f
of skull base, 1699, 1923-1924, 1926f, 2529f
Chorda tympani nerve
anatomy of, 1296f, 1297
in surgical anatomy of lateral skull base, 2436f, 2439f, 2441
in taste, 1208, 1211
Chorda tympani nerve damage, due to small fenestra stapedotomy, 2034
Chordoma(s)
of cerebellopontine angle, 2526-2527, 2527f-2528f
of clivus, 2481f, 2510, 2511f
cranial, 2510, 2511f
of nasopharynx, 1351
of petrous apex, 2511f
of skull base, 1699
Choristoma, salivary gland, of middle ear, 2200-2201
Choroid plexus, 2404f
in surgical anatomy of lateral skull base, 2439f
Choroid plexus papillomas, 2528-2529, 2530f
CHP. *See* Cricohyoidopexy (CHP).
CHQ (Child Health Questionnaire), 57
Chromosomal disorders, 4-5
aneuploidies as, 5
rearrangements as, 4-5
Chromosomal rearrangements, 4-5
Chromosome(s), 3
number of, 2088
segregation of, 2088
Chronic adenotonsillar hypertrophy, in children, 2790-2793
with ADHD, 2791
airway obstruction due to, 2789f-2790f, 2790-2793, 2795
algorithm for evaluation of, 2783f-2784f
cardiopulmonary complications of, 2792, 2792f
craniofacial growth and, 2792-2793
diagnostic assessment of, 2793-2794, 2793f
and enuresis, 2792
etiology of, 2789f-2790f, 2790
and growth problems, 2792
and neurocognitive development, 2791-2792
and obstructive sleep apnea, 2790-2793
Chronic obstructive pulmonary disease (COPD), oral manifestations of, 1250
Chronic otitis media (COM), 1981
bacteriology of, 1981
with cholesteatoma, 1964-1969
acquired, 1964-1966, 1965f-1966f
anterior epitympanic, 1968, 1969f
bone erosion in, 1971-1974, 1972f-1973f
complications of, 1968, 1969b
congenital, 1964-1966, 1966f
diagnosis of, 1965, 1965f-1966f
epidemiology of, 1965
management of, 1968-1969, 1969t, 1970b
pathogenesis of, 1965-1968, 1967f
posterior mesotympanic, 1968, 1968f
sensorineural hearing loss due to, 1974
without cholesteatoma, 1969-1971
diagnosis of, 1969, 1970f
management of, 1971
pathogenesis of, 1970-1971, 1971f, 1971t
complications of, 1981 (*See also* Temporal bone infections, complications of)
defined, 1981
perilymph fistula due to, 2342-2343
suppurative, cochlear implant for, 2221
with tympanostomy tubes, 1970-1971, 1981
Chronic rhinosinusitis (CRS)
acute exacerbation of, 705, 707, 707f
surgical management of, 741
bacterial, 732, 733f
defined, 705, 728-729
frontal, 775-783
fungal, 732-733
allergic, 707
invasive, 711
nonallergic, 715-716, 716t
pathogenesis of, 705-707, 706b, 706f, 742-743
radiologic appearance of, 673-674, 674f-675f, 743, 744t
surgical management of, 741, 760-761
Chronic Sinusitis Survey (CSS), 57
Chronic sniffer, 483-484
Chronic suppurative otitis media (CSOM), cochlear implant for, 2221
Churg-Strauss syndrome (CSS)
nasal manifestations of, 659
otorrhea due to, 2196
Chylothorax, due to neck surgery, 1733
Chylous fistula
due to neck dissection, 1723
due to neck surgery, 1732-1733, 1732f
CI(s). *See* Cochlear implant(s) (CIs).
CI (confidence interval), 65, 66t, 67
Ci (curie), 1031-1032
CIC hearing aid. *See* Completely-in-the-canal (CIC) hearing aid.
Cicatricial membranous stenosis, 951
Cicatricial pemphigoid
esophageal manifestations of, 980
nasal manifestations of, 660
ocular scarring (symblepharon) due to, 1233-1234, 1234f
oral, 1233-1235, 1254
Cicatricial pemphigoid *(Continued)*
clinical differential diagnosis of, 1234, 1234t
clinical features of, 1233-1234, 1233f-1234f
defined, 1233
etiology and pathogenesis of, 1233
histopathologic features of, 1234-1235, 1234f
treatment of, 1235
Ciclopirox olamine antifungal cream or solution (Loprox), for fungal otitis externa, 1954-1955, 1959t-1960t
Cidofovir, for recurrent respiratory papillomatosis, 879
intralesional, 879-880, 2890t, 2892
Cigarette smoking
exposure to, and otitis media, 2767
and Graves' ophthalmopathy, 1807
and skin flap survival, 1075
and squamous cell carcinoma
of head and neck, 1016
of larynx, 1491, 1512-1513
of oral cavity, 1293-1294, 1365
Ciliary dyskinesia, primary, nasal manifestations of, 661
Cimetidine (ranitidine), for recurrent respiratory papillomatosis, 2893
Cinchonism, 2176
Cineradiography
in neurologic evaluation, 835-836
of pharynx and esophagus, 1393
Ciprofloxacin, for rhinosinusitis, 734
Ciprofloxacin with dexamethasone (Ciprodex), for otitis externa, 1946, 1952, 1959t-1960t
Ciprofloxacin with hydrocortisone (Cipro HC Otic), for otitis externa, 1946, 1952, 1959t-1960t
Circadian rhythm sleep disorders, 263-264, 264b
Circulatory disorders, presbycusis due to, 232
Circulatory reflexes, larynx in, 809, 810f
Circumvallate papillae
anatomy of, 1295f, 1359f
taste buds in, 1208
Cirrhosis, oral manifestations of, 1255
CIS (carcinoma in situ)
of larynx, 1486-1491, 1489f-1490f, 1515
treatment of, 1489-1490, 1520-1521
oropharyngeal, 1361
CIS (continuous interleaved sampling), for cochlear implants, 2229-2230
13-*cis* retinoic acid (13-cRA, Accutane)
for cancer chemoprevention, 1018, 1061-1062
laryngeal, 1491
cis-acting elements, 4
Cisapride, for GERD, 970
Cisatracurium, for pediatric anesthesia maintenance, 2593t
Cisplatin
in combination chemotherapy, 1059-1060
for induction chemotherapy, 1052-1053, 1056-1058, 1058f
ototoxicity of, 2171-2173
clinical studies on, 2171-2172
delayed, 2171-2172
experimental studies on, 2172
genetic predisposition to, 2172
histopathology of, 2172
mechanics of, 2172-2173
pharmacokinetics of, 2171
risk factors for, 2172
vestibular, 2172
with radiotherapy, 1041-1042, 1053-1054
in RADPLAT regimen, 1054
for recurrent or metastatic disease, 1059
sensorineural hearing loss due to, 2120
Cisternography, for CSF rhinorrhea
computed tomography, 790, 790f
magnetic resonance, 790-791, 790f
overpressure radionuclide, 790

Citalopram, for neuropathic pain, 245
Civatte bodies, in lichen planus, 1228
CK (CyberKnife) stereotactic radiotherapy
for laryngeal and hypopharyngeal cancer, 1592
for malignant skull base tumors, 1696
c-Kit, in salivary gland neoplasms, 1199
Cl^- (chloride), in saliva, 1139
Clarin-1 *(CLRN1)* gene, in deafness, 2051t-2058t, 2077-2078
Clarinex (desloratadine), for nonallergic rhinitis, 701t
Clarithromycin
for endocarditis prophylaxis, 1249t
for pediatric surgery prophylaxis, 2597t
for rhinosinusitis, 733, 734t
Claritin (loratadine)
for allergic rhinitis, 620
for nonallergic rhinitis, 701t
for rhinosinusitis, 734t
Clark scale, for melanoma, 1111, 1113f
Classic scattering, 1032
Claudin-11 (Cldn11), in perilymphatic-endolymphatic barrier, 2081, 2082f
Claudin-11 *(Cldn11)* gene, in murine deafness, 2058t-2060t
Claudin-14 (Cldn14), in perilymphatic-endolymphatic barrier, 2081, 2082f
Claudin-14 *(CLDN14)* gene, in deafness, 2051t-2058t, 2081
Claudius' cells, 1832, 1832f
CLC (Charcot-Leyden crystal) protein, 604
CLCN7 gene, in osteopetrosis, 2112
Cleaning, for facial trauma, 304-305
Clearance, saliva for, 1141
Cleft lip, 2659-2675
anatomy of, 2665-2666
mucocutaneous junction in, 2665
muscle abnormalities in
bilateral, 2666, 2666f
unilateral, 2665-2666, 2665f-2666f
nasal deformities in
bilateral, 2666
unilateral, 2666, 2666f
premaxillary bone deformity in, 2666, 2666f
classification of, 2659, 2660f
complete, 2659, 2660f
dysphagia due to, 2950
embryology of, 2659-2661, 2661f-2662f, 2661t
epidemiology of, 2664
incomplete, 2659, 2660f
molecular genetics of, 2662-2664
multidisciplinary team for, 2664, 2664b
nursing care for, 2664-2665, 2665f
prenatal diagnosis of, 2661-2662, 2663f
protocol for care of, 2664, 2664t
repair of, 2667-2668
bilateral, 2668, 2669f
definitive unilateral, 2667-2668, 2667f
advancement flap in, 2668, 2668f
closure in, 2668, 2668f
rotation flap in, 2667-2668, 2668f
primary rhinoplasty for, 2668
timing of, 2667
Simonart's band in, 2659, 2660f
Cleft lip nasal deformity, 2692
anatomy of
bilateral, 2666
unilateral, 2666, 2666f
pathogenesis of, 2690
rhinoplasty for, 557-559, 561f, 2692
Abbé flap in, 563f-564f
with bilateral deformity, 557, 559, 561f, 563f-564f
columellar lengthening in, 559, 566f
external approach to, 559, 561f
lateral ala thinning and placement of maxillary implants in, 562f
Cleft lip nasal deformity *(Continued)*
Le Fort I maxillary osteotomies in, 559, 564f-565f
with nasal stenosis, 559, 566f
open approach to, 559, 562f
repositioning and suturing of lower lateral cartilage in, 562f
with severe deformity, 559, 564f-565f
suturing together of medial crura in, 561f-562f
with unilateral deformity, 557, 559, 561f-562f
Cleft palate, 2659-2675
anatomy of, 2666-2667, 2667f
classification of, 2659, 2660f-2661f
complete, 2659, 2660f
embryology of, 2659-2661, 2661t, 2662f-2663f
epidemiology of, 2664
incomplete, 2659, 2661f
molecular genetics of, 2662-2664
multidisciplinary team for, 2664, 2664b
nursing care for, 2664-2665, 2665f
and otitis media, 1872-1873, 1873f, 2674-2675, 2766
palatoplasty for, 2668-2673
basic principles of, 2670
complications of, 2672-2673
and facial growth, 2669
Furlow (double-opposing Z-plasty), 2670
surgical technique for, 2671-2672, 2672f
goals of, 2668
techniques of, 2669-2670
timing of, 2668-2669
two-flap, 2669-2670, 2670f
surgical technique for, 2670-2671, 2670f-2671f
prenatal diagnosis of, 2661-2662
protocol for care of, 2664, 2664t
in Robin sequence, 2673
submucous, 2659, 2661f, 2674
bifid uvula with, 2793, 2793f
in velocardiofacial syndrome, 2673-2674, 2674f
Cleft palate feeders, 2665, 2665f
Cleft rhinoplasty, 2668
Cleidocranial dysplasia, 2641t
parietal foramina with, 2641t
Clemastine (Tavist), for nonallergic rhinitis, 701t
Cl^-/HCO_3^- (chloride/bicarbonate) exchanger, in salivary gland secretion, 1135
Clic5, in stereocilia, 2076f
Clic5 (chloride intracellular channel 5) gene, in murine deafness, 2058t-2060t
Clicks, in auditory brainstem response testing, 1896-1897
condensation and rarefaction, 1899-1901, 1900f
Clindamycin
for endocarditis prophylaxis, 1249t
for pediatric surgery prophylaxis, 2597t
for rhinosinusitis, 734
Clinical Assessment of Musical Perception (CAMP), 57
Clinical importance, *vs.* statistical significance, 66-67
Clinical outcomes, measurement of, 55-56
Clinical practice guidelines, 70
Clinical target volume (CTV), for radiotherapy, 1044
Clinical Test of Sensory Integration and Balance (CTSIB), 2317
Clinical tumor volume (CTV), for radiotherapy, 1036
Clival tumors
chordoma as, 2481f, 2510, 2511f
surgical approaches for, 2509
Clivus
anatomy of, 1823f
approaches to, 2509
radiographic anatomy of, 1399f
Clivus *(Continued)*
in surgical anatomy of anterior skull base, 2474, 2474f
in surgical anatomy of lateral skull base, 2435f
transnasal endoscopic-assisted surgery of, 2479-2481, 2480f-2481f
Closed captioning, 2271
Closure pattern, laryngeal videostroboscopy of, 819, 820f, 848t, 849
Clothesline injury, laryngeal trauma due to, 2914
Clotrimazole (Lotrimin, Mycelex) cream, for fungal otitis externa, 1954-1955, 1959t-1960t
Clouston syndrome, deafness in, 2051t-2058t
Cloverleaf skull, due to craniosynostosis, 2645, 2645f
CLRN1 (clarin-1) gene, in deafness, 2051t-2058t, 2077-2078
Cluster headache, 247-248
CM(s) (cochlear microphonics)
in electrocochleography, 1907-1908
with neural hearing loss, 1899-1901, 1900f
CMAP (compound muscle action potential)
for facial nerve injury, 2041, 2386
for facial nerve monitoring, 2387
after tumor removal, 2545
CME (continuing medical education), and performance measurement, 79, 79t
CMN (congenital melanocytic nevi), and melanoma, 1107-1108
CMS (Centers for Medicare and Medicaid Services), 84t-87t, 87
CMT, in deafness, 2051t-2058t
CMV. *See* Cytomegalovirus (CMV).
CNC (Consonant-Nucleus-Consonant) Monosyllable Word Test, for cochlear implants, 2223, 2244
CNPAS. *See* Congenital nasal pyriform aperture stenosis (CNPAS).
CNS (central nervous system) changes, in Bell's palsy, 2393-2394
CNS (central nervous system) infections, due to cranial base surgery, 2468
CNV (contingent negative variation), 632
CO_2. *See* Carbon dioxide (CO_2).
Coagulation disorders
oral manifestations of, 1256
oral treatment considerations for, 1246t
Coagulation factor C homology *(COCH)* gene, in deafness, 2051t-2058t
Coagulation screening, for adenotonsillectomy, 2794
Coal tar, for eczematoid otitis externa, 1956-1957
Coblation tonsillectomy, 2796
Cobra deformity, after rhytidectomy, 427
COC. *See* Calcifying odontogenic cyst (COC).
Cocaine, as adjunct to induction of anesthesia, 112
Coccidioidomycosis, laryngeal and tracheal manifestations of, 885, 893
COCH (coagulation factor C homology) gene, in deafness, 2051t-2058t
Cochlea
anatomy of, 1825f, 1831-1834, 1840, 1841f, 2050, 2061f
hair cells in, 1832-1834, 1833f
innervation in, 1834, 1834f
membranous labyrinth and inner ear fluids in, 1831-1832, 1832f
osteology in, 1831, 1832f
anomalies of (*See* Cochlear anomaly(ies))
in auditory physiology, 1840, 1841f-1842f, 2050-2060
electrochemical environment of, 1840, 1842f
embryogenesis of, 1852
imaging of, 1920-1921, 1922f
incomplete partition of, 2730-2731
embryogenesis of, 2728f-2729f, 2729t, 2730-2731

Cochlea *(Continued)*
histology of, 2730-2731, 2731f
imaging of, 2730-2731, 2731f
relative incidence of, 2729t
subtypes of, 2730-2731, 2731f
intratympanic delivery of medications to (*See* Intratympanic delivery)
ion transport within, 2081-2082, 2084f
otosclerosis of, 2029, 2030f
physical dimensions of, 2060, 2063f
sound propagation in, 1840-1842, 1842f
in surgical anatomy of lateral skull base, 2437f, 2438
"third window" of, 1842, 1843f
tonotopic map changes after long-term local excitation of, 1880-1881, 1883f
Cochlear agenesis, 2729f
Cochlear anomaly(ies), 2729-2732
cochlear agenesis as, 2729f
cochlear aplasia as, 2728f, 2729-2730, 2729t
cochlear hyperplasia as, 2732
cochlear hypoplasia as, 2730
embryogenesis of, 2728f-2729f, 2730
imaging of, 2730, 2730f
relative incidence of, 2729t
cochlear implantation for, 2739
in combination with other anomalies, 2728, 2738, 2739f
common cavity as, 2728f-2729f, 2729t, 2731-2732
in congenital aural atresia, 2738
embryogenesis of, 2728-2735, 2728f-2729f
incomplete partition as, 2730-2731
embryogenesis of, 2728f-2729f, 2729t, 2730-2731
histology of, 2730-2731, 2731f
imaging of, 2730-2731, 2731f
relative incidence of, 2729t
subtypes of, 2730-2731, 2731f
relative incidence of, 2729t
Cochlear apex, in cochlear transduction, 2061-2062, 2062f
Cochlear aplasia, 2728f, 2729-2730, 2729t
Cochlear aqueduct (CA)
anatomy of, 1822-1823, 1823f
enlargement of, 2734, 2734f
and CSF leakage, 2736
foramen of, 1824f
in surgical anatomy of lateral skull base, 2435f
Cochlear basal turn dysplasia, 2728
Cochlear canaliculus, 2010f
Cochlear conductive presbycusis, 232, 2126
Cochlear damage, in noise-induced hearing loss, 2141-2143, 2143f
Cochlear duct, anatomy of, 1851f, 1853f, 2061f
Cochlear dysplasia, 2235f
Cochlear echoes, 1891
Cochlear efferent system conditioning, for protection from noise-induced hearing loss, 2144
Cochlear hyperplasia, 2732
Cochlear hypoplasia, 2730
and CSF leakage, 2736f
embryogenesis of, 2728f-2729f, 2730
imaging of, 2730, 2730f
relative incidence of, 2729t
Cochlear implant(s) (CIs), 2204f
in adults, 2222-2224
audiologic protocol for, 2223
auditory rehabilitation with, 2254-2255
current trends that affect, 2224, 2224f
outcome expectations for, 2223
recommendations for referral for, 2224
results of, 2244-2245
with hearing preservation, 2245-2246
predictors of, 2245, 2245f
Cochlear implant(s) (CIs) *(Continued)*
quality-of-life studies for, 2251-2252, 2252f, 2252t
selection criteria for, 2222-2223
for asymmetric hearing loss, 2224
auditory evoked potentials with, 1912-1914, 1913f
for auditory neuropathy or dyssynchrony, 2220, 2240
auditory performance with
in adults, 2244-2245
with bilateral implantation, 2247-2251
in children, 2246
early studies of, 2246
measurement of, 2246
more recent studies of, 2246-2247, 2247f
factors related to measurement of, 2244-2247
with hearing preservation, 2245-2246
in infants, 2247
predictors of, 2245, 2245f
tests of, 2244
auditory rehabilitation after, 2253-2257
in adults, 2254-2255
in children, 2254-2255
efficacy of, 2253-2254
binaural (bilateral), 2241
for adults, 2224
for children, 2226
results of, 2247-2251
in children, 2224-2226, 2239-2240
audiologic protocol for, 2225, 2234-2235
auditory performance with, 2246
early studies of, 2246
measurement of, 2246
more recent studies of, 2246-2247, 2247f
auditory rehabilitation with, 2254-2255
binaural (bilateral), 2226
current trends that affect, 2226
ear selection for, 2226
education with, 2251-2253, 2251f, 2255-2257
factors that affect performance of, 2226
and language development, 2239-2240
other evaluations for, 2225
outcome expectations for, 2225-2226
recommendations for referral for, 2226
residual hearing and, 2240
results of, 2246
auditory performance assessments for, 2246
early studies of speech reception in, 2246
for educational placement and support, 2251-2253, 2251f, 2255-2256
for language acquisition, 2249-2251, 2250f
more recent studies of speech reception in, 2246-2247, 2247f
quality-of-life studies for, 2252-2253, 2253f
selection criteria for, 2225-2226, 2235b
surgical techniques for, 2240
with cochlear ossification, 2235f, 2240
with combined electrical and acoustic stimulation, 2224, 2224f
complications of, 2241
with compromised healing, 2241
for congenital inner ear anomalies, 2739
cost effectiveness of, 2251
defined, 2219-2220
device(s) for, 2227-2233
external speech processors for, 2229
size, weight, and aesthetics of, 2232, 2232f
factors that affect choice of, 2231-2233
batteries as, 2233
external speech processor size, weight, and aesthetics as, 2232, 2232f
MRI compatibility as, 2231-2232
need for special electrode arrays as, 2231
technology differences in speech coding strategy and electrode configuration as, 2231
Cochlear implant(s) (CIs) *(Continued)*
internal receiver stimulators and electrode designs in, 2227-2229
HiRes 90K receiver/stimulator as, 2227-2228, 2228f
Med-El PulsarCI100 and SonataTI100 as, 2228-2229, 2228f-2230f
Nucleus Freedom device with Contour Advance electrode as, 2227, 2227f-2228f
maintenance of, 2255
programming of, 2255
signal processing strategies in, 2229-2231
Advanced Combination Encoder for, 2230, 2231f
analog stimulation as, 2230, 2230f
continuous interleaved sampling as, 2229-2230
fine structure, 2230-2231, 2231f-2232f
spectral emphasis, 2230
spectral peak extraction as, 2230, 2230f
temporal, 2229-2230, 2230f
ear selection for, 2235-2236
algorithm for, 2236f
physical characteristics in, 2235-2236
residual hearing level in, 2236
and speech recognition, 2245, 2245f
general background of, 2219-2220
in infants, 2247, 2724
infectious complications of, 2161
for labyrinthine dysplasia, 2240-2241
and language development, 2239-2240, 2249-2251, 2250f
map for, 2255
meningitis vaccination with, 2236-2237, 2237b
for meningitis-induced deafness, 2240
for neural hearing loss, 1899-1901
and neural plasticity
in animal models of deafness, 1881
in infants with hearing loss, 1885, 1885f
in older adults, 233, 2234-2235
and quality of life, 2251-2252, 2252f, 2252t
with otitis media, 2240
patient evaluation for, 2220-2222, 2234-2235
with acquired deafness, 2220-2221
with auditory neuropathy/auditory dyssynchrony, 2220
with chronic suppurative otitis media, 2221
diagnostic therapy in, 2235
with genetic hearing loss, 2220
genetic testing in, 2235
hearing tests in, 2234-2235
imaging in, 2221-2222, 2222f, 2235, 2235f, 2236b
otologic/medical evaluation in, 2220-2222
physical examination in, 2221, 2234
and quality of life, 2251
in adults and elderly, 2251-2252, 2252f, 2252t
in children, 2252-2253, 2253f
with residual hearing
in adults, 2245-2246
in children, 2240
ear selection for, 2236
results of, 2244-2251
in adults, 2244-2245
with hearing preservation, 2245-2246
predictors of, 2245, 2245f
quality-of-life studies for, 2251-2252, 2252f, 2252t
bilateral, 2247-2251
in children, 2246
auditory performance assessments for, 2246
early studies of speech reception in, 2246
for educational placement and support, 2251-2253, 2251f, 2255-2256
for language acquisition, 2249-2251, 2250f

Cochlear implant(s) (CIs) *(Continued)*
more recent studies of speech reception in, 2246-2247, 2247f
quality-of-life studies for, 2252-2253, 2253f
factors related to measurement of, 2244-2247
in infants, 2247
tests for, 2244
revision, 2241
speech perception with, 2244-2245
predictors of, 2245, 2245f
surgical technique for, 2237-2241
bony seat in, 2238, 2239f
in children, 2240
cochleostomy in, 2239
electrode insertion in, 2239
incisions and flap design for, 2237-2238, 2237f-2238f
mastoidectomy in, 2238-2239
preparation and draping in, 2237
receiver stimulator in, 2239
skin flap in, 2238
for tinnitus, 2137
Cochlear lesions, reorganization of central tonotopic maps after, 1877-1878, 1878f-1879f
in adult subjects, 1878-1879, 1881f
in developmental model, 1878, 1880f
Cochlear malformations. *See* Cochlear anomaly(ies).
Cochlear mechanics
active, 2062-2069, 2064f-2065f
conversion of basilar membrane displacement to radial shearing forces in, 2065-2067, 2069f
outer hair cells in, 2063-2064, 2066f-2067f
prestin (SLC26A5) in, 2064-2065, 2068f
radial displacement patterns of basilar membrane in, 2067, 2069f
tectorial membrane pathophysiology and, 2067-2069
passive, 2050-2062, 2061f-2062f
physical dimensions in, 2060, 2063f
traveling wave in, 2060-2069, 2062f-2064f
Cochlear microphonics (CMs)
in electrocochleography, 1907-1908
with neural hearing loss, 1899-1901, 1900f
Cochlear modiolus, in surgical anatomy of lateral skull base, 2439
Cochlear nerve
anatomy of, 1832f, 1854f, 2278f
anomalies of, 2735
in central auditory pathway, 1834-1835
imaging of, 1928-1929, 1929f
intraoperative monitoring of, 2552
direct action potentials for, 2554, 2554f
and outcome, 2554-2555
in surgical anatomy of lateral skull base, 2437f, 2439
Cochlear nerve aplasia, auditory brainstem implants for, 2263-2264
Cochlear nucleus
in auditory physiology, 1845-1846, 1846f
in central auditory pathway, 1835, 1835f
Cochlear ossification, cochlear implant with, 2235f, 2240
Cochlear otosclerosis, imaging of, 1921-1922, 1925f
Cochlear partition
anatomy of, 1840, 2050, 2061f
in auditory physiology, 1840-1842, 1842f
Cochlear promontory, 1825-1826
Cochlear ramus, 1854, 1856f
Cochlear transduction, 2049-2085
active, 2062-2069, 2064f-2065f
conversion of basilar membrane displacement to radial shearing forces in, 2065-2067, 2069f
outer hair cells in, 2063-2064, 2066f-2067f
prestin (SLC26A5) in, 2064-2065, 2068f
Cochlear transduction *(Continued)*
radial displacement patterns of basilar membrane in, 2067, 2069f
tectorial membrane pathophysiology and, 2067-2069
traveling wave in, 2062-2069, 2064f
endolymph homeostasis in, 2081-2083, 2083f-2084f
genetic basis for, 2050, 2051t-2058t
in murine models, 2050, 2058t-2060t
hair cell transduction in, 2070-2081, 2070f
adaptation of mechanoelectrical transduction currents in, 2078-2079, 2079f
and auditory neuropathy, 2081
and defects in cytoskeletal proteins leading to deafness, 2074-2076, 2076f
defects in hair cell–afferent dendrite synapses and, 2080-2081, 2080f
defects of other hair cell channels and, 2079-2080
hair bundle deflections and receptor potentials in, 2069f, 2071, 2072f
myosin VI in, 2078
stereocilia in, 2070-2071
anatomy of, 2070-2071, 2070f, 2072f
composition of, 2074, 2075f-2076f
cross-linkages between, 2076f, 2077-2078
dynamic regulation of length of, 2076-2077
transduction channels in, 2071-2073
effects of deficiencies of, 2079-2080
gating of, 2073-2074
ion selectivity of, 2073, 2073f
structure of, 2076f
passive, 2050-2062, 2061f-2062f
physical dimensions in, 2060, 2063f
traveling wave in, 2060-2062, 2062f-2063f
perilymphatic-endolymphatic barrier in, 2081, 2082f
Cochleariform process, 1826f, 1827
Cochleosaccular dysplasia, 2727-2728
Cochleosacculotomy, for Meniere's disease, 2126, 2362-2363, 2363f
Cochleostomy, for cochlear implant, 2239
Cochleotopic map reorganization. *See* Tonotopic map reorganization.
Cochleovestibular nerve, 1834-1835
Cochleovestibular nerve injury, in lateral skull base surgery, 2512
Cochlin, in deafness, 2051t-2058t
Codeine, for postoperative pain, 241t
in children, 2594
Coding strand, 4
Codman, Ernest, 52
Codons, 4
Coefficient of determination, 64, 72
Cogan's syndrome, 2341
clinical manifestations of, 2341
etiology and pathogenesis of, 2341
historical background of, 2341
inner ear disease in, 2165
sensorineural hearing loss due to, 2123-2124, 2341
serologic tests for, 2327
treatment of, 2341
typical *vs.* atypical, 2341
Cognitive development, sleep-disordered breathing and, 2791-2792
Cognitive expertise, 79t
Cognitive impairment
obstructive sleep apnea and, 2603-2604
pain with, 240
Cognitive-behavioral therapy (CBT), for tinnitus, 2135
Coherent scattering, 1032
Cohort study, 54, 54t
Coiled terminations, 1201
Coiled-coil domain-containing protein 50/Ymer *(CCDC50)* gene, in deafness, 2051t-2058t
COL1A1
in deafness, 2051t-2058t
in osteogenesis imperfecta, 2109
COL1A2, in osteogenesis imperfecta, 2109
COL2A1, in deafness, 2051t-2058t, 2095
COL4A3, in deafness, 2051t-2058t
COL4A4, in deafness, 2051t-2058t
COL4A5, in deafness, 2051t-2058t, 2097
COL9A1, in deafness, 2051t-2058t, 2069
COL11A1, in deafness, 2051t-2058t, 2095
COL11A2, in deafness, 2051t-2058t, 2069, 2092, 2095
Cold
common, pharyngitis due to, 196
dry air provocation test, in nonallergic rhinitis, 696
Cold air–induced rhinitis, 619b
Cold receptors, in nasal obstruction, 641
Cold steel débridement, interventional bronchoscopy for, 1010t
Colectins, in middle ear protection, 1871
Colestipol, for hyperthyroidism, 1739t
Colitis, ulcerative, oral manifestations of, 1254
Collagen
in skin flaps, 1071
for vocal fold medialization, 905-906
Collagen vascular disease
oral manifestations of, 1251-1252
otologic manifestations of, 2114
vertigo due to, 2201
Collagenase, in bone resorption, 1972-1973
Collagenase-I, in wound healing, 1077
Collecting duct, of salivary gland, 1133-1134
Collision kerma, 1033
Colloid bodies, in lichen planus, 1228
Colloid thyroid nodules, ultrasound of, 1644, 1647f
Colonic transposition, for hypopharyngeal and esophageal reconstruction, 1453, 1454f
Colony-forming unit–basophil mast cell (CFU-BM), 605
Colony-forming unit–eosinophil (CFU-Eo), 604
Colony-forming unit–erythroid (CFU-E), 605
Colony-forming unit–granulocyte-macrophage (CFU-GM), 604
Colony-forming units–megakaryocytes (CFU-MEG), 605
Color Doppler sonography, 1644
of salivary glands, 1167-1168
Columella
anatomy of, 509f
surface defects of, 348
hinge flap for, 348, 350f
paramedian forehead flaps for, 348
Columella retraction, correction of, 547-548, 548f
Columellar lengthening, in cleft-lip nose repair, 559, 566f
Columellar strut
for noncaucasian nose, 560f
in revision rhinoplasty, 593, 593f
COM. *See* Chronic otitis media (COM).
Coma, myxedema, 1749
Combination chemotherapy, for recurrent or metastatic disease, 1059-1060
Combined-modality therapy, for head and neck squamous cell carcinoma, 1052-1058
with biologic agents plus radiotherapy, 1054, 1058f
concomitant chemoradiation as, 1052-1056, 1053t-1054t
as adjuvant therapy, 1056
induction chemotherapy in, 1041-1042, 1052-1053
induction chemotherapy in, 1056-1058, 1058f, 1058t-1059t
in concomitant chemoradiation, 1041-1042, 1052-1053
RADPLAT technique for, 1054

Combitube, 109-110, 110f, 114t
Comet-tail artifact, with colloid thyroid nodule, 1644, 1647f
Common canaliculus
 anatomy of, 798f
 in endoscopic dacryocystorhinostomy, 800-801, 801f
Common carotid artery
 anatomy of, 2579, 2579f-2580f
 in extended neck dissection, 1719-1720
Common carotid artery injury, due to penetrating neck trauma
 imaging of, 1632f
 management of, 1632
Common cavity, of inner ear, 2728f-2729f, 2729t, 2731-2732
Common chemical sense
 in olfactory stimulation, 628-629
 of oral cavity, 1202
Common cochlear artery, anatomy of, 1854, 1856f
Common cold, pharyngitis due to, 196
Comorbidity, 53
Comparative genomic hybridization (CGH), for head and neck squamous cell carcinoma, 1019
Complement system, in humoral immune response, 607-608, 608f
Complement system defects, 2114
 otologic manifestations of, 2114
Complementary DNA, 11-12, 12f
Complete strip technique, for nasal tip refinement, 522, 527f-530f
Complete transfixion incisions, for nasal tip projection, 535-536, 536f
Completely-in-the-canal (CIC) hearing aid, 2270, 2270f
 comparison of features of, 2206t
 evolution of, 2267
 in infants, 2723-2724
Complex calyx endings, of hair cells, 1857, 1859f
Complex traits, 8
Complex-motion tomography, of pharynx and esophagus, 1393
Composite grafts, for nasal reconstruction, 368-369, 369f
Composite turnout flap, for nasal defects, 348, 351f
Compound action potential (CAP)
 in Bell's palsy, 2394
 electrically evoked, 1912-1913
  with cochlear implants, 1913f, 1914
Compound melanocytoma, 287
Compound muscle action potential (CMAP)
 for facial nerve injury, 2041, 2386
 for facial nerve monitoring, 2387
  after tumor removal, 2545
Compound nevus, 286
Compound solution of iodine, for hyperthyroidism, 1739t
Compressed analog (CA), for cochlear implants, 2230
Compression, of dynamic range, with traditional hearing aid, 2205-2207
Compression circuitry, for hearing aids, 2268
Compton scattering, 1032f, 1033
Computational fluid dynamics (CFD), CT with, 643
Computed radiography, of pharynx and esophagus, 1393
Computed tomography (CT), 131
 of acoustic neuroma, 2517
 algorithms for, 131, 131f
 applications of, 139-142
 of cervical lymphadenopathy, 139
 combined with PET, 138
 with computational fluid dynamics, 643
Computed tomography (CT) *(Continued)*
 contrast-enhanced, 132, 132f-133f, 139
  of cervical lymphadenopathy, 164
   with extracapsular spread, 164-166, 167f
   inflammatory (reactive), 164
   with invasion of carotid artery, 166-167
   metastatic, 164-165, 167f
   with non-Hodgkin's lymphoma, 165-166, 167f
  of salivary glands
   with AIDS-related parotid cysts, 1146f
   with pleomorphic adenoma, 1144f
   with sialolithiasis, 1148f
 for CSF rhinorrhea, 791, 792f
 of deep neck space infections, 204, 204f-205f
 of facial trauma, 142
 of Graves' ophthalmopathy, 1809, 1811f
 helical
  of laryngeal carcinoma, 1470
  of pharynx and esophagus, 1396
 high-resolution
  for cochlear implant, 2222, 2222f
   with otosclerosis, 2222, 2222f
   in preoperative evaluation, 2235, 2235f, 2236b
  for CSF rhinorrhea, 791, 791f, 2044
  for dizziness, 2326-2327
  for malignant otitis externa, 1947
  of superior canal dehiscence syndrome, 2340-2341, 2340f
  for temporal bone fracture, 2039, 2040f
 for hyperparathyroidism, 1786-1787
 for hypopharyngeal and cervical esophageal cancer, 1424, 1424f
 image display for, 131-132
 with intensity-modulated radiotherapy, 1044
 of laryngeal carcinoma, 1468-1479, 1494
  early glottic, 1516-1517
 of laryngeal trauma, 935-936, 936f
 of larynx and infrahyoid neck, 132f, 140
 of lateral skull base lesions, 2489
 of maxillofacial trauma, 325-326
  of lower third, 325-326
  of middle third, 325, 326f
  of upper third, 325, 325f
 multidetector, 131, 139
 of nasopharyngeal carcinoma, 1354
 of neck masses, 1637, 1637t
 of neck neoplasms, 1656
 of obstructive sleep apnea, 255, 255f
 of oral cancer, 1300
 of oropharyngeal cancer, 1366
 of paranasal sinus tumors, 1124
 of paranasal sinuses, 140-142, 141f, 662-663
  radiation exposure with, 663
  with rhinosinusitis
   diagnostic, 140-142, 141f
   intraoperative, 744, 772
   preoperative, 743, 744t, 763-764, 764f-765f, 764t
   and surgical outcome, 729
  technique for, 662-663, 664f
 patient cooperation for, 132, 132f
 of petrous apicitis, 1986-1987, 1988f
 of pharynx and esophagus, 1396
 radiation exposure from, 132-133, 133t
 of salivary glands, 139, 1148, 1166, 1180
  with AIDS-related parotid cysts, 1146f
  with parotid lipoma, 1166, 1167f
  with pleomorphic adenoma, 1144f, 1148
  with sialadenitis, 1148
  for sialography, 139-140, 1145f
  with sialolithiasis, 1144f, 1148, 1148f
  with Sjögren's syndrome, 1148
  with Warthin's tumor, 1146f
 spiral (helical), of laryngeal carcinoma, 1470
 of suprahyoid neck, 139, 141f
Computed tomography (CT) *(Continued)*
 of temporal bone and skull base, 142
 3D, of laryngeal carcinoma, 1470
 three-dimensional reconstruction from, 138, 140f
 of thyroid and parathyroid glands, 140
 windows for, 131-132, 131f
 xenon blood flow mapping with, 2491
Computed tomography angiography (CTA)
 of anterior skull base, 2475, 2475f
 of neck masses, 1637, 1637t
Computed tomography (CT) cisternography, for CSF rhinorrhea, 790, 790f
Computed tomography–sestamibi (CT-MIBI) fusion, for hyperparathyroidism, 1785-1786, 1786f
 to localize ectopic glands, 1785-1786, 1787f-1788f
 in re-exploration, 1785-1786, 1788f
 to refine minimally invasive approach, 1785-1786, 1786f
Computer imaging
 in facial analysis, 277-280, 279f-280f
 for revision rhinoplasty, 581-582
 prior to rhinoplasty, 514
Computer-aided modeling, in mandibular reconstruction, 1326-1327, 1327f
Computer-assisted navigation, in endoscopic sinus surgery, 772
Computer-assisted voice analysis, for children, 2878, 2878f
Computerized dynamic posturography (CDP), 2324, 2325f
 motor control test in, 2324-2325
 sensory organization test in, 2325-2326, 2325f-2326f
 use of, 2326-2327
Concha, 477
 bullosa, 741
  endoscopic sinus surgery with, 751, 752f
  imaging of, 668, 669f
 cavum, 2742f
 cymba, 2742f
Conchal cartilage grafts, in noncaucasian rhinoplasty, 569
Conchal hypertrophy, 478-479
Conchal-mastoid sutures, 476f, 477-478
Concomitant chemoradiation, 1052-1056, 1053t-1054t
 as adjuvant therapy, 1056
 induction chemotherapy with, 1041-1042, 1052-1053
  with adjuvant therapy, 1056
Condensation and rarefaction clicks, in auditory brainstem response testing, 1899-1901, 1900f
Conditioning activities, in vestibular rehabilitation, 2372-2373, 2379
Conductive hearing loss, 2017-2027
 audiogram of, 1888, 1888f
 in children, 2026-2027, 2200-2201
 diagnostic evaluation of, 2019-2021
  acoustic immittance testing in, 2020
  acoustic reflex testing in, 2020
  history and physical examination in, 2022b
  pure-tone audiometry and speech testing in, 2020, 2020f
  Rinne test in, 2020, 2020t
  tympanometry for, 2020
  Weber test in, 2020
 due to external auditory canal conditions, 2021-2022, 2023f-2024f
 implantable devices for, 2027
 due to measles, 2158
 due to middle ear conditions, 2023-2026
 pathologic conditions leading to, 2018b
 specific lesions of conductive hearing pathway and, 2019, 2019t

Conductive hearing loss *(Continued)*
in superior semicircular canal syndrome, 2020-2021, 2021f
due to temporal bone trauma, 2046
treatment of, 2021-2026
for conditions of external auditory canal, 2021-2022, 2023f-2024f
for conditions of middle ear (*See* Ossiculoplasty)
for conditions of tympanic membrane, 2022-2023
due to tympanic membrane conditions, 2022-2023
Conductive hearing pathway
mechanical properties of, 2017-2019
specific lesions of, 2019, 2019t
Conductive presbycusis, 232, 2126
Condylar agenesis, 1280, 1281t
Condylar fractures, 1280, 1281t
pediatric, 2704, 2706f-2708f
Condylar hyperplasia, 1280, 1281t
Condylar hypoplasia, 1280, 1281t
Condylar process, of mandible, 1319, 1320f
Condylomata acuminata, maternal, and recurrent respiratory papillomatosis, 2886
Confidence interval (CI), 65, 66t, 67
Confounding, 53
vs. efficacy of treatment, 62t
Confusional arousals, 262t, 264
Congenital anomaly(ies)
children with, 2573
of inner ear, 2726-2740
classification of, 2726-2727, 2727b
cochlear, 2729-2732
cochlear agenesis as, 2729f
cochlear aplasia as, 2728f, 2729-2730, 2729t
cochlear aqueduct enlargement as, 2734, 2734f
cochlear hyperplasia as, 2732
cochlear hypoplasia as, 2728f-2730f, 2729t, 2730
cochlear implantation for, 2739
in combination with other anomalies, 2728, 2738, 2739f
common cavity as, 2728f-2729f, 2729t, 2731-2732
embryogenesis of, 2728-2735, 2728f-2729f
incomplete partition as, 2728f-2729f, 2729t, 2730-2731, 2731f
relative incidence of, 2729t
in congenital aural atresia, 2738
CSF leakage and meningitis due to, 2735-2737, 2736f
of eighth nerve, 2735
evaluation and management of, 2738-2739, 2739f
imaging of, 172-173, 174f, 1920-1921, 1923f, 2738
incidence of, 2727
of internal auditory canal, 2735
narrow, 2735, 2735f
wide, 2735, 2735f
labyrinthine, 2732-2733
in combination with other anomalies, 2728, 2738, 2739f
incidence of, 2727
limited to membranous labyrinth, 2727-2728, 2727b
of membranous and osseous labyrinth, 2727b, 2728-2735
semicircular canal aplasia as, 2732-2733, 2732f
semicircular canal dysplasia as, 2732, 2732f-2733f
membranous labyrinthine dysplasia as
complete, 2727
limited, 2727-2728

Congenital anomaly(ies) *(Continued)*
pathogenesis of, 2726
perilymphatic fistula as, 2737-2738, 2737f
syndrome correlations and familial patterns of, 2735
vestibular aqueduct enlargement as, 2727, 2733-2734, 2733f
X-linked stapes gusher syndrome as, 2737
of larynx, 2866-2875
bifid epiglottis as, 2870t, 2874, 2874f
hemangiomas and subglottic cysts as, 2871, 2871f
hypoplastic epiglottis as, 2870t
laryngeal cysts as, 2872-2873, 2872f-2873f
laryngeal webs/atresia as, 2869-2871
anterior, 2869-2870, 2869f-2870f
posterior, 2869, 2869f
subglottic stenosis as, 2870-2871
syndromes associated with, 2870t
laryngeal-laryngotracheoesophageal cleft as, 2873-2874, 2873f
classification of, 2873, 2874f, 2874t
syndromes associated with, 2870t
laryngomalacia as, 2866-2868, 2867f-2868f
syndromes associated with, 2870t
thyroglossal duct cyst as, 2871-2872, 2872f
vocal fold paralysis as, 2868-2869
of nose, 2686-2696
choanal atresia as, 2694-2695
bilateral, 2694-2695, 2694f-2695f
clinical presentation of, 2694
endoscopic evaluation of, 2694, 2695f
epidemiology of, 2694
imaging of, 2694, 2694f
treatment of, 2694-2695, 2695f
unilateral, 2694-2695, 2694f
cleft lip nasal deformity as, 2690, 2692
complete agenesis of nose (arhinia) as, 2690, 2691f
congenital nasal pyriform aperture stenosis as, 2692-2693
clinical presentation of, 2692-2693
diagnosis of, 2693, 2693f
operative management of, 2693, 2693f
pathogenesis of, 2690, 2692
craniofacial clefts as, 2690, 2692
dermal fistula as, 2687f
dermoids as
clinical presentation of, 2689, 2689f
defined, 2687f, 2688-2689
epidemiology of, 2688-2689
histology of, 2689
imaging of, 2689, 2689f
management of, 2689-2690
due to developmental errors of anterior neuropore, 2686-2690, 2687f
due to developmental errors of central midface, 2690-2693, 2691f
due to developmental errors of nasobuccal membrane, 2693-2695
encephaloceles as, 2687-2688
basal, 2687-2688, 2687t, 2688f
classification of, 2687-2688, 2687t
defined, 2687, 2687f
epidemiology of, 2687
vs. gliomas, 2688
histopathology of, 2688
imaging of, 2688, 2688f
management of, 2688
nasoethmoidal, 2687-2688, 2687t
nasofrontal, 2687-2688, 2687t
naso-orbital, 2687-2688, 2687t
sincipital, 2687-2688, 2687f, 2687t
sphenoethmoidal, 2687t
spheno-orbital, 2687t
terminology for, 2687

Congenital anomaly(ies) *(Continued)*
transethmoidal, 2687t
transsphenoidal, 2687t
gliomas as, 2687f, 2688
vs. encephaloceles, 2688
epidemiology of, 2688
extranasal, 2688
histology of, 2688
imaging of, 2688
intranasal, 2688
management of, 2688
intranasal hemangiomas as, 2695
maxillary mega-incisor with, 2690, 2691f
nasolacrimal duct cysts as, 2693, 2694f
nasopharyngeal teratomas as, 2695, 2696f
other mesodermal and germline malformations as, 2695
overview of, 2686
polyrhinia and supernumerary nostril as, 2690-2692
proboscis lateralis as, 2690, 2692, 2692f
of oral cavity, 1287-1288
developmental cysts as, 1287-1288
dermoid, 1287-1288
duplication, 1287-1288, 1288f
nasoalveolar, 1288, 1288f
lingual thyroid as, 1287
torus as, 1287, 1288f
oral manifestations of, 1257
of temporomandibular joint, 1280, 1281t
Congenital aural atresia (CAA), 2752-2760
bone-anchored hearing aid for, 2759
with cholesteatoma, 2754
classification of, 2753-2754, 2753b, 2753t
embryology of, 2753
epidemiology of, 2752-2753
imaging of, 1917, 1917f, 2754, 2754f
initial evaluation of, 2754
inner ear malformations in, 2738
with microtia, 2743
with poor pneumatization, 2754
reconstructive surgery for, 2754-2757
alternatives to, 2759
avoidance of complications of, 2758-2759
candidacy for, 2753, 2753t
contraindications to, 2754
creation of split-thickness skin graft in, 2756, 2756f
dissection of ossicular mass in, 2755-2756, 2756f
drilling for new ear canal in, 2755-2756
ear wick packing in, 2756-2757
facial nerve in, 2754, 2755f, 2759
harvesting of temporalis fascia in, 2755, 2755f
meatoplasty in, 2756-2757
outcomes of, 2754
placement of split-thickness skin graft in, 2756, 2757f-2758f
postauricular incision in, 2755, 2755f
postoperative care after, 2757-2758
preoperative evaluation and patient counseling for, 2754, 2754f-2755f
reconstruction of ossicular chain in, 2756
removal of atretic plate in, 2755-2756, 2755f
Silastic strips in, 2756-2757, 2758f
suturing in, 2756-2757, 2758f
temporal fascia graft in, 2755f, 2756, 2757f
timing of, 2754
Congenital craniofacial anomaly(ies)
in achondroplasia, 2633, 2634f
clinical manifestations of, 2642-2647
acrocephaly as, 2645, 2645f
brachycephaly as, 2644, 2645f
craniosynostosis as, 2642-2645, 2643f
encephalocele as, 2645, 2646f
facial clefts as, 2645
kleeblattschädel as, 2645, 2645f

Congenital craniofacial anomaly(ies) *(Continued)*
plagiocephaly as, 2643-2644, 2644f
scaphocephaly as, 2642, 2643f
syndromic, 2645-2647
trigonocephaly as, 2642-2643, 2643f, 2648f
in Down syndrome (trisomy 21), 2631-2633, 2631f, 2632b
due to abnormal and poor growth, 2633
of ears, 2632
of eyes, 2632-2633
mandibular and oral manifestations of, 2632
of midface, 2632
of skull, 2632
pathophysiology of, 2640-2642
intrauterine causes in, 2640
metabolic disorders in, 2640
molecular genetics in, 2640, 2641t, 2642f
in Robin sequence (Pierre Robin syndrome), 2630-2631, 2630f
surgical management of, 2649-2657
coronal incision in, 2650, 2650f
distraction osteogenesis in, 2654-2657, 2656f
fronto-orbital advancement in, 2650-2653, 2651f-2654f
monobloc advancement in, 2653-2654, 2655f-2656f
for orbital hypertelorism and dystopia, 2654
for sagittal synostosis, 2650, 2650f-2651f
syndromic, 2645-2647
in Apert's syndrome, 2645-2646
in Carpenter's syndrome, 2646
in Crouzon's syndrome, 2641t, 2645
in facio-oculo-auriculo-vertebral spectrum, 2646-2647
in Jackson-Weiss syndrome, 2646
in mandibulofacial dysostosis (Treacher Collins syndrome, Franceschetti syndrome), 2633-2635, 2633b, 2635f, 2646
in Pfeiffer's syndrome, 2641t, 2646
in Saethre-Chotzen syndrome, 2641t, 2646
in Stickler's syndrome, 2646
in velocardiofacial syndrome, 2646
Congenital epulis, of oral cavity, 1290, 1290f
Congenital hearing loss
epidemiology of, 2086
etiology of, 2200, 2200b
evaluation of, 2097-2099
genetic basis for, 2050, 2051t-2058t
in murine model, 2050, 2058t-2060t
due to labyrinthine infections, 2154-2157
with cytomegalovirus, 2154-2156, 2155f
with rubella, 2154, 2156-2157, 2157f
with syphilis, 2161
Congenital heart disease, pediatric anesthesia with, 2596-2597, 2596t-2597t
Congenital hemangioma, 2824, 2825f
Congenital high airway obstruction syndrome (CHAOS), 2869, 2870f, 2904-2905
Congenital hypomyelinating neuropathy, deafness in, 2051t-2058t
Congenital hypothalamic hamartoblastoma syndrome, 2874
Congenital immunodeficiencies, 209-210, 210t
Congenital labyrinthine abnormalities, CSF otorrhea due to, 2197
Congenital laryngeal cysts, 1468, 2872-2873, 2872f-2873f
Congenital laryngeal stenosis
diagnosis of, 2916-2917
etiology and pathophysiology of, 2912-2913, 2913f
management of, 2922
Congenital lesions
of external auditory canal, imaging of, 1917, 1917f
of oral cavity, 154-156
of sublingual space, 156
of submandibular space, 156-157, 158f
Congenital melanocytic nevi (CMN), and melanoma, 1107-1108
Congenital nasal pyriform aperture stenosis (CNPAS), 2692-2693
clinical presentation of, 2692-2693
diagnosis of, 2693, 2693f
operative management of, 2693, 2693f
pathogenesis of, 2690, 2692
Congenital neck mass(es), 1638-1640, 2814-2817
branchial cleft anomalies as, 1639, 2814, 2814f-2815f
dermoid cysts as, 1639, 2816, 2816f-2817f
hemangiomas as, 1640, 2816, 2816f
laryngoceles as, 2816-2817
lymphangiomas as, 1640, 2815, 2815f
sternocleidomastoid tumors of infancy as, 2817, 2817f
teratomas as, 1639-1640, 2816, 2816f
thymic cysts as, 2817
thyroglossal duct cysts as, 1639, 2814-2815, 2815f
vascular malformations as, 2817
Congenital nevi, 287-288
melanocytic, and melanoma, 1107-1108
Congenital salivary gland cysts, 2859
Congenital torticollis, 2817, 2817f
Congenital vascular lesions, of salivary glands, 1172
arteriovenous malformations as, 1172
hemangiomas as, 1172
lymphatic malformations as, 1172
venous malformations as, 1172
Congestion factor, 645
Conjoint tendon, in brow or forehead rejuvenation, 433-434
Conjunctiva, 443f, 444
Conjunctival fornix, 444
Connective tissue diseases, esophageal manifestations of, 978-979, 979f
imaging of, 1400-1401, 1401f
Connective tissue growth factor (CTGF), in formation of granulation tissue, 1077
Connexin(s) (Cx), in endolymph homeostasis, 2083, 2083f
Connexin 26 *(Cx26)* gene
in deafness, 2051t-2058t, 2083
infant screening for, 2723
Connexin 30 *(Cx30)* gene, in deafness, 2051t-2058t, 2083
Connexin 31 *(Cx31),* in deafness, 2051t-2058t
Connexin 32 *(Cx32)* gene, in deafness, 2051t-2058t
Conn's syndrome, preoperative evaluation of, 104-105
Consanguinity, 6
Conscious sedation
for awake fiberoptic nasotracheal intubation, 124
for tracheobronchial endoscopy, 1000
Consecutive sample, 68, 69t
Consensus Auditory Perceptual Evaluation for Voice (CAPE-V), 819, 826
Consent, informed, 102
Conservation laryngeal surgery, 1539-1562
anatomy and physiology and, 1541-1544
anterior commissure tendon in, 1541-1542
cartilage in, 1541
connective tissue barriers in, 1542-1543, 1544f
conus elasticus in, 1541-1542, 1542f
cricothyroid ligament in, 1541-1542
epiglottis in, 1541
hyoid bone in, 1541
hypoepiglottic ligament in, 1541-1542
paraglottic space in, 1542, 1543f
preepiglottic space in, 1542, 1543f
quadrangular membrane in, 1541-1542, 1542f
skeletal structure in, 1541, 1541f
thyrohyoid membrane in, 1541-1542, 1542f
vocal tendon in, 1541-1542
Conservation laryngeal surgery *(Continued)*
current paradigm for, 1558-1559
current state of, 1540-1541
future developments in, 1560-1561
for glottic tumors, 1496, 1547-1549
epiglottic laryngoplasty as, 1549
complications of, 1549
extended procedures for, 1549
functional outcome of, 1549
key surgical points for, 1549
oncologic results of, 1549
surgical technique for, 1549, 1549f
horizontal partial laryngectomies as, 1549
spectrum of, 1557-1560
supracricoid partial laryngectomy with cricohyoidoepiglottopexy, 1549-1550
complications of, 1551
extended procedures for, 1551
functional outcome of, 1551, 1551t-1552t
key surgical points for, 1550-1551
oncologic results of, 1549-1550
surgical technique for, 1550, 1550f-1551f
vertical hemilaryngectomy as, 1547-1549
complications of, 1549
extended, 1548
frontolateral, 1548
functional outcome of, 1548
with imbrication laryngoplasty, 1548, 1548f
key surgical points for, 1549
oncologic results of, 1547-1548, 1547t-1548t
posterolateral, 1548
surgical technique for, 1548
vertical partial laryngectomies for, 1547
history of, 1540
indications for and contraindications to, 1546-1547
intraoperative conversion to total laryngectomy from, 1557-1558
postoperative management issues with, 1560
preoperative evaluation for, 1544-1546
clinical evaluation of primary site in, 1544-1545, 1545f
overall clinical assessment in, 1546
radiologic evaluation of primary site in, 1545-1546
T stage in, 1546
principles of, 1544
and radiotherapy, 1559-1560
spectrum of, 1557-1560, 1558f-1559f
for supraglottic tumors, 1551-1552, 1552t
horizontal partial laryngectomies as, 1553-1554
spectrum of, 1557-1560
supracricoid laryngectomy with cricohyoidopexy as, 1555-1557
complications of, 1557
functional outcome of, 1556-1557, 1557t
key surgical points for, 1556
oncologic results of, 1555
surgical technique for, 1555-1556, 1556f
supraglottic laryngectomy as, 1553-1554
with arytenoid, aryepiglottic fold, or superior medial pyriform involvement, 1554-1555
with base of tongue extension, 1555
complications of, 1555
extended procedures for, 1554
functional outcome of, 1555
key surgical points for, 1554-1555, 1554f
oncologic results of, 1553, 1553t
surgical technique for, 1553-1554, 1554f
Conservative management
of CSF rhinorrhea, 791-792, 792b
of facial nerve injury, 2040, 2042
of laryngeal trauma, 936
of tracheal stenosis, 2927-2928
Consonant-Nucleus-Consonant (CNC) Monosyllable Word Test, for cochlear implants, 2223, 2244

Consumer Assessment of Health Providers and Services (CAHPS), 82, 84t-87t
Contact dermatitis, otitis externa due to, 1945-1946
Contact guidance, in cholesteatoma formation, 1968
Contact inhibition, in cholesteatoma formation, 1968
Contact ulcer or granuloma, of vocal folds, 874-875, 874f
  diagnosis of, 875
    history in, 875
    laryngeal examination in, 875, 875f
    vocal capability battery in, 875
  epidemiology of, 874
  due to extraesophageal reflux, 902, 902f-903f
  management of, 875
  pathophysiology and pathology of, 874
Contingency tables, 71-72
Contingent negative variation (CNV), 632
Continuing medical education (CME), and performance measurement, 79, 79t
Continuous interleaved sampling (CIS), for cochlear implants, 2229-2230
Continuous positive airway pressure (CPAP), for obstructive sleep apnea, 256-257
  in children, 2610-2611
Continuous wave lasers, 33
Contour Advance electrode, 2227, 2227f-2228f
Contour Emboli (polyvinyl alcohol), for embolization, 1933
Contour irregularities
  after liposuction, 459
  after rhytidectomy, 427
Contrast enhancement, for MRI, 134-135, 135f-136f
Contrast-enhanced computed tomography (CECT), 132, 132f-133f, 139
  of cervical lymphadenopathy, 164
    with extracapsular spread, 164-166, 167f
    inflammatory (reactive), 164
    with invasion of carotid artery, 166-167
    metastatic, 164-165, 167f
    with non-Hodgkin's lymphoma, 165-166, 167f
  of salivary glands
    with AIDS-related parotid cysts, 1146f
    with pleomorphic adenoma, 1144f
    with sialolithiasis, 1148f
Control groups, 53
  and data interpretation, 59-61, 60t
Conus elasticus
  in mucosal wave propagation, 848-849
  surgical anatomy of, 1541-1542, 1542f-1544f
Convective flow, across interstitial space, 1066
Convenience sample, 68, 69t
Conventional radiography (CR), 130-131
  of deep neck space infections, 204-205
  of facial bones, 130
  of neck, 131
  of neck masses, 1637, 1637t
  of paranasal sinuses, 130, 662
    Caldwell view in, 662, 663f
    with rhinosinusitis, 729, 729f
    Waters view in, 662, 663f
  of pharynx and esophagus, 1393, 1394f
  radiation exposure from, 132-133, 133t
  for sialography, 139-140, 1149-1150, 1149f, 1155-1156, 1156f
  of temporal bone, 131
Convergence spasm, 2314
COPD (chronic obstructive pulmonary disease), oral manifestations of, 1250
Cor pulmonale
  due to obstructive sleep apnea, 2604, 2604f
  sleep-disordered breathing and, 2792, 2792f
Cordarone (amiodarone)
  dizziness due to, 2310t
  thyrotoxicosis due to, 1744
Cordectomy, for glottic cancer, 1496, 1517t, 1519t
Core competencies, 80, 80b
Core-needle biopsy, of lymphoma, 1676
Coring out, of tracheal tumor, 1619-1621
"Corkscrew" esophagus, 965, 966f
Cornea, in Graves' ophthalmopathy, 1808, 1809t
Corneal protection, for eyelid trauma, 303, 303f, 308
Corniculate cartilage, 1542f
Corniculate tubercle, 1422f, 1543f
Coronal forehead lift, 430, 431t
Coronal incision
  for craniofacial anomalies, 2650, 2650f
  for pediatric facial fracture, 2701-2702, 2703f
Coronal synostosis
  bilateral, 2644, 2645f
  front-orbital advancement for, 2652-2653, 2653f-2654f
  unilateral, 2643-2644, 2644f, 2648f
Coronavirus, pharyngitis due to, 196
Coronoid process, 1319, 1320f
  osteochondroma of, *vs.* myofascial pain dysfunction syndrome, 1285t
Corpuscular radiation, 1031
Correlation coefficient, 64, 64t, 67
Corrugated esophagitis, 967-968, 969f
Corrugator supercilii muscle
  anatomy of, 321f, 441-442, 442f
  contraction of, 442, 442f
Cortical lesions, laryngologic manifestations of, 837-838, 838t
Cortical tonotopic map reorganization
  age-related, 1877, 1879, 1882f
  experimental studies of
    after cochlear lesions, 1877-1878, 1878f-1879f
      in adult subjects, 1878-1879, 1881f
      in developmental model, 1878, 1880f
    after long-term local excitation of cochlea, 1880-1881, 1883f
  mechanisms of
    at cellular level, 1884
      Hebb's postulate for, 1884, 1884f
      long-term potentiation as, 1884
    at systems level
      in adult subjects, 1883-1884
      in developing subject, 1883
  practical issues relating to, 1884-1886
    for hearing loss in infants, 1885, 1885f
    for other hearing disorders, 1885-1886
  time course of, 1877
Corticosporin Otic Solution (polymyxin, neomycin, and hydrocortisone), for otitis externa, 1946, 1952, 1959t-1960t
Corticosteroids
  for acute otitis media, 2770-2771
  for autoimmune inner ear disease, 2166-2167
  for Bell's palsy, 2395, 2409-2410, 2410t
  prior to biopsy of lymphoma, 1676
  for caustic ingestion, 2959
  for croup, 2805-2806
  for facial nerve injury, 2042
  for Graves' ophthalmopathy, 1811
  for hemangioma of infancy, 2826-2828
  for herpes zoster, 2396
  intralesional, for tracheal stenosis, 2928
  intranasal
    for allergic rhinitis, 621
    for nonallergic rhinitis, 700, 700t
    for sinus surgery, 773
  intratympanic, 2183-2185
    dosing of, 2185
    indications for, 2183
    mechanism of action of, 2183
    for Meniere's disease, 2184
Corticosteroids *(Continued)*
    pharmacokinetics of, 2183-2184
    side effects of, 2185
    for sudden sensorineural hearing loss, 2184-2185
  for laryngeal stenosis, 2918
  for obstructive sleep apnea, 2611
  oral sequelae of, 1247t-1248t
  oral treatment considerations with, 1246t
  for otitis media with effusion, 2772
  ototopical
    classes of, 1956, 1956t
    for eczematoid otitis externa, 1955-1956
    hypersensitivity reaction to, 1954
    mechanism of action of, 1951
    ototoxicity of, 1956
  for professional voice disorders, 854, 854b
  for rhinosinusitis
    systemic, 734t, 736
    topical nasal, 734t, 736
  for sarcoidosis, 659
  for scar revision, 299-300, 301f
  for stridulous child, 2906
  for sudden sensorineural hearing loss, 2157
  systemic
    for allergic rhinitis, 621
    for inner ear disorders, 2184
  for tracheal stenosis, 2928
Corynebacterium diphtheriae, pharyngitis due to, 195-196
  in children, 2786-2787
Cosmetic effects, of radiotherapy, 2626t
Cosmetics, for scar camouflage, 301
Cost effectiveness, of cochlear implants, 2251
Costal cartilage grafts
  for laryngeal stenosis, 2919-2920, 2920f
  for noncaucasian rhinoplasty, 569, 570f
    harvesting of, 570, 571f
    results of, 568
  for revision rhinoplasty, 583, 584f
Costal cartilage tracheoplasty, 2930-2931, 2931f
Costocervical trunk, 2581-2582, 2581f
Cost-utility ratio, of cochlear implants, 2251, 2252t
Cottle elevator, for septoplasty, 488-490, 489f
Cottle maneuver, 484, 484f
Cotton-Myers classification, of airway stenosis, 944, 944t
Cough
  due to abnormal swallow, 1217
  due to GERD, 971
  larynx in, 808
  whooping, laryngeal and tracheal manifestations of, 892
Cover-body theory, of vocal fold vibration, 845, 845f
Cowden's disease, oral manifestations of, 1257
COX. *See* Cyclooxygenase (COX).
Coxsackievirus, herpangina due to, 2785, 2786f
CPA. *See* Cerebellopontine angle (CPA).
CPAP (continuous positive airway pressure), for obstructive sleep apnea, 256-257
  in children, 2610-2611
CpG island hypermethylation, in head and neck squamous cell carcinoma, 1020, 1021f
CPIR (cephalic phase insulin release), 1206
CPP (cepstral peak prominence), in acoustic analysis, for voice evaluation, 829t, 830
CR. *See* Conventional radiography (CR).
13-cRA (13-*cis* retinoic acid)
  for cancer chemoprevention, 1018, 1061-1062
    laryngeal, 1491
Cranial base
  anatomy of, 171
  anterior (*See* Anterior cranial base)
  classification of lesions of, 171
  growth and development of, 2617-2619, 2617t, 2619f-2620f

Cranial base *(Continued)*
imaging of, 171, 1929-1930
with benign lesions, 171, 172f
CT for, 142, 171
prior to endoscopic sinus surgery, 764t
with fractures, 171
with inflammatory lesions, 171
with intracerebral neoplastic processes, 171, 174f
with meningiomas, 1929-1930, 1930f
with metastases, 171, 173f
MRI for, 143, 171
normal anatomy in, 171
with paragangliomas, 171, 174f, 1929, 1930f
lateral (*See* Lateral cranial base)
middle (*See* Middle cranial base)
Cranial base defects
endoscopic endonasal techniques for, 763
localization of, for CSF rhinorrhea, 791, 791f
Cranial base disruption, 334-339
Cranial base irradiation, for malignant tumors, 1695-1700
anterior, 1697-1699
with chemotherapy, 1700
chordoma/chondrosarcoma as, 1699
complications after, 1700
CyberKnife, 1696
esthesioneuroblastoma as, 1697-1698, 1698f, 1698t
intensity-modulated, 1696-1697
middle, 1699-1700
nasopharyngeal carcinoma as, 1699-1700, 1699f, 1700t
proton beam, 1696
sinonasal undifferentiated carcinoma as, 1698-1699
stereotactic, 1696, 1700
Cranial base surgery, robotic, 42, 43f-44f
Cranial base tumor(s)
benign, 2446, 2447b
in children, 2647, 2647f
surgical management of, 2657
malignant, 1697-1700
anterior, 1697-1699, 2446, 2447b
esthesioneuroblastoma as, 1697-1698, 1698f, 1698t
sinonasal undifferentiated carcinoma as, 1698-1699
chondrosarcoma as, 1923-1924, 1926f, 2540f
esthesioneuroblastoma as, 1697-1698, 1698f, 1698t
middle, 1699-1700
chordoma/chondrosarcoma as, 1699
nasopharyngeal carcinoma as, 1699-1700, 1699f, 1700t
sinonasal undifferentiated carcinoma as, 1698-1699
preoperative planning for, 2446-2447
Cranial chordomas, 2510, 2511f
Cranial length, 2617t
Cranial nerve I. *See* Olfactory nerve.
Cranial nerve II. *See* Optic nerve.
Cranial nerve III. *See* Oculomotor nerve.
Cranial nerve IV. *See* Trochlear nerve.
Cranial nerve V. *See* Trigeminal nerve.
Cranial nerve VI. *See* Abducens nerve.
Cranial nerve VII. *See* Facial nerve.
Cranial nerve VIII. *See* Cochlear nerve; Vestibular nerve; Vestibulocochlear nerve.
Cranial nerve IX. *See* Glossopharyngeal nerve.
Cranial nerve X. *See* Vagus nerve.
Cranial nerve XI. *See* Spinal accessory nerve.
Cranial nerve XII. *See* Hypoglossal nerve.
Cranial nerve deficits
due to carotid paraganglioma surgery, 1660-1661
due to cranial base surgery, 2469
HIV-associated, 223
Cranial nerve deficits *(Continued)*
after lateral skull base surgery, 2512
due to nasopharyngeal carcinoma, 1353
due to paranasal sinus tumor, 1123-1124
due to penetrating neck trauma, 1629
due to sphenoidotomy, 768t
Cranial nerve monitoring, 2542-2556
anesthesia and, 2544
auditory brainstem response recording for, 2552-2554
interpretation of, 2553-2554, 2553f
and postoperative auditory function, 2553-2554
reducing electrical and acoustic interference in, 2552-2553
stimulus and recording parameters, electrodes, and placement in, 2552
of cochlear nerve, 2552
direct eighth nerve action potentials for, 2554
detection and interpretation of changes in, 2554
placement of electrodes in, 2554
stimulus and recording parameters in, 2554
of facial nerve, 2545-2549
with acoustic neuroma and other cerebellopontine angle tumors, 2545
activity evoked by electrical stimulation in, 2545-2546
for assessment of functional status after tumor removal, 2545-2546
electromyography for, 2545-2548
for intraoperative identification of nervus intermedius, 2546, 2546f
limitations of, 2547-2548, 2548f
during microvascular decompression, 2548-2549, 2549f
during other otologic surgery, 2549
during parotid surgery, 2549
spontaneous and mechanically evoked activity in, 2546-2548, 2547f
future directions in, 2555-2556, 2555f
instrumentation for, 2543
ninth, tenth, eleventh, and twelfth, 2550-2552, 2551f-2552f
and outcome, 2554-2555
for cochlear nerve preservation, 2554-2555
for facial and other motor cranial nerve preservation, 2554
personnel for, 2542-2543
recording electrodes for, 2543-2544, 2543f
stimulating electrodes for, 2544, 2544f
stimulation criteria for, 2544
third, fourth, and sixth, 2549-2550, 2550f
of trigeminal motor branch, 2550
Cranial width, 2617t
Cranialization, of frontal sinus, 782, 783f
Craniocervical junction, osteoma of, 2484f
Craniocervical junction–odontoid approach, for transnasal endoscopic-assisted anterior skull base surgery, 2483-2484, 2484f
Craniofacial anomaly(ies), 2630-2636, 2638-2658
acquired
due to neoplasm, 2647, 2647f
surgical management of, 2657
due to postnatal conditions, 2640-2642
due to trauma, 2647
surgical management of, 2648, 2649f, 2657
classification of, 2638
clinical manifestations of, 2642-2647
congenital, 2642-2647
acrocephaly as, 2645, 2645f
brachycephaly as, 2643f, 2644, 2645f
craniosynostosis as, 2642-2645, 2643f
encephalocele as, 2645, 2646f
facial clefts as, 2645
kleeblattschädel as, 2645, 2645f
plagiocephaly as, 2643-2644, 2643f-2644f
Craniofacial anomaly(ies) *(Continued)*
scaphocephaly as, 2642, 2643f
syndromic, 2645-2647
trigonocephaly as, 2642-2643, 2643f, 2648f
due to neoplasms, 2647, 2647f
due to trauma, 2647
congenital
in achondroplasia, 2633, 2634f
clinical manifestations of, 2642-2647
acrocephaly as, 2645, 2645f
brachycephaly as, 2644, 2645f
craniosynostosis as, 2642-2645, 2643f
encephalocele as, 2645, 2646f
facial clefts as, 2645
kleeblattschädel as, 2645, 2645f
plagiocephaly as, 2643-2644, 2644f
scaphocephaly as, 2642, 2643f
syndromic, 2645-2647
trigonocephaly as, 2642-2643, 2643f, 2648f
in Down syndrome (trisomy 21), 2631-2633, 2631f, 2632b
due to abnormal and poor growth, 2633
of ears, 2632
of eyes, 2632-2633
mandibular and oral manifestations of, 2632
of midface, 2632
of skull, 2632
pathophysiology of, 2640-2642
intrauterine causes in, 2640
metabolic disorders in, 2640
molecular genetics in, 2640, 2641t, 2642f
in Robin sequence (Pierre Robin syndrome), 2630-2631, 2630f
surgical management of, 2649-2657
coronal incision in, 2650, 2650f
distraction osteogenesis in, 2654-2657, 2656f
fronto-orbital advancement in, 2650-2653, 2651f-2654f
monobloc advancement in, 2653-2654, 2655f-2656f
for orbital hypertelorism and dystopia, 2654
for sagittal synostosis, 2650, 2650f-2651f
syndromic, 2645-2647
in Apert's syndrome, 2641t, 2645-2646
in Carpenter's syndrome, 2646
in Crouzon's syndrome, 2641t, 2645
in facio-oculo-auriculo-vertebral spectrum, 2646-2647
in Jackson-Weiss syndrome, 2646
in mandibulofacial dysostosis (Treacher Collins syndrome, Franceschetti syndrome), 2633-2635, 2633b, 2635f, 2646
in Pfeiffer's syndrome, 2641t, 2646
related to branchial arch structures, 2585
in Saethre-Chotzen syndrome, 2641t, 2646
in Stickler's syndrome, 2646
in velocardiofacial syndrome, 2646
defined, 2638
epidemiology of, 2638-2639
mechanisms of postnatal facial growth and, 2639, 2639f
and obstructive sleep apnea, 2605
in other conditions and syndromes, 2635-2636
and otitis media, 2766
pathophysiology of, 2640-2642
acquired, 2640-2642
intrauterine causes in, 2640
metabolic disorders in, 2640
molecular genetics in, 2640, 2641t, 2642f
patient evaluation for, 2647-2649
craniofacial team in, 2647
history and physical examination in, 2647-2648
imaging in, 2648, 2648f-2649f
indications and timing of intervention in, 2648-2649

Craniofacial anomaly(ies) *(Continued)*
surgical management of, 2649-2658
acquired
due to neoplasm, 2657
due to trauma, 2648, 2649f, 2657
biomaterials in skeletal or cartilaginous defect repair in, 2657-2658
congenital, 2649-2657
coronal incision in, 2650, 2650f
distraction osteogenesis in, 2654-2657, 2656f
fronto-orbital advancement in, 2650-2653, 2651f-2654f
monobloc advancement in, 2653-2654, 2655f-2656f
for orbital hypertelorism and dystopia, 2654
for sagittal synostosis, 2650, 2650f-2651f
indications and timing of, 2648-2649
Craniofacial clefts, 2690, 2692
Craniofacial complex, growth and development of. *See* Craniofacial growth and development.
Craniofacial disassembly, 2448
Craniofacial frontoethmoidectomy, 1126, 1126f
Craniofacial growth and development, 2613-2637
abnormal, 2621-2630
functional endoscopic sinus surgery and, 2623-2625
internal fixation and, 2625-2626
nasal obstruction and dentofacial growth in, 2628-2630, 2629f
open mouth posture with, 2628-2629
review of literature on, 2629-2630
due to nasoseptal trauma and surgery, 2626-2628
animal studies on, 2626-2627
human studies on, 2627-2628, 2627f
surgical timing and approach and, 2628
due to radiotherapy, 2622-2623, 2626t
and adenotonsillar hypertrophy, 2792-2793
bone growth concepts in, 2614
osteogenesis as, 2614
endochondral, 2614, 2615f
intramembranous, 2614
remodeling and displacement as, 2614-2615
general facial changes in, 2615, 2615f-2616f
normal, 2615-2621, 2617t
and pediatric facial fractures, 2698-2699
postnatal, 2639, 2639f
regions in, 2615-2621, 2617t
mandible as, 2620-2621, 2623f-2625f
nasomaxillary complex as, 2619-2620, 2621f-2622f
sinuses in, 2619-2620, 2623f
neurocranium as, 2615-2619, 2617t
basicranium of, 2617-2619, 2617t, 2619f-2620f
calvaria of, 2615-2617, 2617t, 2618f
theories of, 2613-2614
cartilage-mediated, 2614
functional matrix, 2614
genetically preprogrammed, 2614
Craniofacial resection
for ethmoid sinus tumors, 1130
extended, 1126-1127, 1127f
supplemental management in, 1126-1127
for maxillary sinus tumor, 1128
Craniofacial surgery, for obstructive sleep apnea, 2610, 2610f
Craniofacial synostosis, 2639
Craniofacial team, 2647
Craniofrontal syndrome, 2641t
Craniolacuna, 2641t
Craniomaxillofacial resorbable plating systems, for pediatric facial fractures, 2700-2701, 2700t-2701t
Craniomaxillofacial trauma. *See* Maxillofacial trauma.
Craniopharyngioma, of nasopharynx, 1349
Craniosynostosis, 2642-2645, 2643f
acrocephaly due to, 2645, 2645f
Boston-type, 2641t
brachycephaly due to, 2643f, 2644, 2645f
front-orbital advancement for, 2652-2653
with deafness, 2051t-2058t
kleeblattschädel as, 2645, 2645f
Muenke-type, 2641t
plagiocephaly due to, 2643-2644, 2643f-2644f
front-orbital advancement for, 2652-2653, 2653f
scaphocephaly due to
clinical manifestations of, 2642, 2643f
surgical management of, 2650f-2651f
trigonocephaly due to, 2642-2643, 2643f, 2648f
front-orbital advancement for, 2645, 2654f
Craniovertebral junction disorder(s), 2354-2356
assimilation of atlas as, 2355
atlantoaxial dissociation as, 2355-2356
basilar impression as, 2355
Chiari malformation as, 2356, 2356f
classification of, 2355-2356
pathophysiology of, 2355
Cranium, size ratio to face of, 2616f, 2617t
Creep, in skin flaps, 1071
Cresylate otic drops, for fungal otitis externa, 1955, 1959t-1960t
Cribriform area
anatomy of, 1822f
in surgical anatomy of anterior cranial base, 2443, 2444f
Cribriform plate
invasive small cell carcinoma of, 170f
lateral lamella of, and CSF rhinorrhea, 787, 787f
surgical anatomy of, 741
in anterior cranial base, 2442-2443, 2443f, 2471, 2472f
in lateral skull base, 2435
Cricoarytenoid joint
in arytenoid adduction, 913
laryngeal carcinoma of, 1545, 1545f
Cricoarytenoid joint fixation, vocal quality disorder due to, 2880
Cricoarytenoid muscle
in arytenoid adduction, 913, 914f
surgical anatomy of, 1543f
Cricoarytenoid unit, in organ-preservation surgery, 1544
Cricohyoidoepiglottopexy (CHEP)
for glottic cancer, 1517t
supracricoid partial laryngectomy with, 1549-1550
complications of, 1551
extended procedures for, 1551
functional outcome of, 1551, 1551t-1552t
key surgical points for, 1550-1551
oncologic results of, 1549-1550
surgical technique for, 1550, 1550f-1551f
vs. total laryngectomy, 1564
Cricohyoidopexy (CHP)
for advanced supraglottic cancer, 1500
supracricoid laryngectomy with, 1555-1557
complications of, 1557
functional outcome of, 1556-1557, 1557t
key surgical points for, 1556
oncologic results of, 1555
partial, 1564
surgical technique for, 1555-1556, 1556f
Cricoid arch
repair of, 939f
surgical anatomy of, 1543f
Cricoid cartilage
anatomy of, 805-806, 1359f, 1422f
radiographic, 1471, 1473f
surgical, 1541, 1542f-1544f
laryngeal carcinoma of, 1541
physical examination of, 95, 96f
Cricoid lamina, surgical anatomy of, 1543f
Cricoid resection with thyrotracheal anastomosis, for laryngeal stenosis, 2921, 2922f
Cricoid ring, radiographic anatomy of, 1473, 1473f
Cricoid split operation, 2908f, 2910f, 2918-2919, 2918f-2919f
Cricoidectomy, for chronic aspiration
partial, 928
subperichondrial, 927-928, 929f
Cricopharyngeal achalasia, 1398-1399, 1400f
Cricopharyngeal chalasia, 1399
Cricopharyngeal dysfunction, 1398-1399, 1400f
Cricopharyngeal muscle
anatomy of, 1422
in arytenoid adduction, 915
delayed opening of, 1399
during swallow, 833
pharyngeal, 1216-1217, 1216f
in Zenker's diverticulum, 987
Cricothyroid (CT) joint
in arytenoid adduction, 915
surgical anatomy of, 1542f
Cricothyroid (CT) ligament, surgical anatomy of, 1541-1542, 1542f-1543f
Cricothyroid membrane (CTM)
anatomy of, 126
dilation of, 127, 128f
palpation and location of, 127, 127f
relocation of, 127, 127f
transverse incision in, 127, 127f
Cricothyroid (CT) muscle
anatomy of
applied, 807, 807f
surgical, 1543f
characteristics of, 918
in professional voice production, 846-847
Cricothyrotomy, 114t, 126-128
anatomic considerations for, 126
complications after, 128, 128f
contraindications for, 126-127
defined, 126
equipment for, 126b
historical perspectives on, 126
indications for, 126-127
percutaneous, 114t, 128
procedure for, 127
cricoid hook in, 127, 128f
dilation of cricothyroid membrane in, 127, 128f
palpation and location of cricothyroid membrane in, 127, 127f
relocation of cricothyroid membrane in, 127, 127f
tracheostomy tube insertion in, 127, 128f
transverse incision in cricothyroid membrane in, 127, 127f
vertical incision over cricoid cartilage in, 127, 127f
rapid five-step technique for, 128
Cricotracheal resection (CTR), for laryngeal stenosis, 2921, 2922f
Cricotracheal separation, management of, 937
Crile clamp, in repair of medial canthal ligaments, 337f
Crile, George, 1702-1703, 1726
Crista ampullaris
anatomy of, 1854, 1856f-1857f
embryogenesis of, 1852
Crista galli, 1124f
aerated, 670
bifid, with nasal dermoid, 2689, 2689f
in surgical anatomy of anterior cranial base, 2442-2443, 2443f, 2471, 2472f
Critical closing pressure, in skin flaps, 1068
Crohn's disease
esophagitis due to, 1405
oral manifestations of, 1254

Cromolyn sodium, for allergic rhinitis, 620
Cronin technique, in cleft-lip nose repair, 559, 566f
Crookes, William, 1031
Cross-face nerve grafting, 2419, 2424-2425
Crossing over, 3
Crossover, in audiologic testing, 1889
Cross-priming, 1024
Croton oil, for deep chemical peel, 394
Croup, 1465, 1465f, 2803-2806
clinical features of, 2803-2804
defined, 2803
diagnosis of, 2804
differential diagnosis of, 2804-2805, 2806t
epidemiology of, 2803
etiology of, 2803
imaging of, 2804, 2804f-2805f
laryngoscopy of, 2804, 2805f
management of, 2805-2806, 2904
membranous (bacterial), 1465, 1465f
pathogenesis of, 2803-2804
postintubation, 2593
pseudo-membranous (*See* Bacterial tracheitis)
spasmodic, 2805
terminology for, 2803
viral, 2803
Crouzonodermoskeletal syndrome, craniofacial anomalies in, 2641t
Crouzon's syndrome, craniofacial anomalies in, 2641t, 2645
Crow's feet, 428
CRS. *See* Chronic rhinosinusitis (CRS).
CRT. *See* Chemoradiation therapy (CRT).
"Crumple zones," of face, 322, 322t
Crus commune, 1851f, 1853f
Crus helicis, 1824f
CRYM, in deafness, 2051t-2058t
Cryoglobulinemia, sensorineural hearing loss due to, 2120
Cryotherapy
interventional bronchoscopy with, 1010t
for skin lesions, 294
for unresectable tracheal tumor, 1621
Cryptococcal meningitis, in HIV, 223-224
Cryptococcosis, laryngeal and tracheal manifestations of, 892-893
μ-Crystallin, in deafness, 2051t-2058t
CS (carotid space)
anatomy of, 203
imaging of, 150-151, 151f-152f
schwannoma of, 1663f
CSD (cat scratch disease)
in children, 2818
deep neck space infections due to, 201
salivary gland involvement in, 1159
CSF. *See* Cerebrospinal fluid (CSF).
CSOM (chronic suppurative otitis media), cochlear implant for, 2221
CSP (cysteine-string protein), 2081
CSS (Chronic Sinusitis Survey), 57
CSS (Churg-Strauss syndrome)
nasal manifestations of, 659
otorrhea due to, 2196
CT. *See* Computed tomography (CT); Cricothyroid (CT).
CTA (computed tomography angiography)
of anterior skull base, 2475, 2475f
of neck masses, 1637, 1637t
CTAP-III (chemokine connective tissue–activating peptide-III), in wound healing, 1076
CTGF (connective tissue growth factor), in formation of granulation tissue, 1077
CTL(s) (cytotoxic T lymphocytes), 601, 602f
CTL2, in autoimmune inner ear disease, 2165
CTM. *See* Cricothyroid membrane (CTM).
CTR (cricotracheal resection), for laryngeal stenosis, 2921, 2922f
CTSIB (Clinical Test of Sensory Integration and Balance), 2317
CTV (clinical target volume), for radiotherapy, 1044
CTV (clinical tumor volume), for radiotherapy, 1036
Cuneiform cartilage, 1542f
Cuneiform tubercle, 1422f, 1543f
Cupula
anatomy of, 1855, 1857f
in vestibular system, 2278f, 2279-2283
torsional pendulum model of, 2279-2283, 2282f
Cupulolithiasis, 2329-2330
of lateral semicircular canal, 2331
Curets, for treatment and biopsy of skin lesions, 293
Curie (Ci), 1031-1032
Curie, Marie, 1031-1032
Curie, Pierre, 1031
Current steering, for cochlear implants, 2231, 2231f
Cushing's disease, oral manifestations of, 1251
Cutaneous branches, of cervical plexus, 2578, 2580f
Cutaneous diseases
esophageal manifestations of, 979-980
nasal manifestations of, 660-661
in Behçet's disease, 660-661
in pemphigoid, 660
in pemphigus vulgaris, 660
in scleroderma, 660
oral manifestations of, 1253-1254
Cutaneous flaps. *See* Skin flap(s).
Cutaneous hemangiomas, and airway involvement, 2899, 2900f
Cutaneous neoplasms
immunosuppression and, 213t, 215
neck dissection for, 1718-1719
definition and rationale for, 1718, 1718f
technique for, 1718-1719
Cuticular plate, 1832-1833, 1833f, 1841f, 1857
CVA (cerebrovascular accident)
chronic aspiration due to, 926b
due to lateral skull base surgery, 2512
oral manifestations of, 1250
Cx. *See* Connexin(s) (Cx).
CXC chemokines, 609t-612t
CXC3C chemokine, 611t-612t
CXCL-14, for head and neck squamous cell carcinoma, 1024
CXCR2 (chemokine receptor 2), in wound healing, 1076
CXCR4 (chemokine receptor 4), in head and neck squamous cell carcinoma, 1060
CXR (chest x-ray)
of early glottic carcinoma, 1516
for imaging of pharynx and esophagus, 1393
for neck masses, 1637
Cyanoacrylates, for embolization, 1933
Cyanotic heart disease, anesthesia with, 2597
CyberKnife (CK) stereotactic radiotherapy
for laryngeal and hypopharyngeal cancer, 1592
for malignant skull base tumors, 1696
Cyclic adenosine monophosphate (cAMP)
in olfactory transduction, 629
in salivary gland secretion, 1137
Cyclin D1, in laryngeal carcinoma, 1505
Cyclin D3, in laryngeal carcinoma, 1505
Cyclin-dependent kinase inhibitor 2D *(Cdkn2d)* gene, in murine deafness, 2058t-2060t
Cyclooxygenase (COX) inhibitors, and skin flap viability, 1074
Cyclooxygenase-1 (COX-1) inhibitors, for head and neck squamous cell carcinoma, 1018
Cyclooxygenase-2 (COX-2), in laryngeal carcinoma, 1505
Cyclooxygenase-2 (COX-2) inhibitors
for chemoprevention of oral cancer, 1315
for head and neck squamous cell carcinoma, 1018
Cyclophosphamide
for autoimmune inner ear disease, 2167
for Wegener's granulomatosis, 658
Cyclosporine, for Graves' ophthalmopathy, 1811
Cylindroma, 288f, 292
Cymba conchae, 476-477, 476f, 1824f
Cymetra. *See* AlloDerm Regenerative Tissue Matrix (Cymetra).
Cyst(s), 289
arachnoid, of cerebellopontine angle, 2523-2524
vs. cholesteatoma (epidermoid), 2519, 2521f
imaging of, 1928, 1929t
benign lymphoepithelial, in HIV, 217-218, 218f
branchial cleft, 2814
in children, 2859
clinical presentation of, 2814, 2814f
embryology of, 2585, 2585f, 2814
imaging of, 131, 158f, 1410, 2814, 2814f
management of, 2814
otorrhea due to infection of, 2195
squamous cell carcinoma arising in, 1671
buccal bifurcation, infected, 1264-1265
of cerebellopontine angle
arachnoid, 2523-2524
vs. cholesteatoma (epidermoid), 2519, 2521f
imaging of, 1928, 1929t
dermoid, 2527
epidermoid, 2518-2519
diagnostic studies of, 2519
differential diagnosis of, 1929t, 2518t, 2519, 2524t
imaging of, 1928, 1928f, 2519, 2520f
signs and symptoms of, 2518-2519
cholesterol, 2508, 2510f
defined, 1260-1262
dermoid, 289
of cerebellopontine angle, 2527
in children, 2859
nasal
clinical presentation of, 2689, 2689f
defined, 2687f, 2688-2689
epidemiology of, 2688-2689
histology of, 2689
imaging of, 2689, 2689f
management of, 2689-2690
of neck, 1639, 2816
clinical appearance of, 2816, 2816f
embryology of, 2586
imaging of, 2816, 2817f
of oral cavity, 1287-1288
developmental, of oral cavity, 1287-1288
dermoid, 1287-1288
duplication, 1287-1288, 1288f
nasoalveolar, 1288, 1288f
dorsal, due to injectable silicone, 578, 579f
ductal
congenital, 2859
of larynx, 869, 869f-870f
duplication
foregut, compression of pharynx and esophagus due to, 1408-1409, 1409f
of oral cavity, 1287-1288, 1288f
epidermoid, 289
of cerebellopontine angle, 2518-2519
diagnostic studies of, 2519
differential diagnosis of, 1929t, 2518t, 2519, 2524t
imaging of, 1928, 1928f, 2519, 2520f
signs and symptoms of, 2518-2519
of cerebellopontine cistern, 2509f
of larynx, 868f-869f, 869
of vocal folds, 2882, 2882f

Cyst(s) *(Continued)*
esophageal
imaging of, 1416, 1416f
retention, 1415-1416, 1415f
intracordal, 869-870
diagnosis of, 869
history in, 869
laryngeal examination in, 869
vocal capability battery in, 869
epidemiology of, 869
epidermoid inclusion, 868f-869f, 869
mucous retention (ductal), 869, 869f-870f
open, 869, 870f
pathophysiology and pathology of, 869
treatment of, 869-870
behavioral, 869-870
medical, 869
surgical, 870, 870f
laryngeal
congenital, 1468, 2872-2873, 2872f-2873f
ductal, 869, 869f-870f
epidermoid inclusion, 868f-869f, 869
mucous retention, 869, 869f-870f
saccular, 2872-2873, 2872f-2873f
milia as, 289
mucous, 289
mucous retention, 289
in children, 2859
imaging of, 676, 677f
of larynx, 869, 869f-870f
of petrous apex, 2525, 2526f
nasal, dermoid
clinical presentation of, 2689, 2689f
defined, 2687f, 2688-2689
epidemiology of, 2688-2689
histology of, 2689
imaging of, 2689, 2689f
management of, 2689-2690
nasoalveolar, of oral cavity, 1288, 1288f
nasolacrimal duct, 2693, 2694f
of neck, dermoid, 1639, 2816
clinical appearance of, 2816, 2816f
embryology of, 2586
imaging of, 2816, 2817f
odontogenic (*See* Odontogenic cysts)
of oral cavity
dermoid, 1287-1288
developmental, 1287-1288
dermoid, 1287-1288
duplication, 1287-1288, 1288f
nasoalveolar, 1288, 1288f
duplication, 1287-1288, 1288f
nasoalveolar, 1288, 1288f
parotid, AIDS-related, 1146, 1146f
of petrous apex, mucous retention, 2525, 2526f
pilar (trichilemmal), 289
saccular, 876-878
anterior, 876f-877f, 877
classification of, 877f
clinical scenario with, 877
defined, 877
diagnosis of, 877
etiology of, 876
of larynx, 2872-2873, 2872f-2873f
lateral, 876f, 877, 878f
treatment of, 877-878
salivary gland, 2859
acquired, 2859
congenital, 2859
in steatocystoma multiplex, 289
subglottic, 2871, 2871f
thymic, 2817
thymopharyngeal, 2585
thyroglossal duct, 2814-2815, 2871-2872
clinical presentation of, 2814-2815, 2815f
vs. ectopic thyroid, 2815
embryology of, 2586, 2814

Cyst(s) *(Continued)*
imaging of, 161-162, 165f
infected, needle aspiration of, 206, 206f
neck masses due to, 1639
Sistrunk operation for, 2815
squamous cell carcinoma arising in, 1671
vallecular, 2871-2872, 2872f
thyroid, 1759-1760
clinical presentation of, 1759-1760
management and prognosis for, 1760
pathology of, 1760
Tornwaldt, 1348-1349
imaging of, 148, 1416, 1416f
vallecular, 1416f
dysphagia due to, 2951-2952
stridor due to, 2898, 2898f
vocal fold, 856, 857f
in children, 2882, 2882f
Cystadenoma, papillary, of salivary glands
lymphomatosum, 1146, 1146f, 1170-1171
oncocytic, 1171
Cysteine-string protein (CSP), 2081
Cystic fibrosis (CF)
gene therapy for, 20
nasal manifestations of, 661
pediatric anesthesia with, 2595
salivary gland enlargement due to, 2864
Cystic hygroma, 156-157, 2815, 2901f
Cystic salivary gland disease, 1647
Cystic thyroid nodules, 1644, 1645f
Cytochrome P-450, in head and neck squamous cell carcinoma, 1016
Cytogenetics, of head and neck squamous cell carcinoma, 1019
Cytokines
in allergic rhinitis, 615
in cisplatin ototoxicity, 2173
in humoral immune response, 608, 609t-610t
in otitis media and cholesteatoma, 1973
in rhinosinusitis, 731
Cytomegalic inclusion disease, 2154-2156, 2155f
Cytomegalovirus (CMV)
labyrinthine infections with
clinical features of, 2154-2155
congenital hearing loss due to, 2154-2156, 2155f
diagnosis of, 2154-2155
experimental, 2156
management and prevention of, 2156
temporal bone pathology due to, 2155-2156, 2155f
Meniere's disease due to, 2163
sensorineural hearing loss due to, 2119
in infants, 2723
Cytomegalovirus (CMV) esophagitis, 976, 977f
Cytoplasmic antineutrophil cytoplasmic antibodies (c-ANCAs), in Wegener's granulomatosis, 658, 2103
Cytoskeletal protein defects, deafness due to, 2074-2076, 2076f
Cytotoxic gene therapy strategies, 16, 21
Cytotoxic hypersensitivity reactions, 608-612
Cytotoxic T lymphocytes (CTLs), 601, 602f

D

da Vinci, Leonardo, 269, 270f
da Vinci Robotic Surgical System, 39-40, 41f
for laryngeal cancer, 1560-1561
Dacryocystoceles, 2693, 2694f
Dacryocystogram (DCG), 798, 798f-799f
Dacryocystorhinostomy (DCR), endoscopic, 763, 797-802
complications of, 801
evaluation for, 797-798
dacryocystogram in, 798, 798f-799f
scintilligraphy in, 798, 799f
nasal preparation for, 798

Dacryocystorhinostomy (DCR), endoscopic *(Continued)*
outcomes of, 801
revision, 801
surgical technique for, 798-801
agger nasi in, 799-800, 800f
bone removal in, 799-800, 800f
common canaliculus in, 800-801, 801f
creation of flap in, 798, 799f
endoscopic septoplasty in, 798, 799f
flap elevation in, 798-799, 800f
flap positioning in, 800, 800f
frontal process and lacrimal bone in, 799-800, 800f
lacrimal probe in, 800
tube stents in, 800-801, 801f
DAG (diacylglycerol), in salivary gland secretion, 1137
DAMES classification, of thyroid cancer, 1754
Danger space No. 4
anatomy of, 202-203
odontogenic infections of, 186, 186f
DART (dynamic adjustable rotational tip) graft, for saddle nose deformity, 555, 559f
Darwinian tubercle, 476-477, 476f, 2742f
excision of, 478f
Data, uncertainty of, 60t, 64-65
Data interpretation, 59-75
censored data in, 63t, 64
coefficient of determination for, 64, 72
common statistical deceptions in, 72-74, 73t
multiple *P* value phenomenon as, 73t, 74
post hoc *P* values as, 73-74, 73t
powerless equalities as, 73t, 74
selective analysis of results as, 73t, 74
small sample whitewash as, 73, 73t
standard error "switcheroo" as, 72, 73t
surgical satisfaction swindle as, 72
confidence intervals in, 65, 66t, 67
correlation coefficient for, 64, 64t, 67
descriptive statistics for, 63, 64t
effect of study design on, 59, 60t
control group in, 59-61
example of, 61-62, 63t
experimental (randomized controlled) *vs.* observational, 59, 61t-62t
prospective *vs.* retrospective, 61
study type and study methodology in, 61, 62t
effect size in, 66-67
explanations other than efficacy in, 61, 61f, 62t
hypothesis testing in, 65, 66t
examples for, 65-66
null hypothesis in, 65, 66t
P value in, 65, 66t
type I and type II errors in, 65, 66t
importance of principles in, 74-75
key habit(s) for, 59-70, 60t
accepting uncertainty of all data as, 60t, 64-65
checking quality before quantity as, 59-62, 60t
describing before analyzing as, 60t, 62-64
measuring error with right statistical test as, 60t, 65-66
putting clinical importance before statistical significance as, 60t, 66-67
seeking sample source as, 60t, 68-69
viewing science as cumulative process as, 60t, 69-70
levels of evidence in, 69-70, 70t
measurement scales for, 63, 63t
meta-analyses in, 70, 71t
odds ratio, relative risk, and rate difference for, 64, 64t
placebo response in, 61
for popular statistical tests, 70-72
analysis of variance (ANOVA) as, 71
contingency tables as, 71-72
multivariate (regression) procedures as, 72

Data interpretation *(Continued)*
nonparametric, 72
survival analysis as, 72
t-test as, 70-71
research integration in, 69-70
sampling methods in, 68-69, 68t-69t
statistical test(s) for
for independent samples, 66, 67t
measuring error with right, 60t, 65-66
for related samples, 66, 67t
survival analysis in, 64
survival curve in, 64
understanding sample size in, 74
validity in, 68, 68t, 69f
Data logging, with hearing aids, 2269
Data-glove, 39, 39f
Daughter cells, 12
Day care, and otitis media, 2767
Daytime somnolence, 263-264
obesity and, 251
dB (decibel), 1839, 2087
dBA (decibel–A) scale, 2140
DCC (deleted in colorectal cancer) gene, in head and neck squamous cell carcinoma, 1020
DCG (dacryocystogram), 798, 798f-799f
DCR. *See* Dacryocystorhinostomy (DCR).
DDP1 (deafness dystonia peptide 1) gene, in deafness, 2051t-2058t
De la Cruz classification, of congenital aural atresia, 2753, 2753b
De Morgan's spots, 290
Deaf culture, 2099
Deafness. *See also* Hearing loss.
autosomal dominant (DFNA), 2050, 2089
autosomal recessive (DFNB), 2050, 2089
X-linked or mitochondrial (DFN), 2050, 2089
Deafness dystonia peptide 1 *(DDP1)* gene, in deafness, 2051t-2058t
Deafwaddler mice, 2080
Débridement
of burns, 315
after endoscopic sinus surgery, 773-774
of tracheal tumor, 1619-1621
Debrox (carbamide peroxide), for cerumen removal, 1958t
Decadron. *See* Dexamethasone (Decadron, Dexacort).
Decannulation, tracheostomy
with laryngeal stenosis, 2923
surgical, 2907-2908
ward, 2907
Decibel(s) (dB), 1839, 2087
Decibel scale, 1839, 2140
Decibel–A (dBA) scale, 2140
Decompression sickness, inner ear, 2343
Decongestant(s)
for otitis media
acute, 2770
with effusion, 2771
for rhinitis
allergic, 620
nonallergic, 700
for rhinosinusitis, 735t, 736
topical
prior to endoscopic sinus surgery, 745
for obstructive sleep apnea, 257
for vocal professionals, 855
Decongestion, for airway obstruction, 655
Deep cervical fascia, 202, 2577-2578, 2578f-2579f
Deep cervical lymph nodes, 2582
Deep jugular nodes, 1298f
Deep lingual artery, 1296f
Deep neck space, anatomy of, 201-202
anterior visceral space in, 203
carotid space in, 203
danger space in, 202-203
Deep neck space, anatomy of *(Continued)*
deep cervical fascia in, 202
masticator space in, 203
parapharyngeal space in, 202
parotid space in, 203
peritonsillar space in, 203
prevertebral space in, 203
retropharyngeal space in, 202
submandibular and sublingual spaces in, 202
superficial cervical fascia in, 202
Deep neck space infections, 201-208
clinical evaluation of, 203
history in, 203
physical examination in, 203
complications of, 207-208
carotid artery pseudoaneurysm or rupture as, 207
cavernous sinus thrombosis as, 207
Lemierre's syndrome as, 207
mediastinitis as, 207-208
necrotizing fasciitis as, 208
etiology of, 201
imaging studies of, 204-205
CT for, 204, 204f-205f
MRI for, 204
plain film radiography for, 204-205
ultrasonography for, 204-205
laboratory evaluation of, 204
microbiology of, 201
of odontogenic origin, 184-187
lateral pharyngeal, 184-185, 186f
prevertebral (danger space No. 4), 186, 186f
retropharyngeal, 185-186, 187f
airway establishment for, 188
normal anatomy and, 186f
surgical drainage and decompression for, 189-190
treatment of, 205-207
airway management in, 205
antibiotic therapy in, 205-206, 206t
fluid resuscitation in, 205
surgical, 206-207
needle aspiration in, 206, 206f
transcervical incision and drainage in, 207
transoral incision and drainage in, 206-207
Deep temporal fascia, 440
Defensins, 599
Deferoxamine
ototoxicity of, 2176-2177
sensorineural hearing loss due to, 2121, 2176-2177
Degenerate code, 4
Degenerative arthritis, of temporomandibular joint, 1281-1282, 1281t
Degenerative neurologic diseases, chronic aspiration due to, 926b
Deglutition, 833, 1215-1221
disorders of (*See* Dysphagia)
inefficient, 1217
physiology of, 954, 955f, 1207
stage(s) of, 1215, 1218f
esophageal, 1217, 2948
oral, 1206f, 1207, 1215, 1216f, 2948
oral preparatory, 1215, 1216f, 2948
pharyngeal, 1216, 2948
airway protection during, 1216-1217
cricopharyngeal (upper esophageal sphincter) opening during, 1217
delayed triggering of, 1215
neuromuscular activities in, 1216, 1216f
pharyngeal pressure generation during, 1217
programmed, 1216-1217
voluntary, 1215
Dehydrating agents, for Meniere's disease, 2337
Deiodinases, 1738
Deiters' cells, 1832, 1832f-1833f
Déjérine-Sottas syndrome, deafness in, 2051t-2058t
Delayed skin flaps, 1072-1073
Delayed sleep phase syndrome, 262t, 263-264
Delayed-type hypersensitivity (DTH) reactions, 601, 608-612
Deleted in colorectal cancer (DCC) gene, in head and neck squamous cell carcinoma, 1020
Deletion, 4-5
Deliverability, of radiotherapy, 1035
Delivery approaches, for nasal tip refinement, 522, 527f
complete strip technique in, 522, 527f-530f
interrupted strip technique in, 522, 532f-533f
suturing in, 522, 530f-531f, 550-551
DeltaSystem, for pediatric facial fractures, 2701t
Deltopectoral flap, for hypopharyngeal and esophageal reconstruction, 1451-1452, 1452f
Dementia
hearing and, 233
HIV-associated, 223
oral manifestations of, 1254-1255
Demineralization, of teeth, 1141
Demyelinating disorders, vertigo due to, 2202
Denaturing high performance liquid chromatography (DHPLC), 9, 10f
Dendritic cell(s), 604
Dendritic cell–based vaccines, for head and neck squamous cell carcinoma, 1024
Dental artifacts
on CT, 139, 141f
on MRI, 134, 134f
Dental care
after radiation therapy, 1333-1337
with conventional 3D conformal radiation therapy, 1333-1335, 1336f
with intensity-modulated radiation therapy, 1335-1337, 1336f-1337f
ipsilateral *vs.* contralateral, 1335
during radiation therapy, 1333
prior to radiation therapy, 1330-1331, 1330b, 1331f
Dental caries, 1252
Dental changes, in geriatric patients, 236
Dental disease
heart disease and, 1248
and stroke, 1250
Dental erosions, due to GERD, 971-972
Dental extractions, prior to radiation therapy, 1330-1331, 1330b, 1579
Dental infection, 1252
Dental lamina, 1259
Dental lamina cyst, 1266, 1266f
microscopic features of, 1266
treatment of, 1266
Dental pain, 1202-1203
Dental papillae, 1276
Dental procedures
cardiac conditions and, 1248-1249, 1249t
with joint replacement, 1253, 1253t
Dental prostheses, and radiation therapy, 1331
Dental rehabilitation, after resection for malignancy, 1087, 1089f
Dental sac, 1276
Dentigerous cyst, 1263-1264
microscopic features of, 1264
neoplastic potential of, 1264
radiographic features of, 1264, 1264f
treatment of, 1264, 1264f
Dentin sialophosphoprotein *(DSPP)* gene, in deafness, 2051t-2058t
Dentinogenesis imperfecta, 1257
Dentinogenic ghost cell tumor, 1275-1276
Dentition, inherited and congenital disorders affecting, 1257
Dentition eruption, 2617t
Dentoalveolar abscess, 1252

Dentoalveolar evaluation, prior to radiation therapy, 1330-1331, 1330b, 1331f
Dentoalveolar fractures, pediatric, 2706-2707, 2710f
Dentofacial growth, nasal obstruction and, 2628-2630, 2629f
  open mouth posture in, 2628-2629
  review of literature on, 2629-2630
Denture sore mouth, 1230, 1230f
Denude method, for tonsillar and pharyngeal wall reconstruction, 1386, 1387f
Deoxyribonucleic acid (DNA), 3
  structure of, 4, 11
Deoxyribonucleic acid (DNA) chips, 9
Deoxyribonucleic acid (DNA) damage, by radiation, 1036-1043, 1037f
Deoxyribonucleic acid (DNA)-mediated transfer, of therapeutic genes, 15-16, 15f
Deoxyribonucleic acid (DNA) methyltransferases (DNMTs), in head and neck squamous cell carcinoma, 1020
Deoxyribonucleic acid (DNA) repair enzyme polymorphisms, in head and neck squamous cell carcinoma, 1027
Deoxyribonucleic acid (DNA) sequencing, 3, 9
Deoxyribonucleic acid (DNA) testing, 8-9
  DNA chips for, 9
  mutation testing as, 9, 10f
  nucleic acid hybridization and Southern blotting for, 9
  polymerase chain reaction for, 8-9
Deoxyribonucleic acid (DNA) vectors, 15-16, 15f
Depakote (divalproex), for migraine, 2350
Department of Defense (DoD), 84t-87t, 87
Department of Veterans Affairs (VA), 84t-87t, 87
Deposition of dose, in radiation, 1033
Deposition of energy, in radiation, 1033
Depression
  palliative care for, 1103-1104
  after rhytidectomy, 427
  subclinical hypothyroidism and, 1748
Depressor anguli oris, 321f
Depressor dysfunction, digastric transposition for, 2431-2432
Depressor labii, 442f
Depressor supercilii muscle, 433f
Depth of focus, of surgical laser, 27-28, 28f
Dermabrasion, 397-399
  complications of, 399
  contraindications to, 397-398
  defined, 397
  equipment for, 398, 398f
  historical background of, 397
  micro-, 402-403
  patient selection and consultation for, 397-398
  postoperative care after, 399, 399f
  for scar revision, 298-299, 300f
  technique of, 398-399, 398f-399f
Dermal matrix, in formation of granulation tissue, 1077
Dermatitis
  contact, otitis externa due to, 1945-1946
  otorrhea due to, 2194
  due to radiotherapy, 1047
Dermatocartilaginous ligament, 496-497
Dermatofibroma, 288f
Dermatofibrosarcoma protuberans (DFSP), 291-292
  in children, 2843, 2843f
Dermatologic diseases
  esophageal manifestations of, 979-980
  nasal manifestations of, 660-661
    in Behçet's disease, 660-661
    in pemphigoid, 660
    in pemphigus vulgaris, 660
    in scleroderma, 660
  oral manifestations of, 1253-1254
Dermatomyositis
  laryngeal hypofunction due to, 842
  oral manifestations of, 1252
Dermatosis papulosa nigra, 282
Dermis, 1065
Dermoid(s). *See* Dermoid cysts.
Dermoid cysts, 289
  of cerebellopontine angle, 2527
  in children, 2859
  nasal
    clinical presentation of, 2689, 2689f
    defined, 2687f, 2688-2689
    epidemiology of, 2688-2689
    histology of, 2689
    imaging of, 2689, 2689f
    management of, 2689-2690
  of neck, 1639, 2816
    clinical appearance of, 2816, 2816f
    embryology of, 2586
    imaging of, 2816, 2817f
  of oral cavity, 1287-1288
Dermoid tumors. *See* Dermoid cysts.
Dermopathy, thyroid, and Graves' ophthalmopathy, 1808
DermOtic Oil (fluticasone acetonide oil), for eczematoid otitis externa, 1956
Descending vestibular nucleus (DVN), 1861, 1862f
  in velocity storage, 2296
Descending "w," in nasal breathing assessment, 644
Descriptive statistics, 63, 64t
Desflurane, for anesthesia, 111
Desipramine, for neuropathic pain, 244-245
Desired sensation level (DSL) method, for hearing aids, 2271
  in infants, 2724
Desloratadine (Clarinex), for nonallergic rhinitis, 701t
Desmoglein 1 (Dsg1), in pemphigus vulgaris, 1231
Desmoglein 3 (Dsg3), in pemphigus vulgaris, 1231
Desmoplastic melanoma (DM), 1108, 1108f
Desmoplastic-neurotropic melanoma (DNM), 1108
  of oral cavity, 1299
Desoxymethasone cream, for eczematoid otitis externa, 1955-1956
Detection bias, *vs.* efficacy of treatment, 62t
Detection threshold tests, for olfaction, 631
Developmental anomalies. *See also* Congenital anomaly(ies).
  sensorineural hearing loss due to, sudden, 2129
  of temporomandibular joint, 1280, 1281t
Developmental cysts, of oral cavity, 1287-1288
  dermoid, 1287-1288
  duplication, 1287-1288, 1288f
  nasoalveolar, 1288, 1288f
Deviated septum, 483f, 484
  endoscopic sinus surgery with, 751
  imaging of, 668, 669f
  in noncaucasian patient, 573, 576f
  rhinitis due to, 619b
  rhinoplasty with, 513-514, 514f, 546, 546f-547f
  septoplasty for (*See* Septoplasty)
  due to trauma, 482, 484
  with twisted nose, 551-552, 552f
Dexamethasone (Decadron, Dexacort)
  during adenotonsillectomy, 2797-2798
  for caustic ingestion, 2957
  with chemical peel, 396
  for croup, 2806
  for hyperthyroidism, 1739t
  intratympanic delivery of
    for cisplatin ototoxicity, 2173
    dosing for, 2185
    for Meniere's disease, 2184, 2339
    pharmacokinetics of, 2183-2184
    for sudden sensorineural hearing loss, 2184-2185
Dexamethasone (Decadron, Dexacort) *(Continued)*
  for nonallergic rhinitis, 700t
  for postintubation croup, 2593
  for postoperative nausea and vomiting, 2593
  for professional voice disorders, 854
  for thyroid storm, 1745
Dextran, after free tissue transfer, 1096-1097
Dextroscope, 48
DFMO. *See* Difluoromethylornithine (DFMO).
DFN (deafness, X-linked or mitochondrial), 2050, 2089
DFN1, 2093
DFN2, 2093t
DFN3, 2051t-2058t, 2083, 2093, 2093t
  infant screening for, 2723
DFN4, 2093t
DFN5, 2093t
DFN6, 2093t
DFN7, 2093t
DFN8, 2093t
DFNA (deafness, autosomal dominant), 2050, 2089
DFNA1, 2051t-2058t, 2092t
DFNA2, 2051t-2058t, 2079, 2083, 2090-2092, 2092t
DFNA3, 2051t-2058t, 2083, 2092t
DFNA4, 2051t-2058t, 2092t
DFNA5, 2051t-2058t, 2090-2091, 2092t
DFNA6, 2051t-2058t, 2092-2093, 2092t, 2098
DFNA8, 2051t-2058t, 2068, 2092, 2092t, 2098
DFNA9, 2051t-2058t, 2090-2091, 2092t
DFNA10, 2051t-2058t, 2092t
DFNA11, 2051t-2058t, 2092t
DFNA12, 2051t-2058t, 2068, 2092, 2092t, 2098
DFNA13, 2051t-2058t, 2069, 2092, 2092t
DFNA14, 2051t-2058t, 2092-2093, 2092t, 2098
DFNA15, 2051t-2058t, 2090-2091, 2092t
DFNA17, 2051t-2058t, 2092t
DFNA20, 2051t-2058t, 2074-2075, 2092t
DFNA22, 2051t-2058t, 2078, 2092t
DFNA25, 2051t-2058t, 2081
DFNA26, 2051t-2058t, 2074-2075, 2092t
DFNA28, 2051t-2058t, 2092t
DFNA36, 2051t-2058t, 2092t
DFNA38, 2051t-2058t, 2092-2093, 2092t, 2098
DFNA39, 2051t-2058t, 2092t
DFNA44, 2051t-2058t
DFNA48, 2051t-2058t, 2092t
DFNAi, 2051t-2058t
DFNB (deafness, autosomal recessive), 2050, 2089
DFNB1, 2051t-2058t, 2083, 2089-2090, 2090t-2091t, 2098
  infant screening for, 2235
DFNB2, 2091t
DFNB3, 2051t-2058t, 2076, 2091t
DFNB4, 2051t-2058t, 2083, 2091t, 2096, 2098
  infant screening for, 2723
DFNB5, 2091t
DFNB6, 2051t-2058t, 2091t
DFNB7, 2051t-2058t, 2091t
DFNB8, 2051t-2058t
DFNB9, 2051t-2058t, 2080-2081
DFNB10, 2051t-2058t
DFNB11, 2051t-2058t, 2091t
DFNB12, 2051t-2058t, 2074
DFNB16, 2051t-2058t, 2077, 2091t
DFNB18, 2051t-2058t, 2091t
DFNB21, 2051t-2058t, 2068, 2091t, 2092
DFNB22, 2051t-2058t, 2091t
DFNB23, 2051t-2058t, 2074, 2091t
DFNB24, 2051t-2058t, 2075-2076
DFNB28, 2051t-2058t, 2091t
DFNB29, 2051t-2058t, 2081, 2091t
DFNB30, 2051t-2058t, 2091t
DFNB31, 2051t-2058t, 2077, 2091t
DFNB35, 2051t-2058t
DFNB36, 2051t-2058t, 2075, 2091t
DFNB37, 2051t-2058t, 2091t

DFNB49, 2051t-2058t, 2081
DFNB53, 2051t-2058t, 2069
DFNB59, 2051t-2058t
DFNB61, 2051t-2058t
DFNB63, 2051t-2058t
DFNB66, 2051t-2058t
DFNB67, 2051t-2058t, 2091t
DFNBi, 2051t-2058t
DFSP (dermatofibrosarcoma protuberans), 291-292
in children, 2843, 2843f
DGER (duodenogastroesophageal reflux), ambulatory 24-hour bile monitoring for, 960-961, 961f
DHE (dihematoporphyrin ether), for recurrent respiratory papillomatosis, 2892
DHPLC (denaturing high performance liquid chromatography), 9, 10f
Diabetes mellitus
and Bell's palsy, 2401
esophageal manifestations of, 979
free tissue transfer with, 1091-1092
oral manifestations of, 1251
and pediatric anesthesia, 2596
preoperative evaluation of, 105
sensorineural hearing loss due to, 2094t, 2097
sudden, 2129
and skin flap survival, 1075
Diabetic angiopathy, presbycusis due to, 232
Diacylglycerol (DAG), in salivary gland secretion, 1137
Diagnostic therapy, in voice evaluation, 831
Diagnostic x-rays, energy for, 1034
Dialysis, oral sequelae of, 1255
Diamox (acetazolamide)
for Meniere's disease, 2337
for migraine, 2350
Diaphanous homolog 1 *(DIAPH1)* gene, in deafness, 2051t-2058t, 2076
Dicer, 13, 14f
Dichotomous scales, 63, 63t
Dickens, Charles, 251
Dieffenbach, Johann Friedrich, 475
Diet
for extraesophageal reflux, 900-901
in children, 2946
and laryngeal cancer, 1492
for Meniere's disease, 2337
for migraine, 2349
for voice professional, 852-853
Difficult airway, 108-129
advances in devices and techniques for, 113-115, 114t
awake fiberoptic nasotracheal intubation for, 122-123
advantages of, 123
avoiding failure in, 125, 126b
bronchoscopy cart for, 123, 123f
conscious sedation for, 124
fiberoptic bronchoscope in, 123-125, 125f
historical perspective on, 122-123
indications for, 123, 123b
keys to successful, 124b
monitoring during, 124
nasal trumpet placement for, 124, 125f
optimal setup for, 125f
patient preparation for, 123-124
technique of, 124-125
topical anesthesia for, 124
blind nasal technique for, 114t
case presentations of, 119
with catastrophic events in operating room, 119-120
classification of, 109, 109f
Combitube for, 109-110, 110f, 114t
consequences of, 110
conventional laryngoscopy for, 114t
critical failed airway as, 122
Difficult airway *(Continued)*
due to difficult laryngoscopy, 121
due to difficult mask ventilation, 121-122
due to difficult tracheal intubation, 121
digital technique for, 114t
education on, 117
institutional systems approach to, 118
ongoing, 118
patient and family, 117-119
physician, 117-118
endotracheal tube guides for, 114t
epidemiology of, 109
evolution of management of, 122, 122b
extubation of, 117
face mask ventilation for, 114t, 115f
fiberoptic bronchoscopy for, 114t
Hollinger anterior commissure laryngoscope for, 122, 122f
Johns Hopkins Airway Management Initiative for, 115-118
Adult Emergency Airway Cart in, 116
advanced monitoring in operating room in, 117
Airway Service resources in, 116
Anesthesia Fiberoptic Cart in, 116
conceptual framework of, 115
education in, 117
institutional systems approach to, 118
ongoing, 118
of patient and family, 117
of physicians, 117-118
extubation locations in, 117
formulation of intraoperative and postoperative plans A, B, and C in, 115-116
identification of "Airway Alert" in, 115
in-hospital wristbands and chart labels in, 117
multispecialty service and joint clinical faculty appointment for, 115
nursing critical pathway in, 117
operating room preparation in, 116
operating room setup in, 117
postoperative considerations in, 117
preoperative evaluation in, 115
staff for, 116-117
standard anesthesia equipment in, 116
laryngeal mask airway for, 109-110, 110f, 113, 122, 122b
legal claims related to, 110
lighted stylet for, 114t
medical records of
electronic, 118-119
previous, 118
monitoring of, 111
as multispecialty problem, 108-111
operative surgical airway options for, 125-126
cricothyrotomy as, 114t, 126-128
anatomic considerations in, 126
complications after, 128, 128f
contraindications for, 126-127
cricoid hook in, 127, 128f
defined, 126
dilation of cricothyroid membrane in, 127, 128f
equipment for, 126b
historical perspectives on, 126
indications for, 126-127
palpation and location of cricothyroid membrane in, 127, 127f
percutaneous, 114t, 128
procedure for, 127
rapid five-step technique for, 128
relocation of cricothyroid membrane in, 127, 127f
tracheostomy tube insertion in, 127, 128f
transverse incision in cricothyroid membrane in, 127, 127f
Difficult airway *(Continued)*
vertical incision over cricoid cartilage in, 127, 127f
historical perspectives on, 125-126
patient identification with, 109-110, 109f-110f
predictors of, 109
retrograde intubation for, 114t
rigid bronchoscopes for, 113f, 114t
rigid fiberoptic laryngoscope for, 114t
rigid laryngoscopy for, 114t
tracheotomy for, 114t
transtracheal jet ventilation for, 114t
transtracheal needle ventilation for, 128-129
Difficult laryngoscopy, 121
Difficult mask ventilation (DMV), 121-122
Difficult tracheal intubation, 121
Diffuse esophageal spasm, 965
esophagogram of, 965, 966f
imaging of, 1400-1401, 1401f
manometric findings with, 959t, 965, 965f
Diffuse infiltrative lymphocytosis syndrome (DILS), 1157-1158
immunosuppression and, 218
Diffuse large B-cell lymphoma (DLBCL), 1677-1678
clinical presentation of, 1674
of paranasal sinus and nasal cavity, 1680
treatment and prognosis for, 1680
of salivary glands, 1191-1192, 1192f
treatment and prognosis for, 1680
of thyroid, 1679
staging of, 1679
treatment and prognosis for, 1679
treatment and prognosis for, 1677-1678
of Waldeyer's ring, 1680
treatment and prognosis for, 1680
Diffusion, across interstitial space, 1066
Difluoromethylornithine (DFMO)
ototoxicity of, 2174
animal studies on, 2174
clinical studies on, 2174
conclusions on, 2174
sensorineural hearing loss due to, 2120-2121
and skin flap viability, 1074
Digastric groove
anatomy of, 1822f, 1824f
in surgical anatomy of lateral skull base, 2436f
Digastric muscle
anatomy of, 1296f, 1320, 2578f
posterior belly of, 1826f
Digastric ridge, 1826f
Digastric sulcus, in surgical anatomy of lateral skull base, 2435-2436, 2435f
Digastric transposition, for depressor dysfunction, 2431-2432
Digenic effect, 8
DiGeorge syndrome, deafness in, 2051t-2058t
Digestion, saliva in, 1141
Digestive enzymes, reflex release of, 1206
Digestive tract evaluation, for penetrating neck trauma, 1633-1634, 1634f-1635f
Digital photography, in facial analysis, 277-280, 279f-280f
Digital radiography, of pharynx and esophagus, 1393
Digital sound processing (DSP), for hearing aids, 2267
Digital technique, for difficult airway, 114t
Dihematoporphyrin ether (DHE), for recurrent respiratory papillomatosis, 2892
1,25-Dihydroxyvitamin D_3, in parathyroid hormone regulation, 1776
Di-iodotyrosine (DIT)
in thyroid hormone release, 1738
in thyroid hormone synthesis, 1738

Dilation
for esophageal strictures, due to caustic ingestion, 2960-2962, 2960f-2961f
for tracheal stenosis, 2928, 2928f
Dilator tubae (DT) muscle
anatomy of, 1869f
development of, 1866-1867
in pressure equalization, 1870
DILS (diffuse infiltrative lymphocytosis syndrome), 1157-1158
immunosuppression and, 218
Diltiazem, for hyperthyroidism, 1739t
Dimorphic vestibular afferent nerve fibers, 2283, 2283f
Diode laser, for facial resurfacing, 403t
Diphenhydramine (Benadryl)
for allergic rhinitis, 620
for nonallergic rhinitis, 701t
Diphtheria, pharyngitis due to, 195-196
in children, 2786-2787
Diplopia, due to paranasal sinus tumor, 1123
Dipyridamole, for rhinosinusitis, 734t
Direct audio input, for hearing aid, 2267
Direct brow lift, 430, 431t
Direct cutaneous arteries, 1065, 1065f
Direct nerve implant, for laryngeal reinnervation, 923-924, 924f
Directional microphones, for hearing aids, 2269
Discontinuity defects, maxillofacial prosthodontics for, 1340-1342, 1342f-1343f
Disease
definition of, 53
severity of, 53
Disease-specific scales, as outcome measures, 55-58, 56t
for head and neck cancer, 56-57, 56t
otologic, 56t, 57
pediatric, 56t, 57
rhinologic, 56t, 57
sleep, 56t, 57
symptom, 56t, 57-58
voice, 56t, 57
Disequilibrium, of aging, 233-234
defined, 233
diagnostic methods for, 233
treatment of, 234
vestibular pathology of, 233
Disk battery, ingestion of, 2941, 2958, 2958f
Dislocation, of temporomandibular joint, 1280
Dispersion, descriptive statistics for, 64t
Distal esophageal pressure, 958f
Distal sensory polyneuropathy (DSP), HIV-associated, 223
Distortion product otoacoustic emissions (DPOAEs), 1891, 1905
and audiometric tests, 1905, 1907f
clinical applications of, 1905-1907
defined, 1891, 1905
distortion product in, 1905
frequencies used in, 1905
with high-frequency hearing loss, 1905, 1907f
in infants, 2720-2721
in noise-induced hearing loss, 2146-2147, 2147f-2150f
with normal hearing, 1892f, 1905, 1907f
procedure for, 1891
Distraction osteogenesis
for craniofacial anomalies, 2654-2657, 2656f
for obstructive sleep apnea, 2610
for Robin sequence, 2673
Distress, palliative care for, 1103-1104
DIT (di-iodotyrosine)
in thyroid hormone release, 1738
in thyroid hormone synthesis, 1738
Diuretics
dizziness due to, 2310t
loop
in noise-induced hearing loss, 2147
ototoxicity of, 2174-2175
sensorineural hearing loss due to, 2120
for Meniere's disease, 2126, 2337
Divalproex (Depakote), for migraine, 2350
Divergence paralysis, 2314
Diverticulectomy, transcervical, 991f
Diverticulopexy technique, 992f
Diverticulostomy
endoscopic diathermic, 993f
endoscopic staple, 992-995
complications of, 995
electrocautery technique for, 993f
instruments for, 994f
laser technique for, 993f
limitations of, 994
positioning for, 993f
recurrence after, 995-997
results of, 994-995
technique of, 995f-996f
Diverticulum(a)
esophageal, 974-975, 974f-975f
classification of, 986
double, 986, 989f
mid-, 1402, 1403f
pseudo-, 975, 975f
imaging of, 1406, 1407f
pulsion, 986
traction, 986
types and sites of, 986, 987f-989f
pharyngeal, 1401-1402, 1402f
dysphagia due to, 2951
Zenker's. *See* Zenker's diverticulum (a).
Dix-Hallpike maneuver, 2315-2316, 2315f, 2330-2331, 2331f
Dizziness. *See also* Vertigo.
classification of, 2346
drug-induced, 2310t
evaluation of, 2305-2327
adaptive capabilities of vestibular system in, 2327
algorithm for differential diagnosis in, 2308, 2309f
audiogram for, 2326
background of, 2305
bedside exam for, 2310-2317
dynamic visual acuity in, 2316
eye movements evoked by sound or changes in middle ear pressure in, 2316, 2316f
eye-head coordination in, 2314
head impulse test in, 2314-2315, 2315f
head-shaking nystagmus in, 2314
hyperventilation in, 2316
low-frequency vestibulo-ocular reflex in, 2314
nystagmus in, 2310-2312, 2310t-2311t, 2312f
optokinetic nystagmus in, 2314
positional testing in, 2315-2316, 2315f
saccades in, 2313, 2313f
sensory integration in, 2317
skew deviation and ocular tilt reaction in, 2312-2313, 2312f
smooth pursuit in, 2313-2314
vergence in, 2314
vestibulo-ocular reflex cancellation in, 2314
vestibulospinal function in, 2316-2317
vibration-induced nystagmus in, 2314
high-resolution temporal bone computed tomography for, 2326-2327
history in, 2308-2310, 2309f, 2310t
MRI for, 2327
quantitative testing for, 2317-2324
active head movement analysis techniques for, 2323-2324, 2324f
Dizziness *(Continued)*
caloric, 2319-2320, 2320f-2321f
electrocochleography in, 2323, 2323f
head impulse, 2323
methods of eye movement recordings for, 2317, 2317f
motor control, 2324-2325
for nystagmus, 2317
optokinetic, 2318-2319
posturography in, 2324, 2325f, 2326-2327
rotatory chair, 2320-2323, 2322f-2323f
for saccades, 2317-2318, 2318f
sensory organization, 2325-2326, 2325f-2326f
for smooth pursuit, 2318, 2319f
subjective visual vertical in, 2323
vestibular evoked myogenic potentials in, 2324, 2325f
serologic tests for, 2327
vestibular function in, 2305-2308
brainstem and cerebellum in, 2308
eye movements in, 2305-2307, 2306f-2307f, 2307t, 2309f
head movements in, 2307-2308
peripheral anatomy and physiology in, 2305
due to migraine, 2347
physiologic, 2357
psychophysiologic, 2346
DLBCL. *See* Diffuse large B-cell lymphoma (DLBCL).
DM (desmoplastic melanoma), 1108, 1108f
DMPO (dorsomedial periolivary nucleus), in auditory pathway, 1834f
DMV (difficult mask ventilation), 121-122
DNA. *See* Deoxyribonucleic acid (DNA).
DNM (desmoplastic-neurotropic melanoma), 1108
of oral cavity, 1299
DNMTs (DNA methyltransferases), in head and neck squamous cell carcinoma, 1020
Docetaxel
with chemoradiation, 1041-1042
for induction chemotherapy, 1057-1058
Doctor's Office Quality–Information Technology (DOQ-IT), 84t-87t
Docusate sodium (Cerumenex), for cerumen removal, 1958t
DoD (Department of Defense), 84t-87t, 87
Dohlman, Gosta, 993f
Domeboro Otic. *See* Acetic acid with aluminum acetate (Domeboro Otic).
Dominant disorders, 6, 6f
Dominant-negative effect, 6, 13
Doppler shift, 1643
Doppler ultrasonography, 137
color, 1644
of salivary glands, 1167-1168
of oropharyngeal cancer, 1366
DOQ-IR (Doctor's Office Quality–Information Technology), 84t-87t
Dorello's canal, 1976
Dorsal acoustic stria, 1835, 1835f
Dorsal augmentation, for noncaucasian nose, 556, 569-570
choice of material for, 569, 570f
concept of, 569
results of, 572f-573f
technical considerations for, 569-570, 571f
Dorsal cochlear nucleus, 1835
Dorsal cyst, due to injectable silicone, 578, 579f
Dorsal deformities, revision rhinoplasty for, 584, 585f
Dorsal draw suture, in septal modification, 548, 549f
Dorsal implant, for saddle nose deformity, 555, 556f-558f
Dorsal lingual artery, 1296f
Dorsal stria, in auditory pathway, 1846

Dorsomedial periolivary nucleus (DMPO), in auditory pathway, 1834f
Dorsonasal flap, for nasal defects, 365-366
Dorsum, low, revision rhinoplasty for, 584, 585f
Dorsum sellae, in surgical anatomy of anterior cranial base, 2472f
Dose deposition, in radiation, 1033
Dose-response curves, with radiation therapy, 1038, 1038f
Dose-volume histograms (DVHs), for radiotherapy, 1043
Double chin, liposuction for. *See* Liposuction.
Double-opposing Z-plasty, 2670
  surgical technique for, 2671-2672, 2672f
  for velopharyngeal dysfunction, 2682-2683
Double-strand breaks, by radiation, 1036, 1038
Down syndrome
  craniofacial abnormalities in, 2631-2633, 2631f, 2632b
    due to abnormal and poor growth, 2633
    of ears, 2632
    of eyes, 2632-2633
    mandibular and oral manifestations of, 2632
    of midface, 2632
    of skull, 2632
  inner ear anomalies in, 2735
  and obstructive sleep apnea, 2605-2606
  oral manifestations of, 1257
Doxycycline, for embolization, 1933
DPOAEs. *See* Distortion product otoacoustic emissions (DPOAEs).
Dressing, after liposuction, 459, 459f
Drooling, 2863-2864
  defined, 2863
  epidemiology of, 2863
  medical management of, 2864
  pathogenesis of, 2863-2864
  surgical management of, 2864
Drop attack, 2300
Droperidol, for postoperative nausea and vomiting, 2593
Drug allergies, 94
Drug toxicity, sensorineural hearing loss due to, 2119-2121
  sudden, 2128
Drug-induced epistaxis, 687
Drug-induced esophagitis, 1406, 1406f
Drug-induced hypercalcemia, 1783-1784, 1783t
Drug-induced hypersensitivity, to ototopical antibiotics, 1954
Drug-induced lymphadenopathy, 2819
Drug-induced olfactory dysfunction, 637, 637t
Drug-induced rhinitis, 619b, 696, 697b
Drug-induced sleep videoendoscopy, of obstructive sleep apnea, 253-255
Dry eyes, 446-447, 447f
Dsg1 (desmoglein 1), in pemphigus vulgaris, 1231
Dsg3 (desmoglein 3), in pemphigus vulgaris, 1231
DSL (desired sensation level) method, for hearing aids, 2271
  in infants, 2724
DSP (digital sound processing), for hearing aids, 2267
DSP (distal sensory polyneuropathy), HIV-associated, 223
DSPP (dentin sialophosphoprotein) gene, in deafness, 2051t-2058t
DT (dilator tubae) muscle
  anatomy of, 1869f
  development of, 1866-1867
  in pressure equalization, 1870
DTH (delayed-type hypersensitivity) reactions, 601, 608-612
Ductal cysts
  congenital, 2859
  of larynx, 869, 869f-870f
Ductal secretion, by salivary glands, 1136
Duct(s) of Rivinus, 2850-2852
Ductus reuniens
  anatomy of, 1851f, 1853f-1854f, 2278f
  embryogenesis of, 1852
Duloxetine, for neuropathic pain, 244-245, 245t
Dumbbell tumor, of salivary glands, 1164-1165, 1165f, 1167f-1168f
Dumon stent, for tracheal stenosis, 2929, 2934f
Duodenogastroesophageal reflux (DGER), ambulatory 24-hour bile monitoring for, 960-961, 961f
Duplication, 4-5
Duplication cysts
  foregut, compression of pharynx and esophagus due to, 1408-1409, 1409f
  of oral cavity, 1287-1288, 1288f
Dura, of semicircular canals, 1853f
DuraGen Dermal Graft Matrix, for CSF rhinorrhea, 792-793
Dura-Guard Dural Repair Patch, for CSF rhinorrhea, 792-793
Dural arteriovenous fistulas, embolization of, 1940-1942, 1940f
Dural defect, after transnasal endoscopic-assisted anterior skull base surgery, 2484
Dural septum, in surgical anatomy of lateral skull base, 2437f
Dural tear, due to mastoidectomy, 2015
Durepair Dural Regeneration Matrix, for CSF rhinorrhea, 792-793
DVA (dynamic visual acuity), 2316
DVA (Dynamic Visual Acuity) testing, 2378
DVHs (dose-volume histograms), for radiotherapy, 1043
DVN (descending vestibular nucleus), 1861, 1862f
  in velocity storage, 2296
Dx-pH Measurement System, 962, 962f
Dying spells, in stridulous child, 2898
Dynamic adjustable rotational tip (DART) graft, for saddle nose deformity, 555, 559f
Dynamic airway assessment, for stridor, 2903
Dynamic compensation, for peripheral vestibular lesions, 2373-2376
Dynamic posturography
  for ablative vestibular surgery, 2365
  for vestibular rehabilitation, 2376-2377
Dynamic range
  of auditory neurons, 1844-1845, 1845f
  with hearing aids, 2268
    compression of, 2205-2207
Dynamic visual acuity (DVA), 2316
Dynamic Visual Acuity (DVA) testing, 2378
Dynamic-range compression, for hearing aids, 2268
Dysgeusia, palliative care for, 1103
Dysphagia, 963-968
  algorithm for evaluation of, 954-955, 955f
  due to chemoradiation, 1219
  in children, 2948-2955
    anatomic site(s) of, 2949-2954, 2951f
      hypopharynx and larynx as, 2950t, 2951-2953, 2953f
      nose and nasopharynx as, 2949, 2950t, 2951f
      oral cavity and oral pharynx as, 2949-2951, 2950t, 2952f
      trachea and esophagus as, 2950t, 2953-2954, 2954f
    evaluation of, 2948-2949
      clinical or bedside, 2948-2949
      instrumental, 2949, 2950t
      other diagnostic tests in, 2949
  defined, 954-955
  differential diagnosis of, 990t
  due to eosinophilic esophagitis, 967-968, 969f
  esophageal, 954-956
    vs. oropharyngeal, 956
  due to esophageal motility abnormalities, 963-965, 963b
Dysphagia *(Continued)*
  achalasia as, 963-965
    defined, 963
    endoscopy of, 964, 964f
    esophageal manometry for, 964, 964f
    esophogram of, 963-964, 963f-964f
    etiology and pathogenesis of, 963
    management of, 964-965
    manometric findings with, 959t
    symptoms of, 963
  nonachalasia, 965, 965f-966f
  evaluation for, 1217-1219
    bedside, 1217
    endoscopic, 1218
      for chronic aspiration, 926
    manometry in, 1219
    ultrasonography in, 1219
    videofluoroscopy in, 1217-1218, 1219f
  in geriatric patients, 237
    diagnostic testing for, 237
    treatment of, 237
  due to hypothyroidism, 979
  imaging of, 1398
    ultrasonography for, 1219
    videofluoroscopy for, 1217-1218, 1219f
  due to laryngeal paralysis, 914
  liquid, 954-955
  vs. odynophagia, 956
  oropharyngeal (transfer), 954-955
    vs. esophageal, 956
    evaluation of, 956
  outcome scales for, 57-58
  palliative care for, 1104
  due to post-treatment complications, 1220
  due to radiotherapy, 1219
  due to rings or webs, 966-967, 967f-968f
  screening for, 1217
  signs and symptoms of, 1217
    aspiration (coughing, choking) as, 1217
  solid food, 954-955
  due to strictures, 965-966
    defined, 965-966
    endoscopy of, 965-966, 967f
    esophagram of, 965-966, 966f
    etiology of, 965-966, 966b
    extrinsic, 965-966, 966b
    intrinsic, 965-966, 966b
    refractory, 966
    treatment of, 966
  due to surgical treatment, 1219
    of larynx, 1220
    of pharynx, 1220
    of posterior oral cavity, 1219-1220
    of tongue, 1219
  due to thyroid disease, 1737
  after total laryngopharyngectomy, 1575
  transnasal esophagoscopy in, 983-984, 984f
Dysphonia
  functional, 851
    in children, 2879
  in geriatric patients, 236
  hyperfunctional, 834
  muscle tension, 842, 853
  postoperative, 873-874, 873f
    diagnosis of, 873-874
      history in, 873
      laryngeal examination in, 874
      vocal capability battery in, 873-874
    epidemiology of, 873
    management of, 874
      behavioral, 874
      medical, 874
    pathophysiology and pathology of, 873, 874f
  in professional voice (*See* Professional voice disorders)
  spasmodic, 839
    botulinum toxin therapy for, 839, 840f-841f
    voice breaks in, 834-835

Dysplasia
of larynx, 1486-1491
of oral cavity, 1299
oropharyngeal, 1360
mild, 1360
moderate, 1360
severe, 1360-1361
Dysplastic nevus, 288, 288f
Dyspnea, due to thyroid disease, 1737
Dystonia
adductor breathing, 839
classification of, 838, 838b
diagnosis of, 838
distribution of, 838, 838b
epidemiology of, 838
family history of, 838-839
focal, 838, 838b
generalized, 838
hemi-, 838
laryngeal, 838-839
primary *vs.* secondary, 838
segmental, 838
spread of, 838
Dystrophic epidermolysis bullosa, esophageal manifestations of, 979

E

Ea (early antigen), of Epstein-Barr virus, 1352, 1354
EABR (electrically evoked auditory brainstem response), 1912-1913, 1913f
EABR (evoked auditory brainstem response). *See* Auditory brainstem response (ABR).
EAC. *See* External auditory canal (EAC).
Eagle's syndrome, *vs.* myofascial pain dysfunction syndrome, 1284t
Ear(s)
aesthetic analysis of, 275, 279f
aging of, 231-234
anatomic landmarks of, 2742f
anatomy of, 476-477, 476f, 2742, 2742f
burns of, 316
in Down syndrome, 2632
embryology of, 476-477, 2741, 2742f, 2753
external (*See* External ear)
growth of, 2742
height of, 2742
inner (*See* Inner ear)
melanoma of, 1114
microscopic examination of, 2574
middle (*See* Middle ear)
physical examination of, 97-98
auricles in, 97
external auditory canal in, 97
hearing assessment in, 97-98, 98t
tympanic membrane in, 97, 98f
physiology of (*See* Auditory physiology)
prosthetic, 1345-1346, 1345t, 1346f
protruding, 2742
embryology of, 476-477
etiology of, 476
incidence of, 476
otoplasty for (*See* Otoplasty)
surfer's, 1918, 1918f
swimmer's, 97
telephone, 479
trauma to, 308f, 310, 310f
width of, 2742
Ear canal volumes, 1890-1891
Ear cartilage grafts, for revision rhinoplasty, 583
Ear disorders, in geriatric patients, 231-234
presbycusis as, 232
etiologies of, 232
treatment of, 233
types of, 232
Ear disorders, in geriatric patients *(Continued)*
presbystasis as, 233-234
diagnostic methods for, 233
treatment of, 234
vestibular pathology of, 233
Ear drainage, chronic, topical therapies for, 1957-1958, 1961f
Ear hygiene, topical therapies for, 1957-1958, 1961f
EAR (Effectiveness of Auditory Rehabilitation) scale, 57
Ear wick, for otitis externa, 1945-1946, 1951, 1951f
Ear wick packing, in atresiaplasty, 2756-2757
Earex (arachis oil, almond oil, rectified camphor oil), for cerumen removal, 1958t
Earex Plus (choline salicylate and glycerol), for cerumen removal, 1958t
Early antigen (Ea), of Epstein-Barr virus, 1352, 1354
Early deblocking, 2385
Early Hearing Detection and Intervention (EHDI) program, 2098-2099
Early interventions, for infant hearing loss, 2724
Early Speech Perception (ESP), for cochlear implant, 2225-2226
Earmuffs, for prevention of noise-induced hearing loss, 2151
EAS (electrical and acoustic stimulation), cochlear implants with, 2224, 2224f
EATT1 (excitatory amino acid transporter 1), 2081
EBERs (Epstein-Barr encoded ribonucleic acids), 1352
EBM (evidence-based medicine) recommendations, grading of, 55, 55t, 69-70, 70t
EBRT. *See* External-beam radiation therapy (EBRT).
EBUS (endobronchial ultrasonography), 1011
EBV. *See* Epstein-Barr virus (EBV).
E-cad, in oral cancer, 1301
ECAP (electrically evoked compound action potential), 1912-1913
with cochlear implants, 1913f, 1914
Ecchymosis, postauricular, 97
Echinacea, for rhinosinusitis, 735t
Echogenicity, in ultrasound, 1643
Echography, orbital, of Graves' ophthalmopathy, 1810
ECHOS1, in deafness, 2051t-2058t
Echosonography, transesophageal, 1396
ECoG. *See* Electrocochleography (ECoG).
ECP (eosinophil cationic protein), 604
in otitis media, 2764
Ectropion, 445-446, 2420-2421, 2421f
after blepharoplasty, 450
Eczema, otorrhea due to, 2194
Eczematoid otitis externa, topical therapies for, 1955-1957
anti-inflammatory and immunosuppressive agents as, 1956-1957
options for, 1955
steroids as, 1955-1956
Edema
cerebral
after lateral skull base surgery, 2513
due to neck dissection, 1723
facial, due to neck dissection, 1723, 1729f
laryngeal, in vocal professional, 854
preseptal orbital, due to rhinosinusitis, 676
pulmonary
after adenotonsillectomy, 2800
postobstructive, 119
EDN (eosinophil-derived neurotoxin), 604
EDN3 (endothelin 3) gene, in deafness, 2051t-2058t, 2095
EDNRB (endothelin receptor type B) gene, in deafness, 2051t-2058t, 2095
Edrophonium test, 963
in neurologic evaluation, 835
Education, with cochlear implant, 2251-2253, 2251f, 2255-2257
Educational Resource Matrix (ERM), with cochlear implants, 2251f, 2253
EEMG (evoked encephalomyography), for facial nerve injury, 2041
EER. *See* Extraesophageal reflux (EER).
Effect size, 66-67
Effective dose equivalent, 133
Effective masking, in audiologic testing, 1889
Effectiveness, 52, 54
Effectiveness of Auditory Rehabilitation (EAR) scale, 57
Efferent auditory system, 1847-1849
middle ear muscle reflex pathways in, 1847, 1848f
olivocochlear reflex pathways in, 1848-1849, 1848f
Efficacy, 53-54
explanations other than, 61, 61f, 62t
Eflornithine, sensorineural hearing loss due to, 2120-2121
EGD (esophagogastroduodenoscopy)
for extraesophageal reflux, 899
for laryngeal stenosis, 2917
EGF (epidermal growth factor)
in saliva, 1140
in wound healing, 1076
EGFR. *See* Epidermal growth factor receptor (EGFR).
EGG (electroglottography)
for measurement of vocal fold vibration, 830, 835
for professional voice, 849
EGM (electrogustometry), 2383-2384
EHDI (Early Hearing Detection and Intervention) program, 2098-2099
EHLL (epithelial hyperplastic laryngeal lesions), 1525
EHR (electronic health record), 84t-87t
EI(s) (entry inhibitors), 211
Eicosanoids, in rhinosinusitis, 731-732, 732f
Einstein, Albert, 1032-1033
Elastin, in skin flaps, 1071
Elderly. *See* Geriatric patients.
Elective lymph node dissection (ELND), for melanoma, 1114-1115
Electric acoustic reflex thresholds, for cochlear implants, 2255
Electric stimulation, for tinnitus, 2136-2137
via cochlear implants, 2137
transcutaneous, 2136-2137
Electrical and acoustic stimulation (EAS), cochlear implants with, 2224, 2224f
Electrically evoked auditory brainstem response (EABR), 1912-1913, 1913f
Electrically evoked auditory potentials, 1912-1914
auditory brainstem response as, 1912-1913, 1913f
clinical applications of, 1914
compound action potential as, 1912-1913
with cochlear implants, 1913f, 1914
middle and long latency response as, 1912-1914, 1913f
Electrically evoked compound action potential (ECAP), 1912-1913
with cochlear implants, 1913f, 1914
Electrically evoked long latency responses (ELLRs), 1913-1914
Electrically evoked middle latency responses (EMLRs), 1912-1914
Electroacoustic characteristics, of hearing aid, 2267-2268, 2268f
Electroacoustic stimulation, cochlear implants with, 2224, 2224f
hearing preservation and, 2245-2246

Electrocautery
interventional bronchoscopy with, 1010t
in otoplasty, 478
Electrocautery tonsillectomy, 2797-2799
Electrocochleography (ECoG), 1892-1896, 1907-1908
and auditory brainstem responses, 1908
clinical applications of, 1908
with cochlear implant, 1913f
cochlear microphonic in, 1907-1908
defined, 1892-1894, 1907
for dizziness, 2323, 2323f
for Meniere's disease, 1892-1896, 1895f, 1908, 2337
with normal hearing, 1894f, 1913f
procedure for, 1894, 1908
for sensorineural hearing loss, in adults, 2117
SP/AP ratio in, 1892-1894
summating potential in, 1892-1894, 1907
whole-nerve action potential in, 1892-1894, 1907
Electrodes, for intraoperative cranial nerve monitoring
recording, 2543-2544, 2543f
stimulating, 2544, 2544f
Electrodiagnostic testing, of facial nerve function, 2385-2387
electromyography in, 2386-2387
electroneuronography in, 2041, 2386, 2387t
maximal stimulation test in, 2040-2041, 2385-2386, 2387t
nerve excitability test in, 2040-2041, 2385, 2387t
Electrodogram, 2230, 2230f
Electroglottography (EGG)
for measurement of vocal fold vibration, 830, 835
for professional voice, 849
Electrogustometry (EGM), 2383-2384
Electrolarynx voice and speech, physiology of, 1596, 1596f
Electrolyte composition, ideal, for infants, 2572t
Electromagnetic (EM) middle ear implantable hearing aids, 2208-2211
Carina as, 2210-2211
clinical results with, 2210-2211
components of, 2210, 2210f
history of, 2210
placement of, 2210, 2211f
Middle Ear Transducer (MET) as, 2027, 2210-2211
clinical results with, 2210-2211
comparison of features of, 2206t
components of, 2210
history of, 2210
indications for, 2210, 2211f
placement of, 2210, 2211f
ossicular coupling in, 2207-2208
sound transduction and coupling to auditory system with, 2205f
transducer design for, 2207
Vibrant Soundbridge as, 2208-2210
clinical data on, 2209
comparison of features of, 2206t
components of, 2208-2209, 2208f
for conductive and mixed hearing loss, 2210
history of, 2208, 2210
implantation of, 2209
indications for, 2209, 2209f
Electromagnetic (EM) radiation, 1031, 1031f
Electromagnetic (EM) stimulation, to assess facial nerve function, 2388-2389
in Bell's palsy, 2394-2395
Electro-mechanical voice devices, after total laryngectomy, 1572
Electromyography (EMG)
artifacts in, 2547-2548, 2548f
for Bell's palsy, 2394
Electromyography (EMG) *(Continued)*
for cranial nerve monitoring
anesthesia and, 2544
of cochlear nerve, 2552
and outcome, 2554-2555
electrodes for
recording, 2543-2544, 2543f
stimulating, 2544, 2544f
of facial nerve, 2387-2388, 2545-2548
for acoustic neuroma and other cerebellopontine angle tumors, 2545
activity evoked by electrical stimulation in, 2545-2546
to assess functional status of nerves after tumor removal, 2545-2546
to identify and map nerves in relation to tumor, 2545
for intraoperative identification of nervus intermedius, 2546, 2546f
limitations of, 2547-2548, 2548f
during microvascular decompression, 2548-2549, 2549f
during other otologic surgery, 2549
and outcome, 2554
during parotid surgery, 2549
spontaneous and mechanically evoked activity in, 2546-2548, 2547f
instrumentation for, 2543
of ninth, tenth, eleventh, and twelfth cranial nerves, 2550-2552, 2551f-2552f
stimulation criteria for, 2544
of third, fourth, and sixth cranial nerves, 2549-2552, 2550f
of trigeminal motor branch, 2550
for facial nerve injury, 2041, 2386-2387
evoked, 2386
laryngeal, 835, 905
for stridor, 2901
Electron beams, in radiotherapy, 1034, 1035f
Electroneuronography/electroneurography (ENoG)
for Bell's palsy, 2394
for facial nerve injury, 2041, 2386, 2387t
for facial nerve neuroma, 2519
Electronic health record (EHR), 84t-87t
Electronic medical record (EMR), 84t-87t
"Electronic nose," for CSF rhinorrhea, 790
Electronic patient record (EPR), of difficult airway, 118-119
Electronic portal imaging devices (EPIDs), with radiotherapy, 1046
Electronystagmography (ENG), 2317
of Meniere's disease, 2337
of saccades, 2318f
of smooth pursuit, 2319f
Electro-oculography (EOG), 2317, 2317f
Electro-olfactogram (EOG), 632
Electrophysiologic hearing assessment, 1904-1915
auditory brainstem response for, 1896, 1908-1911
with acoustic neuroma, 1896, 1898f-1899f, 1911
advantage of, 1908
audiometric thresholds based on
click-evoked, 1909
using more frequency-specific stimuli, 1909-1910, 1910f
with auditory neuropathy or dyssynchrony, 1899-1901, 1900f
click-evoked, 1909
clinical applications of, 1896, 1908-1911
to assess hearing sensitivity, 1909-1910, 1910f
in CHAMP procedure, 1911
for differential diagnosis, 1910-1911
for intraoperative monitoring, 1899f, 1911
Electrophysiologic hearing assessment *(Continued)*
for neurodiagnosis, 1896-1899, 1898f-1899f
otoneurologic, 1910-1911
with cochlear implant, 1913f
defined, 1896, 1908
effect of intensity on, 1908, 1909f
electrically evoked, 1912-1913, 1913f
electrocochleography and, 1908
interpretation of, 1896
maturational changes in, 1908
with normal hearing, 1896, 1896f, 1908, 1909f, 1913f
and otoacoustic emissions, 1891-1892, 1893f
procedure for, 1896, 1908
speech-evoked, 1911
stacked, 1911
tone burst–evoked, 1909-1910
auditory steady-state response for, 1911-1912
clinical applications of, 1910f, 1912
electrically evoked auditory potentials for, 1912-1914
auditory brainstem response as, 1912-1913, 1913f
clinical applications of, 1914
compound action potential as, 1912-1913
with cochlear implants, 1913f, 1914
middle and long latency response as, 1912-1914, 1913f
electrocochleography for, 1892-1896, 1907-1908
auditory brainstem response and, 1908
clinical applications of, 1908
with cochlear implant, 1913f
cochlear microphonic in, 1907-1908
defined, 1892-1894, 1907
for Meniere's disease, 1892-1896, 1895f, 1908
with normal hearing, 1894f, 1913f
procedure for, 1894, 1908
SP/AP ratio in, 1892-1894
summating potential in, 1892-1894, 1907
whole-nerve action potential in, 1892-1894, 1907
middle and long latency evoked potentials for, 1912, 1913f
electronically evoked, 1912-1914
otoacoustic emissions for, 1891-1892, 1904-1907
with acoustic neuroma, 1891-1892, 1893f, 1897
advantages of, 1906
and audiograms, 1905, 1906f
and auditory neuropathy or dyssynchrony, 1907
clinical applications of, 1905-1907
cochlear echoes in, 1891
distortion-product, 1891, 1905
and audiometric tests, 1905, 1907f
clinical applications of, 1905-1907
defined, 1891, 1905
distortion products in, 1905
frequencies used in, 1905
with high-frequency hearing loss, 1905, 1907f
with normal hearing, 1892f, 1905, 1907f
procedure for, 1891
with neural hearing loss, 1899-1901
with normal hearing, 1905, 1906f
procedure for, 1891
with sensorineural hearing loss, 1905, 1906f
spontaneous, 1905
stimulus-frequency, 1891
transient evoked, 1891, 1905
with acoustic neuroma, 1891-1892, 1893f
advantages of, 1891
analysis of, 1905
clinical applications of, 1905-1907
defined, 1891, 1905
with normal hearing, 1892f
types of evoked, 1891, 1905
Electrophysiologic monitoring, during anterior and middle cranial base surgery, 2450

Electrophysiologic testing, of olfactory ability, 632
Electrosurgery, for skin lesions, 294
ELLRs (electrically evoked long latency responses), 1913-1914
ELLRs (evoked long latency responses)
  auditory, 1912, 1913f
  electrically, 1913-1914
ELND (elective lymph node dissection), for melanoma, 1114-1115
EM. *See* Electromagnetic (EM); Erythema multiforme (EM).
Embolic agents, 1933-1934
Embolization
  angiographic catheters for, 1932-1933
  angiographic equipment for, 1932
  embolic agents for, 1933-1934
  for epistaxis, 690, 691f
  of juvenile angiofibroma, 1937-1938, 1938f
    nasopharyngeal, 1351
  of meningiomas, 1938, 1939f
  of paragangliomas, 1934-1937, 1935f
    carotid body tumor as, 1937, 1937f
    glomus jugulare tumor as, 1935-1936, 1936f
    glomus tympanicum tumor as, 1935
    glomus vagale tumor as, 1936-1937, 1936f
  provocative testing to ensure safety of, 1934, 1934f
  of thyroid neoplasms, 1938-1939
  of vascular lesions, 1939-1943
    dural arteriovenous fistulas as, 1940-1942, 1941f
    epistaxis as, 1939-1940, 1940f
    facial arteriovenous fistulas as, 1940, 1940f
    facial vascular malformations as, 1942, 1942f
    hemangiomas of face and neck as, 1942
    pseudoaneurysms as, 1942, 1943f
    tinnitus-producing fibromuscular dysplasia of carotid artery as, 1943
Embosphere Clear, for embolization, 1933
Embryology, of head and neck, 2583-2585, 2583f
  branchial arches in, 2583-2584, 2583f
    craniofacial syndromes related to, 2585
    innervation of, 2584
    muscular derivatives of, 2584
    skeletal derivatives of, 2583-2584, 2583f
  pharyngeal pouch(es) in, 2583-2585, 2583f-2584f
    first, 2584, 2584f-2585f
    fourth through sixth, 2584f-2585f, 2585
    second, 2584, 2584f-2585f
    third, 2584f-2585f, 2585
EMG. *See* Electromyography (EMG).
Emissary vein, in surgical anatomy of lateral skull base, 2436f
EMLA (eutectic mixture of local anesthetics), for premedication of children, 2589
EMLRs (electrically evoked middle latency responses), 1912-1914
EMLRs (evoked middle latency responses)
  auditory, 1912, 1913f
  electrically, 1912-1914
EMP (extramedullary plasmacytoma), of larynx, 1509
Emphysema
  oral manifestations of, 1250
  subcutaneous
    of infrahyoid retropharyngeal space, 161f
    of neck, 1410, 1410f
Empirical Sleepiness and Fatigue Scales, 57
Empty sella syndrome (ESS), CSF rhinorrhea due to, 787
Empyema, subdural, 1994-1995
  epidemiology of, 1980t-1981t, 1994-1995
  imaging of, 1995
  in neonates, 1995
  otitis media and, 2777
  symptoms of, 1995
  treatment of, 1995
EMR (electronic medical record), 84t-87t
ENaCs (epithelial Na⁺ channels), in taste, 1208
Enamel organ, development of, 1259
ENB. *See* Esthesioneuroblastoma (ENB).
Encephalocele(s), 2645, 2646f
  classification of, 2645
  defined, 2645
  imaging of, 670, 671f, 765t
  nasal, 2687-2688
    basal, 2687-2688, 2687t, 2688f
    classification of, 2687-2688, 2687t
    defined, 2687, 2687f
    epidemiology of, 2687
    vs. gliomas, 2688
    histopathology of, 2688
    imaging of, 2688, 2688f
    management of, 2688
    nasoethmoidal, 2687-2688, 2687t
    nasofrontal, 2687-2688, 2687t
    naso-orbital, 2687-2688, 2687t
    sincipital, 2687-2688, 2687f, 2687t
    sphenoethmoidal, 2687t
    spheno-orbital, 2687t
    terminology for, 2687
    transethmoidal, 2687t
    transsphenoidal, 2687t
  due to otitis media, 1992-1993, 1993f
  temporal bone, 2509
    diagnostic evaluation of, 2509
    surgical approach to, 2509
Encephalofacial angiomatosis, 1257
Encephalomyography, evoked, for facial nerve injury, 2041
Enchondral bone formation, 2614, 2615f
End of life care, 1104. *See also* Palliative care.
  for geriatric patients, 231
Endaural approach, in tympanoplasty, 2001-2002, 2001f
End-bulbs of Held, 1845
Endobronchial biopsy, flexible fiberoptic bronchoscopy for, 1004-1005, 1004f
Endobronchial brachytherapy, interventional bronchoscopy with, 1010t
Endobronchial stent placement, interventional bronchoscopy for, 1009
Endobronchial ultrasonography (EBUS), 1011
Endocarditis prophylaxis, 102, 1248, 1249t
  for pediatric surgery, 2596, 2596t-2597t
Endocochlear potential, 1840, 1841f-1842f
Endocrine disorders
  oral manifestations of, 1251
  preoperative evaluation of, 104-105
    of adrenal gland, 104-105
    diabetes mellitus as, 105
    of parathyroid, 104
    of thyroid, 104
  sensorineural hearing loss due to, 2125
Endocrine evaluation, prior to anterior and middle cranial base surgery, 2446
Endolaryngeal stents
  for airway stenosis, 947, 947f
  for chronic aspiration, 928, 930f
  for laryngeal trauma, 937, 939f-940f
Endoluminal stents, for unresectable tracheal tumor, 1621-1622
Endolymph, 1832
  in auditory physiology, 1841f-1842f
  in vestibular system, 1855, 2277, 2278f
Endolymph homeostasis, 2081-2083, 2083f-2084f
Endolymph rotation, ampullopetal and ampullofugal, 2289
Endolymphatic diverticulum, 1852
Endolymphatic duct
  anatomy of, 1832, 1851f, 1853f-1854f, 2278f
  operculum of, 1822, 1823f
Endolymphatic fluid, 1832
Endolymphatic hydrops
  audiogram in, 1895f
  electrocochleography in, 1892-1896, 1895f, 1908
  idiopathic (*See* Meniere's disease)
  otosclerosis with, 2035
  sensorineural hearing loss due to, 2126-2127, 2199
  stacked auditory brainstem response in, 1911
  vertigo due to, 2202
Endolymphatic sac, 1825f, 1832, 1851f, 1853f
Endolymphatic sac surgery
  for congenital inner ear anomalies, 2739
  for Meniere's disease, 2126, 2339, 2363-2364, 2363f
Endolymphatic sac tumor, fluctuating hearing loss due to, 2199
Endolymphatic-perilymphatic barrier, 2081, 2082f
Endoscopes, for visualization of larynx, 813-814
  flexible, 814
  rigid, 813-814
Endoscopic brow lift, 431, 431t
Endoscopic CO_2 laser resection, for hypopharyngeal cancer, 1429-1430, 1442
  outcomes of, 1436-1438
Endoscopic dacryocystorhinostomy, 763, 797-802
  complications of, 801
  evaluation for, 797-798
    dacryocystogram in, 798, 798f-799f
    scintilligraphy in, 798, 799f
  nasal preparation for, 798
  outcomes of, 801
  revision, 801
  surgical technique for, 798-801
    agger nasi in, 799-800, 800f
    bone removal in, 799-800, 800f
    common canaliculus in, 800-801, 801f
    creation of flap in, 798, 799f
    endoscopic septoplasty in, 798, 799f
    flap elevation in, 798-799, 800f
    flap positioning in, 800, 800f
    frontal process and lacrimal bone in, 799-800, 800f
    lacrimal probe in, 800
    tube stents in, 800-801, 801f
Endoscopic diathermic diverticulostomy, 993f
Endoscopic esophagodiverticulostomy, 992
Endoscopic excision, of glottic cancer, 1518, 1520f
Endoscopic frontal sinusotomy, 776-778
  accessing frontal recess in, 777, 777f-778f
  confirming location of instrument in, 777-778, 778f
  contrainidications to, 781, 781f
Endoscopic imaging, of early glottic carcinoma, 1515-1516, 1516f
Endoscopic lung volume reduction, 1011
Endoscopic orbital decompression, for Graves' ophthalmopathy, 1814, 1815f-1816f
  combined with open approach, 1814
  combined with optic nerve decompression, 1815
Endoscopic orbital surgery, 763
Endoscopic parathyroid exploration, 1793-1794
Endoscopic repair, for CSF rhinorrhea, 792-794, 793f-794f
Endoscopic sinus surgery (ESS), 739-758, 759-1
  advances in instrumentation for, 762-763
  complications of, 754-755, 754b
    CSF rhinorrhea as, 787, 788f
    hemorrhage as, 754
    intracranial, 755, 755f
    ophthalmic, 754-755
  failure of, 756
  follow-up after revision, 774
  functional
    abnormal facial growth and development due to, 2623-2625
    extent of, 759-760
    ostiomeatal complex in, 760, 760f

Endoscopic sinus surgery (ESS) *(Continued)*
for pediatric chronic sinusitis, 2779-2781, 2780f-2781f
principles of, 743, 759
radiologic evaluation after, 677-680
expected findings in, 677-679, 679f
operative complications in, 679-680, 680f
historical background of, 739
indications for, 741-742, 741b, 760-761
anterior meningoencephaloceles as, 742
choanal atresia as, 742
CSF rhinorrhea as, 742
expanded utilization of transnasal endoscopic sinus approach as, 742
headache and facial pain as, 742
intractable epistaxis as, 742
mucoceles as, 742, 760f, 761, 762f
removal of foreign body as, 742
rhinosinusitis as
with acute complications, 741, 761
allergic fungal, 761, 762f
chronic, 741, 761
invasive fungal, 742, 761
noninvasive fungal, 742, 761
recurrent acute, 741
sinonasal polyposis as, 741
tumors as, 742, 762-763
medical treatment prior to, 763
results of, 755-756
for rhinosinusitis, 742-756, 759-1
with acute complications, 741, 761
anesthesia for, 744-745
general, 745
local, 744-745
anterior ethmoidectomy in, 747, 748f
antibiotics prior to, 743
chronic, 741-743, 761
complete ethmoidectomy in, 748-749, 749f-750f
complications of, 754-755, 754b
hemorrhage as, 754
intracranial, 755, 755f
ophthalmic, 754-755
computer-assisted navigation in, 772
with concha bullosa, 751, 752f
conclusion of procedure for, 751
failure of, 756
frontal sinusotomy in, 750-751, 768-771
agger nasi cell in, 769, 771f-772f
and causes of frontal sinus disease, 769
challenges of, 768
external approaches as adjunct to, 771, 773f
frontal bullar cell in, 772f
frontal recess dissection in, 769, 770b, 770t, 771f
frontal sinus cells in, 769-770, 772f
image-guided navigation system in, 771f
interfrontal sinus septal cell in, 771, 772f
preoperative evaluation for, 768-769
recessus terminalis in, 771
suprabullar cell in, 772f
supraorbital ethmoid cell in, 770-771, 772f
fungal, 742, 761, 762f
image-guided navigation systems in, 743-744, 745f
intraoperative CT scans during, 744, 772
limited *vs.* extended approaches for, 752-753
maxillary antrostomy in, 747, 747f
failure of, 764-766, 766f
Messerklinger technique for, 746
middle turbinate in, 751, 751f, 771
minimally invasive sinus technique in, 743, 752, 760
with mucoceles, 751
nasal endoscopy in, 746, 763
with nasal septal deviation, 751

Endoscopic sinus surgery (ESS) *(Continued)*
patient preparation and positioning for, 745-746
with polyps, 751-752
posterior ethmoidectomy in, 747-748, 749f
postoperative care after, 753-754, 773-774
preoperative assessment for, 743, 763-764
CT in, 743, 744t, 763-764, 764f-765f, 764t
examination in, 743
history in, 743
MRI in, 764, 765t
nasal endoscopy in, 763
recurrent acute, 741
resection of uncinate process in, 746, 746f
results of, 755-756
sinus balloon catheterization in, 752-753, 753f
sphenoid sinusotomy in, 748, 749f
sphenoidotomy in, 748, 749f
complications of, 767, 768t
for fungus ball, 768f-769f
with image-guided navigation system, 770f
Wigand technique for, 746
simulation of, 46-49
Dextroscope for, 48
ES3 for, 46-48, 46f
curriculum development for, 48
validation studies of, 47-48, 47f, 48t
Nasal Endoscopy Simulator for, 49
Paranasal Sinuses Simulator for, 49
rationale for, 46-49
VR-FESS for, 48
surgical anatomy for, 739-741
anatomic variations in, 741
anterior skull base in, 741
ethmoid complex in, 740
frontal sinus in, 740-741
maxillary sinus in, 740
middle turbinate in, 739-740
ostiomeatal complex in, 739, 740f
sphenoid sinus in, 740, 740f
Endoscopic sinus surgery simulator (ES3), 46-48, 46f
curriculum development for, 48
validation studies of
for discriminant and concurrent validity, 47, 47f
vs. performance on other tests of innate ability, 48, 48t
for predictive validity, 48
Endoscopic sphenopalatine artery ligation (ESPAL), for epistaxis, 689-690, 689f-690f
Endoscopic staple diverticulostomy (ESD), 992-995
complications of, 995
electrocautery technique for, 993f
instruments for, 994f
laser technique for, 993f
limitations of, 994
positioning for, 993f
recurrence after, 995-997
results of, 994-995
technique of, 995f-996f
Endoscopic surgery
of anterior and middle cranial base, 2448-2450
in central compartment, 2457-2458, 2457f
for juvenile nasopharyngeal angiofibroma, 1350-1351
for nasopharyngeal carcinoma, 1355, 1355f
Endoscopic transnasal-transsphenoidal resection, 2457-2458, 2457f
Endoscopic treatment
for GERD, 970
of laryngeal stenosis, 2918
of stridulous child, 2908-2909
balloons in, 2906, 2906f, 2909
endoscopic sutures in, 2909
laser in, 2908-2909, 2908f

Endoscopic treatment *(Continued)*
microdebrider in, 2909
microinstrumentation for, 2908, 2908f
stents, keels, and grafts in, 2909
for topical drug administration, 2909
Endoscopic-assisted anterior skull base surgery, transnasal, 2471-2486
anesthesia for, 2476
combined approaches for, 2484
complications of, 2485
craniocervical junction–odontoid approach for, 2483-2484, 2484f
instrumentation for, 2476
patient preparation for, 2475-2476
pedicled septal flap in, 2476-2477
postoperative care after, 2484-2485
preoperative assessment for, 2475, 2475f
reconstruction after, 2484
surgical anatomy for, 2471-2475
anterior cranial fossa in, 2471, 2472f
clivus in, 2474, 2474f
nasal cavity in, 2471-2473, 2472f-2473f
nasopharynx in, 2474
paranasal sinuses in, 2473-2474, 2473f
retroclival region in, 2474-2475, 2474f-2475f
surgical team setup for, 2476f
transcribriform approach for, 2482
with bilateral access, 2482, 2482f
with unilateral access, 2482
transmaxillary-transpterygoidal-infratemporal approach for, 2482-2483, 2483f
transsellar and parasellar approaches for, 2479, 2480f
transsphenoidal approach for, 2477-2481
with direct transnasal access, 2477, 2477f
with petrous apex access, 2481
with transclival approach, 2479-2481, 2480f-2481f
with transethmoidal access, 2478-2479, 2479f-2480f
with transseptal access, 2477-2478, 2477f-2478f
with transseptal-transnasal access, 2478, 2479f
transtuberculum-transplanum approach for, 2482
Endoscopy
for airway stenosis, 944-945, 945f
for caustic ingestion, 2957-2959, 2958f
for foreign body removal, 2939-2940, 2939t, 2940f
gastroesophageal, 956-957
equipment for, 956
of esophageal varices, 958f
for extraesophageal reflux, 899
of gastroesophageal junction
with Mallory-Weiss tear, 957f
normal, 956-957, 957f
with severe esophagitis, 957f
of squamocolumnar junction, 956-957, 956f-957f
technique of, 956-957
for laryngeal trauma, 936
of larynx (*See* Laryngeal videoendoscopy)
in nasal examination, 642
for oral cancer, 1300
of oropharyngeal cancer, 1366, 1366f
for swallowing disorders, 1218
with chronic aspiration, 926
of tracheal stenosis, 2926-2927
virtual, 138, 140f
ENDOSTITCH autosuture device, 993, 994f-996f
Endothelin 3 *(EDN3)* gene, in deafness, 2051t-2058t, 2095
Endothelin receptor type B *(EDNRB)* gene, in deafness, 2051t-2058t, 2095

Endotracheal intubation (ETT)
for croup, 2806
of difficult airway, Hollinger anterior commissure laryngoscope for, 122, 122f
laryngeal trauma due to, 939
etiology of, 939, 941f
incidence of, 939
with intubation granulomas, 939, 941f
with laryngeal stenosis, 939, 940f, 943
in children, 2914-2915
management of, 939
for supraglottitis, 2808
Endotracheal tube(s) (ETT), for laser surgery, 36-37
Endotracheal tube (ETT) guides, for difficult airway, 114t
Endovascular interventional procedures, 1932-1943
for lesions of vascular etiology, 1939-1943
dural arteriovenous fistulas as, 1940-1942, 1941f
epistaxis as, 1939-1940, 1940f
facial arteriovenous fistulas as, 1940, 1940f
facial vascular malformations as, 1942, 1942f
hemangiomas of face and neck as, 1942
pseudoaneurysms as, 1942, 1943f
tinnitus-producing fibromuscular dysplasia of carotid artery as, 1943
materials and techniques for, 1932-1934
angiographic catheters as, 1932-1933
angiographic equipment as, 1932
embolic agents as, 1933-1934
provocative testing to ensure safety of embolization as, 1934, 1934f
for neoplasms, 1934-1939
inter-arterial chemotherapy as, 1939
juvenile angiofibroma as, 1937-1938, 1938f
meningiomas as, 1938, 1939f
paragangliomas as, 1934-1937, 1935f
carotid body tumor as, 1937, 1937f
glomus jugulare tumor as, 1935-1936, 1935f-1936f
glomus tympanicum tumor as, 1935
glomus vagale tumor as, 1936-1937, 1936f
thyroid, 1938-1939
Energy deposition, in radiation, 1033
ENG. *See* Electronystagmography (ENG).
Enhancers, of gene expression, 19
ENoG (electroneuronography)
for Bell's palsy, 2394
for facial nerve injury, 2041, 2386, 2387t
for facial nerve neuroma, 2519
Enteric transplantation, for hypopharyngeal and esophageal reconstruction, 1455-1457
gastro-omental donor site for, 1457-1458, 1457f
jejunal donor site for, 1455-1457, 1456f
Entropion, 445-446
after blepharoplasty, 450
Entry inhibitors (EIs), 211
Enuresis, 262t
with obstructive sleep apnea, 2603
sleep-disordered breathing and, 2792
Environmental factors
in head and neck squamous cell carcinoma, 1016-1018
and nasopharyngeal carcinoma, 1352
in noise-induced hearing loss, 2147-2148
in otitis media, 2767-2768
in rhinosinusitis, 731
Environmental sleep disorder, 262t
Environmental sound enrichment, for tinnitus, 2133-2134
Environmental tobacco smoke (ETS), and chronic rhinosinusitis, 707
Envoy device, 2206t, 2211-2212, 2212f
EOAEs (evoked otoacoustic emissions), in infants, 2720-2721
EOG (electro-oculography), 2317, 2317f
EOG (electro-olfactogram), 632
EORTC-HN35 (European Organization for Research and Treatment of Cancer Quality of Life Questionnaire), 56
Eosinophil(s)
in adaptive immune system, 604
in allergic rhinitis, 616
Eosinophil cationic protein (ECP), 604
in otitis media, 2764
Eosinophil peroxidase (EPO), 604
Eosinophil-derived neurotoxin (EDN), 604
Eosinophilia
nonallergic rhinitis with, 619b, 696
in rhinosinusitis, 731
Eosinophilic esophagitis, 967-968, 969f
dysphagia due to, 2954
Eosinophilic granuloma, 2100
of oral cavity, 1240, 1257
clinical features of, 1240, 1240f
defined, 1240
differential diagnosis of, 1240
etiology of, 1240
histopathologic features of, 1240, 1240f
treatment of, 1240
otologic manifestations of, 2101f-2102f
otorrhea as, 2196
Eosinophilic inflammation, in chronic rhinosinusitis, 707
Ependymoma, of cerebellopontine angle, 2528-2529, 2531f
EPID(s) (electronic portal imaging devices), with radiotherapy, 1046
Epidemic vertigo, 2332-2333
Epidermal grafts, for airway stenosis, 947
Epidermal growth factor (EGF)
in saliva, 1140
in wound healing, 1076
Epidermal growth factor receptor (EGFR)
in head and neck squamous cell carcinoma, 1022-1023
biology of, 1022, 1025f
as biomarker, 1026
clinical implications of, 1023
oncogene for, 1019
and targeted therapy, 1060-1061
in laryngeal carcinoma, 1505
in salivary gland neoplasms, 1199
Epidermal growth factor receptor (EGFR) inhibitors, for head and neck squamous cell carcinoma, 1018
Epidermal growth factor receptor tyrosine kinase (EGFR-TK), in non–small cell lung cancer, 1023
Epidermal neoplasm(s), 281-286
actinic keratoses as, 283, 284f
basal cell carcinoma as, 283-285, 284f-285f
chondrodermatitis nodularis helicis as, 285, 285f
dermatosis papulosa nigra as, 282
keratoacanthoma as, 284f, 286
seborrheic keratoses as, 281-282, 282f
squamous cell carcinoma as, 285-286, 285f
warts (verruca vulgaris) as, 282-283
filiform, 282, 282f
flat, 282, 283f
due to molluscum contagiosum, 282-283, 283f
Epidermis, 1065
Epidermoid(s). *See* Epidermoid cyst(s).
Epidermoid cyst(s), 289
of cerebellopontine angle, 2518-2519
diagnostic studies of, 2519
imaging of, 1928, 1928f, 2519, 2520f
in differential diagnosis, 1929t, 2518t, 2519, 2524t
signs and symptoms of, 2518-2519
of cerebellopontine cistern, 2509f
of larynx, 868f-869f, 869
of vocal folds, 2882, 2882f
Epidermoid tumor(s). *See* Epidermoid cyst(s).
Epidermolysis bullosa, esophageal manifestations of, 979
imaging of, 1406, 1406f
Epidural abscess, 1995-1996
epidemiology of, 1980t-1981t
Epigenetic profile, in head and neck squamous cell carcinoma, 1022
Epigenetics, of head and neck squamous cell carcinoma, 1020-1022, 1021f-1022f
Epiglottic cartilage, anatomy of
applied, 806
radiographic, 1471
surgical, 1542f-1543f
Epiglottic flap closure, for chronic aspiration, 928, 930f
Epiglottic laryngoplasty, 1549
complications of, 1549
extended procedures for, 1549
functional outcome of, 1549
key surgical points for, 1549
oncologic results of, 1549
surgical technique for, 1549, 1549f
Epiglottis
anatomy of, 1359f
radiographic, 1397, 1399f, 1463f, 1471f, 1473f
surgical, 1541, 1542f-1543f
bifid, 2870t, 2874, 2874f
carcinoma of
anatomic basis for, 1541
imaging of, 1475, 1477f
pre-glottic space extension of, 1485f
hypoplastic, 2870t
omega, 1464
physical examination of, 100
sarcoidosis of, 1465f
during swallowing, 833
Epiglottitis, 883, 1464
in children, 2806-2809
clinical features of, 2807
complications of, 2808-2809
diagnosis of, 2807-2808, 2807f-2808f
differential diagnosis of, 2806t
endoscopy of, 2808, 2808f
epidemiology of, 2806-2807
etiology of, 2807
histology of, 2807, 2807f
historical background of, 2806-2807
imaging of, 2807f, 2808
management of, 2808
clinical presentation of, 2807
defined, 1464
differential diagnosis of, 1464, 1465f, 2806t
imaging of, 159-161, 1406-1407, 1464
in children, 2807f, 2808
CT for, 1406
plain film, 163f, 1406, 1407f, 1464, 1464f
pseudo-, postlaryngectomy, 1416, 1417f
Epiglottopexy, for laryngomalacia, 2867-2868
Epiglottoplasty, for glottic cancer, 1517t
Epilepsy
olfactory auras in, 636
preoperative evaluation of, 106
Epinephrine, racemic, for croup, 2806
postintubation, 2593
Epiphora, 303
after blepharoplasty, 450-451
due to nasal fracture, 498
due to paranasal sinus tumor, 1123
Epiphrenic diverticula, 974-975, 975f
Episodic rhinitis, 617-618
Epistaxis, 682-693
in adults, 686-687, 687f
due to angiofibroma, 686f
anterior *vs.* posterior, 683-684
due to bleeding from anterior ethmoidal artery, 690-691, 691f-692f

Epistaxis *(Continued)*
cautery for, 687-688, 687f
due to cavernous hemangioma, 684f
in children, 686
drug-induced, 687
embolization for, 690, 691f, 1939-1940, 1940f
emergency department "fast tracking" of, 684, 685b
after endoscopic dacryocystorhinostomy, 801
endoscopic sphenopalatine artery ligation for, 689-690, 689f-690f
epidemiology of, 682
etiology of, 684, 685b
external carotid artery ligation for, 689
first aid measures for, 684
headlamp examination of, 686
due to hereditary hemorrhagic telangiectasia, 691-692, 692f
hot water irrigation for, 691
hypertension and, 686-687
initial assessment of, 684
management protocol for, 692, 693f
maxillary artery ligation for, 688
nasal packing for, 688, 688f
due to nasal trauma, 500
postoperative, 685f
due to pyogenic granuloma, 685f
due to septal perforation, 686f
due to squamous cell carcinoma, 686f
surgical management of, 741
topical treatment of, 687
vascular anatomy and, 682-684
anastomoses in, 682-683, 683f
anterior ethmoid artery in, 682, 684f
facial artery in, 682
greater palatine artery in, 682
internal maxillary artery in, 682
posterior ethmoidal artery in, 682-683
sphenopalatine artery in, 682
vidian artery in, 682, 683f
in Wegener's granulomatosis, 685f
Epithelial grafts, for airway stenosis, 947
Epithelial hyperplastic laryngeal lesions (EHLL), 1525
Epithelial invasion theory, of cholesteatoma formation, 1967f, 1968
Epithelial malignancy
of larynx, 878-880
of paranasal sinuses
staging of, 1128f, 1129, 1129b
Epithelial Na^+ channels (ENaCs), in taste, 1208
Epithelial odontogenic ghost cell tumor, 1275-1276
Epithelial precursor lesions, for oropharyngeal cancer, 1360-1361, 1362f
Epithelial resistance factors, in GERD, 895
Epithelial-myoepithelial carcinoma, of salivary glands, 1191
Epithelioid hemangioendothelioma, of neck, 1668-1669
Epithelioid sarcoma, in children, 2843, 2843f
Epitympanum
anatomy of, 1825-1827, 1827f
in mastoidectomy, 2012-2013, 2013f
in surgical anatomy of lateral skull base, 2438
Epley maneuver, for benign paroxysmal positional vertigo, 2331, 2332f
EPO (eosinophil peroxidase), 604
EPR (electronic patient record), of difficult airway, 118-119
EPSPs (excitatory postsynaptic potentials), in vestibular afferent nerve fibers, 2284-2285, 2284f
Epstein-Barr encoded ribonucleic acids (EBERs), 1352
Epstein-Barr virus (EBV), 1352
and lymphoma
Hodgkin's, 217
nasal T-cell, 660
non-Hodgkin's, 216
and nasopharyngeal carcinoma, 1352, 1354
oral hairy leukoplakia due to, 225-226, 1226
pharyngitis due to, 198-199, 198f
in children, 2785-2786, 2786f
salivary gland inflammation due to, 2855
and salivary gland neoplasms, 1163
vestibular neuritis due to, 2162
ePTFE (expanded polytetrafluoroethylene)
for craniofacial defect repair, 2657
for nasal reconstruction, 368
in noncaucasian rhinoplasty, 569, 570f
Epulis
congenital, of oral cavity, 1290, 1290f
gravidarum, 1256
Epworth Sleepiness Scale (ESS), 57, 253, 253f
Equal-energy principle, 2149-2150
Equitest system, 2324, 2325f
Equivalence studies, 73t, 74
ErbB1, in salivary gland neoplasms, 1199
ErbB2, in salivary gland neoplasms, 1194, 1199
Erbitux (cetuximab)
for metastatic squamous cell carcinoma, 1061
with radiotherapy, 1052, 1054
for laryngeal cancer, 1585
Erbium:yttrium-aluminum-garnet (Er:YAG) laser, 33
Erbium:yttrium-aluminum-garnet (Er:YAG) laser resurfacing, 400
Erb's point, in modified radical neck dissection, 1711
Erector spinae muscle, 2579f
Erlotinib, for cancer chemoprevention, 1062
ERN (Educational Resource Matrix), with cochlear implants, 2251f, 2253
Erosive esophagitis, Los Angeles classification of, 969, 969f
Eruption cyst, 1264, 1264f
treatment of, 1264
Er:YAG (erbium:yttrium-aluminum-garnet) laser, 33
Er:YAG (erbium:yttrium-aluminum-garnet) laser resurfacing, 400
Erysipelas, of external ear, 1948, 1949f
Erythema multiforme (EM), of oral cavity, 1239-1240, 1254
clinical features of, 1239, 1239f-1240f
defined, 1239
differential diagnosis of, 1239
etiology and pathogenesis of, 1239
histopathologic features of, 1239-1240
treatment of, 1240
Erythematous candidiasis, 1230, 1230f
in HIV, 225
Erythrocyte(s), in adaptive immune system, 605
Erythrocyte sludging, in skin flaps, 1068-1069
Erythrokeratoderma variabilis, deafness in, 2051t-2058t
Erythromycin
ototoxicity of, 2176
for pediatric chronic sinusitis, 2779
for rhinosinusitis, 733, 734t
sensorineural hearing loss due to, 2120, 2176
Erythroplakia, of oral cavity, 1298, 1360
ES (Ewing's sarcoma)
in children, 2845
malignant, 1671
oral manifestations of, 1253
ES3 (endoscopic sinus surgery simulator), 46-48, 46f
Eschar excision, for burns, 315
ESD. *See* Endoscopic staple diverticulostomy (ESD).
ESFTs (Ewing's sarcoma family of tumors), in children, 2845
Esmolol, intraoperative, 112
Esophageal acid clearance, in GERD, 895
Esophageal adenocarcinoma, 973, 974f
cervical, 1425
GERD and, 899
Esophageal body
manometry of, 958
physiology of, 954, 955f
Esophageal cancer, 973-974
adenocarcinoma as, 973, 974f
cervical, 1425
GERD and, 899
cervical
adenocarcinoma as, 1425
advanced, 1439
chemotherapy for, 1439
quality of life with, 1439
approach to management of, 1426
chemoradiotherapy for, 1434
chemotherapy for, 1433-1434
clinical evaluation of, 1423
physical findings in, 1423
presenting symptoms in, 1423, 1423t
fasciocutaneous free flaps for, 1433
gastric pull-up for, 1432, 1432f
imaging of, 1423-1424
barium swallow for, 1423-1424
CT for, 1424, 1424f
MRI for, 1424
PET/CT for, 1424, 1424f
incidence of, 1423
lymph node metastasis of, 1434-1439
pathology of, 1424-1425
radiation therapy for, 1436
therapeutic outcome of, 1436
staging of, 1426-1434, 1426t-1427t
therapeutic outcomes for, 1435-1436
total pharyngo-laryngo-esophagectomy for, 1430-1431
esophageal strictures due to, 1408, 1408f
imaging of, 1412-1415, 1414f
reconstruction for (*See* Esophageal reconstruction)
squamous cell carcinoma as, 973
due to caustic injury, 978
localized, 1444-1447
definitive chemoradiation for, 1445-1447, 1446t-1447t
postoperative therapy for, 1444-1447
preoperative therapy for, 1444-1445, 1445t
metastatic, 1447
staging of, 973-974, 974b
tracheal invasion by, 1615
varicoid, 1414f
Esophageal defects, classification of, 1450
Esophageal dilation, for strictures, 966
transnasal esophagoscopy in, 984, 984f
Esophageal disease state(s)
causing dysphagia, 963-968
eosinophilic esophagitis as, 967-968, 969f
esophageal motility abnormalities as, 963-965, 963b
achalasia as, 963-965, 963f-964f
nonachalasia, 965, 965f-966f
rings or webs as, 966-967, 967f-968f
strictures as, 965-966
defined, 965-966
endoscopy of, 965-966, 967f
esophagram of, 965-966, 966f
etiology of, 965-966, 966b
extrinsic, 965-966, 966b
intrinsic, 965-966, 966b
refractory, 966
treatment of, 966
due to caustic injury, 977-978, 978f-979f, 978t
chronic aspiration due to, 926b

Esophageal disease state(s) *(Continued)*
due to foreign body (*See* Esophagus, foreign bodies in)
gastroesophageal reflux disease as, 968-973
Barrett's esophagus due to, 972-973, 972f-973f, 973t
defined, 968
diagnosis of, 968-969, 969f
extraesophageal, 970-973, 970f
asthma due to, 971
chest pain due to, 971
chronic cough due to, 971
dental erosions due to, 971-972
laryngitis due to, 970-971
nonerosive, 968
pathogenesis of, 968
reflux esophagitis in, 968
symptoms of, 968
treatment for, 969-970
infectious esophagitis as, 976-977, 976f-978f
neoplastic (*See* Esophageal cancer; Esophageal neoplasm(s))
due to pill-induced injury, 976, 976b
Esophageal diverticulum(a), 974-975, 974f-975f
classification of, 986
double, 986, 989f
mid-, 1402, 1403f
pseudo-, 975, 975f
imaging of, 1406, 1407f
pulsion, 986
traction, 986
types and sites of, 986, 987f-989f
Esophageal duplication, communicating, 1408-1409, 1409f
Esophageal endoscopy, 956-957
equipment for, 956
of esophageal varices, 958f
for extraesophageal reflux, 899
of gastroesophageal junction
with Mallory-Weiss tear, 957f
normal, 956-957, 957f
with severe esophagitis, 957f
of squamocolumnar junction, 956-957, 956f-957f
technique of, 956-957
Esophageal hematoma, 1416
Esophageal imaging, 1393-1420
of benign neoplasms, 1415-1416
of diverticula, 1402, 1403f
of esophageal narrowing, 1407-1409
due to extrinsic compression, 1408-1409
by foregut duplication cysts, 1408-1409, 1409f
by thyroid goiter, 1409, 1409f
by vertebral osteophytes, 1408, 1409f
due to strictures, 1407-1408, 1408f
due to webs, 1407, 1408f
of fistulas, 1409-1411
due to branchial cleft anomaly, 1410, 1410f
congenital, 1409-1410
due to perforation, 1410-1411, 1410f
postoperative, 1411
tracheoesophageal, 1409-1410
of foreign body, 1411, 1412f
of infection/inflammation, 1403-1407
due to alcohol-induced esophagitis, 1406
due to caustic esophagitis, 1404-1405, 1405f
due to drug-induced esophagitis, 1406, 1406f
due to eosinophilic esophagitis, 1406
due to epidermolysis bullosa, 1406, 1406f
due to graft-versus-host disease, 1406
due to granulomatous esophagitides, 1405
due to infectious esophagitis, 1404, 1405f
due to intramural pseudodiverticulosis, 1406, 1407f
due to pemphigoid, 1406
due to peptic esophagitis, 1406
due to radiation esophagitis, 1406
Esophageal imaging *(Continued)*
due to reflux esophagitis, 1403-1404, 1403f-1404f
of malignant neoplasms, 1413-1414, 1414f
with lymphadenopathy, 1414-1415, 1415f
of motility disorder(s), 1399-1401
due to connective tissue diseases, 1400-1401, 1401f
diminished peristalsis as, 1399-1400, 1400f-1401f
esophageal spasm as, 1400-1401, 1401f
post-treatment, 1416-1418
for monitoring and surveillance, 1418
after radiotherapy, 1418, 1418f
radiographic anatomy in, 1397-1398, 1400f
technique(s) for, 1393-1397
conventional radiography as, 1393, 1394f
CT as, 1396
fluoroscopy as, 1393-1394
modified barium swallow as, 1396
MRI as, 1396
oral contrast agents in, 1396
other nuclear medicine as, 1397
PET-CT as, 1396-1397, 1397f
pharyngoesophagram as, 1394, 1394f-1395f
ultrasound as, 1396
of varices, 1411, 1411f
Esophageal leiomyoma, 1415-1416, 1415f
Esophageal manifestations, of systemic disease, 978-980, 979f
cutaneous, 979-980
Esophageal manometry, 957-958, 958f-959f, 959t
for extraesophageal reflux, 899-900
for swallowing disorders, 1219
Esophageal motility, ineffective, 959t, 965
Esophageal motility abnormalities, 963-965, 963b, 1399-1401
achalasia as, 963-965
defined, 963
endoscopy of, 964, 964f
esophageal manometry for, 964, 964f
esophogram of, 963-964, 963f-964f
etiology and pathogenesis of, 963
management of, 964-965
manometric findings with, 959t
symptoms of, 963
due to connective tissue diseases, 1400-1401, 1401f
diminished peristalsis as, 1399-1400, 1400f-1401f
esophageal spasm as, 1400-1401, 1401f
nonachalasia, 965, 965f-966f
Esophageal narrowing, 1407-1409
due to extrinsic compression, 1408-1409
by foregut duplication cysts, 1408-1409, 1409f
by thyroid goiter, 1409, 1409f
by vertebral osteophytes, 1408, 1409f
due to strictures, 1407-1408, 1408f
due to webs, 1407, 1408f
Esophageal neoplasm(s), 973-974
benign
hematoma as, 1416
imaging of, 1415-1416
leiomyoma as, 1415-1416, 1415f
retention cyst as, 1416, 1416f
Tornwaldt cyst as, 1416, 1416f
vs. tortuous internal carotid artery, 1416, 1416f
malignant (*See* Esophageal cancer)
Esophageal perforation
due to foreign body ingestion, 2941
due to penetrating neck trauma, 1633-1634, 1634f
Esophageal peristalsis, 954, 955f
diminished, 1399-1400, 1400f-1401f
Esophageal pH monitoring
ambulatory 24-hour, 958-960, 959f-960f
Bravo wireless pH capsule for, 961, 961f
for GERD-related laryngeal disease in children, 2945
multichannel intraluminal impedance for, 962
Restech Dx-pH Measurement System for, 962, 962f
Esophageal pseudodiverticula, 975, 975f
Esophageal reconstruction, 1448-1461
with circumferential defects, 1431-1432
classification of defects for, 1450
decision making on, 1450, 1451f
free tissue transfer for, 1454, 1454f
enteric, 1455-1457
gastro-omental donor site for, 1457-1458, 1457f
jejunal donor site for, 1455-1457, 1456f
jejunal free flap for, 1432-1433, 1433f
fasciocutaneous, 1433, 1455
antero-lateral thigh donor site for, 1455
other donor sites for, 1455
radial forearm donor site for, 1455
goals and principles of, 1450
local and regional flaps for, 1450-1452, 1452f
myocutaneous flaps for, 1452-1453
patient population for, 1448
perioperative counseling for, 1448-1449
postsurgical complications of, 1458, 1459f
posttreatment speech and swallowing outcomes of, 1459-1460
preoperative evaluation for, 1449-1450
visceral transposition for, 1453
colonic, 1453, 1454f
gastric, 1432, 1432f, 1453
voice rehabilitation after, 1458-1459
Esophageal retention cysts, 1416, 1416f
Esophageal rings, 966-967, 966f, 968f
transnasal esophagoscopy of, 983-984, 984f
Esophageal spasm, diffuse, 965
esophagogram of, 965, 966f
imaging of, 1400-1401, 1401f
manometric findings with, 959t, 965, 965f
Esophageal speech, 1459
physiology of, 1596, 1596f
after total laryngectomy, 1572
Esophageal squamous cell carcinoma, 973
due to caustic injury, 978
Esophageal stage, of deglutition, 1217, 2948
Esophageal stenosis, after hypopharyngeal reconstruction, 1458
Esophageal strictures, 965-966
due to caustic injury, 977-978, 978f-979f
in children, 2960-2962, 2960f-2961f
imaging of, 1405, 1405f
defined, 965-966
dilation of, 966
transnasal esophagoscopy in, 984, 984f
endoscopy of, 965-966, 967f
due to esophageal carcinoma, 1408, 1408f
etiology of, 965-966, 966b
extrinsic, 965-966, 966b
imaging of, 1407-1408
due to caustic injury, 1405, 1405f
due to esophageal carcinoma, 1408, 1408f
esophagram for, 965-966, 966f
inflammatory, 1403, 1404f
inflammatory, 1403, 1404f
intrinsic, 965-966, 966b
postlaryngectomy, 1416
refractory, 966
after total laryngopharyngectomy, 1575
treatment of, 966
mechanical therapy for, 2960-2962, 2960f-2961f
transnasal esophagoscopy in, 984, 984f
Esophageal symptoms, assessment of, 954-956

Esophageal tears, due to penetrating neck trauma, 1633-1634, 1634f
Esophageal testing, 956-963
ambulatory 24-hour bile monitoring for, 960-961, 961f
endoscopy for, 956-957
equipment for, 956
of esophageal varices, 958f
for extraesophageal reflux, 899
of gastroesophageal junction
with Mallory-Weiss tear, 957f
normal, 956-957, 957f
with severe esophagitis, 957f
of squamocolumnar junction, 956-957, 956f-957f
technique of, 956-957
esophageal manometry for, 957-958, 958f-959f, 959t
esophageal pH monitoring for
ambulatory 24-hour, 958-960, 959f-960f
Bravo wireless pH capsule for, 961, 961f
multichannel intraluminal impedance for, 962
Restech Dx-pH Measurement System for, 962, 962f
provocative, 962-963
Esophageal trauma, 941-942
caustic, 942, 977-978
clinical features of, 977
etiology of, 977
grading of, 977, 978t
prognosis for, 977-978
squamous cell carcinoma due to, 978
strictures due to, 977-978, 978f-979f
external, 941-942
mechanisms of injury in, 933, 934f
pill-induced, 976, 976b
Esophageal varices, 958f
imaging of, 1411, 1411f
Esophageal webs, 966-967, 967f
imaging of, 1407, 1408f
Esophageal-bronchial fistulas, 1009
Esophageal-tracheal fistulas, 1009
Esophagectomy, for caustic ingestion, 2961-2962, 2962f
Esophagitis
caustic, 942, 977-978
clinical features of, 977
etiology of, 977
grading of, 977, 978t
imaging of, 1404-1405, 1405f
prognosis for, 977-978
squamous cell carcinoma due to, 978
strictures due to, 977-978, 978f-979f
imaging of, 1405, 1405f
drug-induced, 1406, 1406f
eosinophilic ("ringed," "feline," corrugated), 967-968, 969f
dysphagia due to, 2954
erosive, Los Angeles classification of, 969, 969f
gastroesophageal junction in, 957f
granulomatous, 1405
infectious, 976-977
due to *Candida albicans*, 976, 976f
imaging of, 1404, 1405f
due to cytomegalovirus, 976, 977f
due to herpes simplex virus, 976-977, 977f-978f
imaging of, 1404, 1405f
imaging of, 1404, 1405f
peptic, 1406
radiation, 1406
reflux, 968-969, 969f
imaging of, 1403-1404, 1403f-1404f
tuberculous, 1405
Esophagodiverticulostomy, endoscopic, 992
Esophagogastroduodenoscopy (EGD)
for extraesophageal reflux, 899
for laryngeal stenosis, 2917
Esophagogram, 1394, 1395f
for extraesophageal reflux, 898
mucosal-relief, 1394, 1395f
Esophagoscopy
for foreign body removal, 2939t, 2940
for penetrating neck trauma, 1631t, 1633-1634, 1634f
transnasal (*See* Transnasal esophagoscopy (TNE))
Esophagus
abdominal, 954f
Barrett's
endoscopic appearance of, 967f, 972, 972f
gastroesophageal junction in, 957f
GERD and, 972-973
grading of dysplasia in, 973, 973t
histologic appearance of, 972, 972f-973f
imaging of, 1403-1404, 1404f
long-segment, 972f
short-segment, 972f
surveillance for, 972-973, 973t
transnasal esophagoscopy in, 983, 983f
cancer of (*See* Esophageal cancer)
cervical, 954f
anatomy of, 1421-1422
cancer of (*See* Esophageal cancer, cervical)
congenital anomalies of, dysphagia due to, 2950t, 2953-2954, 2954f
"corkscrew," 965, 966f
defined, 953
food impactions in, 975
foreign bodies in, 975-976, 2935-2943
airway obstruction due to, 1481, 1481f
classification of, 975
complications of, 2942, 2942f
epidemiology of, 2936
due to food impaction, 975
imaging of, 1411, 1412f, 2939
location of, 2936, 2937f
management of, 2939-2941
anesthesia for, 2940
controversies in, 2942
for disk batteries, 2941
equipment for, 2939-2940, 2939t
history of, 2935-2936
for pills, 2941
postoperative, 2941-2942
for sharp objects, 2940-2941
technique for, 2940
perforation due to, 2941
symptoms of, 2938
normal anatomy and physiology of, 953-954, 954f-955f
nutcracker, 959t, 965
imaging of, 1401
presby-, 1400
radiographic anatomy of, 1397-1398, 1398f, 1400f
thoracic, 954f
ESP (Early Speech Perception), for cochlear implant, 2225-2226
ESPAL (endoscopic sphenopalatine artery ligation), for epistaxis, 689-690, 689f-690f
Espin, in stereocilia, 2075, 2076f
Espin *(ESPN)* gene, in deafness, 2051t-2058t
ESRRB (estrogen-related receptor β) gene, in deafness, 2051t-2058t
ESS (Epworth Sleepiness Scale), 57, 253, 253f
ESS (empty sella syndrome), CSF rhinorrhea due to, 787
ESS (endoscopic sinus surgery). *See* Endoscopic sinus surgery (ESS).
Essential tremor, laryngeal hyperfunction due to, 840-841
Esteem-Hearing Implant, 2211-2212, 2212f
Esthesioneuroblastoma (ENB), 1697-1698
epidemiology of, 1697
pathogenesis of, 1697
prognostic factors for, 1697
treatment for
approaches to, 1697-1698
radiation therapy for, 1698, 1698f
results of, 1697, 1698t
Esthetician, for aging skin, 402
Estlander flap, 352, 356f
Estrogen(s), for hyperparathyroidism, 1804
Estrogen-related receptor β *(ESRRB)* gene, in deafness, 2051t-2058t
Etanercept, for autoimmune inner ear disease, 2167
Ethacrynic acid, sensorineural hearing loss due to, 2120, 2175
Ethanol
absolute, for embolization, 1933
percutaneous administration of, for toxic thyroid adenoma, 1744
Ethical issues, with genetics, 9-10
Ethmoid bone, in surgical anatomy of anterior cranial base, 2442-2443, 2443f
Ethmoid bulla
in endoscopic sinus surgery, 747, 748f
normal anatomy of, 666-667, 667f
surgical anatomy of, 740
Ethmoid complex, 740
Ethmoid foramina, in surgical anatomy of anterior cranial base, 2443-2444, 2444f
Ethmoid fractures, naso-orbital, 322
classification of, 326-327, 327f
physical examination of, 324, 324f
repair of, 336-337, 337f
Ethmoid region, in surgical anatomy of anterior cranial base, 2444f
Ethmoid roof
after functional endoscopic sinus surgery, 672f, 679
in surgical anatomy of anterior cranial base, 2443
Ethmoid roof height, asymmetry in, 670-671
Ethmoid sinus(es)
anatomy and physiology of, 320f, 664, 667
growth and development of, 2619-2620
roof of, 1124f
in surgical anatomy of anterior cranial base, 2443, 2472f-2473f, 2473
Ethmoid sinus tumors, 1123, 1130
external ethmoidectomy for, 1124-1125, 1125f
staging of, 1129b
Ethmoid vessels, prior to endoscopic sinus surgery, 764, 764t, 765f
Ethmoidal labyrinth, 1124f
Ethmoidectomy
endoscopic
anterior, 747-748, 748f
complete, 748-749, 749f-750f
failure of, 766-767, 767f
posterior, 747-748, 749f
external, 757, 757f, 1124-1125, 1125f
Lynch-Howarth, 778-779, 779f
intranasal, 756-757
Ethnic differences, in otitis media, 2766
Ethnic noses, rhinoplasty for. *See* Noncaucasian rhinoplasty.
Ethylene oxide polyoxypropylene glycol (Addax), for cerumen removal, 1958t
Etomidate, for induction of anesthesia, 111
ETS (environmental tobacco smoke), and chronic rhinosinusitis, 707
ETT. *See* Endotracheal intubation (ETT).
European Organization for Research and Treatment of Cancer Quality of Life Questionnaire (EORTC-HN35), 56

Eustachian tube, 1866-1875
anatomy of, 1825, 1867-1870, 1867f
anterior pad in, 1869, 1869f
anterior view of, 1868f
arterial supply in, 1870
cartilaginous portion in, 1868-1869, 1869f
dilatory muscles in, 1869-1870, 1869f
histology of lumen of, 1870
junctional portion of, 1868, 1868f
lateral view of, 1868f
in middle cranial base, 1699
mucosa-associated lymphoid tissue in, 1870
in oropharynx, 1360f
osseous portion in, 1867, 1867f
superior view of, 1867f
tubal lumen in, 1867f, 1870
embryology and postnatal development of, 1866-1867
length of, 1866
location of, 1867
in otitis media, 2762-2763, 2763f
patulous, 1872
pharyngeal opening of, in surgical anatomy of anterior cranial base, 2472f, 2474
physiology of, 1870-1872
middle ear protection in, 1871-1872
mucociliary clearance and drainage in, 1871
pressure equalization in, 1870-1871
shape of, 1867
in surgical anatomy of lateral skull base, 2436f-2437f, 2438
Eustachian tube dysfunction, 1872-1874
with abnormalities in lateral wall movement, 1872
aging and, 1872
classic theory of, 1870-1871
with cleft palate, 1872-1873, 1873f
ear pressure and, 1872
with extraesophageal reflux, 1873
hereditary component to, 1873-1874
hypertrophic adenoids and, 1872, 1873f
mucociliary clearance and, 1871
nasal allergy and, 1872
with nasopharyngeal neoplasms, 1873, 1873f
pathophysiology of, 1872
with pressure changes, 1872
respiratory viruses and, 1871
treatment of, 1874
Eustachian tube function, 1867
Eustachian tube function tests, 1874
Eustachian tube opening, in surgical anatomy of lateral skull base, 2436f
Eutectic mixture of local anesthetics (EMLA), for premedication of children, 2589
Euthyrox (levothyroxine, oral synthetic), for hypothyroidism, 1748-1749
Eversion, in wound repair, 306, 306f
Evidence, levels of, 69, 70t
and grade of recommendation, 55, 55t, 69-70, 70t
Evidence-based medicine (EBM) recommendations, grading of, 55, 55t, 69-70, 70t
Evidence-based performance measurement, 76-90
aggregate demand for, 77
anatomy of performance measures in, 82, 83f
definition of quality for, 76-77
engaging in development of, 77-78
implementation of
barriers to, 89
pathway for, 88f
standardization and, 87-89
medical professionalism and, 78-82
board certification and maintenance of certification in, 79-80, 80b-81b
Institute of Medicine in, 81-82
physician education in, 79, 79t
Evidence-based performance measurement *(Continued)*
state medical boards and maintenance of licensure in, 80-81
motivation for, 76
process of building a coherent system of, 77-78
quality-based or value-based purchasing in, 78
stakeholder groups in, 79-89, 84t-87t
surgeon's role in, 89
unifying response to demand for, 77-78
Evoked auditory brainstem response (EABR). *See* Auditory brainstem response (ABR).
Evoked electromyography, 2386
Evoked encephalomyography (EEMG), for facial nerve injury, 2041
Evoked long latency responses (ELLRs)
auditory, 1912, 1913f
electrically, 1913-1914
Evoked middle latency responses (EMLRs)
auditory, 1912, 1913f
electrically, 1912-1914
Evoked otoacoustic emissions (EOAEs), in infants, 2720-2721
Ewald's First Law, 2288
Ewald's Second Law, 2290-2291
Ewing's sarcoma (ES)
in children, 2845
malignant, 1671
oral manifestations of, 1253
Ewing's sarcoma family of tumors (ESFTs), in children, 2845
Ex utero intrapartum treatment (EXIT procedure)
for congenital high airway obstruction syndrome, 2869, 2870f, 2904-2905
for laryngeal atresia, 2869
Ex vivo gene therapy, 18, 19f
Excisional surgery
for scar revision, 295, 297f
expansion with, 296-298
serial, 296
tissue, 296-298, 297f
for skin lesions, 293
Excitation-inhibition asymmetry, of semicircular canals, 2290-2291, 2291f
Excitatory amino acid transporter 1 (EATT1), 2081
Excitatory postsynaptic potentials (EPSPs), in vestibular afferent nerve fibers, 2284-2285, 2284f
Excited state, of atom, 1032
Exclusion criteria, 68
Excretory duct, of salivary gland, 1162, 1163f
Exercise, nasal airflow during, 641
Exercise-induced asthma, in professional singers, 853
EXIT procedure (ex utero intrapartum treatment)
for congenital high airway obstruction syndrome, 2869, 2870f, 2904-2905
for laryngeal atresia, 2869
Exocrine disorders, oral manifestations of, 1251
Exogen phase, 374
Exons, 4, 5f
Exostoses, of external auditory canal
imaging of, 1918, 1918f
management of, 2022, 2024f
Expanded polytetrafluoroethylene (ePTFE)
for craniofacial defect repair, 2657
for nasal reconstruction, 368
in noncaucasian rhinoplasty, 569, 570f
Expansion with excision, for scar revision, 296-298
serial, 296
tissue, 296-298, 297f
Experimental studies, data quality of, 59, 60t-62t
Expert opinion, 52, 54-55, 54t
Expiratory force, in phonation, 811-812
Expiratory resistance, in rhinomanometry, 650-651
Exposure keratitis, after facial nerve injury, 2420, 2420f
Exposure time, of surgical laser, 28
Expression microarrays, in head and neck squamous cell carcinoma, 1025
Expressivity, 7, 7f
Extended craniofacial resection, 1126-1127, 1127f
supplemental management in, 1126-1127
Extended head posture, 2629
Extended maxillotomy, for middle cranial base surgery, 2455t, 2458, 2462f
Extended middle fossa approach, for posterior fossa neoplasms, 2532t, 2538
advantages and disadvantages of, 2532t, 2538
basic features of, 2538
indications for, 2532t, 2538
surgical exposure in, 2538f
technique of, 2538
Extended neck dissection, 1703t, 1719-1721, 1720f
Extended vertical hemilaryngectomy, 1548
External acoustic meatus, 320f, 2010f
External auditory canal (EAC)
anatomy of, 1822f, 1823, 1824f-1825f, 1829
atresia of, 1917, 1917f
benign neoplasms of, 1918, 1918f-1919f
carcinoma of, 2502-2504
imaging of, 1918, 1919f
management of, 2502-2504, 2503f
pertinent anatomy for, 2502
staging of, 2502, 2502f, 2503b
symptoms and signs of, 2502
cholesteatoma of, 1949
imaging of, 1917, 1918f
closure of, in postauricular approach to infratemporal fossa, 2495, 2497f
congenital malformations of (*See* Congenital aural atresia (CAA))
embryogenesis of, 1824
exostoses of
imaging of, 1918, 1918f
management of, 2022, 2024f
foreign bodies in, 2021
imaging of, 172, 1917-1918
with benign neoplasms, 1918, 1918f-1919f
with cholesteatoma, 1917, 1918f
with congenital lesions, 1917, 1917f
with keratosis obturans, 1917, 1918f
with malignant neoplasms, 1918, 1919f
with posinflammatory medial canal fibrosis, 1917-1918, 1918f
with severe infections, 1917, 1917f
keratosis obturans of, 1949
imaging of, 1917, 1918f
management of, 2021
narrowing of, 2021
osteomas of
imaging of, 1918, 1919f
management of, 2022
physical examination of, 97
posinflammatory medial canal fibrosis of, 1917-1918, 1918f
severe infections of, 1917, 1917f
sleeve resection of, 2492
soft tissue stenosis of, 2021-2022, 2023f
in surgical anatomy of lateral skull base, 2435, 2435f
in surgical anatomy of middle cranial base, 2445f
External auditory canal (EAC) stenosis, due to temporal bone trauma, 2038, 2047
External auditory meatus, 320f
embryology of, 2585f, 2753
External carotid artery
anatomy of, 1296f, 1359f, 2579, 2580f
radiographic, 1471f, 1473-1474
injury of, 1632
in parotidectomy, 1195-1196
in surgical anatomy of lateral skull base, 2440f
External carotid artery ligation, for epistaxis, 689

External compression plating, for nasal fractures, 506
External ear
anatomy of, 1823-1825, 1824f-1825f
applied, 1944
tympanic membrane in, 1824-1825, 1825f
in auditory physiology, 1839
embryogenesis of, 1824
imaging of, 172
External ear canal, anatomy of, 1944
External ear disorder(s), topical therapies for, 1950-1962
acidifying agents as
for acute bacterial otitis externa, 1953
for fungal otitis externa, 1954
for acute bacterial otitis externa, 1951-1953
acidifying agents as, 1953
options for, 1951-1953, 1951f
ototopic antibiotics as, 1951-1953
antibiotics as, 1959t-1960t
for acute bacterial otitis externa, 1951-1953
evidence-based data on, 1952
hypersensitivity reaction to, 1954
mechanism of action of, 1951
ototoxicity of, 1953-1954
resistance to, 1951-1953
antifungals as, 1959t-1960t
for fungal otitis externa, 1954-1955
ototoxicity of, 1955
anti-inflammatories as
for eczematoid otitis externa, 1956-1957
mechanism of action of, 1951
antiseptics as, 1955
for fungal otitis externa, 1955
for cerumen impaction, 1957
options for, 1957, 1958t
for ear hygiene and chronic draining ear, 1957-1958, 1961f
for eczematoid otitis externa, 1955-1957
anti-inflammatory and immunosuppressive agents as, 1956-1957
options for, 1955
steroids as, 1955-1956
for fungal otitis externa, 1954-1955
acidifying agents as, 1954
antifungals as, 1954-1955
antiseptics as, 1955
options for, 1954
history of, 1950
immunosuppressive agents as, for eczematoid otitis externa, 1956-1957
mechanism of action of, 1950-1951
for antibiotics, 1951
for anti-inflammatories, 1951
for myringitis, 1955
steroids as
classes of, 1956, 1956t
for eczematoid otitis externa, 1955-1956
hypersensitivity reaction to, 1954
mechanism of action of, 1951
ototoxicity of, 1956
summary of available, 1959t-1960t
for viral infections, 1957, 1957f
options for, 1957
External ear infection(s), 1944-1949
bullous myringitis as, 1948, 1948f
cellulitis as, 1948
due to otitis externa, 1946
erysipelas as, 1948, 1949f
external auditory canal cholesteatoma as, 1949
furunculosis as, 1949, 1949f, 2021
keratosis obturans as, 1949
medial canthal fibrosis due to, 1946-1947, 1946f
otitis externa as, 1944-1947
allergic, 1945-1946
bacterial, 1944
chronic, 1945, 1946f
External ear infection(s) *(Continued)*
clinical manifestations of, 1945
complications of, 1946-1947, 1946f
defined, 1944
fungal, 1944-1946, 1945f
granular, 1945
incidence and epidemiology of, 1944
investigations of, 1945
malignant, 1947-1948
clinical manifestations of, 1947, 1947f
defined, 1947
immunosuppression and, 221-222, 1947
incidence and epidemiology of, 1947
investigations of, 1947
microbiology of, 1947
treatment of, 1947-1948
microbiology of, 1945, 1945t
pathogenesis of, 1944-1945, 1945f
treatment of, 1945-1946
perichondritis and chondritis as, 1948
due to otitis externa, 1946
viral
aural papillomatosis as, 1957, 1957f
management options for, 1957
herpes zoster oticus as, 1948, 1948f
External ethmoidectomy, 1124-1125, 1125f
External expansion surgery, for laryngeal stenosis, 2919-2921
External fixation, of mandibular fracture, 338
External jugular lymph nodes, 1360f
External jugular vein, 1360f
anomalies of, 2817
External nasal nerve, 483f
External nasal splinting, 504
External occipital protuberance, 320f
External otitis. *See* Otitis externa (OE).
External plexiform layer, of olfactory bulb, 628f
External speech processors, 2229
size, weight, and aesthetics of, 2232, 2232f
External validity, 68-69, 68t, 69f
External valve collapse, 493
revision rhinoplasty for, 586-587, 587f
External-beam radiation therapy (EBRT), 1033. *See also* Radiation therapy (RT).
for oral cancer, 1314
for thyroid cancer, 1772
treatment aspects of, 1035-1036
Extracapsular spread, imaging of, 164-166, 167f
Extracorporeal circulation, for flap salvage, 1075
Extracorporeal shock wave lithotripsy, for sialolithiasis, 1156
Extracranial repair, for CSF rhinorrhea, 792-794, 793f-794f
Extraesophageal reflux (EER), 894-903, 970-973
asthma due to, 971
Barrett's esophagus due to, 972-973
grading of dysplasia in, 973, 973t
histologic appearance of, 972, 972f-973f
long-segment, 972f
short-segment, 972f
surveillance for, 972-973, 973t
chest pain due to, 971
in children, 2944-2947
diagnosis of, 2945
disorders due to, 2945-2946, 2945b
evidence of, 2946
history of, 2944
management of, 2946
physiopathology of, 2945
chronic cough due to, 971
contact ulcer due to, 902
defined, 894
dental erosions due to, 971-972
diagnostic evaluation of, 896-900
esophageal endoscopy in, 899
esophagogram in, 898
history in, 896, 896b-897b
Extraesophageal reflux (EER) *(Continued)*
impedance testing in, 900
laryngeal sensory testing in, 898-899
manometry in, 899-900
pH probe monitoring in, 900
physical examination and laryngeal endoscopy in, 896-897, 897t, 898b
voice analysis in, 898
epidemiology of, 894
and head and neck cancer, 902-903
laryngeal granuloma due to, 902, 902f-903f
laryngitis due to, 886, 886f, 901-902, 970-971
and otitis media, 1873
otolaryngologic disorders associated with, 901-903
pathophysiology of, 894-896
epithelial resistance factors in, 895-896
esophageal acid clearance in, 895
lower esophageal sphincter in, 895, 895b
mechanisms of symptoms in, 896
upper esophageal sphincter in, 894-895
professional voice disorders due to, 852
symptoms of, 970
treatment of, 900-901
algorithm for, 970, 970f
behavioral modification for, 900-901
bethanechol for, 901
H_2 blockers for, 901
over-the-counter antacids for, 901
promotility agents for, 901
proton pump inhibitors for, 901
sucralfate for, 901
surgical, 901
Extraglandular parotid lymph node, 1360f
Extramedullary plasmacytoma (EMP), of larynx, 1509
Extranodal marginal cell lymphoma, of thyroid, 1679
Extraocular muscle(s)
in Graves' ophthalmopathy, 1808, 1809t
intraoperative monitoring of, 2549-2550, 2550f
semicircular canal planes and, 2285-2288, 2286f-2288f
Extraocular muscle surgery, for Graves' ophthalmopathy, 1816-1817
Extrapyramidal reaction, *vs.* myofascial pain dysfunction syndrome, 1285t
Extrapyramidal system defects, laryngologic manifestations of, 837-838, 838t
Extrinsic strap muscles, radiographic anatomy of, 1473f
Extubation
of difficult airway, 117
stridor after, 2904, 2904t
Exudative tracheitis, 2809-2810
clinical features of, 2809
complications of, 2810
diagnosis of, 2809, 2809f
differential diagnosis of, 2806t
endoscopy of, 2809, 2809f
epidemiology of, 2809
imaging of, 2809, 2809f
management of, 2809-2810, 2809f
pathogenesis of, 2809
terminology for, 2809
EYA1 gene, in branchio-oto-renal syndrome, 2095
EYA1 (eyes-absent 1 homolog) gene, in deafness, 2051t-2058t
EYA4 (eyes-absent 4 homolog) gene, in deafness, 2051t-2058t
Eye(s)
aesthetic analysis of, 271
in Down syndrome, 2632-2633
effects of radiotherapy on, 2626t
prosthetic, 1345t, 1346-1347, 1347f
trauma to, 303
Eye evaluation, for Graves' ophthalmopathy, 1809

Eye movement(s)
evoked by sound or changes in middle ear pressure, 2316, 2316f
in superior canal dehiscence syndrome, 2339-2340, 2340f
methods of recording, 2317, 2317f
in plane of stimulated semicircular canal, 2285-2289
anatomic and physiologic basis for, 2285-2288, 2286f-2288f
clinical importance of, 2288-2289, 2288f
semicircular canals and, 2306, 2307f
in vestibular function, 2305-2307, 2306f-2307f, 2307t
Eye protection
for facial nerve injury, 2420, 2420f
in laser surgery, 34-35, 35f-36f
Eyebrow(s)
aesthetic proportions of, 428, 429f
anatomy of, 440-442
in Asians *vs.* Occidentals, 442
blood supply in, 442
fascial layers of forehead and temporal region in, 440-441, 441f
motor innervation in, 440, 441f
musculature in, 441-442, 442f
sensory innervation in, 440, 441f
Eyebrow position, aesthetic analysis of, 271, 275f, 445, 445f
Eyebrow shape, aesthetic analysis of, 271, 445, 445f
Eyebrow transplantation, 384, 384f
Eye-head coordination, evaluation of, 2314
Eye-head movements, in vestibular function, 2308
Eyelash transplantation, 384
Eyelid(s)
aesthetic analysis of, 271, 445-447
lower, 445-446, 446f
upper, 445, 446f
anatomy of, 442-444, 443f
anterior lamella in, 442-443, 443f
in Asians *vs.* Caucasians, 443
conjunctiva in, 443f, 444
lower eyelid retractors in, 444
orbital fat pads in, 443-444, 444f
orbital septum in, 443, 443f
posterior lamella in, 442
surface, 442, 443f
tarsus in, 443f, 444
upper eyelid retractors in, 444
biomechanics of, 332
burns of, 316
in Graves' ophthalmopathy, 1808, 1809t
paralysis of
lower, 2420-2421, 2421f
upper, 2421
trauma to, 303, 303f, 307-309, 308f
upper
aesthetic analysis of, 445, 446f
ptosis of
evaluation of, 446-447, 447f
repair of, 447-448, 447f-449f
Eyelid retractors
lower, 444
upper, 444
Eyelid surgery, for Graves' ophthalmopathy, 1817
Eyes-absent 1 homolog *(EYA1)* gene, in deafness, 2051t-2058t
Eyes-absent 4 homolog *(EYA4)* gene, in deafness, 2051t-2058t

F

Fabry's disease, oral manifestations of, 1257
Face
embryology of, 2659-2661, 2661t
postoperative imaging of, 173-174
size ratio of cranium to, 2616f, 2617t
Face, Legs, Activity, Cry, Consolability (FLACC) tool, 240
Face mask ventilation, for difficult airway, 114t, 115f
"Facelift" incision, modified, for parotidectomy, 1172, 1173f
Facelifting. *See* Rhytidectomy.
Faces Pain Scale Revised (FPS-R), 240
Facial analysis, 269-280
aesthetic units in, 269-270, 274f
anatomic landmarks and reference points in, 269
cephalometric, 270b, 272f
Frankfort horizontal plane as, 269, 272f
soft tissue, 270b, 271f
computer imaging and digital photography in, 277-280, 279f-280f
facial proportions in, 269
facial height in, 269, 273f
middle and lower, 269, 273f
facial symmetry through midsagittal plane in, 269, 272f
facial width in, 269, 272f
historical background of, 269
anthropometry in, 269
in antiquity, 269
Renaissance artists in, 269, 270f
relaxed skin tension lines in, 269-270, 274f
for rhinoplasty, 514, 514f
subunit analysis in, 269-275
of chin, 275, 278f
of ears, 275, 279f
of eyes, 271
of forehead, 270-271
eyebrow position in, 271, 275f
eyebrow shape in, 271
nasofrontal angle in, 270, 274f
of lips, 274-275, 278f
of neck, 275, 279f
of nose, 271-272, 275f
alar-columellar complex in, 270f-271f, 274
nasal rotation and projection in, 273-274, 277f
nasofacial angle in, 272-274, 276f
nasofacial relationships in, 272-274
nasofrontal angle in, 270, 272-273, 274f
nasolabial angle in, 272-273, 276f
nasomental angle in, 272-273, 276f
of skin and rhytids, 275, 276b, 279f
Facial anomaly(ies). *See* Craniofacial anomaly(ies).
Facial arteriovenous fistulas, embolization of, 1940, 1940f
Facial artery, 682, 1296, 2579-2580, 2580f
Facial asymmetry, 2621
Facial bipartition, for craniofacial anomalies, 2654, 2656f
Facial bones
conventional radiography of, 130
effects of radiotherapy on, 2626t
Facial changes, during normal growth and development, 2615, 2615f-2616f
Facial clefts, 2645. *See also* Cleft lip; Cleft palate.
molecular genetics of, 2662-2664
Facial defect(s), prosthetic management of, 1344-1345, 1345t
auricular, 1345-1346, 1345t, 1346f
nasal, 1345, 1345t, 1346f
orbital/ocular, 1345t, 1346-1347, 1347f
Facial defect reconstruction, 342-363
algorithm for, 342, 343f
of cheek, 355-359
advancement flaps in, 358
V-Y, 358, 361f
rotation flaps for, 357-358, 359f
sub-superficial musculoaponeurotic system dissection in, 357-358, 360f
Facial defect reconstruction *(Continued)*
transposition flaps for, 358-359, 361f
bilobed, 357, 359f
rhombus shaped, 355
of forehead, 359-363
aesthetic considerations in, 359
central third, 359-360, 362f
goals of, 359
lateral, 360-362
advancement flap for, 360-363, 362f
advancement rotation flap for, 360-362, 362f
O-T or A-T procedure for, 362, 363f
primary wound closure for, 360-362
rotation flaps for, 362
primary wound repair for, 359
tissue expansion in, 363
of lip, 350-353
classification of, 351
greater than two-thirds width, 352
with lateral defect, 352
less than one-half width, 351
primary wound closure in, 351
V-Y musculocutaneous island pedicle flap in, 356f
lower
algorithm for, 351, 355f
midline, 352-353
massive or near-total, 352-353, 357f-358f
melolabial transposition flap for, 353
temporal forehead flap for, 353
from one half to two thirds, 351
Abbé flap for, 352
Estlander flap for, 352, 356f
Karapendzic flap for, 351
lip switch flap for, 351
local *vs.* regional flaps for, 352
upper
algorithm for, 351, 355f
with large defect, 352
V-Y advancement flap in, 347f
local flaps for
advancement, 345-346
bilateral, 345, 346f
island, 345
unipedicle, 345, 345f
V-Y, 345-346, 346f-347f
Y-V, 346
classification of, 342-343, 343b
hinge, 346
pivotal, 343-345
effective length of, 343, 343f
interpolated, 344-345, 344f
rotation, 343-344, 343f
transposition, 344, 344f
of nose, 346-350
aesthetic units in, 346-347, 347f
approach to, 346-347
for defects extending into alar facial sulcus, 348
cheek advancement flap in, 348, 349f
cheek pedicle transposition flap in, 348, 349f
for full-thickness central defects of tip or dorsum, 348
composite turnout flap for, 348, 351f
paramedian forehead flaps for, 348-350, 352f-354f
for full-thickness defects of ala, 347
bipedicle mucosal advancement flap in, 347, 347f
free cartilage grafts in, 348
melolabial interpolated flap in, 348
for surface defects of nasal tip, columella, sidewalls, and dorsum, 348
hinge flap in, 348, 350f
paramedian forehead flaps in, 348
V-Y advancement flap in, 345-346, 346f
Facial dimension, 2617t

Facial edema, due to neck dissection, 1723, 1729f
Facial expression, aging skin and, 439, 440f
Facial fracture(s), 318-341
anatomy, physiology, and pathophysiology of, 319-323, 320f
general, 319
of lower third, 322-323, 323f
of middle third, 319-322
areas of protection in, 322, 322t
infraorbital nerve in, 320, 321f
maxillae in, 320, 321f
nasal bones in, 320
orbits in, 320-321, 322f
zygoma in, 319, 320f-321f
of upper third, 319, 319f
biomechanics of facial skeleton and, 331-333, 331f
in lower third, 332-333, 332f
in middle third, 331-332, 331f
in upper third, 331
bone healing after, 330-331
classification of, 326-327
of lower third, 327
of middle third, 326-327, 327f
of upper third, 326
complications of, 339-340
defined, 318
evaluation and diagnosis of, 323-326
imaging in, 325-326
of lower third, 325-326
of middle third, 325, 326f
of upper third, 325, 325f
physical examination in, 323-325
of lower third, 325
of middle third, 324-325, 324f
of upper third, 324
future directions and new horizons for, 340
historical perspective on, 318-319
management of, 327-330
general, 327-328
surgical access in, 328-330
to lower third, 329-330, 330f
to middle third, 328-329, 329f
to upper third, 328, 328f-329f
pediatric, 2647, 2697-2717
associated injuries with, 2698
clinical and physical evaluation of, 2699
complex, 2698
dentoalveolar, 2706-2707, 2710f
emergency management of, 2698-2699
epidemiology of, 2697-2698
etiology of, 2698
facial growth and, 2698-2699
front sinus, 2711, 2712f
mandibular, 2704-2706
arch and body, 2706, 2709f
complications of, 2704
condylar, 2704, 2706f-2708f
epidemiology of, 2698
symphyseal and parasymphyseal, 2704-2706, 2708f-2709f
mandibular immobilization for, 2701, 2701f
maxillomandibular fixation for, 2701
midface, 2707, 2710f
nasal, 2708-2711, 2711f-2712f
naso-orbitoethmoid, 2714
classification of, 2714, 2716f
evaluation of, 2714, 2716f
repair of, 2714, 2716f
open reduction with internal fixation for, 2701-2702
orbital, 2711-2714
evaluation of, 2712, 2713f
of lateral/medial orbital wall, 2712, 2714, 2716f
of orbital apex, 2712, 2713f
of orbital floor, 2712-2713, 2714f-2715f
Facial fracture(s) *(Continued)*
of orbital roof, 2712-2713, 2716f
patterns of, 2711-2712
permanent *vs.* resorbable plating systems for, 2700-2701, 2700t-2701t
radiologic examination of, 2699
rigid fixation for, 2699-2700
sequencing of procedures for, 2702, 2704, 2706f
surgical approaches for, 2701-2704
bicoronal incision in, 2701-2702, 2703f
lateral cantholysis in, 2704f
maxillary gingivolabial sulcus approach in, 2701-2702, 2703f
midfacial degloving incision in, 2701-2702
subciliary incision in, 2705f
surgical approaches for, 2701-2704
transcaruncular approach in, 2701-2702, 2705f
surgical management of, 2648, 2649f, 2657
surgical reconstruction for, 2704-2714
zygomaticomalar complex, 2707-2708, 2710f
repair of, 333-334
in lower third, 337-339, 338f
with edentulous mandible, 339
in middle third, 334-337
of buttresses, 336
canthal ligament in, 337, 337f
maxillary, 335-336, 335f-336f
naso-orbital ethmoid, 336-337, 337f
orbital, 336
palatal, 335, 335f
of tooth-bearing segments, 334-335, 334f
zygomatic, 336
and occlusion, 330-331, 333-334, 333f
panfacial, 339
secondary, revision, or delayed, 340
in upper third, 333-334, 334f
with CSF rhinorrhea, 334-339
with skull base disruption, 334-339
Facial growth and development. *See* Craniofacial growth and development.
Facial height, 269, 273f, 2617t
middle and lower, 269, 273f
Facial hiatus, 1828
in surgical anatomy of lateral skull base, 2436f, 2437
in surgical anatomy of middle cranial base, 2445f
Facial lipoatrophy, HIV-associated, 227-228, 228f
Facial moulage recording, by maxillofacial prosthodontist, 1331, 1332f
Facial nerve
anatomy of, 1359f, 1827-1829, 2278f
surgical, 2403-2404, 2404f
in congenital aural atresia, 2754, 2755f, 2759
electromagnetic stimulation of, 2394-2395
first genu of, 1826f, 1827-1828
general visceral efferent fibers of, 1827-1828
imaging of, 173, 175f, 1924-1926
to assess function, 2384
with Bell's palsy, 1924, 1927f, 2395
with hemangioma, 1924-1926, 1927f
with meningioma, 175f
with neuroma, 1928
with schwannoma, 1924-1926, 1927f
infratemporal portion of, 1826f, 1828
labyrinthine segment of, 2404, 2404f
mastoid (vertical) segment of, 2404, 2404f
in mastoidectomy, 2012, 2012f
in parotidectomy
anatomy of, 1194, 1194f
involvement of, 1196
main trunk of, 1195, 1195f
marginal mandibular branch of, 1195, 1195f
physical examination of, 95, 95t
rerouting of, 2412, 2412f-2413f
partial, 2412-2413
Facial nerve *(Continued)*
second genu of, 1826f, 1827-1829
small fenestra stapedotomy with exposed or overhanging, 2033
somatic sensory fibers of, 1827-1828
special sensory fibers of, 1827-1828
special visceral efferent fibers of, 1827-1828
in subtotal or total temporal bone resection, 2494-2495
in surgical anatomy
of infratemporal fossa, 2440f
of internal auditory canal, 2437f, 2439
of jugular foramen, 2439f-2440f
of lateral skull base, 2436f
of middle cranial fossa, 2437f, 2438
of posterior cranial fossa, 2438, 2439f
trauma to, 309
tympanic segment of, 1827, 2404, 2404f
in vestibular system, 1852, 1854f
visceral afferent fibers of, 1827-1828
vulnerability to injury of, 1827-1829
Facial nerve decompression, 2041, 2042t
indications for, 2041
middle fossa craniotomy as, 2042-2043
outcome of, 2041, 2042t
supralabyrinthine approach for, 2041-2042, 2043f
timing of, 2041-2042
translabyrinthine approach for, 2041-2042
transmastoid approach for, 2041-2042
Facial nerve disorder(s), 2391-2402
hyperkinetic, 2401
management of, 2432
paralysis as (*See* Facial nerve paralysis)
Facial nerve dissection, in postauricular approach to infratemporal fossa, 2495-2496
Facial nerve function
assessment of, 2381-2390
electrodiagnostic testing in, 2385-2387
electromyography in, 2386-2387
electroneuronography in, 2041, 2386, 2387t
maximal stimulation test in, 2040-2041, 2385-2386, 2387t
nerve excitability test in, 2040-2041, 2385, 2387t
facial nerve monitoring for, 2387-2388
histopathologic classification in, 2384-2385, 2384f
House-Brackmann grading system in, 2381-2382, 2382t, 2383f, 2417-2418, 2417t
imaging in, 2384
physical examination in, 2381-2382
topognostic tests in, 2382-2384
of lacrimal function, 2383
of salivary flow, 2384
of salivary pH, 2384
of stapedius reflex, 2383
of taste, 2383-2384
unconventional tests for, 2388-2389
acoustic reflex evoked potentials as, 2388
antidromic potentials as, 2388
blink reflex as, 2388
magnetic stimulation as, 2388-2389
optical stimulation as, 2389
transcranial electrical stimulation–induced facial motor evoked potentials as, 2389
after stereotactic irradiation, 2563
Facial nerve grafting, 2421-2425
cross-face, 2419, 2424-2425
selection of donor nerve for, 2422
surgical planning for, 2421-2424, 2423f
surgical technique for, 2422-2424, 2424f-2425f
Facial nerve hemangiomas
vs. facial nerve schwannomas, 2507
imaging of, 1924-1926, 1927f

Facial nerve injury
early care of, 2420-2421
eye protection for, 2420, 2420f
histopathologic classification of, 2384-2385, 2384f
iatrogenic, 2399
in lateral skull base surgery, 2512
due to mastoidectomy, 2015-2016
of neck surgery, 1729-1730
due to posterior fossa surgery, 2541
due to rhytidectomy, 422-425, 426f
traumatic, 2039-2044, 2042t, 2398-2399
assessing degree of, 2040
compound muscle action potential in, 2041
electromyography for, 2041
electroneuronography for, 2041
evoked encephalomyography for, 2041
maximal stimulation test for, 2040-2041
nerve excitability test for, 2040-2041
classification of, 2040
conservative treatment of, 2040, 2042
corticosteroids for, 2042
delayed onset of paralysis due to, 2040
epidemiology of, 2039-2040
imaging of, 2398f
observation and symptomatic care for, 2398
outcome of, 2041, 2042t
pathogenesis of, 2398
penetrating, 2399
surgical interventions for, 2041, 2042t, 2398-2399, 2413-2414
indications for, 2041
middle fossa craniotomy as, 2042-2043
outcome of, 2041, 2042t
supralabyrinthine approach for, 2041-2042, 2043f
timing of, 2041-2042
translabyrinthine approach for, 2041-2042
transmastoid approach for, 2041-2042
treatment algorithm for, 2042-2044, 2043f
Facial nerve monitoring, 2387-2388, 2545-2549
for acoustic neuroma and other cerebellopontine angle tumors, 2545
active, 2387
advantages of, 2387
anesthesia and, 2544
electrodes for
recording, 2543-2544, 2543f
stimulating, 2544, 2544f
electromyography for, 2545-2548
activity evoked by electrical stimulation in, 2387, 2545-2546
to assess functional status of nerves after tumor removal, 2545-2546
to identify and map nerves in relation to tumor, 2387, 2545
to identify nerve intermedius, 2546, 2546f
limitations of, 2547-2548, 2548f
spontaneous and mechanically evoked activity in, 2546-2548
patterns of, 2387, 2547, 2547f
in four-channel montage, 2550f
future directions in, 2555-2556, 2555f
instrumentation for, 2405, 2405f, 2543
during microvascular decompression, 2548-2549, 2549f
during other otologic surgery, 2549
and outcome, 2387, 2554
during parotid surgery, 2549
passive, 2387
personnel for, 2542-2543
stimulation criteria for, 2544
Facial nerve neuroma, 2414, 2506-2508
vs. acoustic neuroma, 2414, 2519-2522
of cerebellopontine angle, 2519-2522
Facial nerve neuroma *(Continued)*
diagnostic evaluation of, 2519-2522
imaging of, 2519-2522, 2521f
signs and symptoms of, 2519
diagnostic evaluation of, 2507
imaging of, 1924-1926, 1927f
management and surgical approach for, 2414, 2507-2508
of posterior fossa, 1928
Facial nerve paralysis
assessment of, 2416-2420, 2417b
due to barotrauma, 2400
due to benign intracranial hypertension, 2400-2401
bilateral, 2397-2398
central, 2401
congenital, 2396-2397, 2396b
rehabilitation of, 2420
corticosteroids for, 2409-2410, 2410t
differential diagnosis of, 2392t
familial, 2397
herpes zoster, 2393, 2396
with HIV infection, 2399
iatrogenic, 2399
in Kawasaki disease, 2400
long-standing, 2399
due to Lyme disease, 2106, 2400
management algorithm for, 2392f
due to mastoidectomy, 2015-2016
in Melkersson-Rosenthal syndrome, 2399
due to metabolic disorders, 2401
due to otitis media, 1991, 2400
epidemiology of, 1980t
imaging of, 1991f
treatment for, 1991
due to parotidectomy, 1176-1177
in pregnancy, 2399
progressive, 2398, 2398f
due to tumor, 2413
in Ramsay Hunt syndrome, 2393, 2396
recurrent, 2397
rehabilitation of, 2416-2433
adjunctive procedures in, 2417
for lower third of face, 2431-2432, 2431f
for middle third of face, 2430-2431, 2431f
for upper third of face, 2430
with eyelid dysfunction, 2420-2421
eye protection for, 2420, 2420f
lower (ectropion), 2420-2421, 2421f
upper (lagophthalmos), 2421
facial nerve grafting for, 2421-2425
cross-face, 2419, 2424-2425
selection of donor nerve for, 2422
surgical planning for, 2421-2424, 2423f
surgical technique for, 2422-2424, 2424f-2425f
muscle transfers in, 2427-2430
masseter, 2427, 2428f
microneurovascular, 2429-2430
temporalis, 2427-2429, 2429f
nerve transposition for, 2425-2427
of hypoglossal nerve, 2419, 2424f-2426f, 2425-2426
neurotropic factors in, 2427
of other nerves, 2426-2427
patient assessment for, 2416-2420, 2417b
age in, 2419
with congenital paralysis, 2420
considerations in, 2418-2420
donor consequences in, 2419
health status in, 2419-2420
House-Brackmann grading system in, 2417-2418, 2417t
presence of partial regeneration in, 2418
prior radiotherapy in, 2420
smile pattern in, 2417-2418
status of donor nerves in, 2419
Facial nerve neuroma *(Continued)*
status of proximal and distal facial nerve in, 2418-2419, 2419f
time since transection in, 2418
viability of facial muscles in, 2419
static procedures for, 2430
facial sling as, 2430
with synkinesis, 2432
botulinum A toxin for, 2432
selective myectomy for, 2432
in sarcoidosis, 2400
due to small fenestra stapedotomy, 2030, 2034
spontaneous idiopathic, 2391
auditory symptoms of, 2393-2394
in children, 2397
CNS changes in, 2393-2394
defined, 2391
and diabetes, 2401
differential diagnosis of, 2391, 2392t
electromagnetic stimulation in, 2394-2395
electrophysiology and testing for, 2394
electromyography in, 2394
electroneurography in, 2394
interpretation of electrical tests in, 2394
maximal stimulation test in, 2394
nerve conduction velocity in, 2394
nerve excitability threshold in, 2394
etiology of, 2391-2393
familial, 2397
histopathology of, 2393
imaging in, 1924, 1927f, 2395
incidence of, 2391-2396
management of, 2395-2396
middle cranial fossa decompression for, 2409-2410, 2409t
polyneuropathy in, 2391, 2398f
prognosis and statistics for, 2395
recurrent, 2397
stapedius reflex in, 1891
traumatic, 2398-2399, 2398f
Facial nerve regeneration, partial, 2418
Facial nerve rehabilitation, 2416-2433
adjunctive procedures for, 2417
for lower third of face, 2431-2432, 2431f
for middle third of face, 2430-2431, 2431f
for upper third of face, 2430
with eyelid dysfunction, 2420-2421
eye protection for, 2420, 2420f
lower (ectropion), 2420-2421, 2421f
upper (lagophthalmos), 2421
facial nerve grafting for, 2421-2425
cross-face, 2419, 2424-2425
selection of donor nerve for, 2422
surgical planning for, 2421-2424, 2423f
surgical technique for, 2422-2424, 2424f-2425f
muscle transfers for, 2427-2430
masseter, 2427, 2428f
microneurovascular, 2429-2430
temporalis, 2427-2429, 2429f
nerve transposition for, 2425-2427
of hypoglossal nerve, 2419, 2424f-2426f, 2425-2426
neurotropic factors in, 2427
of other nerves, 2426-2427
patient assessment for, 2416-2420, 2417b
age in, 2419
with congenital paralysis, 2420
considerations in, 2418-2420
donor consequences in, 2419
health status in, 2419-2420
House-Brackmann grading system in, 2417-2418, 2417t
presence of partial regeneration in, 2418
prior radiotherapy in, 2420
smile pattern in, 2417-2418
status of donor nerves in, 2419

Facial nerve rehabilitation *(Continued)*
status of proximal and distal facial nerve in, 2418-2419, 2419f
time since transection in, 2418
viability of facial muscles in, 2419
static procedures for, 2430
facial sling as, 2430
with synkinesis, 2432
botulinum A toxin for, 2432
selective myectomy for, 2432
Facial nerve repair, 2041, 2042t, 2398-2399, 2413-2414
indications for, 2041
middle fossa craniotomy for, 2042-2043
outcome of, 2041, 2042t
supralabyrinthine approach for, 2041-2042, 2043f
timing of, 2041-2042
translabyrinthine approach for, 2041-2042
transmastoid approach for, 2041-2042
Facial nerve schwannomas. *See* Facial nerve neuroma.
Facial nerve surgery, intratemporal, 2403-2415
combination approaches for, 2411-2412
draping for, 2404-2405, 2405f
for facial nerve tumors, 2413-2414, 2414t
general surgical techniques for, 2404-2405
instrumentation for, 2405
intraoperative monitoring for, 2405, 2405f
middle cranial fossa (transtemporal) approach for, 2407-2409
advantages and uses of, 2408-2409
for Bell's palsy, 2409-2410, 2409t-2410t
limitations and potential complications of, 2409
technique of, 2407-2408, 2408f-2409f
nerve repair in, 2413-2414
rerouting in, 2412, 2412f-2413f
partial, 2412-2413
retrolabyrinthine approach for, 2405-2406, 2405f-2406f
retrosigmoid approach for, 2406-2407
advantages and uses of, 2406-2407
limitations and potential complications of, 2407
technique of, 2406, 2407f
surgical anatomy for, 2403-2404, 2404f
translabyrinthine approach for, 2411
advantages and uses of, 2411
limitations and complications of, 2411
technique of, 2411, 2411f-2412f
transmastoid approach for, 2410-2411
advantages and uses of, 2411
limitations and complications of, 2411
technique of, 2410, 2410f
Facial nerve transposition, in postauricular approach to infratemporal fossa, 2497-2498, 2498f
Facial nerve trunk, insults to, 2384-2385
Facial nerve tumors, 2413-2414, 2414t
Facial neuromas. *See* Facial nerve neuroma.
Facial numbness, due to paranasal sinus tumor, 1123
Facial pain, sinus surgery for, 742
Facial palsy. *See* Facial nerve paralysis.
Facial paralysis. *See* Facial nerve paralysis.
Facial processes, fusion of, during embryogenesis, 2639
Facial proportions, 269
facial height in, 269, 273f
middle and lower, 269, 273f
facial symmetry through midsagittal plane in, 269, 272f
facial width in, 269, 272f
Facial recess
in mastoidectomy, 2012, 2012f-2013f
in surgical anatomy of lateral skull base, 2436f
Facial resurfacing
chemical peels for, 391-397
agents for, 392-394
complications of, 396-397
Facial resurfacing *(Continued)*
contraindications to, 391, 392t
in dark-skinned individuals, 392
deep, 394-395
equipment tray for, 393f
histologic changes with, 390-391
indications for, 391, 392t
medium-depth, 393-394, 393f-394f
patient selection and education for, 391-392
and phenol toxicity, 395
postoperative care after, 396, 396f
prepeel preparations for, 392
superficial, 392-393, 403
contraindications to, 391, 392t
dermabrasion for, 397-399
complications of, 399
equipment for, 398, 398f
micro-, 402-403
patient selection and consultation for, 397-398
postoperative care after, 399, 399f
technique of, 398-399, 398f-399f
indications for, 391, 392t
laser, 399-402
CO_2, 400, 400f
Er:YAG, 400
nonablative, 402, 403t
postoperative care after, 401-402, 401f
nonablative, 402, 403t
laser, 402, 403t
microdermabrasion for, 402-403
superficial chemical peels for, 403
Facial schwannomas. *See* Facial nerve neuroma.
Facial skeletal growth, 2615f, 2617t
Facial skeleton
anatomy, physiology, and pathophysiology of, 319-323, 320f
general, 319
of lower third, 322-323, 323f
of middle third, 319-322
areas of protection in, 322, 322t
infraorbital nerve in, 320, 321f
maxillae in, 320, 321f
nasal bones in, 320
orbits in, 320-321, 322f
zygoma in, 319, 320f-321f
of upper third, 319, 319f
biomechanics of, 331-333, 331f
in lower third, 332-333, 332f
in middle third, 331-332, 331f
in upper third, 331
physical examination of, 95
Facial swelling, due to paranasal sinus tumor, 1123
Facial symmetry, through midsagittal plane, 269, 272f
Facial translocation approach, for middle cranial base surgery, 2455t, 2464-2466, 2467f
Facial trauma
due to burns, 314-316
assessment and treatment of, 315-316
classification of, 314-315, 315f
of eyelids, 316
of lips and oral commissure, 316
of nasal and a uricular cartilage, 316
fracture as (*See* Facial fracture(s))
due to frostbite, 316
in geriatric patients, 237
imaging of, 170-171, 170f-171f
CT for, 142
soft tissue, 302-317
approach to, 302-306
anesthesia in, 304
cleaning in, 304-305, 305f
history taking in, 302-303
infection control in, 305
physical examination in, 303-304, 303f
repair in, 305-306, 306f
tetanus prophylaxis for, 303
Facial trauma *(Continued)*
to ears, 308f, 310, 310f
etiology of, 302
to eye, 303
to eyelids, 303, 303f, 307-309, 308f
to facial nerve, 309
to lacrimal apparatus, 307-309, 308f
with large-segment, composite avulsions or amputations, 312, 312f
to lips, 309-310, 309f
to nose, 310-312, 311f
to parotid duct, 312-313, 314f
to salivary glands, 312, 313f
sialocele and salivary fistula due to, 313-314
types of injuries in, 306-307
abrasion as, 306
avulsions as, 307, 308f
laceration as, 307
Facial venous malformations, embolization for, 1942, 1942f
Facial width, 269, 272f
Facies, physical examination of, 95, 95t
Facioauriculovertebral syndrome, 2741
Facio-oculo-auriculo-vertebral spectrum (FOAVS), craniofacial anomalies in, 2646-2647
FACT-HN (Functional Assessment of Cancer Therapy Head and Neck module), 56
Falciform crest
anatomy of, 1822, 1823f
in surgical anatomy of lateral skull base, 2437f, 2439
Fall(s), in elderly, 233
Fallopian canal
anatomy of, 1827-1828
vulnerability to injury of, 1829
False vocal cords, radiographic anatomy of, 1472-1473, 1472f
Falsetto, 811-812, 851
Familial atypical multiple mole-melanoma (FAMMM) syndrome, 1107
Familial episodic ataxia, 2357
Familial facial paralysis, 2397
Familial hemiplegic migraine (FHM), 2349
Familial hyperparathyroidism, 1795-1797
in MEN-I, 1775, 1776f, 1795-1796
in MEN-IIA, 1796
neonatal, 1797
non-MEN, 1796-1797
Familial hypocalciuric hypercalcemia, 1783
Familial hypothyroidism, 1747
Familial vestibulopathy, 2343-2344
FAMMM (familial atypical multiple mole-melanoma) syndrome, 1107
Fanconi's anemia, tumor suppressor gene in, 1020
Farkas, Leslie, 269
Fas, in adaptive immune system, 601
Fascia, of neck, 2577
deep, 2577-2578, 2578f-2579f
superficial, 2577
Fascial layers, of forehead and temporal region, 440-441, 441f
Fascial space involvement, in odontogenic infections, 180-187
cervical (deep neck), 184-187
lateral pharyngeal, 184-185, 186f
prevertebral (danger space No. 4), 186, 186f
retropharyngeal, 185-186, 186f-187f
surgical drainage and decompression for, 189-190
mandibular, 181-184
Ludwig's angina due to, 184, 185f
masseteric, 184, 185f
masticator, 184, 186f
pterygomandibular (medial pterygoid), 184, 185f
secondary, 184
sub-, 183-184, 183f-184f

Fascial space involvement, in odontogenic infections *(Continued)*
sublingual, 183, 183f
submental, 181-183, 183f
temporal, 184, 185f
maxillary, 180-181
buccal, 181, 181f
canine, 180-181, 180f
cavernous sinus thrombosis due to, 181, 182f
orbital cellulitis due to, 181, 182f
natural history of, 179-180
Fasciitis, necrotizing, due to deep neck space infections, 208
Fasciocutaneous free flaps, 1067, 1067f, 1082t, 1083
anterolateral thigh, 1082t, 1083
for hypopharyngeal and esophageal reconstruction, 1455
for oropharyngeal reconstruction, 1379
for hypopharyngeal and esophageal reconstruction, 1433, 1455
anterolateral thigh, 1455
lateral arm, 1455
lateral thigh, 1455
radial forearm, 1455
scapular-parascapular, 1455
lateral arm, 1082t, 1083
for hypopharyngeal and esophageal reconstruction, 1455
for oropharyngeal reconstruction, 1379-1380
lateral thigh, 1082t
for hypopharyngeal and esophageal reconstruction, 1455
for oropharyngeal reconstruction, 1379
for oropharyngeal reconstruction, 1379-1381, 1379f
anterolateral thigh, 1379
lateral arm, 1379-1380
lateral thigh, 1379
radial forearm, 1379, 1379f
radial forearm, 1082t, 1083, 1083f
for hypopharyngeal and esophageal reconstruction, 1455
for oropharyngeal reconstruction, 1379, 1379f
tubed, 1087, 1091f
scapular-parascapular, 1082t
for hypopharyngeal and esophageal reconstruction, 1455
for tongue base reconstruction, 1390-1391
ulnar forearm, 1082t
Fast Fourier Transform (FFT), in acoustic analysis, for voice evaluation, 829t, 830, 830f
Fast neutron, 1034
Fast spin-echo (FSE) imaging, 134
Fasting, prior to anesthesia, 112
in children, 2589, 2590t
Fat(s), dietary, taste of, 1213
Fat saturation, for MRI, 135-136, 136f
Fat suppression methods, for MRI, 135-136, 136f
of laryngeal carcinoma, 1470
FBA. *See* Foreign body aspiration (FBA).
FDG-PET. *See* Fluorodeoxyglucose–positron emission tomography (FDG-PET).
Federation of State Medical Boards (FSMB), 80-81, 84t-87t
Feedback, with traditional hearing aid, 2204
Feedback suppression circuitry, for hearing aids, 2269
FEES (flexible endoscopic evaluation of swallowing), for dysphagia in children, 2949, 2950t
FEES (functional endoscopic evaluation of swallowing)
for chronic aspiration, 926
for laryngeal stenosis, 2917
"Feline" esophagitis, 967-968, 969f
Fenestra, creation of, in small fenestra stapedotomy, 2031-2032, 2032f
Fenestral otosclerosis, 1921-1922, 1925f
Fenretinide, for cancer chemoprevention, 1018, 1061-1062
Fentanyl
as adjunct to induction of anesthesia, 111
for anesthesia maintenance in children, 2591
for postoperative pain, 241t
Fentanyl sublingual spray, for mucositis, 1102
FESS. *See* Functional endoscopic sinus surgery (FESS).
Fever, pharyngoconjunctival, 198
"Fever blisters," in HIV, 226
Fexofenadine (Allegra), for nonallergic rhinitis, 701t
FFB. *See* Flexible fiberoptic bronchoscopy (FFB).
FFL (flexible fiberoptic laryngoscopy), for laryngomalacia, 2867
FFT (Fast Fourier Transform), in acoustic analysis, for voice evaluation, 829t, 830, 830f
FGF(s) (fibroblast growth factors), in wound healing, 1077-1078
FGFR(s) (fibroblast growth factor receptors), in craniofacial anomalies, 2640, 2642f
FGFR3 (fibroblast growth factor receptor 3) gene
in achondroplasia, 2633
in deafness, 2051t-2058t
FHM (familial hemiplegic migraine), 2349
Fiberoptic bronchoscope (FOB)
for awake fiberoptic nasotracheal intubation, 123-125, 125f
for difficult airway, 114t
Fiberoptic intubation (FOI), awake nasotracheal, 122-123
advantages of, 123
avoiding failure in, 125, 126b
bronchoscopy cart for, 123, 123f
conscious sedation for, 124
fiberoptic bronchoscope in, 123-125, 125f
historical perspective on, 122-123
indications for, 123, 123b
keys to successful, 124b
monitoring during, 124
nasal trumpet placement for, 124, 125f
optimal setup for, 125f
patient preparation for, 123-124
technique of, 124-125
topical anesthesia for, 124
Fiberoptic laryngoscope, rigid, for difficult airway, 114t
Fiberoptic nasopharyngoscopy, 101
of obstructive sleep apnea, 253, 254f
Fibrillated ePTFE (Gore-Tex), for chin implants, 465t
Fibrin glue, in intratympanic delivery, 2182
Fibrin sealants, for rhytidectomy, 416-420
Fibroadnexal tumor(s), 291-293
acrochordon as, 291
angiofibroma as, 292
atypical fibroxanthoma as, 292
cylindroma as, 288f, 292
dermatofibroma as, 288f
dermatofibrosarcoma protuberans as, 291-292
fibrous papule as, 288f, 292
hidrocystoma as, 292
keloids and hypertrophic scars as, 291
lipoma as, 293
neurofibromas as, 292
sebaceous hyperplasia as, 288f, 293
syringoma as, 292-293
trichoepithelioma as, 292
xanthelasma as, 293
Fibroblast(s), in formation of granulation tissue, 1077
Fibroblast growth factor(s) (FGFs), in wound healing, 1077-1078
Fibroblast growth factor receptor(s) (FGFRs), in craniofacial anomalies, 2640, 2642f
Fibroblast growth factor receptor 3 *(FGFR3)* gene
in achondroplasia, 2633
in deafness, 2051t-2058t
Fibroepithelial papilloma, 291
Fibroma
ameloblastic, 1274-1275
microscopic findings in, 1274-1275, 1275f
radiographic features of, 1274
treatment of, 1275
irritation, of oral cavity, 1288-1289, 1289f
ossifying, sinonasal, 725-726
subcutaneous, due to neck irradiation, 1695
Fibronectin, in wound contraction, 1078
Fibro-odontoma, ameloblastic, 1275
microscopic findings in, 1275, 1275f
radiographic findings in, 1275
treatment of, 1275
Fibrosarcoma
in children, 2842-2843, 2843f
of larynx, 1508
of neck, 1668
of paranasal sinuses, 1131
Fibrosis, due to radiotherapy, 1048
Fibrous dysplasia, 2110-2111
of anterior skull base, 2647f
cellular and molecular basis of, 2111
clinical manifestations of, 2111
histopathology of, 2111, 2111f
laboratory findings in, 2111
management of, 2111
otologic manifestations of, 2111
radiographic findings in, 2111, 2111f
of sinonasal tract, 718t, 725-726, 726f
Fibrous nonunion, 331, 339-340
Fibrous papule, 288f, 292
Fibrous tumor, solitary, of neck, 1671
Fibrous union, 331, 339-340
Fibroxanthoma, atypical, 292
Fibula flap, for free tissue transfer, 1082t, 1084-1085, 1085f
Fibula osteocutaneous free flap reconstruction
for mandibular defects, 1324-1325, 1325t
for oral cancer, 1316, 1316f
Field cancerization, in head and neck squamous cell carcinoma, 1016, 1061
Filter, in acoustic analysis, for voice evaluation, 830
Finasteride (Propecia), for hair loss, 377-378
Fine structure signal processing, for cochlear implants, 2230-2231, 2231f-2232f
Fine-needle aspiration biopsy (FNAB)
in children, 2574
of salivary glands, 2854
of lymphoma, 1675-1676
of neck masses, 1638
of oropharyngeal cancer, 1366
of salivary glands, 1149, 1149f, 1165-1166, 1180-1181
in children, 2854
of thyroid nodule, 1756-1758
repeat, 1759
ultrasound-guided, 1655f
ultrasound-guided, 1653-1654, 1655f
of parathyroid tumor, 1789
Fine-needle aspiration cytology (FNAC). *See* Fine-needle aspiration biopsy (FNAB).
Fire, in airway, 119
First aid measures, for epistaxis, 684
First bite syndrome
due to carotid paraganglioma surgery, 1660-1661
due to neck surgery, 1732
First branchial cleft cyst, otorrhea due to infection of, 2195
First genu, of facial nerve, 1826f, 1827-1828
FISH (fluorescence in situ hybridization), for head and neck squamous cell carcinoma, 1018-1019

Fissures of Santorini, 1823, 1944
Fistula(s)
arteriovenous, embolization of
dural, 1940-1942, 1940f
facial, 1940, 1940f
branchial cleft, 2585
imaging of, 1410, 1410f
carotid cavernous, due to temporal bone trauma, 2047
cerebrospinal fluid
bacterial meningitis due to, 794
due to cranial base surgery, 2468
CT cisternogram of, 2477f
traumatic, 2044-2046
antibiotic prophylaxis for, 2044-2045
closure of, 2045-2046, 2045f
diagnosis of, 2044
infecting organisms with, 2045
meningitis due to, 2044-2045
pathogenesis of, 2044
signs and symptoms of, 2044
treatment algorithm for, 2045-2046, 2045f
chylous
due to neck dissection, 1723
due to neck surgery, 1732-1733, 1732f
horizontal semicircular canal, due to mastoidectomy, 2015
H-type, 2926
labyrinthine, 1989-1990, 1990f
orocutaneous, 179, 180f
oronasal, after palatoplasty, 2673
perilymph, 2342-2343
categories of, 2342
due to chronic otitis media, 2342-2343
clinical presentation of, 2342
congenital, 2737-2738, 2737f
imaging of, 2342, 2342f
repair of, 2361-2362
sensorineural hearing loss due to, 2122, 2199
fluctuating, 2199
sudden, 2128
due to small fenestra stapedotomy, 2034
due to temporal bone fracture, 2039
due to trauma, 2342
pharyngocutaneous
after hypopharyngeal reconstruction, 1458
due to neck surgery, 1727-1728, 1728f
after total laryngectomy, 1571
after total laryngopharyngectomy, 1575
of pharynx and esophagus
branchial cleft anomaly as, 1410, 1410f
due to perforation, 1410-1411, 1410f
postoperative, 1411, 1411f
tracheoesophageal, 1409-1410
postparotidectomy, 1728
salivary, due to neck surgery, 1727-1728, 1728f
due to sphenoidotomy, 768t
tracheal–innominate artery, 1623
tracheal–pulmonary artery, 1623
tracheoesophageal, 2926
imaging of, 1409-1410
Fistula test
for labyrinthine fistula, 1990
for temporal bone fractures, 2039
Fitting range, of hearing aid, 2271, 2272f
Fitzpatrick sun-reactive skin types, 391, 391t
585-nm pulsed dye laser (PDL), 31t, 33
Fixation eye movements, 2305-2306, 2306f, 2307t
FK-506 (tacrolimus), for eczematoid otitis externa, 1956
FKH10, in deafness, 2051t-2058t
FL (follicular lymphoma), 1678
clinical presentation of, 1674
treatment and prognosis for, 1678
FLACC (Face, Legs, Activity, Cry, Consolability) tool, 240
Flageolet, 851
FLAIR (fluid-attenuated inversion recovery) imaging, of middle ear cholesteatoma, 1919, 1921f
Flap(s), skin. *See* Skin flap(s).
Flash lamp pulsed lasers, 33-34
Flash lamp pumped dye laser, 31t, 33
Flexible endoscopic evaluation of swallowing (FEES), for dysphagia in children, 2949, 2950t
Flexible endoscopy
in children, 2574
for stridor, 2901-2902
Flexible fiberoptic bronchoscopy (FFB), 1001-1007
bronchoscopes for
care of, 1001-1002
range and special features of, 1001, 1002t, 1003f
"therapeutic," 1001, 1003f
ultrathin, 1001, 1003f
diagnostic, 999b, 1003-1007
for bronchial wash, 1003
for bronchoalveolar lavage, 1003-1004
for bronchoscopic brush sampling, 1007
for endobronchial and transbronchial biopsy, 1004-1005, 1004f-1005f
general approaches to, 1003
for transbronchial needle aspiration, 1005-1007, 1005f-1006f
for visual examination, 1003
imaging prior to, 999-1000
indications for, 999, 999b
patient discussion and informed consent for, 1000
patient positioning and route of entry for, 1000
sedation and airway management for, 1000
Flexible fiberoptic laryngoscopy (FFL), for laryngomalacia, 2867
Flexible fiberoptic nasopharyngoscopy, for recurrent respiratory papillomatosis, 2888
Flexible laryngeal mask airway, for children, 2599
Flexible laryngoscopy, 100, 814
advantages of, 814
disadvantages of, 814
in neurologic evaluation, 834
for professional voice disorders, 851-852, 852t
protocols for, 816b, 818b
technique of, 814
troubleshooting for, 814
Floccular lesions, and vestibular function, 2308
Floccular peduncle, 1861
Flocculus, 2404f
Flonase (fluticasone propionate), for nonallergic rhinitis, 700t
Floor of mouth
anatomy of, 1297-1298
carcinoma of, 1307-1308
cervical metastases of, 1308
clinical presentation of, 1294f, 1307
composite resection for, 1307-1308, 1308f, 1315f
coronal partial mandibulectomy for, 1307-1308, 1308f
imaging of, 1307
invasive, 1307
reconstruction for, 1307, 1315f
segmental mandibulectomy for, 1307-1308, 1308f
survival with, 1308
transoral resection for, 1307
vasculature of, 1296
Flow-volume loop, for airway stenosis, 945f
Floxin (ofloxacin) otic solution, for otitis externa, 1946, 1952, 1959t-1960t
Fluence, of surgical laser, 28
Fluid losses, expected, in children, 2572t
Fluid resuscitation
for burns, 315
for deep neck space infections, 205
Fluid secretion, by salivary glands, 1135, 1135f
Fluid utilization, during bed rest, for children, 2572t
Fluid-attenuated inversion recovery (FLAIR) imaging, of middle ear cholesteatoma, 1919, 1921f
Fluids and fluid management, in children, 2572
and expected fluid losses, 2572t
and fluid utilization during bed rest, 2572t
and ideal electrolyte composition for infants, 2572t
Flumazenil, for premedication in children, 2589
Flunisolide (Nasalide, Nasarel)
for nonallergic rhinitis, 700t
for rhinosinusitis, 734t, 736
Fluorescein, intrathecal, for CSF rhinorrhea, 790, 2044
Fluorescence in situ hybridization (FISH), for head and neck squamous cell carcinoma, 1018-1019
Fluorescent tumor markers, for early glottic carcinoma, 1516
Fluoride, in saliva, 1139
Fluoride gel, for dental care during radiation therapy, 1331, 1331f
Fluoride therapy, for otosclerosis, 2034-2035
Fluorodeoxyglucose–positron emission tomography (FDG-PET), 137-138
applications of, 144, 145f
with intensity-modulated radiotherapy, 1044
of laryngeal carcinoma, 1494-1495
early glottic, 1517
of oral cancer, 1300
of salivary glands, 1150, 1168
Fluoroquinolones, for pediatric chronic sinusitis, 2779
Fluoroscopy
of obstructive sleep apnea, 255
of pharynx and esophagus, 1393-1394
5-Fluorouracil (5-FU)
for chemical peels, 392-393
in combination chemotherapy, 1059-1060
for induction chemotherapy, 1056-1058, 1058f
with radiotherapy, 1041-1042, 1052-1054
Fluosol-DA, and skin flap viability, 1073-1074
Fluticasone
for obstructive sleep apnea, 257
for rhinosinusitis, 734t
Fluticasone acetonide oil (DermOtic Oil), for eczematoid otitis externa, 1956
Fluticasone furoate (Veramyst), for nonallergic rhinitis, 700t
Fluticasone propionate (Flonase), for nonallergic rhinitis, 700t
Fluticasone propionate cream, for eczematoid otitis externa, 1955-1956
FM (frequency-modulated) receiver, for hearing aid, 2267
FM (frequency-modulated) system, personal, 2271
fMRI (functional magnetic resonance imaging)
for cerebral blood flow evaluation, 2491
of olfaction, 632
FNAB. *See* Fine-needle aspiration biopsy (FNAB).
FNAC (fine-needle aspiration cytology). *See* Fine-needle aspiration biopsy (FNAB).
F_0. *See* Frequency (F_0).
FOAVS (facio-oculo-auriculo-vertebral spectrum), craniofacial anomalies in, 2646-2647
FOB (fiberoptic bronchoscope)
for awake fiberoptic nasotracheal intubation, 123-125, 125f
for difficult airway, 114t
Focal length, of lens of laser, 28
Focal plane, of surgical laser, 28, 28f
FOI. *See* Fiberoptic intubation (FOI).

Folate deficiency, oral manifestations of, 1254
Foliate papillae, taste buds in, 1208
Follicular cyst, 1263-1264
  microscopic features of, 1264
  neoplastic potential of, 1264
  radiographic features of, 1264, 1264f
  treatment of, 1264, 1264f
Follicular lymphoma (FL), 1678
  clinical presentation of, 1674
  treatment and prognosis for, 1678
Follicular thyroid carcinoma, 1761-1762
  clinical presentation of, 1761-1762
  management and prognosis for, 1762
  pathology of, 1762
Follicular unit extraction (FUE), 384
Follicular-unit hair transplantation, 378, 378f-381f
  completion of procedure for, 383-384
  complications of, 384
  dissection of donor strip in, 382, 382f
  doll's hair appearance with, 378, 378f
  follicular unit extraction for, 384
  graft placement in, 383, 383f
  location of hairline in, 378-379, 381f, 383, 383f
  marking off donor strip of scalp for, 381-382, 382f
  marking out recipient regions for, 379-381, 382f
  micrografts in, 378, 379f-381f
  operative procedure for, 382-384
  postoperative care after, 384
  preoperative evaluation for, 378-382, 381f
  slivers of follicular units in, 382, 383f
  surrounding natural hair growth in, 382-383
Fontaine sign, positive, with carotid paragangliomas, 1659
Fontanelle(s)
  closure of, 2617t
  in newborn, 2615, 2618f
Food impactions, in esophagus, 975
Food sensitivity, and migraines, 2349
Foramen cecum, in surgical anatomy of anterior cranial base, 2442-2443, 2443f, 2471, 2472f
Foramen jugulare, in surgical anatomy of middle cranial base, 2445f
Foramen lacerum
  in surgical anatomy of anterior cranial base, 2472f
  in surgical anatomy of lateral skull base, 2435f, 2436-2437
  in surgical anatomy of middle cranial base, 2444, 2445f
Foramen magnum
  growth and development of, 2617t
  in surgical anatomy of lateral skull base, 2435f
Foramen of Huschke, 1823
Foramen ovale
  anatomy of, 1699
  in surgical anatomy of lateral skull base, 2435f, 2436-2438, 2437f, 2472f
  in surgical anatomy of middle cranial base, 2444, 2445f
Foramen rotundum
  in surgical anatomy of lateral skull base, 2435f, 2438
  in surgical anatomy of middle cranial base, 2444, 2445f
Foramen spinosum
  in surgical anatomy of lateral skull base, 2434, 2435f, 2437-2438, 2441
  in surgical anatomy of middle cranial base, 2444, 2445f
Forced opening test, of eustachian tube function, 1874
Forced oscillation rhinomanometry, 643-644
Fordyce spots, 99
Foregut duplication cysts, compression of pharynx and esophagus due to, 1408-1409, 1409f
Forehead
  aesthetic analysis of, 270-271
    for defect repair, 359
    eyebrow position in, 271, 275f
    eyebrow shape in, 271
    nasofrontal angle in, 270, 274f
  aesthetic proportions of, 428, 429f
  aging, 428-432, 429f
  fascial layers of, 440-441, 441f
Forehead defects, 359-363
  aesthetic considerations with, 359
  central third, 359-360, 362f
  goals of, 359
  lateral, 360-362
    advancement flap for, 360-363, 362f
    advancement rotation flap for, 360-362, 362f
    O-T or A-T procedure for, 362, 363f
    primary wound closure for, 360-362
    rotation flaps for, 362
  primary wound repair for, 359
  tissue expansion for, 363
Forehead feminization, 385, 385f
Forehead flaps, for nasal defects, 366-367, 368f
  paramedian, 348-350, 352f-353f
Forehead lift
  coronal, 430, 431t
  mid-, 430, 431t
  pretrichial, 430, 431t
Forehead rejuvenation, 428-438
  aesthetic proportions for, 428, 429f
  brow muscles in, 431, 433f
  and characteristics of aging brow, 428-432, 429f
  patient selection for, 428-430
    anatomic considerations in, 429-430
    psychological considerations in, 428
  postoperative care after, 434
  results of, 434-438, 436f-438f
  surgical goals of, 430
  surgical technique for, 432-434
    brow elevation and fixation in, 434, 435f
    frontal and parietal bone dissection in, 432-433
    incisions in, 432, 433f
    local anesthesia in, 432
    release of brow depressor muscles in, 434, 434f
    temporal dissection in, 433-434, 433f-434f
  technique(s) for, 430-432, 431t
    browpexy for, 430, 431t, 432f
    coronal forehead lift for, 430, 431t
    direct brow lift for, 430, 431t
    endoscopic brow lift for, 431, 431t
    midforehead brow lift for, 430, 431t
    midforehead lift for, 430, 431t
    pretrichial forehead lift for, 430, 431t
    temporal lift for, 431-432, 431t
  treatment of depressor muscles with botulinum toxin for, 432, 433f
Foreign body(ies)
  in airway, 975-976, 2935-2943
    acute obstruction due to, 2936-2937
    complications of, 2942
    epidemiology of, 2936
    imaging of, 1411, 1412f, 2938-2939
      vs. tonsillar calcifications, 1411, 1412f
    location of, 2936, 2936f
    management of, 2939-2941
      anesthesia for, 2940
      controversies in, 2942
      equipment for, 2939-2940, 2939t, 2940f
      history of, 2935
      postoperative, 2941-2942
      for sharp objects, 2940-2941
      technique for, 2940, 2941f
    symptoms of, 2937-2938
  bronchial
    complications of, 2942
    imaging of, 2938, 2938f-2939f
    location of, 2936, 2936f
Foreign body(ies) *(Continued)*
    management of
      anesthesia for, 2940
      controversies in, 2942
      technique for, 2940
    symptoms of, 2938
  in esophagus, 975-976, 2935-2943
    airway obstruction due to, 1481, 1481f
    classification of, 975
    complications of, 2942, 2942f
    epidemiology of, 2936
    due to food impaction, 975
    imaging of, 1411, 1412f, 2939
    location of, 2936, 2937f
    management of, 2939-2941
      anesthesia for, 2940
      controversies in, 2942
      for disk batteries, 2941
      equipment for, 2939-2940, 2939t
      history of, 2935-2936
      for pills, 2941
      postoperative, 2941-2942
      for sharp objects, 2940-2941
      technique for, 2940
    perforation due to, 2941
    symptoms of, 2938
  in external auditory canal, 2021
  in larynx
    endoscopic removal of, 2904
      anesthesia for, 2940
    imaging of, 1480-1481, 1480f, 2938
      vs. ossification of stylohyoid ligament, 1480, 1481f
    symptoms of, 2937-2938
  rhinitis due to, 619b
  sinonasal, 742
  tracheal
    anesthesia for removal of, 2940
    imaging of, 2938
    symptoms of, 2938
Foreign body aspiration (FBA), 975-976, 2935-2943
  acute obstruction due to, 2936-2937
  complications of, 2942
  epidemiology of, 2936
  imaging of, 1411, 1412f, 2938-2939
    vs. tonsillar calcifications, 1411, 1412f
  interventional bronchoscopy for, 1008
  location of, 2936, 2936f
  management of, 2939-2941
    anesthesia for, 2940
    controversies in, 2942
    equipment for, 2939-2940, 2939t, 2940f
    history of, 2935
    postoperative, 2941-2942
    for sharp objects, 2940-2941
    technique for, 2940, 2941f
  stridor due to, 2898
  symptoms of, 2937-2938
Forked-flap technique, in cleft-lip nose repair, 559, 566f
Forkhead box I1 *(FOXI1)* gene, in deafness, 2051t-2058t, 2096, 2098
Formant(s), 2876
  in acoustic analysis for voice evaluation, 830
  singer's, 847
  in speech, 812
Formant regions, 847
Forward-planning intensity-modulated radiation therapy (FP-IMRT), 1696-1697
Foscan [m-tetra(hydroxyphenyl)chlorin], for recurrent respiratory papillomatosis, 2892
FOSQ (Functional Outcomes of Sleep Questionnaire), 57
Fossa of Rosenmüller, in surgical anatomy of anterior cranial base, 2474
Fossa triangularis, 476-477, 476f, 1824f

Fossa triangularis–temporalis fascia sutures, 476f
Founder effect, 7
Fourth ventricle tumors, 2528-2529, 2530f-2531f
vestibular symptoms of, 2353-2354
Four-vessel arteriography, prior to lateral cranial base surgery, 2489-2490, 2491f
Fovea ethmoidalis, 741, 2472f
FOXI1 (forkhead box I1) gene, in deafness, 2051t-2058t, 2096, 2098
FP-IMRT (forward-planning intensity-modulated radiation therapy), 1696-1697
FPS-R (Faces Pain Scale Revised), 240
Fractional photolysis, for facial resurfacing, 403t
Fracture(s)
condylar and subcondylar, 322-323, 1280, 1281t
pediatric, 2704, 2706f-2708f
dentoalveolar, 2706-2707, 2710f
of frontal bone, 319, 319f
frontal sinus
classification of, 326
imaging of, 325, 325f
management of, 784
pediatric, 2711, 2712f
repair of, 333-334
mandibular, 323
classification of, 327
imaging of, 325-326
pediatric, 2704-2706
arch and body, 2706, 2709f
complications of, 2704
condylar and subcondylar, 2704, 2706f-2708f
epidemiology of, 2698
symphyseal and parasymphyseal, 2704-2706, 2708f-2709f
physical examination of, 325
repair of, 337-339, 338f
surgical access to, 329-330, 330f
teeth in line of, 339
maxillary
classification of, 326, 327f
imaging of, 325
physical examination of, 324-325
repair of, 334-337, 334f-336f
nasal (*See* Nasal fracture(s))
naso-orbitoethmoid, 322
classification of, 326-327, 327f
pediatric, 2714
classification of, 2714, 2716f
evaluation of, 2714, 2716f
repair of, 2714, 2716f
physical examination of, 324, 324f
repair of, 336-337, 337f
orbital
blowout, 170f, 321, 325, 326f
pediatric, 325, 326f
imaging of, 325, 326f
pediatric, 2711-2714
evaluation of, 2712, 2713f
of lateral/medial orbital wall, 2712, 2714, 2716f
of orbital apex, 2712, 2713f
of orbital floor, 2712-2713, 2714f-2715f
of orbital roof, 2712-2713, 2716f
patterns of, 2711-2712
physical examination of, 324
repair of, 336
surgical access to, 328-329, 329f
pediatric
condylar and subcondylar, 2704, 2706f-2708f
dentoalveolar, 2706-2707, 2710f
of frontal sinus, 2711, 2712f
mandibular, 2704-2706
arch and body, 2706, 2709f
complications of, 2704
condylar and subcondylar, 2704, 2706f-2708f
epidemiology of, 2698
Fracture(s) *(Continued)*
symphyseal and parasymphyseal, 2704-2706, 2708f-2709f
naso-orbitoethmoid, 2714
classification of, 2714, 2716f
evaluation of, 2714, 2716f
repair of, 2714, 2716f
orbital, 2711-2714
evaluation of, 2712, 2713f
of lateral/medial orbital wall, 2712, 2714, 2716f
of orbital apex, 2712, 2713f
of orbital floor, 2712-2713, 2714f-2715f
of orbital roof, 2712-2713, 2716f
patterns of, 2711-2712
pterygoid plate, 171f
skull base, 171
temporal bone (*See* Temporal bone fractures)
transverse petrous, 174f
Fracture hematoma, 330
Franceschetti syndrome, craniofacial abnormalities in, 2633-2635, 2633b, 2635f
Francisella tularensis, pharyngitis due to, 195
Frankfort horizontal plane, in facial analysis, 269, 272f
for mentoplasty, 463, 464f
Frechet triple flap repair, for vertical slot defect, 385, 386f
Free cartilage grafts, for nasal defects, 348
Free flap reconstruction, for oral cancer, 1316, 1316f
Free microvascular flaps, 1067
primary ischemia in, 1075
reperfusion period for, 1075
salvage of, 1075
secondary ischemia in, 1068, 1075
vascularity of recipient bed with, 1075
Free radical(s)
in acutely raised skin flaps, 1070-1071, 1071f
in ototoxicity, 2190
in radiation damage, 1036
and skin flap viability, 1074
Free radical scavengers, and skin flap viability, 1074
Free T_3 level, 1740
Free T_4 index, 1740
Free T_4 level, 1740
Free tissue transfer, 1080-1099
advantages of, 1080-1081, 1081b
contraindications to, 1091
costs and outcomes of, 1098
defined, 1080
for dental rehabilitation, 1087, 1089f
with diabetes, 1091-1092
disadvantages of, 1081-1082, 1081b
donor site options for, 1082-1083, 1082t, 1083b
fasciocutaneous (soft tissue) flaps for, 1082t, 1083
anterolateral thigh, 1082t, 1083
for hypopharyngeal and esophageal reconstruction, 1455
for oropharyngeal reconstruction, 1379
for hypopharyngeal and esophageal reconstruction, 1433, 1455
anterolateral thigh, 1455
lateral arm, 1455
lateral thigh, 1455
radial forearm, 1455
lateral arm, 1082t, 1083
for hypopharyngeal and esophageal reconstruction, 1455
for oropharyngeal reconstruction, 1379-1380
lateral thigh, 1082t
for hypopharyngeal and esophageal reconstruction, 1455
for oropharyngeal reconstruction, 1379
for oropharyngeal reconstruction, 1379-1381, 1379f
Free tissue transfer *(Continued)*
anterolateral thigh, 1379
lateral arm, 1379-1380
lateral thigh, 1379
radial forearm, 1379, 1379f
radial forearm, 1082t, 1083, 1083f
for hypopharyngeal and esophageal reconstruction, 1455
for oropharyngeal reconstruction, 1379, 1379f
tubed, 1087, 1091f
scapular-parascapular, 1082t
ulnar forearm, 1082t
future directions in, 1098
historical perspectives on, 1081
for hypopharyngeal and esophageal reconstruction, 1454, 1454f
enteric, 1455-1457
gastro-omental donor site for, 1457-1458, 1457f
jejunal donor site for, 1455-1457, 1456f
fasciocutaneous, 1433, 1455
antero-lateral thigh donor site for, 1455
other donor sites for, 1455
radial forearm donor site for, 1455
indications for, 1081-1087, 1081b-1082b
intraoperative management of, 1092-1093
muscle and myocutaneous flaps for, 1082t, 1083-1084
latissimus dorsi, 1082t, 1083-1084, 1084f
for oropharyngeal reconstruction, 1380
for oropharyngeal reconstruction, 1380
rectus abdominis, 1082t, 1083
for oropharyngeal reconstruction, 1380
for oropharyngeal reconstruction, 1379-1381
fasciocutaneous, 1379-1380
anterolateral thigh, 1379
lateral arm, 1379-1380
lateral thigh, 1379
radial forearm, 1379, 1379f
musculocutaneous, 1380
latissimus dorsi myocutaneous, 1380
rectus abdominis, 1380
osteocutaneous, 1380-1381
of soft palate, 1382
Gehanno method for, 1382
Lacombe and Blackwell's method for, 1382-1383
other groups' experience with, 1383
radial forearm, 1382, 1383f
of tongue base, 1389
lateral arm, 1389
radial forearm, 1389
of tonsils and pharyngeal wall, 1386
with combined lateral and superior defects, 1386, 1387f
lateral arm and thigh, 1386-1387
radial forearm, 1386
visceral, 1380, 1380f
osteocutaneous (vascularized bone) flaps for, 1082t, 1084-1087
fibula, 1082t, 1084-1085, 1085f
iliac crest, 1082t, 1087
for oropharyngeal reconstruction, 1380-1381
radial forearm, 1082t, 1085-1086, 1086f-1087f
scapula, 1082t, 1086-1087, 1088f
other flaps for, 1082t, 1087
jejunum, 1082t, 1087, 1090f
omentum, 1082t
temporal-parietal, 1082t
patient evaluation and preparation for, 1087-1092
history and current illness in, 1087-1088
laboratory and radiologic studies in, 1092
past medical history in, 1091-1092
physical examination in, 1088-1091
surgical treatment planning in, 1092

Free tissue transfer *(Continued)*
postoperative management of, 1096-1098
complications and salvage in, 1097-1098
free flap monitoring in, 1097
pharmacologic, 1096-1097
aspirin in, 1096
dextran in, 1096-1097
heparin in, 1096
surgical techniques for, 1093-1096
drain placement and wound closure in, 1096
free flap harvest in, 1094
free flap inset and microvascular anastomosis in, 1094-1096, 1095f
neck recipient site surgery in, 1094
primary recipient site surgery in, 1093-1094
surgical incisions in, 1093
visceral, for oropharyngeal reconstruction, 1380, 1380f
Freer elevator, for septoplasty, 488, 489f
Frequency (F_0)
in acoustic analysis for voice evaluation, 829, 829t
characteristic, 1844-1845, 1845f
of sound waves, 1838-1839, 1839f
of ultrasound waves, 1643
Frequency distribution, 63, 66
Frequency gain response, for hearing aids, 2267-2268
Frequency response, in vestibular tests, 2302, 2303f
Frequency selective presaturation, for MRI, 135-136, 136f
Frequency-modulated (FM) receiver, for hearing aid, 2267
Frequency-modulated (FM) system, personal, 2271
Frey's syndrome, 2197
after parotidectomy, 1177
Friedreich's ataxia, 2357
Frontal bone
anatomy and physiology of, 319, 319f-320f
fracture of, 319, 319f
imaging of, 325, 325f
repair of, 333-334
surgical access to, 328, 328f-329f
osteomyelitis of, 777f
Paget's disease of, 779-780, 780f
in surgical anatomy of anterior cranial base, 2442-2443
Frontal branch, of facial nerve, 440, 441f
in anterior cranial base surgery, 2451, 2451f
Frontal mucocele, 783
Frontal nerve, 440
Frontal process, in endoscopic dacryocystorhinostomy, 799-800, 800f
Frontal recess
in endoscopic sinus surgery, 750
prior to endoscopic sinus surgery, 764, 764t
after functional endoscopic sinus surgery, 677
normal anatomy of, 665, 665f-667f
reconstruction of lateral wall of, 778-779, 779f
surgical anatomy of, 740-741
Frontal sinus(es)
anatomy of, 319, 319f, 665, 665f
surgical, 740-741
in anterior cranial base, 2442, 2443f, 2473, 2474f
biomechanics of, 331
cranialization of, 782, 783f
prior to endoscopic sinus surgery, 764t
external approaches to, 757
growth and development of, 2619-2620
obliteration of, 779-781
closure in, 780
complications after, 780-781
estimating limit of frontal sinus in, 780, 781f
incision for, 779-780, 780f
materials used for, 780
with Paget's disease, 779-780, 780f
postoperative monitoring after, 780-781
Frontal sinus(es) *(Continued)*
removal of all mucosa in, 780
template for, 779-780
osteoma of, 783-784, 784f
physiology of, 664
pneumosinus dilatans of, 783, 784f
Frontal sinus drainage procedure, median, 779, 779f
Frontal sinus fractures
classification of, 326
imaging of, 325, 325f
management of, 784
pediatric, 2711, 2712f
repair of, 333-334
Frontal sinus surgery
balloon catheter sinusotomy as, 782-783
cranialization of frontal sinus as, 782, 783f
endoscopic frontal sinusotomy as, 776-778
accessing frontal recess in, 777, 777f-778f
confirming location of instrument in, 777-778, 778f
contrainidications to, 781, 781f
history of, 775-776
indications for, 776-783
Lynch-Howarth external ethmoidectomy as, 778-779, 779f
median frontal sinus drainage procedure as, 779, 779f
obliteration of frontal sinuses as, 779-781
closure in, 780
complications after, 780-781
estimating limit of frontal sinus in, 780, 781f
incision for, 779-780, 780f
materials used for, 780
with Paget's disease, 779-780, 780f
postoperative monitoring after, 780-781
removal of all mucosa in, 780
template for, 779-780
Riedel's procedure as, 781-782
indications for, 781-782
postoperative appearance after, 781, 782f
for recurrent infection, 781
Frontal sinus tumors, 1123, 1130
Frontal sinusitis
acute, 775
anatomic variations and, 776
chronic, 775-783
Frontal sinusotomy
balloon catheter, 782-783
in endoscopic sinus surgery, 750-751, 768-771, 776-778
accessing frontal recess in, 777, 777f-778f
agger nasi cell in, 769, 771f-772f
and causes of frontal sinus disease, 769
challenges of, 768
confirming location of instrument in, 777-778, 778f
contrainidications to, 781, 781f
external approaches as adjunct to, 771, 773f
frontal bullar cell in, 772f
frontal recess dissection in, 769, 770b, 770t, 771f
frontal sinus cells in, 769-770, 772f
image-guided navigation system in, 771f
interfrontal sinus septal cell in, 771, 772f
preoperative evaluation for, 768-769
recessus terminalis in, 771
suprabullar cell in, 772f
supraorbital ethmoid cell in, 770-771, 772f
Frontalis muscle, 321f, 433f, 441-442, 444f
Frontobasal meningiomas, embolization of, 1938
Frontoethmoid mucocele, 776f-777f, 783
Frontoethmoid osteoma, 783-784, 784f
Frontoethmoid suture line, in surgical anatomy of anterior cranial base, 2443-2444
Frontoethmoidectomy, craniofacial, 1126, 1126f
Frontofacial monobloc advancement, for craniofacial anomalies, 2653-2654, 2655f-2656f
Frontolateral partial laryngectomy, for glottic cancer, 1517t
Frontolateral vertical hemilaryngectomy, 1548
Frontonasal prominences, in embryology
of lip, 2659-2660, 2661f, 2661t
of nose, 2691f
Fronto-orbital advancement, 2650-2653
bifrontal craniotomy in, 2651-2652, 2651f
for brachycephaly, 2652-2653
closure in, 2653
extent of, 2652-2653, 2653f-2654f
for lambdoid synostosis, 2653
for plagiocephaly, 2652-2653, 2653f
removal of bandeau in, 2651-2652, 2652f
repair of bony defects in, 2653, 2654f
reshaping of bandeau in, 2652, 2652f-2653f
resorbable plates in, 2653
splitting of bandeau in, 2652, 2653f
for trigonocephaly, 2652-2653, 2654f
Frost stitch, 328-329, 329f
Frostbite, 316
Frozen sections, of oropharyngeal cancer, 1366
FSE (fast spin-echo) imaging, 134
FSMB (Federation of State Medical Boards), 80-81, 84t-87t
5-FU. *See* 5-Fluorouracil (5-FU).
FUE (follicular unit extraction), 384
Fugimycin (tacrolimus), for eczematoid otitis externa, 1956
Full denture smile, 2417-2418
Full-thickness skin grafts (FTSGs), for nasal reconstruction, 365
Fully implantable middle ear system, 2027
Function, as outcome measure, 55
Functional Assessment of Cancer Therapy Head and Neck module (FACT-HN), 56
Functional dysphonia, 851
in children, 2879
Functional endoscopic evaluation of swallowing (FEES)
for chronic aspiration, 926
for laryngeal stenosis, 2917
Functional endoscopic sinus surgery (FESS)
abnormal facial growth and development due to, 2623-2625
extent of, 759-760
ostiomeatal complex in, 760, 760f
for pediatric chronic sinusitis, 2779-2781, 2780f-2781f
principles of, 743, 759
radiologic evaluation after, 677-680
expected findings in, 677-679, 679f
operative complications in, 679-680, 680f
Functional hearing loss, evaluation of, 1901
Functional magnetic resonance imaging (fMRI)
for cerebral blood flow evaluation, 2491
of olfaction, 632
Functional matrix hypothesis, of craniofacial growth and development, 2614
Functional Outcomes of Sleep Questionnaire (FOSQ), 57
Functional redundancy, in salivary proteins, 1139
Functional residual capacity, in infants, 2570
Fundamental frequency, 847, 2876
Fundoplication, for extraesophageal reflux, 901
Fungal diseases, 2106
oral manifestations of, 1252
otologic manifestations of, 2106, 2106f
Fungal labyrinthitis, 2160
Fungal laryngitis
acute, 884-885, 884f
chronic, 885
due to blastomycosis, 885
due to coccidioidomycosis, 885

Fungal laryngitis *(Continued)*
due to histoplasmosis, 885
due to paracoccidioidomycosis, 885
Fungal lymphadenopathy, in children, 2818-2819
Fungal otitis externa, 1944-1946, 1945f
otorrhea due to, 2195
topical therapies for, 1954-1955
acidifying agents in, 1954
antifungals in, 1954-1955
ototoxicity of, 1955
antiseptics in, 1955
options for, 1954
Fungal overgrowth, in chronic suppurative otitis media, 2221
Fungal pharyngitis, 199-200
Fungal rhinosinusitis, 709-2
allergic, 707, 712-715
in children, 2778, 2780, 2781f
chronic, 707, 733
classification of, 709
diagnosis of, 707, 712-713
endoscopic sinus surgery for, 761, 762f
epidemiology of, 713-714
imaging of, 706f, 713, 714f
immunochemical staining for, 731, 731f
pathogenesis of, 712-714, 714b
prognosis for, 713
therapy for, 713-715, 715b
chronic, 732-733
allergic, 707
invasive, 711
nonallergic, 715-716, 716t
classification of, 709
fungus balls in, 712, 712f, 714t
in immunocompromised host, 660, 710t
diagnosis of, 220-221, 220f
presentation and pathogenesis of, 220
treatment of, 221
invasive, 705, 709-712
due to *Aspergillus*, 705, 710-711, 712f
in immunocompromised host, 220-221, 220f
due to *Candida*, 711
chronic or indolent, 711
diagnosis of, 711, 711f-712f
due to mucormycosis, 705, 710, 711f
rapidly (fulminant), 709-710, 710f
surgical management of, 742, 761
therapy for, 711-712, 713t
nonallergic eosinophilic, 709, 715-716, 716t
noninvasive, 709
surgical management of, 742, 761
radiologic appearance of, 674-675, 676f
saprophytic, 712
Fungiform papillae, in taste, 1208, 1210, 1212
Fungus balls, of paranasal sinuses, 712, 712f, 714t, 765t
sphenoid, 767, 770f
*N*6-Furfuryladenine (Kinerase), for aging skin, 404
Furlow palatoplasty, 2670
surgical technique for, 2671-2672, 2672f
for velopharyngeal dysfunction, 2682-2683
Furnas suture technique, for otoplasty, 476-477
Furosemide, sensorineural hearing loss due to, 2120, 2175
Furunculosis, of external ear, 1949, 1949f, 2021
Fusiform incisions, for scar revision, 295, 297f
Fusobacterium spp, acute exacerbation of chronic rhinosinusitis due to, 707
F-wave, 2388

G

G protein(s), in salivary gland secretion, 1137
G protein mutations, in thyroid carcinoma, 1752-1753
G protein–coupled receptors
in gustatory transduction, 1208-1209
in olfactory transduction, 629
G1 phase, of cell cycle, 12, 13f
G2 phase, of cell cycle, 12, 13f
GA (genioglossal advancement), for obstructive sleep apnea, 259, 260f
Gabapentin (Neurontin)
for migraine, 2350
for neuropathic pain, 243, 244t
for tinnitus, 2137
GABHS (group A beta hemolytic *Streptococcus pyogenes*), pharyngitis due to, 191-193
in children, 2787
complications of, 2788
Gadolinium enhancement, for MRI, 134-135, 135f-136f
of laryngeal carcinoma, 1470
Gagner, Michel, 39
Gahne, Albert, 1774
Gain
with hearing aids, 2203-2204, 2267-2268
with linear amplification, 2268, 2268f
with nonlinear amplification, 2268, 2268f
target, 2271
vestibuloocular reflex, 2301-2304, 2301f, 2303f
Gait exercises, in vestibular rehabilitation, 2372-2373, 2378-2379
Galanin (GAL), in salivary gland secretion, 1137
Galea aponeurosis, 440
Galectin, in thyroid carcinoma, 1753
Galectin-3, in laryngeal carcinoma, 1505
Gallium-67 citrate scan, for malignant otitis externa, 1947
Gamma Knife radiotherapy, for skull base tumors
benign, 2557, 2558f, 2559t
malignant, 1696
Gamma radiation detection device, for hyperparathyroidism, 1802, 1803f
Gamma rays, 1031-1032
GAN. *See* Greater auricular nerve (GAN).
Ganglioneuroma, 151f
Gap junction(s), 2090f
in endolymph homeostasis, 2081-2083, 2083f-2084f
Gap junction membrane channel protein β1 *(GJB1)* gene, in deafness, 2051t-2058t
Gap junction membrane channel protein β2 *(GJB2)* gene
in deafness, 2051t-2058t, 2083, 2089-2090, 2097
genetic testing for, 2097-2098, 2235
of infants, 2723
Gap junction membrane channel protein β3 *(GJB3)* gene, in deafness, 2051t-2058t, 2083
Gap junction membrane channel protein β6 *(GJB6)* gene
in deafness, 2051t-2058t, 2083
genetic testing for, 2235
Garamycin Ophthalmic (gentamicin), for otitis externa, 1952, 1959t-1960t
Gardasil (human papillomavirus vaccine), 2886-2887, 2890t
Gardner-Robertson scale, for hearing outcomes, after stereotactic irradiation of vestibular schwannoma, 2562, 2562t
Gasserian ganglion, in surgical anatomy of lateral skull base, 2437f, 2438, 2440f
Gastric outlet obstruction, due to caustic ingestion, 2961
Gastric pull-up, for hypopharyngeal and esophageal reconstruction, 1432, 1432f, 1453
Gastric transposition, for hypopharyngeal and esophageal reconstruction, 1432, 1432f, 1453
Gastroesophageal endoscopy, 956-957
equipment for, 956
of esophageal varices, 958f
for extraesophageal reflux, 899
of gastroesophageal junction
Gastroesophageal endoscopy *(Continued)*
with Mallory-Weiss tear, 957f
normal, 956-957, 957f
with severe esophagitis, 957f
of squamocolumnar junction, 956-957, 956f-957f
technique of, 956-957
Gastroesophageal junction (GEJ)
with Barrett's esophagus, 957f
with hiatal hernia, 957f
with Mallory-Weiss tear, 957f
normal anatomy of, 956-957, 957f
with severe esophagitis, 957f
Gastroesophageal reflux (GER)
defined, 2944-2945
physiologic or "functional," 2944
Gastroesophageal reflux disease (GERD), 894-903, 968-973
and airway obstruction, 2905-2906
classification of erosive esophagitis in, 969, 969f
defined, 894, 968, 2944-2945
diagnostic evaluation of, 896-900, 968-969
esophageal endoscopy in, 899, 969, 969f
esophagogram in, 898
history in, 896, 896b-897b
impedance testing in, 900
laryngeal sensory testing in, 898-899
manometry in, 899-900
pH probe monitoring in, 900
physical examination and laryngeal endoscopy in, 896-897, 897t, 898b
voice analysis in, 898
dysphagia due to, 2953
epidemiology of, 894
and esophageal adenocarcinoma, 899
esophageal pH monitoring for
ambulatory 24-hour, 958-960, 959f-960f
Bravo wireless pH capsule for, 961, 961f
multichannel intraluminal impedance for, 962
Restech Dx-pH Measurement System for, 962, 962f
extraeophageal (*See* Extraesophageal reflux (EER))
and head and neck cancer, 902-903
laryngeal stenosis due to, 2915, 2917
and laryngomalacia, 2867
nonerosive, 968
and obstructive sleep apnea, 253
oral manifestations of, 1254
otitis media in, 2765
otolaryngologic disorders associated with, 901-903
chronic laryngitis as, 901-902
contact ulcer and laryngeal granuloma as, 902, 902f-903f
pathophysiology of, 894-896, 968
epithelial resistance factors in, 895-896
esophageal acid clearance in, 895
lower esophageal sphincter in, 895, 895b
mechanisms of symptoms in, 896
upper esophageal sphincter in, 894-895
and pediatric chronic sinusitis, 2778-2779
professional voice disorders due to, 852
reflux esophagitis in, 968
and squamous cell carcinoma of larynx, 1491-1492, 1513
symptoms of, 968
treatment of, 900-901, 969-970
behavioral modification for, 900-901
bethanechol for, 901
H_2 blockers for, 901
over-the-counter antacids for, 901
promotility agents for, 901
proton pump inhibitors for, 901
sucralfate for, 901
surgical, 901
and vocal fold granuloma, 2881

Gastroesophageal reflux disease (GERD)-related laryngeal disease, in children, 2944-2947
  diagnosis of, 2945
  disorders due to, 2945-2946, 2945b
  evidence of, 2946
  history of, 2944
  management of, 2946
  physiopathology of, 2945
Gastrografin swallow, for penetrating neck trauma, 1633
Gastrointestinal disorders
  in hyperparathyroidism, 1781
  oral manifestations of, 1254
Gastrolaryngopharyngeal reflux (GLPR), and laryngeal stenosis, 2917
Gastro-omental flap, for hypopharyngeal and esophageal reconstruction, 1457-1458, 1457f
GATA3, in deafness, 2051t-2058t
Gaucher's disease, oral manifestations of, 1257
Gaze shift, cancellation of vestibulo-ocular reflex in, 2300-2301
Gaze stabilization
  medial vestibulospinal tract in, 1865
  vestibular system in maintaining, 2276-2277
    anatomic and physiologic basis for, 2276-2277
    clinical importance of, 2277
GBI (Glasgow Benefit Inventory), after stereotactic irradiation of vestibular schwannoma, 2564
GBLC (geometric broken line closure), for scar revision, 298, 299f-300f
G-CSF (granulocyte colony-stimulating factor), 604, 609t-610t
GCT (giant cell tumor)
  of larynx, 1510
  malignant, of neck, 1671
  of petrous apex, 2526
GDNF (glial cell–derived neurotrophic factor)
  for facial nerve paralysis, 2427
  in gene therapy of inner ear, 2192
  for prevention of ototoxicity, 2189-2191
GDTF (Guidelines Development Task Force), 89
Gehanno method
  for palatal reconstruction, 1382
  for tonsillar and pharyngeal wall reconstruction, 1386, 1387f
GEJ. *See* Gastroesophageal junction (GEJ).
Gelclair, for mucositis, 1102
Gelfilm, for tympanoplasty, 2000-2001, 2003
Gelfoam
  for embolization, 1933
  in intratympanic delivery, 2182
  for tympanoplasty, 2000-2001, 2003, 2004f
Gender
  and olfactory testing, 633
  and otitis media, 2766
Gene(s), 3
  defined, 4
  liability, 8
  replacing defective, 13
  structure of, 4, 5f
  suicide, 16, 21
Gene expression, 4, 5f, 11-12, 12f
  enhancing, 13
  site-specific, 20
  suppressing, 13, 14f
  therapeutic levels of, 19-20
"Gene gun," 15
Gene mapping, 3
Gene silencing
  direct delivery of RNA for, 16
  RNA interference for, 13, 14f
  therapeutic, 23-24
Gene therapy, 12-15
  advantages of, 20
  applications of, 20-24
Gene therapy *(Continued)*
    for head and neck oncology, 20-22, 21f
      antiangiogenesis in, 22
      conditionally replicating adenovirus therapy in, 22
      cytotoxic or suicide gene therapy strategies in, 21
      direct in vivo stimulation of antitumor immune response in, 21
      genetic modification of tumor-infiltrating lymphocytes in, 20-21
      modifying oncogenes and tumor suppressor genes in, 21-22
    for inherited disease, 20
    for laryngology, 23
    for otology/neurotology, 23
    for plastic and reconstructive surgery, 22-23
      with reconstructive tissue flaps and wound healing, 22-23
      with skin grafting, 23
    for repair and regeneration of irradiated tissue, 23
  basic principle of, 12-13
  enhancing gene expression in, 13
  future of, 23-24
  of inner ear, 2191-2192
    delivery of, 2191
    preclinical applications of, 2192
    safety concerns with, 2192
    vectors for, 2191, 2191t
  methods of delivering, 15-20, 19f
    direct injection of genetic material as, 15-16, 19f
      direct delivery of RNA for gene silencing in, 16
      DNA-mediated transfer of therapeutic genes in, 15-16, 15f
    viral-mediated gene transfer as, 16-18, 18t, 19f
      via adeno-associated virus, 18, 18t
      via adenoviruses, 17-18, 17f, 18t
      via retroviruses, 16, 17f, 18t
  permanent *vs.* temporary, 14-15
  replacing defective genes in, 13
  somatic *vs.* germ cell, 14, 15f
  strategies for administering, 18-19, 19f
    ex vivo, 18, 19f
    in vivo, 18-19, 19f
  suppressing gene expression in, 13, 14f
  therapeutic gene silencing in, 23-24
  therapeutic levels of gene expression in, 19-20
Gene transfer
  DNA-mediated, 15-16, 15f
  viral-mediated, 16-18, 18t, 19f
    via adeno-associated virus, 18, 18t
    via adenoviruses, 17-18, 17f, 18t
    via retroviruses, 16, 17f, 18t
General appearance
  physical examination of, 95
  in voice evaluation, 827
Generalizability, 68-69, 68t, 69f
Generic scales, as outcome measures, 55-56, 56t
Genetic alterations, in head and neck squamous cell carcinoma, 1019-1020
  cytogenetic, 1019
  microsatellites as, 1019
  in oncogenes, 1016, 1019-1020
  single nucleotide polymorphisms as, 1019
  in tumor suppressor genes, 1016, 1020
    and Fanconi's anemia, 1020
Genetic code, 4
Genetic disorders, 4
  chromosomal, 4-5
    aneuploidies as, 4-5
    rearrangements as, 4-5
  oligogenic, 4, 8
    with complex traits, 8
    genetic heterogeneity and, 8
Genetic disorders *(Continued)*
    mitochondrial, 8, 9f
    sporadic cases of, 8
    with X-linkage, 8, 8f
  single-gene, 4, 6
    dominant, 6, 6f
    penetrance and expressivity of, 7, 7f
    recessive, 6-7, 7f
Genetic distance, 3
Genetic factors
  in nasopharyngeal carcinoma, 1352
  presbycusis due to, 233
  in salivary gland neoplasms, 1164
Genetic heterogeneity, 8
Genetic predisposition, to otitis media, 2766-2767
Genetic preprogrammed theory, of craniofacial growth and development, 2614
Genetic progression model, of head and neck squamous cell carcinoma, 1016
Genetic susceptibility, to laryngeal cancer, 1492, 1513
Genetic testing
  for cochlear implants, 2235
  for sensorineural hearing loss, 2098
    in infants, 2722-2723
Genetically determined disease, otologic manifestations of, 2115
Genetics, 3-10
  chromosomal disorders in, 4-5
    aneuploidies as, 4-5
    rearrangements as, 4-5
  DNA structure and genetic code in, 4
  ethical issues in, 9-10
  fundamentals of, 2088
  gene structure and expression in, 4, 5f
  genome in, 9
  historical background of, 2088
  inheritance patterns in, 2088-2089, 2088f
    autosomal dominant, 2088, 2088f
    autosomal recessive, 2088-2089
    mitochondrial, 2089
    molecular basis of, 4
    Punnett squares for, 2088, 2089f
    X-linked, 2089
  oligogenic disorders in, 4, 8
    with complex traits, 8
    genetic heterogeneity and, 8
    mitochondrial, 8, 9f
    sporadic cases of, 8
    with X-linkage, 8, 8f
  single-gene disorders in, 4, 6
    dominant, 6, 6f
    penetrance and expressivity of, 7, 7f
    recessive, 6-7, 7f
  testing human DNA in, 8-9
    DNA chips for, 9
    mutation testing for, 9, 10f
    nucleic acid hybridization and Southern blotting for, 9
    polymerase chain reaction for, 8-9
  utility in otolaryngology of molecular, 10
Geniculate fossa, 1826f, 1828
Geniculate ganglion
  anatomy of, 1826f, 1827-1828
    surgical, 2404f
  surgical, in lateral skull base, 2436f-2437f, 2438
  vulnerability to injury of, 1829
Genioglossal advancement (GA), for obstructive sleep apnea, 259, 260f
Genioglossus (GG) muscle
  anatomy of, 1296f, 1297
  in breathing, 810, 810f
Geniohyoid muscle, anatomy of, 1296f, 1320
Genioplasty, osseous, 465, 467-470
  anesthesia for, 467
  clinical examples of, 470, 472f-473f
  complications after, 470

Genioplasty, osseous *(Continued)*
fixation in, 468-470, 470f
gingivolabial incision for, 467, 468f
inscription of bony midline in, 467-468, 469f
lateral extent of, 468, 469f
measurement of osteotomy site in, 467-468, 469f
subperiosteal dissection in, 467, 468f
three-dimensional movement of chin in, 468
vertical lengthening in, 468-470, 469f
vertical shortening in, 468-470, 470f
wound closure in, 470
Genome, 3-4
Gentamicin
intratympanic, 2185-2189
clinical protocols for, 2187-2188
complications of, 2188-2189
concentration of, 2188
dose of, 2188
indications and contraindications for, 2189
injection interval for, 2188
mechanism of action of, 2185-2186
for Meniere's disease, 2185-2189, 2338-2339, 2338f
number of injections of, 2188
pharmacokinetics of, 2186-2187, 2186f-2187f
practical considerations with, 2188
for rhinosinusitis, 734
vestibulotoxicity of, 2344
Gentamicin ophthalmic (Garamycin Ophthalmic), for otitis externa, 1952, 1959t-1960t
Gentian violet, for fungal otitis externa, 1955, 1959t-1960t
Geometric broken line closure (GBLC), for scar revision, 298, 299f-300f
GER (gastroesophageal reflux)
defined, 2944-2945
physiologic or "functional," 2944
GERD. *See* Gastroesophageal reflux disease (GERD).
Geriatric patients, 230-238
access to medical care by, 231
aging skin in (*See* Aging skin)
basic principles of care for, 230-231
cochlear implants in, 233, 2241
and quality of life, 2251-2252, 2252f, 2252t
demographics of, 230
diagnostic testing for, 231
ear disorders in, 231-234
presbycusis as, 232
etiologies of, 232
treatment of, 233
types of, 232
presbystasis as, 233-234
diagnostic methods for, 233
treatment of, 234
vestibular pathology of, 233
end-of-life care for, 231
facial trauma in, 237
falls in, 233
head and neck oncology in, 237
etiology of, 237
treatment of, 237-238
hearing aids in, 2274
nose in, 234
changes in appearance of, 234
common symptoms of disorders of, 234
intranasal examination of, 234
mucoepithelial changes of, 234
olfactory changes of, 234
treatment of disorders of, 234
olfactory loss in, 635, 635f
olfactory testing in, 632-633
otitis media in, 1872
postoperative pain in, 240-241
preoperative evaluation of, 106-107
Geriatric patients *(Continued)*
presbyphagia in, 237
diagnostic testing for, 237
treatment of, 237
presbyphonia in, 234-237
acoustic changes in, 236
dental/mandibular changes in, 236
factors affecting vocal quality in, 234, 235t
glandular changes in, 236
histologic changes in, 234-235, 235f
laryngoscopic appearance in, 235-236
mucosal changes in, 236
respiratory changes in, 236
and sense of taste, 236
treatment of, 236-237
rhinosinusitis in, 737
salivary gland dysfunction in, 1141-1142, 1141f
treatment of, 231
medical, 231
surgical, 231
Germ cell gene therapy, 14, 15f
Gfi1 (growth factor–independent 1) gene, in murine deafness, 2058t-2060t
GG (genioglossus) muscle
anatomy of, 1296f, 1297
in breathing, 810, 810f
Ghost cell(s), in calcifying odontogenic cyst, 1269, 1269f
Ghost cell tumor, epithelial odontogenic (dentinogenic), 1275-1276
Giant cell tumor (GCT)
of larynx, 1510
malignant, of neck, 1671
of petrous apex, 2526
Gianturco-Z stents, 1009
Gingiva, anatomy of, 1295f
Gingival cyst
of adult, 1266
clinical features of, 1266
radiographic features of, 1266
of newborn, 1266, 1266f
microscopic features of, 1266
treatment of, 1266
Gingival melanoma, 1242f
Gingivitis
in HIV, 227
pregnancy, 1256
Gingivolabial sulcus approach, for pediatric facial fracture, 2701-2702, 2703f
Gingivostomatitis, herpetic, 1235, 1235f
GJB1 (gap junction membrane channel protein β1) gene, in deafness, 2051t-2058t
GJB2 (gap junction membrane channel protein β2) gene
in deafness, 2051t-2058t, 2083, 2089-2090, 2097
genetic testing for, 2097-2098, 2235
of infants, 2723
GJB3 (gap junction membrane channel protein β3) gene, in deafness, 2051t-2058t, 2083
GJB6 (gap junction membrane channel protein β6) gene
in deafness, 2051t-2058t, 2083
genetic testing for, 2235
Glabella, 319, 320f, 509f
Glabellar flaps, for nasal defects, 365-366
Glandular odontogenic cyst, 1267
clinical features of, 1267
microscopic features of, 1267, 1267f
radiographic features of, 1267
treatment of, 1267
Glasgow Benefit Inventory (GBI), after stereotactic irradiation of vestibular schwannoma, 2564
Glasgow Children's Benefit Inventory, 57
GLAST (glutamate-aspartate transporter), 2081
Glenoid fossa
anatomy of, 1822f, 1824f
in surgical anatomy of lateral skull base, 2435f
Glial cell–derived neurotrophic factor (GDNF)
for facial nerve paralysis, 2427
in gene therapy of inner ear, 2192
for prevention of ototoxicity, 2189-2191
Glioma(s)
brainstem
intra-axial, 2528
vestibular symptoms of, 2353
of cerebellum, vestibular symptoms of, 2354
nasal, 2688
vs. encephaloceles, 2688
epidemiology of, 2688
extranasal, 2688
histology of, 2688
imaging of, 2688
intranasal, 2688
management of, 2688
sinonasal, 718t
Glissades, 2308, 2313
Globe, anatomy and physiology of, 319, 321f
Globus, 956
Glogau classification, of photoaging skin, 391, 391t
Glomerulonephritis, poststreptococcal, 2788
Glomus jugulare, 1657
Glomus jugulare tumors, 1934-1935, 1935f
of cerebellopontine angle, 2523f-2524f
endovascular treatment of, 1935-1936, 1936f
paragangliomas as, 2505, 2506f
surgical approach to, 2506, 2507f
stereotactic radiation therapy for, 2565, 2565t
Glomus tumor(s), 1657. *See also* Paragangliomas (PGLs).
of cerebellopontine angle, 2522-2523, 2523f-2524f
of skull base, 171, 174f
Glomus tympanicum, 1657
imaging of, 1919-1920, 1921f
Glomus tympanicum tumors, 1934-1935
endovascular treatment of, 1935
paraganglioma as, 2505-2506
Glomus vagale, 151, 152f
Glomus vagale tumors, 1934-1935, 1935f
endovascular treatment of, 1935f-1936f, 1936-1937
paragangliomas as, 2506f
Glossectomy
laser midline, for obstructive sleep apnea, 259
total or subtotal, tongue base reconstruction after, 1389-1390
innervated free latissimus dorsi musculocutaneous flap for, 1389-1390, 1390f
microvascular reconstruction as, 1390
money pouch–like method for, 1390, 1390f
sensate fasciocutaneous flaps for, 1390-1391
Glossopharyngeal nerve
intraoperative monitoring of, 2550-2552, 2551f
in surgical anatomy
of internal auditory canal, 2437f
of jugular foramen, 2440, 2440f
of lateral skull base, 2436f, 2438
of posterior fossa, 2439f
Glossopharyngeal nerve block, for neuropathic pain, 246t
Glossopharyngeal schwannoma, 2507f
Glossoptosis, in Robin sequence, 2673
Glossotomy, median labiomandibular, for hypopharyngeal cancer, 1429
Glottal closure, laryngeal videostroboscopy of, 819, 820f, 848t, 849
Glottal flow, 818
Glottic cancer
advanced-stage, radiation therapy for, 1497, 1583-1588
balancing cure, organ preservation, and quality of life with, 1583-1584
with chemotherapy, 1584-1586, 1584t

Glottic cancer *(Continued)*
complications of, 1587-1588
dose-fractionation schemes for, 1586, 1586t
general principles of, 1585-1586
mini-mantle field technique for, 1586
outcomes and prognostic factors for, 1586-1587, 1587t
patient setup for, 1586
postoperative (adjuvant), 1584-1585, 1584t
shrinking-field technique for, 1586, 1587f
with targeted biologic agents, 1585
anatomic basis for, 1483-1484, 1483f, 1483t, 1543-1544
cervical metastases of, 1494
chemoradiation for
in advanced stage, 1584-1586, 1584t
with nodal metastases, 1498
optimal dose-fractionation scheme for, 1585-1586
outcomes and prognostic factors with, 1586-1587, 1587t
clinical evaluation of, 1545
clinical presentation of, 1493, 1579
conservation laryngeal surgery for, 1496, 1547-1549
epiglottic laryngoplasty as, 1549
complications of, 1549
extended procedures for, 1549
functional outcome of, 1549
key surgical points for, 1549
oncologic results of, 1549
surgical technique for, 1549, 1549f
horizontal partial laryngectomies as, 1549
spectrum of, 1557-1560
supracricoid partial laryngectomy with cricohyoido-epiglottopexy as, 1549-1550
complications of, 1551
extended procedures for, 1551
functional outcome of, 1551, 1551t-1552t
key surgical points for, 1550-1551
oncologic results of, 1549-1550
surgical technique for, 1550, 1550f-1551f
vertical hemilaryngectomy as, 1547-1549
complications of, 1549
extended, 1548
frontolateral, 1548
functional outcome of, 1548
with imbrication laryngoplasty, 1548, 1548f
key surgical points for, 1549
oncologic results of, 1547-1548, 1547t-1548t
posterolateral, 1548
surgical technique for, 1548
vertical partial laryngectomy as, 1547
early-stage, 1512-1524
biopsy of, 1518
chest x-ray of, 1516
defined, 1515
diagnosis of, 1515-1517, 1516f
endoscopic imaging of, 1515-1516, 1516f
MRI and CT of, 1516-1517
PET of, 1517
radiation therapy for, 1519-1520, 1581
complications of, 1583
local control with, 1519, 1522f
outcome and prognostic factors for, 1581-1583, 1582t-1583t
recurrence after, 1520, 1522t
results of, 1519, 1521t
techniques and dose-fractionation schemes for, 1580-1590, 1581f-1582f
epidemiology of, 1512, 1513f
imaging of, 1474-1475, 1474f, 1691f
with impaired vocal cord mobility, 1496
neck dissection for, 1497-1498
radiation therapy for

Glottic cancer *(Continued)*
with advanced-stage disease, 1497, 1583-1588
balancing cure, organ preservation, and quality of life with, 1583-1584
with chemotherapy, 1584-1586, 1584t
complications of, 1587-1588
dose-fractionation schemes for, 1586, 1586t
general principles of, 1585-1586
mini-mantle field technique for, 1586
outcomes and prognostic factors for, 1586-1587, 1587t
patient setup for, 1586
postoperative (adjuvant), 1584-1585, 1584t
shrinking-field technique for, 1586, 1587f
with targeted biologic agents, 1585
with early-stage disease, 1519-1520, 1581
complications of, 1583
effectiveness of, 1496
local control with, 1519, 1522f
outcome and prognostic factors for, 1581-1583, 1582t-1583t
recurrence after, 1520, 1522t
results of, 1519, 1521t
techniques and dose-fractionation schemes for, 1580-1590, 1581f-1582f
recurrence of, 1521t-1522t, 1522-1523
staging of, 1513-1515
direct laryngoscopy for, 1579-1580, 1580f
stage grouping in, 1515, 1515t
T staging in, 1486, 1488t, 1515t
survival with, 1512, 1514f, 1523
treatment of, 1496-1498, 1517-1520
in advanced stage, 1497
algorithm for, 1588f
with anterior commissure involvement, 1496-1497
for carcinoma in situ, 1520-1521
chemotherapy for, 1520
choice of, 1521-1524
in early stage, 1496
endoscopic excision as, 1518, 1520f
for invasive carcinoma, 1521-1524, 1523t
with nodal metastases, 1497-1498
surgical, 1517-1518, 1517t, 1518f, 1519t
transoral laser microsurgery for, 1531
voice considerations in, 1518-1519
Glottic closure, for chronic aspiration, 929-931, 931f
Glottic lacerations, 1634
Glottic stenosis. *See also* Laryngeal stenosis.
anterior, 948
in children, 2915, 2922
management of, 2922
complete, 949-950
posterior, 948-949, 949f
in children, 2915, 2915f, 2922-2923
management of, 2922-2923
vocal quality with, 2880, 2915
Glottic sulcus, 870-872, 871f
diagnosis of, 870-871
history in, 870
laryngeal examination in, 870-871
vocal capability battery in, 870
epidemiology of, 870
management of, 871-872
behavioral, 871
medical, 871
surgical, 871-872, 872f
mucosal bridge due to, 870, 871f
pathophysiology and pathology of, 869-870
with polypoid nodule, 871f
Glottis, 99, 99f
anatomy of, 1483-1484, 1483f, 1483t, 1578
cartilaginous, 849
embryology of, 1482-1483
physical examination of, 100
during swallowing, 833

Glottis respiratoria, 1464
Glottis vocalis, 1464
Glottography, for voice evaluation, 830, 835
GLPR (gastrolaryngopharyngeal reflux), and laryngeal stenosis, 2917
Glucocorticoids
for allergic rhinitis, 621
for croup, 2805-2806
for otitis media with effusion, 2772
for rhinosinusitis
oral, 734t
topical, 734t, 736
for thyroid storm, 1745
for Wegener's granulomatosis, 658
Glucose, in CSF rhinorrhea, 789, 2044
Glutamate-aspartate transporter (GLAST), 2081
Glutathione *S*-transferase (GST)
in head and neck squamous cell carcinoma, 1016-1017
in oral cancer, 1295
Gluten-sensitive enteropathy, oral manifestations of, 1254
Glycolic acid, for chemical peels, 393
Glycoproteins, in saliva, 1140
Glycopyrrolate, for pediatric premedication, 2589
GM-CSF (granulocyte-macrophage colony-stimulating factor), 604, 609t-610t
Goiter(s)
compression of pharynx and esophagus due to, 1409, 1409f
endemic, 1747
intrathoracic, 1766
tobacco smoke and, 1807
toxic
multinodular, 1744-1745
uninodular, 1744
Gold dust, for ear hygiene or chronic ear drainage, 1958
Gold weights, for lagophthalmos, 2421
Gomphosis joint, 1260
Gonococcal pharyngitis, 193-194
in children, 2786
Gonorrhea, oral manifestations of, 1252
Gonzalez-Ulloa and Stevens analysis, for mentoplasty, 464f
Gore-Tex (fibrillated ePTFE), for chin implants, 465t
Gore-Tex (polytetrafluoroethylene) implant, for saddle nose deformity, 555, 558f
Gore-Tex (polytetrafluoroethylene) strip, for medialization thyroplasty, 908, 910, 911f
Gorlin cyst, 1268-1269
microscopic features of, 1269, 1269f
radiographic features of, 1269
treatment of, 1269
Gorlin syndrome, 1268
treatment of, 1268
Gorlin-Goltz syndrome, 1268
treatment of, 1268
Gout, 2113-2114
otologic manifestations of, 2113-2114
GPR98, in deafness, 2051t-2058t
Grab sample, 68, 69t
Grade(s)
of recommendation, 69-70, 70t
in voice evaluation, 827t
Gradenigo's syndrome, 1829, 1975, 1987
Gradient echo techniques, for MRI, 136-137, 137f
Graft(s)
for airway stenosis
epidermal, 947
epithelial, 947
skin, 946-947
alar batten, 550, 551f
in revision rhinoplasty, 586-587, 587f

Graft(s) *(Continued)*
allo-
for craniofacial defect repair, 2657
for ossiculoplasty, 2006
auto-
for craniofacial defect repair, 2657
for ossiculoplasty, 2006, 2025
autogenous cartilage
for laryngeal stenosis, 2919-2920, 2920f
for nasal reconstruction, 368-369, 369f-370f
in noncaucasian rhinoplasty, 569, 570f
complications of, 578, 579f
bone
in cleft-lip nose repair, 559, 564f
for nasal fractures, 505, 505f
for nasal reconstruction, 369, 370f
buttress
in nasal tip refinement, 576
in revision rhinoplasty, 589
cap
for nasal tip enhancement, 576, 577f
in revision rhinoplasty, 589
cartilage
for nasal reconstruction, 368-369, 369f-370f
for nasal tip projection, 535-536, 537f, 549-550, 550f-551f
for revision rhinoplasty, 583, 584f
for saddle nose deformity, 555, 556f
cartilage plumping, for nasal tip projection, 535-536, 536f
caudal extension
in noncaucasian rhinoplasty, 576, 576f
in revision rhinoplasty, 593
costal cartilage
for laryngeal stenosis, 2919-2920, 2920f
for noncaucasian rhinoplasty, 569, 570f
harvesting of, 570, 571f
results of, 568
for revision rhinoplasty, 583, 584f
for CSF rhinorrhea, 792-794, 793f
in endoscopic treatment of stridulous child, 2909
facial nerve, 2421-2425
cross-face, 2419, 2424-2425
selection of donor nerve for, 2422
surgical planning for, 2421-2424
surgical technique for, 2422-2424, 2424f-2425f
in follicular-unit hair transplantation, 383, 383f
micro-, 378, 379f-381f
free cartilage
for full-thickness alar defects, 348
for nasal defects, 348
full-thickness skin, for nasal reconstruction, 365
homo-
for craniofacial defect repair, 2657
for nasal reconstruction, 368
for ossiculoplasty, 2006, 2025, 2026t
jejunal interposition, after laryngopharyngectomy, 1418, 1418f
for laryngeal stenosis
in children, 2919
skin and mucosal, 946-947
in noncaucasian rhinoplasty
autogenous cartilage, 569, 570f
complications of, 578, 579f
caudal extension, 576, 576f
conchal cartilage, 569, 570f
harvesting of, 570, 571f
results of, 568
septal cartilage, 569
in revision rhinoplasty
alar batten, 586-587, 587f
alar rim, 587, 588f-589f
buttress, 589
cap, 589
ear cartilage, 583
lateral crural, 589-590, 590f

Graft(s) *(Continued)*
septal cartilage, 583
shield, 589, 590f
septal cartilage
in noncaucasian rhinoplasty, 569
for revision rhinoplasty, 583
shield
for nasal tip enhancement, 576, 577f
in revision rhinoplasty, 589, 590f
skin
for airway stenosis, 946-947
for burns, 315
gene therapy with, 23
for nasal reconstruction, 365
for oropharyngeal reconstruction, 1376
of tongue base, 1388
of tonsil and pharyngeal wall, 1384
for pharyngeal wall reconstruction, 1384
in prosthetic maxillary obturation, 1338-1339
for tongue base reconstruction, 1388
for tonsillar reconstruction, 1384
skin and mucosal
for airway stenosis, 946-947
for laryngotracheal stenosis, 946-947
split-thickness skin, in atresiaplasty
creation of, 2756, 2756f
placement of, 2756, 2757f-2758f
suturing of, 2756-2757, 2758f
spreader
for middle vault deformities, 585-586
for saddle nose deformity, 555, 559f
for septal and alar asymmetries, 550, 551f
in septoplasty, 490-491, 491f
for twisted nose, 554, 555f
synthetic hair, 387-388
temporalis fascia
in atresiaplasty, 2755f, 2756, 2757f
for medialization thyroplasty, 910
for saddle nose deformity, 555, 557f
for tympanoplasty, 2000
thyroid alar cartilage, for laryngeal stenosis, 2919, 2921f
in tympanoplasty
lateral, 2002-2003, 2002f
medial, 2003, 2004f
xeno-, for craniofacial defect repair, 2657
Grafting materials, for nasal skeletal reconstruction
alloplastic, 368
autogenous cartilage as, 368-369, 369f-370f
bone as, 369, 370f
homograft tissues as, 368
selection of, 367-368
Graft-versus-host disease (GVHD), chronic, and xerostomia, 218
Grainyhead-like 2 *(GRHL2)* gene, in deafness, 2051t-2058t
Granular cell(s), of olfactory bulb, 628f
Granular cell tumor
of larynx, 882
of oral cavity, 1290, 1290f
of trachea, 1612
Granular myringitis, 1955
otorrhea due to, 2196
Granular otitis externa, 1945
Granulation tissue, formation of, 1077-1078
angiogenesis in, 1077-1078
dermal matrix in, 1077
Granulocyte colony-stimulating factor (G-CSF), 604, 609t-610t
Granulocyte-macrophage colony-stimulating factor (GM-CSF), 604, 609t-610t
Granulocytic sarcoma, 2107
Granuloma(s)
cholesterol
vs. cholesteatoma, 2508, 2510f
of petrous apex, 2524-2525

Granuloma(s) *(Continued)*
differential diagnosis of, 1924t, 2515, 2524t
imaging of, 1923, 1925f-1926f, 2477f, 2526f
of skull base, 171, 172f
transmastoid infralabyrinthine drainage of, 2540f
contact, of vocal folds, 874-875, 874f
diagnosis of, 875
epidemiology of, 874
due to extraesophageal reflux, 902, 902f-903f
management of, 875
pathophysiology and pathology of, 874
eosinophilic, 2100
of oral cavity, 1240, 1257
clinical features of, 1240, 1240f
defined, 1240
differential diagnosis of, 1240
etiology of, 1240
histopathologic features of, 1240, 1240f
traumatic, 1240
treatment of, 1240
otologic manifestations of, 2101f-2102f
otorrhea as, 2196
postintubation, 939, 941f
of vocal folds, 875-876, 875f
diagnosis of, 875-876
epidemiology of, 875
management of, 876
pathophysiology and pathology of, 875
postoperative reparative, after small fenestra stapedotomy, 2034
pyogenic, 290
of oral cavity, 1256, 1289, 1289f
of pregnancy, 1256
on septum, 685f
vocal fold, 2881, 2881f
Granulomatosis, Wegener's. *See* Wegener's granulomatosis (WG).
Granulomatous disease
nasal manifestations of, 657-659
in Churg-Strauss syndrome, 659
in sarcoidosis, 658-659
in Wegener's granulomatosis, 658
neck masses due to, 1638
oral manifestations of, 1251-1252
otologic manifestations of, 2100-2106
in Langerhans' cell histiocytosis, 2100-2101, 2101f-2102f
otorrhea as, 2196
in sarcoidosis, 2104-2105, 2104f
in tuberculosis, 2101-2103, 2102f-2103f
in Wegener's granulomatosis, 2103-2104, 2103f-2104f
of salivary gland, in children, mycobacterial, 2857-2858, 2857f
of salivary glands, 1158-1159
due to actinomycosis, 1159
in children, 2858
due to cat scratch disease, 1159
in children, 2857-2858
due to actinomycosis, 2858
due to sarcoidosis, 2858
mycobacterial
in children, 2857-2858, 2857f
nontuberculous, 1158-1159, 1158f
tuberculous, 1158
due to toxoplasmosis, 1159-1160
Granulomatous esophagitis, 1405
Granulomatous rhinitis, 619b
Granulomatous rhinosinusitis, 675
Graves' disease, 1742-1743
clinical manifestations of, 1742
epidemiology of, 1742
historical background of, 1806
natural history of, 1742
oral manifestations of, 1251
pathology of, 1742

Graves' disease *(Continued)*
pathophysiology of, 1806
and thyroid cancer, 1742
thyroid-stimulating antibody in, 1741
treatment of
pharmacologic
β-blockers for, 1743
cholestyramine for, 1742-1743
inorganic iodine for, 1742-1743
lithium carbonate for, 1742-1743
methimazole for, 1742
propylthiouracil for, 1742
radioactive iodine for, 1743
surgical
indications for, 1743
near-total thyroidectomy for, 1743
postoperative problems after, 1743
preoperative preparation for, 1743
subtotal thyroidectomy for, 1743
Graves' ophthalmopathy, 1806-1818
ancillary procedure(s) for, 1816-1817
extraocular muscle surgery as, 1816-1817
eyelid surgery as, 1817
classification of, 1808, 1808t-1809t
clinical evaluation of, 1809-1810
eye evaluation in, 1809
imaging studies in, 1809-1810, 1811f
thyroid function in, 1809
clinical features of, 1808-1817
differential diagnosis of, 1809-1810, 1810t
epidemiology and etiology of, 1807
eye findings in, 1808-1809, 1809t
genetic predisposition to, 1807
medical therapy for, 1810-1811
local therapy in, 1810
steroid therapy in, 1811
thyroid therapy in, 1810
natural history of, 1807
orbital decompression for, 1811-1816
approaches to, 1811, 1812f
balanced, 1814
without bone removal, 1816
combined endoscopic and open approach to, 1814
combined endoscopic orbital and optic nerve, 1815
endoscopic, 1814, 1815f-1816f
goal of, 1811
indications for, 1811
results of, 1811-1812
three-wall, 1815-1816
transantral, 1812-1814
complications of, 1814
modifications of, 1814
outcome of, 1812-1814, 1813f-1814f
technique for, 1812, 1812f-1813f
two-wall, 1816
pathophysiology of, 1806-1807
pretibial myxedema and, 1808
radiotherapy for, 1811
risk factor(s) for
gender as, 1807
thyroid status as, 1807
tobacco as, 1807
team approach to management of, 1810-1817
thyroid disease and, 1807
Gray (Gy), 132-133, 1033
GRBAS scale, for voice assessment, 826, 827t
Great auricular nerve (GAN)
anatomy of, 2578, 2580f
for facial nerve grafting, 2422
in parotidectomy, 1177, 1195
Great auricular nerve (GAN) injury, due to neck surgery, 1731
Greater palatal nerve, 483f
Greater palatine artery, 682, 1295-1296
Greater palatine foramen, 1297f
Greater palatine nerve, 1297f
Greater superficial petrosal nerve (GSPN)
groove for, 1822f
surgical anatomy of, 2404f
in lateral skull base, 2437f, 2438
in middle cranial base, 2444
vulnerability to injury of, 1829
Greater wing of sphenoid bone
in surgical anatomy of lateral skull base, 2434, 2435f
in surgical anatomy of middle cranial base, 2444, 2445f
Greater zygomatic muscle, reinnervation of, 2423f
GRHL2 (grainyhead-like 2) gene, in deafness, 2051t-2058t
Grieg's cephalopolysyndactyly, craniofacial anomalies in, 2641t
Grisel's syndrome, due to adenotonsillectomy, 2801
GRO-α (growth-related oncogene-α), in wound healing, 1076
Groningen prosthesis, 1598f
Gross tumor volume (GTV), for radiotherapy, 1036, 1044
Group A beta hemolytic *Streptococcus pyogenes* (GABHS), pharyngitis due to, 191-193
in children, 2787
complications of, 2788
Group C streptococci, pharyngitis due to, 193
Group G streptococci, pharyngitis due to, 193
Growth and development, craniofacial. *See* Craniofacial growth and development.
Growth factor–independent 1 *(Gfi1)* gene, in murine deafness, 2058t-2060t
Growth impairment, obstructive sleep apnea and, 2603
Growth problems, sleep-disordered breathing and, 2792
Growth sites, in craniofacial growth and development, 2614
Growth-related oncogene-α (GRO-α), in wound healing, 1076
GSPN. *See* Greater superficial petrosal nerve (GSPN).
GST (glutathione *S*-transferase)
in head and neck squamous cell carcinoma, 1016-1017
in oral cancer, 1295
GTV (gross tumor volume), for radiotherapy, 1036, 1044
Guaifenesin
for rhinosinusitis, 735t, 736
for vocal professionals, 855
Guardian stitch, after tracheal resection, 1618, 1620f
Guidelines Development Task Force (GDTF), 89
Guillain-Barré syndrome, facial paralysis in, 2397
Gull-wing incision
for external ethmoidectomy, 757, 757f
for rhinoplasty, 545-546, 546f
"Gum boil," 179
Gumma, of ear canal or middle ear, 2105
Gunshot injuries, of neck
due to handgun, 1625
due to rifle, 1626, 1626f-1627f
due to shotguns, 1626-1627, 1628t
Gustatory cortex
primary, 1212, 1212f
secondary, 1212, 1212f
Gustatory neurons, 1208
Gustatory otorrhea, 2197
Gustatory pathways, central, 1212-1213, 1212f
Gustatory physiology, 1208
central gustatory pathways and function in, 1212-1213, 1212f
gustatory transduction in, 1208-1210, 1210f
interaction with saliva in, 1141, 1213-1214
peripheral sensitivity in, 1210-1212
Gustatory receptors
individual differences in, 1211-1212
regional differences in, 1210-1211
Gustatory rhinitis, 698
Gustatory sensitivity, 1207-1208
Gustatory structures, 1208
Gustatory sweating, after parotidectomy, 1177
Gustatory thalamus, 1212
Gustatory transduction, 1208-1210, 1210f
Gustducin, 1209-1210
GVHD (graft-versus-host disease), chronic, and xerostomia, 218
Gy (gray), 132-133, 1033

H

"H" angle, in chin analysis, 463, 464f
H_1 blockers (histamine$_1$ receptor antagonists), for allergic rhinitis, 620
H_2 blockers (histamine$_2$ receptor antagonists)
for extraesophageal reflux, 901
for GERD, 970
HAART (highly active antiretroviral therapy), 211
Habenula perforata, anatomy of, 1832f, 1834
Haberman feeder, 2665, 2665f
Habituation
and olfactory testing, 633
in vestibular compensation, 2375
Habituation exercises, in vestibular rehabilitation, 2372-2373, 2378
HAD (HIV-associated dementia), 223
Haemophilus influenzae
with CSF fistula, 2045
otitis media due to, 2763
rhinosinusitis due to
acute, 704, 704f, 732
chronic, 706
acute exacerbation of, 707
Haemophilus influenzae type B (HIB), supraglottitis due to, 2807
Haemophilus influenzae type B (HIB) vaccine
to prevent hearing loss, 2161
to prevent otitis media, 2769
Hair bundle(s), 2070-2071, 2072f
directional sensitivity of, 2072f
Hair bundle deflections
and adaptation of mechanoelectrical transduction currents, 2078, 2079f
in cochlear transduction, 2069f, 2071
Hair cell(s)
auditory
anatomy of, 1832-1834, 1833f
in organ of Corti, 1832, 1832f
arrangement of, 2071, 2072f
in cochlear transduction, 2061f-2062f, 2063-2064, 2064f
defects in afferent dendrite synapses with, 2080-2081, 2080f
innervation of, 1834, 1834f
length of, 2070, 2070f
number and density of, 2070
physiology of
inner, 1841f, 1842, 1844f
outer, 1841f, 1844, 1844f
stereocilia of, 1841f, 1842, 1843f
tip links of, 1841f, 1842, 1843f
tonotopic tuning of, 1844, 1844f
receptor potentials for, 2071, 2072f
scanning electron micrograph of, 1833f
vestibular
anatomy of, 1857, 1858f
arrangement of stereocilia and kinocilium in, 1854-1855, 1856f
embryogenesis of, 1852
morphologic polarization of, 1855, 1856f, 2277-2278, 2279f
on otoconial membrane, 1858f

Hair cell(s) *(Continued)*
sensory transduction by, 2277-2278, 2279f
synaptic morphology and function of, 1857-1859, 1859f-1860f
Hair cell channel deficiencies, effects on hearing of, 2079-2080
Hair cell regeneration and repair, and noise-induced hearing loss, 2144
Hair cell transduction, 2070-2081, 2070f
adaptation of mechanoelectrical transduction currents in, 2078-2079, 2079f
and auditory neuropathy, 2081
and defects in cytoskeletal proteins leading to deafness, 2074-2076, 2076f
defects in hair cell–afferent dendrite synapses and, 2080-2081, 2080f
defects of other hair cell channels and, 2079-2080
hair bundle deflections and receptor potentials in, 2069f, 2071, 2072f
myosin VI in, 2078
stereocilia in, 2070-2071
anatomy of, 2070-2071, 2070f, 2072f
composition of, 2074, 2075f-2076f
cross-linkages between, 2076f, 2077-2078
dynamic regulation of length of, 2076-2077
transduction channels in, 2071-2073
effects of deficiencies of, 2079-2080
gating of, 2073-2074
ion selectivity of, 2073, 2073f
structure of, 2076f
Hair cycle, 374, 374f
Hair follicle(s)
anatomy of, 373-374, 374f
miniaturization of, 375, 375f
regeneration of, 388
Hair grafts. *See* Hair also transplantation.
synthetic, 387-388
Hair loss, 373-389
alternatives and future treatment options for, 387-388
classification of, 376, 377f
counseling on, 376, 378f
epidemiology of, 374
etiology of
alopecia areata as, 376
androgenetic alopecia (male pattern baldness) as, 374-376, 375f
infectious, 376
scarring as, 375-376
telogen effluvium as, 376
evaluation of, 376
in females, 376, 377f
medical management of, 376-378
finasteride for, 377-378
minoxidil for, 376-377
nonsurgical hair restoration for, 387
pathophysiology of, 373-376, 374f
anatomy of hair follicle in, 373-374, 374f
androgenic factors in, 375, 375f
miniaturization of hair follicle in, 375, 375f
phases of hair cycle in, 374, 374f
due to rhytidectomy, 426, 427f
surgical management of
eyebrow, eyelash, and mustache transplantation for, 384, 384f
flap procedures for, 385-387, 387f
complications of, 386-387
follicular-unit hair transplantation for, 378, 378f-381f
completion of procedure for, 383-384
complications of, 384
dissection of donor strip in, 382, 382f
doll's hair appearance with, 378, 378f
follicular unit extraction for, 384
graft placement in, 383, 383f
location of hairline in, 378-379, 381f, 383, 383f

Hair loss *(Continued)*
marking off donor strip of scalp for, 381-382, 382f
marking out recipient regions for, 379-381, 382f
micrografts in, 378, 379f-381f
operative procedure for, 382-384
postoperative care after, 384
preoperative evaluation for, 378-382, 381f
slivers of follicular units in, 382, 383f
surrounding natural hair growth in, 382-383
with reconstructive procedures, 387, 388f
scalp reductions for, 384-385, 385f
complications of, 385, 386f
Hair shaft, 373-374
Hair systems, nonsurgical, 387
Hair transplantation
eyebrow, eyelash, and mustache, 384, 384f
follicular-unit, 378, 378f-381f
completion of procedure for, 383-384
complications of, 384
dissection of donor strip in, 382, 382f
doll's hair appearance with, 378, 378f
follicular unit extraction for, 384
graft placement in, 383, 383f
location of hairline in, 378-379, 381f, 383, 383f
marking off donor strip of scalp for, 381-382, 382f
marking out recipient regions for, 379-381, 382f
micrografts in, 378, 379f-381f
operative procedure for, 382-384
postoperative care after, 384
preoperative evaluation for, 378-382, 381f
slivers of follicular units in, 382, 383f
surrounding natural hair growth in, 382-383
Hair weaves, 387
Hairline lowering, 385, 385f
Hairpieces, 387
Hairstyling, for scar camouflage, 301
Hairy leukoplakia, oral, in HIV, 225-226, 226f
Half-gain rule, for hearing aids, 2271
Haller cells, 668-669, 670f
surgical anatomy of, 740
Hallucinations, olfactory, 636
Halo effect, *vs.* efficacy of treatment, 62t
Halo nevus, 287, 287f
Halo sign, in CSF rhinorrhea, 789
Halothane
for anesthesia, 111
in children, 2590
for premedication in children, 2589
Hamartoma
sinonasal, 718t
tracheal, 1617f
Handgun, neck trauma due to, 1625
Hand-Schüller-Christian disease
oral manifestations of, 1257
otologic manifestations of, 2100-2101
otorrhea as, 2196
Haploinsufficiency, 6
Haptic mentoring, 49, 49f
Haptics. *See* Simulation.
Hard palate
anatomy of, 1295f, 1297f, 1298, 1359f
cancer of, 1309-1310
cervical metastases of, 1310
clinical appearance of, 1310f
epidemiology of, 1309-1310
Kaposi's sarcoma as, 1309-1310
melanoma as, 1242f, 1309-1310
reconstruction for, 1310, 1311f
resection of, 1310, 1310f-1311f
squamous cell carcinoma as, 1310, 1310f
survival with, 1310

Hard palate *(Continued)*
minor salivary gland tumors of, 1310
necrotizing sialometaplasia of, 1309-1310
physical examination of, 99
primary and secondary portions of, 1297f
vasculature of, 1295-1296
Harmonic frequencies, 847, 2876
Harmonic Scalpel, for adenotonsillectomy, 2796-2797
Harmonics, in acoustic analysis for voice evaluation, 830, 834-835
Harmonin
in deafness, 2077-2078
in stereocilia, 2076f
Harmony ear-level speech processor, 2232f
Hartley, Gordon, 2728-2729
Harvard staging system, 53
Hashimoto's thyroiditis, 1747
oral manifestations of, 1251
ultrasound of, 1644
Hasner's valve, 798f
Hawthorne effect, *vs.* efficacy of treatment, 62t
HBO therapy. *See* Hyperbaric oxygen (HBO) therapy.
HC-BPPV (horizontal canal benign paroxysmal positional vertigo)
positional testing for, 2315-2316, 2331
repositioning maneuver for, 2332
HCO_3 (bicarbonate)
in saliva, 1139
in salivary gland secretion, 1135
HDIA1, in deafness, 2051t-2058t
HDR (hypoparathyroidism, sensorineural deafness, and renal dysplasia) syndrome, 2051t-2058t
HDR (high-dose-rate) radiotherapy, 1047
Head & Neck Survey (H&NS), 56
Head and neck cancer (HNC)
outcome scales for, 56-57, 56t
pediatric, 2835-2849
vs. adult, 2835
age and, 2837, 2837t
clinical trials for, 2836
epidemiology of, 2835
histiocytoses as, 2847-2848, 2847t
lymphoma as
Hodgkin's, 2838-2840, 2840f
non-Hodgkin's, 2837, 2838t-2839t, 2839f
neuroectodermal, 2844-2845
neuroblastomas as, 2844-2845, 2844t, 2845f
peripheral primitive, 2845
pathologic evaluation of, 2836-2837, 2836f, 2837t
post-transplantation lymphoprolilferative disorder as, 2840
risk factors for, 2835
salivary gland, 2845-2846, 2846f
sarcoma as, 2840-2843
dermatofibrosarcoma protuberans as, 2843, 2843f
epithelioid, 2843, 2843f
Ewing's, 2845
fibro-, 2842-2843, 2843f
nonrhabdomyosarcoma soft tissue, 2842
rhabdomyo-, 2840-2842, 2841t, 2842f
sequelae of management of, 2848
survival with, 2835-2836
teratomas as, 2846-2847
epidemiology of, 2846
histopathology and molecular biology of, 2847, 2847f
management of, 2846
presentation and evaluation of, 2846, 2846t
thyroglossal duct carcinomas as, 2847
tumorigenesis of, 2836
pre-malignant lesions for, 1061
radiotherapy for (*See* Radiation therapy (RT))

Head and neck cancer (HNC) *(Continued)*
squamous cell carcinoma as (*See* Head and neck squamous cell carcinoma (HNSCC))
transnasal esophagoscopy for, 983
ultrasonography in, 1647-1653
Head and Neck Distress Scale (HNDS), 56
Head and Neck Quality of Life (HNQOL), 56
Head and neck squamous cell carcinoma (HNSCC)
biology of, 1015-9
background of, 1015-1016
chemoprevention of, 1018, 1061-1062
clinical implications of, 1018
chemoradiation for, 1052-1058
concomitant, 1052-1056, 1053t-1054t
as adjuvant therapy, 1056
induction chemotherapy with, 1052-1053
in RADPLAT technique, 1054
chemotherapy for, 1015-9
historical background of, 1051-1052
induction, 1056-1058, 1058f, 1058t-1059t
in comcomitant chemoradiation, 1052-1053
for recurrent or metastatic disease, 1058-1061
combination, 1059-1060
prognostic factors with, 1058-1059
single agents in, 1059
environmental exposures and risk factors for, 1016-1018
alcohol as, 1016
cytochrome P-450 as, 1016
glutathione *S*-transferase as, 1016-1017
human papillomavirus as, 1017-1018
other enzymatic systems as, 1017
tobacco as, 1016
epidermal growth factor receptor in, 1022-1023
biology of, 1022, 1025f
as biomarker, 1026
clinical implications of, 1023
oncogene for, 1019
epigenetics of, 1020-1022, 1021f-1022f
expression microarrays and integrative genomics in, 1025
field cancerization in, 1016
genetic alterations in, 1019-1020
cytogenetic, 1019
microsatellites as, 1019
in oncogenes, 1016, 1019-1020
single nucleotide polymorphisms as, 1019
in tumor suppressor genes, 1016, 1020
and Fanconi's anemia, 1020
genetic progression model of, 1016
human papillomavirus in
as biomarker, 1026
as risk factor, 1017-1018
immunotherapy for, 1023-1024
loss of heterozygosity in, 1019-1020, 1026
metastatic progression of, 1060, 1060f
microRNAs in, 1021, 1022f, 1027-1028
mitochondrial mutations in, 1024-1025, 1028f
molecular biomarkers for, 1026-1027
epidermal growth factor receptor as, 1026
human papillomavirus as, 1026
loss of heterozygosity as, 1026
margin analysis for, 1027
in oral rinses and saliva, 1026
other, 1026-1027
polymorphisms in DNA repair enzymes as, 1027
serum analysis for, 1026-1027
novel fields of research on, 1027-1029
bioinformatics as, 1028-1029
cancer stem cell hypothesis as, 1028
microRNAs as, 1027-1028
proteomics as, 1029
targeted therapy for, 1054, 1055f, 1060-1061, 1060f
Head circumference, in Down syndrome, 2632
Head impulse testing, 2314-2315, 2315f
quantitative, 2323
Head injury. *See* Head trauma.
Head movement(s), in vestibular function, 2307-2308
Head movement analysis techniques, active, 2323-2324, 2324f
Head muscles, effects of radiotherapy on, 2626t
Head rotation
encoding of, 2277-2285
by afferents, 2283-2285, 2283f-2284f
cupula in, 2282f
otoconial membrane in, 2283
sensory transduction in, 2277-2279
anatomy of vestibular end organs in, 2277, 2278f
bidirectional sensitivity in, 2278-2279
cupula in, 2277, 2278f
firing rate in, 2278-2279, 2281f
hair cells in, 2277
otolith organs in, 2278, 2281f
stereocilia in, 2277-2278, 2279f
excitatory and inhibitory responses of semicircular canals to
high-acceleration, 2290-2292
anatomic and physiologic basis for, 2290-2291, 2291f
clinical importance of, 2291-2292, 2291f-2293f
in its plane, 2289
anatomic and physiologic basis for, 2282f, 2289
clinical importance of, 2289
graphical representation of, 2293, 2294f
"Head shadow" effect, 1839, 2248
Head thrust test (HTT), 2291-2292, 2292f, 2346
for Meniere's disease, 2337
with superior semicircular canal dehiscence, 2293f
after unilateral labyrinthectomy, 2291f
Head tilt
encoding of, 2277-2285
by afferents, 2283-2285, 2283f-2284f
cupula in, 2282f
with loss of unilateral utricular function, 2299-2300
anatomic and physiologic basis for, 2299-2300
clinical importance of, 2300, 2300f
otoconial membrane in, 2283
sensory transduction in, 2277-2279
anatomy of vestibular end organs in, 2277, 2278f
bidirectional sensitivity in, 2278-2279
cupula in, 2277, 2278f
firing rate in, 2278-2279, 2281f
hair cells in, 2277
otolith organs in, 2278, 2281f
stereocilia in, 2277-2278, 2279f
vs. translation, 2307, 2307f
with unilateral loss of function of, 2299-2300
anatomic and physiologic basis for, 2299-2300
clinical importance of, 2300, 2300f
Head trauma
CSF otorrhea due to, 2197
hearing loss due to, 2199
olfactory loss after, 634-635
sensorineural hearing loss due to, 2121
sudden, 2128
Head velocity, semicircular canal transfer function relative to, 2303, 2303f
Head voice, 846-847, 851
Headache, 246-248
cluster, 247-248
due to CSF rhinorrhea, 789
diagnosis of, 246, 247f
epidemiology of, 246
Headache *(Continued)*
in hemicrania continua, 248
initial evaluation of, 246
medication overuse (rebound), 248
migraine (*See* Migraine)
primary, 246
secondary, 246
sinus surgery for, 742
tension-type, 247
thunderclap, 248
in trigeminal neuralgia, 248
Healing
cochlear implant with compromised, 2241
of maxillofacial fractures, 330-331
by second intention
for nasal defects, 365
for oropharyngeal defects, 1376
of tongue base, 1387-1388
of tonsil and pharyngeal wall, 1383
for oropharyngeal reconstruction, 1376
for surface defects of nasal tip, columella, sidewalls, and dorsum, 365
Health information technology (HIT), 84t-87t
Health Plan Employer Data and Information Set (HEDIS) measures, 82
Health status, as outcome measure, 55
Health Utilities Index (HUI), 56
Health-related quality of life (HRQOL), as outcome measure, 55
Hearing. *See also* Auditory physiology.
and dementias, 233
in vocal professional, 858
Hearing acuity test(s), 1888, 1888f. *See also* Audiologic test battery (ATB).
auditory brainstem response as, 1909-1910
pure-tone air-conduction testing as, 1888
masking for, 1889-1890
pure-tone bone-conduction testing as, 1888, 1888f-1889f
Hearing aids, 2265-2275
age distribution of, 2265-2266, 2266f
in aging patients, 2274
binaural, 2271
bone-anchored (*See* Bone-anchored hearing aid (BAHA))
conventional (traditional)
vs. implantable, 2204f-2205f, 2206t
implantable adjuncts to, 2204f, 2206t, 2217, 2217f
limitation(s) of, 2203-2207, 2204b
acoustic feedback as, 2204
disorder perception of pitch and sound localization, 2207
distortion of spectral shape and phase shifts as, 2204
human factors as, 2205-2207
insufficient gain as, 2203-2204
nonlinear distortion as, 2204
occlusion effects as, 2204
physical factors as, 2203-2205
poor appearance as, 2204
poor transduction efficiency as, 2204-2205
recruitment and compression of dynamic ranges as, 2205-2207
implantable (*See* Implantable hearing aids)
indications for, 2265-2267
communication disorder and motivation as, 2266
hearing loss considerations in, 2265-2266, 2266f
otologic and other factors in, 2266-2267
in infants and children, 2274, 2723-2724
insertion loss with, 2270
monaural, 2271-2272
occlusion effect with, 2270
for otosclerosis, 2034
outcome measurement for, 2274

Hearing aids *(Continued)*
programmable, 2267, 2269
programming of, 2273
rules of thumb for, 2274-2275
selection and fitting of, 2271-2274
ear considerations in, 2271-2272
fitting process in, 2272-2273
fitting range in, 2271, 2272f
orientation, counseling, and follow-up after, 2273-2274
other considerations in, 2265-2267
target gain in, 2271
verification process in, 2273
sound transduction and coupling to auditory system with, 2205f
styles of, 2269-2270
behind-the-ear, 2269-2270, 2270f
completely-in-the-canal, 2270, 2270f
considerations for, 2270
in-the-canal, 2270, 2270f
in-the-ear, 2270, 2270f
receiver-in-the-canal, 2270
technology of, 2267-2271
amplifier in, 2267, 2267f
analog, 2267
automatic control in, 2269
components in, 2267, 2267f
compression circuitry in, 2268
data logging in, 2269
different acoustic responses or programs in, 2269
digital sound processing in, 2267
directional microphones in, 2269
electroacoustic characteristics in, 2267-2268, 2268f
evolution of, 2267
feedback suppression circuitry in, 2269
input transducer in, 2267, 2267f
direct audio input for, 2267
frequency-modulated (FM) receiver as, 2267
microphone as, 2267
telecoil (t-coil) as, 2267
linear amplification in, 2268, 2268f
noise reduction circuitry in, 2269
nonlinear amplification in, 2268, 2268f
open-fit or open-canal, 2270
other features in, 2269
output transducer in, 2267, 2267f
peak clipping in, 2268
programmability in, 2267, 2269
vent in, 2270
wireless connectivity in, 2267
for tinnitus, 2134
Hearing assessment, 97-98, 98t. *See also* Audiologic test battery (ATB); Electrophysiologic hearing assessment.
with temporal bone fracture, 2039
Hearing assistive technologies, 2270-2271
Hearing conservation program, for noise-induced hearing loss, 2150
Hearing Handicap Inventory in the Elderly (HHIE), 57
Hearing impairment. *See also* Hearing loss.
defined, 2151
Hearing in Noise Test (HINT), for cochlear implants, 2223, 2244
Hearing level (HL), 1839
Hearing loss, 2198-2201, 2198b
acquired, 2097-2098
cochlear implant for, 2220-2221
acute, 2198b, 2199
age-related, 2125-2126, 2126f
genetic basis for, 2074
with tinnitus, 2132
animal models of, and effects of cochlear implant electrical stimulation, 1881
audiograms of, 1888, 1888f-1889f

Hearing loss *(Continued)*
categories of, 1888, 1888f
classification of, 2086-2087, 2087t
conductive, 2017-2027
audiogram of, 1888, 1888f
in children, 2026-2027
diagnostic evaluation of, 2019-2021
acoustic immittance testing in, 2020
acoustic reflex testing in, 2020
history and physical examination in, 2022b
pure-tone audiometry and speech testing in, 2020, 2020f
Rinne test in, 2020, 2020t
Weber test in, 2020
due to external auditory canal conditions, 2021-2022, 2023f-2024f
implantable devices for, 2027
due to measles, 2158
due to middle ear conditions, 2023-2026
pathologic conditions leading to, 2018b
pediatric, 2200-2201
specific lesions of conductive hearing pathway and, 2019, 2019t
in superior semicircular canal syndrome, 2020-2021, 2021f
due to temporal bone trauma, 2046
treatment of, 2021-2026
for conditions of external auditory canal, 2021-2022, 2023f-2024f
for conditions of middle ear (*See* Ossiculoplasty)
for conditions of tympanic membrane, 2022-2023
due to tympanic membrane conditions, 2022-2023
congenital
cochlear implants for, 2220
epidemiology of, 2086
etiology of, 2200, 2200b
evaluation of, 2097-2099
genetic basis for, 2050, 2051t-2058t
in murine model, 2050, 2058t-2060t
due to labyrinthine infections, 2154-2157
with cytomegalovirus, 2154-2156, 2155f
with rubella, 2154, 2156-2157, 2157f
with syphilis, 2161
due to defects in cytoskeletal proteins, 2074-2076, 2076f
due to defects in hair cell–afferent dendrite synapses, 2080-2081, 2080f
diagnosis of, 2087, 2087t
epidemiology of, 2050, 2087
evaluation of, 2198-2199
fluctuating, 2198b, 2199
functional, 1901
genetic basis for, 2050, 2051t-2058t
cochlear implants with, 2220
in murine models, 2050, 2058t-2060t
in geriatric patients, 232
etiologies of, 232
treatment of, 233
types of, 232
gradual, 2198b, 2199
in HIV-positive patients, 223-225, 2161-2162
approach to, 224, 225t
due to cryptococcal meningitis, 223-224
due to otosyphilis, 224
due to hypothyroidism, 1746
in immunocompromised patients, 2161-2162
in infants, 2718-2725
ancillary testing for, 2722-2723
genetic testing in, 2722-2723
laboratory testing in, 2722
screening for connexin 26 mutation in, 2723
screening for maternally transmitted infection in, 2723

Hearing loss *(Continued)*
temporal bone imaging in, 2723
testing for Pendred's syndrome in, 2723
assessment of, 2719-2721
auditory brainstem responses in, 2719-2720
comparison of otoacoustic emissions and auditory brainstem responses in, 2721
evoked otoacoustic emissions in, 2720-2721
testing protocols for, 2719, 2720f
delay in identification of, 2719
diagnosis of, 2721-2722
audiology in, 2722
history in, 2721
middle ear effusions in, 2722
otomicroscopy in, 2722
physical examination in, 2721-2722
vestibular function assessment in, 2722
visual reinforcement audiometry in, 2722
history of screening for, 2718-2719
intervention strategies for, 2723-2724
amplification devices as, 2723-2724
bone conduction amplification as, 2723
cochlear implantation as, 2724
early, 2724
surgical therapy as, 2723
and neural plasticity, 1885, 1885f
prevalence of, 2719
due to intratympanic gentamicin, 2188-2189
due to jugular foramen syndromes, 2199, 2199t
mixed, 1888, 1889f
neural, 1899-1901, 1900f
noise-induced, 2121-2122, 2140-2152
vs. acoustic trauma, 2145-2146
anatomic mechanisms underlying, 2143-2144
clinical course of, 2121, 2121f-2122f, 2141, 2142f
cochlear damage in, 2141-2143, 2143f
diagnosis of, 2199
early detection of, 2146-2147, 2147f-2150f
hair cell regeneration and repair and, 2144
interactive effects in, 2147-2148
irreversible, 2141
legal issues with, 2149-2151
nature of, 2121-2122, 2141
new knowledge about cellular and molecular mechanisms of, 2144-2146
permanent threshold shift in, 2141, 2148
prevention of, 2151
protection from
by conditioning of cochlear efferent system, 2144
pharmacologic, 2144-2145
research on, 2143
resistance to, 2144-2145, 2146f
role of otolaryngologist in, 2150-2151
susceptibility to, 2145-2146, 2146f
temporary threshold shift in, 2141, 2148
with tinnitus, 2131-2132
vestibular disorders in, 2148
vibration and, 2148-2149
due to otitis media, 2776
outcome scales for, 57
due to paranasal sinus tumor, 1123
pediatric
conductive, 2200-2201
sensorineural, 2200, 2200b
quantification of, 2087, 2087t
rapidly progressive, 2198b, 2199-2200
sensorineural (*See* Sensorineural hearing loss (SNHL))
sudden, 2127-2130
clinical features of, 2157
etiology of, 2127-2129, 2195b, 2198-2201
due to labyrinthine infections, 2154, 2154b, 2157
prevalence, natural history, and prognosis for, 2127

Hearing loss *(Continued)*
temporal bone pathology in, 2157
treatment of, 2129-2130, 2157
intratympanic steroids for, 2184-2185
systemic steroids for, 2184
due to temporal bone trauma, 2046-2047, 2046f
in transplant recipients, 224-225
vaccines to prevent, 2161
Hearing preservation, cochlear implants with
in adults, 2245-2246
in children, 2240
ear selection for, 2236
Hearing protection, for prevention of noise-induced hearing loss, 2151
Hearing Satisfaction Scale (HHS), 57
Hearing sensitivity test(s), 1888, 1888f. *See also* Audiologic test battery (ATB).
auditory brainstem response as, 1909-1910
pure-tone air-conduction testing as, 1888
masking for, 1889-1890
pure-tone bone-conduction testing as, 1888, 1888f-1889f
Heart, of newborn, 2571
Heart disease, oral manifestations of, 1246-1249, 1249t
Heart murmur, oral treatment considerations with, 1246t
Heart rate, in children, 2571, 2571t
Heart transplantation, oral sequelae of, 1248
Heartburn, 954
Heat and moisture exchanger (HME), 1599-1600, 1602f
Heat shock protein 27 (HSP-27), in oral cancer, 1295
Hebb's postulate, and neural plasticity, 1882-1884, 1884f
HEDIS (Health Plan Employer Data and Information Set) measures, 82
Heerfordt's disease, facial paralysis in, 2400
Helical crus, 476-477
Helical CT
of laryngeal carcinoma, 1470
of pharynx and esophagus, 1396
Helicobacter pylori, in extraesophageal reflux, 899
Helicotrema
anatomy of, 1831, 1832f, 1840, 1841f, 1853f
in cochlear transduction, 2061-2062, 2062f
Heliox
for croup, 2806
for stridor, 2903
Helix, of ear, 476-477, 476f, 1824f, 2742f
Helix electrode system, 2227-2228, 2228f
Helper T cells, 601-602, 602f
Hemangioblastomas, intra-axial, 2528
Hemangioendothelioma
kaposiform, 2824-2825, 2826f
bone resorption with, 2826
Kasabach-Merritt phenomenon with, 2825
of neck
epithelioid, 1668-1669
spindle cell, 1668-1669
Hemangioma(s)
of airway
assessment and treatment of, 2828-2829, 2829f
complications of, 2825, 2826f
capillary
of cerebellopontine angle, 2524, 2525f
sinonasal, 718t, 725, 725f
cavernous, 290
of cerebellopontine angle, 2524
epistaxis due to, 684f
of cerebellopontine angle, 2524, 2525f
cavernous, 2524
congenital, 2824, 2825f
cutaneous, and airway involvement, 2899, 2900f
Hemangioma(s) *(Continued)*
facial
embolization of, 1942
laser therapy for, 2827f-2828f, 2828
medical therapy for, 2826-2828
principles for management of, 2826-2828
surgical therapy for, 2827f-2828f, 2828
facial nerve
vs. facial nerve schwannomas, 2507
imaging of, 1924-1926, 1927f
intranasal, 2695
laryngeal, 874, 2871, 2871f
of masticator space, 152
neck masses due to, 1640, 2816, 2816f
of oral cavity, 1291
of salivary glands, 1172, 2859-2860, 2860f
spindle cell, 1668-1669
subglottic, 1468, 1468f, 2871, 2871f
dysphagia due to, 2953
stridor due to, 2899, 2900f
of trachea, 1613
Hemangioma of infancy (HOI), 290, 2823-2824
of airway
assessment and treatment of, 2828-2829, 2829f
complications of, 2825, 2826f
clinical presentation of, 2823, 2825f
complications of, 2825, 2826f-2827f
diagnosis of, 2823
focal, 2823, 2825f
imaging of, 2823, 2824f
laser therapy for, 2827f-2828f, 2828
medical therapy for, 2826-2828
natural history of, 2823, 2824f
obstruction of visual axis by, 2825, 2826f
persistent tissue changes due to, 2826, 2827f
in PHACES syndrome, 2824, 2825f
principles for management of, 2826-2828
segmental, 2823, 2824f-2825f
surgical therapy for, 2827f-2828f, 2828
ulceration of, 2825, 2827f
Hemangiopericytoma (HPC), of neck, 1670
Hematocrit, in children, 2571-2572
Hematogenous total joint infection, patients at potential increased risk of, 1253, 1253t
Hematologic disorders
oral manifestations of, 1256
preoperative evaluation of, 105-106
due to anticoagulants, 105
congenital, 105
hemoglobinopathies as, 106
due to liver failure, 105-106
thrombocytopenia as, 106
Hematolymphoid neoplasms
of larynx, 1509
extramedullary plasmacytoma as, 1509
lymphoma as, 1509
mucosal malignant melanoma as, 1509
of oropharynx, 1364, 1364f
Hematoma(s)
auricular, 97, 310, 2038
esophageal, 1416
fracture, 330
after liposuction, 459
due to neck surgery, 1729
after otoplasty, 478-479
due to rhytidectomy, 420-421, 425f
septal, 494
due to nasal fracture, 507
pediatric, 2708-2709, 2712f
due to sphenoidotomy, 768t
after total laryngectomy, 1571
Hematopoietic growth factors, 609t-610t
Hematopoietic tumors, of paranasal sinuses, 1131
Hemicrania continua, 248
Hemidystonia, 838
Hemifacial microsomia, 2585
Hemifacial spasm, 2401
facial nerve monitoring with microvascular decompression for, 2548-2549, 2549f
Hemiglossectomy, for tongue carcinoma, 1305-1306, 1305f
Hemilaryngectomy
for glottic cancer, 1517t, 1519t
extended, 1517t
vertical, 1496, 1518f, 1519t, 1547-1549
with anterior commissure involvement, 1497
swallowing disorders due to, 1220
vertical, 1547-1549
complications of, 1549
extended, 1548
frontolateral, 1548
functional outcome of, 1548
for glottic cancer, 1496, 1518f, 1519t, 1547-1549
with anterior commissure involvement, 1497
historical background of, 1540
with imbrication laryngoplasty, 1548, 1548f
key surgical points for, 1549
oncologic results of, 1547-1548, 1547t-1548t
posterolateral, 1548
radiographic appearance after, 1476, 1479f
surgical technique for, 1548
Hemilaryngopharyngectomy, supracricoid, for hypopharyngeal cancer, 1429, 1436
Hemimandibulectomy
for buccal carcinoma, 1309f
for tongue carcinoma, 1306f
Hemitransfixion incision, for septoplasty, 488, 489f
Hemochromatosis, oral manifestations of, 1257
Hemodialysis, oral sequelae of, 1255
Hemodilution, and skin flap viability, 1073
Hemoglobin level, in children, 2571-2572
Hemoglobinopathies
oral manifestations of, 1256
preoperative evaluation of, 106
Hemophilia, preoperative evaluation of, 105
Hemophilia A, oral manifestations of, 1256
Hemorrhage
after adenotonsillectomy, 2783f-2784f, 2794, 2799-2800, 2800f
cerebellar, 2354f
due to endoscopic sinus surgery, 754
functional, 679
due to neck surgery, 1723
of carotid artery, 1728
of internal jugular vein, 1729, 1729f
due to sphenoidotomy, 768t
due to thyroid surgery, 1770
vocal fold, 867-869
with capillary ectasia, 868f
diagnosis of, 868
history in, 868
laryngeal examination in, 868
vocal capability battery in, 868
epidemiology of, 867
pathophysiology and pathology of, 867-868
treatment of, 868-869
behavioral, 868
medical, 868
surgical, 868-869
Hemotympanum, due to temporal bone fracture, 2038, 2039f, 2046
Hennebert's sign, 2105, 2316, 2329-2330
in otosyphilis, 2341
with perilymph fistula, 2342
Hensen's cells, anatomy of, 1832, 1832f-1833f
Heparin
after free tissue transfer, 1096
preoperative use of, 105
Hepatic disease
oral manifestations of, 1255
preoperative evaluation of, 103-104
Hepatitis, oral manifestations of, 1252

HER1, in head and neck squamous cell carcinoma, 1060
HER2, in head and neck squamous cell carcinoma, 1060
Her2/neu
in oral cancer, 1295
in salivary gland neoplasms, 1199
Hereditary disorders, sensorineural hearing loss due to, in adults, 2117-2118
Hereditary hemorrhagic telangiectasia (HHT), 291
epistaxis in, 691-692, 692f
oral manifestations of, 1257
Hernia, hiatal, gastroesophageal junction in, 957f
Herpangina, 2785, 2786f
Herpes labialis, 1236, 1236f
Herpes simplex virus (HSV)
and Bell's palsy, 2391-2393
and chemical peels, 391-392, 397
deafness due to, 2159-2160
in infants, 2723
esophagitis due to, 976-977, 977f-978f
imaging of, 1404, 1405f
Meniere's disease due to, 2163
oral
in HIV, 226
primary infection with, 1235, 1252
clinical features of, 1235, 1235f, 1252
defined, 1235
diagnosis of, 1235
differential diagnosis of, 1235
etiology and pathogenesis of, 1235
treatment of, 1235, 1252
recurrent infection with, 1235-1236, 1252
clinical features of, 1236, 1236f
defined, 1235
differential diagnosis of, 1236
etiology and pathogenesis of, 1235-1236
histopathology of, 1236, 1237f
vs. recurrent aphthous stomatitis, 1238, 1238t
treatment of, 1236
pharyngitis due to, 199, 199f
vestibular neuritis due to, 2162-2163
Herpes simplex virus-1 (HSV-1) vector, for gene therapy of inner ear, 2191t, 2192
Herpes zoster facial paralysis, 2393, 2396
Herpes zoster ophthalmicus, 2396
Herpes zoster oticus, 1948, 1948f
clinical features of, 2159, 2159f
diagnosis of, 2159
management of, 2159
otorrhea due to, 2195
sensorineural hearing loss due to, 2119, 2159
sudden, 2127
temporal bone pathology in, 2159
Herpesvirus vectors, for gene therapy, 18t
of inner ear, 2191t, 2192
Herpetic gingivostomatitis, 1235, 1235f
Herpetic palsy, imaging of facial nerve in, 1924, 1927f
Herpetiform-type aphthous ulcerations, 1238, 1238f
Hertwig's epithelial root sheath, 1259
Hertz (Hz), 1838-1839, 1839f
Heschl's gyrus, 1847
Heteroduplex testing, 9
Heterogeneity, genetic, 8
Heteroplasmy, 8, 2089
Heterozygosity, 6, 2088
Hexachlorophene and alcohol (Septisol), for deep chemical peel, 394-395
HHIE (Hearing Handicap Inventory in the Elderly), 57
HHT (hereditary hemorrhagic telangiectasia), 291
epistaxis in, 691-692, 692f
oral manifestations of, 1257
HHV. *See* Human herpesvirus (HHV).
Hiatal hernia, gastroesophageal junction in, 957f
Hiatus secondarius, 740
Hiatus semilunaris
normal anatomy of, 667, 667f
surgical anatomy of, 740
HIB (*Haemophilus influenzae* type B), supraglottitis due to, 2807
HIB (*Haemophilus influenzae* type B) vaccine
to prevent hearing loss, 2161
to prevent otitis media, 2769
Hidrocystoma, 292
HIF (hypoxia inducible factor), in Warburg effect, 1028f
HiFocus 1j electrode system, 2227-2228, 2228f
High-density polyethylene (MEDPOR)
for auricular reconstruction, 2744t
for chin implants, 465t
High-dose-rate (HDR) radiotherapy, 1047
Highly active antiretroviral therapy (HAART), 211
High-resolution computed tomography (HRCT)
for cochlear implant, 2222, 2222f
with otosclerosis, 2222, 2222f
in preoperative evaluation, 2235, 2235f, 2236b
for CSF rhinorrhea, 791, 791f, 2044
for dizziness, 2326-2327
for malignant otitis externa, 1947
of superior canal dehiscence syndrome, 2340-2341, 2340f
for temporal bone fracture, 2039, 2040f
High-Risk Registry (HRR), for infant hearing loss, 2718-2719
High-speed digital imaging (HSDI), of larynx, 821-823
applications of, 823
assessment using, 822-823
defined, 813
equipment for, 821
kymography in, 134f, 154, 822f
limitations of, 823
Hilger facial nerve stimulator, for facial nerve injury, 2040-2041
Hillocks of His, embryogenesis of, 1824, 2741, 2742f
Hinge flaps, 346
for nasal defects, 348, 350f, 371-372, 372f
HINT (Hearing in Noise Test), for cochlear implants, 2223, 2244
Hip strategy, 2308
HiRes 90K Bionic Ear device, 2227-2228, 2228f
Histamine provocation test, in nonallergic rhinitis, 695-696
Histamine$_1$ receptor antagonists (H$_1$ blockers), for allergic rhinitis, 620
Histamine$_2$ receptor antagonists (H$_2$ blockers)
for extraesophageal reflux, 901
for GERD, 970
Histiocytoma, malignant fibrous
of larynx, 1508
of neck, 1667
Histiocytosis(es)
in children, 2847-2848
classification of, 2847, 2847t
clinical presentation and evaluation of, 2847-2848
neck masses due to, 2819
pathology of, 2847
treatment of, 2848
Langerhans' cell (*See* Langerhans' cell histiocytosis (LCH))
X (*See* Langerhans' cell histiocytosis (LCH))
Histones, 11
in head and neck squamous cell carcinoma, 1020-1021
Histoplasmosis
laryngeal and tracheal manifestations of, 885, 892
oral, in HIV, 226-227
History, 94, 94b
in assessment of nasal breathing function, 642
for children, 2573
of chronic rhinosinusitis, 743
of facial trauma, 302-303
of nonallergic rhinitis, 699, 699b
of present illness, for disorders of professional voice, 850-851
HIT (health information technology), 84t-87t
HIV. *See* Human immunodeficiency virus (HIV)/HIV infection.
HL. *See* Hodgkin's lymphoma (HL).
HL (hearing level), 1839
HLA (human leukocyte antigen) system, 599
HLA-B7 (human leukocyte antigen-B7), in gene therapy, 21
HM (hyoid myotomy), for obstructive sleep apnea, 259, 261f
HME (heat and moisture exchanger), 1599-1600, 1602f
HNC. *See* Head and neck cancer (HNC).
HNDS (Head and Neck Distress Scale), 56
HNQOL (Head and Neck Quality of Life), 56
H&NS (Head & Neck Survey), 56
HNSCC. *See* Head and neck squamous cell carcinoma (HNSCC).
Hoarseness
gastroesophageal reflux and, 2946
due to hypothyroidism, 1747
due to thyroid disease, 1736-1737
Hockey stick incision, for neck dissection
radical, 1709, 1710f
selective, 1717-1718, 1717f
Hodgkin, Thomas, 2838-2839
Hodgkin's lymphoma (HL), 1676-1677
in children, 2819, 2838-2840
clinical presentation of, 2819, 2839-2840
histopathology and molecular biology of, 2819, 2840, 2840f
imaging of, 2820f
management of, 2840
staging of, 2839-2840
clinical presentation of, 1674, 1674f
complications of, 1677
epidemiology of, 1673-1674
imaging of, 1674, 1674f
immunosuppression and, 213t, 217
staging of, 1676, 1677t
treatment and prognosis for, 1676-1677
HOI. *See* Hemangioma of infancy (HOI).
Holdaway analysis, for mentoplasty, 463, 464f
Hollinger anterior commissure laryngoscope, for difficult airway, 122, 122f
Holmium:YAG (Ho:YAG) laser, 33
Holoprosencephaly, 2690
Homograft(s)
for craniofacial defect repair, 2657
for nasal reconstruction, 368
for ossiculoplasty, 2006, 2025, 2026t
Homoplasmy, 2089
Homozygosity, 6, 2088
Horizontal buttresses, 331-332
Horizontal canal benign paroxysmal positional vertigo (HC-BPPV)
positional testing for, 2315-2316, 2331
repositioning maneuver for, 2332
Horizontal palpebral fissure, 442
Horizontal partial laryngectomy, 1540, 1549
Horizontal phase, of vocal fold vibration, 849
Horizontal semicircular canal (HSCC) fistula, due to mastoidectomy, 2015
Horizontal semicircular duct, 1851f
Hormonal effects, of radiotherapy, 2626t
Horner's syndrome
due to neck surgery, 1732, 1732f
due to thyroid disease, 1736
Hospital Quality Alliance (HQA), 84t-87t, 87

Hospitalization, of children
in dedicated children's hospital, 2575
preparation for, 2574-2575
Hot water irrigation, for epistaxis, 691
Hounsfield units (HU), 131
Hourglass closure, laryngeal videostroboscopy of, 819, 820f
House, William, 2437-2438
House-Brackmann grading system, for facial nerve function, 2381-2382, 2382t, 2383f, 2417-2418, 2417t
Ho:YAG (holmium:YAG) laser, 33
HPC (hemangiopericytoma), of neck, 1670
Hpn, in murine deafness, 2058t-2060t
HPV. *See* Human papillomavirus (HPV).
HQA (Hospital Quality Alliance), 84t-87t, 87
H-ras, in oral cancer, 1294
HRCT. *See* High-resolution computed tomography (HRCT).
HRQOL (health-related quality of life), as outcome measure, 55
HRR (High-Risk Registry), for infant hearing loss, 2718-2719
Hsal1, in deafness, 2051t-2058t
HSCC (horizontal semicircular canal) fistula, due to mastoidectomy, 2015
HSDI. *See* High-speed digital imaging (HSDI).
HSP-27 (heat shock protein 27), in oral cancer, 1295
HSS (Hearing Satisfaction Scale), 57
HSV. *See* Herpes simplex virus (HSV).
HTT. *See* Head thrust test (HTT).
H-type fistula, 2926
HU (Hounsfield units), 131
HUI (Health Utilities Index), 56
Human Genome Project, 2088
Human herpesvirus 1 (HHV-1)
and erythema multiforme, 1239
oral infection with
primary, 1235, 1252
recurrent, 1235-1236, 1252
vs. recurrent aphthous stomatitis, 1238, 1238t
Human herpesvirus 8 (HHV-8), 213
Human immunodeficiency virus (HIV)/HIV infection, 210-212. *See also* Acquired immunodeficiency syndrome (AIDS).
AIDS-defining conditions in, 210-211, 211t
biology and immunology of, 210
diagnosis and classification of, 210-212, 211t
and facial lipoatrophy, 227-228, 228f
facial palsy due to, 2399
and hearing loss, 223-225, 2161-2162
approach to, 224, 225t
due to cryptococcal meningitis, 223-224
due to otosyphilis, 224
highly active antiretroviral therapy for, 211
immune restoration disease in, 211-212
lymphadenopathy due to, in children, 2818
and malignancy, 212-217, 213t
cutaneous neoplasms as, 213t, 215
Hodgkin's lymphoma as, 213t, 217
Kaposi's sarcoma as, 212-215, 213t
epidemiology and pathogenesis of, 212-213
presentation and diagnosis of, 213-214, 214f
treatment of, 214-215
non-Hodgkin's lymphoma as, 213t, 215-216
diagnosis of, 216
epidemiology and presentation of, 216
prognosis and treatment for, 216-217
squamous cell carcinoma as, 213t, 215
and malignant otitis externa, 1947
and neuropathies, 223-225
occupational exposure to, 212, 212t
olfactory loss due to, 636
and oral lesions, 225-227, 1252
aphthous ulcers as, 227, 227f
candidiasis as, 225, 226f
Human immunodeficiency virus (HIV)/HIV infection *(Continued)*
differential diagnosis of, 225t
fungal, 227
gingivitis and periodontal disease as, 227
hairy leukoplakia as, 225-226, 226f
due to herpes simplex virus, 226
histoplasmosis as, 226-227
due to human papillomavirus, 227
otologic and neurotologic manifestations of, 221-223
malignant otitis externa as, 221-222
in middle ear, 222-223
due to *P. jiroveci* and *A. fumigatus*, 222-223
pharyngitis due to, 197
postexposure prophylaxis for, 212, 212t
and salivary gland disease, 217-218
in children, 2856
diffuse infiltrative lymphocytosis syndrome as, 218
parotid lesions as, 217-218, 218f
xerostomia as, 218
and sinonasal infection, 219-221
diagnosis of, 220-221, 220f
presentation and pathogenesis of, 219-220
treatment of, 221
transmission of, 210
Human immunodeficiency virus (HIV)-associated dementia (HAD), 223
Human immunodeficiency virus (HIV) wasting syndrome, 210-211
Human immunodeficiency virus–associated salivary gland disease (HIV-SGD), 1157-1158, 1157f
Human leukocyte antigen (HLA) system, 599
Human leukocyte antigen-B7 (HLA-B7), in gene therapy, 21
Human papillomavirus (HPV)
external ear infection with, 1957, 1957f
management options for, 1957
and oral cancer, 1294, 1365
recurrent respiratory papillomatosis due to, 878, 2884-2886
and squamous cell carcinoma, 215
of head and neck
as biomarker, 1026
as risk factor, 1017-1018
of larynx, 1492, 1513
verrucous, 1505
warts due to, 282
oral, in HIV, 227
Human papillomavirus (HPV) vaccine (Gardasil), 2886-2887, 2890t
Humidified air, for croup, 2806
Humoral immune response, 606-608
antibody-dependent cellular cytotoxicity in, 606
B cells in, 603
T cell–dependent and T cell–independent, 606
chemokines in, 608, 611t-612t
complement system in, 607-608, 608f
cytokines in, 608, 609t-610t
immunoglobulins in, 606-607, 607f
Humoral immunodeficiency disorders, 2114
otologic manifestations of, 2114
Hump reduction, in noncaucasian rhinoplasty, 570-573
concept of, 570-571
results of, 574f-575f
technique for, 571-573, 575f
Hunter's syndrome, 2113
and obstructive sleep apnea in children, 2606
otologic manifestations of, 2113, 2113f
Huntington's disease, saccades in, 2313
Hurler's syndrome, 2113
and obstructive sleep apnea in children, 2606
otologic manifestations of, 2113
Hürthle cell tumor, 1762-1763
clinical presentation of, 1762
management and prognosis for, 1762-1763
pathology of, 1762
Hutchinson's triad, 2341
Hydration
for benign vocal fold mucosal disorders, 862
for voice professional, 852-853
Hydraulic lever, 2018-2019
Hydraulic process, and orbital wall fractures, 2712
Hydrocephalus
normal pressure, vestibular symptoms of, 2357
otitic, 1997
after stereotactic radiation therapy, 2563
Hydrocodone
ototoxicity of, 2175
for postoperative pain, 241t
Hydrocortisone
intratympanic delivery of, 2183
for thyroid storm, 1745
Hydrocortisone butyrate cream, for eczematoid otitis externa, 1955-1956
Hydrocortisone cream (Hytone cream)
after chemical peel, 396
for eczematoid otitis externa, 1955-1956
Hydrocortisone/propylene glycol/acetic acid otic solution (VoSol HC), for otitis externa
bacterial, 1953, 1959t-1960t
fungal, 1954, 1959t-1960t
Hydrodynamic delivery, of siRNA, 16
"Hydrodynamic" theory, of dental pain, 1202-1203
Hydrogen cyanide, in noise-induced hearing loss, 2147-2148
Hydrogen peroxide, for cerumen removal, 1958t
Hydromorphone
as adjunct to induction of anesthesia, 111
for anesthesia maintenance in children, 2592
Hydrops, endolymphatic
audiogram in, 1895f
electrocochleography in, 1892-1896, 1895f, 1908
idiopathic (*See* Meniere's disease)
otosclerosis with, 2035
sensorineural hearing loss due to, 2126-2127, 2199
stacked auditory brainstem response in, 1911
vertigo due to, 2202
Hydrops ex-vacuo model, of eustachian tube dysfunction, 1870
Hydroxyapatite (Bone Source), for chin implants, 465t
Hydroxyapatite cap, for ossiculoplasty, 2026t
Hydroxyapatite (VoCoM) implants, for medialization thyroplasty, 908-910, 908f, 910f
Hydroxychloroquine (Plaquenil)
ototoxicity of, 2176
sensorineural hearing loss due to, 2120
5-Hydroxytryptamine$_3$-receptor antagonists, for postoperative nausea and vomiting in children, 2593
Hydroxyurea, with radiotherapy, 1041
Hygiene hypothesis, of allergic rhinitis, 613-614
Hygroma, cystic, 156-157, 2815, 2901f
Hylan B gel (Hylaform), for vocal fold medialization, 905-906
Hyoepiglottic ligament, 1541-1542, 1542f-1543f
Hyoglossus muscle, 1296f, 1297-1298, 1298f
Hyoid bone
anatomy of, 805-806, 1296f, 1359f
radiographic, 1463f, 1471, 1471f, 1473f
surgical, 1541, 1542f-1543f
in breathing, 810
embryology of, 2583-2584
laryngeal carcinoma of, 1541
palpation of, in voice evaluation, 827, 828f
physical examination of, 95, 96f
Hyoid myotomy (HM), for obstructive sleep apnea, 259, 261f

Hyperacusis, 2138-2139
in Bell's palsy, 2393
defined, 2138
epidemiology of, 2138
evaluation of, 2138-2139
impact of, 2139
vs. recruitment, 2138
treatment of, 2139
Hyperacusis Questionnaire, 2138-2139
Hyperadrenalism, oral manifestations of, 1251
Hyperbaric oxygen (HBO) therapy
for osteoradionecrosis, 1048
with radiotherapy, 1041
for skin flap salvage, 1075
and skin flap viability, 1074
for soft tissue avulsions, 307
Hypercalcemia
due to benign tumors, 1783-1784, 1783t
definition of, 1782
differential diagnosis of, 1782, 1782t-1783t
drug-induced, 1783-1784, 1783t
due to endocrine disease, 1783-1784, 1783t
epidemiology of, 1782
familial hypocalciuric, 1783
due to granulomatous disorders, 1783-1784, 1783t
in hyperparathyroidism
differential diagnosis of, 1782, 1782t
evaluation of, 1782-1784
historical background of, 1774
pathogenesis of, 1781
of malignancy, 1783, 1783t
medical management of, 1804
non–PTH-mediated, nonmalignant, 1783-1784, 1783t
preoperative evaluation of, 104
Hypercalcemic crisis, 1781
Hypercalcemic syndrome, 1781
Hyperdynamic facial lines, 275, 279f
Hyperechoic tissue, 1643
Hyperfractionation, 1040
Hyperfunctional disorders, of larynx, 838-842
botulinum toxin therapy for, 839, 840f-841f
due to dystonia, 838-839, 838b
essential tremor as, 840-841
due to myoclonus, 840
due to pseudobulbar palsy, 839-840
stuttering as, 841-842
Hyperfunctional dysphonia, 834
Hyperkeratosis
of larynx, 1486
leukoplakic-type, 1231, 1231f
Hyperkinetic disorders, of facial nerve, 2401
management of, 2432
Hypermethylation, in head and neck squamous cell carcinoma, 1020-1022, 1021f
Hypernasality
after adenotonsillectomy, 2800
assessment of, 2678-2679, 2679t
in children, 2879
Hyperparathyroidism
asymptomatic, 1781
clinical course of untreated, 1782
clinical manifestations of, 1780-1781
cardiovascular, 1781
gastrointestinal, 1781
hypercalcemic abnormalities as, 1781
neurologic, 1781
neuromuscular, 1781
renal and urinary tract, 1781
skeletal, 1781
diagnosis of, 1784
etiology and pathogenesis of, 1774-1775, 1775f-1776f
familial, 1795-1797
in MEN-I, 1775, 1776f, 1795-1796
in MEN-IIA, 1796
Hyperparathyroidism *(Continued)*
neonatal, 1797
non-MEN (isolated), 1796-1797
historical background of, 1774
hypercalcemia in
evaluation of, 1782-1784, 1782t-1783t
historical background of, 1774
pathogenesis of, 1781
incidence of, 1780
localization study(ies) in, 1784-1789, 1784t
gamma radiation detection device for, 1802, 1803f
intraoperative, 1784t, 1789
invasive preoperative, 1784t, 1788-1789
parathyroid arteriography as, 1788
selective venous sampling for PTH as, 1788-1789
ultrasound-guided fine-needle aspiration as, 1789
mediastinal exploration as, 1801-1802, 1802f
noninvasive preoperative, 1784-1788, 1784t
computed tomography as, 1786-1787
computed tomography–sestamibi fusion as, 1785-1786, 1786f-1788f
magnetic resonance imaging as, 1787-1788, 1789f
pertechnetate (technetium 99m) thallous chloride (thallium 201) imaging as, 1784-1785
sestamibi–technetium 99m scintigraphy as, 1785, 1785f, 1788f, 1794f
technetium 99m sestamibi with single photon emission computed tomography as, 1785
ultrasonography as, 1786, 1788f-1789f
unsuccessful, 1801, 1801f-1802f
medical management of, 1804
oral manifestations of, 1251
due to parathyroid adenoma, 1774-1775, 1778-1779
due to parathyroid carcinoma, 1802-1804, 1803f
during pregnancy, 1804
preoperative evaluation of, 104
re-exploration for recalcitrant, 1798-1800
causes of failed exploration with, 1798
operative risk in, 1798-1799
operative strategy for, 1799-1800, 1799f-1800f
preoperative assessment for, 1798
renal failure–induced, 1797-1798
secondary, 1782-1783
recurrent, 1798
surgical management of, 1789-1804
gamma radiation detection device in, 1802, 1803f
indications for, 1789-1790
intraoperative PTH levels with, 1800-1801
for multiple-gland disease, 1794-1795
due to sporadic hyperplasia, 1794-1795, 1794f
due to true double adenoma, 1794, 1794f
parathyroidectomy as, 1790-1792
anesthesia and preparation for, 1790
closure of incision in, 1792
exploration of neck in, 1790-1792, 1791f
postoperative care after, 1792
for single-gland disease, 1792-1794
directed unilateral cervical exploration as, 1792-1793
endoscopic parathyroid exploration in, 1793-1794
minimally invasive techniques for, 1793
strategy and approach to, 1792
tertiary, 1783
and thyroid disease, 1801, 1801f-1802f
Hyperpigmentation
after chemical peel, 396-397
after rhytidectomy, 427
Hyperplasia
of larynx, 1486-1491
oropharyngeal, 1360
Hyperplastic candidiasis, 1231, 1231f
in HIV, 225
Hyperresponsiveness, in allergic rhinitis, 616-617
nonspecific, 617
specific, 616-617
Hypersensitivity, delayed-type, 601
Hypersensitivity reaction(s), 608-612
to ototopical antibiotics, 1954
Hypersomnia(s)
of central origin, 263-264, 264b
idiopathic, 262t, 264
Hypertension
benign (idiopathic) intracranial
CSF rhinorrhea due to, 787
facial paralysis due to, 2400-2401
sensorineural hearing loss due to, 2123
and epistaxis, 686-687
due to hyperparathyroidism, 1781
malignant, 119
pulmonary, due to obstructive sleep apnea, 2604
Hyperthyroidism. *See also* Graves' disease; Thyrotoxicosis.
antithyroid agents for, 1739t
oral manifestations of, 1251
preoperative evaluation of, 104
with thyroid nodule, 1756
Hypertrophic adenoids, and otitis media, 1872, 1873f
Hypertrophic scars, 291
after otoplasty, 479
due to rhytidectomy, 425-426
Hyperventilation, dizziness due to, 2316
Hypervitaminosis D, hypercalcemia due to, 1784
Hypnotic dependent sleep disorder, 262t
Hypoadrenalism, oral manifestations of, 1251
Hypocalcemia
after hypopharyngeal reconstruction, 1458
after thyroid surgery, 1771
Hypoechoic tissue, 1643
Hypoepiglottic ligament, in laryngeal cancer, 1484, 1484f
Hypofunctional disorders, of larynx, 842-843
due to central causes of vocal fold paresis, 842
due to medullary disorders, 842
due to multiple sclerosis, 843
due to myopathies, 842
due to neuromuscular junction disorders, 842
due to Parkinson's disease, 842-843
due to poliomyelitis, 842
psychogenic, malingering, and mixed causes of, 843
vocal fold paresis as, 843
Hypoglossal canal
anatomy of, 1823f
in surgical anatomy of lateral skull base, 2435f
in surgical anatomy of middle cranial base, 2445f
Hypoglossal nerve
anatomy of, 1295, 1296f, 1297-1298
distribution of, 2580f, 2581
intraoperative monitoring of, 2550-2552, 2552f
in surgical anatomy of lateral skull base, 2439f-2440f
Hypoglossal nerve injury
in lateral skull base surgery, 2512
due to neck surgery, 1730-1731
Hypoglossal nerve transposition, for facial nerve paralysis, 2419, 2424f-2426f, 2425-2426
Hypoglycemic agents, oral sequelae of, 1247t-1248t
Hypomethylation, in head and neck squamous cell carcinoma, 1021-1022
Hyponasality
assessment of, 2678, 2678f, 2678t
in children, 2879

Hypoparathyroidism
oral manifestations of, 1251
preoperative evaluation of, 104
sensorineural deafness, and renal dysplasia (HDR) syndrome, 2051t-2058t
Hypopharnygeal stenosis, 947-948
Hypopharyngeal cancer, 1421-1440
advanced-stage, 1438-1439
chemotherapy for, 1439
conventional treatment modalities for, 1442
quality of life with, 1439
radiation therapy for, 1591-1592
complications of, 1591
CyberKnife stereotactic approach for, 1592
future strategies and directions for, 1592
outcome and prognostic factors for, 1591
RADPLAT approach for, 1592
techniques and dose-fractionation schemes for, 1591
anatomy and, 1421-1422, 1422f
approach to management of, 1426
cervical lymph node metastasis of, 1422, 1422f, 1434-1439
incidence and distribution of, 1686f, 1688t
management of, 1434-1439
radiation therapy for, 1689t
chemoradiotherapy for, 1434, 1442
for advanced disease, 1439
after total laryngectomy, 1442-1443
chemotherapy for, 1433-1434, 1442
for advanced disease, 1439
induction, 1443
for larynx preservation, 1443-1444
clinical evaluation of, 1423
physical findings in, 1423
presenting symptoms in, 1423, 1423t
clinical presentation of, 1579
conventional treatment modalities for, 1441-1442
for advanced disease, 1442
for early disease, 1442
diagnostic evaluation/workup for, 1579
early-stage, radiation therapy for, 1590-1591
complications of, 1591
outcome and prognostic factors for, 1591, 1591t
techniques and dose-fractionation schemes for, 1590-1591
epidemiology of, 1441
etiology and biology of, 1425-1426
imaging of, 1413, 1413f-1414f, 1423-1424, 1579
barium swallow for, 1423-1424
CT for, 1424, 1424f
MRI for, 1424
PET/CT for, 1424, 1424f
incidence of, 1422-1423
location and patterns of spread of, 1425
neck dissection for, 1434-1439, 1716-1718
definition and rationale for, 1716-1717, 1717f
technique for, 1717-1718, 1717f
neck management for, 1580
new treatment modalities for, 1442, 1448, 1449f
overall management of, 1580, 1590
pathology of, 1424-1425
radiation therapy for, 1433, 1443, 1589-1592
with advanced-stage disease, 1591-1592
complications of, 1591
CyberKnife stereotactic approach for, 1592
future strategies and directions for, 1592
outcome and prognostic factors for, 1591
RADPLAT approach for, 1592
techniques and dose-fractionation schemes for, 1591
anatomic considerations in, 1578-1579, 1579f
with early-stage disease, 1590-1591
complications of, 1591
outcome and prognostic factors for, 1591, 1591t
Hypopharyngeal cancer *(Continued)*
techniques and dose-fractionation schemes for, 1590-1591
lymphatic drainage and, 1578-1579, 1579f
overview of, 1578
with recurrent disease, 1591-1592
therapeutic outcomes with, 1436
reconstruction for (*See* Hypopharyngeal reconstruction)
recurrent, radiation therapy for, 1591-1592
squamous cell carcinoma as, intensity-modulated radiotherapy of, 1046
staging of, 1367t, 1426-1434, 1426t-1427t, 1579-1580, 1580f
surgical management of, 1426-1431
endoscopic CO_2 laser resection for, 1429-1430, 1442
outcomes of, 1436-1438
history of, 1426
options for, 1426, 1427t
partial laryngopharyngectomy for, 1429, 1430f
partial pharyngectomy for, 1426-1429
via anterior transhyoid pharyngotomy, 1427-1429, 1428f
via lateral pharyngotomy, 1426-1427
via lateral transthyroid pharyngotomy, 1427, 1428f
via median labiomandibular glossotomy, 1429
supracricoid hemilaryngopharyngectomy for, 1429, 1436
therapeutic outcomes with, 1436-1439, 1437t
total laryngectomy with partial/total pharyngectomy for, 1430, 1431f
total pharyngo-laryngo-esophagectomy for, 1430-1431
therapeutic outcomes of, 1435-1436
with primary radiation therapy, 1436
with primary surgical therapy, 1436-1439, 1437t
Hypopharyngeal lipoma, 1425f
Hypopharyngeal mucosal space, imaging of, 158-159
with lesions, 159, 162f
normal anatomy in, 158-159, 159f-160f
Hypopharyngeal procedures, for obstructive sleep apnea, 258b, 259-260, 260f-261f
Hypopharyngeal reconstruction, 1431-1433, 1448-1461
with circumferential defects, 1431-1432
classification of defects for, 1450
decision making on, 1450, 1451f
free tissue transfer for, 1454, 1454f
enteric, 1455-1457
gastro-omental donor site for, 1457-1458, 1457f
jejunal donor site for, 1455-1457, 1456f
fasciocutaneous, 1433, 1455
antero-lateral thigh donor site for, 1455
other donor sites for, 1455
radial forearm donor site for, 1455
goals and principles of, 1450
jejunal free flap in, 1432-1433, 1433f
local and regional flaps for, 1450-1452, 1452f
myocutaneous flap(s) in, 1452-1453
pectoralis, 1431, 1431f
patient population for, 1448
perioperative counseling for, 1448-1449
postsurgical complications of, 1458, 1459f
posttreatment speech and swallowing outcomes of, 1459-1460
preoperative evaluation for, 1449-1450
visceral transposition for, 1453
colonic, 1453, 1454f
gastric, 1432, 1432f, 1453
voice rehabilitation after, 1458-1459
Hypopharynx
anatomy of, 1359f, 1421-1422, 1422f, 1578
radiographic, 1398f-1399f
dysphagia due to congenital conditions of, 2950t, 2951-2953, 2953f
lymphatic drainage of, 1422, 1422f, 2582
physical examination of, 99-100
Hypopigmentation
after chemical peel, 397
after rhytidectomy, 427
Hypopnea, 251b, 256f
obstructive, in children, 2607
Hypopnea index, 251b
Hypothalamic hypothyroidism, 1747
Hypothesis testing, 65, 66t
examples for, 65-66
null hypothesis in, 65, 66t
P value in, 65, 66t
type I and type II errors in, 65, 66t
Hypothyroidism, 1745-1749
clinical features of, 1745-1746, 1746b
due to endemic goiter, 1747
esophageal manifestations of, 979
etiology of, 1745, 1746b
due to excessive iodine intake, 1747
familial, 1747
goitrous, 1747
hearing loss due to, 1746
hoarseness due to, 1747
hypothalamic, 1747
laboratory diagnosis of, 1748, 1748t
after laryngectomy, 1747
due to lingual thyroid, 1287
management of, 1748-1749
myxedema coma due to, 1749
due to neck irradiation, 1695
nongoitrous, 1747
oral manifestations of, 1251
pituitary, 1747
during pregnancy, 1749
preoperative evaluation of, 104
prevalence of, 1745
after radiation therapy, 1747
due to radiation therapy, 1048
risk factors for, 1745-1746, 1746b
subclinical, 1747-1748
diagnosis of, 1747
effects on lipid, hypothyroid symptoms, and mood of, 1747-1748
natural history of, 1747
prevalence of, 1747
treatment of, 1748
surgery with, 1749
with thyroid nodule, 1756
after total laryngectomy, 1571
transient, 1747
vertigo due to, 1747
Hypotympanum, 1825-1826
Hypoventilation
central alveolar, 262t
obstructive, in children, 2607, 2607f
Hypoventilation syndromes, sleep-related, 263, 263b
Hypovolemic shock, due to pediatric facial fracture, 2699
Hypoxemia
newborn response to, 2571
during sleep in children, 2607
Hypoxemic syndromes, sleep-related, 263, 263b
Hypoxia
newborn response to, 2571
in noise-induced hearing loss, 2144-2145
and radiotherapy, 1041
Hypoxia inducible factor (HIF), in Warburg effect, 1028f
Hypoxic sensitizers, with radiotherapy, 1041
Hyrtl's fissure, 2736

Hysteria, *vs.* myofascial pain dysfunction syndrome, 1285t
Hytone cream (hydrocortisone cream)
after chemical peel, 396
for eczematoid otitis externa, 1955-1956
Hz (hertz), 1838-1839, 1839f

I

^{131}I. *See* Radioactive iodine (^{131}I).
IAC. *See* Internal auditory canal (IAC).
IAR (intermittent allergic rhinitis), 618
IBCA (isobutyl-2-cyanoacrylate), for embolization, 1933
Ibuprofen, and skin flap viability, 1074
I-3-C (indole-3-carbinol), for recurrent respiratory papillomatosis, 879, 2890t, 2892
ICA. *See* Internal carotid artery (ICA).
ICERE-1 protein, in deafness, 2051t-2058t
ICF (International Classification of Functioning), 56
ICP (intracranial pressure), and CSF rhinorrhea, 786-787, 786b
IDEA (Individuals with Disabilities Education Act), 2724
Identification tests, for olfaction, 631
IDL (indirect laryngoscopy), for laryngeal carcinoma, 1494
IFNs. *See* Interferon(s) (IFNs).
IFRS. *See* Invasive fungal rhinosinusitis (IFRS).
Ig(s). *See* Immunoglobulin(s) (Igs).
IGF-I (insulin-like growth factor-I), in wound healing, 1076
IHCs. *See* Inner hair cells (IHCs).
IHI (Institute for Healthcare Improvement), 84t-87t
IJV. *See* Internal jugular vein (IJV).
IL(s). *See* Interleukin(s) (ILs).
Iliac crest flap
for free tissue transfer, 1082t, 1087
for mandibular defects, 1324-1325, 1325t
IM. *See* Infectious mononucleosis (IM).
Image-guided computer-assisted surgery, of anterior and middle cranial base, 2448-2449, 2449f
Image-guided radiotherapy, 1043, 1046-1047
Image-guided surgery (IGS), of paranasal sinuses, 680-681, 743-744, 745f
registration in, 680-681
tracking systems in, 681
Imaging, 130-176
available modalities for, 130-138
computed tomography as, 131, 131f
contrast enhancement for, 132, 133f
image display for, 131-132
patient cooperation for, 132, 132f
radiation exposure from, 132-133, 133t
three-dimensional reconstruction techniques in, 138, 139f
conventional radiography as, 130-131
of facial bones and sinuses, 130
of neck, 131
radiation exposure from, 132-133, 133t
of temporal bone, 131
magnetic resonance angiography as, 137
magnetic resonance imaging as, 133-137
artifacts on, 133-134, 134f
disadvantages of, 137
fat suppression methods for, 135-136, 136f
with frequency (chemical shift) selective presaturation (fat saturation), 135-136, 136f
gadolinium enhancement for, 134-135, 135f-136f
with gradient echo techniques, 136-137, 137f
pulse sequences for, 134-137, 135f-136f
with short T1 inversion recovery (STIR), 135-136, 136f

Imaging *(Continued)*
with spectral presaturation inversion recovery (SPIR), 135-136
T1-weighted, 134, 135f-136f
T2-weighted, 134, 135f-136f
three-dimensional reconstruction techniques in, 138, 139f
in nuclear medicine, 137-138
positron emission tomography as, 137-138
radionuclide imaging as, 138, 139f
ultrasound as, 137
of cochlear implants, 2221-2222, 2222f
of deep neck space infections, 204-205
CT for, 204, 204f-205f
MRI for, 204
plain film radiography for, 204-205
ultrasonography for, 204-205
in differential diagnosis, 144
of Graves' ophthalmopathy, 1809-1810, 1811f
of head and neck, 138-144
computed tomography for, 139-142
with cervical lymphadenopathy, 139
with facial trauma, 142
of larynx and infrahyoid neck, 132f, 140
of paranasal sinuses, 140-142, 141f
of salivary glands, 139
in sialography, 139-140, 1145f, 1150, 1150f
of suprahyoid neck, 139, 141f
of temporal bone and skull base, 142
of thyroid and parathyroid glands, 140
conventional radiography for, in sialography, 139-140, 1149-1150, 1149f
FDG-PET for, 144, 145f
magnetic resonance imaging for, 142-143
of larynx and infrahyoid neck, 142-143
of lymphadenopathy, 142
of paranasal sinuses, 143
of salivary glands, 142
of skull base, 143
of suprahyoid neck, 142
of temporal bone, 143
of thyroid and parathyroid glands, 143
ultrasound for, 143-144
of infrahyoid neck, 143-144
with metastatic lymphadenopathy, 143
of salivary glands, 143
of hypopharyngeal and cervical esophageal cancer, 1413, 1413f-1414f, 1423-1424
barium swallow for, 1423-1424
CT for, 1424, 1424f
MRI for, 1424
PET/CT for, 1424, 1424f
of infrahyoid neck, 157-159
anterior and posterior cervical (lateral cervical) spaces in, 158, 159f-160f, 162f
CT for, 140
hypopharyngeal mucosal space in, 158-159
with lesions, 159, 162f
normal anatomy in, 158-159, 159f-160f
normal anatomy in, 157-159, 159f-160f
prevertebral space in, 158, 159f-160f, 162f
retropharyngeal space in, 158
with lesions, 158, 161f
normal anatomy in, 158, 159f-160f
of larynx, 159-161, 813-824, 1462-1481
with benign mass(es), 1468
congenital cysts as, 1468
laryngocele as, 159-161, 163f, 1468, 1469f
squamous papillomas as, 1468, 1468f
subglottic hemangioma as, 1468, 1468f
with carcinoma, 1494-1495
of anterior commissure, 1474, 1474f
of aryepiglottic fold, 1475, 1478f
with cartilaginous invasion, 1474-1475, 1476f
for conservation laryngeal surgery, 1545-1546
of epiglottis, 1475, 1477f
glottic, 1474-1475, 1474f

Imaging *(Continued)*
with lymph node metastases, 1476, 1479f
normal anatomy and, 1470-1474
paraglottic, 1474
post-therapy, 1476-1479, 1479f
of pyriform sinus, 1475-1476, 1478f
subglottic, 1474, 1475f
supraglottic, 1475-1476
technique for, 1470, 1470f
transglottic, 161, 164f, 1475f, 1476, 1478f
CT for, 132f, 140
flexible endoscopy for, 814
advantages of, 814
disadvantages of, 814
for professional voice disorders, 851-852, 852t
protocols for, 816b, 818b
technique of, 814
troubleshooting for, 814
with foreign bodies, 1480-1481, 1480f-1481f
high-speed digital, 821-823
applications of, 823
assessment using, 822-823
defined, 813
equipment for, 821
kymography in, 134f, 154, 822f
limitations of, 823
with inflammatory disease, 1464-1466
croup as, 1465, 1465f
epiglottis as, 159-161, 163f, 1406-1407, 1407f, 1464, 1464f-1465f
retropharyngeal abscess as, 1465-1466, 1466f
with laryngomalacia, 1466
MRI for, 142-143
with normal airway, 1462-1464
anatomy of, 1462-1464, 1463f-1464f
technique for, 1462
rigid endoscopy for, 813-814
advantages of, 813
disadvantages of, 813-814
for professional voice disorders, 851, 852t
protocols for, 816b, 818b
technique of, 814
troubleshooting for, 814
stroboscopy for, 818-821
of adynamic segments, 820
of amplitude of vibration, 820, 821f, 848, 848t
of closure pattern, 819, 820f, 848t, 849
common problems and solutions for, 815t-816t
defined, 813
flexible endoscopes in, 814
interpretation of, 848t
interval examination in, 847
of mucosal wave, 820, 848-849, 848t
in neurologic examination, 834
of periodicity, 821, 848, 848t
of phase closure, 819-820
for professional voice, 847-849, 848f, 848t
protocol for, 818-819, 818b
of regularity, 821
rigid endoscopes in, 813-814
of symmetry, 820, 847-848, 848t
of vertical closure level, 821
for vocal fold impairment, 905
with trauma, 159, 162f, 1479-1480, 1480f
videoendoscopy for, 814-818
of arytenoid and vocal fold motion, 816
common problems and solutions for, 815t-816t
defined, 813
flexible endoscopes for, 814
of laryngeal structure, 816
of mucous, 816-817
in neurologic examination, 834
protocol for, 814, 816b

Imaging *(Continued)*
rigid endoscopes for, 813-814
of supraglottic activity, 817, 817f
of vascularity, 817
of vocal fold edges, 818
with vocal cord paralysis, 1466-1467, 1467f
of lymph nodes, 164-167
anatomy and classification of, 163-164
with extracapsular spread, 164-166, 167f
inflammatory (reactive), 164
with invasion of carotid artery, 166-167
metastatic
contrast-enhanced CT of, 164-165, 167f
MRI of, 165-166, 168f
with non-Hodgkin's lymphoma, 165-166, 167f
normal anatomy in, 166f
of maxillofacial trauma, 325-326
of lower third, 325-326
of middle third, 325, 326f
of upper third, 325, 325f
of nasal fractures, 500
of nasopharyngeal carcinoma, 148, 149f
for staging, 1354
of neck masses, 1636-1637, 1637t
of neck neoplasms, 1656-1657
of nose, 167-171
with anatomic variations and congenital abnormalities, 167
for facial trauma, 170-171, 170f-171f
MRI for, 143
nasal cavity in, 169, 170f
ostiomeatal complex in, 168f-169f, 169
of oral cancer, 1300
of oropharyngeal cancer, 1366
of paranasal sinus tumors, 1124
of paranasal sinuses, 167-169, 662-2
with anatomic variations and congenital abnormalities, 668-670
aerated crista galli as, 670
asymmetry in ethmoid roof height as, 670
cephalocele as, 670, 671f
of concha bullosa, 668, 669f
extensive pneumatization of sphenoid sinus as, 669, 671f
giant ethmoid bullosa as, 669
Haller or infraorbital cells as, 668-669, 670f
medial deviation or dehiscence of lamina papyracea as, 669
nasal septal deviation as, 668, 669f
Onodi or sphenoethmoidal cells as, 669
paradoxic middle turbinate as, 668, 669f
of uncinate process, 668, 670f
with complications of inflammatory disease, 676-677
inflammatory polyps as, 676, 678f
mucocele as, 676, 678f
mucous retention cyst as, 676, 677f
orbital, 676-677
conventional radiography of, 130, 662
Caldwell view in, 662, 663f
Waters view in, 662, 663f
CT for, 140-142, 141f, 662-663
radiation exposure with, 663
technique of, 662-663, 664f
after functional endoscopic sinus surgery, 677-680
expected findings in, 677-679, 679f
operative complications in, 679-680, 680f
for image-guided surgery, 680-681, 743-744, 745f
registration in, 680-681
tracking systems in, 681
interpretation of, 670-672
evaluation of bony outlines in, 672, 672f
evaluation of critical relationships for surgical planning in, 671-672, 672f

Imaging *(Continued)*
identification and description of important structures in, 671
MRI for, 664, 664f
nasal cycle in, 664, 664f
with normal anatomy, 664-668, 665f
agger nasi cell in, 665-666, 665f-666f
anterior ostiomeatal channels in, 666f
anterior ostiomeatal unit in, 664, 665f
basal lamella and sinus lateralis in, 665f, 667f
frontal recess in, 665, 665f-667f
frontal sinuses in, 664-665, 665f
hiatus semilunaris in, 667, 667f
inferior meatus in, 664
inferior turbinate in, 665f
infundibulum in, 665f, 666-667
maxillary sinuses in, 664, 665f
middle meatus in, 664-665, 665f-667f
middle turbinate in, 667
ostiomeatal channels in, 664
posterior ethmoid sinus in, 667
posterior ostiomeatal unit in, 664
primary ostium in, 665, 665f
retrobullar (suprabullar) recess in, 667
sphenoethmoidal recess in, 667, 668f
sphenoid sinus in, 664, 665f, 667-668, 668f
superior meatus in, 664-665
uncinate process in, 666-667, 666f-667f
ostiomeatal unit in, 664-670
with rhinosinusitis, 167-168, 168f, 672-675
acute, 672-673, 673f
allergic, 675
chronic, 673-674, 674f-675f, 743, 744t
fungal, 674-675, 676f
granulomatous, 675
with sinonasal small cell tumor *vs.* sphenoid pyomucocele, 168-169, 169f
of parathyroid glands, 162-163, 165f
CT for, 140
MRI for, 143
ultrasonography for, 1644-1645, 1650f-1652f
of pharynx and esophagus, 1393-1420
with benign neoplasms, 1415-1416
esophageal hematoma as, 1416
esophageal leiomyoma as, 1415-1416, 1415f
retention cyst as, 1416, 1416f
Tornwaldt cyst as, 1416, 1416f
vs. tortuous internal carotid artery, 1416, 1416f
with diverticula, 1401-1402
laryngoceles as, 1402, 1402f
midesophageal, 1402, 1403f
pharyngeal pouches as, 1401-1402, 1402f
Zenker's, 1401, 1402f
with esophageal narrowing, 1407-1409
due to extrinsic compression, 1408-1409, 1409f
due to strictures, 1407-1408, 1408f
due to webs, 1407, 1408f
with fistulas, 1409-1411
due to branchial cleft anomaly, 1410, 1410f
congenital, 1409-1410
due to perforation, 1410-1411, 1410f
postoperative, 1411, 1411f
tracheoesophageal, 1409-1410
with foreign body, 1411, 1412f
with infection/inflammation, 1403-1407
due to abscess, 1407, 1407f
due to alcohol-induced esophagitis, 1406
due to caustic esophagitis, 1404-1405, 1405f
due to drug-induced esophagitis, 1406, 1406f
due to eosinophilic esophagitis, 1406
due to epidermolysis bullosa, 1406, 1406f
due to graft-versus-host disease, 1406
due to granulomatous esophagitides, 1405
due to infectious esophagitis, 1404, 1405f

Imaging *(Continued)*
due to intramural pseudodiverticulosis, 1406, 1407f
due to pemphigoid, 1406
due to peptic esophagitis, 1406
due to radiation esophagitis, 1406
due to reflux esophagitis, 1403-1404, 1403f-1404f
with malignant neoplasms, 1412-1415
of esophagus, 1413-1414, 1414f
of hypopharynx, 1413, 1413f-1414f
with lymphadenopathy, 1414-1415, 1415f
of nasopharynx, 1412-1413, 1413f
of oropharynx, 1413, 1413f
with motility disorder(s), 1398-1401
abnormal deglutition as, 1398
due to connective tissue diseases, 1400-1401, 1401f
cricopharyngeal dysfunction as, 1398-1399, 1400f
diminished peristalsis as, 1399-1400, 1400f-1401f
esophageal spasm as, 1400-1401, 1401f
of esophagus, 1399-1401
of pharynx, 1398-1399
post-treatment, 1416-1418
after laryngectomy, 1416, 1417f
after laryngopharyngectomy, 1416-1418, 1418f
for monitoring and surveillance, 1418, 1419f-1420f
after radiotherapy, 1418, 1418f
radiographic anatomy in, 1397-1398
of esophagus, 1397-1398, 1400f
of pharynx, 1397, 1398f-1399f
technique(s) for, 1393-1397
computed tomography as, 1396
conventional radiography as, 1393, 1394f
fluoroscopy as, 1393-1394
magnetic resonance imaging as, 1396
modified barium swallow as, 1396
oral contrast agents in, 1396
other nuclear medicine as, 1397
PET-CT as, 1396-1397, 1397f
pharyngoesophagram as, 1394, 1394f-1395f
ultrasound as, 1396
with varices, 1411, 1411f
of postoperative neck and face, 173-174, 175f-176f
principle of interpretation of, 144
of salivary glands, 1143-1150, 1166-1168, 1180
with adenoid cystic carcinoma, 1146-1147, 1146f-1147f, 1180f
with AIDS-related parotid cysts, 1146, 1146f
in children, 2854-2855
CT for, 139, 1148, 1166, 1180
of AIDS-related parotid cysts, 1146f
of parotid lipoma, 1166, 1167f
of pleomorphic adenoma, 1144f, 1148
of sialadenitis, 1148
of sialolithiasis, 1144f, 1148, 1148f
of Sjögren's syndrome, 1148
of Warthin's tumor, 1146f
FDG-PET for, 1150, 1168
minor, 1145
MRI for, 142, 1145-1147, 1166, 1180
of adenoid cystic carcinoma, 1146-1147, 1146f-1147f, 1180f
of glomus tumor, 1169f
of mucoepidermoid carcinoma, 1146, 1147f, 1168f
of pleomorphic adenoma, 1148f, 1167f-1168f, 1180f
of ranula, 1146, 1147f
with mucoepidermoid carcinoma, 1146, 1147f
parotid, 1143-1144, 1145f
with pleomorphic adenomas, 1143

Imaging *(Continued)*
CT for, 1144f, 1148
MRI for, 1148f, 1167f-1168f, 1180f
ultrasound for, 1149, 1149f
with ranula, 1146, 1147f
scintigraphy for, 138, 1150
with sialadenitis, 1148
sialography for, 1149-1150
conventional, 139-140, 1149-1150, 1149f
CT, 139-140, 1145f, 1150, 1150f
MR, 1147
for salivary gland injury, 312
with sialolithiasis, 1143, 1144f, 1148, 1148f
sublingual, 1144-1145
submandibular, 1144
ultrasound for, 143, 1148-1149, 1149f, 1167
color Doppler, 1167-1168
with Warthin's tumor, 1146, 1146f
for sensorineural hearing loss, in adults, 2117
of site-specific lesions, 146-167
of skull base, 171, 1929-1930
with benign lesions, 171, 172f
CT for, 142, 171
prior to endoscopic sinus surgery, 764t
with fractures, 171
with inflammatory lesions, 171
with intracerebral neoplastic processes, 171, 174f
with meningiomas, 1929-1930, 1930f
with metastases, 171, 173f
MRI for, 143, 171
normal anatomy in, 171
with paragangliomas, 171, 174f, 1929, 1930f
of suprahyoid neck, 146-157
carotid space in, 150-151, 151f-152f
CT for, 139, 141f
masticator space in, 151-152
with adenoid cystic carcinoma, 155f
with angiofibroma, 152, 154f
with hemangioma and lymphangioma, 152, 153f
with infection, 151-152, 152f
normal anatomy on, 146f, 151-152
with pseudotumors, 152
with squamous cell carcinoma, 152, 154f
MRI for, 142
normal anatomy in, 146-157, 146f-147f
oral cavity in, 153-156
with abscess, 156f
with congenital lesions, 154-156
with non-Hodgkin's lymphoma, 157f
normal anatomy on, 146f, 153-156
with squamous cell carcinoma, 154, 156f
parapharyngeal space in, 131, 146f
parotid space in, 149-150, 150f-151f
pharyngeal mucosal space in, 148-149
with inflammatory lesions, 148, 148f
with non-Hodgkin's lymphoma, 148-149, 149f
normal anatomy on, 146f, 148-149
with squamous cell carcinoma, 148, 149f
with Thornwaldt cyst, 148
prevertebral space in, 146f, 153
retropharyngeal space in, 146f, 152f, 153, 155f
sublingual space in, 156
with abscess and cellulitis, 156, 157f
with congenital lesions, 156
normal anatomy in, 146f, 154, 156
with ranula, 156, 157f
with squamous cell carcinoma, 156
submandibular space in, 146f, 156-157, 158f
of temporal bone, 171-173, 1916
cerebellopontine angle in, 1926-1928, 1929t
with acoustic schwannoma, 1929t
with arachnoid cyst, 1928, 1929t
with epidermoid tumor, 1928, 1928f, 1929t

Imaging *(Continued)*
with lipoma, 1928, 1929t
with meningioma, 1928, 1928f, 1929t
cochlear nerve in, 1928-1929, 1929f
conventional radiography for, 131
CT for, 142
external auditory canal in, 172, 1917-1918
with benign neoplasms, 1918, 1918f-1919f
with cholesteatoma, 1917, 1918f
with congenital lesions, 1917, 1917f
with keratosis obturans, 1917, 1918f
with malignant neoplasms, 1918, 1919f
with postinflammatory medial canal fibrosis, 1917-1918, 1918f
with severe infections, 1917, 1917f
external ear in, 172
facial nerve in, 173, 1924-1926
with Bell's palsy, 1924, 1927f
with hemangioma, 1924-1926, 1927f
with meningioma, 175f
with neuroma, 1928
with schwannoma, 1924-1926, 1927f
inner ear in, 172-173, 1920-1922
with congenital anomalies, 172-173, 174f, 1920-1921, 1923f
with enlarged vestibular aqueduct, 1921, 1923f
with fenestral and cochlear otosclerosis (otospongiosis), 1921-1922, 1925f
with intravestibular schwannoma, 1921, 1924f
with labyrinthitis ossificans, 1921, 1925f
normal appearance of, 1920-1921, 1922f
with superior semicircular canal dehiscence, 1920-1921, 1922f
internal auditory canal in, 173, 1926-1928
with meningioma, 175f
with vestibular schwannoma, 173, 1928, 1928f
mastoid in, 1918-1920
middle ear in, 172, 1918-1920
with aberrant internal carotid artery, 1919-1920, 1921f-1922f
with cholesteatoma, 174f, 1918-1919
with glomus tympanicum, 1919-1920, 1921f
with transverse petrous fracture with osseous dislocation, 174f
MRI for, 143
petrous apex in, 1922-1924, 1924t
with asymmetric pneumatization, 1922-1923, 1924t, 1925f
with cholesteatoma, 1924t
with cholesterol granuloma, 1923, 1924t, 1925f-1926f
with malignant lesions, 1923-1924, 1926f
with mucocele, 1924t
with retained secretions, 1923, 1924t, 1925f
of thyroid gland, 161-162, 1757
CT for, 140
with follicular carcinoma, 161-162, 165f
lingual, 161-162, 165f
MRI for, 143
normal anatomy in, 161
scintigraphy for, 138, 1757-1758
with thyroglossal duct cyst, 161-162, 165f
ultrasonography for, 1644, 1645f-1647f, 1646b
of tracheal tumors, 1616, 1616f-1617f
of visceral space, 159-163
parathyroid glands in, 162-163, 165f
thyroid gland in, 161-162
CT for, 140
with follicular carcinoma, 161-162, 165f
lingual, 161-162, 165f
MRI for, 143
normal anatomy in, 161
scintigraphy for, 138
with thyroglossal duct cyst, 161-162, 165f

Imbalance, 2308-2310
Imbrication laryngoplasty, 1548, 1548f
IMF (intermaxillary fixation) screws, 330-331, 333f
Imipramine, for neuropathic pain, 245t
Imiquimod (Aldara), for aural papillomatosis, 1957
Imitrex (sumatriptan), for migraine, 2349
Immittance audiometry battery, for otosclerosis, 2030
Immittance testing
of eustachian tube function, 1874
for otitis media, 2762
Immune complex–mediated hypersensitivity reactions, 608-612
Immune reconstitution syndrome, 211-212
Immune response
cell-mediated, 602f
direct in vivo stimulation of antitumoral, 21
Immune restoration disease (IRD), 211-212
cryptococcal meningitis in, 224
Immune system, 597-623
adaptive, 209, 599-605
B cells in, 603
development of, 603
responses by, 603
basophils and mast cells in, 605
eosinophils in, 604
innate *vs.*, 597-598
monocytes and macrophages in, 604
natural killer cells in, 603-604
neutrophils in, 604
overview of, 597-598
platelets and erythrocytes in, 605
stem cells in, 599-600, 600f
T cells in, 600-603
development of, 600-601
effector, 601-603
priming of, 601
toll-like receptors and, 598
antigen presentation in, 606, 606f
humoral, 606-608
antibody-dependent cellular cytotoxicity in, 603-604, 606
B cell responses in, 603
T cell–dependent and T cell–independent, 606
chemokines in, 608, 611t-612t
complement system in, 607-608, 608f
cytokines in, 608, 609t-610t
immunoglobulins in, 606-607, 607f
innate, 209, 598-599
adaptive *vs.*, 597-598
antimicrobial peptides in, 598-599
cathelicidins as, 599
defensins as, 599
tissue distribution of, 599
overview of, 597-598
self and nonself in, 599
Toll-like receptors in, 598
activators of, 598
and adaptive immune response, 598
expression and distribution of, 598
and host, 598
lymphoid organs in, 605
lymph nodes as, 605
mucosal, 605
Peyer's patches and lymphoid follicles in, 605
tonsils in, 605
Immune tolerance, 1023
Immunocompromised patients. *See* Immunosuppression.
Immunodeficiency disorder(s)
acquired, 210, 210t
congenital, 209-210, 210t
nasal manifestations of, 660
otitis media in, 2764-2766

Immunodeficiency disorder(s) *(Continued)*
otologic manifestations of, 2114-2115
in AIDS, 2114-2115
primary of congenital, 2114
sensorineural hearing loss due to, 2123-2124
severe combined, 209-210
Immunoglobulin(s) (Igs)
in humoral immune response, 606-607
structure of, 606, 607f
Immunoglobulin A (IgA)
in humoral immune response, 607
in saliva, 1140
Immunoglobulin D (IgD), in humoral immune response, 607
Immunoglobulin E (IgE)
in allergic rhinitis, 614, 619
in humoral immune response, 607
in nonallergic rhinitis, 696
Immunoglobulin G (IgG), in humoral immune response, 607
Immunoglobulin M (IgM), in humoral immune response, 607
Immunoglobulin M (IgM) testing, for infant hearing impairment, 2723
Immunologic disorders, sudden sensorineural hearing loss due to, 2128
Immunology, and otitis media, 2764-2766
Immunopathology, 608-612
Immunosuppressants
oral sequelae of, 1247t-1248t, 1248
sensorineural hearing loss due to, 2124
topical, for eczematoid otitis externa, 1956-1957
Immunosuppression, 209-229
causes of, 209-210, 210t
and cervical lymphadenopathy, 218-219, 219t
and fungal rhinosinusitis, 660, 710t
diagnosis of, 220-221, 220f
presentation and pathogenesis of, 220
treatment of, 221
for Graves' ophthalmopathy, 1811
and hearing loss, 2161-2162
in HIV-positive patients, 223-225
approach to, 224, 225t
due to cryptococcal meningitis, 223-224
due to otosyphilis, 224
in transplant recipients, 224-225
due to HIV/AIDS, 210-212
biology and immunology of, 210
and cutaneous neoplasms, 213t, 215
diagnosis and classification of, 210-212, 211t
and facial lipoatrophy, 227-228, 228f
and hearing loss, 223-225
approach to, 224, 225t
due to cryptococcal meningitis, 223-224
due to otosyphilis, 224
highly active antiretroviral therapy for, 211
and Hodgkin's lymphoma, 213t, 217
immune restoration disease in, 211-212
and Kaposi's sarcoma, 212-215, 213t
epidemiology and pathogenesis of, 212-213
presentation and diagnosis of, 213-214, 214f
treatment of, 214-215
and malignancy, 212-217, 213t
and neuropathies, 223-225
and non-Hodgkin's lymphoma, 213t, 215-216
diagnosis of, 216
epidemiology and presentation of, 216
prognosis and treatment for, 216-217
occupational exposure to, 212, 212t
and oral lesions, 225-227
aphthous ulcers as, 227, 227f
candidiasis as, 225, 226f
differential diagnosis of, 225t
fungal, 227
gingivitis and periodontal disease as, 227
hairy leukoplakia as, 225-226, 226f
due to herpes simplex virus, 226
Immunosuppression *(Continued)*
histoplasmosis as, 226-227
due to human papillomavirus, 227
otologic and neurotologic manifestations of, 221-223
malignant otitis externa as, 221-222
in middle ear, 222-223
due to *P. jiroveci* and *A. fumigatus,* 222-223
and salivary gland disease, 217-218
diffuse infiltrative lymphocytosis syndrome as, 218
parotid lesions as, 217-218, 218f
xerostomia as, 218
and sinonasal infection, 219-221
diagnosis of, 220-221, 220f
presentation and pathogenesis of, 219-220
treatment of, 221
and squamous cell carcinoma, 213t, 215
and malignancy, 212-217, 213t
basal cell carcinoma as, 213t, 215, 284
cutaneous neoplasms as, 213t, 215
Hodgkin's lymphoma as, 213t, 217
Kaposi's sarcoma as, 212-215, 213t
epidemiology and pathogenesis of, 212-213
presentation and diagnosis of, 213-214, 214f
treatment of, 214-215
non-Hodgkin's lymphoma as, 213t, 215-216
diagnosis of, 216
epidemiology and presentation of, 216
prognosis and treatment for, 216-217
in posttransplantation lymphoproliferative disorder, 213t, 215, 217
squamous cell carcinoma as, 213t, 215
and malignant otitis externa, 221-222, 1947
and neuropathies, 223-225
and oral lesions, 225-227, 1252
aphthous ulcers as, 227, 227f
candidiasis as, 225, 226f
differential diagnosis of, 225t
fungal, 227
gingivitis and periodontal disease as, 227
hairy leukoplakia as, 225-226, 226f
due to herpes simplex virus, 226
histoplasmosis as, 226-227
due to human papillomavirus, 227
oral treatment considerations with, 1246t
otologic and neurotologic manifestations of, 221-223
malignant otitis externa as, 221-222
in middle ear, 222-223
due to *P. jiroveci* and *A. fumigatus,* 222-223
and salivary gland disease, 217-218
diffuse infiltrative lymphocytosis syndrome as, 218
parotid lesions as, 217-218, 218f
xerostomia as, 218
and sinonasal infection, 219-221, 660
diagnosis of, 220-221, 220f
presentation and pathogenesis of, 219-220
treatment of, 221
and sinusitis, 660
spectrum of, 209-210, 210t
Immunotherapy
for allergic fungal rhinosinusitis, 714-715
for allergic rhinitis, 621-622
novel extracts in, 622
subcutaneous, 621
sublingual, 621-622
for head and neck squamous cell carcinoma, 1023-1024
for melanoma, 1118-1119
future investigations on, 1119
interferon in, 1118-1119
interleukin-2 and other cytokines in, 1119
Impact noise, 2121, 2140
Impedance, acoustic, 1839, 2000, 2017-2018
Impedance matching, 1839-1840, 2018
Impedance testing, for extraesophageal reflux, 900
Implant(s)
chin, 465-467
anesthesia for, 465
clinical example of, 470, 471f
complications after, 470
dissection planes for, 465-467, 467f
incision and approach for, 465-467, 467f
intraoral approach for, 467
subperiosteal *vs.* supraperiosteal placement of, 465-467, 467f
surgical procedure for, 465-467
types of, 465, 465t, 467
maxillary, in cleft-lip nose repair, 562f
nasal, for saddle nose deformity, 555, 556f-557f
Implantable adjuncts, to conventional hearing aids, 2204f, 2206t, 2217, 2217f
Implantable hearing aids, 2203-2218
as adjuncts to conventional hearing aids, 2204f, 2206t, 2217, 2217f
bone-conduction (osseointegrated), 2212-2216
background of, 2213
biology and histology of, 2213
biophysical principles of, 2213
comparison of features of, 2206t
complications of, 2215
components of, 2213f
design of, 2213
indications and contraindications for, 2212-2213, 2216t
in infants, 2723-2724
location of, 2204f
materials for, 2213
operative technique for, 2213-2215, 2214f
radiologic implications of, 2213
results of, 2215-2216, 2216t
sound transduction and coupling to auditory system with, 2205f
for unilateral sensorineural hearing loss, 2216
in young children, 2215
conventional (traditional) *vs.,* 2203-2207, 2204b, 2204f-2205f, 2206t
middle ear, 2207-2212
basic design features of, 2207-2208
ossicular coupling as, 2207-2208
transducer design as, 2207
electromagnetic, 2208-2211
Carina as, 2210-2211, 2210f-2211f
Middle Ear Transducer (MET) as, 2206t, 2210-2211, 2211f
sound transduction and coupling to auditory system with, 2205f
Vibrant Soundbridge as, 2206t, 2208-2210, 2208f-2209f
location of, 2204f
piezoelectric, 2211-2212
Esteem-Hearing Implant as, 2211-2212, 2212f
sound transduction and coupling to auditory system with, 2205f
total *vs.* partially, 2208
promise of, 2207
Implantable micropump system, for intratympanic delivery, 2183
Impressions, for prosthetic maxillary obturation, 1338-1339, 1338f
IMPT (intensity-modulated proton therapy), 1046
Impulsive noise, 2121, 2140
IMRT. *See* Intensity-modulated radiation therapy (IMRT).
IMT (inflammatory myofibroblastic tumor), of larynx, 1509-1510
In vivo gene therapy, 18-19, 19f
Incidence, 61
Incision planning, for neck surgery, 1726-1727
Incisive artery, 483

Incisive foramen
  anatomy of, 1297f
  and palate, 2659, 2660f
Incisura anterior, 1824f
Incisura tensoris, 1827f
Inclusion criteria, 68
Incomplete closure, laryngeal videostroboscopy of, 819
Incomplete partition, of cochlea, 2730-2731
  embryogenesis of, 2728f-2729f, 2729t, 2730-2731
  histology of, 2730-2731, 2731f
  imaging of, 2730-2731, 2731f
  relative incidence of, 2729t
  subtypes of, 2730-2731, 2731f
Incudal artery, 1828f
Incudostapedial articulation, 1826
Incus
  anatomy of, 1826
  in auditory physiology, 1839-1840, 1840f
  in cochlear transduction, 2062f
  embryology of, 2583-2584
  ossiculoplasty for absent lenticular process of, 2024, 2024f-2025f
  in surgical anatomy of lateral skull base, 2436f
Incus bridge, with cochlear implant, 2238-2239, 2238f
Incus interposition, in ossiculoplasty, 2024-2025, 2024f
Incus-malleus articulation, in surgical anatomy of lateral skull base, 2436f, 2438
Incus-stapes articulation, in surgical anatomy of lateral skull base, 2436f
Independent samples, statistical tests for, 66, 67t
Inderal (propranolol)
  for hyperthyroidism, 1739t
  for migraine, 2349
  for thyroid storm, 1745
Indirect laryngoscopy (IDL), for laryngeal carcinoma, 1494
Indium-111–labeled leukocyte scans, for malignant otitis externa, 1947
Individuals with Disabilities Education Act (IDEA), 2724
Indole-3-carbinol (I-3-C), for recurrent respiratory papillomatosis, 879, 2890t, 2892
Indomethacin
  for hemicrania continua, 248
  and skin flap viability, 1074
Induction chemotherapy, 1056-1058
  clinical trials of, 1056-1058, 1058f, 1058t-1059t
  in concomitant chemoradiation, 1041-1042, 1052-1053
    with adjuvant therapy, 1056
  defined, 1056
  for hypopharyngeal cancer, 1443
  for laryngeal carcinoma, 1501-1503, 1502f
Infancy
  hemangioma of (*See* Hemangioma of infancy (HOI))
  sternocleidomastoid tumors of, 2817, 2817f
Infant(s)
  cochlear implants in, 2247, 2724
  hearing aids in, 2274, 2723-2724
  hearing loss in, 2718-2725
    ancillary testing for, 2722-2723
      genetic testing in, 2722-2723
      laboratory testing in, 2722
      screening for connexin 26 mutation in, 2723
      screening for maternallyl transmitted infection in, 2723
      temporal bone imaging in, 2723
      testing for Pendred's syndrome in, 2723
    assessment of, 2719-2721
      auditory brainstem responses in, 2719-2720
      comparison of otoacoustic emissions and auditory brainstem responses in, 2721
Infant(s) *(Continued)*
      evoked otoacoustic emissions in, 2720-2721
      testing protocols for, 2719, 2720f
    delay in identification of, 2719
    diagnosis of, 2721-2722
      audiology in, 2722
      history in, 2721
      middle ear effusions in, 2722
      otomicroscopy in, 2722
      physical examination in, 2721-2722
      vestibular function assessment in, 2722
      visual reinforcement audiometry in, 2722
    history of screening for, 2718-2719
    intervention strategies for, 2723-2724
      amplification devices as, 2274, 2723-2724
      bone conduction amplification as, 2723
      cochlear implantation as, 2247, 2724
      early, 2724
      surgical therapy as, 2723
    and neural plasticity, 1885, 1885f
    prevalence of, 2719
  ideal electrolyte composition for, 2572t
  laryngoscopy in, 2866, 2867f
  lung volumes in, 2570
Infantile acute febrile mucocutaneous lymph node syndrome, facial paralysis in, 2400
Infected buccal bifurcation cysts, 1264-1265
Infection(s)
  acute otitis media and otitis media with effusion due to, 2763-2764
  bacterial
    oral manifestations of, 1252
    otitis media due to, 2763, 2764f
    pediatric chronic sinusitis due to, 2779
    of salivary glands, 1151-1153
      in children, 2851t, 2856-2857
  after chemical peel, 397
  deep neck space (*See* Deep neck space infections)
  of external ear (*See* External ear infection(s))
  hair loss due to, 376
  of masticator space, 151-152, 152f
  odontogenic (*See* Odontogenic infections)
  after otoplasty, 479
  of retropharyngeal space, 153, 155f
  of salivary glands, 1151-1161
    acute suppurative sialadenitis as, 1151-1153
      clinical manifestations of, 1152, 1152f
      complications of, 1153, 1154f
      differential diagnosis of, 1152
      epidemiology of, 1151
      laboratory evaluation of, 1152
      pathogenesis of, 1151-1152, 1152f
      treatment of, 1152-1153, 1153f
    bacterial, 1151-1153
    chronic sialadenitis as, 1154, 1155f
    granulomatous, 1158-1159
      due to actinomycosis, 1159
      due to cat scratch disease, 1159
      nontuberculous mycobacterial, 1158-1159, 1158f
      due to toxoplasmosis, 1159-1160
      tuberculous mycobacterial, 1158
    neonatal suppurative parotitis as, 1153
    recurrent parotitis of childhood as, 1153-1154
    sialolithiasis as, 1155-1156, 1155f-1156f
    Sjögren's syndrome as, 1160-1161
    ultrasound of, 1647
    viral, 1156-1158
      due to HIV, 1157-1158, 1157f
      due to mumps, 1156-1157
  after total laryngectomy, 1571
  viral
    of external ear, 1957, 1957f
      topical therapies for, 1957, 1957f
    of labyrinth
      cytomegalovirus as, 2154-2156, 2155f
      herpes simplex virus as, 2159-2160
Infection(s) *(Continued)*
      Lassa fever as, 2158-2159
      measles as, 2158
      mumps as, 2157-2158, 2158f
      rubella as, 2156-2157, 2157f
      varicella-zoster virus as, 2159, 2159f
    oral manifestations of, 1252
    otitis media due to, 2764
    and pediatric chronic sinusitis, 2778
    and rhinosinusitis, 730-731
    of salivary glands, 1156-1158
      due to HIV, 1157-1158, 1157f
      due to mumps, 1156-1157
    sensorineural hearing loss due to, 2119, 2199
      sudden, 2127
  wound, after neck surgery, 1727
Infection control, for facial trauma, 305
Infectious arthritis, of temporomandibular joint, 1281-1282, 1281t
Infectious disease(s)
  oral manifestations of, 1252
  otologic manifestations of, 2100-2106
    in Lyme disease, 2105-2106
    in mycotic diseases, 2106, 2106f
    otorrhea as, 2196
    in syphilis, 2105, 2105f
    in tuberculosis, 2101-2103, 2102f-2103f
  sensorineural hearing loss due to, 2118-2119
    sudden, 2127-2128
Infectious esophagitis, 976-977
  due to *Candida albicans,* 976, 976f
    imaging of, 1404, 1405f
  due to cytomegalovirus, 976, 977f
  due to herpes simplex virus, 976-977, 977f-978f
    imaging of, 1404, 1405f
  imaging of, 1404, 1405f
Infectious mononucleosis (IM)
  adenotonsillar disease in, 2785-2786, 2786f
  pharyngitis due to, 198-199, 198f
  sudden sensorineural hearing loss due to, 2127
  vestibular neuritis due to, 2162
Infectious rhinitis, 619b
Inference, 65
Inferior alveolar artery, 1296, 1359f
Inferior alveolar nerve, 1359f
Inferior alveolar vein, 1359f
Inferior anastomotic vein, 2489
Inferior anulus, of tympanic membrane, 1825-1826
Inferior arcuate line, of vocal folds, in mucosal wave propagation, 848-849
Inferior canaliculus, of lacrimal apparatus, 798f
Inferior cervical sympathetic ganglion, in root of neck, 2582
Inferior colliculus
  in central auditory pathway, 1835f, 1836, 1846
  tonotopic map reorganization in, 1878, 1879f, 1880
Inferior concha, 1359f
Inferior crus, of ear, 476f, 2742f
Inferior deep jugular lymph nodes, 1360f
Inferior hypophyseal arteries, in surgical anatomy of anterior cranial base, 2473f
Inferior incisive muscle, 321f
Inferior medial maxillectomy, 1125, 1125f
Inferior nasal meatus
  normal anatomy of, 664
  in surgical anatomy of anterior cranial base, 2472, 2472f
Inferior oblique muscles, 443f
  in lower eyelid blepharoplasty, 448-449, 450f
  semicircular canal planes and, 2287, 2288f
  in surgical anatomy of lateral skull base, 2439f
Inferior orbital fissure, 322f
  in surgical anatomy of anterior cranial base, 2443-2444, 2444f
  in surgical anatomy of lateral skull base, 2441
  in surgical anatomy of middle cranial base, 2445f

Inferior orbital rims, 319
Inferior petrosal sinus, in surgical anatomy of lateral skull base, 2489
Inferior punctum, of lacrimal apparatus, 798f
Inferior rectus muscles, 443f
semicircular canal planes and, 2287, 2288f
Inferior tarsal muscle, 444
Inferior thyroid artery
anatomy of, 1751, 1752f
and parathyroid glands, 1778
in root of neck, 2581-2582, 2581f
Inferior turbinate
normal anatomy of, 665f, 1124f
in surgical anatomy of anterior cranial base, 2472, 2472f-2473f
Inferior tympanic artery, 1828f
Inferior vestibular ganglion, 1854f, 2278f
Inferior vestibular nerve, in surgical anatomy of lateral skull base, 2437f, 2439
Inferior vestibular nucleus, 1861, 1862f
Inflammation
in acutely raised skin flaps, 1070
and rhinosinusitis, 731, 731f
and skin flap viability, 1074
Inflammatory bowel disease, oral manifestations of, 1254
Inflammatory collateral cyst, 1263, 1263f
Inflammatory condition(s)
of esophagus (*See* Esophagitis)
of larynx, 1464-1466
croup as, 1465, 1465f
epiglottitis as, 159-161, 163f, 1464, 1464f-1465f
laryngeal stenosis due to, 2915
retropharyngeal abscess as, 1465-1466, 1466f
of oral cavity, 1288-1290
amyloidosis as, 1289-1290, 1290f
fibroma as, 1288-1289, 1289f
mucosal ulcerations as, 1289, 1289f
necrotizing sialometaplasia as, 1289, 1299
pyogenic granuloma as, 1289, 1289f
of salivary glands, 1151-1161
acute suppurative sialadenitis as, 1151-1153
in children, 2856, 2856t
clinical manifestations of, 1152, 1152f
complications of, 1153, 1154f
differential diagnosis of, 1152
epidemiology of, 1151
laboratory evaluation of, 1152
pathogenesis of, 1151-1152, 1152f
treatment of, 1152-1153, 1153f
bacterial infections as, 1151-1153
in children, 2856-2857, 2856t
in children, 2855-2858
abscess as, 2856
due to actinomycosis, 2858
acute suppurative sialadenitis as, 2856, 2856t
bacterial, 2856-2857, 2856t
chronic sialadenitis as, 2858
diagnostic algorithm for, 2853, 2854f
differential diagnosis of, 2851t
due to Epstein-Barr virus, 2855
granulomatous, 2857-2858, 2857f
due to HIV, 2856
due to mumps, 2855
mycobacterial, 2857-2858, 2857f
neonatal, 2857
recurrent, 2856-2857
sarcoidosis as, 2858
viral, 2855
chronic sialadenitis as, 1154, 1155f
in children, 2858
granulomatous infections as, 1158-1159
due to actinomycosis, 1159
due to cat scratch disease, 1159
in children, 2857-2858, 2857f
Inflammatory condition(s) *(Continued)*
due to nontuberculous mycobacterial disease, 1158-1159, 1158f
due to toxoplasmosis, 1159-1160
due to tuberculous mycobacterial disease, 1158
neonatal suppurative parotitis as, 1153
noninfectious, 1160-1161
recurrent parotitis of childhood as, 1153-1154
sialolithiasis as, 1155-1156, 1155f-1156f
viral infections as, 1156-1158
in children, 2855
due to Epstein-Barr virus, 2855
due to HIV, 1157-1158, 1157f, 2856
due to mumps, 1156-1157, 2855
Inflammatory lymph nodes, 164
Inflammatory myofibroblastic tumor (IMT), of larynx, 1509-1510
Inflammatory neck masses, 1638
due to granulomatous diseases, 1638
due to lymphadenopathy/lymphadenitis, 1638
due to sialadenitis/sialolithiasis, 1638
Inflammatory phase, of wound healing, 1076
Influenza vaccine, 197
to prevent otitis media, 2769
Influenzavirus, pharyngitis due to, 196-197
Informed consent, 102
Infracochlear approach, for skull base lesions requiring drainage, 2539, 2540f
Infra-frequency sounds, adverse effects of, 2149
Infrahyoid muscles, characteristics of, 918-919
Infrahyoid neck, imaging of, 157-159
anterior and posterior cervical (lateral cervical) spaces in, 158, 159f-160f, 162f
CT for, 140
hypopharyngeal mucosal space in, 158-159
with lesions, 159, 162f
normal anatomy in, 158-159, 159f-160f
MRI for, 142-143
normal anatomy in, 157-159, 159f-160f
prevertebral space in, 158, 159f-160f, 162f
retropharyngeal space in, 158
with lesions, 158, 161f
normal anatomy in, 158, 159f-160f
ultrasound for, 143-144
Infrahyoid prevertebral space, imaging of, 158, 159f-160f, 162f
Infrahyoid retropharyngeal space, imaging of, 158, 159f-161f
Infralabyrinthine approach, for skull base lesions requiring drainage, 2539, 2540f
Infraorbital cells, 668-669, 670f
Infraorbital fissure, 1124f
Infraorbital foramen, 439-440, 1124f
Infraorbital groove, 322f
Infraorbital lymph node, 1360f
Infraorbital nerve, 320, 321f, 497, 497f
Infraorbital nerve block, 242
Infraorbital neurovascular bundle, 439-440
Infraorbital rims, surgical access to, 329
Infraparotid node, 1297f
Infrared video, for recording eye movements, 2317
Infratemporal access, for transnasal endoscopic-assisted anterior skull base surgery, 2483
Infratemporal fossa
in surgical anatomy of lateral skull base, 2440-2441, 2440f
in surgical anatomy of middle cranial base, 2444
Infratemporal fossa approaches, 2495-2501
for middle skull base surgery, 2461-2464, 2464f
postauricular, 2495-2500
cervical dissection in, 2495, 2498f
closure of external auditory canal in, 2495, 2497f
extratemporal facial nerve dissection in, 2495-2496
incisions and skins flaps in, 2495, 2497f
Infratemporal fossa approaches *(Continued)*
radical mastoidectomy in, 2496, 2498f
removal of external auditory canal wall skin and tympanic membrane in, 2495, 2497f
type A, 2497-2499
closure of wound in, 2499, 2499f
exposure of jugular bulb and internal carotid artery in, 2498, 2498f-2499f
facial nerve transposition in, 2497-2498, 2498f
occlusion of sigmoid sinus in, 2498, 2498f
tumor removal in, 2498-2499, 2499f
type B, 2499-2500, 2500f
type C, 2500, 2501f
preauricular, 2500-2501, 2501f
Infratemporal fossa dissection, in subtotal or total temporal bone resection, 2494
Infratip lobule, 509f
Infratrochlear nerve, 321f, 497, 497f
Infundibular cells, 740
Infundibulum, 665f, 666-667
Ingals, E. F., 488
Ingestive sequence, 1206, 1206f
Inhalational agents, in children
for anesthesia induction, 2590
for anesthesia maintenance, 2591
Inheritance, 4
Inheritance patterns, 2088-2089, 2088f
autosomal dominant, 2088, 2088f
autosomal recessive, 2088-2089
mitochondrial, 2089
molecular basis of, 4
Punnett squares for, 2088, 2089f
X-linked, 2089
Inherited disorders
gene therapy for, 20
oral manifestations of, 1257
Inhibitory cutoff, of vestibular hair cells, 2290-2291
Inion, 320f
Injectable filler, with blepharoplasty, 451
Ink4D, in murine deafness, 2058t-2060t
Innate immune system, 209, 598-599
adaptive *vs.,* 597-598
antimicrobial peptides in, 598-599
cathelicidins as, 599
defensins as, 599
tissue distribution of, 599
overview of, 597-598
self and nonself in, 599
toll-like receptors in, 598
activators of, 598
and adaptive immune response, 598
expression and distribution of, 598
and host, 598
Inner border cells, 1833f
Inner ear
anatomy of, 1825f, 1831-1834
hair cells in, 1832-1834, 1833f
innervation in, 1834, 1834f
membranous labyrinth and inner ear fluids in, 1831-1832, 1832f
osteology in, 1831, 1832f
in auditory physiology, 1840-1844
basilar membrane in, 1840-1842, 1841f-1842f
cochlea in, 1841f-1842f
cochlear partition in, 1840-1842, 1842f
endocochlear potential in, 1840, 1841f-1842f
endolymph in, 1841f-1842f
hair cells in
inner, 1841f, 1842, 1844f
outer, 1841f, 1844, 1844f
stereocilia of, 1841f, 1842, 1843f
tip links of, 1841f, 1842, 1843f
tonotopic tuning of, 1844, 1844f
organ of Corti in, 1841f
perilymph in, 1841f-1842f
Reissner's membrane in, 1841f

Inner ear *(Continued)*
scala media in, 1840, 1841f-1842f
scala tympani in, 1841f-1842f
scala vestibuli in, 1841f-1842f
spiral ligament in, 1841f
spiral limbus in, 1841f
stapes footplate in, 1840, 1842f
stria vascularis in, 1840, 1841f
tectorial membrane in, 1841f
"third window" in, 1842, 1843f
congenital malformations of, 2726-2740
classification of, 2726-2727, 2727b
cochlear, 2729-2732
cochlear agenesis as, 2729f
cochlear aplasia as, 2728f, 2729-2730, 2729t
cochlear aqueduct enlargement as, 2734, 2734f
cochlear hyperplasia as, 2732
cochlear hypoplasia as, 2728f-2730f, 2729t, 2730
cochlear implantation for, 2739
in combination with other anomalies, 2728, 2738, 2739f
common cavity as, 2728f-2729f, 2729t, 2731-2732
embryogenesis of, 2728-2735, 2728f-2729f
incomplete partition as, 2728f-2729f, 2729t, 2730-2731, 2731f
relative incidence of, 2729t
complete labyrinthine aplasia as, 2729, 2729f-2730f, 2729t
in congenital aural atresia, 2738
CSF leakage and meningitis due to, 2735-2737, 2736f
of eighth nerve, 2735
evaluation and management of, 2738-2739, 2739f
imaging of, 172-173, 174f, 1920-1921, 1923f, 2738
incidence of, 2727
of internal auditory canal, 2735
narrow, 2735, 2735f
wide, 2735, 2735f
labyrinthine, 2732-2733
in combination with other anomalies, 2728, 2738, 2739f
incidence of, 2727
limited to membranous labyrinth, 2727-2728, 2727b
of membranous and osseous labyrinth, 2727b, 2728-2735
membranous labyrinthine dysplasia as, 2727-2728
semicircular canal aplasia as, 2732-2733, 2732f
semicircular canal dysplasia as, 2732, 2732f-2733f
pathogenesis of, 2726
perilymphatic fistula as, 2737-2738, 2737f
sensorineural hearing loss due to, 2200
syndrome correlations and familial patterns of, 2735
vestibular aqueduct enlargement as, 2727, 2733-2734, 2733f
X-linked stapes gusher syndrome as, 2737
growth and development of, 2617t, 2726
imaging of, 172-173, 1920-1922
with congenital anomalies, 172-173, 174f, 1920-1921, 1923f
with enlarged vestibular aqueduct, 1921, 1923f
with fenestral and cochlear otosclerosis (otospongiosis), 1921-1922, 1925f
with intravestibular schwannoma, 1921, 1924f
with labyrinthitis ossificans, 1921, 1925f
normal appearance of, 1920-1921, 1922f
with superior semicircular canal dehiscence, 1920-1921, 1922f
Inner ear conductive presbycusis, 232
Inner ear decompression sickness (IEDS), 2343
Inner ear disease
autoimmune, 2164-2168
clinical presentation of, 2165-2166
defined, 2164
diagnosis of, 2166, 2167t
differential diagnosis of, 2166
epidemiology of, 2165
future directions for, 2167-2168
pathology and pathogenesis of, 2165
animal studies of, 2165
human temporal bone studies of, 2165
sensorineural hearing loss due to, 2124, 2165
treatment of, 2166-2167
gene therapy for, 2191-2192
delivery of, 2191
preclinical applications of, 2192
safety concerns with, 2192
vectors for, 2191, 2191t
intratympanic delivery of medications for (*See* Intratympanic delivery)
systemic steroids for, 2184
Inner ear fluids, 1831-1832, 1832f
Inner hair cells (IHCs)
anatomy of, 1832-1834, 1833f
in organ of Corti, 1832, 1832f, 1840
arrangement of, 2071, 2072f
in auditory physiology, 1841f, 1842, 1844f
in cochlear transduction, 2061f-2062f, 2066-2067
length of, 2070, 2070f
number and density of, 2070
receptor potentials for, 2071, 2072f
scanning electron micrograph of, 1833f
stereocilia on, 2070f, 2071, 2072f
transduction channels in, 2073f
Inner pillar head plate, 1833f
Inner spiral sulcus, 1832, 1832f
Innominate artery compression, of trachea, 2925-2926
Inorganic iodine
for Graves' disease, 1742-1743
for thyroid storm, 1745
Inosculation, in acutely raised skin flaps, 1069, 1069f
Inositol triphosphate (IP_3)
in olfactory transduction, 629
in salivary gland secretion, 1137-1138
"I-notch," in nasal breathing assessment, 644
INS(s) (intranasal steroids), for allergic rhinitis, 621
Insertion loss, with hearing aids, 2270
Inside-out approach, for pediatric facial fracture repair, 2706f
Insomnia, 262-263, 263b
in children, 263
paradoxical, 263
primary (idiopathic), 262t, 263
psychophysiological, 262t, 263
tinnitus and, 2138
Inspiratory resistance, in rhinomanometry, 650-651
Institute for Healthcare Improvement (IHI), 84t-87t
Institute of Medicine (IOM), 81-82, 84t-87t
Insular thyroid carcinoma, 1764
Insular-opercular region, in gustatory pathway, 1212-1213
Insulin growth factors I and II, for facial nerve paralysis, 2427
Insulin release, cephalic phase, 1206
Insulin-like growth factor-I (IGF-I), in wound healing, 1076
Integrase inhibitors, 211
Integrative genomics, in head and neck squamous cell carcinoma, 1025
Integrin(s), in wound healing, 1077
Integrin α8β1 *(Itga8)* gene, in murine deafness, 2058t-2060t
Intense pulse light laser, for facial resurfacing, 403t
Intensity
in acoustic analysis for voice evaluation, 829, 829t
of sound, 1839
Intensity-modulated proton therapy (IMPT), 1046
Intensity-modulated radiation therapy (IMRT), 1043-1046, 1044f
advantages of, 1043
for cervical metastases, 1691-1692, 1692f
clinical results of, 1045-1046, 1045f
complications of, 1700
defining target in, 1044
dental management after, 1335-1337, 1336f-1337f
forward-planning, 1696-1697
for glottic cancer, 1585-1586
inverse-planning, 1043, 1696-1697
for nasopharyngeal carcinoma, 1045, 1699-1700, 1699f, 1700t
number and directions of beams in, 1045
selection and outlining of targets in, 1044-1045, 1045f
for skull base tumors, 1696-1697
and xerostomia, 1103
Interarytenoid adhesion, 2915, 2915f-2916f
Interarytenoid muscle
applied anatomy of, 806
in professional voice production, 846-847
Interarytenoid web, 2869, 2869f
Interaural attenuation, in audiologic testing, 1889
Intercalated duct, of salivary gland, 1134, 1134f, 1162, 1163f
Intercanthal distances
in aesthetic analysis, 271
in evaluation of maxillofacial trauma, 324, 324f
with nasal fracture, 498
normal, 442
Intercanthal line, 496, 497f
Intercellular secretory canaliculi, of salivary gland, 1134f
Interdental discrimination, 1207
Interdomal ligament, 496-497
Interfascicular nerve repair, 2422-2424
Interferon(s) (IFNs), 609t-610t
for hemangioma of infancy, 2826-2828
for recurrent respiratory papillomatosis, 879, 2890t, 2891-2892
for rhinosinusitis, 734t
Interferon-α (IFN-α), 609t-610t
for recurrent respiratory papillomatosis, 879, 2890t, 2891-2892
thyrotoxicosis due to, 1744
Interferon-α-2b (IFN-α-2β), for melanoma, 1118-1119
Interferon-β (IFN-β), 609t-610t
Interferon-γ (IFN-γ), 609t-610t
Intergroup Rhabdomyosarcoma Study Clinical Grouping Classification (IRSCGC), 2841, 2841t
Interior carotid artery, 2351f
Interleukin(s) (ILs), 609t-610t
in allergic rhinitis, 615
Interleukin-1α (IL-1α), 609t-610t
Interleukin-1β (IL-1β), 609t-610t
Interleukin-2 (IL-2), 609t-610t
in gene therapy, 20-21
for head and neck squamous cell carcinoma, 1023-1024
for melanoma, 1119
Interleukin-3 (IL-3), 609t-610t
Interleukin-4 (IL-4), 609t-610t
Interleukin-5 (IL-5), 609t-610t
Interleukin-6 (IL-6), 609t-610t
Interleukin-7 (IL-7), 609t-610t

Interleukin-8 (IL-8), 609t-610t
in wound healing, 1076
Interleukin-9 (IL-9), 609t-610t
Interleukin-10 (IL-10), 609t-610t
Interleukin-11 (IL-11), 609t-610t
Interleukin-12 (IL-12), 609t-610t
for head and neck squamous cell carcinoma, 1023-1024
Interleukin-13 (IL-13), 609t-610t
Interleukin-14 (IL-14), 609t-610t
Interleukin-15 (IL-15), 609t-610t
Interleukin-16 (IL-16), 609t-610t
Interleukin-17 (IL-17), 609t-610t
Interleukin-18 (IL-18), 609t-610t
Interleukin-19 (IL-19), 609t-610t
Interleukin-20 (IL-20), 609t-610t
Interleukin-21 (IL-21), 609t-610t
Interleukin-22 (IL-22), 609t-610t
Interleukin-23 (IL-23), 609t-610t
Interleukin-24 (IL-24), 609t-610t
Interleukin-25 (IL-25), 609t-610t
Interleukin-26 (IL-26), 609t-610t
Interleukin-27 (IL-27), 609t-610t
Interleukin-28 (IL-28), 609t-610t
Interleukin-29 (IL-29), 609t-610t
Intermaxillary fixation (IMF) screws, 330-331, 333f
Intermaxillary segment, in embryology of palate, 2660-2661, 2662f
Intermaxillary suture, 320f
Intermediate acoustic stria
anatomy of, 1835, 1835f
in auditory pathway, 1846
Intermediate crus, of nose, 496-497, 497f
Intermittent allergic rhinitis (IAR), 618
Intermittent apnea-reintubation anesthesia, with recurrent respiratory papillomatosis, 2891
Internal acoustic meatus, 2010f
Internal acoustic pore, in surgical anatomy of lateral skull base, 2437-2438
Internal auditory artery
anatomy of, 1826f, 1854, 2351f
in surgical anatomy of lateral skull base, 2437f, 2439f
Internal auditory canal (IAC)
anatomy of, 1823f
developmental anomalies of, 2735
and CSF leakage, 2735-2736, 2736f
narrow, 2735, 2735f
wide, 2735, 2735f
imaging of, 173, 1926-1928
with meningioma, 175f
with vestibular schwannoma, 173, 1928, 1928f
lipoma of, 2527, 2529f
narrow, 2735, 2735f
in surgical anatomy of lateral skull base, 2435f-2437f, 2438-2439
wide, 2735, 2735f
Internal auditory meatus, in surgical anatomy of middle cranial base, 2445f
Internal carotid artery (ICA)
aberrant, 1919-1920, 1921f-1922f
anatomy of, 1359f, 2579, 2580f
radiographic, 1471f, 1473-1474
aneurysms of upper cervical and petrous, 2504, 2504f-2505f
in extended neck dissection, 1719-1721, 1720f
injury to, 1632, 1633f
due to carotid paraganglioma surgery, 1661
paranasal sinuses and, 671-672
in postauricular approach to infratemporal fossa, 2498, 2498f-2499f
preoperative embolization of, 2446
preoperative management of, 2445-2446, 2446f, 2489
Internal carotid artery (ICA) *(Continued)*
algorithm for, 2490f, 2491-2492
cerebral blood flow assessment in, 2490-2491, 2490f
four-vessel arteriography in, 2489-2490, 2491f
in surgical anatomy of anterior cranial base, 2442-2443, 2472f-2473f, 2474, 2475f
in surgical anatomy of lateral skull base, 2436f-2437f, 2439f-2440f, 2489
in surgical anatomy of middle cranial base, 2444
tortuous, 1416, 1416f
Internal consistency, 55
Internal fixation, and facial growth, 2625-2626
Internal jugular vein (IJV)
anatomy of, 1359f, 2579f
radiographic, 1471f
in modified radical neck dissection, 1713f-1714f
in neck surgery, 1728-1729, 1729f
Internal jugular vein (IJV) hemorrhage, due to neck surgery, 1729, 1729f
Internal jugular vein (IJV) thrombosis, due to neck surgery, 1728-1729
Internal maxillary artery
anatomy of, 682
in surgical anatomy of lateral skull base, 2440f
Internal plexiform layer, of olfactory bulb, 628f
Internal pterygoid muscle, 1359f
Internal receiver stimulators and electrode designs, for cochlear implants, 2227-2229
HiRes 90K receiver/stimulator as, 2227-2228, 2228f
Med-El PulsarCI100 and SonataTI100 as, 2228-2229, 2228f-2230f
ear-level speech processors for, 2232f
Nucleus Freedom device with Contour Advance electrode as, 2227, 2227f-2228f
external speech processors for, 2232f
Internal thoracic artery, in root of neck, 2581-2582
Internal validity, 68-69, 68t, 69f
Internal valve compromise, nasal obstruction due to, 492, 493f
Internasal suture, 320f
International Classification of Functioning (ICF), 56
International Prognostic Index (IPI), for non-Hodgkin's lymphoma, 216
Interneurons, in neural plasticity, 1884
Interobserver reliability, 55
Interosseous fold, 1827f
Interpeak latencies, in auditory brainstem response, 1897
Interpolated flaps, 344-345, 344f
for nasal defects, 347-348
Interpupillary distances, in evaluation of maxillofacial trauma, 324, 324f
Interquartile range, 64t
Interrupted strip technique, for nasal tip refinement, 522, 532f-533f
Intersphenoid synchondrosis, 2619f
Interstereociliary linkages, 2076f, 2077-2078
Interstitial pressure, of skin flaps, 1068, 1069f
Interstitial system, and skin flaps, 1065-1066, 1065f
Intertragal incisure, 477
Intertragal notch, 2742f
Interval examination, in laryngeal stroboscopy, 847
Interventional neuroradiology, 1932-1943
for lesions of vascular etiology, 1939-1943
dural arteriovenous fistulas as, 1940-1942, 1941f
epistaxis as, 1939-1940, 1940f
facial arteriovenous fistulas as, 1940, 1940f
facial vascular malformations as, 1942, 1942f
hemangiomas of face and neck as, 1942
pseudoaneurysms as, 1942, 1943f
tinnitus-producing fibromuscular dysplasia of carotid artery as, 1943
Interventional neuroradiology *(Continued)*
materials and techniques for, 1932-1934
angiographic catheters as, 1932-1933
angiographic equipment as, 1932
embolic agents as, 1933-1934
provocative testing to ensure safety of embolization as, 1934, 1934f
for neoplasms, 1934-1939
inter-arterial chemotherapy as, 1939
juvenile angiofibroma as, 1937-1938, 1938f
meningiomas as, 1938, 1939f
paragangliomas as, 1934-1937, 1935f
carotid body tumor as, 1937, 1937f
glomus jugulare tumor as, 1935-1936, 1935f-1936f
glomus tympanicum tumor as, 1935
glomus vagale tumor as, 1936-1937, 1936f
thyroid, 1938-1939
Interventional techniques, for chronic pain, 245-246, 246t
In-the-canal (ITC) hearing aid, 2270, 2270f
In-the-ear (ITE) hearing aids, 2270, 2270f
in infants, 2723-2724
selection of, 2266-2267, 2270
Intra-arterial chemotherapy, 1939
Intra-articular disk, anterior displacement of
with reduction, 1280, 1282f
without reduction, 1279-1280, 1282f
Intra-axial tumor(s), 2528-2529
brainstem gliomas as, 2528
hemangioblastomas as, 2528
malignant choroid plexus papillomas and ependymomas of fourth ventricle as, 2528-2529, 2530f-2531f
medulloblastomas as, 2528
Intracapsular disorders, of temporomandibular joint, 1280-1282, 1281t
ankylosis as, 1281t, 1282
anterior disk displacement as
with reduction, 1280, 1282f
without reduction, 1279-1280, 1282f
degenerative joint disease as, 1281-1282, 1281t
Intracapsular subtotal tonsillectomy, for obstructive sleep apnea, 2609
Intracellular pH, in sour taste, 1209
Intracellular space, 1066-1067
Intracerebral injury, due to sphenoidotomy, 768t
Intracochlear membrane rupture, sudden sensorineural hearing loss due to, 2128
Intracordal cysts, 869-870
diagnosis of, 869
history in, 869
laryngeal examination in, 869
vocal capability battery in, 869
epidemiology of, 869
epidermoid inclusion, 868f-869f, 869
mucus retention (ductal), 869, 869f-870f
open, 869, 870f
pathophysiology and pathology of, 869
treatment of, 869-870
behavioral, 869-870
medical, 869
surgical, 870, 870f
Intracordal injection, for vocal fold paralysis, 907, 907f
Intracranial approach, for middle cranial base surgery, 2467
Intracranial complications
of endoscopic sinus surgery, 755, 755f
of otitic infections, 2347
Intracranial hypertension, benign (idiopathic)
CSF rhinorrhea due to, 787
facial paralysis due to, 2400-2401
sensorineural hearing loss due to, 2123
Intracranial paraganglioma, 2499f
Intracranial pressure (ICP), and CSF rhinorrhea, 786-787, 786b

Intracranial sources, of otorrhea, 2195b, 2197
Intradermal nevus, 286, 287f
IntraEar Microcatheter, 2182-2183, 2183f
Intraepithelial lymphocytes, in immune system, 605
Intraglandular parotid lymph node, 1360f
Intralabyrinthine shunt, for Meniere's disease, 2126
Intralesional corticosteroids, for scar revision, 299-300, 301f
Intralymphatic metastasis, of melanoma, 1112
Intramembranous bone formation, 2614
Intramuscular induction, of pediatric anesthesia, 2591
Intranasal dimensions, tests that assess, 643, 643f
Intranasal ethmoidectomy, 756-757
Intranasal hemangiomas, 2695
Intranasal steroids (INSs), for allergic rhinitis, 621
In-transit metastasis (ITM), of melanoma, 1110, 1117
Intraocular pressure, increased, in Graves' ophthalmopathy, 1808
Intraoperative cranial nerve monitoring, 2542-2556
  anesthesia and, 2544
  auditory brainstem response recording for, 2552-2554
    interpretation of, 2553-2554, 2553f
    and postoperative auditory function, 2553-2554
    reducing electrical and acoustic interference in, 2552-2553
    stimulus and recording parameters, electrodes, and placement in, 2552
  of cochlear nerve, 2552
    direct eighth nerve action potentials for, 2554
      detection and interpretation of changes in, 2554
      placement of electrodes in, 2554
      stimulus and recording parameters in, 2554
  electrodes for
    recording, 2543-2544, 2543f
    stimulating, 2544, 2544f
  of facial nerve, 2545-2549
    with acoustic neuroma and other cerebellopontine angle tumors, 2545
    activity evoked by electrical stimulation in, 2545-2546
    for assessment of functional status after tumor removal, 2545-2546
    electromyography for, 2545-2548
    for intraoperative identification of nervus intermedius, 2546, 2546f
    limitations of, 2547-2548, 2548f
    during microvascular decompression, 2548-2549, 2549f
    during other otologic surgery, 2549
    during parotid surgery, 2549
    spontaneous and mechanically evoked activity in, 2546-2548, 2547f
  future directions in, 2555-2556, 2555f
  instrumentation for, 2543
  ninth, tenth, eleventh, and twelfth, 2550-2552, 2551f-2552f
  and outcome, 2554-2555
    for cochlear nerve preservation, 2554-2555
    for facial and other motor cranial nerve preservation, 2554
  personnel for, 2542-2543
  stimulation criteria for, 2544
  third, fourth, and sixth, 2549-2550, 2550f
  of trigeminal motor branch, 2550
Intraoral positioning devices, for radiation therapy, 1331, 1333f
Intratemporal facial nerve surgery, 2403-2415
  combination approaches for, 2411-2412
  draping for, 2404-2405, 2405f
  for facial nerve tumors, 2413-2414, 2414t
  general surgical techniques for, 2404-2405
  instrumentation for, 2405
  intraoperative monitoring for, 2405, 2405f
Intratemporal facial nerve surgery *(Continued)*
  middle cranial fossa (transtemporal) approach for, 2407-2409
    advantages and uses of, 2408-2409
    for Bell's palsy, 2409-2410, 2409t-2410t
    limitations and potential complications of, 2409
    technique of, 2407-2408, 2408f-2409f
  nerve repair in, 2413-2414
  rerouting in, 2412, 2412f-2413f
    partial, 2412-2413
  retrolabyrinthine approach for, 2405-2406, 2405f-2406f
  retrosigmoid approach for, 2406-2407
    advantages and uses of, 2406-2407
    limitations and potential complications of, 2407
    technique of, 2406, 2407f
  surgical anatomy for, 2403-2404, 2404f
  translabyrinthine approach for, 2411
    advantages and uses of, 2411
    limitations and complications of, 2411
    technique of, 2411, 2411f-2412f
  transmastoid approach for, 2410-2411
    advantages and uses of, 2411
    limitations and complications of, 2411
    technique of, 2410, 2410f
Intratemporal fossa approaches, for middle cranial base surgery, 2455t
Intrathecal fluorescein, for CSF rhinorrhea, 790, 2044
Intratympanic delivery
  of gentamicin, 2185-2189
    clinical protocols for, 2187-2188
    complications of, 2188-2189
    concentration of, 2188
    dose of, 2188
    indications and contraindications for, 2189
    injection interval for, 2188
    mechanism of action of, 2185-2186
    for Meniere's disease, 2185-2189, 2338-2339, 2338f
    number of injections of, 2188
    pharmacokinetics of, 2186-2187, 2186f-2187f
    practical considerations with, 2188
  kinetics of, 2181, 2181f
  method of, 2182-2183, 2182f-2183f
    via implantable micropump system, 2183
    via sustained-release devices, 2182-2183, 2182f-2183f
  round window membrane in, 2179-2183
    anatomy of, 2179-2180, 2180f
    kinetics of, 2181, 2181f
    method of, 2182-2183, 2182f-2183f
    obstructive adhesions and, 2181-2182
    permeability of, 2180-2181
    physiology of, 2180, 2181f
  of steroids, 2183-2185
    dosing of, 2185
    indications for, 2183
    mechanism of action of, 2183
    for Meniere's disease, 2184, 2339
    pharmacokinetics of, 2183-2184
    side effects of, 2185
    for sudden sensorineural hearing loss, 2184-2185
Intrauterine causes, of craniofacial anomalies, 2640
Intrauterine infection, infant hearing impairment due to, 2723
Intravenous agents, for pediatric anesthesia
  induction of, 2590
  maintenance of, 2591-2592, 2593t
Intravenous immune globulin (IVIG)
  for pediatric chronic sinusitis, 2779
  for rhinosinusitis, 735t, 737
Intravenous smell testing, 632
Intravestibular schwannoma, imaging of, 1921, 1924f
Intrinsic laryngeal muscles, 806-807, 806f-807f
Introns, 4, 5f
Intubation granuloma(s), 939, 941f
  of vocal folds, 875-876, 875f
    diagnosis of, 875-876
      history in, 875
      vocal capability battery in, 875-876
    epidemiology of, 875
    management of, 876
    pathophysiology and pathology of, 875
Invagination theory, of cholesteatoma formation, 1966, 1967f
Invasive fungal rhinosinusitis (IFRS), 705
  due to *Aspergillus,* 705, 710-711, 712f
    in immunocompromised host, 220-221, 220f
  due to *Candida,* 711
  chronic or indolent, 711
  diagnosis of, 711, 711f-712f
  immunosuppression and
    diagnosis of, 220-221, 220f
    presentation and pathogenesis of, 220
    treatment of, 221
  due to mucormycosis, 705, 710, 711f
  rapidly invasive (fulminant), 709-710, 710f
  surgical management of, 742
  therapy for, 711-712, 713t
Inverse filtered flow, for measurement of vocal fold vibration, 830-831
Inverse-planning intensity-modulated radiation therapy (IP-IMRT), 1043, 1696-1697
Inversion, 4-5
Inversion technique, for Zenker's diverticulum, 992f
Inverted papilloma
  ductal, of salivary glands, 1171-1172
  of nasopharynx, 1349
  sinonasal, 718-720, 1127
    endoscopic appearance of, 718-719, 719f
    epidemiology of, 718
    with frontal sinus involvement, 720, 720f
    histologic appearance of, 718
    human papillomavirus and, 718
    imaging of, 719, 719f
    postoperative surveillance for, 720
    recurrence of, 720
    sites for, 718
    and squamous cell carcinoma, 718
    surgical approach for, 718t, 719-720, 720f, 763, 1127
Inverted V sign, after rhinoplasty, 492, 493f
Investing fascia, 202
  of neck, 2577, 2578f
Iodide, in control of thyroid function, 1739
Iodide transport, in thyroid hormone synthesis, 1737, 1737f
Iodination, in thyroid hormone synthesis, 1737f, 1738
Iodine
  compound solution of, for hyperthyroidism, 1739t
  in control of thyroid function, 1739
  daily intake of, 1737
  excessive intake of, hypothyroidism due to, 1747
  inorganic
    for Graves' disease, 1742-1743
    for thyroid storm, 1745
  radioactive
    for Graves' disease, 1743
    for Graves' ophthalmopathy, 1810
    stunning with, 1771
    after thyroid surgery, 1771-1772
    for toxic multinodular goiter, 1745
    for toxic thyroid adenoma, 1744
  in radioactive iodine uptake test, 1741
  in saliva, 1139
Iodine-induced thyrotoxicosis, 1744
Iodothyronine deiodinases, 1738
IOM (Institute of Medicine), 81-82, 84t-87t

Ionic contrast agents, for imaging of pharynx and esophagus, 1396
Ionizing radiation, 1032, 1036
and parathyroid neoplasm(s), 1775
and thyroid carcinoma, 1753
Iowa Pain Thermometer (IPT), 240
IP_3 (inositol triphosphate)
in olfactory transduction, 629
in salivary gland secretion, 1137-1138
IPI (International Prognostic Index), for non-Hodgkin's lymphoma, 216
IP-IMRT (inverse-planning intensity-modulated radiation therapy), 1043, 1696-1697
Ipodate, for hyperthyroidism, 1739t
Ipratropium bromide
for allergic rhinitis, 620
for nonallergic rhinitis, 701
IPT (Iowa Pain Thermometer), 240
IRD (immune restoration disease), 211-212
cryptococcal meningitis in, 224
Iron deficiency, oral manifestations of, 1254
Iron-dependent pathway, in cisplatin ototoxicity, 2172-2173
Irradiance, of surgical laser, 27
Irradiated tissue, gene therapy for repair and regeneration of, 23
Irradiation. *See* Radiation exposure.
Irregular closure, laryngeal videostroboscopy of, 819
Irregularization, for scar revision, 298
geometric broken line closure in, 298, 299f-300f
W-plasty in, 298, 299f
Z-plasty in, 298, 298f-299f
Irrigation, for pediatric chronic sinusitis, 2779
Irritant rhinitis, 697-698
Irritation fibroma, of oral cavity, 1288-1289, 1289f
IRSCGC (Intergroup Rhabdomyosarcoma Study Clinical Grouping Classification), 2841, 2841t
IRX-2, for head and neck squamous cell carcinoma, 1024
Ischemia-reperfusion injury, in acutely raised skin flaps, 1070, 1074
IsK, in deafness, 2051t-2058t
Island advancement flap, 345
for lip defects, 356f
Isobutyl-2-cyanoacrylate (IBCA), for embolization, 1933
Isoechoic object, 1643
Isoeffect measurements, in radiotherapy, 1039-1040
Isoflurane
for anesthesia, 111
and skin flap viability, 1073
Isotretinoin
for chemoprevention of oral cancer, 1315
for head and neck squamous cell carcinoma, 1018
microtia due to, 2741
Isoxsuprine, and skin flap viability, 1073
Isthmus nasi, in nasal breathing assessment, 644
Isthmus tympani anticus, 1827f
Isthmus tympani oticus, 1827f
ITC (in-the-canal) hearing aid, 2270, 2270f
ITE (in-the-ear) hearing aids, 2270, 2270f
in infants, 2723-2724
selection of, 2266-2267, 2270
Item response theory (IRT), 55
Itga8 (integrin $\alpha 8 \beta 1$) gene, in murine deafness, 2058t-2060t
ITM (in-transit metastasis), of melanoma, 1110, 1117
Itraconazole, for fungal rhinosinusitis, 713t
IVIG (intravenous immune globulin)
for pediatric chronic sinusitis, 2779
for rhinosinusitis, 735t, 737

J

Jackson-Weiss syndrome, craniofacial anomalies in, 2646
Jacobson's organ, 627-628
Jahrsdoerfer grading system, for congenital aural atresia, 2753, 2753t
Jaw, osteoradionecrosis of, 1048
Jaw-closer muscles, 1204
Jaw-closing reflex, 1204, 1204f, 1207
"Jaw-jerk" reflex, 1204
Jaw-opener muscles, 1204
Jaw-opening reflex, 1205, 1205f, 1207
Jaw-tongue reflexes, 1205
JCAHO (Joint Commission on Accreditation of Healthcare Organizations), 82-83, 84t-87t
JCIH (Joint Committee on Infant Hearing), 2718-2719
Jejunal free flap, 1082t, 1087, 1090f
for hypopharyngeal and esophageal reconstruction, 1432-1433, 1433f, 1455-1457, 1456f
for oropharyngeal reconstruction, 1380, 1380f
Jejunal interposition graft, after laryngopharyngectomy, 1418, 1418f
Jensen syndrome, deafness in, 2051t-2058t
Jerker mutation, 2075
Jervell and Lange-Nielsen syndrome (JLNS)
cochlear implant for, 2220
deafness in, 2051t-2058t, 2083, 2094t, 2096
Jessner's solution, for chemical peels, 392-393
Jet lag, 264
Jet ventilation anesthesia, with recurrent respiratory papillomatosis, 2891-2893
Jitter, in acoustic analysis for voice evaluation, 829-830, 834-835
Jitterbug mice, deafness in, 2058t-2060t, 2075-2076
JLNS (Jervell and Lange-Nielsen syndrome)
cochlear implant for, 2220
deafness in, 2051t-2058t, 2083, 2094t, 2096
JNA. *See* Juvenile nasopharyngeal angiofibroma (JNA).
Joint Commission on Accreditation of Healthcare Organizations (JCAHO), 82-83, 84t-87t
Joint Committee on Infant Hearing (JCIH), 2718-2719
Joint replacement, oral treatment considerations with, 1246t
JRP (juvenile recurrent parotitis), 2858
Jugular bulb
anatomy of, 1822-1823
paraganglioma of, 2499f
in postauricular approach to infratemporal fossa, 2498, 2498f-2499f
in subtotal temporal bone resection, 2494-2495
in surgical anatomy of lateral skull base, 2436f-2437f, 2489
Jugular bulb injury, due to mastoidectomy, 2016
Jugular chain lymph nodes, 1578-1579
Jugular foramen
anatomy of, 1822-1823, 1823f
surgical anatomy of, 2439-2440, 2439f-2440f
in lateral skull base, 2435f, 2438
in middle cranial base, 2445f
with temporal bone, 2436f
Jugular foramen meningiomas, imaging of, 1929-1930, 1930f
Jugular foramen schwannomas
imaging of, 1929-1930, 1930f, 2522f
lateral cranial base surgery for, 2504-2505, 2505f
stereotactic radiation therapy for, 2565
Jugular foramen syndromes, hearing loss due to, 2199, 2199t
Jugular foramen tumors, lateral cranial base surgery for, 2504
Jugular fossa, 1824f
Jugular lymph nodes
boundaries and landmarks of, 1705, 1707t-1708t
description of, 1706t
location of, 1704f-1705f
Jugular lymph nodes *(Continued)*
lower, 1704, 1704f-1705f
middle, 1704, 1704f-1705f
upper, 1704, 1704f-1705f
Jugular paragangliomas, 1662f, 2499f
Jugular process
anatomy of, 1823f
in surgical anatomy of lateral skull base, 2435f
Jugular spine, 1822-1823, 1824f
Jugular tuberculum
anatomy of, 1823f
in surgical anatomy of lateral skull base, 2435f
Jugular vein(s)
radiographic anatomy of, 1471f, 1473-1474
in surgical anatomy of lateral skull base, 2436f, 2439f-2440f
Jugulocarotid node, 1298f
Jugulodigastric nodes, 1298f, 2582
Juguloomohyoid nodes, 1298f, 2582
Jump method, for tonsillar and pharyngeal wall reconstruction, 1386, 1387f
Junctional nevus, 286, 287f
Juri flap, for hair loss, 385-387, 387f
complications of, 386-387
Juvenile angiofibroma
endovascular treatment of, 1937-1938, 1943f
sinonasal, 721-722
classification systems for, 722
endoscopic appearance of, 721, 721f
imaging of, 721
natural history of, 721
origin of, 721, 721f
postoperative surveillance for, 722
preoperative embolization for, 721-722
surgical approach for, 718t, 722, 722f-723f, 763
transnasal endoscopic-assisted surgery for, 2483, 2483f
Juvenile melanoma, 287
Juvenile nasopharyngeal angiofibroma (JNA), 152, 154f, 1349-1351
clinical features of, 1349
diagnosis of, 1349-1350, 1350f
growth patterns of, 1349
management of, 1350-1351
pathologic features of, 1349
recurrence of, 1351
staging of, 1350, 1350t
Juvenile recurrent parotitis (JRP), 2858

K

K^+. *See* Potassium (K^+).
Kallikreins, in saliva, 1140
Kallmann's syndrome, anosmia in, 636
Kaposiform hemangioendothelioma (KHE), 2824-2825, 2826f
bone resorption with, 2826
Kasabach-Merritt phenomenon with, 2825
Kaposi's sarcoma (KS)
of hard palate, 1309-1310
immunosuppression and, 212-215, 213t
epidemiology and pathogenesis of, 212-213
presentation and diagnosis of, 213-214, 214f
treatment of, 214-215
of larynx, 1508-1509
of oral cavity, 1299
of oropharynx, 1363-1364, 1364f
Kaposi's sarcoma–associated herpesvirus (KSHV), 213
Karapendzic flap, 351
Karyotype analysis, for head and neck squamous cell carcinoma, 1019
Kasabach-Merritt phenomenon, with vascular tumors, 2825
of salivary glands, 2860

Kawasaki disease
in children, 2819
facial paralysis in, 2400
KayPENTAX HSDI system, 821
Kcc3
in endolymph homeostasis, 2081-2082
in murine deafness, 2058t-2060t
Kcc4
in endolymph homeostasis, 2081-2082
in murine deafness, 2058t-2060t
KCNE1, in deafness, 2051t-2058t, 2083, 2096
Kcnj10, in murine deafness, 2058t-2060t, 2083
KCNQ1, in deafness, 2051t-2058t, 2083
KCNQ4, in deafness, 2051t-2058t, 2079, 2090-2092
Kearns-Sayre (KS) syndrome, deafness in, 2097
Keisselbach's plexus, 483f
Keloid(s), 291
after neck surgery, 1728
after otoplasty, 479
Keratinizing odontogenic cyst, 1266-1267
microscopic features of, 1267
radiographic features of, 1267, 1267f
Keratinocyte migration, in wound healing, 1076-1077
Keratinocyte proliferation, in wound healing, 1077
Keratitis, exposure, after facial nerve injury, 2420, 2420f
Keratitis-ichthyosis-deafness syndrome, 2051t-2058t
Keratoacanthoma, 284f, 286
Keratocystic odontogenic tumor, 1262, 1267-1268
microscopic features of, 1268
radiographic features of, 1267-1268, 1268f
treatment of, 1268
Keratosis(es)
actinic (solar), 283, 284f
obturans, of external auditory canal, 1949
imaging of, 1917, 1918f
management of, 2021
seborrheic, 281-282, 282f
Kerma, 1033
Ketamine
for anesthesia induction, 111
in children, 2591
for premedication in children, 2589
with congenital heart disease, 2596
for prevention of bronchospasm during anesthesia in children, 2595
Ketoconazole, for fungal rhinosinusitis, 713t
Ketoconazole cream (Nizoral, Xolegel), for fungal otitis externa, 1954-1955, 1959t-1960t
Ketorolac, for postoperative pain in children, 2594
Keystone area, of nose, 496, 497f
KHE (kaposiform hemangioendothelioma), 2824-2825, 2826f
bone resorption with, 2826
Kasabach-Merritt phenomenon with, 2825
KHRI-3, in autoimmune inner ear disease, 2165
Ki-67, in salivary gland neoplasms, 1194
Kidney disease
oral manifestations of, 1255
preoperative evaluation of, 103
sensorineural hearing loss with, 2121
Kidney failure, oral manifestations of, 1255
Kidney failure–induced hyperparathyroidism, 1797-1798
Kidney transplantation, oral sequelae of, 1255
Kiesselbach's plexus, 682
in epistaxis, 686-687
Killian incision, for septoplasty, 488, 489f
Killian-Jamieson's triangle, esophageal diverticulum in, 986, 987f
Killian's triangle
anatomy of, 1422
esophageal diverticulum in, 986, 987f
Kilovoltage (kV) x-rays, 1033
Kinerase (*N*6-furfuryladenine), for aging skin, 404
Kinocilium
anatomy of, 1858f
arrangement of, 1854-1855, 1856f
in hair cell transduction, 2070-2071, 2070f
morphologic polarization of, 1855, 1856f, 2279f
Kir4.1, in murine deafness, 2058t-2060t, 2083
Kit, in deafness, 2051t-2058t
Klebsiella rhinoscleromatis, laryngitis due to, 884
Kleeblattschädel, due to craniosynostosis, 2645, 2645f
Klein-Waardenburg syndrome, 2095
Klinefelter's syndrome, 5
Klippel-Trenaunay-Parkes-Weber syndrome, 291
Knife injuries, neck trauma due to, 1627
Körner's septum, 1829
in mastoidectomy, 2012
Krause end bulbs, 1201
KS (Kaposi's sarcoma). *See* Kaposi's sarcoma (KS).
KS (Kearns-Sayre) syndrome, deafness in, 2097
KSHV (Kaposi's sarcoma–associated herpesvirus), 213
KTP (potassium-titanyl-phosphate) laser, 31t, 33
for facial resurfacing, 403t
for recurrent respiratory papillomatosis, 880, 880f, 2891
for stridulous child, 2908
Kupffer cells, 604
Kuttner's tumor, 1154
kV (kilovoltage) x-rays, 1033
KvLQT1, in deafness, 2051t-2058t, 2083, 2096
Kymography, of larynx, 134f, 154, 822f

L

Labetalol, intraoperative, 112
Labial arteries, 1296
Labyrinth, intratympanic gentamicin for chemical ablation of, 2185-2189
clinical protocols for, 2187-2188
complications of, 2188-2189
concentration of, 2188
dose of, 2188
indications and contraindications for, 2189
injection interval for, 2188
mechanism of action of, 2185-2186
number of injections of, 2188
pharmacokinetics of, 2186-2187, 2186f-2187f
practical considerations with, 2188
Labyrinthectomy, 2366-2368
adaptation of vestibular reflexes after, 2300-2302
anatomic and physiologic basis for, 2300-2302, 2301f
clinical implications of, 2302
disadvantages of, 2367-2368
for Meniere's disease, 2339, 2362
chemical, 2185-2189, 2338-2339, 2338f
patient selection for, 2364-2366, 2365b, 2365t
procedure for, 2366-2368, 2367f
transcanal (oval window), 2366, 2367f
transmastoid, 2366-2367, 2367f
Labyrinthine anomalies, 2732-2733
in combination with other anomalies, 2728, 2738, 2739f
CSF otorrhea due to, 2197
incidence of, 2727
semicircular canal aplasia as, 2732-2733, 2732f
semicircular canal dysplasia as, 2732, 2732f-2733f
Labyrinthine aplasia, complete, 2729
imaging of, 2729f-2730f
inherited, 2735
relative incidence of, 2729t
Labyrinthine concussion, 2343
Labyrinthine disease, poor compensation *vs.* unstable, 2364, 2365t
Labyrinthine dysplasia
cochlear implant with, 2240-2241
membranous
complete, 2727
limited, 2727-2728
Labyrinthine fistula, 1989-1990, 1990f
Labyrinthine infections, 2153-2163
acquired sensorineural hearing loss due to, 2157-2161
with herpes simplex virus, 2159-2160
with Lassa fever, 2158-2159
with measles, 2158
with meningitis, 2160-2161
with mumps, 2157-2158, 2158f
sudden, 2154, 2154b, 2157
with varicella-zoster virus, 2159, 2159f
bacterial and fungal, 2160
with cochlear implant, 2161
congenital hearing loss due to, 2154-2157
with cytomegalovirus, 2154-2156, 2155f
with rubella, 2156-2157, 2157f
with syphilis, 2161
with cytomegalovirus
clinical features of, 2154-2155
congenital hearing loss due to, 2154-2156, 2155f
diagnosis of, 2154-2155
experimental, 2156
management and prevention of, 2156
temporal bone pathology due to, 2155-2156, 2155f
diagnosis of, 2153-2154, 2154b
with herpes simplex virus, 2159-2160
in immunocompromised patients, 2161-2162
with Lassa fever, 2158
with measles, 2158
Meniere's disease due to, 2163
with mumps, 2119, 2157-2158, 2158f
clinical features of, 2157
diagnosis of, 2157
experimental, 2158
sudden, 2127
temporal bone pathology in, 2158, 2158f
with rubella, 2156-2157, 2157f
syphilitic, 2161
vaccines to prevent hearing loss due to, 2161
with varicella-zoster virus, 2159, 2159f
vestibular neuritis due to, 2162-2163, 2162f
viral
cytomegalovirus as, 2154-2156, 2155f
herpes simplex virus as, 2159-2160
Lassa fever as, 2158-2159
measles as, 2158
mumps as, 2157-2158, 2158f
rubella as, 2156-2157, 2157f
varicella-zoster virus as, 2159, 2159f
Labyrinthine segment
anatomy of, 1826f, 1828
surgical, 2404, 2404f
vulnerability to injury of, 1829
Labyrinthine upset, acute chemical, due to intratympanic gentamicin, 2189
Labyrinthine vertigo, 2201-2202
Labyrinthitis
acute (*See* Vestibular neuritis)
suppurative, 1991-1992, 2118
diagnosis of, 1991-1992
epidemiology of, 1980t
etiology of, 1991
imaging of, 1991f-1992f
bacterial and fungal, 2160
diagnosis of, 2118
ossificans, imaging of, 1921, 1925f
in evaluation for cochlear implant, 2222
sensorineural hearing loss due to, 2118
serous, 2118
after small fenestra stapedotomy, 2034
viral, vertigo due to, 2201

Lacerations, 307
Lacrimal apparatus
anatomy of, 798f
obstruction of, 797
anatomic *vs.* functional, 797-798, 798f-799f
trauma to, 307-309, 308f
Lacrimal bone
anatomy and physiology of, 320-321, 320f, 798f
in endoscopic dacryocystorhinostomy, 799-800, 800f
Lacrimal crest, 320-321, 322f
Lacrimal duct, 798f
Lacrimal foramen, 322f
Lacrimal fossa, 439, 1124f
anatomy and physiology of, 320-321, 322f
in surgical anatomy of anterior cranial base, 2444f
Lacrimal function, assessment of, 2383
Lacrimal gland, 321f
pleomorphic adenoma of, 1169, 1170f
in upper eyelid blepharoplasty, 448
Lacrimal nerve, 321f, 440
Lacrimal obstruction
anatomic *vs.* functional, 797-798, 798f-799f
endoscopic dacryocystorhinostomy for (*See* Endoscopic dacryocystorhinostomy)
pathophysiology of, 797, 798f
Lacrimal puncta, in endoscopic dacryocystorhinostomy, 800
Lacrimal sac, 439, 798f
Lactate dehydrogenase (LDH), with melanoma, 1109-1110, 1113
Lactobacillus spp, dental caries due to, 1252
Lactoferrin
in middle ear protection, 1871
in saliva, 1140-1141
LactoSorb plating system, for pediatric facial fractures, 2700, 2701t
Lag screw fixation, of mandibular fracture, 338, 338f
Lagophthalmos, 446, 2421
after blepharoplasty, 449-450
Laimer's triangle, esophageal diverticulum in, 986, 987f
LAIV (live-attenuated influenza vaccine), to prevent otitis media, 2769
Lambda, 320f
Lambdoid synostosis, 2643-2644
front-orbital advancement for, 2653
Lamina papyracea
in endoscopic sinus surgery, 748-749, 750f
after functional endoscopic sinus surgery, 679, 679f-680f
medial deviation or dehiscence of, 669, 671-672
Lamina propria, in immune system, 605
Lamotrigine, for neuropathic pain, 243, 244t
Langerhans cell(s), 604, 2100
in allergic rhinitis, 616
Langerhans' cell eosinophilic granuloma, oral manifestations of, 1257
Langerhans' cell histiocytosis (LCH), 2100-2101
oral manifestations of, 1257
otologic manifestations of, 2101
eosinophilic granulomas as
of external ear, 2102f
multiple, 2101f
unifocal, 2102f
in Letterer-Siwe disease, 2102f
otorrhea as, 2196
Language, defined, 2248
Language development, 2248-2249, 2248f-2249f
cochlear implants and, 2239-2240, 2249-2251, 2250f
otitis media and, 2776
Lano classification, of airway stenosis, 944t
Laplace transform, 2303
LAR (laryngeal adductor reflex), in laryngomalacia, 2866-2867
Large clear cell adenoma, of parathyroid gland, 1778
Large granular lymphocytes, in adaptive immune system, 603-604
Large vestibular aqueduct syndrome, sensorineural hearing loss in, 2118, 2118f
sudden, 2129
LARP (left anterior–right posterior) semicircular canal plane, 2285, 2286f, 2287, 2288f
Laryngeal adductor muscles, during breathing, 809, 809f
Laryngeal adductor reflex (LAR), in laryngomalacia, 2866-2867
Laryngeal aditus, 1359f
Laryngeal airway resistance (R_{law}), in voice evaluation, 828-829, 828t
Laryngeal appendix, 876
Laryngeal atresia, 2869, 2869f-2870f, 2913
management of, 2922
Laryngeal biopsy, for benign vocal fold mucosal disorders, 862
Laryngeal cancer, 1482-1511
adenoid cystic carcinoma as, 1507
adenosquamous carcinoma as, 1506
advanced, 1526
new treatment protocols for, 1448, 1449f
transoral laser microsurgery for, 1531-1532, 1532f-1533f
anatomy and, 1483-1486, 1483f, 1483t
anterior commissure in, 1486
glottis in, 1483-1484, 1483f, 1483t
mucosal lining in, 1484
paraglottic space in, 1484-1485, 1484f-1485f
pre-epiglottic space in, 1484, 1484f
subglottis in, 1483-1484, 1483f, 1483t
supraglottis in, 1483-1484, 1483f, 1483t
of anterior commissure, 1486
anatomic basis for, 1486
imaging of, 161, 1474, 1474f
treatment of, 1496-1497
transoral laser microsurgery for, 1531
of aryepiglottic fold, 1475, 1478f
carcinoma in situ as, 1486-1491, 1489f-1490f, 1515
treatment of, 1489-1490, 1520-1521
carcinosarcoma as, 1506
cartilaginous invasion by, 161, 1474
CT of, 1474, 1476f, 1495
contrast-enhanced, 161, 164f
MRI of, 161, 1474-1475, 1476f, 1495
chemoprevention of, 1491
in children, 2881
classification of, 1487t, 1525-1526
clinical presentation of, 1579
concomitant chemoradiation for, 1052-1056, 1053t
conservation laryngeal surgery for (*See* Conservation laryngeal surgery)
diagnostic evaluation/workup for, 1579
early, 1526
transoral laser microsurgery for, 1530-1531
embryology and, 1482-1483
of epiglottis, 1475, 1477f
glottic (*See* Glottic cancer)
hematolymphoid, 1509
extramedullary plasmacytoma as, 1509
lymphoma as, 1509
mucosal malignant melanoma as, 1509
histopathology of, 1512, 1514f
imaging of, 161, 1494-1495, 1579
of anterior commissure, 161, 1474, 1474f
of aryepiglottic fold, 1475, 1478f
with cartilaginous invasion, 161, 1474
contrast-enhanced CT for, 161, 164f
CT for, 1474, 1476f, 1495
MRI for, 161, 1474-1475, 1476f, 1495
Laryngeal cancer *(Continued)*
for conservation laryngeal surgery, 1545-1546
CT for, 1468-1479
with cartilaginous invasion, 1474, 1476f, 1495
contrast-enhanced, 161, 164f
of epiglottis, 1475, 1477f
glottic, 1474-1475, 1474f
with lymph node metastases, 1476, 1479f
MRI for, 1468-1479
with cartilaginous invasion, 161, 1474-1475, 1476f, 1495
normal anatomy and, 1470-1474
of paraglottic space, 1474
PET/CT for, 1470, 1470f
post-therapy, 1476-1479, 1479f
of pyriform sinus, 1475-1476, 1478f
subglottic, 1474, 1475f
supraglottic, 1475-1476
technique for, 1470, 1470f
transglottic, 161, 164f, 1475f, 1476, 1478f
intermediate, 1526
transoral laser microsurgery for, 1531
mucoepidermoid carcinoma as, 1506-1507
neck dissection for, 1716-1718
definition and rationale for, 1716-1717, 1717f
glottic, 1497-1498
after nonsurgical organ preservation treatment, 1502-1503
supraglottic, 1500-1501
technique for, 1717-1718, 1717f
with transoral laser microsurgery, 1532
neck management for, 1580
neuroendocrine, 1507-1508
carcinoid as
atypical, 1507
typical, 1507
paraganglioma as, 1508
small cell carcinoma as, 1507-1508
nodal metastases of, 1493-1494, 1493f
embryology and, 1482-1483
glottic, 1497-1498
imaging of, 1476, 1479f
radiation therapy for, 1690t
subglottic, 1501, 1501f
supraglottic, 1500-1501
incidence and distribution of, 1686f, 1688t
organ preservation treatment for, 1501-1503, 1502f (*See also* Conservation laryngeal surgery)
current paradigm for, 1558-1559
glottic, 1497
chemoradiation as, 1584-1585
targeted biologic agents with radiation therapy as, 1585
management of neck after, 1502-1503
recurrence after, 1503-1504
supraglottic, 1500
overall management of, 1580
of paraglottic space, 1484-1485, 1484f-1485f
anatomic basis for, 1484-1485, 1484f-1485f
imaging of, 1474
of preepiglottic space, 1484, 1485f
anatomic basis for, 1484, 1484f
imaging of, 1495
premalignant lesions for, 1486-1491, 1489f-1490f
of pyriform sinus, 1475-1476, 1478f
radiation therapy for, 1577-1593
advanced glottic, 1497, 1583-1588
balancing cure, organ preservation, and quality of life with, 1583-1584
with chemotherapy, 1584-1586, 1584t
complications of, 1587-1588
dose-fractionation schemes for, 1586, 1586t
general principles of, 1585-1586
mini-mantle field technique for, 1586

Laryngeal cancer *(Continued)*
outcomes and prognostic factors for, 1586-1587, 1587t
patient setup for, 1586
postoperative (adjuvant), 1584-1585, 1584t
shrinking-field technique for, 1586, 1587f
with targeted biologic agents, 1585
advanced supraglottic, 1589
outcomes and prognostic factors for, 1589, 1590t
techniques and dose-fractionation schemes for, 1589
anatomic considerations with, 1578-1579, 1578f
with anterior commissure involvement, 1496-1497
CyberKnife stereotactic approach for, 1592
early glottic, 1519-1520, 1581
complications of, 1583
effectiveness of, 1496
local control with, 1519, 1522f
outcome and prognostic factors for, 1581-1583, 1582t-1583t
recurrence after, 1522t
results of, 1519, 1521t
techniques and dose-fractionation schemes for, 1580-1590, 1581f-1582f
early supraglottic, 1496, 1588-1589
complications of, 1589
outcomes and prognostic factors for, 1589, 1589t
techniques and dose-fractionation schemes for, 1588-1589
future strategies and directions for, 1592
lymphatic drainage and, 1578-1579, 1579f
with nodal metastases, 1498
overview of, 1578
RADPLAT approach for, 1592
recurrence after, 1476-1479, 1522, 1522t
with recurrent disease, 1591-1592
subglottic, 1589-1590
with transoral laser microsurgery, 1532-1533
recurrence of, 1476-1479
after radiation therapy, 1476-1479, 1522, 1522t
radiation therapy for, 1591-1592
salivary gland type, 1506-1508
sarcoma as, 1508-1509
chondro-, 1508
fibro-, 1508
Kaposi, 1508-1509
lipo-, 1508
malignant fibrous histiocytoma as, 1508
pseudo-, 1506
sarcomatoid carcinoma as, 1506
second primary tumors in, 1492, 1510
spindle cell carcinoma as, 1506
squamous cell carcinoma as, 1491
acantholytic, 1506
adenoid, 1506
basaloid, 1506
cervical nodal metastases of, 1493-1494, 1493f
embryology and, 1482-1483
glottic, 1497-1498
imaging of, 1476, 1479f
subglottic, 1501, 1501f
supraglottic, 1500-1501
chemoprevention of, 1491
clinical presentation of, 1493-1494
diagnosis and evaluation of, 1494-1495
differential diagnosis of, 1495
history and physical examination in, 1494
imaging in, 1494-1495
operative endoscopic examination in, 1495
distant metastases of, 1494-1495
epidemiology of, 1491-1492, 1512, 1513f
etiology of, 1512-1513

Laryngeal cancer *(Continued)*
follow-up for, 1505
grading of, 1492-1493
human papillomavirus and, 1492, 2887-2888
imaging of, 161, 164f
in situ, 1493
microinvasive, 1493
molecular biology of, 1492
papillary, 1506
pathology of, 1492-1493
prognosis and prognostic predictors for, 1504-1505
clinical features as, 1504
disease factors as, 1504-1505
histopathologic characteristics as, 1504-1505
molecular markers as, 1493, 1505
patient factors as, 1505
radiologic characteristics as, 1504
recurrence of, 1503-1504
stomal, 1504, 1504f
recurrent respiratory papillomatosis and, 2887-2888
risk factor(s) for, 1491-1492, 1512-1513
diet as, 1492
exposure to toxins as, 1492, 1513
genetic susceptibility as, 1492, 1513
human papillomavirus as, 1492, 1513
laryngopharyngeal reflux as, 1491-1492, 1513
second primary tumors as, 1492
tobacco and alcohol as, 1491, 1512-1513
staging of, 1486, 1488t-1489t
radiology in, 1495
transition zones of, 1489, 1490f
treatment of, 1495
acronyms for, 1526-1527
background of, 1512-1515, 1513f-1514f
CO_2 laser for, 33
goals of, 1495
intensity-modulated radiotherapy for, 1046
intensity-modulated radiotherapy of, 1046
nonsurgical organ preservation, 1501-1503, 1502f
options for, 1495, 1496t
prognostic factors in, 1495, 1496t
for recurrence, 1503-1504, 1504f
for subglottic tumors, 1501-1503, 1501f
for supraglottic tumors, 1498-1501, 1498f
therapeutic decision making for, 1495
variants of, 1505-1506
acantholytic, 1506
adenosquamous, 1506
basaloid, 1506
papillary, 1506
spindle cell, 1506
verrucous, 1505-1506, 1505f
staging of, 1486, 1488t-1489t, 1579-1580
laryngoscopy in, 1579-1580, 1580f
radiology in, 1495
and transoral laser microsurgery, 1526
subglottic
anatomic basis for, 1483-1484, 1483f, 1483t
cervical metastases of, 1494
clinical presentation of, 1493, 1579
imaging of, 1474, 1475f
staging of, 1488t, 1580f
treatment of, 1501-1503, 1501f
supraglottic, 1484, 1484f-1485f
anatomic basis for, 1483-1484, 1483f, 1483t
cervical metastases of, 1493-1494
clinical presentation of, 1493, 1579
imaging of, 1475-1476
neck dissection for, 1500-1501
staging of, 1488t, 1580f
treatment of, 1498-1501
in advanced stage, 1500
in early stage, 1498-1500, 1498f

Laryngeal cancer *(Continued)*
with nodal metastases, 1500-1501
transoral laser microsurgery for, 1531
transglottic, 1486
imaging of, 161, 164f, 1475f, 1476, 1478f
transoral laser microsurgery for, 1525-1538
with advanced tumors, 1531-1532, 1532f-1533f
with anterior commissure involvement, 1497
complications of, 1533-1534, 1534f
conclusions on, 1536-1537
contraindications to, 1534
with early tumors, 1496, 1498-1500, 1530-1531
with glottic tumors, 1496
historical background of, 1527
instruments for, 1528-1529
with intermediate tumors, 1531
and neck dissection, 1532
vs. open conservation surgery, 1528
pathology issues with, 1530
and radiotherapy, 1532-1533
results of, 1534-1536
with supraglottic tumors, 1498-1500
techniques for, 1529-1530
theoretical basis of, 1527-1528
with very advanced tumors, 1532
with very early tumors, 1530
due to tumors from continuous sites, 1510
types of local, 1526
verrucous carcinoma as, 1505-1506, 1505f
very advanced, 1526
transoral laser microsurgery for, 1532
very early, 1526
transoral laser microsurgery for, 1530
Laryngeal cartilage
calcification of, in geriatric patients, 235, 235f
invasive carcinoma of, 161, 1474
CT of, 1474, 1476f, 1495
contrast-enhanced, 161, 164f
MRI of, 161, 1474-1475, 1476f, 1495
repair of, 939f
Laryngeal chemoreflex (LCR), 2570
Laryngeal cleft (LC), 2873-2874, 2873f, 2910f
classification of, 2873, 2874f, 2874t
dysphagia due to, 2952-2953
syndromes associated with, 2870t
Laryngeal cysts, congenital, 1468, 2872-2873, 2872f-2873f
Laryngeal denervation
effects of, 919
reinnervation for (*See* Laryngeal reinnervation)
Laryngeal diadochokinesis, 814
Laryngeal edema, in vocal professional, 854
Laryngeal electromyography, 835, 905
for stridor, 2901
Laryngeal examination
for benign vocal fold mucosal disorders, 862, 862f
bilateral diffuse polyposis as, 872
capillary ectasia as, 866-867
contact ulcer or granuloma as, 875
glottic sulcus as, 870-871
intracordal cysts as, 869
postoperative dysphonia as, 874
tools for, 862, 862f
vocal fold hemorrhage and unilateral (hemorrhagic) vocal fold polyp as, 868
vocal nodules as, 865
for disorders of professional voice, 851-852, 852t
Laryngeal hemangiomas, 874, 2871, 2871f
Laryngeal hygiene, in voice professional, 852-853
Laryngeal image biofeedback, for benign vocal fold mucosal disorders, 863, 864f
Laryngeal inlet obliteration, due to trauma, 940f
Laryngeal instillations, for mucosal inflammation, 863

Laryngeal invasion, by tumors from contiguous sites, 1510
Laryngeal lesions, epithelial hyperplastic, 1525
Laryngeal mask airway (LMA), 110f
for difficult airway, 109-110, 113, 114t, 122, 122b
flexible, for children, 2599
Laryngeal mass, differential diagnosis of, 1487t
Laryngeal motion, 805-807, 806f-807f
Laryngeal mucosal lacerations, 1634
Laryngeal muscles, characteristics of, 918
Laryngeal musculoskeletal tension, in voice evaluation, 827-831, 828f
Laryngeal nerve, recurrent. *See* Recurrent laryngeal nerve (RLN).
Laryngeal obstruction, in neonate, 2905
Laryngeal open repair, for laryngeal trauma, 936-937, 939f
Laryngeal papillomatosis, stridor due to, 2898, 2899f
Laryngeal paralysis
arytenoid adduction for (*See* Arytenoid adduction)
clinical impact of, 912
dysphagia due to, 914
pathophysiology of, 912-913
"posterior gap" in, 912, 913f
variation in symptoms of, 912
vocal fold positions in, 912-913
vocal process in, 913-914
Laryngeal preservation surgery, 1501-1503, 1502f
for glottic tumors, 1497
management of neck after, 1502-1503
recurrence after, 1503-1504
for supraglottic tumors, 1500
Laryngeal reinnervation, 917-924
ansa cervicalis–recurrent laryngeal nerve anastomosis for, 922-923
advantages of, 922
clinical results of, 923
disadvantage of, 922
history of, 917-918
surgical indications and contraindications for, 922
surgical technique for, 922-923, 923f
direct nerve implant for, 923-924, 924f
effects of denervation and, 919
history of, 917
neuromuscular pedicle for, 919-922
for bilateral paralysis, 920
complications of, 922
future of, 922
history of, 917
indications for, 920
laboratory investigations of, 919-920
rationale for, 919
reported results of, 920-921
technique for, 920, 921f
for unilateral paralysis, 920
physiologic and anatomic issues in, 918-919
infrahyoid muscles as, 918-919
laryngeal muscles as, 918
muscle fibers in general as, 918
nerve characteristics as, 918
principles of, 919-924
Laryngeal release procedures, for laryngotracheal stenosis, 952
Laryngeal sensory testing, for extraesophageal reflux, 898-899
Laryngeal skeleton, anatomy of
radiographic, 1471
surgical, 1541, 1541f
Laryngeal stenosis, 943-952
in children, 2912-2924
anterior glottic, 2922
anterior subglottic, 2923
due to atresia and webs, 2922
diagnosis of, 2916-2917
Laryngeal stenosis *(Continued)*
endoscopic examination in, 2916-2917
esophagogastroduodenoscopy and biopsy in, 2917
evaluation of GERD and GLPRD in, 2917
functional endoscopic evaluation of swallowing in, 2917
history and physical examination in, 2916
pulmonary function tests in, 2917
radiologic evaluation in, 2916
voice assessment in, 2917
etiology and pathophysiology of, 2912-2916
acquired, 2914-2915
congenital, 2912-2913, 2913f
grading of, 2917, 2917t
management of, 2917-2921
algorithm for, 2913f
anterior cricoid split operation for, 2918-2919, 2918f-2919f
autogenous costal cartilage reconstruction in, 2919-2920, 2920f-2921f
combined laryngofissure and posterior cricoid division for, 2919, 2919f
cricoid resection with thyrotracheal anastomosis for, 2921, 2922f
decannulation after, 2923
endoscopic, 2918
external expansion surgery for, 2919-2921
grafts in, 2919
postoperative, 2923
single-stage laryngotracheal reconstruction for, 2920-2921
stents in, 2920
posterior glottic, 2922-2923
prevention of, 2916
types of, 2915, 2915f-2916f
with vocal cord paralysis, 2922
due to chronic infection, 2915
due to chronic inflammatory disease, 2915
classification of, 944, 944t
CO_2 laser for, 32
congenital
diagnosis of, 2916-2917
etiology and pathophysiology of, 2912-2913, 2913f
management of, 2922
due to GERD, 2915, 2917
local application of mitomycin C for, 946
pathophysiology of, 943-944, 944b
surgical management of, 943-952
for chronic disease, 947-952
anterior glottic, 948
due to anterior wall collapse, 951
complete glottic, 949-950
laryngeal release procedures in, 952
posterior glottic, 948-949, 949f
subglottic, 945f, 950-951
supraglottic, 947-948
endoscopic *vs.* open, 945
goals and assessment in, 944, 945f
microsurgical débridement in, 946, 946b, 946f
planning for, 946-947
skin and mucosal grafts in, 946-947
stent placement in, 947, 947f
due to trauma, 937-939, 939f-940f, 943
in children
external, 2914
internal, 2914-2915
Laryngeal stroboscopy, 818-821
of adynamic segments, 820
of amplitude of vibration, 820, 821f, 848, 848t
in children, 2877
of closure pattern, 819, 820f, 848t, 849
common problems and solutions for, 815t-816t
defined, 813
of early glottic carcinoma, 1515-1516
Laryngeal stroboscopy *(Continued)*
flexible endoscope for, 814
advantages of, 814
disadvantages of, 814
protocol for, 818b
technique of, 814
troubleshooting for, 814
interpretation of, 848t
interval examination in, 847
of mucosal wave, 820, 848-849, 848t
in neurologic examination, 834
of periodicity, 821, 848, 848t
of phase closure, 819-820
of professional voice, 847-849, 848f, 848t
protocol for, 818-819, 818b
of regularity, 821
rigid endoscopes for, 813-814
advantages of, 813
disadvantages of, 813-814
protocol for, 818b
technique of, 814
troubleshooting for, 814
of symmetry, 820, 847-848, 848t
of vertical closure level, 821
for vocal fold impairment, 905
Laryngeal structure, videoendoscopy of, 816
Laryngeal surgery
anesthesia for, in children, 2599-2600
conservation (*See* Conservation laryngeal surgery)
swallowing disorders due to, 1220
in vocal professional, 855-857
Laryngeal trauma, 933-941, 1479-1480
caustic or thermal, 939-941
etiology of, 940-941
incidence of, 939-940
management of, 941
external, 933-938
anterior cervical, 933-934, 934f
blunt *vs.* penetrating, 933-934, 934f
in children, 938
classification of, 936, 936t-937t
cricotracheal separation due to, 937
diagnosis of, 934-935
etiology of, 933-934, 934f
examination and initial management of, 935, 935t
incidence of, 933
laryngeal inlet obliteration due to, 940f
laryngeal stenosis due to, 937-939, 939f-940f, 943
in children, 2914
management of, 936-937
airway management in, 936
choice of therapy for, 936
conservative, 936
for cricotracheal separation, 937
diagnostic or therapeutic endoscopy in, 936
endolaryngeal stenting for, 937, 939f-940f
open laryngeal repair in, 936-937, 939f
partial or total laryngectomy for, 937, 940f
postoperative care in, 937
protocol for, 938f
surgical, 936-937
for vocal cord immobility, 937
mechanism of injury in, 934-935
outcome of, 938, 941f, 941t
sequelae of, 937-938, 940f
symptoms of, 934-935, 935t
vocal cord immobility due to, 937-938
iatrogenic, 939
etiology of, 939, 941f
incidence of, 939
with intubation granulomas, 939, 941f
with laryngeal stenosis, 939, 940f, 943
in children, 2914-2915
management of, 939

Laryngeal trauma *(Continued)*
imaging of, 159, 162f, 1479-1480
CT for, 935-936, 936f, 1480f
NEXUS criteria for, 935-936, 935b
internal, laryngeal stenosis due to, 2914
mechanisms of injury in, 933, 934f
Laryngeal ventricle, radiographic anatomy of, 1463f, 1472-1473
Laryngeal videoendoscopy, 814-818
of arytenoid and vocal fold motion, 816
common problems and solutions for, 815t-816t
defined, 813
flexible endoscope for, 814
advantages of, 814
disadvantages of, 814
protocol for, 816b
technique of, 814
troubleshooting for, 814
of laryngeal structure, 816
of mucous, 816-817
in neurologic examination, 834
protocol for, 814, 816b
rigid endoscopes for, 813-814
advantages of, 813
disadvantages of, 813-814
protocol for, 816b
technique of, 814
troubleshooting for, 814
of supraglottic activity, 817, 817f
of vascularity, 817
of vocal fold edges, 818
Laryngeal videoendoscopy and stroboscopy (LVES). *See* Laryngeal stroboscopy; Laryngeal videoendoscopy.
Laryngeal webs, 2869-2871, 2913
anterior, 2869-2870, 2869f
in congenital high airway obstruction syndrome, 2869, 2870f
dysphagia due to, 2952
epidemiology of, 2913
etiology and pathophysiology of, 2913
in laryngeal atresia, 2869, 2869f-2870f
posterior, 2869, 2869f
stridor due to, 2899, 2900f
syndromes associated with, 2869, 2870t
treatment of, 2922
vocal quality disorder due to, 2880, 2880f
Laryngectomy
for chronic aspiration, 927, 928f
for glottic cancer
in advanced stage
near-total, 1497
partial, 1497
total, 1497
anterior partial, 1517t
frontolateral partial, 1517t
partial, 1496
subtotal, 1517t
horizontal partial, 1540, 1549
hypothyroidism after, 1747
for laryngeal trauma, 937, 940f
near-total, 1564
olfactory dysfunction after, 637
supracricoid
with cricohyoidopexy, 1555-1557
complications of, 1557
functional outcome of, 1556-1557, 1557t
key surgical points for, 1556
oncologic results of, 1555
surgical technique for, 1555-1556, 1556f
historical background of, 1540
supracricoid partial
with cricohyoido-epiglottopexy, 1549-1550
complications of, 1551
extended procedures for, 1551
functional outcome of, 1551, 1551t-1552t
key surgical points for, 1550-1551
Laryngectomy *(Continued)*
oncologic results of, 1549-1550
surgical technique for, 1550, 1550f-1551f
for laryngeal cancer
with anterior commissure involvement, 1497
historical background of, 1540
intermediate, 1531
supraglottic, 1500
supraglottic, 1553-1554
with arytenoid, aryepiglottic fold, or superior medial pyriform involvement, 1554-1555
with base of tongue extension, 1555
complications of, 1555
extended procedures for, 1554
functional outcome of, 1555
historical background of, 1540
key surgical points for, 1554-1555, 1554f
oncologic results of, 1553, 1553t
surgical technique for, 1553-1554, 1554f
for supraglottic cancer, in early stage
open supraglottic, 1498-1500, 1498f
supraglottic partial, 1498-1500, 1498f
supraglottic subtotal, recurrence after, 1476
swallowing disorders due to, 1220
total, 1563-1572
chemotherapy after, 1442-1443
complication(s) of, 1570-1571
drain failure as, 1571
early, 1571
hematoma as, 1571
hypothyroidism as, 1571
infection as, 1571
late, 1571
pharyngocutaneous fistula as, 1571
stomal stenosis as, 1571
wound dehiscence as, 1571
historical development of, 1563-1564
indications for, 1564-1565
intraoperative conversion from conservation laryngeal surgery to, 1557-1558
vs. organ preservation surgery, 1564
with partial/total pharyngectomy, for hypopharyngeal cancer, 1430, 1431f
patient selection and workup for, 1565
pharyngeal reconstruction after, 1569-1570, 1570f
postoperative management of, 1570-1571
radiographic appearance after, 1416, 1417f-1418f
recurrence after, 1476
rehabilitation after, 1572
of swallowing, 1572
of voice (*See* Voice rehabilitation)
repair and reconstruction after, 1569-1570
for subglottic cancer, 1501
for supraglottic cancer, in advanced stage, 1500
technique for, 1565-1569
access to larynx in, 1566
airway management in, 1565-1566, 1565f
entry into larynx in, 1566, 1568f
entry into trachea in, 1566
incision in, 1565-1566, 1565f
inspection of specimen in, 1566-1568, 1569f
patient positioning in, 1565-1566
skeletonization of larynx in, 1566, 1567f
thyroid gland in, 1566
tracheoesophageal puncture in, 1568-1569, 1569f
tracheotomy in, 1566-1568
wound closure in, 1568-1569, 1569f
tracheal stoma after, 1570, 1571f
tumor recurrence after, 1416, 1417f
vertical partial, 1540, 1547
voice rehabilitation after (*See* Voice rehabilitation)
wide-field, 1568-1569, 1570f
Laryngitis, 883-888
acute, 883-885
bacterial, 884
fungal, 884-885, 884f
due to phonotrauma, 883-884, 884f
viral, 884
chronic, 885-886
due to autoimmune disorders, 887, 887f
bacterial, 885
due to extraesophageal reflux, 901-902
fungal, 885
due to blastomycosis, 885
due to coccidioidomycosis, 885
due to histoplasmosis, 885
due to paracoccidioidomycosis, 885
mycobacterial, 885-886, 886f
noninfectious, 886
and malignant transformation, 883
reflux, 886, 886f, 901-902, 970-971
in voice professional, 852
significance of, 883
in vocal professional, 853-854
due to reflux, 852
Laryngocele, 876-878, 1402, 2816-2817, 2872-2873
classification of, 877, 1402, 1468
clinical scenario with, 877, 2816-2817
defined, 877, 1468, 2816
diagnosis of, 877
etiology of, 159-161, 876
external, 159-161, 1468, 2816
imaging of, 159-161, 1402, 1468
CT for, 163f, 1402f, 1468, 1469f
plain films for, 1468, 1469f
internal, 159-161, 163f, 1402f, 1468, 1469f, 2816
mixed, 159-161, 1468, 1469f
treatment of, 877-878
types of, 876f
Laryngofissure, with posterior cricoid division, for laryngeal stenosis, 2919, 2919f
Laryngofissure approach, for glottic cancer, 1517t, 1519t
Laryngologic manifestations, of neurologic diseases, 837-838, 838t
Laryngology, gene therapy in, 23
Laryngomalacia, 1466, 2866-2868
bronchoscopy for, 2867
classification of, 2867
clinical presentation of, 2866
dysphagia due to, 2952
flexible fiberoptic laryngoscopy for, 2867
gastroesophageal reflux and, 2946
GERD with, 2867
in older children and adults, 2868
pathophysiology of, 2866-2867, 2867f
stridor due to, 2866
surgical intervention for, 2867-2868, 2868f
Laryngopathia praemenstrualis, 850
Laryngopharyngeal cancer, advanced, 1438-1439
chemotherapy for, 1439
quality of life with, 1439
Laryngopharyngeal reflux (LPR), 886, 886f, 901-902, 970-971
defined, 894
diagnostic evaluation of, 896-900
esophageal endoscopy in, 899
esophagogram in, 898
history in, 896, 896b-897b
impedance testing in, 900
laryngeal sensory testing in, 898-899
manometry in, 899-900
pH probe monitoring in, 900
physical examination and laryngeal endoscopy in, 896-897, 897t, 898b
voice analysis in, 898

Laryngopharyngeal reflux (LPR) *(Continued)*
dysphagia due to, 2953
epidemiology of, 894
and head and neck cancer, 902-903
laryngitis due to, 886, 886f
otolaryngologic disorders associated with, 901-903
chronic laryngitis as, 901-902
contact ulcer and laryngeal granuloma as, 902, 902f-903f
pathophysiology of, 894-896
epithelial resistance factors in, 895-896
esophageal acid clearance in, 895
lower esophageal sphincter in, 895, 895b
mechanisms of symptoms in, 896
upper esophageal sphincter in, 894-895
professional voice disorders due to, 852
and rhinosinusitis, 732
and squamous cell carcinoma of larynx, 1491-1492, 1513
treatment of, 900-901, 971
behavioral modification for, 900-901
bethanechol for, 901
H_2 blockers for, 901
over-the-counter antacids for, 901
promotility agents for, 901
proton pump inhibitors for, 901, 971
sucralfate for, 901
surgical, 901
Laryngopharyngeal Reflux Disease Index, 897, 898b
Laryngopharyngectomy
jejunal interposition graft after, 1418, 1418f
partial, for hypopharyngeal cancer, 1429, 1430f
radiographic appearance after, 1416-1418, 1418f
total, 1572-1575
complication(s) of
early, 1575
functional swallowing problems as, 1575
late, 1575
stricture as, 1575
defined, 1572
historical development of, 1572
incision for, 1565f
indications for, 1573
patient selection and workup for, 1573
postoperative management of, 1574-1575
reconstruction after, 1574, 1574f-1575f
rehabilitation after, 1575
technique for, 1573-1574, 1573f
entry into pharynx in, 1573-1574
initial steps in, 1573-1574
neck dissection in, 1573
patient positioning and anesthetic considerations in, 1573
with superior mediastinal adenopathy, 1574, 1574f
thyroid gland in, 1574
voice after, 1575
voice rehabilitation after, 1458-1459
Laryngopharyngitis, acid reflux, 863, 863f
Laryngopharyngoesophagectomy, total, 1574, 1574f
for cervical esophageal cancer, 1430-1431
Laryngoplasty
epiglottic, 1549
complications of, 1549
extended procedures for, 1549
functional outcome of, 1549
key surgical points for, 1549
oncologic results of, 1549
surgical technique for, 1549, 1549f
imbrication, 1548, 1548f
vertical, for chronic aspiration, 928-929, 930f
Laryngopyocele, 877
Laryngoscope(s), 864, 864f
Hollinger anterior commissure, for difficult airway, 122, 122f
for transoral laser microsurgery, 1529
Laryngoscopic appearance, in geriatric patients, 235-236
Laryngoscopic injection, for vocal fold medialization, 906-907, 907f
Laryngoscopy, 100
for airway stenosis, 944
for benign vocal fold mucosal disorders, 862
for difficult airway, 121
conventional, 114t
rigid, 114t
fiberoptic, 114t
direct
for laryngeal carcinoma, 1495
microscopic, for glottic cancer, 1519t
for penetrating neck trauma, 1631t, 1634
equipment for, 864, 864f
for extraesophageal reflux, 896-897, 897t, 898b
transnasal fiberoptic, 898
fiberoptic flexible, for laryngomalacia, 2867
flexible, 100, 814
advantages of, 814
disadvantages of, 814
in neurologic evaluation, 834
for professional voice disorders, 851-852, 852t
protocols for, 816b, 818b
technique of, 814
troubleshooting for, 814
for foreign body removal, 2939t, 2940
indirect, for laryngeal carcinoma, 1494
in infants, 2866, 2867f
for laryngeal carcinoma
direct, 1495
indirect, 1494
rigid, 813-814
advantages of, 813
disadvantages of, 813-814
for professional voice disorders, 851, 852t
protocols for, 816b, 818b
technique of, 814
troubleshooting for, 814
virtual, 138, 140f, 1464, 1464f
Laryngospasm
in children, 2570
recurrent paroxysmal, 808
Laryngotracheal cleft, 2873-2874, 2873f
classification of, 2873, 2874f, 2874t
syndromes associated with, 2870t
Laryngotracheal injury, due to penetrating neck trauma, 1634
Laryngotracheal reconstruction, single-stage, for laryngeal stenosis, 2920-2921
Laryngotracheal separation, for chronic aspiration, 931-932, 931f
Laryngotracheal stenosis, 943-952
classification of, 944, 944t
CO_2 laser for, 32
local application of mitomycin C for, 946
pathophysiology of, 943-944, 944b
surgical management of, 943-952
for chronic disease, 947-952
anterior glottic, 948
due to anterior wall collapse, 951
cervical tracheal, 951, 951b, 951f
cicatricial membranous, 951
complete glottic, 949-950
complete tracheal, 951-952, 952f
laryngeal release procedures in, 952
posterior glottic, 948-949, 949f
subglottic, 945f, 950-951
supraglottic, 947-948
endoscopic *vs.* open, 945
goals and assessment in, 944, 945f
microsurgical débridement in, 946, 946b, 946f
planning for, 946-947
skin and mucosal grafts in, 946-947
Laryngotracheal stenosis *(Continued)*
stent placement in, 947, 947f
timing of, 945
due to trauma, 937-939, 939f-940f, 943
Laryngotracheitis, 1465, 1465f, 2803-2806
clinical features of, 2803-2804
defined, 2803
diagnosis of, 2804
differential diagnosis of, 2804-2805, 2806t
epidemiology of, 2803
etiology of, 2803
imaging of, 2804, 2804f-2805f
laryngoscopy of, 2804, 2805f
management of, 2805-2806, 2904
membranous (bacterial), 1465, 1465f
pathogenesis of, 2803-2804
postintubation, 2593
spasmodic, 2805
terminology for, 2803
Laryngotracheobronchitis. *See* Laryngotracheitis.
bacterial (membranous) (*See* Bacterial tracheitis)
Laryngotracheobronchoscopy, for stridor, 2902
anesthetic considerations for, 2902
bronchoscopy technique for, 2903, 2903f
complications of, 2903
dynamic airway assessment during, 2903
equipment for, 2902-2903, 2902f
microlaryngoscopy technique for, 2902-2903
postoperative car after, 2903
preparation and positioning for, 2902
Laryngotracheoesophageal clefts (LTECs), 2873-2874, 2873f
classification of, 2873, 2874f, 2874t
syndromes associated with, 2870t
Laryngovideostroboscopy. *See* Laryngeal stroboscopy.
Larynx
anatomy of, 1578
applied, 805, 806f-807f
cartilage in, 805-806, 806f
mucosa in, 807
musculature in, 806-807, 806f-807f
nerve supply in, 807
post-therapy, 1476-1479, 1479f
radiographic, 1462-1464, 1578f
aryepiglottic folds in, 1471, 1471f
arytenoid cartilage in, 1471, 1473f
coronal plane in, 1473f
cricoid cartilage in, 1471, 1473f
cricoid ring in, 1473, 1473f
epiglottic cartilage in, 1471
epiglottis in, 1471f, 1473f
external carotid artery in, 1471f, 1473-1474
extrinsic strap muscles in, 1473f
false vocal cords in, 1472-1473, 1472f
hyoid bone in, 1471, 1471f, 1473f
internal carotid artery in, 1471f, 1473-1474
jugular veins in, 1471f, 1473-1474
laryngeal skeleton in, 1471
laryngeal ventricle in, 1472-1473
median glossoepiglottic fold in, 1471f
midsagittal plane in, 1473f
paralaryngeal (paraglottic) space in, 1471f, 1473
preepiglottic space in, 1471f, 1473, 1473f
pyriform sinuses in, 1471f, 1472
soft tissue structures in, 1471
sternocleidomastoid muscle in, 1471f
subglottic, 1473f
superior thyroid notch in, 1472f
supraglottic, 1471f
thyroid cartilage in, 1471, 1473f
true vocal cords in, 1472, 1472f-1473f
valleculae in, 1471f
surgical, 1541-1544
anterior commissure tendon in, 1541-1542
cartilage in, 1541

Larynx *(Continued)*
connective tissue barriers in, 1542-1543, 1544f
conus elasticus in, 1541-1542, 1542f
cricothyroid ligament in, 1541-1542
epiglottis in, 1541
hyoid bone in, 1541
hypoepiglottic ligament in, 1541-1542
paraglottic space in, 1542, 1543f
preepiglottic space in, 1542, 1543f
quadrangular membrane in, 1541-1542, 1542f
skeletal structure in, 1541, 1541f
thyrohyoid membrane in, 1541-1542, 1542f
vocal tendon in, 1541-1542
artificial (*See* Voice prosthesis(es))
benign mass(es) of, 1468
congenital cysts as, 1468
laryngocele as, 159-161, 163f, 1468, 1469f
squamous papillomas as, 1468, 1468f
subglottic hemangioma as, 1468, 1468f
benign mesenchymal neoplasms of, 878-882
chondroma as, 881-882
granular cell, 882
lipoma as, 881
mixed, 881
neurilemmoma as, 882
neurofibroma as, 882
oncocytic, 881
recurrent respiratory papillomatosis as, 868f-869f, 878-880
adult-onset, 879
epidemiology of, 878
etiology of, 878-879
juvenile form of, 879
treatment of, 879, 880f
rhabdomyoma as, 881
vascular, 880-881
laryngeal hemangiomas as, 880-881
polypoid granulation tissue as, 880
benign vocal fold mucosal disorders of (*See* Benign vocal fold mucosal disorder(s))
congenital disorder(s) of, 2866-2875
bifid epiglottis as, 2870t, 2874, 2874f
dysphagia due to, 2950t, 2951-2953, 2953f
hemangiomas and subglottic cysts as, 2871, 2871f
hypoplastic epiglottis as, 2870t
laryngeal cysts as, 2872-2873, 2872f-2873f
laryngeal webs/atresia as, 2869-2871
anterior, 2869-2870, 2869f-2870f
posterior, 2869, 2869f
subglottic stenosis as, 2870-2871
syndromes associated with, 2870t
laryngeal-laryngotracheoesophageal cleft as, 2873-2874, 2873f
classification of, 2873, 2874f, 2874t
syndromes associated with, 2870t
laryngomalacia as, 2866-2868, 2867f-2868f
syndromes associated with, 2870t
thyroglossal duct cyst as, 2871-2872, 2872f
vocal fold paralysis as, 2868-2869
connective tissue barriers within, 1542-1543, 1544f
electrical artificial, 1459
embryology of, 1482-1483
epiglottic flap closure of, for chronic aspiration, 928, 930f
foreign bodies in
endoscopic removal of, 2904
anesthesia for, 2940
imaging of, 1480-1481, 1480f-1481f
vs. ossification of stylohyoid ligament, 1480, 1481f
symptoms of, 2937-2938

Larynx *(Continued)*
functions of, 807-809, 833
in circulatory reflexes, 809, 810f
in control of ventilation, 808-809, 808f-809f
in cough, 808
as immune organ, 886-887, 887f
in protection, 808, 833
sensory receptors in, 809
in speech, 810-812, 811b, 811f, 833
GERD-related disease of, in children, 2944-2947
diagnosis of, 2945
disorders due to, 2945-2946, 2945b
evidence of, 2946
history of, 2944
management of, 2946
pathophysiology of, 2945
in geriatric patients, 234-237
acoustic changes in, 236
dental/mandibular changes in, 236
factors affecting vocal quality in, 234, 235t
glandular changes in, 236
histologic changes in, 234-235, 235f
laryngoscopic appearance in, 235-236
mucosal changes in, 236
respiratory changes in, 236
and sense of taste, 236
treatment of, 236-237
giant cell tumor of, 1510
imaging of, 159-161, 813-824, 1462-1481
with benign mass(es), 1468
congenital cysts as, 1468
laryngocele as, 159-161, 163f, 1468, 1469f
squamous papillomas as, 1468, 1468f
subglottic hemangioma as, 1468, 1468f
with carcinoma, 161, 164f
of anterior commissure, 1474, 1474f
of aryepiglottic fold, 1475, 1478f
with cartilaginous invasion, 1474-1475, 1476f
of epiglottis, 1475, 1477f
glottic, 1474-1475, 1474f
with lymph node metastases, 1476, 1479f
normal anatomy and, 1470-1474
paraglottic, 1474
post-therapy, 1476-1479, 1479f
of pyriform sinus, 1475-1476, 1478f
subglottic, 1474, 1475f
supraglottic, 1475-1476
technique for, 1470, 1470f
transglottic, 161, 164f, 1475f, 1476, 1478f
CT for, 132f, 140
flexible endoscopy for, 814
advantages of, 814
disadvantages of, 814
for professional voice disorders, 851-852, 852t
protocols for, 816b, 818b
technique of, 814
troubleshooting for, 814
with foreign bodies, 1480-1481, 1480f-1481f
high-speed digital, 821-823
applications of, 823
assessment using, 822-823
defined, 813
equipment for, 821
kymography in, 134f, 154, 822f
limitations of, 823
with inflammatory disease, 1464-1466
croup as, 1465, 1465f
epiglottitis as, 159-161, 163f, 1406-1407, 1407f, 1464, 1464f-1465f
retropharyngeal abscess as, 1465-1466, 1466f
with laryngomalacia, 1466
MRI for, 142-143
narrow-band, 813, 823-824, 823f-824f
with normal airway, 1462-1464
anatomy of, 1462-1464, 1463f-1464f
technique for, 1462

Larynx *(Continued)*
rigid endoscopy for, 813-814
advantages of, 813
disadvantages of, 813-814
for professional voice disorders, 851, 852t
protocols for, 816b, 818b
technique of, 814
troubleshooting for, 814
stroboscopy for, 818-821
of adynamic segments, 820
of amplitude of vibration, 820, 821f, 848, 848t
of closure pattern, 819, 820f, 848t, 849
common problems and solutions for, 815t-816t
defined, 813
flexible endoscopes in, 814
interpretation of, 848t
interval examination in, 847
of mucosal wave, 820, 848-849, 848t
in neurologic examination, 834
of periodicity, 821, 848, 848t
of phase closure, 819-820
for professional voice, 847-849, 848f, 848t
protocol for, 818-819, 818b
of regularity, 821
rigid endoscopes in, 813-814
of symmetry, 820, 847-848, 848t
of vertical closure level, 821
for vocal fold impairment, 905
with trauma, 159, 162f, 1479-1480, 1480f
videoendoscopy for, 814-818
of arytenoid and vocal fold motion, 816
common problems and solutions for, 815t-816t
defined, 813
flexible endoscopes for, 814
of laryngeal structure, 816
of mucous, 816-817
in neurologic examination, 834
protocol for, 814, 816b
rigid endoscopes for, 813-814
of supraglottic activity, 817, 817f
of vascularity, 817
of vocal fold edges, 818
with vocal cord paralysis, 1466-1467, 1467f
inflammatory disease of, 1464-1466
croup as, 1465, 1465f
epiglottitis as, 159-161, 163f, 1406-1407, 1407f, 1464, 1464f-1465f
retropharyngeal abscess as, 1465-1466, 1466f
inflammatory myofibroblastic tumor of, 1509-1510
lymphatic drainage of, 1578-1579, 1579f, 2582
metastases to, 1510
mucosal lining of, 1484
mucous in, videoendoscopy of, 816-817
necrotizing sialometaplasia of, 1493
neoplasms of uncertain behavior of, 1509-1510
neurologic disorders of, 837-843
hyperfunctional, 838-842
botulinum toxin therapy for, 839, 840f-841f
due to dystonia, 838-839, 838b
essential tremor as, 840-841
due to myoclonus, 840
due to pseudobulbar palsy, 839-840
stuttering as, 841-842
hypofunctional, 842-843
due to central causes of vocal fold paresis, 842
due to medullary disorders, 842
due to multiple sclerosis, 843
due to myopathies, 842
due to neuromuscular junction disorders, 842
due to Parkinson's disease, 842-843
due to poliomyelitis, 842

Larynx *(Continued)*
psychogenic, malingering, and mixed causes of, 843
vocal fold paresis as, 843
laryngologic manifestations of neurologic diseases as, 837-838, 838t
neurologic evaluation of, 832-836
acoustic analysis in, 834-835
aerodynamic assessment in, 835
cineradiography in, 835-836
edrophonium test in, 835
electromyography in, 835, 905
flexible laryngoscopy in, 834
glottography in, 835
indications for, 832-833, 833b
normal function and, 833
performance measures in, 835-836
rating scales in, 834
sensory assessment in, 836
during pharyngeal swallow, 1216-1217, 1216f
physical examination of, 99-100, 99f-100f
flexible endoscopy in, 100
postnasal descent of, 805, 806f
premalignant lesions and carcinoma in situ of, 1486-1491, 1489f-1490f, 1515
treatment of, 1489-1490, 1490t
in-office, 1490-1491
pseudoepitheliomatous hyperplasia of, 1493
pseudoretropharyngeal mass of, 1462, 1463f
saccular disorders of, 876-878
classification of, 876f, 877
clinical scenario with, 877
diagnosis of, 877
etiology of, 876
laryngocele as, 876f, 877
laryngopyocele as, 877
saccular cysts as, 877, 877f
anterior, 876f-877f, 877
lateral, 876f, 877, 878f
treatment of, 877-878
sensory receptors in, 807, 809
during swallowing, 833
systemic medicines that may affect, 863
taste buds in, 1208
vascularity of, videoendoscopy of, 817
Laser(s)
argon (Ar), 30, 31t
argon tunable (pumped) dye, 30, 31t
beam pattern of, 27
beam waist of, 27-28, 28f
carbon dioxide, 31t, 32-33
cavity dumped, 34
continuous wave, 33
control of, 26-28
exposure time in, 28
power in, 27, 29f
spot size in, 27-28, 28f-29f
defined, 26
depth of focus of, 27-28, 28f
erbium:YAG, 33
flash lamp pulsed, 33-34
flash lamp pumped dye, 31t, 33
fluence of, 28
focal length of lens of, 28
focal plane of, 28, 28f
history of, 25-26
holmium:YAG, 33
irradiance of, 27
KTP, 31t, 33
mode-locked, 34
neodymium:YAG, 31t, 32
pulse structure of, 33-34
pulsed, 30
pulsed dye, 31t, 33
Q-switched, 34
quantum physics of, 26, 26f
safety considerations with, 34-37

Laser(s) *(Continued)*
anesthesia and risk of intraoperative fire as, 36-37
education on, 34
eye protection as, 34-35, 35f-36f
protocol for, 34
effectiveness of, 37
skin protection as, 35
smoke evacuation as, 35
tissue effects of, 28-30, 30f
types and applications of, 30-33, 31t
wound created by, 29-30, 30f
Laser ablation, 30
interventional bronchoscopy with, 1010t
Laser device, 26, 27f
Laser Doppler velocimetry, for assessment of nasal airway, 643-644
Laser midline glossectomy (LMG), for obstructive sleep apnea, 259
Laser resurfacing, 399-402
CO_2, 400, 400f
complications of, 402
Er:YAG, 400
nonablative, 402, 403t
postoperative care after, 401-402, 401f
results of, 401f-402f
Laser surgery, 25-37
endotracheal tubes for, 36-37
for hemangioma of infancy, 2827f-2828f, 2828
history of, 25-26
for laryngeal stenosis, 2918
for recurrent respiratory papillomatosis
with carbon dioxide laser, 879, 2889-2891
pulsed dye laser for, 880, 880f, 2891
for skin lesions, 294
for stridulous child, 2908-2909, 2908f
for tracheal stenosis, 2928, 2929f
Laser vaporization, for unresectable tracheal tumor, 1619-1621
Laser-assisted uvulopalatoplasty, in vocal professional, 858
"Laser-safe" endotracheal tube, with recurrent respiratory papillomatosis, 2891
Lassa fever, sensorineural hearing loss due to, 2158-2159
sudden, 2127
LAT (lidocaine-adrenaline-tetracaine) anesthesia, for facial trauma, 304
Lateral ala, thinning of, in cleft-lip nose repair, 562f
Lateral alar angle, 509f
Lateral ampullary nerve, 1854f, 2278f
Lateral arm flap, 1082t, 1083
for hypopharyngeal and esophageal reconstruction, 1455
for oropharyngeal reconstruction, 1379-1380
of tongue base, 1389
of tonsils and pharyngeal wall, 1386-1387
Lateral arteriorrhaphy, for vascular repair, 1632-1633, 1634f
Lateral canal benign paroxysmal positional vertigo
positional testing for, 2315-2316, 2331
repositioning maneuver for, 2332
Lateral canthal angle, 442
Lateral canthal tendon, 439
Lateral cantholysis, for pediatric facial fracture, 2704f
Lateral canthoplasty, 2420-2421
Lateral canthus, in brow or forehead rejuvenation, 434, 434f
Lateral cephalometric radiograph, for mentoplasty, 463, 463f
Lateral cervical space, 158, 162f
Lateral cranial base, surgical anatomy of, 2434-2438, 2442, 2443f, 2488-2489
abducens nerve in, 2439f
anterior clinoid process in, 2435f
anterior cranial fossa in, 2435f

Lateral cranial base, surgical anatomy of *(Continued)*
anterior division in, 2442-2444
anterior boundaries of, 2442, 2443f
boundaries in, 2442, 2443f
craniofacial junction in, 2442, 2443f
extracranial structures related to, 2443, 2444f
superior boundaries of, 2442-2443, 2443f
and surgical landmarks of orbital skeleton, 2443-2444, 2444f
anterior inferior cerebellar artery in, 2437f, 2439f
arcuate eminence in, 2436f, 2437
Bill's bar (vertical crest) in, 2437-2439
brainstem in, 2439f
bulbopontine sulcus in, 2439f
carotid artery canal in, 2435f-2436f, 2438
carotid artery in, 2436f, 2438
cerebellar floccules in, 2439f
cerebellar hemispheres in, 2439f
cerebellar horizontal fissure in, 2439f
cerebellar olive in, 2439f
cerebellopontine angle in, 2438
chorda tympani nerve in, 2436f, 2439f, 2441
choroid plexus in, 2439f
clivus in, 2435f
cochlea in, 2437f, 2438
cochlear aqueduct in, 2435f
cochlear modiolus in, 2439
cochlear nerve in, 2437f, 2439
craniofacial junction in, 2442, 2443f
cribriform plate in, 2435
digastric groove in, 2436f
digastric sulcus in, 2435-2436, 2435f
dural septum in, 2437f
emissary vein in, 2436f
epitympanum in, 2438
eustachian tube in, 2436f-2437f, 2438
eustachian tube opening in, 2436f
external auditory canal in, 2435, 2435f
external carotid artery in, 2440f
facial hiatus in, 2436f, 2437
facial nerve in, 2436f-2437f, 2438-2439, 2439f-2440f
facial recess in, 2436f
foramen lacerum in, 2435f, 2436-2437
foramen magnum in, 2435f
foramen ovale in, 2435f, 2436-2438, 2437f
foramen rotundum in, 2435f, 2438
foramen spinosum in, 2434, 2435f, 2437-2438, 2441
gasserian ganglion in, 2437f, 2438, 2440f
geniculate ganglion in, 2436f-2437f, 2438
glenoid fossa in, 2435f
glossopharyngeal nerve in, 2436f-2437f, 2438, 2439f-2440f, 2440
greater superficial petrosal nerve in, 2437f, 2438
greater wing of sphenoid bone in, 2434, 2435f
hypoglossal nerve canal in, 2435f
hypoglossal nerve in, 2439f-2440f
incus in, 2436f
incus-malleus articulation in, 2436f, 2438
incus-stapes articulation in, 2436f
inferior oblique muscle in, 2439f
inferior orbital fissure in, 2441
inferior vestibular nerve in, 2437f, 2439
infratemporal cranial fossa in, 2440-2441, 2440f
internal acoustic pore (porus acusticus) in, 2437-2438
internal auditory artery in, 2437f, 2439f
internal auditory canal in, 2435f-2437f, 2438-2439
internal carotid artery in, 2436f-2437f, 2439f-2440f
internal maxillary artery in, 2440f
jugular bulb in, 2436f-2437f
jugular foramen in, 2435f-2436f, 2438-2440, 2439f-2440f
jugular process in, 2435f

Lateral cranial base, surgical anatomy of *(Continued)*
jugular tuberculum in, 2435f
jugular vein in, 2436f, 2439f-2440f
lateral pterygoid muscle in, 2441
lateral pterygoid process in, 2435f
lateral semicircular canal in, 2436f, 2439f
mandible in, 2440f
mandibular division of trigeminal nerve in, 2437f, 2438, 2440f, 2441
masseter muscle in, 2440f
mastoid antrum in, 2438
mastoid bone in, 2435, 2435f
mastoid process in, 2435
mastoid tegmen in, 2435f
mastoid tip in, 2435f
maxillary artery in, 2441
maxillary division of trigeminal nerve in, 2437f, 2438, 2440f
medial pterygoid muscle in, 2441
medial pterygoid process in, 2435f
middle cranial fossa in, 2434, 2435f-2437f, 2438
middle division in, 2444
boundaries in, 2442, 2443f
craniofacial junction in, 2442, 2443f
extracranial view of, 2444, 2445f
foramina along floor of, 2444, 2445f
intracranial view of, 2444, 2445f
lateral pterygoid plate in, 2444, 2445f
lateral view of, 2444, 2445f
sphenoid spine in, 2444
superomedial boundary of, 2444
middle meningeal artery in, 2437f, 2438, 2440f
middle meningeal artery sulcus in, 2436f
nervus intermedius (of Wrisberg) in, 2437f
occipital bone in, 2435f
occipitomastoid suture in, 2435, 2435f
oculomotor nerve in, 2439f
ophthalmic division of trigeminal nerve in, 2437f, 2438
ossicular chain in, 2436f
parietal bone in, 2434
parietomastoid suture in, 2435, 2435f
parotid gland in, 2439f-2440f
petroclival sutures in, 2436
petro-occipital sulcus in, 2435f, 2438
petro-occipital suture in, 2438
petrosphenoid suture in, 2435f
petrosquamous suture in, 2434, 2436f
petrotympanic suture in, 2435
petrous apex in, 2435f, 2436
petrous bone in, 2436, 2437f
petrous bone projection in, 2435f
pons in, 2439f
pontine-mesencephalic sulcus in, 2439f
posterior clinoid process in, 2435f
posterior cranial fossa in, 2435f, 2438-2440, 2439f
posterior division in, 2442, 2443f
posterior semicircular canal in, 2436f, 2439f
pteroygoid venous plexus in, 2441
pteroygomaxillary fissure in, 2441
pteroygomaxillary fossa in, 2435f
pyramidal eminence in, 2436f
quadrangular cerebellar lobule in, 2439f
rectus capitis major muscle in, 2439f
rectus lateralis muscle in, 2439f
round window niche in, 2436f
sella in, 2435f
semicanal of tensor tympani muscle in, 2436f
sigmoid sinus impression in, 2435f
sigmoid sinus in, 2436f, 2439f-2440f
sphenoid bone in, 2435f
sphenopalatine foramen in, 2435f
spinal accessory nerve in, 2436f, 2438, 2439f-2440f, 2440
squamosa in, 2434, 2435f-2436f
stapes in, 2436f

Lateral cranial base, surgical anatomy of *(Continued)*
stapes tendon in, 2436f
styloid process in, 2435, 2435f
stylomastoid foramen in, 2435
subarcuate artery in, 2439f
subarcuate fossa in, 2435f, 2438
superior laryngeal nerve in, 2440f
superior oblique muscle in, 2439f
superior orbital fissure in, 2435f, 2438
superior petrosal sinus impression in, 2435f
superior petrosal (petrous) sinus in, 2436f, 2438
superior petrosal vein in, 2439f
superior semicircular canal in, 2436f-2437f, 2439f
superior vestibular nerve in, 2437f, 2438-2439
suprameatal spine in, 2435f
tegmen mastoideum in, 2438
tegmen tympani in, 2438
temporal bone in, 2434, 2436f
temporis muscle in, 2440f
tensor tympani muscle in, 2437f, 2438
transverse (falciform) crest in, 2437f, 2439
transverse sinus in, 2436f, 2439f
Trautmann's triangle in, 2436f
trigeminal depression (Meckel's cave) in, 2435f, 2436-2437
trigeminal impression in, 2435f
trigeminal nerve in, 2439f
trochlear nerve in, 2439f
tympanic bone in, 2434-2435, 2435f, 2439f
tympanic membrane in, 2436f
tympanic sulcus in, 2435
tympanomastoid suture in, 2434-2435, 2435f
tympanosquamous suture in, 2434, 2435f
vagus nerve in, 2436f-2437f, 2438, 2439f-2440f, 2440
vertebral artery in, 2439f
vestibular aqueduct in, 2435f
vestibulocochlear nerve in, 2438, 2439f
zygoma in, 2435f-2436f
Lateral cranial base lesion(s)
aneurysms of upper cervical and petrous internal carotid artery as, 2504, 2504f-2505f
evaluation of, 2489-2492
carotid management algorithms in, 2491-2492
cerebral blood flow assessment in, 2490-2491, 2490f
qualitative, 2490-2491
quantitative, 2491
CT and MRI for, 2489
four-vessel arteriography in, 2489-2490, 2491f
preoperative carotid artery management in, 2489
algorithm for, 2490f, 2491-2492
cerebral blood flow assessment in, 2490-2491, 2490f
four-vessel arteriography in, 2489-2490, 2491f
postsurgical and postinfectious encephalocele and CSF leaks as, 2509
Lateral cranial base neoplasm(s)
carcinoma as, 2502-2504
management of, 2502-2504, 2503f
pertinent anatomy for, 2502
staging of, 2502, 2502f, 2503b
symptoms and signs of, 2502
of cavernous sinus, 2509-2510
choice of surgical approach for, 2492-2501
chordoma as, 2510, 2511f
of clivus, 2509
evaluation of, 2489-2492
carotid management algorithms in, 2491-2492
cerebral blood flow assessment in, 2490-2491, 2490f
qualitative, 2490-2491
quantitative, 2491
CT and MRI for, 2489

Lateral cranial base neoplasm(s) *(Continued)*
four-vessel arteriography in, 2489-2490, 2491f
preoperative carotid artery assessment in, 2489, 2490f
facial nerve schwannomas as, 2506-2508
diagnostic evaluation of, 2507
management and surgical approach to, 2507-2508
of jugular foramen, 2504
schwannomas as, 2504-2505, 2505f
paragangliomas as, 2505-2506
diagnostic evaluation of, 2505, 2506f-2507f
preoperative evaluation of, 2491f
radiotherapy for, 2506
surgical approach to, 2505-2506, 2507f
symptoms of, 2505
of parapharyngeal space, 2510, 2512f
of petrous apex, 2508, 2508f
sleeve resection of external auditory canal for, 2492
Lateral cranial base surgery, 2487-2513
choice of approach for, 2492-2501
complications of, 2511-2513
intraoperative, 2511
postoperative, 2512-2513
cerebrovascular, 2512-2513
cranial nerve deficits as, 2512
encephalocele and CSF leaks as, 2509
infratemporal fossa approaches for, 2495-2501
postauricular, 2495-2500
cervical dissection in, 2495, 2498f
closure of external auditory canal in, 2495, 2497f
closure of wound in, 2499, 2499f
exposure of jugular bulb and internal carotid artery in, 2498, 2498f-2499f
extratemporal facial nerve dissection in, 2495-2496
facial nerve transposition in, 2497-2498, 2498f
incisions and skins flaps in, 2495, 2497f
occlusion of sigmoid sinus in, 2498, 2498f
radical mastoidectomy in, 2496, 2498f
removal of external auditory canal wall skin and tympanic membrane in, 2495, 2497f
tumor removal in, 2498-2499, 2499f
type A, 2497-2499, 2498f-2499f
type B, 2499-2500, 2500f
type C, 2500, 2501f
preauricular, 2500-2501, 2501f
for nasopharyngeal tumors, 2510-2511
postsurgical encephalocele and CSF leaks with
diagnostic evaluation of, 2509
surgical approach to, 2509
Lateral cricoarytenoid (LCA) muscle
applied anatomy of, 806
characteristics of, 918
in professional voice production, 846-847
Lateral cricothyroid muscle, applied anatomy of, 806
Lateral crural grafts, in revision rhinoplasty, 589-590, 590f
Lateral crus(crura), of alar cartilage, 496-497, 497f, 509f
in cleft-lip nose repair, 562f
transposition of, 551
Lateral facial approach, for middle cranial base surgery, 2462, 2465f
Lateral lamella of cribriform plate (LLCP), and CSF rhinorrhea, 787, 787f
Lateral lemniscal nuclei, in central auditory pathway, 1835-1836, 1835f
Lateral lemniscus, in central auditory pathway, 1835-1836, 1835f, 1846
Lateral medullary syndrome, 2313, 2352f, 2354f

Lateral nasal prominences, in embryology
of lip, 2660, 2661f-2662f, 2661t
of nose, 2691f
Lateral nasal wall, in surgical anatomy of anterior cranial base, 2472, 2472f-2473f
Lateral nasal wall deformities, revision rhinoplasty for, 586
Lateral neck dissection, 1716-1718
definition and rationale for, 1716-1717, 1717f
technique for, 1717-1718, 1717f
Lateral olfactory tract, 628f
Lateral olivocochlear (LOC) reflex pathways, in efferent auditory system, 1848-1849
Lateral orbital rim, surgical access to, 328-329, 329f
Lateral orbital tubercle, 439
Lateral orbital wall, 439
Lateral orbital wall fractures, pediatric, 2712, 2714
Lateral periapical cyst, 1263
Lateral periodontal cyst, 1265-1266
microscopic features of, 1265-1266, 1265f
radiographic features of, 1265
treatment of, 1266
Lateral pharyngeal node, 1298f
Lateral pharyngeal space
anatomy of, 202
odontogenic infections of, 184-185, 186f
Lateral pharyngotomy approach
for hypopharyngeal cancer, 1426-1427
for oropharyngeal cancer, 1371, 1371f
Lateral pontomedullary syndrome, 2353f
Lateral process, 1824, 1825f, 1826-1827
Lateral pterygoid muscle
anatomy of, 1320
in surgical anatomy of lateral skull base, 2441
Lateral pterygoid plate, in surgical anatomy of middle cranial base, 2444, 2445f
Lateral pterygoid process, in surgical anatomy of lateral skull base, 2435f
Lateral radicular cyst, 1263
Lateral rectus muscle(s)
semicircular canal planes and, 2285-2287, 2286f-2287f
in surgical anatomy of anterior cranial base, 2472f
Lateral retropharyngeal nodes, 1422
Lateral rhinotomy
for middle cranial base surgery, 2455t, 2458, 2458f
for nasopharyngeal carcinoma, 1355-1356, 1355f
Lateral semicircular canal (LSSC)
anatomy of, 1826f, 1827, 1851f, 1854f, 2278f
dysplasia of, 2732, 2732f-2733f
imaging of, 1922f
in surgical anatomy of lateral skull base, 2436f, 2439f
Lateral sinus thrombosis
epidemiology of, 1980t-1981t
imaging of, 1996f-1997f, 1997
otitis media and, 2777
pathogenesis of, 1996
signs and symptoms of, 1996-1997
treatment of, 1997
Lateral skull base. *See* Lateral cranial base.
Lateral superior olive (LSO), in auditory pathway, 1834-1835, 1834f, 1846
Lateral thigh flap(s), 1082t
for hypopharyngeal and esophageal reconstruction, 1455
for oropharyngeal reconstruction, 1379
of tongue base, 1390-1391
of tonsils and pharyngeal wall, 1386-1387
Lateral transtemporal sphenoid approach, for middle cranial base surgery, 2462, 2465f
Lateral transthyroid pharyngotomy, for hypopharyngeal cancer, 1427, 1428f
Lateral vertical buttress, 319, 331, 331f
Lateral vestibular nucleus (of Dieters), 1860-1861, 1862f
Lateral vestibulospinal tract, in postural balance, 1865
Lateral view, of facial bones and sinuses, 130
Lateralized radicular cyst, 1263
Latex, adverse reactions to, 102
Lathyrogenic drugs, for caustic ingestion, 2959
Latissimus dorsi musculocutaneous flap, for oropharyngeal reconstruction, 1378, 1378f
of tongue base, 1389
Latissimus dorsi myocutaneous free flap, 1082t, 1083-1084, 1084f
for hypopharyngeal and esophageal reconstruction, 1452
for oropharyngeal reconstruction, 1380
of tongue base, 1389-1390, 1390f
LATS (long-acting thyroid stimulator), 1741
LC. *See* Laryngeal cleft (LC).
LCA (lateral cricoarytenoid) muscle
applied anatomy of, 806
characteristics of, 918
in professional voice production, 846-847
LCH. *See* Langerhans' cell histiocytosis (LCH).
LCR (laryngeal chemoreflex), 2570
LDH (lactate dehydrogenase), with melanoma, 1109-1110, 1113
LDL (low-density lipoprotein) cholesterol, subclinical hypothyroidism and, 1747
Leapfrog Group, 84t-87t, 87
Learning problems, obstructive sleep apnea and, 2603-2604
Leeches, medicinal, for flap salvage, 1075, 1098
LeFort I fractures, 326, 327f
pediatric, 2707
repair of, 334-335, 334f
LeFort I osteotomy(ies)
in cleft-lip nose repair, 559, 564f-565f
for juvenile nasopharyngeal angiofibroma, 1350-1351
for middle cranial base surgery, 2455t, 2458, 2460f
LeFort II fractures, 326, 327f
pediatric, 2707
repair of, 335-336, 335f-336f
LeFort III fractures, 326, 327f
pediatric, 2707
Left anterior–right posterior (LARP) semicircular canal plane, 2285, 2286f, 2287, 2288f
Legal issues
with difficult airway, 110
with noise-induced hearing loss, 2149-2151
Leiomyoma
esophageal, 1415-1416, 1415f
of trachea, 1613
Leiomyosarcoma, of neck, 1670
Leksell, Lars, 1696
Lemierre's syndrome, due to deep neck space infections, 207
Length-to-width ratio, of skin flaps, 1068, 1068f
Lentigo, solar (actinic, senilis), 288
Lentigo maligna (LM), 1108
surgical excision of, 1114
Lentigo maligna melanoma (LMM), 287f, 1108
surgical excision of, 1114
Lentiviral vectors, for gene transfer, 16, 18t
Leprosy, laryngitis due to, 885
Leptomeningeal nevus flammeus, 291
LES. *See* Lower esophageal sphincter (LES).
Leser-Trélat sign, 282
Lesser occipital nerve, 2578, 2580f
Lesser palatine nerve, 1297f
Lesser wing of sphenoid bone, in surgical anatomy of middle cranial base, 2444, 2445f
Lesser zygomatic muscle, reinnervation of, 2423f
Letterer-Siwe disease, 2100-2101
oral manifestations of, 1257
otologic manifestations of, 2102f
otorrhea as, 2196
Leucine-rich transmembrane *O*-methyltransferase *(LRTOMT)* gene, in deafness, 2051t-2058t
Leucovorin, for induction chemotherapy, 1056
Leukemia
oral manifestations of, 1256
otologic manifestations of, 2107, 2108f
otorrhea as, 2197
sensorineural hearing loss due to, 2123
Leukocytosis, in deep neck infections, 204
Leukoedema, oral, 1222-1223
clinical features of, 1222, 1223f
defined, 1222
etiology and pathogenesis of, 1222
histopathologic features of, 1222, 1223f
management of, 1223
Leukoencephalopathy, progressive multifocal, HIV-associated, 223
Leukoplakia
candidal, 1231, 1231f
oral, 1223-1225
chemoprevention of, 1225
clinical features of, 1224-1225, 1224f
defined, 1223
etiology of, 1223-1224, 1223f-1224f
hairy, 1226, 1226f
in HIV, 225-226, 226f
histopathologic features of, 1225, 1226f
malignant transformation of, 1223, 1298
proliferative verrucous, 1225, 1225f
thin, 1224f, 1225
of tongue, 1362f
treatment of, 1225
Leukoplakic-type hyperkeratosis, 1231, 1231f
Leukotriene modifiers
for allergic rhinitis, 620-621
for rhinosinusitis, 735t, 736
Levator anguli oris, 321f
Levator aponeurosis, 443f, 444
in upper eyelid blepharoplasty, 448
Levator labii, 442f
Levator labii superioris, reinnervation of, 2423f
Levator nasi, 442f
Levator palpebrae, 321f
Levator palpebrae superioris, 444
Levator repositioning, for velopharyngeal dysfunction, 2682
Levator scapulae muscle, 2579f
Levator veli palatini (LVP) muscle
anatomy of, 1360f, 1868f, 1870
in cleft palate, 2666-2667
development of, 1866
in pressure equalization, 1870
in velopharyngeal function, 2676, 2677t
Levels of evidence, 69-70, 70t
Lever ratio, in auditory physiology, 1840, 1840f
Levetiracetam, for neuropathic pain, 244t
Levocetirizine (Xyzal), for nonallergic rhinitis, 701t
Levothyroxine, oral synthetic (Euthyrox, Levothroid, Levoxyl, Synthroid, Unithroid), for hypothyroidism, 1748-1749
Lexical Neighborhood Test (LNT), for cochlear implant, 2225-2226
Lhermitte's sign, due to radiotherapy, 1049
LHFPL5 (lipoma HMGIC fusion partner-like 5) gene, in deafness, 2051t-2058t
Liability genes, 8
Licensure, maintenance of, 80-81
Lichen planus
esophageal manifestations of, 980
oral, 1226-1229, 1253-1254
atrophic or erythematous, 1227, 1227f
bullous variant of, 1227-1228
clinical differential diagnosis of, 1228
clinical features of, 1227-1228
erosive, 1227, 1228f
etiology and pathogenesis of, 1227
histopathologic features of, 1228, 1228f

Lichen planus *(Continued)*
and oral carcinoma, 1229, 1298-1299
plaque form of, 1227
reticular-type, 1227, 1227f
systemic diseases and, 1228
treatment of, 1228
Lichenoid dysplasia, 1229
Lichenoid lesion, oral, 1229
Lid crease, 442, 443f
Lid lag, in Graves' ophthalmopathy, 1808
Lid shortening procedure, 449
Lidocaine (Xylocaine)
with anesthesia induction, 111-112
in children, 2590
for facial trauma, 304
for prevention of bronchospasm during anesthesia, in children, 2595
and skin flap viability, 1073
Lidocaine (Xylocaine) block, for neuropathic pain, 245
Lidocaine (Xylocaine) provocation test, for embolization, 1934
Lidocaine-adrenaline-tetracaine (LAT) anesthesia, for facial trauma, 304
LIFE (lung imaging fluorescence endoscope) system, for early glottic carcinoma, 1516
Lifelong learning, 79t
Lifestyle modifications, for GERD, 969-970
Lighted stylet, for difficult airway, 114t
Lightheadedness, 2308-2310
Limbus, 1832f
Limen nasi, 641
Limen vestibuli, 641
LINACs. *See* Linear accelerator(s) (LINACs).
Lindbergh Operation, 39
Linear acceleration, encoding of, 2277-2285
by afferents in, 2283-2285, 2283f-2284f
cupula in, 2282f
otoconial membrane in, 2283
sensory transduction in, 2277-2279
anatomy of vestibular end organs in, 2277, 2278f
bidirectional sensitivity in, 2278-2279
cupula in, 2277, 2278f
firing rate in, 2278-2279, 2281f
hair cells in, 2277
otolith organs in, 2278, 2281f
stereocilia in, 2277-2278, 2279f
Linear accelerator(s) (LINACs), 1034
block diagram of, 1034f
megavoltage x-rays produced by, 1034
orthovoltage x-rays produced by, 1034
photograph of, 1035f
radiation production from, 1032-1033
in stereotactic radiation therapy, 2557-2558, 2560t
Linear accelerator (LINAC)-based stereotactic irradiation, for malignant skull base tumors, 1696
Linear amplification, for hearing aids, 2268, 2268f
Linear jerk, 2284
Linear predictive coding (LPC) spectrum, in acoustic analysis for voice evaluation, 829t, 830, 830f
Linear tomography, of pharynx and esophagus, 1393
Lingual artery, 1295, 1296f, 2579-2580, 2580f
Lingual frenulum, 1297-1298
Lingual muscles, 1205
Lingual nerve, 1296f, 1297-1298
Lingual nerve injury, due to neck surgery, 1731
Lingual reflexes, 1205
Lingual thyroid gland, 161-162, 165f, 1287, 1736
Lingual tonsil(s), in immune system, 605
Lingual tonsillectomy, for obstructive sleep apnea, 259
Lingual veins, 1295
Lingualplasty, for obstructive sleep apnea, 259
Lip(s)
aesthetic analysis of, 274-275, 278f
anatomy of, 1296-1297
burns of, 316
cancer of, 1302
lymphatic drainage of, 1296-1297, 1297f
neurologic examination of, 833-834
physical examination of, 98
squamous cell carcinoma of, 1302-1304
clinical findings in, 1294f, 1302, 1302f
epidemiology of, 1302
neck metastases of, 1303-1304
prognostic features of, 1303
resection and reconstruction of, 1303-1304, 1303f
Abbe-Estlander flap in, 1303-1304, 1303f
Karapandzic fan flap in, 1303-1304, 1303f
survival with, 1304
trauma to, 309-310, 309f
Lip defects, 350-353
classification of, 351
greater than two-thirds width, 352
lateral, 352
less than one-half width, 351
primary wound closure for, 351
V-Y musculocutaneous island pedicle flap for, 356f
lower
algorithm for, 351, 355f
midline, 352-353
massive or near-total, 352-353, 357f-358f
melolabial transposition flap for, 353
temporal forehead flap for, 353
from one half to two thirds, 351
Abbé flap for, 352
Estlander flap for, 352, 356f
Karapendzic flap for, 351
lip switch flap for, 351
local *vs.* regional flaps for, 352
upper
algorithm for, 351, 355f
large, 352
V-Y advancement flap for, 347f
Lip switch flap, 351
Lip wedge excision, 2431, 2431f
Lipectomy
submental, 456
suction, 452, 456
Lipid(s), subclinical hypothyroidism and, 1747
Lipid-lowering drugs, sensorineural hearing loss due to, 2121
Lipoadenoma, of parathyroid gland, 1778
Lipoatrophy, facial, HIV-associated, 227-228, 228f
Lipocontouring. *See* Liposuction.
Lipofection, 15
Lipoma(s), 293
of cerebellopontine angle, 2527, 2529f-2530f
imaging of, 1928, 1929t
in children, 2819
hypopharyngeal, 1425f
of internal auditory canal, 2527, 2529f
of larynx, 881
of neck, 1663
atypical, 1670
neck masses due to, 1641
in children, 2819
of oral cavity, 1291
parotid, 1166, 1167f
Lipoma HMGIC fusion partner-like 5 *(LHFPL5)* gene, in deafness, 2051t-2058t
Lipopeptides, and toll-like receptors, 598
Lipopolysaccharides (LPSs), and Toll-like receptors, 598
Lipoproteins
subclinical hypothyroidism and, 1747
and Toll-like receptors, 598
Liposarcoma, of neck, 1670
Liposarcoma of the larynx (LSL), 1508
Liposhaving, 452, 456, 458f
Liposome vector, for gene therapy, 16, 19f
of inner ear, 2191t
Liposuction, 452-460
adipocyte hyperplasia and, 452
anesthesia for, 456
common pitfalls in, 453, 455f
complications of, 459
defined, 452
instrumentation for, 453, 455f
integration into facial plastic and reconstructive surgery of, 452, 453f
patient preparation for, 455, 455f
patient selection for, 452-453, 454f
postsurgical dressing after, 459, 459f
recovery phase after, 459
results of, 459, 460f
surgical technique for, 456-459
determining depth of dissection in, 456, 457f
developing subcutaneous tunnels in, 456, 456f
distal feathering in, 456, 457f
identification of plane of dissection in, 456, 456f
incisions in, 456
liposhaving in, 456, 458f
multiple distal tunneling in, 456, 457f
open, 456-459
with other cosmetic procedures, 456-459
sites that can be approached in, 456, 458f
submental lipectomy in, 456
suction lipectomy in, 456
ultrasonic, 452
Lithium, for hyperthyroidism, 1739t
Lithium carbonate, for Graves' disease, 1742-1743
Lithium compounds, hypercalcemia due to, 1784
Little's area, 682
in epistaxis, 686-687
Live-attenuated influenza vaccine (LAIV), to prevent otitis media, 2769
Liver disease, oral manifestations of, 1255
Liver failure, preoperative evaluation of, 103-106
LL. *See* Lymphoblastic lymphoma (LL).
LL-37, 599
LLCP (lateral lamella of cribriform plate), and CSF rhinorrhea, 787, 787f
LLR (long latency response)
auditory evoked, 1912, 1913f
electrically evoked, 1913-1914, 1913f
LM (lentigo maligna), 1108
surgical excision of, 1114
LMG (laser midline glossectomy), for obstructive sleep apnea, 259
LMM (lentigo maligna melanoma), 287f, 1108
surgical excision of, 1114
LNT (Lexical Neighborhood Test), for cochlear implant, 2225-2226
Lobes, of lung, 998
Lobular capillary hemangioma, sinonasal, 718t, 725, 725f
Lobule(s)
of ear, 476-477, 476f, 1824f, 2742f
reduction of, 478f
of lung, 998
Lobule transfer, in microtia reconstruction, 2746, 2747f
LOC (lateral olivocochlear) reflex pathways, in efferent auditory system, 1848-1849
Local anesthetic(s), 112
oral sequelae of, 1247t-1248t
Local anesthetic blocks, for neuropathic pain, 245
Local flap(s)
advancement, 345-346
bilateral, 345, 346f
island, 345
unipedicle, 345, 345f

Local flap(s) *(Continued)*
V-Y, 345-346, 346f-347f
Y-V, 346
classification of, 342-343, 343b
complications of, 366
hinge, 346
for hypopharyngeal and esophageal reconstruction, 1450-1452
for oropharyngeal reconstruction, 1376-1377
palatal island, 1376-1377, 1376f
of soft palate, 1381
buccinator musculomucosal, 1381-1382, 1381f
palatal island mucosal, 1382
Superior Constrictor Rotation-Advancement Flap (SCARF) as, 1382, 1382f
uvulopalatal, 1377f, 1381
tongue, 1376
of tonsils and pharyngeal wall, 1384-1385
uvulopalatal, 1377, 1377f
pivotal, 343-345
effective length of, 343, 343f
interpolated, 344-345, 344f
rotation, 343-344, 343f
transposition, 344, 344f
Local overpressure therapy, for Meniere's disease, 2338
Localization study(ies), for hyperparathyroidism, 1784-1789, 1784t
gamma radiation detection device for, 1802, 1803f
intraoperative, 1784t, 1789
invasive preoperative, 1784t, 1788-1789
parathyroid arteriography as, 1788
selective venous sampling for PTH as, 1788-1789
ultrasound-guided fine-needle aspiration as, 1789
mediastinal exploration as, 1801-1802, 1802f
noninvasive preoperative, 1784-1788, 1784t
computed tomography as, 1786-1787
computed tomography–sestamibi fusion as, 1785-1786, 1786f-1788f
magnetic resonance imaging as, 1787-1788, 1789f
pertechnetate (technetium 99m) thallous chloride (thallium 201) imaging as, 1784-1785
sestamibi–technetium 99m scintigraphy as, 1785, 1785f, 1788f, 1794f
technetium 99m sestamibi with single photon emission computed tomography as, 1785
ultrasonography as, 1786, 1789f
unsuccessful, 1801, 1801f-1802f
Lockwood's ligament, 439
LOH (loss of heterozygosity), in head and neck squamous cell carcinoma, 1019-1020, 1026
Long latency response (LLR)
auditory evoked, 1912, 1913f
electrically evoked, 1913-1914, 1913f
Long process incus, anatomy of, 1825f
Long-acting thyroid stimulator (LATS), 1741
Long-term average spectra (LTAS), in acoustic analysis for voice evaluation, 829t, 830
Long-term potentiation (LTP), in neural plasticity, 1882-1884
Longus capitis muscle, 2579f
Longus colli muscle, 2579f
Longus colli muscle flap, for lateral pharyngeal wall defects, 1384-1385
Loop diuretics
in noise-induced hearing loss, 2147
ototoxicity of, 2174-2175
sensorineural hearing loss due to, 2120
Loprox (ciclopirox olamine antifungal cream or solution), for fungal otitis externa, 1954-1955, 1959t-1960t
Loratadine (Claritin)
for allergic rhinitis, 620
for nonallergic rhinitis, 701t
for rhinosinusitis, 734t
Los Angeles classification, of erosive esophagitis, 969, 969f
Loss of heterozygosity (LOH), in head and neck squamous cell carcinoma, 1019-1020, 1026
Lotrimin (clotrimazole) cream, for fungal otitis externa, 1954-1955, 1959t-1960t
Lou Gehrig's disease, laryngeal hypofunction due to, 842
Low-density lipoprotein (LDL) cholesterol, subclinical hypothyroidism and, 1747
Lower esophageal sphincter (LES)
anatomy of, 953, 954f
in GERD, 895, 895b
impairment of, 1400
manometry of, 958, 958f
physiology of, 954, 955f
Lower esophageal sphincter (LES) pressure, 958f
Lower esophageal sphincter (LES) relaxation, transient, 954, 968
Lower eyelid
aesthetic analysis of, 445-446, 446f
paralysis of, 2420-2421, 2421f
Lower eyelid blepharoplasty, 448-449
subciliary approach to, 449, 450f-451f
transconjunctival approach to, 448-449, 450f
Lower eyelid retractors, 444
Lower jugular lymph nodes, in neck dissection, 1704, 1704f, 1706t
Lower lateral cartilage, of nose, 497f
in cleft-lip nose repair, 562f-564f
reshaping of, 577
Lower lip, of vocal folds, in mucosal wave propagation, 848-849
Lower lip defects
algorithm for, 351, 355f
midline, 352-353
LPC (linear predictive coding) spectrum, in acoustic analysis for voice evaluation, 829t, 830, 830f
LPR. *See* Laryngopharyngeal reflux (LPR).
LPSs (lipopolysaccharides), and toll-like receptors, 598
LRTOMT (leucine-rich transmembrane *O*-methyltransferase) gene, in deafness, 2051t-2058t
LSL (liposarcoma of the larynx), 1508
LSO (lateral superior olive), in auditory pathway, 1834-1835, 1834f, 1846
LSSC. *See* Lateral semicircular canal (LSSC).
L-strut, in septoplasty, 489-490, 490f
LTα (lymphotoxin α), 609t-610t
LTαβ (lymphotoxin αβ), 609t-610t
LTAS (long-term average spectra), in acoustic analysis for voice evaluation, 829t, 830
LTECs (laryngotracheoesophageal clefts), 2873-2874, 2873f
classification of, 2873, 2874f, 2874t
syndromes associated with, 2870t
LTP (long-term potentiation), in neural plasticity, 1882-1884
Lubrication, saliva in, 1140-1141
Ludwig classification, of hair loss, 376, 377f
Ludwig's angina
airway establishment for, 188
due to mandibular space infections, 184, 185f
Lugol's solution
for Graves' disease, 1742-1743
for hyperthyroidism, 1739t
Lumbar drains, for CSF rhinorrhea, 792
Lumbar puncture, for meningitis due to temporal bone infection, 1982
Lund-MacKay scoring system, 53
for chronic sinusitis, 674
Lung, anatomy of, 998-999
Lung carcinoma, tracheal invasion by, 1615
Lung function tests, for stridor, 2901
Lung imaging fluorescence endoscope (LIFE) system, for early glottic carcinoma, 1516
Lung volume(s), in children, 2570
Lung volume reduction, endoscopic/bronchoscopic, 1011
LVES (laryngeal videoendoscopy and stroboscopy). *See* Laryngeal stroboscopy; Laryngeal videoendoscopy.
LVP muscle. *See* Levator veli palatini (LVP) muscle.
Lyme disease, 2105-2106, 2400
diagnosis of, 2400
facial paralysis in, 2106, 2400
head and neck symptoms of, 2400
otologic manifestations of, 2106
sensorineural hearing loss due to, 2119
sudden, 2128
stages of, 2400
treatment of, 2400
Lymph node(s)
anatomy and classification in, 163-164
imaging of, 164-167
with extracapsular spread, 164-166, 167f
inflammatory (reactive), 164
with invasion of carotid artery, 166-167
metastatic
contrast-enhanced CT of, 164-165, 167f
MRI of, 165-166, 168f
with non-Hodgkin's lymphoma, 165-166, 167f
normal anatomy in, 166f
in immune system, 605
number of positive, in melanoma, 1111
Lymph node biopsy, sentinel. *See* Sentinel lymph node biopsy (SLNB).
Lymph node dissection
for melanoma
elective, 1114-1115
therapeutic, 1114, 1116
for salivary gland tumors, 1196-1197
Lymph node metastasis(es). *See* Cervical lymph node metastasis(es).
Lymph node regions, physical examination of, 96-97, 96f
Lymphadenitis, neck masses due to, 1638
Lymphadenopathy
in children
bacterial, 2818, 2818f-2819f
drug-induced, 2819
fungal, 2818-2819
reactive, 2818
suppurative, 2818, 2818f
viral, 2817-2818
imaging of, 164-167
CT of, 139
with extracapsular spread, 164-166, 167f
inflammatory (reactive), 164
with invasion of carotid artery, 166-167
metastatic
contrast-enhanced CT of, 164-165, 167f
MRI of, 165-166, 168f
MRI of, 142
with non-Hodgkin's lymphoma, 165-166, 167f
ultrasound imaging of, 143
in immunosuppressed patients, 218-219, 219t
neck masses due to, 1638
in children
bacterial, 2818, 2818f-2819f
fungal, 2818-2819
viral, 2817-2818
Lymphangiomas
of masticator space, 152, 153f
neck masses due to, 1640, 2815, 2815f
of posterior cervical space, 158, 162f
with salivary gland involvement, 2861f
Lymphatic clinical target volumes, selection and delineation of, 1044

Lymphatic drainage
of larynx and hypopharynx, 1578-1579, 1579f, 2582
of skin flaps, 1068
Lymphatic malformations, 2829-2830
associated conditions with, 2829-2830, 2831f
clinical assessment and behavior of, 2829, 2830f
diagnostic evaluation of, 2829
imaging of, 2824f, 2829
macrocystic, 2860-2861
mandibular overgrowth with, 2823f
of neck, 1640, 2815, 2815f
of salivary glands, 1172, 2860-2861, 2861f
sclerotherapy for, 2830-2831
spontaneous resolution of, 2830, 2831f
surgery for, 2831, 2832f
Lymphatic system
of neck, 1683, 1683f, 2582-2583
classification of cervical lymphatics in, 2582-2583
deep cervical lymph nodes in, 2582
for pharynx and larynx, 2582
superficial lymph nodes in, 2582
of oropharynx, 1359-1360, 1360f-1361f, 1361t
Lymphoblastic lymphoma (LL), 1679
clinical presentation of, 1674
fine-needle aspiration of, 1675
treatment and prognosis for, 1679
Lymphocytes
in allergic rhinitis, 616
B, 602f, 603
development of, 603
responses by, 603
T cell–dependent and T cell–independent, 606
in Graves' ophthalmopathy, 1807
intraepithelial, 605
large granular, 603-604
T, 600-603
cytotoxic, 601, 602f
development of, 600-601
effector, 601-603
helper, 601-602, 602f
priming of, 601
regulatory, 602-603
in wound healing, 1076
Lymphocytoma, due to Lyme disease, 2106
Lymphoepithelial carcinoma, of oropharynx, 1362
Lymphoepithelial cyst, benign, in HIV, 217-218, 218f
Lymphoepitheliomas, of hypopharynx and cervical esophagus, 1425
Lymphoid follicles, in immune system, 605
Lymphoid organs, 605
lymph nodes as, 605
Lymphoid stem cells, 599-600, 600f
Lymphoid tumors, of paranasal sinuses, 1131
Lymphoma(s)
biopsy of
core-needle, 1676
corticosteroids prior to, 1676
fine-needle aspiration, 1675-1676
open, 1676
Burkitt's, 1679
in children, 2838, 2839f
clinical presentation of, 1674
treatment and prognosis for, 1679
in children, 2819-2820, 2837
Burkitt's, 2838, 2839f
Hodgkin's, 2819, 2838-2840
clinical presentation of, 2819, 2839-2840
histopathology and molecular biology of, 2819, 2840, 2840f
imaging of, 2820f
management of, 2840
staging of, 2839-2840
neck masses due to, 2819-2820, 2820f

Lymphoma(s) *(Continued)*
non-Hodgkin's, 2819-2820, 2837
epidemiology of, 2837
histopathology and molecular biology of, 2838, 2839f
management of, 2838
presentation and evaluation of, 2837-2838, 2838t
staging of, 2838, 2839t
diffuse large B-cell, 1677-1678
clinical presentation of, 1674
of paranasal sinus and nasal cavity, 1680
treatment and prognosis for, 1680
of salivary glands, 1191-1192, 1192f
treatment and prognosis for, 1680
of thyroid, 1679
staging of, 1679
treatment and prognosis for, 1679
treatment and prognosis for, 1677-1678
of Waldeyer's ring, 1680
treatment and prognosis for, 1680
follicular, 1678
clinical presentation of, 1674
treatment and prognosis for, 1678
of head and neck, 1673-1681
biopsy of, 1674-1676
core-needle, 1676
corticosteroids prior to, 1676
fine-needle aspiration, 1675-1676
open, 1676
classification of, 1675, 1675t
clinical presentation of, 1674, 1674f
epidemiology of, 1673-1674
Hodgkin's, 1676-1677
clinical presentation of, 1674, 1674f
complications of, 1677
epidemiology of, 1673-1674
treatment and prognosis for, 1676-1677
nodal, 1676-1679
non-Hodgkin's
Burkitt's, 1674
clinical presentation of, 1674, 1674f
diffuse large B-cell, 1677-1678
epidemiology of, 1673
follicular, 1674, 1678
highly aggressive, 1674, 1679
indolent, 1674, 1678
lymphoblastic, 1674-1675
MALT, 1674, 1679-1680
mantle cell, 1678-1679
paranasal sinus and nasal cavity, 1680
salivary gland, 1679-1680
small lymphocytic, 1674, 1674f, 1678
thyroid, 1679
highly aggressive, 1679
clinical presentation of, 1674
treatment and prognosis for, 1679
Hodgkin's, 1676-1677
in children, 2819, 2838-2840, 2840f
clinical presentation of, 2819, 2839-2840
histopathology and molecular biology of, 2819, 2840, 2840f
imaging of, 2820f
management of, 2840
staging of, 2839-2840
clinical presentation of, 1674, 1674f
complications of, 1677
epidemiology of, 1673-1674
imaging of, 1674, 1674f
immunosuppression and, 213t, 217
staging of, 1676, 1677t
treatment and prognosis for, 1676-1677
of hypopharynx and cervical esophagus, 1424-1425
indolent, 1678
clinical presentation of, 1674
treatment and prognosis for, 1678

Lymphoma(s) *(Continued)*
lymphoblastic, 1679
clinical presentation of, 1674
fine-needle aspiration of, 1675
treatment and prognosis for, 1679
MALT, 1679-1680
clinical presentation of, 1674
of salivary glands, 1191-1192, 1192f, 1679-1680
treatment and prognosis for, 1680
of thyroid, 1679
staging of, 1679
treatment and prognosis for, 1679
mantle cell, 1678-1679
treatment and prognosis for, 1678-1679
mediastinal mass ratio for, 1676
of nasal cavity, 1680
therapy and prognosis for, 1680
of neck, 1671
neck masses due to, 1640
in children, 2819-2820, 2820f
NK/T, of nasal cavity, 1680
therapy and prognosis for, 1680
non-Hodgkin's
Burkitt's, 1674
in children, 2819-2820, 2837
epidemiology of, 2837
histopathology and molecular biology of, 2838, 2839f
management of, 2838
presentation and evaluation of, 2837-2838, 2838t
staging of, 2838, 2839t
clinical presentation of, 1674, 1674f
diffuse large B-cell, 1677-1678
epidemiology of, 1673
follicular, 1674, 1678
highly aggressive, 1674, 1679
imaging of, 148-149, 149f
immunosuppression and, 213t, 215-216
diagnosis of, 216
epidemiology and presentation of, 216
prognosis and treatment for, 216-217
indolent, 1674, 1678
of larynx, 1509
lymphoblastic, 1674-1675
MALT, 1674, 1679-1680
mantle cell, 1678-1679
nodal involvement by, 165-166, 167f
of oral cavity, 157f
of oropharynx, 1364, 1364f
paranasal sinus and nasal cavity, 1680
of salivary glands, 1191-1192, 1192f, 1679-1680
small lymphocytic, 1674, 1674f, 1678
staging of, 1676, 1677t
thyroid, 1679
of paranasal sinuses, 1131, 1680
therapy and prognosis for, 1680
plasmablastic, 216
salivary gland, 1191-1192, 1192f, 1679-1680
treatment and prognosis for, 1680
sensorineural hearing loss due to, 2123
small lymphocytic, 1678
clinical presentation of, 1674
imaging of, 1674, 1674f
treatment and prognosis for, 1678
staging of, 1676, 1677t
T-cell, nasal manifestations of, 659-660
thyroid, 1679, 1764
diffuse large B-cell, 1679
staging of, 1679
treatment and prognosis for, 1679
extranodal marginal cell, 1679
MALT, 1679
staging of, 1679
treatment and prognosis for, 1679

Lymphoma(s) *(Continued)*
marginal zone, 1679
non-Hodgkin's, 1679
staging of, 1679
treatment and prognosis for, 1679
Waldeyer's ring, 1680
treatment and prognosis for, 1680
Lymphoproliferative disorder, posttransplantation, 213t, 215, 217
in children, 2818, 2840
Lymphoscintigraphy
for oral cancer, 1313
with sentinel lymph node biopsy, 1115-1117, 1116f
Lymphoscintigraphy-directed neck dissection, 1721-1722
Lymphotoxin α (LTα), 609t-610t
Lymphotoxin αβ (LTαβ), 609t-610t
Lynch-Howarth external ethmoidectomy, 778-779, 779f
Lyre's sign, for paraganglioma, 1641
Lysozyme, 598
in middle ear protection, 1871
in saliva, 1140
Lytic antigens, of Epstein-Barr virus, 1352

M

M (metastatic) classification, for melanoma, 1111t, 1113
M phase, of cell cycle, 12, 13f
MAC (membrane attack complex), 608
Macewen's triangle, 1822f
MACIS classification, of thyroid cancer, 1754, 1756t
Macrocirculatory system, and skin flaps, 1064-1066, 1065f
Macrogenia, 463
Macroglobulinemia, Waldenström's, sensorineural hearing loss due to, 2123
Macroglossia, dysphagia due to, 2951
Macrolide antibiotics
for acute otitis media, 2770
long-term, for rhinosinusitis, 733, 734t
ototoxicity of, 2176
Macromolecule secretion, by salivary glands, 1135-1136
Macrophage(s)
in adaptive immune system, 604
in wound healing, 1076
Macrophage colony-stimulating factor (M-CSF), 604, 609t-610t
Macropore plating system, for pediatric facial fractures, 2701t
Macula sacculi, 2278
arrangement of otoliths in, 1855, 1858f, 2278, 2280f
embryogenesis of, 1852
morphologic polarization of, 1855, 1856f, 2278, 2280f
orientation of, 1855, 1857f
Macula utriculi, 2278
arrangement of otoliths in, 1855, 1858f, 2278, 2280f
embryogenesis of, 1852
morphologic polarization of, 1855, 1856f, 2278, 2280f
orientation of, 1855, 1857f
MAGE (melanoma antigen E) tumor–associated antigen, in head and neck squamous cell carcinoma, 1024
Magnesium, for migraine, 2349
Magnetic resonance angiography (MRA), 137
of anterior skull base, 2475
of neck masses, 1637, 1637t
of petrous apicitis, 1989f
Magnetic resonance (MR) cisternography, for CSF rhinorrhea, 790-791, 790f
Magnetic resonance imaging (MRI), 133-137
of acoustic neuroma, 2517
applications of, 142-143
artifacts on, 133-134, 134f
and cochlear implants, 2231-2232, 2236b
for CSF rhinorrhea, 791, 791f
of deep neck space infections, 204
disadvantages of, 137
for dizziness, 2327
effect on hearing of, 2149
of facial nerve, 2384
fast spin-echo, 134
fat suppression methods for, 135-136, 136f
with frequency (chemical shift) selective presaturation (fat saturation), 135-136, 136f
functional
for cerebral blood flow evaluation, 2491
of olfaction, 632
gadolinium enhancement for, 134-135, 135f-136f
with gradient echo techniques, 136-137, 137f
of Graves' ophthalmopathy, 1810
for hyperparathyroidism, 1787-1788, 1789f
for hypopharyngeal and cervical esophageal cancer, 1424
with intensity-modulated radiotherapy, 1044
of laryngeal carcinoma, 1468-1479, 1494
early glottic, 1516-1517
of larynx and infrahyoid neck, 142-143
of lymphadenopathy, 142
metastatic, 165-166, 168f
magnetic field strengths of, 133
of malignant otitis externa, 1947
of nasopharyngeal carcinoma, 1354
of neck masses, 1637, 1637t
of neck neoplasms, 1656-1657
of obstructive sleep apnea, 255
of oral cancer, 1300
of oropharyngeal cancer, 1366
of paranasal sinus tumors, 1124
of paranasal sinuses, 143, 664, 664f
prior to endoscopic sinus surgery, 764, 765t
permanent *vs.* superconducting magnets in, 133
of petrous apicitis, 1986-1987, 1988f-1989f
of pharynx and esophagus, 1396
pulse sequences for, 133-137, 135f-136f
of salivary glands, 142, 1145-1147, 1166, 1180
with adenoid cystic carcinoma, 1146-1147, 1146f-1147f
with glomus tumor, 1169f
with mucoepidermoid carcinoma, 1146, 1147f, 1168f
with pleomorphic adenoma, 1148f, 1167f-1168f, 1180f
with ranula, 1146, 1147f
for sensorineural hearing loss in adults, 2117
with short T1 inversion recovery (STIR), 135-136, 136f
of skull base, 143
anterior, 2475
lateral, 2489
slice thickness in, 133
with spectral presaturation inversion recovery (SPIR), 135-136
spin density–weighted, 134, 136f
for stereotactic radiation therapy, 2558
of suprahyoid neck, 142
surface coils in, 133
T1-weighted, 134, 135f-136f
T2-weighted, 134, 135f-136f
of temporal bone, 143
three-dimensional reconstruction from, 138, 140f
of thyroid and parathyroid glands, 143
Magnetic resonance (MR) sialography, 1147
Magnetic resonance (MR) spectroscopy, of laryngeal carcinoma, 1470
Magnetic search coil technique, for recording eye movements, 2317
Magnetic stimulation, to assess facial nerve function, 2388-2389
in Bell's palsy, 2394-2395
Maintenance activities, in vestibular rehabilitation, 2372-2373, 2379
Maintenance of certification (MOC), 80, 81b
MAIS (Meaningful Auditory Integration Scale), for cochlear implant, 2225
Major basic protein (MBP), 604
in allergic rhinitis, 616
Major histocompatibility complex (MHC) molecules, 599
Major histocompatibility complex (MHC)-restricted cytotoxicity, 603-604
Major histocompatibility complex (MHC) restriction, 603-604
Mal de débarquement (MDD) syndrome, 2357
Malabsorption diseases, oral manifestations of, 1254
Malar eminence
anatomy and physiology of, 319
biomechanics of, 332
Malar prominences, with aging, 444
MALDI-TOF (matrix-assisted laser desorption-ionization–time-of-flight), in head and neck squamous cell carcinoma, 1029
Male-pattern baldness, 374-376, 375f
Malignancy(ies)
in geriatric patients, 237-238
etiology of, 237
treatment of, 237-238
hypercalcemia of, 1783, 1783t
immunosuppression and, 212-217, 213t
cutaneous neoplasms in, 213t, 215
Hodgkin's lymphoma in, 213t, 217
Kaposi's sarcoma in, 212-215, 213t
epidemiology and pathogenesis of, 212-213
presentation and diagnosis of, 213-214, 214f
treatment of, 214-215
non-Hodgkin's lymphoma in, 213t, 215-216
diagnosis of, 216
epidemiology and presentation of, 216
prognosis and treatment for, 216-217
in posttransplantation lymphoproliferative disorder, 213t, 215, 217
squamous cell carcinoma in, 213t, 215
Malignant fibrous histiocytoma (MFH)
of larynx, 1508
of neck, 1667
Malignant giant cell tumor (MGCT), 1671
Malignant hypertension (MH), 119
Malignant melanoma (MM). *See* Melanoma.
Malignant mixed tumors, of salivary glands, 1186-1189
carcinoma ex pleomorphic adenoma as, 1187-1189, 1188f
metastasizing, 1189
true (carcinosarcoma), 1187, 1188f
Malignant otitis externa (MOE), 1947-1948
clinical manifestations of, 1947, 1947f
conductive hearing loss due to, 2021, 2023f
defined, 1947
immunosuppression and, 221-222, 1947
incidence and epidemiology of, 1947
investigations of, 1947
microbiology of, 1947
otorrhea due to, 2195
treatment of, 1947-1948
Malignant peripheral nerve sheath tumor (MPNST), 1670-1671
Mallear stria, 1824, 1825f
Malleolar artery, 1828f
Malleus, 97, 98f
anatomy of, 1826
in auditory physiology, 1839-1840, 1840f, 2018
in cochlear transduction, 2062f

Malleus fixation, 2024-2025
small fenestra stapedotomy with, 2033
Mallory-Weiss syndrome, 1410-1411
Mallory-Weiss tear, gastroesophageal junction in, 957f
Malnutrition, palliative care for, 1104
Malocclusion
after maxillofacial trauma, 339
due to paranasal sinus tumor, 1123
Maloney bougies, for esophageal strictures, 966
MALT. *See* Mucosa-associated lymphoid tissue (MALT).
Malunion, after maxillofacial trauma, 339
Mammillary bodies, in surgical anatomy of anterior cranial base, 2481f
Mandible
anatomy of, 320f, 322-323, 1319, 1320f
alveolar canal in, 1319-1320
alveolar process in, 1319, 1320f
body of mandible in, 1319, 1320f
coronoid and condylar processes in, 1319, 1320f
dentulous *vs.* edentulous, 1319, 1320f
mandibular notch in, 1319, 1320f
mental foramen in, 1319, 1320f
rami in, 1319, 1320f
biomechanics of, 332-333, 332f
body of, 1319, 1320f
dentulous, *vs.* edentulous, 1319, 1320f
in Down syndrome, 2632
edentulous
vs. dentulous, 1319, 1320f
repair of, 339
growth and development of, 2620-2621
downward translation in, 2621, 2624f
mandibular arch in, 2621, 2624f
Meckel's cartilage in, 2620-2621, 2623f
rotational changes in, 2621, 2625f
size in, 2621, 2624f
surface remodeling in, 2621, 2623f
odontogenic tumors of, 1270-1271, 1271f
osteoradionecrosis of, 1048
physiology of, 320f, 322-323
reconstruction of (*See* Mandibular reconstruction)
in surgical anatomy of lateral skull base, 2440f
surgical treatment of, 1310-1312
with oral cancer
for access, 1311
mandible-sparing procedures in, 1311
marginal mandibulectomy for, 1311, 1312f
paramedian mandibulotomy in, 1311
pull-through technique for, 1311, 1312f-1313f
segmental mandibulectomy for, 1311-1312, 1312t
tension and compression areas in, 331-332, 331f-332f
vasculature of, 1296
Mandible-sparing procedures, 1311
Mandibular advancement, for obstructive sleep apnea, 257f
in children, 2610
Mandibular ameloblastomas, 1274
Mandibular arch, in embryology of nose, 2691f
Mandibular branch, of facial nerve, 1194f
Mandibular changes, in geriatric patients, 236
Mandibular condylar fossa, in surgical anatomy of middle cranial base, 2444, 2445f
Mandibular discontinuity defects, maxillofacial prosthodontics for, 1340-1342, 1342f-1343f
Mandibular distraction, 2656, 2656f
for obstructive sleep apnea in children, 2610, 2610f
for Robin sequence, 2673
Mandibular division, of trigeminal nerve, in surgical anatomy of lateral skull base, 2437f, 2438, 2440f, 2441
Mandibular fix-bridge system, with free tissue transfer, 1093-1094
Mandibular fossa, 2011f
Mandibular fractures, 323
classification of, 327
imaging of, 325-326
pediatric, 2704-2706
arch and body, 2706, 2709f
complications of, 2704
condylar and subcondylar, 2704, 2706f-2708f
epidemiology of, 2698
symphyseal and parasymphyseal, 2704-2706, 2708f-2709f
physical examination of, 325
repair of, 337-339, 338f
surgical access to, 329-330, 330f
teeth in line of, 339
Mandibular hypoplasia, obstructive sleep apnea due to, 2610, 2610f
Mandibular movement, nonarticular conditions producing limitation of, 1285t
Mandibular nerve block
for neuropathic pain, 246t
for postoperative pain, 242
Mandibular notch, 1319, 1320f
Mandibular overgrowth, with lymphatic malformation, 2823f
Mandibular prominences, in embryology
of lip, 2661f-2662f, 2661t
of nose, 2691f
Mandibular prosthesis, 1340, 1341f-1342f
with discontinuity defects, 1340-1342, 1342f-1343f
Mandibular reconstruction, 1315-1316, 1319-1328
anatomy of mandible and, 1319, 1320f
alveolar canal in, 1319-1320
alveolar process in, 1319, 1320f
body of mandible in, 1319, 1320f
coronoid and condylar processes in, 1319, 1320f
dentulous *vs.* edentulous, 1319, 1320f
mandibular notch in, 1319, 1320f
mental foramen in, 1319, 1320f
rami in, 1319, 1320f
background and history of, 1319, 1320f, 1322-1324
classification of defects for, 1321-1322, 1323f
computer-assisted modeling for, 1326-1327, 1327f
current method(s) of, 1324-1326
fibular free flap, 1316, 1316f
future approaches to, 1327-1328, 1328f
goals of, 1320, 1322
location of defect and, 1316
after mandibulectomy
with anterior defect, 1321, 1321f
with lateral defect, 1321, 1322f
marginal, 1320
segmental, 1321
movement of mandible and, 1320
outcomes of, 1326
reconstruction plate alone for, 1324
reconstruction plate with osseous free tissue transfer for, 1324
advantages and disadvantages of, 1324
flap inset in, 1324f, 1325
flap options for, 1324, 1325t
planning and harvesting of flaps in, 1324-1325, 1324f
reconstruction plate with soft tissue flap for, 1325
advantages and disadvantages of, 1325
plate extrusion with, 1325, 1326f
plate fracture with, 1325-1326, 1326f
volume-based, 1325, 1326f
Mandibular reconstruction plate (MRP), 337-338, 1324
with osseous free tissue transfer, 1324
advantages and disadvantages of, 1324
flap inset in, 1324f, 1325
flap options for, 1324, 1325t
planning and harvesting of flaps in, 1324-1325, 1324f
with soft tissue flap, 1325
advantages and disadvantages of, 1325
plate extrusion with, 1325, 1326f
plate fracture with, 1325-1326, 1326f
volume-based, 1325, 1326f
Mandibular resection prosthesis, 1340, 1341f-1342f
Mandibular space involvement, in odontogenic infections, 181-184
Ludwig's angina due to, 184, 185f
masseteric, 184, 185f
masticator, 184, 186f
pterygomandibular (medial pterygoid), 184, 185f
secondary, 184
sub-, 183-184, 183f-184f
sublingual, 183, 183f
submental, 181-183, 183f
temporal, 184, 185f
Mandibular splint, acrylic, for pediatric facial fractures, 2701, 2701f
Mandibular swing approach, for oropharyngeal cancer, 1371-1372, 1372f
Mandibulectomy
for alveolar ridge carcinoma, 1304, 1304f-1305f, 1307f
for excision of tumors in parapharyngeal space, 1176, 1176f
mandibular resection prosthesis with, 1340, 1341f-1342f
marginal, 1311, 1312f
defect from, 1320, 1321f
for retromolar trigone carcinoma, 1307, 1307f
segmental, 1311-1312, 1312t
defect from, 1321, 1321f
free tissue transfer after, 1093-1094
Mandibulofacial dysostosis (MFD), 2585
craniofacial abnormalities in, 2633-2635, 2633b, 2635f, 2646
Mandibulotomy
for middle cranial base surgery, 2455t, 2458, 2460f
paramedian, 1311
Mannequins, for difficult airway management, 118
Manometric rhinometry, 643-644
Manometry, esophageal, 957-958, 958f-959f, 959t
for extraesophageal reflux, 899-900
for swallowing disorders, 1219
Mantle cell lymphoma (MCL), 1678-1679
treatment and prognosis for, 1678-1679
MAPK (mitogen-activated protein kinase) pathway, in thyroid carcinoma, 1753
Marble bone disease, 2112
Marcel Proust syndrome, 636
Marescaux, Jacques, 39
Marfanoid syndrome, craniofacial anomalies in, 2641t
Marfan's syndrome, oral manifestations of, 1257
Margin analysis, for biomarkers, in head and neck squamous cell carcinoma, 1027
Marginal cells, of taste buds, 1208
Marginal mandibular branch, of facial nerve, 2418-2419
"Marginal mandibular lip," 2431
Marginal zone lymphoma, of thyroid, 1679
Margin-reflex-distance (MRD), 446
Market accountability, 82
Marshall syndrome, deafness in, 2051t-2058t
Martell, Charles, 1774
MARVELD2, in deafness, 2051t-2058t

Marx hyperbaric oxygen regimen, after radiation therapy, 1333
Maser, 25
MASH (Multiple-Activity Scale for Hyperacusis), 2138-2139
Mask ventilation, difficult, 121-122
Masking, in audiologic testing, 1889-1890
  effective, 1889
  errors in, 1901-1902
Masking dilemma, 1890
Masking therapy, for tinnitus, 2134
MASS1, in deafness, 2051t-2058t
Masseter muscle
  anatomy of, 321f, 1320, 1359f, 1821
  in surgical anatomy of lateral skull base, 2440f
Masseter transfer, for facial nerve paralysis, 2427, 2428f
Masseteric space involvement, in odontogenic infections, 184, 185f
Mast cell(s)
  in adaptive immune system, 605
  in allergic rhinitis, 616
  in wound healing, 1078
Mast cell–mediated hypersensitivity reactions, 608-612
Mastication, 1206-1207, 1206f
  muscles and reflex control of, 1204-1205, 1204f-1205f
Masticator space (MS)
  anatomy of, 203
  imaging of, 151-152
    with adenoid cystic carcinoma, 155f
    with angiofibroma, 152, 154f
    with hemangioma and lymphangioma, 152, 153f
    with infection, 151-152, 152f
    normal anatomy on, 146f, 151-152
    with pseudotumors, 152
    with squamous cell carcinoma, 152, 154f
  odontogenic infections of, 184, 186f
Masticatory rhythm, 1206-1207
Mastoid abscess, due to temporal bone infection, 1980t
Mastoid air cell system, in pressure equalization, 1870-1871
Mastoid antrum, in surgical anatomy of lateral skull base, 2438
Mastoid bone
  anatomy of, 1823f
  imaging of, 1918-1920
  in surgical anatomy of lateral skull base, 2435, 2435f
Mastoid emissary vein, foramen for, 1822f
Mastoid foramen, 2010f
Mastoid obliteration, 2011
Mastoid part, of temporal bone, 1821-1822, 1822f, 1829
  anatomy of, 2009-2010, 2010f
Mastoid pneumatization, otitis media with effusion and, 1963-1964
Mastoid powder, for ear hygiene or chronic ear drainage, 1958
Mastoid process
  anatomy of, 2010f
  in craniofacial skeleton, 320f
  in osteology of temporal bone, 1821-1822, 1822f, 1824f
  in surgical anatomy of lateral skull base, 2435
  in surgical anatomy of middle cranial base, 2445f
Mastoid segment
  anatomy of, 1826f
    surgical, 2404, 2404f
  vulnerability to injury of, 1826f
Mastoid sources, of otorrhea, 2195-2196, 2195b
Mastoid tegmen, in surgical anatomy of lateral skull base, 2435f
Mastoid tip
  anatomy of, 1821-1822, 1822f
    in infants, 2010
  in surgical anatomy of lateral skull base, 2435f
Mastoidectomy, 2009-2016
  anatomic basis for, 2009-2010, 2010f
  canal wall down, 2010-2011
    for chronic otitis media with cholesteatoma, 1969, 1970t
    intact canal wall *vs.,* 2014
      indications for, 2014-2015, 2015f
    operative procedure for, 2013-2014, 2014f
  canal wall up (intact canal wall), 2010
    vs. canal wall down procedure, 2014
    for chronic otitis media with cholesteatoma, 1969, 1970t
  indications for, 2014-2015
  for cholesteatoma, 1969, 1970t, 2014-2015
  for cochlear implant, 2238-2239
  complication(s) of, 2015-2016
    dural tear as, 2015
    facial nerve injury as, 2015-2016
    horizontal semicircular fistula as, 2015
    sigmoid sinus and jugular bulb injury as, 2016
  history of, 2009
  nomenclature for, 2010-2011, 2010b
  operative procedure for, 2011-2014
    bur selection for, 2011
    facial nerve in, 2012, 2012f
    incision in, 2011, 2011f
    initial bur cuts in, 2011, 2011f
    irrigation in, 2011
    Körner's septum in, 2012
    location of antrum in, 2011-2012
    opening of epitympanum in, 2012-2013, 2013f
    opening of facial recess in, 2012, 2012f-2013f
    saucerization in, 2011-2012
    surgical site preparation in, 2011
    tegmen plate in, 2011-2012
    thinning of posterior wall in, 2011-2012
  radical, 2011
    modified, 2011
    in postauricular approach to infratemporal fossa, 2496, 2498f
  simple, 2010
Mastoiditis
  acute, 1983, 1983f
    otorrhea due to, 2196
  chronic, 1984-1985, 1985f
    otorrhea due to, 2196
  coalescent, 1983-1984
    diagnosis of, 1984, 1984f
    etiology of, 1983
    otorrhea due to, 2196
    pathology of, 1983-1984
    pathophysiology of, 1984
    treatment of, 1984
  masked, 1985
  mycobacterial, 2196
  otitis media and, 2776
Matas test, for cerebral blood flow evaluation, 2490
Matched samples, statistical tests for, 66, 67t
Math1
  in hair cell regeneration and repair, 2144
  in murine deafness, 2058t-2060t
Matrix metalloproteinase(s) (MMPs)
  in bone resorption, 1972
  in head and neck squamous cell carcinoma, 1019-1020
Matrix metalloproteinase-1 (MMP-1), in head and neck squamous cell carcinoma, 1077
Matrix-assisted laser desorption-ionization–time-of-flight (MALDI-TOF), in head and neck squamous cell carcinoma, 1029
Maxilla(e)
  anatomy and physiology of, 320, 320f-321f
  biomechanics of, 332
  frontal process of, 509f
  growth and development of, 2619-2620, 2621f-2622f
  odontogenic tumors of, 1270-1271
Maxillary ameloblastomas, 1274
Maxillary antrostomy, in endoscopic sinus surgery, 747, 747f
  failure of, 764-766, 766f
Maxillary antrum
  height of, 2617t
  malignant neoplasms of, 1122-1123
Maxillary artery
  anatomy of, 2580f
  in surgical anatomy of lateral skull base, 2441
Maxillary artery ligation, for epistaxis, 688
Maxillary crest, in septoplasty, 490, 490f
Maxillary division, of trigeminal nerve, in surgical anatomy of lateral skull base, 2437f, 2438, 2440f
Maxillary fractures
  classification of, 326, 327f
  imaging of, 325
  physical examination of, 324-325
  repair of, 334-337, 334f-336f
Maxillary gingivolabial sulcus approach, for pediatric facial fracture, 2701-2702, 2703f
Maxillary implants, in cleft-lip nose repair, 562f
Maxillary incisors, in chin analysis, 464, 464f
Maxillary lymph node, 1360f
Maxillary mega-incisor, 2690, 2691f
Maxillary nerve block
  for neuropathic pain, 246t
  for postoperative pain, 242
Maxillary obturation, prosthetic, 1338
  definitive, 1339-1340
    for dentate patients, 1339-1340, 1340f
    for edentulous patients, 1340, 1340f-1341f
  interim, 1339, 1339f
  surgical, 1338-1339
    abutments in, 1338-1339
    impressions for diagnostic casts in, 1338-1339, 1338f
    postoperative radiograph of, 1338, 1338f
    preoperative assessment for, 1338, 1338f
    preservation of support structures in, 1338
    removal of packing material and prosthesis in, 1339, 1339f
    securing of prosthesis in, 1338-1339, 1339f
    skin graft in, 1338-1339
Maxillary osteotomies, in cleft-lip nose repair, 559, 564f-565f
Maxillary process, in embryology of palate, 2662f
Maxillary prominences, in embryology
  of lip, 2659-2660, 2661f-2662f, 2661t
  of nose, 2691f
  of palate, 2660-2661
Maxillary prosthesis, 1338
  definitive, 1339-1340
    for dentate patients, 1339-1340, 1340f
    for edentulous patients, 1340, 1340f-1341f
  interim, 1339, 1339f
  surgical, 1338-1339
    abutments in, 1338-1339
    impressions for diagnostic casts in, 1338-1339, 1338f
    postoperative radiograph of, 1338, 1338f
    preoperative assessment for, 1338, 1338f
    preservation of support structures in, 1338
    removal of packing material and prosthesis in, 1339, 1339f
    securing of prosthesis in, 1338-1339, 1339f
    skin graft in, 1338-1339

Maxillary sinus(es)
anatomy and physiology of, 319f, 320, 664, 665f
growth and development of, 2619-2620, 2623f
medial wall of, prior to endoscopic sinus surgery, 764t
pneumatization of, prior to endoscopic sinus surgery, 764
surgical anatomy of, 740
in anterior cranial base, 2474
Maxillary sinus defect, reconstruction of, 1128
Maxillary sinus tumors, 1128-1130
chemoradiotherapy for, 1130
combined irradiation and surgery for, 1128
inoperable, 1130
radiotherapy for, 1128-1130
staging of, 1129b
surgery alone for, 1128
Maxillary space involvement, in odontogenic infections, 180-181
buccal, 181, 181f
canine, 180-181, 180f
cavernous sinus thrombosis due to, 181, 182f
orbital cellulitis due to, 181, 182f
Maxillary swing, for nasopharyngeal carcinoma, 1356, 1356f
Maxillectomy
alone, 1128
for hard palate malignancy, 1310, 1310f
medial, 1125, 1125f
inferior, 1125, 1125f
for nasopharyngeal carcinoma, 1355-1356, 1355f
with orbital exenteration, 1125-1126
partial, for buccal carcinoma, 1309f
prosthetic maxillary obturation with (*See* Maxillary obturation, prosthetic)
radical, 1125-1126, 1125f
with radiotherapy, 1128
Maxillofacial prosthodontics, 1329-1347
for acquired facial defects, 1344-1345, 1345t
auricular, 1345-1346, 1345t, 1346f
nasal, 1345, 1345t, 1346f
orbital/ocular, 1345t, 1346-1347, 1347f
prosthetic maxillary obturation in, 1338
definitive, 1339-1340
for dentate patients, 1339-1340, 1340f
for edentulous patients, 1340, 1340f-1341f
interim, 1339, 1339f
surgical, 1338-1339
abutments in, 1338-1339
impressions for diagnostic casts in, 1338-1339, 1338f
postoperative radiograph of, 1338, 1338f
preoperative assessment for, 1338, 1338f
preservation of support structures in, 1338
removal of packing material and prosthesis in, 1339, 1339f
securing of prosthesis in, 1338-1339, 1339f
skin graft in, 1338-1339
and radiation therapy, 1330
dental diagnoses and oral surgical management prior to, 1330-1331, 1330b, 1331f
dental management after, 1333-1337
with conventional 3D conformal radiation therapy, 1333-1335, 1336f
with intensity-modulated radiation therapy, 1335-1337, 1336f-1337f
ipsilateral *vs.* contralateral, 1335
dental management during, 1333
overview of interactions of, 1337-1344
prosthodontic support of radiation oncologist in, 1331-1332
with brachytherapy, 1332, 1335f
for facial moulage recording and bolus fabrication, 1331, 1332f
intraoral positioning devices in, 1331, 1333f
Maxillofacial prosthodontics *(Continued)*
for portals and shielding devices, 1331-1332, 1334f
shelf for tissue-equivalent material in, 1332, 1335f
for tumor-ablative surgical defects, 1337-1338
of mandible, 1340, 1341f-1342f
discontinuity, 1340-1342, 1342f-1343f
of maxilla, 1338
of soft palate, 1343-1344, 1344f
of tongue, 1342-1343, 1344f
Maxillofacial trauma, 318-341
anatomy, physiology, and pathophysiology of, 319-323, 320f
general, 319
of lower third, 322-323, 323f
of middle third, 319-322
areas of protection in, 322, 322t
infraorbital nerve in, 320, 321f
maxillae in, 320, 321f
nasal bones in, 320
orbits in, 320-321, 322f
zygoma in, 319, 320f-321f
of upper third, 319, 319f
biomechanics of facial skeleton and, 331-333, 331f
in lower third, 332-333, 332f
in middle third, 331-332, 331f
in upper third, 331
bone healing after, 330-331
classification of, 326-327
of lower third, 327
of middle third, 326-327, 327f
of upper third, 326
complications of, 339-340
defined, 318
evaluation and diagnosis of, 323-326
imaging in, 325-326
of lower third, 325-326
of middle third, 325, 326f
of upper third, 325, 325f
physical examination in, 323-325
of lower third, 325
of middle third, 324-325, 324f
of upper third, 324
fracture repair for, 333-334
in lower third, 337-339, 338f
with edentulous mandible, 339
in middle third, 334-337
of buttresses, 336
canthal ligament in, 337, 337f
maxillary, 335-336, 335f-336f
naso-orbital ethmoid, 336-337, 337f
orbital, 336
palatal, 335, 335f
of tooth-bearing segments, 334-335, 334f
zygomatic, 336
and occlusion, 330-331, 333-334, 333f
panfacial, 339
secondary, revision, or delayed, 340
in upper third, 333-334, 334f
with CSF rhinorrhea, 334-339
with skull base disruption, 334-339
future directions and new horizons for, 340
historical perspective on, 318-319
management of, 327-330
general, 327-328
surgical access in, 328-330
to lower third, 329-330, 330f
to middle third, 328-329, 329f
to upper third, 328, 328f-329f
pediatric, 2647, 2697-2717
associated injuries with, 2698
clinical and physical evaluation of, 2699
complex, 2698
dentoalveolar fracture due to, 2706-2707, 2710f
Maxillofacial trauma *(Continued)*
emergency management of, 2698-2699
epidemiology of, 2697-2698
etiology of, 2698
facial growth and, 2698-2699
front sinus fracture due to, 2711, 2712f
mandibular fracture due to, 2704-2706
arch and body, 2706, 2709f
complications of, 2704
condylar and subcondylar, 2704, 2706f-2708f
epidemiology of, 2698
symphyseal and parasymphyseal, 2704-2706, 2708f-2709f
mandibular immobilization for, 2701, 2701f
maxillomandibular fixation for, 2701
midface fracture due to, 2707, 2710f
nasal fractures due to, 2708-2711, 2711f-2712f
naso-orbitoethmoid, 2714
classification of, 2714, 2716f
evaluation of, 2714, 2716f
repair of, 2714, 2716f
open reduction with internal fixation for, 2701-2702
orbital fracture due to, 2711-2714
evaluation of, 2712, 2713f
of lateral/medial orbital wall, 2712, 2714, 2716f
of orbital apex, 2712, 2713f
of orbital floor, 2712-2713, 2714f-2715f
of orbital roof, 2712-2713, 2716f
patterns of, 2711-2712
permanent *vs.* resorbable plating systems for, 2700-2701, 2700t-2701t
radiologic examination of, 2699
rigid fixation for, 2699-2700
sequencing of procedures for, 2702, 2704, 2706f
surgical approaches for, 2701-2704
bicoronal incision in, 2701-2702, 2703f
lateral cantholysis in, 2704f
maxillary gingivolabial sulcus approach in, 2701-2702, 2703f
midfacial degloving incision in, 2701-2702
subciliary incision in, 2705f
transcaruncular approach in, 2701-2702, 2705f
surgical management of, 2648, 2649f, 2657
surgical reconstruction for, 2704-2714
zygomaticomalar complex fractures due to, 2707-2708, 2710f
Maxillomandibular advancement (MMA), for obstructive sleep apnea, 260, 261f
Maxillomandibular fixation (MMF), 335-336, 335f-336f
avoiding need for, 328, 330-331
biomechanics with, 332
with free tissue transfer, 1093-1094
and occlusion, 333, 335-336
pediatric, 2701
for subcondylar fractures, 338-339
Maxillotomy, extended, for middle cranial base surgery, 2455t, 2458, 2462f
Maximal stimulation test (MST)
for Bell's palsy, 2394
for facial nerve injury, 2040-2041, 2382t, 2385-2386
Maximum interincisal opening (MIO), 1280
Maximum phonation time (MPT)
in tracheoesophageal speech, 1597
in voice evaluation, 828, 849
Maximum phonational frequency range (MPFR), 829
Maximum resistance, in rhinomanometry, 650
MBP (major basic protein), 604
in allergic rhinitis, 616

MBS (modified barium swallow), 1394, 1396
for swallowing disorders, 1217-1218, 1219f
in children, 2949, 2950t
MCA (minimal cross-sectional area), in rhinomanometry and acoustic rhinometry, 643f, 644
anatomic, 644
physiologic, 644
McCaffrey classification, of airway stenosis, 944, 944t
McFee incision, for radical neck dissection, 1709, 1710f
mCi (millicurie), 1031-1032
MCL (mantle cell lymphoma), 1678-1679
treatment and prognosis for, 1678-1679
Mcoln3, in murine deafness, 2058t-2060t
MCP-1 (monocyte chemoattractant protein-1), in wound healing, 1076
M-CSF (macrophage colony-stimulating factor), 604, 609t-610t
M.D. Anderson Dysphagia Inventory (MDADI), 57-58
M.D. Anderson Symptom Inventory, Head and Neck Module, 56
MDD (mal de débarquement) syndrome, 2357
Mead-Johnson feeder, 2665, 2665f
Mean, 63-64, 64t
regression to, *vs.* efficacy of treatment, 62t
Mean airflow rate, in voice evaluation, 849
Meaningful Auditory Integration Scale (MAIS), for cochlear implant, 2225
Measles
conductive hearing loss due to, 2158
diagnosis of, 2158
sensorineural hearing loss due to, 2119, 2158
sudden, 2127
Measurement scales, for describing and analyzing data, 63, 63t
Meatal foramen
anatomy of, 1826f
surgical, 2403-2404, 2404f
in Bell's palsy, 2393
vulnerability to injury of, 1829
Meatoplasty, in atresiaplasty, 2756-2757
MEC. *See* Mucoepidermoid carcinoma (MEC).
Mechanical débridement, of tracheal tumor, 1619-1621
Mechanical presbycusis, 232, 2126
Mechanoelectrical transduction (MET) channel, in hair cell transduction, 2072f
Mechanoelectrical transduction (MET) currents, adaptation of, in hair cell transduction, 2078-2079, 2079f
Mechanoreceptors, of oral cavity, 1201-1202, 1201f
Meckel's cartilage, 2583, 2583f, 2620-2621, 2623f
Meckel's cave, in surgical anatomy of lateral skull base, 2435f, 2436-2437
Med-El PulsarCI100, 2228-2229, 2228f-2230f
ear-level speech processors for, 2232f
Med-El Sonata TI100, 2228-2229, 2228f-2230f
ear-level speech processors for, 2232f
Medial antebrachial cutaneous nerve, for facial nerve grafting, 2422
Medial canal fibrosis
due to otitis externa, 1946-1947, 1946f
postinflammatory, 1917-1918, 1918f
Medial canthal ligaments
anatomy and physiology of, 320-321, 322f
of lacrimal apparatus, 798f
repair of, 336-337, 337f
Medial canthal relationships, in evaluation of maxillofacial trauma, 324, 324f
Medial crural footplate, 509f
Medial crus(crura), of alar cartilage, 496-497, 497f, 509f
in cleft-lip nose repair, 561f-562f
Medial geniculate body
in central auditory pathway, 1835f, 1836, 1846-1847
tonotopic map reorganization in, 1879-1880
Medial incudal fold, 1827f
Medial maxillectomy, 1125, 1125f
for nasopharyngeal carcinoma, 1355-1356, 1355f
Medial nasal prominences, in embryology
of lip, 2660, 2661f-2662f, 2661t
of nose, 2691f
of palate, 2660-2661
Medial nucleus of trapezoid body (MNTB), in auditory pathway, 1834f
Medial olfactory tract, 628f
Medial olivocochlear (MOC) reflex pathways, in efferent auditory system, 1848-1849, 1848f
Medial olivocochlear (MOC) "unmasking," 1849
Medial orbital wall, 439
prior to endoscopic sinus surgery, 764, 764f, 764t
Medial orbital wall fractures, pediatric, 2712, 2714, 2716f
Medial pterygoid involvement, in odontogenic infections, 184, 185f
Medial pterygoid muscle, in surgical anatomy of lateral skull base, 2441
Medial pterygoid process, in surgical anatomy of lateral skull base, 2435f
Medial rectus muscle(s)
semicircular canal planes and, 2285-2287, 2286f-2287f
in surgical anatomy of anterior cranial base, 2472f
Medial superior olive (MSO), in auditory pathway, 1834-1835, 1834f, 1846
Medial vertical buttress, 331, 331f
Medial vestibular nucleus (MVN) (of Schwalbe), 1861, 1862f
in velocity storage, 2296
Medial vestibulospinal tract, in gaze stabilization, 1865
Medialization thyroplasty, 904-911
advantages of, 908
arytenoid adduction *vs.*, 912-913
autologous temporalis fascia grafts for, 910
complications of, 911
disadvantages of, 908
factors affecting outcome of, 908
with Gore-Tex strip, 908, 910, 911f
historical aspects of, 904-905
implant placement in, 909-910, 910f
indications for, 905, 908
limitations of, 910
outcome measures for, 910
patient evaluation and selection for, 905
prefabricated implants for, 908, 908f, 910
prosthesis templates in, 909-910, 910f
technique for, 908-911, 909f
Median, 63-64, 64t
Median frontal sinus drainage procedure, 779, 779f
Median glossoepiglottic fold, radiographic anatomy of, 1471f
Median hyoepiglottic ligament, 1359f
Median labiomandibular glossotomy, for hypopharyngeal cancer, 1429
Mediastinal exploration, for hyperparathyroidism, 1801-1802, 1802f
Mediastinal mass ratio (MMR), for lymphomas, 1676
Mediastinitis, due to deep neck space infections, 207-208
Medical history, 94, 94b
for disorders of professional voice, 850
Medical Outcomes Study Short Form-36 (SF-36), 56, 642
Medical professionalism, 78-82
board certification and maintenance of certification in, 79-80, 80b-81b
Institute of Medicine in, 81-82
Medical professionalism *(Continued)*
physician education in, 79, 79t
state medical boards and maintenance of licensure in, 80-81
Medical records, of difficult airway
electronic, 118-119
previous, 118
Medication(s), for systemic diseases, oral sequelae of, 1246, 1247t-1248t
Medication history, 94
Medication overuse headache, 248
MEDPOR (high-density polyethylene)
for auricular reconstruction, 2744t
for chin implants, 465t
Medulla, in surgical anatomy of anterior cranial base, 2474f
Medullary disorders, laryngeal hypofunction due to, 842
Medullary thyroid carcinoma (MTC), 1763-1764
clinical presentation of, 1763
management and prognosis for, 1763-1764
nodal metastasis of, 1766
pathology of, 1763
Medulloblastomas
intra-axial, 2528
vestibular symptoms of, 2353-2354
MEE (middle ear effusion)
collection vehicle for aspiration of, 2773-2774, 2774f
and hearing loss in infants, 2722
otitis media with (*See* Otitis media with effusion (OME))
Megaelectron volts (MeV), 1033
Mega-incisor, maxillary, 2690, 2691f
Megalin, and cisplatin ototoxicity, 2172
Megavoltage (MV) electrons, 1033
Megavoltage (MV) x-rays, 1033-1034
Meissner corpuscles, 1201
Meissner's plexus, 953, 954f
Melanocytic neoplasm(s), 286-289
blue nevus as, 286-287, 287f
compound nevus as, 286
congenital nevi as, 287-288
dysplastic nevus as, 288, 288f
halo nevus as, 287, 287f
intradermal nevus as, 286, 287f
junctional nevus as, 286, 287f
lentigo maligna melanoma as, 287f
nevocellular nevus as, 286
nevus sebaceus as, 287f, 289
solar (actinic) lentigo as, 288
Spitz nevus as, 287
superficial spreading melanoma as, 285f
Melanocytic nevus(i)
blue, 286-287, 287f
compound, 286
congenital, 287-288
and melanoma, 1107-1108
dysplastic, 288, 288f
halo, 287, 287f
intradermal, 286, 287f
junctional, 286, 287f
nevocellular, 286
of oral mucosa
clinical features of, 1241
histopathologic features of, 1242
treatment of, 1243
sebaceus, 287f, 289
Spitz, 287
Melanocytoma, compound, 287
Melanoma, 1106-1120
ABCD checklist for, 1109
chemotherapy for, 1118
classification of, 1108-1109
congenital melanocytic nevi and, 1107-1108
desmoplastic, 1108, 1108f

Melanoma *(Continued)*
desmoplastic-neurotropic, 1108
of oral cavity, 1299
diagnostic workup for, 1109-1110
biopsy in, 1109
history in, 1109
metastatic workup in, 1109-1110, 1110b, 1110t
physical examination in, 1109
differential diagnosis for, 1109
of ear, 1114
epidemiology of, 1107
etiology of, 1107-1108
follow-up and surveillance for, 1119
genetics of, 1107, 1107b
of hard palate, 1242f, 1309-1310
immunotherapy for, 1118-1119
future investigations on, 1119
interferon in, 1118-1119
interleukin-2 and other cytokines in, 1119
in-transit metastasis with, 1110, 1117
juvenile, 287
lentigo maligna, 287f, 1108
surgical excision of, 1114
mucosal, 1108-1109
of larynx, 1509
of oral cavity, 1242-1243
clinical features of, 1242, 1242f
differential diagnosis of, 1242
etiology and pathogenesis of, 1241, 1241t
histopathologic features of, 1242-1243, 1242f-1243f
treatment of, 1243
of oropharynx, 1364-1365, 1364f-1365f
of neck, 1671
nodular, 1108
of paranasal sinuses, 1131-1132
prognostic factors for, 1110-1113
anatomic site as, 1113
intralymphatic metastasis as, 1112
lactate dehydrogenase as, 1109-1110, 1113
number of positive lymph nodes as, 1111
and predictors of survival, 1112b
tumor burden as, 1111-1112
tumor ulceration as, 1111-1112
radiation therapy for, 1118
risk factors for, 1107, 1107b
signs and symptoms of, 1109
staging of, 1110-1113
Breslow microstaging in, 1113f
Clark scale in, 1111, 1113f
clinical and pathologic groupings in, 1112t
molecular, 1118
summary of revisions in, 1111, 1112b
TNM classification for, 1111, 1111t
metastatic (M) classification (distant metastases) in, 1111t, 1113
nodal (N) classification (regional disease) in, 1111-1113, 1111t
tumor (T) classification (localized disease) in, 1111, 1111t, 1113f
superficial spreading, 285f, 1108
surgical management of distant metastases of, 1118
surgical management of primary tumor in, 1113-1114
closure and reconstruction in, 1114
of ear, 1114
wide local excision and surgical margins in, 1113-1114, 1114t
surgical management of regional lymph nodes in, 1114-1118
elective lymph node dissection in, 1114-1115
sentinel lymph node biopsy in, 1115-1118
complexity in head and neck region of, 1117
excision of primary tumor prior to, 1115, 1116f

Melanoma *(Continued)*
future investigations on, 1117-1118
histologic evaluation of, 1116
indications for, 1115, 1115b
inflammation and fibrosis due to, 1117
injury to facial nerve due to, 1117
intraoperative lymphatic mapping for, 1115, 1116f
learning curve for, 1116
lymphoscintigraphy with, 1115-1117, 1116f
and overall survival, 1117
potential therapeutic benefits of, 1117
as prognostic factor, 1117
risk of in-transit metastasis with, 1117
technique for, 1115-1116
therapeutic lymph node dissection after, 1116
therapeutic lymph node dissection in, 1114, 1116
of unknown primary, 1109
Melanoma antigen E (MAGE) tumor–associated antigen, in head and neck squamous cell carcinoma, 1024
Melanosis, focal ("smoker's"), of oral mucosa, 1241f
Melanotic macules, of oral mucosa, 1241
clinical features of, 1241, 1241f
defined, 1241
differential diagnosis of, 1242
etiology and pathogenesis of, 1241, 1241t
histopathologic features of, 1242, 1242f
treatment of, 1243
MELAS (mitochondrial encephalopathy, lactic acidosis, and strokelike episodes) syndrome, sensorineural hearing loss in, 2094t, 2097
Melkersson-Rosenthal syndrome, 2399
facial paralysis in, 2399
oral manifestations of, 1257
Melolabial flap
for lip defects, 353
for nasal defects, 366, 367f, 371f
Melolabial fold, in aging, 406, 406f
Melolabial interpolated flap, for nasal defects, 348
Membrane attack complex (MAC), 608
Membranous labyrinth
anatomy of, 1831-1832, 1832f, 1852, 1853f
embryogenesis of, 1852
malformations limited to, 2727-2728, 2727b
malformations of osseous and, 2727b, 2728-2735
ruptures in, in Meniere's disease, 2334
Membranous labyrinthine dysplasia
complete, 2727
limited, 2727-2728
Membranous laryngotracheobronchitis. *See* Bacterial tracheitis.
MEN. *See* Multiple endocrine neoplasia (MEN).
MEN-1 tumor suppressor gene, in parathyroid neoplasm(s), 1775, 1776f
Meniere, Prosper, 2329, 2333
Meniere's disease, 2333-2339
atypical, 2335
bilateral, 2333
clinical course of, 2335
clinical features of, 2333, 2335, 2335t
sensorineural hearing loss as, 2126-2127, 2335t
fluctuating, 2199
history of, 2337
sudden, 2129
severity of, 2335, 2336t
tinnitus as, 2335t, 2337
vertigo as, 2202, 2335t
cochlear, 2335
diagnosis of, 2335-2337
AAO-HNS criteria for, 2335, 2335t
audiogram in, 1895f
clinical presentation in, 2335, 2335t
defined, 2333
dehydrating agents in, 2337

Meniere's disease *(Continued)*
electrocochleography in, 1892-1896, 1895f, 1908, 2337
electronystagmography in, 2337
hearing loss and tinnitus in, 2337
heat thrust testing in, 2337
history in, 2335-2337
imaging studies in, 2333-2334, 2334f
stacked auditory brainstem response in, 1911
vestibular evoked myopotentials in, 2337
endolymphatic hydrops in, 2333-2334, 2334f
etiology of, 2334-2335
infectious, 2163, 2335
familial, 2333
historical background of, 2329, 2333
imaging studies in, 2333-2334, 2334f
incidence of, 2333
and migraine, 2350
otosclerosis with, 2035
pathogenesis of, 2333-2334, 2334f
ruptures in membranous labyrinth in, 2334
severity of, 2335, 2336t
treatment of, 2126, 2337-2339
dietary modification and diuretics in, 2337
historical background of, 2329
intratympanic gentamicin for, 2185-2189, 2338-2339, 2338f
clinical protocols for, 2187-2188
complications of, 2188-2189
concentration of, 2188
dose of, 2188
indications and contraindications for, 2189
injection interval for, 2188
mechanism of action of, 2185-2186
number of injections of, 2188
pharmacokinetics of, 2186-2187, 2186f-2187f
practical considerations with, 2188
intratympanic steroids for, 2184, 2339
local overpressure therapy for, 2338
surgical, 2362-2364
cochleosacculotomy for, 2126, 2362-2363, 2363f
endolymphatic sac surgery for, 2126, 2339, 2363-2364, 2364f
labyrinthectomy for, 2339, 2362
vestibular nerve section for, 2339, 2362
symptomatic, 2338
vasodilators in, 2337-2338
vestibular, 2335
Meniett device, 2338
Meningioma(s)
of cerebellopontine angle, 2517-2518
diagnostic studies of, 2518
imaging of, 1928, 1928f, 2518, 2519f
in differential diagnosis, 1929t, 2518t
with intracanalicular extension, 2520f
sensorineural hearing loss due to, 2125, 2125f
signs and symptoms of, 2518
endovascular treatment of, 1938, 1938f
of internal auditory canal, 175f
jugular foramen, 1929-1930, 1930f
of posterior fossa
embolization of, 1938
with petrous apex involvement, 2508f
Meningitis
bacterial, hearing loss due to, 2160-2161
due to cranial base surgery, 2468
cryptococcal, in HIV, 223-224
due to CSF fistulas, 794, 2044
delayed, due to temporal bone fracture, 2037-2038, 2038f
hearing loss due to
cochlear implants for, 2240
sudden, 2127
due to inner ear anomalies, 2736f, 2737, 2739
due to otitis media, 1993-1994, 2777

Meningitis *(Continued)*
diagnosis of, 1993
imaging in, 1993-1994, 1994f
lumbar puncture for, 1982
epidemiology of, 1980t-1981t, 1993
pathogenesis of, 1993
pathology of, 1993
symptoms of, 1993
treatment of, 1993-1994
due to posterior fossa surgery, 2541
Meningitis vaccination, with cochlear implants, 2236-2237, 2237b
Meningocele
with CSF rhinorrhea, 787
defined, 2645, 2687
imaging of, 765t
Meningoencephalocele
anterior, surgical management of, 742
with CSF rhinorrhea, 787, 791f-792f
defined, 2645, 2687
endoscopic view of, 2646f
due to otitis media, 1992-1993, 1993f
Meningoencephalocystocele, defined, 2645
Menopause, oral health during and after, 1256-1257
Menstrual cycle
oral changes during, 1256
and professional voice, 850
Menstrual cycle synchrony, olfaction in, 630
Mental foramen, of mandible, 1319, 1320f
Mental nerve, in osseous genioplasty, 467, 470
Mental protuberance, 320f
Mental tubercle, 320f
Mentalis muscle, 442f
Mentalis strain, 461, 462f
Menthol, for vocal professionals, 855
Menthol-sensitive receptors, in nasal mucosa, 641-642
Mentocervical angle, in aesthetic analysis, 275, 279f
Mentoplasty, 461-474
chin implants in, 465-467
anesthesia for, 465
clinical example of, 470, 471f
complications after, 470
dissection planes for, 465-467, 467f
incision and approach for, 465-467, 467f
intraoral approach for, 467
subperiosteal *vs.* supraperiosteal placement of, 465-467, 467f
surgical procedure for, 465-467
types of, 465, 465t, 467
clinical examples of, 470, 471f-473f
complications after, 470
correction of soft tissue ptosis in, 465
osseous genioplasty in, 465, 467-470
anesthesia for, 467
clinical examples of, 470, 473f
complications after, 470
fixation in, 468-470, 470f
gingivolabial incision for, 467, 468f
inscription of bony midline in, 467-468, 469f
lateral extent of, 468, 469f
measurement of osteotomy site in, 467-468, 469f
subperiosteal dissection in, 467, 468f
three-dimensional movement of chin in, 468
vertical lengthening in, 468-470, 469f
vertical shortening in, 468-470, 470f
wound closure in, 470
patient evaluation for, 461-465
Burstone analysis in, 463, 463f
Gonzalez-Ulloa and Stevens analysis in, 464f
history in, 461
Holdaway "H" angle in, 463, 464f
horizontal relationships in, 463, 464f
lateral cephalometric radiograph in, 463, 463f
Mentoplasty *(Continued)*
panoramic radiograph (Panorex) in, 462-463, 462f
photography in, 461-462, 462f
physical examination in, 461, 462f
Ricketts analysis in, 463, 463f
Steiner analysis in, 463, 463f
symmetry in sagittal plane in, 464-465
vertical relationships in, 463-464, 464f
procedure selection for, 461, 462t, 465
MEP(s) (motor evoked potentials), transcranial electrical stimulation–induced, to assess facial nerve function, 2389
Meperidine
for pediatric anesthesia, 2592
for postoperative pain, 241t
Merbromin (Mercurochrome), for fungal otitis externa, 1955
Merkel cells, 1201
Merocel wicks, in atresiaplasty, 2756-2757
MERRF (myoclonic epilepsy and red ragged fibers) syndrome, sensorineural hearing loss in, 2094t, 2097
Mesotympanum, 1825-1826, 1827f
Messenger RNA, 11-12, 12f
Messerklinger technique, for endoscopic sinus surgery, 746
MET (D-methionine), for noise-induced hearing loss, 2145
MET (Middle Ear Transducer). *See* Middle Ear Transducer (MET).
MET (mechanoelectrical transduction) channel, in hair cell transduction, 2072f
MET (mechanoelectrical transduction) currents, adaptation of, in hair cell transduction, 2078-2079, 2079f
Meta-analyses, 70, 71t
Metabolic disorders
craniofacial anomalies due to, 2640
facial paralysis due to, 2401
otologic manifestations of, 2112-2114
in gout, 2113-2114
in mucopolysaccharidoses, 2112-2113, 2113f
in ochronosis, 2114
presbycusis due to, 232
sensorineural hearing loss due to, 2125
vertigo due to, 2201
Metabolic manipulation, and skin flap viability, 1074-1075
Metabolic myopathies, laryngeal hypofunction due to, 842
Metabolic presbycusis, 232
Metachronous lesion, in oral cancer, 1301-1302
Metallic artifacts
on CT, 139, 141f
on MRI, 134, 134f
Metallic coils, for embolization, 1933
Metastasis(es)
cervical lymph node (*See* Cervical lymph node metastasis(es))
to larynx, 1510
rapidly progressive hearing loss due to, 2200
to salivary glands, 1191
to skull base, 171, 173f
to trachea, 1615-1616
Metastasizing mixed tumor, of salivary glands, 1189
Metastatic (M) classification, for melanoma, 1111t, 1113
Metastatic disease, systemic chemotherapy for, 1058-1061
combination, 1059-1060
prognostic factors with, 1058-1059
single agent, 1059
Metastatic lesions
of cerebellopontine angle, 2526
of ear, 2107-2108, 2108f
otorrhea due to, 2196-2197
Metastatic lesions *(Continued)*
of neck, 1664
from distant tumor, 1664-1666
from regional tumor, 1664
from unknown primary, 1664, 1665f
Metastatic lymphadenopathy
CT of, 139
MRI of, 142
ultrasound of, 143
Metastatic workup, for melanoma, 1109-1110, 1110b, 1110t
Methacholine challenge test, in nonallergic rhinitis, 695
Methacrylates, for craniofacial defect repair, 2657
Methadone, for postoperative pain, 241t
Methicillin-resistant *Streptococcus aureus* (MRSA), rhinosinusitis due to
acute, 704, 732
chronic, 732, 733f
Methimazole
adverse reactions to, 1742
for Graves' disease, 1742
for hyperthyroidism, 1739t
D-Methionine (MET), for noise-induced hearing loss, 2145
Methotrexate (Rheumatrex)
for autoimmune inner ear disease, 2167
in combination chemotherapy, 1059-1060
dizziness due to, 2310t
for induction chemotherapy, 1056-1057
for recurrent or metastatic disease, 1059
for recurrent respiratory papillomatosis, 879
for sarcoidosis, 659
for Wegener's granulomatosis, 658
Methoxyisobutyl isonitrile (MIBI). *See* Sestamibi.
Methylation, in head and neck squamous cell carcinoma, 1020-1022, 1021f
Methylprednisolone
with chemical peel, 396
intratympanic delivery of
dosing for, 2185
pharmacokinetics of, 2183-2184
for sudden sensorineural hearing loss, 2184-2185
for vestibular neuritis, 2162
Methylprednisone, for rhinosinusitis, 734t
Metoclopramide
for extraesophageal reflux, 901
for GERD, 970
Metopic suture, 320f
Metopic synostosis, 2642-2643, 2643f
Metoprolol, intraoperative, 112
Metrizamide powder (Nycomed), for embolization, 1933
MeV (megaelectron volts), 1033
MFD (mandibulofacial dysostosis), 2585
craniofacial abnormalities in, 2633-2635, 2633b, 2635f, 2646
MFH (malignant fibrous histiocytoma)
of larynx, 1508
of neck, 1667
MGCT (malignant giant cell tumor), 1671
MH (malignant hypertension), 119
MHC (myosin heavy chain) isoforms
in lingual muscles, 1205
in muscles of mastication, 1204
MHC (major histocompatibility complex) molecules, 599
MHC (major histocompatibility complex)-restricted cytotoxicity, 603-604
MHC (major histocompatibility complex) restriction, 603-604
MIBI (methoxyisobutyl isonitrile). *See* Sestamibi.
MIBI-SPECT (technetium-99m sestamibi scintigraphy with single photon emission computed tomography), for hyperparathyroidism, 1785

Michel's aplasia, 2200, 2729
imaging of, 2729f-2730f
inherited, 2735
relative incidence of, 2729t
Miconazole cream (Micatin, Monistat), for fungal otitis externa, 1954-1955, 1959t-1960t
Micro Retin A (tretinoin)
for aging skin, 403-404
with chemical peels, 392-393
for chemoprevention of oral cancer, 1315
Microcirculatory changes, in acutely raised skin flaps, 1068-1069
Microcirculatory impairment, of skin flaps, 1071f
Microdebrider
for adenoidectomy, 2797-2798
for recurrent respiratory papillomatosis, 2891
for stridulous child, 2909
Microdeletion chromosome 22 syndrome, cleft lip and palate in, 2673-2674, 2674f
Microdermabrasion, 402-403
Microfibrillar collagen (Avitene), for embolization, 1933
Microgenia, 463
Microglial cells, 604
Micrognathia
dysphagia due to, 2950-2951
and obstructive sleep apnea, 2610
Microlaryngoscopy, 864, 864f
Microlaryngoscopy partial cordectomy, for glottic cancer, 1517t
Microneurovascular muscle transfer, for facial nerve paralysis, 2429-2430
Microphone, for hearing aid, 2267
directional, 2269
Microphthalmia transcription factor *(MITF)* gene, in deafness, 2051t-2058t, 2095
MicroRNAs (miRNAs, miRs), in head and neck squamous cell carcinoma, 1021, 1022f, 1027-1028
Microsatellite repeats, in head and neck squamous cell carcinoma, 1019
Microscopic direct laryngoscopy, for glottic cancer, 1519t
Microscopic examination, of ear, in children, 2574
Microsurgical débridement, for airway stenosis, 946, 946b, 946f
Microtia, 2741-2751
atypical, 2742, 2743f
reconstruction for, 2747-2748, 2749f-2750f
classic, 2742, 2743f
classification of, 2742
ear anatomy and, 2742, 2742f
embryology of, 2741, 2742f
epidemiology of, 2741
evaluation of, 2742-2743
reconstruction for
advantages and disadvantages of, 2744t
atypical, 2747-2748, 2749f-2750f
autogenous costochondral, 2744, 2744t
classic, 2744-2747
cartilage implantation in, 2744-2746
carving of framework and helix in, 2746, 2746f
construction of implant in, 2746, 2746f
creation of postauricular sulcus in, 2746, 2748f
donor site in, 2745, 2745f
incision in, 2745-2746
lobule transfer in, 2746, 2747f
placement of implant in, 2746, 2747f
templates in, 2744-2745, 2745f
tragus reconstruction in, 2747, 2748f
complications of, 2748-2751
planning for, 2743-2744, 2744t
treatment options for, 2744t
type I, 2742, 2742f
Microtia *(Continued)*
type II, 2742, 2743f
type III, 2742, 2743f
Microvarices, of larynx, 817
Microvascular decompression, facial nerve monitoring with, 2548-2549, 2549f
Microvascular reconstruction, total glossectomy with, 1390
Microvillar cells, of olfactory epithelium, 626, 627f
Microwaves, effect on hearing of, 2149
Midazolam
for adenotonsillectomy, 2797
as adjunct to induction of anesthesia, 111
for premedication in children, 2589
with congenital heart disease, 2596
Middle cerebral artery, 2351f
Middle cervical sympathetic ganglion, in root of neck, 2582
Middle constrictor muscle, 1296f
Middle cranial base
anatomy of, 1699
central and lateral compartments of, 2454-2455, 2455f
surgical anatomy of, 2444
boundaries in, 2442, 2443f
craniofacial junction in, 2442, 2443f
extracranial view of, 2444, 2445f
foramina along floor of, 2444, 2445f
intracranial view of, 2444, 2445f
lateral pterygoid plate in, 2444, 2445f
lateral view of, 2444, 2445f
sphenoid spine in, 2444
superomedial boundary of, 2444
Middle cranial base irradiation, 1699-1700
Middle cranial base surgery
anesthesia for, 2447-2448
complications of, 2468-2469, 2469t
electrophysiologic monitoring during, 2450
goals of, 2448, 2448b
intraoperative imaging during, 2449
operative approaches for, 2454-2467
for central compartment, 2455-2461, 2455t
endoscopic, 2457-2458, 2457f
extended maxillotomy, 2455t, 2458, 2462f
facial translocation, 2455t, 2464-2466, 2467f
intratemporal fossa, 2455t
lateral rhinotomy, 2455t, 2458, 2458f
Le Fort I osteotomy as, 2455t, 2458, 2460f
mandibulotomy, 2455t, 2458, 2460f
midfacial degloving, 2455t, 2458, 2459f
midfacial split, 2455t, 2458-2461, 2463f
transantral, 2455t, 2458, 2459f
transethmoidal sphenoidotomy, 2455-2457, 2455t, 2456f
transoral, 2455t, 2458, 2461f
transpalatal, 2455t, 2458, 2461f
transseptal sphenoidotomy, 2455-2457, 2455t, 2456f
division into central and lateral compartments in, 2454-2455, 2455f
endoscopic, 2449-2450
for central compartment, 2457-2458, 2457f
functional and aesthetic considerations in choice of, 2450
general considerations with, 2448-2450
image-guided computer-assisted, 2448-2449, 2449f
for lateral compartment, 2461-2467
infratemporal, 2461-2464, 2464f
intracranial, 2467
lateral facial, 2462, 2465f
lateral transtemporal sphenoid, 2462, 2465f
subtemporal-preauricular infratemporal approach, 2462, 2466f
transfacial, 2464-2467, 2467f
transtemporal, 2461
Middle cranial base surgery *(Continued)*
overview of, 2448
planning of, 2448-2450
robotic, 2450
outcomes of, 2469-2470
pathology and management planning for, 2446-2447, 2447b
postoperative care after, 2468
preoperative embolization for, 2446
preoperative evaluation for, 2444-2448
angiography in, 2444-2445
of cerebral blood flow, 2445-2446, 2446f
other evaluations in, 2446-2447
reconstruction after, 2467-2468
Middle cranial base tumors, malignant, 1699-1700
chordoma/chondrosarcoma as, 1699
nasopharyngeal carcinoma as, 1699-1700, 1699f, 1700t
Middle cranial fossa, in surgical anatomy of lateral skull base, 2434, 2435f-2437f, 2438
Middle cranial fossa approach
for intratemporal facial nerve surgery, 2407-2409
advantages and uses of, 2408-2409
for Bell's palsy, 2409-2410, 2409t-2410t
limitations and potential complications of, 2409
technique of, 2407-2408, 2408f-2409f
for skull base lesions requiring drainage, 2539
Middle ear
anatomy of, 1825-1827, 1825f-1827f
in auditory physiology, 1839-1840, 1840f
bidirectional gas exchange in, 1870-1871
effects of radiotherapy on, 2626t
embryogenesis of, 1825
imaging of, 172, 1918-1920
with aberrant internal carotid artery, 1919-1920, 1921f-1922f
with cholesteatoma
acquired, 1919, 1920f
congenital, 1918-1919, 1919f-1920f
with CT, 174f, 1919f-1920f
with MRI, 1919, 1920f-1921f
with glomus tympanicum, 1919-1920, 1921f
with transverse petrous fracture with osseous dislocation, 174f
infection of (*See* Otitis media (OM))
mucociliary clearance and drainage of, 1871
protection of, 1871-1872
salivary gland choristoma of, 2200-2201
sound transfer in, 2017-2019
Middle ear aeration, in sound transmission, 2000
Middle ear atelectasis, 1964, 1964f-1965f
tympanoplasty with, 2003-2004
Middle ear cavity, 1825-1826
Middle ear effusion (MEE)
collection vehicle for aspiration of, 2773-2774, 2774f
and hearing loss in infants, 2722
otitis media with (*See* Otitis media with effusion (OME))
Middle ear function, tests to evaluate, 1890-1891, 1890f
Middle ear implants, 2207-2212
basic design features of, 2207-2208
ossicular coupling as, 2207-2208
transducer design as, 2207
electromagnetic, 2208-2211
Carina as, 2210-2211
clinical results with, 2210-2211
components of, 2210, 2210f
history of, 2210
placement of, 2210, 2211f
Middle Ear Transducer (MET) as, 2027, 2210-2211
clinical results with, 2210-2211
comparison of features of, 2206t
components of, 2210
history of, 2210

Middle ear implants *(Continued)*
indications for, 2210, 2211f
placement of, 2210, 2211f
ossicular coupling in, 2207-2208
sound transduction and coupling to auditory system with, 2205f
transducer design for, 2207
Vibrant Soundbridge as, 2208-2210
clinical data on, 2209
comparison of features of, 2206t
components of, 2208-2209, 2208f
for conductive and mixed hearing loss, 2210
history of, 2208, 2210
implantation of, 2209
indications for, 2209, 2209f
location of, 2204f
piezoelectric, 2211-2212
Esteem-Hearing Implant as, 2211-2212, 2212f
ossicular coupling in, 2207-2208
sound transduction and coupling to auditory system with, 2205f
transducer design for, 2207
total *vs.* partial, 2208
Middle ear muscle reflex pathways, in efferent auditory system, 1847, 1848f
Middle ear pressure changes, eye movements evoked by, 2316, 2316f
Middle ear sources, of otorrhea, 2195-2196, 2195b
Middle Ear Transducer (MET), 2027, 2210-2211
clinical results with, 2210-2211
comparison of features of, 2206t
components of, 2210
history of, 2210
indications for, 2210, 2211f
placement of, 2210, 2211f
Middle Eastern patient, hump reduction in, 570-573
concept of, 570-571
results of, 574f-575f
technique for, 571-573, 575f
Middle fossa approach
for middle cranial base surgery, 2467
for posterior fossa neoplasms, 2532t, 2534-2536
advantages and disadvantages of, 2532t, 2536
basic features of, 2534
extended, 2532t, 2538
advantages and disadvantages of, 2532t, 2538
basic features of, 2538
indications for, 2532t, 2538
surgical exposure in, 2538f
technique of, 2538
indications for, 2532t, 2534-2535
surgical exposure in, 2535f
technique of, 2535-2536, 2535f
Middle fossa craniotomy, for facial nerve decompression, 2042-2043
Middle jugular lymph nodes, in neck dissection, 1704, 1704f, 1706t-1708t
Middle latency response (MLR)
auditory evoked, 1912, 1913f
electrically evoked, 1912-1914
Middle meningeal artery
groove for, 1822f
in surgical anatomy of lateral skull base, 2437f, 2438, 2440f
Middle meningeal artery sulcus, in surgical anatomy of lateral skull base, 2436f
Middle nasal meatus
normal anatomy of, 664-665, 665f-667f
in surgical anatomy of anterior cranial base, 2472, 2472f
Middle skull base. *See* Middle cranial base.
Middle temporal artery, sulcus for, 2010f
Middle turbinate
in endoscopic sinus surgery, 751, 751f, 771
normal anatomy of, 667
paradoxic, 668, 669f
surgical anatomy of, 739-740
in anterior cranial base, 2472, 2472f-2473f
Middle vault deformities, revision rhinoplasty for, 585-586, 586f
Midesophageal diverticula, 974, 974f
imaging of, 1402, 1403f
Midface
aesthetic ideals for, 447
aging of, 444, 444f
congenital malformations of nose due to developmental errors of, 2690-2693, 2691f
in Down syndrome, 2632
Midface fractures, pediatric, 2707, 2710f
Midface lift, 2431
Midface soft tissue laxity and sagging, after facial paralysis, 2431
Midfacial clefting, 2690, 2692
Midfacial degloving approach
for middle cranial base surgery, 2455t, 2458, 2459f
for pediatric facial fracture, 2701-2702
Midfacial split approach, for middle cranial base surgery, 2455t, 2458-2461, 2463f
Midforehead brow lift, 430, 431t
Midforehead flap, 344-345
Midforehead lift, 430, 431t
Midline cleft, 2586
Midline lesions, of neck, 2586
Midline malignant reticulosis, 659-660
Migraine, 246-247, 2347-2350
auditory symptoms of, 2348-2349
distortion as, 2349
hearing loss as, 2123, 2348-2349
phonophobia as, 2349
tinnitus as, 2349
without aura, 2347b
aura with, 2347, 2347b
basilar, 2349
diagnosis and classification of, 2347, 2347b
epidemiology of, 2347
etiology of, 2349
familial hemiplegic, 2349
familial vestibulopathy with, 2344
family history of, 2349
without headache, 2349
management of, 2349-2350, 2350f
with neurotologic symptoms, 2349
vestibular disorders associated with, 2350
benign paroxysmal positional vertigo as, 2350
Meniere's disease as, 2350
vestibular disorders related to, 2350-2351
benign paroxysmal vertigo of childhood as, 2350-2351
paroxysmal torticollis as, 2351
vestibular symptoms of, 2347-2348
motion sickness as, 2348
nonspecific dizziness as, 2347
vertigo as, 2202, 2347-2348, 2348f
Migraine accompaniments, 2349
Migraine equivalent, 2349
MII (multichannel intraluminal impedance), 962
Milia, 289
after skin resurfacing, 451
Millard forked-flap technique, in cleft-lip nose repair, 559, 566f
Millard rotation advancement closure, for cleft lip, 2667-2668, 2667f
advancement flap in, 2668, 2668f
closure in, 2668, 2668f
rotation flap in, 2667-2668, 2668f
Millicurie (mCi), 1031-1032
Mineral oil, for cerumen removal, 1958t
Mini Rhinoconjunctivitis QoL Questionnaire, 57
Minimal cross-sectional area (MCA), in rhinomanometry and acoustic rhinometry, 643f, 644
anatomic, 644
physiologic, 644
Minimally invasive sinus technique (MIST), 743, 752, 760
Minimally invasive techniques, for parathyroid surgery, 1793
Minimally invasive thyroidectomy, 1769, 1769f
Mini-mantle field technique, for glottic cancer, 1586
Minimum Speech Test Battery for Adult Cochlear Implant Users (MSTB), 2223, 2244
Miniplate, for mandibular fracture, 338
MinK, in deafness, 2051t-2058t
Minoxidil, for hair loss, 376-377
MIO (maximum interincisal opening), 1280
miR(s) (microRNAs), in head and neck squamous cell carcinoma, 1021, 1022f, 1027-1028
miRNAs (microRNAs), in head and neck squamous cell carcinoma, 1021, 1022f, 1027-1028
MirrorSuite, 279-280
MIST (minimally invasive sinus technique), 743, 752, 760
MIT (monoiodotyrosine)
in thyroid hormone release, 1738
in thyroid hormone synthesis, 1738
MITF (microphthalmia transcription factor) gene, in deafness, 2051t-2058t, 2095
Mitochondrial disorders, 8, 8f, 2088f, 2089
Mitochondrial DNA (mtDNA), 2089
Mitochondrial encephalopathy, lactic acidosis, and strokelike episodes (MELAS) syndrome, sensorineural hearing loss in, 2094t, 2097
Mitochondrial mutations, in head and neck squamous cell carcinoma, 1024-1025, 1028f
Mitochondrial sensorineural hearing loss
nonsyndromic, 2093, 2093t
screening for, 2090t
syndromic, 2094t, 2097
Mitogen-activated protein kinase (MAPK) pathway, in thyroid carcinoma, 1753
Mitomycin C
for airway stenosis, 946, 2918
for caustic ingestion, 2960
with radiotherapy, 1041
Mitotic death, due to radiation, 1037
Mitral cell, of olfactory bulb, 628f
Mivacurium, for pediatric anesthesia, 2593t
Mixed acinus, 1134, 1134t
Mixed apnea index, 251b
Mixed sleep apnea, 251b
MLC (multileaf collimator), in radiotherapy, 1035-1036
MLR (middle latency response)
auditory evoked, 1912, 1913f
electrically evoked, 1912-1914
MM (malignant melanoma). *See* Melanoma.
MMA (maxillomandibular advancement), for obstructive sleep apnea, 260, 261f
MMF. *See* Maxillomandibular fixation (MMF).
MMP. *See* Mucous membrane pemphigoid (MMP).
MMP(s) (matrix metalloproteinases)
in bone resorption, 1972
in head and neck squamous cell carcinoma, 1019-1020
MMP-1 (matrix metalloproteinase-1), in head and neck squamous cell carcinoma, 1077
MMR (mediastinal mass ratio), for lymphomas, 1676
MNTB (medial nucleus of trapezoid body), in auditory pathway, 1834f
Möbius syndrome, facial paralysis in, 2397
MOC (maintenance of certification), 80, 81b
MOC (medial olivocochlear) reflex pathways, in efferent auditory system, 1848-1849, 1848f

MOC (medial olivocochlear) "unmasking," 1849
Modafinil, for obstructive sleep apnea, 257
Modal register, of voice production, 850-851
Mode, 64t
Mode-locked lasers, 34
Modified barium swallow (MBS), 1394, 1396
for swallowing disorders, 1217-1218, 1219f
in children, 2949, 2950t
Modified radical neck dissection (MRND), 1711-1712
definition of, 1703t, 1711, 1712f
historical perspective on, 1703
indications for, 1711
for oral cancer, 1313
results of, 1721
technique for, 1711-1712, 1713f-1714f
Modified Schobinger incision, for radical neck dissection, 1709, 1710f
Modified voice use, for vocal abuse, 853
Modiolus, anatomy of, 1831, 1832f, 1834, 1840, 1841f, 2049-2050
MOE. *See* Malignant otitis externa (MOE).
Mohr-Tranebjaerg syndrome, deafness in, 2051t-2058t, 2094t, 2097
Mole(s), 286
atypical, 1107
Molecular biology, 11-12
cell division in, 12, 13f
gene expression in, 11-12, 12f
of laryngeal cancer, 1492
Molecular biomarkers
for head and neck squamous cell carcinoma, 1026-1027
epidermal growth factor receptor as, 1026
human papillomavirus as, 1026
loss of heterozygosity as, 1026
margin analysis for, 1027
in oral rinses and saliva, 1026
other, 1026-1027
polymorphisms in DNA repair enzymes as, 1027
serum analysis for, 1026-1027
for laryngeal squamous cell carcinoma, 1493, 1505
for salivary gland neoplasms, 1194
Molecular genetics, of orofacial clefts, 2662-2664
Molecular staging, of melanoma, 1118
Molluscum contagiosum, 282-283, 283f
Mometasone, for otitis media with effusion, 2772
Mometasone furoate nasal spray (Nasonex)
for nonallergic rhinitis, 700t
for rhinosinusitis, 734t, 736
"Mona Lisa" smile, 2417-2418
Mondini, Carlo, 2728-2729
Mondini malformation, 172-173, 174f
congenital hearing loss due to, 2200
CSF otorrhea due to, 2197
Mondini's dysplasia, 2730-2731
embryogenesis of, 2728f-2729f, 2729t, 2730-2731
familial, 2735
histology of, 2730-2731, 2731f
historical background of, 2728-2729
imaging of, 2730-2731, 2731f
relative incidence of, 2729t
subtypes of, 2730-2731, 2731f
Monistat (miconazole cream), for fungal otitis externa, 1954-1955, 1959t-1960t
Monobloc advancement, for craniofacial anomalies, 2653-2654, 2655f-2656f
Monocyte(s)
in adaptive immune system, 604
in allergic rhinitis, 616
in wound healing, 1076
Monocyte chemoattractant protein-1 (MCP-1), in wound healing, 1076
Monoiodotyrosine (MIT)
in thyroid hormone release, 1738
in thyroid hormone synthesis, 1738
Mononucleosis, infectious
adenotonsillar disease in, 2785-2786, 2786f
pharyngitis due to, 198-199, 198f
sudden sensorineural hearing loss due to, 2127
vestibular neuritis due to, 2162
Monosodium glutamate (MSG), taste of, 1213
Monostotic fibrous dysplasia, of paranasal sinuses, 1132
Montelukast
for allergic rhinitis, 620-621
for rhinosinusitis, 735t, 736
Montgomery T-tube, 1009
Moraxella catarrhalis
otitis media due to, 2763
rhinosinusitis due to
acute, 704, 704f, 732
acute exacerbation of chronic, 707
Moraxella catarrhalis vaccine, to prevent otitis media, 2769
Morphine
as adjunct to induction of anesthesia, 111
for pediatric anesthesia maintenance, 2591-2592
for postoperative pain, 241t
topical, for mucositis, 1102
Morquio's syndrome, 2113
Morsicatio, 1223
Mosaicism, 5
Motion artifacts, on MRI, 133-134, 134f
Motion sickness, 2357
and migraine, 2348
Motor control test, 2324-2325
Motor evoked potentials (MEPs), transcranial electrical stimulation–induced, to assess facial nerve function, 2389
Motor function, oral, 1203-1207
autonomic reflexes in, 1205-1206
jaw-tongue reflexes in, 1205
lingual muscles and reflexes in, 1205
mastication as, 1206-1207, 1206f
muscles of mastication and reflex control in, 1204-1205, 1204f-1205f
oral phase of deglutition as, 1206f, 1207
Motor nerve complications, of neck surgery, 1729-1731
facial, 1729-1730
hypoglossal, 1730-1731
phrenic, 1731, 1731f
spinal accessory, 1730, 1731f
vagus, 1730
Motor vehicle collisions
laryngeal trauma due to, 2914
pediatric facial fractures due to, 2698
Mouth. *See* Oral cavity.
Mouth breathing, 809, 2628-2629
and craniofacial growth, 2792-2793
Movement disorders, sleep-related, 265, 265b
MPD syndrome. *See* Myofascial pain dysfunction (MPD) syndrome.
MPFR (maximum phonational frequency range), 829
M-plasty, for forehead defects, 359-360, 362f
MPNST (malignant peripheral nerve sheath tumor), of neck, 1670-1671
MPS. *See* Mucopolysaccharidoses (MPS).
MPT (maximum phonation time)
in tracheoesophageal speech, 1597
in voice evaluation, 828, 849
MPZ (myelin protein zero) gene, in deafness, 2051t-2058t, 2081
MR (magnetic resonance) cisternography, for CSF rhinorrhea, 790-791, 790f
MR (magnetic resonance) sialography, 1147
MR (magnetic resonance) spectroscopy, of laryngeal carcinoma, 1470
MRA. *See* Magnetic resonance angiography (MRA).
MRD (margin-reflex-distance), 446
MRI. *See* Magnetic resonance imaging (MRI).
MRND. *See* Modified radical neck dissection (MRND).
MRP. *See* Mandibular reconstruction plate (MRP).
MRSA (methicillin-resistant *Streptococcus aureus*), rhinosinusitis due to
acute, 704, 732
chronic, 732, 733f
MS. *See* Masticator space (MS); Multiple sclerosis (MS).
MSG (monosodium glutamate), taste of, 1213
MSLT (multiple sleep latency test), 263-264
MSO (medial superior olive), in auditory pathway, 1834-1835, 1834f, 1846
MST (maximal stimulation test)
for Bell's palsy, 2394
for facial nerve injury, 2040-2041, 2382t, 2385-2386
MSTB (Minimum Speech Test Battery for Adult Cochlear Implant Users), 2223, 2244
M&T (myringotomy with tympanostomy tube insertion)
for acute otitis media, 2771
for otitis media with effusion, 2772
MTC. *See* Medullary thyroid carcinoma (MTC).
mtDNA (mitochondrial DNA), 2089
m-tetra(hydroxyphenyl)chlorin (Foscan), for recurrent respiratory papillomatosis, 2892
MTRNR1, 2093t
MTTS1, 2093t
MUC5AC gene, in otitis media, 1871
Mucins, in saliva, 1140-1141
Mucoceles, 289
in children, 2859
endoscopic sinus surgery for, 742, 760f, 761, 762f
frontoethmoid, 776f-777f, 783
imaging of, 169, 169f, 676, 678f, 765t
of petrous apex, 2524t, 2525, 2527f
surgical management of, 742
Mucociliary diseases, nasal manifestations of, 661
in cystic fibrosis, 661
in primary ciliary dyskinesia, 661
Mucocutaneous end organs, 1201
Mucocutaneous junction, in cleft lip, 2665
Mucocutaneous lymph node syndrome, in children, 2819
Mucoepidermoid carcinoma (MEC)
of larynx, 1506-1507
of salivary glands
in children, 2820, 2846, 2846f, 2862-2863
differential diagnosis of, 1183
grading of, 1183, 1184t
histopathology of, 1182-1183, 1183f
imaging of, 1146, 1147f, 1168f
minor, 1363
of trachea, 1615
Mucoepithelial changes, with aging, 234
Mucolytic agents
for rhinosinusitis, 735t, 736
for vocal professionals, 855
Mucoperichondrium, in rhinoplasty, 539-540, 546
Mucopolysaccharidoses (MPS), 2112-2113
craniofacial anomalies due to, 2640
and obstructive sleep apnea, 2606
otologic manifestations of, 2113, 2113f
Mucormycosis
otologic manifestation of, 2106f
rhinosinusitis due to, 705, 710, 711f
Mucosa, effects of radiotherapy on, 2626t
Mucosa-associated lymphoid tissue (MALT)
in eustachian tube, 1870
in middle ear protection, 1871

Mucosa-associated lymphoid tissue (MALT) lymphoma, 1679-1680
clinical presentation of, 1674
of salivary glands, 1191-1192, 1192f, 1679-1680
treatment and prognosis for, 1680
of thyroid, 1679
staging of, 1679
treatment and prognosis for, 1679
Mucosal changes, in geriatric patients, 236
Mucosal edema, olfactory dysfunction due to, 625, 635f
Mucosal grafts, for airway stenosis, 946-947
Mucosal immune system, 605
Peyer's patches and lymphoid follicles in, 605
tonsils in, 605
Mucosal lesions, oral. *See* Oral mucosal lesions.
Mucosal melanocytic nevi, of oral cavity
clinical features of, 1241
histopathologic features of, 1242
treatment of, 1243
Mucosal melanoma, 1108-1109
of larynx, 1509
of oropharynx, 1364-1365, 1364f-1365f
Mucosal ulcerations, of oral cavity, 1289, 1289f
Mucosal wave, laryngeal videostroboscopy of, 820, 848-849, 848t
Mucosal-relief esophagogram, 1394, 1395f
Mucositis
palliative care for, 1101-1102
due to radiotherapy, 1047, 1047f, 1102
Mucotrol, for mucositis, 1102
Mucous acinus, 1134, 1134f, 1134t
Mucous cysts, 289
Mucous membrane pemphigoid (MMP)
esophageal manifestations of, 980
nasal manifestations of, 660
ocular scarring (symblepharon) due to, 1233-1234, 1234f
oral, 1233-1235, 1254
clinical differential diagnosis of, 1234, 1234t
clinical features of, 1233-1234, 1233f-1234f
defined, 1233
etiology and pathogenesis of, 1233
histopathologic features of, 1234-1235, 1234f
treatment of, 1235
Mucous retention cysts, 289
in children, 2859
imaging of, 676, 677f
of larynx, 869, 869f-870f
of petrous apex, 2525, 2526f
Muenke syndrome, deafness in, 2051t-2058t
Muenke-type craniosynostosis, 2641t
Müller maneuver, in obstructive sleep apnea, 253, 254f
Müller's muscle
anatomy of, 443f, 444
in upper eyelid blepharoplasty, 448, 449f
Multicellular theory, of salivary gland tumorigenesis, 1163
Multichannel intraluminal impedance (MII), 962
Multifactorial traits, 8
MULTIFIRE ENDO GIA 30 stapler, 993-994
Multileaf collimator (MLC), in radiotherapy, 1035-1036
Multinodular thyroid gland, ultrasound imaging of, 1644
Multiple endocrine adenomatosis type 3, oral manifestations of, 1257
Multiple endocrine neoplasia type I (MEN-I)
defined, 1795
epidemiology of, 1795
familial hyperparathyroidism in, 1795-1796
genetic basis for, 1775, 1776f, 1795
Multiple endocrine neoplasia type IIA (MEN-IIA)
defined, 1773
familial hyperparathyroidism in, 1796
genetic basis for, 1796
and medullary thyroid carcinoma, 1763-1764
Multiple endocrine neoplasia type IIB (MEN-IIB), and medullary thyroid carcinoma, 1763-1764
Multiple myeloma, 2106-2107
otologic manifestations of, 2107, 2107f
Multiple sclerosis (MS)
laryngeal hypofunction due to, 843
oral manifestations of, 1255
preoperative evaluation of, 106
sensorineural hearing loss due to, 2122-2123
sudden, 2129
vertigo due to, 2202
vestibular symptoms of, 2356, 2356f
Multiple sleep latency test (MSLT), 263-264
Multiple system atrophy, laryngeal hypofunction due to, 843
Multiple-Activity Scale for Hyperacusis (MASH), 2138-2139
Multivariate analysis, 72
Mumps
salivary gland involvement in, 1156-1157
in children, 2855
sensorineural hearing loss due to, 2119, 2157-2158, 2158f
clinical features of, 2157
diagnosis of, 2157
experimental, 2158
sudden, 2127
temporal bone pathology in, 2158, 2158f
vestibular neuritis due to, 2162
Mumps vaccine, for recurrent respiratory papillomatosis, 2890t, 2892-2893
Mupirocin, for rhinosinusitis, 734, 735t
Murine removal kit (carbamide peroxide), for cerumen removal, 1958t
Muscarinic receptors, in salivary gland secretion, 1136-1137
Muscle fibers, characteristics of, 918
Muscle flaps, for free tissue transfer, 1082t, 1083-1084
latissimus, 1082t, 1083-1084, 1084f
rectus abdominis, 1082t, 1083
Muscle neoplasms, of larynx, 881
Muscle relaxants
oral sequelae of, 1247t-1248t
for pediatric anesthesia, 2592, 2593t
Muscle tension dysphonia, 842, 853
Muscle transfers, for facial nerve paralysis, 2427-2430
masseter, 2427, 2428f
microneurovascular, 2429-2430
temporalis, 2427-2429, 2429f
Muscle weakness, due to hyperparathyroidism, 1781
Muscular disorders, chronic aspiration due to, 926b
Muscular dystrophy(ies)
laryngeal hypofunction due to, 842
myotonic, oral manifestations of, 1255
Muscular tension dysphonia, 842, 853
Muscular triangle, of neck, 96, 96f, 2578f
Muscularis uvulae
in cleft palate, 2666-2667
in velopharyngeal function, 2676, 2677t
Musculocutaneous arteries, 1065, 1065f
Musculocutaneous flaps, 1067, 1067f
for free tissue transfer, 1082t, 1083-1084
latissimus, 1082t, 1083-1084, 1084f
for oropharyngeal reconstruction, 1380
for oropharyngeal reconstruction, 1380
rectus abdominis, 1082t, 1083
for oropharyngeal reconstruction, 1380
Musculoskeletal tension, in voice evaluation, 827-831, 828f
Mustache transplantation, 384
Mustarde suture technique, for otoplasty, 475-478, 476f-477f
Mutation testing, 9, 9f-10f
MV (megavoltage) electrons, 1033
MV (megavoltage) x-rays, 1033-1034
MVN (medial vestibular nucleus), 1861, 1862f
in velocity storage, 2296
M-wave, 2388
MX350-1, for head and neck squamous cell carcinoma, 1018
Myasthenia gravis
abnormal pharyngeal motility due to, 1398
edrophonium test for, 835
laryngeal hypofunction due to, 842
oral manifestations of, 1255
Mycelex (clotrimazole) cream, for fungal otitis externa, 1954-1955, 1959t-1960t
Mycobacterial infection
lymphadenopathy due to, 2818, 2819f
of salivary glands
in children, 2857-2858, 2857f
nontuberculous, 1158-1159, 1158f
tuberculous, 1158
Mycobacterial laryngitis, 885-886, 886f
Mycobacterial mastoiditis, 2196
Mycobacterium tuberculosis. See Tuberculosis (TB).
Mycophenolate mofetil, microtia due to, 2741
Mycoplasma pneumoniae, pharyngitis due to, 194-195
Mycoplasma spp, bullous myringitis due to, 1948
Mycostatin (nystatin cream), for fungal otitis externa, 1954-1955, 1959t-1960t
Mycotic diseases. *See* Fungal diseases.
Myectomy, selective, for synkinesis, 2432
Myelin protein zero *(MPZ)* gene, in deafness, 2051t-2058t, 2081
Myeloid stem cells, 600, 600f
Myeloma, multiple, 2106-2107
otologic manifestations of, 2107, 2107f
Myelopathy, due to radiotherapy, 1049
Myenteric plexus, 953, 954f
Myers-Cotton classification, of airway stenosis, 944, 944t
MYH9 (myosin heavy chain IX) gene, in deafness, 2051t-2058t
MYH14 (myosin heavy chain XIV) gene, in deafness, 2051t-2058t
Mylohyoid muscle, anatomy of, 1296f-1297f, 1297-1298, 1320, 2578f
MYO. *See* Myosin.
Myocardium, of newborn, 2571
Myoclonic epilepsy and red ragged fibers (MERRF) syndrome, sensorineural hearing loss in, 2094t, 2097
Myoclonus, oculopalatolaryngopharyngeal, 840
Myocutaneous flaps, 1067, 1067f
for free tissue transfer, 1082t, 1083-1084
latissimus, 1082t, 1083-1084, 1084f
for oropharyngeal reconstruction, 1380
for oropharyngeal reconstruction, 1380
rectus abdominis, 1082t, 1083
for oropharyngeal reconstruction, 1380
for hypopharyngeal and esophageal reconstruction, 1452-1453
Myoepithelial carcinoma, of salivary glands, 1191
Myoepithelial cells, of salivary glands, 1134, 1134f, 1163f
Myoepithelioma, of salivary glands, 1171
Myofascial pain dysfunction (MPD) syndrome, of temporomandibular joint, 1283-1285
clinical features of, 1283-1284
defined, 1283
differential diagnosis of, 1284t-1285t
epidemiology of, 1283
etiology of, 1283, 1283f
treatment of, 1284-1285, 1286f
Myopathies, laryngeal hypofunction due to, 842
Myosin(s), in stereocilia, 2076f
Myosin 1A *(MYO1A)* gene, in deafness, 2051t-2058t
Myosin 1c, in adaptation of mechanoelectrical transduction currents, 2079, 2079f

Myosin heavy chain (MHC) isoforms
in lingual muscles, 1205
in muscles of mastication, 1204
Myosin heavy chain IX *(MYH9)* gene, in deafness, 2051t-2058t
Myosin heavy chain XIV *(MYH14)* gene, in deafness, 2051t-2058t
Myosin IIIA, in stereocilia, 2077
Myosin IIIA *(MYO3A)* gene, in deafness, 2051t-2058t
Myosin VI, in stereocilia, 2078
Myosin VI *(MYO6)* gene, in deafness, 2051t-2058t, 2078
Myosin VIIA *(MYO7A)* gene, in deafness, 2051t-2058t, 2077-2078, 2096
Myosin XVA, in hair bundle development, 2077
Myosin XVA *(MYO15A)* gene, in deafness, 2051t-2058t, 2076
Myositis, *vs.* myofascial pain dysfunction syndrome, 1285t
Myositis ossificans, *vs.* myofascial pain dysfunction syndrome, 1285t
Myotomy, surgical, for achalasia, 964-965
Myotonic muscular dystrophy, oral manifestations of, 1255
Myringitis
bullous, 1948, 1948f
defined, 1955
granular, 1955
otorrhea due to, 2196
topical therapies for, 1955
Myringotomy
for acute otitis media, 2771
with tympanostomy tube insertion, 2771
for eustachian tube dysfunction, 1874
for otitis media with effusion, 2772
with tympanostomy tube insertion, 2772
Myringotomy with tympanostomy tube insertion (M&T)
for acute otitis media, 2771
for otitis media with effusion, 2772
Myxedema, pretibial, and Graves' ophthalmopathy, 1808
Myxedema coma, 1749
Myxoma, odontogenic, 1276-1277, 1276f
microscopic findings in, 1276
radiographic findings in, 1276
treatment and prognosis for, 1276-1277, 1277f

N

N (nodal) classification, for melanoma, 1111-1113, 1111t
*N*6-furfuryladenine (Kinerase), for aging skin, 404
Na⁺. *See* Sodium (Na⁺).
NaCl (sodium chloride), gustatory response to, 1208-1209
NADP-regulated thyroid hormone–binding protein, in deafness, 2051t-2058t
NA-EFRS (nonallergic eosinophilic fungal rhinosinusitis), 709, 715-716, 716t
Na^+,K^+ (sodium-potassium) pump, ATPase-driven, in salivary gland secretion, 1135
NAP-2 (neutrophil-activating peptide-2), in wound healing, 1076
Napoleon I, 251
NAR. *See* Nonallergic rhinitis (NAR).
Narcolepsy, 262t, 264
Narcotic analgesics. *See* Opioids.
NARES (nonallergic rhinitis with eosinophilia syndrome), 619b, 696
Narrow-band imaging (NBI), of larynx, 813, 823-824, 823f-824f
Nasacort (triamcinolone), for nonallergic rhinitis, 700t
Nasal airflow, 485-487
during exercise, 641
peak, 643
physical factors affecting, 643
in rhinomanometry
measurement of, 647
and transnasal pressure, 643
with rhinosinusitis, 730
and transnasal pressure, 643
Nasal allergy, and otitis media, 1872
Nasal base sculpting, for noncaucasian nose, 556-557, 559f-560f
Nasal block, 501-502
Nasal bones, anatomy and physiology of, 320
Nasal breathing function, 640-642
anatomy of, 641-642
septum and turbinates in, 641
nasal valve in, 641, 641f
site of sensation of obstruction in, 641-642
assessment of, 642-644
acoustic rhinometry for, 643-645
in allergic rhinitis, 651
to assess effect of treatment, 651-652
equipment for, 486-487, 486f, 644
interpretation of results of, 645
intranasal dimensions and cross-sectional area in, 643, 643f
intranasal sites assessed by, 644
reporting results of, 645
rhinogram generated by, 486-487, 487f, 645
vs. rhinomanometry, 644
for snoring and sleep apnea, 651
sources of variability in, 651
technical concerns and testing pitfalls with, 645
technique of, 644-645
nasal examination in, 642
objective testing of nasal airway in, 642-644
air stream through nose in, 643
to assess effects of treatment, 651-652
for challenge testing in allergic rhinitis, 651
in clinical evaluation of patient with nasal obstruction, 652-656
complementary information in, 656
correlation between results and symptoms with, 654
criteria for, 642
history of, 642
in identifying site of pathology affecting airflow, 655-656
intranasal dimensions and cross-sectional area in, 643, 643f
laser Doppler velocimetry for, 643-644
for normal nasal airway, 652t-653t, 654f
other methods of, 643-644
role of, 651-652
for snoring and sleep apnea, 651
sources of variability in, 651
and threshold level at which patient feels airway restriction, 655
when results do not match physical findings or symptoms, 653-654
when symptoms are not due to airway restriction, 653
patient history in, 642
rhinomanometry for, 643-651
vs. acoustic rhinometry, 644
active *vs.* passive, 647-648
in allergic rhinitis, 651
anterior *vs.* posterior, 645-647, 648f-649f
to assess effect of treatment, 651-652
for children, 645
defined, 642
equipment for, 645
examining pressure-flow curve in, 648-649, 649f-650f
inspiratory or expiratory values in, 650-651
Nasal breathing function *(Continued)*
intranasal sites assessed by, 644
maximum (vertex) resistance in, 650
measurement of nasal airflow in, 647
measurement of transnasal pressure in, 645-647, 648f
nasal airflow and transnasal pressure in, 643
nasal resistance in, 649-650, 650f
parameters in, 649-651, 650f
reporting results of, 648-651
sources of variability in, 651
technical concerns and testing pitfalls with, 645-648
technique of, 645, 645f-648f
unilateral *vs.* bilateral measurements in, 648, 649f
pathologic conditions affecting, 642
physiologic factors affecting, 640-641
Nasal bridge length, 2617t
Nasal cartilage, burns of, 316
Nasal cavity
bony outlines of, 672, 672f
imaging of, 169, 170f
lymphoma of, 1680
therapy and prognosis for, 1680
in surgical anatomy of anterior cranial base, 2443, 2471-2473, 2472f-2473f
Nasal challenge testing, objective measurement methods in, 651
Nasal clefts, 2690, 2692
Nasal cycle, 486, 641
MRI of, 664, 664f
Nasal defects, 346-350, 364-372
aesthetic units and, 346-347, 347f, 364
approach to, 346-347
extending into alar facial sulcus, 348
cheek advancement flap for, 348, 349f
cheek pedicle transposition flap for, 348, 349f
full-thickness alar, 347, 371-372
bipedicle mucosal advancement flap for, 347, 347f
free cartilage grafts for, 348
melolabial interpolated flap for, 348
full-thickness central defects of tip or dorsum as, 348
composite turnout flap for, 348, 351f
paramedian forehead flaps for, 348-350, 352f-354f
involving skeletal supporting structures, 367-371
grafting material for
alloplastic, 368
autogenous cartilage as, 368-369, 369f-370f
bone as, 369, 370f
homograft tissues as, 368
selection of, 367-368
prosthetic management of, 1345, 1345t, 1346f
reconstruction of, 364-372
external covering layer in, 364-367
framework in, 367-371
internal lining in, 371-372
surface defects of nasal tip, columella, sidewalls, and dorsum as, 348, 364-367
bilobed flaps for, 365-366, 365f
complications of local flaps for, 366
dorsonasal (Rieger) flap for, 365-366
forehead flap for, 366-367, 368f
full-thickness skin grafts for, 365
glabellar flaps for, 365-366
healing by second intention for, 365
hinge flap for, 348, 350f
melolabial flap for, 366, 367f
paramedian forehead flaps for, 348
primary closure for, 365, 365f
retroauricular flap for, 365-366
transposition flaps for, 365-366, 366f
vestibular lining reconstruction for, 371-372, 371f-372f
V-Y advancement flap for, 345-346, 346f

Nasal depth, anterior and posterior, 2617t
Nasal dilator strips, for obstructive sleep apnea, 257
Nasal dorsum
  cartilaginous, 509f
  full-thickness central defects of, 348
    composite turnout flap for, 348, 351f
    paramedian forehead flaps for, 348-350, 352f-354f
  growth and development of, 2617t
  reconstruction of, 371
  surface defects of, 348
    hinge flap for, 348, 350f
    paramedian forehead flaps for, 348
Nasal endoscopy, 100
  for CSF rhinorrhea, 791
  in endoscopic sinus surgery, 746, 763
Nasal Endoscopy Simulator, 49
Nasal examination
  in assessment of nasal breathing function, 642
  for professional voice disorders, 851
Nasal fracture(s), 496-507
  acute intervention for, 500
  algorithm for management of, 501, 502f
  cantilever bone graft for, 505, 505f
  classification of, 498-499, 498f-499f
  complications of, 507
  diagnostic assessment of, 499-500
    history in, 499
    physical examination in, 499-500
    radiography in, 325, 500
  external compression plating for, 506
  external nasal splinting for, 504
  injuries associated with, 498
  mucoperiosteal tunnel dissection and wire for, 506, 506f
  nasal anatomy and, 496-497, 497f
  "open-book", 2708, 2711f
  pathophysiology of, 497-498
  pediatric, 506-507, 2708-2711, 2711f-2712f
  percutaneous Kirschner wire for, 506, 506f
  reduction of
    alternative methods for, 506, 506f
    in children, 2628
    closed
      anesthesia for, 501-502
      care after, 504
      equipment and medications for, 503, 503f
      vs. open, 500-501, 501f
      technique for, 502-504, 503f-504f
    open
      vs. closed, 500-501, 501f
      failed, 503-504
      technique for, 504-506, 505f
    timing of, 500
  septal splints for, 504
Nasal function, and nonallergic rhinitis, 695
Nasal height, 2617t
Nasal implant, for saddle nose deformity, 555, 556f-558f
Nasal innervation, and nonallergic rhinitis, 695
Nasal lymphoma, 1680
  therapy and prognosis for, 1680
Nasal manifestations, of systemic diseases, 657-661
  cutaneous, 660-661
    Behçet's disease as, 660-661
    pemphigoid as, 660
    pemphigus vulgaris as, 660
    scleroderma as, 660
  granulomatous, 657-659
    Churg-Strauss syndrome as, 659
    in sarcoidosis, 658-659
    Wegener's granulomatosis as, 658
  immunodeficiency, 660
    AIDS as, 660
    sinusitis in immunocompromised patient as, 660
Nasal manifestations, of systemic diseases *(Continued)*
  mucociliary, 661
    cystic fibrosis as, 661
    primary ciliary dyskinesia as, 661
  neoplastic, 659-660
    T-cell lymphoma as, 659-660
Nasal meatuses
  normal anatomy of, 664-665
  in surgical anatomy of anterior cranial base, 2472, 2472f
"Nasal neurotic," 483-484
Nasal obstruction
  and dentofacial growth, 2628-2630, 2629f
    open mouth posture in, 2628-2629
    review of literature on, 2629-2630
  evaluation of, 483-485, 642-644
    acoustic rhinometry for, 643-645
      in allergic rhinitis, 651
      to assess effect of treatment, 651-652
      equipment for, 486-487, 486f, 644
      interpretation of results of, 645
      intranasal dimensions and cross-sectional area in, 643, 643f
      intranasal sites assessed by, 644
      reporting results of, 645
      rhinogram generated by, 486-487, 487f, 645
      vs. rhinomanometry, 644
      for snoring and sleep apnea, 651
      sources of variability in, 651
      technical concerns and testing pitfalls with, 645
      technique of, 644-645
    anterior rhinoscopy for, 484
    Cottle maneuver in, 484, 484f
    with deviated nasal septum, 483f, 484
    during forced inspiration, 483-484, 484f
    nasal airflow and nasal resistance in, 485-487
    nasal examination in, 642
    nasal valve angle and nasal valve area in, 485, 485f
    objective testing of nasal airway in, 642-644
      air stream through nose in, 643
      to assess effects of treatment, 651-652
      for challenge testing in allergic rhinitis, 651
      in clinical evaluation, 652-656
      complementary information in, 656
      correlation between results and symptoms with, 654
      criteria for, 642
      history of, 642
      in identifying site of pathology affecting airflow, 655-656
      intranasal dimensions and cross-sectional area in, 643, 643f
      laser Doppler velocimetry for, 643-644
      for normal nasal airway, 651-653, 652t-653t, 654f
      other methods of, 643-644
      role of, 651-652
      for snoring and sleep apnea, 651
      sources of variability in, 651
      and threshold level at which patient feels airway restriction, 655
      when results do not match physical findings or symptoms, 653-654
      when symptoms are not due to airway restriction, 653
    patient history in, 642
    rhinomanometry for, 643-651
      vs. acoustic rhinometry, 644
      active *vs.* passive, 647-648
      in allergic rhinitis, 651
      anterior *vs.* posterior, 645-647, 648f-649f
      to assess effect of treatment, 651-652
      for children, 645
Nasal obstruction *(Continued)*
      defined, 642
      equipment for, 645
      examining pressure-flow curve in, 648-649, 649f-650f
      inspiratory or expiratory values in, 650-651
      intranasal sites assessed by, 644
      maximum (vertex) resistance in, 650
      measurement of nasal airflow in, 647
      measurement of transnasal pressure in, 645-647, 648f
      nasal airflow and transnasal pressure in, 643
      nasal resistance in, 649-650, 650f
      parameters in, 649-651, 650f
      reporting results of, 648-651
      sources of variability in, 651
      technical concerns and testing pitfalls with, 645-648
      technique of, 645, 645f-648f
      unilateral *vs.* bilateral measurements in, 648, 649f
    with tip ptosis, 484, 485f
  due to external valve collapse, 493
  after facial paralysis, 2430-2431
  due to internal valve compromise, 492, 493f
  measurement of, 486-487, 486f-487f
  olfactory dysfunction due to, 633, 634f-635f
  paradoxic, 484, 486
  septal
    evaluation of, 483f, 484
    vs. turbinate, 486
  sites of sensation of, 641-642
  symptoms of, with open airway, 653
Nasal Obstruction Symptom Evaluation (NOSE), 57
Nasal ocular reflex, in allergic rhinitis, 614-615
Nasal packing, for epistaxis, 688, 688f
Nasal passageways, in olfactory stimulation, 624-625, 625f
Nasal peak inspiratory flowmeter, 643
Nasal pits, 482, 2660, 2661f, 2691f
Nasal placodes, 482, 2659-2660, 2661f, 2691f
Nasal polyp(s)
  endoscopic sinus surgery for, 751-752
  olfactory dysfunction due to, 625, 634f
  surgical management of, 741
Nasal polyposis
  in aspirin-exacerbated respiratory disease, 732f
  with methicillin-resistant *Staphylococcus aureus* infection, 733f
  surgical management of, 741
Nasal pressure-flow curves
  normal range for, 652, 654f
  in rhinomanometry, 648-649, 649f-650f
Nasal projection, in aesthetic analysis, 273-274, 277f
Nasal prosthesis, 1345, 1345t, 1346f
Nasal provocation testing
  in nonallergic rhinitis, 695-696
  objective measurement methods in, 651
Nasal reconstruction, 364-372. *See also* Nasal defects.
  of external covering layer, 364-367
    aesthetic units in, 364
    full-thickness skin grafts for, 365
    healing by secondary intention in, 365
    local flaps in, 365-366, 365f
      advantages of, 365-366
      bilobed, 365-366, 365f
      complications of, 366
      dorsonasal (Rieger), 365-366
      forehead, 366-367, 368f
      glabellar, 365-366
      melolabial, 366, 367f
      retroauricular, 365-366
      transposition, 365-366, 366f

Nasal reconstruction *(Continued)*
primary closure in, 365, 365f
skin texture and thickness in, 364-365
of framework, 367-371
grafting material for
alloplastic, 368
autogenous cartilage as, 368-369, 369f-370f
bone as, 369, 370f
homograft tissues as, 368
selection of, 367-368
of internal lining, 371-372, 371f-372f
Nasal reflex arc, 695
Nasal resistance, 485-487
in normal individuals *vs.* those with nasal obstruction, 653, 654f
in rhinomanometry, 649-650, 650f
total normal, 652, 653t
unilateral normal mean and median, 652, 652t
Nasal rotation, in aesthetic analysis, 273-274, 277f
Nasal saline lavage, for rhinosinusitis, 734t, 736
Nasal septal mucosal flap, 2478, 2479f
Nasal septum, 481-495
anatomy and embryology of, 482-483, 482f, 497, 1359f
blood supply and innvervation of, 483, 483f
caudal
repositioning of, 547, 547f
in septoplasty, 491-492, 491f-492f
overaggressive resection of, 492, 492f
shortening of, 547-548, 547f-548f
deviated, 483f, 484
endoscopic sinus surgery with, 751
imaging of, 668, 669f
in noncaucasian patient, 573, 576f
rhinitis due to, 619b
rhinoplasty with, 513-514, 514f, 546, 546f-547f
due to trauma, 482, 484
with twisted nose, 551-552, 552f
examination of, 483-485
fracture of, 498, 501, 501f
closed reduction of, 503, 503f
open reduction of, 505-506
functions of, 482
growth centers of, 2627, 2627f
and nasal breathing function, 641
perforation of, epistaxis due to, 686f
pyogenic granuloma on, 685f
radiographic anatomy of, 1398f
surgery on (*See* Septoplasty)
in surgical anatomy of anterior cranial base, 2471-2472, 2472f
tension, 492, 493f
variations in, 482, 482f
Nasal sidewalls, surface defects of, 348
hinge flap for, 348, 350f
paramedian forehead flaps for, 348
Nasal skeletal reconstruction, 367-371
grafting material for
alloplastic, 368
autogenous cartilage as, 368-369, 369f-370f
bone as, 369, 370f
homograft tissues as, 368
selection of, 367-368
Nasal skin, texture and thickness of, 364-365
Nasal splints, after septoplasty, 494
Nasal stenosis, in cleft-lip nose repair, 559, 566f
Nasal surgery, for obstructive sleep apnea, 258, 258b
Nasal tip
anatomy of, 509f
asymmetrical, in newborn, 2709-2711
overrotation of, revision rhinoplasty for, 590, 590f-591f
persistently wide or bulbous, revision rhinoplasty for, 589-590, 590f
pinched, revision rhinoplasty for, 590, 591f-592f
Nasal tip *(Continued)*
ptosis of, 484, 485f
caudal extension graft for, 576, 576f
due to overaggressive resection of caudal septum, 492, 492f
revision rhinoplasty for, 590-593, 593f
after rhinoplasty, 519, 520f
Nasal tip bossae, revision rhinoplasty for, 588-589, 590f
Nasal tip defects
full-thickness central, 348
composite turnout flap for, 348, 351f
paramedian forehead flaps for, 348-350, 352f-354f
surface, 348
hinge flap for, 348, 350f
paramedian forehead flaps for, 348
primary closure of, 365, 365f
Nasal tip deformities, revision rhinoplasty for, 588
irregularities and bossae as, 588-589, 590f
overrotation (short nose) as, 590, 590f-591f
persistently wide or bulbous tip as, 589-590, 590f
pinched tip as, 590, 591f-592f
ptotic tip as, 590-593, 593f
Nasal tip projection, 520, 535-536, 549-551
autogenous cartilage struts for, 535-536, 536f
cephalic rotation for, 519, 536, 549-550, 551f
onlay tip cartilage grafts for, 535-536, 537f, 549-550, 550f-551f
partial-transfixion *vs.* complete-transfixion incisions for, 535-536, 536f
plumping grafts for, 535-536, 536f
transdomal sutures for, 536
Nasal tip protrusion, 2617t
Nasal tip refinement, 519-536
considerations in, 520, 522f
delivery approaches for, 522, 527f
complete strip technique in, 522, 527f-530f
interrupted strip technique in, 522, 532f-533f
suturing in, 522, 530f-531f, 550-551
incisions, approaches, and techniques for, 520, 521f, 521t
in noncaucasian patients, 573-577
cap graft in, 576, 577f
caudal extension graft in, 576, 576f
concept of, 573-576
reshaping of lower lateral cartilage in, 577
shield graft in, 576, 577f
technique for, 576-577
thinning of subcutaneous tissue in, 577, 577f
nondelivery (cartilage-splitting, retrograde-eversion) approaches for, 522, 523f-526f
objective of, 519
open approach for, 522-535, 534f-535f
indications for, 521b
preservation of lateral crus and strip of alar cartilage in, 520-522, 522f
tip projection in, 520, 535-536, 549-551
autogenous cartilage struts for, 535-536, 536f
cephalic rotation for, 519, 536, 549-550, 551f
onlay tip cartilage grafts for, 535-536, 537f, 549-550, 550f-551f
partial-transfixion *vs.* complete-transfixion incisions for, 535-536, 536f
plumping grafts for, 535-536, 536f
transdomal sutures for, 536
tip ptosis after, 519, 520f
tip support mechanisms and, 519, 520f
Nasal tip support mechanisms, 519, 520f
Nasal trumpet, for awake fiberoptic nasotracheal intubation, 124, 125f
Nasal turbinates
anatomy and embryology of, 482-483
hypertrophy of, 486
and nasal breathing function, 641
in surgical anatomy of anterior cranial base, 2472, 2472f
Nasal valve
defined, 641
external, collapse of, 493
internal, compromise of, 492, 493f
and nasal breathing function, 641, 641f
vs. nasal valve area, 641
septoplasty with correction of, 493
Nasal valve angle, 485, 485f
Nasal valve area, 485, 485f
defined, 641
description of, 641, 641f
Nasalance, in acoustic analysis, for voice evaluation, 829t, 830
Nasalide (flunisolide)
for nonallergic rhinitis, 700t
for rhinosinusitis, 734t, 736
Nasarel (flunisolide)
for nonallergic rhinitis, 700t
for rhinosinusitis, 734t, 736
Nascher, I. L., 230
Nasion, 320f, 509f
growth and development of, 2617t
Nasoalveolar cysts, of oral cavity, 1288, 1288f
Nasobuccal membrane, 482
congenital malformations of nose due to developmental errors of, 2693-2695
Nasoethmoid complex (NEC) fractures, 322
classification of, 326-327, 327f
physical examination of, 324, 324f
repair of, 336-337, 337f
Nasoethmoidal encephalocele, 2687-2688, 2687t
Nasofacial angle, in aesthetic analysis, 272-274, 276f
Nasofacial relationships, in aesthetic analysis, 272-274
nasofacial angle in, 272-274, 276f
nasofrontal angle in, 270, 272-273, 274f
nasolabial angle in, 272-273, 276f
nasomental angle in, 272-273, 276f
Nasofrontal angle
in aesthetic analysis, 270, 272-273, 274f
in rhinoplasty, 514
Nasofrontal angle modifications, rhinoplasty for, 548-549, 550f
Nasofrontal encephalocele, 2687-2688, 2687t
Nasofrontal suture, 497f
Nasogastric tube, for caustic ingestion, 2960
Nasolabial angle
in aesthetic analysis, 272-273, 276f
anatomy of, 509f
in rhinoplasty, 514
with tip ptosis, 485f
Nasolacrimal duct cysts, 2693, 2694f
Nasolacrimal duct injury, in functional endoscopic sinus surgery, 679
Nasolacrimal groove
in embryology of lip, 2661f-2662f
in embryology of nose, 2691f
Nasolaryngoscopy, flexible fiberoptic, for recurrent respiratory papillomatosis, 2888
Nasomaxillary complex, growth and development of, 2619-2620, 2621f-2622f
sinuses in, 2619-2620, 2623f
Nasomental angle, in aesthetic analysis, 272-273, 276f
Nasometry, for velopharyngeal dysfunction, 2679, 2679f
Nasonex (mometasone furoate nasal spray)
for nonallergic rhinitis, 700t
for rhinosinusitis, 734t, 736
Naso-orbital encephalocele, 2687-2688, 2687t
Naso-orbitoethmoid (NOE) fractures, 322
classification of, 326-327, 327f
pediatric, 2714, 2716f

Naso-orbitoethmoid (NOE) fractures *(Continued)*
pediatric, 2714
classification of, 2714, 2716f
evaluation of, 2714, 2716f
repair of, 2714, 2716f
physical examination of, 324, 324f
repair of, 336-337, 337f
pediatric, 2714, 2716f
Nasopalatine nerve, 483f, 1297f
Nasopharyngeal biopsy, 1353
Nasopharyngeal carcinoma (NPC), 1351-1357, 1699-1700
audiogram and tympanogram for, 1354
cervical lymph node metastasis of, 1352-1353, 1353f
incidence and distribution of, 1687f
radiation therapy for, 1690, 1690t
in children, 2820
classification of, 1353-1354, 1354t
clinical presentation of, 1352-1353, 1353f
endoscopic appearance in, 1353, 1354f
nodal metastases in, 1352-1353, 1353f
diagnosis of, 1353-1354
epidemiology of, 1350-1351, 1699
Epstein-Barr virus and, 1352, 1354
etiology of, 1352
environmental factors in, 1352
Epstein-Barr virus in, 1352, 1354
genetic factors in, 1352
imaging of, 148, 149f, 1412-1413, 1413f
for staging, 1354
vs. myofascial pain dysfunction syndrome, 1284t
prognosis for, 1356-1357
recurrences of
local, 1355
regional, 1356, 1357f
staging of, 1354
imaging in, 1354
treatment of, 1354-1355
approach to, 1354-1355, 1699
chemoradiation for, 1355
pretreatment planning for, 1354
radiation therapy for, 1354-1355
intensity-modulated, 1045, 1699-1700, 1699f, 1700t
surgical, 1355
endoscopic approach for, 1355, 1355f
lateral rhinotomy and medial maxillectomy approach for, 1355-1356, 1356f
for local recurrences, 1355
maxillary swing for, 1356, 1356f
other approaches to, 1356
of regional recurrences, 1356, 1357f
VEGF in, 1700
Nasopharyngeal lymphoma, 149f
Nasopharyngeal stenosis, after adenotonsillectomy, 2800-2801, 2801f
Nasopharyngeal teratomas, 2695, 2696f
Nasopharyngeal tumor(s), 1348-1357
adenoid cystic carcinoma as, 1351
angiofibroma as, 152, 154f, 1349-1351
clinical features of, 1349
diagnosis of, 1349-1350, 1350f
growth patterns of, 1349
management of, 1350-1351
pathologic features of, 1349
recurrence of, 1351
staging of, 1350, 1350t
chordoma as, 1351
classification of, 1349t
craniopharyngioma as, 1349
diagnostic approach for, 1348-1349
lateral skull base approach for, 2510-2511
nasopharyngeal carcinoma as (*See* Nasopharyngeal carcinoma (NPC))
and otitis media, 1873, 1873f
squamous papilloma as, 1349
Tornwaldt cyst/bursa as, 1348-1349
Nasopharyngoscopy
in children, 2574
fiberoptic, 101
of obstructive sleep apnea, 253, 254f
Nasopharynx
anatomy of, 1359f
radiographic, 1398f-1399f
dysphagia due to congenital anomalies of, 2949, 2950t, 2951f
physical examination of, 100-101
in surgical anatomy of anterior skull base, 2474
Nasoseptal surgery, effects on craniofacial growth and development of, 2627-2628
Nasoseptal trauma, abnormal facial growth and development due to, 2626-2628
animal studies on, 2626-2627
human studies on, 2627-2628, 2627f
surgical timing and approach and, 2628
Nasotracheal intubation
awake fiberoptic, 122-123
advantages of, 123
avoiding failure in, 125, 126b
bronchoscopy cart for, 123, 123f
conscious sedation for, 124
fiberoptic bronchoscope in, 123-125, 125f
historical perspective on, 122-123
indications for, 123, 123b
keys to successful, 124b
monitoring during, 124
nasal trumpet placement for, 124, 125f
optimal setup for, 125f
patient preparation for, 123-124
technique of, 124-125
topical anesthesia for, 124
for stridor, 2904
National Business Group on Health (NBGH), 84t-87t, 87
National Committee for Quality Assurance (NCQA), 82, 84t-87t
National Emergency X-Radiography Utilization Study (NEXUS) criteria, for laryngeal trauma, 935-936, 935b
National Guidelines Clearinghouse (NGC), 84t-87t
National Quality Forum (NQF), 84t-87t, 87
National Quality Measures Clearinghouse (NQMC), 84t-87t
National Surgical Quality Improvement Program (NSQIP), 84t-87t
Natural history, *vs.* efficacy of treatment, 62t
Natural killer (NK) cells, in adaptive immune system, 603-604
Nausea, postoperative, in children, 2593
Nbc3, in murine deafness, 2058t-2060t
NBGH (National Business Group on Health), 84t-87t, 87
NBI (narrow-band imaging), of larynx, 813, 823-824, 823f-824f
N-butyl-2-cyanoacrylate (NBCA), for embolization, 1933
NCQA (National Committee for Quality Assurance), 82, 84t-87t
ND (Norrie disease) gene, in deafness, 2051t-2058t
Nd:YAG (neodymium:yttrium-aluminum-garnet) laser, 31t, 32
for facial resurfacing, 403t
Near-total laryngectomy (NTL), 1564
for advanced glottic cancer, 1497
Near-total thyroidectomy, for Graves' disease, 1743
NEC fractures. *See* Nasoethmoid complex (NEC) fractures.
Neck
aesthetic analysis of, 275, 279f
anatomy of, 2577-2586
anterior triangle of, 2578f, 2579-2581
ansa cervicalis in, 2580f, 2581
carotid triangle in, 2578f, 2579-2580, 2580f
Neck *(Continued)*
conventional radiography of, 131
embryology of, 2583-2585, 2583f
branchial arches in, 2583-2584, 2583f
craniofacial syndromes related to, 2585
innervation of, 2584
muscular derivatives of, 2584
skeletal derivatives of, 2583-2584, 2583f
pharyngeal pouch(es) in, 2583-2585, 2583f-2584f
first, 2584, 2584f-2585f
fourth through sixth, 2584f-2585f, 2585
second, 2584, 2584f-2585f
third, 2584f-2585f, 2585
lymphatic system of, 1683, 1683f, 2582-2583
classification of cervical lymphatics in, 2582-2583
deep cervical lymph nodes in, 2582
for pharynx and larynx, 2582
superficial lymph nodes in, 2582
midline lesions of, 2586
physical examination of, 95, 96f
adenopathy in, 95-96
lymph node regions in, 96-97, 96f
thyroid gland in, 95
triangles of, 96-97, 96f
posterior triangle of, 2577-2579, 2578f-2579f
accessory nerve in, 2578-2579, 2580f
arterial branches in, 2579
cutaneous branches of cervical plexus in, 2578, 2580f
fascia in, 2577
deep, 2577-2578, 2578f-2579f
superficial, 2577
postoperative changes in, 173-174, 175f
postradiation changes in, 1476-1479
radiation changes in, 173-174, 176f
root of, 2581-2582, 2581f
subcutaneous emphysema of, 1410, 1410f
Neck abscess, 1407, 1407f
Neck control
with N0 status, 1688, 1690, 1692, 1692t
with N1-N3 status, 1692-1695
postoperative irradiation or chemo-irradiation for, 1693-1694, 1694t
after primary radiotherapy, 1692-1693, 1693t
Neck dissection, 1702-1725
algorithm for, 1724, 1724f
anterior, 1703
central compartment, 1719
defined, 1719, 1719f
technique for, 1719, 1720f
for cancer of midline structures of anterior lower neck, 1719
definition and rationale for, 1719, 1719f
technique for, 1719, 1720f
for cervical esophageal cancer, 1434-1439
cervical lymph node groups in, 1703-1705
levels of, 1703-1705, 1704f, 1706t
radiologic anatomic markers for, 1705, 1707t-1708t
sublevels of, 1704-1705, 1705f, 1706t
after chemoradiation, 1724
classification of, 1705-1721
complication(s) of, 1722-1724
air leaks as, 1722-1723
bleeding as, 1723
blindness as, 1723
carotid artery rupture as, 1723-1724
chylous fistula as, 1723
facial/cerebral edema as, 1723
for cutaneous malignancies, 1718-1719
definition and rationale for, 1718, 1718f
technique for, 1718-1719
defined, 1702
elective, 1702
extended, 1703t, 1719-1721, 1720f

Neck dissection *(Continued)*
historical perspective on, 1702-1703
for hypopharyngeal cancer, 1434-1439, 1716-1718
definition and rationale for, 1716-1717, 1717f
technique for, 1717-1718, 1717f
for laryngeal cancer, 1716-1718
definition and rationale for, 1716-1717, 1717f
glottic, 1497-1498
after nonsurgical organ preservation treatment, 1502-1503
supraglottic, 1500-1501
technique for, 1717-1718, 1717f
with trasoral laser microsurgery, 1532
lateral, 1716-1718
definition and rationale for, 1716-1717, 1717f
technique for, 1717-1718, 1717f
lymphoscintigraphy-directed, 1721-1722
with N0 status, 1692
for nasopharyngeal carcinoma, 1356
for oral cavity cancer, 1312-1314, 1313f, 1713-1716
definition and rationale for, 1713, 1714f
technique for, 1713-1716, 1715f-1716f
for oropharyngeal cancer, 1716-1718
definition and rationale for, 1716-1717, 1717f
technique for, 1717-1718, 1717f
posterolateral, 1718-1719
after radiation therapy, 1694, 1721
radical, 1705-1709
anterior triangle dissection in, 1709-1710
defined, 1703t, 1705, 1709f
dissection of upper neck compartments in, 1710-1711
flap elevation in, 1709, 1711f
historical perspective on, 1702-1703
incision planning for, 1709, 1710f
indications for, 1705
modified, 1711-1712
definition of, 1703t, 1711, 1712f
historical perspective on, 1703
indications for, 1711
results of, 1721
technique for, 1711-1712, 1713f-1714f
nodular masses at site of, 1476
for oral cancer, 1313
positioning for, 1709
posterior triangle dissection in, 1709
results of, 1721
results of, 1721-1722
for salivary gland tumors, 1196-1197
selective, 1712-1713
for cancer of midline structures of anterior lower neck, 1719
definition and rationale for, 1719, 1719f
technique for, 1719, 1720f
for cutaneous malignancies, 1718-1719
definition and rationale for, 1718, 1718f
technique for, 1718-1719
definition of, 1703t, 1712
historical perspective on, 1703
for oral cavity cancer, 1313, 1713-1716
definition and rationale for, 1713, 1714f
technique for, 1713-1716, 1715f-1716f
for oropharyngeal, hypopharyngeal, and laryngeal cancer, 1716-1718
definition and rationale for, 1716-1717, 1717f
technique for, 1717-1718, 1717f
rationale for, 1712-1713
results of, 1721
for thyroid cancer, 1719, 1719f-1720f
sequelae of, 1722
supraomohyoid, 1313-1314, 1703
for oral cancer, 1313-1314, 1713
definition and rationale for, 1713, 1714f
technique for, 1713-1716, 1715f-1716f

Neck dissection *(Continued)*
terminology of, 1703, 1703t
therapeutic, 1702
Neck injury. *See* Neck trauma.
Neck irradiation
indications for neck node dissection after, 1694
late complications after, 1694-1695
with N0 status, 1688, 1690, 1692, 1692t
with N1-N3 status, 1692-1695
neck control after, 1692-1693, 1693t
postoperative, 1693-1694, 1694t
of retropharyngeal nodes, 1688
for salivary gland neoplasms, 1198
target volumes for, 1688-1690
delineation of, 1690-1691, 1691f
for hypopharyngeal tumors, 1689t
for laryngeal tumors, 1690t
for nasopharyngeal tumors, 1690, 1690t
for oral cavity tumors, 1689t
for oropharyngeal tumors, 1689t
techniques for, 1691, 1692f
Neck lump, in nasopharyngeal carcinoma, 1352-1353, 1353f
Neck management, for laryngeal and hypopharyngeal cancer, 1580
Neck mass(es)
in children, 2812-2821
acquired, 2817-2819
bacterial lymphadenopathy as, 2818, 2818f-2819f
benign neoplasms as, 2819
drug-induced lymphadenopathy as, 2819
due to fungal infections, 2818-2819
in Kawasaki disease, 2819
malignant neoplasms as, 2819-2820, 2820f
in sarcoidosis, 2819
sialadenitis as, 2819
in sinus histiocytosis, 2819
viral lymphadenopathy as, 2817-2818
algorithm for differential diagnosis of, 2813f
biopsy of, 2814
congenital, 2814-2817
branchial cleft cysts as, 2814, 2814f-2815f
dermoid cysts as, 2816, 2816f-2817f
hemangiomas as, 2816, 2816f
laryngoceles as, 2816-2817
lymphatic malformations (lymphangiomas) as, 2815, 2817f
sternocleidomastoid tumors of infancy as, 2817, 2817f
teratomas as, 2816, 2816f
thymic cysts as, 2817
thyroglossal duct cysts as, 2814-2815, 2815f
vascular malformations as, 2817
history of, 2812
imaging of, 2813-2814
laboratory studies for, 2814
physical examination of, 2812-2813
congenital, 1638-1640, 2814-2817
branchial cleft anomalies as, 1639, 2814, 2814f-2815f
dermoid cysts as, 1639, 2816, 2816f-2817f
hemangiomas as, 1640, 2816, 2816f
laryngoceles as, 2816-2817
lymphangiomas as, 1640, 2815, 2815f
sternocleidomastoid tumors of infancy as, 2817, 2817f
teratomas as, 1639-1640, 2816, 2816f
thymic cysts as, 2817
thyroglossal duct cysts as, 1639, 2814-2815, 2815f
vascular malformations as, 2817
diagnostic imaging of, 1636-1637, 1637t
epidemiology of, 1636, 1637f
history and physical examination for, 1636, 1637f

Neck mass(es) *(Continued)*
inflammatory, 1638
due to granulomatous diseases, 1638
due to lymphadenopathy/lymphadenitis, 1638
due to sialadenitis/sialolithiasis, 1638
due to paranasal sinus tumor, 1123
due to primary neoplasms, 1640-1641
lipomas as, 1641
lymphoma as, 1640
neurogenic, 1640-1641
paragangliomas as, 1641
of salivary glands, 1640
thyroid, 1640
unknown
differential diagnosis of, 1638-1640
initial workup of, 1637-1638, 1638f
unknown primary squamous cell carcinoma as, 1641-1642, 1641t
Neck muscles, effects of radiotherapy on, 2626t
Neck neoplasm(s), 1656-1672
benign, 1657-1664
in children, 2819
lipomas as, 2819
neurofibromas as, 2819
pleomorphic adenomas as, 2819
thyroid adenomas as, 2819
lipomas as, 1663
in children, 2819
neurofibromas as, 1663, 1664f
in children, 2819
of parapharyngeal space, 1663-1664, 1665f
of peripheral nerves, 1663
neurofibromas as, 1663, 1664f
schwannomas as, 1663, 1663f
pleomorphic adenomas as, 2819
thyroid adenomas as, 2819
vascular, 1657
arteriovenous malformations as, 1662-1663
carotid paragangliomas as, 1657-1658, 1658f, 1659t
epidemiology of, 1657-1659
jugular paragangliomas as, 1662f
nomenclature for, 1657
pathology of, 1657, 1658f
vagal paragangliomas as, 1661-1662
in children
benign, 2819
lipomas as, 2819
neurofibromas as, 2819
pleomorphic adenomas as, 2819
thyroid adenomas as, 2819
malignant, 2819-2820
lymphomas as, 2819-2820, 2820f
nasopharyngeal carcinoma as, 2820
neuroblastomas as, 2820, 2844-2845, 2844t, 2845f
rhabdomyosarcomas as, 2820
of salivary gland, 2820, 2845-2846, 2846f
thyroid carcinoma as, 2820
diagnostic evaluation of, 1656
malignant, 1664-1671
carcinoma arising within thyroglossal duct cyst as, 1671
in children, 2819-2820
lymphomas as, 2819-2820, 2820f
nasopharyngeal carcinoma as, 2820
neuroblastomas as, 2820, 2844-2845, 2844t, 2845f
rhabdomyosarcomas as, 2820
of salivary gland, 2820, 2845-2846, 2846f
thyroid carcinoma as, 2820
lymphoma as, 1671
in children, 2819-2820, 2820f
melanoma as, 1671
metastatic, 1664

Neck neoplasm(s) *(Continued)*
from distant tumor, 1664-1666
from regional tumor, 1664
from unknown primary, 1664, 1665f
nasopharyngeal carcinoma as, in children, 2820
neuroblastomas as, in children, 2820, 2844-2845, 2844t, 2845f
of parapharyngeal space, 1666
primary, 1664-1666
of salivary gland, in children, 2820, 2845-2846, 2846f
sarcomas as, 1666
alveolar soft part, 1668
angio-, 1668
bone, 1666, 1667t
chondro-, 1669-1670
classification and staging of, 1666, 1666t-1667t
epithelioid hemangioendothelioma as, 1668-1669
Ewing's, 1671
fibro-, 1668
hemangiopericytoma as, 1670
leiomyo-, 1670
lipo-, 1670
malignant fibrous histiocytoma as, 1667
malignant giant cell tumor as, 1671
malignant peripheral nerve sheath tumor as, 1670-1671
osteo-, 1668
rhabdomyo-, 1667-1668, 1668f, 1669t, 2820
soft tissue, 1666, 1666t
synovial, 1670
solitary fibrous tumor as, 1671
squamous cell carcinoma arising in branchial cleft cyst as, 1671
thyroid carcinoma as, in children, 2820
radiologic studies of, 1656-1657
Neck node metastasis. *See* Cervical lymph node metastasis(es).
Neck spaces, 202-203
anterior visceral, 203
carotid, 203
danger, 202-203
masticator, 203
parapharyngeal, 202
parotid, 203
peritonsillar, 203
prevertebral, 203
retropharyngeal, 202
submandibular and sublingual, 202
Neck surgery, complication(s) of, 1726-1734
chyle/chest, 1732-1733
chylothorax as, 1733
chylous fistula as, 1732-1733, 1732f
pneumothorax as, 1733
nerve, 1729-1732
cervical sensory, 1731-1732
facial, 1729-1730
greater auricular, 1731
hypoglossal, 1730-1731
lingual, 1731
motor, 1729-1731
phrenic, 1731, 1731f
sensory, 1731-1732
spinal accessory, 1730, 1731f
sympathetic, 1732, 1732f
vagus, 1730
vascular, 1728-1729
carotid artery hemorrhage as, 1728
hematoma as, 1729
of internal jugular vein, 1728-1729, 1729f
wound, 1726-1728
incision planning and, 1726-1727
infection as, 1727
salivary fistula as, 1727-1728, 1728f
scar formation as, 1728, 1729f
Neck surgery, complication(s) of *(Continued)*
seroma as, 1727, 1727f
wound dehiscence and flap necrosis as, 1727
Neck trauma, 1625-1635
blunt, 1634-1635
penetrating
airway management for, 1629
algorithmic approach to, 1631f
angiography for, 1630-1632, 1631t, 1632f-1633f
barium swallow for, 1631t, 1633
classification of, 1628-1629, 1630f
cranial nerve injury due to, 1629
diagnostic evaluation of, 1630
digestive tract evaluation for, 1633-1634, 1634f-1635f
direct laryngoscopy and bronchoscopy for, 1631t, 1634
esophagoscopy for, 1631t, 1633-1634, 1634f
imaging of, 1629-1630
initial management of, 1629
management of laryngotracheal injury due to, 1634
mandatory *vs.* selective exploration of, 1627-1630, 1629t, 1630f, 1631t
mortality from, 1627-1628, 1629t
physical properties of objects causing, 1625-1627
due to handgun, 1625
due to knife and stab injuries, 1627
due to rifle, 1626, 1626f-1627f
due to shotguns, 1626-1627, 1628t
signs and symptoms of, 1626b
vascular injury due to
imaging of, 1630-1632, 1631t, 1632f-1633f
management of, 1632-1633, 1633f-1634f
Necrotizing fasciitis, due to deep neck space infections, 208
Necrotizing otitis externa. *See* Malignant otitis externa (MOE).
Necrotizing sialometaplasia
in children, 2857
of hard palate, 1309-1310
of larynx, 1493
of oral cavity, 1289, 1299
Needle aspiration, for deep neck space infections, 206, 206f
Needle biopsy, in children, 2574
Negative plasticity, 1881
Negatron, 1031-1032
Neisseria gonorrhoeae
oral manifestations of, 1252
pharyngitis due to, 193-194, 194f
in children, 2786
Neoadjuvant chemotherapy, for laryngeal carcinoma, 1501-1503, 1502f
Neodymium:yttrium-aluminum-garnet (Nd:YAG) laser, 31t, 32
for facial resurfacing, 403t
Neonatal familial hyperparathyroidism, 1797
Neonatal sialadenitis, 2857
Neonatal suppurative parotitis (NSP), 1153
Neonate(s). *See* Newborn(s).
Neopharynx, postlaryngectomy, 1415f, 1416
Neoplastic disease
nasal manifestations of, 659-660
in T-cell lymphoma, 659-660
olfactory loss due to, 636
otologic manifestations of, 2106-2108
in leukemia, 2107, 2108f
metastatic, 2107-2108, 2108f
in multiple myeloma, 2106-2107, 2107f
otorrhea as, 2196-2197
sensorineural hearing loss due to, 2124-2125, 2125f
sudden, 2128
Neoplastic rhinitis, 619b
Neovascularization
in acutely raised skin flaps, 1069, 1069f
and skin flap viability, 1073
Nerve blocks
for neuropathic pain, 245-246, 246t
for postoperative pain control, 241-242
Nerve complication(s), of neck surgery, 1729-1732
motor, 1729-1731
facial, 1729-1730
hypoglossal, 1730-1731
phrenic, 1731, 1731f
spinal accessory, 1730, 1731f
vagus, 1730
sensory, 1731-1732
cervical, 1731-1732
greater auricular, 1731
lingual, 1731
sympathetic, 1732, 1732f
Nerve conduction velocity, in Bell's palsy, 2394
Nerve excitability test (NET)
for Bell's palsy, 2394
for facial nerve injury, 2040-2041, 2385, 2387t
Nerve growth factor (NGF)
for facial nerve paralysis, 2427
for prevention of ototoxicity, 2189-2190
in submandibular gland, 1140
Nerve injury, due to rhytidectomy, 422-425, 426f
Nerve regeneration, 919-924
Nerve section, in acutely raised skin flaps, 1069-1070
Nerve sheath neoplasms, of facial nerve, 2414
Nerve transection, complete, 2384-2385
Nervus intermedius (of Wrisberg), 2403-2404
intraoperative identification of, 2546, 2546f
in surgical anatomy of lateral skull base, 2437f
NET (nerve excitability test)
for Bell's palsy, 2394
for facial nerve injury, 2040-2041, 2385, 2387t
Neural hearing loss, neurodiagnostic studies with, 1899-1901, 1900f
Neural integrator, in vestibular function, 2308
Neural origin, laryngeal neoplasms of, 882
Neural plasticity, in otology, 1876-1886
age-related, 1877, 1879, 1882f
basic mechanisms of, 1881-1884
for cortical map plasticity in adult subjects, 1883-1884
at systems physiology level, 1882-1883
for tonotopic map reorganization in developing subject, 1883
cellular level mechanisms of, 1884
Hebb's postulate for, 1884, 1884f
long-term potentiation in, 1884
definition of, 1876-1877
experiments showing, 1877-1881
on adult *vs.* developmental plasticity of sensory systems, 1879, 1882f
on animal models of deafness and effects of cochlear implant electrical stimulation, 1881
on conditions for plasticity in adult cortex, 1881
on cortical frequency map reorganization in adult subjects, 1878-1879, 1881f
developmental *vs.* adult, 1879, 1882f
historical background of, 1877
on reorganization of central tonotopic maps after cochlear lesions, 1877-1878, 1878f-1879f
on tonotopic map changes after long-term local excitation of cochlea, 1880-1881, 1883f
on tonotopic map reorganization at subcortical levels, 1879-1880
on tonotopic reorganization in a developmental model, 1878, 1880f
negative, 1881

Neural plasticity, in otology *(Continued)*
practical issues relating to, 1884-1886
for hearing loss in infants, 1885, 1885f
for other hearing disorders, 1885-1886
for tinnitus, 1886
time course of, 1877
and tinnitus treatment strategies, 2133
Neural presbycusis, 232, 2126
Neural Response Imaging (NRI), 2255
Neural Response Telemetry (NRT), 2255
Neurapraxia, 2384-2385
Neurilemmomas. *See* Schwannoma(s).
Neuroblastoma(s)
in children, 2844-2845
epidemiology of, 2844
histopathology and molecular biology of, 2845, 2845f
management of, 2844-2845
neck masses due to, 2820
presentation and evaluation of, 2844, 2844t
neck masses due to, 1640
in children, 2820
Neurocognitive development, sleep-disordered breathing and, 2791-2792
Neurocranium, 2443f
growth and development of, 2615-2619, 2617t
basicranium in, 2617-2619, 2617t, 2619f-2620f
calvaria in, 2615-2617, 2617t, 2618f
size ratio to face of, 2616f, 2617t
Neurodiagnosis
with auditory brainstem response, 1896-1899, 1898f-1899f
with auditory neuropathy or dyssynchrony, 1899-1901, 1900f
Neuroectodermal tumors, in children, 2844-2845
neuroblastomas as, 2844-2845
epidemiology of, 2844
histopathology and molecular biology of, 2845, 2845f
management of, 2844-2845
neck masses due to, 2820
presentation and evaluation of, 2844, 2844t
peripheral primitive, 2845
Neuroendocrine carcinoma, high-grade, of salivary glands, 1190-1191, 1190f
Neuroendocrine tumor of the larynx (NTL), 1507-1508
carcinoid as
atypical, 1507
typical, 1507
paraganglioma as, 1508
small cell carcinoma as, 1507-1508
Neurofibroma(s), 292
of carotid space, 150-151
in children, 2819
of infrahyoid prevertebral space, 162f
of larynx, 882
of neck, 1663, 1664f
neck masses due to, 1640
in children, 2819
of oral cavity, 1290-1291
Neurofibromatosis type 1 (NF1), acoustic neuromas in, 2515
Neurofibromatosis type 2 (NF2)
acoustic neuromas in, 2515
stereotactic radiation therapy for, 2563
central neural auditory prosthesis for (*See* Central neural auditory prosthesis)
cochlear implant for, 2220
sensorineural hearing loss in, 2094t, 2095
Neurogenic neoplasms, neck masses due to, 1640-1641
Neurologic complications, of radiotherapy, 1049
Neurologic disorders
in HIV, 223-225
of larynx, 837-843
hyperfunctional, 838-842
botulinum toxin therapy for, 839, 840f-841f
due to dystonia, 838-839, 838b
essential tremor as, 840-841
due to myoclonus, 840
due to pseudobulbar palsy, 839-840
stuttering as, 841-842
hypofunctional, 842-843
due to central causes of vocal fold paresis, 842
due to medullary disorders, 842
due to multiple sclerosis, 843
due to myopathies, 842
due to neuromuscular junction disorders, 842
due to Parkinson's disease, 842-843
due to poliomyelitis, 842
psychogenic, malingering, and mixed causes of, 843
vocal fold paresis as, 843
laryngologic manifestations of neurologic diseases as, 837-838, 838t
oral manifestations of, 1254-1255
preoperative evaluation of, 106
sensorineural hearing loss due to, 2122-2123
Neurologic dysfunction, in voice evaluation, 827
Neurologic evaluation, 101, 101t
of larynx and pharynx, 832-836
acoustic analysis in, 834-835
aerodynamic assessment in, 835
cineradiography in, 835-836
edrophonium test in, 835
electromyography in, 835, 905
flexible laryngoscopy in, 834
glottography in, 835
indications for, 832-833, 833b
normal function and, 833
performance measures in, 835-836
rating scales in, 834
sensory assessment in, 836
of mouth, larynx, and pharynx, 833-834
for pediatric facial fracture, 2699
Neurologic impairment, of upper airway, diagnosis of, 832-833, 833b
Neurologic manifestations, of hyperparathyroidism, 1781
Neurolytic blocks, for neuropathic pain, 245-246
Neuroma(s)
acoustic (*See* Acoustic neuroma(s))
amputation, due to neck surgery, 1731-1732
facial nerve (*See* Facial nerve neuroma)
neck masses due to, 1640
Neuromuscular blockers (NMBs), intraoperative, 111-112
Neuromuscular disorders
chronic aspiration due to, 926b
and obstructive sleep apnea in children, 2605-2606
Neuromuscular junction disorders, laryngeal hypofunction due to, 842
Neuromuscular pedicle (NMP)
for facial nerve paralysis, 2426-2427
for laryngeal reinnervation, 919-922
for bilateral paralysis, 920
complications of, 922
future of, 922
history of, 917
indications for, 920
laboratory investigations of, 919-920
rationale for, 919
reported results of, 920-921
technique for, 920, 921f
for unilateral paralysis, 920
Neuromuscular symptoms, of hyperparathyroidism, 1781
Neuronal control, of salivary gland secretion, 1136
neurotransmitters and receptors in, 1136-1137, 1136f, 1137t
signal transduction in, 1137-1138
adenylate cyclase system in, 1137
G proteins in, 1137
phospholipase C system in, 1137-1138
Neurontin (gabapentin)
for migraine, 2350
for neuropathic pain, 243, 244t
for tinnitus, 2137
Neuropathic pain
anticonvulsant agents for, 243-244, 244t
antidepressants for, 244-245, 245t
interventional techniques for, 245-246, 246t
palliative care for, 1103
Neuropathies, in HIV, 223-225
Neuropeptide(s), in allergic rhinitis, 615
Neuropeptide Y (NPY), in salivary gland secretion, 1137
Neuropraxia, of facial nerve, 2040
Neurotmesis, 2384-2385
of facial nerve, 2040
Neurotologic examination, for temporal bone fracture, 2038-2039
Neurotologic manifestations, of immunosuppression, 221-223
malignant otitis externa as, 221-222
in middle ear, 222-223
due to *P. jiroveci* and *A. fumigatus,* 222-223
Neurotologic surgery, cranial nerve monitoring in, 2542-2556
anesthesia and, 2544
auditory brainstem response recording for, 2552-2554
interpretation of, 2553-2554, 2553f
and postoperative auditory function, 2553-2554
reducing electrical and acoustic interference in, 2552-2553
stimulus and recording parameters, electrodes, and placement in, 2552
of cochlear nerve, 2552
direct eighth nerve action potentials for, 2554
detection and interpretation of changes in, 2554
placement of electrodes in, 2554
stimulus and recording parameters in, 2554
of facial nerve, 2545-2549
with acoustic neuroma and other cerebellopontine angle tumors, 2545
activity evoked by electrical stimulation in, 2545-2546
for assessment of functional status after tumor removal, 2545-2546
electromyography for, 2545-2548
for intraoperative identification of nervus intermedius, 2546, 2546f
limitations of, 2547-2548, 2548f
during microvascular decompression, 2548-2549, 2549f
during other otologic surgery, 2549
during parotid surgery, 2549
spontaneous and mechanically evoked activity in, 2546-2548, 2547f
future directions in, 2555-2556, 2555f
instrumentation for, 2543
ninth, tenth, eleventh, and twelfth, 2550-2552, 2551f-2552f
and outcome, 2554-2555
for cochlear nerve preservation, 2554-2555
for facial and other motor cranial nerve preservation, 2554
personnel for, 2542-2543
recording electrodes for, 2543-2544, 2543f
stimulating electrodes for, 2544, 2544f
stimulation criteria for, 2544
third, fourth, and sixth, 2549-2550, 2550f
of trigeminal motor branch, 2550

Neurotologic symptoms, migraine with, 2349
Neurotology, gene therapy in, 23
Neurotransmitters, in salivary gland secretion, 1136-1137, 1136f, 1137t
Neurotrophic factors, for facial nerve paralysis, 2427
Neurotrophic tyrosine receptor kinase type 1, in thyroid carcinoma, 1753
Neurotrophin(s) (NTs)
  in gene therapy of inner ear, 2192
  for prevention of ototoxicity, 2189-2191
Neurotrophin-3 (NT-3)
  in gene therapy of inner ear, 2192
  for prevention of ototoxicity, 2190
Neutron, fast, 1034
Neutron beam radiotherapy, for salivary gland neoplasms, 1198-1199
Neutron therapy, 1046
Neutrophil(s)
  in adaptive immune system, 604
  in wound healing, 1076
Neutrophil-activating peptide-2 (NAP-2), in wound healing, 1076
Nevocellular nevus, 286
Nevoid basal cell carcinoma syndrome, 1268
  treatment of, 1268
Nevus(i)
  araneus, 291
  blue, 286-287, 287f
  compound, 286
  congenital, 287-288
    melanocytic, and melanoma, 1107-1108
  dysplastic, 288, 288f
  flammeus, 291
  halo, 287, 287f
  intradermal, 286, 287f
  junctional, 286, 287f
  melanocytic
    congenital, and melanoma, 1107-1108
    of oral mucosa
      clinical features of, 1241
      histopathologic features of, 1242
      treatment of, 1243
  nevocellular, 286
  salmon patch, 290-291
  sebaceus of Jadassohn, 287f, 289
  Spitz, 287
Newborn(s)
  airway obstruction in
    expected, 2904-2905
    unexpected, 2905
      laryngeal, 2905
      supralaryngeal, 2905, 2905f
      tracheobronchial, 2905
  asymmetrical nasal tip deformities in, 2709-2711
  blood volume of, 2571
  control of ventilation in, 2569-2570
  gingival (dental lamina, alveolar) cyst of, 1266, 1266f
    microscopic features of, 1266
    treatment of, 1266
  hearing loss in, 2718-2725
    ancillary testing for, 2722-2723
      genetic testing in, 2722-2723
      laboratory testing in, 2722
      screening for connexin 26 mutation in, 2723
      screening for maternally transmitted infection in, 2723
      temporal bone imaging in, 2723
      testing for Pendred's syndrome in, 2723
    assessment of, 2719-2721
      auditory brainstem responses in, 2719-2720
      comparison of otoacoustic emissions and auditory brainstem responses in, 2721
      evoked otoacoustic emissions in, 2720-2721
      testing protocols for, 2719, 2720f
Newborn(s) *(Continued)*
    diagnosis of, 2721-2722
      audiology in, 2722
      history in, 2721
      middle ear effusions in, 2722
      otomicroscopy in, 2722
      physical examination in, 2721-2722
      vestibular function assessment in, 2722
      visual reinforcement audiometry in, 2722
    history of screening for, 2718-2719
    intervention strategies for, 2723-2724
      amplification devices as, 2274, 2723-2724
      bone conduction amplification as, 2723
      cochlear implantation as, 2247, 2724
      early, 2724
      surgical therapy as, 2723
  heart and cardiac output of, 2571, 2571t
  oxygen transport in, 2571-2572
  respiratory rate in, 2570
  response to hypoxia in, 2571
  subdural empyema in, 1995
  ventilation-perfusion relationships in, 2570, 2571t
NEXUS (National Emergency X-Radiography Utilization Study) criteria, for laryngeal trauma, 935-936, 935b
NF. *See* Neurofibromatosis (NF).
NGC (National Guidelines Clearinghouse), 84t-87t
NGF (nerve growth factor)
  for facial nerve paralysis, 2427
  for prevention of ototoxicity, 2189-2190
  in submandibular gland, 1140
NHL. *See* Non-Hodgkin's lymphoma (NHL).
Niacin deficiency, oral manifestations of, 1254
NICH (non-involuting congenital hemangioma), 2824, 2825f
Nicotinamide, with radiotherapy, 1041
NIDDM (non–insulin-dependent diabetes mellitus), sensorineural hearing loss in, 2094t, 2097
Nifedipine, and skin flap viability, 1073
Nightmares, 262t, 264-265
NIHL. *See* Noise-induced hearing loss (NIHL).
Nijmegen Cochlear Implant Questionnaire, 57
Nine-step inflation-deflation tympanometric test, 1874
NIS (sodium/iodide symporter), in thyroid hormone synthesis, 1737
Nissen fundoplication, for extraesophageal reflux, 901
Nitinol stent, for tracheal stenosis, 2930
Nitrates, for achalasia, 965
Nitric oxide (NO)
  and rhinosinusitis, 732
  and skin flap viability, 1074
  in wound healing, 1076-1077
Nitric oxide synthases (NOSs), in wound healing, 1076-1077
Nitrogen mustards, sensorineural hearing loss due to, 2120
Nitroglycerin, and skin flap viability, 1073
Nitrous oxide, for pediatric anesthesia, 2590
Nizoral (ketoconazole cream), for fungal otitis externa, 1954-1955, 1959t-1960t
NK (natural killer) cells, in adaptive immune system, 603-604
Nkcc1, in murine deafness, 2058t-2060t, 2083
NKCC2 protein, in deafness, 2051t-2058t
NK/T lymphoma, of nasal cavity, 1680
  therapy and prognosis for, 1680
NMBs (neuromuscular blockers), intraoperative, 111-112
N-methyl-D-aspartate (NMDA) glutamate receptors, in central sensitization, 1203
N-methyl-D-aspartate (NMDA) receptor, in neural plasticity, 1884
NMP. *See* Neuromuscular pedicle (NMP).
NMSC (nonmelanoma skin cancer), immunosuppression and, 213t, 215
NNRTs (non-nucleoside reverse transcriptase inhibitors), 211
NO (nitric oxide)
  and rhinosinusitis, 732
  and skin flap viability, 1074
  in wound healing, 1076-1077
Nocturnal oxygen supplementation, for obstructive sleep apnea in children, 2611
Nocturnal polysomnography, of obstructive sleep apnea, 255, 255b, 256f
Nocturnal Rhinoconjunctivitis Questionnaire, 57
Nodal (N) classification, for melanoma, 1111-1113, 1111t
Nodal involvement, of salivary gland tumors, 1196-1197
Nodal metastasis(es). *See* Cervical lymph node metastasis(es).
Nodes of Rouvière, 1422
Nodular melanoma, 1108
NOE fractures. *See* Naso-orbitoethmoid (NOE) fractures.
Noise, 1838-1839
  continuous or steady-state, 2140
  defined, 2121, 2140
  fluctuating, 2140
  impulsive or impact, 2121, 2140
  intermittent, 2140
  measurement of, 2140-2141
  other adverse effects caused by, 2148-2149
  presbycusis due to, 232-233
Noise dosimeter, personal, 2140-2141
Noise reduction circuitry, for hearing aids, 2269
Noise-induced hearing loss (NIHL), 2121-2122, 2140-2152
  vs. acoustic trauma, 2141, 2145-2146
  anatomic mechanisms underlying, 2143-2144
  clinical course of, 2121, 2121f-2122f
  cochlear damage in, 2141-2143, 2143f
  diagnosis of, 2199
  early detection of, 2146-2147, 2147f-2150f
  hair cell regeneration and repair and, 2144
  interactive effects in, 2147-2148
  irreversible, 2141
  legal issues with, 2149-2151
  nature of, 2121-2122, 2141
  new knowledge about cellular and molecular mechanisms of, 2144-2146
  pattern of, 2141, 2142f
  permanent threshold shift in, 2141, 2148
  prevention of, 2151
  protection from
    by conditioning of cochlear efferent system, 2144
    pharmacologic, 2144-2145
  research on, 2143
  resistance to, 2144-2145, 2146f
  role of otolaryngologist in, 2150-2151
  susceptibility to, 2145-2146, 2146f
  temporary threshold shift in, 2141, 2148
  with tinnitus, 2131-2132
  vestibular disorders in, 2148
  vibration and, 2148-2149
Nominal scales, 63, 63t
Nonadrenergic, noncholinergic secretory response, in salivary glands, 1137
Nonallergic eosinophilic fungal rhinosinusitis (NA-EFRS), 709, 715-716, 716t
Nonallergic rhinitis (NAR), 619b, 694-2
  atrophic, 696-697
  classification of, 696-699, 697b
  defined, 695
  diagnosis of, 699
    diagnostic testing for, 699
    history of, 699, 699b
    physical examination for, 699

Nonallergic rhinitis (NAR) *(Continued)*
economic impact of, 695
epidemiology of, 695
gustatory, 698
hormonal, 696
idiopathic, 619b, 695, 698
irritant, 697-698
local factors associated with, 698-699, 698b
medication-induced, 619b, 696, 697b
occupational, 698
pathophysiology of, 695-696
allergic component in, 696
nasal function and innervation in, 695
perennial, 695
during pregnancy, 696, 702
problems resulting from, 695
provocation testing in, 695-696
systemic conditions associated with, 698-699, 698b
terminology for, 695
treatment of, 699-702
anticholinergics for, 701
antihistamines for, 700-701, 701t
avoidance for, 699-700
general considerations in, 702
surgical, 701-702
topical nasal corticosteroids for, 700, 700t
vasomotor, 619b, 695, 698
Nonallergic rhinitis with eosinophilia syndrome (NARES), 619b, 696
Noncaucasian rhinoplasty, 556-557, 568-579
aesthetic considerations in, 569
alar base modification in, 577-578, 578f
alar soft tissue sculpting in, 557, 561f
anatomic considerations in, 568-569, 569f, 569t
complications of, 578, 578f-579f
for correction of deviated nose, 573, 576f
dorsal augmentation in, 556, 569-570
choice of material for, 569, 570f
concept of, 569
results of, 572f-573f
technical considerations for, 569-570, 571f
hump reduction in, 570-573
concept of, 570-571
results of, 574f-575f
technique for, 571-573, 575f
nasal base sculpting in, 556-557, 559f-560f
objective of, 568
tip surgery in, 573-577
cap graft in, 576, 577f
caudal extension graft in, 576, 576f
concept of, 573-576
reshaping of lower lateral cartilage in, 577
shield graft in, 576, 577f
technique for, 576-577
thinning of subcutaneous tissue in, 577, 577f
Nonchromaffin tumors, 1657
Nonconductive hearing loss, neurodiagnostic studies with, 1899-1901, 1900f
Nondelivery approaches, for nasal tip refinement, 522, 523f-526f
Nonerosive reflux disease, 968
Non–group A beta hemolytic streptococcal infections, pharyngitis due to, 193
Non-Hodgkin's lymphoma (NHL)
Burkitt's, 1674
in children, 2819-2820, 2837
epidemiology of, 2837
histopathology and molecular biology of, 2838, 2839f
management of, 2838
presentation and evaluation of, 2837-2838, 2838t
staging of, 2838, 2839t
clinical presentation of, 1674, 1674f
diffuse large B-cell, 1677-1678
epidemiology of, 1673
Non-Hodgkin's lymphoma (NHL) *(Continued)*
follicular, 1674, 1678
highly aggressive, 1674, 1679
imaging of, 148-149, 149f
immunosuppression and, 213t, 215-216
diagnosis of, 216
epidemiology and presentation of, 216
prognosis and treatment for, 216-217
indolent, 1674, 1678
of larynx, 1509
lymphoblastic, 1674-1675
MALT, 1674, 1679-1680
mantle cell, 1678-1679
nodal involvement by, 165-166, 167f
of oral cavity, 157f
of oropharynx, 1364, 1364f
paranasal sinus and nasal cavity, 1680
of salivary glands, 1191-1192, 1192f, 1679-1680
small lymphocytic, 1674, 1674f, 1678
staging of, 1676, 1677t
thyroid, 1679
Noninferiority studies, 73t, 74
Non–insulin-dependent diabetes mellitus (NIDDM), sensorineural hearing loss in, 2094t, 2097
Non-involuting congenital hemangioma (NICH), 2824, 2825f
Nonlinear amplification, for hearing aids, 2268, 2268f
Nonlinear distortion, with traditional hearing aid, 2204
Nonmelanoma skin cancer (NMSC), immunosuppression and, 213t, 215
Non-nucleoside reverse transcriptase inhibitors (NNRTs), 211
Nonodontogenic infection, *vs.* myofascial pain dysfunction syndrome, 1285t
Nonparametric tests, 72
Nonpenetrance, 7, 7f
Nonpolarizing muscle relaxants, for pediatric anesthesia, 2592, 2593t
Non–rapid eye movement (NREM) sleep, 261-262
Nonrhabdomyosarcoma soft tissue sarcoma (NRSTS), 2842
Nonself, *vs.* self, in immune system, 599
Non–small cell lung cancer (NSCLC), epidermal growth factor receptor tyrosine kinase in, 1023
Nonsteroidal anti-inflammatory drugs (NSAIDs)
for postoperative pain, 241
sensorineural hearing loss due to, 2120
Nonsurgical organ preservation treatment, for laryngeal carcinoma, 1501-1503, 1502f
glottic, 1497
management of neck after, 1502-1503
recurrence after, 1503-1504
supraglottic, 1500
Nontuberculous mycobacteria (NTM), salivary gland infection with, 1158-1159, 1158f
in children, 2857-2858, 2857f
Nonunion, 331, 339-340
No-reflow phenomenon, in acutely raised skin flaps, 1070-1071
Norian CRS (carbonated apatite), for chin implants, 465t
Normal flora, of mouth, 177, 179f
Normal standard dose (NSD), in radiotherapy, 1039-1040
Norrie disease, sensorineural hearing loss in, 2094t
Norrie disease *(ND)* gene, in deafness, 2051t-2058t
Norrin, in deafness, 2051t-2058t
Nortriptyline, for neuropathic pain, 244-245, 245t
Norwood classification, of hair loss, 376, 377f
NOS(s) (nitric oxide synthases), in wound healing, 1076-1077
Nose
aesthetic analysis of, 271-272, 275f
alar-columellar complex in, 270f-271f, 274
for defect repair, 346-347, 347f, 364
nasal rotation and projection in, 273-274, 277f
nasofacial relationships in, 272-274
nasofacial angle in, 272-274, 276f
nasofrontal angle in, 270, 272-273, 274f
nasolabial angle in, 272-273, 276f
nasomental angle in, 272-273, 276f
air stream through, tests that assess, 643
anatomy of, 167-171, 322, 482-483
and nasal fractures, 496-497, 497f
surgical, 509f
vascular, 497, 682-684
anastomoses in, 682-683, 683f
anterior ethmoid artery in, 682, 684f
facial artery in, 682
greater palatine artery in, 682
internal maxillary artery in, 682
posterior ethmoidal artery in, 682-683
sphenopalatine artery in, 682
vidian artery in, 682, 683f
bridge of, 509f
burns of, 316
congenital malformations of, 2686-2696
choanal atresia as, 2694-2695
bilateral, 2694-2695, 2694f-2695f
clinical presentation of, 2694
endoscopic evaluation of, 2694, 2695f
epidemiology of, 2694
imaging of, 2694, 2694f
treatment of, 2694-2695, 2695f
unilateral, 2694-2695, 2694f
cleft lip nasal deformity as, 2690, 2692
complete agenesis of nose (arhinia) as, 2690, 2691f
congenital nasal pyriform aperture stenosis as, 2692-2693
clinical presentation of, 2692-2693
diagnosis of, 2693, 2693f
operative management of, 2693, 2693f
pathogenesis of, 2690, 2692
craniofacial clefts as, 2690, 2692
dermal fistula as, 2687f
dermoids as
clinical presentation of, 2689, 2689f
defined, 2687f, 2688-2689
epidemiology of, 2688-2689
histology of, 2689
imaging of, 2689, 2689f
management of, 2689-2690
due to developmental errors of anterior neuropore, 2686-2690, 2687f
due to developmental errors of central midface, 2690-2693, 2691f
due to developmental errors of nasobuccal membrane, 2693-2695
dysphagia due to, 2949, 2950t, 2951f
encephaloceles as, 2687-2688
basal, 2687-2688, 2687t, 2688f
classification of, 2687-2688, 2687t
defined, 2687, 2687f
epidemiology of, 2687
vs. gliomas, 2688
histopathology of, 2688
imaging of, 2688, 2688f
management of, 2688
nasoethmoidal, 2687-2688, 2687t
nasofrontal, 2687-2688, 2687t
naso-orbital, 2687-2688, 2687t
sincipital, 2687-2688, 2687f, 2687t
sphenoethmoidal, 2687t
spheno-orbital, 2687t
terminology for, 2687
transethmoidal, 2687t
transsphenoidal, 2687t

Nose *(Continued)*
gliomas as, 2687f, 2688
vs. encephaloceles, 2688
epidemiology of, 2688
extranasal, 2688
histology of, 2688
imaging of, 2688
intranasal, 2688
management of, 2688
intranasal hemangiomas as, 2695
maxillary mega-incisor with, 2690, 2691f
nasolacrimal duct cysts as, 2693, 2694f
nasopharyngeal teratomas as, 2695, 2696f
other mesodermal and germline malformations as, 2695
overview of, 2686
polyrhinia and supernumerary nostril as, 2690-2692
proboscis lateralis as, 2690, 2692, 2692f
cross-sectional area of, tests that assess, 643, 643f
double, 2690-2692
embryology of, 482-483, 496, 2660, 2690, 2691f
in geriatric patients, 234
changes in appearance of, 234
common symptoms of disorders of, 234
intranasal examination of, 234
mucoepithelial changes of, 234
olfactory changes of, 234
treatment of disorders of, 234
imaging of, 167-171
for facial trauma, 170-171, 170f-171f
nasal cavity in, 169, 170f
ostiomeatal complex in, 168f-169f, 169
paranasal sinuses in, 167-169, 168f-169f
keystone area of, 496, 497f
physical examination of, 100
physiology of, 322, 485-487
prosthetic, 1345, 1345t, 1346f
root of, 509f
sensory innervation of, 497, 497f
trauma to, 310-312, 311f
twisted
rhinoplasty for, 551-554
in noncaucasian patient, 573, 576f
osteotomies in, 551-554, 552f-554f
preoperative examination of, 551, 552f
results of, 511f-512f, 553f-554f
septal reconstruction in, 551
spreader grafts in, 554, 555f
varieties of, 552f
NOSE (Nasal Obstruction Symptom Evaluation), 57
Nostril
supernumerary (accessory), 2690-2692
in surgical anatomy of anterior cranial base, 2472f
Nostril sill excision, 577-578, 578f
Notch of Rivinus, 1826-1827
Nothing-by-mouth orders, for pediatric anesthesia, 2589, 2590t
NOX-3, in cisplatin ototoxicity, 2172
NPC. *See* Nasopharynageal carcinoma (NPC).
NPY (neuropeptide Y), in salivary gland secretion, 1137
NQF (National Quality Forum), 84t-87t, 87
NQMC (National Quality Measures Clearinghouse), 84t-87t
NR3B2, in deafness, 2051t-2058t
NREM (non–rapid eye movement) sleep, 261-262
NRI (Neural Response Imaging), 2255
NRS (Numeric Rating Scale), 240
NRSTS (nonrhabdomyosarcoma soft tissue sarcoma), 2842
NRT (Neural Response Telemetry), 2255
NRTIs (nucleoside/nucleotide reverse transcriptase inhibitors), 211
NSAIDs (nonsteroidal anti-inflammatory drugs)
for postoperative pain, 241
sensorineural hearing loss due to, 2120
NSCLC (non–small cell lung cancer), epidermal growth factor receptor tyrosine kinase in, 1023
NSD (normal standard dose), in radiotherapy, 1039-1040
NSP (neonatal suppurative parotitis), 1153
NSQIP (National Surgical Quality Improvement Program), 84t-87t
NST (nucleus of the solitary tract), in gustatory pathway, 1212-1213
NT(s). *See* Neurotrophin(s) (NTs).
NTL. *See* Neuroendocrine tumor of the larynx (NTL).
NTL (near-total laryngectomy), 1564
for advanced glottic cancer, 1497
NTM (nontuberculous mycobacteria), salivary gland infection with, 1158-1159, 1158f
in children, 2857-2858, 2857f
Nuclear antigens, of Epstein-Barr virus, 1352
Nuclear imaging, 137-138
of pharynx and esophagus, 1397
positron emission tomography as, 137-138
applications of, 144, 145f
radionuclide, 138, 139f
of salivary glands, 138, 1150
Nucleic acid hybridization, 9
Nucleoside/nucleotide reverse transcriptase inhibitors (NRTIs), 211
Nucleotide(s), 4
wobble, 4
Nucleus basalis, in neural plasticity, 1881
Nucleus Contour Advance electrode, 2227, 2227f-2228f
Nucleus Freedom device, 2227, 2227f-2228f
external speech processors for, 2232f
Nucleus Hybrid device, 2224, 2224f
Nucleus of the solitary tract (NST), in gustatory pathway, 1212-1213
Nuel's spaces, 1832, 1832f
Null hypothesis, 65, 66t
Numeric Rating Scale (NRS), 240
Numerical scales, 63, 63t
Nutcracker esophagus, 959t, 965
imaging of, 1401
Nutrition
and migraine, 2349
in palliative care, 1104
Nutritional support, vascular supply of skin in, 1064
Nycomed (metrizamide powder), for embolization, 1933
Nystagmus, 2310-2312
anatomic and physiologic basis for, 2289
Bruns', 2312
during caloric testing, 2290
"centripetal," 2310t-2311t
"convergence-retraction," 2310t-2311t
defined, 2289, 2307t
"dissociated," 2310t-2311t
downbeat, 2310t-2311t
evaluation of
in bedside exam, 2310-2312
recording methods for, 2317
gaze-evoked, 2310t-2311t
head-shaking, 2296-2297, 2314
hyperventilation-induced, 2316
"infantile" or "congenital," 2310t-2311t
irritative, 2294
jerk, 2310-2312
optokinetic, 2277, 2314
"pendular," 2310t-2311t
"perverted," 2310t-2311t
positional and positioning, 2315-2316, 2315f
pre- and post-rotatory, 2296, 2298f, 2329
purely torsional, 2310t-2311t
Nystagmus *(Continued)*
quick phases of, 2289
"seesaw," 2310t-2311t
sensitivity axes of semicircular canals and, 2294-2295, 2295f
slow phases of, 2289
spontaneous, of vestibular origin, 2312
in superior canal dehiscence syndrome, 2339-2340, 2340f
due to temporal bone fracture, 2039
types of, 2310t-2311t
upbeat, 2310t-2311t
vibration-induced, 2314
Nystatin cream (Mycostatin), for fungal otitis externa, 1954-1955, 1959t-1960t

O

O_2. *See* Oxygen.
O_2^- (superoxide anion radical), in acutely raised skin flaps, 1070-1071, 1071f
OA (osteoarthritis)
oral manifestations of, 1253
of temporomandibular joint, 1281t, 1282
OAEs. *See* Otoacoustic emissions (OAEs).
Obesity
and gustatory physiology, 1213
and obstructive sleep apnea, 251-253
in children, 2605
and otitis media, 2768
Oblique arytenoid muscle, surgical anatomy of, 1542f
Oblique rectus muscle, in surgical anatomy of anterior cranial base, 2472f
Obliteration, of frontal sinuses, 779-781
closure in, 780
complications after, 780-781
estimating limit of frontal sinus in, 780, 781f
incision for, 779-780, 780f
materials used for, 780
with Paget's disease, 779-780, 780f
postoperative monitoring after, 780-781
removal of all mucosa in, 780
template for, 779-780
Observation
for acute otitis media, 2770
for carotid paragangliomas, 1661-1662
for otitis media with effusion, 2771
Observational studies, 54, 54t
data quality of, 59, 60t-62t
Obstructive apnea, in children, 2607
Obstructive hypopnea, in children, 2607
Obstructive hypoventilation, in children, 2607, 2607f
Obstructive sleep apnea (OSA), 250-266
in children, 2602-2612
acute-onset or rapidly progressive, 2606
vs. adults, 2603, 2603t
anesthesia with, 2598, 2599b
complications of, 2603-2604
behavior and learning problems as, 2603-2604
cardiopulmonary, 2604, 2604f
growth impairment as, 2603
diagnosis of, 2606-2608
history in, 2606
other studies in, 2607-2608
physical examination in, 2606
polysomnography in, 2606-2607, 2607f, 2607t
epidemiology of, 2603
nonsurgical management of, 2610-2611
pathophysiology of, 2604-2605
polysomnography in, 2606-2607, 2607f, 2607t
indications for, 2608
risk factors for, 2605-2606, 2605t
adenotonsillar hypertrophy as, 2604-2606, 2790-2793

Obstructive sleep apnea (OSA) *(Continued)*
craniofacial abnormalities as, 2605
mucopolysaccharidoses as, 2606
neuromuscular disease as, 2605-2606
obesity as, 2605
surgical management of, 2608-2610
craniofacial surgery in, 2610, 2610f
other pharyngeal surgery in, 2609-2610
other types of, 2610
tonsillectomy or adenoidectomy in, 2608-2609
tracheotomy in, 2610
symptoms and signs of, 2603, 2603t
concomitant sleep disorders with, 261, 262t
consequences of untreated, 252-253
defined, 251b, 252
diagnosis of, 253-255
cephalometric radiography in, 255, 255f
with comorbid conditions, 253
computed tomography in, 255, 255f
differential, 253, 253b
drug-induced sleep videoendoscopy in, 253-255
Epworth Sleepiness Scale in, 253, 253f
fiberoptic nasopharyngoscopy in, 253, 254f
fluoroscopy in, 255
MRI in, 255
Müller maneuver in, 253, 254f
nocturnal polysomnography in, 255, 255b, 256f
physical examination in, 253, 254b
in women, 253
gastroesophageal reflux and, 253, 2946
historical perspectives on, 251
obesity and, 251-253
in children, 2605
outcome scales for, 56t, 57
parasomnias associated with, 265, 265b
pathophysiology of, 252
symptoms of, 252, 252b
treatment of, 255-261
medical, 256-257
CPAP for, 256-257
nasal dilator strips for, 257
oral appliances for, 257, 257f
pharmacologic, 257
weight loss for, 256
surgical, 257-261
endoscopic studies prior to, 258
hypopharyngeal procedures for, 258b, 259-260, 260f-261f
indications for, 257, 257b
nasal procedures for, 258, 258b
palatal procedures for, 251t, 258-259, 258b, 258f, 260f
postoperative management after, 261
preoperative planning for, 257
stepwise protocol for, 257-258, 258b
tongue base procedures for, 259
tracheotomy for, 260-261
Obstructive sleep apnea syndrome (OSAS). *See* Obstructive sleep apnea (OSA).
Obstructive sleep-related breathing disorders, classification of, 251-252, 251b
Obturatoria stapedis, 1827f
Occipital artery, 2580, 2580f
sulcus for, 1824f
Occipital bone, in surgical anatomy of lateral skull base, 2435f
Occipital lymph node, 1360f, 2582
Occipital triangle, of neck, 96, 96f, 2578f
Occipitalization, of atlas, 2355
Occipitofrontalis muscle, 442f
Occipitomastoid suture, in surgical anatomy of lateral skull base, 2435, 2435f
Occlusion
anatomy and physiology of, 323
after maxillofacial trauma, 330-331, 333-334, 333f
Occlusion effects, with hearing aids, 2204, 2270
Occlusive bubble, for facial nerve injury, 2420, 2420f
Occult metastases, of salivary gland tumors, 1196-1197
Occupational exposure
to HIV infection, 212, 212t
to noise, sensorineural hearing loss due to (*See* Noise-induced hearing loss (NIHL))
to toxins, and laryngeal squamous cell carcinoma, 1492, 1513
Occupational rhinitis, 698
Ochronosis, 2114
otologic manifestations of, 2114
OCT (optical coherence tomography), for premalignant lesions of larynx, 1489, 1490f
Octopus cells, in cochlear nucleus, 1835, 1845
Octreotide, for hyperthyroidism, 1739t
Octyl-2-cyanoacrylate, in otoplasty, 478
Ocular defects, prosthetic management of, 1345t, 1346-1347, 1347f
Ocular flutter, 2313
Ocular hypotelorism, in Down syndrome, 2632-2633
Ocular motor apraxia, 2314
Ocular motor nerve injury, in lateral skull base surgery, 2512
Ocular scarring, due to cicatricial pemphigoid, 1233-1234, 1234f
Ocular tilt reaction, 2300, 2300f, 2312-2313, 2312f
Oculofacial prosthesis, 1345t, 1346-1347, 1347f
Oculomotor nerve, 2351f
intraoperative monitoring of, 2549-2550, 2550f
in surgical anatomy of anterior skull base, 2481f
in surgical anatomy of lateral skull base, 2439f
Oculopalatolaryngopharyngeal myoclonus, 840
Odds ratio, 64, 64t
Odontoameloblastoma, 1278
Odontogenesis, 1259-1260
enamel organ in, 1259
root development in, 1260
stages of, 1260
Odontogenic cysts, 1260-1269
in basal cell nevus syndrome, 1268
treatment of, 1268
botryoid, 1265-1266
radiographic features of, 1266
treatment of, 1266
calcifying (Gorlin), 1268-1269
microscopic features of, 1269, 1269f
radiographic features of, 1269
treatment of, 1269
classification of, 1260-1262, 1261b
common, 1262, 1265
defined, 1260-1262
dentigerous (follicular), 1263-1264
microscopic features of, 1264
neoplastic potential of, 1264
radiographic features of, 1264, 1264f
treatment of, 1264, 1264f
eruption, 1264, 1264f
treatment of, 1264
gingival
of adult, 1266
clinical features of, 1266
radiographic features of, 1266
of newborn (dental lamina, alveolar), 1266, 1266f
microscopic features of, 1266
treatment of, 1266
Odontogenic cysts *(Continued)*
glandular (sialo-), 1267
clinical features of, 1267
microscopic features of, 1267, 1267f
radiographic features of, 1267
treatment of, 1267
infected buccal bifurcation, 1264-1265
inflammatory collateral, 1263, 1263f
keratinizing (orthokeratinizing), 1266-1267
microscopic features of, 1267
radiographic features of, 1267, 1267f
kerato- (parakeratinizing, keratocystic), 1262, 1267-1268
in basal cell nevus syndrome, 1268
microscopic features of, 1268
radiographic features of, 1267-1268, 1268f
treatment of, 1268
lateral periodontal, 1265-1266
microscopic features of, 1265-1266, 1265f
radiographic features of, 1265
treatment of, 1266
lateralized radicular (lateral radicular, lateral periapical), 1263
malignancies arising in, 1269, 1270b
paradental, 1264-1265
radiographic features of, 1265
pathogenesis of, 1262
periapical (radicular, periradicular), 1262-1263
microscopic features of, 1262-1263, 1262f
radiographic features of, 1262, 1262f
treatment of, 1263, 1263f
primordial, 1265
residual, 1263
of undetermined origin, 1265
defined, 1265, 1265f
Odontogenic ghost cell tumor, 1275-1276
Odontogenic infections, 177-190
direction of spread of, 179-180, 179f-180f
fascial space involvement in, 180-187
cervical (deep neck), 184-187
lateral pharyngeal, 184-185, 186f
prevertebral (danger space No. 4), 186, 186f
retropharyngeal, 185-186, 186f-187f
surgical drainage and decompression for, 189-190
mandibular, 181-184
Ludwig's angina due to, 184, 185f
masseteric, 184, 185f
masticator, 184, 186f
pterygomandibular (medial pterygoid), 184, 185f
secondary, 184
sub-, 183-184, 183f-184f
sublingual, 183, 183f
submental, 181-183, 183f
temporal, 184, 185f
maxillary, 180-181
buccal, 181, 181f
canine, 180-181, 180f
cavernous sinus thrombosis due to, 181, 182f
orbital cellulitis due to, 181, 182f
natural history of, 179-180
management of, 180, 187-190
airway establishment in, 188
assessment and support of hose defenses in, 188
choice of antibiotic in, 178, 188
history and physical examination in, 187-188
identification of bacteria in, 188
surgical drainage and decompression in, 188-190
for deep neck space infections, 189-190
for jaw space infections, 189, 189f
for vestibular infections, 188-189
microbiology of, 177-178, 178t, 188
and implications for antibiotics, 178
vs. myofascial pain dysfunction syndrome, 1285t
natural history of, 178

Odontogenic keratocyst (OKC), 1262, 1267-1268
in basal cell nevus syndrome, 1268
microscopic features of, 1268
orthokeratinizing, 1266-1267
microscopic features of, 1267
radiographic features of, 1267, 1267f
parakeratinizing, 1262, 1267-1268
in basal cell nevus syndrome, 1268
microscopic features of, 1268
radiographic features of, 1267-1268, 1268f
treatment of, 1268
radiographic features of, 1267-1268, 1268f
treatment of, 1268
Odontogenic myxoma, 1276-1277, 1276f
microscopic findings in, 1276
radiographic findings in, 1276
treatment and prognosis for, 1276-1277, 1277f
Odontogenic tumors, 1270-1274
adenomatoid, 1277
microscopic features of, 1277
radiographic features of, 1277
treatment of, 1277
ameloblastic carcinoma as, 1274
ameloblastic fibroma as, 1274-1275
microscopic findings in, 1274-1275, 1275f
radiographic features of, 1274
treatment of, 1275
ameloblastic fibro-odontoma, 1275
microscopic findings in, 1275, 1275f
radiographic findings in, 1275
treatment of, 1275
ameloblastoma as
intraosseous type, 1273-1274
defined, 1273
mandibular, 1274
maxillary, 1274
microscopic features of, 1273, 1273f
natural history and treatment of, 1273-1274
radiographic findings in, 1273, 1273f
malignant, 1274-1275
odonto-, 1278
peripheral (extraosseous), 1274
unicystic, 1271-1272
definitions, clarifications, and treatment for, 1272, 1272f
microscopic features of, 1271, 1271f
vs. multicystic or multilocular, 1272
radiographic features of, 1271
"simple," 1272
calcifying epithelial (Pindborg) as, 1276
microscopic findings in, 1276
radiographic findings in, 1276, 1276f
classification of, 1270, 1270b
epithelial (dentinogenic) ghost cell, 1275-1276
malignant, 1269, 1270b
in mandible, 1270-1271, 1271f
in maxilla, 1270-1271
odontogenic myxoma as, 1276-1277, 1276f
microscopic findings in, 1276
radiographic findings in, 1276
treatment and prognosis for, 1276-1277, 1277f
odontomas as, 1277
microscopic findings in, 1277
radiographic findings in, 1277
treatment of, 1277
squamous, 1278
treatment of, 1276
Odontomas, 1277
microscopic findings in, 1277
radiographic findings in, 1277
treatment of, 1277
Odor aversion, 630
Odor memory, 630-631, 631b
Odorant-binding proteins, 629
Odynophagia, 956
OE. *See* Otitis externa (OE).
Office of the National Coordinator for Health Information Technology (ONC-HIT), 84t-87t, 89
Ofloxacin (Floxin) otic solution, for otitis externa, 1946, 1952, 1959t-1960t
OHCs. *See* Outer hair cell(s) (OHCs).
Ohngren's line, 1127, 1128f
OI. *See* Osteogenesis imperfecta (OI).
OKAN (optokinetic afternystagmus), 2319
OKC. *See* Odontogenic keratocyst (OKC).
OKN (optokinetic nystagmus), 2277, 2314
Old age dependency ratio, 230
Older patients. *See* Geriatric patients.
Olfaction, 624-639
with rhinosinusitis, 730
stimulation and measurement of, 631-632
Olfactometer, 631
Olfactory auras, in epilepsy, 636
Olfactory bulb, in olfactory stimulation, 628, 628f
Olfactory changes, with aging, 234
Olfactory coding, 629-630, 629f
Olfactory cognition, 630-631, 631b
Olfactory connections, in brain, 628
Olfactory cross-adaptation, and olfactory testing, 633
Olfactory dysfunction(s), 633-639
congenital, 636
decreased olfaction as, 633
diagnostic assessment of, 637-638
distorted olfaction (parosmia and phantosmia) as, 633, 636, 639
epidemiology of, 633, 634t
etiology of
aging as, 635, 635f
epilepsy as, 636
head trauma as, 634-635
HIV infection as, 636
medications as, 637, 637t
neoplasms as, 636
obstructive nasal and sinus disease as, 633, 634f-635f
psychiatric disorders as, 636
surgery as, 637
toxic exposure as, 636
upper respiratory infection as, 633-637
idiopathic, 637
management of, 638-639, 638f
Olfactory ensheathing cells, 626
Olfactory epithelium
cell types in, 626, 626f
basal cells as, 626f, 627
microvillar cells as, 626, 627f
olfactory ensheathing cells as, 626
olfactory receptor neuron as, 626, 626f-627f
supporting or sustentacular cells as, 626-627, 626f
and lamina propria, 626, 626f
in olfactory stimulation, 625-627
and respiratory epithelium, 625, 625f
Olfactory glomeruli, 628, 628f
Olfactory hallucinations, 636
Olfactory knob, 626, 627f
Olfactory map, 628, 630
Olfactory mucus, in olfactory stimulation, 625
Olfactory receptor neuron, 626, 626f-627f
Olfactory reference syndrome, 636
Olfactory stimulation, 624-629
common chemical sense in, 628-629
nasal passageways in, 624-625, 625f
olfactory bulb in, 628, 628f
olfactory connection to brain in, 628
olfactory epithelium in, 625-627
cell types of, 626, 626f
basal cells as, 626f, 627
microvillar cells as, 626, 627f
olfactory ensheathing cells as, 626
olfactory receptor neuron as, 626, 626f-627f
Olfactory stimulation *(Continued)*
supporting or sustentacular cells as, 626-627, 626f
and lamina propria, 626, 626f
and respiratory epithelium, 625, 625f
olfactory mucus in, 625
orthonasal, 631
retronasal, 631
vomeronasal organ in, 627-628, 627f
Olfactory testing, 631-632
factors affecting, 632-633
adaptation and habituation as, 633
age as, 632-633
gender as, 633
Olfactory transduction, 629-630, 629f
Olfactory-evoked potentials, 632
Oligogenic disorders, 4, 8
with complex traits, 8
genetic heterogeneity and, 8
mitochondrial, 8, 9f
sporadic cases of, 8
with X-linkage, 8, 8f
Oligonucleotides, 9
Olive oil, for cerumen removal, 1958t
Olivocochlear bundle, in auditory pathway, 1834-1835, 1834f
Olivocochlear reflex pathways, in efferent auditory system, 1848-1849, 1848f
Olopatadine hydrochloride
for allergic rhinitis, 620
for rhinosinusitis, 734t, 737
OM. *See* Otitis media (OM).
OM-6 scale, 57
Omalizumab, for rhinosinusitis, 735t, 737
allergic fungal, 715
OMC (ostiomeatal complex)
in functional endoscopic sinus surgery, 760, 760f
imaging of, 168f-169f, 169
surgical anatomy of, 739, 740f
OME. *See* Otitis media with effusion (OME).
Omega epiglottis, 1464
Omentum flaps, for free tissue transfer, 1082t
Omeprazole, for extraesophageal reflux, 901
Omohyoid muscle
anatomy of, 2578f
in neuromuscular pedicle procedure, 920, 921f
OMU (ostiomeatal unit)
in chronic sinusitis, 674, 674f
after functional endoscopic sinus surgery, 677-679
and sinus physiology, 664-670
ONC-HIT (Office of the National Coordinator for Health Information Technology), 84t-87t, 89
Oncocytic adenoma, of parathyroid gland, 1778
Oncocytic neoplasms, of larynx, 881
Oncocytic papillary cystadenoma, of salivary glands, 1171
Oncocytoma, of salivary glands, 1171
Oncogenes, 12
in head and neck squamous cell carcinoma, 1016, 1019-1020
modification of, 21-22
in thyroid carcinoma, 1752-1753
Ondansetron, for postoperative nausea and vomiting in children, 2593
Onlay tip cartilage grafts, for nasal tip projection, 535-536, 537f, 549-550, 550f-551f
Onodi cells, 669, 740, 749f
in surgical anatomy of anterior cranial base, 2473
Onyx, for embolization, 1933
Onyx-015 vector, in gene therapy, 22
OOPS (operation on placental support), for congenital high airway obstruction syndrome, 2904-2905
OPC. *See* Oropharyngeal candidiasis (OPC).

Open approach, for nasal tip refinement, 522-535, 534f-535f
 indications for, 521b
Open bite deformities, 461, 462f
Open laryngeal surgery
 for laryngeal trauma, 936-937, 939f
 for stridulous child, 2909-2910, 2910f
Open mouth posture (OMP), 2628-2630, 2629f
Open quotient, in measurement of vocal fold vibration, 830-831
Open reduction, for subcondylar fractures, 338-339
Open reduction with internal fixation (ORIF), for pediatric facial fractures, 2701-2702
Open sky incision, for nasal fracture repair, 505, 505f
Open supraglottic laryngectomy (OSGL), for early supraglottic cancer, 1498-1500, 1498f
"Open-book" fracture, of nose, 2708, 2711f
Open-canal fittings, for hearing aids, 2270
Open-fit technology, for hearing aids, 2270
Operation on placental support (OOPS), for congenital high airway obstruction syndrome, 2904-2905
OPGL (osteoprotegerin ligand), 609t-610t
Ophthalmic artery(ies), in surgical anatomy of anterior cranial base, 2472f-2473f
Ophthalmic complications, of endoscopic sinus surgery, 754-755
Ophthalmic division, of trigeminal nerve, 440
 in surgical anatomy of lateral skull base, 2437f, 2438
Ophthalmic division block, 242
Ophthalmologic considerations, with posterior fossa surgery, 2541
Ophthalmopathy, Graves'. *See* Graves' ophthalmopathy.
Opioids
 addiction *vs.* tolerance to, 240, 242
 as adjuncts to induction of anesthesia, 111
 in children
  for anesthesia maintenance, 2591-2592
  for pain, 2572
   postoperative, 2594
 chronic use of, and postoperative pain control, 241
 for noncancer chronic pain, 243
 via patient-controlled analgesia, 240, 241t
Opsoclonus, 2313
Optic canal(s), 322f, 335f
 fracture of, 2479, 2479f
 in surgical anatomy of anterior cranial base, 2442-2444, 2443f, 2472f, 2473-2474
 in surgical anatomy of middle cranial base, 2444, 2445f
Optic chiasm, in surgical anatomy of anterior cranial base, 2475f
Optic foramen, 320-321, 440, 1124f
 in surgical anatomy of anterior cranial base, 2444f
Optic nerve(s)
 paranasal sinuses and, 672, 672f
 in surgical anatomy of anterior cranial base, 2473f-2475f
Optic nerve decompression, combined endoscopic orbital and, for Graves' ophthalmopathy, 1815
Optic nerve injury, in functional endoscopic sinus surgery, 679, 680f
Optic nerve involvement, in Graves' ophthalmopathy, 1808-1809, 1809t
Optical coherence tomography (OCT), for premalignant lesions of larynx, 1489, 1490f
Optical resonating chamber, of carbon dioxide laser, 26, 27f
Optical stimulation, to assess facial nerve function, 2389
Opticocarotid recess, in surgical anatomy of anterior cranial base, 2473-2474
Optokinetic afternystagmus (OKAN), 2319
Optokinetic nystagmus (OKN), 2277, 2314
Optokinetic testing, 2318-2319
Optokinetic tracking, 2306f, 2307t, 2318-2319
Oral appliances, for obstructive sleep apnea, 257, 257f
Oral breathing, 809
Oral cancer, 1249-1250, 1293-1318
 adenoid cystic carcinoma as, 1299
 adjunctive chemotherapy for, 1314-1315
 of alveolar ridge, 1304-1305
  clinical presentation of, 1304, 1304f
  epidemiology of, 1304
  mandibulectomy for, 1304, 1304f-1305f, 1307f
  maxillary, 1304
  neck dissection for, 1304
  survival with, 1304-1305
 anatomic basis for, 1295-1298, 1295f
  alveolar ridge in, 1297-1298
  arteriovenous, 1295-1296, 1296f-1297f
  buccal mucosa in, 1295f, 1298
  floor of mouth in, 1297-1298
  hard palate in, 1295f, 1298
  lips in, 1296-1297, 1297f
  retromolar trigone in, 1295f, 1297, 1298f
  tongue in, 1297, 1298f
 of buccal mucosa, 1308-1309
  clinical appearance of, 1308f
  epidemiology of, 1308
  radiation and chemoradiation for, 1309
  reconstruction for, 1308-1309, 1309f
  squamous cell, 1308, 1308f
  surgical treatment of, 1308-1309, 1309f
  survival with, 1309
  verrucous, 1308
 cervical lymph node metastasis of
  incidence and distribution of, 1685f, 1688t
  radiation therapy for, 1689t
 chemoprevention of, 1315
 desmoplastic-neurotropic melanoma as, 1299
 diagnostic evaluation of, 1299-1300
  endoscopy for, 1300
  history and physical examination in, 1299-1300, 1300f
 epidemiology of, 1295
 etiology of, 1293-1295, 1294f
 of floor of mouth, 1307-1308
  cervical metastases of, 1308
  clinical presentation of, 1294f, 1307
  composite resection for, 1307-1308, 1308f, 1315f
  coronal partial mandibulectomy for, 1307-1308, 1308f
  imaging of, 1307
  invasive, 1307
  reconstruction for, 1307, 1315f
  segmental mandibulectomy for, 1307-1308, 1308f
  survival with, 1308
  transoral resection for, 1307
 of hard palate, 1309-1310
  cervical metastases of, 1310
  clinical appearance of, 1310f
  epidemiology of, 1309-1310
  Kaposi's sarcoma of, 1309-1310
  melanoma of, 1242f, 1309-1310
  reconstruction for, 1310, 1311f
  resection of, 1310, 1310f-1311f
  squamous cell carcinoma as, 1310, 1310f
  survival with, 1310
 imaging of, 1300
 of lip, 1302-1304
  clinical findings in, 1294f, 1302, 1302f
  epidemiology of, 1302
  neck metastases of, 1303-1304
  prognostic features of, 1303
  resection and reconstruction of, 1303-1304, 1303f
Oral cancer *(Continued)*
   Abbe-Estlander flap in, 1303-1304, 1303f
   Karapandzic fan flap in, 1303-1304, 1303f
  survival with, 1304
 long-term management and rehabilitation for, 1316-1317
  follow-up in, 1317, 1317t
  pain management in, 1316
  palliative care in, 1316
  for speech and swallowing, 1316
 molecular biology of, 1294-1295
 neck dissection for, 1312-1314, 1313f, 1713-1716
  definition and rationale for, 1713, 1714f
  technique for, 1713-1716, 1715f-1716f
 organ preservation protocols for, 1315
 pathology of, 1298-1299
 photodynamic therapy for, 1315
 premalignant lesions and, 1298-1299
 preoperative assessment of, 1300
 preoperative interventions for, 1300
 prognosis for, 1300-1302, 1301t
 radiation therapy for, 1314
  brachytherapy as, 1314, 1314f
  external beam, 1314
  package time for, 1314
 of retromolar trigone, 1306-1307
  clinical presentation of, 1306
  resection for, 1307, 1307f
  survival with, 1307
 sarcomas as, 1299, 1299f
 second primary tumors with, 1301-1302
 squamous cell carcinoma as, 1299
  of alveolar ridge–retromolar trigone, 1307f
  basaloid, 1299
  of buccal mucosa, 1308f
  epidemiology of, 1295
  etiology of, 1293-1295, 1294f
  of floor of mouth, 1294f, 1315f
  of hard palate, 1310f
  of lip, 1294f, 1302f-1303f
  sarcomatoid, 1299
  of tongue, 1306f
  verrucous, 1299
 staging of, 1300, 1301t
 surgical treatment of, 1302-1315
  of alveolar ridge, 1304-1305, 1304f-1305f
  approaches for, 1302
  of buccal mucosa, 1308-1309, 1308f-1309f
  complications of, 1317
  of floor of mouth, 1307-1308, 1308f
  of hard palate, 1309-1310, 1310f-1311f
  of lip, 1302-1304, 1302f-1303f
  of mandible, 1310-1312, 1312f-1313f, 1312t
  of neck, 1312-1314, 1313f
  perioperative antibiotics with, 1302
  preoperative assessment for, 1300
  reconstruction after, 1315-1316, 1315f-1316f
  of retromolar trigone, 1306-1307, 1307f
  of tongue, 1305-1306, 1305f-1306f
 of tongue, 1305-1306
  advanced-stage, 1306
  cervical lymph node metastases of, 1306
  clinical presentation of, 1305
  composite resection of, 1305, 1305f-1306f
  differential diagnosis of, 1305
  epidemiology of, 1295, 1305
  etiology of, 1305
  gross pathology of, 1305f
  hemiglossectomy for, 1305-1306, 1305f
  hemimandibulectomy for, 1306f
  local invasion by, 1305, 1305f-1306f
  reconstruction for, 1305-1306
  survival with, 1306
  wide local excision for, 1305
 treatment considerations for, 1302

Oral candidiasis, 199-200, 1229-1231, 1252
acute, 1230, 1230f, 1230t
angular cheilitis due to, 1230, 1230f
chronic, 1230, 1230t
clinical features of, 1230-1231
defined, 1229
differential diagnosis of, 1231
erythematous, 1230, 1230f
etiology and pathogenesis of, 1229-1230
histopathologic/diagnostic features of, 1231, 1231f
in HIV, 225, 226f
hyperplastic, 1231, 1231f
pseudomembranous, 1230, 1230f
risk factors for, 1229, 1230t
treatment of, 1231
Oral cavity
anatomy of, 1295-1298, 1295f, 1359f
alveolar ridge in, 1297-1298
arteriovenous, 1295-1296, 1296f-1297f
buccal mucosa in, 1295f, 1298
floor of mouth in, 1297-1298
hard palate in, 1295f, 1298
lips in, 1296-1297, 1297f
retromolar trigone in, 1295f, 1297, 1298f
tongue in, 1297, 1298f
benign neoplasm(s) of, 1290-1292
ameloblastoma as, 1291, 1291f
congenital epulis as, 1290, 1290f
granular cell tumor as, 1290, 1290f
hemangioma as, 1291
lipoma as, 1291
neurofibroma as, 1290-1291
papilloma as, 1290, 1290f
pleomorphic adenoma as, 1291-1292, 1292f
congenital condition(s) of, 1287-1288
developmental cysts as, 1287-1288
dermoid, 1287-1288
duplication, 1287-1288, 1288f
nasoalveolar, 1288, 1288f
dysphagia due to, 2949-2951, 2950t, 2952f
lingual thyroid as, 1287
torus as, 1287, 1288f
dysplasia of, 1299
erythroplakia of, 1298
imaging of, 153-156
with abscess, 156f
with congenital lesions, 154-156
with non-Hodgkin's lymphoma, 157f
normal anatomy on, 146f, 153-156
with squamous cell carcinoma, 154, 156f
inflammatory/traumatic condition(s) of, 1288-1290
amyloidosis as, 1289-1290, 1290f
fibroma as, 1288-1289, 1289f
mucosal ulcerations as, 1289, 1289f
necrotizing sialometaplasia as, 1289, 1299
pyogenic granuloma as, 1289, 1289f
malignant neoplasms of (*See* Oral cancer)
neurologic examination of, 833-834
normal flora of, 177, 179f
physical examination of, 98-99
physiology of, 1200-1214
motor function in, 1203-1207
autonomic reflexes in, 1205-1206
jaw-tongue reflexes in, 1205
lingual muscles and reflexes in, 1205
mastication as, 1206-1207, 1206f
muscles of mastication and reflex control in, 1204-1205, 1204f-1205f
oral phase of deglutition as, 1206f, 1207
sensory function in, 1201-1203
central projections of trigeminal system in, 1203
common chemical sense in, 1202
dental pain in, 1202-1203
oral somesthesia in, 1201-1202, 1201f-1202f
Oral cavity *(Continued)*
specialized sensory system of taste in, 1207-1214
central gustatory pathways and function in, 1212-1213, 1212f
gustatory physiology in, 1208
gustatory sensitivity in, 1207-1208
gustatory structures in, 1208
gustatory transduction in, 1208-1210, 1210f
interaction between saliva and taste in, 1213-1214
peripheral sensitivity in, 1210-1212
posterior, swallowing disorders due to surgery of, 1219-1220
premalignant lesions of, 1298-1299
somatosensory innvervation of, 1201
sublingual space of (*See* Sublingual space (SLS))
submandibular space of (*See* Submandibular space (SMS))
tuberculosis of, 1250-1251
verrucous hyperplasia of, 1299
Oral commissure, burns of, 316
Oral contrast agents, for imaging of pharynx and esophagus, 1396
Oral hairy leukoplakia, 1226, 1226f
in HIV infection, 225-226, 226f
Oral health, women's, 1256-1257
during and after menopause, 1256-1257
during menses, 1256
during pregnancy, 1256
during puberty, 1256
Oral histoplasmosis, in HIV infection, 226-227
Oral hygiene, in palliative care, 1101
Oral lesions, in HIV infection, 225-227, 1252
aphthous ulcers as, 227, 227f
candidiasis as, 225, 226f
differential diagnosis of, 225t
fungal, 227
gingivitis and periodontal disease as, 227
hairy leukoplakia as, 225-226, 226f
due to herpes simplex virus, 226
histoplasmosis as, 226-227
due to human papillomavirus, 227
Oral leukoplakia, 1223-1225
chemoprevention of, 1225
clinical features of, 1224-1225, 1224f
defined, 1223
etiology of, 1223-1224, 1223f-1224f
hairy, 1226, 1226f
in HIV infection, 225-226, 226f
histopathologic features of, 1225, 1226f
malignant transformation of, 1223, 1298
proliferative verrucous, 1225, 1225f
thin, 1224f, 1225
treatment of, 1225
Oral lichen planus, 1226-1229, 1253-1254
atrophic or erythematous, 1227, 1227f
bullous variant of, 1227-1228
clinical differential diagnosis of, 1228
clinical features of, 1227-1228
erosive, 1227, 1228f
etiology and pathogenesis of, 1227
histopathologic features of, 1228, 1228f
and oral carcinoma, 1229, 1298-1299
plaque form of, 1227
reticular-type, 1227, 1227f
systemic diseases and, 1228
treatment of, 1228
Oral lichenoid lesion, 1229
Oral manifestations
of Down syndrome, 2632
of systemic diseases, 1245-1258
arthritides and bone disorders as, 1253
Ewing's sarcoma as, 1253
osteoarthritis as, 1253
Paget's disease as, 1253
Oral manifestations *(Continued)*
Reiter's syndrome as, 1253
rheumatoid arthritis as, 1253, 1253t
cerebrovascular, 1250
collagen-vascular and granulomatous, 1251-1252
dermatomyositis-polymyositis as, 1252
sarcoidosis as, 1252
scleroderma as, 1252
Sjögren's syndrome as, 1251
systemic lupus erythematosus as, 1251-1252
Wegener's granulomatosis as, 1252
dermatologic, 1253-1254
erythema multiforme as, 1254
lichen planus as, 1253-1254
mucous membrane pemphigoid as, 1254
pemphigus vulgaris as, 1254
endocrine and exocrine, 1251
adrenal, 1251
diabetes mellitus as, 1251
parathyroid, 1251
pituitary, 1251
thyroid, 1251
gastrointestinal, 1254
Behçet's syndrome as, 1254
Crohn's disease and ulcerative colitis as, 1254
gastroesophageal reflux disease as, 1254
malabsorption diseases as, 1254
of heart, 1246-1249, 1249t
hematologic, 1256
bleeding disorders as, 1256
hemoglobin problems as, 1256
white blood cell disorders as, 1256
infectious, 1252
bacterial, 1252
fungal, 1252
viral, 1252
inherited and congenital, 1257
of liver, 1255
malignant neoplasms as, 1249-1250
neurologic, 1254-1255
Bell's palsy as, 1255
dementias (including Alzheimer's disease) as, 1254-1255
multiple sclerosis as, 1255
myasthenia gravis as, 1255
myotonic muscular dystrophy as, 1255
Parkinson's disease as, 1255
pulmonary, 1250-1251
renal, 1255
Oral motor function, 1203-1207
autonomic reflexes in, 1205-1206
jaw-tongue reflexes in, 1205
lingual muscles and reflexes in, 1205
mastication as, 1206-1207, 1206f
muscles of mastication and reflex control in, 1204-1205, 1204f-1205f
oral phase of deglutition as, 1206f, 1207
Oral mucosal lesions, 1222-1244
pigmented, 1241-1243
amalgam tattoo as, 1243
clinical features of, 1243, 1243f
defined, 1243
differential diagnosis of, 1243
etiology of, 1243
histopathologic features of, 1243, 1243f
treatment of, 1243
melanoma as, 1242-1243
clinical features of, 1242, 1242f
differential diagnosis of, 1242
etiology and pathogenesis of, 1241, 1241t
histopathologic features of, 1242-1243, 1242f-1243f
treatment of, 1243
melanotic macules as, 1241
clinical features of, 1241, 1241f
defined, 1241

Oral mucosal lesions *(Continued)*
differential diagnosis of, 1242
etiology and pathogenesis of, 1241, 1241t
histopathologic features of, 1242, 1242f
treatment of, 1243
mucosal melanocytic nevi as
clinical features of, 1241
histopathologic features of, 1242
treatment of, 1243
red/white, 1222-1231
candidiasis as, 199-200, 1229-1231, 1252
acute, 1230, 1230f, 1230t
angular cheilitis due to, 1230, 1230f
chronic, 1230, 1230t
clinical features of, 1230-1231
defined, 1229
differential diagnosis of, 1231
erythematous, 1230, 1230f
etiology and pathogenesis of, 1229-1230
histopathologic/diagnostic features of, 1231, 1231f
hyperplastic, 1231, 1231f
pseudomembranous, 1230, 1230f
risk factors for, 1229, 1230t
treatment of, 1231
leukoedema as, 1222-1223
clinical features of, 1222, 1223f
defined, 1222
etiology and pathogenesis of, 1222
histopathologic features of, 1222, 1223f
management of, 1223
leukoplakia as, 1223-1225
chemoprevention of, 1225
clinical features of, 1224-1225, 1224f
defined, 1223
etiology of, 1223-1224, 1223f-1224f
hairy, 1226, 1226f
histopathologic features of, 1225, 1226f
malignant transformation of, 1223, 1298
proliferative verrucous, 1225, 1225f
thin, 1224f, 1225
treatment of, 1225
lichen planus as, 1226-1229, 1253-1254
atrophic or erythematous, 1227, 1227f
bullous variant of, 1227-1228
clinical differential diagnosis of, 1228
clinical features of, 1227-1228
erosive, 1227, 1228f
etiology and pathogenesis of, 1227
histopathologic features of, 1228, 1228f
and oral carcinoma, 1229, 1298-1299
plaque form of, 1227
reticular-type, 1227, 1227f
systemic diseases and, 1228
treatment of, 1228
submucous fibrosis as, 1229, 1295
clinical features of, 1229
defined, 1229
etiology and pathogenesis of, 1229
histologic/diagnostic features of, 1229
treatment of, 1229
verruciform xanthoma as, 1229
clinical features of, 1229
defined, 1229
etiology and pathogenesis of, 1229
histopathologic/diagnostic features of, 1229
treatment of, 1229
vesiculobullous/ulcerative, 1231-1240
erythema multiforme as, 1239-1240, 1254
clinical features of, 1239, 1239f-1240f
defined, 1239
differential diagnosis of, 1239
etiology and pathogenesis of, 1239
histopathologic features of, 1239-1240
treatment of, 1240

Oral mucosal lesions *(Continued)*
mucous membrane (cicatricial) pemphigoid as, 1233-1235, 1254
clinical differential diagnosis of, 1234, 1234t
clinical features of, 1233-1234, 1233f-1234f
defined, 1233
etiology and pathogenesis of, 1233
histopathologic features of, 1234-1235, 1234f
treatment of, 1235
pemphigus vulgaris as, 1231-1233, 1254
clinical differential diagnosis of, 1232
clinical presentation of, 1232, 1232f
defined, 1231-1232
etiology/pathogenesis of, 1232
histopathologic features of, 1232-1233, 1232f-1233f
treatment of, 1233
primary herpes simplex infection as, 1235, 1252
clinical features of, 1235, 1235f, 1252
defined, 1235
diagnosis of, 1235
differential diagnosis of, 1235
etiology and pathogenesis of, 1235
treatment of, 1235, 1252
recurrent aphthous stomatitis as, 1236-1239
clinical features of, 1237-1238
defined, 1236-1237
differential diagnosis of, 1238, 1238t
etiology and pathogenesis of, 1237, 1237t
herpetiform-type, 1238, 1238f
histopathologic features of, 1239
major, 1237-1238, 1238f
minor, 1237, 1238f
treatment of, 1239
recurrent herpes simplex infection as, 1235-1236, 1252
clinical features of, 1236, 1236f
defined, 1235
differential diagnosis of, 1236
etiology and pathogenesis of, 1235-1236
histopathology of, 1236, 1237f
vs. recurrent aphthous stomatitis, 1238, 1238t
treatment of, 1236
traumatic (eosinophilic) granuloma as, 1240
clinical features of, 1240, 1240f
defined, 1240
differential diagnosis of, 1240
etiology of, 1240
histopathologic features of, 1240, 1240f
treatment of, 1240
Oral mucosal pigmentation, inherited and congenital disorders affecting, 1257
Oral phosphate salts, for hyperparathyroidism, 1804
Oral preparatory stage, of deglutition, 1215, 1216f, 2948
Oral preservation treatment, *vs.* total laryngectomy, 1564
Oral rinses, biomarkers in, for head and neck squamous cell carcinoma, 1026
Oral sequelae, of medications for systemic diseases, 1246, 1247t-1248t
Oral somesthesia, 1201-1202, 1201f-1202f
Oral stage, of deglutition, 1206f, 1207, 1215, 1216f, 2948
Oral treatment considerations, due to systemic conditions, 1246, 1246t
Oral warts, in HIV, 227
Oral-facial-digital syndrome, 1257
Orbicularis muscle, in aging, 406, 406f
Orbicularis oculi muscle
with aging, 444
anatomy of, 433f, 441-443, 442f-443f
botulinum toxin for, 432, 433f
in lower eyelid blepharoplasty, 448-449, 450f
origin of, 443
paralysis of, 2420, 2420f, 2423f

Orbicularis oculi muscle *(Continued)*
sphincter mechanism of, 443, 443f
in upper eyelid blepharoplasty, 448
Orbicularis oris muscle, 442f
in cleft lip, 2665-2666, 2665f-2666f
Orbit(s)
anatomy and physiology of, 320-321, 322f, 439-444
biomechanics of, 332
effects of radiotherapy on, 2626t
endoscopic surgery of, 763
growth and development of, 2617t
invasive small cell carcinoma of, 170f
in surgical anatomy of anterior cranial base, 2443-2444, 2444f
Orbital apex, 320-321
Orbital apex fractures, pediatric, 2712, 2713f
Orbital blowout fractures, 170f, 321, 325, 326f
pediatric, 325, 326f
Orbital cellulitis, due to odontogenic infections, 181, 182f
Orbital complications
of functional endoscopic sinus surgery, 679, 680f
of rhinosinusitis, 676-677
Orbital decompression, for Graves' ophthalmopathy, 1811-1816
approaches to, 1811, 1812f
balanced, 1814
without bone removal, 1816
combined endoscopic and open approach to, 1814
combined endoscopic orbital and optic nerve, 1815
endoscopic, 1814, 1815f-1816f
goal of, 1811
indications for, 1811
results of, 1811-1812
three-wall, 1815-1816
transantral, 1812-1814
complications of, 1814
modifications of, 1814
outcome of, 1812-1814, 1813f-1814f
technique for, 1812, 1812f-1813f
two-wall, 1816
Orbital defects, prosthetic management of, 1345t, 1346-1347, 1347f
Orbital dystopia, surgical correction of, 2654
Orbital echography, of Graves' ophthalmopathy, 1810
Orbital edema, preseptal, due to rhinosinusitis, 676
Orbital enucleation, prosthesis for, 1346
Orbital evisceration, prosthesis for, 1346
Orbital exenteration
prosthesis for, 1346-1347
radial maxillectomy with, 1125-1126
Orbital fat pads, 443-444, 444f
Orbital floor, 439-440
surgical access to, 328-329
Orbital floor fractures, pediatric, 2712-2713, 2714f-2715f
Orbital fractures
blowout, 170f, 321, 325, 326f
pediatric, 325, 326f
imaging of, 325, 326f
pediatric, 2711-2714
evaluation of, 2712, 2713f
of lateral/medial orbital wall, 2712, 2714, 2716f
of orbital apex, 2712, 2713f
of orbital floor, 2712-2713, 2714f-2715f
of orbital roof, 2712-2713, 2716f
patterns of, 2711-2712
physical examination of, 324
repair of, 336
surgical access to, 328-329, 329f
Orbital hemorrhage, after blepharoplasty, 449
Orbital hypertelorism, surgical correction of, 2654

Orbital periosteum, 439
Orbital rim, lateral, surgical access to, 328-329, 329f
Orbital roof, in surgical anatomy of anterior cranial base, 2443
Orbital roof fractures, pediatric, 2712-2713, 2716f
Orbital septum
anatomy of, 443, 443f
in lower eyelid blepharoplasty
with subciliary approach, 449, 450f
transconjunctival, 448-449, 450f
in upper eyelid blepharoplasty, 448, 449f
Orbital wall(s), 439
Orbital wall fractures, pediatric, 2712, 2714, 2716f
Ordinal scales, 63, 63t
ORFFF (osteocutaneous radial forearm free flap), 1082t, 1085-1086, 1086f-1087f
Organ of Corti
anatomy of, 1832, 1832f, 1840, 1841f
in auditory physiology, 1841f
in cochlear transduction, 2061f, 2067f, 2069f
embryogenesis of, 1852
in noise-induced hearing loss, 2142-2143, 2142f
Organ preservation treatment
for laryngeal carcinoma, 1501-1503, 1502f
(*See also* Conservation laryngeal surgery)
current paradigm for, 1558-1559
glottic, 1497
chemoradiation as, 1584-1585
targeted biologic agents with radiation therapy as, 1585
management of neck after, 1502-1503
recurrence after, 1503-1504
supraglottic, 1500
for oral cancer, 1315
principles of, 1544
Orientation, hearing aid, 2273-2274
ORIF (open reduction with internal fixation), for pediatric facial fractures, 2701-2702
ORN (osteoradionecrosis), 1048, 1314, 1317, 1478-1479
ORNC (overpressure radionuclide cisternography), for CSF rhinorrhea, 790
Orocutaneous fistula, 179, 180f
Orodigitofacial dysostosis, 1257
Orofacial clefts. *See also* Cleft lip; Cleft palate.
molecular genetics of, 2662-2664
Oromotor reflexes
autonomic, 1205-1206
jaw-tongue, 1205
lingual, 1205
of muscles of mastication, 1204-1205, 1204f-1205f
Oronasal fistula, after palatoplasty, 2673
Oropharyngeal cancer, 1249-1250, 1358-1374
anatomy of oropharynx and, 1358-1360, 1359f
base of tongue in, 1359, 1359f
lymphatics in, 1359-1360, 1360f-1361f, 1361t
oropharyngeal wall in, 1359, 1360f
soft palate in, 1359
tonsillar fossae in, 1359
of base of tongue, 1369-1370
carcinoma in-situ as, 1361
cervical lymph node metastasis of, 1360f, 1361t
incidence and distribution of, 1685f, 1688t
radiation therapy for, 1689t
classification of, 1360-1365, 1362t
complications of, 1372-1373
diagnostic evaluation of, 1365-1372
anamnesis in, 1365-1366
endoscopy, biopsy, and frozen section in, 1366, 1366f
imaging in, 1366
physical examination in, 1366
epithelial precursor lesions for, 1360-1361, 1362f
follow-up for, 1372, 1373f
hematolymphoid, 1364, 1364f
Oropharyngeal cancer *(Continued)*
imaging of, 1366, 1413, 1413f
intensity-modulated radiotherapy for, 1046
Kaposi's sarcoma as, 1363-1364, 1364f
lymphatic spread of, 1359-1360, 1360f-1361f, 1361t
lymphoepithelial, 1362
management algorithm for, 1368, 1368f
mucosal malignant melanoma as, 1364-1365, 1364f-1365f
neck dissection for, 1716-1718
definition and rationale for, 1716-1717, 1717f
technique for, 1717-1718, 1717f
of oropharyngeal wall, 1370
prognostic factors for, 1373
quality of life with, 1373
reconstruction for (*See* Oropharyngeal reconstruction)
salivary gland tumors as, 1362-1363
of soft palate, 1368-1369, 1368f
soft tissue tumors as, 1363-1364, 1364f
special treatment considerations for, 1372
squamous cell carcinoma as, 1361-1362, 1365
clinical presentation of, 1361, 1362f, 1365
etiology of, 1365
grading of, 1361-1362, 1363t
imaging of, 149f
pathology of, 1361
staging of, 1366-1367, 1367t
surgical approach(es) for, 1370
lateral and transhyoid pharyngotomy as, 1371, 1371f-1372f
mandibular swing, 1371-1372, 1372f
transoral, 1370-1371, 1370f-1371f
of tonsillar fossae, 1369, 1369f
Oropharyngeal candidiasis (OPC), 199-200, 1229-1231, 1252
acute, 1230, 1230f, 1230t
angular cheilitis due to, 1230, 1230f
chronic, 1230, 1230t
clinical features of, 1230-1231
defined, 1229
differential diagnosis of, 1231
erythematous, 1230, 1230f
etiology and pathogenesis of, 1229-1230
histopathologic/diagnostic features of, 1231, 1231f
in HIV, 225, 226f
hyperplastic, 1231, 1231f
pseudomembranous, 1230, 1230f
risk factors for, 1229, 1230t
treatment of, 1231
Oropharyngeal reconstruction, 1375-1392
considerations for, 1375
cost of, 1375-1376
historical background of, 1375
option(s) for, 1376-1379, 1376f
free tissue transfer as, 1379-1381
anterolateral thigh, 1379
fasciocutaneous, 1379-1380, 1379f
lateral arm, 1379-1380
lateral thigh, 1379
latissimus dorsi myocutaneous, 1380
musculocutaneous, 1380
osteocutaneous, 1380-1381
radial forearm, 1379, 1379f
rectus abdominis, 1380
visceral, 1380, 1380f
healing by second intention as, 1376
local flap(s) as, 1376-1377
palatal island, 1376-1377, 1376f
tongue, 1376
uvulopalatal, 1377, 1377f
primary closure as, 1376
regional flaps as, 1377-1379
latissimus dorsi musculocutaneous, 1378, 1378f
Oropharyngeal reconstruction *(Continued)*
pectoralis major, 1377, 1377f
platysmal myocutaneous, 1377, 1378f
temporalis, 1377-1378
temporoparietal fascial, 1377-1378, 1378f
trapezius musculocutaneous, 1378-1379
skin grafts as, 1376
preoperative evaluation for, 1375
of soft palate, 1381-1383
algorithm for, 1384f
free flaps for, 1382
Gehanno method for, 1382
Lacombe and Blackwell's method for, 1382-1383
other groups' experience with, 1383
radial forearm, 1382, 1383f
local flaps for, 1381
buccinator musculomucosal, 1381-1382, 1381f
palatal island mucosal, 1382
Superior Constrictor Rotation-Advancement Flap (SCARF) as, 1382, 1382f
uvulopalatal, 1377f, 1381
prosthetic obturation for, 1381
speech function after, 1383
of tongue base, 1387-1391
algorithm for, 1391f
free flaps for, 1389
lateral arm, 1389
radial forearm, 1389
goals of, 1387
healing by second intention for, 1387-1388
local flaps for, 1388
primary closure for, 1387-1388
regional flaps for
latissimus dorsi, 1389
pectoralis major myocutaneous, 1388-1389
platysmal myocutaneous, 1389
skin grafting for, 1388
after total or subtotal glossectomy, 1389-1390
innervated free latissimus dorsi musculocutaneous flap for, 1389-1390, 1390f
microvascular reconstruction as, 1390
money pouch–like method for, 1390, 1390f
sensate fasciocutaneous flaps for, 1390-1391
of tonsil and pharyngeal wall, 1383-1387
algorithm for, 1388f
free flaps for, 1386
with combined lateral and superior defects, 1386, 1387f
lateral arm and thigh, 1386-1387
radial forearm, 1386
healing by second intention for, 1383
local flaps for, 1384-1385
primary closure for, 1383-1384
regional flaps for
pectoralis major, 1385, 1385f
platysmal myocutaneous, 1385
sternocleidomastoid myocutaneous, 1385-1386
temporalis, 1386
temporoparietal fascia, 1386
skin grafting for, 1384
Oropharyngeal surgery, robotic, 42-43
Oropharyngeal wall
anatomy of, 1359, 1360f
cancer of
cervical lymph node metastasis of, 1361t
clinical presentation of, 1365
management of, 1370
Oropharyngeal wall reconstruction, 1383-1387
algorithm for, 1388f
free flaps for, 1386
with combined lateral and superior defects, 1386, 1387f

Oropharyngeal wall reconstruction *(Continued)*
lateral arm and thigh, 1386-1387
radial forearm, 1386
healing by second intention for, 1383
local flaps for, 1384-1385
primary closure for, 1383-1384
regional flaps for
pectoralis major, 1385, 1385f
platysmal myocutaneous, 1385
sternocleidomastoid myocutaneous, 1385-1386
temporalis, 1386
temporoparietal fascia, 1386
skin grafting for, 1384
Oropharyngocutaneous fistula, due to radiotherapy, 1048
Oropharynx
anatomy of, 1358-1360, 1359f
base of tongue in, 1359, 1359f
lymphatics in, 1359-1360, 1360f-1361f, 1361t
oropharyngeal wall in, 1359, 1360f
radiographic, 1398f
soft palate in, 1359
tonsillar fossae in, 1359
dysphagia due to congenital conditions of, 2949-2951, 2950t, 2952f
lymphatics of, 1359-1360, 1360f-1361f, 1361t
physical examination of, 99, 99f
Orotracheal intubation, with pediatric facial fractures, 2698-2699
Orthodontic devices, for obstructive sleep apnea in children, 2611
Orthokeratinizing odontogenic cyst, 1266-1267
microscopic features of, 1267
radiographic features of, 1267, 1267f
Orthokeratinizing odontogenic keratocyst, 1266-1267
microscopic features of, 1267
radiographic features of, 1267, 1267f
Orthonasal stimulation, 631
Orthopedic joint patients, antibiotic prophylaxis for, 1253, 1253t
Orthovoltage x-rays, 1034
OSA. *See* Obstructive sleep apnea (OSA).
OSA-18 scale, 57
OSAS (obstructive sleep apnea syndrome). *See* Obstructive sleep apnea (OSA).
Oscillopsia, 2277, 2309, 2344
OSD-6 scale, 57
OSGL (open supraglottic laryngectomy), for early supraglottic cancer, 1498-1500, 1498f
OSMED (otospondylomegaepiphyseal dysplasia) syndrome, deafness in, 2051t-2058t
Osseointegrated implantable hearing aids, 2212-2216
background of, 2213
biology and histology of, 2213
biophysical principles of, 2213
comparison of features of, 2206t
complications of, 2215
components of, 2213f
design of, 2213
indications and contraindications for, 2212-2213, 2216t
in infants, 2723-2724
location of, 2204f
materials for, 2213
operative technique for, 2213-2215, 2214f
radiologic implications of, 2213
results of, 2215-2216, 2216t
sound transduction and coupling to auditory system with, 2205f
for unilateral sensorineural hearing loss, 2216
in young children, 2215
Osseous free tissue transfer, mandibular reconstruction plate with, 1324
advantages and disadvantages of, 1324
flap inset in, 1324f, 1325
flap options for, 1324, 1325t
planning and harvesting of flaps in, 1324-1325, 1324f
Osseous genioplasty, 465, 467-470
anesthesia for, 467
clinical examples of, 470, 472f-473f
complications after, 470
fixation in, 468-470, 470f
gingivolabial incision for, 467, 468f
inscription of bony midline in, 467-468, 469f
lateral extent of, 468, 469f
measurement of osteotomy site in, 467-468, 469f
subperiosteal dissection in, 467, 468f
three-dimensional movement of chin in, 468
vertical lengthening in, 468-470, 469f
vertical shortening in, 468-470, 470f
wound closure in, 470
Osseous labyrinth
anatomy of, 1831, 1852, 1853f
embryogenesis of, 1852
malformations of membranous and, 2727b, 2728-2735
Osseous spiral lamina, 1831, 1832f, 1834
Ossicles
anatomy of, 1826
blood supply of, 1828f
in cochlear transduction, 2050-2060, 2062f
hearing loss due to total loss of, 2019, 2019t
Ossicular branch, 1828f
Ossicular chain
anatomy of, 1825f, 1826, 1827f
in auditory physiology, 1839, 1840f, 2017-2019
blood supply of, 1828f
in cochlear transduction, 2050-2060, 2062f
reconstruction of (*See* Ossiculoplasty)
in surgical anatomy of lateral skull base, 2436f
Ossicular coupling, 1839, 2000
in middle ear implants, 2207-2208
Ossicular discontinuity
audiometric correlates of, 2005-2006
ossiculoplasty for, 2008
pathophysiology of, 2005
Ossicular dislocation, 174f
Ossicular disruption, hearing loss due to
with closure of oval window, 2019, 2019t
with intact tympanic membrane, 2019, 2019t
with tympanic membrane perforation, 2019, 2019t
Ossicular fixation
audiometric correlates of, 2005-2006
ossiculoplasty with, 2007-2008, 2024-2025
pathophysiology of, 2005
Ossicular lever, 2018
Ossicular prosthesis(es), 2006
causes of failure of, 2008
hydroxyapatite cap for, 2026t
length of, 2025
materials for, 2006
Cervital as, 2026t
choice of, 2007, 2007f
comparison of, 2026, 2026t
Plastipore as, 2026t
titanium as, 2006, 2025-2026, 2026t
for otosclerosis
measurement of, 2031, 2031f-2032f
placement of, 2031-2032, 2032f
partial, 2006
with absent lenticular process of incus, 2024, 2025f
factors affecting success of, 2023
with ossicular discontinuity, 2008
results with, 2006
Ossicular prosthesis(es) *(Continued)*
total, 2006
with absent stapes superstructure, 2024, 2025f
factors affecting success of, 2023
with ossicular discontinuity, 2008
results with, 2006
Ossicular reconstruction. *See* Ossiculoplasty.
Ossiculoplasty, 2005-2008, 2023-2026
for absent lenticular process of incus, 2024, 2024f-2025f
for absent stapes superstructure, 2024, 2025f
autografts for, 2006, 2025
causes of failure of, 2008
factors affecting surgical decisions in, 2006-2007, 2007f
goal of, 2006-2007
homografts for, 2006, 2025, 2026t
length of prosthesis in, 2025
materials for, 2006
choice of, 2007, 2007f
comparison of, 2026, 2026t
with ossicular fixation, 2007-2008, 2024-2025
partial ossicular replacement prosthesis (PORP) for, 2006
with absent lenticular process of incus, 2024, 2025f
factors affecting success of, 2023
with ossicular discontinuity, 2008
results with, 2006
pathophysiology and, 2005
audiometric correlates of, 2005-2006
ossicular discontinuity in, 2005
ossicular fixation in, 2005
patient selection for, 2023, 2024b
surgical techniques for, 2007-2008
with ossicular discontinuity, 2008
with ossicular fixation, 2007-2008
for temporal bone trauma, 2046-2047
timing of, 2007
titanium prostheses for, 2006, 2025-2026, 2026t
total ossicular replacement prosthesis (TORP) for, 2006
with absent stapes superstructure, 2024, 2025f
factors affecting success of, 2023
with ossicular discontinuity, 2008
results with, 2006
with tympanosclerosis, 2007-2008, 2024-2025
Ossifying fibroma, sinonasal, 725-726
Osteitis
deformans (*See* Paget's disease)
fibrosa cystica, 1774, 1782
with laryngeal involvement, 882
oral manifestations of, 1257
otologic manifestations of, 2112
of paranasal sinus walls, 672, 672f
of skull base, 171
Osteoarthritis (OA)
oral manifestations of, 1253
of temporomandibular joint, 1281t, 1282
Osteochondroma, of coronoid process, *vs.* myofascial pain dysfunction syndrome, 1285t
Osteocutaneous flaps, for free tissue transfer, 1082t, 1084-1087
fibula, 1082t, 1084-1085, 1085f
iliac crest, 1082t, 1087
for oropharyngeal reconstruction, 1380-1381
radial forearm, 1082t, 1085-1086, 1086f-1087f
scapula, 1082t, 1086-1087, 1088f
Osteocutaneous radial forearm free flap (ORFFF), 1082t, 1085-1086, 1086f-1087f
Osteogenesis, 2614
distraction
for craniofacial anomalies, 2654-2657, 2656f
for obstructive sleep apnea, 2610
for Robin sequence, 2673
endochondral, 2614, 2615f
intramembranous, 2614

Osteogenesis imperfecta (OI), 2109-2110
clinical features of, 2109-2110
deafness in, 2051t-2058t, 2109-2110
genetic basis for, 2109-2110
management of, 2110
oral manifestations of, 1257
otologic manifestations of, 2110, 2110f
radiographic imaging of, 2109-2110, 2110f
Osteogenic sarcomas, of paranasal sinuses, 1131
Osteohypertrophic nevus flammeus, 291
Osteoma(s)
of craniocervical junction, 2484f
of external auditory canal
imaging of, 1918, 1919f
management of, 2022
sinonasal, 723-725
classification of, 723
endoscopic appearance of, 723
epidemiology of, 723
ethmoid, 724f
frontal, 724-725, 724f
frontoethmoid, 783-784, 784f
imaging of, 723-725, 723f-724f
ivory ("eburnated"), 723, 723f-724f
mature (spongiosum), 723
microscopic appearance of, 723
mixed, 723, 724f
pathogenesis of, 723
postoperative surveillance for, 725
spongiosum variant of, 724f
surgical approach for, 718t, 724-725
symptoms of, 723
Osteomyelitis
of frontal bone, 777f
of skull base, 171
Osteopetrosis(es), 2111-2112
autosomal dominant
type I, 2112
type II, 2112
otologic manifestations of, 2112, 2113f
autosomal recessive, 2112
otologic manifestations of, 2112, 2112f
malignant, 2112
oral manifestations of, 1257
otologic manifestations of, 2112, 2112f-2113f
Osteophytes, vertebral, compression of pharynx and esophagus due to, 1408, 1409f
Osteoprotegerin ligand (OPGL), 609t-610t
Osteoradionecrosis (ORN), 1048, 1314, 1317, 1478-1479
Osteosarcoma
of neck, 1668
of oral cavity, 1299f
Osteotomy(ies)
maxillary, in cleft-lip nose repair, 559, 564f-565f
for narrowing of nose, 541-542
double, 542, 542f-543f
lateral, 541, 542f
medial-oblique, 541, 541f
for twisted nose, 551-554
intermediate, 553, 554f
lateral, 552-554, 553f
medial, 552-553, 552f-553f
Ostiomeatal channels, 664
Ostiomeatal complex (OMC)
in functional endoscopic sinus surgery, 760, 760f
imaging of, 168f-169f, 169
surgical anatomy of, 739, 740f
Ostiomeatal unit (OMU)
in chronic sinusitis, 674, 674f
after functional endoscopic sinus surgery, 677-679
and sinus physiology, 664-670
Ostmann's fatty tissue
anatomy of, 1869, 1869f
in pressure equalization, 1870
O-T procedure, for forehead repair, 362, 363f
Otalgia, 2197-2198
with bloody or serous otorrhea, 2195-2196
primary, 2197
referred, 2197-2198
Otic capsule, 1840
Otic pit, 1851-1852
Otic placode, 477, 1851-1852
Otic vesicle, 1851-1852
Otitic hydrocephalus, 1997
Otitic infections, intracranial complications of, 2347
Otitis externa (OE), 97, 1944-1947
allergic, 1945-1946
bacterial, 1944
ear wick for, 1945-1946, 1951, 1951f
otorrhea due to, 2194-2195
systemic antibiotics for, 1953
topical therapies for, 1951-1953
acidifying agents as, 1953
failure to respond to, 1953, 1953t
options for, 1951-1953, 1951f
ototopic antibiotics as, 1951-1953
chronic, 1945, 1946f, 1953
clinical manifestations of, 1945
complications of, 1946-1947, 1946f
conductive hearing loss due to, 2021, 2023f
defined, 1944
eczematoid, topical therapies for, 1955-1957
anti-inflammatory and immunosuppressive agents as, 1956-1957
options for, 1955
steroids as, 1955-1956
fungal, 1944-1946, 1945f
otorrhea due to, 2195
topical therapies for, 1954-1955
acidifying agents as, 1954
antifungals as, 1954-1955
antiseptics as, 1955
options for, 1954
ototoxicity of, 1955
granular, 1945
immunosuppression and, 221-223
incidence and epidemiology of, 1944
investigations of, 1945
malignant or necrotizing, 1947-1948
clinical manifestations of, 1947, 1947f
conductive hearing loss due to, 2021, 2023f
defined, 1947
imaging of, 1917, 1917f
immunosuppression and, 221-222, 1947
incidence and epidemiology of, 1947
investigations of, 1947
microbiology of, 1947
otorrhea due to, 2195
treatment of, 1947-1948
microbiology of, 1945, 1945t
otorrhea due to, 2194-2195
pathogenesis of, 1944-1945, 1945f
treatment of, 1945-1946
Otitis media (OM), 1963-1978
acute, 1979-1981
in children, 2761-2777
complications and sequelae of, 2776-2777
diagnosis of, 2761-2762
epidemiology of, 2765-2768
pathophysiology and pathogenesis of, 2762-2765, 2762f
prevention of, 2768-2769
recurrent, 2771
treatment of, 2770-2771
clinical features of, 1980
complication(s) of, 1963, 1979-1981 (*See also* Temporal bone infections, complications of)
otitis media with effusion as, 1963
tympanosclerosis as, 1974
Otitis media (OM) *(Continued)*
epidemiology of, 1979-1980
immunosuppression and, 222-223
otorrhea due to, 2196
pathogenesis of, 1980-1981
treatment of, 1980-1981
adenoidectomy for, 2796
adhesive, 1964, 1965f
chronic, 1981
bacteriology of, 1981
with cholesteatoma, 1964-1969
acquired, 1964-1966, 1965f-1966f
anterior epitympanic, 1968, 1969f
bone erosion in, 1971-1974, 1972f-1973f
complications of, 1968, 1969b
congenital, 1964-1966, 1966f
diagnosis of, 1965, 1965f-1966f
epidemiology of, 1965
management of, 1968-1969, 1969t, 1970b
pathogenesis of, 1965-1968, 1967f
posterior mesotympanic, 1968, 1968f
sensorineural hearing loss due to, 1974
without cholesteatoma, 1969-1971
diagnosis of, 1969, 1970f
management of, 1971
pathogenesis of, 1970-1971, 1971f, 1971t
complications of, 1981 (*See also* Temporal bone infections, complications of)
defined, 1981
otorrhea due to, 2195-2196
perilymph fistula due to, 2342-2343
suppurative, cochlear implant for, 2221
with tympanostomy tubes, 1970-1971, 1981
and cleft palate, 1872-1873, 1873f, 2674-2675
and cochlear implants, 2240
with effusion (*See* Otitis media with effusion (OME))
eustachian tube dysfunction and
aging and, 1872
with cleft palate, 1872-1873, 1873f
ear pressure and, 1872
with extraesophageal reflux, 1873
hereditary component to, 1873-1874
hypertrophic adenoids and, 1872, 1873f
mucociliary clearance and, 1871
nasal allergy and, 1872
with nasopharyngeal neoplasms, 1873, 1873f
pathophysiology of, 1872
respiratory viruses and, 1871
facial nerve paralysis due to, 1991, 2400
epidemiology of, 1980t
imaging of, 1991f
treatment for, 1991
immunosuppression and, 222-223
middle ear atelectasis due to, 1964, 1964f-1965f
mucociliary clearance and, 1871
vs. myofascial pain dysfunction syndrome, 1284t
petrositis due to, 1975-1977
anatomic basis for, 1975-1976, 1976f-1977f
diagnostic tests for, 1977, 1977f
historical notes on, 1975
management of, 1977
symptoms of, 1976-1977, 1976t
respiratory viruses and, 1871
sensorineural hearing loss due to, 2118-2119
serous, immunosuppression and, 222-223
tuberculous, 2101-2103, 2102f-2103f
tympanosclerosis due to, 1974-1975
diagnosis of, 1974, 1974f
epidemiology of, 1974
management of, 1975, 1975f
pathogenesis of, 1974-1975, 1975f
Otitis media with effusion (OME)
in children, 2761-2777
complications and sequelae of, 2776-2777
intracranial, 2776-2777
intratemporal, 2776

Otitis media with effusion (OME) *(Continued)*
diagnosis of, 2761-2762
audiometry in, 2762
immittance testing (tympanometry) in, 2762
physical examination in, 2761-2762
symptoms and signs in, 2761
epidemiology of, 2765-2768
incidence and prevalence of, 2765
risk factors in, 2766-2768
trend over time in, 2765-2766
guidelines for, 2773
pathophysiology and pathogenesis of, 2762-2765, 2762f
allergy and immunology in, 2764-2765
eustachian tube function in, 2762-2763, 2763f
gastroesophageal reflux in, 2765
infection in, 2763-2764, 2764f
prevention of, 2768-2769
antibiotic prophylaxis for, 2771
management of environmental factors in, 2768
vaccines in, 2768-2769
quality of life assessment for, 2773
recurrent, 2771
treatment of, 2771-2773
medical, 2771-2772
observation in, 2771
for recurrent disease, 2771
surgical, 2772-2776
clinical course of, 1963
etiology of, 1963
and mastoid pneumatization, 1963-1964
middle ear atelectasis due to, 1964, 1964f-1965f
sensorineural hearing loss due to, 1974
tympanosclerosis due to, 1974
OTOA (otoancorin) gene, in deafness, 2051t-2058t
Otoacoustic emissions (OAEs), 1891-1892, 1904-1907
with acoustic neuroma, 1891-1892, 1893f, 1897
advantages of, 1906
and audiograms, 1905, 1906f
and auditory neuropathy or dyssynchrony, 1907
clinical applications of, 1905-1907
cochlear echoes in, 1891
distortion product, 1891, 1905
and audiometric tests, 1905, 1907f
clinical applications of, 1905-1907
defined, 1891, 1905
distortion products in, 1905
frequencies used in, 1905
with high-frequency hearing loss, 1905, 1907f
in infants, 2720-2721
with normal hearing, 1892f, 1905, 1907f
procedure for, 1891
evoked
in infants, 2720-2721
types of, 1891, 1905
with neural hearing loss, 1899-1901
for noise-induced hearing loss
early detection of, 2146-2147, 2147f-2150f
susceptibility to, 2144
with normal hearing, 1905, 1906f
with otitis media, 2762
procedure for, 1891
with sensorineural hearing loss, 1905, 1906f, 2117
spontaneous, 1905
stimulus-frequency, 1891
transient evoked, 1891, 1905
with acoustic neuroma, 1891-1892, 1893f
advantages of, 1891
analysis of, 1905
clinical applications of, 1905-1907
defined, 1891, 1905
in infants, 2720-2721
with normal hearing, 1892f
Otoancorin *(OTOA)* gene, in deafness, 2051t-2058t
Otocadherin, in deafness, 2051t-2058t
Otocerol (arachis oil, almond oil, rectified camphor oil), for cerumen removal, 1958t
Otoconia. *See* Otolith(s).
Otoconial membrane
response to head acceleration by, 2283
in vestibular system, 1855, 1858f
Otocyst, 1851-1852, 1851f
Otoferlin *(OTOF)* gene, in deafness, 2051t-2058t, 2080-2081
Otogelin, 2067
Otogelin *(Otog)* gene, in murine deafness, 2058t-2060t, 2067-2069
Otolith(s), in vestibular system, 1855, 1858f
anatomy of, 2277, 2278f
arrangement of, 2278, 2280f
estimated patterns of excitation and inhibition for, 2278, 2281f
morphologic polarizations of stereociliary bundles in, 2278, 2280f
Otolith membrane
response to head acceleration by, 2283
in vestibular system, 1855, 1858f
Otolithic crisis of Tumarkin, 2300
Otologic disease, outcome scales for, 56t, 57
Otologic manifestations
of immunosuppression, 221-223
malignant otitis externa as, 221-222
in middle ear, 222-223
due to *P. jiroveci* and *A. fumigatus,* 222-223
of systemic diseases, 2100-2115, 2101t
of bone, 2108-2112
in fibrous dysplasia, 2110-2111, 2111f
in osteitis fibrosa cystica, 2112
in osteogenesis imperfecta, 2109-2110, 2110f
in osteopetroses, 2111-2112, 2112f-2113f
in Paget's disease, 2108-2109, 2109f
collagen vascular and autoimmune, 2114
genetically determined, 2115
granulomatous and infectious, 2100-2106
in Langerhans' cell histiocytosis, 2100-2101, 2101f-2102f
in Lyme disease, 2105-2106
in mycotic diseases, 2106, 2106f
in sarcoidosis, 2104-2105, 2104f
in syphilis, 2105, 2105f
in tuberculosis, 2101-2103, 2102f-2103f
in Wegener's granulomatosis, 2103-2104, 2103f-2104f
immunodeficiency, 2114-2115
in AIDS, 2114-2115
primary or congenital, 2114
neoplastic, 2106-2108
in leukemia, 2107, 2108f
metastatic, 2107-2108, 2108f
in multiple myeloma, 2106-2107, 2107f
storage and metabolic, 2112-2114
in gout, 2113-2114
in mucopolysaccharidoses, 2112-2113, 2113f
in ochronosis, 2114
Otologic symptoms and syndromes, 2194-2202
aural fullness as, 2198
hearing loss as, 2198-2201, 2198b
acute, 2198b, 2199
fluctuating, 2198b, 2199
gradual, 2198b, 2199
due to jugular foramen syndromes, 2199, 2199t
pediatric
conductive, 2200-2201
sensorineural, 2200, 2200b
rapidly progressive, 2198b, 2199-2200
otalgia as, 2197-2198
primary, 2197
referred, 2197-2198
Otologic symptoms and syndromes *(Continued)*
otorrhea as, 2194-2197, 2195b
external ear sources of, 2194-2197, 2195b
intracranial sources of, 2195b, 2197
neoplastic disease causing, 2196-2197
systemic disease associated with, 2196
infectious, 2196
noninfectious, 2196
tympanic membrane, middle ear, and mastoid sources of, 2195-2196, 2195b
vertigo as, 2201-2202
labyrinthine, 2201-2202
retrocochlear, 2202
time course of, 2201, 2201b
Otologics fully implantable middle ear system, 2027
Otology, gene therapy in, 23
Otomastoiditis, immunosuppression and, 222
Otomicroscopy
in children, 2574
in infants, 2722
Otomycosis, 1944-1945, 1945f
otorrhea due to, 2195
Otoplasty, 475-480
cartilage-cutting *vs.* cartilage-sparing techniques of, 477, 477f
complications of, 478-479
electrocautery in, 478
graduated-approach, 477-478, 478f
history of, 475-476, 476f
incisionless, 478
octyl-2-cyanoacrylate in, 478
other techniques of, 478
results of, 479-480, 479f-480f
suture techniques in, 477-478, 477f
complications of, 479
history of, 475-476, 476f
Mustarde, 475-476, 476f
Otoprotective agents, 2189-2191
Otorrhea, 97, 2194-2197
bloody or serous, otalgia with, 2195-2196
CSF, 788, 2197
gustatory, 2197
purulent
due to chronic dermatitis or eczema, 2194
due to infection of first branchial cleft cyst, 2195
due to otitis externa, 2194
sources of, 2194-2197, 2195b
external ear, 2194-2197, 2195b
intracranial, 2195b, 2197
neoplastic, 2196-2197
systemic, 2196
infectious, 2196
noninfectious, 2196
tympanic membrane, middle ear, and mastoid, 2195-2196, 2195b
topical therapies for, 1957-1958
with tympanostomy tubes, 1971, 2774-2775
Otos (otospiralin) gene, in murine deafness, 2058t-2060t
Otosclerosis, 2028-2035
alternative treatment of, 2034-2035
fluoride therapy as, 2034-2035
hearing aids as, 2034
clinical course of, 2028-2029
clinical presentation of, 2028
defined, 2028
evaluation of, 2029-2030
audiometry in, 2030, 2030f
history in, 2029-2030
physical examination in, 2030
far-advanced, 2035
fenestral and cochlear, imaging of, 1921-1922, 1925f
histopathology of, 2028-2029, 2029f-2030f
inheritance of, 2028-2030

Otosclerosis *(Continued)*
with Meniere's disease, 2035
prevalence of, 2028, 2029t
sensorineural hearing loss due to, 2124
small fenestra stapedotomy for, 2030-2032
with laser minus prosthesis, 2033
laser *vs.* microdrill in, 2033
postoperative care after, 2032-2033
postoperative complication(s) of, 2030, 2034
facial paralysis as, 2030, 2034
perilymph fistula as, 2034
reparative granuloma as, 2034
sensorineural hearing loss as, 2030, 2034
serous labyrinthitis as, 2034
taste disturbance as, 2034
tinnitus as, 2034
tympanic membrane perforation as, 2034
vertigo as, 2030, 2034
procedure for, 2030-2032
anesthesia for, 2030
creation of fenestra in, 2031-2032, 2032f
flap elevation in, 2031, 2031f
incisions for, 2031
measurement of distance from incus to footplate in, 2031, 2031f-2032f
placement of prosthesis in, 2031-2032, 2032f
positioning for, 2031, 2031f
removal of posterior superior bony wall in, 2031, 2031f
stapedectomy *vs.*, 2030
surgical problems in, 2033-2034
chorda tympani nerve damage as, 2034
exposed, overhanging facial nerve as, 2033
fixed malleus as, 2033
floating footplate as, 2033
intraoperative vertigo as, 2034
perilymph gusher as, 2034
solid or obliterated footplate as, 2033
tympanic membrane perforation as, 2034
stapedectomy for
in children, 2035
revision, 2035
vs. stapedotomy, 2030
Otoscopy
in children, 2574
pneumatic, for otitis media, 2761-2762
for temporal bone fractures, 2038f-2039f
Otospiralin *(Otos)* gene, in murine deafness, 2058t-2060t
Otospondylomegaepiphyseal dysplasia (OSMED) syndrome, deafness in, 2051t-2058t
Otospongiosis, 2028
imaging of, 1921-1922, 1925f
Otosyphilis, 2105, 2105f, 2341-2342
early *vs.* late, 2341
in HIV, 224
treatment for, 2341-2342
Ototopical agents
acidifying, 1959t-1960t
for acute bacterial otitis externa, 1953
for fungal otitis externa, 1954
for acute bacterial otitis externa, 1951-1953
acidifying agents as, 1953
antibiotics as, 1951-1953
failure to respond to, 1953, 1953t
options for, 1951-1953, 1951f
antibiotics as, 1959t-1960t
for acute bacterial otitis externa, 1951-1953
evidence-based data on, 1952
hypersensitivity reaction to, 1954
mechanism of action of, 1951
ototoxicity of, 1953-1954
resistance to, 1953
antifungals as, 1959t-1960t
for fungal otitis externa, 1954-1955
ototoxicity of, 1955

Ototopical agents *(Continued)*
anti-inflammatories as
for eczematoid otitis externa, 1956-1957
mechanism of action of, 1951
antiseptics as, 1955
for fungal otitis externa, 1955
for cerumen impaction, 1957
options for, 1957, 1958t
for ear hygiene and chronic draining ear, 1957-1958, 1961f
for eczematoid otitis externa, 1955-1957
anti-inflammatory and immunosuppressive agents as, 1956-1957
options for, 1955
steroids as, 1955-1956
for fungal otitis externa, 1954-1955
acidifying agents as, 1954
antifungals as, 1954-1955
antiseptics as, 1955
options for, 1954
history of, 1950
immunosuppressive, for eczematoid otitis externa, 1956-1957
mechanism of action of, 1950-1951
for antibiotics, 1951
for anti-inflammatories, 1951
for myringitis, 1955
defined, 1955
options for, 1955
sensorineural hearing loss due to, 2119-2120
steroids as
classes of, 1956, 1956t
for eczematoid otitis externa, 1955-1956
hypersensitivity reaction to, 1954
mechanism of action of, 1951
ototoxicity of, 1956
summary of available, 1959t-1960t
for viral infections, 1957, 1957f
options for, 1957
Ototoxicity, 2169-2178
of aminoglycoside antibiotics, 1953-1954, 2169
clinical manifestations of, 2170
delayed, 2170
histopathology of, 2170
mechanisms of, 2170-2171
monitoring for, 2170
in noise-induced hearing loss, 2147
pharmacokinetics of, 2169-2170
risk factors for, 2170
sensorineural hearing loss due to, 2119-2120, 2170
with topical preparations, 2119-2120
susceptibility to, 2097, 2170
vertigo due to, 2201
vestibular, 2170
of analgesics, 2175-2176
hydrocodone as, 2175
salicylates as, 2175-2176
of antineoplastic agent(s), 2171-2174
carboplatin as, 2173-2174
cisplatin as, 2171-2173
clinical studies on, 2171-2172
delayed, 2171-2172
experimental studies on, 2172
genetic predisposition to, 2172
histopathology of, 2172
mechanics of, 2172-2173
pharmacokinetics of, 2171
risk factors for, 2172
vestibular, 2172
difluoromethylornithine as, 2174
animal studies on, 2174
clinical studies on, 2174
conclusions on, 2174
of deferoxamine, 2176-2177
of erythromycin and related macrolide antibiotics, 2176

Ototoxicity *(Continued)*
of loop diuretics, 2174-2175
monitoring for, 2177
in noise-induced hearing loss, 2147
of quinine and related drugs, 2176
sensorineural hearing loss due to, 2119-2121
sudden, 2128
of topical antibiotics, 1953-1954
of topical antifungals, 1955
of topical steroids, 1956
of vancomycin, 2177
Outcome(s)
assessment of, 53-54
categories of, 55-56
descriptive statistics for, 64t
Outcome measures, with rhinosinusitis, 730, 730t
Outcomes research, 52-58
defined, 52
future directions for, 58
history of, 52-53
key terms and concepts in, 53-54
assessment of baseline as, 53
comorbidity in, 53
definition of disease in, 53
disease severity in, 53
assessment of outcomes as, 53-54
effectiveness in, 52, 54
efficacy in, 53-54
assessment of treatment as, 53
control groups in, 53
biasing and confounding in, 53
measurement of clinical outcomes in, 55-56
categories of outcomes for, 55-56
psychometric validation for, 55
outcome measures in, 56, 56t
disease-specific scales as, 55-58, 56t
for head and neck cancer, 56-57, 56t
otologic, 56t, 57
pediatric, 56t, 57
rhinologic, 56t, 57
sleep, 56t, 57
symptom, 56t, 57-58
voice, 56t, 57
generic scales as, 55-56, 56t
study design for, 54-55, 54t
case series as, 54-55, 54t
case-control, 54, 54t
expert opinion as, 52, 54-55, 54t
grading of evidence-based medicine recommendations as, 55, 55t
observational (cohort), 54, 54t
other types of, 55
randomized trial as, 52, 54, 54t
Outer hair cell(s) (OHCs)
anatomy of, 1832-1834, 1832f-1833f, 1840
arrangement of, 2071, 2072f
in auditory physiology, 1841f, 1844, 1844f
in cochlear transduction
active, 2063-2064, 2064f, 2066f-2067f
passive, 2061f-2062f
length of, 2070, 2070f
in noise-induced hearing loss, 2141-2142, 2142f
number and density of, 2070
and otoacoustic emissions, 1904-1906
receptor potentials for, 2071, 2072f
stereocilia on, 2070f, 2071, 2072f
transduction channels in, 2073f
Outer hair cell (OHC) motility, prestin (SLC26A5) and, 2064-2065, 2068f
Oval window
anatomy of, 1831, 1840, 1853f
atresia of, 1917, 1917f
in cochlear transduction, 2062f
hearing loss due to ossicular disruption with closure of, 2019, 2019t
in sound transmission, 2019

Overbite, 323, 323f
Overjet, 323, 323f
Overpressure radionuclide cisternography (ORNC), for CSF rhinorrhea, 790
Overpressure therapy, local, 2338
Overrotation, of nasal tip, revision rhinoplasty for, 590, 590f-591f
Oxcarbazepine, for neuropathic pain, 243, 244t
Oxidative stress, in noise-induced hearing loss, 2144-2145
Oxycephaly, synostotic, 2645, 2645f
Oxycodone, for postoperative pain, 241t
Oxygen free radicals, in acutely raised skin flaps, 1070-1071, 1071f
Oxygen saturation monitoring, for stridor, 2900
Oxygen supplementation
  nocturnal, for obstructive sleep apnea in children, 2611
  for stridor, 2903
Oxygen transport, in children, 2571-2572
Oxymetazoline
  for obstructive sleep apnea, 257
  for rhinosinusitis, 735t, 736
Oxyphil cells, 1778

P

P values, 65, 66t
  multiple, 73t, 74
  post hoc, 73-74, 73t
P_0, in deafness, 2051t-2058t
p16, in head and neck squamous cell carcinoma, 1020-1021
p53
  in head and neck squamous cell carcinoma, 1020, 1024
  in laryngeal carcinoma, 1505
  in oral cancer, 1295
  in thyroid carcinoma, 1753
Pa (pascal), 1839
PABI (penetrating auditory brainstem implant), 2262, 2262f
Pacemaker, pediatric anesthesia with, 2587
Pacific Business Group on Health (PBGH), 84t-87t, 87
Pacifier use, and otitis media, 2767
Package time, for oral cancer, 1314
Paclitaxel
  in combination chemotherapy, 1060
  with radiotherapy, 1041-1042
PACS (picture archival and communication systems), 138
Paget, James, 1223
Paget's disease, 2108-2109
  clinical manifestations of, 2108
  epidemiology of, 2108
  etiology of, 2108
  of frontal bone, 779-780, 780f
  genetic basis for, 2108
  oral manifestations of, 1253
  otologic manifestations of, 2109, 2109f
  radiographic findings in, 2108, 2109f
  sensorineural hearing loss due to, 2124
Pain, 239-249
  acute postoperative, 240-242
    defined, 239
    epidemiology of, 240
    management of
      with chronic opioid therapy, 241
      NSAIDs for, 241
      in older adults, 240-241
      opioid addiction *vs.* tolerance in, 240
      patient satisfaction with, 240
      patient-controlled analgesia for, 240, 241t
      preemptive analgesia for, 241
      regional anesthesia for, 241-242
Pain *(Continued)*
  chronic, 242-246
    adjuvant analgesics for, 243-244
      anticonvulsant agents as, 243-244, 244t
      antidepressants as, 244-245, 245t
    analgesic ladder for, 242-243
    ceiling of efficacy and/or safety with, 243
    defined, 239, 242-243
    first-line agents for, 243
    guidelines for opioid use for, 243
    interventional techniques for, 245-246, 246t
    types of, 242-243
  with cognitive impairment, 240
  defined, 239
  due to headache, 246-248
    cluster, 247-248
    diagnosis of, 246, 247f
    epidemiology of, 246
    in hemicrania continua, 248
    initial evaluation of, 246
    medication overuse (rebound), 248
    migraine, 246-247
    primary, 246
    secondary, 246
    tension-type, 247
    thunderclap, 248
    in trigeminal neuralgia, 248
  measurement of, 239-240
  neuropathic
    anticonvulsant agents for, 243-244, 244t
    antidepressants for, 244-245, 245t
    interventional techniques for, 245-246, 246t
    palliative care for, 1103
  palliative care for, 1103
Pain management
  in children, 2572
    postoperative, 2594
  postoperative
    in children, 2594
    after surgical resection of oral cancer, 1316
Pair production, 1032f, 1033
Paired box gene 2 *(PAX2),* in deafness, 2051t-2058t
Paired box gene 3 *(PAX3),* in deafness, 2051t-2058t, 2095
Paired samples, statistical tests for, 66, 67t
Palatal augmentation prosthesis, 1342-1343, 1344f
Palatal bulb obturator, for velopharyngeal dysfunction, 2681, 2682f
Palatal fracture, repair of, 335, 335f
Palatal implant, for obstructive sleep apnea, 258-259
Palatal island mucosal flap, for oropharyngeal reconstruction, 1376-1377, 1376f
  of soft palate, 1382
  of tonsils and pharyngeal wall, 1385
Palatal lift, for velopharyngeal dysfunction, 2681, 2681f
Palatal lift prosthesis, 1343-1344
Palatal reconstruction, 1381-1383
  algorithm for, 1384f
  free flaps for, 1382
    Gehanno method for, 1382
    Lacombe and Blackwell's method for, 1382-1383
    other groups' experience with, 1383
    radial forearm, 1382, 1383f
  jejunal flaps for, 1380, 1380f
  local flaps for, 1381
    buccinator musculomucosal, 1381-1382, 1381f
    palatal island mucosal, 1382
    Superior Constrictor Rotation-Advancement Flap (SCARF) as, 1382, 1382f
    uvulopalatal, 1377f, 1381
  prosthetic obturation for, 1381
  speech function after, 1383
Palatal surgery, for obstructive sleep apnea, 251t, 258-259, 258b, 258f, 260f
Palate
  inherited and congenital disorders affecting, 1257
  non-Hodgkin's lymphoma of, 1364f
  pleomorphic adenoma of, 1169, 1169f
  primary *vs.* secondary, 2659, 2660f
Palatine shelves, 2661, 2662f-2663f
Palatine tonsil(s)
  anatomy of, 1359f, 2783-2784
    radiographic, 1463f-1464f
  embryology of, 2585f
  in immune system, 605
Palatoglossal arch, 1359f
Palatoglossus muscle
  anatomy of, 1297, 1359f-1360f
  in velopharyngeal function, 2676, 2677t
Palatopharyngeal arch, 1359f
Palatopharyngeus muscle
  anatomy of, 1360f
  in velopharyngeal function, 2676, 2677t
Palatoplasty, 2668-2673
  basic principles of, 2670
  complications of, 2672-2673
  and facial growth, 2669
  Furlow (double-opposing Z-plasty), 2670
    surgical technique for, 2671-2672, 2672f
    for velopharyngeal dysfunction, 2682-2683
  goals of, 2668
  techniques of, 2669-2670
  timing of, 2668-2669
  two-flap, 2669-2670, 2670f
    surgical technique for, 2670-2671, 2670f-2671f
Palifermin, for mucositis, 1102
Palindromic sequence, 9
Palliative care, 1100-1105
  for dysphagia and speech dysfunction, 1104
  for end of life, 1104
  for mucositis, 1101-1102
  for nutrition, 1104
  for oral cancer, 1316
  oral hygiene in, 1101
  for pain, 1103
  pretreatment management in, 1101
  for psychological distress, 1103-1104
  for taste dysfunction, 1103
  for xerostomia, 1102-1103
Palliative treatment, for tracheal tumors, 1619-1624
Pallister-Hall syndrome (PHS), 2874
Palmaz stent, for tracheal stenosis, 2929-2930
Palmoplantar hyperkeratosis, deafness in, 2051t-2058t
Palmoplantar keratoderma, deafness in, 2051t-2058t
Palpebral conjunctiva, 444
Palpebral fissure, 442, 445
Palpebral opening, in aesthetic analysis, 271
Palpebral springs, for lagophthalmos, 2421
Pancuronium, for pediatric anesthesia, 2593t
Panfacial fractures, 339
Panje prosthesis, 1598f
Panoramic radiograph (Panorex), for mentoplasty, 462-463, 462f
Pansynostosis, 2641t
PaO_2 (arterial oxygen tension), in children, 2570, 2571t
Papillary cystadenoma, of salivary glands
  lymphomatosum, 1170-1171
    imaging of, 1146, 1146f
  oncocytic, 1171
Papillary dermis, 1065
Papillary squamous cell carcinoma (PSCC), of larynx, 1506
Papillary thyroid carcinoma, 1760-1761
  clinical presentation of, 1760
  management and prognosis for, 1760-1761
  pathology of, 1760
  ultrasound of, 1646f
    metastatic, 1648f-1649f

Papilloma(s)
choroid plexus, 2528-2529, 2530f
fibroepithelial, 291
inverted (Schneiderian, inverted type)
ductal, of salivary glands, 1171-1172
of nasopharynx, 1349
sinonasal, 718-720, 1127
endoscopic appearance of, 718-719, 719f
epidemiology of, 718
with frontal sinus involvement, 720, 720f
histologic appearance of, 718
human papillomavirus and, 718
imaging of, 719, 719f
postoperative surveillance for, 720
recurrence of, 720
sites for, 718
and squamous cell carcinoma, 718
surgical approach for, 718t, 719-720, 720f, 763, 1127
of oral cavity, 1290, 1290f
squamous
of larynx, 1468, 1468f
of nasopharynx, 1349
of oral cavity, 1290, 1290f
of trachea, 1612
Papillomatosis
aural, 1957, 1957f
management options for, 1957
laryngeal, stridor due to, 2898, 2899f
recurrent respiratory (*See* Recurrent respiratory papillomatosis (RRP))
PAR (perennial allergic rhinitis), 617-618
and pediatric chronic sinusitis, 2778
Parabrachial nucleus, in gustatory pathway, 1212-1213
Paracoccidioidomycosis, laryngitis due to, 885
Paradental cyst, 1264-1265
radiographic features of, 1265
Paradoxic nasal obstruction, 484, 486
Paragangliomas (PGLs), 1657
carotid, 1657-1658, 2506f
anatomy and physiology of, 1658-1659
classification of, 1660
clinical presentation and diagnosis of, 1659-1660
endovascular treatment of, 1937, 1937f
etiology of, 1659, 1659t
history of, 1657-1658
imaging of, 1658f, 1660-1661
malignancy of, 1660
multicentricity of, 1660-1661
observation for, 1661-1662
radiation therapy for, 1661
surgical management of, 1660-1661
of cerebellopontine angle, 2522-2523, 2523f-2524f
endovascular treatment of, 1934-1937, 1935f
for carotid body tumor, 1937, 1937f
for glomus jugulare tumor, 1935-1936, 1935f-1936f
for glomus tympanicum tumor, 1935
for glomus vagale tumor, 1936-1937, 1936f
epidemiology of, 1657-1659
familial syndromes of, 1659, 1659t, 2506f
glomus jugulare, 2505, 2506f
endovascular treatment of, 1935-1936, 1935f-1936f
surgical approach to, 2506, 2507f
glomus tympanicum, 2505-2506
endovascular treatment of, 1935
glomus vagale, 2506f
endovascular treatment of, 1936-1937, 1936f
imaging of, 151, 152f
intracranial, 2499f
jugular, 1662f, 2499f
of larynx, 1508
neck masses due to, 1641
Paragangliomas (PGLs) *(Continued)*
nomenclature for, 1657
pathology of, 1657, 1658f
of skull base, 171, 174f, 1929, 1930f
stereotactic radiation therapy for, 2565, 2565t
of temporal bone, 2505-2506
diagnostic evaluation of, 2505, 2506f-2507f
preoperative evaluation of, 2491f
radiotherapy for, 2506
surgical approach to, 2505-2506, 2507f
symptoms of, 2505
vagal, 1661-1662
clinical presentation and diagnosis of, 1662
management of, 1662-1663
Paraglottic space (PGS)
anatomy of, 1484-1485, 1484f-1485f
radiographic, 1471f, 1473
surgical, 1542, 1543f-1544f
laryngeal cancer of
anatomic basis for, 1484-1485, 1484f-1485f
imaging of, 1474
Parainfluenza virus, pharyngitis due to, 196
Parakeratinizing odontogenic keratocyst, 1262, 1267-1268
in basal cell nevus syndrome, 1268
microscopic features of, 1268
radiographic features of, 1267-1268, 1268f
treatment of, 1268
Parakeratosis, of larynx, 1486
Paralaryngeal space, radiographic anatomy of, 1471f, 1473
Paralytic agents, intraoperative, 111-112
Paramedian forehead flaps, for nasal defects, 348, 352f-353f
Paramedian mandibulotomy, 1311
Paramedian pontine reticular formation (PPRF), in velocity-to-position integration, 2296, 2297f
Paranasal sinus(es)
anatomy of
normal, 167, 664-668, 665f
agger nasi cell in, 665-666, 665f-666f
anterior ostiomeatal channels in, 666f
anterior ostiomeatal unit in, 664, 665f
basal lamella and sinus lateralis in, 665f, 667f
ethmoid bulla in, 666-667, 667f
ethmoid sinuses in, 664, 667
frontal recess in, 665, 665f-667f
frontal sinuses in, 664-665, 665f
hiatus semilunaris in, 667, 667f
inferior meatus in, 664
inferior turbinate in, 665f
infundibulum in, 665f, 666-667
maxillary sinuses in, 664, 665f
middle meatus in, 664-665, 665f-667f
middle turbinate in, 667
ostiomeatal channels in, 664
ostiomeatal unit in, 664-670
posterior ostiomeatal unit in, 664
primary ostium in, 665, 665f
retrobullar (suprabullar) recess in, 667
sphenoethmoidal recess in, 667, 668f
sphenoid sinus in, 664, 665f, 667-668, 668f
superior meatus in, 664-665
uncinate process in, 666-667, 666f-667f
variations in, 741
surgical, 739-741, 1124f
anatomic variations in, 741
anterior skull base in, 741
ethmoid complex in, 740
frontal sinus in, 740-741
maxillary sinus in, 740
middle turbinate in, 739-740
ostiomeatal complex in, 739, 740f
sphenoid sinus in, 740, 740f
in transnasal endoscopic-assisted anterior skull base surgery, 2473-2474, 2473f
Paranasal sinus(es) *(Continued)*
bony outlines of, 672, 672f
effects of radiotherapy on, 2626t
growth and development of, 2619-2620, 2623f
imaging of, 167-169, 662-2
with anatomic variations and congenital abnormalities, 668-670
aerated crista galli as, 670
asymmetry in ethmoid roof height as, 670
cephalocele as, 670, 671f
of concha bullosa, 668, 669f
extensive pneumatization of sphenoid sinus as, 669, 671f
giant ethmoid bullosa as, 669
Haller or infraorbital cells as, 668-669, 670f
medial deviation or dehiscence of lamina papyracea as, 669
nasal septal deviation as, 668, 669f
Onodi or sphenoethmoidal cells as, 669
paradoxic middle turbinate as, 668, 669f
of uncinate process, 668, 670f
with complications of inflammatory disease, 676-677
inflammatory polyps as, 676, 678f
mucocele as, 676, 678f
mucous retention cyst as, 676, 677f
orbital, 676-677
with congenital and developmental anomalies, 167
conventional radiography for, 130, 662
Caldwell view in, 662, 663f
Waters view in, 662, 663f
CT for, 140-142, 141f, 662-663
radiation exposure with, 663
technique of, 662-663, 664f
after functional endoscopic sinus surgery, 677-680
expected findings in, 677-679, 679f
operative complications in, 679-680, 680f
for image-guided surgery, 680-681, 743-744, 745f
registration in, 680-681
tracking systems in, 681
with inflammatory disease, 167-168, 168f, 672-675
acute rhinosinusitis as, 672-673, 673f
allergic rhinosinusitis as, 675
chronic rhinosinusitis as, 673-674, 674f-675f
fungal rhinosinusitis as, 674-675, 676f
granulomatous rhinosinusitis as, 675
interpretation of, 670-672
evaluation of bony outlines in, 672, 672f
evaluation of critical relationships for surgical planning in, 671-672, 672f
identification and description of important structures in, 671
MRI for, 143, 664, 664f
nasal cycle in, 664, 664f
with normal anatomy, 664-668, 665f
agger nasi cell in, 665-666, 665f-666f
anterior ostiomeatal channels in, 666f
anterior ostiomeatal unit in, 664, 665f
basal lamella and sinus lateralis in, 665f, 667f
ethmoid bulla in, 666-667, 667f
ethmoid sinuses in, 664, 667
frontal recess in, 665, 665f-667f
frontal sinuses in, 664-665, 665f
hiatus semilunaris in, 667, 667f
inferior meatus in, 664
inferior turbinate in, 665f
infundibulum in, 665f, 666-667
maxillary sinuses in, 664, 665f
middle meatus in, 664-665, 665f-667f
middle turbinate in, 667
ostiomeatal channels in, 664
posterior ostiomeatal unit in, 664

Paranasal sinus(es) *(Continued)*
primary ostium in, 665, 665f
retrobullar (suprabullar) recess in, 667
sphenoethmoidal recess in, 667, 668f
sphenoid sinus in, 664, 665f, 667-668, 668f
superior meatus in, 664-665
uncinate process in, 666-667, 666f-667f
with sinonasal small cell tumor *vs.* sphenoid pyomucocele, 168-169, 169f
intensity-modulated radiotherapy of, 1045-1046, 1045f
and optic nerve, 672, 672f
physiology of, 664-670
Paranasal sinus tumor(s), 1121-1132
anatomic basis of, 1122-1123
ethmoid sinus in, 1123
frontal sinus in, 1123
lymphatics in, 1123
maxillary antrum in, 1122-1123
sphenoid sinus in, 1123
benign, 717-727, 718t
diagnosis of, 717-718
fibrous dysplasia as, 718t, 725-726, 726f
glioma as, 718t
hamartoma as, 718t
inverted papilloma (Schneiderian papilloma, inverted type) as, 718-720
endoscopic appearance of, 718-719, 719f
epidemiology of, 718
with frontal sinus involvement, 720, 720f
histologic appearance of, 718
human papillomavirus and, 718
imaging of, 719, 719f
postoperative surveillance for, 720
recurrence of, 720
sites for, 718
and squamous cell carcinoma, 718
surgical approach for, 718t, 719-720, 720f, 763
juvenile angiofibroma as, 721-722
classification systems for, 722
endoscopic appearance of, 721, 721f
imaging of, 721
natural history of, 721
origin of, 721, 721f
postoperative surveillance for, 722
preoperative embolization for, 721-722
surgical approach for, 718t, 722, 722f-723f, 763
lobular capillary hemangioma as, 718t, 725, 725f
ossifying fibroma as, 725-726
osteoma as, 723-725
classification of, 723
endoscopic appearance of, 723
epidemiology of, 723
ethmoid, 724f
frontal, 724-725, 724f
imaging of, 723-725, 723f-724f
ivory ("eburnated"), 723, 723f-724f
mature (spongiosum), 723
microscopic appearance of, 723
mixed, 723, 724f
pathogenesis of, 723
postoperative surveillance for, 725
spongiosum variant of, 724f
surgical approach for, 718t, 724-725
symptoms of, 723
pleomorphic adenoma as, 718t
schwannoma as, 726-727, 726f
surgical approach for, 718, 718t, 763
cervical lymph node metastasis of, 1130
in children, 1132
complications of, 1131
diagnostic assessment of, 1124
biopsy in, 1124
imaging studies for, 1124

Paranasal sinus tumor(s) *(Continued)*
angiography, 1124
CT, 1124
MRI, 1124
PET, 1124
intermediate, 1127
inverted papillomas as, 1127
malignant, 1127-1128
adenocarcinoma as, 1131
adenoid cystic carcinoma as, 1131
algorithm for evaluation and management of, 1122f
epidemiology and survival with, 1121-1122, 1123t
epithelial
staging of, 1127-1128, 1128f, 1129b
ethmoid, sphenoid, and frontal, 1130
staging of, 1129b
hematopoietic and lymphoid, 1131
involvement of cervical lymph nodes in, 1130
lymphoma as, 1131, 1680
therapy and prognosis for, 1680
maxillary, 1128-1130
chemoradiotherapy for, 1130
combined irradiation and surgery for, 1128
inoperable, 1130
radiotherapy for, 1128-1130
staging of, 1129b
surgery alone for, 1128
melanoma as, 1131-1132
sarcomas as, 1131
staging of, 1127-1128, 1128f, 1129b
therapeutic decision-making for, 1131
physical findings with, 1123-1124
surgical options for, 1124-1127
anatomic reference for, 1124f
classical "open" procedures as, 1124-1127
craniofacial frontoethmoidectomy as, 1126, 1126f
extended craniofacial resection as, 1126-1127, 1127f
external ethmoidectomy as, 1124-1125, 1125f
inferior medial maxillectomy as, 1125, 1125f
medial maxillectomy as, 1125, 1125f
radical maxillectomy as, 1125-1126, 1125f
minimally invasive approaches as, 1127
symptoms of, 1123
Paranasal sinus walls, evaluation of, 672, 672f
Paranasal Sinuses Simulator, 49
Paraneoplastic cerebellar degeneration (PCD), 2357
Paraneoplastic pemphigus, 1231-1232
Paraneoplastic syndromes
sensorineural hearing loss due to, 2124
vertigo due to, 2202
Parapharyngeal space (PPS)
anatomy of, 202
lymph nodes in, 1422f
imaging of, 131, 146f
Parapharyngeal space (PPS) abscess, in children, 2788-2789
Parapharyngeal space (PPS) tumor(s), 2510, 2512f
benign, 1663-1664, 1665f
of salivary glands, 1174-1176
mandibulectomy approach for, 1176, 1176f
transcervical approach for, 1174-1176, 1175f
malignant, 1664-1666
of salivary glands, 1195-1196, 1196f
of salivary glands
benign, 1174-1176
mandibulectomy approach for, 1176, 1176f
transcervical approach for, 1174-1176, 1175f
malignant, 1195-1196, 1196f
Parasellar approach, for transnasal endoscopic-assisted anterior skull base surgery, 2479, 2480f

Parasomnias, 264-265, 265b
Parasympathetic control, of salivary gland secretion, 1136
Parathyroid adenoma, 1774-1775, 1778-1779
atypical, 1778-1779
double, 1785f, 1794, 1794f, 1798
ectopic
within carotid sheath, 1800f
intrathymic, 1800f
intrathyroidal, 1789f
mediastinal, 1787f, 1802f
missed, 1798
re-exploration for, 1799-1800, 1800f
superior, 1786f, 1800f
imaging of, 162-163, 165f
CT for, 1786-1787
CT-MIBI fusion, 1785-1786, 1786f-1788f
MRI for, 1787-1788, 1789f, 1802f
scintigraphy for, 138, 139f
sestamibi–technetium 99m scintigraphy for, 1785, 1785f, 1802f
technetium 99m sestamibi with SPECT for, 1785
technetium 99m thallium 201, 162-163, 165f
ultrasonography for, 1644-1645, 1650f-1652f, 1786, 1789f
inferior, 1802f
intraoperative photograph of, 1788f
large clear cell, 1778
lipoadenoma as, 1778
localization of
cervical exploration for, 1792-1793
CT for, 1786-1787
CT-MIBI fusion imaging of, 1785-1786, 1786f-1788f
endoscopic exploration for, 1793-1794
gamma radiation detection device for, 1802, 1803f
intraoperative, 1789
mediastinal exploration for, 1801-1802, 1802f
minimally invasive techniques for, 1793
missed, 1798
MRI for, 1787-1788, 1789f, 1802f
with multiple-gland disease, 1794-1795
parathyroid arteriography for, 1788
re-exploration for, 1799-1800, 1800f
scintigraphy for, 138, 139f
selective venous sampling for PTH for, 1788-1789
sestamibi–technetium 99m scintigraphy for, 1785, 1785f, 1802f
with sporadic hyperplasia, 1794-1795, 1794f
technetium 99m sestamibi with SPECT for, 1785
technetium 99m thallium 201 imaging for, 1784-1785
ultrasonography for, 1644-1645, 1650f-1652f, 1786, 1789f
ultrasound-guided fine needle aspiration for, 1789
unsuccessful, 1801, 1801f-1802f
oncocytic, 1778
superior
ectopic, 1786f
pseudo-intrathyroidal, 1800f
undescended, 1789f
water clear cell, 1778
Parathyroid adenomatosis 1 oncogene *(PRAD1)*, in hyperparathyroidism, 1774-1775, 1775f
Parathyroid arteriography, 1788
Parathyroid carcinoma, 1779, 1802-1804, 1803f
Parathyroid disorder(s), 1773-1805
historical background of, 1774
hyperparathyroidism as (*See* Hyperparathyroidism)
oral manifestations of, 1251

Parathyroid exploration
causes of failed, 1798
endoscopic, 1793-1794
indications for, 1789-1790
minimally invasive techniques for, 1793
for multiple-gland disease, 1794-1795
repeat, 1798-1800
causes of failed exploration with, 1798
operative risk in, 1798-1799
operative strategy for, 1799-1800, 1799f-1800f
preoperative assessment for, 1798
for single-gland disease, 1792-1794
surgical strategy and approach to, 1792
technique for, 1790-1792, 1791f
Parathyroid gland(s)
anatomy of, normal, 1777
vascular, 1778
ectopic
CT-MIBI fusion imaging of, 1786f-1787f
intraoperative photograph of, 1788f
intrathyroidal, 1777, 1788f
mediastinal, 1802, 1803f
technetium-99 sestamibi imaging of, 1774
ultrasound of, 1645
embryology of, 1780, 1780f, 2585f
enlargement of
multiple glandular, 1779
single glandular, 1778-1779
histopathology of, 1778
imaging of, 162-163, 165f
CT for, 140
MRI for, 143
ultrasound imaging for, 1644-1645, 1650f-1652f
inferior, 1777
location of, 1777
morphologic characteristics of, 1777-1778
preoperative evaluation of, 104
superior, 1777
supernumerary, 1777
CT-MIBI fusion imaging of, 1787f
mediastinal, 1802, 1803f
in MEN-I, 1795-1796
during thyroid surgery, 1752, 1765f, 1766
Parathyroid gland hyperplasia, 1779
chief cell, 1779
sporadic, 1794-1795, 1794f
ultrasound of, 1645
water clear cell, 1779
Parathyroid hormone (PTH)
in calcium homeostasis, 1775-1777
functions of, 1775
historical background of, 1774
immunometric "sandwich" assays of, 1776-1777
intraoperative levels of, 1792-1793, 1800-1801
metabolism of, 1776
secretion and regulation of, 1775-1777
selective venous sampling for, 1788-1789
Parathyroid hormone (*PTH*) gene, in hyperparathyroidism, 1774-1775, 1775f
Parathyroid hyperplasia, 1779
chief cell, 1779
sporadic, 1794-1795, 1794f
ultrasound of, 1645
water clear cell, 1779
Parathyroid neoplasm(s), etiology and pathogenesis of, 1775, 1776f
Parathyroid surgery, 1789-1804
gamma radiation detection device in, 1802, 1803f
indications for, 1789-1790
intraoperative PTH levels with, 1792-1793, 1800-1801
for multiple-gland disease, 1794-1795
due to sporadic hyperplasia, 1794-1795, 1794f
due to true double adenoma, 1794, 1794f
parathyroidectomy as, 1790-1792
anesthesia and preparation for, 1790
closure of incision in, 1792
Parathyroid surgery *(Continued)*
exploration of neck in, 1790-1792, 1791f
postoperative care after, 1792
for single-gland disease, 1792-1794
directed unilateral cervical exploration as, 1792-1793
endoscopic parathyroid exploration in, 1793-1794
minimally invasive techniques for, 1793
strategy and approach to, 1792
Parathyroidectomy, 1790-1792
anesthesia and preparation for, 1790
with autotransplantation
for MEN-I, 1795
for renal failure–induced hyperparathyroidism, 1797-1798
closure of incision in, 1792
exploration of neck in, 1790-1792, 1791f
postoperative care after, 1792
radiation-guided, 1793
subtotal, for renal failure–induced hyperparathyroidism, 1797-1798
Parent(s), of child as patient, 2573
Parental presence, during anesthesia induction, in children, 2590
Parietal bone, 320f
in surgical anatomy of lateral skull base, 2434
Parietal foramina, 2641t
with cleidocranial dysplasia, 2641t
Parietal incisura, 2010f
Parietomastoid suture, in surgical anatomy of lateral skull base, 2435, 2435f
Parkinsonism, preoperative evaluation of, 106
Parkinson's disease
laryngeal hypofunction due to, 842-843
olfactory dysfunction in, 635
oral manifestations of, 1255
Parkinson's-plus syndromes, laryngeal hypofunction due to, 843
Parosmia, 633, 636
Parotid cysts, AIDS-related, 1146, 1146f
Parotid duct, trauma to, 312-313, 314f
Parotid gland(s)
accessory, 2850
anatomy of, 1133-1134, 1359f
in children, 2850-2853
radiographic, 1143-1144, 1144f
contributions to saliva of, 1134t
hemangioma of, 2859-2860, 2860f
neuronal control of, 1136
physical examination of, 95
salivary flow rate and composition of saliva in, 1138t
sialolithiasis of, 1155-1156
in surgical anatomy of lateral skull base, 2439f-2440f
trauma to, 312, 313f
in children, 2863
Parotid gland abscess, 1152f-1153f
Parotid gland neoplasm(s)
acinic cell tumor as, 151f
benign
basal cell adenomas as, 1170
clinical features of, 1164-1165, 1165f-1166f
oncocytic papillary cystadenoma as, 1171
oncocytoma as, 1171
pleomorphic adenoma as, 1169
imaging of, 150, 150f
malignant, physical examination of, 1179
Parotid injury, due to rhytidectomy, 426-427
Parotid lesions, in HIV, 217-218, 218f
Parotid lipoma, 1166, 1167f
Parotid lymph node(s), 2582
extraglandular, 1360f
Parotid mass, ultrasonography of, 1654f
Parotid space (PS)
anatomy of, 203
imaging of, 149-150, 150f-151f
Parotid surgery, facial nerve monitoring during, 2549
Parotidectomy
for benign neoplasms, 1172-1174, 1173f
complication(s) of, 1176-1177
facial nerve paresis or paralysis as, 1176-1177
gustatory sweating ("Frey's syndrome") as, 1177
salivary fistula as, 1177
sensory abnormalities as, 1177
facial nerve monitoring during, 2549
fistula after, 1728
for malignant neoplasms, 1194-1196
elevation of skin flap in, 1195
external carotid artery in, 1195-1196
facial nerve in
anatomy of, 1194, 1194f
involvement of, 1196
main trunk of, 1195, 1195f
marginal mandibular branch of, 1195, 1195f
greater auricular nerve in, 1195
modified Blair incision for, 1195, 1195f
partial deep, 1194-1196, 1196f
retromandibular (posterior facial) vein in, 1195-1196, 1195f
superficial, 1194-1195
total, 1194-1196
Parotitis
chronic, 1154, 1155f
vs. myofascial pain dysfunction syndrome, 1284t
recurrent
of childhood, 1153-1154
juvenile, 2858
suppurative
acute, 1151-1153
clinical manifestations of, 1152, 1152f
complications of, 1153, 1154f
defined, 1151
differential diagnosis of, 1152
epidemiology of, 1151
laboratory evaluation of, 1152
pathogenesis of, 1151-1152, 1152f
sialolithiasis and, 1151-1152, 1155, 1155f
treatment of, 1152-1153, 1153f
neonatal, 1153
viral, 1156-1158
in children
due to Epstein-Barr virus, 2855
due to HIV, 2856
due to mumps, 2855
HIV-associated, 1157-1158, 1157f
in children, 2856
due to mumps, 1156-1157
in children, 2855
Paroxetine, for neuropathic pain, 245
Paroxysmal torticollis, and migraine, 2351
Pars flaccida
anatomy of, 1824, 1825f
of tympanic membrane, 97, 98f
Pars flaccida cholesteatoma, 174f
Pars tensa, 1825f
Partial cricoidectomy, for chronic aspiration, 928
Partial dynamic-range compression, for hearing aids, 2268
Partial laryngectomy, for glottic cancer, 1496
in advanced stage, 1497
Partial ossicular replacement prosthesis (PORP), 2006
with absent lenticular process of incus, 2024, 2025f
factors affecting success of, 2023
with ossicular discontinuity, 2008
results with, 2006
Partial-transfixion incisions, for nasal tip projection, 535-536, 536f

Particle beams, in radiotherapy, 1034-1035, 1035f
Particulate radiation, 1031
Parulis, 179
Pascal (Pa), 1839
Passagio, 851
Passavant's ridge, 2676
Past pointing, 2316-2317
Patch method, for tonsillar and pharyngeal wall reconstruction, 1386, 1387f
Paterson-Brown-Kelly syndrome, and postcricoid carcinoma, 1425-1426
Paterson-Kelly syndrome, 967
Patient education
  on difficult airway, 117-119
  for nonallergic rhinitis, 699-700
Patient history, 94, 94b
Patient Outcomes of Surgery–Head/Neck (POS-Head/Neck), 57
Patient Questionnaire of Vocal Performance (VPQ), 826, 826t
Patient scales, for voice evaluation, 825-826, 826t, 834
  Patient Questionnaire of Vocal Performance as, 826, 826t
  Reflux Symptom Index as, 826, 826t
  Voice Activity and Participation Profile as, 826, 826t
  Voice Handicap Index as, 826, 826t, 834
  Voice Outcome Survey as, 826, 826t
  Voice Symptom Scale as, 826, 826t
  Voice-Related Quality of Life scale as, 826, 826t, 834
Patient verification, for radiotherapy, 1035
Patient-controlled analgesia (PCA), 240, 241t
  for oral cancer, 1316
  for postoperative pain in children, 2594
PAX2 (paired box gene 2), in deafness, 2051t-2058t
PAX3 (paired box gene 3), in deafness, 2051t-2058t, 2095
PAX8/PPARγγ1 rearrangement, in thyroid carcinoma, 1753
"Pay for performance," 78
PBGH (Pacific Business Group on Health), 84t-87t, 87
PBK (Phonetically Balanced Kindergarten) Test, for cochlear implant, 2225
PBL (plasmablastic lymphoma), 216
PBP (progressive bulbar palsy), laryngeal disorders due to, 839-840, 842
PBP (pseudobulbar palsy), laryngeal disorders due to, 839-840, 842
PC (posterior cervical) space, 158, 159f-160f, 162f
PCA. *See* Posterior cricoarytenoid (PCA).
PCA (patient-controlled analgesia), 240, 241t
  for oral cancer, 1316
  for postoperative pain in children, 2594
P-cad, in oral cancer, 1301
PC-BPPV. *See* Posterior canal benign paroxysmal positional vertigo (PC-BPPV).
PCD (paraneoplastic cerebellar degeneration), 2357
PCDH15 (protocadherin-15), in tip links, 2074
PCDH15 (protocadherin-15) gene, in deafness, 2051t-2058t, 2074
PCNA (proliferating cell nuclear antigen), in salivary gland neoplasms, 1194
PCPI (Physician Consortium for Performance Improvement), 82-87, 84t-87t
PCR (polymerase chain reaction), 8-9
PCV7 (pneumococcal conjugate vaccine)
  with cochlear implants, 2237, 2237b
  to prevent otitis media, 2763, 2768
    maternal immunization with, 2768-2769
PDGF (platelet-derived growth factor), in wound healing, 1076
PDL (periodontal ligament)
  in interdental discrimination, 1207
  tactile sensitivity of, 1201-1202, 1202f
PDL (pulsed dye laser). *See* Pulsed dye laser (PDL).
PDLA (poly D-lactic acid), in resorbable plating system, for pediatric facial fractures, 2700, 2700t
PDS (polydioxanone), in resorbable plating system, for pediatric facial fractures, 2700, 2700t
PDS (pendrin) gene, in deafness, 2051t-2058t, 2083
PDT. *See* Photodynamic therapy (PDT).
PE (pharyngoesophageal) segment, in alaryngeal speech
  physiology of, 1596
  prevention of hypertonicity of, 1599-1600, 1599f
Peak clipping, with hearing aids, 2268
Peak inspiratory flowmeter, nasal, 643
Pectoralis major flap
  for buccal carcinoma, 1309f
  for hypopharyngeal and esophageal reconstruction, 1452
  for hypopharyngeal cancer, 1431, 1431f
  for oral cancer, 1316
  for oropharyngeal reconstruction, 1377, 1377f
    of tongue base, 1388-1389
    of tonsils and pharyngeal wall, 1385, 1385f
Pediatric diseases, outcome scales for, 56t, 57
Pediatric patients. *See* Children.
Pediatric Quality of Life Inventory (PedQL), 57
Pediatric Voice Handicap Index (pVHI), 2876
Pediatric Voice Outcomes Survey (PVOS), 57, 2876
Pediatric Voice-Related Quality-of-Life survey (PVQOL), 57, 2876
Pedicle flaps. *See also* Free tissue transfer.
  salvage of, 1075
Pedigree(s), 2088, 2088f
  of dominantly inherited trait, 6, 6f, 2088f
  of mitochondrial disorder, 8, 8f, 2086
  of recessively inherited trait, 2086
  variable expression and nonpenetrance in, 7, 7f
  of X-linked recessive disorder, 7, 7f, 2086
PedQL (Pediatric Quality of Life Inventory), 57
PEH (pseudoepitheliomatous hyperplasia), of larynx, 1493
Pejvakin *(PJVK)* gene, in deafness, 2051t-2058t
Pellagra, oral manifestations of, 1254
Pellets, shotgun, 1626, 1628t
Pemberton's sign, in thyroid disease, 1736, 1754-1756
Pemphigoid
  bullous, esophageal manifestations of, 980
  esophageal manifestations of, 980
    imaging of, 1406
  laryngeal involvement in, 887
  mucous membrane (cicatricial)
    esophageal manifestations of, 980
    nasal manifestations of, 660
    ocular scarring (symblepharon) due to, 1233-1234, 1234f
    oral, 1233-1235, 1254
      clinical differential diagnosis of, 1234, 1234t
      clinical features of, 1233-1234, 1233f-1234f
      defined, 1233
      etiology and pathogenesis of, 1233
      histopathologic features of, 1234-1235, 1234f
      treatment of, 1235
  nasal manifestations of, 660
Pemphigus
  paraneoplastic, 1231-1232
  vulgaris
    esophageal manifestations of, 980
    laryngeal and tracheal manifestations of, 887, 887f, 891-892, 892f
    nasal manifestations of, 660
    oral, 1231-1233, 1254
      clinical differential diagnosis of, 1232
      clinical presentation of, 1232, 1232f
      defined, 1231-1232
Pemphigus *(Continued)*
      etiology/pathogenesis of, 1232
      histopathologic features of, 1232-1233, 1232f-1233f
      treatment of, 1233
Pendred syndrome (PS)
  cochlear implant for, 2220
  deafness in, 2051t-2058t, 2083, 2094t, 2096
  genetic testing for, 2098
    in infants, 2723
  inner ear anomalies in, 2735
Pendrin, in thyroid hormone synthesis, 1737
Pendrin *(PDS)* gene, in deafness, 2051t-2058t, 2083
Penetrance, 7, 7f
Penetrating auditory brainstem implant (PABI), 2262, 2262f
Penetrating auditory midbrain implant, 2262-2263, 2263f
Penetrating facial nerve injuries, 2399
Penetrating neck trauma
  airway management for, 1629
  algorithmic approach to, 1631f
  angiography for, 1630-1632, 1631t, 1632f-1633f
  barium swallow for, 1631t, 1633
  classification of, 1628-1629, 1630f
  cranial nerve injury due to, 1629
  diagnostic evaluation of, 1630
  digestive tract evaluation for, 1633-1634, 1634f-1635f
  direct laryngoscopy and bronchoscopy for, 1631t, 1634
  esophagoscopy for, 1631t, 1633-1634, 1634f
  imaging of, 1629-1630
  initial management of, 1629
  management of laryngotracheal injury due to, 1634
  mandatory *vs.* selective exploration of, 1627-1630, 1629t, 1630f, 1631t
  mortality from, 1627-1628, 1629t
  physical properties of objects causing, 1625-1627
    with handgun, 1625
    for knife and stab injuries, 1627
    with rifle, 1626, 1626f-1627f
    with shotguns, 1626-1627, 1628t
  signs and symptoms of, 1626b
  vascular injury due to, 1630-1632, 1631t, 1632f-1633f
    management of, 1632-1633, 1633f-1634f
Penicillin
  adverse reactions to, 102
  for otosyphilis, 2341-2342
  for streptococcal pharyngitis, 2787
Pentoxifylline, and skin flap viability, 1073-1074
PEP (postexposure prophylaxis), for HIV infection, 212, 212t
Pepsin
  in GERD, 896
  in reflux laryngitis, 886, 886f
Peptic esophagitis, 1406
Peptic strictures, 1403, 1404f
Peptostreptococcus spp, acute exacerbation of chronic rhinosinusitis due to, 707
PER (persistent allergic rhinitis), 618
Percentile, 64t
Perceptual evaluation, of voice, 826-831
  auditory, 826-831
    CAPE-V for, 826
    GRBAS for, 826, 827t
    other aspects of, 826-827
    for professional voice, 850
  tactile, 827-831, 828f
  visual, 827
Perchlorate, for hyperthyroidism, 1739t
Percutaneous cricothyrotomy, 114t, 128
Percutaneous injection, for vocal fold medialization, 906, 906f-907f

Perennial allergic rhinitis (PAR), 617-618
and pediatric chronic sinusitis, 2778
Perennial nonallergic rhinitis, 695
Perennial rhinitis, 619b, 695
nonallergic, noninfectious, 695
Performance cancellation, professional voice disorders requiring, 854, 854b
Performance measurement, 76-90
aggregate demand for, 77
anatomy of performance measures in, 82, 83f
definition of quality for, 76-77
engaging in development of, 77-78
implementation of
barriers to, 89
pathway for, 88f
standardization and, 87-89
medical professionalism and, 78-82
board certification and maintenance of certification in, 79-80, 80b-81b
Institute of Medicine in, 81-82
physician education in, 79, 79t
state medical boards and maintenance of licensure in, 80-81
motivation for, 76
process of building coherent system of, 77-78
quality-based or value-based purchasing in, 78
stakeholders in, 79-89, 84t-87t
surgeon's role in, 89
unifying response to demand for, 77-78
Performance Status Scale, 56
Performers, voice disorders in. *See* Professional voice disorders.
Perfusion washout, for flap salvage, 1075
Perfusion zones, 1064-1065, 1065f
Periapical cyst, 1262-1263
lateral, 1263
microscopic features of, 1262-1263, 1262f
radiographic features of, 1262, 1262f
treatment of, 1263, 1263f
Pericardial patch, for tracheal stenosis, 2930, 2931f
Perichondritis
of external ear, 1946, 1948
after otoplasty, 479
Perichondrium, anatomy of, 1944
Pericoronitis, *vs.* myofascial pain dysfunction syndrome, 1284t
Pericranial flap, for cochlear implant, 2238
Periesophageal nodes, anatomy of, 1422f
Perigeniculate region, vulnerability to injury of, 1826f
Perilymph, 1832, 1840
in auditory physiology, 1841f-1842f
Perilymph fistula, 2342-2343
categories of, 2342
due to chronic otitis media, 2342-2343
clinical presentation of, 2342
congenital, 2737-2738, 2737f
imaging of, 2342, 2342f
repair of, 2361-2362
sensorineural hearing loss due to, 2122, 2199
fluctuating, 2199
sudden, 2128
due to small fenestra stapedotomy, 2034
due to temporal bone fracture, 2039
due to trauma, 2342
Perilymph gusher
in evaluation for cochlear implant, 2221-2222
during small fenestra stapedotomy, 2034
Perilymphatic duct, 1853f
Perilymphatic fistula. *See* Perilymph fistula.
Perilymphatic fluid, 1832
Perilymphatic-endolymphatic barrier, 2081, 2082f
Perineurial disruption, 2384-2385
Period, of sound waves, 1838-1839, 1839f
Periodic limb movement disorder (PLMD), 262t, 265
Periodicity, laryngeal videostroboscopy of, 821, 848, 848t
Periodontal cyst, lateral, 1265-1266
microscopic features of, 1265-1266, 1265f
radiographic features of, 1265
treatment of, 1266
Periodontal disease
alcoholism and, 1255
bacterial infections and, 1252
diabetes mellitus and, 1251
heart disease and, 1248
in HIV, 227
during pregnancy, 1256
and stroke, 1250
Periodontal ligament (PDL)
in interdental discrimination, 1207
tactile sensitivity of, 1201-1202, 1202f
Periorbita, 439
Periorbital area, aesthetic considerations and ideals in, 444-447
for brow position, 445, 445f
for eyelids, 445-447, 446f
and upper eyelid ptosis, 446-447, 447f
for midface, 447
Periotic tissue, 1852
Periparotid node, 1298f
Peripheral myelin protein 22 *(PMP22)* gene, in deafness, 2051t-2058t, 2081
Peripheral nerve disorders, chronic aspiration due to, 926b
Peripheral nerve injury, histopathologic classification of, 2384-2385, 2384f
Peripheral nerve sheath tumor, malignant, of neck, 1670-1671
Peripheral nerves neoplasms, of neck, 1663
neurofibromas as, 1663, 1664f
schwannomas as, 1663, 1663f
Peripheral neuropathy, HIV-associated, 223
Peripheral primitive neuroectodermal tumor (PPNET), 2845
Peripheral sensitivity, in gustatory physiology, 1210-1212
Peripheral vestibular apparatus
autonomic supply of, 1854
efferent innervation of, 1854, 1855f
Peripheral vestibular disorder(s), 2328-2345
benign paroxysmal positional vertigo as, 2330-2332
diagnosis of, 2330-2331
findings on examination in, 2330-2331, 2331f
history in, 2330
test results in, 2331
etiology of, 2330
incidence of, 2330
mechanism of, 2330-2332
treatment of
with repositioning, 2331-2332, 2332f
surgical, 2332, 2360-2361, 2360f-2361f
bilateral vestibular hypofunction as, 2344
central *vs.*, 2346, 2347t
clinical relevance of, 2329
Cogan's syndrome as, 2341
compensation for, 2373-2374
dynamic, 2373-2376
static, 2373-2374
enlarged vestibular aqueduct as, 2344, 2344f
epidemiology of, 2329
familial vestibulopathy as, 2343-2344
historical background of, 2329-2330
Meniere's disease as, 2333-2339
diagnosis of, 2335-2337
AAO-HNS criteria for, 2335, 2335t
clinical presentation in, 2335, 2336t
dehydrating agents in, 2337
electrocochleography in, 2337
electronystagmography in, 2337
Peripheral vestibular disorder(s) *(Continued)*
hearing loss and tinnitus in, 2337
heat thrust testing in, 2337
history in, 2335-2337
vestibular evoked myopotentials in, 2337
etiology of, 2334-2335
historical background of, 2333
incidence of, 2333
pathogenesis of, 2333-2334, 2334f
severity of, 2335, 2336t
treatment of, 2337-2339
dietary modification and diuretics in, 2337
endolymphatic sac surgery for, 2126, 2339, 2363-2364, 2364f
intratympanic injection for, 2338-2339, 2338f
labyrinthectomy for, 2339
local overpressure therapy for, 2338
nerve section for, 2339
symptomatic, 2338
vasodilators in, 2337-2338
otosyphilis as, 2341-2342
perilymph fistulas as, 2342-2343, 2342f
superior canal dehiscence syndrome as, 2339-2341, 2339f-2340f
due to trauma, 2343
baro-, 2343
nonpenetrating, 2343
blast, 2343
labyrinthine concussion as, 2343
penetrating, 2343
vestibular neuritis as, 2332-2333
Peripheral vestibular physiology, 2328-2329
Periradicular cyst, 1262-1263
microscopic features of, 1262-1263, 1262f
radiographic features of, 1262, 1262f
treatment of, 1263, 1263f
Peristalsis
esophageal, 954, 955f
diminished, 1399-1400, 1400f-1401f
during pharyngeal swallow, 1216f
Peritoneal dialysis, oral sequelae of, 1255
Peritonsillar abscess, 1407, 1407f
in children, 2788, 2789f
Peritonsillar infections, in children, 2788, 2789f
Peritonsillar space
anatomy of, 203
infections of, 206-207
Permanent threshold shift (PTS), 2121, 2141
Peroxisome proliferator-activated receptor (PPAR), for chemoprevention of oral cancer, 1315
Persistent allergic rhinitis (PER), 618
Personal FM system, 2271
Personal listening devices
in noise-induced hearing loss, 2150-2151
for tinnitus, 2134
Personal noise dosimeter, 2140-2141
Pertechnetate scanning. *See* Technetium-99m (^{99m}Tc) scanning.
PES. *See* Preepiglottic space (PES).
Pes anserinus, 2418-2419, 2419f
PET. *See* Positron emission tomography (PET).
Petroclival fissure, in surgical anatomy of anterior cranial base, 2474
Petroclival sutures, in surgical anatomy of lateral skull base, 2436
Petro-occipital sulcus
anatomy of, 1823f
in surgical anatomy of lateral skull base, 2435f, 2438
Petro-occipital suture, in surgical anatomy of lateral skull base, 2438
Petrosal approach, for posterior fossa neoplasms, 2532t, 2539
advantages and disadvantages of, 2532t, 2539
basic features of, 2539
indications for, 2532t, 2539
technique of, 2539, 2539f

Petrositis, 1975-1977, 1986-1989
anatomic basis for, 1975-1976, 1976f-1977f, 1986-1989
defined, 1986
diagnostic tests for, 1977, 1977f
epidemiology of, 1980t
historical note on, 1975
imaging of, 1986-1987
CT for, 1986-1987, 1988f
MR angiography for, 1989f
MRI for, 1986-1987, 1988f-1989f
management of, 1977
pathogenesis of, 1986
pathology of, 1986-1987
symptoms of, 1976-1977, 1976t, 1987
treatment of, 1987-1989
Petrosphenoid suture, in surgical anatomy of lateral skull base, 2435f
Petrosquamous suture, in surgical anatomy of lateral skull base, 2434, 2436f
Petrotympanic fissure, 1828f, 2010f
Petrotympanic suture, in surgical anatomy of lateral skull base, 2435
Petrotympanic suture line, 1823
Petrous apex
anatomy of, 1822f, 1831, 1975-1976
anterior, 1975-1976, 1976f
carotid artery aneurysms of, 2525, 2527f
and foramen magnum, 1976f
imaging of, 1922-1924, 1924t
with asymmetric pneumatization, 1922-1923, 1924t, 1925f
with cholesteatoma, 1924t
with cholesterol granuloma, 1923, 1924t, 1925f-1926f
with malignant lesions, 1923-1924, 1926f
with mucocele, 1924t
with retained secretions, 1923, 1924t, 1925f
pneumatic, 1976, 1977f
pneumatization of, 1867, 1986
asymmetric, 1922-1923, 1924t, 1925f
vs. neoplasms, 2525, 2526f
via infralabyrinthine cell tract, 1988f
via retrolabyrinthine cell tract, 1988f
via supralabyrinthine cell tract, 1987f
posterior, 1975-1976, 1976f
retained secretions in, 1923, 1924t, 1925f
in surgical anatomy of lateral skull base, 2435f, 2436
transcochlear approach to, 2499-2500, 2500f
Petrous apex access
for lateral cranial base neoplasms, 2508, 2508f
for transnasal endoscopic-assisted anterior skull base surgery, 2481
Petrous apex effusion, 2525
Petrous apex tumor(s), 2524-2526
cephalocele as, 2508
cholesteatoma as, 1924t
drainage of, 2508
cholesterol granuloma as, 2524-2525
differential diagnosis of, 1924t, 2515, 2524t
imaging of, 1923, 1925f-1926f, 2477f, 2526f
chondrosarcoma as, 2528f
chordoma as, 2511f
giant cell tumors as, 2526
malignant, 1923-1924, 1926f
mucocele, mucous retention cysts, and petrous apex effusion as, 1924t, 2524t, 2525, 2526f-2527f
surgical access for
for lateral cranial base neoplasms, 2508, 2508f
for transnasal endoscopic-assisted anterior skull base surgery, 2481
Petrous apicitis, 1975-1977, 1986-1989
anatomic basis for, 1975-1976, 1976f-1977f, 1986-1989
defined, 1986
diagnostic tests for, 1977, 1977f
epidemiology of, 1980t
history of, 1975
imaging of, 1986-1987
CT for, 1986-1987, 1988f
MR angiography for, 1989f
MRI for, 1986-1987, 1988f-1989f
management of, 1977
pathogenesis of, 1986
pathology of, 1986-1987
symptoms of, 1976-1977, 1976t, 1987
treatment of, 1987-1989
Petrous bone, in surgical anatomy of lateral skull base, 2436, 2437f
Petrous bone projection, in surgical anatomy of lateral skull base, 2435f
Petrous fracture, transverse, 174f
Petrous part, of temporal bone, 2010f
anterior surface of, 1822, 1822f
inferior surface of, 1822-1823, 1824f
posterior surface of, 1822, 1823f
Peutz-Jeghers syndrome, oral manifestations of, 1257
PEX7 gene, in Refsum disease, 2096
Peyer's patches, in immune system, 605
Pfeiffer's syndrome, craniofacial anomalies in, 2641t, 2646
PG(s) (prostaglandins)
in acutely raised skin flaps, 1070, 1070f
in bone remodeling, 1973
and skin flap viability, 1073
PGA (polyglycolic acid), in resorbable plating system, for pediatric facial fractures, 2700, 2700t-2701t
PGLs. *See* Paragangliomas (PGLs).
PGS. *See* Paraglottic space (PGS).
pH
intracellular, in sour taste, 1209
salivary, 2384
pH monitoring, esophageal
ambulatory 24-hour, 958-960, 959f-960f
Bravo wireless pH capsule for, 961, 961f
for GERD-related laryngeal disease in children, 2945
multichannel intraluminal impedance for, 962
Restech Dx-pH Measurement System for, 962, 962f
pH probe monitoring, for extraesophageal reflux, 900
PHACES syndrome, 290
hemangioma of infancy in, 2824, 2825f
Phagocyte function disorders, 2114
otologic manifestations of, 2114
Phagocytosis
by monocytes and macrophages, 604
by neutrophils, 604
Phalangeal cells, 1832
Phalangeal processes, 1832, 1832f-1833f
Phantosmia, 633, 636, 639
Pharmacologic toxicity, sensorineural hearing loss due to, 2119-2121
sudden, 2128
Pharyngeal arches, 2659-2660, 2661f
in embryology of nose, 2691f
Pharyngeal cancer, 1412-1415
carcinoma as, 1412-1415
of hypopharynx, 1413, 1413f-1414f
with lymphadenopathy, 1414-1415, 1415f
of nasopharynx, 1412-1413, 1413f
of oropharynx, 1413, 1413f
Pharyngeal constrictors, in breathing, 809
Pharyngeal contraction, during pharyngeal swallow, 1217
Pharyngeal defects, classification of, 1450
Pharyngeal dilators, in breathing, 810, 810f
Pharyngeal disorders, chronic aspiration due to, 926b
Pharyngeal diverticula, 1401-1402, 1402f
dysphagia due to, 2951
Pharyngeal flap, for velopharyngeal dysfunction, 2683
Pharyngeal flap surgery, for obstructive sleep apnea, 2609-2610
Pharyngeal fossa, 1359f
Pharyngeal function, in breathing, 809-810, 810f
Pharyngeal imaging, 1393-1420
with benign neoplasms, 1415-1416
retention cyst as, 1416, 1416f
Tornwaldt cyst as, 1416, 1416f
vs. tortuous internal carotid artery, 1416, 1416f
with diverticula, 1401-1402
laryngoceles as, 1402, 1402f
pharyngeal pouches as, 1401-1402, 1402f
Zenker's, 1401, 1402f
with fistulas, 1409-1411
due to perforation, 1410-1411, 1410f
postoperative, 1411, 1411f
with foreign body, 1411, 1412f
with infection/inflammation, 1403-1407
due to abscess, 1407, 1407f
due to epiglottitis, 1406-1407, 1407f
with malignant neoplasms, 1412-1415
carcinoma as, 1412-1415
of hypopharynx, 1413, 1413f-1414f
with lymphadenopathy, 1414-1415, 1415f
of nasopharynx, 1412-1413, 1413f
of oropharynx, 1413, 1413f
with motility disorder(s), 1398-1399
abnormal deglutition as, 1398
cricopharyngeal dysfunction as, 1398-1399, 1400f
post-treatment, 1416-1418
after laryngectomy, 1416, 1417f
after laryngopharyngectomy, 1416-1418, 1418f
for monitoring and surveillance, 1418, 1419f-1420f
after radiotherapy, 1418, 1418f
radiographic anatomy in, 1397, 1398f-1399f
technique(s) for, 1393-1397
conventional radiography as, 1393, 1394f
CT as, 1396
fluoroscopy as, 1393-1394
modified barium swallow as, 1396
MRI as, 1396
oral contrast agents in, 1396
other nuclear medicine as, 1397
PET-CT as, 1396-1397, 1397f
pharyngoesophagram as, 1394, 1394f-1395f
ultrasound as, 1396
Pharyngeal leak, postoperative, 1411, 1411f
Pharyngeal mucosal space (PMS), imaging of, 148-149
with inflammatory lesions, 148, 148f
with non-Hodgkin's lymphoma, 148-149, 149f
normal anatomy on, 146f, 148-149
with squamous cell carcinoma, 148, 149f
with Tornwaldt cyst, 148
Pharyngeal neoplasm(s)
benign, 1415-1416
esophageal hematoma as, 1416
esophageal leiomyoma as, 1415-1416, 1415f
retention cyst as, 1416, 1416f
Tornwaldt cyst as, 1416, 1416f
vs. tortuous internal carotid artery, 1416, 1416f
malignant, 1412-1415
carcinoma as, 1412-1415
of hypopharynx, 1413, 1413f-1414f
with lymphadenopathy, 1414-1415, 1415f
of nasopharynx, 1412-1413, 1413f
of oropharynx, 1413, 1413f

Pharyngeal nerve, 1297f
Pharyngeal obturator prosthesis, 1343, 1344f
Pharyngeal palsy, unilateral, 1398
Pharyngeal pouch(es)
embryology of, 2583-2585, 2583f-2584f
first, 2584, 2584f-2585f
fourth through sixth, 2584f-2585f, 2585
second, 2584, 2584f-2585f
third, 2584f-2585f, 2585
imaging of, 1401-1402, 1402f
Pharyngeal pressure generation, during pharyngeal swallow, 1217
Pharyngeal recess, in surgical anatomy of anterior cranial base, 2474
Pharyngeal reconstruction, after total laryngectomy, 1569-1570, 1570f
Pharyngeal swallow, 1216, 2948
airway protection during, 1216-1217
cricopharyngeal (upper esophageal sphincter) opening during, 1217
delayed triggering of, 1215
neuromuscular activities in, 1216, 1216f
pharyngeal pressure generation during, 1217
Pharyngeal tonsils, 1359f, 2784
Pharyngeal tubercle, in surgical anatomy of anterior cranial base, 2474
Pharyngeal wall
anatomy of, 1359, 1360f
cancer of
cervical lymph node metastasis of, 1361t
clinical presentation of, 1365
management of, 1370
Pharyngeal wall reconstruction, 1383-1387
algorithm for, 1388f
free flaps for, 1386
with combined lateral and superior defects, 1386, 1387f
lateral arm and thigh, 1386-1387
radial forearm, 1386
healing by second intention for, 1383
local flaps for, 1384-1385
primary closure for, 1383-1384
regional flaps for
pectoralis major, 1385, 1385f
platysmal myocutaneous, 1385
sternocleidomastoid myocutaneous, 1385-1386
temporalis, 1386
temporoparietal fascia, 1386
skin grafting for, 1384
Pharyngectomy, for hypopharyngeal cancer
partial, 1426-1429
via anterior transhyoid pharyngotomy, 1427-1429, 1428f
via lateral pharyngotomy, 1426-1427
via lateral transthyroid pharyngotomy, 1427, 1428f
via median labiomandibular glossotomy, 1429
with total laryngectomy, 1430, 1431f
total, 1430, 1431f
Pharyngitis, 191-200
bacterial, 191-196
due to *Arcanobacterium haemolyticum,* 193
due to *Chlamydia pneumoniae,* 194
due to *Corynebacterium diphtheriae,* 195-196
in children, 2786-2787
due to *Francisella tularensis,* 195
due to group A beta hemolytic *Streptococcus pyogenes,* 191-193
in children, 2787
due to *Mycobacterium tuberculosis,* 195
due to *Mycoplasma pneumoniae,* 194-195
due to *Neisseria gonorrhoeae* (gonococcal), 193-194, 194f
in children, 2786
due to non–group A beta hemolytic streptococcal infections, 193
Pharyngitis *(Continued)*
in children, 2787
complications of, 2788
due to *Treponema pallidum,* 194
in children, 2786
due to *Yersinia enterocolitica,* 196
in children, 2782, 2783f-2784f
due to *Corynebacterium diphtheriae,* 2786-2787
due to *Neisseria gonorrhoeae,* 2786
streptococcal, 2787
due to syphilis, 2786
due to Vincent's angina, 2786
viral, 2785-2786
defined, 191
differential diagnosis of, 191
epidemiology of, 191
etiologies for, 191, 192t
fungal, 199-200
due to *Candida* spp, 199-200
in children, 2786
traumatic, 194, 194f
viral, 196-199
due to adenovirus, 198
in children, 2785-2786
due to common cold (rhinovirus, coronavirus, parainfluenza virus), 196
due to Epstein-Barr virus, 198-199, 198f
due to herpes simplex virus, 199, 199f
due to HIV, 197
due to influenzavirus, 196-197
Pharyngobasilar fascia retropharyngeal, 1359f
Pharyngocele, lateral, 986, 987f-988f
Pharyngoconjunctival fever, 198
Pharyngocutaneous fistula
after hypopharyngeal reconstruction, 1458
due to neck surgery, 1727-1728, 1728f
after total laryngectomy, 1571
after total laryngopharyngectomy, 1575
Pharyngoesophageal defects, classification of, 1450
Pharyngoesophageal (PE) segment, in alaryngeal speech
physiology of, 1596
prevention of hypertonicity of, 1599-1600, 1599f
Pharyngoesophageal webs, 966-967, 967f
imaging of, 1407, 1408f
Pharyngoesophagography, postlaryngectomy, 1416, 1417f-1418f
Pharyngoesophagram, 1394, 1394f-1395f
Pharyngogram, 1394, 1394f
air-contrast, 1394, 1395f
Pharyngo-laryngo-esophagectomy, total, 1574, 1574f
for cervical esophageal cancer, 1430-1431
Pharyngomaxillary space, anatomy of, 202
Pharyngoplasty
transpalatal advancement, for obstructive sleep apnea, 258, 260f
for velopharyngeal dysfunction, 2683
Pharyngostomy, after hypopharyngeal reconstruction, 1458, 1459f
Pharyngotomy
for hypopharyngeal cancer
anterior transhyoid, 1427-1429, 1428f
lateral, 1426-1427
lateral transthyroid, 1427, 1428f
for oropharyngeal cancer
lateral, 1371, 1371f
transhyoid, 1371, 1372f
Pharyngotympanic tube, 2585f. *See also* Eustachian tube.
Pharynx
bacteriology of, 2785-2788
lymphatic drainage of, 2582
motility disorder(s) of, 1398-1399
abnormal deglutition as, 1398
cricopharyngeal dysfunction as, 1398-1399, 1400f
Pharynx *(Continued)*
neurologic evaluation of, 832-836
radiographic anatomy of, 1397, 1398f-1399f
in swallowing, 833
swallowing disorders due to surgery of, 1220
taste buds in, 1208
Phase closure, laryngeal videostroboscopy of, 819-820
Phase shifts, with traditional hearing aid, 2204
Phelps, Peter, 2728-2729
Phenol
structure and function of, 394-395
toxicity of, 395
Phenol block, for neuropathic pain, 245-246
Phenol chemical peels, 394-395
agent for, 394-395
complications of, 396-397
occluded *vs.* nonoccluded, 395
patient preparation and education for, 395
patient selection for, 395
postoperative care after, 396
results of, 396f
technique of, 395
toxicity of, 395
Phenotype, 2088
Phenoxybenzamine, and skin flap viability, 1073
Phentolamine, and skin flap viability, 1073
Phenylephrine
for allergic rhinitis, 620
for rhinosinusitis, 736
Phenylpropanolamine, for rhinosinusitis, 735t, 736
Phenylthiocarbamide (PTC), taste sensitivity to, 1211-1212
Phenytoin, for neuropathic pain, 243
Pheochromocytoma, 120, 1657
preoperative evaluation of, 105
Pheromones, 624, 627-628, 630, 631b
Philtrum, embryology of, 2660, 2662f
Phonation
defined, 833
in geriatric patients, 234-237
acoustic changes in, 236
dental/mandibular changes in, 236
factors affecting vocal quality in, 234, 235t
glandular changes in, 236
histologic changes in, 234-235, 235f
laryngoscopic appearance in, 235-236
mucosal changes in, 236
respiratory changes in, 236
and sense of taste, 236
treatment of, 236-237
process of, 833
in speech, 810-811, 811b, 811f
Phonation threshold pressure, in voice evaluation, 828, 828t
Phoneme-specific velopharyngeal dysfunction, 2679
Phonetically Balanced Kindergarten (PBK) Test, for cochlear implant, 2225
Phonetogram, in acoustic analysis for voice evaluation, 829, 829f, 829t
Phonophobia, with migraine, 2349
Phonotrauma, laryngitis due to, 883-884, 884f
Phosphatase and tensin homolog (PTEN) gene, in thyroid carcinoma, 1753
Phosphate, in saliva, 1139
Phosphate salts, oral, for hyperparathyroidism, 1804
Phospholipase C system, in salivary gland secretion, 1137-1138
Photoaging skin types, 275, 276b, 391, 391t
Photodisintegration, 1033
Photodynamic therapy (PDT)
interventional bronchoscopy with, 1010t
for oral cancer, 1315
for premalignant lesions of larynx, 1491
for recurrent respiratory papillomatosis, 2890t, 2892
for unresectable tracheal tumor, 1621

Photoelectric effect, 1032-1033, 1032f
Photoglottography, for voice evaluation, 835
Photography, prior to rhinoplasty, 514, 515f
Photolysis, fractional, for facial resurfacing, 403t
Photon, 1031
  absorption of, 26, 26f
  spontaneous emission of, 26, 26f
  stimulated emission of, 26, 26f
Photon beams, in radiotherapy, 1033-1034, 1035f
Phrenic ampulla, 1397-1398, 1400f
Phrenic nerve, 2579f
Phrenic nerve injury, 1731, 1731f
Phrenic nerve paralysis, due to neck surgery, 1731
Phrenic nerve paresis, due to neck surgery, 1731, 1731f
Phrenic nerve reinnervation, 917
PHS (Pallister-Hall syndrome), 2874
PHYH gene, in Refsum disease, 2096
Physical examination, 94-101
  of children, 2574
  for chronic rhinosinusitis, 743
  for disorders of professional voice, 851-852, 852t
  of ears, 97-98
    auricles in, 97
    external auditory canal in, 97
    hearing assessment in, 97-98, 98t
    tympanic membrane in, 97, 98f
  of facial skeleton, 95
  of facial trauma, 303-304, 303f
  of facies, 95, 95t
  of general appearance, 95
  of larynx and hypopharynx, 99-100, 99f-100f
    flexible endoscopy in, 100
  of maxillofacial trauma, 323-325
    of lower third, 325
    of middle third, 324-325, 324f
    of upper third, 324
  of nasopharynx, 100-101
  of neck, 95, 96f
    adenopathy in, 95-96
    lymph node regions in, 96-97, 96f
    thyroid gland in, 95
    triangles of, 96-97, 96f
  for nonallergic rhinitis, 699
  of nose, 100
  of oral cavity, 98-99
  of oropharynx, 99, 99f
  of parotid gland, 95
  of skin, 95
Physician Consortium for Performance Improvement (PCPI), 82-87, 84t-87t
Physician education, and performance measurement, 79, 79t
Physician-patient relationship, 78-82
PI(s) (protease inhibitors), 211
Pickwickian syndrome, 251
Picture archival and communication systems (PACS), 138
Piebald syndrome, deafness in, 2051t-2058t
Pierre Robin syndrome, craniofacial abnormalities in, 2630-2631, 2630f
Piezoelectric middle ear implantable hearing aids, 2211-2212
  Esteem-Hearing Implant as, 2211-2212, 2212f
  ossicular coupling in, 2207-2208
  sound transduction and coupling to auditory system with, 2205f
  transducer design for, 2207
Pigeon feeder, 2665, 2665f
Pigmentation changes
  after blepharoplasty, 451
  after chemical peel, 396-397
  after liposuction, 459
  after rhytidectomy, 427
  after skin resurfacing, 451
Pigmented oral mucosal lesions, 1241-1243
  amalgam tattoo as, 1243
    clinical features of, 1243, 1243f
    defined, 1243
    differential diagnosis of, 1243
    etiology of, 1243
    histopathologic features of, 1243, 1243f
    treatment of, 1243
  melanoma as, 1242-1243
    clinical features of, 1242, 1242f
    differential diagnosis of, 1242
    etiology and pathogenesis of, 1241, 1241t
    histopathologic features of, 1242-1243, 1242f-1243f
    treatment of, 1243
  melanotic macules as, 1241
    clinical features of, 1241, 1241f
    defined, 1241
    differential diagnosis of, 1242
    etiology and pathogenesis of, 1241, 1241t
    histopathologic features of, 1242, 1242f
    treatment of, 1243
  mucosal melanocytic nevi as
    clinical features of, 1241
    histopathologic features of, 1242
    treatment of, 1243
Pilar cysts, 289
Pillars
  of Corti, 1832, 1832f
  of facial skeleton, 331, 331f
Pill-induced esophageal injury, 976, 976b, 2941
Pilocarpine, for xerostomia due to radiotherapy, 1048
Pimecrolimus cream, for eczematoid otitis externa, 1956
Pinch test, 445, 446f, 447-448, 448f
Pinched nasal tip, revision rhinoplasty for, 590, 591f-592f
Pincushioning, with local flaps, 366
Pindborg tumor, 1276
  microscopic findings in, 1276
  radiographic findings in, 1276, 1276f
Pinna(e)
  anatomy of, 476-477, 476f
  in sound transmission, 2019
Piriform sinus. *See* Pyriform sinus(es).
Pistol, neck trauma due to, 1625
Piston prosthesis, for otosclerosis
  measurement of, 2031, 2031f-2032f
  placement of, 2031-2032, 2032f
Pitch
  in computed tomography, 131
  disordered perception of, with traditional hearing aid, 2207
Pitch control, 812
Pituitary diseases, oral manifestations of, 1251
Pituitary fossa
  in surgical anatomy of anterior cranial base, 2443f
  in surgical anatomy of middle cranial base, 2445f
Pituitary gland, in surgical anatomy of anterior cranial base, 2473f-2475f
Pituitary hypothyroidism, 1747
Pituitary stalk, in surgical anatomy of anterior cranial base, 2474-2475, 2475f
Pivotal flaps, 343-345
  effective length of, 343, 343f
  interpolated, 344-345, 344f
  rotation, 343-344, 343f
  transposition, 344, 344f
PJVK (pejvakin) gene, in deafness, 2051t-2058t
PLA (polylactic acid), in resorbable plating system, for pediatric facial fractures, 2700, 2700t-2701t
Placebo effect, 61, 62t
Plagiocephaly, synostotic, 2643-2644, 2643f-2644f
  anterior, 2643f
  deformational, 2643f-2644f, 2644
  front-orbital advancement for, 2652-2653, 2653f
  posterior, 2643f
Plain film radiography. *See* Conventional radiography (CR).
Planning tumor volume (PTV), for radiotherapy, 1036, 1044-1045, 1045f
Planum sphenoidale, in surgical anatomy of anterior cranial base, 2442-2443, 2443f, 2471, 2472f
Plaquenil (hydroxychloroquine)
  ototoxicity of, 2176
  sensorineural hearing loss due to, 2120
Plasmablastic lymphoma (PBL), 216
Plasmacytoma
  extramedullary, 2107
    of larynx, 1509
  solitary bone, 2107
Plasmid(s), 15-16, 15f
Plasmid vector, for gene therapy of inner ear, 2191t
Plasmin, in wound healing, 1077
Plasminogen activator, in bone resorption, 1972-1973
Plastic surgery, gene therapy for, 22-23
  with reconstructive tissue flaps and wound healing, 22-23
  with skin grafting, 23
Plasticity, neural. *See* Neural plasticity.
Plastipore, for ossiculoplasty, 2026t
Platelet(s), in adaptive immune system, 605
Platelet count, preoperative evaluation of, 106
Platelet disorders, oral manifestations of, 1256
Platelet glycoprotein IIb/IIIa inhibitor, and skin flap viability, 1074
Platelet-derived growth factor (PDGF), in wound healing, 1076
Plating systems, permanent *vs.* resorbable, for pediatric facial fractures, 2700-2701, 2700t-2701t
Platinum derivatives, in noise-induced hearing loss, 2147
Platybasia, 2355
Platysma, 321f, 442f
Platysmal myocutaneous flap, for oropharyngeal reconstruction, 1377, 1378f
  of tongue base, 1389
  of tonsils and pharyngeal wall, 1385
Play audiometry, for otitis media, 2762
Pleconaril, for rhinosinusitis, 734t
Pleiotropism, 7
Pleomorphic adenoma(s)
  in children, 2819
  of larynx, 881
  of oral cavity, 1291-1292, 1292f
  of parapharyngeal space, 1663-1664, 1665f
  of salivary gland, 1168-1169
    carcinoma ex, 1187-1189, 1188f
    in children, 2861-2862
    clinical features of, 1166f, 1169
    histopathology of, 1169
    imaging of, 1143
      CT for, 1144f, 1148
      MRI for, 1148f, 1167f-1168f, 1180f
      parotid, 150, 150f
      ultrasound imaging, 1149, 1149f
    of lacrimal gland, 1169, 1170f
    malignant transformation of, 1169
    metastasizing, 1189
    of palate, 1169, 1169f
    pathogenesis of, 1168-1169
    recurrent, 1169, 1170f
    sites of, 1169, 1169f-1170f
    submandibular, 1653f
  sinonasal, 718t
PLGA (polymorphous low-grade adenocarcinoma), of salivary glands, 1184-1185, 1186f

Plica aryepiglottica, 1543f
Plica interarytaenoidea, 1543f
Plica stapedis, 1827f
Plica ventricularis, 815t-816t, 853
surgical anatomy of, 1543f
Plica vocalis, 1543f
PLLA (poly L-lactic acid), in resorbable plating system, for pediatric facial fractures, 2700, 2700t-2701t
PLMD (periodic limb movement disorder), 262t, 265
Plummer-Vinson syndrome, 967
and postcricoid carcinoma, 1425-1426
Plumping grafts, for nasal tip projection, 535-536, 536f
Pluripotent stem cells, in adaptive immune system, 599-600, 600f
PMCA2, in deafness, 2051t-2058t, 2080
PML (progressive multifocal leukoencephalopathy), HIV-associated, 223
PMMML (primary mucosal malignant melanoma of the larynx), 1509
PMP22 (peripheral myelin protein 22) gene, in deafness, 2051t-2058t, 2081
PMS. *See* Pharyngeal mucosal space (PMS).
Pneumatic dilation
for achalasia, 964-965
for tracheal stenosis, 2928, 2928f
Pneumatic otoscopy, for acute otitis media, 2761-2762
Pneumatization
of petrous apex, 1867, 1986
asymmetric, 1922-1923, 1924t, 1925f
vs. neoplasms, 2525, 2526f
via infralabyrinthine cell tract, 1988f
via retrolabyrinthine cell tract, 1988f
via supralabyrinthine cell tract, 1987f
of sphenoid sinus, 669, 670f
Pneumocephalus, due to cranial base surgery, 2468
Pneumococcal capsular polysaccharide vaccine (PPV23, Pneumovax), with cochlear implants, 2236-2237, 2237b
Pneumococcal conjugate vaccine (PCV7, Prevnar)
with cochlear implants, 2237, 2237b
to prevent otitis media, 2763, 2768
maternal immunization with, 2768-2769
Pneumococcal polysaccharide–meningococcal outer membrane protein complex conjugate (PncOMPC) vaccine, to prevent otitis media, 2768
Pneumococcal vaccine
to prevent hearing loss, 2161
to prevent otitis media, 2768
maternal immunization with, 2768-2769
Pneumocystis jiroveci
otologic manifestations of, 2114-2115
otomastoiditis due to, immunosuppression and, 222
Pneumolabyrinth, 2737, 2737f
Pneumomediastinum, 1410, 1410f
Pneumonia, aspiration, 1250
Pneumosinus dilatans, 783, 784f
Pneumothorax
due to neck surgery, 1733
tension, *vs.* anaphylactic reaction, 119
Pneumovax (pneumococcal capsular polysaccharide vaccine), with cochlear implants, 2236-2237, 2237b
PNH (polymyxin, neomycin, and hydrocortisone), for otitis externa, 1946, 1952, 1959t-1960t
PnoOMPC (pneumococcal polysaccharide–meningococcal outer membrane protein complex conjugate) vaccine, to prevent otitis media, 2768
Pogonion, in chin analysis, 463, 463f-464f
Point estimate, 65
Point of equilibrium, in radiation, 1033
Poiseuille's equation, 1073, 2897
Poliomyelitis, laryngeal hypofunction due to, 842
Politzer test, of eustachian tube function, 1874
Politzerization, 1870
Pollybeak deformity, 512, 512f, 539, 539f
revision rhinoplasty for, 584-585, 586f
Poly D-lactic acid (PDLA), in resorbable plating system, for pediatric facial fractures, 2700, 2700t
Poly L-lactic acid (PLLA), in resorbable plating system, for pediatric facial fractures, 2700, 2700t-2701t
Polyamide mesh, for nasal reconstruction, 368
Polyarteritis nodosa, sensorineural hearing loss due to, 2124, 2166
Polychondritis, relapsing
laryngeal and tracheal manifestations of, 890
sensorineural hearing loss due to, 2124
Polyclitus, 269
Polydimethylsiloxane. *See* Silicone (polydimethylsiloxane, Silastic).
Polydioxanone (PDS), in resorbable plating system, for pediatric facial fractures, 2700, 2700t
Polyethylene, high-density
for auricular reconstruction, 2744t
for chin implants, 465t
Polyethylene implant, for nasal reconstruction, 368
Polygenic traits, 8
Polyglycolic acid (PGA), in resorbable plating system, for pediatric facial fractures, 2700, 2700t-2701t
Polylactic acid (PLA), in resorbable plating system, for pediatric facial fractures, 2700, 2700t-2701t
Polymer(s), for craniofacial defect repair, 2657
Polymer allografts, for ossiculoplasty, 2006
Polymerase chain reaction (PCR), 8-9
Polymorphic reticulosis, 659-660
Polymorphisms, in DNA repair enzymes, in head and neck squamous cell carcinoma, 1027
Polymorphous low-grade adenocarcinoma (PLGA), of salivary glands, 1184-1185, 1186f
Polymyositis, oral manifestations of, 1252
Polymyxin, neomycin, and hydrocortisone (PNH, Cortisporin Otic Solution), for otitis externa, 1946, 1952, 1959t-1960t
Polyneuropathy, in Bell's palsy, 2391, 2392t
Polyostotic fibrous dysplasia, oral manifestations of, 1257
Polyp(s)
aural, 1965
nasal
endoscopic sinus surgery for, 751-752
olfactory dysfunction due to, 625, 634f
surgical management of, 741
in paranasal sinuses, 676, 678f
vocal fold, 867-869
with capillary ectasia, 868f
in children, 2882
diagnosis of, 868
history in, 868
laryngeal examination in, 868
vocal capability battery in, 868
epidemiology of, 867
pathophysiology and pathology of, 867-868
treatment of, 868-869
behavioral, 868
medical, 868
surgical, 868-869
in vocal professional, 846
Polypeptides, in saliva, 1140
Polypoid granulation tissue, of larynx, 880
Polyposis
sinonasal
in aspirin-exacerbated respiratory disease, 732f
endoscopic sinus surgery for, 751-752
Polyposis *(Continued)*
with methicillin-resistant *Staphylococcus aureus* infection, 733f
surgical management of, 741
vocal fold, 872-873, 872f
diagnosis of, 872
history in, 872
laryngeal examination in, 872
vocal capability battery in, 872
epidemiology of, 872
management of, 872-873
behavioral, 872
medical, 872
surgical, 872-873, 873f
pathophysiology and pathology of, 872
Polyrhinia, 2690-2692
Polysomnography (PSG), for obstructive sleep apnea, 255, 255b, 256f
in children, 2606-2607, 2607f, 2607t, 2794
indications for, 2608
Polytef injection, for vocal fold paralysis in children, 2879
Polytetrafluoroethylene (Teflon), for vocal fold medialization
history of, 905
by injection, 905-906
complications of, 907, 908f
Polytetrafluoroethylene carbon, for nasal reconstruction, 368
Polytetrafluoroethylene (Gore-Tex) implant, for saddle nose deformity, 555, 558f
Polytetrafluoroethylene (Gore-Tex) strip, for medialization thyroplasty, 908, 910, 911f
Polyvinyl alcohol (PVA, PVA Foam, Trufill, Contour Emboli), for embolization, 1933
Pons
in surgical anatomy of anterior cranial base, 2474f
in surgical anatomy of lateral skull base, 2439f
Pontine arteries, 2351f
Pontine-mesencephalic sulcus, in surgical anatomy of lateral skull base, 2439f
PONV (postoperative nausea and vomiting), in children, 2593
Popcorn activity, in facial nerve monitoring, 2547f
Population
accessible, 68, 68t
target, 68, 68t
Porous high-density polyethylene implant, for nasal reconstruction, 368
PORP. *See* Partial ossicular replacement prosthesis (PORP).
Porphyromonas gingivalis, 1252
PORT (postoperative radiation therapy), 1042-1043
Port wine stain, 291, 2832-2833
Porus acusticus
anatomy of, 1822
in surgical anatomy of lateral skull base, 2437-2438
Posaconazole, for fungal rhinosinusitis, 712, 713t
POS-Head/Neck (Patient Outcomes of Surgery–Head/Neck), 57
Positional testing, 2315-2316, 2315f
after vestibular rehabilitation, 2373f-2374f
Positioning template, in microtia reconstruction, 2744-2745, 2745f
Positron, 1031-1032
Positron emission tomography (PET), 137-138
applications of, 144, 145f
for cerebral blood flow evaluation, 2491
with intensity-modulated radiotherapy, 1044
of laryngeal carcinoma, 1494-1495
early glottic, 1517
of nasopharyngeal carcinoma, 1354
of neck masses, 1637, 1637t
of neck neoplasms, 1656-1657
of olfaction, 632

Positron emission tomography (PET) *(Continued)*
of oral cancer, 1300
of oropharyngeal cancer, 1366
of paranasal sinus tumors, 1124
of salivary glands, 1150, 1168
Positron emission tomography/computed tomography (PET/CT), 138
for hypopharyngeal and cervical esophageal cancer, 1424, 1424f
of laryngeal carcinoma, 1470, 1470f, 1494-1495
of neck neoplasms, 1656-1657
of pharynx and esophagus, 1396-1397, 1397f
for tumor recurrence, 1418, 1419f-1420f
Postauricular abscess, 1985, 1985f-1986f
Postauricular approach(es)
to infratemporal fossa, 2495-2500
cervical dissection in, 2495, 2498f
closure of external auditory canal in, 2495, 2497f
extratemporal facial nerve dissection in, 2495-2496
incisions and skin flaps in, 2495, 2497f
radical mastoidectomy in, 2496, 2498f
removal of external auditory canal wall skin and tympanic membrane in, 2495, 2497f
type A, 2497-2499
closure of wound in, 2499, 2499f
exposure of jugular bulb and internal carotid artery in, 2498, 2498f-2499f
facial nerve transposition in, 2497-2498, 2498f
occlusion of sigmoid sinus in, 2498, 2498f
tumor removal in, 2498-2499, 2499f
type B, 2499-2500, 2500f
type C, 2500, 2501f
for mastoidectomy, 2011, 2011f
for tympanoplasty, 2001-2002
Postauricular ecchymosis, 97
Postauricular lymph node, 1360f
Postauricular sulcus, in microtia reconstruction, 2746, 2748f
Postcricoid carcinoma
Plummer-Vinson syndrome and, 1425-1426
total laryngopharyngectomy for, 1573
Postcricoid region, 1421
Posterior ampullary nerve, 1854f, 2278f
Posterior auricular artery, 2580, 2580f
Posterior canal benign paroxysmal positional vertigo (PC-BPPV)
anatomic and physiologic basis for, 2288-2289, 2288f
conversion of, 2332
positional testing for, 2315, 2315f, 2331, 2331f
repositioning maneuver for, 2331-2332, 2332f
surgical treatment of, 2332
Posterior cerebral artery(ies), 2351f
in surgical anatomy of anterior skull base, 2481f
Posterior cervical (PC) space, 158, 159f-160f, 162f
Posterior clinoid process, in surgical anatomy of lateral skull base, 2435f
Posterior commissure scar, 2915, 2916f
Posterior commissure stenosis, 948
Posterior communicating artery, 2351f
Posterior cranial fossa. *See* Posterior fossa.
Posterior cricoarytenoid (PCA) ligament, 1542f
Posterior cricoarytenoid (PCA) muscle
anatomy of
applied, 806, 806f
surgical, 1542f
botulinum toxic injection of, for spasmodic dysphonia, 841f
in breathing, 808-809, 808f
characteristics of, 918
compartmentalization of, 806-807, 807f
reinnervation of, 917-918
Posterior cricoid division, laryngofissure with, for laryngeal stenosis, 2919, 2919f
Posterior ethmoid, prior to endoscopic sinus surgery, 764t
Posterior ethmoid air cells, and internal carotid artery, 671-672
Posterior ethmoid branch, 483f
Posterior ethmoidal artery
anatomy of, 682-683, 1124f
in surgical anatomy of anterior cranial base, 2471-2473, 2472f
Posterior ethmoidal foramen, 322f, 439
Posterior ethmoidectomy, in endoscopic sinus surgery, 747-748, 749f
Posterior facial vein
anatomy of, 1359f
in parotidectomy, 1195-1196, 1195f
Posterior fontanelle, 2618f
Posterior fossa
in surgical anatomy of anterior cranial base, 2475f
in surgical anatomy of lateral skull base, 2435f, 2438-2440, 2439f
Posterior fossa neoplasm(s), 2514-2541
of cerebellopontine angle
acoustic neuroma as, 2514-2517
diagnostic studies of, 2516-2517
imaging of, 2517, 2517t-2518t
natural history of, 2515, 2515f-2516f
signs and symptoms of, 2515-2516
arachnoid cysts as, 2523-2524
chondrosarcomas as, 2527, 2528f-2529f
chordomas as, 2526-2527, 2527f-2528f
common, 2514-2524, 2515b
dermoid tumors as, 2527
differential diagnosis of, 2517t-2518t
facial nerve neuroma as, 2519-2522
diagnostic studies of, 2519-2522
imaging of, 2519-2522, 2521f
signs and symptoms of, 2519
glomus tumors as, 2522-2523, 2523f-2524f
hemangiomas as, 2524, 2525f
lipomas as, 2527, 2529f-2530f
meningiomas as, 2517-2518
diagnostic studies of, 2518
imaging of, 1928, 1928f, 1929t, 2518, 2518t, 2519f-2520f
signs and symptoms of, 2518
metastatic, 2526
other cranial nerve neuromas as, 2522, 2522f
primary cholesteatomas as, 2518-2519
diagnostic studies of, 2519
imaging of, 2519, 2520f-2521f
signs and symptoms of, 2518-2519
teratomas as, 2527
uncommon, 2515b, 2526-2527
differential diagnosis of, 2514, 2515b
intra-axial, 2528-2529
brainstem gliomas as, 2528
hemangioblastomas as, 2528
malignant choroid plexus papillomas and ependymomas of fourth ventricle as, 2528-2529, 2530f-2531f
medulloblastomas as, 2528
meningiomas as
embolization of, 1938
with petrous apex involvement, 2508f
of petrous apex, 2524-2526
vs. asymmetrical pneumatization, 2525, 2526f
vs. carotid artery aneurysms, 2525, 2527f
cholesterol granulomas as, 2524-2525, 2524t, 2526f
giant cell tumors as, 2526
mucocele, mucus retention cysts, and petrous apex effusion as, 2524t, 2525, 2526f-2527f
requiring drainage, surgical approaches for, 2539
infralabyrinthine, 2539, 2540f
middle cranial fossa, 2539
Posterior fossa neoplasm(s) *(Continued)*
transcanal intracochlear, 2539, 2540f
translabyrinthine, 2539
surgical approaches for, 2529-2539, 2532t
combined (petrosal), 2532t, 2539
advantages and disadvantages of, 2532t, 2539
basic features of, 2539
indications for, 2532t, 2539
technique of, 2539, 2539f
complications of, 2540-2541
CSF leaks as, 2540
facial nerve injury as, 2541
involving anteroinferior cerebellar artery, 2540
meningitis as, 2541
ophthalmologic, 2541
with drainage, 2539
infralabyrinthine, 2539, 2540f
middle cranial fossa, 2539
transcanal intracochlear, 2539, 2540f
translabyrinthine, 2539
experimental, 2539
extended middle fossa, 2532t, 2538
advantages and disadvantages of, 2532t, 2538
basic features of, 2538
indications for, 2532t, 2538
surgical exposure in, 2538f
technique of, 2538
middle fossa, 2532t, 2534-2536
advantages and disadvantages of, 2532t, 2536
basic features of, 2534
indications for, 2532t, 2534-2535
surgical exposure in, 2535f
technique of, 2535-2536, 2535f
patient management with, 2540-2541
intraoperative, 2540
postoperative, 2540
preoperative, 2540
retrolabyrinthine, 2532t, 2536
advantages and disadvantages of, 2532t, 2536
basic features of, 2536
indications for, 2532t, 2536
surgical exposure in, 2536f
technique of, 2536, 2536f
retrosigmoid (suboccipital), 2532t, 2533-2534
advantages and disadvantages of, 2532t, 2534
basic features of, 2533
indications for, 2532t, 2533
surgical exposure in, 2533f
technique of, 2534, 2534f
selection of, 2539-2540
transcochlear, 2532t, 2537
advantages and disadvantages of, 2532t, 2537
basic features of, 2537
indications for, 2532t, 2537
surgical exposure in, 2537f
technique of, 2537, 2537f
translabyrinthine, 2530-2533, 2532t
advantages and disadvantages of, 2532t, 2533
basic features of, 2530
indications for, 2530, 2532t
requiring drainage, 2539
surgical exposure in, 2531f
technique of, 2530-2532, 2533f
tumor removal in, 2532-2533
transotic, 2532t, 2537-2538
advantages and disadvantages of, 2532t, 2538
basic features of, 2537
indications for, 2532t, 2537-2538
technique for, 2538, 2538f
vestibular symptoms of, 2354
Posterior glottic gap, laryngeal videostroboscopy of, 819, 820f
Posterior hypopharyngeal wall, 1421
Posterior hypopharyngeal wall carcinoma, total laryngopharyngectomy for, 1573

Posterior incudal ligament, anatomy of, 1827f
Posterior inferior cerebellar artery, 2351f
Posterior lamella, of eyelid, 442
Posterior laryngeal clefts, dysphagia due to, 2952-2953
Posterior lateral nasal artery, in surgical anatomy of anterior cranial base, 2473f
Posterior mallear fold, 1825f
Posterior medial scalene muscle, 2579f
Posterior nasal depth, 2617t
Posterior ostiomeatal unit, 664
Posterior petrous apex (PPA), 1975-1976, 1976f
  pneumatic, 1976, 1977f
Posterior pole, 320f
Posterior semicircular canal
  anatomy of, 2278f
  in surgical anatomy of lateral skull base, 2436f, 2439f
Posterior semicircular canal occlusion, 2360-2361, 2361f
Posterior semicircular duct, 1851f, 1854f
Posterior spiral vein, 1856f
Posterior suspensory ligament, 1751
Posterior triangle, of neck, 2577-2579, 2578f-2579f
  accessory nerve in, 2578-2579, 2580f
  arterial branches in, 2579
  cutaneous branches of cervical plexus in, 2578, 2580f
  fascia in, 2577
    deep, 2577-2578, 2578f-2579f
    superficial, 2577
Posterior triangle dissection, 96, 96f, 1709
Posterior triangle lymph nodes, 1704, 1704f, 1706t-1708t
Posterior vestibular artery, 1854, 1856f
Posterior vestibular vein, 1856f
Posterior wall augmentation, for velopharyngeal dysfunction, 2683-2684
Posterolateral fontanelle, 2618f
Posterolateral neck dissection, 1718-1719
Posterolateral vertical hemilaryngectomy, 1548
Postexposure prophylaxis (PEP), for HIV infection, 212, 212t
Postintubation croup, in children, 2593
Postintubation granuloma(s), 939, 941f
  of vocal folds, 875-876, 875f
    diagnosis of, 875-876
      history in, 875
      vocal capability battery in, 875-876
    epidemiology of, 875
    management of, 876
    pathophysiology and pathology of, 875
Postobstructive pulmonary edema, 119
Postoperative dysphonia, 873-874, 873f
  diagnosis of, 873-874
    history in, 873
    laryngeal examination in, 874
    vocal capability battery in, 873-874
  epidemiology of, 873
  management of, 874
    behavioral, 874
    medical, 874
  pathophysiology and pathology of, 873, 874f
Postoperative epistaxis, 685f
Postoperative management, for children, 2575
Postoperative nausea and vomiting (PONV), in children, 2593
Postoperative neck and face, imaging of, 173-174, 175f-176f
Postoperative radiation therapy (PORT), 1042-1043
Postparotidectomy fistula, 1728
Postpolio syndrome, laryngeal hypofunction due to, 842
Postsaccadic drift, 2308, 2313
Poststreptococcal glomerulonephritis, 2788
Post-styloid compartment, 202
Poststyloid space, 1699
Post-tetanic potentiation, 1884
Posttransplantation lymphoproliferative disorder (PTLD), 213t, 215, 217
  in children, 2818, 2840
Postural balance, lateral vestibulospinal tract in, 1865
Postural control exercises, in vestibular rehabilitation, 2372-2373, 2378-2379
Postural rehabilitation, posturography in, 2326
Postural tone, sudden changes in saccular activity and changes in, 2300
  anatomic and physiologic basis for, 2300
  clinical importance of, 2300
Posture
  in vestibular function, 2308
  vestibular system in maintaining stability of, 2276-2277
    anatomic and physiologic basis for, 2276-2277
    clinical importance of, 2277
  in voice evaluation, 827
Posturography, 2324, 2325f
  dynamic
    for ablative vestibular surgery, 2365
    for vestibular rehabilitation, 2376-2377
  motor control test in, 2324-2325
  sensory organization test in, 2325-2326, 2325f-2326f
  use of, 2326-2327
Potassium (K^+)
  in endolymph homeostasis, 2081-2082, 2084f
  in saliva, 1139
Potassium (K^+) channels, in hair cell transduction, 2073, 2073f
  effects of deficiencies of, 2079-2080
Potassium iodide, saturated solution of
  for Graves' disease, 1742-1743
  for hyperthyroidism, 1739t
Potassium-titanyl-phosphate (KTP) laser, 31t, 33
  for facial resurfacing, 403t
  for recurrent respiratory papillomatosis, 880, 880f, 2891
  for stridulous child, 2908
POU3F4, in deafness, 2051t-2058t, 2083
POU4F3, in deafness, 2051t-2058t
Povidone-iodine (Betadine), for embolization, 1933
Powder insufflator, for ear hygiene or chronic ear drainage, 1958, 1961f
Power
  of statistical test, 65, 66t
  of surgical laser, 27, 29f
Powered microsurgical debrider, interventional bronchoscopy with, 1010t
PPA (posterior petrous apex), 1975-1976, 1976f
  pneumatic, 1976, 1977f
PPAR (peroxisome proliferator-activated receptor), for chemoprevention of oral cancer, 1315
PPIs. *See* Proton pump inhibitors (PPIs).
PPNET (peripheral primitive neuroectodermal tumor), 2845
PPRF (paramedian pontine reticular formation), in velocity-to-position integration, 2296, 2297f
PPS. *See* Parapharyngeal space (PPS).
PPV23 (pneumococcal capsular polysaccharide vaccine), with cochlear implants, 2236-2237, 2237b
Practice performance assessment, 79t
PRAD1 (parathyroid adenomatosis 1 oncogene), in hyperparathyroidism, 1774-1775, 1775f
Pramoxine hydrochloride and hydrocortisone (Pramosone steroid cream), after chemical peel, 396
Preauricular infratemporal approach, 2500-2501, 2501f
Preauricular node, 1297f
Precapillary sphincter, 1066
Precision, 65
Prednisolone, for hemangioma of infancy, 2826-2828
Prednisone
  for autoimmune inner ear disease, 2166
  for Graves' ophthalmopathy, 1811
  for herpes zoster oticus, 1948
  for hyperthyroidism, 1739t
  for otosyphilis, 2341-2342
  for rhinosinusitis, 734t
  for sarcoidosis, 659
  for Wegener's granulomatosis, 658
Preeclampsia, and facial palsy, 2399
Preemptive analgesia, 241
Preepiglottic space (PES)
  anatomy of, 1484, 1484f
    radiographic, 1471f, 1473, 1473f
    surgical, 1542, 1543f
  laryngeal cancer of
    anatomic basis for, 1484, 1484f
    imaging of, 1495
Pregabalin (isobutyl-GABA), for neuropathic pain, 243, 244t
Preglandular node, 1298f
Pregnancy
  facial paralysis in, 2399
  hyperparathyroidism during, 1804
  hypothyroidism during, 1749
  oral health during, 1256
  rhinitis during, 696, 702
  rhinosinusitis during, 737
  thyroid neoplasms during, 1770
Pregnancy gingivitis, 1256
Pregnancy granuloma, 1256
Pregnancy tumor, 1256
Premalignant lesions
  for head and neck cancer, 1061
  of larynx, 1486-1491, 1489f-1490f
    treatment of, 1489-1490, 1490t
      in-office, 1490-1491
  of oral cavity, 1298-1299
Premature infants, anesthesia for, 2595
Prematurity, and otitis media, 2766
Premaxillary bone deformity, in cleft lip, 2666, 2666f
Premedication, for anesthesia in children, 2589
  with congenital heart disease, 2596
Prenatal diagnosis, of cleft lip and palate, 2661-2662, 2663f
Prenatal testing, for sensorineural hearing loss, 2098
Preoperative embolization, for juvenile nasopharyngeal angiofibroma, 1351
Preoperative evaluation, 101-107
  of allergy, 102
  of cardiovascular system, 102
  consent in, 102
  of endocrine disorders, 104-105
    of adrenal gland, 104-105
    diabetes mellitus as, 105
    of parathyroid, 104
    of thyroid, 104
  of hematologic disorders, 105-106
    due to anticoagulants, 105
    congenital, 105
    hemoglobinopathies as, 106
    due to liver failure, 105-106
    thrombocytopenia as, 106
  of hepatic disorders, 103-104
  of neurologic disorders, 106
  of older patients, 106-107
  of renal system, 103
  of respiratory system, 102-103
  routine screening tests in, 101
PRES, in deafness, 2051t-2058t

Presbycusis, 232
  defined, 232
  etiologies of, 232
  inner ear conductive (mechanical), 232, 2126
  neural, 232, 2126
  sensorineural hearing loss due to, 2125-2126, 2126f
  sensory, 232, 2126
  strial (metabolic), 232, 2126
  with tinnitus, 2132
  treatment of, 233
  types of, 232
Presbyesophagus, 1400
Presbyphagia, 237
  diagnostic testing for, 237
  treatment of, 237
Presbyphonia, 234-237
  acoustic changes in, 236
  dental/mandibular changes in, 236
  factors affecting vocal quality in, 234, 235t
  glandular changes in, 236
  histologic changes in, 234-235, 235f
  laryngoscopic appearance in, 235-236
  mucosal changes in, 236
  respiratory changes in, 236
  and sense of taste, 236
  treatment of, 236-237
Presbystasis, 233-234
  defined, 233
  diagnostic methods for, 233
  treatment of, 234
  vestibular pathology of, 233
Preseptal orbital edema, due to rhinosinusitis, 676
Preshunt sphincters, 1066
Pressure changes, and eustachian tube dysfunction, 1872
Pressure flow measurement, for velopharyngeal dysfunction, 2679
Prestin
  in hair cells, 1844
  and outer hair cell motility, 2064-2065, 2068f
Prestyloid compartment, 202
Presyncope, 2346
Pretibial myxedema, and Graves' ophthalmopathy, 1808
Pretrichial forehead lift, 430, 431t
Prevalence, 61
Prevascular node, 1298f
Prevertebral fascia, 202, 2577-2578, 2578f, 2580f
Prevertebral layer, 202
Prevertebral space (PVS)
  anatomy of, 203
  infrahyoid, 158, 159f-160f, 162f
  odontogenic infections of, 186, 186f
  suprahyoid, 146f, 153
Prevnar (pneumococcal conjugate vaccine)
  with cochlear implants, 2237, 2237b
  to prevent otitis media, 2763, 2768
    maternal immunization with, 2768-2769
Primary auditory cortex, 1847
Primary autoimmune inner ear disease, sensorineural hearing loss due to, 2124
Primary ciliary dyskinesia, nasal manifestations of, 661
Primary closure
  of forehead defects, 359-362
  of lip defects, 351
  of nasal defects, 365, 365f
  for oropharyngeal reconstruction, 1376
    of tongue base, 1387-1388
    of tonsil and pharyngeal wall, 1383-1384
Primary mucosal malignant melanoma of the larynx (PMMML), 1509
Primary ostium, of maxilla, 665, 665f
Primo passagio, 851
Primordial cyst, 1265
Probe therapy, in voice evaluation, 831
Proboscis lateralis, 2690, 2692, 2692f
Procerus muscle, 321f, 433f, 441-442, 442f
Processus vocalis, 1543f
Professional accountability, 82
Professional standing, 79t
Professional voice disorders, 844-858
  anatomic considerations with, 845-846
    basement membrane and lamina propria in, 846, 846f
    blood vessels in, 845-846
    cover-body theory of vocal fold vibration in, 845, 845f
  causes of, 852-854
    anxiety as, 853
    extraesophageal reflux as, 852
    laryngeal hygiene as, 852-853
    laryngitis as, 853
    pulmonary disease as, 853
    vocal abuse and misuse as, 853
    vocal fold varices as, 853-854
  evaluation of, 850-852
    history of present illness in, 850-851
    medical history in, 850
    physical examination in, 851-852, 852t
  laryngeal stroboscopy for, 847-849, 848f, 848t
  management of, 854-857
    medical therapy for, 854-855, 854b
    speech language pathologist and vocal pedagogue in, 852, 855
    surgical therapy for, 855-857, 856f-857f
      postoperative care after, 856-857, 858t
  performance cancellation due to, 854, 854b
  types of
    cysts as, 856, 857f
    superficial vocal cord lesions as, 855-856, 856f
    vocal fold varices as, 846-847, 856, 857f
  voice analysis for, 849-850
    acoustic measures in, 849
    aerodynamic measures in, 849
    electroglottography in, 849
    perceptual analysis in, 850
    spectrometry in, 849
    voice outcomes in, 850
  voice production and, 846-847
Professional voice patients, related surgical procedures in, 857-858
Professional voice production, 846-847
Programmable hearing aids, 2267, 2269
  programming of, 2273
Progressive bulbar palsy (PBP), laryngeal disorders due to, 839-840, 842
Progressive multifocal leukoencephalopathy (PML), HIV-associated, 223
Progressive spinal muscular atrophy (PSMA), laryngeal hypofunction due to, 842
Progressive supranuclear palsy (PSP), laryngeal hypofunction due to, 843
Progressive systemic sclerosis (PSS), esophageal manifestations of, 979, 979f
Prokinetic agents
  for extraesophageal reflux in children, 2946
  for GERD, 970
Proliferating cell nuclear antigen (PCNA), in salivary gland neoplasms, 1194
Proliferation phase, of wound healing, 1076-1078
  formation of granulation tissue in, 1077-1078
    angiogenesis in, 1077-1078
    dermal matrix in, 1077
  reepithelialization in, 1076-1077
    keratinocyte migration in, 1076-1077
    keratinocyte proliferation in, 1077
  wound contraction in, 1078
Proliferative verrucous leukoplakia, 1225, 1225f
Promoter(s), of gene expression, 19
Promoter hypermethylation, in head and neck squamous cell carcinoma, 1021
Promotility agents, for extraesophageal reflux, 901
PROP (propylthiouracil), taste sensitivity to, 1211-1212
Propecia (finasteride), for hair loss, 377-378
Proper cochlear artery, 1854, 1856f
Prophylaxis
  antibiotic
    for acute otitis media, 2771
    for burns, 315
    for orthopedic joint patients, 1253, 1253t
    for sinus surgery, 743, 773
    for temporal bone fractures, 2044-2045
  for cluster headaches, 248
  for CSF fistulas, 794
  for migraines, 247
  postexposure, for HIV infection, 212, 212t
  subacute bacterial endocarditis, for pediatric surgery, 2596, 2596t-2597t
  for trigeminal neuralgia, 248
Propofol, for anesthesia induction, 111
  in children, 2590
Propoxyphene, for postoperative pain, 241t
Propranolol (Inderal)
  for hyperthyroidism, 1739t
  for migraine, 2349
  for thyroid storm, 1745
Proptosis
  in Graves' ophthalmopathy, 1808, 1809t
  due to paranasal sinus tumor, 1123-1124
Propylene glycol, for cerumen removal, 1958t
Propylene glycol and acetic acid otic solution (VoSol), for otitis externa, 1946, 1953, 1959t-1960t
Propylthiouracil (PROP), taste sensitivity to, 1211-1212
Propylthiouracil (PTU)
  adverse reactions to, 1742
  for Graves' disease, 1742
  for hyperthyroidism, 1739t
Prosody, in voice evaluation, 826-827
Prospective studies, 61
Prostaglandins (PGs)
  in acutely raised skin flaps, 1070, 1070f
  in bone remodeling, 1973
  and skin flap viability, 1073
Prostate carcinoma, skull base metastases of, 173f
Prosthesis(es)
  ossicular (*See* Ossicular prosthesis(es))
  for velopharyngeal dysfunction, 2681-2682, 2681f-2682f
  voice (*See* Voice prosthesis(es))
Prosthetic ear, 1345-1346, 1345t, 1346f
Prosthetic eye, 1345t, 1346-1347, 1347f
Prosthetic management
  of acquired facial defects, 1344-1345, 1345t
    auricular, 1345-1346, 1345t, 1346f
    nasal, 1345, 1345t, 1346f
    orbital/ocular, 1345t, 1346-1347, 1347f
  of head and neck defects (*See* Maxillofacial prosthodontics)
  of tumor-ablative surgical defects, 1337-1338
    of mandible, 1340, 1341f-1342f
      discontinuity, 1340-1342, 1342f-1343f
    of maxilla, 1338
    of soft palate, 1343-1344, 1344f
    of tongue, 1342-1343, 1344f
Prosthetic maxillary obturation, 1338
  definitive, 1339-1340
    for dentate patients, 1339-1340, 1340f
    for edentulous patients, 1340, 1340f-1341f
  interim, 1339, 1339f
  surgical, 1338-1339
    abutments in, 1338-1339
    impressions for diagnostic casts in, 1338-1339, 1338f
    postoperative radiograph of, 1338, 1338f
    preoperative assessment for, 1338, 1338f
    preservation of support structures in, 1338

Prosthetic maxillary obturation *(Continued)*
removal of packing material and prosthesis in, 1339, 1339f
securing of prosthesis in, 1338-1339, 1339f
skin graft in, 1338-1339
Prosthetic nose, 1345, 1345t, 1346f
Prosthetic obturation
maxillary (*See* Prosthetic maxillary obturation)
for soft palate reconstruction, 1381
Protease inhibitors (PIs), 211
Protection, saliva in, 1140-1141
Protein(s)
formation of, 4, 5f, 11-12, 12f
salivary, 1139-1140, 1139t-1140t
Protein tyrosine phosphatase receptor Q (Ptprq)
and interstereociliary linkages, 2077
in stereocilia, 2076f
Protein tyrosine phosphatase receptor Q *(Ptprq)* gene, in murine deafness, 2058t-2060t
Proteomics, in head and neck squamous cell carcinoma, 1029
Protocadherin-15 (PCDH15), in tip links, 2074
Protocadherin-15 *(PCDH15)* gene, in deafness, 2051t-2058t, 2074
Proton beam radiotherapy, for malignant skull base tumors, 1696
Proton pump inhibitors (PPIs)
for extraesophageal reflux, 901
in children, 2946
for GERD, 970
for laryngoesophageal reflux, 901, 971
for rhinosinusitis, 735t
Proton therapy, 1046
Proto-oncogenes, in head and neck squamous cell carcinoma, 1016, 1019-1020
Protopic (tacrolimus), for eczematoid otitis externa, 1956
Provocation testing
in nonallergic rhinitis, 695-696
objective measurement methods in, 651
Provocative testing, of esophagus, 962-963
Provox 2 anterograde replacement system, 1598f
Provox voice rehabilitation system, 1598f
Proximal esophageal pressure, 958f
Prussak's space, anatomy of, 1826-1827
PS (Pendred syndrome). *See* Pendred syndrome (PS).
PS (parotid space)
anatomy of, 203
imaging of, 149-150, 150f-151f
P_s (subglottic air pressure)
in professional voice production, 846
in voice evaluation, 828, 828t, 849
PSCC (papillary squamous cell carcinoma), of larynx, 1506
Pseudallescheria boydii, invasive fungal rhinosinusitis due to, 705
Pseudoaneurysms
embolization of, 1942, 1943f
due to radiotherapy, 1049
Pseudoarthrosis, 331, 339-340
Pseudobulbar palsy (PBP), laryngeal disorders due to, 839-840, 842
Pseudodiverticula, esophageal, 975, 975f
imaging of, 1406, 1407f
Pseudoephedrine, for rhinosinusitis, 736
Pseudoepiglottitis, postlaryngectomy, 1416, 1417f
Pseudoepitheliomatous hyperplasia (PEH), of larynx, 1493
Pseudohypoacusis
evaluation of, 1901
sensorineural hearing loss due to, 2125
Pseudohypoparathyroidism, oral manifestations of, 1251
Pseudomembranous candidiasis, 1230, 1230f
in HIV, 225, 226f
Pseudo-membranous croup. *See* Bacterial tracheitis.
Pseudomonas aeruginosa, otitis externa due to, 1945, 2194-2195
malignant, 1947
Pseudoretropharyngeal mass, 1462, 1463f
Pseudosarcoma, of larynx, 1506
Pseudosulcus, due to extraesophageal reflux, 897
Pseudotumor(s)
cerebri, CSF rhinorrhea due to, 787
of masticator space, 152
Pseudovallecula, prevention of formation of, 1599-1600, 1601f
PSG (polysomnography), for obstructive sleep apnea, 255, 255b, 256f
in children, 2606-2607, 2607f, 2607t, 2794
indications for, 2608
PSMA (progressive spinal muscular atrophy), laryngeal hypofunction due to, 842
PSP (progressive supranuclear palsy), laryngeal hypofunction due to, 843
PSS (progressive systemic sclerosis), esophageal manifestations of, 979, 979f
Psychiatric disorders, olfactory dysfunctions in, 636
Psychogenic disorders, sensorineural hearing loss due to, 2129
Psychological distress, palliative care for, 1103-1104
Psychological effects, of radiotherapy, 2626t
Psychometric validation, 55
Psychotherapeutic agents, oral sequelae of, 1247t-1248t
Psychotropic medications, in palliative care, 1104
PTA (pure-tone average), 1888-1889
PTC (phenylthiocarbamide), taste sensitivity to, 1211-1212
PTEN (phosphatase and tensin homolog) gene, in thyroid carcinoma, 1753
Pterygoid hamulus, 1297f, 1360f
Pterygoid muscle, 1320
Pterygoid plate, 1124f
Pterygoid plate fractures, 171f
Pterygoid process, 2445f
Pterygoid venous plexus, 2441
Pterygomandibular involvement, in odontogenic infections, 184, 185f
Pterygomaxillary fissure, 2441
Pterygomaxillary fossa, 2435f
Pterygopalatine fossa
anatomy of, 1699
in surgical anatomy of anterior cranial base, 2473
Pterygopalatine ganglion
anatomy of, 1297f
in surgical anatomy of anterior cranial base, 2473
PTH. *See* Parathyroid hormone (PTH).
PTLD (posttransplantation lymphoproliferative disorder), 213t, 215, 217
in children, 2818, 2840
Ptosis
brow, 445, 445f
of chin, 465, 466f
of nasal tip, 484, 485f
caudal extension graft for, 576, 576f
due to overaggressive resection of caudal septum, 492, 492f
revision rhinoplasty for, 590-593, 593f
after rhinoplasty, 519, 520f
of upper eyelid
evaluation of, 446-447, 447f
repair of, 447-448, 447f-449f
Ptprq (protein tyrosine phosphatase receptor Q)
and interstereociliary linkages, 2077
in stereocilia, 2076f
Ptprq (protein tyrosine phosphatase receptor Q) gene, in murine deafness, 2058t-2060t
PTS (permanent threshold shift), 2121, 2141
PTU (propylthiouracil)
adverse reactions to, 1742
for Graves' disease, 1742
for hyperthyroidism, 1739t
PTV (planning tumor volume), for radiotherapy, 1036, 1044-1045, 1045f
Puberty, oral health during, 1256
Pull-through technique, as mandible-sparing procedure, 1311, 1312f-1313f
Pulmonary artery anomalies, tracheal compression due to, 2926
Pulmonary diseases
oral manifestations of, 1250-1251
professional voice disorders due to, 853
Pulmonary edema
after adenotonsillectomy, 2800
postobstructive, 119
Pulmonary function, in geriatric patients, 236
Pulmonary function testing
for airway stenosis, 944, 945f
in children, 2917
preoperative, 103
for tracheal neoplasms, 1616
Pulmonary hypertension, due to obstructive sleep apnea, in children, 2604
Pulmonary vascular resistance, factors influencing, 2597, 2597t
Pulpitis, *vs.* myofascial pain dysfunction syndrome, 1284t
Pulse sequences, for MRI, 133-137, 135f-136f
Pulsed dye laser (PDL), 30
585-nm, 31t, 33
for facial resurfacing, 403t
for premalignant lesions of larynx, 1490-1491
for recurrent respiratory papillomatosis, 880, 880f, 2891
for stridulous child, 2908
Pulsion diverticula, 986
Punch biopsy, for skin lesions, 293
Punnett squares, 2088, 2089f
Pure tone, 1838-1839
Pure-tone audiometry, 1888, 1888f
air-conduction testing in, 1888
masking for, 1889-1890
errors in, 1901-1902
bone-conduction testing in, 1888, 1888f-1889f
for conductive hearing loss, 2020, 2020f
for sensorineural hearing loss, in adults, 2117
Pure-tone average (PTA), 1888-1889
Pure-tone Stenger test, 1901
Purkinje cells, in modification of vestibuloocular reflex, 2301, 2301f
Purkinje, Jan E., 2329
PVA (polyvinyl alcohol), for embolization, 1933
PVA Foam (polyvinyl alcohol), for embolization, 1933
pVHI (Pediatric Voice Handicap Index), 2876
PVOS (Pediatric Voice Outcomes Survey), 57, 2876
PVQOL (Pediatric Voice-Related Quality-of-Life survey), 57, 2876
PVS. *See* Prevertebral space (PVS).
Pyogenic granuloma, 290
of oral cavity, 1256, 1289, 1289f
on septum, 685f
Pyramidal eminence
anatomy of, 1825-1829, 1827f
in surgical anatomy of lateral skull base, 2436f
Pyramidal lobe, of thyroid gland, 1751, 1751f
Pyriform aperture, 641f
edge of, 509f
Pyriform aperture stenosis, congenital nasal, 2692-2693
clinical presentation of, 2692-2693
diagnosis of, 2693, 2693f
operative management of, 2693, 2693f
pathogenesis of, 2690, 2692
Pyriform sinus(es)
anatomy of, 1421, 1422f
radiographic, 1397, 1463f, 1471f, 1472
lymphatic drainage from, 1422, 1422f

Pyriform sinus carcinoma, 162f
advanced, 1438-1439
chemotherapy for, 1439
quality of life with, 1439
imaging of, 1413f, 1423-1424, 1424f, 1475-1476, 1478f
surgical management of
endoscopic CO_2 laser resection for, 1429-1430, 1442
outcomes of, 1436-1438
partial laryngopharyngectomy for, 1429, 1430f
partial pharyngectomy for, 1426-1429
via anterior transhyoid pharyngotomy, 1427-1429, 1428f
via lateral pharyngotomy, 1426-1427
via lateral transthyroid pharyngotomy, 1427, 1428f
via median labiomandibular glossotomy, 1429
supracricoid hemilaryngopharyngectomy for, 1429, 1436
total laryngectomy with partial/total pharyngectomy for, 1430, 1431f
total laryngopharyngectomy for, 1573-1574
Pyriform sinus mucosa, in arytenoid adduction, 915
Pyrosis, 954

Q

Q (quality factor), of radiation, 133
QALY (quality-adjusted life-year), costs per, for cochlear implants
in adults, 2251, 2252t
in children, 2252-2253, 2253f
QASC (Quality Alliance Steering Committee), 84t-87t
QIOs (quality improvement organizations), 84t-87t
QOL. *See* Quality of life (QOL).
QOLRAD (Quality of Life in Reflux and Dyspepsia), 57-58
QSQ (Quebec Sleep Questionnaire), 57
Q-switched laser, 34
Q-switched Nd:YAG laser, for facial resurfacing, 403t
Quadrangular cartilage, of nose, 496
reduction of overlong caudal, 513f
Quadrangular cerebellar lobule, in surgical anatomy of lateral skull base, 2439f
Quadrangular membrane, surgical anatomy of, 1541-1542, 1542f-1544f
Quadratus, 321f
Quadrilateral cartilage, 482
in septoplasty, 490
Quality, definition of, 76-77
Quality Alliance Steering Committee (QASC), 84t-87t
Quality factor (Q), of radiation, 133
Quality improvement. *See* Performance measurement.
Quality improvement organizations (QIOs), 84t-87t
Quality of life (QOL)
cochlear implants and, 2251
in adults and elderly, 2251-2252, 2252f, 2252t
in children, 2252-2253, 2253f
with hypopharyngeal or cervical esophageal cancer, 1439
with otitis media, 2773
as outcome measure, 55
with rhinosinusitis, 730, 730t
after stereotactic irradiation of vestibular schwannoma, 2564-2565
Quality of Life in Reflux and Dyspepsia (QOLRAD), 57-58
Quality of Well Being (QWB), 56
Quality-adjusted life-year (QALY), costs per, for cochlear implants
in adults, 2251, 2252t
in children, 2252-2253, 2253f
Quality-based purchasing, 78
Quebec Sleep Questionnaire (QSQ), 57
Quid, and oral cancer, 1294, 1365
Quinine
ototoxicity of, 2176
sensorineural hearing loss due to, 2120, 2176
Quinolones, for rhinosinusitis, 734t, 736
Quivering mutation, 2081
QWB (Quality of Well Being), 56

R

RA (rheumatoid arthritis)
laryngeal and tracheal manifestations of, 891, 891f
oral manifestations of, 1253, 1253t
of temporomandibular joint, 1281t, 1282
Racemic epinephrine, for croup, 2806
postintubation, 2593
Racial differences, in otitis media, 2766
Rad, 132-133, 1031, 1033
Radial forearm free flap (RFFF)
fasciocutaneous, 1082t, 1083, 1083f
for hypopharyngeal and esophageal reconstruction, 1433, 1455
for oropharyngeal reconstruction, 1379, 1379f
tubed, 1087, 1091f
for oral cancer, 1316
for oropharyngeal reconstruction, 1379, 1379f
of soft palate, 1382, 1383f
of tongue base, 1389
of tonsils and pharyngeal wall, 1386
osteocutaneous, 1082t, 1085-1086, 1086f-1087f
for mandibular defects, 1324-1325, 1325t
after total laryngopharyngectomy, 1574, 1574f-1575f
Radiation
characteristics of, 1031, 1031f-1032f
defined, 1031
electromagnetic, 1031, 1031f
ionizing, 1032, 1036
particulate (corpuscular), 1031
spontaneous emission of, 26, 26f
stimulated emission of, 26, 26f
Radiation absorbed dose, 132-133
Radiation damage
gene therapy for, 23
mechanisms of, 1036-1043, 1037f
Radiation dose, 1033
Radiation dose equivalent, 133
Radiation esophagitis, 1406
Radiation exposure, 132-133, 133t
and parathyroid neoplasms, 1775
and salivary gland neoplasms, 1163
sensorineural hearing loss due to, 2122
and skin flap survival, 1075
and thyroid carcinoma, 1753
Radiation fractionation, 1040
Radiation physics, 1031-1033
characteristics of radiation in, 1031, 1031f
deposition of dose in, 1033
deposition of energy in, 1033
interactions of x-rays with matter in, 1032-1033, 1032f
coherent scattering as, 1032
Compton scattering as, 1032f, 1033
pair production as, 1032f, 1033
photodisintegration as, 1033
photoelectric effect as, 1032-1033, 1032f
radiation production in
from linear accelerators, 1032-1033
by radioactive decay, 1031-1032
Radiation production
from linear accelerators, 1032-1033
by radioactive decay, 1031-1032
Radiation therapy (RT), 1030-1050
abnormal facial growth and development due to, 2622-2623, 2626t
adjuvant
for advanced-stage glottic cancer, 1584-1585, 1584t
for salivary gland neoplasms, 1197-1198, 1198t
advanced technologies in, 1043-1047
brachytherapy as, 1047
imaging-guided, 1043, 1046-1047
intensity-modulated, 1043-1046, 1044f
advantages of, 1043
clinical results of, 1045-1046, 1045f
defining target in, 1044
inverse planning in, 1043
number and directions of beams in, 1045
selection and outlining of targets in, 1044-1045, 1045f
neutron and carbon ion therapy as, 1046
proton therapy as, 1046
basic physics of, 1031-1033
characteristics of radiation in, 1031, 1031f
deposition of dose in, 1033
deposition of energy in, 1033
interactions of x-rays with matter in, 1032-1033, 1032f
coherent scattering as, 1032
Compton scattering as, 1032f, 1033
pair production as, 1032f, 1033
photodisintegration as, 1033
photoelectric effect as, 1032-1033, 1032f
radiation production in
from linear accelerators, 1032-1033
by radioactive decay, 1031-1032
brachytherapy for, 1036, 1047
interventional bronchoscopy with endobronchial, 1010t
maxillofacial prosthodontics in, 1332, 1335f
for oral cancer, 1314, 1314f
for unresectable tracheal tumor, 1621
for carotid paragangliomas, 1661
for cervical lymph node metastases
of hypopharyngeal tumors, 1689t
indications for neck node dissection after, 1694
of laryngeal tumors, 1690t
late complications of, 1694-1695
with N0 status, 1688, 1690, 1692, 1692t
with N1-N3 status, 1692-1695
of nasopharyngeal tumors, 1690, 1690t
neck control after, 1692-1693, 1693t
of oral cavity tumors, 1689t
of oropharyngeal tumors, 1689t
postoperative, 1693-1694, 1694t
retropharyngeal, 1688
target volumes for, 1688-1690
delineation of, 1690-1691, 1691f
for hypopharyngeal tumors, 1689t
for laryngeal tumors, 1690t
for nasopharyngeal tumors, 1690, 1690t
for oral cavity tumors, 1689t
for oropharyngeal tumors, 1689t
techniques for, 1691, 1692f
with chemotherapy (*See* Chemoradiation therapy (CRT))
conservation laryngeal surgery and, 1559-1560
in conventional medicine, 1033-1036
brachytherapy for, 1036
energy of x-rays used in, 1033-1036
external beam radiation for, 1033
treatment aspects of, 1035-1036
linear accelerators in, 1034
block diagram of, 1034f
megavoltage x-rays produced by, 1034
orthovoltage x-rays produced by, 1034
photograph of, 1035f
particle beams in, 1034-1035, 1035f
treatment planning for, 1036

Radiation therapy (RT) *(Continued)*
for cranial base tumors, 1695-1700
anterior, 1697-1699
benign, 2557-2566
cystic schwannomas as, 2563
dose selection for, 2558
facial nerve outcomes with, 2563
fractionation *vs.* nonfractionation of, 2558-2559, 2561t
gamma knife–based, 2559t
hearing outcomes with, 2562-2563, 2562t
hydrocephalus due to, 2563
imaging for, 2558
jugular foramen schwannomas as, 2565
LINAC-based, 2560t
neurofibromatosis 2–related vestibular schwannoma as, 2563
outcome assessment with, 2559-2563
paraganglioma as, 2565, 2565t
principles of, 2557-2558, 2558f
quality of life with, 2564-2565
radiobiology of, 2558
treatment of failures of, 2564
trigeminal nerve outcomes with, 2563
tumor control with, 2562
vestibular schwannomas as, 2558, 2560f
with chemotherapy, 1700
complications after, 1700
malignant, 1695-1700
anterior, 1697-1699
with chemotherapy, 1700
chordoma/chondrosarcoma as, 1699
complications after, 1700
CyberKnife, 1696
esthesioneuroblastoma as, 1697-1698, 1698f, 1698t
intensity-modulated, 1696-1697
middle, 1699-1700
nasopharyngeal carcinoma as, 1699-1700, 1699f, 1700t
proton beam, 1696
sinonasal undifferentiated carcinoma as, 1698-1699
stereotactic, 1696, 1700
middle, 1699-1700
dental management after, 1333-1337
with conventional 3D conformal radiation therapy, 1333-1335, 1336f
with intensity-modulated radiation therapy, 1335-1337, 1336f-1337f
ipsilateral *vs.* contralateral, 1335
dental management during, 1333
dental management prior to, 1330-1331, 1330b, 1331f, 1579
for esophageal carcinoma, preoperative, 1444
facial moulage recording and bolus fabrication for, 1331, 1332f
and facial nerve rehabilitation, 2420
four Rs of, 1039-1040, 1039f
for Graves' ophthalmopathy, 1811
for hard palate malignancy, 1310
high-dose-rate, 1047
historical background of, 1031
for hypopharyngeal cancer, 1433, 1443, 1589-1592
advanced-stage, 1591-1592
complications of, 1591
CyberKnife stereotactic approach for, 1592
future strategies and directions for, 1592
outcome and prognostic factors for, 1591
RADPLAT approach for, 1592
techniques and dose-fractionation schemes for, 1591
anatomic considerations in, 1578-1579, 1579f

Radiation therapy (RT) *(Continued)*
early-stage, 1590-1591
complications of, 1591
outcome and prognostic factors for, 1591, 1591t
techniques and dose-fractionation schemes for, 1590-1591
lymphatic drainage and, 1578-1579, 1579f
overview of, 1578
recurrent, 1591-1592
therapeutic outcome of, 1436
hypothyroidism after, 1747
imaging-guided, 1043, 1046-1047
intensity-modulated, 1043-1046, 1044f
advantages of, 1043
for cervical metastases, 1691-1692, 1692f
clinical results of, 1045-1046, 1045f
complications of, 1700
defining target in, 1044
dental management after, 1335-1337, 1336f-1337f
forward-planning, 1696-1697
for glottic cancer, 1585-1586
inverse-planning, 1043, 1696-1697
for malignant skull base tumors, 1696-1697
for nasopharyngeal carcinoma, 1045, 1699-1700, 1699f, 1700t
number and directions of beams in, 1045
selection and outlining of targets in, 1044-1045, 1045f
and xerostomia, 1103
intraoral positioning devices for, 1331, 1333f
for laryngeal cancer, 1577-1593
advanced glottic, 1497, 1583-1588
balancing cure, organ preservation, and quality of life with, 1583-1584
with chemotherapy, 1584-1586, 1584t
complications of, 1587-1588
dose-fractionation schemes for, 1586, 1586t
general principles of, 1585-1586
mini-mantle field technique for, 1586
outcomes and prognostic factors for, 1586-1587, 1587t
patient setup for, 1586
postoperative (adjuvant), 1584-1585, 1584t
shrinking-field technique for, 1586, 1587f
with targeted biologic agents, 1585
advanced supraglottic, 1589
outcomes and prognostic factors for, 1589, 1590t
techniques and dose-fractionation schemes for, 1589
anatomic considerations with, 1578-1579, 1578f
with anterior commissure involvement, 1496-1497
CyberKnife stereotactic approach for, 1592
early glottic, 1519-1520, 1581
complications of, 1583
effectiveness of, 1496
local control with, 1519, 1522f
outcome and prognostic factors for, 1581-1583, 1582t-1583t
recurrence after, 1522t
results of, 1519, 1521t
techniques and dose-fractionation schemes for, 1580-1590, 1581f-1582f
early supraglottic, 1496, 1588-1589
complications of, 1589
outcomes and prognostic factors for, 1589, 1589t
techniques and dose-fractionation schemes for, 1588-1589
future strategies and directions for, 1592
lymphatic drainage and, 1578-1579, 1579f
with nodal metastases, 1498
overview of, 1578

Radiation therapy (RT) *(Continued)*
RADPLAT approach for, 1592
recurrence after, 1476-1479, 1522, 1522t
recurrent, 1591-1592
subglottic, 1589-1590
with trasoral laser microsurgery, 1532-1533
laryngeal stenosis due to, 2915
Marx hyperbaric oxygen regimen after, 1333
for maxillary sinus tumor, 1128-1130
with maxillectomy, 1128
maxillofacial prosthetics and, 1330
dental diagnoses and oral surgical management prior to, 1330-1331, 1330b, 1331f
dental management after, 1333-1337
with conventional 3D conformal radiation therapy, 1333-1335, 1336f
with intensity-modulated radiation therapy, 1335-1337, 1336f-1337f
ipsilateral *vs.* contralateral, 1335
dental management during, 1333
overview of interactions of, 1337-1344
prosthodontic support of radiation oncologist in, 1331-1332
with brachytherapy, 1332, 1335f
for facial moulage recording and bolus fabrication, 1331, 1332f
intraoral positioning devices in, 1331, 1333f
for portals and shielding devices, 1331-1332, 1334f
shelf for tissue-equivalent material in, 1332, 1335f
for melanoma, 1118
for nasopharyngeal carcinoma, 1354-1355
intensity-modulated, 1045, 1699-1700, 1699f, 1700t
of neck
radiographic appearance after, 1476-1479
for salivary gland neoplasms, 1198
neck after, 173-174, 176f
neck dissection after, 1694, 1721
neutron beam, for salivary gland neoplasms, 1198-1199
for oral cancer, 1314
brachytherapy as, 1314, 1314f
external beam, 1314
package time for, 1314
oral treatment considerations with, 1246t
postoperative, 1042-1043
for premalignant lesions of larynx, 1490
prosthetic voice rehabilitation and, 1600, 1602b
proton beam, for malignant skull base tumors, 1696
radiobiology in, 1036-1043, 1037f
cell cycle arrest in, 1037, 1037f
cell survival in, 1037-1039, 1038f
clinical applications of, 1040-1043
with concomitant chemotherapy, 1041-1043
hypoxia in, 1041
radiation fractionation as, 1040
radiosensitizers as, 1040-1043
mitotic death in, 1037
radiosensitivity in, 1037
tissue-radiation characterizations in, 1039-1040, 1039f
radiographic appearance of pharynx and esophagus after, 1418, 1418f
for rhabdomyosarcoma, 2841-2842
and salivary gland neoplasms, 1163
for salivary gland neoplasms, 1197-1199
adjuvant, 1197-1198, 1198t
in children, 2863
of neck, 1198
neutron beam, 1198-1199
shelf for tissue-equivalent material in, 1332, 1335f
shielding devices for, 1331-1332, 1334f
side effects of, 1047-1049

Radiation therapy (RT) *(Continued)*
acute, 1047
dermatitis as, 1047
mucositis as, 1047, 1047f
xerostomia as, 1047
late toxicities as, 1048-1049
fibrosis as, 1048
neurologic complications as, 1049
osteoradionecrosis as, 1048
thyroid dysfunction as, 1048
vascular complications as, 1048-1049
xerostomia as, 1048
and skin flap survival, 1075
stereotactic
for benign skull base tumors, 2557-2566
cystic schwannomas as, 2563
dose selection for, 2558
facial nerve outcomes with, 2563
fractionation *vs.* nonfractionation of, 2558-2559, 2561t
gamma knife–based, 2559t
hearing outcomes with, 2562-2563, 2562t
hydrocephalus due to, 2563
imaging for, 2558
jugular foramen schwannomas as, 2565
LINAC-based, 2560t
neurofibromatosis 2–related vestibular schwannoma as, 2563
outcome assessment with, 2559-2563
paraganglioma as, 2565, 2565t
principles of, 2557-2558, 2558f
quality of life with, 2564-2565
radiobiology of, 2558
treatment of failures of, 2564
trigeminal nerve outcomes with, 2563
tumor control with, 2562
vestibular schwannomas as, 2558, 2560f
CyberKnife
for laryngeal and hypopharyngeal cancer, 1592
for malignant skull base tumors, 1696
defined, 1696, 2557
dose selection for, 2558
history of, 1696
imaging for, 2558
for malignant skull base tumors, 1696, 1700
principles of, 2557-2558, 2558f
radiobiology of, 2558
swallowing disorders due to, 1219
with targeted biologic agents, 1054, 1055f
for laryngeal cancer, 1585
and taste, 1214
three-dimensional conformal, 1043
for cervical metastases, 1691-1692
for glottic cancer
advanced-stage, 1585-1586
early-stage, 1581, 1581f-1582f
for thyroid cancer, 1772
Radiation-guided parathyroidectomy. 1793
Radiation-induced fibrosis (RIF), 1048
Radiation-induced thyroid follicular necrosis, 1744
Radical maxillectomy, 1125-1126, 1125f
Radical neck dissection (RND), 1705-1709
anterior triangle dissection in, 1709-1710
defined, 1703t, 1705, 1709f
dissection of upper neck compartments in, 1710-1711
flap elevation in, 1709, 1711f
historical perspective on, 1702-1703
incision planning for, 1709, 1710f
indications for, 1705
modified, 1711-1712
definition of, 1703t, 1711, 1712f
historical perspective on, 1703
indications for, 1711
for oral cancer, 1313
Radical neck dissection (RND) *(Continued)*
results of, 1721
technique for, 1711-1712, 1713f-1714f
nodular masses at site of, 1476
for oral cancer, 1313
positioning for, 1709
posterior triangle dissection in, 1709
results of, 1721
Radicular cyst, 1262-1263
lateralized (lateral), 1263
microscopic features of, 1262-1263, 1262f
radiographic features of, 1262, 1262f
treatment of, 1263, 1263f
Radiesse dermal filler (calcium hydroxyapatite), for vocal fold medialization, 906
Radioactive decay, radiation production by, 1031-1032
Radioactive iodine (^{131}I)
for Graves' disease, 1743
for Graves' ophthalmopathy, 1810
stunning with, 1771
after thyroid surgery, 1771-1772
for toxic multinodular goiter, 1745
for toxic thyroid adenoma, 1744
Radioactive iodine uptake test, 1741
Radioactivity, 1031-1032
Radiobiology, 1036-1043, 1037f
cell cycle arrest in, 1037, 1037f
cell survival in, 1037-1039, 1038f
clinical applications of, 1040-1043
with concomitant chemotherapy, 1041-1043
hypoxia in, 1041
radiation fractionation as, 1040
radiosensitizers as, 1040-1043
defined, 1036
mechanisms of damage in, 1036-1043, 1037f
mitotic death in, 1037
radiosensitivity in, 1037
of stereotactic radiation therapy, 2558
tissue-radiation characterizations in, 1039-1040, 1039f
Radiofrequency neurotomy, for neuropathic pain, 246
Radiofrequency tongue base ablation (RFA), for obstructive sleep apnea, 259
Radiofrequency tonsil reduction, for obstructive sleep apnea, 2609
Radionuclide scintigraphy, 138, 139f
for CSF rhinorrhea, 790
of neck masses, 1637, 1637t
of salivary glands, 138, 1150
of thyroid nodule, 1757-1758
Radiosensitivity, 1037
Radiosensitizers, 1040-1043
Radiotherapy. *See* Radiation therapy (RT).
Radix graft, improperly placed, revision rhinoplasty for, 584
Radixin, in stereocilia, 2075-2076, 2076f
Radixin *(RDX)* gene, in deafness, 2051t-2058t, 2075-2076
RADPLAT regimen, 1054
for laryngeal and hypopharyngeal cancer, 1592
RALP (right anterior–left posterior) semicircular canal plane, 2285, 2286f, 2287
Ramsay Hunt syndrome, 1948. *See also* Herpes zoster oticus.
facial nerve paralysis in, 2393, 2396
Ramus(i), 320f
of mandible, anatomy of, 1319, 1320f, 1359f
Random cutaneous flaps, 1067, 1067f
Random sample, 68, 69t
Randomized clinical trials (RCTs), 52, 54, 54t
data quality of, 59, 60t-62t
Range, 64t
Ranitidine (Cimetidine), for recurrent respiratory papillomatosis, 2893
RANKL (receptor activator of NF-κB ligand), in bone resorption, 1972
RANTES, in otitis media, 2764
Ranula(s)
in children, 2850-2852, 2859
imaging of, 1146, 1147f
of sublingual space, 156, 157f
of submandibular space, 157
Rapid eye movement (REM) sleep, 261-262
Rapid eye movement (REM) sleep behavior disorder (RBD), 264-265
Rapid maxillary expansion (RME)
for nasal obstruction, 2630
for obstructive sleep apnea in children, 2611
Rapidly involuting congenital hemangioma (RICH), 2824
Rapid-sequence induction (RSI), 112-113
in children, 2590
RARS (recurrent acute rhinosinusitis), 705
RAS. *See* Recurrent aphthous stomatitis (RAS).
Rate difference, 64, 64t
RB tumor suppressor gene, in parathyroid neoplasm(s), 1776f
RBD (REM sleep behavior disorder), 264-265
RCTs (randomized clinical trials), 52, 54, 54t
data quality of, 59, 60t-62t
RDX (radixin) gene, in deafness, 2051t-2058t, 2075-2076
Reactive lymph nodes, 164
Reactive lymphadenopathy, 2818
Reactive oxygen species (ROS), in ototoxicity
of aminoglycosides, 2171
of carboplatin, 2173-2174
of cisplatin, 2172
Real-ear aided response or gain (REAR/G), 2273
Real-ear insertion gain (REIG), 2273
Real-ear unaided response or gain (REUR/G), 2273
Real-ear-to-coupler difference (RECD), in infants, 2724
Rearrangements, chromosomal, 4-5
Rebound headache, 248
Receiver-in-the-canal (RIC) fitting, for hearing aids, 2270
Receptor activator of NF-κB ligand (RANKL), in bone resorption, 1972
Receptor potentials, in hair cell transduction, 2071, 2072f
Recessive disorders, 6-7, 7f
Recommendation, grades of, 69-70, 70t
Reconstruction
for congenital aural atresia, 2754-2757
alternatives to, 2759
avoidance of complications of, 2758-2759
candidacy for, 2753, 2753t
contraindications to, 2754
creation of split-thickness skin graft in, 2756, 2756f
dissection of ossicular mass in, 2755-2756, 2756f
drilling for new ear canal in, 2755-2756
ear wick packing in, 2756-2757
facial nerve in, 2754, 2755f, 2759
harvesting of temporalis fascia in, 2755, 2755f
meatoplasty in, 2756-2757
outcomes of, 2754
placement of split-thickness skin graft in, 2756, 2757f-2758f
postauricular incision in, 2755, 2755f
postoperative care after, 2757-2758
preoperative evaluation and patient counseling for, 2754, 2754f-2755f
reconstruction of ossicular chain in, 2756
removal of atretic plate in, 2755-2756, 2755f
Silastic strips in, 2756-2757, 2758f
suturing in, 2756-2757, 2758f
temporal fascia graft in, 2755f, 2756, 2757f
timing of, 2754

Reconstruction *(Continued)*
for hypopharyngeal cancer, 1431-1433
with circumferential defects, 1431-1432
fasciocutaneous free flaps in, 1433
gastric pull-up in, 1432, 1432f
jejunal free flap in, 1432-1433, 1433f
pectoralis myocutaneous flap in, 1431, 1431f
mandibular (*See* Mandibular reconstruction)
for microtia
advantages and disadvantages of, 2744t
atypical, 2747-2748, 2749f-2750f
autogenous costochondral, 2744, 2744t
classic, 2744-2747
cartilage implantation in, 2744-2746
carving of framework and helix in, 2746, 2746f
construction of implant in, 2746, 2746f
creation of postauricular sulcus in, 2746, 2748f
donor site in, 2745, 2745f
incision in, 2745-2746
lobule transfer in, 2746, 2747f
placement of implant in, 2746, 2747f
templates in, 2744-2745, 2745f
tragus reconstruction in, 2747, 2748f
complications of, 2748-2751
planning for, 2743-2744, 2744t
for oral cancer, 1315-1316
of alveolar ridge, 1304
of buccal mucosa, 1308-1309, 1309f
of floor of mouth, 1307, 1315f
free flap, 1316, 1316f
of hard palate, 1310, 1311f
of lip, 1303-1304, 1303f
of tongue, 1305-1306
oropharyngeal (*See* Oropharyngeal reconstruction)
for skull base defects, 2467-2468
after subtotal or total temporal bone resection, 2495
after total laryngopharyngectomy, 1574, 1574f-1575f
after transnasal endoscopic-assisted anterior skull base surgery, 2484
Reconstructive procedures, hair loss with, 387, 388f
Reconstructive surgery, gene therapy for, 22-23
with reconstructive tissue flaps and wound healing, 22-23
with skin grafting, 23
Recording electrodes, for intraoperative cranial nerve monitoring, 2543-2544, 2543f
Recruitment
vs. hyperacusis, 2138
with traditional hearing aid, 2205-2207
Rectus abdominis free flap, 1082t, 1083
for oropharyngeal reconstruction, 1082t, 1083
of tongue base, 1390, 1390f
of tonsils and pharyngeal wall, 1386
Rectus capitis major muscle, 2439f
Rectus lateralis muscle, 2439f
Recurrent acute rhinosinusitis (RARS), 705
Recurrent aphthous stomatitis (RAS), 1236-1239
clinical features of, 1237-1238
defined, 1236-1237
differential diagnosis of, 1238, 1238t
etiology and pathogenesis of, 1237, 1237t
herpetiform-type, 1238, 1238f
histopathologic features of, 1239
major, 1237-1238, 1238f
minor, 1237, 1238f
treatment of, 1239
Recurrent laryngeal nerve (RLN)
applied anatomy of, 807
characteristics of, 918
denervation of
effects of, 919
reinnervation for (*See* Laryngeal reinnervation)
in root of neck, 2582
Recurrent laryngeal nerve (RLN) *(Continued)*
and thyroid gland, 1752, 1752f
in thyroid surgery
identification of, 1765, 1765f
injury of, 1770-1771
invasive carcinoma of, 1766
reoperative, 1767
Recurrent laryngeal nerve (RLN) injury
electromyography of, 835
due to thyroid surgery, 1770-1771
Recurrent parotitis of childhood (RPC), 1153-1154
Recurrent paroxysmal laryngospasm, 808
Recurrent respiratory papillomatosis (RRP), 878-880, 2884-2895
adult-onset, 879
clinical features of, 2887-2888, 2887f-2888f
CO_2 laser for, 32
epidemiology of, 878, 2884-2885
etiology of, 878-879, 2885-2886
extralaryngeal spread of, 2887, 2887f-2888f
gastroesophageal reflux and, 2946
gross appearance of, 868f-869f, 2885f
histopathology of, 2885-2886, 2885f
juvenile form of, 879
malignant transformation of, 2887-2888
other considerations with, 2894
patient assessment for, 2888, 2889f
airway endoscopy in, 2888
history in, 2888
physical examination in, 2888
practice pathway for, 2889f
prevention of, 2886-2887, 2890t
registry and task force initiatives for, 2894
staging severity of, 2893-2894, 2893f-2894f
support groups for, 2894
tracheostomy and, 2887
transmission of, 2886
treatment of, 2890t
adjuvant modality(ies) for, 2891-2893
acyclovir as, 2890t, 2892
antireflux therapy as, 2893
celecoxib as, 2892
cidofovir as, 879-880, 2890t
indole-3-carbinol as, 879, 2890t, 2892
interferon as, 879, 2890t., 2891-2892
methotrexate as, 879
mumps vaccine as, 2890t, 2892-2893
photodynamic therapy as, 2890t, 2892
retinoids as, 2890t, 2892
ribavirin as, 2892
vaccines for, 2890t
surgical, 2888-2891
anesthetic techniques for, 2891
carbon dioxide laser for, 879, 2889-2891
emerging technologies for, 2891
microdebrider for, 2891
pulsed dye laser for, 880, 880f, 2891
virology of, 2885-2886
vocal quality disorder due to, 2880-2881
Recurrent Respiratory Papillomatosis Foundation, 2894
Redistribution, in radiotherapy, 1039, 1039f
Reduced penetrance, 7
Reed-Sternberg cells, 2838-2839
Reepithelialization, 1076-1077
keratinocyte migration in, 1076-1077
keratinocyte proliferation in, 1077
Reexcision, for scar revision, 295, 297f
Referral sources, for children, 2572-2573
Referred pain, trigeminal system in, 1203
Refixation saccade, 2292
Reflection, of laser energy, 28-29, 29f
Reflux. *See also* Gastroesophageal reflux disease (GERD).
outcome scales for, 57-58
Reflux esophagitis, 968-969, 969f, 1403-1404, 1403f-1404f
Reflux Finding Score (RFS), 897, 897t
Reflux laryngitis, 886, 886f
in voice professional, 852
Reflux laryngopharyngitis, 863, 863f
Reflux Symptom Index (RSI), 826, 826t, 896, 897b
Refsum disease
biochemical defect in, 7
sensorineural hearing loss in, 2094t, 2096
Region of transient electronic equilibrium, in radiation, 1033
Regional anesthesia, for postoperative pain control, 241-242
Regional flaps
for hypopharyngeal and esophageal reconstruction, 1450-1452
for oropharyngeal reconstruction, 1377-1379
latissimus dorsi musculocutaneous, 1378, 1378f
pectoralis major, 1377, 1377f
platysmal myocutaneous, 1377, 1378f
temporalis, 1377-1378
temporoparietal fascial, 1377-1378, 1378f
of tongue base
latissimus dorsi, 1389
pectoralis major myocutaneous, 1388-1389
platysmal myocutaneous, 1389
of tonsils and pharyngeal wall
pectoralis major, 1385, 1385f
platysmal myocutaneous, 1385
sternocleidomastoid myocutaneous, 1385-1386
temporalis, 1386
temporoparietal fascia, 1386
trapezius musculocutaneous, 1378-1379
Register shifts, 851
Registration, for image-guided sinus surgery, 680-681
Regression procedures, 72
Regression to the mean, *vs.* efficacy of treatment, 62t
Regularity, laryngeal videostroboscopy of, 821
Regulatory accountability, 82
Regulatory T cells (Tregs), 602-603
Regurgitation, 956
Rehabilitation
after cochlear implantation, 2253-2257
in adults, 2254-2255
in children, 2254-2255
efficacy of, 2253-2254
facial nerve (*See* Facial nerve rehabilitation)
after total laryngectomy, 1572
for swallowing, 1572
for voice, 1572
after total laryngopharyngectomy, 1575
vestibular (*See* Vestibular and balance rehabilitation therapy (VBRT))
voice (*See* Voice rehabilitation)
Reicher's cartilage, 2583-2584
Reinke's space, 812, 845
surgical anatomy of, 1544f
Reissner's membrane
anatomy of, 1831-1832, 1832f, 2050, 2061f
in auditory physiology, 1841f
Reiter's syndrome, oral manifestations of, 1253
Relapsing polychondritis
laryngeal and tracheal manifestations of, 890
sensorineural hearing loss due to, 2124
Related samples, statistical tests for, 66, 67t
Relative risk, 64, 64t
Relaxed skin tension lines (RSTLs), 269-270, 274f
and scars, 295, 296f
Release maneuvers, with tracheal resection, 1618-1619, 1620f
Reliability, in psychometric validation, 55
rem (Roentgen equivalent for man), 133
REM (rapid eye movement) sleep, 261-262
REM (rapid eye movement) sleep behavior disorder (RBD), 264-265

Remifentanil
for anesthesia induction, 111
for anesthesia maintenance in children, 2592
Remineralization, of teeth, 1141
Remodeling phase, of wound healing, 1078
Renal disease
oral manifestations of, 1255
preoperative evaluation of, 103
sensorineural hearing loss with, 2121
Renal failure, oral manifestations of, 1255
Renal failure–induced hyperparathyroidism, 1797-1798
Renal symptoms, of hyperparathyroidism, 1781-1782
Renal transplantation, oral sequelae of, 1255
Renal-coloboma syndrome, deafness in, 2051t-2058t
Rendu-Osler-Weber syndrome, 291
oral manifestations of, 1257
Renin, in saliva, 1140
Renova (tretinoin)
for aging skin, 403-404
with chemical peels, 392-393
for chemoprevention of oral cancer, 1315
Reoxygenation, in radiotherapy, 1039, 1039f
Repair, in radiotherapy, 1039
Repaired Facial Nerve Recovery Scale (RFNRS), 2414, 2414t
Repeated samples, statistical tests for, 66, 67t
Reperfusion injury, in acutely raised skin flaps, 1070, 1074
Repopulation, in radiotherapy, 1039
Repose tongue suspension procedure, for obstructive sleep apnea, 259-260
Repositioning maneuvers, for benign paroxysmal positional vertigo, 2331-2332, 2332f
RERA (respiratory effort–related arousals), 251-252, 251b
RERA (respiratory effort–related arousal) index, 251b
Rerouting, of facial nerve, 2412, 2412f-2413f
partial, 2412-2413
Research integration, 69-70
Residual cyst, 1263
Residual hearing
cochlear implants with
in adults, 2245-2246
in children, 2240
ear selection for, 2236
in patient selection for ablative vestibular surgery, 2366
Reskeletonization, in septoplasty, 491
Resonance
in speech, 810-812, 833
speech therapy for, with velopharyngeal dysfunction, 2681
in voice evaluation, 826-827
Resonance disorders, in children, 2879
Resorbable Fixation System, for pediatric facial fractures, 2701t
Resorbable plating systems, for pediatric facial fractures, 2700-2701, 2700t-2701t
Respiratory changes, in geriatric patients, 236
Respiratory disturbance index, 251b
Respiratory effort–related arousal(s) (RERA), 251-252, 251b
Respiratory effort–related arousal (RERA) index, 251b
Respiratory epithelium, in olfactory area, 625, 625f
Respiratory rate, in children, 2570
Respiratory syncytial virus (RSV) vaccine, to prevent otitis media, 2769
Respiratory system
of children, 2569-2570
and control of ventilation, 2569-2570
and laryngospasm, 2570
and lung volumes, 2570
Respiratory system *(Continued)*
and respiratory rate, 2570
and ventilation-perfusion relationships, 2570, 2571t
preoperative evaluation of, 102-103
Respiratory viruses, and otitis media, 1871
Responsiveness, in psychometric validation, 55
Restech Dx-pH Measurement System, 962, 962f
Restless leg syndrome (RLS), 265
Restriction enzymes, 9
Restriction sites, 9
Rests of Malassez, 1259
Resurfacing, facial. *See* Facial resurfacing.
RET oncogene
suppression of expression of, 13
in thyroid carcinoma, 1753
Retention cysts, esophageal, 1415-1416, 1415f
Reticular dermis, 1065
Reticular lamina
anatomy of, 1832-1833, 1832f
in cochlear transduction, 2065-2066, 2069f
scanning electron micrograph of, 1833, 1833f
Reticulosis, midline malignant (polymorphic), 659-660
Retin A (tretinoin)
for aging skin, 403-404
with chemical peels, 392-393
for chemoprevention of oral cancer, 1315
Retinal slip velocity, 2277
Retinoic acid (Retin A)
after chemical peel, 396
for head and neck squamous cell carcinoma, 1018
Retinoids
for cancer chemoprevention, 1018, 1061-1062
for recurrent respiratory papillomatosis, 2890t, 2892
Retinol, for cancer chemoprevention, 1018, 1061-1062
Retinyl palmitate, for cancer chemoprevention, 1061-1062
Retroauricular flap, for nasal defects, 365-366, 371f
Retroauricular lymph nodes
anatomy of, 1718f, 2582
dissection of, 1718-1719
Retrobulbar fibroblast, in Graves' ophthalmopathy, 1807
Retrobulbar recess
normal anatomy of, 667
surgical anatomy of, 740
Retroclival region
in surgical anatomy of anterior skull base, 2474-2475, 2474f-2475f
transnasal endoscopic-assisted surgery of, 2479-2481, 2480f-2481f
Retrocochlear neoplasm, in cerebellopontine angle, hearing loss due to, 2199
Retrocochlear vertigo, 2202
Retrognathia, dysphagia due to, 2950-2951
Retrograde dilators, for esophageal strictures, due to caustic ingestion, 2960-2962, 2960f-2961f
Retrograde intubation, for difficult airway, 114t
Retrograde-eversion approaches, for nasal tip refinement, 522, 523f-526f
Retrolabyrinthine approach
for intratemporal facial nerve surgery, 2405-2406, 2405f-2406f
for posterior fossa neoplasms, 2532t, 2536
advantages and disadvantages of, 2532t, 2536
basic features of, 2536
indications for, 2532t, 2536
surgical exposure in, 2536f
technique of, 2536, 2536f
Retromandibular vein, in parotidectomy, 1195-1196, 1195f
Retromolar trigone
anatomy of, 1295f, 1297, 1298f
carcinoma of, 1306-1307
clinical presentation of, 1306
resection for, 1307, 1307f
survival with, 1307
lymphatic drainage of, 1297, 1298f
melanoma of, 1364f
vasculature of, 1296
Retronasal stimulation, 631
Retropharyngeal abscess, 1407, 1465-1466
in children, 2789-2790, 2789f, 2810-2811
anatomy of, 2810
clinical features of, 2810
complications of, 2811
diagnosis of, 2810-2811, 2810f-2811f
differential diagnosis of, 2806t
epidemiology of, 2810
historical background of, 2810
imaging of, 2810-2811, 2810f-2811f
management of, 2811
imaging of, 1465-1466, 1466f
infrahyoid, 134
suprahyoid, 153, 155f
Retropharyngeal cellulitis, 2810-2811, 2810f
Retropharyngeal lymph node(s), in hypopharyngeal and cervical esophageal cancer, 1434-1435
Retropharyngeal lymph node metastasis, 1687-1688
Retropharyngeal lymphadenopathy, 1414, 1415f
Retropharyngeal space (RPS)
anatomy of, 202
infections of, 207
in children, 2789-2790, 2789f
odontogenic, 185-186, 187f
airway establishment for, 188
normal anatomy and, 186f
of infrahyoid neck, imaging of, 158
with lesions, 158, 161f
normal anatomy in, 158, 159f-160f
of suprahyoid neck, imaging of, 146f, 152f, 153, 155f
Retrosigmoid approach
for intratemporal facial nerve surgery, 2406-2407
advantages and uses of, 2406-2407
limitations and potential complications of, 2407
technique of, 2406, 2407f
for posterior fossa neoplasms, 2532t, 2533-2534
advantages and disadvantages of, 2532t, 2534
basic features of, 2533
indications for, 2532t, 2533
surgical exposure in, 2533f
technique of, 2534, 2534f
Retrospective studies, 61
Retrovascular node, 1298f
Retroviral vectors
for gene therapy of inner ear, 2191t
for gene transfer, 16, 17f, 18t
RetroX, 2204f, 2206t, 2217, 2217f
REUR/G (real-ear unaided response or gain), 2273
Revascularization, of acutely raised skin flaps, 1069, 1069f
Review of systems, 94, 94b
Revision rhinoplasty, 580-594
for alar pinching and retraction, 587, 587f-589f
for caudal septal deviation, 593
for caudal septal excision (short nose), 593
computer imaging for, 581-582
for dorsal irregularity, 584
due to errors of omission, 582, 582t
due to excessive excision, 582, 582t, 583f
due to failure to restabilize, 582, 582t
general considerations with, 582-583, 582t, 583f
grafting material for, 583, 584f
due to gross errors of judgment, 582-583, 582t, 583f
for improperly placed radix graft, 584
for lateral nasal wall deformities, 586

Revision rhinoplasty *(Continued)*
for low dorsum/saddle deformity, 584, 585f
for middle vault deformities, 585-586, 586f
due to minor errors of technique, 582, 582t
for nasal tip deformities, 588
irregularities and bossae as, 588-589, 590f
overrotation (short nose) as, 590, 590f-591f
persistently wide or bulbous tip as, 589-590, 590f
pinched tip as, 590, 591f-592f
ptotic tip as, 590-593, 593f
for overly narrowed alar base, 593-594, 594f
patient interview for, 580-581
photography for, 581
physical examination for, 581
for pollybeak deformity, 584-585, 586f
of skin–soft tissue envelope, 581, 594
for supra-alar and external valve collapse, 586-587, 587f
Reynell Developmental Language Scale, 2249-2250
RFA (radiofrequency tongue base ablation), for obstructive sleep apnea, 259
RFFF. *See* Radial forearm free flap (RFFF).
RFNRS (Repaired Facial Nerve Recovery Scale), 2414, 2414t
RFS (Reflux Finding Score), 897, 897t
Rhabdomyoma, of larynx, 881
Rhabdomyosarcoma (RMS)
in children, 2820, 2840-2842
epidemiology of, 2820, 2840
histopathology and molecular biology of, 2842, 2842f
management of, 2820, 2841-2842
presentation and evaluation of, 2840-2841, 2841t
sites of, 2820
survival with, 2840
of middle ear or mastoid, 2501-2502
of neck, 1667-1668, 1668f, 1669t
of paranasal sinuses, 1132
Rheologic disorders, sensorineural hearing loss due to, 2123
Rheology, and skin flap viability, 1073-1074
Rheumatic fever, acute, 2788
Rheumatoid arthritis (RA)
laryngeal and tracheal manifestations of, 891, 891f
oral manifestations of, 1253, 1253t
of temporomandibular joint, 1281t, 1282
Rheumatrex. *See* Methotrexate (Rheumatrex).
Rhinion, 496, 497f
Rhinitis
allergic (*See* Allergic rhinitis (AR))
atrophic, 696-697
chronic (*See* Nonallergic rhinitis (NAR))
cold air–induced, 619b
drug-induced, 619b, 696, 697b
granulomatous, 619b
gustatory, 698
idiopathic, 695
in immunocompromised patient, 660
infectious, 619b
irritant, 697-698
due to mechanical obstruction, 619b
medicamentosa, 862-863
neoplastic, 619b
nonallergic (*See* Nonallergic rhinitis (NAR))
occupational, 698
perennial, 619b, 695
nonallergic, noninfectious, 695
during pregnancy, 696, 702
vasomotor, 619b, 695, 698
Rhinitis Outcome Questionnaire, 57
Rhinitis Quality of Life Questionnaire (RQLQ), 642
Rhinoconjunctivitis, allergic, 622
Rhinocort (budesonide nasal spray)
for nonallergic rhinitis, 700t
for rhinosinusitis, 734t, 736
Rhinohygrometry, 642
Rhinologic disease, outcome scales for, 56t, 57
Rhinomanometry, 643-651
vs. acoustic rhinometry, 644
active *vs.* passive, 647-648
in allergic rhinitis, 651
anterior
placement of pressure tubing for, 645-646, 648f
vs. posterior, 645-647
technique of, 645
baseline collection in, 645f
dilating devices in, 648f
for left nasal airway, 647f-648f
positioning in, 645f
for right nasal airway, 646f-647f
to assess effect of treatment, 651-652
for children, 645
defined, 642
equipment for, 645
examining pressure-flow curve in, 648-649, 649f-650f
forced oscillation, 643-644
inspiratory or expiratory values in, 650-651
intranasal sites assessed by, 644
maximum (vertex) resistance in, 650
nasal airflow in
measurement of, 647
and transnasal pressure, 643
nasal resistance in, 649-650, 650f
parameters in, 649-651, 650f
posterior (peroral)
vs. anterior, 645-647
placement of pressure tubing for, 645-646, 649f
postnasal (pernasal), placement of pressure tubing for, 645-646, 649f
reporting results of, 648-651
sources of variability in, 651
technical concerns and testing pitfalls with, 645-648
technique of, 645
baseline collection in, 645f
dilating devices in, 648f
for left nasal airway, 647f-648f
positioning in, 645f
for right nasal airway, 646f-647f
transnasal pressure in
measurement of, 645-647, 648f
nasal airflow and, 643
unilateral *vs.* bilateral measurements in, 648, 649f
Rhinometry
acoustic, 486-487, 643-645
in allergic rhinitis, 651
to assess effect of treatment, 651-652
equipment for, 486-487, 486f, 644
interpretation of results of, 645
intranasal sites assessed by, 644
reporting results of, 645
rhinogram generated by, 486-487, 487f, 645
vs. rhinomanometry, 644
for snoring and sleep apnea, 651
sources of variability in, 651
technical concerns and testing pitfalls with, 645
technique of, 644-645
airflow, 487
manometric, 643-644
Rhinoplasty, 508-544
anesthesia for, 515-519, 518f
and surgical planes, 516-517, 516f-517f
anosmia after, 637
of bony vault, 540-542
for bony profile reduction, 540-541, 540f
for narrowing of nose, 541-542
double osteotomies in, 542, 542f-543f
lateral osteotomies in, 541, 542f
medial-oblique osteotomies in, 541, 541f
Rhinoplasty *(Continued)*
of cartilaginous vault, 536-540
access to nasal skeleton in, 537-539, 539f
aesthetic improvement after, 537, 538f
factors to consider in, 537
incremental cartilaginous profile alignment in, 539
mucoperichondrium in, 539-540
pollybeak deformity due to, 512, 512f, 539, 539f
for reduction of overlong caudal quadrangular cartilage, 513f
with traumatic or iatrogenic avulsion of upper lateral cartilage, 539-540, 540f
for cleft-lip nose, 557-559, 561f
Abbé flap in, 563f-564f
with bilateral deformity, 557, 559, 561f, 563f-564f
columellar lengthening in, 559, 566f
external approach to, 559, 561f
lateral ala thinning and placement of maxillary implants in, 562f
Le Fort I maxillary osteotomies in, 559, 564f-565f
with nasal stenosis, 559, 566f
open approach to, 559, 562f
repositioning and suturing lower lateral cartilage in, 562f
with severe deformity, 559, 564f-565f
suturing together medial crura in, 561f-562f
with unilateral deformity, 557, 559, 561f-562f
complications of
noncaucasian, 578, 578f-579f
revision rhinoplasty for (*See* Rhinoplasty, revision)
components of successful, 516f
inverted V sign after, 492, 493f
of nasal tip, 519-536
considerations in, 520, 522f
delivery approaches to, 522, 527f
complete strip technique in, 522, 527f-530f
interrupted strip technique in, 522, 532f-533f
suturing in, 522, 530f-531f, 550-551
incisions, approaches, and techniques for, 520, 521f, 521t
in noncaucasian patients, 573-577
cap graft in, 576, 577f
caudal extension graft in, 576, 576f
concept of, 573-576
reshaping of lower lateral cartilage in, 577
shield graft in, 576, 577f
technique for, 576-577
thinning of subcutaneous tissue in, 577, 577f
nondelivery (cartilage-splitting, retrograde-eversion) approaches to, 522, 523f-526f
objective of, 519
open approach to, 522-535, 534f-535f
indications for, 521b
preservation of lateral crus and strip of alar cartilage in, 520-522, 522f
tip projection in, 520, 535-536, 549-551
autogenous cartilage struts for, 535-536, 536f
cephalic rotation for, 519, 536, 549-550, 551f
onlay tip cartilage grafts for, 535-536, 537f, 549-550, 550f-551f
partial-transfixion *vs.* complete-transfixion incisions for, 535-536, 536f
plumping grafts for, 535-536, 536f
transdomal sutures for, 536
tip ptosis after, 519, 520f
tip support mechanisms and, 519, 520f
for nasofrontal angle modifications, 548-549, 550f
noncaucasian, 556-557, 568-579
aesthetic considerations in, 569
alar base modification in, 577-578, 578f

Rhinoplasty *(Continued)*
alar soft tissue sculpting in, 557, 561f
anatomic considerations in, 568-569, 569f, 569t
complications of, 578, 578f-579f
for correction of deviated nose, 573, 576f
dorsal augmentation in, 556, 569-570
choice of material for, 569, 570f
concept of, 569
results of, 572f-573f
technical considerations for, 569-570, 571f
hump reduction in, 570-573
concept of, 570-571
results of, 574f-575f
technique for, 571-573, 575f
nasal base sculpting in, 556-557, 559f-560f
objective of, 568
tip surgery in, 573-577
cap graft in, 576, 577f
caudal extension graft in, 576, 576f
concept of, 573-576
reshaping of lower lateral cartilage in, 577
shield graft in, 576, 577f
technique for, 576-577
thinning of subcutaneous tissue in, 577, 577f
postsurgical considerations after, 542-543
preoperative patient assessment for, 508-519
anatomic evaluation in, 508-514
aesthetic analysis in, 514, 514f
with major deformities, 508-512, 511f-512f
with minimal deformities, 508-512, 509f-510f
normal nasal surgical anatomy and, 509f
palpation of internal vestibules in, 513, 513f
rhinoscopy in, 513-514, 514f
skin quality in, 512-513, 512f
tip recoil in, 513, 513f
laboratory evaluation in, 514-515
photography and imaging in, 514, 515f
revision, 580-594
for alar pinching and retraction, 587, 587f-589f
for caudal septal deviation, 593
for caudal septal excision (short nose), 593
computer imaging for, 581-582
for dorsal irregularity, 584
due to errors of omission, 582, 582t
due to excessive excision, 582, 582t, 583f
due to failure to restabilize, 582, 582t
general considerations with, 582-583, 582t, 583f
grafting material for, 583, 584f
due to gross errors of judgment, 582-583, 582t, 583f
for improperly placed radix graft, 584
for lateral nasal wall deformities, 586
for low dorsum/saddle deformity, 584, 585f
for middle vault deformities, 585-586, 586f
due to minor errors of technique, 582, 582t
for nasal tip deformities, 588
irregularities and bossae as, 588-589, 590f
overrotation (short nose) as, 590, 590f-591f
persistently wide or bulbous tip as, 589-590, 590f
pinched tip as, 590, 591f-592f
ptotic tip as, 590-593, 593f
for overly narrowed alar base, 593-594, 594f
patient interview for, 580-581
photography for, 581
physical examination for, 581
for pollybeak deformity, 584-585, 586f
of skin–soft tissue envelope, 581, 594
for supra-alar and external valve collapse, 586-587, 587f
for saddle nose deformity, 554-555
dynamic adjustable rotational tip graft in, 555, 559f
implant material in, 555, 556f-557f
indications for, 555, 558f

Rhinoplasty *(Continued)*
for septal and columella modifications, 546-548, 546f-547f
caudal repositioning in, 547, 547f
dorsal draw suture in, 548, 549f
making final septal assessment in, 548, 549f
septocolumellar complex in, 548, 549f-550f
shortening of caudal septum in, 547-548, 547f-548f
with septal deviation, 513-514, 514f, 546, 546f-547f
special techniques in, 545-567
for cleft-lip nose, 557-559, 561f
Abbé flap in, 563f-564f
with bilateral deformity, 559, 561f, 563f-564f, 566
columellar lengthening in, 559, 566f
external approach to, 559, 561f
lateral ala thinning and placement of maxillary implants in, 562f
Le Fort I maxillary osteotomies in, 559, 564f-565f
with nasal stenosis, 559, 566f
open approach to, 559, 562f
repositioning and suturing lower lateral cartilage in, 562f
with severe deformity, 559, 564f-565f
suturing together medial crura in, 561f-562f
with unilateral deformity, 557, 559, 561f-562f
external approach for, 545-546, 546f
incisions and soft tissue elevation for, 545-546, 546f
for nasofrontal angle modifications, 548-549, 550f
for noncaucasian nose (*See* Rhinoplasty, noncaucasian)
open approach for, 545-546
preoperative analysis for, 545-546
for saddle nose deformity, 554-555
dynamic adjustable rotational tip graft in, 555, 559f
implant material in, 555, 556f-557f
indications for, 555, 558f
for septal and columella modifications, 546-548, 546f-547f
caudal repositioning in, 547, 547f
dorsal draw suture in, 548, 549f
making final septal assessment in, 548, 549f
septocolumellar complex in, 548, 549f-550f
shortening of caudal septum in, 547-548, 547f-548f
for tip and alar asymmetries, 549-551
alar batten grafts in, 550, 551f
suture techniques in, 550-551
tip grafts in, 549-550, 550f-551f
transposition techniques in, 551
for twisted nose, 551-554, 552f
osteotomies in, 551-554, 552f-554f
septal reconstruction in, 551
spreader grafts in, 554, 555f
surgical landmarks in, 519, 519f
surgical philosophy of, 508
for tip and alar asymmetries, 549-551
alar batten grafts in, 550, 551f
suture techniques in, 550-551
tip grafts in, 549-550, 550f-551f
transposition techniques in, 551
for twisted nose, 551-554
in noncaucasian patient, 573, 576f
osteotomies in, 551-554
intermediate, 553, 554f
lateral, 552-554, 553f
medial, 552-553, 552f-553f
preoperative examination of, 551, 552f
results of, 511f-512f, 553f-554f

Rhinoplasty *(Continued)*
septal reconstruction in, 551
spreader grafts in, 554, 555f
RhinoQOL (Rhinosinusitis Quality of Life survey), 57
Rhinorrhea, cerebrospinal fluid. *See* Cerebrospinal fluid (CSF) rhinorrhea.
Rhinoscleroma, laryngitis due to, 884
Rhinoscopy
anterior, 100, 484
prior to rhinoplasty, 513-514, 514f
of rhinosinusitis, 730
Rhinosinusitis
abbreviations used in, 729t
acute
bacterial, 703-705, 704f, 732
endoscopic sinus surgery for, 761
frontal, 775
pathogenesis of, 704-705, 704f
radiologic appearance of, 672-673, 673f
recurrent, 705
surgical management of, 741
allergic
fungal, 712-715
in children, 2778, 2780, 2781f
chronic, 707, 733
classification of, 709
diagnosis of, 707, 712-713
epidemiology of, 713-714
imaging of, 706f, 713, 714f
immunochemical staining for, 731, 731f
pathogenesis of, 712-714, 714b
prognosis for, 713
therapy for, 713-715, 715b
radiologic appearance of, 675
in athletes, 737
bacterial
acute, 703-705, 704f, 732
chronic, 732, 733f
in children, 737
chronic
acute exacerbation of, 705, 707, 707f
surgical management of, 741
bacterial, 732, 733f
defined, 705, 728-729
frontal, 775-783
fungal, 732-733
allergic, 707, 733
invasive, 711
nonallergic, 715-716, 716t
pathogenesis of, 705-707, 706b, 706f, 742-743
radiologic appearance of, 673-674, 674f-675f
surgical management of, 741, 760-761
classification of, 703-704
complications of, 676-677
inflammatory polyps as, 676, 678f
mucocele as, 676, 678f
mucous retention cyst as, 676, 677f
orbital, 676-677
defined, 703-704
diagnosis of, 728-730
imaging in, 729, 729f
rhinoscopy in, 730
smell and nasal airflow in, 730
in elderly, 737
endoscopic sinus surgery for, 742-756
with acute complications, 741
anesthesia for, 744-745
general, 745
local, 744-745
antibiotics prior to, 743
chronic, 741-743
complications of, 754-755, 754b
hemorrhage as, 754
intracranial, 755, 755f
ophthalmic, 754-755

Rhinosinusitis *(Continued)*
computer-assisted navigation in, 772
with concha bullosa, 751, 752f
conclusion of procedure for, 751
ethmoidectomy in
anterior, 747, 748f
complete, 748-749, 749f-750f
failure of, 766-767, 767f
posterior, 747-748, 749f
failure of, 756
frontal sinusotomy in, 750-751, 768-771
agger nasi cell in, 769, 771f-772f
and causes of frontal sinus disease, 769
challenges of, 768
external approaches as adjunct to, 771, 773f
frontal bullar cell in, 772f
frontal recess dissection in, 769, 770b, 770t, 771f
frontal sinus cells in, 769-770, 772f
image-guided navigation system in, 771f
interfrontal sinus septal cell in, 771, 772f
preoperative evaluation for, 768-769
recessus terminalis in, 771
suprabullar cell in, 772f
supraorbital ethmoid cell in, 770-771, 772f
fungal
invasive, 742
noninvasive, 742
image-guided navigation systems in, 743-744, 745f
intraoperative CT scans during, 744, 772
limited *vs.* extended approaches for, 752-753
maxillary antrostomy in, 747, 747f
failure of, 764-766, 766f
Messerklinger technique for, 746
minimally invasive sinus technique in, 743, 752, 760
with mucoceles, 751
nasal endoscopy in, 746, 763
with nasal septal deviation, 751
patient preparation and positioning for, 745-746
with polyps, 751-752
postoperative care after, 753-754, 773-774
preoperative assessment for, 743
examination in, 743
history in, 743
imaging in, 743, 744t
recurrent acute, 741
resection of uncinate process in, 746, 746f
results of, 755-756
sinus balloon catheterization in, 752-753, 753f
sphenoid sinusotomy in, 748, 749f
sphenoidotomy in, 748, 749f
complications of, 767, 768t
for fungus ball, 768f-769f
with image-guided navigation system, 770f
treatment of middle turbinate in, 751, 751f, 771
Wigand technique for, 746
epidemiology of, 728
frontal
acute, 775
anatomic variations and, 776
chronic, 775-783
fungal, 709-2
allergic, 712-715
chronic, 707
classification of, 709
diagnosis of, 707, 712-713
endoscopic sinus surgery for, 761, 762f
epidemiology of, 713-714
imaging of, 706f, 713, 714f
immunochemical staining for, 731, 731f
pathogenesis of, 712-714, 714b
prognosis for, 713
therapy for, 713-715, 715b

Rhinosinusitis *(Continued)*
chronic, 732-733
allergic, 707
invasive, 711
nonallergic, 715-716, 716t
classification of, 709
endoscopic sinus surgery for, 761, 762f
fungus balls in, 712, 712f, 714t
in immunocompromised host, 660, 710t
diagnosis of, 220-221, 220f
presentation and pathogenesis of, 220
treatment of, 221
invasive, 705, 709-712
due to *Aspergillus,* 220-221, 220f, 705, 710-711, 712f
due to *Candida,* 711
chronic or indolent, 711
diagnosis of, 711, 711f-712f
due to mucormycosis, 705, 710, 711f
rapidly (fulminant), 709-710, 710f
surgical management of, 742, 761
therapy for, 711-712, 713t
nonallergic eosinophilic, 709, 715-716, 716t
noninvasive, 709
surgical management of, 742, 761
radiologic appearance of, 674-675, 676f
saprophytic, 712
granulomatous, 675
immunosuppression and, 219-221, 660
diagnosis of, 220-221, 220f
presentation and pathogenesis of, 219-220
treatment of, 221
medical treatment of, 733-737
alternative, 731, 735t
antibiotics for, 733-735
intravenous, 733-734, 735t
long-term macrolide, 733, 734t
oral, 733
short-term, 734t
topical, 734-735, 735t
antifungals for
systemic, 735, 735t
topical, 735-736, 735t
antihistamines for, 734t, 737
anti-IgE (omalizumab) for, 735t, 737
anti-reflux therapy for, 735t, 737
antivirals for, 731, 734t
aspirin desensitization therapy for, 734t, 737
in athletes, 737
in children, 737
decongestants for, 735t, 736
in elderly, 737
intravenous immune globulin for, 735t, 737
issues with antimicrobials for, 736
leukotriene modifiers for, 735t, 736
mucolytics for, 735t, 736
nasal saline lavage for, 734t, 736
during pregnancy, 737
with proven benefit in comparative trials, 734t
without proven benefit in comparative trials, 735t
steroids for
systemic, 734t, 736
topical nasal, 734t, 736
outcome measures and quality of life with, 730, 730t
pathogenesis of, 703-708
predisposing factor(s) for, 730-733
allergy as, 731
bacteria as, 732
eicosanoids and aspirin sensitivity triad as, 731-732, 732f
environmental irritants as, 731
fungi as, 732-733
inflammation as, 731, 731f
laryngopharyngeal reflux as, 732
nitric oxide as, 732

Rhinosinusitis *(Continued)*
superantigens as, 706, 732
viral illness as, 730-731
during pregnancy, 737
radiologic appearances of, 167-168, 672-675, 729
acute, 672-673, 673f
allergic, 675
chronic, 673-674, 674f-675f
with complications, 676-677
inflammatory polyps as, 676, 678f
mucocele as, 676, 678f
mucous retention cyst as, 676, 677f
orbital, 676-677
on CT, 140-142, 141f, 729
granulomatous, 675
on plain radiographs, 729, 729f
recurrent, 728
signs and symptoms of, 703, 704b
Rhinosinusitis Disability Index (RSDI), 642
Rhinosinusitis Outcome Measure, 57
Rhinosinusitis Quality of Life survey (RhinoQOL), 57
Rhinostereometry, 643
Rhinotomy, lateral
for middle cranial base surgery, 2455t, 2458, 2458f
for nasopharyngeal carcinoma, 1355-1356, 1355f
Rhinovirus, pharyngitis due to, 196
Rhizopus oryzae, rhinosinusitis due to, 710
Rhytid(s), 275, 279f
Rhytidectomy, 405-427
complication(s) of, 420-427
contour deformities as, 427
depression as, 427
hair loss as, 426, 427f
hematoma as, 420-421, 425f
nerve injury as, 422-425, 426f
parotid injury as, 426-427
pigmentary changes as, 427
scars as, 425-426, 425f, 427f
skin flap necrosis as, 421-422, 425f-426f
composite, 406
deep-plane, 406, 407f, 409
hair restoration after, 387, 388f
historical perspective on, 405-408
melolabial fold in, 406, 406f
orbicularis muscle in, 406, 406f
postoperative care after, 420
results of, 414f-415f, 417f-418f, 423f-424f
SMAS-, 409
extended, 409
SMAS flap for, 405-406, 409
SMAS in, 405, 406f
strip SMAS-ectomy for, 409
subcutaneous, 408-409
subperiosteal, 410
advantages and disadvantages of, 407-408, 408t
defined, 410
historical perspective on, 407
surgical approaches for, 408, 410
combined, 408, 410
transoral, 408, 410
transorbital, 408, 410, 410f
transtemporal, 407f, 408, 410
sub-SMAS, 406
supra-SMAS, 409-410
advantages and disadvantages of, 408, 408t
defined, 409
extended, 406, 408-410
historical perspective on, 406
surgical approaches to, 408-410, 409t
surgical technique for, 410-420
drain insertion and wound closure in, 420
fibrin sealants in, 416-420
incisions in, 410-411

Rhytidectomy *(Continued)*
for men, 411, 412f
for women, 410-411, 411f
mid-facelift in, 413
procedure for, 413, 415f-416f
results of, 413, 417f-418f
skin flap elevation in, 413-416
extent of skin undermining in, 413, 418f
over parotid gland in preauricular area, 413-416, 419f
posterior neck dissection in, 413-416
subplatysmal dissection in, 413-416, 420f
superior musculoaponeurotic system in, 413-416, 419f
suturing in, 413-416, 421f
in temple, 413
trimming of cervical skin flap in, 413-416, 421f
skin trimming in, 416-420, 422f-423f
submentoplasty in, 411-413
aesthetic considerations for, 411, 412f
procedure for, 411-413, 413f
results of, 414f-415f
Rib cartilage, for auricular reconstruction, 2744, 2744t
Ribavirin, for recurrent respiratory papillomatosis, 2892
Ribbon synapse, with hair cells, 2080, 2080f
Riboflavin, for migraine, 2349
Riboflavin deficiency, oral manifestations of, 1254
Ribonucleic acid (RNA), direct delivery of, for gene silencing, 16
Ribonucleic acid (RNA)-induced silencing complex (RISC), 13, 14f
Ribonucleic acid interference (RNAi), 13, 14f
therapeutic applications of, 23-24
RIC (receiver-in-the-canal) fitting, for hearing aids, 2270
RICH (rapidly involuting congenital hemangioma), 2824
Ricketts analysis, for mentoplasty, 463, 463f
Rickettsia rickettsii, sensorineural hearing loss due to, 2119
Riedel's procedure, 781-782
indications for, 781-782
postoperative appearance after, 781, 782f
for recurrent infection, 781
Rieger flap, for nasal defects, 365-366
RIF (radiation-induced fibrosis), 1048
Rifle, neck trauma due to, 1626, 1626f-1627f
Right anterior–left posterior (RALP) semicircular canal plane, 2285, 2286f, 2287
Right hilar release, with tracheal resection, 1618-1619, 1620f
Right-hand rule, for head rotation, 2293, 2294f
Rigid bronchoscopy, 1000-1001
for difficult airway, 113f, 114t
pediatric anesthesia for, 2597-2598, 2597t
Rigid fixation, for pediatric facial fracture, 2699-2700
Rigid laryngoscopy, 813-814
advantages of, 813
disadvantages of, 813-814
for professional voice disorders, 851, 852t
protocols for, 816b, 818b
technique of, 814
troubleshooting for, 814
Rima glottidis, 1464
surgical anatomy of, 1543f
Rima vestibuli, 1543f
Ring-down artifact, with colloid thyroid nodule, 1644
"Ringed" esophagitis, 967-968, 969f
Rinne test, 98, 98t, 2020, 2020t
for otosclerosis, 2030
RISC (RNA-induced silencing complex), 13, 14f
Rising "w," in nasal breathing assessment, 644
Risk factors, in medical history, 94, 94b
R_{law} (laryngeal airway resistance), in voice evaluation, 828-829, 828t
RLN. *See* Recurrent laryngeal nerve (RLN).
RLS (restless legs syndrome), 265
RME (rapid maxillary expansion)
for nasal obstruction, 2630
for obstructive sleep apnea in children, 2611
RMS. *See* Rhabdomyosarcoma (RMS).
RNA (ribonucleic acid), direct delivery of, for gene silencing, 16
RNA (ribonucleic acid)-induced silencing complex (RISC), 13, 14f
RNAi (ribonucleic acid interference), 13, 14f
therapeutic applications of, 23-24
RND. *See* Radical neck dissection (RND).
Robbins classification, of cervical lymph nodes, 1683, 1683f, 1684t
Robert's syndrome, 2690
Robin, Pierre, 2673
Robin sequence
cleft lip and palate in, 2673
craniofacial abnormalities in, 2630-2631, 2630f
Robodoc, 39
Robotic surgery
of anterior and middle cranial base, 2450
defined, 38-39
history of, 39, 39f-40f
instruments for, 40, 42f
for laryngeal cancer, 1560-1561
in otolaryngology, 39-43
clinical applications of, 41
for oropharyngeal surgery, 42-43
for skull base surgery, 42, 43f-44f
for thyroidectomy, 41-42
experimental origins of, 40-41
articulated instruments in, 40, 42f
in cadaver, 40-41, 43f
da Vinci surgical system in, 40, 41f
in mannequin, 41
operating room orientation in, 41, 43f
in porcine model, 40, 41f
for submandibular gland resection, 40-41, 42f-43f
future directions for, 43-44
procedural times for, 40, 42f
Robotics, 38-44
active, 38-39
definitions for, 38-39
history of, 38, 39f
passive, 38-39
semiactive, 38-39
Rocky Mountain spotted fever, sensorineural hearing loss in, 2119
Rocuronium
in children
for anesthesia maintenance, 2593t
for rapid-sequence anesthesia induction, 2590
intraoperative, 112
Roentgen, 1031
Roentgen equivalent for man (rem), 133
Roentgen, Wilhelm, 1031
Romano-Ward syndrome, deafness in, 2096
Romberg test, 2316-2317
ROS (reactive oxygen species), in ototoxicity
of aminoglycosides, 2171
of carboplatin, 2173-2174
of cisplatin, 2172
Rosai-Dorfman disease, 2819
Rosenmüller's fossa, anatomy of, 1359f
radiographic, 1398f-1399f
Rosenthal's canal, 1832f, 1834
Rose's position, for adenotonsillectomy, 2798, 2798f
Rotation advancement closure, for cleft lip, 2667-2668, 2667f
advancement flap in, 2668, 2668f
closure in, 2668, 2668f
rotation flap in, 2667-2668, 2668f
Rotation flaps, 343-344, 343f
for cheek defects, 357-358, 359f
in cleft lip repair, 2667-2668, 2668f
for forehead repair, 362
advancement, 360-362, 362f
Rotatory chair testing, 2320-2323
bias velocity in, 2322
with cerebellar abnormalities, 2322
directionally dependent asymmetries in, 2322
interpretation of, 2297-2299
protocol for, 2320-2322
step changes in head velocity in, 2322-2323, 2323f
with unilateral vestibular loss, 2322, 2322f
for vestibular rehabilitation, 2377
Roughness, in voice evaluation, 827t
Round window
anatomy of, 1826f, 1831, 1840
in cochlear transduction, 2062f
Round window membrane (RWM), 2179-2183
with aging, 2180
anatomy of, 2179-2180, 2180f
delivery of therapeutic agents across
kinetics of, 2181, 2181f
method of, 2182-2183, 2182f-2183f
"false," 2180
obstructive adhesions of, 2181-2182
permeability of, 2180-2181
physiology of, 2180, 2181f
Round window niche, in surgical anatomy of lateral skull base, 2436f
Rowe midfacial disimpacters, 335-336
Roxithromycin, for rhinosinusitis, 733, 734t
RPC (recurrent parotitis of childhood), 1153-1154
RPS. *See* Retropharyngeal space (RPS).
RQLQ (Rhinitis Quality of Life Questionnaire), 642
RRP. *See* Recurrent respiratory papillomatosis (RRP).
RSDI (Rhinosinusitis Disability Index), 642
RSI (Reflux Symptom Index), 826, 826t, 896, 897b
RSI (rapid-sequence induction), 112-113
in children, 2590
RSTLs (relaxed skin tension lines), 269-270, 274f
and scars, 295, 296f
RSV (respiratory syncytial virus) vaccine, to prevent otitis media, 2769
RT. *See* Radiation therapy (RT).
Rubella, congenital deafness due to, 2154, 2156-2157, 2157f, 2723
Rubeola. *See* Measles.
Rubin osteotome, for rhinoplasty, 540, 540f
with hump reduction, 573
Ruffini's endings, 1202
RWM. *See* Round window membrane (RWM).

S

S phase, of cell cycle, 12, 13f
Saccade(s), 2305-2306, 2306f, 2307t, 2313
anticipatory or corrective, in vestibular compensation, 2375
evaluation of
in bedside exam, 2313
testing for, 2317-2318, 2318f
main sequence of, 2313
neural signal for, 2313, 2313f
normal latency of, 2313
refixation, 2292
Saccular activity, changes in postural tone due to sudden changes in, 2300
anatomic and physiologic basis for, 2300
clinical importance of, 2300

Saccular cysts, 876-878
anterior, 876f-877f, 877
classification of, 877f
clinical scenario with, 877
defined, 877
diagnosis of, 877
etiology of, 876
of larynx, 2872-2873, 2872f-2873f
lateral, 876f, 877, 878f
treatment of, 877-878
Saccular disorders, of larynx, 876-878
classification of, 876f, 877
clinical scenario with, 877
diagnosis of, 877
etiology of, 876
laryngocele as, 876f, 877
laryngopyocele as, 877
saccular cysts as, 877, 877f
anterior, 876f-877f, 877
lateral, 876f, 877, 878f
treatment of, 877-878
Saccular macula. *See* Macula sacculi.
Saccular nerve, 1854f, 2278f
Saccule
anatomy of, 1851f, 1853f-1854f, 2278f
embryogenesis of, 1852
of larynx, 876
in vestibular system
arrangement of, 2278, 2280f
estimated patterns of excitation and inhibition for, 2278, 2281f
morphologic polarizations of stereociliary bundles in, 2278, 2280f
Sacculus. *See* Saccule.
Saddle nose deformity, rhinoplasty for, 554-555
dynamic adjustable rotational tip graft in, 555, 559f
implant material in, 555, 556f-557f
indications for, 555, 558f
revision, 584, 585f
Saethre-Chotzen syndrome, craniofacial anomalies in, 2641t, 2646
Safety considerations, with lasers, 34-37
anesthesia and risk of intraoperative fire as, 36-37
education on, 34
eye protection as, 34-35, 35f-36f
protocol for, 34
effectiveness of, 37
skin protection as, 35
smoke evacuation as, 35
Safety pins, in airway or esophagus, 2941
Sagittal synostosis, 2642, 2643f
surgical management of, 2650, 2650f-2651f
Salicylates
in noise-induced hearing loss, 2147
ototoxicity of, 2175-2176
sensorineural hearing loss due to, 2120, 2176
Salicylic acid
for chemical peels, 392-393
after free tissue transfer, 1096
Saline, for cerumen removal, 1958t
Saline spray, after endoscopic sinus surgery, 773
Saliva
biomarkers in, for head and neck squamous cell carcinoma, 1026
composition of, 1138-1139, 1138t
inorganic component in, 1138t, 1139
organic components in, 1138t-1140t, 1139-1140
variability in, 1138-1139
contribution by salivary glands to, 1134t
flow rate of, 1133, 1138, 1138t
control of, 1138
factors influencing, 1138
intraoral variations in, 1138
Saliva *(Continued)*
functions of, 1133, 1140-1141
antibacterial activity as, 1141
buffering and clearance as, 1141
lubrication and protection as, 1140-1141
maintenance of tooth integrity as, 1141
taste and digestion as, 1141, 1213-1214
osmolarity of, 1138-1139
pH of, 1138-1139
reflex release of, 1205-1206
relative viscosities of, 1134t
Salivary duct carcinoma (SDC), 1189-1190, 1189f
Salivary fistula
due to neck surgery, 1727-1728, 1728f
after parotidectomy, 1177
posttraumatic, 313-314
Salivary flow test, 2384
Salivary gland(s)
aberrant, 2864, 2864f
anatomy of, 1162, 1163f
in children, 2850-2853
contribution to saliva by, 1134t
embryology of, 1162
fine-needle aspiration biopsy of, 1149, 1149f, 1165-1166, 1180-1181
in children, 2854
in geriatric patients, 236
histology of, 1179, 1182f
imaging of, 1143-1150
with adenoid cystic carcinoma, 1146-1147, 1146f-1147f, 1180f
with AIDS-related parotid cysts, 1146, 1146f
anatomic basis for, 1143-1145
in children, 2854-2855
CT for, 139, 1148, 1166, 1180
of AIDS-related parotid cysts, 1146f
of parotid lipoma, 1166, 1167f
of pleomorphic adenoma, 1144f, 1148
of sialadenitis, 1148
of sialolithiasis, 1144f, 1148, 1148f
of Sjögren's syndrome, 1148
of Warthin's tumor, 1146f
FDG-PET for, 1150, 1168
with malignant neoplasms, 1180
minor, 1145
MRI for, 142, 1145-1147, 1166, 1180
of adenoid cystic carcinoma, 1146-1147, 1146f-1147f, 1180f
of glomus tumor, 1169f
of mucoepidermoid carcinoma, 1146, 1147f, 1168f
of pleomorphic adenoma, 1148f, 1167f-1168f, 1180f
of ranula, 1146, 1147f
with mucoepidermoid carcinoma, 1146, 1147f, 1168f
parotid, 1143-1144, 1145f
with pleomorphic adenomas, 1143
CT for, 1144f, 1148
MRI for, 1148f, 1167f-1168f, 1188f
ultrasound for, 1149, 1149f
with ranula, 1146, 1147f
scintigraphy for, 138, 1150
with sialadenitis, 1148
sialography for, 1149-1150
conventional, 139-140, 1149-1150, 1149f, 1155-1156, 1156f
CT, 139-140, 1145f, 1150, 1150f
MR, 1147, 1155-1156
for salivary gland injury, 312
with sialolithiasis, 1143, 1144f, 1148, 1148f
sublingual, 1144-1145
submandibular, 1144
ultrasound for, 143, 1148-1149, 1149f, 1167, 1645-1647
Salivary gland(s) *(Continued)*
with acute infections, 1647
with calculous lesions, 1647
color Doppler, 1167-1168
with cystic salivary gland disease, 1647
with parotid mass, 1654f
with Sjögren's syndrome, 1647
with submandibular pleomorphic adenoma, 1653f
with Warthin's tumor, 1146, 1146f
major, 1133
minor, 1133
anatomy of, 1133-1134
in children, 2850-2852
benign neoplasms of, 1165
basal cell adenomas as, 1170
canalicular cell adenomas as, 1170
oncocytomas as, 1171
pleomorphic adenoma as, 1169, 1170f
contributions to saliva of, 1134t
imaging of, 1145
malignant neoplasms of
adenoid cystic carcinoma as, 1362-1363
excision of, 1196
of hard palate, 1310
of larynx, 1506-1508
mucoepidermoid carcinoma as, 1363
physical examination of, 1179
physiology of, 1133-1142
in children, 2853
secretory unit of, 1133-1134, 1134f
Salivary gland calculi. *See* Sialolithiasis.
Salivary gland choristoma, of middle ear, 2200-2201
Salivary gland cysts, 2859
acquired, 2859
congenital, 2859
Salivary gland disease
benign lymphoepithelial, 1154
in children, 2858
in children, 2850-2865
aberrant salivary glands as, 2864, 2864f
due to allergic reactions, 2864
anatomy and, 2850-2853
autoimmune, 2858-2863
benign lymphoepithelial, 2858
biopsy for, 2855
congenital, differential diagnosis of, 2851t
in cystic fibrosis, 2864
cysts and mucoceles as, 2859
acquired, 2859
congenital, 2859
differential diagnosis of, 2850, 2851t, 2852f-2853f
history and physical examination for, 2853
imaging of, 2854-2855
inflammatory, 2855-2858
abscess as, 2856
due to actinomycosis, 2858
bacterial, 2856-2857, 2856t
diagnostic algorithm for, 2853, 2854f
differential diagnosis of, 2851t
due to Epstein-Barr virus, 2855
granulomatous, 2857-2858, 2857f
due to HIV, 2856
due to mumps, 2855
mycobacterial, 2857-2858, 2857f
sarcoidosis as, 2858
viral, 2855
juvenile recurrent parotitis as, 2858
laboratory studies for, 2853-2854
due to medications, 2864-2865
necrotizing sialometaplasia as, 2857
neoplastic, 1192, 2861-2862, 2862t
benign, 2861-2862
differential diagnosis of, 2851t
malignant, 2862-2863

Salivary gland disease *(Continued)*
sialadenitis as, 2819
acute suppurative, 2856, 2856t
bacterial, 2856-2857, 2856t
chronic, 2858
neonatal, 2857
recurrent, 2856-2857
viral, 2855
sialadenoscopy for, 2855
sialolithiasis as, 2858-2859
sialorrhea as, 2863-2864
in systemic conditions, 2864-2865
traumatic, 2863-2865
vascular anomalies as, 2859
hemangiomas as, 2859-2860, 2860f
lymphatic malformations as, 2860-2861, 2861f
cysts and mucoceles as, 2859
acquired, 2859
congenital, 2859
ultrasound imaging of, 1647
HIV-associated, 1157-1158, 1157f
immunosuppression and, 217-218
diffuse infiltratrive lymphocytosis syndrome as, 218
parotid lesions as, 217-218, 218f
xerostomia as, 218
inflammatory, 1151-1161
bacterial infections as, 1151-1153
in children, 2856-2857, 2856t
in children, 2855-2858
abscess as, 2856
due to actinomycosis, 2858
bacterial, 2856-2857, 2856t
diagnostic algorithm for, 2853, 2854f
differential diagnosis of, 2851t
due to Epstein-Barr virus, 2855
granulomatous, 2857-2858, 2857f
due to HIV, 2856
due to mumps, 2855
mycobacterial, 2857-2858, 2857f
sarcoidosis as, 2858
viral, 2855
chronic sialadenitis as, 1154, 1155f
granulomatous infections as, 1158-1159
due to actinomycosis, 1159
due to cat scratch disease, 1159
in children, 2857-2858, 2857f
due to nontuberculous mycobacterial disease, 1158-1159, 1158f
due to toxoplasmosis, 1159-1160
due to tuberculous mycobacterial disease, 1158
neonatal suppurative parotitis as, 1153
noninfectious, 1160-1161
recurrent parotitis of childhood as, 1153-1154
sialolithiasis as, 1155-1156, 1155f-1156f
viral infections as, 1156-1158
in children, 2855
due to Epstein-Barr virus, 2855
due to HIV, 1157-1158, 1157f, 2856
due to mumps, 1156-1157, 2855
necrotizing sialometaplasia as, 2857
neoplastic (*See* Salivary gland neoplasm(s))
sialadenitis as
acute suppurative, 1151-1153
in children, 2856, 2856t
clinical manifestations of, 1152, 1152f
complications of, 1153, 1154f
differential diagnosis of, 1152
epidemiology of, 1151
laboratory evaluation of, 1152
pathogenesis of, 1151-1152, 1152f
treatment of, 1152-1153, 1153f
in children
acute suppurative, 2856, 2856t
bacterial, 2856-2857, 2856t

Salivary gland disease *(Continued)*
chronic, 2858
neonatal, 2857
recurrent, 2856-2857
viral, 2855
chronic, 1154, 1155f
in children, 2858
sialolithiasis as
in children, 2858-2859
ultrasound of, 1647
in Sjögren's syndrome, 1160-1161
in children, 2858
traumatic, 312, 313f
in children, 2863-2865
sialocele and salivary fistula due to, 313-314
vascular anomalies as, 2859
hemangiomas as, 2859-2860, 2860f
lymphatic malformations as, 1172, 2860-2861, 2861f
Salivary gland dysfunction, aging and, 1141-1142, 1141f
Salivary gland hypofunction, 1138
Salivary gland neoplasm(s)
benign, 1162-1177
basal cell adenomas as, 1170
canalicular adenomas as, 1170
in children, 2861-2862
complications of, 1176-1177
facial nerve paresis or paralysis as, 1176-1177
gustatory sweating ("Frey's syndrome") as, 1177
salivary fistula as, 1177
sensory abnormalities as, 1177
congenital vascular, 1172
arteriovenous malformations as, 1172
hemangiomas as, 1172
lymphatic malformations as, 1172
venous malformations as, 1172
dumbbell, 1164-1165, 1165f, 1167f-1168f
glomus tumors as, 1169f
incidence of, 1164
by histologic type, 1164, 1164t
by site of origin, 1164, 1164f
inverted ductal papilloma as, 1171-1172
management of, 1172-1176
excision of parapharyngeal salivary gland tumors in, 1174-1176, 1176f
parotidectomy for, 1172-1174, 1173f
submandibular gland excision for, 1174, 1174f
myoepithelioma as, 1171
oncocytoma as, 1171
papillary cystadenoma as
lymphomatosum (Warthin's tumors), 1170-1171
oncocytic, 1171
parapharyngeal, excision of, 1174-1176, 1175f
parotid lipoma as, 1166, 1167f
patient evaluation for, 1164-1168
clinical features in, 1164-1165, 1165f-1166f
fine-needle aspiration biopsy in, 1165-1166
imaging in, 1166-1168, 1167f-1169f
pleomorphic adenoma as, 1168-1169
carcinoma ex, 1187-1189, 1188f
in children, 2861-2862
clinical features of, 1166f, 1169
histopathology of, 1169
imaging of, 1167f-1168f
of lacrimal gland, 1169, 1170f
malignant transformation of, 1169
metastasizing, 1189
of palate, 1169, 1169f
pathogenesis of, 1168-1169
recurrent, 1169, 1170f
sites of, 1169, 1169f-1170f
sialadenoma papilliferum as, 1171
Warthin's tumor as, 2862

Salivary gland neoplasm(s) *(Continued)*
biomarkers for, 1163
in children, 1192, 2861-2862, 2862t
benign, 2861-2862
differential diagnosis of, 2851t
malignant, 2845-2846, 2862-2863
epidemiology of, 2845
histopathology and molecular biology of, 2846, 2846f
management of, 2845-2846
neck mass due to, 2820
presentation and evaluation of, 2845
embryology of, 1162, 1163f
Epstein-Barr virus and, 1163
etiology of, 1163-1164
genetic factors in, 1164
other factors in, 1163-1164
radiation in, 1163
viral, 1163
fine-needle aspiration biopsy of, 1149, 1149f, 1165-1166, 1180-1181
histogenesis of, 1163
malignant, 1178-1199
acinic cell carcinoma as, 1185-1186, 1187f
in children, 2820, 2846, 2846f, 2863
adenocarcinoma as
basal cell, 1191
NOS, 1191
polymorphous low-grade, 1184-1185, 1186f
adenoid cystic carcinoma as
histopathology of, 1183-1184, 1185f
imaging of, 1146-1147, 1146f-1147f, 1180f
cervical lymph node metastasis of, 1196-1197
chemotherapy for, 1199
in children, 1192, 2845-2846, 2862-2863
epidemiology of, 2845
histopathology and molecular biology of, 2846, 2846f
management of, 2845-2846
neck mass due to, 2820
presentation and evaluation of, 2845
epidemiology of, 1143, 1178
by histologic type, 1178, 1179t
by site, 1178, 1179t
epithelial-myoepithelial carcinomas as, 1191
histopathology of, 1181-1192, 1182f, 1182t
lymphoma as, 1191-1192, 1192f, 1679-1680
treatment and prognosis for, 1680
metastatic, 1191
minor salivary gland excision for, 1196
mixed, 1186-1189
carcinoma ex pleomorphic adenoma as, 1187-1189, 1188f
metastasizing, 1189
true (carcinosarcoma), 1187, 1188f
molecular markers for, 1194
mucoepidermoid carcinoma as
in children, 2820, 2846, 2846f, 2862-2863
differential diagnosis of, 1183
grading of, 1183, 1184t
histopathology of, 1182-1183, 1183f
imaging of, 1146, 1147f, 1168f
with N+ neck, 1197
with N0 neck, 1196-1197
of oropharynx, 1362-1363
other, 1191
parotidectomy for, 1194-1196
branches of facial nerve in, 1194, 1194f
elevation of skin flap in, 1195
external carotid artery in, 1195-1196
with facial nerve involvement, 1196
greater auricular nerve in, 1195
main trunk of facial nerve in, 1195, 1195f
marginal mandibular branch of facial nerve in, 1195, 1195f
modified Blair incision for, 1195, 1195f
partial deep, 1194-1196, 1196f

Salivary gland neoplasm(s) *(Continued)*
retromandibular (posterior facial) vein in, 1195-1196, 1195f
superficial, 1194-1195
total, 1194-1196
patient evaluation for, 1178-1181
biopsy in, 1180-1181
physical examination in, 1178-1179
radiologic studies in, 1180, 1180f
staging in, 1181, 1181t
prognostic variables for, 1192-1194, 1193t
clinical, 1192-1193
histologic, 1193-1194
molecular markers as, 1194
radiation therapy for, 1197-1199
adjuvant, 1197-1198, 1198t
in children, 2863
of neck, 1198
neutron beam, 1198-1199
salivary duct carcinoma as, 1189-1190, 1189f
small cell carcinoma as, 1190-1191, 1190f
squamous cell carcinoma as, 1190
sublingual gland excision for, 1196
submandibular gland excision for, 1196
surgical treatment of, 1194-1197
neck masses due to, 1640
radiation and, 1163
ultrasonography of, 1645-1647, 1653f-1654f
Salivary gland secretion, 1133-1136
anatomy of secretory unit in, 1133-1134, 1134f
neuronal control of, 1136
neurotransmitters and receptors in, 1136-1137, 1136f, 1137t
signal transduction in, 1137-1138
adenylate cyclase system in, 1137
G proteins in, 1137
phospholipase C system in, 1137-1138
process of, 1134-1136
ductal, 1136
fluid, 1135, 1135f
macromolecule, 1135-1136
Salivary gland unit, 1162, 1163f
Salivary pH, 2384
Salivation, reflex, 1205-1206
Sal-like 1 *(SALL1)* gene, in deafness, 2051t-2058t
Salmon patch, 290-291
Salpingopharyngeal fold, 1359f
Salpingopharyngeus muscle
anatomy of, 1870
development of, 1866
Salt restriction, for Meniere's disease, 2337
Salty taste
individual differences in, 1211-1212
peripheral sensitivity to, 1211
transduction of, 1208-1209
Sample size
calculation of, 74
determination of, 68t
small, 73, 73t
Sampling methods, 68-69, 68t-69t
SAN. *See* Spinal accessory nerve (SAN).
Sanguinaria, oral leukoplakia due to, 1223-1224, 1224f
SANS, in deafness, 2051t-2058t, 2077-2078
Saphenous vein repair, for aneurysms of upper cervical and petrous internal carotid artery, 2504, 2505f
Saprophytic fungal rhinosinusitis, 712
SAQLI (Sleep Apnea Quality of Life Index), 57
SAR (seasonal allergic rhinitis), 617-618
and pediatric chronic sinusitis, 2778
Sarcoidosis, 2104-2105
in children, 2819
salivary gland involvement in, 2858
clinical course of, 659
clinical presentation of, 2104
diagnosis of, 659
Sarcoidosis *(Continued)*
epidemiology of, 658-659, 2104
of epiglottis, 1465f
etiology of, 658
facial paralysis in, 2400
laboratory findings in, 2104, 2104f
laryngeal and tracheal manifestations of, 890-891, 890f
nasal manifestations of, 658-659
oral manifestations of, 1252
otologic manifestations of, 2105
pathology of, 659, 2104f
sudden sensorineural hearing loss due to, 2129
treatment of, 659, 2104
Sarcoma(s)
alveolar soft part, 1668
angio-, 1668
bone, 1666, 1667t
in children, 2840-2843
dermatofibrosarcoma protuberans as, 2843, 2843f
epithelioid, 2843, 2843f
Ewing's, 2845
fibro-, 2842-2843, 2843f
nonrhabdomyosarcoma soft tissue, 2842
rhabdomyo-, 2820, 2840-2842
epidemiology of, 2820, 2840
histopathology and molecular biology of, 2842, 2842f
management of, 2820, 2841-2842
presentation and evaluation of, 2840-2841, 2841t
sites of, 2820
survival with, 2840
chondro-
of cerebellopontine angle, 2527, 2528f-2529f
of larynx, 1508
of neck, 1669-1670
of paranasal sinuses, 1131
of petrous apex, 2528f
of skull base, 1699, 1923-1924, 1926f, 2529f
dermatofibrosarcoma protuberans as, 2843, 2843f
epithelioid
in children, 2843, 2843f
of neck, 1668-1669
Ewing's
in children, 2845
of neck, 1671
of oral cavity, 1253
fibro-
in children, 2842-2843, 2843f
of larynx, 1508
of neck, 1668
of paranasal sinuses, 1131
granulocytic, 2107
hemangiopericytoma as, 1670
Kaposi's
of hard palate, 1309-1310
immunosuppression and, 212-215, 213t
epidemiology and pathogenesis of, 212-213
presentation and diagnosis of, 213-214, 214f
treatment of, 214-215
of larynx, 1508-1509
of oral cavity, 1299
of oropharynx, 1363-1364, 1364f
of larynx, 1508-1509
chondro-, 1508
fibro-, 1508
Kaposi, 1508-1509
lipo-, 1508
malignant fibrous histiocytoma as, 1508
pseudo-, 1506
leiomyo-, 1670
lipo-
of larynx, 1508
of neck, 1670
Sarcoma(s) *(Continued)*
malignant fibrous histiocytoma as
of larynx, 1508
of neck, 1667
malignant giant cell tumor as, 1671
malignant peripheral nerve sheath tumor as, 1670-1671
of neck, 1666
alveolar soft part, 1668
angio-, 1668
bone, 1666, 1667t
chondro-, 1669-1670
classification and staging of, 1666, 1666t-1667t
epithelioid hemangioendothelioma as, 1668-1669
Ewing's, 1671
fibro-, 1668
hemangiopericytoma as, 1670
leiomyo-, 1670
lipo-, 1670
malignant fibrous histiocytoma as, 1667
malignant giant cell tumor as, 1671
malignant peripheral nerve sheath tumor as, 1670-1671
osteo-, 1668
rhabdomyo-, 1667-1668, 1668f, 1669t
soft tissue, 1666, 1666t
synovial, 1670
nonrhabdomyosarcoma soft tissue, 2842
of oral cavity, 1299, 1299f
osteo-
of neck, 1668
of oral cavity, 1299f
of paranasal sinuses, 1131
postradiation, 1479
pseudo-, of larynx, 1506
rhabdomyo-
in children, 2820, 2840-2842
epidemiology of, 2820, 2840
histopathology and molecular biology of, 2842, 2842f
management of, 2820, 2841-2842
presentation and evaluation of, 2840-2841, 2841t
sites of, 2820
survival with, 2840
of middle ear or mastoid, 2501-2502
of neck, 1667-1668, 1668f, 1669t
of paranasal sinuses, 1132
soft tissue, 1666, 1666t
synovial, 1670
Sarcomatoid carcinoma, of larynx, 1506
Sarcomatoid squamous cell carcinoma, of oral cavity, 1299
SAS (Simultaneous Analog Stimulation), for cochlear implants, 2230, 2230f
Satisfaction surveys, 72
Saturated solution of potassium iodide (SSKI)
for Graves' disease, 1742-1743
for hyperthyroidism, 1739t
Saturation, of auditory neurons, 1844-1845, 1845f
Saucer fracture, of orbital floor, pediatric, 2712-2713, 2715f
Savage, Terry, 2086
Savary-Guillard dilator, for esophageal strictures, 966
SBE (subacute bacterial endocarditis) prophylaxis, for pediatric surgery, 2596, 2596t-2597t
Scala media
anatomy of, 1831-1832, 1832f, 1840, 1841f
in auditory physiology, 1840, 1841f-1842f
in cochlear transduction, 2050, 2061f-2062f
Scala tympani
anatomy of, 1831, 1832f, 1840, 1841f, 1853f
in auditory physiology, 1841f-1842f
in cochlear transduction, 2050, 2061f-2062f

Scala vestibuli
anatomy of, 1831, 1832f, 1840, 1841f, 1853f
in auditory physiology, 1841f-1842f
in cochlear transduction, 2050, 2061f-2062f
Scales, for psychometric validation, 55
Scalp, 440, 441f
Scalp extenders, for hair loss, 384, 385f
Scalp reductions, for hair loss, 384-385, 385f
complications of, 385, 386f
Scanning speech, 837-838
Scapha, 476-477, 476f, 1824f
Scapha-conchal sutures, 476f-477f
Scaphal reduction, 478f
Scaphocephaly, synostotic
clinical manifestations of, 2642, 2643f, 2650f
surgical management of, 2650f-2651f
Scaphoid fossa, 2742f
Scapula composite flap, for oral cancer, 1316
Scapula free flap, 1082t, 1086-1087, 1088f
Scapular flap, for hypopharyngeal and esophageal reconstruction, 1455
Scapular osteocutaneous free flap, for mandibular defects, 1324-1325, 1324f, 1325t
Scapular-parascapular flaps, for free tissue transfer, 1082t
Scar(s)
hypertrophic, 291
after neck surgery, 1728, 1729f
after otoplasty, 479
due to rhytidectomy, 425-426
after neck surgery, 1728, 1729f
and relaxed skin tension lines, 295, 296f
due to rhytidectomy, 425-426, 425f, 427f
Scar revision and camouflage, 295-301
cosmetics and hairstyling for, 301
dermabrasion for, 298-299, 300f
excision for, 295, 297f
expansion with excision for, 296-298
serial, 296
tissue, 296-298, 297f
indications for, 295
irregularization for, 298
geometric broken line closure in, 298, 299f-300f
W-plasty in, 298, 299f
Z-plasty in, 298, 298f-299f
silicone sheeting for, 300-301
steroids for, 299-300, 301f
techniques for, 295
SCARF (Superior Constrictor Rotation-Advancement Flap), for reconstruction of soft palate, 1382, 1382f
Scarlet fever, 2788
Scarpa's fascia, 2577
Scarpa's ganglion, 1851f, 1852-1854
Scarring alopecia, 375-376
Scattering, of laser energy, 28-29, 29f
SCC. *See* Squamous cell carcinoma (SCC).
SCC(s) (semicircular canals). *See* Semicircular canal(s) (SCCs).
SCCHN (squamous cell carcinoma of the head and neck). *See* Head and neck squamous cell carcinoma (HNSCC).
SCCNET (small cell carcinoma, neuroendocrine type), of larynx, 1507-1508
SCDS (superior canal dehiscence syndrome). *See* Superior semicircular canal dehiscence (SSCD) syndrome.
SCF (stem cell factor), 609t-610t
Schaefer-Fuhrman classification, of laryngeal trauma, 936, 936t
Schatzki's ring, 966f, 967, 968f
transnasal esophagoscopy of, 984f
Scheibe aplasia, 2200
Scheibe dysplasia, 2727-2728
Schirmer test, 446-447, 447f, 2383
SCHLP (supracricoid hemilaryngopharyngectomy), for hypopharyngeal cancer, 1429, 1436
Schneiderian papilloma, inverted type
of nasopharynx, 1349
sinonasal, 718-720
endoscopic appearance of, 718-719, 719f
epidemiology of, 718
with frontal sinus involvement, 720, 720f
histologic appearance of, 718
human papillomavirus and, 718
imaging of, 719, 719f
postoperative surveillance for, 720
recurrence of, 720
sites for, 718
and squamous cell carcinoma, 718
surgical approach for, 718t, 719-720, 720f, 763
Schobinger incision, modified, for radical neck dissection, 1709, 1710f
Schüller projection, of temporal bone, 131
Schwabach test, 98
Schwannoma(s)
acoustic (*See* Acoustic neuroma(s))
of ethmoid region, 2479, 2480f
facial nerve (*See* Facial nerve neuroma)
glossopharyngeal, 2507f
imaging of, 150-151
of jugular foramen
imaging of, 1929-1930, 1930f, 2522f
lateral cranial base surgery for, 2504-2505, 2505f
stereotactic radiation therapy for, 2565
of larynx, 882
of neck, 1663, 1663f
neck masses due to, 1640
sinonasal, 726-727, 726f
trigeminal, 2512f
vestibular (*See* Acoustic neuroma(s))
Schwartze sign, 2030
SCID (severe combined immunodeficiency), 209-210
Scintigraphy, 138, 139f
for CSF rhinorrhea, 790
of neck masses, 1637, 1637t
of salivary glands, 138, 1150
of thyroid nodule, 1757-1758
Scintillations, in migraine, 247
Scintilligraphy, of lacrimal obstruction, 798, 799f
Scissors excision, for skin lesions, 293
SCIT (subcutaneous immunotherapy), for allergic rhinitis, 621
SCJ. *See* Squamocolumnar junction (SCJ).
Scleroderma
esophageal manifestations of, 979, 979f
imaging of, 1400, 1401f
vs. myofascial pain dysfunction syndrome, 1285t
nasal manifestations of, 660
oral manifestations of, 1252
Sclerotherapy, for lymphatic malformations, 2830-2831
Scoring systems, 53
Scotoma, in migraine, 247
SCPL. *See* Supracricoid partial laryngectomy (SCPL).
Screening, for infant hearing loss, 2718-2719
Scrofula, imaging of, 166f
Scurvy, oral manifestations of, 1254
SD (standard deviation), 63, 64t
vs. standard error, 73, 73t
SDB. *See* Sleep-disordered breathing (SDB).
SDC (salivary duct carcinoma), 1189-1190, 1189f
SDF-1 (stromal cell–derived factor), in head and neck squamous cell carcinoma, 1060
SDH (succinate-dehydrogenase), in familial paraganglioma syndromes, 1659, 1659t
SDT (speech detection threshold), 1888-1889
SE (standard error), *vs.* standard deviation, 73, 73t
Seasonal allergic rhinitis (SAR), 617-618
and pediatric chronic sinusitis, 2778
Seasonality, of otitis media, 2767
Sebaceous hyperplasia, 288f, 293
Seborrheic keratoses, 281-282, 282f
Second genu, of facial nerve, 1826f, 1827-1829
Second intention healing
of oropharyngeal defects, 1376
of tongue base, 1387-1388
of tonsil and pharyngeal wall, 1383
of surface defects of nasal tip, columella, sidewalls, and dorsum as, 365
with trasoral laser microsurgery, 1533
Second malignancy
with pediatric head and neck malignancies, 2848
radiation therapy and, 2626t
Second primary tumors (SPTs)
of larynx, 1492, 1510
in oral cancer, 1301-1302
Secretory duct, of salivary gland, 1133-1135
Secretory endpiece, of salivary gland, 1133-1134
Secretory proteins, in salivary gland secretion, 1135-1136
Secretory unit, of salivary gland, 1134-1135
Secundum passagio, 851
Sedation
of children, 2572, 2594
for tracheobronchial endoscopy, 1000
Sedatives, as adjuncts to induction of anesthesia, 111
Segmental resection, for tracheal stenosis, 2931-2932, 2932f
Segregation, of chromosomes, 2088
Seizures
focal, vestibular symptoms of, 2357
preoperative evaluation of, 106
SELDI-TOF (surface-enhanced laser desorption-ionization–time-of-flight), in head and neck squamous cell carcinoma, 1029
Selection bias, 53, 68t
Selection criteria, 68
Selective neck dissection (SND), 1712-1713
for cancer of midline structures of anterior lower neck, 1719
definition and rationale for, 1719, 1719f
technique for, 1719, 1720f
for cutaneous malignancies, 1718-1719
definition and rationale for, 1718, 1718f
technique for, 1718-1719
definition of, 1703t, 1712
historical perspective on, 1703
for oral cancer, 1313, 1713-1716
definition and rationale for, 1713, 1714f
technique for, 1713-1716, 1715f-1716f
for oropharyngeal, hypopharyngeal, and laryngeal cancer, 1716-1718
definition and rationale for, 1716-1717, 1717f
technique for, 1717-1718, 1717f
rationale for, 1712-1713
results of, 1721
for thyroid cancer, 1719, 1719f-1720f
Selective serotonin reuptake inhibitors (SSRIs)
for migraine, 2350
for tinnitus, 2137
Self, *vs.* nonself, in immune system, 599
Self-assessment, 79t
Sella
anatomy of, 1823f
in surgical anatomy of lateral skull base, 2435f
Sella turcica, 1699
Sellick maneuver, during rapid-sequence anesthesia induction, in children, 2590
Semicanal, of tensor tympani muscle, 2436f
Semicircular canal(s) (SCCs)
anatomy of, 1825f, 1831, 1850-1851, 1851f, 1853f, 2278f
in cochlear transduction, 2062f

Semicircular canal(s) (SCCs) *(Continued)*
congenital anomalies of, 2732-2733
in combination with other anomalies, 2728, 2738, 2739f
in congenital aural atresia, 2738
incidence of, 2727
semicircular canal aplasia as, 2732-2733, 2732f
semicircular canal dysplasia as, 2732, 2732f-2733f
embryogenesis of, 1851-1852, 1851f
encoding of head rotation, linear acceleration, and tilt by, 2277-2285
afferents in, 2283-2285, 2283f-2284f
cupula in, 2282f
otoconial membrane in, 2283
sensory transduction in, 2277-2279
anatomy of vestibular end organs in, 2277, 2278f
bidirectional sensitivity in, 2278-2279
cupula in, 2277, 2278f
firing rate in, 2278-2279, 2281f
hair cells in, 2277
otolith organs in, 2278, 2281f
stereocilia in, 2277-2278, 2279f
excitation-inhibition asymmetry of, 2290-2291, 2291f
excitatory and inhibitory responses to head rotation by
high-acceleration, 2290-2292
anatomic and physiologic basis for, 2290-2291, 2291f
clinical importance of, 2291-2292, 2291f-2293f
in its plane, 2289
anatomic and physiologic basis for, 2282f, 2289
clinical importance of, 2289
and eye movements, 2306, 2307f
imaging of, 1920-1921, 1922f
interpretation of any stimulus that excites afferents as excitatory rotation in plane of, 2289
anatomic and physiologic basis for, 2289
clinical importance of, 2289-2290
for nystagmus during caloric testing, 2290
in posterior canal benign paroxysmal positional vertigo, 2289-2290
in superior canal dehiscence syndrome, 2290, 2290f
orientation of, 1852, 1852f
and stimulation of eye movements, 2285-2289
anatomic and physiologic basis for, 2285-2288, 2286f-2288f
clinical importance of, 2288-2289, 2288f
response to simultaneous stimuli of, 2292-2294
anatomic and physiologic basis for, 2292-2294, 2294f-2295f
clinical implications of, 2294
sensitivity axis(es) of, 2293-2294, 2294f
and nystagmus, 2294-2295, 2295f
stimulation of, eyes movements in plane of canal produced by, 2285-2289
anatomic and physiologic basis for, 2285-2288, 2286f-2288f
clinical importance of, 2288-2289, 2288f
transfer function relative to head velocity for, 2303, 2303f
Semicircular canal (SCC) aplasia, 2732-2733, 2732f
Semicircular canal (SCC) dysplasia, 2732, 2732f-2733f
Semont maneuver, for benign paroxysmal positional vertigo, 2331
Semprex D (acrivastine), for nonallergic rhinitis, 701t
Senile angiomas, 290-291
Senile sebaceous hyperplasia, 293
Sensitivity axis(es), of semicircular canals, 2293-2294, 2294f
and nystagmus, 2294-2295, 2295f
Sensitization, in allergic rhinitis, 614
Sensorineural hearing loss (SNHL)
due to acoustic neuroma, 2124-2125, 2125f, 2515-2516
sudden, 2128
in adults, 2116-2130
clinical evaluation of, 2116-2117
audiometric testing in, 2117
history in, 2116
laboratory testing in, 2117
physical examination in, 2116
radiographic testing in, 2117
vestibular testing in, 2117
cochlear *vs.* retrocochlear, 2117
etiology of, 2117-2127
bone disorders as, 2124
endocrine and metabolic, 2125
hereditary disorders as, 2117-2118, 2118f
immune, 2123-2124
infectious, 2118-2119
inner ear anomalies as, 2118, 2118f
neoplastic, 2124-2125, 2125f
neurologic, 2122-2123
paraneoplastic, 2124
pharmacologic toxicity as, 2119-2121
pseudohypacusis as, 2125
renal, 2121
traumatic, 2121-2122, 2121f-2122f
unknown, 2125-2127, 2126f
vascular and hematologic, 2123
sudden, 2127-2130
etiology of, 2127-2129
prevalence, natural history, and prognosis of, 2127
treatment of, 2129-2130
audiogram of, 1888, 1889f, 1906f-1907f
in children, 2200, 2200b
prevalence of, 2719
due to cholesteatoma, 1974
congenital
due to congenital anomalies of inner ear, 2727
due to labyrinthine infections, 2154-2157
with cytomegalovirus, 2154-2156, 2155f
with rubella, 2154, 2156-2157, 2157f
with syphilis, 2161
epidemiology of, 2087
genetic, 2086-2099, 2200
autosomal dominant
nonsyndromic, 2090-2093, 2092t
syndromic, 2093-2096, 2094t
autosomal recessive
nonsyndromic, 2089-2090, 2090f, 2091t
syndromic, 2094t, 2096
background of, 2086-2089
cultural considerations with, 2099
diagnosis of, 2097-2098
epidemiology of, 2089t
genetic testing for, 2098
mitochondrial
nonsyndromic, 2093, 2093t
screening for, 2090t
syndromic, 2094t, 2097
nonsyndromic, 2089-2093
adult-onset, 2117
autosomal dominant, 2090-2093, 2092t
autosomal recessive, 2089-2090, 2090f, 2091t
epidemiology of, 2089, 2089t
high-frequency, 2090-2092
low-frequency, 2092-2093
midfrequency, 2092
mitochondrial, 2093, 2093t
screening for, 2090t
X-linked, 2093, 2093t
Sensorineural hearing loss (SNHL) *(Continued)*
patient management with, 2097-2099
prenatal testing for, 2098
prevention of, 2099
syndromic, 2093-2097, 2094t, 2200, 2200b
in Alport syndrome, 2094t, 2096-2097
autosomal dominant, 2093-2096, 2094t
autosomal recessive, 2094t, 2096
in biotinidase deficiency, 2094t, 2096
in branchio-oto-renal syndrome, 2093-2095, 2094t
epidemiology of, 2089t
in Jervell and Lange-Nielsen syndrome, 2094t, 2096
in MELAS, 2094t, 2097
in MERRF, 2094t, 2097
mitochondrial, 2094t, 2097
in Mohr-Tranebjaerg syndrome, 2094t, 2097
in neurofibromatosis type 2, 2094t, 2095
in non–insulin-dependent diabetes mellitus, 2094t, 2097
in Norrie's disease, 2094t
in Pendred syndrome, 2094t, 2096
in Refsum disease, 2094t, 2096
screening for, 2090t
in Stickler syndrome, 2094t, 2095
in Treacher Collins syndrome, 2094t, 2096
in Usher syndrome, 2094t, 2096
in Waardenburg syndrome, 2094t, 2095-2096
X-linked, 2094t, 2096-2097
treatment of, 2098-2099
X-linked
nonsyndromic, 2093, 2093t
syndromic, 2094t, 2096-2097
in HIV-positive patients, 223-225
approach to, 224, 225t
due to cryptococcal meningitis, 223-224
due to otosyphilis, 224
in infants, 2718-2725
ancillary testing for, 2722-2723
genetic testing in, 2722-2723
laboratory testing in, 2722
screening for connexin 26 mutation in, 2723
screening for maternally transmitted infection in, 2723
temporal bone imaging in, 2723
testing for Pendred's syndrome in, 2723
assessment of, 2719-2721
auditory brainstem responses in, 2719-2720
comparison of otoacoustic emissions and auditory brainstem responses in, 2721
evoked otoacoustic emissions in, 2720-2721
testing protocols for, 2719, 2720f
delay in identification of, 2719
diagnosis of, 2721-2722
audiology in, 2722
history in, 2721
middle ear effusions in, 2722
otomicroscopy in, 2722
physical examination in, 2721-2722
vestibular function assessment in, 2722
visual reinforcement audiometry in, 2722
history of screening for, 2718-2719
intervention strategies for, 2723-2724
amplification devices as, 2723-2724
bone conduction amplification as, 2723
cochlear implantation as, 2724
early, 2724
surgical therapy as, 2723
due to labyrinthine infections, 2118-2119, 2153-2163
acquired, 2157-2161
with herpes simplex virus, 2159-2160
with Lassa fever, 2158-2159
with measles, 2158
with meningitis, 2160-2161

Sensorineural hearing loss (SNHL) *(Continued)*
with mumps, 2157-2158, 2158f
sudden, 2154, 2154b, 2157
with varicella-zoster virus, 2159, 2159f
bacterial and fungal, 2160
with cochlear implant, 2161
congenital, 2154-2157
with cytomegalovirus, 2154-2156, 2155f
with rubella, 2156-2157, 2157f
in immunocompromised patients, 2161-2162
syphilitic, 2161
vaccines to prevent hearing loss due to, 2161
vestibular neuritis due to, 2162-2163, 2162f
due to Lassa fever, 2158-2159
sudden, 2127
in Meniere's disease, 2126-2127, 2335t
fluctuating, 2199
history of, 2337
sudden, 2129
with migraine, 2123, 2348-2349
noise-induced, 2121-2122, 2121f-2122f
otoacoustic emissions with
distortion product, 1905, 1907f
transient evoked, 1905, 1906f
due to small fenestra stapedotomy, 2030, 2034
sudden, 2127-2130
due to acoustic neuroma, 2128
clinical features of, 2157
etiology of, 2127-2129, 2195b, 2198-2201
due to labyrinthine infections, 2154, 2154b, 2157
prevalence, natural history, and prognosis of, 2127
temporal bone pathology in, 2157
treatment of, 2129-2130, 2157
intratympanic steroids for, 2184-2185
systemic steroids for, 2184
due to temporal bone trauma, 2047
in transplant recipients, 224-225
unilateral, bone-anchored hearing aid for, 2216
Sensory abnormalities, after parotidectomy, 1177
Sensory assessment, laryngopharyngeal, 836
Sensory integration, evaluation of, 2317
Sensory nerve complications, of neck surgery, 1731-1732
cervical, 1731-1732
greater auricular, 1731
lingual, 1731
Sensory organization test (SOT), 2325-2326, 2325f-2326f
Sensory presbycusis, 232, 2126
Sensory substitution, in vestibular compensation, 2375
Sensory substitution exercises, in vestibular rehabilitation, 2372-2373, 2378
"Sensory-specific" satiety, 1212-1213
Sentences-in-noise (SIN), for cochlear implants, 2223
Sentinel lymph node biopsy (SLNB)
for melanoma, 1115-1118
complexity in head and neck region of, 1117
excision of primary tumor prior to, 1115, 1116f
future investigations on, 1117-1118
histologic evaluation of, 1116
indications for, 1115, 1115b
inflammation and fibrosis due to, 1117
injury to facial nerve due to, 1117
intraoperative lymphatic mapping for, 1115, 1116f
learning curve for, 1116
lymphoscintigraphy with, 1115-1117, 1116f
and overall survival, 1117
potential therapeutic benefits of, 1117
as prognostic factor, 1117
risk of in-transit metastasis with, 1117
technique of, 1115-1116
therapeutic lymph node dissection after, 1116
for oral cancer, 1313-1314
Sentinel lymph node mapping, 1115, 1116f
Sentinel vein, in brow or forehead rejuvenation, 433-434, 433f
Septal abscess, 2627, 2627f
Septal artery, in surgical anatomy of anterior cranial base, 2473, 2473f
Septal branch
of anterior ethmoid artery, 483f
of sphenopalatal artery, 483f
Septal cartilage grafts
in noncaucasian rhinoplasty, 569
in revision rhinoplasty, 583
Septal deviation, 483f, 484
endoscopic sinus surgery with, 751
imaging of, 668, 669f
in noncaucasian patient, 573, 576f
rhinitis due to, 619b
rhinoplasty with, 513-514, 514f, 546, 546f-547f
septoplasty for (*See* Septoplasty)
due to trauma, 482, 484
with twisted nose, 551-552, 552f
Septal fracture, 498, 501, 501f
closed reduction of, 503, 503f
open reduction of, 505-506
Septal hematoma, 494
due to nasal fracture, 507
pediatric, 2708-2709, 2712f
Septal modifications, rhinoplasty for, 546-548, 546f-547f
caudal repositioning in, 547, 547f
dorsal draw suture in, 548, 549f
making final septal assessment in, 548, 549f
septocolumellar complex in, 548, 549f-550f
shortening of caudal septum in, 547-548, 547f-548f
Septal mucoperichondrial flap, for nasal reconstruction, 371-372, 372f
Septal nerve, 483f
Septal perforation, 493-494, 493f
epistaxis due to, 686f
Septal splints, after nasal fractures, 504
Septal spur, 482, 482f, 489, 494, 669f
Septisol (hexachlorophene and alcohol), for deep chemical peel, 394-395
Septocolumellar complex, in rhinoplasty, 548, 549f-550f
Septocutaneous arteries, 1065, 1065f
Septolabial angle, correction of acute, 547-548, 548f
Septomaxillary ligament, in craniofacial growth and development, 2614
Septoplasty, 488-494
adjuncts to, 494
alar deformity due to, 491, 491f
anesthesia and analgesia for, 488
bony deflection or spur in, 482, 482f, 489, 494
with caudal absence and tip collapse, 492, 492f
caudal septum in, 491-492, 491f-492f
complications of, 494
Cottle and Freer elevators in, 488, 489f
with crooked nose, 494
defined, 488
effects on craniofacial growth and development of, 2627-2628
elevation of mucoperiosteum in, 488-489
endoscopic, with endoscopic dacryocystorhinostomy, 798, 799f
evolution of technique for, 487-488
incisions and planes of dissection for, 488, 489f
L-strut in, 489-490, 490f
maxillary crest in, 490, 490f
with nasal valve correction, 493
postoperative care after, 494, 494f
of previously fractured nose, 483-484
reoperation after, 492-493, 493f
reskeletonization in, 491
with septal perforation repair, 493-494, 493f
Septoplasty *(Continued)*
spreader graft placement in, 490-491, 491f
suturing in, 491, 491f
in vocal professional, 858
wedge excision in, 490-491, 490f
Septum, nasal. *See* Nasal septum.
Sequencing, 3, 9
Serial excision, for scar revision, 296
Serologic tests, for dizziness, 2327
Seroma
after liposuction, 459
after neck surgery, 1727, 1727f
Serotonin (5-hydroxytryptamine$_3$)-receptor antagonists, for postoperative nausea and vomiting in children, 2593
Serotonin-norepinephrine reuptake inhibitors, for neuropathic pain, 244
Serous acinus, 1134, 1134f, 1134t
Serous demilune, 1134, 1134f
Serous labyrinthitis, after small fenestra stapedotomy, 2034
Serous otitis media (SOM), immunosuppression and, 222-223
Sertraline, for tinnitus, 2137
Serum analysis, for biomarkers, for head and neck squamous cell carcinoma, 1026-1027
Sesamoid cartilages, 497f
Sestamibi–technetium 99m scintigraphy, for hyperparathyroidism, 1785
due to double parathyroid adenoma, 1785, 1785f
due to mediastinal supernumerary thyroid gland, 1802, 1803f
and multinodular thyroid disease, 1801, 1801f
due to multiple-gland hyperplasia, 1794, 1794f
due to parathyroid carcinoma, 1803, 1803f
Severe combined immunodeficiency (SCID), 209-210
Severity, of disease, 53
Sevoflurane, for anesthesia, 111
in children, 2590
Sexually transmitted diseases, oral manifestations of, 1252
SF-36 (Medical Outcomes Study Short Form-36), 56, 642
SGL (supraglottic partial laryngectomy), for early-stage supraglottic cancer, 1498-1500, 1498f
SGNs (spiral ganglion neurons), salvage of, 2189-2191
SGS. *See* Subglottic stenosis (SGS).
Shaker 2 mutant mouse, 2076
Shave biopsy, for skin lesions, 293
Shield graft
for nasal tip enhancement, 576, 577f
in revision rhinoplasty, 589, 590f
Shielding devices, for radiation therapy, 1331-1332, 1334f
Shift worker disorder, 262t, 264
Shimmer, in acoustic analysis for voice evaluation, 829-830, 834-835
Short nose, revision rhinoplasty for
due to excessive caudal septal excision, 591f, 593
due to overrotation, 590, 590f-591f
Short T1 inversion recovery (STIR), MRI with, 135-136, 136f
Short-hairpin RNA (shRNA), 14f, 16
Short-interfering RNA (siRNA)
direct delivery of, 16
in RNA interference, 13, 14f
Shotgun(s), neck trauma due to, 1626-1627, 1628t
Shotgun shells, 1626, 1628t
Shoulder dysfunction, after neck dissection, 1722
Shoulder region, of cell survival curve, 1037-1038, 1038f

Shprintzen-Goldberg syndrome, craniofacial anomalies in, 2641t
Shrapnell's membrane, 1824, 1825f
Shrinking field technique, for radiation therapy for glottic cancer, 1586, 1587f
shRNA (short-hairpin RNA), 14f, 16
Shy-Drager syndrome, laryngeal hypofunction due to, 843
Sialadenitis
acute suppurative, 1151-1153
in children, 2856, 2856t
clinical manifestations of, 1152, 1152f
complications of, 1153, 1154f
defined, 1151
differential diagnosis of, 1152
epidemiology of, 1151
laboratory evaluation of, 1152
pathogenesis of, 1151-1152, 1152f
sialolithiasis and, 1151-1152, 1155, 1155f
treatment of, 1152-1153, 1153f
in children, 2819
acute suppurative, 2856, 2856t
bacterial, 2856-2857, 2856t
chronic, 2858
neonatal, 2857
recurrent, 2856-2857
viral, 2855
chronic, 1154, 1155f
in children, 2858
neck masses due to, 1638
in children, 2819
of parotid gland, 150
Sialadenoma papilliferum, 1171
Sialadenoscopy, in children, 2855
Sialectasis, in children, 2858
Sialocele, posttraumatic, 313-314
Sialoendoscopy, for sialolithiasis, 1156
Sialogogues, for xerostomia due to radiotherapy, 1048
Sialography, 1149-1150
in children, 2854
conventional, 139-140, 1149-1150, 1149f, 1155-1156, 1156f
CT, 139-140, 1145f, 1150, 1150f
MR, 1147
for salivary gland injury, 312
Sialolithiasis, 1155-1156, 1156f
and acute suppurative sialadenitis, 1151-1152, 1155, 1155f
in children, 2858-2859
clinical manifestations of, 1155
defined, 1155
epidemiology of, 1155
etiology of, 1155
imaging of, 1143, 1155-1156
conventional sialography for, 1155-1156, 1156f
CT for, 1143, 1148, 1148f
MR sialography for, 1155-1156
of submandibular gland, 1144f, 1154, 1157f
management of
extracorporeal shock wave lithotripsy for, 1156
nonsurgical, 1156
of parotid gland, 1156
sialendoscopy for, 1156
surgical, 1156, 1156f
neck masses due to, 1638
of parotid gland, 1155-1156
stone composition in, 1155
of submandibular gland, 1155
imaging of, 1144f, 1154, 1157f
surgical management of, 1156, 1156f
ultrasound imaging of, 1647
Sialometaplasia, necrotizing
in children, 2857
of hard palate, 1309-1310
of larynx, 1493
of oral cavity, 1289, 1299
Sialo-odontogenic cyst, 1267
clinical features of, 1267
microscopic features of, 1267, 1267f
radiographic features of, 1267
treatment of, 1267
Sialoperoxidase, in saliva, 1140
Sialorrhea, 2863-2864
defined, 2863
epidemiology of, 2863
medical management of, 2864
pathogenesis of, 2863-2864
surgical management of, 2864
Sick euthyroid syndrome, 1748
Sickle cell anemia, preoperative evaluation of, 106
Sickle cell disease, sensorineural hearing loss due to, 2120
Sickness Impact Profile, 56
SIDS (sudden infant death syndrome), 2570
Sievert (Sv), 133
Sigmoid sinus
in subtotal temporal bone resection, 2494-2495
in surgical anatomy of lateral skull base, 2436f, 2439f-2440f
Sigmoid sinus impression
anatomy of, 1823f
in surgical anatomy of lateral skull base, 2435f
Sigmoid sinus injury, due to mastoidectomy, 2016
Sigmoid sinus occlusion, in postauricular approach to infratemporal fossa, 2498, 2498f
Sigmoid sulcus, 1823f, 2010f
Signal processing strategies, for cochlear implants, 2229-2231
Advanced Combination Encoder as, 2230, 2231f
analog stimulation as, 2230, 2230f
continuous interleaved sampling as, 2229-2230
fine structure, 2230-2231, 2231f-2232f
spectral emphasis, 2230
spectral peak extraction as, 2230, 2230f
temporal, 2229-2230, 2230f
Signal transduction, in salivary gland secretion, 1137-1138
adenylate cyclase system in, 1137
G proteins in, 1137
phospholipase C system in, 1137-1138
Silastic. *See* Silicone (polydimethylsiloxane, Silastic).
Silicone (polydimethylsiloxane, Silastic)
for chin implants, 465t
injectable, dorsal cyst due to, 578, 579f
for medialization thyroplasty, 908-910, 910f
in noncaucasian rhinoplasty, 569, 570f
Silicone (polydimethylsiloxane, Silastic) rubber, for nasal reconstruction, 368
Silicone (polydimethylsiloxane, Silastic) sheeting, for scar revision, 300-301
Silicone (polydimethylsiloxane, Silastic) slings, for lagophthalmos, 2421
Silicone (polydimethylsiloxane, Silastic) strips, in atresiaplasty, 2756-2757, 2758f
Silver nitrate gel, for fungal otitis externa, 1955
Silverstein MicroWick, 2182, 2182f
Simonart's band, 2659, 2660f
Simple calyx endings, of hair cells, 1857, 1859f
Simple harmonic motion, 1838-1839, 1839f
Simulation, 45-51
advantages of, 45
for difficult airway management, 118
of endoscopic sinus surgery, 46-49
Dextroscope for, 48
ES3 for, 46-48, 46f
curriculum development for, 48
validation studies of, 47-48, 47f, 48t
Nasal Endoscopy Simulator for, 49
Paranasal Sinuses Simulator for, 49
rationale for, 46-49
VR-FESS for, 48
of temporal bone surgery, 49-50, 49f-50f
virtual reality, 45-46
Simultaneous Analog Stimulation (SAS), for cochlear implants, 2230, 2230f
SIN (sentences-in-noise), for cochlear implants, 2223
Sincipital encephaloceles, of nose, 2687-2688, 2687f, 2687t
Singers, voice disorders in. *See* Professional voice disorders.
Singer's formant, 847
Singing Voice Handicap Index, 57
Single nucleotide polymorphisms (SNPs), 9
in head and neck squamous cell carcinoma, 1019
Single photon emission computed tomography (SPECT)
of Graves' ophthalmopathy, 1810
of malignant otitis externa, 1947
of oral cancer, 1300
technetium 99m scintigraphy with, for hyperparathyroidism, 1785
Single strand conformation polymorphism (SSCP), 9
Single-gene disorders, 4, 6
dominant, 6, 6f
penetrance and expressivity of, 7, 7f
recessive, 6-7, 7f
Single-stage laryngotracheal reconstruction (SSLTR), for laryngeal stenosis, 2920-2921
Single-strand breaks, by radiation, 1036
Singular neurectomy, 2360, 2360f
Sinonasal infection, immunosuppression and, 219-221
diagnosis of, 220-221, 220f
presentation and pathogenesis of, 219-220
treatment of, 221
Sinonasal management, for benign vocal fold mucosal disorders, 862-863
Sinonasal neoplasm(s)
benign, 717-727, 718t
diagnosis of, 717-718
fibrous dysplasia as, 718t, 725-726, 726f
glioma as, 718t
hamartoma as, 718t
inverted papilloma (Schneiderian papilloma, inverted type) as, 718-720
endoscopic appearance of, 718-719, 719f
epidemiology of, 718
with frontal sinus involvement, 720, 720f
histologic appearance of, 718
human papillomavirus and, 718
imaging of, 719, 719f
postoperative surveillance for, 720
recurrence of, 720
sites for, 718
and squamous cell carcinoma, 718
surgical approach for, 718t, 719-720, 720f, 763
juvenile angiofibroma as, 721-722
classification systems for, 722
endoscopic appearance of, 721, 721f
imaging of, 721
natural history of, 721
origin of, 721, 721f
postoperative surveillance for, 722
preoperative embolization for, 721-722
surgical approach for, 718t, 722, 722f-723f, 763
lobular capillary hemangioma as, 718t, 725, 725f
ossifying fibroma as, 725-726
osteoma as, 723-725
classification of, 723
endoscopic appearance of, 723
epidemiology of, 723
ethmoid, 724f
frontal, 724-725, 724f
imaging of, 723-725, 723f-724f
ivory ("eburnated"), 723, 723f-724f

Sinonasal neoplasm(s) *(Continued)*
mature (spongiosum), 723
microscopic appearance of, 723
mixed, 723, 724f
pathogenesis of, 723
postoperative surveillance for, 725
spongiosum variant of, 724f
surgical approach for, 718t, 724-725
symptoms of, 723
pleomorphic adenoma as, 718t
schwannoma as, 726-727, 726f
surgical approach for, 718, 718t, 763
malignant, 1127-1128
adenocarcinoma as, 1131
adenoid cystic carcinoma as, 1131
algorithm for evaluation and management of, 1122f
epidemiology and survival with, 1121-1122, 1123t
epithelial
management of
staging of, 1127-1128, 1128f, 1129b
ethmoid, sphenoid, and frontal, 1130
staging of, 1129b
hematopoietic and lymphoid, 1131
involvement of cervical lymph nodes in, 1130
lymphoma as, 1131, 1680
therapy and prognosis for, 1680
maxillary, 1128-1130
chemoradiotherapy for, 1130
combined irradiation and surgery for, 1128
inoperable, 1130
radiotherapy for, 1128-1130
staging of, 1129b
surgery alone for, 1128
melanoma as, 1131-1132
sarcomas as, 1131
staging of, 1127-1128, 1128f, 1129b
therapeutic decision-making for, 1131
Sinonasal Outcome Test (SNOT-20), 57, 642, 730
Sinonasal polyp(s), endoscopic sinus surgery for, 751-752
Sinonasal polyposis
in aspirin-exacerbated respiratory disease, 732f
with methicillin-resistant *Staphylococcus aureus* infection, 733f
surgical management of, 741
Sinonasal undifferentiated carcinoma (SNUC), 1698-1699
Sinus(es). *See* Paranasal sinus(es).
Sinus balloon catheterization, 752-753, 753f
Sinus disease, olfactory dysfunction due to, 633
Sinus histiocytosis, in children, 2819
Sinus lateralis, 665f, 667f
Sinus mucocele, 676, 678f
Sinus surgery, 739-758
endoscopic (*See* Endoscopic sinus surgery (ESS))
external procedures for, 756-757
Caldwell-Luc procedure as, 756, 756f
external ethmoidectomy as, 757, 757f
for frontal sinus, 757
intranasal ethmoidectomy as, 756-757
for sphenoid sinus, 757
historical background of, 739
indications for, 741-742, 741b
anterior meningoencephaloceles as, 742
choanal atresia as, 742
CSF rhinorrhea as, 742
endoscopic transnasal approach as, 742
headache and facial pain as, 742
intractable epistaxis as, 742
mucoceles as, 742
removal of foreign body as, 742
rhinosinusitis as
with acute complications, 741
chronic, 741
invasive fungal, 742
Sinus surgery *(Continued)*
noninvasive fungal, 742
recurrent acute, 741
sinonasal polyposis as, 741
tumors as, 742
minimally invasive, 743, 752, 760
surgical anatomy for, 739-741
anatomic variations in, 741
anterior skull base in, 741
ethmoid complex in, 740
frontal sinus in, 740-741
maxillary sinus in, 740
middle turbinate in, 739-740
ostiomeatal complex in, 739, 740f
sphenoid sinus in, 740, 740f
in vocal professional, 858
Sinus tympani
anatomy of, 1825-1826
in mastoidectomy, 2015, 2015f
Sinusitis. *See also* Rhinosinusitis.
acute
frontal, 775
radiologic appearance of, 672-673, 673f
allergic, 675
chronic
frontal, 775-783
pediatric, 2778-2781
cultures for, 2779
etiology of, 2778-2779
imaging of, 2779
irrigation for, 2779
medical management of, 2779
surgical management of, 2779-2781, 2780f-2781f
radiologic appearance of, 673-674, 674f-675f
complications of, 676-677
inflammatory polyps as, 676, 678f
mucocele as, 676, 678f
mucous retention cyst as, 676, 677f
orbital, 676-677
frontal
acute, 775
anatomic variations and, 776
chronic, 775-783
granulomatous, 675
immunosuppression and, 219-221, 660
diagnosis of, 220-221, 220f
presentation and pathogenesis of, 219-220
treatment of, 221
vs. myofascial pain dysfunction syndrome, 1284t
radiologic appearance of, 167-168, 168f, 672-675
acute, 672-673, 673f
allergic, 675
chronic, 673-674, 674f-675f
with complications, 676-677
inflammatory polyps as, 676, 678f
mucocele as, 676, 678f
mucous retention cyst as, 676, 677f
orbital, 676-677
on CT, 140-142, 141f
granulomatous, 675
rhino- (*See* Rhinosinusitis)
use of term, 729
siRNA (short-interfering RNA)
direct delivery of, 16
in RNA interference, 13, 14f
Sistrunk operation, for thyroglossal duct cyst, 2815
SIX1 gene
in branchio-oto-renal syndrome, 2095
in deafness, 2051t-2058t
SIX5 gene
in branchio-oto-renal syndrome, 2095
in deafness, 2051t-2058t
Sizing template, in microtia reconstruction, 2744-2745, 2745f
Sjögren's syndrome (SS)
autoantibodies in, 1160
clinical presentation of, 1160
defined, 1160
diagnostic criteria for, 1160
differential diagnosis of, 1160
etiology of, 1160
and malignant lymphoproliferative disorders, 1160
ocular findings in, 1160
oral manifestations of, 1251
physical examination for, 1160
primary, 1160
salivary gland involvement in, 1160-1161
in children, 2858
imaging of, 1148, 1647
secondary, 1160
systemic manifestations of, 1160
treatment of, 1160-1161
SJS (Stevens-Johnson syndrome), 1239
SK2 channel defects, and hearing, 2079-2080
Skeletal abnormalities, due to hyperparathyroidism, 1781
Skeletal defect repair, biomaterials in, 2657-2658
Skeletal dysplasias, and obstructive sleep apnea, 2605
Skew deviation, 2312-2313
Skewing quotient, in measurement of vocal fold vibration, 830-831
Skin
aesthetic analysis of, 275, 276b, 279f
aging (*See* Aging skin)
anatomy and physiology of, 1065-1067
angiosomes in, 1064
capillary system in, 1066
cellular systems in, 1066-1067
interstitial system in, 1066
macrocirculatory system in, 1065-1066, 1065f
zones of perfusion in, 1064-1065, 1065f
effects of radiotherapy on, 2626t
physical examination of, 95
vascular supply to, 1064
Skin cancer, immunosuppression and, 213t, 215
Skin Cancer Index, 57
Skin diseases
esophageal manifestations of, 979-980
nasal manifestations of, 660-661
in Behçet's disease, 660-661
in pemphigoid, 660
in pemphigus vulgaris, 660
in scleroderma, 660
oral manifestations of, 1253-1254
Skin erythema dose, 1031
Skin flap(s), 1064-1079
acutely raised, 1067-1071
capillary obstruction (no-reflow phenomenon) in, 1070-1071
critical closing pressure in, 1068
free radical formation in, 1070-1071, 1071f
impairment of vascular supply in, 1067-1068
increased interstitial pressure in, 1068, 1069f
inflammation and prostaglandins in, 1070, 1070f
length-to-width ratio in, 1068, 1068f
microcirculatory changes in, 1068-1069
neovascularization in, 1069, 1069f
nerve section in, 1069-1070
reperfusion injury in, 1070
vascular territories in, 1067, 1068f
advancement, 345-346
bilateral, 345, 346f
island, 345
unipedicle, 345, 345f
V-Y, 345-346, 346f-347f
Y-V, 346

Skin flap(s) *(Continued)*
anatomy and physiology of skin and, 1065-1067
angiosomes in, 1064
capillary system in, 1065-1066, 1065f
cellular systems in, 1065-1067, 1065f
interstitial system in, 1065-1066, 1065f
macrocirculatory system in, 1064-1066, 1065f
zones of perfusion in, 1064-1065, 1065f
arterial (axial pattern), 1067, 1067f
attempts to alter viability of, 1072-1074
delay as, 1072-1073
with increased blood supply, 1072, 1072f, 1072t
inflammation as, 1074
neovascularization as, 1073
rheology as, 1073-1074
tissue expansion as, 1074
vasodilators in, 1073
direct, 1073
indirect, 1073
biomechanics of, 1071-1072, 1071f
classification of, 342-343, 343b, 1067, 1067f
complications of, 366
delayed, 1072-1073
free microvascular, 1067
primary ischemia in, 1075
reperfusion period for, 1075
salvage of, 1075
secondary ischemia in, 1068, 1075
vascularity of recipient bed with, 1075
for hair loss, 385-387, 387f
complications of, 386-387
hinge, 346
impaired, 1075
salvage of, 1075
myocutaneous and fasciocutaneous, 1067, 1067f
necrosis of, 1068
after neck surgery, 1727
with rhytidectomy, 421-422, 425f-426f
pedicled, salvage of, 1075
pivotal, 343-345
effective length of, 343, 343f
interpolated, 344-345, 344f
rotation, 343-344, 343f
transposition, 344, 344f
prolonged viability of, 1074-1075
hyperbaric oxygen and, 1074
metabolic manipulation and, 1074-1075
protection against harmful agents and, 1074
random, 1067, 1067f
cutaneous, 1067, 1067f
stresses due to, 1064
undermining of, 1071-1072
Skin grafting
for airway stenosis, 946-947
for burns, 315
gene therapy for, 23
for nasal reconstruction, 365
for oropharyngeal reconstruction, 1376
of tongue base, 1388
of tonsil and pharyngeal wall, 1384
Skin lesion(s), 281-294
cysts as, 289
dermoid, 289
epidermoid, 289
milia as, 289
mucous, 289
pilar, 289
in steatocystoma multiplex, 289
epidermal, 281-286
actinic keratoses as, 283, 284f
basal cell carcinoma as, 283-285, 284f-285f
chondrodermatitis nodularis helicis as, 285, 285f
dermatosis papulosa nigra as, 282
keratoacanthoma as, 284f, 286
seborrheic keratoses as, 281-282, 282f
Skin lesion(s) *(Continued)*
squamous cell carcinoma as, 285-286, 285f
warts (verruca vulgaris) as, 282-283
filiform, 282, 282f
flat, 282, 283f
due to molluscum contagiosum, 282-283, 283f
fibroadnexal, 291-293
acrochordon as, 291
angiofibroma as, 292
atypical fibroxanthoma as, 292
cylindroma as, 288f, 292
dermatofibroma as, 288f
dermatofibrosarcoma protuberans as, 291-292
fibrous papule as, 288f, 292
hidrocystoma as, 292
keloids and hypertrophic scars as, 291
lipoma as, 293
neurofibromas as, 292
sebaceous hyperplasia as, 288f, 293
syringoma as, 292-293
trichoepithelioma as, 292
xanthelasma as, 293
melanocytic, 286-289
blue nevus as, 286-287, 287f
compound nevus as, 286
congenital nevi as, 287-288
dysplastic nevus as, 288, 288f
halo nevus as, 287, 287f
intradermal nevus as, 286, 287f
junctional nevus as, 286, 287f
lentigo maligna melanoma as, 287f
nevocellular nevus as, 286
nevus sebaceus as, 287f, 289
solar (actinic) lentigo as, 288
Spitz nevus as, 287
superficial spreading melanoma as, 285f
telangiectasia as, 291
hereditary hemorrhagic, 291
spider angioma as, 291
venous lakes as, 288f, 291
treatment methods and biopsy techniques for, 293-294
chemical or abrasive surgery as, 294
cryosurgery as, 294
electrosurgery as, 294
excisional surgery as, 293
laser surgery as, 294
vascular, 290-291
cherry angiomas as, 290
infantile hemangiomas as, 290
port wine stain as, 291
pyogenic granuloma as, 290
salmon patch as, 290-291
Skin protection, in laser surgery, 35
Skin quality, in rhinoplasty, 512-513, 512f
Skin resurfacing, with blepharoplasty, 451
Skin sparing, in radiotherapy, 1033-1034
Skin tag, 291
Skin tension lines, relaxed, 269-270, 274f
Skin testing, for allergic rhinitis, 619
Skin types, sun-reactive (photoaging), 275, 276b
Skin–soft tissue envelope (SSTE), revision rhinoplasty of, 581, 594
Skipped generation, 2089
Skull
cloverleaf, due to craniosynostosis, 2645, 2645f
in Down syndrome, 2632
Skull base. *See* Cranial base.
SKY (spectral karyotyping), for head and neck squamous cell carcinoma, 1019
Slc. See Solute carrier family *entries.*
SLE (systemic lupus erythematosus), oral manifestations of, 1251-1252
Sleep apnea
acoustic rhinometry for, 651
central, 251b, 256f, 263, 263b
mixed, 251b
obstructive (*See* Obstructive sleep apnea (OSA))
Sleep Apnea Quality of Life Index (SAQLI), 57
Sleep disorder(s), 261-266
circadian rhythm, 264, 264b
classification of, 261-266, 262b
hypersomnias of central origin as, 263-264, 264b
insomnia as, 262-263, 263b
isolated symptoms, apparently normal variants, and unresolved issues with, 265-266, 265b
with obstructive sleep apnea, 261, 262t
obstructive sleep apnea as (*See* Obstructive sleep apnea (OSA))
outcome scales for, 56t, 57
parasomnias as, 264-265, 265b
sleep-related breathing disorders as, 263, 263b
sleep-related movement disorders, 265, 265b
Sleep hygiene, inadequate, 262t, 263
Sleep onset REM periods (SOREMPs), 263-264
Sleep paralysis, 264-265
Sleep stages, 261-262
Sleep study, for stridor, 2901
Sleep talking, 262t
Sleep terrors, 262t, 264
Sleep videoendoscopy, drug-induced, of obstructive sleep apnea, 253-255
Sleep-disordered breathing (SDB), 263, 263b
in children, 2602-2612
and ADHD, 2791
cardiopulmonary complications of, 2792
classification of, 2602
and enuresis, 2792
and growth problems, 2792
and neurocognitive development, 2791-2792
obstructive sleep apnea as (*See* Obstructive sleep apnea (OSA))
primary snoring as, 2602-2603
upper airway resistance syndrome as, 2602-2603
classification of, 251-252, 251b
indices of, 251b
symptoms of, 252b
Sleepiness, daytime, 263-264
obesity and, 251
Sleep-related breathing disorders, 263, 263b
classification of, 251-252, 251b
indices of, 251b
symptoms of, 252b
Sleep-related hypoventilation/hypoxemic syndromes, 263, 263b
Sleep-related movement disorders (SRMDs), 265, 265b
Sleep-related upper airway obstruction, 2607
Sleepwalking, 262t, 264
Slide tracheoplasty, 2932-2933, 2933f
SLIT (sublingual immunotherapy), for allergic rhinitis, 621-622
SLL. *See* Small lymphocytic lymphoma (SLL).
SLN. *See* Superior laryngeal nerve (SLN).
SLNB. *See* Sentinel lymph node biopsy (SLNB).
Slow-wave sleep, 261-262
SLS. *See* Sublingual space (SLS).
SLUG, in deafness, 2051t-2058t
Small cell carcinoma
invasive, of cribriform plate and orbits, 170f
neuroendocrine type (SCCNET), of larynx, 1507-1508
of salivary glands, 1190-1191, 1190f
Small fenestra stapedotomy, 2030-2032
with laser minus prosthesis, 2033
laser *vs.* microdrill in, 2033
postoperative care after, 2032-2033
postoperative complication(s) of, 2030, 2034

Small fenestra stapedotomy *(Continued)*
facial paralysis as, 2030, 2034
perilymph fistula as, 2034
reparative granuloma as, 2034
sensorineural hearing loss as, 2030, 2034
serous labyrinthitis as, 2034
taste disturbance as, 2034
tinnitus as, 2034
tympanic membrane perforation as, 2034
vertigo as, 2030, 2034
procedure for, 2030-2032
anesthesia for, 2030
creation of fenestra in, 2031-2032, 2032f
flap elevation in, 2031, 2031f
incisions for, 2031
measurement of distance from incus to footplate in, 2031, 2031f-2032f
placement of prosthesis in, 2031-2032, 2032f
positioning for, 2031, 2031f
removal of posterior superior bony wall in, 2031, 2031f
stapedectomy *vs.*, 2030
surgical problems in, 2033-2034
chorda tympani nerve damage as, 2034
exposed, overhanging facial nerve as, 2033
fixed malleus as, 2033
floating footplate as, 2033
intraoperative vertigo as, 2034
perilymph gusher as, 2034
solid or obliterated footplate as, 2033
tympanic membrane perforation as, 2034
Small lymphocytic lymphoma (SLL), 1678
clinical presentation of, 1674
imaging of, 1674, 1674f
treatment and prognosis for, 1678
Small round blue cell (SRBC) tumors, 2836
SMAS. *See* Superficial musculoaponeurotic system (SMAS).
SMCP (submucous cleft palate), 2659, 2661f, 2674
bifid uvula with, 2793, 2793f
Smell. *See* Olfaction.
Smell Identification Test, 637-638
Smile pattern, in facial nerve assessment, 2417-2418
Smith, Will, 38
Smith-Magenis syndrome, deafness in, 2051t-2058t
Smoke evacuation, in laser surgery, 35
"Smoker's melanosis," 1241f
Smoking
exposure to, and otitis media, 2767
and Graves' ophthalmopathy, 1807
and skin flap survival, 1075
and squamous cell carcinoma
of head and neck, 1016
of larynx, 1491, 1512-1513
of oral cavity, 1293-1294, 1365
Smooth pursuit, 2277, 2306f, 2307t
evaluation of
in bedside exam, 2313-2314
testing for, 2318, 2319f
Smooth pursuit tracking system, in vestibular compensation, 2375
SMS (submandibular space)
anatomy of, 202
imaging of, 146f, 156-157, 158f
odontogenic infections of, 183-184, 183f-184f
SMV (submentovertex) view, of facial bones and sinuses, 130
SNAI2, in deafness, 2051t-2058t, 2095
Snap test, 445, 446f
SND. *See* Selective neck dissection (SND).
Snell's waltzer mice, 2078
SNHL. *See* Sensorineural hearing loss (SNHL).
Sniffer, chronic, 483-484
Sniffin' Sticks, 631
Sniffing, in olfaction, 625
SNORE-25 (Symptoms of Nocturnal Obstruction and Respiratory Events), 57
Snoring, 251, 266
acoustic rhinometry for, 651
in children
due to obstructive sleep apnea. *See* Obstructive sleep apnea (OSA).
primary, 2602-2603
due to upper airway resistance syndrome, 2602-2603
SNOT-20 (Sinonasal Outcome Test), 57, 642, 730
SNPs (single nucleotide polymorphisms), 9
in head and neck squamous cell carcinoma, 1019
SNUC (sinonasal undifferentiated carcinoma), 1698-1699
SOC (superior olivary complex), in central auditory pathway, 1835, 1835f, 1846
Social history, 94
Socioeconomic status, and otitis media, 2767
SOD (superoxide dismutase), and skin flap viability, 1074
Sodium (Na^+)
in saliva, 1139
in taste, 1208
Sodium bicarbonate, for cerumen removal, 1958t
Sodium channels, in taste, 1208
Sodium chloride (NaCl), gustatory response to, 1208-1209
Sodium restriction, for Meniere's disease, 2126
Sodium salts, gustatory response to, 1208-1209
Sodium tetradecyl sulfate (Sotradecol), for embolization, 1933
Sodium/hydrogen (Na^+,H^+) exchanger, in salivary gland secretion, 1135
Sodium/iodide symporter (NIS), in thyroid hormone synthesis, 1737
Sodium-potassium (Na^+,K^+) pump, ATPase-driven, in salivary gland secretion, 1135
Sodium-potassium-chloride (Na^+,K^+-$2Cl^-$) cotransporter, in salivary gland secretion, 1135
Soft palate
anatomy of, 1295f, 1359f, 1366
cancers of
cervical lymph node metastasis of, 1361t
clinical presentation of, 1365
management of, 1368-1369, 1368f
neurologic evaluation of, 834
during pharyngeal swallow, 1216, 1216f
taste buds on, 1208, 1211
Soft palate reconstruction, 1381-1383
algorithm for, 1384f
free flaps for, 1382
Gehanno method for, 1382
Lacombe and Blackwell's method for, 1382-1383
other groups' experience with, 1383
radial forearm, 1382, 1383f
local flaps for, 1381
buccinator musculomucosal, 1381-1382, 1381f
palatal island mucosal, 1382
Superior Constrictor Rotation-Advancement Flap (SCARF) as, 1382, 1382f
uvulopalatal, 1377f, 1381
prosthetic obturation for, 1381
speech function after, 1383
Soft palate resection, prostheses for, 1343-1344, 1344f
Soft tissue(s), effects of radiotherapy on, 2626t
Soft tissue avulsions, 307, 308f
Soft tissue flap(s)
for free tissue transfer, 1082t, 1083
anterolateral thigh, 1082t, 1083
lateral arm, 1082t, 1083
lateral thigh, 1082t
radial forearm, 1082t, 1083, 1083f
tubed, 1087, 1091f
scapular-parascapular, 1082t
ulnar forearm, 1082t
Soft tissue flap(s) *(Continued)*
mandibular reconstruction plate with, 1325
advantages and disadvantages of, 1325
plate extrusion with, 1325, 1326f
plate fracture with, 1325-1326, 1326f
volume-based, 1325, 1326f
Soft tissue landmarks and reference points, in facial analysis, 270b, 271f
Soft tissue sarcomas, 1666, 1666t
Soft tissue stenosis, of external auditory canal, 2021-2022, 2023f
Soft tissue trauma, 302-317
approach to, 302-306
anesthesia in, 304
cleaning in, 304-305, 305f
history taking in, 302-303
infection control in, 305
physical examination in, 303-304, 303f
repair in, 305-306, 306f
tetanus prophylaxis for, 303
to ears, 308f, 310, 310f
etiology of, 302
to eye, 303
to eyelids, 303, 303f, 307-309, 308f
to facial nerve, 309
to lacrimal apparatus, 307-309, 308f
with large-segment, composite avulsions or amputations, 312, 312f
to lips, 309-310, 309f
to nose, 310-312, 311f
to parotid duct, 312-313, 314f
to salivary glands, 312, 313f
sialocele and salivary fistula due to, 313-314
types of injuries in, 306-307
abrasion as, 306
avulsions as, 307, 308f
laceration as, 307
Soft tissue tumors, of oropharynx, 1363-1364, 1364f
SOHND. *See* Supraomohyoid neck dissection (SOHND).
Solar cheilitis, 283
Solar keratoses, 283, 284f
Solar (actinic) lentigo, 288
Solitary fibrous tumor, 1671
Solute carrier family 4 member 7 *(Slc4a7)* gene, in murine deafness, 2058t-2060t
Solute carrier family 12 member 2 *(Slc12a2)* gene, in murine deafness, 2058t-2060t
Solute carrier family 12 member 6 *(Slc12a6)* gene, in murine deafness, 2058t-2060t
Solute carrier family 12 member 7 *(Slc12a7)* gene, in murine deafness, 2058t-2060t
Solute carrier family 17 member 8 *(SLC17A8)* gene, in deafness, 2051t-2058t, 2081
Solute carrier family 19 member 2 *(SLC19A2)* gene, in deafness, 2051t-2058t
Solute carrier family 26 member 4 *(SLC26A4)* gene, in deafness, 2051t-2058t, 2096, 2098
Solute carrier family 26 member 5 (SLC26A5), and outer hair cell motility, 2064-2065, 2068f
Solute carrier family 26 member 5 *(SLC26A5)* gene, in deafness, 2051t-2058t
SOM (serous otitis media), immunosuppression and, 222-223
Somatic gene therapy, 14, 15f
Somatic tinnitus, 2132-2133, 2132t
Somesthesia, oral, 1201-1202, 1201f-1202f
Somnolence, daytime, 263-264
obesity and, 251
Sonotubometry, for eustachian tube assessment, 1874
SOOF (suborbicularis oculi fat), 444, 447
after facial paralysis, 2431
Sore throat. *See* Pharyngitis.
SOREMPs (sleep onset REM periods), 263-264

SOT (sensory organization test), 2325-2326, 2325f-2326f
Sotradecol (sodium tetradecyl sulfate), for embolization, 1933
Sound, 1838-1839, 1839f
defined, 2017
eye movements evoked by, 2316, 2339-2340, 2340f
Sound enrichment, for tinnitus, 2133-2134
Sound localization
in binaural processing, 2248
external ear in, 1839
with traditional hearing aid, 2207
Sound pressure, 1839
Sound pressure level (SPL), 1839, 2140
in acoustic analysis for voice evaluation, 829, 829t
Sound protection, eustachian tube in, 1871-1872
Sound stimulation, for tinnitus, 2133-2134
Sound transduction, with hearing aids, 2205f
Sound transfer, in middle ear, 2017-2019
Sound transmission, 2000, 2017-2019, 2050-2060, 2062f
Sour taste
peripheral sensitivity to, 1211
transduction of, 1209
Source-filter hypothesis, of speech, 812
Southern blotting, 9
SOX2, in deafness, 2051t-2058t
SOX10, in Waardenburg syndrome, 2095
SP (substance P), in salivary gland secretion, 1137
SP (summating potential), in electrocochleography, 1892-1894, 1907
in Meniere's disease, 2337
Space-frequency map, 2060-2061, 2063f
SP/AP (summating potential/action potential) ratio, 1892-1894
in Meniere's disease, 2337
Spasmodic dysphonia, 839
botulinum toxin therapy for, 839, 840f-841f
voice breaks in, 834-835
Spatial coherence, 26, 27f
SPCC (spindle cell carcinoma), of larynx, 1506
SPEAK (spectral peak extraction), for cochlear implants, 2230, 2230f
Speaking tasks, in pediatric voice evaluation, 2877-2878
SPECT. *See* Single photon emission computed tomography (SPECT).
Spectral displays, in acoustic analysis for voice evaluation, 829t, 830, 830f
of professional voice, 849
Spectral emphasis strategies, for cochlear implants, 2230
Advanced Combination Encoder as, 2230, 2231f
spectral peak extraction as, 2230, 2230f
Spectral karyotyping (SKY), for head and neck squamous cell carcinoma, 1019
Spectral peak extraction (SPEAK), for cochlear implants, 2230, 2230f
Spectral presaturation inversion recovery (SPIR), MRI with, 135-136
Spectral shape, distortion of, with traditional hearing aid, 2204
Spectral tilt, in acoustic analysis for voice evaluation, 830
β-Spectrin 4 *(Spnb4)* gene, in murine deafness, 2058t-2060t, 2081
Spectrogram, in acoustic analysis for voice evaluation, 830, 830f
Spectrometry, for voice analysis of professional voice, 849
Speech
alaryngeal (*See* Alaryngeal voice and speech)
defined, 833
effects of radiotherapy on, 2626t
Speech *(Continued)*
esophageal, 1459
physiology of, 1596, 1596f
after total laryngectomy, 1572
after hypopharyngeal and esophageal reconstruction, 1459-1460
laryngeal function in, 810-812, 811b, 811f, 833
scanning, 837-838
after surgical resection of oral cancer, 1316
tracheoesophageal
physiology of, 1597, 1597f
after total laryngectomy, 1572
Speech aid, for soft palate resection, 1343, 1344f
Speech analysis, for velopharyngeal dysfunction, 2678-2679, 2678f, 2678t-2679t
Speech bulb prosthesis, for velopharyngeal dysfunction, 2681, 2682f
Speech control, sensory input to, 812
Speech detection threshold (SDT), 1888-1889
Speech discrimination testing, 1889
for sensorineural hearing loss in adults, 2117
Speech dysfunction, palliative care for, 1104
Speech endoscopy, for velopharyngeal dysfunction, 2680, 2680f
Speech language pathologist, for professional voice disorders, 855
Speech mapping, with hearing aid, 2273
Speech pathologist, for benign vocal fold mucosal disorders, 863, 864f
Speech perception, with cochlear implants
in adults, 2244-2245
predictors of, 2245, 2245f
in children
early studies of, 2246
more recent studies of, 2246-2247, 2247f
tests for, 2246
Speech reception, with cochlear implants
in adults, 2244-2245
predictors of, 2245, 2245f
in children
early studies of, 2246
more recent studies of, 2246-2247, 2247f
tests for, 2246
Speech reception threshold (SRT), 1888-1889
masking for, 1889
Speech recognition, with cochlear implants
in adults, 2244-2245
predictors of, 2245, 2245f
in children
early studies of, 2246
more recent studies of, 2246-2247, 2247f
tests for, 2246
Speech recognition tests, for cochlear implants, 2223
Speech rehabilitation, after laryngectomy. *See* Voice rehabilitation.
Speech testing, in audiologic test battery, 1888-1889
Speech therapy, for velopharyngeal dysfunction, 2680-2681
articulation in, 2681
compensatory strategies in, 2681
resonance in, 2681
Speech videofluoroscopy, for velopharyngeal dysfunction, 2679-2680
Speech-language development, otitis media and, 2776
Sphenoethmoid synchondrosis, 2619f
Sphenoethmoidal cells, 669, 740, 749f
in surgical anatomy of anterior cranial base, 2473
Sphenoethmoidal encephalocele, 2687t
Sphenoethmoidal recess(es)
normal anatomy of, 667, 668f
in surgical anatomy of anterior cranial base, 2472
Sphenoid bone, 320f
lesser and greater wings of, 322f, 335f
in surgical anatomy of anterior cranial base, 2442-2443, 2443f
in surgical anatomy of lateral skull base, 2435f
Sphenoid ostium(ia), 740, 741f, 2472, 2473f
Sphenoid sinus(es)
anatomy of
normal, 664, 665f, 667-668, 668f
surgical, 740, 741f
in anterior cranial base, 2443, 2472f-2474f, 2473
prior to endoscopic sinus surgery, 764, 764t
extensive pneumatization of, 669, 670f
external approaches to, 757
after functional endoscopic sinus surgery, 679
growth and development of, 2619-2620
and internal carotid artery, 671-672
and optic nerve, 672, 672f
Sphenoid sinus tumors, 1123, 1130
Sphenoid spine, in surgical anatomy of middle cranial base, 2444, 2445f
Sphenoidotomy
in endoscopic sinus surgery, 748, 749f
complications of, 767, 768t
for fungus ball, 768f-769f
with image-guided navigation system, 770f
in middle cranial base surgery
transethmoidal, 2455-2457, 2455t, 2456f
transseptal, 2455-2457, 2455t, 2456f
Spheno-occipital synchondrosis, 2617-2619, 2619f-2620f
Spheno-orbital encephalocele, 2687t
Sphenopalatine artery
anatomy of, 682
septal branch of, 483f
Sphenopalatine artery ligation, endoscopic, for epistaxis, 689-690, 689f-690f
Sphenopalatine foramen
in surgical anatomy of anterior cranial base, 2473f
in surgical anatomy of lateral skull base, 2435f
Sphenopalatine ganglion, 497
Sphincter pharyngoplasty, for velopharyngeal dysfunction, 2683
Spider angioma, 291
Spin density–weighted image, 134, 135f-136f
Spinal accessory lymph nodes
anatomy of, 1360f
in neck dissection, 1705f
Spinal accessory nerve (SAN)
intraoperative monitoring of, 2550-2552, 2550f
in modified radical neck dissection, 1712, 1713f-1714f, 1730
in neck dissection, 1722
in posterior triangle, 2578-2579, 2579f-2580f
in surgical anatomy of lateral skull base, 2436f, 2438, 2439f-2440f, 2440
Spinal accessory nerve (SAN) injury
in lateral skull base surgery, 2512
due to neck surgery, 1730, 1731f
Spinal accessory nerve (SAN) transposition, for facial nerve paralysis, 2426
Spinal cord input, to vestibular nuclei, 1864
Spinal nerve, posterior ramus of, 2579f
Spindle cell carcinoma (SPCC), of larynx, 1506
Spindle cell hemangioendothelioma, 1668-1669
Spindle cell hemangioma, 1668-1669
Spindle-shaped gap, laryngeal videostroboscopy of, 819, 820f
Spine of Henle, anatomy of, 1822f, 2009-2010
Spinocerebellar atrophy, 2357
SPIR (spectral presaturation inversion recovery), MRI with, 135-136
Spiral CT, of laryngeal carcinoma, 1470
Spiral ganglion, anatomy of, 1832f, 1834, 1854f, 2278f

Spiral ganglion cells, in auditory physiology, 1844, 1845f
Spiral ganglion neurons (SGNs), salvage of, 2189-2191
Spiral lamina, 1831, 1832f, 1834
Spiral ligament
  anatomy of, 1832f
  in auditory physiology, 1841f
  in cochlear transduction, 2061f
Spiral limbus
  anatomy of, 1832
  in auditory physiology, 1841f
Spiral modiolar artery, 1854, 1856f
Spirochaeta denticulata, Vincent's angina due to, 2786
Spitz nevus, 287
SPL (sound pressure level), 1839, 2140
  in acoustic analysis for voice evaluation, 829, 829t
Spleen, in immune system, 605
Splenius muscle, 2579f
Splice sites, 4, 5f
Split bridge, for cochlear implant, 2238-2239, 2238f
Split-thickness skin graft (STSG), in atresiaplasty
  creation of, 2756, 2757f
  placement of, 2756, 2757f-2758f
  suturing of, 2756-2757, 2758f
Spnb4 (β-spectrin 4) gene, in murine deafness, 2058t-2060t, 2081
Spontaneous emission, of radiation, 26, 26f
Spontaneous ventilation anesthesia
  in children, 2599-2600
  with recurrent respiratory papillomatosis, 2891
Spot size, of surgical laser, 27-28, 28f-29f
Spreader grafts
  in revision rhinoplasty for middle vault deformities, 585-586
  for saddle nose deformity, 555, 559f
  for septal and alar asymmetries, 550, 551f
  in septoplasty, 490-491, 491f
  for twisted nose, 554, 555f
SPTs (second primary tumors)
  of larynx, 1492, 1510
  in oral cancer, 1301-1302
Spurring, nasal septal deviation with, 482, 482f, 489, 494, 669f
SQA (Surgical Quality Alliance), 84t-87t, 88
Squamocolumnar junction (SCJ), of esophagus
  with Barrett's esophagus, 957f, 972
  with hiatal hernia, 957f
  normal anatomy of, 956-957, 956f-957f
  in transnasal esophagoscopy, 982-983, 983f
Squamosa, in surgical anatomy of lateral skull base, 2434, 2435f-2436f
Squamous cell carcinoma (SCC), 285-286
  basaloid
    of hypopharynx and cervical esophagus, 1425
    of larynx, 1506
  cervical lymph node metastasis of (*See* Cervical lymph node metastasis(es))
  clinical presentation of, 285f, 286
  cutaneous, immunosuppression and, 213t, 215
  defined, 1361
  epidemiology of, 285
  epistaxis due to, 686f
  esophageal, 973
    due to caustic injury, 978
    cervical, 1425
      imaging of, 1414f, 1424f
    imaging of, 1412-1415
    localized, 1444-1447
      definitive chemoradiation for, 1445-1447, 1446t-1447t
      postoperative therapy for, 1444-1447
      preoperative therapy for, 1444-1445, 1445t
    metastatic, 1447
Squamous cell carcinoma (SCC) *(Continued)*
  of external auditory canal and temporal bone
    computed tomography of, 2502f
    imaging of, 1918, 1919f
    symptoms and signs of, 2502
  extraesophageal reflux and, 902-903
  head and neck (*See* Head and neck squamous cell carcinoma (HNSCC))
  of hypopharynx, 1425
    chemoradiation for, 1442-1444
    chemotherapy for, 1442
      induction, 1443
      after total laryngectomy, 1442-1443
    conventional treatment modalities for, 1441-1442
      for advanced disease, 1442
      for early disease, 1442
    epidemiology of, 1441
    imaging of, 1414f, 1424f
    new treatment modalities for, 1442
    radiation therapy for, 1443
      intensity-modulated, 1046
  laryngeal, 1491
    acantholytic, 1506
    adenoid, 1506
    basaloid, 1506
    cervical nodal metastases of, 1493-1494, 1493f
      embryology and, 1482-1483
      glottic, 1497-1498
      imaging of, 1476, 1479f
      subglottic, 1501, 1501f
      supraglottic, 1500-1501
    chemoprevention of, 1491
    clinical presentation of, 1493-1494
    diagnosis and evaluation of, 1494-1495
      differential diagnosis in, 1495
      history and physical examination in, 1494
      imaging in, 1494-1495
      operative endoscopic examination in, 1495
    distant metastases of, 1494
    epidemiology of, 1491-1492, 1512, 1513f
    etiology of, 1512-1513
    follow-up for, 1505
    grading of, 1492-1493
    human papillomavirus and, 1492, 2887-2888
    imaging of, 161, 164f
    in situ, 1493
    microinvasive, 1493
    molecular biology of, 1492
    papillary, 1506
    pathology of, 1492-1493
    prognosis and prognostic predictors for, 1504-1505
      clinical features as, 1504
      disease factors as, 1504-1505
      histopathologic characteristics as, 1504-1505
      molecular markers as, 1493, 1505
      patient factors as, 1505
      radiologic characteristics as, 1504
    recurrence of, 1503-1504
      stomal, 1504, 1504f
    recurrent respiratory papillomatosis and, 2887-2888
    risk factor(s) for, 1491-1492, 1512-1513
      diet as, 1492
      exposure to toxins as, 1492, 1513
      genetic susceptibility as, 1492, 1513
      human papillomavirus as, 1492, 1513
      laryngeal reflux as, 1491-1492, 1513
      second primary tumors as, 1492
      tobacco and alcohol as, 1491, 1512-1513
    staging of, 1486, 1488t-1489t
      radiology in, 1495
    transition zones of, 1489, 1490f
    treatment of, 1495
      background of, 1512-1515, 1513f-1514f
      CO_2 laser for, 33
Squamous cell carcinoma (SCC) *(Continued)*
      goals of, 1495
      intensity-modulated radiotherapy for, 1046
      nonsurgical organ preservation, 1501-1503, 1502f
      options for, 1495, 1496t
      prognostic factors in, 1495, 1496t
      for recurrence, 1503-1504, 1504f
      for subglottic tumors, 1501-1503, 1501f
      for supraglottic tumors, 1498-1501, 1498f
      therapeutic decision making for, 1495
    variants of, 1505-1506
      acantholytic, 1506
      adenosquamous, 1506
      basaloid, 1506
      papillary, 1506
      spindle cell, 1506
      verrucous, 1505-1506, 1505f
  of masticator space, 152, 154f
  of neck
    arising in branchial cleft cyst, 1671
    arising in thyroglossal duct cyst, 1671
    with unknown primary, 1641-1642, 1641t, 1664, 1665f
  noncutaneous, immunosuppression and, 213t, 215
  of oral cavity, 154, 156f, 1299
    of alveolar ridge–retromolar trigone, 1307f
    basaloid, 1299
    of buccal mucosa, 1308f
    epidemiology of, 1295
    etiology of, 1293-1295, 1294f
    of floor of mouth, 1294f, 1315f
    of hard palate, 1310, 1310f
    lichen planus and, 1229
    of lip, 1302-1304
      clinical findings in, 1294f, 1302, 1302f
      epidemiology of, 1302
      neck metastases of, 1303-1304
      prognostic features of, 1303
      reconstruction for, 1303-1304, 1303f
      resection of, 1303, 1303f
      survival with, 1304
    sarcomatoid, 1299
    of tongue, 1306f
    verrucous, 1299
  oropharyngeal, 1361-1362, 1365
    clinical presentation of, 1361, 1362f, 1365
    etiology of, 1365
    grading of, 1361-1362, 1363t
    imaging of, 149f, 1413f
    pathology of, 1361
    of tonsil, 1362f, 1369f
    transnasal esophagoscopy in, 983
    of uvula, 1368f
  pharyngeal, imaging of, 1412-1415
  of pharyngeal mucosal space, 148, 149f
  pigmented, 285f, 286
  of pyriform sinus, 162f, 1424f
  recurrence or metastasis of, 285-286
  risk factors for, 285
  of salivary glands, 1190
  of sublingual space, 156
  of thyroid gland, 1764
  of trachea, 1613-1614, 1614f
Squamous cell carcinoma of the head and neck (SCCHN). *See* Head and neck squamous cell carcinoma (HNSCC).
Squamous cell dysplasia, of larynx, 1486
Squamous metaplasia theory, of cholesteatoma formation, 1967f, 1968
Squamous odontogenic tumor, 1278
Squamous papilloma(s)
  of larynx, 1468, 1468f
  of nasopharynx, 1349
  of oral cavity, 1290, 1290f
  of trachea, 1612

Squamous part, of temporal bone, 1821, 1822f
Square-wave jerks, 2313
Squelch, in binaural processing, 1846, 2248
SRBC (small round blue cell) tumors, 2836
SRMDs (sleep-related movement disorders), 265, 265b
SRT. *See* Stereotactic radiation therapy (SRT).
SRT (speech reception threshold), 1888-1889
  masking for, 1889
SS (Sjögren's syndrome). *See* Sjögren's syndrome (SS).
SS (Stickler syndrome)
  craniofacial anomalies in, 2646
  deafness in, 2051t-2058t, 2094t, 2095
SS (synovial sarcoma), 1670
SSCD syndrome. *See* Superior semicircular canal dehiscence (SSCD) syndrome.
SSCP (single strand conformation polymorphism), 9
SSKI (saturated solution of potassium iodide)
  for Graves' disease, 1742-1743
  for hyperthyroidism, 1739t
SSLTR (single-stage laryngotracheal reconstruction), for laryngeal stenosis, 2920-2921
SSRIs (selective serotonin reuptake inhibitors)
  for migraine, 2350
  for tinnitus, 2137
SSTE (skin–soft tissue envelope), revision rhinoplasty of, 581, 594
Stabbing, neck trauma due to, 1627
Staging, FDG-PET for, 144
Staging systems, 53
Stakeholders, in performance measurement, 79-89, 84t-87t
Standard deviation (SD), 63, 64t
  vs. standard error, 73, 73t
Standard error (SE), *vs.* standard deviation, 73, 73t
Standardization, 87-89
Stapedectomy
  in children, 2035
  for far-advanced otosclerosis, 2035
  for Meniere's disease, 2035
  in ossiculoplasty, 2007, 2024-2025
  revision, 2035
  vs. stapedotomy, 2030
Stapedial fixation
  acoustic reflex testing for, 2030, 2030f
  due to otosclerosis, 2028-2029, 2029f
Stapedial reflex measures, 1890-1891
Stapedius reflex, assessment of, 2383
Stapedius reflex pathways, in efferent auditory system, 1847, 1848f
Stapedotomy
  in ossiculoplasty, 2024-2025
  small fenestra (*See* Small fenestra stapedotomy)
Stapes
  absent superstructure of, ossiculoplasty for, 2024, 2025f
  anatomy of, 1853f
  in auditory physiology, 1839, 1840f
  in cochlear transduction, 2050-2060, 2062f
  embryology of, 2583-2584, 2583f
  in surgical anatomy of lateral skull base, 2436f
Stapes footplate
  in auditory physiology, 1839-1840, 1840f, 1842f, 2018-2019
  embryology of, 2583-2584
  floating, small fenestra stapedotomy with, 2033
  solid or obliterated, small fenestra stapedotomy with, 2033
Stapes footplate fixation, 2024-2025
Stapes gusher syndrome, X-linked, 2737
Stapes tendon, in surgical anatomy of lateral skull base, 2436f
Staphylococcus aureus
  furunculosis of external ear due to, 1949
  laryngitis due to, 885
  otitis externa due to, 2194-2195
    malignant, 1947
  rhinosinusitis due to
    acute, 704, 704f, 732
    chronic, 706, 732
  salivary gland infections due to, 1252
Staphylococcus spp, otitis externa due to, 1945
Stare, in Graves' ophthalmopathy, 1808
Starling equation, 1066
STAT1 activation, in oral cancer, 1301
State medical boards, 80-81
State migration, 53
Statherin, in saliva, 1140
Static compensation, for peripheral vestibular lesions, 2373-2374
Static facial sling, for facial nerve paralysis, 2430
Statistical significance, 66-67
  based on subgroup comparisons, 73t, 74
Statistical tests, 65-66, 66t
  for independent samples, 66, 67t
  for related samples, 66, 67t
  used by otolaryngologists, 70-72
    analysis of variance (ANOVA) as, 71
    contingency tables as, 71-72
    multivariate (regression) procedures as, 72
    nonparametric, 72
    survival analysis as, 72
    t-test as, 70-71
Statoacoustic receptor cell potentials, in hair cell transduction, 2071, 2072f
Steatocystoma multiplex, 289
Steiner analysis, for mentoplasty, 463, 463f
Stellate lacerations, 307
Stellate neurons, in cochlear nucleus, 1835
Stem cell(s), in adaptive immune system, 599-600, 600f
Stem cell factor (SCF), 609t-610t
Stenbeck, Thor, 1031
Stenger test, pure-tone, 1901
Stenosis.
  laryngeal. *See* Laryngeal stenosis.
  subglottic. *See* Subglottic stenosis.
  supraglottic, 947-948
  upper airway. *See* Upper airway stenosis.
Stensen's duct
  anatomy of, 2850-2852
  sialography of, 1150
  trauma to, in children, 2863
Stents
  for caustic ingestion, 2960
  endolaryngeal
    for airway stenosis, 947, 947f
    for chronic aspiration, 928, 930f
    for laryngeal trauma, 937, 939f-940f
  for laryngeal stenosis, 2920
  for tracheal stenosis, 2928-2930, 2930f
Stenvers projection, of temporal bone, 131
Stepping test, 2316-2317
Stereocilia
  in auditory system
    anatomy of, 1832-1833, 1833f, 1840, 1841f
    arrangement of, 2071, 2072f
    in auditory physiology, 1841f, 1842, 1843f
    in cochlear transduction, 2061f, 2065-2067, 2069f
    composition of, 2074, 2075f-2076f
    cross-linkages between, 2076f, 2077-2078
    in hair cell transduction, 2070-2071
      anatomy of, 2070-2071, 2070f, 2072f
      composition of, 2074, 2075f-2076f
      cross-linkages between, 2076f, 2077-2078
      dynamic regulation of length of, 2076-2077
    lengths of, 2070f, 2071
      dynamic regulation of, 2076-2077
Stereocilia *(Continued)*
    number of, 2071
    in waltzer mice, 2074
  in vestibular system
    anatomy of, 1857, 1858f
    arrangement of, 1854-1855, 1856f
    morphologic polarization of, 1855, 1856f, 2279f
    sensory transduction by, 2277-2278, 2279f
Stereociliary bundles, in vestibular system, morphologic polarizations of, 2278, 2280f
Stereocilin (STRC), and interstereociliary linkages, 2077
Stereocilin *(STRC)* gene, in deafness, 2051t-2058t
Stereolithographic modeling, in mandibular reconstruction, 1326-1327, 1327f
Stereotactic computer-assisted surgery, of anterior and middle cranial base, 2448-2449, 2449f
Stereotactic radiation therapy (SRT)
  for benign skull base tumors, 2557-2566
    dose selection for, 2558
    gamma knife–based, 2559t
    imaging for, 2558
    jugular foramen schwannomas as, 2565
    LINAC-based, 2560t
    paraganglioma as, 2565, 2565t
    principles of, 2557-2558, 2558f
    radiobiology of, 2558
    vestibular schwannomas as, 2558, 2560f
      cystic, 2563
      facial nerve outcomes with, 2563
      fractionation *vs.* nonfractionation of, 2558-2559, 2561t
      hearing outcomes with, 2562-2563, 2562t
      hydrocephalus due to, 2563
      neurofibromatosis 2–related, 2563
      outcome assessment with, 2559-2563
      quality of life with, 2564-2565
      treatment of failures of, 2564
      trigeminal nerve outcomes with, 2563
      tumor control with, 2562
  CyberKnife
    for laryngeal and hypopharyngeal cancer, 1592
    for malignant skull base tumors, 1696
  defined, 1696, 2557
  dose selection for, 2558
  Gamma Knife, 2557, 2558f, 2559t
  history of, 1696
  imaging for, 2558
  linear accelerator (LINAC)-based, 2557-2558, 2560t
  for malignant skull base tumors, 1696, 1700
  principles of, 2557-2558, 2558f
  radiobiology of, 2558
Sternocleidomastoid muscle
  anatomy of, 1359f, 1821-1822, 2578f
    radiographic, 1471f
  in modified radical neck dissection, 1712, 1713f
Sternocleidomastoid myocutaneous flap, for reconstruction of tonsils and pharyngeal wall, 1385-1386
Sternocleidomastoid tumors, of infancy, 2817, 2817f
Sternohyoid muscle, 2578f
Sternomastoid muscle, 2579f
Sternothyroid muscle
  characteristics of, 918-919
  surgical anatomy of, 1543f
Steroids. *See* Corticosteroids.
Stertor, defined, 2896-2897
Stevens-Johnson syndrome (SJS), 1239
Stickler syndrome (SS)
  craniofacial anomalies in, 2646
  deafness in, 2051t-2058t, 2094t, 2095
Stimulated emission, of radiation, 26, 26f
Stimulating electrodes, for intraoperative cranial nerve monitoring, 2544, 2544f
Stimulus-frequency otoacoustic emissions, 1891

STIR (short T1 inversion recovery), MRI with, 135-136, 136f
Stoma, for voice prosthesis, 1597, 1597f
  creation of optimally contoured, 1599-1600, 1600f
  postoperative care for, 1600, 1602f
  prevention of excessively deep, 1599-1600, 1600f
Stomal recurrences, of laryngeal carcinoma, 1504, 1504f
Stomal stenosis, after total laryngectomy, 1571
Stomatitis
  aphthous, 1289, 1289f
    in HIV, 227, 227f
    recurrent, 1236-1239
      clinical features of, 1237-1238
      defined, 1236-1237
      differential diagnosis of, 1238, 1238t
      etiology and pathogenesis of, 1237, 1237t
      herpetiform-type, 1238, 1238f
      histopathologic features of, 1239
      major, 1237-1238, 1238f
      minor, 1237, 1238f
      treatment of, 1239
  uremic, 1255
Stomodeum, 2661f, 2691f
Stop codons, 4
Storage diseases, otologic manifestations of, 2112-2114
  in gout, 2113-2114
  in mucopolysaccharidoses, 2112-2113, 2113f
  in ochronosis, 2114
"Stork bite," 290-291
Strain, in voice evaluation, 827t
Strangulation injuries, 934-935
Stratum intermedium, in tooth development, 1259
Strawberry angioma, 290
STRC (stereocilin), and interstereociliary linkages, 2077
STRC (stereocilin) gene, in deafness, 2051t-2058t
Streptococcal tonsillitis-pharyngitis, 193
  in children, 2787
  complications of, 2788
Streptococcus mutans, dental caries due to, 1252
Streptococcus pneumonia, otitis media due to, 2763
Streptococcus pneumoniae
  with CSF fistula, 2045
  rhinosinusitis due to
    acute, 704-705, 704f, 732
    chronic, 706, 732
      acute exacerbation of, 707
Streptococcus pneumoniae vaccine
  to prevent hearing loss, 2161
  to prevent otitis media, 2763, 2768
    maternal immunization with, 2768-2769
Streptococcus pyogenes
  group A beta hemolytic, pharyngitis due to, 191-193
    in children, 2787
    complications of, 2788
  otitis media due to, 2763
Streptococcus viridans, salivary gland infections due to, 1252
Streptokinase, for free flap salvage, 1098
Stress relaxation, in skin flaps, 1071
Stress-strain curve, for skin flaps, 1071
Stria of Held, in auditory pathway, 1846
Stria of Monaco, in auditory pathway, 1846
Stria vascularis
  anatomy of, 1831-1832, 1832f
  in auditory physiology, 1840, 1841f
  in cochlear transduction, 2061f
Strial presbycusis, 232, 2126
Striated duct, of salivary gland, 1134, 1134f, 1162, 1163f
Strictures, esophageal. *See* Esophageal strictures.
Stridor
  biphasic, 2900
  in child (*See* Stridulous child)
  defined, 2896-2897
  expiratory, 2900
  inspiratory, 2900
  postextubation, 2904, 2904t
Stridulous child, 2896-2911
  with acute airway obstruction, 2903-2905
    emergency tracheotomy for, 2904
    endoscopic removal of foreign bodies for, 2904
    medical management for, 2903-2904
    therapeutic intubation for, 2904
  due to airway hemangiomas, 2899, 2899f-2900f
  due to anterior glottic web, 2899, 2900f
  assessment of, 2897-2901
    examination in, 2899-2900, 2899t
    flexible endoscopy in, 2901-2902
    history in, 2897t, 2898-2899
    imaging in, 2901, 2901f
    laryngotracheobronchoscopy in, 2902
      anesthetic considerations for, 2902
      bronchoscopy technique for, 2903, 2903f
      complications of, 2903
      dynamic airway assessment during, 2903
      equipment for, 2902-2903, 2902f
      microlaryngoscopy technique for, 2902-2903
      postoperative car after, 2903
      preparation and positioning for, 2902
    other investigations in, 2901
    oxygen saturation monitoring in, 2900
  with chronic airway obstruction, 2905-2910
    endoscopic treatment of, 2908-2909
      balloons in, 2906, 2906f, 2909
      endoscopic sutures in, 2909
      laser in, 2908-2909, 2908f
      microdébrider in, 2909
      microinstrumentation for, 2908, 2908f
      stents, keels, and grafts in, 2909
      for topical drug administration, 2909
    medical management for, 2905-2906
    open laryngeal surgery for, 2909-2910, 2910f
    tracheotomy for, 2906
      complications of, 2907
      indications for, 2906, 2906t
      patient positioning for, 2906, 2907f
      preoperative planning for, 2906
      surgical decannulation of, 2907-2908
      surgical procedure for, 2906-2908, 2907f
      techniques to avoid, 2906, 2906f
      ward decannulation of, 2907
  definition of, 2896-2897
  differential diagnosis of, 2897t
  future developments for, 2910
  due to laryngeal papillomatosis, 2898, 2899f
  due to laryngomalacia, 2866
  physical principles of airway narrowing in, 2897, 2898f
  postextubation, 2904, 2904t
  postpartum
    expected airway obstruction in, 2904-2905
    unexpected airway obstruction in, 2905
      laryngeal, 2905
      supralaryngeal, 2905, 2905f
      tracheobronchial, 2905
  due to subglottic stenosis, 2900f
  due to vallecular cyst, 2898, 2898f
  due to vocal fold paralysis, 2868
Striola, in vestibular system, 1855, 1858f, 2278, 2280f
Stroboscope, defined, 818
Stroboscopy, laryngeal, 818-821
  of adynamic segments, 820
  of amplitude of vibration, 820, 821f, 848, 848t
  of closure pattern, 819, 820f, 848t, 849
  common problems and solutions for, 815t-816t
  defined, 813
Stroboscopy, laryngeal *(Continued)*
  of early glottic carcinoma, 1515-1516
  flexible endoscope for, 814
    advantages of, 814
    disadvantages of, 814
    protocol for, 818b
    technique of, 814
    troubleshooting for, 814
  interpretation of, 848t
  interval examination in, 847
  of mucosal wave, 820, 848-849, 848t
  in neurologic examination, 834
  of periodicity, 821, 848, 848t
  of phase closure, 819-820
  for professional voice, 847-849, 848f, 848t
  protocol for, 818-819, 818b
  of regularity, 821
  rigid endoscopes for, 813-814
    advantages of, 813
    disadvantages of, 813-814
    protocol for, 818b
    technique of, 814
    troubleshooting for, 814
  of symmetry, 820, 847-848, 848t
  of vertical closure level, 821
  for vocal fold impairment, 905
Stroke
  due to lateral skull base surgery, 2512
  oral manifestations of, 1250
Stromal cell–derived factor (SDF-1), in head and neck squamous cell carcinoma, 1060
STSG (split-thickness skin graft), in atresiaplasty
  creation of, 2756, 2757f
  placement of, 2756, 2757f-2758f
  suturing of, 2756-2757, 2758f
Student's *t*-test, 70-71
Study design, 54-55, 54t
  case series as, 54-55, 54t
  case-control, 54, 54t
  and data interpretation, 59-61, 60t-61t
  and data quality, 59, 60t
  expert opinion as, 52, 54-55, 54t
  grading of evidence-based medicine recommendations as, 55, 55t
  observational (cohort), 54, 54t
  other types of, 55
  randomized trial as, 52, 54, 54t
Study sample, 68t
Stunning, with radioactive iodine, 1771
Sturge-Weber syndrome, 291
  oral manifestations of, 1257
Stuttering, 841-842
Styloglossus muscle, 1296f, 1297, 1359f
Stylohyoid ligament
  embryology of, 2583-2584
  ossification of, 1480, 1481f
Stylohyoid muscle, 1296f, 1359f
Styloid foramen, 2404f
Styloid ligament, 2583f
Styloid process
  anatomy of, 320f, 1296f, 1822-1823, 1822f, 1824f, 1826f, 2010f
    radiographic, 1398f
  elongated, *vs.* myofascial pain dysfunction syndrome, 1284t
  embryology of, 2583-2584, 2583f
  in surgical anatomy of lateral skull base, 2435, 2435f
  in surgical anatomy of middle cranial base, 2445f
Stylomastoid artery, 1826f
Stylomastoid foramen
  anatomy of, 1822-1823, 1824f
  annular ligament of, 1826f
  in surgical anatomy of lateral skull base, 2435
  in surgical anatomy of middle cranial base, 2445f
Stylopharyngeus muscle, 1296f, 1359f

Subacute bacterial endocarditis (SBE) prophylaxis, for pediatric surgery, 2596, 2596t-2597t
Subarcuate artery, in surgical anatomy of lateral skull base, 2439f
Subarcuate fossa
anatomy of, 1823f, 2010f
in surgical anatomy of lateral skull base, 2435f, 2438
Subciliary approach
for lower eyelid blepharoplasty, 449, 450f-451f
for pediatric facial fracture, 2705f
Subclavian artery, root of neck and, 2581-2582, 2581f
Subclavian steal syndrome, 2351
Subclavian triangle, of neck, 2578f
Subcondylar fractures, 322-323, 1280, 1281t
pediatric, 2704, 2706f-2708f
physical examination of, 325
repair of, 338-339
Subcranial approach, for anterior cranial base surgery, 2454, 2454f
Subcutaneous emphysema
of infrahyoid retropharyngeal space, 161f
of neck, 1410, 1410f
Subcutaneous fibroma, due to neck irradiation, 1695
Subcutaneous immunotherapy (SCIT), for allergic rhinitis, 621
Subcutaneous layer, 1065
Subcutaneous tissue, thinning of, in nasal tip refinement, 577, 577f
Subcutaneous tunnels, in liposuction, 456, 456f
Subdural abscess, otitis media and, 2777
Subdural empyema, 1994-1995
epidemiology of, 1980t-1981t, 1994-1995
imaging of, 1995
in neonates, 1995
otitis media and, 2777
symptoms of, 1995
treatment of, 1995
Subglottal resections, for tracheal tumors, 1619, 1620f
Subglottic air pressure (P_s)
in professional voice production, 846
in voice evaluation, 828, 828t, 849
Subglottic airway, radiographic anatomy of, 1463f
Subglottic cancer
anatomic basis for, 1483-1484, 1483f, 1483t
cervical metastases of, 1494
clinical presentation of, 1493, 1579
imaging of, 1474, 1475f
staging of, 1488t, 1580f
treatment of, 1501-1503, 1501f
radiation therapy for, 1589-1590
Subglottic cyst, 2871, 2871f
Subglottic hemangioma, 1468, 1468f, 2871, 2871f
dysphagia due to, 2953
stridor due to, 2899, 2900f
Subglottic stenosis (SGS), 945f, 950-951. *See also* Laryngeal stenosis.
anterior, in children, 2923
balloon dilatation for, 2906, 2906f
congenital, 2870-2871, 2913-2914
dysphagia due to, 2953
gastroesophageal reflux and, 2945
due to internal laryngeal trauma, 2914-2915
stridor due to, 2899, 2900f
Subglottis, 99, 99f
anatomy of, 1483-1484, 1483f, 1483t, 1578
surgical, 1544f
embryology of, 1482
physical examination of, 100
Subharmonic frequencies, 847
Subjective visual horizontal (SVH), perceptual test of, 2300
Subjective visual vertical (SVV), perceptual test of, 2300, 2323
Sublingual artery, 1296f
Sublingual gland(s)
anatomy of, 1133-1134
in children, 2850-2853
radiographic, 1144-1145
contributions to saliva of, 1134t
malignant neoplasms of
excision of, 1196
physical examination of, 1179
Sublingual immunotherapy (SLIT), for allergic rhinitis, 621-622
Sublingual lymph nodes, 2582
Sublingual space (SLS)
anatomy of, 202
imaging of, 156
with abscess and cellulitis, 156, 157f
with congenital lesions, 156
normal anatomy in, 146f, 154, 156
with ranula, 156, 157f
with squamous cell carcinoma, 156
odontogenic infections of, 183, 183f
Submandibular fossa, 1296f
Submandibular gland(s)
anatomy of, 1133-1134, 1296f
in children, 2850-2853
radiographic, 1144, 1399f
contributions to saliva of, 1134t
CT of, 139
neuronal control of, 1136
physical examination of, 96f
pleomorphic adenoma of, 1653f
salivary flow rate and composition of saliva in, 1138t
sialolithiasis of, 1155
imaging of, 1144f, 1154, 1157f
surgical management of, 1156, 1156f
sialolithiasis promoting factors in, 1140
trauma to, 312
Submandibular gland neoplasm(s)
benign
clinical features of, 1165
excision of, 1174, 1174f
malignant
excision of, 1196
physical examination of, 1179
Submandibular gland resection, robotic surgery for, 40-41, 42f-43f
Submandibular lymph nodes
anatomy of, 1297f-1298f, 1360f, 2582
in neck dissection, 1704-1705, 1704f-1705f, 1706t-1708t
Submandibular region, musculature of, 1296f
Submandibular space (SMS)
anatomy of, 202
imaging of, 146f, 156-157, 158f
odontogenic infections of, 183-184, 183f-184f
Submandibular triangle, of neck, 96, 96f, 2578f
Submental lipectomy, 456
Submental lymph nodes
anatomy of, 1297f-1298f, 1360f
in neck dissection, 1704, 1704f-1705f, 1706t-1708t
Submental space involvement, in odontogenic infections, 181-183, 183f
Submental triangle, 2578f
Submentoplasty, 411-413
aesthetic considerations for, 411, 412f
procedure for, 411-413, 413f
results of, 414f-415f
Submentovertex (SMV) view, of facial bones and sinuses, 130
Submucous cleft palate (SMCP), 2659, 2661f, 2674
bifid uvula with, 2793, 2793f
Submucous fibrosis, oral, 1229, 1298
clinical features of, 1229
defined, 1229
etiology and pathogenesis of, 1229
Submucous fibrosis, oral *(Continued)*
histologic/diagnostic features of, 1229
treatment of, 1229
Submuscular recess lymph nodes, in neck dissection, 1707t-1708t
Suboccipital approach, for posterior fossa neoplasms, 2532t, 2533-2534
advantages and disadvantages of, 2532t, 2534
basic features of, 2533
indications for, 2532t, 2533
surgical exposure in, 2533f
technique of, 2534, 2534f
Suboccipital lymph nodes
anatomy of, 1718f
dissection of, 1718-1719
Suborbicularis oculi fat (SOOF), 444, 447
after facial paralysis, 2431
Subparotid node, 1298f
Subperichondrial cricoidectomy, for chronic aspiration, 927-928, 929f
Substance P (SP), in salivary gland secretion, 1137
Substitution, in vestibular compensation, 2375
Substitution exercises, in vestibular rehabilitation, 2372-2373, 2378
Sub-superficial musculoaponeurotic system dissection, for cheek defects, 357-358, 360f
Subtemporal craniectomy, for middle cranial base surgery, 2465f, 2467, 2467f
Subtemporal-preauricular infratemporal approach, for middle cranial base surgery, 2462, 2466f
Subtilisin, and interstereociliary linkages, 2077
Subtotal laryngectomy, for glottic cancer, 1517t
Subtotal thyroidectomy, for Graves' disease, 1743
Succinate-dehydrogenase (SDH), in familial paraganglioma syndromes, 1659, 1659t
Succinylcholine
in children
for anesthesia maintenance, 2592
for rapid-sequence anesthesia induction, 2590
intraoperative, 111-112
Sucralfate
for caustic ingestion, 2959-2960
for extraesophageal reflux, 901
for GERD, 970
Suction lipectomy, 452, 456
Sudden infant death syndrome (SIDS), 2570
Sufentanil, as adjunct to induction of anesthesia, 111
Suicide genes, 16, 21
Sulcus vocalis, 2882
Sulindac, for head and neck squamous cell carcinoma, 1018
Sullivan, Colin, 251
Sumatriptan (Imitrex), for migraine, 2349
Summating potential (SP), in electrocochleography, 1892-1894, 1907
in Meniere's disease, 2337
Summating potential/action potential (SP/AP) ratio, 1892-1894
in Meniere's disease, 2337
Summation, in auditory processing, 1846, 2248
Sun-reactive skin types, 275, 276b, 391, 391t
Superantigens, in chronic rhinosinusitis, 706, 732
Superficial cervical fascia, 202, 2577
Superficial cervical lymph nodes, 2582
Superficial cervical plexus block, 242
Superficial musculoaponeurotic system (SMAS), 405, 406f
in deep-plane rhytidectomy, 406, 407f
and temporoparietal fascia, 440-441, 441f
Superficial musculoaponeurotic system (SMAS) flap, 405-406, 409
Superficial petrosal artery, 1826f, 1828f
Superficial petrosal nerve, 1826f
Superficial spreading carcinoma, 285f
Superficial spreading melanoma, 285f, 1108
Superficial temporal artery, 2580f

Superficial vocal fold lesions, in vocal professional, 855-856, 856f
Superficial x-rays, energy for, 1034
Superior alveolar arteries, 1295-1296
Superior ampullary nerve, 1854f, 2278f
Superior canal benign paroxysmal positional vertigo
positional testing for, 2331
repositioning maneuver for, 2332
Superior canal dehiscence syndrome (SCDS). *See* Superior semicircular canal dehiscence (SSCD) syndrome.
Superior canaliculus, of lacrimal apparatus, 798f
Superior cerebellar artery, 2351f
in surgical anatomy of anterior skull base, 2481f
Superior cervical sympathetic ganglion, in root of neck, 2582
Superior constrictor muscle
anatomy of, 1359f
in velopharyngeal function, 2676, 2677t
Superior Constrictor Rotation-Advancement Flap (SCARF), for reconstruction of soft palate, 1382, 1382f
Superior crus, of ear, 476f, 2742f
Superior deep jugular lymph nodes, 1360f
Superior incudal fold, 1827f
Superior laryngeal nerve, in surgical anatomy of lateral skull base, 2440f
Superior laryngeal nerve (SLN)
anatomy of, 807, 1422
injury during thyroid surgery of, 1770
in taste, 1211
and thyroid gland, 1751-1752
Superior malleolar fold, 1827f
Superior malleolar ligament, 1827f
Superior medial pyriform involvement, supraglottic laryngectomy for laryngeal cancer with, 1554-1555
Superior mediastinal adenopathy, total laryngopharyngectomy with, 1574, 1574f
Superior mediastinal lymph nodes, in neck dissection, 1704, 1704f, 1706t-1708t
Superior nasal meatus
normal anatomy of, 664-665
in surgical anatomy of anterior cranial base, 2472, 2472f
Superior oblique muscles
semicircular canal planes and, 2287, 2288f
in surgical anatomy of lateral skull base, 2439f
Superior olivary complex (SOC), in central auditory pathway, 1835, 1835f, 1846
Superior ophthalmic vein thrombosis, due to rhinosinusitis, 676
Superior orbital fissure, anatomy of, 322f, 440, 1823f
surgical
in anterior cranial base, 2443-2444, 2444f
in lateral skull base, 2435f, 2438
in middle cranial base, 2444, 2445f
Superior orbital fissure syndrome, 320-321
Superior petrosal sinus, in surgical anatomy of lateral skull base, 2436f, 2438, 2489
Superior petrosal sinus impression
anatomy of, 1823f
in surgical anatomy of lateral skull base, 2435f
Superior petrosal sulcus, 1823f
Superior petrosal vein, in surgical anatomy of lateral skull base, 2439f
Superior pharyngeal constrictor muscle, 1360f
Superior punctum, of lacrimal apparatus, 798f
Superior rectus muscle(s), 443f
semicircular canal planes and, 2287, 2288f
in surgical anatomy of anterior cranial base, 2472f
Superior saccular nerve, 1854f, 2278f
Superior semicircular canal
anatomy of, 1827, 1854f, 2278f
in surgical anatomy of lateral skull base, 2436f-2437f, 2439f
Superior semicircular canal dehiscence (SSCD) syndrome, 1842, 1843f, 2339-2341
anatomic and physiologic basis for, 2290, 2290f
auditory manifestations of, 2341
clinical features of, 2339
eye movements evoked by pressure changes in, 2316f
hearing loss due to, 2020-2021, 2021f
imaging of, 1920-1921, 1922f
high-resolution CT for, 2340-2341, 2340f, 2362f
ocular responses to sound in, 2339-2340, 2340f
pathophysiology of, 2339-2340, 2339f-2340f
severity of, 2340
treatment of, 2341
surgical, 2361
vestibular evoked myogenic potentials in, 2341
Superior semicircular duct, 1851f
Superior tarsal muscle, 443f, 444
Superior tarsal plate, 321f
Superior thyroid artery
anatomy of, 1751-1752, 2579-2580, 2580f
and parathyroid glands, 1778
Superior thyroid notch, radiographic anatomy of, 1472f
Superior turbinate, in surgical anatomy of anterior cranial base, 2472, 2472f
Superior tympanic artery, 1828f
Superior vestibular ganglion, 1854f, 2278f
Superior vestibular nerve, 2404f
in surgical anatomy of lateral skull base, 2437f, 2438-2439
Superior vestibular nucleus (of Bechterew), 1860, 1862f
Supernumerary nostril, 2690-2692
Superoxide anion radical (O_2^-), in acutely raised skin flaps, 1070-1071, 1071f
Superoxide dismutase (SOD), and skin flap viability, 1074
Supervoltage x-rays, 1034
Supporting cells
of olfactory epithelium, 626-627, 626f
in vestibular system, 1854-1855, 1858f
Suppurative lymphadenopathy, in children, 2818, 2818f
Supra-alar collapse, revision rhinoplasty for, 586-587, 587f
Supra-alar pinching, revision rhinoplasty for, 585-586, 586f
Suprabullar cells, in endoscopic sinus surgery, 749, 750f
Suprabullar recess
normal anatomy of, 667
surgical anatomy of, 740
Supraclavicular lymph nodes, in neck dissection, 1705f
Supraclavicular nerve, 2578, 2580f
Supraclavicular triangle, of neck, 96, 96f
Supracricoid hemilaryngopharyngectomy (SCHLP), for hypopharyngeal cancer, 1429, 1436
Supracricoid laryngectomy
with cricohyoidopexy, 1555-1557
complications of, 1557
functional outcome of, 1556-1557, 1557t
key surgical points for, 1556
oncologic results of, 1555
surgical technique for, 1555-1556, 1556f
historical background of, 1540
Supracricoid partial laryngectomy (SCPL)
with anterior commissure involvement, 1497
historical background of, 1540
intermediate, 1531
supraglottic, in advanced stage, 1500
Supracricoid partial laryngectomy with cricohyoidoepiglottopexy (SCPL-CHEP), 1549-1550
complications of, 1551
extended procedures for, 1551
functional outcome of, 1551, 1551t-1552t
key surgical points for, 1550-1551
oncologic results of, 1549-1550
surgical technique for, 1550, 1550f-1551f
vs. total laryngectomy, 1564
Supracricoid partial laryngectomy with cricohyoidopexy (SCPL-CHP), 1564
Supraglottic activity, videoendoscopy of, 817, 817f
Supraglottic cancer
advanced-stage
chemoradiation for, 1500, 1589
radiation therapy for, 1589
outcomes and prognostic factors for, 1589, 1590t
techniques and dose-fractionation schemes for, 1589
anatomic basis for, 1483-1484, 1483f, 1483t, 1542-1543
cervical metastases of, 1493-1494
chemoradiation for, 1500, 1589
clinical evaluation of, 1545
clinical presentation of, 1493, 1579
conservation laryngeal surgery for, 1551-1552, 1552t
horizontal partial laryngectomies as, 1553-1554
spectrum of, 1557-1560
supracricoid laryngectomy with cricohyoidopexy as, 1555-1557
complications of, 1557
functional outcome of, 1556-1557, 1557t
key surgical points for, 1556
oncologic results of, 1555
surgical technique for, 1555-1556, 1556f
supraglottic laryngectomy as, 1553-1554
with arytenoid, aryepiglottic fold, or superior medial pyriform involvement, 1554-1555
with base of tongue extension, 1555
complications of, 1555
extended procedures for, 1554
functional outcome of, 1555
key surgical points for, 1554-1555, 1554f
oncologic results of, 1553, 1553t
surgical technique for, 1553-1554, 1554f
early-stage, radiation therapy for, 1496, 1588-1589
complications of, 1589
outcomes and prognostic factors for, 1589, 1589t
techniques and dose-fractionation schemes for, 1588-1589
imaging of, 1475-1476
of aryepiglottic folds, 1475, 1478f
of epiglottis, 1475, 1477f
of pyriform sinuses, 1475-1476, 1478f
neck dissection for, 1500-1501
radiation therapy for
with advanced-stage disease, 1589
outcomes and prognostic factors for, 1589, 1590t
techniques and dose-fractionation schemes for, 1589
with early-stage disease, 1496, 1588-1589
complications of, 1589
outcomes and prognostic factors for, 1589, 1589t
techniques and dose-fractionation schemes for, 1588-1589
staging of, 1488t, 1580f
treatment of, 1498-1501
in advanced stage, 1500
in early stage, 1498-1500, 1498f

Supraglottic cancer *(Continued)*
with nodal metastases, 1500-1501
transoral laser microsurgery for, 1531
Supraglottic jet ventilation, for pediatric anesthesia, 2600
Supraglottic lacerations, 1634
Supraglottic laryngectomy, 1553-1554
with arytenoid, aryepiglottic fold, or superior medial pyriform involvement, 1554-1555
with base of tongue extension, 1555
complications of, 1555
extended procedures for, 1554
functional outcome of, 1555
historical background of, 1540
key surgical points for, 1554-1555, 1554f
oncologic results of, 1553, 1553t
surgical technique for, 1553-1554, 1554f
swallowing disorders due to, 1220
Supraglottic partial laryngectomy (SGL), for early-stage supraglottic cancer, 1498-1500, 1498f
Supraglottic stenosis, 947-948
Supraglottic subtotal laryngectomy, recurrence after, 1476
Supraglottis, 99, 99f
anatomy of, 1483-1484, 1483f, 1483t, 1578
surgical, 1542-1543, 1544f
embryology of, 1482
innervation of, 1544
Supraglottitis, 883, 1464
in children, 2806-2809
clinical features of, 2807
complications of, 2808-2809
diagnosis of, 2807-2808, 2807f-2808f
differential diagnosis of, 2806t
endoscopy of, 2808, 2808f
epidemiology of, 2806-2807
etiology of, 2807
histology of, 2807, 2807f
historical background of, 2806-2807
imaging of, 2807f, 2808
management of, 2808
clinical presentation of, 2807
defined, 1464
differential diagnosis of, 1464, 1465f, 2806t
imaging of, 159-161, 1406-1407, 1464
in children, 2807f, 2808
CT for, 1406
plain film, 163f, 1406, 1407f, 1464, 1464f
pseudo-, postlaryngectomy, 1416, 1417f
Supraglottoplasty, for laryngomalacia, 2867, 2868f
Suprahyoid musculature, palpation of, in voice evaluation, 827, 828f
Suprahyoid neck, imaging of, 146-157
carotid space in, 150-151, 151f-152f
CT for, 139, 141f
masticator space in, 151-152
with adenoid cystic carcinoma, 155f
with angiofibroma, 152, 154f
with hemangioma and lymphangioma, 152, 153f
with infection, 151-152, 152f
normal anatomy on, 146f, 151-152
with pseudotumors, 152
with squamous cell carcinoma, 152, 154f
MRI for, 142
normal anatomy in, 146-157, 146f-147f
oral cavity in, 153-156
with abscess, 156f
with congenital lesions, 154-156
with non-Hodgkin's lymphoma, 157f
normal anatomy on, 146f, 153-156
with squamous cell carcinoma, 154, 156f
parapharyngeal space in, 131, 146f
parotid space in, 149-150, 150f-151f
Suprahyoid neck, imaging of *(Continued)*
pharyngeal mucosal space in, 148-149
with inflammatory lesions, 148, 148f
with non-Hodgkin's lymphoma, 148-149, 149f
normal anatomy on, 146f, 148-149
with squamous cell carcinoma, 148, 149f
with Tornwaldt cyst, 148
prevertebral space in, 146f, 153
retropharyngeal space in, 146f, 152f, 153, 155f
sublingual space in, 156
with abscess and cellulitis, 156, 157f
with congenital lesions, 156
normal anatomy in, 146f, 154, 156
with ranula, 156, 157f
with squamous cell carcinoma, 156
submandibular space in, 146f, 156-157, 158f
Suprainfundibular cell, surgical anatomy of, 740
Supralabyrinthine approach, for facial nerve decompression, 2041-2042, 2043f
Supralaryngeal obstruction, in neonate, 2905, 2905f
Supramandibular lymph node, 1360f
Supramarginal gyrus, in central auditory pathway, 1837
Suprameatal spine, 2010f
in surgical anatomy of lateral skull base, 2435f
Supraomohyoid neck dissection (SOHND), 1703
for oral cancer, 1313-1314, 1713-1716
definition and rationale for, 1713, 1714f
technique for, 1713-1716, 1715f-1716f
Supraorbital artery, 439
Supraorbital bandeau, in fronto-orbital advancement
removal of, 2651-2652, 2652f
reshaping of, 2652, 2652f-2653f
splitting of, 2652, 2653f
Supraorbital cells, in frontal sinusitis, 776
Supraorbital ethmoid cells, surgical anatomy of, 741
Supraorbital foramina, in surgical anatomy of anterior cranial base, 2442, 2443f
Supraorbital nerve, 321f, 439-440, 441f
Supraorbital neurovascular pedicle, technique for preserving, 2451, 2451f
Supraorbital notch, 322f
in surgical anatomy of anterior cranial base, 2442, 2443f
Supraorbital rims, 319
Suprascapular artery
anatomy of, 2579
in root of neck, 2581-2582, 2581f
Suprascapular vein, 2579
Supratrochlear nerve, 321f, 440, 441f, 497, 497f
Supratubal recess
anatomy of, 1826f, 1827
in mastoidectomy, 2012-2013, 2013f
Sural nerve, for facial nerve grafting, 2422
Surface-enhanced laser desorption-ionization–time-of-flight (SELDI-TOF), in head and neck squamous cell carcinoma, 1029
Surfactant, in middle ear protection, 1871
Surfer's ear, imaging of, 1918, 1918f
Surgical decompression, for Bell's palsy, 2395
Surgical drainage and decompression, of odontogenic infections, 188-190
of deep neck space, 189-190
of jaw space, 189, 189f
vestibular, 188-189
Surgical history, 94
Surgical margins, with melanoma, 1113-1114, 1114t
Surgical myotomy, for achalasia, 964-965
Surgical Quality Alliance (SQA), 84t-87t, 88
Surrogate endpoints, biomarkers as, 1026
Surveillance, after surgical resection of oral cancer, 1317, 1317t
Survival analysis, 64, 72
Survival curve, 64
Survival rate, 64t
Susceptibility bias, *vs.* efficacy of treatment, 62t
Sushruta, 475
Sustained-release devices, for intratympanic delivery, 2182-2183, 2182f-2183f
Sustentacular cells, of olfactory epithelium, 626-627, 626f
Sutton's disease, in HIV, 227, 227f
Suturing
for facial trauma, 305-306, 306f
for nasal tip refinement, 522, 530f-531f, 550-551
for otoplasty, 477-478, 477f
complications of, 479
history of, 475-476, 476f
Mustarde technique for, 475-478, 476f-477f
for septoplasty, 491, 491f
Sv (sievert), 133
SVH (subjective visual horizontal), perceptual test of, 2300
SVV (subjective visual vertical), perceptual test of, 2300, 2323
Swallowing, 833, 1215-1221
functional endoscopic evaluation
for chronic aspiration, 926
for laryngeal stenosis, 2917
functions of, 2948
after hypopharyngeal and esophageal reconstruction, 1459-1460
inefficient, 1217
maturation of, 2948
physiology of, 954, 955f, 1207
stage(s) of, 1215, 1218f, 2948
esophageal, 1217, 2948
oral, 1206f, 1207, 1215, 1216f, 2948
oral preparatory, 1215, 1216f, 2948
pharyngeal, 1216, 2948
airway protection during, 1216-1217
cricopharyngeal (upper esophageal sphincter) opening during, 1217
delayed triggering of, 1215
neuromuscular activities in, 1216, 1216f
pharyngeal pressure generation during, 1217
programmed, 1216-1217
voluntary, 1215
after surgical resection of oral cancer, 1316
after total laryngectomy, 1572
Swallowing disorder(s). *See* Dysphagia.
Sweet taste
individual differences in, 1211-1212
peripheral sensitivity to, 1211
transduction of, 1209
Swimmer's ear, 97
Symblepharon, due to cicatricial pemphigoid, 1233-1234, 1234f
Symmetry, laryngeal videostroboscopy of, 820, 847-848, 848t
Sympathetic control, of salivary gland secretion, 1136
Sympathetic nerve injury, due to neck surgery, 1732, 1732f
Sympathetic trunk, in root of neck, 2582
Sympathomimetics, oral sequelae of, 1247t-1248t
Symphyseal region, anatomy and physiology of, 322-323
Symphysis
anatomy and physiology of, 322-323
menti, 320f
Symptoms, outcome scales for, 56t, 57-58
Symptoms of Nocturnal Obstruction and Respiratory Events (SNORE-25), 57
Synaptic bars, of hair cells, 1833-1834, 1833f, 1857, 1859f
Synaptic plasticity, 1884, 1884f
Synaptic ribbons, of hair cells, 1833-1834, 1833f, 1857, 1859f
Synaptic strengthening, Hebb's postulate for, 1884, 1884f
Synaptobrevin, 2080-2081

Synchondroses, in craniofacial growth and development, 2617-2619, 2619f-2620f
Synchronous lesion, in oral cancer, 1301-1302
Synergistic effect, of chemoradiation, 1041
Synkinesis, 904, 2384-2385
with Bell's palsy, 2396
management of, 2432
botulinum A toxin for, 2432
selective myectomy for, 2432
Synostosis
coronal
bilateral, 2644, 2645f
fronto-orbital advancement for, 2652-2653, 2653f-2654f
unilateral, 2643-2644, 2644f, 2648f
craniofacial, 2639
imaging of, 2648, 2648f
lambdoid, 2643-2644
fronto-orbital advancement for, 2653
metopic, 2642-2643, 2643f
pan-, 2641t
sagittal, 2642, 2643f
surgical management of, 2650, 2650f-2651f
Synovial sarcoma (SS), 1670
Synthetic biomimetic materials, for craniofacial defect repair, 2658
Synthroid (levothyroxine, oral synthetic), for hypothyroidism, 1748-1749
Syphilis
diagnosis of, 2341
HIV and, 224
oral manifestations of, 1252, 1257
otologic manifestations of, 2105, 2105f, 2341-2342
early *vs.* late, 2341
treatment for, 2341-2342
pharyngitis due to, 194
in children, 2786
sensorineural hearing loss due to, 2119, 2161
fluctuating, 2199
in infants, 2723
sudden, 2127-2128
Syringoma, 292-293
Systematic sample, 68, 69t
Systemic disease(s)
laryngeal and tracheal manifestations of, 889-893
in actinomycosis, 893
in amyloidosis, 891, 891f
in blastomycosis, 885, 892
in candidiasis, 884-885, 884f, 893
in coccidioidomycosis, 885, 893
in cryptococcosis, 892-893
in histoplasmosis, 885, 892
in pemphigus, 887, 887f, 891-892, 892f
in relapsing polychondritis, 890
in rheumatoid arthritis, 891, 891f
in sarcoidosis, 890-891, 890f
in tuberculosis, 885-886, 886f, 892
in Wegener's granulomatosis, 889-890, 890f
in whooping cough, 892
nasal manifestations of, 657-1
cutaneous, 660-661
in Behçet's disease, 660-661
in pemphigoid, 660
in pemphigus vulgaris, 660
in scleroderma, 660
granulomatous, 657-659
in Churg-Strauss syndrome, 659
in sarcoidosis, 658-659
in Wegener's granulomatosis, 658
immunodeficiency, 660
in AIDS, 660
sinusitis in immunocompromised patient as, 660
mucociliary, 661
in cystic fibrosis, 661
in primary ciliary dyskinesia, 661
Systemic disease(s) *(Continued)*
neoplastic, 659-660
in T-cell lymphoma, 659-660
oral manifestations of, 1245-1258
arthritides and bone disorders as, 1253
Ewing's sarcoma as, 1253
osteoarthritis as, 1253
Paget's disease as, 1253
Reiter's syndrome as, 1253
rheumatoid arthritis as, 1253, 1253t
cerebrovascular, 1250
collagen-vascular and granulomatous, 1251-1252
dermatomyositis-polymyositis as, 1252
sarcoidosis as, 1252
scleroderma as, 1252
Sjögren's syndrome as, 1251
systemic lupus erythematosus as, 1251-1252
Wegener's granulomatosis as, 1252
dermatologic, 1253-1254
erythema multiforme as, 1254
lichen planus as, 1253-1254
mucous membrane pemphigoid as, 1254
pemphigus vulgaris as, 1254
endocrine and exocrine, 1251
adrenal, 1251
diabetes mellitus as, 1251
parathyroid, 1251
pituitary, 1251
thyroid, 1251
gastrointestinal, 1254
Behçet's syndrome as, 1254
Crohn's disease and ulcerative colitis as, 1254
gastroesophageal reflux disease as, 1254
malabsorption diseases as, 1254
of heart, 1246-1249, 1249t
hematologic, 1256
bleeding disorders as, 1256
hemoglobin problems as, 1256
white blood cell disorders as, 1256
infectious, 1252
bacterial, 1252
fungal, 1252
viral, 1252
inherited and congenital, 1257
of liver, 1255
malignant neoplasms as, 1249-1250
neurologic, 1254-1255
Bell's palsy as, 1255
dementias (including Alzheimer's disease) as, 1254-1255
multiple sclerosis as, 1255
myasthenia gravis as, 1255
myotonic muscular dystrophy as, 1255
Parkinson's disease as, 1255
pulmonary, 1250-1251
renal, 1255
oral sequelae of medications for, 1246, 1247t-1248t
oral treatment considerations due to, 1246, 1246t
otologic manifestations of, 2100-2115, 2101t
of bone, 2108-2112
in fibrous dysplasia, 2110-2111, 2111f
in osteitis fibrosa cystica, 2112
in osteogenesis imperfecta, 2109-2110, 2110f
in osteopetroses, 2111-2112, 2112f-2113f
in Paget's disease, 2108-2109, 2109f
collagen vascular and autoimmune, 2114
genetically determined, 2115
granulomatous and infectious, 2100-2106
in Langerhans' cell histiocytosis, 2100-2101, 2101f-2102f
in Lyme disease, 2105-2106
in mycotic diseases, 2106, 2106f
otorrhea as, 2196
in sarcoidosis, 2104-2105, 2104f
in syphilis, 2105, 2105f
Systemic disease(s) *(Continued)*
in tuberculosis, 2101-2103, 2102f-2103f
in Wegener's granulomatosis, 2103-2104, 2103f-2104f
immunodeficiency, 2114-2115
in AIDS, 2114-2115
primary of congenital, 2114
neoplastic, 2106-2108
in leukemia, 2107, 2108f
metastatic, 2107-2108, 2108f
in multiple myeloma, 2106-2107, 2107f
otorrhea as, 2196
storage and metabolic, 2112-2114
in gout, 2113-2114
in mucopolysaccharidoses, 2112-2113, 2113f
in ochronosis, 2114
with rhinitis, 698-699, 698b
Systemic lupus erythematosus (SLE), oral manifestations of, 1251-1252
Systemic vascular resistance, factors influencing, 2597, 2597t

T

T & T olfactometer, 631
T cell(s), 600-603
cytotoxic, 601, 602f
development of, 600-601
effector, 601-603
in head and neck squamous cell carcinoma, 1023-1024
helper, 601-602, 602f
priming of, 601
regulatory, 602-603
T cell–dependent (TD) B cell responses, 606
T cell–independent B cell responses, 606
T cell–mediated hypersensitivity reactions, 601, 608-612
T (tumor) classification, for melanoma, 1111, 1111t, 1113f
T1 receptors (T1Rs), in gustatory transduction, 1209, 1210f
T1-weighted images (T1WI), 134, 135f-136f
T2 receptors (T2Rs), in gustatory transduction, 1209, 1210f
T2-weighted images (T2WI), 134, 135f-136f
T_3. *See* 3,5,3′-Triiodothyronine (T_3).
T_4. *See* Thyroxine (T_4).
TA (tufted angioma), 2824-2825
Kasabach-Merritt phenomenon with, 2825
TA muscle. *See* Thyroarytenoid (TA) muscle.
TAARs (trace amine–associated receptors), 630-631
TAC (tetracaine-adrenaline-cocaine) anesthesia, for facial trauma, 304
Tacrolimus (FK-506, Fugimycin, Protopic), for eczematoid otitis externa, 1956
Tactile perceptual evaluation, in voice assessment, 827-831, 828f
Tactile sensitivity, of oral cavity, 1201-1202, 1201f-1202f
Taft, William Howard, 251
Tailchaser mice, 2078
Talbot's law, 818, 847
Talkativeness profile, 861
Tandem walking, 2316-2317
Tangier disease, oral manifestations of, 1257
TARA, in deafness, 2051t-2058t
Target population, 68, 68t
Targeted therapy
historical background of, 1052
with radiotherapy, 1054, 1055f
for laryngeal cancer, 1585
for salivary gland neoplasms, 1199
Tarsal plates, 444
Tarsorrhaphy, 2420, 2421f
Tarsus
anatomy of, 443f, 444
in lower eyelid blepharoplasty, 448-449, 450f

Taste, 1207-1214
assessment of, 2383-2384
categories of, 1207
of dietary fats, 1213
in geriatric patients, 236
gustatory sensitivity in, 1207-1208
gustatory structures in, 1208
hedonic attribute of, 1207-1208
individual differences in, 1211-1212
physiology of, 1208
central gustatory pathways and function in, 1212-1213, 1212f
gustatory transduction in, 1208-1210, 1210f
interaction with saliva in, 1141, 1213-1214
with obesity, 1213
peripheral sensitivity in, 1210-1212
"sensory-specific" satiety in, 1212-1213
radiation therapy and, 1214
of umami, 1207, 1209, 1213
Taste buds, 1208
Taste disturbance, due to small fenestra stapedotomy, 2034
Taste dysfunction, palliative care for, 1103
Taste-odor tests, 632
Tattoos
amalgam (*See* Amalgam tattoo)
traumatic, 305, 305f
Tavist (clemastine), for nonallergic rhinitis, 701t
Tazarotene cream, for aging skin, 403-404
TB. *See* Tuberculosis (TB).
TBBX (transbronchial biopsy), flexible fiberoptic bronchoscopy for, 1004-1005, 1004f-1005f
TBG (thyroxine-binding globulin), 1738
TBII (thyroid binding inhibitory immunoglobulins), 1741
TBNA (transbronchial needle aspiration), flexible fiberoptic bronchoscopy for, 1005-1007, 1005f-1006f
T-box 1 *(TBX1)* gene, in deafness, 2051t-2058t
T-box transcription factor 18 *(Tbx18)* gene, in murine deafness, 2058t-2060t
TBP (thyroxine-binding protein), 1738
^{99m}Tc. *See* Technetium-99m (^{99m}Tc).
TC (typical carcinoid), of larynx, 1507
TCA(s) (tricyclic antidepressants)
for migraine, 2350
for neuropathic pain, 244-245
TCA (trichloroacetic acid). *See* Trichloroacetic acid (TCA).
T-cell lymphoma, nasal manifestations of, 659-660
tcMEP (transcranial motor evoked potential), for intraoperative monitoring, 2555, 2555f
TCOF1
in deafness, 2051t-2058t
in mandibulofacial dysostosis, 2633
T-coil (telecoil), for hearing aid, 2267
$TcPCO_2$ (transcutaneous carbon dioxide pressure), in skin flaps, 1068
$TcPO_2$ (transcutaneous oxygen pressure), in skin flaps, 1068
TD (T cell–dependent) B cell responses, 606
TE. *See* Tracheoesophageal (TE).
Technetium-99m (^{99m}Tc) scanning, 138, 139f
for malignant otitis externa, 1947
for thyroid nodule, 1757-1758
Technetium-99m (^{99m}Tc) sestamibi scintigraphy, for hyperparathyroidism, 1785
due to double parathyroid adenoma, 1785, 1785f
due to mediastinal supernumerary thyroid gland, 1802, 1803f
and multinodular thyroid disease, 1801, 1801f
due to multiple-gland hyperplasia, 1794, 1794f
due to parathyroid carcinoma, 1803, 1803f
Technetium-99m (^{99m}Tc) sestamibi scintigraphy with single photon emission computed tomography (MIBI-SPECT), for hyperparathyroidism, 1785
Technetium-99m (^{99m}Tc) thallous chloride imaging, for hyperparathyroidism, 1784-1785
TECTA (α-tectorin) gene
in deafness, 2051t-2058t, 2067-2068, 2092
genetic testing for, 2098
Tectb (β-tectorin) gene, in murine deafness, 2058t-2060t, 2067-2069.
Tectorial membrane
anatomy of, 1832, 1832f, 2067
in auditory physiology, 1841f
in cochlear transduction, 2050, 2061f, 2065-2066, 2069f
mass and stiffness of, 2067
pathophysiology of, 2067-2069
in surgical anatomy of anterior cranial base, 2474
α-Tectorin, 2067
α-Tectorin *(TECTA)* gene
in deafness, 2051t-2058t, 2067-2068, 2092
genetic testing for, 2098
β-Tectorin, 2067
β-Tectorin *(Tectb)* gene, in murine deafness, 2058t-2060t, 2067-2069.
Teeth
anatomy and physiology of, 323
development of, 1259-1260
enamel organ in, 1259
root development in, 1260
stages of, 1260
effects of radiotherapy on, 2626t
eruption of, 2617t
extraction of, prior to radiation therapy, 1330-1331, 1330b
in geriatric patients, 236
infections of (*See* Odontogenic infections)
maintaining integrity of, saliva in, 1141
physical examination of, 98
tactile sensitivity of, 1201-1202
TEF (tracheoesophageal fistula), 2926
imaging of, 1409-1410
Teflon (polytetrafluoroethylene), for vocal fold medialization
history of, 905
by injection, 905-906
complications of, 907, 908f
Tegmen mastoideum, in surgical anatomy of lateral skull base, 2438
Tegmen plate, in mastoidectomy, 2011-2012
Tegmen tympani
anatomy of, 1827
in surgical anatomy of lateral skull base, 2438
Telangiectasia, 291
hereditary hemorrhagic, 291
epistaxis in, 691-692, 692f
oral manifestations of, 1257
spider angioma as, 291
venous lakes as, 288f, 291
Telecanthus, in evaluation of maxillofacial trauma, 324, 324f
Telecoil (t-coil), for hearing aid, 2267
Telementoring, 38-39
Telephone ear deformity, 479
Telepresence, 38-39
Telerobotic surgery, 38-39
transatlantic, 39
Telogen effluvium, 376, 382, 426
Telogen phase, 374, 374f
TEM (transverse electromagnetic mode), 27, 28f
Template(s), in microtia) reconstruction, 2744-2745, 2745f
Template strand, 4
Temporal arteritis, *vs.* myofascial pain dysfunction syndrome, 1284t
Temporal bone, 320f
anatomy of, 2009-2010, 2010f
in infants, 2010
in autoimmune inner ear disease, 2165
in bacterial labyrinthitis, 2160
Temporal bone *(Continued)*
congenital rubella infection of, 2156-2157, 2157f
cytomegalic inclusion disease of, 2155-2156, 2155f
in herpes zoster oticus, 2159
imaging of, 171-173, 1916
cerebellopontine angle in, 1926-1928, 1929t
with acoustic schwannoma, 1929t
with arachnoid cyst, 1928, 1929t
with epidermoid tumor, 1928, 1928f, 1929t
with lipoma, 1928, 1929t
with meningioma, 1928, 1928f, 1929t
cochlear nerve in, 1928-1929, 1929f
conventional radiography for, 131
CT for, 142
external auditory canal in, 172, 1917-1918
with benign neoplasms, 1918, 1918f-1919f
with cholesteatoma, 1917, 1918f
with congenital lesions, 1917, 1917f
with keratosis obturans, 1917, 1918f
with malignant neoplasms, 1918, 1919f
with postinflammatory medial canal fibrosis, 1917-1918, 1918f
with severe infections, 1917, 1917f
external ear in, 172
facial nerve in, 173, 1924-1926
with Bell's palsy, 1924, 1927f
with hemangioma, 1924-1926, 1927f
with meningioma, 175f
with neuroma, 1928
with schwannoma, 1924-1926, 1927f
for infant hearing impairment, 2723
inner ear in, 172-173, 1920-1922
with congenital anomalies, 172-173, 174f, 1920-1921, 1923f
with enlarged vestibular aqueduct, 1921, 1923f
with fenestral and cochlear otosclerosis (otospongiosis), 1921-1922, 1925f
with intravestibular schwannoma, 1921, 1924f
with labyrinthitis ossificans, 1921, 1925f
normal appearance of, 1920-1921, 1922f
with superior semicircular canal dehiscence, 1920-1921, 1922f
internal auditory canal in, 173, 1926-1928
with meningioma, 175f
with vestibular schwannoma, 173, 1928, 1928f
mastoid in, 1918-1920
middle ear in, 172, 1918-1920
with aberrant internal carotid artery, 1919-1920, 1921f-1922f
with cholesteatoma, 174f, 1918-1919
with glomus tympanicum, 1919-1920, 1921f
with transverse petrous fracture with osseous dislocation, 174f
MRI for, 143
petrous apex in, 1922-1924, 1924t
with asymmetric pneumatization, 1922-1923, 1924t, 1925f
with cholesteatoma, 1924t
with cholesterol granuloma, 1923, 1924t, 1925f-1926f
with malignant lesions, 1923-1924, 1926f
with mucocele, 1924t
with retained secretions, 1923, 1924t, 1925f
in measles, 2158
multiple myeloma of, 2107, 2107f
in mumps, 2158, 2158f
osteology of, 1821-1823
lateral view of, 1822f
mastoid part in, 1821-1822, 1822f, 1829
anatomy of, 2009-2010, 2010f

Temporal bone *(Continued)*
petrous part in, 2010f
anterior surface of, 1822, 1822f
inferior surface of, 1822-1823, 1824f
posterior surface of, 1822, 1823f
squamous part in, 1821, 1822f
superior view of, 1822f
tympanic part in, 320f, 1822f, 1823, 2010f
pneumatization of, 1829
secondary mycosis of, 2195
in sudden sensorineural hearing loss, 2157
in surgical anatomy of lateral skull base, 2434, 2436f
in surgical anatomy of middle cranial base, 2445f
syphilis of, 2161
in vestibular neuritis, 2162, 2162f
Temporal bone fractures, 2036-2048
bilateral, 2036
classification of, 2036-2038
longitudinally oriented, 2036-2037, 2037f
mixed-oriented, 2037f
otic capsule–disrupting, 2037-2038
otic capsule–sparing, 2037-2038
transverse-oriented, 2036-2037, 2037f
cochlear implant for, 2221
complications of, 2039-2047
carotid artery injury as, 2039, 2040f, 2047
cholesteatoma as, 2038, 2047
CSF fistulas as, 2044-2046
closure of, 2045-2046, 2045f
treatment algorithm for, 2045-2046, 2045f
delayed meningitis as, 2037-2038, 2038f
external auditory canal stenosis as, 2038, 2047
facial nerve injury as, 2039-2044, 2042t, 2398-2399
assessing degree of, 2040
classification of, 2040
compound muscle action potential in, 2041
conservative treatment of, 2040, 2042
corticosteroids for, 2042
delayed onset of paralysis due to, 2040
electromyography for, 2041
electroneuronography for, 2041
epidemiology of, 2039-2040
evoked encephalomyography for, 2041
imaging of, 2398f
maximal stimulation test for, 2040-2041
middle fossa craniotomy for, 2042-2043
nerve excitability test for, 2040-2041
observation and symptomatic care for, 2398
outcome of, 2041, 2042t
pathogenesis of, 2398
supralabyrinthine approach for, 2042, 2043f
surgical interventions for, 2041, 2042t, 2398-2399
translabyrinthine approach for, 2041-2042
transmastoid approach for, 2042
treatment algorithm for, 2042-2044, 2043f
hearing loss as, 2046-2047, 2046f
hemotympanum as, 2038, 2039f, 2046
nystagmus as, 2039
perilymph fistula as, 2039
profuse hemorrhage as, 2038
vertigo as, 2039, 2201
epidemiology of, 2036, 2037f
evaluation of, 2038-2039
fistula test in, 2039
hearing assessment in, 2039
imaging in, 2039, 2040f
neurotologic examination in, 2038-2039
otoscopy in, 2038f-2039f
physical examination in, 2038
tympanic membrane in, 2038
open, 2036
pathophysiology of, 2036
severe, 2038-2039
Temporal bone infections, complications of, 1979-1998
diagnosis of, 1981-1982
history in, 1981-1982
imaging in, 1982
lumbar puncture in, 1982
physical examination in, 1982
epidemiology of, 1979-1981
age distribution in, 1979, 1980t
extracranial, 1979, 1980t
intracranial, 1979, 1980t-1981t
extracranial (intratemporal), 1983-1993
acute mastoiditis as, 1983, 1983f
acute suppurative labyrinthitis as, 1991-1992, 1991f-1992f
age distribution of, 1979, 1980t
Bezold abscess as, 1985-1986, 1986f-1987f
chronic mastoiditis as, 1984-1985, 1985f
coalescent mastoiditis as, 1983-1984, 1984f
encephalocele and CSF leakage as, 1992-1993, 1993f
facial nerve paralysis as, 1991, 1991f
labyrinthine fistula as, 1989-1990, 1990f
masked mastoiditis as, 1985
petrous apicitis as, 1986-1989, 1988f-1989f
postauricular abscess as, 1985, 1985f-1986f
temporal root abscess as, 1986
general considerations for, 1979
intracranial, 1993-1997
age distribution in, 1979, 1980t
brain abscess as, 1994, 1994f-1995f
epidemiology of, 1979, 1980t
epidural abscess as, 1995-1996
interrelationship of, 1979, 1981t
lateral sinus thrombosis as, 1996-1997, 1996f-1997f
meningitis as, 1993-1994, 1994f
otitic hydrocephalus as, 1997
subdural empyema as, 1994-1995
otitis media and
acute, 1979-1981
chronic, 1981
pathophysiology of, 1981
treatment of, 1982-1983
Temporal bone neoplasm(s), 2488b
carcinoma as, 2502-2504
management of, 2502-2504, 2503f
pertinent anatomy for, 2502
staging of, 2502, 2502f, 2503b
symptoms and signs of, 2502
choice of surgical approach for, 2492-2501
complications of, 2511-2513
intraoperative, 2511
postoperative, 2512-2513
cerebrovascular, 2512-2513
cranial nerve deficits as, 2512
congenital cholesteatoma as, 2508-2509
diagnostic evaluation of, 2508, 2509f-2510f
surgical approach to, 2508-2509
evaluation of, 2489-2492
carotid management algorithms in, 2491-2492
cerebral blood flow assessment in, 2490-2491, 2490f
qualitative, 2490-2491
quantitative, 2491
CT and MRI for, 2489
four-vessel arteriography in, 2489-2490, 2491f
preoperative carotid artery management in, 2489
algorithm for, 2490f, 2491-2492
cerebral blood flow assessment in, 2490-2491, 2490f
four-vessel arteriography in, 2489-2490, 2491f
facial nerve schwannomas as, 2506-2508
diagnostic evaluation of, 2507
management and surgical approach to, 2507-2508
Temporal bone neoplasm(s) *(Continued)*
infratemporal fossa approaches for, 2495-2501
postauricular, 2495-2500
cervical dissection in, 2495, 2498f
closure of external auditory canal in, 2495, 2497f
closure of wound in, 2499, 2499f
exposure of jugular bulb and internal carotid artery in, 2498, 2498f-2499f
extratemporal facial nerve dissection in, 2495-2496
facial nerve transposition in, 2497-2498, 2498f
incisions and skins flaps in, 2495, 2497f
occlusion of sigmoid sinus in, 2498, 2498f
radical mastoidectomy in, 2496, 2498f
removal of external auditory canal wall skin and tympanic membrane in, 2495, 2497f
tumor removal in, 2498-2499, 2499f
type A, 2497-2499, 2498f-2499f
type B, 2499-2500, 2500f
type C, 2500, 2501f
preauricular, 2500-2501, 2501f
lateral (partial) temporal bone resection for, 2492-2493
for carcinoma, 2503-2504
closure in, 2493, 2493f
incisions for, 2492-2493, 2493f
margins of resection for, 2492f
mastoidectomy and facial recess approach in, 2493, 2493f
removal of specimen in, 2493, 2493f
paragangliomas as, 2505-2506
diagnostic evaluation of, 2505, 2506f-2507f
preoperative evaluation of, 2491f
radiotherapy for, 2506
surgical approach to, 2505-2506, 2507f
symptoms of, 2505
postsurgical encephalocele and CSF leaks with
diagnostic evaluation of, 2509
surgical approach to, 2509
rhabdomyosarcoma as, 2501-2502
subtotal temporal bone resection for, 2494
for carcinoma, 2503-2504
defined, 2493
delineation of sigmoid sinus and jugular bulb in, 2494-2495
facial nerve management in, 2494-2495
incision for, 2494, 2494f
indications for, 2493
infratemporal fossa dissection in, 2494
margins of resection for, 2492f
neck dissection in, 2494
osteotomy in, 2495
proximal vascular control in, 2494
reconstruction after, 2495
temporal craniotomy in, 2494, 2494f
total temporal bone resection for, 2495
for carcinoma, 2504
defined, 2493-2494
facial nerve management in, 2494
incision for, 2494
indications for, 2493-2494
infratemporal fossa dissection in, 2494
margins of resection for, 2492f
neck dissection in, 2494
proximal vascular control in, 2494
reconstruction after, 2495
temporal craniotomy in, 2494
Temporal bone resection
lateral (partial), 2492-2493
for carcinoma, 2503-2504
closure in, 2493, 2493f
incisions for, 2492-2493, 2493f
margins of resection for, 2492f

Temporal bone resection *(Continued)*
mastoidectomy and facial recess approach in, 2493, 2493f
removal of specimen in, 2493, 2493f
subtotal, 2494
for carcinoma, 2503-2504
defined, 2493
delineation of sigmoid sinus and jugular bulb in, 2494-2495
facial nerve management in, 2494-2495
incision for, 2494, 2494f
indications for, 2493
infratemporal fossa dissection in, 2494
margins of resection for, 2492f
neck dissection in, 2494
osteotomy in, 2495
proximal vascular control in, 2494
reconstruction after, 2495
temporal craniotomy in, 2494, 2494f
total, 2495
for carcinoma, 2504
defined, 2493-2494
facial nerve management in, 2494
incision for, 2494
indications for, 2493-2494
infratemporal fossa dissection in, 2494
margins of resection for, 2492f
neck dissection in, 2494
proximal vascular control in, 2494
reconstruction after, 2495
temporal craniotomy in, 2494
Temporal bone surgery
CSF otorrhea due to, 2197
simulation of, 49-50, 49f-50f
surgical anatomy for, 2488-2489
Temporal branch, of facial nerve, 440, 441f, 1194f
Temporal coherence, 26, 27f
Temporal craniotomy
for middle cranial base surgery, 2467
in subtotal or total temporal bone resection, 2494, 2494f
Temporal fascia, 440
in brow or forehead rejuvenation, 433-434, 433f
Temporal fat pad, 440
Temporal forehead flap, for lip defects, 353
Temporal fossa, 320f
Temporal lift, 431-432, 431t
Temporal line, 320f, 1821, 1822f, 2009, 2010f
Temporal region, fascial layers of, 440-441, 441f
Temporal root abscess, 1986
Temporal signal processing strategies, for cochlear implants, 2229-2230, 2230f
analog stimulation as, 2230, 2230f
continuous interleaved sampling as, 2229-2230
Temporal space involvement, in odontogenic infections, 184, 185f
Temporal squama, 1822f-1823f, 2010f
Temporalis fascia graft
in atresiaplasty, 2755f, 2756, 2757f
for medialization thyroplasty, 910
for saddle nose deformity, 555, 557f
for tympanoplasty, 2000
Temporalis flap, for oropharyngeal reconstruction, 1377-1378
of tonsils and pharyngeal wall, 1386
Temporalis muscle
anatomy of, 1320, 1821
in surgical anatomy of lateral skull base, 2440f
Temporalis transfer, for facial nerve paralysis, 2427-2429, 2429f
Temporary threshold shift (TTS), 2121, 2141
Temporomandibular disorders (TMDs), 1279-1286
agenesis as, 1281t
ankylosis as, 1281t, 1282
anterior disk displacement as, 1281t
with reduction, 1280, 1282f
without reduction, 1280-1281, 1282f
Temporomandibular disorders (TMDs) *(Continued)*
arthritis as, 1281-1282
degenerative, 1281, 1281t
infectious, 1281-1282, 1281t
rheumatoid, 1253, 1281t, 1282
traumatic, 1281, 1281t
clinical presentation of, 1279
condylar and subcondylar fractures as, 1280
condylar hyperplasia as, 1281t
condylar hypoplasia as, 1281t
congenital and developmental, 1280
defined, 1279
differential diagnosis of, 1281t
dislocation as, 1280
intracapsular, 1280-1282
myofascial pain dysfunction syndrome as, 1283-1285
clinical features of, 1283-1284
defined, 1283
differential diagnosis of, 1284t-1285t
epidemiology of, 1283
etiology of, 1283, 1283f
treatment of, 1284-1285, 1286f
neoplasms as, 1280, 1281t
vs. myofascial pain dysfunction syndrome, 1285t
Temporomandibular joint (TMJ)
anatomy and physiology of, 322-323, 1279-1280
in geriatric patients, 236
in interdental discrimination, 1207
physical examination of, 95
Temporomandibular joint (TMJ) dysfunction, tinnitus with, 2132-2133
Temporomandibular joint (TMJ) surgery, 1282-1283
arthrocentesis as, 1283
arthroscopy as, 1283
arthrotomy as, 1283
Temporoparietal fascia, 440
Temporoparietal fascial flap, for oropharyngeal reconstruction, 1377-1378, 1378f
of tonsils and pharyngeal wall, 1386
Temporoparietal flaps, for free tissue transfer, 1082t
Temporoparietal-occipital (TPO) pedicle flaps, for hair loss, 385-387, 387f
complications of, 386-387
TEN (toxic epidermal necrolysis), 1239
Tension pneumothorax, *vs.* anaphylactic reaction, 119
Tension septum, 492, 493f
Tension-type headache (TTH), 247
Tensor fold, anatomy of, 1827f
Tensor tympani (TT) muscle
anatomy of
in eustachian tube, 1867, 1867f-1868f
in middle ear, 1825-1826
tensor veli palatini and, 1869-1870
in efferent auditory system, 1847
in pressure equalization, 1870
in surgical anatomy of lateral skull base, 2437f, 2438
Tensor tympani (TT) tendon, anatomy of, 1827f
Tensor veli palatini (TVP) muscle
anatomy of
in eustachian tube, 1869-1870, 1869f
in middle ear, 1825
in oral cavity, 1297f
in oropharynx, 1360f
in cleft palate, 2666-2667
development of, 1866
in pressure equalization, 1870
in velopharyngeal function, 2677t
TEOAEs. *See* Transient evoked otoacoustic emissions (TEOAEs).
TEP. *See* Tracheoesophageal puncture (TEP).
Teratomas
of cerebellopontine angle, 2527
in children, 2846-2847
epidemiology of, 2846
histopathology and molecular biology of, 2847, 2847f
management of, 2846
presentation and evaluation of, 2846, 2846t
nasopharyngeal, 2695, 2696f
neck masses due to, 1639-1640, 2816, 2816f
Terbinafine, for rhinosinusitis, 713t, 735t
Terminal cell, surgical anatomy of, 740
Tessier, Paul, 318
Test-retest reliability, 55
Tetanus prophylaxis, for facial trauma, 303
Tetracaine-adrenaline-cocaine (TAC) anesthesia, for facial trauma, 304
Tetracycline, for embolization, 1933
3,5,3′,5′-Tetraiodothyronine (T_4), 1737. *See also* Thyroid hormone(s).
oral synthetic, for hypothyroidism, 1748-1749
serum free, 1740
in thyrotoxicosis, 1742
Tetraspan membrane protein of hair cell stereocilia *(TMHS)* gene, in deafness, 2051t-2058t
TFCP2L3 (transcription factor cellular promotor 2-like 3) gene, in deafness, 2051t-2058t
TG. *See* Thyroglobulin (TG).
TGF (transforming growth factor), 609t-610t
TGF-α (transforming growth factor α), in wound healing, 1076
TGF-β (transforming growth factor β), 609t-610t
in wound healing, 1076
TH1 cells, 601
in otitis media, 2764
TH2 cells, 601
in otitis media, 2764
TH17 cells, 601-602
Thalamus, in auditory pathway, 1846-1847
Thalassemia
oral manifestations of, 1256
preoperative evaluation of, 106
Thalidomide, microtia due to, 2741
Thallium 201 (Tl 201) imaging, for hyperparathyroidism, 1784-1785
Thallous chloride imaging, for hyperparathyroidism, 1784-1785
Thanatophoric dysplasia, craniofacial anomalies in, 2641t
Therapeutic lymph node dissection (TLND), for melanoma, 1114, 1116
Thermal ablation, interventional bronchoscopy with, 1010t
Thermal laryngeal trauma, 939-941
etiology of, 940-941
incidence of, 939-940
management of, 941
Thermal sensitivity, of oral cavity, 1201
Thermoregulation, vascular supply of skin in, 1064
θ-defensins, 599
THI (Tinnitus Handicap Inventory), 2135, 2138
Thiamine-responsive megaloblastic anemia syndrome, deafness in, 2051t-2058t
Thiazide diuretics, hypercalcemia due to, 1784
Thiopental, for anesthesia induction, 111
in children, 2590
Third "mobile window," in superior canal dehiscence syndrome, 2339-2340
Third-gain rule, for hearing aids, 2271
Thoracic duct, anatomy of, 2582
Thornwaldt cyst. *See* Tornwaldt cyst.
THRB (thyroid hormone receptor β) gene, in deafness, 2051t-2058t

Three-dimensional conformal radiotherapy (3DCRT), 1043
for cervical metastases, 1691-1692
for glottic cancer
advanced-stage, 1585-1586
early-stage, 1581, 1581f-1582f
Three-dimensional (3D) CT, of laryngeal carcinoma, 1470
Three-dimensional reconstruction, from CT or MRI, 138, 140f
Three-field technique, for radiation therapy, for glottic cancer, 1586, 1587f
Three-wall orbital decompression, for Graves' ophthalmopathy, 1815-1816
Threshold, of auditory neurons, 1839-1840, 1844-1845, 1845f
Throat, sore. *See* Pharyngitis.
Throat cultures, 2787
Thrombocytopenia
oral manifestations of, 1256
preoperative evaluation of, 106
Thromboxane synthetase, in acutely raised skin flaps, 1070, 1070f
"Through-and-through" resection, for buccal carcinoma, 1308-1309, 1309f
Through-the-scope (TTS) balloons, for esophageal strictures, 966
Thrush, 1230, 1230f
in HIV, 225, 226f
Thulium laser, for stridulous child, 2908
Thunderclap headache, 248
Thymic cysts, 2817
Thymopharyngeal cysts, 2585
Thyroarytenoid (TA) muscle
anatomy of
applied, 806-807, 807f
surgical, 1543f
botulinum toxin injection of, for spasmodic dysphonia, 840f
in breathing, 810f
characteristics of, 918
in pitch control, 812
in professional voice production, 846-847
Thyrocervical trunk, in root of neck, 2581-2582
Thyroepiglottic ligament, surgical anatomy of, 1542f-1543f
Thyroglobulin (TG)
serum measurement of, 1740
with thyroid nodule, 1756
in thyroid hormone storage and release, 1737f, 1738
in thyroid hormone synthesis
iodination of, 1737f, 1738
synthesis of, 1737-1738, 1737f
Thyroglossal duct carcinomas, 2847
Thyroglossal duct cyst(s), 2814-2815, 2871-2872
clinical presentation of, 2814-2815, 2815f
vs. ectopic thyroid, 2815
embryology of, 2586, 2814
imaging of, 161-162, 165f
infected, needle aspiration of, 206, 206f
neck masses due to, 1639
Sistrunk operation for, 2815
squamous cell carcinoma arising in, 1671
vallecular, 2871-2872, 2872f
Thyrohyoid ligament, surgical anatomy of, 1542f
Thyrohyoid membrane, surgical anatomy of, 1541-1542, 1542f-1543f
Thyrohyoid muscle, characteristics of, 918-919
Thyrohyoid space, palpation of, in voice evaluation, 827, 828f
Thyroid adenoma, 1758-1759
autonomously functioning, 1759
in children, 2819
clinical presentation of, 1758
Thyroid adenoma *(Continued)*
management and prognosis for, 1759
pathology of, 1758-1759
sestamibi–technetium 99m scintigraphy of, 1785f
toxic, 1744
Thyroid alar cartilage graft, for laryngeal stenosis, 2919, 2921f
Thyroid antibody status, 1740-1741
Thyroid binding inhibitory immunoglobulins (TBII), 1741
Thyroid cancer
anaplastic, 1764
clinical presentation of, 1764
management and prognosis for, 1764
pathology of, 1764
in children, 1769-1770, 2820
clinical presentation of, 1751
epidemiology of, 1751
etiology of, 1753
follicular, 1761-1762
clinical presentation of, 1761-1762
imaging of, 161-162, 165f
management and prognosis for, 1762
pathology of, 1762
follow-up for, 1772
in geriatric patients, 238
Graves' disease and, 1742
Hürthle cell, 1762-1763
clinical presentation of, 1762
management and prognosis for, 1762-1763
pathology of, 1762
insular, 1764
with laryngeal invasion, 1510
lymphoma as, 1764
medullary, 1763-1764
clinical presentation of, 1763
management and prognosis for, 1763-1764
nodal metastasis of, 1766
pathology of, 1763
metastatic, 1764
ultrasound imaging of, 1644, 1648f-1649f
molecular basis for, 1752-1753
papillary, 1760-1761
clinical presentation of, 1760
management and prognosis for, 1760-1761
pathology of, 1760
during pregnancy, 1770
risk factors for, 1753
with aggressive behavior, 1756, 1756t
selective neck dissection for, 1719, 1719f-1720f
squamous cell, 1764
staging and classification of, 1753-1754
AGES and MACIS, 1754
AMES, 1754, 1756t
TNM, 1754, 1755t
surgical management of (*See* Thyroid surgery)
tracheal invasion by, 1615
ultrasound of, 1644, 1646b, 1646f
metastatic, 1644, 1648f-1649f
Thyroid capsule, anatomy of, 1751
Thyroid cartilage
anatomy of, 805-806, 1359f
radiographic, 1471, 1473f
surgical, 1541, 1542f-1544f
laryngeal carcinoma of, 1541
imaging of, 1474-1475, 1476f
palpation of, in voice evaluation, 827, 828f
physical examination of, 95, 96f
repair of, 936-937
Thyroid cyst, 1759-1760
clinical presentation of, 1759-1760
management and prognosis for, 1760
pathology of, 1760
Thyroid dermopathy, and Graves' ophthalmopathy, 1808
Thyroid disorder(s), 1735-1749
history and review of symptoms for, 1736
hyperparathyroidism and, 1801, 1801f-1802f
hypothyroidism as, 1745-1749
clinical features of, 1745-1746, 1746b
due to endemic goiter, 1747
etiology of, 1745, 1746b
due to excessive iodine intake, 1747
familial, 1747
goitrous, 1747
hearing loss due to, 1746
hoarseness due to, 1747
hypothalamic, 1747
laboratory diagnosis of, 1748, 1748t
after laryngectomy, 1747
management of, 1748-1749
myxedema coma due to, 1749
nongoitrous, 1747
pituitary, 1747
prevalence of, 1745
after radiation therapy, 1747
risk factors for, 1745-1746, 1746b
subclinical, 1747-1748
diagnosis of, 1747
effects on lipid, hypothyroid symptoms, and mood of, 1747-1748
natural history of, 1747
prevalence of, 1747
treatment of, 1748
surgery with, 1749
transient, 1747
vertigo due to, 1747
oral manifestations of, 1251
physical examination for, 1736-1737
due to radiotherapy, 1048
thyrotoxicosis as, 1741-1745
defined, 1741
ectopic, 1745
epidemiology of, 1741
etiology of, 1742, 1742t
exogenous, 1744
due to Graves' disease, 1742-1743
overt, 1741
pathophysiology of, 1742
subclinical, 1741, 1745
thyroid storm in, 1745
due to thyroiditis, 1744
due to toxic multinodular goiter, 1744-1745
due to toxic thyroid adenoma, 1744
Thyroid eye disease. *See* Graves' ophthalmopathy.
Thyroid follicular necrosis, radiation-induced, 1744
Thyroid function
control of, 1738-1739
in Graves' ophthalmopathy, 1809
Thyroid function study(ies), 1739-1741
circulating thyroid hormone measurement as, 1739-1740
in hypothyroidism, 1748, 1748t
radioactive iodine uptake test as, 1741
serum thyroglobulin measurement as, 1740
serum thyrotropin measurement as, 1740, 1741f
thyroid antibody status as, 1740-1741
thyroid-stimulating antibody measurement as, 1741
Thyroid gland, 1735-1749
anatomy of, 1359f, 1736
surgical, 1751-1752, 1751f-1752f
blood supply to and from, 1751-1752, 1752f
ectopic
lingual, 161-162, 165f, 1287, 1736
median, 1639
vs. thyroglossal duct cyst, 2815
embryology of, 1751
imaging of, 161-162
CT for, 140
with follicular carcinoma, 161-162, 165f
lingual, 161-162, 165f

Thyroid gland *(Continued)*
MRI for, 143
normal anatomy in, 161
scintigraphy for, 138
with thyroglossal duct cyst, 161-162, 165f
ultrasonography for, 1644, 1645f-1647f, 1646b
multinodular, ultrasound imaging of, 1644
physical examination of, 95, 1736-1737
physiology of, 1737-1739, 1737f
control of function in, 1738-1739
iodide transport in, 1737, 1737f
iodination and thyroperoxidase in, 1737f, 1738
thyroglobulin in, 1737-1738, 1737f
thyroid hormones in, 1737
and antithyroid agents, 1739, 1739t
circulating, 1737f, 1738-1740
mechanism of action of, 1739
metabolism of, 1737f, 1738
storage and release of, 1737f, 1738
synthesis of, 1737f, 1738
during pregnancy, 1770
preoperative evaluation of, 104
Thyroid goiter
compression of pharynx and esophagus due to, 1409, 1409f
endemic, 1747
intrathoracic, 1766
tobacco smoke and, 1807
toxic
multinodular, 1744-1745
uninodular, 1744
Thyroid hormonal status, and Graves' ophthalmopathy, 1807
Thyroid hormone(s), 1737
and antithyroid agents, 1739, 1739t
circulating, 1737f, 1738
measurement of, 1739-1740
free *vs.* bound, 1738
mechanism of action of, 1739
metabolism of, 1737f, 1738
storage and release of, 1737f, 1738
synthesis of, 1737f, 1738
iodide transport in, 1737, 1737f
iodination and thyroperoxidase in, 1737f, 1738
thyroglobulin in, 1737-1738, 1737f
in thyrotoxicosis, 1742
thyrotoxicosis due to, 1744
Thyroid hormone receptor β *(THRB)* gene, in deafness, 2051t-2058t
Thyroid hormone replacement, after thyroid surgery, 1771
Thyroid hormone resistance, and deafness, 2051t-2058t
Thyroid isotope scanning, 1757-1758
Thyroid lobe(s), 1751, 1751f
Thyroid lobectomy, for thyroid adenoma, 1759
Thyroid lymphomas, 1679
staging of, 1679
treatment and prognosis for, 1679
Thyroid neoplasm(s), 1750-1772
in children, 1769-1770
classification of, 1759t
embolization of, 1938-1939
epidemiology of, 1750
Hürthle cell tumor as, 1762-1763
clinical presentation of, 1762
management and prognosis for, 1762-1763
pathology of, 1762
malignant (*See* Thyroid cancer)
molecular basis for, 1752-1753
neck masses due to, 1640
during pregnancy, 1770
surgical management of (*See* Thyroid surgery)
thyroid adenoma as, 1758-1759
autonomously functioning, 1759
in children, 2819
Thyroid neoplasm(s) *(Continued)*
clinical presentation of, 1758
management and prognosis for, 1759
pathology of, 1758-1759
sestamibi–technetium 99m scintigraphy of, 1785f
toxic, 1744
thyroid cyst as, 1759-1760
clinical presentation of, 1759-1760
management and prognosis for, 1760
pathology of, 1760
Thyroid nodule(s)
algorithm for management of, 1758, 1758f
in children, 1769-1770
"cold," 1758
colloid, 1644, 1647f
cystic, 1644, 1645f
epidemiology of, 1750-1751
evaluation of, 1754-1758
fine-needle aspiration cytology for, 1756-1758
history and physical examination for, 1754-1756
imaging for, 1757
laboratory studies for, 1756
thyroid isotope scanning for, 1757-1758
fine-needle aspiration biopsy of, 1756-1758
repeat, 1759
ultrasound-guided, 1655f
"hot," 1758
imaging of, 1757
CT and MRI for, 1757
thyroid isotope scanning for, 1757-1758
ultrasound for, 1644, 1757
colloid, 1644, 1647f
cystic, 1644, 1645f
malignant, 1644, 1646b, 1646f
with multiple nodules, 1644
solid hyperfunctioning, 1644
malignant, 1644, 1646b, 1646f
multiple, 1644
neck masses due to, 1640
during pregnancy, 1770
solid hyperfunctioning, 1644
Thyroid storm, 104, 1745
Thyroid surgery, 1764-1771
approach to, 1764-1766
exposure of thyroid gland in, 1765
incision for, 1764-1765
parathyroid glands in, 1752, 1765f, 1766
positioning for, 1764-1765
recurrent laryngeal nerve in, 1765, 1765f
strap muscles in, 1765
thyroid dissection in, 1765, 1765f
transection of isthmus in, 1766
in children, 1769-1770
complication(s) of, 1770-1771
bleeding as, 1770
hypocalcemia as, 1771
recurrent laryngeal nerve injury as, 1770-1771
superior laryngeal nerve injury as, 1770
extended, 1766, 1767f-1768f
extent of, 1768-1769
follow-up after, 1772
with intrathoracic goiter, 1766
management of regional lymphatics in, 1766
minimally invasive, 1769, 1769f
parathyroid glands during, 1752
postoperative management after, 1771-1772
external-beam radiotherapy and chemotherapy in, 1772
radioactive iodine treatment in, 1771-1772
thyroid hormone replacement in, 1771
during pregnancy, 1770
with recurrent laryngeal nerve invasion, 1766
reoperative, 1767-1768
Thyroidectomy
for Graves' disease
near-total, 1743
subtotal, 1743
minimally invasive, 1769, 1769f
robotic, 41-42
with total laryngectomy, 1566
with total laryngopharyngectomy, 1574
Thyroiditis, 1744
acute suppurative, 1744
Hashimoto's (autoimmune), 1747
oral manifestations of, 1251
ultrasound imaging of, 1644
painless or silent, 1744
subacute, 1743-1744
lymphocytic, 1744
Thyroid-stimulating antibody, 1741
Thyroid-stimulating hormone (TSH). *See* Thyrotropin (TSH).
Thyrometabolic status, measurement of, 1739-1740
Thyroperoxidase (TPO), in thyroid hormone synthesis, 1737f, 1738
Thyropharyngeal muscle, surgical anatomy of, 1543f
Thyroplasty, medialization, 904-911
advantages of, 908
arytenoid adduction *vs.*, 912-913
autologous temporalis fascia grafts for, 910
complications of, 911
disadvantages of, 908
factors affecting outcome of, 908
with Gore-Tex strip, 908, 910, 911f
historical aspects of, 904-905
implant placement in, 909-910, 910f
indications for, 905, 908
limitations of, 910
outcome measures for, 910
patient evaluation and selection for, 905
prefabricated implants for, 908, 908f, 910
prosthesis templates in, 909-910, 910f
technique for, 908-911, 909f
Thyrotoxicosis, 1741-1745
defined, 1741
ectopic, 1745
epidemiology of, 1741
etiology of, 1742, 1742t
exogenous, 1744
due to Graves' disease, 1742-1743
with Graves' ophthalmopathy, 1810
oral manifestations of, 1251
overt, 1741
pathophysiology of, 1742
subclinical, 1741, 1745
thyroid storm in, 1745
due to thyroiditis, 1744
due to toxic multinodular goiter, 1744-1745
due to toxic thyroid adenoma, 1744
Thyrotracheal anastomosis, cricoid resection with, for laryngeal stenosis, 2921, 2922f
Thyrotropin (TSH)
in control of thyroid function, 1738-1739
elevation of, due to nonthyroidal illness, 1748
and Graves' ophthalmopathy, 1807, 1809
serum measurement of, 1740, 1741f
for thyroid nodule, 1758
Thyrotropin (TSH) receptor, in thyroid carcinoma, 1752-1753
Thyrotropin-releasing hormone (TRH), in control of thyroid function, 1739
Thyroxine (T_4), 1737. *See also* Thyroid hormone(s).
oral synthetic, for hypothyroidism, 1748-1749
serum free, 1740
in thyrotoxicosis, 1742
Thyroxine-binding globulin (TBG), 1738
Thyroxine-binding protein (TBP), 1738
Tic douloureux, 248

Tidal volume, in infants, 2570
Tietz syndrome, deafness in, 2051t-2058t
Tight junctions, in perilymphatic-endolymphatic barrier, 2081, 2082f
TIL (tumor-infiltrating lymphocytes), genetic modification of, 13, 20-21
Times 1 adaptation exercise, 2375f, 2378
Times 2 adaptation exercise, 2375f, 2378
TIMM8A (translocase of mitochondrial inner membrane 8A) gene
  in deafness, 2051t-2058t
  in Mohr-Tranebjaerg syndrome, 2097
Tinactin (tolnaftate), for fungal otitis externa, 1954-1955, 1959t-1960t
Tinnitus, 2131-2138
  clinical evaluation of, 2137-2138
  comorbidities with, 2138
  deafferentation–loss-of-inhibition hypothesis of, 2133
  defined, 2131
  due to erythromycin, 2176
  and insomnia, 2138
  in Meniere's disease, 2335t, 2337
  with migraine, 2349
  neural plasticity and, 1886
  objective, 2131, 2132t
    pulsatile, 2131, 2132t
  due to quinine, 2176
  due to salicylates, 2175-2176
  due to small fenestra stapedotomy, 2034
  standardized outcome measures for, 2138
  subjective, 2132t
    defined, 2131
    epidemiology of, 2131
    idiopathic, 2131-2133
    patterns of hearing loss in, 2131-2132, 2132t
    somatic, 2132-2133, 2132t
    typewriter, 2133
  treatment strategies for, 2133-2137
    acoustic-based, 2133
      acoustic desensitization protocol as, 2135
      ambient stimulation as, 2133-2134
      combined with education and counseling, 2134-2135
      personal listening devices as, 2134
      total masking therapy as, 2134
    cognitive-behavioral, 2135
    electric stimulation as, 2136-2137
      via cochlear implants, 2137
      transcutaneous, 2136-2137
    pharmacologic, 2137
    transcranial magnetic stimulation as, 2135-2136
Tinnitus Handicap Inventory (THI), 2135, 2138
Tinnitus retraining therapy (TRT), 2134-2135
  for hyperacusis, 2139
Tinnitus-producing fibromuscular dysplasia, of carotid artery, endovascular treatment for, 1943
Tip links
  in auditory physiology, 1841f, 1842, 1843f
  composition of, 2072f, 2074
  in hair cell transduction, 2072f, 2073-2074
  in vestibular physiology, 2277-2278, 2279f
Tip projection, 520, 535-536
  in aesthetic analysis, 273-274, 277f
  autogenous cartilage struts for, 535-536, 536f
  cephalic rotation for, 519, 536, 549-550, 551f
  onlay tip cartilage grafts for, 535-536, 537f, 549-550, 550f-551f
  partial-transfixion *vs.* complete-transfixion incisions for, 535-536, 536f
  plumping grafts for, 535-536, 536f
  transdomal sutures for, 536
Tip ptosis, 484, 485f
  caudal extension graft for, 576, 576f
  due to overaggressive resection of caudal septum, 492, 492f
  revision rhinoplasty for, 590-593, 593f
  after rhinoplasty, 519, 520f
Tip recoil, 513, 513f
Tip rotation, in aesthetic analysis, 273-274, 277f
Tip support mechanisms, 519, 520f
Tirapazamine, with radiotherapy, 1041
Tissue adhesives, for facial trauma, 306
Tissue débridement, interventional bronchoscopy for, 1008-1009, 1010t
Tissue effects, of surgical laser, 28-30, 30f
Tissue engineering, in mandibular reconstruction, 1327-1328, 1328f
Tissue expansion
  for forehead repair, 363
  for hair loss, 384, 385f
  for scar revision, 296-298, 297f
  and skin flap viability, 1074
Tissue flaps, gene therapy for, 22-23
Tissue-radiation characterizations, 1039-1040, 1039f
Titanium, for craniofacial defect repair, 2657
Titanium chain link implants, for lagophthalmos, 2421
Titanium prostheses, for ossiculoplasty, 2006, 2025-2026, 2026t
TIV (trivalent inactivated influenza vaccine), to prevent otitis media, 2769
TIVA (total intravenous anesthesia), in children, 2592
Tl 201 (thallium 201) imaging, for hyperparathyroidism, 1784-1785
TLESR (transient lower esophageal sphincter relaxation), 954, 968
TLM. *See* Transoral laser microsurgery (TLM).
TLND (therapeutic lymph node dissection), for melanoma, 1114, 1116
TLRs. *See* Toll-like receptors (TLRs).
TM. *See* Tympanic membrane (TM).
TMC1 (transmembrane channel-like gene 1), in deafness, 2051t-2058t
TMDs. *See* Temporomandibular disorders (TMDs).
TMHS (tetraspan membrane protein of hair cell stereocilia) gene, in deafness, 2051t-2058t
TMIE (transmembrane inner ear expressed gene), in deafness, 2051t-2058t
TMJ. *See* Temporomandibular joint (TMJ).
Tmprss1 (transmembrane protease serine 1) gene, in murine deafness, 2058t-2060t
TMPRSS3 (transmembrane protease serine 3) gene, in deafness, 2051t-2058t
TMS (transcranial magnetic stimulation), for tinnitus, 2135-2136
TNE. *See* Transnasal esophagoscopy (TNE).
TNF (transnasal fiberoptic laryngoscopy), for extraesophageal reflux, 898
TNF (tumor necrosis factor), 609t-610t
TNF-α (tumor necrosis factor α), in gene therapy, 21
TNF-β (tumor necrosis factor β), 609t-610t
TNFerade, in gene therapy, 21
TNM classification. *See* Tumor-node-metastasis (TNM) classification.
TOAE (transitory otoacoustic emission), for otitis media, 2762
Tobacco
  and Graves' ophthalmopathy, 1807
  and skin flap survival, 1075
  and squamous cell carcinoma
    of head and neck, 1016
    of larynx, 1491, 1512-1513
    of oral cavity, 1293-1294, 1365
Tobacco smoke exposure, and otitis media, 2767
Tobramycin, for rhinosinusitis, 734-735, 735t
Tobramycin with dexamethasone (Tobradex), for otitis externa, 1952, 1959t-1960t
Tolerance, immune, 1023
Toll-like receptors (TLRs), 598
  activators of, 598
  and adaptive immune response, 598
  expression and distribution of, 598
  and host, 598
Tolnaftate (Tinactin), for fungal otitis externa, 1954-1955, 1959t-1960t
Tone(s), 1838-1839
Tone-pips, in auditory brainstem response testing, 1896-1897
Tongue
  anatomy of, 1297
  fungiform papillae on, 1208
  leukoplakia of, 1362f
  lymphatic drainage of, 1297, 1298f
  muscles and reflexes of, 1205
  neurologic examination of, 833
  physical examination of, 98
  in swallowing
    in oral preparatory stage, 1215, 1216f
    in oral stage, 1215, 1216f
  tactile sensitivity of, 1201, 1201f
  taste buds on, 1208
Tongue base
  anatomy of, 1359, 1359f
    radiographic, 1399f
  lymphatics of, 1361f
Tongue base cancer
  cervical lymph node metastasis of, 1361t
  clinical presentation of, 1365
  management of, 1369-1370
Tongue base extension, laryngeal cancer with, supraglottic laryngectomy for, 1555
Tongue base procedures, for obstructive sleep apnea, 259
Tongue base reconstruction, 1387-1391
  algorithm for, 1391f
  free flaps for, 1389
    lateral arm, 1389
    radial forearm, 1389
  goals of, 1387
  healing by second intention for, 1387-1388
  local flaps for, 1388
  primary closure for, 1387-1388
  regional flaps for
    latissimus dorsi, 1389
    pectoralis major myocutaneous, 1388-1389
    platysmal myocutaneous, 1389
  skin grafting for, 1388
  after total or subtotal glossectomy, 1389-1390
    innervated free latissimus dorsi musculocutaneous flap for, 1389-1390, 1390f
    microvascular reconstruction as, 1390
    money pouch–like method for, 1390, 1390f
    sensate fasciocutaneous flaps for, 1390-1391
Tongue base retraction, during pharyngeal swallow, 1217
Tongue carcinoma, 1305-1306
  advanced-stage, 1306
  cervical lymph node metastases of, 1306
  clinical presentation of, 1305
  composite resection of, 1305, 1305f-1306f
  differential diagnosis of, 1305
  epidemiology of, 1295, 1305
  etiology of, 1305
  gross pathology of, 1305f
  hemiglossectomy for, 1305-1306, 1305f
  hemimandibulectomy for, 1306f
  local invasion by, 1305, 1305f-1306f
  palatal augmentation prosthesis for, 1342-1343, 1344f

Tongue carcinoma *(Continued)*
reconstruction for, 1305-1306
survival with, 1306
wide local excision for, 1305
Tongue flaps, for oropharyngeal reconstruction, 1376
Tongue prosthesis, 1342-1343, 1344f
Tongue reduction surgery, for obstructive sleep apnea in children, 2609
Tongue resection, palatal augmentation prosthesis for, 1342-1343, 1344f
Tongue surgery, swallowing disorders due to, 1219
Tongue suspension, for obstructive sleep apnea in children, 2610
Tonic activity, in facial nerve monitoring, 2387, 2547, 2547f
Tonotopic map, 2060-2061, 2063f
Tonotopic map reorganization
age-related, 1877, 1879, 1882f
experimental studies of
after cochlear lesions, 1877-1878, 1878f-1879f
in adult subjects, 1878-1879, 1881f
in developmental model, 1878, 1880f
after long-term local excitation of cochlea, 1880-1881, 1883f
at subcortical levels, 1879-1880
mechanisms of
at cellular level, 1884
Hebb's postulate for, 1884, 1884f
long-term potentiation as, 1884
at systems level of
in adult subjects, 1883-1884
in developing subject, 1883
practical issues relating to, 1884-1886
for hearing loss in infants, 1885, 1885f
for other hearing disorders, 1885-1886
time course of, 1877
Tonotopic tuning
of afferent auditory neurons, 1845
of basilar membrane, 1840-1842, 1844f
of hair cells, 1844, 1844f
Tonsil(s)
anatomy of, 2783-2784
bacteriology of, 2785-2788
diagnostic assessment of, 2793-2794
in immune system, 605
immunology of, 2784-2785
lymphoma of, 1364f
physical examination of, 99
radiographic anatomy of, 1462-1463, 1464f
squamous cell carcinoma of, 1362f, 1369f
Tonsillar abscess, imaging of, 148, 148f
Tonsillar calcifications, 1411, 1412f
Tonsillar capsule, 2783
Tonsillar concretions, 2787-2788, 2788f
Tonsillar crypts, 2783-2784
Tonsillar fossae
anatomy of, 1359, 2784
cancer of
cervical lymph node metastasis of, 1361t
clinical presentation of, 1365
management of, 1369, 1369f
melanoma as, 1365f
Tonsillar hypertrophy, due to Epstein-Barr virus, 2786f
Tonsillar pillars, radiographic anatomy of, 1398f
Tonsillar reconstruction, 1383-1387
algorithm for, 1388f
free flaps for, 1386
with combined lateral and superior defects, 1386, 1387f
lateral arm and thigh, 1386-1387
radial forearm, 1386
healing by second intention for, 1383
local flaps for, 1384-1385
primary closure for, 1383-1384
pectoralis major, 1385, 1385f
platysmal myocutaneous, 1385
Tonsillar reconstruction *(Continued)*
regional flaps for
sternocleidomastoid myocutaneous, 1385-1386
temporalis, 1386
temporoparietal fascia, 1386
skin grafting for, 1384
Tonsillectomy
for acute otitis media, 2771
Coblation, 2796
electrocautery, 2797-2799
hemorrhage after, 2783f-2784f, 2794, 2799-2800, 2800f
hemostasis after, 2798-2799
history of, 2782
immunologic consequences of, 2785
indications for, 2794b, 2795
for obstructive sleep apnea
in children, 2608-2609
lingual, 259
subtotal, 2797
in vocal professional, 857
Tonsillitis, 1464f
chronic recurrent, 2795
complication(s) of, 2788-2790
nonsuppurative, 2788
parapharyngeal space abscess as, 2788-2789
peritonsillar infections as, 2788, 2789f
retropharyngeal space infections as, 2789-2790, 2789f
suppurative, 2788-2790
streptococcal, 2787
Tonsilloliths, 99, 2787-2788, 2788f
Tonsillopharyngitis, due to group A beta hemolytic *Streptococcus pyogenes,* 192
Tooth buds, 1259
Tooth development, 1259-1260
enamel organ in, 1259
root development in, 1260
stages of, 1260
Tooth eruption, 2617t
Tooth extractions, prior to radiation therapy, 1330-1331, 1330b
Tooth infections. *See* Odontogenic infections.
Tooth integrity, maintenance of, saliva in, 1141
Tooth pain, 1202-1203
Tooth root, development of, 1260
"Toothy" smile, 2417-2418
Topical anesthesia
for awake fiberoptic nasotracheal intubation, 124
for tracheobronchial endoscopy, 1000
for vocal professionals, 855
Topical decongestants, for obstructive sleep apnea, 257
Topical nasal corticosteroids, for nonallergic rhinitis, 700, 700t
Topical therapies, for external ear disorders, 1950-1962
acidifying agents as, 1959t-1960t
for acute bacterial otitis externa, 1953
for fungal otitis externa, 1954
for acute bacterial otitis externa, 1951-1953
acidifying agents as, 1953
antibiotics as, 1951-1953
failure to respond to, 1953, 1953t
options for, 1951-1953, 1951f
antibiotics as, 1959t-1960t
for acute bacterial otitis externa, 1951-1953
evidence-based data on, 1952
hypersensitivity reaction to, 1954
mechanism of action of, 1951
ototoxicity of, 1953-1954
resistance to, 1953
antifungals as, 1959t-1960t
for fungal otitis externa, 1954-1955
ototoxicity of, 1955
Topical therapies, for external ear disorders *(Continued)*
anti-inflammatories as
for eczematoid otitis externa, 1956-1957
mechanism of action of, 1951
antiseptics as, 1955
for fungal otitis externa, 1955
for cerumen impaction, 1957
options for, 1957, 1958t
for ear hygiene and chronic draining ear, 1957-1958, 1961f
for eczematoid otitis externa, 1955-1957
anti-inflammatory and immunosuppressive agents as, 1956-1957
options for, 1955
steroids as, 1955-1956
for fungal otitis externa, 1954-1955
acidifying agents as, 1954
antifungals as, 1954-1955
antiseptics as, 1955
options for, 1954
history of, 1950
immunosuppressive agents as, for eczematoid otitis externa, 1956-1957
mechanism of action of, 1950-1951
for antibiotics, 1951
for anti-inflammatories, 1951
for myringitis, 1955
steroids as
classes of, 1956, 1956t
for eczematoid otitis externa, 1955-1956
hypersensitivity reaction to, 1954
mechanism of action of, 1951
ototoxicity of, 1956
summary of available, 1959t-1960t
for viral infections, 1957, 1957f
options for, 1957
Topiramate, for neuropathic pain, 244t
Topognostic tests, for assessment of facial nerve function, 2382-2384
of lacrimal function, 2383
of salivary flow, 2384
of salivary pH, 2384
of stapedius reflex, 2383
of taste, 2383-2384
Torcular Herophili, 2489
Tornwaldt cyst, 1348-1349
imaging of, 148, 1416, 1416f
TORP. *See* Total ossicular replacement prosthesis (TORP).
TORS (transoral robotic surgery), for laryngeal cancer, 1560-1561
Torsemide, ototoxicity of, 2175
Torsional pendulum model, of cupular displacement, 2279-2283, 2282f
Torticollis
congenital, 2817, 2817f
paroxysmal, and migraine, 2351
Torus
of oral cavity, 1287, 1288f
mandibularis, 1287
palatinus, 99, 1287, 1288f
tubarius
of eustachian tube, 1869, 1869f
anatomy of, 1825
of oropharynx
anatomy of, 1359f
radiographic anatomy of, 1398f-1399f
of tube, 1359f
Total intravenous anesthesia (TIVA), in children, 2592
Total laryngectomy, 1563-1572
for advanced glottic cancer, 1497
for advanced supraglottic cancer, 1500
complication(s) of, 1570-1571
drain failure as, 1571
early, 1571

Total laryngectomy *(Continued)*
hematoma as, 1571
hypothyroidism as, 1571
infection as, 1571
late, 1571
pharyngocutaneous fistula as, 1571
stomal stenosis as, 1571
wound dehiscence as, 1571
historical development of, 1563-1564
indications for, 1564-1565
intraoperative conversion from conservation laryngeal surgery to, 1557-1558
vs. organ preservation surgery, 1564
with partial/total pharyngectomy, for hypopharyngeal cancer, 1430, 1431f
patient selection and workup for, 1565
pharyngeal reconstruction after, 1569-1570, 1570f
postoperative management of, 1570-1571
recurrence after, 1476
rehabilitation after, 1572
of swallowing, 1572
of voice (*See* Voice rehabilitation)
for subglottic cancer, 1501
technique for, 1565-1569
access to larynx in, 1566
airway management in, 1565-1566, 1565f
entry into larynx in, 1566, 1568f
entry into trachea in, 1566
incision in, 1565-1566, 1565f
inspection of specimen in, 1566-1568, 1569f
patient positioning in, 1565-1566
skeletonization of larynx in, 1566, 1567f
thyroid gland in, 1566
tracheoesophageal puncture in, 1568-1569, 1569f
tracheotomy in, 1566-1568
wound closure in, 1568-1569, 1569f
tracheal stoma after, 1570, 1571f
Total laryngopharyngectomy, 1572-1575
complication(s) of
early, 1575
functional swallowing problems as, 1575
late, 1575
stricture as, 1575
defined, 1572
historical development of, 1572
incision for, 1565f
indications for, 1573
patient selection and workup for, 1573
postoperative management of, 1574-1575
reconstruction after, 1574, 1574f-1575f
rehabilitation after, 1575
technique for, 1573-1574, 1573f
entry into pharynx in, 1573-1574
initial steps in, 1573-1574
neck dissection in, 1573
patient positioning and anesthetic considerations in, 1573
with superior mediastinal adenopathy, 1574, 1574f
thyroid gland in, 1574
voice after, 1575
Total laryngopharyngoesophagectomy, 1574, 1574f
for cervical esophageal cancer, 1430-1431
Total masking therapy, for tinnitus, 2134
Total ossicular replacement prosthesis (TORP), 2006
with absent stapes superstructure, 2024, 2025f
factors affecting success of, 2023
with ossicular discontinuity, 2008
results with, 2006
Total pharyngo-laryngo-esophagectomy, 1574, 1574f
for cervical esophageal cancer, 1430-1431
Townes-Brocks syndrome, deafness in, 2051t-2058t
Toxic epidermal necrolysis (TEN), 1239
Toxic exposure, olfactory loss due to, 636
Toxic multinodular goiter, 1744-1745
Toxic thyroid adenoma, 1744
Toxin dependent sleep disorder, 262t
Toxoplasma gondii infection
of brain, 223
of salivary glands, 1159-1160
Toxoplasmosis
lymphadenopathy due to, in children, 2818
salivary gland involvement in, 1159-1160
Toynbee maneuver, 1870
Toynbee test, of eustachian tube function, 1874
TPO (thyroperoxidase), in thyroid hormone synthesis, 1737f, 1738
TPO (temporoparietal-occipital) pedicle flaps, for hair loss, 385-387, 387f
complications of, 386-387
T1R(s) (T1 receptors), in gustatory transduction, 1209, 1210f
T2R(s) (T2 receptors), in gustatory transduction, 1209, 1210f
Trace amine–associated receptors (TAARs), 630-631
Trachea
anatomy of, 998-999, 999f
embryology of, 2925-2926
vascular compression of, 2925-2926
Tracheal anomaly(ies)
arterial compression as, 2925-2926
dysphagia due to, 2950t, 2953-2954, 2954f
tracheoesophageal fistula as, 2926
tracheomalacia as, 2925
vascular rings as, 2925
Tracheal foreign bodies
anesthesia for removal of, 2940
imaging of, 2938
symptoms of, 2938
Tracheal homograft transplantation, 2933, 2934f
Tracheal intubation, difficult, 121
Tracheal lacerations, 1634
Tracheal neoplasm(s), 1611-1624
anesthetic management with, 1617
classification of, 1611, 1612t-1613t
diagnosis of, 1616-1617
bronchoscopy in, 1616-1617
pulmonary function testing in, 1616
radiographic evaluation in, 1616, 1616f-1617f
symptoms, signs, and physical examination in, 1616
historical review of, 1611-1612
overview of, 1611
primary, 1611-1612
benign, 1612-1613, 1612t-1613t
chondroma as, 1612-1613
granular cell tumor as, 1612
hamartoma as, 1617f
hemangioma as, 1613
leiomyoma as, 1613
miscellaneous, 1613
squamous papilloma as, 1612
treatment of, 1619
classification of, 1612, 1612t
epidemiology of, 1612, 1613t
malignant, 1612t-1613t, 1613-1615
adenoid cystic carcinoma as, 1614, 1614f
carcinoid tumors as, 1615, 1615f
carinal resections for, 1619, 1621f-1623f
mucoepidermoid carcinoma as, 1615
other, 1614-1615
palliative treatment for, 1619-1624
release maneuvers for, 1618-1619, 1620f
squamous cell carcinoma as, 1613-1614, 1614f
subglottal resections for, 1619, 1620f
therapeutic bronchoscopy for, 1619-1622
tracheal resection and primary reconstruction for, 1617-1618, 1618f-1620f
Tracheal neoplasm(s) *(Continued)*
treatment of, 1617
unresectable, 1619-1624
staging of, 1612
secondary, 1611, 1612t, 1615-1616
treatment of, 1617-1619
for benign tumors, 1619
complications of, 1623-1624
for primary malignant tumors, 1617
anesthetic management in, 1617
carinal resections in, 1619, 1621f-1623f
release maneuvers in, 1618-1619, 1620f
subglottal resections in, 1619, 1620f
tracheal resection and primary reconstruction in, 1617-1618, 1618f-1620f
results of, 1622
for unresectable tumors, 1619-1624
therapeutic bronchoscopy in, 1619-1622
Tracheal prostheses, synthetic, for tracheal stenosis, 2934, 2934f
Tracheal resection, 1617-1618, 1618f-1620f
release maneuvers with, 1618-1619, 1620f
Tracheal stenosis, 943-952
due to anterior wall collapse, 951
cervical, 951, 951b, 951f
in children, 2925-2934
anomalies associated with, 2927
due to arterial compression, 2925-2926
classification of, 2927, 2927t
conservative management of, 2927-2928
diagnosis of, 2926-2927
dilation for, 2928, 2928f
embryology of, 2925-2926
endoscopic evaluation of, 2926-2927
imaging of, 2927
laser therapy for, 2928, 2929f
long-segment, 2926, 2926f
treatment of, 2934
open repair for, 2930-2934
complications of, 2934
costal cartilage tracheoplasty in, 2930-2931, 2931f
granulation at graft site with, 2931
long-segment, 2934
partial tracheal resection, posterior end-to-end anastomosis, and anterior repair with resected trachea in, 2933-2934
pericardial patch in, 2930, 2931f
segmental resection in, 2931-2932, 2932f
short-segment, 2934
slide tracheoplasty in, 2932-2933, 2933f
synthetic tracheal prostheses in, 2934, 2934f
tracheal homograft transplantation in, 2933, 2934f
wedge resection in, 2931, 2931f
short-segment, 2926, 2926f
treatment of, 2934
stents for, 2928-2930, 2930f
due to vascular rings, 2925
cicatricial membranous, 951
classification of, 944, 944t
complete, 951-952, 952f
diagnosis of, 2926-2927
dysphagia due to, 2954
local application of mitomycin C for, 946
long-segment, 2926, 2926f
pathophysiology of, 943-944, 944b
short-segment, 2926, 2926f
surgical management of, 943-952
for chronic disease, 947-952
endoscopic *vs.* open, 945
goals and assessment in, 944, 945f
planning for, 946-947
skin and mucosal grafts in, 946-947
timing of, 945
Tracheal stoma, after total laryngectomy, 1570, 1571f

Tracheal–innominate artery fistula, 1623
Tracheal–pulmonary artery fistula, 1623
Tracheitis, bacterial (exudative), 2809-2810
clinical features of, 2809
complications of, 2810
diagnosis of, 2809, 2809f
differential diagnosis of, 2806t
endoscopy of, 2809, 2809f
epidemiology of, 2809
imaging of, 2809, 2809f
management of, 2809-2810, 2809f
pathogenesis of, 2809
terminology for, 2809
Tracheobronchial endoscopy, 998-1012
airway anatomy and nomenclature for, 998-999, 999f
flexible fiberoptic, 1001-1007
care of bronchoscopes for, 1001-1002
diagnostic, 999b, 1003-1007
for bronchial wash, 1003
for bronchoalveolar lavage, 1003-1004
for bronchoscopic brush sampling, 1007
for endobronchial and transbronchial biopsy, 1004-1005, 1004f-1005f
general approaches to, 1003
for transbronchial needle aspiration, 1005-1007, 1005f-1006f
for visual examination, 1003
range and special features of bronchoscopes for, 1001, 1002t, 1003f
imaging prior to, 999-1000
indications for, 999, 999b
innovations and future developments in, 1009-1011
autofluorescence bronchoscopy as, 1009
endobronchial ultrasonography as, 1011
endoscopic/bronchoscopic lung volume reduction as, 1011
interventional, 999b, 1007-1009
for balloon bronchoplasty, 1009
for endobronchial stent placement, 1009
for foreign body removal, 1008
general principles of, 1007-1008
patient preparation and instrument selection for, 1008
for tissue débridement, 1008-1009, 1010t
patient discussion and informed consent for, 1000
patient positioning and route of entry for, 1000
rigid, 1000-1001
sedation and airway management for, 1000
Tracheobronchial obstruction, in neonate, 2905
Tracheobronchoscopy. *See* Tracheobronchial endoscopy.
Tracheoesophageal diversion, for chronic aspiration, 931-932, 931f-932f
Tracheoesophageal fistula (TEF), 2926
imaging of, 1409-1410
Tracheoesophageal puncture (TEP)
in total laryngectomy, 1568-1569, 1569f, 1572
transnasal esophagoscopy in, 984
for voice prosthesis, 1459, 1599
and radiation therapy, 1600, 1602b
secondary, 1600
Tracheoesophageal (TE) speech
physiology of, 1597, 1597f
after total laryngectomy, 1572
Tracheoesophageal voice prosthesis, 1459
Tracheomalacia, 2925
dysphagia due to, 2954
Tracheoplasty, 2930-2934
balloon, 2928, 2928f
complications of, 2934
costal cartilage, 2930-2931, 2931f
granulation at graft site with, 2931
long-segment, 2934
Tracheoplasty *(Continued)*
partial tracheal resection, posterior end-to-end anastomosis, and anterior repair with resected trachea in, 2933-2934
pericardial patch in, 2930, 2931f
segmental resection in, 2931-2932, 2932f
short-segment, 2934
slide, 2932-2933, 2933f
synthetic tracheal prostheses in, 2934, 2934f
tracheal homograft transplantation in, 2933, 2934f
wedge resection in, 2931, 2931f
Tracheostoma, after total laryngectomy, 1570, 1571f
Tracheostomy, 125-126
for deep neck space infections, 205
and recurrent respiratory papillomatosis, 2887
for Robin sequence, 2673
Tracheostomy tube, for children, 2906-2907
Tracheostomy tube insertion, in cricothyrotomy, 127, 128f
Tracheotomy
for chronic aspiration, 927
for difficult airway, 114t
for obstructive sleep apnea, 260-261
in children, 2610
for stridulous child, 2906
complications of, 2907
emergency, 2904
indications for, 2906, 2906t
patient positioning for, 2906, 2907f
preoperative planning for, 2906
surgical decannulation of, 2907-2908
surgical procedure for, 2906-2908, 2907f
techniques to avoid, 2906, 2906f
ward decannulation of, 2907
Tracking systems, for image-guided sinus surgery, 681
Traction diverticula, 986
Tragus, 476-477, 476f
anatomy of, 1824f, 2742f
Tragus reconstruction, in microtia reconstruction, 2747, 2748f
"Train" activity, in facial nerve monitoring, 2387, 2547, 2547f
Tranquilizers, dizziness due to, 2310t
trans elements, 5f
Transantral approach, for middle cranial base surgery, 2455t, 2458, 2459f
Transantral orbital decompression, for Graves' ophthalmopathy, 1812-1814
complications of, 1814
modifications of, 1814
outcome of, 1812-1814, 1813f-1814f
technique for, 1812
ethmoidectomy in, 1812, 1812f
incisions into periorbital fascia in, 1812, 1813f
removal of orbital floor in, 1812, 1813f
sublabial buccogingival incision in, 1812, 1812f
Transantrosphenoidal approach, for middle cranial base surgery, 2455t, 2458, 2459f
Transbasal approach, for anterior cranial base surgery, 2453-2454, 2454f
Transbronchial biopsy (TBBX), flexible fiberoptic bronchoscopy for, 1004-1005, 1004f-1005f
Transbronchial needle aspiration (TBNA), flexible fiberoptic bronchoscopy for, 1005-1007, 1005f-1006f
Transcanal approach, for tympanoplasty, 2001, 2001f
Transcanal infracochlear approach, for skull base lesions requiring drainage, 2539, 2540f
Transcartilaginous approaches, for nasal tip refinement, 522, 523f-526f
Transcaruncular approach, for pediatric facial fracture, 2701-2702, 2705f
Transcervical approach, for excision of tumors in parapharyngeal space, 1174-1176, 1175f
Transcervical diverticulectomy, 991f
Transcervical incision and drainage, for deep neck space infections, 207
Transclival approach, for transnasal endoscopic-assisted anterior skull base surgery, 2479-2481, 2480f-2481f
Transcochlear approach
to petrous apex, 2499-2500, 2500f
for posterior fossa neoplasms, 2532t, 2537
advantages and disadvantages of, 2532t, 2537
basic features of, 2537
indications for, 2532t, 2537
surgical exposure in, 2537f
technique of, 2537, 2537f
Transconjunctival blepharoplasty, 448-449, 450f
Transcranial electrical stimulation–induced facial motor evoked potentials, to assess facial nerve function, 2389
Transcranial magnetic stimulation (TMS), for tinnitus, 2135-2136
Transcranial motor evoked potential (tcMEP), for intraoperative monitoring, 2555, 2555f
Transcranial repair, for CSF rhinorrhea, 792
Transcribriform approach, for transnasal endoscopic-assisted anterior skull base surgery, 2482
with bilateral access, 2482, 2482f
with unilateral access, 2482
Transcription, of genes, 4, 5f, 11-12, 12f
Transcription factor cellular promotor 2-like 3 *(TFCP2L3)* gene, in deafness, 2051t-2058t
Transcutaneous carbon dioxide pressure (TcPCO$_2$), in skin flaps, 1068
Transcutaneous electric stimulation, for tinnitus, 2136-2137
Transcutaneous oxygen pressure (TcPO$_2$), in skin flaps, 1068
Transdomal suturing
for nasal tip projection, 536
for nasal tip refinement, 522, 530f-531f
Transduction channels, in hair cell transduction, 2071-2073
effects of deficiencies of, 2079-2080
gating of, 2073-2074
ion selectivity of, 2073, 2073f
structure of, 2076f
Transduction efficiency, with traditional hearing aid, 2204-2205
Transesophageal echosonography, 1396
Transethmoidal access, for transnasal endoscopic-assisted anterior skull base surgery, 2478-2479, 2479f-2480f
Transethmoidal encephalocele, 2687t
Transethmoidal sphenoidotomy, for middle cranial base surgery, 2455-2457, 2455t, 2456f
Transfacial approach, for middle cranial base surgery, 2464-2467, 2467f
Transfection, 15-16, 15f
Transfixion incision, for septoplasty, 488, 489f
Transforming growth factor (TGF), 609t-610t
Transforming growth factor α (TGF-α), in wound healing, 1076
Transforming growth factor β (TGF-β), 609t-610t
in wound healing, 1076
Transglottic cancer
anatomic basis for, 1486
imaging of, 161, 164f, 1475f, 1476, 1478f
Transhyoid pharyngotomy approach, for oropharyngeal cancer, 1371, 1372f
Transient evoked otoacoustic emissions (TEOAEs), 1891, 1905
with acoustic neuroma, 1891-1892, 1893f
advantages of, 1891
analysis of, 1905
clinical applications of, 1905-1907

Transient evoked otoacoustic emissions (TEOAEs) *(Continued)*
defined, 1891, 1905
in infants, 2720-2721
in noise-induced hearing loss, 2146-2147, 2147f-2150f
with normal hearing, 1892f
Transient lower esophageal sphincter relaxation (TLESR), 954, 968
Transient receptor potential (TRP) channel, in gustatory transduction, 1209-1210
Transition register, 851
Transition voice, 851
Transition zones, of laryngeal carcinoma, 1489, 1490f
Transitory otoacoustic emission (TOAE), for otitis media, 2762
Translabyrinthine approach
for facial nerve decompression, 2041-2042
for intratemporal facial nerve surgery, 2411
advantages and uses of, 2411
limitations and complications of, 2411
technique of, 2411, 2411f-2412f
for posterior fossa neoplasms, 2530-2533, 2532t
advantages and disadvantages of, 2532t, 2533
basic features of, 2530
indications for, 2530, 2532t
requiring drainage, 2539
surgical exposure in, 2531f
technique of, 2530-2532, 2533f
tumor removal in, 2532-2533
Translation
of DNA, 4, 11-12, 12f
vs. head tilt, 2307, 2307f
with unilateral loss of function of, 2299-2300
anatomic and physiologic basis for, 2299-2300
clinical importance of, 2300, 2300f
Translational vestibulo-ocular reflexes, 2306-2307, 2309f
Translocase of mitochondrial inner membrane 8A *(TIMM8A)* gene
in deafness, 2051t-2058t
in Mohr-Tranebjaerg syndrome, 2097
Translocation, 4-5
Transmandibular approach, for middle cranial base surgery, 2455t, 2458, 2460f
Transmastoid approach
for facial nerve decompression, 2041-2042, 2411
for intratemporal facial nerve surgery, 2410-2411
advantages and uses of, 2411
limitations and complications of, 2411
technique of, 2410, 2410f
Transmastoid labyrinthine drainage, of cholesterol granuloma, 2540f
Transmaxillary approach, for transnasal endoscopic-assisted anterior skull base surgery, 2482-2483, 2483f
Transmembrane channel-like gene 1 *(TMC1),* in deafness, 2051t-2058t
Transmembrane inner ear expressed gene *(TMIE),* in deafness, 2051t-2058t
Transmembrane protease serine 1 *(Tmprss1)* gene, in murine deafness, 2058t-2060t
Transmembrane protease serine 3 *(TMPRSS3)* gene, in deafness, 2051t-2058t
Transmission, of laser energy, 28-29, 29f
Transnasal access, direct, for transnasal endoscopic-assisted anterior skull base surgery, 2477, 2477f
Transnasal endoscopic sinus approach, 742
Transnasal endoscopic-assisted anterior skull base surgery, 2471-2486
anesthesia for, 2476
combined approaches for, 2484
complications of, 2485
Transnasal endoscopic-assisted anterior skull base surgery *(Continued)*
craniocervical junction–odontoid approach for, 2483-2484, 2484f
instrumentation for, 2476
patient preparation for, 2475-2476
pedicled septal flap in, 2476-2477
postoperative care after, 2484-2485
preoperative assessment for, 2475, 2475f
reconstruction after, 2484
surgical anatomy for, 2471-2475
anterior cranial fossa in, 2471, 2472f
clivus in, 2474, 2474f
nasal cavity in, 2471-2473, 2472f-2473f
nasopharynx in, 2474
paranasal sinuses in, 2473-2474, 2473f
retroclival region in, 2474-2475, 2474f-2475f
surgical team setup for, 2476f
transcribriform approach for, 2482
with bilateral access, 2482, 2482f
with unilateral access, 2482
transmaxillary-transpterygoidal-infratemporal approach for, 2482-2483, 2483f
transsellar and parasellar approaches for, 2479, 2480f
transsphenoidal approach for, 2477-2481
with direct transnasal access, 2477, 2477f
with petrous apex access, 2481
with transclival access, 2479-2481, 2480f-2481f
with transethmoidal access, 2478-2479, 2479f-2480f
with transseptal access, 2477-2478, 2477f-2478f
with transseptal-transnasal access, 2478, 2479f
transtuberculum-transplanum approach for, 2482
Transnasal esophagoscopy (TNE), 981-985
accuracy of, 982
in Barrett's esophagitis, 983, 983f
complications of, 984
in dysphagia, 983-984, 984f
of early glottic carcinoma, 1516, 1516f
equipment for, 981, 982f
for extraesophageal reflux, 899
in head and neck oncology, 983
history of, 981
indications for, 983-984
normal findings in, 982-983, 983f
in stricture dilation, 984, 984f
technique for, 982, 982f
therapeutic applications of, 984
tolerance of unsedated examination in, 981-982
in transesophageal puncture, 984
Transnasal fiberoptic laryngoscopy (TFL), for extraesophageal reflux, 898
Transnasal pressure, in rhinomanometry
measurement of, 645-647, 648f
nasal airflow and, 643
Transoral approach
for middle cranial base surgery, 2455t, 2458, 2461f
for oropharyngeal cancer, 1370-1371, 1370f-1371f
Transoral esophagoscopy, for extraesophageal reflux, 899
Transoral incision and drainage, for deep neck space infections, 206-207
Transoral injection, for vocal fold medialization, 906
Transoral laser microsurgery (TLM)
for hypopharyngeal cancer, 1429-1430, 1442
outcomes of, 1436-1438
for laryngeal cancer, 1525-1538
advanced, 1531-1532, 1532f-1533f
complications of, 1533-1534, 1534f
conclusions on, 1536-1537
contraindications to, 1534
costs of, 1534
Transoral laser microsurgery (TLM) *(Continued)*
early, 1530-1531
glottic, 1496
supraglottic, 1498-1500
glottic
with anterior commissure involvement, 1497
in early stage, 1496
historical background of, 1527
instruments for, 1528-1529
intermediate, 1531
and neck dissection, 1532
vs. open conservation surgery, 1528
pathology issues with, 1530
and radiotherapy, 1532-1533
results of, 1534-1535
Gottingen Group, 1535-1536
supraglottic, in early stage, 1498-1500
techniques for, 1529-1530
theoretical basis of, 1527-1528
very advanced, 1532
very early, 1530
terms and definitions for, 1525-1526
Transoral robotic surgery (TORS), for laryngeal cancer, 1560-1561
Transorbital projection, of temporal bone, 131
Transotic approach, for posterior fossa neoplasms, 2532t, 2537-2538
advantages and disadvantages of, 2532t, 2538
basic features of, 2537
indications for, 2532t, 2537-2538
technique for, 2538, 2538f
Transpalatal advancement pharyngoplasty, for obstructive sleep apnea, 258, 260f
Transpalatal approach, for middle cranial base surgery, 2455t, 2458, 2461f
Transplantation
and cervical lymphadenopathy, 219
and hearing loss, 224-225
and non-Hodgkin's lymphoma, 213t, 215-216
posttransplantation lymphoproliferative disorder after, 213t, 215, 217
and sinonasal infection, 219-221
diagnosis of, 220-221, 220f
presentation and pathogenesis of, 219-220
treatment of, 221
and squamous cell carcinoma, 215
and xerostomia, 218
Transposition flaps, 344, 344f
for cheek defects, 358-359, 361f
bilobed, 357, 359f
rhombus shaped, 355
for lip defects, 353
for nasal defects, 348, 349f, 365-366, 366f
Transpterygoid approach, for transnasal endoscopic-assisted anterior skull base surgery, 2483
Transsellar approach, for transnasal endoscopic-assisted anterior skull base surgery, 2479, 2480f
Transseptal access, for transnasal endoscopic-assisted anterior skull base surgery, 2477-2478, 2477f-2478f
Transseptal coaptation sutures, 546-547, 547f
Transseptal sphenoidotomy, for middle cranial base surgery, 2455-2457, 2455t, 2456f
Transseptal-transnasal access, for transnasal endoscopic-assisted anterior skull base surgery, 2478, 2479f
Transsphenoidal approach, for transnasal endoscopic-assisted anterior skull base surgery, 2477-2481
with direct transnasal access, 2477, 2477f
with petrous apex access, 2481
with transclival access, 2479-2481, 2480f-2481f
with transethmoidal access, 2478-2479, 2479f-2480f
with transseptal access, 2477-2478, 2477f-2478f
with transseptal-transnasal access, 2478, 2479f

Transsphenoidal encephalocele, 2687t
Transsphenoidal-transclival approach, for transnasal endoscopic-assisted anterior skull base surgery, 2479-2481, 2480f-2481f
Transtemporal approach
for intratemporal facial nerve surgery, 2407-2409
advantages and uses of, 2408-2409
for Bell's palsy, 2409-2410, 2409t-2410t
limitations and potential complications of, 2409
technique of, 2407-2408, 2408f-2409f
for middle cranial base surgery, 2461
Transtracheal jet ventilation, for difficult airway, 114t
Transtracheal needle ventilation, 128-129
Transtuberculum-transplanum approach, for transnasal endoscopic-assisted anterior skull base surgery, 2482
Transverse arytenoid cartilage, 1542f
Transverse arytenoid muscle, 1359f
Transverse cervical artery
anatomy of, 2579
in root of neck, 2581-2582, 2581f
Transverse cervical lymph nodes
anatomy of, 1360f
in neck dissection, 1705f
Transverse cervical vein, 2579
Transverse crest, in surgical anatomy of lateral skull base, 2437f, 2439
Transverse electromagnetic mode (TEM), 27, 28f
Transverse sinus, in surgical anatomy of lateral skull base, 2436f, 2439f
Trapdoor flaps, 346
for tracheal stenosis, 2928, 2929f
Trapdoor fracture, of orbital floor, pediatric, 2712, 2714f
Trapezius muscle, anatomy of, 2578f-2579f
Trapezius musculocutaneous flap, for oropharyngeal reconstruction, 1378-1379
Trapezoid body, in auditory pathway, 1846
Trauma
acoustic, 2121-2122, 2121f-2122f, 2141
chronic aspiration due to, 926b
CSF rhinorrhea due to, 786b, 794-795
esophageal, 941-942
caustic, 942, 977-978
clinical features of, 977
etiology of, 977
grading of, 977, 978t
prognosis for, 977-978
squamous cell carcinoma due to, 978
strictures due to, 977-978, 978f-979f
external, 941-942
mechanisms of injury in, 933, 934f
facial (*See* Facial trauma)
laryngeal (*See* Laryngeal trauma)
neck (*See* Neck trauma)
peripheral vestibular disorders due to, 2343
baro-, 2343
nonpenetrating, 2343
blast, 2343
labyrinthine concussion as, 2343
penetrating, 2343
to salivary glands, 312, 313f
in children, 2863-2865
sialocele and salivary fistula due to, 313-314
sensorineural hearing loss due to, 2121-2122, 2121f-2122f
sudden, 2128
soft tissue, 302-317
approach to, 302-306
anesthesia in, 304
cleaning in, 304-305, 305f
history taking in, 302-303
infection control in, 305
physical examination in, 303-304, 303f
repair in, 305-306, 306f
tetanus prophylaxis for, 303
Trauma *(Continued)*
to ears, 308f, 310, 310f
etiology of, 302
to eye, 303
to eyelids, 303, 303f, 307-309, 308f
to facial nerve, 309
to lacrimal apparatus, 307-309, 308f
with large-segment, composite avulsions or amputations, 312, 312f
to lips, 309-310, 309f
to nose, 310-312, 311f
to parotid duct, 312-313, 314f
to salivary glands, 312, 313f
sialocele and salivary fistula due to, 313-314
types of injuries in, 306-307
abrasion as, 306
avulsions as, 307, 308f
laceration as, 307
temporal bone (*See* Temporal bone fractures)
vertigo due to, 2039, 2201
Traumatic condition(s), of oral cavity, 1288-1290
amyloidosis as, 1289-1290, 1290f
fibroma as, 1288-1289, 1289f
mucosal ulcerations as, 1289, 1289f
necrotizing sialometaplasia as, 1289, 1299
pyogenic granuloma as, 1289, 1289f
Traumatic facial paralysis, 2398-2399, 2398f
Traumatic granuloma, of oral cavity, 1240
clinical features of, 1240, 1240f
defined, 1240
differential diagnosis of, 1240
etiology of, 1240
histopathologic features of, 1240, 1240f
treatment of, 1240
Traumatic pharyngitis, 194, 194f
Traumatic tattoos, 305, 305f
Trautmann's triangle, in surgical anatomy of lateral skull base, 2436f
Traveling wave, in cochlear transduction
active, 2062-2069, 2064f
passive, 2060-2062, 2062f-2063f
Treacher Collins syndrome
branchial arch structures in, 2585
craniofacial abnormalities in, 2633-2635, 2633b, 2635f, 2646
deafness in, 2051t-2058t, 2094t, 2096
TREACLE gene, in mandibulofacial dysostosis, 2633
Treacle protein, in deafness, 2051t-2058t
Treatment, assessment of, 53
Treatment bias, 53
Tregs (regulatory T cells), 602-603
Tremor
defined, 840
essential, laryngeal hyperfunction due to, 840-841
voice (vocal), 840-841
Treponema denticola, 1252
Treponema pallidum
oral manifestations of, 1252
pharyngitis due to, 194
in children, 2786
Treponema vincentii, Vincent's angina due to, 2786
Tretinoin (Retin A, Renova, Micro Retin A, Avita)
for aging skin, 403-404
with chemical peels, 392-393
for chemoprevention of oral cancer, 1315
TRH (thyrotropin-releasing hormone), in control of thyroid function, 1739
Triamcinolone (Nasacort), for nonallergic rhinitis, 700t
Triangular fossa, of ear, 2742f
Triangularis muscle, 321f
Tricellulin *(TRIC)* gene, in deafness, 2051t-2058t, 2081
Trichilemmal cysts, 289
Trichion, 378-379
Trichloroacetic acid (TCA)
for chemical peels, 392-393
history of, 391, 393
Jessner's solution before, 393
postoperative care after, 394
results of, 394f
technique of, 393-394, 393f-394f
for ear hygiene or chronic ear drainage, 1958
Trichoepithelioma, 292
Tricyclic antidepressants (TCAs)
for migraine, 2350
for neuropathic pain, 244-245
Trigeminal depression
anatomy of, 1822, 1822f
in surgical anatomy of lateral skull base, 2435f, 2436-2437
Trigeminal gasserian ganglion block, for neuropathic pain, 246t
Trigeminal impression
anatomy of, 1823f
in surgical anatomy of lateral skull base, 2435f
Trigeminal nerve
intraoperative monitoring of, 2550, 2550f
in olfactory stimulation, 628-629
in surgical anatomy of anterior cranial base, 2473f
in surgical anatomy of lateral skull base, 2439f
Trigeminal nerve block, 242
Trigeminal nerve toxicity, due to stereotactic irradiation, 2563
Trigeminal nerve transposition, for facial nerve paralysis, 2419
Trigeminal neuralgia, 248
microvascular decompression for, facial nerve monitoring with, 2548-2549
vs. myofascial pain dysfunction syndrome, 1284t
Trigeminal neuromas, 2522, 2522f
Trigeminal pain, 1203
Trigeminal schwannoma, 2512f
Trigeminal system, central projections of, 1203
Trigonocephaly, synostotic, 2642-2643, 2643f, 2648f
front-orbital advancement for, 2645, 2654f
3,5,3′-Triiodothyronine (T_3), 1737. *See also* Thyroid hormone(s).
serum free, 1740
in thyrotoxicosis, 1742
TRIOBP, in deafness, 2051t-2058t, 2076
Trismus
due to deep neck space infection, 185-186
due to masticator space infection, 184, 186f
due to paranasal sinus tumor, 1123
Trisomies, 5
Trisomy 21. *See* Down syndrome.
Trisomy E, inner ear anomalies in, 2735
Triticeal cartilage, 1542f
Trivalent inactivated influenza vaccine (TIV), to prevent otitis media, 2769
Trochlear nerve
intraoperative monitoring of, 2549-2550, 2550f
in surgical anatomy of lateral skull base, 2439f
Trochlear notch, 322f
Trolamine polypeptide oleate-condensate (Cerumenex), for cerumen removal, 1958t
Tropomycin–receptor kinase A, in thyroid carcinoma, 1753
Trotter's syndrome, *vs.* myofascial pain dysfunction syndrome, 1284t
TRP (transient receptor potential) channel, in gustatory transduction, 1209-1210
Trpm13, in murine deafness, 2058t-2060t
TRT (tinnitus retraining therapy), 2134-2135
for hyperacusis, 2139
True vocal folds
anatomy of, 1359f
radiographic, 1472, 1472f-1473f
carcinoma of, imaging of, 1474-1475, 1474f
physical examination of, 100

Trufill (polyvinyl alcohol), for embolization, 1933
Tryptans, for migraines, 247
TSGs. *See* Tumor suppressor genes (TSGs).
TSH. *See* Thyrotropin (TSH).
TT. *See* Tensor tympani (TT).
t-test, 70-71
TTH (tension-type headache), 247
TTS (temporary threshold shift), 2121, 2141
TTS (through-the-scope) balloons, for esophageal strictures, 966
Tubal artery, 1870
Tubal lumen, of eustachian tube, 1867f, 1870
Tuberculosis (TB)
cervical lymphadenopathy due to
in children, 2818, 2819f
in HIV-positive patients, 219
deep neck space infections due to, 201
laryngeal and tracheal manifestations of, 885-886, 886f, 892
of oral cavity, 1250-1251
otologic manifestations of, 2101-2103, 2102f-2103f
otorrhea as, 2196
pharyngitis due to, 195
of salivary glands, 1158
in children, 2858
Tuberculous esophagitis, 1405
Tuberculous nodal mass, 166f
Tuberculous otitis media, 2101-2103, 2102f-2103f
Tuberculous salivary gland infection, 1158
Tuberous sclerosis, oral manifestations of, 1257
Tubulotympanic recess, 1866
Tufted angioma (TA), 2824-2825
Kasabach-Merritt phenomenon with, 2825
Tufted cell, of olfactory bulb, 628f
Tularemia, pharyngitis due to, 195
Tullio phenomenon, 2316
due to acquired cholesteatoma, 2196
with labyrinthine fistula, 1989
in superior canal dehiscence syndrome, 2290, 2329-2330, 2339
Tumarkin attacks, due to intratympanic gentamicin, 2189
Tumor burden, in melanoma, 1111-1112
Tumor (T) classification, for melanoma, 1111, 1111t, 1113f
Tumor necrosis factor (TNF), 609t-610t
Tumor necrosis factor α (TNF-α), in gene therapy, 21
Tumor necrosis factor β (TNF-β), 609t-610t
Tumor suppressor genes (TSGs), 12
in Fanconi's anemia, 1020
in head and neck squamous cell carcinoma, 1016, 1020
modification of, 21-22
Tumor ulceration, with melanoma, 1111-1112
Tumor vaccines, for head and neck squamous cell carcinoma, 1023-1024
Tumor-infiltrating lymphocytes (TIL), genetic modification of, 13, 20-21
Tumor-node-metastasis (TNM) classification
for melanoma, 1111, 1111t
metastatic (M) classification (distant metastases) in, 1111t, 1113
nodal (N) classification (regional disease) in, 1111-1113, 1111t
tumor (T) classification (localized disease) in, 1111, 1111t, 1113f
for thyroid cancer, 1754, 1755t-1756t
Tuning, tonotopic
of afferent auditory neurons, 1845
of basilar membrane, 1840-1842, 1844f
of hair cells, 1844, 1844f
Tuning curves, of basilar membrane, 1844, 1844f
Tuning fork testing, 97-98, 98t
Tunnel of Corti, 1832, 1832f
Turbinates
anatomy and embryology of, 482-483
hypertrophy of, 486
and nasal breathing function, 641
in surgical anatomy of anterior cranial base, 2472, 2472f
Turbinectomy, in vocal professional, 858
Turn-down flaps, 346
Turner's syndrome, 5
oral manifestations of, 1257
Turn-in flaps, 346
Turricephaly, synostotic, 2645, 2645f
TVP muscle. *See* Tensor veli palatini (TVP) muscle.
TW (tympanometric width), with otitis media, 2762
T1WI (T1-weighted images), 134, 135f-136f
T2WI (T2-weighted images), 134, 135f-136f
Twisted nose
rhinoplasty for, 551-554
in noncaucasian patient, 573, 576f
osteotomies in, 551-554
intermediate, 553, 554f
lateral, 552-554, 553f
medial, 552-553, 552f-553f
preoperative examination of, 551, 552f
results of, 511f-512f, 553f-554f
septal reconstruction in, 551
spreader grafts in, 554, 555f
varieties of, 552f
Two-flap palatoplasty, 2669-2670, 2670f
surgical technique for, 2670-2671, 2670f-2671f
Two-hit effect, 6
Two-mass model, of phonation, 811
Two-thirds tumor, 1277
Two-wall decompression, of superior-lateral orbit, for Graves' ophthalmopathy, 1816
Tympanic anulus, 1825-1826, 1825f
Tympanic bone, 2434-2435, 2435f, 2439f
Tympanic canaliculus, 1822-1823
Tympanic cavity, 2585f
Tympanic cover layer, 2050
Tympanic membrane (TM)
anatomy of, 1824-1825, 1825f
in auditory physiology, 1839-1840, 1840f, 2018-2019
in cochlear transduction, 2050-2060, 2062f
hearing loss due to total loss of, 2019, 2019t
in otitis media, 2761-2762
physical examination of, 97, 98f
in surgical anatomy of lateral skull base, 2436f
tympanoplasty with atrophic and atelectatic, 2003-2004
Tympanic membrane perforation, 1969-1971
diagnosis of, 1969, 1970f
hearing loss due to, 2000, 2019, 2019t
management of, 2022-2023
management of, 1971
with ossicular disruption, hearing loss due to, 2019, 2019t
due to otitis externa, 1947
pathogenesis of, 1970-1971, 1971f, 1971t
repair of (*See* Tympanoplasty)
due to small fenestra stapedotomy, 2034
traumatic, 2038
Tympanic membrane sources, of otorrhea, 2195-2196, 2195b
Tympanic membrane surface electrode, electrocochleography with, 1894, 1894f
Tympanic part, of temporal bone, 320f, 1822f, 1823, 2010f
Tympanic segment
anatomy of, 1826f
surgical, 2404, 2404f
vulnerability to injury of, 1826f, 1829
Tympanic sulcus, 2435
Tympanocentesis, for acute otitis media, 2771
Tympanogram, for nasopharyngeal carcinoma, 1354
Tympanomastoid fissure, 2010f
Tympanomastoid suture, 2434-2435, 2435f
Tympanomastoid suture line, 1822f, 1823
Tympanomeatal flap, in tympanoplasty, 2001, 2001f
with lateral graft technique, 2002
with medial graft technique, 2003, 2004f
Tympanomeningeal fissure, 2736
Tympanometric test, nine-step inflation-deflation, 1874
Tympanometric width (TW), with otitis media, 2762
Tympanometry, 1890-1891, 1890f
for conductive hearing loss, 2020
for eustachian tube assessment, 1874
for otitis media, 2762
for sensorineural hearing loss, 2117
Tympanoplasty, 1999-2005
with atrophic and atelectatic tympanic membrane, 2003-2004
cartilage, 2004-2005
classification of, 1999
defined, 1999
formal procedure for, 2001
anesthesia in, 2001
approaches and incisions in, 2001-2002, 2001f
graft placement in, 2002
lateral graft (overlay) technique for, 2002-2003, 2002f
medial graft technique for, 2003, 2004f
functional considerations with, 1999-2000
graft materials for, 2000
minimalist techniques for, 2000-2002
pediatric, 2005
preoperative evaluation for, 2000
with tympanosclerosis, 2003
Tympanosclerosis, 1974-1975
audiometric correlates of, 2005-2006
diagnosis of, 1974, 1974f
epidemiology of, 1974
management of, 1975, 1975f
ossiculoplasty for, 2007-2008, 2024-2025
pathogenesis of, 1974-1975, 1975f
pathophysiology of, 2005
tympanoplasty with, 2003
with tympanostomy tubes, 2775
Tympanosquamous suture, 2434, 2435f
Tympanosquamous suture line, 1822f, 1823, 1824f
Tympanostomy tubes, 2773-2776
blockage of, 2775
chronic otitis media with, 1970-1971, 1981
complications and sequelae of, 2774-2776
cholesteatoma as, 2775
displacement into middle ear as, 2775
early extrusion as, 2775
otorrhea as, 1971, 2774-2775
persistent perforation as, 2775
retained tubes as, 2775
tube blockage as, 2775
tube displacement into middle ear as, 2775
tympanosclerosis, atrophy, and retraction pockets as, 2775
indications for, 2774
for otitis media
acute, 2771
with effusion, 2772
placement of, 2773-2774
aspiration of effusions during, 2773-2774, 2774f
perioperative and postoperative ototopical drops for, 2774
postsurgical follow-up after, 2774
rationale for, 2773
selection of, 2774
water precautions with, 2775-2776
Tympanum, congenital malformations of. *See* Congenital aural atresia (CAA).

Type I error, 65, 66t
Type II error, 65, 66t
Typewriter tinnitus, 2133
Typical carcinoid (TC), of larynx, 1507

U

UARS (upper airway resistance syndrome), 251-252
in children, 2602-2603
UDPGT (uridine diphosphate-glucuronosyl transferase), in head and neck squamous cell carcinoma, 1017
UES. *See* Upper esophageal sphincter (UES).
UGI (upper gastrointestinal) series, for dysphagia in children, 2949
ULC (upper lateral cartilage), of nose, 496, 497f, 509f
revision rhinoplasty for collapse of, 585-586, 586f
Ulcer(s), contact, of vocal folds, 874-875, 874f
diagnosis of, 875
epidemiology of, 874
due to extraesophageal reflux, 902, 902f-903f
management of, 875
pathophysiology and pathology of, 874
Ulceration(s)
aphthous, 1289, 1289f
in HIV, 227, 227f
recurrent, 1236-1239
clinical features of, 1237-1238
defined, 1236-1237
differential diagnosis of, 1238, 1238t
etiology and pathogenesis of, 1237, 1237t
herpetiform-type, 1238, 1238f
histopathologic features of, 1239
major, 1237-1238, 1238f
minor, 1237, 1238f
treatment of, 1239
of melanoma, 1111-1112
Ulcerative colitis, oral manifestations of, 1254
Ulcerative oral mucosal lesions, 1231-1240
erythema multiforme as, 1239-1240, 1254
clinical features of, 1239, 1239f-1240f
defined, 1239
differential diagnosis of, 1239
etiology and pathogenesis of, 1239
histopathologic features of, 1239-1240
treatment of, 1240
herpes simplex infection as
primary, 1235, 1252
clinical features of, 1235, 1235f, 1252
defined, 1235
diagnosis of, 1235
differential diagnosis of, 1235
etiology and pathogenesis of, 1235
treatment of, 1235, 1252
recurrent, 1235-1236, 1252
clinical features of, 1236, 1236f
defined, 1235
differential diagnosis of, 1236
etiology and pathogenesis of, 1235-1236
histopathology of, 1236, 1237f
vs. recurrent aphthous stomatitis, 1238, 1238t
treatment of, 1236
mucous membrane (cicatricial) pemphigoid as, 1233-1235, 1254
clinical differential diagnosis of, 1234, 1234t
clinical features of, 1233-1234, 1233f-1234f
defined, 1233
etiology and pathogenesis of, 1233
histopathologic features of, 1234-1235, 1234f
treatment of, 1235
pemphigus vulgaris as, 1231-1233, 1254
clinical differential diagnosis of, 1232
clinical presentation of, 1232, 1232f
defined, 1231-1232
etiology/pathogenesis of, 1232
Ulcerative oral mucosal lesions *(Continued)*
histopathologic features of, 1232-1233, 1232f-1233f
treatment of, 1233
recurrent aphthous stomatitis as, 1236-1239
clinical features of, 1237-1238
defined, 1236-1237
differential diagnosis of, 1238, 1238t
etiology and pathogenesis of, 1237, 1237t
herpetiform-type, 1238, 1238f
histopathologic features of, 1239
major, 1237-1238, 1238f
minor, 1237, 1238f
treatment of, 1239
traumatic (eosinophilic) granuloma as, 1240
clinical features of, 1240, 1240f
defined, 1240
differential diagnosis of, 1240
etiology of, 1240
histopathologic features of, 1240, 1240f
treatment of, 1240
Ulnar forearm flap, for free tissue transfer, 1082t
Ultimobranchial body, 2584f-2585f
Ultra-frequency sounds, adverse effects of, 2149
Ultrasonic liposuction, 452
Ultrasonography (US), 137
applications of, 143-144
basics of, 1643-1644
B-mode, 1643
of deep neck space infections, 204-205
Doppler, 137
color, 1644
of salivary glands, 1167-1168
of oropharyngeal cancer, 1366
endobronchial, 1011
for fine-needle aspiration biopsy, 1653-1654, 1655f
of parathyroid tumor, 1789
of Graves' ophthalmopathy, 1810
of head and neck cancer, 1647-1653
for hyperparathyroidism, 1786, 1789f
of infrahyoid neck, 143-144
of metastatic lymphadenopathy, 143
of neck masses, 1636-1637, 1637t
of neck neoplasms, 1657
parathyroid, 1644-1645, 1650f-1652f
of pharynx and esophagus, 1396
of salivary glands, 143, 1148-1149, 1149f, 1167, 1645-1647
with acute infections, 1647
with calculous lesions, 1647
color Doppler, 1167-1168
with cystic disease, 1647
with parotid mass, 1654f
in Sjögren's syndrome, 1647
with submandibular pleomorphic adenoma, 1653f
for swallowing disorders, 1219
technique of, 1643-1644, 1645f
terminology for, 1643
of thyroid gland, 1644, 1757
with colloid nodule with comet-tail or ring-down artifact, 1644, 1647f
with cystic nodule, 1644, 1645f
with lymph node metastases, 1644, 1648f-1649f
with malignant tumor, 1644, 1646b, 1646f
multinodular, 1644
with recurrent thyroid carcinoma, 1644
with solid hyperfunctioning nodule, 1644
with solitary nodule, 1644
utility and limitations of, 1644
vocal cord, for stridor, 2901
Ultraviolet light exposure, and oral cancer, 1294, 1294f
Ultravoice, after total laryngectomy, 1572
Umami, 1207, 1209, 1213
Umbo, of tympanic membrane, 97, 98f, 1824, 1825f
Uncertainty, of all data, 60t, 64-65
Uncinate process
anatomy of
normal, 666-667, 666f-667f
surgical, 739, 740f
atelectatic, 668, 670f
in endoscopic sinus surgery, 746, 746f, 750-751
variations in, 668, 670f
Unimate, 38
Unipedicle advancement flaps, 345, 345f
Unithroid (levothyroxine, oral synthetic), for hypothyroidism, 1748-1749
Universal Newborn Hearing Screening (UNHS), 2719
University of Washington Quality of Life scale (UW-QOL), 56
Unknown primary
melanoma of, 1109
squamous cell carcinoma metastatic to neck from, 1641-1642, 1641t, 1664, 1665f
Unloading reflex, 1204, 1204f
Unrestricted toxicity, 603-604
Upper aerodigestive tract, in geriatric patients
presbyphagia of, 237
diagnostic testing for, 237
treatment of, 237
presbyphonia of, 234-237
acoustic changes in, 236
dental/mandibular changes in, 236
factors affecting vocal quality in, 234, 235t
glandular changes in, 236
histologic changes in, 234-235, 235f
laryngoscopic appearance in, 235-236
mucosal changes in, 236
respiratory changes in, 236
and sense of taste, 236
treatment of, 236-237
Upper airway obstruction
after adenotonsillectomy, 2800
in children (*See* Stridulous child)
due to chronic adenotonsillar hypertrophy, 2789f-2790f, 2790-2793, 2795
decongestion for, 655
due to foreign body, 2936-2937
in neonate
expected, 2904-2905
unexpected, 2905
laryngeal, 2905
supralaryngeal, 2905, 2905f
tracheobronchial, 2905
posterior to valve area, 655-656
in Robin sequence, 2673
sleep-related, 2607
valve area stenting for, 655
Upper airway resistance syndrome (UARS), 251-252
in children, 2602-2603
Upper airway stenosis, 943-952
classification of, 944, 944t
local application of mitomycin C for, 946
pathophysiology of, 943-944, 944b
surgical management of, 943-952
for chronic disease, 947-952
anterior glottic, 948
due to anterior wall collapse, 951
cervical tracheal, 951, 951b, 951f
cicatricial membranous, 951
complete glottic, 949-950
complete tracheal, 951-952, 952f
laryngeal release procedures in, 952
posterior glottic, 948-949, 949f
subglottic, 945f, 950-951
supraglottic, 947-948
endoscopic *vs.* open, 945
goals and assessment in, 944, 945f

Upper airway stenosis *(Continued)*
microsurgical débridement in, 946, 946b, 946f
planning for, 946-947
skin and mucosal grafts in, 946-947
stent placement in, 947, 947f
timing of, 945
Upper deep cervical node, 1297f
Upper esophageal sphincter (UES)
anatomy of, 953, 954f
in GERD, 894-895
incompetence of, 1399
manometry of, 958, 959f
during pharyngeal swallow, 1216-1217, 1216f
physiology of, 954, 955f
Upper eyelid
aesthetic analysis of, 445, 446f
paralysis of, 2421
Upper eyelid blepharoplasty, 447-448, 447f-449f
Upper eyelid blepharoplasty incision, 328-329, 329f
Upper eyelid crease, 442, 443f
Upper eyelid ptosis
evaluation of, 446-447, 447f
repair of, 447-448, 447f-449f
Upper eyelid retractors, 444
Upper gastrointestinal (UGI) series, for dysphagia in children, 2949
Upper jugular lymph nodes, in neck dissection, 1704, 1704f-1705f, 1706t
Upper lateral cartilage (ULC), of nose, 496, 497f, 509f
revision rhinoplasty for collapse of, 585-586, 586f
Upper lip, of vocal folds, in mucosal wave propagation, 848-849
Upper lip defects
algorithm for, 351, 355f
large, 352
Upper motor neuron diseases, preoperative evaluation of, 106
Upper respiratory infection (URI)
olfactory loss after, 633-637
and otitis media, 2767
pediatric anesthesia with, 2594-2595
UPPP (uvulopalatopharyngoplasty), for obstructive sleep apnea, 251, 258, 258f, 259t
in children, 2609
Uremic stomatitis, 1255
Uridine diphosphate-glucuronosyl transferase (UDPGT), in head and neck squamous cell carcinoma, 1017
Urinary tract symptoms, of hyperparathyroidism, 1781
Urokinase, for flap salvage, 1075
US. *See* Ultrasonography (US).
USH1C, in deafness, 2051t-2058t
USH2A, in deafness, 2051t-2058t
USH3A, in deafness, 2051t-2058t
Usher syndrome (US)
clinical variants of, 2096
cochlear implant for, 2220
epidemiology of, 2096
genetic basis for, 2051t-2058t, 2074, 2077-2078, 2094t, 2096
genetic testing for, 2098
inheritance pattern of, 6, 8
inner ear anomalies in, 2735
interstereociliary linkages in, 2077
sensorineural hearing loss in, 2077-2078, 2096
adult-onset, 2118
Usherin
and deafness, 2051t-2058t, 2077
in stereocilia, 2076f
Utricle
anatomy of, 1851f, 1853f-1854f, 2278f
embryogenesis of, 1852
Utricle *(Continued)*
sensing of head tilt and translation with unilateral loss of function of, 2299-2300
anatomic and physiologic basis for, 2299-2300
clinical importance of, 2300, 2300f
in vestibular system
arrangement of, 2278, 2280f
estimated patterns of excitation and inhibition for, 2278, 2281f
morphologic polarizations of stereociliary bundles in, 2278, 2280f
Utricular macula. *See* Macula utriculi.
Utriculosaccular chamber, 1852
Utriculus. *See* Utricle.
Uveoparotid fever, facial paralysis in, 2400
Uvula
bifid, 2793, 2793f
physical examination of, 99
radiographic anatomy of, 1398f
squamous cell carcinoma of, 1368f
Uvulopalatal flap, for oropharyngeal reconstruction, 1377, 1377f
of soft palate, 1377f, 1381
Uvulopalatopharyngoplasty (UPPP), for obstructive sleep apnea, 251, 258, 258f, 259t
in children, 2609
Uvuolpalatoplasty, laser-assisted, in vocal professional, 858
UW-QOL (University of Washington Quality of Life scale), 56

V

VA. *See* Vestibular aqueduct (VA).
Vaccine(s)
for head and neck squamous cell carcinoma, 1023-1024
human papillomavirus, 1023-1024
to prevent hearing loss, 2161
to prevent otitis media, 2768-2769
for recurrent respiratory papillomatosis, 2890t
Vacuum-assisted closure (VAC) device, 307
and skin flap viability, 1074-1075
Vagal paragangliomas, 1661-1662
clinical presentation and diagnosis of, 1662
management of, 1662-1663
Vagus nerve
in deep cervical fascia, 2579f
intraoperative monitoring of, 2550-2552, 2551f
in root of neck, 2581f, 2582
surgical anatomy of
auricular branch in, 2440
in brainstem and cerebellum, 2439f
in infratemporal region, 2440f
in internal auditory canal, 2437f
in jugular foramen, 2438, 2439f-2440f
in posterior fossa, 2439f
in temporal bone, 2436f
Vagus nerve injury
in lateral skull base surgery, 2512
due to neck surgery, 1730
Valacyclovir (Valtrex)
with chemical peels, 392, 397
for herpes zoster oticus, 1948
Validation, psychometric, 55
Validation studies, for endoscopic sinus surgery simulator
for discriminant and concurrent validity, 47, 47f
vs. performance on other tests of innate ability, 48, 48t
for predictive validity, 48
Validity
external, 68-69, 68t, 69f
internal, 68-69, 68t, 69f
in psychometric validation, 55
Vallecula(e)
anatomy of
radiographic, 1397, 1463f, 1471f
surgical, 1543f
pseudo-, prevention of formation of, 1599-1600, 1601f
Vallecular cyst(s)
dysphagia due to, 2951-2952
imaging of, 1416f
stridor due to, 2898, 2898f
Valproic acid derivatives, for migraine, 2350
Valsalva maneuver, eye movements evoked by, 2316, 2316f
Valsalva test, of eustachian tube function, 1874
Value-based purchasing, 78
Valve area stenting, for airway obstruction, 655
Valvular damage, oral treatment considerations with, 1246t
Valvular disease, antibiotic prophylaxis with, 1248, 1249t
VAMP (vesicle-associated membrane protein), 2080-2081
van der Hoeve–de Kleyn syndrome. *See* Osteogenesis imperfecta (OI).
Vancenase (beclomethasone nasal), for nonallergic rhinitis, 700t
Vancomycin
ototoxicity of, 2177
sensorineural hearing loss due to, 2120
VAPP (Voice Activity and Participation Profile), 826, 826t
Variability measures, in acoustic analysis for voice evaluation, 829-830, 829t
Variable closure, laryngeal videostroboscopy of, 819
Variable expressivity, 7, 7f, 2088
Variance, analysis of, 71
Varicella vaccine (Zostavax), 2159
Varicella-zoster oticus, 1948, 1948f
clinical features of, 2159, 2159f
diagnosis of, 2159
management of, 2159
sensorineural hearing loss due to, 2119, 2159
sudden, 2127
temporal bone pathology in, 2159
vestibular neuritis due to, 2162
Varicella-zoster virus (VZV)
and Bell's palsy, 2391-2393
deafness and vertigo due to, 2159, 2159f
Meniere's disease due to, 2163
oral manifestations of, 1252
Ramsay Hunt syndrome due to, 2396
Vascular anatomy, of nose, 497, 682-684
anastomoses in, 682-683, 683f
anterior ethmoid artery in, 682, 684f
facial artery in, 682
greater palatine artery in, 682
internal maxillary artery in, 682
posterior ethmoidal artery in, 682-683
sphenopalatine artery in, 682
vidian artery in, 682, 683f
Vascular anomaly(ies), 2822-2834
arteriovenous malformations as, 2832, 2833f
capillary malformations as, 2832-2833, 2834f
classification of, 2823t
lymphatic malformations as, 2829-2830
associated conditions with, 2829-2830, 2831f
clinical assessment and behavior of, 2829, 2830f
diagnostic evaluation of, 2829
imaging of, 2824f, 2829
mandibular overgrowth with, 2823f
of salivary glands, 2861f
sclerotherapy for, 2830-2831
spontaneous resolution of, 2830, 2831f
surgery for, 2831, 2832f

Vascular anomaly(ies) *(Continued)*
neoplastic (*See* Vascular neoplasm(s))
of salivary glands, 2858
hemangiomas as, 2859-2860, 2860f
lymphatic malformations as, 2861f
venous malformations as, 2832
clinical presentation of, 2832, 2833f
imaging of, 2824f
treatment of, 2832, 2833f
Vascular complication(s)
of deep neck space infections, 207-208
of neck surgery, 1728-1729
carotid artery hemorrhage as, 1728
hematoma as, 1729
of internal jugular vein, 1728-1729, 1729f
of radiotherapy, 1048-1049
Vascular compression, of trachea, 2925-2926
Vascular disorder(s)
presbycusis due to, 232
sensorineural hearing loss due to, 2123, 2166
sudden, 2128-2129, 2199
vertigo due to, 2201-2202
with vestibular symptoms, 2351-2353, 2351f
cerebellar hemorrhage as, 2354f
cerebellar infarction as, 2353f
evaluation and management of, 2354f-2355f
lateral medullary syndrome as, 2352f, 2354f
lateral pontomedullary syndrome as, 2353f
vertebrobasilar insufficiency as, 2355f
Vascular endothelial growth factor(s) (VEGFs)
in head and neck squamous cell carcinoma, 1060
in laryngeal carcinoma, 1505
in nasopharyngeal carcinoma, 1700
and skin flap viability, 1073
in wound healing, 1077-1078
Vascular endothelial growth factor (VEGF) inhibitors, for head and neck squamous cell carcinoma, 1060
Vascular injury, due to penetrating neck trauma, 1630-1632, 1631t, 1632f-1633f
management of, 1632-1633, 1633f-1634f
Vascular lesions, endovascular therapy for, 1939-1943
dural arteriovenous fistulas as, 1940-1942, 1941f
epistaxis as, 1939-1940, 1940f
facial arteriovenous fistulas as, 1940, 1940f
facial vascular malformations as, 1942, 1942f
hemangiomas of face and neck as, 1942
pseudoaneurysms as, 1942, 1943f
tinnitus-producing fibromuscular dysplasia of carotid artery as, 1943
Vascular loops, sensorineural hearing loss due to, 2120
Vascular malformations. *See* Vascular anomaly(ies).
Vascular neoplasm(s), 290-291, 2823-2826
and bone resorption, 2826
cherry angiomas as, 290
complications of, 2825, 2826f-2827f
facial nerve involvement in, 2414
hemangioma as (*See* Hemangioma(s))
of salivary glands, 2859-2860, 2860f
kaposiform hemangioendothelioma as, 2824-2825, 2826f
and Kasabach-Merritt phenomenon, 2825
of larynx, 880-881
of neck, 1657
arteriovenous malformations as, 1662-1663
carotid paragangliomas as, 1657-1658
anatomy and physiology of, 1658-1659
classification of, 1660
clinical presentation and diagnosis of, 1659-1660
etiology of, 1659, 1659t
history of, 1657-1658
imaging of, 1658f, 1660-1661
malignancy of, 1660
multicentricity of, 1660-1661

Vascular neoplasm(s) *(Continued)*
observation for, 1661-1662
radiation therapy for, 1661
surgical management of, 1660-1661
epidemiology of, 1657-1659
jugular paragangliomas as, 1662f
nomenclature for, 1657
pathology of, 1657, 1658f
vagal paragangliomas as, 1661-1662
neck mass due to, 2817
port wine stain as, 291
pyogenic granuloma as, 290
salmon patch as, 290-291
tufted angioma as, 2824-2825
Vascular neuralgia, *vs.* myofascial pain dysfunction syndrome, 1284t
Vascular rings, 2925
Vascular supply
impairment of, in acutely raised skin flaps, 1067-1068, 1068f-1069f
to skin, purposes of, 1064
Vascular territories, in skin flaps, 1067-1068, 1068f
Vascularized bone flaps, for free tissue transfer, 1082t, 1084-1087
fibula, 1082t, 1084-1085, 1085f
iliac crest, 1082t, 1087
radial forearm, 1082t, 1085-1086, 1086f-1087f
scapula, 1082t, 1086-1087, 1088f
Vasoactive intestinal peptide (VIP), in salivary gland secretion, 1137
Vasodilation, in salivary glands, 1137
Vasodilators
for Meniere's disease, 2337-2338
oral sequelae of, 1247t-1248t
and skin flap viability, 1073
Vasomotor rhinitis, 619b, 695, 698
VBRT. *See* Vestibular and balance rehabilitation therapy (VBRT).
VC (verrucous carcinoma)
of larynx, 1505-1506, 1505f
of oral cavity, 1299
VCA (viral capsid antigen), of Epstein-Barr virus, 1352, 1354
VCFS (velocardiofacial syndrome)
anterior glottic web in, 2899, 2900f, 2913
cleft lip and palate in, 2673-2674, 2674f
craniofacial anomalies in, 2646
VCR (vestibulocollic reflex), 1851, 2276, 2307-2308
VDS (Verbal Descriptor Scale), 240
Vectors
DNA, 15-16, 15f
nonviral, 16, 19f
viral, 16-18, 18t, 19f
adeno-associated virus as, 18, 18t
adenoviruses as, 17-18, 17f, 18t
retroviruses as, 16, 17f, 18t
Vecuronium, for pediatric anesthesia maintenance, 2593t
VEGFs. *See* Vascular endothelial growth factor(s) (VEGFs).
Vein of cochlear aqueduct, 1856f
Vein of Labbé, 2489
Vein of round window, 1856f
Vein of vestibular aqueduct, 1856f
Velar port, 2676
Velocardiofacial syndrome (VCFS)
anterior glottic web in, 2899, 2900f, 2913
cleft lip and palate in, 2673-2674, 2674f
craniofacial anomalies in, 2646
Velocity storage, brainstem in, 2296, 2308
Velocity-to-position integration, brainstem in, 2296, 2297f-2298f
Velopharyngeal closure, during pharyngeal swallow, 1216
Velopharyngeal closure pattern, 2680, 2680f

Velopharyngeal dysfunction (VPD), 2676-2685
approaches to diagnosis and management of, 2678
assessment of, 2678-2680
general speech analysis in, 2678-2679, 2678f, 2678t-2679t
imaging studies in, 2679
nasometry in, 2679, 2679f
pressure flow in, 2679
speech endoscopy in, 2680, 2680f
speech videofluoroscopy in, 2679-2680
causes of, 2678
defined, 2678
phoneme-specific, 2679
treatment of, 2680-2684
prosthetics for, 2681-2682, 2681f-2682f
speech therapy for, 2680-2681
articulation in, 2681
compensatory strategies in, 2681
resonance in, 2681
surgical intervention(s) for, 2682-2684
choice of, 2684
double-opposing Z-plasty palatoplasty as, 2682-2683
levator repositioning as, 2682
pharyngeal flap as, 2683
pharyngoplasty as, 2683
posterior wall augmentation as, 2683-2684
Velopharyngeal function, 2676
acoustic assessment of, 830
aerodynamic assessment of, 828t, 829
anatomic basis for, 2676, 2677t
Velopharyngeal inadequacy, defined, 2678
Velopharyngeal insufficiency
after adenotonsillectomy, 2800
defined, 2678
impact of, 2679
after palatoplasty, 2673
Velopharyngeal mislearning, 2678-2679
Velopharyngeal port, 2676
Velopharyngeal sphincter, in cleft palate, 2666-2667
Velopharynx
functional anatomy of, 2676, 2677t
muscles of, 2676, 2677t
VEMPs (vestibular evoked myogenic potentials), 2300, 2324, 2325f
in Meniere's disease, 2337
in superior canal dehiscence syndrome, 2341
Venlafaxine, for neuropathic pain, 244-245, 245t
Venous lakes, 288f, 291
Venous malformations, 2832
clinical presentation of, 2832, 2833f
imaging of, 2824f
of neck, 2817
of salivary glands, 1172
treatment of, 2832, 2833f
embolization for, 1942, 1942f
Venous outflow, of skin flaps, 1068
Venous stroke, due to lateral skull base surgery, 2513
Vent, for hearing aids, 2270
Ventilating bronchoscope, 2903, 2903f
Ventilation
control of, in children, 2569-2570
difficult (*See* Difficult airway)
larynx in, 808-809, 808f-809f
Ventilation tubes, for otitis media, with cleft palate, 2675
Ventilation-perfusion relationships, in children, 2570, 2571t
Ventral acoustic stria, 1835, 1835f
Ventral cochlear nucleus, 1835, 1845
Ventral nucleus of trapezoid body (VNTB), in auditory pathway, 1834f
Ventral stria, in auditory pathway, 1846
Ventricular ligament, surgical anatomy of, 1544f

Veramyst (fluticasone furoate), for nonallergic rhinitis, 700t
Verapamil, and skin flap viability, 1073
Verbal Descriptor Scale (VDS), 240
Vergence eye movements, 2305-2306, 2306f, 2307t
  evaluation of, 2314
Verification, of hearing aids, 2273
Vermilion border, 1295f, 1296-1297
Verocay bodies, in schwannomas, 1663
Verruca vulgaris, 282-283
  filiform, 282, 282f
  flat, 282, 283f
  due to molluscum contagiosum, 282-283, 283f
Verruciform xanthoma, oral, 1229
  clinical features of, 1229
  defined, 1229
  etiology and pathogenesis of, 1229
  histopathologic/diagnostic features of, 1229
  treatment of, 1229
Verrucous carcinoma (VC)
  of larynx, 1505-1506, 1505f
  of oral cavity, 1299
Verrucous hyperplasia, of oral cavity, 1299
Verrucous leukoplakia, proliferative, 1225, 1225f
Vertebral artery, 2351f
  in root of neck, 2581-2582, 2581f
  in surgical anatomy of anterior skull base, 2481f
  in surgical anatomy of lateral skull base, 2439f
Vertebral osteophytes, compression of pharynx and esophagus due to, 1408, 1409f
Vertebrobasilar arterial occlusion, sensorineural hearing loss due to, 2123
Vertebrobasilar insufficiency, 2355f
Vertex resistance, in rhinomanometry, 650
Vertical buttresses, 331, 331f
Vertical closure level, laryngeal videostroboscopy of, 821
Vertical crest, in surgical anatomy of lateral skull base, 2437-2439
Vertical hemilaryngectomy, 1547-1549
  complications of, 1549
  extended, 1548
  frontolateral, 1548
  functional outcome of, 1548
  with imbrication laryngoplasty, 1548, 1548f
  key surgical points for, 1549
  oncologic results of, 1547-1548, 1547t-1548t
  posterolateral, 1548
  surgical technique for, 1548
Vertical hemilaryngectomy (VHL)
  for glottic cancer, 1496, 1518f, 1519t, 1547-1549
    with anterior commissure involvement, 1497
  historical background of, 1540
  radiographic appearance after, 1476, 1479f
Vertical laryngoplasty, for chronic aspiration, 928-929, 930f
Vertical partial laryngectomy, 1540, 1547
Vertical phase, of vocal fold vibration, 848-849
Vertical ramus, biomechanics of, 333
Vertical slot defect, after scalp reductions, 385, 386f
  Frechet triple flap repair for, 385, 386f
Vertical transmission, 2088
Vertico-ocular reflex, in vestibular compensation, 2375
Vertigo, 2201-2202. *See also* Dizziness.
  ablative surgery for
    labyrinthectomy as, 2366-2368, 2367f
    patient selection for, 2364-2366
      clinical history in, 2364-2365
      consideration of other potential treatments in, 2366
      identification of intracranial pathology in, 2366
      identification of offending labyrinth in, 2365-2366
      poor compensation *vs.* unstable labyrinthine disease in, 2364, 2365t
Vertigo *(Continued)*
      residual hearing and selection of procedure in, 2366
      therapeutic trial of vestibular rehabilitation in, 2365
      vestibular testing in, 2365, 2365b
    vestibular compensation after, 2370
    vestibular nerve section as, 2368-2370, 2368f-2369f
  acute vestibular, systemic steroids for, 2184
  alternobaric, 2343
  anatomic and physiologic basis for, 2289
  benign paroxysmal of childhood, and migraine, 2350-2351
  benign paroxysmal positional, 2330-2332
    diagnosis of, 2330-2331
      findings on examination in, 2330-2331, 2331f
      history in, 2330
      test results in, 2331
    etiology of, 2330
    historical background of, 2329-2330
    horizontal canal
      positional testing for, 2315-2316, 2331
      repositioning maneuver for, 2332
    incidence of, 2330
    mechanism of, 2330-2332
    and migraine, 2350
    posterior canal
      anatomic and physiologic basis for, 2288-2289, 2288f
      conversion of, 2332
      positional testing for, 2315, 2315f, 2331, 2331f
      repositioning maneuver for, 2331-2332, 2332f
      surgical treatment of, 2332
    superior canal
      positional testing for, 2331
      repositioning maneuver for, 2332
    treatment of
      with repositioning, 2331-2332, 2332f
      surgical, 2332, 2360-2361, 2360f-2361f
      vestibular rehabilitation for, 2376, 2378t
  central (*See* Central vestibular disorder(s))
  cervical, 2354
  defined, 2308-2310, 2329, 2346
  duration of, 2329
  epidemic, 2332-2333 (*See also* Vestibular neuritis)
  etiology of, 2201-2202, 2201b
  history of, 2329
  due to hypothyroidism, 1747
  intractable, intratympanic gentamicin for, 2185-2189
    clinical protocols for, 2187-2188
    complications of, 2188-2189
    concentration of, 2188
    dose of, 2188
    indications and contraindications for, 2189
    injection interval for, 2188
    mechanism of action of, 2185-2186
    number of injections of, 2188
    pharmacokinetics of, 2186-2187, 2186f-2187f
    practical considerations with, 2188
  labyrinthine, 2201-2202
  in Meniere's disease, 2202, 2335t
  migrainous, 2202, 2347-2348, 2348f
  peripheral (*See* Peripheral vestibular disorder(s))
  retrocochlear, 2202
  due to small fenestra stapedotomy
    intraoperative, 2034
    postoperative, 2030, 2034
  due to temporal bone fracture, 2039
  time course of, 2201, 2201b
  due to varicella-zoster virus, 2159, 2159f
Very large G-protein–coupled receptor 1 *(VLGR1)* gene, in deafness, 2051t-2058t, 2077
Vesicle-associated membrane protein (VAMP), 2080-2081
Vesicular glutamate transporter-1 *(VGLUT1)* gene, in deafness, 2081
Vesicular glutamate transporter-3 *(VGLUT3)* gene, in deafness, 2051t-2058t, 2081
Vesiculobullous oral mucosal lesions, 1231-1240
  erythema multiforme as, 1239-1240, 1254
    clinical features of, 1239, 1239f-1240f
    defined, 1239
    differential diagnosis of, 1239
    etiology and pathogenesis of, 1239
    histopathologic features of, 1239-1240
    treatment of, 1240
  herpes simplex infection as
    primary, 1235, 1252
      clinical features of, 1235, 1235f, 1252
      defined, 1235
      diagnosis of, 1235
      differential diagnosis of, 1235
      etiology and pathogenesis of, 1235
      treatment of, 1235, 1252
    recurrent, 1235-1236, 1252
      clinical features of, 1236, 1236f
      defined, 1235
      differential diagnosis of, 1236
      etiology and pathogenesis of, 1235-1236
      histopathology of, 1236, 1237f
      vs. recurrent aphthous stomatitis, 1238, 1238t
      treatment of, 1236
  mucous membrane (cicatricial) pemphigoid as, 1233-1235, 1254
    clinical differential diagnosis of, 1234, 1234t
    clinical features of, 1233-1234, 1233f-1234f
    defined, 1233
    etiology and pathogenesis of, 1233
    histopathologic features of, 1234-1235, 1234f
    treatment of, 1235
  pemphigus vulgaris as, 1231-1233, 1254
    clinical differential diagnosis of, 1232
    clinical presentation of, 1232, 1232f
    defined, 1231-1232
    etiology/pathogenesis of, 1232
    histopathologic features of, 1232-1233, 1232f-1233f
    treatment of, 1233
  recurrent aphthous stomatitis as, 1236-1239
    clinical features of, 1237-1238
    defined, 1236-1237
    differential diagnosis of, 1238, 1238t
    etiology and pathogenesis of, 1237, 1237t
    herpetiform-type, 1238, 1238f
    histopathologic features of, 1239
    major, 1237-1238, 1238f
    minor, 1237, 1238f
    treatment of, 1239
  traumatic (eosinophilic) granuloma as, 1240
    clinical features of, 1240, 1240f
    defined, 1240
    differential diagnosis of, 1240
    etiology of, 1240
    histopathologic features of, 1240, 1240f
    treatment of, 1240
Vestibular ablation
  intratympanic gentamicin for, 2185-2189
    clinical protocols for, 2187-2188
    complications of, 2188-2189
    concentration of, 2188
    dose of, 2188
    indications and contraindications for, 2189
    injection interval for, 2188
    mechanism of action of, 2185-2186
    number of injections of, 2188
    pharmacokinetics of, 2186-2187, 2186f-2187f
    practical considerations with, 2188
  labyrinthectomy for, 2366-2368, 2367f
  patient selection for, 2364-2366

Vestibular ablation *(Continued)*
clinical history in, 2364-2365
consideration of other potential treatments in, 2366
identification of intracranial pathology in, 2366
identification of offending labyrinth in, 2365-2366
poor compensation *vs.* unstable labyrinthine disease in, 2364, 2365t
residual hearing and selection of procedure in, 2366
therapeutic trial of vestibular rehabilitation in, 2365
vestibular testing in, 2365, 2365b
vestibular compensation after, 2370
vestibular nerve section for, 2368-2370, 2368f-2369f
Vestibular afferent nerve fibers
encoding by, 2283-2285, 2284f
firing rate of, 2278-2279, 2281f
interpretation of excitation of, 2289
anatomic and physiologic basis for, 2289
clinical importance of, 2289-2290
for nystagmus during caloric testing, 2290
in posterior canal benign paroxysmal positional vertigo, 2289-2290
in superior canal dehiscence syndrome, 2290, 2290f
irregular, 2284-2285, 2284f
morphology of, 2283, 2283f
regular, 2283-2285, 2284f
synaptic morphology and function of, 1857-1859, 1859f-1860f
Vestibular and balance rehabilitation therapy (VBRT), 2372-2
adaptive capabilities and, 2327
as adjunctive modality, 2377
assessment for, 2376
clinical history in, 2376
vestibular testing in, 2376
basis of, 2302
expected results of, 2379
goals of, 2372, 2373f-2374f
history of, 2372
patient education on, 2379
patient selection criteria for, 2376-2377
as adjunctive modality, 2377
balance function studies in, 2376-2377
inappropriate candidates in, 2377
as primary treatment modality, 2376-2377
as therapeutic trial, 2377
physiologic rationale for, 2373-2376
dynamic compensation in, 2374-2376
static compensation in, 2374
positional testing after, 2373f-2374f
posturography in, 2326
as primary treatment modality, 2376-2377
techniques for, 2372-2373, 2378-2379, 2378t
adaptation exercises as, 2372-2373, 2375f, 2378
balance and postural control exercises as, 2372-2373, 2378-2379
conditioning activities as, 2372-2373, 2379
gait exercises as, 2372-2373, 2378-2379
habituation exercises as, 2372-2373, 2378
maintenance activities as, 2372-2373, 2379
sensory substitution exercises as, 2372-2373, 2378
therapeutic trial of, 2365, 2377
for uncompensated vestibular neuritis, 2365t
videonystagmography after, 2373f-2374f
Vestibular apparatus
embryology of, 1851-1852, 1851f
peripheral
autonomic supply of, 1854
efferent innervation of, 1854, 1855f

Vestibular aqueduct (VA)
anatomy of, 1823f, 1832, 2010f
enlarged, 2733-2734
in adults, 2344, 2344f
clinical manifestations of, 2734
in combination with other anomalies, 2728, 2738, 2739f
and CSF leakage, 2735-2736, 2736f
embryology of, 2733-2734
imaging of, 1921, 2733
CT for, 1921, 1923f, 2733, 2733f
MRI for, 1921, 1923f, 2733, 2733f
incidence of, 2727, 2733
treatment of, 2734, 2739
in surgical anatomy of lateral skull base, 2435f
Vestibular Autorotation Test, 2323-2324, 2324f
Vestibular cecum, 1853f
Vestibular commissural system, 1863, 1863f
Vestibular compensation, 2300-2302
anatomic and physiologic basis for, 2300-2302, 2301f
assessment of, 2376
clinical history in, 2376
vestibular testing in, 2376
clinical implications of, 2302
defined, 2373-2374
dynamic, 2373-2376
effect of suppressive drugs on, 2302
postoperative, 2370
static, 2373-2374
with static *vs.* fluctuating loss of vestibular function, 2302
and vestibular rehabilitation, 2302
Vestibular deafferentation syndrome, acute, due to intratympanic gentamicin, 2189
Vestibular decompensation, 2370
Vestibular deficits, static *vs.* fluctuating, 2302
Vestibular destructive therapy, for Meniere's disease, 2126
Vestibular disorder(s)
associated with migraine, 2350
benign paroxysmal positional vertigo as, 2350
Meniere's disease as, 2350
central (*See* Central vestibular disorder(s))
due to noise, 2148
peripheral (*See* Peripheral vestibular disorder(s))
related to migraine, 2350-2351
benign paroxysmal vertigo of childhood as, 2350-2351
paroxysmal torticollis as, 2351
Vestibular efferent nerve fibers, 2285
Vestibular end organ(s)
anatomy of, 1853f, 1854-1855, 2277, 2278f
ampulla in, 1851f-1852f, 1854
crista ampullaris in, 1854, 1856f-1857f
cupula in, 1855, 1857f
endolymph in, 1855
hair cells in, 1854-1855, 1856f
kinocilium in, 1854-1855, 1856f
macula sacculi in, 1855, 1856f-1858f
macula utriculi in, 1855, 1856f-1858f
otolith membrane in, 1855, 1858f
otoliths in, 1855, 1858f
stereocilia in, 1854-1855, 1856f
striola in, 1855, 1858f
supporting cells in, 1854-1855
blood supply to, 1854, 1856f
Vestibular evoked myogenic potentials (VEMPs), 2300, 2324, 2325f
in Meniere's disease, 2337
in superior canal dehiscence syndrome, 2341
Vestibular eye movements, 2307t
Vestibular function, 2305-2308
assessment of, in infants, 2722
bilateral loss of, 2344
brainstem and cerebellum in, 2308

Vestibular function *(Continued)*
eye movements in, 2305-2307, 2306f-2307f, 2307t, 2309f
head movements in, 2307-2308
peripheral anatomy and physiology in, 2305
unilateral loss of, adaptation of vestibular reflexes with, 2300-2302
anatomic and physiologic basis for, 2300-2302, 2301f
clinical implications of, 2302
Vestibular ganglion, 1852-1854
Vestibular ganglionitis. *See* Vestibular neuritis.
Vestibular hair cells, excitation-inhibition asymmetry of, 2290-2291, 2291f
Vestibular labyrinth, intratympanic delivery of medications to. *See* Intratympanic delivery.
Vestibular ligament, 1542f
Vestibular nerve
anatomy of
in auditory system, 1832f
in vestibular system, 1851f, 1852-1854, 1854f, 2278f
distribution to end organs of, 1852, 1854f
organization of inputs to vestibular nuclei from, 1861-1863, 1863f
projections to cerebellum from, 1860
terminations in brainstem of, 1858f, 1859-1860
Vestibular nerve section, 2368-2370
for Meniere's disease, 2339, 2362
results of, 2370
selective, 2368
infralabyrinthine approach for, 2370
lateral suboccipital craniotomy approach for, 2370
middle fossa approach for, 2368-2369, 2369f
retrolabyrinthine, 2369-2370, 2369f
retrosigmoid approach for, 2370
transcochlear, 2368, 2368f
translabyrinthine, 2368
transmastoid, 2368f
for uncompensated vestibular neuritis, 2365t
Vestibular neural plasticity. *See* Neural plasticity, in otology.
Vestibular neuritis, 2162-2163, 2332-2333
clinical features of, 2159, 2332-2333
diagnostic testing for, 2333
etiology of, 2333
infectious causes of, 2159
management of, 2159
pathophysiology of, 2294
with sudden sensorineural hearing loss, 2333
temporal bone pathology in, 2159, 2162f, 2333
treatment of, 2333
vestibular nerve section *vs.* vestibular rehabilitation for, 2365t
Vestibular neuropathy. *See* Vestibular neuritis.
Vestibular nuclei
anatomic subdivisions of, 1860-1861, 1862f
efferent projection pathways from, 1864-1865, 1864f
organization of vestibular nerve inputs to, 1861-1863, 1863f
other inputs to, 1863-1864, 1864f
pathways from cerebellum to, 1864
spinal cord afferents to, 1864
terminations of vestibular nerve in, 1859-1860, 1861f
visual inputs to, 1863-1864
Vestibular ototoxicity
of aminoglycoside antibiotics, 2170
of cisplatin, 2172
Vestibular paralysis. *See* Vestibular neuritis.
Vestibular ramus, 1854, 1856f

Vestibular reflexes, adaptation to unilateral loss of vestibular function of, 2300-2302
anatomic and physiologic basis for, 2300-2302, 2301f
clinical implications of, 2302
for effect of suppressive drugs, 2302
with static *vs.* fluctuating loss, 2302
for vestibular rehabilitation, 2302
Vestibular rehabilitation. *See* Vestibular and balance rehabilitation therapy (VBRT).
Vestibular schwannoma. *See* Acoustic neuroma(s).
Vestibular sensory epithelium
cellular morphology of, 1855-1857, 1856f, 1858f
specialized subregions of, 1858-1859, 1859f-1860f
Vestibular skin, in sensation of nasal obstruction, 641-642
Vestibular surgery, 2359-2371
for ablative control of vertigo
labyrinthectomy as, 2366-2368, 2367f
patient selection for, 2364-2366
clinical history in, 2364-2365
consideration of other potential treatments in, 2366
identification of intracranial pathology in, 2366
identification of offending labyrinth in, 2365-2366
poor compensation *vs.* unstable labyrinthine disease in, 2364, 2365t
residual hearing and selection of procedure in, 2366
therapeutic trial of vestibular rehabilitation in, 2365
vestibular testing in, 2365, 2365b
vestibular compensation after, 2370
vestibular nerve section as, 2368-2370, 2368f-2369f
for benign paroxysmal positional vertigo, 2360-2361
posterior semicircular canal occlusion as, 2360-2361, 2361f
singular neurectomy as, 2360, 2360f
for Meniere's disease, 2362-2364
cochleosacculotomy as, 2126, 2362-2363, 2363f
endolymphatic sac surgery as, 2126, 2339, 2363-2364, 2364f
rationale for, 2359-2360
for repair of perilymphatic fistula, 2361-2362
for superior semicircular canal dehiscence, 2361, 2362f
Vestibular symptoms, of migraine, 2347-2348
motion sickness as, 2348
nonspecific dizziness as, 2347
vertigo as, 2202, 2347-2348, 2348f
Vestibular system, 1850-1865
adaptive capabilities of, 2327
age-related degeneration of, 233
bidirectional sensitivity of, 2278-2279
cellular morphology of vestibular sensory epithelium in, 1855-1857, 1858f
central pathways of, 1859-1865
anatomic subdivisions of vestibular nuclei in, 1860-1861, 1862f
efferent projection pathways from vestibular nuclei in, 1864-1865, 1864f
organization of vestibular nerve inputs to vestibular nuclei in, 1861-1863, 1863f
other inputs to vestibular nuclei in, 1863-1864, 1864f
projections of vestibular nerve to cerebellum in, 1860
terminations of vestibular nerve in brainstem in, 1858f, 1859-1860
dynamic disturbance of, 2327
embryology of, 1851-1852, 1851f
Vestibular system *(Continued)*
experimental viral infections of, 2163
in maintaining stable vision and posture, 2276-2277
anatomic and physiologic basis for, 2276-2277
clinical importance of, 2277
overall organization of labyrinth in, 1852-1854
facial nerve in, 1852
membranous labyrinth and bony labyrinth in, 1852, 1853f
orientation of semicircular canals in, 1852, 1852f
vestibular (Scarpa's) ganglion in, 1852-1854
vestibular nerve in, 1852-1854, 1854f
vestibule in, 1852
vestibulocochlear nerve in, 1852, 1853f
peripheral vestibular apparatus in
autonomic supply of, 1854
efferent innervation of, 1854, 1855f
principles of applied physiology of, 2276-2304
static imbalance of, 2327
synaptic morphology and function of vestibular afferents in, 1857-1859, 1859f-1860f
vestibular end organs in
anatomy of, 1853f, 1854-1855
ampulla in, 1851f-1852f, 1854
crista ampullaris in, 1854, 1856f-1857f
cupula in, 1855, 1857f
endolymph in, 1855
hair cells in, 1854-1855, 1856f
kinocilium in, 1854-1855, 1856f
macula sacculi in, 1855, 1856f-1858f
macula utriculi in, 1855, 1856f-1858f
otolith membrane in, 1855, 1858f
otoliths in, 1855, 1858f
stereocilia in, 1854-1855, 1856f
striola in, 1855, 1858f
supporting cells in, 1854-1855
blood supply to, 1854, 1856f
Vestibular testing
for ablative vestibular surgery, 2365, 2365b
with acoustic neuroma, 2517
in assessment of vestibular compensation, 2376
gain, phase, and time constant in, 2302-2304, 2303f
for sensorineural hearing loss, 2117
Vestibule, 1825f, 1831
anatomy of, 1852
imaging of, 1920-1921, 1922f
Vestibulocochlear anastomosis of Oort, 1835
Vestibulocochlear artery, 1854, 1856f
Vestibulocochlear nerve
anatomy of, 1852, 1853f
in surgical anatomy of lateral skull base, 2438, 2439f
Vestibulocollic reflex (VCR), 1851, 2276, 2307-2308
Vestibulo-ocular reflex (VOR), 1851, 2276
active head movement analysis techniques for, 2323-2324, 2324f
adaptation exercises and, 2378
angular, 2306, 2307f
after labyrinthectomy, 2291-2292, 2291f-2293f
brainstem circuitry in, 2296-2297
anatomic and physiologic basis for, 2296
velocity storage in, 2296
velocity-to-position integration in, 2296, 2297f-2298f
clinical implications of, 2296-2297
for Alexander's law, 2297, 2299f
for head-shake nystagmus, 2296-2297
for interpreting rotary chair tests, 2297-2299
for pre- and post-rotatory nystagmus, 2296, 2298f
efferent projection pathways from vestibular nuclei in, 1865
eye movements in, 2306, 2306f
Vestibulo-ocular reflex (VOR) *(Continued)*
head movements in, 2308
after labyrinthectomy, 2291-2292, 2291f-2293f
low-frequency, 2314
orientation of semicircular canals and, 2285-2287, 2286f-2287f
in patient selection for ablative vestibular surgery, 2365
translational, 2306-2307, 2309f
Vestibulo-ocular reflex (VOR) cancellation, 2300-2301, 2306f, 2314
Vestibulo-ocular reflex (VOR) gain, 2301-2304, 2301f, 2303f
Vestibulopathy
familial, 2343-2344
recurrent, 2335
Vestibulospinal reflexes (VSRs), 1851, 2276
evaluation of, 2316-2317
Vestibulothalamic pathways, 1865
Vestibulotoxicity, 2344
Vezatin, in stereocilia, 2078
VFP. *See* Vocal fold paralysis (VFP).
VFSS (videofluoroscopic swallow study), for dysphagia in children, 2949, 2950t
VGLUT1 (vesicular glutamate transporter-1) gene, in deafness, 2081
VGLUT3 (vesicular glutamate transporter-3) gene, in deafness, 2051t-2058t, 2081
VHL. *See* Vertical hemilaryngectomy (VHL).
VHL (von Hippel–Lindau) protein, in Warburg effect, 1028f
Viadent-related leukoplakia, 1223-1224, 1224f
Vibrant Soundbridge semi-implantable hearing aid, 2208-2210
clinical data on, 2209
comparison of features of, 2206t
components of, 2208-2209, 2208f
for conductive and mixed hearing loss, 2210
history of, 2208, 2210
implantation of, 2209
indications for, 2209, 2209f
Vibrating ossicular prosthesis (VORP), 2208, 2208f
Vibration, and noise-induced hearing loss, 2148-2149
Vickers and Gorlin criteria, for unicystic ameloblastoma, 1271
Videoendoscopy
drug-induced, of obstructive sleep apnea, 253-255
of early glottic carcinoma, 1515-1516
laryngeal, 814-818
of arytenoid and vocal fold motion, 816
common problems and solutions for, 815t-816t
defined, 813
endoscopes for, 813-814
of laryngeal structure, 816
of mucus, 816-817
in neurologic examination, 834
protocol for, 814, 816b
of supraglottic activity, 817, 817f
of vascularity, 817
of vocal fold edges, 818
Videofluoroscopic swallow study (VFSS), for dysphagia in children, 2949, 2950t
Videofluoroscopy
speech, for velopharyngeal dysfunction, 2679-2680
for stridor, 2901
for swallowing disorders, 1217-1218, 1219f
Videonystagmography (VNG), and vestibular rehabilitation, 2373f-2374f, 2376-2377
Videostroboscopy, laryngeal, 818-821
of adynamic segments, 820
of amplitude of vibration, 820, 821f, 848, 848t
of closure pattern, 819, 820f, 848t, 849
common problems and solutions for, 815t-816t
defined, 813
of early glottic carcinoma, 1515-1516

Videostroboscopy, laryngeal *(Continued)*
flexible endoscope for, 814
advantages of, 814
disadvantages of, 814
protocol for, 818b
technique of, 814
troubleshooting for, 814
interpretation of, 848t
interval examination in, 847
of mucosal wave, 820, 848-849, 848t
in neurologic examination, 834
of periodicity, 821, 848, 848t
of phase closure, 819-820
for professional voice, 847-849, 848f, 848t
protocol for, 818-819, 818b
of regularity, 821
rigid endoscopes for, 813-814
advantages of, 813
disadvantages of, 813-814
protocol for, 818b
technique of, 814
troubleshooting for, 814
of symmetry, 820, 847-848, 848t
of vertical closure level, 821
for vocal fold impairment, 905
Vidian artery, 682, 683f
Vinblastine
for induction chemotherapy, 1056
sensorineural hearing loss due to, 2120
Vincent's angina, 2786
Vincristine
for hemangioma of infancy, 2826-2828
for induction chemotherapy, 1056-1057
sensorineural hearing loss due to, 2120
VIP (vasoactive intestinal peptide), in salivary gland secretion, 1137
Viral capsid antigen (VCA), of Epstein-Barr virus, 1352, 1354
Viral infection(s)
of external ear, 1957, 1957f
topical therapies for, 1957, 1957f
options for, 1957
of labyrinth
cytomegalovirus as, 2154-2156, 2155f
herpes simplex virus as, 2159-2160
Lassa fever as, 2158-2159
measles as, 2158
mumps as, 2157-2158, 2158f
rubella as, 2156-2157, 2157f
varicella-zoster virus as, 2159, 2159f
oral manifestations of, 1252
otitis media due to, 2764
and pediatric chronic sinusitis, 2778
and rhinosinusitis, 730-731
of salivary glands, 1156-1158
in children, 2855
due to Epstein-Barr virus, 2855
due to HIV, 2856
due to mumps, 2855
due to HIV, 1157-1158, 1157f
in children, 2856
due to mumps, 1156-1157
in children, 2855
sensorineural hearing loss due to, 2119, 2199
sudden, 2127
Viral labyrinthitis, vertigo due to, 2201
Viral laryngitis, 884
Viral lymphadenopathy, in children, 2817-2818
Viral parotitis, 1156-1158
in children, 2855
due to Epstein-Barr virus, 2855
due to HIV, 2856
due to mumps, 2855
due to HIV, 1157-1158, 1157f
in children, 2856
due to mumps, 1156-1157
in children, 2855
Viral pharyngitis, 196-199
due to adenovirus, 198
in children, 2785-2786
due to common cold (rhinovirus, coronavirus, parainfluenza virus), 196
due to Epstein-Barr virus, 198-199, 198f
due to herpes simplex virus, 199, 199f
due to HIV, 197
due to influenza virus, 196-197
Viral vaccines, to prevent otitis media, 2769
Viral vectors, 16-18, 18t, 19f
adeno-associated virus as, 18, 18t
adenoviruses as, 17-18, 17f, 18t
conditionally replicating, 22
retroviruses as, 16, 17f, 18t
Viral-mediated gene transfer, 16-18, 18t, 19f
via adeno-associated virus, 18, 18t
via adenoviruses, 17-18, 17f, 18t
via retroviruses, 16, 17f, 18t
Virtual endoscopy, 138, 140f
Virtual laryngoscopy, 1464, 1464f
Virtual reality (VR) headset, 39, 39f
Virtual reality (VR) simulator, 45-46
Visceral fascia, 202, 2577, 2578f
Visceral space, imaging of, 159-163
with abscess, 161f
larynx in, 159-161
with epiglottitis, 159-161, 163f
with laryngoceles, 159-161, 163f
with squamous cell carcinoma, 161, 164f
with trauma, 159, 162f
parathyroid glands in, 162-163, 165f
thyroid gland in, 161-162
CT for, 140
with follicular carcinoma, 161-162, 165f
lingual, 161-162, 165f
MRI for, 143
normal anatomy in, 161
scintigraphy for, 138
with thyroglossal duct cyst, 161-162, 165f
Visceral tissue free flaps, for oropharyngeal reconstruction, 1380, 1380f
Visceral transposition, for hypopharyngeal and esophageal reconstruction, 1453
colonic, 1453, 1454f
gastric, 1453
Viscerocranium, 2443f
Viscerovertebral angle, 1799, 1799f
Vision, vestibular system in maintaining stability of, 2276-2277
anatomic and physiologic basis for, 2276-2277
clinical importance of, 2277
Vision loss, due to paranasal sinus tumor, 1123
Visual acuity, dynamic, 2316
Visual acuity examination, prior to anterior and middle cranial base surgery, 2446
Visual analog pain scale, 239
Visual fixation, 2305-2306, 2306f, 2307t
Visual input, to vestibular nuclei, 1863-1864
Visual perceptual examination, in voice assessment, 827
Visual reinforcement audiometry (VRA)
in infants, 2722
for otitis media, 2762
Visual vestibular mismatch, due to intratympanic gentamicin, 2189
Vitamin A
for cancer chemoprevention, 1018, 1061-1062
for olfactory dysfunction, 639
Vitamin A deficiency, oral manifestations of, 1254
Vitamin B_2, for migraine, 2349
Vitamin B_2 deficiency, oral manifestations of, 1254
Vitamin B_{12} deficiency, oral manifestations of, 1254
Vitamin C
for aging skin, 404
with chemical peel, 396
for rhinosinusitis, 731, 735t
Vitamin C deficiency, oral manifestations of, 1254
Vitamin D
and allergic rhinitis, 613
in calcium homeostasis, 1775
hypercalcemia due to excessive intake of, 1784
Vitamin D deficiency, oral manifestations of, 1254
Vitamin E, for chemoprevention of oral cancer, 1315
Vitamin K deficiency, oral manifestations of, 1254
Vitruvian man, 269, 270f
VLGR1 (very large G-protein–coupled receptor 1) gene, in deafness, 2051t-2058t, 2077
VNG (videonystagmography), and vestibular rehabilitation, 2373f-2374f, 2376-2377
VNTB (ventral nucleus of trapezoid body), in auditory pathway, 1834f
Vocal abuse
laryngitis due to, 883-884, 884f
by voice professional, 853
Vocal capability battery, for benign vocal fold mucosal disorders, 861-862
bilateral diffuse polyposis as, 872
capillary ectasia as, 866
contact ulcer or granuloma as, 875
glottic sulcus as, 870
intracordal cysts as, 869
intubation granuloma as, 875-876
postoperative dysphonia as, 873-874
vocal fold hemorrhage and unilateral (hemorrhagic) vocal fold polyp as, 868
vocal nodules as, 865
Vocal commitments, assessment of, 861
Vocal cord(s). *See* Vocal fold(s).
Vocal fold(s)
applied anatomy of, 805-806
false, radiographic anatomy of, 1472-1473, 1472f
microarchitecture of, 860, 860f
movement of, 805, 806f
neurologic evaluation of, 834
in phonation, 811, 811f, 833
positioning of, 812
shape of, 812
vibratory capacity of, 812
physiology of, 860, 860f
in pitch control, 812
superficial lesions of, in vocal professional, 855-856, 856f
true
anatomy of, 1359f
radiographic, 1472, 1472f-1473f
carcinoma of, imaging of, 1474-1475, 1474f
physical examination of, 100
vibratory cycle of, 860, 861f
videoendoscopy of, 816, 817f
edges in, 818
Vocal fold angle, in laryngeal paralysis, 912, 913f
Vocal fold atrophy, in geriatric patients, 234-235
Vocal fold cysts, 856, 857f
in children, 2882, 2882f
Vocal fold granuloma, 2881, 2881f
Vocal fold hemorrhage, 854, 867-869
with capillary ectasia, 868f
diagnosis of, 868
history in, 868
laryngeal examination in, 868
vocal capability battery in, 868
epidemiology of, 867
pathophysiology and pathology of, 867-868
treatment of, 868-869
behavioral, 868
medical, 868
surgical, 868-869

Vocal fold immobility, 843
CO$_2$ laser for, 33
due to trauma, 937
Vocal fold injection, 905-907
vs. arytenoid adduction, 912-913
complications of, 907, 908f
laryngoscopic, 906-907, 907f
materials used in, 905-906
percutaneous, 906, 906f-907f
transoral, 906
Vocal fold medialization, 904-911
in children, 2879
for chronic aspiration, 927
historical aspects of, 904-905
by injection, 905-907
vs. arytenoid adduction, 912-913
complications of, 907, 908f
laryngoscopic, 906-907, 907f
materials used in, 905-906
percutaneous, 906, 906f-907f
transoral, 906
medialization thyroplasty for, 908-911
advantages of, 908
arytenoid adduction *vs.*, 912-913
disadvantages of, 908
factors affecting outcome of, 908
with Gore-Tex strip, 908, 910, 911f
implant placement in, 909-910, 910f
indications for, 905, 908
prefabricated implants for, 908, 908f, 910
prosthesis templates in, 909-910, 910f
technique for, 908-911, 909f
patient evaluation and selection for, 905
Vocal fold mobility
clinical evaluation of, 1545
glottic cancer with impaired, 1496
Vocal fold mucosal disorders, benign. *See* Benign vocal fold mucosal disorder(s).
Vocal fold nodules. *See* Vocal nodules.
Vocal fold paralysis (VFP), 843
in children, 2879-2880
dysphagia due to, 2952
chronic aspiration due to, 927
congenital, 2868-2869
etiology of, 1466-1467
iatrogenic left, 2868
imaging of, 1466-1467, 1467f
laryngeal reinnervation for (*See* Laryngeal reinnervation)
laryngeal stenosis and, 2922
due to laryngeal trauma, 937-938
due to thyroid disease, 1737
vocal fold medialization for (*See* Vocal fold medialization)
Vocal fold paresis, 843
causes of, 843
central, 842
clinical presentation of, 843
diagnosis of, 843
vocal fold positioning in, 843
Vocal fold polyp(s)
in children, 2882
unilateral (hemorrhagic), 867-869
with capillary ectasia, 868f
diagnosis of, 868
history in, 868
laryngeal examination in, 868
vocal capability battery in, 868
epidemiology of, 867
pathophysiology and pathology of, 867-868
treatment of, 868-869
behavioral, 868
medical, 868
surgical, 868-869
in vocal professional, 846
Vocal fold polyposis, bilateral diffuse, 872-873, 872f
diagnosis of, 872
history in, 872
laryngeal examination in, 872
vocal capability battery in, 872
epidemiology of, 872
management of, 872-873
behavioral, 872
medical, 872
surgical, 872-873, 873f
pathophysiology and pathology of, 872
Vocal fold positions, in laryngeal paralysis, 912-913
Vocal fold reinnervation. *See* Laryngeal reinnervation.
Vocal fold stripping, 872-873, 873f
for premalignant lesions of larynx, 1490
Vocal fold ultrasound, for stridor, 2901
Vocal fold varix(ices), 846-847, 856, 857f
Vocal fold vibration
cover-body theory of, 845, 845f
horizontal phase of, 849
measures of, 830-831
electroglottography for, 830, 835
for professional voice, 849
inverse filtered flow for, 830-831
videostroboscopy for, 818-821
adynamic segments in, 820
amplitude of vibration in, 820, 821f, 848, 848t
closure patterns in, 819, 820f, 848t, 849
interpretation of, 848t
interval examination in, 847
mucosal wave in, 820, 848-849, 848t
of periodicity, 821, 848, 848t
phase closure in, 819-820
for professional voice, 847-849, 848f, 848t
protocol for, 818-819, 818b
regularity in, 821
symmetry in, 820, 847-848, 848t
vertical closure level in, 821
for vocal fold impairment, 905
vertical phase of, 848-849
Vocal ligament
anatomy of, 860, 860f, 1484f
surgical, 1542f-1544f
in vocal fold vibration, 845
Vocal misuse
laryngitis due to, 883-884, 884f
by voice professional, 853
Vocal muscle, 1543f
Vocal nodules, 865-866
with capillary ectasia, 867f
in children, 2881-2882, 2882f
defined, 865
diagnosis of, 865
history in, 865
laryngeal examination in, 865
vocal capability battery in, 865
epidemiology of, 865
gastroesophageal reflux and, 2946
management of, 865-866
behavioral, 865
medical, 865
surgical, 865-866, 866f, 867t
pathophysiology and pathology of, 865
in vocal professionals, 846, 853, 855
voice therapy for, 863
Vocal output, objective measures of, for benign vocal fold mucosal disorders, 862
"Vocal overdoer" syndrome, 861
Vocal overuse
acute mucosal swelling of, 863
laryngitis due to, 883-884, 884f
Vocal pedagogue, for professional voice disorders, 852, 855
Vocal Performance Questionnaire (VPQ), 57, 826, 826t
Vocal process
in arytenoid adduction, 913-914, 913f-914f
in laryngeal paralysis, 913-914
Vocal professionals. *See* Professional voice disorders.
Vocal quality disorders, in children
due to cricoarytenoid joint fixation, 2880
due to epidermoid cysts, 2882, 2882f
due to granuloma, 2881, 2881f
due to laryngeal web, 2880, 2880f
due to malignant tumors, 2881
medical management of, 2881
due to posterior glottic stenosis, 2880
due to recurrent respiratory papillomatosis, 2880-2881
due to sulcus vocalis, 2882
surgical management of, 2879-2881
due to vocal fold paralysis, 2879-2880
due to vocal fold polyps, 2882
due to vocal nodules, 2881-2882, 2882f
voice therapy for, 2881-2882
Vocal rehabilitation, after laryngectomy. *See* Voice rehabilitation.
Vocal tendon, 1541-1542
Vocal tremor, 840-841
Vocalization, 846-847
VoCoM (hydroxyapatite) implants, for medialization thyroplasty, 908-910, 908f, 910f
Vogt-Koyanagi-Harada syndrome, inner ear disease in, 2165
Voice
alaryngeal (*See* Alaryngeal voice and speech)
chest, 846-847, 851
head, 846-847, 851
outcome scales for, 56t, 57
transition, 851
Voice Activity and Participation Profile (VAPP), 826, 826t
Voice analysis
computer-assisted, for children, 2878, 2878f
for extraesophageal reflux, 898
Voice breaks, 846-847
in professional voice, 851
in spasmodic dysphonia, 834-835
Voice considerations, with early glottic cancer, 1518-1519
Voice disorder(s)
in children, 2876-2883
evaluation of, 2876-2878
aerodynamic analysis in, 2878
algorithm for, 2877f
computer-assisted voice analysis for, 2878, 2878f
history in, 2876
physical examination in, 2876-2877
for social and functional impact, 2876
speaking tasks in, 2877-2878
stroboscopic examination in, 2877
voice profile in, 2878
functional, 2876, 2879
incidence of, 2876
organic, 2876, 2879
of resonance, 2879
of vocal quality
due to cricoarytenoid joint fixation, 2880
due to epidermoid cysts, 2882, 2882f
due to granuloma, 2881, 2881f
due to laryngeal web, 2880, 2880f
due to malignant tumors, 2881
medical management of, 2881
due to posterior glottic stenosis, 2880
due to recurrent respiratory papillomatosis, 2880-2881
due to sulcus vocalis, 2882
surgical management of, 2879-2881
due to vocal fold paralysis, 2879-2880

Voice disorder(s) *(Continued)*
due to vocal fold polyps, 2882
due to vocal nodules, 2881-2882, 2882f
voice therapy for, 2881-2882
voice therapy for, 2878-2879, 2881-2882
in singers (*See* Professional voice disorders)
Voice evaluation, 825-831
diagnostic (probe) therapy for, 831
for laryngeal stenosis, 2917
measurements in, 827-831
acoustic analysis for, 829t, 834-835
cepstral peak prominence in, 829t, 830
combined frequency and intensity in, 829, 829f, 829t
Fast Fourier Transform in, 829t, 830, 830f
frequency in, 829, 829t
intensity (sound pressure level) in, 829, 829t
linear predictive coding in, 829t, 830, 830f
long-term average spectrum in, 829t, 830
nasalance in, 829t, 830
phonetogram (voice range profile) in, 829, 829f, 829t
for professional voice, 849
spectral displays in, 829t, 830, 830f
variability in, 829-830, 829t
of velopharyngeal function, 829t, 830
aerodynamic, 828-829, 828t, 835
airflow as, 828, 828t
laryngeal airway resistance as, 828-829, 828t
maximum phonation time as, 828
phonation threshold pressure as, 828, 828t
of professional voice, 849
subglottic air pressure as, 828, 828t
of velopharyngeal function, 828t, 829
of chest wall displacement, 828
of vocal fold vibration, 830-831
electroglottography for, 830, 835
inverse filtered flow for, 830-831
patient scales for, 825-826, 826t, 834
Patient Questionnaire of Vocal Performance as, 826, 826t
Reflux Symptom Index as, 826, 826t
Voice Activity and Participation Profile as, 826, 826t
Voice Handicap Index as, 826, 826t, 834
Voice Outcome Survey as, 826, 826t
Voice Symptom Scale as, 826, 826t
Voice-Related Quality of Life scale as, 826, 826t, 834
perceptual, 826-831
auditory, 826-831
CAPE-V for, 826
GRBAS for, 826, 827t
other aspects of, 826-827
for professional voice, 850
tactile, 827-831, 828f
visual, 827
for professional voice, 849-850
Voice Handicap Index, 57, 826, 826t, 834
Voice Outcome Survey (VOS), 826, 826t
Voice production, 846-847, 2876
modal register of, 850-851
Voice profile, for children, 2878
Voice prosthesis(es), 1597, 1597f
history of, 1594-1595, 1595f
indwelling *vs.* nonindwelling, 1597-1598, 1598f
physiology of, 1595-1597, 1596f
postoperative management of, 1600
alimentary care in, 1600
pulmonary care in, 1600, 1602f
and radiotherapy, 1600, 1602b
replacement of, 1601
indications for, 1601
nonindwelling, 1602
for valve discrepancy (periprosthetic leakage), 1602
Voice prosthesis(es) *(Continued)*
for valve incompetence (transprosthetic leakage), 1601-1602
secondary, 1600
surgical aspects of, 1598-1600, 1599f-1600f
creation of optimally contoured stoma as, 1599-1600, 1600f
pharyngeal mucosa closure as, 1599-1600, 1601f
prevention of excessively deep stoma as, 1599-1600, 1600f
prevention of hypertonicity of PE segment as, 1599-1600, 1599f
timing of insertion of, 1597-1599
troubleshooting with, 1603-1605
types of, 1597-1598, 1598f
Voice quality
assessment of, 826-831
CAPE-V for, 826
GRBAS for, 826, 827t
other aspects of, 826-827
in geriatric patients, 234-237
acoustic changes and, 236
dental/mandibular changes and, 236
factors affecting, 234, 235t
glandular changes and, 236
histologic changes and, 234-235, 235f
laryngoscopic appearance and, 235-236
mucosal changes and, 236
respiratory changes and, 236
and sense of taste, 236
treatment of, 236-237
Voice quality disorders, in children
due to cricoarytenoid joint fixation, 2880
due to epidermoid cysts, 2882, 2882f
due to granuloma, 2881, 2881f
due to laryngeal web, 2880, 2880f
due to malignant tumors, 2881
medical management of, 2881
due to posterior glottic stenosis, 2880
due to recurrent respiratory papillomatosis, 2880-2881
due to sulcus vocalis, 2882
surgical management of, 2879-2881
due to vocal fold paralysis, 2879-2880
due to vocal fold polyps, 2882
due to vocal nodules, 2881-2882, 2882f
voice therapy for, 2881-2882
Voice range profile (VRP), in acoustic analysis for voice evaluation, 829, 829f, 829t
Voice rehabilitation, 1594-1610
electrolarynx voice and speech for, 1596, 1596f
esophageal voice and speech for, 1596, 1596f
history of, 1594-1595, 1595f
after laryngopharyngectomy, 1458-1459
physiology of, 1595-1597, 1596f
after total laryngectomy, 1572
after total laryngopharyngectomy, 1575
tracheoesophageal voice and speech for, 1597, 1597f
voice prosthesis(es) for, 1597, 1597f
indwelling *vs.* nonindwelling, 1597-1598, 1598f
postoperative management of, 1600
alimentary care in, 1600
pulmonary care in, 1600, 1602f
and radiotherapy, 1600, 1602b
replacement of, 1601
indications for, 1601
nonindwelling, 1602
for valve discrepancy (periprosthetic leakage), 1602
for valve incompetence (transprosthetic leakage), 1601-1602
secondary, 1600
surgical aspects of, 1598-1600, 1599f-1600f
creation of optimally contoured stoma as, 1599-1600, 1600f
Voice rehabilitation *(Continued)*
pharyngeal mucosa closure as, 1599-1600, 1601f
prevention of excessively deep stoma as, 1599-1600, 1600f
prevention of hypertonicity of PE segment as, 1599-1600, 1599f
timing of insertion of, 1597-1599
troubleshooting with, 1603-1605
types of, 1597-1598, 1598f
Voice Symptoms Scale (VoiSS), 57, 826, 826t
Voice therapy
for benign vocal fold mucosal disorders, 863, 864f
for children, 2878-2879, 2881-2882
for postoperative dysphonia, 874
Voice tremor, 840-841
Voice-Related Quality of Life (V-RQOL) Instrument, 57, 826, 826t
in neurologic evaluation, 834
pediatric, 57
VoiSS (Voice Symptoms Scale), 57, 826, 826t
Voit's anastomosis, 1852-1854
Volatile anesthetic agents, 111
Volume correction, for hyperparathyroidism, 1804
Vomer, 320f
Vomeronasal cartilage, 482
Vomeronasal organ, 482
in olfactory stimulation, 627-628, 627f
Vomiting, pediatric postoperative, 2593
von Békésy, Georg, 2050
von Hippel–Lindau (VHL) protein, in Warburg effect, 1028f
von Recklinghausen's disease, 1774, 1782
acoustic neuromas in, 2515
with laryngeal involvement, 882
oral manifestations of, 1257
otologic manifestations of, 2112
von Willebrand's disease
oral manifestations of, 1256
preoperative evaluation of, 105
VOR. *See* Vestibulo-ocular reflex (VOR).
Voriconazole, for rhinosinusitis, 712, 713t, 735, 735t
VORP (vibrating ossicular prosthesis), 2208, 2208f
VOS (Voice Outcome Survey), 826, 826t
VoSol (propylene glycol and acetic acid otic solution), for otitis externa, 1946, 1953, 1959t-1960t
VoSol HC (hydrocortisone/propylene glycol/acetic acid otic solution), for otitis externa
bacterial, 1953, 1959t-1960t
fungal, 1954, 1959t-1960t
VOXEL-MAN TempoSurg simulator, 50
VPD. *See* Velopharyngeal dysfunction (VPD).
VPQ (Patient Questionnaire of Vocal Performance), 826, 826t
VPQ (Vocal Performance Questionnaire), 57, 826, 826t
VR (virtual reality) headset, 39, 39f
VR (virtual reality) simulator, 45-46
VRA (visual reinforcement audiometry)
in infants, 2722
for otitis media, 2762
VR-FESS, 48
VRP (voice range profile), in acoustic analysis for voice evaluation, 829, 829f, 829t
V-RQOL (Voice-Related Quality of Life) Instrument, 57, 826, 826t
in neurologic evaluation, 834
pediatric, 57
VSRs (vestibulospinal reflexes), 1851, 2276
evaluation of, 2316-2317
V-Y advancement flap, 345-346, 346f-347f
for cheek defects, 358, 361f
for lip defects, 356f
VZV. *See* Varicella-zoster virus (VZV).

W

Waardenburg-Hirschsprung disease, deafness in, 2051t-2058t, 2095
Waardenburg syndrome (WS)
inner ear anomalies in, 2735
sensorineural hearing loss in, 2051t-2058t, 2094t, 2095-2096
adult-onset, 2117-2118, 2118f
types of, 2095
variable expression and nonpenetrance in, 7, 7f
Waardenburg-Shah syndrome, 2095
Wagner-Grossman hypothesis, for vocal fold paralysis, 912
Waldenström's macroglobulinemia, sensorineural hearing loss due to, 2123
Waldeyer's ring
anatomy of, 2783
infections of, 2785
Waldeyer's ring lymphomas, 1680
treatment and prognosis for, 1680
Wallenberg's syndrome, 2313, 2352f, 2354f
Wallerian degeneration, 2384-2385
Walsh scoring system, for GABHS pharyngitis, 192-193
Walsh-Ogura operation. *See* Transantral orbital decompression.
Waltzer mouse, deafness in, 2074
Warburg effect, 1024-1025, 1028f
Warfarin
epistaxis due to, 687
preoperative use of, 105
Wart(s), 282-283
filiform, 282, 282f
flat, 282, 283f
due to molluscum contagiosum, 282-283, 283f
oral, in HIV, 227
Warthin, Aldred, 1170-1171
Warthin's tumors, 1170-1171
in children, 2862
imaging of, 1146, 1146f
Water brash, 956
Water clear cell adenoma, of parathyroid gland, 1778
Water clear cell hyperplasia, of parathyroid gland, 1779
Water precautions, with tympanostomy tubes, 2775-2776
Waters view, 130, 662, 663f
Watson, Patrick, 1563
Web(s)
esophageal, 966-967, 967f
imaging of, 1407, 1408f
laryngeal, 2869-2871, 2913
anterior, 2869-2870, 2869f
in congenital high airway obstruction syndrome, 2869, 2870f
dysphagia due to, 2952
epidemiology of, 2913
etiology and pathophysiology of, 2913
in laryngeal atresia, 2869, 2869f-2870f
posterior, 2869, 2869f
stridor due to, 2899, 2900f
syndromes associated with, 2869, 2870t
treatment of, 2922
vocal quality disorder due to, 2880, 2880f
Web formation, after neck surgery, 1728, 1729f
Weber test, 97-98, 98t, 2020
for otosclerosis, 2030
Wedge excision biopsy, for skin lesions, 293
Wedge resection, for tracheal stenosis, 2931, 2931f
Wegener, Friedrich, 658
Wegener's granulomatosis (WG), 2103-2104
clinical presentation of, 2103
diagnosis of, 658, 2103
epidemiology of, 658
epistaxis due to, 685f
etiology and pathogenesis of, 2103
Wegener's granulomatosis (WG) *(Continued)*
inner ear disease in, 2165-2166
laboratory findings in, 2103
laryngeal and tracheal manifestations of, 889-890, 890f
nasal manifestations of, 658
oral manifestations of, 1252
otologic manifestations of, 2103f, 2104
otorrhea as, 2196
pathology of, 658, 2104f
prognosis for, 2103-2104
sensorineural hearing loss due to, 2124
treatment of, 658
type 1, 658
type 2, 658
type 3, 658
Weight loss, for obstructive sleep apnea, 256
Weir procedure, for noncaucasian nose, 556
Wens, 289
Wernicke's area, in central auditory pathway, 1836-1837, 1847
WFS1 (Wolfram syndrome gene 1), in deafness, 2051t-2058t, 2092-2093, 2098
WG. *See* Wegener's granulomatosis (WG).
Wharton's duct
anatomy of, 2850-2852
sialography of, 1149-1150
Whirler mice, 2077
Whirlin, in stereocilia, 2076f, 2078
Whirlin *(WHRN)* gene, in deafness, 2051t-2058t, 2077
Whistletone register, 851
White blood cell disorders, oral manifestations of, 1256
Whitnall's ligament, 439, 444
Whitnall's tubercle, 439
Whooping cough, laryngeal and tracheal manifestations of, 892
WHO-QOL (World Health Organization quality of life scale), 56
WHRN (whirlin) gene, in deafness, 2051t-2058t, 2077
Wide dynamic-range compression, for hearing aids, 2268
Wide local excision (WLE), of melanoma, 1113-1114
Wide-field laryngectomy, 1568-1569, 1570f
Wig(s), 387
Wigand technique, for endoscopic sinus surgery, 746
Williams, Frand, 1031
Williams, Robin, 38
Witch's chin, 465, 466f
WLE (wide local excision), of melanoma, 1113-1114
Wobble nucleotide, 4
Wolf High Speed Endocam, 821
Wolff's law, 330, 2613
Wolfram syndrome gene 1 *(WFS1),* in deafness, 2051t-2058t, 2092-2093, 2098
Wolframin, and deafness, 2051t-2058t
Women
hair loss in, 376, 377f
oral health of, 1256-1257
during and after menopause, 1256-1257
during menses, 1256
during pregnancy, 1256
during puberty, 1256
World Health Organization quality of life scale (WHO-QOL), 56
Wormian bone, in osteogenesis imperfecta, 2109-2110, 2110f
Wound, created by laser, 29-30, 30f
Wound closure, for facial trauma, 305-306, 306f
Wound complication(s), of neck surgery, 1726-1728
incision planning and, 1726-1727
infection as, 1727
salivary fistula as, 1727-1728, 1728f
scar formation as, 1728, 1729f
seroma as, 1727, 1727f
wound dehiscence and flap necrosis as, 1727
Wound contraction, 1078
Wound dehiscence
after neck surgery, 1727
after total laryngectomy, 1571
Wound healing, 1075-1078
cell types in, 1076t
gene therapy for, 22-23
inflammatory phase of, 1076
proliferation phase of, 1076-1078
formation of granulation tissue in, 1077-1078
angiogenesis in, 1077-1078
dermal matrix in, 1077
reepithelialization in, 1076-1077
keratinocyte migration in, 1076-1077
keratinocyte proliferation in, 1077
wound contraction in, 1078
remodeling phase of, 1078
Wound infection, after neck surgery, 1727
Wound tension, in skin flaps, 1071
W-plasty
for forehead defects, 359-360, 362f
for scar revision, 298, 299f
Wrapped endotracheal tube, with recurrent respiratory papillomatosis, 2891
Wrinkle(s), 275, 279f. *See also* Aging skin.
rhytidectomy for (*See* Rhytidectomy)
Wrinkle cream products, 403
WS. *See* Waardenburg syndrome (WS).

X

X inactivation, 8
X linkage, 8
Xanthelasma, 293
Xanthine oxidase, in acutely raised skin flaps, 1070-1071, 1071f
Xanthine oxidase inhibitor, and skin flap viability, 1074
Xanthoma, oral verruciform, 1229
clinical features of, 1229
defined, 1229
etiology and pathogenesis of, 1229
histopathologic/diagnostic features of, 1229
treatment of, 1229
XCL chemokines, 611t-612t
Xenografts, for craniofacial defect repair, 2657
Xenon CT blood flow mapping, for cerebral blood flow evaluation, 2491
Xeroderma pigmentosa, and melanoma, 1107
Xeroradiography, of pharynx and esophagus, 1393
Xerostomia
with aging, 1141-1142, 1141f
immunosuppression and, 218
palliative care for, 1102-1103
due to radiotherapy, 1047-1048, 1102-1103
X-linked dominant disorder, 6, 2089
X-linked inhibitor of apoptosis (XIAP), in aminoglycoside ototoxicity, 2171
X-linked recessive disorders, 7, 7f, 2088f, 2089
X-linked sensorineural hearing loss
nonsyndromic, 2093, 2093t
syndromic, 2094t, 2096-2097
X-linked stapes gusher syndrome, 2737
Xolegel (ketoconazole cream), for fungal otitis externa, 1954-1955, 1959t-1960t
X-rays
interaction with matter of, 1032-1033, 1032f
interactions with DNA of, 1036-1043, 1037f
Xylocaine. *See* Lidocaine (Xylocaine).
Xyzal (levocetirizine), for nonallergic rhinitis, 701t

Y

Yersinia enterocolitica, pharyngitis due to, 196
Yodel, 846-847
Y-V advancement flaps, 346

Z

Zafirlukast
  for allergic rhinitis, 620-621
  for rhinosinusitis, 735t, 736
Zellballen, in paragangliomas, 1657, 1658f
Zenker, Friedrich Albert von, 987
Zenker's diverticulum(a), 974, 986-997
  classification of, 987, 991t
  defined, 986
  diagnosis of, 986-987, 989f-990f
  differential diagnosis of, 986-987, 990t
  epidemiology of, 986
  history of, 986-987, 987f
  imaging of, 1401, 1402f
  management of, 987-997
    algorithm for, 997, 997f
    endoscopic techniques for, 992-997
      complications of, 995
      electrocautery technique in, 993f
      equipment for, 994f
      history of, 992, 993f
      laser technique in, 993f
      positioning for, 993f
      procedure for, 992-995, 995f-996f
      results of, 994-995
Zenker's diverticulum(a) *(Continued)*
    external techniques for, 988-992
      complications of, 992
      diverticulopexy technique as, 992f
      history of, 988-990
      inversion technique as, 992f
      procedure for, 990-992
      transcervical diverticulectomy as, 991f
    recurrence after, 995-997
  pathophysiology of, 986-987
  presentation of, 986-987
Zeus telerobotic system, 39, 40f
Zileuton
  for allergic rhinitis, 620-621
  for rhinosinusitis, 735t, 736
Zinc, for olfactory dysfunction, 639
Zinc deficiency, oral manifestations of, 1254
Zinc gluconate, for rhinosinusitis, 731, 735t
Z-line, in transnasal esophagoscopy, 982
Zones of perfusion, 1064-1065, 1065f
Zonisamide, for neuropathic pain, 244t
Zostavax (varicella vaccine), 2159
Zovirax (acyclovir)
  with chemical peels, 397
  for herpes zoster, 2396
  for recurrent respiratory papillomatosis, 2890t, 2892
Z-palatoplasty, for obstructive sleep apnea, 258, 260f
Z-plasty, for scar revision, 298, 298f-299f
Zygoma
  anatomy and physiology of, 319, 320f-321f
  biomechanics of, 332
  in surgical anatomy of lateral skull base, 2435f-2436f
Zygomatic arch(es)
  anatomy and physiology of, 319, 320f
  biomechanics of, 332
  depressed, *vs.* myofascial pain dysfunction syndrome, 1285t
Zygomatic bone, 320f
Zygomatic branch, of facial nerve, 1194f
Zygomatic fractures
  imaging of, 325
  repair of, 336
  surgical access to, 328-329
Zygomatic injury, physical examination of, 324
Zygomatic process
  anatomy of, 1821, 1822f-1823f, 2010f
  articular tubercle of, 1822f
Zygomatic root, 1822f, 1824f
Zygomatic "tripod," biomechanics of, 332
Zygomaticofacial nerve, 321f
Zygomaticomalar complex fractures, pediatric, 2707-2708, 2710f
Zygomaticus major muscle, 321f, 442f, 444
Zygomaticus minor muscle, 442f, 444
Zyrtec (cetirizine)
  for nonallergic rhinitis, 701t
  for rhinosinusitis, 734t